2018

ICD-10-CM

INCLUDES NETTER'S ANATOMY ART

Carol J. Buck
MS, CPC, CCS-P

Former Program Director
Medical Secretary Programs
Northwest Technical College
East Grand Forks, Minnesota

ELSEVIER

ELSEVIER

3251 Riverport Lane
St. Louis, Missouri 63043

2018 ICD-10-CM STANDARD EDITION

ISBN: 978-0-323-43070-8

Content Strategist: Brandi Graham
Content Development Manager: Luke Held
Associate Content Development Specialist: Anna Miller
Publishing Services Manager: Jeffrey Patterson
Project Manager: Lisa A. P. Bushey
Designer: Maggie Reid

Printed in the United States of America

Last digit is the print number: 9 8 7 6 5 4 3 2 1

 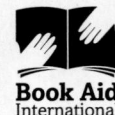

Working together
to grow libraries in
developing countries

www.elsevier.com • www.bookaid.org

DEDICATION

To all the brave medical coders who transitioned the nation into a new coding system. Decades of waiting finally concluded with the implementation of I-10, and you have been the pioneers leading the way.

With greatest appreciations for your efforts!

Carol J. Buck, MS, CPC, CCS-P

DEVELOPMENT OF THIS EDITION

Query Team

Patricia Cordy Henricksen, MS, CHCA, CPC-I, CPC, CCP-P, ASC-PM
Auditing and Coding Educator
Soterion Medical Services
Lexington, Kentucky

Jackie Grass Koesterman, CPC
Coding and Reimbursement Specialist
Grand Forks, North Dakota

Kathleen Buchda, CPC, CPMA
Revenue Recognition
New Richmond, Wisconsin

Editorial Consultant

Jenna Price, CPC
President
Price Editorial Services, LLC
St. Louis, Missouri

Elsevier/MC Strategies Revenue Cycle, Coding and Compliance Staff

"Experts in providing e-learning on revenue cycle, coding and compliance."

Deborah Neville, RHIA, CCS-P
Director

Lynn-Marie D. Wozniak, MS, RHIT
Content Manager

Sandra L. Macica, MS, RHIA, CCS, ROCC
Content Manager

CONTENTS

ICD-1 0-CM

GUIDE TO USING THE 2018 ICD-10-CM STANDARD

Medical coding has long been a part of the health care profession. Through the years medical coding systems have become more complex and extensive. Today, medical coding is an intricate and immense process that is present in every health care setting. The increased use of electronic submissions for health care services only increases the need for coders who understand the coding process.

2018 ICD-10-CM Standard Edition was developed to help meet the needs of coding professionals at all levels by offering a comprehensive coding text at a reasonable price.

All material strictly adheres to the latest government versions available at the time of printing. Updates from the *Definitions of Medicare Code Edits* (MCE) will be posted to the companion website (www. codingupdates.com) when available.

Illustrations and Items

The ICD-10-CM Tabular List contains illustrations, pictures, and items to assist you in understanding difficult terminology, diseases/conditions, or coding in a specific category. Items are always printed in ▬▬▬ ink so that the added material is not mistaken for official notations or instructions. ▬▬▬ ink is used for other annotations in the text. Your ideas on what other descriptions or illustrations should be in future editions of this text are always appreciated.

Instructional Notations

Includes Notes

Includes

The word 'Includes' appears immediately under certain categories to further define, or give examples of, the content of the category.

Excludes Notes

The ICD-10-CM has two types of excludes notes. Each note has a different definition for use, but they are both similar in that they indicate that codes excluded from each other are independent of each other.

Excludes1

A type 1 Excludes note is a pure excludes. It means "NOT CODED HERE!" An Excludes1 note indicates that the code excluded should never be used at the same time as the code above the Excludes1 note. An Excludes1 is for use when two conditions cannot occur together, such as a congenital form versus an acquired form of the same condition.

Excludes2

A type 2 Excludes note represents "NOT INCLUDED HERE." An Excludes2 note indicates that the condition excluded is not part of the condition it is excluded from but a patient may have both conditions at the same time. When an Excludes2 note appears under a code, it is acceptable to use both the code and the excluded code together.

Code First/Use Additional Code notes (etiology/manifestation paired codes)

Certain conditions have both an underlying etiology and multiple body system manifestations due to the underlying etiology. For such conditions the ICD-10-CM has a coding convention that requires the underlying condition be sequenced first, followed by the manifestation. Wherever such a combination exists, there is a "use additional code" note at the etiology code, and a "code first" note at the manifestation code. These instructional notes indicate the proper sequencing order of the codes, etiology followed by manifestation.

In most cases the manifestation codes will have in the code title, "in diseases classified elsewhere." Codes with this title are a component of the etiology/manifestation convention. The code title indicates that it is a manifestation code. "In diseases classified elsewhere" codes are never permitted to be used as first-listed or principal diagnosis codes. They must be used in conjunction with an underlying condition code, and they must be listed following the underlying condition.

Use additional

The words indicate an instructional note that another code may be needed.

Code first

The words indicate an instructional note that directs the coder to sequence the underlying condition before the manifestation.

Code also

A "code also" note instructs that two codes may be required to fully describe a condition, but the sequencing of the two codes is discretionary, depending on the severity of the conditions and the reason for the encounter.

7th characters and placeholder X

For codes less than 6 characters that require a 7th character a placeholder X should be assigned for all characters less than 6. The 7th character must always be the 7th character of a code.

Annotated

Throughout the manual, revisions, additions, and deleted codes or words are indicated by the following symbols:

⇒ **Revised:** Revisions within the line or code from the previous edition are indicated by the arrow.
▶ **New:** Additions to the previous edition are indicated by the triangle.
~~deleted~~ **Deleted:** Deletions from the previous edition are struck through.

ICD-10-CM Tabular List Symbols

● **Use Additional Character(s):** The red stop sign cautions that the code requires additional character(s) to ensure the greatest specificity.

X   For codes less than 6 characters that require a 7th character, a placeholder X should be assigned for all characters less than 6. The 7th character must always be the 7th character of a code.

OGCR   The *Official Guidelines for Coding and Reporting* symbol includes the placement of a portion of a guideline as that guideline pertains to the code by which it is located. The complete OGCR are located in Part I.

Key words
Highlight identifies key words within similar code descriptions in a particular category.

SYMBOLS AND CONVENTIONS

ICD-10-CM Tabular

Use Additional Character(s): The stop sign cautions you that the code requires additional character(s) to ensure greatest specificity.

Volume 1, Tabular List

● **K22   Other diseases of esophagus**

     Excludes2   esophageal varices (I85.-)

X ● **V00.01   Pedestrian on foot injured in collision with roller-skater**

A02.20   Localized salmonella infection, unspecified

A48.3   Toxic shock syndrome
     Use additional code to identify the organism (B95, B96)

B39   Histoplasmosis
     Code first associated AIDS (B20)

E34.0   Carcinoid syndrome
     Note: May be used as an additional code to identify functional activity associated with a carcinoid tumor.

Placeholder X: The X reminds you that for codes less than 6 characters that require a 7th character, a placeholder X should be assigned to all characters less than 6.

Unspecified: These codes are for use when the information in the medical record is insufficient to assign a more specific code. For those categories for which an unspecified code is not provided, the "other specified" code may represent both other and unspecified.

Use additional code: Located at the etiology code and directs you to assign a manifestation code.

Code first indicates the etiology code is to be first-listed before the manifestation code.

Notes define terms or give coding instructions.

Codes or index entries are for purposes of illustration only and may not be current.

OGCR Section I.C.6.B.5.

Neoplasm Related Pain Code G89.3 is assigned to pain documented as being related, associated or due to cancer, primary or secondary malignancy, or tumor. This code is assigned regardless of whether the pain is acute or chronic.

OGCR: The *Official Guidelines for Coding and Reporting* are placed near the codes to which they refer and are highlighted.

I70.2 **Atherosclerosis of native arteries of the extremities**
Mönckeberg's (medial) sclerosis

Use additional code, if applicable, to identify chronic total occlusion of artery of extremity (I70.92)

code, if applicable, directs the coder to other conditions that may be appropriate to report.

The word "and" should be interpreted to mean either "and" or "or" when it appears in a statement.

I74   **Arterial embolism and thrombosis**
Includes   embolic infarction
embolic occlusion
thrombotic infarction
thrombotic occlusion

Bold typeface is used on all codes and titles.

I83.001 **Varicose veins of unspecified lower extremity with ulcer of thigh**

"with" should be interpreted to mean "associated with" or "due to."

K73.2 **Chronic active hepatitis, not elsewhere classified**

"not elsewhere classified" or **NEC** identifies a code that is assigned only when the information at hand specifies a condition for which no more specific code is available.

"not otherwise specified" or **NOS** is equivalent to unspecified.

W13.9 **Fall from, out of or through building, not otherwise specified**

M19 **Other and unspecified osteoarthritis**

Excludes1 means "NOT CODED HERE!" An Excludes1 note indicates that the code excluded should never be assigned at the same time as the code above the Excludes1 note.

Excludes1   polyarthritis (M15.-)
Excludes2   arthrosis of spine (M47.-)
hallux rigidus (M20.2)
osteoarthritis of spine (M47.-)

Excludes2 represents "NOT INCLUDED HERE." An Excludes2 note indicates that the condition excluded is not part of the condition represented by the code, but a patient may have both conditions at the same time and it is acceptable to use both the code and the excluded code together, when appropriate.

Includes: This note appears immediately under a three-character code title to further define, or give examples of, the content.

A06 **Amebiasis**
Includes   infection due to Entamoeba histolytica

Codes or index entries are for purposes of illustration only and may not be current.

E26.Ø1   Conn's syndrome
         Code also adrenal adenoma (D35.Ø)

Code also instructs that two codes may be required to fully describe a condition, but this note does not provide sequencing direction.

Codes titled "other" or "other specified" are for use when the information in the medical record provides detail for which a specific code does not exist.

E25.8   Other adrenogenital disorders

F10.21   Alcohol dependence, in remission

Key Term Highlight identifies key words within similar code descriptions in a particular category.

Alphabetic Index

Main terms are in **bold** typeface.

Aberrant (congenital) —*see also* Malposition, congenital
   adrenal gland Q89.1

Etiology code first followed by the manifestation code in **brackets**. The code in brackets is always to be sequenced second.

Amyloid heart (disease) E85.4 *[I43]*

Amylophagia —*see* Pica

"see" indicates another term should be referenced.

Angiofibroma —*see also* Neoplasm, benign, by site

"see also" follows a main term and instructs that there is another main term that may also be referenced.

Appendicitis (pneumococcal) (retrocecal) K37
   with
      perforation or rupture K35.2
      peritoneal abscess K35.3

Use Additional Character(s): The red stop sign cautions you that the code requires additional character(s) to ensure greatest specificity.

Abrasion T14.8
   ankle S90.51-•

A default code is listed next to the main term and represents that condition most commonly associated with the main term. If a condition is documented in a medical record without any additional information, such as acute or chronic, the default code should be assigned.

Codes or index entries are for purposes of illustration only and may not be current.

CHAPTER 1

CERTAIN INFECTIOUS AND PARASITIC DISEASES (A00-B99)

INTESTINAL INFECTIOUS DISEASES (A00-A09)

A04.7 Enterocolitis due to Clostridium difficile

New   **A04.71 Enterocolitis due to Clostridium difficile, recurrent**

New   **A04.72 Enterocolitis due to Clostridium difficile, not specified as recurrent**

A05 Other bacterial foodborne intoxications, not elsewhere classified

Revised   **Excludes1**   Clostridium difficile foodborne intoxication and infection (A04.7-)

HELMINTHIASES (B65-B83)

B81 Other intestinal helminthiases, not elsewhere classified

Revised   **Excludes1**   angiostrongyliasis due to:
New   Angiostrongylus cantonensis (B83.2)
New   Parastrongylus cantonensis (B83.2)

B81.3 Intestinal angiostrongyliasis
Revised   Angiostrongyliasis due to:
New   Angiostrongylus costaricensis (B83.2)
New   Parastrongylus costaricensis (B83.2)

CHAPTER 2

NEOPLASMS (C00-D49)

MALIGNANT NEOPLASMS OF ILL-DEFINED, OTHER SECONDARY AND UNSPECIFIED SITES (C76-C80)

C79 Secondary malignant neoplasm of other and unspecified sites
Deleted   **Excludes2**   lymph node metastases (C77.0)

     C79.11 Secondary malignant neoplasm of bladder
New   **Excludes2**   lymph node metastases (C77.0)

C86.4 Blastic NK-cell lymphoma
New   Blastic plasmacytoid dendritic cell neoplasm (BPDCN)

Revised   **C96.2 Malignant mast cell neoplasm**
Deleted   Aggressive systemic mastocytosis
Deleted   Mast cell sarcoma
Revised   **Excludes1**   indolent mastocytosis (D47.02)
New   **C96.20 Malignant mast cell neoplasm, unspecified**
New   **C96.21 Aggressive systemic mastocytosis**
New   **C96.22 Mast cell sarcoma**
New   **C96.29 Other malignant mast cell neoplasm**

NEOPLASMS OF UNCERTAIN BEHAVIOR, POLYCYTHEMIA VERA AND MYELODYSPLASTIC SYNDROMES (D37-D48)

Revised   **D47.0 Mast cell neoplasms of uncertain behavior**
Deleted   Indolent systemic mastocytosis
Deleted   Mast cell tumor NOS
Deleted   Mastocytoma NOS
     Excludes1
Deleted   malignant mast cell tumor (C96.2)
Deleted   mastocytosis (congenital) (cutaneous) (Q82.2)
New   congenital cutaneous mastocytosis (Q82.2-)
New   histiocytic neoplasms of uncertain behavior (D47.Z9)
New   malignant mast cell neoplasm (C96.2-)

New   **D47.01 Cutaneous mastocytosis**
New   Diffuse cutaneous mastocytosis
New   Maculopapular cutaneous mastocytosis
New   Solitary mastocytoma
New   Telangiectasia macularis eruptiva perstans
New   Urticaria pigmentosa
New   **Excludes1**   congenital (diffuse) (maculopapular) cutaneous mastocytosis (Q82.2)
New   congenital urticaria pigmentosa (Q82.2)
New   extracutaneous mastocytoma (D47.09)

New   **D47.02 Systemic mastocytosis**
New   Indolent systemic mastocytosis
New   Isolated bone marrow mastocytosis
New   Smoldering systemic mastocytosis
New   Systemic mastocytosis, with an associated hematological non-mast cell lineage disease (SM-AHNMD)
New   Code also if applicable, any associated hematological non-mast cell lineage disease, such as:
New   acute myeloid leukemia (C92.6-, C92.A-)
New   chronic myelomonocytic leukemia (C93.1-)
New   essential thrombocytosis (D47.3)
New   hypereosinophilic syndrome (D72.1)
New   myelodysplastic syndrome (D46.9)
New   myeloproliferative syndrome (D47.1)
New   non-Hodgkin lymphoma (C82-C85)
New   plasma cell myeloma (C90.0-)
New   polycythemia vera (D45)
New   **Excludes1**   aggressive systemic mastocytosis (C96.21)
New   mast cell leukemia (C94.3-)

New   **D47.09 Other mast cell neoplasms of uncertain behavior**
New   Extracutaneous mastocytoma
New   Mast cell tumor NOS
New   Mastocytoma NOS
New   Mastocytosis NOS

CHAPTER 3

DISEASES OF THE BLOOD AND BLOOD-FORMING ORGANS AND CERTAIN DISORDERS INVOLVING THE IMMUNE MECHANISM (D50-D89)

APLASTIC AND OTHER ANEMIAS AND OTHER BONE MARROW FAILURE SYNDROMES (D60-D64)

D63.0 **Anemia in neoplastic disease**

Deleted   **Excludes1** anemia due to antineoplastic chemotherapy (D64.81)

New   **Excludes2** anemia due to antineoplastic chemotherapy (D64.81)

CERTAIN DISORDERS INVOLVING THE IMMUNE MECHANISM (D80-D89)

D89.4 **Mast cell activation syndrome and related disorders**

Revised   **Excludes1** aggressive systemic mastocytosis (C96.21)

Revised   congenital cutaneous mastocytosis (Q82.2)

Deleted   indolent systemic mastocytosis (D47.0)

Deleted   malignant mastocytoma (C96.2)

New   (non-congenital) cutaneous mastocytosis (D47.01)

New   (indolent) systemic mastocytosis (D47.02)

New   malignant mast cell neoplasm (C96.2-)

New   malignant mastocytoma (C96.29)

Deleted   mastocytoma (D47.0)

Deleted   systemic mastocytosis associated with a clonal hematologic non-mast cell lineage disease (SM-AHNMD) (D47.0)

New   mast cell sarcoma (C96.22)

New   mastocytoma NOS (D47.09)

New   other mast cell neoplasms of uncertain behavior (D47.09)

New   systemic mastocytosis associated with a clonal hematologic non-mast cell lineage disease (SM-AHNMD) (D47.02)

CHAPTER 4

ENDOCRINE, NUTRITIONAL AND METABOLIC DISEASES (E00-E89)

DIABETES MELLITUS (E08-E13)

New   E11.1 **Type 2 diabetes mellitus with ketoacidosis**

New   E11.10 **Type 2 diabetes mellitus with ketoacidosis without coma**

New   E11.11 **Type 2 diabetes mellitus with ketoacidosis with coma**

E13 **Other specified diabetes mellitus**

Deleted   **Excludes1** type 2 diabetes mellitus (E11.-)

E13.00 **Other specified diabetes mellitus with hyperosmolarity without nonketotic hyperglycemic-hyperosmolar coma (NKHHC)**

New   **Excludes2** type 2 diabetes mellitus (E11.-)

OTHER DISORDERS OF GLUCOSE REGULATION AND PANCREATIC INTERNAL SECRETION (E15-E16)

E16.0 **Drug-induced hypoglycemia without coma**

Revised   **Excludes1** diabetes with hypoglycemia without coma (E09.649)

METABOLIC DISORDERS (E70-E88)

E78.00 **Pure hypercholesterolemia, unspecified**

New   (Pure) hypercholesterolemia NOS

E83.11 **Hemochromatosis**

New   **Excludes1** GALD (P78.84)

New   Gestational alloimmune liver disease (P78.84)

New   Neonatal hemochromatosis (P78.84)

E85 **Amyloidosis**

Deleted   **Excludes1** Alzheimer's disease (G30.0-)

New   **Excludes2** Alzheimer's disease (G30.0-)

E85.0 **Non-neuropathic heredofamilial amyloidosis**

New   Code also associated disorders, such as:

New   autoinflammatory syndromes (M04.-)

New   **Excludes2** Transthyretin-related (ATTR) familial amyloid cardiomyopathy (E85.4)

E85.1 **Neuropathic heredofamilial amyloidosis**

New   Transthyretin-related (ATTR) familial amyloid polyneuropathy

E85.4 **Organ-limited amyloidosis**

New   Transthyretin-related (ATTR) familial amyloid cardiomyopathy

E85.8 **Other amyloidosis**

New   E85.81 **Light chain (AL) amyloidosis**

New   E85.82 **Wild-type transthyretin-related (ATTR) amyloidosis**

New   Senile systemic amyloidosis (SSA)

New   E85.89 **Other amyloidosis**

CHAPTER 5

MENTAL, BEHAVIORAL AND NEURODEVELOPMENTAL DISORDERS (F01-F99)

MENTAL DISORDERS DUE TO KNOWN PHYSIOLOGICAL CONDITIONS (F01-F09)

F06.31 **Mood disorder due to known physiological condition with depressive features**

New   Depressive disorder due to known physiological condition, with depressive features

F06.32 **Mood disorder due to known physiological condition with major depressive-like episode**

New   Depressive disorder due to known physiological condition, with major depressive-like episode

F06.33 **Mood disorder due to known physiological condition with manic features**

New   Bipolar and related disorder due to a known physiological condition, with manic features

New   Bipolar and related disorder due to known physiological condition, with manic- or hypomanic-like episodes

F06.34 **Mood disorder due to known physiological condition with mixed features**

New   Bipolar and related disorder due to known physiological condition, with mixed features

New   Depressive disorder due to known physiological condition, with mixed features

F06.8 **Other specified mental disorders due to known physiological condition**

New   Obsessive-compulsive and related disorder due to a known physiological condition

MENTAL AND BEHAVIORAL DISORDERS DUE TO PSYCHOACTIVE SUBSTANCE USE (F10-F19)

New	**F10.11**	**Alcohol abuse, in remission**
New		Alcohol use disorder, mild, in early remission
New		Alcohol use disorder, mild, in sustained remission
	F10.21	**Alcohol dependence, in remission**
New		Alcohol use disorder, moderate, in early remission
New		Alcohol use disorder, moderate, in sustained remission
New		Alcohol use disorder, severe, in early remission
New		Alcohol use disorder, severe, in sustained remission
New	**F11.11**	**Opioid abuse, in remission**
New		Opioid use disorder, mild, in early remission
New		Opioid use disorder, mild, in sustained remission
	F11.21	**Opioid dependence, in remission**
New		Opioid use disorder, moderate, in early remission
New		Opioid use disorder, moderate, in sustained remission
New		Opioid use disorder, severe, in early remission
New		Opioid use disorder, severe, in sustained remission
New	**F12.11**	**Cannabis abuse, in remission**
New		Cannabis use disorder, mild, in early remission
		Cannabis use disorder, mild, in sustained remission
	F12.21	**Cannabis dependence, in remission**
New		Cannabis use disorder, moderate, in early remission
New		Cannabis use disorder, moderate, in sustained remission
New		Cannabis use disorder, severe, in early remission
New		Cannabis use disorder, severe, in sustained remission
New	**F13.11**	**Sedative, hypnotic or anxiolytic abuse, in remission**
New		Sedative, hypnotic or anxiolytic use disorder, mild, in early remission
New		Sedative, hypnotic or anxiolytic use disorder, mild, in sustained remission
	F13.14	**Sedative, hypnotic or anxiolytic abuse with sedative, hypnotic or anxiolytic-induced mood disorder**
Revised		Sedative, hypnotic, or anxiolytic use disorder, mild, with sedative, hypnotic, or anxiolytic-induced bipolar or related disorder
Revised		Sedative, hypnotic, or anxiolytic use disorder, mild, with sedative, hypnotic, or anxiolytic-induced depressive disorder
	F13.21	**Sedative, hypnotic or anxiolytic dependence, in remission**
New		Sedative, hypnotic or anxiolytic use disorder, moderate, in early remission
New		Sedative, hypnotic or anxiolytic use disorder, moderate, in sustained remission
New		Sedative, hypnotic or anxiolytic use disorder, severe, in early remission
New		Sedative, hypnotic or anxiolytic use disorder, severe, in sustained remission

	F13.24	**Sedative, hypnotic or anxiolytic dependence with sedative, hypnotic or anxiolytic-induced mood disorder**
Revised		Sedative, hypnotic, or anxiolytic use disorder, moderate, with sedative, hypnotic, or anxiolytic-induced bipolar or related disorder
Revised		Sedative, hypnotic, or anxiolytic use disorder, moderate, with sedative, hypnotic, or anxiolytic-induced depressive disorder
Revised		Sedative, hypnotic, or anxiolytic use disorder, severe, with sedative, hypnotic, or anxiolytic-induced depressive disorder
	F13.27	**Sedative, hypnotic or anxiolytic dependence with sedative, hypnotic or anxiolytic-induced persisting dementia**
Revised		Sedative, hypnotic, or anxiolytic use disorder, moderate, with sedative, hypnotic, or anxiolytic-induced major neurocognitive disorder
	F13.288	**Sedative, hypnotic or anxiolytic dependence with other sedative, hypnotic or anxiolytic-induced disorder**
Revised		Sedative, hypnotic, or anxiolytic use disorder, moderate, with sedative, hypnotic, or anxiolytic-induced mild neurocognitive disorder
Revised		Sedative, hypnotic, or anxiolytic use disorder, severe, with sedative, hypnotic, or anxiolytic-induced mild neurocognitive disorder
	F13.959	**Sedative, hypnotic or anxiolytic use, unspecified with sedative, hypnotic or anxiolytic-induced psychotic disorder, unspecified**
Revised		Sedative, hypnotic, or anxiolytic-induced psychotic disorder, without use disorder
	F13.97	**Sedative, hypnotic or anxiolytic use, unspecified with sedative, hypnotic or anxiolytic-induced persisting dementia**
Revised		Sedative, hypnotic, or anxiolytic-induced major neurocognitive disorder, without use disorder
	F13.980	**Sedative, hypnotic or anxiolytic use, unspecified with sedative, hypnotic or anxiolytic-induced anxiety disorder**
Revised		Sedative, hypnotic, or anxiolytic-induced anxiety disorder, without use disorder
	F13.981	**Sedative, hypnotic or anxiolytic use, unspecified with sedative, hypnotic or anxiolytic-induced sexual dysfunction**
Revised		Sedative, hypnotic, or anxiolytic-induced sexual dysfunction disorder, without use disorder
	F13.982	**Sedative, hypnotic or anxiolytic use, unspecified with sedative, hypnotic or anxiolytic-induced sleep disorder**
Revised		Sedative, hypnotic, or anxiolytic-induced sleep disorder, without use disorder
	F13.988	**Sedative, hypnotic or anxiolytic use, unspecified with other sedative, hypnotic or anxiolytic-induced disorder**
Revised		Sedative, hypnotic, or anxiolytic-induced mild neurocognitive disorder

New   **F14.11**   **Cocaine abuse, in remission**
New   Cocaine use disorder, mild, in early remission
New   Cocaine use disorder, mild, in sustained remission

New   **F14.21**   **Cocaine dependence, in remission**
New   Cocaine use disorder, moderate, in early remission
New   Cocaine use disorder, moderate, in sustained remission
New   Cocaine use disorder, severe, in early remission
New   Cocaine use disorder, severe, in sustained remission

New   **F15.11**   **Other stimulant abuse, in remission**
New   Amphetamine type substance use disorder, mild, in early remission
New   Amphetamine type substance use disorder, mild, in sustained remission
New   Other or unspecified stimulant use disorder, mild, in early remission
New   Other or unspecified stimulant use disorder, mild, in sustained remission

F15.21   **Other stimulant dependence, in remission**
New   Amphetamine type substance use disorder, moderate, in early remission
New   Amphetamine type substance use disorder, moderate, in sustained remission
New   Amphetamine type substance use disorder, severe, in early remission
New   Amphetamine type substance use disorder, severe, in sustained remission
New   Other or unspecified stimulant use disorder, moderate, in early remission
New   Other or unspecified stimulant use disorder, moderate, in sustained remission
New   Other or unspecified stimulant use disorder, severe, in early remission
New   Other or unspecified stimulant use disorder, severe, in sustained remission

F15.288   **Other stimulant dependence with other stimulant-induced disorder**
Revised   Amphetamine or other stimulant use disorder, moderate, with amphetamine or other stimulant-induced obsessive-compulsive or related disorder
Revised   Amphetamine or other stimulant use disorder, severe, with amphetamine or other stimulant-induced obsessive-compulsive or related disorder

F15.959   **Other stimulant use, unspecified with stimulant-induced psychotic disorder, unspecified**
Revised   Amphetamine or other stimulant-induced psychotic disorder, without use disorder

New   **F16.11**   **Hallucinogen abuse, in remission**
New   Other hallucinogen use disorder, mild, in early remission
New   Other hallucinogen use disorder, mild, in sustained remission
New   Phencyclidine use disorder, mild, in early remission
New   Phencyclidine use disorder, mild, in sustained remission

New   **F16.21**   **Hallucinogen dependence, in remission**
New   Other hallucinogen use disorder, moderate, in early remission
New   Other hallucinogen use disorder, moderate, in sustained remission
New   Other hallucinogen use disorder, severe, in early remission
New   Other hallucinogen use disorder, severe, in sustained remission
New   Phencyclidine use disorder, moderate, in early remission
New   Phencyclidine use disorder, moderate, in sustained remission
New   Phencyclidine use disorder, severe, in early remission
New   Phencyclidine use disorder, severe, in sustained remission

F17.201   **Nicotine dependence, unspecified, in remission**
New   Tobacco use disorder, mild, in early remission
New   Tobacco use disorder, mild, in sustained remission
New   Tobacco use disorder, moderate, in early remission
New   Tobacco use disorder, moderate, in sustained remission
New   Tobacco use disorder, severe, in early remission
New   Tobacco use disorder, severe, in sustained remission

F17.211   **Nicotine dependence, cigarettes, in remission**
New   Tobacco use disorder, cigarettes, mild, in early remission
New   Tobacco use disorder, cigarettes, mild, in sustained remission
New   Tobacco use disorder, cigarettes, moderate, in early remission
New   Tobacco use disorder, cigarettes, moderate, in sustained remission
New   Tobacco use disorder, cigarettes, severe, in early remission
New   Tobacco use disorder, cigarettes, severe, in sustained remission

F17.221   **Nicotine dependence, chewing tobacco, in remission**
New   Tobacco use disorder, chewing tobacco, mild, in early remission
New   Tobacco use disorder, chewing tobacco, mild, in sustained remission
New   Tobacco use disorder, chewing tobacco, moderate, in early remission
New   Tobacco use disorder, chewing tobacco, moderate, in sustained remission
New   Tobacco use disorder, chewing tobacco, severe, in early remission
New   Tobacco use disorder, chewing tobacco, severe, in sustained remission

	F17.291	**Nicotine dependence, other tobacco product, in remission**
New		Tobacco use disorder, other tobacco product, mild, in early remission
New		Tobacco use disorder, other tobacco product, mild, in sustained remission
New		Tobacco use disorder, other tobacco product, moderate, in early remission
New		Tobacco use disorder, other tobacco product, moderate, in sustained remission
New		Tobacco use disorder, other tobacco product, severe, in early remission
New		Tobacco use disorder, other tobacco product, severe, in sustained remission
New	**F18.11**	**Inhalant abuse, in remission**
New		Inhalant use disorder, mild, in early remission
New		Inhalant use disorder, mild, in sustained remission
	F18.21	**Inhalant dependence, in remission**
New		Inhalant use disorder, moderate, in early remission
New		Inhalant use disorder, moderate, in sustained remission
New		Inhalant use disorder, severe, in early remission
New		Inhalant use disorder, severe, in sustained remission
New	**F19.11**	**Other psychoactive substance abuse, in remission**
New		Other (or unknown) substance use disorder, mild, in early remission
New		Other (or unknown) substance use disorder, mild, in sustained remission
	F19.21	**Other psychoactive substance dependence, in remission**
New		Other (or unknown) substance use disorder, moderate, in early remission
New		Other (or unknown) substance use disorder, moderate, in sustained remission
New		Other (or unknown) substance use disorder, severe, in early remission
New		Other (or unknown) substance use, severe, in sustained remission

SCHIZOPHRENIA, SCHIZOTYPAL, DELUSIONAL, AND OTHER NON-MOOD PSYCHOTIC DISORDERS (F20-F29)

	F25.0	**Schizoaffective disorder, bipolar type**
Deleted		Schizophreniform psychosis, manic type
	F25.1	**Schizoaffective disorder, depressive type**
Deleted		Schizophreniform psychosis, depressive type
	F28	**Other psychotic disorder not due to a substance or known physiological condition**
New		Other specified schizophrenia spectrum and other psychotic disorder
	F29	**Unspecified psychosis not due to a substance or known physiological condition**
New		Unspecified schizophrenia spectrum and other psychotic disorder

MOOD [AFFECTIVE] DISORDERS (F30-F39)

	F31	**Bipolar disorder**
New		**Includes** bipolar I disorder
New		bipolar type I disorder
	F31.2	**Bipolar disorder, current episode manic severe with psychotic features**
New		Bipolar I disorder, current or most recent episode manic with psychotic features
	F31.5	**Bipolar disorder, current episode depressed, severe, with psychotic features**
New		Bipolar I disorder, current or most recent episode depressed, with psychotic features
	F31.8	**Other bipolar disorders**
	F31.81	**Bipolar II disorder**
New		Bipolar disorder, type 2
	F31.9	**Bipolar disorder, unspecified**
New		Manic depression
	F33.3	**Major depressive disorder, recurrent, severe with psychotic symptoms**
New		Major depressive disorder, recurrent, with psychotic features

ANXIETY, DISSOCIATIVE, STRESS-RELATED, SOMATOFORM AND OTHER NONPSYCHOTIC MENTAL DISORDERS (F40-F48)

	F40.1	**Social phobias**
New		Social anxiety disorder
Revised	**F41.0**	**Panic disorder [episodic paroxysmal anxiety]**
	F44.4	**Conversion disorder with motor symptom or deficit**
New		Conversion disorder with abnormal movement
New		Conversion disorder with speech symptoms
New		Conversion disorder with swallowing symptoms
New		Conversion disorder with weakness/paralysis
	F44.5	**Conversion disorder with seizures or convulsions**
New		Conversion disorder with attacks or seizures
	F44.6	**Conversion disorder with sensory symptom or deficit**
New		Conversion disorder with anesthesia or sensory loss
New		Conversion disorder with special sensory symptoms

BEHAVIORAL SYNDROMES ASSOCIATED WITH PHYSIOLOGICAL DISTURBANCES AND PHYSICAL FACTORS (F50-F59)

	F50	**Eating disorders**
New		**Excludes1** feeding problems of newborn (P92.-)
	F50.8	**Other eating disorders**
New		**F50.82** **Avoidant/restrictive food intake disorder**
	F50.9	**Eating disorder, unspecified**
New		Feeding or eating disorder, unspecified
New		Other specified feeding disorder
	F51.3	**Sleepwalking [somnambulism]**
New		Non-rapid eye movement sleep arousal disorders, sleepwalking type
	F51.4	**Sleep terrors [night terrors]**
New		Non-rapid eye movement sleep arousal disorders, sleep terror type
	F52.0	**Hypoactive sexual desire disorder**
New		Male hypoactive sexual desire disorder
	F52.21	**Male erectile disorder**
New		Erectile disorder
	F52.22	**Female sexual arousal disorder**
New		Female sexual interest/arousal disorder

DISORDERS OF ADULT PERSONALITY AND BEHAVIOR (F60-F69)

	F63.0	**Pathological gambling**
New		Gambling disorder

	F64.8	**Other gender identity disorders**
New		Other specified gender dysphoria
New	**F64.9**	**Gender identity disorder, unspecified**
		Gender dysphoria, unspecified

	F65.0	**Fetishism**
New		Fetishistic disorder
New	**F65.1**	**Transvestic fetishism**
		Transvestic disorder
New	**F65.2**	**Exhibitionism**
		Exhibitionistic disorder
New	**F65.3**	**Voyeurism**
		Voyeuristic disorder
New	**F65.4**	**Pedophilia**
		Pedophilic disorder

		F65.51	**Sexual masochism**
New			Sexual masochism disorder
New		**F65.52**	**Sexual sadism**
			Sexual sadism disorder
New		**F65.81**	**Frotteurism**
			Frotteuristic disorder
New		**F65.89**	**Other paraphilias**
			Other specified paraphilic disorder
New	**F65.9**	**Paraphilia, unspecified**
		Paraphilic disorder, unspecified

PERVASIVE AND SPECIFIC DEVELOPMENTAL DISORDERS (F80-F89)

	F81.0	**Specific reading disorder**
New		Specific learning disorder, with impairment in reading
New	**F81.2**	**Mathematics disorder**
		Specific learning disorder, with impairment in mathematics

		F81.81	**Disorder of written expression**
New			Specific learning disorder, with impairment in written expression

BEHAVIORAL AND EMOTIONAL DISORDERS WITH ONSET USUALLY OCCURRING IN CHILDHOOD AND ADOLESCENCE (F90-F98)

	F90.0	**Attention-deficit hyperactivity disorder, predominantly inattentive type**
New		Attention-deficit/hyperactivity disorder, predominantly inattentive presentation
	F90.1	**Attention-deficit hyperactivity disorder, predominantly hyperactive type**
New		Attention-deficit/hyperactivity disorder, predominantly hyperactive impulsive presentation
	F90.2	**Attention-deficit hyperactivity disorder, combined type**
New		Attention-deficit/hyperactivity disorder, combined presentation

CHAPTER 6

DISEASES OF THE NERVOUS SYSTEM (G00-G99)

INFLAMMATORY DISEASES OF THE CENTRAL NERVOUS SYSTEM (G00-G09)

	G00	**Bacterial meningitis, not elsewhere classified**
Revised		**Excludes1** bacterial meningoencephalitis (G04.2)
Revised		bacterial meningomyelitis (G04.2)
Deleted		meningomyelitis (G04.2)

SYSTEMIC ATROPHIES PRIMARILY AFFECTING THE CENTRAL NERVOUS SYSTEM (G10-G14)

	G10	**Huntington's disease**
New		Code also dementia in other diseases classified elsewhere without behavioral disturbance (F02.80)

	G12.21	**Amyotrophic lateral sclerosis**
Deleted		Progressive spinal muscle atrophy
New	**G12.23**	**Primary lateral sclerosis**
New	**G12.24**	**Familial motor neuron disease**
New	**G12.25**	**Progressive spinal muscle atrophy**
	G12.29	**Other motor neuron disease**
Deleted		Familial motor neuron disease
Deleted		Primary lateral sclerosis

EXTRAPYRAMIDAL AND MOVEMENT DISORDERS (G20-G26)

	G21.19	**Other drug induced secondary parkinsonism**
New		Other medication-induced parkinsonism
	G25.71	**Drug induced akathisia**
New		Tardive akathisia

OTHER DEGENERATIVE DISEASES OF THE NERVOUS SYSTEM (G30-G32)

	G31.84	**Mild cognitive impairment, so stated**
New		Mild neurocognitive disorder

EPISODIC AND PAROXYSMAL DISORDERS (G40-G47)

	G47.24	**Circadian rhythm sleep disorder, free running type**
New		Circadian rhythm sleep disorder, non-24-hour sleep-wake type
	G47.31	**Primary central sleep apnea**
New		Idiopathic central sleep apnea
	G47.33	**Obstructive sleep apnea (adult) (pediatric)**
New		Obstructive sleep apnea hypopnea
	G47.61	**Periodic limb movement disorder**
Deleted		Periodic limb movement disorder
	G47.8	**Other sleep disorders**
New		Other specified sleep-wake disorder
	G47.9	**Sleep disorder, unspecified**
New		Unspecified sleep-wake disorder

OTHER DISORDERS OF THE NERVOUS SYSTEM (G89-G99)

	G92	**Toxic encephalopathy**
New		*Code first if applicable, drug induced (T36-T50)*
	G93.7	**Reye's syndrome**
New		*Code first* (poisoning due to salicylates, if applicable (T39.0-, with sixth character 1-4)
Deleted		(T39.0-), if salicylates-induced
New		Use additional code for adverse effect due to salicylates, if applicable (T39.0-, with sixth character 5)

CHAPTER 7

DISEASES OF THE EYE AND ADNEXA (H00-H59)

DISORDERS OF EYELID, LACRIMAL SYSTEM AND ORBIT (H00-H05)

	H02.05	**Trichiasis without entropion**
Revised		
Revised	**H02.051**	**Trichiasis without entropion right upper eyelid**
Revised	**H02.052**	**Trichiasis without entropion right lower eyelid**
Revised	**H02.053**	**Trichiasis without entropion right eye, unspecified eyelid**
Revised	**H02.054**	**Trichiasis without entropion left upper eyelid**
Revised	**H02.055**	**Trichiasis without entropion left lower eyelid**
Revised	**H02.056**	**Trichiasis without entropion left eye, unspecified eyelid**
Revised	**H02.059**	**Trichiasis without entropion unspecified eye, unspecified eyelid**

GLAUCOMA (H40-H42)

H42   **Glaucoma in diseases classified elsewhere**
Code first underlying condition, such as:

New   glaucoma (in) diabetes mellitus (E08.39, E09.39, E10.39, E11.39, E13.39)

Deleted   Excludes2 glaucoma (in) diabetes mellitus (E08.39, E09.39, E10.39, E11.39, E13.39)

DISORDERS OF VITREOUS BODY AND GLOBE (H43-H44)

New   H44.2A   **Degenerative myopia with choroidal neovascularization**

New   Use Additional code for any associated choroid disorders (H31.-)

New   H44.2A1   **Degenerative myopia with choroidal neovascularization, right eye**

New   H44.2A2   **Degenerative myopia with choroidal neovascularization, left eye**

New   H44.2A3   **Degenerative myopia with choroidal neovascularization, bilateral eye**

New   H44.2A9   **Degenerative myopia with choroidal neovascularization, unspecified eye**

New   H44.2B   **Degenerative myopia with macular hole**

New   H44.2B1   **Degenerative myopia with macular hole, right eye**

New   H44.2B2   **Degenerative myopia with macular hole, left eye**

New   H44.2B3   **Degenerative myopia with macular hole, bilateral eye**

New   H44.2B9   **Degenerative myopia with macular hole, unspecified eye**

New   H44.2C   **Degenerative myopia with retinal detachment**

New   Use Additional code to identify the retinal detachment (H33.-)

New   H44.2C1   **Degenerative myopia with retinal detachment, right eye**

New   H44.2C2   **Degenerative myopia with retinal detachment, left eye**

New   H44.2C3   **Degenerative myopia with retinal detachment, bilateral eye**

New   H44.2C9   **Degenerative myopia with retinal detachment, unspecified eye**

New   H44.2D   **Degenerative myopia with foveoschisis**

New   H44.2D1   **Degenerative myopia with foveoschisis, right eye**

New   H44.2D2   **Degenerative myopia with foveoschisis, left eye**

New   H44.2D3   **Degenerative myopia with foveoschisis, bilateral eye**

New   H44.2D9   **Degenerative myopia with foveoschisis, unspecified eye**

New   H44.2E   **Degenerative myopia with other maculopathy**

New   H44.2E1   **Degenerative myopia with other maculopathy, right eye**

New   H44.2E2   **Degenerative myopia with other maculopathy, left eye**

New   H44.2E3   **Degenerative myopia with other maculopathy, bilateral eye**

New   H44.2E9   **Degenerative myopia with other maculopathy, unspecified eye**

VISUAL DISTURBANCES AND BLINDNESS (H53-H54)

New   H54.0X   **Blindness, both eyes, different category levels**

New   H54.0X3   **Blindness right eye, category 3**

New   H54.0X33   **Blindness right eye category 3, blindness left eye category 3**

New   H54.0X34   **Blindness right eye category 3, blindness left eye category 4**

New   H54.0X35   **Blindness right eye category 3, blindness left eye category 5**

New   H54.0X4   **Blindness right eye, category 4**

New   H54.0X43   **Blindness right eye category 4, blindness left eye category 3**

New   H54.0X44   **Blindness right eye category 4, blindness left eye category 4**

New   H54.0X45   **Blindness right eye category 4, blindness left eye category 5**

New   H54.0X5   **Blindness right eye, category 5**

New   H54.0X53   **Blindness right eye category 5, blindness left eye category 3**

New   H54.0X54   **Blindness right eye category 5, blindness left eye category 4**

New   H54.0X55   **Blindness right eye category 5, blindness left eye category 5**

New   H54.113   **Blindness right eye category 3, low vision left eye**

New   H54.1131   **Blindness right eye category 3, low vision left eye category 1**

New   H54.1132   **Blindness right eye category 3, low vision left eye category 2**

New   H54.114   **Blindness right eye category 4, low vision left eye**

New   H54.1141   **Blindness right eye category 4, low vision left eye category 1**

New   H54.1142   **Blindness right eye category 4, low vision left eye category 2**

New   H54.115   **Blindness right eye category 5, low vision left eye**

New   H54.1151   **Blindness right eye category 5, low vision left eye category 1**

New   H54.1152   **Blindness right eye category 5, low vision left eye category 2**

New		H54.121	Low vision right eye category 1, blindness left eye
New			H54.1213 Low vision right eye category 1, blindness left eye category 3
New			H54.1214 Low vision right eye category 1, blindness left eye category 4
New			H54.1215 Low vision right eye category 1, blindness left eye category 5
New		H54.122	Low vision right eye category 2, blindness left eye
New			H54.1223 Low vision right eye category 2, blindness left eye category 3
New			H54.1224 Low vision right eye category 2, blindness left eye category 4
New			H54.1225 Low vision right eye category 2, blindness left eye category 5
New	H54.2X		Low vision, both eyes, different category levels
New		H54.2X1	Low vision, right eye, category 1
New			H54.2X11 Low vision right eye category 1, low vision left eye category 1
New			H54.2X12 Low vision right eye category 1, low vision left eye category 2
New		H54.2X2	Low vision, right eye, category 2
New			H54.2X21 Low vision right eye category 2, low vision left eye category 1
New			H54.2X22 Low vision right eye category 2, low vision left eye category 2
New		H54.413	Blindness, right eye, category 3
New			H54.413A Blindness right eye category 3, normal vision left eye
New		H54.414	Blindness, right eye, category 4
New			H54.414A Blindness right eye category 4, normal vision left eye
New		H54.415	Blindness, right eye, category 5
New			H54.415A Blindness right eye category 5, normal vision left eye
New		H54.42A	Blindness, left eye, category 3-5
New			H54.42A3 Blindness left eye category 3, normal vision right eye
New			H54.42A4 Blindness left eye category 4, normal vision right eye
New			H54.42A5 Blindness left eye category 5, normal vision right eye

New		H54.511	Low vision, right eye, category 1-2
New			H54.511A Low vision right eye category 1, normal vision left eye
New			H54.512A Low vision right eye category 2, normal vision left eye
New		H54.52A	Low vision, left eye, category 1-2
New			H54.52A1 Low vision left eye category 1, normal vision right eye
New			H54.52A2 Low vision left eye category 2, normal vision right eye

CHAPTER 9

DISEASES OF THE CIRCULATORY SYSTEM (I00–I99)

HYPERTENSIVE DISEASES (I10–I16)

	I11	Hypertensive heart disease
Revised		**Includes** any condition in I50.-, I51.4-I51.9 due to hypertension

ISCHEMIC HEART DISEASES (I20–I25)

Revised	I21	Acute myocardial infarction
Revised		**Excludes2** subsequent type 1 myocardial infarction (I22.-)
	I21.0	ST elevation (STEMI) myocardial infarction of anterior wall
New		Type 1 ST elevation myocardial infarction of anterior wall
	I21.1	ST elevation (STEMI) myocardial infarction of inferior wall
New		Type 1 ST elevation myocardial infarction of inferior wall
	I21.2	ST elevation (STEMI) myocardial infarction of other sites
New		Type 1 ST elevation myocardial infarction of other sites
	I21.3	ST elevation (STEMI) myocardial infarction of unspecified site
Deleted		Myocardial infarction (acute) NOS
New		Type 1 ST elevation myocardial infarction of unspecified site
	I21.4	Non-ST elevation (NSTEMI) myocardial infarction
New		Type 1 non-ST elevation myocardial infarction
New	I21.9	Acute myocardial infarction, unspecified
New		Myocardial infarction (acute) NOS
New	I21.A	Other type of myocardial infarction
New	I21.A1	Myocardial infarction type 2
New		Myocardial infarction due to demand ischemia
New		Myocardial infarction secondary to ischemic imbalance
New		Code also the underlying cause, if known and applicable, such as:
New		anemia (D50.0-D64.9)
New		chronic obstructive pulmonary disease (J44.-)
New		heart failure (I50.-)
New		paroxysmal tachycardia (I47.0-I47.9)
New		renal failure (N17.0-N19)
New		shock (R57.0-R57.9)

New	**I21.A9**	**Other myocardial infarction type**
New		Myocardial infarction associated with revascularization procedure
New		Myocardial infarction type 3
New		Myocardial infarction type 4a
New		Myocardial infarction type 4b
New		Myocardial infarction type 4c
New		Myocardial infarction type 5
New		Code first, *if applicable, postprocedural myocardial infarction following cardiac surgery (I97.190), or postprocedural myocardial infarction during cardiac surgery (I97.790)*
New		Code also *complication, if known and applicable, such as:*
New		(acute) stent occlusion (T82.897-)
New		(acute) stent stenosis (T82.857-)
New		(acute) stent thrombosis (T82.867-)
New		cardiac arrest due to underlying cardiac condition (I46.2)
New		complication of percutaneous coronary intervention (PCI) (I97.89)
New		occlusion of coronary artery bypass graft (T82.218-)

	I22	**Subsequent ST elevation (STEMI) and non-ST elevation (NSTEMI) myocardial infarction**
New		**Includes** subsequent type 1 myocardial infarction
New		**Excludes1** subsequent myocardial infarction, type 2 (I21.A1)
New		subsequent myocardial infarction of other type (type 3) (type 4) (type 5) (I21.A9)

	I24.8	**Other forms of acute ischemic heart disease**
New		**Excludes1** myocardial infarction due to demand ischemia (I21.A1)

	I25.7	**Atherosclerosis of coronary artery bypass graft(s) and coronary artery of transplanted heart with angina pectoris**
Deleted		**Excludes1** embolism or thrombus of coronary artery bypass graft(s) (T82.8-)
	I25.710	**Atherosclerosis of autologous vein coronary artery bypass graft(s) with unstable angina pectoris**
New		**Excludes2** embolism or thrombus of coronary artery by-pass graft(s) (T82.8-)

	I25.82	**Chronic total occlusion of coronary artery**
Revised		**Excludes1** acute coronary occlusion with myocardial infarction (I21.0-I21.9, I22.-)
Revised		acute coronary occlusion without myocardial infarction (I24.0)

PULMONARY HEART DISEASE AND DISEASES OF PULMONARY CIRCULATION (I26-I28)

	I27.0	**Primary pulmonary hypertension**
New		Heritable pulmonary arterial hypertension
New		Idiopathic pulmonary arterial hypertension
New		Primary group 1 pulmonary hypertension
New		Primary pulmonary arterial hypertension
		Excludes1
Deleted		pulmonary hypertension NOS (I27.2)
Deleted		secondary pulmonary hypertension (I27.2)
New		persistent pulmonary hypertension of newborn (P29.30)
New		pulmonary hypertension NOS (I27.20)
New		secondary pulmonary arterial hypertension (I27.21)
New		secondary pulmonary hypertension (I27.29)

	I27.2	**Other secondary pulmonary hypertension**
Deleted		Pulmonary hypertension NOS
New		**Excludes1** Eisenmenger's syndrome (I27.83)
New	**I27.20**	**Pulmonary hypertension, unspecified**
New		Pulmonary hypertension NOS
New	**I27.21**	**Secondary pulmonary arterial hypertension**
New		(Associated) (drug-induced) (toxin-induced) pulmonary arterial hypertension NOS
New		(Associated) (drug-induced) (toxin-induced) (secondary) group 1 pulmonary hypertension
New		Code also *associated conditions if applicable, or adverse effects of drugs or toxins, such as:*
New		adverse effect of appetite depressants (T50.5X5)
New		congenital heart disease (Q20-Q28)
New		human immunodeficiency virus [HIV] disease (B20)
New		polymyositis (M33.2-)
New		portal hypertension (K76.6)
New		rheumatoid arthritis (M05.-)
New		schistosomiasis (B65.-)
New		Sjögren syndrome (M35.0-)
New		systemic sclerosis (M34.-)
New	**I27.22**	**Pulmonary hypertension due to left heart disease**
New		Group 2 pulmonary hypertension
New		Code also *associated left heart disease, if known, such as:*
New		multiple valve disease (I08.-)
New		rheumatic mitral valve diseases (I05.-)
New		rheumatic aortic valve diseases (I06.-)
New	**I27.23**	**Pulmonary hypertension due to lung diseases and hypoxia**
New		Group 3 pulmonary hypertension
New		Code also *associated lung disease, if known, such as:*
New		bronchiectasis (J47.-)
New		cystic fibrosis with pulmonary manifestations (E84.0)
New		interstitial lung disease (J84.-)
New		pleural effusion (J90)
New		sleep apnea (G47.3-)
New	**I27.24**	**Chronic thromboembolic pulmonary hypertension**
New		Group 4 pulmonary hypertension
New		Code also *associated pulmonary embolism, if applicable (I26.-, I27.82)*
New	**I27.29**	**Other secondary pulmonary hypertension**
New		Group 5 pulmonary hypertension
New		Pulmonary hypertension with unclear multifactorial mechanisms
New		Pulmonary hypertension due to hematologic disorders
New		Pulmonary hypertension due to metabolic disorders
New		Pulmonary hypertension due to other systemic disorders
New		Code also *other associated disorders, if known, such as:*
New		chronic myeloid leukemia (C92.10-C92.22)
New		essential thrombocythemia (D47.3)
New		Gaucher disease (E75.22)
New		hypertensive chronic kidney disease with end stage renal disease (I12.0, I12.11, I13.2)
New		hyperthyroidism (E05.-)
New		hypothyroidism (E00-E03)
New		polycythemia vera (D45)
New		sarcoidosis (D86.-)

New   I27.83   **Eisenmenger's syndrome**
New   Eisenmenger's complex
New   (Irreversible) Eisenmenger's disease
New   Pulmonary hypertension with right
                    to left shunt related to congenital
                    heart disease
New   Code also underlying heart defect, if
                    known, such as:
New   atrial septal defect (Q21.1)
New   Eisenmenger's defect (Q21.8)
New   patent ductus arteriosus (Q25.0)
New   ventricular septal defect (Q21.0)
           I27.89   **Other specified pulmonary heart diseases**
Deleted   Eisenmenger's complex
Deleted   Eisenmenger's syndrome
Deleted   Excludes1 Eisenmenger's defect
                                 (Q21.8)

OTHER FORMS OF HEART DISEASE (I30-I52)

           I30   **Acute pericarditis**
New   Excludes1 viral pericarditis due to Coxsakie virus
                                 (B33.23)

           I34   **Nonrheumatic mitral valve disorders**
Revised   Excludes1 mitral valve disorder specified as
                                 congenital (Q23.2, Q23.9)

           I49   **Other cardiac arrhythmias**
Deleted   Excludes1 bradycardia NOS (R00.1)
New   Excludes2 bradycardia NOS (R00.1)
           I49.8   **Other specified cardiac arrhythmias**
New   Brugada syndrome

           I50   **Heart failure**
Revised   I50.1   **Left ventricular failure, unspecified**
             I50.2   **Systolic (congestive) heart failure**
New   Heart failure with reduced ejection fraction
                     [HFrEF]
New   Systolic left ventricular heart failure
New   Code also end stage heart failure, if applicable
                     (I50.84)
             I50.3   **Diastolic (congestive) heart failure**
New   Diastolic left ventricular heart failure
New   Heart failure with normal ejection fraction
New   Heart failure with preserved ejection fraction
                     [HFpEF]
New   Code also end stage heart failure, if applicable
                     (I50.84)
             I50.4   **Combined systolic (congestive) and diastolic (congestive) heart failure**
New   Combined systolic and diastolic left ventricular
                     heart failure
New   Heart failure with reduced ejection fraction and
                     diastolic dysfunction
New   Code also end stage heart failure, if applicable
                     (I50.84)
New   I50.8   **Other heart failure**
New   I50.81   **Right heart failure**
New   Right ventricular failure
New   I50.810   **Right heart failure, unspecified**
New   Right heart failure without
                           mention of left heart
                           failure
                           Right ventricular failure NOS
New   I50.811   **Acute right heart failure**
New   Acute isolated right heart
                           failure
New   Acute (isolated) right
                           ventricular failure
New   I50.812   **Chronic right heart failure**
New   Chronic isolated right heart
                           failure
New   Chronic (isolated) right
                           ventricular failure

New   I50.813   **Acute on chronic right heart failure**
New   Acute on chronic isolated
                           right heart failure
New   Acute on chronic (isolated)
                           right ventricular failure
New   Acute decompensation of
                           chronic (isolated) right
                           ventricular failure
New   Acute exacerbation of
                           chronic (isolated) right
                           ventricular failure
New   I50.814   **Right heart failure due to left heart failure**
New   Right ventricular failure
                           secondary to left
                           ventricular failure
New   Code also the type of left
                           ventricular failure, if
                           known (I50.2-I50.43)
New   Excludes1 Right heart fail-
                                        ure with but
                                        not due to
                                        left heart fail-
                                        ure (I50.82)

New   I50.82   **Biventricular heart failure**
New   Code also the type of left ventricular
                      failure as systolic, diastolic, or
                      combined, if known (I50.2-I50.43)
New   I50.83   **High output heart failure**
New   I50.84   **End stage heart failure**
New   Stage D heart failure
New   Code also the type of heart failure as
                      systolic, diastolic, or combined, if
                      known (I50.2-I50.43)
New   I50.89   **Other heart failure**
             I50.9   **Heart failure, unspecified**
Deleted   Biventricular (heart) failure NOS
Deleted   Right ventricular failure (secondary to left heart
                     failure)

CEREBROVASCULAR DISEASES (I60-I69)

Deleted   Excludes1 transient cerebral ischemic attacks and
                                 related syndromes (G45.-)

           I60   **Nontraumatic subarachnoid hemorrhage**
Deleted   Includes ruptured cerebral aneurysm

Revised   I63.211   **Cerebral infarction due to unspecified occlusion or stenosis of right vertebral artery**
Revised   I63.212   **Cerebral infarction due to unspecified occlusion or stenosis of left vertebral artery**
Revised   I63.22   **Cerebral infarction due to unspecified occlusion or stenosis of basilar artery**
Revised   I63.323   **Cerebral infarction due to thrombosis of bilateral anterior cerebral arteries**
Revised   I63.333   **Cerebral infarction to thrombosis of bilateral posterior cerebral arteries**
Revised   I63.513   **Cerebral infarction due to unspecified occlusion or stenosis of bilateral middle cerebral arteries**
Revised   I63.523   **Cerebral infarction due to unspecified occlusion or stenosis of bilateral anterior cerebral arteries**
Revised   I63.533   **Cerebral infarction due to unspecified occlusion or stenosis of bilateral posterior cerebral arteries**

I63.9   Cerebral infarction, unspecified
New   Excludes2 transient cerebral ischemic attacks
                              and related syndromes (G45.-)

I67.4   Hypertensive encephalopathy
New   Excludes2 insufficiency, NOS, of precerebral
                              arteries (G45.2)

I69   Sequelae of cerebrovascular disease
Deleted   Excludes1 transient ischemic attack (TIA) (G45.9)

        I69.322 Dysarthria following cerebral
                 infarction
New   Excludes2 transient
                                       ischemic
                                       attack (TIA)
                                       (G45.9)

        I69.351 Hemiplegia and hemiparesis
                 following cerebral infarction
                 affecting right dominant side
New   Excludes2 transient
                                       ischemic
                                       attack (TIA)
                                       (G45.9)

DISEASES OF ARTERIES, ARTERIOLES AND CAPILLARIES (I70-I79)

I72   Other aneurysm
New   Excludes2 precerebral artery, congenital (nonruptured)
                              (Q28.1)

DISEASES OF VEINS, LYMPHATIC VESSELS AND LYMPH NODES, NOT ELSEWHERE CLASSIFIED (I80-I89)

Revised   I82.811 Embolism and thrombosis of
                      superficial veins of right lower
                      extremity

Revised   I82.812 Embolism and thrombosis of
                      superficial veins of left lower
                      extremity

Revised   I82.819 Embolism and thrombosis of
                      superficial veins of unspecified
                      lower extremity

Revised   I83.811 Varicose veins of right lower
                      extremity with pain

Revised   I83.812 Varicose veins of left lower
                      extremity with pain

Revised   I83.819 Varicose veins of unspecified
                      lower extremity with pain

Revised   I83.891 Varicose veins of right
                      lower extremity with other
                      complications

Revised   I83.892 Varicose veins of left
                      lower extremity with other
                      complications

Revised   I83.899 Varicose veins of unspecified
                      lower extremity with other
                      complications

OTHER AND UNSPECIFIED DISORDERS OF THE CIRCULATORY SYSTEM (I95-I99)

I96   Gangrene, not elsewhere classified
Deleted   Excludes1 gangrene in diabetes mellitus
                              (E08-E13 with .52)
New   Excludes2 gangrene in diabetes mellitus (E08-E13
                              with .52)

        I97.190 Other postprocedural cardiac
                 functional disturbances
                 following cardiac surgery
New   Use Additional code, if
                 applicable, for type 4
                 or type 5 myocardial
                 infarction, to further
                 specify disorder

CHAPTER 10

DISEASES OF THE RESPIRATORY SYSTEM (J00-J99)

INFLUENZA AND PNEUMONIA (J09-J18)

J09   Influenza due to certain identified influenza viruses
New   Excludes1 influenza A/H1N1 (J10.-)

Revised J15.6   Pneumonia due to other Gram-negative bacteria
New   Pneumonia due to other aerobic Gram-negative
                   bacteria

CHRONIC LOWER RESPIRATORY DISEASES (J40-J47)

J44   Other chronic obstructive pulmonary disease
Deleted   Excludes2 lung diseases due to external agents
                              (J60-J70)

        J44.0   Chronic obstructive pulmonary disease with
                 acute lower respiratory infection
Deleted   Use additional code to identify the infection
New   Code also to identify the infection

        J44.1   Chronic obstructive pulmonary disease with
                 (acute) exacerbation
New   Excludes2 lung diseases due to external
                                       agents (J60-J70)

        J44.9   Chronic obstructive pulmonary disease,
                 unspecified
New   Excludes2 lung diseases due to external
                                       agents (J60-J70)

J45   Asthma
Deleted   Excludes1 lung diseases due to external agents
                              (J60-J70)

        J45.909 Unspecified asthma,
                 uncomplicated
New   Excludes2 lung diseases
                                       due to exter-
                                       nal agents
                                       (J60-J70)

OTHER RESPIRATORY DISEASES PRINCIPALLY AFFECTING THE INTERSTITIUM (J80-J84)

J84   Other interstitial pulmonary diseases
Deleted   Excludes1 lung diseases due to external agents
                              (J60-J70)
New   Excludes2 lung diseases due to external agents
                              (J60-J70)

INTRAOPERATIVE AND POSTPROCEDURAL COMPLICATIONS AND DISORDERS OF RESPIRATORY SYSTEM, NOT ELSEWHERE CLASSIFIED (J95)

        J95.02   Infection of tracheostomy stoma
                 Use additional code to identify type of
                 infection, such as:
Revised   cellulitis of neck (L03.221)

CHAPTER 11

DISEASES OF THE DIGESTIVE SYSTEM (K00-K95)

DISEASES OF ORAL CAVITY AND SALIVARY GLANDS (K00-K14)

        K04.7   Periapical abscess without sinus
Deleted   Periapical abscess without sinus

        K06.0   Gingival recession
Revised   Gingival recession (postinfective)
                 (postprocedural)
New   K06.01   Gingival recession, localized
New   K06.010 Localized gingival recession,
                                   unspecified
                                   Localized gingival recession,
                                   NOS
New   K06.011 Localized gingival recession,
                                   minimal

New	K06.012	Localized gingival recession, moderate
New	K06.013	Localized gingival recession, severe
New	K06.02	Gingival recession, generalized
New	K06.020	Generalized gingival recession, unspecified
		Generalized gingival recession, NOS
New	K06.021	Generalized gingival recession, minimal
New	K06.022	Generalized gingival recession, moderate
New	K06.023	Generalized gingival recession, severe

OTHER DISEASES OF INTESTINES (K55-K64)

	K55.3	Necrotizing enterocolitis
Revised		Excludes2 necrotizing enterocolitis due to Clostridium difficile (A04.7-)
	K56	Paralytic ileus and intestinal obstruction without hernia
Revised		Excludes1 postprocedural intestinal obstruction (K91.3-)
Deleted		intestinal obstruction with hernia (K40-K46)
	K56.0	Paralytic ileus
Revised		Excludes1 obstructive ileus NOS (K56.69-)
Revised	K56.5	Intestinal adhesions [bands] with obstruction (postinfection)
Revised		Peritoneal adhesions [bands] with intestinal obstruction (postinfection)
New	K56.50	Intestinal adhesions [bands], unspecified as to partial versus complete obstruction
New		Intestinal adhesions with obstruction NOS
New	K56.51	Intestinal adhesions [bands], with partial obstruction
New		Intestinal adhesions with incomplete obstruction
New	K56.52	Intestinal adhesions [bands] with complete obstruction
	K56.60	Unspecified intestinal obstruction
Deleted		Intestinal obstruction NOS
New	K56.600	Partial intestinal obstruction, unspecified as to cause
New		Incomplete intestinal obstruction, NOS
New	K56.601	Complete intestinal obstruction, unspecified as to cause
New	K56.609	Unspecified intestinal obstruction, unspecified as to partial versus complete obstruction
New		Intestinal obstruction NOS
New	K56.690	Other partial intestinal obstruction
New		Other incomplete intestinal obstruction
New	K56.691	Other complete intestinal obstruction
New	K56.699	Other intestinal obstruction unspecified as to partial versus complete obstruction
New		Other intestinal obstruction, NEC
	K56.7	Ileus, unspecified
Revised		Excludes1 obstructive ileus (K56.69-)
New		Excludes2 intestinal obstruction with hernia (K40-K46)
	K59.3	Megacolon, not elsewhere classified
Revised		Excludes1 megacolon (due to) (in) Clostridium difficile (A04.7-)

DISEASES OF PERITONEUM AND RETROPERITONEUM (K65-K68)

	K66.0	Peritoneal adhesions (postprocedural) (postinfection)
Revised		Excludes1 peritoneal adhesions with intestinal obstruction (K56.5-)

OTHER DISEASES OF THE DIGESTIVE SYSTEM (K90-K95)

	K90.0	Celiac disease
Revised		Celiac gluten-sensitive enteropathy
	K90.4	Other malabsorption due to intolerance
Revised		Excludes2 celiac gluten-sensitive enteropathy (K90.0)
New	K91.30	Postprocedural intestinal obstruction, unspecified as to partial versus complete
New		Postprocedural intestinal obstruction NOS
New	K91.31	Postprocedural partial intestinal obstruction
New		Postprocedural incomplete intestinal obstruction
New	K91.32	Postprocedural complete intestinal obstruction

CHAPTER 12

DISEASES OF THE SKIN AND SUBCUTANEOUS TISSUE (L00-L99)

RADIATION-RELATED DISORDERS OF THE SKIN AND SUBCUTANEOUS TISSUE (L55-L59)

	L57	Skin changes due to chronic exposure to nonionizing radiation
Revised		Use additional code to identify the source of the ultraviolet radiation (W89)

OTHER DISORDERS OF THE SKIN AND SUBCUTANEOUS TISSUE (L80-L99)

	L89.019	Pressure ulcer of right elbow, unspecified stage
Revised		Healing pressure ulcer of right elbow, unspecified stage
	L89.029	Pressure ulcer of left elbow, unspecified stage
Revised		Healing pressure ulcer of left elbow, unspecified stage
	L89.619	Pressure ulcer of right heel, unspecified stage
Revised		Healing pressure ulcer of right heel, unspecified stage
	L92.9	Granulomatous disorder of the skin and subcutaneous tissue, unspecified
New		Excludes2 umbilical granuloma (P83.81)
New	L97.105	Non-pressure chronic ulcer of unspecified thigh with muscle involvement without evidence of necrosis
New	L97.106	Non-pressure chronic ulcer of unspecified thigh with bone involvement without evidence of necrosis
New	L97.108	Non-pressure chronic ulcer of unspecified thigh with other specified severity
New	L97.115	Non-pressure chronic ulcer of right thigh with muscle involvement without evidence of necrosis
New	L97.116	Non-pressure chronic ulcer of right thigh with bone involvement without evidence of necrosis

New	L97.118	Non-pressure chronic ulcer of right thigh with other specified severity	*New*	L97.326	Non-pressure chronic ulcer of left ankle with bone involvement without evidence of necrosis
New	L97.125	Non-pressure chronic ulcer of left thigh with muscle involvement without evidence of necrosis	*New*	L97.328	Non-pressure chronic ulcer of left ankle with other specified severity
New	L97.126	Non-pressure chronic ulcer of left thigh with bone involvement without evidence of necrosis	*New*	L97.405	Non-pressure chronic ulcer of unspecified heel and midfoot with muscle involvement without evidence of necrosis
New	L97.128	Non-pressure chronic ulcer of left thigh with other specified severity	*New*	L97.406	Non-pressure chronic ulcer of unspecified heel and midfoot with bone involvement without evidence of necrosis
New	L97.205	Non-pressure chronic ulcer of unspecified calf with muscle involvement without evidence of necrosis	*New*	L97.408	Non-pressure chronic ulcer of unspecified heel and midfoot with other specified severity
New	L97.206	Non-pressure chronic ulcer of unspecified calf with bone involvement without evidence of necrosis	*New*	L97.415	Non-pressure chronic ulcer of right heel and midfoot with muscle involvement without evidence of necrosis
New	L97.208	Non-pressure chronic ulcer of unspecified calf with other specified severity	*New*	L97.416	Non-pressure chronic ulcer of right heel and midfoot with bone involvement without evidence of necrosis
New	L97.215	Non-pressure chronic ulcer of right calf with muscle involvement without evidence of necrosis	*New*	L97.418	Non-pressure chronic ulcer of right heel and midfoot with other specified severity
New	L97.216	Non-pressure chronic ulcer of right calf with bone involvement without evidence of necrosis	*New*	L97.425	Non-pressure chronic ulcer of left heel and midfoot with muscle involvement without evidence of necrosis
New	L97.218	Non-pressure chronic ulcer of right calf with other specified severity	*New*	L97.426	Non-pressure chronic ulcer of left heel and midfoot with bone involvement without evidence of necrosis
New	L97.225	Non-pressure chronic ulcer of left calf with muscle involvement without evidence of necrosis	*New*	L97.428	Non-pressure chronic ulcer of left heel and midfoot with other specified severity
New	L97.226	Non-pressure chronic ulcer of left calf with bone involvement without evidence of necrosis	*New*	L97.505	Non-pressure chronic ulcer of other part of unspecified foot with muscle involvement without evidence of necrosis
New	L97.228	Non-pressure chronic ulcer of left calf with other specified severity	*New*	L97.506	Non-pressure chronic ulcer of other part of unspecified foot with bone involvement without evidence of necrosis
New	L97.305	Non-pressure chronic ulcer of unspecified ankle with muscle involvement without evidence of necrosis	*New*	L97.508	Non-pressure chronic ulcer of other part of unspecified foot with other specified severity
New	L97.306	Non-pressure chronic ulcer of unspecified ankle with bone involvement without evidence of necrosis	*New*	L97.515	Non-pressure chronic ulcer of other part of right foot with muscle involvement without evidence of necrosis
New	L97.308	Non-pressure chronic ulcer of unspecified ankle with other specified severity	*New*	L97.516	Non-pressure chronic ulcer of other part of right foot with bone involvement without evidence of necrosis
New	L97.315	Non-pressure chronic ulcer of right ankle with muscle involvement without evidence of necrosis	*New*	L97.518	Non-pressure chronic ulcer of other part of right foot with other specified severity
New	L97.316	Non-pressure chronic ulcer of right ankle with bone involvement without evidence of necrosis	*New*	L97.525	Non-pressure chronic ulcer of other part of left foot with muscle involvement without evidence of necrosis
New	L97.318	Non-pressure chronic ulcer of right ankle with other specified severity	*New*	L97.526	Non-pressure chronic ulcer of other part of left foot with bone involvement without evidence of necrosis
New	L97.325	Non-pressure chronic ulcer of left ankle with muscle involvement without evidence of necrosis	*New*	L97.528	Non-pressure chronic ulcer of other part of left foot with other specified severity

New	L97.805	Non-pressure chronic ulcer of other part of unspecified lower leg with muscle involvement without evidence of necrosis
New	L97.806	Non-pressure chronic ulcer of other part of unspecified lower leg with bone involvement without evidence of necrosis
New	L97.808	Non-pressure chronic ulcer of other part of unspecified lower leg with other specified severity
New	L97.815	Non-pressure chronic ulcer of other part of right lower leg with muscle involvement without evidence of necrosis
New	L97.816	Non-pressure chronic ulcer of other part of right lower leg with bone involvement without evidence of necrosis
New	L97.818	Non-pressure chronic ulcer of other part of right lower leg with other specified severity
New	L97.825	Non-pressure chronic ulcer of other part of left lower leg with muscle involvement without evidence of necrosis
New	L97.826	Non-pressure chronic ulcer of other part of left lower leg with bone involvement without evidence of necrosis
New	L97.828	Non-pressure chronic ulcer of other part of left lower leg with other specified severity
New	L97.905	Non-pressure chronic ulcer of unspecified part of unspecified lower leg with muscle involvement without evidence of necrosis
New	L97.906	Non-pressure chronic ulcer of unspecified part of unspecified lower leg with bone involvement without evidence of necrosis
New	L97.908	Non-pressure chronic ulcer of unspecified part of unspecified lower leg with other specified severity
New	L97.915	Non-pressure chronic ulcer of unspecified part of right lower leg with muscle involvement without evidence of necrosis
New	L97.916	Non-pressure chronic ulcer of unspecified part of right lower leg with bone involvement without evidence of necrosis
New	L97.918	Non-pressure chronic ulcer of unspecified part of right lower leg with other specified severity
New	L97.925	Non-pressure chronic ulcer of unspecified part of left lower leg with muscle involvement without evidence of necrosis
New	L97.926	Non-pressure chronic ulcer of unspecified part of left lower leg with bone involvement without evidence of necrosis
New	L97.928	Non-pressure chronic ulcer of unspecified part of left lower leg with other specified severity

New	L98.415	Non-pressure chronic ulcer of buttock with muscle involvement without evidence of necrosis
New	L98.416	Non-pressure chronic ulcer of buttock with bone involvement without evidence of necrosis
New	L98.418	Non-pressure chronic ulcer of buttock with other specified severity
New	L98.425	Non-pressure chronic ulcer of back with muscle involvement without evidence of necrosis
New	L98.426	Non-pressure chronic ulcer of back with bone involvement without evidence of necrosis
New	L98.428	Non-pressure chronic ulcer of back with other specified severity
New	L98.495	Non-pressure chronic ulcer of other sites with muscle involvement without evidence of necrosis
New	L98.496	Non-pressure chronic ulcer of other sites with bone involvement without evidence of necrosis
New	L98.498	Non-pressure chronic ulcer of other sites with other specified severity

CHAPTER 13

DISEASES OF THE MUSCULOSKELETAL SYSTEM AND CONNECTIVE TISSUE (M00-M99)

This chapter contains the following blocks:

Deleted	M04	Autoinflammatory syndromes
Deleted	M97	Periprosthetic fracture around internal prosthetic joint

SYSTEMIC CONNECTIVE TISSUE DISORDERS (M30-M36)

Revised	M33.0	Juvenile dermatomyositis
Revised	M33.00	Juvenile dermatomyositis, organ involvement unspecified
Revised	M33.01	Juvenile dermatomyositis with respiratory involvement
Revised	M33.02	Juvenile dermatomyositis with myopathy
New	M33.03	Juvenile dermatomyositis without myopathy
Revised	M33.09	Juvenile dermatomyositis with other organ involvement
Revised	M33.1	Other dermatomyositis
New		Adult dermatomyositis
Revised	M33.10	Other dermatomyositis, organ involvement unspecified
Revised	M33.11	Other dermatomyositis with respiratory involvement
Revised	M33.12	Other dermatomyositis with myopathy
New	M33.13	Other dermatomyositis without myopathy
New		Dermatomyositis NOS
Revised	M33.19	Other dermatomyositis with other organ involvement
New	M33.93	Dermatopolymyositis, unspecified without myopathy

SPONDYLOPATHIES (M45-M49)

New   M48.061 Spinal stenosis, lumbar region without neurogenic claudication

New   Spinal stenosis, lumbar region NOS

New   M48.062 Spinal stenosis, lumbar region with neurogenic claudication

DISORDERS OF MUSCLES (M60-M63)

M62.5 Muscle wasting and atrophy, not elsewhere classified

Revised   Excludes1 progressive muscular atrophy (G12.21)

CHAPTER 14

DISEASES OF THE GENITOURINARY SYSTEM (N00-N99)

RENAL TUBULO-INTERSTITIAL DISEASES (N10-N16)

N13 Obstructive and reflux uropathy

Revised   Excludes2 hydronephrosis with ureteropelvic junction obstruction (Q62.11)

ACUTE KIDNEY FAILURE AND CHRONIC KIDNEY DISEASE (N17-N19)

N18.9 Chronic kidney disease, unspecified

Revised   Chronic uremia NOS

New   Diffuse sclerosing glomerulonephritis NOS

OTHER DISORDERS OF KIDNEY AND URETER (N25-N29)

N25 Disorders resulting from impaired renal tubular function

Deleted   Excludes1 metabolic disorders classifiable to E70-E88

N25.0 Renal osteodystrophy

New   Excludes2 metabolic disorders classifiable to E70-E88

N25.81 Secondary hyperparathyroidism of renal origin

New   Excludes2 metabolic disorders classifiable to E70-E88

N28.1 Cyst of kidney, acquired

Revised   Cyst (multiple) (solitary) of kidney, (acquired)

OTHER DISEASES OF THE URINARY SYSTEM (N30-N39)

Revised   N35.112 Postinfective bulbous urethral stricture, not elsewhere classified, male

Revised   N35.113 Postinfective membranous urethral stricture, not elsewhere classified, male

Revised   N35.114 Postinfective anterior urethral stricture, not elsewhere classified, male

DISORDERS OF BREAST (N60-N65)

New   N63.0 Unspecified lump in unspecified breast

New   N63.1 Unspecified lump in the right breast

New   N63.10 Unspecified lump in the right breast, unspecified quadrant

New   N63.11 Unspecified lump in the right breast, upper outer quadrant

New   N63.12 Unspecified lump in the right breast, upper inner quadrant

New   N63.13 Unspecified lump in the right breast, lower outer quadrant

New   N63.14 Unspecified lump in the right breast, lower inner quadrant

New   N63.2 Unspecified lump in the left breast

New   N63.20 Unspecified lump in the left breast, unspecified quadrant

New   N63.21 Unspecified lump in the left breast, upper outer quadrant

New   N63.22 Unspecified lump in the left breast, upper inner quadrant

New   N63.23 Unspecified lump in the left breast, lower outer quadrant

New   N63.24 Unspecified lump in the left breast, lower inner quadrant

New   N63.3 Unspecified lump in axillary tail

New   N63.31 Unspecified lump in axillary tail of the right breast

New   N63.32 Unspecified lump in axillary tail of the left breast

New   N63.4 Unspecified lump in breast, subareolar

New   N63.41 Unspecified lump in right breast, subareolar

New   N63.42 Unspecified lump in left breast, subareolar

NONINFLAMMATORY DISORDERS OF FEMALE GENITAL TRACT (N80-N98)

N80.8 Other endometriosis

New   Endometriosis of thorax

N81.2 Incomplete uterovaginal prolapse

Revised   Excludes1 cervical stump prolapse (N81.85)

N94.3 Premenstrual tension syndrome

Deleted   Premenstrual dysphoric disorder

INTRAOPERATIVE AND POSTPROCEDURAL COMPLICATIONS AND DISORDERS OF GENITOURINARY SYSTEM, NOT ELSEWHERE CLASSIFIED (N99)

Revised   N99.111 Postprocedural bulbous urethral stricture, male

Revised   N99.112 Postprocedural membranous urethral stricture, male

Revised   N99.113 Postprocedural anterior bulbous urethral stricture, male

CHAPTER 15

PREGNANCY, CHILDBIRTH AND THE PUERPERIUM (O00-O9A)

PREGNANCY WITH ABORTIVE OUTCOME (O00-O08)

O00.10 Tubal pregnancy without intrauterine pregnancy

New   O00.101 Right tubal pregnancy without intrauterine pregnancy

New   O00.102 Left tubal pregnancy without intrauterine pregnancy

New   O00.109 Unspecified tubal pregnancy without intrauterine pregnancy

New   O00.111 Right tubal pregnancy with intrauterine pregnancy

New   O00.112 Left tubal pregnancy with intrauterine pregnancy

New   O00.119 Unspecified tubal pregnancy with intrauterine pregnancy

New   O00.201 Right ovarian pregnancy without intrauterine pregnancy

New   O00.202 Left ovarian pregnancy without intrauterine pregnancy

New   O00.209 Unspecified ovarian pregnancy without intrauterine pregnancy

New   O00.211 Right ovarian pregnancy with intrauterine pregnancy

New   O00.212 Left ovarian pregnancy with intrauterine pregnancy

New   O00.219 Unspecified ovarian pregnancy with intrauterine pregnancy

MATERNAL CARE RELATED TO THE FETUS AND AMNIOTIC CAVITY AND POSSIBLE DELIVERY PROBLEMS (O30–O48)

New   O36.83   Maternal care for abnormalities of the fetal heart rate or rhythm

New   O36.831   Maternal care for abnormalities of the fetal heart rate or rhythm, first trimester

New   O36.832   Maternal care for abnormalities of the fetal heart rate or rhythm, second trimester

New   O36.833   Maternal care for abnormalities of the fetal heart rate or rhythm, third trimester

New   O36.839   Maternal care for abnormalities of the fetal heart rate or rhythm, unspecified trimester

OTHER OBSTETRIC CONDITIONS, NOT ELSEWHERE CLASSIFIED (O94–O9A)

O99.1   Other diseases of the blood and blood-forming organs and certain disorders involving the immune mechanism complicating pregnancy, childbirth and the puerperium

New   **Excludes1**   hemorrhage with coagulation defects (O45.-, O46.0-, O67.0, O72.3)

Deleted   **Excludes2**   hemorrhage with coagulation defects (O45.-, O46.0-, O67.0, O72.3)

CHAPTER 16

CERTAIN CONDITIONS ORIGINATING IN THE PERINATAL PERIOD (P00-P96)

NEWBORN AFFECTED BY MATERNAL FACTORS AND BY COMPLICATIONS OF PREGNANCY, LABOR, AND DELIVERY (P00–P04)

P00.2   Newborn affected by maternal infectious and parasitic diseases

Deleted   **Excludes1**   infections specific to the perinatal period (P35-P39)

New   **Excludes2**   infections specific to the perinatal period (P35-P39)

RESPIRATORY AND CARDIOVASCULAR DISORDERS SPECIFIC TO THE PERINATAL PERIOD (P19-P29)

P24.01   Meconium aspiration with respiratory symptoms

Revised   Use additional code to identify any secondary pulmonary hypertension, if applicable (I27.2-)

P24.11   Neonatal aspiration of (clear) amniotic fluid and mucus with respiratory symptoms

Revised   Use additional code to identify any secondary pulmonary hypertension, if applicable (I27.2-)

P24.21   Neonatal aspiration of blood with respiratory symptoms

Revised   Use additional code to identify any secondary pulmonary hypertension, if applicable (I27.2-)

P24.31   Neonatal aspiration of milk and regurgitated food with respiratory symptoms

Revised   Use additional code to identify any secondary pulmonary hypertension, if applicable (I27.2-)

P24.81   Other neonatal aspiration with respiratory symptoms

Revised   Use additional code to identify any secondary pulmonary hypertension, if applicable (I27.2-)

P27   Chronic respiratory disease originating in the perinatal period

Deleted   **Excludes1**   respiratory distress of newborn (P22.0-P22.9)

New   **Excludes2**   respiratory distress of newborn (P22.0-P22.9)

P29.3   Persistent fetal circulation

Deleted   Delayed closure of ductus arteriosus

Deleted   (Persistent) pulmonary hypertension of newborn

New   P29.30   Pulmonary hypertension of newborn

New   Persistent pulmonary hypertension of newborn

New   P29.38   Other persistent fetal circulation

New   Delayed closure of ductus arteriosus

DIGESTIVE SYSTEM DISORDERS OF NEWBORN (P76-P78)

New   P78.84   Gestational alloimmune liver disease

New   GALD

New   Neonatal hemochromatosis

New   **Excludes1**   hemochromatosis (E83.11-)

CONDITIONS INVOLVING THE INTEGUMENT AND TEMPERATURE REGULATION OF NEWBORN (P80-P83)

P83.8   Other specified conditions of integument specific to newborn

Deleted   Bronze baby syndrome

Deleted   Neonatal scleroderma

Deleted   Urticaria neonatorum

New   P83.81   Umbilical granuloma

New   **Excludes2**   Granulomatous disorder of the skin and subcutaneous tissue, unspecified (L92.9)

New   P83.88   Other specified conditions of integument specific to newborn

New   Bronze baby syndrome

New   Neonatal scleroderma

New   Urticaria neonatorum

OTHER DISORDERS ORIGINATING IN THE PERINATAL PERIOD (P90-P96)

P91.6   Hypoxic ischemic encephalopathy [HIE]

New   **Excludes1**   Neonatal cerebral depression (P91.4)

New   Neonatal cerebral irritability (P91.3)

New   Neonatal coma (P91.5)

New   P91.81   Neonatal encephalopathy

New   P91.811   Neonatal encephalopathy in diseases classified elsewhere

New   *Code first underlying condition, if known, such as:*

New   congenital cirrhosis (of liver) (P78.71)

New   intracranial nontraumatic hemorrhage of newborn (P52.-)

New   kernicterus (P57.-)

New   P91.819   Neonatal encephalopathy, unspecified

New   P91.88   Other specified disturbances of cerebral status of newborn

P92   Feeding problems of newborn

New   **Excludes1**   eating disorders (F50.-)

CHAPTER 17

CONGENITAL MALFORMATIONS, DEFORMATIONS AND CHROMOSOMAL ABNORMALITIES (Q00-Q99)

CONGENITAL MALFORMATIONS OF THE CIRCULATORY SYSTEM (Q20-Q28)

	Q21.8	Other congenital malformations of cardiac septa
Deleted		Excludes1 Eisenmenger's complex (I27.8)
Deleted		Eisenmenger's syndrome (I27.8)
New		Code also if applicable:
New		Eisenmenger's complex (I27.83)
New		Eisenmenger's syndrome (I27.83)
	Q25.49	Other congenital malformations of aorta
New		Aortic arch
New		Bovine arch

CONGENITAL MALFORMATIONS OF GENITAL ORGANS (Q50-Q56)

New	Q53.111	Unilateral intraabdominal testis
New	Q53.112	Unilateral inguinal testis
New	Q53.13	Unilateral high scrotal testis
New	Q53.211	Bilateral intraabdominal testes
New	Q53.212	Bilateral inguinal testes
New	Q53.23	Bilateral high scrotal testes

CONGENITAL MALFORMATIONS OF THE URINARY SYSTEM (Q60-Q64)

Revised	Q64.12	Cloacal exstrophy of urinary bladder

OTHER CONGENITAL MALFORMATIONS (Q80-Q89)

Revised	Q82.2	Congenital cutaneous mastocytosis
Deleted		Urticaria pigmentosa
New		Congenital diffuse cutaneous mastocytosis
New		Congenital maculopapular cutaneous mastocytosis
New		Congenital urticaria pigmentosa
		Excludes1
Deleted		malignant mastocytosis (C96.2)
New		cutaneous mastocytosis NOS (D47.01)
New		diffuse cutaneous mastocytosis (with onset after newborn period) (D47.01)
New		malignant mastocytosis (C96.2-)
New		systemic mastocytosis (D47.02)
New		urticaria pigmentosa (non-congenital) (with onset after newborn period) (D47.01)

CHAPTER 18

SYMPTOMS, SIGNS AND ABNORMAL CLINICAL AND LABORATORY FINDINGS, NOT ELSEWHERE CLASSIFIED (R00-R99)

SYMPTOMS AND SIGNS INVOLVING THE CIRCULATORY AND RESPIRATORY SYSTEMS (R00-R09)

New	R06.03	Acute respiratory distress
	R09.0	Asphyxia and hypoxemia
Deleted		Excludes1 hypercapnia (R06.4)
New		Excludes2 hypercapnia (R06.89)

SYMPTOMS AND SIGNS INVOLVING THE GENITOURINARY SYSTEM (R30-R39)

New	R39.83	Unilateral non-palpable testicle
New	R39.84	Bilateral non-palpable testicles

SYMPTOMS AND SIGNS INVOLVING COGNITION, PERCEPTION, EMOTIONAL STATE AND BEHAVIOR (R40-R46)

	R40.222	Coma scale, best verbal response, incomprehensible words
New		Incomprehensible sounds (2-5 years of age)
New		Moans/grunts to pain; restless (<2 years old)
	R40.223	Coma scale, best verbal response, inappropriate words
New		Inappropriate crying or screaming (< 2 years of age)
New		Screaming (2-5 years of age)
	R40.224	Coma scale, best verbal response, confused conversation
New		Inappropriate words (2-5 years of age)
New		Irritable cries (< 2 years of age)
	R40.225	Coma scale, best verbal response, oriented
New		Cooing or babbling or crying appropriately (< 2 years of age)
New		Uses appropriate words (2- 5 years of age)
	R40.232	Coma scale, best motor response, extension
New		Abnormal extensor posturing to pain or noxious stimuli (< 2 years of age)
New		Extensor posturing to pain or noxious stimuli (2-5 years of age)
	R40.233	Coma scale, best motor response, abnormal
New		Abnormal flexure posturing to pain or noxious stimuli (0-5 years of age)
New		Flexion/decorticate posturing (< 2 years of age)
	R40.234	Coma scale, best motor response, flexion withdrawal
New		Withdraws from pain or noxious stimuli (0-5 years of age)
	R40.235	Coma scale, best motor response, localizes pain
New		Localizes pain (2-5 years of age)
New		Withdraws to touch (< 2 years of age)
	R40.236	Coma scale, best motor response, obeys commands
New		Normal or spontaneous movement (< 2 years of age)
New		Obeys commands (2-5 years of age)
	R41.9	Unspecified symptoms and signs involving cognitive functions and awareness
New		Unspecified neurocognitive disorder

GENERAL SYMPTOMS AND SIGNS (R50-R69)

	R53.8	Other malaise and fatigue
Deleted		Excludes1 exhaustion and fatigue due to depressive episode (F32.-)
	R53.83	Other fatigue
New		Excludes2 exhaustion and fatigue due to depressive episode (F32.-)

R57   Shock, not elsewhere classified

Deleted   **Excludes1**   septic shock (R65.21)

R57.0   Cardiogenic shock

New   **Excludes2**   septic shock (R65.21)

R60   Edema, not elsewhere classified

Deleted   **Excludes1**   nutritional edema (E40-E46)

R60.1   Generalized edema

New   **Excludes2**   nutritional edema (E40-E46)

R63.3   Feeding difficulties

New   Picky eater

New   **Excludes1**   eating disorders (F50.-)

R68.13   Apparent life threatening event in infant (ALTE)

New   Brief resolved unexplained event (BRUE)

ABNORMAL FINDINGS ON EXAMINATION OF BLOOD, WITHOUT DIAGNOSIS (R70-R79)

R79   Other abnormal findings of blood chemistry

Deleted   **Excludes1**   abnormality of fluid, electrolyte or acid-base balance (E86-E87)

R79.1   Abnormal coagulation profile

New   **Excludes2**   abnormality of fluid, electrolyte or acid-base balance (E86-E87)

CHAPTER 19

INJURY, POISONING AND CERTAIN OTHER CONSEQUENCES OF EXTERNAL CAUSES (S00-T88)

This chapter contains the following blocks:

Deleted   T20-T32   Burns and corrosions

INJURIES TO THE HEAD (S00-S09)

S00.531   Contusion of lip

Revised   Hematoma of lip

S00.532   Contusion of oral cavity

Revised   Bruise of oral cavity

S01.85   Open bite of other part of head

Revised   **Excludes1**   superficial bite of other part of head (S00.87)

S04.0   Injury of optic nerve and pathways

Revised   Use additional code to identify any visual field defect or blindness (H53.4-, H54.-)

Revised   S04.031   Injury of optic tract and pathways, right side

Revised   S04.032   Injury of optic tract and pathways, left side

Revised   S04.039   Injury of optic tract and pathways, unspecified side

Revised   S04.041   Injury of visual cortex, right side

Revised   S04.042   Injury of visual cortex, left side

Revised   S04.049   Injury of visual cortex, unspecified side

S06   Intracranial injury

New   Note: 7th characters D and S do not apply to codes in category S06 with 6th character 7 - death due to brain injury prior to regaining consciousness, or 8 - death due to other cause prior to regaining consciousness.

INJURIES TO THE WRIST, HAND AND FINGERS (S60-S69)

Revised   S62.311   Displaced fracture of base of second metacarpal bone, left hand

Revised   S62.317   Displaced fracture of base of fifth metacarpal bone, left hand

Revised   S62.341   Nondisplaced fracture of base of second metacarpal bone, left hand

Revised   S62.347   Nondisplaced fracture of base of fifth metacarpal bone, left hand

Revised   S62.62   Displaced fracture of middle phalanx of finger

Revised   S62.620   Displaced fracture of middle phalanx of right index finger

Revised   S62.621   Displaced fracture of middle phalanx of left index finger

Revised   S62.622   Displaced fracture of middle phalanx of right middle finger

Revised   S62.623   Displaced fracture of middle phalanx of left middle finger

Revised   S62.624   Displaced fracture of middle phalanx of right ring finger

Revised   S62.625   Displaced fracture of middle phalanx of left ring finger

Revised   S62.65   Nondisplaced fracture of middle phalanx of finger

Revised   S62.650   Nondisplaced fracture of middle phalanx of right index finger

Revised   S62.651   Nondisplaced fracture of middle phalanx of left index finger

Revised   S62.652   Nondisplaced fracture of middle phalanx of right middle finger

Revised   S62.653   Nondisplaced fracture of middle phalanx of left middle finger

Revised   S63.12   Subluxation and dislocation of interphalangeal joint of thumb

Revised   S63.121   Subluxation of interphalangeal joint of right thumb

Revised   S63.122   Subluxation of interphalangeal joint of left thumb

Revised   S63.123   Subluxation of interphalangeal joint of unspecified thumb

Revised   S63.124   Dislocation of interphalangeal joint of right thumb

Revised   S63.125   Dislocation of interphalangeal joint of left thumb

Revised   S63.126   Dislocation of interphalangeal joint of unspecified thumb

Deleted   S63.13   Subluxation and dislocation of proximal interphalangeal joint of thumb

Deleted   S63.131   Subluxation of proximal interphalangeal joint of right thumb

Deleted   S63.132   Subluxation of proximal interphalangeal joint of left thumb

Deleted   S63.133   Subluxation of proximal interphalangeal joint of unspecified thumb

Deleted   S63.134   Dislocation of proximal interphalangeal joint of right thumb

Deleted		S63.135 Dislocation of proximal interphalangeal joint of left thumb
Deleted		S63.136 Dislocation of proximal interphalangeal joint of unspecified thumb
Deleted	S63.14	Subluxation and dislocation of distal interphalangeal joint of thumb
Deleted		S63.141 Subluxation of distal interphalangeal joint of right thumb
Deleted		S63.142 Subluxation of distal interphalangeal joint of left thumb
Deleted		S63.143 Subluxation of distal interphalangeal joint of unspecified thumb
Deleted		S63.144 Dislocation of distal interphalangeal joint of right thumb
Deleted		S63.145 Dislocation of distal interphalangeal joint of left thumb
Deleted		S63.146 Dislocation of distal interphalangeal joint of unspecified thumb
		S63.259 Unspecified dislocation of unspecified finger
Revised		Unspecified dislocation of unspecified finger with unspecified laterality
		S63.279 Dislocation of unspecified interphalangeal joint of unspecified finger
Revised		Dislocation of unspecified interphalangeal joint of unspecified finger without specified laterality

INJURIES TO THE HIP AND THIGH (S70-S79)

	S72	Fracture of femur
Revised		**Excludes2** periprosthetic fracture of prosthetic implant of hip (M97.0-)
Revised	S73.03	Other anterior subluxation and dislocation of hip
Revised	S73.04	Central subluxation and dislocation of hip

INJURIES TO THE KNEE AND LOWER LEG (S80-S89)

	S82	Fracture of lower leg, including ankle
Revised		**Excludes2** periprosthetic fracture of prosthetic implant of knee (M97.0-)

INJURIES TO THE ANKLE AND FOOT (S90-S99)

Revised	S92.52	Fracture of middle phalanx of lesser toe(s)
Revised		S92.521 Displaced fracture of middle phalanx of right lesser toe(s)
Revised		S92.522 Displaced fracture of middle phalanx of left lesser toe(s)
Revised		S92.523 Displaced fracture of middle phalanx of unspecified lesser toe(s)
Revised		S92.524 Nondisplaced fracture of middle phalanx of right lesser toe(s)
Revised		S92.525 Nondisplaced fracture of middle phalanx of left lesser toe(s)
Revised		S92.526 Nondisplaced fracture of middle phalanx of unspecified lesser toe(s)

INJURIES INVOLVING MULTIPLE BODY REGIONS (T07)

	T07	Unspecified multiple injuries
New		The appropriate 7th character is to be added to code T07
New		A initial encounter
New		D subsequent encounter
New		S sequela
Revised		**Excludes1** injury NOS (T14.90)

INJURY OF UNSPECIFIED BODY REGION (T14)

	T14	Injury of unspecified body region
New		The appropriate 7th character is to be added to each code from category T14
New		A initial encounter
New		D subsequent encounter
New		S sequela
	T14.8	Other injury of unspecified body region
New		Wound NOS

BURNS AND CORROSIONS CONFINED TO EYE AND INTERNAL ORGANS (T26-T28)

	T27.3	Burn of respiratory tract, part unspecified
Deleted		*Code first (T51-T65) to identify chemical and intent for codes T27.4-T27.7*
	T27.4	Corrosion of larynx and trachea
New		*Code first (T51-T65) to identify chemical and intent*
	T27.6	Corrosion of other parts of respiratory tract
New		*Code first (T51-T65) to identify chemical and intent*
	T27.7	Corrosion of respiratory tract, part unspecified
New		*Code first (T51-T65) to identify chemical and intent*
	T28.4	Burns of other and unspecified internal organs
New		*Code first (T51-T65) to identify chemical and intent*
		T28.49 Burn of other internal organ
Deleted		*Code first (T51-T65) to identify chemical and intent for T28.5-T28.9-*
	T28.5	Corrosion of mouth and pharynx
New		*Code first (T51-T65) to identify chemical and intent*
	T28.6	Corrosion of esophagus
New		*Code first (T51-T65) to identify chemical and intent*
	T28.7	Corrosion of other parts of alimentary tract
New		*Code first (T51-T65) to identify chemical and intent*
	T28.8	Corrosion of internal genitourinary organs
New		*Code first (T51-T65) to identify chemical and intent*
	T28.9	Corrosions of other and unspecified internal organs
New		*Code first (T51-T65) to identify chemical and intent*

POISONING BY, ADVERSE EFFECTS OF AND UNDERDOSING OF DRUGS, MEDICAMENTS AND BIOLOGICAL SUBSTANCES (T36-T50)

	T43.205	Adverse effect of unspecified antidepressants
New		Antidepressant discontinuation syndrome

OTHER AND UNSPECIFIED EFFECTS OF EXTERNAL CAUSES (T66-T78)

	T76.2	Sexual abuse, suspected
Deleted		Sexual abuse, suspected

COMPLICATIONS OF SURGICAL AND MEDICAL CARE NOT ELSEWHERE CLASSIFIED (T80-T88)

	T80.69	Other serum reaction due to other serum
New		Code also, if applicable, arthropathy in hypersensitivity reactions classified elsewhere (M36.4)
	T84.01	Broken internal joint prosthesis
Revised		**Excludes1** periprosthetic joint implant fracture (M97-)
	T85.623	Displacement of artificial skin graft and decellularized allodermis
Deleted		Displacement of artificial skin graft and decellularized allodermis

CHAPTER 20

EXTERNAL CAUSES OF MORBIDITY (V00-Y99)

This chapter contains the following blocks:

Deleted	X50	Overexertion and strenuous or repetitive movements

OTHER LAND TRANSPORT ACCIDENTS (V80-V89)

New	V86.05	Driver of 3- or 4-wheeled all-terrain vehicle (ATV) injured in traffic accident
New	V86.06	Driver of dirt bike or motor/cross bike injured in traffic accident
New	V86.15	Passenger of 3- or 4-wheeled all-terrain vehicle (ATV) injured in traffic accident
New	V86.16	Passenger of dirt bike or motor/cross bike injured in traffic accident
New	V86.25	Person on outside of 3- or 4-wheeled all-terrain vehicle (ATV) injured in traffic accident
New	V86.26	Person on outside of dirt bike or motor/cross bike injured in traffic accident
New	V86.35	Unspecified occupant of 3- or 4-wheeled all-terrain vehicle (ATV) injured in traffic accident
New	V86.36	Unspecified occupant of dirt bike or motor/cross bike injured in traffic accident
New	V86.45	Person injured while boarding or alighting from a 3- or 4-wheeled all-terrain vehicle (ATV)
New	V86.46	Person injured while boarding or alighting from a dirt bike or motor/cross bike
New	V86.55	Driver of 3- or 4-wheeled all-terrain vehicle (ATV) injured in nontraffic accident
New	V86.56	Driver of dirt bike or motor/cross bike injured in nontraffic accident
New	V86.65	Passenger of 3- or 4-wheeled all-terrain vehicle (ATV) injured in nontraffic accident
New	V86.66	Passenger of dirt bike or motor/cross bike injured in nontraffic accident
New	V86.75	Person on outside of 3- or 4-wheeled all-terrain vehicle (ATV) injured in nontraffic accident
New	V86.76	Person on outside of dirt bike or motor/cross bike injured in nontraffic accident

New	V86.95	Unspecified occupant of 3- or 4-wheeled all-terrain vehicle (ATV) injured in nontraffic accident
New	V86.96	Unspecified occupant of dirt bike or motor/cross bike injured in nontraffic accident
	V86.99	Unspecified occupant of other special all-terrain or other off-road motor vehicle injured in nontraffic accident
Deleted		All-terrain motor-vehicle accident NOS
Deleted		Unspecified occupant of dirt bike injured in nontraffic accident

SLIPPING, TRIPPING, STUMBLING AND FALLS (W00-W19)

Revised	**Excludes2** fall into fire (X00-X04, X08)

EXPOSURE TO INANIMATE MECHANICAL FORCES (W20-W49)

Revised	W29.8	Contact with other powered hand tools and household machinery

CONTACT WITH HEAT AND HOT SUBSTANCES (X10-X19)

Revised	**Excludes1** exposure to fire and flames (X00-X08)

	X19	Contact with other heat and hot substances
Revised		**Excludes1** objects that are not normally hot, e.g., an object made hot by a house fire (X00-X08)

EXPOSURE TO FORCES OF NATURE (X30-X39)

	X32	Exposure to sunlight
New		**Excludes2** radiation-related disorders of the skin and subcutaneous tissue (L55-L59)

CHAPTER 21

FACTORS INFLUENCING HEALTH STATUS AND CONTACT WITH HEALTH SERVICES (Z00-Z99)

This chapter contains the following blocks:

Deleted	Z19	Hormone sensitivity malignancy status

PERSONS ENCOUNTERING HEALTH SERVICES FOR EXAMINATIONS (Z00-Z13)

	Z03	Encounter for medical observation for suspected diseases and conditions ruled out
New		**Excludes1** encounter for observation and evaluation of newborn for suspected diseases and conditions ruled out (Z05.0-)
Deleted		newborn observation for suspected condition, ruled out (P00-P04)
	Z05	Encounter for observation and evaluation of newborn for suspected diseases and conditions ruled out
Revised		This category is to be used for newborns, within the neonatal period (the first 28 days of life), who are suspected of having an abnormal condition, but without signs or symptoms, and which, after examination and observation, is ruled out.
Deleted		**Excludes2** newborn observation for suspected condition, related to exposure from the mother or birth process (P00-P04)

RESISTANCE TO ANTIMICROBIAL DRUGS (Z16)

	Z16	Resistance to antimicrobial drugs
Deleted		**Excludes1** Methicillin resistant Staphylococcus aureus infection in diseases classified elsewhere (B95.62)
	Z16.12	Extended spectrum beta lactamase (ESBL) resistance
New		**Excludes2** Methicillin resistant Staphylococcus aureus infection in diseases classified elsewhere (B95.62)

PERSONS ENCOUNTERING HEALTH SERVICES IN CIRCUMSTANCES RELATED TO REPRODUCTION (Z30-Z39)

Revised   **Z31.5**   **Encounter for procreative genetic counseling**

Z36   **Encounter for antenatal screening of mother**

New   **Includes**   Encounter for placental sample (taken vaginally)

New   Screening is the testing for disease or disease precursors in asymptomatic individuals so that early detection and treatment can be provided for those who test positive for the disease.

Deleted   **Excludes1**   abnormal findings on antenatal screening of mother (O28.-)

New   **Excludes2**   abnormal findings on antenatal screening of mother (O28.-)

New   **Z36.0**   **Encounter for antenatal screening for chromosomal anomalies**

New   **Z36.1**   **Encounter for antenatal screening for raised alphafetoprotein level**

New   Encounter for antenatal screening for elevated maternal serum alphafetoprotein level

New   **Z36.2**   **Encounter for other antenatal screening follow-up**

New   Non-visualized anatomy on a previous scan

New   **Z36.3**   **Encounter for antenatal screening for malformations**

New   Screening for a suspected anomaly

New   **Z36.4**   **Encounter for antenatal screening for fetal growth retardation**

New   Intrauterine growth restriction (IUGR)/ small-for-dates

New   **Z36.5**   **Encounter for antenatal screening for isoimmunization**

New   **Z36.8**   **Encounter for other antenatal screening**

New   **Z36.81**   **Encounter for antenatal screening for hydrops fetalis**

New   **Z36.82**   **Encounter for antenatal screening for nuchal translucency**

New   **Z36.83**   **Encounter for fetal screening for congenital cardiac abnormalities**

New   **Z36.84**   **Encounter for antenatal screening for fetal lung maturity**

New   **Z36.85**   **Encounter for antenatal screening for Streptococcus B**

New   **Z36.86**   **Encounter for antenatal screening for cervical length**

New   Screening for risk of pre-term labor

New   **Z36.87**   **Encounter for antenatal screening for uncertain dates**

New   **Z36.88**   **Encounter for antenatal screening for fetal macrosomia**

New   Screening for large-for-dates

New   **Z36.89**   **Encounter for other specified antenatal screening**

New   **Z36.8A**   **Encounter for antenatal screening for other genetic defects**

New   **Z36.9**   **Encounter for antenatal screening, unspecified**

Z3A   **Weeks of gestation**

Revised   *Code first* complications of pregnancy, childbirth and the puerperium (O09-O9A)

ENCOUNTERS FOR OTHER SPECIFIC HEALTH CARE (Z40-Z53)

Revised   **Z40.02**   **Encounter for prophylactic removal of ovary(s)**

New   Encounter for prophylactic removal of ovary(s) and fallopian tube(s)

New   **Z40.03**   **Encounter for prophylactic removal of fallopian tube(s)**

Z43   **Encounter for attention to artificial openings**

Deleted   **Excludes1**   artificial opening status only, without need for care (Z93.-)

Z43.1   **Encounter for attention to gastrostomy**

New   **Excludes2**   artificial opening status only, without need for care (Z93.-)

Z45   **Encounter for adjustment and management of implanted device**

Deleted   **Excludes1**   presence of prosthetic and other devices (Z95-Z97)

Z45.018   **Encounter for adjustment and management of other part of cardiac pacemaker**

New   **Excludes2**   presence of prosthetic and other devices (Z95-Z97)

Z48   **Encounter for other postprocedural aftercare**

New   **Excludes1**   encounter for aftercare following injury - code to Injury, by site, with appropriate 7th character for subsequent encounter

PERSONS WITH POTENTIAL HEALTH HAZARDS RELATED TO SOCIOECONOMIC AND PSYCHOSOCIAL CIRCUMSTANCES (Z55-Z65)

Z63.0   **Problems in relationship with spouse or partner**

New   Relationship distress with spouse or intimate partner

Z65.8   **Other specified problems related to psychosocial circumstances**

New   Religious or spiritual problem

BODY MASS INDEX [BMI] (Z68)

Revised   **Z68.1**   **Body mass index (BMI) 19.9 or less, adult**

PERSONS ENCOUNTERING HEALTH SERVICES IN OTHER CIRCUMSTANCES (Z69-Z76)

Z69.010   **Encounter for mental health services for victim of parental child abuse**

New   Encounter for mental health services for victim of child abuse by parent

New   Encounter for mental health services for victim of child neglect by parent

New   Encounter for mental health services for victim of child psychological abuse by parent

New   Encounter for mental health services for victim of child sexual abuse by parent

Z69.011   **Encounter for mental health services for perpetrator of parental child abuse**

New   Encounter for mental health services for perpetrator of parental child neglect

New   Encounter for mental health services for perpetrator of parental child psychological abuse

New   Encounter for mental health services for perpetrator of parental child sexual abuse

	Z69.020	**Encounter for mental health services for victim of non-parental child abuse**
New		Encounter for mental health services for victim of non-parental child neglect
New		Encounter for mental health services for victim of non-parental child psychological abuse
New		Encounter for mental health services for victim of non-parental child sexual abuse
	Z69.021	**Encounter for mental health services for perpetrator of non-parental child abuse**
New		Encounter for mental health services for perpetrator of non-parental child neglect
New		Encounter for mental health services for perpetrator of non-parental child psychological abuse
New		Encounter for mental health services for perpetrator of non-parental child sexual abuse
	Z69.11	**Encounter for mental health services for victim of spousal or partner abuse**
New		Encounter for mental health services for victim of spouse or partner neglect
New		Encounter for mental health services for victim of spouse or partner psychological abuse
New		Encounter for mental health services for victim of spouse or partner violence, physical
	Z69.12	**Encounter for mental health services for perpetrator of spousal or partner abuse**
New		Encounter for mental health services for perpetrator of spouse or partner neglect
New		Encounter for mental health services for perpetrator of spouse or partner psychological abuse
New		Encounter for mental health services for perpetrator of spouse or partner violence, physical
New		Encounter for mental health services for perpetrator of spouse or partner violence, sexual
	Z69.81	**Encounter for mental health services for victim of other abuse**
New		Encounter for mental health services for perpetrator of non-spousal adult abuse
New		Encounter for mental health services for victim of non-spousal adult abuse
New		Encounter for mental health services for victim of spouse or partner violence, sexual

	Z71.8		**Other specified counseling**
Deleted	Excludes2		counseling for genetics (Z31.5)
Deleted			counseling for procreative management (Z31.6-)
New	**Z71.82**		**Exercise counseling**
New	**Z71.83**		**Encounter for nonprocreative genetic counseling**
New	Excludes1		counseling for procreative genetics (Z31.5)
New			counseling for procreative management (Z31.6)

PERSONS WITH POTENTIAL HEALTH HAZARDS RELATED TO FAMILY AND PERSONAL HISTORY AND CERTAIN CONDITIONS INFLUENCING HEALTH STATUS (Z77-Z99)

	Z79.81		**Long term (current) use of agents affecting estrogen receptors and estrogen levels**
Revised	Excludes1		hormone replacement therapy (Z79.890)
Revised	**Z79.890**		**Hormone replacement therapy**
	Z83.71		**Family history of colonic polyps**
Deleted	Excludes1		family history of malignant neoplasm of digestive organs (Z80.0)
New	Excludes2		family history of malignant neoplasm of digestive organs (Z80.0)
	Z87.41		**Personal history of dysplasia of the female genital tract**
Revised	Excludes1		personal history of intraepithelial neoplasia III of female genital tract (Z86.001, Z86.008)
	Z91		**Personal risk factors, not elsewhere classified**
New	Excludes2		female genital mutilation status (N90.81-)
	Z91.19		**Patient's noncompliance with other medical treatment and regimen**
New			Nonadherence to medical treatment
New	**Z91.84**		**Oral health risk factors**
New		**Z91.841**	**Risk for dental caries, low**
New		**Z91.842**	**Risk for dental caries, moderate**
New		**Z91.843**	**Risk for dental caries, high**
New		**Z91.849**	**Unspecified risk for dental caries**
	Z95		**Presence of cardiac and vascular implants and grafts**
Deleted	Excludes1		complications of cardiac and vascular devices, implants and grafts (T82.-)
New	Excludes2		complications of cardiac and vascular devices, implants and grafts (T82.-)

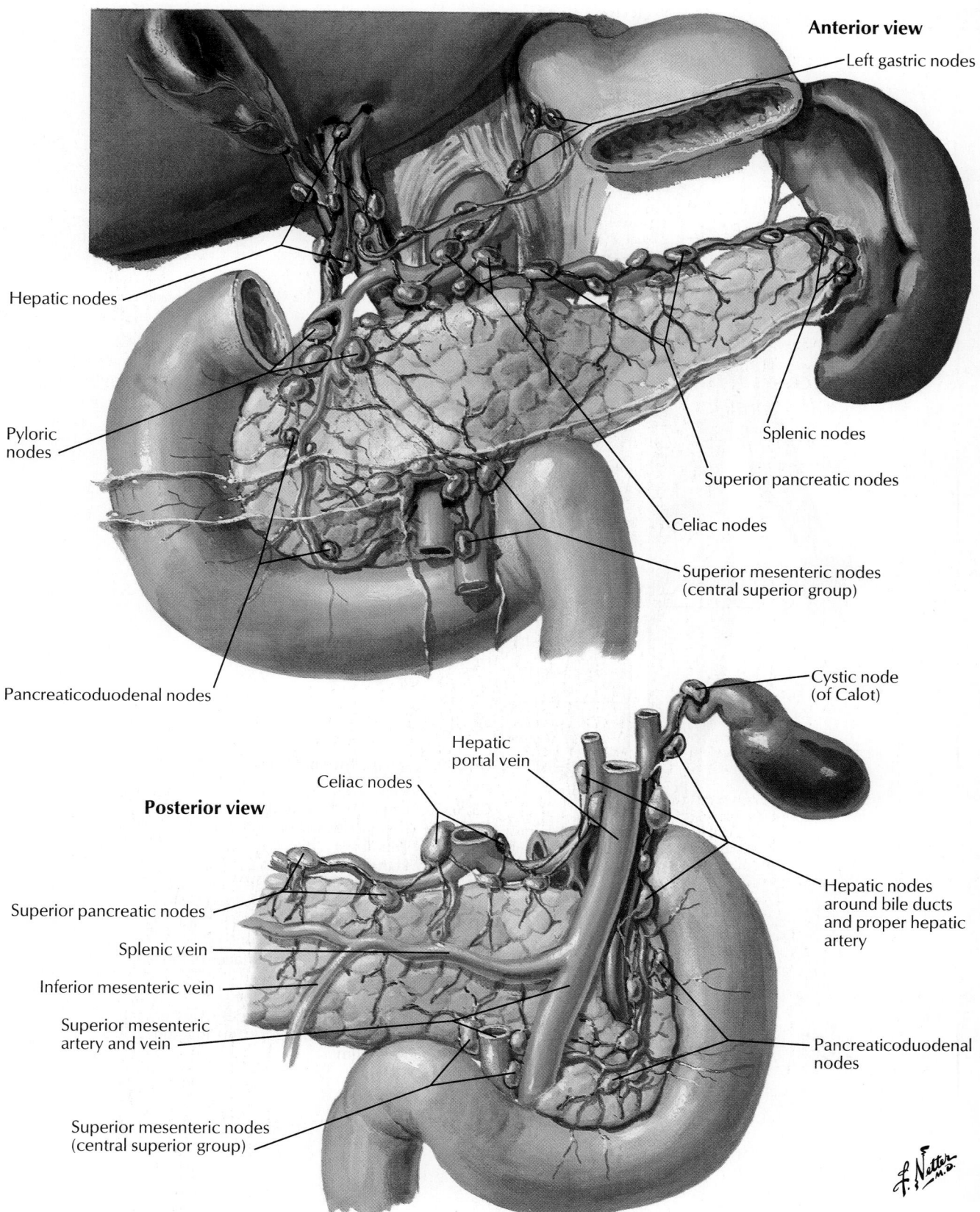

Anterior view

Left gastric nodes

Hepatic nodes

Pyloric nodes

Pancreaticoduodenal nodes

Splenic nodes

Superior pancreatic nodes

Celiac nodes

Superior mesenteric nodes (central superior group)

Posterior view

Celiac nodes

Hepatic portal vein

Cystic node (of Calot)

Superior pancreatic nodes

Splenic vein

Inferior mesenteric vein

Superior mesenteric artery and vein

Hepatic nodes around bile ducts and proper hepatic artery

Pancreaticoduodenal nodes

Superior mesenteric nodes (central superior group)

Plate 315 Lymph Vessels and Nodes of Pancreas. (Netter: Atlas of Human Anatomy, 4 ed, 2006, Saunders.)

Dermatome pattern

C2
C3
C4
C5
C6
C7
C8
T1
T2
T3
T4
T5
T6
T7
T8
T9
T10
T11
T12
L1
L2
L3
L4
L5
S1
S2
S3
S4
S5

C2
C3
C4
C5
C6
C7
C8
T1
T2
T3
T4
T5
T6
T7
T8
T9
T10
T11
T12
L1
L2
L3
L4
L5
S1
S2
S3

C6
C5
C8
C6
C7
C8
C7
S2–3
L1
L2
L3
L4
L5
S1

C6
C8
C7
C6
C8
S3
S4
S5
L1
L5
L2
L3
S1
S2
S2
S1
L4
S1
L5
L5
L4

Levels of principal dermatomes

C5	Clavicles
C5, 6, 7	Lateral parts of upper limbs
C8; T1	Medial sides of upper limbs
C6	Thumb
C6, 7, 8	Hand
C8	Ring and little fingers
T4	Level of nipples
T10	Level of umbilicus
T12	Inguinal or groin regions
L1, 2, 3, 4	Anterior and inner surfaces of lower limbs
L4, 5; S1	Foot
L4	Medial side of great toe
L5; S1, 2	Outer and posterior sides of lower limbs
S1	Lateral margin of foot and little toe
S2, 3, 4	Perineum

Plate 164   Dermatomes. (Netter: Atlas of Human Anatomy, 4 ed, 2006, Saunders.)

NAP-2

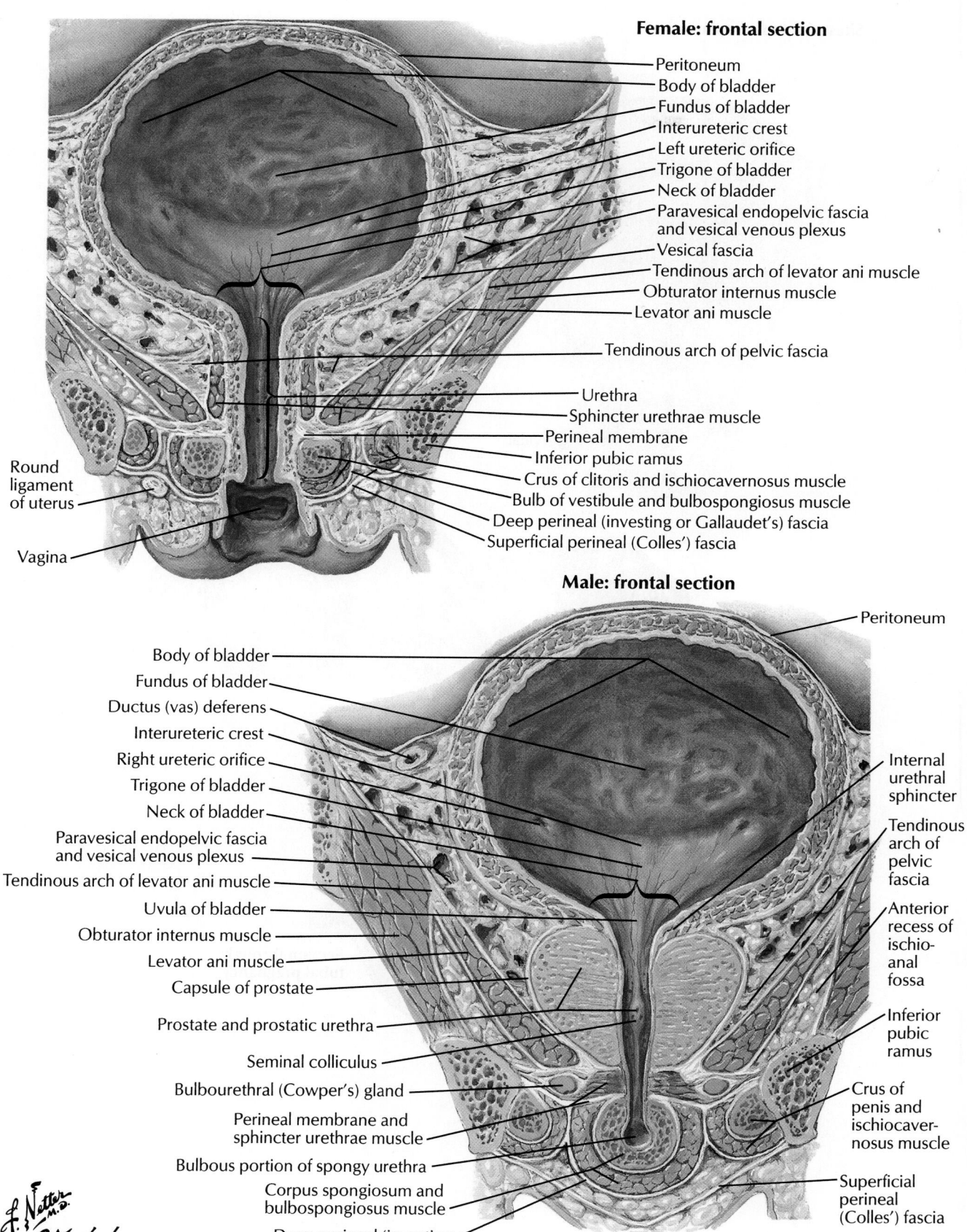

Female: frontal section

Peritoneum
Body of bladder
Fundus of bladder
Interureteric crest
Left ureteric orifice
Trigone of bladder
Neck of bladder
Paravesical endopelvic fascia
and vesical venous plexus
Vesical fascia
Tendinous arch of levator ani muscle
Obturator internus muscle
Levator ani muscle

Tendinous arch of pelvic fascia

Urethra
Sphincter urethrae muscle
Perineal membrane
Inferior pubic ramus
Crus of clitoris and ischiocavernosus muscle
Bulb of vestibule and bulbospongiosus muscle
Deep perineal (investing or Gallaudet's) fascia
Superficial perineal (Colles') fascia

Round
ligament
of uterus

Vagina

Male: frontal section

Peritoneum

Body of bladder
Fundus of bladder
Ductus (vas) deferens
Interureteric crest
Right ureteric orifice
Trigone of bladder
Neck of bladder
Paravesical endopelvic fascia
and vesical venous plexus
Tendinous arch of levator ani muscle
Uvula of bladder
Obturator internus muscle
Levator ani muscle
Capsule of prostate
Prostate and prostatic urethra
Seminal colliculus
Bulbourethral (Cowper's) gland
Perineal membrane and
sphincter urethrae muscle
Bulbous portion of spongy urethra
Corpus spongiosum and
bulbospongiosus muscle
Deep perineal (investing
or Gallaudet's) fascia

Internal
urethral
sphincter

Tendinous
arch of
pelvic
fascia

Anterior
recess of
ischio-
anal
fossa

Inferior
pubic
ramus

Crus of
penis and
ischiocaver-
nosus muscle

Superficial
perineal
(Colles')
fascia

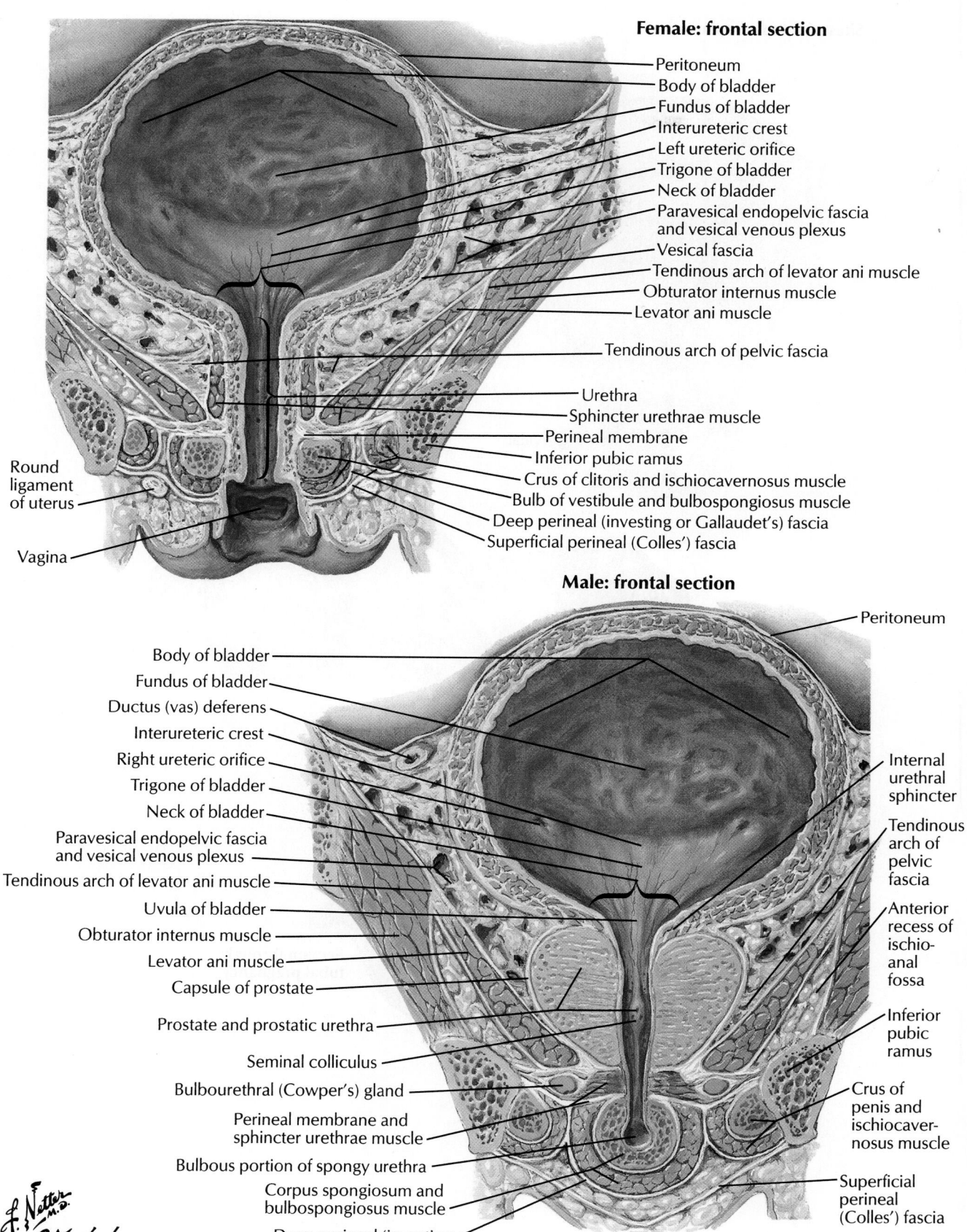

Plate 366 Urinary Bladder: Female and Male. (Netter: Atlas of Human Anatomy, 4 ed, 2006, Saunders.)

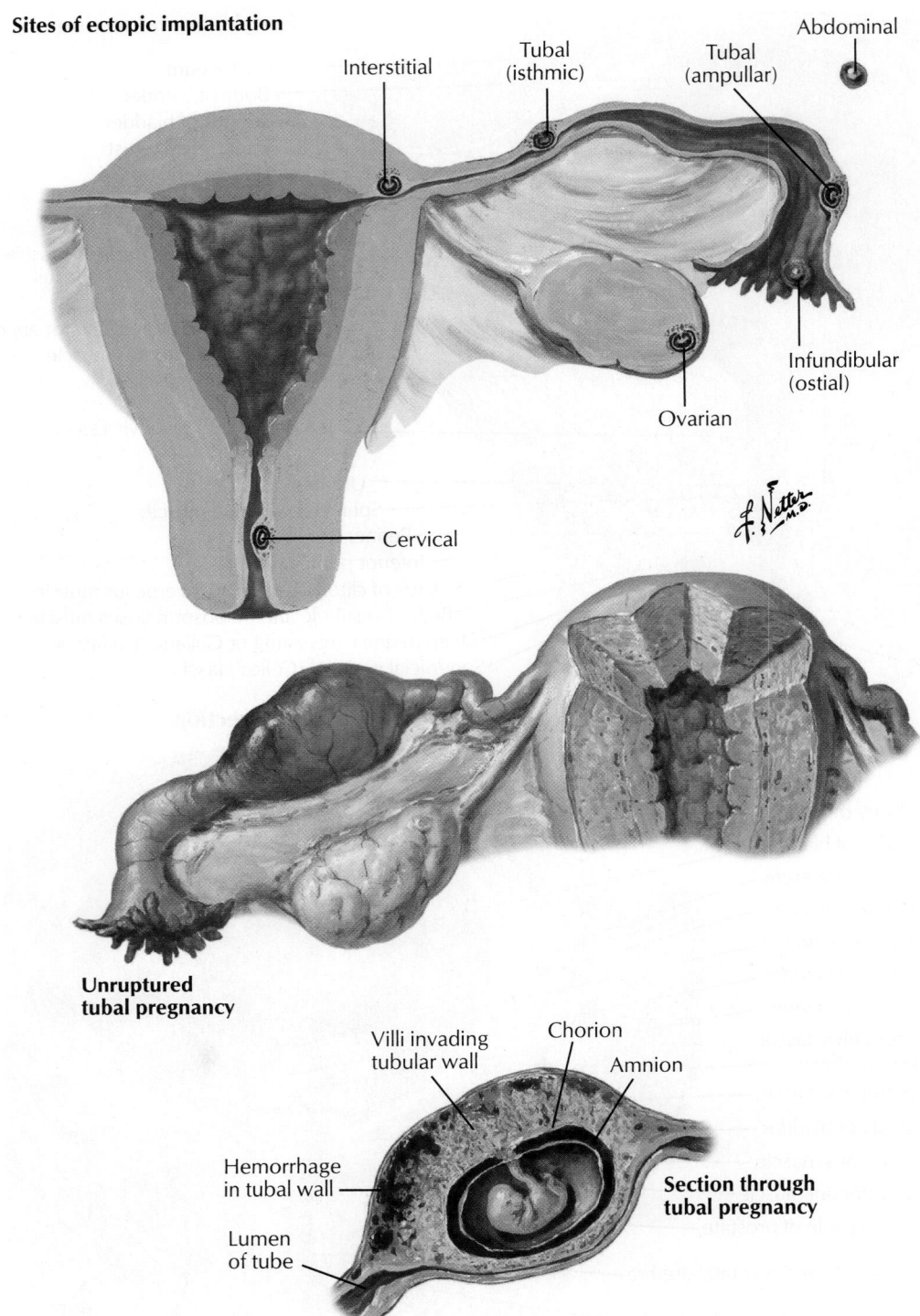

Sites of ectopic implantation

Interstitial

Tubal (isthmic)

Tubal (ampullar)

Abdominal

Infundibular (ostial)

Ovarian

Cervical

Unruptured tubal pregnancy

Villi invading tubular wall

Chorion

Amnion

Hemorrhage in tubal wall

Section through tubal pregnancy

Lumen of tube

Plate 375 Ectopic Pregnancy. (Netter: Atlas of Human Anatomy, 4 ed, 2006, Saunders.)

Skin of penis

Superficial fascia of penis (Colles' fascia)

Deep (Buck's) fascia of penis

Testicular artery

Ductus deferens

Artery to ductus deferens

Genital branch of genitofemoral nerve

Pampiniform (venous) plexus

Epididymis

Appendix of epididymis

Appendix of testis

Testis (covered by visceral layer of tunica vaginalis)

Parietal layer of tunica vaginalis

Superficial inguinal ring

External spermatic fascia

Cremaster muscle and fascia

Septum of scrotum (formed by dartos fascia)

Superficial (dartos) fascia of scrotum

Skin of scrotum

Superficial (dartos) fascia of scrotum

External spermatic fascia

Cremaster muscle and fascia

Internal spermatic fascia

Parietal layer of tunica vaginalis

Epididymis

Testis (covered by visceral layer of tunica vaginalis)

Skin of scrotum

Plate 387   Scrotum and Contents. (Netter: Atlas of Human Anatomy, 4 ed, 2006, Saunders.)

NAP-5

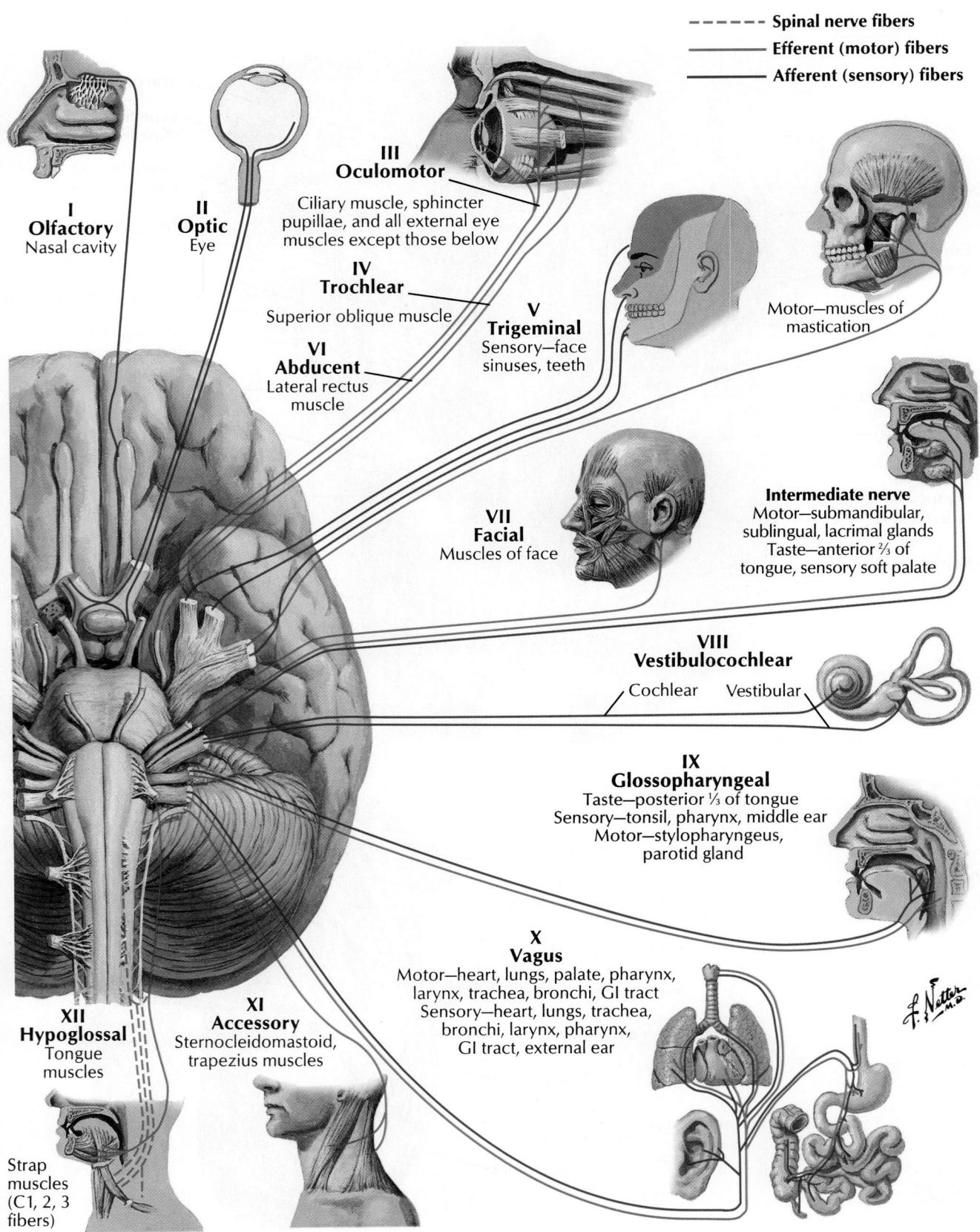

------ Spinal nerve fibers
——— Efferent (motor) fibers
——— Afferent (sensory) fibers

I Olfactory
Nasal cavity

II Optic
Eye

III Oculomotor
Ciliary muscle, sphincter pupillae, and all external eye muscles except those below

IV Trochlear
Superior oblique muscle

VI Abducent
Lateral rectus muscle

V Trigeminal
Sensory—face sinuses, teeth

Motor—muscles of mastication

VII Facial
Muscles of face

Intermediate nerve
Motor—submandibular, sublingual, lacrimal glands
Taste—anterior ⅔ of tongue, sensory soft palate

VIII Vestibulocochlear
Cochlear   Vestibular

IX Glossopharyngeal
Taste—posterior ⅓ of tongue
Sensory—tonsil, pharynx, middle ear
Motor—stylopharyngeus, parotid gland

X Vagus
Motor—heart, lungs, palate, pharynx, larynx, trachea, bronchi, GI tract
Sensory—heart, lungs, trachea, bronchi, larynx, pharynx, GI tract, external ear

XII Hypoglossal
Tongue muscles

Strap muscles (C1, 2, 3 fibers)

XI Accessory
Sternocleidomastoid, trapezius muscles

NETTER'S ANATOMY ILLUSTRATIONS

Plate 118 Cranial Nerves (Motor and Sensory Distribution): Schema. (Netter: Atlas of Human Anatomy, 4 ed, 2006, Saunders.)

Superior view

Supratrochlear nerve

Medial rectus muscle

Superior oblique muscle

Infratrochlear nerve

Nasociliary nerve

Trochlear nerve (IV)

Common tendinous ring

Ophthalmic nerve (V₁)

Optic nerve (II)

Internal carotid artery and nerve plexus

Oculomotor nerve (III)

Trochlear nerve (IV)

Abducent nerve (VI)

Tentorium cerebelli

Medial branch
Lateral branch } Supraorbital nerve

Levator palpebrae superioris muscle

Superior rectus muscle

Lacrimal gland

Lacrimal nerve

Lateral rectus muscle

Frontal nerve

Maxillary nerve (V₂)

Meningeal branch of maxillary nerve

Mandibular nerve (V₃)

Lesser petrosal nerve

Meningeal branch of mandibular nerve

Greater petrosal nerve

Trigeminal (semilunar) ganglion

Tentorial (meningeal) branch of ophthalmic nerve

Superior view:
levator palpebrae superioris, superior rectus, and superior oblique muscles partially cut away

Supratrochlear nerve *(cut)*

Supraorbital nerve branches *(cut)*

Infratrochlear nerve

Anterior ethmoidal nerve

Optic nerve (II)

Posterior ethmoidal nerve

Superior branch of oculomotor nerve (III) *(cut)*

Nasociliary nerve

Internal carotid plexus

Trochlear nerve (IV) *(cut)*

Oculomotor nerve (III)

Abducent nerve (VI)

Long ciliary nerves

Short ciliary nerves

Lacrimal nerve

Ciliary ganglion

Parasympathetic root of ciliary ganglion (from inferior branch of oculomotor nerve)

Sympathetic root of ciliary ganglion (from internal carotid plexus)

Sensory root of ciliary ganglion (from nasociliary nerve)

Branches to inferior and medial rectus muscles

Abducent nerve (VI)

Inferior branch of oculomotor nerve (III)

Lacrimal nerve

Frontal nerve *(cut)*

Ophthalmic nerve (V₁)

f. Netter m.d.

Plate 86 Nerves of Orbit. (Netter: Atlas of Human Anatomy, 4 ed, 2006, Saunders.)

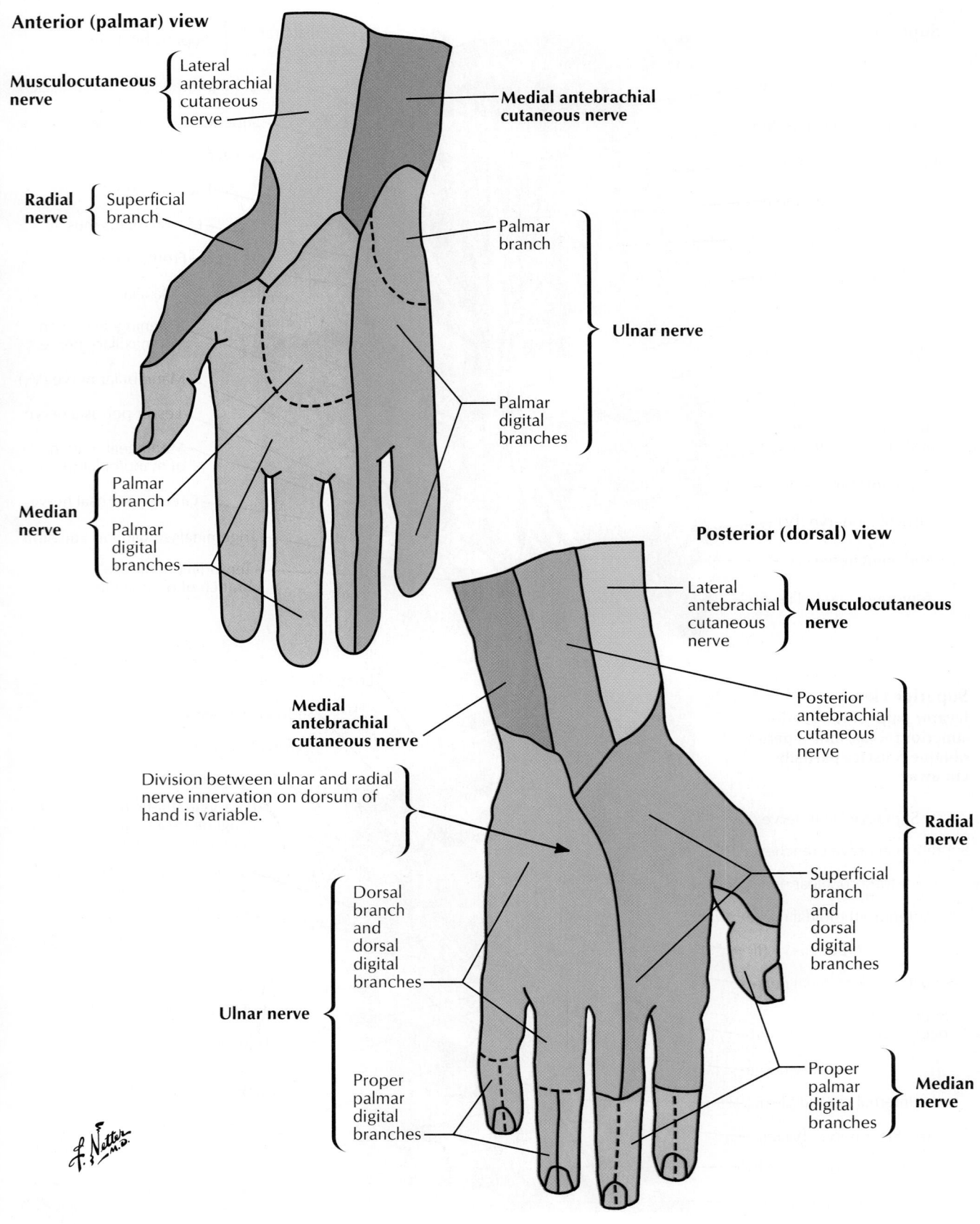

Anterior (palmar) view

Musculocutaneous nerve { Lateral antebrachial cutaneous nerve

Medial antebrachial cutaneous nerve

Radial nerve { Superficial branch

Palmar branch

Ulnar nerve

Palmar digital branches

Median nerve { Palmar branch

Palmar digital branches

Posterior (dorsal) view

Lateral antebrachial cutaneous nerve **Musculocutaneous nerve**

Medial antebrachial cutaneous nerve

Posterior antebrachial cutaneous nerve

Division between ulnar and radial nerve innervation on dorsum of hand is variable.

Radial nerve

Superficial branch and dorsal digital branches

Ulnar nerve

Dorsal branch and dorsal digital branches

Proper palmar digital branches

Proper palmar digital branches **Median nerve**

f. Netter
M.D.

Plate 472   Cutaneous Innervation of Wrist and Hand. (Netter: Atlas of Human Anatomy, 4 ed, 2006, Saunders.)

Anterior view

Deltoid muscle

Coracobrachialis muscle

Biceps brachii muscle { Short head (*cut*)

Long head (*cut*)

Musculocutaneous nerve

Brachialis muscle

Biceps brachii muscle (*cut*) and tendon

Lateral antebrachial cutaneous nerve (from musculocutaneous nerve)

Radial nerve { Deep branch

Superficial branch

Supinator muscle

Brachioradialis muscle

Radial artery

Pronator teres muscle (*partially cut*)

Median nerve

Flexor pollicis longus muscle

Flexor carpi radialis tendon (*cut*)

Flexor retinaculum (transverse carpal ligament)

Superficial branch of radial nerve

Recurrent (motor) branch of median nerve to thenar muscles

Common palmar digital branches of median nerve

Proper palmar digital branches of median nerve

Intercostobrachial nerve

Medial brachial cutaneous nerve

Radial nerve

Ulnar nerve

Medial antebrachial cutaneous nerve

Median nerve

Brachial artery

Bicipital aponeurosis

Humeral head (*cut*) } Pronator teres muscle

Ulnar head

Flexor carpi radialis muscle (*cut*)

Humeroulnar head } Flexor digitorum superficialis muscle (*cut*)

Radial head

Flexor digitorum profundus muscle

Flexor carpi ulnaris muscle

Ulnar artery and nerve

Dorsal branch of ulnar nerve

Flexor digitorum superficialis tendons (*cut*)

Deep palmar branch of ulnar artery and deep branch of ulnar nerve

Superficial branch of ulnar nerve

Superficial palmar arch (*cut*)

Common palmar digital branch of ulnar nerve

Communicating branch of median nerve with ulnar nerve

Proper palmar digital branches of ulnar nerve

Plate 473 Arteries and Nerves of Upper Limb. (Netter: Atlas of Human Anatomy, 4 ed, 2006, Saunders.)

NAP-9

Lateral cutaneous branch of subcostal nerve

Inguinal ligament (Poupart's)

Superficial circumflex iliac vein

Femoral branches of genitofemoral nerve

Lateral femoral cutaneous nerve

Saphenous opening (fossa ovalis)

Fascia lata

Anterior cutaneous branches of femoral nerve

Patellar nerve plexus

Branches of lateral sural cutaneous nerve (from common fibular [peroneal] nerve)

Deep fascia of leg (crural fascia)

Superficial fibular (peroneal) nerve
Medial dorsal cutaneous branch

Intermediate dorsal cutaneous branch

Small saphenous vein and lateral dorsal cutaneous nerve (from sural nerve)

Lateral dorsal digital nerve and vein of 5th toe

Dorsal metatarsal veins

Dorsal digital nerves and veins

Superficial epigastric vein

Ilioinguinal nerve (scrotal branch) (usually passes through superficial inguinal ring)

Genital branch of genitofemoral nerve

Femoral vein

Superficial external pudendal vein

Accessory saphenous vein

Great saphenous vein

Cutaneous branches of obturator nerve

Infrapatellar branch of saphenous nerve

Saphenous nerve (terminal branch of femoral nerve)

Great saphenous vein

Dorsal digital nerves

Dorsal venous arch

Dorsal digital nerve and vein of medial side of great toe

Dorsal digital branch of deep fibular (peroneal) nerve

Plate 544 Superficial Nerves and Veins of Lower Limb: Anterior View. (Netter: Atlas of Human Anatomy, 4 ed, 2006, Saunders.)

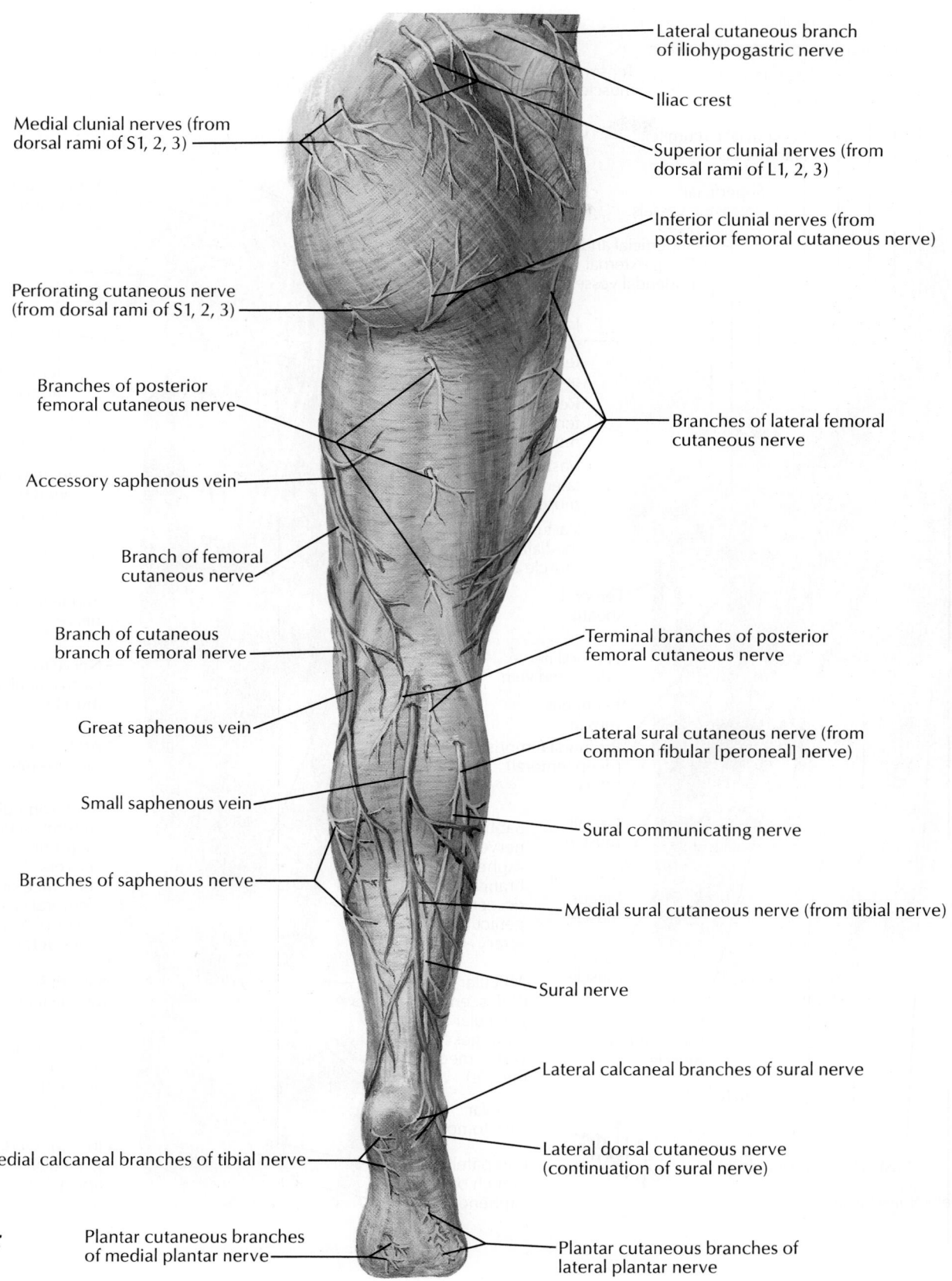

Lateral cutaneous branch
of iliohypogastric nerve

Iliac crest

Medial clunial nerves (from
dorsal rami of S1, 2, 3)

Superior clunial nerves (from
dorsal rami of L1, 2, 3)

Inferior clunial nerves (from
posterior femoral cutaneous nerve)

Perforating cutaneous nerve
(from dorsal rami of S1, 2, 3)

Branches of posterior
femoral cutaneous nerve

Branches of lateral femoral
cutaneous nerve

Accessory saphenous vein

Branch of femoral
cutaneous nerve

Branch of cutaneous
branch of femoral nerve

Terminal branches of posterior
femoral cutaneous nerve

Great saphenous vein

Lateral sural cutaneous nerve (from
common fibular [peroneal] nerve)

Small saphenous vein

Sural communicating nerve

Branches of saphenous nerve

Medial sural cutaneous nerve (from tibial nerve)

Sural nerve

Lateral calcaneal branches of sural nerve

Lateral dorsal cutaneous nerve
(continuation of sural nerve)

Medial calcaneal branches of tibial nerve

Plantar cutaneous branches
of medial plantar nerve

Plantar cutaneous branches of
lateral plantar nerve

Plate 545 Superficial Nerves and Veins of Lower Limb: Posterior View. (Netter: Atlas of Human Anatomy, 4 ed, 2006, Saunders.)

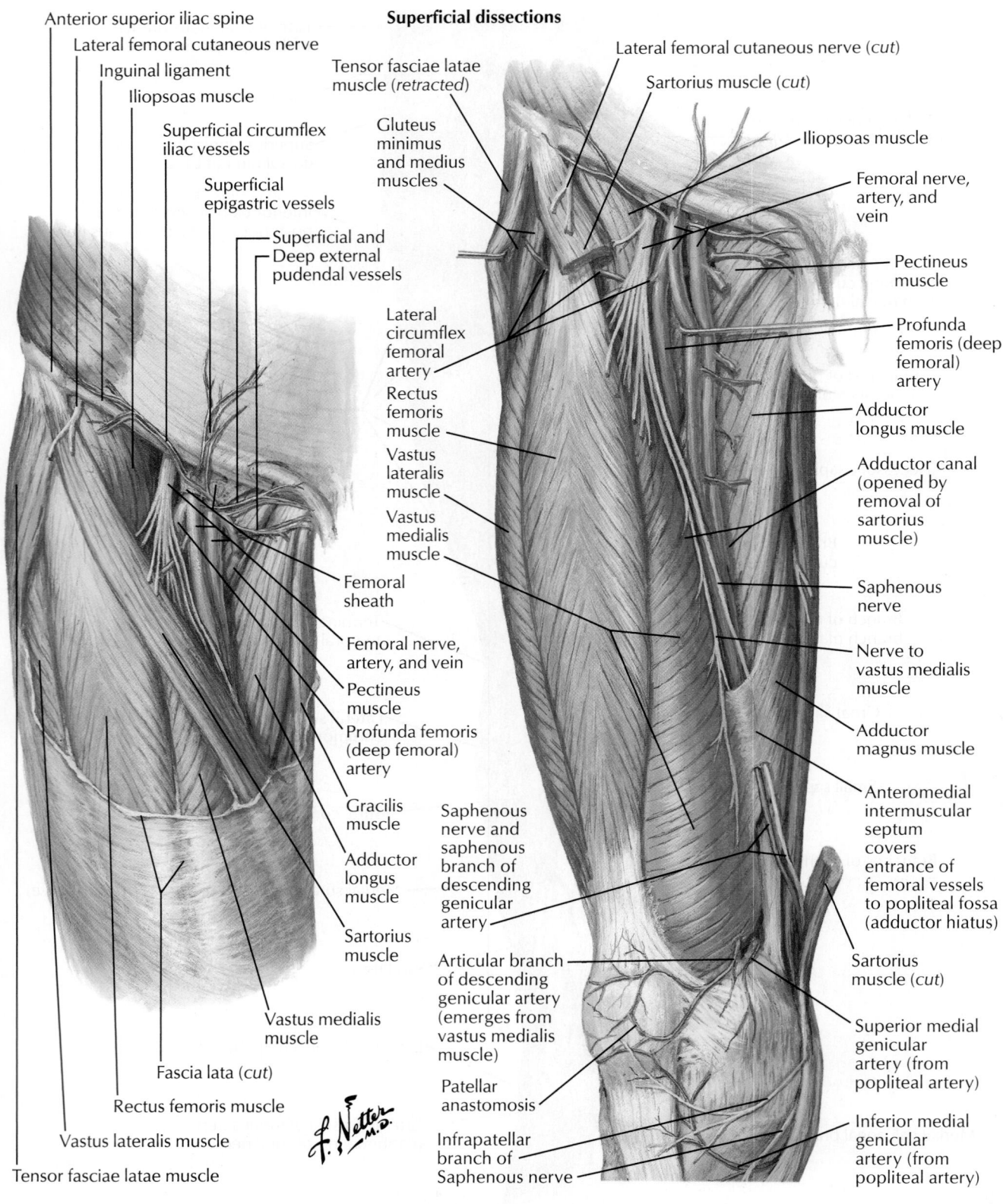

Anterior superior iliac spine

Lateral femoral cutaneous nerve

Inguinal ligament

Iliopsoas muscle

Superficial circumflex iliac vessels

Superficial epigastric vessels

Superficial and Deep external pudendal vessels

Superficial dissections

Tensor fasciae latae muscle (*retracted*)

Gluteus minimus and medius muscles

Lateral circumflex femoral artery

Rectus femoris muscle

Vastus lateralis muscle

Vastus medialis muscle

Femoral sheath

Femoral nerve, artery, and vein

Pectineus muscle

Profunda femoris (deep femoral) artery

Gracilis muscle

Adductor longus muscle

Sartorius muscle

Saphenous nerve and saphenous branch of descending genicular artery

Articular branch of descending genicular artery (emerges from vastus medialis muscle)

Patellar anastomosis

Infrapatellar branch of Saphenous nerve

Vastus medialis muscle

Fascia lata (*cut*)

Rectus femoris muscle

Vastus lateralis muscle

Tensor fasciae latae muscle

Lateral femoral cutaneous nerve (*cut*)

Sartorius muscle (*cut*)

Iliopsoas muscle

Femoral nerve, artery, and vein

Pectineus muscle

Profunda femoris (deep femoral) artery

Adductor longus muscle

Adductor canal (opened by removal of sartorius muscle)

Saphenous nerve

Nerve to vastus medialis muscle

Adductor magnus muscle

Anteromedial intermuscular septum covers entrance of femoral vessels to popliteal fossa (adductor hiatus)

Sartorius muscle (*cut*)

Superior medial genicular artery (from popliteal artery)

Inferior medial genicular artery (from popliteal artery)

f. Netter
M.D.

Plate 500   Arteries and Nerves of Thigh: Anterior Views. (Netter: Atlas of Human Anatomy, 4 ed, 2006, Saunders.)

NETTER'S ANATOMY ILLUSTRATIONS

Deep dissection

Deep circumflex iliac artery

Lateral femoral cutaneous nerve

Sartorius muscle (*cut*)

Iliopsoas muscle

Tensor fasciae latae muscle (*retracted*)

Gluteus medius and minimus muscles

Femoral nerve

Rectus femoris muscle (*cut*)

Ascending, transverse and descending branches of Lateral circumflex femoral artery

Medial circumflex femoral artery

Pectineus muscle (*cut*)

Profunda femoris (deep femoral) artery

Perforating branches

Adductor longus muscle (*cut*)

Vastus lateralis muscle

Vastus intermedius muscle

Rectus femoris muscle (*cut*)

Saphenous nerve

Anteromedial intermuscular septum (*opened*)

Vastus medialis muscle

Quadriceps femoris tendon

Patella and patellar anastomosis

Medial patellar retinaculum

Patellar ligament

External iliac artery and vein

Inguinal ligament (Poupart's)

Femoral artery and vein (*cut*)

Pectineus muscle (*cut*)

Obturator canal

Obturator externus muscle

Adductor longus muscle (*cut*)

Anterior branch and Posterior branch of obturator nerve

Quadratus femoris muscle

Adductor brevis muscle

Branches of posterior branch of obturator nerve

Adductor magnus muscle

Gracilis muscle

Cutaneous branch of obturator nerve

Femoral artery and vein (*cut*)

Descending genicular artery
Articular branch
Saphenous branch

Adductor hiatus

Sartorius muscle (*cut*)

Adductor magnus tendon

Adductor tubercle on medial epicondyle of femur

Superior medial genicular artery (from popliteal artery)

Infrapatellar branch of Saphenous nerve

Inferior medial genicular artery (from popliteal artery)

Plate 5Ø1 Arteries and Nerves of Thigh: Posterior View. (Netter: Atlas of Human Anatomy, 4 ed, 2006, Saunders.)

NAP-13

NETTER'S ANATOMY ILLUSTRATIONS

Deep dissection

Superior clunial nerves

Gluteus maximus muscle (cut)

Medial clunial nerves

Inferior gluteal artery and nerve

Pudendal nerve

Nerve to obturator internus (and superior gemellus)

Posterior femoral cutaneous nerve

Sacrotuberous ligament

Ischial tuberosity

Inferior clunial nerves (cut)

Adductor magnus muscle

Gracilis muscle

Sciatic nerve

Muscular branches of sciatic nerve

Semitendinosus muscle (retracted)

Semimembranosus muscle

Sciatic nerve

Articular branch

Adductor hiatus

Popliteal vein and artery

Superior medial genicular artery

Medial epicondyle of femur

Tibial nerve

Gastrocnemius muscle (medial head)

Medial sural cutaneous nerve

Small saphenous vein

Iliac crest

Gluteal aponeurosis and gluteus medius muscle (cut)

Superior gluteal artery and nerve

Gluteus minimus muscle

Tensor fasciae latae muscle

Piriformis muscle

Gluteus medius muscle (cut)

Superior gemellus muscle

Greater trochanter of femur

Obturator internus muscle

Inferior gemellus muscle

Gluteus maximus muscle (cut)

Quadratus femoris muscle

Medial circumflex femoral artery

Vastus lateralis muscle and iliotibial tract

Adductor minimus part of adductor magnus muscle

1st perforating artery (from profunda femoris artery)

Adductor magnus muscle

2nd and 3rd perforating arteries (from profunda femoris artery)

4th perforating artery (from profunda femoris artery)

Long head (retracted)
Short head   } Biceps femoris muscle

Superior lateral genicular artery

Common fibular (peroneal) nerve

Plantaris muscle

Gastrocnemius muscle (lateral head)

Lateral sural cutaneous nerve

NETTER'S ANATOMY ILLUSTRATIONS

Plate 502   Arteries and Nerves of Thigh: Posterior View. (Netter: Atlas of Human Anatomy, 4 ed, 2006, Saunders.)

Horizontal section

Zonular fibers
(suspensory ligament of lens)

Scleral venous sinus
(canal of Schlemm)

Scleral spur

Ciliary body and ciliary muscle

Ciliary part of retina

Tendon of
lateral rectus
muscle

Iris

Capsule of lens

Lens

Cornea

Anterior chamber

Posterior chamber

Iridocorneal angle

Ciliary processes

Bulbar conjunctiva

Ora serrata

Tendon of
medial rectus
muscle

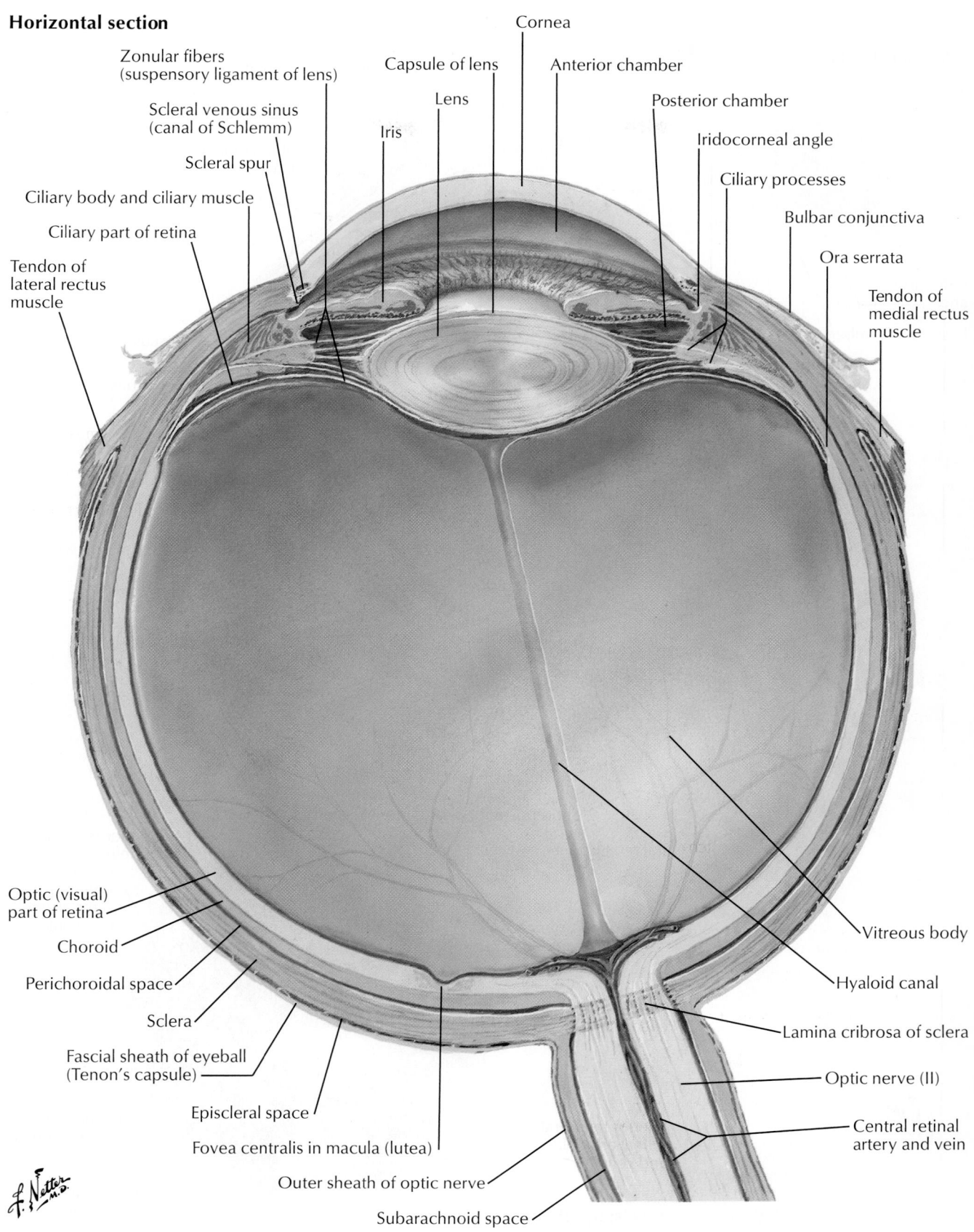

Optic (visual)
part of retina

Choroid

Perichoroidal space

Sclera

Fascial sheath of eyeball
(Tenon's capsule)

Episcleral space

Fovea centralis in macula (lutea)

Outer sheath of optic nerve

Subarachnoid space

Vitreous body

Hyaloid canal

Lamina cribrosa of sclera

Optic nerve (II)

Central retinal
artery and vein

Plate 87   Eyeball. (Netter: Atlas of Human Anatomy, 4 ed, 2006, Saunders.)

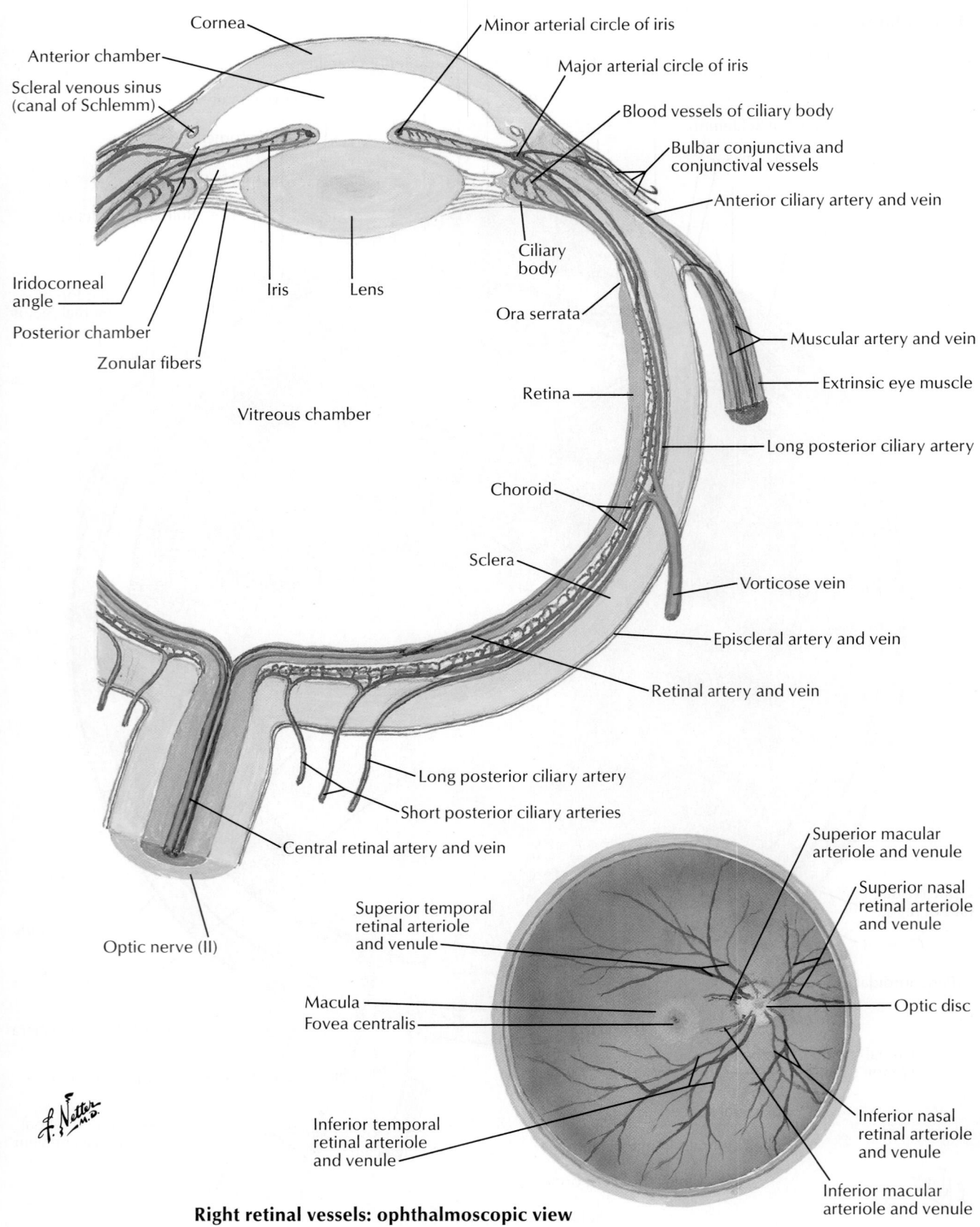

Cornea

Anterior chamber

Scleral venous sinus (canal of Schlemm)

Minor arterial circle of iris

Major arterial circle of iris

Blood vessels of ciliary body

Bulbar conjunctiva and conjunctival vessels

Anterior ciliary artery and vein

Iridocorneal angle

Iris

Lens

Ciliary body

Posterior chamber

Zonular fibers

Ora serrata

Muscular artery and vein

Extrinsic eye muscle

Vitreous chamber

Retina

Long posterior ciliary artery

Choroid

Sclera

Vorticose vein

Episcleral artery and vein

Retinal artery and vein

Long posterior ciliary artery

Short posterior ciliary arteries

Central retinal artery and vein

Optic nerve (II)

Superior temporal retinal arteriole and venule

Superior macular arteriole and venule

Superior nasal retinal arteriole and venule

Optic disc

Macula

Fovea centralis

Inferior temporal retinal arteriole and venule

Inferior nasal retinal arteriole and venule

Inferior macular arteriole and venule

Right retinal vessels: ophthalmoscopic view

Plate 90   Intrinsic Arteries and Veins of Eye. (Netter: Atlas of Human Anatomy, 4 ed, 2006, Saunders.)

NAP-16

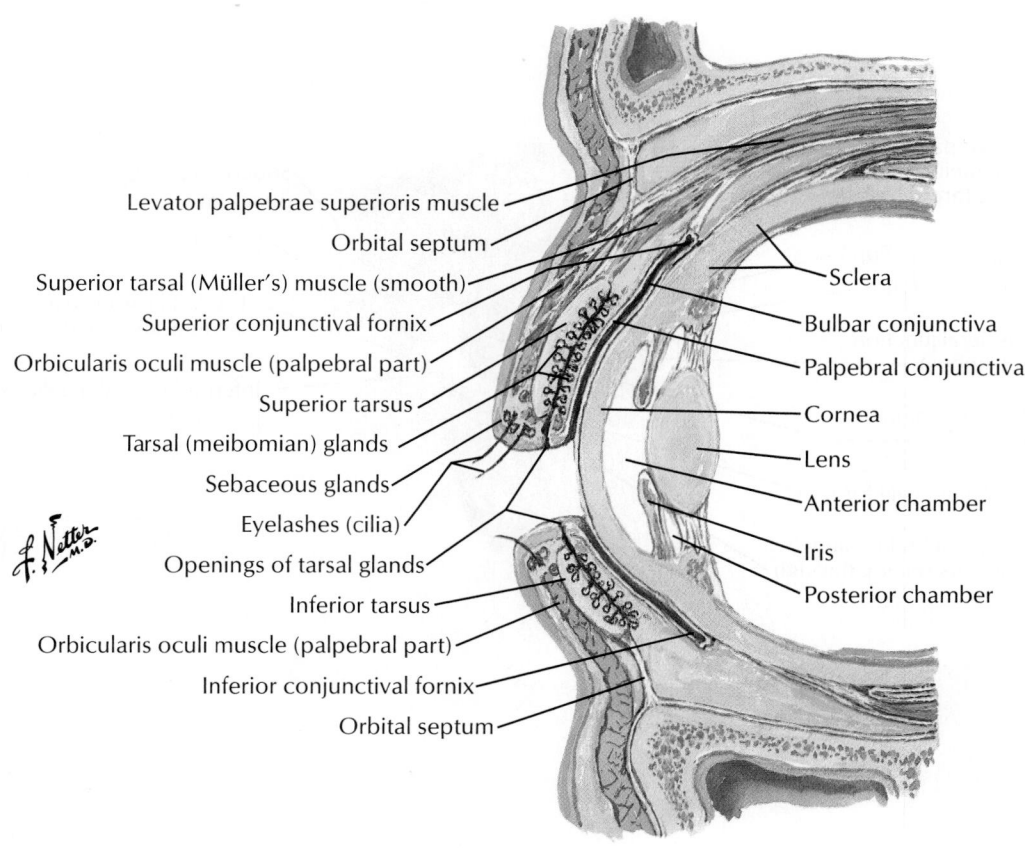

Levator palpebrae superioris muscle
Orbital septum
Superior tarsal (Müller's) muscle (smooth)
Superior conjunctival fornix
Orbicularis oculi muscle (palpebral part)
Superior tarsus
Tarsal (meibomian) glands
Sebaceous glands
Eyelashes (cilia)
Openings of tarsal glands
Inferior tarsus
Orbicularis oculi muscle (palpebral part)
Inferior conjunctival fornix
Orbital septum

Sclera
Bulbar conjunctiva
Palpebral conjunctiva
Cornea
Lens
Anterior chamber
Iris
Posterior chamber

Plate 81, Middle Eyelids. (Netter: Atlas of Human Anatomy, 4 ed, 2006, Saunders.)

Superior palpebral conjunctiva:
tarsal (meibomian) glands
shining through

Superior lacrimal papilla and
punctum

Seen through { Pupil
cornea { Iris

Plica semilunaris

Lacrimal caruncle in
lacrimal lake (lacus lacrimalis)

Corneoscleral junction
(corneal limbus)

Bulbar conjunctiva
over sclera

Inferior lacrimal papilla and
punctum

Inferior conjunctival fornix

Inferior palpebral conjunctiva:
tarsal glands shining through

Plate 81, Upper Eyelid. (Netter: Atlas of Human Anatomy, 4 ed, 2006, Saunders.)

Orbital part of lacrimal gland

Palpebral part of lacrimal gland

Excretory ducts of lacrimal gland

Plica semilunaris

Lacrimal caruncle

Inferior lacrimal papilla and punctum

Superior lacrimal papilla and punctum

Lacrimal canaliculi

Lacrimal sac

Nasolacrimal duct

Opening of nasolacrimal duct

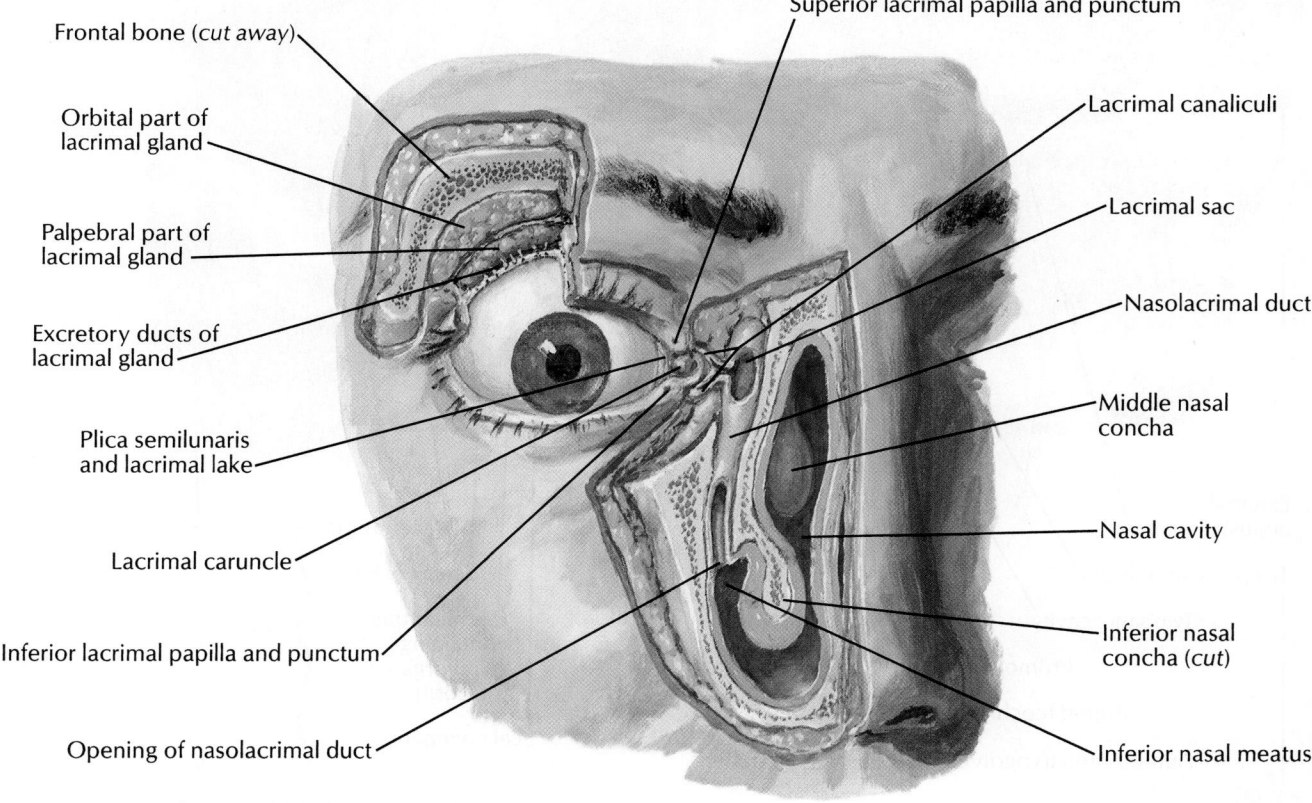

Frontal bone (cut away)

Orbital part of lacrimal gland

Palpebral part of lacrimal gland

Excretory ducts of lacrimal gland

Plica semilunaris and lacrimal lake

Lacrimal caruncle

Inferior lacrimal papilla and punctum

Opening of nasolacrimal duct

Superior lacrimal papilla and punctum

Lacrimal canaliculi

Lacrimal sac

Nasolacrimal duct

Middle nasal concha

Nasal cavity

Inferior nasal concha (cut)

Inferior nasal meatus

Plate 82 Lacrimal Apparatus. (Netter: Atlas of Human Anatomy, 4 ed, 2006, Saunders.)

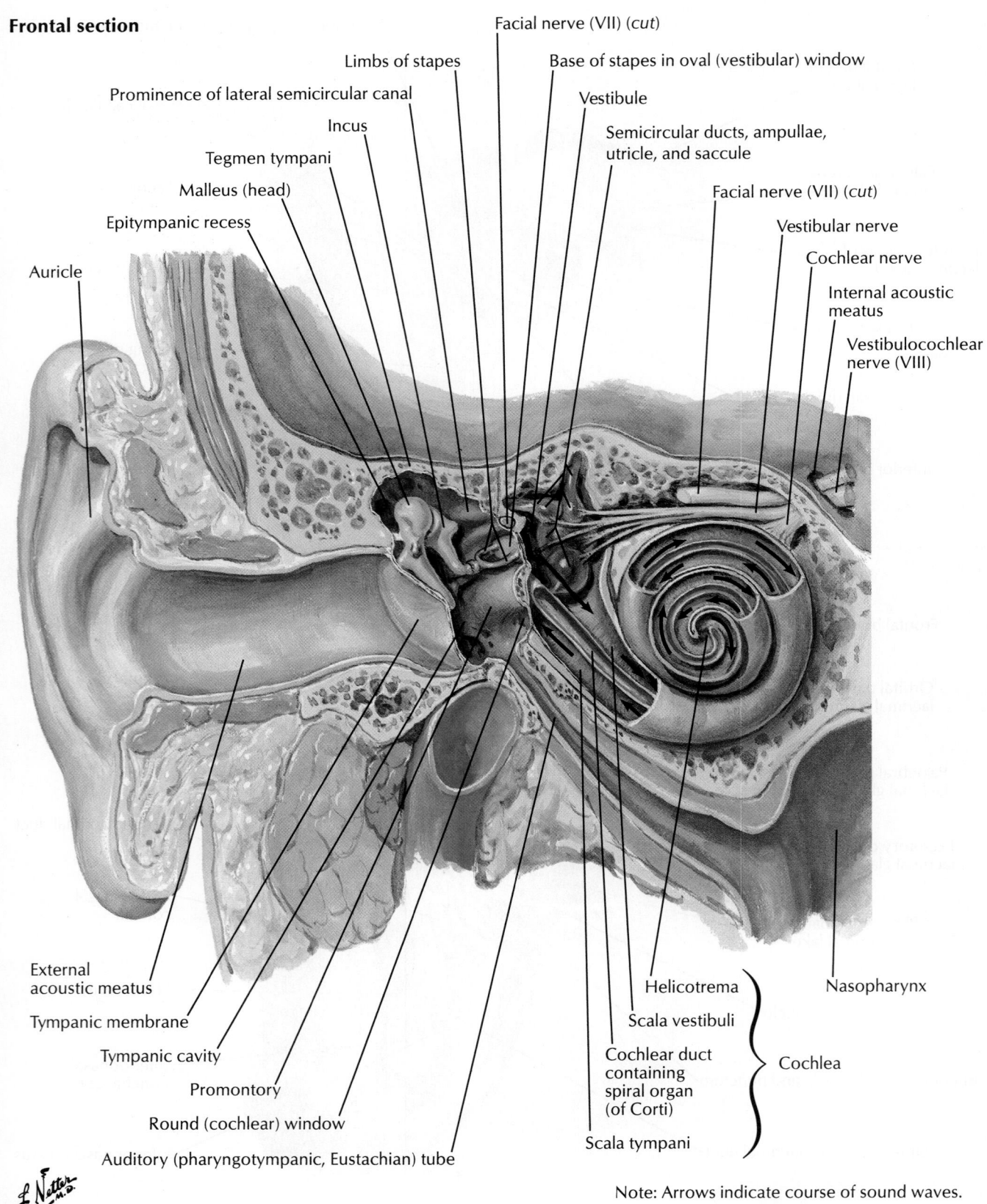

Facial nerve (VII) (*cut*)

Limbs of stapes

Base of stapes in oval (vestibular) window

Prominence of lateral semicircular canal

Vestibule

Incus

Semicircular ducts, ampullae, utricle, and saccule

Tegmen tympani

Malleus (head)

Facial nerve (VII) (*cut*)

Epitympanic recess

Vestibular nerve

Cochlear nerve

Auricle

Internal acoustic meatus

Vestibulocochlear nerve (VIII)

External acoustic meatus

Tympanic membrane

Tympanic cavity

Promontory

Round (cochlear) window

Auditory (pharyngotympanic, Eustachian) tube

Helicotrema

Scala vestibuli

Cochlear duct containing spiral organ (of Corti)

Scala tympani

Cochlea

Nasopharynx

Note: Arrows indicate course of sound waves.

Plate 92 Pathway of Sound Reception. (Netter: Atlas of Human Anatomy, 4 ed, 2006, Saunders.)

NAP-20

Medial wall of tympanic cavity: lateral view

Mastoid antrum

Prominence of lateral semicircular canal

Prominence of facial canal

Geniculum (geniculate ganglion) of facial nerve

Greater petrosal nerve

Base of stapes in fossa of oval (vestibular) window

Limbs of stapes

Pyramidal eminence

Chorda tympani nerve (cut)

Mastoid cells

Tendon of stapedius muscle

Fossa of round (cochlear) window

Facial nerve (VII) in stylomastoid foramen

Jugular fossa

Tympanic cells

Tensor tympani muscle (tendon cut)

Auditory (pharyngotympanic, Eustachian) tube

Levator veli palatini muscle

Promontory with tympanic nerve (of Jacobson) and plexus under mucosa

Internal carotid artery

Plate 94 Tympanic Cavity. (Netter: Atlas of Human Anatomy, 4 ed, 2006, Saunders.)

Otoscopic view of right tympanic membrane

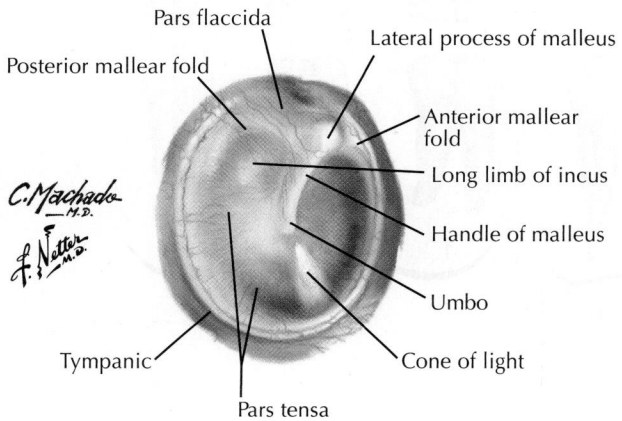

Pars flaccida

Posterior mallear fold

Lateral process of malleus

Anterior mallear fold

Long limb of incus

Handle of malleus

Umbo

Cone of light

Tympanic

Pars tensa

Plate 93 Tympanic Cavity. (Netter: Atlas of Human Anatomy, 4 ed, 2006, Saunders.)

Dissected right bony labyrinth (otic capsule): membranous labyrinth removed

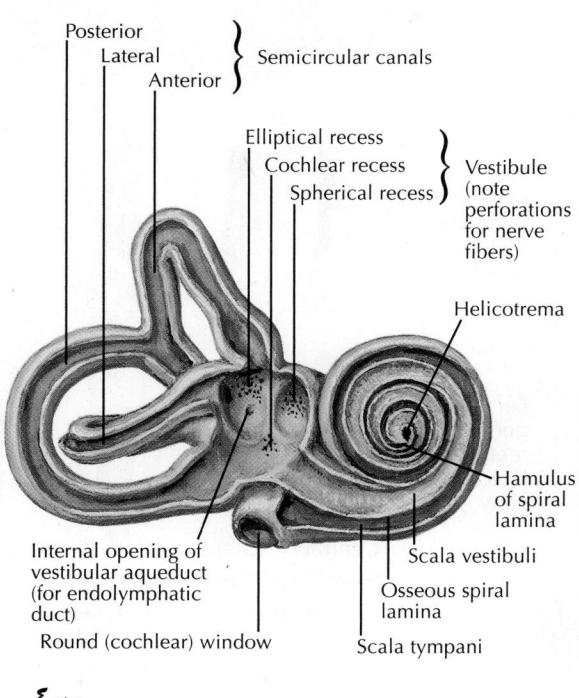

Posterior

Lateral

Anterior

Semicircular canals

Elliptical recess

Cochlear recess

Spherical recess

Vestibule (note perforations for nerve fibers)

Helicotrema

Internal opening of vestibular aqueduct (for endolymphatic duct)

Round (cochlear) window

Hamulus of spiral lamina

Scala vestibuli

Osseous spiral lamina

Scala tympani

Plate 95 Bony Membranous Labyrinth. (Netter: Atlas of Human Anatomy, 4 ed, 2006, Saunders.)

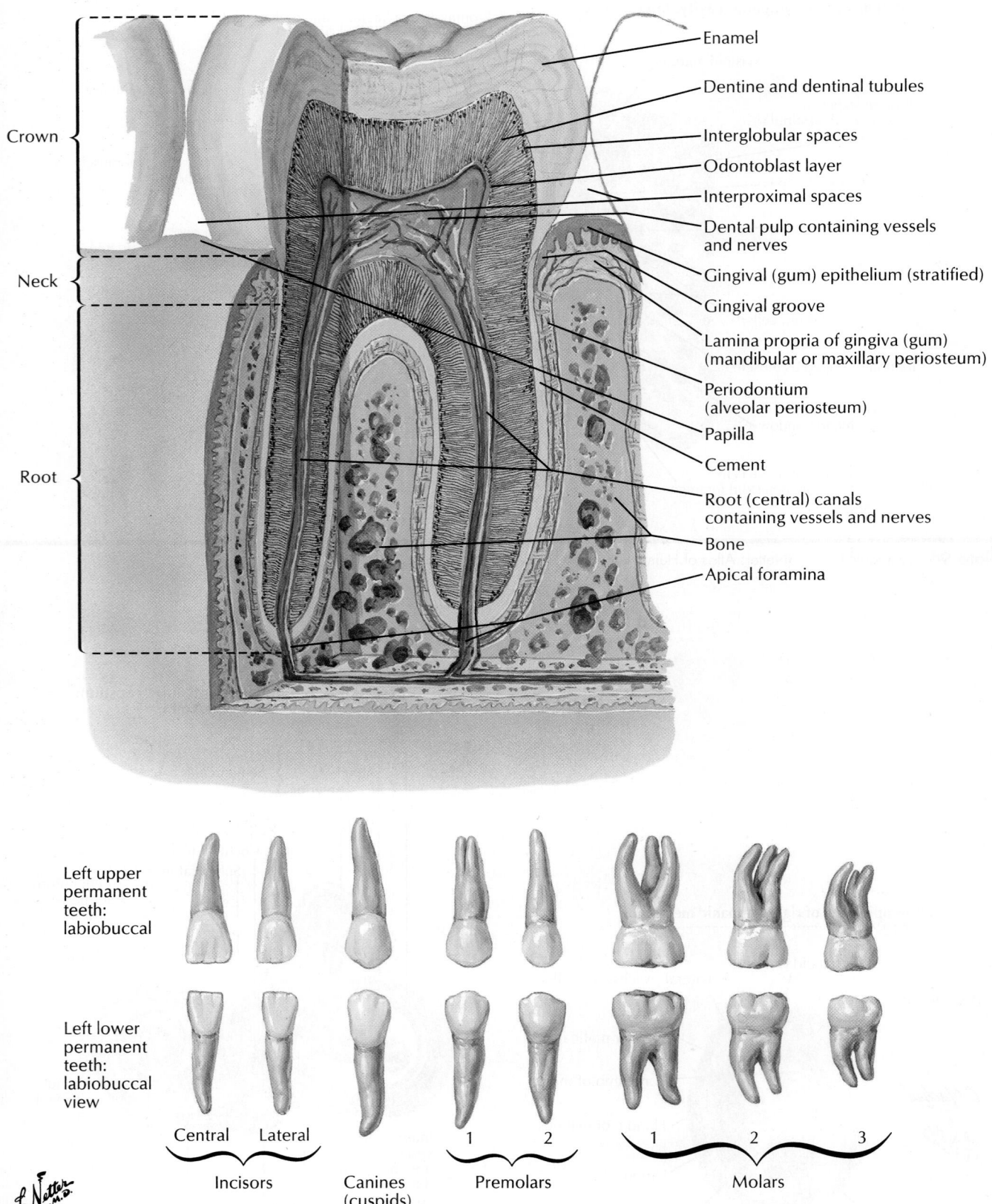

Crown

Neck

Root

Enamel

Dentine and dentinal tubules

Interglobular spaces

Odontoblast layer

Interproximal spaces

Dental pulp containing vessels and nerves

Gingival (gum) epithelium (stratified)

Gingival groove

Lamina propria of gingiva (gum) (mandibular or maxillary periosteum)

Periodontium (alveolar periosteum)

Papilla

Cement

Root (central) canals containing vessels and nerves

Bone

Apical foramina

Left upper permanent teeth: labiobuccal

Left lower permanent teeth: labiobuccal view

Central   Lateral

Incisors

Canines (cuspids)

1   2

Premolars

1   2   3

Molars

Plate 57   Teeth. (Netter: Atlas of Human Anatomy, 4 ed, 2006, Saunders.)

Tongue

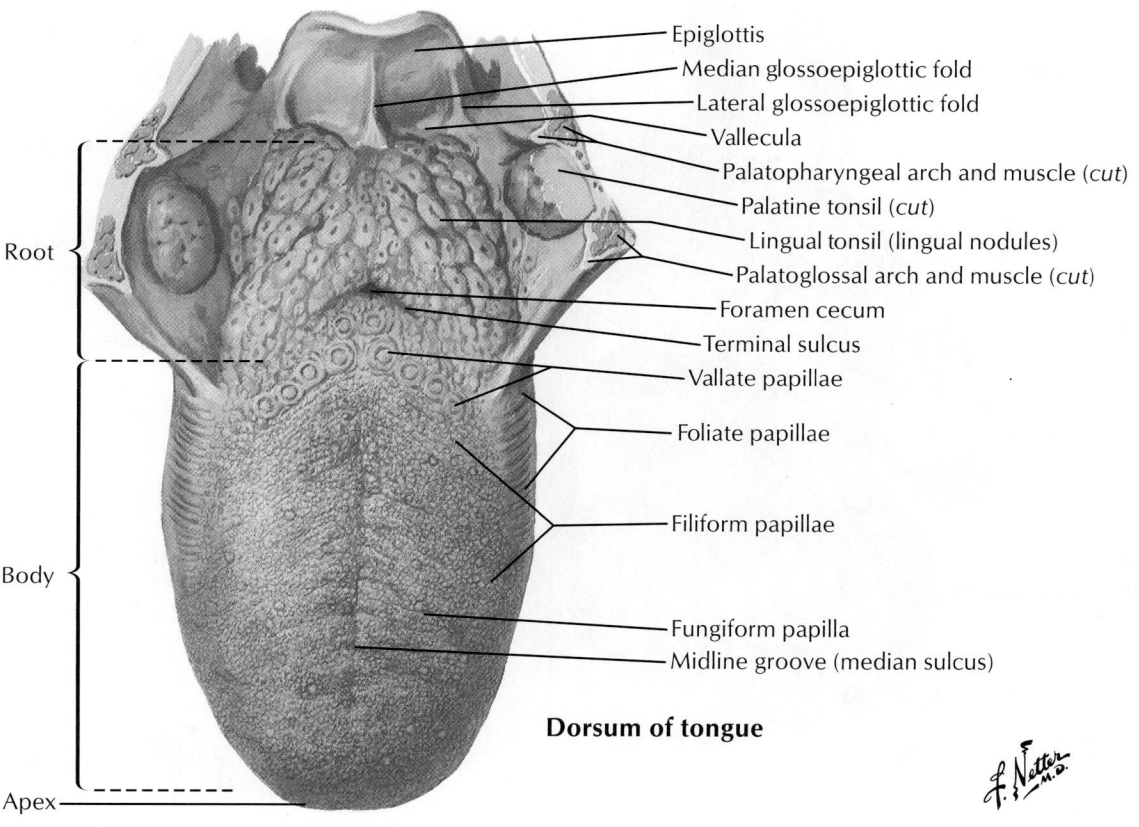

Epiglottis
Median glossoepiglottic fold
Lateral glossoepiglottic fold
Vallecula
Palatopharyngeal arch and muscle (*cut*)
Palatine tonsil (*cut*)
Lingual tonsil (lingual nodules)
Palatoglossal arch and muscle (*cut*)
Foramen cecum
Terminal sulcus
Vallate papillae
Foliate papillae
Filiform papillae
Fungiform papilla
Midline groove (median sulcus)

Root

Body

Apex

Dorsum of tongue

Plate 58   Tongue. (Netter: Atlas of Human Anatomy, 4 ed, 2006, Saunders.)

NAP-23

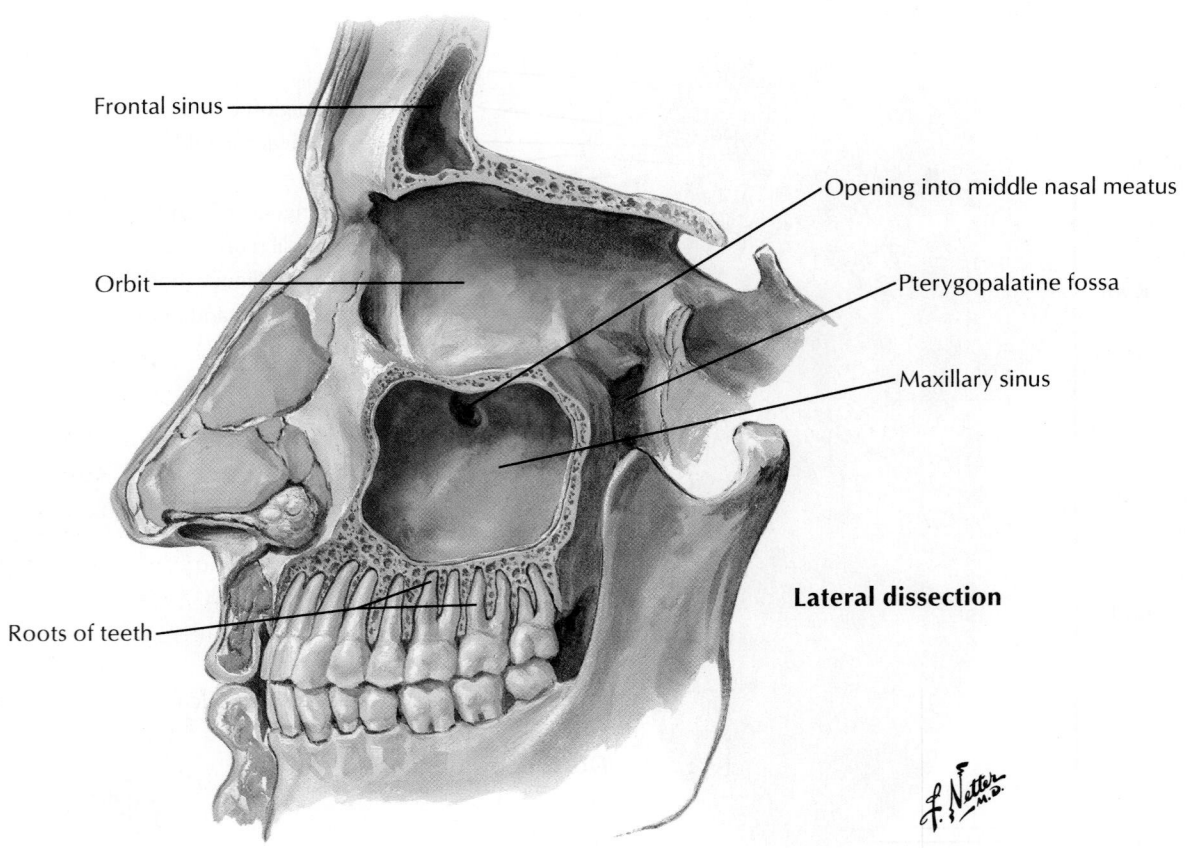

Frontal sinus

Opening into middle nasal meatus

Orbit

Pterygopalatine fossa

Maxillary sinus

Lateral dissection

Roots of teeth

Plate 49 Paranasal Sinuses. (Netter: Atlas of Human Anatomy, 4 ed, 2006, Saunders.)

NAP-24

Superficial temporal artery and vein and auriculotemporal nerve

Branches of facial nerve

Transverse facial artery

Accessory parotid gland

Parotid duct

Buccinator muscle (*cut*)

Masseter muscle

Lingual nerve

Submandibular ganglion

Tongue

Frenulum of tongue

Sublingual fold with openings of sublingual ducts

Sublingual caruncle with opening of submandibular duct

Sublingual gland

Submandibular duct

Sublingual artery and vein

Mylohyoid muscle (*cut*)

Digastric muscle (anterior belly)

Submandibular gland

Facial artery and vein

Parotid gland

Retromandibular vein (anterior and posterior branches)

Digastric muscle (posterior belly)

Stylohyoid muscle

External jugular vein

Sternocleidomastoid muscle

Common trunk receiving facial, anterior branch of retromandibular, and lingual veins (common facial vein)

Internal jugular vein

External carotid artery

Hyoid bone

Parotid gland: totally serous

Submandibular gland: mostly serous, partially mucous

Sublingual gland: almost completely mucous

Plate 61   Salivary Glands. (Netter: Atlas of Human Anatomy, 4 ed, 2006, Saunders.)

Coronary Arteries: Arteriographic Views

Right coronary artery: left anterior oblique view

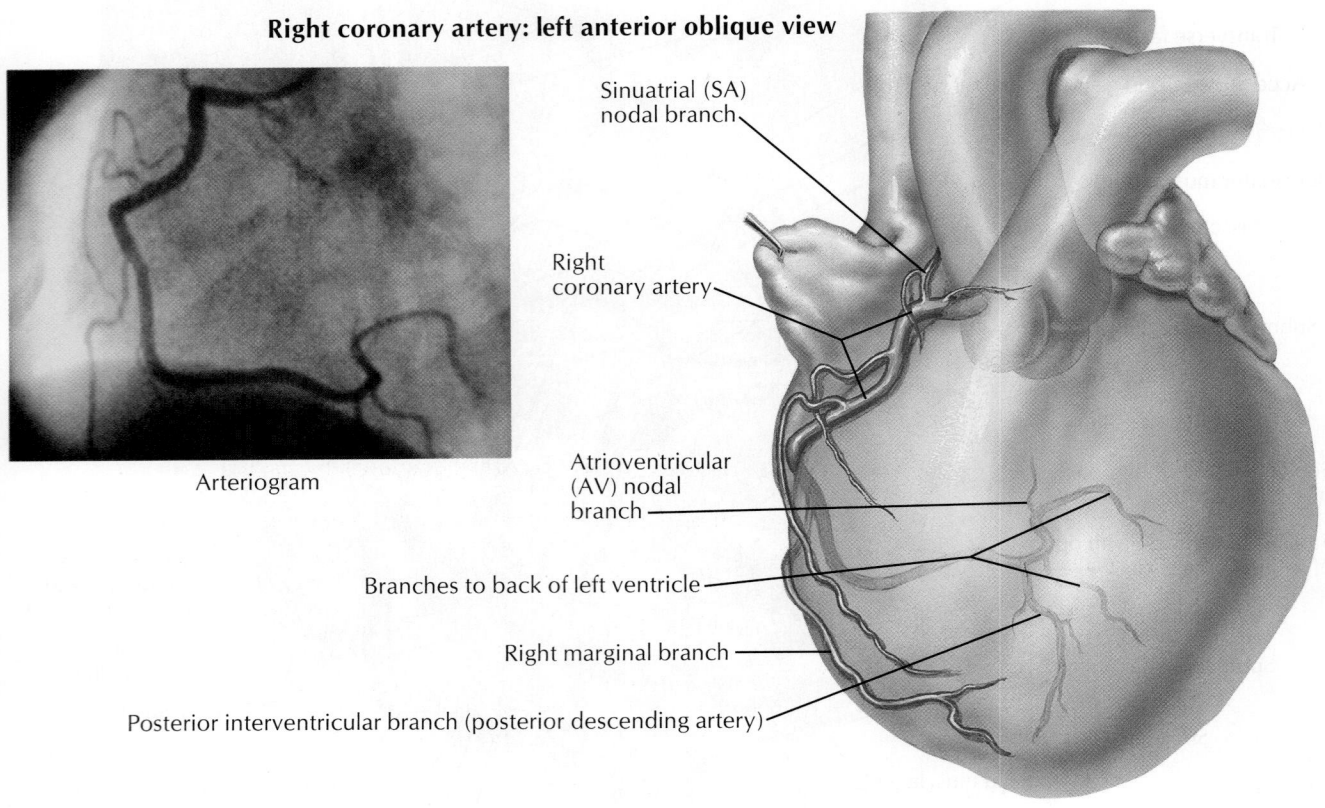

Sinuatrial (SA) nodal branch

Right coronary artery

Atrioventricular (AV) nodal branch

Branches to back of left ventricle

Right marginal branch

Posterior interventricular branch (posterior descending artery)

Arteriogram

Right coronary artery: right anterior oblique view

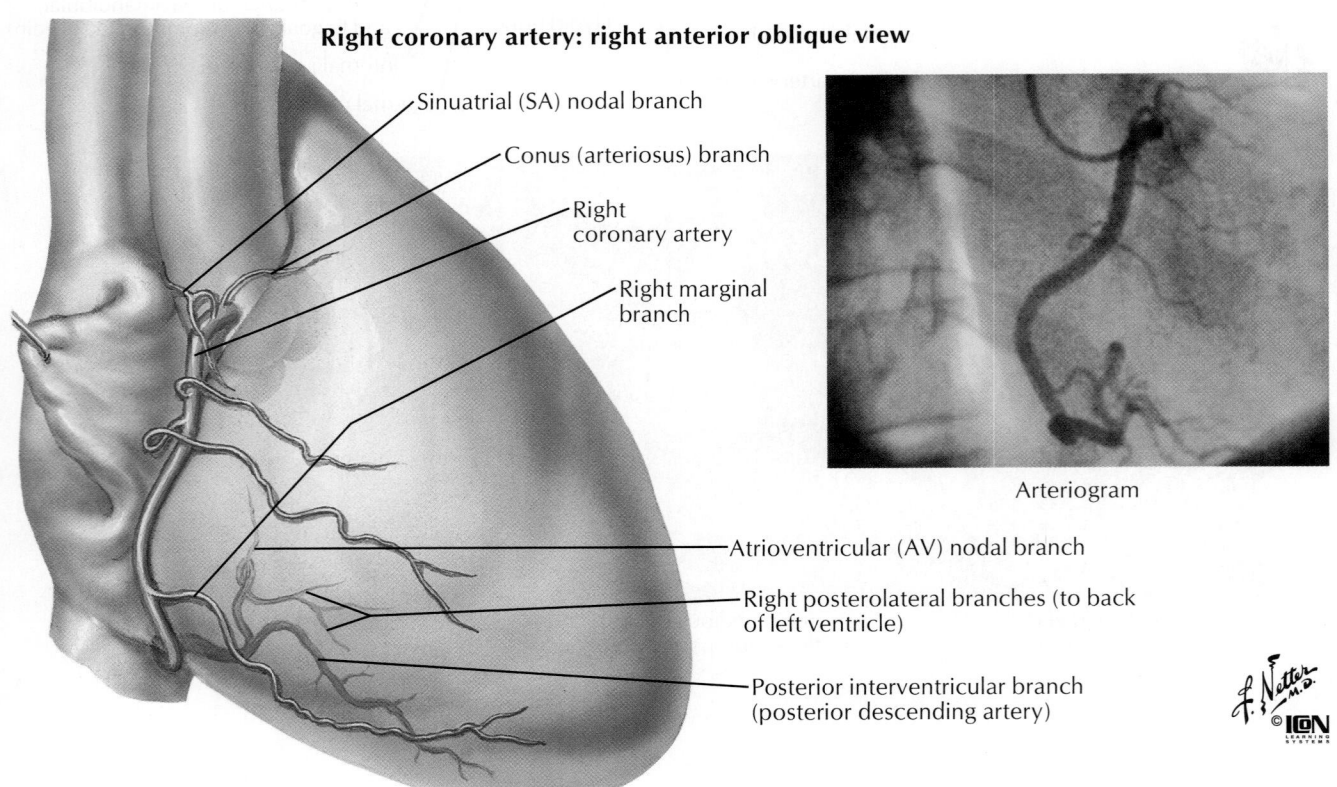

Sinuatrial (SA) nodal branch

Conus (arteriosus) branch

Right coronary artery

Right marginal branch

Arteriogram

Atrioventricular (AV) nodal branch

Right posterolateral branches (to back of left ventricle)

Posterior interventricular branch (posterior descending artery)

Plate 218 Coronary Arteries: Arteriographic Views. (Netter: Atlas of Human Anatomy, 4 ed, 2006, Saunders.)

NAP-26

Left coronary artery: left anterior oblique view

Left coronary artery

Circumflex branch

Arteriogram

Anterior interventricular branch (left anterior descending)

Diagonal branches of anterior interventricular branch

Atrioventricular branch of circumflex branch

Left (obtuse) marginal branch

Posterolateral branches

(Perforating) interventricular septal branches

Left coronary artery: right anterior oblique view

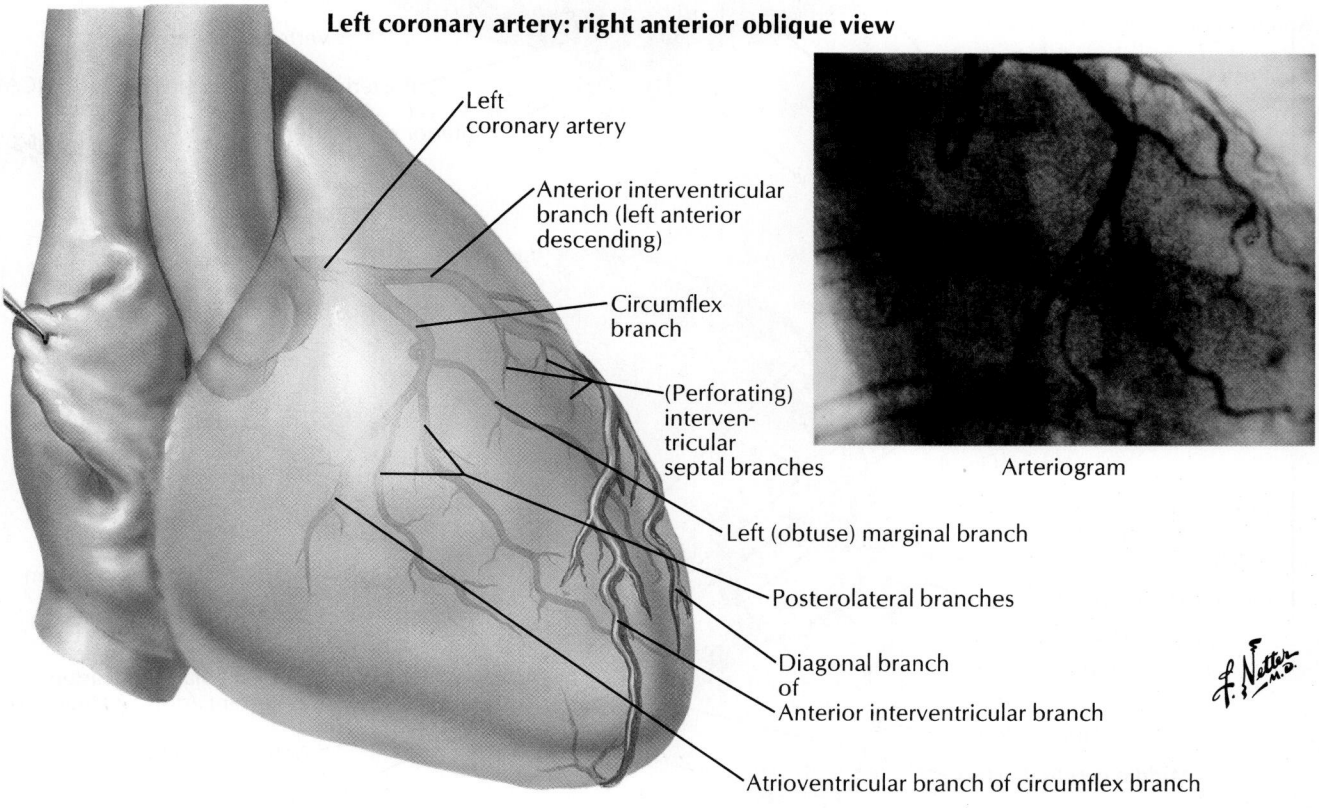

Left coronary artery

Anterior interventricular branch (left anterior descending)

Circumflex branch

(Perforating) interventricular septal branches

Arteriogram

Left (obtuse) marginal branch

Posterolateral branches

Diagonal branch of Anterior interventricular branch

Atrioventricular branch of circumflex branch

Plate 219   Coronary Arteries: Arteriographic Views. (Netter: Atlas of Human Anatomy, 4 ed, 2006, Saunders.)

NAP-27

NETTER'S ANATOMY ILLUSTRATIONS

Corpus callosum

Anterolateral central (lenticulostriate) arteries

Lateral frontobasal (orbitofrontal) artery

Prefrontal artery

Precentral (pre-Rolandic) and central (Rolandic) sulcal arteries

Anterior parietal (postcentral sulcal) artery

Posterior parietal artery

Branch to angular gyrus

Temporal branches (anterior, middle, and posterior)

Middle cerebral artery and branches (deep in lateral cerebral [Sylvian] sulcus)

Anterior communicating artery

Posterior communicating artery

Anterior inferior cerebellar artery (AICA)

Posterior spinal artery

Paracentral artery

Medial frontal branches

Pericallosal artery

Callosomarginal artery

Polar frontal artery

Anterior cerebral arteries

Medial frontobasal (orbitofrontal) artery

Distal medial striate artery (recurrent artery of Heubner)

Internal carotid artery

Anterior choroidal artery

Posterior cerebral artery

Superior cerebellar artery

Basilar and pontine arteries

Labyrinthine (internal acoustic) artery

Vertebral artery

Posterior inferior cerebellar artery (PICA)

Anterior spinal artery

Corpus striatum (caudate and lentiform nuclei)

Anterolateral central (lenticulostriate) arteries

Insula (island of Reil)

Limen of insula

Precentral (pre-Rolandic), central (Rolandic) sulcal, and parietal arteries

Lateral cerebral (Sylvian) sulcus

Temporal branches of middle cerebral artery

Temporal lobe

Middle cerebral artery

Internal carotid artery

Falx cerebri

Callosomarginal arteries and Pericallosal arteries (branches of anterior cerebral arteries)

Trunk of corpus callosum

Internal capsule

Septum pellucidum

Rostrum of corpus callosum

Anterior cerebral arteries

Distal medial striate artery (recurrent artery of Heubner)

Anterior communicating artery

Optic chiasm

Plate 141 Arteries of Brain: Frontal View and Section. (Netter: Atlas of Human Anatomy, 4 ed, 2006, Saunders.)

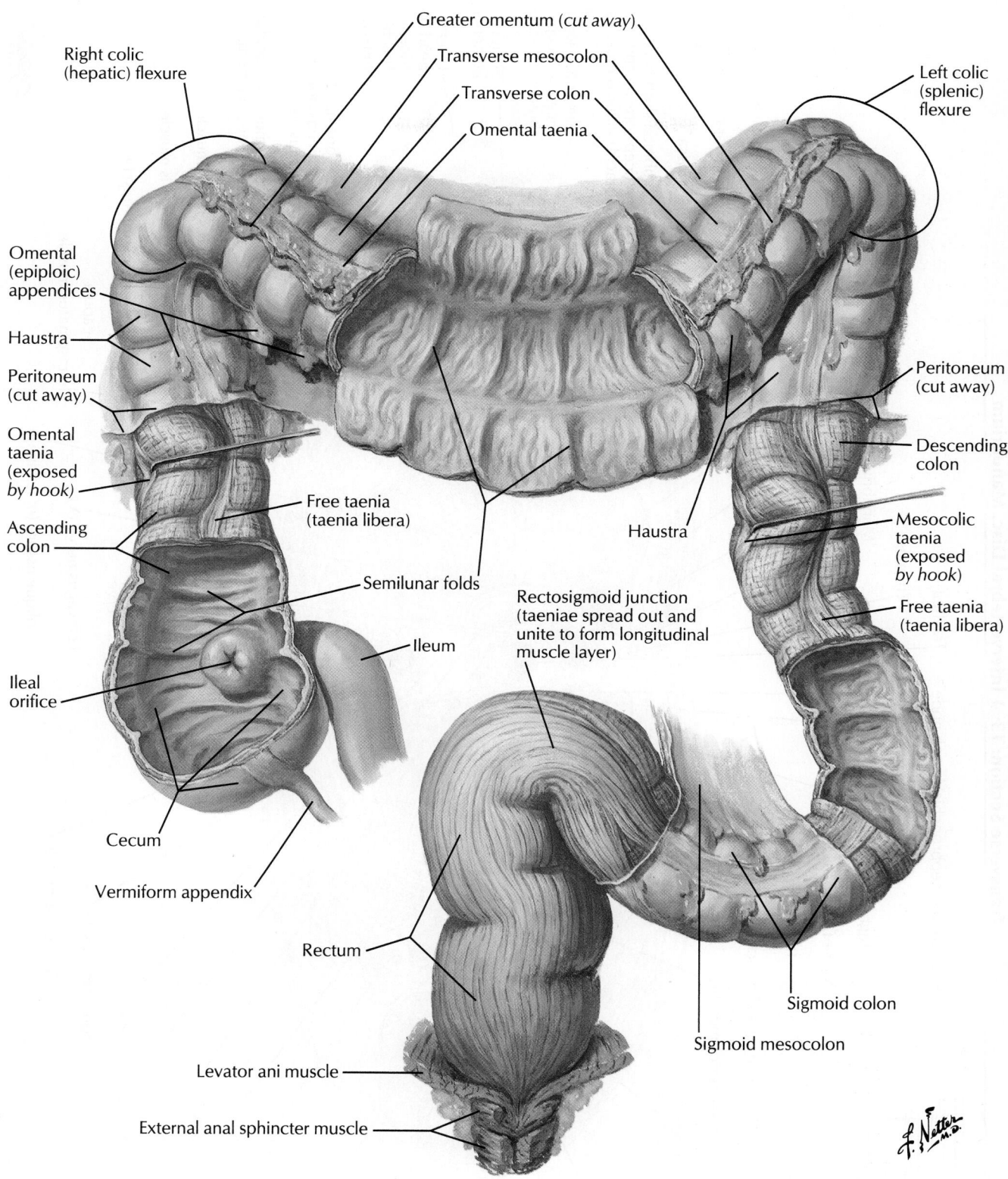

Right colic (hepatic) flexure

Greater omentum (*cut away*)

Transverse mesocolon

Transverse colon

Omental taenia

Left colic (splenic) flexure

Omental (epiploic) appendices

Haustra

Peritoneum (cut away)

Omental taenia (exposed *by hook*)

Ascending colon

Ileal orifice

Cecum

Vermiform appendix

Rectum

Levator ani muscle

External anal sphincter muscle

Free taenia (taenia libera)

Semilunar folds

Ileum

Rectosigmoid junction (taeniae spread out and unite to form longitudinal muscle layer)

Haustra

Peritoneum (cut away)

Descending colon

Mesocolic taenia (exposed *by hook*)

Free taenia (taenia libera)

Sigmoid colon

Sigmoid mesocolon

Plate 284   Mucosa and Musculature of Large Intestine. (Netter: Atlas of Human Anatomy, 4 ed, 2006, Saunders.)

NAP-29

Transverse Section: T3–4 Intervertebral Disc, Manubrium

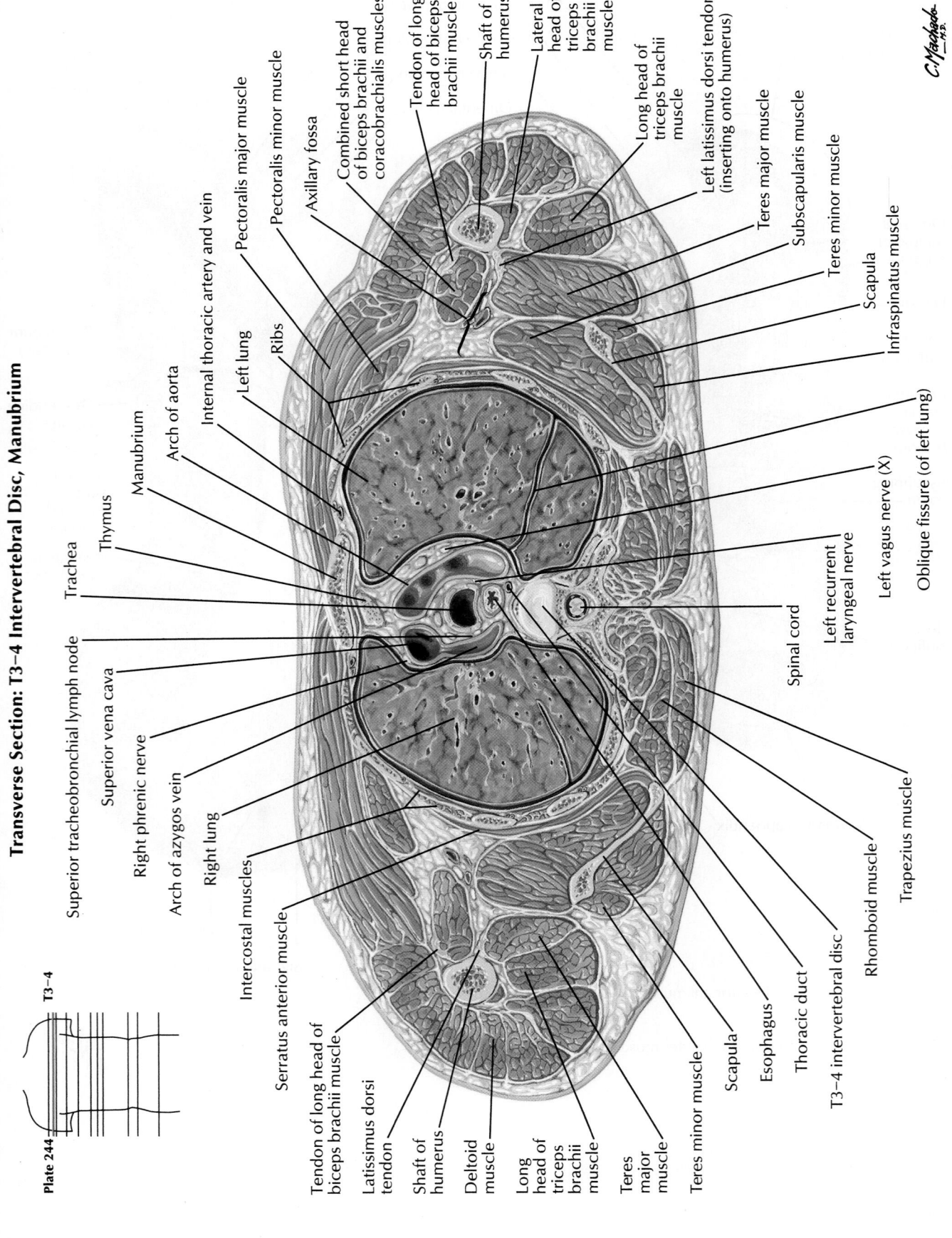

Superior tracheobronchial lymph node

Superior vena cava

Right phrenic nerve

Arch of azygos vein

Right lung

Intercostal muscles

Serratus anterior muscle

Trachea

Thymus

Manubrium

Arch of aorta

Internal thoracic artery and vein

Left lung

Ribs

Axillary fossa

Pectoralis minor muscle

Pectoralis major muscle

Combined short head of biceps brachii and coracobrachialis muscles

Tendon of long head of biceps brachii muscle

Shaft of humerus

Lateral head of triceps brachii muscle

Long head of triceps brachii muscle

Left latissimus dorsi tendon (inserting onto humerus)

Teres major muscle

Subscapularis muscle

Teres minor muscle

Scapula

Infraspinatus muscle

Oblique fissure (of left lung)

Left vagus nerve (X)

Left recurrent laryngeal nerve

Spinal cord

Tendon of long head of biceps brachii muscle

Latissimus dorsi tendon

Shaft of humerus

Deltoid muscle

Long head of triceps brachii muscle

Teres major muscle

Teres minor muscle

Scapula

Esophagus

Thoracic duct

T3–4 intervertebral disc

Rhomboid muscle

Trapezius muscle

Plate 244 Cross Section of Thorax at T3–4 Disc Level. (Netter: Atlas of Human Anatomy, 4 ed, 2006, Saunders.)

T3–4

Plate 244

Right knee in extension: posterior view

Posterior cruciate ligament

Anterior cruciate ligament

Posterior meniscofemoral ligament

Adductor tubercle on medial epicondyle of femur

Medial condyle of femur (articular surface)

Lateral condyle of femur (articular surface)

Medial meniscus

Popliteus tendon

Tibial collateral ligament

Fibular collateral ligament

Medial condyle of tibia

Lateral meniscus

Head of fibula

Plate 509   Knee: Cruciate and Collateral Ligaments. (Netter: Atlas of Human Anatomy, 4 ed, 2006, Saunders.)

NAP-31

NETTER'S ANATOMY ILLUSTRATIONS

Paramedian (sagittal) dissection

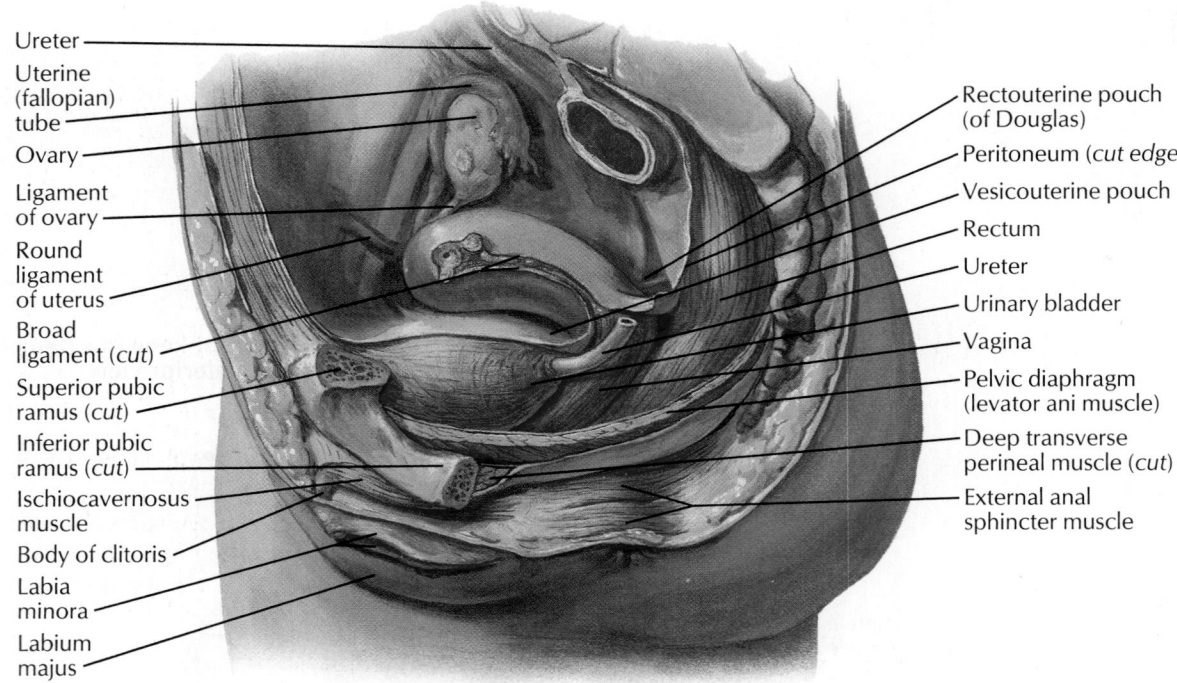

Ureter

Uterine (fallopian) tube

Ovary

Ligament of ovary

Round ligament of uterus

Broad ligament (*cut*)

Superior pubic ramus (*cut*)

Inferior pubic ramus (*cut*)

Ischiocavernosus muscle

Body of clitoris

Labia minora

Labium majus

Rectouterine pouch (of Douglas)

Peritoneum (*cut edge*)

Vesicouterine pouch

Rectum

Ureter

Urinary bladder

Vagina

Pelvic diaphragm (levator ani muscle)

Deep transverse perineal muscle (*cut*)

External anal sphincter muscle

Median (sagittal) section

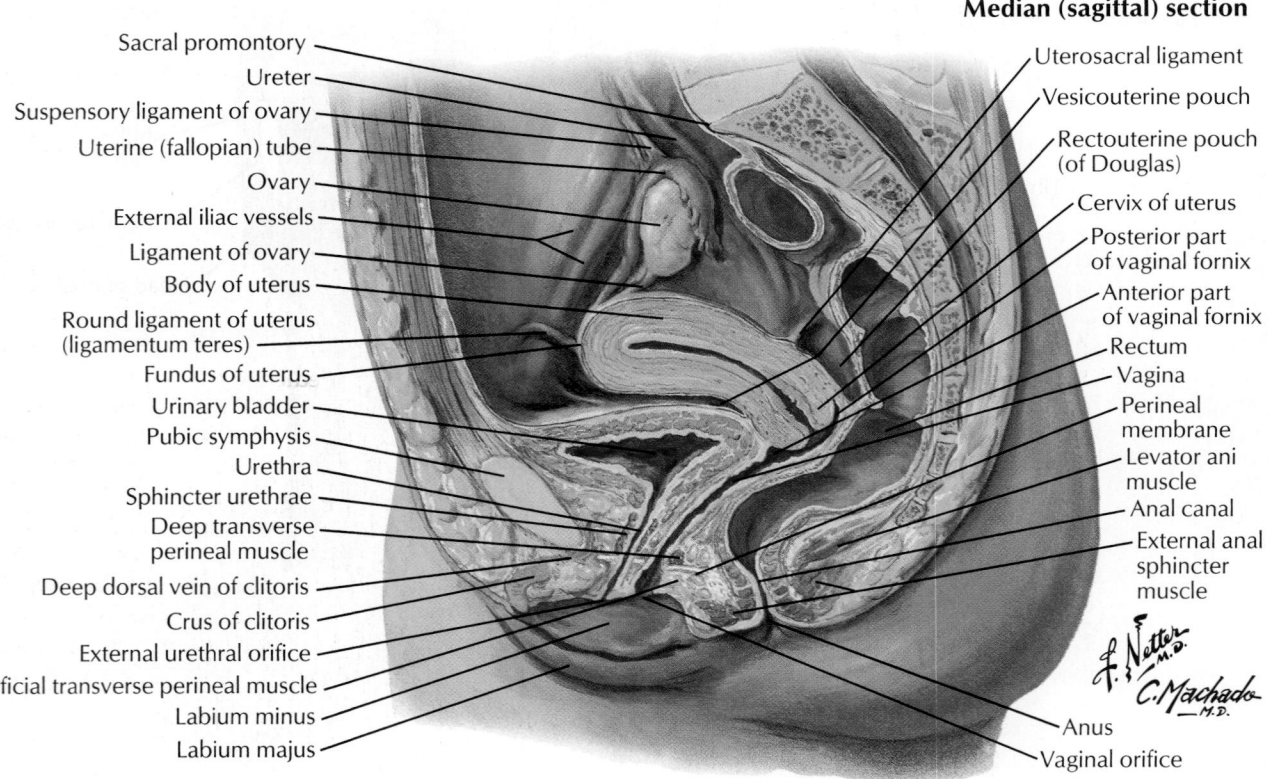

Sacral promontory

Ureter

Suspensory ligament of ovary

Uterine (fallopian) tube

Ovary

External iliac vessels

Ligament of ovary

Body of uterus

Round ligament of uterus (ligamentum teres)

Fundus of uterus

Urinary bladder

Pubic symphysis

Urethra

Sphincter urethrae

Deep transverse perineal muscle

Deep dorsal vein of clitoris

Crus of clitoris

External urethral orifice

Superficial transverse perineal muscle

Labium minus

Labium majus

Uterosacral ligament

Vesicouterine pouch

Rectouterine pouch (of Douglas)

Cervix of uterus

Posterior part of vaginal fornix

Anterior part of vaginal fornix

Rectum

Vagina

Perineal membrane

Levator ani muscle

Anal canal

External anal sphincter muscle

Anus

Vaginal orifice

Plate 360 Pelvic Viscera and Perineum: Female. (Netter: Atlas of Human Anatomy, 4 ed, 2006, Saunders.)

NAP-32

NETTER'S ANATOMY ILLUSTRATIONS

Introduction

ICD-10-CM Official Guidelines for Coding and Reporting 2018
Narrative changes appear in **bold** text
Items <u>underlined</u> have been moved within the guidelines since the 2017 version
Italics are used to indicate revisions to heading changes

The Centers for Medicare and Medicaid Services (CMS) and the National Center for Health Statistics (NCHS), two departments within the U.S. Federal Government's Department of Health and Human Services (DHHS) provide the following guidelines for coding and reporting using the International Classification of Diseases, 10th Revision, Clinical Modification (ICD-10-CM). These guidelines should be used as a companion document to the official version of the ICD-10-CM as published on the NCHS website. The ICD-10-CM is a morbidity classification published by the United States for classifying diagnoses and reason for visits in all health care settings. The ICD-10-CM is based on the ICD-10, the statistical classification of disease published by the World Health Organization (WHO).

These guidelines have been approved by the four organizations that make up the Cooperating Parties for the ICD-10-CM: the American Hospital Association (AHA), the American Health Information Management Association (AHIMA), CMS, and NCHS.

These guidelines are a set of rules that have been developed to accompany and complement the official conventions and instructions provided within the ICD-10-CM itself. The instructions and conventions of the classification take precedence over guidelines. These guidelines are based on the coding and sequencing instructions in the Tabular List and Alphabetic Index of ICD-10-CM, but provide additional instruction. Adherence to these guidelines when assigning ICD-10-CM diagnosis codes is required under the Health Insurance Portability and Accountability Act (HIPAA). The diagnosis codes (Tabular List and Alphabetic Index)

have been adopted under HIPAA for all healthcare settings. A joint effort between the healthcare provider and the coder is essential to achieve complete and accurate documentation, code assignment, and reporting of diagnoses and procedures. These guidelines have been developed to assist both the healthcare provider and the coder in identifying those diagnoses that are to be reported. The importance of consistent, complete documentation in the medical record cannot be overemphasized. Without such documentation accurate coding cannot be achieved. The entire record should be reviewed to determine the specific reason for the encounter and the conditions treated.

The term encounter is used for all settings, including hospital admissions. In the context of these guidelines, the term provider is used throughout the guidelines to mean physician or any qualified health care practitioner who is legally accountable for establishing the patient's diagnosis. Only this set of guidelines, approved by the Cooperating Parties, is official.

The guidelines are organized into sections. Section I includes the structure and conventions of the classification and general guidelines that apply to the entire classification, and chapter-specific guidelines that correspond to the chapters as they are arranged in the classification. Section II includes guidelines for selection of principal diagnosis for non-outpatient settings. Section III includes guidelines for reporting additional diagnoses in non-outpatient settings. Section IV is for outpatient coding and reporting. It is necessary to review all sections of the guidelines to fully understand all of the rules and instructions needed to code properly.

ICD-10-CM Official Guidelines for Coding and Reporting

Section I. Conventions, general coding guidelines and chapter specific guidelines

A. Conventions for the ICD-10-CM
 1. The Alphabetic Index and Tabular List
 2. Format and Structure:
 3. Use of codes for reporting purposes
 4. Placeholder character
 5. 7th Characters
 6. Abbreviations
  a. Alphabetic Index abbreviations
  b. Tabular List abbreviations
 7. Punctuation
 8. Use of "and"
 9. Other and Unspecified codes
  a. "Other" codes
  b. "Unspecified" codes
 10. Includes Notes
 11. Inclusion terms
 12. Excludes Notes
  a. Excludes1
  b. Excludes2
 13. Etiology/manifestation convention ("code first", "use additional code" and "in diseases classified elsewhere" notes)
 14. "And"
 15. "With"
 16. "See" and "See Also"
 17. "Code also note"
 18. Default codes
 19. Code assignment and Clinical Criteria
B. General Coding Guidelines
 1. Locating a code in the ICD-10-CM
 2. Level of Detail in Coding
 3. Code or codes from A00.0 through T88.9, Z00-Z99.8
 4. Signs and symptoms
 5. Conditions that are an integral part of a disease process
 6. Conditions that are not an integral part of a disease process
 7. Multiple coding for a single condition
 8. Acute and Chronic Conditions
 9. Combination Code
 10. Sequela (Late Effects)
 11. Impending or Threatened Condition
 12. Reporting Same Diagnosis Code More than Once
 13. Laterality
 14. Documentation for BMI, Depth of Non-pressure ulcers, Pressure Ulcer Stages, Coma Scale, and NIH Stroke Scale
 15. Syndromes
 16. Documentation of Complications of Care
 17. Borderline Diagnosis
 18. Use of Sign/Symptom/Unspecified Codes
C. Chapter-Specific Coding Guidelines
 1. Chapter 1: Certain Infectious and Parasitic Diseases (A00-B99)
  a. Human Immunodeficiency Virus (HIV) Infections
  b. Infectious agents as the cause of diseases classified to other chapters
  c. Infections resistant to antibiotics

  d. Sepsis, Severe Sepsis, and Septic Shock
  e. Methicillin Resistant *Staphylococcus aureus* (MRSA) Conditions
  f. Zika virus infection
 2. Chapter 2: Neoplasms (C00-D49)
  a. Treatment directed at the malignancy
  b. Treatment of secondary site
  c. Coding and sequencing of complications
  d. Primary malignancy previously excised
  e. Admissions/Encounters involving chemotherapy, immunotherapy and radiation therapy
  f. Admission/encounter to determine extent of malignancy
  g. Symptoms, signs, and abnormal findings listed in Chapter 18 associated with neoplasms
  h. Admission/encounter for pain control/management
  i. Malignancy in two or more noncontiguous sites
  j. Disseminated malignant neoplasm, unspecified
  k. Malignant neoplasm without specification of site
  l. Sequencing of neoplasm codes
  m. Current malignancy versus personal history of malignancy
  n. Leukemia, Multiple Myeloma, and Malignant Plasma Cell Neoplasms in remission versus personal history
  o. Aftercare following surgery for neoplasm
  p. Follow-up care for completed treatment of a malignancy
  q. Prophylactic organ removal for prevention of malignancy
  r. Malignant neoplasm associated with transplanted organ
 3. Chapter 3: Disease of the blood and blood-forming organs and certain disorders involving the immune mechanism (D50-D89)
 4. Chapter 4: Endocrine, Nutritional, and Metabolic Diseases (E00-E89)
  a. Diabetes mellitus
 5. Chapter 5: Mental, Behavioral and Neurodevelopmental disorders (F01 – F99)
  a. Pain disorders related to psychological factors
  b. Mental and behavioral disorders due to psychoactive substance use
 6. Chapter 6: Diseases of the Nervous System (G00-G99)
  a. Dominant/nondominant side
  b. Pain - Category G89
 7. Chapter 7: Diseases of the Eye and Adnexa (H00-H59)
  a. Glaucoma
  b. Blindness
 8. Chapter 8: Diseases of the Ear and Mastoid Process (H60-H95)
 9. Chapter 9: Diseases of the Circulatory System (I00-I99)
  a. Hypertension
  b. Atherosclerotic Coronary Artery Disease and Angina
  c. Intraoperative and Postprocedural Cerebrovascular Accident
  d. Sequelae of Cerebrovascular Disease
  e. Acute myocardial infarction (AMI)

Section II. Selection of Principal Diagnosis

A. Codes for symptoms, signs, and ill-defined conditions
B. Two or more interrelated conditions, each potentially meeting the definition for principal diagnosis
C. Two or more diagnoses that equally meet the definition for principal diagnosis
D. Two or more comparative or contrasting conditions
E. A symptom(s) followed by contrasting/comparative diagnoses
F. Original treatment plan not carried out
G. Complications of surgery and other medical care
H. Uncertain Diagnosis

Section I. Conventions, general coding guidelines and chapter specific guidelines

The conventions, general guidelines and chapter-specific guidelines are applicable to all health care settings unless otherwise indicated. The conventions and instructions of the classification take precedence over guidelines.

A. Conventions for the ICD-10-CM

The conventions for the ICD-10-CM are the general rules for use of the classification independent of the guidelines. These conventions are incorporated within the Alphabetic Index and Tabular List of the ICD-10-CM as instructional notes.

1. **The Alphabetic Index and Tabular List**
   The ICD-10-CM is divided into the Alphabetic Index, an alphabetical list of terms and their corresponding code, and the Tabular List, a structured list of codes divided into chapters based on body system or condition. The Alphabetic Index consists of the following parts: the Index of Diseases and Injury, the Index of External Causes of Injury, the Table of Neoplasms and the Table of Drugs and Chemicals.
   See Section I.C2. General guidelines
   See Section I.C.19. Adverse effects, poisoning, underdosing and toxic effects

2. **Format and Structure:**
   The ICD-10-CM Tabular List contains categories, subcategories and codes. Characters for categories, subcategories and codes may be either a letter or a number. All categories are 3 characters. A three-character category that has no further subdivision is equivalent to a code. Subcategories are either 4 or 5 characters. Codes may be 3, 4, 5, 6 or 7 characters. That is, each level of subdivision after a category is a subcategory. The final level of subdivision is a code. Codes that have applicable 7th characters are still referred to as codes, not subcategories. A code that has an applicable 7th character is considered invalid without the 7th character.
   The ICD-10-CM uses an indented format for ease in reference

3. **Use of codes for reporting purposes**
   For reporting purposes only codes are permissible, not categories or subcategories, and any applicable 7th character is required.

4. **Placeholder character**
   The ICD-10-CM utilizes a placeholder character "X". The "X" is used as a placeholder at certain codes to allow for future expansion. An example of this is at the poisoning, adverse effect and underdosing codes, categories T36-T50. Where a placeholder exists, the X must be used in order for the code to be considered a valid code.

5. **7th Characters**
   Certain ICD-10-CM categories have applicable 7th characters. The applicable 7th character is required for all codes within the category, or as the notes in the Tabular List instruct. The 7th character must always be the 7th character in the data field. If a code that requires a 7th character is not 6 characters, a placeholder X must be used to fill in the empty characters.

6. **Abbreviations**
   a. **Alphabetic Index abbreviations**
      NEC "Not elsewhere classifiable"
         This abbreviation in the Alphabetic Index represents "other specified". When a specific code is not available for a condition the Alphabetic Index directs the coder to the "other specified" code in the Tabular List.
      NOS "Not otherwise specified"
         This abbreviation is the equivalent of unspecified.

GUIDELINES (ICD-10-CM)

b. **Tabular List abbreviations**

NEC "Not elsewhere classifiable"
This abbreviation in the Tabular List represents "other specified". When a specific code is not available for a condition, the Tabular List includes an NEC entry under a code to identify the code as the "other specified" code.

NOS "Not otherwise specified"
This abbreviation is the equivalent of unspecified.

7. **Punctuation**

[ ] Brackets are used in the Tabular List to enclose synonyms, alternative wording or explanatory phrases. Brackets are used in the Alphabetic Index to identify manifestation codes.

( ) Parentheses are used in both the Alphabetic Index and Tabular List to enclose supplementary words that may be present or absent in the statement of a disease or procedure without affecting the code number to which it is assigned. The terms within the parentheses are referred to as nonessential modifiers. The nonessential modifiers in the Alphabetic Index to Diseases apply to subterms following a main term except when a nonessential modifier and a subentry are mutually exclusive, the subentry takes precedence. For example, in the ICD-10-CM Alphabetic Index under the main term Enteritis, "acute" is a nonessential modifier and "chronic" is a subentry. In this case, the nonessential modifier "acute" does not apply to the subentry "chronic".

: Colons are used in the Tabular List after an incomplete term which needs one or more of the modifiers following the colon to make it assignable to a given category.

8. **Use of "and".**
See Section I.A.14. Use of the term "And"

9. **Other and Unspecified codes**

a. **"Other" codes**
Codes titled "other" or "other specified" are for use when the information in the medical record provides detail for which a specific code does not exist. Alphabetic Index entries with NEC in the line designate "other" codes in the Tabular List. These Alphabetic Index entries represent specific disease entities for which no specific code exists so the term is included within an "other" code.

b. **"Unspecified" codes**
Codes titled "unspecified" are for use when the information in the medical record is insufficient to assign a more specific code. For those categories for which an unspecified code is not provided, the "other specified" code may represent both other and unspecified.
See Section I.B.18 Use of Signs/Symptom/Unspecified Codes

10. **Includes Notes**
This note appears immediately under a three-character code title to further define, or give examples of, the content of the category.

11. **Inclusion terms**
List of terms is included under some codes. These terms are the conditions for which that code is to be used. The terms may be synonyms of the code title, or, in the case of "other specified" codes, the terms are a list of the various conditions assigned to that code. The inclusion terms are not necessarily exhaustive. Additional terms found only in the Alphabetic Index may also be assigned to a code.

12. **Excludes Notes**
The ICD-10-CM has two types of excludes notes. Each type of note has a different definition for use but they are all similar in that they indicate that codes excluded from each other are independent of each other.

a. **Excludes1**
A type 1 Excludes note is a pure excludes note. It means "NOT CODED HERE!" An Excludes1 note indicates that the code excluded should never be used at the same time as the code above the Excludes1 note. An Excludes1 is used when two conditions cannot occur together, such as a congenital form versus an acquired form of the same condition.

An exception to the Excludes1 definition is the circumstance when the two conditions are unrelated to each other. If it is not clear whether the two conditions involving an Excludes1 note are related or not, query the provider. For example, code F45.8, Other somatoform disorders, has an Excludes1 note for "sleep related teeth grinding (G47.63)," because "teeth grinding" is an inclusion term under F45.8. Only one of these two codes should be assigned for teeth grinding. However psychogenic dysmenorrhea is also an inclusion term under F45.8, and a patient could have both this condition and sleep related teeth grinding. In this case, the two conditions are clearly unrelated to each other, and so it would be appropriate to report F45.8 and G47.63 together.

b. **Excludes2**
A Type 2 Excludes note represents "Not included here." An excludes2 note indicates that the condition excluded is not part of the condition represented by the code, but a patient may have both conditions at the same time. When an Excludes2 note appears under a code, it is acceptable to use both the code and the excluded code together, when appropriate.

13. **Etiology/manifestation convention ("code first", "use additional code" and "in diseases classified elsewhere" notes)**
Certain conditions have both an underlying etiology and multiple body system manifestations

due to the underlying etiology. For such conditions, the ICD-10-CM has a coding convention that requires the underlying condition be sequenced first, if applicable, followed by the manifestation. Wherever such a combination exists, there is a "use additional code" note at the etiology code, and a "code first" note at the manifestation code. These instructional notes indicate the proper sequencing order of the codes, etiology followed by manifestation.

In most cases the manifestation codes will have in the code title, "in diseases classified elsewhere." Codes with this title are a component of the etiology/ manifestation convention. The code title indicates that it is a manifestation code. "In diseases classified elsewhere" codes are never permitted to be used as first-listed or principal diagnosis codes. They must be used in conjunction with an underlying condition code and they must be listed following the underlying condition. See category F02, Dementia in other diseases classified elsewhere, for an example of this convention.

There are manifestation codes that do not have "in diseases classified elsewhere" in the title. For such codes, there is a "use additional code" note at the etiology code and a "code first" note at the manifestation code and the rules for sequencing apply.

In addition to the notes in the Tabular List, these conditions also have a specific Alphabetic Index entry structure. In the Alphabetic Index both conditions are listed together with the etiology code first followed by the manifestation codes in brackets. The code in brackets is always to be sequenced second.

An example of the etiology/manifestation convention is dementia in Parkinson's disease. In the Alphabetic Index, code G20 is listed first, followed by code F02.80 or F02.81 in brackets. Code G20 represents the underlying etiology, Parkinson's disease, and must be sequenced first, whereas code F02.80 and F02.81 represent the manifestation of dementia in diseases classified elsewhere, with or without behavioral disturbance.

"Code first" and "Use additional code" notes are also used as sequencing rules in the classification for certain codes that are not part of an etiology/manifestation combination.

See Section I.B.7. Multiple coding for a single condition.

14. **"And"**
The word "and" should be interpreted to mean either "and" or "or" when it appears in a title.

For example, cases of "tuberculosis of bones", "tuberculosis of joints" and "tuberculosis of bones and joints" are classified to subcategory A18.0, Tuberculosis of bones and joints.

15. **"With"**
The word "with" **or "in"** should be interpreted to mean "associated with" or "due to" when it appears in a code title, the Alphabetic Index, or an instructional note in the Tabular List. The classification presumes a causal relationship

between the two conditions linked by these terms in the Alphabetic Index or Tabular List. These conditions should be coded as related even in the absence of provider documentation explicitly linking them, unless the documentation clearly states the conditions are unrelated **or when another guideline exists that specifically requires a documented linkage between two conditions (e.g., sepsis guideline for "acute organ dysfunction that is not clearly associated with the sepsis").**

For conditions not specifically linked by these relational terms in the classification **or when a guideline requires that a linkage between two conditions be explicitly documented** provider documentation must link the conditions in order to code them as related.

The word "with" in the Alphabetic Index is sequenced immediately following the main term, not in alphabetical order.

16. **"See" and "See Also"**
The "see" instruction following a main term in the Alphabetic Index indicates that another term should be referenced. It is necessary to go to the main term referenced with the "see" note to locate the correct code.

A "see also" instruction following a main term in the Alphabetic Index instructs that there is another main term that may also be referenced that may provide additional Alphabetic Index entries that may be useful. It is not necessary to follow the "see also" note when the original main term provides the necessary code.

17. **"Code also" note**
A "code also" note instructs that two codes may be required to fully describe a condition, but this note does not provide sequencing direction. **The sequencing depends on the circumstances of the encounter.**

18. **Default codes**
A code listed next to a main term in the ICD-10-CM Alphabetic Index is referred to as a default code. The default code represents that condition that is most commonly associated with the main term, or is the unspecified code for the condition. If a condition is documented in a medical record (for example, appendicitis) without any additional information, such as acute or chronic, the default code should be assigned.

19. **Code assignment and Clinical Criteria**
The assignment of a diagnosis code is based on the provider's diagnostic statement that the condition exists. The provider's statement that the patient has a particular condition is sufficient. Code assignment is not based on clinical criteria used by the provider to establish the diagnosis.

B. **General Coding Guidelines**

1. **Locating a code in the ICD-10-CM**
To select a code in the classification that corresponds to a diagnosis or reason for visit documented in a medical record, first locate the

term in the Alphabetic Index, and then verify the code in the Tabular List. Read and be guided by instructional notations that appear in both the Alphabetic Index and the Tabular List.

It is essential to use both the Alphabetic Index and Tabular List when locating and assigning a code. The Alphabetic Index does not always provide the full code. Selection of the full code, including laterality and any applicable 7th character can only be done in the Tabular List. A dash (-) at the end of an Alphabetic Index entry indicates that additional characters are required. Even if a dash is not included at the Alphabetic Index entry, it is necessary to refer to the Tabular List to verify that no 7th character is required.

2. Level of Detail in Coding
Diagnosis codes are to be used and reported at their highest number of characters available.

ICD-10-CM diagnosis codes are composed of codes with 3, 4, 5, 6 or 7 characters. Codes with three characters are included in ICD-10-CM as the heading of a category of codes that may be further subdivided by the use of fourth and/or fifth characters and/or sixth characters, which provide greater detail.

A three-character code is to be used only if it is not further subdivided. A code is invalid if it has not been coded to the full number of characters required for that code, including the 7th character, if applicable.

3. Code or codes from A00.0 through T88.9, Z00-Z99.8
The appropriate code or codes from A00.0 through T88.9, Z00-Z99.8 must be used to identify diagnoses, symptoms, conditions, problems, complaints or other reason(s) for the encounter/visit.

4. Signs and symptoms
Codes that describe symptoms and signs, as opposed to diagnoses, are acceptable for reporting purposes when a related definitive diagnosis has not been established (confirmed) by the provider. Chapter 18 of ICD-10-CM, Symptoms, Signs, and Abnormal Clinical and Laboratory Findings, Not Elsewhere Classified (codes R00.0 - R99) contains many, but not all codes for symptoms.

See Section I.B.18 Use of Signs/Symptom/ Unspecified Codes

5. Conditions that are an integral part of a disease process
Signs and symptoms that are associated routinely with a disease process should not be assigned as additional codes, unless otherwise instructed by the classification.

6. Conditions that are not an integral part of a disease process
Additional signs and symptoms that may not be associated routinely with a disease process should be coded when present.

7. Multiple coding for a single condition
In addition to the etiology/manifestation convention that requires two codes to fully describe a single condition that affects multiple body systems, there are other single conditions that also require more than one code. "Use additional code" notes are found in the Tabular List at codes that are not part of an etiology/manifestation pair where a secondary code is useful to fully describe a condition. The sequencing rule is the same as the etiology/manifestation pair, "use additional code" indicates that a secondary code should be added, **if known.**

For example, for bacterial infections that are not included in chapter 1, a secondary code from category B95, Streptococcus, Staphylococcus, and Enterococcus, as the cause of diseases classified elsewhere, or B96, Other bacterial agents as the cause of diseases classified elsewhere, may be required to identify the bacterial organism causing the infection. A "use additional code" note will normally be found at the infectious disease code, indicating a need for the organism code to be added as a secondary code.

"Code first" notes are also under certain codes that are not specifically manifestation codes but may be due to an underlying cause. When there is a "code first" note and an underlying condition is present, the underlying condition should be sequenced first, **if known.**

"Code, if applicable, any causal condition first," notes indicate that this code may be assigned as a principal diagnosis when the causal condition is unknown or not applicable. If a causal condition is known, then the code for that condition should be sequenced as the principal or first-listed diagnosis.

Multiple codes may be needed for sequela, complication codes and obstetric codes to more fully describe a condition. See the specific guidelines for these conditions for further instruction.

8. Acute and Chronic Conditions
If the same condition is described as both acute (subacute) and chronic, and separate subentries exist in the Alphabetic Index at the same indentation level, code both and sequence the acute (subacute) code first.

9. Combination Code
A combination code is a single code used to classify:
Two diagnoses, or
A diagnosis with an associated secondary process (manifestation)
A diagnosis with an associated complication
Combination codes are identified by referring to subterm entries in the Alphabetic Index and by reading the inclusion and exclusion notes in the Tabular List.

Assign only the combination code when that code fully identifies the diagnostic conditions involved or when the Alphabetic Index so directs. Multiple coding should not be used when the classification provides a combination code that clearly identifies all of the elements documented in the diagnosis. When the combination code lacks necessary specificity in describing the manifestation or complication, an additional code should be used as a secondary code.

10. Sequela (Late Effects)

A sequela is the residual effect (condition produced) after the acute phase of an illness or injury has terminated. There is no time limit on when a sequela code can be used. The residual may be apparent early, such as in cerebral infarction, or it may occur months or years later, such as that due to a previous injury. Examples of sequela include: scar formation resulting from a burn, deviated septum due to a nasal fracture, and infertility due to tubal occlusion from old tuberculosis. Coding of sequela generally requires two codes sequenced in the following order: the condition or nature of the sequela is sequenced first. The sequela code is sequenced second.

An exception to the above guidelines are those instances where the code for the sequela is followed by a manifestation code identified in the Tabular List and title, or the sequela code has been expanded (at the fourth, fifth or sixth character levels) to include the manifestation(s). The code for the acute phase of an illness or injury that led to the sequela is never used with a code for the late effect.

See Section I.C.9. Sequelae of cerebrovascular disease
See Section I.C.15. Sequelae of complication of pregnancy, childbirth and the puerperium
See Section I.C.19. Application of 7th characters for Chapter 19

11. Impending or Threatened Condition

Code any condition described at the time of discharge as "impending" or "threatened" as follows:

If it did occur, code as confirmed diagnosis.

If it did not occur, reference the Alphabetic Index to determine if the condition has a subentry term for "impending" or "threatened" and also reference main term entries for "Impending" and for "Threatened."

If the subterms are listed, assign the given code.

If the subterms are not listed, code the existing underlying condition(s) and not the condition described as impending or threatened.

12. Reporting Same Diagnosis Code More than Once

Each unique ICD-10-CM diagnosis code may be reported only once for an encounter. This applies to bilateral conditions when there are no distinct codes identifying laterality or two different conditions classified to the same ICD-10-CM diagnosis code.

13. Laterality

Some ICD-10-CM codes indicate laterality, specifying whether the condition occurs on the left, right or is bilateral. If no bilateral code is provided and the condition is bilateral, assign separate codes for both the left and right side. If the side is not identified in the medical record, assign the code for the unspecified side.

When a patient has a bilateral condition and each side is treated during separate encounters, assign the "bilateral" code (as the condition still exists on both sides), including for the encounter to treat the first side. For the second encounter for treatment after one side has previously been treated and the condition no longer exists on that side, assign the appropriate unilateral code for the side where the condition still exists (e.g., cataract surgery performed on each eye in separate encounters). The bilateral code would not be assigned for the subsequent encounter, as the patient no longer has the condition in the previously-treated site. If the treatment on the first side did not completely resolve the condition, then the bilateral code would still be appropriate.

14. Documentation for BMI, Depth of Non-pressure ulcers, Pressure Ulcer Stages, Coma Scale, and NIH Stroke Scale

For the Body Mass Index (BMI), depth of non-pressure chronic ulcers, pressure ulcer stage, coma scale, and NIH stroke scale (NIHSS) codes, code assignment may be based on medical record documentation from clinicians who are not the patient's provider (i.e., physician or other qualified healthcare practitioner legally accountable for establishing the patient's diagnosis), since this information is typically documented by other clinicians involved in the care of the patient (e.g., a dietitian often documents the BMI, a nurse often documents the pressure ulcer stages, and an emergency medical technician often documents the coma scale). However, the associated diagnosis (such as overweight, obesity, acute stroke, or pressure ulcer) must be documented by the patient's provider. If there is conflicting medical record documentation, either from the same clinician or different clinicians, the patient's attending provider should be queried for clarification.

The BMI, coma scale, and NIHSS codes should only be reported as secondary diagnoses.

15. Syndromes

Follow the Alphabetic Index guidance when coding syndromes. In the absence of Alphabetic Index guidance, assign codes for the documented manifestations of the syndrome. Additional codes for manifestations that are not an integral part of the disease process may also be assigned when the condition does not have a unique code.

16. Documentation of Complications of Care

Code assignment is based on the provider's documentation of the relationship between the condition and the care or procedure, unless otherwise instructed by the classification. The guideline extends to any complications of care, regardless of the chapter the code is located in. It is important to note that not all conditions that occur during or following medical care or surgery are classified as complications. There must be a cause-and-effect relationship between the care provided and the condition, and an indication in the documentation that it is a complication. Query the provider for clarification, if the complication is not clearly documented.

17. Borderline Diagnosis

If the provider documents a "borderline" diagnosis at the time of discharge, the diagnosis is coded as confirmed, unless the classification provides a specific entry (e.g., borderline diabetes). If a borderline condition has a specific index entry in ICD-10-CM, it should be coded as such. Since borderline conditions are not uncertain diagnoses, no distinction is made between the care setting (inpatient versus outpatient). Whenever the documentation is unclear regarding a borderline condition, coders are encouraged to query for clarification.

18. **Use of Sign/Symptom/Unspecified Codes**
Sign/symptom and "unspecified" codes have acceptable, even necessary, uses. While specific diagnosis codes should be reported when they are supported by the available medical record documentation and clinical knowledge of the patient's health condition, there are instances when signs/symptoms or unspecified codes are the best choices for accurately reflecting the healthcare encounter. Each healthcare encounter should be coded to the level of certainty known for that encounter.

If a definitive diagnosis has not been established by the end of the encounter, it is appropriate to report codes for sign(s) and/or symptom(s) in lieu of a definitive diagnosis. When sufficient clinical information isn't known or available about a particular health condition to assign a more specific code, it is acceptable to report the appropriate "unspecified" code (e.g., a diagnosis of pneumonia has been determined, but not the specific type). Unspecified codes should be reported when they are the codes that most accurately reflect what is known about the patient's condition at the time of that particular encounter. It would be inappropriate to select a specific code that is not supported by the medical record documentation or conduct medically unnecessary diagnostic testing in order to determine a more specific code.

C. **Chapter-Specific Coding Guidelines**
In addition to general coding guidelines, there are guidelines for specific diagnoses and/or conditions in the classification. Unless otherwise indicated, these guidelines apply to all health care settings. Please refer to Section II for guidelines on the selection of principal diagnosis.

1. **Chapter 1: Certain Infectious and Parasitic Diseases (A00-B99)**

   a. **Human Immunodeficiency Virus (HIV) Infections**

   1) **Code only confirmed cases**
   Code only confirmed cases of HIV infection/illness. This is an exception to the hospital inpatient guideline Section II, H.

   In this context, "confirmation" does not require documentation of positive serology or culture for HIV; the provider's diagnostic statement that the patient is HIV positive, or has an HIV-related illness is sufficient.

   2) **Selection and sequencing of HIV codes**

   (a) **Patient admitted for HIV-related condition**
   If a patient is admitted for an HIV-related condition, the principal diagnosis should be B20, Human immunodeficiency virus [HIV] disease followed by additional diagnosis codes for all reported HIV-related conditions.

   (b) **Patient with HIV disease admitted for unrelated condition**
   If a patient with HIV disease is admitted for an unrelated condition (such as a traumatic injury), the code for the unrelated condition (e.g., the nature of injury code) should be the principal diagnosis. Other diagnoses would be B20 followed by additional diagnosis codes for all reported HIV-related conditions.

   (c) **Whether the patient is newly diagnosed**
   Whether the patient is newly diagnosed or has had previous admissions/encounters for HIV conditions is irrelevant to the sequencing decision.

   (d) **Asymptomatic human immunodeficiency virus**
   Z21, Asymptomatic human immunodeficiency virus [HIV] infection status, is to be applied when the patient without any documentation of symptoms is listed as being "HIV positive," "known HIV," "HIV test positive," or similar terminology. Do not use this code if the term "AIDS" is used or if the patient is treated for any HIV-related illness or is described as having any condition(s) resulting from his/her HIV positive status; use B20 in these cases.

   (e) **Patients with inconclusive HIV serology**
   Patients with inconclusive HIV serology, but no definitive diagnosis or manifestations of the illness, may be assigned code R75, Inconclusive laboratory evidence of human immunodeficiency virus [HIV].

   (f) **Previously diagnosed HIV-related illness**
   Patients with any known prior diagnosis of an HIV-related illness should be coded to B20. Once a patient has developed an HIV-related illness, the patient should always be assigned code B20 on every subsequent admission/encounter. Patients previously diagnosed with any HIV illness (B20) should never be assigned to R75 or Z21, Asymptomatic human immunodeficiency virus [HIV] infection status.

   (g) **HIV Infection in Pregnancy, Childbirth and the Puerperium**
   During pregnancy, childbirth or the puerperium, a patient admitted (or presenting for a health care encounter) because of an HIV-related illness should receive a principal diagnosis code of O98.7-, Human immunodeficiency [HIV] disease complicating pregnancy, childbirth and the puerperium, followed by B20 and the code(s) for the HIV-related illness(es). Codes from Chapter 15 always take sequencing priority.

Patients with asymptomatic HIV infection status admitted (or presenting for a health care encounter) during pregnancy, childbirth, or the puerperium should receive codes of O98.7- and Z21.

(h) Encounters for testing for HIV

If a patient is being seen to determine his/her HIV status, use code Z11.4, Encounter for screening for human immunodeficiency virus [HIV]. Use additional codes for any associated high risk behavior.

If a patient with signs or symptoms is being seen for HIV testing, code the signs and symptoms. An additional counseling code Z71.7, Human immunodeficiency virus [HIV] counseling, may be used if counseling is provided during the encounter for the test.

When a patient returns to be informed of his/her HIV test results and the test result is negative, use code Z71.7, Human immunodeficiency virus [HIV] counseling.

If the results are positive, see previous guidelines and assign codes as appropriate.

b. Infectious agents as the cause of diseases classified to other chapters

Certain infections are classified in chapters other than Chapter 1 and no organism is identified as part of the infection code. In these instances, it is necessary to use an additional code from Chapter 1 to identify the organism. A code from category B95, Streptococcus, Staphylococcus, and Enterococcus as the cause of diseases classified to other chapters, B96, Other bacterial agents as the cause of diseases classified to other chapters, or B97, Viral agents as the cause of diseases classified to other chapters, is to be used as an additional code to identify the organism. An instructional note will be found at the infection code advising that an additional organism code is required.

c. Infections resistant to antibiotics

Many bacterial infections are resistant to current antibiotics. It is necessary to identify all infections documented as antibiotic resistant. Assign a code from category Z16, Resistance to antimicrobial drugs, following the infection code only if the infection code does not identify drug resistance.

d. Sepsis, Severe Sepsis, and Septic Shock

1) Coding of Sepsis and Severe Sepsis

(a) Sepsis

For a diagnosis of sepsis, assign the appropriate code for the underlying systemic infection. If the type of infection or causal organism is not further specified, assign code A41.9, Sepsis, unspecified organism.

A code from subcategory R65.2, Severe sepsis, should not be assigned unless severe sepsis or an associated acute organ dysfunction is documented.

(i) Negative or inconclusive blood cultures and sepsis
Negative or inconclusive blood cultures do not preclude a diagnosis of sepsis in patients with clinical evidence of the condition, however, the provider should be queried.

(ii) Urosepsis
The term urosepsis is a nonspecific term. It is not to be considered synonymous with sepsis. It has no default code in the Alphabetic Index. Should a provider use this term, he/she must be queried for clarification.

(iii) Sepsis with organ dysfunction
If a patient has sepsis and associated acute organ dysfunction or multiple organ dysfunction (MOD), follow the instructions for coding severe sepsis.

(iv) Acute organ dysfunction that is not clearly associated with the sepsis
If a patient has sepsis and an acute organ dysfunction, but the medical record documentation indicates that the acute organ dysfunction is related to a medical condition other than the sepsis, do not assign a code from subcategory R65.2, Severe sepsis. An acute organ dysfunction must be associated with the sepsis in order to assign the severe sepsis code. If the documentation is not clear as to whether an acute organ dysfunction is related to the sepsis or another medical condition, query the provider.

(b) Severe sepsis

The coding of severe sepsis requires a minimum of 2 codes: first a code for the underlying systemic infection, followed by a code from subcategory R65.2, Severe sepsis. If the causal organism is not documented, assign code A41.9, Sepsis, unspecified organism, for the infection. Additional code(s) for the associated acute organ dysfunction are also required.

Due to the complex nature of severe sepsis, some cases may require querying the provider prior to assignment of the codes.

2) Septic shock

(a) Septic shock generally refers to circulatory failure associated with severe sepsis, and therefore, it represents a type of acute organ dysfunction.

For all cases of septic shock, the code for the systemic infection should be sequenced first, followed by code R65.21, Severe sepsis with septic shock or code T81.12, Postprocedural septic shock. Any additional codes for the other acute organ dysfunctions should also be assigned. As noted in the sequencing instructions in the Tabular List, the code for septic shock cannot be assigned as a principal diagnosis.

3) Sequencing of severe sepsis

If severe sepsis is present on admission, and meets the definition of principal diagnosis, the underlying systemic infection should be assigned as principal diagnosis followed by the appropriate code from subcategory R65.2 as required by the sequencing rules in the Tabular List. A code from subcategory R65.2 can never be assigned as a principal diagnosis.

When severe sepsis develops during an encounter (it was not present on admission) the underlying systemic infection and the appropriate code from subcategory R65.2 should be assigned as secondary diagnoses.

Severe sepsis may be present on admission but the diagnosis may not be confirmed until sometime after admission. If the documentation is not clear whether severe sepsis was present on admission, the provider should be queried.

4) Sepsis and severe sepsis with a localized infection

If the reason for admission is both sepsis or severe sepsis and a localized infection, such as pneumonia or cellulitis, a code(s) for the underlying systemic infection should be assigned first and the code for the localized infection should be assigned as a secondary diagnosis. If the patient has severe sepsis, a code from subcategory R65.2 should also be assigned as a secondary diagnosis. If the patient is admitted with a localized infection, such as pneumonia, and sepsis/severe sepsis doesn't develop until after admission, the localized infection should be assigned first, followed by the appropriate sepsis/severe sepsis codes.

5) Sepsis due to a postprocedural infection

(a) Documentation of causal relationship

As with all postprocedural complications, code assignment is based on the provider's documentation of the relationship between the infection and the procedure.

(b) Sepsis due to a postprocedural infection

For such cases, the postprocedural infection code, such as, T80.2, Infections following infusion, transfusion, and therapeutic injection, T81.4, Infection following a procedure, T88.0, Infection following immunization, or O86.0, Infection of obstetric surgical wound, should be coded first, followed by the code for the specific infection. If the patient has severe sepsis the appropriate code from subcategory R65.2 should also be assigned with the additional code(s) for any acute organ dysfunction.

(c) Postprocedural infection and postprocedural septic shock

In cases where a postprocedural infection has occurred and has resulted in severe sepsis the code for the precipitating complication such as code T81.4, Infection following a procedure, or O86.0, Infection of obstetrical surgical wound should be coded first followed by code R65.20, Severe sepsis

without septic shock. A Code for the systemic infection should also be assigned.

If a postprocedural infection has resulted in postprocedural septic shock, the code for the precipitating complication such as code T81.4, Infection following a procedure, or O86.0, Infection of obstetrical surgical wound should be coded first followed by code T81.12-, Postprocedural septic shock. A code for the systemic infection should also be assigned.

6) Sepsis and severe sepsis associated with a noninfectious process (condition)

In some cases a noninfectious process (condition), such as trauma, may lead to an infection which can result in sepsis or severe sepsis. If sepsis or severe sepsis is documented as associated with a noninfectious condition, such as a burn or serious injury, and this condition meets the definition for principal diagnosis, the code for the noninfectious condition should be sequenced first, followed by the code for the resulting infection. If severe sepsis is present, a code from subcategory R65.2 should also be assigned with any associated organ dysfunction(s) codes. It is not necessary to assign a code from subcategory R65.1, Systemic inflammatory response syndrome (SIRS) of non-infectious origin, for these cases.

If the infection meets the definition of principal diagnosis it should be sequenced before the non-infectious condition. When both the associated non-infectious condition and the infection meet the definition of principal diagnosis either may be assigned as principal diagnosis.

Only one code from category R65, Symptoms and signs specifically associated with systemic inflammation and infection, should be assigned. Therefore, when a non-infectious condition leads to an infection resulting in severe sepsis, assign the appropriate code from subcategory R65.2, Severe sepsis. Do not additionally assign a code from subcategory R65.1, Systemic inflammatory response syndrome (SIRS) of non-infectious origin.

See Section I.C.18. SIRS due to non-infectious process

7) Sepsis and septic shock complicating abortion, pregnancy, childbirth, and the puerperium

See Section I.C.15. Sepsis and septic shock complicating abortion, pregnancy, childbirth and the puerperium

8) Newborn sepsis

See Section I.C.16. f. Bacterial sepsis of Newborn

e. Methicillin Resistant Staphylococcus aureus (MRSA) Conditions

1) Selection and sequencing of MRSA codes

(a) Combination codes for MRSA infection

When a patient is diagnosed with an infection that is due to methicillin resistant *Staphylococcus aureus* (MRSA), and that infection has a combination code that includes the causal organism (e.g., sepsis, pneumonia) assign the appropriate combination code for the condition (e.g., code A41.02, Sepsis due to Methicillin resistant Staphylococcus aureus or code J15.212, Pneumonia due to Methicillin resistant Staphylococcus aureus). Do not assign code B95.62, Methicillin resistant Staphylococcus aureus infection as the cause of diseases classified elsewhere, as an additional code because the combination code includes the type of infection and the MRSA organism. Do not assign a code from subcategory Z16.11, Resistance to penicillins, as an additional diagnosis.

See Section C.1. for instructions on coding and sequencing of sepsis and severe sepsis.

(b) Other codes for MRSA infection

When there is documentation of a current infection (e.g., wound infection, stitch abscess, urinary tract infection) due to MRSA, and that infection does not have a combination code that includes the causal organism, assign the appropriate code to identify the condition along with code B95.62, Methicillin resistant Staphylococcus aureus infection as the cause of diseases classified elsewhere for the MRSA infection. Do not assign a code from subcategory Z16.11, Resistance to penicillins.

(c) Methicillin susceptible Staphylococcus aureus (MSSA) and MRSA colonization

The condition or state of being colonized or carrying MSSA or MRSA is called colonization or carriage, while an individual person is described as being colonized or being a carrier. Colonization means that MSSA or MSRA is present on or in the body without necessarily causing illness. A positive MRSA colonization test might be documented by the provider as "MRSA screen positive" or "MRSA nasal swab positive".

Assign code Z22.322, Carrier or suspected carrier of Methicillin resistant Staphylococcus aureus, for patients documented as having MRSA colonization. Assign code Z22.321, Carrier or suspected carrier of Methicillin susceptible Staphylococcus aureus, for patient documented as having MSSA colonization. Colonization is not necessarily indicative of a disease process or as the cause of a specific condition the patient may have unless documented as such by the provider.

(d) MRSA colonization and infection

If a patient is documented as having both MRSA colonization and infection during a hospital admission, code Z22.322, Carrier or suspected carrier of Methicillin resistant Staphylococcus aureus, and a code for the MRSA infection may both be assigned.

f. Zika virus infections

1) Code only confirmed cases

Code only a confirmed diagnosis of Zika virus (A92.5, Zika virus disease) as documented by the provider. This is an exception to the hospital inpatient guideline Section II, H.

In this context, "confirmation" does not require documentation of the type of test performed; the physician's diagnostic statement that the condition is confirmed is sufficient. This code should be assigned regardless of the stated mode of transmission.

If the provider documents "suspected", "possible" or "probable" Zika, do not assign code A92.5. Assign a code(s) explaining the reason for encounter (such as fever, rash, or joint pain) or Z20.828, Contact with and (suspected) exposure to other viral communicable diseases.

2. Chapter 2: Neoplasms (C00-D49)

General guidelines

Chapter 2 of the ICD-10-CM contains the codes for most benign and all malignant neoplasms. Certain benign neoplasms, such as prostatic adenomas, may be found in the specific body system chapters. To properly code a neoplasm it is necessary to determine from the record if the neoplasm is benign, in-situ, malignant, or of uncertain histologic behavior. If malignant, any secondary (metastatic) sites should also be determined.

Primary malignant neoplasms overlapping site boundaries

A primary malignant neoplasm that overlaps two or more contiguous (next to each other) sites should be classified to the subcategory/ code .8 ('overlapping lesion'), unless the combination is specifically indexed elsewhere. For multiple neoplasms of the same site that are not contiguous such as tumors in different quadrants of the same breast, codes for each site should be assigned.

Malignant neoplasm of ectopic tissue

Malignant neoplasms of ectopic tissue are to be coded to the site of origin mentioned, e.g., ectopic pancreatic malignant neoplasms involving the stomach are coded to **malignant neoplasm of** pancreas, unspecified (C25.9).

The neoplasm table in the Alphabetic Index should be referenced first. However, if the histological term is documented, that term should be referenced first, rather than going immediately to the Neoplasm Table, in order to determine which column in the Neoplasm Table is appropriate. For example, if the documentation indicates "adenoma," refer to the term in the Alphabetic Index to review the entries under this term and the instructional note to "see also neoplasm, by site, benign." The table provides the proper code based on the type of neoplasm and the site. It is important to select the proper column in the table that corresponds to the type of neoplasm. The Tabular List should then be referenced to verify that the correct code has been selected from the table and that a more specific site code does not exist.

See Section I.C.21. Factors influencing health status and contact with health services, Status, for information regarding Z15.0, codes for genetic susceptibility to cancer.

a. Treatment directed at the malignancy

If the treatment is directed at the malignancy, designate the malignancy as the principal diagnosis.

The only exception to this guideline is if a patient admission/encounter is solely for the administration of chemotherapy, immunotherapy or **external beam** radiation therapy, assign the appropriate Z51.— code as the first-listed or principal diagnosis, and the diagnosis or problem for which the service is being performed as a secondary diagnosis.

b. Treatment of secondary site

When a patient is admitted because of a primary neoplasm with metastasis and treatment is directed toward the secondary site only, the secondary neoplasm is designated as the principal diagnosis even though the primary malignancy is still present.

c. Coding and sequencing of complications

Coding and sequencing of complications associated with the malignancies or with the therapy thereof are subject to the following guidelines:

1) Anemia associated with malignancy

When admission/encounter is for management of an anemia associated with the malignancy, and the treatment is only for anemia, the appropriate code for the malignancy is sequenced as the principal or first-listed diagnosis followed by the appropriate code for the anemia (such as code D63.0, Anemia in neoplastic disease).

2) Anemia associated with chemotherapy, immunotherapy and radiation therapy

When the admission/encounter is for management of an anemia associated with an adverse effect of the administration of chemotherapy or immunotherapy and the only treatment is for the anemia, the anemia code is sequenced first followed by the appropriate codes for the neoplasm and the adverse effect (T45.1X5, Adverse effect of antineoplastic and immunosuppressive drugs).

When the admission/encounter is for management of an anemia associated with an adverse effect of radiotherapy, the anemia code should be sequenced first, followed by the appropriate neoplasm code and code Y84.2, Radiological procedure and radiotherapy as the cause of abnormal reaction of the patient, or of later complication, without mention of misadventure at the time of the procedure.

3) Management of dehydration due to the malignancy

When the admission/encounter is for management of dehydration due to the malignancy and only the dehydration is being treated (intravenous rehydration), the dehydration is sequenced first, followed by the code(s) for the malignancy.

4) Treatment of a complication resulting from a surgical procedure

When the admission/encounter is for treatment of a complication resulting from a surgical procedure, designate the complication as the principal or first-listed diagnosis if treatment is directed at resolving the complication.

d. Primary malignancy previously excised

When a primary malignancy has been previously excised or eradicated from its site and there is no further treatment directed to that site and there is no evidence of any existing primary malignancy, a code from category Z85, Personal history of malignant neoplasm, should be used to indicate the former site of the malignancy. Any mention of extension, invasion, or metastasis to another site is coded as a secondary malignant neoplasm to that site. The secondary site may be the principal or first-listed with the Z85 code used as a secondary code.

e. Admissions/Encounters involving chemotherapy, immunotherapy and radiation therapy

1) Episode of care involves surgical removal of neoplasm

When an episode of care involves the surgical removal of a neoplasm, primary or secondary site, followed by adjunct chemotherapy or radiation treatment during the same episode of care, the code for the neoplasm should be assigned as principal or first-listed diagnosis.

2) Patient admission/encounter solely for administration of chemotherapy, immunotherapy and radiation therapy

If a patient admission/encounter is solely for the administration of chemotherapy, immunotherapy or **external beam** radiation therapy assign code Z51.0, Encounter for antineoplastic radiation therapy, or Z51.11, Encounter for antineoplastic chemotherapy, or Z51.12, Encounter for antineoplastic immunotherapy as the first-listed or principal diagnosis. If a patient receives more than one of these therapies during the same admission more than one of these codes may be assigned, in any sequence.

The malignancy for which the therapy is being administered should be assigned as a secondary diagnosis.

If a patient admission/encounter is for the insertion or implantation of radioactive elements (e.g., brachytherapy) the appropriate code for the malignancy is sequenced as the principal or first-listed diagnosis. Code Z51.0 should not be assigned.

3) Patient admitted for radiation therapy, chemotherapy or immunotherapy and develops complications

When a patient is admitted for the purpose of **external beam** radiotherapy, immunotherapy or chemotherapy and develops complications such as uncontrolled nausea and vomiting or dehydration, the principal or first-listed diagnosis is Z51.0, Encounter for antineoplastic radiation therapy, or Z51.11, Encounter for antineoplastic chemotherapy, or Z51.12, Encounter for antineoplastic immunotherapy followed by any codes for the complications.

When a patient is admitted for the purpose of insertion or implantation of radioactive elements (e.g., brachytherapy) and develops complications such as uncontrolled nausea and vomiting or dehydration, the principal or first-listed diagnosis is the appropriate code for the malignancy followed by any codes for the complications.

f. Admission/encounter to determine extent of malignancy

When the reason for admission/encounter is to determine the extent of the malignancy, or for a procedure such as paracentesis or thoracentesis, the primary malignancy or appropriate metastatic site is designated as the principal or first-listed diagnosis, even though chemotherapy or radiotherapy is administered.

g. Symptoms, signs, and abnormal findings listed in Chapter 18 associated with neoplasms

Symptoms, signs, and ill-defined conditions listed in Chapter 18 characteristic of, or associated with, an existing primary or secondary site malignancy cannot be used to replace the malignancy as principal or first-listed diagnosis, regardless of the number of admissions or encounters for treatment and care of the neoplasm.

See section I.C.21. Factors influencing health status and contact with health services, Encounter for prophylactic organ removal.

h. Admission/encounter for pain control/management

See Section I.C.6. for information on coding admission/encounter for pain control/management.

i. Malignancy in two or more noncontiguous sites

A patient may have more than one malignant tumor in the same organ. These tumors may represent different primaries or metastatic disease, depending on the site. Should the documentation be unclear, the provider should be queried as to the status of each tumor so that the correct codes can be assigned.

j. Disseminated malignant neoplasm, unspecified

Code C80.0, Disseminated malignant neoplasm, unspecified, is for use only in those cases where the patient has advanced metastatic disease and no known primary or secondary sites are specified. It should not be used in place of assigning codes for the primary site and all known secondary sites.

k. Malignant neoplasm without specification of site

Code C80.1, Malignant (primary) neoplasm, unspecified, equates to Cancer, unspecified. This code should only be used when no determination can be made as to the primary site of a malignancy. This code should rarely be used in the inpatient setting.

l. Sequencing of neoplasm codes

1) Encounter for treatment of primary malignancy

If the reason for the encounter is for treatment of a primary malignancy, assign the malignancy as the principal/first-listed diagnosis. The primary site is to be sequenced first, followed by any metastatic sites.

2) Encounter for treatment of secondary malignancy

When an encounter is for a primary malignancy with metastasis and treatment is directed toward the metastatic (secondary) site(s) only, the metastatic site(s) is designated as the principal/

first-listed diagnosis. The primary malignancy is coded as an additional code.

3) Malignant neoplasm in a pregnant patient

When a pregnant woman has a malignant neoplasm, a code from subcategory O9A.1-, Malignant neoplasm complicating pregnancy, childbirth, and the puerperium, should be sequenced first, followed by the appropriate code from Chapter 2 to indicate the type of neoplasm.

4) Encounter for complication associated with a neoplasm

When an encounter is for management of a complication associated with a neoplasm, such as dehydration, and the treatment is only for the complication, the complication is coded first, followed by the appropriate code(s) for the neoplasm.

The exception to this guideline is anemia. When the admission/encounter is for management of an anemia associated with the malignancy, and the treatment is only for anemia, the appropriate code for the malignancy is sequenced as the principal or first-listed diagnosis followed by code D63.0, Anemia in neoplastic disease.

5) Complication from surgical procedure for treatment of a neoplasm

When an encounter is for treatment of a complication resulting from a surgical procedure performed for the treatment of the neoplasm, designate the complication as the principal/first-listed diagnosis. See guideline regarding the coding of a current malignancy versus personal history to determine if the code for the neoplasm should also be assigned.

6) Pathologic fracture due to a neoplasm

When an encounter is for a pathological fracture due to a neoplasm, and the focus of treatment is the fracture, a code from subcategory M84.5, Pathological fracture in neoplastic disease, should be sequenced first, followed by the code for the neoplasm.

If the focus of treatment is the neoplasm with an associated pathological fracture, the neoplasm code should be sequenced first, followed by a code from M84.5 for the pathological fracture.

m. Current malignancy versus personal history of malignancy

When a primary malignancy has been excised but further treatment, such as an additional surgery for the malignancy, radiation therapy or chemotherapy is directed to that site, the primary malignancy code should be used until treatment is completed.

When a primary malignancy has been previously excised or eradicated from its site, there is no further treatment (of the malignancy) directed to that site, and there is no evidence of any existing primary malignancy, a code from category Z85, Personal history of malignant neoplasm, should be used to indicate the former site of the malignancy.

See Section I.C.21. Factors influencing health status and contact with health services, History (of)

n. **Leukemia, Multiple Myeloma, and Malignant Plasma Cell Neoplasms in remission versus personal history**

The categories for leukemia, and category C90, Multiple myeloma and malignant plasma cell neoplasms, have codes indicating whether or not the leukemia has achieved remission. There are also codes Z85.6, Personal history of leukemia, and Z85.79, Personal history of other malignant neoplasms of lymphoid, hematopoietic and related tissues. If the documentation is unclear, as to whether the leukemia has achieved remission, the provider should be queried.

See Section I.C.21. Factors influencing health status and contact with health services, History (of)

o. **Aftercare following surgery for neoplasm**
See Section I.C.21. Factors influencing health status and contact with health services, Aftercare

p. **Follow-up care for completed treatment of a malignancy**
See Section I.C.21. Factors influencing health status and contact with health services, Follow-up

q. **Prophylactic organ removal for prevention of malignancy**
See Section I.C. 21, Factors influencing health status and contact with health services, Prophylactic organ removal

r. **Malignant neoplasm associated with transplanted organ**

A malignant neoplasm of a transplanted organ should be coded as a transplant complication. Assign first the appropriate code from category T86.-, Complications of transplanted organs and tissue, followed by code C80.2, Malignant neoplasm associated with transplanted organ. Use an additional code for the specific malignancy.

3. **Chapter 3: Disease of the blood and blood-forming organs and certain disorders involving the immune mechanism (D50-D89)**
Reserved for future guideline expansion

4. **Chapter 4: Endocrine, Nutritional, and Metabolic Diseases (E00-E89)**

a. **Diabetes mellitus**

The diabetes mellitus codes are combination codes that include the type of diabetes mellitus, the body system affected, and the complications affecting that body system. As many codes within a particular category as are necessary to describe all of the complications of the disease may be used. They should be sequenced based on the reason for a particular encounter. Assign as many codes from categories E08 – E13 as needed to identify all of the associated conditions that the patient has.

1) **Type of diabetes**
The age of a patient is not the sole determining factor, though most type 1 diabetics develop the condition before reaching puberty. For this reason type 1 diabetes mellitus is also referred to as juvenile diabetes.

2) **Type of diabetes mellitus not documented**
If the type of diabetes mellitus is not documented in the medical record the default is E11.-, Type 2 diabetes mellitus.

3) **Diabetes mellitus and the use of insulin oral hypoglycemics**
If the documentation in a medical record does not indicate the type of diabetes but does indicate that the patient uses insulin, code E11, Type 2 diabetes mellitus, should be assigned. **An additional code should be assigned from category Z79 to identify the long-term (current) use of insulin or oral hypoglycemic drugs. If the patient is treated with both oral medications and insulin, only the code for long-term (current) use of insulin should be assigned. Code Z79.4 should not be assigned if insulin is given temporarily to bring a type 2 patient's blood sugar under control during an encounter.**

4) **Diabetes mellitus in pregnancy and gestational diabetes**
See Section I.C.15. Diabetes mellitus in pregnancy.
See Section I.C.15. Gestational (pregnancy induced) diabetes

5) **Complications due to insulin pump malfunction**

(a) **Underdose of insulin due to insulin pump failure**
An underdose of insulin due to an insulin pump failure should be assigned to a code from subcategory T85.6, Mechanical complication of other specified internal and external prosthetic devices, implants and grafts, that specifies the type of pump malfunction, as the principal or first-listed code, followed by code T38.3X6-, Underdosing of insulin and oral hypoglycemic [antidiabetic] drugs. Additional codes for the type of diabetes mellitus and any associated complications due to the underdosing should also be assigned.

(b) **Overdose of insulin due to insulin pump failure**
The principal or first-listed code for an encounter due to an insulin pump malfunction resulting in an overdose of insulin, should also be T85.6-, Mechanical complication of other specified internal and external prosthetic devices, implants and grafts, followed by code T38.3X1-, Poisoning by insulin and oral hypoglycemic [antidiabetic] drugs, accidental (unintentional).

6) **Secondary diabetes mellitus**
Codes under categories E08, Diabetes mellitus due to underlying condition, E09, Drug or chemical induced diabetes mellitus and E13, Other specified diabetes mellitus, identify complications/manifestations associated with secondary diabetes mellitus. Secondary diabetes is always caused by another condition or event (e.g., cystic fibrosis, malignant neoplasm of pancreas, pancreatectomy, adverse effect of drug, or poisoning).

GUIDELINES (ICD-10-CM)

15

(a) Secondary diabetes mellitus and the use of insulin or hypoglycemic drugs
For patients with secondary diabetes mellitus who routinely use insulin or oral hypoglycemic drugs, an additional code from category Z79 should be assigned to identify the long-term (current) use of insulin or oral hypoglycemic drugs. If the patient is treated with both oral medications and insulin, only the code for long-term (current) use of insulin should be assigned. Code Z79.4 should not be assigned if insulin is given temporarily to bring a secondary diabetic patient's blood sugar under control during an encounter.

(b) Assigning and sequencing secondary diabetes codes and its causes
The sequencing of the secondary diabetes codes in relationship to codes for the cause of the diabetes is based on the Tabular List instructions for categories E08, E09 and E13.

(i) Secondary diabetes mellitus due to pancreatectomy For postpancreatectomy diabetes mellitus (lack of insulin due to the surgical removal of all or part of the pancreas), assign code E89.1, Postprocedural hypoinsulinemia. Assign a code from category E13 and a code from subcategory Z90.41-, Acquired absence of pancreas, as additional codes.

(ii) Secondary diabetes due to drugs Secondary diabetes may be caused by an adverse effect of correctly administered medications, poisoning or sequela of poisoning.

See section I.C.19.e for coding of adverse effects and poisoning, and section I.C.20 for external cause code reporting.

5. **Chapter 5: Mental, Behavioral and Neurodevelopmental disorders (F01 – F99)**

a. Pain disorders related to psychological factors
Assign code F45.41, for pain that is exclusively related to psychological disorders. As indicated by the Excludes 1 note under category G89, a code from category G89 should not be assigned with code F45.41

Code F45.42, Pain disorders with related psychological factors, should be used with a code from category G89, Pain, not elsewhere classified, if there is documentation of a psychological component for a patient with acute or chronic pain.
See Section I.C.6. Pain

c. Mental and behavioral disorders due to psychoactive substance use

1) In Remission
Selection of codes for "in remission" for categories F10-F19, Mental and behavioral disorders due to psychoactive substance use (categories F10-F19 with **-11, -.21**) requires the provider's clinical judgment. The appropriate codes for "in remission" are assigned only on the basis of

provider documentation (as defined in the Official Guidelines for Coding and Reporting), **unless otherwise instructed by the classification.**

Mild substance use disorders in early or sustained remission are classified to the appropriate codes for substance abuse in remission, and moderate or severe substance use disorders in early or sustained remission are classified to the appropriate codes for substance dependence in remission.

2) Psychoactive Substance Use, Abuse and Dependence
When the provider documentation refers to use, abuse and dependence of the same substance (e.g. alcohol, opioid, cannabis, etc.), only one code should be assigned to identify the pattern of use based on the following hierarchy:
- If both use and abuse are documented, assign only the code for abuse
- If both abuse and dependence are documented, assign only the code for dependence
- If use, abuse and dependence are all documented, assign only the code for dependence
- If both use and dependence are documented, assign only the code for dependence.

3) Psychoactive Substance Use *Disorders*
As with all other diagnoses, the codes for psychoactive substance use **disorders** (F10.9-, F11.9-, F12.9-, F13.9-, F14.9-, F15.9-, F16.9-) should only be assigned based on provider documentation and when they meet the definition of a reportable diagnosis (see Section III, Reporting Additional Diagnoses). The codes are to be used only when the psychoactive substance use is associated with a **physical,** mental or behavioral disorder, and such a relationship is documented by the provider.

6. **Chapter 6: Diseases of the Nervous System (G00-G99)**

a. Dominant/nondominant side
Codes from category G81, Hemiplegia and hemiparesis, and subcategories, G83.1, Monoplegia of lower limb, G83.2, Monoplegia of upper limb, and G83.3, Monoplegia, unspecified, identify whether the dominant or nondominant side is affected. Should the affected side be documented, but not specified as dominant or nondominant, and the classification system does not indicate a default, code selection is as follows:
- For ambidextrous patients, the default should be dominant.
- If the left side is affected, the default is nondominant.
- If the right side is affected, the default is dominant.

b. Pain - Category G89

1) General coding information
Codes in category G89, Pain, not elsewhere classified, may be used in conjunction with codes from other categories and chapters to provide more detail about acute or chronic pain and neoplasm-related pain, unless otherwise indicated below.

If the pain is not specified as acute or chronic, post-thoracotomy, postprocedural, or neoplasm-related, do not assign codes from category G89.

A code from category G89 should not be assigned if the underlying (definitive) diagnosis is known, unless the reason for the encounter is pain control/management and not management of the underlying condition.

When an admission or encounter is for a procedure aimed at treating the underlying condition (e.g., spinal fusion, kyphoplasty), a code for the underlying condition (e.g., vertebral fracture, spinal stenosis) should be assigned as the principal diagnosis. No code from category G89 should be assigned.

(a) Category G89 Codes as Principal or First-Listed Diagnosis

Category G89 codes are acceptable as principal diagnosis or the first-listed code:

- When pain control or pain management is the reason for the admission/encounter (e.g., a patient with displaced intervertebral disc, nerve impingement and severe back pain presents for injection of steroid into the spinal canal). The underlying cause of the pain should be reported as an additional diagnosis, if known.
- When a patient is admitted for the insertion of a neurostimulator for pain control, assign the appropriate pain code as the principal or first-listed diagnosis. When an admission or encounter is for a procedure aimed at treating the underlying condition and a neurostimulator is inserted for pain control during the same admission/encounter, a code for the underlying condition should be assigned as the principal diagnosis and the appropriate pain code should be assigned as a secondary diagnosis.

(b) Use of Category G89 Codes in Conjunction with Site Specific Pain Codes

(i) Assigning Category G89 and Site-Specific Pain Codes

Codes from category G89 may be used in conjunction with codes that identify the site of pain (including codes from chapter 18) if the category G89 code provides additional information. For example, if the code describes the site of the pain, but does not fully describe whether the pain is acute or chronic, then both codes should be assigned.

(ii) Sequencing of Category G89 Codes with Site-Specific Pain Codes

The sequencing of category G89 codes with site-specific pain codes (including chapter 18 codes), is dependent on the circumstances of the encounter/admission as follows:

- If the encounter is for pain control or pain management, assign the code from category G89 followed by the code identifying the specific site of pain (e.g., encounter for pain management for acute neck pain from trauma is assigned code G89.11, Acute pain due to trauma, followed by code M54.2, Cervicalgia, to identify the site of pain).
- If the encounter is for any other reason except pain control or pain management, and a related definitive diagnosis has not been established (confirmed) by the provider, assign the code for the specific site of pain first, followed by the appropriate code from category G89.

2) Pain due to devices, implants and grafts
See Section I.C.19. Pain due to medical devices

3) Postoperative Pain
The provider's documentation should be used to guide the coding of postoperative pain, as well as Section III. Reporting Additional Diagnoses and Section IV. Diagnostic Coding and Reporting in the Outpatient Setting.

The default for post-thoracotomy and other postoperative pain not specified as acute or chronic is the code for the acute form.

Routine or expected postoperative pain immediately after surgery should not be coded.

(a) Postoperative pain not associated with specific postoperative complication
Postoperative pain not associated with a specific postoperative complication is assigned to the appropriate postoperative pain code in category G89.

(b) Postoperative pain associated with specific postoperative complication
Postoperative pain associated with a specific postoperative complication (such as painful wire sutures) is assigned to the appropriate code(s) found in Chapter 19, Injury, poisoning, and certain other consequences of external causes. If appropriate, use additional code(s) from category G89 to identify acute or chronic pain (G89.18 or G89.28).

4) Chronic pain
Chronic pain is classified to subcategory G89.2. There is no time frame defining when pain becomes chronic pain. The provider's documentation should be used to guide use of these codes.

5) Neoplasm Related Pain
Code G89.3 is assigned to pain documented as being related, associated or due to cancer, primary or secondary malignancy, or tumor. This code is assigned regardless of whether the pain is acute or chronic.

This code may be assigned as the principal or first-listed code when the stated reason for the admission/encounter is documented as pain control/pain management. The underlying neoplasm should be reported as an additional diagnosis.

When the reason for the admission/encounter is management of the neoplasm and the pain associated with the neoplasm is also documented, code G89.3 may be assigned as an additional diagnosis. It is not necessary to assign an additional code for the site of the pain.

See Section I.C.2 for instructions on the sequencing of neoplasms for all other stated reasons for the admission/ encounter (except for pain control/pain management).

6) Chronic pain syndrome

Central pain syndrome (G89.0) and chronic pain syndrome (G89.4) are different than the term "chronic pain," and therefore codes should only be used when the provider has specifically documented this condition.

See Section I.C.5. Pain disorders related to psychological factors

7. Chapter 7: Diseases of the Eye and Adnexa (H00-H59)

a. Glaucoma

1) Assigning Glaucoma Codes

Assign as many codes from category H40, Glaucoma, as needed to identify the type of glaucoma, the affected eye, and the glaucoma stage.

2) Bilateral glaucoma with same type and stage

When a patient has bilateral glaucoma and both eyes are documented as being the same type and stage, and there is a code for bilateral glaucoma, report only the code for the type of glaucoma, bilateral, with the seventh character for the stage.

When a patient has bilateral glaucoma and both eyes are documented as being the same type and stage, and the classification does not provide a code for bilateral glaucoma (i.e. subcategories H40.10, H40.11 and H40.20) report only one code for the type of glaucoma with the appropriate seventh character for the stage.

3) Bilateral glaucoma stage with different types or stages

When a patient has bilateral glaucoma and each eye is documented as having a different type or stage, and the classification distinguishes laterality, assign the appropriate code for each eye rather than the code for bilateral glaucoma.

When a patient has bilateral glaucoma and each eye is documented as having a different type, and the classification does not distinguish laterality (i.e. subcategories H40.10, H40.11 and H40.20), assign one code for each type of glaucoma with the appropriate seventh character for the stage.

When a patient has bilateral glaucoma and each eye is documented as having the same type, but different stage, and the classification does not distinguish laterality (i.e. subcategories H40.10, H40.11 and H40.20), assign a code for the type of glaucoma for each eye with the seventh character for the specific glaucoma stage documented for each eye.

4) Patient admitted with glaucoma and stage evolves during the admission

If a patient is admitted with glaucoma and the stage progresses during the admission, assign the code for highest stage documented.

5) Indeterminate stage glaucoma

Assignment of the seventh character "4" for "indeterminate stage" should be based on the clinical documentation. The seventh character "4" is used for glaucomas whose stage cannot be clinically determined. This seventh character should not be confused with the seventh character "0", unspecified, which should be assigned when there is no documentation regarding the stage of the glaucoma.

b. Blindness

If "blindness" or "low vision" of both eyes is documented but the visual impairment category is not documented, assign code H54.3, Unqualified visual loss, both eyes. If "blindness" or "low vision" in one eye is documented but the visual impairment category is not documented, assign a code from H54.6-, Unqualified visual loss, one eye. If "blindness" or "visual loss" is documented without any information about whether one or both eyes are affected, assign code H54.7, Unspecified visual loss.

8. Chapter 8: Diseases of the Ear and Mastoid Process (H60-H95)

Reserved for future guideline expansion

9. Chapter 9: Diseases of the Circulatory System (I00-I99)

a. Hypertension

The classification presumes a causal relationship between hypertension and heart involvement and between hypertension and kidney involvement, as the two conditions are linked by the term "with" in the Alphabetic Index. These conditions should be coded as related even in the absence of provider documentation explicitly linking them, unless the documentation clearly states the conditions are unrelated.

For hypertension and conditions not specifically linked by relational terms such as "with," "associated with" or "due to" in the classification, provider documentation must link the conditions in order to code them as related.

1) Hypertension with Heart Disease

Hypertension with heart conditions classified to I50.- or I51.4-I51.9, are assigned to, a code from category I11, Hypertensive heart disease. Use additional code(s) from category I50, Heart failure, to identify the type(s) of heart failure in those patients with heart failure.

The same heart conditions (I50.-, I51.4-I51.9) with hypertension are coded separately if the provider has specifically documented a different cause. Sequence according to the circumstances of the admission/encounter.

2) Hypertensive Chronic Kidney Disease

Assign codes from category I12, Hypertensive chronic kidney disease, when both hypertension and a condition classifiable to category N18, Chronic kidney disease (CKD), are present. CKD should not be coded as hypertensive if the physician has specifically documented a different cause.

The appropriate code from category N18 should be used as a secondary code with a code from category I12 to identify the stage of chronic kidney disease.

See Section I.C.14. Chronic kidney disease.

If a patient has hypertensive chronic kidney disease and acute renal failure, an additional code for the acute renal failure is required.

3) Hypertensive Heart and Chronic Kidney Disease

Assign codes from combination category I13, Hypertensive heart and chronic kidney disease, when there is hypertension with both heart and kidney involvement. If heart failure is present, assign an additional code from category I50 to identify the type of heart failure.

The appropriate code from category N18, Chronic kidney disease, should be used as a secondary code with a code from category I13 to identify the stage of chronic kidney disease.

See Section I.C.14. Chronic kidney disease.

The codes in category I13, Hypertensive heart and chronic kidney disease, are combination codes that include hypertension, heart disease and chronic kidney disease. The Includes note at I13 specifies that the conditions included at I11 and I12 are included together in I13. If a patient has hypertension, heart disease and chronic kidney disease then a code from I13 should be used, not individual codes for hypertension, heart disease and chronic kidney disease, or codes from I11 or I12.

For patients with both acute renal failure and chronic kidney disease an additional code for acute renal failure is required.

4) Hypertensive Cerebrovascular Disease

For hypertensive cerebrovascular disease, first assign the appropriate code from categories I60-I69, followed by the appropriate hypertension code.

5) Hypertensive Retinopathy

Subcategory H35.0, Background retinopathy and retinal vascular changes, should be used with a code from category I10 – I15, Hypertensive disease to include the systemic hypertension. The sequencing is based on the reason for the encounter.

6) Hypertension, Secondary

Secondary hypertension is due to an underlying condition. Two codes are required: one to identify the underlying etiology and one from category I15 to identify the hypertension. Sequencing of codes is determined by the reason for admission/encounter.

7) Hypertension, Transient

Assign code R03.0, Elevated blood pressure reading without diagnosis of hypertension, unless patient has an established diagnosis of hypertension. Assign code O13.-, Gestational [pregnancy-induced] hypertension without

significant proteinuria, or O14.-, Pre-eclampsia, for transient hypertension of pregnancy.

8) Hypertension, Controlled

This diagnostic statement usually refers to an existing state of hypertension under control by therapy. Assign the appropriate code from categories I10-I15, Hypertensive diseases.

9) Hypertension, Uncontrolled

Uncontrolled hypertension may refer to untreated hypertension or hypertension not responding to current therapeutic regimen. In either case, assign the appropriate code from categories I10-I15, Hypertensive diseases.

10) Hypertensive Crisis

Assign a code from category I16, Hypertensive crisis, for documented hypertensive urgency, hypertensive emergency or unspecified hypertensive crisis. Code also any identified hypertensive disease (I10-I15). The sequencing is based on the reason for the encounter.

11) Pulmonary Hypertension

Pulmonary hypertension is classified to category I27, Other pulmonary heart diseases. For secondary pulmonary hypertension (I27.1, I27.2-), code also any associated conditions or adverse effects of drugs or toxins. The sequencing is based on the reason for the encounter.

b. Atherosclerotic Coronary Artery Disease and Angina

ICD-10-CM has combination codes for atherosclerotic heart disease with angina pectoris. The subcategories for these codes are I25.11, Atherosclerotic heart disease of native coronary artery with angina pectoris and I25.7, Atherosclerosis of coronary artery bypass graft(s) and coronary artery of transplanted heart with angina pectoris.

When using one of these combination codes it is not necessary to use an additional code for angina pectoris. A causal relationship can be assumed in a patient with both atherosclerosis and angina pectoris, unless the documentation indicates the angina is due to something other than the atherosclerosis.

If a patient with coronary artery disease is admitted due to an acute myocardial infarction (AMI), the AMI should be sequenced before the coronary artery disease.

See Section I.C.9. Acute myocardial infarction (AMI)

c. Intraoperative and Postprocedural Cerebrovascular Accident

Medical record documentation should clearly specify the cause-and-effect relationship between the medical intervention and the cerebrovascular accident in order to assign a code for intraoperative or postprocedural cerebrovascular accident.

Proper code assignment depends on whether it was an infarction or hemorrhage and whether it occurred intraoperatively or postoperatively. If it was a cerebral hemorrhage, code assignment depends on the type of procedure performed.

d. Sequelae of Cerebrovascular Disease

1) Category I69, Sequelae of Cerebrovascular disease

Category I69 is used to indicate conditions classifiable to categories I60-I67 as the causes of sequela (neurologic deficits), themselves classified elsewhere. These "late effects" include neurologic deficits that persist after initial onset of conditions classifiable to categories I60-I67. The neurologic deficits caused by cerebrovascular disease may be present from the onset or may arise at any time after the onset of the condition classifiable to categories I60-I67.

Codes from category I69, Sequelae of cerebrovascular disease, that specify hemiplegia, hemiparesis and monoplegia identify whether the dominant or nondominant side is affected. Should the affected side be documented, but not specified as dominant or nondominant, and the classification system does not indicate a default, code selection is as follows:

- For ambidextrous patients, the default should be dominant.
- If the left side is affected, the default is non-dominant.
- If the right side is affected, the default is dominant.

2) Codes from category I69 with codes from I60-I67

Codes from category I69 may be assigned on a health care record with codes from I60-I67, if the patient has a current cerebrovascular disease and deficits from an old cerebrovascular disease.

3) Codes from category I69 and Personal history of transient ischemic attack (TIA) and cerebral infarction (Z86.73)

Codes from category I69 should not be assigned if the patient does not have neurologic deficits.

See Section I.C.21. 4. History (of) for use of personal history codes

e. Acute myocardial infarction (AMI)

1) Type 1 ST elevation myocardial infarction (STEMI) and non ST elevation myocardial infarction (NSTEMI)

The ICD-10-CM codes for **type 1** acute myocardial infarction (AMI) identify the site, such as anterolateral wall or true posterior wall. Subcategories I21.0-I21.2 and code I21.3 are used for **type 1** ST elevation myocardial infarction (STEMI). Code I21.4, Non-ST elevation (NSTEMI) myocardial infarction, is used for **type 1** non ST elevation myocardial infarction (NSTEMI) and nontransmural MIs.

If **a type 1** NSTEMI evolves to STEMI, assign the STEMI code. If **a type 1** STEMI converts to NSTEMI due to thrombolytic therapy, it is still coded as STEMI.

For encounters occurring while the myocardial infarction is equal to, or less than, four weeks old, including transfers to another acute setting or a postacute setting, and the myocardial infarction meets the definition for "other diagnoses" (see Section III, Reporting Additional Diagnoses), codes from category I21 may continue to be reported. For encounters after the 4 week time frame and the patient is still receiving care related to the myocardial infarction, the appropriate aftercare code should be assigned, rather than a code from category I21. For old or healed myocardial infarctions not requiring further care, code I25.2, Old myocardial infarction, may be assigned.

2) Acute myocardial infarction, unspecified

Code **I21.9, Acute myocardial infarction, unspecified,** is the default for unspecified acute myocardial infarction **or unspecified type**. If only **type 1** STEMI or transmural MI without the site is documented, assign code I21.3, **ST elevation (STEMI) myocardial infarction of unspecified site**.

3) AMI documented as nontransmural or subendocardial but site provided

If an AMI is documented as nontransmural or subendocardial, but the site is provided, it is still coded as a subendocardial AMI.

See Section I.C.21.3 for information on coding status post administration of tPA in a different facility within the last 24 hours.

4) Subsequent acute myocardial infarction

A code from category I22, Subsequent ST elevation (STEMI) and non ST elevation (NSTEMI) myocardial infarction, is to be used when a patient who has suffered **a type 1 or unspecified** AMI has a new AMI within the 4 week time frame of the initial AMI. A code from category I22 must be used in conjunction with a code from category I21. The sequencing of the I22 and I21 codes depends on the circumstances of the encounter.

Do not assign code I22 for subsequent myocardial infarctions other than type 1 or unspecified. For subsequent type 2 AMI assign only code I21.A1. For subsequent type 4 or type 5 AMI, assign only code I21.A9.

5) Other Types of Myocardial Infarction

The ICD-10-CM provides codes for different types of myocardial infarction. Type 1 myocardial infarctions are assigned to codes I21.0-I21.4.

Type 2 myocardial infarction, and myocardial infarction due to demand ischemia or secondary to ischemic balance, is assigned to code I21.A1, Myocardial infarction type 2 with a code for the underlying cause. Do not assign code I24.8, Other forms of acute ischemic heart disease for the demand ischemia. Sequencing of type 2 AMI or the underlying cause is dependent on the circumstances of admission. When a type 2 AMI code is described as NSTEMI or STEMI, only assign code I21.A1. Codes I21.01-I21.4 should only be assigned for type 1 AMIs.

Acute myocardial infarctions type 3, 4a, 4b, 4c and 5 are assigned to code I21.A9, Other myocardial infarction type.

The "Code also" and "Code first" notes should be followed related to complications, and for coding of postprocedural myocardial infarctions during or following cardiac surgery.

10. Chapter 10: Diseases of the Respiratory System (J00-J99)

  a. Chronic Obstructive Pulmonary Disease [COPD] and Asthma

   1) Acute exacerbation of chronic obstructive bronchitis and asthma

The codes in categories J44 and J45 distinguish between uncomplicated cases and those in acute exacerbation. An acute exacerbation is a worsening or a decompensation of a chronic condition. An acute exacerbation is not equivalent to an infection superimposed on a chronic condition, though an exacerbation may be triggered by an infection.

  b. Acute Respiratory Failure

   1) Acute respiratory failure as principal diagnosis

A code from subcategory J96.0, Acute respiratory failure, or subcategory J96.2, Acute and chronic respiratory failure, may be assigned as a principal diagnosis when it is the condition established after study to be chiefly responsible for occasioning the admission to the hospital, and the selection is supported by the Alphabetic Index and Tabular List. However, chapter-specific coding guidelines (such as obstetrics, poisoning, HIV, newborn) that provide sequencing direction take precedence.

   2) Acute respiratory failure as secondary diagnosis

Respiratory failure may be listed as a secondary diagnosis if it occurs after admission, or if it is present on admission, but does not meet the definition of principal diagnosis.

   3) Sequencing of acute respiratory failure and another acute condition

When a patient is admitted with respiratory failure and another acute condition, (e.g., myocardial infarction, cerebrovascular accident, aspiration pneumonia), the principal diagnosis will not be the same in every situation. This applies whether the other acute condition is a respiratory or nonrespiratory condition. Selection of the principal diagnosis will be dependent on the circumstances of admission. If both the respiratory failure and the other acute condition are equally responsible for occasioning the admission to the hospital, and there are no chapter-specific sequencing rules, the guideline regarding two or more diagnoses that equally meet the definition for principal diagnosis (*Section II, C.*) may be applied in these situations.

If the documentation is not clear as to whether acute respiratory failure and another condition are equally responsible for occasioning the admission, query the provider for clarification.

  c. Influenza due to certain identified influenza viruses

Code only confirmed cases of influenza due to certain identified influenza viruses (category J09), and due to other identified influenza virus (category J10). This is an exception to the hospital inpatient guideline Section II, H. (Uncertain Diagnosis).

In this context, "confirmation" does not require documentation of positive laboratory testing specific for avian or other novel influenza A or other identified influenza virus. However, coding should be based on the provider's diagnostic statement that the patient has avian influenza, or other novel influenza A, for category J09, or has another particular identified strain of influenza, such as H1N1 or H3N2, but not identified as novel or variant, for category J10.

If the provider records "suspected" or "possible" or "probable" avian influenza, or novel influenza, or other identified influenza, then the appropriate influenza code from category J11, Influenza due to unidentified influenza virus, should be assigned. A code from category J09, Influenza due to certain identified influenza viruses, should not be assigned nor should a code from category J10, Influenza due to other identified influenza virus.

  d. Ventilator associated Pneumonia

   1) Documentation of Ventilator associated Pneumonia

As with all procedural or postprocedural complications, code assignment is based on the provider's documentation of the relationship between the condition and the procedure.

Code J95.851, Ventilator associated pneumonia, should be assigned only when the provider has documented ventilator associated pneumonia (VAP). An additional code to identify the organism (e.g., Pseudomonas aeruginosa, code B96.5) should also be assigned. Do not assign an additional code from categories J12-J18 to identify the type of pneumonia.

Code J95.851 should not be assigned for cases where the patient has pneumonia and is on a mechanical ventilator and the provider has not specifically stated that the pneumonia is ventilator-associated pneumonia. If the documentation is unclear as to whether the patient has a pneumonia that is a complication attributable to the mechanical ventilator, query the provider.

   2) Ventilator associated Pneumonia Develops after Admission

A patient may be admitted with one type of pneumonia (e.g., code J13, Pneumonia due to Streptococcus pneumonia) and subsequently develop VAP. In this instance, the principal diagnosis would be the appropriate code from categories J12-J18 for the pneumonia diagnosed at the time of admission. Code J95.851, Ventilator associated pneumonia, would be assigned as an additional diagnosis when the provider has also documented the presence of ventilator associated pneumonia.

11. Chapter 11: Diseases of the Digestive System (K00-K95)
Reserved for future guideline expansion

12. **Chapter 12: Diseases of the Skin and Subcutaneous Tissue (L00-L99)**

   a. **Pressure ulcer stage codes**

      1) **Pressure ulcer stages**

Codes from category L89, Pressure ulcer, identify the site of the pressure ulcer as well as the stage of the ulcer.

The ICD-10-CM classifies pressure ulcer stages based on severity, which is designated by stages 1-4, unspecified stage and unstageable.

Assign as many codes from category L89 as needed to identify all the pressure ulcers the patient has, if applicable.

      2) **Unstageable pressure ulcers**

Assignment of the code for unstageable pressure ulcer (L89.--0) should be based on the clinical documentation. These codes are used for pressure ulcers whose stage cannot be clinically determined (e.g., the ulcer is covered by eschar or has been treated with a skin or muscle graft) and pressure ulcers that are documented as deep tissue injury but not documented as due to trauma. This code should not be confused with the codes for unspecified stage (L89.--9). When there is no documentation regarding the stage of the pressure ulcer, assign the appropriate code for unspecified stage (L89.--9).

      3) **Documented pressure ulcer stage**

Assignment of the pressure ulcer stage code should be guided by clinical documentation of the stage or documentation of the terms found in the Alphabetic Index. For clinical terms describing the stage that are not found in the Alphabetic Index, and there is no documentation of the stage, the provider should be queried.

      4) **Patients admitted with pressure ulcers documented as healed**

No code is assigned if the documentation states that the pressure ulcer is completely healed.

      5) **Patients admitted with pressure ulcers documented as healing**

Pressure ulcers described as healing should be assigned the appropriate pressure ulcer stage code based on the documentation in the medical record. If the documentation does not provide information about the stage of the healing pressure ulcer, assign the appropriate code for unspecified stage.

If the documentation is unclear as to whether the patient has a current (new) pressure ulcer or if the patient is being treated for a healing pressure ulcer, query the provider.

For ulcers that were present on admission but healed at the time of discharge, assign the code for the site and stage of the pressure ulcer at the time of admission.

      6) **Patient admitted with pressure ulcer evolving into another stage during the admission**

If a patient is admitted **to an inpatient hospital** with a pressure ulcer at one stage and it progresses to a higher stage, two separate codes should be assigned: one code for the site and stage of the ulcer on admission and a second code for the same ulcer site and the highest stage reported during the stay.

   b. **Non-Pressure Chronic Ulcers**

      1) **Patients admitted with non-pressure ulcers documented as healed**

No code is assigned if the documentation states that the non-pressure ulcer is completely healed.

      2) **Patients admitted with non-pressure ulcers documented as healing**

Non-pressure ulcers described as healing should be assigned the appropriate non-pressure ulcer code based on the documentation in the medical record. If the documentation does not provide information about the severity of the healing non-pressure ulcer, assign the appropriate code for unspecified severity.

If the documentation is unclear as to whether the patient has a current (new) non-pressure ulcer or if the patient is being treated for a healing non-pressure ulcer, query the provider.

For ulcers that were present on admission but healed at the time of discharge, assign the code for the site and severity of the non-pressure ulcer at the time of admission.

      3) **Patient admitted with non-pressure ulcer that progresses to another severity level during the admission**

If a patient is admitted to an inpatient hospital with a non-pressure ulcer at one severity level and it progresses to a higher severity level, two separate codes should be assigned: one code for the site and severity level of the ulcer on admission and a second code for the same ulcer site and the highest severity level reported during the stay.

13. **Chapter 13: Diseases of the Musculoskeletal System and Connective Tissue (M00-M99)**

   a. **Site and laterality**

Most of the codes within Chapter 13 have site and laterality designations. The site represents the bone, joint or the muscle involved. For some conditions where more than one bone, joint or muscle is usually involved, such as osteoarthritis, there is a "multiple sites" code available. For categories where no multiple site code is provided and more than one bone, joint or muscle is involved, multiple codes should be used to indicate the different sites involved.

      1) **Bone versus joint**

For certain conditions, the bone may be affected at the upper or lower end, (e.g., avascular necrosis of bone, M87, Osteoporosis, M80, M81). Though the portion of the bone affected may be at the joint, the site designation will be the bone, not the joint.

   b. **Acute traumatic versus chronic or recurrent musculoskeletal conditions**

Many musculoskeletal conditions are a result of previous injury or trauma to a site, or are recurrent conditions. Bone, joint or muscle conditions that are the result of a healed injury are usually found in chapter 13. Recurrent bone, joint or muscle conditions are also usually found in chapter 13. Any current, acute injury should be coded to the appropriate injury code from chapter 19. Chronic or recurrent conditions should generally be coded with a code from chapter 13. If it is difficult to determine from the documentation in the record which code is best to describe a condition, query the provider.

c. Coding of Pathologic Fractures

7th character A is for use as long as the patient is receiving active treatment for the fracture. While the patient may be seen by a new or different provider over the course of treatment for a pathological fracture, assignment of the 7th character is based on whether the patient is undergoing active treatment and not whether the provider is seeing the patient for the first time.

7th character, D is to be used for encounters after the patient has completed active treatment **for the fracture and is receiving routine care for the fracture during the healing or recovery phase**. The other 7th characters, listed under each subcategory in the Tabular List, are to be used for subsequent encounters for treatment of problems associated with the healing, such as malunions, nonunions, and sequelae.

Care for complications of surgical treatment for fracture repairs during the healing or recovery phase should be coded with the appropriate complication codes.

See Section I.C.19. Coding of traumatic fractures.

d. Osteoporosis

Osteoporosis is a systemic condition, meaning that all bones of the musculoskeletal system are affected. Therefore, site is not a component of the codes under category M81, Osteoporosis without current pathological fracture. The site codes under category M80, Osteoporosis with current pathological fracture, identify the site of the fracture, not the osteoporosis.

1) Osteoporosis without pathological fracture

Category M81, Osteoporosis without current pathological fracture, is for use for patients with osteoporosis who do not currently have a pathologic fracture due to the osteoporosis, even if they have had a fracture in the past. For patients with a history of osteoporosis fractures, status code Z87.310, Personal history of (healed) osteoporosis fracture, should follow the code from M81.

2) Osteoporosis with current pathological fracture

Category M80, Osteoporosis with current pathological fracture, is for patients who have a current pathologic fracture at the time of an encounter. The codes under M80 identify the site of the fracture. A code from category M80, not a traumatic fracture code, should be used for any patient with known osteoporosis who suffers a fracture, even if the patient had a minor fall or trauma, if that fall or trauma would not usually break a normal, healthy bone.

14. Chapter 14: Diseases of Genitourinary System (N00-N99)

a. Chronic kidney disease

1) Stages of chronic kidney disease (CKD)

The ICD-10-CM classifies CKD based on severity. The severity of CKD is designated by stages 1-5. Stage 2, code N18.2, equates to mild CKD; stage 3, code N18.3, equates to moderate CKD; and stage 4, code N18.4, equates to severe CKD. Code N18.6, End stage renal disease (ESRD), is assigned when the provider has documented end-stage-renal disease (ESRD).

If both a stage of CKD and ESRD are documented, assign code N18.6 only.

2) Chronic kidney disease and kidney transplant status

Patients who have undergone kidney transplant may still have some form of chronic kidney disease CKD because the kidney transplant may not fully restore kidney function. Therefore, the presence of CKD alone does not constitute a transplant complication. Assign the appropriate N18 code for the patient's stage of CKD and code Z94.0, Kidney transplant status. If a transplant complication such as failure or rejection or other transplant complication is documented, see section I.C.19.g for information on coding complications of a kidney transplant. If the documentation is unclear as to whether the patient has a complication of the transplant, query the provider.

3) Chronic kidney disease with other conditions

Patients with CKD may also suffer from other serious conditions, most commonly diabetes mellitus and hypertension. The sequencing of the CKD code in relationship to codes for other contributing conditions is based on the conventions in the Tabular List.

See I.C.9. Hypertensive chronic kidney disease.
See I.C.19. Chronic kidney disease and kidney transplant complications.

15. Chapter 15: Pregnancy, Childbirth, and the Puerperium (O00-O9A)

a. General Rules for Obstetric Cases

1) Codes from chapter 15 and sequencing priority

Obstetric cases require codes from chapter 15, codes in the range O00-O9A, Pregnancy, Childbirth, and the Puerperium. Chapter 15 codes have sequencing priority over codes from other chapters. Additional codes from other chapters may be used in conjunction with chapter 15 codes to further specify conditions. Should the provider document that the pregnancy is incidental to the encounter, then code Z33.1, Pregnant state, incidental, should be used in place of any chapter 15 codes. It is the provider's responsibility to state that the condition being treated is not affecting the pregnancy.

2) Chapter 15 codes used only on the maternal record

Chapter 15 codes are to be used only on the maternal record, never on the record of the newborn.

3) Final character for trimester

The majority of codes in Chapter 15 have a final character indicating the trimester of pregnancy. The timeframes for the trimesters are indicated at the beginning of the chapter. If trimester is not a component of a code it is because the condition always occurs in a specific trimester, or the concept of trimester of pregnancy is not applicable. Certain codes have characters for only certain trimesters because the condition does not occur in all trimesters, but it may occur in more than just one.

Assignment of the final character for trimester should be based on the provider's documentation of the trimester (or number of weeks) for the current admission/encounter. This applies to the assignment of trimester for pre-existing conditions as well as those that develop during or are due to the pregnancy. The provider's documentation of the number of weeks may be used to assign the appropriate code identifying the trimester.

Whenever delivery occurs during the current admission, and there is an "in childbirth" option for the obstetric complication being coded, the "in childbirth" code should be assigned.

4) Selection of trimester for inpatient admissions that encompass more than one trimester

In instances when a patient is admitted to a hospital for complications of pregnancy during one trimester and remains in the hospital into a subsequent trimester, the trimester character for the antepartum complication code should be assigned on the basis of the trimester when the complication developed, not the trimester of the discharge. If the condition developed prior to the current admission/encounter or represents a pre-existing condition, the trimester character for the trimester at the time of the admission/encounter should be assigned.

5) Unspecified trimester

Each category that includes codes for trimester has a code for "unspecified trimester." The "unspecified trimester" code should rarely be used, such as when the documentation in the record is insufficient to determine the trimester and it is not possible to obtain clarification.

6) 7th character for Fetus Identification

Where applicable, a 7th character is to be assigned for certain categories (O31, O32, O33.3 - O33.6, O35, O36, O40, O41, O60.1, O60.2, O64, and O69) to identify the fetus for which the complication code applies.

Assign 7th character "0":
- For single gestations
- When the documentation in the record is insufficient to determine the fetus affected and it is not possible to obtain clarification.
- When it is not possible to clinically determine which fetus is affected.

b. Selection of OB Principal or First-listed Diagnosis

1) Routine outpatient prenatal visits

For routine outpatient prenatal visits when no complications are present, a code from category Z34, Encounter for supervision of normal pregnancy, should be used as the first-listed diagnosis. These codes should not be used in conjunction with chapter 15 codes.

2) Supervision of High-Risk Pregnancy

Codes from category O09, Supervision of high-risk pregnancy, are intended for use only during the prenatal period. For complications during the labor or delivery episode as a result of a high-risk pregnancy, assign the applicable complication codes from Chapter 15. If there are no complications during the labor or delivery episode, assign code O80, Encounter for full-term uncomplicated delivery.

For routine prenatal outpatient visits for patients with high-risk pregnancies, a code from category O09, Supervision of high-risk pregnancy, should be used as the first-listed diagnosis. Secondary chapter 15 codes may be used in conjunction with these codes if appropriate.

3) Episodes when no delivery occurs

In episodes when no delivery occurs, the principal diagnosis should correspond to the principal complication of the pregnancy which necessitated the encounter. Should more than one complication exist, all of which are treated or monitored, any of the complications codes may be sequenced first.

4) When a delivery occurs

When an obstetric patient is admitted and delivers during that admission, the condition that prompted the admission should be sequenced as the principal diagnosis. If multiple conditions prompted the admission, sequence the one most related to the delivery as the principal diagnosis. A code for any complication of the delivery should be assigned as an additional diagnosis. In cases of cesarean delivery, if the patient was admitted with a condition that resulted in the performance of a cesarean procedure, that condition should be selected as the principal diagnosis. If the reason for the admission was unrelated to the condition resulting in the cesarean delivery, the condition related to the reason for the admission should be selected as the principal diagnosis.

5) Outcome of delivery

A code from category Z37, Outcome of delivery, should be included on every maternal record when a delivery has occurred. These codes are not to be used on subsequent records or on the newborn record.

c. Pre-existing conditions versus conditions due to the pregnancy

Certain categories in Chapter 15 distinguish between conditions of the mother that existed prior to pregnancy (pre-existing) and those that are a direct result of pregnancy. When assigning codes from Chapter 15, it is important to assess if a condition was pre-existing prior to pregnancy or developed during or due to the pregnancy in order to assign the correct code.

Categories that do not distinguish between pre-existing and pregnancy-related conditions may be used for either. It is acceptable to use codes specifically for the puerperium with codes complicating pregnancy and childbirth if a condition arises postpartum during the delivery encounter.

d. Pre-existing hypertension in pregnancy
Category O10, Pre-existing hypertension complicating pregnancy, childbirth and the puerperium, includes codes for hypertensive heart and hypertensive chronic kidney disease. When assigning one of the O10 codes that includes hypertensive heart disease or hypertensive chronic kidney disease, it is necessary to add a secondary code from the appropriate hypertension category to specify the type of heart failure or chronic kidney disease.

See Section I.C.9. Hypertension.

e. Fetal Conditions Affecting the Management of the Mother

1) Codes from categories O35 and O36
Codes from categories O35, Maternal care for known or suspected fetal abnormality and damage, and O36, Maternal care for other fetal problems, are assigned only when the fetal condition is actually responsible for modifying the management of the mother, i.e., by requiring diagnostic studies, additional observation, special care, or termination of pregnancy. The fact that the fetal condition exists does not justify assigning a code from this series to the mother's record.

2) In utero surgery
In cases when surgery is performed on the fetus, a diagnosis code from category O35, Maternal care for known or suspected fetal abnormality and damage, should be assigned identifying the fetal condition. Assign the appropriate procedure code for the procedure performed.

No code from Chapter 16, the perinatal codes, should be used on the mother's record to identify fetal conditions. Surgery performed in utero on a fetus is still to be coded as an obstetric encounter.

f. HIV Infection in Pregnancy, Childbirth and the Puerperium
During pregnancy, childbirth or the puerperium, a patient admitted because of an HIV-related illness should receive a principal diagnosis from subcategory O98.7-, Human immunodeficiency [HIV] disease complicating pregnancy, childbirth and the puerperium, followed by the code(s) for the HIV-related illness(es).

Patients with asymptomatic HIV infection status admitted during pregnancy, childbirth, or the puerperium should receive codes of O98.7- and Z21, Asymptomatic human immunodeficiency virus [HIV] infection status.

g. Diabetes mellitus in pregnancy
Diabetes mellitus is a significant complicating factor in pregnancy. Pregnant women who are diabetic should be assigned a code from category O24, Diabetes mellitus in pregnancy, childbirth, and the puerperium, first, followed by the appropriate diabetes code(s) (E08-E13) from Chapter 4.

h. Long term use of insulin and oral hypoglycemics
See section I.C.4.a.3 for information on the long term use of insulin and oral hypoglycemic.

i. Gestational (pregnancy induced) diabetes
Gestational (pregnancy induced) diabetes can occur during the second and third trimester of pregnancy in women who were not diabetic prior to pregnancy. Gestational diabetes can cause complications in the pregnancy similar to those of pre-existing diabetes mellitus. It also puts the woman at greater risk of developing diabetes after the pregnancy. Codes for gestational diabetes are in subcategory O24.4, Gestational diabetes mellitus. No other code from category O24, Diabetes mellitus in pregnancy, childbirth, and the puerperium, should be used with a code from O24.4.

The codes under subcategory O24.4 include diet controlled, insulin controlled, and controlled by oral hypoglycemic drugs. If a patient with gestational diabetes is treated with both diet and insulin, only the code for insulin-controlled is required. If a patient with gestational diabetes is treated with both diet and oral hypoglycemic medications, only the code for "controlled by oral hypoglycemic drugs" is required. Code Z79.4, Long-term (current) use of insulin or code Z79.84, Long-term (current) use of oral hypoglycemic drugs, should not be assigned with codes from subcategory O24.4.

An abnormal glucose tolerance in pregnancy is assigned a code from subcategory O99.81, Abnormal glucose complicating pregnancy, childbirth, and the puerperium.

j. Sepsis and septic shock complicating abortion, pregnancy, childbirth and the puerperium
When assigning a chapter 15 code for sepsis complicating abortion, pregnancy, childbirth, and the puerperium, a code for the specific type of infection should be assigned as an additional diagnosis. If severe sepsis is present, a code from subcategory R65.2, Severe sepsis, and code(s) for associated organ dysfunction(s) should also be assigned as additional diagnoses.

k. Puerperal sepsis
Code O85, Puerperal sepsis, should be assigned with a secondary code to identify the causal organism (e.g., for a bacterial infection, assign a code from category B95-B96, Bacterial infections in conditions classified elsewhere). A code from category A40, Streptococcal sepsis, or A41, Other sepsis, should not be used for puerperal sepsis. If

applicable, use additional codes to identify severe sepsis (R65.2-) and any associated acute organ dysfunction.

l. Alcohol and tobacco use during pregnancy, childbirth and the puerperium

1) Alcohol use during pregnancy, childbirth and the puerperium

Codes under subcategory O99.31, Alcohol use complicating pregnancy, childbirth, and the puerperium, should be assigned for any pregnancy case when a mother uses alcohol during the pregnancy or postpartum. A secondary code from category F10, Alcohol related disorders, should also be assigned to identify manifestations of the alcohol use.

2) Tobacco use during pregnancy, childbirth and the puerperium

Codes under subcategory O99.33, Smoking (tobacco) complicating pregnancy, childbirth, and the puerperium, should be assigned for any pregnancy case when a mother uses any type of tobacco product during the pregnancy or postpartum. A secondary code from category F17, Nicotine dependence, should also be assigned to identify the type of nicotine dependence.

m. Poisoning, toxic effects, adverse effects and underdosing in a pregnant patient

A code from subcategory O9A.2, Injury, poisoning and certain other consequences of external causes complicating pregnancy, childbirth, and the puerperium, should be sequenced first, followed by the appropriate injury, poisoning, toxic effect, adverse effect or underdosing code, and then the additional code(s) that specifies the condition caused by the poisoning, toxic effect, adverse effect or underdosing.

See Section I.C.19. Adverse effects, poisoning, underdosing and toxic effects.

n. Normal Delivery, Code O80

1) Encounter for full term uncomplicated delivery

Code O80 should be assigned when a woman is admitted for a full-term normal delivery and delivers a single, healthy infant without any complications antepartum, during the delivery, or postpartum during the delivery episode. Code O80 is always a principal diagnosis. It is not to be used if any other code from chapter 15 is needed to describe a current complication of the antenatal, delivery, or perinatal period. Additional codes from other chapters may be used with code O80 if they are not related to or are in any way complicating the pregnancy.

2) Uncomplicated delivery with resolved antepartum complication

Code O80 may be used if the patient had a complication at some point during the pregnancy, but the complication is not present at the time of the admission for delivery.

3) Outcome of delivery for O80

Z37.0, Single live birth, is the only outcome of delivery code appropriate for use with O80.

o. The Peripartum and Postpartum Periods

1) Peripartum and Postpartum periods

The postpartum period begins immediately after delivery and continues for six weeks following delivery. The peripartum period is defined as the last month of pregnancy to five months postpartum.

2) Peripartum and postpartum complication

A postpartum complication is any complication occurring within the six-week period.

3) Pregnancy-related complications after 6 week period

Chapter 15 codes may also be used to describe pregnancy-related complications after the peripartum or postpartum period if the provider documents that a condition is pregnancy related.

4) Admission for routine postpartum care following delivery outside hospital

When the mother delivers outside the hospital prior to admission and is admitted for routine postpartum care and no complications are noted, code Z39.0, Encounter for care and examination of mother immediately after delivery, should be assigned as the principal diagnosis.

5) Pregnancy associated cardiomyopathy

Pregnancy associated cardiomyopathy, code O90.3, is unique in that it may be diagnosed in the third trimester of pregnancy but may continue to progress months after delivery. For this reason, it is referred to as peripartum cardiomyopathy. Code O90.3 is only for use when the cardiomyopathy develops as a result of pregnancy in a woman who did not have pre-existing heart disease.

p. Code O94, Sequelae of complication of pregnancy, childbirth, and the puerperium

1) Code O94

Code O94, Sequelae of complication of pregnancy, childbirth, and the puerperium, is for use in those cases when an initial complication of a pregnancy develops a sequelae requiring care or treatment at a future date.

2) After the initial postpartum period

This code may be used at any time after the initial postpartum period.

3) Sequencing of Code O94

This code, like all sequela codes, is to be sequenced following the code describing the sequelae of the complication.

q. Termination of Pregnancy and Spontaneous abortions

1) Abortion with Liveborn Fetus

When an attempted termination of pregnancy results in a liveborn fetus assign code Z33.2, Encounter for elective termination of pregnancy and a code from category Z37, Outcome of Delivery.

2) Retained Products of Conception following an abortion

Subsequent encounters for retained products of conception following a spontaneous abortion or elective termination of pregnancy, **without**

complications are assigned O03.**4, Incomplete spontaneous,** abortion **without complication** or codes O07.4, Failed attempted termination of pregnancy without complication. This advice is appropriate even when the patient was discharged previously with a discharge diagnosis of complete abortion. **If the patient has a specific complication associated with the spontaneous abortion or elective termination of pregnancy in addition to retained products of conception, assign the appropriate complication in category O03 or O07 instead of code O03.4 or O07.4**

3) Complications leading to abortion

Codes from Chapter 15 may be used as additional codes to identify any documented complications of the pregnancy in conjunction with codes in categories in **O04,** O07 and O08.

r. Abuse in a pregnant patient

For suspected or confirmed cases of abuse of a pregnant patient, a code(s) from subcategories O9A.3, Physical abuse complicating pregnancy, childbirth, and the puerperium, O9A.4, Sexual abuse complicating pregnancy, childbirth, and the puerperium, and O9A.5, Psychological abuse complicating pregnancy, childbirth, and the puerperium, should be sequenced first, followed by the appropriate codes (if applicable) to identify any associated current injury due to physical abuse, sexual abuse, and the perpetrator of abuse.

See Section I.C.19. Adult and child abuse, neglect and other maltreatment.

16. Chapter 16: Certain Conditions Originating in the Perinatal Period (P00-P96)

For coding and reporting purposes the perinatal period is defined as before birth through the 28th day following birth. The following guidelines are provided for reporting purposes

a. General Perinatal Rules

1) Use of Chapter 16 Codes

Codes in this chapter are never for use on the maternal record. Codes from Chapter 15, the obstetric chapter, are never permitted on the newborn record. Chapter 16 codes may be used throughout the life of the patient if the condition is still present.

2) Principal Diagnosis for Birth Record

When coding the birth episode in a newborn record, assign a code from category Z38, Liveborn infants according to place of birth and type of delivery, as the principal diagnosis. A code from category Z38 is assigned only once, to a newborn at the time of birth. If a newborn is transferred to another institution, a code from category Z38 should not be used at the receiving hospital.

A code from category Z38 is used only on the newborn record, not on the mother's record.

3) Use of Codes from other Chapters with Codes from Chapter 16

Codes from other chapters may be used with codes from chapter 16 if the codes from the other chapters provide more specific detail. Codes for

signs and symptoms may be assigned when a definitive diagnosis has not been established. If the reason for the encounter is a perinatal condition, the code from chapter 16 should be sequenced first.

4) Use of Chapter 16 Codes after the Perinatal Period

Should a condition originate in the perinatal period, and continue throughout the life of the patient, the perinatal code should continue to be used regardless of the patient's age.

5) Birth process or community acquired conditions

If a newborn has a condition that may be either due to the birth process or community acquired and the documentation does not indicate which it is, the default is due to the birth process and the code from Chapter 16 should be used. If the condition is community-acquired, a code from Chapter 16 should not be assigned.

6) Code all clinically significant conditions

All clinically significant conditions noted on routine newborn examination should be coded. A condition is clinically significant if it requires:
- clinical evaluation; or
- therapeutic treatment; or
- diagnostic procedures; or
- extended length of hospital stay; or
- increased nursing care and/or monitoring; or
- has implications for future health care needs

Note: The perinatal guidelines listed above are the same as the general coding guidelines for "additional diagnoses", except for the final point regarding implications for future health care needs. Codes should be assigned for conditions that have been specified by the provider as having implications for future health care needs.

b. Observation and Evaluation of Newborns for Suspected Conditions not Found

1) *Use of Z05 codes*

Assign a code from category Z05, Observation and evaluation of newborns and infants for suspected conditions ruled out, to identify those instances when a healthy newborn is evaluated for a suspected condition that is determined after study not to be present. Do not use a code from category Z05 when the patient has identified signs or symptoms of a suspected problem; in such cases code the sign or symptom.

2) *Z05 on Other than the Birth Record*

A code from category Z05 may also be assigned as a principal or first-listed code for readmissions or encounters when the code from category Z38 code no longer applies. Codes from category Z05 are for use only for healthy newborns and infants for which no condition after study is found to be present.

3) Z05 on a birth record

A code from category Z05 is to be used as a secondary code after the code from category Z38, Liveborn infants according to place of birth and type of delivery.

c. Coding Additional Perinatal Diagnoses

1) Assigning codes for conditions that require treatment

Assign codes for conditions that require treatment or further investigation, prolong the length of stay, or require resource utilization.

2) Codes for conditions specified as having implications for future health care needs

Assign codes for conditions that have been specified by the provider as having implications for future health care needs.

Note: This guideline should not be used for adult patients.

d. Prematurity and Fetal Growth Retardation

Providers utilize different criteria in determining prematurity. A code for prematurity should not be assigned unless it is documented. Assignment of codes in categories P05, Disorders of newborn related to slow fetal growth and fetal malnutrition, and P07, Disorders of newborn related to short gestation and low birth weight, not elsewhere classified, should be based on the recorded birth weight and estimated gestational age.

When both birth weight and gestational age are available, two codes from category P07 should be assigned, with the code for birth weight sequenced before the code for gestational age.

e. Low birth weight and immaturity status

Codes from category P07, Disorders of newborn related to short gestation and low birth weight, not elsewhere classified, are for use for a child or adult who was premature or had a low birth weight as a newborn and this is affecting the patient's current health status.

See Section I.C.21. Factors influencing health status and contact with health services, Status.

f. Bacterial Sepsis of Newborn

Category P36, Bacterial sepsis of newborn, includes congenital sepsis. If a perinate is documented as having sepsis without documentation of congenital or community acquired, the default is congenital and a code from category P36 should be assigned. If the P36 code includes the causal organism, an additional code from category B95, Streptococcus, Staphylococcus, and Enterococcus as the cause of diseases classified elsewhere, or B96, Other bacterial agents as the cause of diseases classified elsewhere, should not be assigned. If the P36 code does not include the causal organism, assign an additional code from category B96. If applicable, use additional codes to identify severe sepsis (R65.2-) and any associated acute organ dysfunction.

g. Stillbirth

Code P95, Stillbirth, is only for use in institutions that maintain separate records for stillbirths. No other code should be used with P95. Code P95 should not be used on the mother's record.

17. Chapter 17: Congenital malformations, deformations, and chromosomal abnormalities (Q00-Q99)

Assign an appropriate code(s) from categories Q00-Q99, Congenital malformations, deformations, and chromosomal abnormalities when a malformation/deformation or chromosomal abnormality is documented. A malformation/ deformation/or chromosomal abnormality may be the principal/first-listed diagnosis on a record or a secondary diagnosis.

When a malformation/deformation/or chromosomal abnormality does not have a unique code assignment, assign additional code(s) for any manifestations that may be present.

When the code assignment specifically identifies the malformation/deformation/or chromosomal abnormality, manifestations that are an inherent component of the anomaly should not be coded separately. Additional codes should be assigned for manifestations that are not an inherent component.

Codes from Chapter 17 may be used throughout the life of the patient. If a congenital malformation or deformity has been corrected, a personal history code should be used to identify the history of the malformation or deformity. Although present at birth, malformation/deformation/or chromosomal abnormality may not be identified until later in life. Whenever the condition is diagnosed by the physician, it is appropriate to assign a code from codes Q00-Q99.

For the birth admission, the appropriate code from category Z38, Liveborn infants, according to place of birth and type of delivery, should be sequenced as the principal diagnosis, followed by any congenital anomaly codes, Q00-Q99.

18. Chapter 18: Symptoms, signs, and abnormal clinical and laboratory findings, not elsewhere classified (R00-R99)

Chapter 18 includes symptoms, signs, abnormal results of clinical or other investigative procedures, and ill-defined conditions regarding which no diagnosis classifiable elsewhere is recorded. Signs and symptoms that point to a specific diagnosis have been assigned to a category in other chapters of the classification.

a. Use of symptom codes

Codes that describe symptoms and signs are acceptable for reporting purposes when a related definitive diagnosis has not been established (confirmed) by the provider.

b. Use of a symptom code with a definitive diagnosis code

Codes for signs and symptoms may be reported in addition to a related definitive diagnosis when the sign or symptom is not routinely associated with that diagnosis, such as the various signs and symptoms associated with complex syndromes. The definitive diagnosis code should be sequenced before the symptom code.

Signs or symptoms that are associated routinely with a disease process should not be assigned as additional codes, unless otherwise instructed by the classification.

c. Combination codes that include symptoms

ICD-10-CM contains a number of combination codes that identify both the definitive diagnosis and common symptoms of that diagnosis. When using one of these combination codes, an additional code should not be assigned for the symptom.

d. Repeated falls
Code R29.6, Repeated falls, is for use for encounters when a patient has recently fallen and the reason for the fall is being investigated.

Code Z91.81, History of falling, is for use when a patient has fallen in the past and is at risk for future falls. When appropriate, both codes R29.6 and Z91.81 may be assigned together.

e. Coma scale
The coma scale codes (R40.2-) can be used in conjunction with traumatic brain injury codes, acute cerebrovascular disease or sequelae of cerebrovascular disease codes. These codes are primarily for use by trauma registries, but they may be used in any setting where this information is collected. The coma scale may also be used to assess the status of the central nervous system for other non-trauma conditions, such as monitoring patients in the intensive care unit regardless of medical condition. The coma scale codes should be sequenced after the diagnosis code(s).

These codes, one from each subcategory, are needed to complete the scale. The 7th character indicates when the scale was recorded. The 7th character should match for all three codes.

At a minimum, report the initial score documented on presentation at your facility. This may be a score from the emergency medicine technician (EMT) or in the emergency department. If desired, a facility may choose to capture multiple coma scale scores.

Assign code R40.24, Glasgow coma scale, total score, when only the total score is documented in the medical record and not the individual score(s).

f. Functional quadriplegia
GUIDELINE HAS BEEN DELETED EFFECTIVE OCTOBER 1, 2017

g. SIRS due to Non-Infectious Process
The systemic inflammatory response syndrome (SIRS) can develop as a result of certain non-infectious disease processes, such as trauma, malignant neoplasm, or pancreatitis. When SIRS is documented with a noninfectious condition, and no subsequent infection is documented, the code for the underlying condition, such as an injury, should be assigned, followed by code R65.10, Systemic inflammatory response syndrome (SIRS) of non-infectious origin without acute organ dysfunction, or code R65.11, Systemic inflammatory response syndrome (SIRS) of non-infectious origin with acute organ dysfunction. If an associated acute organ dysfunction is documented, the appropriate code(s) for the specific type of organ dysfunction(s) should be assigned in addition to code R65.11. If acute organ dysfunction is documented, but it cannot be determined if the acute organ dysfunction is associated with SIRS or due to another condition (e.g., directly due to the trauma), the provider should be queried.

h. Death NOS
Code R99, Ill-defined and unknown cause of mortality, is only for use in the very limited circumstance when a patient who has already died is brought into an emergency department or other healthcare facility and is pronounced dead upon arrival. It does not represent the discharge disposition of death.

i. NIHSS Stroke Scale
The NIH stroke scale (NIHSS) codes (R29.7- -) can be used in conjunction with acute stroke codes (I63) to identify the patient's neurological status and the severity of the stroke. The stroke scale codes should be sequenced after the acute stroke diagnosis code(s).

At a minimum, report the initial score documented. If desired, a facility may choose to capture multiple stroke scale scores.

See Section I.B.14. for information concerning the medical record documentation that may be used for assignment of the NIHSS codes.

19. **Chapter 19: Injury, poisoning, and certain other consequences of external causes (S00-T88)**

a. Application of 7th Characters in Chapter 19
Most categories in chapter 19 have a 7th character requirement for each applicable code. Most categories in this chapter have three 7th character values (with the exception of fractures): A, initial encounter, D, subsequent encounter and S, sequela. Categories for traumatic fractures have additional 7th character values. While the patient may be seen by a new or different provider over the course of treatment for an injury, assignment of the 7th character is based on whether the patient is undergoing active treatment and not whether the provider is seeing the patient for the first time.

For complication codes, active treatment refers to treatment for the condition described by the code, even though it may be related to an earlier precipitating problem. For example, code T84.50XA, Infection and inflammatory reaction due to unspecified internal joint prosthesis, initial encounter, is used when active treatment is provided for the infection, even though the condition relates to the prosthetic device, implant or graft that was placed at a previous encounter.

7th character "A", initial encounter is used for each encounter where the patient is receiving active treatment for the condition.

7th character "D" subsequent encounter is used for encounters after the patient has completed active treatment of the condition and is receiving routine care for the condition during the healing or recovery phase.

The aftercare Z codes should not be used for aftercare for conditions such as injuries or poisonings, where 7th characters are provided to identify subsequent care. For example, for aftercare of an injury, assign the acute injury code with the 7th character "D" (subsequent encounter).

7th character "S", sequela, is for use for complications or conditions that arise as a direct result of a condition, such as scar formation after a burn. The scars are sequelae of the burn. When using 7th character "S", it is necessary to use both

GUIDELINES (ICD-10-CM)

the injury code that precipitated the sequela and the code for the sequela itself. The "S" is added only to the injury code, not the sequela code. The 7th character "S" identifies the injury responsible for the sequela. The specific type of sequela (e.g. scar) is sequenced first, followed by the injury code.

See Section I.B.10. Sequelae, (Late Effects)

b. Coding of Injuries

When coding injuries, assign separate codes for each injury unless a combination code is provided, in which case the combination code is assigned. **Codes from category T07,** Unspecified multiple injuries should not be assigned in the inpatient setting unless information for a more specific code is not available. Traumatic injury codes (S00-T14.9) are not to be used for normal, healing surgical wounds or to identify complications of surgical wounds.

The code for the most serious injury, as determined by the provider and the focus of treatment, is sequenced first.

1) Superficial injuries

Superficial injuries such as abrasions or contusions are not coded when associated with more severe injuries of the same site.

2) Primary injury with damage to nerves/ blood vessels

When a primary injury results in minor damage to peripheral nerves or blood vessels, the primary injury is sequenced first with additional code(s) for injuries to nerves and spinal cord (such as category S04), and/or injury to blood vessels (such as category S15). When the primary injury is to the blood vessels or nerves, that injury should be sequenced first.

c. Coding of Traumatic Fractures

The principles of multiple coding of injuries should be followed in coding fractures. Fractures of specified sites are coded individually by site in accordance with both the provisions within categories S02, S12, S22, S32, S42, S49, S52, S59, S62, S72, S79, S82, S89, S92 and the level of detail furnished by medical record content.

A fracture not indicated as open or closed should be coded to closed. A fracture not indicated whether displaced or not displaced should be coded to displaced.

More specific guidelines are as follows:

1) Initial vs. Subsequent Encounter for Fractures

Traumatic fractures are coded using the appropriate 7th character for initial encounter (A, B, C) for each encounter where the patient is receiving active treatment for the fracture. The appropriate 7th character for initial encounter should also be assigned for a patient who delayed seeking treatment for the fracture or nonunion.

Fractures are coded using the appropriate 7th character for subsequent care for encounters after the patient has completed active treatment of the fracture and is receiving routine care for the fracture during the healing or recovery phase.

Care for complications of surgical treatment for fracture repairs during the healing or recovery phase should be coded with the appropriate complication codes.

Care of complications of fractures, such as malunion and nonunion, should be reported with the appropriate 7th character for subsequent care with nonunion (K, M, N,) or subsequent care with malunion (P, Q, R).

Malunion/nonunion: The appropriate 7th character for initial encounter should also be assigned for a patient who delayed seeking treatment for the fracture or nonunion.

The open fracture designations in the assignment of the 7th character for fractures of the forearm, femur and lower leg, including ankle are based on the Gustilo open fracture classification. When the Gustilo classification type is not specified for an open fracture, the 7th character for open fracture type I or II should be assigned (B, E, H, M, Q).

A code from category M80, not a traumatic fracture code, should be used for any patient with known osteoporosis who suffers a fracture, even if the patient had a minor fall or trauma, if that fall or trauma would not usually break a normal, healthy bone.

See Section I.C.13. Osteoporosis.

The aftercare Z codes should not be used for aftercare for traumatic fractures. For aftercare of a traumatic fracture, assign the acute fracture code with the appropriate 7th character.

2) Multiple fractures sequencing

Multiple fractures are sequenced in accordance with the severity of the fracture.

d. Coding of Burns and Corrosions

The ICD-10-CM makes a distinction between burns and corrosions. The burn codes are for thermal burns, except sunburns, that come from a heat source, such as a fire or hot appliance. The burn codes are also for burns resulting from electricity and radiation. Corrosions are burns due to chemicals. The guidelines are the same for burns and corrosions.

Current burns (T20-T25) are classified by depth, extent and by agent (X code). Burns are classified by depth as first degree (erythema), second degree (blistering), and third degree (full-thickness involvement). Burns of the eye and internal organs (T26-T28) are classified by site, but not by degree.

1) Sequencing of burn and related condition codes

Sequence first the code that reflects the highest degree of burn when more than one burn is present.

   a. When the reason for the admission or encounter is for treatment of external multiple burns, sequence first the code that reflects the burn of the highest degree.

   b. When a patient has both internal and external burns, the circumstances of admission govern the selection of the principal diagnosis or first-listed diagnosis.

c. When a patient is admitted for burn injuries and other related conditions such as smoke inhalation and/or respiratory failure, the circumstances of admission govern the selection of the principal or first-listed diagnosis.

2) Burns of the same local site
Classify burns of the same local site (three-character category level, T20-T28) but of different degrees to the subcategory identifying the highest degree recorded in the diagnosis.

3) Non-healing burns
Non-healing burns are coded as acute burns.
   Necrosis of burned skin should be coded as a non-healed burn.

4) Infected Burn
For any documented infected burn site, use an additional code for the infection.

5) Assign separate codes for each burn site
When coding burns, assign separate codes for each burn site. Category T30, Burn and corrosion, body region unspecified is extremely vague and should rarely be used.

6) Burns and Corrosions Classified According to Extent of Body Surface Involved
Assign codes from category T31, Burns classified according to extent of body surface involved, or T32, Corrosions classified according to extent of body surface involved, when the site of the burn is not specified or when there is a need for additional data. It is advisable to use category T31 as additional coding when needed to provide data for evaluating burn mortality, such as that needed by burn units. It is also advisable to use category T31 as an additional code for reporting purposes when there is mention of a third-degree burn involving 20 percent or more of the body surface.

   Categories T31 and T32 are based on the classic "rule of nines" in estimating body surface involved: head and neck are assigned nine percent, each arm nine percent, each leg 18 percent, the anterior trunk 18 percent, posterior trunk 18 percent, and genitalia one percent. Providers may change these percentage assignments where necessary to accommodate infants and children who have proportionately larger heads than adults, and patients who have large buttocks, thighs, or abdomen that involve burns.

7) Encounters for treatment of sequela of burns
Encounters for the treatment of the late effects of burns or corrosions (i.e., scars or joint contractures) should be coded with a burn or corrosion code with the 7th character "S" for sequela.

8) Sequelae with a late effect code and current burn
When appropriate, both a code for a current burn or corrosion with 7th character "A" or "D" and a burn or corrosion code with 7th character "S" may be assigned on the same record (when both a current burn and sequelae of an old burn exist).

Burns and corrosions do not heal at the same rate and a current healing wound may still exist with sequela of a healed burn or corrosion.
   See Section I.B.10. Sequela, (Late Effects)

9) Use of an external cause code with burns and corrosions
An external cause code should be used with burns and corrosions to identify the source and intent of the burn, as well as the place where it occurred.

e. Adverse Effects, Poisoning, Underdosing and Toxic Effects
Codes in categories T36-T65 are combination codes that include the substance that was taken as well as the intent. No additional external cause code is required for poisonings, toxic effects, adverse effects and underdosing codes.

1) Do not code directly from the Table of Drugs
Do not code directly from the Table of Drugs and Chemicals. Always refer back to the Tabular List.

2) Use as many codes as necessary to describe
Use as many codes as necessary to describe completely all drugs, medicinal or biological substances.

3) If the same code would describe the causative agent
If the same code would describe the causative agent for more than one adverse reaction, poisoning, toxic effect or underdosing, assign the code only once.

4) If two or more drugs, medicinal or biological substances
If two or more drugs, medicinal or biological substances are reported, code each individually unless a combination code is listed in the Table of Drugs and Chemicals.

5) The occurrence of drug toxicity is classified in ICD-10-CM as follows:
   (a) Adverse Effect
When coding an adverse effect of a drug that has been correctly prescribed and properly administered, assign the appropriate code for the nature of the adverse effect followed by the appropriate code for the adverse effect of the drug (T36-T50). The code for the drug should have a 5th or 6th character "5" (for example T36.0X5-) Examples of the nature of an adverse effect are tachycardia, delirium, gastrointestinal hemorrhaging, vomiting, hypokalemia, hepatitis, renal failure, or respiratory failure.

   (b) Poisoning
When coding a poisoning or reaction to the improper use of a medication (e.g., overdose, wrong substance given or taken in error, wrong route of administration), first assign the appropriate code from categories T36-T50. The poisoning codes have an associated intent as their 5th or 6th character (accidental, intentional self-harm, assault and undetermined). If the intent of the poisoning is unknown or unspecified, code the intent as accidental intent. The undetermined

intent is only for use if the documentation in the record specifies that the intent cannot be determined. Use additional code(s) for all manifestations of poisonings.

If there is also a diagnosis of abuse or dependence of the substance, the abuse or dependence is assigned as an additional code.

Examples of poisoning include:

(i) Error was made in drug prescription Errors made in drug prescription or in the administration of the drug by provider, nurse, patient, or other person.

(ii) Overdose of a drug intentionally taken If an overdose of a drug was intentionally taken or administered and resulted in drug toxicity, it would be coded as a poisoning.

(iii) Nonprescribed drug taken with correctly prescribed and properly administered drug.
If a nonprescribed drug or medicinal agent was taken in combination with a correctly prescribed and properly administered drug, any drug toxicity or other reaction resulting from the interaction of the two drugs would be classified as a poisoning.

(iv) Interaction of drug(s) and alcohol. When a reaction results from the interaction of a drug(s) and alcohol, this would be classified as poisoning.

See Section I.C.4. if poisoning is the result of insulin pump malfunctions.

(c) Underdosing

Underdosing refers to taking less of a medication than is prescribed by a provider or a manufacturer's instruction. For underdosing, assign the code from categories T36-T50 (fifth or sixth character "6").

Codes for underdosing should never be assigned as principal or first-listed codes. If a patient has a relapse or exacerbation of the medical condition for which the drug is prescribed because of the reduction in dose, then the medical condition itself should be coded.

Noncompliance (Z91.12-, Z91.13-) or complication of care (Y63.6-Y63.9) codes are to be used with an underdosing code to indicate intent, if known.

(d) Toxic Effects

When a harmful substance is ingested or comes in contact with a person, this is classified as a toxic effect. The toxic effect codes are in categories T51-T65.

Toxic effect codes have an associated intent: accidental, intentional self-harm, assault and undetermined.

f. Adult and child abuse, neglect and other maltreatment

Sequence first the appropriate code from categories T74 (Adult and child abuse, neglect and other maltreatment, confirmed) or T76 (Adult and child abuse, neglect and other maltreatment, suspected) for abuse, neglect and other maltreatment, followed by any accompanying mental health or injury code(s).

If the documentation in the medical record states abuse or neglect it is coded as confirmed (T74.-). It is coded as suspected if it is documented as suspected (T76.-).

For cases of confirmed abuse or neglect an external cause code from the assault section (X92-Y09) should be added to identify the cause of any physical injuries. A perpetrator code (Y07) should be added when the perpetrator of the abuse is known. For suspected cases of abuse or neglect, do not report external cause or perpetrator code.

If a suspected case of abuse, neglect or mistreatment is ruled out during an encounter code Z04.71, Encounter for examination and observation following alleged physical adult abuse, ruled out, or code Z04.72, Encounter for examination and observation following alleged child physical abuse, ruled out, should be used, not a code from T76.

If a suspected case of alleged rape or sexual abuse is ruled out during an encounter code Z04.41, Encounter for examination and observation following alleged adult rape or code Z04.42, Encounter for examination and observation following alleged child rape, should be used, not a code from T76.

See Section I.C.15. Abuse in a pregnant patient.

g. Complications of care

1) General guidelines for complications of care

(a) Documentation of complications of care

See Section I.B.16. for information on documentation of complications of care.

2) Pain due to medical devices

Pain associated with devices, implants or grafts left in a surgical site (for example painful hip prosthesis) is assigned to the appropriate code(s) found in Chapter 19, Injury, poisoning, and certain other consequences of external causes. Specific codes for pain due to medical devices are found in the T code section of the ICD-10-CM. Use additional code(s) from category G89 to identify acute or chronic pain due to presence of the device, implant or graft (G89.18 or G89.28).

3) Transplant complications

(a) Transplant complications other than kidney

Codes under category T86, Complications of transplanted organs and tissues, are for use for both complications and rejection of transplanted organs. A transplant complication code is only assigned if the complication affects the function of the transplanted organ. Two codes are required to fully describe a transplant complication: the appropriate code from category T86 and a secondary code that identifies the complication.

Pre-existing conditions or conditions that develop after the transplant are not coded as complications unless they affect the function of the transplanted organs.

See I.C.21. for transplant organ removal status
See I.C.2. for malignant neoplasm associated with transplanted organ.

(b) Kidney transplant complications

Patients who have undergone kidney transplant may still have some form of chronic kidney disease (CKD) because the kidney transplant may not fully restore kidney function. Code T86.1- should be assigned for documented complications of a kidney transplant, such as transplant failure or rejection or other transplant complication. Code T86.1- should not be assigned for post kidney transplant patients who have chronic kidney (CKD) unless a transplant complication such as transplant failure or rejection is documented. If the documentation is unclear as to whether the patient has a complication of the transplant, query the provider.

Conditions that affect the function of the transplanted kidney, other than CKD, should be assigned a code from subcategory T86.1, Complications of transplanted organ, Kidney, and a secondary code that identifies the complication.

For patients with CKD following a kidney transplant, but who do not have a complication such as failure or rejection, *see section I.C.14. Chronic kidney disease and kidney transplant status.*

4) Complication codes that include the external cause

As with certain other T codes, some of the complications of care codes have the external cause included in the code. The code includes the nature of the complication as well as the type of procedure that caused the complication. No external cause code indicating the type of procedure is necessary for these codes.

5) Complications of care codes within the body system chapters

Intraoperative and postprocedural complication codes are found within the body system chapters with codes specific to the organs and structures of that body system. These codes should be sequenced first, followed by a code(s) for the specific complication, if applicable.

20. Chapter 20: External Causes of Morbidity (V00-Y99)

The external causes of morbidity codes should never be sequenced as the first-listed or principal diagnosis.

External cause codes are intended to provide data for injury research and evaluation of injury prevention strategies. These codes capture how the injury or health condition happened (cause), the intent (unintentional or accidental; or intentional, such as suicide or assault), the place where the event occurred the activity of the patient at the time of the event, and the person's status (e.g., civilian, military).

There is no national requirement for mandatory ICD-10-CM external cause code reporting. Unless a provider is subject to a state-based external cause code reporting mandate or these codes are required by a particular payer, reporting of ICD-10-CM codes in Chapter 20, External Causes of Morbidity, is not required. In the absence of a mandatory reporting requirement, providers are encouraged to voluntarily report external cause codes, as they provide valuable data for injury research and evaluation of injury prevention strategies.

a. General External Cause Coding Guidelines

1) Used with any code in the range of A00.0-T88.9, Z00-Z99

An external cause code may be used with any code in the range of A00.0-T88.9, Z00-Z99, classification that **represents** a health condition due to an external cause. Though they are most applicable to injuries, they are also valid for use with such things as infections or diseases due to an external source, and other health conditions, such as a heart attack that occurs during strenuous physical activity.

2) External cause code used for length of treatment

Assign the external cause code, with the appropriate 7th character (initial encounter, subsequent encounter or sequela) for each encounter for which the injury or condition is being treated.

Most categories in chapter 20 have a 7th character requirement for each applicable code. Most categories in this chapter have three 7th character values: A, initial encounter, D, subsequent encounter and S, sequela. While the patient may be seen by a new or different provider over the course of treatment for an injury or condition, assignment of the 7th character for external cause should match the 7th character of the code assigned for the associated injury or condition for the encounter.

3) Use the full range of external cause codes

Use the full range of external cause codes to completely describe the cause, the intent, the place of occurrence and if applicable, the activity of the patient at the time of the event, and the patient's status, for all injuries, and other health conditions due to an external cause.

4) Assign as many external cause codes as necessary

Assign as many external cause codes as necessary to fully explain each cause. If only one external code can be recorded, assign the code most related to the principal diagnosis.

5) The selection of the appropriate external cause code

The selection of the appropriate external cause code is guided by the Alphabetic Index of External Causes and by Inclusion and Exclusion notes in the Tabular List.

6) External cause code can never be a principal diagnosis

An external cause code can never be a principal (first-listed) diagnosis.

7) Combination external cause codes

Certain of the external cause codes are combination codes that identify sequential events that result in an injury, such as a fall which results in striking against an object. The injury may be due to either event or both. The combination external cause code used should correspond to the sequence of events regardless of which caused the most serious injury.

8) No external cause code needed in certain circumstances

No external cause code from Chapter 20 is needed if the external cause and intent are included in a code from another chapter (e.g. T36.0X1- Poisoning by penicillins, accidental (unintentional)).

b. Place of Occurrence Guideline

Codes from category Y92, Place of occurrence of the external cause, are secondary codes for use after other external cause codes to identify the location of the patient at the time of injury or other condition.

Generally, a place of occurrence code is assigned only once, at the initial encounter for treatment. However, in the rare instance that a new injury occurs during hospitalization, an additional place of occurrence code may be assigned. No 7th characters are used for Y92. Only one code from Y92 should be recorded on a medical record.

Do not use place of occurrence code Y92.9 if the place is not stated or is not applicable.

c. Activity Code

Assign a code from category Y93, Activity code, to describe the activity of the patient at the time the injury or other health condition occurred.

An activity code is used only once, at the initial encounter for treatment. Only one code from Y93 should be recorded on a medical record.

The activity codes are not applicable to poisonings, adverse effects, misadventures or sequela.

Do not assign Y93.9, Unspecified activity, if the activity is not stated.

A code from category Y93 is appropriate for use with external cause and intent codes if identifying the activity provides additional information about the event.

d. Place of Occurrence, Activity, and Status Codes Used with other External Cause Code

When applicable, place of occurrence, activity, and external cause status codes are sequenced after the main external cause code(s). Regardless of the number of external cause codes assigned, there should be only one place of occurrence code, one activity code, and one external cause status code assigned to an encounter.

e. If the Reporting Format Limits the Number of External Cause Codes

If the reporting format limits the number of external cause codes that can be used in reporting clinical data, report the code for the cause/intent most related to the principal diagnosis. If the format permits capture of additional external cause codes, the cause/intent, including medical misadventures, of the additional events should be reported rather than the codes for place, activity, or external status.

f. Multiple External Cause Coding Guidelines

More than one external cause code is required to fully describe the external cause of an illness or injury. The assignment of external cause codes should be sequenced in the following priority:

If two or more events cause separate injuries, an external cause code should be assigned for each cause. The first-listed external cause code will be selected in the following order:

External codes for child and adult abuse take priority over all other external cause codes. *See Section I.C.19., Child and Adult abuse guidelines.*

External codes for terrorism events take priority over all other external cause codes except child and adult abuse.

External cause codes for cataclysmic events take priority over all other external cause codes except child and adult abuse and terrorism.

External cause codes for transport accidents take priority over all other external cause codes except cataclysmic events, child and adult abuse and terrorism.

Activity and external cause status codes are assigned following all causal (intent) external cause codes.

The first-listed external cause code should correspond to the cause of the most serious diagnosis due to an assault, accident, or self-harm, following the order of hierarchy listed above.

g. Child and Adult Abuse Guideline

Adult and child abuse, neglect and maltreatment are classified as assault. Any of the assault codes may be used to indicate the external cause of any injury resulting from the confirmed abuse.

For confirmed cases of abuse, neglect and maltreatment, when the perpetrator is known, a code from Y07, Perpetrator of maltreatment and neglect, should accompany any other assault codes. *See Section I.C.19. Adult and child abuse, neglect and other maltreatment*

h. Unknown or Undetermined Intent Guideline

If the intent (accident, self-harm, assault) of the cause of an injury or other condition is unknown or unspecified, code the intent as accidental intent. All transport accident categories assume accidental intent.

1) Use of undetermined intent

External cause codes for events of undetermined intent are only for use if the documentation in the record specifies that the intent cannot be determined.

i. Sequelae (Late Effects) of External Cause Guidelines

1) Sequelae external cause codes

Sequela are reported using the external cause code with the 7th character "S" for sequela. These codes

should be used with any report of a late effect or sequela resulting from a previous injury.
See Section I.B.10. Sequela, (Late Effects)

2) Sequela external cause code with a related current injury

A sequela external cause code should never be used with a related current nature of injury code.

3) Use of sequela external cause codes for subsequent visits

Use a late effect external cause code for subsequent visits when a late effect of the initial injury is being treated. Do not use a late effect external cause code for subsequent visits for follow-up care (e.g., to assess healing, to receive rehabilitative therapy) of the injury when no late effect of the injury has been documented.

j. Terrorism Guidelines

1) Cause of injury identified by the Federal Government (FBI) as terrorism

When the cause of an injury is identified by the Federal Government (FBI) as terrorism, the first-listed external cause code should be a code from category Y38, Terrorism. The definition of terrorism employed by the FBI is found at the inclusion note at the beginning of category Y38. Use additional code for place of occurrence (Y92.-). More than one Y38 code may be assigned if the injury is the result of more than one mechanism of terrorism.

2) Cause of an injury is suspected to be the result of terrorism

When the cause of an injury is suspected to be the result of terrorism a code from category Y38 should not be assigned. Suspected cases should be classified as assault.

3) Code Y38.9, Terrorism, secondary effects

Assign code Y38.9, Terrorism, secondary effects, for conditions occurring subsequent to the terrorist event. This code should not be assigned for conditions that are due to the initial terrorist act.

It is acceptable to assign code Y38.9 with another code from Y38 if there is an injury due to the initial terrorist event and an injury that is a subsequent result of the terrorist event.

k. External cause status

A code from category Y99, External cause status, should be assigned whenever any other external cause code is assigned for an encounter, including an Activity code, except for the events noted below. Assign a code from category Y99, External cause status, to indicate the work status of the person at the time the event occurred. The status code indicates whether the event occurred during military activity, whether a non-military person was at work, whether an individual including a student or volunteer was involved in a non-work activity at the time of the causal event.

A code from Y99, External cause status, should be assigned, when applicable, with other external cause codes, such as transport accidents and falls. The external cause status codes are not applicable to poisonings, adverse effects, misadventures or late effects.

Do not assign a code from category Y99 if no other external cause codes (cause, activity) are applicable for the encounter.

An external cause status code is used only once, at the initial encounter for treatment. Only one code from Y99 should be recorded on a medical record.

Do not assign code Y99.9, Unspecified external cause status, if the status is not stated.

21. Chapter 21: Factors influencing health status and contact with health services (Z00-Z99)

Note: The chapter specific guidelines provide additional information about the use of Z codes for specified encounters.

a. Use of Z codes in any healthcare setting

Z codes are for use in any healthcare setting. Z codes may be used as either a first-listed (principal diagnosis code in the inpatient setting) or secondary code, depending on the circumstances of the encounter. Certain Z codes may only be used as first-listed or principal diagnosis.

b. Z Codes indicate a reason for an encounter

Z codes are not procedure codes. A corresponding procedure code must accompany a Z code to describe any procedure performed.

c. Categories of Z Codes

1) Contact/Exposure

Category Z20 indicates contact with, and suspected exposure to, communicable diseases. These codes are for patients who do not show any sign or symptom of a disease but are suspected to have been exposed to it by close personal contact with an infected individual or are in an area where a disease is epidemic.

Category Z77, Other contact with and (suspected) exposures hazardous to health, indicates contact with and suspected exposures hazardous to health.

Contact/exposure codes may be used as a first-listed code to explain an encounter for testing, or, more commonly, as a secondary code to identify a potential risk.

2) Inoculations and vaccinations

Code Z23 is for encounters for inoculations and vaccinations. It indicates that a patient is being seen to receive a prophylactic inoculation against a disease. Procedure codes are required to identify the actual administration of the injection and the type(s) of immunizations given. Code Z23 may be used as a secondary code if the inoculation is given as a routine part of preventive health care, such as a well-baby visit.

3) Status

Status codes indicate that a patient is either a carrier of a disease or has the sequelae or residual of a past disease or condition. This includes such things as the presence of prosthetic or mechanical devices resulting from past treatment. A status code is informative, because the status may affect the course of treatment and its outcome. A status code is distinct from a history code. The history code indicates that the patient no longer has the condition.

A status code should not be used with a diagnosis code from one of the body system chapters, if the diagnosis code includes the information provided by the status code. For example, code Z94.1, Heart transplant status, should not be used with a code from subcategory T86.2, Complications of heart transplant. The status code does not provide additional information. The complication code indicates that the patient is a heart transplant patient.

For encounters for weaning from a mechanical ventilator, assign a code from subcategory J96.1, Chronic respiratory failure, followed by code Z99.11, Dependence on respirator [ventilator] status.

The status Z codes/categories are:

Z14   Genetic carrier
Genetic carrier status indicates that a person carries a gene, associated with a particular disease, which may be passed to offspring who may develop that disease. The person does not have the disease and is not at risk of developing the disease.

Z15   Genetic susceptibility to disease Genetic susceptibility indicates that a person has a gene that increases the risk of that person developing the disease.

Codes from category Z15 should not be used as principal or first-listed codes. If the patient has the condition to which he/she is susceptible, and that condition is the reason for the encounter, the code for the current condition should be sequenced first. If the patient is being seen for follow-up after completed treatment for this condition, and the condition no longer exists, a follow-up code should be sequenced first, followed by the appropriate personal history and genetic susceptibility codes. If the purpose of the encounter is genetic counseling associated with procreative management, code Z31.5, Encounter for genetic counseling, should be assigned as the first-listed code, followed by a code from category Z15. Additional codes should be assigned for any applicable family or personal history.

Z16   Resistance to antimicrobial drugs
This code indicates that a patient has a condition that is resistant to antimicrobial drug treatment. Sequence the infection code first.

Z17   Estrogen receptor status
Z18   Retained foreign body fragments
Z19   Hormone sensitivity malignancy status
Z21   Asymptomatic HIV infection status This code indicates that a patient has tested positive for HIV but has manifested no signs or symptoms of the disease.

Z22   Carrier of infectious disease Carrier status indicates that a person harbors the specific organisms of a disease without manifest symptoms and is capable of transmitting the infection.

Z28.3   Underimmunization status
Z33.1   Pregnant state, incidental This code is a secondary code only for use when the pregnancy is in no way complicating the reason for visit. Otherwise, a code from the obstetric chapter is required.

Z66   Do not resuscitate
This code may be used when it is documented by the provider that a patient is on do not resuscitate status at any time during the stay.

Z67   Blood type
Z68   Body mass index (BMI)
As with all other secondary diagnosis codes, the BMI codes should only be assigned when they meet the definition of a reportable diagnosis (see Section III, Reporting Additional Diagnoses).

Z74.01   Bed confinement status
Z76.82   Awaiting organ transplant status
Z78   Other specified health status
Code Z78.1, Physical restraint status, may be used when it is documented by the provider that a patient has been put in restraints during the current encounter. Please note that this code should not be reported when it is documented by the provider that a patient is temporarily restrained during a procedure.

Z79   Long-term (current) drug therapy
Codes from this category indicate a patient's continuous use of a prescribed drug (including such things as aspirin therapy) for the long-term treatment of a condition or for prophylactic use. It is not for use for patients who have addictions to drugs. This subcategory is not for use of medications for detoxification or maintenance programs to prevent withdrawal symptoms in patients with drug dependence (e.g., methadone maintenance for opiate dependence). Assign the appropriate code for the drug dependence instead.

Assign a code from Z79 if the patient is receiving a medication for an extended period as a prophylactic measure (such as for the prevention of deep vein thrombosis) or as treatment of a chronic condition (such as arthritis) or a disease requiring a lengthy course of treatment (such as cancer). Do not assign a code from category Z79 for medication being administered for a brief period of time to treat an acute illness or injury (such as a course of antibiotics to treat acute bronchitis).

Z88   Allergy status to drugs, medicaments and biological substances Except: Z88.9, Allergy status to unspecified drugs, medicaments and biological substances status

Z89   Acquired absence of limb
Z90   Acquired absence of organs, not elsewhere classified
Z91.0-   Allergy status, other than to drugs and biological substances
Z92.82   Status post administration of tPA (rtPA) in a different facility within the last 24 hours prior to admission to a current

facility Assign code Z92.82, Status post administration of tPA (rtPA) in a different facility within the last 24 hours prior to admission to current facility, as a secondary diagnosis when a patient is received by transfer into a facility and documentation indicates they were administered tissue plasminogen activator (tPA) within the last 24 hours prior to admission to the current facility. This guideline applies even if the patient is still receiving the tPA at the time they are received into the current facility. The appropriate code for the condition for which the tPA was administered (such as cerebrovascular disease or myocardial infarction) should be assigned first. Code Z92.82 is only applicable to the receiving facility record and not to the transferring facility record.

Z93   Artificial opening status
Z94   Transplanted organ and tissue status
Z95   Presence of cardiac and vascular implants and grafts
Z96   Presence of other functional implants
Z97   Presence of other devices
Z98   Other postprocedural states

Assign code Z98.85, Transplanted organ removal status, to indicate that a transplanted organ has been previously removed. This code should not be assigned for the encounter in which the transplanted organ is removed. The complication necessitating removal of the transplant organ should be assigned for that encounter.

See section I.C.19. for information on the coding of organ transplant complications.

Z99   Dependence on enabling machines and devices, not elsewhere classified

Note: Categories Z89-Z9Ø and Z93-Z99 are for use only if there are no complications or malfunctions of the organ or tissue replaced, the amputation site or the equipment on which the patient is dependent.

4) History (of)

There are two types of history Z codes, personal and family. Personal history codes explain a patient's past medical condition that no longer exists and is not receiving any treatment, but that has the potential for recurrence, and therefore may require continued monitoring.

Family history codes are for use when a patient has a family member(s) who has had a particular disease that causes the patient to be at higher risk of also contracting the disease.

Personal history codes may be used in conjunction with follow-up codes and family history codes may be used in conjunction with screening codes to explain the need for a test or procedure. History codes are also acceptable on any medical record regardless of the reason for visit. A history of an illness, even if no longer present, is important information that may alter the type of treatment ordered.

The history Z code categories are:
Z8Ø   Family history of primary malignant neoplasm
Z81   Family history of mental and behavioral disorders
Z82   Family history of certain disabilities and chronic diseases (leading to disablement)
Z83   Family history of other specific disorders
Z84   Family history of other conditions
Z85   Personal history of malignant neoplasm
Z86   Personal history of certain other diseases
Z87   Personal history of other diseases and conditions
Z91.4-   Personal history of psychological trauma, not elsewhere classified
Z91.5   Personal history of self-harm
Z91.81   History of falling
Z91.82   Personal history of military deployment
Z92   Personal history of medical treatment Except: Z92.Ø, Personal history of contraception Except: Z92.82, Status post administration of tPA (rtPA) in a different facility within the last 24 hours prior to admission to a current facility

5) Screening

Screening is the testing for disease or disease precursors in seemingly well individuals so that early detection and treatment can be provided for those who test positive for the disease (e.g., screening mammogram).

The testing of a person to rule out or confirm a suspected diagnosis because the patient has some sign or symptom is a diagnostic examination, not a screening. In these cases, the sign or symptom is used to explain the reason for the test.

A screening code may be a first-listed code if the reason for the visit is specifically the screening exam. It may also be used as an additional code if the screening is done during an office visit for other health problems. A screening code is not necessary if the screening is inherent to a routine examination, such as a pap smear done during a routine pelvic examination.

Should a condition be discovered during the screening then the code for the condition may be assigned as an additional diagnosis.

The Z code indicates that a screening exam is planned. A procedure code is required to confirm that the screening was performed.

The screening Z codes/categories:
Z11   Encounter for screening for infectious and parasitic diseases
Z12   Encounter for screening for malignant neoplasms
Z13   Encounter for screening for other diseases and disorders Except: Z13.9, Encounter for screening, unspecified
Z36   Encounter for antenatal screening for mother

6) Observation

There are three observation Z code categories. They are for use in very limited circumstances when a person is being observed for a suspected condition that is ruled out. The observation codes are not for use if an injury or illness or any signs or symptoms related to the suspected condition are present. In such cases the diagnosis/symptom code is used with the corresponding external cause code.

The observation codes are to be used as principal diagnosis only. The only exception to this is when the principal diagnosis is required to be a code from category Z38, Liveborn infants according to place of birth and type of delivery. Then a code from category Z05, Encounter for observation and evaluation of newborn for suspected diseases and conditions ruled out, is sequenced after the Z38 code. Additional codes may be used in addition to the observation code, but only if they are unrelated to the suspected condition being observed.

Codes from subcategory Z03.7 Encounter for suspected maternal and fetal conditions ruled out, may either be used as a first-listed or as an additional code assignment depending on the case. They are for use in very limited circumstances on a maternal record when an encounter is for a suspected maternal or fetal condition that is ruled out during that encounter (for example, a maternal or fetal condition may be suspected due to an abnormal test result). These codes should not be used when the condition is confirmed. In those cases, the confirmed condition should be coded. In addition, these codes are not for use if an illness or any signs or symptoms related to the suspected condition or problem are present. In such cases the diagnosis/symptom code is used.

Additional codes may be used in addition to the code from subcategory Z03.7, but only if they are unrelated to the suspected condition being evaluated.

Codes from subcategory Z03.7 may not be used for encounters for antenatal screening of mother. *See Section I.C.21. Screening.*

For encounters for suspected fetal condition that are inconclusive following testing and evaluation, assign the appropriate code from category O35, O36, O40 or O41.

The observation Z code categories:

Z03	Encounter for medical observation for suspected diseases and conditions ruled out
Z04	Encounter for examination and observation for other reasons Except: Z04.9, Encounter for examination and observation for unspecified reason
Z05	Encounter for observation and evaluation of newborn for suspected diseases and conditions ruled out

7) Aftercare

Aftercare visit codes cover situations when the initial treatment of a disease has been performed and the patient requires continued care during the healing or recovery phase, or for the long-term consequences of the disease. The aftercare Z code should not be used if treatment is directed at a current, acute disease. The diagnosis code is to be used in these cases.

Exceptions to this rule are codes Z51.0, Encounter for antineoplastic radiation therapy, and codes from subcategory Z51.1, Encounter for antineoplastic chemotherapy and immunotherapy. These codes are to be first-listed, followed by the diagnosis code when a patient's encounter is solely to receive radiation therapy, chemotherapy, or immunotherapy for the treatment of a neoplasm. If the reason for the encounter is more than one type of antineoplastic therapy, code Z51.0 and a code from subcategory Z51.1 may be assigned together, in which case one of these codes would be reported as a secondary diagnosis.

The aftercare Z codes should also not be used for aftercare for injuries. For aftercare of an injury, assign the acute injury code with the appropriate 7th character (for subsequent encounter).

The aftercare codes are generally first-listed to explain the specific reason for the encounter. An aftercare code may be used as an additional code when some type of aftercare is provided in addition to the reason for admission and no diagnosis code is applicable. An example of this would be the closure of a colostomy during an encounter for treatment of another condition.

Aftercare codes should be used in conjunction with other aftercare codes or diagnosis codes to provide better detail on the specifics of an aftercare encounter visit, unless otherwise directed by the classification. Should a patient receive multiple types of antineoplastic therapy during the same encounter, code Z51.0, Encounter for antineoplastic radiation therapy, and codes from subcategory Z51.1, Encounter for antineoplastic chemotherapy and immunotherapy, may be used together on a record. The sequencing of multiple aftercare codes depends on the circumstances of the encounter.

Certain aftercare Z code categories need a secondary diagnosis code to describe the resolving condition or sequelae. For others, the condition is included in the code title.

Additional Z code aftercare category terms include fitting and adjustment, and attention to artificial openings.

Status Z codes may be used with aftercare Z codes to indicate the nature of the aftercare. For example code Z95.1, Presence of aortocoronary bypass graft, may be used with code Z48.812, Encounter for surgical aftercare following surgery on the circulatory system, to indicate the surgery for which the aftercare is being performed. A status code should not be used when the aftercare code indicates the type of status, such as using Z43.0, Encounter for attention to tracheostomy, with Z93.0, Tracheostomy status.

The aftercare Z category/codes:

Z42 Encounter for plastic and reconstructive surgery following medical procedure or healed injury

Z43 Encounter for attention to artificial openings

Z44 Encounter for fitting and adjustment of external prosthetic device

Z45 Encounter for adjustment and management of implanted device

Z46 Encounter for fitting and adjustment of other devices

Z47 Orthopedic aftercare

Z48 Encounter for other postprocedural aftercare

Z49 Encounter for care involving renal dialysis

Z51 Encounter for other aftercare and medical care

8) Follow-up

The follow-up codes are used to explain continuing surveillance following completed treatment of a disease, condition, or injury. They imply that the condition has been fully treated and no longer exists. They should not be confused with aftercare codes, or injury codes with a 7th character for subsequent encounter, that explain ongoing care of a healing condition or its sequelae. Follow-up codes may be used in conjunction with history codes to provide the full picture of the healed condition and its treatment. The follow-up code is sequenced first, followed by the history code.

A follow-up code may be used to explain multiple visits. Should a condition be found to have recurred on the follow-up visit, then the diagnosis code for the condition should be assigned in place of the follow-up code.

The follow-up Z code categories:

Z08 Encounter for follow-up examination after completed treatment for malignant neoplasm

Z09 Encounter for follow-up examination after completed treatment for conditions other than malignant neoplasm

Z39 Encounter for maternal postpartum care and examination

9) Donor

Codes in category Z52, Donors of organs and tissues, are used for living individuals who are donating blood or other body tissue. These codes are only for individuals donating for others, not for self-donations. They are not used to identify cadaveric donations.

10) Counseling

Counseling Z codes are used when a patient or family member receives assistance in the aftermath of an illness or injury, or when support is required in coping with family or social problems.

The counseling Z codes/categories:

Z30.0- Encounter for general counseling and advice on contraception

Z31.5 Encounter for **procreative** genetic counseling

Z31.6- Encounter for general counseling and advice on procreation

Z32.2 Encounter for childbirth instruction

Z32.3 Encounter for childcare instruction

Z69 Encounter for mental health services for victim and perpetrator of abuse

Z70 Counseling related to sexual attitude, behavior and orientation

Z71 Persons encountering health services for other counseling and medical advice, not elsewhere classified

Z76.81 Expectant mother prebirth pediatrician visit

11) Encounters for Obstetrical and Reproductive Services

See Section I.C.15. Pregnancy, Childbirth, and the Puerperium, for further instruction on the use of these codes.

Z codes for pregnancy are for use in those circumstances when none of the problems or complications included in the codes from the Obstetrics chapter exist (a routine prenatal visit or postpartum care). Codes in category Z34, Encounter for supervision of normal pregnancy, are always first listed and are not to be used with any other code from the OB chapter.

Codes in category Z3A, Weeks of gestation, may be assigned to provide additional information about the pregnancy. Category Z3A codes should not be assigned for pregnancies with abortive outcomes (categories O00-O08), elective termination of pregnancy (code **Z33.2**), nor for postpartum conditions, as category Z3A is not applicable to these conditions. The date of the admission should be used to determine weeks of gestation for inpatient admissions that encompass more than one gestational week.

The outcome of delivery, category Z37, should be included on all maternal delivery records. It is always a secondary code. Codes in category Z37 should not be used on the newborn record.

Z codes for family planning (contraceptive) or procreative management and counseling should be included on an obstetric record either during the pregnancy or the postpartum stage, if applicable.

Z codes/categories for obstetrical and reproductive services:

Z30 Encounter for contraceptive management

Z31 Encounter for procreative management

Z32.2 Encounter for childbirth instruction

Z32.3 Encounter for childcare instruction

Z33 Pregnant state

Z34 Encounter for supervision of normal pregnancy

Z36 Encounter for antenatal screening of mother

Z3A Weeks of gestation

Z37 Outcome of delivery

Z39 Encounter for maternal postpartum care and examination

Z76.81 Expectant mother prebirth pediatrician visit

12) Newborns and Infants

See Section I.C.16. Newborn (Perinatal) Guidelines, for further instruction on the use of these codes.

Newborn Z codes/categories:

Z76.1 Encounter for health supervision and care of foundling

Z00.1- Encounter for routine child health examination

Z38 Liveborn infants according to place of birth and type of delivery

13) Routine and administrative examinations

The Z codes allow for the description of encounters for routine examinations, such as, a general check-up, or, examinations for administrative purposes, such as, a pre-employment physical. The codes are not to be used if the examination is for diagnosis of a suspected condition or for treatment purposes. In such cases the diagnosis code is used. During a routine exam, should a diagnosis or condition be discovered, it should be coded as an additional code. Pre-existing and chronic conditions and history codes may also be included as additional codes as long as the examination is for administrative purposes and not focused on any particular condition.

Some of the codes for routine health examinations distinguish between "with" and "without" abnormal findings. Code assignment depends on the information that is known at the time the encounter is being coded. For example, if no abnormal findings were found during the examination, but the encounter is being coded before test results are back, it is acceptable to assign the code for "without abnormal findings." When assigning a code for "with abnormal findings," additional code(s) should be assigned to identify the specific abnormal finding(s).

Pre-operative examination and pre-procedural laboratory examination Z codes are for use only in those situations when a patient is being cleared for a procedure or surgery and no treatment is given.

The Z codes/categories for routine and administrative examinations:

Z00 Encounter for general examination without complaint, suspected or reported diagnosis

Z01 Encounter for other special examination without complaint, suspected or reported diagnosis

Z02 Encounter for administrative examination
Except: Z02.9, Encounter for administrative examinations, unspecified

Z32.0- Encounter for pregnancy test

14) Miscellaneous Z codes

The miscellaneous Z codes capture a number of other health care encounters that do not fall into one of the other categories. Certain of these codes identify the reason for the encounter; others are for use as additional codes that provide useful information on circumstances that may affect a patient's care and treatment.

Prophylactic Organ Removal

For encounters specifically for prophylactic removal of an organ (such as prophylactic removal of breasts due to a genetic susceptibility to cancer or a family history of cancer), the principal or first-listed code should be a code from category Z40, Encounter for prophylactic surgery, followed by the appropriate codes to identify the associated risk factor (such as genetic susceptibility or family history).

If the patient has a malignancy of one site and is having prophylactic removal at another site to prevent either a new primary malignancy or metastatic disease, a code for the malignancy should also be assigned in addition to a code from subcategory Z40.0, Encounter for prophylactic surgery for risk factors related to malignant neoplasms. A Z40.0 code should not be assigned if the patient is having organ removal for treatment of a malignancy, such as the removal of the testes for the treatment of prostate cancer.

Miscellaneous Z codes/categories:

Z28 Immunization not carried out
Except: Z28.3, Underimmunization status

Z29 Encounter for other prophylactic measures

Z40 Encounter for prophylactic surgery

Z41 Encounter for procedures for purposes other than remedying health state
Except: Z41.9, Encounter for procedure for purposes other than remedying health state, unspecified

Z53 Persons encountering health services for specific procedures and treatment, not carried out

Z55 Problems related to education and literacy

Z56 Problems related to employment and unemployment

Z57 Occupational exposure to risk factors

Z58 Problems related to physical environment

Z59 Problems related to housing and economic circumstances

Z60 Problems related to social environment

Z62 Problems related to upbringing

Z63 Other problems related to primary support group, including family circumstances

Z64 Problems related to certain psychosocial circumstances

Z65 Problems related to other psychosocial circumstances

Z72 Problems related to lifestyle
Note: These codes should be assigned only when the documentation specifies that the patient has an associated problem

Z73 Problems related to life management difficulty

Z74 Problems related to care provider dependency Except: Z74.01, Bed confinement status

Z75	Problems related to medical facilities and other health care
Z76.0	Encounter for issue of repeat prescription
Z76.3	Healthy person accompanying sick person
Z76.4	Other boarder to healthcare facility
Z76.5	Malingerer [conscious simulation]
Z91.1-	Patient's noncompliance with medical treatment and regimen
Z91.83	Wandering in diseases classified elsewhere
Z91.84-	**Oral health risk factors**
Z91.89	Other specified personal risk factors, not elsewhere classified

15) Nonspecific Z codes

Certain Z codes are so non-specific, or potentially redundant with other codes in the classification, that there can be little justification for their use in the inpatient setting. Their use in the outpatient setting should be limited to those instances when there is no further documentation to permit more precise coding. Otherwise, any sign or symptom or any other reason for visit that is captured in another code should be used.

Nonspecific Z codes/categories:

Z02.9	Encounter for administrative examinations, unspecified
Z04.9	Encounter for examination and observation for unspecified reason
Z13.9	Encounter for screening, unspecified
Z41.9	Encounter for procedure for purposes other than remedying health state, unspecified
Z52.9	Donor of unspecified organ or tissue
Z86.59	Personal history of other mental and behavioral disorders
Z88.9	Allergy status to unspecified drugs, medicaments and biological substances status
Z92.0	Personal history of contraception

16) Z Codes That May Only be Principal/First-Listed Diagnosis

The following Z codes/categories may only be reported as the principal/first-listed diagnosis, except when there are multiple encounters on the same day and the medical records for the encounters are combined:

Z00	Encounter for general examination without complaint, suspected or reported diagnosis Except: Z00.6
Z01	Encounter for other special examination without complaint, suspected or reported diagnosis
Z02	Encounter for administrative examination
Z03	Encounter for medical observation for suspected diseases and conditions ruled out
Z04	Encounter for examination and observation for other reasons
Z33.2	Encounter for elective termination of pregnancy

Z31.81	Encounter for male factor infertility in female patient
Z31.83	Encounter for assisted reproductive fertility procedure cycle
Z31.84	Encounter for fertility preservation procedure
Z34	Encounter for supervision of normal pregnancy
Z39	Encounter for maternal postpartum care and examination
Z38	Liveborn infants according to place of birth and type of delivery
Z40	**Encounter for prophylactic surgery**
Z42	Encounter for plastic and reconstructive surgery following medical procedure or healed injury
Z51.0	Encounter for antineoplastic radiation therapy
Z51.1-	Encounter for antineoplastic chemotherapy and immunotherapy
Z52	Donors of organs and tissues Except: Z52.9, Donor of unspecified organ or tissue
Z76.1	Encounter for health supervision and care of foundling
Z76.2	Encounter for health supervision and care of other healthy infant and child
Z99.12	Encounter for respirator [ventilator] dependence during power failure

Section II. Selection of Principal Diagnosis

The circumstances of inpatient admission always govern the selection of principal diagnosis. The principal diagnosis is defined in the Uniform Hospital Discharge Data Set (UHDDS) as "that condition established after study to be chiefly responsible for occasioning the admission of the patient to the hospital for care."

The UHDDS definitions are used by hospitals to report inpatient data elements in a standardized manner. These data elements and their definitions can be found in the July 31, 1985, Federal Register (Vol. 50, No, 147), pp. 31038-40.

Since that time the application of the UHDDS definitions has been expanded to include all nonoutpatient settings (acute care, short term, long term care and psychiatric hospitals; home health agencies; rehab facilities; nursing homes, etc). The UHDDS definitions also apply to hospice services (all levels of care).

In determining principal diagnosis, coding conventions in the ICD-10-CM, the Tabular List and Alphabetic Index take precedence over these official coding guidelines.

(See Section I.A., Conventions for the ICD-10-CM)

The importance of consistent, complete documentation in the medical record cannot be overemphasized. Without such documentation the application of all coding guidelines is a difficult, if not impossible, task.

A. Codes for symptoms, signs, and ill-defined conditions

Codes for symptoms, signs, and ill-defined conditions from Chapter 18 are not to be used as principal diagnosis when a related definitive diagnosis has been established.

B. Two or more interrelated conditions, each potentially meeting the definition for principal diagnosis.

When there are two or more interrelated conditions (such as diseases in the same ICD-10-CM chapter or manifestations characteristically associated with a certain disease) potentially meeting the definition of principal diagnosis, either condition may be sequenced first, unless the circumstances of the admission, the therapy provided, the Tabular List, or the Alphabetic Index indicate otherwise.

C. Two or more diagnoses that equally meet the definition for principal diagnosis

In the unusual instance when two or more diagnoses equally meet the criteria for principal diagnosis as determined by the circumstances of admission, diagnostic workup and/or therapy provided, and the Alphabetic Index, Tabular List, or another coding guidelines does not provide sequencing direction, any one of the diagnoses may be sequenced first.

D. Two or more comparative or contrasting conditions.

In those rare instances when two or more contrasting or comparative diagnoses are documented as "either/or" (or similar terminology), they are coded as if the diagnoses were confirmed and the diagnoses are sequenced according to the circumstances of the admission. If no further determination can be made as to which diagnosis should be principal, either diagnosis may be sequenced first.

E. A symptom(s) followed by contrasting/comparative diagnoses

GUIDELINE HAS BEEN DELETED EFFECTIVE OCTOBER 1, 2014

F. Original treatment plan not carried out

Sequence as the principal diagnosis the condition, which after study occasioned the admission to the hospital, even though treatment may not have been carried out due to unforeseen circumstances.

G. Complications of surgery and other medical care

When the admission is for treatment of a complication resulting from surgery or other medical care, the complication code is sequenced as the principal diagnosis. If the complication is classified to the T80-T88 series and the code lacks the necessary specificity in describing the complication, an additional code for the specific complication should be assigned.

H. Uncertain Diagnosis

If the diagnosis documented at the time of discharge is qualified as "probable", "suspected", "likely", "questionable", "possible", or "still to be ruled out", or other similar terms indicating uncertainty, code the condition as if it existed or was established. The bases for these guidelines are the diagnostic workup, arrangements for further workup or observation, and initial therapeutic approach that correspond most closely with the established diagnosis.

Note: This guideline is applicable only to inpatient admissions to short-term, acute, long-term care and psychiatric hospitals.

I. Admission from Observation Unit

1. Admission Following Medical Observation

When a patient is admitted to an observation unit for a medical condition, which either worsens or does not improve, and is subsequently admitted as an inpatient of the same hospital for this same medical condition, the principal diagnosis would be the medical condition which led to the hospital admission.

2. Admission Following Post-Operative Observation

When a patient is admitted to an observation unit to monitor a condition (or complication) that develops following outpatient surgery, and then is subsequently admitted as an inpatient of the same hospital, hospitals should apply the Uniform Hospital Discharge Data Set (UHDDS) definition of principal diagnosis as "that condition established after study to be chiefly responsible for occasioning the admission of the patient to the hospital for care."

J. Admission from Outpatient Surgery

When a patient receives surgery in the hospital's outpatient surgery department and is subsequently admitted for continuing inpatient care at the same hospital, the following guidelines should be followed in selecting the principal diagnosis for the inpatient admission:

• If the reason for the inpatient admission is a complication, assign the complication as the principal diagnosis.
• If no complication, or other condition, is documented as the reason for the inpatient admission, assign the reason for the outpatient surgery as the principal diagnosis.
• If the reason for the inpatient admission is another condition unrelated to the surgery, assign the unrelated condition as the principal diagnosis.

K. Admissions/Encounters for Rehabilitation

When the purpose for the admission/encounter is rehabilitation, sequence first the code for the condition for which the service is being performed. For example, for an admission/encounter for rehabilitation for right-sided dominant hemiplegia following a cerebrovascular infarction, report code I69.351, Hemiplegia and hemiparesis following cerebral infarction affecting right dominant side, as the first-listed or principal diagnosis.

If the condition for which the rehabilitation service is being provided is no longer present, report the appropriate aftercare code **as the first-listed or principal diagnosis, unless the rehabilitation service is being provided following an injury. For rehabilitation services following active treatment of an injury, assign the injury code with the appropriate seventh character for subsequent encounter** as the first-listed or principal diagnosis. For example, if a patient with severe degenerative osteoarthritis of the hip, underwent hip replacement and the current encounter/ admission is for rehabilitation, report code Z47.1, Aftercare following joint replacement surgery, as the first-listed or principal diagnosis. **If the patient requires rehabilitation post hip replacement for right intertrochanteric femur fracture, report code S72.141D, Displaced intertrochanteric fracture of right femur, subsequent encounter for closed fracture with routine healing, as the first-listed or principal diagnosis.**

See Section I.C.21.c.7, Factors influencing health states and contact with health services, Aftercare.

See Section I.C.19.a for additional information about the use of 7th characters for injury codes.

Section III. Reporting Additional Diagnoses

GENERAL RULES FOR OTHER (ADDITIONAL) DIAGNOSES

For reporting purposes the definition for "other diagnoses" is interpreted as additional conditions that affect patient care in terms of requiring:

clinical evaluation; or
therapeutic treatment; or
diagnostic procedures; or
extended length of hospital stay; or
increased nursing care and/or monitoring.

The UHDDS item #11-b defines Other Diagnoses as "all conditions that coexist at the time of admission, that develop subsequently, or that affect the treatment received and/or the length of stay. Diagnoses that relate to an earlier episode which have no bearing on the current hospital stay are to be excluded." UHDDS definitions apply to inpatients in acute care, short-term, long term care and psychiatric hospital setting. The UHDDS definitions are used by acute care short-term hospitals to report inpatient data elements in a standardized manner. These data elements and their definitions can be found in the July 31, 1985, Federal Register (Vol. 50, No, 147), pp. 31038-40.

Since that time the application of the UHDDS definitions has been expanded to include all nonoutpatient settings (acute care, short term, long term care and psychiatric hospitals; home health agencies; rehab facilities; nursing homes, etc). The UHDDS definitions also apply to hospice services (all levels of care).

The following guidelines are to be applied in designating "other diagnoses" when neither the Alphabetic Index nor the Tabular List in ICD-10-CM provide direction. The listing of the diagnoses in the patient record is the responsibility of the attending provider.

A. Previous conditions

If the provider has included a diagnosis in the final diagnostic statement, such as the discharge summary or the face sheet, it should ordinarily be coded. Some providers include in the diagnostic statement resolved conditions or diagnoses and status-post procedures from previous admission that have no bearing on the current stay. Such conditions are not to be reported and are coded only if required by hospital policy.

However, history codes (categories Z80-Z87) may be used as secondary codes if the historical condition or family history has an impact on current care or influences treatment.

B. Abnormal findings

Abnormal findings (laboratory, x-ray, pathologic, and other diagnostic results) are not coded and reported unless the provider indicates their clinical significance. If the findings are outside the normal range and the attending provider has ordered other tests to evaluate the condition or prescribed treatment, it is appropriate to ask the provider whether the abnormal finding should be added.

Please note: This differs from the coding practices in the outpatient setting for coding encounters for diagnostic tests that have been interpreted by a provider.

C. Uncertain Diagnosis

If the diagnosis documented at the time of discharge is qualified as "probable", "suspected", "likely", "questionable", "possible", or "still to be ruled out" or other similar terms indicating uncertainty, code the condition as if it existed or was established. The bases for these guidelines are the diagnostic workup, arrangements for further workup or observation, and initial therapeutic approach that correspond most closely with the established diagnosis.

Note: This guideline is applicable only to inpatient admissions to short-term, acute, long-term care and psychiatric hospitals.

Section IV. Diagnostic Coding and Reporting Guidelines for Outpatient Services

These coding guidelines for outpatient diagnoses have been approved for use by hospitals/ providers in coding and reporting hospital-based outpatient services and provider-based office visits. Guidelines in Section I, Conventions, general coding guidelines and chapter-specific guidelines, should also be applied for outpatient services and office visits.

Information about the use of certain abbreviations, punctuation, symbols, and other conventions used in the ICD-10-CM Tabular List (code numbers and titles), can be found in Section IA of these guidelines, under "Conventions Used in the Tabular List." Section I.B. contains general guidelines that apply to the entire classification. Section I.C. contains chapter-specific guidelines that correspond to the chapters as they are arranged in the classification. Information about the correct sequence to use in finding a code is also described in Section I.

The terms encounter and visit are often used interchangeably in describing outpatient service contacts and, therefore, appear together in these guidelines without distinguishing one from the other.

Though the conventions and general guidelines apply to all settings, coding guidelines for outpatient and provider reporting of diagnoses will vary in a number of instances from those for inpatient diagnoses, recognizing that:

The Uniform Hospital Discharge Data Set (UHDDS) definition of principal diagnosis does not apply to hospital-based outpatient services and provider-based office visits.

Coding guidelines for inconclusive diagnoses (probable, suspected, rule out, etc.) were developed for inpatient reporting and do not apply to outpatients.

A. Selection of first-listed condition

In the outpatient setting, the term first-listed diagnosis is used in lieu of principal diagnosis.

In determining the first-listed diagnosis the coding conventions of ICD-10-CM, as well as the general and disease specific guidelines take precedence over the outpatient guidelines.

Diagnoses often are not established at the time of the initial encounter/visit. It may take two or more visits before the diagnosis is confirmed.

The most critical rule involves beginning the search for the correct code assignment through the Alphabetic Index. Never begin searching initially in the Tabular List as this will lead to coding errors.

1. Outpatient Surgery

When a patient presents for outpatient surgery (same day surgery), code the reason for the surgery as the first-listed diagnosis (reason for the encounter), even if the surgery is not performed due to a contraindication.

2. Observation Stay

When a patient is admitted for observation for a medical condition, assign a code for the medical condition as the first-listed diagnosis.

When a patient presents for outpatient surgery and develops complications requiring admission to observation, code the reason for the surgery as the first reported diagnosis (reason for the encounter), followed by codes for the complications as secondary diagnoses.

B. Codes from A00.0 through T88.9, Z00-Z99

The appropriate code(s) from A00.0 through T88.9, Z00-Z99 must be used to identify diagnoses, symptoms, conditions, problems, complaints, or other reason(s) for the encounter/visit.

C. Accurate reporting of ICD-10-CM diagnosis codes

For accurate reporting of ICD-10-CM diagnosis codes, the documentation should describe the patient's condition, using terminology which includes specific diagnoses as well as symptoms, problems, or reasons for the encounter. There are ICD-10-CM codes to describe all of these.

D. Codes that describe symptoms and signs

Codes that describe symptoms and signs, as opposed to diagnoses, are acceptable for reporting purposes when a diagnosis has not been established (confirmed) by the provider. Chapter 18 of ICD-10-CM, Symptoms, Signs, and Abnormal Clinical and Laboratory Findings Not Elsewhere Classified (codes R00-R99) contain many, but not all codes for symptoms.

E. Encounters for circumstances other than a disease or injury

ICD-10-CM provides codes to deal with encounters for circumstances other than a disease or injury. The Factors Influencing Health Status and Contact with Health Services codes (Z00-Z99) are provided to deal with occasions when circumstances other than a disease or injury are recorded as diagnosis or problems.

See Section I.C.21. Factors influencing health status and contact with health services.

F. Level of Detail in Coding

1. ICD-10-CM codes with 3, 4, 5, 6 or 7 characters

ICD-10-CM is composed of codes with 3, 4, 5, 6 or 7 characters. Codes with three characters are included in ICD-10-CM as the heading of a category of codes that may be further subdivided by the use of fourth, fifth, sixth or seventh characters to provide greater specificity.

2. Use of full number of characters required for a code

A three-character code is to be used only if it is not further subdivided. A code is invalid if it has not been coded to the full number of characters required for that code, including the 7th character, if applicable.

G. ICD-10-CM code for the diagnosis, condition, problem, or other reason for encounter/visit

List first the ICD-10-CM code for the diagnosis, condition, problem, or other reason for encounter/visit shown in the medical record to be chiefly responsible for the services provided. List additional codes that describe any coexisting conditions. In some cases the first-listed diagnosis may be a symptom when a diagnosis has not been established (confirmed) by the physician.

H. Uncertain diagnosis

Do not code diagnoses documented as "probable", "suspected," "questionable," "rule out," or "working diagnosis" or other similar terms indicating uncertainty. Rather, code the condition(s) to the highest degree of certainty for that encounter/visit, such as symptoms, signs, abnormal test results, or other reason for the visit.

Please note: This differs from the coding practices used by short-term, acute care, long-term care and psychiatric hospitals.

I. Chronic diseases

Chronic diseases treated on an ongoing basis may be coded and reported as many times as the patient receives treatment and care for the condition(s)

J. Code all documented conditions that coexist

Code all documented conditions that coexist at the time of the encounter/visit, and require or affect patient care treatment or management. Do not code conditions that were previously treated and no longer exist. However, history codes (categories Z80-Z87) may be used as secondary codes if the historical condition or family history has an impact on current care or influences treatment.

K. Patients receiving diagnostic services only

For patients receiving diagnostic services only during an encounter/visit, sequence first the diagnosis, condition, problem, or other reason for encounter/visit shown in the medical record to be chiefly responsible for the outpatient services provided during the encounter/visit. Codes for other diagnoses (e.g., chronic conditions) may be sequenced as additional diagnoses.

For encounters for routine laboratory/radiology testing in the absence of any signs, symptoms, or associated diagnosis, assign Z01.89, Encounter for other specified special examinations. If routine testing is performed during the same encounter as a test to evaluate a sign, symptom, or diagnosis, it is appropriate to assign both the Z code and the code describing the reason for the non-routine test.

For outpatient encounters for diagnostic tests that have been interpreted by a physician, and the final report is available at the time of coding, code any confirmed or definitive diagnosis(es) documented in the interpretation. Do not code related signs and symptoms as additional diagnoses.

Please note: This differs from the coding practice in the hospital inpatient setting regarding abnormal findings on test results.

L. Patients receiving therapeutic services only

For patients receiving therapeutic services only during an encounter/visit, sequence first the diagnosis, condition, problem, or other reason for encounter/visit shown in the medical record to be chiefly responsible for the outpatient services provided during the encounter/visit. Codes for other diagnoses (e.g., chronic conditions) may be sequenced as additional diagnoses.

The only exception to this rule is that when the primary reason for the admission/encounter is chemotherapy or radiation therapy, the appropriate Z code for the service is listed first, and the diagnosis or problem for which the service is being performed listed second.

M. Patients receiving preoperative evaluations only

For patients receiving preoperative evaluations only, sequence first a code from subcategory Z01.81, Encounter for pre-procedural examinations, to describe the pre-op consultations. Assign a code for the condition to describe the reason for the surgery as an additional diagnosis. Code also any findings related to the pre-op evaluation.

N. Ambulatory surgery

For ambulatory surgery, code the diagnosis for which the surgery was performed. If the postoperative diagnosis is known to be different from the preoperative diagnosis at the time the diagnosis is confirmed, select the postoperative diagnosis for coding, since it is the most definitive.

O. Routine outpatient prenatal visits

See Section I.C.15. Routine outpatient prenatal visits.

P. Encounters for general medical examinations with abnormal findings

The subcategories for encounters for general medical examinations, Z00.0- **and encounter for routine child health examination, Z00.12-,** provide codes for with and without abnormal findings. Should a general medical examination result in an abnormal finding, the code for general medical examination with abnormal finding should be assigned as the first-listed diagnosis. An examination with abnormal findings refers to a condition/diagnosis that is newly identified or a change in severity of a chronic condition (such as uncontrolled hypertension, or an acute exacerbation of chronic obstructive pulmonary disease) during a routine physical examination. A secondary code for the abnormal finding should also be coded.

Q. Encounters for routine health screenings

See Section I.C.21. Factors influencing health status and contact with health services, Screening

GUIDELINES (ICD-10-CM)

Appendix I
Present on Admission Reporting Guidelines

Introduction

These guidelines are to be used as a supplement to the *ICD-10-CM Official Guidelines for Coding and Reporting* to facilitate the assignment of the Present on Admission (POA) indicator for each diagnosis and external cause of injury code reported on claim forms (UB-04 and 837 Institutional).

These guidelines are not intended to replace any guidelines in the main body of the *ICD-10-CM Official Guidelines for Coding and Reporting*. The POA guidelines are not intended to provide guidance on when a condition should be coded, but rather, how to apply the POA indicator to the final set of diagnosis codes that have been assigned in accordance with Sections I, II, and III of the official coding guidelines. Subsequent to the assignment of the ICD-10-CM codes, the POA indicator should then be assigned to those conditions that have been coded.

As stated in the Introduction to the ICD-10-CM Official Guidelines for Coding and Reporting, a joint effort between the healthcare provider and the coder is essential to achieve complete and accurate documentation, code assignment, and reporting of diagnoses and procedures. The importance of consistent, complete documentation in the medical record cannot be overemphasized. Medical record documentation from any provider involved in the care and treatment of the patient may be used to support the determination of whether a condition was present on admission or not. In the context of the official coding guidelines, the term "provider" means a physician or any qualified healthcare practitioner who is legally accountable for establishing the patient's diagnosis.

These guidelines are not a substitute for the provider's clinical judgment as to the determination of whether a condition was/was not present on admission. The provider should be queried regarding issues related to the linking of signs/symptoms, timing of test results, and the timing of findings.

Please see the CDC website for the detailed list of ICD-10-CM codes that do not require the use of a POA indicator **(https://www.cdc.gov/nchs/icd/icd10cm.htm) (https://www.cms.gov/Medicare/Coding/ICD10/2018-ICD-10-CM-and-GEMs.html)**. The **codes and categories** on this exempt list **are** for circumstances regarding the healthcare encounter or factors influencing health status that do not represent a current disease or injury or **that describe conditions that** are always present on admission.

General Reporting Requirements

All claims involving inpatient admissions to general acute care hospitals or other facilities that are subject to a law or regulation mandating collection of present on admission information.

Present on admission is defined as present at the time the order for inpatient admission occurs—conditions that develop during an outpatient encounter, including emergency department, observation, or outpatient surgery, are considered as present on admission.

POA indicator is assigned to principal and secondary diagnoses (as defined in Section II of the Official Guidelines for Coding and Reporting) and the external cause of injury codes.

Issues related to inconsistent, missing, conflicting or unclear documentation must still be resolved by the provider.

If a condition would not be coded and reported based on UHDDS definitions and current official coding guidelines, then the POA indicator would not be reported.

Reporting Options

Y - Yes

N - No

U - Unknown

W - Clinically undetermined

Unreported/Not used - (Exempt from POA reporting)

Reporting Definitions

Y = present at the time of inpatient admission

N = not present at the time of inpatient admission

U = documentation is insufficient to determine if condition is present on admission

W = provider is unable to clinically determine whether condition was present on admission or not

Timeframe for POA Identification and Documentation

There is no required timeframe as to when a provider (per the definition of "provider" used in these guidelines) must identify or document a condition to be present on admission. In some clinical situations, it may not be possible for a provider to make a definitive diagnosis (or a condition may not be recognized or reported by the patient) for a period of time after admission. In some cases it may be several days before the provider arrives at a definitive diagnosis. This does not mean that the condition was not present on admission. Determination of whether the condition was present on admission or not will be based on the applicable POA guideline as identified in this document, or on the provider's best clinical judgment.

If at the time of code assignment the documentation is unclear as to whether a condition was present on admission or not, it is appropriate to query the provider for clarification.

Assigning the POA Indicator

Condition is on the "Exempt from Reporting" list

Leave the "present on admission" field blank if the condition is on the list of ICD-10-CM codes for which this field is not applicable. This is the only circumstance in which the field may be left blank.

POA Explicitly Documented

Assign Y for any condition the provider explicitly documents as being present on admission.

Assign N for any condition the provider explicitly documents as not present at the time of admission.

Conditions diagnosed prior to inpatient admission

Assign "Y" for conditions that were diagnosed prior to admission (example: hypertension, diabetes mellitus, asthma)

Conditions diagnosed during the admission but clearly present before admission

Assign "Y" for conditions diagnosed during the admission that were clearly present but not diagnosed until after admission occurred.

Diagnoses subsequently confirmed after admission are considered present on admission if at the time of admission they are documented as suspected, possible, rule out, differential diagnosis, or constitute an underlying cause of a symptom that is present at the time of admission.

Condition develops during outpatient encounter prior to inpatient admission

Assign Y for any condition that develops during an outpatient encounter prior to a written order for inpatient admission.

Documentation does not indicate whether condition was present on admission

Assign "U" when the medical record documentation is unclear as to whether the condition was present on admission. "U" should not be routinely assigned and used only in very limited circumstances. Coders are encouraged to query the providers when the documentation is unclear.

Documentation states that it cannot be determined whether the condition was or was not present on admission

Assign "W" when the medical record documentation indicates that it cannot be clinically determined whether or not the condition was present on admission.

Chronic condition with acute exacerbation during the admission

If a single code identifies both the chronic condition and the acute exacerbation, see POA guidelines pertaining to codes that contain multiple clinical concepts.

If a single code only identifies the chronic condition and not the acute exacerbation (e.g., acute exacerbation of chronic leukemia), assign "Y."

Conditions documented as possible, probable, suspected, or rule out at the time of discharge

If the final diagnosis contains a possible, probable, suspected, or rule out diagnosis, and this diagnosis was based on signs, symptoms or clinical findings suspected at the time of inpatient admission, assign "Y."

If the final diagnosis contains a possible, probable, suspected, or rule out diagnosis, and this diagnosis was based on signs, symptoms or clinical findings that were not present on admission, assign "N".

Conditions documented as impending or threatened at the time of discharge

If the final diagnosis contains an impending or threatened diagnosis, and this diagnosis is based on symptoms or clinical findings that were present on admission, assign "Y".

If the final diagnosis contains an impending or threatened diagnosis, and this diagnosis is based on symptoms or clinical findings that were not present on admission, assign "N".

Acute and Chronic Conditions

Assign "Y" for acute conditions that are present at time of admission and N for acute conditions that are not present at time of admission.

Assign "Y" for chronic conditions, even though the condition may not be diagnosed until after admission.

If a single code identifies both an acute and chronic condition, see the POA guidelines for codes that contain multiple clinical concepts.

Codes That Contain Multiple Clinical Concepts

Assign "N" if at least one of the clinical concepts included in the code was not present on admission (e.g., COPD with acute exacerbation and the exacerbation was not present on admission; gastric ulcer that does not start bleeding until after admission; asthma patient develops status asthmaticus after admission).

Assign "Y" if all of the clinical concepts included in the code were present on admission (e.g., duodenal ulcer that perforates prior to admission).

For infection codes that include the causal organism, assign "Y" if the infection (or signs of the infection) were present on admission, even though the culture results may not be known until after admission (e.g., patient is admitted with pneumonia and the provider documents Pseudomonas as the causal organism a few days later).

Same Diagnosis Code for Two or More Conditions

When the same ICD-10-CM diagnosis code applies to two or more conditions during the same encounter (e.g. two separate conditions classified to the same ICD-10-CM diagnosis code):

Assign "Y" if all conditions represented by the single ICD-10-CM code were present on admission (e.g. bilateral unspecified age-related cataracts).

Assign "N" if any of the conditions represented by the single ICD-10-CM code was not present on admission (e.g. traumatic secondary and recurrent hemorrhage and seroma is assigned to a single code T79.2, but only one of the conditions was present on admission).

Obstetrical conditions

Whether or not the patient delivers during the current hospitalization does not affect assignment of the POA indicator. The determining factor for POA assignment is whether the pregnancy complication or obstetrical condition described by the code was present at the time of admission or not.

If the pregnancy complication or obstetrical condition was present on admission (e.g., patient admitted in preterm labor), assign "Y".

If the pregnancy complication or obstetrical condition was not present on admission (e.g., 2nd degree laceration during delivery, postpartum hemorrhage that occurred during current hospitalization, fetal distress develops after admission), assign "N".

If the obstetrical code includes more than one diagnosis and any of the diagnoses identified by the code were not present on admission assign "N".

(e.g., Category O11, Pre-existing hypertension with pre-eclampsia)

Perinatal conditions

Newborns are not considered to be admitted until after birth. Therefore, any condition present at birth or that developed in utero is considered present at admission and should be assigned "Y". This includes conditions that occur during delivery (e.g., injury during delivery, meconium aspiration, exposure to streptococcus B in the vaginal canal).

Congenital conditions and anomalies

Assign "Y" for congenital conditions and anomalies except for categories Q00-Q99, Congenital anomalies, which are on the exempt list. Congenital conditions are always considered present on admission.

External cause of injury codes

Assign "Y" for any external cause code representing an external cause of morbidity that occurred prior to inpatient admission (e.g., patient fell out of bed at home, patient fell out of bed in emergency room prior to admission).

Assign "N" for any external cause code representing an external cause of morbidity that occurred during inpatient hospitalization (e.g., patient fell out of hospital bed during hospital stay, patient experienced an adverse reaction to a medication administered after inpatient admission).

PART II

Alphabetic Index

A

Aarskog's syndrome Q87.1
Abandonment —see Maltreatment
Abasia (-astasia) (hysterical) F44.4
Abderhalden-Kaufmann-Lignac syndrome
    (cystinosis) E72.04
Abdomen, abdominal —see also condition
    acute R10.0
    angina K55.1
    muscle deficiency syndrome Q79.4
Abdominalgia —see Pain, abdominal
Abduction contracture, hip or other joint —see
    Contraction, joint
Aberrant (congenital) —see also Malposition,
    congenital
    adrenal gland Q89.1
    artery (peripheral) Q27.8
        basilar NEC Q28.1
        cerebral Q28.3
        coronary Q24.5
        digestive system Q27.8
        eye Q15.8
        lower limb Q27.8
        precerebral Q28.1
        pulmonary Q25.79
        renal Q27.2
        retina Q14.1
        specified site NEC Q27.8
        subclavian Q27.8
        upper limb Q27.8
        vertebral Q28.1
    breast Q83.8
    endocrine gland NEC Q89.2
    hepatic duct Q44.5
    pancreas Q45.3
    parathyroid gland Q89.2
    pituitary gland Q89.2
    sebaceous glands, mucous membrane,
        mouth, congenital Q38.6
    spleen Q89.09
    subclavian artery Q27.8
    thymus (gland) Q89.2
    thyroid gland Q89.2
    vein (peripheral) NEC Q27.8
        cerebral Q28.3
        digestive system Q27.8
        lower limb Q27.8
        precerebral Q28.1
        specified site NEC Q27.8
        upper limb Q27.8
Aberration
    distantial —see Disturbance, visual
    mental F99
Abetalipoproteinemia E78.6
Abiotrophy R68.89
Ablatio, ablation
    retinae —see Detachment, retina
Ablepharia, ablepharon Q10.3
Abnormal, abnormality, abnormalities —see
    also Anomaly
    acid-base balance (mixed) E87.4
    albumin R77.0
    alphafetoprotein R77.2
    alveolar ridge K08.9
    anatomical relationship Q89.9
    apertures, congenital, diaphragm
        Q79.1
    auditory perception H93.29-●
        diplacusis —see Diplacusis
        hyperacusis —see Hyperacusis
        recruitment —see Recruitment, auditory
        threshold shift —see Shift, auditory
            threshold
    autosomes Q99.9
        fragile site Q95.5
    basal metabolic rate R94.8
    biosynthesis, testicular androgen
        E29.1
    bleeding time R79.1

Abnormal, abnormality, abnormalities —
    (Continued)
    blood level (of)
        cobalt R79.0
        copper R79.0
        iron R79.0
        lithium R78.89
        magnesium R79.0
        mineral NEC R79.0
        zinc R79.0
    blood pressure
        elevated R03.0
        low reading (nonspecific) R03.1
    blood sugar R73.09
    blood-gas level R79.81
    bowel sounds R19.15
        absent R19.11
        hyperactive R19.12
    brain scan R94.02
    breathing R06.9
    caloric test R94.138
    cerebrospinal fluid R83.9
        cytology R83.6
        drug level R83.2
        enzyme level R83.0
        hormones R83.1
        immunology R83.4
        microbiology R83.5
        nonmedicinal level R83.3
        specified type NEC R83.8
    chemistry, blood R79.9
        C-reactive protein R79.82
        drugs —see Findings, abnormal, in blood
        gas level R79.81
        minerals R79.0
        pancytopenia D61.818
        PTT R79.1
        specified NEC R79.89
        toxins —see Findings, abnormal, in
            blood
    chest sounds (friction) (rales) R09.89
    chromosome, chromosomal Q99.9
        with more than three X chromosomes,
            female Q97.1
        analysis result R89.8
            bronchial washings R84.8
            cerebrospinal fluid R83.8
            cervix uteri NEC R87.89
            nasal secretions R84.8
            nipple discharge R89.8
            peritoneal fluid R85.89
            pleural fluid R84.8
            prostatic secretions R86.8
            saliva R85.89
            seminal fluid R86.8
            sputum R84.8
            synovial fluid R89.8
            throat scrapings R84.8
            vagina R87.89
            vulva R87.89
            wound secretions R89.8
        dicentric replacement Q93.2
        ring replacement Q93.2
        sex Q99.8
            female phenotype Q97.9
                specified NEC Q97.8
            male phenotype Q98.9
                specified NEC Q98.8
            structural male Q98.6
        specified NEC Q99.8
    clinical findings NEC R68.89
    coagulation D68.9
        newborn, transient P61.6
        profile R79.1
        time R79.1
    communication —see Fistula
    conjunctiva, vascular H11.41-●
    coronary artery Q24.5
    cortisol-binding globulin E27.8
    course, eustachian tube Q17.8

Abnormal, abnormality, abnormalities —
    (Continued)
    creatinine clearance R94.4
    cytology
        anus R85.619
            atypical squamous cells cannot
                exclude high grade squamous
                intraepithelial lesion (ASC-H)
                R85.611
            atypical squamous cells of undetermined
                significance (ASC-US) R85.610
            cytologic evidence of malignancy
                R85.614
            high grade squamous intraepithelial
                lesion (HGSIL) R85.613
            human papillomavirus (HPV) DNA test
                high risk positive R85.81
                low risk postive R85.82
            inadequate smear R85.615
            low grade squamous intraepithelial
                lesion (LGSIL) R85.612
            satisfactory anal smear but lacking
                transformation zone R85.616
            specified NEC R85.618
            unsatisfactory smear R85.615
        female genital organs —see Abnormal,
            Papanicolaou (smear)
    dark adaptation curve H53.61
    dentofacial NEC —see Anomaly, dentofacial
    development, developmental Q89.9
        central nervous system Q07.9
    diagnostic imaging
        abdomen, abdominal region NEC R93.5
        biliary tract R93.2
        bladder R93.41
        breast R92.8
        central nervous system NEC R90.89
        cerebrovascular NEC R90.89
        coronary circulation R93.1
        digestive tract NEC R93.3
        gastrointestinal (tract) R93.3
        genitourinary organs R93.8
        head R93.0
        heart R93.1
        intrathoracic organ NEC R93.8
        kidney R93.42-●
        limbs R93.6
        liver R93.2
        lung (field) R91.8
        musculoskeletal system NEC R93.7
        renal pelvis R93.41
        retroperitoneum R93.5
        site specified NEC R93.8
        skin and subcutaneous tissue R93.8
        skull R93.0
        urinary organs specified NEC R93.49
        ureter R93.41
    direction, teeth, fully erupted M26.30
    ear ossicles, acquired NEC H74.39-●
        ankylosis —see Ankylosis, ear ossicles
        discontinuity —see Discontinuity, ossicles,
            ear
        partial loss —see Loss, ossicles, ear (partial)
    Ebstein Q22.5
    echocardiogram R93.1
    echoencephalogram R90.81
    echogram —see Abnormal, diagnostic
        imaging
    electrocardiogram [ECG] [EKG] R94.31
    electroencephalogram [EEG] R94.01
    electrolyte —see Imbalance, electrolyte
    electromyogram [EMG] R94.131
    electro-oculogram [EOG] R94.110
    electrophysiological intracardiac studies
        R94.39
    electroretinogram [ERG] R94.111
    erythrocytes
        congenital, with perinatal jaundice
            D58.9
    feces (color) (contents) (mucus) R19.5

Abnormal, abnormality, abnormalities —
  (Continued)
  finding —see Findings, abnormal, without
    diagnosis
  fluid
    amniotic —see Abnormal, specimen,
      specified
    cerebrospinal —see Abnormal,
      cerebrospinal fluid
    peritoneal —see Abnormal, specimen,
      digestive organs
    pleural —see Abnormal, specimen,
      respiratory organs
    synovial —see Abnormal, specimen,
      specified
    thorax (bronchial washings) (pleural
      fluid) —see Abnormal, specimen,
      respiratory organs
    vaginal —see Abnormal, specimen, female
      genital organs
  form
    teeth K00.2
    uterus —see Anomaly, uterus
  function studies
    auditory R94.120
    bladder R94.8
    brain R94.09
    cardiovascular R94.30
    ear R94.128
    endocrine NEC R94.7
    eye NEC R94.118
    kidney R94.4
    liver R94.5
    nervous system
      central NEC R94.09
      peripheral NEC R94.138
    pancreas R94.8
    placenta R94.8
    pulmonary R94.2
    special senses NEC R94.128
    spleen R94.8
    thyroid R94.6
    vestibular R94.121
  gait —see Gait
    hysterical F44.4
  gastrin secretion E16.4
  globulin R77.1
    cortisol-binding E27.8
    thyroid-binding E07.89
  glomerular, minor —see also N00-N07 with
    fourth character .0 N05.0
  glucagon secretion E16.3
  glucose tolerance (test) (non-fasting)
    R73.09
  gravitational (G) forces or states (effect of)
    T75.81
  hair (color) (shaft) L67.9
    specified NEC L67.8
  hard tissue formation in pulp (dental)
    K04.3
  head movement R25.0
  heart
    rate R00.9
      specified NEC R00.8
    shadow R93.1
    sounds NEC R01.2
  hemoglobin (disease) —see also Disease,
    hemoglobin D58.2
    trait —see Trait, hemoglobin, abnormal
  histology NEC R89.7
  immunological findings R89.4
    in serum R76.9
      specified NEC R76.8
  increase in appetite R63.2
  involuntary movement —see Abnormal,
    movement, involuntary
  jaw closure M26.51
  karyotype R89.8
  kidney function test R94.4
  knee jerk R29.2
  leukocyte (cell) (differential) NEC D72.9

Abnormal, abnormality, abnormalities —
  (Continued)
  ~~liver~~
▶ liver function test R94.5
  loss of
    height R29.890
    weight R63.4
  mammogram NEC R92.8
    calcification (calculus) R92.1
    microcalcification R92.0
  Mantoux test R76.11
  movement (disorder) —see also Disorder,
    movement
    head R25.0
    involuntary R25.9
      fasciculation R25.3
      of head R25.0
      spasm R25.2
      specified type NEC R25.8
      tremor R25.1
  myoglobin (Aberdeen) (Annapolis) R89.7
  neonatal screening P09
  oculomotor study R94.113
  palmar creases Q82.8
  Papanicolaou (smear)
    anus R85.619
      atypical squamous cells cannot
        exclude high grade squamous
        intraepithelial lesion (ASC-H)
        R85.611
      atypical squamous cells of undetermined
        significance (ASC-US) R85.610
      cytologic evidence of malignancy
        R85.614
      high grade squamous intraepithelial
        lesion (HGSIL) R85.613
      human papillomavirus (HPV)
        DNA test
        high risk positive R85.81
        low risk postive R85.82
      inadequate smear R85.615
      low grade squamous intraepithelial
        lesion (LGSIL) R85.612
      satisfactory anal smear but lacking
        transformation zone R85.616
      specified NEC R85.618
      unsatisfactory smear R85.615
    bronchial washings R84.6
    cerebrospinal fluid R83.6
    cervix R87.619
      atypical squamous cells cannot
        exclude high grade squamous
        intraepithelial lesion (ASC-H)
        R87.611
      atypical squamous cells of undetermined
        significance (ASC-US) R87.610
      cytologic evidence of malignancy
        R87.614
      high grade squamous intraepithelial
        lesion (HGSIL) R87.613
      inadequate smear R87.615
      low grade squamous intraepithelial
        lesion (LGSIL) R87.612
      non-atypical endometrial cells R87.618
      satisfactory cervical smear but
        lacking transformation zone
        R87.616
      specified NEC R87.618
      thin preparaton R87.619
      unsatisfactory smear R87.615
    nasal secretions R84.6
    nipple discharge R89.6
    peritoneal fluid R85.69
    pleural fluid R84.6
    prostatic secretions R86.6
    saliva R85.69
    seminal fluid R86.6
    sites NEC R89.6
    sputum R84.6
    synovial fluid R89.6
    throat scrapings R84.6

Abnormal, abnormality, abnormalities —
  (Continued)
  Papanicolaou (smear) (Continued)
    vagina R87.629
      atypical squamous cells cannot
        exclude high grade squamous
        intraepithelial lesion (ASC-H)
        R87.621
      atypical squamous cells of
        undetermined significance
        (ASC-US) R87.620
      cytologic evidence of malignancy
        R87.624
      high grade squamous intraepithelial
        lesion (HGSIL) R87.623
      inadequate smear R87.625
      low grade squamous intraepithelial
        lesion (LGSIL) R87.622
      specified NEC R87.628
      thin preparation R87.629
      unsatisfactory smear R87.625
    vulva R87.69
    wound secretions R89.6
  partial thromboplastin time (PTT) R79.1
  pelvis (bony) —see Deformity, pelvis
  percussion, chest (tympany) R09.89
  periods (grossly) —see Menstruation
  phonocardiogram R94.39
  plantar reflex R29.2
  plasma
    protein R77.9
      specified NEC R77.8
    viscosity R70.1
  pleural (folds) Q34.0
  posture R29.3
  product of conception O02.9
    specified type NEC O02.89
  prothrombin time (PT) R79.1
  pulmonary
    artery, congenital Q25.79
    function, newborn P28.89
    test results R94.2
  pulsations in neck R00.2
  pupillary H21.56-●
    function (reaction) (reflex) —see Anomaly,
      pupil, function
  radiological examination —see Abnormal,
    diagnostic imaging
  red blood cell(s) (morphology) (volume)
    R71.8
  reflex —see Reflex
  renal function test R94.4
  response to nerve stimulation R94.130
  retinal correspondence H53.31
  retinal function study R94.111
  rhythm, heart —see also Arrhythmia
  saliva —see Abnormal, specimen, digestive
    organs
  scan
    kidney R94.4
    liver R93.2
    thyroid R94.6
  secretion
    gastrin E16.4
    glucagon E16.3
  semen, seminal fluid —see Abnormal,
    specimen, male genital organs
  serum level (of)
    acid phosphatase R74.8
    alkaline phosphatase R74.8
    amylase R74.8
    enzymes R74.9
      specified NEC R74.8
    lipase R74.8
    triacylglycerol lipase R74.8
  shape
    gravid uterus —see Anomaly, uterus
  sinus venosus Q21.1
  size, tooth, teeth K00.2
  spacing, tooth, teeth, fully erupted
    M26.30

Abnormal, abnormality, abnormalities —
(Continued)
specimen
digestive organs (peritoneal fluid) (saliva)
R85.9
cytology R85.69
drug level R85.2
enzyme level R85.0
histology R85.7
hormones R85.1
immunology R85.4
microbiology R85.5
nonmedicinal level R85.3
specified type NEC R85.89
female genital organs (secretions) (smears)
R87.9
cytology R87.69
cervix R87.619
human papillomavirus (HPV) DNA
test
high risk positive R87.810
low risk positive R87.820
inadequate (unsatisfactory) smear
R87.615
non-atypical endometrial cells
R87.618
specified NEC R87.618
vagina R87.629
human papillomavirus (HPV) DNA
test
high risk positive R87.811
low risk positive R87.821
inadequate (unsatisfactory) smear
R87.625
vulva R87.69
drug level R87.2
enzyme level R87.0
histological R87.7
hormones R87.1
immunology R87.4
microbiology R87.5
nonmedicinal level R87.3
specified type NEC R87.89
male genital organs (prostatic secretions)
(semen) R86.9
cytology R86.6
drug level R86.2
enzyme level R86.0
histological R86.7
hormones R86.1
immunology R86.4
microbiology R86.5
nonmedicinal level R86.3
specified type NEC R86.8
nipple discharge —see Abnormal,
specimen, specified
respiratory organs (bronchial washings)
(nasal secretions) (pleural fluid)
(sputum) R84.9
cytology R84.6
drug level R84.2
enzyme level R84.0
histology R84.7
hormones R84.1
immunology R84.4
microbiology R84.5
nonmedicinal level R84.3
specified type NEC R84.8
specified organ, system and tissue NOS
R89.9
cytology R89.6
drug level R89.2
enzyme level R89.0
histology R89.7
hormones R89.1
immunology R89.4
microbiology R89.5
nonmedicinal level R89.3
specified type NEC R89.8
synovial fluid —see Abnormal, specimen,
specified

Abnormal, abnormality, abnormalities —
(Continued)
specimen (Continued)
thorax (bronchial washings) (pleural
fluids) —see Abnormal, specimen,
respiratory organs
vagina (secretion) (smear) R87.629
vulva (secretion) (smear) R87.69
wound secretion —see Abnormal,
specimen, specified
spermatozoa —see Abnormal, specimen, male
genital organs
sputum (amount) (color) (odor) R09.3
stool (color) (contents) (mucus) R19.5
bloody K92.1
guaiac positive R19.5
synchondrosis Q78.8
thermography —see also Abnormal,
diagnostic imaging R93.8
thyroid-binding globulin E07.89
tooth, teeth (form) (size) K00.2
toxicology (findings) R78.9
transport protein E88.09
tumor marker NEC R97.8
ultrasound results —see Abnormal, diagnostic
imaging
umbilical cord complicating delivery O69.9
urination NEC R39.198
urine (constituents) R82.90
bile R82.2
cytological examination R82.8
drugs R82.5
fat R82.0
glucose R81
heavy metals R82.6
hemoglobin R82.3
histological examination R82.8
ketones R82.4
microbiological examination (culture)
R82.79
myoglobin R82.1
positive culture R82.79
protein —see Proteinuria
specified substance NEC R82.99
chromoabnormality NEC R82.91
substances nonmedical R82.6
uterine hemorrhage —see Hemorrhage,
uterus
vectorcardiogram R94.39
visually evoked potential (VEP) R94.112
white blood cells D72.9
specified NEC D72.89
X-ray examination —see Abnormal,
diagnostic imaging
Abnormity (any organ or part) —see Anomaly
Abocclusion M26.29
hemolytic disease (newborn) P55.1
incompatibility reaction ABO —see
Complication(s), transfusion,
incompatibility reaction, ABO
Abolition, language R48.8
Aborter, habitual or recurrent —see Loss (of),
pregnancy, recurrent
Abortion (complete) (spontaneous) O03.9
with
retained products of conception —see
Abortion, incomplete
attempted (elective) (failed) O07.4
complicated by O07.30
afibrinogenemia O07.1
cardiac arrest O07.36
chemical damage of pelvic organ(s)
O07.34
circulatory collapse O07.31
cystitis O07.38
defibrination syndrome O07.1
electrolyte imbalance O07.33
embolism (air) (amniotic fluid) (blood
clot) (fat) (pulmonary) (septic)
(soap) O07.2
endometritis O07.0

Abortion (Continued)
attempted (Continued)
complicated by (Continued)
genital tract and pelvic infection O07.0
hemolysis O07.1
hemorrhage (delayed) (excessive) O07.1
infection
genital tract or pelvic O07.0
urinary tract tract O07.38
intravascular coagulation O07.1
laceration of pelvic organ(s) O07.34
metabolic disorder O07.33
oliguria O07.32
oophoritis O07.0
parametritis O07.0
pelvic peritonitis O07.0
perforation of pelvic organ(s) O07.34
renal failure or shutdown O07.32
salpingitis or salpingo-oophoritis O07.0
sepsis O07.37
shock O07.31
specified condition NEC O07.39
tubular necrosis (renal) O07.32
uremia O07.32
urinary tract infection O07.38
venous complication NEC O07.35
embolism (air) (amniotic fluid) (blood
clot) (fat) (pulmonary) (septic)
(soap) O07.2
complicated (by) (following) O03.80
afibrinogenemia O03.6
cardiac arrest O03.86
chemical damage of pelvic organ(s) O03.84
circulatory collapse O03.81
cystitis O03.88
defibrination syndrome O03.6
electrolyte imbalance O03.83
embolism (air) (amniotic fluid) (blood clot)
(fat) (pulmonary) (septic) (soap) O03.7
endometritis O03.5
genital tract and pelvic infection O03.5
hemolysis O03.6
hemorrhage (delayed) (excessive) O03.6
infection
genital tract or pelvic O03.5
urinary tract O03.88
intravascular coagulation O03.6
laceration of pelvic organ(s) O03.84
metabolic disorder O03.83
oliguria O03.82
oophoritis O03.5
parametritis O03.5
pelvic peritonitis O03.5
perforation of pelvic organ(s) O03.84
renal failure or shutdown O03.82
salpingitis or salpingo-oophoritis
O03.5
sepsis O03.87
shock O03.81
specified condition NEC O03.89
tubular necrosis (renal) O03.82
uremia O03.82
urinary tract infection O03.88
venous complication NEC O03.85
embolism (air) (amniotic fluid) (blood
clot) (fat) (pulmonary) (septic)
(soap) O03.7
failed —see Abortion, attempted
habitual or recurrent N96
with current abortion —see categories
O03-O04
without current pregnancy N96
care in current pregnancy O26.2-•
incomplete (spontaneous) O03.4
complicated (by) (following) O03.30
afibrinogenemia O03.1
cardiac arrest O03.36
chemical damage of pelvic organ(s)
O03.34
circulatory collapse O03.31
cystitis O03.38

Abortion (Continued)
  incomplete (Continued)
    complicated (Continued)
      defibrination syndrome O03.1
      electrolyte imbalance O03.33
      embolism (air) (amniotic fluid) (blood clot) (fat) (pulmonary) (septic) (soap) O03.2
      endometritis O03.0
      genital tract and pelvic infection O03.0
      hemolysis O03.1
      hemorrhage (delayed) (excessive) O03.1
      infection
        genital tract or pelvic O03.0
        urinary tract O03.38
      intravascular coagulation O03.1
      laceration of pelvic organ(s) O03.34
      metabolic disorder O03.33
      oliguria O03.32
      oophoritis O03.0
      parametritis O03.0
      pelvic peritonitis O03.0
      perforation of pelvic organ(s) O03.34
      renal failure or shutdown O03.32
      salpingitis or salpingo-oophoritis O03.0
      sepsis O03.37
      shock O03.31
      specified condition NEC O03.39
      tubular necrosis (renal) O03.32
      uremia O03.32
      urinary infection O03.38
      venous complication NEC O03.35
        embolism (air) (amniotic fluid) (blood clot) (fat) (pulmonary) (septic) (soap) O03.2
  induced (encounter for) Z33.2
    complicated by O04.80
      afibrinogenemia O04.6
      cardiac arrest O04.86
      chemical damage of pelvic organ(s) O04.84
      circulatory collapse O04.81
      cystitis O04.88
      defibrination syndrome O04.6
      electrolyte imbalance O04.83
      embolism (air) (amniotic fluid) (blood clot) (fat) (pulmonary) (septic) (soap) O04.7
      endometritis O04.5
      genital tract and pelvic infection O04.5
      hemolysis O04.6
      hemorrhage (delayed) (excessive) O04.6
      infection
        genital tract or pelvic O04.5
        urinary tract O04.88
      intravascular coagulation O04.6
      laceration of pelvic organ(s) O04.84
      metabolic disorder O04.83
      oliguria O04.82
      oophoritis O04.5
      parametritis O04.5
      pelvic peritonitis O04.5
      perforation of pelvic organ(s) O04.84
      renal failure or shutdown O04.82
      salpingitis or salpingo-oophoritis O04.5
      sepsis O04.87
      shock O04.81
      specified condition NEC O04.89
      tubular necrosis (renal) O04.82
      uremia O04.82
      urinary tract infection O04.88
      venous complication NEC O04.85
        embolism (air) (amniotic fluid) (blood clot) (fat) (pulmonary) (septic) (soap) O04.7
  missed O02.1
  spontaneous —see Abortion (complete) (spontaneous)
    threatened O20.0
  threatened (spontaneous) O20.0

Abortion (Continued)
  tubal O00.10-
    with intrauterine pregnancy O00.11-
Abortus fever A23.1
Aboulomania F60.7
Abrami's disease D59.8
Abramov-Fiedler myocarditis (acute isolated myocarditis) I40.1
Abrasion T14.8
  abdomen, abdominal (wall) S30.811
  alveolar process S00.512
  ankle S90.51-●
  antecubital space —see Abrasion, elbow
  anus S30.817
  arm (upper) S40.81-●
  auditory canal —see Abrasion, ear
  auricle —see Abrasion, ear
  axilla —see Abrasion, arm
  back, lower S30.810
  breast S20.11-●
  brow S00.81
  buttock S30.810
  calf —see Abrasion, leg
  canthus —see Abrasion, eyelid
  cheek S00.81
    internal S00.512
  chest wall —see Abrasion, thorax
  chin S00.81
  clitoris S30.814
  cornea S05.0-●
  costal region —see Abrasion, thorax
  dental K03.1
  digit(s)
    foot —see Abrasion, toe
    hand —see Abrasion, finger
  ear S00.41-●
  elbow S50.31-●
  epididymis S30.813
  epigastric region S30.811
  epiglottis S10.11
  esophagus (thoracic) S27.818
    cervical S10.11
  eyebrow —see Abrasion, eyelid
  eyelid S00.21-●
  face S00.81
  finger(s) S60.41-●
    index S60.41-●
    little S60.41-●
    middle S60.41-●
    ring S60.41-●
  flank S30.811
  foot (except toe(s) alone) S90.81-●
    toe —see Abrasion, toe
  forearm S50.81-●
    elbow only —see Abrasion, elbow
  forehead S00.81
  genital organs, external
    female S30.816
    male S30.815
  groin S30.811
  gum S00.512
  hand S60.51-●
  head S00.91
    ear —see Abrasion, ear
    eyelid —see Abrasion, eyelid
    lip S00.511
    nose S00.31
    oral cavity S00.512
    scalp S00.01
    specified site NEC S00.81
  heel —see Abrasion, foot
  hip S70.21-●
  inguinal region S30.811
  interscapular region S20.419
  jaw S00.81
  knee S80.21-●
  labium (majus) (minus) S30.814
  larynx S10.11
  leg (lower) S80.81-●
    knee —see Abrasion, knee
    upper —see Abrasion, thigh

Abrasion (Continued)
  lip S00.511
  lower back S30.810
  lumbar region S30.810
  malar region S00.81
  mammary —see Abrasion, breast
  mastoid region S00.81
  mouth S00.512
  nail
    finger —see Abrasion, finger
    toe —see Abrasion, toe
  nape S10.81
  nasal S00.31
  neck S10.91
    specified site NEC S10.81
    throat S10.11
  nose S00.31
  occipital region S00.01
  oral cavity S00.512
  orbital region —see Abrasion, eyelid
  palate S00.512
  palm —see Abrasion, hand
  parietal region S00.01
  pelvis S30.810
  penis S30.812
  perineum
    female S30.814
    male S30.810
  periocular area —see Abrasion, eyelid
  phalanges
    finger —see Abrasion, finger
    toe —see Abrasion, toe
  pharynx S10.11
  pinna —see Abrasion, ear
  popliteal space —see Abrasion, knee
  prepuce S30.812
  pubic region S30.810
  pudendum
    female S30.816
    male S30.815
  sacral region S30.810
  scalp S00.01
  scapular region —see Abrasion, shoulder
  scrotum S30.813
  shin —see Abrasion, leg
  shoulder S40.21-●
  skin NEC T14.8
  sternal region S20.319
  submaxillary region S00.81
  submental region S00.81
  subungual
    finger(s) —see Abrasion, finger
    toe(s) —see Abrasion, toe
  supraclavicular fossa S10.81
  supraorbital S00.81
  temple S00.81
  temporal region S00.81
  testis S30.813
  thigh S70.31-●
  thorax, thoracic (wall) S20.91
    back S20.41-●
    front S20.31-●
  throat S10.11
  thumb S60.31-●
  toe(s) (lesser) S90.416
    great S90.41-●
  tongue S00.512
  tooth, teeth (dentifrice) (habitual) (hard tissues) (occupational) (ritual) (traditional) K03.1
  trachea S10.11
  tunica vaginalis S30.813
  tympanum, tympanic membrane —see Abrasion, ear
  uvula S00.512
  vagina S30.814
  vocal cords S10.11
  vulva S30.814
  wrist S60.81-●
Abrism —see Poisoning, food, noxious, plant

Abruptio placentae O45.9-●
  with
    afibrinogenemia O45.01-●
    coagulation defect O45.00-●
      specified NEC O45.09-●
    disseminated intravascular coagulation
      O45.02-●
    hypofibrinogenemia O45.01-●
  specified NEC O45.8-●
Abruption, placenta —see Abruptio placentae
Abscess (connective tissue) (embolic) (fistulous)
    (infective) (metastatic) (multiple)
    (pernicious) (pyogenic) (septic) L02.91
  with
    diverticular disease (intestine) K57.80
      with bleeding K57.81
      large intestine K57.20
        with
          bleeding K57.21
          small intestine K57.40
            with bleeding K57.41
      small intestine K57.00
        with
          bleeding K57.01
          large intestine K57.40
            with bleeding K57.41
    lymphangitis - code by site under
      Abscess
  abdomen, abdominal
    cavity K65.1
    wall L02.211
  abdominopelvic K65.1
  accessory sinus —see Sinusitis
  adrenal (capsule) (gland) E27.8
  alveolar K04.7
    with sinus K04.6
  amebic A06.4
    brain (and liver or lung abscess) A06.6
    genitourinary tract A06.82
    liver (without mention of brain or lung
      abscess) A06.4
    lung (and liver) (without mention of brain
      abscess) A06.5
    specified site NEC A06.89
    spleen A06.89
  anerobic A48.0
  ankle —see Abscess, lower limb
  anorectal K61.2
  antecubital space —see Abscess, upper limb
  antrum (chronic) (Highmore) —see Sinusitis,
    maxillary
  anus K61.0
  apical (tooth) K04.7
    with sinus (alveolar) K04.6
  appendix K35.3
  areola (acute) (chronic) (nonpuerperal)
    N61.1
    puerperal, postpartum or gestational —see
      Infection, nipple
  arm (any part) —see Abscess, upper limb
  artery (wall) I77.89
  atheromatous I77.2
  auricle, ear —see Abscess, ear, external
  axilla (region) L02.41-●
    lymph gland or node L04.2
  back (any part, except buttock) L02.212
  Bartholin's gland N75.1
    with
      abortion —see Abortion, by type
        complicated by, sepsis
      ectopic or molar pregnancy O08.0
    following ectopic or molar pregnancy O08.0
  Bezold's —see Mastoiditis, acute
  bilharziasis B65.1
  bladder (wall) —see Cystitis, specified type
    NEC
  bone (subperiosteal) —see also Osteomyelitis,
    specified type NEC
    accessory sinus (chronic) —see Sinusitis
    chronic or old —see Osteomyelitis, chronic
    jaw (lower) (upper) M27.2

Abscess (Continued)
  bone (Continued)
    mastoid —see Mastoiditis, acute,
      subperiosteal
    petrous —see Petrositis
    spinal (tuberculous) A18.01
      nontuberculous —see Osteomyelitis,
        vertebra
  bowel K63.0
  brain (any part) (cystic) (otogenic) G06.0
    amebic (with abscess of any other site) A06.6
    gonococcal A54.82
    pheomycotic (chromomycotic) B43.1
    tuberculous A17.81
  breast (acute) (chronic) (nonpuerperal)
    N61.1
    newborn P39.0
    puerperal, postpartum, gestational —see
      Mastitis, obstetric, purulent
  broad ligament N73.2
    acute N73.0
    chronic N73.1
  Brodie's (localized) (chronic) M86.8X-●
  bronchi J98.09
  buccal cavity K12.2
  bulbourethral gland N34.0
  bursa M71.00
    ankle M71.07-●
    elbow M71.02-●
    foot M71.07-●
    hand M71.04-●
    hip M71.05-●
    knee M71.06-●
    multiple sites M71.09
    pharyngeal J39.1
    shoulder M71.01-●
    specified site NEC M71.08
    wrist M71.03-●
  buttock L02.31
  canthus —see Blepharoconjunctivitis
  cartilage —see Disorder, cartilage, specified
    type NEC
  cecum K35.3
  cerebellum, cerebellar G06.0
    sequelae G09
  cerebral (embolic) G06.0
    sequelae G09
  cervical (meaning neck) L02.11
    lymph gland or node L04.0
  cervix (stump) (uteri) —see Cervicitis
  cheek (external) L02.01
    inner K12.2
  chest J86.9
    with fistula J86.0
    wall L02.213
  chin L02.01
  choroid —see Inflammation, chorioretinal
  circumtonsillar J36
  cold (lung) (tuberculous) —see also
      Tuberculosis, abscess, lung
    articular —see Tuberculosis, joint
  colon (wall) K63.0
  colostomy K94.02
  conjunctiva —see Conjunctivitis, acute
  cornea H16.31-●
  corpus
    cavernosum N48.21
    luteum —see Oophoritis
  Cowper's gland N34.0
  cranium G06.0
  cul-de-sac (Douglas') (posterior) —see
      Peritonitis, pelvic, female
  cutaneous —see Abscess, by site
  dental K04.7
    with sinus (alveolar) K04.6
  dentoalveolar K04.7
    with sinus K04.6
  diaphragm, diaphragmatic K65.1
  Douglas' cul-de-sac or pouch —see
      Peritonitis, pelvic, female
  Dubois A50.59

Abscess (Continued)
  ear (middle) —see also Otitis, media,
      suppurative
    acute —see Otitis, media, suppurative,
      acute
    external H60.0-●
  entamebic —see Abscess, amebic
  enterostomy K94.12
  epididymis N45.4
  epidural G06.2
    brain G06.0
    spinal cord G06.1
  epiglottis J38.7
  epiploon, epiploic K65.1
  erysipelatous —see Erysipelas
  esophagus K20.8
  ethmoid (bone) (chronic) (sinus) J32.2
  external auditory canal —see Abscess, ear,
    external
  extradural G06.2
    brain G06.0
      sequelae G09
    spinal cord G06.1
  extraperitoneal K68.19
  eye —see Endophthalmitis, purulent
  eyelid H00.03-●
  face (any part, except ear, eye and nose)
    L02.01
  fallopian tube —see Salpingitis
  fascia M72.8
  fauces J39.1
  fecal K63.0
  femoral (region) —see Abscess, lower limb
  filaria, filarial —see Infestation, filarial
  finger (any) —see also Abscess, hand
    nail —see Cellulitis, finger
  foot L02.61-●
  forehead L02.01
  frontal sinus (chronic) J32.1
  gallbladder K81.0
  genital organ or tract
    female (external) N76.4
    male N49.9
      multiple sites N49.8
      specified NEC N49.8
  gestational mammary O91.11-●
  gestational subareolar O91.11-●
  gingival —see Peridontitis, aggressive,
    localized
  gland, glandular (lymph) (acute) —see
      Lymphadenitis, acute
  gluteal (region) L02.31
  gonorrheal —see Gonococcus
  groin L02.214
  gum —see Peridontitis, aggressive, localized
  hand L02.51-●
  head NEC L02.811
    face (any part, except ear, eye and nose)
      L02.01
  heart —see Carditis
  heel —see Abscess, foot
  helminthic —see Infestation, helminth
  hepatic (cholangitic) (hematogenic)
    (lymphogenic) (pylephlebitic) K75.0
    amebic A06.4
  hip (region) —see Abscess, lower limb
  ileocecal K35.3
  ileostomy (bud) K94.12
  iliac (region) L02.214
    fossa K35.3
  infraclavicular (fossa) —see Abscess, upper
    limb
  inguinal (region) L02.214
    lymph gland or node L04.1
  intestine, intestinal NEC K63.0
    rectal K61.1
  intra-abdominal —see also Abscess,
    peritoneum K65.1
  ➧postprocedural T81.4
    retroperitoneal K68.11
  intra-muscular, postprocedural T81.42

▶ New   ➧ Revised   ~~deleted~~ Deleted   ● Use Additional Character(s)

Abscess (Continued)
  intracranial G06.0
  intramammary —see Abscess, breast
  intraorbital —see Abscess, orbit
  intraperitoneal K65.1
  intrasphincteric (anus) K61.4
  intraspinal G06.1
  intratonsillar J36
  ischiorectal (fossa) K61.3
  jaw (bone) (lower) (upper) M27.2
  joint —see Arthritis, pyogenic or pyemic
    spine (tuberculous) A18.01
      nontuberculous —see Spondylopathy,
        infective
  kidney N15.1
    with calculus N20.0
      with hydronephrosis N13.6
    puerperal (postpartum) O86.21
  knee —see also Abscess, lower limb
    joint M00.9
  labium (majus) (minus) N76.4
  lacrimal
    caruncle —see Inflammation, lacrimal,
      passages, acute
    gland —see Dacryoadenitis
    passages (duct) (sac) —see Inflammation,
      lacrimal, passages, acute
  lacunar N34.0
  larynx J38.7
  lateral (alveolar) K04.7
    with sinus K04.6
  leg (any part) —see Abscess, lower limb
  lens H27.8
  lingual K14.0
    tonsil J36
  lip K13.0
  Littre's gland N34.0
  liver (cholangitic) (hematogenic)
    (lymphogenic) (pylephlebitic) (pyogenic)
    K75.0
    amebic (due to Entamoeba histolytica)
      (dysenteric) (tropical) A06.4
      with
        brain abscess (and liver or lung
          abscess) A06.6
        lung abscess A06.5
  loin (region) L02.211
  lower limb L02.41-●
  lumbar (tuberculous) A18.01
    nontuberculous L02.212
  lung (miliary) (putrid) J85.2
    with pneumonia J85.1
      due to specified organism (see
        Pneumonia, in (due to))
    amebic (with liver abscess) A06.5
      with
        brain abscess A06.6
        pneumonia A06.5
  lymph, lymphatic, gland or node (acute) —see
    also Lymphadenitis, acute
    mesentery I88.0
  malar M27.2
  mammary gland —see Abscess, breast
  marginal, anus K61.0
  mastoid —see Mastoiditis, acute
  maxilla, maxillary M27.2
    molar (tooth) K04.7
      with sinus K04.6
    premolar K04.7
    sinus (chronic) J32.0
  mediastinum J85.3
  meibomian gland —see Hordeolum
  meninges G06.2
  mesentery, mesenteric K65.1
  mesosalpinx —see Salpingitis
  mons pubis L02.215
  mouth (floor) K12.2
  muscle —see Myositis, infective
  myocardium I40.0
  nabothian (follicle) —see Cervicitis
  nasal J32.9
  nasopharyngeal J39.1

Abscess (Continued)
  navel L02.216
    newborn P38.9
      with mild hemorrhage P38.1
      without hemorrhage P38.9
  neck (region) L02.11
    lymph gland or node L04.0
  nephritic —see Abscess, kidney
  nipple N61.1
    associated with
      lactation —see Pregnancy, complicated by
      pregnancy —see Pregnancy, complicated
        by
  nose (external) (fossa) (septum) J34.0
    sinus (chronic) —see Sinusitis
  omentum K65.1
  ⇨operative wound T81.4
  orbit, orbital —see Cellulitis, orbit
  otogenic G06.0
  ovary, ovarian (corpus luteum) —see
    Oophoritis
  oviduct —see Oophoritis
  palate (soft) K12.2
    hard M27.2
  palmar (space) —see Abscess, hand
  pancreas (duct) —see Pancreatitis, acute
  parafrenal N48.21
  parametric, parametrium N73.2
    acute N73.0
    chronic N73.1
  paranephric N15.1
  parapancreatic —see Pancreatitis, acute
  parapharyngeal J39.0
  pararectal K61.1
  parasinus —see Sinusitis
  parauterine (see also Disease, pelvis,
    inflammatory) N73.2
  paravaginal —see Vaginitis
  parietal region (scalp) L02.811
  parodontal —see Peridontitis, aggressive,
    localized
  parotid (duct) (gland) K11.3
    region K12.2
  pectoral (region) L02.213
  pelvis, pelvic
    female —see Disease, pelvis, inflammatory
    male, peritoneal K65.1
  penis N48.21
    gonococcal (accessory gland) (periurethral)
      A54.1
  perianal K61.0
  periapical K04.7
    with sinus (alveolar) K04.6
  periappendicular K35.3
  pericardial I30.1
  pericecal K35.3
  pericemental —see Peridontitis, aggressive,
    localized
  pericholecystic —see Cholecystitis, acute
  pericoronal —see Peridontitis, aggressive,
    localized
  peridental —see Peridontitis, aggressive,
    localized
  perimetric —see also Disease, pelvis,
    inflammatory N73.2
  perinephric, perinephritic —see Abscess,
    kidney
  perineum, perineal (superficial) L02.215
    urethra N34.0
  periodontal (parietal) —see Peridontitis,
    aggressive, localized
    apical K04.7
  periosteum, periosteal —see also
    Osteomyelitis, specified type NEC
    with osteomyelitis —see also Osteomyelitis,
      specified type NEC
    acute —see Osteomyelitis, acute
    chronic —see Osteomyelitis, chronic
  peripharyngeal J39.0
  peripleuritic J86.9
    with fistula J86.0

Abscess (Continued)
  periprostatic N41.2
  perirectal K61.1
  perirenal (tissue) —see Abscess, kidney
  perisinuous (nose) —see Sinusitis
  peritoneum, peritoneal (perforated)
    (ruptured) K65.1
    with appendicitis K35.3
    pelvic
      female —see Peritonitis, pelvic, female
      male K65.1
    ⇨postoperative T81.4
    puerperal, postpartum, childbirth O85
    tuberculous A18.31
  peritonsillar J36
  perityphlic K35.3
  periureteral N28.89
  periurethral N34.0
    gonococcal (accessory gland) (periurethral)
      A54.1
  periuterine —see also Disease, pelvis,
    inflammatory N73.2
  perivesical —see Cystitis, specified type NEC
  petrous bone —see Petrositis
  phagedenic NOS L02.91
    chancroid A57
  pharynx, pharyngeal (lateral) J39.1
  pilonidal L05.01
  pituitary (gland) E23.6
  pleura J86.9
    with fistula J86.0
  popliteal —see Abscess, lower limb
  postcecal K35.3
  postlaryngeal J38.7
  postnasal J34.0
  ⇨postoperative (any site) T81.4
    retroperitoneal K68.11
  postpharyngeal J39.0
  posttonsillar J36
  post-typhoid A01.09
  pouch of Douglas —see Peritonitis, pelvic,
    female
  premammary —see Abscess, breast
  prepatellar —see Abscess, lower limb
  prostate N41.2
    gonococcal (acute) (chronic) A54.22
  psoas muscle K68.12
  puerperal - code by site under Puerperal,
    abscess
  pulmonary —see Abscess, lung
  pulp, pulpal (dental) K04.01
    irreversible K04.02
    reversible K04.01
  rectovaginal septum K63.0
  rectovesical —see Cystitis, specified type NEC
  rectum K61.1
  renal —see Abscess, kidney
  retina —see Inflammation, chorioretinal
  retrobulbar —see Abscess, orbit
  retrocecal K65.1
  retrolaryngeal J38.7
  retromammary —see Abscess, breast
  retroperitoneal NEC K68.19
    postprocedural K68.11
  retropharyngeal J39.0
  retrouterine —see Peritonitis, pelvic, female
  retrovesical —see Cystitis, specified type NEC
  root, tooth K04.7
    with sinus (alveolar) K04.6
  round ligament —see also Disease, pelvis,
    inflammatory N73.2
  rupture (spontaneous) NOS L02.91
  sacrum (tuberculous) A18.01
    nontuberculous M46.28
  salivary (duct) (gland) K11.3
  scalp (any part) L02.811
  scapular —see Osteomyelitis, specified type
    NEC
  sclera —see Scleritis
  scrofulous (tuberculous) A18.2
  scrotum N49.2

Abscess *(Continued)*
seminal vesicle N49.0
septal, dental K04.7
  with sinus (alveolar) K04.6
serous —*see* Periostitis
shoulder (region) —*see* Abscess, upper limb
sigmoid K63.0
sinus (accessory) (chronic) (nasal) —*see also*
  Sinusitis
  intracranial venous (any) G06.0
Skene's duct or gland N34.0
skin —*see* Abscess, by site
specified site NEC L02.818
spermatic cord N49.1
sphenoidal (sinus) (chronic) J32.3
spinal cord (any part) (staphylococcal) G06.1
  tuberculous A17.81
spine (column) (tuberculous) A18.01
  epidural G06.1
  nontuberculous —*see* Osteomyelitis,
    vertebra
spleen D73.3
  amebic A06.89
▶stitch T81.4
subarachnoid G06.2
  brain G06.0
  spinal cord G06.1
subareolar —*see* Abscess, breast
subcecal K35.3
subcutaneous —*see also* Abscess, by site
  pheomycotic (chromomycotic) B43.2
  ~~postprocedural T81.41~~
subdiaphragmatic K65.1
subdural G06.2
  brain G06.0
    sequelae G09
  spinal cord G06.1
subgaleal L02.811
subhepatic K65.1
sublingual K12.2
  gland K11.3
submammary —*see* Abscess, breast
submandibular (region) (space) (triangle) K12.2
  gland K11.3
submaxillary (region) L02.01
  gland K11.3
submental L02.01
  gland K11.3
subperiosteal —*see* Osteomyelitis, specified
  type NEC
subphrenic K65.1
▶postoperative T81.4
suburethral N34.0
sudoriparous L75.8
supraclavicular (fossa) —*see* Abscess, upper
  limb
suprapelvic, acute N73.0
suprarenal (capsule) (gland) E27.8
sweat gland L74.8
tear duct —*see* Inflammation, lacrimal,
  passages, acute
temple L02.01
temporal region L02.01
temporosphenoidal G06.0
tendon (sheath) M65.00
  ankle M65.07-●
  foot M65.07-●
  forearm M65.03-●
  hand M65.04-●
  lower leg M65.06-●
  pelvic region M65.05-●
  shoulder region M65.01-●
  specified site NEC M65.08
  thigh M65.05-●
  upper arm M65.02-●
testis N45.4
thigh —*see* Abscess, lower limb
thorax J86.9
  with fistula J86.0
throat J39.1
thumb —*see also* Abscess, hand
  nail —*see* Cellulitis, finger

Abscess *(Continued)*
thymus (gland) E32.1
thyroid (gland) E06.0
toe (any) —*see also* Abscess, foot
  nail —*see* Cellulitis, toe
tongue (staphylococcal) K14.0
tonsil(s) (lingual) J36
tonsillopharyngeal J36
tooth, teeth (root) K04.7
  with sinus (alveolar) K04.6
  supporting structures NEC —*see*
    Peridontitis, aggressive, localized
trachea J39.8
trunk L02.219
  abdominal wall L02.211
  back L02.212
  chest wall L02.213
  groin L02.214
  perineum L02.215
  umbilicus L02.216
tubal —*see* Salpingitis
tuberculous —*see* Tuberculosis, abscess
tubo-ovarian —*see* Salpingo-oophoritis
tunica vaginalis N49.1
umbilicus L02.216
upper
  limb L02.41-●
  respiratory J39.8
urethral (gland) N34.0
urinary N34.0
uterus, uterine (wall) —*see also* Endometritis
  ligament —*see also* Disease, pelvis,
    inflammatory N73.2
  neck —*see* Cervicitis
uvula K12.2
vagina (wall) —*see* Vaginitis
vaginorectal —*see* Vaginitis
vas deferens N49.1
vermiform appendix K35.3
vertebra (column) (tuberculous) A18.01
  nontuberculous —*see* Osteomyelitis,
    vertebra
vesical —*see* Cystitis, specified type NEC
vesico-uterine pouch —*see* Peritonitis, pelvic,
  female
vitreous (humor) —*see* Endophthalmitis,
  purulent
vocal cord J38.3
von Bezold's —*see* Mastoiditis, acute
vulva N76.4
vulvovaginal gland N75.1
web space —*see* Abscess, hand
▶wound T81.4
wrist —*see* Abscess, upper limb
Absence (of) (organ or part) (complete or
  partial)
adrenal (gland) (congenital) Q89.1
  acquired E89.6
albumin in blood E88.09
alimentary tract (congenital) Q45.8
  upper Q40.8
alveolar process (acquired) —*see* Anomaly,
  alveolar
ankle (acquired) Z89.44-●
anus (congenital) Q42.3
  with fistula Q42.2
aorta (congenital) Q25.41
appendix, congenital Q42.8
arm (acquired) Z89.20-●
  above elbow Z89.22-●
    congenital (with hand present) —*see*
      Agenesis, arm, with hand present
      and hand —*see* Agenesis, forearm,
      and hand
  below elbow Z89.21-●
    congenital (with hand present) —*see*
      Agenesis, arm, with hand present
      and hand —*see* Agenesis, forearm,
      and hand
  congenital —*see* Defect, reduction, upper
    limb

Absence *(Continued)*
arm *(Continued)*
  shoulder (following explantation of
    shoulder joint prosthesis) (joint) (with
    or without presence of antibiotic-
    impregnated cement spacer) Z89.23-●
  congenital (with hand present) —*see*
    Agenesis, arm, with hand present
artery (congenital) (peripheral) Q27.8
  brain Q28.3
  coronary Q24.5
  pulmonary Q25.79
  specified NEC Q27.8
  umbilical Q27.0
atrial septum (congenital) Q21.1
auditory canal (congenital) (external) Q16.1
auricle (ear), congenital Q16.0
bile, biliary duct, congenital Q44.5
bladder (acquired) Z90.6
  congenital Q64.5
bowel sounds R19.11
brain Q00.0
  part of Q04.3
breast(s) (and nipple(s)) (acquired) Z90.1-●
  congenital Q83.8
broad ligament Q50.6
bronchus (congenital) Q32.4
canaliculus lacrimalis, congenital Q10.4
cerebellum (vermis) Q04.3
cervix (acquired) (with uterus) Z90.710
  with remaining uterus Z90.712
  congenital Q51.5
chin, congenital Q18.8
cilia (congenital) Q10.3
  acquired —*see* Madarosis
clitoris (congenital) Q52.6
coccyx, congenital Q76.49
cold sense R20.8
congenital
  lumen —*see* Atresia
  organ or site NEC —*see* Agenesis
  septum —*see* Imperfect, closure
corpus callosum Q04.0
cricoid cartilage, congenital Q31.8
diaphragm (with hernia), congenital Q79.1
digestive organ(s) or tract, congenital Q45.8
  acquired NEC Z90.49
  upper Q40.8
ductus arteriosus Q28.8
duodenum (acquired) Z90.49
  congenital Q41.0
ear, congenital Q16.9
  acquired H93.8-●
  auricle Q16.0
  external Q16.0
  inner Q16.5
  lobe, lobule Q17.8
  middle, except ossicles Q16.4
    ossicles Q16.3
  ossicles Q16.3
ejaculatory duct (congenital) Q55.4
endocrine gland (congenital) NEC Q89.2
  acquired E89.89
epididymis (congenital) Q55.4
  acquired Z90.79
epiglottis, congenital Q31.8
esophagus (congenital) Q39.8
  acquired (partial) Z90.49
eustachian tube (congenital) Q16.2
extremity (acquired) Z89.9
  congenital Q73.0
  knee (following explantation of knee joint
    prosthesis) (joint) (with or without
    presence of antibiotic-impregnated
    cement spacer) Z89.52-●
  lower (above knee) Z89.619
    below knee Z89.51-●
  upper —*see* Absence, arm
eye (acquired) Z90.01
  congenital Q11.1
  muscle (congenital) Q10.3

Absence (Continued)
  eyeball (acquired) Z90.01
  eyelid (fold) (congenital) Q10.3
    acquired Z90.01
  face, specified part NEC Q18.8
  fallopian tube(s) (acquired) Z90.79
    congenital Q50.6
  family member (causing problem in home)
    NEC —see also Disruption, family Z63.32
  femur, congenital —see Defect, reduction,
    lower limb, longitudinal, femur
  fibrinogen (congenital) D68.2
    acquired D65
  finger(s) (acquired) Z89.02-●
    congenital —see Agenesis, hand
  foot (acquired) Z89.43-●
    congenital —see Agenesis, foot
  forearm (acquired) —see Absence, arm, below
    elbow
  gallbladder (acquired) Z90.49
    congenital Q44.0
  gamma globulin in blood D80.1
    hereditary D80.0
  genital organs
    acquired (female) (male) Z90.79
    female, congenital Q52.8
      external Q52.71
      internal NEC Q52.8
    male, congenital Q55.8
  genitourinary organs, congenital NEC
    female Q52.8
    male Q55.8
  globe (acquired) Z90.01
    congenital Q11.1
  glottis, congenital Q31.8
  hand and wrist (acquired) Z89.11-●
    congenital —see Agenesis, hand
  head, part (acquired) NEC Z90.09
  heat sense R20.8
  hip (following explantation of hip joint
    prosthesis) (joint) (with or without
    presence of antibiotic-impregnated
    cement spacer) Z89.62-●
  hymen (congenital) Q52.4
  ileum (acquired) Z90.49
    congenital Q41.2
  immunoglobulin, isolated NEC D80.3
    IgA D80.2
    IgG D80.3
    IgM D80.4
  incus (acquired) —see Loss, ossicles, ear
    congenital Q16.3
  inner ear, congenital Q16.5
  intestine (acquired) (small) Z90.49
    congenital Q41.9
      specified NEC Q41.8
    large Z90.49
      congenital Q42.9
        specified NEC Q42.8
  iris, congenital Q13.1
  jejunum (acquired) Z90.49
    congenital Q41.1
  joint
    acquired
      hip (following explantation of hip joint
        prosthesis) (with or without
        presence of antibiotic-impregnated
        cement spacer) Z89.62-●
      knee (following explantation of knee
        joint prosthesis) (with or without
        presence of antibiotic-impregnated
        cement spacer) Z89.52-●
      shoulder (following explantation of
        shoulder joint prosthesis) (with or
        without presence of antibiotic-
        impregnated cement spacer)
        Z89.23-●
    congenital NEC Q74.8
  kidney(s) (acquired) Z90.5
    congenital Q60.2
      bilateral Q60.1
      unilateral Q60.0

Absence (Continued)
  knee (following explantation of knee joint
    prosthesis) (joint) (with or without
    presence of antibiotic-impregnated
    cement spacer) Z89.52-●
  labyrinth, membranous Q16.5
  larynx (congenital) Q31.8
    acquired Z90.02
  leg (acquired) (above knee) Z89.61-●
    below knee (acquired) Z89.51-●
    congenital —see Defect, reduction, lower
      limb
  lens (acquired) —see also Aphakia
    congenital Q12.3
    post cataract extraction Z98.4-●
  limb (acquired) —see Absence, extremity
  lip Q38.6
  liver (congenital) Q44.7
  lung (fissure) (lobe) (bilateral) (unilateral)
    (congenital) Q33.3
    acquired (any part) Z90.2
  menstruation —see Amenorrhea
  muscle (congenital) (pectoral) Q79.8
    ocular Q10.3
  neck, part Q18.8
  neutrophil —see Agranulocytosis
  nipple(s) (with breast(s)) (acquired) Z90.1-●
    congenital Q83.2
  nose (congenital) Q30.1
    acquired Z90.09
  organ
    of Corti, congenital Q16.5
    or site, congenital NEC Q89.8
      acquired NEC Z90.89
  osseous meatus (ear) Q16.4
  ovary (acquired)
    bilateral Z90.722
    congenital
      bilateral Q50.02
      unilateral Q50.01
    unilateral Z90.721
  oviduct (acquired)
    bilateral Z90.722
    congenital Q50.6
    unilateral Z90.721
  pancreas (congenital) Q45.0
    acquired Z90.410
      complete Z90.410
      partial Z90.411
      total Z90.410
  parathyroid gland (acquired) E89.2
    congenital Q89.2
  patella, congenital Q74.1
  penis (congenital) Q55.5
    acquired Z90.79
  pericardium (congenital) Q24.8
  pituitary gland (congenital) Q89.2
    acquired E89.3
  prostate (acquired) Z90.79
    congenital Q55.4
  pulmonary valve Q22.0
  punctum lacrimale (congenital) Q10.4
  radius, congenital —see Defect, reduction,
    upper limb, longitudinal, radius
  rectum (congenital) Q42.1
    with fistula Q42.0
    acquired Z90.49
  respiratory organ NOS Q34.9
  rib (acquired) Z90.89
    congenital Q76.6
  sacrum, congenital Q76.49
  salivary gland(s), congenital Q38.4
  scrotum, congenital Q55.29
  seminal vesicles (congenital) Q55.4
    acquired Z90.79
  septum
    atrial (congenital) Q21.1
    between aorta and pulmonary artery Q21.4
    ventricular (congenital) Q20.4
  sex chromosome
    female phenotype Q97.8
    male phenotype Q98.8

Absence (Continued)
  skull bone (congenital) Q75.8
    with
      anencephaly Q00.0
      encephalocele —see Encephalocele
      hydrocephalus Q03.9
        with spina bifida —see Spina
          bifida, by site, with
          hydrocephalus
      microcephaly Q02
  spermatic cord, congenital Q55.4
  spine, congenital Q76.49
  spleen (congenital) Q89.01
    acquired Z90.81
  sternum, congenital Q76.7
  stomach (acquired) (partial) Z90.3
    congenital Q40.2
  superior vena cava, congenital
    Q26.8
  teeth, tooth (congenital) K00.0
    acquired (complete) K08.109
      class I K08.101
      class II K08.102
      class III K08.103
      class IV K08.104
      due to
        caries K08.139
          class I K08.131
          class II K08.132
          class III K08.133
          class IV K08.134
        periodontal disease K08.129
          class I K08.121
          class II K08.122
          class III K08.123
          class IV K08.124
        specified NEC K08.199
          class I K08.191
          class II K08.192
          class III K08.193
          class IV K08.194
        trauma K08.119
          class I K08.111
          class II K08.112
          class III K08.113
          class IV K08.114
    partial K08.409
      class I K08.401
      class II K08.402
      class III K08.403
      class IV K08.404
      due to
        caries K08.439
          class I K08.431
          class II K08.432
          class III K08.433
          class IV K08.434
        periodontal disease K08.429
          class I K08.421
          class II K08.422
          class III K08.423
          class IV K08.424
        specified NEC K08.499
          class I K08.491
          class II K08.492
          class III K08.493
          class IV K08.494
        trauma K08.419
          class I K08.411
          class II K08.412
          class III K08.413
          class IV K08.414
  tendon (congenital) Q79.8
  testis (congenital) Q55.0
    acquired Z90.79
  thumb (acquired) Z89.01-●
    congenital —see Agenesis, hand
  thymus gland Q89.2
  thyroid (gland) (acquired) E89.0
    cartilage, congenital Q31.8
    congenital E03.1

Absence *(Continued)*
   toe(s) (acquired) Z89.42-●
      with foot —*see* Absence, foot and
         ankle
      congenital —*see* Agenesis, foot
      great Z89.41-●
   tongue, congenital Q38.3
   trachea (cartilage), congenital Q32.1
   transverse aortic arch, congenital
      Q25.49
   tricuspid valve Q22.4
   umbilical artery, congenital Q27.0
   upper arm and forearm with hand present,
      congenital —*see* Agenesis, arm, with
      hand present
   ureter (congenital) Q62.4
      acquired Z90.6
   urethra, congenital Q64.5
   uterus (acquired) Z90.710
      with cervix Z90.710
      with remaining cervical stump
         Z90.711
      congenital Q51.0
   uvula, congenital Q38.5
   vagina, congenital Q52.0
   vas deferens (congenital) Q55.4
      acquired Z90.79
   vein (peripheral) congenital NEC
      Q27.8
      cerebral Q28.3
      digestive system Q27.8
      great Q26.8
      lower limb Q27.8
      portal Q26.5
      precerebral Q28.1
      specified site NEC Q27.8
      upper limb Q27.8
   vena cava (inferior) (superior), congenital
      Q26.8
   ventricular septum Q20.4
   vertebra, congenital Q76.49
   vulva, congenital Q52.71
   wrist (acquired) Z89.12-●
Absorbent system disease I87.8
Absorption
   carbohydrate, disturbance K90.49
   chemical —*see* Table of Drugs and
      Chemicals
      through placenta (newborn) P04.9
         environmental substance P04.6
         nutritional substance P04.5
         obstetric anesthetic or analgesic drug
            P04.0
   drug NEC —*see* Table of Drugs and
      Chemicals
      addictive
         through placenta (newborn) P04.49
            cocaine P04.41
      medicinal
         through placenta (newborn) P04.1
      through placenta (newborn) P04.1
         obstetric anesthetic or analgesic drug
            P04.0
   fat, disturbance K90.49
      pancreatic K90.3
   noxious substance —*see* Table of Drugs and
      Chemicals
   protein, disturbance K90.49
   starch, disturbance K90.49
   toxic substance —*see* Table of Drugs and
      Chemicals
   uremic —*see* Uremia
Abstinence symptoms, syndrome
   alcohol F10.239
      with delirium F10.231
   cocaine F14.23
   neonatal P96.1
   nicotine —*see* Dependence, drug, nicotine,
      with, withdrawal
   opioid F11.93
      with dependence F11.23

Abstinence symptoms, syndrome *(Continued)*
   psychoactive NEC F19.939
      with
         delirium F19.931
         dependence F19.239
            with
               delirium F19.231
               perceptual disturbance F19.232
            uncomplicated F19.230
         perceptual disturbance F19.932
      uncomplicated F19.930
   sedative F13.939
      with
         delirium F13.931
         dependence F13.239
            with
               delirium F13.231
               perceptual disturbance F13.232
            uncomplicated F13.230
         perceptual disturbance F13.932
      uncomplicated F13.930
   stimulant NEC F15.93
      with dependence F15.23
Abulia R68.89
Abulomania F60.7
Abuse
   adult —*see* Maltreatment, adult
      as reason for
         couple seeking advice (including
            offender) Z63.0
   alcohol (non-dependent) F10.10
      with
         anxiety disorder F10.180
         intoxication F10.129
            with delirium F10.121
            uncomplicated F10.120
         mood disorder F10.14
         other specified disorder F10.188
         psychosis F10.159
            delusions F10.150
            hallucinations F10.151
         sexual dysfunction F10.181
         sleep disorder F10.182
         unspecified disorder F10.19
      counseling and surveillance Z71.41
   ▶in remission (early) (sustained) F10.11
   amphetamine (or related substance) —*see*
      Abuse, drug, stimulant NEC
   analgesics (non-prescribed) (over the counter)
      F55.8
   antacids F55.0
   antidepressants —*see* Abuse, drug,
      psychoactive NEC
   anxiolytic —*see* Abuse, drug, sedative
   barbiturates —*see* Abuse, drug, sedative
   caffeine —*see* Abuse, drug, stimulant NEC
   cannabis, cannabinoids —*see* Abuse, drug,
      cannabis
   child —*see* Maltreatment, child
   cocaine —*see* Abuse, drug, cocaine
   drug NEC (non-dependent) F19.10
      with sleep disorder F19.182
      amphetamine type —*see* Abuse, drug,
         stimulant NEC
      analgesics (non-prescribed) (over the
         counter) F55.8
      antacids F55.0
      antidepressants —*see* Abuse, drug,
         psychoactive NEC
      anxiolytics —*see* Abuse, drug, sedative
      barbiturates —*see* Abuse, drug, sedative
      caffeine —*see* Abuse, drug, stimulant NEC
      cannabis F12.10
         with
            anxiety disorder F12.180
            intoxication F12.129
               with
                  delirium F12.121
                  perceptual disturbance F12.122
               uncomplicated F12.120
            other specified disorder F12.188

Abuse *(Continued)*
   drug NEC *(Continued)*
      cannabis *(Continued)*
         with *(Continued)*
            psychosis F12.159
               delusions F12.150
               hallucinations F12.151
            unspecified disorder F12.19
        ▶in remission (early) (sustained) F12.11
      cocaine F14.10
         with
            anxiety disorder F14.180
            intoxication F14.129
               with
                  delirium F14.121
                  perceptual disturbance F14.122
               uncomplicated F14.120
            mood disorder F14.14
            other specified disorder F14.188
            psychosis F14.159
               delusions F14.150
               hallucinations F14.151
            sexual dysfunction F14.181
            sleep disorder F14.182
            unspecified disorder F14.19
        ▶in remission (early) (sustained) F14.11
      counseling and surveillance Z71.51
      hallucinogen F16.10
         with
            anxiety disorder F16.180
            flashbacks F16.183
            intoxication F16.129
               with
                  delirium F16.121
                  perceptual disturbance F16.122
               uncomplicated F16.120
            mood disorder F16.14
            other specified disorder F16.188
            perception disorder, persisting
               F16.183
            psychosis F16.159
               delusions F16.150
               hallucinations F16.151
            unspecified disorder F16.19
        ▶in remission (early) (sustained) F16.11
      hashish —*see* Abuse, drug, cannabis
      herbal or folk remedies F55.1
      hormones F55.3
      hypnotics —*see* Abuse, drug, sedative
      inhalant F18.10
         with
            anxiety disorder F18.180
            dementia, persisting F18.17
            intoxication F18.129
               with delirium F18.121
               uncomplicated F18.120
            mood disorder F18.14
            other specified disorder F18.188
            psychosis F18.159
               delusions F18.150
               hallucinations F18.151
            unspecified disorder F18.19
        ▶in remission (early) (sustained) F18.11
      ▶in remission (early) (sustained) F19.11
      laxatives F55.2
      LSD —*see* Abuse, drug, hallucinogen
      marihuana —*see* Abuse, drug, cannabis
      morphine type (opioids) —*see* Abuse, drug,
         opioid
      opioid F11.10
         with
            intoxication F11.129
               with
                  delirium F11.121
                  perceptual disturbance F11.122
               uncomplicated F11.120
            mood disorder F11.14
            other specified disorder F11.188
            psychosis F11.159
               delusions F11.150
               hallucinations F11.151

   ▶ New   ➡ Revised   ~~deleted~~ Deleted   ● Use Additional Character(s)

Abuse *(Continued)*
  drug NEC *(Continued)*
    opioid *(Continued)*
      with *(Continued)*
        sexual dysfunction F11.181
        sleep disorder F11.182
        unspecified disorder F11.19
      ▶in remission (early) (sustained) F11.11
      PCP (phencyclidine) (or related substance) —
        see Abuse, drug, hallucinogen
      psychoactive NEC F19.10
        with
          amnestic disorder F19.16
          anxiety disorder F19.180
          dementia F19.17
          intoxication F19.129
            with
              delirium F19.121
              perceptual disturbance F19.122
            uncomplicated F19.120
          mood disorder F19.14
          other specified disorder F19.188
          psychosis F19.159
            delusions F19.150
            hallucinations F19.151
          sexual dysfunction F19.181
          sleep disorder F19.182
          unspecified disorder F19.19
    sedative, hypnotic or anxiolytic F13.10
      with
        anxiety disorder F13.180
        intoxication F13.129
          with delirium F13.121
          uncomplicated F13.120
        mood disorder F13.14
        other specified disorder F13.188
        psychosis F13.159
          delusions F13.150
          hallucinations F13.151
        sexual dysfunction F13.181
        sleep disorder F13.182
        unspecified disorder F13.19
    ▶in remission (early) (sustained) F13.11
    solvent —*see* Abuse, drug, inhalant
    steroids F55.3
    stimulant NEC F15.10
      with
        anxiety disorder F15.180
        intoxication F15.129
          with
            delirium F15.121
            perceptual disturbance F15.122
          uncomplicated F15.120
        mood disorder F15.14
        other specified disorder F15.188
        psychosis F15.159
          delusions F15.150
          hallucinations F15.151
        sexual dysfunction F15.181
        sleep disorder F15.182
        unspecified disorder F15.19
    ▶in remission (early) (sustained) F15.11
    tranquilizers —*see* Abuse, drug, sedative
    vitamins F55.4
  hallucinogens —*see* Abuse, drug, hallucinogen
  hashish —*see* Abuse, drug, cannabis
  herbal or folk remedies F55.1
  hormones F55.3
  hypnotic —*see* Abuse, drug, sedative
  inhalant —*see* Abuse, drug, inhalant
  laxatives F55.2
  LSD —*see* Abuse, drug, hallucinogen
  marihuana —*see* Abuse, drug, cannabis
  morphine type (opioids) —*see* Abuse, drug,
    opioid
  non-psychoactive substance NEC F55.8
    antacids F55.0
    folk remedies F55.1
    herbal remedies F55.1
    hormones F55.3
    laxatives F55.2

Abuse *(Continued)*
  non-psychoactive substance NEC *(Continued)*
    steroids F55.3
    vitamins F55.4
  opioids —*see* Abuse, drug, opioid
  PCP (phencyclidine) (or related substance) —
    see Abuse, drug, hallucinogen
  physical (adult) (child) —*see* Maltreatment
  psychoactive substance —*see* Abuse, drug,
    psychoactive NEC
  psychological (adult) (child) —*see* Maltreatment
  sedative —*see* Abuse, drug, sedative
  sexual —*see* Maltreatment
  solvent —*see* Abuse, drug, inhalant
  steroids F55.3
  vitamins F55.4
Acalculia R48.8
  developmental F81.2
Acanthamebiasis (with) B60.10
  conjunctiva B60.12
  keratoconjunctivitis B60.13
  meningoencephalitis B60.11
  other specified B60.19
Acanthocephaliasis B83.8
Acanthocheilonemiasis B74.4
Acanthocytosis E78.6
Acantholysis L11.9
Acanthosis (acquired) (nigricans) L83
  benign Q82.8
  congenital Q82.8
  seborrheic L82.1
    inflamed L82.0
  tongue K14.3
Acapnia E87.3
Acarbia E87.2
Acardia, acardius Q89.8
Acardiacus amorphus Q89.8
Acardiotrophia I51.4
Acariasis B88.0
  scabies B86
Acarodermatitis (urticarioides) B88.0
Acarophobia F40.218
Acatalasemia, acatalasia E80.3
Acathisia (drug induced) G25.71
Accelerated atrioventricular conduction I45.6
Accentuation of personality traits (type A) Z73.1
Accessory (congenital)
  adrenal gland Q89.1
  anus Q43.4
  appendix Q43.4
  atrioventricular conduction I45.6
  auditory ossicles Q16.3
  auricle (ear) Q17.0
  biliary duct or passage Q44.5
  bladder Q64.79
  blood vessels NEC Q27.9
    coronary Q24.5
  bone NEC Q79.8
  breast tissue, axilla Q83.1
  carpal bones Q74.0
  cecum Q43.4
  chromosome(s) NEC (nonsex) Q92.9
    with complex rearrangements NEC Q92.5
      seen only at prometaphase Q92.8
    13 —*see* Trisomy, 13
    18 —*see* Trisomy, 18
    21 —*see* Trisomy, 21
    partial Q92.9
    sex
      female phenotype Q97.8
  coronary artery Q24.5
  cusp(s), heart valve NEC Q24.8
    pulmonary Q22.3
  cystic duct Q44.5
  digit(s) Q69.9
  ear (auricle) (lobe) Q17.0
  endocrine gland NEC Q89.2
  eye muscle Q10.3
  eyelid Q10.3
  face bone(s) Q75.8
  fallopian tube (fimbria) (ostium) Q50.6

Accessory *(Continued)*
  finger(s) Q69.0
  foreskin N47.8
  frontonasal process Q75.8
  gallbladder Q44.1
  genital organ(s)
    female Q52.8
      external Q52.79
      internal NEC Q52.8
    male Q55.8
  genitourinary organs NEC Q89.8
    female Q52.8
    male Q55.8
  hallux Q69.2
  heart Q24.8
    valve NEC Q24.8
      pulmonary Q22.3
  hepatic ducts Q44.5
  hymen Q52.4
  intestine (large) (small) Q43.4
  kidney Q63.0
  lacrimal canal Q10.6
  leaflet, heart valve NEC Q24.8
  ligament, broad Q50.6
  liver Q44.7
    duct Q44.5
  lobule (ear) Q17.0
  lung (lobe) Q33.1
  muscle Q79.8
  navicular of carpus Q74.0
  nervous system, part NEC Q07.8
  nipple Q83.3
  nose Q30.8
  organ or site not listed —*see* Anomaly, by site
  ovary Q50.31
  oviduct Q50.6
  pancreas Q45.3
  parathyroid gland Q89.2
  parotid gland (and duct) Q38.4
  pituitary gland Q89.2
  preauricular appendage Q17.0
  prepuce N47.8
  renal arteries (multiple) Q27.2
  rib Q76.6
    cervical Q76.5
  roots (teeth) K00.2
  salivary gland Q38.4
  sesamoid bones Q74.8
    foot Q74.2
    hand Q74.0
  skin tags Q82.8
  spleen Q89.09
  sternum Q76.7
  submaxillary gland Q38.4
  tarsal bones Q74.2
  teeth, tooth K00.1
  tendon Q79.8
  thumb Q69.1
  thymus gland Q89.2
  thyroid gland Q89.2
  toes Q69.2
  tongue Q38.3
  tooth, teeth K00.1
  tragus Q17.0
  ureter Q62.5
  urethra Q64.79
  urinary organ or tract NEC Q64.8
  uterus Q51.2
  vagina Q52.10
  valve, heart NEC Q24.8
    pulmonary Q22.3
  vertebra Q76.49
  vocal cords Q31.8
  vulva Q52.79
Accident
  birth —*see* Birth, injury
  cardiac —*see* Infarct, myocardium
  cerebral I63.9
  cerebrovascular (embolic) (ischemic)
    (thrombotic) I63.9
    aborted I63.9

Accident *(Continued)*
  cerebrovascular *(Continued)*
    hemorrhagic —*see* Hemorrhage,
      intracranial, intracerebral
    old (without sequelae) Z86.73
      with sequelae (of) —*see* Sequelae,
        infarction, cerebral
    coronary —*see* Infarct, myocardium
    craniovascular I63.9
    vascular, brain I63.9
Accidental —*see* condition
Accommodation (disorder) —*see also* condition
  hysterical paralysis of F44.89
  insufficiency of H52.4
  paresis —*see* Paresis, of accommodation
  spasm —*see* Spasm, of accommodation
Accouchement —*see* Delivery
Accreta placenta O43.21-•
Accretio cordis (nonrheumatic) I31.0
Accretions, tooth, teeth K03.6
Acculturation difficulty Z60.3
Accumulation secretion, prostate N42.89
Acephalia, acephalism, acephalus, acephaly
  Q00.0
Acephalobrachia monster Q89.8
Acephalochirus monster Q89.8
Acephalogaster Q89.8
Acephalostomus monster Q89.8
Acephalothorax Q89.8
Acerophobia F40.298
Acetonemia R79.89
  in Type 1 diabetes E10.10
    with coma E10.11
Acetonuria R82.4
Achalasia (cardia) (esophagus) K22.0
  congenital Q39.5
  pylorus Q40.0
  sphincteral NEC K59.8
Ache(s) —*see* Pain
Acheilia Q38.6
Achillobursitis —*see* Tendinitis, Achilles
Achillodynia —*see* Tendinitis, Achilles
Achlorhydria, achlorhydric (neurogenic) K31.83
  anemia D50.8
  diarrhea K31.83
  psychogenic F45.8
  secondary to vagotomy K91.1
Achluophobia F40.228
Acholia K82.8
Acholuric jaundice (familial)
  (splenomegalic) —*see also* Spherocytosis
  acquired D59.8
Achondrogenesis Q77.0
Achondroplasia (osteosclerosis congenita) Q77.4
Achroma, cutis L80
Achromat (ism), achromatopsia (acquired)
  (congenital) H53.51
Achromia, congenital —*see* Albinism
Achromia parasitica B36.0
Achylia gastrica K31.89
  psychogenic F45.8
Acid
  burn —*see* Corrosion
  deficiency
    amide nicotinic E52
    ascorbic E54
    folic E53.8
    nicotinic E52
    pantothenic E53.8
  intoxication E87.2
  peptic disease K30
  phosphatase deficiency E83.39
  stomach K30
    psychogenic F45.8
Acidemia E87.2
  argininosuccinic E72.22
  isovaleric E71.110
  metabolic (newborn) P19.9
    first noted before onset of labor P19.0
    first noted during labor P19.1
    noted at birth P19.2

Acidemia *(Continued)*
  methylmalonic E71.120
  pipecolic E72.3
  propionic E71.121
Acidity, gastric (high) K30
  psychogenic F45.8
Acidocytopenia —*see* Agranulocytosis
Acidocytosis D72.1
Acidopenia —*see* Agranulocytosis
Acidosis (lactic) (respiratory) E87.2
  in Type 1 diabetes E10.10
    with coma E10.11
  kidney, tubular N25.89
  lactic E87.2
  metabolic NEC E87.2
    with respiratory acidosis E87.4
    late, of newborn P74.0
  mixed metabolic and respiratory,
    newborn P84
  newborn P84
  renal (hyperchloremic) (tubular)
    N25.89
  respiratory E87.2
    complicated by
      metabolic
        acidosis E87.4
        alkalosis E87.4
Aciduria
  argininosuccinic E72.22
  glutaric (type I) E72.3
    type II E71.313
    type III E71.5-•
  orotic (congenital) (hereditary) (pyrimidine
    deficiency) E79.8
    anemia D53.0
Acladiosis (skin) B36.0
Aclasis, diaphyseal Q78.6
Acleistocardia Q21.1
Aclusion —*see* Anomaly, dentofacial,
  malocclusion
Acne L70.9
  artificialis L70.8
  atrophica L70.2
  cachecticorum (Hebra) L70.8
  conglobata L70.1
  cystic L70.0
  decalvans L66.2
  excoriée (des jeunes filles) L70.5
  frontalis L70.2
  indurata L70.0
  infantile L70.4
  keloid L73.0
  lupoid L70.2
  necrotic, necrotica (miliaris) L70.2
  neonatal L70.4
  nodular L70.0
  occupational L70.8
  picker's L70.5
  pustular L70.0
  rodens L70.2
  rosacea L71.9
  specified NEC L70.8
  tropica L70.3
  varioliformis L70.2
  vulgaris L70.0
Acnitis (primary) A18.4
Acosta's disease T70.29
Acoustic —*see* condition
Acousticophobia F40.298
Acquired —*see also* condition
  immunodeficiency syndrome (AIDS)
    B20
Acrania Q00.0
Acroangiodermatitis I78.9
Acroasphyxia, chronic I73.89
Acrobystitis N47.7
Acrocephalopolysyndactyly Q87.0
Acrocephalosyndactyly Q87.0
Acrocephaly Q75.0
Acrochondrohyperplasia —*see* Syndrome,
  Marfan's

Acrocyanosis I73.8
  newborn P28.2
    meaning transient blue hands and feet -
      omit code
Acrodermatitis L30.8
  atrophicans (chronica) L90.4
  continua (Hallopeau) L40.2
  enteropathica (hereditary) E83.2
  Hallopeau's L40.2
  infantile papular L44.4
  perstans L40.2
  pustulosa continua L40.2
  recalcitrant pustular L40.2
Acrodynia —*see* Poisoning, mercury
Acromegaly, acromegalia E22.0
Acromelalgia I73.81
Acromicria, acromikria Q79.8
Acronyx L60.0
Acropachy, thyroid —*see* Thyrotoxicosis
Acroparesthesia (simple) (vasomotor) I73.89
Acropathy, thyroid —*see* Thyrotoxicosis
Acrophobia F40.241
Acroposthitis N47.7
Acroscleriasis, acroscleroderma,
  acrosclerosis —*see* Sclerosis, systemic
Acrosphacelus I96
Acrospiroma, eccrine —*see* Neoplasm, skin,
  benign
Acrostealgia —*see* Osteochondropathy
Acrotrophodynia —*see* Immersion
ACTH ectopic syndrome E24.3
Actinic —*see* condition
Actinobacillosis, actinobacillus A28.8
  mallei A24.0
  muris A25.1
Actinomyces israelii (infection) —*see*
  Actinomycosis
Actinomycetoma (foot) B47.1
Actinomycosis, actinomycotic A42.9
  with pneumonia A42.0
  abdominal A42.1
  cervicofacial A42.2
  cutaneous A42.89
  gastrointestinal A42.1
  pulmonary A42.0
  sepsis A42.7
  specified site NEC A42.89
Actinoneuritis G62.82
Action, heart
  disorder I49.9
  irregular I49.9
    psychogenic F45.8
Activated protein C resistance D68.51
Activation
  mast cell (disorder) (syndrome) D89.40
    idiopathic D89.42
    monoclonal D89.41
    secondary D89.43
    specified type NEC D89.49
Active —*see* condition
Acute —*see also* condition
  abdomen R10.0
  gallbladder —*see* Cholecystitis, acute
Acyanotic heart disease (congenital) Q24.9
Acystia Q64.5
Adair-Dighton syndrome (brittle bones and
  blue sclera, deafness) Q78.0
Adamantinoblastoma —*see* Ameloblastoma
Adamantinoma —*see also* Cyst, calcifying
  odontogenic
  long bones C40.90
    lower limb C40.2-•
    upper limb C40.0-•
  malignant C41.1
    jaw (bone) (lower) C41.1
      upper C41.0
  tibial C40.2-•
Adamantoblastoma —*see* Ameloblastoma
Adams-Stokes (-Morgagni) disease or
  syndrome I45.9
Adaption reaction —*see* Disorder, adjustment

▶ New   ⇒ Revised   ~~deleted~~ Deleted   • Use Additional Character(s)

Addiction —*see also* Dependence F19.20
  alcohol, alcoholic (ethyl) (methyl) (wood)
      (without remission) F10.20
    with remission F10.21
  drug —*see* Dependence, drug
  ethyl alcohol (without remission) F10.20
    with remission F10.21
  heroin —*see* Dependence, drug, opioid
  methyl alcohol (without remission) F10.20
    with remission F10.21
  methylated spirit (without remission) F10.20
    with remission F10.21
  morphine(-like substances) —*see*
      Dependence, drug, opioid
  nicotine —*see* Dependence, drug, nicotine
  opium and opioids —*see* Dependence, drug,
      opioid
  tobacco —*see* Dependence, drug, nicotine
Addisonian crisis E27.2
Addison's
  anemia (pernicious) D51.0
  disease (bronze) or syndrome E27.1
    tuberculous A18.7
  keloid L94.0
Addison-Biermer anemia (pernicious) D51.0
Addison-Schilder complex E71.528
Additional —*see also* Accessory
  chromosome(s) Q99.8
    21 —*see* Trisomy, 21
    sex —*see* Abnormal, chromosome, sex
Adduction contracture, hip or other joint —*see*
    Contraction, joint
Adenitis —*see also* Lymphadenitis
  acute, unspecified site L04.9
  axillary I88.9
    acute L04.2
    chronic or subacute I88.1
  Bartholin's gland N75.8
  bulbourethral gland —*see* Urethritis
  cervical I88.9
    acute L04.0
    chronic or subacute I88.1
  chancroid (Hemophilus ducreyi) A57
  chronic, unspecified site I88.1
  Cowper's gland —*see* Urethritis
  due to Pasteurella multocida (P. septica)
      A28.0
  epidemic, acute B27.09
  gangrenous L04.9
  gonorrheal NEC A54.89
  groin I88.9
    acute L04.1
    chronic or subacute I88.1
  infectious (acute) (epidemic) B27.09
  inguinal I88.9
    acute L04.1
    chronic or subacute I88.1
  lymph gland or node, except mesenteric I88.9
    acute —*see* Lymphadenitis, acute
    chronic or subacute I88.1
  mesenteric (acute) (chronic) (nonspecific)
      (subacute) I88.0
  parotid gland (suppurative) —*see* Sialoadenitis
  salivary gland (any) (suppurative) —*see*
      Sialoadenitis
  scrofulous (tuberculous) A18.2
  Skene's duct or gland —*see* Urethritis
  strumous, tuberculous A18.2
  subacute, unspecified site I88.1
  sublingual gland (suppurative) —*see*
      Sialoadenitis
  submandibular gland (suppurative) —*see*
      Sialoadenitis
  submaxillary gland (suppurative) —*see*
      Sialoadenitis
  tuberculous —*see* Tuberculosis, lymph gland
  urethral gland —*see* Urethritis
  Wharton's duct (suppurative) —*see*
      Sialoadenitis
Adenoacanthoma —*see* Neoplasm, malignant,
    by site

Adenoameloblastoma —*see* Cyst, calcifying
    odontogenic
Adenocarcinoid (tumor) —*see* Neoplasm,
    malignant, by site
Adenocarcinoma —*see also* Neoplasm,
    malignant, by site
  acidophil
    specified site —*see* Neoplasm, malignant,
        by site
    unspecified site C75.1
  adrenal cortical C74.0-●
  alveolar —*see* Neoplasm, lung, malignant
  apocrine
    breast —*see* Neoplasm, breast, malignant
    in situ
      breast D05.8-●
      specified site NEC —*see* Neoplasm, skin,
          in situ
      unspecified site D04.9
    specified site NEC —*see* Neoplasm, skin,
        malignant
    unspecified site C44.99
  basal cell
    specified site —*see* Neoplasm, skin,
        malignant
    unspecified site C08.9
  basophil
    specified site —*see* Neoplasm, malignant,
        by site
    unspecified site C75.1
  bile duct type C22.1
    liver C22.1
    specified site NEC —*see* Neoplasm,
        malignant, by site
    unspecified site C22.1
  bronchiolar —*see* Neoplasm, lung, malignant
  bronchioloalveolar —*see* Neoplasm, lung,
      malignant
  ceruminous C44.29-●
  cervix, in situ (*see also* Carcinoma, cervix
      uteri, in situ) D06.9
  chromophobe
    specified site —*see* Neoplasm, malignant,
        by site
    unspecified site C75.1
  diffuse type
    specified site —*see* Neoplasm, malignant,
        by site
    unspecified site C16.9
  duct
    infiltrating
      with Paget's disease —*see* Neoplasm,
          breast, malignant
      specified site —*see* Neoplasm,
          malignant, by site
      unspecified site (female) C50.91-●
        male C50.92-●
    specified site —*see* Neoplasm, malignant,
        by site
    unspecified site
      female C56.9
      male C61
  eosinophil
    specified site —*see* Neoplasm, malignant,
        by site
    unspecified site C75.1
  follicular
    with papillary C73
    moderately differentiated C73
    specified site —*see* Neoplasm, malignant,
        by site
    trabecular C73
    unspecified site C73
    well differentiated C73
  Hurthle cell C73
  in
    adenomatous
      polyposis coli C18.9
  infiltrating duct
    with Paget's disease —*see* Neoplasm,
        breast, malignant

Adenocarcinoma (*Continued*)
  infiltrating duct (*Continued*)
    specified site —*see* Neoplasm, malignant,
        by site
    unspecified site (female) C50.91-●
      male C50.92-●
  inflammatory
    specified site —*see* Neoplasm, malignant,
        by site
    unspecified site (female) C50.91-●
      male C50.92-●
  intestinal type
    specified site —*see* Neoplasm, malignant,
        by site
    unspecified site C16.9
  intracystic papillary
  intraductal
    breast D05.1-●
    noninfiltrating
      breast D05.1-●
      papillary
        with invasion
          specified site —*see* Neoplasm,
              malignant, by site
          unspecified site (female) C50.91-●
            male C50.92-●
        breast D05.1-●
        specified site NEC —*see* Neoplasm, in
            situ, by site
        unspecified site D05.1-●
    specified site NEC —*see* Neoplasm, in
        situ, by site
    unspecified site D05.1-●
    papillary
      with invasion
        specified site —*see* Neoplasm,
            malignant, by site
        unspecified site (female) C50.91-●
          male C50.92-●
      breast D05.1-●
      specified site —*see* Neoplasm, in situ,
          by site
      unspecified site D05.1-●
    specified site NEC —*see* Neoplasm, in situ,
        by site
    unspecified site D05.1-●
  islet cell
    with exocrine, mixed
      specified site —*see* Neoplasm,
          malignant, by site
      unspecified site C25.9
    pancreas C25.4
    specified site NEC —*see* Neoplasm,
        malignant, by site
    unspecified site C25.4
  lobular
    in situ
      breast D05.0-●
      specified site NEC —*see* Neoplasm, in
          situ, by site
      unspecified site D05.0-●
    specified site —*see* Neoplasm, malignant,
        by site
    unspecified site (female) C50.91-●
      male C50.92-●
  mucoid —*see also* Neoplasm, malignant, by site
    cell
      specified site —*see* Neoplasm,
          malignant, by site
      unspecified site C75.1
  nonencapsulated sclerosing C73
  papillary
    with follicular C73
    follicular variant C73
    intraductal (noninfiltrating)
      with invasion
        specified site —*see* Neoplasm,
            malignant, by site
        unspecified site (female) C50.91-●
          male C50.92-●
      breast D05.1-●

Adenocarcinoma *(Continued)*
 papillary *(Continued)*
  intraductal *(Continued)*
   specified site NEC —*see* Neoplasm, in situ, by site
   unspecified site D05.1-●
  serous
   specified site —*see* Neoplasm, malignant, by site
   unspecified site C56.9
  papillocystic
   specified site —*see* Neoplasm, malignant, by site
   unspecified site C56.9
  pseudomucinous
   specified site —*see* Neoplasm, malignant, by site
   unspecified site C56.9
  renal cell C64-●
  sebaceous —*see* Neoplasm, skin, malignant, by site
  serous —*see also* Neoplasm, malignant, by site
   papillary
    specified site —*see* Neoplasm, malignant, by site
    unspecified site C56.9
  sweat gland —*see* Neoplasm, skin, malignant
  water-clear cell C75.0
Adenocarcinoma-in-situ —*see also* Neoplasm, in situ, by site
 breast D05.9-●
Adenofibroma
 clear cell —*see* Neoplasm, benign, by site
 endometrioid D27.9
  borderline malignancy D39.10
  malignant C56-●
 mucinous
  specified site —*see* Neoplasm, benign, by site
  unspecified site D27.9
 papillary
  specified site —*see* Neoplasm, benign, by site
  unspecified site D27.9
 prostate —*see* Enlargement, enlarged, prostate
 serous
  specified site —*see* Neoplasm, benign, by site
  unspecified site D27.9
 specified site —*see* Neoplasm, benign, by site
 unspecified site D27.9
Adenofibrosis
 breast —*see* Fibroadenosis, breast
 endometrioid N80.0
Adenoiditis (chronic) J35.02
 with tonsillitis J35.03
 acute J03.90
  recurrent J03.91
  specified organism NEC J03.80
   recurrent J03.81
  staphylococcal J03.80
   recurrent J03.81
  streptococcal J03.00
   recurrent J03.01
Adenoids —*see* condition
Adenolipoma —*see* Neoplasm, benign, by site
Adenolipomatosis, Launois-Bensaude E88.89
Adenolymphoma
 specified site —*see* Neoplasm, benign, by site
 unspecified site D11.9
Adenoma —*see also* Neoplasm, benign, by site
 acidophil
  specified site —*see* Neoplasm, benign, by site
  unspecified site D35.2
 acidophil-basophil, mixed
  specified site —*see* Neoplasm, benign, by site
  unspecified site D35.2

Adenoma *(Continued)*
 adrenal (cortical) D35.00
  clear cell D35.00
  compact cell D35.00
  glomerulosa cell D35.00
  heavily pigmented variant D35.00
  mixed cell D35.00
 alpha-cell
  pancreas D13.7
  specified site NEC —*see* Neoplasm, benign, by site
  unspecified site D13.7
 alveolar D14.30
 apocrine
  breast D24-●
  specified site NEC —*see* Neoplasm, skin, benign, by site
  unspecified site D23.9
 basal cell D11.9
 basophil
  specified site —*see* Neoplasm, benign, by site
  unspecified site D35.2
 basophil-acidophil, mixed
  specified site —*see* Neoplasm, benign, by site
  unspecified site D35.2
 beta-cell
  pancreas D13.7
  specified site NEC —*see* Neoplasm, benign, by site
  unspecified site D13.7
 bile duct D13.4
  common D13.5
  extrahepatic D13.5
  intrahepatic D13.4
  specified site NEC —*see* Neoplasm, benign, by site
  unspecified site D13.4
 black D35.00
 bronchial D38.1
  cylindroid type —*see* Neoplasm, lung, malignant
 ceruminous D23.2-●
 chief cell D35.1
 chromophobe
  specified site —*see* Neoplasm, benign, by site
  unspecified site D35.2
 colloid
  specified site —*see* Neoplasm, benign, by site
  unspecified site D34
 duct
 eccrine, papillary —*see* Neoplasm, skin, benign
 endocrine, multiple
  single specified site —*see* Neoplasm, uncertain behavior, by site
  two or more specified sites D44-●
  unspecified site D44.9
 endometrioid —*see also* Neoplasm, benign
  borderline malignancy —*see* Neoplasm, uncertain behavior, by site
 eosinophil
  specified site —*see* Neoplasm, malignant, by site
  unspecified site D35.2
 fetal
  specified site —*see* Neoplasm, benign, by site
  unspecified site D34
 follicular
  specified site —*see* Neoplasm, benign, by site
  unspecified site D34
 hepatocellular D13.4
 Hurthle cell D34
 islet cell
  pancreas D13.7
  specified site NEC —*see* Neoplasm, benign, by site
  unspecified site D13.7

Adenoma *(Continued)*
 liver cell D13.4
 macrofollicular
  specified site —*see* Neoplasm, benign, by site
  unspecified site D34
 malignant, malignum —*see* Neoplasm, malignant, by site
 microcystic
  pancreas D13.6
  specified site NEC —*see* Neoplasm, benign, by site
  unspecified site D13.6
 microfollicular
  specified site —*see* Neoplasm, benign, by site
  unspecified site D34
 mucoid cell
  specified site —*see* Neoplasm, benign, by site
  unspecified site D35.2
 multiple endocrine
  single specified site —*see* Neoplasm, uncertain behavior, by site
  two or more specified sites D44-●
  unspecified site D44.9
 nipple D24-●
 papillary —*see also* Neoplasm, benign, by site
  eccrine —*see* Neoplasm, skin, benign, by site
 Pick's tubular
  specified site —*see* Neoplasm, benign, by site
  unspecified site
   female D27.9
   male D29.20
 pleomorphic
  carcinoma in —*see* Neoplasm, salivary gland, malignant
   specified site —*see* Neoplasm, malignant, by site
   unspecified site C08.9
 polypoid —*see also* Neoplasm, benign
  adenocarcinoma in —*see* Neoplasm, malignant, by site
  adenocarcinoma in situ —*see* Neoplasm, in situ, by site
 prostate —*see* Neoplasm, benign, prostate
 rete cell D29.20
 sebaceous —*see* Neoplasm, skin, benign
 Sertoli cell
  specified site —*see* Neoplasm, benign, by site
  unspecified site
   female D27.9
   male D29.20
 skin appendage —*see* Neoplasm, skin, benign
 sudoriferous gland —*see* Neoplasm, skin, benign
 sweat gland —*see* Neoplasm, skin, benign
 testicular
  specified site —*see* Neoplasm, benign, by site
  unspecified site
   female D27.9
   male D29.20
 tubular —*see also* Neoplasm, benign, by site
  adenocarcinoma in —*see* Neoplasm, malignant, by site
  adenocarcinoma in situ —*see* Neoplasm, in situ, by site
  Pick's
   specified site —*see* Neoplasm, benign
   unspecified site
    female D27.9
    male D29.20
 tubulovillous —*see also* Neoplasm, benign, by site
  adenocarcinoma in —*see* Neoplasm, malignant, by site
  adenocarcinoma in situ —*see* Neoplasm, in situ, by site

► New ⇒ Revised ~~deleted~~ Deleted ● Use Additional Character(s)

Adenoma *(Continued)*
  villous —*see* Neoplasm, uncertain behavior,
    by site
    adenocarcinoma in —*see* Neoplasm,
      malignant, by site
    adenocarcinoma in situ —*see* Neoplasm, in
      situ, by site
  water-clear cell D35.1
Adenomatosis
  endocrine (multiple) E31.20
    single specified site —*see* Neoplasm,
      uncertain behavior, by site
  erosive of nipple D24-●
  pluriendocrine —*see* Adenomatosis,
    endocrine
  pulmonary D38.1
    malignant —*see* Neoplasm, lung,
      malignant
  specified site —*see* Neoplasm, benign, by site
  unspecified site D12.6
Adenomatous
  goiter (nontoxic) E04.9
    with hyperthyroidism —*see* Hyper-
      thyroidism, with, goiter, nodular
    toxic —*see* Hyperthyroidism, with, goiter,
      nodular
Adenomyoma —*see also* Neoplasm, benign, by
  site
  prostate —*see* Enlarged, prostate
Adenomyometritis N80.0
Adenomyosis N80.0
Adenopathy (lymph gland) R59.9
  generalized R59.1
  inguinal R59.0
  localized R59.0
  mediastinal R59.0
  mesentery R59.0
  syphilitic (secondary) A51.49
  tracheobronchial R59.0
    tuberculous A15.4
      primary (progressive) A15.7
  tuberculous —*see also* Tuberculosis, lymph
    gland
    tracheobronchial A15.4
      primary (progressive) A15.7
Adenosalpingitis —*see* Salpingitis
Adenosarcoma —*see* Neoplasm, malignant, by
  site
Adenosclerosis I88.8
Adenosis (sclerosing) **breast** —*see*
  Fibroadenosis, breast
Adenovirus, as cause of disease classified
  elsewhere B97.0
Adentia (complete) (partial) —*see* Absence,
  teeth
Adherent —*see also* Adhesions
  labia (minora) N90.89
  pericardium (nonrheumatic) I31.0
    rheumatic I09.2
  placenta (with hemorrhage) O72.0
    without hemorrhage O73.0
  prepuce, newborn N47.0
  scar (skin) L90.5
  tendon in scar L90.5
Adhesions, adhesive (postinfective) K66.0
  ⇒with intestinal obstruction K56.50
    ▶complete K56.52
    ▶incomplete K56.51
    ▶partial K56.51
  abdominal (wall) —*see* Adhesions, peritoneum
  appendix K38.8
  bile duct (common) (hepatic) K83.8
  bladder (sphincter) N32.89
  bowel —*see* Adhesions, peritoneum
  cardiac I31.0
    rheumatic I09.2
  cecum —*see* Adhesions, peritoneum
  cervicovaginal N88.1
    congenital Q52.8
    postpartal O90.89
      old N88.1

Adhesions, adhesive *(Continued)*
  cervix N88.1
  ciliary body NEC —*see* Adhesions, iris
  clitoris N90.89
  colon —*see* Adhesions, peritoneum
  common duct K83.8
  congenital —*see also* Anomaly, by site
    fingers —*see* Syndactylism, complex, fingers
    omental, anomalous Q43.3
    peritoneal Q43.3
    tongue (to gum or roof of mouth) Q38.3
  conjunctiva (acquired) H11.21-●
    congenital Q15.8
  cystic duct K82.8
  diaphragm —*see* Adhesions, peritoneum
  due to foreign body —*see* Foreign body
  duodenum —*see* Adhesions, peritoneum
  ear
    middle H74.1-●
  epididymis N50.89
  epidural —*see* Adhesions, meninges
  epiglottis J38.7
  eyelid H02.59
  female pelvis N73.6
  gallbladder K82.8
  globe H44.89
  heart I31.0
    rheumatic I09.2
  ileocecal (coil) —*see* Adhesions, peritoneum
  ileum —*see* Adhesions, peritoneum
  intestine —*see also* Adhesions, peritoneum
  ⇒with obstruction K56.50
    ▶complete K56.52
    ▶incomplete K56.51
    ▶partial K56.51
  intra-abdominal —*see* Adhesions, peritoneum
  iris H21.50-●
    anterior H21.51-●
    goniosynechiae H21.52-●
    posterior H21.54-●
    to corneal graft T85.898
  joint —*see* Ankylosis
    knee M23.8X
    temporomandibular M26.61-●
  labium (majus) (minus), congenital Q52.5
  liver —*see* Adhesions, peritoneum
  lung J98.4
  mediastinum J98.59
  meninges (cerebral) (spinal) G96.12
    congenital Q07.8
    tuberculous (cerebral) (spinal) A17.0
  mesenteric —*see* Adhesions, peritoneum
  nasal (septum) (to turbinates) J34.89
  ocular muscle —*see* Strabismus, mechanical
  omentum —*see* Adhesions, peritoneum
  ovary N73.6
    congenital (to cecum, kidney or omentum)
      Q50.39
  paraovarian N73.6
  pelvic (peritoneal)
    female N73.6
      postprocedural N99.4
    male —*see* Adhesions, peritoneum
    postpartal (old) N73.6
    tuberculous A18.17
  penis to scrotum (congenital) Q55.8
  periappendiceal —*see also* Adhesions,
    peritoneum
  pericardium (nonrheumatic) I31.0
    focal I31.8
    rheumatic I09.2
    tuberculous A18.84
  pericholecystic K82.8
  perigastric —*see* Adhesions, peritoneum
  periovarian N73.6
  periprostatic N42.89
  perirectal —*see* Adhesions, peritoneum
  perirenal N28.89
  ⇒peritoneum, peritoneal (postinfective)
  ⇒with obstruction (intestinal) K56.50
    ▶complete K56.52

Adhesions, adhesive *(Continued)*
  peritoneum, peritoneal *(Continued)*
    with obstruction *(Continued)*
      ▶incomplete K56.51
      ▶partial K56.51
    congenital Q43.3
    pelvic, female N73.6
      postprocedural N99.4
    postpartal, pelvic N73.6
    ▶postprocedural K66.0
    to uterus N73.6
  peritubal N73.6
  periureteral N28.89
  periuterine N73.6
  perivesical N32.89
  perivesicular (seminal vesicle) N50.89
  pleura, pleuritic J94.8
    tuberculous NEC A15.6
  pleuropericardial J94.8
  postoperative (gastrointestinal tract) K66.0
  ⇒with obstruction —*see also* Obstruction,
    intestine, postoperative K91.30
    due to foreign body accidentally left
      in wound —*see* Foreign body,
      accidentally left during a procedure
    pelvic peritoneal N99.4
    urethra —*see* Stricture, urethra,
      postprocedural
    vagina N99.2
  postpartal, old (vulva or perineum) N90.89
  preputial, prepuce N47.5
  pulmonary J98.4
  pylorus —*see* Adhesions, peritoneum
  sciatic nerve —*see* Lesion, nerve, sciatic
  seminal vesicle N50.89
  shoulder (joint) —*see* Capsulitis, adhesive
  sigmoid flexure —*see* Adhesions, peritoneum
  spermatic cord (acquired) N50.89
    congenital Q55.4
  spinal canal G96.12
  stomach —*see* Adhesions, peritoneum
  subscapular —*see* Capsulitis, adhesive
  temporomandibular M26.61-●
  tendinitis —*see also* Tenosynovitis, specified
    type NEC
    shoulder —*see* Capsulitis, adhesive
  testis N44.8
  tongue, congenital (to gum or roof of mouth)
    Q38.3
    acquired K14.8
  trachea J39.8
  tubo-ovarian N73.6
  tunica vaginalis N44.8
  uterus N73.6
    internal N85.6
    to abdominal wall N73.6
  vagina (chronic) N89.5
    postoperative N99.2
  vitreomacular H43.82-●
  vitreous H43.89
  vulva N90.89
Adiaspiromycosis B48.8
Adie (-Holmes) pupil or syndrome —*see*
  Anomaly, pupil, function, tonic pupil
⇒**Adiponecrosis neonatorum** P83.88
Adiposis —*see also* Obesity
  cerebralis E23.6
  dolorosa E88.2
Adiposity —*see also* Obesity
  heart —*see* Degeneration, myocardial
  localized E65
Adiposogenital dystrophy E23.6
Adjustment
  disorder —*see* Disorder, adjustment
  implanted device —*see* Encounter (for),
    adjustment (of)
  prosthesis, external —*see* Fitting
  reaction —*see* Disorder, adjustment
Administration of tPA (rtPA) in a different
  facility within the last 24 hours prior to
  admission to current facility Z92.82

▶ New   ⇒ Revised   ~~deleted~~ Deleted   ● Use Additional Character(s)

Admission (for) —*see also* Encounter (for)
  adjustment (of)
    artificial
      arm Z44.00-•
        complete Z44.01-•
        partial Z44.02-•
      eye Z44.2
      leg Z44.10-•
        complete Z44.11-•
        partial Z44.12-•
    brain neuropacemaker Z46.2
      implanted Z45.42
    breast
      implant Z45.81
      prosthesis (external) Z44.3
    colostomy belt Z46.89
    contact lenses Z46.0
    cystostomy device Z46.6
    dental prosthesis Z46.3
    device NEC
      abdominal Z46.89
      implanted Z45.89
        cardiac Z45.09
          defibrillator (with synchronous
            cardiace pacemaker) Z45.02
          pacemaker (cardiac
            resynchronization therapy
            (CRT-P)) Z45.018
            pulse generator Z45.010
          resynchronization therapy
            defibrillator (CRT-D) Z45.02
        hearing device Z45.328
          bone conduction Z45.320
          cochlear Z45.321
        infusion pump Z45.1
        nervous system Z45.49
          CSF drainage Z45.41
          hearing device —*see* Admission,
            adjustment, device, implanted,
            hearing device
          neuropacemaker Z45.42
          visual substitution Z45.31
        specified NEC Z45.89
        vascular access Z45.2
        visual substitution Z45.31
      nervous system Z46.2
        implanted —*see* Admission,
          adjustment, device, implanted,
          nervous system
    orthodontic Z46.4
    prosthetic Z44.9
      arm —*see* Admission, adjustment,
        artificial, arm
      breast Z44.3
      dental Z46.3
      eye Z44.2
      leg —*see* Admission, adjustment,
        artificial, leg
      specified type NEC Z44.8
    substitution
      auditory Z46.2
        implanted —*see* Admission,
          adjustment, device, implanted,
          hearing device
      nervous system Z46.2
        implanted —*see* Admission,
          adjustment, device, implanted,
          nervous system
      visual Z46.2
        implanted Z45.31
    urinary Z46.6
    hearing aid Z46.1
      implanted —*see* Admission, adjustment,
        device, implanted, hearing device
    ileostomy device Z46.89
    intestinal appliance or device NEC Z46.89
    neuropacemaker (brain) (peripheral nerve)
      (spinal cord) Z46.2
      implanted Z45.42
    orthodontic device Z46.4
    orthopedic (brace) (cast) (device) (shoes)
      Z46.89

Admission (*Continued*)
  adjustment (*Continued*)
    pacemaker (cardiac resynchronization
      therapy (CRT-P))
      cardiac Z45.018
        pulse generator Z45.010
      nervous system Z46.2
        implanted Z45.42
    portacath (port-a-cath) Z45.2
    prosthesis Z44.9
      arm —*see* Admission, adjustment,
        artificial, arm
      breast Z44.3
      dental Z46.3
      eye Z44.2
      leg —*see* Admission, adjustment,
        artificial, leg
      specified NEC Z44.8
    spectacles Z46.0
  aftercare (*see also* Aftercare) Z51.89
    postpartum
      immediately after delivery Z39.0
      routine follow-up Z39.2
    radiation therapy (antineoplastic) Z51.0
  attention to artificial opening (of) Z43.9
    artificial vagina Z43.7
    colostomy Z43.3
    cystostomy Z43.5
    enterostomy Z43.4
    gastrostomy Z43.1
    ileostomy Z43.2
    jejunostomy Z43.4
    nephrostomy Z43.6
    specified site NEC Z43.8
      intestinal tract Z43.4
      urinary tract Z43.6
    tracheostomy Z43.0
    ureterostomy Z43.6
    urethrostomy Z43.6
  breast augmentation or reduction Z41.1
  breast reconstruction following mastectomy
    Z42.1
  change of
    dressing (nonsurgical) Z48.00
    neuropacemaker device (brain) (peripheral
      nerve) (spinal cord) Z46.2
      implanted Z45.42
    surgical dressing Z48.01
  circumcision, ritual or routine (in absence of
    diagnosis) Z41.2
  clinical research investigation (control)
    (normal comparison) (participant) Z00.6
  contraceptive management Z30.9
  cosmetic surgery NEC Z41.1
  counseling (*see also* Counseling)
    dietary Z71.3
    gestational carrier Z31.7
    HIV Z71.7
    human immunodeficiency virus Z71.7
    nonattending third party Z71.0
    procreative management NEC Z31.69
  delivery, full-term, uncomplicated O80
    cesarean, without indication O82
  desensitization to allergens Z51.6
  dietary surveillance and counseling Z71.3
  ear piercing Z41.3
  examination at health care facility (adult) —
    see also Examination Z00.00
    with abnormal findings Z00.01
    clinical research investigation (control)
      (normal comparison) (participant)
      Z00.6
    dental Z01.20
      with abnormal findings Z01.21
    donor (potential) Z00.5
    ear Z01.10
      with abnormal findings NEC Z01.118
    eye Z01.00
      with abnormal findings Z01.01
    general, specified reason NEC Z00.8
    hearing Z01.10
      with abnormal findings NEC Z01.118

Admission (*Continued*)
  examination at health care facility (*Continued*)
    postpartum checkup Z39.2
    psychiatric (general) Z00.8
      requested by authority Z04.6
    vision Z01.00
      with abnormal findings Z01.01
  fitting (of)
    artificial
      arm —*see* Admission, adjustment,
        artificial, arm
      eye Z44.2
      leg —*see* Admission, adjustment,
        artificial, leg
    brain neuropacemaker Z46.2
      implanted Z45.42
    breast prosthesis (external) Z44.3
    colostomy belt Z46.89
    contact lenses Z46.0
    cystostomy device Z46.6
    dental prosthesis Z46.3
    dentures Z46.3
    device NEC
      abdominal Z46.89
      nervous system Z46.2
        implanted —*see* Admission,
          adjustment, device, implanted,
          nervous system
    orthodontic Z46.4
    prosthetic Z44.9
      breast Z44.3
      dental Z46.3
      eye Z44.2
    substitution
      auditory Z46.2
        implanted —*see* Admission,
          adjustment, device, implanted,
          hearing device
      nervous system Z46.2
        implanted —*see* Admission,
          adjustment, device, implanted,
          nervous system
      visual Z46.2
        implanted Z45.31
    hearing aid Z46.1
    ileostomy device Z46.89
    intestinal appliance or device NEC Z46.89
    neuropacemaker (brain) (peripheral nerve)
      (spinal cord) Z46.2
      implanted Z45.42
    orthodontic device Z46.4
    orthopedic device (brace) (cast) (shoes)
      Z46.89
    prosthesis Z44.9
      arm —*see* Admission, adjustment,
        artificial, arm
      breast Z44.3
      dental Z46.3
      eye Z44.2
      leg —*see* Admission, adjustment,
        artificial, leg
      specified type NEC Z44.8
    spectacles Z46.0
  follow-up examination Z09
  intrauterine device management Z30.431
    initial prescription Z30.014
  mental health evaluation Z00.8
    requested by authority Z04.6
  observation —*see* Observation
  Papanicolaou smear, cervix Z12.4
    for suspected malignant neoplasm Z12.4
  plastic and reconstructive surgery following
    medical procedure or healed injury NEC
    Z42.8
  plastic surgery, cosmetic NEC Z41.1
  postpartum observation
    immediately after delivery Z39.0
    routine follow-up Z39.2
  poststerilization (for restoration) Z31.0
    aftercare Z31.42
  procreative management Z31.9
  prophylactic (measure) —*see also* Encounter,
    prophylactic measures

► New   ⮞ Revised   ~~deleted~~ Deleted   • Use Additional Character(s)

Admission *(Continued)*
  prophylactic *(Continued)*
    organ removal Z40.00
      breast Z40.01
      ▶fallopian tube(s) Z40.03
        ▶with ovary(s) Z40.02
      ⇛ovary(s) Z40.02
      specified organ NEC Z40.09
      testes Z40.09
    vaccination Z23
  psychiatric examination (general) Z00.8
    requested by authority Z04.6
  radiation therapy (antineoplastic) Z51.0
  reconstructive surgery following medical
      procedure or healed injury NEC Z42.8
  removal of
    cystostomy catheter Z43.5
    drains Z48.03
    dressing (nonsurgical) Z48.00
    implantable subdermal contraceptive Z30.46
    intrauterine contraceptive device Z30.432
    neuropacemaker (brain) (peripheral nerve)
        (spinal cord) Z46.2
      implanted Z45.42
    staples Z48.02
    surgical dressing Z48.01
    sutures Z48.02
    ureteral stent Z46.6
  respirator [ventilator] use during power
      failure Z99.12
  restoration of organ continuity
      (poststerilization) Z31.0
    aftercare Z31.42
  sensitivity test —*see also* Test, skin
    allergy NEC Z01.82
    Mantoux Z11.1
  tuboplasty following previous sterilization
      Z31.0
    aftercare Z31.42
  vasoplasty following previous sterilization
      Z31.0
    aftercare Z31.42
  vision examination Z01.00
    with abnormal findings Z01.01
  waiting period for admission to other facility
      Z75.1
Adnexitis (suppurative) —*see* Salpingo-oophoritis
Adolescent X-linked adrenoleukodystrophy
    E71.521
Adrenal (gland) —*see* condition
Adrenalism, tuberculous A18.7
Adrenalitis, adrenitis E27.8
  autoimmune E27.1
  meningococcal, hemorrhagic A39.1
Adrenarche, premature E27.0
Adrenocortical syndrome —*see* Cushing's,
    syndrome
Adrenogenital syndrome E25.9
  acquired E25.8
  congenital E25.0
  salt loss E25.0
Adrenogenitalism, congenital E25.0
Adrenoleukodystrophy E71.529
  neonatal E71.511
  X-linked E71.529
    Addison only phenotype E71.528
    Addison-Schilder E71.528
    adolescent E71.521
    adrenomyeloneuropathy E71.522
    childhood cerebral E71.520
    other specified E71.528
Adrenomyeloneuropathy E71.522
Adventitious bursa —*see* Bursopathy, specified
    type NEC
Adverse effect —*see* Table of Drugs and
    Chemicals, categories T36-T50, with 6th
    character 5
Advice —*see* Counseling
Adynamia (episodica) (hereditary) (periodic)
    G72.3
Aeration lung imperfect, newborn —*see*
    Atelectasis

Aerobullosis T70.3
Aerocele —*see* Embolism, air
Aerodermectasia
  subcutaneous (traumatic) T79.7
Aerodontalgia T70.29
Aeroembolism T70.3
Aerogenes capsulatus infection A48.0
Aero-otitis media T70.0
Aerophagy, aerophagia (psychogenic) F45.8
Aerophobia F40.228
Aerosinusitis T70.1
Aerotitis T70.0
Affection —*see* Disease
Afibrinogenemia —*see also* Defect, coagulation
    D68.8
  acquired D65
  congenital D68.2
  following ectopic or molar pregnancy
    O08.1
  in abortion —*see* Abortion, by type,
      complicated by, afibrinogenemia
  puerperal O72.3
African
  sleeping sickness B56.9
  tick fever A68.1
  trypanosomiasis B56.9
    gambian B56.0
    rhodesian B56.1
Aftercare —*see also* Care Z51.89
  following surgery (for) (on)
    amputation Z47.81
    attention to
      drains Z48.03
      dressings (nonsurgical) Z48.00
        surgical Z48.01
      sutures Z48.02
    circulatory system Z48.812
    delayed (planned) wound closure Z48.1
    digestive system Z48.815
    explantation of joint prosthesis (staged
        procedure)
      hip Z47.32
      knee Z47.33
      shoulder Z47.31
    genitourinary system Z48.816
    joint replacement Z47.1
    neoplasm Z48.3
    nervous system Z48.811
    oral cavity Z48.814
    organ transplant
      bone marrow Z48.290
      heart Z48.21
      heart-lung Z48.280
      kidney Z48.22
      liver Z48.23
      lung Z48.24
      multiple organs NEC Z48.288
      specified NEC Z48.298
    orthopedic NEC Z47.89
    planned wound closure Z48.1
    removal of internal fixation device
        Z47.2
    respiratory system Z48.813
    scoliosis Z47.82
    sense organs Z48.810
    skin and subcutaneous tissue Z48.817
    specified body system
      circulatory Z48.812
      digestive Z48.815
      genitourinary Z48.816
      nervous Z48.811
      oral cavity Z48.814
      respiratory Z48.813
      sense organs Z48.810
      skin and subcutaneous tissue Z48.817
      teeth Z48.814
    specified NEC Z48.89
  ⇛spinal Z47.89
    teeth Z48.814
  fracture — code to fracture with seventh
      character D

Aftercare *(Continued)*
  involving
    removal of
      drains Z48.03
      dressings (nonsurgical) Z48.00
      staples Z48.02
      surgical dressings Z48.01
      sutures Z48.02
    neuropacemaker (brain) (peripheral nerve)
        (spinal cord) Z46.2
      implanted Z45.42
  orthopedic NEC Z47.89
  postprocedural —*see* Aftercare, following
      surgery
After-cataract —*see* Cataract, secondary
Agalactia (primary) O92.3
  elective, secondary or therapeutic O92.5
Agammaglobulinemia (acquired (secondary))
    (nonfamilial) D80.1
  with
    immunoglobulin-bearing B-lymphocytes
        D80.1
    lymphopenia D81.9
  autosomal recessive (Swiss type) D80.0
  Bruton's X-linked D80.0
  common variable (CVAgamma) D80.1
  congenital sex-linked D80.0
  hereditary D80.0
  lymphopenic D81.9
  Swiss type (autosomal recessive) D80.0
  X-linked (with growth hormone deficiency)
      (Bruton) D80.0
Aganglionosis (bowel) (colon) Q43.1
Age (old) —*see* Senility
Agenesis
  adrenal (gland) Q89.1
  alimentary tract (complete) (partial) NEC
      Q45.8
    upper Q40.8
  anus, anal (canal) Q42.3
    with fistula Q42.2
  aorta Q25.41
  appendix Q42.8
  arm (complete) Q71.0-●
    with hand present Q71.1-●
  artery (peripheral) Q27.9
    brain Q28.3
    coronary Q24.5
    pulmonary Q25.79
    specified NEC Q27.8
    umbilical Q27.0
  auditory (canal) (external) Q16.1
  auricle (ear) Q16.0
  bile duct or passage Q44.5
  bladder Q64.5
  bone Q79.9
  brain Q00.0
    part of Q04.3
  breast (with nipple present) Q83.8
    with absent nipple Q83.0
  bronchus Q32.4
  canaliculus lacrimalis Q10.4
  carpus —*see* Agenesis, hand
  cartilage Q79.9
  cecum Q42.8
  cerebellum Q04.3
  cervix Q51.5
  chin Q18.8
  cilia Q10.3
  circulatory system, part NOS Q28.9
  clavicle Q74.0
  clitoris Q52.6
  coccyx Q76.49
  colon Q42.9
    specified NEC Q42.8
  corpus callosum Q04.0
  cricoid cartilage Q31.8
  diaphragm (with hernia) Q79.1
  digestive organ(s) or tract (complete) (partial)
      NEC Q45.8
    upper Q40.8

Agenesis (Continued)
ductus arteriosus Q28.8
duodenum Q41.0
ear Q16.9
   auricle Q16.0
   lobe Q17.8
ejaculatory duct Q55.4
endocrine (gland) NEC Q89.2
epiglottis Q31.8
esophagus Q39.8
eustachian tube Q16.2
eye Q11.1
   adnexa Q15.8
eyelid (fold) Q10.3
face
   bones NEC Q75.8
   specified part NEC Q18.8
fallopian tube Q50.6
femur —see Defect, reduction, lower limb,
   longitudinal, femur
fibula —see Defect, reduction, lower limb,
   longitudinal, fibula
finger (complete) (partial) —see Agenesis,
   hand
foot (and toes) (complete) (partial) Q72.3-●
forearm (with hand present) —see Agenesis,
   arm, with hand present
   and hand Q71.2-●
gallbladder Q44.0
gastric Q40.2
genitalia, genital (organ(s))
   female Q52.8
      external Q52.71
      internal NEC Q52.8
   male Q55.8
glottis Q31.8
hair Q84.0
hand (and fingers) (complete) (partial) Q71.3-●
heart Q24.8
   valve NEC Q24.8
      pulmonary Q22.0
hepatic Q44.7
humerus —see Defect, reduction, upper limb
hymen Q52.4
ileum Q41.2
incus Q16.3
intestine (small) Q41.9
   large Q42.9
      specified NEC Q42.8
iris (dilator fibers) Q13.1
jaw M26.09
jejunum Q41.1
kidney(s) (partial) Q60.2
   bilateral Q60.1
   unilateral Q60.0
labium (majus) (minus) Q52.71
labyrinth, membranous Q16.5
lacrimal apparatus Q10.4
larynx Q31.8
leg (complete) Q72.0-●
   with foot present Q72.1-●
   lower leg (with foot present) —see
      Agenesis, leg, with foot present
      and foot Q72.2-●
lens Q12.3
limb (complete) Q73.0
   lower —see Agenesis, leg
   upper —see Agenesis, arm
lip Q38.0
liver Q44.7
lung (fissure) (lobe) (bilateral) (unilateral)
   Q33.3
mandible, maxilla M26.09
metacarpus —see Agenesis, hand
metatarsus —see Agenesis, foot
muscle Q79.8
   eyelid Q10.3
   ocular Q15.8
musculoskeletal system NEC Q79.8
nail(s) Q84.3
neck, part Q18.8

Agenesis (Continued)
nerve Q07.8
nervous system, part NEC Q07.8
nipple Q83.2
nose Q30.1
nuclear Q07.8
organ
   of Corti Q16.5
   or site not listed —see Anomaly, by site
osseous meatus (ear) Q16.1
ovary
   bilateral Q50.02
   unilateral Q50.01
oviduct Q50.6
pancreas Q45.0
parathyroid (gland) Q89.2
parotid gland(s) Q38.4
patella Q74.1
pelvic girdle (complete) (partial) Q74.2
penis Q55.5
pericardium Q24.8
pituitary (gland) Q89.2
prostate Q55.4
punctum lacrimale Q10.4
radioulnar —see Defect, reduction, upper limb
radius —see Defect, reduction, upper limb,
   longitudinal, radius
rectum Q42.1
   with fistula Q42.0
renal Q60.2
   bilateral Q60.1
   unilateral Q60.0
respiratory organ NEC Q34.8
rib Q76.6
roof of orbit Q75.8
round ligament Q52.8
sacrum Q76.49
salivary gland Q38.4
scapula Q74.0
scrotum Q55.29
seminal vesicles Q55.4
septum
   atrial Q21.1
   between aorta and pulmonary artery Q21.4
   ventricular Q20.4
shoulder girdle (complete) (partial) Q74.0
skull (bone) Q75.8
   with
      anencephaly Q00.0
      encephalocele —see Encephalocele
      hydrocephalus Q03.9
         with spina bifida —see Spina bifida, by
            site, with hydrocephalus
      microcephaly Q02
spermatic cord Q55.4
spinal cord Q06.0
spine Q76.49
spleen Q89.01
sternum Q76.7
stomach Q40.2
submaxillary gland(s) (congenital) Q38.4
tarsus —see Agenesis, foot
tendon Q79.8
testicle Q55.0
thymus (gland) Q89.2
thyroid (gland) E03.1
   cartilage Q31.8
tibia —see Defect, reduction, lower limb,
   longitudinal, tibia
tibiofibular —see Defect, reduction, lower
   limb, specified type NEC
toe (and foot) (complete) (partial) —see
   Agenesis, foot
tongue Q38.3
trachea (cartilage) Q32.1
ulna —see Defect, reduction, upper limb,
   longitudinal, ulna
upper limb —see Agenesis, arm
ureter Q62.4
urethra Q64.5
urinary tract NEC Q64.8

Agenesis (Continued)
uterus Q51.0
uvula Q38.5
vagina Q52.0
vas deferens Q55.4
vein(s) (peripheral) Q27.9
   brain Q28.3
   great NEC Q26.8
   portal Q26.5
vena cava (inferior) (superior) Q26.8
vermis of cerebellum Q04.3
vertebra Q76.49
vulva Q52.71
Ageusia R43.2
Agitated —see condition
Agitation R45.1
Aglossia (congenital) Q38.3
Aglossia-adactylia syndrome Q87.0
Aglycogenosis E74.00
Agnosia (body image) (other senses) (tactile)
   R48.1
developmental F88
verbal R48.1
   auditory R48.1
      developmental F80.2
   developmental F80.2
visual (object) R48.3
Agoraphobia F40.00
   with panic disorder F40.01
   without panic disorder F40.02
Agrammatism R48.8
Agranulocytopenia —see Agranulocytosis
Agranulocytosis (chronic) (cyclical) (genetic)
   (infantile) (periodic) (pernicious) (see also
   Neutropenia) D70.9
congenital D70.0
cytoreductive cancer chemotherapy sequela
   D70.1
drug-induced D70.2
   due to cytoreductive cancer chemotherapy
      D70.1
due to infection D70.3
secondary D70.4
   drug-induced D70.2
      due to cytoreductive cancer
         chemotherapy D70.1
Agraphia (absolute) R48.8
   with alexia R48.0
developmental F81.81
Ague (dumb) —see Malaria
Agyria Q04.3
Ahumada-del Castillo syndrome E23.0
Aichmophobia F40.298
AIDS (related complex) B20
Ailment heart —see Disease, heart
Ailurophobia F40.218
Ainhum (disease) L94.6
AIN —see Neoplasia, intraepithelial, anal
AIPHI (acute idiopathic pulmonary hemorrhage
   in infants (over 28 days old)) R04.81
Air
anterior mediastinum J98.2
compressed, disease T70.3
conditioner lung or pneumonitis J67.7
embolism (artery) (cerebral) (any site) T79.0
   with ectopic or molar pregnancy O08.2
   due to implanted device NEC —see
      Complications, by site and type,
      specified NEC
   following
      abortion —see Abortion by type,
         complicated by, embolism
      ectopic or molar pregnancy O08.2
      infusion, therapeutic injection or
         transfusion T80.0
   in pregnancy, childbirth or puerperium —
      see Embolism, obstetric
   traumatic T79.0
hunger, psychogenic F45.8
rarefied, effects of —see Effect, adverse, high
   altitude
sickness T75.3

▶ New   ⇒ Revised   ~~deleted~~ Deleted   ● Use Additional Character(s)

Airplane sickness T75.3
Akathisia (drug-induced) (treatment- induced)
  G25.71
  neuroleptic induced (acute) G25.71
  ▶tardive G25.71
Akinesia R29.898
Akinetic mutism R41.89
Akureyri's disease G93.3
Alactasia, congenital E73.0
Alagille's syndrome Q44.7
Alastrim B03
Albers-Schönberg syndrome Q78.2
Albert's syndrome —see Tendinitis, Achilles
Albinism, albino E70.30
  with hematologic abnormality E70.339
    Chédiak-Higashi syndrome E70.330
    Hermansky-Pudlak syndrome E70.331
    other specified E70.338
  I E70.320
  II E70.321
  ocular E70.319
    autosomal recessive E70.311
    other specified E70.318
    X-linked E70.310
  oculocutaneous E70.329
    other specified E70.328
    tyrosinase (ty) negative E70.320
    tyrosinase (ty) positive E70.321
  other specified E70.39
Albinismus E70.30
Albright (-McCune)(-Sternberg) syndrome
  Q78.1
Albuminous —see condition
Albuminuria, albuminuric (acute) (chronic)
  (subacute) —see also Proteinuria R80.9
  complicating pregnancy —see Proteinuria,
    gestational
    with
      gestational hypertension —see
        Pre-eclampsia
      pre-existing hypertension —see
        Hypertension, complicating
        pregnancy, pre-existing, with,
        pre-eclampsia
  gestational —see Proteinuria, gestational
    with
      gestational hypertension —see
        Pre-eclampsia
      pre-existing hypertension —see
        Hypertension, complicating
        pregnancy, pre-existing, with,
        pre-eclampsia
  orthostatic R80.2
  postural R80.2
  pre-eclamptic —see Pre-eclampsia
  scarlatinal A38.8
Albuminurophobia F40.298
Alcaptonuria E70.29
Alcohol, alcoholic, alcohol-induced
  addiction (without remission) F10.20
    with remission F10.21
  amnestic disorder, persisting F10.96
    with dependence F10.26
  anxiety disorder F10.980
  bipolar and related disorder F10.94
  brain syndrome, chronic F10.97
    with dependence F10.27
  cardiopathy I42.6
  counseling and surveillance Z71.41
    family member Z71.42
  delirium (acute) (tremens) (withdrawal)
    F10.231
    with intoxication F10.921
      in
        abuse F10.121
        dependence F10.221
  dementia F10.97
    with dependence F10.27
  depressive disorder F10.94
  deterioration F10.97
    with dependence F10.27

Alcohol, alcoholic, alcohol-induced (Continued)
  hallucinosis (acute) F10.951
    in
      abuse F10.151
      dependence F10.251
  insanity F10.959
  intoxication (acute) (without dependence)
    F10.129
    with
      delirium F10.121
      dependence F10.229
        with delirium F10.221
        uncomplicated F10.220
      uncomplicated F10.120
  jealousy F10.988
  Korsakoff's, Korsakov's, Korsakow's
    F10.26
  liver K70.9
    acute —see Disease, liver, alcoholic,
      hepatitis
  major neurocognitive disorder, amnestic-
    confabulatory type F10.96
  major neurocognitive disorder, nonamnestic-
    confabulatory type F10.97
  mania (acute) (chronic) F10.959
  mild neurocognitive disorder F10.988
  paranoia, paranoid (type) psychosis F10.950
  pellagra E52
  poisoning, accidental (acute) NEC —see
    Table of Drugs and Chemicals, alcohol,
    poisoning
  psychosis —see Psychosis, alcoholic
  psychotic disorder F10.959
  sexual dysfunction F10.981
  sleep disorder F10.982
  withdrawal (without convulsions) F10.239
    with delirium F10.231
Alcoholism (chronic) (without remission)
  F10.20
  with
    psychosis —see Psychosis, alcoholic
    remission F10.21
  Korsakov's F10.96
    with dependence F10.26
Alder (-Reilly) anomaly or syndrome
  (leukocyte granulation) D72.0
Aldosteronism E26.9
  familial (type I) E26.02
  glucocorticoid-remediable E26.02
  primary (due to (bilateral) adrenal
    hyperplasia) E26.09
  primary NEC E26.09
  secondary E26.1
  specified NEC E26.89
Aldosteronoma D44.10
Aldrich(-Wiskott) syndrome (eczema-
  thrombocytopenia) D82.0
Alektorophobia F40.218
Aleppo boil B55.1
Aleukemic —see condition Aleukia
  congenital D70.0
  hemorrhagica D61.9
    congenital D61.09
  splenica D73.1
Alexia R48.0
  developmental F81.0
  secondary to organic lesion R48.0
Algoneurodystrophy M89.00
  ankle M89.07-●
  foot M89.07-●
  forearm M89.03-●
  hand M89.04-●
  lower leg M89.06-●
  multiple sites M89.0-●
  shoulder M89.01-●
  specified site NEC M89.08
  thigh M89.05-●
  upper arm M89.02-●
Algophobia F40.298
Alienation, mental —see Psychosis
Alkalemia E87.3

Alkalosis E87.3
  metabolic E87.3
    with respiratory acidosis E87.4
  respiratory E87.3
Alkaptonuria E70.29
Allen-Masters syndrome N83.8
Allergy, allergic (reaction) (to) T78.40
  air-borne substance NEC (rhinitis) J30.89
  alveolitis (extrinsic) J67.9
    due to
      Aspergillus clavatus J67.4
      Cryptostroma corticale J67.6
      organisms (fungal, thermophilic
        actinomycete) growing in
        ventilation (air conditioning)
        systems J67.7
      specified type NEC J67.8
  anaphylactic reaction or shock T78.2
  angioneurotic edema T78.3
  animal (dander) (epidermal) (hair) (rhinitis)
    J30.81
  bee sting (anaphylactic shock) —see Toxicity,
    venom, arthropod, bee
  biological —see Allergy, drug
  colitis —see also Colitis, allergic K52.29
  dander (animal) (rhinitis) J30.81
  dandruff (rhinitis) J30.81
  dental restorative material (existing) K08.55
  dermatitis —see Dermatitis, contact, allergic
  diathesis —see History, allergy
  drug, medicament & biological (any)
    (external) (internal) T78.40
    correct substance properly administered —
      see Table of Drugs and Chemicals, by
      drug, adverse effect
    wrong substance given or taken NEC (by
      accident) —see Table of Drugs and
      Chemicals, by drug, poisoning
  due to pollen J30.1
  dust (house) (stock) (rhinitis) J30.89
    with asthma —see Asthma, allergic extrinsic
  eczema —see Dermatitis, contact, allergic
  epidermal (animal) (rhinitis) J30.81
  feathers (rhinitis) J30.89
  food (any) (ingested) NEC T78.1
    anaphylactic shock —see Shock,
      anaphylactic, due to food
    dermatitis —see Dermatitis, due to, food
    dietary counseling and surveillance Z71.3
    in contact with skin L23.6
    rhinitis J30.5
    status (without reaction) Z91.018
      eggs Z91.012
      milk products Z91.011
      peanuts Z91.010
      seafood Z91.013
      specified NEC Z91.018
  gastrointestinal —see also specific type of
    allergic reaction
    meaning colitis —see also Colitis, allergic)
      K52.29
    meaning gastroenteritis —see also
      Gastroenteritis, allergic) K52.29
    meaning other adverse food reaction not
      elsewhere classified T78.1
  grain J30.1
  grass (hay fever) (pollen) J30.1
    asthma —see Asthma, allergic extrinsic
  hair (animal) (rhinitis) J30.81
  history (of) —see History, allergy
  horse serum —see Allergy, serum
  inhalant (rhinitis) J30.89
    pollen J30.1
  kapok (rhinitis) J30.89
  medicine —see Allergy, drug
  milk protein —see also Allergy, food Z91.011
    anaphylactic reaction T78.07
    dermatitis L27.2
    enterocolitis syndrome K52.21
    enteropathy K52.22
    gastroenteritis K52.29

A

Allergy, allergic *(Continued)*
  milk protein *(Continued)*
    gastroesophageal reflux —*see also* Reaction,
        adverse, food) K21.9
      with esophagitis K21.0
    proctocolitis K52.82   ]
  nasal, seasonal due to pollen J30.1
  pneumonia J82
  pollen (any) (hay fever) J30.1
    asthma —*see* Asthma, allergic extrinsic
  primrose J30.1
  primula J30.1
  proctocolitis K52.82
  purpura D69.0
  ragweed (hay fever) (pollen) J30.1
    asthma —*see* Asthma, allergic extrinsic
  rose (pollen) J30.1
  seasonal NEC J30.2
  Senecio jacobae (pollen) J30.1
  serum —*see also* Reaction, serum T80.69
    anaphylactic shock T80.59
  shock (anaphylactic) T78.2
    due to
      administration of blood and blood
          products T80.51
      adverse effect of correct medicinal
          substance properly administered
          T88.6
      immunization T80.52
      serum NEC T80.59
      vaccination T80.52
    specific NEC T78.49
  tree (any) (hay fever) (pollen) J30.1
    asthma —*see* Asthma, allergic extrinsic
  upper respiratory J30.9
  urticaria L50.0
  vaccine —*see* Allergy, serum
  wheat —*see* Allergy, food
Allescheriasis B48.2
Alligator skin disease Q80.9
Allocheiria, allochiria R20.8
Almeida's disease —*see*
    Paracoccidioidomycosis
Alopecia (hereditaria) (seborrheica)
    L65.9
  androgenic L64.9
    drug-induced L64.0
    specified NEC L64.8
  areata L63.9
    ophiasis L63.2
    specified NEC L63.8
    totalis L63.0
    universalis L63.1
  cicatricial L66.9
    specified NEC L66.8
  circumscripta L63.9
  congenital, congenitalis Q84.0
  due to cytotoxic drugs NEC L65.8
  mucinosa L65.2
  postinfective NEC L65.8
  postpartum L65.0
  premature L64.8
  specific (syphilitic) A51.32
  specified NEC L65.8
  syphilitic (secondary) A51.32
  totalis (capitis) L63.0
  universalis (entire body) L63.1
  X-ray L58.1
Alpers' disease G31.81
Alpine sickness T70.29
Alport syndrome Q87.81
ALTE (apparent life threatening event) in
    newborn and infant R68.13
Alteration (of), Altered
  awareness
    transient R40.4
    unintended under general anesthesia,
        during procedure T88.53
  mental status R41.82
  pattern of family relationships affecting child
      Z62.898

Alteration (of), Altered *(Continued)*
  sensation
    following
      cerebrovascular disease I69.998
        cerebral infarction I69.398
        intracerebral hemorrhage I69.198
        nontraumatic intracranial hemorrhage
            NEC I69.298
        specified disease NEC I69.898
        subarachnoid hemorrhage I69.098
Alternating —*see* condition
Altitude, high (effects) —*see* Effect, adverse,
    high altitude
Aluminosis (of lung) J63.0
Alveolitis
  allergic (extrinsic) —*see* Pneumonitis,
      hypersensitivity
  due to
    Aspergillus clavatus J67.4
    Cryptostroma corticale J67.6
  fibrosing (cryptogenic) (idiopathic) J84.112
  jaw M27.3
  sicca dolorosa M27.3
Alveolus, alveolar —*see* condition
Alymphocytosis D72.810
  thymic (with immunodeficiency) D82.1
Alymphoplasia, thymic D82.1
Alzheimer's disease or sclerosis —*see* Disease,
    Alzheimer's
Amastia (with nipple present) Q83.8
  with absent nipple Q83.0
Amathophobia F40.228
Amaurosis (acquired) (congenital) —*see also*
    Blindness
  fugax G45.3
  hysterical F44.6
  Leber's congenital H35.50
  uremic —*see* Uremia
Amaurotic idiocy (infantile) (juvenile) (late) E75.4
Amaxophobia F40.248
Ambiguous genitalia Q56.4
Amblyopia (congenital) (ex anopsia) (partial)
    (suppression) H53.00-●
  anisometropic —*see* Amblyopia, refractive
  deprivation H53.01-●
  hysterical F44.6
  nocturnal —*see also* Blindness, night
    vitamin A deficiency E50.5
  refractive H53.02-●
  strabismic H53.03-●
  suspect H53.04-●
  tobacco H53.8
  toxic NEC H53.8
  uremic —*see* Uremia
Ameba, amebic (histolytica) —*see also* Amebiasis
  abscess (liver) A06.4
Amebiasis A06.9
  with abscess —*see* Abscess, amebic
  acute A06.0
  chronic (intestine) A06.1
    with abscess —*see* Abscess, amebic
  cutaneous A06.7
  cutis A06.7
  cystitis A06.81
  genitourinary tract NEC A06.82
  hepatic —*see* Abscess, liver, amebic
  intestine A06.0
  nondysenteric colitis A06.2
  skin A06.7
  specified site NEC A06.89
Ameboma (of intestine) A06.3
Amelia Q73.0
  lower limb —*see* Agenesis, leg
  upper limb —*see* Agenesis, arm
Ameloblastoma —*see also* Cyst, calcifying
    odontogenic
  long bones C40.9-●
    lower limb C40.2-●
    upper limb C40.0-●
  malignant C41.1
    jaw (bone) (lower) C41.1
      upper C41.0
  tibial C40.2-●

Amelogenesis imperfecta K00.5
  nonhereditaria (segmentalis) K00.4
Amenorrhea N91.2
  hyperhormonal E28.8
  primary N91.0
  secondary N91.1
Amentia —*see* Disability, intellectual
  Meynert's (nonalcoholic) F04
American
  leishmaniasis B55.2
  mountain tick fever A93.2
Ametropia —*see* Disorder, refraction
AMH (asymptomatic microscopic hematuria)
    R31.21
Amianthosis J61
Amimia R48.8
Amino-acid disorder E72.9
  anemia D53.0
Aminoacidopathy E72.9
Aminoaciduria E72.9
Amnes (t)ic syndrome (post-traumatic) F04
  induced by
    alcohol F10.96
      with dependence F10.26
    psychoactive NEC F19.96
      with
        abuse F19.16
        dependence F19.26
    sedative F13.96
      with dependence F13.26
Amnesia R41.3
  anterograde R41.1
  auditory R48.8
  dissociative F44.0
    with dissociative fugue F44.1
  hysterical F44.0
  postictal in epilepsy —*see* Epilepsy
  psychogenic F44.0
  retrograde R41.2
  transient global G45.4
Amnion, amniotic —*see* condition
Amnionitis —*see* Pregnancy, complicated by
Amok F68.8
Amoral traits F60.89
Amphetamine (or other stimulant) —
    induced
  anxiety disorder F15.980
  bipolar and related disorder F15.94
  delirium F15.921
  depressive disorder F15.94
  obsessive-compulsive and related disorder
      F15.988
  psychotic disorder F15.959
  sexual dysfunction F15.981
  sleep disorder F15.982
  stimulant withdrawal F15.23
Ampulla
  lower esophagus K22.8
  phrenic K22.8
Amputation —*see also* Absence, by site,
    acquired
  neuroma (postoperative) (traumatic) —*see*
      Complications, amputation stump,
      neuroma
  stump (surgical)
    abnormal, painful, or with complication
        (late) —*see* Complications, amputation
        stump
    healed or old NOS Z89.9
  traumatic (complete) (partial)
    arm (upper) (complete) S48.91-●
      at
        elbow S58.01-●
          partial S58.02-●
        shoulder joint (complete) S48.01-●
          partial S48.02-●
      between
        elbow and wrist (complete) S58.11-●
          partial S58.12-●
        shoulder and elbow (complete)
            S48.11-●
          partial S48.12-●
      partial S48.92-●

Amputation *(Continued)*
  traumatic *(Continued)*
    breast (complete) S28.21-●
      partial S28.22-●
    clitoris (complete) S38.211
      partial S38.212
    ear (complete) S08.11-●
      partial S08.12-●
    finger (complete) (metacarpophalangeal)
        S68.11-●
      index S68.11-●
      little S68.11-●
      middle S68.11-●
      partial S68.12-●
        index S68.12-●
        little S68.12-●
        middle S68.12-●
        ring S68.12-●
      ring S68.11-●
      thumb —*see* Amputation, traumatic,
          thumb
      transphalangeal (complete) S68.61-●
        index S68.61-●
        little S68.61-●
        middle S68.61-●
        partial S68.62-●
          index S68.62-●
          little S68.62-●
          middle S68.62-●
          ring S68.62-●
        ring S68.61-●
    foot (complete) S98.91-●
      at ankle level S98.01-●
        partial S98.02-●
      midfoot S98.31-●
        partial S98.32-●
      partial S98.92-●
    forearm (complete) S58.91-●
      at elbow level (complete) S58.01-●
        partial S58.02-●
      between elbow and wrist (complete)
          S58.11-●
        partial S58.12-●
      partial S58.92-●
    genital organ(s) (external)
      female (complete) S38.211
        partial S38.212
      male
        penis (complete) S38.221
          partial S38.222
        scrotum (complete) S38.231
          partial S38.232
        testes (complete) S38.231
          partial S38.232
    hand (complete) (wrist level) S68.41-●
      finger(s) alone —*see* Amputation,
          traumatic, finger
      partial S68.42-●
      thumb alone —*see* Amputation,
          traumatic, thumb
      transmetacarpal (complete) S68.71-●
        partial S68.72-●
    head
      ear —*see* Amputation, traumatic, ear
      nose (partial) S08.812
        complete S08.811
      part S08.89
        scalp S08.0
    hip (and thigh) (complete) S78.91-●
      at hip joint (complete) S78.01-●
        partial S78.02-●
      between hip and knee (complete) S78.11-●
        partial S78.12-●
      partial S78.92-●
    labium (majus) (minus) (complete) S38.21-●
      partial S38.21-●
    leg (lower) S88.91-●
      at knee level S88.01-●
        partial S88.02-●
      between knee and ankle S88.11-●
        partial S88.12-●
      partial S88.92-●

Amputation *(Continued)*
  traumatic *(Continued)*
    nose (partial) S08.812
      complete S08.811
    penis (complete) S38.221
      partial S38.222
    scrotum (complete) S38.231
      partial S38.232
    shoulder —*see* Amputation, traumatic, arm
      at shoulder joint —*see* Amputation,
          traumatic, arm, at shoulder joint
    testes (complete) S38.231
      partial S38.232
    thigh —*see* Amputation, traumatic, hip
    thorax, part of S28.1
      breast —*see* Amputation, traumatic,
          breast
    thumb (complete) (metacarpophalangeal)
        S68.01-●
      partial S68.02-●
      transphalangeal (complete) S68.51-●
        partial S68.52-●
    toe (lesser) S98.13-●
      great S98.11-●
        partial S98.12-●
      more than one S98.21-●
        partial S98.22-●
      partial S98.14-●
    vulva (complete) S38.211
      partial S38.212
Amputee (bilateral) (old) Z89.9
Amsterdam dwarfism Q87.1
Amusia R48.8
  developmental F80.89
Amyelencephalus, amyelencephaly Q00.0
Amyelia Q06.0
Amygdalitis —*see* Tonsillitis
Amygdalolith J35.8
Amyloid heart (disease) E85.4 *[I43]*
Amyloidosis (generalized) (primary) E85.9
  with lung involvement E85.4 *[J99]*
  familial E85.2
  genetic E85.2
  heart E85.4 *[I43]*
  hemodialysis-associated E85.3
▶ light chain (AL) E85.81
  liver E85.4 *[K77]*
  localized E85.4
  neuropathic heredofamilial E85.1
  non-neuropathic heredofamilial E85.0
  organ limited E85.4
  Portuguese E85.1
  pulmonary E85.4 *[J99]*
  secondary systemic E85.3
▶ senile systemic (SSA) E85.82
  skin (lichen) (macular) E85.4 *[L99]*
⟹ specified NEC E85.89
  subglottic E85.4 *[J99]*
▶ wild-type transthyretin-related (ATTR)
      E85.82
Amylopectinosis (brancher enzyme deficiency)
    E74.03
Amylophagia —*see* Pica
Amyoplasia congenita Q79.8
Amyotonia M62.89
  congenita G70.2
Amyotrophia, amyotrophy, amyotrophic G71.8
  congenita Q79.8
  diabetic —*see* Diabetes, amyotrophy
  lateral sclerosis G12.21
  neuralgic G54.5
⟹ spinal progressive G12.25
Anacidity, gastric K31.83
  psychogenic F45.8
Anaerosis of newborn P28.89
Analbuminemia E88.09
Analgesia —*see* Anesthesia
Analphalipoproteinemia E78.6
Anaphylactic
  purpura D69.0
  shock or reaction —*see* Shock, anaphylactic

Anaphylactoid shock or reaction —*see* Shock,
    anaphylactic
Anaphylactoid syndrome of pregnancy O88.01-●
Anaphylaxis —*see* Shock, anaphylactic
Anaplasia cervix —*see also* Dysplasia, cervix
    N87.9
Anaplasmosis, human A77.49
Anarthria R47.1
Anasarca R60.1
  cardiac —*see* Failure, heart, congestive
  lung J18.2
  newborn P83.2
  nutritional E43
  pulmonary J18.2
  renal N04.9
Anastomosis
  aneurysmal —*see* Aneurysm
  arteriovenous ruptured brain I60.8
  intestinal K63.89
    complicated NEC K91.89
      involving urinary tract N99.89
  retinal and choroidal vessels (congenital) Q14.8
Anatomical narrow angle H40.03-●
Ancylostoma, ancylostomiasis (braziliense)
    (caninum) (ceylanicum) (duodenale) B76.0
  Necator americanus B76.1
Andersen's disease (glycogen storage) E74.09
Anderson-Fabry disease E75.21
Andes disease T70.29
Andrews' disease (bacterid) L08.89
Androblastoma
  benign
    specified site —*see* Neoplasm, benign, by
        site
    unspecified site
      female D27.9
      male D29.20
  malignant
    specified site —*see* Neoplasm, malignant,
        by site
    unspecified site
      female C56.9
      male C62.90
  specified site —*see* Neoplasm, uncertain
      behavior, by site
  tubular
    with lipid storage
      specified site —*see* Neoplasm, benign,
          by site
      unspecified site
        female D27.9
        male D29.20
    specified site —*see* Neoplasm, benign,
        by site
    unspecified site
      female D27.9
      male D29.20
  unspecified site
    female D39.10
    male D40.10
Androgen insensitivity syndrome —*see also*
    Syndrome, androgen insensitivity E34.50
Androgen resistance syndrome —*see also*
    Syndrome, androgen insensitivity E34.50
Android pelvis Q74.2
  with disproportion (fetopelvic) O33.3
    causing obstructed labor O65.3
Androphobia F40.290
Anectasis, pulmonary (newborn) —*see*
    Atelectasis
Anemia (essential) (general) (hemoglobin
    deficiency) (infantile) (primary) (profound)
    D64.9
  with (due to) (in)
    disorder of
      anaerobic glycolysis D55.2
      pentose phosphate pathway D55.1
    koilonychia D50.9
  achlorhydric D50.8
  achrestic D53.1
  Addison (-Biermer) (pernicious) D51.0

Anemia (*Continued*)
agranulocytic —*see* Agranulocytosis
amino-acid-deficiency D53.0
aplastic D61.9
  congenital D61.09
  drug-induced D61.1
  due to
    drugs D61.1
    external agents NEC D61.2
    infection D61.2
    radiation D61.2
  idiopathic D61.3
  red cell (pure) D60.9
    chronic D60.0
    congenital D61.01
    specified type NEC D60.8
    transient D60.1
  specified type NEC D61.89
  toxic D61.2
aregenerative
  congenital D61.09
asiderotic D50.9
atypical (primary) D64.9
Baghdad spring D55.0
Balantidium coli A07.0
Biermer's (pernicious) D51.0
blood loss (chronic) D50.0
  acute D62
bothriocephalus B70.0 [*D63.8*]
brickmaker's B76.9 [*D63.8*]
cerebral I67.89
childhood D58.9
chlorotic D50.8
chronic
  blood loss D50.0
  hemolytic D58.9
    idiopathic D59.9
  simple D53.9
chronica congenita aregenerativa D61.09
combined system disease NEC D51.0 [*G32.0*]
  due to dietary vitamin B12 deficiency
    D51.3 [*G32.0*]
complicating pregnancy, childbirth
  or puerperium —*see* Pregnancy,
  complicated by (management affected
  by), anemia
congenital P61.4
  aplastic D61.09
  due to isoimmunization NOS P55.9
  dyserythropoietic, dyshematopoietic D64.4
  following fetal blood loss P61.3
  Heinz body D58.2
  hereditary hemolytic NOS D58.9
  pernicious D51.0
  spherocytic D58.0
Cooley's (erythroblastic) D56.1
cytogenic D51.0
deficiency D53.9
  2, 3 diphosphoglycurate mutase D55.2
  2, 3 PG D55.2
  6 phosphogluconate dehydrogenase D55.1
  6-PGD D55.1
  amino-acid D53.0
  combined B12 and folate D53.1
  enzyme D55.9
    drug-induced (hemolytic) D59.2
    glucose-6-phosphate dehydrogenase
      (G6PD) D55.0
    glycolytic D55.2
    nucleotide metabolism D55.3
    related to hexose monophosphate
      (HMP) shunt pathway NEC D55.1
    specified type NEC D55.8
  erythrocytic glutathione D55.1
  folate D52.9
    dietary D52.0
    drug-induced D52.1
  folic acid D52.9
    dietary D52.0
    drug-induced D52.1
  G SH D55.1

Anemia (*Continued*)
deficiency (*Continued*)
  G6PD D55.0
  GGS-R D55.1
  glucose-6-phosphate dehydrogenase D55.0
  glutathione reductase D55.1
  glyceraldehyde phosphate dehydrogenase
    D55.2
  hexokinase D55.2
  iron D50.9
    secondary to blood loss (chronic) D50.0
  nutritional D53.9
    with
      poor iron absorption D50.8
      specified deficiency NEC D53.8
  phosphofructo-aldolase D55.2
  phosphoglycerate kinase D55.2
  PK D55.2
  protein D53.0
  pyruvate kinase D55.2
  transcobalamin II D51.2
  triose-phosphate isomerase D55.2
  vitamin B12 NOS D51.9
    dietary D51.3
    due to
      intrinsic factor deficiency D51.0
      selective vitamin B12 malabsorption
        with proteinuria D51.1
    pernicious D51.0
    specified type NEC D51.8
Diamond-Blackfan (congenital hypoplastic)
  D61.01
dibothriocephalus B70.0 [*D63.8*]
dimorphic D53.1
diphasic D53.1
Diphyllobothrium (Dibothriocephalus) B70.0
  [*D63.8*]
due to (in) (with)
  antineoplastic chemotherapy D64.81
  blood loss (chronic) D50.0
    acute D62
  chemotherapy, antineoplastic D64.81
  chronic disease classified elsewhere NEC
    D63.8
  chronic kidney disease D63.1
  deficiency
    amino-acid D53.0
    copper D53.8
    folate (folic acid) D52.9
      dietary D52.0
      drug-induced D52.1
    molybdenum D53.8
    protein D53.0
    zinc D53.8
  dietary vitamin B12 deficiency D51.3
  disorder of
    glutathione metabolism D55.1
    nucleotide metabolism D55.3
  drug —*see* Anemia, by type —*see also* Table
    of Drugs and Chemicals
  end stage renal disease D63.1
  enzyme disorder D55.9
  fetal blood loss P61.3
  fish tapeworm (D latum) infestation B70.0
    [*D63.8*]
  hemorrhage (chronic) D50.0
    acute D62
  impaired absorption D50.9
  loss of blood (chronic) D50.0
    acute D62
  myxedema E03.9 [*D63.8*]
  Necator americanus B76.1 [*D63.8*]
  prematurity P61.2
  selective vitamin B12 malabsorption with
    proteinuria D51.1
  transcobalamin II deficiency D51.2
Dyke-Young type (secondary) (symptomatic)
  D59.1
dyserythropoietic (congenital) D64.4
dyshematopoietic (congenital) D64.4
Egyptian B76.9 [*D63.8*]

Anemia (*Continued*)
elliptocytosis —*see* Elliptocytosis
enzyme-deficiency, drug-induced D59.2
epidemic —*see also* Ancylostomiasis B76.9
  [*D63.8*]
erythroblastic
  familial D56.1
  newborn —*see also* Disease, hemolytic P55.9
  of childhood D56.1
erythrocytic glutathione deficiency D55.1
erythropoietin-resistant anemia (EPO
  resistant anemia) D63.1
Faber's (achlorhydric anemia) D50.9
factitious (self-induced blood letting) D50.0
familial erythroblastic D56.1
Fanconi's (congenital pancytopenia) D61.09
favism D55.0
fish tapeworm (D. latum) infestation B70.0
  [*D63.8*]
folate (folic acid) deficiency D52.9
glucose-6-phosphate dehydrogenase (G6PD)
  deficiency D55.0
glutathione-reductase deficiency D55.1
goat's milk D52.0
granulocytic —*see* Agranulocytosis
Heinz body, congenital D58.2
hemolytic D58.9
  acquired D59.9
    with hemoglobinuria NEC D59.6
    autoimmune NEC D59.1
    infectious D59.4
    specified type NEC D59.8
    toxic D59.4
  acute D59.9
    due to enzyme deficiency specified type
      NEC D55.8
    Lederer's D59.1
  autoimmune D59.1
    drug-induced D59.0
  chronic D58.9
    idiopathic D59.9
  cold type (secondary) (symptomatic) D59.1
  congenital (spherocytic) —*see* Spherocytosis
  due to
    cardiac conditions D59.4
    drugs (nonautoimmune) D59.2
      autoimmune D59.0
    enzyme disorder D55.9
      drug-induced D59.2
    presence of shunt or other internal
      prosthetic device D59.4
  familial D58.9
  hereditary D58.9
    due to enzyme disorder D55.9
      specified type NEC D55.8
    specified type NEC D58.8
  idiopathic (chronic) D59.9
  mechanical D59.4
  microangiopathic D59.4
  nonautoimmune D59.4
    drug-induced D59.2
  nonspherocytic
    congenital or hereditary NEC D55.8
      glucose-6-phosphate dehydrogenase
        deficiency D55.0
      pyruvate kinase deficiency D55.2
      type
        I D55.1
        II D55.2
    type
      I D55.1
      II D55.2
  secondary D59.4
    autoimmune D59.1
  specified (hereditary) type NEC D58.8
  Stransky-Regala type —*see also*
    Hemoglobinopathy D58.8
  symptomatic D59.4
    autoimmune D59.1
  toxic D59.4
  warm type (secondary) (symptomatic) D59.1

Anemia *(Continued)*
  hemorrhagic (chronic) D50.0
    acute D62
  Herrick's D57.1
  hexokinase deficiency D55.2
  hookworm B76.9 *[D63.8]*
  hypochromic (idiopathic) (microcytic)
      (normoblastic) D50.9
    due to blood loss (chronic) D50.0
      acute D62
    familial sex-linked D64.0
    pyridoxine-responsive D64.3
    sideroblastic, sex-linked D64.0
  hypoplasia, red blood cells D61.9
    congenital or familial D61.01
  hypoplastic (idiopathic) D61.9
    congenital or familial (of childhood)
        D61.01
  hypoproliferative (refractive) D61.9
  idiopathic D64.9
    aplastic D61.3
    hemolytic, chronic D59.9
  in (due to) (with)
    chronic kidney disease D63.1
    end stage renal disease D63.1
    failure, kidney (renal) D63.1
    neoplastic disease —*see also* Neoplasm
        D63.0
  intertropical —*see also* Ancylostomiasis D63.8
  iron deficiency D50.9
    secondary to blood loss (chronic) D50.0
      acute D62
    specified type NEC D50.8
  Joseph-Diamond-Blackfan (congenital
      hypoplastic) D61.01
  Lederer's (hemolytic) D59.1
  leukoerythroblastic D61.82
  macrocytic D53.9
    nutritional D52.0
    tropical D52.8
  malarial (*see also* Malaria) B54 *[D63.8]*
  malignant (progressive) D51.0
  malnutrition D53.9
  marsh (*see also* Malaria) B54 *[D63.8]*
  Mediterranean (with other
      hemoglobinopathy) D56.9
  megaloblastic D53.1
    combined B12 and folate deficiency
        D53.1
    hereditary D51.1
    nutritional D52.0
    orotic aciduria D53.0
    refractory D53.1
    specified type NEC D53.1
  megalocytic D53.1
  microcytic (hypochromic) D50.9
    due to blood loss (chronic) D50.0
      acute D62
    familial D56.8
  microdrepanocytosis D57.40
  microelliptopoikilocytic (Rietti-Greppi-
      Micheli) D56.9
  miner's B76.9 *[D63.8]*
  myelodysplastic D46.9
  myelofibrosis D75.81
  myelogenous D64.89
  myelopathic D64.89
  myelophthisic D61.82
  myeloproliferative D47.Z9
  newborn P61.4
    due to
      ABO (antibodies, isoimmunization,
          maternal/fetal incompatibility)
          P55.1
      Rh (antibodies, isoimmunization,
          maternal/fetal incompatibility)
          P55.0
    following fetal blood loss P61.3
    posthemorrhagic (fetal) P61.3
  nonspherocytic hemolytic —*see* Anemia,
      hemolytic, nonspherocytic

Anemia *(Continued)*
  normocytic (infectional) D64.9
    due to blood loss (chronic) D50.0
      acute D62
    myelophthisic D61.82
  nutritional (deficiency) D53.9
    with
      poor iron absorption D50.8
      specified deficiency NEC D53.8
    megaloblastic D52.0
  of prematurity P61.2
  orotaciduric (congenital) (hereditary) D53.0
  osteosclerotic D64.89
  ovalocytosis (hereditary) —*see* Elliptocytosis
  paludal —*see also* Malaria B54 *[D63.8]*
  pernicious (congenital) (malignant)
      (progressive) D51.0
  pleochromic D64.89
    of sprue D52.8
  posthemorrhagic (chronic) D50.0
    acute D62
    newborn P61.3
  postoperative (postprocedural)
    due to (acute) blood loss D62
      chronic blood loss D50.0
    specified NEC D64.9
  postpartum O90.81
  pressure D64.89
  progressive D64.9
    malignant D51.0
    pernicious D51.0
  protein-deficiency D53.0
  pseudoleukemica infantum D64.89
  pure red cell D60.9
    congenital D61.01
  pyridoxine-responsive D64.3
  pyruvate kinase deficiency D55.2
  refractory D46.4
    with
      excess of blasts D46.20
        1 (RAEB 1) D46.21
        2 (RAEB 2) D46.22
        in transformation (RAEB T) —*see*
            Leukemia, acute myeloblastic
      hemochromatosis D46.1
      sideroblasts (ring) (RARS) D46.1
    without ring sideroblasts, so stated D46.0
    without sideroblasts without excess of
        blasts D46.0
    megaloblastic D53.1
    sideroblastic D46.1
    sideropenic D50.9
  Rietti-Greppi-Micheli D56.9
  scorbutic D53.2
  secondary to
    blood loss (chronic) D50.0
      acute D62
    hemorrhage (chronic) D50.0
      acute D62
  semiplastic D61.89
  sickle-cell —*see* Disease, sickle-cell
  sideroblastic D64.3
    hereditary D64.0
    hypochromic, sex-linked D64.0
    pyridoxine-responsive NEC D64.3
    refractory D46.1
    secondary (due to)
      disease D64.1
      drugs and toxins D64.2
    specified type NEC D64.3
  sideropenic (refractory) D50.9
    due to blood loss (chronic) D50.0
      acute D62
  simple chronic D53.9
  specified type NEC D64.89
  spherocytic (hereditary) —*see* Spherocytosis
  splenic D64.89
  splenomegalic D64.89
  stomatocytosis D58.8
  syphilitic (acquired) (late) A52.79 *[D63.8]*
  target cell D64.89

Anemia *(Continued)*
  thalassemia D56.9
  thrombocytopenic —*see* Thrombocytopenia
  toxic D61.2
  tropical B76.9 *[D63.8]*
    macrocytic D52.8
  tuberculous A18.89 *[D63.8]*
  vegan D51.3
  vitamin
    B6-responsive D64.3
    B12 deficiency (dietary) pernicious D51.0
  von Jaksch's D64.89
  Witts' (achlorhydric anemia) D50.8
Anemophobia F40.228
Anencephalus, anencephaly Q00.0
Anergasia —*see* Psychosis, organic
Anesthesia, anesthetic R20.0
  complication or reaction NEC —*see also*
      Complications, anesthesia T88.59
    due to
      correct substance properly
          administered —*see* Table of Drugs
          and Chemicals, by drug, adverse
          effect
      overdose or wrong substance given —*see*
          Table of Drugs and Chemicals, by
          drug, poisoning
      unintended awareness under general
          anesthesia during procedure
          T88.53
      personal history of Z92.84
  cornea H18.81-●
  dissociative F44.6
  functional (hysterical) F44.6
  hyperesthetic, thalamic G89.0
  hysterical F44.6
  local skin lesion R20.0
  sexual (psychogenic) F52.1
  shock (due to) T88.2
  skin R20.0
  testicular N50.9
Anetoderma (maculosum) (of) L90.8
  Jadassohn-Pellizzari L90.2
  Schweniger-Buzzi L90.1
Aneurin deficiency E51.9
Aneurysm (anastomotic) (artery) (cirsoid)
    (diffuse) (false) (fusiform) (multiple)
    (saccular) I72.9
  abdominal (aorta) I71.4
    ruptured I71.3
    syphilitic A52.01
  aorta, aortic (nonsyphilitic) I71.9
    abdominal I71.4
      ruptured I71.3
    arch I71.2
      ruptured I71.1
    arteriosclerotic I71.9
      ruptured I71.8
    ascending I71.2
      ruptured I71.1
    congenital Q25.43
    descending I71.9
      abdominal I71.4
        ruptured I71.3
      ruptured I71.8
      thoracic I71.2
        ruptured I71.1
    root Q25.43
    ruptured I71.8
    sinus, congenital Q25.43
    syphilitic A52.01
    thoracic I71.2
      ruptured I71.1
    thoracoabdominal I71.6
      ruptured I71.5
    thorax, thoracic (arch) I71.2
      ruptured I71.1
    transverse I71.2
      ruptured I71.1
    valve (heart) —*see also* Endocarditis, aortic
        I35.8

Aneurysm (Continued)
  arteriosclerotic I72.9
    cerebral I67.1
      ruptured —see Hemorrhage, intracranial,
        subarachnoid
  arteriovenous (congenital) —see also
    Malformation, arteriovenous
    acquired I77.0
      brain I67.1
      coronary I25.41
      pulmonary I28.0
    brain Q28.2
      ruptured I60.8
    peripheral —see Malformation,
      arteriovenous, peripheral
    precerebral vessels Q28.0
    specified site NEC —see also Malformation,
      arteriovenous
      acquired I77.0
  basal —see Aneurysm, brain
  basilar (trunk) I72.5
  berry (congenital) (nonruptured) I67.1
    ruptured I60.7
  brain I67.1
    arteriosclerotic I67.1
      ruptured —see Hemorrhage, intracranial,
        subarachnoid
    arteriovenous (congenital) (nonruptured)
      Q28.2
      acquired I67.1
        ruptured I60.8
      ruptured I60.8
    berry (congenital) (nonruptured) I67.1
      ruptured —see also Hemorrhage,
        intracranial, subarachnoid I60.7
    congenital Q28.3
      aorta (root) (sinus) Q25.43
        ruptured I60.7
    meninges I67.1
      ruptured I60.8
    miliary (congenital) (nonruptured) I67.1
      ruptured —see also Hemorrhage,
        intracranial, subarachnoid I60.7
    mycotic I33.0
    ruptured —see Hemorrhage, intracranial,
      subarachnoid
    syphilitic (hemorrhage) A52.05
  cardiac (false) —see also Aneurysm, heart
    I25.3
  carotid artery (common) (external) I72.0
    internal (intracranial) I67.1
      extracranial portion I72.0
    ruptured into brain I60.0- ●
    syphilitic A52.09
      intracranial A52.05
  cavernous sinus I67.1
    arteriovenous (congenital) (nonruptured)
      Q28.3
      ruptured I60.8
  celiac I72.8
  central nervous system, syphilitic A52.05
  cerebral —see Aneurysm, brain
  chest —see Aneurysm, thorax
  circle of Willis I67.1
    congenital Q28.3
      ruptured I60.6
    ruptured I60.6
  common iliac artery I72.3
  congenital (peripheral) Q27.8
    aorta (root) (sinus) Q25.43
    brain Q28.3
      ruptured I60.7
    coronary Q24.5
    digestive system Q27.8
    lower limb Q27.8
    pulmonary Q25.79
    retina Q14.1
    specified site NEC Q27.8
    upper limb Q27.8
  conjunctiva —see Abnormality, conjunctiva,
    vascular

Aneurysm (Continued)
  conus arteriosus —see Aneurysm, heart
  coronary (arteriosclerotic) (artery) I25.41
    arteriovenous, congenital Q24.5
    congenital Q24.5
    ruptured —see Infarct, myocardium
    syphilitic A52.06
    vein I25.89
  cylindroid (aorta) I71.9
    ruptured I71.8
    syphilitic A52.01
  ductus arteriosus Q25.0
  endocardial, infective (any valve) I33.0
  femoral (artery) (ruptured) I72.4
  gastroduodenal I72.8
  gastroepiploic I72.8
  heart (wall) (chronic or with a stated duration
    of over 4 weeks) I25.3
    valve —see Endocarditis
  hepatic I72.8
  iliac (common) (artery) (ruptured) I72.3
  infective I72.9
    endocardial (any valve) I33.0
  innominate (nonsyphilitic) I72.8
    syphilitic A52.09
  interauricular septum —see Aneurysm,
    heart
  interventricular septum —see Aneurysm,
    heart
  intrathoracic (nonsyphilitic) I71.2
    ruptured I71.1
    syphilitic A52.01
  lower limb I72.4
  lung (pulmonary artery) I28.1
  mediastinal (nonsyphilitic) I72.8
    syphilitic A52.09
  miliary (congenital) I67.1
    ruptured —see Hemorrhage, intracerebral,
      subarachnoid, intracranial
  mitral (heart) (valve) I34.8
  mural —see Aneurysm, heart
  mycotic I72.9
    endocardial (any valve) I33.0
    ruptured, brain —see Hemorrhage,
      intracerebral, subarachnoid
  myocardium —see Aneurysm, heart
  neck I72.0
  pancreaticoduodenal I72.8
  patent ductus arteriosus Q25.0
  peripheral NEC I72.8
    congenital Q27.8
      digestive system Q27.8
      lower limb Q27.8
      specified site NEC Q27.8
      upper limb Q27.8
  popliteal (artery) (ruptured) I72.4
  precerebral
    congenital (nonruptured) Q28.1
    specified site, NEC I72.5
  pulmonary I28.1
    arteriovenous Q25.72
      acquired I28.0
    syphilitic A52.09
    valve (heart) —see Endocarditis,
      pulmonary
  racemose (peripheral) I72.9
    congenital —see Aneurysm,
      congenital
  radial I72.1
  Rasmussen NEC A15.0
  renal (artery) I72.2
  retina —see also Disorder, retina,
    microaneurysms
    congenital Q14.1
    diabetic —see Diabetes, microaneurysms,
      retinal
  sinus of Valsalva Q25.49
  specified NEC I72.8
  spinal (cord) I72.8
    syphilitic (hemorrhage) A52.09
  splenic I72.8

Aneurysm (Continued)
  subclavian (artery) (ruptured) I72.8
    syphilitic A52.09
  superior mesenteric I72.8
  syphilitic (aorta) A52.01
    central nervous system A52.05
    congenital (late) A50.54 [I79.0]
    spine, spinal A52.09
  thoracoabdominal (aorta) I71.6
    ruptured I71.5
    syphilitic A52.01
  thorax, thoracic (aorta) (arch) (nonsyphilitic)
    I71.2
    ruptured I71.1
    syphilitic A52.01
  traumatic (complication) (early), specified
    site —see Injury, blood vessel
  tricuspid (heart) (valve) I07.8
  ulnar I72.1
  upper limb (ruptured) I72.1
  valve, valvular —see Endocarditis
  visceral NEC I72.8
  venous —see also Varix I86.8
    congenital Q27.8
      digestive system Q27.8
      lower limb Q27.8
      specified site NEC Q27.8
      upper limb Q27.8
  ventricle —see Aneurysm, heart
  vertebral artery I72.6
  visceral NEC I72.8
Angelman syndrome Q93.5
Anger R45.4
Angiectasis, angiectopia I99.8
Angiitis I77.6
  allergic granulomatous M30.1
  hypersensitivity M31.0
  necrotizing M31.9
    specified NEC M31.8
  nervous system, granulomatous I67.7
Angina (attack) (cardiac) (chest) (heart)
    (pectoris) (syndrome) (vasomotor) I20.9
  with
    atherosclerotic heart disease —see
      Arteriosclerosis, coronary (artery)
    documented spasm I20.1
  abdominal K55.1
  accelerated —see Angina, unstable
  agranulocytic —see Agranulocytosis
  angiospastic —see Angina, with documented
    spasm
  aphthous B08.5
  crescendo —see Angina, unstable
  croupous J05.0
  cruris I73.9
  de novo effort —see Angina, unstable
  diphtheritic, membranous A36.0
  equivalent I20.8
  exudative, chronic J37.0
  following acute myocardial infarction
    I23.7
  gangrenous diphtheritic A36.0
  intestinal K55.1
  Ludovici K12.2
  Ludwig's K12.2
  malignant diphtheritic A36.0
  membranous J05.0
    diphtheritic A36.0
    Vincent's A69.1
  mesenteric K55.1
  monocytic —see Mononucleosis, infectious
  of effort —see Angina, specified NEC
  phlegmonous J36
    diphtheritic A36.0
  post-infarctional I23.7
  pre-infarctional —see Angina, unstable
  Prinzmetal —see Angina, with documented
    spasm
  progressive —see Angina, unstable
  pseudomembranous A69.1
  pultaceous, diphtheritic A36.0

▶ New   ⇒ Revised   ~~deleted~~ Deleted   ● Use Additional Character(s)

Angina (Continued)
spasm-induced —see Angina, with
documented spasm
specified NEC I20.8
stable I20.8
stenocardia —see Angina, specified NEC
stridulous, diphtheritic A36.2
tonsil J36
trachealis J05.0
unstable I20.0
variant —see Angina, with documented
spasm
Vincent's A69.1
worsening effort —see Angina, unstable
Angioblastoma —see Neoplasm, connective
tissue, uncertain behavior
Angiocholecystitis —see Cholecystitis, acute
Angiocholitis —see also Cholecystitis, acute
K83.0
Angiodysgenesis spinalis G95.19
Angiodysplasia (cecum) (colon) K55.20
with bleeding K55.21
duodenum (and stomach) K31.819
with bleeding K31.811
stomach (and duodenum) K31.819
with bleeding K31.811
Angioedema (allergic) (any site) (with urticaria)
T78.3
hereditary D84.1
Angioendothelioma —see Neoplasm, uncertain
behavior, by site
benign D18.00
intra-abdominal D18.03
intracranial D18.02
skin D18.01
specified site NEC D18.09
bone —see Neoplasm, bone, malignant
Ewing's —see Neoplasm, bone, malignant
Angioendotheliomatosis C85.8-●
Angiofibroma —see also Neoplasm, benign, by
site
juvenile
specified site —see Neoplasm, benign, by
site
unspecified site D10.6
Angiohemophilia (A) (B) D68.0
Angioid streaks (choroid) (macula) (retina)
H35.33
Angiokeratoma —see Neoplasm, skin,
benign
corporis diffusum E75.21
Angioleiomyoma —see Neoplasm, connective
tissue, benign
Angiolipoma —see also Lipoma
infiltrating —see Lipoma
Angioma —see also Hemangioma, by site
capillary I78.1
hemorrhagicum hereditaria I78.0
intra-abdominal D18.03
intracranial D18.02
malignant —see Neoplasm, connective tissue,
malignant
plexiform D18.00
intra-abdominal D18.03
intracranial D18.02
skin D18.01
specified site NEC D18.09
senile I78.1
serpiginosum L81.7
skin D18.01
specified site NEC D18.09
spider I78.1
stellate I78.1
venous Q28.3
Angiomatosis Q82.8
bacillary A79.89
encephalotrigeminal Q85.8
hemorrhagic familial I78.0
hereditary familial I78.0
liver K76.4
Angiomyolipoma —see Lipoma

Angiomyoliposarcoma —see Neoplasm,
connective tissue, malignant
Angiomyoma —see Neoplasm, connective
tissue, benign
Angiomyosarcoma —see Neoplasm, connective
tissue, malignant
Angiomyxoma —see Neoplasm, connective
tissue, uncertain behavior
Angioneurosis F45.8
Angioneurotic edema (allergic) (any site) (with
urticaria) T78.3
hereditary D84.1
Angiopathia, angiopathy I99.9
cerebral I67.9
amyloid E85.4 [I68.0]
diabetic (peripheral) —see Diabetes,
angiopathy
peripheral I73.9
diabetic —see Diabetes, angiopathy
specified type NEC I73.89
retinae syphilitica A52.05
retinalis (juvenilis)
diabetic —see Diabetes, retinopathy
proliferative —see Retinopathy,
proliferative
Angiosarcoma —see also Neoplasm, connective
tissue, malignant
liver C22.3
Angiosclerosis —see Arteriosclerosis
Angiospasm (peripheral) (traumatic) (vessel)
I73.9
brachial plexus G54.0
cerebral G45.9
cervical plexus G54.2
nerve
arm —see Mononeuropathy, upper limb
axillary G54.0
median —see Lesion, nerve, median
ulnar —see Lesion, nerve, ulnar
axillary G54.0
leg —see Mononeuropathy, lower limb
median —see Lesion, nerve, median
plantar —see Lesion, nerve, plantar
ulnar —see Lesion, nerve, ulnar
Angiospastic disease or edema I73.9
Angiostrongyliasis
due to
Parastrongylus
cantonensis B83.2
costaricensis B81.3
intestinal B81.3
Anguillulosis —see Strongyloidiasis
Angulation
cecum —see Obstruction, intestine
coccyx (acquired) —see also subcategory
M43.8
congenital NEC Q76.49
femur (acquired) —see also Deformity, limb,
specified type NEC, thigh
congenital Q74.2
intestine (large) (small) —see Obstruction,
intestine
sacrum (acquired) —see also subcategory
M43.8
congenital NEC Q76.49
sigmoid (flexure) —see Obstruction,
intestine
spine —see Dorsopathy, deforming,
specified NEC
tibia (acquired) —see also Deformity, limb,
specified type NEC, lower leg
congenital Q74.2
ureter N13.5
with infection N13.6
wrist (acquired) —see also Deformity,
limb, specified type NEC, forearm
congenital Q74.0
Angulus infectiosus (lips) K13.0
Anhedonia R45.84
sexual F52.0
Anhidrosis L74.4

Anhydration E86.0
Anhydremia E86.0
Anidrosis L74.4
Aniridia (congenital) Q13.1
Anisakiasis (infection) (infestation) B81.0
Anisakis larvae infestation B81.0
Aniseikonia H52.32
Anisocoria (pupil) H57.02
congenital Q13.2
Anisocytosis R71.8
Anisometropia (congenital) H52.31
Ankle —see condition
Ankyloblepharon (eyelid) (acquired) —see also
Blepharophimosis
filiforme (adnatum) (congenital) Q10.3
total Q10.3
Ankyloglossia Q38.1
Ankylosis (fibrous) (osseous) (joint) M24.60
ankle M24.67-●
arthrodesis status Z98.1
cricoarytenoid (cartilage) (joint) (larynx)
J38.7
dental K03.5
ear ossicles H74.31-●
elbow M24.62-●
foot M24.67-●
hand M24.64-●
hip M24.65-●
incostapedial joint (infectional) —see
Ankylosis, ear ossicles
jaw (temporomandibular) M26.61-●
knee M24.66-●
lumbosacral (joint) M43.27
postoperative (status) Z98.1
produced by surgical fusion, status Z98.1
sacro-iliac (joint) M43.28
shoulder M24.61-●
spine (joint) —see also Fusion, spine
spondylitic —see Spondylitis, ankylosing
surgical Z98.1
temporomandibular M26.61-●
tooth, teeth (hard tissues) K03.5
wrist M24.63-●
Ankylostoma —see Ancylostoma
Ankylostomiasis —see Ancylostomiasis
Ankylurethria —see Stricture, urethra
Annular —see also condition
detachment, cervix N88.8
organ or site, congenital NEC —see Distortion
pancreas (congenital) Q45.1
Anodontia (complete) (partial) (vera) K00.0
acquired K08.10
Anomaly, anomalous (congenital) (unspecified
type) Q89.9
abdominal wall NEC Q79.59
acoustic nerve Q07.8
adrenal (gland) Q89.1
Alder (-Reilly) (leukocyte granulation)
D72.0
alimentary tract Q45.9
upper Q40.9
alveolar M26.70
hyperplasia M26.79
mandibular M26.72
maxillary M26.71
hypoplasia M26.79
mandibular M26.74
maxillary M26.73
ridge (process) M26.79
specified NEC M26.79
ankle (joint) Q74.2
anus Q43.9
aorta (arch) NEC Q25.40
coarctation (preductal) (postductal)
Q25.1
aortic cusp or valve Q23.9
appendix Q43.8
apple peel syndrome Q41.1
aqueduct of Sylvius Q03.0
with spina bifida —see Spina bifida, with
hydrocephalus

Anomaly, anomalous (Continued)
arm Q74.0
arteriovenous NEC
  coronary Q24.5
  gastrointestinal Q27.33
  acquired —see Angiodysplasia
artery (peripheral) Q27.9
  basilar NEC Q28.1
  cerebral Q28.3
  coronary Q24.5
  digestive system Q27.8
  eye Q15.8
  great Q25.9
    specified NEC Q25.8
  lower limb Q27.8
  peripheral Q27.9
    specified NEC Q27.8
  pulmonary NEC Q25.79
  renal Q27.2
  retina Q14.1
  specified site NEC Q27.8
  subclavian Q27.8
    origin Q25.48
  umbilical Q27.0
  upper limb Q27.8
  vertebral NEC Q28.1
aryteno-epiglottic folds Q31.8
atrial
  bands or folds Q20.8
  septa Q21.1
atrioventricular
  excitation I45.6
  septum Q21.0
auditory canal Q17.8
auricle
  ear Q17.8
    causing impairment of hearing
      Q16.9
  heart Q20.8
Axenfeld's Q15.0
back Q89.9
band
  atrial Q20.8
  heart Q24.8
  ventricular Q24.8
Bartholin's duct Q38.4
biliary duct or passage Q44.5
bladder Q64.70
  absence Q64.5
  diverticulum Q64.6
  exstrophy Q64.10
    cloacal Q64.12
    extroversion Q64.19
    specified type NEC Q64.19
    supravesical fissure Q64.11
  neck obstruction Q64.31
  specified type NEC Q64.79
bone Q79.9
  arm Q74.0
  face Q75.9
  leg Q74.2
  pelvic girdle Q74.2
  shoulder girdle Q74.0
  skull Q75.9
    with
      anencephaly Q00.0
      encephalocele —see Encephalocele
      hydrocephalus Q03.9
        with spina bifida —see Spina bifida,
          by site, with hydrocephalus
      microcephaly Q02
brain (multiple) Q04.9
  vessel Q28.3
breast Q83.9
broad ligament Q50.6
bronchus Q32.4
bulbus cordis Q21.9
bursa Q79.9
canal of Nuck Q52.4
canthus Q10.3
capillary Q27.9

Anomaly, anomalous (Continued)
cardiac Q24.9
  chambers Q20.9
    specified NEC Q20.8
  septal closure Q21.9
    specified NEC Q21.8
  valve NEC Q24.8
    pulmonary Q22.3
cardiovascular system Q28.8
carpus Q74.0
caruncle, lacrimal Q10.6
cascade stomach Q40.2
cauda equina Q06.3
cecum Q43.9
cerebral Q04.9
  vessels Q28.3
cervix Q51.9
Chédiak-Higashi(-Steinbrinck) (congenital
    gigantism of peroxidase granules)
    E70.330
cheek Q18.9
chest wall Q67.8
  bones Q76.9
chin Q18.9
chordae tendineae Q24.8
choroid Q14.3
  plexus Q07.8
chromosomes, chromosomal Q99.9
  D (1) —see condition, chromosome 13
  E (3) —see condition, chromosome 18
  G —see condition, chromosome 21
  sex
    female phenotype Q97.8
    gonadal dysgenesis (pure) Q99.1
    Klinefelter's Q98.4
    male phenotype Q98.9
    Turner's Q96.9
    specified NEC Q99.8
cilia Q10.3
circulatory system Q28.9
clavicle Q74.0
clitoris Q52.6
coccyx Q76.49
colon Q43.9
common duct Q44.5
communication
  coronary artery Q24.5
  left ventricle with right atrium Q21.0
concha (ear) Q17.3
connection
  portal vein Q26.5
  pulmonary venous Q26.4
    partial Q26.3
    total Q26.2
  renal artery with kidney Q27.2
cornea (shape) Q13.4
coronary artery or vein Q24.5
cranium —see Anomaly, skull
cricoid cartilage Q31.8
cystic duct Q44.5
dental
  alveolar —see Anomaly, alveolar
  arch relationship M26.20
    specified NEC M26.29
dentofacial M26.9
  alveolar —see Anomaly, alveolar
  dental arch relationship M26.20
    specified NEC M26.29
  functional M26.50
    specified NEC M26.59
  jaw-cranial base relationship M26.10
    asymmetry M26.12
      maxillary M26.11
    specified type NEC M26.19
  jaw size M26.00
    macrogenia M26.05
    mandibular
      hyperplasia M26.03
      hypoplasia M26.04
    maxillary
      hyperplasia M26.01
      hypoplasia M26.02

Anomaly, anomalous (Continued)
dentofacial (Continued)
  jaw size (Continued)
    microgenia M26.06
    specified type NEC M26.09
  malocclusion M26.4
    dental arch relationship NEC M26.29
    jaw-cranial base relationship —see
      Anomaly, dentofacial, jaw-cranial
      base relationship
    jaw size —see Anomaly, dentofacial, jaw
      size
  specified type NEC M26.89
  temporomandibular joint M26.60-●
    adhesions M26.61-●
    ankylosis M26.61-●
    arthralgia M26.62-●
    articular disc M26.63-●
    specified type NEC M26.69
  tooth position, fully erupted M26.30
    specified NEC M26.39
dermatoglyphic Q82.8
diaphragm (apertures) NEC Q79.1
digestive organ(s) or tract Q45.9
  lower Q43.9
  upper Q40.9
distance, interarch (excessive) (inadequate)
    M26.25
distribution, coronary artery Q24.5
ductus
  arteriosus Q25.0
  botalli Q25.0
duodenum Q43.9
dura (brain) Q04.9
  spinal cord Q06.9
ear (external) Q17.9
  causing impairment of hearing Q16.9
  inner Q16.5
  middle (causing impairment of hearing)
    Q16.4
    ossicles Q16.3
Ebstein's (heart) (tricuspid valve) Q22.5
ectodermal Q82.9
Eisenmenger's (ventricular septal defect)
    Q21.8
ejaculatory duct Q55.4
elbow Q74.0
endocrine gland NEC Q89.2
epididymis Q55.4
epiglottis Q31.8
esophagus Q39.9
eustachian tube Q17.8
eye Q15.9
  anterior segment Q13.9
    specified NEC Q13.89
  posterior segment Q14.9
    specified NEC Q14.8
  ptosis (eyelid) Q10.0
  specified NEC Q15.8
eyebrow Q18.8
eyelid Q10.3
  ptosis Q10.0
face Q18.9
  bone(s) Q75.9
fallopian tube Q50.6
fascia Q79.9
femur NEC Q74.2
fibula NEC Q74.2
finger Q74.0
fixation, intestine Q43.3
flexion (joint) NOS Q74.9
  hip or thigh Q65.89
foot NEC Q74.2
  varus (congenital) Q66.3
foramen
  Botalli Q21.1
  ovale Q21.1
forearm Q74.0
forehead Q75.8
form, teeth K00.2
fovea centralis Q14.1

▶ New   ⇒ Revised   ~~deleted~~ Deleted   ● Use Additional Character(s)

Anomaly, anomalous *(Continued)*
  frontal bone —*see* Anomaly, skull
  gallbladder (position) (shape) (size) Q44.1
  Gartner's duct Q52.4
  gastrointestinal tract Q45.9
  genitalia, genital organ(s) or system
    female Q52.9
      external Q52.70
      internal NOS Q52.9
    male Q55.9
      hydrocele P83.5
      specified NEC Q55.8
  genitourinary NEC
    female Q52.9
    male Q55.9
  Gerbode Q21.0
  glottis Q31.8
  granulation or granulocyte, genetic
      (constitutional) (leukocyte) D72.0
  gum Q38.6
  gyri Q07.9
  hair Q84.2
  hand Q74.0
  hard tissue formation in pulp K04.3
  head —*see* Anomaly, skull
  heart Q24.9
    auricle Q20.8
    bands or folds Q24.8
    fibroelastosis cordis I42.4
    obstructive NEC Q22.6
    patent ductus arteriosus (Botalli) Q25.0
    septum Q21.9
      auricular Q21.1
      interatrial Q21.1
      interventricular Q21.0
        with pulmonary stenosis or atresia,
            dextraposition of aorta and
            hypertrophy of right ventricle
            Q21.3
      specified NEC Q21.8
      ventricular Q21.0
        with pulmonary stenosis or atresia,
            dextraposition of aorta and
            hypertrophy of right ventricle
            Q21.3
    tetralogy of Fallot Q21.3
    valve NEC Q24.8
      aortic
        bicuspid valve Q23.1
        insufficiency Q23.1
        stenosis Q23.0
          subaortic Q24.4
      mitral
        insufficiency Q23.3
        stenosis Q23.2
      pulmonary Q22.3
        atresia Q22.0
        insufficiency Q22.2
        stenosis Q22.1
          infundibular Q24.3
          subvalvular Q24.3
      tricuspid
        atresia Q22.4
        stenosis Q22.4
    ventricle Q20.8
  heel NEC Q74.2
  Hegglin's D72.0
  hemianencephaly Q00.0
  hemicephaly Q00.0
  hemicrania Q00.0
  hepatic duct Q44.5
  hip NEC Q74.2
  hourglass stomach Q40.2
  humerus Q74.0
  hydatid of Morgagni
    female Q50.5
    male (epididymal) Q55.4
      testicular Q55.29
  hymen Q52.4
  hypersegmentation of neutrophils, hereditary
      D72.0

Anomaly, anomalous *(Continued)*
  hypophyseal Q89.2
  ileocecal (coil) (valve) Q43.9
  ileum Q43.9
  ilium NEC Q74.2
  integument Q84.9
    specified NEC Q84.8
  interarch distance (excessive) (inadequate)
      M26.25
  intervertebral cartilage or disc Q76.49
  intestine (large) (small) Q43.9
    with anomalous adhesions, fixation or
        malrotation Q43.3
  iris Q13.2
  ischium NEC Q74.2
  jaw —*see* Anomaly, dentofacial
    alveolar —*see* Anomaly, alveolar
  jaw-cranial base relationship —*see*
      Anomaly, dentofacial, jaw-cranial
      base relationship
  jejunum Q43.8
  joint Q74.9
    specified NEC Q74.8
  Jordan's D72.0
  kidney(s) (calyx) (pelvis) Q63.9
    artery Q27.2
    specified NEC Q63.8
  Klippel-Feil (brevicollis) Q76.1
  knee Q74.1
  labium (majus) (minus) Q52.70
  labyrinth, membranous Q16.5
  lacrimal apparatus or duct Q10.6
  larynx, laryngeal (muscle) Q31.9
    web (bed) Q31.0
  lens Q12.9
  leukocytes, genetic D72.0
    granulation (constitutional) D72.0
  lid (fold) Q10.3
  ligament Q79.9
    broad Q50.6
    round Q52.8
  limb Q74.9
    lower NEC Q74.2
      reduction deformity —*see* Defect,
          reduction, lower limb
    upper Q74.0
  lip Q38.0
  liver Q44.7
    duct Q44.5
  lower limb NEC Q74.2
  lumbosacral (joint) (region) Q76.49
    kyphosis —*see* Kyphosis, congenital
    lordosis —*see* Lordosis, congenital
  lung (fissure) (lobe) Q33.9
  mandible —*see* Anomaly, dentofacial
  maxilla —*see* Anomaly, dentofacial
  May (-Hegglin) D72.0
  meatus urinarius NEC Q64.79
  meningeal bands or folds Q07.9
    constriction of Q07.8
    spinal Q06.9
  meninges Q07.9
    cerebral Q04.8
    spinal Q06.9
  meningocele Q05.9
  mesentery Q45.9
  metacarpus Q74.0
  metatarsus NEC Q74.2
  middle ear Q16.4
    ossicles Q16.3
  mitral (leaflets) (valve) Q23.9
    insufficiency Q23.3
    specified NEC Q23.8
    stenosis Q23.2
  mouth Q38.6
  Müllerian —*see also* Anomaly, by site
    uterus NEC Q51.818
  multiple NEC Q89.7
  muscle Q79.9
    eyelid Q10.3
  musculoskeletal system, except limbs Q79.9

Anomaly, anomalous *(Continued)*
  myocardium Q24.8
  nail Q84.6
  narrowness, eyelid Q10.3
  nasal sinus (wall) Q30.8
  neck (any part) Q18.9
  nerve Q07.9
    acoustic Q07.8
    optic Q07.8
  nervous system (central) Q07.9
  nipple Q83.9
  nose, nasal (bones) (cartilage) (septum)
      (sinus) Q30.9
    specified NEC Q30.8
  ocular muscle Q15.8
  omphalomesenteric duct Q43.0
  opening, pulmonary veins Q26.4
  optic
    disc Q14.2
    nerve Q07.8
  opticociliary vessels Q13.2
  orbit (eye) Q10.7
  organ Q89.9
    of Corti Q16.5
  origin
    artery
      innominate Q25.8
      pulmonary Q25.79
      renal Q27.2
      subclavian Q25.48
  osseous meatus (ear) Q16.1
  ovary Q50.39
  oviduct Q50.6
  palate (hard) (soft) NEC Q38.5
  pancreas or pancreatic duct Q45.3
  papillary muscles Q24.8
  parathyroid gland Q89.2
  paraurethral ducts Q64.79
  parotid (gland) Q38.4
  patella Q74.1
  Pelger-Huët (hereditary hyposegmentation)
      D72.0
  pelvic girdle NEC Q74.2
  pelvis (bony) NEC Q74.2
    rachitic E64.3
  penis (glans) Q55.69
  pericardium Q24.8
  peripheral vascular system Q27.9
  Peter's Q13.4
  pharynx Q38.8
  pigmentation L81.9
    congenital Q82.8
  pituitary (gland) Q89.2
  pleural (folds) Q34.0
  portal vein Q26.5
    connection Q26.5
  position, tooth, teeth, fully erupted M26.30
    specified NEC M26.39
  precerebral vessel Q28.1
  prepuce Q55.69
  prostate Q55.4
  pulmonary Q33.9
    artery NEC Q25.79
    valve Q22.3
      atresia Q22.0
      insufficiency Q22.2
      specified type NEC Q22.3
      stenosis Q22.1
        infundibular Q24.3
        subvalvular Q24.3
    venous connection Q26.4
      partial Q26.3
      total Q26.2
  pupil Q13.2
    function H57.00
      anisocoria H57.02
      Argyll Robertson pupil H57.01
      miosis H57.03
      mydriasis H57.04
      specified type NEC H57.09
      tonic pupil H57.05-●

Anomaly, anomalous *(Continued)*
pylorus Q40.3
radius Q74.0
rectum Q43.9
reduction (extremity) (limb)
  femur (longitudinal) —*see* Defect, reduction, lower limb, longitudinal, femur
  fibula (longitudinal) —*see* Defect, reduction, lower limb, longitudinal, fibula
  lower limb —*see* Defect, reduction, lower limb
  radius (longitudinal) —*see* Defect, reduction, upper limb, longitudinal, radius
  tibia (longitudinal) —*see* Defect, reduction, lower limb, longitudinal, tibia
  ulna (longitudinal) —*see* Defect, reduction, upper limb, longitudinal, ulna
  upper limb —*see* Defect, reduction, upper limb
refraction —*see* Disorder, refraction
renal Q63.9
  artery Q27.2
  pelvis Q63.9
    specified NEC Q63.8
respiratory system Q34.9
  specified NEC Q34.8
retina Q14.1
rib Q76.6
  cervical Q76.5
Rieger's Q13.81
rotation —*see* Malrotation
  hip or thigh Q65.89
round ligament Q52.8
sacroiliac (joint) NEC Q74.2
sacrum NEC Q76.49
  kyphosis —*see* Kyphosis, congenital
  lordosis —*see* Lordosis, congenital
saddle nose, syphilitic A50.57
salivary duct or gland Q38.4
scapula Q74.0
scrotum —*see* Malformation, testis and scrotum
sebaceous gland Q82.9
seminal vesicles Q55.4
sense organs NEC Q07.8
sex chromosomes NEC —*see also* Anomaly, chromosomes
  female phenotype Q97.8
  male phenotype Q98.9
shoulder (girdle) (joint) Q74.0
sigmoid (flexure) Q43.9
simian crease Q82.8
sinus of Valsalva Q25.49
skeleton generalized Q78.9
skin (appendage) Q82.9
skull Q75.9
  with
    anencephaly Q00.0
    encephalocele —*see* Encephalocele
    hydrocephalus Q03.9
      with spina bifida —*see* Spina bifida, by site, with hydrocephalus
    microcephaly Q02
specified organ or site NEC Q89.8
spermatic cord Q55.4
spine, spinal NEC Q76.49
  column NEC Q76.49
    kyphosis —*see* Kyphosis, congenital
    lordosis —*see* Lordosis, congenital
  cord Q06.9
  nerve root Q07.8
spleen Q89.09
  agenesis Q89.01
stenonian duct Q38.4
sternum NEC Q76.7
stomach Q40.3
submaxillary gland Q38.4
tarsus NEC Q74.2

Anomaly, anomalous *(Continued)*
tendon Q79.9
testis —*see* Malformation, testis and scrotum
thigh NEC Q74.2
thorax (wall) Q67.8
  bony Q76.9
throat Q38.8
thumb Q74.0
thymus gland Q89.2
thyroid (gland) Q89.2
  cartilage Q31.8
tibia NEC Q74.2
  saber A50.56
toe Q74.2
tongue Q38.3
tooth, teeth K00.9
  eruption K00.6
  position, fully erupted M26.30
  spacing, fully erupted M26.30
trachea (cartilage) Q32.1
tragus Q17.9
tricuspid (leaflet) (valve) Q22.9
  atresia or stenosis Q22.4
  Ebstein's Q22.5
Uhl's (hypoplasia of myocardium, right ventricle) Q24.8
ulna Q74.0
umbilical artery Q27.0
union
  cricoid cartilage and thyroid cartilage Q31.8
  thyroid cartilage and hyoid bone Q31.8
  trachea with larynx Q31.8
upper limb Q74.0
urachus Q64.4
ureter Q62.8
  obstructive NEC Q62.39
    cecoureterocele Q62.32
    orthotopic ureterocele Q62.31
urethra Q64.70
  absence Q64.5
  double Q64.74
  fistula to rectum Q64.73
  obstructive Q64.39
    stricture Q64.32
  prolapse Q64.71
  specified type NEC Q64.79
urinary tract Q64.9
uterus Q51.9
  with only one functioning horn Q51.4
uvula Q38.5
vagina Q52.4
valleculae Q31.8
valve (heart) NEC Q24.8
  coronary sinus Q24.5
  inferior vena cava Q24.8
  pulmonary Q22.3
  sinus coronario Q24.5
  venae cavae inferioris Q24.8
vas deferens Q55.4
vascular Q27.9
  brain Q28.3
  ring Q25.45
vein(s) (peripheral) Q27.9
  brain Q28.3
  cerebral Q28.3
  coronary Q24.5
  developmental Q28.3
  great Q26.9
    specified NEC Q26.8
vena cava (inferior) (superior) Q26.9
venous —*see* Anomaly, vein(s)
venous return Q26.8
ventricular
  bands or folds Q24.8
  septa Q21.0
vertebra Q76.49
  kyphosis —*see* Kyphosis, congenital
  lordosis —*see* Lordosis, congenital

Anomaly, anomalous *(Continued)*
vesicourethral orifice Q64.79
vessel(s) Q27.9
  optic papilla Q14.2
  precerebral Q28.1
vitelline duct Q43.0
vitreous body or humor Q14.0
vulva Q52.70
wrist (joint) Q74.0
Anomia R48.8
Anonychia (congenital) Q84.3
  acquired L60.8
Anophthalmos, anophthalmus (congenital) (globe) Q11.1
  acquired Z90.01
Anopia, anopsia H53.46-●
  quadrant H53.46-●
Anorchia, anorchism, anorchidism Q55.0
Anorexia R63.0
  hysterical F44.89
  nervosa F50.00
    atypical F50.9
    binge-eating type F50.2
      with purging F50.02
    restricting type F50.01
Anorgasmy, psychogenic (female) F52.31
  male F52.32
Anosmia R43.0
  hysterical F44.6
  postinfectional J39.8
Anosognosia R41.89
Anosteoplasia Q78.9
Anovulatory cycle N97.0
Anoxemia R09.02
  newborn P84
Anoxia (pathological) R09.02
  altitude T70.29
  cerebral G93.1
    complicating
      anesthesia (general) (local) or other sedation T88.59
        in labor and delivery O74.3
        in pregnancy O29.21-●
        postpartum, puerperal O89.2
      delivery (cesarean) (instrumental) O75.4
    during a procedure G97.81
    newborn P84
    resulting from a procedure G97.82
  due to
    drowning T75.1
    high altitude T70.29
  heart —*see* Insufficiency, coronary
  intrauterine P84
  myocardial —*see* Insufficiency, coronary
  newborn P84
  spinal cord G95.11
  systemic (by suffocation) (low content in atmosphere) —*see* Asphyxia, traumatic
Anteflexion —*see* Anteversion
Antenatal
  care (normal pregnancy) Z34.90
  screening (encounter for) of mother —*see also* Encounter, antenatal screening Z36.9
Antepartum —*see* condition
Anterior —*see* condition
Antero-occlusion M26.220
Anteversion
  cervix —*see* Anteversion, uterus
  femur (neck), congenital Q65.89
  uterus, uterine (cervix) (postinfectional) (postpartal, old) N85.4
    congenital Q51.818
    in pregnancy or childbirth —*see* Pregnancy, complicated by
Anthophobia F40.228
Anthracosilicosis J60
Anthracosis (lung) (occupational) J60
  lingua K14.3

▶ New   ⇒ Revised   ~~deleted~~ Deleted   ● Use Additional Character(s)

Anthrax A22.9
  with pneumonia A22.1
  cerebral A22.8
  colitis A22.2
  cutaneous A22.0
  gastrointestinal A22.2
  inhalation A22.1
  intestinal A22.2
  meningitis A22.8
  pulmonary A22.1
  respiratory A22.1
  sepsis A22.7
  specified manifestation NEC A22.8
Anthropoid pelvis Q74.2
  with disproportion (fetopelvic) O33.0
Anthropophobia F40.10
  generalized F40.11
Antibodies, maternal (blood group) —see
    Isoimmunization, affecting management of
    pregnancy
  anti-D —see Isoimmunization, affecting
    management of pregnancy, Rh
    newborn P55.0
Antibody
  anticardiolipin R76.0
    with
      hemorrhagic disorder D68.312
      hypercoagulable state D68.61
  antiphosphatidylglycerol R76.0
    with
      hemorrhagic disorder D68.312
      hypercoagulable state D68.61
  antiphosphatidylinositol R76.0
    with
      hemorrhagic disorder D68.312
      hypercoagulable state D68.61
  antiphosphatidylserine R76.0
    with
      hemorrhagic disorder D68.312
      hypercoagulable state D68.61
  antiphospholipid R76.0
    with
      hemorrhagic disorder D68.312
      hypercoagulable state D68.61
Anticardiolipin syndrome D68.61
Anticoagulant, circulating (intrinsic) —see also -
    Disorder, hemorrhagic D68.318
  drug-induced (extrinsic) —see also - Disorder,
    hemorrhagic D68.32
  iatrogenic D68.32
Antidiuretic hormone syndrome E22.2
Antimonial cholera —see Poisoning,
    antimony
Antiphospholipid
  antibody
    with hemorrhagic disorder D68.312
    syndrome D68.61
Antisocial personality F60.2
Antithrombinemia —see Circulating
    anticoagulants
Antithromboplastinemia D68.318
Antithromboplastinogenemia D68.318
Antitoxin complication or reaction —see
    Complications, vaccination
Antlophobia F40.228
Antritis J32.0
  maxilla J32.0
    acute J01.00
      recurrent J01.01
  stomach K29.60
    with bleeding K29.61
Antrum, antral —see condition
Anuria R34
  calculus (impacted) (recurrent) —see also
    Calculus, urinary N20.9
  following
    abortion —see Abortion by type
      complicated by, renal failure
    ectopic or molar pregnancy O08.4
  newborn P96.0
  postprocedural N99.0

Anuria (Continued)
  postrenal N13.8
  traumatic (following crushing) T79.5
Anus, anal —see condition
Anusitis K62.89
Anxiety F41.9
  depression F41.8
  episodic paroxysmal F41.0
  generalized F41.1
  hysteria F41.8
  neurosis F41.1
  panic type F41.0
  reaction F41.1
  separation, abnormal (of childhood) F93.0
  specified NEC F41.8
  state F41.1
Aorta, aortic —see condition
Aortectasia —see Ectasia, aorta
  with aneurysm —see Aneurysm, aorta
Aortitis (nonsyphilitic) (calcific) I77.6
  arteriosclerotic I70.0
  Doehle-Heller A52.02
  luetic A52.02
  rheumatic —see Endocarditis, acute,
    rheumatic
  specific (syphilitic) A52.02
  syphilitic A52.02
    congenital A50.54 [I79.1]
Apathetic thyroid storm —see Thyrotoxicosis
Apathy R45.3
Apeirophobia F40.228
Apepsia K30
  psychogenic F45.8
Aperistalsis, esophagus K22.0
Apertognathia M26.29
Apert's syndrome Q87.0
Aphagia R13.0
  psychogenic F50.9
Aphakia (acquired) (postoperative) H27.0-●
  congenital Q12.3
Aphasia (amnestic) (global) (nominal)
    (semantic) (syntactic) R47.01
  acquired, with epilepsy (Landau-Kleffner
    syndrome) —see Epilepsy, specified
    NEC
  auditory (developmental) F80.2
  developmental (receptive type) F80.2
    expressive type F80.1
    Wernicke's F80.2
  following
    cerebrovascular disease I69.920
      cerebral infarction I69.320
      intracerebral hemorrhage I69.120
      nontraumatic intracranial hemorrhage
        NEC I69.220
      specified disease NEC I69.820
      subarachnoid hemorrhage I69.020
  primary progressive G31.01 [F02.80]
    with behavioral disturbance G31.01
      [F02.81]
  progressive isolated G31.01 [F02.80]
    with behavioral disturbance G31.01
      [F02.81]
  sensory F80.2
  syphilis, tertiary A52.19
  Wernicke's (developmental) F80.2
Aphonia (organic) R49.1
  hysterical F44.4
  psychogenic F44.4
Aphthae, aphthous —see also condition
  Bednar's K12.0
  cachectic K14.0
  epizootic B08.8
  fever B08.8
  oral (recurrent) K12.0
  stomatitis (major) (minor) K12.0
  thrush B37.0
  ulcer (oral) (recurrent) K12.0
    genital organ(s) NEC
      female N76.6
      male N50.89
    larynx J38.7

Apical —see condition
Apiphobia F40.218
Aplasia —see also Agenesis
  abdominal muscle syndrome Q79.4
  alveolar process (acquired) —see Anomaly,
    alveolar
    congenital Q38.6
  aorta (congenital) Q25.41
  axialis extracorticalis (congenita) E75.29
  bone marrow (myeloid) D61.9
    congenital D61.01
  brain Q00.0
    part of Q04.3
  bronchus Q32.4
  cementum K00.4
  cerebellum Q04.3
  cervix (congenital) Q51.5
  congenital pure red cell D61.01
  corpus callosum Q04.0
  cutis congenita Q84.8
  erythrocyte congenital D61.01
  extracortical axial E75.29
  eye Q11.1
  fovea centralis (congenital) Q14.1
  gallbladder, congenital Q44.0
  iris Q13.1
  labyrinth, membranous Q16.5
  limb (congenital) Q73.8
    lower —see Defect, reduction, lower limb
    upper —see Agenesis, arm
  lung, congenital (bilateral) (unilateral) Q33.3
  pancreas Q45.0
  parathyroid-thymic D82.1
  Pelizaeus-Merzbacher E75.29
  penis Q55.5
  prostate Q55.4
  red cell (with thymoma) D60.9
    acquired D60.9
      due to drugs D60.9
    adult D60.9
    chronic D60.0
    congenital D61.01
    constitutional D61.01
    due to drugs D60.9
    hereditary D61.01
    of infants D61.01
    primary D61.01
    pure D61.01
      due to drugs D60.9
    specified type NEC D60.8
    transient D60.1
  round ligament Q52.8
  skin Q84.8
  spermatic cord Q55.4
  spleen Q89.01
  testicle Q55.0
  thymic, with immunodeficiency D82.1
  thyroid (congenital) (with myxedema) E03.1
  uterus Q51.0
  ventral horn cell Q06.1
Apnea, apneic (of) (spells) R06.81
  newborn NEC P28.4
    obstructive P28.4
    sleep (central) (obstructive) (primary) P28.3
  prematurity P28.4
  sleep G47.30
    central (primary) G47.31
    ▶idiopathic G47.31
      in conditions classified elsewhere
        G47.37
    obstructive (adult) (pediatric) G47.33
    ▶hypopnea G47.33
    primary central G47.31
    specified NEC G47.39
Apneumatosis, newborn P28.0
Apocrine metaplasia (breast) —see Dysplasia,
    mammary, specified type NEC
Apophysitis (bone) —see also
    Osteochondropathy
  calcaneus M92.8
  juvenile M92.9

Apoplectiform convulsions (cerebral ischemia) I67.82

Apoplexia, apoplexy, apoplectic
adrenal A39.1
heart (auricle) (ventricle) —see Infarct, myocardium
heat T67.0
hemorrhagic (stroke) —see Hemorrhage, intracranial
meninges, hemorrhagic —see Hemorrhage, intracranial, subarachnoid
uremic N18.9 [I68.8]

Appearance
bizarre R46.1
specified NEC R46.89
very low level of personal hygiene R46.0

Appendage
epididymal (organ of Morgagni) Q55.4
intestine (epiploic) Q43.8
preauricular Q17.0
testicular (organ of Morgagni) Q55.29

Appendicitis (pneumococcal) (retrocecal) K37
with
perforation or rupture K35.2
peritoneal abscess K35.3
peritonitis NEC K35.3
generalized (with perforation or rupture) K35.2
localized (with perforation or rupture) K35.3
acute (catarrhal) (fulminating) (gangrenous) (obstructive) (retrocecal) (suppurative) K35.80
with
peritoneal abscess K35.3
peritonitis NEC K35.3
generalized (with perforation or rupture) K35.2
localized (with perforation or rupture) K35.3
specified NEC K35.89
amebic A06.89
chronic (recurrent) K36
exacerbation —see Appendicitis, acute
gangrenous —see Appendicitis, acute
healed (obliterative) K36
interval K36
neurogenic K36
obstructive K36
recurrent K36
relapsing K36
subacute (adhesive) K36
subsiding K36
suppurative —see Appendicitis, acute
tuberculous A18.32

Appendicopathia oxyurica B80

Appendix, appendicular —see also condition
epididymis Q55.4
Morgagni
female Q50.5
male (epididymal) Q55.4
testicular Q55.29
testis Q55.29

Appetite
depraved —see Pica
excessive R63.2
lack or loss —see also Anorexia R63.0
nonorganic origin F50.89
psychogenic F50.89
perverted (hysterical) —see Pica

Apple peel syndrome Q41.1

Apprehension state F41.1

Apprehensiveness, abnormal F41.9

Approximal wear K03.0

Apraxia (classic) (ideational) (ideokinetic) (ideomotor) (motor) (verbal) R48.2
following
cerebrovascular disease I69.990
cerebral infarction I69.390
intracerebral hemorrhage I69.190

Apraxia (Continued)
following (Continued)
cerebrovascular disease (Continued)
nontraumatic intracranial hemorrhage NEC I69.290
specified disease NEC I69.890
subarachnoid hemorrhage I69.090
oculomotor, congenital H51.8

Aptyalism K11.7

Apudoma —see Neoplasm, uncertain behavior, by site

Aqueous misdirection H40.83-●

Arabicum elephantiasis —see Infestation, filarial

Arachnitis —see Meningitis

Arachnodactyly —see Syndrome, Marfan's

Arachnoiditis (acute) (adhesive) (basal) (brain) (cerebrospinal) —see Meningitis

Arachnophobia F40.210

Arboencephalitis, Australian A83.4

Arborization block (heart) I45.5

ARC (AIDS-related complex) B20

▶Arch
▶aortic Q25.49
▶bovine Q25.49

Arches —see condition

Arcuate uterus Q51.810

Arcuatus uterus Q51.810

Arcus (cornea) senilis —see Degeneration, cornea, senile

Arc-welder's lung J63.4

Areflexia R29.2

Areola —see condition

Argentaffinoma —see also Neoplasm, uncertain behavior, by site
malignant —see Neoplasm, malignant, by site
syndrome E34.0

Argininemia E72.21

Arginosuccinic aciduria E72.22

Argyll Robertson phenomenon, pupil or syndrome (syphilitic) A52.19
atypical H57.09
nonsyphilitic H57.09

Argyria, argyriasis
conjunctival H11.13-●
from drug or medicament —see Table of Drugs and Chemicals, by substance

Argyrosis, conjunctival H11.13-●

Arhinencephaly Q04.1

Ariboflavinosis E53.0

Arm —see condition

Arnold-Chiari disease, obstruction or syndrome (type II) Q07.00
with
hydrocephalus Q07.02
with spina bifida Q07.03
spina bifida Q07.01
with hydrocephalus Q07.03
type III —see Encephalocele
type IV Q04.8

Aromatic amino-acid metabolism disorder E70.9
specified NEC E70.8

Arousals, confusional G47.51

Arrest, arrested
cardiac I46.9
complicating
abortion —see Abortion, by type, complicated by, cardiac arrest
anesthesia (general) (local) or other sedation —see Table of Drugs and Chemicals, by drug
in labor and delivery O74.2
in pregnancy O29.11-●
postpartum, puerperal O89.1
delivery (cesarean) (instrumental) O75.4
due to
cardiac condition I46.2
specified condition NEC I46.8
intraoperative I97.71-●
newborn P29.81
▶personal history, successfully resuscitated Z86.74

Arrest, arrested (Continued)
cardiac (Continued)
postprocedural I97.12-●
obstetric procedure O75.4
cardiorespiratory —see Arrest, cardiac
circulatory —see Arrest, cardiac
deep transverse O64.0
development or growth
bone —see Disorder, bone, development or growth
child R62.50
tracheal rings Q32.1
epiphyseal
complete
femur M89.15-●
humerus M89.12-●
tibia M89.16-●
ulna M89.13-●
forearm M89.13-●
specified NEC M89.13-●
ulna —see Arrest, epiphyseal, by type, ulna
lower leg M89.16-●
specified NEC M89.168
tibia —see Arrest, epiphyseal, by type, tibia
partial
femur M89.15-●
humerus M89.12-●
tibia M89.16-●
ulna M89.13-●
specified NEC M89.18
granulopoiesis —see Agranulocytosis
growth plate —see Arrest, epiphyseal
heart —see Arrest, cardiac
legal, anxiety concerning Z65.3
physeal —see Arrest, epiphyseal
respiratory R09.2
newborn P28.81
sinus I45.5
spermatogenesis (complete) —see Azoospermia
incomplete —see Oligospermia
transverse (deep) O64.0

Arrhenoblastoma
benign
specified site —see Neoplasm, benign, by site
unspecified site
female D27.9
male D29.20
malignant
specified site —see Neoplasm, malignant, by site
unspecified site
female C56.9
male C62.90
specified site —see Neoplasm, uncertain behavior, by site
unspecified site
female D39.10
male D40.10

Arrhythmia (auricle)(cardiac) (juvenile)(nodal) (reflex)(sinus)(supraventricular)(transitory) (ventricle) I49.9
block I45.9
extrasystolic I49.49
newborn
bradycardia P29.12
occurring before birth P03.819
before onset of labor P03.810
during labor P03.811
tachycardia P29.11
psychogenic F45.8
specified NEC I49.8
vagal R55
ventricular re-entry I47.0

Arrillaga-Ayerza syndrome (pulmonary sclerosis with pulmonary hypertension) I27.0

Arsenical pigmentation L81.8
from drug or medicament —see Table of Drugs and Chemicals

Arsenism —see Poisoning, arsenic

Arterial —*see* condition
Arteriofibrosis —*see* Arteriosclerosis
Arteriolar sclerosis —*see* Arteriosclerosis
Arteriolith —*see* Arteriosclerosis
Arteriolitis I77.6
  necrotizing, kidney I77.5
  renal —*see* Hypertension, kidney
Arteriolosclerosis —*see* Arteriosclerosis
Arterionephrosclerosis —*see* Hypertension,
    kidney
Arteriopathy I77.9
Arteriosclerosis, arteriosclerotic (diffuse)
    (obliterans) (of) (senile) (with calcification)
    I70.90
  aorta I70.0
  arteries of extremities —*see* Arteriosclerosis,
    extremities
  brain I67.2
  bypass graft
    coronary —*see* Arteriosclerosis, coronary,
      bypass graft
    extremities —*see* Arteriosclerosis,
      extremities, bypass graft
  cardiac —*see* Disease, heart, ischemic,
    atherosclerotic
  cardiopathy —*see* Disease, heart, ischemic,
    atherosclerotic
  cardiorenal —*see* Hypertension, cardiorenal
  cardiovascular —*see* Disease, heart, ischemic,
    atherosclerotic
  carotid —*see also* Occlusion, artery, carotid
    I65.2-●
  central nervous system I67.2
  cerebral I67.2
  cerebrovascular I67.2
  coronary (artery) I25.10
    bypass graft I25.810
      with
        angina pectoris I25.709
          with documented spasm I25.701
          specified type NEC I25.708
          unstable I25.700
        ischemic chest pain I25.709
      autologous artery I25.810
        with
          angina pectoris I25.729
            with documented spasm I25.721
            specified type I25.728
            unstable I25.720
          ischemic chest pain I25.729
      autologous vein I25.810
        with
          angina pectoris I25.719
            with documented spasm I25.711
            specified type I25.718
            unstable I25.710
          ischemic chest pain I25.719
      nonautologous biological I25.810
        with
          angina pectoris I25.739
            with documented spasm I25.731
            specified type I25.738
            unstable I25.730
          ischemic chest pain I25.739
      specified type NEC I25.810
        with
          angina pectoris I25.799
            with documented spasm I25.791
            specified type I25.798
            unstable I25.790
          ischemic chest pain I25.799
    due to
      calcified coronary lesion (severely) I25.84
      lipid rich plaque I25.83
    native vessel
      with
        angina pectoris I25.119
          with documented spasm I25.111
          specified type NEC I25.118
          unstable I25.110
        ischemic chest pain I25.119

Arteriosclerosis, arteriosclerotic (Continued)
  coronary (Continued)
    transplanted heart I25.811
      bypass graft I25.812
        with
          angina pectoris I25.769
            with documented spasm
              I25.761
            specified type I25.768
            unstable I25.760
          ischemic chest pain I25.769
      native coronary artery I25.811
        with
          angina pectoris I25.759
            with documented spasm I25.751
            specified type I25.758
            unstable I25.750
          ischemic chest pain I25.759
  extremities (native arteries) I70.209
    bypass graft I70.309
      autologous vein graft I70.409
        leg I70.409
          with
            gangrene (and intermittent
              claudication, rest pain and
              ulcer) I70.469
            intermittent claudication
              I70.419
            rest pain (and intermittent
              claudication) I70.429
          bilateral I70.403
            with
              gangrene (and intermittent
                claudication, rest pain and
                ulcer) I70.463
              intermittent claudication
                I70.413
              rest pain (and intermittent
                claudication) I70.423
            specified type NEC I70.493
          left I70.402
            with
              gangrene (and intermittent
                claudication, rest pain and
                ulcer) I70.462
              intermittent claudication
                I70.412
              rest pain (and intermittent
                claudication) I70.422
              ulceration (and intermittent
                claudication and rest
                pain) I70.449
              ankle I70.443
              calf I70.442
              foot site NEC I70.445
              heel I70.444
              lower leg NEC I70.448
              midfoot I70.444
              thigh I70.441
            specified type NEC I70.492
          right I70.401
            with
              gangrene (and intermittent
                claudication, rest pain and
                ulcer) I70.461
              intermittent claudication
                I70.411
              rest pain (and intermittent
                claudication) I70.421
              ulceration (and intermittent
                claudication and rest
                pain) I70.439
              ankle I70.433
              calf I70.432
              foot site NEC I70.435
              heel I70.434
              lower leg NEC I70.438
              midfoot I70.434
              thigh I70.431
            specified type NEC I70.491
        specified type NEC I70.499

Arteriosclerosis, arteriosclerotic (Continued)
  extremities (Continued)
    bypass graft (Continued)
      autologous vein graft (Continued)
        specified NEC I70.408
          with
            gangrene (and intermittent
              claudication, rest pain and
              ulcer) I70.468
            intermittent claudication I70.418
            rest pain (and intermittent
              claudication) I70.428
            ulceration (and intermittent
              claudication and rest pain)
              I70.45
          specified type NEC I70.498
      leg I70.309
        with
          gangrene (and intermittent
            claudication, rest pain and
            ulcer) I70.369
          intermittent claudication I70.319
          rest pain (and intermittent
            claudication) I70.329
        bilateral I70.303
          with
            gangrene (and intermittent
              claudication, rest pain and
              ulcer) I70.363
            intermittent claudication I70.313
            rest pain (and intermittent
              claudication) I70.323
          specified type NEC I70.393
        left I70.302
          with
            gangrene (and intermittent
              claudication, rest pain and
              ulcer) I70.362
            intermittent claudication I70.312
            rest pain (and intermittent
              claudication) I70.322
            ulceration (and intermittent
              claudication and rest pain)
              I70.349
            ankle I70.343
            calf I70.342
            foot site NEC I70.345
            heel I70.344
            lower leg NEC I70.348
            midfoot I70.344
            thigh I70.341
          specified type NEC I70.392
        right I70.301
          with
            gangrene (and intermittent
              claudication, rest pain and
              ulcer) I70.361
            intermittent claudication I70.311
            rest pain (and intermittent
              claudication) I70.321
            ulceration (and intermittent
              claudication and rest pain)
              I70.339
            ankle I70.333
            calf I70.332
            foot site NEC I70.335
            heel I70.334
            lower leg NEC I70.338
            midfoot I70.334
            thigh I70.331
          specified type NEC I70.391
        specified type NEC I70.399
      nonautologous biological graft I70.509
        leg I70.509
          with
            gangrene (and intermittent
              claudication, rest pain and
              ulcer) I70.569
            intermittent claudication I70.519
            rest pain (and intermittent
              claudication) I70.529

Arteriosclerosis, arteriosclerotic (Continued)
  extremities (Continued)
    bypass graft (Continued)
     nonautologous biological graft
      (Continued)
      leg (Continued)
       bilateral I70.503
        with
         gangrene (and intermittent
          claudication, rest pain and
          ulcer) I70.563
         intermittent claudication
          I70.513
         rest pain (and intermittent
          claudication) I70.523
        specified type NEC I70.593
       left I70.502
        with
         gangrene (and intermittent
          claudication, rest pain and
          ulcer) I70.562
         intermittent claudication
          I70.512
         rest pain (and intermittent
          claudication)
          I70.522
         ulceration (and intermittent
          claudication and rest
          pain) I70.549
          ankle I70.543
          calf I70.542
          foot site NEC I70.545
          heel I70.544
          lower leg NEC I70.548
          midfoot I70.544
          thigh I70.541
        specified type NEC I70.592
       right I70.501
        with
         gangrene (and intermittent
          claudication, rest pain and
          ulcer) I70.561
         intermittent claudication
          I70.511
         rest pain (and intermittent
          claudication) I70.521
         ulceration (and intermittent
          claudication and rest
          pain) I70.539
          ankle I70.533
          calf I70.532
          foot site NEC I70.535
          heel I70.534
          lower leg NEC I70.538
          midfoot I70.534
          thigh I70.531
        specified type NEC I70.591
       specified type NEC I70.599
      specified NEC I70.508
       with
        gangrene (and intermittent
         claudication, rest pain and
         ulcer) I70.568
        intermittent claudication
         I70.518
        rest pain (and intermittent
         claudication) I70.528
        ulceration (and intermittent
         claudication and rest pain)
         I70.55
        specified type NEC I70.598
     nonbiological graft I70.609
      leg I70.609
       with
        gangrene (and intermittent
         claudication, rest pain and
         ulcer) I70.669
        intermittent claudication
         I70.619
        rest pain (and intermittent
         claudication) I70.629

Arteriosclerosis, arteriosclerotic (Continued)
  extremities (Continued)
    bypass graft (Continued)
     nonbiological graft (Continued)
      leg (Continued)
       bilateral I70.603
        with
         gangrene (and intermittent
          claudication, rest
          pain and ulcer)
          I70.663
         intermittent claudication
          I70.613
         rest pain (and intermittent
          claudication) I70.623
        specified type NEC I70.693
       left I70.602
        with
         gangrene (and intermittent
          claudication, rest
          pain and ulcer)
          I70.662
         intermittent claudication
          I70.612
         rest pain (and intermittent
          claudication) I70.622
         ulceration (and intermittent
          claudication and rest
          pain) I70.649
          ankle I70.643
          calf I70.642
          foot site NEC I70.645
          heel I70.644
          lower leg NEC I70.648
          midfoot I70.644
          thigh I70.641
        specified type NEC I70.692
       right I70.601
        with
         gangrene (and intermittent
          claudication, rest pain and
          ulcer) I70.661
         intermittent claudication
          I70.611
         rest pain (and intermittent
          claudication) I70.621
         ulceration (and intermittent
          claudication and rest
          pain) I70.639
          ankle I70.633
          calf I70.632
          foot site NEC I70.635
          heel I70.634
          lower leg NEC I70.638
          midfoot I70.634
          thigh I70.631
        specified type NEC I70.691
      specified NEC I70.608
       with
        gangrene (and intermittent
         claudication, rest pain and
         ulcer) I70.668
        intermittent claudication
         I70.618
        rest pain (and intermittent
         claudication) I70.628
        ulceration (and intermittent
         claudication and rest pain)
         I70.65
        specified type NEC I70.698
     specified graft NEC I70.709
      leg I70.709
       with
        gangrene (and intermittent
         claudication, rest pain and
         ulcer) I70.769
        intermittent claudication
         I70.719
        rest pain (and intermittent
         claudication) I70.729

Arteriosclerosis, arteriosclerotic (Continued)
  extremities (Continued)
    bypass graft (Continued)
     specified graft NEC (Continued)
      leg (Continued)
       bilateral I70.703
        with
         gangrene (and intermittent
          claudication, rest pain and
          ulcer) I70.763
         intermittent claudication
          I70.713
         rest pain (and intermittent
          claudication) I70.723
        specified type NEC I70.793
       left I70.702
        with
         gangrene (and intermittent
          claudication, rest pain and
          ulcer) I70.762
         intermittent claudication
          I70.712
         rest pain (and intermittent
          claudication) I70.722
         ulceration (and intermittent
          claudication and rest
          pain) I70.749
          ankle I70.743
          calf I70.742
          foot site NEC I70.745
          heel I70.744
          lower leg NEC I70.748
          midfoot I70.744
          thigh I70.741
        specified type NEC I70.792
       right I70.701
        with
         gangrene (and intermittent
          claudication, rest pain and
          ulcer) I70.761
         intermittent claudication
          I70.711
         rest pain (and intermittent
          claudication) I70.721
         ulceration (and intermittent
          claudication and rest
          pain) I70.739
          ankle I70.733
          calf I70.732
          foot site NEC I70.735
          heel I70.734
          lower leg NEC I70.738
          midfoot I70.734
          thigh I70.731
        specified type NEC I70.791
       specified type NEC I70.799
      specified NEC I70.708
       with
        gangrene (and intermittent
         claudication, rest pain and
         ulcer) I70.768
        intermittent claudication
         I70.718
        rest pain (and intermittent
         claudication) I70.728
        ulceration (and intermittent
         claudication and rest pain)
         I70.75
        specified type NEC I70.798
    specified NEC I70.308
     with
      gangrene (and intermittent
       claudication, rest pain and
       ulcer) I70.368
      intermittent claudication I70.318
      rest pain (and intermittent
       claudication) I70.328
      ulceration (and intermittent
       claudication and rest pain)
       I70.35
     specified type NEC I70.398

▶ New ⇒ Revised ~~deleted~~ Deleted ● Use Additional Character(s)

Arteriosclerosis, arteriosclerotic (Continued)
  extremities (Continued)
    leg I70.209
      with
        gangrene (and intermittent
          claudication, rest pain and ulcer)
          I70.269
        intermittent claudication I70.219
        rest pain (and intermittent
          claudication) I70.229
    bilateral I70.203
      with
        gangrene (and intermittent
          claudication, rest pain and
          ulcer) I70.263
        intermittent claudication I70.213
        rest pain (and intermittent
          claudication) I70.223
      specified type NEC I70.293
    left I70.202
      with
        gangrene (and intermittent
          claudication, rest pain and
          ulcer) I70.262
        intermittent claudication I70.212
        rest pain (and intermittent
          claudication) I70.222
        ulceration (and intermittent
          claudication and rest pain)
          I70.249
          ankle I70.243
          calf I70.242
          foot site NEC I70.245
          heel I70.244
          lower leg NEC I70.248
          midfoot I70.244
          thigh I70.241
      specified type NEC I70.292
    right I70.201
      with
        gangrene (and intermittent
          claudication, rest pain and
          ulcer) I70.261
        intermittent claudication I70.211
        rest pain (and intermittent
          claudication) I70.221
        ulceration (and intermittent
          claudication and rest pain)
          I70.239
          ankle I70.233
          calf I70.232
          foot site NEC I70.235
          heel I70.234
          lower leg NEC I70.238
          midfoot I70.234
          thigh I70.231
      specified type NEC I70.291
    specified type NEC I70.299
    specified site NEC I70.208
      with
        gangrene (and intermittent
          claudication, rest pain and ulcer)
          I70.268
        intermittent claudication I70.218
        rest pain (and intermittent
          claudication) I70.228
        ulceration (and intermittent
          claudication and rest pain) I70.25
      specified type NEC I70.298
  generalized I70.91
  heart (disease) —see Arteriosclerosis,
    coronary (artery)
  kidney —see Hypertension, kidney
  medial —see Arteriosclerosis, extremities
  mesenteric (artery) K55.1
  Mönckeberg's —see Arteriosclerosis,
    extremities
  myocarditis I51.4
  peripheral (of extremities) —see
    Arteriosclerosis, extremities
  pulmonary (idiopathic) I27.0

Arteriosclerosis, arteriosclerotic (Continued)
  renal (arterioles) —see also Hypertension,
    kidney
    artery I70.1
  retina (vascular) I70.8 [H35.0-•]
  specified artery NEC I70.8
  spinal (cord) G95.19
  vertebral (artery) I67.2
Arteriospasm I73.9
Arteriovenous —see condition
Arteritis I77.6
  allergic M31.0
  aorta (nonsyphilitic) I77.6
    syphilitic A52.02
  aortic arch M31.4
  brachiocephalic M31.4
  brain I67.7
    syphilitic A52.04
  cerebral I67.7
    in
      diseases classified elsewhere I68.2
      systemic lupus erythematosus M32.19
    listerial A32.89
    syphilitic A52.04
    tuberculous A18.89
  coronary (artery) I25.89
    rheumatic I01.8
      chronic I09.89
    syphilitic A52.06
  cranial (left) (right), giant cell M31.6
  deformans —see Arteriosclerosis
  giant cell NEC M31.6
    with polymyalgia rheumatica M31.5
  necrosing or necrotizing M31.9
    specified NEC M31.8
  nodosa M30.0
  obliterans —see Arteriosclerosis
  pulmonary I28.8
  rheumatic —see Fever, rheumatic
  senile —see Arteriosclerosis
  suppurative I77.2
  syphilitic (general) A52.09
    brain A52.04
    coronary A52.06
    spinal A52.09
  temporal, giant cell M31.6
  young female aortic arch syndrome M31.4
Artery, arterial —see also condition
  abscess I77.89
  single umbilical Q27.0
Arthralgia (allergic) —see also Pain, joint
  in caisson disease T70.3
  temporomandibular M26.62
Arthritis, arthritic (acute) (chronic)
  (nonpyogenic) (subacute) M19.90
  allergic —see Arthritis, specified form NEC
  ankylosing (crippling) (spine) —see also
    Spondylitis, ankylosing
    sites other than spine —see Arthritis,
      specified form NEC
  atrophic —see Osteoarthritis
    spine —see Spondylitis, ankylosing
  back —see Spondylopathy, inflammatory
  blennorrhagic (gonococcal) A54.42
  Charcot's —see Arthropathy, neuropathic
    diabetic —see Diabetes, arthropathy,
      neuropathic
    syringomyelic G95.0
  chylous (filarial) —see also category M01
    B74.9
  climacteric (any site) NEC —see Arthritis,
    specified form NEC
  crystal (-induced) —see Arthritis, in, crystals
  deformans —see Osteoarthritis
  degenerative —see Osteoarthritis
  due to or associated with
    acromegaly E22.0
    brucellosis —see Brucellosis
    caisson disease T70.3
    diabetes —see Diabetes, arthropathy
    dracontiasis —see also category M01 B72

Arthritis, arthritic (Continued)
  due to or associated with (Continued)
    enteritis NEC
      regional —see Enteritis, regional
    erysipelas —see also category M01 A46
    erythema
      epidemic A25.1
      nodosum L52
    filariasis NOS B74.9
    glanders A24.0
    helminthiasis —see also category M01 B83.9
    hemophilia D66 [M36.2]
    Henoch-(Schönlein) purpura D69.0 [M36.4]
    human parvovirus —see also category M01
      B97.6
    infectious disease NEC —see category M01
    leprosy (see also category M01) —see also
      Leprosy A30.9
    Lyme disease A69.23
    mycobacteria —see also category M01
      A31.8
    parasitic disease NEC —see also category
      M01 B89
    paratyphoid fever (see also category M01)
      —see also Fever, paratyphoid A01.4
    rat bite fever —see also category M01
      A25.1
    regional enteritis —see Enteritis, regional
    respiratory disorder NOS J98.9
    serum sickness —see also Reaction, serum
      T80.69
    syringomyelia G95.0
    typhoid fever A01.04
  epidemic erythema A25.1
  febrile —see Fever, rheumatic
  gonococcal A54.42
  gouty (acute) —see Gout
  in (due to)
    acromegaly —see also subcategory
      M14.8-• E22.0
    amyloidosis —see also subcategory
      M14.8-• E85.4
    bacterial disease —see also subcategory
      M01 A49.9
    Behçet's syndrome M35.2
    caisson disease —see also subcategory
      M14.8-• T70.3
    coliform bacilli (Escherichia coli) —see
      Arthritis, in, pyogenic organism NEC
    crystals M11.9
      dicalcium phosphate —see Arthritis, in,
        crystals, specified type NEC
      hydroxyapatite M11.0-•
      pyrophosphate —see Arthritis, in,
        crystals, specified type NEC
      specified type NEC M11.80
        ankle M11.87-•
        elbow M11.82-•
        foot joint M11.87-•
        hand joint M11.84-•
        hip M11.85-•
        knee M11.86-•
        multiple sites M11.8-•
        shoulder M11.81-•
        vertebrae M11.88
        wrist M11.83-•
    dermatoarthritis, lipoid E78.81
    dracontiasis (dracunculiasis) —see also
      category M01 B72
    endocrine disorder NEC —see also
      subcategory M14.8-• E34.9
    enteritis, infectious NEC —see also category
      M01 A09
      specified organism NEC —see also
        category M01 A08.8
    erythema
      multiforme —see also subcategory
        M14.8-• L51.9
      nodosum —see also subcategory M14.8-•
        L52
    gout —see Gout

Arthritis, arthritic (Continued)
  in (Continued)
    helminthiasis NEC —see also category M01
      B83.9
    hemochromatosis —see also subcategory
      M14.8-• E83.118
    hemoglobinopathy NEC D58.2 [M36.3]
    hemophilia NEC D66 [M36.2]
    Hemophilus influenzae M00.8-• [B96.3]
    Henoch(-Schönlein) purpura D69.0 [M36.4]
    hyperparathyroidism NEC —see also
      subcategory M14.8-• E21.3
    hypersensitivity reaction NEC T78.49
      [M36.4]
    hypogammaglobulinemia —see also
      subcategory M14.8-• D80.1
    hypothyroidism NEC —see also
      subcategory M14.8-• E03.9
    infection —see Arthritis, pyogenic or
      pyemic
      spine —see Spondylopathy, infective
    infectious disease NEC —see category M01
    leprosy —see also category M01 A30.9
    leukemia NEC C95.9-• [M36.1]
    lipoid dermatoarthritis E78.81
    Lyme disease A69.23
    Mediterranean fever, familial —see also
      subcategory M14.8-• M04.1
    Meningococcus A39.83
    metabolic disorder NEC —see also
      subcategory M14.8-• E88.9
    multiple myelomatosis C90.0-• [M36.1]
    mumps B26.85
    mycosis NEC —see also category M01 B49
    myelomatosis (multiple) C90.0-• [M36.1]
    neurological disorder NEC G98.0
    ochronosis —see also subcategory M14.8-•
      E70.29
    O'nyong-nyong —see also category M01
      A92.1
    parasitic disease NEC —see also category
      M01 B89
    paratyphoid fever —see also category M01
      A01.4
    Pseudomonas —see Arthritis, pyogenic,
      bacterial NEC
    psoriasis L40.50
    pyogenic organism NEC —see Arthritis,
      pyogenic, bacterial NEC
    Reiter's disease —see Reiter's disease
    respiratory disorder NEC —see also
      subcategory M14.8-• J98.9
    reticulosis, malignant —see also
      subcategory M14.8-• C86.0
    rubella B06.82
    Salmonella (arizonae) (cholerae-suis)
      (enteritidis) (typhimurium)
      A02.23
    sarcoidosis D86.86
    specified bacteria NEC —see Arthritis,
      pyogenic, bacterial NEC
    sporotrichosis B42.82
    syringomyelia G95.0
    thalassemia NEC D56.9 [M36.3]
    tuberculosis —see Tuberculosis, arthritis
    typhoid fever A01.04
    urethritis, Reiter's —see Reiter's disease
    viral disease NEC —see also category M01
      B34.9
  infectious or infective —see also Arthritis,
    pyogenic or pyemic
    spine —see Spondylopathy, infective
  juvenile M08.90
    with systemic onset —see Still's disease
    ankle M08.97-•
    elbow M08.92-•
    foot joint M08.97-•
    hand joint M08.94-•
    hip M08.95-•
    knee M08.96-•
    multiple site M08.99

Arthritis, arthritic (Continued)
  juvenile (Continued)
    pauciarticular M08.40
      ankle M08.47-•
      elbow M08.42-•
      foot joint M08.47-•
      hand joint M08.44-•
      hip M08.45-•
      knee M08.46-•
      shoulder M08.41-•
      vertebrae M08.48
      wrist M08.43-•
    psoriatic L40.54
    rheumatoid —see Arthritis, rheumatoid,
      juvenile
    shoulder M08.91-•
    specified type NEC M08.80
      ankle M08.87-•
      elbow M08.82-•
      foot joint M08.87-•
      hand joint M08.84-•
      hip M08.85-•
      knee M08.86-•
      multiple site M08.89
      shoulder M08.81-•
      specified joint NEC M08.88
      vertebrae M08.88
      wrist M08.83-•
    vertebra M08.98
    wrist M08.93-•
  meaning osteoarthritis —see Osteoarthritis
  meningococcal A39.83
  menopausal (any site) NEC —see Arthritis,
    specified form NEC
  mutilans (psoriatic) L40.52
  mycotic NEC —see also category M01 B49
  neuropathic (Charcot) —see Arthropathy,
    neuropathic
    diabetic —see Diabetes, arthropathy,
      neuropathic
    nonsyphilitic NEC G98.0
    syringomyelic G95.0
  ochronotic —see also subcategory M14.8-•
    E70.29
  palindromic (any site) —see Rheumatism,
    palindromic
  pneumococcal M00.10
    ankle M00.17-•
    elbow M00.12-•
    foot joint —see Arthritis, pneumococcal,
      ankle
    hand joint M00.14-•
    hip M00.15-•
    knee M00.16-•
    multiple site M00.19
    shoulder M00.11-•
    vertebra M00.18
    wrist M00.13-•
  postdysenteric —see Arthropathy,
    postdysenteric
  postmeningococcal A39.84
  postrheumatic, chronic —see Arthropathy,
    postrheumatic, chronic
  primary progressive —see also Arthritis,
    specified form NEC
    spine —see Spondylitis, ankylosing
  psoriatic L40.50
  purulent (any site except spine) —see
    Arthritis, pyogenic or pyemic
    spine —see Spondylopathy, infective
  pyogenic or pyemic (any site except spine)
    M00.9
    bacterial NEC M00.80
      ankle M00.87-•
      elbow M00.82-•
      foot joint —see Arthritis, pyogenic,
        bacterial NEC, ankle
      hand joint M00.84-•
      hip M00.85-•
      knee M00.86-•
      multiple site M00.89

Arthritis, arthritic (Continued)
  pyogenic or pyemic (Continued)
    bacterial NEC (Continued)
      shoulder M00.81-•
      vertebra M00.88
      wrist M00.83-•
    pneumococcal —see Arthritis,
      pneumococcal
    spine —see Spondylopathy, infective
    staphylococcal —see Arthritis,
      staphylococcal
    streptococcal —see Arthritis, streptococcal
      NEC
      pneumococcal —see Arthritis,
        pneumococcal
  reactive —see Reiter's disease
  rheumatic —see also Arthritis, rheumatoid
    acute or subacute —see Fever, rheumatic
  rheumatoid M06.9
    with
      carditis —see Rheumatoid, carditis
      endocarditis —see Rheumatoid, carditis
      heart involvement NEC —see
        Rheumatoid, carditis
      lung involvement —see Rheumatoid,
        lung
      myocarditis —see Rheumatoid, carditis
      myopathy —see Rheumatoid, myopathy
      pericarditis —see Rheumatoid, carditis
      polyneuropathy —see Rheumatoid,
        polyneuropathy
      rheumatoid factor —see Arthritis,
        rheumatoid, seropositive
      splenoadenomegaly and leukopenia —
        see Felty's syndrome
      vasculitis —see Rheumatoid, vasculitis
      visceral involvement NEC —see
        Rheumatoid, arthritis, with
        involvement of organs NEC
    juvenile (with or without rheumatoid
      factor) M08.00
      ankle M08.07-•
      elbow M08.02-•
      foot joint M08.07-•
      hand joint M08.04-•
      hip M08.05-•
      knee M08.06-•
      multiple site M08.09
      shoulder M08.01-•
      vertebra M08.08
      wrist M08.03-•
    seronegative M06.00
      ankle M06.07-•
      elbow M06.02-•
      foot joint M06.07-•
      hand joint M06.04-•
      hip M06.05-•
      knee M06.06-•
      multiple sites M06.09
      shoulder M06.01-•
      vertebra M06.08
      wrist M06.03-•
    seropositive M05.9
      without organ involvement M05.70
        ankle M05.77-•
        elbow M05.72-•
        foot joint M05.77-•
        hand joint M05.74-•
        hip M05.75-•
        knee M05.76-•
        multiple sites M05.79
        shoulder M05.71-•
        vertebra —see Spondylitis, ankylosing
        wrist M05.73-•
    specified NEC M05.80
      ankle M05.87-•
      elbow M05.82-•
      foot joint M05.87-•
      hand joint M05.84-•
      hip M05.85-•
      knee M05.86-•

▶ New   ⇒ Revised   ~~deleted~~ Deleted   • Use Additional Character(s)

Arthritis, arthritic *(Continued)*
  rheumatoid *(Continued)*
    specified NEC *(Continued)*
      multiple sites M05.89
      shoulder M05.81-●
      vertebra —*see* Spondylitis, ankylosing
      wrist M05.83-●
    specified type NEC M06.80
      ankle M06.87-●
      elbow M06.82-●
      foot joint M06.87-●
      hand joint M06.84-●
      hip M06.85-●
      knee M06.86-●
      multiple site M06.89
      shoulder M06.81-●
      vertebra M06.88
      wrist M06.83-●
    spine —*see* Spondylitis, ankylosing
  rubella B06.82
  scorbutic —*see also* subcategory M14.8-● E54
  senile or senescent —*see* Osteoarthritis
  septic (any site except spine) —*see* Arthritis,
      pyogenic or pyemic
    spine —*see* Spondylopathy, infective
  serum (nontherapeutic) (therapeutic) —*see*
      Arthropathy, postimmunization
  specified form NEC M13.80
    ankle M13.87-●
    elbow M13.82-●
    foot joint M13.87-●
    hand joint M13.84-●
    hip M13.85-●
    knee M13.86-●
    multiple site M13.89
    shoulder M13.81-●
    specified joint NEC M13.88
    wrist M13.83-●
  spine —*see also* Spondylopathy,
      inflammatory
    infectious or infective NEC —*see*
      Spondylopathy, infective
    Marie-Strümpell —*see* Spondylitis,
      ankylosing
    pyogenic —*see* Spondylopathy, infective
    rheumatoid —*see* Spondylitis, ankylosing
    traumatic (old) —*see* Spondylopathy,
      traumatic
    tuberculous A18.01
  staphylococcal M00.00
    ankle M00.07-●
    elbow M00.02-●
    foot joint —*see* Arthritis, staphylococcal,
      ankle
    hand joint M00.04-●
    hip M00.05-●
    knee M00.06-●
    multiple site M00.09
    shoulder M00.01-●
    vertebra M00.08
    wrist M00.03-●
  streptococcal NEC M00.20
    ankle M00.27-●
    elbow M00.22-●
    foot joint —*see* Arthritis, streptococcal,
      ankle
    hand joint M00.24-●
    hip M00.25-●
    knee M00.26-●
    multiple site M00.29
    shoulder M00.21-●
    vertebra M00.28
    wrist M00.23-●
  suppurative —*see* Arthritis, pyogenic or
      pyemic
  syphilitic (late) A52.16
    congenital A50.55 [M12.80]
  syphilitica deformans (Charcot) A52.16
  temporomandibular M26.69
  toxic of menopause (any site) —*see* Arthritis,
      specified form NEC

Arthritis, arthritic *(Continued)*
  transient —*see* Arthropathy, specified form
      NEC
  traumatic (chronic) —*see* Arthropathy,
      traumatic
  tuberculous A18.02
    spine A18.01
  uratic —*see* Gout
  urethritica (Reiter's) —*see* Reiter's disease
  vertebral —*see* Spondylopathy, inflammatory
  villous (any site) —*see* Arthropathy, specified
      form NEC
Arthrocele —*see* Effusion, joint
Arthrodesis status Z98.1
Arthrodynia —*see also* Pain, joint
Arthrodysplasia Q74.9
Arthrofibrosis, joint —*see* Ankylosis
Arthrogryposis (congenital) Q68.8
  multiplex congenita Q74.3
Arthrokatadysis M24.7
Arthropathy (*see also* Arthritis) M12.9
  Charcot's —*see* Arthropathy, neuropathic
    diabetic —*see* Diabetes, arthropathy,
      neuropathic
    syringomyelic G95.0
  cricoarytenoid J38.7
  crystal(-induced) —*see* Arthritis, in, crystals
  diabetic NEC —*see* Diabetes, arthropathy
  distal interphalangeal, psoriatic L40.51
  enteropathic M07.60
    ankle M07.67-●
    elbow M07.62-●
    foot joint M07.67-●
    hand joint M07.64-●
    hip M07.65-●
    knee M07.66-●
    multiple site M07.69
    shoulder M07.61-●
    vertebra M07.68
    wrist M07.63-●
  following intestinal bypass M02.00
    ankle M02.07-●
    elbow M02.02-●
    foot joint M02.07-●
    hand joint M02.04-●
    hip M02.05-●
    knee M02.06-●
    multiple site M02.09
    shoulder M02.01-●
    vertebra M02.08
    wrist M02.03-●
  gouty —*see also* Gout
    in (due to)
      Lesch-Nyhan syndrome E79.1 [M14.8-●]
      sickle-cell disorders D57-● [M14.8-●]
  hemophilic NEC D66 [M36.2]
    in (due to)
      hyperparathyroidism NEC E21.3
        [M14.8-●]
      metabolic disease NOS E88.9 [M14.8-●]
  in (due to)
    acromegaly E22.0 [M14.8-●]
    amyloidosis E85.4 [M14.8-●]
    blood disorder NOS D75.9 [M36.3]
    diabetes —*see* Diabetes, arthropathy
    endocrine disease NOS E34.9 [M14.8-●]
    erythema
      multiforme L51.9 [M14.8-●]
      nodosum L52 [M14.8-●]
    hemochromatosis E83.118 [M14.8-●]
    hemoglobinopathy NEC D58.2 [M36.3]
    hemophilia NEC D66 [M36.2]
    Henoch-Schönlein purpura D69.0 [M36.4]
    hyperthyroidism E05.90 [M14.8-●]
    hypothyroidism E03.9 [M14.8-●]
    infective endocarditis I33.0 [M12.80]
    leukemia NEC C95.9-● [M36.1]
    malignant histiocytosis C96.A [M36.1]
    metabolic disease NOS E88.9 [M14.8-●]
    multiple myeloma C90.0-● [M36.1]
    neoplastic disease NOS (*see also* Neoplasm)
      D49.9 [M36.1]

Arthropathy *(Continued)*
  hemochromatosis *(Continued)*
    nutritional deficiency —*see also*
      subcategory M14.8-● E63.9
    psoriasis NOS L40.50
    sarcoidosis D86.86
    syphilis (late) A52.77
      congenital A50.55 [M12.80]
    thyrotoxicosis —*see also* subcategory
      M14.8-● E05.90
    ulcerative colitis K51.90 [M07.60]
    viral hepatitis (postinfectious) NEC B19.9
      [M12.80]
    Whipple's disease —*see also* subcategory
      M14.8-● K90.81
  Jaccoud —*see* Arthropathy, postrheumatic,
      chronic
  juvenile —*see* Arthritis, juvenile
    psoriatic L40.54
  mutilans (psoriatic) L40.52
  neuropathic (Charcot) M14.60
    ankle M14.67-●
    diabetic —*see* Diabetes, arthropathy,
      neuropathic
    elbow M14.62-●
    foot joint M14.67-●
    hand joint M14.64-●
    hip M14.65-●
    knee M14.66-●
    multiple site M14.69
    nonsyphilitic NEC G98.0
    shoulder M14.61-●
    syringomyelic G95.0
    vertebra M14.68
    wrist M14.63-●
  osteopulmonary —*see* Osteoarthropathy,
      hypertrophic, specified NEC
  postdysenteric M02.10
    ankle M02.17-●
    elbow M02.12-●
    foot joint M02.17-●
    hand joint M02.14-●
    hip M02.15-●
    knee M02.16-●
    multiple site M02.19
    shoulder M02.11-●
    vertebra M02.18
    wrist M02.13-●
  postimmunization M02.20
    ankle M02.27-●
    elbow M02.22-●
    foot joint M02.27-●
    hand joint M02.24-●
    hip M02.25-●
    knee M02.26-●
    multiple site M02.29
    shoulder M02.21-●
    vertebra M02.28
    wrist M02.23-●
  postinfectious NEC B99 [M12.80]
    in (due to)
      enteritis due to Yersinia enterocolitica
        A04.6 [M12.80]
      syphilis A52.77
      viral hepatitis NEC B19.9
        [M12.80]
  postrheumatic, chronic (Jaccoud)
      M12.00
    ankle M12.07-●
    elbow M12.02-●
    foot joint M12.07-●
    hand joint M12.04-●
    hip M12.05-●
    knee M12.06-●
    multiple site M12.09
    shoulder M12.01-●
    specified joint NEC M12.08
    vertebrae M12.08
    wrist M12.03-●
  psoriatic NEC L40.59
    interphalangeal, distal L40.51

▶ New   ⇒ Revised   ~~deleted~~ Deleted   ● Use Additional Character(s)   83

Arthropathy (Continued)
  reactive M02.9
    in (due to)
      infective endocarditis I33.0 [M02.9]
    specified type NEC M02.80
      ankle M02.87-●
      elbow M02.82-●
      foot joint M02.87-●
      hand joint M02.84-●
      hip M02.85-●
      knee M02.86-●
      multiple site M02.89
      shoulder M02.81-●
      vertebra M02.88
      wrist M02.83-●
  specified form NEC M12.80
    ankle M12.87-●
    elbow M12.82-●
    foot joint M12.87-●
    hand joint M12.84-●
    hip M12.85-●
    knee M12.86-●
    multiple site M12.89
    shoulder M12.81-●
    specified joint NEC M12.88
    vertebrae M12.88
    wrist M12.83-●
  syringomyelic G95.0
  tabes dorsalis A52.16
  tabetic A52.16
  transient —*see* Arthropathy, specified form
    NEC
  traumatic M12.50
    ankle M12.57-●
    elbow M12.52-●
    foot joint M12.57-●
    hand joint M12.54-●
    hip M12.55-●
    knee M12.56-●
    multiple site M12.59
    shoulder M12.51-●
    specified joint NEC M12.58
    vertebrae M12.58
    wrist M12.53-●
Arthropyosis —*see* Arthritis, pyogenic or pyemic
Arthrosis (deformans) (degenerative)
  (localized) —*see also* Osteoarthritis
  M19.90
  spine —*see* Spondylosis
Arthus' phenomenon or reaction T78.41
  due to
    drug —*see* Table of Drugs and Chemicals,
      by drug
Articular —*see* condition
Articulation, reverse (teeth) M26.24
Artificial
  insemination complication —*see*
    Complications, artificial, fertilization
  opening status (functioning) (without
    complication) Z93.9
    anus (colostomy) Z93.3
    colostomy Z93.3
    cystostomy Z93.50
      appendico-vesicostomy Z93.52
      cutaneous Z93.51
      specified NEC Z93.59
    enterostomy Z93.4
    gastrostomy Z93.1
    ileostomy Z93.2
    intestinal tract NEC Z93.4
    jejunostomy Z93.4
    nephrostomy Z93.6
    specified site NEC Z93.8
    tracheostomy Z93.0
    ureterostomy Z93.6
    urethrostomy Z93.6
    urinary tract NEC Z93.6
    vagina Z93.8
  vagina status Z93.8
Arytenoid —*see* condition
Asbestosis (occupational) J61

ASC-H (atypical squamous cells cannot exclude
  high grade squamous intraepithelial lesion
  on cytologic smear)
  anus R85.611
  cervix R87.611
  vagina R87.621
ASC-US (atypical squamous cells of
  undetermined significance on cytologic
  smear)
  anus R85.610
  cervix R87.610
  vagina R87.620
Ascariasis B77.9
  with
    complications NEC B77.89
    intestinal complications B77.0
    pneumonia, pneumonitis B77.81
Ascaridosis, ascaridiasis —*see* Ascariasis
Ascaris (infection) (infestation)
  (lumbricoides) —*see* Ascariasis
Ascending —*see* condition
Aschoff's bodies —*see* Myocarditis,
  rheumatic
Ascites (abdominal) R18.8
➡ cardiac —*see also* Failure, heart, right
    I50.810
  chylous (nonfilarial) I89.8
    filarial —*see* Infestation, filarial
  due to
    cirrhosis, alcoholic K70.31
    hepatitis
      alcoholic K70.11
      chronic active K71.51
    S. japonicum B65.2
➡ heart —*see also* Failure, heart, right I50.810
  malignant R18.0
  pseudochylous R18.8
  syphilitic A52.74
  tuberculous A18.31
Aseptic —*see* condition
Asherman's syndrome N85.6
Asialia K11.7
Asiatic cholera —*see* Cholera
Asimultagnosia (simultanagnosia) R48.3
Askin's tumor —*see* Neoplasm, connective
  tissue, malignant
Asocial personality F60.2
Asomatognosia R41.4
Aspartylglucosaminuria E77.1
Asperger's disease or syndrome F84.5
Aspergilloma —*see* Aspergillosis
Aspergillosis (with pneumonia) B44.9
  bronchopulmonary, allergic B44.81
  disseminated B44.7
  generalized B44.7
  pulmonary NEC B44.1
    allergic B44.81
    invasive B44.0
  specified NEC B44.89
  tonsillar B44.2
Aspergillus (flavus) (fumigatus) (infection)
  (terreus) —*see* Aspergillosis
Aspermatogenesis —*see* Azoospermia
Aspermia (testis) —*see* Azoospermia
Asphyxia, asphyxiation (by) R09.01
  antenatal P84
  birth P84
  bunny bag —*see* Asphyxia, due to,
    mechanical threat to breathing, trapped
    in bed clothes
  crushing S28.0
  drowning T75.1
  gas, fumes, or vapor —*see* Table of Drugs and
    Chemicals
  inhalation —*see* Inhalation
  intrauterine P84
  local I73.00
    with gangrene I73.01
  mucus —*see also* Foreign body, respiratory
    tract, causing asphyxia
  newborn P84

Asphyxia, asphyxiation (Continued)
  pathological R09.01
  postnatal P84
    mechanical —*see* Asphyxia, due to,
      mechanical threat to breathing
  prenatal P84
  reticularis R23.1
  strangulation —*see* Asphyxia, due to,
    mechanical threat to breathing
  submersion T75.1
  traumatic T71.9
    due to
      crushed chest S28.0
      foreign body (in) —*see* Foreign body,
        respiratory tract, causing asphyxia
    low oxygen content of ambient air T71.20
      due to
        being trapped in
          low oxygen environment T71.29
          in car trunk T71.221
            circumstances undetermined
              T71.224
            done with intent to harm by
              another person T71.223
              self T71.222
          in refrigerator T71.231
            circumstances undetermined
              T71.234
            done with intent to harm by
              another person T71.233
              self T71.232
      cave-in T71.21
    mechanical threat to breathing
      (accidental) T71.191
      circumstances undetermined T71.194
      done with intent to harm by
        another person T71.193
      self T71.192
      hanging T71.161
        circumstances undetermined
          T71.164
        done with intent to harm by
          another person T71.163
        self T71.162
      plastic bag T71.121
        circumstances undetermined
          T71.124
        done with intent to harm by
          another person T71.123
        self T71.122
      smothering
        in furniture T71.151
          circumstances undetermined
            T71.154
          done with intent to harm by
            another person T71.153
          self T71.152
        under
          another person's body T71.141
            circumstances undetermined
              T71.144
            done with intent to harm
              T71.143
          pillow T71.111
            circumstances undetermined
              T71.114
            done with intent to harm by
              another person T71.113
              self T71.112
      trapped in bed clothes T71.131
        circumstances undetermined
          T71.134
        done with intent to harm by
          another person T71.133
        self T71.132
  vomiting, vomitus —*see* Foreign body,
    respiratory tract, causing asphyxia
Aspiration
  amniotic (clear) fluid (newborn) P24.10
    with
      pneumonia (pneumonitis) P24.11
      respiratory symptoms P24.11

▶ New   ⇒ Revised   ~~deleted~~ Deleted   ● Use Additional Character(s)

Aspiration *(Continued)*
  blood
    newborn (without respiratory symptoms)
        P24.20
      with
        pneumonia (pneumonitis) P24.21
        respiratory symptoms P24.21
    specified age NEC —*see* Foreign body,
        respiratory tract
  bronchitis J69.0
  food or foreign body (with asphyxiation) —
      see Asphyxia, food
  liquor (amnii) (newborn) P24.10
    with
      pneumonia (pneumonitis) P24.11
      respiratory symptoms P24.11
  meconium (newborn) (without respiratory
      symptoms) P24.00
    with
      pneumonitis (pneumonitis) P24.01
      respiratory symptoms P24.01
  milk (newborn) (without respiratory
      symptoms) P24.30
    with
      pneumonia (pneumonitis) P24.31
      respiratory symptoms P24.31
  specified age NEC —*see* Foreign body,
      respiratory tract
  mucus —*see also* Foreign body, by site,
      causing asphyxia
    newborn P24.10
      with
        pneumonia (pneumonitis) P24.11
        respiratory symptoms P24.11
  neonatal P24.9
    specific NEC (without respiratory
        symptoms) P24.80
      with
        pneumonia (pneumonitis) P24.81
        respiratory symptoms P24.81
  newborn P24.9
    specific NEC (without respiratory
        symptoms) P24.80
      with
        pneumonia (pneumonitis) P24.81
        respiratory symptoms P24.81
  pneumonia J69.0
  pneumonitis J69.0
  syndrome of newborn —*see* Aspiration, by
      substance, with pneumonia
  vernix caseosa (newborn) P24.80
    with
      pneumonia (pneumonitis) P24.81
      respiratory symptoms P24.81
  vomitus —*see also* Foreign body, respiratory
      tract
    newborn (without respiratory symptoms)
        P24.30
      with
        pneumonia (pneumonitis) P24.31
        respiratory symptoms P24.31
Asplenia (congenital) Q89.01
  postsurgical Z90.81
Assam fever B55.0
Assault, sexual —*see* Maltreatment
Assmann's focus NEC A15.0
Astasia (-abasia) (hysterical) F44.4
Asteatosis cutis L85.3
Astereognosia, astereognosis R48.1
Asterixis R27.8
  in liver disease K71.3
Asteroid hyalitis —*see* Deposit, crystalline
Asthenia, asthenic R53.1
  cardiac —*see also* Failure, heart I50.9
    psychogenic F45.8
  cardiovascular —*see also* Failure, heart
      I50.9
    psychogenic F45.8
  heart —*see also* Failure, heart I50.9
    psychogenic F45.8
  hysterical F44.4

Asthenia, asthenic *(Continued)*
  myocardial —*see also* Failure, heart I50.9
    psychogenic F45.8
  nervous F48.8
  neurocirculatory F45.8
  neurotic F48.8
  psychogenic F48.8
  psychoneurotic F48.8
  psychophysiologic F48.8
  reaction (psychophysiologic) F48.8
  senile R54
Asthenopia —*see also* Discomfort, visual
  hysterical F44.6
  psychogenic F44.6
Asthenospermia —*see* Abnormal, specimen,
    male genital organs
Asthma, asthmatic (bronchial) (catarrh)
    (spasmodic) J45.909
  with
    chronic obstructive bronchitis J44.9
      with
        acute lower respiratory infection J44.0
        exacerbation (acute) J44.1
    chronic obstructive pulmonary disease
        J44.9
      with
        acute lower respiratory infection J44.0
        exacerbation (acute) J44.1
    exacerbation (acute) J45.901
    hay fever —*see* Asthma, allergic extrinsic
    rhinitis, allergic —*see* Asthma, allergic
        extrinsic
    status asthmaticus J45.902
  allergic extrinsic J45.909
    with
      exacerbation (acute) J45.901
      status asthmaticus J45.902
  atopic —*see* Asthma, allergic extrinsic
  cardiac —*see* Failure, ventricular, left
  cardiobronchial I50.1
  childhood J45.909
    with
      exacerbation (acute) J45.901
      status asthmaticus J45.902
  chronic obstructive J44.9
    with
      acute lower respiratory infection J44.0
      exacerbation (acute) J44.1
  collier's J60
  cough variant J45.991
  detergent J69.8
  due to
    detergent J69.8
    inhalation of fumes J68.3
  eosinophilic J82
  extrinsic, allergic —*see* Asthma, allergic
      extrinsic
  grinder's J62.8
  hay —*see* Asthma, allergic extrinsic
  heart I50.1
  idiosyncratic —*see* Asthma, nonallergic
  intermittent (mild) J45.20
    with
      exacerbation (acute) J45.21
      status asthmaticus J45.22
  intrinsic, nonallergic —*see* Asthma, nonallergic
  Kopp's E32.8
  late-onset J45.909
    with
      exacerbation (acute) J45.901
      status asthmaticus J45.902
  mild intermittent J45.20
    with
      exacerbation (acute) J45.21
      status asthmaticus J45.22
  mild persistent J45.30
    with
      exacerbation (acute) J45.31
      status asthmaticus J45.32
  Millar's (laryngismus stridulus) J38.5
  miner's J60

Asthma, asthmatic *(Continued)*
  mixed J45.909
    with
      exacerbation (acute) J45.901
      status asthmaticus J45.902
  moderate persistent J45.40
    with
      exacerbation (acute) J45.41
      status asthmaticus J45.42
  nervous —*see* Asthma, nonallergic
  nonallergic (intrinsic) J45.909
    with
      exacerbation (acute) J45.901
      status asthmaticus J45.902
  persistent
    mild J45.30
      with
        exacerbation (acute) J45.31
        status asthmaticus J45.32
    moderate J45.40
      with
        exacerbation (acute) J45.41
        status asthmaticus J45.42
    severe J45.50
      with
        exacerbation (acute) J45.51
        status asthmaticus J45.52
  platinum J45.998
  pneumoconiotic NEC J64
  potter's J62.8
  predominantly allergic J45.909
  psychogenic F54
  pulmonary eosinophilic J82
  red cedar J67.8
  Rostan's I50.1
  sandblaster's J62.8
  sequoiosis J67.8
  severe persistent J45.50
    with
      exacerbation (acute) J45.51
      status asthmaticus J45.52
  specified NEC J45.998
  stonemason's J62.8
  thymic E32.8
  tuberculous —*see* Tuberculosis, pulmonary
  Wichmann's (laryngismus stridulus) J38.5
  wood J67.8
Astigmatism (compound) (congenital)
    H52.20-●
  irregular H52.21-●
  regular H52.22-●
Astraphobia F40.220
Astroblastoma
  specified site —*see* Neoplasm, malignant, by
      site
  unspecified site C71.9
Astrocytoma (cystic)
  anaplastic
    specified site —*see* Neoplasm, malignant,
        by site
    unspecified site C71.9
  fibrillary
    specified site —*see* Neoplasm, malignant,
        by site
    unspecified site C71.9
  fibrous
    specified site —*see* Neoplasm, malignant,
        by site
    unspecified site C71.9
  gemistocytic
    specified site —*see* Neoplasm, malignant,
        by site
    unspecified site C71.9
  juvenile
    specified site —*see* Neoplasm, malignant,
        by site
    unspecified site C71.9
  pilocytic
    specified site —*see* Neoplasm, malignant,
        by site
    unspecified site C71.9

Astrocytoma (Continued)
  piloid
    specified site —see Neoplasm, malignant,
      by site
    unspecified site C71.9
  protoplasmic
    specified site —see Neoplasm, malignant,
      by site
    unspecified site C71.9
  specified site NEC —see Neoplasm,
    malignant, by site
  subependymal D43.2
    giant cell
      specified site —see Neoplasm, uncertain
        behavior, by site
      unspecified site D43.2
    specified site —see Neoplasm, uncertain
      behavior, by site
    unspecified site D43.2
  unspecified site C71.9
Astroglioma
  specified site —see Neoplasm, malignant, by
    site
  unspecified site C71.9
Asymbolia R48.8
Asymmetry —see also Distortion
  between native and reconstructed breast N65.1
  face Q67.0
  jaw (lower) —see Anomaly, dentofacial, jaw-
    cranial base relationship, asymmetry
Asynergia, asynergy R27.8
  ventricular I51.89
Asystole (heart) —see Arrest, cardiac
At risk
  ~~for falling Z91.81~~
  ▶for
    ▶dental caries Z91.849
      ▶high Z91.843
      ▶low Z91.841
      ▶moderate Z91.842
    ▶falling Z91.81
Ataxia, ataxy, ataxic R27.0
  acute R27.8
  brain (hereditary) G11.9
  cerebellar (hereditary) G11.9
    with defective DNA repair G11.3
    alcoholic G31.2
    early-onset G11.1
    in
      alcoholism G31.2
      myxedema E03.9 [G13.2]
      neoplastic disease —see also Neoplasm
        D49.9 [G32.81]
      specified disease NEC G32.81
    late-onset (Marie's) G11.2
  cerebral (hereditary) G11.9
  congenital nonprogressive G11.0
  family, familial —see Ataxia, hereditary
  following
    cerebrovascular disease I69.993
      cerebral infarction I69.393
      intracerebral hemorrhage I69.193
      nontraumatic intracranial hemorrhage
        NEC I69.293
      specified disease NEC I69.893
      subarachnoid hemorrhage I69.093
  Friedreich's (heredofamilial) (cerebellar)
    (spinal) G11.1
  gait R26.0
    hysterical F44.4
  general R27.8
  gluten M35.9 [G32.81]
    with celiac disease K90.0 [G32.81]
  hereditary G11.9
    with neuropathy G60.2
    cerebellar —see Ataxia, cerebellar
    spastic G11.4
    specified NEC G11.8
    spinal (Friedreich's) G11.1
  heredofamilial —see Ataxia, hereditary
  Hunt's G11.1

Ataxia, ataxy, ataxic (Continued)
  hysterical F44.4
  locomotor (progressive) (syphilitic) (partial)
    (spastic) A52.11
    diabetic —see Diabetes, ataxia
  Marie's (cerebellar) (heredofamilial)
    (late- onset) G11.2
  nonorganic origin F44.4
  nonprogressive, congenital G11.0
  psychogenic F44.4
  Roussy-Lévy G60.0
  Sanger-Brown's (hereditary) G11.2
  spastic hereditary G11.4
  spinal
    hereditary (Friedreich's) G11.1
    progressive (syphilitic) A52.11
  spinocerebellar, X-linked recessive G11.1
  telangiectasia (Louis-Bar) G11.3
Ataxia-telangiectasia (Louis-Bar) G11.3
Atelectasis (massive) (partial) (pressure)
  (pulmonary) J98.11
  newborn P28.10
    due to resorption P28.11
    partial P28.19
    primary P28.0
    secondary P28.19
  primary (newborn) P28.0
  tuberculous —see Tuberculosis, pulmonary
Atelocardia Q24.9
Atelomyelia Q06.1
Atheroembolism
  of
    extremities
      lower I75.02-●
      upper I75.01-●
    kidney I75.81
    specified NEC I75.89
Atheroma, atheromatous —see also
  Arteriosclerosis I70.90
  aorta, aortic I70.0
    valve —see also Endocarditis, aortic I35.8
  aorto-iliac I70.0
  artery —see Arteriosclerosis
  basilar (artery) I67.2
  carotid (artery) (common) (internal) I67.2
  cerebral (arteries) I67.2
  coronary (artery) I25.10
    with angina pectoris —see Arteriosclerosis,
      coronary (artery)
  degeneration —see Arteriosclerosis
  heart, cardiac —see Disease, heart, ischemic,
    atherosclerotic
  mitral (valve) I34.8
  myocardium, myocardial —see Disease, heart,
    ischemic, atherosclerotic
  pulmonary valve (heart) —see also
    Endocarditis, pulmonary I37.8
  tricuspid (heart) (valve) I36.8
  valve, valvular —see Endocarditis
  vertebral (artery) I67.2
Atheromatosis —see Arteriosclerosis
Atherosclerosis —see also Arteriosclerosis
  coronary
    artery I25.10
      with angina pectoris —see
        Arteriosclerosis, coronary (artery),
      due to
        calcified coronary lesion (severely)
          I25.84
        lipid rich plaque I25.83
    transplanted heart I25.811
      bypass graft I25.812
        with angina pectoris —see
          Arteriosclerosis, coronary (artery)
      native coronary artery I25.811
        with angina pectoris —see
          Arteriosclerosis, coronary (artery)
Athetosis (acquired) R25.8
  bilateral (congenital) G80.3
  congenital (bilateral) (double) G80.3
  double (congenital) G80.3
  unilateral R25.8

Athlete's
  foot B35.3
  heart I51.7
Athrepsia E41
Athyrea (acquired) —see also Hypothyroidism
  congenital E03.1
Atonia, atony, atonic
  bladder (sphincter) (neurogenic) N31.2
  capillary I78.8
  cecum K59.8
    psychogenic F45.8
  colon —see Atony, intestine
  congenital P94.2
  esophagus K22.8
  intestine K59.8
    psychogenic F45.8
  stomach K31.89
    neurotic or psychogenic F45.8
  uterus (during labor) O62.2
    with hemorrhage (postpartum) O72.1
    postpartum (with hemorrhage) O72.1
      without hemorrhage O75.89
Atopy —see History, allergy
Atransferrinemia, congenital E88.09
Atresia, atretic
  alimentary organ or tract NEC Q45.8
    upper Q40.8
  ani, anus, anal (canal) Q42.3
    with fistula Q42.2
  aorta (ring) Q25.29
  aortic (orifice) (valve) Q23.0
    arch Q25.21
    congenital with hypoplasia of ascending
      aorta and defective development of
      left ventricle (with mitral stenosis)
      Q23.4
    in hypoplastic left heart syndrome Q23.4
  aqueduct of Sylvius Q03.0
    with spina bifida —see Spina bifida, with
      hydrocephalus
  artery NEC Q27.8
    cerebral Q28.3
    coronary Q24.5
    digestive system Q27.8
    eye Q15.8
    lower limb Q27.8
    pulmonary Q25.5
    specified site NEC Q27.8
    umbilical Q27.0
    upper limb Q27.8
  auditory canal (external) Q16.1
  bile duct (common) (congenital) (hepatic)
    Q44.2
    acquired —see Obstruction, bile duct
  bladder (neck) Q64.39
    obstruction Q64.31
  bronchus Q32.4
  cecum Q42.8
  cervix (acquired) N88.2
    congenital Q51.828
    in pregnancy or childbirth —see Anomaly,
      cervix, in pregnancy or childbirth
      causing obstructed labor O65.5
  choana Q30.0
  colon Q42.9
    specified NEC Q42.8
  common duct Q44.2
  cricoid cartilage Q31.8
  cystic duct Q44.2
    acquired K82.8
      with obstruction K82.0
  digestive organs NEC Q45.8
  duodenum Q41.0
  ear canal Q16.1
  ejaculatory duct Q55.4
  epiglottis Q31.8
  esophagus Q39.0
    with tracheoesophageal fistula Q39.1
  eustachian tube Q17.8
  fallopian tube (congenital) Q50.6
    acquired N97.1

Atresia, atretic (Continued)
follicular cyst N83.0-●
foramen of
Luschka Q03.1
with spina bifida —see Spina bifida, with
hydrocephalus
Magendie Q03.1
with spina bifida —see Spina bifida, with
hydrocephalus
gallbladder Q44.1
genital organ
external
female Q52.79
male Q55.8
internal
female Q52.8
male Q55.8
glottis Q31.8
gullet Q39.0
with tracheoesophageal fistula Q39.1
heart valve NEC Q24.8
pulmonary Q22.0
tricuspid Q22.4
hymen Q52.3
acquired (postinfective) N89.6
ileum Q41.2
intestine (small) Q41.9
large Q42.9
specified NEC Q42.8
iris, filtration angle Q15.0
jejunum Q41.1
lacrimal apparatus Q10.4
larynx Q31.8
meatus urinarius Q64.33
mitral valve Q23.2
in hypoplastic left heart syndrome
Q23.4
nares (anterior) (posterior) Q30.0
nasopharynx Q34.8
nose, nostril Q30.0
acquired J34.89
organ or site NEC Q89.8
osseous meatus (ear) Q16.1
oviduct (congenital) Q50.6
acquired N97.1
parotid duct Q38.4
acquired K11.8
pulmonary (artery) Q25.5
valve Q22.0
pulmonic Q22.0
pupil Q13.2
rectum Q42.1
with fistula Q42.0
salivary duct Q38.4
acquired K11.8
sublingual duct Q38.4
acquired K11.8
submandibular duct Q38.4
acquired K11.8
submaxillary duct Q38.4
acquired K11.8
thyroid cartilage Q31.8
trachea Q32.1
tricuspid valve Q22.4
ureter Q62.10
pelvic junction Q62.11
vesical orifice Q62.12
ureteropelvic junction Q62.11
ureterovesical orifice Q62.12
urethra (valvular) Q64.39
stricture Q64.32
urinary tract NEC Q64.8
uterus Q51.818
acquired N85.8
vagina (congenital) Q52.4
acquired (postinfectional) (senile)
N89.5
vas deferens Q55.3
vascular NEC Q27.8
cerebral Q28.3
digestive system Q27.8

Atresia, atretic (Continued)
vascular NEC (Continued)
lower limb Q27.8
specified site NEC Q27.8
upper limb Q27.8
vein NEC Q27.8
digestive system Q27.8
great Q26.8
lower limb Q27.8
portal Q26.5
➥pulmonary Q26.4
▶partial Q26.3
▶total Q26.2
specified site NEC Q27.8
upper limb Q27.8
vena cava (inferior) (superior) Q26.8
vesicourethral orifice Q64.31
vulva Q52.79
acquired N90.5
Atrichia, atrichosis —see Alopecia
Atrophia —see also Atrophy
cutis senilis L90.8
due to radiation L57.8
gyrata of choroid and retina H31.23
senilis R54
dermatological L90.8
due to radiation (nonionizing) (solar)
L57.8
unguium L60.3
congenita Q84.6
Atrophie blanche (en plaque) (de Milian) L95.0
Atrophoderma, atrophodermia (of) L90.9
diffusum (idiopathic) L90.4
maculatum L90.8
et striatum L90.8
due to syphilis A52.79
syphilitic A51.39
neuriticum L90.8
Pasini and Pierini L90.3
pigmentosum Q82.1
reticulatum symmetricum faciei L66.4
senile L90.8
due to radiation (nonionizing) (solar) L57.8
vermiculata (cheeks) L66.4
Atrophy, atrophic (of)
adrenal (capsule) (gland) E27.49
primary (autoimmune) E27.1
alveolar process or ridge (edentulous) K08.20
anal sphincter (disuse) N81.84
appendix K38.8
arteriosclerotic —see Arteriosclerosis
bile duct (common) (hepatic) K83.8
bladder N32.89
neurogenic N31.8
blanche (en plaque) (of Milian) L95.0
bone (senile) NEC —see also Disorder, bone,
specified type NEC
due to
tabes dorsalis (neurogenic) A52.11
brain (cortex) (progressive) G31.9
frontotemporal circumscribed G31.01
[F02.80]
with behavioral disturbance G31.01
[F02.81]
senile NEC G31.1
breast N64.2
obstetric —see Disorder, breast, specified
type NEC
buccal cavity K13.79
cardiac —see Degeneration, myocardial
cartilage (infectional) (joint) —see Disorder,
cartilage, specified NEC
cerebellar —see Atrophy, brain
cerebral —see Atrophy, brain
cervix (mucosa) (senile) (uteri) N88.8
menopausal N95.8
Charcot-Marie-Tooth G60.0
choroid (central) (macular) (myopic) (retina)
H31.10-●
diffuse secondary H31.12-●
gyrate H31.23
senile H31.11-●

Atrophy, atrophic (Continued)
ciliary body —see Atrophy, iris
conjunctiva (senile) H11.89
corpus cavernosum N48.89
cortical —see Atrophy, brain
cystic duct K82.8
Déjérine-Thomas G23.8
disuse NEC —see Atrophy, muscle
Duchenne-Aran G12.21
ear H93.8-●
edentulous alveolar ridge K08.20
endometrium (senile) N85.8
cervix N88.8
enteric K63.89
epididymis N50.89
eyeball —see Disorder, globe, degenerated
condition, atrophy
eyelid (senile) —see Disorder, eyelid,
degenerative
facial (skin) L90.9
fallopian tube (senile) N83.32-●
with ovary N83.33-●
fascioscapulohumeral (Landouzy-Déjérine)
G71.0
fatty, thymus (gland) E32.8
gallbladder K82.8
gastric K29.40
with bleeding K29.41
gastrointestinal K63.89
glandular I89.8
globe H44.52-●
➥gum —see Recession, gingival
hair L67.8
heart (brown) —see Degeneration, myocardial
hemifacial Q67.4
Romberg G51.8
infantile E41
paralysis, acute —see Poliomyelitis,
paralytic
intestine K63.89
iris (essential) (progressive) H21.26-●
specified NEC H21.29
kidney (senile) (terminal) —see also Sclerosis,
renal N26.1
congenital or infantile Q60.5
bilateral Q60.4
unilateral Q60.3
hydronephrotic —see Hydronephrosis
lacrimal gland (primary) H04.14-●
secondary H04.15-●
Landouzy-Déjérine G71.0
laryngitis, infective J37.0
larynx J38.7
Leber's optic (hereditary) H47.22
lip K13.0
liver (yellow) K72.90
with coma K72.91
acute, subacute K72.00
with coma K72.01
chronic K72.10
with coma K72.11
lung (senile) J98.4
macular (dermatological) L90.8
syphilitic, skin A51.39
striated A52.79
mandible (edentulous) K08.20
minimal K08.21
moderate K08.22
severe K08.23
maxilla K08.20
minimal K08.24
moderate K08.25
severe K08.26
muscle, muscular (diffuse) (general)
(idiopathic) (primary) M62.50
ankle M62.57-●
Duchenne-Aran G12.21
foot M62.57-●
forearm M62.53-●
hand M62.54-●
infantile spinal G12.0
lower leg M62.56-●

Atrophy, atrophic *(Continued)*
  muscle, muscular *(Continued)*
    multiple sites M62.59
    myelopathic —*see* Atrophy, muscle,
      spinal
    myotonic G71.11
    neuritic G58.9
    neuropathic (peroneal) (progressive)
      G60.0
    pelvic (disuse) N81.84
    peroneal G60.0
    progressive (bulbar) G12.21
      adult G12.1
      infantile (spinal) G12.0
    ➡spinal G12.25
      adult G12.1
      infantile G12.0
    pseudohypertrophic G71.0
    shoulder region M62.51-●
    specified site NEC M62.58
    spinal G12.9
      adult form G12.1
      Aran-Duchenne G12.21
      childhood form, type II G12.1
      distal G12.1
      hereditary NEC G12.1
      infantile, type I (Werdnig-Hoffmann)
        G12.0
      juvenile form, type III (Kugelberg-
        Welander) G12.1
      ➡progressive G12.25
      scapuloperoneal form G12.1
      specified NEC G12.8
    syphilitic A52.78
    thigh M62.55-●
    upper arm M62.52-●
  myocardium —*see* Degeneration,
    myocardial
  myometrium (senile) N85.8
    cervix N88.8
  myopathic NEC —*see* Atrophy, muscle
  myotonia G71.11
  nail L60.3
  nasopharynx J31.1
  nerve —*see also* Disorder, nerve
    abducens —*see* Strabismus, paralytic, sixth
      nerve
    accessory G52.8
    acoustic or auditory —*see* subcategory
      H93.3
    cranial G52.9
      eighth (auditory) —*see* subcategory
        H93.3
      eleventh (accessory) G52.8
      fifth (trigeminal) G50.8
      first (olfactory) G52.0
      fourth (trochlear) —*see* Strabismus,
        paralytic, fourth nerve
      second (optic) H47.20
      sixth (abducens) —*see* Strabismus,
        paralytic, sixth nerve
      tenth (pneumogastric) (vagus) G52.2
      third (oculomotor) —*see* Strabismus,
        paralytic, third nerve
      twelfth (hypoglossal) G52.3
    hypoglossal G52.3
    oculomotor —*see* Strabismus, paralytic,
      third nerve
    olfactory G52.0
    optic (papillomacular bundle)
      syphilitic (late) A52.15
      congenital A50.44
    pneumogastric G52.2
    trigeminal G50.8
    trochlear —*see* Strabismus, paralytic,
      fourth nerve
    vagus (pneumogastric) G52.2
  neurogenic, bone, tabetic A52.11
  nutritional E41
  old age R54
  olivopontocerebellar G23.8

Atrophy, atrophic *(Continued)*
  optic (nerve) H47.20
    glaucomatous H47.23-●
    hereditary H47.22
    primary H47.21-●
    specified type NEC H47.29-●
    syphilitic (late) A52.15
      congenital A50.44
  orbit H05.31-●
  ovary (senile) N83.31-●
    with fallopian tube N83.33-●
  oviduct (senile) —*see* Atrophy, fallopian tube
  palsy, diffuse (progressive) G12.22
  pancreas (duct) (senile) K86.89
  parotid gland K11.0
  pelvic muscle N81.84
  penis N48.89
  pharynx J39.2
  pluriglandular E31.8
    autoimmune E31.0
  polyarthritis M15.9
  prostate N42.89
  pseudohypertrophic (muscle) G71.0
  renal —*see also* Sclerosis, renal N26.1
  retina, retinal (postinfectional) H35.89
  rhinitis J31.0
  salivary gland K11.0
  scar L90.5
  sclerosis, lobar (of brain) G31.09 *[F02.80]*
    with behavioral disturbance G31.09
      [F02.81]
  scrotum N50.89
  seminal vesicle N50.89
  senile R54
    due to radiation (nonionizing) (solar) L57.8
  skin (patches) (spots) L90.9
    degenerative (senile) L90.8
    due to radiation (nonionizing) (solar) L57.8
    senile L90.8
  spermatic cord N50.89
  spinal (acute) (cord) G95.89
    muscular —*see* Atrophy, muscle, spinal
    paralysis G12.20
      acute —*see* Poliomyelitis, paralytic
      meaning progressive muscular atrophy
        G12.21
  spine (column) —*see* Spondylopathy,
    specified NEC
  spleen (senile) D73.0
  stomach K29.40
    with bleeding K29.41
  striate (skin) L90.6
    syphilitic A52.79
  subcutaneous L90.9
  sublingual gland K11.0
  submandibular gland K11.0
  submaxillary gland K11.0
  Sudeck's —*see* Algoneurodystrophy
  suprarenal (capsule) (gland) E27.49
    primary E27.1
  systemic affecting central nervous system
    in
      myxedema E03.9 *[G13.2]*
      neoplastic disease —*see also* Neoplasm
        D49.9 *[G13.1]*
      specified disease NEC G13.8
  tarso-orbital fascia, congenital Q10.3
  testis N50.0
  thenar, partial —*see* Syndrome, carpal tunnel
  thymus (fatty) E32.8
  thyroid (gland) (acquired) E03.4
    with cretinism E03.1
    congenital (with myxedema) E03.1
  tongue (senile) K14.8
    papillae K14.4
  trachea J39.8
  tunica vaginalis N50.89
  turbinate J34.89
  tympanic membrane (nonflaccid) H73.82-●
    flaccid H73.81-●
  upper respiratory tract J39.8

Atrophy, atrophic *(Continued)*
  uterus, uterine (senile) N85.8
    cervix N88.8
    due to radiation (intended effect)
      N85.8
      adverse effect or misadventure
        N99.89
  vagina (senile) N95.2
  vas deferens N50.89
  vascular I99.8
  vertebra (senile) —*see* Spondylopathy,
    specified NEC
  vulva (senile) N90.5
  Werdnig-Hoffmann G12.0
  yellow —*see* Failure, hepatic
Attack, attacks
  with alteration of consciousness (with
    automatisms) —*see* Epilepsy,
    localization-related, symptomatic, with
    complex partial seizures
  without alteration of consciousness —
    see Epilepsy, localization-related,
    symptomatic, with simple partial seizures
  Adams-Stokes I45.9
  akinetic —*see* Epilepsy, generalized, specified
    NEC
  angina —*see* Angina
  atonic —*see* Epilepsy, generalized, specified
    NEC
  benign shuddering G25.83
  cataleptic —*see* Catalepsy
  coronary —*see* Infarct, myocardium
  cyanotic, newborn P28.2
  drop NEC R55
  epileptic —*see* Epilepsy
  heart —*see* infarct, myocardium
  hysterical F44.9
  jacksonian —*see* Epilepsy, localization-
    related, symptomatic, with simple
    partial seizures
  myocardium, myocardial —*see* Infarct,
    myocardium
  myoclonic —*see* Epilepsy, generalized,
    specified NEC
  panic F41.0
  psychomotor —*see* Epilepsy, localization-
    related, symptomatic, with complex
    partial seizures
  salaam —*see* Epilepsy, spasms
  schizophreniform, brief F23
  shuddering, benign G25.83
  Stokes-Adams I45.9
  syncope R55
  transient ischemic (TIA) G45.9
    specified NEC G45.8
  unconsciousness R55
    hysterical F44.89
  vasomotor R55
  vasovagal (paroxysmal) (idiopathic) R55
Attention (to)
  artificial
    opening (of) Z43.9
      digestive tract NEC Z43.4
        colon Z43.3
        ilium Z43.2
        stomach Z43.1
      specified NEC Z43.8
      trachea Z43.0
      urinary tract NEC Z43.6
        cystostomy Z43.5
        nephrostomy Z43.6
        ureterostomy Z43.6
        urethrostomy Z43.6
      vagina Z43.7
  colostomy Z43.3
  cystostomy Z43.5
  deficit disorder or syndrome F98.8
    with hyperactivity —*see* Disorder,
      attention-deficit hyperactivity
  gastrostomy Z43.1
  ileostomy Z43.2

Attention (Continued)
  jejunostomy Z43.4
  nephrostomy Z43.6
  surgical dressings Z48.01
  sutures Z48.02
  tracheostomy Z43.0
  ureterostomy Z43.6
  urethrostomy Z43.6
Attrition
  gum —see Recession, gingival
  tooth, teeth (excessive) (hard tissues) K03.0
Atypical, atypism —see also condition
  cells (on cytolgocial smear) (endocervical)
    (endometrial) (glandular)
     cervix R87.619
     vagina R87.629
  cervical N87.9
  endometrium N85.9
    hyperplasia N85.00
  parenting situation Z62.9
Auditory —see condition
Aujeszky's disease B33.8
Aurantiasis, cutis E67.1
Auricle, auricular —see also condition
  cervical Q18.2
Auriculotemporal syndrome G50.8
Austin Flint murmur (aortic insufficiency)
  I35.1
Australian
  Q fever A78
  X disease A83.4
Autism, autistic (childhood) (infantile) F84.0
  atypical F84.9
  spectrum disorder F84.0
Autodigestion R68.89
Autoerythrocyte sensitization (syndrome)
  D69.2
Autographism L50.3
Autoimmune
  disease (systemic) M35.9
  inhibitors to clotting factors D68.311
  lymphoproliferative syndrome [ALPS]
    D89.82
  thyroiditis E06.3
Autointoxication R68.89
Automatism G93.89
  with temporal sclerosis G93.81
  epileptic —see Epilepsy, localization- related,
    symptomatic, with complex partial
    seizures

Automatism (Continued)
  paroxysmal, idiopathic —see Epilepsy,
    localization-related, symptomatic, with
    complex partial seizures
Autonomic, autonomous
  bladder (neurogenic) N31.2
  hysteria seizure F44.5
Autosensitivity, erythrocyte D69.2
Autosensitization, cutaneous L30.2
Autosome —see condition by chromosome
  involved
Autotopagnosia R48.1
Autotoxemia R68.89
Autumn —see condition
Avellis' syndrome G46.8
Aversion
  oral R63.3
    newborn P92.-●
    nonorganic origin F98.2
  sexual F52.1
Aviator's
  disease or sickness —see Effect, adverse, high
    altitude
  ear T70.0
Avitaminosis (multiple) —see also Deficiency,
    vitamin E56.9
  B E53.9
    with
      beriberi E51.11
      pellagra E52
  B2 E53.0
  B6 E53.1
  B12 E53.8
  D E55.9
    with rickets E55.0
  G E53.0
  K E56.1
  nicotinic acid E52
AVNRT (atrioventricular nodal re-entrant
  tachycardia) I47.1
AVRT (atrioventricular nodal re-entrant
  tachycardia) I47.1
Avulsion (traumatic)
  blood vessel —see Injury, blood vessel
  bone —see Fracture, by site
  cartilage —see also Dislocation, by site
    symphyseal (inner), complicating delivery
     O71.6
  external site other than limb —see Wound,
    open, by site

Avulsion (Continued)
  eye S05.7-●
  head (intracranial)
    external site NEC S08.89
    scalp S08.0
  internal organ or site —see Injury, by site
  joint —see also Dislocation, by site
    capsule —see Sprain, by site
  kidney S37.06-●
  ligament —see Sprain, by site
  limb —see also Amputation, traumatic,
    by site
    skin and subcutaneous tissue —see Wound,
     open, by site
  muscle —see Injury, muscle
  nerve (root) —see Injury, nerve
  scalp S08.0
  skin and subcutaneous tissue —see Wound,
    open, by site
  spleen S36.032
  symphyseal cartilage (inner), complicating
    delivery O71.6
  tendon —see Injury, muscle
  tooth S03.2
Awareness of heart beat R00.2
Axenfeld's
  anomaly or syndrome Q15.0
  degeneration (calcareous) Q13.4
Axilla, axillary —see also condition
  breast Q83.1
Axonotmesis —see Injury, nerve
Ayerza's disease or syndrome (pulmonary
  artery sclerosis with pulmonary
  hypertension) I27.0
Azoospermia (organic) N46.01
  due to
    drug therapy N46.021
    efferent duct obstruction N46.023
    infection N46.022
    radiation N46.024
    specified cause NEC N46.029
    systemic disease N46.025
Azotemia R79.89
  meaning uremia N19
Aztec ear Q17.3
Azygos
  continuation inferior vena cava Q26.8
  lobe (lung) Q33.1

B

Baastrup's disease —see Kissing spine
Babesiosis B60.0
Babington's disease (familial hemorrhagic telangiectasia) I78.0
Babinski's syndrome A52.79
Baby
  crying constantly R68.11
  floppy (syndrome) P94.2
Bacillary —see condition
Bacilluria R82.71
Bacillus —see also Infection, bacillus
  abortus infection A23.1
  anthracis infection A22.9
  coli infection —see also Escherichia coli B96.20
  Flexner's A03.1
  mallei infection A24.0
  Shiga's A03.0
  suipestifer infection —see Infection, salmonella
Back —see condition
Backache (postural) M54.9
  sacroiliac M53.3
  specified NEC M54.89
Backflow —see Reflux
Backward reading (dyslexia) F81.0
Bacteremia R78.81
  with sepsis —see Sepsis
Bactericholia —see Cholecystitis, acute
Bacterid, bacteride (pustular) L40.3
Bacterium, bacteria, bacterial
  agent NEC, as cause of disease classified elsewhere B96.89
  in blood —see Bacteremia
  in urine —see Bacteriuria
Bacteriuria, bacteruria R82.71
  asymptomatic R82.71
Bacteroides
  fragilis, as cause of disease classified elsewhere B96.6
Bad
  heart —see Disease, heart
. trip
    due to drug abuse —see Abuse, drug, hallucinogen
    due to drug dependence —see Dependence, drug, hallucinogen
Baelz's disease (cheilitis glandularis apostematosa) K13.0
Baerensprung's disease (eczema marginatum) B35.6
Bagasse disease or pneumonitis J67.1
Bagassosis J67.1
Baker's cyst —see Cyst, Baker's
Bakwin-Krida syndrome (metaphyseal dysplasia) Q78.5
Balancing side interference M26.56
Balanitis (circinata) (erosiva) (gangrenosa) (phagedenic) (vulgaris) N48.1
  amebic A06.82
  candidal B37.42
  due to Haemophilus ducreyi A57
  gonococcal (acute) (chronic) A54.09
  xerotica obliterans N48.0
Balanoposthitis N47.6
  gonococcal (acute) (chronic) A54.09
  ulcerative (specific) A63.8
Balanorrhagia —see Balanitis
Balantidiasis, balantidiosis A07.0
Bald tongue K14.4
Baldness —see also Alopecia
  male-pattern —see Alopecia, androgenic
Balkan grippe A78
Balloon disease —see Effect, adverse, high altitude
Balo's disease (concentric sclerosis) G37.5
Bamberger-Marie disease —see Osteoarthropathy, hypertrophic, specified type NEC
Bancroft's filariasis B74.0

Band(s)
  adhesive —see Adhesions, peritoneum
  anomalous or congenital —see also Anomaly, by site
    heart (atrial) (ventricular) Q24.8
    intestine Q43.3
    omentum Q43.3
  cervix N88.1
  constricting, congenital Q79.8
  gallbladder (congenital) Q44.1
  intestinal (adhesive) —see Adhesions, peritoneum
  obstructive
➡️   intestine K56.50
▶   complete K56.52
▶   incomplete K56.51
▶   partial K56.51
➡️   peritoneum K56.50
▶   complete K56.52
▶   incomplete K56.51
▶   partial K56.51
  periappendiceal, congenital Q43.3
  peritoneal (adhesive) —see Adhesions, peritoneum
  uterus N73.6
    internal N85.6
  vagina N89.5
Bandemia D72.825
Bandl's ring (contraction), complicating delivery O62.4
Bangkok hemorrhagic fever A91
Bang's disease (brucella abortus) A23.1
Bankruptcy, anxiety concerning Z59.8
Bannister's disease T78.3
  hereditary D84.1
Banti's disease or syndrome (with cirrhosis) (with portal hypertension) K76.6
Bar, median, prostate —see Enlargement, enlarged, prostate
Barcoo disease or rot —see Ulcer, skin
Barlow's disease E54
Barodontalgia T70.29
Baron Münchausen syndrome —see Disorder, factitious
Barosinusitis T70.1
Barotitis T70.0
Barotrauma T70.29
  odontalgia T70.29
  otitic T70.0
  sinus T70.1
Barraquer (-Simons) disease or syndrome (progressive lipodystrophy) E88.1
Barré-Guillain disease or syndrome G61.0
Barré-Liéou syndrome (posterior cervical sympathetic) M53.0
Barrel chest M95.4
Barrett's
  disease —see Barrett's, esophagus
  esophagus K22.70
    with dysplasia K22.719
      high grade K22.711
      low grade K22.710
    without dysplasia K22.70
  syndrome —see Barrett's, esophagus
  ulcer K22.10
    with bleeding K22.11
    without bleeding K22.10
Barth syndrome E78.71
Bársony (-Polgár) (-Teschendorf) syndrome (corkscrew esophagus) K22.4
Bartholinitis (suppurating) N75.8
  gonococcal (acute) (chronic) (with abscess) A54.1
Bartonellosis A44.9
  cutaneous A44.1
  mucocutaneous A44.1
  specified NEC A44.8
  systemic A44.0
Barton's fracture S52.56-●
Bartter's syndrome E26.81
Basal —see condition

Basan's (hidrotic) ectodermal dysplasia Q82.4
Baseball finger —see Dislocation, finger
Basedow's disease (exophthalmic goiter) —see Hyperthyroidism, with, goiter
Basic —see condition
Basilar —see condition
Bason's (hidrotic) ectodermal dysplasia Q82.4
Basopenia —see Agranulocytosis
Basophilia D72.824
Basophilism (cortico-adrenal) (Cushing's) (pituitary) E24.0
Bassen-Kornzweig disease or syndrome E78.6
Bat ear Q17.5
Bateman's
  disease B08.1
  purpura (senile) D69.2
Bathing cramp T75.1
Bathophobia F40.248
Batten (-Mayou) disease E75.4
  retina E75.4 [H36]
Batten-Steinert syndrome G71.11
Battered —see Maltreatment
Battey Mycobacterium infection A31.0
Battle exhaustion F43.0
Battledore placenta O43.19-●
Baumgarten-Cruveilhier cirrhosis, disease or syndrome K74.69
Bauxite fibrosis (of lung) J63.1
Bayle's disease (general paresis) A52.17
Bazin's disease (primary) (tuberculous) A18.4
Beach ear —see Swimmer's, ear
Beaded hair (congenital) Q84.1
Béal conjunctivitis or syndrome B30.2
Beard's disease (neurasthenia) F48.8
Beat(s)
  atrial, premature I49.1
  ectopic I49.49
  elbow —see Bursitis, elbow
  escaped, heart I49.49
  hand —see Bursitis, hand
  knee —see Bursitis, knee
  premature I49.40
    atrial I49.1
    auricular I49.1
    supraventricular I49.1
Beau's
  disease or syndrome —see Degeneration, myocardial
  lines (transverse furrows on fingernails) L60.4
Bechterev's syndrome —see Spondylitis, ankylosing
Beck's syndrome (anterior spinal artery occlusion) I65.8
Becker's
  cardiomyopathy I42.8
  disease
    idiopathic mural endomyocardial disease I42.3
    myotonia congenita, recessive form G71.12
  dystrophy G71.0
  pigmented hairy nevus D22.5
Beckwith-Wiedemann syndrome Q87.3
Bed confinement status Z74.01
Bed sore —see Ulcer, pressure, by site
Bedbug bite(s) —see Bite(s), by site, superficial, insect
Bedclothes, asphyxiation or suffocation by —see Asphyxia, traumatic, due to, mechanical, trapped
Bednar's
  aphthae K12.0
  tumor —see Neoplasm, malignant, by site
Bedridden Z74.01
Bedsore —see Ulcer, pressure, by site
Bedwetting —see Enuresis
Bee sting (with allergic or anaphylactic shock) —see Toxicity, venom, arthropod, bee
Beer drinker's heart (disease) I42.6
Begbie's disease (exophthalmic goiter) —see Hyperthyroidism, with, goiter

▶ New   ➡️ Revised   ~~deleted~~ Deleted   ● Use Additional Character(s)

Behavior
antisocial
adult Z72.811
child or adolescent Z72.810
disorder, disturbance —see Disorder, conduct
disruptive —see Disorder, conduct
drug seeking Z76.5
inexplicable R46.2
marked evasiveness R46.5
obsessive-compulsive R46.81
overactivity R46.3
poor responsiveness R46.4
self-damaging (life-style) Z72.89
sleep-incompatible Z72.821
slowness R46.4
specified NEC R46.89
strange (and inexplicable) R46.2
suspiciousness R46.5
type A pattern Z73.1
undue concern or preoccupation with stressful events R46.6
verbosity and circumstantial detail obscuring reason for contact R46.7
Behcet's disease or syndrome M35.2
Behr's disease —see Degeneration, macula
Beigel's disease or morbus (white piedra) B36.2
Bejel A65
Bekhterev's syndrome —see Spondylitis, ankylosing
Belching —see Eructation
Bell's
mania F30.8
palsy, paralysis G51.0
infant or newborn P11.3
spasm G51.3
Bence Jones albuminuria or proteinuria NEC R80.3
Bends T70.3
Benedikt's paralysis or syndrome G46.3
Benign (see also condition)
prostatic hyperplasia —see Hyperplasia, prostate
Bennett's fracture (displaced) S62.21-●
Benson's disease —see Deposit, crystalline
Bent
back (hysterical) F44.4
nose M95.0
congenital Q67.4
Bereavement (uncomplicated) Z63.4
Bergeron's disease (hysterical chorea) F44.4
Berger's disease —see Nephropathy, IgA
Beriberi (dry) E51.11
heart (disease) E51.12
polyneuropathy E51.11
wet E51.12
involving circulatory system E51.11
Berlin's disease or edema (traumatic) S05.8X-●
Berlock (berloque) dermatitis L56.2
Bernard-Horner syndrome G90.2
Bernard-Soulier disease or thrombopathia D69.1
Bernhardt (-Roth) disease —see Mononeuropathy, lower limb, meralgia paresthetica
Bernheim's syndrome —see Failure, heart, right
Bertielliasis B71.8
Berylliosis (lung) J63.2
Besnier-Boeck (-Schaumann) disease —see Sarcoidosis
Besnier's
lupus pernio D86.3
prurigo L20.0
Bestiality F65.89
Best's disease H35.50
Beta-mercaptolactate-cysteine disulfiduria E72.09
Betalipoproteinemia, broad or floating E78.2
Betting and gambling Z72.6
pathological (compulsive) F63.0

Bezoar T18.9
intestine T18.3
stomach T18.2
Bezold's abscess —see Mastoiditis, acute
Bianchi's syndrome R48.8
Bicornate or bicornis uterus Q51.3
in pregnancy or childbirth O34.00
causing obstructed labor O65.5
Bicuspid aortic valve Q23.1
Biedl-Bardet syndrome Q87.89
Bielschowsky (-Jansky) disease E75.4
Biermer's (pernicious) anemia or disease D51.0
Biett's disease L93.0
Bifid (congenital)
apex, heart Q24.8
clitoris Q52.6
kidney Q63.8
nose Q30.2
patella Q74.1
scrotum Q55.29
toe NEC Q74.2
tongue Q38.3
ureter Q62.8
uterus Q51.3
uvula Q35.7
Biforis uterus (suprasimplex) Q51.3
Bifurcation (congenital)
gallbladder Q44.1
kidney pelvis Q63.8
renal pelvis Q63.8
rib Q76.6
tongue, congenital Q38.3
trachea Q32.1
ureter Q62.8
urethra Q64.74
vertebra Q76.49
Big spleen syndrome D73.1
Bigeminal pulse R00.8
Bilateral —see condition
Bile
duct —see condition
pigments in urine R82.2
Bilharziasis —see also Schistosomiasis
chyluria B65.0
cutaneous B65.3
galacturia B65.0
hematochyluria B65.0
intestinal B65.1
lipemia B65.9
lipuria B65.0
oriental B65.2
piarhemia B65.9
pulmonary NOS B65.9 [J99]
pneumonia B65.9 [J17]
tropical hematuria B65.0
vesical B65.0
Biliary —see condition
Bilirubin metabolism disorder E80.7
specified NEC E80.6
Bilirubinemia, familial nonhemolytic E80.4
Bilirubinuria R82.2
Biliuria R82.2
Bilocular stomach K31.2
Binswanger's disease I67.3
Biparta, bipartite
carpal scaphoid Q74.0
patella Q74.1
vagina Q52.10
Bird
face Q75.8
fancier's disease or lung J67.2
Birt-Hogg-Dube syndrome Q87.89
Birth
complications in mother —see Delivery, complicated
compression during NOS P15.9
defect —see Anomaly
immature (less than 37 completed weeks) —see Preterm, newborn
extremely (less than 28 completed weeks) —see Immaturity, extreme

Birth (Continued)
inattention, at or after —see Maltreatment, child, neglect
injury NOS P15.9
basal ganglia P11.1
brachial plexus NEC P14.3
brain (compression) (pressure) P11.2
central nervous system NOS P11.9
cerebellum P11.1
cerebral hemorrhage P10.1
external genitalia P15.5
eye P15.3
face P15.4
fracture
bone P13.9
specified NEC P13.8
clavicle P13.4
femur P13.2
humerus P13.3
long bone, except femur P13.3
radius and ulna P13.3
skull P13.0
spine P11.5
tibia and fibula P13.3
intracranial P11.2
laceration or hemorrhage P10.9
specified NEC P10.8
intraventricular hemorrhage P10.2
laceration
brain P10.1
by scalpel P15.8
peripheral nerve P14.9
liver P15.0
meninges
brain P11.1
spinal cord P11.5
nerve
brachial plexus P14.3
cranial NEC (except facial) P11.4
facial P11.3
peripheral P14.9
phrenic (paralysis) P14.2
paralysis
facial nerve P11.3
spinal P11.5
penis P15.5
rupture
spinal cord P11.5
scalp P12.9
scalpel wound P15.8
scrotum P15.5
skull NEC P13.1
fracture P13.0
specified type NEC P15.8
spinal cord P11.5
spine P11.5
spleen P15.1
sternomastoid (hematoma) P15.2
subarachnoid hemorrhage P10.3
subcutaneous fat necrosis P15.6
subdural hemorrhage P10.0
tentorial tear P10.4
testes P15.5
vulva P15.5
lack of care, at or after —see Maltreatment, child, neglect
neglect, at or after —see Maltreatment, child, neglect
palsy or paralysis, newborn, NOS (birth injury) P14.9
premature (infant) —see Preterm, newborn
shock, newborn P96.89
trauma —see Birth, injury
weight
4000 grams to 4499 grams P08.1
4500 grams or more P08.0
low (2499 grams or less) —see Low, birthweight
extremely (999 grams or less) —see Low, birthweight, extreme
Birthmark Q82.5

Bisalbuminemia E88.09
Biskra's button B55.1
Bite(s) (animal) (human)
  abdomen, abdominal
    wall S31.159
      with penetration into peritoneal cavity
        S31.659
      epigastric region S31.152
        with penetration into peritoneal cavity
          S31.652
      left
        lower quadrant S31.154
          with penetration into peritoneal
            cavity S31.654
        upper quadrant S31.151
          with penetration into peritoneal
            cavity S31.651
      periumbilic region S31.155
        with penetration into peritoneal cavity
          S31.655
      right
        lower quadrant S31.153
          with penetration into peritoneal
            cavity S31.653
        upper quadrant S31.150
          with penetration into peritoneal
            cavity S31.650
      superficial NEC S30.871
        insect S30.861
  alveolar (process) —see Bite, oral cavity
  amphibian (venomous) —see Venom, bite,
    amphibian
  animal —see also Bite, by site
    venomous —see Venom
  ankle S91.05-•
    superficial NEC S90.57-•
      insect S90.56-•
  antecubital space —see Bite, elbow
  anus S31.835
    superficial NEC S30.877
      insect S30.867
  arm (upper) S41.15-•
    lower —see Bite, forearm
    superficial NEC S40.87-•
      insect S40.86-•
  arthropod NEC —see Venom, bite, arthropod
  auditory canal (external) (meatus) —
    see Bite, ear
  auricle, ear —see Bite, ear
  axilla —see Bite, arm
  back —see also Bite, thorax, back
    lower S31.050
      with penetration into retroperitoneal
        space S31.051
      superficial NEC S30.870
        insect S30.860
  bedbug —see Bite(s), by site, superficial,
    insect
  breast S21.05-•
    superficial NEC S20.17-•
      insect S20.16-•
  brow —see Bite, head, specified site NEC
  buttock S31.805
    left S31.825
    right S31.815
    superficial NEC S30.870
      insect S30.860
  calf —see Bite, leg
  canaliculus lacrimalis —see Bite, eyelid
  canthus, eye —see Bite, eyelid
  centipede —see Toxicity, venom, arthropod,
    centipede
  cheek (external) S01.45-•
    internal —see Bite, oral cavity
    superficial NEC S00.87
      insect S00.86
  chest wall —see Bite, thorax
  chigger B88.0
  chin —see Bite, head, specified site NEC
  clitoris —see Bite, vulva
  costal region —see Bite, thorax

Bite (Continued)
  digit(s)
    hand —see Bite, finger
    toe —see Bite, toe
  ear (canal) (external) S01.35-•
    superficial NEC S00.47-•
      insect S00.46-•
  elbow S51.05-•
    superficial NEC S50.37-•
      insect S50.36-•
  epididymis —see Bite, testis
  epigastric region —see Bite, abdomen
  epiglottis —see Bite, neck, specified site
    NEC
  esophagus, cervical S11.25
    superficial NEC S10.17
      insect S10.16
  eyebrow —see Bite, eyelid
  eyelid S01.15-•
    superficial NEC S00.27-•
      insect S00.26-•
  face NEC —see Bite, head, specified site
    NEC
  finger(s) S61.259
    with
      damage to nail S61.359
    index S61.258
      with
        damage to nail S61.358
      left S61.251
        with
          damage to nail S61.351
      right S61.250
        with
          damage to nail S61.350
      superficial NEC S60.478
        insect S60.46-•
    little S61.25-•
      with
        damage to nail S61.35-•
      superficial NEC S60.47-•
        insect S60.46-•
    middle S61.25-•
      with
        damage to nail S61.35-•
      superficial NEC S60.47-•
        insect S60.46-•
    ring S61.25-•
      with
        damage to nail S61.35-•
      superficial NEC S60.47-•
        insect S60.46-•
    superficial NEC S60.479
      insect S60.469
    thumb —see Bite, thumb
  flank —see Bite, abdomen, wall
  flea —see Bite, by site, superficial,
    insect
  foot (except toe(s) alone) S91.35-•
    superficial NEC S90.87-•
      insect S90.86-•
    toe —see Bite, toe
  forearm S51.85-•
    elbow only —see Bite, elbow
    superficial NEC S50.87-•
      insect S50.86-•
  forehead —see Bite, head, specified site
    NEC
  genital organs, external
    female S31.552
      superficial NEC S30.876
        insect S30.866
      vagina and vulva —see Bite, vulva
    male S31.551
      penis —see Bite, penis
      scrotum —see Bite, scrotum
      superficial NEC S30.875
        insect S30.865
      testes —see Bite, testis
  groin —see Bite, abdomen, wall
  gum —see Bite, oral cavity

Bite (Continued)
  hand S61.45-•
    finger —see Bite, finger
    superficial NEC S60.57-•
      insect S60.56-•
    thumb —see Bite, thumb
  head S01.95
    cheek —see Bite, cheek
    ear —see Bite, ear
    eyelid —see Bite, eyelid
    lip —see Bite, lip
    nose —see Bite, nose
    oral cavity —see Bite, oral cavity
    scalp —see Bite, scalp
    specified site NEC S01.85
      superficial NEC S00.87
        insect S00.86
    superficial NEC S00.97
      insect S00.96
    temporomandibular area —see Bite, cheek
  heel —see Bite, foot
  hip S71.05-•
    superficial NEC S70.27-•
      insect S70.26-•
  hymen S31.45
  hypochondrium —see Bite, abdomen, wall
  hypogastric region —see Bite, abdomen, wall
  inguinal region —see Bite, abdomen, wall
  insect —see Bite, by site, superficial, insect
  instep —see Bite, foot
  interscapular region —see Bite, thorax, back
  jaw —see Bite, head, specified site NEC
  knee S81.05-•
    superficial NEC S80.27-•
      insect S80.26-•
  labium (majus) (minus) —see Bite, vulva
  lacrimal duct —see Bite, eyelid
  larynx S11.015
    superficial NEC S10.17
      insect S10.16
  leg (lower) S81.85-•
    ankle —see Bite, ankle
    foot —see Bite, foot
    knee —see Bite, knee
    superficial NEC S80.87-•
      insect S80.86-•
    toe —see Bite, toe
    upper —see Bite, thigh
  lip S01.551
    superficial NEC S00.571
      insect S00.561
  lizard (venomous) —see Venom, bite, reptile
  loin —see Bite, abdomen, wall
  lower back —see Bite, back, lower
  lumbar region —see Bite, back, lower
  malar region —see Bite, head, specified site
    NEC
  mammary —see Bite, breast
  marine animals (venomous) —see Toxicity,
    venom, marine animal
  mastoid region —see Bite, head, specified site
    NEC
  mouth —see Bite, oral cavity
  nail
    finger —see Bite, finger
    toe —see Bite, toe
  nape —see Bite, neck, specified site NEC
  nasal (septum) (sinus) —see Bite, nose
  nasopharynx —see Bite, head, specified site
    NEC
  neck S11.95
    involving
      cervical esophagus —see Bite,
        esophagus, cervical
      larynx —see Bite, larynx
      pharynx —see Bite, pharynx
      thyroid gland S11.15
      trachea —see Bite, trachea
    specified site NEC S11.85
      superficial NEC S10.87
        insect S10.86

▶ New   ⇒ Revised   ~~deleted~~ Deleted   • Use Additional Character(s)

Bite *(Continued)*
  neck *(Continued)*
    superficial NEC S10.97
      insect S10.96
    throat S11.85
      superficial NEC S10.17
        insect S10.16
  nose (septum) (sinus) S01.25
    superficial NEC S00.37
      insect S00.36
  occipital region —*see* Bite, scalp
  oral cavity S01.552
    superficial NEC S00.572
      insect S00.562
  orbital region —*see* Bite, eyelid
  palate —*see* Bite, oral cavity
  palm —*see* Bite, hand
  parietal region —*see* Bite, scalp
  pelvis S31.050
    with penetration into retroperitoneal space
      S31.051
    superficial NEC S30.870
      insect S30.860
  penis S31.25
    superficial NEC S30.872
      insect S30.862
  perineum
    female —*see* Bite, vulva
    male —*see* Bite, pelvis
  periocular area (with or without lacrimal
      passages) —*see* Bite, eyelid
  phalanges
    finger —*see* Bite, finger
    toe —*see* Bite, toe
  pharynx S11.25
    superficial NEC S10.17
      insect S10.16
  pinna —*see* Bite, ear
  poisonous —*see* Venom
  popliteal space —*see* Bite, knee
  prepuce —*see* Bite, penis
  pubic region —*see* Bite, abdomen, wall
  rectovaginal septum —*see* Bite, vulva
  red bug B88.0
  reptile NEC —*see also* Venom, bite,
      reptile
    nonvenomous —*see* Bite, by site
    snake —*see* Venom, bite, snake
  sacral region —*see* Bite, back, lower
  sacroiliac region —*see* Bite, back, lower
  salivary gland —*see* Bite, oral cavity
  scalp S01.05
    superficial NEC S00.07
      insect S00.06
  scapular region —*see* Bite, shoulder
  scrotum S31.35
    superficial NEC S30.873
      insect S30.863
  sea-snake (venomous) —*see* Toxicity, venom,
      snake, sea snake
  shin —*see* Bite, leg
  shoulder S41.05-●
    superficial NEC S40.27-●
      insect S40.26-●
  snake —*see also* Venom, bite, snake
    nonvenomous —*see* Bite, by site
  spermatic cord —*see* Bite, testis
  spider (venomous) —*see* Toxicity, venom,
      spider
    nonvenomous —*see* Bite, by site,
        superficial, insect
  sternal region —*see* Bite, thorax, front
  submaxillary region —*see* Bite, head,
      specified site NEC
  submental region —*see* Bite, head, specified
      site NEC
  subungual
    finger(s) —*see* Bite, finger
    toe —*see* Bite, toe
  superficial —*see* Bite, by site, superficial
  supraclavicular fossa S11.85

Bite *(Continued)*
  supraorbital —*see* Bite, head, specified site
      NEC
  temple, temporal region —*see* Bite, head,
      specified site NEC
  temporomandibular area —*see* Bite, cheek
  testis S31.35
    superficial NEC S30.873
      insect S30.863
  thigh S71.15-●
    superficial NEC S70.37-●
      insect S70.36-●
  thorax, thoracic (wall) S21.95
    back S21.25-●
      with penetration into thoracic cavity
        S21.45-●
    breast —*see* Bite, breast
    front S21.15-●
      with penetration into thoracic cavity
        S21.35-●
    superficial NEC S20.97
      back S20.47-●
      front S20.37-●
      insect S20.96
        back S20.46-●
        front S20.36-●
  throat —*see* Bite, neck, throat
  thumb S61.05-●
    with
      damage to nail S61.15-●
    superficial NEC S60.37-●
      insect S60.36-●
  thyroid S11.15
    superficial NEC S10.87
      insect S10.86
  toe(s) S91.15-●
    with
      damage to nail S91.25-●
    great S91.15-●
      with
        damage to nail S91.25-●
    lesser S91.15-●
      with
        damage to nail S91.25-●
    superficial NEC S90.47-●
      great S90.47-●
      insect S90.46-●
        great S90.46-●
  tongue S01.552
  trachea S11.025
    superficial NEC S10.17
      insect S10.16
  tunica vaginalis —*see* Bite, testis
  tympanum, tympanic membrane —*see* Bite,
      ear
  umbilical region S31.155
  uvula —*see* Bite, oral cavity
  vagina —*see* Bite, vulva
  venomous —*see* Venom
  vocal cords S11.035
    superficial NEC S10.17
      insect S10.16
  vulva S31.45
    superficial NEC S30.874
      insect S30.864
  wrist S61.55-●
    superficial NEC S60.87-●
      insect S60.86-●
Biting, cheek or lip K13.1
▶ Biventricular failure (heart) I50.82
Björck (-Thorson) syndrome (malignant
    carcinoid) E34.0
Black
  death A20.9
  eye S00.1-●
  hairy tongue K14.3
  heel (foot) S90.3-●
  lung (disease) J60
  palm (hand) S60.22-●
Blackfan-Diamond anemia or syndrome
    (congenital hypoplastic anemia) D61.01

Blackhead L70.0
Blackout R55
Bladder —*see* condition
Blast (air) (hydraulic) (immersion) (underwater)
  blindness S05.8X-●
  injury
    abdomen or thorax —*see* Injury, by site
    ear (acoustic nerve trauma) —*see* Injury,
        nerve, acoustic, specified type NEC
  syndrome NEC T70.8
Blastoma —*see* Neoplasm, malignant, by site
  pulmonary —*see* Neoplasm, lung, malignant
Blastomycosis, blastomycotic B40.9
  Brazilian —*see* Paracoccidioidomycosis
  cutaneous B40.3
  disseminated B40.7
  European —*see* Cryptococcosis
  generalized B40.7
  keloidal B48.0
  North American B40.9
  primary pulmonary B40.0
  pulmonary B40.2
    acute B40.0
    chronic B40.1
  skin B40.3
  South American —*see*
      Paracoccidioidomycosis
  specified NEC B40.89
Bleb(s) R23.8
  emphysematous (lung) (solitary) J43.9
  endophthalmitis H59.43
  filtering (vitreous), after glaucoma surgery
      Z98.83
  inflammed (infected), postprocedural H59.40
    stage 1 H59.41
    stage 2 H59.42
    stage 3 H59.43
  lung (ruptured) J43.9
    congenital —*see* Atelectasis
    newborn P25.8
  subpleural (emphysematous) J43.9
Blebitis, postprocedural H59.40
  stage 1 H59.41
  stage 2 H59.42
  stage 3 H59.43
Bleeder (familial) (hereditary) —*see* Hemophilia
Bleeding —*see also* Hemorrhage
  anal K62.5
  anovulatory N97.0
  atonic, following delivery O72.1
  capillary I78.8
    puerperal O72.2
  contact (postcoital) N93.0
  due to uterine subinvolution N85.3
  ear —*see* Otorrhagia
  excessive, associated with menopausal onset
      N92.4
  familial —*see* Defect, coagulation
  following intercourse N93.0
  gastrointestinal K92.2
  hemorrhoids —*see* Hemorrhoids
  intermenstrual (regular) N92.3
    irregular N92.1
  intraoperative —*see* Complication,
      intraoperative, hemorrhage
  irregular N92.6
  menopausal N92.4
  newborn, intraventricular —*see* Newborn,
      affected by, hemorrhage, intraventricular
  nipple N64.59
  nose R04.0
  ovulation N92.3
  postclimacteric N95.0
  postcoital N93.0
  postmenopausal N95.0
  postoperative —*see* Complication,
      postprocedural, hemorrhage
  preclimacteric N92.4
  pre-pubertal vaginal N93.1
  puberty (excessive, with onset of menstrual
      periods) N92.2

B

Bleeding (Continued)
  rectum, rectal K62.5
    newborn P54.2
  tendencies —see Defect, coagulation
  throat R04.1
  tooth socket (post-extraction) K91.840
  umbilical stump P51.9
  uterus, uterine NEC N93.9
    climacteric N92.4
  ▸ dysfunctional or functional N93.8
    menopausal N92.4
    preclimacteric or premenopausal N92.4
    unrelated to menstrual cycle N93.9
  vagina, vaginal (abnormal) N93.9
    dysfunctional or functional N93.8
    newborn P54.6
    pre-pubertal N93.1
  vicarious N94.89
Blennorrhagia, blennorrhagic —see Gonorrhea
Blennorrhea (acute) (chronic) —see also
    Gonorrhea
  inclusion (neonatal) (newborn) P39.1
  lower genitourinary tract (gonococcal)
    A54.00
  neonatorum (gonococcal ophthalmia)
    A54.31
Blepharelosis —see Entropion
Blepharitis (angularis) (ciliaris) (eyelid)
    (marginal) (nonulcerative) H01.009
  herpes zoster B02.39
  left H01.006
    lower H01.005
    upper H01.004
  right H01.003
    lower H01.002
    upper H01.001
  squamous H01.029
    left H01.026
      lower H01.025
      upper H01.024
    right H01.023
      lower H01.022
      upper H01.021
  ulcerative H01.019
    left H01.016
      lower H01.015
      upper H01.014
    right H01.013
      lower H01.012
      upper H01.011
Blepharochalasis H02.30
  congenital Q10.0
  left H02.36
    lower H02.35
    upper H02.34
  right H02.33
    lower H02.32
    upper H02.31
Blepharoclonus H02.59
Blepharoconjunctivitis H10.50-●
  angular H10.52-●
  contact H10.53-●
  ligneous H10.51-●
Blepharophimosis (eyelid) H02.529
  congenital Q10.3
  left H02.526
    lower H02.525
    upper H02.524
  right H02.523
    lower H02.522
    upper H02.521
Blepharoptosis H02.40-●
  congenital Q10.0
  mechanical H02.41-●
  myogenic H02.42-●
  neurogenic H02.43-●
  paralytic H02.43-●
Blepharopyorrhea, gonococcal A54.39
Blepharospasm G24.5
  drug induced G24.01
Blighted ovum O02.0

Blind —see also Blindness
  bronchus (congenital) Q32.4
  loop syndrome K90.2
    congenital Q43.8
  sac, fallopian tube (congenital) Q50.6
  spot, enlarged —see Defect, visual field,
    localized, scotoma, blind spot area
  tract or tube, congenital NEC —see Atresia,
    by site
▸**Blindness** (acquired) (congenital) (both eyes)
    H54.0X-●
  blast S05.8X-●
  color —see Deficiency, color vision
  concussion S05.8X-●
  cortical H47.619
    left brain H47.612
    right brain H47.611
  day H53.11
  due to injury (current episode) S05.9-●
    sequelae — code to injury with seventh
      character S
  eclipse (total) —see Retinopathy, solar
  emotional (hysterical) F44.6
  face H53.16
  hysterical F44.6
  legal (both eyes) (USA definition) H54.8
  mind R48.8
  night H53.60
    abnormal dark adaptation curve H53.61
    acquired H53.62
    congenital H53.63
    specified type NEC H53.69
    vitamin A deficiency E50.5
  one eye (other eye normal) H54.40
  ⇛ left (normal vision on right) H54.42-●
    ⇛ low vision on right H54.12-●
    low vision, other eye H54.10
  ⇛ right (normal vision on left) H54.41-●
    ⇛ low vision on left H54.11-●
  psychic R48.8
  river B73.01
  snow —see Photokeratitis
  sun, solar —see Retinopathy, solar
  transient —see Disturbance, vision, subjective,
    loss, transient
  traumatic (current episode) S05.9-●
  word (developmental) F81.0
    acquired R48.0
    secondary to organic lesion R48.0
Blister (nonthermal)
  abdominal wall S30.821
  alveolar process S00.522
  ankle S90.52-●
  antecubital space —see Blister, elbow
  anus S30.827
  arm (upper) S40.82-●
  auditory canal —see Blister, ear
  auricle —see Blister, ear
  axilla —see Blister, arm
  back, lower S30.820
  beetle dermatitis L24.89
  breast S20.12-●
  brow S00.82
  calf —see Blister, leg
  canthus —see Blister, eyelid
  cheek S00.82
    internal S00.522
  chest wall —see Blister, thorax
  chin S00.82
  costal region —see Blister, thorax
  digit(s)
    foot —see Blister, toe
    hand —see Blister, finger
  due to burn —see Burn, by site, second degree
  ear S00.42-●
  elbow S50.32-●
  epiglottis S10.12
  esophagus, cervical S10.12
  eyebrow —see Blister, eyelid
  eyelid S00.22-●
  face S00.82

Blister (Continued)
  fever B00.1
  finger(s) S60.429
    index S60.42-●
    little S60.42-●
    middle S60.42-●
    ring S60.42-●
  foot (except toe(s) alone) S90.82-●
    toe —see Blister, toe
  forearm S50.82-●
    elbow only —see Blister, elbow
  forehead S00.82
  fracture - omit code
  genital organ
    female S30.826
    male S30.825
  gum S00.522
  hand S60.52-●
  head S00.92
    ear —see Blister, ear
    eyelid —see Blister, eyelid
    lip S00.521
    nose S00.32
    oral cavity S00.522
    scalp S00.02
    specified site NEC S00.82
  heel —see Blister, foot
  hip S70.22-●
  interscapular region S20.429
  jaw S00.82
  knee S80.22-●
  larynx S10.12
  leg (lower) S80.82-●
    knee —see Blister, knee
    upper —see Blister, thigh
  lip S00.521
  malar region S00.82
  mammary —see Blister, breast
  mastoid region S00.82
  mouth S00.522
  multiple, skin, nontraumatic R23.8
  nail
    finger —see Blister, finger
    toe —see Blister, toe
  nasal S00.32
  neck S10.92
    specified site NEC S10.82
    throat S10.12
  nose S00.32
  occipital region S00.02
  oral cavity S00.522
  orbital region —see Blister, eyelid
  palate S00.522
  palm —see Blister, hand
  parietal region S00.02
  pelvis S30.820
  penis S30.822
  periocular area —see Blister, eyelid
  phalanges
    finger —see Blister, finger
    toe —see Blister, toe
  pharynx S10.12
  pinna —see Blister, ear
  popliteal space —see Blister, knee
  scalp S00.02
  scapular region —see Blister, shoulder
  scrotum S30.823
  shin —see Blister, leg
  shoulder S40.22-●
  sternal region S20.329
  submaxillary region S00.82
  submental region S00.82
  subungual
    finger(s) —see Blister, finger
    toe(s) —see Blister, toe
  supraclavicular fossa S10.82
  supraorbital S00.82
  temple S00.82
  temporal region S00.82
  testis S30.823
  thermal —see Burn, second degree, by site

Blister *(Continued)*
  thigh S70.32-●
  thorax, thoracic (wall) S20.92
    back S20.42-●
    front S20.32-●
  throat S10.12
  thumb S60.32-●
  toe(s) S90.42-●
    great S90.42-●
  tongue S00.522
  trachea S10.12
  tympanum, tympanic membrane —*see* Blister, ear
  upper arm —*see* Blister, arm (upper)
  uvula S00.522
  vagina S30.824
  vocal cords S10.12
  vulva S30.824
  wrist S60.82-●
Bloating R14.0
Bloch-Sulzberger disease or syndrome Q82.3
Block, blocked
  alveolocapillary J84.10
  arborization (heart) I45.5
  arrhythmic I45.9
  atrioventricular (incomplete) (partial) I44.30
    with atrioventricular dissociation I44.2
    complete I44.2
      congenital Q24.6
    congenital Q24.6
    first degree I44.0
    second degree (types I and II) I44.1
    specified NEC I44.39
    third degree I44.2
    types I and II I44.1
  auriculoventricular —*see* Block, atrioventricular
  bifascicular (cardiac) I45.2
  bundle-branch (complete) (false) (incomplete) I45.4
    bilateral I45.2
    left I44.7
      with right bundle branch block I45.2
      hemiblock I44.60
        anterior I44.4
        posterior I44.5
      incomplete I44.7
        with right bundle branch block I45.2
    right I45.10
      with
        left bundle branch block I45.2
        left fascicular block I45.2
      specified NEC I45.19
    Wilson's type I45.19
  cardiac I45.9
  conduction I45.9
    complete I44.2
  fascicular (left) I44.60
    anterior I44.4
    posterior I44.5
    right I45.0
    specified NEC I44.69
  foramen Magendie (acquired) G91.1
    congenital Q03.1
      with spina bifida —*see* Spina bifida, by site, with hydrocephalus
  heart I45.9
    bundle branch I45.4
      bilateral I45.2
    complete (atrioventricular) I44.2
    congenital Q24.6
    first degree (atrioventricular) I44.0
    second degree (atrioventricular) I44.1
    specified type NEC I45.5
    third degree (atrioventricular) I44.2
  hepatic vein I82.0
  intraventricular (nonspecific) I45.4
    bundle branch
      bilateral I45.2
  kidney N28.9
    postcystoscopic or postprocedural N99.0

Block, blocked *(Continued)*
  Mobitz (types I and II) I44.1
  myocardial —*see* Block, heart
  nodal I45.5
  organ or site, congenital NEC —*see* Atresia, by site
  portal (vein) I81
  second degree (types I and II) I44.1
  sinoatrial I45.5
  sinoauricular I45.5
  third degree I44.2
  trifascicular I45.3
  tubal N97.1
  vein NOS I82.90
  Wenckebach (types I and II) I44.1
Blockage —*see* Obstruction
Blocq's disease F44.4
Blood
  constituents, abnormal R78.9
  disease D75.9
  donor —*see* Donor, blood
  dyscrasia D75.9
    with
      abortion —*see* Abortion, by type, complicated by, hemorrhage
      ectopic pregnancy O08.1
      molar pregnancy O08.1
      following ectopic or molar pregnancy O08.1
      newborn P61.9
      puerperal, postpartum O72.3
  flukes NEC —*see* Schistosomiasis
  in
    feces K92.1
      occult R19.5
    urine —*see* Hematuria
  mole O02.0
  occult in feces R19.5
  pressure
    decreased, due to shock following injury T79.4
    examination only Z01.30
    fluctuating I99.8
    high —*see* Hypertension
      borderline R03.0
      incidental reading, without diagnosis of hypertension R03.0
    low —*see also* Hypotension
      incidental reading, without diagnosis of hypotension R03.1
  spitting —*see* Hemoptysis
  staining cornea —*see* Pigmentation, cornea, stromal
  transfusion
    reaction or complication —*see* Complications, transfusion
  type
    A (Rh positive) Z67.10
      Rh negative Z67.11
    AB (Rh positive) Z67.30
      Rh negative Z67.31
    B (Rh positive) Z67.20
      Rh negative Z67.21
    O (Rh positive) Z67.40
      Rh negative Z67.41
    Rh (positive) Z67.90
      negative Z67.91
  vessel rupture —*see* Hemorrhage
  vomiting —*see* Hematemesis
Blood-forming organs, disease D75.9
Bloodgood's disease —*see* Mastopathy, cystic
Bloom (-Machacek)(-Torre) syndrome Q82.8
Blount's disease or osteochondrosis —*see* Osteochondrosis, juvenile, tibia
Blue
  baby Q24.9
  diaper syndrome E72.09
  dome cyst (breast) —*see* Cyst, breast
  dot cataract Q12.0
  nevus D22.9

Blue *(Continued)*
  sclera Q13.5
    with fragility of bone and deafness Q78.0
  toe syndrome I75.02-●
Blueness —*see* Cyanosis
Blues, postpartal O90.6
  baby O90.6
Blurring, visual H53.8
Blushing (abnormal) (excessive) R23.2
BMI —*see* Body, mass index
Boarder, hospital NEC Z76.4
  accompanying sick person Z76.3
  healthy infant or child Z76.2
    foundling Z76.1
Bochart's impetigo L01.02
Bodechtel-Guttman disease (subacute sclerosing panencephalitis) A81.1
Boder-Sedgwick syndrome (ataxia-telangiectasia) G11.3
Body, bodies
  Aschoff's —*see* Myocarditis, rheumatic
  asteroid, vitreous —*see* Deposit, crystalline
  cytoid (retina) —*see* Occlusion, artery, retina
  drusen (degenerative) (macula) (retinal) —*see also* Degeneration, macula, drusen
    optic disc —*see* Drusen, optic disc
  foreign —*see* Foreign body
  loose
    joint, except knee —*see* Loose, body, joint
      knee M23.4-●
    sheath, tendon —*see* Disorder, tendon, specified type NEC
  mass index (BMI)
    adult
      ~~19 or less Z68.1~~
      ▶ 19.9 or less Z68.1
      20.0-20.9 Z68.20
      21.0-21.9 Z68.21
      22.0-22.9 Z68.22
      23.0-23.9 Z68.23
      24.0-24.9 Z68.24
      25.0-25.9 Z68.25
      26.0-26.9 Z68.26
      27.0-27.9 Z68.27
      28.0-28.9 Z68.28
      29.0-29.9 Z68.29
      30.0-30.9 Z68.30
      31.0-31.9 Z68.31
      32.0-32.9 Z68.32
      33.0-33.9 Z68.33
      34.0-34.9 Z68.34
      35.0-35.9 Z68.35
      36.0-36.9 Z68.36
      37.0-37.9 Z68.37
      38.0-38.9 Z68.38
      39.0-39.9 Z68.39
      40.0-44.9 Z68.41
      45.0-49.9 Z68.42
      50.0-59.9 Z68.43
      60.0-69.9 Z68.44
      70 and over Z68.45
    pediatric
      5th percentile to less than 85th percentile for age Z68.52
      85th percentile to less than 95th percentile for age Z68.53
      greater than or equal to ninety-fifth percentile for age Z68.54
      less than fifth percentile for age Z68.51
  Mooser's A75.2
  rice —*see also* Loose, body, joint
    knee M23.4-●
  rocking F98.4
Boeck's
  disease or sarcoid —*see* Sarcoidosis
  lupoid (miliary) D86.3
Boerhaave's syndrome (spontaneous esophageal rupture) K22.3
Boggy
  cervix N88.8
  uterus N85.8

Boil —*see also* Furuncle, by site
 Aleppo B55.1
 Baghdad B55.1
 Delhi B55.1
 lacrimal
  gland —*see* Dacryoadenitis
  passages (duct) (sac) —*see* Inflammation,
   lacrimal, passages, acute
 Natal B55.1
 orbit, orbital —*see* Abscess, orbit
 tropical B55.1
Bold hives —*see* Urticaria
Bombé, iris —*see* Membrane, pupillary
Bone —*see* condition
Bonnevie-Ullrich syndrome —*see also* Turner's
 syndrome Q87.1
Bonnier's syndrome —*see* subcategory H81.8
Bonvale dam fever T73.3
Bony block of joint —*see* Ankylosis
BOOP (bronchiolitis obliterans organized
 pneumonia) J84.89
Borderline
 diabetes mellitus R73.03
 hypertension R03.0
 osteopenia M85.8-●
 pelvis, with obstruction during labor O65.1
 personality F60.3
Borna disease A83.9
Bornholm disease B33.0
Boston exanthem A88.0
Botalli, ductus (patent) (persistent) Q25.0
Bothriocephalus latus infestation B70.0
Botulism (foodborne intoxication) A05.1
 infant A48.51
 non-foodborne A48.52
 wound A48.52
Bouba —*see* Yaws
Bouchard's nodes (with arthropathy) M15.2
Bouffée délirante F23
Bouillaud's disease or syndrome (rheumatic
 heart disease) I01.9
Bourneville's disease Q85.1
Boutonniere deformity (finger) —*see*
 Deformity, finger, boutonniere
Bouveret (-Hoffmann) syndrome (paroxysmal
 tachycardia) I47.9
Bovine heart —*see* Hypertrophy, cardiac
Bowel —*see* condition
Bowen's
 dermatosis (precancerous) —*see* Neoplasm,
  skin, in situ
 disease —*see* Neoplasm, skin, in situ
 epithelioma —*see* Neoplasm, skin, in situ
 type
  epidermoid carcinoma-in-situ —*see*
   Neoplasm, skin, in situ
  intraepidermal squamous cell carcinoma —
   see Neoplasm, skin, in situ
Bowing
 femur —*see also* Deformity, limb, specified
  type NEC, thigh
  congenital Q68.3
 fibula —*see also* Deformity, limb, specified
  type NEC, lower leg
  congenital Q68.4
 forearm —*see* Deformity, limb, specified type
  NEC, forearm
 leg(s), long bones, congenital Q68.5
 radius —*see* Deformity, limb, specified type
  NEC, forearm
 tibia —*see also* Deformity, limb, specified type
  NEC, lower leg
  congenital Q68.4
Bowleg(s) (acquired) M21.16-●
 congenital Q68.5
 rachitic E64.3
Boyd's dysentery A03.2
Brachial —*see* condition
Brachycardia R00.1
Brachycephaly Q75.0
Bradley's disease A08.19

Bradyarrhythmia, cardiac I49.8
Bradycardia (sinoatrial) (sinus) (vagal) R00.1
 neonatal P29.12
 reflex G90.09
 tachycardia syndrome I49.5
Bradykinesia R25.8
Bradypnea R06.89
Bradytachycardia I49.5
Brailsford's disease or osteochondrosis —*see*
 Osteochondrosis, juvenile, radius
Brain —*see also* condition
 death G93.82
 syndrome —*see* Syndrome, brain
Branched-chain amino-acid disorder E71.2
Branchial —*see* condition
 cartilage, congenital Q18.2
Branchiogenic remnant (in neck) Q18.0
Brandt's syndrome (acrodermatitis
 enteropathica) E83.2
Brash (water) R12
Bravais-jacksonian epilepsy —*see* Epilepsy,
 localization-related, symptomatic, with
 simple partial seizures
Braxton Hicks contractions —*see* False, labor
Brazilian leishmaniasis B55.2
BRBPR K62.5
Break, retina (without detachment) H33.30-●
 with retinal detachment —*see* Detachment,
  retina
 horseshoe tear H33.31-●
 multiple H33.33-●
 round hole H33.32-●
Breakdown
 device, graft or implant —*see also*
  Complications, by site and type,
  mechanical T85.618
  arterial graft NEC —*see* Complication,
   cardiovascular device, mechanical,
   vascular
  breast (implant) T85.41
  catheter NEC T85.618
   cystostomy T83.010
   dialysis (renal) T82.41
    intraperitoneal T85.611
   Hopkins T83.018
   ileostomy T83.018
   infusion NEC T82.514
    cranial T85.610
    epidural T85.610
    intrathecal T85.610
    spinal T85.610
    subarachnoid T85.610
    subdural T85.610
   nephrostomy T83.012
   urethral indwelling T83.011
   urinary NEC T83.018
   urostomy T83.018
  electronic (electrode) (pulse generator)
   (stimulator)
   bone T84.310
   cardiac T82.119
    electrode T82.110
    pulse generator T82.111
    specified type NEC T82.118
   nervous system —*see* Complication,
    prosthetic device, mechanical,
    electronic nervous system stimulator
   urinary —*see* Complication,
    genitourinary, device, urinary,
    mechanical
  fixation, internal (orthopedic) NEC —
   see Complication, fixation device,
   mechanical
  gastrointestinal —*see* Complications,
   prosthetic device, mechanical,
   gastrointestinal device
  genital NEC T83.418
   intrauterine contraceptive device T83.31
   penile prosthesis (cylinder) (implanted)
    (pump) (resevoir) T83.410
   testicular prosthesis T83.411

Breakdown *(Continued)*
 device, graft or implant *(Continued)*
  heart NEC —*see* Complication,
   cardiovascular device, mechanical
  intrathecal infusion pump T85.615
  joint prosthesis —*see* Complications..., joint
   prosthesis,internal, mechanical, by site
  nervous system, specified device NEC
   T85.615
  ocular NEC —*see* Complications, prosthetic
   device, mechanical, ocular device
  orthopedic NEC —*see* Complication,
   orthopedic, device, mechanical
  specified NEC T85.618
  subcutaneous device pocket
   nervous system prosthetic device,
    implant, or graft T85.890
   other internal prosthetic device, implant,
    or graft T85.898
  sutures, permanent T85.612
   used in bone repair —*see* Complications,
    fixation device, internal
    (orthopedic), mechanical
  urinary NEC T83.118
   graft T83.21
   sphincter, implanted T83.111
   stent (ileal conduit) (nephroureteral)
    T83.113
   ureteral indwelling T83.112
  vascular NEC —*see* Complication,
   cardiovascular device, mechanical
  ventricular intracranial shunt T85.01
 nervous F48.8
 perineum O90.1
 respirator J95.850
  specified NEC J95.859
 ventilator J95.850
  specified NEC J95.859
Breast —*see also* condition
 buds E30.1
  in newborn P96.89
 dense R92.2
 nodule —*see also* Lump, breast N63.0
Breath
 foul R19.6
 holder, child R06.89
 holding spell R06.89
 shortness R06.02
Breathing
 labored —*see* Hyperventilation
 mouth R06.5
  causing malocclusion M26.5
 periodic R06.3
  high altitude G47.32
Breathlessness R06.81
Breda's disease —*see* Yaws
Breech presentation (mother) O32.1
 causing obstructed labor O64.1
 footling O32.8
  causing obstructed labor O64.8
 incomplete O32.8
  causing obstructed labor O64.8
Breisky's disease N90.4
Brennemann's syndrome I88.0
Brenner
 tumor (benign) D27.9
  borderline malignancy D39.1-●
  malignant C56
  proliferating D39.1
Bretonneau's disease or angina A36.0
Breus' mole O02.0
Brevicollis Q76.49
Brickmakers' anemia B76.9 [D63.8]
Bridge, myocardial Q24.5
Bright red blood per rectum (BRBPR) K62.5
Bright's disease —*see also* Nephritis
 arteriosclerotic —*see* Hypertension, kidney
Brill (-Zinsser) disease (recrudescent typhus)
 A75.1
 flea-borne A75.2
 louse-borne A75.1

▶ New   ⇒ Revised   ~~deleted~~ Deleted   ● Use Additional Character(s)

Brill-Symmers' disease C82.90
Brion-Kayser disease —*see* Fever, parathyroid
Briquet's disorder or syndrome F45.0
Brissaud's
  infantilism or dwarfism E23.0
  motor-verbal tic F95.2
Brittle
  bones disease Q78.0
  nails L60.3
    congenital Q84.6
Broad —*see also* condition
  beta disease E78.2
  ligament laceration syndrome N83.8
Broad- or floating-betalipoproteinemia E78.2
Brock's syndrome (atelectasis due to enlarged
    lymph nodes) J98.19
Brocq-Duhring disease (dermatitis
    herpetiformis) L13.0
Brodie's abscess or disease M86.8X- •
Broken
  arches —*see also* Deformity, limb, flat foot
  arm (meaning upper limb) —*see* Fracture, arm
  back —*see* Fracture, vertebra
  bone —*see* Fracture
  implant or internal device —*see*
    Complications, by site and type,
    mechanical
  leg (meaning lower limb) —*see* Fracture, leg
  nose S02.2
  tooth, teeth —*see* Fracture, tooth
Bromhidrosis, bromidrosis L75.0
Bromidism, bromism G92
  chronic (dependence) F13.20
  due to
    correct substance properly administered —
      see Table of Drugs and Chemicals, by
      drug, adverse effect
    overdose or wrong substance given
      or taken —*see* Table of Drugs and
      Chemicals, by drug, poisoning
Bromidrosiphobia F40.298
Bronchi, bronchial —*see* condition
Bronchiectasis (cylindrical) (diffuse) (fusiform)
    (localized) (saccular) J47.9
  with
    acute
      bronchitis J47.0
      lower respiratory infection J47.0
    exacerbation (acute) J47.1
  congenital Q33.4
  tuberculous NEC —*see* Tuberculosis,
    pulmonary
Bronchiolectasis —*see* Bronchiectasis
Bronchiolitis (acute) (infective) (subacute) J21.9
  with
    bronchospasm or obstruction J21.9
    influenza, flu or grippe —*see* Influenza,
      with, respiratory manifestations NEC
  chemical (chronic) J68.4
    acute J68.0
  chronic (fibrosing) (obliterative) J44.9
  due to
    external agent —*see* Bronchitis, acute, due to
    human metapneumovirus J21.1
    respiratory syncytial virus J21.0
    specified organism NEC J21.8
  fibrosa obliterans J44.9
  influenzal —*see* Influenza, with, respiratory
    manifestations NEC
  obliterans J42
    with organizing pneumonia (BOOP) J84.89
  obliterative (chronic) (subacute) J44.9
    due to chemicals, gases, fumes or vapors
      (inhalation) J68.4
    due to fumes or vapors J68.4
  respiratory, interstitial lung disease J84.115
Bronchitis (diffuse) (fibrinous) (hypostatic)
    (infective) (membranous) J40
  with
    influenza, flu or grippe —*see* Influenza,
      with, respiratory manifestations NEC

Bronchitis (*Continued*)
  with (*Continued*)
    obstruction (airway) (lung) J44.9
    tracheitis (15 years of age and above) J40
      acute or subacute J20.9
      chronic J42
      under 15 years of age J20.9
  acute or subacute (with bronchospasm or
    obstruction) J20.9
    with
      bronchiectasis J47.0
      chronic obstructive pulmonary disease
        J44.0
    chemical (due to gases, fumes or vapors)
      J68.0
    due to
      fumes or vapors J68.0
      Haemophilus influenzae J20.1
      Mycoplasma pneumoniae J20.0
      radiation J70.0
      specified organism NEC J20.8
      Streptococcus J20.2
      virus
        coxsackie J20.3
        echovirus J20.7
        parainfluenzae J20.4
        respiratory syncytial J20.5
        rhinovirus J20.6
    viral NEC J20.8
  allergic (acute) J45.909
    with
      exacerbation (acute) J45.901
      status asthmaticus J45.902
  arachidic T17.528
  aspiration (due to fumes or vapors) J68.0
  asthmatic J45.9
    chronic J44.9
      with
        acute lower respiratory infection J44.0
        exacerbation (acute) J44.1
  capillary —*see* Pneumonia, broncho
  caseous (tuberculous) A15.5
  Castellani's A69.8
  catarrhal (15 years of age and above) J40
    acute —*see* Bronchitis, acute
    chronic J41.0
    under 15 years of age J20.9
  chemical (acute) (subacute) J68.0
    chronic J68.4
    due to fumes or vapors J68.0
      chronic J68.4
  chronic J42
    with
      airways obstruction J44.9
      tracheitis (chronic) J42
    asthmatic (obstructive) J44.9
    catarrhal J41.0
    chemical (due to fumes or vapors) J68.4
    due to
      chemicals, gases, fumes or vapors
        (inhalation) J68.4
      radiation J70.1
      tobacco smoking J41.0
    emphysematous J44.9
    mucopurulent J41.1
    non-obstructive J41.0
    obliterans J44.9
    obstructive J44.9
    purulent J41.1
    simple J41.0
  croupous —*see* Bronchitis, acute
  due to gases, fumes or vapors (chemical)
    J68.0
  emphysematous (obstructive) J44.9
  exudative —*see* Bronchitis, acute
  fetid J41.1
  grippal —*see* Influenza, with, respiratory
    manifestations NEC
  in those under 15 years age —*see* Bronchitis,
    acute
    chronic —*see* Bronchitis, chronic

Bronchitis (*Continued*)
  influenzal —*see* Influenza, with, respiratory
    manifestations NEC
  mixed simple and mucopurulent J41.8
  moulder's J62.8
  mucopurulent (chronic) (recurrent) J41.1
    acute or subacute J20.9
    simple (mixed) J41.8
  obliterans (chronic) J44.9
  obstructive (chronic) (diffuse) J44.9
  pituitous J41.1
  pneumococcal, acute or subacute J20.2
  pseudomembranous, acute or subacute —*see*
    Bronchitis, acute
  purulent (chronic) (recurrent) J41.1
    acute or subacute —*see* Bronchitis, acute
  putrid J41.1
  senile (chronic) J42
  simple and mucopurulent (mixed) J41.8
  smokers' J41.0
  spirochetal NEC A69.8
  subacute —*see* Bronchitis, acute
  suppurative (chronic) J41.1
    acute or subacute —*see* Bronchitis, acute
  tuberculous A15.5
  under 15 years of age —*see* Bronchitis, acute
    chronic —*see* Bronchitis, chronic
  viral NEC, acute or subacute —*see also*
    Bronchitis, acute J20.8
Bronchoalveolitis J18.0
Bronchoaspergillosis B44.1
Bronchocele meaning goiter E04.0
Broncholithiasis J98.09
  tuberculous NEC A15.5
Bronchomalacia J98.09
  congenital Q32.2
Bronchomycosis NOS B49 [*J99*]
  candidal B37.1
Bronchopleuropneumonia —*see* Pneumonia,
  broncho
Bronchopneumonia —*see* Pneumonia, broncho
Bronchopneumonitis —*see* Pneumonia,
  broncho
Bronchopulmonary —*see* condition
Bronchopulmonitis —*see* Pneumonia, broncho
Bronchorrhagia (*see* Hemoptysis)
Bronchorrhea J98.09
  acute J20.9
  chronic (infective) (purulent) J42
Bronchospasm (acute) J98.01
  with
    bronchiolitis, acute J21.9
    bronchitis, acute (conditions in J20) —*see*
      Bronchitis, acute
  due to external agent —*see* condition,
    respiratory, acute, due to
  exercise induced J45.990
Bronchospirochetosis A69.8
  Castellani A69.8
Bronchostenosis J98.09
Bronchus —*see* condition
Brontophobia F40.220
➡ Bronze baby syndrome P83.88
Brooke's tumor —*see* Neoplasm, skin, benign
Brown enamel of teeth (hereditary) K00.5
Brown's sheath syndrome H50.61- •
Brown-Séquard disease, paralysis or
  syndrome G83.81
Bruce sepsis A23.0
Brucellosis (infection) A23.9
  abortus A23.1
  canis A23.3
  dermatitis A23.9
  melitensis A23.0
  mixed A23.8
  sepsis A23.9
    melitensis A23.0
    specified NEC A23.8
  suis A23.2
Bruck-de Lange disease Q87.1
Bruck's disease —*see* Deformity, limb

▶ BRUE (brief resolved unexplained event) R68.13
Brugsch's syndrome Q82.8
Bruise (skin surface intact) —see also Contusion
with
⟶ open wound —see Wound, open
internal organ —see Injury, by site
newborn P54.5
scalp, due to birth injury, newborn P12.3
umbilical cord O69.5
Bruit (arterial) R09.89
cardiac R01.1
Brush burn —see Abrasion, by site
Bruton's X-linked agammaglobulinemia D80.0
Bruxism
psychogenic F45.8
sleep related G47.63
Bubbly lung syndrome P27.0
Bubo I88.8
blennorrhagic (gonococcal) A54.89
chancroidal A57
climatic A55
due to Haemophilus ducreyi A57
gonococcal A54.89
indolent (nonspecific) I88.8
inguinal (nonspecific) I88.8
chancroidal A57
climatic A55
due to H. ducreyi A57
infective I88.8
scrofulous (tuberculous) A18.2
soft chancre A57
suppurating —see Lymphadenitis, acute
syphilitic (primary) A51.0
congenital A50.07
tropical A55
virulent (chancroidal) A57
Bubonic plague A20.0
Bubonocele —see Hernia, inguinal
Buccal —see condition
Buchanan's disease or osteochondrosis M91.0
Buchem's syndrome (hyperostosis corticalis)
M85.2
Bucket-handle fracture or tear (semilunar
cartilage) —see Tear, meniscus
Budd-Chiari syndrome (hepatic vein
thrombosis) I82.0
Budgerigar fancier's disease or lung
J67.2
Buds
breast E30.1
in newborn P96.89
Buerger's disease (thromboangiitis obliterans)
I73.1
Bulbar —see condition
Bulbus cordis (left ventricle) (persistent) Q21.8
Bulimia (nervosa) F50.2
atypical F50.9
normal weight F50.9
Bulky
stools R19.5
uterus N85.2
Bulla (e) R23.8
lung (emphysematous) (solitary) J43.9
newborn P25.8
Bullet wound —see also Wound, open
fracture - code as Fracture, by site
internal organ —see Injury, by site
Bundle
branch block (complete) (false)
(incomplete) —see Block, bundle-branch
of His —see condition
Bunion M21.61-●
tailor's M21.62-●
Bunionette M21.62-●
Buphthalmia, buphthalmos (congenital) Q15.0
Burdwan fever B55.0
Bürger-Grütz disease or syndrome E78.3
Buried
penis (congenital) Q55.64
acquired N48.83
roots K08.3

Burke's syndrome K86.89
Burkitt
cell leukemia C91.0-●
lymphoma (malignant) C83.7-●
small noncleaved, diffuse C83.7-●
spleen C83.77
undifferentiated C83.7-●
tumor C83.7-●
type
acute lymphoblastic leukemia C91.0-●
undifferentiated C83.7-●
Burn (electricity) (flame) (hot gas, liquid or hot
object) (radiation) (steam) (thermal) T30.0
abdomen, abdominal (muscle) (wall)
T21.02
first degree T21.12
second degree T21.22
third degree T21.32
above elbow T22.039
first degree T22.139
left T22.032
first degree T22.132
second degree T22.232
third degree T22.332
right T22.031
first degree T22.131
second degree T22.231
third degree T22.331
second degree T22.239
third degree T22.339
acid (caustic) (external) (internal) —see
Corrosion, by site
alimentary tract NEC T28.2
esophagus T28.1
mouth T28.0
pharynx T28.0
alkaline (caustic) (external) (internal) —see
Corrosion, by site
ankle T25.019
first degree T25.119
left T25.012
first degree T25.112
second degree T25.212
third degree T25.312
multiple with foot —see Burn, lower, limb,
multiple, ankle and foot
right T25.011
first degree T25.111
second degree T25.211
third degree T25.311
second degree T25.219
third degree T25.319
anus —see Burn, buttock
arm (lower) (upper) —see Burn, upper,
limb
axilla T22.049
first degree T22.149
left T22.042
first degree T22.142
second degree T22.242
third degree T22.342
right T22.041
first degree T22.141
second degree T22.241
third degree T22.341
second degree T22.249
third degree T22.349
back (lower) T21.04
first degree T21.14
second degree T21.24
third degree T21.34
upper T21.03
first degree T21.13
second degree T21.23
third degree T21.33
blisters - code as Burn, second degree, by site
breast(s) —see Burn, chest wall
buttock(s) T21.05
first degree T21.15
second degree T21.25
third degree T21.35

Burn (Continued)
calf T24.039
first degree T24.139
left T24.032
first degree T24.132
second degree T24.232
third degree T24.332
right T24.031
first degree T24.131
second degree T24.231
third degree T24.331
second degree T24.239
third degree T24.339
canthus (eye) —see Burn, eyelid
caustic acid or alkaline —see Corrosion, by
site
cervix T28.3
cheek T20.06
first degree T20.16
second degree T20.26
third degree T20.36
chemical (acids) (alkalines) (caustics) (external)
(internal) —see Corrosion, by site
chest wall T21.01
first degree T21.11
second degree T21.21
third degree T21.31
chin T20.03
first degree T20.13
second degree T20.23
third degree T20.33
colon T28.2
conjunctiva (and cornea) —see Burn, cornea
cornea (and conjunctiva) T26.1-●
chemical —see Corrosion, cornea
corrosion (external) (internal) —see
Corrosion, by site
deep necrosis of underlying tissue - code as
Burn, third degree, by site
dorsum of hand T23.069
first degree T23.169
left T23.062
first degree T23.162
second degree T23.262
third degree T23.362
right T23.061
first degree T23.161
second degree T23.261
third degree T23.361
second degree T23.269
third degree T23.369
due to ingested chemical agent —see
Corrosion, by site
ear (auricle) (external) (canal) T20.01
first degree T20.11
second degree T20.21
third degree T20.31
elbow T22.029
first degree T22.129
left T22.022
first degree T22.122
second degree T22.222
third degree T22.322
right T22.021
first degree T22.121
second degree T22.221
third degree T22.321
second degree T22.229
third degree T22.329
epidermal loss - code as Burn, second degree,
by site
erythema, erythematous - code as Burn, first
degree, by site
esophagus T28.1
extent (percentage of body surface)
less than 10 percent T31.0
10-19 percent T31.10
with 0-9 percent third degree burns
T31.10
with 10-19 percent third degree burns
T31.11

▶ New ⟹ Revised deleted Deleted ● Use Additional Character(s)

Burn (Continued)
extent (Continued)
20-29 percent T31.20
with 0-9 percent third degree burns T31.20
with 10-19 percent third degree burns T31.21
with 20-29 percent third degree burns T31.22
30-39 percent T31.30
with 0-9 percent third degree burns T31.30
with 10-19 percent third degree burns T31.31
with 20-29 percent third degree burns T31.32
with 30-39 percent third degree burns T31.33
40-49 percent T31.40
with 0-9 percent third degree burns T31.40
with 10-19 percent third degree burns T31.41
with 20-29 percent third degree burns T31.42
with 30-39 percent third degree burns T31.43
with 40-49 percent third degree burns T31.44
50-59 percent T31.50
with 0-9 percent third degree burns T31.50
with 10-19 percent third degree burns T31.51
with 20-29 percent third degree burns T31.52
with 30-39 percent third degree burns T31.53
with 40-49 percent third degree burns T31.54
with 50-59 percent third degree burns T31.55
60-69 percent T31.60
with 0-9 percent third degree burns T31.60
with 10-19 percent third degree burns T31.61
with 20-29 percent third degree burns T31.62
with 30-39 percent third degree burns T31.63
with 40-49 percent third degree burns T31.64
with 50-59 percent third degree burns T31.65
with 60-69 percent third degree burns T31.66
70-79 percent T31.70
with 0-9 percent third degree burns T31.70
with 10-19 percent third degree burns T31.71
with 20-29 percent third degree burns T31.72
with 30-39 percent third degree burns T31.73
with 40-49 percent third degree burns T31.74
with 50-59 percent third degree burns T31.75
with 60-69 percent third degree burns T31.76
with 70-79 percent third degree burns T31.77
80-89 percent T31.80
with 0-9 percent third degree burns T31.80
with 10-19 percent third degree burns T31.81
with 20-29 percent third degree burns T31.82
with 30-39 percent third degree burns T31.83
with 40-49 percent third degree burns T31.84

Burn (Continued)
extent (Continued)
80-89 percent T31.80 (Continued)
with 50-59 percent third degree burns T31.85
with 60-69 percent third degree burns T31.86
with 70-79 percent third degree burns T31.87
with 80-89 percent third degree burns T31.88
90 percent or more T31.90
with 0-9 percent third degree burns T31.90
with 10-19 percent third degree burns T31.91
with 20-29 percent third degree burns T31.92
with 30-39 percent third degree burns T31.93
with 40-49 percent third degree burns T31.94
with 50-59 percent third degree burns T31.95
with 60-69 percent third degree burns T31.96
with 70-79 percent third degree burns T31.97
with 80-89 percent third degree burns T31.98
with 90 percent or more third degree burns T31.99
extremity —see Burn, limb
eye(s) and adnexa T26.4-●
with resulting rupture and destruction of eyeball T26.2-●
conjunctival sac —see Burn, cornea
cornea —see Burn, cornea
lid —see Burn, eyelid
periocular area —see Burn, eyelid
specified site NEC T26.3-●
eyeball —see Burn, eye
eyelid(s) T26.0-●
chemical —see Corrosion, eyelid
face —see Burn, head
finger T23.029
first degree T23.129
left T23.022
first degree T23.122
second degree T23.222
third degree T23.322
multiple sites (without thumb) T23.039
with thumb T23.049
first degree T23.149
left T23.042
first degree T23.142
second degree T23.242
third degree T23.342
right T23.041
first degree T23.141
second degree T23.241
third degree T23.341
second degree T23.249
third degree T23.349
first degree T23.139
left T23.032
first degree T23.132
second degree T23.232
third degree T23.332
right T23.031
first degree T23.131
second degree T23.231
third degree T23.331
second degree T23.239
third degree T23.339
right T23.021
first degree T23.121
second degree T23.221
third degree T23.321
second degree T23.229
third degree T23.329
flank —see Burn, abdominal wall

Burn (Continued)
foot T25.029
first degree T25.129
left T25.022
first degree T25.122
second degree T25.222
third degree T25.322
multiple with ankle —see Burn, lower, limb, multiple, ankle and foot
right T25.021
first degree T25.121
second degree T25.221
third degree T25.321
second degree T25.229
third degree T25.329
forearm T22.019
first degree T22.119
left T22.012
first degree T22.112
second degree T22.212
third degree T22.312
right T22.011
first degree T22.111
second degree T22.211
third degree T22.311
second degree T22.219
third degree T22.319
forehead T20.06
first degree T20.16
second degree T20.26
third degree T20.36
fourth degree - code as Burn, third degree, by site
friction —see Burn, by site
from swallowing caustic or corrosive substance NEC —see Corrosion, by site
full thickness skin loss - code as Burn, third degree, by site
gastrointestinal tract NEC T28.2
from swallowing caustic or corrosive substance T28.7
genital organs
external
female T21.07
first degree T21.17
second degree T21.27
third degree T21.37
male T21.06
first degree T21.16
second degree T21.26
third degree T21.36
internal T28.3
from caustic or corrosive substance T28.8
groin —see Burn, abdominal wall
hand(s) T23.009
back —see Burn, dorsum of hand
finger —see Burn, finger
first degree T23.109
left T23.002
first degree T23.102
second degree T23.202
third degree T23.302
multiple sites with wrist T23.099
first degree T23.199
left T23.092
first degree T23.192
second degree T23.292
third degree T23.392
right T23.091
first degree T23.191
second degree T23.291
third degree T23.391
second degree T23.299
third degree T23.399
palm —see Burn, palm
right T23.001
first degree T23.101
second degree T23.201
third degree T23.301

Burn (Continued)
  hand (Continued)
    second degree T23.209
    third degree T23.309
    thumb —see Burn, thumb
  head (and face) (and neck) T20.00
    cheek —see Burn, cheek
    chin —see Burn, chin
    ear —see Burn, ear
    eye(s) only —see Burn, eye
    first degree T20.10
    forehead —see Burn, forehead
    lip —see Burn, lip
    multiple sites T20.09
      first degree T20.19
      second degree T20.29
      third degree T20.39
    neck —see Burn, neck
    nose —see Burn, nose
    scalp —see Burn, scalp
    second degree T20.20
    third degree T20.30
  hip(s) —see Burn, thigh
  inhalation —see Burn, respiratory tract
    caustic or corrosive substance (fumes) —see
      Corrosion, respiratory tract
  internal organ(s) T28.40
    alimentary tract T28.2
      esophagus T28.1
    eardrum T28.41
    esophagus T28.1
    from caustic or corrosive substance
      (swallowing) NEC —see Corrosion,
      by site
    genitourinary T28.3
    mouth T28.0
    pharynx T28.0
    respiratory tract —see Burn, respiratory
      tract
    specified organ NEC T28.49
  interscapular region —see Burn, back,
    upper
  intestine (large) (small) T28.2
  knee T24.029
    first degree T24.129
    left T24.022
      first degree T24.122
      second degree T24.222
      third degree T24.322
    right T24.021
      first degree T24.121
      second degree T24.221
      third degree T24.321
    second degree T24.229
    third degree T24.329
  labium (majus) (minus) —see Burn, genital
    organs, external, female
  lacrimal apparatus, duct, gland or sac —see
    Burn, eye, specified site NEC
  larynx T27.0
    with lung T27.1
  leg(s) (lower) (upper) —see Burn, lower,
    limb
  lightning —see Burn, by site
  limb(s)
    lower (except ankle or foot alone) —see
      Burn, lower, limb
    upper —see Burn, upper limb
  lip(s) T20.02
    first degree T20.12
    second degree T20.22
    third degree T20.32
  lower
    back —see Burn, back
    limb T24.009
      ankle —see Burn, ankle
      calf —see Burn, calf
      first degree T24.109
      foot —see Burn, foot
      hip —see Burn, thigh
      knee —see Burn, knee

Burn (Continued)
  lower (Continued)
    limb (Continued)
      left T24.002
        first degree T24.102
        second degree T24.202
        third degree T24.302
      multiple sites, except ankle and foot
        T24.099
        ankle and foot T25.099
          first degree T25.199
          left T25.092
            first degree T25.192
            second degree T25.292
            third degree T25.392
          right T25.091
            first degree T25.191
            second degree T25.291
            third degree T25.391
          second degree T25.299
          third degree T25.399
        first degree T24.199
        left T24.092
          first degree T24.192
          second degree T24.292
          third degree T24.392
        right T24.091
          first degree T24.191
          second degree T24.291
          third degree T24.391
        second degree T24.299
        third degree T24.399
      right T24.001
        first degree T24.101
        second degree T24.201
        third degree T24.301
      second degree T24.209
      thigh —see Burn, thigh
      third degree T24.309
      toe —see Burn, toe
  lung (with larynx and trachea) T27.1
  mouth T28.0
  neck T20.07
    first degree T20.17
    second degree T20.27
    third degree T20.37
  nose (septum) T20.04
    first degree T20.14
    second degree T20.24
    third degree T20.34
  ocular adnexa —see Burn, eye
  orbit region —see Burn, eyelid
  palm T23.059
    first degree T23.159
    left T23.052
      first degree T23.152
      second degree T23.252
      third degree T23.352
    right T23.051
      first degree T23.151
      second degree T23.251
      third degree T23.351
    second degree T23.259
    third degree T23.359
  partial thickness - code as Burn, unspecified
    degree, by site
  pelvis —see Burn, trunk
  penis —see Burn, genital organs, external,
    male
  perineum
    female —see Burn, genital organs, external,
      female
    male —see Burn, genital organs, external,
      male
  periocular area —see Burn, eyelid
  pharynx T28.0
  rectum T28.2
  respiratory tract T27.3
    larynx —see Burn, larynx
    specified part NEC T27.2
    trachea —see Burn, trachea

Burn (Continued)
  sac, lacrimal —see Burn, eye, specified site
    NEC
  scalp T20.05
    first degree T20.15
    second degree T20.25
    third degree T20.35
  scapular region T22.069
    first degree T22.169
    left T22.062
      first degree T22.162
      second degree T22.262
      third degree T22.362
    right T22.061
      first degree T22.161
      second degree T22.261
      third degree T22.361
    second degree T22.269
    third degree T22.369
  sclera —see Burn, eye, specified site NEC
  scrotum —see Burn, genital organs, external,
    male
  shoulder T22.059
    first degree T22.159
    left T22.052
      first degree T22.152
      second degree T22.252
      third degree T22.352
    right T22.051
      first degree T22.151
      second degree T22.251
      third degree T22.351
    second degree T22.259
    third degree T22.359
  stomach T28.2
  temple —see Burn, head
  testis —see Burn, genital organs, external, male
  thigh T24.019
    first degree T24.119
    left T24.012
      first degree T24.112
      second degree T24.212
      third degree T24.312
    right T24.011
      first degree T24.111
      second degree T24.211
      third degree T24.311
    second degree T24.219
    third degree T24.319
  thorax (external) —see Burn, trunk
  throat (meaning pharynx) T28.0
  thumb(s) T23.019
    first degree T23.119
    left T23.012
      first degree T23.112
      second degree T23.212
      third degree T23.312
    multiple sites with fingers T23.049
      first degree T23.149
      left T23.042
        first degree T23.142
        second degree T23.242
        third degree T23.342
      right T23.041
        first degree T23.141
        second degree T23.241
        third degree T23.341
      second degree T23.249
      third degree T23.349
    right T23.011
      first degree T23.111
      second degree T23.211
      third degree T23.311
    second degree T23.219
    third degree T23.319
  toe T25.039
    first degree T25.139
    left T25.032
      first degree T25.132
      second degree T25.232
      third degree T25.332

▶ New   ⇒ Revised   ~~deleted~~ Deleted   ● Use Additional Character(s)

Burn (Continued)
  toe (Continued)
    right T25.031
      first degree T25.131
      second degree T25.231
      third degree T25.331
    second degree T25.239
    third degree T25.339
  tongue T28.0
  tonsil(s) T28.0
  trachea T27.0
    with lung T27.1
  trunk T21.00
    abdominal wall —see Burn, abdominal
      wall
    anus —see Burn, buttock
    axilla —see Burn, upper limb
    back —see Burn, back
    breast —see Burn, chest wall
    buttock —see Burn, buttock
    chest wall —see Burn, chest wall
    first degree T21.10
    flank —see Burn, abdominal wall
    genital
      female —see Burn, genital organs,
        external, female
      male —see Burn, genital organs, external,
        male
    groin —see Burn, abdominal wall
    interscapular region —see Burn, back,
      upper
    labia —see Burn, genital organs, external,
      female
    lower back —see Burn, back
    penis —see Burn, genital organs, external,
      male
    perineum
      female —see Burn, genital organs,
        external, female
      male —see Burn, genital organs, external,
        male
    scapula region —see Burn, scapular
      region
    scrotum —see Burn, genital organs,
      external, male
    second degree T21.20
    specified site NEC T21.09
      first degree T21.19
      second degree T21.29
      third degree T21.39
    testes —see Burn, genital organs, external,
      male
    third degree T21.30
    upper back —see Burn, back, upper
    vulva —see Burn, genital organs, external,
      female
  unspecified site with extent of body surface
    involved specified
    ➡ less than 10 percent T31.0
    ➡ 10-19 percent (0-9 percent third degree)
      T31.10
      with 10-19 percent third degree
        T31.11
    ➡ 20-29 percent (0-9 percent third degree)
      T31.20
      with
        10-19 percent third degree T31.21
        20-29 percent third degree T31.22
    ➡ 30-39 percent (0-9 percent third degree)
      T31.30
      with
        10-19 percent third degree T31.31
        20-29 percent third degree T31.32
        30-39 percent third degree T31.33
    ➡ 40-49 percent (0-9 percent third degree)
      T31.40
      with
        10-19 percent third degree T31.41
        20-29 percent third degree T31.42
        30-39 percent third degree T31.43
        40-49 percent third degree T31.44

Burn (Continued)
  unspecified site with extent of body surface
    involved specified (Continued)
    ➡ 50-59 percent (0-9 percent third degree)
      T31.50
      with
        10-19 percent third degree T31.51
        20-29 percent third degree T31.52
        30-39 percent third degree T31.53
        40-49 percent third degree T31.54
        50-59 percent third degree T31.55
    ➡ 60-69 percent (0-9 percent third degree)
      T31.60
      with
        10-19 percent third degree T31.61
        20-29 percent third degree T31.62
        30-39 percent third degree T31.63
        40-49 percent third degree T31.64
        50-59 percent third degree T31.65
        60-69 percent third degree T31.66
    ➡ 70-79 percent (0-9 percent third degree)
      T31.70
      with
        10-19 percent third degree T31.71
        20-29 percent third degree T31.72
        30-39 percent third degree T31.73
        40-49 percent third degree T31.74
        50-59 percent third degree T31.75
        60-69 percent third degree T31.76
        70-79 percent third degree T31.77
    ➡ 80-89 percent (0-9 percent third degree)
      T31.80
      with
        10-19 percent third degree T31.81
        20-29 percent third degree T31.82
        30-39 percent third degree T31.83
        40-49 percent third degree T31.84
        50-59 percent third degree T31.85
        60-69 percent third degree T31.86
        70-79 percent third degree T31.87
        80-89 percent third degree T31.88
    ➡ 90 percent or more (0-9 percent third
      degree) T31.90
      with
        10-19 percent third degree T31.91
        20-29 percent third degree T31.92
        30-39 percent third degree T31.93
        40-49 percent third degree T31.94
        50-59 percent third degree T31.95
        60-69 percent third degree T31.96
        70-79 percent third degree T31.97
        80-89 percent third degree T31.98
        90-99 percent third degree T31.99
  upper limb T22.00
    above elbow —see Burn, above elbow
    axilla —see Burn, axilla
    elbow —see Burn, elbow
    first degree T22.10
    forearm —see Burn, forearm
    hand —see Burn, hand
    interscapular region —see Burn, back,
      upper
    multiple sites T22.099
      first degree T22.199
      left T22.092
        first degree T22.192
        second degree T22.292
        third degree T22.392
      right T22.091
        first degree T22.191
        second degree T22.291
        third degree T22.391
      second degree T22.299
      third degree T22.399
    scapular region —see Burn, scapular region
    second degree T22.20
    shoulder —see Burn, shoulder
    third degree T22.30
    wrist —see Burn, wrist
  uterus T28.3
  vagina T28.3

Burn (Continued)
  vulva —see Burn, genital organs, external,
    female
  wrist T23.079
    first degree T23.179
    left T23.072
      first degree T23.172
      second degree T23.272
      third degree T23.372
    multiple sites with hand T23.099
      first degree T23.199
      left T23.092
        first degree T23.192
        second degree T23.292
        third degree T23.392
      right T23.091
        first degree T23.191
        second degree T23.291
        third degree T23.391
      second degree T23.299
      third degree T23.399
    right T23.071
      first degree T23.171
      second degree T23.271
      third degree T23.371
    second degree T23.279
    third degree T23.379
Burnett's syndrome E83.52
Burning
  feet syndrome E53.9
  sensation R20.8
  tongue K14.6
Burn-out (state) Z73.0
Burns' disease or osteochondrosis —see
  Osteochondrosis, juvenile, ulna
Bursa —see condition
Bursitis M71.9
  Achilles —see Tendinitis, Achilles
  adhesive —see Bursitis, specified NEC
  ankle —see Enthesopathy, lower limb, ankle,
    specified type NEC
  calcaneal —see Enthesopathy, foot, specified
    type NEC
  collateral ligament, tibial —see Bursitis, tibial
    collateral
  due to use, overuse, pressure —see also
    Disorder, soft tissue, due to use,
    specified type NEC
    specified NEC —see Disorder, soft tissue,
      due to use, specified NEC
  Duplay's M75.0
  elbow NEC M70.3-●
    olecranon M70.2-●
  finger —see Disorder, soft tissue, due to use,
    specified type NEC, hand
  foot —see Enthesopathy, foot, specified type
    NEC
  gonococcal A54.49
  gouty —see Gout
  hand M70.1-●
  hip NEC M70.7-●
    trochanteric M70.6-●
  infective NEC M71.10
    abscess —see Abscess, bursa
    ankle M71.17-●
    elbow M71.12-●
    foot M71.17-●
    hand M71.14-●
    hip M71.15-●
    knee M71.16-●
    multiple sites M71.19
    shoulder M71.11-●
    specified site NEC M71.18
    wrist M71.13-●
  ischial —see Bursitis, hip
  knee NEC M70.5-●
    prepatellar M70.4-●
  occupational NEC —see also Disorder, soft
    tissue, due to, use
  olecranon —see Bursitis, elbow, olecranon
  pharyngeal J39.1

Bursitis *(Continued)*
  popliteal —*see* Bursitis, knee
  prepatellar M70.4-●
  radiohumeral M77.8
  rheumatoid M06.20
    ankle M06.27-●
    elbow M06.22-●
    foot joint M06.27-●
    hand joint M06.24-●
    hip M06.25-●
    knee M06.26-●
    multiple site M06.29
    shoulder M06.21-●
    vertebra M06.28
    wrist M06.23-●
  scapulohumeral —*see* Bursitis, shoulder
  semimembranous muscle (knee) —*see*
    Bursitis, knee
  shoulder M75.5-●
    adhesive —*see* Capsulitis, adhesive
  specified NEC M71.50
    ankle M71.57-●
    due to use, overuse or pressure —*see*
      Disorder, soft tissue, due to, use
    elbow M71.52-●
    foot M71.57-●
    hand M71.54-●

Bursitis *(Continued)*
  specified NEC *(Continued)*
    hip M71.55-●
    knee M71.56-●
    shoulder —*see* Bursitis, shoulder
    specified site NEC M71.58
    tibial collateral M76.4-●
    wrist M71.53-●
  subacromial —*see* Bursitis, shoulder
  subcoracoid —*see* Bursitis, shoulder
  subdeltoid —*see* Bursitis, shoulder
  syphilitic A52.78
  Thornwaldt, Tornwaldt J39.2
  tibial collateral M76.4-●
  toe —*see* Enthesopathy, foot, specified type
    NEC
  trochanteric (area) —*see* Bursitis, hip,
    trochanteric
  wrist —*see* Bursitis, hand
Bursopathy M71.9
  specified type NEC M71.80
    ankle M71.87-●
    elbow M71.82-●
    foot M71.87-●
    hand M71.84-●
    hip M71.85-●
    knee M71.86-●

Bursopathy *(Continued)*
  specified type NEC *(Continued)*
    multiple sites M71.89
    shoulder M71.81-●
    specified site NEC M71.88
    wrist M71.83-●
Burst stitches or sutures (complication of
    surgery) T81.31
  external operation wound T81.31
  internal operation wound T81.32
Buruli ulcer A31.1
Bury's disease L95.1
Buschke's
  disease B45.3
  scleredema —*see* Sclerosis, systemic
Busse-Buschke disease B45.3
Buttock —*see* condition
Button
  Biskra B55.1
  Delhi B55.1
  oriental B55.1
Buttonhole deformity (finger) —*see* Deformity,
  finger, boutonniere
Bwamba fever A92.8
Byssinosis J66.0
Bywaters' syndrome T79.5

▶ New   ➡ Revised   ~~deleted~~ Deleted   ● Use Additional Character(s)

C

Cachexia R64
  cancerous R64
  cardiac —see Disease, heart
  dehydration E86.0
  due to malnutrition R64
  exophthalmic —see Hyperthyroidism
  heart —see Disease, heart
  hypophyseal E23.0
  hypopituitary E23.0
  lead —see Poisoning, lead
  malignant R64
  marsh —see Malaria
  nervous F48.8
  old age R54
  paludal —see Malaria
  pituitary E23.0
  renal N28.9
  saturnine —see Poisoning, lead
  senile R54
  Simmonds' E23.0
  splenica D73.0
  strumipriva E03.4
  tuberculous NEC —see Tuberculosis
Café au lait spots L81.3
Caffeine-induced
  anxiety disorder F15.980
  sleep disorder F15.982
Caffey's syndrome Q78.8
Caisson disease T70.3
Cake kidney Q63.1
Caked breast (puerperal, postpartum)
    O92.79
Calabar swelling B74.3
Calcaneal spur —see Spur, bone, calcaneal
Calcaneo-apophysitis M92.8
Calcareous —see condition
Calcicosis J62.8
Calciferol (vitamin D) deficiency E55.9
  with rickets E55.0
Calcification
  adrenal (capsule) (gland) E27.49
    tuberculous E35 [B90.8]
  aorta I70.0
  artery (annular) —see Arteriosclerosis
  auricle (ear) —see Disorder, pinna, specified
      type NEC
  basal ganglia G23.8
  bladder N32.89
    due to Schistosoma hematobium
        B65.0
  brain (cortex) —see Calcification, cerebral
  bronchus J98.09
  bursa M71.40
    ankle M71.47-●
    elbow M71.42-●
    foot M71.47-●
    hand M71.44-●
    hip M71.45-●
    knee M71.46-●
    multiple sites M71.49
    shoulder M75.3-●
    specified site NEC M71.48
    wrist M71.43-●
  cardiac —see Degeneration, myocardial
  cerebral (cortex) G93.89
    artery I67.2
  cervix (uteri) N88.8
  choroid plexus G93.89
  conjunctiva —see Concretion, conjunctiva
  corpora cavernosa (penis) N48.89
  cortex (brain) —see Calcification, cerebral
  dental pulp (nodular) K04.2
  dentinal papilla K00.4
  fallopian tube N83.8
  falx cerebri G96.19
  gallbladder K82.8
  general E83.59
  heart —see also Degeneration, myocardial
    valve —see Endocarditis

Calcification (Continued)
  idiopathic infantile arterial (IIAC) Q28.8
  intervertebral cartilage or disc
      (postinfective) —see Disorder, disc,
      specified NEC
  intracranial —see Calcification, cerebral
  joint —see Disorder, joint, specified type
      NEC
  kidney N28.89
    tuberculous N29 [B90.1]
  larynx (senile) J38.7
  lens —see Cataract, specified NEC
  lung (active) (postinfectional) J98.4
    tuberculous B90.9
  lymph gland or node (postinfectional) I89.8
    tuberculous —see also Tuberculosis, lymph
        gland B90.8
  mammographic R92.1
  massive (paraplegic) —see Myositis,
      ossificans, in, quadriplegia
  medial —see Arteriosclerosis, extremities
  meninges (cerebral) (spinal) G96.19
  metastatic E83.59
  Mönckeberg's —see Arteriosclerosis,
      extremities
  muscle M61.9
    due to burns —see Myositis, ossificans, in,
        burns
    paralytic —see Myositis, ossificans, in,
        quadriplegia
    specified type NEC M61.40
      ankle M61.47-●
      foot M61.47-●
      forearm M61.43-●
      hand M61.44-●
      lower leg M61.46-●
      multiple sites M61.49
      pelvic region M61.45-●
      shoulder region M61.41-●
      specified site NEC M61.48
      thigh M61.45-●
      upper arm M61.42-●
  myocardium, myocardial —see Degeneration,
      myocardial
  ovary N83.8
  pancreas K86.89
  penis N48.89
  periarticular —see Disorder, joint, specified
      type NEC
  pericardium —see also Pericarditis I31.1
  pineal gland E34.8
  pleura J94.8
    postinfectional J94.8
    tuberculous NEC B90.9
  pulpal (dental) (nodular) K04.2
  sclera H15.89
  spleen D73.89
  subcutaneous L94.2
  suprarenal (capsule) (gland) E27.49
  tendon (sheath) —see also Tenosynovitis,
      specified type NEC
    with bursitis, synovitis or tenosynovitis —
        see Tendinitis, calcific
  trachea J39.8
  ureter N28.89
  vitreous —see Deposit, crystalline
Calcified —see Calcification
Calcinosis (interstitial) (tumoral) (universalis)
    E83.59
  with Raynaud's phenomenon, esophageal
      dysfunction, sclerodactyly, telangiectasia
      (CREST syndrome) M34.1
  circumscripta (skin) L94.2
  cutis L94.2
Calciphylaxis —see also Calcification, by site
    E83.59
Calcium
  deposits —see Calcification, by site
  metabolism disorder E83.50
  salts or soaps in vitreous —see Deposit,
      crystalline

Calciuria R82.99
Calculi —see Calculus
Calculosis, intrahepatic —see Calculus, bile
    duct
Calculus, calculi, calculous
  ampulla of Vater —see Calculus, bile duct
  anuria (impacted) (recurrent) —see also
      Calculus, urinary N20.9
  appendix K38.1
  bile duct (common) (hepatic) K80.50
    with
      calculus of gallbladder —see Calculus,
          gallbladder and bile duct
      cholangitis K80.30
        with
          cholecystitis —see Calculus, bile
              duct, with cholecystitis
          obstruction K80.31
        acute K80.32
          with
            chronic cholangitis K80.36
              with obstruction K80.37
            obstruction K80.33
        chronic K80.34
          with
            acute cholangitis K80.36
              with obstruction K80.37
            obstruction K80.35
      cholecystitis (with cholangitis) K80.40
        with obstruction K80.41
        acute K80.42
          with
            chronic cholecystitis K80.46
              with obstruction K80.47
            obstruction K80.43
        chronic K80.44
          with
            acute cholecystitis K80.46
              with obstruction K80.47
            obstruction K80.45
      obstruction K80.51
    biliary —see also Calculus, gallbladder
      specified NEC K80.80
        with obstruction K80.81
    bilirubin, multiple —see Calculus,
        gallbladder
    bladder (encysted) (impacted) (urinary)
        (diverticulum) N21.0
    bronchus J98.09
    calyx (kidney) (renal) —see Calculus, kidney
    cholesterol (pure) (solitary) —see Calculus,
        gallbladder
    common duct (bile) —see Calculus, bile duct
    conjunctiva —see Concretion, conjunctiva
    cystic N21.0
      duct —see Calculus, gallbladder
    dental (subgingival) (supragingival)
        K03.6
    diverticulum
      bladder N21.0
      kidney N20.0
    epididymis N50.89
    gallbladder K80.20
      with
        bile duct calculus —see Calculus,
            gallbladder and bile duct
        cholecystitis K80.10
          with obstruction K80.11
          acute K80.00
            with
              chronic cholecystitis K80.12
                with obstruction K80.13
              obstruction K80.01
          chronic K80.10
            with
              acute cholecystitis K80.12
                with obstruction K80.13
              obstruction K80.11
        specified NEC K80.18
          with obstruction K80.19
      obstruction K80.21

Calculus, calculi, calculous *(Continued)*
  gallbladder and bile duct K80.70
    with
      cholecystitis K80.60
        with obstruction K80.61
        acute K80.62
          with
            chronic cholecystitis K80.66
              with obstruction K80.67
            obstruction K80.63
        chronic K80.64
          with
            acute cholecystitis K80.66
              with obstruction K80.67
            obstruction K80.65
      obstruction K80.71
  hepatic (duct) —*see* Calculus, bile duct
  hepatobiliary K80.80
    with obstruction K80.81
  ileal conduit N21.8
  intestinal (impaction) (obstruction) K56.49
  kidney (impacted) (multiple) (pelvis)
      (recurrent) (staghorn) N20.0
    with calculus, ureter N20.2
    congenital Q63.8
  lacrimal passages —*see* Dacryolith
  liver (impacted) —*see* Calculus, bile duct
  lung J98.4
  mammographic R92.1
  nephritic (impacted) (recurrent) —*see*
      Calculus, kidney
  nose J34.89
  pancreas (duct) K86.89
  parotid duct or gland K11.5
  pelvis, encysted —*see* Calculus, kidney
  prostate N42.0
  pulmonary J98.4
  pyelitis (impacted) (recurrent) N20.0
    with hydronephrosis N13.2
  pyelonephritis (impacted) (recurrent) —*see*
      category N20
    with hydronephrosis N13.2
  renal (impacted) (recurrent) —*see* Calculus,
      kidney
  salivary (duct) (gland) K11.5
  seminal vesicle N50.89
  staghorn —*see* Calculus, kidney
  Stensen's duct K11.5
  stomach K31.89
  sublingual duct or gland K11.5
    congenital Q38.4
  submandibular duct, gland or region K11.5
  submaxillary duct, gland or region K11.5
  suburethral N21.8
  tonsil J35.8
  tooth, teeth (subgingival) (supragingival)
      K03.6
  tunica vaginalis N50.89
  ureter (impacted) (recurrent) N20.1
    with calculus, kidney N20.2
      with hydronephrosis N13.2
        with infection N13.6
  urethra (impacted) N21.1
  urinary (duct) (impacted) (passage) (tract)
      N20.9
    with hydronephrosis N13.2
      with infection N13.6
    in (due to)
    lower N21.9
      specified NEC N21.8
  vagina N89.8
  vesical (impacted) N21.0
  Wharton's duct K11.5
  xanthine E79.8 *[N22]*
Calicectasis N28.89
Caliectasis N28.89
California
  disease B38.9
  encephalitis A83.5
Caligo cornea —*see* Opacity, cornea, central
Callositas, callosity (infected) L84

Callus (infected) L84
  bone —*see* Osteophyte
    excessive, following fracture - code as
        Sequelae of fracture
CALME (childhood asymmetric labium majus
    enlargement) N90.61
Calorie deficiency or malnutrition —*see also*
    Malnutrition E46
Calvé-Perthes disease —*see* Legg-Calve-Perthes
    disease
Calvé's disease —*see* Osteochondrosis, juvenile,
    spine
Calvities —*see* Alopecia, androgenic
Cameroon fever —*see* Malaria
Camptocormia (hysterical) F44.4
Camurati-Engelmann syndrome Q78.3
Canal —*see also* condition
  atrioventricular common Q21.2
Canaliculitis (lacrimal) (acute) (subacute)
    H04.33- •
  Actinomyces A42.89
  chronic H04.42- •
Canavan's disease E75.29
Canceled procedure (surgical) Z53.9
  because of
    contraindication Z53.09
      smoking Z53.01
    left against medical advice (AMA) Z53.21
    patient's decision Z53.20
      for reasons of belief or group pressure
          Z53.1
      specified reason NEC Z53.29
    specified reason NEC Z53.8
Cancer —*see also* Neoplasm, by site, malignant
  bile duct type, liver C22.1
  blood —*see* Leukemia
  breast —*see also* Neoplasm, breast, malignant
      C50.91- •
  hepatocellular C22.0
  lung —*see also* Neoplasm, lung, malignant
      C34.90- •
  ovarian —*see also* Neoplasm, ovary,
      malignant C56.9- •
  unspecified site (primary) C80.1
Cancer (o)phobia F45.29
Cancerous —*see* Neoplasm, malignant, by site
Cancrum oris A69.0
Candidiasis, candidal B37.9
  balanitis B37.42
  bronchitis B37.1
  cheilitis B37.83
  congenital P37.5
  cystitis B37.41
  disseminated B37.7
  endocarditis B37.6
  enteritis B37.82
  esophagitis B37.81
  intertrigo B37.2
  lung B37.1
  meningitis B37.5
  mouth B37.0
  nails B37.2
  neonatal P37.5
  onychia B37.2
  oral B37.0
  osteomyelitis B37.89
  otitis externa B37.84
  paronychia B37.2
  perionyxis B37.2
  pneumonia B37.1
  proctitis B37.82
  pulmonary B37.1
  pyelonephritis B37.49
  sepsis B37.7
  skin B37.2
  specified site NEC B37.89
  stomatitis B37.0
  systemic B37.7
  urethritis B37.41
  urogenital site NEC B37.49
  vagina B37.3
  vulva B37.3
  vulvovaginitis B37.3

Candidid L30.2
Candidosis —*see* Candidiasis
Candiru infection or infestation B88.8
Canities (premature) L67.1
  congenital Q84.2
Canker (mouth) (sore) K12.0
  rash A38.9
Cannabinosis J66.2
Cannabis induced
  anxiety disorder F12.980
  psychotic disorder F12.959
  sleep disorder F12.988
Canton fever A75.9
Cantrell's syndrome Q87.89
Capillariasis (intestinal) B81.1
  hepatic B83.8
Capillary —*see* condition
Caplan's syndrome —*see* Rheumatoid, lung
Capsule —*see* condition
Capsulitis (joint) —*see also* Enthesopathy
  adhesive (shoulder) M75.0- •
  hepatic K65.8
  labyrinthine —*see* Otosclerosis, specified NEC
  thyroid E06.9
Caput
  crepitus Q75.8
  medusae I86.8
  succedaneum P12.81
Car sickness T75.3
Carapata (disease) A68.0
Carate —*see* Pinta
Carbon lung J60
Carbuncle L02.93
  abdominal wall L02.231
  anus K61.0
  auditory canal, external —*see* Abscess, ear,
      external
  auricle ear —*see* Abscess, ear, external
  axilla L02.43- •
  back (any part) L02.232
  breast N61.1
  buttock L02.33
  cheek (external) L02.03
  chest wall L02.233
  chin L02.03
  corpus cavernosum N48.21
  ear (any part) (external) (middle) —*see*
      Abscess, ear, external
  external auditory canal —*see* Abscess, ear,
      external
  eyelid —*see* Abscess, eyelid
  face NEC L02.03
  femoral (region) —*see* Carbuncle, lower limb
  finger —*see* Carbuncle, hand
  flank L02.231
  foot L02.63- •
  forehead L02.03
  genital —*see* Abscess, genital
  gluteal (region) L02.33
  groin L02.234
  hand L02.53- •
  head NEC L02.831
  heel —*see* Carbuncle, foot
  hip —*see* Carbuncle, lower limb
  kidney —*see* Abscess, kidney
  knee —*see* Carbuncle, lower limb
  labium (majus) (minus) N76.4
  lacrimal
    gland —*see* Dacryoadenitis
    passages (duct) (sac) —*see* Inflammation,
        lacrimal, passages, acute
  leg —*see* Carbuncle, lower limb
  lower limb L02.43- •
  malignant A22.0
  navel L02.236
  neck L02.13
  nose (external) (septum) J34.0
  orbit, orbital —*see* Abscess, orbit
  palmar (space) —*see* Carbuncle, hand
  partes posteriores L02.33
  pectoral region L02.233
  penis N48.21

C

▶ New   ⇒ Revised   ~~deleted~~ Deleted   • Use Additional Character(s)

Carbuncle *(Continued)*
  perineum L02.235
  pinna —*see* Abscess, ear, external
  popliteal —*see* Carbuncle, lower limb
  scalp L02.831
  seminal vesicle N49.0
  shoulder —*see* Carbuncle, upper limb
  specified site NEC L02.838
  temple (region) L02.03
  thumb —*see* Carbuncle, hand
  toe —*see* Carbuncle, foot
  trunk L02.239
    abdominal wall L02.231
    back L02.232
    chest wall L02.233
    groin L02.234
    perineum L02.235
    umbilicus L02.236
  umbilicus L02.236
  upper limb L02.43-●
  urethra N34.0
  vulva N76.4
Carbunculus —*see* Carbuncle
Carcinoid (tumor) —*see* Tumor, carcinoid
Carcinoidosis E34.0
Carcinoma (malignant) —*see also* Neoplasm,
  by site, malignant
  acidophil
    specified site —*see* Neoplasm, malignant,
      by site
    unspecified site C75.1
  acidophil-basophil, mixed
    specified site —*see* Neoplasm, malignant,
      by site
    unspecified site C75.1
  adnexal (skin) —*see* Neoplasm, skin, malignant
  adrenal cortical C74.0-●
  alveolar —*see* Neoplasm, lung, malignant
    cell —*see* Neoplasm, lung, malignant
  ameloblastic C41.1
    upper jaw (bone) C41.0
  apocrine
    breast —*see* Neoplasm, breast, malignant
    specified site NEC —*see* Neoplasm, skin,
      malignant
    unspecified site C44.99
  basal cell (pigmented) (*see also* Neoplasm,
    skin, malignant) C44.91
    fibro-epithelial —*see* Neoplasm, skin,
      malignant
    morphea —*see* Neoplasm, skin, malignant
    multicentric —*see* Neoplasm, skin,
      malignant
  basaloid
  basal-squamous cell, mixed —*see* Neoplasm,
    skin, malignant
  basophil
    specified site —*see* Neoplasm, malignant,
      by site
    unspecified site C75.1
  basophil-acidophil, mixed
    specified site —*see* Neoplasm, malignant,
      by site
    unspecified site C75.1
  basosquamous —*see* Neoplasm, skin, malignant
  bile duct
    with hepatocellular, mixed C22.0
    liver C22.1
    specified site NEC —*see* Neoplasm,
      malignant, by site
    unspecified site C22.1
  branchial or branchiogenic C10.4
  bronchial or bronchogenic —*see* Neoplasm,
    lung, malignant
  bronchiolar —*see* Neoplasm, lung, malignant
  bronchioloalveolar —*see* Neoplasm, lung,
    malignant
  C cell
    specified site —*see* Neoplasm, malignant,
      by site
    unspecified site C73
  ceruminous C44.29-●

Carcinoma *(Continued)*
  cervix uteri
    in situ D06.9
      endocervix D06.0
      exocervix D06.1
      specified site NEC D06.7
  chorionic
    specified site —*see* Neoplasm, malignant,
      by site
    unspecified site
      female C58
      male C62.90
  chromophobe
    specified site —*see* Neoplasm, malignant,
      by site
    unspecified site C75.1
  cloacogenic
    specified site —*see* Neoplasm, malignant,
      by site
    unspecified site C21.2
  diffuse type
    specified site —*see* Neoplasm, malignant,
      by site
    unspecified site C16.9
  duct (cell)
    with Paget's disease —*see* Neoplasm,
      breast, malignant
    infiltrating
      with lobular carcinoma (in situ)
        specified site —*see* Neoplasm,
          malignant, by site
        unspecified site (female) C50.91-●
          male C50.92-●
      specified site —*see* Neoplasm,
        malignant, by site
      unspecified site (female) C50.91-●
        male C50.92-●
  ductal
    with lobular
      specified site —*see* Neoplasm,
        malignant, by site
      unspecified site (female) C50.91-●
        male C50.92-●
  ductular, infiltrating
    specified site —*see* Neoplasm, malignant,
      by site
    unspecified site (female) C50.91-●
      male C50.92-●
  embryonal
    liver C22.7
  endometrioid
    specified site —*see* Neoplasm, malignant,
      by site
    unspecified site
      female C56.9
      male C61
  eosinophil
    specified site —*see* Neoplasm, malignant,
      by site
    unspecified site C75.1
  epidermoid —*see also* Neoplasm, skin
    malignant
    in situ, Bowen's type —*see* Neoplasm, skin,
      in situ
  fibroepithelial, basal cell —*see* Neoplasm,
    skin, malignant
  follicular
    with papillary (mixed) C73
    moderately differentiated C73
    pure follicle C73
    specified site —*see* Neoplasm, malignant,
      by site
    trabecular C73
    unspecified site C73
    well differentiated C73
  generalized, with unspecified primary site
    C80.0
  glycogen-rich —*see* Neoplasm, breast,
    malignant
  granulosa cell C56-●
  hepatic cell C22.0

Carcinoma *(Continued)*
  hepatocellular C22.0
    with bile duct, mixed C22.0
    fibrolamellar C22.0
  hepatocholangiolitic C22.0
  Hurthle cell C73
  in
    adenomatous
      polyposis coli C18.9
    pleomorphic adenoma —*see* Neoplasm,
      salivary glands, malignant
    situ —*see* Carcinoma-in-situ
  infiltrating
    duct
      with lobular
        specified site —*see* Neoplasm,
          malignant, by site
        unspecified site (female) C50.91-●
          male C50.92-●
      with Paget's disease —*see* Neoplasm,
        breast, malignant
      specified site —*see* Neoplasm,
        malignant
      unspecified site (female) C50.91-●
        male C50.92-●
    ductular
      specified site —*see* Neoplasm,
        malignant
      unspecified site (female) C50.91-●
        male C50.92-●
    lobular
      specified site —*see* Neoplasm,
        malignant
      unspecified site (female) C50.91-●
        male C50.92-●
  inflammatory
    specified site —*see* Neoplasm, malignant
    unspecified site (female) C50.91-●
      male C50.92-●
  intestinal type
    specified site —*see* Neoplasm, malignant,
      by site
    unspecified site C16.9
  intracystic
    noninfiltrating —*see* Neoplasm, in situ,
      by site
  intraductal (noninfiltrating)
    with Paget's disease —*see* Neoplasm,
      breast, malignant
    breast D05.1-●
    papillary
      with invasion
        specified site —*see* Neoplasm,
          malignant, by site
        unspecified site (female) C50.91-●
          male C50.92-●
      breast D05.1-●
      specified site NEC —*see* Neoplasm,
        in situ, by site
      unspecified site (female) D05.1-●
    specified site NEC —*see* Neoplasm,
      in situ, by site
    unspecified site (female) D05.1-●
  intraepidermal —*see* Neoplasm, in situ
    squamous cell, Bowen's type —*see*
      Neoplasm, skin, in situ
  intraepithelial —*see* Neoplasm, in situ,
    by site
    squamous cell —*see* Neoplasm, in situ,
      by site
  intraosseous C41.1
    upper jaw (bone) C41.0
  islet cell
    with exocrine, mixed
      specified site —*see* Neoplasm,
        malignant, by site
      unspecified site C25.9
    pancreas C25.4
    specified site NEC —*see* Neoplasm,
      malignant, by site
    unspecified site C25.4

Carcinoma *(Continued)*
   juvenile, breast —*see* Neoplasm, breast,
      malignant
   large cell
     small cell
       specified site —*see* Neoplasm,
         malignant, by site
       unspecified site C34.90
   Leydig cell (testis)
     specified site —*see* Neoplasm, malignant,
       by site
     unspecified site
      female C56.9
      male C62.90
   lipid-rich (female) C50.91-●
     male C50.92-●
   liver cell C22.0
   liver NEC C22.7
   lobular (infiltrating)
     with intraductal
       specified site —*see* Neoplasm,
         malignant, by site
       unspecified site (female) C50.91-●
        male C50.92-●
     noninfiltrating
       breast D05.0-●
       specified site NEC —*see* Neoplasm, in
         situ, by site
       unspecified site D05.0-●
     specified site —*see* Neoplasm, malignant,
       by site
     unspecified site (female) C50.91-●
      male C50.92-●
   medullary
     with
      amyloid stroma
       specified site —*see* Neoplasm,
         malignant, by site
       unspecified site C73
      lymphoid stroma
       specified site —*see* Neoplasm,
         malignant, by site
       unspecified site (female) C50.91-●
        male C50.92-●
   Merkel cell C4A.9
     anal margin C4A.51
     anal skin C4A.51
     canthus C4A.1-●
     ear and external auricular canal C4A.2-●
     external auricular canal C4A.2-●
     eyelid, including canthus C4A.1-●
     face C4A.30
      specified NEC C4A.39
     hip C4A.7-●
     lip C4A.0
     lower limb, including hip C4A.7-●
     neck C4A.4
     nodal presentation C7B.1
     nose C4A.31
     overlapping sites C4A.8
     perianal skin C4A.51
     scalp C4A.4
     secondary C7B.1
     shoulder C4A.6-●
     skin of breast C4A.52
     trunk NEC C4A.59
     upper limb, including shoulder C4A.6-●
     visceral metastatic C7B.1
   metastatic —*see* Neoplasm, secondary
   metatypical —*see* Neoplasm, skin, malignant
   morphea, basal cell —*see* Neoplasm, skin,
     malignant
   mucoid
     cell
      specified site —*see* Neoplasm,
        malignant, by site
      unspecified site C75.1
   neuroendocrine —*see also* Tumor,
     neuroendocrine
     high grade, any site C7A.1
     poorly differentiated, any site C7A.1

Carcinoma *(Continued)*
   nonencapsulated sclerosing C73
   noninfiltrating
     intracystic —*see* Neoplasm, in situ, by site
     intraductal
      breast D05.1-●
      papillary
       breast D05.1-●
       specified site NEC —*see* Neoplasm, in
         situ, by site
       unspecified site D05.1-●
      specified site —*see* Neoplasm, in situ,
       by site
      unspecified site D05.1-●
     lobular
      breast D05.0-●
      specified site NEC —*see* Neoplasm, in
        situ, by site
      unspecified site (female) D05.0-●
   oat cell
     specified site —*see* Neoplasm, malignant,
      by site
     unspecified site C34.90
   odontogenic C41.1
     upper jaw (bone) C41.0
   papillary
     with follicular (mixed) C73
     follicular variant C73
     intraductal (noninfiltrating)
      with invasion
       specified site —*see* Neoplasm,
         malignant, by site
       unspecified site (female) C50.91-●
        male C50.92-●
      breast D05.1-●
      specified site NEC —*see* Neoplasm, in
        situ, by site
      unspecified site D05.1-●
     serous
      specified site —*see* Neoplasm,
        malignant, by site
      surface
       specified site —*see* Neoplasm,
        malignant, by site
       unspecified site C56.9
      unspecified site C56.9
   papillocystic
     specified site —*see* Neoplasm, malignant,
      by site
     unspecified site C56.9
   parafollicular cell
     specified site —*see* Neoplasm, malignant,
      by site
     unspecified site C73
   pilomatrix —*see* Neoplasm, skin, malignant
   pseudomucinous
     specified site —*see* Neoplasm, malignant,
      by site
     unspecified site C56.9
   renal cell C64-●
   Schmincke —*see* Neoplasm, nasopharynx,
     malignant
   Schneiderian
     specified site —*see* Neoplasm, malignant,
      by site
     unspecified site C30.0
   sebaceous —*see* Neoplasm, skin, malignant
   secondary —*see also* Neoplasm, secondary,
     by site
     Merkel cell C7B.1
   secretory, breast —*see* Neoplasm, breast,
     malignant
   serous
     papillary
      specified site —*see* Neoplasm,
        malignant, by site
      unspecified site C56.9
     surface, papillary
      specified site —*see* Neoplasm,
        malignant, by site
      unspecified site C56.9

Carcinoma *(Continued)*
   Sertoli cell
     specified site —*see* Neoplasm, malignant,
      by site
     unspecified site C62.90
      female C56.9
      male C62.90
   skin appendage —*see* Neoplasm, skin,
     malignant
   small cell
     fusiform cell
      specified site —*see* Neoplasm,
        malignant, by site
      unspecified site C34.90
     intermediate cell
      specified site —*see* Neoplasm,
        malignant, by site
      unspecified site C34.90
     large cell
      specified site —*see* Neoplasm,
        malignant, by site
      unspecified site C34.90
   solid
     with amyloid stroma
      specified site —*see* Neoplasm,
        malignant, by site
      unspecified site C73
     microinvasive
      specified site —*see* Neoplasm,
        malignant, by site
      unspecified site C53.9
   sweat gland —*see* Neoplasm, skin,
     malignant
   theca cell C56.-●
   thymic C37
   unspecified site (primary) C80.1
   water-clear cell C75.0
Carcinoma-in-situ —*see also* Neoplasm, in situ,
   by site
   breast NOS D05.9-●
     specified type NEC D05.8-●
   epidermoid —*see also* Neoplasm, in situ, by
     site
     with questionable stromal invasion
      cervix D06.9
      specified site NEC —*see* Neoplasm, in
        situ, by site
      unspecified site D06.9
     Bowen's type —*see* Neoplasm, skin,
      in situ
   intraductal
     breast D05.1-●
     specified site NEC —*see* Neoplasm, in situ,
      by site
     unspecified site D05.1-●
   lobular
     with
      infiltrating duct
       breast (female) C50.91-●
        male C50.92-●
       specified site NEC —*see* Neoplasm,
        malignant
       unspecified site (female) C50.91-●
        male C50.92-●
      intraductal
       breast D05.8-●
       specified site NEC —*see* Neoplasm, in
        situ, by site
       unspecified site (female) D05.8-●
     breast D05.0-●
     specified site NEC —*see* Neoplasm, in situ,
      by site
     unspecified site D05.0-●
   squamous cell —*see also* Neoplasm, in situ,
     by site
     with questionable stromal invasion
      cervix D06.9
      specified site NEC —*see* Neoplasm, in
        situ, by site
      unspecified site D06.9
Carcinomaphobia F45.29

▶ New   ⇒ Revised   ~~deleted~~ Deleted   ● Use Additional Character(s)

Carcinomatosis C80.0
  peritonei C78.6
  unspecified site (primary) (secondary) C80.0
Carcinosarcoma —see Neoplasm, malignant,
    by site
  embryonal —see Neoplasm, malignant, by
    site
Cardia, cardial —see condition
Cardiac —see also condition
  death, sudden —see Arrest, cardiac
  pacemaker
    in situ Z95.0
    management or adjustment Z45.018
  tamponade I31.4
Cardialgia —see Pain, precordial
Cardiectasis —see Hypertrophy, cardiac
Cardiochalasia K21.9
Cardiomalacia I51.5
Cardiomegalia glycogenica diffusa E74.02 [143]
Cardiomegaly —see also Hypertrophy, cardiac
  congenital Q24.8
  glycogen E74.02 [143]
  idiopathic I51.7
Cardiomyoliposis I51.5
Cardiomyopathy (familial) (idiopathic) I42.9
  alcoholic I42.6
  amyloid E85.4 [143]
  ▶transthyretin-related (ATTR) familial E85.4
  arteriosclerotic —see Disease, heart, ischemic,
    atherosclerotic
  beriberi E51.12
  cobalt-beer I42.6
  congenital I42.4
  congestive I42.0
  constrictive NOS I42.5
  dilated I42.0
  due to
    alcohol I42.6
    beriberi E51.12
    cardiac glycogenosis E74.02 [143]
    drugs I42.7
    external agents NEC I42.7
    Friedreich's ataxia G11.1
    myotonia atrophica G71.11 [143]
  ⇒progressive muscular dystrophy G71.0 [143]
  glycogen storage E74.02 [143]
  hypertensive —see Hypertension, heart
  hypertrophic (nonobstructive) I42.2
    obstructive I42.1
      congenital Q24.8
  in
    Chagas' disease (chronic) B57.2
      acute B57.0
    sarcoidosis D86.85
  ischemic I25.5
  metabolic E88.9 [143]
    thyrotoxic E05.90 [143]
      with thyroid storm E05.91 [143]
  newborn I42.8
    congenital I42.4
  nutritional E63.9 [143]
    beriberi E51.12
  obscure of Africa I42.8
  peripartum O90.3
  postpartum O90.3
  restrictive NEC I42.5
  rheumatic I09.0
  secondary I42.9
  stress induced I51.81
  takotsubo I51.81
  thyrotoxic E05.90 [143]
    with thyroid storm E05.91 [143]
  toxic NEC I42.7
  ▶transthyretin-related (ATTR) familial amyloid
    E85.4
  tuberculous A18.84
  viral B33.24
Cardionephritis —see Hypertension,
    cardiorenal
Cardionephropathy —see Hypertension,
    cardiorenal

Cardionephrosis —see Hypertension, cardiorenal
Cardiopathia nigra I27.0
Cardiopathy —see also Disease, heart I51.9
  idiopathic I42.9
  mucopolysaccharidosis E76.3 [152]
Cardiopericarditis —see Pericarditis
Cardiophobia F45.29
Cardiorenal —see condition
Cardiorrhexis —see Infarct, myocardium
Cardiosclerosis —see Disease, heart, ischemic,
    atherosclerotic
Cardiosis —see Disease, heart
Cardiospasm (esophagus) (reflex) (stomach)
    K22.0
  congenital Q39.5
    with megaesophagus Q39.5
Cardiostenosis —see Disease, heart
Cardiosymphysis I31.0
Cardiovascular —see condition
Carditis (acute) (bacterial) (chronic) (subacute)
    I51.89
  meningococcal A39.50
  rheumatic —see Disease, heart, rheumatic
  rheumatoid —see Rheumatoid, carditis
  viral B33.20
Care (of) (for) (following)
  child (routine) Z76.2
  family member (handicapped) (sick)
    creating problem for family Z63.6
    provided away from home for holiday
      relief Z75.5
    unavailable, due to
      absence (person rendering care)
        (sufferer) Z74.2
      inability (any reason) of person
        rendering care Z74.2
  foundling Z76.1
  holiday relief Z75.5
  improper —see Maltreatment
  lack of (at or after birth) (infant) —see
    Maltreatment, child, neglect
  lactating mother Z39.1
  palliative Z51.5
  postpartum
    immediately after delivery Z39.0
    routine follow-up Z39.2
  respite Z75.5
  unavailable, due to
    absence of person rendering care Z74.2
    inability (any reason) of person rendering
      care Z74.2
  well-baby Z76.2
Caries
  bone NEC A18.03
  dental (dentino enamel junction) (early
      childhood) (of dentine) (pre-eruptive)
      (recurrent) (to the pulp) K02.9
    arrested (coronal) (root) K02.3
    chewing surface
      limited to enamel K02.51
      penetrating into dentin K02.52
      penetrating into pulp K02.53
    coronal surface
      chewing surface
        limited to enamel K02.51
        penetrating into dentin K02.52
        penetrating into pulp K02.53
      pit and fissure surface
        limited to enamel K02.51
        penetrating into dentin K02.52
        penetrating into pulp K02.53
      smooth surface
        limited to enamel K02.61
        penetrating into dentin K02.62
        penetrating into pulp K02.63
    pit and fissure surface
      limited to enamel K02.51
      penetrating into dentin K02.52
      penetrating into pulp K02.53
    primary, cervical origin K02.52
    root K02.7

Caries (Continued)
  dental (Continued)
    smooth surface
      limited to enamel K02.61
      penetrating into dentin K02.62
      penetrating into pulp K02.63
    external meatus —see Disorder, ear, external,
      specified type NEC
  hip (tuberculous) A18.02
  initial (tooth)
    chewing surface K02.51
    pit and fissure surface K02.51
    smooth surface K02.61
  knee (tuberculous) A18.02
  labyrinth —see subcategory H83.8
  limb NEC (tuberculous) A18.03
  mastoid process (chronic) —see Mastoiditis,
    chronic
    tuberculous A18.03
  middle ear —see subcategory H74.8
  nose (tuberculous) A18.03
  orbit (tuberculous) A18.03
  ossicles, ear —see Abnormal, ear ossicles
  petrous bone —see Petrositis
  root (dental) (tooth) K02.7
  sacrum (tuberculous) A18.01
  spine, spinal (column) (tuberculous) A18.01
  syphilitic A52.77
    congenital (early) A50.02 [M90.80]
  tooth, teeth —see Caries, dental
  tuberculous A18.03
  vertebra (column) (tuberculous) A18.01
Carious teeth —see Caries, dental
Carneous mole O02.0
Carnitine insufficiency E71.40
Carotid body or sinus syndrome G90.01
Carotidynia G90.01
Carotinemia (dietary) E67.1
Carotinosis (cutis) (skin) E67.1
Carpal tunnel syndrome —see Syndrome,
    carpal tunnel
Carpenter's syndrome Q87.0
Carpopedal spasm —see Tetany
Carr-Barr-Plunkett syndrome Q97.1
Carrier (suspected) of
  amebiasis Z22.1
  bacterial disease NEC Z22.39
    diphtheria Z22.2
    intestinal infectious NEC Z22.1
      typhoid Z22.0
    meningococcal Z22.31
    sexually transmitted Z22.4
    specified NEC Z22.39
    staphylococcal (Methicillin susceptible)
      Z22.321
      Methicillin resistant Z22.322
    streptococcal Z22.338
      group B Z22.330
        complicating pregnancy or delivery
          O99.82-•
    typhoid Z22.0
  cholera Z22.1
  diphtheria Z22.2
  gastrointestinal pathogens NEC Z22.1
  genetic Z14.8
    cystic fibrosis Z14.1
    hemophilia A (asymptomatic) Z14.01
      symptomatic Z14.02
  gestational, pregnant Z33.1
  gonorrhea Z22.4
  HAA (hepatitis Australian-antigen) B18.8
  HB (c)(s)-AG B18.1
  hepatitis (viral) B18.9
    Australia-antigen (HAA) B18.8
    B surface antigen (HBsAg) B18.1
      with acute delta- (super)infection
        B17.0
    C B18.2
    specified NEC B18.8
  human T-cell lymphotropic virus type-1
    (HTLV-1) infection Z22.6

Carrier of (Continued)
  infectious organism Z22.9
    specified NEC Z22.8
  meningococci Z22.31
  Salmonella typhosa Z22.0
  serum hepatitis —see Carrier, hepatitis
  staphylococci (Methicillin susceptible) Z22.321
    Methicillin resistant Z22.322
  streptococci Z22.338
    group B Z22.330
      complicating pregnancy or delivery
        O99.82-●
  syphilis Z22.4
  typhoid Z22.0
  venereal disease NEC Z22.4
Carrion's disease A44.0
Carter's relapsing fever (Asiatic) A68.1
Cartilage —see condition
Caruncle (inflamed)
  conjunctiva (acute) —see Conjunctivitis, acute
  labium (majus) (minus) N90.89
  lacrimal —see Inflammation, lacrimal,
    passages
  myrtiform N89.8
  urethral (benign) N36.2
Cascade stomach K31.2
Caseation lymphatic gland (tuberculous) A18.2
Cassidy (-Scholte) syndrome (malignant
    carcinoid) E34.0
Castellani's disease A69.8
Castration, traumatic, male S38.231
Casts in urine R82.99
Cat
  cry syndrome Q93.4
  ear Q17.3
  eye syndrome Q92.8
Catabolism, senile R54
Catalepsy (hysterical) F44.2
  schizophrenic F20.2
Cataplexy (idiopathic) —see - Narcolepsy
Cataract (cortical) (immature) (incipient) H26.9
  with
    neovascularization —see Cataract,
      complicated
  age-related —see Cataract, senile
  anterior
    and posterior axial embryonal Q12.0
    pyramidal Q12.0
  associated with
    galactosemia E74.21 [H28]
    myotonic disorders G71.19 [H28]
  blue Q12.0
  central Q12.0
  cerulean Q12.0
  complicated H26.20
    with
      neovascularization H26.21-●
      ocular disorder H26.22-●
      glaucomatous flecks H26.23-●
  congenital Q12.0
  coraliform Q12.0
  coronary Q12.0
  crystalline Q12.0
  diabetic —see Diabetes, cataract
  drug-induced H26.3-●
  due to
    ocular disorder —see Cataract, complicated
    radiation H26.8
  electric H26.8
  extraction status Z98.4-●
  glass-blower's H26.8
  heat ray H26.8
  heterochromic —see Cataract, complicated
  hypermature —see Cataract, senile,
    morgagnian type
  in (due to)
    chronic iridocyclitis —see Cataract,
      complicated
    diabetes —see Diabetes, cataract
    endocrine disease E34.9 [H28]
    eye disease —see Cataract, complicated

Cataract (Continued)
  in (due to) (Continued)
    hypoparathyroidism E20.9 [H28]
    malnutrition-dehydration E46 [H28]
    metabolic disease E88.9 [H28]
    myotonic disorders G71.19 [H28]
    nutritional disease E63.9 [H28]
  infantile —see Cataract, presenile
  irradiational —see Cataract, specified NEC
  juvenile —see Cataract, presenile
  malnutrition-dehydration E46 [H28]
  morgagnian —see Cataract, senile,
    morgagnian type
  myotonic G71.19 [H28]
  myxedema E03.9 [H28]
  nuclear
    embryonal Q12.0
    sclerosis —see Cataract, senile, nuclear
  presenile H26.00-●
    combined forms H26.06-●
    cortical H26.01-●
    lamellar —see Cataract, presenile, cortical
    nuclear H26.03-●
    specified NEC H26.09
    subcapsular polar (anterior) H26.04-●
      posterior H26.05-●
    zonular —see Cataract, presenile, cortical
  secondary H26.40
    Soemmering's ring H26.41-●
    specified NEC H26.49-●
  to eye disease —see Cataract, complicated
  senile H25.9
    brunescens —see Cataract, senile, nuclear
    combined forms H25.81-●
    coronary —see Cataract, senile, incipient
    cortical H25.01-●
    hypermature —see Cataract, senile,
      morgagnian type
    incipient (mature) (total) H25.09-●
      cortical —see Cataract, senile, cortical
      subcapsular —see Cataract, senile,
        subcapsular
    morgagnian type (hypermature) H25.2-●
    nuclear (sclerosis) H25.1-●
    polar subcapsular (anterior) (posterior) —
      see Cataract, senile, incipient
    punctate —see Cataract, senile, incipient
    specified NEC H25.89
    subcapsular polar (anterior) H25.03-●
      posterior H25.04-●
  snowflake —see Diabetes, cataract
  specified NEC H26.8
  toxic —see Cataract, drug-induced
  traumatic H26.10-●
    localized H26.11-●
    partially resolved H26.12-●
    total H26.13-●
  zonular (perinuclear) Q12.0
Cataracta —see also Cataract
  brunescens —see Cataract, senile, nuclear
  centralis pulverulenta Q12.0
  cerulea Q12.0
  complicata —see Cataract, complicated
  congenita Q12.0
  coralliformis Q12.0
  coronaria Q12.0
  diabetic —see Diabetes, cataract
  membranacea
    accreta —see Cataract, secondary
    congenita Q12.0
  nigra —see Cataract, senile, nuclear
  sunflower —see Cataract, complicated
Catarrh, catarrhal (acute) (febrile) (infectious)
    (inflammation) (see also condition) J00
  bronchial —see Bronchitis
  chest —see Bronchitis
  chronic J31.0
  due to congenital syphilis A50.03
  enteric —see Enteritis
  eustachian H68.009
  fauces —see Pharyngitis

Catarrh, catarrhal (Continued)
  gastrointestinal —see Enteritis
  gingivitis K05.00
    nonplaque induced K05.01
    plaque induced K05.00
  hay —see Fever, hay
  intestinal —see Enteritis
  larynx, chronic J37.0
  liver B15.9
    with hepatic coma B15.0
  lung —see Bronchitis
  middle ear, chronic —see Otitis, media,
    nonsuppurative, chronic, serous
  mouth K12.1
  nasal (chronic) —see Rhinitis
  nasobronchial J31.1
  nasopharyngeal (chronic) J31.1
    acute J00
  pulmonary —see Bronchitis
  spring (eye) (vernal) —see Conjunctivitis,
    acute, atopic
  summer (hay) —see Fever, hay
  throat J31.2
  tubotympanal —see also Otitis, media,
    nonsuppurative
    chronic —see Otitis, media,
      nonsuppurative, chronic, serous
Catatonia (schizophrenic) F20.2
Catatonic
  disorder due to known physiologic condition
    F06.1
  schizophrenia F20.2
  stupor R40.1
Cat-scratch —see also Abrasion
  disease or fever A28.1
Cauda equina —see condition
Cauliflower ear M95.1-●
Causalgia (upper limb) G56.4-●
  lower limb G57.7-●
Cause
  external, general effects T75.89
Caustic burn —see Corrosion, by site
Cavare's disease (familial periodic paralysis)
    G72.3
Cave-in, injury
  crushing (severe) —see Crush
  suffocation —see Asphyxia, traumatic, due to
    low oxygen, due to cave-in
Cavernitis (penis) N48.29
Cavernositis N48.29
Cavernous —see condition
Cavitation of lung —see also Tuberculosis,
    pulmonary
  nontuberculous J98.4
Cavities, dental —see Caries, dental
Cavity
  lung —see Cavitation of lung
  optic papilla Q14.2
  pulmonary —see Cavitation of lung
Cavovarus foot, congenital Q66.1
Cavus foot (congenital) Q66.7
  acquired —see Deformity, limb, foot, specified
    NEC
Cazenave's disease L10.2
Cecitis K52.9
  with perforation, peritonitis, or rupture K65.8
Cecum —see condition
Celiac
  artery compression syndrome I77.4
  disease (with steatorrhea) K90.0
  infantilism K90.0
Cell(s), cellular —see also condition
  in urine R82.99
Cellulitis (diffuse) (phlegmonous) (septic)
    (suppurative) L03.90
  abdominal wall L03.311
  anaerobic A48.0
  ankle —see Cellulitis, lower limb
  anus K61.0
  arm —see Cellulitis, upper limb
  auricle (ear) —see Cellulitis, ear

▶ New   ➡ Revised   ~~deleted~~ Deleted   ● Use Additional Character(s)

Cellulitis (Continued)
  axilla L03.11-●
  back (any part) L03.312
  breast (acute) (nonpuerperal) (subacute)
      N61.0
    nipple N61.0
  broad ligament
    acute N73.0
  buttock L03.317
  cervical (meaning neck) L03.221
  cervix (uteri) —see Cervicitis
  cheek (external) L03.211
    internal K12.2
  chest wall L03.313
  chronic L03.90
  clostridial A48.0
  corpus cavernosum N48.22
  digit
    finger —see Cellulitis, finger
    toe —see Cellulitis, toe
  Douglas' cul-de-sac or pouch
    acute N73.0
➡ drainage site (following operation) T81.4
  ear (external) H60.1-●
  eosinophilic (granulomatous) L98.3
  erysipelatous —see Erysipelas
  external auditory canal —see Cellulitis, ear
  eyelid —see Abscess, eyelid
  face NEC L03.211
  finger (intrathecal) (periosteal)
      (subcutaneous) (subcuticular) L03.01-●
  foot —see Cellulitis, lower limb
  gangrenous —see Gangrene
  genital organ NEC
    female (external) N76.4
    male N49.9
      multiple sites N49.8
      specified NEC N49.8
  gluteal (region) L03.317
  gonococcal A54.89
  groin L03.314
  hand —see Cellulitis, upper limb
  head NEC L03.811
    face (any part, except ear, eye and nose)
        L03.211
  heel —see Cellulitis, lower limb
  hip —see Cellulitis, lower limb
  jaw (region) L03.211
  knee —see Cellulitis, lower limb
  labium (majus) (minus) —see Vulvitis
  lacrimal passages —see Inflammation,
      lacrimal, passages
  larynx J38.7
  leg —see Cellulitis, lower limb
  lip K13.0
  lower limb L03.11-●
    toe —see Cellulitis, toe
  mouth (floor) K12.2
  multiple sites, so stated L03.90
  nasopharynx J39.1
  navel L03.316
    newborn P38.9
      with mild hemorrhage P38.1
      without hemorrhage P38.9
  neck (region) L03.221
  nipple (acute) (nonpuerperal) (subacute)
      N61.0
  nose (septum) (external) J34.0
  orbit, orbital H05.01-●
  palate (soft) K12.2
  pectoral (region) L03.313
  pelvis, pelvic (chronic)
    female —see also Disease, pelvis,
        inflammatory N73.2
      acute N73.0
    following ectopic or molar pregnancy
        O08.0
    male K65.0
  penis N48.22
  perineal, perineum L03.315
  periorbital L03.213

Cellulitis (Continued)
  perirectal K61.1
  peritonsillar J36
  periurethral N34.0
  periuterine —see also Disease, pelvis,
      inflammatory N73.2
    acute N73.0
  pharynx J39.1
  preseptal L03.213
  rectum K61.1
  retroperitoneal K68.9
  round ligament
    acute N73.0
  scalp (any part) L03.811
  scrotum N49.2
  seminal vesicle N49.0
  shoulder —see Cellulitis, upper limb
  specified site NEC L03.818
  submandibular (region) (space) (triangle)
      K12.2
    gland K11.3
  submaxillary (region) K12.2
    gland K11.3
  thigh —see Cellulitis, lower limb
  thumb (intrathecal) (periosteal)
      (subcutaneous) (subcuticular) —see
      Cellulitis, finger
  toe (intrathecal) (periosteal) (subcutaneous)
      (subcuticular) L03.03-●
  tonsil J36
  trunk L03.319
    abdominal wall L03.311
    back (any part) L03.312
    buttock L03.317
    chest wall L03.313
    groin L03.314
    perineal, perineum L03.315
    umbilicus L03.316
  tuberculous (primary) A18.4
  umbilicus L03.316
  upper limb L03.11-●
    axilla —see Cellulitis, axilla
    finger —see Cellulitis, finger
    thumb —see Cellulitis, finger
  vaccinal T88.0
  vocal cord J38.3
  vulva —see Vulvitis
  wrist —see Cellulitis, upper limb
Cementoblastoma, benign —see Cyst,
    calcifying odontogenic
Cementoma —see Cyst, calcifying odontogenic
Cementoperiostitis —see Periodontitis
Cementosis K03.4
Central auditory processing disorder H93.25
Central pain syndrome G89.0
Cephalematocele, cephal (o)hematocele
  newborn P52.8
    birth injury P10.8
  traumatic —see Hematoma, brain
Cephalematoma, cephalhematoma (calcified)
  newborn (birth injury) P12.0
  traumatic —see Hematoma, brain
Cephalgia, cephalalgia —see also Headache
  histamine G44.009
    intractable G44.001
    not intractable G44.009
  trigeminal autonomic (TAC) NEC G44.099
    intractable G44.091
    not intractable G44.099
Cephalic —see condition
Cephalitis —see Encephalitis
Cephalocele —see Encephalocele
Cephalomenia N94.89
Cephalopelvic —see condition
Cerclage (with cervical incompetence) in
    pregnancy —see Incompetence, cervix, in
    pregnancy
Cerebellitis —see Encephalitis
Cerebellum, cerebellar —see condition
Cerebral —see condition
Cerebritis —see Encephalitis

Cerebro-hepato-renal syndrome Q87.89
Cerebromalacia —see Softening, brain
  sequelae of cerebrovascular disease I69.398
Cerebroside lipidosis E75.22
Cerebrospasticity (congenital) G80.1
Cerebrospinal —see condition
Cerebrum —see condition
Ceroid-lipofuscinosis, neuronal E75.4
Cerumen (accumulation) (impacted) H61.2-●
Cervical —see also condition
  auricle Q18.2
  dysplasia in pregnancy —see Abnormal,
      cervix, in pregnancy or childbirth
  erosion in pregnancy —see Abnormal, cervix,
      in pregnancy or childbirth
  fibrosis in pregnancy —see Abnormal, cervix,
      in pregnancy or childbirth
  fusion syndrome Q76.1
  rib Q76.5
  shortening (complicating pregnancy)
      O26.87-●
Cervicalgia M54.2
Cervicitis (acute) (chronic) (nonvenereal)
    (senile (atrophic)) (subacute) (with
    ulceration) N72
  with
    abortion —see Abortion, by type
      complicated by genital tract and
        pelvic infection
    ectopic pregnancy O08.0
    molar pregnancy O08.0
  chlamydial A56.09
  gonococcal A54.03
  herpesviral A60.03
  puerperal (postpartum) O86.11
  syphilitic A52.76
  trichomonal A59.09
  tuberculous A18.16
Cervicocolpitis (emphysematosa) (see also
    Cervicitis) N72
Cervix —see condition
Cesarean delivery, previous, affecting
    management of pregnancy O34.219
  classical (vertical) scar O34.212
  low transverse scar O34.211
Céstan (-Chenais) paralysis or syndrome G46.3
Céstan-Raymond syndrome I65.8
Cestode infestation B71.9
  specified type NEC B71.8
Cestodiasis B71.9
Chabert's disease A22.9
Chacaleh E53.8
Chafing L30.4
Chagas' (-Mazza) disease (chronic) B57.2
  with
    cardiovascular involvement NEC B57.2
    digestive system involvement B57.30
      megacolon B57.32
      megaesophagus B57.31
      other specified B57.39
    megacolon B57.32
    megaesophagus B57.31
    myocarditis B57.2
    nervous system involvement B57.40
      meningitis B57.41
      meningoencephalitis B57.42
      other specified B57.49
    specified organ involvement NEC B57.5
  acute (with) B57.1
    cardiovascular NEC B57.0
    myocarditis B57.0
Chagres fever B50.9
Chairridden Z74.09
Chalasia (cardiac sphincter) K21.9
Chalazion H00.19
  left H00.16
    lower H00.15
    upper H00.14
  right H00.13
    lower H00.12
    upper H00.11

Chalcosis —see also Disorder, globe,
   degenerative, chalcosis
  cornea —see Deposit, cornea
  crystalline lens —see Cataract, complicated
  retina H35.89
Chalicosis (pulmonum) J62.8
Chancre (any genital site) (hard) (hunterian)
   (mixed) (primary) (seronegative)
   (seropositive) (syphilitic) A51.0
  congenital A50.07
  conjunctiva NEC A51.2
  Ducrey's A57
  extragenital A51.2
  eyelid A51.2
  lip A51.2
  nipple A51.2
  Nisbet's A57
  of
    carate A67.0
    pinta A67.0
    yaws A66.0
  palate, soft A51.2
  phagedenic A57
  simple A57
  soft A57
    bubo A57
    palate A51.2
  urethra A51.0
  yaws A66.0
Chancroid (anus) (genital) (penis) (perineum)
   (rectum) (urethra) (vulva) A57
Chandler's disease (osteochondritis dissecans,
   hip) —see Osteochondritis, dissecans,
   hip
Change(s) (in) (of) —see also Removal
  arteriosclerotic —see Arteriosclerosis
  bone —see also Disorder, bone
    diabetic —see Diabetes, bone change
  bowel habit R19.4
  cardiorenal (vascular) —see Hypertension,
    cardiorenal
  cardiovascular —see Disease, cardiovascular
  circulatory I99.9
  cognitive (mild) (organic) R41.89
  color, tooth, teeth
    during formation K00.8
    posteruptive K03.7
  contraceptive device Z30.433
  corneal membrane H18.30
    Bowman's membrane fold or rupture
      H18.31- •
    Descemet's membrane
      fold H18.32- •
      rupture H18.33- •
  coronary —see Disease, heart, ischemic
  degenerative, spine or vertebra —see
    Spondylosis
  dental pulp, regressive K04.2
  dressing (nonsurgical) Z48.00
    surgical Z48.01
  heart —see Disease, heart
  hip joint —see Derangement, joint, hip
  hyperplastic larynx J38.7
  hypertrophic
    nasal sinus J34.89
    turbinate, nasal J34.3
    upper respiratory tract J39.8
  indwelling catheter Z46.6
  inflammatory —see also Inflammation
    sacroiliac M46.1
  job, anxiety concerning Z56.1
  joint —see Derangement, joint
  life —see Menopause
  mental status R41.82
  minimal (glomerular) —see also N00-N07
    with fourth character .0 N05.0
  myocardium, myocardial —see also
    Degeneration, myocardial - of life —see
    Menopause
  pacemaker Z45.018
    pulse generator Z45.010

Change (Continued)
  personality (enduring) F68.8
    due to (secondary to)
      general medical condition F07.0
      secondary (nonspecific) F60.89
  regressive, dental pulp K04.2
  renal —see Disease, renal
  retina H35.9
  ⮕myopic —see also Myopia, degenerative
      H44.2- •
  sacroiliac joint M53.3
  senile —see also condition R54
  sensory R20.8
  skin R23.9
    acute, due to ultraviolet radiation L56.9
      specified NEC L56.8
    chronic, due to nonionizing radiation L57.9
      specified NEC L57.8
    cyanosis R23.0
    flushing R23.2
    pallor R23.1
    petechiae R23.3
    specified change NEC R23.8
    swelling —see Mass, localized
    texture R23.4
  trophic
    arm —see Mononeuropathy, upper limb
    leg —see Mononeuropathy, lower limb
  vascular I99.9
  vasomotor I73.9
  voice R49.9
    psychogenic F44.4
    specified NEC R49.8
Changing sleep-work schedule, affecting sleep
   G47.26
Changuinola fever A93.1
Chapping skin T69.8
Charcot-Marie-Tooth disease, paralysis or
   syndrome G60.0
Charcot's
  arthropathy —see Arthropathy, neuropathic
  cirrhosis K74.3
  disease (tabetic arthropathy) A52.16
  joint (disease) (tabetic) A52.16
    diabetic —see Diabetes, with, arthropathy
    syringomyelic G95.0
  syndrome (intermittent claudication) I73.9
CHARGE association Q89.8
Charley-horse (quadriceps) M62.831
  traumatic (quadriceps) S76.11- •
Charlouis' disease —see Yaws
Cheadle's disease E54
Checking (of)
  cardiac pacemaker (battery) (electrode(s))
    Z45.018
    pulse generator Z45.010
  implantable subdermal contraceptive Z30.46
  intrauterine contraceptive device Z30.431
 ▶wound Z48.0- •
   ▶due to injury - code to Injury, by site, using
     appropriate seventh character for
     subsequent encounter
Check-up —see Examination
Chédiak-Higashi (-Steinbrinck) syndrome
   (congenital gigantism of peroxidase
   granules) E70.330
Cheek —see condition
Cheese itch B88.0
Cheese-washer's lung J67.8
Cheese-worker's lung J67.8
Cheilitis (acute) (angular) (catarrhal) (chronic)
   (exfoliative) (gangrenous) (glandular)
   (infectional) (suppurative) (ulcerative)
   (vesicular) K13.0
  actinic (due to sun) L56.8
    other than from sun L59.8
  candidal B37.83
Cheilodynia K13.0
Cheiloschisis —see Cleft, lip
Cheilosis (angular) K13.0
  with pellagra E52
  due to
    vitamin B2 (riboflavin) deficiency E53.0

Cheiromegaly M79.89
Cheiropompholyx L30.1
Cheloid —see Keloid
Chemical burn —see Corrosion, by site
Chemodectoma —see Paraganglioma,
   nonchromaffin
Chemosis, conjunctiva —see Edema,
   conjunctiva
Chemotherapy (session) (for)
  cancer Z51.11
  neoplasm Z51.11
Cherubism M27.8
Chest —see condition
Cheyne-Stokes breathing (respiration) R06.3
Chiari's
  disease or syndrome (hepatic vein
    thrombosis) I82.0
  malformation
    type I G93.5
    type II —see Spina bifida
  net Q24.8
Chicago disease B40.9
Chickenpox —see Varicella
Chiclero ulcer or sore B55.1
Chigger (infestation) B88.0
Chignon (disease) B36.8
  newborn (from vacuum extraction) (birth
    injury) P12.1
Chilaiditi's syndrome (subphrenic
   displacement, colon) Q43.3
Chilblain(s) (lupus) T69.1
Child
  custody dispute Z65.3
Childbirth —see Delivery
Childhood
  cerebral X-linked adrenoleukodystrophy
    E71.520
  period of rapid growth Z00.2
Chill(s) R68.83
  with fever R50.9
  without fever R68.83
  congestive in malarial regions B54
Chilomastigiasis A07.8
Chimera 46,XX/46,XY Q99.0
Chin —see condition
Chinese dysentery A03.9
Chionophobia F40.228
Chitral fever A93.1
Chlamydia, chlamydial A74.9
  cervicitis A56.09
  conjunctivitis A74.0
  cystitis A56.01
  endometritis A56.11
  epididymitis A56.19
  female
    pelvic inflammatory disease A56.11
    pelviperitonitis A56.11
  orchitis A56.19
  peritonitis A74.81
  pharyngitis A56.4
  proctitis A56.3
  psittaci (infection) A70
  salpingitis A56.11
  sexually-transmitted infection NEC A56.8
  specified NEC A74.89
  urethritis A56.01
  vulvovaginitis A56.02
Chlamydiosis —see Chlamydia
Chloasma (skin) (idiopathic) (symptomatic)
   L81.1
  eyelid H02.719
    hyperthyroid E05.90 [H02.719]
      with thyroid storm E05.91 [H02.719]
    left H02.716
      lower H02.715
      upper H02.714
    right H02.713
      lower H02.712
      upper H02.711
Chloroma C92.3- •
Chlorosis D50.9
  Egyptian B76.9 [D63.8]
  miner's B76.9 [D63.8]

▶ New   ⮕ Revised   ~~deleted~~ Deleted   • Use Additional Character(s)

Chlorotic anemia D50.8
Chocolate cyst (ovary) N80.1
Choked
   disc or disk —see Papilledema
   on food, phlegm, or vomitus NOS —see
      Foreign body, by site
   while vomiting NOS —see Foreign body, by
      site
Chokes (resulting from bends) T70.3
Choking sensation R09.89
Cholangiectasis K83.8
Cholangiocarcinoma
   with hepatocellular carcinoma, combined
      C22.0
   liver C22.1
   specified site NEC —see Neoplasm,
      malignant, by site
   unspecified site C22.1
Cholangiohepatitis K83.8
   due to fluke infestation B66.1
Cholangiohepatoma C22.0
Cholangiolitis (acute) (chronic) (extrahepatic)
      (gangrenous) (intrahepatic) K83.0
   paratyphoidal —see Fever, paratyphoid
   typhoidal A01.09
Cholangioma D13.4
   malignant —see Cholangiocarcinoma
Cholangitis (ascending) (primary) (recurrent)
      (sclerosing) (secondary) (stenosing)
      (suppurative) K83.0
   with calculus, bile duct —see Calculus, bile
      duct, with cholangitis
   chronic nonsuppurative destructive K74.3
Cholecystectasia K82.8
Cholecystitis K81.9
   with
      calculus, stones in
         bile duct (common) (hepatic) —
            see Calculus, bile duct, with
            cholecystitis
         cystic duct —see Calculus, gallbladder,
            with cholecystitis
         gallbladder —see Calculus, gallbladder,
            with cholecystitis
         choledocholithiasis —see Calculus, bile
            duct, with cholecystitis
         cholelithiasis —see Calculus, gallbladder,
            with cholecystitis
      acute (emphysematous) (gangrenous)
         (suppurative) K81.0
         with
            calculus, stones in
               cystic duct —see Calculus, gallbladder,
                  with cholecystitis, acute
               gallbladder —see Calculus,
                  gallbladder, with cholecystitis,
                  acute
            choledocholithiasis —see Calculus, bile
               duct, with cholecystitis, acute
            cholelithiasis —see Calculus, gallbladder,
               with cholecystitis, acute
         chronic cholecystitis K81.2
            with gallbladder calculus K80.12
               with obstruction K80.13
      chronic K81.1
         with acute cholecystitis K81.2
            with gallbladder calculus K80.12
               with obstruction K80.13
      emphysematous (acute) —see Cholecystitis,
         acute
      gangrenous —see Cholecystitis, acute
      paratyphoidal, current A01.4
      suppurative —see Cholecystitis, acute
      typhoidal A01.09
Cholecystolithiasis —see Calculus, gallbladder
Choledochitis (suppurative) K83.0
Choledocholith —see Calculus, bile duct
Choledocholithiasis (common duct) (hepatic
      duct) —see Calculus, bile duct
   cystic —see Calculus, gallbladder
   typhoidal A01.09

Cholelithiasis (cystic duct) (gallbladder)
      (impacted) (multiple) —see Calculus,
      gallbladder
   bile duct (common) (hepatic) —see Calculus,
      bile duct
   hepatic duct —see Calculus, bile duct
   specified NEC K80.80
      with obstruction K80.81
Cholemia —see also Jaundice
   familial (simple) (congenital) E80.4
   Gilbert's E80.4
Choleperitoneum, choleperitonitis K65.3
Cholera (Asiatic) (epidemic) (malignant) A00.9
   antimonial —see Poisoning, antimony
   classical A00.0
   due to Vibrio cholerae 01 A00.9
      biovar cholerae A00.0
      biovar eltor A00.1
      el tor A00.1
   el tor A00.1
Cholerine —see Cholera
Cholestasis NEC K83.1
   with hepatocyte injury K71.0
   due to total parenteral nutrition (TPN) K76.89
   pure K71.0
Cholesteatoma (ear) (middle) (with reaction)
      H71.9-•
   attic H71.0-•
   external ear (canal) H60.4-•
   mastoid H71.2-•
   postmastoidectomy cavity (recurrent) —see
      Complications, postmastoidectomy,
      recurrent cholesteatoma
   recurrent (postmastoidectomy) —see
      Complications, postmastoidectomy,
      recurrent cholesteatoma
   tympanum H71.1-•
Cholesteatosis, diffuse H71.3-•
Cholesteremia E78.00
Cholesterin in vitreous —see Deposit, crystalline
Cholesterol
   deposit
      retina H35.89
      vitreous —see Deposit, crystalline
   elevated (high) E78.00
      with elevated (high) triglycerides E78.2
      screening for Z13.220
   imbibition of gallbladder K82.4
Cholesterolemia (essential) (pure) E78.00
   familial E78.01
   hereditary E78.01
Cholesterolosis, cholesterosis (gallbladder)
      K82.4
   cerebrotendinous E75.5
Cholocolic fistula K82.3
Choluria R82.2
Chondritis M94.8X9
   aurical H61.03-•
   costal (Tietze's) M94.0
   external ear H61.03-•
   patella, posttraumatic —see Chondromalacia,
      patella
   pinna H61.03-•
   purulent M94.8X-•
   tuberculous NEC A18.02
      intervertebral A18.01
Chondroblastoma —see also Neoplasm, bone,
      benign
   malignant —see Neoplasm, bone, malignant
Chondrocalcinosis M11.20
   ankle M11.27-•
   elbow M11.22-•
   familial M11.10
      ankle M11.17-•
      elbow M11.12-•
      foot joint M11.17-•
      hand joint M11.14-•
      hip M11.15-•
      knee M11.16-•
      multiple site M11.19
      shoulder M11.11-•

Chondrocalcinosis (Continued)
   familial (Continued)
      vertebrae M11.18
      wrist M11.13-•
   foot joint M11.27-•
   hand joint M11.24-•
   hip M11.25-•
   knee M11.26-•
   multiple site M11.29
   shoulder M11.21-•
   specified type NEC M11.20
      ankle M11.27-•
      elbow M11.22-•
      foot joint M11.27-•
      hand joint M11.24-•
      hip M11.25-•
      knee M11.26-•
      multiple site M11.29
      shoulder M11.21-•
      vertebrae M11.28
      wrist M11.23-•
   vertebrae M11.28
   wrist M11.23-•
Chondrodermatitis nodularis helicis or
      anthelicis —see Perichondritis, ear
Chondrodysplasia Q78.9
   with hemangioma Q78.4
   calcificans congenita Q77.3
   fetalis Q77.4
   metaphyseal (Jansen's) (McKusick's)
      (Schmid's) Q78.8
   punctata Q77.3
Chondrodystrophy, chondrodystrophia
      (familial) (fetalis) (hypoplastic) Q78.9
   calcificans congenita Q77.3
   myotonic (congenital) G71.13
   punctata Q77.3
Chondroectodermal dysplasia Q77.6
Chondrogenesis imperfecta Q77.4
Chondrolysis M94.35-•
Chondroma —see also Neoplasm, cartilage,
      benign
   juxtacortical —see Neoplasm, bone, benign
   periosteal —see Neoplasm, bone, benign
Chondromalacia (systemic) M94.20
   acromioclavicular joint M94.21-•
   ankle M94.27-•
   elbow M94.22-•
   foot joint M94.27-•
   glenohumeral joint M94.21-•
   hand joint M94.24-•
   hip M94.25-•
   knee M94.26-•
      patella M22.4-•
   multiple sites M94.29
   patella M22.4-•
   rib M94.28
   sacroiliac joint M94.259
   shoulder M94.21-•
   sternoclavicular joint M94.21-•
   vertebral joint M94.28
   wrist M94.23-•
Chondromatosis —see also Neoplasm, cartilage,
      uncertain behavior
   internal Q78.4
Chondromyxosarcoma —see Neoplasm,
      cartilage, malignant
Chondro-osteodysplasia (Morquio-Brailsford
      type) E76.219
Chondro-osteodystrophy E76.29
Chondro-osteoma —see Neoplasm, bone, benign
Chondropathia tuberosa M94.0
Chondrosarcoma —see Neoplasm, cartilage,
      malignant
   juxtacortical —see Neoplasm, bone, malignant
   mesenchymal —see Neoplasm, connective
      tissue, malignant
   myxoid —see Neoplasm, cartilage, malignant
Chordee (nonvenereal) N48.89
   congenital Q54.4
   gonococcal A54.09

Chorditis (fibrinous) (nodosa) (tuberosa) J38.2
Chordoma —see Neoplasm, vertebral (column),
   malignant
Chorea (chronic) (gravis) (posthemiplegic)
   (senile) (spasmodic) G25.5
   with
      heart involvement I02.0
         active or acute (conditions in I01-•) I02.0
         rheumatic I02.9
            with valvular disorder I02.0
         rheumatic heart disease (chronic) (inactive)
            (quiescent) — code to rheumatic heart
            condition involved
   drug-induced G25.4
   habit F95.8
   hereditary G10
   Huntington's G10
   hysterical F44.4
   minor I02.9
      with heart involvement I02.0
   progressive G25.5
      hereditary G10
   rheumatic (chronic) I02.9
      with heart involvement I02.0
   Sydenham's I02.9
      with heart involvement —see Chorea, with
         rheumatic heart disease
      nonrheumatic G25.5
Choreoathetosis (paroxysmal) G25.5
Chorioadenoma (destruens) D39.2
Chorioamnionitis O41.12-•
Chorioangioma D26.7
Choriocarcinoma —see Neoplasm, malignant,
   by site
   combined with
      embryonal carcinoma —see Neoplasm,
         malignant, by site
      other germ cell elements —see Neoplasm,
         malignant, by site
      teratoma —see Neoplasm, malignant, by
         site
   specified site —see Neoplasm, malignant, by
      site
   unspecified site
      female C58
      male C62.90
Chorioencephalitis (acute) (lymphocytic)
   (serous) A87.2
Chorioepithelioma —see Choriocarcinoma
Choriomeningitis (acute) (lymphocytic)
   (serous) A87.2
Chorionepithelioma —see Choriocarcinoma
Chorioretinitis —see also Inflammation,
   chorioretinal
   disseminated —see also Inflammation,
      chorioretinal, disseminated
      in neurosyphilis A52.19
   Egyptian B76.9 [D63.8]
   focal —see also Inflammation, chorioretinal,
      focal
   histoplasmic B39.9 [H32]
   in (due to)
      histoplasmosis B39.9 [H32]
      syphilis (secondary) A51.43
         late A52.71
      toxoplasmosis (acquired) B58.01
         congenital (active) P37.1 [H32]
      tuberculosis A18.53
   juxtapapillary, juxtapapillaris —see
      Inflammation, chorioretinal, focal,
      juxtapapillary
   leprous A30.9 [H32]
   miner's B76.9 [D63.8]
➡ progressive myopia (degeneration) —see also
      Myopia, degenerative H44.2-•
   syphilitic (secondary) A51.43
      congenital (early) A50.01 [H32]
         late A50.32
      late A52.71
   tuberculous A18.53
Chorioretinopathy, central serous H35.71-•

Choroid —see condition
Choroideremia H31.21
Choroiditis —see Chorioretinitis
Choroidopathy —see Disorder, choroid
Choroidoretinitis —see Chorioretinitis
Choroidoretinopathy, central serous —see
      Chorioretinopathy, central serous
Christian-Weber disease M35.6
Christmas disease D67
Chromaffinoma —see also Neoplasm, benign,
      by site
   malignant —see Neoplasm, malignant, by site
Chromatopsia —see Deficiency, color vision
Chromhidrosis, chromidrosis L75.1
Chromoblastomycosis —see Chromomycosis
Chromoconversion R82.91
Chromomycosis B43.9
   brain abscess B43.1
   cerebral B43.1
   cutaneous B43.0
   skin B43.0
   specified NEC B43.8
   subcutaneous abscess or cyst B43.2
Chromophytosis B36.0
Chromosome —see condition by chromosome
      involved
   D (1) —see condition, chromosome 13
   E (3) —see condition, chromosome 18
   G —see condition, chromosome 21
Chromotrichomycosis B36.8
Chronic —see condition
   fracture —see Fracture, pathological
Churg-Strauss syndrome M30.1
Chyle cyst, mesentery I89.8
Chylocele (nonfilarial) I89.8
   filarial —see also Infestation, filarial B74.9
      [N51]
   tunica vaginalis N50.89
      filarial —see also Infestation, filarial B74.9
         [N51]
Chylomicronemia (fasting) (with
      hyperprebetalipoproteinemia) E78.3
Chylopericardium I31.3
   acute I30.9
Chylothorax (nonfilarial) I89.8
   filarial —see also Infestation, filarial B74.9 [J91.8]
Chylous —see condition
Chyluria (nonfilarial) R82.0
   due to
      bilharziasis B65.0
      Brugia (malayi) B74.1
         timori B74.2
      schistosomiasis (bilharziasis) B65.0
      Wuchereria (bancrofti) B74.0
   filarial —see Infestation, filarial
Cicatricial (deformity) —see Cicatrix
Cicatrix (adherent) (contracted) (painful)
      (vicious) —see also Scar L90.5
   adenoid (and tonsil) J35.8
   alveolar process M26.79
   anus K62.89
   auricle —see Disorder, pinna, specified type
      NEC
   bile duct (common) (hepatic) K83.8
   bladder N32.89
   bone —see Disorder, bone, specified type
      NEC
   brain G93.89
   cervix (postoperative) (postpartal) N88.1
   common duct K83.8
   cornea H17.9
      tuberculous A18.59
   duodenum (bulb), obstructive K31.5
   esophagus K22.2
   eyelid —see Disorder, eyelid function
   hypopharynx J39.2
   lacrimal passages —see Obstruction, lacrimal
   larynx J38.7
   lung J98.4
   middle ear —see subcategory H74.8
   mouth K13.79

Cicatrix (Continued)
   muscle M62.89
      with contracture —see Contraction, muscle
         NEC
   nasopharynx J39.2
   palate (soft) K13.79
   penis N48.89
   pharynx J39.2
   prostate N42.89
   rectum K62.89
   retina —see Scar, chorioretinal
   semilunar cartilage —see Derangement,
      meniscus
   seminal vesicle N50.89
   skin L90.5
      infected L08.89
      postinfective L90.5
      tuberculous B90.8
   specified site NEC L90.5
   throat J39.2
   tongue K14.8
   tonsil (and adenoid) J35.8
   trachea J39.8
   tuberculous NEC B90.9
   urethra N36.8
   uterus N85.8
   vagina N89.8
      postoperative N99.2
   vocal cord J38.3
   wrist, constricting (annular) L90.5
CIDP (chronic inflammatory demyelinating
      polyneuropathy) G61.81
CIN —see Neoplasia, intraepithelial, cervix
CINCA (chronic infantile neurological,
      cutaneous and articular syndrome)
      M04.2
Cinchonism —see Deafness, ototoxic
   correct substance properly administered —see
      Table of Drugs and Chemicals, by drug,
      adverse effect
   overdose or wrong substance given
      or taken —see Table of Drugs and
      Chemicals, by drug, poisoning
Circle of Willis —see condition
Circular —see condition
Circulating anticoagulants —see also - Disorder,
      hemorrhagic D68.318
   due to drugs —see also - Disorder,
      hemorrhagic D68.32
   following childbirth O72.3
Circulation
   collateral, any site I99.8
➡ defective (lower extremity) I99.9
      congenital Q28.9
   embryonic Q28.9
   failure (peripheral) R57.9
      newborn P29.89
➡ fetal, persistent P29.38
   heart, incomplete Q28.9
Circulatory system —see condition
Circulus senilis (cornea) —see Degeneration,
      cornea, senile
Circumcision (in absence of medical indication)
      (ritual) (routine) Z41.2
Circumscribed —see condition
Circumvallate placenta O43.11-•
Cirrhosis, cirrhotic (hepatic) (liver) K74.60
   alcoholic K70.30
      with ascites K70.31
   atrophic —see Cirrhosis, liver
   Baumgarten-Cruveilhier K74.69
   biliary (cholangiolitic) (cholangitic)
         (hypertrophic) (obstructive)
         (pericholangiolitic) K74.5
      due to
         Clonorchiasis B66.1
         flukes B66.3
      primary K74.3
      secondary K74.4
   cardiac (of liver) K76.1
   Charcot's K74.3

Cirrhosis, cirrhotic *(Continued)*
  cholangiolitic, cholangitic, cholostatic
    (primary) K74.3
  congestive K76.1
  Cruveilhier-Baumgarten K74.69
  cryptogenic (liver) K74.69
  due to
    hepatolenticular degeneration E83.01
    Wilson's disease E83.01
    xanthomatosis E78.2
  fatty K76.0
    alcoholic K70.0
  Hanot's (hypertrophic) K74.3
  hepatic —*see* Cirrhosis, liver
  hypertrophic K74.3
  Indian childhood K74.69
  kidney —*see* Sclerosis, renal
  Laennec's K70.30
    with ascites K70.31
    alcoholic K70.30
      with ascites K70.31
    nonalcoholic K74.69
  liver K74.60
    alcoholic K70.30
      with ascites K70.31
      fatty K70.0
    congenital P78.81
    syphilitic A52.74
  lung (chronic) J84.10
  macronodular K74.69
    alcoholic K70.30
      with ascites K70.31
  micronodular K74.69
    alcoholic K70.30
      with ascites K70.31
  mixed type K74.69
  monolobular K74.3
  nephritis —*see* Sclerosis, renal
  nutritional K74.69
    alcoholic K70.30
      with ascites K70.31
  obstructive —*see* Cirrhosis, biliary
  ovarian N83.8
  pancreas (duct) K86.89
  pigmentary E83.110
  portal K74.69
    alcoholic K70.30
      with ascites K70.31
  postnecrotic K74.69
    alcoholic K70.30
      with ascites K70.31
  pulmonary J84.10
  renal —*see* Sclerosis, renal
  spleen D73.2
  stasis K76.1
  Todd's K74.3
  unilobar K74.3
  xanthomatous (biliary) K74.5
    due to xanthomatosis (familial) (metabolic)
    (primary) E78.2
Cistern, subarachnoid R93.0
Citrullinemia E72.23
Citrullinuria E72.23
Civatte's disease or poikiloderma L57.3
Clam digger's itch B65.3
Clammy skin R23.1
Clap —*see* Gonorrhea
Clarke-Hadfield syndrome (pancreatic
  infantilism) K86.89
Clark's paralysis G80.9
Clastothrix L67.8
Claude Bernard-Horner syndrome G90.2
  traumatic —*see* Injury, nerve, cervical
    sympathetic
Claude's disease or syndrome G46.3
Claudicatio venosa intermittens I87.8
Claudication (intermittent) I73.9
  cerebral (artery) G45.9
  spinal cord (arteriosclerotic) G95.19
    syphilitic A52.09
  venous (axillary) I87.8

Claustrophobia F40.240
Clavus (infected) L84
Clawfoot (congenital) Q66.89
  acquired —*see* Deformity, limb, clawfoot
Clawhand (acquired) —*see also* Deformity, limb,
  clawhand
  congenital Q68.1
Clawtoe (congenital) Q66.89
  acquired —*see* Deformity, toe, specified NEC
Clay eating —*see* Pica
Cleansing of artificial opening —*see* Attention
  to, artificial, opening
Cleft (congenital) —*see also* Imperfect, closure
  alveolar process M26.79
▶ branchial (persistent) Q18.2
▶ cyst Q18.0
  ▶ fistula Q18.0
  ▶ sinus Q18.0
  cricoid cartilage, posterior Q31.8
  foot Q72.7
  hand Q71.6
  lip (unilateral) Q36.9
    with cleft palate Q37.9
      hard Q37.1
        with soft Q37.5
      soft Q37.3
        with hard Q37.5
    bilateral Q36.0
      with cleft palate Q37.8
        hard Q37.0
          with soft Q37.4
        soft Q37.2
          with hard Q37.4
    median Q36.1
  nose Q30.2
  palate Q35.9
    with cleft lip (unilateral) Q37.9
      bilateral Q37.8
    hard Q35.1
      with
        cleft lip (unilateral) Q37.1
          bilateral Q37.0
        soft Q35.5
          with cleft lip (unilateral) Q37.5
            bilateral Q37.4
    medial Q35.5
    soft Q35.3
      with
        cleft lip (unilateral) Q37.3
          bilateral Q37.2
        hard Q35.5
          with cleft lip (unilateral) Q37.5
            bilateral Q37.4
  penis Q55.69
  scrotum Q55.29
  thyroid cartilage Q31.8
  uvula Q35.7
Cleidocranial dysostosis Q74.0
Cleptomania F63.2
Clicking hip (newborn) R29.4
Climacteric (female) —*see also* Menopause
  arthritis (any site) NEC —*see* Arthritis,
    specified form NEC
  depression (single episode) F32.89
    recurrent episode F33.8
  male (symptoms) (syndrome) NEC N50.89
  melancholia (single episode) F32.89
    recurrent episode F33.8
  paranoid state F22
  polyarthritis NEC —*see* Arthritis, specified
    form NEC
  symptoms (female) N95.1
Clinical research investigation (clinical trial)
  (control subject) (normal comparison)
  (participant) Z00.6
Clitoris —*see* condition Cloaca (persistent)
  Q43.7
Clonorchiasis, clonorchis infection (liver)
  B66.1
Clonus R25.8
Closed bite M26.29

Clostridium (C.) perfringens, as cause of
  disease classified elsewhere B96.7
Closure
  congenital, nose Q30.0
  cranial sutures, premature Q75.0
  defective or imperfect NEC —*see* Imperfect,
    closure
  fistula, delayed —*see* Fistula
  foramen ovale, imperfect Q21.1
  hymen N89.6
  interauricular septum, defective Q21.1
  interventricular septum, defective Q21.0
  lacrimal duct —*see also* Stenosis, lacrimal,
    duct
    congenital Q10.5
  nose (congenital) Q30.0
    acquired M95.0
  of artificial opening —*see* Attention to,
    artificial, opening
  primary angle, without glaucoma damage
    H40.06-●
  vagina N89.5
  valve —*see* Endocarditis
  vulva N90.5
Clot (blood) —*see also* Embolism
  artery (obstruction) (occlusion) —*see*
    Embolism
  bladder N32.89
  brain (intradural or extradural) —*see*
    Occlusion, artery, cerebral
  circulation I74.9
  heart —*see also* Infarct, myocardium
    not resulting in infarction I51.3
  vein —*see* Thrombosis
Clouded state R40.1
  epileptic —*see* Epilepsy, specified NEC
  paroxysmal —*see* Epilepsy, specified NEC
Cloudy antrum, antra J32.0
Clouston's (hidrotic) ectodermal dysplasia
  Q82.4
Clubbed nail pachydermoperiostosis M89.40
  [L62]
Clubbing of finger(s) (nails) R68.3
Clubfinger R68.3
  congenital Q68.1
Clubfoot (congenital) Q66.89
  acquired —*see* Deformity, limb, clubfoot
  equinovarus Q66.0
  paralytic —*see* Deformity, limb, clubfoot
Clubhand (congenital) (radial) Q71.4-●
  acquired —*see* Deformity, limb, clubhand
Clubnail R68.3
  congenital Q84.6
Clump, kidney Q63.1
Clumsiness, clumsy child syndrome F82
Cluttering F98.81
Clutton's joints A50.51 [M12.80]
Coagulation, intravascular (diffuse)
  (disseminated) —*see also* Defibrination
    syndrome
  complicating abortion —*see* Abortion, by
    type, complicated by, intravascular
    coagulation
  following ectopic or molar pregnancy
    O08.1
Coagulopathy —*see also* Defect, coagulation
  consumption D65
  intravascular D65
  newborn P60
Coalition
  calcaneo-scaphoid Q66.89
  tarsal Q66.89
Coalminer's
  elbow —*see* Bursitis, elbow, olecranon
  lung or pneumoconiosis J60
Coalworker's lung or pneumoconiosis
  J60
Coarctation
  aorta (preductal) (postductal) Q25.1
  pulmonary artery Q25.71
Coated tongue K14.3

Coats' disease (exudative retinopathy) —see
  Retinopathy, exudative
Cocaine-induced
  anxiety disorder F14.980
  bipolar and related disorder F14.94
  depressive disorder F14.94
  obsessive-compulsive and related disorder
    F14.988
  psychotic disorder F14.959
  sleep disorder F14.982
  sexual dysfunction F14.981
Cocainism —see Disorder, cocaine use
Coccidioidomycosis B38.9
  cutaneous B38.3
  disseminated B38.7
  generalized B38.7
  meninges B38.4
  prostate B38.81
  pulmonary B38.2
    acute B38.0
    chronic B38.1
  skin B38.3
  specified NEC B38.89
Coccidioidosis —see Coccidioidomycosis
Coccidiosis (intestinal) A07.3
Coccydynia, coccygodynia M53.3
Coccyx —see condition
Cochin-China diarrhea K90.1
Cockayne's syndrome Q87.1
Cocked up toe —see Deformity, toe, specified
  NEC
Cock's peculiar tumor L72.3
Codman's tumor —see Neoplasm, bone, benign
Coenurosis B71.8
Coffee-worker's lung J67.8 •
Cogan's syndrome H16.32- •
  oculomotor apraxia H51.8
Coitus, painful (female) N94.10
  male N53.12
  psychogenic F52.6
Cold J00
  with influenza, flu, or grippe —see Influenza,
    with, respiratory manifestations NEC
  agglutinin disease or hemoglobinuria
    (chronic) D59.1
  bronchial —see Bronchitis
  chest —see Bronchitis
  common (head) J00
  effects of T69.9
    specified effect NEC T69.8
  excessive, effects of T69.9
    specified effect NEC T69.8
  exhaustion from T69.8
  exposure to T69.9
    specified effect NEC T69.8
  head J00
  injury syndrome (newborn) P80.0
  on lung —see Bronchitis
  rose J30.1
  sensitivity, auto-immune D59.1
  ▶symptoms J00
  virus J00
Coldsore B00.1
Colibacillosis A49.8
  as the cause of other disease (see also
    Escherichia coli) B96.20
  generalized A41.50
Colic (bilious) (infantile) (intestinal) (recurrent)
  (spasmodic) R10.83
  abdomen R10.83
    psychogenic F45.8
  appendix, appendicular K38.8
  bile duct —see Calculus, bile duct
  biliary —see Calculus, bile duct
  common duct —see Calculus, bile duct
  cystic duct —see Calculus, gallbladder
  Devonshire NEC —see Poisoning, lead
  gallbladder —see Calculus, gallbladder
  gallstone —see Calculus, gallbladder
    gallbladder or cystic duct —see Calculus,
      gallbladder

Colic (Continued)
  hepatic (duct) —see Calculus, bile duct
  hysterical F45.8
  kidney N23
  lead NEC —see Poisoning, lead
  mucous K58.9
    with diarrhea K58.0
    psychogenic F54
  nephritic N23
  painter's NEC —see Poisoning, lead
  pancreas K86.89
  psychogenic F45.8
  renal N23
  saturnine NEC —see Poisoning, lead
  ureter N23
  urethral N36.8
    due to calculus N21.1
  uterus NEC N94.89
    menstrual —see Dysmenorrhea
  worm NOS B83.9
Colicystitis —see Cystitis
Colitis (acute) (catarrhal) (chronic)
    (noninfective) (hemorrhagic) (see also
    Enteritis) K52.9
  allergic K52.29
    with
      food protein-induced enterocolitis
        syndrome K52.21
      proctocolitis K52.82
  amebic (acute) —see also Amebiasis A06.0
    nondysenteric A06.2
  anthrax A22.2
  bacillary —see Infection, Shigella
  balantidial A07.0
  ▸Clostridium difficile
    ▶not specified as recurrent A04.72
    ▶recurrent A04.71
  coccidial A07.3
  collagenous K52.831
  cystica superficialis K52.89
  dietary counseling and surveillance (for) Z71.3
  dietetic —see also Colitis, allergic K52.29
  drug-induced K52.1
  due to radiation K52.0
  eosinophilic K52.82
  food hypersensitivity —see also Colitis,
    allergic K52.29
  giardial A07.1
  granulomatous —see Enteritis, regional, large
    intestine
  infectious —see Enteritis, infectious
  indeterminate, so stated K52.3
  ischemic K55.9
    acute (subacute) —see also Ischemia,
      intestine, acute K55.039
    chronic K55.1
    due to mesenteric artery insufficiency K55.1
    fulminant (acute) —see also Ischemia,
      intestine, acute K55.039
  left sided K51.50
    with
      abscess K51.514
      complication K51.519
        specified NEC K51.518
      fistula K51.513
      obstruction K51.512
      rectal bleeding K51.511
  lymphocytic K52.832
  membranous
    psychogenic F54
  microscopic K52.839
    specified NEC K52.838
  mucous —see Syndrome, irritable, bowel
    psychogenic F54
  noninfective K52.9
    specified NEC K52.89
  polyposa —see Polyp, colon, inflammatory
  protozoal A07.9
  ▸pseudomembranous
    ▶not specified as recurrent A04.72
    ▶recurrent A04.71

Colitis (Continued)
  pseudomucinous —see Syndrome, irritable,
    bowel
  regional —see Enteritis, regional, large intestine
    ▶infectious A09
  segmental —see Enteritis, regional, large
    intestine
  septic —see Enteritis, infectious
  spastic K58.9
    with diarrhea K58.0
    psychogenic F54
  staphylococcal A04.8
    foodborne A05.0
  subacute ischemic —see also Ischemia,
    intestine, acute K55.039
  thromboulcerative —see also Ischemia,
    intestine, acute K55.039
  toxic NEC K52.1
  ▸due to Clostridium difficile
    ▶not specified as recurrent A04.72
    ▶recurrent A04.71
  transmural —see Enteritis, regional, large
    intestine
  trichomonal A07.8
  tuberculous (ulcerative) A18.32
  ulcerative (chronic) K51.90
    with
      complication K51.919
        abscess K51.914
        fistula K51.913
        obstruction K51.912
        rectal bleeding K51.911
        specified complication NEC K51.918
    enterocolitis —see Enterocolitis, ulcerative
    ileocolitis —see Ileocolitis, ulcerative
    mucosal proctocolitis —see Proctocolitis,
      mucosal
    proctitis —see Proctitis, ulcerative
    pseudopolyposis —see Polyp, colon,
      inflammatory
    psychogenic F54
    rectosigmoiditis —see Rectosigmoiditis,
      ulcerative
    specified type NEC K51.80
      with
        complication K51.819
          abscess K51.814
          fistula K51.813
          obstruction K51.812
          rectal bleeding K51.811
          specified complication NEC K51.818
Collagenosis, collagen disease (nonvascular)
    (vascular) M35.9
  cardiovascular I42.8
  reactive perforating L87.1
  specified NEC M35.8
Collapse R55
  adrenal E27.2
  cardiorespiratory R57.0
  cardiovascular R57.0
    newborn P29.89
  circulatory (peripheral) R57.9
    during or after labor and delivery O75.1
    following ectopic or molar pregnancy O08.3
    newborn P29.89
  during or
    after labor and delivery O75.1
    resulting from a procedure, not elsewhere
      classified T81.10
  external ear canal —see Stenosis, external ear
    canal
  general R55
  heart —see Disease, heart
  heat T67.1
  hysterical F44.89
  labyrinth, membranous (congenital) Q16.5
  lung (massive) —see also Atelectasis J98.19
    pressure due to anesthesia (general) (local)
      or other sedation T88.2
      during labor and delivery O74.1
      in pregnancy O29.02- •
      postpartum, puerperal O89.09

▶ New   ▦ Revised   ~~deleted~~ Deleted   • Use Additional Character(s)

Collapse *(Continued)*
  myocardial —*see* Disease, heart
  nervous F48.8
  neurocirculatory F45.8
  nose M95.0
  postoperative T81.10
  pulmonary —*see also* Atelectasis J98.19
    newborn —*see* Atelectasis
  trachea J39.8
  tracheobronchial J98.09
  valvular —*see* Endocarditis
  vascular (peripheral) R57.9
    during or after labor and delivery O75.1
    following ectopic or molar pregnancy O08.3
    newborn P29.89
  vertebra M48.50-●
    cervical region M48.52-●
    cervicothoracic region M48.53-●
    in (due to)
      metastasis —*see* Collapse, vertebra, in,
        specified disease NEC
      osteoporosis —*see also* Osteoporosis
        M80.88
        cervical region M80.88
        cervicothoracic region M80.88
        lumbar region M80.88
        lumbosacral region M80.88
        multiple sites M80.88
        occipito-atlanto-axial region M80.88
        sacrococcygeal region M80.88
        thoracic region M80.88
        thoracolumbar region M80.88
      specified disease NEC M48.50-●
        cervical region M48.52-●
        cervicothoracic region M48.53-●
        lumbar region M48.56-●
        lumbosacral region M48.57-●
        occipito-atlanto-axial region M48.51-●
        sacrococcygeal region M48.58-●
        thoracic region M48.54-●
        thoracolumbar region M48.55-●
    lumbar region M48.56-●
    lumbosacral region M48.57-●
    occipito-atlanto-axial region M48.51-●
    sacrococcygeal region M48.58-●
    thoracic region M48.54-●
    thoracolumbar region M48.55-●
Collateral —*see also* condition
  circulation (venous) I87.8
  dilation, veins I87.8
Colles' fracture S52.53-●
Collet (-Sicard) syndrome G52.7
Collier's asthma or lung J60
Collodion baby Q80.2
Colloid nodule (of thyroid) (cystic) E04.1
Coloboma (iris) Q13.0
  eyelid Q10.3
  fundus Q14.8
  lens Q12.2
  optic disc (congenital) Q14.2
    acquired H47.31-●
Coloenteritis —*see* Enteritis
Colon —*see* condition
Colonization
  MRSA (Methicillin resistant Staphylococcus
    aureus) Z22.322
  MSSA (Methicillin susceptible
    Staphylococcus aureus) Z22.321
  status —*see* Carrier (suspected) of
Coloptosis K63.4
Color blindness —*see* Deficiency, color vision
Colostomy
  attention to Z43.3
  fitting or adjustment Z46.89
  malfunctioning K94.03
  status Z93.3
Colpitis (acute) —*see* Vaginitis
Colpocele N81.5
Colpocystitis —*see* Vaginitis
Colpospasm N94.2
Column, spinal, vertebral —*see* condition

Coma R40.20
  with
    motor response (none) R40.231
      abnormal R40.233
    ▶abnormal extensor posturing to pain or
      noxious stimuli (<2 years of age)
      R40.232
    ▶abnormal flexure posturing to pain or
      noxious stimuli (0-5 years of age)
      R40.233
      extension R40.232
    ▶extensor posturing to pain or noxious
      stimuli (2-5 years of age) R40.232
    ▶flexion/decorticate posturing
      (<2 years of age) R40.233
      flexion withdrawal R40.234
    ⇒localizes pain (2-5 years of age) R40.235
    ▶normal or spontaneous movement
      (<2 years of age) R40.236
    ⇒obeys commands (2-5 years of age)
      R40.236
    ▶withdraws from pain or noxious stimuli
      (0-5 years of age) R40.234
    ▶withdraws to touch (<2 years of age)
      R40.235
    opening of eyes (never) R40.211
      in response to
        pain R40.212
        sound R40.213
      spontaneous R40.214
    verbal response (none) R40.221
      confused conversation R40.224
    ▶cooing or babbling or crying
        appropriately (<2 years of age)
        R40.225
    ▶inappropriate crying or screaming
        (<2 years of age) R40.223
      inappropriate words R40.223
    ⇒inappropriate words (2-5 years of age)
        R40.224
    ▶incomprehensible sounds (2-5 years of
        age) R40.222
      incomprehensible words R40.222
    ▶irritable cries (<2 years of age) R40.224
    ▶moans/grunts to pain; restless
        (<2 years old) R40.222
      oriented R40.225
    ▶screaming (2-5 years of age) R40.223
    ▶uses appropriate words (2-5 years of
        age) R40.225
  eclamptic —*see* Eclampsia
  epileptic —*see* Epilepsy
  Glasgow, scale score —*see* Glasgow coma scale
  hepatic —*see* Failure, hepatic, by type, with
    coma
  hyperglycemic (diabetic) —*see* Diabetes, by
    type, with hyperosmolarity, with coma
  hyperosmolar (diabetic) —*see* Diabetes, by
    type, with hyperosmolarity, with coma
  hypoglycemic (diabetic) —*see* Diabetes, by
    type, with hypoglycemia, with coma
  nondiabetic E15
  in diabetes —*see* Diabetes, coma
  insulin-induced —*see* Coma, hypoglycemic
  ▶ketoacidotic (diabetic) —*see* Diabetes, by
    type, with ketoacidosis, with coma
  myxedematous E03.5
  newborn P91.5
  persistent vegetative state R40.3
  specified NEC, without documented
    Glasgow coma scale score, or with
    partial Glasgow coma scale score
    reported R40.244
Comatose —*see* Coma
Combat fatigue F43.0
Combined —*see* condition
Comedo, comedones (giant) L70.0
Comedocarcinoma —*see also* Neoplasm, breast,
  malignant
  noninfiltrating
    breast D05.8-●
    specified site —*see* Neoplasm, in situ, by site
    unspecified site D05.8-●

Comedomastitis —*see* Ectasia, mammary duct
Comminuted fracture - code as Fracture, closed
Common
  arterial trunk Q20.0
  atrioventricular canal Q21.2
  atrium Q21.1
  cold (head) J00
  truncus (arteriosus) Q20.0
  variable immunodeficiency —*see*
    Immunodeficiency, common variable
  ventricle Q20.4
Commotio, commotion (current)
  brain —*see* Injury, intracranial, concussion
  cerebri —*see* Injury, intracranial, concussion
  retinae S05.8X-●
  spinal cord —*see* Injury, spinal cord,
    by region
  spinalis —*see* Injury, spinal cord, by region
Communication
  between
    base of aorta and pulmonary artery
      Q21.4
    left ventricle and right atrium Q20.5
    pericardial sac and pleural sac Q34.8
    pulmonary artery and pulmonary vein,
      congenital Q25.72
  congenital between uterus and digestive or
    urinary tract Q51.7
Compartment syndrome (deep) (posterior)
  (traumatic) T79.A0
  abdomen T79.A3
  lower extremity (hip, buttock, thigh, leg, foot,
    toes) T79.A2
  nontraumatic
    abdomen M79.A3
    lower extremity (hip, buttock, thigh, leg,
      foot, toes) M79.A2-●
    specified site NEC M79.A9
    upper extremity (shoulder, arm, forearm,
      wrist, hand, fingers) M79.A1-●
  specified site NEC T79.A9
  upper extremity (shoulder, arm, forearm,
    wrist, hand, fingers) T79.A1
Compensation
  failure —*see* Disease, heart
  neurosis, psychoneurosis —*see* Disorder,
    factitious
Complaint —*see also* Disease
  bowel, functional K59.9
    psychogenic F45.8
  intestine, functional K59.9
    psychogenic F45.8
  kidney —*see* Disease, renal
  miners' J60
Complete —*see* condition
Complex
  Addison-Schilder E71.528
  cardiorenal —*see* Hypertension, cardiorenal
  Costen's M26.69
  disseminated mycobacterium avium-
    intracellulare (DMAC) A31.2
  ⇒Eisenmenger's (ventricular septal defect)
    I27.83
  hypersexual F52.8
  jumped process, spine —*see* Dislocation,
    vertebra
  primary, tuberculous A15.7
  Schilder-Addison E71.528
  subluxation (vertebral) M99.19
    abdomen M99.19
    acromioclavicular M99.17
    cervical region M99.11
    cervicothoracic M99.11
    costochondral M99.18
    costovertebral M99.18
    head region M99.10
    hip M99.15
    lower extremity M99.16
    lumbar region M99.13
    lumbosacral M99.13
    occipitocervical M99.10
    pelvic region M99.15
    pubic M99.15

Complex *(Continued)*
  subluxation (vertebral) *(Continued)*
    rib cage M99.18
    sacral region M99.14
    sacrococcygeal M99.14
    sacroiliac M99.14
    specified NEC M99.19
    sternochondral M99.18
    sternoclavicular M99.17
    thoracic region M99.12
    thoracolumbar M99.12
    upper extremity M99.17
  Taussig-Bing (transposition, aorta and
    overriding pulmonary artery) Q20.1
Complication(s) (from) (of)
  accidental puncture or laceration during
    a procedure (of) —*see* Complications,
    intraoperative (intraprocedural),
    puncture or laceration
  amputation stump (surgical) (late) NEC T87.9
    dehiscence T87.81
    infection or inflammation T87.40
      lower limb T87.4-●
      upper limb T87.4-●
    necrosis T87.50
      lower limb T87.5-●
      upper limb T87.5-●
    neuroma T87.30
      lower limb T87.3-●
      upper limb T87.3-●
    specified type NEC T87.89
  anastomosis (and bypass) —*see also*
    Complications, prosthetic device or
    implant
    intestinal (internal) NEC K91.89
      involving urinary tract N99.89
    urinary tract (involving intestinal tract)
      N99.89
    vascular —*see* Complications,
      cardiovascular device or implant
  anesthesia, anesthetic —*see also* Anesthesia,
    complication T88.59
    brain, postpartum, puerperal O89.2
    cardiac
      in
        labor and delivery O74.2
        pregnancy O29.19-●
      postpartum, puerperal O89.1
    central nervous system
      in
        labor and delivery O74.3
        pregnancy O29.29-●
      postpartum, puerperal O89.2
    difficult or failed intubation T88.4
      in pregnancy O29.6-●
    failed sedation (conscious) (moderate)
      during procedure T88.52
    general, unintended awareness during
      procedure T88.53
    hyperthermia, malignant T88.3
    hypothermia T88.51
    intubation failure T88.4
    malignant hyperthermia T88.3
    pulmonary
      in
        labor and delivery O74.1
        pregnancy NEC O29.09-●
      postpartum, puerperal O89.09
    shock T88.2
    spinal and epidural
      in
        labor and delivery NEC O74.6
          headache O74.5
        pregnancy NEC O29.5X-●
      postpartum, puerperal NEC O89.5
        headache O89.4
    unintended awareness under general
      anesthesia during procedure T88.53
  anti-reflux device —*see* Complications,
    esophageal anti-reflux device
  aortic (bifurcation) graft —*see* Complications,
    graft, vascular

Complication *(Continued)*
  aortocoronary (bypass) graft —*see*
    Complications, coronary artery (bypass)
    graft
  aortofemoral (bypass) graft —*see*
    Complications, extremity artery (bypass)
    graft
  arteriovenous
    fistula, surgically created T82.9
      embolism T82.818
      fibrosis T82.828
      hemorrhage T82.838
      infection or inflammation T82.7
      mechanical
        breakdown T82.510
        displacement T82.520
        leakage T82.530
        malposition T82.520
        obstruction T82.590
        perforation T82.590
        protrusion T82.590
      pain T82.848
      specified type NEC T82.898
      stenosis T82.858
      thrombosis T82.868
    shunt, surgically created T82.9
      embolism T82.818
      fibrosis T82.828
      hemorrhage T82.838
      infection or inflammation T82.7
      mechanical
        breakdown T82.511
        displacement T82.521
        leakage T82.531
        malposition T82.521
        obstruction T82.591
        perforation T82.591
        protrusion T82.591
      pain T82.848
      specified type NEC T82.898
      stenosis T82.858
      thrombosis T82.868
  arthroplasty —*see* Complications, joint
    prosthesis
  artificial
    fertilization or insemination N98.9
      attempted introduction (of)
        embryo in embryo transfer N98.3
        ovum following in vitro fertilization
          N98.2
      hyperstimulation of ovaries N98.1
      infection N98.0
      specified NEC N98.8
    heart T82.9
      embolism T82.817
      fibrosis T82.827
      hemorrhage T82.837
      infection or inflammation T82.7
      mechanical
        breakdown T82.512
        displacement T82.522
        leakage T82.532
        malposition T82.522
        obstruction T82.592
        perforation T82.592
        protrusion T82.592
      pain T82.847
      specified type NEC T82.897
      stenosis T82.857
      thrombosis T82.867
    opening
      cecostomy —*see* Complications,
        colostomy
      colostomy —*see* Complications,
        colostomy
      cystostomy —*see* Complications,
        cystostomy
      enterostomy —*see* Complications,
        enterostomy
      gastrostomy —*see* Complications,
        gastrostomy
      ileostomy —*see* Complications,
        enterostomy

Complication *(Continued)*
  artificial *(Continued)*
    opening *(Continued)*
      jejunostomy —*see* Complications,
        enterostomy
      nephrostomy —*see* Complications,
        stoma, urinary tract
      tracheostomy —*see* Complications,
        tracheostomy
      ureterostomy —*see* Complications,
        stoma, urinary tract
      urethrostomy —*see* Complications,
        stoma, urinary tract
  balloon implant or device
    gastrointestinal T85.9
      embolism T85.818
      fibrosis T85.828
      hemorrhage T85.838
      infection and inflammation T85.79
      pain T85.848
      specified type NEC T85.898
      stenosis T85.858
      thrombosis T85.868
    vascular (counterpulsation) T82.9
      embolism T82.818
      fibrosis T82.828
      hemorrhage T82.838
      infection or inflammation T82.7
      mechanical
        breakdown T82.513
        displacement T82.523
        leakage T82.533
        malposition T82.523
        obstruction T82.593
        perforation T82.593
        protrusion T82.593
      pain T82.848
      specified type NEC T82.898
      stenosis T82.858
      thrombosis T82.868
  bariatric procedure
    gastric band procedure K95.09
      infection K95.01
    specified procedure NEC K95.89
      infection K95.81
  bile duct implant (prosthetic) T85.9
    embolism T85.818
    fibrosis T85.828
    hemorrhage T85.838
    infection and inflammation T85.79
    mechanical
      breakdown T85.510
      displacement T85.520
      malfunction T85.510
      malposition T85.520
      obstruction T85.590
      perforation T85.590
      protrusion T85.590
      specified NEC T85.590
    pain T85.848
    specified type NEC T85.898
    stenosis T85.858
    thrombosis T85.868
  bladder device (auxiliary) —*see*
    Complications, genitourinary, device or
    implant, urinary system
  bleeding (postoperative) —*see* Complication,
    postoperative, hemorrhage
    intraoperative —*see* Complication,
      intraoperative, hemorrhage
  blood vessel graft —*see* Complications, graft,
    vascular
  bone
    device NEC T84.9
      embolism T84.81
      fibrosis T84.82
      hemorrhage T84.83
      infection or inflammation T84.7
      mechanical
        breakdown T84.318
        displacement T84.328
        malposition T84.328

▶ New   ⟹ Revised   ~~deleted~~ Deleted   ● Use Additional Character(s)

Complication *(Continued)*
  bone *(Continued)*
    device *(Continued)*
      mechanical *(Continued)*
        obstruction T84.398
        perforation T84.398
        protrusion T84.398
      pain T84.84
      specified type NEC T84.89
      stenosis T84.85
      thrombosis T84.86
    graft —*see* Complications, graft, bone
    growth stimulator (electrode) —*see*
      Complications, electronic stimulator
      device, bone
    marrow transplant —*see* Complications,
      transplant, bone, marrow
  brain neurostimulator (electrode) —*see*
    Complications, electronic stimulator
    device, brain
  breast implant (prosthetic) T85.9
    capsular contracture T85.44
    embolism T85.818
    fibrosis T85.828
    hemorrhage T85.838
    infection and inflammation T85.79
    mechanical
      breakdown T85.41
      displacement T85.42
      leakage T85.43
      malposition T85.42
      obstruction T85.49
      perforation T85.49
      protrusion T85.49
      specified NEC T85.49
    pain T85.848
    specified type NEC T85.898
    stenosis T85.858
    thrombosis T85.868
  bypass —*see also* Complications, prosthetic
    device or implant
    aortocoronary —*see* Complications,
      coronary artery (bypass) graft
    arterial —*see also* Complications, graft,
      vascular
      extremity —*see* Complications, extremity
        artery (bypass) graft
  cardiac —*see also* Disease, heart
    device, implant or graft T82.9
      embolism T82.817
      fibrosis T82.827
      hemorrhage T82.837
      infection or inflammation T82.7
        valve prosthesis T82.6
      mechanical
        breakdown T82.519
          specified device NEC T82.518
        displacement T82.529
          specified device NEC T82.528
        leakage T82.539
          specified device NEC T82.538
        malposition T82.529
          specified device NEC T82.528
        obstruction T82.599
          specified device NEC T82.598
        perforation T82.599
          specified device NEC T82.598
        protrusion T82.599
          specified device NEC T82.598
      pain T82.847
      specified type NEC T82.897
      stenosis T82.857
      thrombosis T82.867
  cardiovascular device, graft or implant T82.9
    aortic graft —*see* Complications, graft,
      vascular
    arteriovenous
      fistula, artificial —*see* Complication,
        arteriovenous, fistula, surgically
        created
      shunt —*see* Complication, arteriovenous,
        shunt, surgically created

Complication *(Continued)*
  cardiovascular device, graft or implant
    (Continued)
    artificial heart —*see* Complication,
      artificial, heart
    balloon (counterpulsation) device —*see*
      Complication, balloon implant,
      vascular
    carotid artery graft —*see* Complications,
      graft, vascular
    coronary bypass graft —*see* Complication,
      coronary artery (bypass) graft
    dialysis catheter (vascular) —*see*
      Complication, catheter, dialysis
    electronic T82.9
      electrode T82.9
        embolism T82.817
        fibrosis T82.827
        hemorrhage T82.837
        infection T82.7
        mechanical
          breakdown T82.110
          displacement T82.120
          leakage T82.190
          obstruction T82.190
          perforation T82.190
          protrusion T82.190
          specified type NEC T82.190
        pain T82.847
        specified NEC T82.897
        stenosis T82.857
        thrombosis T82.867
      embolism T82.817
      fibrosis T82.827
      hemorrhage T82.837
      infection T82.7
      mechanical
        breakdown T82.119
        displacement T82.129
        leakage T82.199
        obstruction T82.199
        perforation T82.199
        protrusion T82.199
        specified type NEC T82.199
      pain T82.847
      pulse generator T82.9
        embolism T82.817
        fibrosis T82.827
        hemorrhage T82.837
        infection T82.7
        mechanical
          breakdown T82.111
          displacement T82.121
          leakage T82.191
          obstruction T82.191
          perforation T82.191
          protrusion T82.191
          specified type NEC T82.191
        pain T82.847
        specified NEC T82.897
        stenosis T82.857
        thrombosis T82.867
      specified condition NEC T82.897
      specified device NEC T82.9
        embolism T82.817
        fibrosis T82.827
        hemorrhage T82.837
        infection T82.7
        mechanical
          breakdown T82.118
          displacement T82.128
          leakage T82.198
          obstruction T82.198
          perforation T82.198
          protrusion T82.198
          specified type NEC T82.198
        pain T82.847
        specified NEC T82.897
        stenosis T82.857
        thrombosis T82.867
      stenosis T82.857
      thrombosis T82.867

Complication *(Continued)*
  cardiovascular device, graft or implant
    (Continued)
    extremity artery graft —*see* Complication,
      extremity artery (bypass) graft
    femoral artery graft —*see* Complication,
      extremity artery (bypass) graft
    heart
      transplant —*see* Complication,
        transplant, heart
      valve —*see* Complication, prosthetic
        device, heart valve
        graft —*see* Complication, heart, valve,
          graft
    heart-lung transplant —*see* Complication,
      transplant, heart, with lung
    infection or inflammation T82.7
    umbrella device —*see* Complication,
      umbrella device, vascular
    vascular graft (or anastomosis) —*see*
      Complication, graft, vascular
  carotid artery (bypass) graft —*see*
    Complications, graft, vascular
  catheter (device) NEC —*see also*
    Complications, prosthetic device or
    implant
    cranial infusion
      infection and inflammation T85.735
      mechanical
        breakdown T85.610
        displacement T85.620
        leakage T85.630
        malfunction T85.690
        malposition T85.620
        obstruction T85.690
        perforation T85.690
        protrusion T85.690
        specified NEC T85.690
    cystostomy T83.9
      embolism T83.81
      fibrosis T83.82
      hemorrhage T83.83
      infection and inflammation T83.510
      mechanical
        breakdown T83.010
        displacement T83.020
        leakage T83.030
        malposition T83.020
        obstruction T83.090
        perforation T83.090
        protrusion T83.090
        specified NEC T83.090
      pain T83.84
      specified type NEC T83.89
      stenosis T83.85
      thrombosis T83.86
    dialysis (vascular) T82.9
      embolism T82.818
      fibrosis T82.828
      hemorrhage T82.838
      infection and inflammation T82.7
      intraperitoneal —*see* Complications,
        catheter, intraperitoneal
      mechanical
        breakdown T82.41
        displacement T82.42
        leakage T82.43
        malposition T82.42
        obstruction T82.49
        perforation T82.49
        protrusion T82.49
      pain T82.848
      specified type NEC T82.898
      stenosis T82.858
      thrombosis T82.868
    epidural infusion T85.9
      embolism T85.810
      fibrosis T85.820
      hemorrhage T85.830
      infection and inflammation T85.735
      mechanical
        breakdown T85.610
        displacement T85.620

Complication (Continued)
  catheter NEC (Continued)
    epidural infusion (Continued)
      mechanical (Continued)
        leakage T85.630
        malfunction T85.610
        malposition T85.620
        obstruction T85.690
        perforation T85.690
        protrusion T85.690
        specified NEC T85.690
      pain T85.840
      specified type NEC T85.890
      stenosis T85.850
      thrombosis T85.860
    intraperitoneal dialysis T85.9
      embolism T85.818
      fibrosis T85.828
      hemorrhage T85.838
      infection and inflammation T85.71
      mechanical
        breakdown T85.611
        displacement T85.621
        leakage T85.631
        malfunction T85.611
        malposition T85.621
        obstruction T85.691
        perforation T85.691
        protrusion T85.691
        specified NEC T85.691
      pain T85.848
      specified type NEC T85.898
      stenosis T85.858
      thrombosis T85.868
    intrathecal infusion
      infection and inflammation T85.735
      mechanical
        breakdown T85.610
        displacement T85.620
        leakage T85.630
        malfunction T85.690
        malposition T85.620
        obstruction T85.690
        perforation T85.690
        protrusion T85.690
        specified NEC T85.690
    intravenous infusion T82.9
      embolism T82.818
      fibrosis T82.828
      hemorrhage T82.838
      infection or inflammation T82.7
      mechanical
        breakdown T82.514
        displacement T82.524
        leakage T82.534
        malposition T82.524
        obstruction T82.594
        perforation T82.594
        protrusion T82.594
      pain T82.848
      specified type NEC T82.898
      stenosis T82.858
      thrombosis T82.868
    spinal infusion
      infection and inflammation T85.735
      mechanical
        breakdown T85.610
        displacement T85.620
        leakage T85.630
        malfunction T85.690
        malposition T85.620
        obstruction T85.690
        perforation T85.690
        protrusion T85.690
        specified NEC T85.690
    subarachnoid infusion
      infection and inflammation
        T85.735
      mechanical
        breakdown T85.610
        displacement T85.620

Complication (Continued)
  catheter NEC (Continued)
    subarachnoid infusion (Continued)
      mechanical (Continued)
        leakage T85.630
        malfunction T85.690
        malposition T85.620
        obstruction T85.690
        perforation T85.690
        protrusion T85.690
        specified NEC T85.690
    subdural infusion T85.9
      embolism T85.810
      fibrosis T85.820
      hemorrhage T85.830
      infection and inflammation T85.735
      mechanical
        breakdown T85.610
        displacement T85.620
        leakage T85.630
        malfunction T85.610
        malposition T85.620
        obstruction T85.690
        perforation T85.690
        protrusion T85.690
        specified NEC T85.690
      pain T85.840
      specified type NEC T85.890
      stenosis T85.850
      thrombosis T85.860
    urethral T83.9
      displacement T83.028
      embolism T83.81
      fibrosis T83.82
      hemorrhage T83.83
      indwelling
        breakdown T83.011
        displacement T83.021
        infection and inflammation
          T83.511
        leakage T83.031
        specified complication NEC
          T83.091
      infection and inflammation
        T83.511
      leakage T83.038
      malposition T83.028
      mechanical
        breakdown T83.011
      obstruction (mechanical) T83.091
      pain T83.84
      perforation T83.091
      protrusion T83.091
      specified type NEC T83.091
      stenosis T83.85
      thrombosis T83.86
    urinary NEC
      breakdown T83.018
      displacement T83.028
      infection and inflammation T83.518
      leakage T83.038
      specified complication NEC T83.098
  cecostomy (stoma) —see Complications,
      colostomy
  cesarean delivery wound NEC O90.89
    disruption O90.0
    hematoma O90.2
    infection (following delivery) O86.0
  chemotherapy (antineoplastic) NEC T88.7
  chin implant (prosthetic) —see Complication,
      prosthetic device or implant, specified
      NEC
  circulatory system I99.8
    intraoperative I97.88
    postprocedural I97.89
    ⟼following cardiac surgery —see also
        Infarct, myocardium, associated
        with revascularization procedure
        I97.19-●
      postcardiotomy syndrome I97.0
    hypertension I97.3
    lymphedema after mastectomy I97.2

Complication (Continued)
  circulatory system (Continued)
    postprocedural (Continued)
      postcardiotomy syndrome I97.0
      specified NEC I97.89
  colostomy (stoma) K94.00
    hemorrhage K94.01
    infection K94.02
    malfunction K94.03
    mechanical K94.03
    specified complication NEC K94.09
  contraceptive device, intrauterine —
      see Complications, intrauterine,
      contraceptive device
  cord (umbilical) —see Complications,
      umbilical cord
  corneal graft —see Complications, graft, cornea
  coronary artery (bypass) graft T82.9
    atherosclerosis —see Arteriosclerosis,
        coronary (artery)
    embolism T82.818
    fibrosis T82.828
    hemorrhage T82.838
    infection and inflammation T82.7
    mechanical
      breakdown T82.211
      displacement T82.212
      leakage T82.213
      malposition T82.212
      obstruction T82.218
      perforation T82.218
      protrusion T82.218
      specified NEC T82.218
    pain T82.848
    specified type NEC T82.898
    stenosis T82.858
    thrombosis T82.868
  counterpulsation device (balloon), intra-
      aortic —see Complications, balloon
      implant, vascular
  cystostomy (stoma) N99.518
    catheter —see Complications, catheter,
        cystostomy
    hemorrhage N99.510
    infection N99.511
    malfunction N99.512
    specified type NEC N99.518
  delivery —see also Complications, obstetric
      O75.9
    procedure (instrumental) (manual)
        (surgical) O75.4
    specified NEC O75.89
  dialysis (peritoneal) (renal) —see also
      Complications, infusion
    catheter (vascular) —see Complication,
        catheter, dialysis
    peritoneal, intraperitoneal —see
        Complications, catheter,
        intraperitoneal
  dorsal column (spinal) neurostimulator —see
      Complications, electronic stimulator
      device, spinal cord
  drug NEC T88.7
  ear procedure —see also Disorder, ear
    intraoperative H95.88-●
      hematoma —see Complications,
          intraoperative, hematoma (of), ear
      hemorrhage —see Complications,
          intraoperative, hemorrhage (of), ear
      laceration —see Complications,
          intraoperative, puncture or
          laceration..., ear
      seroma —see Complications,
          postprocedural, seroma (of),
          mastoid process
      specified NEC H95.88-●
    postoperative H95.89-●
      external ear canal stenosis H95.81-●
      hematoma —see Complications,
          postprocedural, hemorrhage
          (hematoma) (of), ear

▶ New   ⟼ Revised   ~~deleted~~ Deleted   ● Use Additional Character(s)

Complication *(Continued)*
ear procedure *(Continued)*
postoperative *(Continued)*
hemorrhage —*see* Complications, postprocedural, hemorrhage (hematoma) (of), ear
postmastoidectomy —*see* Complications, postmastoidectomy
specified NEC H95.89-•
ectopic pregnancy O08.9
damage to pelvic organs O08.6
embolism O08.2
genital infection O08.0
hemorrhage (delayed) (excessive) O08.1
metabolic disorder O08.5
renal failure O08.4
shock O08.3
specified type NEC O08.0
venous complication NEC O08.7
electronic stimulator device
bladder (urinary) —*see* Complications, electronic stimulator device, urinary
bone T84.9
breakdown T84.310
displacement T84.320
embolism T84.81
fibrosis T84.82
hemorrhage T84.83
infection or inflammation T84.7
malfunction T84.310
malposition T84.320
mechanical NEC T84.390
obstruction T84.390
pain T84.84
perforation T84.390
protrusion T84.390
specified type NEC T84.89
stenosis T84.85
thrombosis T84.86
brain T85.9
embolism T85.810
fibrosis T85.820
hemorrhage T85.830
infection and inflammation T85.731
mechanical
breakdown T85.110
displacement T85.120
leakage T85.190
malposition T85.120
obstruction T85.190
perforation T85.190
protrusion T85.190
specified NEC T85.190
pain T85.840
specified type NEC T85.890
stenosis T85.850
thrombosis T85.860
cardiac (defibrillator) (pacemaker) —*see* Complications, cardiovascular device or implant, electronic
generator (brain) (gastric) (peripheral) (sacral) (spinal)
breakdown T85.113
displacement T85.123
leakage T85.193
malposition T85.123
obstruction T85.193
perforation T85.193
protrusion T85.193
specified type NEC T85.193
muscle T84.9
breakdown T84.418
displacement T84.428
embolism T84.81
fibrosis T84.82
hemorrhage T84.83
infection or inflammation T84.7
mechanical NEC T84.498
pain T84.84
specified type NEC T84.89
stenosis T84.85
thrombosis T84.86

Complication *(Continued)*
electronic stimulator device *(Continued)*
nervous system T85.9
brain —*see* Complications, electronic stimulator device, brain
cranial nerve —*see* Complications, electronic stimulator device, peripheral nerve
embolism T85.810
fibrosis T85.820
gastric nerve —*see* Complications, electronic stimulator device, peripheral nerve
hemorrhage T85.830
infection and inflammation T85.738
mechanical
breakdown T85.118
displacement T85.128
leakage T85.199
malposition T85.128
obstruction T85.199
perforation T85.199
protrusion T85.199
specified NEC T85.199
pain T85.840
peripheral nerve —*see* Complications, electronic stimulator device, peripheral nerve
sacral nerve —*see* Complications, electronic stimulator device, peripheral nerve
specified type NEC T85.890
spinal cord —*see* Complications, electronic stimulator device, spinal cord
stenosis T85.850
thrombosis T85.860
vagal nerve —*see* Complications, electronic stimulator device, peripheral nerve
peripheral nerve T85.9
embolism T85.810
fibrosis T85.820
hemorrhage T85.830
infection and inflammation T85.732
mechanical
breakdown T85.111
displacement T85.121
leakage T85.191
malposition T85.121
obstruction T85.191
perforation T85.191
protrusion T85.191
specified NEC T85.191
pain T85.840
specified type NEC T85.890
stenosis T85.850
thrombosis T85.860
spinal cord T85.9
embolism T85.810
fibrosis T85.820
hemorrhage T85.830
infection and inflammation T85.733
mechanical
breakdown T85.112
displacement T85.122
leakage T85.192
malposition T85.122
obstruction T85.192
perforation T85.192
protrusion T85.192
specified NEC T85.192
pain T85.840
specified type NEC T85.890
stenosis T85.850
thrombosis T85.860
urinary T83.9
embolism T83.81
fibrosis T83.82
hemorrhage T83.83
infection and inflammation T83.598

Complication *(Continued)*
electronic stimulator device *(Continued)*
urinary *(Continued)*
mechanical
breakdown T83.110
displacement T83.120
malposition T83.120
perforation T83.190
protrusion T83.190
specified NEC T83.190
pain T83.84
specified type NEC T83.89
stenosis T83.85
thrombosis T83.86
electroshock therapy T88.9
specified NEC T88.8
endocrine E34.9
postprocedural
adrenal hypofunction E89.6
hypoinsulinemia E89.1
hypoparathyroidism E89.2
hypopituitarism E89.3
hypothyroidism E89.0
ovarian failure E89.40
asymptomatic E89.40
symptomatic E89.41
specified NEC E89.89
testicular hypofunction E89.5
endodontic treatment NEC M27.59
enterostomy (stoma) K94.10
hemorrhage K94.11
infection K94.12
malfunction K94.13
mechanical K94.13
specified complication NEC K94.19
episiotomy, disruption O90.1
esophageal anti-reflux device T85.9
embolism T85.818
fibrosis T85.828
hemorrhage T85.838
infection and inflammation T85.79
mechanical
breakdown T85.511
displacement T85.521
malfunction T85.511
malposition T85.521
obstruction T85.591
perforation T85.591
protrusion T85.591
specified NEC T85.591
pain T85.848
specified type NEC T85.898
stenosis T85.858
thrombosis T85.868
esophagostomy K94.30
hemorrhage K94.31
infection K94.32
malfunction K94.33
mechanical K94.33
specified complication NEC K94.39
extracorporeal circulation T80.90
extremity artery (bypass) graft T82.9
arteriosclerosis —*see* Arteriosclerosis, extremities, bypass graft
embolism T82.818
fibrosis T82.828
hemorrhage T82.838
infection and inflammation T82.7
mechanical
breakdown T82.318
femoral artery T82.312
displacement T82.328
femoral artery T82.322
leakage T82.338
femoral artery T82.332
malposition T82.328
femoral artery T82.322
obstruction T82.398
femoral artery T82.392
perforation T82.398
femoral artery T82.392
protrusion T82.398
femoral artery T82.392

Complication (Continued)

extremity artery (bypass) graft (Continued)
- pain T82.848
- specified type NEC T82.898
- stenosis T82.858
- thrombosis T82.868

eye H57.9
- corneal graft —see Complications, graft, cornea
- implant (prosthetic) T85.9
  - embolism T85.818
  - fibrosis T85.828
  - hemorrhage T85.838
  - infection and inflammation T85.79
  - mechanical
    - breakdown T85.318
    - displacement T85.328
    - leakage T85.398
    - malposition T85.328
    - obstruction T85.398
    - perforation T85.398
    - protrusion T85.398
    - specified NEC T85.398
  - pain T85.848
  - specified type NEC T85.898
  - stenosis T85.858
  - thrombosis T85.868
- intraocular lens —see Complications, intraocular lens
- orbital prosthesis —see Complications, orbital prosthesis

female genital N94.9
- device, implant or graft NEC —see Complications, genitourinary, device or implant, genital tract

femoral artery (bypass) graft —see Complication, extremity artery (bypass) graft

fixation device, internal (orthopedic) T84.9
- infection and inflammation T84.60
  - arm T84.61-●
    - humerus T84.61-●
    - radius T84.61-●
    - ulna T84.61-●
  - leg T84.629
    - femur T84.62-●
    - fibula T84.62-●
    - tibia T84.62-●
  - specified site NEC T84.69
  - spine T84.63
- mechanical
  - breakdown
    - limb T84.119
      - carpal T84.210
      - femur T84.11-●
      - fibula T84.11-●
      - humerus T84.11-●
      - metacarpal T84.210
      - metatarsal T84.213
      - phalanx
        - foot T84.213
        - hand T84.210
      - radius T84.11-●
      - tarsal T84.213
      - tibia T84.11-●
      - ulna T84.11-●
    - specified bone NEC T84.218
    - spine T84.216
  - displacement
    - limb T84.129
      - carpal T84.220
      - femur T84.12-●
      - fibula T84.12-●
      - humerus T84.12-●
      - metacarpal T84.220
      - metatarsal T84.223
      - phalanx
        - foot T84.223
        - hand T84.220
      - radius T84.12-●
      - tarsal T84.223

Complication (Continued)

fixation device, internal (Continued)
- mechanical (Continued)
  - displacement (Continued)
    - limb (Continued)
      - tibia T84.12-●
      - ulna T84.12-●
    - specified bone NEC T84.228
    - spine T84.226
  - malposition —see Complications, fixation device, internal, mechanical, displacement
  - obstruction —see Complications, fixation device, internal, mechanical, specified type NEC
  - perforation —see Complications, fixation device, internal, mechanical, specified type NEC
  - protrusion —see Complications, fixation device, internal, mechanical, specified type NEC
  - specified type NEC
    - limb T84.199
      - carpal T84.290
      - femur T84.19-●
      - fibula T84.19-●
      - humerus T84.19-●
      - metacarpal T84.290
      - metatarsal T84.293
      - phalanx
        - foot T84.293
        - hand T84.290
      - radius T84.19-●
      - tarsal T84.293
      - tibia T84.19-●
      - ulna T84.19-●
    - specified bone NEC T84.298
    - vertebra T84.296
- specified type NEC T84.89
  - embolism T84.81
  - fibrosis T84.82
  - hemorrhage T84.83
  - pain T84.84
  - specified complication NEC T84.89
  - stenosis T84.85
  - thrombosis T84.86

following
- acute myocardial infarction NEC I23.8
  - aneurysm (false) (of cardiac wall) (of heart wall) (ruptured) I23.3
  - angina I23.7
  - atrial
    - septal defect I23.1
    - thrombosis I23.6
  - cardiac wall rupture I23.3
  - chordae tendinae rupture I23.4
  - defect
    - septal
      - atrial (heart) I23.1
      - ventricular (heart) I23.2
  - hemopericardium I23.0
  - papillary muscle rupture I23.5
  - rupture
    - cardiac wall I23.3
      - with hemopericardium I23.0
    - chordae tendineae I23.4
    - papillary muscle I23.5
  - specified NEC I23.8
  - thrombosis
    - atrium I23.6
    - auricular appendage I23.6
    - ventricle (heart) I23.6
  - ventricular
    - septal defect I23.2
    - thrombosis I23.6
- ectopic or molar pregnancy O08.9
  - cardiac arrest O08.81
  - sepsis O08.82
  - specified type NEC O08.89
  - urinary tract infection O08.83
- termination of pregnancy —see Abortion

Complication (Continued)

gastrointestinal K92.9
- bile duct prosthesis —see Complications, bile duct implant
- esophageal anti-reflux device —see Complications, esophageal anti-reflux device
- postoperative
  - colostomy —see Complications, colostomy
  - dumping syndrome K91.1
  - enterostomy —see Complications, enterostomy
  - gastrostomy —see Complications, gastrostomy
  - malabsorption NEC K91.2
  - ➡obstruction —see also Obstruction, intestine, postoperative K91.30
  - postcholecystectomy syndrome K91.5
  - specified NEC K91.89
  - vomiting after GI surgery K91.0
- prosthetic device or implant
  - bile duct prosthesis —see Complications, bile duct implant
  - esophageal anti-reflux device —see Complications, esophageal anti-reflux device
  - specified type NEC
    - embolism T85.818
    - fibrosis T85.828
    - hemorrhage T85.838
    - mechanical
      - breakdown T85.518
      - displacement T85.528
      - malfunction T85.518
      - malposition T85.528
      - obstruction T85.598
      - perforation T85.598
      - protrusion T85.598
      - specified NEC T85.598
    - pain T85.848
    - specified complication NEC T85.898
    - stenosis T85.858
    - thrombosis T85.868

gastrostomy (stoma) K94.20
- hemorrhage K94.21
- infection K94.22
- malfunction K94.23
- mechanical K94.23
- specified complication NEC K94.29

genitourinary
- device or implant T83.9
  - genital tract T83.9
    - infection or inflammation T83.69
    - intrauterine contraceptive device —see Complications, intrauterine, contraceptive device
    - mechanical —see Complications, by device, mechanical
    - mesh —see Complications, mesh
    - penile prosthesis —see Complications, prosthetic device, penile
    - specified type NEC T83.89
      - embolism T83.81
      - fibrosis T83.82
      - hemorrhage T83.83
      - pain T83.84
      - specified complication NEC T83.89
      - stenosis T83.85
      - thrombosis T83.86
    - vaginal mesh —see Complications, mesh
  - urinary system T83.9
    - cystostomy catheter —see Complication, catheter, cystostomy
    - electronic stimulator —see Complications, electronic stimulator device, urinary
    - indwelling urethral catheter —see Complications, catheter, urethral, indwelling

▶ New   ➡ Revised   ~~deleted~~ Deleted   ● Use Additional Character(s)

Complication (Continued)
  genitourinary (Continued)
    device or implant (Continued)
      urinary system (Continued)
        infection or inflammation T83.598
          indwelling urethral catheter
            T83.511
        kidney transplant —see Complication,
          transplant, kidney
        organ graft —see Complication, graft,
          urinary organ
        specified type NEC T83.89
          embolism T83.81
          fibrosis T83.82
          hemorrhage T83.83
          mechanical T83.198
            breakdown T83.118
            displacement T83.128
            malfunction T83.118
            malposition T83.128
            obstruction T83.198
            perforation T83.198
            protrusion T83.198
            specified NEC T83.198
          sphincter, implanted T83.191
          stent (ileal conduit) (nephroureteral)
            T83.193
            ureteral indwelling T83.192
          pain T83.84
          specified complication NEC
            T83.89
          stenosis T83.85
          thrombosis T83.86
        sphincter implant —see
          Complications, implant, urinary
          sphincter
    postprocedural
      pelvic peritoneal adhesions N99.4
      renal failure N99.0
      specified NEC N99.89
      stoma —see Complications, stoma,
        urinary tract
      urethral stricture —see Stricture, urethra,
        postprocedural
      vaginal
        adhesions N99.2
        vault prolapse N99.3
  graft (bypass) (patch) —see also
    Complications, prosthetic device or
    implant
    aorta —see Complications, graft, vascular
    arterial —see Complication, graft,
      vascular
    bone T86.839
      failure T86.831
      infection T86.832
      mechanical T84.318
        breakdown T84.318
        displacement T84.328
        protrusion T84.398
        specified type NEC T84.398
      rejection T86.830
      specified type NEC T86.838
    carotid artery —see Complications, graft,
      vascular
    cornea T86.849
      failure T86.841
      infection T86.842
      mechanical T85.398
        breakdown T85.318
        displacement T85.328
        protrusion T85.398
        specified type NEC T85.398
      rejection T86.840
      retroprosthetic membrane T85.398
      specified type NEC T86.848
    femoral artery (bypass) —see Complication,
      extremity artery (bypass) graft
    genital organ or tract —see Complications,
      genitourinary, device or implant,
      genital tract

Complication (Continued)
  graft (Continued)
    muscle T84.9
      breakdown T84.410
      displacement T84.420
      embolism T84.81
      fibrosis T84.82
      hemorrhage T84.83
      infection and inflammation
        T84.7
      mechanical NEC T84.490
      pain T84.84
      specified type NEC T84.89
      stenosis T84.85
      thrombosis T84.86
    nerve —see Complication, prosthetic device
      or implant, specified NEC
    skin —see Complications, prosthetic device
      or implant, skin graft
    tendon T84.9
      breakdown T84.410
      displacement T84.420
      embolism T84.81
      fibrosis T84.82
      hemorrhage T84.83
      infection and inflammation T84.7
      mechanical NEC T84.490
      pain T84.84
      specified type NEC T84.89
      stenosis T84.85
      thrombosis T84.86
    urinary organ T83.9
      embolism T83.81
      fibrosis T83.82
      hemorrhage T83.83
      infection and inflammation
        T83.598
        indwelling urethral catheter
          T83.511
      mechanical
        breakdown T83.21
        displacement T83.22
        erosion T83.24
        exposure T83.25
        leakage T83.23
        malposition T83.22
        obstruction T83.29
        perforation T83.29
        protrusion T83.29
        specified NEC T83.29
      pain T83.84
      specified type NEC T83.89
      stenosis T83.85
      thrombosis T83.86
    vascular T82.9
      embolism T82.818
      femoral artery —see Complication,
        extremity artery (bypass) graft
      fibrosis T82.828
      hemorrhage T82.838
      mechanical
        breakdown T82.319
          aorta (bifurcation) T82.310
          carotid artery T82.311
          specified vessel NEC T82.318
        displacement T82.329
          aorta (bifurcation) T82.320
          carotid artery T82.321
          specified vessel NEC T82.328
        leakage T82.339
          aorta (bifurcation) T82.330
          carotid artery T82.331
          specified vessel NEC T82.338
        malposition T82.329
          aorta (bifurcation) T82.320
          carotid artery T82.321
          specified vessel NEC T82.328
        obstruction T82.399
          aorta (bifurcation) T82.390
          carotid artery T82.391
          specified vessel NEC T82.398

Complication (Continued)
  graft (Continued)
    vascular (Continued)
      mechanical (Continued)
        perforation T82.399
          aorta (bifurcation) T82.390
          carotid artery T82.391
          specified vessel NEC T82.398
        protrusion T82.399
          aorta (bifurcation) T82.390
          carotid artery T82.391
          specified vessel NEC T82.398
      pain T82.848
      specified complication NEC
        T82.898
      stenosis T82.858
      thrombosis T82.868
  heart I51.9
    assist device
      infection and inflammation T82.7
    following acute myocardial infarction —
      see Complications, following, acute
      myocardial infarction
    postoperative —see Complications,
      circulatory system
    transplant —see Complication, transplant,
      heart
      and lung(s) —see Complications,
        transplant, heart, with lung
    valve
      graft (biological) T82.9
        embolism T82.817
        fibrosis T82.827
        hemorrhage T82.837
        infection and inflammation T82.7
        mechanical T82.228
          breakdown T82.221
          displacement T82.222
          leakage T82.223
          malposition T82.222
          obstruction T82.228
          perforation T82.228
          protrusion T82.228
        pain T82.847
        specified type NEC T82.897
        stenosis T82.857
        thrombosis T82.867
      prosthesis T82.9
        embolism T82.817
        fibrosis T82.827
        hemorrhage T82.837
        infection or inflammation T82.6
        mechanical T82.09
          breakdown T82.01
          displacement T82.02
          leakage T82.03
          malposition T82.02
          obstruction T82.09
          perforation T82.09
          protrusion T82.09
        pain T82.847
        specified type NEC T82.897
          mechanical T82.09
        stenosis T82.857
        thrombosis T82.867
  hematoma
    intraoperative —see Complication,
      intraoperative, hemorrhage
    postprocedural —see Complication,
      postprocedural, hematoma
  hemodialysis —see Complications,
    dialysis
  hemorrhage
    intraoperative —see Complication,
      intraoperative, hemorrhage
    postprocedural —see Complication,
      postprocedural, hemorrhage
  ileostomy (stoma) —see Complications,
    enterostomy
  immunization (procedure) —see
    Complications, vaccination

Complication *(Continued)*
  implant —*see also* Complications, by site and type
    urinary sphincter T83.9
      embolism T83.81
      fibrosis T83.82
      hemorrhage T83.83
      infection and inflammation T83.591
      mechanical
        breakdown T83.111
        displacement T83.121
        leakage T83.191
        malposition T83.121
        obstruction T83.191
        perforation T83.191
        protrusion T83.191
        specified NEC T83.191
      pain T83.84
      specified type NEC T83.89
      stenosis T83.85
      thrombosis T83.86
  infusion (procedure) T80.90
    air embolism T80.0
    blood —*see* Complications, transfusion
    catheter —*see* Complications, catheter
    infection T80.29
    pump —*see* Complications, cardiovascular, device or implant
    sepsis T80.29
    serum reaction —*see also* Reaction, serum T80.69
      anaphylactic shock —*see also* Shock, anaphylactic T80.59
    specified type NEC T80.89
  inhalation therapy NEC T81.81
  injection (procedure) T80.90
    drug reaction —*see* Reaction, drug
    infection T80.29
    sepsis T80.29
    serum (prophylactic) (therapeutic) —*see* Complications, vaccination
    specified type NEC T80.89
    vaccine (any) —*see* Complications, vaccination
  inoculation (any) —*see* Complications, vaccination
  insulin pump
    infection and inflammation T85.72
    mechanical
      breakdown T85.614
      displacement T85.624
      leakage T85.633
      malposition T85.624
      obstruction T85.694
      perforation T85.694
      protrusion T85.694
      specified NEC T85.694
  intestinal pouch NEC K91.858
  intraocular lens (prosthetic) T85.9
    embolism T85.818
    fibrosis T85.828
    hemorrhage T85.838
    infection and inflammation T85.79
    mechanical
      breakdown T85.21
      displacement T85.22
      malposition T85.22
      obstruction T85.29
      perforation T85.29
      protrusion T85.29
      specified NEC T85.29
    pain T85.848
    specified type NEC T85.898
    stenosis T85.858
    thrombosis T85.868
  intraoperative (intraprocedural)
    cardiac arrest —*see also* Infarct, myocardium, associated with revascularization procedure
      during cardiac surgery I97.710
      during other surgery I97.711

Complication *(Continued)*
  intraoperative (intraprocedural) *(Continued)*
    cardiac functional disturbance NEC —*see also* Infarct, myocardium, associated with revascularization procedure
      during cardiac surgery I97.790
      during other surgery I97.791
    hemorrhage (hematoma) (of)
      circulatory system organ or structure
        during cardiac bypass I97.411
        during cardiac catheterization I97.410
        during other circulatory system procedure I97.418
        during other procedure I97.42
      digestive system organ
        during procedure on digestive system K91.61
        during procedure on other organ K91.62
      ear
        during procedure on ear and mastoid process H95.21
        during procedure on other organ H95.22
      endocrine system organ or structure
        during procedure on endocrine system organ or structure E36.01
        during procedure on other organ E36.02
      eye and adnexa
        during ophthalmic procedure H59.11-•
        during other procedure H59.12-•
      genitourinary organ or structure
        during procedure on genitourinary organ or structure N99.61
        during procedure on other organ N99.62
      mastoid process
        during procedure on ear and mastoid process H95.21
        during procedure on other organ H95.22
      musculoskeletal structure
        during musculoskeletal surgery M96.810
        during non-orthopedic surgery M96.811
        during orthopedic surgery M96.810
      nervous system
        during a nervous system procedure G97.31
        during other procedure G97.32
      respiratory system
        during other procedure J95.62
        during procedure on respiratory system organ or structure J95.61
      skin and subcutaneous tissue
        during a dermatologic procedure L76.01
        during a procedure on other organ L76.02
      spleen
        during a procedure on other organ D78.02
        during a procedure on the spleen D78.01
    puncture or laceration (accidental) (unintentional) (of)
    brain
      during a nervous system procedure G97.48
      during other procedure G97.49
    circulatory system organ or structure
      during circulatory system procedure I97.51
      during other procedure I97.52
    digestive system
      during procedure on digestive system K91.71
      during procedure on other organ K91.72

Complication *(Continued)*
  intraoperative *(Continued)*
    puncture or laceration *(Continued)*
      ear
        during procedure on ear and mastoid process H95.31
        during procedure on other organ H95.32
      endocrine system organ or structure
        during procedure on endocrine system organ or structure E36.11
        during procedure on other organ E36.12
      eye and adnexa
        during ophthalmic procedure H59.21-•
        during other procedure H59.22-•
      genitourinary organ or structure
        during procedure on genitourinary organ or structure N99.71
        during procedure on other organ N99.72
      mastoid process
        during procedure on ear and mastoid process H95.31
        during procedure on other organ H95.32
      musculoskeletal structure
        during musculoskeletal surgery M96.820
        during non-orthopedic surgery M96.821
        during orthopedic surgery M96.820
      nervous system
        during a nervous system procedure G97.48
        during other procedure G97.49
      respiratory system
        during other procedure J95.72
        during procedure on respiratory system organ or structure J95.71
      skin and subcutaneous tissue
        during a dermatologic procedure L76.11
        during a procedure on other organ L76.12
      spleen
        during a procedure on other organ D78.12
        during a procedure on the spleen D78.11
    specified NEC
      circulatory system I97.88
      digestive system K91.81
      ear H95.88
      endocrine system E36.8
      eye and adnexa H59.88
      genitourinary system N99.81
      mastoid process H95.88
      musculoskeletal structure M96.89
      nervous system G97.81
      respiratory system J95.88
      skin and subcutaneous tissue L76.81
      spleen D78.81
  intraperitoneal catheter (dialysis) (infusion) —*see* Complications, catheter, intraperitoneal
  intrathecal infusion pump
    infection and inflammation T85.738
    mechanical
      breakdown T85.615
      displacement T85.625
      leakage T85.635
      malfunction T85.695
      malposition T85.625
      obstruction T85.695
      perforation T85.695
      protrusion T85.695
      specified NEC T85.695

Complication *(Continued)*
  intrauterine
    contraceptive device
      embolism T83.81
      fibrosis T83.82
      hemorrhage T83.83
      infection and inflammation T83.69
      mechanical
        breakdown T83.31
        displacement T83.32
        malposition T83.32
        obstruction T83.39
        perforation T83.39
        protrusion T83.39
        specified NEC T83.39
      pain T83.84
      specified type NEC T83.89
      stenosis T83.85
      thrombosis T83.86
    procedure (fetal), to newborn P96.5
  jejunostomy (stoma) —*see* Complications,
      enterostomy
  joint prosthesis, internal T84.9
    breakage (fracture) T84.01-●
    dislocation T84.02-●
    fracture T84.01-●
    infection or inflammation T84.50
      hip T84.5-●
      knee T84.5-●
      specified joint NEC T84.59
    instability T84.02-●
    malposition —*see* Complications, joint
        prosthesis, mechanical, displacement
    mechanical
      breakage, broken T84.01-●
      dislocation T84.02-●
      fracture T84.01-●
      instability T84.02-●
      leakage —*see* Complications, joint
          prosthesis, mechanical, specified
          NEC
      loosening T84.039
        hip T84.03-●
        knee T84.03-●
        specified joint NEC T84.038
      obstruction —*see* Complications, joint
          prosthesis, mechanical, specified
          NEC
      perforation —*see* Complications, joint
          prosthesis, mechanical, specified
          NEC
      osteolysis T84.059
        hip T84.05-●
        knee T84.05-●
        other specified joint T84.058
      protrusion —*see* Complications, joint
          prosthesis, mechanical, specified
          NEC
    specified complication NEC T84.099
      hip T84.09-●
      knee T84.09-●
      other specified joint T84.098
    subluxation T84.02-●
    wear of articular bearing surface
        T84.069
      hip T84.06-●
      knee T84.06-●
      other specified joint T84.068
  specified joint NEC T84.89
    embolism T84.81
    fibrosis T84.82
    hemorrhage T84.83
    pain T84.84
    specified complication NEC T84.89
    stenosis T84.85
    thrombosis T84.86
    subluxation T84.02-●
  kidney transplant —*see* Complications,
      transplant, kidney
  labor O75.9
    specified NEC O75.89

Complication *(Continued)*
  liver transplant (immune or nonimmune) —
      see Complications, transplant,
      liver
  lumbar puncture G97.1
    cerebrospinal fluid leak G97.0
    headache or reaction G97.1
  lung transplant —*see* Complications,
      transplant, lung
    and heart —*see* Complications, transplant,
        lung, with heart
  male genital N50.9
    device, implant or graft —*see*
        Complications, genitourinary,
        device or implant, genital tract
    postprocedural or postoperative —*see*
        Complications, genitourinary,
        postprocedural
    specified NEC N99.89
  mastoid (process) procedure
    intraoperative H95.88-●
      hematoma —*see* Complications,
          intraoperative, hemorrhage
          (hematoma) (of), mastoid
          process
      hemorrhage —*see* Complications,
          intraoperative, hemorrhage
          (hematoma) (of), mastoid
          process
      laceration —*see* Complications,
          intraoperative, puncture or
          laceration..., mastoid
          process
      specified NEC H95.88-●
    postmastoidectomy —*see* Complications,
        postmastoidectomy
    postoperative H95.89-●
      external ear canal stenosis H95.81-●
      hematoma —*see* Complications...,
          postprocedural, hematoma (of),
          mastoid process
      hemorrhage —*see* Complications...,
          postprocedural, hemorrhage (of),
          mastoid process
      postmastoidectomy —*see* Complications,
          postmastoidectomy
      seroma —*see* Complications,
          postprocedural, seroma (of),
          mastoid process
      specified NEC H95.89-●
  mastoidectomy cavity —*see* Complications,
      postmastoidectomy
  mechanical —*see* Complications, by site and
      type, mechanical
  medical procedures (*see also* Complication(s),
      intraoperative) T88.9
  metabolic E88.9
    postoperative E89.89
      specified NEC E89.89
  molar pregnancy NOS O08.9
    damage to pelvic organs O08.6
    embolism O08.2
    genital infection O08.0
    hemorrhage (delayed) (excessive)
        O08.1
    metabolic disorder O08.5
    renal failure O08.4
    shock O08.3
    specified type NEC O08.0
    venous complication NEC O08.7
  musculoskeletal system —*see also*
      Complication, intraoperative
      (intraprocedural), by site
    device, implant or graft NEC —*see*
        Complications, orthopedic, device or
        implant
    internal fixation (nail) (plate) (rod) —*see*
        Complications, fixation device,
        internal
    joint prosthesis —*see* Complications, joint
        prosthesis

Complication *(Continued)*
  musculoskeletal system *(Continued)*
    postoperative (postprocedural) M96.89
      with osteoporosis —*see* Osteoporosis
      fracture following insertion of device —
          see Fracture, following insertion of
          orthopedic implant, joint prosthesis
          or bone plate
      joint instability after prosthesis removal
          M96.89
      lordosis M96.4
      postlaminectomy syndrome NEC M96.1
        kyphosis M96.2
      pseudarthrosis M96.0
      specified complication NEC M96.89
    post radiation M96.89
      kyphosis M96.3
      scoliosis M96.5
      specified complication NEC M96.89
  nephrostomy (stoma) —*see* Complications,
      stoma, urinary tract, external NEC
  nervous system G98.8
    central G96.9
    device, implant or graft —*see also*
        Complication, prosthetic device or
        implant, specified NEC
      electronic stimulator (electrode(s)) —*see*
          Complications, electronic stimulator
          device
      specified NEC
        infection and inflammation T85.738
        mechanical T85.695
          breakdown T85.615
          displacement T85.625
          leakage T85.635
          malfunction T85.695
          malposition T85.625
          obstruction T85.695
          perforation T85.695
          protrusion T85.695
          specified NEC T85.695
      ventricular shunt —*see* Complications,
          ventricular shunt
    electronic stimulator (electrode(s)) —*see*
        Complications, electronic stimulator
        device
    postprocedural G97.82
      intracranial hypotension G97.2
      specified NEC G97.82
      spinal fluid leak G97.0
  newborn, due to intrauterine (fetal)
      procedure P96.5
  nonabsorbable (permanent) sutures —*see*
      Complication, sutures, permanent
  obstetric O75.9
    procedure (instrumental) (manual)
        (surgical) specified NEC O75.4
    specified NEC O75.89
    surgical wound NEC O90.89
      hematoma O90.2
      infection O86.0
  ocular lens implant —*see* Complications,
      intraocular lens
  ophthalmologic
    postprocedural bleb —*see* Blebitis
  orbital prosthesis T85.9
    embolism T85.818
    fibrosis T85.828
    hemorrhage T85.838
    infection and inflammation T85.79
    mechanical
      breakdown T85.31-●
      displacement T85.32-●
      malposition T85.32-●
      obstruction T85.39-●
      perforation T85.39-●
      protrusion T85.39-●
      specified NEC T85.39-●
    pain T85.848
    specified type NEC T85.898
    stenosis T85.858
    thrombosis T85.868

Complication (*Continued*)
organ or tissue transplant (partial) (total) —
   see Complications, transplant
orthopedic —*see also* Disorder, soft tissue
  device or implant T84.9
    bone
      device or implant —*see* Complication,
        bone, device NEC
      graft —*see* Complication, graft, bone
    breakdown T84.418
    displacement T84.428
    electronic bone stimulator —*see*
      Complications, electronic stimulator
      device, bone
    embolism T84.81
    fibrosis T84.82
    fixation device —*see* Complication,
      fixation device, internal
    hemorrhage T84.83
    infection or inflammation T84.7
    joint prosthesis —*see* Complication, joint
      prosthesis, internal
    malfunction T84.418
    malposition T84.428
    mechanical NEC T84.498
    muscle graft —*see* Complications, graft,
      muscle
    obstruction T84.498
    pain T84.84
    perforation T84.498
    protrusion T84.498
    specified complication NEC T84.89
    stenosis T84.85
    tendon graft —*see* Complications, graft,
      tendon
    thrombosis T84.86
  fracture (following insertion of device) —
    see Fracture, following insertion of
    orthopedic implant, joint prosthesis or
    bone plate
  postprocedural M96.89
    fracture —*see* Fracture, following
      insertion of orthopedic implant,
      joint prosthesis or bone plate
    postlaminectomy syndrome NEC M96.1
      kyphosis M96.3
      lordosis M96.4
    postradiation
      kyphosis M96.2
      scoliosis M96.5
    pseudarthrosis post-fusion M96.0
    specified type NEC M96.89
pacemaker (cardiac) —*see* Complications,
  cardiovascular device or implant,
  electronic
pancreas transplant —*see* Complications,
  transplant, pancreas
penile prosthesis (implant) —*see*
  Complications, prosthetic device, penile
perfusion NEC T80.90
perineal repair (obstetrical) NEC O90.89
  disruption O90.1
  hematoma O90.2
  infection (following delivery) O86.0
phototherapy T88.9
  specified NEC T88.8
postmastoidectomy NEC H95.19-●
  cyst, mucosal H95.13-●
  granulation H95.12-●
  inflammation, chronic H95.11-●
  recurrent cholesteatoma H95.0-●
postoperative —*see* Complications,
  postprocedural
  circulatory —*see* Complications, circulatory
    system
  ear —*see* Complications, ear
  endocrine —*see* Complications,
    endocrine
  eye —*see* Complications, eye
  lumbar puncture G97.1
    cerebrospinal fluid leak G97.0

Complication (*Continued*)
postoperative (*Continued*)
  nervous system (central) (peripheral) —*see*
    Complications, nervous system
  respiratory system —*see* Complications,
    respiratory system
postprocedural —*see also* Complications,
  surgical procedure
➡cardiac arrest —*see also* Infarct,
  myocardium, associated with
  revascularization procedure
  following cardiac surgery I97.120
  following other surgery I97.121
➡cardiac functional disturbance NEC —*see
  also* Infarct, myocardium, associated
  with revascularization procedure
  following cardiac surgery I97.190
  following other surgery I97.191
cardiac insufficiency
  following cardiac surgery I97.110
  following other surgery I97.111
chorioretinal scars following retinal
  surgery H59.81-●
following cataract surgery
  cataract (lens) fragments H59.02-●
  cystoid macular edema H59.03-●
  specified NEC H59.09-●
  vitreous (touch) syndrome H59.01-●
heart failure
  following cardiac surgery I97.130
  following other surgery I97.131
hematoma (of)
  circulatory system organ or structure
    following cardiac bypass I97.631
    following cardiac catheterization
      I97.630
    following other circulatory system
      procedure I97.638
    following other procedure I97.621
  digestive system
    following procedure on digestive
      system K91.870
    following procedure on other organ
      K91.871
  ear
    following other procedure H95.52
    following procedure on ear and
      mastoid process H95.51
  endocrine system
    following endocrine system procedure
      E89.820
    following other procedure E89.821
  eye and adnexa
    following ophthalmic procedure
      H59.33-●
    following other procedure H59.34-●
  genitourinary organ or structure
    following procedure on genitourinary
      organ or structure N99.840
    following procedure on other organ
      N99.841
  mastoid process
    following other procedure H95.52
    following procedure on ear and
      mastoid process H95.51
  musculoskeletal structure
    following musculoskeletal surgery
      M96.840
    following non-orthopedic surgery
      M96.841
    following orthopedic surgery M96.840
  nervous system
    following nervous system procedure
      G97.61
    following other procedure G97.62
  respiratory system
    following other procedure J95.861
    following procedure on respiratory
      system organ or structure J95.860
  skin and subcutaneous tissue
    following dermatologic procedure
      L76.31

Complication(s) (*Continued*)
postprocedural (*Continued*)
  hematoma (*Continued*)
    skin and subcutaneous tissue (*Continued*)
      following procedure on other organ
        L76.32
    spleen
      following procedure on other organ
        D78.32
      following procedure on the spleen
        D78.31
  hemorrhage (of)
    circulatory system organ or structure
      following cardiac bypass I97.611
      following cardiac catheterization
        I97.610
      following other circulatory system
        procedure I97.618
      following other procedure I97.620
    digestive system
      following procedure on digestive
        system K91.840
      following procedure on other organ
        K91.841
    ear
      following other procedure H95.42
      following procedure on ear and
        mastoid process H95.41
    endocrine system
      following endocrine system procedure
        E89.810
      following other procedure E89.811
    eye and adnexa
      following ophthalmic procedure
        H59.31-●
      following other procedure H59.32-●
    genitourinary organ or structure
      following procedure on genitourinary
        organ or structure N99.820
      following procedure on other organ
        N99.821
    mastoid process
      following other procedure H95.42
      following procedure on ear and
        mastoid process H95.41
    musculoskeletal structure
      following musculoskeletal surgery
        M96.830
      following non-orthopedic surgery
        M96.831
      following orthopedic surgery M96.830
    nervous system
      following nervous system procedure
        G97.51
      following other procedure G97.52
    respiratory system
      following other procedure J95.831
      following procedure on respiratory
        system organ or structure J95.830
    skin and subcutaneous tissue
      following dermatologic procedure
        L76.21
      following a procedure on other organ
        L76.22
    spleen
      following procedure on other organ
        D78.22
      following procedure on the spleen
        D78.21
  seroma (of)
    circulatory system organ or structure
      following cardiac bypass I97.641
      following cardiac catheterization
        I97.640
      following other circulatory system
        procedure I97.648
      following other procedure I97.622
    digestive system
      following procedure on digestive
        system K91.872
      following procedure on other organ
        K91.873

▶ New   ➡ Revised   ~~deleted~~ Deleted   ● Use Additional Character(s)

Complication *(Continued)*
  postprocedural *(Continued)*
    seroma *(Continued)*
      ear
        following other procedure H95.54
        following procedure on ear and
          mastoid process H95.53
      endocrine system
        following endocrine system procedure
          E89.822
        following other procedure E89.823
      eye and adnexa
        following ophthalmic procedure
          H59.35-●
        following other procedure H59.36-●
      genitourinary organ or structure
        following procedure on genitourinary
          organ or structure N99.842
        following procedure on other organ
          N99.843
      mastoid process
        following other procedure H95.54
        following procedure on ear and
          mastoid process H95.53
      musculoskeletal structure
        following musculoskeletal surgery
          M96.842
        following non-orthopedic surgery
          M96.843
        following orthopedic surgery M96.842
      nervous system
        following nervous system procedure
          G97.63
        following other procedure G97.64
      respiratory system
        following other procedure J95.863
        following procedure on respiratory
          system organ or structure J95.862
      skin and subcutaneous tissue
        following dermatologic procedure
          L76.33
        following procedure on other organ
          L76.34
      spleen
        following procedure on other organ
          D78.34
        following procedure on the spleen
          D78.33
    specified NEC
      circulatory system I97.89
      digestive K91.89
      ear H95.89
      endocrine E89.89
      eye and adnexa H59.89
      genitourinary N99.89
      mastoid process H95.89
      metabolic E89.89
      musculoskeletal structure M96.89
      nervous system G97.82
      respiratory system J95.89
      skin and subcutaneous tissue L76.82
      spleen D78.89
  pregnancy NEC —*see* Pregnancy,
    complicated by
  prosthetic device or implant T85.9
    bile duct —*see* Complications, bile duct
      implant
    breast —*see* Complications, breast
      implant
    bulking agent
      ureteral
        erosion T83.714
        exposure T83.724
      urethral
        erosion T83.713
        exposure T83.723
    cardiac and vascular NEC —*see*
      Complications, cardiovascular device
      or implant
    corneal transplant —*see* Complications,
      graft, cornea

Complication *(Continued)*
  prosthetic device or implant *(Continued)*
    electronic nervous system stimulator —*see*
      Complications, electronic stimulator
      device
    epidural infusion catheter —*see*
      Complications, catheter, epidural
    esophageal anti-reflux device —*see*
      Complications, esophageal anti-reflux
      device
    genital organ or tract —*see* Complications,
      genitourinary, device or implant,
      genital tract
      specified NEC T83.79
    heart valve —*see* Complications, heart,
      valve, prosthesis
    infection or inflammation T85.79
      intestine transplant T86.892
      liver transplant T86.43
      lung transplant T86.812
      pancreas transplant T86.892
      skin graft T86.822
    intraocular lens —*see* Complications,
      intraocular lens
    intraperitoneal (dialysis) catheter —
      see Complications, catheter,
      intraperitoneal
    joint —*see* Complications, joint prosthesis,
      internal
    mechanical NEC T85.698
      dialysis catheter (vascular) —*see also*
        Complication, catheter, dialysis,
        mechanical
        peritoneal —*see* Complication, catheter,
          intraperitoneal, mechanical
      gastrointestinal device T85.598
      ocular device T85.398
      subdural (infusion) catheter T85.690
      suture, permanent T85.692
        that for bone repair —*see*
          Complications, fixation device,
          internal (orthopedic), mechanical
      ventricular shunt
        breakdown T85.01
        displacement T85.02
        leakage T85.03
        malposition T85.02
        obstruction T85.09
        perforation T85.09
        protrusion T85.09
        specified NEC T85.09
    mesh
      ➡ erosion (to surrounding organ or tissue)
        T83.718
        urethral (into pelvic floor muscles)
          T83.712
        vaginal (into pelvic floor muscles)
          T83.711
      ➡ exposure (into surrounding organ or
        tissue) T83.728
        urethral (through urethral wall)
          T83.722
        vaginal (into vagina) (through vaginal
          wall) T83.721
    orbital —*see* Complications, orbital
      prosthesis
    penile T83.9
      embolism T83.81
      fibrosis T83.82
      hemorrhage T83.83
      infection and inflammation T83.61
      mechanical
        breakdown T83.410
        displacement T83.420
        leakage T83.490
        malposition T83.420
        obstruction T83.490
        perforation T83.490
        protrusion T83.490
        specified NEC T83.490
      pain T83.84

Complication *(Continued)*
  prosthetic device or implant *(Continued)*
    penile *(Continued)*
      specified type NEC T83.89
      stenosis T83.85
      thrombosis T83.86
    prosthetic materials NEC
      erosion (to surrounding organ or tissue)
        T83.718
      exposure (into surrounding organ or
        tissue) T83.728
    skin graft T86.829
      artificial skin or decellularized
        allodermis
        embolism T85.818
        fibrosis T85.828
        hemorrhage T85.838
        infection and inflammation T85.79
        mechanical
          breakdown T85.613
          displacement T85.623
          malfunction T85.613
          malposition T85.623
          obstruction T85.693
          perforation T85.693
          protrusion T85.693
          specified NEC T85.693
        pain T85.848
        specified type NEC T85.898
        stenosis T85.858
        thrombosis T85.868
      failure T86.821
      infection T86.822
      rejection T86.820
      specified NEC T86.828
    sling
      urethral (female) (male)
        erosion T83.712
        exposure T83.722
    specified NEC T85.9
      embolism T85.818
      fibrosis T85.828
      hemorrhage T85.838
      infection and inflammation T85.79
      mechanical
        breakdown T85.618
        displacement T85.628
        leakage T85.638
        malfunction T85.618
        malposition T85.628
        obstruction T85.698
        perforation T85.698
        protrusion T85.698
        specified NEC T85.698
      pain T85.848
      specified type NEC T85.898
      stenosis T85.858
      thrombosis T85.868
    subdural infusion catheter —*see*
      Complications, catheter, subdural
    sutures —*see* Complications, sutures
    urinary organ or tract NEC —*see*
      Complications, genitourinary, device
      or implant, urinary system
    vascular —*see* Complications,
      cardiovascular device or implant
    ventricular shunt —*see* Complications,
      ventricular shunt (device)
  puerperium —*see* Puerperal
  puncture, spinal G97.1
    cerebrospinal fluid leak G97.0
    headache or reaction G97.1
  pyelogram N99.89
  radiation
    kyphosis M96.2
    scoliosis M96.5
  reattached
    extremity (infection) (rejection)
      lower T87.1X-●
      upper T87.0X-●
    specified body part NEC T87.2

Complication *(Continued)*
  reconstructed breast
    asymmetry between native and
      reconstructed breast N65.1
    deformity N65.0
    disproportion between native and
      reconstructed breast N65.1
    excess tissue N65.0
    misshappen N65.0
  reimplant NEC *—see also* Complications,
    prosthetic device or implant
    limb (infection) (rejection) *—see*
      Complications, reattached,
      extremity
    organ (partial) (total) *—see* Complications,
      transplant
    prosthetic device NEC *—see* Complications,
      prosthetic device
  renal N28.9
    allograft *—see* Complications, transplant,
      kidney
    dialysis *—see* Complications, dialysis
  respirator
    mechanical J95.850
      specified NEC J95.859
  respiratory system J98.9
    device, implant or graft *—see*
      Complication, prosthetic device or
      implant, specified NEC
    lung transplant *—see* Complications,
      prosthetic device or implant, lung
      transplant
    postoperative J95.89
      air leak J95.812
      Mendelson's syndrome (chemical
        pneumonitis) J95.4
      pneumothorax J95.811
      pulmonary insufficiency (acute) (after
        nonthoracic surgery) J95.2
        chronic J95.3
        following thoracic surgery J95.1
      respiratory failure (acute) J95.821
        acute and chronic J95.822
      specified NEC J95.89
      subglottic stenosis J95.5
      tracheostomy complication *—see*
        Complications, tracheostomy
    therapy T81.89
  sedation during labor and delivery O74.9
    cardiac O74.2
    central nervous system O74.3
    pulmonary NEC O74.1
  shunt *—see also* Complications, prosthetic
    device or implant
    arteriovenous *—see* Complications,
      arteriovenous, shunt
    ventricular (communicating) *—see*
      Complications, ventricular shunt
  skin
    graft T86.829
      failure T86.821
      infection T86.822
      rejection T86.820
      specified type NEC T86.828
  spinal
    anesthesia *—see* Complications, anesthesia,
      spinal
    catheter (epidural) (subdural) *—see*
      Complications, catheter
    puncture or tap G97.1
      cerebrospinal fluid leak G97.0
      headache or reaction G97.1
  stent
    bile duct *—see* Complications, bile duct
      prosthesis
    ureteral indwelling
      breakdown T83.112
      displacement T83.122
      leakage T83.192
      malposition T83.122

Complication *(Continued)*
  stent *(Continued)*
    ureteral indwelling *(Continued)*
      obstruction T83.192
      perforation T83.192
      protrusion T83.192
      specified NEC T83.192
    urinary (ileal conduit) (nephroureteral)
      T83.193
      embolism T83.81
      fibrosis T83.82
      hemorrhage T83.83
      infection and inflammation T83.593
      mechanical
        breakdown T83.113
        displacement T83.123
        leakage T83.193
        malposition T83.123
        obstruction T83.193
        perforation T83.193
        protrusion T83.193
        specified NEC T83.193
      pain T83.84
      specified type NEC T83.89
      stenosis T83.85
      thrombosis T83.86
    vascular
      end stent stenosis *—see* Restenosis,
        stent
      in stent stenosis *—see* Restenosis, stent
  stoma
    digestive tract
      colostomy *—see* Complications,
        colostomy
      enterostomy *—see* Complications,
        enterostomy
      esophagostomy *—see* Complications,
        esophagostomy
      gastrostomy *—see* Complications,
        gastrostomy
    urinary tract N99.528
      continent N99.538
        hemorrhage N99.530
        herniation N99.533
        infection N99.531
        malfunction N99.532
        specified type NEC N99.538
        stenosis N99.534
      cystostomy *—see* Complications,
        cystostomy
      external NOS N99.528
      hemorrhage N99.520
      herniation N99.523
      incontinent N99.528
        hemorrhage N99.520
        herniation N99.523
        infection N99.521
        malfunction N99.522
        specified type NEC N99.528
        stenosis N99.524
      infection N99.521
      malfunction N99.522
      specified type NEC N99.528
      stenosis N99.524
  stomach banding *—see* Complication(s),
    bariatric procedure
  stomach stapling *—see* Complication(s),
    bariatric procedure
  surgical material, nonabsorbable *—see*
    Complication, suture, permanent
  surgical procedure (on) T81.9
    amputation stump (late) *—see*
      Complications, amputation stump
    cardiac *—see* Complications, circulatory
      system
    cholesteatoma, recurrent *—see*
      Complications, postmastoidectomy,
      recurrent cholesteatoma
    circulatory (early) *—see* Complications,
      circulatory system

Complication *(Continued)*
  surgical procedure *(Continued)*
    digestive system *—see* Complications,
      gastrointestinal
    dumping syndrome (postgastrectomy)
      K91.1
    ear *—see* Complications, ear
    elephantiasis or lymphedema I97.89
      postmastectomy I97.2
    emphysema (surgical) T81.82
    endocrine *—see* Complications, endocrine
    eye *—see* Complications, eye
    fistula (persistent postoperative) T81.83
    foreign body inadvertently left in wound
      (sponge) (suture) (swab) *—see* Foreign
      body, accidentally left during a
      procedure
    gastrointestinal *—see* Complications,
      gastrointestinal
    genitourinary NEC N99.89
    hematoma
      intraoperative *—see* Complication,
        intraoperative, hemorrhage
      postprocedural *—see* Complication,
        postprocedural, hematoma
    hemorrhage
      intraoperative *—see* Complication,
        intraoperative, hemorrhage
      postprocedural *—see* Complication,
        postprocedural, hemorrhage
    hepatic failure K91.82
    hyperglycemia (postpancreatectomy) E89.1
    hypoinsulinemia (postpancreatectomy)
      E89.1
    hypoparathyroidism
      (postparathyroidectomy) E89.2
    hypopituitarism (posthypophysectomy)
      E89.3
    hypothyroidism (post-thyroidectomy)
      E89.0
    ➨intestinal obstruction *—see also*
      Obstruction, intestine, postoperative
      K91.30
    intracranial hypotension following
      ventricular shunting
      (ventriculostomy) G97.2
    lymphedema I97.89
      postmastectomy I97.2
    malabsorption (postsurgical) NEC K91.2
      osteoporosis *—see* Osteoporosis,
        postsurgical malabsorption
    mastoidectomy cavity NEC *—see*
      Complications, postmastoidectomy
    metabolic E89.89
      specified NEC E89.89
    musculoskeletal *—see* Complications,
      musculoskeletal system
    nervous system (central) (peripheral) *—see*
      Complications, nervous system
    ovarian failure E89.40
      asymptomatic E89.40
      symptomatic E89.41
    peripheral vascular *—see* Complications,
      surgical procedure, vascular
    postcardiotomy syndrome I97.0
    postcholecystectomy syndrome K91.5
    postcommissurotomy syndrome I97.0
    postgastrectomy dumping syndrome K91.1
    postlaminectomy syndrome NEC M96.1
      kyphosis M96.3
    postmastectomy lymphedema syndrome
      I97.2
    postmastoidectomy cholesteatoma *—see*
      Complications, postmastoidectomy,
      recurrent cholesteatoma
    postvagotomy syndrome K91.1
    postvalvulotomy syndrome I97.0
    pulmonary insufficiency (acute) J95.2
      chronic J95.3
      following thoracic surgery J95.1

▶ New   ➠ Revised   ~~deleted~~ Deleted   ● Use Additional Character(s)

Complication *(Continued)*
  surgical procedure *(Continued)*
    reattached body part —*see* Complications,
      reattached
    respiratory —*see* Complications,
      respiratory system
    shock (hypovolemic) T81.19
    spleen (postoperative) D78.89
      intraoperative D78.81
  ⇒stitch abscess T81.4
    subglottic stenosis (postsurgical) J95.5
    testicular hypofunction E89.5
    transplant —*see* Complications, organ or
      tissue transplant
    urinary NEC N99.89
    vaginal vault prolapse (posthysterectomy)
      N99.3
    vascular (peripheral)
      artery T81.719
        mesenteric T81.710
        renal T81.711
        specified NEC T81.718
      vein T81.72
  ⇒wound infection T81.4
  suture, permanent (wire) NEC T85.9
    with repair of bone —*see* Complications,
      fixation device, internal
    embolism T85.818
    fibrosis T85.828
    hemorrhage T85.838
    infection and inflammation T85.79
    mechanical
      breakdown T85.612
      displacement T85.622
      malfunction T85.612
      malposition T85.622
      obstruction T85.692
      perforation T85.692
      protrusion T85.692
      specified NEC T85.692
    pain T85.848
    specified type NEC T85.898
    stenosis T85.858
    thrombosis T85.868
  tracheostomy J95.00
    granuloma J95.09
    hemorrhage J95.01
    infection J95.02
    malfunction J95.03
    mechanical J95.03
    obstruction J95.03
    specified type NEC J95.09
    tracheo-esophageal fistula J95.04
  transfusion (blood) (lymphocytes) (plasma)
    T80.92
    air embolism T80.0
    circulatory overload E87.71
    febrile nonhemolytic transfusion reaction
      R50.84
    hemochromatosis E83.111
    hemolysis T80.89
    hemolytic reaction (antigen unspecified)
      T80.919
    incompatibility reaction (antigen
      unspecified) T80.919
      ABO T80.30
        delayed serologic (DSTR) T80.39
        hemolytic transfusion reaction
          (HTR) (unspecified time after
          transfusion) T80.319
          acute (AHTR) (less than 24 hours
            after transfusion) T80.310
          delayed (DHTR) (24 hours or
            more after transfusion)
            T80.311
        specified NEC T80.39
      acute (antigen unspecified) T80.910
      delayed (antigen unspecified)
        T80.911
      delayed serologic (DSTR) T80.89

Complication *(Continued)*
  transfusion *(Continued)*
    incompatibility reaction *(Continued)*
      Non-ABO (minor antigens (Duffy) (Kell)
        (Kidd) (Lewis) (M) (N) (P) (S))
        T80.A0
        delayed serologic (DSTR) T80.A9
        hemolytic transfusion reaction
          (HTR) (unspecified time after
          transfusion) T80.A19
          acute (AHTR) (less than 24 hours
            after transfusion) T80.A10
          delayed (DHTR) (24 hours or more
            after transfusion) T80.A11
        specified NEC T80.A9
      Rh (antigens (C) (c) (D) (E) (e)) (factor)
        T80.40
        delayed serologic (DSTR) T80.49
        hemolytic transfusion reaction
          (HTR) (unspecified time after
          transfusion) T80.419
          acute (AHTR) (less than 24 hours
            after transfusion) T80.410
          delayed (DHTR) (24 hours or more
            after transfusion) T80.411
        specified NEC T80.49
    infection T80.29
      acute T80.22
    reaction NEC T80.89
    sepsis T80.29
    shock T80.89
  transplant T86.90
    bone T86.839
      failure T86.831
      infection T86.832
      rejection T86.830
      specified type NEC T86.838
    bone marrow T86.00
      failure T86.02
      infection T86.03
      rejection T86.01
      specified type NEC T86.09
    cornea T86.849
      failure T86.841
      infection T86.842
      rejection T86.840
      specified type NEC T86.848
    failure T86.92
    heart T86.20
      with lung T86.30
      cardiac allograft vasculopathy T86.290
        failure T86.32
        infection T86.33
        rejection T86.31
        specified type NEC T86.39
      failure T86.22
      infection T86.23
      rejection T86.21
      specified type NEC T86.298
    infection T86.93
    intestine T86.859
      failure T86.851
      infection T86.852
      rejection T86.850
      specified type NEC T86.858
    kidney T86.10
      failure T86.12
      infection T86.13
      rejection T86.11
      specified type NEC T86.19
    liver T86.40
      failure T86.42
      infection T86.43
      rejection T86.41
      specified type NEC T86.49
    lung T86.819
      with heart T86.30
        failure T86.32
        infection T86.33
        rejection T86.31
        specified type NEC T86.39

Complication *(Continued)*
  transplant *(Continued)*
    lung *(Continued)*
      failure T86.811
      infection T86.812
      rejection T86.810
      specified type NEC T86.818
    malignant neoplasm C80.2
    pancreas T86.899
      failure T86.891
      infection T86.892
      rejection T86.890
      specified type NEC T86.898
    peripheral blood stem cells T86.5
    post-transplant lymphoproliferative
      disorder (PTLD) D47.Z1
    rejection T86.91
    skin T86.829
      failure T86.821
      infection T86.822
      rejection T86.820
      specified type NEC T86.828
    specified
      tissue T86.899
        failure T86.891
        infection T86.892
        rejection T86.890
        specified type NEC T86.898
      type NEC T86.99
    stem cell (from peripheral blood) (from
      umbilical cord) T86.5
    umbilical cord stem cells T86.5
  trauma (early) T79.9
    specified NEC T79.8
  ultrasound therapy NEC T88.9
  umbilical cord NEC
    complicating delivery O69.9
      specified NEC O69.89
  umbrella device, vascular T82.9
    embolism T82.818
    fibrosis T82.828
    hemorrhage T82.838
    infection or inflammation T82.7
    mechanical
      breakdown T82.515
      displacement T82.525
      leakage T82.535
      malposition T82.525
      obstruction T82.595
      perforation T82.595
      protrusion T82.595
    pain T82.848
    specified type NEC T82.898
    stenosis T82.858
    thrombosis T82.868
  urethral catheter —*see* Complications,
    catheter, urethral, indwelling
  vaccination T88.1
    anaphylaxis NEC T80.52
    arthropathy —*see* Arthropathy,
      postimmunization
    cellulitis T88.0
    encephalitis or encephalomyelitis
      G04.02
    infection (general) (local) NEC T88.0
    meningitis G03.8
    myelitis G04.02
    protein sickness T80.62
    rash T88.1
    reaction (allergic) T88.1
      serum T80.62
    sepsis T88.0
    serum intoxication, sickness, rash, or other
      serum reaction NEC T80.62
      anaphylactic shock T80.52
    shock (allergic) (anaphylactic) T80.52
    vaccinia (generalized) (localized) T88.1
  vas deferens device or implant —*see*
    Complications, genitourinary, device or
    implant, genital tract

Complication *(Continued)*
  vascular I99.9
    device or implant T82.9
      embolism T82.818
      fibrosis T82.828
      hemorrhage T82.838
      infection or inflammation T82.7
      mechanical
        breakdown T82.519
          specified device NEC T82.518
        displacement T82.529
          specified device NEC T82.528
        leakage T82.539
          specified device NEC T82.538
        malposition T82.529
          specified device NEC T82.528
        obstruction T82.599
          specified device NEC T82.598
        perforation T82.599
          specified device NEC T82.598
        protrusion T82.599
          specified device NEC T82.598
      pain T82.848
      specified type NEC T82.898
      stenosis T82.858
      thrombosis T82.868
    dialysis catheter —*see* Complication, catheter, dialysis
    following infusion, therapeutic injection or transfusion T80.1
    graft T82.9
      embolism T82.818
      fibrosis T82.828
      hemorrhage T82.838
      mechanical
        breakdown T82.319
          aorta (bifurcation) T82.310
          carotid artery T82.311
          specified vessel NEC T82.318
        displacement T82.329
          aorta (bifurcation) T82.320
          carotid artery T82.321
          specified vessel NEC T82.328
        leakage T82.339
          aorta (bifurcation) T82.330
          carotid artery T82.331
          specified vessel NEC T82.338
        malposition T82.329
          aorta (bifurcation) T82.320
          carotid artery T82.321
          specified vessel NEC T82.328
        obstruction T82.399
          aorta (bifurcation) T82.390
          carotid artery T82.391
          specified vessel NEC T82.398
        perforation T82.399
          aorta (bifurcation) T82.390
          carotid artery T82.391
          specified vessel NEC T82.398
        protrusion T82.399
          aorta (bifurcation) T82.390
          carotid artery T82.391
          specified vessel NEC T82.398
      pain T82.848
      specified complication NEC T82.898
      stenosis T82.858
      thrombosis T82.868
    postoperative —*see* Complications, postoperative, circulatory
    vena cava device (filter) (sieve) (umbrella) — *see* Complications, umbrella device, vascular
  ventilation therapy NEC T81.81
  ventilator
    mechanical J95.850
      specified NEC J95.859
  ventricular (communicating) shunt (device) T85.9
    embolism T85.810
    fibrosis T85.820
    hemorrhage T85.830

Complication *(Continued)*
  ventricular shunt *(Continued)*
    infection and inflammation T85.730
    mechanical
      breakdown T85.01
      displacement T85.02
      leakage T85.03
      malposition T85.02
      obstruction T85.09
      perforation T85.09
      protrusion T85.09
      specified NEC T85.09
    pain T85.840
    specified type NEC T85.890
    stenosis T85.850
    thrombosis T85.860
  wire suture, permanent (implanted) —*see* Complications, suture, permanent
Compressed air disease T70.3
Compression
  with injury - code by Nature of injury
  artery I77.1
    celiac, syndrome I77.4
  brachial plexus G54.0
  brain (stem) G93.5
    due to
      contusion (diffuse) —*see* Injury, intracranial, diffuse
        focal —*see* Injury, intracranial, focal
      injury NEC —*see* Injury, intracranial, diffuse
      traumatic —*see* Injury, intracranial, diffuse
  bronchus J98.09
  cauda equina G83.4
  celiac (artery) (axis) I77.4
  cerebral —*see* Compression, brain
  cervical plexus G54.2
  cord
    spinal —*see* Compression, spinal
    umbilical —*see* Compression, umbilical cord
  cranial nerve G52.9
    eighth —*see* subcategory H93.3
    eleventh G52.8
    fifth G50.8
    first G52.0
    fourth —*see* Strabismus, paralytic, fourth nerve
    ninth G52.1
    second —*see* Disorder, nerve, optic
    ➡seventh G51.8
    sixth —*see* Strabismus, paralytic, sixth nerve
    tenth G52.2
    third —*see* Strabismus, paralytic, third nerve
    twelfth G52.3
  diver's squeeze T70.3
  during birth (newborn) P15.9
  esophagus K22.2
  eustachian tube —*see* Obstruction, eustachian tube, cartilaginous
  facies Q67.1
  fracture
    nontraumatic NOS —*see* Collapse, vertebra
    pathological —*see* Fracture, pathological
    traumatic —*see* Fracture, traumatic
  heart —*see* Disease, heart
  intestine —*see* Obstruction, intestine
  laryngeal nerve, recurrent G52.2
    with paralysis of vocal cords and larynx J38.00
      bilateral J38.02
      unilateral J38.01
  lumbosacral plexus G54.1
  lung J98.4
  lymphatic vessel I89.0
  medulla —*see* Compression, brain
  nerve —*see also* Disorder, nerve G58.9
    arm NEC —*see* Mononeuropathy, upper limb

Compression *(Continued)*
  nerve *(Continued)*
    axillary G54.0
    cranial —*see* Compression, cranial nerve
    leg NEC —*see* Mononeuropathy, lower limb
    median (in carpal tunnel) —*see* Syndrome, carpal tunnel
    optic —*see* Disorder, nerve, optic
    plantar —*see* Lesion, nerve, plantar
    posterior tibial (in tarsal tunnel) —*see* Syndrome, tarsal tunnel
    root or plexus NOS (in) G54.9
      intervertebral disc disorder NEC — *see* Disorder, disc, with, radiculopathy
      with myelopathy —*see* Disorder, disc, with, myelopathy
    neoplastic disease —*see also* Neoplasm D49.9 *[G55]*
    spondylosis —*see* Spondylosis, with radiculopathy
    sciatic (acute) —*see* Lesion, nerve, sciatic
    sympathetic G90.8
    traumatic —*see* Injury, nerve
    ulnar —*see* Lesion, nerve, ulnar
    upper extremity NEC —*see* Mononeuropathy, upper limb
  spinal (cord) G95.20
    by displacement of intervertebral disc NEC —*see also* Disorder, disc, with, myelopathy
    nerve root NOS G54.9
      due to displacement of intervertebral disc NEC —*see* Disorder, disc, with, radiculopathy
      with myelopathy —*see* Disorder, disc, with, myelopathy
    specified NEC G95.29
    spondylogenic (cervical) (lumbar, lumbosacral) (thoracic) —*see* Spondylosis, with myelopathy NEC
    anterior —*see* Syndrome, anterior, spinal artery, compression
    traumatic —*see* Injury, spinal cord, by region
  subcostal nerve (syndrome) —*see* Mononeuropathy, upper limb, specified NEC
  sympathetic nerve NEC G90.8
  syndrome T79.5
  trachea J39.8
  ulnar nerve (by scar tissue) —*see* Lesion, nerve, ulnar
  umbilical cord
    complicating delivery O69.2
      cord around neck O69.1
      prolapse O69.0
      specified NEC O69.2
  ureter N13.5
  vein I87.1
  vena cava (inferior) (superior) I87.1
Compulsion, compulsive
  gambling F63.0
  neurosis F42.8
  personality F60.5
  states F42.8
  swearing F42.8
    in Gilles de la Tourette's syndrome F95.2
  tics and spasms F95.9
Concato's disease (pericardial polyserositis) A19.9
  nontubercular I31.1
  pleural —*see* Pleurisy, with effusion
Concavity chest wall M95.4
Concealed penis Q55.69
Concern (normal) about sick person in family Z63.6
Concrescence (teeth) K00.2
Concretio cordis I31.1
  rheumatic I09.2

▶ New   ➡ Revised   ~~deleted~~ Deleted   ● Use Additional Character(s)

Concretion —*see also* Calculus
  appendicular K38.1
  canaliculus —*see* Dacryolith
  clitoris N90.89
  conjunctiva H11.12-●
  eyelid —*see* Disorder, eyelid, specified type
    NEC
  lacrimal passages —*see* Dacryolith
  prepuce (male) N47.8
  salivary gland (any) K11.5
  seminal vesicle N50.89
  tonsil J35.8
Concussion (brain) (cerebral) (current)
  S06.0X9
  with
    loss of consciousness of 30 minutes or less
      S06.0X1
    loss of consciousness of unspecified
      duration S06.0X9
  blast (air) (hydraulic) (immersion)
    (underwater)
    abdomen or thorax —*see* Injury, blast, by
      site
    ear with acoustic nerve injury —*see* Injury,
      nerve, acoustic, specified type NEC
  cauda equina S34.3
  conus medullaris S34.02
  ocular S05.8X-●
  spinal (cord)
    cervical S14.0
    lumbar S34.01
    sacral S34.02
    thoracic S24.0
  syndrome F07.81
  Without loss of consciousness S06.0X0
Condition —*see* Disease
Conditions arising in the perinatal period —
  see Newborn, affected by
Conduct disorder —*see* Disorder, conduct
Condyloma A63.0
  acuminatum A63.0
  gonorrheal A54.09
  latum A51.31
  syphilitic A51.31
    congenital A50.07
  venereal, syphilitic A51.31
Conflagration —*see also* Burn
  asphyxia (by inhalation of gases, fumes or
    vapors) —*see also* Table of Drugs and
    Chemicals T59.9-●
Conflict (with) —*see also* Discord
  family Z73.9
  marital Z63.0
    involving divorce or estrangement Z63.5
  parent-child Z62.820
    parent-adopted child Z62.821
    parent-biological child Z62.820
    parent-foster child Z62.822
  social role NEC Z73.5
Confluent —*see* condition
Confusion, confused R41.0
  epileptic F05
  mental state (psychogenic) F44.89
  psychogenic F44.89
  reactive (from emotional stress, psychological
    trauma) F44.89
Confusional arousals G47.51
Congelation T69.9
Congenital —*see also* condition
  aortic septum Q25.49
  intrinsic factor deficiency D51.0
  malformation —*see* Anomaly
Congestion, congestive
  bladder N32.89
  bowel K63.89
  brain G93.89
  breast N64.59
  bronchial J98.09
  catarrhal J31.0
  chest R09.89
  chill, malarial —*see* Malaria

Congestion, congestive *(Continued)*
  circulatory NEC I99.8
  duodenum K31.89
  eye —*see* Hyperemia, conjunctiva
  facial, due to birth injury P15.4
  general R68.89
  glottis J37.0
  heart —*see* Failure, heart, congestive
  hepatic K76.1
  hypostatic (lung) —*see* Edema, lung
  intestine K63.89
  kidney N28.89
  labyrinth —*see* subcategory H83.8
  larynx J37.0
  liver K76.1
  lung R09.89
    active or acute —*see* Pneumonia
  malaria, malarial —*see* Malaria
  nasal R09.81
  nose R09.81
  orbit, orbital —*see also* Exophthalmos
    inflammatory (chronic) —*see* Inflammation,
      orbit
  ovary N83.8
  pancreas K86.89
  pelvic, female N94.89
  pleural J94.8
  prostate (active) N42.1
  pulmonary —*see* Congestion, lung
  renal N28.89
  retina H35.81
  seminal vesicle N50.1
  spinal cord G95.19
  spleen (chronic) D73.2
  stomach K31.89
  trachea —*see* Tracheitis
  urethra N36.8
  uterus N85.8
    with subinvolution N85.3
  venous (passive) I87.8
  viscera R68.89
Congestive —*see* Congestion
Conical
  cervix (hypertrophic elongation) N88.4
  cornea —*see* Keratoconus
  teeth K00.2
Conjoined twins Q89.4
Conjugal maladjustment Z63.0
  involving divorce or estrangement Z63.5
Conjunctiva —*see* condition
Conjunctivitis (staphylococcal) (streptococcal)
  NOS H10.9
  Acanthamoeba B60.12
  acute H10.3-●
    atopic H10.1-●
    chemical —*see also* Corrosion, cornea
      H10.21-●
    mucopurulent H10.02-●
      follicular H10.01-●
    pseudomembranous H10.22-●
    serous except viral H10.23-●
      viral —*see* Conjunctivitis, viral
    toxic H10.21-●
  adenoviral (acute) (follicular) B30.1
  allergic (acute) —*see* Conjunctivitis, acute,
    atopic
    chronic H10.45
      vernal H10.44
  anaphylactic —*see* Conjunctivitis, acute,
    atopic
  Apollo B30.3
  atopic (acute) —*see* Conjunctivitis, acute,
    atopic
  Béal's B30.2
  blennorrhagic (gonococcal) (neonatorum)
    A54.31
  chemical (acute) —*see also* Corrosion, cornea
    H10.21-●
  chlamydial A74.0
    due to trachoma A71.1
    neonatal P39.1

Conjunctivitis *(Continued)*
  chronic (nodosa) (petrificans) (phlyctenular)
    H10.40-●
    allergic H10.45
      vernal H10.44
    follicular H10.43-●
    giant papillary H10.41-●
    simple H10.42-●
    vernal H10.44
  coxsackievirus 24 B30.3
  diphtheritic A36.86
  due to
    dust —*see* Conjunctivitis, acute, atopic
    filariasis B74.9
    mucocutaneous leishmaniasis B55.2
  enterovirus type 70 (hemorrhagic) B30.3
  epidemic (viral) B30.9
    hemorrhagic B30.3
  gonococcal (neonatorum) A54.31
  granular (trachomatous) A71.1
    sequelae (late effect) B94.0
  hemorrhagic (acute) (epidemic) B30.3
  herpes zoster B02.31
  in (due to)
    Acanthamoeba B60.12
    adenovirus (acute) (follicular) B30.1
    Chlamydia A74.0
    coxsackievirus 24 B30.3
    diphtheria A36.86
    enterovirus type 70 (hemorrhagic) B30.3
    filariasis B74.9
    gonococci A54.31
    herpes (simplex) virus B00.53
      zoster B02.31
    infectious disease NEC B99
    meningococci A39.89
    mucocutaneous leishmaniasis B55.2
    rosacea L71.9
    syphilis (late) A52.71
    zoster B02.31
  inclusion A74.0
  infantile P39.1
    gonococcal A54.31
  Koch-Weeks' —*see* Conjunctivitis, acute,
    mucopurulent
  light —*see* Conjunctivitis, acute, atopic
  ligneous —*see* Blepharoconjunctivitis,
    ligneous
  meningococcal A39.89
  mucopurulent —*see* Conjunctivitis, acute,
    mucopurulent
  neonatal P39.1
    gonococcal A54.31
  Newcastle B30.8
  of Béal B30.2
  parasitic
    filariasis B74.9
    mucocutaneous leishmaniasis B55.2
  Parinaud's H10.89
  petrificans H10.89
  rosacea L71.9
  specified NEC H10.89
  swimming-pool B30.1
  trachomatous A71.1
    acute A71.0
    sequelae (late effect) B94.0
  traumatic NEC H10.89
  tuberculous A18.59
  tularemic A21.1
  tularensis A21.1
  viral B30.9
    due to
      adenovirus B30.1
      enterovirus B30.3
      specified NEC B30.8
Conjunctivochalasis H11.82-●
Connective tissue —*see* condition
Conn's syndrome E26.01
Conradi (-Hunermann) disease Q77.3
Consanguinity Z84.3
  counseling Z71.89

Conscious simulation (of illness) Z76.5
Consecutive —see condition
Consolidation lung (base) —see Pneumonia, lobar
Constipation (atonic) (neurogenic) (simple) (spastic) K59.00
  chronic K59.09
    idiopathic K59.04
  drug-induced K59.03
  functional K59.04
  outlet dysfunction K59.02
  psychogenic F45.8
  slow transit K59.01
  specified NEC K59.09
Constitutional —see also condition
  substandard F60.7
Constitutionally substandard F60.7
Constriction —see also Stricture
  auditory canal —see Stenosis, external ear canal
  bronchial J98.09
  duodenum K31.5
  esophagus K22.2
  external
    abdomen, abdominal (wall) S30.841
    alveolar process S00.542
    ankle S90.54-●
    antecubital space —see Constriction, external, forearm
    arm (upper) S40.84-●
    auricle —see Constriction, external, ear
    axilla —see Constriction, external, arm
    back, lower S30.840
    breast S20.14-●
    brow S00.84
    buttock S30.840
    calf —see Constriction, external, leg
    canthus —see Constriction, external, eyelid
    cheek S00.84
      internal S00.542
    chest wall —see Constriction, external, thorax
    chin S00.84
    clitoris S30.844
    costal region —see Constriction, external, thorax
    digit(s)
      foot —see Constriction, external, toe
      hand —see Constriction, external, finger
    ear S00.44-●
    elbow S50.34-●
    epididymis S30.843
    epigastric region S30.841
    esophagus, cervical S10.14
    eyebrow —see Constriction, external, eyelid
    eyelid S00.24-●
    face S00.84
    finger(s) S60.44-●
      index S60.44-●
      little S60.44-●
      middle S60.44-●
      ring S60.44-●
    flank S30.841
    foot (except toe(s) alone) S90.84-●
      toe —see Constriction, external, toe
    forearm S50.84-●
      elbow only —see Constriction, external, elbow
    forehead S00.84
    genital organs, external
      female S30.846
      male S30.845
    groin S30.841
    gum S00.542
    hand S60.54-●
    head S00.94
      ear —see Constriction, external, ear
      eyelid —see Constriction, external, eyelid
      lip S00.541
      nose S00.34
      oral cavity S00.542

Constriction (Continued)
  external (Continued)
    head (Continued)
      scalp S00.04
      specified site NEC S00.84
    heel —see Constriction, external, foot
    hip S70.24-●
    inguinal region S30.841
    interscapular region S20.449
    jaw S00.84
    knee S80.24-●
    labium (majus) (minus) S30.844
    larynx S10.14
    leg (lower) S80.84-●
      knee —see Constriction, external, knee
      upper —see Constriction, external, thigh
    lip S00.541
    lower back S30.840
    lumbar region S30.840
    malar region S00.84
    mammary —see Constriction, external, breast
    mastoid region S00.84
    mouth S00.542
    nail
      finger —see Constriction, external, finger
      toe —see Constriction, external, toe
    nasal S00.34
    neck S10.94
      specified site NEC S10.84
      throat S10.14
    nose S00.34
    occipital region S00.04
    oral cavity S00.542
    orbital region —see Constriction, external, eyelid
    palate S00.542
    palm —see Constriction, external, hand
    parietal region S00.04
    pelvis S30.840
    penis S30.842
    perineum
      female S30.844
      male S30.840
    periocular area —see Constriction, external, eyelid
    phalanges
      finger —see Constriction, external, finger
      toe —see Constriction, external, toe
    pharynx S10.14
    pinna —see Constriction, external, ear
    popliteal space —see Constriction, external, knee
    prepuce S30.842
    pubic region S30.840
    pudendum
      female S30.846
      male S30.845
    sacral region S30.840
    scalp S00.04
    scapular region —see Constriction, external, shoulder
    scrotum S30.843
    shin —see Constriction, external, leg
    shoulder S40.24-●
    sternal region S20.349
    submaxillary region S00.84
    submental region S00.84
    subungual
      finger(s) —see Constriction, external, finger
      toe(s) —see Constriction, external, toe
    supraclavicular fossa S10.84
    supraorbital S00.84
    temple S00.84
    temporal region S00.84
    testis S30.843
    thigh S70.34-●
    thorax, thoracic (wall) S20.94
      back S20.44-●
      front S20.34-●

Constriction (Continued)
  external (Continued)
    throat S10.14
    thumb S60.34-●
    toe(s) (lesser) S90.44-●
      great S90.44-●
    tongue S00.542
    trachea S10.14
    tunica vaginalis S30.843
    uvula S00.542
    vagina S30.844
    vulva S30.844
    wrist S60.84-●
  gallbladder —see Obstruction, gallbladder
  intestine —see Obstruction, intestine
  larynx J38.6
    congenital Q31.8
      specified NEC Q31.8
      subglottic Q31.1
  organ or site, congenital NEC —see Atresia, by site
  prepuce (acquired) (congenital) N47.1
  pylorus (adult hypertrophic) K31.1
    congenital or infantile Q40.0
    newborn Q40.0
  ring dystocia (uterus) O62.4
  spastic —see also Spasm
    ureter N13.5
  ureter N13.5
    with infection N13.6
  urethra —see Stricture, urethra
  visual field (peripheral) (functional) —see Defect, visual field
Constrictive —see condition
Consultation
  without complaint or sickness Z71.9
    feared complaint unfounded Z71.1
    specified reason NEC Z71.89
  medical —see Counseling, medical
  religious Z71.81
  specified reason NEC Z71.89
  spiritual Z71.81
Consumption —see Tuberculosis
Contact (with) —see also Exposure (to)
  acariasis Z20.7
  AIDS virus Z20.6
  air pollution Z77.110
  algae and algae toxins Z77.121
  algae bloom Z77.121
  anthrax Z20.810
  aromatic (hazardous) compounds NEC Z77.028
  aromatic amines Z77.020
  aromatic dyes NOS Z77.028
  arsenic Z77.010
  asbestos Z77.090
  bacterial disease NEC Z20.818
  benzene Z77.021
  blue-green algae bloom Z77.121
  body fluids (potentially hazardous) Z77.21
  brown tide Z77.121
  chemicals (chiefly nonmedicinal) (hazardous) NEC Z77.098
  cholera Z20.09
  chromium compounds Z77.018
  communicable disease Z20.9
    bacterial NEC Z20.818
    specified NEC Z20.89
    viral NEC Z20.828
  cyanobacteria bloom Z77.121
  dyes Z77.098
  Escherichia coli (E. coli) Z20.01
  fiberglass —see Table of Drugs and Chemicals, fiberglass
  German measles Z20.4
  gonorrhea Z20.2
  hazardous metals NEC Z77.018
  hazardous substances NEC Z77.29
  hazards in the physical environment NEC Z77.128
  hazards to health NEC Z77.9

▶ New   ⇒ Revised   ~~deleted~~ Deleted   ● Use Additional Character(s)

Contact *(Continued)*
HIV Z20.6
HTLV-III/LAV Z20.6
human immunodeficiency virus (HIV) Z20.6
infection Z20.9
 specified NEC Z20.89
infestation (parasitic) NEC Z20.7
intestinal infectious disease NEC Z20.09
 Escherichia coli (E. coli) Z20.01
lead Z77.011
meningococcus Z20.811
mold (toxic) Z77.120
nickel dust Z77.018
noise Z77.122
parasitic disease Z20.7
pediculosis Z20.7
pfiesteria piscicida Z77.121
poliomyelitis Z20.89
pollution
 air Z77.110
 environmental NEC Z77.118
 soil Z77.112
 water Z77.111
polycyclic aromatic hydrocarbons Z77.028
rabies Z20.3
radiation, naturally occurring NEC Z77.123
radon Z77.123
red tide (Florida) Z77.121
rubella Z20.4
sexually-transmitted disease Z20.2
smallpox (laboratory) Z20.89
syphilis Z20.2
tuberculosis Z20.1
uranium Z77.012
varicella Z20.820
venereal disease Z20.2
viral disease NEC Z20.828
viral hepatitis Z20.5
water pollution Z77.111
Contamination, food —*see* Intoxication, foodborne
Contraception, contraceptive
advice Z30.09
counseling Z30.09
device (intrauterine) (in situ) Z97.5
 causing menorrhagia T83.83
 checking Z30.431
 complications —*see* Complications, intrauterine, contraceptive device
 in place Z97.5
 initial prescription Z30.014
 reinsertion Z30.433
 removal Z30.432
 replacement Z30.433
emergency (postcoital) Z30.012
initial prescription Z30.019
 barrier Z30.018
 diaphragm Z30.018
 injectable Z30.013
 intrauterine device Z30.014
 pills Z30.011
 postcoital (emergency) Z30.012
 specified type NEC Z30.018
 subdermal implantable Z30.017
 transdermal patch hormonal Z30.016
 vaginal ring hormonal Z30.015
maintenance Z30.40
 barrier Z30.49
 diaphragm Z30.49
 examination Z30.8
 injectable Z30.42
 intrauterine device Z30.431
 pills Z30.41
 specified type NEC Z30.49
 subdermal implantable Z30.46
 transdermal patch hormonal Z30.45
 vaginal ring hormonal Z30.44
management Z30.9
 specified NEC Z30.8
postcoital (emergency) Z30.012
prescription Z30.019
 repeat Z30.40

Contraception, contraceptive *(Continued)*
sterilization Z30.2
surveillance (drug) —*see* Contraception, maintenance
Contraction(s), contracture, contracted
Achilles tendon —*see also* Short, tendon, Achilles
 congenital Q66.89
amputation stump (surgical) (flexion) (late) next proximal joint T87.89
anus K59.8
bile duct (common) (hepatic) K83.8
bladder N32.89
 neck or sphincter N32.0
bowel, cecum, colon or intestine, any part —*see* Obstruction, intestine
Braxton Hicks —*see* False, labor
breast implant, capsular T85.44
bronchial J98.09
burn (old) —*see* Cicatrix
cervix —*see* Stricture, cervix
cicatricial —*see* Cicatrix
conjunctiva, trachomatous, active A71.1
 sequelae (late effect) B94.0
Dupuytren's M72.0
eyelid —*see* Disorder, eyelid function
fascia (lata) (postural) M72.8
 Dupuytren's M72.0
 palmar M72.0
 plantar M72.2
finger NEC —*see also* Deformity, finger
 congenital Q68.1
 joint —*see* Contraction, joint, hand
flaccid —*see* Contraction, paralytic
gallbladder K82.0
heart valve —*see* Endocarditis
hip —*see* Contraction, joint, hip
hourglass
 bladder N32.89
 congenital Q64.79
 gallbladder K82.0
 congenital Q44.1
 stomach K31.89
 congenital Q40.2
 psychogenic F45.8
 uterus (complicating delivery) O62.4
hysterical F44.4
internal os —*see* Stricture, cervix
joint (abduction) (acquired) (adduction) (flexion) (rotation) M24.50
 ankle M24.57-●
 congenital NEC Q68.8
 hip Q65.89
 elbow M24.52-●
 foot joint M24.57-●
 hand joint M24.54-●
 hip M24.55-●
 congenital Q65.89
 hysterical F44.4
 knee M24.56-●
 shoulder M24.51-●
 wrist M24.53-●
kidney (granular) (secondary) N26.9
 congenital Q63.8
 hydronephritic —*see* Hydronephrosis Page N26.2
 pyelonephritic —*see* Pyelitis, chronic
 tuberculous A18.11
ligament —*see also* Disorder, ligament
 congenital Q79.8
muscle (postinfective) (postural) NEC M62.40
 with contracture of joint —*see* Contraction, joint
 ankle M62.47-●
 congenital Q79.8
 sternocleidomastoid Q68.0
 extraocular —*see* Strabismus
 eye (extrinsic) —*see* Strabismus
 foot M62.47-●
 forearm M62.43-●
 hand M62.44-●

Contraction, contracture, contracted *(Continued)*
muscle *(Continued)*
 hysterical F44.4
 ischemic (Volkmann's) T79.6
 lower leg M62.46-●
 multiple sites M62.49
 pelvic region M62.45-●
 posttraumatic —*see* Strabismus, paralytic
 psychogenic F45.8
 conversion reaction F44.4
 shoulder region M62.41-●
 specified site NEC M62.48
 thigh M62.45-●
 upper arm M62.42-●
neck —*see* Torticollis
ocular muscle —*see* Strabismus
organ or site, congenital NEC —*see* Atresia, by site
outlet (pelvis) —*see* Contraction, pelvis
palmar fascia M72.0
paralytic
 joint —*see* Contraction, joint
 muscle —*see also* Contraction, muscle NEC
 ocular —*see* Strabismus, paralytic
pelvis (acquired) (general) M95.5
 with disproportion (fetopelvic) O33.1
 causing obstructed labor O65.1
 inlet O33.2
 mid-cavity O33.3
 outlet O33.3
plantar fascia M72.2
premature
 atrium I49.1
 auriculoventricular I49.49
 heart I49.49
 junctional I49.2
 supraventricular I49.1
 ventricular I49.3
prostate N42.89
pylorus NEC —*see also* Pylorospasm
 psychogenic F45.8
rectum, rectal (sphincter) K59.8
ring (Bandl's) (complicating delivery) O62.4
scar —*see* Cicatrix
spine —*see* Dorsopathy, deforming
sternocleidomastoid (muscle), congenital Q68.0
stomach K31.89
 hourglass K31.89
 congenital Q40.2
 psychogenic F45.8
 psychogenic F45.8
tendon (sheath) M62.40
 with contracture of joint —*see* Contraction, joint
 Achilles —*see* Short, tendon, Achilles
 ankle M62.47-●
 Achilles —*see* Short, tendon, Achilles
 foot M62.47-●
 forearm M62.43-●
 hand M62.44-●
 lower leg M62.46-●
 multiple sites M62.49
 neck M62.48
 pelvic region M62.45-●
 shoulder region M62.41-●
 specified site NEC M62.48
 thigh M62.45-●
 thorax M62.48
 trunk M62.48
 upper arm M62.42-●
toe —*see* Deformity, toe, specified NEC
ureterovesical orifice (postinfectional) N13.5
 with infection N13.6
urethra —*see also* Stricture, urethra
 orifice N32.0
uterus N85.8
 abnormal NEC O62.9
 clonic (complicating delivery) O62.4
 dyscoordinate (complicating delivery) O62.4

▶ New ⇒ Revised ~~deleted~~ Deleted ● Use Additional Character(s) 131

Contraction, contracture, contracted
  (Continued)
  uterus *(Continued)*
    hourglass (complicating delivery) O62.4
    hypertonic O62.4
    hypotonic NEC O62.2
    inadequate
      primary O62.0
      secondary O62.1
    incoordinate (complicating delivery) O62.4
    poor O62.2
    tetanic (complicating delivery) O62.4
  vagina (outlet) N89.5
  vesical N32.89
    neck or urethral orifice N32.0
  visual field —*see* Defect, visual field,
    generalized
  Volkmann's (ischemic) T79.6
Contusion (skin surface intact) T14.8
  abdomen, abdominal (muscle) (wall) S30.1
  adnexa, eye NEC S05.8X-●
  adrenal gland S37.812
  alveolar process S00.532
  ankle S90.0-●
  antecubital space —*see* Contusion, forearm
  anus S30.3
  arm (upper) S40.02-●
    lower (with elbow) —*see* Contusion,
      forearm
  auditory canal —*see* Contusion, ear
  auricle —*see* Contusion, ear
  axilla —*see* Contusion, arm, upper
  back —*see also* Contusion, thorax, back
    lower S30.0
  bile duct S36.13
  bladder S37.22
  bone NEC T14.8
  brain (diffuse) —*see* Injury, intracranial, diffuse
    focal —*see* Injury, intracranial, focal
  brainstem S06.38-●
  breast S20.0-●
  broad ligament S37.892
  brow S00.83
  buttock S30.0
  canthus, eye S00.1-●
  cauda equina S34.3
  cerebellar, traumatic S06.37-●
  cerebral S06.33-●
    left side S06.32-●
    right side S06.31-●
  cheek S00.83
    internal S00.532
  chest (wall) —*see* Contusion, thorax
  chin S00.83
  clitoris S30.23
  colon —*see* Injury, intestine, large, contusion
  common bile duct S36.13
  conjunctiva S05.1-●
    with foreign body (in conjunctival sac) —
      see Foreign body, conjunctival sac
  conus medullaris (spine) S34.139
  cornea —*see* Contusion, eyeball
    with foreign body —*see* Foreign body,
      cornea
  corpus cavernosum S30.21
  cortex (brain) (cerebral) —*see* Injury,
    intracranial, diffuse
    focal —*see* Injury, intracranial, focal
  costal region —*see* Contusion, thorax
  cystic duct S36.13
  diaphragm S27.802
  duodenum S36.420
  ear S00.43-●
  elbow S50.0-●
    with forearm —*see* Contusion, forearm
  epididymis S30.22
  epigastric region S30.1
  epiglottis S10.0
  esophagus (thoracic) S27.812
    cervical S10.0
  eyeball S05.1-●

Contusion *(Continued)*
  eyebrow S00.1-●
  eyelid (and periocular area) S00.1-●
  face NEC S00.83
  fallopian tube S37.529
    bilateral S37.522
    unilateral S37.521
  femoral triangle S30.1
  finger(s) S60.00
    with damage to nail (matrix) S60.10
    index S60.02-●
      with damage to nail S60.12-●
    little S60.05-●
      with damage to nail S60.15-●
    middle S60.03-●
      with damage to nail S60.13-●
    ring S60.04-●
      with damage to nail S60.14-●
    thumb —*see* Contusion, thumb
  flank S30.1
  foot (except toe(s) alone) S90.3-●
    toe —*see* Contusion, toe
  forearm S50.1-●
    elbow only —*see* Contusion, elbow
  forehead S00.83
  gallbladder S36.122
  genital organs, external
    female S30.202
    male S30.201
  globe (eye) —*see* Contusion, eyeball
  groin S30.1
  gum S00.532
  hand S60.22-●
    finger(s) —*see* Contusion, finger
    wrist —*see* Contusion, wrist
  head S00.93
    ear —*see* Contusion, ear
    eyelid —*see* Contusion, eyelid
    lip S00.531
    nose S00.33
    oral cavity S00.532
    scalp S00.03
    specified part NEC S00.83
  heart —*see also* Injury, heart S26.91
  heel —*see* Contusion, foot
  hepatic duct S36.13
  hip S70.0-●
  ileum S36.428
  iliac region S30.1
  inguinal region S30.1
  interscapular region S20.229
  intra-abdominal organ S36.92
    colon —*see* Injury, intestine, large, contusion
    liver S36.112
    pancreas —*see* Contusion, pancreas
    rectum S36.62
    small intestine —*see* Injury, intestine, small,
      contusion
    specified organ NEC S36.892
    spleen —*see* Contusion, spleen
    stomach S36.32
  iris (eye) —*see* Contusion, eyeball
  jaw S00.83
  jejunum S36.428
  kidney S37.01-●
    major (greater than 2 cm) S37.02-●
    minor (less than 2 cm) S37.01-●
  knee S80.0-●
  labium (majus) (minus) S30.23
  lacrimal apparatus, gland or sac S05.8X-●
  larynx S10.0
  leg (lower) S80.1-●
    knee —*see* Contusion, knee
  lens —*see* Contusion, eyeball
  lip S00.531
  liver S36.112
  lower back S30.0
  lumbar region S30.0
  lung S27.329
    bilateral S27.322
    unilateral S27.321

Contusion *(Continued)*
  malar region S00.83
  mastoid region S00.83
  membrane, brain —*see* Injury, intracranial,
    diffuse
    focal —*see* Injury, intracranial, focal
  mesentery S36.892
  mesosalpinx S37.892
  mouth S00.532
  muscle —*see* Contusion, by site
  nail
    finger —*see* Contusion, finger, with
      damage to nail
    toe —*see* Contusion, toe, with damage to
      nail
  nasal S00.33
  neck S10.93
    specified site NEC S10.83
    throat S10.0
  nerve —*see* Injury, nerve
  newborn P54.5
  nose S00.33
  occipital
    lobe (brain) —*see* Injury, intracranial,
      diffuse
      focal —*see* Injury, intracranial,
        focal
    region (scalp) S00.03
  orbit (region) (tissues) S05.1-●
  ovary S37.429
    bilateral S37.422
    unilateral S37.421
  palate S00.532
  pancreas S36.229
    body S36.221
    head S36.220
    tail S36.222
  parietal
    lobe (brain) —*see* Injury, intracranial,
      diffuse
      focal —*see* Injury, intracranial, focal
    region (scalp) S00.03
  pelvic organ S37.92
    adrenal gland S37.812
    bladder S37.22
    fallopian tube —*see* Contusion, fallopian
      tube
    kidney —*see* Contusion, kidney
    ovary —*see* Contusion, ovary
    prostate S37.822
    specified organ NEC S37.892
    ureter S37.12
    urethra S37.32
    uterus S37.62
  pelvis S30.0
  penis S30.21
  perineum
    female S30.23
    male S30.0
  periocular area S00.1-●
  peritoneum S36.81
  periurethral tissue —*see* Contusion,
    urethra
  pharynx S10.0
  pinna —*see* Contusion, ear
  popliteal space —*see* Contusion, knee
  prepuce S30.21
  prostate S37.822
  pubic region S30.1
  pudendum
    female S30.202
    male S30.201
  quadriceps femoris —*see* Contusion, thigh
  rectum S36.62
  retroperitoneum S36.892
  round ligament S37.892
  sacral region S30.0
  scalp S00.03
    due to birth injury P12.3
  scapular region —*see* Contusion, shoulder
  sclera —*see* Contusion, eyeball

▶ New   ⇒ Revised   ~~deleted~~ Deleted   ● Use Additional Character(s)

Contusion (Continued)
scrotum S30.22
seminal vesicle S37.892
shoulder S40.01-•
skin NEC T14.8
small intestine —see Injury, intestine, small,
   contusion
spermatic cord S30.22
spinal cord —see Injury, spinal cord,
   by region
   cauda equina S34.3
   conus medullaris S34.139
spleen S36.029
   major S36.021
   minor S36.020
sternal region S20.219
stomach S36.32
subconjunctival S05.1-•
subcutaneous NEC T14.8
submaxillary region S00.83
submental region S00.83
subperiosteal NEC T14.8
subungual
   finger —see Contusion, finger, with
      damage to nail
   toe —see Contusion, toe, with damage to
      nail
supraclavicular fossa S10.83
supraorbital S00.83
suprarenal gland S37.812
temple (region) S00.83
temporal
   lobe (brain) —see Injury, intracranial,
      diffuse
   focal —see Injury, intracranial, focal
   region S00.83
testis S30.22
thigh S70.1-•
thorax (wall) S20.20
   back S20.22-•
   front S20.21-•
throat S10.0
thumb S60.01-•
   with damage to nail S60.11-•
toe(s) (lesser) S90.12-•
   with damage to nail S90.22-•
   great S90.11-•
      with damage to nail S90.21-•
      specified type NEC S90.221
tongue S00.532
trachea (cervical) S10.0
   thoracic S27.52
tunica vaginalis S30.22
tympanum, tympanic membrane —see
   Contusion, ear
ureter S37.12
urethra S37.32
urinary organ NEC S37.892
uterus S37.62
uvula S00.532
vagina S30.23
vas deferens S37.892
vesical S37.22
vocal cord(s) S10.0
vulva S30.23
wrist S60.21-•
Conus (congenital) (any type) Q14.8
   cornea —see Keratoconus
   medullaris syndrome G95.81
Conversion hysteria, neurosis or reaction
   F44.9
Converter, tuberculosis (test reaction) R76.11
Conviction (legal), anxiety concerning Z65.0
   with imprisonment Z65.1
Convulsions (idiopathic) —see also Seizure(s)
   R56.9
   apoplectiform (cerebral ischemia) I67.82
   dissociative F44.5
   epileptic —see Epilepsy
   epileptiform, epileptoid —see Seizure,
      epileptiform

Convulsions (Continued)
   ether (anesthetic) —see Table of Drugs and
      Chemicals, by drug
   febrile R56.00
      with status epilepticus G40.901
      complex R56.01
         with status epilepticus G40.901
      simple R56.00
   hysterical F44.5
   infantile P90
      epilepsy —see Epilepsy
   jacksonian —see Epilepsy, localization-
      related, symptomatic, with simple
      partial seizures
   myoclonic G25.3
   newborn P90
   obstetrical (nephritic) (uremic) —see
      Eclampsia
   paretic A52.17
   post traumatic R56.1
   psychomotor —see Epilepsy, localization-
      related, symptomatic, with complex
      partial seizures
   recurrent R56.9
   reflex R25.8
   scarlatinal A38.8
   tetanus, tetanic —see Tetanus
   thymic E32.8
Convulsive —see also Convulsions
Cooley's anemia D56.1
Coolie itch B76.9
Cooper's
   disease —see Mastopathy, cystic
   hernia —see Hernia, abdomen, specified site
      NEC
Copra itch B88.0
Coprophagy F50.89
Coprophobia F40.298
Coproporphyria, hereditary E80.29
Cor
   biloculare Q20.8
   bovis, bovinum —see Hypertrophy,
      cardiac
   pulmonale (chronic) I27.81
      acute I26.09
   triatriatum, triatrium Q24.2
   triloculare Q20.8
      biatrium Q20.4
      biventriculare Q21.1
Corbus' disease (gangrenous balanitis) N48.1
Cord —see also condition
➠around neck
   ➠complicating delivery O69.81
      ▶with compression O69.1
   bladder G95.89
      tabetic A52.19
Cordis ectopia Q24.8
Corditis (spermatic) N49.1
Corectopia Q13.2
Cori's disease (glycogen storage) E74.03
Corkhandler's disease or lung J67.3
Corkscrew esophagus K22.4
Corkworker's disease or lung J67.3
Corn (infected) L84
Cornea —see also condition
   donor Z52.5
   plana Q13.4
Cornelia de Lange syndrome Q87.1
Cornu cutaneum L85.8
Cornual gestation or pregnancy O00.80
   with intrauterine pregnancy O00.81
Coronary (artery) —see condition
Coronavirus, as cause of disease classified
   elsewhere B97.29
   SARS-associated B97.21
Corpora —see also condition
   amylacea, prostate N42.89
   cavernosa —see condition
Corpulence —see Obesity
Corpus —see condition
Corrected transposition Q20.5

Corrosion (injury) (acid) (caustic) (chemical)
   (lime) (external) (internal) T30.4
   abdomen, abdominal (muscle) (wall) T21.42
      first degree T21.52
      second degree T21.62
      third degree T21.72
   above elbow T22.439
      first degree T22.539
      left T22.432
         first degree T22.532
         second degree T22.632
         third degree T22.732
      right T22.431
         first degree T22.531
         second degree T22.631
         third degree T22.731
      second degree T22.639
      third degree T22.739
   alimentary tract NEC T28.7
   ankle T25.419
      first degree T25.519
      left T25.412
         first degree T25.512
         second degree T25.612
         third degree T25.712
      multiple with foot —see Corrosion, lower,
         limb, multiple, ankle and foot
      right T25.411
         first degree T25.511
         second degree T25.611
         third degree T25.711
      second degree T25.619
      third degree T25.719
   anus —see Corrosion, buttock
   arm(s) (meaning upper limb(s)) —see
      Corrosion, upper limb
   axilla T22.449
      first degree T22.549
      left T22.442
         first degree T22.542
         second degree T22.642
         third degree T22.742
      right T22.441
         first degree T22.541
         second degree T22.641
         third degree T22.741
      second degree T22.649
      third degree T22.749
   back (lower) T21.44
      first degree T21.54
      second degree T21.64
      third degree T21.74
      upper T21.43
         first degree T21.53
         second degree T21.63
         third degree T21.73
   blisters - code as Corrosion, second degree,
      by site
   breast(s) —see Corrosion, chest wall
   buttock(s) T21.45
      first degree T21.55
      second degree T21.65
      third degree T21.75
   calf T24.439
      first degree T24.539
      left T24.432
         first degree T24.532
         second degree T24.632
         third degree T24.732
      right T24.431
         first degree T24.531
         second degree T24.631
         third degree T24.731
      second degree T24.639
      third degree T24.739
   canthus (eye) —see Corrosion, eyelid
   cervix T28.8
   cheek T20.46
      first degree T20.56
      second degree T20.66
      third degree T20.76

▶ New   ➡ Revised   ~~deleted~~ Deleted   ● Use Additional Character(s)

Corrosion (Continued)
  hand(s) (Continued)
    multiple sites (Continued)
      right T23.491
        first degree T23.591
        second degree T23.691
        third degree T23.791
      second degree T23.699
      third degree T23.799
    palm —see Corrosion, palm
    right T23.401
      first degree T23.501
      second degree T23.601
      third degree T23.701
    second degree T23.609
    third degree T23.709
    thumb —see Corrosion, thumb
  head (and face) (and neck) T20.40
    cheek —see Corrosion, cheek
    chin —see Corrosion, chin
    ear —see Corrosion, ear
    eye(s) only —see Corrosion, eye
    first degree T20.50
    forehead —see Corrosion, forehead
    lip —see Corrosion, lip
    multiple sites T20.49
      first degree T20.59
      second degree T20.69
      third degree T20.79
    neck —see Corrosion, neck
    nose —see Corrosion, nose
    scalp —see Corrosion, scalp
    second degree T20.60
    third degree T20.70
  hip(s) —see Corrosion, lower, limb
  inhalation —see Corrosion, respiratory
      tract
  internal organ(s) (see also Corrosion, by site)
      T28.90
    alimentary tract T28.7
      esophagus T28.6
    esophagus T28.6
    genitourinary T28.8
    mouth T28.5
    pharynx T28.5
    specified organ NEC T28.99
  interscapular region —see Corrosion, back,
      upper
  intestine (large) (small) T28.7
  knee T24.429
    first degree T24.529
    left T24.422
      first degree T24.522
      second degree T24.622
      third degree T24.722
    right T24.421
      first degree T24.521
      second degree T24.621
      third degree T24.721
    second degree T24.629
    third degree T24.729
  labium (majus) (minus) —see Corrosion,
      genital organs, external, female
  lacrimal apparatus, duct, gland or sac —see
      Corrosion, eye, specified site NEC
  larynx T27.4
    with lung T27.5
  leg(s) (meaning lower limb(s)) —see
      Corrosion, lower limb
  limb(s)
    lower —see Corrosion, lower, limb
    upper —see Corrosion, upper limb
  lip(s) T20.42
    first degree T20.52
    second degree T20.62
    third degree T20.72
  lower
    back —see Corrosion, back
    limb T24.409
      ankle —see Corrosion, ankle
      calf —see Corrosion, calf

Corrosion (Continued)
  lower (Continued)
    limb (Continued)
      first degree T24.509
      foot —see Corrosion, foot
      hip —see Corrosion, thigh
      knee —see Corrosion, knee
      left T24.402
        first degree T24.502
        second degree T24.602
        third degree T24.702
      multiple sites, except ankle and foot
          T24.499
        ankle and foot T25.499
          first degree T25.599
          left T25.492
            first degree T25.592
            second degree T25.692
            third degree T25.792
          right T25.491
            first degree T25.591
            second degree T25.691
            third degree T25.791
          second degree T25.699
          third degree T25.799
        first degree T24.599
        left T24.492
          first degree T24.592
          second degree T24.692
          third degree T24.792
        right T24.491
          first degree T24.591
          second degree T24.691
          third degree T24.791
        second degree T24.699
        third degree T24.799
      right T24.401
        first degree T24.501
        second degree T24.601
        third degree T24.701
      second degree T24.609
      third degree T24.709
      thigh —see Corrosion, thigh
  lung (with larynx and trachea)
      T27.5
  mouth T28.5
  neck T20.47
    first degree T20.57
    second degree T20.67
    third degree T20.77
  nose (septum) T20.44
    first degree T20.54
    second degree T20.64
    third degree T20.74
  ocular adnexa —see Corrosion, eye
  orbit region —see Corrosion, eyelid
  palm T23.459
    first degree T23.559
    left T23.452
      first degree T23.552
      second degree T23.652
      third degree T23.752
    right T23.451
      first degree T23.551
      second degree T23.651
      third degree T23.751
    second degree T23.659
    third degree T23.759
  partial thickness - code as Corrosion,
      unspecified degree, by site
  pelvis —see Corrosion, trunk
  penis —see Corrosion, genital organs,
      external, male
  perineum
    female —see Corrosion, genital organs,
        external, female
    male —see Corrosion, genital organs,
        external, male
  periocular area —see Corrosion, eyelid
  pharynx T28.5
  rectum T28.7

Corrosion (Continued)
  respiratory tract T27.7
    larynx —see Corrosion, larynx
    specified part NEC T27.6
    trachea —see Corrosion, larynx
  sac, lacrimal —see Corrosion, eye,
      specified site NEC
  scalp T20.45
    first degree T20.55
    second degree T20.65
    third degree T20.75
  scapular region T22.469
    first degree T22.569
    left T22.462
      first degree T22.562
      second degree T22.662
      third degree T22.762
    right T22.461
      first degree T22.561
      second degree T22.661
      third degree T22.761
    second degree T22.669
    third degree T22.769
  sclera —see Corrosion, eye, specified site
      NEC
  scrotum —see Corrosion, genital organs,
      external, male
  shoulder T22.459
    first degree T22.559
    left T22.452
      first degree T22.552
      second degree T22.652
      third degree T22.752
    right T22.451
      first degree T22.551
      second degree T22.651
      third degree T22.751
    second degree T22.659
    third degree T22.759
  stomach T28.7
  temple —see Corrosion, head
  testis —see Corrosion, genital organs,
      external, male
  thigh T24.419
    first degree T24.519
    left T24.412
      first degree T24.512
      second degree T24.612
      third degree T24.712
    right T24.411
      first degree T24.511
      second degree T24.611
      third degree T24.711
    second degree T24.619
    third degree T24.719
  thorax (external) —see Corrosion, trunk
  throat (meaning pharynx) T28.5
  thumb(s) T23.419
    first degree T23.519
    left T23.412
      first degree T23.512
      second degree T23.612
      third degree T23.712
    multiple sites with fingers T23.449
      first degree T23.549
      left T23.442
        first degree T23.542
        second degree T23.642
        third degree T23.742
      right T23.441
        first degree T23.541
        second degree T23.641
        third degree T23.741
      second degree T23.649
      third degree T23.749
    right T23.411
      first degree T23.511
      second degree T23.611
      third degree T23.711
    second degree T23.619
    third degree T23.719

Corrosion *(Continued)*
  toe T25.439
    first degree T25.539
    left T25.432
      first degree T25.532
      second degree T25.632
      third degree T25.732
    right T25.431
      first degree T25.531
      second degree T25.631
      third degree T25.731
    second degree T25.639
    third degree T25.739
  tongue T28.5
  tonsil(s) T28.5
  total body —*see* Corrosion, multiple body
    regions
  trachea T27.4
    with lung T27.5
  trunk T21.40
    abdominal wall —*see* Corrosion,
      abdominal wall
    anus —*see* Corrosion, buttock
    axilla —*see* Corrosion, upper limb
    back —*see* Corrosion, back
    breast —*see* Corrosion, chest wall
    buttock —*see* Corrosion, buttock
    chest wall —*see* Corrosion, chest wall
    first degree T21.50
    flank —*see* Corrosion, abdominal wall
    genital
      female —*see* Corrosion, genital organs,
        external, female
      male —*see* Corrosion, genital organs,
        external, male
    groin —*see* Corrosion, abdominal wall
    interscapular region —*see* Corrosion, back,
      upper
    labia —*see* Corrosion, genital organs,
      external, female
    lower back —*see* Corrosion, back
    penis —*see* Corrosion, genital organs,
      external, male
    perineum
      female —*see* Corrosion, genital organs,
        external, female
      male —*see* Corrosion, genital organs,
        external, male
    scapular region —*see* Corrosion, upper
      limb
    scrotum —*see* Corrosion, genital organs,
      external, male
    second degree T21.60
    shoulder —*see* Corrosion, upper limb
    specified site NEC T21.49
      first degree T21.59
      second degree T21.69
      third degree T21.79
    testes —*see* Corrosion, genital organs,
      external, male
    third degree T21.70
    upper back —*see* Corrosion, back, upper
    vagina T28.8
    vulva —*see* Corrosion, genital organs,
      external, female
  unspecified site with extent of body surface
    involved specified
    ▉▶less than 10 percent T32.0
    ▉▶10-19 percent (0-9 percent third degree)
      T32.10
      with 10-19 percent third degree T32.11
    ▉▶20-29 percent (0-9 percent third degree)
      T32.20
      with
        10-19 percent third degree T32.21
        20-29 percent third degree T32.22
    ▉▶30-39 percent (0-9 percent third degree)
      T32.30
      with
        10-19 percent third degree T32.31
        20-29 percent third degree T32.32
        30-39 percent third degree T32.33

Corrosion *(Continued)*
  unspecified site with extent of body surface
    involved specified *(Continued)*
    ▉▶40-49 percent (0-9 percent third degree)
      T32.40
      with
        10-19 percent third degree T32.41
        20-29 percent third degree T32.42
        30-39 percent third degree T32.43
        40-49 percent third degree T32.44
    ▉▶50-59 percent (0-9 percent third degree)
      T32.50
      with
        10-19 percent third degree T32.51
        20-29 percent third degree T32.52
        30-39 percent third degree T32.53
        40-49 percent third degree T32.54
        50-59 percent third degree T32.55
    ▉▶60-69 percent (0-9 percent third degree)
      T32.60
      with
        10-19 percent third degree T32.61
        20-29 percent third degree T32.62
        30-39 percent third degree T32.63
        40-49 percent third degree T32.64
        50-59 percent third degree T32.65
        60-69 percent third degree T32.66
    ▉▶70-79 percent (0-9 percent third degree)
      T32.70
      with
        10-19 percent third degree T32.71
        20-29 percent third degree T32.72
        30-39 percent third degree T32.73
        40-49 percent third degree T32.74
        50-59 percent third degree T32.75
        60-69 percent third degree T32.76
        70-79 percent third degree T32.77
    ▉▶80-89 percent (0-9 percent third degree)
      T32.80
      with
        10-19 percent third degree T32.81
        20-29 percent third degree T32.82
        30-39 percent third degree T32.83
        40-49 percent third degree T32.84
        50-59 percent third degree T32.85
        60-69 percent third degree T32.86
        70-79 percent third degree T32.87
        80-89 percent third degree T32.88
    ▉▶90 percent or more (0-9 percent third
      degree) T32.90
      with
        10-19 percent third degree T32.91
        20-29 percent third degree T32.92
        30-39 percent third degree T32.93
        40-49 percent third degree T32.94
        50-59 percent third degree T32.95
        60-69 percent third degree T32.96
        70-79 percent third degree T32.97
        80-89 percent third degree T32.98
        90-99 percent third degree T32.99
  upper limb (axilla) (scapular region) T22.40
    above elbow —*see* Corrosion, above elbow
    axilla —*see* Corrosion, axilla
    elbow —*see* Corrosion, elbow
    first degree T22.50
    forearm —*see* Corrosion, forearm
    hand —*see* Corrosion, hand
    interscapular region —*see* Corrosion, back,
      upper
    multiple sites T22.499
      first degree T22.599
      left T22.492
        first degree T22.592
        second degree T22.692
        third degree T22.792
      right T22.491
        first degree T22.591
        second degree T22.691
        third degree T22.791
      second degree T22.699
      third degree T22.799

Corrosion *(Continued)*
  upper limb (axilla) (scapular region)
    (Continued)
    scapular region —*see* Corrosion, scapular
      region
    second degree T22.60
    shoulder —*see* Corrosion, shoulder
    third degree T22.70
    wrist —*see* Corrosion, hand
  uterus T28.8
  vagina T28.8
  vulva —*see* Corrosion, genital organs,
    external, female
  wrist T23.479
    first degree T23.579
    left T23.472
      first degree T23.572
      second degree T23.672
      third degree T23.772
    multiple sites with hand T23.499
      first degree T23.599
      left T23.492
        first degree T23.592
        second degree T23.692
        third degree T23.792
      right T23.491
        first degree T23.591
        second degree T23.691
        third degree T23.791
      second degree T23.699
      third degree T23.799
    right T23.471
      first degree T23.571
      second degree T23.671
      third degree T23.771
    second degree T23.679
    third degree T23.779
Corrosive burn —*see* Corrosion
Corsican fever —*see* Malaria
Cortical —*see* condition
Cortico-adrenal —*see* condition
Coryza (acute) J00
  with grippe or influenza —*see* Influenza,
    with, respiratory manifestations
    NEC
  syphilitic
    congenital (chronic) A50.05
Costen's syndrome or complex M26.69
Costiveness —*see* Constipation
Costochondritis M94.0
Cot death R99
Cotard's syndrome F22
Cotia virus B08.8
Cotton wool spots (retinal) H35.81
Cotungo's disease —*see* Sciatica
Cough (affected) (chronic) (epidemic) (nervous)
  R05
  with hemorrhage —*see* Hemoptysis
  bronchial R05
    with grippe or influenza —*see* Influenza,
      with, respiratory manifestations
      NEC
  functional F45.8
  hysterical F45.8
  laryngeal, spasmodic R05
  psychogenic F45.8
  smokers' J41.0
  tea taster's B49
Counseling (for) Z71.9
  abuse NEC
    perpetrator Z69.82
    victim Z69.81
  alcohol abuser Z71.41
    family Z71.42
  child abuse
    nonparental
      perpetrator Z69.021
      victim Z69.020
    parental
      perpetrator Z69.011
      victim Z69.010

▶ New   ▉▶ Revised   ~~deleted~~ Deleted   ● Use Additional Character(s)

Counseling (Continued)
  consanguinity Z71.89
  contraceptive Z30.09
  dietary Z71.3
  drug abuser Z71.51
    family member Z71.52
▶ exercise Z71.82
  family Z71.89
  fertility preservation (prior to cancer therapy)
      (prior to removal of gonads) Z31.62
  for non-attending third party Z71.0
    related to sexual behavior or orientation
        Z70.2
  ~~genetic NEC Z31.5~~
▶ genetic
  ▶ nonprocreative Z71.83
  ▶ procreative NEC Z31.5
  gestational carrier Z31.7
  health (advice) (education) (instruction) —see
      Counseling, medical
  human immunodeficiency virus (HIV) Z71.7
  impotence Z70.1
  insulin pump use Z46.81
  medical (for) Z71.9
    boarding school resident Z59.3
    consanguinity Z71.89
    feared complaint and no disease found Z71.1
    human immunodeficiency virus (HIV) Z71.7
    institutional resident Z59.3
    on behalf of another Z71.0
      related to sexual behavior or orientation
          Z70.2
    person living alone Z60.2
    specified reason NEC Z71.89
  natural family planning
    procreative Z31.61
    to avoid pregnancy Z30.02
  perpetrator (of)
    abuse NEC Z69.82
    child abuse
      non-parental Z69.021
      parental Z69.011
    rape NEC Z69.82
    spousal abuse Z69.12
  procreative NEC Z31.69
    fertility preservation (prior to cancer
        therapy) (prior to removal of
        gonads) Z31.62
    using natural family planning Z31.61
  promiscuity Z70.1
  rape victim Z69.81
  religious Z71.81
  sex, sexual (related to) Z70.9
    attitude(s) Z70.0
    behavior or orientation Z70.1
    combined concerns Z70.3
    non-responsiveness Z70.1
    on behalf of third party Z70.2
    specified reason NEC Z70.8
  specified reason NEC Z71.89
  spiritual Z71.81
  spousal abuse (perpetrator) Z69.12
    victim Z69.11
  substance abuse Z71.89
    alcohol Z71.41
    drug Z71.51
    tobacco Z71.6
  tobacco use Z71.6
  use (of)
    insulin pump Z46.81
  victim (of)
    abuse Z69.81
    child abuse
      by parent Z69.010
      non-parental Z69.020
    rape NEC Z69.81
Coupled rhythm R00.8
Couvelaire syndrome or uterus (complicating
    delivery) O45.8X-●
Cowperitis —see Urethritis
Cowper's gland —see condition

Cowpox B08.010
  due to vaccination T88.1
Coxa
  magna M91.4-●
  plana M91.2-●
  valga (acquired) —see also Deformity, limb,
      specified type NEC, thigh
    congenital Q65.81
    sequelae (late effect) of rickets E64.3
  vara (acquired) —see also Deformity, limb,
      specified type NEC, thigh
    congenital Q65.82
    sequelae (late effect) of rickets E64.3
Coxalgia, coxalgic (nontuberculous) —see also
    Pain, joint, hip
  tuberculous A18.02
Coxitis —see Monoarthritis, hip
Coxsackie (virus) (infection) B34.1
  as cause of disease classified elsewhere B97.11
  carditis B33.20
  central nervous system NEC A88.8
  endocarditis B33.21
  enteritis A08.39
  meningitis (aseptic) A87.0
  myocarditis B33.22
  pericarditis B33.23
  pharyngitis B08.5
  pleurodynia B33.0
  specific disease NEC B33.8
Crabs, meaning pubic lice B85.3
Crack baby P04.41
Cracked nipple N64.0
  associated with
    lactation O92.13
      pregnancy O92.11-●
      puerperium O92.12
Cracked tooth K03.81
Cradle cap L21.0
Craft neurosis F48.8
Cramp(s) R25.2
  abdominal —see Pain, abdominal
  bathing T75.1
  colic R10.83
    psychogenic F45.8
  due to immersion T75.1
  fireman T67.2
  heat T67.2
  immersion T75.1
  intestinal —see Pain, abdominal
    psychogenic F45.8
  leg, sleep related G47.62
  limb (lower) (upper) NEC R25.2
    sleep related G47.62
  linotypist's F48.8
    organic G25.89
  muscle (limb) (general) R25.2
    due to immersion T75.1
    psychogenic F45.8
  occupational (hand) F48.8
    organic G25.89
  salt-depletion E87.1
  sleep related, leg G47.62
  stoker's T67.2
  swimmer's T75.1
  telegrapher's F48.8
    organic G25.89
  typist's F48.8
    organic G25.89
  uterus N94.89
    menstrual —see Dysmenorrhea
  writer's F48.8
    organic G25.89
Cranial —see condition
Craniocleidodysostosis Q74.0
Craniofenestria (skull) Q75.8
Craniolacunia (skull) Q75.8
Craniopagus Q89.4
Craniopathy, metabolic M85.2
Craniopharyngeal —see condition
Craniopharyngioma D44.4
Craniorachischisis (totalis) Q00.1

Cranioschisis Q75.8
Craniostenosis Q75.0
Craniosynostosis Q75.0
Craniotabes (cause unknown) M83.8
  neonatal P96.3
  rachitic E64.3
  syphilitic A50.56
Cranium —see condition
Craw-craw —see Onchocerciasis
Creaking joint —see Derangement, joint,
    specified type NEC
Creeping
  eruption B76.9
  palsy or paralysis G12.22
Crenated tongue K14.8
Creotoxism A05.9
Crepitus
  caput Q75.8
  joint —see Derangement, joint, specified type
      NEC
Crescent or conus choroid, congenital Q14.3
CREST syndrome M34.1
Cretin, cretinism (congenital) (endemic)
    (nongoitrous) (sporadic) E00.9
  pelvis
    with disproportion (fetopelvic) O33.0
      causing obstructed labor O65.0
  type
    hypothyroid E00.1
    mixed E00.2
    myxedematous E00.1
    neurological E00.0
Creutzfeldt-Jakob disease or syndrome (with
    dementia) A81.00
  familial A81.09
  iatrogenic A81.09
  specified NEC A81.09
  sporadic A81.09
  variant (vCJD) A81.01
Crib death R99
Cribriform hymen Q52.3
Cri-du-chat syndrome Q93.4
Crigler-Najjar disease or syndrome E80.5
Crime, victim of Z65.4
Crimean hemorrhagic fever A98.0
Criminalism F60.2
Crisis
  abdomen R10.0
  acute reaction F43.0
  addisonian E27.2
  adrenal (cortical) E27.2
  celiac K90.0
  Dietl's N13.8
  emotional —see also Disorder, adjustment
    acute reaction to stress F43.0
    specific to childhood and adolescence F93.8
  glaucomatocyclitic —see Glaucoma,
      secondary, inflammation
  heart —see Failure, heart
  nitritoid I95.2
    correct substance properly administered —
        see Table of Drugs and Chemicals, by
        drug, adverse effect
    overdose or wrong substance given
        or taken —see Table of Drugs and
        Chemicals, by drug, poisoning
  oculogyric H51.8
    psychogenic F45.8
  Pel's (tabetic) A52.11
  psychosexual identity F64.2
  renal N28.0
  sickle-cell D57.00
    with
      acute chest syndrome D57.01
      splenic sequestration D57.02
  state (acute reaction) F43.0
  tabetic A52.11
  thyroid —see Thyrotoxicosis with thyroid
      storm
  thyrotoxic —see Thyrotoxicosis with thyroid
      storm

Crocq's disease (acrocyanosis) I73.89
Crohn's disease —see Enteritis, regional
Crooked septum, nasal J34.2
Cross syndrome E70.328
Crossbite (anterior) (posterior) M26.24
Cross-eye —see Strabismus, convergent
    concomitant
Croup, croupous (catarrhal) (infectious)
    (inflammatory) (nondiphtheritic) J05.0
  bronchial J20.9
  diphtheritic A36.2
  false J38.5
  spasmodic J38.5
    diphtheritic A36.2
  stridulous J38.5
    diphtheritic A36.2
Crouzon's disease Q75.1
Crowding, tooth, teeth, fully erupted M26.31
CRST syndrome M34.1
Cruchet's disease A85.8
Cruelty in children —see also Disorder, conduct
Crural ulcer —see Ulcer, lower limb
Crush, crushed, crushing T14.8
  abdomen S38.1
  ankle S97.0-●
  arm (upper) (and shoulder) S47.-●
  axilla —see Crush, arm
  back, lower S38.1
  buttock S38.1
  cheek S07.0
  chest S28.0
  cranium S07.1
  ear S07.0
  elbow S57.0-●
  extremity
    lower
      ankle —see Crush, ankle
      below knee —see Crush, leg
      foot —see Crush, foot
      hip —see Crush, hip
      knee —see Crush, knee
      thigh —see Crush, thigh
      toe —see Crush, toe
    upper
      below elbow S67.9-●
      elbow —see Crush, elbow
      finger —see Crush, finger
      forearm —see Crush, forearm
      hand —see Crush, hand
      thumb —see Crush, thumb
      upper arm —see Crush, arm
      wrist —see Crush, wrist
  face S07.0
  finger(s) S67.1-●
    with hand (and wrist) —see Crush, hand,
      specified site NEC
    index S67.19-●
    little S67.19-●
    middle S67.19-●
    ring S67.19-●
    thumb —see Crush, thumb
  foot S97.8-●
    toe —see Crush, toe
  forearm S57.8-●
  genitalia, external
    female S38.002
      vagina S38.03
      vulva S38.03
    male S38.001
      penis S38.01
      scrotum S38.02
      testis S38.02
  hand (except fingers alone) S67.2-●
    with wrist S67.4-●
  head S07.9
    specified NEC S07.8
  heel —see Crush, foot
  hip S77.0-●
    with thigh S77.2-●
  internal organ (abdomen, chest, or pelvis)
    NEC T14.8

Crush, crushed, crushing (Continued)
  knee S87.0-●
  labium (majus) (minus) S38.03
  larynx S17.0
  leg (lower) S87.8-●
    knee —see Crush, knee
  lip S07.0
  lower
    back S38.1
    leg —see Crush, leg
  neck S17.9
  nerve —see Injury, nerve
  nose S07.0
  pelvis S38.1
  penis S38.01
  scalp S07.8
  scapular region —see Crush, arm
  scrotum S38.02
  severe, unspecified site T14.8
  shoulder (and upper arm) —see Crush, arm
  skull S07.1
  syndrome (complication of trauma) T79.5
  testis S38.02
  thigh S77.1-●
    with hip S77.2-●
  throat S17.8
  thumb S67.0-●
    with hand (and wrist) —see Crush, hand,
      specified site NEC
  toe(s) S97.10-●
    great S97.11-●
    lesser S97.12-●
  trachea S17.0
  vagina S38.03
  vulva S38.03
  wrist S67.3-●
    with hand S67.4-●
Crusta lactea L21.0
Crusts R23.4
Crutch paralysis —see Injury, brachial plexus
Cruveilhier-Baumgarten cirrhosis, disease or
    syndrome K74.69
Cruveilhier's atrophy or disease G12.8
Crying (constant) (continuous) (excessive)
  child, adolescent, or adult R45.83
  infant (baby) (newborn) R68.11
Cryofibrinogenemia D89.2
Cryoglobulinemia (essential) (idiopathic)
    (mixed) (primary) (purpura) (secondary)
    (vasculitis) D89.1
  with lung involvement D89.1 [J99]
Cryptitis (anal) (rectal) K62.89
Cryptococcosis, cryptococcus (infection)
    (neoformans) B45.9
  bone B45.3
  cerebral B45.1
  cutaneous B45.2
  disseminated B45.7
  generalized B45.7
  meningitis B45.1
  meningocerebralis B45.1
  osseous B45.3
  pulmonary B45.0
  skin B45.2
  specified NEC B45.8
Cryptopapillitis (anus) K62.89
Cryptophthalmos Q11.2
  syndrome Q87.0
Cryptorchid, cryptorchism, cryptorchidism
    Q53.9
  bilateral Q53.20
    ➠abdominal Q53.211
    perineal Q53.22
  unilateral Q53.10
    ➠abdominal Q53.111
    perineal Q53.12
Cryptosporidiosis A07.2
  hepatobiliary B88.8
  respiratory B88.8
Cryptostromosis J67.6
Crystalluria R82.99

Cubitus
  congenital Q68.8
  valgus (acquired) M21.0-●
    congenital Q68.8
    sequelae (late effect) of rickets E64.3
  varus (acquired) M21.1-●
    congenital Q68.8
    sequelae (late effect) of rickets E64.3
Cultural deprivation or shock Z60.3
Curling esophagus K22.4
Curling's ulcer —see Ulcer, peptic, acute
Curschmann (-Batten) (-Steinert) disease or
    syndrome G71.11
Curse, Ondine's —see Apnea, sleep
Curvature
  organ or site, congenital NEC —see Distortion
  penis (lateral) Q55.61
  Pott's (spinal) A18.01
  radius, idiopathic, progressive (congenital)
    Q74.0
  spine (acquired) (angular) (idiopathic)
    (incorrect) (postural) —see Dorsopathy,
    deforming
    congenital Q67.5
    due to or associated with
      Charcot-Marie-Tooth disease —see also
        subcategory M49.8 G60.0
      osteitis
        deformans M88.88
        fibrosa cystica —see also subcategory
          M49.8 E21.0
      tuberculosis (Pott's curvature) A18.01
    sequelae (late effect) of rickets E64.3
    tuberculous A18.01
Cushingoid due to steroid therapy E24.2
  correct substance properly administered —see
    Table of Drugs and Chemicals, by drug,
    adverse effect
  overdose or wrong substance given
    or taken —see Table of Drugs and
    Chemicals, by drug, poisoning
Cushing's
  syndrome or disease E24.9
    drug-induced E24.2
    iatrogenic E24.2
    pituitary-dependent E24.0
    specified NEC E24.8
  ulcer —see Ulcer, peptic, acute
Cusp, Carabelli - omit code
Cut (external) —see also Laceration
  muscle —see Injury, muscle
Cutaneous —see also condition
  hemorrhage R23.3
  larva migrans B76.9
Cutis —see also condition
  hyperelastica Q82.8
    acquired L57.4
  laxa (hyperelastica) —see Dermatolysis
  marmorata R23.8
  osteosis L94.2
  pendula —see Dermatolysis
  rhomboidalis nuchae L57.2
  verticis gyrata Q82.8
    acquired L91.8
Cyanosis R23.0
  due to
    patent foramen botalli Q21.1
    persistent foramen ovale Q21.1
  enterogenous D74.8
  paroxysmal digital —see Raynaud's disease
    with gangrene I73.01
  retina, retinal H35.89
Cyanotic heart disease I24.9
  congenital Q24.9
Cycle
  anovulatory N97.0
  menstrual, irregular N92.6
Cyclencephaly Q04.9
Cyclical vomiting (see also Vomiting, cyclical)
    G43.A0
  psychogenic F50.89

Cyclitis —*see also* Iridocyclitis H20.9
  chronic —*see* Iridocyclitis, chronic
  Fuchs' heterochromic H20.81-●
  granulomatous —*see* Iridocyclitis, chronic
  lens-induced —*see* Iridocyclitis, lens-induced
  posterior H30.2-●
Cycloid personality F34.0
Cyclophoria H50.54
Cyclopia, cyclops Q87.0
Cyclopism Q87.0
Cyclosporiasis A07.4
Cyclothymia F34.0
Cyclothymic personality F34.0
Cyclotropia H50.41-●
Cylindroma —*see also* Neoplasm, malignant, by site
  eccrine dermal —*see* Neoplasm, skin, benign
  skin —*see* Neoplasm, skin, benign
Cylindruria R82.99
Cynanche
  diphtheritic A36.2
  tonsillaris J36
Cynophobia F40.218
Cynorexia R63.2
Cyphosis —*see* Kyphosis
Cyprus fever —*see* Brucellosis
Cyst (colloid) (mucous) (simple) (retention)
  adenoid (infected) J35.8
  adrenal gland E27.8
    congenital Q89.1
  air, lung J98.4
  allantoic Q64.4
  alveolar process (jaw bone) M27.40
  amnion, amniotic O41.8X-●
  aneurysmal M27.49
  anterior
    chamber (eye) —*see* Cyst, iris
    nasopalatine K09.1
  antrum J34.1
  anus K62.89
  apical (tooth) (periodontal) K04.8
  appendix K38.8
  arachnoid, brain (acquired) G93.0
    congenital Q04.6
  arytenoid J38.7
  Baker's M71.2-●
    ruptured M66.0
    tuberculous A18.02
  Bartholin's gland N75.0
  bile duct (common) (hepatic) K83.5
  bladder (multiple) (trigone) N32.89
  blue dome (breast) —*see* Cyst, breast
  bone (local) NEC M85.60
    aneurysmal M85.50
      ankle M85.57-●
      foot M85.57-●
      forearm M85.53-●
      hand M85.54-●
      jaw M27.49
      lower leg M85.56-●
      multiple site M85.59
      neck M85.58
      rib M85.58
      shoulder M85.51-●
      skull M85.58
      specified site NEC M85.58
      thigh M85.55-●
      toe M85.57-●
      upper arm M85.52-●
      vertebra M85.58
    solitary M85.40
      ankle M85.47-●
      fibula M85.46-●
      foot M85.47-●
      hand M85.44-●
      humerus M85.42-●
      jaw M27.49
      neck M85.48
      pelvis M85.45-●

Cyst (Continued)
  bone NEC (Continued)
    solitary (Continued)
      radius M85.43-●
      rib M85.48
      shoulder M85.41-●
      skull M85.48
      specified site NEC M85.48
      tibia M85.46-●
      toe M85.47-●
      ulna M85.43-●
      vertebra M85.48
    specified type NEC M85.60
      ankle M85.67-●
      foot M85.67-●
      forearm M85.63-●
      hand M85.64-●
      jaw M27.40
        developmental (nonodontogenic) K09.1
        odontogenic K09.0
        latent M27.0
      lower leg M85.66-●
      multiple site M85.69
      neck M85.68
      rib M85.68
      shoulder M85.61-●
      skull M85.68
      specified site NEC M85.68
      thigh M85.65-●
      toe M85.67-●
      upper arm M85.62-●
      vertebra M85.68
  brain (acquired) G93.0
    congenital Q04.6
    hydatid B67.99 [G94]
    third ventricle (colloid), congenital Q04.6
  branchial (cleft) Q18.0
  branchiogenic Q18.0
  breast (benign) (blue dome) (pedunculated) (solitary) N60.0-●
    involution —*see* Dysplasia, mammary, specified type NEC
    sebaceous —*see* Dysplasia, mammary, specified type NEC
  broad ligament (benign) N83.8
  bronchogenic (mediastinal) (sequestration) J98.4
    congenital Q33.0
  buccal K09.8
  bulbourethral gland N36.8
  bursa, bursal NEC M71.30
    with rupture —*see* Rupture, synovium
    ankle M71.37-●
    elbow M71.32-●
    foot M71.37-●
    hand M71.34-●
    hip M71.35-●
    multiple sites M71.39
    pharyngeal J39.2
    popliteal space —*see* Cyst, Baker's
    shoulder M71.31-●
    specified site NEC M71.38
    wrist M71.33-●
  calcifying odontogenic D16.5
    upper jaw (bone) (maxilla) D16.4
  canal of Nuck (female) N94.89
    congenital Q52.4
  canthus —*see* Cyst, conjunctiva
  carcinomatous —*see* Neoplasm, malignant, by site
  cauda equina G95.89
  cavum septi pellucidi —*see* Cyst, brain
  celomic (pericardium) Q24.8
  cerebellopontine (angle) —*see* Cyst, brain
  cerebellum —*see* Cyst, brain
  cerebral —*see* Cyst, brain
  cervical lateral Q18.0
  cervix NEC N88.8
    embryonic Q51.6
    nabothian N88.8

Cyst (Continued)
  chiasmal optic NEC —*see* Disorder, optic, chiasm
  chocolate (ovary) N80.1
  choledochus, congenital Q44.4
  chorion O41.8X-●
  choroid plexus G93.0
  ciliary body —*see* Cyst, iris
  clitoris N90.7
  colon K63.89
  common (bile) duct K83.5
  congenital NEC Q89.8
    adrenal gland Q89.1
    epiglottis Q31.8
    esophagus Q39.8
    fallopian tube Q50.4
    kidney Q61.00
      more than one (multiple) Q61.02
        specified as polycystic Q61.3
          adult type Q61.2
          infantile type NEC Q61.19
            collecting duct dilation Q61.11
      solitary Q61.01
    larynx Q31.8
    liver Q44.6
    lung Q33.0
    mediastinum Q34.1
    ovary Q50.1
    oviduct Q50.4
    periurethral (tissue) Q64.79
    prepuce Q55.69
    salivary gland (any) Q38.4
    sublingual Q38.6
    submaxillary gland Q38.6
    thymus (gland) Q89.2
    tongue Q38.3
    ureterovesical orifice Q62.8
    vulva Q52.79
  conjunctiva H11.44-●
  cornea H18.89-●
  corpora quadrigemina G93.0
  corpus
    albicans N83.29-●
    luteum (hemorrhagic) (ruptured) N83.1-●
  Cowper's gland (benign) (infected) N36.8
  cranial meninges G93.0
  craniobuccal pouch E23.6
  craniopharyngeal pouch E23.6
  cystic duct K82.8
  Cysticercus —*see* Cysticercosis
  Dandy-Walker Q03.1
    with spina bifida —*see* Spina bifida
  dental (root) K04.8
    developmental K09.0
    eruption K09.0
    primordial K09.0
  dentigerous (mandible) (maxilla) K09.0
  dermoid —*see* Neoplasm, benign, by site
    with malignant transformation C56.-●
    implantation
      external area or site (skin) NEC L72.0
      iris —*see* Cyst, iris, implantation
      vagina N89.8
      vulva N90.7
    mouth K09.8
    oral soft tissue K09.8
    sacrococcygeal —*see* Cyst, pilonidal
  developmental K09.1
    odontogenic K09.0
    oral region (nonodontogenic) K09.1
    ovary, ovarian Q50.1
  dura (cerebral) G93.0
    spinal G96.19
  ear (external) Q18.1
  echinococcal —*see* Echinococcus
  embryonic
    cervix uteri Q51.6
    fallopian tube Q50.4
  ▶vagina Q52.4
  endometrium, endometrial (uterus) N85.8
    ectopic —*see* Endometriosis

Cyst *(Continued)*
  enterogenous Q43.8
  epidermal, epidermoid (inclusion) *(see also*
      Cyst, skin) L72.0
    mouth K09.8
    oral soft tissue K09.8
  epididymis N50.3
  epiglottis J38.7
  epiphysis cerebri E34.8
  epithelial (inclusion) L72.0
  epoophoron Q50.5
  eruption K09.0
  esophagus K22.8
  ethmoid sinus J34.1
  external female genital organs NEC N90.7
  eye NEC H57.8
    congenital Q15.8
  eyelid (sebaceous) H02.829
    infected —*see* Hordeolum
    left H02.826
      lower H02.825
      upper H02.824
    right H02.823
      lower H02.822
      upper H02.821
  fallopian tube N83.8
    congenital Q50.4
  fimbrial (twisted) Q50.4
  fissural (oral region) K09.1
  follicle (graafian) (hemorrhagic) N83.0-•
    nabothian N88.8
  follicular (atretic) (hemorrhagic) (ovarian)
      N83.0-•
    dentigerous K09.0
    odontogenic K09.0
    skin L72.9
      specified NEC L72.8
  frontal sinus J34.1
  gallbladder K82.8
  ganglion —*see* Ganglion
  Gartner's duct Q52.4
  gingiva K09.0
  gland of Moll —*see* Cyst, eyelid
  globulomaxillary K09.1
  graafian follicle (hemorrhagic) N83.0-•
  granulosal lutein (hemorrhagic) N83.1-•
  hemangiomatous D18.00
    intra-abdominal D18.03
    intracranial D18.02
    skin D18.01
    specified site NEC D18.09
  hemorrhagic M27.49
  hydatid —*see also* Echinococcus B67.90
    brain B67.99 [G94]
    liver —*see also* Cyst, liver, hydatid B67.8
    lung NEC B67.99 [J99]
    Morgagni
      female Q50.5
      male (epididymal) Q55.4
        testicular Q55.29
    specified site NEC B67.99
  hymen N89.8
    embryonic Q52.4
  hypopharynx J39.2
  hypophysis, hypophyseal (duct) (recurrent)
      E23.6
    cerebri E23.6
  implantation (dermoid)
    external area or site (skin) NEC L72.0
    iris —*see* Cyst, iris, implantation
    vagina N89.8
    vulva N90.7
  incisive canal K09.1
  inclusion (epidermal) (epithelial)
      (epidermoid) (squamous) L72.0
    not of skin - code under Cyst, by site
  intestine (large) (small) K63.89
  intracranial —*see* Cyst, brain
  intraligamentous —*see also* Disorder,
      ligament
    knee —*see* Derangement, knee

Cyst *(Continued)*
  intrasellar E23.6
  iris H21.309
    exudative H21.31-•
    idiopathic H21.30-•
    implantation H21.32-•
    parasitic H21.33-•
    pars plana (primary) H21.34-•
      exudative H21.35-•
  jaw (bone) M27.40
    aneurysmal M27.49
    developmental (odontogenic) K09.0
    fissural K09.1
    hemorrhagic M27.49
    traumatic M27.49
  joint NEC —*see* Disorder, joint, specified type
      NEC
  kidney (acquired) N28.1
    calyceal —*see* Hydronephrosis
    congenital Q61.00
    more than one (multiple) Q61.02
      specified as polycystic Q61.3
        adult type (autosomal dominant)
          Q61.2
        infantile type (autosomal recessive)
          NEC Q61.19
          collecting duct dilation Q61.11
    pyelogenic —*see* Hydronephrosis
    simple N28.1
    solitary (single) Q61.01
      acquired N28.1
  labium (majus) (minus) N90.7
    sebaceous N90.7
  lacrimal —*see also* Disorder, lacrimal system,
      specified NEC
    gland H04.13-•
    passages or sac —*see* Disorder, lacrimal
      system, specified NEC
  larynx J38.7
  lateral periodontal K09.0
  lens H27.8
    congenital Q12.8
  lip (gland) K13.0
  liver (idiopathic) (simple) K76.89
    congenital Q44.6
    hydatid B67.8
      granulosus B67.0
      multilocularis B67.5
  lung J98.4
    congenital Q33.0
    giant bullous J43.9
  lutein N83.1-•
  lymphangiomatous D18.1
  lymphoepithelial, oral soft tissue K09.8
  macula —*see* Degeneration, macula, hole
  malignant —*see* Neoplasm, malignant, by site
  mammary gland —*see* Cyst, breast
  mandible M27.40
    dentigerous K09.0
    radicular K04.8
  maxilla M27.40
    dentigerous K09.0
    radicular K04.8
  medial, face and neck Q18.8
  median
    anterior maxillary K09.1
    palatal K09.1
  mediastinum, congenital Q34.1
  meibomian (gland) —*see* Chalazion
    infected —*see* Hordeolum
  membrane, brain G93.0
  meninges (cerebral) G93.0
    spinal G96.19
  meniscus, knee —*see* Derangement, knee,
      meniscus, cystic
  mesentery, mesenteric K66.8
    chyle I89.8
  mesonephric duct
    female Q50.5
    male Q55.4
  milk N64.89

Cyst *(Continued)*
  Morgagni (hydatid)
    female Q50.5
    male (epididymal) Q55.4
      testicular Q55.29
  mouth K09.8
  Müllerian duct Q50.4
    appendix testis Q55.29
    cervix Q51.6
    fallopian tube Q50.4
    female Q50.4
    male Q55.29
    prostatic utricle Q55.4
    vagina (embryonal) Q52.4
  multilocular (ovary) D39.10
    benign —*see* Neoplasm, benign, by site
  myometrium N85.8
  nabothian (follicle) (ruptured) N88.8
  nasoalveolar K09.1
  nasolabial K09.1
  nasopalatine (anterior) (duct) K09.1
  nasopharynx J39.2
  neoplastic —*see* Neoplasm, uncertain
      behavior, by site
    benign —*see* Neoplasm, benign, by site
  nervous system NEC G96.8
  neuroenteric (congenital) Q06.8
  nipple —*see* Cyst, breast
  nose (turbinates) J34.1
    sinus J34.1
  odontogenic, developmental K09.0
  omentum (lesser) K66.8
    congenital Q45.8
  ora serrata —*see* Cyst, retina, ora serrata
  oral
    region K09.9
      developmental (nonodontogenic) K09.1
      specified NEC K09.8
    soft tissue K09.9
      specified NEC K09.8
  orbit H05.81-•
  ovary, ovarian (twisted) N83.20-•
    adherent N83.20-•
    chocolate N80.1
    corpus
      albicans N83.29-•
      luteum (hemorrhagic) N83.1-•
    dermoid D27.9
    developmental Q50.1
    due to failure of involution NEC N83.20-•
    endometrial N80.1
    follicular (graafian) (hemorrhagic) N83.0-•
    hemorrhagic N83.20-•
    in pregnancy or childbirth O34.8-•
      with obstructed labor O65.5
    multilocular D39.10
    pseudomucinous D27.9
    retention N83.29-•
    serous N83.20-•
    specified NEC N83.29-•
    theca lutein (hemorrhagic) N83.1-•
    tuberculous A18.18
  oviduct N83.8
  palate (median) (fissural) K09.1
  palatine papilla (jaw) K09.1
  pancreas, pancreatic (hemorrhagic) (true) K86.2
    congenital Q45.2
    false K86.3
  paralabral
    hip M24.85-•
    shoulder S43.43-•
  paramesonephric duct Q50.4
    female Q50.4
    male Q55.29
  paranephric N28.1
  paraphysis, cerebri, congenital Q04.6
  parasitic B89
  parathyroid (gland) E21.4
  paratubal N83.8
  paraurethral duct N36.8
  paroophoron Q50.5

▶ New   ⇒ Revised   ~~deleted~~ Deleted   • Use Additional Character(s)

Cyst *(Continued)*
  parotid gland K11.6
  parovarian Q50.5
  pelvis, female N94.89
    in pregnancy or childbirth O34.8-●
      causing obstructed labor O65.5
  penis (sebaceous) N48.89
  periapical K04.8
  pericardial (congenital) Q24.8
    acquired (secondary) I31.8
  pericoronal K09.0
  periodontal K04.8
    lateral K09.0
  peripelvic (lymphatic) N28.1
  peritoneum K66.8
    chylous I89.8
  periventricular, acquired, newborn P91.1
  pharynx (wall) J39.2
  pilar L72.11
  pilonidal (infected) (rectum) L05.91
    with abscess L05.01
    malignant C44.59-●
  pituitary (duct) (gland) E23.6
  placenta O43.19-●
  pleura J94.8
  popliteal —*see* Cyst, Baker's
  porencephalic Q04.6
    acquired G93.0
  postanal (infected) —*see* Cyst, pilonidal
  postmastoidectomy cavity (mucosal) —*see*
    Complications, postmastoidectomy, cyst
  preauricular Q18.1
  prepuce N47.4
    congenital Q55.69
  primordial (jaw) K09.0
  prostate N42.83
  pseudomucinous (ovary) D27.9
  pupillary, miotic H21.27-●
  radicular (residual) K04.8
  radiculodental K04.8
  ranular K11.8
  Rathke's pouch E23.6
  rectum (epithelium) (mucous) K62.89
  renal —*see* Cyst, kidney
  residual (radicular) K04.8
  retention (ovary) N83.29-●
    salivary gland K11.6
  retina H33.19-●
    ora serrata H33.11-●
    parasitic H33.12-●
  retroperitoneal K68.9
  sacrococcygeal (dermoid) —*see* Cyst,
    pilonidal
  salivary gland or duct (mucous extravasation
    or retention) K11.6
  Sampson's N80.1
  sclera H15.89
  scrotum L72.9
    sebaceous L72.3
  sebaceous (duct) (gland) L72.3
    breast —*see* Dysplasia, mammary, specified
      type NEC
    eyelid —*see* Cyst, eyelid
    genital organ NEC
      female N94.89
      male N50.89
    scrotum L72.3
  semilunar cartilage (knee) (multiple) —*see*
    Derangement, knee, meniscus, cystic
  seminal vesicle N50.89
  serous (ovary) N83.20-●
  sinus (accessory) (nasal) J34.1
  Skene's gland N36.8
  skin L72.9
    breast —*see* Dysplasia, mammary, specified
      type NEC
    epidermal, epidermoid L72.0
    epithelial L72.0
    eyelid —*see* Cyst, eyelid
    genital organ NEC
      female N90.7
      male N50.89

Cyst *(Continued)*
  skin *(Continued)*
    inclusion L72.0
    scrotum L72.9
    sebaceous L72.3
    sweat gland or duct L74.8
  solitary
    bone —*see* Cyst, bone, solitary
    jaw M27.40
    kidney N28.1
  spermatic cord N50.89
  sphenoid sinus J34.1
  spinal meninges G96.19
  spleen NEC D73.4
    congenital Q89.09
    hydatid —*see also* Echinococcus B67.99 [D77]
  Stafne's M27.0
  subarachnoid intrasellar R93.0
  subcutaneous, pheomycotic (chromomycotic)
    B43.2
  subdural (cerebral) G93.0
    spinal cord G96.19
  sublingual gland K11.6
  submandibular gland K11.6
  submaxillary gland K11.6
  suburethral N36.8
  suprarenal gland E27.8
  suprasellar —*see* Cyst, brain
  sweat gland or duct L74.8
  synovial —*see also* Cyst, bursa
    ruptured —*see* Rupture, synovium
  tarsal —*see* Chalazion
  tendon (sheath) —*see* Disorder, tendon,
    specified type NEC
  testis N44.2
    tunica albuginea N44.1
  theca lutein (ovary) N83.1-●
  Thornwaldt's J39.2
  thymus (gland) E32.8
  thyroglossal duct (infected) (persistent)
    Q89.2
  thyroid (gland) E04.1
  thyrolingual duct (infected) (persistent)
    Q89.2
  tongue K14.8
  tonsil J35.8
  tooth —*see* Cyst, dental
  Tornwaldt's J39.2
  trichilemmal (proliferating) L72.12
  trichodermal L72.12
  tubal (fallopian) N83.8
    inflammatory —*see* Salpingitis, chronic
  tubo-ovarian N83.8
    inflammatory N70.13
  tunica
    albuginea testis N44.1
    vaginalis N50.89
  turbinate (nose) J34.1
  Tyson's gland N48.89
  urachus, congenital Q64.4
  ureter N28.89
  ureterovesical orifice N28.89
  urethra, urethral (gland) N36.8
  uterine ligament N83.8
  uterus (body) (corpus) (recurrent)
    N85.8
    embryonic Q51.818
      cervix Q51.6
  vagina, vaginal (implantation) (inclusion)
    (squamous cell) (wall) N89.8
    embryonic Q52.4
  vallecula, vallecular (epiglottis) J38.7
  vesical (orifice) N32.89
  vitreous body H43.89
  vulva (implantation) (inclusion) N90.7
    congenital Q52.79
    sebaceous gland N90.7
  vulvovaginal gland N90.7
  wolffian
    female Q50.5
    male Q55.4

Cystadenocarcinoma —*see* Neoplasm,
  malignant, by site
  bile duct C22.1
  endometrioid —*see* Neoplasm, malignant,
    by site
  specified site —*see* Neoplasm, malignant,
    by site
  unspecified site
    female C56.9
    male C61
  mucinous
    papillary
      specified site —*see* Neoplasm,
        malignant, by site
      unspecified site C56.9
    specified site —*see* Neoplasm, malignant,
      by site
    unspecified site C56.9
  papillary
    mucinous
      specified site —*see* Neoplasm,
        malignant, by site
      unspecified site C56.9
    pseudomucinous
      specified site —*see* Neoplasm,
        malignant, by site
      unspecified site C56.9
    serous
      specified site —*see* Neoplasm,
        malignant, by site
      unspecified site C56.9
    specified site —*see* Neoplasm, malignant,
      by site
    unspecified site C56.9
  pseudomucinous
    papillary
      specified site —*see* Neoplasm,
        malignant, by site
      unspecified site C56.9
    specified site —*see* Neoplasm, malignant,
      by site
    unspecified site C56.9
  serous
    papillary
      specified site —*see* Neoplasm,
        malignant, by site
      unspecified site C56.9
    specified site —*see* Neoplasm, malignant,
      by site
    unspecified site C56.9
Cystadenofibroma
  clear cell —*see* Neoplasm, benign, by site
  endometrioid D27.9
    borderline malignancy D39.1-●
    malignant C56.-●
  mucinous
    specified site —*see* Neoplasm, benign, by site
    unspecified site D27.9
  serous
    specified site —*see* Neoplasm, benign, by site
    unspecified site D27.9
  specified site —*see* Neoplasm, benign, by site
  unspecified site D27.9
Cystadenoma —*see also* Neoplasm, benign, by
  site
  bile duct D13.4
  endometrioid —*see* Neoplasm, benign, by site
    borderline malignancy —*see* Neoplasm,
      uncertain behavior, by site
    malignant —*see* Neoplasm, malignant, by site
  mucinous
    borderline malignancy
      ovary C56.-●
      specified site NEC —*see* Neoplasm,
        uncertain behavior, by site
      unspecified site C56.9
    papillary
      borderline malignancy
        ovary C56.-●
        specified site NEC —*see* Neoplasm,
          uncertain behavior, by site
        unspecified site C56.9

Cystadenoma *(Continued)*
  mucinous *(Continued)*
    papillary *(Continued)*
      specified site —*see* Neoplasm, benign,
        by site
      unspecified site D27.9
    specified site —*see* Neoplasm, benign, by site
    unspecified site D27.9
  papillary
    borderline malignancy
      ovary C56-●
      specified site NEC —*see* Neoplasm,
        uncertain behavior, by site
      unspecified site C56.9
    lymphomatosum
      specified site —*see* Neoplasm, benign,
        by site
      unspecified site D11.9
    mucinous
      borderline malignancy
        ovary C56.-●
        specified site NEC —*see* Neoplasm,
          uncertain behavior, by site
        unspecified site C56.9
      specified site —*see* Neoplasm, benign,
        by site
      unspecified site D27.9
    pseudomucinous
      borderline malignancy
        ovary C56.-●
        specified site NEC —*see* Neoplasm,
          uncertain behavior, by site
        unspecified site C56.9
      specified site —*see* Neoplasm, benign,
        by site
      unspecified site D27.9
    serous
      borderline malignancy
        ovary C56.-●
        specified site NEC —*see* Neoplasm,
          uncertain behavior, by site
        unspecified site C56.9
      specified site —*see* Neoplasm, benign,
        by site
      unspecified site D27.9
    specified site —*see* Neoplasm, benign, by site
    unspecified site D27.9
  pseudomucinous
    borderline malignancy
      ovary C56.-●
      specified site NEC —*see* Neoplasm,
        uncertain behavior, by site
      unspecified site C56.9
    papillary
      borderline malignancy
        ovary C56.-●
        specified site NEC —*see* Neoplasm,
          uncertain behavior, by site
        unspecified site C56.9
      specified site —*see* Neoplasm, benign,
        by site
      unspecified site D27.9
    specified site —*see* Neoplasm, benign, by site
    unspecified site D27.9
  serous
    borderline malignancy
      ovary C56.-●
      specified site NEC —*see* Neoplasm,
        uncertain behavior, by site
      unspecified site C56.9
    papillary
      borderline malignancy
        ovary C56.-●
        specified site NEC —*see* Neoplasm,
          uncertain behavior, by site
        unspecified site C56.9
      specified site —*see* Neoplasm, benign,
        by site
      unspecified site D27.9
    specified site —*see* Neoplasm, benign, by site
    unspecified site D27.9

Cystathionine synthase deficiency E72.11
Cystathioninemia E72.19
Cystathioninuria E72.19
Cystic —*see also* condition
  breast (chronic) —*see* Mastopathy, cystic
  corpora lutea (hemorrhagic) N83.1-●
  duct —*see* condition
  eyeball (congenital) Q11.0
  fibrosis —*see* Fibrosis, cystic
  kidney (congenital) Q61.9
    adult type Q61.2
    infantile type NEC Q61.19
      collecting duct dilatation Q61.11
    medullary Q61.5
  liver, congenital Q44.6
  lung disease J98.4
    congenital Q33.0
  mastitis, chronic —*see* Mastopathy, cystic
  medullary, kidney Q61.5
  meniscus —*see* Derangement, knee,
    meniscus, cystic
  ovary N83.20-●
Cysticercosis, cysticerciasis B69.9
  with
    epileptiform fits B69.0
    myositis B69.81
  brain B69.0
  central nervous system B69.0
  cerebral B69.0
  ocular B69.1
  specified NEC B69.89
Cysticercus cellulose infestation —*see*
  Cysticercosis
Cystinosis (malignant) E72.04
Cystinuria E72.01
Cystitis (exudative) (hemorrhagic) (septic)
    (suppurative) N30.90
  with
    fibrosis —*see* Cystitis, chronic, interstitial
    hematuria N30.91
    leukoplakia —*see* Cystitis, chronic,
      interstitial
    malakoplakia —*see* Cystitis, chronic,
      interstitial
    metaplasia —*see* Cystitis, chronic, interstitial
    prostatitis N41.3
  acute N30.00
    with hematuria N30.01
    of trigone N30.30
      with hematuria N30.31
  allergic —*see* Cystitis, specified type NEC
  amebic A06.81
  bilharzial B65.9 [N33]
  blennorrhagic (gonococcal) A54.01
  bullous —*see* Cystitis, specified type NEC
  calculous N21.0
  chlamydial A56.01
  chronic N30.20
    with hematuria N30.21
    interstitial N30.10
      with hematuria N30.11
    of trigone N30.30
      with hematuria N30.31
    specified NEC N30.20
      with hematuria N30.21
  cystic (a) —*see* Cystitis, specified type NEC
  diphtheritic A36.85
  echinococcal
    granulosus B67.39
    multilocularis B67.69
  emphysematous —*see* Cystitis, specified type
    NEC
  encysted —*see* Cystitis, specified type NEC
  eosinophilic —*see* Cystitis, specified type
    NEC
  follicular —*see* Cystitis, of trigone
  gangrenous —*see* Cystitis, specified type
    NEC
  glandularis —*see* Cystitis, specified type
    NEC

Cystitis *(Continued)*
  gonococcal A54.01
  incrusted —*see* Cystitis, specified type
    NEC
  interstitial (chronic) —*see* Cystitis, chronic,
    interstitial
  irradiation N30.40
    with hematuria N30.41
  irritation —*see* Cystitis, specified type
    NEC
  malignant —*see* Cystitis, specified type
    NEC
  of trigone N30.30
    with hematuria N30.31
  panmural —*see* Cystitis, chronic, interstitial
  polyposa —*see* Cystitis, specified type NEC
  prostatic N41.3
  puerperal (postpartum) O86.22
  radiation —*see* Cystitis, irradiation
  specified type NEC N30.80
    with hematuria N30.81
  subacute —*see* Cystitis, chronic
  submucous —*see* Cystitis, chronic, interstitial
  syphilitic (late) A52.76
  trichomonal A59.03
  tuberculous A18.12
  ulcerative —*see* Cystitis, chronic, interstitial
Cystocele (-urethrocele)
  female N81.10
    with prolapse of uterus —*See* Prolapse,
      uterus
    lateral N81.12
    midline N81.11
    paravaginal N81.12
  in pregnancy or childbirth O34.8-●
    causing obstructed labor O65.5
  male N32.89
Cystolithiasis N21.0
Cystoma —*see also* Neoplasm, benign, by site
  endometrial, ovary N80.1
  mucinous
    specified site —*see* Neoplasm, benign, by site
    unspecified site D27.9
  serous
    specified site —*see* Neoplasm, benign, by site
    unspecified site D27.9
  simple (ovary) N83.29-●
Cystoplegia N31.2
Cystoptosis N32.89
Cystopyelitis —*see* Pyelonephritis
Cystorrhagia N32.89
Cystosarcoma phyllodes D48.6-●
  benign D24-●
  malignant —*see* Neoplasm, breast, malignant
Cystostomy
  attention to Z43.5
  complication —*see* Complications, cystostomy
  status Z93.50
    appendico-vesicostomy Z93.52
    cutaneous Z93.51
    specified NEC Z93.59
Cystourethritis —*see* Urethritis
Cystourethrocele —*see also* Cystocele
  female N81.10
    with uterine prolapse —*see* Prolapse,
      uterus
    lateral N81.12
    midline N81.11
    paravaginal N81.12
  male N32.89
Cytomegalic inclusion disease
  congenital P35.1
Cytomegalovirus infection B25.9
Cytomycosis (reticuloendothelial) B39.4
Cytopenia D75.9
  refractory
    with multilineage dysplasia D46.A
      and ring sideroblasts (RCMD RS) D46.B
Czerny's disease (periodic hydrarthrosis of the
    knee) —*see* Effusion, joint, knee

▶ New ⇒ Revised ~~deleted~~ Deleted ● Use Additional Character(s)

D

Daae (-Finsen) disease (epidemic pleurodynia) B33.0
Dabney's grip B33.0
Da Costa's syndrome F45.8
Dacryoadenitis, dacryadenitis H04.00-●
acute H04.01-●
chronic H04.02-●
Dacryocystitis H04.30-●
acute H04.32-●
chronic H04.41-●
neonatal P39.1
phlegmonous H04.31-●
syphilitic A52.71
congenital (early) A50.01
trachomatous, active A71.1
sequelae (late effect) B94.0
Dacryocystoblenorrhea —see Inflammation, lacrimal, passages, chronic
Dacryocystocele —see Disorder, lacrimal system, changes
Dacryolith, dacryolithiasis H04.51-●
Dacryoma —see Disorder, lacrimal system, changes
Dacryopericystitis —see Dacryocystitis
Dacryops H04.11-●
Dacryostenosis —see also Stenosis, lacrimal
congenital Q10.5
Dactylitis
bone —see Osteomyelitis
sickle-cell D57.00
Hb C D57.219
Hb SS D57.00
specified NEC D57.819
skin L08.9
syphilitic A52.77
tuberculous A18.03
Dactylolysis spontanea (ainhum) L94.6
Dactylosymphysis Q70.9
fingers —see Syndactylism, complex, fingers
toes —see Syndactylism, complex, toes
Damage
arteriosclerotic —see Arteriosclerosis
brain (nontraumatic) G93.9
anoxic, hypoxic G93.1
resulting from a procedure G97.82
child NEC G80.9
due to birth injury P11.2
cardiorenal (vascular) —see Hypertension, cardiorenal
cerebral NEC —see Damage, brain
coccyx, complicating delivery O71.6
coronary —see Disease, heart, ischemic
eye, birth injury P15.3
liver (nontraumatic) K76.9
alcoholic K70.9
due to drugs —see Disease, liver, toxic
toxic —see Disease, liver, toxic
medication T88.7
pelvic
joint or ligament, during delivery O71.6
organ NEC
during delivery O71.5
following ectopic or molar pregnancy O08.6
renal —see Disease, renal
subendocardium, subendocardial —see Degeneration, myocardial
vascular I99.9
Dana-Putnam syndrome (subacute combined sclerosis with pernicious anemia) —see Degeneration, combined
Danbolt (-Cross) syndrome (acrodermatitis enteropathica) E83.2
Dandruff L21.0
Dandy-Walker syndrome Q03.1
with spina bifida —see Spina bifida
Danlos' syndrome Q79.6

Darier (-White) disease (congenital) Q82.8
meaning erythema annulare centrifugum L53.1
Darier-Roussy sarcoid D86.3
Darling's disease or histoplasmosis B39.4
Darwin's tubercle Q17.8
Dawson's (inclusion body) encephalitis A81.1
De Beurmann (-Gougerot) disease B42.1
De la Tourette's syndrome F95.2
De Lange's syndrome Q87.1
De Morgan's spots (senile angiomas) I78.1
De Quervain's
disease (tendon sheath) M65.4
syndrome E34.51
thyroiditis (subacute granulomatous thyroiditis) E06.1
De Toni-Fanconi (-Debré) syndrome E72.09
with cystinosis E72.04
Dead
fetus, retained (mother) O36.4
early pregnancy O02.1
labyrinth —see subcategory H83.2
ovum, retained O02.0
Deaf nonspeaking NEC H91.3
Deafmutism (acquired) (congenital) NEC H91.3
hysterical F44.6
syphilitic, congenital —see also subcategory H94.8 A50.09
Deafness (acquired) (complete) (hereditary) (partial) H91.9-●
with blue sclera and fragility of bone Q78.0
auditory fatigue —see Deafness, specified type NEC
aviation T70.0
nerve injury —see Injury, nerve, acoustic, specified type NEC
boilermaker's —see subcategory H83.3
central —see Deafness, sensorineural
conductive H90.2
and sensorineural
mixed H90.8
bilateral H90.6
bilateral H90.0
unilateral H90.1-●
with restricted hearing on the contralateral side H90.A-●
congenital H90.5
with blue sclera and fragility of bone Q78.0
due to toxic agents —see Deafness, ototoxic
emotional (hysterical) F44.6
functional (hysterical) F44.6
high frequency H91.9-●
hysterical F44.6
low frequency H91.9-●
mental R48.8
mixed conductive and sensorineural H90.8
bilateral H90.6
unilateral H90.7-●
nerve —see Deafness, sensorineural
neural —see Deafness, sensorineural
noise-induced —see also subcategory H83.3
nerve injury —see Injury, nerve, acoustic, specified type NEC
nonspeaking H91.3
ototoxic —see subcategory H91.0
perceptive —see Deafness, sensorineural
psychogenic (hysterical) F44.6
sensorineural H90.5
and conductive
mixed H90.8
bilateral H90.6
bilateral H90.3
unilateral H90.4-●
with restricted hearing on the contralateral side H90.A-●
sensory —see Deafness, sensorineural
specified type NEC —see subcategory H91.8
sudden (idiopathic) H91.2-●

Deafness (Continued)
syphilitic A52.15
transient ischemic H93.01-●
traumatic —see Injury, nerve, acoustic, specified type NEC
word (developmental) H93.25
Death (cause unknown) (of) (unexplained) (unspecified cause) R99
brain G93.82
cardiac (sudden) (with successful resuscitation) — code to underlying disease
family history of Z82.41
personal history of Z86.74
family member (assumed) Z63.4
Debility (chronic) (general) (nervous) R53.81
congenital or neonatal NOS P96.9
nervous R53.81
old age R54
senile R54
Débove's disease (splenomegaly) R16.1
Decalcification
bone —see Osteoporosis
teeth K03.89
Decapsulation, kidney N28.89
Decay
dental —see Caries, dental
senile R54
tooth, teeth —see Caries, dental
Deciduitis (acute)
following ectopic or molar pregnancy O08.0
Decline (general) —see Debility
cognitive, age-associated R41.81
Decompensation
cardiac (acute) (chronic) —see Disease, heart
cardiovascular —see Disease, cardiovascular
heart —see Disease, heart
hepatic —see Failure, hepatic
myocardial (acute) (chronic) —see Disease, heart
respiratory J98.8
Decompression sickness T70.3
Decrease (d)
absolute neutrophile count —see Neutropenia
blood
platelets —see Thrombocytopenia
pressure R03.1
due to shock following
injury T79.4
operation T81.19
estrogen E28.39
postablative E89.40
asymptomatic E89.40
symptomatic E89.41
fragility of erythrocytes D58.8
function
lipase (pancreatic) K90.3
ovary in hypopituitarism E23.0
parenchyma of pancreas K86.89
pituitary (gland) (anterior) (lobe) E23.0
posterior (lobe) E23.0
functional activity R68.89
glucose R73.09
hematocrit R71.0
hemoglobin R71.0
leukocytes D72.819
specified NEC D72.818
libido R68.82
lymphocytes D72.810
platelets D69.6
respiration, due to shock following injury T79.4
sexual desire R68.82
tear secretion NEC —see Syndrome, dry eye
tolerance
fat K90.49
glucose R73.09
pancreatic K90.3
salt and water E87.8
vision NEC H54.7
white blood cell count D72.819
specified NEC D72.818

Decubitus (ulcer) —*see* Ulcer, pressure, by site
  cervix N86
Deepening acetabulum —*see* Derangement,
    joint, specified type NEC, hip
Defect, defective Q89.9
  3-beta-hydroxysteroid dehydrogenase E25.0
  11-hydroxylase E25.0
  21-hydroxylase E25.0
  abdominal wall, congenital Q79.59
  antibody immunodeficiency D80.9
  aorticopulmonary septum Q21.4
  atrial septal (ostium secundum type) Q21.1
    following acute myocardial infarction
        (current complication) I23.1
    ostium primum type Q21.2
  atrioventricular
    canal Q21.2
    septum Q21.2
  auricular septal Q21.1
  bilirubin excretion NEC E80.6
  biosynthesis, androgen (testicular) E29.1
  bulbar septum Q21.0
  catalase E80.3
  cell membrane receptor complex (CR3) D71
  circulation I99.9
    congenital Q28.9
    newborn Q28.9
  coagulation (factor) —*see also* Deficiency,
      factor D68.9
    with
      ectopic pregnancy O08.1
      molar pregnancy O08.1
    acquired D68.4
    antepartum with hemorrhage —*see*
        Hemorrhage, antepartum, with
        coagulation defect
    due to
      liver disease D68.4
      vitamin K deficiency D68.4
    hereditary NEC D68.2
    intrapartum O67.0
    newborn, transient P61.6
  ⟹postpartum O99.13
    ▶with hemorrhage O72.3
    specified type NEC D68.8
  complement system D84.1
  conduction (heart) I45.9
    bone —*see* Deafness, conductive
  congenital, organ or site not listed —*see*
      Anomaly, by site
  coronary sinus Q21.1
  cushion, endocardial Q21.2
  degradation, glycoprotein E77.1
  dental bridge, crown, fillings —*see* Defect,
      dental restoration
  dental restoration K08.50
    specified NEC K08.59
  dentin (hereditary) K00.5
  Descemet's membrane, congenital Q13.89
  developmental —*see also* Anomaly
    cauda equina Q06.3
  diaphragm
    with elevation, eventration or hernia —*see*
        Hernia, diaphragm
    congenital Q79.1
      with hernia Q79.0
      gross (with hernia) Q79.0
  ectodermal, congenital Q82.9
  Eisenmenger's Q21.8
  enzyme
    catalase E80.3
    peroxidase E80.3
  esophagus, congenital Q39.9
  extensor retinaculum M62.89
  fibrin polymerization D68.2
  filling
    bladder R93.41
    kidney R93.42-●
    renal pelvis R93.41
    stomach R93.3
    ureter R93.41
    urinary organs, specified NEC R93.49

Defect, defective *(Continued)*
  Gerbode Q21.0
  glycoprotein degradation E77.1
  Hageman (factor) D68.2
  hearing —*see* Deafness
  high grade F70
  interatrial septal Q21.1
  interauricular septal Q21.1
  interventricular septal Q21.0
    with dextroposition of aorta, pulmonary
        stenosis and hypertrophy of right
        ventricle Q21.3
    in tetralogy of Fallot Q21.3
  learning (specific) —*see* Disorder, learning
  lymphocyte function antigen-1 (LFA-1) D84.0
  lysosomal enzyme, post-translational
      modification E77.0
  major osseous M89.70
    ankle M89.77-●
    carpus M89.74-●
    clavicle M89.71-●
    femur M89.75-●
    fibula M89.76-●
    fingers M89.74-●
    foot M89.77-●
    forearm M89.73-●
    hand M89.74-●
    humerus M89.72-●
    lower leg M89.76-●
    metacarpus M89.74-●
    metatarsus M89.77-●
    multiple sites M89.79
    pelvic region M89.75-●
    pelvis M89.75-●
    radius M89.73-●
    scapula M89.71-●
    shoulder region M89.71-●
    specified NEC M89.78
    tarsus M89.77-●
    thigh M89.75-●
    tibia M89.76-●
    toes M89.77-●
    ulna M89.73-●
  mental —*see* Disability, intellectual
  modification, lysosomal enzymes, post-
      translational E77.0
  obstructive, congenital
    renal pelvis Q62.39
    ureter Q62.39
      atresia —*see* Atresia, ureter
      cecoureterocele Q62.32
      megaureter Q62.2
      orthotopic ureterocele Q62.31
  osseous, major M89.70
    ankle M89.77-●
    carpus M89.74-●
    clavicle M89.71-●
    femur M89.75-●
    fibula M89.76-●
    fingers M89.74-●
    foot M89.77-●
    forearm M89.73-●
    hand M89.74-●
    humerus M89.72-●
    lower leg M89.76-●
    metacarpus M89.74-●
    metatarsus M89.77-●
    multiple sites M89.9
    pelvic region M89.75-●
    pelvis M89.75-●
    radius M89.73-●
    scapula M89.71-●
    shoulder region M89.71-●
    specified NEC M89.78
    tarsus M89.77-●
    thigh M89.75-●
    tibia M89.76-●
    toes M89.77-●
    ulna M89.73-●
  osteochondral NEC —*see also* Deformity
      M95.8-●

Defect, defective *(Continued)*
  ostium
    primum Q21.2
    secundum Q21.1
  peroxidase E80.3
  placental blood supply —*see* Insufficiency,
      placental
  platelets, qualitative D69.1
    constitutional D68.0
  postural NEC, spine —*see* Dorsopathy,
      deforming
  reduction
    limb Q73.8
      lower Q72.9-●
        absence —*see* Agenesis, leg
        foot —*see* Agenesis, foot
        longitudinal
          femur Q72.4-●
          fibula Q72.6-●
          tibia Q72.5-●
        specified type NEC Q72.89-●
        split foot Q72.7-●
      specified type NEC Q73.8
      upper Q71.9-●
        absence —*see* Agenesis, arm
          forearm —*see* Agenesis, forearm
          hand —*see* Agenesis, hand
        lobster-claw hand Q71.6-●
        longitudinal
          radius Q71.4-●
          ulna Q71.5-●
        specified type NEC Q71.89-●
  renal pelvis Q63.8
    obstructive Q62.39
  respiratory system, congenital Q34.9
  restoration, dental K08.50
    specified NEC K08.59
  retinal nerve bundle fibers H35.89
  septal (heart) NOS Q21.9
    acquired (atrial) (auricular) (ventricular)
        (old) I51.0
    atrial Q21.1
      concurrent with acute myocardial
          infarction —*see* Infarct,
          myocardium
      following acute myocardial infarction
          (current complication) I23.1
    ventricular —*see also* Defect, ventricular
        septal Q21.0
  sinus venosus Q21.1
  speech R47.9
    developmental F80.9
    specified NEC R47.89
  Taussig-Bing (aortic transposition and
      overriding pulmonary artery) Q20.1
  teeth, wedge K03.1
  vascular (local) I99.9
    congenital Q27.9
  ventricular septal Q21.0
    concurrent with acute myocardial
        infarction —*see* Infarct, myocardium
    following acute myocardial infarction
        (current complication) I23.2
    in tetralogy of Fallot Q21.3
  vision NEC H54.7
  visual field H53.40
    bilateral
      heteronymous H53.47
      homonymous H53.46-●
    generalized contraction H53.48-●
    localized
      arcuate H53.43-●
      scotoma (central area) H53.41-●
        blind spot area H53.42-●
      sector H53.43-●
    specified type NEC H53.45-●
  voice R49.9
    specified NEC R49.8
  wedge, tooth, teeth (abrasion) K03.1
Deferentitis N49.1
  gonorrheal (acute) (chronic) A54.23

Defibrination (syndrome) D65
  antepartum —*see* Hemorrhage, antepartum,
      with coagulation defect, disseminated
      intravascular coagulation
  following ectopic or molar pregnancy O08.1
  intrapartum O67.0
  newborn P60
  postpartum O72.3
Deficiency, deficient
  3-beta hydroxysteroid dehydrogenase E25.0
  11-hydroxylase E25.0
  21-hydroxylase E25.0
  5-alpha reductase (with male
      pseudohermaphroditism) E29.1
  abdominal muscle syndrome Q79.4
  AC globulin (congenital) (hereditary) D68.2
      acquired D68.4
  accelerator globulin (Ac G) (blood) D68.2
  acid phosphatase E83.39
  activating factor (blood) D68.2
  adenosine deaminase (ADA) D81.3
  aldolase (hereditary) E74.19
  alpha-1-antitrypsin E88.01
  amino-acids E72.9
  anemia —*see* Anemia
  aneurin E51.9
  antibody with
      hyperimmunoglobulinemia D80.6
      near-normal immunoglobins D80.6
  antidiuretic hormone E23.2
  anti-hemophilic
      factor (A) D66
          B D67
          C D68.1
      globulin (AHG) NEC D66
  antithrombin (antithrombin III) D68.59
  ascorbic acid E54
  attention (disorder) (syndrome) F98.8
      with hyperactivity —*see* Disorder,
          attention-deficit hyperactivity
  autoprothrombin
      I D68.2
      II D67
      C D68.2
  beta-glucuronidase E76.29
  biotin E53.8
  biotin-dependent carboxylase D81.819
  biotinidase D81.810
  brancher enzyme (amylopectinosis) E74.03
  C1 esterase inhibitor (C1-INH) D84.1
  calciferol E55.9
      with
          adult osteomalacia M83.8
          rickets —*see* Rickets
  calcium (dietary) E58
  calorie, severe E43
      with marasmus E41
          and kwashiorkor E42
  cardiac —*see* Insufficiency, myocardial
  carnitine E71.40
      due to
          hemodialysis E71.43
          inborn errors of metabolism E71.42
          Valproic acid therapy E71.43
      iatrogenic E71.43
      muscle palmityltransferase E71.314
      primary E71.41
      secondary E71.448
  carotene E50.9
  central nervous system G96.8
  ceruloplasmin (Wilson) E83.01
  choline E53.8
  Christmas factor D67
  chromium E61.4
  clotting (blood) —*see also* Deficiency,
      coagulation factor D68.9
  clotting factor NEC (hereditary) —*see also*
      Deficiency, factor D68.2
  coagulation NOS D68.9
      with
          ectopic pregnancy O08.1
          molar pregnancy O08.1

Deficiency, deficient (*Continued*)
  coagulation NOS (*Continued*)
      acquired (any) D68.4
      antepartum hemorrhage —*see*
          Hemorrhage, antepartum, with
          coagulation defect
      clotting factor NEC —*see also* Deficiency,
          factor D68.2
      due to
          hyperprothrombinemia D68.4
          liver disease D68.4
          vitamin K deficiency D68.4
      newborn, transient P61.6
      postpartum O72.3
      specified NEC D68.8
  cognitive F09
  color vision H53.50
      achromatopsia H53.51
      acquired H53.52
      deuteranomaly H53.53
      protanomaly H53.54
      specified type NEC H53.59
      tritanomaly H53.55
  combined glucocorticoid and
      mineralocorticoid E27.49
  contact factor D68.2
  copper (nutritional) E61.0
  corticoadrenal E27.40
      primary E27.1
  craniofacial axis Q75.0
  cyanocobalamin E53.8
  debrancher enzyme (limit dextrinosis) E74.03
  dehydrogenase
      long chain/very long chain acyl CoA
          E71.310
      medium chain acyl CoA E71.311
      short chain acyl CoA E71.312
  diet E63.9
  dihydropyrimidine dehydrogenase (DPD)
      E88.89
  disaccharidase E73.9
  edema —*see* Malnutrition, severe
  endocrine E34.9
  energy-supply —*see* Malnutrition
  enzymes, circulating NEC E88.09
  ergosterol E55.9
      with
          adult osteomalacia M83.8
          rickets —*see* Rickets
  essential fatty acid (EFA) E63.0
  factor —*see also* Deficiency, coagulation
      Hageman D68.2
      I (congenital) (hereditary) D68.2
      II (congenital) (hereditary) D68.2
      IX (congenital) (functional) (hereditary)
          (with functional defect) D67
      multiple (congenital) D68.8
          acquired D68.4
      V (congenital) (hereditary) D68.2
      VII (congenital) (hereditary) D68.2
      VIII (congenital) (functional) (hereditary)
          (with functional defect) D66
          with vascular defect D68.0
      X (congenital) (hereditary) D68.2
      XI (congenital) (hereditary) D68.1
      XII (congenital) (hereditary) D68.2
      XIII (congenital) (hereditary) D68.2
  femoral, proximal focal (congenital) —
      see Defect, reduction, lower limb,
      longitudinal, femur
  fibrin-stabilizing factor (congenital)
      (hereditary) D68.2
      acquired D68.4
  fibrinase D68.2
  fibrinogen (congenital) (hereditary) D68.2
      acquired D65
  folate E53.8
  folic acid E53.8
  foreskin N47.3
  fructokinase E74.11
  fructose 1,6-diphosphatase E74.19

Deficiency, deficient (*Continued*)
  fructose-1-phosphate aldolase E74.19
  galactokinase E74.29
  galactose-1-phosphate uridyl transferase
      E74.29
  gammaglobulin in blood D80.1
      hereditary D80.0
  glass factor D68.2
  glucocorticoid E27.49
      mineralocorticoid E27.49
  glucose-6-phosphatase E74.01
  glucose-6-phosphate dehydrogenase anemia
      D55.0
  glucuronyl transferase E80.5
  glycogen synthetase E74.09
  gonadotropin (isolated) E23.0
  growth hormone (idiopathic) (isolated) E23.0
  Hageman factor D68.2
  hemoglobin D64.9
  hepatophosphorylase E74.09
  homogentisate 1,2-dioxygenase E70.29
  hormone
      anterior pituitary (partial) NEC E23.0
          growth E23.0
      growth (isolated) E23.0
      pituitary E23.0
      testicular E29.1
  hypoxanthine-(guanine)-
      phosphoribosyltransferase (HG-PRT)
      (total HG-PRT) E79.1
  immunity D84.9
      cell-mediated D84.8
          with thrombocytopenia and eczema
              D82.0
      combined D81.9
      humoral D80.9
      IgA (secretory) D80.2
      IgG D80.3
      IgM D80.4
  immuno —*see* Immunodeficiency
  immunoglobulin, selective
      A (IgA) D80.2
      G (IgG) (subclasses) D80.3
      M (IgM) D80.4
  inositol (B complex) E53.8
  intrinsic
      factor (congenital) D51.0
      sphincter N36.42
          with urethral hypermobility N36.43
  iodine E61.8
      congenital syndrome —*see* Syndrome,
          iodine-deficiency, congenital
  iron E61.1
      anemia D50.9
  kalium E87.6
  kappa-light chain D80.8
  labile factor (congenital) (hereditary) D68.2
      acquired D68.4
  lacrimal fluid (acquired) —*see also* Syndrome,
      dry eye
      congenital Q10.6
  lactase
      congenital E73.0
      secondary E73.1
  Laki-Lorand factor D68.2
  lecithin cholesterol acyltransferase E78.6
  lipocaic K86.89
  lipoprotein (familial) (high density) E78.6
  liver phosphorylase E74.09
  lysosomal alpha-1, 4 glucosidase E74.02
  magnesium E61.2
  major histocompatibility complex
      class I D81.6
      class II D81.7
  manganese E61.3
  menadione (vitamin K) E56.1
      newborn P53
  mental (familial) (hereditary) —*see* Disability,
      intellectual
  methylenetetrahydrofolate reductase
      (MTHFR) E72.12

Deficiency, deficient *(Continued)*
  mevalonate kinase M04.1
  mineral NEC E61.8
  mineralocorticoid E27.49
    with glucocorticoid E27.49
  molybdenum (nutritional) E61.5
  moral F60.2
  multiple nutrient elements E61.7
  muscle
    carnitine (palmityltransferase) E71.314
    phosphofructokinase E74.09
  myoadenylate deaminase E79.2
  myocardial —*see* Insufficiency, myocardial
  myophosphorylase E74.04
  NADH diaphorase or reductase (congenital)
      D74.0
  NADH-methemoglobin reductase
      (congenital) D74.0
  natrium E87.1
  niacin (amide) (-tryptophan) E52
  nicotinamide E52
  nicotinic acid E52
  number of teeth —*see* Anodontia
  nutrient element E61.9
    multiple E61.7
    specified NEC E61.8
  nutrition, nutritional E63.9
    sequelae —*see* Sequelae, nutritional
        deficiency
    specified NEC E63.8
  of interleukin 1 receptor antagonist [DIRA]
      M04.8
  ornithine transcarbamylase E72.4
  ovarian E28.39
  oxygen —*see* Anoxia
  pantothenic acid E53.8
  parathyroid (gland) E20.9
  perineum (female) N81.89
  phenylalanine hydroxylase E70.1
  phosphoenolpyruvate carboxykinase E74.4
  phosphofructokinase E74.19
  phosphomannomutuse E74.8
  phosphomannose isomerase E74.8
  phosphomannosyl mutase E74.8
  phosphorylase kinase, liver E74.09
  pituitary hormone (isolated) E23.0
  plasma thromboplastin
    antecedent (PTA) D68.1
    component (PTC) D67
  platelet NEC D69.1
    constitutional D68.0
  polyglandular E31.8
    autoimmune E31.0
  potassium (K) E87.6
  prepuce N47.3
  proaccelerin (congenital) (hereditary) D68.2
    acquired D68.4
  proconvertin factor (congenital) (hereditary)
      D68.2
    acquired D68.4
  protein —*see also* Malnutrition E46
    anemia D53.0
    C D68.59
    S D68.59
  prothrombin (congenital) (heredItary) D68.2
    acquired D68.4
  Prower factor D68.2
  pseudocholinesterase E88.09
  PTA (plasma thromboplastin antecedent)
      D68.1
  PTC (plasma thromboplastin component)
      D67
  purine nucleoside phosphorylase (PNP) D81.5
  pyracin (alpha) (beta) E53.1
  pyridoxal E53.1
  pyridoxamine E53.1
  pyridoxine (derivatives) E53.1
  pyruvate
    carboxylase E74.4
    dehydrogenase E74.4
  riboflavin (vitamin B2) E53.0

Deficiency, deficient *(Continued)*
  salt E87.1
  secretion
    ovary E28.39
    salivary gland (any) K11.7
    urine R34
  selenium (dietary) E59
  serum antitrypsin, familial E88.01
  short stature homeobox gene (SHOX)
    with
        dyschondrosteosis Q78.8
        short stature (idiopathic) E34.3
        Turner's syndrome Q96.9
  sodium (Na) E87.1
  SPCA (factor VII) D68.2
  sphincter, intrinsic N36.42
    with urethral hypermobility N36.43
  stable factor (congenital) (hereditary)
      D68.2
    acquired D68.4
  Stuart-Prower (factor X) D68.2
  sucrase E74.39
  sulfatase E75.29
  sulfite oxidase E72.19
  thiamin, thiaminic (chloride) E51.9
    beriberi (dry) E51.11
    wet E51.12
  thrombokinase D68.2
    newborn P53
  thyroid (gland) —*see* Hypothyroidism
  tocopherol E56.0
  tooth bud K00.0
  transcobalamine II (anemia) D51.2
  vanadium E61.6
  vascular I99.9
  vasopressin E23.2
  vertical ridge K06.8
  viosterol —*see* Deficiency, calciferol
  vitamin (multiple) NOS E56.9
    A E50.9
      with
          Bitot's spot (corneal) E50.1
          follicular keratosis E50.8
          keratomalacia E50.4
          manifestations NEC E50.8
          night blindness E50.5
          scar of cornea, xerophthalmic
              E50.6
          xeroderma E50.8
          xerophthalmia E50.7
          xerosis
              conjunctival E50.0
                and Bitot's spot E50.1
              cornea E50.2
                and ulceration E50.3
      sequelae E64.1
    B (complex) NOS E53.9
      with
          beriberi (dry) E51.11
            wet E51.12
          pellagra E52
    B1 NOS E51.9
      beriberi (dry) E51.11
        with circulatory system
            manifestations E51.11
        wet E51.12
    B12 E53.8
    B2 (riboflavin) E53.0
    B6 E53.1
    C E54
      sequelae E64.2
    D E55.9
      with
          adult osteomalacia M83.8
          rickets —*see* Rickets
      25-hydroxylase E83.32
    E E56.0
    folic acid E53.8
    G E53.0
    group B E53.9
      specified NEC E53.8

Deficiency, deficient *(Continued)*
  vitamin *(Continued)*
    H (biotin) E53.8
    K E56.1
      of newborn P53
    nicotinic E52
    P E56.8
    PP (pellagra-preventing) E52
    specified NEC E56.8
    thiamin E51.9
      beriberi —*see* Beriberi
    zinc, dietary E60
Deficit —*see also* Deficiency
  attention and concentration R41.840
    following
        cerebral infarction I69.310
        cerebrovascular disease I69.910
          specified disease NEC I69.810
        nontraumatic
            intracerebral hemorrhage I69.110
            specified intracranial hemorrhage
                NEC I69.210
            subarachnoid hemorrhage I69.010
  disorder —*see* Attention, deficit
  cognitive
    communication R41.841
    emotional
      following
          cerebral infarction I69.315
          cerebrovascular disease I69.915
            specified disease NEC I69.815
          nontraumatic
              intracerebral hemorrhage I69.115
              specified intracranial hemorrhage
                  NEC I69.215
              subarachnoid hemorrhage I69.015
    following
        cerebral infarction I69.319
        cerebrovascular disease I69.919
          specified disease NEC I69.819
        nontraumatic
            intracerebral hemorrhage I69.119
            specified intracranial hemorrhage
                NEC I69.219
            subarachnoid hemorrhage I69.019
    social
      following
          cerebral infarction I69.315
          cerebrovascular disease I69.915
            specified disease NEC I69.815
          nontraumatic
              intracerebral hemorrhage I69.115
              specified intracranial hemorrhage
                  NEC I69.215
              subarachnoid hemorrhage I69.015
  cognitive NEC R41.89
    following
        cerebral infarction I69.318
        cerebrovascular disease I69.918
          specified disease NEC I69.818
        nontraumatic
            intracerebral hemorrhage I69.118
            specified intracranial hemorrhage
                NEC I69.218
            subarachnoid hemorrhage I69.018
  concentration R41.840
  executive function R41.844
    following
        cerebral infarction I69.314
        cerebrovascular disease I69.914
          specified disease NEC I69.814
        nontraumatic
            intracerebral hemorrhage I69.114
            specified intracranial hemorrhage
                NEC I69.214
            subarachnoid hemorrhage I69.014
  frontal lobe R41.844
    following
        cerebral infarction I69.314
        cerebrovascular disease I69.914
          specified disease NEC I69.814

Deficit *(Continued)*
  frontal lobe *(Continued)*
    following *(Continued)*
      nontraumatic
        intracerebral hemorrhage I69.114
        specified intracranial hemorrhage
          NEC I69.214
        subarachnoid hemorrhage I69.014
  memory
    following
      cerebral infarction I69.311
      cerebrovascular disease I69.911
        specified disease NEC I69.811
      nontraumatic
        intracerebral hemorrhage I69.111
        specified intracranial hemorrhage
          NEC I69.211
        subarachnoid hemorrhage I69.011
  neurologic NEC R29.818
    ischemic
      reversible (RIND) I63.9
        prolonged (PRIND) I63.9
  oxygen R09.02
  prolonged reversible ischemic neurologic
    (PRIND) I63.9
  psychomotor R41.843
    following
      cerebral infarction I69.313
      cerebrovascular disease I69.913
        specified disease NEC I69.813
      nontraumatic
        intracerebral hemorrhage I69.113
        specified intracranial hemorrhage
          NEC I69.213
        subarachnoid hemorrhage
          I69.013
  visuospatial R41.842
    following
      cerebral infarction I69.312
      cerebrovascular disease I69.912
        specified disease NEC I69.812
      nontraumatic
        intracerebral hemorrhage I69.112
        specified intracranial hemorrhage
          NEC I69.212
        subarachnoid hemorrhage I69.012
Deflection
  radius —*see* Deformity, limb, specified type
    NEC, forearm
  septum (acquired) (nasal) (nose) J34.2
  spine —*see* Curvature, spine
  turbinate (nose) J34.2
Defluvium
  capillorum —*see* Alopecia
  ciliorum —*see* Madarosis
  unguium L60.8
Deformity Q89.9
  abdomen, congenital Q89.9
  abdominal wall
    acquired M95.8
    congenital Q79.59
  acquired (unspecified site) M95.9
  adrenal gland Q89.1
  alimentary tract, congenital Q45.9
    upper Q40.9
  ankle (joint) (acquired) —*see also* Deformity,
    limb, lower leg
    abduction —*see* Contraction, joint, ankle
    congenital Q68.8
    contraction —*see* Contraction, joint, ankle
    specified type NEC —*see* Deformity, limb,
      foot, specified NEC
  anus (acquired) K62.89
    congenital Q43.9
  aorta (arch) (congenital) Q25.40
    acquired I77.89
  aortic
    arch, acquired I77.89
    cusp or valve (congenital) Q23.8
      acquired —*see also* Endocarditis, aortic
        I35.8

Deformity *(Continued)*
  arm (acquired) (upper) —*see also* Deformity,
    limb, upper arm
    congenital Q68.8
    forearm —*see* Deformity, limb, forearm
  artery (congenital) (peripheral) NOS Q27.9
    acquired I77.89
    coronary (acquired) I25.9
      congenital Q24.5
    umbilical Q27.0
  atrial septal Q21.1
  auditory canal (external) (congenital) —*see*
    also Malformation, ear, external
    acquired —*see* Disorder, ear, external,
      specified type NEC
  auricle
    ear (congenital) —*see also* Malformation,
      ear, external
      acquired —*see* Disorder, pinna,
        deformity
  back —*see* Dorsopathy, deforming
  bile duct (common) (congenital) (hepatic)
    Q44.5
    acquired K83.8
  biliary duct or passage (congenital) Q44.5
    acquired K83.8
  bladder (neck) (trigone) (sphincter)
    (acquired) N32.89
    congenital Q64.79
  bone (acquired) NOS M95.9
    congenital Q79.9
    turbinate M95.0
  brain (congenital) Q04.9
    acquired G93.89
    reduction Q04.3
  breast (acquired) N64.89
    congenital Q83.9
    reconstructed N65.0
  bronchus (congenital) Q32.4
    acquired NEC J98.09
  bursa, congenital Q79.9
  canaliculi (lacrimalis) (acquired) —*see also*
    Disorder, lacrimal system, changes
    congenital Q10.6
  canthus, acquired —*see* Disorder, eyelid,
    specified type NEC
  capillary (acquired) I78.8
  cardiovascular system, congenital Q28.9
  caruncle, lacrimal (acquired) —*see also*
    Disorder, lacrimal system, changes
    congenital Q10.6
  cascade, stomach K31.2
  cecum (congenital) Q43.9
    acquired K63.89
  cerebral, acquired G93.89
    congenital Q04.9
  cervix (uterus) (acquired) NEC N88.8
    congenital Q51.9
  cheek (acquired) M95.2
    congenital Q18.9
  chest (acquired) (wall) M95.4
    congenital Q67.8
    sequelae (late effect) of rickets E64.3
  chin (acquired) M95.2
    congenital Q18.9
  choroid (congenital) Q14.3
    acquired H31.8
    plexus Q07.8
      acquired G96.19
  cicatricial —*see* Cicatrix
  cilia, acquired —*see* Disorder, eyelid,
    specified type NEC
  clavicle (acquired) M95.8
    congenital Q68.8
  clitoris (congenital) Q52.6
    acquired N90.89
  clubfoot —*see* Clubfoot
  coccyx (acquired) —*see* subcategory
    M43.8
  colon (congenital) Q43.9
    acquired K63.89

Deformity *(Continued)*
  concha (ear), congenital —*see also*
    Malformation, ear, external
    acquired —*see* Disorder, pinna, deformity
  cornea (acquired) H18.70
    congenital Q13.4
    descemetocele —*see* Descemetocele
    ectasia —*see* Ectasia, cornea
    specified NEC H18.79-•
    staphyloma —*see* Staphyloma, cornea
  coronary artery (acquired) I25.9
    congenital Q24.5
  cranium (acquired) —*see* Deformity,
    skull
  cricoid cartilage (congenital) Q31.8
    acquired J38.7
  cystic duct (congenital) Q44.5
    acquired K82.8
  Dandy-Walker Q03.1
    with spina bifida —*see* Spina bifida
  diaphragm (congenital) Q79.1
    acquired J98.6
  digestive organ NOS Q45.9
  ductus arteriosus Q25.0
  duodenal bulb K31.89
  duodenum (congenital) Q43.9
    acquired K31.89
  dura —*see* Deformity, meninges
  ear (acquired) —*see also* Disorder, pinna,
    deformity
    congenital (external) Q17.9
      internal Q16.5
      middle Q16.4
        ossicles Q16.3
      ossicles Q16.3
  ectodermal (congenital) NEC Q84.9
  ejaculatory duct (congenital) Q55.4
    acquired N50.89
  elbow (joint) (acquired) —*see also* Deformity,
    limb, upper arm
    congenital Q68.8
    contraction —*see* Contraction, joint,
      elbow
  endocrine gland NEC Q89.2
  epididymis (congenital) Q55.4
    acquired N50.89
  epiglottis (congenital) Q31.8
    acquired J38.7
  esophagus (congenital) Q39.9
    acquired K22.8
  eustachian tube (congenital) NEC Q17.8
  eye, congenital Q15.9
  eyebrow (congenital) Q18.8
  eyelid (acquired) —*see also* Disorder, eyelid,
    specified type NEC
    congenital Q10.3
  face (acquired) M95.2
    congenital Q18.9
  fallopian tube, acquired N83.8
  femur (acquired) —*see* Deformity, limb,
    specified type NEC, thigh
  fetal
    with fetopelvic disproportion O33.7
    causing obstructed labor O66.3
  finger (acquired) M20.00-•
    boutonniere M20.02-•
    congenital Q68.1
    flexion contracture —*see* Contraction, joint,
      hand
    mallet finger M20.01-•
    specified NEC M20.09-•
    swan-neck M20.03-•
  flexion (joint) (acquired) —*see also* Deformity,
    limb, flexion M21.20
    congenital NOS Q74.9
      hip Q65.89
  foot (acquired) —*see also* Deformity, limb,
    lower leg
    cavovarus (congenital) Q66.1
    congenital NOS Q66.9
      specified type NEC Q66.89

Deformity (*Continued*)
foot (*Continued*)
    specified type NEC —*see* Deformity, limb,
        foot, specified NEC
    valgus (congenital) Q66.6
        acquired —*see* Deformity, valgus, ankle
    varus (congenital) NEC Q66.3
        acquired —*see* Deformity, varus, ankle
forearm (acquired) —*see also* Deformity, limb,
    forearm
    congenital Q68.8
forehead (acquired) M95.2
    congenital Q75.8
frontal bone (acquired) M95.2
    congenital Q75.8
gallbladder (congenital) Q44.1
    acquired K82.8
gastrointestinal tract (congenital) NOS
    Q45.9
    acquired K63.89
genitalia, genital organ(s) or system NEC
    female (congenital) Q52.9
        acquired N94.89
        external Q52.70
    male (congenital) Q55.9
        acquired N50.89
globe (eye) (congenital) Q15.8
    acquired H44.89
gum, acquired NEC K06.8
hand (acquired) —*see* Deformity, limb,
    hand
    congenital Q68.1
head (acquired) M95.2
    congenital Q75.8
heart (congenital) Q24.9
    septum Q21.9
        auricular Q21.1
        ventricular Q21.0
    valve (congenital) NEC Q24.8
        acquired —*see* Endocarditis
heel (acquired) —*see* Deformity, foot
hepatic duct (congenital) Q44.5
    acquired K83.8
hip (joint) (acquired) —*see also* Deformity,
    limb, thigh
    congenital Q65.9
    due to (previous) juvenile
        osteochondrosis —*see* Coxa, plana
    flexion —*see* Contraction, joint, hip
hourglass —*see* Contraction, hourglass
humerus (acquired) M21.82-●
    congenital Q74.0
hypophyseal (congenital) Q89.2
ileocecal (coil) (valve) (acquired) K63.89
    congenital Q43.9
ileum (congenital) Q43.9
    acquired K63.89
ilium (acquired) M95.5
    congenital Q74.2
integument (congenital) Q84.9
intervertebral cartilage or disc (acquired) —
    see Disorder, disc, specified NEC
intestine (large) (small) (congenital) NOS
    Q43.9
    acquired K63.89
intrinsic minus or plus (hand) —*see*
    Deformity, limb, specified type NEC,
    forearm
iris (acquired) H21.89
    congenital Q13.2
ischium (acquired) M95.5
    congenital Q74.2
jaw (acquired) (congenital) M26.9
joint (acquired) NEC M21.90
    congenital Q68.8
    elbow M21.92-●
    hand M21.94-●
    hip M21.95-●
    knee M21.96-●
    shoulder M21.92-●
    wrist M21.93-●

Deformity (*Continued*)
kidney(s) (calyx) (pelvis) (congenital) Q63.9
    acquired N28.89
    artery (congenital) Q27.2
        acquired I77.89
Klippel-Feil (brevicollis) Q76.1
knee (acquired) NEC —*see also* Deformity,
    limb, lower leg
    congenital Q68.2
labium (majus) (minus) (congenital) Q52.79
    acquired N90.89
lacrimal passages or duct (congenital) NEC
    Q10.6
    acquired —*see* Disorder, lacrimal system,
        changes
larynx (muscle) (congenital) Q31.8
    acquired J38.7
    web (glottic) Q31.0
leg (upper) (acquired) NEC —*see also*
    Deformity, limb, thigh
    congenital Q68.8
    lower leg —*see* Deformity, limb, lower leg
lens (acquired) H27.8
    congenital Q12.9
lid (fold) (acquired) —*see also* Disorder,
    eyelid, specified type NEC
    congenital Q10.3
ligament (acquired) —*see* Disorder, ligament
    congenital Q79.9
limb (acquired) M21.90
    clawfoot M21.53-●
    clawhand M21.51-●
    clubfoot M21.54-●
    clubhand M21.52-●
    congenital, except reduction deformity
        Q74.9
    flat foot M21.4-●
    flexion M21.20
        ankle M21.27-●
        elbow M21.22-●
        finger M21.24-●
        hip M21.25-●
        knee M21.26-●
        shoulder M21.21-●
        toe M21.27-●
        wrist M21.23-●
    foot
        claw —*see* Deformity, limb, clawfoot
        club —*see* Deformity, limb, clubfoot
        drop M21.37-●
        flat —*see* Deformity, limb, flat foot
        specified type NEC M21.6X-●
    forearm M21.93-●
    hand M21.94-●
    lower leg M21.96-●
    specified type NEC M21.80
        forearm M21.83-●
        lower leg M21.86-●
        thigh M21.85-●
        upper arm M21.82-●
    thigh M21.95-●
    unequal length M21.70
        short site is
            femur M21.75-●
            fibula M21.76-●
            humerus M21.72-●
            radius M21.73-●
            tibia M21.76-●
            ulna M21.73-●
    upper arm M21.92-●
    valgus —*see* Deformity, valgus
    varus —*see* Deformity, varus
    wrist drop M21.33-●
lip (congenital) NEC K13.0
    congenital Q38.0
liver (congenital) Q44.7
    acquired K76.89
lumbosacral (congenital) (joint) (region) Q76.49
    acquired —*see* subcategory M43.8
    kyphosis —*see* Kyphosis, congenital
    lordosis —*see* Lordosis, congenital

Deformity (*Continued*)
lung (congenital) Q33.9
    acquired J98.4
lymphatic system, congenital Q89.9
Madelung's (radius) Q74.0
mandible (acquired) (congenital) M26.9
maxilla (acquired) (congenital) M26.9
meninges or membrane (congenital) Q07.9
    cerebral Q04.8
        acquired G96.19
    spinal cord (congenital) G96.19
        acquired G96.19
metacarpus (acquired) —*see* Deformity, limb,
    forearm
    congenital Q74.0
metatarsus (acquired) —*see* Deformity,
    foot
    congenital Q66.9
middle ear (congenital) Q16.4
    ossicles Q16.3
mitral (leaflets) (valve) I05.8
    parachute Q23.2
    stenosis, congenital Q23.2
mouth (acquired) K13.79
    congenital Q38.6
multiple, congenital NEC Q89.7
muscle (acquired) M62.89
    congenital Q79.9
        sternocleidomastoid Q68.0
musculoskeletal system (acquired) M95.9
    congenital Q79.9
    specified NEC M95.8
nail (acquired) L60.8
    congenital Q84.6
nasal —*see* Deformity, nose
neck (acquired) M95.3
    congenital Q18.9
    sternocleidomastoid Q68.0
nervous system (congenital) Q07.9
nipple (congenital) Q83.9
    acquired N64.89
nose (acquired) (cartilage) M95.0
    bone (turbinate) M95.0
    congenital Q30.9
        bent or squashed Q67.4
    saddle M95.0
        syphilitic A50.57
    septum (acquired) J34.2
        congenital Q30.8
    sinus (wall) (congenital) Q30.8
        acquired M95.0
    syphilitic (congenital) A50.57
        late A52.73
ocular muscle (congenital) Q10.3
    acquired —*see* Strabismus, mechanical
opticociliary vessels (congenital) Q13.2
orbit (eye) (acquired) H05.30
    atrophy —*see* Atrophy, orbit
    congenital Q10.7
    due to
        bone disease NEC H05.32-●
        trauma or surgery H05.33-●
    enlargement —*see* Enlargement, orbit
    exostosis —*see* Exostosis, orbit
organ of Corti (congenital) Q16.5
ovary (congenital) Q50.39
    acquired N83.8
oviduct, acquired N83.8
palate (congenital) Q38.5
    acquired M27.8
    cleft (congenital) —*see* Cleft, palate
pancreas (congenital) Q45.3
    acquired K86.89
parathyroid (gland) Q89.2
parotid (gland) (congenital) Q38.4
    acquired K11.8
patella (acquired) —*see* Disorder, patella,
    specified NEC
pelvis, pelvic (acquired) (bony) M95.5
    with disproportion (fetopelvic) O33.0
        causing obstructed labor O65.0

    ▶ New   ⇒ Revised   ~~deleted~~ Deleted   ● Use Additional Character(s)

Deformity (*Continued*)
pelvis, pelvic (*Continued*)
congenital Q74.2
rachitic sequelae (late effect) E64.3
penis (glans) (congenital) Q55.69
acquired N48.89
pericardium (congenital) Q24.8
acquired —*see* Pericarditis
pharynx (congenital) Q38.8
acquired J39.2
pinna, acquired —*see also* Disorder, pinna, deformity
congenital Q17.9
pituitary (congenital) Q89.2
posture —*see* Dorsopathy, deforming
prepuce (congenital) Q55.69
acquired N47.8
prostate (congenital) Q55.4
acquired N42.89
pupil (congenital) Q13.2
acquired —*see* Abnormality, pupillary
pylorus (congenital) Q40.3
acquired K31.89
rachitic (acquired), old or healed E64.3
radius (acquired) —*see also* Deformity, limb, forearm
congenital Q68.8
rectum (congenital) Q43.9
acquired K62.89
reduction (extremity) (limb), congenital (*see also* condition and site) Q73.8
brain Q04.3
lower —*see* Defect, reduction, lower limb
upper —*see* Defect, reduction, upper limb
renal —*see* Deformity, kidney
respiratory system (congenital) Q34.9
rib (acquired) M95.4
congenital Q76.6
cervical Q76.5
rotation (joint) (acquired) —*see* Deformity, limb, specified site NEC
congenital Q74.9
hip —*see* Deformity, limb, specified type NEC, thigh
congenital Q65.89
sacroiliac joint (congenital) Q74.2
acquired —*see* subcategory M43.8
sacrum (acquired) —*see* subcategory M43.8
saddle
back —*see* Lordosis
nose M95.0
syphilitic A50.57
salivary gland or duct (congenital) Q38.4
acquired K11.8
scapula (acquired) M95.8
congenital Q68.8
scrotum (congenital) —*see also* Malformation, testis and scrotum
acquired N50.89
seminal vesicles (congenital) Q55.4
acquired N50.89
septum, nasal (acquired) J34.2
shoulder (joint) (acquired) —*see* Deformity, limb, upper arm
congenital Q74.0
contraction —*see* Contraction, joint, shoulder
sigmoid (flexure) (congenital) Q43.9
acquired K63.89
skin (congenital) Q82.9
skull (acquired) M95.2
congenital Q75.8
with
anencephaly Q00.0
encephalocele —*see* Encephalocele
hydrocephalus Q03.9
with spina bifida —*see* Spina bifida, by site, with hydrocephalus
microcephaly Q02

Deformity (*Continued*)
soft parts, organs or tissues (of pelvis)
in pregnancy or childbirth NEC O34.8-•
causing obstructed labor O65.5
spermatic cord (congenital) Q55.4
acquired N50.89
torsion —*see* Torsion, spermatic cord
spinal —*see* Dorsopathy, deforming
column (acquired) —*see* Dorsopathy, deforming
congenital Q67.5
cord (congenital) Q06.9
acquired G95.89
nerve root (congenital) Q07.9
spine (acquired) —*see also* Dorsopathy, deforming
congenital Q67.5
rachitic E64.3
specified NEC —*see* Dorsopathy, deforming, specified NEC
spleen
acquired D73.89
congenital Q89.09
Sprengel's (congenital) Q74.0
sternocleidomastoid (muscle), congenital Q68.0
sternum (acquired) M95.4
congenital NEC Q76.7
stomach (congenital) Q40.3
acquired K31.89
submandibular gland (congenital) Q38.4
submaxillary gland (congenital) Q38.4
acquired K11.8
talipes —*see* Talipes
testis (congenital) —*see also* Malformation, testis and scrotum
acquired N44.8
torsion —*see* Torsion, testis
thigh (acquired) —*see also* Deformity, limb, thigh
congenital NEC Q68.8
thorax (acquired) (wall) M95.4
congenital Q67.8
sequelae of rickets E64.3
thumb (acquired) —*see also* Deformity, finger
congenital NEC Q68.1
thymus (tissue) (congenital) Q89.2
thyroid (gland) (congenital) Q89.2
cartilage Q31.8
acquired J38.7
tibia (acquired) —*see also* Deformity, limb, specified type NEC, lower leg
congenital NEC Q68.8
saber (syphilitic) A50.56
toe (acquired) M20.6-•
congenital Q66.9
hallux rigidus M20.2-•
hallux valgus M20.1-•
hallux varus M20.3-•
hammer toe M20.4-•
specified NEC M20.5X-•
tongue (congenital) Q38.3
acquired K14.8
tooth, teeth K00.2
trachea (rings) (congenital) Q32.1
acquired J39.8
transverse aortic arch (congenital) Q25.49
tricuspid (leaflets) (valve) I07.8
atresia or stenosis Q22.4
Ebstein's Q22.5
trunk (acquired) M95.8
congenital Q89.9
ulna (acquired) —*see also* Deformity, limb, forearm
congenital NEC Q68.8
urachus, congenital Q64.4
ureter (opening) (congenital) Q62.8
acquired N28.89
urethra (congenital) Q64.79
acquired N36.8

Deformity (*Continued*)
urinary tract (congenital) Q64.9
urachus Q64.4
uterus (congenital) Q51.9
acquired N85.8
uvula (congenital) Q38.5
vagina (acquired) N89.8
congenital Q52.4
valgus NEC M21.00
ankle M21.07-•
elbow M21.02-•
hip M21.05-•
knee M21.06-•
valve, valvular (congenital) (heart) Q24.8
acquired —*see* Endocarditis
varus NEC M21.10
ankle M21.17-•
elbow M21.12-•
hip M21.15
knee M21.16-•
tibia —*see* Osteochondrosis, juvenile, tibia
vas deferens (congenital) Q55.4
acquired N50.89
vein (congenital) Q27.9
great Q26.9
vertebra —*see* Dorsopathy, deforming
vertical talus (congenital) Q66.80
left foot Q66.82
right foot Q66.81
vesicourethral orifice (acquired) N32.89
congenital NEC Q64.79
vessels of optic papilla (congenital) Q14.2
visual field (contraction) —*see* Defect, visual field
vitreous body, acquired H43.89
vulva (congenital) Q52.79
acquired N90.89
wrist (joint) (acquired) —*see also* Deformity, limb, forearm
congenital Q68.8
contraction —*see* Contraction, joint, wrist
Degeneration, degenerative
adrenal (capsule) (fatty) (gland) (hyaline) (infectional) E27.8
amyloid —*see also* Amyloidosis E85.9
anterior cornua, spinal cord G12.29
anterior labral S43.49-•
aorta, aortic I70.0
fatty I77.89
aortic valve (heart) —*see* Endocarditis, aortic
arteriovascular —*see* Arteriosclerosis
artery, arterial (atheromatous) (calcareous) — *see also* Arteriosclerosis
cerebral, amyloid E85.4 [I68.0]
medial —*see* Arteriosclerosis, extremities
articular cartilage NEC —*see* Derangement, joint, articular cartilage, by site
atheromatous —*see* Arteriosclerosis
basal nuclei or ganglia G23.9
specified NEC G23.8
bone NEC —*see* Disorder, bone, specified type NEC
brachial plexus G54.0
brain (cortical) (progressive) G31.9
alcoholic G31.2
arteriosclerotic I67.2
childhood G31.9
specified NEC G31.89
cystic G31.89
congenital Q04.6
in
alcoholism G31.2
beriberi E51.2
cerebrovascular disease I67.9
congenital hydrocephalus Q03.9
with spina bifida —*see also* Spina bifida
Fabry-Anderson disease E75.21
Gaucher's disease E75.22
Hunter's syndrome E76.1

Degeneration, degenerative *(Continued)*
  brain *(Continued)*
    in *(Continued)*
      lipidosis
        cerebral E75.4
        generalized E75.6
      mucopolysaccharidosis —*see*
        Mucopolysaccharidosis
      myxedema E03.9 *[G32.89]*
      neoplastic disease —*see also* Neoplasm
        D49.6 *[G32.89]*
      Niemann-Pick disease E75.249 *[G32.89]*
      sphingolipidosis E75.3 *[G32.89]*
      vitamin B12 deficiency E53.8 *[G32.89]*
    senile NEC G31.1
  breast N64.89
  Bruch's membrane —*see* Degeneration,
    choroid
  capillaries (fatty) I78.8
➡ amyloid E85.89 *[I79.8]*
  cardiac —*see also* Degeneration, myocardial
    valve, valvular —*see* Endocarditis
  cardiorenal —*see* Hypertension, cardiorenal
  cardiovascular —*see also* Disease,
    cardiovascular
    renal —*see* Hypertension, cardiorenal
  cerebellar NOS G31.9
    alcoholic G31.2
    primary (hereditary) (sporadic) G11.9
  cerebral —*see* Degeneration, brain
  cerebrovascular I67.9
    due to hypertension I67.4
  cervical plexus G54.2
  cervix N88.8
    due to radiation (intended effect) N88.8
      adverse effect or misadventure N99.89
  chamber angle H21.21-●
  changes, spine or vertebra —*see* Spondylosis
  chorioretinal —*see also* Degeneration, choroid
    hereditary H31.20
  choroid (colloid) (drusen) H31.10-●
    atrophy —*see* Atrophy, choroidal
    hereditary —*see* Dystrophy, choroidal,
      hereditary
  ciliary body H21.22-●
  cochlear —*see* subcategory H83.8
  combined (spinal cord) (subacute) E53.8
    [G32.0]
    with anemia (pernicious) D51.0 *[G32.0]*
      due to dietary vitamin B12 deficiency
        D51.3 *[G32.0]*
    in (due to)
      vitamin B12 deficiency E53.8 *[G32.0]*
        anemia D51.9 *[G32.0]*
  conjunctiva H11.10
    concretions —*see* Concretion, conjunctiva
    deposits —*see* Deposit, conjunctiva
    pigmentations —*see* Pigmentation,
      conjunctiva
    pinguecula —*see* Pinguecula
    xerosis —*see* Xerosis, conjunctiva
  cornea H18.40
    calcerous H18.43
      band keratopathy H18.42-●
    familial, hereditary —*see* Dystrophy, cornea
    hyaline (of old scars) H18.49
    keratomalacia —*see* Keratomalacia
    nodular H18.45-●
    peripheral H18.46-●
    senile H18.41-●
    specified type NEC H18.49
  cortical (cerebellar) (parenchymatous)
    G31.89
    alcoholic G31.2
    diffuse, due to arteriopathy I67.2
  corticobasal G31.85
  cutis L98.8
    amyloid E85.4 *[L99]*
  dental pulp K04.2
  disc disease —*see* Degeneration,
    intervertebral disc NEC

Degeneration, degenerative *(Continued)*
  dorsolateral (spinal cord) —*see* Degeneration,
    combined
  extrapyramidal G25.9
  eye, macular —*see also* Degeneration, macula
    congenital or hereditary —*see* Dystrophy,
      retina
  facet joints —*see* Spondylosis
  fatty
    liver NEC K76.0
      alcoholic K70.0
  grey matter (brain) (Alpers') G31.81
  heart —*see also* Degeneration, myocardial
    amyloid E85.4 *[I43]*
    atheromatous —*see* Disease, heart,
      ischemic, atherosclerotic
    ischemic —*see* Disease, heart, ischemic
  hepatolenticular (Wilson's) E83.01
  hepatorenal K76.7
  hyaline (diffuse) (generalized)
    localized —*see* Degeneration, by site
  infrapatellar fat pad M79.4
  intervertebral disc NOS
    with
      myelopathy —*see* Disorder, disc, with,
        myelopathy
      radiculitis or radiculopathy —*see*
        Disorder, disc, with, radiculopathy
    cervical, cervicothoracic —*see* Disorder,
      disc, cervical, degeneration
    with
      myelopathy —*see* Disorder, disc,
        cervical, with myelopathy
      neuritis, radiculitis or
        radiculopathy —*see* Disorder,
        disc, cervical, with neuritis
    lumbar region M51.36
      with
        myelopathy M51.06
        neuritis, radiculitis, radiculopathy or
          sciatica M51.16
    lumbosacral region M51.37
      with
        neuritis, radiculitis, radiculopathy or
          sciatica M51.17
    sacrococcygeal region M53.3
    thoracic region M51.34
      with
        myelopathy M51.04
        neuritis, radiculitis, radiculopathy
          M51.14
    thoracolumbar region M51.35
      with
        myelopathy M51.05
        neuritis, radiculitis, radiculopathy
          M51.15
  intestine, amyloid E85.4
  iris (pigmentary) H21.23-●
  ischemic —*see* Ischemia
  joint disease —*see* Osteoarthritis
  kidney N28.89
    amyloid E85.4 *[N29]*
    cystic, congenital Q61.9
    fatty N28.89
    polycystic Q61.3
      adult type (autosomal dominant)
        Q61.2
      infantile type (autosomal recessive) NEC
        Q61.19
        collecting duct dilatation Q61.11
  Kuhnt-Junius —*see also* Degeneration, macula
    H35.32-●
  lens —*see* Cataract
  lenticular (familial) (progressive) (Wilson's)
    (with cirrhosis of liver) E83.01
  liver (diffuse) NEC K76.89
    amyloid E85.4 *[K77]*
    cystic K76.89
      congenital Q44.6
    fatty NEC K76.0
      alcoholic K70.0

Degeneration, degenerative *(Continued)*
  liver *(Continued)*
    hypertrophic K76.89
    parenchymatous, acute or subacute
      K72.00
      with coma K72.01
    pigmentary K76.89
    toxic (acute) K71.9
  lung J98.4
  lymph gland I89.8
    hyaline I89.8
  macula, macular (acquired) (age-related)
    (senile) H35.30
    angioid streaks H35.33
    atrophic age-related H35.31-●
    congenital or hereditary —*see* Dystrophy,
      retina
    cystoid H35.35-●
    drusen H35.36-●
    dry age-related H35.31-●
    exudative H35.32-●
    hole H35.34-●
    nonexudative H35.31-●
    puckering H35.37-●
    toxic H35.38-●
    wet age-related H35.32-●
  membranous labyrinth, congenital (causing
    impairment of hearing) Q16.5
  meniscus —*see* Derangement, meniscus
  mitral —*see* Insufficiency, mitral
  Mönckeberg's —*see* Arteriosclerosis,
    extremities
  motor centers, senile G31.1
  multi-system G90.3
  mural —*see* Degeneration, myocardial
  muscle (fatty) (fibrous) (hyaline)
    (progressive) M62.89
    heart —*see* Degeneration, myocardial
  myelin, central nervous system G37.9
  myocardial, myocardium (fatty) (hyaline)
    (senile) I51.5
    with rheumatic fever (conditions in I00)
      I09.0
      active, acute or subacute I01.2
        with chorea I02.0
      inactive or quiescent (with chorea) I09.0
    hypertensive —*see* Hypertension, heart
    rheumatic —*see* Degeneration, myocardial,
      with rheumatic fever
    syphilitic A52.06
  nasal sinus (mucosa) J32.9
    frontal J32.1
    maxillary J32.0
  nerve —*see* Disorder, nerve
  nervous system G31.9
    alcoholic G31.2
    amyloid E85.4 *[G99.8]*
    autonomic G90.9
    fatty G31.89
    specified NEC G31.89
  nipple N64.89
  olivopontocerebellar (hereditary) (familial)
    G23.8
  osseous labyrinth —*see* subcategory H83.8
  ovary N83.8
    cystic N83.20-●
    microcystic N83.20-●
  pallidal pigmentary (progressive) G23.0
  pancreas K86.89
    tuberculous A18.83
  penis N48.89
  pigmentary (diffuse) (general)
    localized —*see* Degeneration, by site
    pallidal (progressive) G23.0
  pineal gland E34.8
  pituitary (gland) E23.6
  popliteal fat pad M79.4
  posterolateral (spinal cord) —*see*
    Degeneration, combined
  pulmonary valve (heart) I37.8
  pulp (tooth) K04.2

▶ New   ➡ Revised   ~~deleted~~ Deleted   ● Use Additional Character(s)

Degeneration, degenerative (Continued)
  pupillary margin H21.24-●
  renal —see Degeneration, kidney
  retina H35.9
    hereditary (cerebroretinal) (congenital)
        (juvenile) (macula) (peripheral)
        (pigmentary) —see Dystrophy, retina
    Kuhnt-Junius —see also Degeneration,
        macula H35.32-●
    macula (cystic) (exudative) (hole)
        (nonexudative) (pseudohole) (senile)
        (toxic) —see Degeneration, macula
    peripheral H35.40
      lattice H35.41-●
      microcystoid H35.42-●
      paving stone H35.43-●
      secondary
        pigmentary H35.45-●
        vitreoretinal H35.46-●
      senile reticular H35.44-●
    pigmentary (primary) —see also Dystrophy,
        retina
      secondary —see Degeneration, retina,
        peripheral, secondary
    posterior pole —see Degeneration, macula
  saccule, congenital (causing impairment of
        hearing) Q16.5
  senile R54
    brain G31.1
    cardiac, heart or myocardium —see
        Degeneration, myocardial
    motor centers G31.1
    vascular —see Arteriosclerosis
  sinus (cystic) —see also Sinusitis
    polypoid J33.1
  skin L98.8
    amyloid E85.4 [L99]
    colloid L98.8
  spinal (cord) G31.89
    amyloid E85.4 [G32.89]
    combined (subacute) —see Degeneration,
        combined
    dorsolateral —see Degeneration, combined
    familial NEC G31.89
    fatty G31.89
    funicular —see Degeneration, combined
    posterolateral —see Degeneration,
        combined
    subacute combined —see Degeneration,
        combined
    tuberculous A17.81
  spleen D73.0
    amyloid E85.4 [D77]
  stomach K31.89
  striatonigral G23.2
  suprarenal (capsule) (gland) E27.8
  synovial membrane (pulpy) —see Disorder,
        synovium, specified type NEC
  tapetoretinal —see Dystrophy, retina
  thymus (gland) E32.8
    fatty E32.8
  thyroid (gland) E07.89
  tricuspid (heart) (valve) I07.9
  tuberculous NEC —see Tuberculosis
  turbinate J34.89
  uterus (cystic) N85.8
  vascular (senile) —see Arteriosclerosis
    hypertensive —see Hypertension
  vitreoretinal, secondary —see Degeneration,
        retina, peripheral, secondary, vitreoretinal
  vitreous (body) H43.81-●
  Wallerian —see Disorder, nerve
  Wilson's hepatolenticular E83.01
Deglutition
  paralysis R13.0
    hysterical F44.4
  pneumonia J69.0
Degos' disease I77.89
Dehiscence (of)
  amputation stump T87.81
  cesarean wound O90.0

Dehiscence (Continued)
  closure of
    cornea T81.31
    craniotomy T81.32
    fascia (muscular) (superficial) T81.32
    internal organ or tissue T81.32
    laceration (external) (internal) T81.33
    ligament T81.32
    mucosa T81.31
    muscle or muscle flap T81.32
    ribs or rib cage T81.32
    skin and subcutaneous tissue (full-
        thickness) (superficial) T81.31
    skull T81.32
    sternum (sternotomy) T81.32
    tendon T81.32
    traumatic laceration (external) (internal)
        T81.33
  episiotomy O90.1
  operation wound NEC T81.31
    external operation wound (superficial)
        T81.31
    internal operation wound (deep)
        T81.32
  perineal wound (postpartum) O90.1
  traumatic injury wound repair T81.33
  wound T81.30
    traumatic repair T81.33
Dehydration E86.0
  newborn P74.1
Déjérine-Roussy syndrome G93.89
Déjérine-Sottas disease or neuropathy
    (hypertrophic) G60.0
Déjérine-Thomas atrophy G23.8
Delay, delayed
  any plane in pelvis
    complicating delivery O66.9
  birth or delivery NOS O63.9
➠closure, ductus arteriosus (Botalli) P29.38
  coagulation —see Defect, coagulation
  conduction (cardiac) (ventricular) I45.9
  delivery, second twin, triplet, etc O63.2
  development R62.50
    global F88
    intellectual (specific) F81.9
    language F80.9
      due to hearing loss F80.4
    learning F81.9
    pervasive F84.9
    physiological R62.50
      specified stage NEC R62.0
    reading F81.0
    sexual E30.0
    speech F80.9
      due to hearing loss F80.4
    spelling F81.81
  ejaculation F52.32
  gastric emptying K30
  menarche E30.0
  menstruation (cause unknown) N91.0
  milestone R62.0
  passage of meconium (newborn)
      P76.0
  primary respiration P28.9
  puberty (constitutional) E30.0
  separation of umbilical cord P96.82
  sexual maturation, female E30.0
  sleep phase syndrome G47.21
  union, fracture —see Fracture, by site
  vaccination Z28.9
Deletion(s)
  autosome Q93.9
    identified by fluorescence in situ
        hybridization (FISH) Q93.89
    identified by in situ hybridization (ISH)
        Q93.89
  chromosome
    with complex rearrangements NEC
        Q93.7
    part of NEC Q93.5
    seen only at prometaphase Q93.89

Deletion (Continued)
  chromosome (Continued)
    short arm
      4 Q93.3
      5p Q93.4
      22q11.2 Q93.81
      specified NEC Q93.89
    long arm chromosome 18 or 21 Q93.89
      with complex rearrangements NEC
          Q93.7
    microdeletions NEC Q93.88
Delhi boil or button B55.1
Delinquency (juvenile) (neurotic) F91.8
  group Z72.810
Delinquent immunization status Z28.3
Delirium, delirious (acute or subacute) (not
    alcohol or drug-induced) (with dementia)
    R41.0
  alcoholic (acute) (tremens) (withdrawal)
      F10.921
    with intoxication F10.921
    in
      abuse F10.121
      dependence F10.221
  due to (secondary to)
    alcohol
      intoxication F10.921
      in
        abuse F10.121
        dependence F10.221
      withdrawal F10.231
    amphetamine intoxication F15.921
      in
        abuse F15.121
        dependence F15.221
    anxiolytic
      intoxication F13.921
      in
        abuse F13.121
        dependence F13.221
      withdrawal F13.231
    cannabis intoxication (acute) F12.921
      in
        abuse F12.121
        dependence F12.221
    cocaine intoxication (acute) F14.921
      in
        abuse F14.121
        dependence F14.221
    general medical condition F05
    hallucinogen intoxication F16.921
      in
        abuse F16.121
        dependence F16.221
    hypnotic
      intoxication F13.921
      in
        abuse F13.121
        dependence F13.221
      withdrawal F13.231
    inhalant intoxication (acute) F18.921
      in
        abuse F18.121
        dependence F18.221
    multiple etiologies F05
    opioid intoxication (acute) F11.921
      in
        abuse F11.121
        dependence F11.221
    other (or unknown) substance
        F19.921
    phencyclidine intoxication (acute)
        F16.921
      in
        abuse F16.121
        dependence F16.221
    psychoactive substance NEC intoxication
        (acute) F19.921
      in
        abuse F19.121
        dependence F19.221

Delirium, delirious *(Continued)*
  due to *(Continued)*
    sedative
      intoxication F13.921
        in
          abuse F13.121
          dependence F13.221
      withdrawal F13.231
    unknown etiology F05
  exhaustion F43.0
  hysterical F44.89
  postprocedural (postoperative) F05
  puerperal F05
  thyroid —*see* Thyrotoxicosis with thyroid
    storm
  traumatic —*see* Injury, intracranial
  tremens (alcohol-induced) F10.231
    sedative-induced F13.231
Delivery (childbirth) (labor)
  arrested active phase O62.1
  cesarean (for)
    without indication O82
    abnormal
      pelvis (bony) (deformity) (major) NEC
        with disproportion (fetopelvic)
          O33.0
          with obstructed labor O65.0
        presentation or position O32.9
    abruptio placentae —*see also* Abruptio
      placentae 045.9-●
    acromion presentation O32.2
    atony, uterus O62.2
    breech presentation O32.1
      incomplete O32.8
    brow presentation O32.3
    cephalopelvic disproportion O33.9
    cerclage O34.3-●
    chin presentation O32.3
    cicatrix of cervix O34.4-●
    contracted pelvis (general)
      inlet O33.2
      outlet O33.3
    cord presentation or prolapse O69.0
    cystocele O34.8-●
    deformity (acquired) (congenital)
      pelvic organs or tissues NEC O34.8-●
      pelvis (bony) NEC O33.0
    disproportion NOS O33.9
    eclampsia —*see* Eclampsia
    face presentation O32.3
    failed
      forceps O66.5
      induction of labor O61.9
        instrumental O61.1
        mechanical O61.1
        medical O61.0
        specified NEC O61.8
        surgical O61.1
      trial of labor NOS O66.40
        following previous cesarean delivery
          O66.41
      vacuum extraction O66.5
      ventouse O66.5
    fetal-maternal hemorrhage O43.01-●
    hemorrhage (intrapartum) O67.9
      with coagulation defect O67.0
      specified cause NEC O67.8
    high head at term O32.4
    hydrocephalic fetus O33.6
    incarceration of uterus O34.51-●
    incoordinate uterine action O62.4
    increased size, fetus O33.5
    inertia, uterus O62.2
      primary O62.0
      secondary O62.1
    lateroversion, uterus O34.59-●
    mal lie O32.9
    malposition
      fetus O32.9
      pelvic organs or tissues NEC O34.8-●
      uterus NEC O34.59-●

Delivery *(Continued)*
  cesarean *(Continued)*
    malpresentation NOS O32.9
    oblique presentation O32.2
    occurring after 37 completed weeks of
      gestation but before 39 completed
      weeks gestation due to (spontaneous)
      onset of labor O75.82
    oversize fetus O33.5
    pelvic tumor NEC O34.8-●
    placenta previa O44.0-●
      complete O44.0-●
        with hemorrhage O44.1-●
    placental insufficiency O36.51-●
    planned, occurring after 37 completed
      weeks of gestation but before 39
      completed weeks gestation due to
      (spontaneous) onset of labor O75.82
    polyp, cervix O34.4-●
      causing obstructed labor O65.5
    poor dilatation, cervix O62.0
    pre-eclampsia O14.94
      mild O14.04
      moderate O14.04
      severe O14.14
        with hemolysis, elevated liver
          enzymes and low platelet count
          (HELLP) O14.24
    previous
      cesarean delivery O34.219
        classical (vertical) scar O34.212
        low transverse scar O34.211
      surgery (to)
        cervix O34.4-●
        gynecological NEC O34.8-●
        rectum O34.7-●
        uterus O34.29
        vagina O34.6-●
    prolapse
      arm or hand O32.2
      uterus O34.52-●
    prolonged labor NOS O63.9
    rectocele O34.8-●
    retroversion
      uterus O34.53-●
    rigid
      cervix O34.4-●
      pelvic floor O34.8-●
      perineum O34.7-●
      vagina O34.6-●
      vulva O34.7-●
    sacculation, pregnant uterus O34.59-●
    scar(s)
      cervix O34.4-●
      cesarean delivery O34.219
        classical (vertical) O34.212
        low transverse O34.211
      transmural uterine O34.29
      uterus O34.29
    Shirodkar suture in situ O34.3-●
    shoulder presentation O32.2
    stenosis or stricture, cervix O34.4-●
    streptococcus group B (GBS) carrier state
      O99.824
    transmural uterine scar O34.29
    transverse presentation or lie O32.2
    tumor, pelvic organs or tissues NEC
      O34.8-●
      cervix O34.4-●
    umbilical cord presentation or prolapse
      O69.0
  completely normal case O80
  complicated O75.9
    by
      abnormal, abnormality (of)
        forces of labor O62.9
          specified type NEC O62.8
        glucose O99.814
        uterine contractions NOS O62.9
      abruptio placentae —*see also* Abruptio
        placentae O45.9-●

Delivery *(Continued)*
  complicated *(Continued)*
    by *(Continued)*
      abuse
        physical O9A.32
        psychological O9A.52
        sexual O9A.42
      adherent placenta O72.0
        without hemorrhage O73.0
      alcohol use O99.314
      anemia (pre-existing) O99.02
      anesthetic death O74.8
      annular detachment of cervix O71.3
      atony, uterus O62.2
      attempted vacuum extraction and
        forceps O66.5
      Bandl's ring O62.4
      bariatric surgery status O99.844
      biliary tract disorder O26.62
      bleeding —*see* Delivery, complicated by,
        hemorrhage
      blood disorder NEC O99.12
      cervical dystocia (hypotonic) O62.2
        primary O62.0
        secondary O62.1
      circulatory system disorder O99.42
      compression of cord (umbilical) NEC
        O69.2
      condition NEC O99.89
      contraction, contracted ring O62.4
      cord (umbilical)
        around neck
          with compression O69.1
          without compression O69.81
        bruising O69.5
        complication O69.9
          specified NEC O69.89
        compression NEC O69.2
        entanglement O69.2
          without compression O69.82
        hematoma O69.5
        presentation O69.0
        prolapse O69.0
        short O69.3
        thrombosis (vessels) O69.5
        vascular lesion O69.5
      Couvelaire uterus O45.8X-●
      damage to (injury to) NEC
        perineum O71.82
        periurethral tissue O71.82
        vulva O71.82
      delay following rupture of membranes
        (spontaneous) —*see* Pregnancy,
        complicated by, premature rupture
        of membranes
      depressed fetal heart tones O76
      diabetes O24.92
        gestational O24.429
          diet controlled O24.420
          insulin controlled O24.424
          oral drug controlled (antidiabetic)
            (hypoglycemic) O24.425
        pre-existing O24.32
          specified NEC O24.82
          type 1 O24.02
          type 2 O24.12
      diastasis recti (abdominis) O71.89
      dilatation
        bladder O66.8
        cervix incomplete, poor or slow O62.0
      disease NEC O99.89
      disruptio uteri —*see* Delivery,
        complicated by, rupture, uterus
      drug use O99.324
      dysfunction, uterus NOS O62.9
        hypertonic O62.4
        hypotonic O62.2
          primary O62.0
          secondary O62.1
        incoordinate O62.4
      eclampsia O15.1

▶ New   ⇒ Revised   ~~deleted~~ Deleted   ● Use Additional Character(s)

Delivery *(Continued)*
  complicated *(Continued)*
    by *(Continued)*
      embolism (pulmonary) —*see* Embolism, obstetric
      endocrine, nutritional or metabolic disease NEC O99.284
      failed
        attempted vaginal birth after previous cesarean delivery O66.41
        induction of labor O61.9
          instrumental O61.1
          mechanical O61.1
          medical O61.0
          specified NEC O61.8
          surgical O61.1
        trial of labor O66.40
      female genital mutilation O65.5
      fetal
        abnormal acid-base balance O68
        acidemia O68
        acidosis O68
        alkalosis O68
        death, early O02.1
        deformity O66.3
        heart rate or rhythm (abnormal) (non-reassuring) O76
        hypoxia O77.8
        stress O77.9
          due to drug administration O77.1
          electrocardiographic evidence of O77.8
          specified NEC O77.8
          ultrasound evidence of O77.8
      fever during labor O75.2
      gastric banding status O99.844
      gastric bypass status O99.844
      gastrointestinal disease NEC O99.62
      gestational
        diabetes O24.429
          diet controlled O24.420
          insulin (and diet) controlled O24.424
          oral drug controlled (antidiabetic) (hypoglycemic) O24.425
        edema O12.04
          with proteinuria O12.24
        proteinuria O12.14
      gonorrhea O98.22
      hematoma O71.7
        ischial spine O71.7
        pelvic O71.7
        vagina O71.7
        vulva or perineum O71.7
      hemorrhage (uterine) O67.9
        associated with
          afibrinogenemia O67.0
          coagulation defect O67.0
          hyperfibrinolysis O67.0
          hypofibrinogenemia O67.0
        due to
          low implantation of placenta O44.5-●
          low-lying placenta O44.5-●
          placenta previa O44.1-●
            marginal O44.3-●
            partial O44.3-●
          premature separation of placenta (normally implanted) *(see also* Abruptio placentae) O45.9-●
          retained placenta O72.0
          uterine leiomyoma O67.8
        placenta NEC O67.8
        postpartum NEC (atonic) (immediate) O72.1
          with retained or trapped placenta O72.0
          delayed O72.2
          secondary O72.2
          third stage O72.0

Delivery *(Continued)*
  complicated *(Continued)*
    by *(Continued)*
      hourglass contraction, uterus O62.4
      hypertension, hypertensive (pre-existing) —*see* Hypertension, complicated by, childbirth (labor)
      hypotension O26.5-●
      incomplete dilatation (cervix) O62.0
      incoordinate uterus contractions O62.4
      inertia, uterus O62.2
        during latent phase of labor O62.0
        primary O62.0
        secondary O62.1
      infection (maternal) O98.92
        carrier state NEC O99.834
        gonorrhea O98.22
        human immunodeficiency virus (HIV) O98.72
        sexually transmitted NEC O98.32
        specified NEC O98.82
        syphilis O98.12
        tuberculosis O98.02
        viral hepatitis O98.42
        viral NEC O98.52
      injury (to mother) *(see also* Delivery, complicated, by, damage to) O71.9
        nonobstetric O9A.22
          caused by abuse —*see* Delivery, complicated by, abuse
      intrauterine fetal death, early O02.1
      inversion, uterus O71.2
      laceration (perineal) O70.9
        anus (sphincter) O70.4
          with third degree laceration —*see also* Delivery, complicated, by, laceration, perineum, third degree O70.20
          with mucosa O70.3
          without third degree laceration O70.4
        bladder (urinary) O71.5
        bowel O71.5
        cervix (uteri) O71.3
        fourchette O70.0
        hymen O70.0
        labia O70.0
        pelvic
          floor O70.1
          organ NEC O71.5
        perineum, perineal O70.9
          first degree O70.0
          fourth degree O70.3
          muscles O70.1
          second degree O70.1
          skin O70.0
          slight O70.0
          third degree O70.20
            with
              both external anal sphincter (EAS) and internal anal sphincter (IAS) torn (IIIc) O70.23
              less than 50% of external anal sphincter (EAS) thickness torn (IIIa) O70.21
              more than 50% external anal sphincter (EAS) thickness torn (IIIb) O70.22
            IIIa O70.21
            IIIb O70.22
            IIIc O70.23
        peritoneum (pelvic) O71.5
        rectovaginal (septum) (without perineal laceration) O71.4
          with perineum —*see also* Delivery, complicated, by, laceration, perineum, third degree O70.20
          with anal or rectal mucosa O70.3

Delivery *(Continued)*
  complicated *(Continued)*
    by *(Continued)*
      laceration *(Continued)*
        specified NEC O71.89
        sphincter ani —*see* Delivery, complicated, by, laceration, anus (sphincter)
        urethra O71.5
        uterus O71.81
          before labor O71.81
        vagina, vaginal (deep) (high) (without perineal laceration) O71.4
          with perineum O70.0
          muscles, with perineum O70.1
        vulva O70.0
      liver disorder O26.62
      malignancy O9A.12
      malnutrition O25.2
      malposition, malpresentation
        without obstruction O32.9 —*see also* Delivery, complicated by, obstruction
        breech O32.1
        compound O32.6
        face (brow) (chin) O32.3
        footling O38.8
        high head O32.4
        oblique O32.2
        specified NEC O32.8
        transverse O32.2
        unstable lie O32.0
        placenta O44.0-●
          with hemorrhage O44.1-●
        uterus or cervix O65.5
      meconium in amniotic fluid O77.0
      mental disorder NEC O99.344
      metrorrhexis —*see* Delivery, complicated by, rupture, uterus
      nervous system disorder O99.354
      obesity (pre-existing) O99.214
      obesity surgery status O99.844
      obstetric trauma O71.9
        specified NEC O71.89
      obstructed labor
        due to
          breech (complete) (frank) presentation O64.1
            incomplete O64.8
          brow presenation O64.3
          buttock presentation O64.1
          chin presentation O64.2
          compound presentation O64.5
          contracted pelvis O65.1
          deep transverse arrest O64.0
          deformed pelvis O65.0
          dystocia (fetal) O66.9
            due to
              conjoined twins O66.3
              fetal
                abnormality NEC O66.3
                ascites O66.3
                hydrops O66.3
                meningomyelocele O66.3
                sacral teratoma O66.3
                tumor O66.3
             hydrocephalic fetus O66.3
            shoulder O66.0
          face presentation O64.2
          fetopelvic disproportion O65.4
          footling presentation O64.8
          impacted shoulders O66.0
          incomplete rotation of fetal head O64.0
          large fetus O66.2
          locked twins O66.1
          malposition O64.9
            specified NEC O64.8
          malpresentation O64.9
            specified NEC O64.8

Delivery *(Continued)*
  complicated *(Continued)*
    by *(Continued)*
      obstructed labor *(Continued)*
        due to *(Continued)*
          multiple fetuses NEC O66.6
          pelvic
            abnormality (maternal) O65.9
              organ O65.5
              specified NEC O65.8
            contraction
              inlet O65.2
              mid-cavity O65.3
              outlet O65.3
          persistent (position)
            occipitoiliac O64.0
            occipitoposterior O64.0
            occipitosacral O64.0
            occipitotransverse O64.0
          prolapsed arm O64.4
          shoulder presentation O64.4
        specified NEC O66.8
      pathological retraction ring, uterus
          O62.4
      penetration, pregnant uterus by
          instrument O71.1
      perforation —*see* Delivery, complicated
          by, laceration
      placenta, placental
        ablatio —*see also* Abruptio placentae
            O45.9-●
        abnormality O43.9-●
          specified NEC O43.89-●
        abruptio —*see also* Abruptio placentae
            O45.9-●
        accreta O43.21-●
        adherent (with hemorrhage) O72.0
          without hemorrhage O73.0
        detachment (premature) —*see also*
            Abruptio placentae O45.9-●
        disorder O43.9-●
          specified NEC O43.89-●
        hemorrhage NEC O67.8
        increta O43.22-●
        low (implantation) (lying) O44.4-●
          with hemorrhage O44.5-●
        malformation O43.10-●
        malposition O44.0-●
          without hemorrhage O44.1-●
        percreta O43.23-●
        previa (central) (complete) (lateral)
            (total) O44.0-●
          with hemorrhage O44.1-●
            marginal O44.2-●
              with hemorrhage O44.3-●
            partial O44.2-●
              with hemorrhage O44.3-●
        retained (with hemorrhage) O72.0
          without hemorrhage O73.0
        separation (premature) O45.9-●
          specified NEC O45.8X-●
        vicious insertion O44.1-●
      precipitate labor O62.3
      premature rupture, membranes (*see
          also* Pregnancy, complicated by,
          premature rupture of membranes)
          O42.90
      prolapse
        arm or hand O32.2
        cord (umbilical) O69.0
        foot or leg O32.8
        uterus O34.52-●
      prolonged labor O63.9
        first stage O63.0
        second stage O63.1
      protozoal disease (maternal) O98.62
      respiratory disease NEC O99.52
      retained membranes or portions of
          placenta O72.2
        without hemorrhage O73.1
      retarded birth O63.9

Delivery *(Continued)*
  complicated *(Continued)*
    by *(Continued)*
      retention of secundines (with
          hemorrhage) O72.0
        without hemorrhage O73.0
        partial O72.2
          without hemorrhage O73.1
      rupture
        bladder (urinary) O71.5
        cervix O71.3
        pelvic organ NEC O71.5
        urethra O71.5
        uterus (during or after labor) O71.1
          before labor O71.0-●
      separation, pubic bone (symphysis
          pubis) O71.6
      shock O75.1
      shoulder presentation O64.4
      skin disorder NEC O99.72
      spasm, cervix O62.4
      stenosis or stricture, cervix O65.5
      streptococcus group B (GBS) carrier state
          O99.824
      subluxation of symphysis (pubis)
          O26.72
      syphilis (maternal) O98.12
      tear —*see* Delivery, complicated by,
          laceration
      tetanic uterus O62.4
      trauma (obstetrical) —*see also* Delivery,
          complicated, by, damage to O71.9
        non-obstetric O9A.22
        periurethral O71.82
        specified NEC O71.89
      tuberculosis (maternal) O98.02
      tumor, pelvic organs or tissues NEC
          O65.5
      umbilical cord around neck
        with compression O69.1
        without compression O69.81
      uterine inertia O62.2
        during latent phase of labor O62.0
        primary O62.0
        secondary O62.1
      vasa previa O69.4
      velamentous insertion of cord O43.12-●
    specified complication NEC O75.89
  delayed NOS O63.9
    following rupture of membranes
        artificial O75.5
    second twin, triplet, etc. O63.2
  forceps, low following failed vacuum
      extraction O66.5
  missed (at or near term) O36.4
  normal O80
  ⇒obstructed —*see* Delivery, complicated by,
      obstructed labor
  precipitate O62.3
  preterm —*see also* Pregnancy, complicated by,
      preterm labor O60.10
  spontaneous O80
  term pregnancy NOS O80
  uncomplicated O80
  vaginal, following previous cesarean delivery
      O34.219
    classical (vertical) scar O34.212
    low transverse scar O34.211
Delusions (paranoid) —*see* Disorder, delusional
Dementia (degenerative (primary)) (old age)
    (persisting) F03.90
  with
    aggressive behavior F03.91
    behavioral disturbance F03.91
    combative behavior F03.91
    Lewy bodies G31.83 *[F02.80]*
      with behavioral disturbance G31.83
          [F02.81]
    Parkinson's disease G20 *[F02.80]*
      with behavioral disturbance G20
          [F02.81]

Dementia *(Continued)*
  with *(Continued)*
    Parkinsonism G31.83 *[F02.80]*
      with behavioral disturbance G31.83
          [F02.81]
    violent behavior F03.91
  alcoholic F10.97
    with dependence F10.27
  Alzheimer's type —*see* Disease, Alzheimer's
  arteriosclerotic —*see* Dementia, vascular
  atypical, Alzheimer's type —*see* Disease,
      Alzheimer's, specified NEC
  congenital —*see* Disability, intellectual
  frontal (lobe) G31.09 *[F02.80]*
    with behavioral disturbance G31.09
        [F02.81]
  frontotemporal G31.09 *[F02.80]*
    with behavioral disturbance G31.09 *[F02.81]*
    specified NEC G31.09 *[F02.80]*
      with behavioral disturbance G31.09
          [F02.81]
  in (due to)
    alcohol F10.97
      with dependence F10.27
    Alzheimer's disease —*see* Disease,
        Alzheimer's
    arteriosclerotic brain disease —*see*
        Dementia, vascular
    cerebral lipidoses E75.-● *[F02.80]*
      with behavioral disturbance
          E75.-● *[F02.81]*
    Creutzfeldt-Jakob disease —*see also*
        Creutzfeldt-Jakob disease or
        syndrome (with dementia) A81.00
    epilepsy G40.-● *[F02.80]*
      with behavioral disturbance
          G40.-● *[F02.81]*
    hepatolenticular degeneration E83.01
        [F02.80]
      with behavioral disturbance E83.01
          [F02.81]
    human immunodeficiency virus (HIV)
        disease B20 *[F02.80]*
      with behavioral disturbance B20 *[F02.81]*
    ⇒Huntington's disease or chorea G10 *[F02.80]*
      ▶with behavioral disturbance G10 *[F02.81]*
    hypercalcemia E83.52 *[F02.80]*
      with behavioral disturbance E83.52
          [F02.81]
    hypothyroidism, acquired E03.9 *[F02.80]*
      with behavioral disturbance E03.9
          [F02.81]
      due to iodine deficiency E01.8 *[F02.80]*
        with behavioral disturbance E01.8
            [F02.81]
    inhalants F18.97
      with dependence F18.27
    multiple
      etiologies F03
      sclerosis G35 *[F02.80]*
        with behavioral disturbance G35
            [F02.81]
    neurosyphilis A52.17 *[F02.80]*
      with behavioral disturbance A52.17
          [F02.81]
      juvenile A50.49 *[F02.80]*
        with behavioral disturbance A50.49
            [F02.81]
    niacin deficiency E52 *[F02.80]*
      with behavioral disturbance E52 *[F02.81]*
    paralysis agitans G20 *[F02.80]*
      with behavioral disturbance G20 *[F02.81]*
    Parkinson's disease G20 *[F02.80]*
    pellagra E52 *[F02.80]*
      with behavioral disturbance E52 *[F02.81]*
    Pick's G31.01 *[F02.80]*
      with behavioral disturbance G31.01
          [F02.81]
    polyarteritis nodosa M30.0 *[F02.80]*
      with behavioral disturbance M30.0
          [F02.81]

Dementia *(Continued)*
  in *(Continued)*
    psychoactive drug F19.97
      with dependence F19.27
      inhalants F18.97
        with dependence F18.27
      sedatives, hypnotics or anxiolytics
        F13.97
        with dependence F13.27
    sedatives, hypnotics or anxiolytics F13.97
      with dependence F13.27
    systemic lupus erythematosus
      M32.-● *[F02.80]*
      with behavioral disturbance
        M32.-● *[F02.81]*
    trypanosomiasis
      African B56.9 *[F02.80]*
        with behavioral disturbance B56.9
          [F02.81]
    unknown etiology F03
    vitamin B12 deficiency E53.8 *[F02.80]*
      with behavioral disturbance E53.8
        [F02.81]
    volatile solvents F18.97
      with dependence F18.27
  infantile, infantilis F84.3
  Lewy body G31.83 *[F02.80]*
    with behavioral disturbance G31.83
      [F02.81]
  multi-infarct —*see* Dementia, vascular
  paralytica, paralytic (syphilitic) A52.17
    [F02.80]
    with behavioral disturbance A52.17
      [F02.81]
    juvenilis A50.45
  paretic A52.17
  praecox —*see* Schizophrenia
  presenile F03
    Alzheimer's type —*see* Disease,
      Alzheimer's, early onset
  primary degenerative F03
  progressive, syphilitic A52.17
  senile F03
    with acute confusional state F05
    Alzheimer's type —*see* Disease,
      Alzheimer's, late onset
    depressed or paranoid type F03
  vascular (acute onset) (mixed) (multi-infarct)
    (subcortical) F01.50
    with behavioral disturbance F01.51
Demineralization, bone —*see* Osteoporosis
Demodex folliculorum (infestation) B88.0
Demophobia F40.248
Demoralization R45.3
Demyelination, demyelinization
  central nervous system G37.9
    specified NEC G37.8
  corpus callosum (central) G37.1
  disseminated, acute G36.9
    specified NEC G36.8
  global G35
  in optic neuritis G36.0
Dengue (classical) (fever) A90
  hemorrhagic A91
  sandfly A93.1
Dennie-Marfan syphilitic syndrome
  A50.45
Dens evaginatus, in dente or invaginatus
  K00.2
Dense breasts R92.2
Density
  increased, bone (disseminated) (generalized)
    (spotted) —*see* Disorder, bone, density
    and structure, specified type NEC
  lung (nodular) J98.4
Dental —*see also* condition
  examination Z01.20
    with abnormal findings Z01.21
  restoration
    aesthetically inadequate or displeasing
      K08.56

Dental *(Continued)*
  restoration *(Continued)*
    defective K08.50
      specified NEC K08.59
    failure of marginal integrity K08.51
    failure of periodontal anatomical integrity
      K08.54
Dentia praecox K00.6
Denticles (pulp) K04.2
Dentigerous cyst K09.0
Dentin
  irregular (in pulp) K04.3
  opalescent K00.5
  secondary (in pulp) K04.3
  sensitive K03.89
Dentinogenesis imperfecta K00.5
Dentinoma —*see* Cyst, calcifying odontogenic
Dentition (syndrome) K00.7
  delayed K00.6
  difficult K00.7
  precocious K00.6
  premature K00.6
  retarded K00.6
Dependence (on) (syndrome) F19.20
  with remission F19.21
  alcohol (ethyl) (methyl) (without remission)
    F10.20
    with
      amnestic disorder, persisting F10.26
      anxiety disorder F10.280
      dementia, persisting F10.27
      intoxication F10.229
        with delirium F10.221
        uncomplicated F10.220
      mood disorder F10.24
      psychotic disorder F10.259
        with
          delusions F10.250
          hallucinations F10.251
      remission F10.21
      sexual dysfunction F10.281
      sleep disorder F10.282
      specified disorder NEC F10.288
      withdrawal F10.239
        with
          delirium F10.231
          perceptual disturbance F10.232
        uncomplicated F10.230
    counseling and surveillance Z71.41
  amobarbital —*see* Dependence, drug,
    sedative
  amphetamine(s) (type) —*see* Dependence,
    drug, stimulant NEC
  amytal (sodium) —*see* Dependence, drug,
    sedative
  analgesic NEC F55.8
  anesthetic (agent) (gas) (general) (local)
    NEC —*see* Dependence, drug,
    psychoactive NEC
  anxiolytic NEC —*see* Dependence, drug,
    sedative
  barbital(s) —*see* Dependence, drug, sedative
  barbiturate(s) (compounds) (drugs
    classifiable to T42) —*see* Dependence,
    drug, sedative
  benzedrine —*see* Dependence, drug,
    stimulant NEC
  bhang —*see* Dependence, drug, cannabis
  bromide(s) NEC —*see* Dependence, drug,
    sedative
  caffeine —*see* Dependence, drug, stimulant
    NEC
  cannabis (sativa) (indica) (resin) (derivatives)
    (type) —*see* Dependence, drug, cannabis
  chloral (betaine) (hydrate) —*see* Dependence,
    drug, sedative
  chlordiazepoxide —*see* Dependence, drug,
    sedative
  coca (leaf) (derivatives) —*see* Dependence,
    drug, cocaine
  cocaine —*see* Dependence, drug, cocaine

Dependence *(Continued)*
  codeine —*see* Dependence, drug, opioid
  combinations of drugs F19.20
  dagga —*see* Dependence, drug, cannabis
  demerol —*see* Dependence, drug, opioid
  dexamphetamine —*see* Dependence, drug,
    stimulant NEC
  dexedrine —*see* Dependence, drug, stimulant
    NEC
  dextromethorphan —*see* Dependence, drug,
    opioid
  dextromoramide —*see* Dependence, drug,
    opioid
  dextro-nor-pseudo-ephedrine —*see*
    Dependence, drug, stimulant NEC
  dextrorphan —*see* Dependence, drug, opioid
  diazepam —*see* Dependence, drug, sedative
  dilaudid —*see* Dependence, drug, opioid
  D-lysergic acid diethylamide —*see*
    Dependence, drug, hallucinogen
  drug NEC F19.20
    with sleep disorder F19.282
    cannabis F12.20
      with
        anxiety disorder F12.280
        intoxication F12.229
          with
            delirium F12.221
            perceptual disturbance F12.222
          uncomplicated F12.220
        other specified disorder F12.288
        psychosis F12.259
          delusions F12.250
          hallucinations F12.251
        unspecified disorder F12.29
      in remission F12.21
    cocaine F14.20
      with
        anxiety disorder F14.280
        intoxication F14.229
          with
            delirium F14.221
            perceptual disturbance F14.222
          uncomplicated F14.220
        mood disorder F14.24
        other specified disorder F14.288
        psychosis F14.259
          delusions F14.250
          hallucinations F14.251
        sexual dysfunction F14.281
        sleep disorder F14.282
        unspecified disorder F14.29
        withdrawal F14.23
      in remission F14.21
      withdrawal symptoms in newborn P96.1
    counseling and surveillance Z71.51
    hallucinogen F16.20
      with
        anxiety disorder F16.280
        flashbacks F16.283
        intoxication F16.229
          with delirium F16.221
          uncomplicated F16.220
        mood disorder F16.24
        other specified disorder F16.288
        perception disorder, persisting F16.283
        psychosis F16.259
          delusions F16.250
          hallucinations F16.251
        unspecified disorder F16.29
      in remission F16.21
    in remission F19.21
    inhalant F18.20
      with
        anxiety disorder F18.280
        dementia, persisting F18.27
        intoxication F18.229
          with delirium F18.221
          uncomplicated F18.220
        mood disorder F18.24
        other specified disorder F18.288

Dependence *(Continued)*
  drug NEC *(Continued)*
    inhalant *(Continued)*
      with *(Continued)*
        psychosis F18.259
          delusions F18.250
          hallucinations F18.251
        unspecified disorder F18.29
      in remission F18.21
    nicotine F17.200
      with disorder F17.209
        ~~remission F17.201~~
        ▶in remission F17.201
        specified disorder NEC F17.208
        withdrawal F17.203
      chewing tobacco F17.220
        with disorder F17.229
          ~~remission F17.221~~
          ▶in remission F17.221
          specified disorder NEC F17.228
          withdrawal F17.223
      cigarettes F17.210
        with disorder F17.219
          ~~remission F17.211~~
          ▶in remission F17.211
          specified disorder NEC F17.218
          withdrawal F17.213
      specified product NEC F17.290
        with disorder F17.299
          remission F17.291
          specified disorder NEC F17.298
          withdrawal F17.293
    opioid F11.20
      with
        intoxication F11.229
          with
            delirium F11.221
            perceptual disturbance F11.222
          uncomplicated F11.220
        mood disorder F11.24
        other specified disorder F11.288
        psychosis F11.259
          delusions F11.250
          hallucinations F11.251
        sexual dysfunction F11.281
        sleep disorder F11.282
        unspecified disorder F11.29
        withdrawal F11.23
      in remission F11.21
    psychoactive NEC F19.20
      with
        amnestic disorder F19.26
        anxiety disorder F19.280
        dementia F19.27
        intoxication F19.229
          with
            delirium F19.221
            perceptual disturbance F19.222
          uncomplicated F19.220
        mood disorder F19.24
        other specified disorder F19.288
        psychosis F19.259
          delusions F19.250
          hallucinations F19.251
        sexual dysfunction F19.281
        sleep disorder F19.282
        unspecified disorder F19.29
        withdrawal F19.239
          with
            delirium F19.231
            perceptual disturbance F19.232
          uncomplicated F19.230
    sedative, hypnotic or anxiolytic F13.20
      with
        amnestic disorder F13.26
        anxiety disorder F13.280
        dementia, persisting F13.27
        intoxication F13.229
          with delirium F13.221
          uncomplicated F13.220
        mood disorder F13.24
        other specified disorder F13.288

Dependence *(Continued)*
  drug NEC *(Continued)*
    sedative, hypnotic or anxiolytic *(Continued)*
      with *(Continued)*
        psychosis F13.259
          delusions F13.250
          hallucinations F13.251
        sexual dysfunction F13.281
        sleep disorder F13.282
        unspecified disorder F13.29
        withdrawal F13.239
          with
            delirium F13.231
            perceptual disturbance F13.232
          uncomplicated F13.230
      in remission F13.21
    stimulant NEC F15.20
      with
        anxiety disorder F15.280
        intoxication F15.229
          with
            delirium F15.221
            perceptual disturbance F15.222
          uncomplicated F15.220
        mood disorder F15.24
        other specified disorder F15.288
        psychosis F15.259
          delusions F15.250
          hallucinations F15.251
        sexual dysfunction F15.281
        sleep disorder F15.282
        unspecified disorder F15.29
        withdrawal F15.23
      in remission F15.21
  ethyl
    alcohol (without remission) F10.20
      with remission F10.21
    bromide —*see* Dependence, drug, sedative
    carbamate F19.20
    chloride F19.20
    morphine —*see* Dependence, drug, opioid
  ganja —*see* Dependence, drug, cannabis
  glue (airplane) (sniffing) —*see* Dependence, drug, inhalant
  glutethimide —*see* Dependence, drug, sedative
  hallucinogenics —*see* Dependence, drug, hallucinogen
  hashish —*see* Dependence, drug, cannabis
  hemp —*see* Dependence, drug, cannabis
  heroin (salt) (any) —*see* Dependence, drug, opioid
  hypnotic NEC —*see* Dependence, drug, sedative
  Indian hemp —*see* Dependence, drug, cannabis
  inhalants —*see* Dependence, drug, inhalant
  khat —*see* Dependence, drug, stimulant NEC
  laudanum —*see* Dependence, drug, opioid
  LSD (-25) (derivatives) —*see* Dependence, drug, hallucinogen
  luminal —*see* Dependence, drug, sedative
  lysergic acid —*see* Dependence, drug, hallucinogen
  maconha —*see* Dependence, drug, cannabis
  marihuana —*see* Dependence, drug, cannabis
  meprobamate —*see* Dependence, drug, sedative
  mescaline —*see* Dependence, drug, hallucinogen
  methadone —*see* Dependence, drug, opioid
  methamphetamine(s) —*see* Dependence, drug, stimulant NEC
  methaqualone —*see* Dependence, drug, sedative
  methyl
    alcohol (without remission) F10.20
      with remission F10.21
    bromide —*see* Dependence, drug, sedative
    morphine —*see* Dependence, drug, opioid

Dependence *(Continued)*
  methyl *(Continued)*
    phenidate —*see* Dependence, drug, stimulant NEC
    sulfonal —*see* Dependence, drug, sedative
  morphine (sulfate) (sulfite) (type) —*see* Dependence, drug, opioid
  narcotic (drug) NEC —*see* Dependence, drug, opioid
  nembutal —*see* Dependence, drug, sedative
  neraval —*see* Dependence, drug, sedative
  neravan —*see* Dependence, drug, sedative
  neurobarb —*see* Dependence, drug, sedative
  nicotine —*see* Dependence, drug, nicotine
  nitrous oxide F19.20
  nonbarbiturate sedatives and tranquilizers with similar effect —*see* Dependence, drug, sedative
  on
    artificial heart (fully implantable) (mechanical) Z95.812
    aspirator Z99.0
    care provider (because of) Z74.9
      impaired mobility Z74.09
      need for
        assistance with personal care Z74.1
        continuous supervision Z74.3
      no other household member able to render care Z74.2
      specified reason NEC Z74.8
    machine Z99.89
      enabling NEC Z99.89
      specified type NEC Z99.89
    renal dialysis (hemodialysis) (peritoneal) Z99.2
    respirator Z99.11
    ventilator Z99.11
    wheelchair Z99.3
  opiate —*see* Dependence, drug, opioid
  opioids —*see* Dependence, drug, opioid
  opium (alkaloids) (derivatives) (tincture) —*see* Dependence, drug, opioid
  oxygen (long-term) (supplemental) Z99.81
  paraldehyde —*see* Dependence, drug, sedative
  paregoric —*see* Dependence, drug, opioid
  PCP (phencyclidine) (or related substance) —*see* Dependence, drug, hallucinogen
  pentobarbital —*see* Dependence, drug, sedative
  pentobarbitone (sodium) —*see* Dependence, drug, sedative
  pentothal —*see* Dependence, drug, sedative
  peyote —*see* Dependence, drug, hallucinogen
  phencyclidine (PCP) (or related substance) —*see* Dependence, drug, hallucinogen
  phenmetrazine —*see* Dependence, drug, stimulant NEC
  phenobarbital —*see* Dependence, drug, sedative
  polysubstance F19.20
  psilocibin, psilocin, psilocyn, psilocyline —*see* Dependence, drug, hallucinogen
  psychostimulant NEC —*see* Dependence, drug, stimulant NEC
  secobarbital —*see* Dependence, drug, sedative
  seconal —*see* Dependence, drug, sedative
  sedative NEC —*see* Dependence, drug, sedative
  specified drug NEC —*see* Dependence, drug
  stimulant NEC —*see* Dependence, drug, stimulant NEC
  substance NEC —*see* Dependence, drug
  supplemental oxygen Z99.81
  tobacco —*see* Dependence, drug, nicotine
    counseling and surveillance Z71.6
  tranquilizer NEC —*see* Dependence, drug, sedative
  vitamin B6 E53.1
  volatile solvents —*see* Dependence, drug, inhalant

Dependency
  care-provider Z74.9
  passive F60.7
  reactions (persistent) F60.7
Depersonalization (in neurotic state) (neurotic)
    (syndrome) F48.1
Depletion
  extracellular fluid E86.9
  plasma E86.1
  potassium E87.6
    nephropathy N25.89
  salt or sodium E87.1
    causing heat exhaustion or prostration T67.4
    nephropathy N28.9
  volume NOS E86.9
Deployment (current) (military) status Z56.82
  in theater or in support of military war,
      peacekeeping and humanitarian
      operations Z56.82
  personal history of Z91.82
    military war, peacekeeping and
        humanitarian deployment (current or
        past conflict) Z91.82
  returned from Z91.82
Depolarization, premature I49.40
  atrial I49.1
  junctional I49.2
  specified NEC I49.49
  ventricular I49.3
Deposit
  bone in Boeck's sarcoid D86.89
  calcareous, calcium —see Calcification
  cholesterol
    retina H35.89
    vitreous (body) (humor) —see Deposit,
        crystalline
  conjunctiva H11.11-●
  cornea H18.00-●
    argentous H18.02-●
    due to metabolic disorder H18.03-●
    Kayser-Fleischer ring H18.04-●
    pigmentation —see Pigmentation, cornea
  crystalline, vitreous (body) (humor) H43.2-●
  hemosiderin in old scars of cornea —see
      Pigmentation, cornea, stromal
  metallic in lens —see Cataract, specified NEC
  skin R23.8
  tooth, teeth (betel) (black) (green) (materia
      alba) (orange) (tobacco) K03.6
  urate, kidney —see Calculus, kidney
Depraved appetite —see Pica
Depressed
  HDL cholesterol E78.6
Depression (acute) (mental) F32.9
  agitated (single episode) F32.2
  anaclitic —see Disorder, adjustment
  anxiety F41.8
    persistent F34.1
  arches —see also Deformity, limb, flat foot
  atypical (single episode) F32.89
    recurrent episode F33.8
  basal metabolic rate R94.8
  bone marrow D75.89
  central nervous system R09.2
  cerebral R29.818
    newborn P91.4
  cerebrovascular I67.9
  chest wall M95.4
  climacteric (single episode) F32.89
    recurrent episode F33.8
  endogenous (without psychotic symptoms)
      F33.2
    with psychotic symptoms F33.3
  functional activity R68.89
  hysterical F44.89
  involutional (single episode) F32.89
    recurrent episode F33.8
  major F32.9
    with psychotic symptoms F32.3
    recurrent —see Disorder, depressive,
        recurrent

Depression (Continued)
  manic-depressive —see Disorder, depressive,
      recurrent
  masked (single episode) F32.89
  medullary G93.89
  menopausal (single episode) F32.89
    recurrent episode F33.8
  metatarsus —see Depression, arches
  monopolar F33.9
  nervous F34.1
  neurotic F34.1
  nose M95.0
  postnatal F53
  postpartum F53
  post-psychotic of schizophrenia F32.89
  post-schizophrenic F32.89
  psychogenic (reactive) (single episode) F32.9
  psychoneurotic F34.1
  psychotic (single episode) F32.3
    recurrent F33.3
  reactive (psychogenic) (single episode) F32.9
    psychotic (single episode) F32.3
  recurrent —see Disorder, depressive,
      recurrent
  respiratory center G93.89
  seasonal —see Disorder, depressive, recurrent
  senile F03
  severe, single episode F32.2
  situational F43.21
  skull Q67.4
  specified NEC (single episode) F32.89
  sternum M95.4
  visual field —see Defect, visual field
  vital (recurrent) (without psychotic
      symptoms) F33.2
    with psychotic symptoms F33.3
    single episode F32.2
Deprivation
  cultural Z60.3
  effects NOS T73.9
    specified NEC T73.8
  emotional NEC Z65.8
    affecting infant or child —see
        Maltreatment, child, psychological
  food T73.0
  protein —see Malnutrition
  sleep Z72.820
  social Z60.4
    affecting infant or child —see
        Maltreatment, child, psychological
  specified NEC T73.8
  vitamins —see Deficiency, vitamin
  water T73.1
Derangement
  ankle (internal) —see Derangement, joint,
      ankle
  cartilage (articular) NEC —see Derangement,
      joint, articular cartilage, by site
    recurrent —see Dislocation, recurrent
  cruciate ligament, anterior, current injury —
      see Sprain, knee, cruciate, anterior
  elbow (internal) —see Derangement, joint,
      elbow
  hip (joint) (internal) (old) —see Derangement,
      joint, hip
  joint (internal) M24.9
    ankylosis —see Ankylosis
    articular cartilage M24.10
      ankle M24.17-●
      elbow M24.12-●
      foot M24.17-●
      hand M24.14-●
      hip M24.15-●
      knee NEC M23.9-●
      loose body —see Loose, body
      shoulder M24.11-●
      wrist M24.13-●
    contracture —see Contraction, joint
    current injury —see also Dislocation
      knee, meniscus or cartilage —see Tear,
          meniscus

Derangement (Continued)
  joint (Continued)
    dislocation
      pathological —see Dislocation,
          pathological
      recurrent —see Dislocation, recurrent
    knee —see Derangement, knee
    ligament —see Disorder, ligament
    loose body —see Loose, body
    recurrent —see Dislocation, recurrent
    specified type NEC M24.80
      ankle M24.87-●
      elbow M24.82-●
      foot joint M24.87-●
      hand joint M24.84-●
      hip M24.85-●
      shoulder M24.81-●
      wrist M24.83-●
    temporomandibular M26.69
  knee (recurrent) M23.9-●
    ligament disruption, spontaneous
        M23.60-●
      anterior cruciate M23.61-●
      capsular M23.67-●
      instability, chronic M23.5-●
      lateral collateral M23.64-●
      medial collateral M23.63-●
      posterior cruciate M23.62-●
    loose body M23.4-●
    meniscus M23.30-●
      cystic M23.00-●
        lateral M23.002
          anterior horn M23.04-●
          posterior horn M23.05-●
          specified NEC M23.06-●
        medial M23.005
          anterior horn M23.01-●
          posterior horn M23.02-●
          specified NEC M23.03-●
      degenerate —see Derangement, knee,
          meniscus, specified NEC
      detached —see Derangement, knee,
          meniscus, specified NEC
      due to old tear or injury M23.20-●
        lateral M23.20-●
          anterior horn M23.24-●
          posterior horn M23.25-●
          specified NEC M23.26-●
        medial M23.20-●
          anterior horn M23.21-●
          posterior horn M23.22-●
          specified NEC M23.23-●
      retained —see Derangement, knee,
          meniscus, specified NEC
      specified NEC M23.30-●
        lateral M23.30-●
          anterior horn M23.34-●
          posterior horn M23.35-●
          specified NEC M23.36-●
        medial M23.30-●
          anterior horn M23.31-●
          posterior horn M23.32-●
          specified NEC M23.33-●
    old M23.8X-●
    specified NEC —see subcategory M23.8
  low back NEC —see Dorsopathy, specified
      NEC
  meniscus —see Derangement, knee,
      meniscus
  mental —see Psychosis
  patella, specified NEC —see Disorder,
      patella, derangement NEC
  semilunar cartilage (knee) —see
      Derangement, knee, meniscus,
      specified NEC
  shoulder (internal) —see Derangement,
      joint, shoulder
Dercum's disease E88.2
Derealization (neurotic) F48.1
Dermal —see condition
Dermaphytid —see Dermatophytosis

Dermatitis (eczematous) L30.9
  ab igne L59.0
  acarine B88.0
  actinic (due to sun) L57.8
    other than from sun L59.8
  allergic —see Dermatitis, contact, allergic
  ambustionis, due to burn or scald —see Burn
  amebic A06.7
  ammonia L22
  arsenical (ingested) L27.8
  artefacta L98.1
    psychogenic F54
  atopic L20.9
    psychogenic F54
    specified NEC L20.89
  autoimmune progesterone L30.8
  berlock, berloque L56.2
  blastomycotic B40.3
  blister beetle L24.89
  bullous, bullosa L13.9
    mucosynechial, atrophic L12.1
    seasonal L30.8
    specified NEC L13.8
  calorica L59.0
    due to burn or scald —see Burn
  caterpillar L24.89
  cercarial B65.3
  combustionis L59.0
    due to burn or scald —see Burn
  congelationis T69.1
  contact (occupational) L25.9
    allergic L23.9
      due to
        adhesives L23.1
        cement L23.5
        chemical products NEC L23.5
        chromium L23.0
        cosmetics L23.2
        dander (cat) (dog) L23.81
        drugs in contact with skin L23.3
        dyes L23.4
        food in contact with skin L23.6
        hair (cat) (dog) L23.81
        insecticide L23.5
        metals L23.0
        nickel L23.0
        plants, non-food L23.7
        plastic L23.5
        rubber L23.5
        specified agent NEC L23.89
    due to
      cement L25.3
      chemical products NEC L25.3
      cosmetics L25.0
      dander (cat) (dog) L23.81
      drugs in contact with skin L25.1
      dyes L25.2
      food in contact with skin L25.4
      hair (cat) (dog) L23.81
      plants, non-food L25.5
      specified agent NEC L25.8
    irritant L24.9
      due to
        cement L24.5
        chemical products NEC L24.5
        cosmetics L24.3
        detergents L24.0
        drugs in contact with skin L24.4
        food in contact with skin L24.6
        oils and greases L24.1
        plants, non-food L24.7
        solvents L24.2
        specified agent NEC L24.89
  contusiformis L52
  diabetic —see E08-E13 with .620
  diaper L22
  diphtheritica A36.3
  dry skin L85.3
  due to
    acetone (contact) (irritant) L24.2
    acids (contact) (irritant) L24.5

Dermatitis (Continued)
  due to (Continued)
    adhesive(s) (allergic) (contact) (plaster)
        L23.1
      irritant L24.5
    alcohol (irritant) (skin contact) (substances
        in category T51) L24.2
      taken internally L27.8
    alkalis (contact) (irritant) L24.5
    arsenic (ingested) L27.8
    carbon disulfide (contact) (irritant) L24.2
    caustics (contact) (irritant) L24.5
    cement (contact) L25.3
    cereal (ingested) L27.2
    chemical(s) NEC L25.3
      taken internally L27.8
    chlorocompounds L24.2
    chromium (contact) (irritant) L24.81
    coffee (ingested) L27.2
    cold weather L30.8
    cosmetics (contact) L25.0
      allergic L23.2
      irritant L24.3
    cyclohexanes L24.2
    dander (cat) (dog) L23.81
    Demodex species B88.0
    Dermanyssus gallinae B88.0
    detergents (contact) (irritant) L24.0
    dichromate L24.81
    drugs and medicaments (generalized)
        (internal use) L27.0
      external —see Dermatitis, due to, drugs,
          in contact with skin
      in contact with skin L25.1
        allergic L23.3
        irritant L24.4
      localized skin eruption L27.1
      specified substance —see Table of Drugs
          and Chemicals
    dyes (contact) L25.2
      allergic L23.4
      irritant L24.89
    epidermophytosis —see Dermatophytosis
    esters L24.2
    external irritant NEC L24.9
    fish (ingested) L27.2
    flour (ingested) L27.2
    food (ingested) L27.2
      in contact with skin L25.4
    fruit (ingested) L27.2
    furs (allergic) (contact) L23.81
    glues —see Dermatitis, due to, adhesives
    glycols L24.2
    greases NEC (contact) (irritant) L24.1
    hair (cat) (dog) L23.81
    hot
      objects and materials —see Burn
      weather or places L59.0
    hydrocarbons L24.2
    infrared rays L59.8
    ingestion, ingested substance L27.9
      chemical NEC L27.8
      drugs and medicaments —see
          Dermatitis, due to, drugs
      food L27.2
      specified NEC L27.8
    insecticide in contact with skin L24.5
    internal agent L27.9
      drugs and medicaments (generalized) —
          see Dermatitis, due to, drugs
      food L27.2
    irradiation —see Dermatitis, due to,
        radioactive substance
    ketones L24.2
    lacquer tree (allergic) (contact) L23.7
    light (sun) NEC L57.8
      acute L56.8
      other L59.8
    Liponyssoides sanguineus B88.0
    low temperature L30.8
    meat (ingested) L27.2

Dermatitis (Continued)
  due to (Continued)
    metals, metal salts (contact) (irritant)
        L24.81
    milk (ingested) L27.2
    nickel (contact) (irritant) L24.81
    nylon (contact) (irritant) L24.5
    oils NEC (contact) (irritant) L24.1
    paint solvent (contact) (irritant) L24.2
    petroleum products (contact) (irritant)
        (substances in T52) L24.2
    plants NEC (contact) L25.5
      allergic L23.7
      irritant L24.7
    plasters (adhesive) (any) (allergic) (contact)
        L23.1
      irritant L24.5
    plastic (contact) L25.3
    preservatives (contact) —see Dermatitis,
        due to, chemical, in contact with
        skin
    primrose (allergic) (contact) L23.7
    primula (allergic) (contact) L23.7
    radiation L59.8
      nonionizing (chronic exposure) L57.8
      sun NEC L57.8
        acute L56.8
    radioactive substance L58.9
      acute L58.0
      chronic L58.1
    radium L58.9
      acute L58.0
      chronic L58.1
    ragweed (allergic) (contact) L23.7
    Rhus (allergic) (contact) (diversiloba)
        (radicans) (toxicodendron) (venenata)
        (verniciflua) L23.7
    rubber (contact) L24.5
    Senecio jacobaea (allergic) (contact)
        L23.7
    solvents (contact) (irritant) (substances in
        categories T52) L24.2
    specified agent NEC (contact) L25.8
      allergic L23.89
      irritant L24.89
    sunshine NEC L57.8
      acute L56.8
    tetrachlorethylene (contact) (irritant)
        L24.2
    toluene (contact) (irritant) L24.2
    turpentine (contact) L24.2
    ultraviolet rays (sun NEC) (chronic
        exposure) L57.8
      acute L56.8
    vaccine or vaccination L27.0
      specified substance —see Table of Drugs
          and Chemicals
    varicose veins —see Varix, leg, with,
        inflammation
    X-rays L58.9
      acute L58.0
      chronic L58.1
  dyshydrotic L30.1
  dysmenorrheica N94.6
  escharotica —see Burn
  exfoliative, exfoliativa (generalized) L26
    neonatorum L00
  eyelid —see also Dermatosis, eyelid
    allergic H01.119
      left H01.116
        lower H01.115
        upper H01.114
      right H01.113
        lower H01.112
        upper H01.111
    contact —see Dermatitis, eyelid,
        allergic
    due to
      Demodex species B88.0
      herpes (zoster) B02.39
        simplex B00.59

▶ New   ⇒ Revised   ~~deleted~~ Deleted   ● Use Additional Character(s)

Dermatitis (Continued)
eyelid (Continued)
eczematous H01.139
left H01.136
lower H01.135
upper H01.134
right H01.133
lower H01.132
upper H01.131
facta, factitia, factitial L98.1
psychogenic F54
flexural NEC L20.82
friction L30.4
fungus B36.9
specified type NEC B36.8
gangrenosa, gangrenous infantum L08.0
harvest mite B88.0
heat L59.0
herpesviral, vesicular (ear) (lip) B00.1
herpetiformis (bullous) (erythematous)
(pustular) (vesicular) L13.0
juvenile L12.2
senile L12.0
hiemalis L30.8
hypostatic, hypostatica —see Varix, leg, with,
inflammation
infectious eczematoid L30.3
infective L30.3
irritant —see Dermatitis, contact, irritant
Jacquet's (diaper dermatitis) L22
Leptus B88.0
lichenified NEC L28.0
medicamentosa (generalized) (internal
use) —see Dermatitis, due to drugs
mite B88.0
multiformis L13.0
juvenile L12.2
napkin L22
neurotica L13.0
nummular L30.0
papillaris capillitii L73.0
pellagrous E52
perioral L71.0
photocontact L56.2
polymorpha dolorosa L13.0
pruriginosa L13.0
pruritic NEC L30.8
psychogenic F54
purulent L08.0
pustular
contagious B08.02
subcorneal L13.1
pyococcal L08.0
pyogenica L08.0
repens L40.2
Ritter's (exfoliativa) L00
Schamberg's L81.7
schistosome B65.3
seasonal bullous L30.8
seborrheic L21.9
infantile L21.1
specified NEC L21.8
sensitization NOS L23.9
septic L08.0
solare L57.8
specified NEC L30.8
stasis I87.2
with
varicose ulcer —see Varix, leg, with ulcer,
with inflammation
varicose veins —see Varix, leg, with,
inflammation
due to postthrombotic syndrome —see
Syndrome, postthrombotic
suppurative L08.0
traumatic NEC L30.4
trophoneurotica L13.0
ultraviolet (sun) (chronic exposure) L57.8
acute L56.8
varicose —see Varix, leg, with, inflammation
vegetans L10.1

Dermatitis (Continued)
verrucosa B43.0
vesicular, herpesviral B00.1
Dermatoarthritis, lipoid E78.81
Dermatochalasis, eyelid H02.839
left H02.836
lower H02.835
upper H02.834
right H02.833
lower H02.832
upper H02.831
Dermatofibroma (lenticulare) —see Neoplasm,
skin, benign
protuberans —see Neoplasm, skin, uncertain
behavior
Dermatofibrosarcoma (pigmented)
(protuberans) —see Neoplasm, skin,
malignant
Dermatographia L50.3
Dermatolysis (exfoliativa) (congenital) Q82.8
acquired L57.4
eyelids —see Blepharochalasis
palpebrarum —see Blepharochalasis
senile L57.4
Dermatomegaly NEC Q82.8
Dermatomucosomyositis M33.10
with
myopathy M33.12
respiratory involvement M33.11
specified organ involvement NEC M33.19
Dermatomycosis B36.9
furfuracea B36.0
specified type NEC B36.8
Dermatomyositis (acute) (chronic) —see also
Dermatopolymyositis
▶adult —see also Dermatomyositis, specified
NEC M33.10
in (due to) neoplastic disease —see also
Neoplasm D49.9 [M36.0]
▶juvenile M33.00
▶with
▶myopathy M33.02
▶respiratory involvement M33.01
▶specified organ involvement NEC
M33.09
▶without myopathy M33.03
▶specified NEC M33.10
▶with
▶myopathy M33.12
▶respiratory involvement M33.11
▶specified organ involvement NEC M33.19
▶without myopathy M33.13
Dermatoneuritis of children —see Poisoning,
mercury
Dermatophilosis A48.8
Dermatophytid L30.2
Dermatophytide —see Dermatophytosis
Dermatophytosis (epidermophyton) (infection)
(Microsporum) (tinea) (Trichophyton)
B35.9
beard B35.0
body B35.4
capitis B35.0
corporis B35.4
deep-seated B35.8
disseminated B35.8
foot B35.3
granulomatous B35.8
groin B35.6
hand B35.2
nail B35.1
perianal (area) B35.6
scalp B35.0
specified NEC B35.8
Dermatopolymyositis M33.90
with
myopathy M33.92
respiratory involvement M33.91
specified organ involvement NEC M33.99
in neoplastic disease (see also Neoplasm)
D49.9 [M36.0]

Dermatopolymyositis (Continued)
juvenile M33.00
with
myopathy M33.02
respiratory involvement M33.01
specified organ involvement NEC M33.09
specified NEC M33.10
myopathy M33.12
respiratory involvement M33.11
specified organ involvement NEC M33.19
▶without myopathy M33.93
Dermatopolyneuritis —see Poisoning, mercury
Dermatorrhexis Q79.6
acquired L57.4
Dermatosclerosis —see also Scleroderma
localized L94.0
Dermatosis L98.9
Andrews' L08.89
Bowen's —see Neoplasm, skin, in situ
bullous L13.9
specified NEC L13.8
exfoliativa L26
eyelid (noninfectious)
dermatitis —see Dermatitis, eyelid
discoid lupus erythematosus —see Lupus,
erythematosus, eyelid
xeroderma —see Xeroderma, acquired,
eyelid
factitial L98.1
febrile neutrophilic L98.2
gonococcal A54.89
herpetiformis L13.0
juvenile L12.2
linear IgA L13.8
menstrual NEC L98.8
neutrophilic, febrile L98.2
occupational —see Dermatitis, contact
papulosa nigra L82.1
pigmentary L81.9
progressive L81.7
Schamberg's L81.7
psychogenic F54
purpuric, pigmented L81.7
pustular, subcorneal L13.1
transient acantholytic L11.1
Dermographia, dermographism L50.3
Dermoid (cyst) —see also Neoplasm, benign,
by site
with malignant transformation C56-●
due to radiation (nonionizing) L57.8
Dermopathy
infiltrative with thyrotoxicosis —see
Thyrotoxicosis
nephrogenic fibrosing L90.8
Dermophytosis —see Dermatophytosis
Descemetocele H18.73-●
Descemet's membrane —see condition
Descending —see condition
Descensus uteri —see Prolapse, uterus
Desert
rheumatism B38.0
sore —see Ulcer, skin
Desertion (newborn) —see Maltreatment
Desmoid (extra-abdominal) (tumor) —see
Neoplasm, connective tissue, uncertain
behavior
abdominal D48.1
Despondency F32.9
Desquamation, skin R23.4
Destruction, destructive —see also Damage
articular facet —see also Derangement, joint,
specified type NEC
knee M23.8X-●
vertebra —see Spondylosis
bone —see also Disorder, bone, specified type
NEC
syphilitic A52.77
joint —see also Derangement, joint, specified
type NEC
sacroiliac M53.3
rectal sphincter K62.89

Destruction, destructive *(Continued)*
  septum (nasal) J34.89
  tuberculous NEC —*see* Tuberculosis
  tympanum, tympanic membrane
    (nontraumatic) —*see* Disorder, tympanic
    membrane, specified NEC
  vertebral disc —*see* Degeneration,
    intervertebral disc
Destructiveness —*see also* Disorder, conduct
  adjustment reaction —*see* Disorder,
    adjustment
Desultory labor O62.2
Detachment
  cartilage —*see* Sprain
  cervix, annular N88.8
    complicating delivery O71.3
  choroid (old) (postinfectional) (simple)
    (spontaneous) H31.40-•
    hemorrhagic H31.41-•
    serous H31.42-•
  ligament —*see* Sprain
  meniscus (knee) —*see also* Derangement,
    knee, meniscus, specified NEC
    current injury —*see* Tear, meniscus
    due to old tear or injury —*see*
      Derangement, knee, meniscus, due to
      old tear
  retina (without retinal break) (serous)
    H33.2-•
    with retinal:
      break H33.00-•
        giant H33.03-•
        multiple H33.02-•
        single H33.01-•
      dialysis H33.04-•
    pigment epithelium —*see* Degeneration,
      retina, separation of layers, pigment
      epithelium detachment
    rhegmatogenous —*see* Detachment, retina,
      with retinal, break
    specified NEC H33.8
    total H33.05-•
    traction H33.4-•
  vitreous (body) H43.81
Detergent asthma J69.8
Deterioration
  epileptic F06.8
  general physical R53.81
  heart, cardiac —*see* Degeneration,
    myocardial
  mental —*see* Psychosis
  myocardial, myocardium —*see* Degeneration,
    myocardial
  senile (simple) R54
Deuteranomaly (anomalous trichromat) H53.53
Deuteranopia (complete) (incomplete) H53.53
Development
  abnormal, bone Q79.9
  arrested R62.50
    bone —*see* Arrest, development or growth,
      bone
    child R62.50
    due to malnutrition E45
  defective, congenital —*see also* Anomaly, by
    site
    cauda equina Q06.3
    left ventricle Q24.8
      in hypoplastic left heart syndrome Q23.4
    valve Q24.8
    pulmonary Q22.3
  delayed *(see also* Delay, development) R62.50
    arithmetical skills F81.2
    language (skills) (expressive) F80.1
    learning skill F81.9
    mixed skills F88
    motor coordination F82
    reading F81.0
    specified learning skill NEC F81.89
    speech F80.9
    spelling F81.81
    written expression F81.81

Development *(Continued)*
  imperfect, congenital —*see also* Anomaly, by
    site
    heart Q24.9
    lungs Q33.6
  incomplete
    bronchial tree Q32.4
    organ or site not listed —*see* Hypoplasia,
      by site
    respiratory system Q34.9
  sexual, precocious NEC E30.1
  tardy, mental *(see also* Disability, intellectual)
    F79
Developmental —*see* condition
  testing, infant or child —*see* Examination,
    child
Devergie's disease (pityriasis rubra pilaris)
  L44.0
Deviation (in)
  conjugate palsy (eye) (spastic) H51.0
  esophagus (acquired) K22.8
  eye, skew H51.8
  midline (jaw) (teeth) (dental arch) M26.29
    specified site NEC —*see* Malposition
  nasal septum J34.2
    congenital Q67.4
  opening and closing of the mandible M26.53
  organ or site, congenital NEC —*see*
    Malposition, congenital
  septum (nasal) (acquired) J34.2
    congenital Q67.4
  sexual F65.9
    bestiality F65.89
    erotomania F52.8
    exhibitionism F65.2
    fetishism, fetishistic F65.0
      transvestism F65.1
    frotteurism F65.81
    masochism F65.51
    multiple F65.89
    necrophilia F65.89
    nymphomania F52.8
    pederosis F65.4
    pedophilia F65.4
    sadism, sadomasochism F65.52
    satyriasis F52.8
    specified type NEC F65.89
    transvestism F64.1
    voyeurism F65.3
  teeth, midline M26.29
  trachea J39.8
  ureter, congenital Q62.61
Device
  cerebral ventricle (communicating) in situ
    Z98.2
  contraceptive —*see* Contraceptive, device
  drainage, cerebrospinal fluid, in situ Z98.2
Devic's disease G36.0
Devil's
  grip B33.0
  pinches (purpura simplex) D69.2
Devitalized tooth K04.99
Devonshire colic —*see* Poisoning, lead
Dextraposition, aorta Q20.3
  in tetralogy of Fallot Q21.3
Dextrinosis, limit (debrancher enzyme
  deficiency) E74.03
Dextrocardia (true) Q24.0
  with
    complete transposition of viscera Q89.3
    situs inversus Q89.3
Dextrotransposition, aorta Q20.3
d-glycericacidemia E72.59
Dhat syndrome F48.8
Dhobi itch B35.6
Di George's syndrome D82.1
Di Guglielmo's disease C94.0-•
Diabetes, diabetic (mellitus) (sugar) E11.9
  with
    amyotrophy E11.44
    arthropathy NEC E11.618

Diabetes, diabetic *(Continued)*
  with *(Continued)*
    autonomic (poly)neuropathy E11.43
    cataract E11.36
    Charcot's joints E11.610
    chronic kidney disease E11.22
    circulatory complication NEC E11.59
    complication E11.8
      specified NEC E11.69
    dermatitis E11.620
    foot ulcer E11.621
    gangrene E11.52
    gastroparalysis E11.43
    gastroparesis E11.43
    glomerulonephrosis, intracapillary E11.21
    glomerulosclerosis, intercapillary E11.21
    hyperglycemia E11.65
    hyperosmolarity E11.00
      with coma E11.01
    hypoglycemia E11.649
      with coma E11.641
  ▶ketoacidosis E11.10
    ▶with coma E11.11
    kidney complications NEC E11.29
    Kimmelstiel-Wilson disease E11.21
    loss of protective sensation (LOPS) —*see*
      Diabetes, by type, with neuropathy
    mononeuropathy E11.41
    myasthenia E11.44
    necrobiosis lipoidica E11.620
    nephropathy E11.21
    neuralgia E11.42
    neurologic complication NEC E11.49
    neuropathic arthropathy E11.610
    neuropathy E11.40
    ophthalmic complication NEC E11.39
    oral complication NEC E11.638
    osteomyelitis E11.69
    periodontal disease E11.630
    peripheral angiopathy E11.51
      with gangrene E11.52
    polyneuropathy E11.42
    renal complication NEC E11.29
    renal tubular degeneration E11.29
    retinopathy E11.319
      with macular edema E11.311
        resolved following treatment
          E11.37
      nonproliferative E11.329
        with macular edema E11.321
        mild E11.329
          with macular edema E11.321
        moderate E11.339
          with macular edema E11.331
        severe E11.349
          with macular edema E11.341
      proliferative E11.359
        with
          combined traction retinal
            detachment and
            rhegmatogenous retinal
            detachment E11.354
          macular edema E11.351
          stable proliferative diabetic
            retinopathy E11.355
          traction retinal detachment
            involving the macula E11.352
          traction retinal detachment not
            involving the macula E11.353
    skin complication NEC E11.628
    skin ulcer NEC E11.622
  brittle —*see* Diabetes, type 1
  bronzed E83.110
  complicating pregnancy —*see* Pregnancy,
    complicated by, diabetes
  dietary counseling and surveillance Z71.3
  due to
    autoimmune process —*see* Diabetes, type 1
    immune mediated pancreatic islet
      beta-cell destruction —*see* Diabetes,
        type 1

▶ New   ⮕ Revised   ~~deleted~~ Deleted   • Use Additional Character(s)

Diabetes, diabetic *(Continued)*
  due to drug or chemical E09.9
    with
      amyotrophy E09.44
      arthropathy NEC E09.618
      autonomic (poly)neuropathy E09.43
      cataract E09.36
      Charcot's joints E09.610
      chronic kidney disease E09.22
      circulatory complication NEC E09.59
      complication E09.8
        specified NEC E09.69
      dermatitis E09.620
      foot ulcer E09.621
      gangrene E09.52
      gastroparalysis E09.43
      gastroparesis E09.43
      glomerulonephrosis, intracapillary E09.21
      glomerulosclerosis, intercapillary E09.21
      hyperglycemia E09.65
      hyperosmolarity E09.00
        with coma E09.01
      hypoglycemia E09.649
        with coma E09.641
      ketoacidosis E09.10
        with coma E09.11
      kidney complications NEC E09.29
      Kimmelstein-Wilson disease E09.21
      mononeuropathy E09.41
      myasthenia E09.44
      necrobiosis lipoidica E09.620
      nephropathy E09.21
      neuralgia E09.42
      neurologic complication NEC E09.49
      neuropathic arthropathy E09.610
      neuropathy E09.40
      ophthalmic complication NEC E09.39
      oral complication NEC E09.638
      periodontal disease E09.630
      peripheral angiopathy E09.51
        with gangrene E09.52
      polyneuropathy E09.42
      renal complication NEC E09.29
      renal tubular degeneration E09.29
      retinopathy E09.319
        with macular edema E09.311
          resolved following treatment E09.37
        nonproliferative E09.329
          with macular edema E09.321
          mild E09.329
            with macular edema E09.321
          moderate E09.339
            with macular edema E09.331
          severe E09.349
            with macular edema E09.341
        proliferative E09.359
          with
            combined traction retinal detachment and rhegmatogenous retinal detachment E09.354
            macular edema E09.351
            stable proliferative diabetic retinopathy E09.355
            traction retinal detachment involving the macula E09.352
            traction retinal detachment not involving the macula E09.353
      skin complication NEC E09.628
      skin ulcer NEC E09.622
  due to underlying condition E08.9
    with
      amyotrophy E08.44
      arthropathy NEC E08.618
      autonomic (poly)neuropathy E08.43
      cataract E08.36
      Charcot's joints E08.610

Diabetes, diabetic *(Continued)*
  due to underlying condition *(Continued)*
    with *(Continued)*
      chronic kidney disease E08.22
      circulatory complication NEC E08.59
      complication E08.8
        specified NEC E08.69
      dermatitis E08.620
      foot ulcer E08.621
      gangrene E08.52
      gastroparalysis E08.43
      gastroparesis E08.43
      glomerulonephrosis, intracapillary E08.21
      glomerulosclerosis, intercapillary E08.21
      hyperglycemia E08.69
      hyperosmolarity E08.00
        with coma E08.01
      hypoglycemia E08.649
        with coma E08.641
      ketoacidosis E08.10
        with coma E08.11
      kidney complications NEC E08.29
      Kimmelsteil-WIlson disease E08.21
      mononeuropathy E08.41
      myasthenia E08.44
      necrobiosis lipoidica E08.620
      nephropathy E08.21
      neuralgia E08.42
      neurologic complication NEC E08.49
      neuropathic arthropathy E08.610
      neuropathy E08.40
      ophthalmic complication NEC E08.39
      oral complication NEC E08.638
      periodontal disease E08.630
      peripheral angiopathy E08.51
        with gangrene E08.52
      polyneuropathy E08.42
      renal complication NEC E08.29
      renal tubular degeneration E08.29
      retinopathy E08.319
        with macular edema E08.311
          resolved following treatment E08.37
        nonproliferative E08.329
          with macular edema E08.321
          mild E08.329
            with macular edema E08.321
          moderate E08.339
            with macular edema E08.331
          severe E08.349
            with macular edema E08.341
        proliferative E08.359
          with
            combined traction retinal detachment and rhegmatogenous retinal detachment E08.354
            macular edema E08.351
            stable proliferative diabetic retinopathy E08.355
            traction retinal detachment involving the macula E08.352
            traction retinal detachment not involving the macula E08.353
      skin complication NEC E08.628
      skin ulcer NEC E08.622
  gestational (in pregnancy) O24.419
    affecting newborn P70.0
    diet-controlled O24.410
    in childbirth O24.429
      diet-controlled O24.420
      insulin (and diet) controlled O24.424
      oral drug controlled (antidiabetic) (hypoglycemic) O24.425
    insulin (and diet) controlled O24.414
    oral drug controlled (antidiabetic) (hypoglycemic) O24.415

Diabetes, diabetic *(Continued)*
  gestational (in pregnancy) *(Continued)*
    puerperal O24.439
      diet-controlled O24.430
      insulin (and diet) controlled O24.434
      oral drug controlled (antidiabetic) (hypoglycemic) O24.435
  hepatogenous E13.9
  idiopathic —*see* Diabetes, type 1
  inadequately controlled — code to Diabetes, by type, with hyperglycemia
  insipidus E23.2
    nephrogenic N25.1
    pituitary E23.2
    vasopressin resistant N25.1
  insulin dependent — code to type of diabetes
  juvenile-onset —*see* Diabetes, type 1
  ketosis-prone —*see* Diabetes, type 1
  latent R73.03
  neonatal (transient) P70.2
  non-insulin dependent — code to type of diabetes
  out of control — code to Diabetes, by type, with hyperglycemia
  phosphate E83.39
  poorly controlled — code to Diabetes, by type, with hyperglycemia
  postpancreatectomy —*see* Diabetes, specified type NEC
  postprocedural —*see* Diabetes, specified type NEC
  secondary diabetes mellitus NEC —*see* Diabetes, specified type NEC
  specified type NEC E13.9
    with
      amyotrophy E13.44
      arthropathy NEC E13.618
      autonomic (poly)neuropathy E13.43
      cataract E13.36
      Charcot's joints E13.610
      chronic kidney disease E13.22
      circulatory complication NEC E13.59
      complication E13.8
        specified NEC E13.69
      dermatitis E13.620
      foot ulcer E13.621
      gangrene E13.52
      gastroparalysis E13.43
      gastroparesis E13.43
      glomerulonephrosis, intracapillary E13.21
      glomerulosclerosis, intercapillary E13.21
      hyperglycemia E13.65
      hyperosmolarity E13.00
        with coma E13.01
      hypoglycemia E13.649
        with coma E13.641
      ketoacidosis E13.10
        with coma E13.11
      kidney complications NEC E13.29
      Kimmelsteil-Wilson disease E13.21
      mononeuropathy E13.41
      myasthenia E13.44
      necrobiosis lipoidica E13.620
      nephropathy E13.21
      neuralgia E13.42
      neurologic complication NEC E13.49
      neuropathic arthropathy E13.610
      neuropathy E13.40
      ophthalmic complication NEC E13.39
      oral complication NEC E13.638
      periodontal disease E13.630
      peripheral angiopathy E13.51
        with gangrene E13.52
      polyneuropathy E13.42
      renal complication NEC E13.29
      renal tubular degeneration E13.29
      retinopathy E13.319
        with macular edema E13.311
          resolved following treatment E13.37

▶ New   ➡ Revised   ~~deleted~~ Deleted   ● Use Additional Character(s)

Diabetes, diabetic *(Continued)*
  specified type NEC *(Continued)*
    with *(Continued)*
      retinopathy *(Continued)*
        nonproliferative E13.329
          with macular edema E13.321
          mild E13.329
            with macular edema E13.321
          moderate E13.339
            with macular edema E13.331
          severe E13.349
            with macular edema E13.341
        proliferative E13.359
          with
            combined traction retinal
              detachment and
              rhegmatogenous retinal
              detachment E13.354
            macular edema E13.351
            stable proliferative diabetic
              retinopathy E13.355
            traction retinal detachment
              involving the macula
              E13.352
            traction retinal detachment not
              involving the macula
              E13.353
      skin complication NEC E13.628
      skin ulcer NEC E13.622
    steroid-induced —*see* Diabetes, due to, drug
      or chemical
  type 1 E10.9
    with
      amyotrophy E10.44
      arthropathy NEC E10.618
      autonomic (poly)neuropathy E10.43
      cataract E10.36
      Charcot's joints E10.610
      chronic kidney disease E10.22
      circulatory complication NEC E10.59
      complication E10.8
        specified NEC E10.69
      dermatitis E10.620
      foot ulcer E10.621
      gangrene E10.52
      gastroparalysis E10.43
      gastroparesis E10.43
      glomerulonephrosis, intracapillary E10.21
      glomerulosclerosis, intercapillary E10.21
      hyperglycemia E10.65
      hypoglycemia E10.649
        with coma E10.641
      ketoacidosis E10.10
        with coma E10.11
      kidney complications NEC E10.29
      Kimmelstiel-Wilson disease E10.21
      mononeuropathy E10.41
      myasthenia E10.44
      necrobiosis lipoidica E10.620
      nephropathy E10.21
      neuralgia E10.42
      neurologic complication NEC E10.49
      neuropathic arthropathy E10.610
      neuropathy E10.40
      ophthalmic complication NEC E10.39
      oral complication NEC E10.638
      ▶osteomyelitis E10.69
      periodontal disease E10.630
      peripheral angiopathy E10.51
        with gangrene E10.52
      polyneuropathy E10.42
      renal complication NEC E10.29
      renal tubular degeneration E10.29
      retinopathy E10.319
        with macular edema E10.311
          resolved following treatment E10.37
        nonproliferative E10.329
          with macular edema E10.321
          mild E10.329
            with macular edema E10.321
          moderate E10.339
            with macular edema E10.331

Diabetes, diabetic *(Continued)*
  type 1 *(Continued)*
    with *(Continued)*
      retinopathy *(Continued)*
        nonproliferative *(Continued)*
          severe E10.349
            with macular edema E10.341
        proliferative E10.359
          with
            combined traction retinal
              detachment and
              rhegmatogenous retinal
              detachment E13.354
            macular edema E13.351
            stable proliferative diabetic
              retinopathy E13.355
            traction retinal detachment
              involving the macula E13.352
            traction retinal detachment not
              involving the macula E13.353
      skin complication NEC E10.628
      skin ulcer NEC E10.622
  type 2 E11.9
    with
      amyotrophy E11.44
      arthropathy NEC E11.618
      autonomic (poly)neuropathy E11.43
      cataract E11.36
      Charcot's joints E11.610
      chronic kidney disease E11.22
      circulatory complication NEC E11.59
      complication E11.8
        specified NEC E11.69
      dermatitis E11.620
      foot ulcer E11.621
      gangrene E11.52
      gastroparalysis E11.43
      gastroparesis E11.43
      glomerulonephrosis, intracapillary E11.21
      glomerulosclerosis, intercapillary E11.21
      hyperglycemia E11.65
      hyperosmolarity E11.00
        with coma E11.01
      hypoglycemia E11.649
        with coma E11.641
      ▶ketoacidosis E11.10
        ▶with coma E11.11
      kidney complications NEC E11.29
      Kimmelstiel-Wilson disease E11.21
      mononeuropathy E11.41
      myasthenia E11.44
      necrobiosis lipoidica E11.620
      nephropathy E11.21
      neuralgia E11.42
      neurologic complication NEC E11.49
      neuropathic arthropathy E11.610
      neuropathy E11.40
      ophthalmic complication NEC E11.39
      oral complication NEC E11.638
      ▶osteomyelitis E11.69
      periodontal disease E11.630
      peripheral angiopathy E11.51
        with gangrene E11.52
      polyneuropathy E11.42
      renal complication NEC E11.29
      renal tubular degeneration E11.29
      retinopathy E11.319
        with macular edema E11.311
          resolved following treatment E11.37
        nonproliferative E11.329
          with macular edema E11.321
          mild E11.329
            with macular edema E11.321
          moderate E11.339
            with macular edema E11.331
          severe E11.349
            with macular edema E11.341
        proliferative E11.359
          with
            combined traction retinal
              detachment and
              rhegmatogenous retinal
              detachment E11.354

Diabetes, diabetic *(Continued)*
  type 2 *(Continued)*
    with *(Continued)*
      retinopathy *(Continued)*
        proliferative *(Continued)*
          with *(Continued)*
            macular edema E11.351
            stable proliferative diabetic
              retinopathy E11.355
            traction retinal detachment
              involving the macula E11.352
            traction retinal detachment not
              involving the macula E11.353
      skin complication NEC E11.628
      skin ulcer NEC E11.622
    uncontrolled
      meaning
        hyperglycemia —*see* Diabetes, by type,
          with, hyperglycemia
        hypoglycemia —*see* Diabetes, by type,
          with, hypoglycemia
Diacyclothrombopathia D69.1
Diagnosis deferred R69
Dialysis (intermittent) (treatment)
  noncompliance (with) Z91.15
  renal (hemodialysis) (peritoneal), status Z99.2
  retina, retinal —*see* Detachment, retina, with
    retinal, dialysis
Diamond-Blackfan anemia (congenital
  hypoplastic) D61.01
Diamond-Gardener syndrome
  (autoerythrocyte sensitization) D69.2
Diaper rash L22
Diaphoresis (excessive) R61
Diaphragm —*see* condition
Diaphragmalgia R07.1
Diaphragmatitis, diaphragmitis J98.6
Diaphysial aclasis Q78.6
Diaphysitis —*see* Osteomyelitis, specified type
  NEC
Diarrhea, diarrheal (disease) (infantile)
  (inflammatory) R19.7
  achlorhydric K31.83
  allergic K52.29
  due to
    colitis —*see* Colitis, allergic
    enteritis —*see* Enteritis, allergic
  amebic —*see also* Amebiasis A06.0
    with abscess —*see* Abscess, amebic
    acute A06.0
    chronic A06.1
    nondysenteric A06.2
  bacillary —*see* Dysentery, bacillary
  balantidial A07.0
  cachectic NEC K52.89
  Chilomastix A07.8
  choleriformis A00.1
  chronic (noninfectious) K52.9
  coccidial A07.3
  Cochin-China K90.1
    strongyloidiasis B78.0
  Dientamoeba A07.8
  dietetic —*see also* Diarrhea, allergic K52.29
  drug-induced K52.1
  due to
    bacteria A04.9
      specified NEC A04.8
    Campylobacter A04.5
    Capillaria philippinensis B81.1
    ⟹Clostridium difficile
      ▶not specified as recurrent A04.72
      ▶recurrent A04.71
    Clostridium perfringens (C) (F) A04.8
    Cryptosporidium A07.2
    drugs K52.1
    Escherichia coli A04.4
      enteroaggregative A04.4
      enterohemorrhagic A04.3
      enteroinvasive A04.2
      enteropathogenic A04.0
      enterotoxigenic A04.1
      specified NEC A04.4

▶ New   ⟹ Revised   ~~deleted~~ Deleted   ● Use Additional Character(s)

Diarrhea, diarrheal *(Continued)*
  due to *(Continued)*
    food hypersensitivity —*see also* Diarrhea,
      allergic K52.29
    Necator americanus B76.1
    S. japonicum B65.2
    specified organism NEC A08.8
      bacterial A04.8
      viral A08.39
    Staphylococcus A04.8
    Trichuris trichiuria B79
    virus —*see* Enteritis, viral
    Yersinia enterocolitica A04.6
  dysenteric A09
  endemic A09
  epidemic A09
  flagellate A07.9
  Flexner's (ulcerative) A03.1
  functional K59.1
    following gastrointestinal surgery
      K91.89
    psychogenic F45.8
  Giardia lamblia A07.1
  giardial A07.1
  hill K90.1
  infectious A09
  malarial —*see* Malaria
  mite B88.0
  mycotic NEC B49
  neonatal (noninfectious) P78.3
  nervous F45.8
  neurogenic K59.1
  noninfectious K52.9
  postgastrectomy K91.1
  postvagotomy K91.1
  protozoal A07.9
    specified NEC A07.8
  psychogenic F45.8
  specified
    bacterium NEC A04.8
    virus NEC A08.39
  strongyloidiasis B78.0
  toxic K52.1
  trichomonal A07.8
  tropical K90.1
  tuberculous A18.32
  viral —*see* Enteritis, viral
Diastasis
  cranial bones M84.88
    congenital NEC Q75.8
  joint (traumatic) —*see* Dislocation
  muscle M62.00
    ankle M62.07-●
    congenital Q79.8
    foot M62.07-●
    forearm M62.03-●
    hand M62.04-●
    lower leg M62.06-●
    pelvic region M62.05-●
    shoulder region M62.01-●
    specified site NEC M62.08
    thigh M62.05-●
    upper arm M62.02-●
  recti (abdomen)
    complicating delivery O71.89
    congenital Q79.59
Diastema, tooth, teeth, fully erupted
  M26.32
Diastematomyelia Q06.2
Diataxia, cerebral G80.4
Diathesis
  allergic —*see* History, allergy
  bleeding (familial) D69.9
  cystine (familial) E72.00
  gouty —*see* Gout
  hemorrhagic (familial) D69.9
    newborn NEC P53
  spasmophilic R29.0
Diaz's disease or osteochondrosis (juvenile)
  (talus) —*see* Osteochondrosis, juvenile,
  tarsus

Dibothriocephalus, dibothriocephaliasis
  (latus) (infection) (infestation) B70.0
  larval B70.1
Dicephalus, dicephaly Q89.4
Dichotomy, teeth K00.2
Dichromat, dichromatopsia (congenital) —*see*
  Deficiency, color vision
Dichuchwa A65
Dicroceliasis B66.2
Didelphia, didelphys —*see* Double uterus
Didymitis N45.1
  with orchitis N45.3
Dietary
  inadequacy or deficiency E63.9
  surveillance and counseling Z71.3
Dietl's crisis N13.8
Dieulafoy lesion (hemorrhagic)
  duodenum K31.82
  esophagus K22.8
  intestine (colon) K63.81
  stomach K31.82
Difficult, difficulty (in)
  acculturation Z60.3
  feeding R63.3
    newborn P92.9
      breast P92.5
      specified NEC P92.8
    nonorganic (infant or child) F98.29
  intubation, in anesthesia T88.4
  mechanical, gastroduodenal stoma K91.89
  ➡causing obstruction —*see also* Obstruction,
      intestine, postoperative K91.30
  micturition
    need to immediately re-void R39.191
    position dependent R39.192
    specified NEC R39.198
  reading (developmental) F81.0
    secondary to emotional disorders F93.9
  spelling (specific) F81.81
    with reading disorder F81.89
    due to inadequate teaching Z55.8
  swallowing —*see* Dysphagia
  walking R26.2
  work
    conditions NEC Z56.5
    schedule Z56.3
Diffuse —*see* condition
DiGeorge's syndrome (thymic hypoplasia)
  D82.1
Digestive —*see* condition
Dihydropyrimidine dehydrogenase disease
  (DPD) E88.89
Diktyoma —*see* Neoplasm, malignant, by site
Dilaceration, tooth K00.4
Dilatation
  anus K59.8
    venule —*see* Hemorrhoids
  aorta (focal) (general) —*see* Ectasia, aorta
    with aneurysm —*see* Aneurysm, aorta
    congenital Q25.44
  artery —*see* Aneurysm
  bladder (sphincter) N32.89
    congenital Q64.79
  blood vessel I99.8
  bronchial J47.9
    with
      exacerbation (acute) J47.1
      lower respiratory infection J47.0
  calyx (due to obstruction) —*see*
    Hydronephrosis
  capillaries I78.8
  cardiac (acute) (chronic) —*see also*
    Hypertrophy, cardiac
    congenital Q24.8
      valve NEC Q24.8
        pulmonary Q22.3
    valve —*see* Endocarditis
  cavum septi pellucidi Q06.8
  cervix (uteri) —*see also* Incompetency, cervix
    incomplete, poor, slow complicating
      delivery O62.0

Dilatation *(Continued)*
  colon K59.39
    congenital Q43.1
    psychogenic F45.8
    toxic K59.31
  common duct (acquired) K83.8
    congenital Q44.5
  cystic duct (acquired) K82.8
    congenital Q44.5
  duct, mammary —*see* Ectasia, mammary duct
  duodenum K59.8
  esophagus K22.8
    congenital Q39.5
    due to achalasia K22.0
  eustachian tube, congenital Q17.8
  gallbladder K82.8
  gastric —*see* Dilatation, stomach
  heart (acute) (chronic) —*see also* Hypertrophy,
    cardiac
    congenital Q24.8
    valve —*see* Endocarditis
  ileum K59.8
    psychogenic F45.8
  jejunum K59.8
    psychogenic F45.8
  kidney (calyx) (collecting structures) (cystic)
    (parenchyma) (pelvis) (idiopathic)
    N28.89
  lacrimal passages or duct —*see* Disorder,
    lacrimal system, changes
  lymphatic vessel I89.0
  mammary duct —*see* Ectasia, mammary
    duct
  Meckel's diverticulum (congenital) Q43.0
    malignant —*see* Table of Neoplasms, small
      intestine, malignant
  myocardium (acute) (chronic) —*see*
    Hypertrophy, cardiac organ or site,
      congenital NEC —*see* Distortion
  pancreatic duct K86.89
  pericardium —*see* Pericarditis
  pharynx J39.2
  prostate N42.89
  pulmonary
    artery (idiopathic) I28.8
    valve, congenital Q22.3
  pupil H57.04
  rectum K59.39
  saccule, congenital Q16.5
  salivary gland (duct) K11.8
  sphincter ani K62.89
  stomach K31.89
    acute K31.0
    psychogenic F45.8
  submaxillary duct K11.8
  trachea, congenital Q32.1
  ureter (idiopathic) N28.82
    congenital Q62.2
    due to obstruction N13.4
  urethra (acquired) N36.8
  vasomotor I73.9
  vein I86.8
  ventricular, ventricle (acute) (chronic) —*see*
    also Hypertrophy, cardiac
    cerebral, congenital Q04.8
  venule NEC I86.8
  vesical orifice N32.89
Dilated, dilation —*see* Dilatation
Diminished, diminution
  hearing (acuity) —*see* Deafness
  sense or sensation (cold) (heat) (tactile)
    (vibratory) R20.8
  vision NEC H54.7
  vital capacity R94.2
Diminuta taenia B71.0
Dimitri-Sturge-Weber disease Q85.8
Dimple
  congenital sacral Q82.6
  parasacral Q82.6
  pilonidal or postanal —*see* Cyst,
    pilonidal

Dioctophyme renalis (infection) (infestation)
  B83.8
Dipetalonemiasis B74.4
Diphallus Q55.69
Diphtheria, diphtheritic (gangrenous)
    (hemorrhagic) A36.9
  carrier (suspected) Z22.2
  cutaneous A36.3
  faucial A36.0
  infection of wound A36.3
  laryngeal A36.2
  myocarditis A36.81
  nasal, anterior A36.89
  nasopharyngeal A36.1
  neurological complication A36.89
  pharyngeal A36.0
  specified site NEC A36.89
  tonsillar A36.0
Diphyllobothriasis (intestine) B70.0
  larval B70.1
Diplacusis H93.22-●
Diplegia (upper limbs) G83.0
  congenital (cerebral) G80.8
  facial G51.0
  lower limbs G82.20
  spastic G80.1
Diplococcus, diplococcal —see condition
Diplopia H53.2
Dipsomania F10.20
  with
    psychosis —see Psychosis, alcoholic
    remission F10.21
Dipylidiasis B71.1
DIRA (deficiency of interleukin 1 receptor
    antagonist) M04.8
Direction, teeth, abnormal, fully erupted
    M26.30
Dirofilariasis B74.8
Dirt-eating child F98.3
Disability, disabilities
  heart —see Disease, heart
  intellectual F79
    with
      autistic features F84.9
    mild (I.Q. 50-69) F70
    moderate (I.Q. 35-49) F71
    profound (I.Q. under 20) F73
    severe (I.Q. 20-34) F72
    specified level NEC F78
  knowledge acquisition F81.9
  learning F81.9
  limiting activities Z73.6
  spelling, specific F81.81
Disappearance of family member Z63.4
Disarticulation —see Amputation
  meaning traumatic amputation —see
    Amputation, traumatic
Discharge (from)
  abnormal finding in —see Abnormal,
    specimen
  breast (female) (male) N64.52
  diencephalic autonomic idiopathic —see
    Epilepsy, specified NEC
  ear —see also Otorrhea
    blood —see Otorrhagia
  excessive urine R35.8
  nipple N64.52
  penile R36.9
  postnasal R09.82
  prison, anxiety concerning Z65.2
  urethral R36.9
    without blood R36.0
    hematospermia R36.1
  vaginal N89.8
Discitis, diskitis M46.40
  cervical region M46.42
  cervicothoracic region M46.43
  lumbar region M46.46
  lumbosacral region M46.47
  multiple sites M46.49
  occipito-atlanto-axial region M46.41

Discitis, diskitis (Continued)
  pyogenic —see Infection, intervertebral
    disc, pyogenic
  sacrococcygeal region M46.48
  thoracic region M46.44
  thoracolumbar region M46.45
Discoid
  meniscus (congenital) Q68.6
  semilunar cartilage (congenital) —see
    Derangement, knee, meniscus,
    specified NEC
Discoloration
  nails L60.8
  teeth (posteruptive) K03.7
    during formation K00.8
Discomfort
  chest R07.89
  visual H53.14-●
Discontinuity, ossicles, ear H74.2-●
Discord (with)
  boss Z56.4
  classmates Z55.4
  counselor Z64.4
  employer Z56.4
  family Z63.8
  fellow employees Z56.4
  in-laws Z63.1
  landlord Z59.2
  lodgers Z59.2
  neighbors Z59.2
  probation officer Z64.4
  social worker Z64.4
  teachers Z55.4
  workmates Z56.4
Discordant connection
  atrioventricular (congenital)
    Q20.5
  ventriculoarterial Q20.3
Discrepancy
  centric occlusion maximum intercuspation
    M26.55
  leg length (acquired) —see Deformity, limb,
    unequal length
    congenital —see Defect, reduction, lower
      limb
  uterine size date O26.84-●
Discrimination
  ethnic Z60.5
  political Z60.5
  racial Z60.5
  religious Z60.5
  sex Z60.5
Disease, diseased —see also Syndrome
  absorbent system I87.8
  acid-peptic K30
  Acosta's T70.29
  Adams-Stokes (-Morgagni) (syncope with
    heart block) I45.9
  Addison's anemia (pernicious) D51.0
  adenoids (and tonsils) J35.9
  adrenal (capsule) (cortex) (gland) (medullary)
    E27.9
    hyperfunction E27.0
    specified NEC E27.8
  ainhum L94.6
  airway
    obstructive, chronic J44.9
      due to
        cotton dust J66.0
        specific organic dusts NEC J66.8
    reactive —see Asthma
  akamushi (scrub typhus) A75.3
  Albers-Schönberg (marble bones)
    Q78.2
  Albert's —see Tendinitis, Achilles
  alimentary canal K63.9
  alligator-skin Q80.9
    acquired L85.0
  alpha heavy chain C88.3
  alpine T70.29
  altitude T70.20

Disease, diseased (Continued)
  alveolar ridge
    edentulous K06.9
    specified NEC K06.8
  alveoli, teeth K08.9
  Alzheimer's G30.9 [F02.80]
    with behavioral disturbance G30.9 [F02.81]
    early onset G30.0 [F02.80]
      with behavioral disturbance G30.0
        [F02.81]
    late onset G30.1 [F02.80]
      with behavioral disturbance G30.1
        [F02.81]
    specified NEC G30.8 [F02.80]
      with behavioral disturbance G30.8
        [F02.81]
  amyloid —see Amyloidosis
  Andersen's (glycogenosis IV) E74.09
  Andes T70.29
  Andrews' (bacterid) L08.89
  angiospastic I73.9
    cerebral G45.9
    vein I87.8
  anterior
    chamber H21.9
    horn cell G12.29
  antiglomerular basement membrane (anti-
    GBM) antibody M31.0
    tubulo-interstitial nephritis N12
  antral —see Sinusitis, maxillary
  anus K62.9
    specified NEC K62.89
  aorta (nonsyphilitic) I77.9
    syphilitic NEC A52.02
  aortic (heart) (valve) I35.9
    rheumatic I06.9
  Apollo B30.3
  aponeuroses —see Enthesopathy
  appendix K38.9
    specified NEC K38.8
  aqueous (chamber) H21.9
  Arnold-Chiari —see Arnold-Chiari disease
  arterial I77.9
    occlusive —see Occlusion, by site
      due to stricture or stenosis I77.1
  arteriocardiorenal —see Hypertension,
    cardiorenal
  arteriolar (generalized) (obliterative)
    I77.9
  arteriorenal —see Hypertension, kidney
  arteriosclerotic —see also Arteriosclerosis
    cardiovascular —see Disease, heart,
      ischemic, atherosclerotic
    coronary (artery) —see Disease, heart,
      ischemic, atherosclerotic
    heart —see Disease, heart, ischemic,
      atherosclerotic
  artery I77.9
    cerebral I67.9
    coronary I25.10
      with angina pectoris —see
        Arteriosclerosis, coronary
        (artery),
  arthropod-borne NOS (viral) A94
    specified type NEC A93.8
  atticoantral, chronic H66.20
    left H66.22
      with right H66.23
    right H66.21
      with left H66.23
  auditory canal —see Disorder, ear, external
  auricle, ear NEC —see Disorder, pinna
  Australian X A83.4
  autoimmune (systemic) NOS M35.9
    hemolytic (cold type) (warm type)
      D59.1
      drug-induced D59.0
    thyroid E06.3
  aviator's —see Effect, adverse, high altitude
  Ayerza's (pulmonary artery sclerosis with
    pulmonary hypertension) I27.0

▶ New   ⇒ Revised   ~~deleted~~ Deleted   ● Use Additional Character(s)

Disease, diseased *(Continued)*
  Babington's (familial hemorrhagic
    telangiectasia) I78.0
  bacterial A49.9
    specified NEC A48.8
    zoonotic A28.9
      specified type NEC A28.8
  Baelz's (cheilitis glandularis apostematosa)
    K13.0
  bagasse J67.1
  balloon —*see* Effect, adverse, high altitude
  Bang's (brucella abortus) A23.1
  Bannister's T78.3
  barometer makers' —*see* Poisoning, mercury
  Barraquer (-Simons') (progressive
    lipodystrophy) E88.1
  Barrett's —*see* Barrett's, esophagus
  Bartholin's gland N75.9
  basal ganglia G25.9
    degenerative G23.9
      specified NEC G23.8
    specified NEC G25.89
  Basedow's (exophthalmic goiter) —*see*
    Hyperthyroidism, with, goiter (diffuse)
  Bateman's B08.1
  Batten-Steinert G71.11
  Battey A31.0
  Beard's (neurasthenia) F48.8
  Becker
    idiopathic mural endomyocardial I42.3
    myotonia congenita G71.12
  Begbie's (exophthalmic goiter) —*see*
    Hyperthyroidism, with, goiter (diffuse)
  behavioral, organic F07.9
  Beigel's (white piedra) B36.2
  Benson's —*see* Deposit, crystalline
  Bernard-Soulier (thrombopathy) D69.1
  Bernhardt (-Roth) —*see* Mononeuropathy,
    lower limb, meralgia paresthetica
  Biermer's (pernicious anemia) D51.0
  bile duct (common) (hepatic) K83.9
    with calculus, stones —*see* Calculus, bile
      duct
    specified NEC K83.8
  biliary (tract) K83.9
    specified NEC K83.8
  Billroth's —*see* Spina bifida
  bird fancier's J67.2
  black lung J60
  bladder N32.9
    in (due to)
      schistosomiasis (bilharziasis) B65.0 [N33]
    specified NEC N32.89
  bleeder's D66
  blood D75.9
    forming organs D75.9
    vessel I99.9
  Bloodgood's —*see* Mastopathy, cystic
  Bodechtel-Guttmann (subacute sclerosing
    panencephalitis) A81.1
  bone —*see also* Disorder, bone
    aluminum M83.4
    fibrocystic NEC
      jaw M27.49
  bone-marrow D75.9
  Borna A83.9
  Bornholm (epidemic pleurodynia) B33.0
  Bouchard's (myopathic dilatation of the
    stomach) K31.0
  Bouillaud's (rheumatic heart disease) I01.9
  Bourneville (-Brissaud) (tuberous sclerosis)
    Q85.1
  Bouveret (-Hoffmann) (paroxysmal
    tachycardia) I47.9
  bowel K63.9
    functional K59.9
      psychogenic F45.8
  brain G93.9
    arterial, artery I67.9
    arteriosclerotic I67.2
    congenital Q04.9

Disease, diseased *(Continued)*
  brain *(Continued)*
    degenerative —*see* Degeneration, brain
    inflammatory —*see* Encephalitis
    organic G93.9
      arteriosclerotic I67.2
    parasitic NEC B71.9 [G94]
    senile NEC G31.1
    specified NEC G93.89
  breast (*see also* Disorder, breast) N64.9
    cystic (chronic) —*see* Mastopathy, cystic
    fibrocystic —*see* Mastopathy, cystic
    Paget's
      female, unspecified side C50.91-●
      male, unspecified side C50.92-●
    specified NEC N64.89
  Breda's —*see* Yaws
  Bretonneau's (diphtheritic malignant angina)
    A36.0
  Bright's —*see* Nephritis
    arteriosclerotic —*see* Hypertension, kidney
  Brill's (recrudescent typhus) A75.1
  Brill-Zinsser (recrudescent typhus) A75.1
  Brion-Kayser —*see* Fever, paratyphoid
  broad
    beta E78.2
    ligament (noninflammatory) N83.9
      inflammatory —*see* Disease, pelvis,
        inflammatory
      specified NEC N83.8
  Brocq-Duhring (dermatitis herpetiformis)
    L13.0
  Brocq's
    meaning
      dermatitis herpetiformis L13.0
      prurigo L28.2
  bronchopulmonary J98.4
  bronchus NEC J98.09
  bronze Addison's E27.1
    tuberculous A18.7
  budgerigar fancier's J67.2
  Buerger's (thromboangiitis obliterans)
    I73.1
  bullous L13.9
    chronic of childhood L12.2
    specified NEC L13.8
  Bürger-Grütz (essential familial
    hyperlipemia) E78.3
  bursa —*see* Bursopathy
  caisson T70.3
  California —*see* Coccidioidomycosis
  capillaries I78.9
    specified NEC I78.8
  Carapata A68.0
  cardiac —*see* Disease, heart
  cardiopulmonary, chronic I27.9
  cardiorenal (hepatic) (hypertensive)
    (vascular) —*see* Hypertension,
    cardiorenal
  cardiovascular (atherosclerotic) I25.10
    with angina pectoris —*see* Arteriosclerosis,
      coronary (artery),
    congenital Q28.9
    hypertensive —*see* Hypertension, heart
    newborn P29.9
      specified NEC P29.89
    renal (hypertensive) —*see* Hypertension,
      cardiorenal
    syphilitic (asymptomatic) A52.00
  cartilage —*see* Disorder, cartilage
  Castellani's A69.8
  Castleman (unicentric) (multicentric)
    D47.Z2
    HHV-8-associated —*see also* Herpesvirus,
      human, 8 D47.Z2
  cat-scratch A28.1
  Cavare's (familial periodic paralysis) G72.3
  cecum K63.9
  celiac (adult) (infantile) (with steatorrhea)
    K90.0
  cellular tissue L98.9

Disease, diseased *(Continued)*
  central core G71.2
  cerebellar, cerebellum —*see* Disease, brain
  cerebral —*see also* Disease, brain
    degenerative —*see* Degeneration, brain
  cerebrospinal G96.9
  cerebrovascular I67.9
    acute I67.89
      embolic I63.4-●
      thrombotic I63.3-●
    arteriosclerotic I67.2
    specified NEC I67.89
  cervix (uteri) (noninflammatory) N88.9
    inflammatory —*see* Cervicitis
    specified NEC N88.8
  Chabert's A22.9
  Chandler's (osteochondritis dissecans, hip) —
    see Osteochondritis, dissecans, hip
  Charlouis —*see* Yaws
  Chédiak-Steinbrinck (-Higashi) (congenital
    gigantism of peroxidase granules)
    E70.330
  chest J98.9
  Chiari's (hepatic vein thrombosis) I82.0
  Chicago B40.9
  Chignon B36.8
  chigo, chigoe B88.1
  childhood granulomatous D71
  Chinese liver fluke B66.1
  chlamydial A74.9
    specified NEC A74.89
  cholecystic K82.9
  choroid H31.9
    specified NEC H31.8
  Christmas D67
  chronic bullous of childhood L12.2
  chylomicron retention E78.3
  ciliary body H21.9
    specified NEC H21.89
  circulatory (system) NEC I99.8
    newborn P29.9
    syphilitic A52.00
      congenital A50.54
  coagulation factor deficiency (congenital) —
    see Defect, coagulation
  coccidioidal —*see* Coccidioidomycosis
  cold
    agglutinin or hemoglobinuria D59.1
      paroxysmal D59.6
    hemagglutinin (chronic) D59.1
  collagen NOS (nonvascular) (vascular) M35.9
    specified NEC M35.8
  colon K63.9
    functional K59.9
      congenital Q43.2
    ischemic —*see also* Ischemia, intestine,
      acute K55.039
  colonic inflammatory bowel, unclassified
    (IBDU) K52.3
  combined system —*see* Degeneration,
    combined
  compressed air T70.3
  Concato's (pericardial polyserositis) A19.9
    nontubercular I31.1
    pleural —*see* Pleurisy, with effusion
  conjunctiva H11.9
    chlamydial A74.0
    specified NEC H11.89
    viral B30.9
      specified NEC B30.8
  connective tissue, systemic (diffuse) M35.9
    in (due to)
      hypogammaglobulinemia D80.1 [M36.8]
      ochronosis E70.29 [M36.8]
    specified NEC M35.8
  Conor and Bruch's (boutonneuse fever) A77.1
  Cooper's —*see* Mastopathy, cystic
  Cori's (glycogenosis III) E74.03
  corkhandler's or corkworker's J67.3
  cornea H18.9
    specified NEC H18.89-●

Disease, diseased *(Continued)*
  coronary (artery) —*see* Disease, heart,
      ischemic, atherosclerotic
    congenital Q24.5
    ostial, syphilitic (aortic) (mitral)
      (pulmonary) A52.03
  corpus cavernosum N48.9
    specified NEC N48.89
  Cotugno's —*see* Sciatica
  coxsackie (virus) NEC B34.1
  cranial nerve NOS G52.9
  Creutzfeldt-Jakob —*see* Creutzfeldt-Jakob
    disease or syndrome
  Crocq's (acrocyanosis) I73.89
  Crohn's —*see* Enteritis, regional
  Curschmann G71.11
  cystic
    breast (chronic) —*see* Mastopathy, cystic
    kidney, congenital Q61.9
    liver, congenital Q44.6
    lung J98.4
      congenital Q33.0
  cytomegalic inclusion (generalized) B25.9
    with pneumonia B25.0
    congenital P35.1
  cytomegaloviral B25.9
    specified NEC B25.8
  Czerny's (periodic hydrarthrosis of the
    knee) —*see* Effusion, joint, knee
  Daae (-Finsen) (epidemic pleurodynia) B33.0
  Darling's —*see* Histoplasmosis capsulati
  Débove's (splenomegaly) R16.1
  deer fly —*see* Tularemia
  Degos' I77.8
  demyelinating, demyelinizating (nervous
    system) G37.9
    multiple sclerosis G35
    specified NEC G37.8
  dense deposit —*see also* N00-N07 with fourth
    character .6 N05.6
  deposition, hydroxyapatite —*see* Disease,
    hydroxyapatite deposition
  de Quervain's (tendon sheath) M65.4
    thyroid (subacute granulomatous
      thyroiditis) E06.1
  Devergie's (pityriasis rubra pilaris) L44.0
  Devic's G36.0
  diaphorase deficiency D74.0
  diaphragm J98.6
  diarrheal, infectious NEC A09
  digestive system K92.9
    specified NEC K92.89
  disc, degenerative —*see* Degeneration,
    intervertebral disc
  discogenic —*see also* Displacement,
    intervertebral disc NEC
    with myelopathy —*see* Disorder, disc, with,
      myelopathy
  diverticular —*see* Diverticula
  Dubois (thymus) A50.59 *[E35]*
  Duchenne-Griesinger G71.0
  Duchenne's
    muscular dystrophy G71.0
    pseudohypertrophy, muscles G71.0
  ductless glands E34.9
  Duhring's (dermatitis herpetiformis) L13.0
  duodenum K31.9
    specified NEC K31.89
  Dupré's (meningism) R29.1
  Dupuytren's (muscle contracture) M72.0
  Durand-Nicholas-Favre (climatic bubo) A55
  Duroziez's (congenital mitral stenosis) Q23.2
  ear —*see* Disorder, ear
  Eberth's —*see* Fever, typhoid
  Ebola (virus) A98.4
  Ebstein's heart Q22.5
  Echinococcus —*see* Echinococcus
  echovirus NEC B34.1
  Eddowes' (brittle bones and blue sclera) Q78.0
  edentulous (alveolar) ridge K06.9
    specified NEC K06.8

Disease, diseased *(Continued)*
  Edsall's T67.2
  Eichstedt's (pityriasis versicolor) B36.0
  ▶ Eisenmenger's (irreversible) I27.83
  Ellis-van Creveld (chondroectodermal
    dysplasia) Q77.6
  end stage renal (ESRD) N18.6
    due to hypertension I12.0
  endocrine glands or system NEC E34.9
  endomyocardial (eosinophilic) I42.3
  English (rickets) E55.0
  enteroviral, enterovirus NEC B34.1
    central nervous system NEC A88.8
  epidemic B99.9
    specified NEC B99.8
  epididymis N50.9
  Erb (-Landouzy) G71.0
  Erdheim-Chester (ECD) E88.89
  esophagus K22.9
    functional K22.4
    psychogenic F45.8
    specified NEC K22.8
  Eulenburg's (congenital paramyotonia) G71.19
  eustachian tube —*see* Disorder, eustachian tube
  external
    auditory canal —*see* Disorder, ear, external
    ear —*see* Disorder, ear, external
  extrapyramidal G25.9
    specified NEC G25.89
  eye H57.9
    anterior chamber H21.9
    inflammatory NEC H57.8
    muscle (external) —*see* Strabismus
    specified NEC H57.8
    syphilitic —*see* Oculopathy, syphilitic
  eyeball H44.9
    specified NEC H44.89
  eyelid —*see* Disorder, eyelid
    specified NEC —*see* Disorder, eyelid,
      specified type NEC
  eyeworm of Africa B74.3
  facial nerve (seventh) G51.9
    newborn (birth injury) P11.3
  Fahr (of brain) G23.8
  Fahr Volhard (of kidney) I12.-●
  fallopian tube (noninflammatory) N83.9
    inflammatory —*see* Salpingo-oophoritis
    specified NEC N83.8
  familial periodic paralysis G72.3
  Fanconi's (congenital pancytopenia) D61.09
  fascia NEC —*see also* Disorder, muscle
    inflammatory —*see* Myositis
    specified NEC M62.89
  Fauchard's (periodontitis) —*see* Periodontitis
  Favre-Durand-Nicolas (climatic bubo) A55
  Fede's K14.0
  Feer's —*see* Poisoning, mercury
  female pelvic inflammatory —*see also* Disease,
    pelvis, inflammatory N73.9
    syphilitic (secondary) A51.42
    tuberculous A18.17
  Fernels' (aortic aneurysm) I71.9
  fibrocaseous of lung —*see* Tuberculosis,
    pulmonary
  fibrocystic —*see* Fibrocystic disease
  Fiedler's (leptospiral jaundice) A27.0
  fifth B08.3
  file-cutter's —*see* Poisoning, lead
  fish-skin Q80.9
    acquired L85.0
  Flajani (-Basedow) (exophthalmic goiter) —
    see Hyperthyroidism, with, goiter
    (diffuse)
  flax-dresser's J66.1
  fluke —*see* Infestation, fluke
  foot and mouth B08.8
  foot process N04.9
  Forbes' (glycogenosis III) E74.03
  Fordyce-Fox (apocrine miliaria) L75.2
  Fordyce's (ectopic sebaceous glands) (mouth)
    Q38.6

Disease, diseased *(Continued)*
  Forestier's (rhizomelic pseudopolyarthritis)
    M35.3
    meaning ankylosing hyperostosis —*see*
      Hyperostosis, ankylosing
  Fothergill's
    neuralgia —*see* Neuralgia, trigeminal
    scarlatina anginosa A38.9
  Fournier (gangrene) N49.3
    female N76.89
  fourth B08.8
  Fox (-Fordyce) (apocrine miliaria) L75.2
  Francis' —*see* Tularemia
  Franklin C88.2
  Frei's (climatic bubo) A55
  Friedreich's
    combined systemic or ataxia G11.1
    myoclonia G25.3
  frontal sinus —*see* Sinusitis, frontal
  fungus NEC B49
  Gaisböck's (polycythemia hypertonica) D75.1
  gallbladder K82.9
    calculus —*see* Calculus, gallbladder
    cholecystitis —*see* Cholecystitis
    cholesterolosis K82.4
    fistula —*see* Fistula, gallbladder
    hydrops K82.1
    obstruction —*see* Obstruction, gallbladder
    perforation K82.2
    specified NEC K82.8
  gamma heavy chain C88.2
  Gamna's (siderotic splenomegaly) D73.2
  Gamstorp's (adynamia episodica hereditaria)
    G72.3
  Gandy-Nanta (siderotic splenomegaly) D73.2
  ganister J62.8
  gastric —*see* Disease, stomach
  gastroesophageal reflux (GERD) K21.9
    with esophagitis K21.0
  gastrointestinal (tract) K92.9
    amyloid E85.4
    functional K59.9
      psychogenic F45.8
    specified NEC K92.89
  Gee (-Herter) (-Heubner) (-Thaysen)
    (nontropical sprue) K90.0
  genital organs
    female N94.9
    male N50.9
  Gerhardt's (erythromelalgia) I73.81
  Gibert's (pityriasis rosea) L42
  Gierke's (glycogenosis I) E74.01
  Gilles de la Tourette's (motor-verbal tic) F95.2
  gingiva K06.9
    plaque induced K05.00
    specified NEC K06.8
  gland (lymph) I89.9
  Glanzmann's (hereditary hemorrhagic
    thrombasthenia) D69.1
  glass-blower's (cataract) —*see* Cataract,
    specified NEC
    salivary gland hypertrophy K11.1
  Glisson's —*see* Rickets
  globe H44.9
    specified NEC H44.89
  glomerular —*see also* Glomerulonephritis
    with edema —*see* Nephrosis
    acute —*see* Nephritis, acute
    chronic —*see* Nephritis, chronic
    minimal change N05.0
    rapidly progressive N01.9
  glycogen storage E74.00
    Andersen's E74.09
    Cori's E74.03
    Forbes' E74.03
    generalized E74.00
    glucose-6-phosphatase deficiency E74.01
    heart E74.02 *[143]*
    hepatorenal E74.09
    Hers' E74.09
    liver and kidney E74.09

Disease, diseased *(Continued)*
  glycogen storage *(Continued)*
    McArdle's E74.04
    muscle phosphofructokinase E74.09
    myocardium E74.02 *[143]*
    Pompe's E74.02
    Tauri's E74.09
    type Ø E74.09
    type I E74.01
    type II E74.02
    type III E74.03
    type IV E74.09
    type V E74.04
    type VI-XI E74.09
    Von Gierke's E74.01
  Goldstein's (familial hemorrhagic
      telangiectasia) I78.0
  gonococcal NOS A54.9
  graft-versus-host (GVH) D89.813
    acute D89.810
    acute on chronic D89.812
    chronic D89.811
  grainhandler's J67.8
  granulomatous (childhood) (chronic) D71
  Graves' (exophthalmic goiter) —*see*
      Hyperthyroidism, with, goiter
      (diffuse)
  Griesinger's —*see* Ancylostomiasis
  Grisel's M43.6
  Gruby's (tinea tonsurans) B35.0
  Guillain-Barré G61.0
  Guinon's (motor-verbal tic) F95.2
  gum K06.9
  gynecological N94.9
  H (Hartnup's) E72.02
  Haff —*see* Poisoning, mercury
  Hageman (congenital factor XII deficiency)
      D68.2
  hair (color) (shaft) L67.9
    follicles L73.9
      specified NEC L73.8
  Hamman's (spontaneous mediastinal
      emphysema) J98.2
  hand, foot and mouth B08.4
  Hansen's —*see* Leprosy
  Hantavirus, with pulmonary manifestations
      B33.4
    with renal manifestations A98.5
  Harada's H30.81-•
  Hartnup (pellagra-cerebellar ataxia-renal
      aminoaciduria) E72.02
  Hart's (pellagra-cerebellar ataxia-renal
      aminoaciduria) E72.02
  Hashimoto's (struma lymphomatosa) E06.3
  Hb —*see* Disease, hemoglobin
  heart (organic) I51.9
    with
      pulmonary edema (acute) —*see also*
          Failure, ventricular, left I50.1
      rheumatic fever (conditions in I00)
        active I01.9
          with chorea I02.0
          specified NEC I01.8
        inactive or quiescent (with chorea)
            I09.9
          specified NEC I09.89
    amyloid E85.4 *[143]*
    aortic (valve) I35.9
    arteriosclerotic or sclerotic (senile) —
        see Disease, heart, ischemic,
        atherosclerotic
    artery, arterial —*see* Disease, heart,
        ischemic, atherosclerotic
    beer drinkers' I42.6
    beriberi (wet) E51.12
    black I27.0
    congenital Q24.9
      cyanotic Q24.9
      specified NEC Q24.8
    coronary —*see* Disease, heart, ischemic
    cryptogenic I51.9

Disease, diseased *(Continued)*
  heart *(Continued)*
    fibroid —*see* Myocarditis
    functional I51.89
      psychogenic F45.8
    glycogen storage E74.02 *[143]*
    gonococcal A54.83
    hypertensive —*see* Hypertension, heart
    hyperthyroid —*see also* Hyperthyroidism
        E05.90 *[143]*
      with thyroid storm E05.91 *[143]*
    ischemic (chronic or with a stated duration
        of over 4 weeks) I25.9
      atherosclerotic (of) I25.10
        with angina pectoris —*see*
            Arteriosclerosis, coronary (artery)
        coronary artery bypass graft —*see*
            Arteriosclerosis, coronary
            (artery),
      cardiomyopathy I25.5
      diagnosed on ECG or other special
          investigation, but currently
          presenting no symptoms I25.6
      silent I25.6
      specified form NEC I25.89
    kyphoscoliotic I27.1
    meningococcal A39.50
      endocarditis A39.51
      myocarditis A39.52
      pericarditis A39.53
    mitral I05.9
      specified NEC I05.8
    muscular —*see* Degeneration, myocardial
    psychogenic (functional) F45.8
    pulmonary (chronic) I27.9
      in schistosomiasis B65.9 *[152]*
      specified NEC I27.89
    rheumatic (chronic) (inactive) (old)
        (quiescent) (with chorea) I09.9
      active or acute I01.9
        with chorea (acute) (rheumatic)
            (Sydenham's) I02.0
      specified NEC I09.89
    senile —*see* Myocarditis
    syphilitic A52.06
      aortic A52.03
        aneurysm A52.01
      congenital A50.54 *[152]*
    thyrotoxic —*see also* Thyrotoxicosis E05.90
        [143]
      with thyroid storm E05.91 *[143]*
    valve, valvular (obstructive)
        (regurgitant) —*see also* Endocarditis
      congenital NEC Q24.8
      pulmonary Q22.3
    vascular —*see* Disease, cardiovascular
  heavy chain NEC C88.2
    alpha C88.3
    gamma C88.2
    mu C88.2
  Hebra's
    pityriasis
      maculata et circinata L42
      rubra pilaris L44.0
    prurigo L28.2
  hematopoietic organs D75.9
  hemoglobin or Hb
    abnormal (mixed) NEC D58.2
      with thalassemia D56.9
    AS genotype D57.3
    Bart's D56.0
    C (Hb-C) D58.2
      with other abnormal hemoglobin NEC
          D58.2
      elliptocytosis D58.1
      Hb-S D57.2-•
      sickle-cell D57.2-•
      thalassemia D56.8
    Constant Spring D58.2
    D (Hb-D) D58.2
    E (Hb-E) D58.2

Disease, diseased *(Continued)*
  hemoglobin or Hb *(Continued)*
    E-beta thalassemia D56.5
    elliptocytosis D58.1
    H (Hb-H) (thalassemia) D56.0
      with other abnormal hemoglobin NEC
          D56.9
      Constant Spring D56.0
    I thalassemia D56.9
    M D74.0
    S or SS D57.1
    SC D57.2-•
    SD D57.8-•
    SE D57.8-•
    spherocytosis D58.0
    unstable, hemolytic D58.2
  hemolytic (newborn) P55.9
    autoimmune (cold type) (warm type) D59.1
    drug-induced D59.0
    due to or with
      incompatibility
        ABO (blood group) P55.1
        blood (group) (Duffy) (K(ell)) (Kidd)
            (Lewis) (M) (S) NEC P55.8
        Rh (blood group) (factor) P55.0
      Rh negative mother P55.0
    specified type NEC P55.8
    unstable hemoglobin D58.2
  hemorrhagic D69.9
    newborn P53
  Henoch (-Schönlein) (purpura nervosa) D69.0
  hepatic —*see* Disease, liver
  hepatobiliary K83.9
    toxic K71.9
  hepatolenticular E83.01
  heredodegenerative NEC
    spinal cord G95.89
  herpesviral, disseminated B00.7
  Hers' (glycogenosis VI) E74.09
  Herter (-Gee) (-Heubner) (nontropical sprue)
      K90.0
  Heubner-Herter (nontropical sprue) K90.0
  high fetal gene or hemoglobin thalassemia
      D56.9
  Hildenbrand's —*see* Typhus
  hip (joint) M25.9
    congenital Q65.89
    suppurative M00.9
    tuberculous A18.02
  His (-Werner) (trench fever) A79.0
  Hodgson's I71.2
    ruptured I71.1
  Holla —*see* Spherocytosis
  hookworm B76.9
    specified NEC B76.8
  host-versus-graft D89.813
    acute D89.810
    acute on chronic D89.812
    chronic D89.811
  human immunodeficiency virus (HIV) B20
  Huntington's G10
  ▶with dementia G10 *[F02.80]*
  Hutchinson's (cheiropompholyx) —*see*
      Hutchinson's disease
  hyaline (diffuse) (generalized)
    membrane (lung) (newborn) P22.0
      adult J80
  hydatid —*see* Echinococcus
  hydroxyapatite deposition M11.00
    ankle M11.07-•
    elbow M11.02-•
    foot joint M11.07-•
    hand joint M11.04-•
    hip M11.05-•
    knee M11.06-•
    multiple site M11.09
    shoulder M11.01-•
    vertebra M11.08
    wrist M11.03-•
  hyperkinetic —*see* Hyperkinesia
  hypertensive —*see* Hypertension

Disease, diseased *(Continued)*
  hypophysis E23.7
  Iceland G93.3
  I-cell E77.0
  immune D89.9
  immunoproliferative (malignant) C88.9
    small intestinal C88.3
    specified NEC C88.8
  inclusion B25.9
    salivary gland B25.9
  infectious, infective B99.9
    congenital P37.9
      specified NEC P37.8
      viral P35.9
        specified type NEC P35.8
    specified NEC B99.8
  inflammatory
    penis N48.29
      abscess N48.21
      cellulitis N48.22
    prepuce N47.7
      balanoposthitis N47.6
    tubo-ovarian —*see* Salpingo-oophoritis
  intervertebral disc —*see also* Disorder, disc
    with myelopathy —*see* Disorder, disc, with, myelopathy
    cervical, cervicothoracic —*see* Disorder, disc, cervical
      with
        myelopathy —*see* Disorder, disc, cervical, with myelopathy
        neuritis, radiculitis or radiculopathy —*see* Disorder, disc, cervical, with neuritis
        specified NEC —*see* Disorder, disc, cervical, specified type NEC
    lumbar (with)
      myelopathy M51.06
      neuritis, radiculitis, radiculopathy or sciatica M51.16
      specified NEC M51.86
    lumbosacral (with)
      neuritis, radiculitis, radiculopathy or sciatica M51.17
      specified NEC M51.87
    specified NEC —*see* Disorder, disc, specified NEC
    thoracic (with)
      myelopathy M51.04
      neuritis, radiculitis or radiculopathy M51.14
      specified NEC M51.84
    thoracolumbar (with)
      myelopathy M51.05
      neuritis, radiculitis or radiculopathy M51.15
      specified NEC M51.85
  intestine K63.9
    functional K59.9
      psychogenic F45.8
      specified NEC K59.8
    organic K63.9
    protozoal A07.9
    specified NEC K63.89
  iris H21.9
    specified NEC H21.89
  iron metabolism or storage E83.10
  island (scrub typhus) A75.3
  itai-itai —*see* Poisoning, cadmium
  Jakob-Creutzfeldt —*see* Creutzfeldt-Jakob disease or syndrome
  jaw M27.9
    fibrocystic M27.49
    specified NEC M27.8
  jigger B88.1
  joint —*see also* Disorder, joint
    Charcot's —*see* Arthropathy, neuropathic (Charcot)
    degenerative —*see* Osteoarthritis
      multiple M15.9
      spine —*see* Spondylosis

Disease, diseased *(Continued)*
  joint *(Continued)*
    hypertrophic —*see* Osteoarthritis
    sacroiliac M53.3
    specified NEC —*see* Disorder, joint, specified type NEC
    spine NEC —*see* Dorsopathy
    suppurative —*see* Arthritis, pyogenic or pyemic
  Jourdain's (acute gingivitis) K05.00
    nonplaque induced K05.01
    plaque induced K05.00
  Kaschin-Beck (endemic polyarthritis) M12.10
    ankle M12.17-●
    elbow M12.12-●
    foot joint M12.17-●
    hand joint M12.14-●
    hip M12.15-●
    knee M12.16-●
    multiple site M12.19
    shoulder M12.11-●
    vertebra M12.18
    wrist M12.13-●
  Katayama B65.2
  Kedani (scrub typhus) A75.3
  Keshan E59
  kidney (functional) (pelvis) N28.9
    chronic N18.9
      hypertensive —*see* Hypertension, kidney
      stage 1 N18.1
      stage 2 (mild) N18.2
      stage 3 (moderate) N18.3
      stage 4 (severe) N18.4
      stage 5 N18.5
    complicating pregnancy —*see* Pregnancy, complicated by, renal disease
    cystic (congenital) Q61.9
    diabetic —*see* E08-E13 with .22
    fibrocystic (congenital) Q61.8
    hypertensive —*see* Hypertension, kidney
    in (due to)
      schistosomiasis (bilharziasis) B65.9 *[N29]*
    multicystic Q61.4
    polycystic Q61.3
      adult type Q61.2
      childhood type NEC Q61.19
        collecting duct dilatation Q61.11
  Kimmelstiel (-Wilson) (intercapillary polycystic (congenital) glomerulosclerosis) —*see* E08-E13 with .21
  Kimura D21.9
    specified site (see Neoplasm, connective tissue benign)
  Kinnier Wilson's (hepatolenticular degeneration) E83.01
  kissing —*see* Mononucleosis, infectious
  Klebs' —*see also* Glomerulonephritis N05.-●
  Klippel-Feil (brevicollis) Q76.1
  Köhler-Pellegrini-Stieda (calcification, knee joint) —*see* Bursitis, tibial collateral
  Kok Q89.8
  König's (osteochondritis dissecans) —*see* Osteochondritis, dissecans
  Korsakoff's (nonalcoholic) F04
    alcoholic F10.96
      with dependence F10.26
  Kostmann's (infantile genetic agranulocytosis) D70.0
  kuru A81.81
  Kyasanur Forest A98.2
  labyrinth, ear —*see* Disorder, ear, inner
  lacrimal system —*see* Disorder, lacrimal system
  Lafora's —*see* Epilepsy, generalized, idiopathic
  Lancereaux-Mathieu (leptospiral jaundice) A27.0
  Landry's G61.0
  Larrey-Weil (leptospiral jaundice) A27.0
  larynx J38.7

Disease, diseased *(Continued)*
  legionnaires' A48.1
    nonpneumonic A48.2
  Lenegre's I44.2
  lens H27.9
    specified NEC H27.8
  Lev's (acquired complete heart block) I44.2
  Lewy body (dementia) G31.83 *[F02.80]*
    with behavioral disturbance G31.83 *[F02.81]*
  Lichtheim's (subacute combined sclerosis with pernicious anemia) D51.0
  Lightwood's (renal tubular acidosis) N25.89
  Lignac's (cystinosis) E72.04
  lip K13.0
  lipid-storage E75.6
    specified NEC E75.5
  Lipschütz's N76.6
  liver (chronic) (organic) K76.9
    alcoholic (chronic) K70.9
      acute —*see* Disease, liver, alcoholic, hepatitis
      cirrhosis K70.30
        with ascites K70.31
      failure K70.40
        with coma K70.41
      fatty liver K70.0
      fibrosis K70.2
      hepatitis K70.10
        with ascites K70.11
      sclerosis K70.2
    cystic, congenital Q44.6
    drug-induced (idiosyncratic) (toxic) (predictable) (unpredictable) —*see* Disease, liver, toxic
    end stage K72.90
      due to hepatitis —*see* Hepatitis
    fatty, nonalcoholic (NAFLD) K76.0
      alcoholic K70.0
    fibrocystic (congenital) Q44.6
    fluke
      Chinese B66.1
      oriental B66.1
      sheep B66.3
    ▶gestational alloimmune (GALD) P78.84
    glycogen storage E74.09 *[K77]*
    in (due to)
      schistosomiasis (bilharziasis) B65.9 *[K77]*
    inflammatory K75.9
      alcoholic K70.1
      specified NEC K75.89
    polycystic (congenital) Q44.6
    toxic K71.9
      with
        cholestasis K71.0
        cirrhosis (liver) K71.7
        fibrosis (liver) K71.7
        focal nodular hyperplasia K71.8
        hepatic granuloma K71.8
        hepatic necrosis K71.10
          with coma K71.11
        hepatitis NEC K71.6
          acute K71.2
          chronic
            active K71.50
              with ascites K71.51
            lobular K71.4
            persistent K71.3
          lupoid K71.50
            with ascites K71.51
        peliosis hepatis K71.8
        veno-occlusive disease (VOD) of liver K71.8
    veno-occlusive K76.5
  Lobo's (keloid blastomycosis) B48.0
  Lobstein's (brittle bones and blue sclera) Q78.0
  Ludwig's (submaxillary cellulitis) K12.2
  lumbosacral region M53.87
  lung J98.4
    black J60
    congenital Q33.9
    cystic J98.4
      congenital Q33.0

▶ New   ➡ Revised   ~~deleted~~ Deleted   ● Use Additional Character(s)

Disease, diseased *(Continued)*
  lung *(Continued)*
    fibroid (chronic) —*see* Fibrosis, lung
    fluke B66.4
      oriental B66.4
    in
      amyloidosis E85.4 *[J99]*
      sarcoidosis D86.0
      Sjögren's syndrome M35.02
      systemic
        lupus erythematosus M32.13
        sclerosis M34.81
    interstitial J84.9
      of childhood, specified NEC J84.848
      respiratory bronchiolitis J84.115
      specified NEC J84.89
    obstructive (chronic) J44.9
      with
        acute
          bronchitis J44.0
          exacerbation NEC J44.1
          lower respiratory infection J44.0
        alveolitis, allergic J67.9
        asthma J44.9
        bronchiectasis J47.9
          with
            exacerbation (acute) J47.1
            lower respiratory infection J47.0
        bronchitis J44.9
          with
            exacerbation (acute) J44.1
            lower respiratory infection J44.0
        ➠emphysema J43.9
        hypersensitivity pneumonitis J67.9
      decompensated J44.1
        with
          exacerbation (acute) J44.1
    polycystic J98.4
      congenital Q33.0
    rheumatoid (diffuse) (interstitial) —*see*
      Rheumatoid, lung
  Lutembacher's (atrial septal defect with
    mitral stenosis) Q21.1
  Lyme A69.20
  lymphatic (gland) (system) (channel) (vessel)
    I89.9
  lymphoproliferative D47.9
    specified NEC D47.Z9
    T-gamma D47.Z9
    X-linked D82.3
  Magitot's M27.2
  malarial —*see* Malaria
  malignant —*see also* Neoplasm, malignant,
    by site
  Manson's B65.1
  maple bark J67.6
  maple-syrup-urine E71.0
  Marburg (virus) A98.3
  Marion's (bladder neck obstruction) N32.0
  Marsh's (exophthalmic goiter) —*see*
    Hyperthyroidism, with, goiter (diffuse)
  mastoid (process) —*see* Disorder, ear, middle
  Mathieu's (leptospiral jaundice) A27.0
  Maxcy's A75.2
  McArdle (-Schmid-Pearson) (glycogenosis
    V) E74.04
  mediastinum J98.59
  medullary center (idiopathic) (respiratory)
    G93.89
  Meige's (chronic hereditary edema) Q82.0
  meningococcal —*see* Infection, meningococcal
  mental F99
    organic F09
  mesenchymal M35.9
  mesenteric embolic —*see also* Ischemia,
    intestine, acute K55.039
  metabolic, metabolism E88.9
    bilirubin E80.7
  metal-polisher's J62.8
  metastatic —*see also* Neoplasm, secondary, by
    site C79.9

Disease, diseased *(Continued)*
  microvascular — code to condition
  microvillus
    atrophy Q43.8
    inclusion (MVD) Q43.8
  middle ear —*see* Disorder, ear, middle
  Mikulicz' (dryness of mouth, absent or
    decreased lacrimation) K11.8
  Milroy's (chronic hereditary edema) Q82.0
  Minamata —*see* Poisoning, mercury
  minicore G71.2
  Minor's G95.19
  Minot's (hemorrhagic disease, newborn) P53
  Minot-von Willebrand-Jürgens
    (angiohemophilia) D68.0
  Mitchell's (erythromelalgia) I73.81
  mitral (valve) I05.9
    nonrheumatic I34.9
  mixed connective tissue M35.1
  moldy hay J67.0
  Monge's T70.29
  Morgagni-Adams-Stokes (syncope with heart
    block) I45.9
  Morgagni's (syndrome) (hyperostosis
    frontalis interna) M85.2
  Morton's (with metatarsalgia) —*see* Lesion,
    nerve, plantar
  Morvan's G60.8
  ➠motor neuron (bulbar) (mixed type) (spinal)
    G12.20
    amyotrophic lateral sclerosis G12.21
    ▶familial G12.24
    progressive bulbar palsy G12.22
    specified NEC G12.29
  moyamoya I67.5
  mu heavy chain disease C88.2
  multicore G71.2
  muscle —*see also* Disorder, muscle
    inflammatory —*see* Myositis
    ocular (external) —*see* Strabismus
  musculoskeletal system, soft tissue —*see also*
    Disorder, soft tissue
    specified NEC —*see* Disorder, soft tissue,
      specified type NEC
  mushroom workers' J67.5
  mycotic B49
  myelodysplastic, not classified C94.6
  myeloproliferative, not classified C94.6
    chronic D47.1
  myocardium, myocardial —*see also*
    Degeneration, myocardial I51.5
    primary (idiopathic) I42.9
  myoneural G70.9
  Naegeli's D69.1
  nails L60.9
    specified NEC L60.8
  Nairobi (sheep virus) A93.8
  nasal J34.9
  nemaline body G71.2
  nerve —*see* Disorder, nerve
  nervous system G98.8
    autonomic G90.9
    central G96.9
      specified NEC G96.8
    congenital Q07.9
    parasympathetic G90.9
    specified NEC G98.8
    sympathetic G90.9
    vegetative G90.9
  neuromuscular system G70.9
  Newcastle B30.8
  Nicolas (-Durand)-Favre (climatic bubo) A55
  nipple N64.9
    Paget's C50.01-●
      female C50.01-●
      male C50.02-●
  Nishimoto (-Takeuchi) I67.5
  nonarthropod-borne NOS (viral) B34.9
    enterovirus NEC B34.1
  nonautoimmune hemolytic D59.4
    drug-induced D59.2

Disease, diseased *(Continued)*
  Nonne-Milroy-Meige (chronic hereditary
    edema) Q82.0
  nose J34.9
  nucleus pulposus —*see* Disorder, disc
  nutritional E63.9
  oast-house-urine E72.19
    ocular
      herpesviral B00.50
      zoster B02.30
  obliterative vascular I77.1
  Ohara's —*see* Tularemia
  Opitz's (congestive splenomegaly)
    D73.2
  Oppenheim-Urbach (necrobiosis lipoidica
    diabeticorum) —*see* E08-E13 with .620
  optic nerve NEC —*see* Disorder, nerve, optic
    orbit —*see* Disorder, orbit
  Oriental liver fluke B66.1
  Oriental lung fluke B66.4
  Ormond's N13.5
  Oropouche virus A93.0
  Osler-Rendu (familial hemorrhagic
    telangiectasia) I78.0
  osteofibrocystic E21.0
  Otto's M24.7
  outer ear —*see* Disorder, ear, external
  ovary (noninflammatory) N83.9
    cystic N83.20-●
    inflammatory —*see* Salpingo-oophoritis
    polycystic E28.2
    specified NEC N83.8
  Owren's (congenital) —*see* Defect,
    coagulation
  pancreas K86.9
    cystic K86.2
    fibrocystic E84.9
    specified NEC K86.89
  panvalvular I08.9
    specified NEC I08.8
  parametrium (noninflammatory) N83.9
  parasitic B89
    cerebral NEC B71.9 *[G94]*
    intestinal NOS B82.9
    mouth B37.0
    skin NOS B88.9
    specified type —*see* Infestation
    tongue B37.0
  parathyroid (gland) E21.5
    specified NEC E21.4
  Parkinson's G20
  parodontal K05.6
  Parrot's (syphilitic osteochondritis) A50.02
  Parry's (exophthalmic goiter) —*see*
    Hyperthyroidism, with, goiter (diffuse)
  Parson's (exophthalmic goiter) —*see*
    Hyperthyroidism, with, goiter (diffuse)
  Paxton's (white piedra) B36.2
  pearl-worker's —*see* Osteomyelitis, specified
    type NEC
  Pellegrini-Stieda (calcification, knee joint) —
    see Bursitis, tibial collateral
  pelvis, pelvic
    female NOS N94.9
      specified NEC N94.89
    gonococcal (acute) (chronic) A54.24
    inflammatory (female) N73.9
      acute N73.0
      chlamydial A56.11
      chronic N73.1
      specified NEC N73.8
      syphilitic (secondary) A51.42
        late A52.76
      tuberculous A18.17
    organ, female N94.9
    peritoneum, female NEC N94.89
  penis N48.9
    inflammatory N48.29
      abscess N48.21
      cellulitis N48.22
      specified NEC N48.89

Disease, diseased (Continued)

periapical tissues NOS K04.90
periodontal K05.6
  specified NEC K05.5
periosteum —see Disorder, bone, specified
  type NEC
peripheral
  arterial I73.9
  autonomic nervous system G90.9
  nerves —see Polyneuropathy
  vascular NOS I73.9
peritoneum K66.9
  pelvic, female NEC N94.89
  specified NEC K66.8
persistent mucosal (middle ear) H66.20
  left H66.22
    with right H66.23
  right H66.21
    with left H66.23
Petit's —see Hernia, abdomen, specified site
  NEC
pharynx J39.2
  specified NEC J39.2
Phocas' —see Mastopathy, cystic
photochromogenic (acid-fast bacilli)
  (pulmonary) A31.0
  nonpulmonary A31.9
Pick's G31.01 [F02.80]
  with behavioral disturbance G31.01
    [F02.81]
  brain G31.01 [F02.80]
    with behavioral disturbance G31.01
      [F02.81]
  of pericardium (pericardial pseudocirrhosis
    of liver) I31.1
pigeon fancier's J67.2
pineal gland E34.8
pink —see Poisoning, mercury
Pinkus' (lichen nitidus) L44.1
pinworm B80
Piry virus A93.8
pituitary (gland) E23.7
pituitary-snuff-taker's J67.8
pleura (cavity) J94.9
  specified NEC J94.8
pneumatic drill (hammer) T75.21
Pollitzer's (hidradenitis suppurativa)
  L73.2
polycystic
  kidney or renal Q61.3
    adult type Q61.2
    childhood type NEC Q61.19
      collecting duct dilatation Q61.11
  liver or hepatic Q44.6
  lung or pulmonary J98.4
    congenital Q33.0
  ovary, ovaries E28.2
  spleen Q89.09
polyethylene T84.05-●
Pompe's (glycogenosis II) E74.02
Posadas-Wernicke B38.9
Potain's (pulmonary edema) —see Edema,
  lung
prepuce N47.8
  inflammatory N47.7
    balanoposthitis N47.6
Pringle's (tuberous sclerosis) Q85.1
prion, central nervous system A81.9
  specified NEC A81.89
prostate N42.9
  specified NEC N42.89
protozoal B64
  acanthamebiasis —see Acanthamebiasis
  African trypanosomiasis —see African
    trypanosomiasis
  babesiosis B60.0
  Chagas disease —see Chagas disease
  intestine, intestinal A07.9
  leishmaniasis —see Leishmaniasis
  malaria —see Malaria
  naegleriasis B60.2

Disease, diseased (Continued)

protozoal (Continued)
  pneumocystosis B59
  specified organism NEC B60.8
  toxoplasmosis —see Toxoplasmosis
pseudo-Hurler's E77.0
psychiatric F99
psychotic —see Psychosis
Puente's (simple glandular cheilitis) K13.0
puerperal —see also Puerperal O90.89
pulmonary —see also Disease, lung
  artery I28.9
  chronic obstructive J44.9
    with
      acute bronchitis J44.0
      exacerbation (acute) J44.1
      lower respiratory infection (acute)
        J44.0
    decompensated J44.1
      with
        exacerbation (acute) J44.1
  heart I27.9
    specified NEC I27.89
➡hypertensive (vascular) —see also
    Hypertension, pulmonary I27.20
  ▶primary (idiopathic) I27.0
  valve I37.9
    rheumatic I09.89
pulp (dental) NOS K04.90
pulseless M31.4
Putnam's (subacute combined sclerosis with
  pernicious anemia) D51.0
Pyle (-Cohn) (metaphyseal dysplasia) Q78.5
ragpicker's or ragsorter's A22.1
Raynaud's —see Raynaud's disease
reactive airway —see Asthma
Reclus' (cystic) —see Mastopathy, cystic
rectum K62.9
  specified NEC K62.89
Refsum's (heredopathia atactica
  polyneuritiformis) G60.1
renal (functional) (pelvis) —see also Disease,
  kidney N28.9
  with
    edema —see Nephrosis
    glomerular lesion —see
      Glomerulonephritis
      with edema —see Nephrosis
    interstitial nephritis N12
  acute N28.9
  chronic —see also Disease, kidney, chronic
    N18.9
  cystic, congenital Q61.9
  diabetic —see E08-E13 with .22
  end-stage (failure) N18.6
    due to hypertension I12.0
  fibrocystic (congenital) Q61.8
  hypertensive —see Hypertension,
    kidney
  lupus M32.14
  phosphate-losing (tubular) N25.0
  polycystic (congenital) Q61.3
    adult type Q61.2
    childhood type NEC Q61.19
      collecting duct dilatation Q61.11
  rapidly progressive N01.9
  subacute N01.9
Rendu-Osler-Weber (familial hemorrhagic
  telangiectasia) I78.0
renovascular (arteriosclerotic) —see
  Hypertension, kidney
respiratory (tract) J98.9
  acute or subacute NOS J06.9
    due to
      chemicals, gases, fumes or vapors
        (inhalation) J68.3
      external agent J70.9
        specified NEC J70.8
      radiation J70.0
      smoke inhalation J70.5
  noninfectious J39.8

Disease, diseased (Continued)

respiratory (Continued)
  chronic NOS J98.9
    due to
      chemicals, gases, fumes or vapors
        J68.4
      external agent J70.9
        specified NEC J70.8
      radiation J70.1
  newborn P27.9
    specified NEC P27.8
  due to
    chemicals, gases, fumes or vapors J68.9
      acute or subacute NEC J68.3
      chronic J68.4
    external agent J70.9
      specified NEC J70.8
  newborn P28.9
    specified type NEC P28.89
  upper J39.9
    acute or subacute J06.9
    noninfectious NEC J39.8
    specified NEC J39.8
    streptococcal J06.9
retina, retinal H35.9
  Batten's or Batten-Mayou E75.4 [H36]
  specified NEC H35.89
rheumatoid —see Arthritis, rheumatoid
rickettsial NOS A79.9
  specified type NEC A79.89
Riga (-Fede) (cachectic aphthae) K14.0
Riggs' (compound periodontitis) —see
  Periodontitis
Ritter's L00
Rivalta's (cervicofacial actinomycosis)
  A42.2
Robles' (onchocerciasis) B73.01
Roger's (congenital interventricular septal
  defect) Q21.0
Rosenthal's (factor XI deficiency) D68.1
Ross River B33.1
Rossbach's (hyperchlorhydria) K30
Rotes Quérol —see Hyperostosis, ankylosing
Roth (-Bernhardt) —see Mononeuropathy,
  lower limb, meralgia paresthetica
Runeberg's (progressive pernicious anemia)
  D51.0
sacroiliac NEC M53.3
salivary gland or duct K11.9
  inclusion B25.9
  specified NEC K11.8
  virus B25.9
sandworm B76.9
Schimmelbusch's —see Mastopathy, cystic
Schmorl's —see Schmorl's disease or nodes
Schönlein (-Henoch) (purpura rheumatica)
  D69.0
Schottmüller's —see Fever, paratyphoid
Schultz's (agranulocytosis) —see
  Agranulocytosis
Schwalbe-Ziehen-Oppenheim G24.1
Schwartz-Jampel G71.13
sclera H15.9
  specified NEC H15.89
scrofulous (tuberculous) A18.2
scrotum N50.9
sebaceous glands L73.9
semilunar cartilage, cystic —see also
  Derangement, knee, meniscus, cystic
seminal vesicle N50.9
serum NEC —see also Reaction, serum T80.69
sexually transmitted A64
  anogenital
    herpesviral infection —see Herpes,
      anogenital
    warts A63.0
  chancroid A57
  chlamydial infection —see Chlamydia
  gonorrhea —see Gonorrhea
  granuloma inguinale A58
  specified organism NEC A63.8

▶ New   ➡ Revised   ~~deleted~~ Deleted   ● Use Additional Character(s)

Disease, diseased *(Continued)*
  sexually transmitted *(Continued)*
    syphilis —*see* Syphilis
    trichomoniasis —*see* Trichomoniasis
  Sézary C84.1-●
  shimamushi (scrub typhus) A75.3
  shipyard B30.0
  sickle-cell D57.1
    with crisis (vasoocclusive pain) D57.00
      with
        acute chest syndrome D57.01
        splenic sequestration D57.02
    elliptocytosis D57.8-●
    Hb-C D57.20
      with crisis (vasoocclusive pain) D57.219
        with
          acute chest syndrome D57.211
          splenic sequestration D57.212
      without crisis D57.20
    Hb-SD D57.80
      with crisis D57.819
        with
          acute chest syndrome D57.811
          splenic sequestration D57.812
    Hb-SE D57.80
      with crisis D57.819
        with
          acute chest syndrome D57.811
          splenic sequestration D57.812
    specified NEC D57.80
      with crisis D57.819
        with
          acute chest syndrome D57.811
          splenic sequestration D57.812
    spherocytosis D57.80
      with crisis D57.819
        with
          acute chest syndrome D57.811
          splenic sequestration D57.812
    thalassemia D57.40
      with crisis (vasoocclusive pain) D57.419
        with
          acute chest syndrome D57.411
          splenic sequestration D57.412
      without crisis D57.40
  silo-filler's J68.8
    bronchitis J68.0
    pneumonitis J68.0
    pulmonary edema J68.1
  simian B B00.4
  Simons' (progressive lipodystrophy) E88.1
  sin nombre virus B33.4
  sinus —*see* Sinusitis
  Sirkari's B55.0
  sixth B08.20
    due to human herpesvirus 6 B08.21
    due to human herpesvirus 7 B08.22
  skin L98.9
    due to metabolic disorder NEC E88.9
      [L99]
    specified NEC L98.8
  slim (HIV) B20
  small vessel I73.9
  Sneddon-Wilkinson (subcorneal pustular
    dermatosis) L13.1
  South African creeping B88.0
  spinal (cord) G95.9
    congenital Q06.9
    specified NEC G95.89
  spine —*see also* Spondylopathy
    joint —*see* Dorsopathy
    tuberculous A18.01
  spinocerebellar (hereditary) G11.9
    specified NEC G11.8
  spleen D73.9
    amyloid E85.4 *[D77]*
    organic D73.9
    polycystic Q89.09
    postinfectional D73.89
  sponge-diver's —*see* Toxicity, venom, marine
    animal, sea anemone

Disease, diseased *(Continued)*
  Startle Q89.8
  Steinert's G71.11
  Sticker's (erythema infectiosum) B08.3
  Stieda's (calcification, knee joint) —*see*
    Bursitis, tibial collateral
  Stokes' (exophthalmic goiter) —*see*
    Hyperthyroidism, with, goiter (diffuse)
  Stokes-Adams (syncope with heart block)
    I45.9
  stomach K31.9
    functional, psychogenic F45.8
    specified NEC K31.89
  stonemason's J62.8
  storage
    glycogen —*see* Disease, glycogen storage
    mucopolysaccharide —*see*
      Mucopolysaccharidosis
  striatopallidal system NEC G25.89
  Stuart-Prower (congenital factor X deficiency)
    D68.2
  Stuart's (congenital factor X deficiency) D68.2
  subcutaneous tissue —*see* Disease, skin
  supporting structures of teeth K08.9
    specified NEC K08.89
  suprarenal (capsule) (gland) E27.9
    hyperfunction E27.0
    specified NEC E27.8
  sweat glands L74.9
    specified NEC L74.8
  Sweeley-Klionsky E75.21
  Swift (-Feer) —*see* Poisoning, mercury
  swimming-pool granuloma A31.1
  Sylvest's (epidemic pleurodynia) B33.0
  sympathetic nervous system G90.9
  synovium —*see* Disorder, synovium
  syphilitic —*see* Syphilis
⇒ systemic tissue mast cell C96.20
  tanapox (virus) B08.71
  Tangier E78.6
  Tarral-Besnier (pityriasis rubra pilaris) L44.0
  Tauri's E74.09
  tear duct —*see* Disorder, lacrimal system
  tendon, tendinous —*see also* Disorder, tendon
    nodular —*see* Trigger finger
  terminal vessel I73.9
  testis N50.9
  thalassemia Hb-S —*see* Disease, sickle-cell,
    thalassemia
  Thaysen-Gee (nontropical sprue) K90.0
  Thomsen G71.12
  throat J39.2
    septic J02.0
  thromboembolic —*see* Embolism
  thymus (gland) E32.9
    specified NEC E32.8
  thyroid (gland) E07.9
    heart —*see also* Hyperthyroidism E05.90
      [I43]
      with thyroid storm E05.91 *[I43]*
    specified NEC E07.8
  Tietze's M94.0
  tongue K14.9
    specified NEC K14.89
  tonsils, tonsillar (and adenoids) J35.9
  tooth, teeth K08.9
    hard tissues K03.9
      specified NEC K03.89
    pulp NEC K04.99
    specified NEC K08.89
  Tourette's F95.2
  trachea NEC J39.8
  tricuspid I07.9
    nonrheumatic I36.9
  triglyceride-storage E75.5
  trophoblastic —*see* Mole, hydatidiform
  tsutsugamushi A75.3
  tube (fallopian) (noninflammatory) N83.9
    inflammatory —*see* Salpingitis
    specified NEC N83.8
  tuberculous NEC —*see* Tuberculosis

Disease, diseased *(Continued)*
  tubo-ovarian (noninflammatory) N83.9
    inflammatory —*see* Salpingo-oophoritis
    specified NEC N83.8
  tubotympanic, chronic —*see* Otitis, media,
    suppurative, chronic, tubotympanic
  tubulo-interstitial N15.9
    specified NEC N15.8
  tympanum —*see* Disorder, tympanic
    membrane
  Uhl's Q24.8
  Underwood's (sclerema neonatorum) P83.0
  Unverricht (-Lundborg) —*see* Epilepsy,
    generalized, idiopathic
  Urbach-Oppenheim (necrobiosis lipoidica
    diabeticorum) —*see* E08-E13 with .620
  ureter N28.9
    in (due to)
      schistosomiasis (bilharziasis) B65.0 *[N29]*
  urethra N36.9
    specified NEC N36.8
  urinary (tract) N39.9
    bladder N32.9
      specified NEC N32.89
    specified NEC N39.8
  uterus (noninflammatory) N85.9
    infective —*see* Endometritis
    inflammatory —*see* Endometritis
    specified NEC N85.8
  uveal tract (anterior) H21.9
    posterior H31.9
  vagabond's B85.1
  vagina, vaginal (noninflammatory) N89.9
    inflammatory NEC N76.89
    specified NEC N89.8
  valve, valvular I38
    multiple I08.9
      specified NEC I08.8
  van Creveld-von Gierke (glycogenosis I)
    E74.01
  vas deferens N50.9
  vascular I99.9
    arteriosclerotic —*see* Arteriosclerosis
    ciliary body NEC —*see* Disorder, iris,
      vascular
    hypertensive —*see* Hypertension
    iris NEC —*see* Disorder, iris, vascular
    obliterative I77.1
      peripheral I73.9
    occlusive I99.8
    peripheral (occlusive) I73.9
      in diabetes mellitus —*see* E08-E13 with .51
  vasomotor I73.9
  vasospastic I73.9
  vein I87.9
  venereal —*see also* Disease, sexually
    transmitted A64
    chlamydial NEC A56.8
      anus A56.3
      genitourinary NOS A56.2
      pharynx A56.4
      rectum A56.3
    fifth A55
    sixth A55
    specified nature or type NEC A63.8
  vertebra, vertebral —*see also* Spondylopathy
    disc —*see* Disorder, disc
  vibration —*see* Vibration, adverse effects
  viral, virus —*see also* Disease, by type of virus
    B34.9
    arbovirus NOS A94
    arthropod-borne NOS A94
    congenital P35.9
      specified NEC P35.8
    Hanta (with renal manifestations)
      (Dobrava) (Puumala) (Seoul) A98.5
      with pulmonary manifestations (Andes)
        (Bayou) (Bermejo) (Black Creek
        Canal) (Choclo) (Juquitiba) (Laguna
        negra) (Lechiguanas) (New York)
        (Oran) (Sin nombre) B33.4

Disease, diseased *(Continued)*
  viral, virus *(Continued)*
    Hantaan (Korean hemorrhagic fever) A98.5
    human immunodeficiency (HIV) B20
    Kunjin A83.4
    nonarthropod-borne NOS B34.9
    Powassan A84.8
    Rocio (encephalitis) A83.6
    Sin nombre (Hantavirus) (cardio)-
        pulmonary syndrome B33.4
    Tahyna B33.8
    vesicular stomatitis A93.8
  vitreous H43.9
    specified NEC H43.89
  vocal cord J38.3
  Volkmann's, acquired T79.6
  von Eulenburg's (congenital paramyotonia)
      G71.19
  von Gierke's (glycogenosis I) E74.01
  von Graefe's —*see* Strabismus, paralytic,
      ophthalmoplegia, progressive
  von Willebrand (-Jürgens) (angiohemophilia)
      D68.0
  Vrolik's (osteogenesis imperfecta) Q78.0
  vulva (noninflammatory) N90.9
    inflammatory NEC N76.89
    specified NEC N90.89
  Wallgren's (obstruction of splenic vein with
      collateral circulation) I87.8
  Wassilieff's (leptospiral jaundice) A27.0
  wasting NEC R64
    due to malnutrition E41
  Waterhouse-Friderichsen A39.1
  Wegner's (syphilitic osteochondritis) A50.02
  Weil's (leptospiral jaundice of lung) A27.0
  Weir Mitchell's (erythromelalgia) I73.81
  Werdnig-Hoffmann G12.0
  Wermer's E31.21
  Werner-His (trench fever) A79.0
  Werner-Schultz (neutropenic splenomegaly)
      D73.81
  Wernicke-Posadas B38.9
  whipworm B79
  white blood cells D72.9
    specified NEC D72.89
  white matter R90.82
  white-spot, meaning lichen sclerosus et
      atrophicus L90.0
    penis N48.0
    vulva N90.4
  Wilkie's K55.1
  Wilkinson-Sneddon (subcorneal pustular
      dermatosis) L13.1
  Willis' —*see* Diabetes
  Wilson's (hepatolenticular degeneration)
      E83.01
  woolsorter's A22.1
  yaba monkey tumor B08.72
  yaba pox (virus) B08.72
  Zika virus A92.5
  zoonotic, bacterial A28.9
    specified type NEC A28.8
Disfigurement (due to scar) L90.5
Disgerminoma —*see* Dysgerminoma
DISH (diffuse idiopathic skeletal
    hyperostosis) —*see* Hyperostosis,
    ankylosing
Disinsertion, retina —*see* Detachment, retina
Dislocatable hip, congenital Q65.6
Dislocation (articular)
  with fracture —*see* Fracture
  acromioclavicular (joint) S43.10-●
    with displacement
      100%-200% S43.12-●
      more than 200% S43.13-●
    inferior S43.14-●
    posterior S43.15-●
  ankle S93.0-●
  astragalus —*see* Dislocation, ankle
  atlantoaxial S13.121
  atlantooccipital S13.111

Dislocation *(Continued)*
  atloidooccipital S13.111
  breast bone S23.29
  capsule, joint code by site under Dislocation
  carpal (bone) —*see* Dislocation, wrist
  carpometacarpal (joint) NEC S63.05-●
    thumb S63.04-●
  cartilage (joint) - code by site under
    Dislocation
  cervical spine (vertebra) —*see* Dislocation,
    vertebra, cervical
  chronic —*see* Dislocation, recurrent
  clavicle —*see* Dislocation, acromioclavicular
    joint
  coccyx S33.2
  congenital NEC Q68.8
  coracoid —*see* Dislocation, shoulder
  costal cartilage S23.29
  costochondral S23.29
  cricoarytenoid articulation S13.29
  cricothyroid articulation S13.29
  dorsal vertebra —*see* Dislocation, vertebra,
    thoracic
  ear ossicle —*see* Discontinuity, ossicles, ear
  elbow S53.10-●
    congenital Q68.8
    pathological —*see* Dislocation, pathological
      NEC, elbow
    radial head alone —*see* Dislocation, radial
      head
    recurrent —*see* Dislocation, recurrent,
      elbow
    traumatic S53.10-●
      anterior S53.11-●
      lateral S53.14-●
      medial S53.13-●
      posterior S53.12-●
      specified type NEC S53.19-●
  eye, nontraumatic —*see* Luxation, globe
  eyeball, nontraumatic —*see* Luxation, globe
  femur
    distal end —*see* Dislocation, knee
    proximal end —*see* Dislocation, hip
  fibula
    distal end —*see* Dislocation, ankle
    proximal end —*see* Dislocation, knee
  finger S63.25-●
    index S63.25-●
    interphalangeal S63.27-●
      distal S63.29-●
        index S63.29-●
        little S63.29-●
        middle S63.29-●
        ring S63.29-●
      index S63.27-●
      little S63.27-●
      middle S63.27-●
      proximal S63.28-●
        index S63.28-●
        little S63.28-●
        middle S63.28-●
        ring S63.28-●
      ring S63.27-●
    little S63.25-●
    metacarpophalangeal S63.26-●
      index S63.26-●
      little S63.26-●
      middle S63.26-●
      ring S63.26-●
    middle S63.25-●
    recurrent —*see* Dislocation, recurrent,
      finger
    ring S63.25-●
    thumb —*see* Dislocation, thumb
  foot S93.30-●
    recurrent —*see* Dislocation, recurrent,
      foot
    specified site NEC S93.33-●
    tarsal joint S93.31-●
    tarsometatarsal joint S93.32-●
    toe —*see* Dislocation, toe

Dislocation *(Continued)*
  fracture —*see* Fracture
  glenohumeral (joint) —*see* Dislocation,
    shoulder
  glenoid —*see* Dislocation, shoulder
  habitual —*see* Dislocation, recurrent
  hip S73.00-●
    anterior S73.03-●
      obturator S73.02-●
    central S73.04-●
    congenital (total) Q65.2
      bilateral Q65.1
      partial Q65.5
        bilateral Q65.4
        unilateral Q65.3-●
      unilateral Q65.0-●
    developmental M24.85-●
    pathological —*see* Dislocation, pathological
      NEC, hip
    posterior S73.01-●
    recurrent —*see* Dislocation, recurrent,
      hip
  humerus, proximal end —*see* Dislocation,
    shoulder
  incomplete —*see* Subluxation, by site
  incus —*see* Discontinuity, ossicles, ear
  infracoracoid —*see* Dislocation, shoulder
  innominate (pubic junction) (sacral junction)
    S33.39
    acetabulum —*see* Dislocation, hip
  interphalangeal (joint(s))
    finger S63.279
      distal S63.29-●
        index S63.29-●
        little S63.29-●
        middle S63.29-●
        ring S63.29-●
      index S63.27-●
      little S63.27-●
      middle S63.27-●
      proximal S63.28-●
        index S63.28-●
        little S63.28-●
        middle S63.28-●
        ring S63.28-●
      ring S63.27-●
    foot or toe —*see* Dislocation, toe
    thumb S63.12-●
      distal joint S63.14-●
      proximal joint S63.13-●
  jaw (cartilage) (meniscus) S03.0-●
  joint prosthesis —*see* Complications, joint
    prosthesis, mechanical, displacement,
    by site
  knee S83.106
    cap —*see* Dislocation, patella
    congenital Q68.2
    old M23.8X-●
    patella —*see* Dislocation, patella
    pathological —*see* Dislocation, pathological
      NEC, knee
    proximal tibia
      anteriorly S83.11-●
      laterally S83.14-●
      medially S83.13-●
      posteriorly S83.12-●
    recurrent —*see also* Derangement, knee,
      specified NEC
    specified type NEC S83.19-●
  lacrimal gland H04.16-●
  lens (complete) H27.10-●
    anterior H27.12-●
    congenital Q12.1
    ocular implant —*see* Complications,
      intraocular lens
    partial H27.11-●
    posterior H27.13-●
    traumatic S05.8X-●
  ligament code by site under Dislocation
  lumbar (vertebra) —*see* Dislocation, vertebra,
    lumbar

Dislocation *(Continued)*
  lumbosacral (vertebra) —*see also* Dislocation,
    vertebra, lumbar
    congenital Q76.49
  mandible S03.0-●
  meniscus (knee) —*see* Tear, meniscus
    other sites code by site under Dislocation
  metacarpal (bone)
    distal end —*see* Dislocation, finger
    proximal end S63.06-●
  metacarpophalangeal (joint)
    finger S63.26-●
      index S63.26-●
      little S63.26-●
      middle S63.26-●
      ring S63.26-●
      thumb S63.11-●
  metatarsal (bone) —*see* Dislocation, foot
  metatarsophalangeal (joint(s)) —*see*
    Dislocation, toe
  midcarpal (joint) S63.03-●
  midtarsal (joint) —*see* Dislocation, foot
  neck S13.20
    specified site NEC S13.29
    vertebra —*see* Dislocation, vertebra,
      cervical
  nose (septal cartilage) S03.1
  occipitoatloid S13.111
  old —*see* Derangement, joint, specified type
    NEC
  ossicles, ear —*see* Discontinuity, ossicles, ear
  partial —*see* Subluxation, by site
  patella S83.006
    congenital Q74.1
    lateral S83.01-●
    recurrent (nontraumatic) M22.0-●
      incomplete M22.1-●
    specified type NEC S83.09-●
  pathological NEC M24.30
    ankle M24.37-●
    elbow M24.32-●
    foot joint M24.37-●
    hand joint M24.34-●
    hip M24.35-●
    knee M24.36-●
    lumbosacral joint —*see* subcategory M53.2
    pelvic region —*see* Dislocation,
      pathological, hip
    sacroiliac —*see* subcategory M53.2
    shoulder M24.31-●
    wrist M24.33-●
  pelvis NEC S33.30
    specified NEC S33.39
  phalanx
    finger or hand —*see* Dislocation, finger
    foot or toe —*see* Dislocation, toe
  prosthesis, internal —*see* Complications,
    prosthetic device, by site, mechanical
  radial head S53.006
    anterior S53.01-●
    posterior S53.02-●
    specified type NEC S53.09-●
  radiocarpal (joint) S63.02-●
  radiohumeral (joint) —*see* Dislocation, radial
    head
  radioulnar (joint)
    distal S63.01-●
    proximal —*see* Dislocation, elbow
  radius
    distal end —*see* Dislocation, wrist
    proximal end —*see* Dislocation, radial head
  recurrent M24.40
    ankle M24.47-●
    elbow M24.42-●
    finger M24.44-●
    foot joint M24.47-●
    hand joint M24.44-●
    hip M24.45-●
    knee M24.46-●
      patella —*see* Dislocation, patella,
        recurrent

Dislocation *(Continued)*
  recurrent *(Continued)*
    patella —*see* Dislocation, patella, recurrent
    sacroiliac —*see* subcategory M53.2
    shoulder M24.41-●
    toe M24.47-●
    vertebra —*see also* subcategory M43.5
      atlantoaxial M43.4
        with myelopathy M43.3
    wrist M24.43-●
  rib (cartilage) S23.29
  sacrococcygeal S33.2
  sacroiliac (joint) (ligament) S33.2
    congenital Q74.2
    recurrent —*see* subcategory M53.2
  sacrum S33.2
  scaphoid (bone) (hand) (wrist) —*see*
    Dislocation, wrist
    foot —*see* Dislocation, foot
  scapula —*see* Dislocation, shoulder, girdle,
    scapula
  semilunar cartilage, knee —*see* Tear, meniscus
  septal cartilage (nose) S03.1
  septum (nasal) (old) J34.2
  sesamoid bone code by site under Dislocation
  shoulder (blade) (ligament) (joint) (traumatic)
    S43.006
    acromioclavicular —*see* Dislocation,
      acromioclavicular
    chronic —*see* Dislocation, recurrent,
      shoulder
    congenital Q68.8
    girdle S43.30-●
      scapula S43.31-●
      specified site NEC S43.39-●
    humerus S43.00-●
      anterior S43.01-●
      inferior S43.03-●
      posterior S43.02-●
    pathological —*see* Dislocation, pathological
      NEC, shoulder
    recurrent —*see* Dislocation, recurrent,
      shoulder
    specified type NEC S43.08-●
  spine
    cervical —*see* Dislocation, vertebra, cervical
    congenital Q76.49
    due to birth trauma P11.5
    lumbar —*see* Dislocation, vertebra, lumbar
    thoracic —*see* Dislocation, vertebra,
      thoracic
  spontaneous —*see* Dislocation, pathological
  sternoclavicular (joint) S43.206
    anterior S43.21-●
    posterior S43.22-●
  sternum S23.29
  subglenoid —*see* Dislocation, shoulder
  symphysis pubis S33.4
  talus —*see* Dislocation, ankle
  tarsal (bone(s)) (joint(s)) —*see* Dislocation,
    foot
  tarsometatarsal (joint(s)) —*see* Dislocation,
    foot
  temporomandibular (joint) S03.0-●
  thigh, proximal end —*see* Dislocation, hip
  thorax S23.20
    specified site NEC S23.29
    vertebra —*see* Dislocation, vertebra
  thumb S63.10-●
    interphalangeal joint —*see* Dislocation,
      interphalangeal (joint), thumb
    metacarpophalangeal joint —*see*
      Dislocation, metacarpophalangeal
      (joint), thumb
  thyroid cartilage S13.29
  tibia
    distal end —*see* Dislocation, ankle
    proximal end —*see* Dislocation, knee
  tibiofibular (joint)
    distal —*see* Dislocation, ankle
    superior —*see* Dislocation, knee

Dislocation *(Continued)*
  toe(s) S93.106
    great S93.10-●
      interphalangeal joint S93.11-●
      metatarsophalangeal joint S93.12-●
    interphalangeal joint S93.119
    lesser S93.106
      interphalangeal joint S93.11-●
      metatarsophalangeal joint S93.12-●
    metatarsophalangeal joint S93.12-●
  tooth S03.2
  trachea S23.29
  ulna
    distal end S63.07-●
    proximal end —*see* Dislocation, elbow
  ulnohumeral (joint) —*see* Dislocation, elbow
  vertebra (articular process) (body)
    (traumatic)
    cervical S13.101
      atlantoaxial joint S13.121
      atlantooccipital joint S13.111
      atloidooccipital joint S13.111
      joint between
        C0 and C1 S13.111
        C1 and C2 S13.121
        C2 and C3 S13.131
        C3 and C4 S13.141
        C4 and C5 S13.151
        C5 and C6 S13.161
        C6 and C7 S13.171
        C7 and T1 S13.181
      occipitoatloid joint S13.111
    congenital Q76.49
    lumbar S33.101
      joint between
        L1 and L2 S33.111
        L2 and L3 S33.121
        L3 and L4 S33.131
        L4 and L5 S33.141
    nontraumatic —*see* Displacement,
      intervertebral disc
    partial —*see* Subluxation, by site
    recurrent NEC —*see* subcategory
      M43.5
    thoracic S23.101
      joint between
        T1 and T2 S23.111
        T2 and T3 S23.121
        T3 and T4 S23.123
        T4 and T5 S23.131
        T5 and T6 S23.133
        T6 and T7 S23.141
        T7 and T8 S23.143
        T8 and T9 S23.151
        T9 and T10 S23.153
        T10 and T11 S23.161
        T11 and T12 S23.163
        T12 and L1 S23.171
  wrist (carpal bone) S63.006
    carpometacarpal joint —*see* Dislocation,
      carpometacarpal (joint)
    distal radioulnar joint —*see* Dislocation,
      radioulnar (joint), distal
    metacarpal bone, proximal —*see*
      Dislocation, metacarpal (bone),
      proximal end
    midcarpal —*see* Dislocation, midcarpal
      (joint)
    radiocarpal joint —*see* Dislocation,
      radiocarpal (joint)
    recurrent —*see* Dislocation, recurrent,
      wrist
    specified site NEC S63.09-●
    ulna —*see* Dislocation, ulna, distal end
  xiphoid cartilage S23.29
Disorder (of) —*see also* Disease
  acantholytic L11.9
    specified NEC L11.8
  acute
    psychotic —*see* Psychosis, acute
    stress F43.0

▶ New   ⟹ Revised   ~~deleted~~ Deleted   ● Use Additional Character(s)

Disorder (*Continued*)
  avoidant
    child or adolescent F40.10
    ⇒restrictive food intake F50.82
  balance
    acid-base E87.8
      mixed E87.4
    electrolyte E87.8
    fluid NEC E87.8
  behavioral (disruptive) —*see* Disorder,
      conduct
  beta-amino-acid metabolism E72.8
  bile acid and cholesterol metabolism E78.70
    Barth syndrome E78.71
    other specified E78.79
    Smith-Lemli-Opitz syndrome E78.72
  bilirubin excretion E80.6
  binge eating F50.81
  binocular
    movement H51.9
      convergence
        excess H51.12
        insufficiency H51.11
      internuclear ophthalmoplegia —*see*
        Ophthalmoplegia, internuclear
      palsy of conjugate gaze H51.0
      specified type NEC H51.8
    vision NEC —*see* Disorder, vision, binocular
  ⇒bipolar (I) (type 1) F31.9
    ~~current episode~~
      ~~depressed F31.9~~
        ~~with psychotic features F31.5~~
        ~~without psychotic features~~
          ~~F31.30~~
          ~~mild F31.31~~
          ~~moderate F31.32~~
          ~~severe (without psychotic features)~~
            ~~F31.4~~
            ~~with psychotic features F31.5~~
      ~~hypomanic F31.0~~
      ~~manic F31.9~~
        ~~with psychotic features F31.2~~
        ~~without psychotic features F31.10~~
          ~~mild F31.11~~
          ~~moderate F31.12~~
          ~~severe (without psychotic features)~~
            ~~F31.13~~
            ~~with psychotic features F31.2~~
      ~~mixed F31.60~~
        ~~mild F31.61~~
        ~~moderate F31.62~~
        ~~severe (without psychotic features)~~
          ~~F31.63~~
          ~~with psychotic features F31.64~~
        ~~severe depression (without psychotic~~
          ~~features) F31.4~~
          ~~with psychotic features F31.5~~
    ▶and related due to a known physiological
        condition
      ▶with
        ▶manic features F06.33
        ▶manic- or hypomanic-like episodes
          F06.33
        ▶mixed features F06.34
    ▶current (or most recent) episode
      ▶depressed F31.9
        ▶with psychotic features F31.5
        ▶without psychotic features F31.30
          ▶mild F31.31
          ▶moderate F31.32
          ▶severe (without psychotic features)
            F31.4
            ▶with psychotic features F31.5
      ▶hypomanic F31.0
      ▶manic F31.9
        ▶with psychotic features F31.2
        ▶without psychotic features F31.10
          ▶mild F31.11
          ▶moderate F31.12
          ▶severe (without psychotic features)
            F31.13
            ▶with psychotic features F31.2

Disorder (*Continued*)
  bipolar (I) (type 1) (*Continued*)
    current (or most recent) episode (*Continued*)
      ▶mixed F31.60
        ▶mild F31.61
        ▶moderate F31.62
        ▶severe (without psychotic features)
          F31.63
          ▶with psychotic features F31.64
        ▶severe depression (without psychotic
          features) F31.4
          ▶with psychotic features F31.5
    ⇒II (type 2) F31.81
    in remission (currently) F31.70
      in full remission
        most recent episode
          depressed F31.76
          hypomanic F31.72
          manic F31.74
          mixed F31.78
      in partial remission
        most recent episode
          depressed F31.75
          hypomanic F31.71
          manic F31.73
          mixed F31.77
    organic F06.30
    single manic episode F30.9
      mild F30.11
      moderate F30.12
      hhsevere (without psychotic symptoms)
        F30.13
        with psychotic symptoms F30.2
    specified NEC F31.89
  bladder N32.9
    functional NEC N31.9
    in schistosomiasis B65.0 [*N33*]
    specified NEC N32.89
  bleeding D68.9
  blood D75.9
    in congenital early syphilis A50.09 [*D77*]
  body dysmorphic F45.22
  bone M89.9
    continuity M84.9
      specified type NEC M84.80
        ankle M84.87-●
        fibula M84.86-●
        foot M84.87-●
        hand M84.84-●
        humerus M84.82-●
        neck M84.88
        pelvis M84.859
        radius M84.83-●
        rib M84.88
        shoulder M84.81-●
        skull M84.85
        thigh M84.85-●
        tibia M84.86-●
        ulna M84.83-●
        vertebra M84.88
    density and structure M85.9
      cyst —*see also* Cyst, bone, specified type
          NEC
        aneurysmal —*see* Cyst, bone,
            aneurysmal
        solitary —*see* Cyst, bone, solitary
      diffuse idiopathic skeletal
          hyperostosis —*see* Hyperostosis,
          ankylosing
      fibrous dysplasia (monostotic) —*see*
          Dysplasia, fibrous, bone
      fluorosis —*see* Fluorosis, skeletal
      hyperostosis of skull M85.2
      osteitis condensans —*see* Osteitis,
          condensans
      specified type NEC M85.8-●
        ankle M85.87-●
        foot M85.87-●
        forearm M85.83-●
        hand M85.84-●
        lower leg M85.86-●

Disorder (*Continued*)
  bone (*Continued*)
    density and structure (*Continued*)
      specified type NEC (*Continued*)
        multiple sites M85.89
        neck M85.88
        rib M85.88
        shoulder M85.81-●
        skull M85.88
        thigh M85.85-●
        upper arm M85.82-●
        vertebra M85.88
    development and growth NEC M89.20
      carpus M89.24-●
      clavicle M89.21-●
      femur M89.25-●
      fibula M89.26-●
      finger M89.24-●
      humerus M89.22-●
      ilium M89.259
      ischium M89.259
      metacarpus M89.24-●
      metatarsus M89.27-●
      multiple sites M89.29
      neck M89.28
      radius M89.23-●
      rib M89.28
      scapula M89.21-●
      skull M89.28
      tarsus M89.27-●
      tibia M89.26-●
      toe M89.27-●
      ulna M89.23-●
      vertebra M89.28
    specified type NEC M89.8X-●
  brachial plexus G54.0
  branched-chain amino-acid metabolism E71.2
    specified NEC E71.19
  breast N64.9
    agalactia —*see* Agalactia
    associated with
      lactation O92.70
        specified NEC O92.79
      pregnancy O92.20
        specified NEC O92.29
      puerperium O92.20
        specified NEC O92.29
    cracked nipple —*see* Cracked nipple
    galactorrhea —*see* Galactorrhea
    hypogalactia O92.4
    lactation disorder NEC O92.79
    mastitis —*see* Mastitis
    nipple infection —*see* Infection, nipple
    retracted nipple —*see* Retraction, nipple
    specified type NEC N64.89
  Briquet's F45.0
  bullous, in diseases classified elsewhere L14
  caffeine use
    mild
      with
        caffeine-induced
          anxiety disorder F15.180
          sleep disorder F15.182
    moderate or severe
      with
        caffeine-induced
          anxiety disorder F15.280
          sleep disorder F15.282
  cannabis use
    mild F12.10
      with
        cannabis-induced
          anxiety disorder F12.180
          psychotic disorder F12.159
          sleep disorder F12.188
        cannabis intoxication delirium F12.121
          with perceptual disturbances
            F12.122
          without perceptual disturbances
            F12.129
      ▶in remission (early) (sustained) F12.11

Disorder *(Continued)*
  cannabis use *(Continued)*
    moderate or severe F12.20
      with
        cannabis-induced
          anxiety disorder F12.280
          psychotic disorder F12.259
          sleep disorder F12.288
        cannabis intoxication
          with perceptual disturbances F12.222
          without perceptual disturbances F12.229
        delirium F12.221
      ▶in remission (early) (sustained) F12.21
  carbohydrate
    absorption, intestinal NEC E74.39
    metabolism (congenital) E74.9
      specified NEC E74.8
  cardiac, functional I51.89
  carnitine metabolism E71.40
  cartilage M94.9
    articular NEC —*see* Derangement, joint, articular cartilage
    chondrocalcinosis —*see* Chondrocalcinosis
    specified type NEC M94.8X-●
      articular —*see* Derangement, joint, articular cartilage
      multiple sites M94.8X0
  catatonia (due to known physiological condition) (with another mental disorder) F06.1
  catatonic
    due to (secondary to) known physiological condition F06.1
    organic F06.1
  central auditory processing H93.25
  cervical
    region NEC M53.82
    root (nerve) NEC G54.2
  character NOS F60.9
  childhood disintegrative NEC F84.3
  cholesterol and bile acid metabolism E78.70
    Barth syndrome E78.71
    other specified E78.79
    Smith-Lemli-Opitz syndrome E78.72
  choroid H31.9
    atrophy —*see* Atrophy, choroid
    degeneration —*see* Degeneration, choroid
    detachment —*see* Detachment, choroid
    dystrophy —*see* Dystrophy, choroid
    hemorrhage —*see* Hemorrhage, choroid
    rupture —*see* Rupture, choroid
    scar —*see* Scar, chorioretinal
    solar retinopathy —*see* Retinopathy, solar
    specified type NEC H31.8
  ciliary body —*see* Disorder, iris
    degeneration —*see* Degeneration, ciliary body
  coagulation (factor) (*see also* Defect, coagulation) D68.9
    newborn, transient P61.6
  cocaine use
    mild F14.10
      with
        amphetamine, cocaine, or other stimulant intoxication
          with perceptual disturbances F14.122
          without perceptual disturbances F14.129
        cocaine-induced
          anxiety disorder F14.180
          bipolar and related disorder F14.14
          depressive disorder F14.14
          obsessive-compulsive and related disorder F14.188
          psychotic disorder F14.159
          sexual dysfunction F14.181
          sleep disorder F14.182
        cocaine intoxication delirium F14.121
    ▶in remission (early) (sustained) F14.11

Disorder *(Continued)*
  cocaine use *(Continued)*
    moderate or severe F14.20
      with
        amphetamine, cocaine, or other stimulant intoxication
          with perceptual disturbances F14.222
          without perceptual disturbances F14.229
        cocaine-induced
          anxiety disorder F14.280
          bipolar and related disorder F14.24
          depressive disorder F14.24
          obsessive-compulsive and related disorder F14.288
          psychotic disorder F14.259
          sexual dysfunction F14.281
          sleep disorder F14.282
        cocaine intoxication delirium F14.221
    ▶in remission (early) (sustained) F14.21
  coccyx NEC M53.3
  cognitive F09
    due to (secondary to) general medical condition F09
    persisting R41.89
      due to
        alcohol F10.97
          with dependence F10.27
        anxiolytics F13.97
          with dependence F13.27
        hypnotics F13.97
          with dependence F13.27
        sedatives F13.97
          with dependence F13.27
        specified substance NEC F19.97
          with
            abuse F19.17
            dependence F19.27
  communication F80.9
    social pragmatic F80.82
  conduct (childhood) F91.9
    adjustment reaction —*see* Disorder, adjustment
    adolescent onset type F91.2
    childhood onset type F91.1
    compulsive F63.9
    confined to family context F91.0
    depressive F91.8
    group type F91.2
    hyperkinetic —*see* Disorder, attention-deficit hyperactivity
    oppositional defiance F91.3
    socialized F91.2
    solitary aggressive type F91.1
    specified NEC F91.8
    unsocialized (aggressive) F91.1
  conduction, heart I45.9
  congenital glycosylation (CDG) E74.8
  conjunctiva H11.9
    infection —*see* Conjunctivitis
  connective tissue, localized L94.9
    specified NEC L94.8
  conversion (functional neurological symptom disorder)
    with
      abnormal movement F44.4
      anesthesia or sensory loss F44.6
      attacks or seizures F44.5
      mixed symptoms F44.7
      special sensory symptoms F44.6
      speech symptoms F44.4
      swallowing symptoms F44.4
      weakness or paralysis F44.4
  convulsive (secondary) —*see* Convulsions
  cornea H18.9
    deformity —*see* Deformity, cornea
    degeneration —*see* Degeneration, cornea
    deposits —*see* Deposit, cornea
    due to contact lens H18.82-●
      specified as edema —*see* Edema, cornea
    edema —*see* Edema, cornea

Disorder *(Continued)*
  cornea *(Continued)*
    keratitis —*see* Keratitis
    keratoconjunctivitis —*see* Keratoconjunctivitis
    membrane change —*see* Change, corneal membrane
    neovascularization —*see* Neovascularization, cornea
    scar —*see* Opacity, cornea
    specified type NEC H18.89-●
    ulcer —*see* Ulcer, cornea
  corpus cavernosum N48.9
  cranial nerve —*see* Disorder, nerve, cranial
  cyclothymic F34.0
  defiant oppositional F91.3
  delusional (persistent) (systematized) F22
    induced F24
  depersonalization F48.1
  depressive F32.9
  ▶due to known physiological condition
    ▶with
      ▶depressive features F06.31
      ▶major depressive-like episode F06.32
      ▶mixed features F06.34
    major F32.9
      with psychotic symptoms F32.3
      in remission (full) F32.5
        partial F32.4
      recurrent F33.9
      ▶with psychotic features F33.3
      single episode F32.9
        mild F32.0
        moderate F32.1
        severe (without psychotic symptoms) F32.2
          with psychotic symptoms F32.3
    organic F06.31
    persistent F34.1
    recurrent F33.9
      current episode
        mild F33.0
        moderate F33.1
        severe (without psychotic symptoms) F33.2
          with psychotic symptoms F33.3
      in remission F33.40
        full F33.42
        partial F33.41
      specified NEC F33.8
    single episode —*see* Episode, depressive
    specified NEC F32.89
  developmental F89
    arithmetical skills F81.2
    coordination (motor) F82
    expressive writing F81.81
    language F80.9
      expressive F80.1
      mixed receptive and expressive F80.2
      receptive type F80.2
      specified NEC F80.89
    learning F81.9
      arithmetical F81.2
      reading F81.0
    mixed F88
    motor coordination or function F82
    pervasive F84.9
      specified NEC F84.8
    phonological F80.0
    reading F81.0
    scholastic skills —*see also* Disorder, learning
      mixed F81.89
    specified NEC F88
    speech F80.9
      articulation F80.0
      specified NEC F80.89
    written expression F81.81
  diaphragm J98.6

▶ New   ⇒ Revised   ~~deleted~~ Deleted   ● Use Additional Character(s)

Disorder (Continued)
  digestive (system) K92.9
    newborn P78.9
      specified NEC P78.89
    postprocedural —see Complication, gastrointestinal
    psychogenic F45.8
  disc (intervertebral) M51.9
    with
      myelopathy
        cervical region M50.00
        cervicothoracic region M50.03
        high cervical region M50.01
        lumbar region M51.06
        mid-cervical region M50.020
        sacrococcygeal region M53.3
        thoracic region M51.04
        thoracolumbar region M51.05
      radiculopathy
        cervical region M50.10
        cervicothoracic region M50.13
        high cervical region M50.11
        lumbar region M51.16
        lumbosacral region M51.17
        mid-cervical region M50.120
        sacrococcygeal region M53.3
        thoracic region M51.14
        thoracolumbar region M51.15
    cervical M50.90
      with
        myelopathy M50.00
          C2-C3 M50.01
          C3-C4 M50.01
          C4-C5 M50.021
          C5-C6 M50.022
          C6-C7 M50.023
          C7-T1 M50.03
          cervicothoracic region M50.03
          high cervical region M50.01
          mid-cervical region M50.020
        neuritis, radiculitis or radiculopathy M50.10
          C2-C3 M50.11
          C3-C4 M50.11
          C4-C5 M50.121
          C5-C6 M50.122
          C6-C7 M50.123
          C7-T1 M50.13
          cervicothoracic region M50.13
          high cervical region M50.11
          mid-cervical region M50.120
      C2-C3 M50.91
      C3-C4 M50.91
      C4-C5 M50.921
      C5-C6 M50.922
      C6-C7 M50.923
      C7-T1 M50.93
      cervicothoracic region M50.93
      degeneration M50.30
        C2-C3 M50.31
        C3-C4 M50.31
        C4-C5 M50.321
        C5-C6 M50.322
        C6-C7 M50.323
        C7-T1 M50.33
        cervicothoracic region M50.33
        high cervical region M50.31
        mid-cervical region M50.320
      displacement M50.20
        C2-C3 M50.21
        C3-C4 M50.21
        C4-C5 M50.221
        C5-C6 M50.222
        C6-C7 M50.223
        C7-T1 M50.23
        cervicothoracic region M50.23
        high cervical region M50.21
        mid-cervical region M50.220
      high cervical region M50.91
      mid-cervical region M50.920
      specified type NEC M50.80
        C2-C3 M50.81
        C3-C4 M50.81

Disorder (Continued)
  disc (intervertebral) (Continued)
    cervical (Continued)
      specified type NEC (Continued)
        C4-C5 M50.821
        C5-C6 M50.822
        C6-C7 M50.823
        C7-T1 M50.83
        cervicothoracic region M50.83
        high cervical region M50.81
        mid-cervical region M50.820
    specified NEC
      lumbar region M51.86
      lumbosacral region M51.87
      sacrococcygeal region M53.3
      thoracic region M51.84
      thoracolumbar region M51.85
  disinhibited attachment (childhood) F94.2
  disintegrative, childhood NEC F84.3
  disruptive F91.9
    mood dysregulation F34.81
    specified NEC F91.8
  ➡ disruptive behavior —see Disorder, conduct
  dissocial personality F60.2
  dissociative F44.9
    affecting
      motor function F44.4
        and sensation F44.7
      sensation F44.6
        and motor function F44.7
    brief reactive F43.0
    due to (secondary to) general medical condition F06.8
    mixed F44.7
    organic F06.8
    other specified NEC F44.89
  double heterozygous sickling —see Disease, sickle-cell
  dream anxiety F51.5
  drug induced hemorrhagic D68.32
  drug related F19.99
    abuse —see Abuse, drug
    dependence —see Dependence, drug
  dysmorphic body F45.22
  dysthymic F34.1
  ear H93.9-●
    bleeding —see Otorrhagia
    deafness —see Deafness
    degenerative H93.09-●
    discharge —see Otorrhea
    external H61.9-●
      auditory canal stenosis —see Stenosis, external ear canal
      exostosis —see Exostosis, external ear canal
      impacted cerumen —see Impaction, cerumen
      otitis —see Otitis, externa
      perichondritis —see Perichondritis, ear
      pinna —see Disorder, pinna
      specified type NEC H61.89-●
        in diseases classified elsewhere H62.8X-●
    inner H83.9-●
      vestibular dysfunction —see Disorder, vestibular function
    middle H74.9-●
      adhesive H74.1-●
      ossicle —see Abnormal, ear ossicles
      polyp —see Polyp, ear (middle)
      specified NEC, in diseases classified elsewhere H75.8-●
    postprocedural —see Complications, ear, procedure
    specified NEC, in diseases classified elsewhere H94.8-●
  eating (adult) (psychogenic) F50.9
    anorexia —see Anorexia
    binge F50.81
    bulimia F50.2
    child F98.29
      pica F98.3
      rumination disorder F98.21

Disorder (Continued)
  eating (Continued)
    pica F50.89
      childhood F98.3
  electrolyte (balance) NEC E87.8
    with
      abortion —see Abortion by type complicated by specified condition NEC
      ectopic pregnancy O08.5
      molar pregnancy O08.5
    acidosis (metabolic) (respiratory) E87.2
    alkalosis (metabolic) (respiratory) E87.3
  elimination, transepidermal L87.9
    specified NEC L87.8
  emotional (persistent) F34.9
    of childhood F93.9
      specified NEC F93.8
  endocrine E34.9
    postprocedural E89.89
    specified NEC E89.89
  erectile (male) (organic) —see also Dysfunction, sexual, male, erectile N52.9
    nonorganic F52.21
  erythematous —see Erythema
  esophagus K22.9
    functional K22.4
    psychogenic F45.8
  eustachian tube H69.9-●
    infection —see Salpingitis, eustachian
    obstruction —see Obstruction, eustachian tube
    patulous —see Patulous, eustachian tube
    specified NEC H69.8-●
  ▶ exhibitionistic F65.2
  extrapyramidal G25.9
    in diseases classified elsewhere —see category G26
    specified type NEC G25.89
  eye H57.9
    postprocedural —see Complication, postprocedural, eye
  eyelid H02.9
    cyst —see Cyst, eyelid
    degenerative H02.70
      chloasma —see Chloasma, eyelid
      madarosis —see Madarosis
      specified type NEC H02.79
      vitiligo —see Vitiligo, eyelid
      xanthelasma —see Xanthelasma
    dermatochalasis —see Dermato-chalasis
    edema —see Edema, eyelid
    elephantiasis —see Elephantiasis, eyelid
    foreign body, retained —see Foreign body, retained, eyelid
    function H02.59
      abnormal innervation syndrome —see Syndrome, abnormal innervation
      blepharochalasis —see Blepharochalasis
      blepharoclonus —see Blepharoclonus
      blepharophimosis —see Blepharophimosis
      blepharoptosis —see Blepharoptosis
      lagophthalmos —see Lagophthalmos
      lid retraction —see Retraction, lid
    hypertrichosis —see Hypertrichosis, eyelid
    specified type NEC H02.89
    vascular H02.879
      left H02.876
        lower H02.875
        upper H02.874
      right H02.873
        lower H02.872
        upper H02.871
  factitious F68.10
    with predominantly
      physical symptoms F68.12
        with psychological symptoms F68.13
      psychological symptoms F68.11
        with physical symptoms F68.13
  factor, coagulation —see Defect, coagulation

Disorder *(Continued)*
  fatty acid
    metabolism E71.30
      specified NEC E71.39
    oxidation
      LCAD E71.310
      MCAD E71.311
      SCAD E71.312
      specified deficiency NEC E71.318
  feeding (infant or child) —*see also* Disorder,
      eating R63.3-●
  ▶or eating disorder F50.9
  ▶specified NEC F50.9
  feigned (with obvious motivation) Z76.5
    without obvious motivation —*see* Disorder,
      factitious
  female
    hypoactive sexual desire F52.0
    orgasmic F52.31
    ~~sexual arousal F52.22~~
  ▶sexual interest/arousal F52.22
  ▶fetishistic F65.0
  fibroblastic M72.9
    specified NEC M72.8
  fluency
    adult onset F98.5
    childhood onset F80.81
    following
      cerebral infarction I69.323
      cerebrovascular disease I69.923
        specified disease NEC I69.823
      intracerebral hemorrhage I69.123
      nontraumatic intracranial hemorrhage
        NEC I69.223
      subarachnoid hemorrhage I69.023
    in conditions classified elsewhere R47.82
  fluid balance E87.8
  follicular (skin) L73.9
    specified NEC L73.8
  ▶frotteuristic F65.81
  fructose metabolism E74.10
    essential fructosuria E74.11
    fructokinase deficiency E74.11
    fructose-1, 6-diphosphatase deficiency
      E74.19
    hereditary fructose intolerance E74.12
    other specified E74.19
  functional polymorphonuclear neutrophils D71
  gallbladder, biliary tract and pancreas in
      diseases classified elsewhere K87
  ▶gambling F63.0
  gamma-glutamyl cycle E72.8
  gastric (functional) K31.9
    motility K30
    psychogenic F45.8
    secretion K30
  gastrointestinal (functional) NOS K92.9
    newborn P78.9
    psychogenic F45.8
  gender-identity or -role F64.9
    childhood F64.2
    effect on relationship F66
    of adolescence or adulthood F64.0
      nontranssexual F64.8
    specified NEC F64.8
    uncertainty F66
  genito-pelvic pain penetration F52.6
  genitourinary system
    female N94.9
    male N50.9
    psychogenic F45.8
  globe H44.9
    degenerated condition H44.50
      absolute glaucoma H44.51-●
      atrophy H44.52-●
      leucocoria H44.53-●
    degenerative H44.30
      chalcosis H44.31-●
    ⇒myopia —*see also* Myopia, degenerative
        H44.2-●
      siderosis H44.32-●
      specified type NEC H44.39-●

Disorder *(Continued)*
  globe *(Continued)*
    endophthalmitis —*see* Endophthalmitis
    foreign body, retained —*see* Foreign body,
        intraocular, old, retained
    hemophthalmos —*see* Hemophthalmos
    hypotony H44.40
      due to
        ocular fistula H44.42-●
        specified disorder NEC H44.43-●
      flat anterior chamber H44.41-●
      primary H44.44-●
    luxation —*see* Luxation, globe
    specified type NEC H44.89
  glomerular (in) N05.9
    amyloidosis E85.4 *[N08]*
    cryoglobulinemia D89.1 *[N08]*
    disseminated intravascular coagulation
        D65 *[N08]*
    Fabry's disease E75.21 *[N08]*
    familial lecithin cholesterol acyltransferase
        deficiency E78.6 *[N08]*
    Goodpasture's syndrome M31.0
    hemolytic-uremic syndrome D59.3
    Henoch (-Schönlein) purpura D69.0 *[N08]*
    malariae malaria B52.0
    microscopic polyangiitis M31.7 *[N08]*
    multiple myeloma C90.0-● *[N08]*
    mumps B26.83
    schistosomiasis B65.9 *[N08]*
    sepsis NEC A41.-● *[N08]*
      streptococcal A40.-● *[N08]*
    sickle-cell disorders D57.-● *[N08]*
    strongyloidiasis B78.9 *[N08]*
    subacute bacterial endocarditis I33.0 *[N08]*
    syphilis A52.75
    systemic lupus erythematosus M32.14
    thrombotic thrombocytopenic purpura
        M31.1 *[N08]*
    Waldenström macroglobulinemia C88.0
        [N08]
    Wegener's granulomatosis M31.31
  gluconeogenesis E74.4
  glucosaminoglycan metabolism —
      see Disorder, metabolism,
      glucosaminoglycan
  glycine metabolism E72.50
    d-glycericacidemia E72.59
    hyperhydroxyprolinemia E72.59
    hyperoxaluria E72.53
    hyperprolinemia E72.59
    non-ketotic hyperglycinemia E72.51
    oxalosis E72.53
    oxaluria E72.53
    sarcosinemia E72.59
    trimethylaminuria E72.52
  glycoprotein metabolism E77.9
    specified NEC E77.8
  habit (and impulse) F63.9
    involving sexual behavior NEC F65.9
    specified NEC F63.89
  hallucinogen use
    mild F16.10
      with
        hallucinogen-induced
          anxiety disorder F16.180
          bipolar and related disorder F16.14
          depressive disorder F16.14
          psychotic disorder F16.159
        hallucinogen intoxication delirium
          F16.121
        other hallucinogen intoxication
          F16.129
      ▶in remission (early) (sustained) F16.11
    moderate or severe F16.20
      with
        hallucinogen-induced
          anxiety disorder F16.280
          bipolar and related disorder F16.24
          depressive disorder F16.24
          psychotic disorder F16.259

Disorder *(Continued)*
  hallucinogen use *(Continued)*
    moderate or severe *(Continued)*
      with *(Continued)*
        hallucinogen intoxication delirium
          F16.221
        other hallucinogen intoxication F16.229
      ▶in remission (early) (sustained) F16.21
  heart action I49.9
  hematological D75.9
    newborn (transient) P61.9
      specified NEC P61.8
  hematopoietic organs D75.9
  hemorrhagic NEC D69.9
    drug-induced D68.32
    due to
      extrinsic circulating anticoagulants
          D68.32
        increase in
          anti-IIa D68.32
          anti-Xa D68.32
      intrinsic
        circulating anticoagulants D68.318
          increase in
            antithrombin D68.318
            anti-VIIIa D68.318
            anti-IXa D68.318
            anti-XIa D68.318
    following childbirth O72.3
  hemostasis —*see* Defect, coagulation
  histidine metabolism E70.40
    histidinemia E70.41
    other specified E70.49
  hoarding F42.3
  hyperkinetic —*see* Disorder, attention-deficit
      hyperactivity
  hyperleucine-isoleucinemia E71.19
  hypervalinemia E71.19
  hypoactive sexual desire F52.0
  hypochondriacal F45.20
    body dysmorphic F45.22
    neurosis F45.21
    other specified F45.29
  identity
    dissociative F44.81
    illness anxiety F45.21
    of childhood F93.8
  immune mechanism (immunity) D89.9
    specified type NEC D89.89
  impaired renal tubular function N25.9
    specified NEC N25.89
  impulse (control) F63.9
  inflammatory
    pelvic, in diseases classified elsewhere —
        see category N74
    penis N48.29
      abscess N48.21
      cellulitis N48.22
  inhalant use
    mild F18.10
      with
        inhalant-induced
          anxiety disorder F18.180
          depressive disorder F18.14
          major neurocognitive disorder
            F18.17
          mild neurocognitive disorder
            F18.188
          psychotic disorder F18.159
        inhalant intoxication F18.129
        inhalant intoxication delirium F18.121
      ▶in remission (early) (sustained) F18.11
    moderate or severe F18.20
      with
        inhalant-induced
          anxiety disorder F18.280
          depressive disorder F18.24
          major neurocognitive disorder F18.27
          mild neurocognitive disorder F18.288
          psychotic disorder F18.259
        inhalant intoxication F18.229
        inhalant intoxication delirium F18.221
      ▶in remission (early) (sustained) F18.21

▶ New   ⇒ Revised   ~~deleted~~ Deleted   ● Use Additional Character(s)

Disorder (*Continued*)
  integument, newborn P83.9
  ➠specified NEC P83.88
  intermittent explosive F63.81
  internal secretion pancreas —*see* Increased,
      secretion, pancreas, endocrine
  intestine, intestinal
    carbohydrate absorption NEC E74.39
      postoperative K91.2
    functional NEC K59.9
      postoperative K91.89
    psychogenic F45.8
    vascular K55.9
      chronic K55.1
      specified NEC K55.8
  intraoperative (intraprocedural) —*see*
      Complications, intraoperative
  involuntary emotional expression (IEED) F48.2
  iris H21.9
    adhesions —*see* Adhesions, iris
    atrophy —*see* Atrophy, iris
    chamber angle recession —*see* Recession,
        chamber angle
    cyst —*see* Cyst, iris
    degeneration —*see* Degeneration, iris
    in diseases classified elsewhere H22
    iridodialysis —*see* Iridodialysis
    iridoschisis —*see* Iridoschisis
    miotic pupillary cyst —*see* Cyst, pupillary
    pupillary
      abnormality —*see* Abnormality,
          pupillary
      membrane —*see* Membrane, pupillary
    specified type NEC H21.89
    vascular NEC H21.1X-●
  iron metabolism E83.10
    specified NEC E83.19
  isovaleric acidemia E71.110
  jaw, developmental M27.0
    temporomandibular —*see also* Anomaly,
        dentofacial, temporomandibular joint
        M26.60-●
  joint M25.9
    derangement —*see* Derangement, joint
    effusion —*see* Effusion, joint
    fistula —*see* Fistula, joint
    hemarthrosis —*see* Hemarthrosis
    instability —*see* Instability, joint
    osteophyte —*see* Osteophyte
    pain —*see* Pain, joint
    psychogenic F45.8
    specified type NEC M25.80
      ankle M25.87-●
      elbow M25.82-●
      foot joint M25.87-●
      hand joint M25.84-●
      hip M25.85-●
      knee M25.86-●
      shoulder M25.81-●
      wrist M25.83-●
    stiffness —*see* Stiffness, joint
  ketone metabolism E71.32
  kidney N28.9
    functional (tubular) N25.9
    in
      schistosomiasis B65.9 [*N29*]
    tubular function N25.9
      specified NEC N25.89
  lacrimal system H04.9
    changes H04.69
    fistula —*see* Fistula, lacrimal
    gland H04.19
      atrophy —*see* Atrophy, lacrimal gland
      cyst —*see* Cyst, lacrimal, gland
      dacryops —*see* Dacryops
      dislocation —*see* Dislocation, lacrimal
          gland
      dry eye syndrome —*see* Syndrome, dry
          eye
      infection —*see* Dacryoadenitis
      granuloma —*see* Granuloma, lacrimal

Disorder (*Continued*)
  lacrimal system (*Continued*)
    inflammation —*see* Inflammation, lacrimal
    obstruction —*see* Obstruction, lacrimal
    specified NEC H04.89
  lactation NEC O92.79
  language (developmental) F80.9
    expressive F80.1
    mixed receptive and expressive F80.2
    receptive F80.2
  late luteal phase dysphoric N94.89
  learning (specific) F81.9
    acalculia R48.8
    alexia R48.0
    mathematics F81.2
    reading F81.0
    ▶specified
      ▶with impairment in
        ▶mathematics F81.2
        ▶reading F81.0
        ▶written expression F81.81
    specified NEC F81.89
    spelling F81.81
    written expression F81.81
  lens H27.9
    aphakia —*see* Aphakia
    cataract —*see* Cataract
    dislocation —*see* Dislocation, lens
    specified type NEC H27.8
  ligament M24.20
    ankle M24.27-●
    attachment, spine —*see* Enthesopathy,
        spinal
    elbow M24.22-●
    foot joint M24.27-●
    hand joint M24.24-●
    hip M24.25-●
    knee —*see* Derangement, knee, specified
        NEC
    shoulder M24.21-●
    vertebra M24.28
    wrist M24.23-●
  ligamentous attachments —*see also*
      Enthesopathy
    spine —*see* Enthesopathy, spinal
  lipid
    metabolism, congenital E78.9
    storage E75.6
      specified NEC E75.5
  lipoprotein
    deficiency (familial) E78.6
    metabolism E78.9
      specified NEC E78.89
  liver K76.9
    malarial B54 [*K77*]
  low back —*see also* Dorsopathy, specified NEC
  lumbosacral
    plexus G54.1
    root (nerve) NEC G54.4
  lung, interstitial, drug-induced J70.4
    acute J70.2
    chronic J70.3
  lymphoproliferative, post-transplant (PTLD)
      D47.Z1
  lysine and hydroxylysine metabolism E72.3
  major neurocognitive —*see* Dementia, in (due
      to)
  male
    erectile (organic) —*see also* Dysfunction,
        sexual, male, erectile N52.9
      nonorganic F52.21
    hypoactive sexual desire F52.0
    orgasmic F52.32
  manic F30.9
    organic F06.33
  mast cell activation —*see* Activation, mast
      cell
  mastoid —*see also* Disorder, ear, middle
    postprocedural —*see* Complications, ear,
        procedure
  meniscus —*see* Derangement, knee, meniscus

Disorder (*Continued*)
  menopausal N95.9
    specified NEC N95.8
  menstrual N92.6
    psychogenic F45.8
    specified NEC N92.5
  mental (or behavioral) (nonpsychotic) F99
    due to (secondary to)
      amphetamine
        due to drug abuse —*see* Abuse, drug,
            stimulant
        due to drug dependence —*see*
            Dependence, drug, stimulant
      brain disease, damage and dysfunction
          F09
      caffeine use
        due to drug abuse —*see* Abuse, drug,
            stimulant
        due to drug dependence —*see*
            Dependence, drug, stimulant
      cannabis use
        due to drug abuse —*see* Abuse, drug,
            cannabis
        due to drug dependence —*see*
            Dependence, drug, cannabis
      general medical condition F09
      sedative or hypnotic use
        due to drug abuse —*see* Abuse, drug,
            sedative
        due to drug dependence —*see*
            Dependence, drug, sedative
      tobacco (nicotine) use —*see* Dependence,
          drug, nicotine
    following organic brain damage F07.9
      frontal lobe syndrome F07.0
      personality change F07.0
      postconcussional syndrome F07.81
      specified NEC F07.89
    infancy, childhood or adolescence F98.9
    neurotic —*see* Neurosis
    organic or symptomatic F09
    presenile, psychotic F03
    problem NEC
    psychoneurotic —*see* Neurosis
    psychotic —*see* Psychosis
    puerperal F53
    senile, psychotic NEC F03
  metabolic, amino acid, transitory, newborn
      P74.8
  metabolism NOS E88.9
    amino-acid E72.9
      aromatic E70.9
        albinism —*see* Albinism
        histidine E70.40
          histidinemia E70.41
          other specified E70.49
        hyperphenylalaninemia E70.1
          classical phenylketonuria E70.0
        other specified E70.8
        tryptophan E70.5
        tyrosine E70.20
          hypertyrosinemia E70.21
          other specified E70.29
      branched chain E71.2
        3-methylglutaconic aciduria E71.111
        hyperleucine-isoleucinemia E71.19
        hypervalinemia E71.19
        isovaleric acidemia E71.110
        maple syrup urine disease E71.0
        methylmalonic acidemia E71.120
        organic aciduria NEC E71.118
        other specified E71.19
        proprionate NEC E71.128
        proprionic acidemia E71.121
      glycine E72.50
        d-glycericacidemia E72.59
        hyperhydroxyprolinemia E72.59
        hyperoxaluria E72.53
        hyperprolinemia E72.59
        non-ketotic hyperglycinemia E72.51
        other specified E72.59
        sarcosinemia E72.59
        trimethylaminuria E72.52

Disorder (Continued)
  metabolism (Continued)
    amino-acid (Continued)
      hydroxylysine E72.3
      lysine E72.3
      ornithine E72.4
      other specified E72.8
        beta-amino acid E72.8
        gamma-glutamyl cycle E72.8
      straight-chain E72.8
      sulfur-bearing E72.10
        homocystinuria E72.11
        methylenetetrahydrofolate reductase
          deficiency E72.12
        other specified E72.19
    bile acid and cholesterol metabolism E78.70
    bilirubin E80.7
      specified NEC E80.6
    calcium E83.50
      hypercalcemia E83.52
      hypocalcemia E83.51
      other specified E83.59
    carbohydrate E74.9
      specified NEC E74.8
    cholesterol and bile acid metabolism
      E78.70
    congenital E88.9
    copper E83.00
      specified type NEC E83.09
      Wilson's disease E83.01
    cystinuria E72.01
    fructose E74.10
    galactose E74.20
    glucosaminoglycan E76.9
      mucopolysaccharidosis —see
        Mucopolysaccharidosis
      specified NEC E76.8
    glutamine E72.8
    glycine E72.50
    glycogen storage (hepatorenal) E74.09
    glycoprotein E77.9
      specified NEC E77.8
    glycosaminoglycan E76.9
      specified NEC E76.8
    in labor and delivery O75.89
    iron E83.10
    isoleucine E71.19
    leucine E71.19
    lipoid E78.9
    lipoprotein E78.9
      specified NEC E78.89
    magnesium E83.40
      hypermagnesemia E83.41
      hypomagnesemia E83.42
      other specified E83.49
    mineral E83.9
      specified NEC E83.89
    mitochondrial E88.40
      MELAS syndrome E88.41
      MERRF syndrome (myoclonic epilepsy
        associated with ragged-red fibers)
        E88.42
      other specified E88.49
    ornithine E72.4
    phosphatases E83.30
    phosphorus E83.30
      acid phosphatase deficiency E83.39
      hypophosphatasia E83.39
      hypophosphatemia E83.39
        familial E83.31
      other specified E83.39
      pseudovitamin D deficiency E83.32
    plasma protein NEC E88.09
    porphyrin —see Porphyria
    postprocedural E89.89
      specified NEC E89.89
    purine E79.9
      specified NEC E79.8
    pyrimidine E79.9
      specified NEC E79.8
    pyruvate E74.4

Disorder (Continued)
  metabolism (Continued)
    serine E72.8
    sodium E87.8
    specified NEC E88.89
    threonine E72.8
    valine E71.19
    zinc E83.2
  methylmalonic acidemia E71.120
  micturition NEC —see also Difficulty,
    micturition R39.198
    feeling of incomplete emptying R39.14
    hesitancy R39.11
    poor stream R39.12
    psychogenic F45.8
    split stream R39.13
    straining R39.16
    urgency R39.15
  mild neurocognitive G31.84
  mitochondrial metabolism E88.40
  mitral (valve) —see Endocarditis, mitral
  mixed
    anxiety and depressive F41.8
    of scholastic skills (developmental) F81.89
    receptive expressive language F80.2
  mood F39
    bipolar —see Disorder, bipolar
    depressive —see Disorder, depressive
    due to (secondary to)
      alcohol F10.94
      amphetamine F15.94
        in
          abuse F15.14
          dependence F15.24
      anxiolytic F13.94
        in
          abuse F13.14
          dependence F13.24
      cocaine F14.94
        in
          abuse F14.14
          dependence F14.24
      general medical condition F06.30
      hallucinogen F16.94
        in
          abuse F16.14
          dependence F16.24
      hypnotic F13.94
        in
          abuse F13.14
          dependence F13.24
      inhalant F18.94
        in
          abuse F18.14
          dependence F18.24
      opioid F11.94
        in
          abuse F11.14
          dependence F11.24
      phencyclidine (PCP) F16.94
        in
          abuse F16.14
          dependence F16.24
      physiological condition F06.30
        with
          depressive features F06.31
          major depressive-like episode
            F06.32
          manic features F06.33
          mixed features F06.34
      psychoactive substance NEC F19.94
        in
          abuse F19.14
          dependence F19.24
      sedative F13.94
        in
          abuse F13.14
          dependence F13.24
      volatile solvents F18.94
        in
          abuse F18.14
          dependence F18.24

Disorder (Continued)
  mood (Continued)
    manic episode F30.9
      with psychotic symptoms F30.2
      without psychotic symptoms F30.10
        mild F30.11
        moderate F30.12
        severe F30.13
      in remission (full) F30.4
        partial F30.3
      specified type NEC F30.8
    organic F06.30
      right hemisphere F07.89
    persistent F34.9
      cyclothymia F34.0
      dysthymia F34.1
      specified type NEC F34.89
    recurrent F39
    right hemisphere organic F07.89
  movement G25.9
    drug-induced G25.70
      akathisia G25.71
      specified NEC G25.79
    hysterical F44.4
    in diseases classified elsewhere —see
      category G26
    periodic limb G47.61
      sleep related G47.61
    sleep related NEC G47.69
    specified NEC G25.89
    stereotyped F98.4
    treatment-induced G25.9
  multiple personality F44.81
  muscle M62.9
    attachment, spine —see Enthesopathy,
      spinal
    in trichinellosis —see Trichinellosis, with
      muscle disorder
    psychogenic F45.8
    specified type NEC M62.89
    tone, newborn P94.9
      specified NEC P94.8
  muscular
    attachments —see also Enthesopathy
      spine —see Enthesopathy, spinal
    urethra N36.44
  musculoskeletal system, soft tissue —see
    Disorder, soft tissue
    postprocedural M96.89
    psychogenic F45.8
  myoneural G70.9
    due to lead G70.1
    specified NEC G70.89
    toxic G70.1
  myotonic NEC G71.19
  nail, in diseases classified elsewhere L62
  neck region NEC —see Dorsopathy, specified
    NEC
  neonatal onset multisystemic inflammatory
    (NOMID) M04.2
  nerve G58.9
    abducent NEC —see Strabismus, paralytic,
      sixth nerve
    accessory G52.8
    acoustic —see subcategory H93.3
    auditory —see subcategory H93.3
    auriculotemporal G50.8
    axillary G54.0
    cerebral —see Disorder, nerve, cranial
    cranial G52.9
      eighth —see subcategory H93.3
      eleventh G52.8
      fifth G50.9
      first G52.0
      fourth NEC —see Strabismus, paralytic,
        fourth nerve
      multiple G52.7
      ninth G52.1
      second NEC —see Disorder, nerve, optic
      seventh NEC G51.8
      sixth NEC —see Strabismus, paralytic,
        sixth nerve

▶ New   ⇒ Revised   ~~deleted~~ Deleted   ● Use Additional Character(s)

Disorder (Continued)
  nerve (Continued)
    cranial (Continued)
      specified NEC G52.8
      tenth G52.2
      third NEC —see Strabismus, paralytic,
        third nerve
      twelfth G52.3
    entrapment —see Neuropathy, entrapment
    facial G51.9
      specified NEC G51.8
    femoral —see Lesion, nerve, femoral
    glossopharyngeal NEC G52.1
    hypoglossal G52.3
    intercostal G58.0
    lateral
      cutaneous of thigh —see
        Mononeuropathy, lower limb,
        meralgia paresthetica
      popliteal —see Lesion, nerve, popliteal
    lower limb —see Mononeuropathy, lower
      limb
    medial popliteal —see Lesion, nerve,
      popliteal, medial
    median NEC —see Lesion, nerve, median
    multiple G58.7
    oculomotor NEC —see Strabismus,
      paralytic, third nerve
    olfactory G52.0
    optic NEC H47.09-●
      hemorrhage into sheath —see
        Hemorrhage, optic nerve
      ischemic H47.01-●
    peroneal —see Lesion, nerve, popliteal
    phrenic G58.8
    plantar —see Lesion, nerve, plantar
    pneumogastric G52.2
    posterior tibial —see Syndrome, tarsal
      tunnel
    radial —see Lesion, nerve, radial
    recurrent laryngeal G52.2
    root G54.9
      cervical G54.2
      lumbosacral G54.1
      specified NEC G54.8
      thoracic G54.3
    sciatic NEC —see Lesion, nerve, sciatic
    specified NEC G58.8
      lower limb —see Mononeuropathy,
        lower limb, specified NEC
      upper limb —see Mononeuropathy,
        upper limb, specified NEC
    sympathetic G90.9
    tibial —see Lesion, nerve, popliteal, medial
    trigeminal G50.9
      specified NEC G50.8
    trochlear NEC —see Strabismus, paralytic,
      fourth nerve
    ulnar —see Lesion, nerve, ulnar
    upper limb —see Mononeuropathy, upper
      limb
    vagus G52.2
  nervous system G98.8
    autonomic (peripheral) G90.9
      specified NEC G90.8
    central G96.9
      specified NEC G96.8
    parasympathetic G90.9
    specified NEC G98.8
    sympathetic G90.9
    vegetative G90.9
  neurocognitive R41.9
    major
      with
        aggressive behavior F01.51
        combative behavior F01.51
        violent behavior F01.51
      due to vascular disease, with behavioral
        disturbance F01.51
      in (due to) (other diseases classified
        elsewhere) —see also Dementia, in
        (due to) F02.80

Disorder (Continued)
  neurocognitive (Continued)
    major (Continued)
      in (Continued)
        with
          aggressive behavior F02.81
          combative behavior F02.81
          violent behavior F02.81
        without behavioral disturbance F01.50
    mild G31.84
    neurodevelopmental F89
      specified NEC F88
    neurohypophysis NEC E23.3
    neurological NEC R29.818
    neuromuscular G70.9
      hereditary NEC G71.9
      specified NEC G70.89
      toxic G70.1
    neurotic F48.9
      specified NEC F48.8
    neutrophil, polymorphonuclear D71
    nicotine use —see Dependence, drug, nicotine
    nightmare F51.5
  ▶non-rapid eye movement sleep arousal
    ▶sleep terror type F51.4
    ▶sleepwalking type F51.3
    nose J34.9
      specified NEC J34.89
    obsessive-compulsive F42.9
  ▶and related disorder due to a known
      physiological condition F06.8
    odontogenesis NOS K00.9
    opioid use
      with
        opioid-induced psychotic disorder F11.959
          with
            delusions F11.950
            hallucinations F11.951
      due to drug abuse —see Abuse, drug,
        opioid
      due to drug dependence —see Dependence,
        drug, opioid
      mild F11.10
        with
          opioid-induced
            anxiety disorder F11.188
            depressive disorder F11.14
            sexual dysfunction F11.181
          opioid intoxication
            with perceptual disturbances F11.122
            delirium F11.121
            without perceptual disturbances
              F11.129
  ▶in remission (early) (sustained) F11.11
      moderate or severe F11.20
        with
          opioid-induced
            anxiety disorder F11.288
            anxiety disorder F11.988
            depressive disorder F11.24
            depressive disorder F11.94
            sexual dysfunction F11.281
            sexual dysfunction F11.981
          opioid intoxication
            with perceptual disturbances F11.222
            delirium F11.221
            without perceptual disturbances
              F11.229
  ▶in remission (early) (sustained) F11.21
    oppositional defiant F91.3
    optic
      chiasm H47.49
        due to
          inflammatory disorder H47.41
          neoplasm H47.42
          vascular disorder H47.43
      disc H47.39-●
        coloboma —see Coloboma, optic disc
        drusen —see Drusen, optic disc
        pseudopapilledema —see
          Pseudopapilledema

Disorder (Continued)
  optic (Continued)
    radiations —see Disorder, visual, pathway
    tracts —see Disorder, visual, pathway
    orbit H05.9
      cyst —see Cyst, orbit
      deformity —see Deformity, orbit
      edema —see Edema, orbit
      enophthalmos —see Enophthalmos
      exophthalmos —see Exophthalmos
      hemorrhage —see Hemorrhage, orbit
      inflammation —see Inflammation, orbit
      myopathy —see Myopathy, extraocular
        muscles
      retained foreign body —see Foreign body,
        orbit, old
      specified type NEC H05.89
  organic
    anxiety F06.4
    catatonic F06.1
    delusional F06.2
    dissociative F06.8
    emotionally labile (asthenic) F06.8
    mood (affective) F06.30
    schizophrenia-like F06.2
  orgasmic (female) F52.31
    male F52.32
  ornithine metabolism E72.4
  overanxious F41.1
    of childhood F93.8
  pain
    with related psychological factors F45.42
    exclusively related to psychological factors
      F45.41
    genito-pelvic penetration disorder F52.6
  pancreatic internal secretion E16.9
    specified NEC E16.8
  panic F41.0
    with agoraphobia F40.01
  papulosquamous L44.9
    in diseases classified elsewhere L45
    specified NEC L44.8
  paranoid F22
    induced F24
    shared F24
  ▶paraphilic F65.9
  ▶specified NEC F65.89
  parathyroid (gland) E21.5
    specified NEC E21.4
  parietoalveolar NEC J84.09
  paroxysmal, mixed R56.9
  patella M22.9-●
    chondromalacia —see Chondromalacia,
      patella
    derangement NEC M22.3X-●
    recurrent
      dislocation —see Dislocation, patella,
        recurrent
      subluxation —see Dislocation, patella,
        recurrent, incomplete
    specified NEC M22.8X-●
  patellofemoral M22.2X-●
  ▶pedophilic F65.4
  pentose phosphate pathway with anemia
    D55.1
  perception, due to hallucinogens F16.983
    in
      abuse F16.183
      dependence F16.283
  peripheral nervous system NEC G64
  peroxisomal E71.50
    biogenesis
      neonatal adrenoleukodystrophy E71.511
      specified disorder NEC E71.518
      Zellweger syndrome E71.510
    rhizomelic chondrodysplasia punctata
      E71.540
    specified form NEC E71.548
      group 1 E71.518
      group 2 E71.53
      group 3 E71.542

Disorder *(Continued)*
  peroxisomal *(Continued)*
    X-linked adrenoleukodystrophy E71.529
      adolescent E71.521
      adrenomyeloneuropathy E71.522
      childhood E71.520
      specified form NEC E71.528
    Zellweger-like syndrome E71.541
  persistent
    (somatoform) pain F45.41
    affective (mood) F34.9
  personality —*see also* Personality F60.9
    affective F34.0
    aggressive F60.3
    amoral F60.2
    anankastic F60.5
    antisocial F60.2
    anxious F60.6
    asocial F60.2
    asthenic F60.7
    avoidant F60.6
    borderline F60.3
    change (secondary) due to general medical
        condition F07.0
    compulsive F60.5
    cyclothymic F34.0
    dependent (passive) F60.7
    depressive F34.1
    dissocial F60.2
    emotional instability F60.3
    expansive paranoid F60.0
    explosive F60.3
    following organic brain damage F07.9
    histrionic F60.4
    hyperthymic F34.0
    hypothymic F34.1
    hysterical F60.4
    immature F60.89
    inadequate F60.7
    labile F60.3
    mixed (nonspecific) F60.89
    moral deficiency F60.2
    narcissistic F60.81
    negativistic F60.89
    obsessional F60.5
    obsessive (-compulsive) F60.5
    organic F07.9
    overconscientious F60.5
    paranoid F60.0
    passive (-dependent) F60.7
    passive-aggressive F60.89
    pathological NEC F60.9
    pseudosocial F60.2
    psychopathic F60.2
    schizoid F60.1
    schizotypal F21
    self-defeating F60.7
    specified NEC F60.89
    type A F60.5
    unstable (emotional) F60.3
  pervasive, developmental F84.9
  phencyclidine use
    mild F16.10
      with
        phencyclidine-induced
          anxiety disorder F16.180
          bipolar and related disorder F16.14
          depressive disorder F16.14
          psychotic disorder F16.159
        phencyclidine intoxication F16.129
        phencyclidine intoxication delirium
            F16.121
      ▶in remission (early) (sustained) F16.11
    moderate or severe F16.20
      with
        phencyclidine-induced
          anxiety disorder F16.280
          bipolar and related disorder F16.24
          depressive disorder F16.24
          psychotic disorder F16.259
        phencyclidine intoxication F16.229

Disorder *(Continued)*
  phencyclidine use *(Continued)*
    moderate or severe *(Continued)*
      with *(Continued)*
        phencyclidine intoxication delirium
            F16.221
      ▶in remission (early) (sustained) F16.21
  phobic anxiety, childhood F40.8
  phosphate-losing tubular N25.0
  pigmentation L81.9
    choroid, congenital Q14.3
    diminished melanin formation L81.6
    iron L81.8
    specified NEC L81.8
  pinna (noninfective) H61.10-●
    deformity, acquired H61.11-●
    hematoma H61.12-●
    perichondritis —*see* Perichondritis, ear
    specified type NEC H61.19-●
  pituitary gland E23.7
    iatrogenic (postprocedural) E89.3
    specified NEC E23.6
  platelets D69.1
  plexus G54.9
    specified NEC G54.8
  polymorphonuclear neutrophils D71
  porphyrin metabolism —*see* Porphyria
  postconcussional F07.81
  posthallucinogen perception F16.983
    in
      abuse F16.183
      dependence F16.283
  postmenopausal N95.9
    specified NEC N95.8
  postprocedural (postoperative) —*see*
      Complications, postprocedural
  post-transplant lymphoproliferative D47.z1
  post-traumatic stress (PTSD) F43.10
    acute F43.11
    chronic F43.12
  premenstrual dysphoric (PMDD) F32.81
  prepuce N47.8
  propionic acidemia E71.121
  prostate N42.9
    specified NEC N42.89
  psychogenic NOS —*see also* condition F45.9
    anxiety F41.8
    appetite F50.9
    asthenic F48.8
    cardiovascular (system) F45.8
    compulsive F42.8
    cutaneous F54
    depressive F32.9
    digestive (system) F45.8
    dysmenorrheic F45.8
    dyspneic F45.8
    endocrine (system) F54
    eye NEC F45.8
    feeding —*see* Disorder, eating
    functional NEC F45.8
    gastric F45.8
    gastrointestinal (system) F45.8
    genitourinary (system) F45.8
    heart (function) (rhythm) F45.8
    hyperventilatory F45.8
    hypochondriacal —*see* Disorder,
        hypochondriacal
    intestinal F45.8
    joint F45.8
    learning F81.9
    limb F45.8
    lymphatic (system) F45.8
    menstrual F45.8
    micturition F45.8
    monoplegic NEC F44.4
    motor F44.4
    muscle F45.8
    musculoskeletal F45.8
    neurocirculatory F45.8
    obsessive F42.8
    occupational F48.8
    organ or part of body NEC F45.8

Disorder *(Continued)*
  psychogenic NOS *(Continued)*
    paralytic NEC F44.4
    phobic F40.9
    physical NEC F45.8
    rectal F45.8
    respiratory (system) F45.8
    rheumatic F45.8
    sexual (function) F52.9
    skin (allergic) (eczematous) F54
    sleep F51.9
    specified part of body NEC F45.8
    stomach F45.8
  psychological F99
    associated with
      disease classified elsewhere F54
      sexual
        development F66
        relationship F66
      uncertainty about gender identity F64.9
  psychomotor NEC F44.4
    hysterical F44.4
  psychoneurotic —*see also* Neurosis
    mixed NEC F48.8
  psychophysiologic —*see* Disorder,
      somatoform
  psychosexual F65.9
    development F66
    identity of childhood F64.2
  psychosomatic NOS —*see* Disorder,
      somatoform
    multiple F45.0
    undifferentiated F45.1
  psychotic —*see* Psychosis
    transient (acute) F23
  puberty E30.9
    specified NEC E30.8
  pulmonary (valve) —*see* Endocarditis,
      pulmonary
  purine metabolism E79.9
  pyrimidine metabolism E79.9
  pyruvate metabolism E74.4
  reactive attachment (childhood) F94.1
  reading R48.0
    developmental (specific) F81.0
  receptive language F80.2
  receptor, hormonal, peripheral —*see also*
      Syndrome, androgen insensitivity E34.50
  recurrent brief depressive F33.8
  reflex R29.2
  refraction H52.7
    aniseikonia H52.32
    anisometropia H52.31
    astigmatism —*see* Astigmatism
    hypermetropia —*see* Hypermetropia
    myopia —*see* Myopia
    presbyopia H52.4
    specified NEC H52.6
  relationship F68.8
    due to sexual orientation F66
  REM sleep behavior G47.52
  renal function, impaired (tubular) N25.9
  resonance R49.9
    specified NEC R49.8
  respiratory function, impaired —*see also*
      Failure, respiration
    postprocedural —*see* Complication,
        postoperative, respiratory system
    psychogenic F45.8
  retina H35.9
    angioid streaks H35.33
    changes in vascular appearance H35.01-●
    degeneration —*see* Degeneration, retina
    dystrophy (hereditary) —*see* Dystrophy,
        retina
    edema H35.81
    hemorrhage —*see* Hemorrhage, retina
    ischemia H35.82
    macular degeneration —*see* Degeneration,
        macula
    microaneurysms H35.04-●
    microvascular abnormality NEC H35.09

▶ New   ⮕ Revised   ~~deleted~~ Deleted   ● Use Additional Character(s)

Disorder *(Continued)*
  retina *(Continued)*
    neovascularization —*see*
      Neovascularization, retina
    retinopathy —*see* Retinopathy
    separation of layers H35.70
      central serous chorioretinopathy H35.71-●
      pigment epithelium detachment (serous)
        H35.72-●
      hemorrhagic H35.73-●
    specified type NEC H35.89
    telangiectasis —*see* Telangiectasis, retina
    vasculitis —*see* Vasculitis, retina
  retroperitoneal K68.9
  right hemisphere organic affective F07.89
  rumination (infant or child) F98.21
  sacrum, sacrococcygeal NEC M53.3
  schizoaffective F25.9
    bipolar type F25.0
    depressive type F25.1
    manic type F25.0
    mixed type F25.0
    specified NEC F25.8
  schizoid of childhood F84.5
  ►schizophrenia spectrum and other psychotic
      disorder F29
  ►specified NEC F28
  schizophreniform F20.81
    brief F23
  schizotypal (personality) F21
  secretion, thyrocalcitonin E07.0
  sedative, hypnotic, or anxiolytic use
    mild F13.10
      with
        sedative, hypnotic, or
          anxiolytic-induced
          anxiety disorder F13.180
          bipolar and related disorder F13.14
          depressive disorder F13.14
          psychotic disorder F13.159
          sexual dysfunction F13.181
          sedative, hypnotic, or anxiolytic
            intoxication F13.129
          sedative, hypnotic, or anxiolytic
            intoxication delirium F13.121
      ►in remission (early) (sustained) F13.11
    moderate or severe F13.20
      with
        sedative, hypnotic, or
          anxiolytic-induced
          anxiety disorder F13.280
          bipolar and related disorder F13.24
          depressive disorder F13.24
          major neurocognitive disorder F13.27
          mild neurocognitive disorder F13.288
          psychotic disorder F13.259
          sexual dysfunction F13.281
          sedative, hypnotic, or anxiolytic
            intoxication F13.229
          sedative, hypnotic, or anxiolytic
            intoxication delirium F13.221
      ►in remission (early) (sustained) F13.21
  seizure —*see also* Epilepsy G40.909
    intractable G40.919
      with status epilepticus G40.911
  semantic pragmatic F80.89
    with autism F84.0
  sense of smell R43.1
    psychogenic F45.8
  separation anxiety, of childhood F93.0
  sexual
    arousal, female F52.22
    aversion F52.1
    function, psychogenic F52.9
    ►interest/arousal, female F52.22
    ►masochism F65.51
    maturation F66
    nonorganic F52.9
    preference —*see also* Deviation, sexual F65.9
      fetishistic transvestism F65.1
    relationship F66
    ►sadism F65.52

Disorder *(Continued)*
  shyness, of childhood and adolescence F40.10
  sibling rivalry F93.8
  sickle-cell (sickling) (homozygous) —*see*
      Disease, sickle-cell
    heterozygous D57.3
    specified type NEC D57.8-●
    trait D57.3
  sinus (nasal) J34.9
    specified NEC J34.89
  skin L98.9
    atrophic L90.9
      specified NEC L90.8
    granulomatous L92.9
      specified NEC L92.8
    hypertrophic L91.9
      specified NEC L91.8
    infiltrative NEC L98.6
    newborn P83.9
      ⇒specified NEC P83.88
    picking F42.4
    psychogenic (allergic) (eczematous) F54
  sleep G47.9
    breathing-related —*see* Apnea, sleep
    circadian rhythm G47.20
      advance sleep phase type G47.22
      delayed sleep phase type G47.21
      due to
        alcohol
          abuse F10.182
          dependence F10.282
          use F10.982
        amphetamines
          abuse F15.182
          dependence F15.282
          use F15.982
        caffeine
          abuse F15.182
          dependence F15.282
          use F15.982
        cocaine
          abuse F14.182
          dependence F14.282
          use F14.982
        drug NEC
          abuse F19.182
          dependence F19.282
          use F19.982
        opioid
          abuse F11.182
          dependence F11.282
          use F11.982
        psychoactive substance NEC
          abuse F19.182
          dependence F19.282
          use F19.982
        sedative, hypnotic, or anxiolytic
          abuse F13.182
          dependence F13.282
          use F13.982
        stimulant NEC
          abuse F15.182
          dependence F15.282
          use F15.982
      free running type G47.24
      in conditions classified elsewhere
        G47.27
      irregular sleep wake type G47.23
      jet lag type G47.25
      ►non-24-hour sleep-wake type G47.24
      shift work type G47.26
      specified NEC G47.29
    due to
      alcohol
        abuse F10.182
        dependence F10.282
        use F10.982
      amphetamine
        abuse F15.182
        dependence F15.282
        use F15.982

Disorder *(Continued)*
  sleep *(Continued)*
    due to *(Continued)*
      anxiolytic
        abuse F13.182
        dependence F13.282
        use F13.982
      caffeine
        abuse F15.182
        dependence F15.282
        use F15.982
      cocaine
        abuse F14.182
        dependence F14.282
        use F14.982
      drug NEC
        abuse F19.182
        dependence F19.282
        use F19.982
      hypnotic
        abuse F13.182
        dependence F13.282
        use F13.982
      opioid
        abuse F11.182
        dependence F11.282
        use F11.982
      psychoactive substance NEC
        abuse F19.182
        dependence F19.282
        use F19.982
      sedative
        abuse F13.182
        dependence F13.282
        use F13.982
      stimulant NEC
        abuse F15.182
        dependence F15.282
        use F15.982
    emotional F51.9
    excessive somnolence —*see* Hypersomnia
    hypersomnia type —*see* Hypersomnia
    initiating or maintaining —*see* Insomnia
    nightmares F51.5
    nonorganic F51.9
      specified NEC F51.8
    parasomnia type G47.50
    specified NEC G47.8
    terrors F51.4
    walking F51.3
  ⇒sleep-wake pattern or schedule —*see also*
      Disorder, sleep, circadian rhythm G47.9
  ►specified NEC G47.8
  social
    ~~anxiety of childhood F40.10~~
    ►anxiety (of childhood) F40.10
      ►generalized F40.11
    functioning in childhood F94.9
      specified NEC F94.8
    pragmatic F80.82
  soft tissue M79.9
    ankle M79.9
    due to use, overuse and pressure M70.90
      ankle M70.97-●
      bursitis —*see* Bursitis
      foot M70.97-●
      forearm M70.93-●
      hand M70.94-●
      lower leg M70.96-●
      multiple sites M70.99
      pelvic region M70.95-●
      shoulder region M70.91-●
      specified site NEC M70.98
      specified type NEC M70.80
        ankle M70.87-●
        foot M70.87-●
        forearm M70.83-●
        hand M70.84-●
        lower leg M70.86-●
        multiple sites M70.89
        pelvic region M70.85-●

Disorder *(Continued)*
  soft tissue *(Continued)*
    due to use, overuse and pressure
        (Continued)
      specified type NEC *(Continued)*
        shoulder region M70.81-●
        specified site NEC M70.88
        thigh M70.85-●
        upper arm M70.82-●
      thigh M70.95-●
      upper arm M70.92-●
    foot M79.9
    forearm M79.9
    hand M79.9
    lower leg M79.9
    multiple sites M79.9
    occupational —*see* Disorder, soft tissue,
        due to use, overuse and pressure
    pelvic region M79.9
    shoulder region M79.9
    specified type NEC M79.89
    thigh M79.9
    upper arm M79.9
  somatic symptom F45.1
  somatization F45.0
  somatoform F45.9
    pain (persistent) F45.41
    somatization (multiple) (long-lasting) F45.0
    specified NEC F45.8
    undifferentiated F45.1
  somnolence, excessive —*see* Hypersomnia
  specific
    arithmetical F81.2
    developmental, of motor F82
    reading F81.0
    speech and language F80.9
    spelling F81.81
    written expression F81.81
  speech R47.9
    articulation (functional) (specific) F80.0
    developmental F80.9
    specified NEC R47.89
  speech-sound F80.0
  spelling (specific) F81.81
  spine —*see also* Dorsopathy
    ligamentous or muscular attachments,
        peripheral —*see* Enthesopathy, spinal
    specified NEC —*see* Dorsopathy, specified
        NEC
  stereotyped, habit or movement F98.4
  stimulant use (other) (unspecified)
    mild F15.10
    ▶in remission (early) (sustained) F15.11
    moderate or severe F15.20
    ▶in remission (early) (sustained) F15.21
  stomach (functional) —*see* Disorder, gastric
  stress F43.9
    acute F43.0
    post-traumatic F43.10
      acute F43.11
      chronic F43.12
  substance use (other) (unknown)
    mild F19.10
      with substance-induced
        anxiety disorder F19.180
        bipolar and related disorder F19.14
        depressive disorder F19.14
        major neurocognitive disorder F19.17
        mild neurocognitive disorder F19.188
        obsessive-compulsive and related
            disorder F19.188
        sexual dysfunction F19.181
      substance intoxication F19.129
      substance intoxication delirium F19.121
    moderate or severe F19.20
      with substance-induced
        anxiety disorder F19.280
        bipolar and related disorder F19.24
        depressive disorder F19.24
        major neurocognitive disorder F19.27
        mild neurocognitive disorder F19.288

Disorder *(Continued)*
  substance use (other) (unknown) *(Continued)*
    moderate or severe *(Continued)*
      with substance-induced anxiety disorder
          (Continued)
        obsessive-compulsive and related
            disorder F19.288
        sexual dysfunction F19.281
    ▶in remission (early) (sustained) F19.21
      substance intoxication F19.229
      substance intoxication delirium F19.221
  sulfur-bearing amino-acid metabolism E72.10
  sweat gland (eccrine) L74.9
    apocrine L75.9
      specified NEC L75.8
    specified NEC L74.8
  synovium M67.90
    acromioclavicular M67.91-●
    ankle M67.97-●
    elbow M67.92-●
    foot M67.97-●
    forearm M67.93-●
    hand M67.94-●
    hip M67.95-●
    knee M67.96-●
    multiple sites M67.99
    rupture —*see* Rupture, synovium
    shoulder M67.91-●
    specified type NEC M67.80
      acromioclavicular M67.81-●
      ankle M67.87-●
      elbow M67.82-●
      foot M67.87-●
      hand M67.84-●
      hip M67.85-●
      knee M67.86-●
      multiple sites M67.89
      wrist M67.83-●
    synovitis —*see* Synovitis
    upper arm M67.92-●
    wrist M67.93-●
  temperature regulation, newborn P81.9
    specified NEC P81.8
  temporomandibular joint M26.60-●
  tendon M67.90
    acromioclavicular M67.91-●
    ankle M67.97-●
    contracture —*see* Contracture, tendon
    elbow M67.92-●
    foot M67.97-●
    forearm M67.93-●
    hand M67.94-●
    hip M67.95-●
    knee M67.96-●
    multiple sites M67.99
    rupture —*see* Rupture, tendon
    shoulder M67.91-●
    specified type NEC M67.80
      acromioclavicular M67.81-●
      ankle M67.87-●
      elbow M67.82-●
      foot M67.87-●
      hand M67.84-●
      hip M67.85-●
      knee M67.86-●
      multiple sites M67.89
      trunk M67.88
      wrist M67.83-●
    synovitis —*see* Synovitis
    tendinitis —*see* Tendinitis
    tenosynovitis —*see* Tenosynovitis
    trunk M67.98
    upper arm M67.92-●
    wrist M67.93-●
  thoracic root (nerve) NEC G54.3
  thyrocalcitonin hypersecretion E07.0
  thyroid (gland) E07.9
    function NEC, neonatal, transitory P72.2
    iodine-deficiency related E01.8
    specified NEC E07.89
  tic —*see* Tic

Disorder *(Continued)*
  tobacco use
    ▶chewing tobacco (mild) (moderate) (severe)
      ▶in remission (early) (sustained) F17.221
    ▶cigarettes (mild) (moderate) (severe)
      ▶in remission (early) (sustained) F17.211
    mild Z72.0
      ▶in remission (early) (sustained) F17.201
    moderate F17.200
      ▶in remission (early) (sustained) F17.201
    severe F17.200
      ▶in remission (early) (sustained) F17.201
    ▶specified product NEC (mild) (moderate)
        (severe)
      ▶in remission (early) (sustained) F17.291
  tooth K08.9
    development K00.9
      specified NEC K00.8
    eruption K00.6
  Tourette's F95.2
  trance and possession F44.89
  ▶transvestic F65.1
  trauma and stressor-related F43.9
    other specified F43.8
  tricuspid (valve) —*see* Endocarditis, tricuspid
  tryptophan metabolism E70.5
  tubular, phosphate-losing N25.0
  tubulo-interstitial (in)
    brucellosis A23.9 *[N16]*
    cystinosis E72.04
    diphtheria A36.84
    glycogen storage disease E74.00 *[N16]*
    leukemia NEC C95.9-● *[N16]*
    lymphoma NEC C85.9-● *[N16]*
    mixed cryoglobulinemia D89.1 *[N16]*
    multiple myeloma C90.0-● *[N16]*
    Salmonella infection A02.25
    sarcoidosis D86.84
    sepsis A41.9 *[N16]*
      streptococcal A40.9 *[N16]*
    systemic lupus erythematosus M32.15
    toxoplasmosis B58.83
    transplant rejection T86.91 *[N16]*
    Wilson's disease E83.01 *[N16]*
  tubulo-renal function, impaired N25.9
    specified NEC N25.89
  tympanic membrane H73.9-●
    atrophy —*see* Atrophy, tympanic membrane
    infection —*see* Myringitis
    perforation —*see* Perforation, tympanum
    specified NEC H73.89-●
  unsocialized aggressive F91.1
  urea cycle metabolism E72.20
    argininemia E72.21
    arginosuccinic aciduria E72.22
    citrullinemia E72.23
    ornithine transcarbamylase deficiency E72.4
    other specified E72.29
  ureter (in) N28.9
    schistosomiasis B65.0 *[N29]*
    tuberculosis A18.11
  urethra N36.9
    specified NEC N36.8
  urinary system N39.9
    specified NEC N39.8
  valve, heart
    aortic —*see* Endocarditis, aortic
    mitral —*see* Endocarditis, mitral
    pulmonary —*see* Endocarditis, pulmonary
    rheumatic
      aortic —*see* Endocarditis, aortic,
          rheumatic
      mitral —*see* Endocarditis, mitral
      pulmonary —*see* Endocarditis,
          pulmonary, rheumatic
      tricuspid —*see* Endocarditis, tricuspid
    tricuspid —*see* Endocarditis, tricuspid
  vestibular function H81.9-●
    specified NEC —*see* subcategory H81.8
      in diseases classified elsewhere H82.-●
  vertigo —*see* Vertigo

▶ New   ⇒ Revised   ~~deleted~~ Deleted   ● Use Additional Character(s)

Disorder *(Continued)*
  vision, binocular H53.30
    abnormal retinal correspondence H53.31
    diplopia H53.2
    fusion with defective stereopsis H53.32
    simultaneous perception H53.33
    suppression H53.34
  visual
    cortex
      blindness H47.619
        left brain H47.612
        right brain H47.611
        due to
          inflammatory disorder H47.629
            left brain H47.622
            right brain H47.621
          neoplasm H47.639
            left brain H47.632
            right brain H47.631
          vascular disorder H47.649
            left brain H47.642
            right brain H47.641
      pathway H47.9
        due to
          inflammatory disorder H47.51-•
          neoplasm H47.52-•
          vascular disorder H47.53-•
      optic chiasm —*see* Disorder, optic, chiasm
  vitreous body H43.9
    crystalline deposits —*see* Deposit,
        crystalline
    degeneration —*see* Degeneration, vitreous
    hemorrhage —*see* Hemorrhage, vitreous
    opacities —*see* Opacity, vitreous
    prolapse —*see* Prolapse, vitreous
    specified type NEC H43.89
  voice R49.9
    specified type NEC R49.8
  volatile solvent use
    due to drug abuse —*see* Abuse, drug,
        inhalant
    due to drug dependence —*see* Dependence,
        drug, inhalant
▶voyeuristic F65.3
  white blood cells D72.9
    specified NEC D72.89
  withdrawing, child or adolescent
      F40.10
Disorientation R41.0
Displacement, displaced
  acquired traumatic of bone, cartilage, joint,
      tendon NEC —*see* Dislocation
  adrenal gland (congenital) Q89.1
  appendix, retrocecal (congenital) Q43.8
  auricle (congenital) Q17.4
  bladder (acquired) N32.89
    congenital Q64.19
  brachial plexus (congenital) Q07.8
  brain stem, caudal (congenital) Q04.8
  canaliculus (lacrimalis), congenital Q10.6
  cardia through esophageal hiatus (congenital)
      Q40.1
  cerebellum, caudal (congenital) Q04.8
  cervix —*see* Malposition, uterus
  colon (congenital) Q43.3
  device, implant or graft —*see also*
      Complications, by site and type,
      mechanical T85.628
    arterial graft NEC —*see* Complication,
        cardiovascular device, mechanical,
        vascular
    breast (implant) T85.42
    catheter NEC T85.628
      dialysis (renal) T82.42
        intraperitoneal T85.621
      infusion NEC T82.524
        spinal (epidural) (subdural) T85.620
      urinary
        cystostomy T83.020
        Hopkins T83.028
        ileostomy T83.028

Displacement, displaced *(Continued)*
  device, implant or graft *(Continued)*
    catheter NEC *(Continued)*
      urinary *(Continued)*
        indwelling T83.021
        nephrostomy T83.022
        specified NEC T83.028
        urostomy T83.028
    electronic (electrode) (pulse generator)
        (stimulator) —*see* Complication,
        electronic stimulator
    fixation, internal (orthopedic) NEC —
        see Complication, fixation device,
        mechanical
    gastrointestinal —*see* Complications,
        prosthetic device, mechanical,
        gastrointestinal device
    genital NEC T83.428
      intrauterine contraceptive device (string)
          T83.32
      penile prosthesis (cylinder) (implanted)
          (pump) (resevoir) T83.420
      testicular prosthesis T83.421
    heart NEC —*see* Complication,
        cardiovascular device, mechanical
    joint prosthesis —*see* Complications, joint
        prosthesis, mechanical
    ocular —*see* Complications, prosthetic
        device, mechanical, ocular device
    orthopedic NEC —*see* Complication,
        orthopedic, device or graft,
        mechanical
    specified NEC T85.628
    urinary NEC T83.128
      graft T83.22
      sphincter, implanted T83.121
      stent (ileal conduit) (nephroureteral)
          T83.123
      ureteral indwelling T83.122
    vascular NEC —*see* Complication,
        cardiovascular device, mechanical
    ventricular intracranial shunt T85.02
  electronic stimulator
    bone T84.320
    cardiac —*see* Complications, cardiac
        device, electronic
    nervous system —*see* Complication,
        prosthetic device, mechanical,
        electronic nervous system
        stimulator
    urinary —*see* Complications, electronic
        stimulator, urinary
  esophageal mucosa into cardia of stomach,
      congenital Q39.8
  esophagus (acquired) K22.8
    congenital Q39.8
  eyeball (acquired) (lateral) (old) —*see*
      Displacement, globe
    congenital Q15.8
    current —*see* Avulsion, eye
  fallopian tube (acquired) N83.4-•
    congenital Q50.6
    opening (congenital) Q50.6
  gallbladder (congenital) Q44.1
  gastric mucosa (congenital) Q40.2
  globe (acquired) (old) (lateral) H05.21-•
    current —*see* Avulsion, eye
  heart (congenital) Q24.8
    acquired I51.89
  hymen (upward) (congenital) Q52.4
  intervertebral disc NEC
    with myelopathy —*see* Disorder, disc, with,
        myelopathy
    cervical, cervicothoracic (with)
        M50.20
      myelopathy —*see* Disorder, disc,
          cervical, with myelopathy
      neuritis, radiculitis or radiculopathy —
          see Disorder, disc, cervical, with
          neuritis
    due to trauma —*see* Dislocation, vertebra

Displacement, displaced *(Continued)*
  intervertebral disc NEC *(Continued)*
    lumbar region M51.26
      with
        neuritis, radiculitis, radiculopathy or
            sciatica M51.16
    lumbosacral region M51.27
      with
        myelopathy M51.07
        neuritis, radiculitis, radiculopathy or
            sciatica M51.17
    sacrococcygeal region M53.3
    thoracic region M51.24
      with
        myelopathy M51.04
        neuritis, radiculitis, radiculopathy
            M51.14
    thoracolumbar region M51.25
      with
        myelopathy M51.05
        neuritis, radiculitis, radiculopathy
            M51.15
  intrauterine device (string) T83.32
  kidney (acquired) N28.83
    congenital Q63.2
  lachrymal, lacrimal apparatus or duct
      (congenital) Q10.6
  lens, congenital Q12.1
  macula (congenital) Q14.1
  Meckel's diverticulum Q43.0
    malignant —*see* Table of Neoplasms, small
        intestine, malignant
  nail (congenital) Q84.6
    acquired L60.8
  opening of Wharton's duct in mouth Q38.4
  organ or site, congenital NEC —*see*
      Malposition, congenital
  ovary (acquired) N83.4-•
    congenital Q50.39
    free in peritoneal cavity (congenital)
        Q50.39
    into hernial sac N83.4-•
  oviduct (acquired) N83.4-•
    congenital Q50.6
  parathyroid (gland) E21.4
  parotid gland (congenital) Q38.4
  punctum lacrimale (congenital) Q10.6
  sacro-iliac (joint) (congenital) Q74.2
    current injury S33.2
    old —*see* subcategory M53.2
  salivary gland (any) (congenital) Q38.4
  spleen (congenital) Q89.09
  stomach, congenital Q40.2
  sublingual duct Q38.4
  tongue (downward) (congenital) Q38.3
  tooth, teeth, fully erupted M26.30
    horizontal M26.33
    vertical M26.34
  trachea (congenital) Q32.1
  ureter or ureteric opening or orifice
      (congenital) Q62.62
  uterine opening of oviducts or fallopian tubes
      Q50.6
  uterus, uterine —*see* Malposition, uterus
  ventricular septum Q21.0
    with rudimentary ventricle Q20.4
Disproportion
  between native and reconstructed breast N65.1
  fiber-type G71.2
Disruptio uteri —*see* Rupture, uterus
Disruption (of)
  ciliary body NEC H21.89
  closure of
    cornea T81.31
    craniotomy T81.32
    fascia (muscular) (superficial) T81.32
    internal organ or tissue T81.32
    laceration (external) (internal) T81.33
    ligament T81.32
    mucosa T81.31
    muscle or muscle flap T81.32

Disruption *(Continued)*
  closure of *(Continued)*
    ribs or rib cage T81.32
    skin and subcutaneous tissue (full-thickness) (superficial) T81.31
    skull T81.32
    sternum (sternotomy) T81.32
    tendon T81.32
    traumatic laceration (external) (internal) T81.33
  family Z63.8
    due to
      absence of family member due to military deployment Z63.31
      absence of family member NEC Z63.32
      alcoholism and drug addiction in family Z63.72
      bereavement Z63.4
      death (assumed) or disappearance of family member Z63.4
      divorce or separation Z63.5
      drug addiction in family Z63.72
      return of family member from military deployment (current or past conflict) Z63.71
      stressful life events NEC Z63.79
  iris NEC H21.89
  ligament(s) —*see also* Sprain
    knee
      current injury —*see* Dislocation, knee
      old (chronic) —*see* Derangement, knee, ligament, instability, chronic
      spontaneous NEC —*see* Derangement, knee, disruption ligament
  ossicular chain —*see* Discontinuity, ossicles, ear
  pelvic ring (stable) S32.810
    unstable S32.811
  traumatic injury wound repair T81.33
  wound T81.30
    episiotomy O90.1
    operation T81.31
      cesarean O90.0
      external operation wound (superficial) T81.31
      internal operation wound (deep) T81.32
    perineal (obstetric) O90.1
  traumatic injury repair T81.33
Dissatisfaction with
  employment Z56.9
  school environment Z55.4
Dissecting —*see* condition
Dissection
  aorta I71.00
    abdominal I71.02
    thoracic I71.01
    thoracoabdominal I71.03
  artery I77.70
    basilar (trunk) I77.75
    carotid I77.71
    cerebral (nonruptured) I67.0
      ruptured —*see* Hemorrhage, intracranial, subarachnoid
    coronary I25.42
    extremity
      lower I77.77
      upper I77.76
    iliac I77.72
    precerebral
      congenital (nonruptured) Q28.1
      specified site NEC I77.75
    renal I77.73
    specified NEC I77.79
    vertebral I77.74
  ▶precerebral artery, congenital (nonruptured) Q28.1
  ▶Heartland A93.8
  traumatic —*see* Wound, open, by site
  vascular I99.8
  wound —*see* Wound, open
Disseminated —*see* condition

Dissociation
  auriculoventricular or atrioventricular (AV) (any degree) (isorhythmic) I45.89
    with heart block I44.2
  interference I45.89
Dissociative reaction, state F44.9
Dissolution, vertebra —*see* Osteoporosis
Distension, distention
  abdomen R14.0
  bladder N32.89
  cecum K63.89
  colon K63.89
  gallbladder K82.8
  intestine K63.89
  kidney N28.89
  liver K76.89
  seminal vesicle N50.89
  stomach K31.89
    acute K31.0
    psychogenic F45.8
  ureter —*see* Dilatation, ureter
  uterus N85.8
Distoma hepaticum infestation B66.3
Distomiasis B66.9
  bile passages B66.3
  hemic B65.9
  hepatic B66.3
    due to Clonorchis sinensis B66.1
  intestinal B66.5
  liver B66.3
    due to Clonorchis sinensis B66.1
  lung B66.4
  pulmonary B66.4
Distomolar (fourth molar) K00.1
Disto-occlusion (Division I) (Division II) M26.212
Distortion(s) (congenital)
  adrenal (gland) Q89.1
  arm NEC Q68.8
  bile duct or passage Q44.5
  bladder Q64.79
  brain Q04.9
  cervix (uteri) Q51.9
  chest (wall) Q67.8
    bones Q76.8
  clavicle Q74.0
  clitoris Q52.6
  coccyx Q76.49
  common duct Q44.5
  coronary Q24.5
  cystic duct Q44.5
  ear (auricle) (external) Q17.3
    inner Q16.5
    middle Q16.4
      ossicles Q16.3
  endocrine NEC Q89.2
  eustachian tube Q17.8
  eye (adnexa) Q15.8
  face bone(s) NEC Q75.8
  fallopian tube Q50.6
  femur NEC Q68.8
  fibula NEC Q68.8
  finger(s) Q68.1
  foot Q66.9
  genitalia, genital organ(s)
    female Q52.8
      external Q52.79
      internal NEC Q52.8
  gyri Q04.8
  hand bone(s) Q68.1
  heart (auricle) (ventricle) Q24.8
    valve (cusp) Q24.8
  hepatic duct Q44.5
  humerus NEC Q68.8
  hymen Q52.4
  intrafamilial communications Z63.8
  jaw NEC M26.89
  labium (majus) (minus) Q52.79
  leg NEC Q68.8
  lens Q12.8
  liver Q44.7

Distortion *(Continued)*
  lumbar spine Q76.49
    with disproportion O33.8
      causing obstructed labor O65.0
  lumbosacral (joint) (region) Q76.49
    kyphosis —*see* Kyphosis, congenital
    lordosis —*see* Lordosis, congenital
  nerve Q07.8
  nose Q30.8
  organ
    of Corti Q16.5
    or site not listed —*see* Anomaly, by site
      ossicles, ear Q16.3
  oviduct Q50.6
  pancreas Q45.3
  parathyroid (gland) Q89.2
  pituitary (gland) Q89.2
  radius NEC Q68.8
  sacroiliac joint Q74.2
  sacrum Q76.49
  scapula Q74.0
  shoulder girdle Q74.0
  skull bone(s) NEC Q75.8
    with
      anencephalus Q00.0
      encephalocele —*see* Encephalocele
      hydrocephalus Q03.9
        with spina bifida —*see* Spina bifida, with hydrocephalus
      microcephaly Q02
  spinal cord Q06.8
  spine Q76.49
    kyphosis —*see* Kyphosis, congenital
    lordosis —*see* Lordosis, congenital
  spleen Q89.09
  sternum NEC Q76.7
  thorax (wall) Q67.8
    bony Q76.8
  thymus (gland) Q89.2
  thyroid (gland) Q89.2
  tibia NEC Q68.8
  toe(s) Q66.9
  tongue Q38.3
  trachea (cartilage) Q32.1
  ulna NEC Q68.8
  ureter Q62.8
  urethra Q64.79
    causing obstruction Q64.39
  uterus Q51.9
  vagina Q52.4
  vertebra Q76.49
    kyphosis —*see* Kyphosis, congenital
    lordosis —*see* Lordosis, congenital
  visual —*see also* Disturbance, vision
    shape and size H53.15
  vulva Q52.79
  wrist (bones) (joint) Q68.8
Distress
  abdomen —*see* Pain, abdominal
  ➠acute respiratory R06.03
    syndrome (adult) (child) J80
  epigastric R10.13
  fetal P84
    complicating pregnancy —*see* Stress, fetal
  gastrointestinal (functional) K30
    psychogenic F45.8
  intestinal (functional) NOS K59.9
    psychogenic F45.8
  maternal, during labor and delivery O75.0
  ▶relationship, with spouse or intimate partner Z63.0
  ➠respiratory (adult) (child) R06.03
    newborn P22.9
      specified NEC P22.8
    orthopnea R06.01
    psychogenic F45.8
    shortness of breath R06.02
    specified type NEC R06.09
Distribution vessel, atypical Q27.9
  coronary artery Q24.5
  precerebral Q28.1

▶ New   ➠ Revised   ~~deleted~~ Deleted   ● Use Additional Character(s)

Districhiasis L68.8
Disturbance(s) —see also Disease
  absorption K90.9
    calcium E58
    carbohydrate K90.49
    fat K90.49
      pancreatic K90.3
    protein K90.49
    starch K90.49
    vitamin —see Deficiency, vitamin
  acid-base equilibrium E87.8
    mixed E87.4
  activity and attention (with hyperkinesis) —
      see Disorder, attention-deficit
      hyperactivity
  amino acid transport E72.00
  assimilation, food K90.9
  auditory nerve, except deafness —see
      subcategory H93.3
  behavior —see Disorder, conduct
  blood clotting (mechanism) —see also Defect,
      coagulation D68.9
  cerebral
    nerve —see Disorder, nerve, cranial
    status, newborn P91.9
    ➠specified NEC P91.88
  circulatory I99.9
  conduct —see also Disorder, conduct F91.9
    adjustment reaction —see Disorder,
        adjustment
    compulsive F63.9
    disruptive F91.9
    hyperkinetic —see Disorder, attention-
        deficit hyperactivity
    socialized F91.2
    specified NEC F91.8
    unsocialized F91.1
  coordination R27.8
  cranial nerve —see Disorder, nerve, cranial
  deep sensibility —see Disturbance, sensation
  digestive K30
    psychogenic F45.8
  electrolyte —see also Imbalance, electrolyte
    newborn, transitory P74.4
      hyperammonemia P74.6
      potassium balance P74.3
      sodium balance P74.2
      specified type NEC P74.4
  emotions specific to childhood and
      adolescence F93.9
    with
      anxiety and fearfulness NEC F93.8
      elective mutism F94.0
      oppositional disorder F91.3
      sensitivity (withdrawal) F40.10
      shyness F40.10
      social withdrawal F40.10
    involving relationship problems
        F93.8
    mixed F93.8
    specified NEC F93.8
  endocrine (gland) E34.9
    neonatal, transitory P72.9
      specified NEC P72.8
  equilibrium R42
  fructose metabolism E74.10
  gait —see Gait
    hysterical F44.4
    psychogenic F44.4
  gastrointestinal (functional) K30
    psychogenic F45.8
  habit, child F98.9
  hearing, except deafness and tinnitus —see
      Abnormal, auditory perception
  heart, functional (conditions in I44-I50)
    due to presence of (cardiac) prosthesis
        I97.19-●
    postoperative I97.89
    ➠cardiac surgery —see also Infarct,
        myocardium, associated with
        revascularization procedure I97.19-●

Disturbance (Continued)
  hormones E34.9
  innervation uterus (parasympathetic)
      (sympathetic) N85.8
  keratinization NEC
    gingiva K05.10
      nonplaque induced K05.11
      plaque induced K05.10
    lip K13.0
    oral (mucosa) (soft tissue) K13.29
    tongue K13.29
  learning (specific) —see Disorder, learning
  memory —see Amnesia
    mild, following organic brain damage
        F06.8
  mental F99
    associated with diseases classified
        elsewhere F54
  metabolism E88.9
    with
      abortion —see Abortion, by type with
          other specified complication
      ectopic pregnancy O08.5
      molar pregnancy O08.5
    amino-acid E72.9
      aromatic E70.9
      branched-chain E71.2
      straight-chain E72.8
      sulfur-bearing E72.10
    ammonia E72.20
    arginine E72.21
    arginosuccinic acid E72.22
    carbohydrate E74.9
    cholesterol E78.9
    citrulline E72.23
    cystathionine E72.19
    general E88.9
    glutamine E72.8
    histidine E70.40
    homocystine E72.19
    hydroxylysine E72.3
    in labor or delivery O75.89
    iron E83.10
    lipoid E78.9
    lysine E72.3
    methionine E72.19
    neonatal, transitory P74.9
      calcium and magnesium P71.9
        specified type NEC P71.8
      carbohydrate metabolism P70.9
        specified type NEC P70.8
      specified NEC P74.8
    ornithine E72.4
    phosphate E83.39
    sodium NEC E87.8
    threonine E72.8
    tryptophan E70.5
    tyrosine E70.20
    urea cycle E72.20
  motor R29.2
  nervous, functional R45.0
  neuromuscular mechanism (eye), due to
      syphilis A52.15
  nutritional E63.9
    nail L60.3
  ocular motion H51.9
    psychogenic F45.8
  oculogyric H51.8
    psychogenic F45.8
  oculomotor H51.9
    psychogenic F45.8
  olfactory nerve R43.1
  optic nerve NEC —see Disorder, nerve, optic
  oral epithelium, including tongue NEC
      K13.29
  perceptual due to
    alcohol withdrawal F10.232
    amphetamine intoxication F15.922
    in
      abuse F15.122
      dependence F15.222

Disturbance (Continued)
  perceptual due to (Continued)
    anxiolytic withdrawal F13.232
    cannabis intoxication (acute) F12.922
      in
        abuse F12.122
        dependence F12.222
    cocaine intoxication (acute) F14.922
      in
        abuse F14.122
        dependence F14.222
    hypnotic withdrawal F13.232
    opioid intoxication (acute) F11.922
      in
        abuse F11.122
        dependence F11.222
    phencyclidine intoxication (acute)
        F16.122
    sedative withdrawal F13.232
  personality (pattern) (trait) —see also
      Disorder, personality F60.9
    following organic brain damage
        F07.9
  polyglandular E31.9
    specified NEC E31.8
  potassium balance, newborn P74.3
  psychogenic F45.9
  psychomotor F44.4
  psychophysical visual H53.16
  pupillary —see Anomaly, pupil, function
  reflex R29.2
  rhythm, heart I49.9
  salivary secretion K11.7
  sensation (cold) (heat) (localization) (tactile
      discrimination) (texture) (vibratory)
      NEC R20.9
    hysterical F44.6
    skin R20.9
      anesthesia R20.0
      hyperesthesia R20.3
      hypoesthesia R20.1
      paresthesia R20.2
      specified type NEC R20.8
    smell R43.9
      and taste (mixed) R43.8
      anosmia R43.0
      parosmia R43.1
      specified NEC R43.8
    taste R43.9
      and smell (mixed) R43.8
      parageusia R43.2
      specified NEC R43.8
  sensory —see Disturbance, sensation
  situational (transient) —see also Disorder,
      adjustment
    acute F43.0
  sleep G47.9
    nonorganic origin F51.9
  smell —see Disturbance, sensation, smell
  sociopathic F60.2
  sodium balance, newborn P74.2
  speech R47.9
    developmental F80.9
    specified NEC R47.89
  stomach (functional) K31.9
  sympathetic (nerve) G90.9
  taste —see Disturbance, sensation, taste
  temperature
    regulation, newborn P81.9
      specified NEC P81.8
    sense R20.8
      hysterical F44.6
  tooth
    eruption K00.6
    formation K00.4
    structure, hereditary NEC K00.5
  touch —see Disturbance, sensation
  vascular I99.9
    arteriosclerotic —see Arteriosclerosis
  vasomotor I73.9
  vasospastic I73.9

▶ New   ➠ Revised   ~~deleted~~ Deleted   ● Use Additional Character(s)

▶ New   ⇒ Revised   ~~deleted~~ Deleted   ● Use Additional Character(s)

Double (Continued)
  vagina Q52.10
    with doubling of uterus (and cervix)
        Q51.10
      with obstruction Q51.11
  vision H53.2
  vulva Q52.79
Douglas' pouch, cul-de-sac —see condition
Down syndrome Q90.9
  meiotic nondisjunction Q90.0
  mitotic nondisjunction Q90.1
  mosaicism Q90.1
  translocation Q90.2
DPD (dihydropyrimidine dehydrogenase
    deficiency) E88.89
Dracontiasis B72
Dracunculiasis, dracunculosis B72
Dream state, hysterical F44.89
Drepanocytic anemia —see Disease, sickle-cell
Dresbach's syndrome (elliptocytosis) D58.1
Dreschlera (hawaiiensis) (infection) B43.8
Dressler's syndrome I24.1
Drift, ulnar —see Deformity, limb, specified
    type NEC, forearm
Drinking (alcohol)
  excessive, to excess NEC (without
      dependence) F10.10
    habitual (continual) (without remission)
        F10.20
      with remission F10.21
Drip, postnasal (chronic) R09.82
  due to
    allergic rhinitis —see Rhinitis, allergic
    common cold J00
    gastroesophageal reflux —see Reflux,
        gastroesophageal
    nasopharyngitis —see Nasopharyngitis
    other known condition — code to
        condition
    sinusitis —see Sinusitis
Droop
  facial R29.810
    cerebrovascular disease I69.992
      cerebral infarction I69.392
      intracerebral hemorrhage I69.192
      nontraumatic intracranial hemorrhage
          NEC I69.292
      specified disease NEC I69.892
      subarachnoid hemorrhage I69.092
Drop (in)
  attack NEC R55
  finger —see Deformity, finger
  foot —see Deformity, limb, foot, drop
  hematocrit (precipitous) R71.0
  hemoglobin R71.0
  toe —see Deformity, toe, specified NEC
  wrist —see Deformity, limb, wrist drop
Dropped heart beats I45.9
Dropsy, dropsical —see also Hydrops
  abdomen R18.8
  brain —see Hydrocephalus
  cardiac, heart —see Failure, heart, congestive
  gangrenous —see Gangrene
  heart —see Failure, heart, congestive
  kidney —see Nephrosis
  lung —see Edema, lung
  newborn due to isoimmunization P56.0
  pericardium —see Pericarditis
Drowned, drowning (near) T75.1
Drowsiness R40.0
Drug
  abuse counseling and surveillance Z71.51
  addiction —see Dependence
  dependence —see Dependence
  habit —see Dependence
  harmful use —see Abuse, drug
  induced fever R50.2
  overdose —see Table of Drugs and Chemicals,
      by drug, poisoning
  poisoning —see Table of Drugs and
      Chemicals, by drug, poisoning

Drug (Continued)
  resistant organism infection —see also
      Resistant, organism, to, drug Z16.30
  therapy
    long term (current) (prophylactic) —see
        Therapy, drug long-term (current)
        (prophylactic)
    short term - omit code
  wrong substance given or taken in error —see
      Table of Drugs and Chemicals, by drug,
      poisoning
Drunkenness (without dependence) F10.129
  acute in alcoholism F10.229
  chronic (without remission) F10.20
    with remission F10.21
  pathological (without dependence) F10.129
    with dependence F10.229
  sleep F51.9
Drusen
  macula (degenerative) (retina) —see
      Degeneration, macula, drusen
  optic disc H47.32-●
Dry, dryness —see also condition
  larynx J38.7
  mouth R68.2
    due to dehydration E86.0
  nose J34.89
  socket (teeth) M27.3
  throat J39.2
DSAP L56.5
Duane's syndrome H50.81-●
Dubin-Johnson disease or syndrome E80.6
Dubois' disease (thymus gland) A50.59 [E35]
Dubowitz' syndrome Q87.1
Duchenne-Aran muscular atrophy G12.21
Duchenne-Griesinger disease G71.0
Duchenne's
  disease or syndrome
    motor neuron disease G12.22
    muscular dystrophy G71.0
  locomotor ataxia (syphilitic) A52.11
  paralysis
    birth injury P14.0
    due to or associated with
      motor neuron disease G12.22
      muscular dystrophy G71.0
Ducrey's chancre A57
Duct, ductus —see condition
Duhring's disease (dermatitis herpetiformis)
    L13.0
Dullness, cardiac (decreased) (increased) R01.2
Dumb ague —see Malaria
Dumbness —see Aphasia
Dumdum fever B55.0
Dumping syndrome (postgastrectomy) K91.1
Duodenitis (nonspecific) (peptic) K29.80
  with bleeding K29.81
Duodenocholangitis —see Cholangitis
Duodenum, duodenal —see condition
Duplay's bursitis or periarthritis —see
    Tendinitis, calcific, shoulder
Duplication, duplex —see also Accessory
  alimentary tract Q45.8
  anus Q43.4
  appendix (and cecum) Q43.4
  biliary duct (any) Q44.5
  bladder Q64.79
  cecum (and appendix) Q43.4
  cervix Q51.820
  chromosome NEC
    with complex rearrangements NEC
        Q92.5
    seen only at prometaphase Q92.8
  cystic duct Q44.5
  digestive organs Q45.8
  esophagus Q39.8
  frontonasal process Q75.8
  intestine (large) (small) Q43.4
  kidney Q63.0
  liver Q44.7
  pancreas Q45.3

Duplication, duplex (Continued)
  penis Q55.69
  respiratory organs NEC Q34.8
  salivary duct Q38.4
  spinal cord (incomplete) Q06.2
  stomach Q40.2
Dupré's disease (meningism) R29.1
Dupuytren's contraction or disease M72.0
Durand-Nicolas-Favre disease A55
Durotomy (inadvertent) (incidental) G97.41
Duroziez's disease (congenital mitral stenosis)
    Q23.2
Dutton's relapsing fever (West African) A68.1
Dwarfism E34.3
  achondroplastic Q77.4
  congenital E34.3
  constitutional E34.3
  hypochondroplastic Q77.4
  hypophyseal E23.0
  infantile E34.3
  Laron-type E34.3
  Lorain (-Levi) type E23.0
  metatropic Q77.8
  nephrotic-glycosuric (with
      hypophosphatemic rickets) E72.09
  nutritional E45
  pancreatic K86.89
  pituitary E23.0
  renal N25.0
  thanatophoric Q77.1
Dyke-Young anemia (secondary)
    (symptomatic) D59.1
Dysacusis —see Abnormal, auditory
    perception
Dysadrenocortism E27.9
  hyperfunction E27.0
Dysarthria R47.1
  following
    cerebral infarction I69.322
    cerebrovascular disease I69.922
      specified disease NEC I69.822
    intracerebral hemorrhage I69.122
    nontraumatic intracranial hemorrhage
        NEC I69.222
    subarachnoid hemorrhage I69.022
Dysautonomia (familial) G90.1
Dysbarism T70.3
Dysbasia R26.2
  angiosclerotica intermittens I73.9
  hysterical F44.4
  lordotica (progressiva) G24.1
  nonorganic origin F44.4
  psychogenic F44.4
Dysbetalipoproteinemia (familial) E78.2
Dyscalculia R48.8
  developmental F81.2
Dyschezia K59.00
Dyschondroplasia (with hemangiomata) Q78.4
Dyschromia (skin) L81.9
Dyscollagenosis M35.9
Dyscranio-pygo-phalangy Q87.0
Dyscrasia
  blood (with) D75.9
    antepartum hemorrhage —see
        Hemorrhage, antepartum, with
        coagulation defect
    intrapartum hemorrhage O67.0
    newborn P61.9
      specified type NEC P61.8
    puerperal, postpartum O72.3
  polyglandular, pluriglandular E31.9
Dysendocrinism E34.9
Dysentery, dysenteric (catarrhal) (diarrhea)
    (epidemic) (hemorrhagic) (infectious)
    (sporadic) (tropical) A09
  abscess, liver A06.4
  amebic —see also Amebiasis A06.0
    with abscess —see Abscess, amebic
    acute A06.0
    chronic A06.1
  arthritis —see also category M01 A09
  bacillary —see also category M01 A03.9

Dysentery, dysenteric *(Continued)*
  bacillary A03.9
    arthritis —*see also* category M01 A03.9
    Boyd A03.2
    Flexner A03.1
    Schmitz (-Stutzer) A03.0
    Shiga (-Kruse) A03.0
    Shigella A03.9
      boydii A03.2
      dysenteriae A03.0
      flexneri A03.1
      group A A03.0
      group B A03.1
      group C A03.2
      group D A03.3
      sonnei A03.3
      specified type NEC A03.8
    Sonne A03.3
    specified type NEC A03.8
  balantidial A07.0
  Balantidium coli A07.0
  Boyd's A03.2
  candidal B37.82
  Chilomastix A07.8
  Chinese A03.9
  coccidial A07.3
  Dientamoeba (fragilis) A07.8
  Embadomonas A07.8
  Entamoeba, entamebic —*see* Dysentery,
    amebic
  Flexner-Boyd A03.2
  Flexner's A03.1
  Giardia lamblia A07.1
  Hiss-Russell A03.1
  Lamblia A07.1
  leishmanial B55.0
  malarial —*see* Malaria
  metazoal B82.0
  monilial B37.82
  protozoal A07.9
  Salmonella A02.0
  schistosomal B65.1
  Schmitz (-Stutzer) A03.0
  Shiga (-Kruse) A03.0
  Shigella NOS —*see* Dysentery, bacillary
  Sonne A03.3
  strongyloidiasis B78.0
  trichomonal A07.8
  viral —*see also* Enteritis, viral A08.4
Dysequilibrium R42
Dysesthesia R20.8
  hysterical F44.6
Dysfibrinogenemia (congenital) D68.2
Dysfunction
  adrenal E27.9
    hyperfunction E27.0
  autonomic
    due to alcohol G31.2
    somatoform F45.8
  bladder N31.9
    neurogenic NOS —*see* Dysfunction,
      bladder, neuromuscular
    neuromuscular NOS N31.9
      atonic (motor) (sensory) N31.2
      autonomous N31.2
      flaccid N31.2
      nonreflex N31.2
      reflex N31.1
      specified NEC N31.8
      uninhibited N31.0
  bleeding, uterus N93.8
  cerebral G93.89
  colon K59.9
    psychogenic F45.8
  colostomy K94.03
  cystic duct K82.8
  cystostomy (stoma) —*see* Complications,
    cystostomy
  ejaculatory N53.19
    anejaculatory orgasm N53.13
    painful N53.12

Dysfunction *(Continued)*
  ejaculatory *(Continued)*
    premature F52.4
    retarded N53.11
  endocrine NOS E34.9
  endometrium N85.8
  enterostomy K94.13
  erectile —*see* Dysfunction, sexual, male, erectile
  gallbladder K82.8
  gastrostomy (stoma) K94.23
  gland, glandular NOS E34.9
  heart I51.89
  hemoglobin D75.89
  hepatic K76.89
  hypophysis E23.7
  hypothalamic NEC E23.3
  ileostomy (stoma) K94.13
  jejunostomy (stoma) K94.13
  kidney —*see* Disease, renal
  labyrinthine —*see* subcategory H83.2
  left ventricular, following sudden emotional
    stress I51.81
  liver K76.89
  male —*see* Dysfunction, sexual, male
  orgasmic (female) F52.31
    male F52.32
  ovary E28.9
    specified NEC E28.8
  papillary muscle I51.89
  parathyroid E21.4
  physiological NEC R68.89
    psychogenic F59
  pineal gland E34.8
  pituitary (gland) E23.3
  platelets D69.1
  polyglandular E31.9
    specified NEC E31.8
  psychophysiologic F59
  psychosexual F52.9
    with
      dyspareunia F52.6
      premature ejaculation F52.4
      vaginismus F52.5
  pylorus K31.9
  rectum K59.9
    psychogenic F45.8
  reflex (sympathetic) —*see* Syndrome, pain,
    complex regional I
  segmental —*see* Dysfunction, somatic
  senile R54
  sexual (due to) R37
    alcohol F10.981
    amphetamine F15.981
      in
        abuse F15.181
        dependence F15.281
    anxiolytic F13.981
      in
        abuse F13.181
        dependence F13.281
    cocaine F14.981
      in
        abuse F14.181
        dependence F14.281
    excessive sexual drive F52.8
    failure of genital response (male) F52.21
      female F52.22
    female N94.9
      aversion F52.1
      dyspareunia N94.10
        psychogenic F52.6
      frigidity F52.22
      nymphomania F52.8
      orgasmic F52.31
      psychogenic F52.9
        aversion F52.1
        dyspareunia F52.6
        frigidity F52.22
        nymphomania F52.8
        orgasmic F52.31
        vaginismus F52.5

Dysfunction *(Continued)*
  sexual *(Continued)*
    female *(Continued)*
      vaginismus N94.2
        psychogenic F52.5
    hypnotic F13.981
      in
        abuse F13.181
        dependence F13.281
    inhibited orgasm (female) F52.31
      male F52.32
    lack
      of sexual enjoyment F52.1
      or loss of sexual desire F52.0
    male N53.9
      anejaculatory orgasm N53.13
      ejaculatory N53.19
        painful N53.12
        premature F52.4
        retarded N53.11
      erectile N52.9
        drug induced N52.2
        due to
          disease classified elsewhere N52.1
          drug N52.2
        postoperative (postprocedural) N52.39
          following
            cryotherapy N52.37
            interstitial seed therapy N52.36
            prostate ablative therapy N52.37
            prostatectomy N52.34
              radical N52.31
            radiation therapy N52.35
            radical cystectomy N52.32
            ultrasound ablative therapy
              N52.37
            urethral surgery N52.33
        psychogenic F52.21
        specified cause NEC N52.8
        vasculogenic
          arterial insufficiency N52.01
            with corporo-venous occlusive
              N52.03
          corporo-venous occlusive N52.02
            with arterial insufficiency N52.03
      impotence —*see* Dysfunction, sexual,
        male, erectile
      psychogenic F52.9
        aversion F52.1
        erectile F52.21
        orgasmic F52.32
        premature ejaculation F52.4
        satyriasis F52.8
        specified type NEC F52.8
      specified type NEC N53.8
    nonorganic F52.9
      specified NEC F52.8
    opioid F11.981
      in
        abuse F11.181
        dependence F11.281
    orgasmic dysfunction (female) F52.31
      male F52.32
    premature ejaculation F52.4
    psychoactive substances NEC F19.981
      in
        abuse F19.181
        dependence F19.281
    psychogenic F52.9
    sedative F13.981
      in
        abuse F13.181
        dependence F13.281
    sexual aversion F52.1
    vaginismus (nonorganic) (psychogenic)
      F52.5
  sinoatrial node I49.5
  somatic M99.09
    abdomen M99.09
    acromioclavicular M99.07
    cervical region M99.01

▶ New   ⇒ Revised   ~~deleted~~ Deleted   ● Use Additional Character(s)

Dysfunction *(Continued)*
  somatic *(Continued)*
    cervicothoracic M99.01
    costochondral M99.08
    costovertebral M99.08
    head region M99.00
    hip M99.05
    lower extremity M99.06
    lumbar region M99.03
    lumbosacral M99.03
    occipitocervical M99.00
    pelvic region M99.05
    pubic M99.05
    rib cage M99.08
    sacral region M99.04
    sacrococcygeal M99.04
    sacroiliac M99.04
    specified NEC M99.09
    sternochondral M99.08
    sternoclavicular M99.07
    thoracic region M99.02
    thoracolumbar M99.02
    upper extremity M99.07
  somatoform autonomic F45.8
  stomach K31.89
    psychogenic F45.8
  suprarenal E27.9
    hyperfunction E27.0
  symbolic R48.9
    specified type NEC R48.8
  temporomandibular (joint) M26.69
    joint-pain syndrome M26.62-•
  testicular (endocrine) E29.9
    specified NEC E29.8
  thymus E32.9
  thyroid E07.9
  ureterostomy (stoma) —*see* Complications, stoma, urinary tract
  urethrostomy (stoma) —*see* Complications, stoma, urinary tract
  uterus, complicating delivery O62.9
    hypertonic O62.4
    hypotonic O62.2
      primary O62.0
      secondary O62.1
  ventricular I51.9
    ~~with congestive heart failure I50.9-•~~
    ~~left, reversible, following sudden emotional stress I51.81~~
    ▶with congestive heart failure —*see also* Failure, heart I50.9
    ▶left, reversible, following sudden emotional stress I51.81
Dysgenesis
  gonadal (due to chromosomal anomaly) Q96.9
    pure Q99.1
  renal Q60.5
    bilateral Q60.4
    unilateral Q60.3
  reticular D72.0
  tidal platelet D69.3
Dysgerminoma
  specified site —*see* Neoplasm, malignant, by site
  unspecified site
    female C56.9
    male C62.90
Dysgeusia R43.2
Dysgraphia R27.8
Dyshidrosis, dysidrosis L30.1
Dyskaryotic cervical smear R87.619
Dyskeratosis L85.8
  cervix —*see* Dysplasia, cervix
  congenital Q82.8
  uterus NEC N85.8
Dyskinesia G24.9
  biliary (cystic duct or gallbladder) K82.8
  drug induced
    orofacial G24.01
  esophagus K22.4

Dyskinesia *(Continued)*
  hysterical F44.4
  intestinal K59.8
  nonorganic origin F44.4
  orofacial (idiopathic) G24.4
    drug induced G24.01
  psychogenic F44.4
  subacute, drug induced G24.01
  tardive G24.01
    neuroleptic induced G24.01
  trachea J39.8
  tracheobronchial J98.09
Dyslalia (developmental) F80.0
Dyslexia R48.0
  developmental F81.0
Dyslipidemia E78.5
  depressed HDL cholesterol E78.6
  elevated fasting triglycerides E78.1
Dysmaturity —*see also* Light for dates
  pulmonary (newborn) (Wilson-Mikity) P27.0
Dysmenorrhea (essential) (exfoliative) N94.6
  congestive (syndrome) N94.6
  primary N94.4
  psychogenic F45.8
  secondary N94.5
Dysmetabolic syndrome X E88.81
Dysmetria R27.8
Dysmorphism (due to)
  alcohol Q86.0
  exogenous cause NEC Q86.8
  hydantoin Q86.1
  warfarin Q86.2
Dysmorphophobia (nondelusional) F45.22
  delusional F22
Dysnomia R47.01
Dysorexia R63.0
  psychogenic F50.89
Dysostosis
  cleidocranial, cleidocranialis Q74.0
  craniofacial Q75.1
  Fairbank's (idiopathic familial generalized osteophytosis) Q78.9
  mandibulofacial (incomplete) Q75.4
  multiplex E76.01
  oculomandibular Q75.5
Dyspareunia (female) N94.10
  deep N94.12
  male N53.12
  nonorganic F52.6
  psychogenic F52.6
  secondary N94.19
  specified NEC N94.19
  superficial (introital) N94.11
Dyspepsia R10.13
  atonic K30
  functional (allergic) (congenital) (gastrointestinal) (occupational) (reflex) K30
  intestinal K59.8
  nervous F45.8
  neurotic F45.8
  psychogenic F45.8
Dysphagia R13.10
  cervical R13.19
  following
    cerebral infarction I69.391
    cerebrovascular disease I69.991
      specified NEC I69.891
    intracerebral hemorrhage I69.191
    nontraumatic intracranial hemorrhage NEC I69.291
    specified disease NEC I69.891
    subarachnoid hemorrhage I69.091
  functional (hysterical) F45.8
  hysterical F45.8
  nervous (hysterical) F45.8
  neurogenic R13.19
  oral phase R13.11
  oropharyngeal phase R13.12
  ~~pharyneal phase R13.13~~
  ▶pharyngeal phase R13.13

Dysphagia *(Continued)*
  pharyngoesophageal phase R13.14
  psychogenic F45.8
  sideropenic D50.1
  spastica K22.4
  specified NEC R13.19
Dysphagocytosis, congenital D71
Dysphasia R47.02
  developmental
    expressive type F80.1
    receptive type F80.2
  following
    cerebrovascular disease I69.921
      cerebral infarction I69.321
      intracerebral hemorrhage I69.121
    nontraumatic intracranial hemorrhage NEC I69.221
      specified disease NEC I69.821
      subarachnoid hemorrhage I69.021
Dysphonia R49.0
  functional F44.4
  hysterical F44.4
  psychogenic F44.4
  spastica J38.3
Dysphoria
  ⇒gender F64.9
    in
      adolescence and adulthood F64.0
      children F64.2
    ▶specified NEC F64.8
    postpartal O90.6
Dyspituitarism E23.3
Dysplasia —*see also* Anomaly
  acetabular, congenital Q65.89
  alveolar capillary, with vein misalignment J84.843
  anus (histologically confirmed) (mild) (moderate) K62.82
    severe D01.3
  arrhythmogenic right ventricular I42.8
  arterial, fibromuscular I77.3
  asphyxiating thoracic (congenital) Q77.2
  brain Q07.9
  bronchopulmonary, perinatal P27.1
  cervix (uteri) N87.9
    mild N87.0
    moderate N87.1
    severe D06.9
  chondroectodermal Q77.6
  colon D12.6
  craniometaphyseal Q78.58
  dentinal K00.5
  diaphyseal, progressive Q78.3
  dystrophic Q77.5
  ectodermal (anhidrotic) (congenital) (hereditary) Q82.4
    hydrotic Q82.8
  epithelial, uterine cervix —*see* Dysplasia, cervix
  eye (congenital) Q11.2
  fibrous
    bone NEC (monostotic) M85.00
      ankle M85.07-•
      foot M85.07-•
      forearm M85.03-•
      hand M85.04-•
      lower leg M85.06-•
      multiple site M85.09
      neck M85.08
      rib M85.08
      shoulder M85.01-•
      skull M85.08
      specified site NEC M85.08
      thigh M85.05-•
      toe M85.07-•
      upper arm M85.02-•
      vertebra M85.08
    diaphyseal, progressive Q78.3
    jaw M27.8
    polyostotic Q78.1
  florid osseous —*see also* Cyst, calcifying odontogenic

Dysplasia (*Continued*)
  high grade, focal D12.6
  hip, congenital Q65.89
  joint, congenital Q74.8
  kidney Q61.4
    multicystic Q61.4
  leg Q74.2
  lung, congenital (not associated with short
      gestation) Q33.6
  mammary (gland) (benign) N60.9- •
    cyst (solitary) —*see* Cyst, breast
    cystic —*see* Mastopathy, cystic
    duct ectasia —*see* Ectasia, mammary
        duct
    fibroadenosis —*see* Fibroadenosis, breast
    fibrosclerosis —*see* Fibrosclerosis, breast
    specified type NEC N60.8- •
  metaphyseal Q78.5
  muscle Q79.8
  oculodentodigital Q87.0
  periapical (cemental) (cemento-osseous) —*see*
      Cyst, calcifying odontogenic
  periosteum —*see* Disorder, bone, specified
      type NEC
  polyostotic fibrous Q78.1
  prostate —*see also* Neoplasia, intraepithelial,
      prostate N42.30
    severe D07.5
    specified NEC N42.39
  renal Q61.4
    multicystic Q61.4
  retinal, congenital Q14.1
  right ventricular, arrhythmogenic I42.8
  septo-optic Q04.4
  skin L98.8
  spinal cord Q06.1
  spondyloepiphyseal Q77.7
  thymic, with immunodeficiency D82.1
  vagina N89.3
    mild N89.0
    moderate N89.1
    severe NEC D07.2
  vulva N90.3
    mild N90.0
    moderate N90.1
    severe NEC D07.1
Dyspnea (nocturnal) (paroxysmal) R06.00
  asthmatic (bronchial) J45.909
    with
      bronchitis J45.909
        with
          exacerbation (acute) J45.901
          status asthmaticus J45.902
        chronic J44.9
        exacerbation (acute) J45.901
        status asthmaticus J45.902
    cardiac —*see* Failure, ventricular, left
  cardiac —*see* Failure, ventricular, left
  functional F45.8
  hyperventilation R06.4
  hysterical F45.8
  newborn P28.89
  psychogenic F45.8
  shortness of breath R06.02
  specified type NEC R06.09
Dyspraxia R27.8
  developmental (syndrome) F82
Dysproteinemia E88.09
Dysreflexia, autonomic G90.4

Dysrhythmia
  cardiac I49.9
    newborn
      bradycardia P29.12
        occurring before birth P03.819
          before onset of labor P03.810
          during labor P03.811
      tachycardia P29.11
    postoperative I97.89
  cerebral or cortical —*see* Epilepsy
Dyssomnia —*see* Disorder, sleep
Dyssynergia
  biliary K83.8
  bladder sphincter N36.44
  cerebellaris myoclonica (Hunt's ataxia)
      G11.1
Dysthymia F34.1
Dysthyroidism E07.9
Dystocia O66.9
  affecting newborn P03.1
  cervical (hypotonic) O62.2
    affecting newborn P03.6
    primary O62.0
    secondary O62.1
  contraction ring O62.4
  fetal O66.9
    abnormality NEC O66.3
    conjoined twins O66.3
    oversize O66.2
  maternal O66.9
  positional O64.9
  shoulder (girdle) O66.0
    causing obstructed labor O66.0
  uterine NEC O62.4
Dystonia G24.9
  deformans progressiva G24.1
  drug induced NEC G24.09
    acute G24.02
    specified NEC G24.09
  familial G24.1
  idiopathic G24.1
    familial G24.1
    nonfamilial G24.2
    orofacial G24.4
  lenticularis G24.8
  musculorum deformans G24.1
  neuroleptic induced (acute) G24.02
  orofacial (idiopathic) G24.4
  oromandibular G24.4
    due to drug G24.01
  specified NEC G24.8
  torsion (familial) (idiopathic) G24.1
    acquired G24.8
    genetic G24.1
  symptomatic (nonfamilial) G24.2
Dystonic movements R25.8
Dystrophy, dystrophia
  adiposogenital E23.6
  Becker's type G71.0
  cervical sympathetic G90.2
  choroid (hereditary) H31.20
    central areolar H31.22
    choroideremia H31.21
    gyrate atrophy H31.23
    specified type NEC H31.29
  cornea (hereditary) H18.50
    endothelial H18.51
    epithelial H18.52
    granular H18.53

Dystrophy, dystrophia (*Continued*)
  cornea (*Continued*)
    lattice H18.54
    macular H18.55
    specified type NEC H18.59
  Duchenne's type G71.0
  due to malnutrition E45
  Erb's G71.0
  Fuchs' H18.51
  Gower's muscular G71.0
  hair L67.8
  infantile neuraxonal G31.89
  Landouzy-Déjérine G71.0
  Leyden-Möbius G71.0
  muscular G71.0
    benign (Becker type) G71.0
    congenital (hereditary) (progressive) (with
        specific morphological abnormalities
        of the muscle fiber) G71.0
      myotonic G71.11
    distal G71.0
    Duchenne type G71.0
    Emery-Dreifuss G71.0
    Erb type G71.0
    facioscapulohumeral G71.0
    Gower's G71.0
    hereditary (progressive) G71.0
    Landouzy-Déjérine type G71.0
    limb-girdle G71.0
    myotonic G71.11
    progressive (hereditary) G71.0
      Charcot-Marie (-Tooth) type G60.0
    pseudohypertrophic (infantile) G71.0
    severe (Duchenne type) G71.0
  myocardium, myocardial —*see*
      Degeneration, myocardial
  nail L60.3
    congenital Q84.6
  nutritional E45
  ocular G71.0
  oculocerebrorenal E72.03
  oculopharyngeal G71.0
  ovarian N83.8
  polyglandular E31.8
  reflex (neuromuscular) (sympathetic) —
      see Syndrome, pain, complex regional I
  retinal (hereditary) H35.50
    in
      lipid storage disorders E75.6 [*H36*]
      systemic lipidoses E75.6 [*H36*]
    involving
      pigment epithelium H35.54
      sensory area H35.53
    pigmentary H35.52
    vitreoretinal H35.51
  Salzmann's nodular —*see* Degeneration,
      cornea, nodular
  scapuloperoneal G71.0
  skin NEC L98.8
  sympathetic (reflex) —*see* Syndrome, pain,
      complex regional I
    cervical G90.2
  tapetoretinal H35.54
  thoracic, asphyxiating Q77.2
  unguium L60.3
    congenital Q84.6
  vitreoretinal H35.51
  vulva N90.4
  yellow (liver) —*see* Failure, hepatic
Dysuria R30.0
  psychogenic F45.8

▶ New   ⇒ Revised   ~~deleted~~ Deleted   • Use Additional Character(s)

E

Eales' disease H35.06-●
Ear —*see also* condition
 piercing Z41.3
 tropical NEC B36.9 *[H62.40]*
 in
  aspergillosis B44.89
  candidiasis B37.84
  moniliasis B37.84
 wax (impacted) H61.20
  left H61.22
   with right H61.23
  right H61.21
   with left H61.23
Earache —*see* subcategory H92.0
Early satiety R68.81
Eaton-Lambert syndrome—*see* Syndrome,
 Lambert-Eaton
Eberth's disease (typhoid fever) A01.00
Ebola virus disease A98.4
Ebstein's anomaly or syndrome (heart) Q22.5
Eccentro-osteochondrodysplasia E76.29
Ecchondroma —*see* Neoplasm, bone, benign
Ecchondrosis D48.0
Ecchymosis R58
 conjunctiva —*see* Hemorrhage, conjunctiva
 eye (traumatic) —*see* Contusion, eyeball
 eyelid (traumatic) —*see* Contusion, eyelid
 newborn P54.5
 spontaneous R23.3
 traumatic —*see* Contusion
Echinococciasis —*see* Echinococcus
Echinococcosis —*see* Echinococcus
Echinococcus (infection) B67.90
 granulosus B67.4
  bone B67.2
  liver B67.0
  lung B67.1
  multiple sites B67.32
  specified site NEC B67.39
  thyroid B67.31
 liver NOS B67.8
  granulosus B67.0
  multilocularis B67.5
 lung NEC B67.99
  granulosus B67.1
  multilocularis B67.69
 multilocularis B67.7
  liver B67.5
  multiple sites B67.61
  specified site NEC B67.69
 specified site NEC B67.99
  granulosus B67.39
  multilocularis B67.69
 thyroid NEC B67.99
  granulosus B67.31
  multilocularis B67.69 *[E35]*
Echinorhynchiasis B83.8
Echinostomiasis B66.8
Echolalia R48.8
Echovirus, as cause of disease classified
 elsewhere B97.12
Eclampsia, eclamptic (coma) (convulsions)
 (delirium) (with hypertension) NEC O15.9
 complicating
  labor and delivery O15.1
  postpartum O15.2
  pregnancy O15.0-●
  puerperium O15.2
Economic circumstances affecting care Z59.9
Economo's disease A85.8
Ectasia, ectasis
 annuloaortic I35.8
 aorta I77.819
  with aneurysm —*see* Aneurysm, aorta
  abdominal I77.811
  thoracic I77.810
  thoracoabdominal I77.812
 breast —*see* Ectasia, mammary duct

Ectasia, ectasis *(Continued)*
 capillary I78.8
 cornea H18.71-●
 gastric antral vascular (GAVE) K31.819
  with hemorrhage K31.811
  without hemorrhage K31.819
 mammary duct N60.4-●
 salivary gland (duct) K11.8
 sclera —*see* Sclerectasia
Ecthyma L08.0
 contagiosum B08.02
 gangrenosum L08.0
 infectiosum B08.02
Ectocardia Q24.8
Ectodermal dysplasia (anhidrotic) Q82.4
Ectodermosis erosiva pluriorificialis
 L51.1
Ectopic, ectopia (congenital)
 abdominal viscera Q45.8
  due to defect in anterior abdominal wall
   Q79.59
 ACTH syndrome E24.3
 adrenal gland Q89.1
 anus Q43.5
 atrial beats I49.1
 beats I49.49
  atrial I49.1
  ventricular I49.3
 bladder Q64.10
 bone and cartilage in lung Q33.5
 brain Q04.8
 breast tissue Q83.8
 cardiac Q24.8
 cerebral Q04.8
 cordis Q24.8
 endometrium —*see* Endometriosis
 gastric mucosa Q40.2
 gestation —*see* Pregnancy, by site
 heart Q24.8
 hormone secretion NEC E34.2
 kidney (crossed) (pelvis) Q63.2
 lens, lentis Q12.1
 mole —*see* Pregnancy, by site
 organ or site NEC —*see* Malposition,
  congenital
 pancreas Q45.3
 pregnancy —*see* Pregnancy, ectopic
 pupil —*see* Abnormality, pupillary
 renal Q63.2
 sebaceous glands of mouth Q38.6
 spleen Q89.09
 testis Q53.00
  bilateral Q53.02
  unilateral Q53.01
 thyroid Q89.2
 tissue in lung Q33.5
 ureter Q62.63
 ventricular beats I49.3
 vesicae Q64.10
Ectromelia Q73.8
 lower limb —*see* Defect, reduction, limb,
  lower, specified type NEC
 upper limb —*see* Defect, reduction, limb,
  upper, specified type NEC
Ectropion H02.109
 cervix N86
  with cervicitis N72
 congenital Q10.1
 eyelid (paralytic) H02.109
  cicatricial H02.119
   left H02.116
    lower H02.115
    upper H02.114
   right H02.113
    lower H02.112
    upper H02.111
  congenital Q10.1
  left H02.106
   lower H02.105
   upper H02.104

Ectropion *(Continued)*
 eyelid *(Continued)*
  mechanical H02.129
   left H02.126
    lower H02.125
    upper H02.124
   right H02.123
    lower H02.122
    upper H02.121
  right H02.103
   lower H02.102
   upper H02.101
  senile H02.139
   left H02.136
    lower H02.135
    upper H02.134
   right H02.133
    lower H02.132
    upper H02.131
  spastic H02.149
   left H02.146
    lower H02.145
    upper H02.144
   right H02.143
    lower H02.142
    upper H02.141
 iris H21.89
 lip (acquired) K13.0
  congenital Q38.0
 urethra N36.8
 uvea H21.89
Eczema (acute) (chronic) (erythematous)
 (fissum) (rubrum) (squamous) (*see also*
 Dermatitis) L30.9
 contact —*see* Dermatitis, contact
 dyshydrotic L30.1
 external ear —*see* Otitis, externa, acute,
  eczematoid
 flexural L20.82
 herpeticum B00.0
 hypertrophicum L28.0
 hypostatic —*see* Varix, leg, with,
  inflammation
 impetiginous L01.1
 infantile (due to any substance) L20.83
  intertriginous L21.1
  seborrheic L21.1
 intertriginous NEC L30.4
  infantile L21.1
 intrinsic (allergic) L20.84
 lichenified NEC L28.0
 marginatum (hebrae) B35.6
 pustular L30.3
 stasis I87.2
  with varicose veins —*see* Varix, leg, with,
   inflammation
 vaccination, vaccinatum T88.1
 varicose —*see* Varix, leg, with, inflammation
Eczematid L30.2
Eddowes (-Spurway) syndrome Q78.0
Edema, edematous (infectious) (pitting)
 (toxic) R60.9
 with nephritis —*see* Nephrosis
 allergic T78.3
 amputation stump (surgical) (sequelae
  (late effect)) T87.89
 angioneurotic (allergic) (any site) (with
  urticaria) T78.3
  hereditary D84.1
 angiospastic I73.9
 Berlin's (traumatic) S05.8X-●
 brain (cytotoxic) (vasogenic) G93.6
  due to birth injury P11.0
  newborn (anoxia or hypoxia) P52.4
   birth injury P11.0
  traumatic —*see* Injury, intracranial,
   cerebral edema
 cardiac —*see* Failure, heart, congestive
 cardiovascular —*see* Failure, heart, congestive
 cerebral —*see* Edema, brain

Edema, edematous *(Continued)*
- cerebrospinal —*see* Edema, brain
- cervix (uteri) (acute) N88.8
  - puerperal, postpartum O90.89
- chronic hereditary Q82.0
- circumscribed, acute T78.3
  - hereditary D84.1
- conjunctiva H11.42-●
- cornea H18.2-●
  - idiopathic H18.22-●
  - secondary H18.23-●
    - due to contact lens H18.21-●
- due to
  - lymphatic obstruction I89.0
  - salt retention E87.0
- epiglottis —*see* Edema, glottis
- essential, acute T78.3
  - hereditary D84.1
- extremities, lower —*see* Edema, legs
- eyelid NEC H02.849
  - left H02.846
    - lower H02.845
    - upper H02.844
  - right H02.843
    - lower H02.842
    - upper H02.841
- familial, hereditary Q82.0
- famine —*see* Malnutrition, severe
- generalized R60.1
- glottis, glottic, glottidis (obstructive) (passive) J38.4
  - allergic T78.3
    - hereditary D84.1
- heart —*see* Failure, heart, congestive
- heat T67.7
- hereditary Q82.0
- inanition —*see* Malnutrition, severe
- intracranial G93.6
- iris H21.89
- joint —*see* Effusion, joint
- larynx —*see* Edema, glottis
- legs R60.0
  - due to venous obstruction I87.1
  - hereditary Q82.0
- localized R60.0
  - due to venous obstruction I87.1
- lower limbs —*see* Edema, legs
- lung J81.1
  - with heart condition or failure —*see* Failure, ventricular, left
  - acute J81.0
  - chemical (acute) J68.1
    - chronic J68.1
  - chronic J81.1
    - due to
      - chemicals, gases, fumes or vapors (inhalation) J68.1
      - external agent J70.9
        - specified NEC J70.8
      - radiation J70.1
  - due to
    - chemicals, fumes or vapors (inhalation) J68.1
    - external agent J70.9
      - specified NEC J70.8
    - high altitude T70.29
    - near drowning T75.1
    - radiation J70.0
  - meaning failure, left ventricle I50.1
- lymphatic I89.0
  - due to mastectomy I97.2
- macula H35.81
  - cystoid, following cataract surgery —*see* Complications, postprocedural, following cataract surgery
  - diabetic —*see* Diabetes, by type, with, retinopathy, with macular edema
- malignant —*see* Gangrene, gas
- Milroy's Q82.0

Edema, edematous *(Continued)*
- nasopharynx J39.2
- newborn P83.30
  - hydrops fetalis —*see* Hydrops, fetalis
  - specified NEC P83.39
- nutritional —*see also* Malnutrition, severe
  - with dyspigmentation, skin and hair E40
- optic disc or nerve —*see* Papilledema
- orbit H05.22-●
- pancreas K86.89
- papilla, optic —*see* Papilledema
- penis N48.89
- periodic T78.3
  - hereditary D84.1
- pharynx J39.2
- pulmonary —*see* Edema, lung
- Quincke's T78.3
  - hereditary D84.1
- renal —*see* Nephrosis
- retina H35.81
  - diabetic —*see* Diabetes, by type, with, retinopathy, with macular edema
- salt E87.0
- scrotum N50.89
- seminal vesicle N50.89
- spermatic cord N50.89
- spinal (cord) (vascular) (nontraumatic) G95.19
- starvation —*see* Malnutrition, severe
- stasis —*see* Hypertension, venous, (chronic)
- subglottic —*see* Edema, glottis
- supraglottic —*see* Edema, glottis
- testis N44.8
- tunica vaginalis N50.89
- vas deferens N50.89
- vulva (acute) N90.89

Edentulism —*see* Absence, teeth, acquired
Edsall's disease T67.2
Educational handicap Z55.9
- specified NEC Z55.8
Edward's syndrome —*see* Trisomy, 18
Effect, adverse
- abnormal gravitational (G) forces or states T75.81
- abuse —*see* Maltreatment
- air pressure T70.9
  - specified NEC T70.8
- altitude (high) —*see* Effect, adverse, high altitude
- anesthesia —*see also* Anesthesia T88.59
  - in labor and delivery O74.9
  - local, toxic
    - in labor and delivery O74.4-●
    - in pregnancy NEC O29.3-●
    - postpartum, puerperal O89.3
  - postpartum, puerperal O89.9
  - specified NEC T88.59
    - in labor and delivery O74.8
    - postpartum, puerperal O89.8
  - spinal and epidural T88.59
    - headache T88.59
      - in labor and delivery O74.5
      - postpartum, puerperal O89.4
    - specified NEC
      - in labor and delivery O74.6
      - postpartum, puerperal O89.5
- antitoxin —*see* Complications, vaccination
- atmospheric pressure T70.9
  - due to explosion T70.8
  - high T70.3
  - low —*see* Effect, adverse, high altitude
  - specified effect NEC T70.8
- biological, correct substance properly administered —*see* Effect, adverse, drug
- blood (derivatives) (serum) (transfusion) — *see* Complications, transfusion
- chemical substance —*see* Table of Drugs and Chemicals
- cold (temperature) (weather) T69.9
  - chilblains T69.1
  - frostbite —*see* Frostbite
  - specified effect NEC T69.8

Effect, adverse *(Continued)*
- drugs and medicaments T88.7
  - specified drug —*see* Table of Drugs and Chemicals, by drug, adverse effect
  - specified effect — code to condition
- electric current, electricity (shock) T75.4
  - burn —*see* Burn
- exertion (excessive) T73.3
- exposure —*see* Exposure
- external cause NEC T75.89
- foodstuffs T78.1
  - allergic reaction —*see* Allergy, food
    - causing anaphylaxis —*see* Shock, anaphylactic, due to food
  - noxious —*see* Poisoning, food, noxious
- gases, fumes, or vapors T59.9-●
  - specified agent —*see* Table of Drugs and Chemicals
- glue (airplane) sniffing
  - due to drug abuse —*see* Abuse, drug, inhalant
  - due to drug dependence —*see* Dependence, drug, inhalant
- heat —*see* Heat
- high altitude NEC T70.29
  - anoxia T70.29
  - on
    - ears T70.0
    - sinuses T70.1
  - polycythemia D75.1
- high pressure fluids T70.4
- hot weather —*see* Heat
- hunger T73.0
- immersion, foot —*see* Immersion
- immunization —*see* Complications, vaccination
- immunological agents —*see* Complications, vaccination
- infrared (radiation) (rays) NOS T66
  - dermatitis or eczema L59.8
- infusion —*see* Complications, infusion
- lack of care of infants —*see* Maltreatment, child
- lightning —*see* Lightning
- medical care T88.9
  - specified NEC T88.8
- medicinal substance, correct, properly administered —*see* Effect, adverse, drug
- motion T75.3
- noise, on inner ear —*see* subcategory H83.3
- overheated places —*see* Heat
- psychosocial, of work environment Z56.5
- radiation (diagnostic) (infrared) (natural source) (therapeutic) (ultraviolet) (X-ray) NOS T66
  - dermatitis or eczema —*see* Dermatitis, due to, radiation
  - fibrosis of lung J70.1
  - pneumonitis J70.0
  - pulmonary manifestations
    - acute J70.0
    - chronic J70.1
  - skin L59.9
- radioactive substance NOS
  - dermatitis or eczema —*see* Radiodermatitis
- reduced temperature T69.9
  - immersion foot or hand —*see* Immersion
  - specified effect NEC T69.8
- serum NEC (*see also* Reaction, serum) T80.69
- specified NEC T78.8
  - external cause NEC T75.89
- strangulation —*see* Asphyxia, traumatic
- submersion T75.1
- thirst T73.1
- toxic —*see* Toxicity
- transfusion —*see* Complications, transfusion
- ultraviolet (radiation) (rays) NOS T66
  - burn —*see* Burn
  - dermatitis or eczema —*see* Dermatitis, due to, ultraviolet rays
    - acute L56.8

▶ New   ⇒ Revised   ~~deleted~~ Deleted   ● Use Additional Character(s)

Effect, adverse *(Continued)*
vaccine (any) —*see* Complications, vaccination
vibration —*see* Vibration, adverse effects
water pressure NEC T70.9
specified NEC T70.8
weightlessness T75.82
whole blood —*see* Complications, transfusion
work environment Z56.5
Effect(s) (of) (from) —*see* Effect, adverse NEC
Effects, late —*see* Sequelae
Effluvium
anagen L65.1
telogen L65.0
Effort syndrome (psychogenic) F45.8
Effusion
amniotic fluid —*see* Pregnancy, complicated
by, prematue rupture of membranes
brain (serous) G93.6
bronchial —*see* Bronchitis
cerebral G93.6
cerebrospinal —*see also* Meningitis
vessel G93.6
chest —*see* Effusion, pleura
chylous, chyliform (pleura) J94.0
intracranial G93.6
joint M25.40
ankle M25.47-●
elbow M25.42-●
foot joint M25.47-●
hand joint M25.44-●
hip M25.45-●
knee M25.46-●
shoulder M25.41-●
specified joint NEC M25.48
wrist M25.43-●
malignant pleural J91.0
meninges —*see* Meningitis
pericardium, pericardial (noninflammatory)
I31.3
acute —*see* Pericarditis, acute
peritoneal (chronic) R18.8
pleura, pleurisy, pleuritic, pleuropericardial
J90
chylous, chyliform J94.0
due to systemic lupus erythematosis
M32.13
▶in conditions classified elsewhere J91.8
influenzal —*see* Influenza, with, respiratory
manifestations NEC
malignant J91.0
newborn P28.89
tuberculous NEC A15.6
primary (progressive) A15.7
spinal —*see* Meningitis
thorax, thoracic —*see* Effusion, pleura
Egg shell nails L60.3
congenital Q84.6
Egyptian splenomegaly B65.1
Ehlers-Danlos syndrome Q79.6
Ehrlichiosis A77.40
due to
E. chafeensis A77.41
E. sennetsu A79.81
specified organism NEC A77.49
Eichstedt's disease B36.0
Eisenmenger's
⟹complex or syndrome I27.83
defect Q21.8
Ejaculation
delayed F52.32
painful N53.12
premature F52.4
retarded N53.11
retrograde N53.14
semen, painful N53.12
psychogenic F52.6
Ekbom's syndrome (restless legs) G25.81
Ekman's syndrome (brittle bones and blue
sclera) Q78.0
Elastic skin Q82.8
acquired L57.4

Elastofibroma —*see* Neoplasm, connective
tissue, benign
Elastoma (juvenile) Q82.8
Miescher's L87.2
Elastomyofibrosis I42.4
Elastosis
actinic, solar L57.8
atrophicans (senile) L57.4
perforans serpiginosa L87.2
senilis L57.4
Elbow —*see* condition
Electric current, electricity, effects (concussion)
(fatal) (nonfatal) (shock) T75.4
burn —*see* Burn
Electric feet syndrome E53.8
Electrocution T75.4
from electroshock gun (taser) T75.4
Electrolyte imbalance E87.8
with
abortion —*see* Abortion by type,
complicated by, electrolyte imbalance
ectopic pregnancy O08.5
molar pregnancy O08.5
Elephantiasis (nonfilarial) I89.0
arabicum —*see* Infestation, filarial
bancroftian B74.0
congenital (any site) (hereditary) Q82.0
due to
Brugia (malayi) B74.1
timori B74.2
mastectomy I97.2
Wuchereria (bancrofti) B74.0
eyelid H02.859
left H02.856
lower H02.855
upper H02.854
right H02.853
lower H02.852
upper H02.851
filarial, filariensis —*see* Infestation, filarial
glandular I89.0
graecorum A30.9
lymphangiectatic I89.0
lymphatic vessel I89.0
due to mastectomy I97.2
scrotum (nonfilarial) I89.0
streptococcal I89.0
surgical I97.89
postmastectomy I97.2
telangiectodes I89.0
vulva (nonfilarial) N90.89
Elevated, elevation
antibody titer R76.0
basal metabolic rate R94.8
blood pressure —*see also* Hypertension
reading (incidental) (isolated) (nonspecific),
no diagnosis of hypertension R03.0
blood sugar R73.9
body temperature (of unknown origin) R50.9
C-reactive protein (CRP) R79.82
cancer antigen 125 [CA 125] R97.1
carcinoembryonic antigen [CEA] R97.0
cholesterol E78.00
with high triglycerides E78.2
conjugate, eye H51.0
diaphragm, congenital Q79.1
erythrocyte sedimentation rate R70.0
fasting glucose R73.01
fasting triglycerides E78.1
finding on laboratory examination —*see*
Findings, abnormal, inconclusive,
without diagnosis, by type of exam
GFR (glomerular filtration rate) —*see*
Findings, abnormal, inconclusive,
without diagnosis, by type of exam
glucose tolerance (oral) R73.02
immunoglobulin level R76.8
indoleacetic acid R82.5
lactic acid dehydrogenase (LDH) level R74.0
leukocytes D72.829
lipoprotein a level E78.8

Elevated, elevation *(Continued)*
liver function
study R94.5
test R79.89
alkaline phosphatase R74.8
aminotransferase R74.0
bilirubin R17
hepatic enzyme R74.8
lactate dehydrogenase R74.0
lymphocytes D72.820
prostate specific antigen [PSA] R97.20
Rh titer —*see* Complication(s), transfusion,
incompatibility reaction, Rh (factor)
scapula, congenital Q74.0
sedimentation rate R70.0
SGOT R74.0
SGPT R74.0
transaminase level R74.0
triglycerides E78.1
with high cholesterol E78.2
tumor associated antigens [TAA] NEC R97.8
tumor specific antigens [TSA] NEC R97.8
urine level of
17-ketosteroids R82.5
catecholamine R82.5
indoleacetic acid R82.5
steroids R82.5
vanillylmandelic acid (VMA) R82.5
venous pressure I87.8
white blood cell count D72.829
specified NEC D72.828
Elliptocytosis (congenital) (hereditary) D58.1
Hb C (disease) D58.1
hemoglobin disease D58.1
sickle-cell (disease) D57.8-●
trait D57.3
Ellison-Zollinger syndrome E16.4
Ellis-van Creveld syndrome
(chondroectodermal dysplasia) Q77.6
Elongated, elongation (congenital) —*see also*
Distortion
bone Q79.9
cervix (uteri) Q51.828
acquired N88.4
hypertrophic N88.4
colon Q43.8
common bile duct Q44.5
cystic duct Q44.5
frenulum, penis Q55.69
labia minora (acquired) N90.69
ligamentum patellae Q74.1
petiolus (epiglottidis) Q31.8
tooth, teeth K00.2
uvula Q38.6
Eltor cholera A00.1
Emaciation (due to malnutrition) E41
Embadomoniasis A07.8
Embedded tooth, teeth K01.0
root only K08.3
Embolic —*see* condition
Embolism (multiple) (paradoxical) I74.9
air (any site) (traumatic) T79.0
following
abortion —*see* Abortion by type
complicated by embolism
ectopic pregnancy O08.2
infusion, therapeutic injection or
transfusion T80.0
molar pregnancy O08.2
procedure NEC
artery T81.719
mesenteric T81.710
renal T81.711
specified NEC T81.718
vein T81.72
in pregnancy, childbirth or puerperium —
see Embolism, obstetric
amniotic fluid (pulmonary) —*see also*
Embolism, obstetric
following
abortion —*see* Abortion by type
complicated by embolism

Embolism *(Continued)*
  amniotic fluid *(Continued)*
    following *(Continued)*
      ectopic pregnancy O08.2
      molar pregnancy O08.2
  aorta, aortic I74.10
    abdominal I74.09
      saddle I74.01
    bifurcation I74.09
    saddle I74.01
    thoracic I74.11
  artery I74.9
    auditory, internal I65.8
    basilar —*see* Occlusion, artery, basilar
    carotid (common) (internal) —*see*
      Occlusion, artery, carotid
    cerebellar (anterior inferior) (posterior
      inferior) (superior) I66.3
    cerebral —*see* Occlusion, artery, cerebral
    ➡choroidal (anterior) I65.8
    ➡communicating posterior I65.8
    coronary —*see also* Infarct, myocardium
      not resulting in infarction I24.0
    extremity I74.4
      lower I74.3
      upper I74.2
    ➡hypophyseal I65.8
    iliac I74.5
    limb I74.4
      lower I74.3
      upper I74.2
    mesenteric (with gangrene) —*see also*
      Ischemia, intestine, acute K55.09
    ophthalmic —*see* Occlusion, artery, retina
    peripheral I74.4
    ➡pontine I65.8
    precerebral —*see* Occlusion, artery,
      precerebral
    pulmonary —*see* Embolism, pulmonary
    renal N28.0
    retinal —*see* Occlusion, artery, retina
    septic I76
    specified NEC I74.8
    vertebral —*see* Occlusion, artery, vertebral
  basilar (artery) I65.1
  blood clot
    following
      abortion —*see* Abortion by type
        complicated by embolism
      ectopic or molar pregnancy O08.2
    in pregnancy, childbirth or puerperium —
      see Embolism, obstetric
  brain —*see also* Occlusion, artery, cerebral
    following
      abortion —*see* Abortion by type
        complicated by embolism
      ectopic or molar pregnancy O08.2
    puerperal, postpartum, childbirth —*see*
      Embolism, obstetric
  capillary I78.8
  cardiac —*see also* Infarct, myocardium
    not resulting in infarction I51.3
  carotid (artery) (common) (internal) —*see*
    Occlusion, artery, carotid
  cavernous sinus (venous) —*see* Embolism,
    intracranial venous sinus
  cerebral —*see* Occlusion, artery, cerebral
  cholesterol —*see* Atheroembolism
  coronary (artery or vein) (systemic) —*see*
    Occlusion, coronary
  due to device, implant or graft —*see also*
    Complications, by site and type,
    specified NEC
    arterial graft NEC T82.818
    breast (implant) T85.818
    catheter NEC T85.818
      dialysis (renal) T82.818
        intraperitoneal T85.818
      infusion NEC T82.818
        spinal (epidural) (subdural) T85.810
      urinary (indwelling) T83.81

Embolism *(Continued)*
  due to device, implant or graft *(Continued)*
    electronic (electrode) (pulse generator)
      (stimulator)
      bone T84.81
      cardiac T82.817
      nervous system (brain) (peripheral
        nerve) (spinal) T85.810
      urinary T83.81
    fixation, internal (orthopedic) NEC T84.81
    gastrointestinal (bile duct) (esophagus)
      T85.818
    genital NEC T83.81
    heart (graft) (valve) T82.817
    joint prosthesis T84.81
    ocular (corneal graft) (orbital implant)
      T85.818
    orthopedic (bone graft) NEC T86.838
    specified NEC T85.818
    urinary (graft) NEC T83.81
    vascular NEC T82.818
    ventricular intracranial shunt T85.810
  extremities
    lower —*see* Embolism, vein, lower
      extremity
      arterial I74.3
    upper I74.2
  eye H34.9
  fat (cerebral) (pulmonary) (systemic) T79.1
    complicating delivery —*see* Embolism,
      obstetric
    following
      abortion —*see* Abortion by type
        complicated by embolism
      ectopic or molar pregnancy O08.2
  following
    abortion —*see* Abortion by type
      complicated by embolism
    ectopic or molar pregnancy O08.2
    infusion, therapeutic injection or
      transfusion
      air T80.0
  heart (fatty) —*see also* Infarct, myocardium
    not resulting in infarction I51.3
  hepatic (vein) I82.0
  in pregnancy, childbirth or puerperium —*see*
    Embolism, obstetric
  intestine (artery) (vein) (with gangrene) —*see*
    also Ischemia, intestine, acute K55.039
  intracranial —*see also* Occlusion, artery,
    cerebral
    venous sinus (any) G08
      nonpyogenic I67.6
  intraspinal venous sinuses or veins G08
    nonpyogenic G95.19
  kidney (artery) N28.0
  lateral sinus (venous) —*see* Embolism,
    intracranial, venous sinus
  leg —*see* Embolism, vein, lower extremity
    arterial I74.3
  longitudinal sinus (venous) —*see* Embolism,
    intracranial, venous sinus
  lung (massive) —*see* Embolism, pulmonary
  meninges I66.8
  mesenteric (artery) (vein) (with gangrene) —
    see also Ischemia, intestine, acute
    K55.059
  obstetric (in) (pulmonary)
    childbirth O88.22
      air O88.02
      amniotic fluid O88.12
      blood clot O88.22
      fat O88.82
      pyemic O88.32
      septic O88.32
      specified type NEC O88.82
    pregnancy O88.21-●
      air O88.01-●
      amniotic fluid O88.11-●
      blood clot O88.21-●
      fat O88.81-●

Embolism *(Continued)*
  obstetric *(Continued)*
    pregnancy *(Continued)*
      pyemic O88.31-●
      septic O88.31-●
      specified type NEC O88.81-●
    puerperal O88.23
      air O88.03
      amniotic fluid O88.13
      blood clot O88.23
      fat O88.83
      pyemic O88.33
      septic O88.33
      specified type NEC O88.83
  ophthalmic —*see* Occlusion, artery, retina
  penis N48.81
  peripheral artery NOS I74.4
  pituitary E23.6
  popliteal (artery) I74.3
  portal (vein) I81
  postoperative, postprocedural
    artery T81.719
      mesenteric T81.710
      renal T81.711
      specified NEC T81.718
    vein T81.72
  precerebral artery —*see* Occlusion, artery,
    precerebral
  puerperal —*see* Embolism, obstetric
  pulmonary (acute) (artery) (vein) I26.99
    with acute cor pulmonale I26.09
    chronic I27.82
    following
      abortion —*see* Abortion by type
        complicated by embolism
      ectopic or molar pregnancy O08.2
    healed or old Z86.711
    in pregnancy, childbirth or puerperium —
      see Embolism, obstetric
    personal history of Z86.711
    saddle I26.92
      with acute cor pulmonale I26.02
    septic I26.90
      with acute cor pulmonale I26.01
  pyemic (multiple) I76
    following
      abortion —*see* Abortion by type
        complicated by embolism
      ectopic or molar pregnancy O08.2
    Hemophilus influenzae A41.3
    pneumococcal A40.3
      with pneumonia J13
    puerperal, postpartum, childbirth (any
      organism) —*see* Embolism, obstetric
    specified organism NEC A41.89
    staphylococcal A41.2
    streptococcal A40.9
  renal (artery) N28.0
    vein I82.3
  retina, retinal —*see* Occlusion, artery,
    retina
  saddle
    abdominal aorta I74.01
    pulmonary artery I26.92
      with acute cor pulmonale I26.02
  septic (arterial) I76
    complicating abortion —*see* Abortion, by
      type, complicated by, embolism
  sinus —*see* Embolism, intracranial, venous
    sinus
  soap complicating abortion —*see* Abortion,
    by type, complicated by, embolism
  spinal cord G95.19
    pyogenic origin G06.1
  spleen, splenic (artery) I74.8
  upper extremity I74.2
  vein (acute) I82.90
    antecubital I82.61-●
      chronic I82.71-●
    axillary I82.A1-●
      chronic I82.A2-●

▶ New   ➡ Revised   ~~deleted~~ Deleted   ● Use Additional Character(s)

Embolism *(Continued)*
  vein *(Continued)*
    basilic I82.61-●
      chronic I82.71-●
    brachial I82.62-●
      chronic I82.72-●
    brachiocephalic (innominate) I82.290
      chronic I82.291
    cephalic I82.61-●
      chronic I82.71-●
    chronic I82.91
    deep (DVT) I82.40-●
      calf I82.4Z-●
        chronic I82.5Z-●
      lower leg I82.4Z-●
        chronic I82.5Z-●
      thigh I82.4Y-●
        chronic I82.5Y-●
      upper leg I82.4Y
        chronic I82.5y--●
    femoral I82.41-●
      chronic I82.51-●
    iliac (iliofemoral) I82.42-●
      chronic I82.52-●
    innominate I82.290
      chronic I82.291
    internal jugular I82.C1-●
      chronic I82.C2-●
    lower extremity
      deep I82.40-●
        chronic I82.50-●
          specified NEC I82.49-●
            chronic NEC I82.59-●
      distal
        deep I82.4Z-●
      proximal
        deep I82.4Y-●
          chronic I82.5Y-●
      superficial I82.81-●
    popliteal I82.43-●
      chronic I82.53-●
    radial I82.62-●
      chronic I82.72-●
    renal I82.3
    saphenous (greater) (lesser) I82.81-●
    specified NEC I82.890
      chronic NEC I82.891
    subclavian I82.B1-●
      chronic I82.B2-●
    thoracic NEC I82.290
      chronic I82.291
    tibial I82.44-●
      chronic I82.54-●
    ulnar I82.62-●
      chronic I82.72-●
    upper extremity I82.60-●
      chronic I82.70-●
      deep I82.62-●
        chronic I82.72-●
      superficial I82.61-●
        chronic I82.71-●
  vena cava
    inferior (acute) I82.220
      chronic I82.221
    superior (acute) I82.210
      chronic I82.211
  venous sinus G08
  vessels of brain —*see* Occlusion, artery,
    cerebral
Embolus —*see* Embolism
Embryoma —*see also* Neoplasm, uncertain
  behavior, by site
  benign —*see* Neoplasm, benign, by site
  kidney C64.-●
  liver C22.0
  malignant —*see also* Neoplasm, malignant,
    by site
    kidney C64.-●
    liver C22.0
    testis C62.9-●
      descended (scrotal) C62.1-●
      undescended C62.0-●

Embryoma *(Continued)*
  testis C62.9-●
    descended (scrotal) C62.1-●
    undescended C62.0-●
Embryonic
  circulation Q28.9
  heart Q28.9
  vas deferens Q55.4
Embryopathia NOS Q89.9
Embryotoxon Q13.4
Emesis —*see* Vomiting
Emotional lability R45.86
Emotionality, pathological F60.3
Emotogenic disease —*see* Disorder,
  psychogenic
Emphysema (atrophic) (bullous) (chronic)
  (interlobular) (lung) (obstructive)
  (pulmonary) (senile) (vesicular)
  J43.9
  cellular tissue (traumatic) T79.7
    surgical T81.82
  centrilobular J43.2
  compensatory J98.3
  congenital (interstitial) P25.0
  conjunctiva H11.89
  connective tissue (traumatic) T79.7
    surgical T81.82
  due to chemicals, gases, fumes or vapors
    J68.4
  eyelid(s) —*see* Disorder, eyelid, specified type
    NEC
    surgical T81.82
    traumatic T79.7
  interstitial J98.2
    congenital P25.0
    perinatal period P25.0
  laminated tissue T79.7
    surgical T81.82
  mediastinal J98.2
    newborn P25.2
  orbit, orbital —*see* Disorder, orbit, specified
    type NEC
  panacinar J43.1
  panlobular J43.1
  specified NEC J43.8
  subcutaneous (traumatic) T79.7
    nontraumatic J98.2
    postprocedural T81.82
    surgical T81.82
  surgical T81.82
  thymus (gland) (congenital) E32.8
  traumatic (subcutaneous) T79.7
  unilateral J43.0
Empty nest syndrome Z60.0
Empyema (acute) (chest) (double) (pleura)
  (supradiaphragmatic) (thorax) J86.9
  with fistula J86.0
  accessory sinus (chronic) —*see* Sinusitis
  antrum (chronic) —*see* Sinusitis, maxillary
  brain (any part) —*see* Abscess, brain
  ethmoidal (chronic) (sinus) —*see* Sinusitis,
    ethmoidal
  extradural —*see* Abscess, extradural
  frontal (chronic) (sinus) —*see* Sinusitis,
    frontal
  gallbladder K81.0
  mastoid (process) (acute) —*see* Mastoiditis,
    acute
  maxilla, maxillary M27.2
    sinus (chronic) —*see* Sinusitis,
      maxillary
  nasal sinus (chronic) —*see* Sinusitis
  sinus (accessory) (chronic) (nasal) —*see*
    Sinusitis
  sphenoidal (sinus) (chronic) —*see* Sinusitis,
    sphenoidal
  subarachnoid —*see* Abscess, extradural
  subdural —*see* Abscess, subdural
  tuberculous A15.6
  ureter —*see* Ureteritis
  ventricular —*see* Abscess, brain

En coup de sabre lesion L94.1
Enamel pearls K00.2
Enameloma K00.2
Enanthema, viral B09
Encephalitis (chronic) (hemorrhagic)
  (idiopathic) (nonepidemic) (spurious)
  (subacute) G04.90
  acute —*see also* Encephalitis, viral A86
    disseminated G04.00
      infectious G04.01
      noninfectious G04.81
      postimmunization (postvaccination)
        G04.02
      postinfectious G04.01
    inclusion body A85.8
    necrotizing hemorrhagic G04.30
      postimmunization G04.32
      postinfectious G04.31
      specified NEC G04.39
  arboviral, arbovirus NEC A85.2
  arthropod-borne NEC (viral) A85.2
  Australian A83.4
  California (virus) A83.5
  Central European (tick-borne) A84.1
  Czechoslovakian A84.1
  Dawson's (inclusion body) A81.1
  diffuse sclerosing A81.1
  disseminated, acute G04.00
  due to
    cat scratch disease A28.1
    human immunodeficiency virus (HIV)
      disease B20 *[G05.3]*
    malaria —*see* Malaria
    rickettsiosis —*see* Rickettsiosis
    smallpox inoculation G04.02
    typhus —*see* Typhus
  Eastern equine A83.2
  endemic (viral) A86
  epidemic NEC (viral) A86
  equine (acute) (infectious) (viral) A83.9
    Eastern A83.2
    Venezuelan A92.2
    Western A83.1
  Far Eastern (tick-borne) A84.0
  following vaccination or other immunization
    procedure G04.02
  herpes zoster B02.0
  herpesviral B00.4
    due to herpesvirus 6 B10.01
    due to herpesvirus 7 B10.09
    specified NEC B10.09
  Ilheus (virus) A83.8
  in (due to)
    actinomycosis A42.82
    adenovirus A85.1
    African trypanosomiasis B56.9 *[G05.3]*
    Chagas' disease (chronic) B57.42
    cytomegalovirus B25.8
    enterovirus A85.0
    herpes (simplex) virus B00.4
      due to herpesvirus 6 B10.01
      due to herpesvirus 7 B10.09
      specified NEC B10.09
    infectious disease NEC B99 *[G05.3]*
    influenza —*see* Influenza, with,
      encephalopathy
    listeriosis A32.12
    measles B05.0
    mumps B26.2
    naegleriasis B60.2
    parasitic disease NEC B89 *[G05.3]*
    poliovirus A80.9 *[G05.3]*
    rubella B06.01
    syphilis
      congenital A50.42
      late A52.14
    systemic lupus erythematosus M32.19
    toxoplasmosis (acquired) B58.2
      congenital P37.1
    tuberculosis A17.82
    zoster B02.0

Encephalitis (Continued)
inclusion body A81.1
infectious (acute) (virus) NEC A86
Japanese (B type) A83.0
La Crosse A83.5
lead —see Poisoning, lead
lethargica (acute) (infectious) A85.8
louping ill A84.8
lupus erythematosus, systemic M32.19
lymphatica A87.2
Mengo A85.8
meningococcal A39.81
Murray Valley A83.4
otitic NEC H66.40 [G05.3]
parasitic NOS B71.9
periaxial G37.0
periaxialis (concentrica) (diffuse) G37.5
postchickenpox B01.11
postexanthematous NEC B09
postimmunization G04.02
postinfectious NEC G04.01
postmeasles B05.0
postvaccinal G04.02
postvaricella B01.11
postviral NEC A86
Powassan A84.8
Rasmussen G04.81
Rio Bravo A85.8
Russian
    autumnal A83.0
    spring-summer (taiga) A84.0
saturnine —see Poisoning, lead
specified NEC G04.81
St. Louis A83.3
subacute sclerosing A81.1
summer A83.0
suppurative G04.81
tick-borne A84.9
Torula, torular (cryptococcal) B45.1
toxic NEC G92
trichinosis B75 [G05.3]
type
    B A83.0
    C A83.3
van Bogaert's A81.1
Venezuelan equine A92.2
Vienna A85.8
viral, virus A86
    arthropod-borne NEC A85.2
        mosquito-borne A83.9
            Australian X disease A83.4
            California virus A83.5
            Eastern equine A83.2
            Japanese (B type) A83.0
            Murray Valley A83.4
            specified NEC A83.8
            St. Louis A83.3
            type B A83.0
            type C A83.3
            Western equine A83.1
        tick-borne A84.9
            biundulant A84.1
            central European A84.1
            Czechoslovakian A84.1
            diphasic meningoencephalitis A84.1
            Far Eastern A84.0
            Russian spring-summer (taiga)
                A84.0
            specified NEC A84.8
        specified type NEC A85.8
    Western equine A83.1
Encephalocele Q01.9
frontal Q01.0
nasofrontal Q01.1
occipital Q01.2
specified NEC Q01.8
Encephalocystocele —see Encephalocele
Encephaloduroarteriomyosynangiosis
    (EDAMS) I67.5
Encephalomalacia (brain) (cerebellar)
    (cerebral) —see Softening, brain

Encephalomeningitis —see
    Meningoencephalitis
Encephalomeningocele —see Encephalocele
Encephalomeningomyelitis —see
    Meningoencephalitis
Encephalomyelitis —see also Encephalitis
    G04.90
acute disseminated G04.00
    infectious G04.01
    noninfectious G04.81
    postimmunization G04.02
    postinfectious G04.01
acute necrotizing hemorrhagic G04.30
    postimmunization G04.32
    postinfectious G04.31
    specified NEC G04.39
benign myalgic G93.3
equine A83.9
    Eastern A83.2
    Venezuelan A92.2
    Western A83.1
in diseases classified elsewhere G05.3
myalgic, benign G93.3
postchickenpox B01.11
postinfectious NEC G04.01
postmeasles B05.0
postvaccinal G04.02
postvaricella B01.11
rubella B06.01
specified NEC G04.81
Venezuelan equine A92.2
Encephalomyelocele —see Encephalocele
Encephalomyelomeningitis —see
    Meningoencephalitis
Encephalomyelopathy G96.9
Encephalomyeloradiculitis (acute) G61.0
Encephalomyeloradiculoneuritis (acute)
    (Guillain-Barré) G61.0
Encephalomyeloradiculopathy G96.9
Encephalopathia hyperbilirubinemica,
    newborn P57.9
due to isoimmunization (conditions in P55)
    P57.0
Encephalopathy (acute) G93.40
acute necrotizing hemorrhagic G04.30
    postimmunization G04.32
    postinfectious G04.31
    specified NEC G04.39
alcoholic G31.2
anoxic —see Damage, brain, anoxic
arteriosclerotic I67.2
centrolobar progressive (Schilder) G37.0
congenital Q07.9
degenerative, in specified disease NEC
    G32.89
due to
    drugs (see also Table of Drugs and
        Chemicals) G92
demyelinating callosal G37.1
hepatic —see Failure, hepatic
hyperbilirubinemic, newborn P57.9
    due to isoimmunization (conditions in P55)
        P57.0
hypertensive I67.4
hypoglycemic E16.2
hypoxic —see Damage, brain, anoxic
hypoxic ischemic P91.60
    mild P91.61
    moderate P91.62
    severe P91.63
in (due to) (with)
    birth injury P11.1
    hyperinsulinism E16.1 [G94]
    influenza —see Influenza, with,
        encephalopathy
    lack of vitamin (see also Deficiency, vitamin)
        E56.9 [G32.89]
    neoplastic disease (see also Neoplasm)
        D49.9 [G13.1]
    serum (see also Reaction, serum) T80.69
    syphilis A52.17

Encephalopathy (Continued)
in (Continued)
    trauma (postconcussional) F07.81
        current injury —see Injury, intracranial
    vaccination G04.02
lead —see Poisoning, lead
metabolic G93.41
    drug induced G92
    toxic G92
myoclonic, early, symptomatic —see Epilepsy,
    generalized, specified NEC
necrotizing, subacute (Leigh) G31.82
▶neonatal P91.819
    ▶in diseases classified elsewhere P91.811
pellagrous E52 [G32.89]
portosystemic —see Failure, hepatic
postcontusional F07.81
    current injury —see Injury, intracranial,
        diffuse
posthypoglycemic (coma) E16.1 [G94]
postradiation G93.89
saturnine —see Poisoning, lead
septic G93.41
specified NEC G93.49
spongiform, subacute (viral) A81.09
toxic G92
    metabolic G92
traumatic (postconcussional) F07.81
    current injury —see Injury, intracranial
vitamin B deficiency NEC E53.9 [G32.89]
    vitamin B1 E51.2
Wernicke's E51.2
Encephalorrhagia —see Hemorrhage,
    intracranial, intracerebral
Encephalosis, posttraumatic F07.81
Enchondroma —see also Neoplasm, bone,
    benign
Enchondromatosis (cartilaginous) (multiple)
    Q78.4
Encopresis R15.9
functional F98.1
nonorganic origin F98.1
psychogenic F98.1
Encounter (with health service) (for) Z76.89
adjustment and management (of)
    breast implant Z45.81
    implanted device NEC Z45.89
    myringotomy device (stent) (tube) Z45.82
administrative purpose only Z02.9
    examination for
        adoption Z02.82
        armed forces Z02.3
        disability determination Z02.71
        driving license Z02.4
        employment Z02.1
        insurance Z02.6
        medical certificate NEC Z02.79
        paternity testing Z02.81
        residential institution admission Z02.2
        school admission Z02.0
        sports Z02.5
    specified reason NEC Z02.89
aftercare —see Aftercare
➡antenatal screening Z36.9
    ▶cervical length Z36.86
    ▶chromosomal anomalies Z36.0
    ▶congenital cardiac abnormalities Z36.83
    ▶elevated maternal serum alphafetoprotein
        level Z36.1
    ▶fetal growth retardation Z36.4
    ▶fetal lung maturity Z36.84
    ▶fetal macrosomia Z36.88
    ▶hydrops fetalis Z36.81
    ▶intrauterine growth restriction (IUGR)/
        small-for-dates Z36.4
    ▶isoimmunization Z36.5
    ▶large-for-dates Z36.88
    ▶malformations Z36.3
    ▶non-visualized anatomy on a previous scan
        Z36.2
    ▶nuchal translucency Z36.82

Encounter *(Continued)*
  antenatal screening *(Continued)*
    ▶raised alphafetoprotein level Z36.1
    ▶risk of pre-term labor Z36.86
    ▶specified type NEC Z36.89
    ▶specified follow-up NEC Z36.2
    ▶specified genetic defects NEC Z36.8A
    ▶Streptococcus B Z36.85
    ▶suspected anomaly Z36.3
    ▶uncertain dates Z36.87
  assisted reproductive fertility procedure cycle Z31.83
  blood typing Z01.83
    Rh typing Z01.83
  breast augmentation or reduction Z41.1
  breast implant exchange (different material) (different size) Z45.81
  breast reconstruction following mastectomy Z42.1
  check-up —*see* Examination
  chemotherapy for neoplasm Z51.11
  colonoscopy, screening Z12.11
  counseling —*see* Counseling
  delivery, full-term, uncomplicated O80
    cesarean, without indication O82
  desensitization to allergens Z51.6
  ear piercing Z41.3
  examination —*see* Examination
  expectant parent(s) (adoptive) pre-birth pediatrician visit Z76.81
  fertility preservation procedure (prior to cancer therapy) (prior to removal of gonads) Z31.84
  fitting (of) —*see* Fitting (and adjustment) (of)
  genetic
  ⇒counseling
    ▶nonprocreative Z71.83
    ▶procreative Z31.5
    testing —*see* Test, genetic
  hearing conservation and treatment Z01.12
  immunotherapy for neoplasm Z51.12
  in vitro fertilization cycle Z31.83
  instruction (in)
    child care (postpartal) (prenatal) Z32.3
    childbirth Z32.2
    natural family planning
      procreative Z31.61
      to avoid pregnancy Z30.02
  insulin pump titration Z46.81
  joint prosthesis insertion following prior explantation of joint prosthesis (staged procedure)
    hip Z47.32
    knee Z47.33
    shoulder Z47.31
  laboratory (as part of a general medical examination) Z00.00
    with abnormal findings Z00.01
  mental health services (for)
    abuse NEC
      perpetrator Z69.82
      victim Z69.81
    child abuse
      nonparental
        perpetrator Z69.021
        victim Z69.020
      parental
        perpetrator Z69.011
        victim Z69.010
      ~~spousal or partner abuse~~
      ~~perpetrator Z69.12~~
      ~~victim Z69.11~~
    ▶child neglect
    ▶nonparental
      ▶perpetrator Z69.021
      ▶victim Z69.020
    ▶parental
      ▶perpetrator Z69.011
      ▶victim Z69.010
    ▶child psychological abuse
    ▶nonparental
      ▶perpetrator Z69.021
      ▶victim Z69.020

Encounter *(Continued)*
  mental health services *(Continued)*
    child psychological abuse *(Continued)*
    ▶parental
      ▶perpetrator Z69.011
      ▶victim Z69.010
    ▶child sexual abuse
    ▶nonparental
      ▶perpetrator Z69.021
      ▶victim Z69.020
    ▶parental
      ▶perpetrator Z69.011
      ▶victim Z69.010
    ▶non-spousal adult abuse (perpetrator) (victim) Z69.81
    ▶spousal or partner
    ▶abuse
      ▶perpetrator Z69.12
      ▶victim Z69.11
    ▶neglect
      ▶perpetrator Z69.12
      ▶victim Z69.11
    ▶psychological abuse
      ▶perpetrator Z69.12
      ▶victim Z69.11
    ▶violence
      ▶perpetrator (physical) (sexual) Z69.12
      ▶victim (physical) Z69.11
      ▶sexual Z69.81
  observation (for) (ruled out)
    exposure to (suspected)
      anthrax Z03.810
      biological agent NEC Z03.818
  pediatrician visit, by expectant parent(s) (adoptive) Z76.81
  ▶placental sample (taken vaginally) —*see also* Encounter, antenatal screening Z36.9
  plastic and reconstructive surgery following medical procedure or healed injury NEC Z42.8
  pregnancy
    supervision of —*see* Pregnancy, supervision of
    test Z32.00
      result negative Z32.02
      result positive Z32.01
  procreative management and counseling for gestational carrier Z31.7
  prophylactic measures Z29.9
    antivenin Z29.12
    fluoride administration Z29.3
    immunotherapy for respiratory syncytial virus (RSV) Z29.11
    rabies immune globin Z29.14
    Rho (D) immune globulin Z29.13
    specified NEC Z29.8
  radiation therapy (antineoplastic) Z51.0
  radiological (as part of a general medical examination) Z00.00
    with abnormal findings Z00.01
  reconstructive surgery following medical procedure or healed injury NEC Z42.8
  removal (of) —*see also* Removal
    artificial
      arm Z44.00-●
        complete Z44.01-●
        partial Z44.02-●
      eye Z44.2-●
      leg Z44.10-●
        complete Z44.11-●
        partial Z44.12-●
    breast implant Z45.81
      tissue expander (without synchronous insertion of permanent implant) Z45.81
    device Z46.9
      specified NEC Z46.89
    external
      fixation device — code to fracture with seventh character D

Encounter *(Continued)*
  removal *(Continued)*
    external *(Continued)*
      prosthesis, prosthetic device Z44.9
        breast Z44.3-●
        specified NEC Z44.8
    implanted device NEC Z45.89
    insulin pump Z46.81
    internal fixation device Z47.2
    myringotomy device (stent) (tube) Z45.82
    nervous system device NEC Z46.2
      brain neuropacemaker Z46.2
      visual substitution device Z46.2
        implanted Z45.31
    non-vascular catheter Z46.82
    orthodontic device Z46.4
    stent
      ureteral Z46.6
    urinary device Z46.6
  repeat cervical smear to confirm findings of recent normal smear following initial abnormal smear Z01.42
  respirator [ventilator] use during power failure (Z99.12)
  Rh typing Z01.83
  screening —*see* Screening
  specified NEC Z76.89
  sterilization Z30.2
  suspected condition, ruled out
    amniotic cavity and membrane Z03.71
    cervical shortening Z03.75
    fetal anomaly Z03.73
    fetal growth Z03.74
    maternal and fetal conditions NEC Z03.79
    oligohydramnios Z03.71
    placental problem Z03.72
    polyhydramnios Z03.71
  suspected exposure (to), ruled out
    anthrax Z03.810
    biological agents NEC Z03.818
  termination of pregnancy, elective Z33.2
  testing —*see* Test
  therapeutic drug level monitoring Z51.81
  titration, insulin pump Z46.81
  to determine fetal viability of pregnancy O36.80
  training
    insulin pump Z46.81
  X-ray of chest (as part of a general medical examination Z00.00)
    with abnormal findings Z00.01
Encystment —*see* Cyst
Endarteritis (bacterial, subacute) (infective) I77.6
  brain I67.7
  cerebral or cerebrospinal I67.7
  deformans —*see* Arteriosclerosis
  embolic —*see* Embolism
  obliterans —*see also* Arteriosclerosis
    pulmonary I28.8
  pulmonary I28.8
  retina —*see* Vasculitis, retina
  senile —*see* Arteriosclerosis
  syphilitic A52.09
    brain or cerebral A52.04
    congenital A50.54 *[I79.8]*
  tuberculous A18.89
Endemic —*see* condition
Endocarditis (chronic) (marantic) (nonbacterial) (thrombotic) (valvular) I38
  with rheumatic fever (conditions in I00)
    active —*see* Endocarditis, acute, rheumatic
    inactive or quiescent (with chorea) I09.1
  acute or subacute I33.9
    infective I33.0
    rheumatic (aortic) (mitral) (pulmonary) (tricuspid) I01.1
      with chorea (acute) (rheumatic) (Sydenham's) I02.0

Endocarditis *(Continued)*
  aortic (heart) (nonrheumatic) (valve) I35.8
    with
      mitral disease I08.0
        with tricuspid (valve) disease I08.3
        active or acute I01.1
          with chorea (acute) (rheumatic)
            (Sydenham's) I02.0
      rheumatic fever (conditions in I00)
        active —*see* Endocarditis, acute,
          rheumatic
        inactive or quiescent (with chorea)
          I06.9
      tricuspid (valve) disease I08.2
        with mitral (valve) disease I08.3
    acute or subacute I33.9
    arteriosclerotic I35.8
    rheumatic I06.9
      with mitral disease I08.0
        with tricuspid (valve) disease I08.3
        active or acute I01.1
          with chorea (acute) (rheumatic)
            (Sydenham's) I02.0
      active or acute I01.1
        with chorea (acute) (rheumatic)
          (Sydenham's) I02.0
      specified NEC I06.8
    specified cause NEC I35.8
    syphilitic A52.03
  arteriosclerotic I38
  atypical verrucous (Libman-Sacks) M32.11
  bacterial (acute) (any valve) (subacute) I33.0
  candidal B37.6
  congenital Q24.8
  constrictive I33.0
  Coxiella burnetii A78 *[I39]*
  Coxsackie B33.21
  due to
    prosthetic cardiac valve T82.6
    Q fever A78 *[I39]*
    Serratia marcescens I33.0
    typhoid (fever) A01.02
  gonococcal A54.83
  infectious or infective (acute) (any valve)
    (subacute) I33.0
  lenta (acute) (any valve) (subacute) I33.0
  Libman-Sacks M32.11
  listerial A32.82
  Löffler's I42.3
  malignant (acute) (any valve) (subacute) I33.0
  meningococcal A39.51
  mitral (chronic) (double) (fibroid) (heart)
    (inactive) (valve) (with chorea) I05.9
    with
      aortic (valve) disease I08.0
        with tricuspid (valve) disease I08.3
        active or acute I01.1
          with chorea (acute) (rheumatic)
            (Sydenham's) I02.0
      rheumatic fever (conditions in I00)
        active —*see* Endocarditis, acute,
          rheumatic
        inactive or quiescent (with chorea)
          I05.9
      tricuspid (valve) disease I08.1
        with aortic (valve) disease I08.3
    active or acute I01.1
      with chorea (acute) (rheumatic)
        (Sydenham's) I02.0
      bacterial I33.0
    arteriosclerotic I34.8
    nonrheumatic I34.8
      acute or subacute I33.9
    specified NEC I05.8
  monilial B37.6
  multiple valves I08.9
    specified disorders I08.8
  mycotic (acute) (any valve) (subacute) I33.0
  pneumococcal (acute) (any valve) (subacute)
    I33.0
  pulmonary (chronic) (heart) (valve) I37.8

Endocarditis *(Continued)*
  pulmonary *(Continued)*
    with rheumatic fever (conditions in I00)
      active —*see* Endocarditis, acute,
        rheumatic
      inactive or quiescent (with chorea) I09.89
        with aortic, mitral or tricuspid disease
          I08.8
    acute or subacute I33.9
      rheumatic I01.1
        with chorea (acute) (rheumatic)
          (Sydenham's) I02.0
    arteriosclerotic I37.8
    congenital Q22.2
    rheumatic (chronic) (inactive) (with chorea)
      I09.89
      active or acute I01.1
        with chorea (acute) (rheumatic)
          (Sydenham's) I02.0
    syphilitic A52.03
  purulent (acute) (any valve) (subacute) I33.0
  Q fever A78 *[I39]*
  rheumatic (chronic) (inactive) (with chorea)
    I09.1
    active or acute (aortic) (mitral)
      (pulmonary) (tricuspid) I01.1
      with chorea (acute) (rheumatic)
        (Sydenham's) I02.0
  rheumatoid —*see* Rheumatoid, carditis
  septic (acute) (any valve) (subacute) I33.0
  streptococcal (acute) (any valve) (subacute)
    I33.0
  subacute —*see* Endocarditis, acute
  suppurative (acute) (any valve) (subacute)
    I33.0
  syphilitic A52.03
  toxic I33.9
  tricuspid (chronic) (heart) (inactive)
    (rheumatic) (valve) (with chorea) I07.9
    with
      aortic (valve) disease I08.2
        mitral (valve) disease I08.3
      mitral (valve) disease I08.1
        aortic (valve) disease I08.3
      rheumatic fever (conditions in I00)
        active —*see* Endocarditis, acute,
          rheumatic
        inactive or quiescent (with chorea)
          I07.8
    active or acute I01.1
      with chorea (acute) (rheumatic)
        (Sydenham's) I02.0
    arteriosclerotic I36.8
    nonrheumatic I36.8
      acute or subacute I33.9
    specified cause, except rheumatic I36.8
  tuberculous —*see* Tuberculosis, endocarditis
  typhoid A01.02
  ulcerative (acute) (any valve) (subacute) I33.0
  vegetative (acute) (any valve) (subacute) I33.0
  verrucous (atypical) (nonbacterial)
    (nonrheumatic) M32.11
Endocardium, endocardial —*see also* condition
  cushion defect Q21.2
Endocervicitis —*see also* Cervicitis
  due to intrauterine (contraceptive) device
    T83.69
  hyperplastic N72
Endocrine —*see* condition
Endocrinopathy, pluriglandular E31.9
Endodontic
  overfill M27.52
  underfill M27.53
Endodontitis K04.01
  irreversible K04.02
  reversible K04.01
Endomastoiditis —*see* Mastoiditis
Endometrioma N80.9
Endometriosis N80.9
  appendix N80.5
  bladder N80.8

Endometriosis *(Continued)*
  bowel N80.5
  broad ligament N80.3
  cervix N80.0
  colon N80.5
  cul-de-sac (Douglas') N80.3
  exocervix N80.0
  fallopian tube N80.2
  female genital organ NEC N80.8
  gallbladder N80.8
  in scar of skin N80.6
  internal N80.0
  intestine N80.5
  lung N80.8
  myometrium N80.0
  ovary N80.1
  parametrium N80.3
  pelvic peritoneum N80.3
  peritoneal (pelvic) N80.3
  rectovaginal septum N80.4
  rectum N80.5
  round ligament N80.3
  skin (scar) N80.6
  specified site NEC N80.8
  stromal D39.0
▶ thorax N80.8
  umbilicus N80.8
  uterus (internal) N80.0
  vagina N80.4
  vulva N80.8
Endometritis (decidual) (nonspecific) (purulent)
  (senile (atrophic) (suppurative) N71.9
  with ectopic pregnancy O08.0
  acute N71.0
  blenorrhagic (gonococcal) (acute) (chronic)
    A54.24
  cervix, cervical (with erosion or ectropion) —
    see also Cervicitis
    hyperplastic N72
  chlamydial A56.11
  chronic N71.1
  following
    abortion —*see* Abortion by type
      complicated by genital infection
    ectopic or molar pregnancy O08.0
  gonococcal, gonorrheal (acute) (chronic) A54.24
  hyperplastic —*see also* Hyperplasia,
    endometrial N85.00-●
    cervix N72
  puerperal, postpartum, childbirth O86.12
  subacute N71.0
  tuberculous A18.17
Endometrium —*see* condition
Endomyocardiopathy, South African I42.3
Endomyocarditis —*see* Endocarditis
Endomyofibrosis I42.3
Endomyometritis —*see* Endometritis
Endopericarditis —*see* Endocarditis
Endoperineuritis —*see* Disorder, nerve
Endophlebitis —*see* Phlebitis
Endophthalmia —*see* Endophthalmitis,
  purulent
Endophthalmitis (acute) (infective) (metastatic)
  (subacute) H44.009
  bleb associated H59.4 —*see also* Bleb,
    inflammed (infected), postprocedural
  gonorrheal A54.39
  in (due to)
    cysticercosis B69.1
    onchocerciasis B73.01
    toxocariasis B83.0
  panuveitis —*see* Panuveitis
  parasitic H44.12-●
  purulent H44.00-●
    panophthalmitis —*see* Panophthalmitis
    vitreous abscess H44.02-●
  specified NEC H44.19
  sympathetic —*see* Uveitis, sympathetic
Endosalpingioma D28.2
Endosalpingiosis N94.89
Endosteitis —*see* Osteomyelitis

Endothelioma, bone —*see* Neoplasm, bone, malignant
Endotheliosis (hemorrhagic infectional) D69.8
Endotoxemia — code to condition
Endotrachelitis —*see* Cervicitis
Engelmann (-Camurati) syndrome Q78.3
English disease —*see* Rickets
Engman's disease L30.3
Engorgement
  breast N64.59
    newborn P83.4
    puerperal, postpartum O92.79
  lung (passive) —*see* Edema, lung
  pulmonary (passive) —*see* Edema, lung
  stomach K31.89
  venous, retina —*see* Occlusion, retina, vein, engorgement
Enlargement, enlarged —*see also* Hypertrophy
  adenoids J35.2
    with tonsils J35.3
  alveolar ridge K08.89
    congenital —*see* Anomaly, alveolar
  apertures of diaphragm (congenital) Q79.1
  gingival K06.1
  heart, cardiac —*see* Hypertrophy, cardiac
  labium majus, childhood asymmetric (CALME) N90.61
  lacrimal gland, chronic H04.03-•
  liver —*see* Hypertrophy, liver
  lymph gland or node R59.9
    generalized R59.1
    localized R59.0
  orbit H05.34-•
  organ or site, congenital NEC —*see* Anomaly, by site
  parathyroid (gland) E21.0
  pituitary fossa R93.0
  prostate N40.0
    with lower urinary tract symptoms (LUTS) N40.1
    without lower urinary tract symptoms (LUTS) N40.0
  sella turcica R93.0
  spleen —*see* Splenomegaly
  thymus (gland) (congenital) E32.0
  thyroid (gland) —*see* Goiter
  tongue K14.8
  tonsils J35.1
    with adenoids J35.3
  uterus N85.2
  ▶vestibular aqueduct Q16.5
Enophthalmos H05.40-•
  due to
    orbital tissue atrophy H05.41-•
    trauma or surgery H05.42-•
Enostosis M27.8
Entamebic, entamebiasis —*see* Amebiasis
Entanglement
  ⇒umbilical cord(s) O69.82
    with compression O69.2
      ~~without compression O69.82~~
    ⇒around neck (with compression) O69.81
      ▶with compression O69.1
      without compression O69.81
    of twins in monoamniotic sac O69.2
    ▶without compression O69.82
Enteralgia —*see* Pain, abdominal
Enteric —*see* condition
Enteritis (acute) (diarrheal) (hemorrhagic) (noninfective) K52.9
  adenovirus A08.2
  aertrycke infection A02.0
  allergic K52.29
    with
      eosinophilic gastritis or gastroenteritis K52.81
      food protein-induced enterocolitis syndrome K52.21
      food protein-induced enteropathy K52.22

Enteritis *(Continued)*
  amebic (acute) A06.0
    with abscess —*see* Abscess, amebic
    chronic A06.1
      with abscess —*see* Abscess, amebic
      nondysenteric A06.2
    nondysenteric A06.2
  astrovirus A08.32
  bacillary NOS A03.9
  bacterial A04.9
    specified NEC A04.8
  calicivirus A08.31
  candidal B37.82
  Chilomastix A07.8
  choleriformis A00.1
  chronic (noninfectious) K52.9
    ulcerative —*see* Colitis, ulcerative
  cicatrizing (chronic) —*see* Enteritis, regional, small intestine
  Clostridium
    botulinum (food poisoning) A05.1
  ⇒difficile
    ▶not specified as recurrent A04.72
    ▶recurrent A04.71
  coccidial A07.3
  coxsackie virus A08.39
  dietetic —*see also* Enteritis, allergic K52.29
  drug-induced K52.1
  due to
    astrovirus A08.32
    calicivirus A08.31
    coxsackie virus A08.39
    drugs K52.1
    echovirus A08.39
    enterovirus NEC A08.39
    food hypersensitivity —*see also* Enteritis, allergic K52.29
    infectious organism (bacterial) (viral) —*see* Enteritis, infectious
    torovirus A08.39
    Yersinia enterocolitica A04.6
  echovirus A08.39
  eltor A00.1
  enterovirus NEC A08.39
  eosinophilic K52.81
  epidemic (infectious) A09
  fulminant —*see also* Ischemia, intestine, acute K55.019
  gangrenous —*see* Enteritis, infectious
  giardial A07.1
  infectious NOS A09
    due to
      adenovirus A08.2
      Aerobacter aerogenes A04.8
      Arizona (bacillus) A02.0
      bacteria NOS A04.9
        specified NEC A04.8
      Campylobacter A04.5
    ⇒Clostridium difficile
      ▶not specified as recurrent A04.72
      ▶recurrent A04.71
      Clostridium perfringens A04.8
      Enterobacter aerogenes A04.8
      enterovirus A08.39
      Escherichia coli A04.4
        enteroaggregative A04.4
        enterohemorrhagic A04.3
        enteroinvasive A04.2
        enteropathogenic A04.0
        enterotoxigenic A04.1
        specified NEC A04.4
      specified
        bacteria NEC A04.8
        virus NEC A08.39
      Staphylococcus A04.8
      virus NEC A08.4
        specified type NEC A08.39
      Yersinia enterocolitica A04.6
    specified organism NEC A08.8
  influenzal —*see* Influenza, with, digestive manifestations

Enteritis *(Continued)*
  ischemic K55.9
    acute —*see also* Ischemia, intestine, acute K55.019
    chronic K55.1
  microsporidial A07.8
  mucomembranous, myxomembranous —*see* Syndrome, irritable bowel
  mucous —*see* Syndrome, irritable bowel
  necroticans A05.2
  necrotizing of newborn —*see* Enterocolitis, necrotizing, in newborn
  neurogenic —*see* Syndrome, irritable bowel
  newborn necrotizing —*see* Enterocolitis, necrotizing, in newborn
  noninfectious K52.9
  norovirus A08.11
  parasitic NEC B82.9
  paratyphoid (fever) —*see* Fever, paratyphoid
  protozoal A07.9
    specified NEC A07.8
  radiation K52.0
  regional (of) K50.90
    with
      complication K50.919
        abscess K50.914
        fistula K50.913
        intestinal obstruction K50.912
        rectal bleeding K50.911
        specified complication NEC K50.918
    colon —*see* Enteritis, regional, large intestine
    duodenum —*see* Enteritis, regional, small intestine
    ileum —*see* Enteritis, regional, small intestine
    jejunum —*see* Enteritis, regional, small intestine
    large bowel —*see* Enteritis, regional, large intestine
    large intestine (colon) (rectum) K50.10
      with
        complication K50.119
          abscess K50.114
          fistula K50.113
          intestinal obstruction K50.112
          rectal bleeding K50.111
          small intestine (duodenum) (ileum) (jejunum) involvement K50.80
            with
              complication K50.819
                abscess K50.814
                fistula K50.813
                intestinal obstruction K50.812
                rectal bleeding K50.811
                specified complication NEC K50.818
          specified complication NEC K50.118
    rectum —*see* Enteritis, regional, large intestine
    small intestine (duodenum) (ileum) (jejunum) K50.00
      with
        complication K50.019
          abscess K50.014
          fistula K50.013
          intestinal obstruction K50.012
          large intestine (colon) (rectum) involvement K50.80
            with
              complication K50.819
                abscess K50.814
                fistula K50.813
                intestinal obstruction K50.812
                rectal bleeding K50.811
                specified complication NEC K50.818
          rectal bleeding K50.011
          specified complication NEC K50.018
  rotaviral A08.0

Enteritis *(Continued)*
  Salmonella, salmonellosis (arizonae)
      (cholerae-suis) (enteritidis)
      (typhimurium) A02.0
  segmental —*see* Enteritis, regional
  septic A09
  Shigella —*see* Infection, Shigella
  small round structured NEC A08.19
  spasmodic, spastic —*see* Syndrome, irritable
      bowel
  staphylococcal A04.8
    due to food A05.0
  torovirus A08.39
  toxic NEC K52.1
    ⟹due to Clostridium difficile
      ▶not specified as recurrent A04.72
      ▶recurrent A04.71
  trichomonal A07.8
  tuberculous A18.32
  typhosa A01.00
  ulcerative (chronic) —*see* Colitis, ulcerative
  viral A08.4
    adenovirus A08.2
    enterovirus A08.39
    Rotavirus A08.0
    small round structured NEC A08.19
    specified NEC A08.39
    virus specified NEC A08.39
Enterobiasis B80
Enterobius vermicularis (infection) (infestation)
    B80
Enterocele —*see also* Hernia, abdomen
  pelvic, pelvis (acquired) (congenital) N81.5
  vagina, vaginal (acquired) (congenital)
      NEC N81.5
Enterocolitis —*see also* Enteritis K52.9
  ⟹due to Clostridium difficile
    ▶not specified as recurrent A04.72
    ▶recurrent A04.71
  fulminant ischemic —*see also* Ischemia,
      intestine, acute K55.059
  granulomatous —*see* Enteritis, regional
  hemorrhagic (acute) —*see also* Ischemia,
      intestine, acute K55.059
    chronic K55.1
  infectious NEC A09
  ischemic K55.9
  necrotizing K55.30
    with
      perforation K55.33
      pneumatosis K55.32
      and perforation K55.33
    ⟹due to Clostridium difficile
      ▶not specified as recurrent A04.72
      ▶recurrent A04.71
    in non-newborn K55.30
      stage 1 (without pneumatosis, without
          perforation) K55.31
      stage 2 (with pneumatosis, without
          perforation) K55.32
      stage 3 (with pneumatosis, with
          perforation) K55.33
    in newborn P77.9
      stage 1 (without pneumatosis, without
          perforation) P77.1
      stage 2 (with pneumatosis, without
          perforation) P77.2
      stage 3 (with pneumatosis, with
          perforation) P77.3
    without pneumatosis or perforation K55.31
  noninfectious K52.9
    newborn —*see* Enterocolitis, necrotizing, in
        newborn
  ⟹pseudomembranous (newborn)
    ▶not specified as recurrent A04.72
    ▶recurrent A04.71
  radiation K52.0
    newborn —*see* Enterocolitis, necrotizing, in
        newborn
  ulcerative (chronic) —*see* Pancolitis,
      ulcerative (chronic)

Enterogastritis —*see* Enteritis
Enteropathy K63.9
  celiac-gluten-sensitive K90.0
    ▶non-celiac K90.41
  food protein-induced enterocolitis K52.22
  gluten-sensitive K90.0
    non-celiac K90.41
  hemorrhagic, terminal —*see also* Ischemia,
      intestine, acute K55.059
  protein-losing K90.49
Enteroperitonitis —*see* Peritonitis
Enteroptosis K63.4
Enterorrhagia K92.2
Enterospasm —*see also* Syndrome, irritable,
    bowel
  psychogenic F45.8
⟹Enterostenosis —*see also* Obstruction, intestine,
    specified NEC K56.699
Enterostomy
  complication —*see* Complication,
      enterostomy
  status Z93.4
Enterovirus, as cause of disease classified
    elsewhere B97.10
  coxsackievirus B97.11
  echovirus B97.12
  other specified B97.19
Enthesopathy (peripheral) M77.9
  Achilles tendinitis —*see* Tendinitis, Achilles
  ankle and tarsus M77.9
    specified type NEC —*see* Enthesopathy,
        foot, specified type NEC
  anterior tibial syndrome M76.81-●
  calcaneal spur —*see* Spur, bone, calcaneal
  elbow region M77.8
    lateral epicondylitis —*see* Epicondylitis,
        lateral
    medial epicondylitis —*see* Epicondylitis,
        medial
  foot NEC M77.9
    metatarsalgia —*see* Metatarsalgia
    specified type NEC M77.5-●
  forearm M77.9
  gluteal tendinitis —*see* Tendinitis, gluteal
  hand M77.9
  hip —*see* Enthesopathy, lower limb, specified
      type NEC
  iliac crest spur —*see* Spur, bone, iliac crest
  iliotibial band syndrome —*see* Syndrome,
      iliotibial band
  knee —*see* Enthesopathy, lower limb, lower
      leg, specified type NEC
  lateral epicondylitis —*see* Epicondylitis,
      lateral
  lower limb (excluding foot) M76.9
    Achilles tendinitis —*see* Tendinitis, Achilles
    anterior tibial syndrome M76.81-●
    gluteal tendinitis —*see* Tendinitis, gluteal
    iliac crest spur —*see* Spur, bone, iliac crest
    iliotibial band syndrome —*see* Syndrome,
        iliotibial band
    patellar tendinitis —*see* Tendinitis, patellar
    pelvic region —*see* Enthesopathy, lower
        limb, specified type NEC
    peroneal tendinitis —*see* Tendinitis,
        peroneal
    posterior tibial syndrome M76.82-●
    psoas tendinitis —*see* Tendinitis, psoas
  shoulder M77.9
    specified type NEC M76.89-●
    tibial collateral bursitis —*see* Bursitis, tibial
        collateral
  medial epicondylitis —*see* Epicondylitis,
      medial
  multiple sites M77.9
  patellar tendinitis —*see* Tendinitis, patellar
  pelvis M77.9
  periarthritis of wrist —*see* Periarthritis, wrist
  peroneal tendinitis —*see* Tendinitis, peroneal
  posterior tibial syndrome M76.82-●
  psoas tendinitis —*see* Tendinitis, psoas

Enthesopathy *(Continued)*
  shoulder region —*see* Lesion, shoulder
  specified site NEC M77.9
  specified type NEC M77.8
  spinal M46.00
    cervical region M46.02
    cervicothoracic region M46.03
    lumbar region M46.06
    lumbosacral region M46.07
    multiple sites M46.09
    occipito-atlanto-axial region M46.01
    sacrococcygeal region M46.08
    thoracic region M46.04
    thoracolumbar region M46.05
  tibial collateral bursitis —*see* Bursitis, tibial
      collateral
  upper arm M77.9
  wrist and carpus NEC M77.8
    calcaneal spur —*see* Spur, bone, calcaneal
    periarthritis of wrist —*see* Periarthritis,
        wrist
Entomophobia F40.218
Entomophthoromycosis B46.8
Entrance, air into vein —*see* Embolism, air
Entrapment, nerve —*see* Neuropathy,
    entrapment
Entropion (eyelid) (paralytic) H02.009
  cicatricial H02.019
    left H02.016
      lower H02.015
      upper H02.014
    right H02.013
      lower H02.012
      upper H02.011
  congenital Q10.2
  left H02.006
    lower H02.005
    upper H02.004
  mechanical H02.029
    left H02.026
      lower H02.025
      upper H02.024
    right H02.023
      lower H02.022
      upper H02.021
  right H02.003
    lower H02.002
    upper H02.001
  senile H02.039
    left H02.036
      lower H02.035
      upper H02.034
    right H02.033
      lower H02.032
      upper H02.031
  spastic H02.049
    left H02.046
      lower H02.045
      upper H02.044
    right H02.043
      lower H02.042
      upper H02.041
Enucleated eye (traumatic, current) S05.7-●
Enuresis R32
  functional F98.0
  habit disturbance F98.0
  nocturnal N39.44
    psychogenic F98.0
  nonorganic origin F98.0
  psychogenic F98.0
Eosinopenia —*see* Agranulocytosis
Eosinophilia (allergic) (hereditary) (idiopathic)
    (secondary) D72.1
  with
    angiolymphoid hyperplasia (ALHE)
        D18.01
  infiltrative J82
  Löffler's J82
  peritoneal —*see* Peritonitis, eosinophilic
  pulmonary NEC J82
  tropical (pulmonary) J82

Eosinophilia-myalgia syndrome M35.8
Ependymitis (acute) (cerebral) (chronic)
   (granular) —*see* Encephalomyelitis
Ependymoblastoma
  specified site —*see* Neoplasm, malignant, by
    site
  unspecified site C71.9
Ependymoma (epithelial) (malignant)
  anaplastic
    specified site —*see* Neoplasm, malignant,
      by site
    unspecified site C71.9
  benign
    specified site —*see* Neoplasm, benign, by
      site
    unspecified site D33.2
  myxopapillary D43.2
    specified site —*see* Neoplasm, uncertain
      behavior, by site
    unspecified site D43.2
  papillary D43.2
    specified site —*see* Neoplasm, uncertain
      behavior, by site
    unspecified site D43.2
  specified site —*see* Neoplasm, malignant, by
    site
  unspecified site C71.9
Ependymopathy G93.89
Ephelis, ephelides L81.2
Epiblepharon (congenital) Q10.3
Epicanthus, epicanthic fold (eyelid)
  (congenital) Q10.3
Epicondylitis (elbow)
  lateral M77.1-•
  medial M77.0-•
Epicystitis —*see* Cystitis
Epidemic —*see* condition
Epidermidalization, cervix —*see* Dysplasia,
  cervix
Epidermis, epidermal —*see* condition
Epidermodysplasia verruciformis B07.8
Epidermolysis
  bullosa (congenital) Q81.9
    acquired L12.30
      drug-induced L12.31
      specified cause NEC L12.35
    dystrophica Q81.2
    letalis Q81.1
    simplex Q81.0
    specified NEC Q81.8
  necroticans combustiformis L51.2
    due to drug —*see* Table of Drugs and
      Chemicals, by drug
Epidermophytid —*see* Dermatophytosis
Epidermophytosis (infected) —*see*
  Dermatophytosis
Epididymis —*see* condition
Epididymitis (acute) (nonvenereal) (recurrent)
  (residual) N45.1
  with orchitis N45.3
  blennorrhagic (gonococcal) A54.23
  caseous (tuberculous) A18.15
  chlamydial A56.19
  filarial —*see also* Infestation, filarial B74.9
    [N51]
  gonococcal A54.23
  syphilitic A52.76
  tuberculous A18.15
Epididymo-orchitis —*see also* Epididymitis
  N45.3
Epidural —*see* condition
Epigastrium, epigastric —*see* condition
Epigastrocele —*see* Hernia, ventral
Epiglottis —*see* condition
Epiglottitis, epiglottiditis (acute) J05.10
  with obstruction J05.11
  chronic J37.0
Epignathus Q89.4
Epilepsia partialis continua —*see also*
  Kozhevnikof's epilepsy G40.1-•

Epilepsy, epileptic, epilepsia (attack) (cerebral)
  (convulsion) (fit) (seizure) G40.909

> Note: the following terms are to be
> considered equivalent to intractable:
> pharmacoresistant (pharmacologically
> resistant), treatment resistant, refractory
> (medically) and poorly controlled

with
  complex partial seizures —*see* Epilepsy,
    localization-related, symptomatic,
    with complex partial seizures
  grand mal seizures on awakening —
    see Epilepsy, generalized, specified
    NEC
  myoclonic absences —*see* Epilepsy,
    generalized, specified NEC
  myoclonic-astatic seizures —*see* Epilepsy,
    generalized, specified NEC
  simple partial seizures —*see* Epilepsy,
    localization-related, symptomatic,
    with simple partial seizures
akinetic —*see* Epilepsy, generalized, specified
  NEC
benign childhood with centrotemporal EEG
  spikes —*see* Epilepsy, localization-
  related, idiopathic
benign myoclonic in infancy G40.80-•
Bravais-jacksonian —*see* Epilepsy,
  localization-related, symptomatic,
  with simple partial seizures
childhood
  with occipital EEG paroxysms —*see*
    Epilepsy, localization-related,
    idiopathic
  absence G40.A09
    intractable G40.A19
      with status epilepticus G40.A11
      without status epilepticus G40.A19
    not intractable G40.A09
      with status epilepticus G40.A01
      without status epilepticus G40.A09
climacteric —*see* Epilepsy, specified NEC
cysticercosis B69.0
deterioration (mental) F06.8
due to syphilis A52.19
focal —*see* Epilepsy, localization-related,
  symptomatic, with simple partial
  seizures
generalized
  idiopathic G40.309
    intractable G40.319
      with status epilepticus G40.311
      without status epilepticus G40.319
    not intractable G40.309
      with status epilepticus G40.301
      without status epilepticus G40.309
  specified NEC G40.409
    intractable G40.419
      with status epilepticus G40.411
      without status epilepticus G40.419
    not intractable G40.409
      with status epilepticus G40.401
      without status epilepticus G40.409
impulsive petit mal —*see* Epilepsy, juvenile
  myoclonic
intractable G40.919
  with status epilepticus G40.911
  without status epilepticus G40.919
juvenile absence G40.A09
  intractable G40.A19
    with status epilepticus G40.A11
    without status epilepticus G40.A19
  not intractable G40.A09
    with status epilepticus G40.A01
    without status epilepticus G40.A09
juvenile myoclonic G40.B11
  intractable G40.B19
    with status epilepticus G40.B11
    without status epilepticus G40.B19

Epilepsy, epileptic, epilepsia (Continued)
  juvenile myoclonic (Continued)
    not intractable G40.B09
      with status epilepticus G40.B01
      without status epilepticus G40.B09
  localization-related (focal) (partial)
    idiopathic G40.009
      with seizures of localized onset G40.009
        intractable G40.019
          with status epilepticus G40.011
          without status epilepticus G40.019
        not intractable G40.009
          with status epilepticus G40.001
          without status epilepticus G40.009
    symptomatic
      with complex partial seizures G40.209
        intractable G40.219
          with status epilepticus G40.211
          without status epilepticus G40.219
        not intractable G40.209
          with status epilepticus G40.201
          without status epilepticus
            G40.209
      with simple partial seizures G40.109
        intractable G40.119
          with status epilepticus G40.111
          without status epilepticus
            G40.119
        not intractable G40.109
          with status epilepticus G40.101
          without status epilepticus G40.109
  myoclonus, myoclonic —*see* Epilepsy,
    generalized, specified NEC
  progressive —*see* Epilepsy, generalized,
    idiopathic
  not intractable G40.909
    with status epilepticus G40.901
    without status epilepticus G40.909
  on awakening —*see* Epilepsy, generalized,
    specified NEC
  parasitic NOS B71.9 [G94]
  partialis continua —*see also* Kozhevnikof's
    epilepsy G40.1-•
  peripheral —*see* Epilepsy, specified NEC
  procursiva —*see* Epilepsy, localization-
    related, symptomatic, with simple
    partial seizures
  progressive (familial) myoclonic —*see*
    Epilepsy, generalized, idiopathic
  reflex —*see* Epilepsy, specified NEC
  related to
    alcohol G40.509
      not intractable G40.509
        with status epilepticus G40.501
        without status epliepticus G40.509
    drugs G40.509
      not intractable G40.509
        with status epilepticus G40.501
        without status epliepticus G40.509
    external causes G40.509
      not intractable G40.509
        with status epilepticus G40.501
        without status epilepticus G40.509
    hormonal changes G40.509
      not intractable G40.509
        with status epilepticus G40.501
        without status epliepticus G40.509
    sleep deprivation G40.509
      not intractable G40.509
        with status epilepticus G40.501
        without status epliepticus G40.509
    stress G40.509
      not intractable G40.509
        with status epilepticus G40.501
        without status epliepticus G40.509
  somatomotor —*see* Epilepsy, localization-
    related, symptomatic, with simple
    partial seizures
  somatosensory —*see* Epilepsy, localization-
    related, symptomatic, with simple
    partial seizures

Epilepsy, epileptic, epilepsia *(Continued)*
  spasms G40.822
    intractable G40.824
      with status epilepticus G40.823
      without status epilepticus G40.824
    not intractable G40.822
      with status epilepticus G40.821
      without status epilepticus G40.822
  specified NEC G40.802
    intractable G40.804
      with status epilepticus G40.803
      without status epilepticus G40.804
    not intractable G40.802
      with status epilepticus G40.801
      without status epilepticus G40.802
  syndromes
    generalized
      idiopathic G40.309
        intractable G40.319
          with status epilepticus G40.311
          without status epilepticus G40.319
        not intractable G40.309
          with status epilepticus G40.301
          without status epilepticus G40.309
      specified NEC G40.409
        intractable G40.419
          with status epilepticus G40.411
          without status epilepticus G40.419
        not intractable G40.409
          with status epilepticus G40.401
          without status epilepticus G40.409
    localization-related (focal) (partial)
      idiopathic G40.009
        with seizures of localized onset
          G40.009
          intractable G40.019
            with status epilepticus G40.011
            without status epilepticus
              G40.019
          not intractable G40.009
            with status epilepticus G40.001
            without status epilepticus
              G40.009
      symptomatic
        with complex partial seizures G40.209
          intractable G40.219
            with status epilepticus G40.211
            without status epilepticus G40.219
          not intractable G40.209
            with status epilepticus G40.201
            without status epilepticus G40.209
        with simple partial seizures G40.109
          intractable G40.119
            with status epilepticus G40.111
            without status epilepticus G40.119
          not intractable G40.109
            with status epilepticus G40.101
            without status epilepticus G40.109
      specified NEC G40.802
        intractable G40.804
          with status epilepticus G40.803
          without status epilepticus G40.804
        not intractable G40.802
          with status epilepticus G40.801
          without status epilepticus G40.802
  tonic (-clonic) —*see* Epilepsy, generalized,
    specified NEC
  twilight F05
  uncinate (gyrus) —*see* Epilepsy, localization-
    related, symptomatic, with complex
    partial seizures
  Unverricht (-Lundborg) (familial myoclonic) —
    see Epilepsy, generalized, idiopathic
  visceral —*see* Epilepsy, specified NEC
  visual —*see* Epilepsy, specified NEC
Epiloia Q85.1
Epimenorrhea N92.0
Epipharyngitis —*see* Nasopharyngitis
Epiphora H04.20-●
  due to
    excess lacrimation H04.21-●
    insufficient drainage H04.22-●

Epiphyseal arrest —*see* Arrest, epiphyseal
Epiphyseolysis, epiphysiolysis —*see*
  Osteochondropathy
Epiphysitis —*see also* Osteochondropathy
  juvenile M92.9
  syphilitic (congenital) A50.02
Epiplocele —*see* Hernia, abdomen
Epiploitis —*see* Peritonitis
Epiplosarcomphalocele —*see* Hernia, umbilicus
Episcleritis (suppurative) H15.10-●
  in (due to)
    syphilis A52.71
    tuberculosis A18.51
  nodular H15.12-●
  periodica fugax H15.11-●
    angioneurotic —*see* Edema, angioneurotic
  syphilitic (late) A52.71
  tuberculous A18.51
Episode
  affective, mixed F39
  depersonalization (in neurotic state) F48.1
  depressive F32.9
    major F32.9
      mild F32.0
      moderate F32.1
      severe (without psychotic symptoms)
        F32.2
        with psychotic symptoms F32.3
    recurrent F33.9
      brief F33.8
    specified NEC F32.89
  hypomanic F30.8
  manic F30.9
    with
      psychotic symptoms F30.2
      remission (full) F30.4
        partial F30.3
    without psychotic symptoms F30.10
      mild F30.11
      moderate F30.12
      severe (without psychotic symptoms)
        F30.13
        with psychotic symptoms F30.2
    other specified F30.8
    recurrent F31.89
  psychotic F23
    organic F06.8
  schizophrenic (acute) NEC, brief F23
Epispadias (female) (male) Q64.0
Episplenitis D73.89
Epistaxis (multiple) R04.0
  hereditary I78.0
  vicarious menstruation N94.89
Epithelioma (malignant) —*see also* Neoplasm,
  malignant, by site
  adenoides cysticum —*see* Neoplasm, skin,
    benign
  basal cell —*see* Neoplasm, skin, malignant
  benign —*see* Neoplasm, benign, by site
  Bowen's —*see* Neoplasm, skin, in situ
  calcifying, of Malherbe —*see* Neoplasm, skin,
    benign
  external site —*see* Neoplasm, skin, malignant
  intraepidermal, Jadassohn —*see* Neoplasm,
    skin, benign
  squamous cell —*see* Neoplasm, malignant,
    by site
Epitheliomatosis pigmented Q82.1
Epitheliopathy, multifocal placoid pigment
  H30.14-●
Epithelium, epithelial —*see* condition
Epituberculosis (with atelectasis) (allergic)
  A15.7
Eponychia Q84.6
Epstein's
  nephrosis or syndrome —*see* Nephrosis
  pearl K09.8
Epulis (gingiva) (fibrous) (giant cell) K06.8
Equinia A24.0
Equinovarus (congenital) (talipes) Q66.0
  acquired —*see* Deformity, limb, clubfoot

Equivalent
  convulsive (abdominal) —*see* Epilepsy,
    specified NEC
  epileptic (psychic) —*see* Epilepsy,
    localization-related, symptomatic, with
    complex partial seizures
Erb (-Duchenne) **paralysis** (birth injury)
  (newborn) P14.0
Erb's
  disease G71.0
  palsy, paralysis (brachial) (birth) (newborn)
    P14.0
    spinal (spastic) syphilitic A52.17
  pseudohypertrophic muscular dystrophy
    G71.0
Erb-Goldflam disease or syndrome G70.00
  with exacerbation (acute) G70.01
  in crisis G70.01
Erdheim's syndrome (acromegalic
  macrospondylitis) E22.0
Erection, painful (persistent) —*see* Priapism
Ergosterol deficiency (vitamin D) E55.9
  with
    adult osteomalacia M83.8
    rickets —*see* Rickets
Ergotism —*see also* Poisoning, food, noxious,
  plant
  from ergot used as drug (migraine
    therapy) —*see* Table of Drugs and
    Chemicals
Erosio interdigitalis blastomycetica B37.2
Erosion
  artery I77.2
    without rupture I77.89
  bone —*see* Disorder, bone, density and
    structure, specified NEC
  bronchus J98.09
  cartilage (joint) —*see* Disorder, cartilage,
    specified type NEC
  cervix (uteri) (acquired) (chronic) (congenital)
    N86
    with cervicitis N72
  cornea (nontraumatic) —*see* Ulcer, cornea
    recurrent H18.83-●
    traumatic —*see* Abrasion, cornea
  dental (idiopathic) (occupational) (due to
    diet, drugs or vomiting) K03.2
  duodenum, postpyloric —*see* Ulcer,
    duodenum
  esophagus K22.10
    with bleeding K22.11
  gastric —*see* Ulcer, stomach
  gastrojejunal —*see* Ulcer, gastrojejunal
  implanted mesh —*see* Complications, mesh
  intestine K63.3
  lymphatic vessel I89.8
  pylorus, pyloric (ulcer) —*see* Ulcer, stomach
  spine, aneurysmal A52.09
  stomach —*see* Ulcer, stomach
  subcutaneous device pocket
    nervous system prosthetic device, implant,
      or graft T85.890
    other internal prosthetic device, implant, or
      graft T85.898
  teeth (idiopathic) (occupational) (due to diet,
    drugs or vomiting) K03.2
  urethra N36.8
  uterus N85.8
Erotomania F52.8
Error
  metabolism, inborn —*see* Disorder, metabolism
  refractive —*see* Disorder, refraction
Eructation R14.2
  nervous or psychogenic F45.8
Eruption
  creeping B76.9
  drug (generalized) (taken internally) L27.0
    fixed L27.1
    in contact with skin —*see* Dermatitis, due
      to drugs
    localized L27.1

▶ New   ⇒ Revised   ~~deleted~~ Deleted   ● Use Additional Character(s)

Eruption (Continued)
  Hutchinson, summer L56.4
  Kaposi's varicelliform B00.0
  napkin L22
  polymorphous light (sun) L56.4
  recalcitrant pustular L13.8
  ringed R23.8
  skin (nonspecific) R21
    creeping (meaning hookworm) B76.9
    due to inoculation/vaccination
      (generalized) —see also Dermatitis,
        due to, vaccine L27.0
      localized L27.1
    erysipeloid A26.0
    feigned L98.1
    Kaposi's varicelliform B00.0
    lichenoid L28.0
    meaning dermatitis —see Dermatitis
    toxic NEC L53.0
  tooth, teeth, abnormal (incomplete) (late)
    (premature) (sequence) K00.6
  vesicular R23.8
Erysipelas (gangrenous) (infantile) (newborn)
    (phlegmonous) (suppurative) A46
  external ear A46 [H62.40]
  puerperal, postpartum O86.89
Erysipeloid A26.9
  cutaneous (Rosenbach's) A26.0
  disseminated A26.8
  sepsis A26.7
  specified NEC A26.8
Erythema, erythematous (infectional)
    (inflammation) L53.9
  ab igne L59.0
  annulare (centrifugum) (rheumaticum) L53.1
  arthriticum epidemicum A25.1
  brucellum —see Brucellosis
  chronic figurate NEC L53.3
  chronicum migrans (Borrelia burgdorferi)
    A69.20
  diaper L22
  due to
    chemical NEC L53.0
      in contact with skin L24.5
    drug (internal use) —see Dermatitis, due
      to, drugs
  elevatum diutinum L95.1
  endemic E52
  epidemic, arthritic A25.1
  figuratum perstans L53.3
  gluteal L22
  heat - code by site under Burn, first degree
  ichthyosiforme congenitum bullous Q80.3
  in diseases classified elsewhere L54
  induratum (nontuberculous) L52
    tuberculous A18.4
  infectiosum B08.3
  intertrigo L30.4
  iris L51.9
  marginatum L53.2
    in (due to) acute rheumatic fever I00
  medicamentosum —see Dermatitis, due to,
    drugs
  migrans A26.0
    chronicum A69.20
    tongue K14.1
  multiforme (major) (minor) L51.9
    bullous, bullosum L51.1
    conjunctiva L51.1
    nonbullous L51.0
    pemphigoides L12.0
    specified NEC L51.8
  napkin L22
  neonatorum P83.88
    toxic P83.1
  nodosum L52
    tuberculous A18.4
  palmar L53.8
  pernio T69.1
  rash, newborn P83.88
  scarlatiniform (recurrent) (exfoliative) L53.8

Erythema, erythematous (Continued)
  solare L55.0
  specified NEC L53.8
  toxic, toxicum NEC L53.0
    newborn P83.1
  tuberculous (primary) A18.4
Erythematous, erythematosus —see condition
Erythermalgia (primary) I73.81
Erythralgia I73.81
Erythrasma L08.1
Erythredema (polyneuropathy) —see Poisoning,
    mercury
Erythremia (acute) C94.0-●
  chronic D45
  secondary D75.1
Erythroblastopenia —see also Aplasia, red cell
    D60.9
  congenital D61.01
Erythroblastophthisis D61.09
Erythroblastosis (fetalis) (newborn) P55.9
  due to
    ABO (antibodies) (incompatibility)
      (isoimmunization) P55.1
    Rh (antibodies) (incompatibility)
      (isoimmunization) P55.0
Erythrocyanosis (crurum) I73.89
Erythrocythemia —see Erythremia
Erythrocytosis (megalosplenic) (secondary)
    D75.1
  familial D75.0
  oval, hereditary —see Elliptocytosis
  secondary D75.1
  stress D75.1
Erythroderma (secondary) —see also Erythema
    L53.9
  bullous ichthyosiform, congenital Q80.3
  desquamativum L21.1
  ichthyosiform, congenital (bullous) Q80.3
  neonatorum P83.88
  psoriaticum L40.8
Erythrodysesthesia, palmar plantar (PPE) L27.1
Erythrogenesis imperfecta D61.09
Erythroleukemia C94.0-●
Erythromelalgia I73.81
Erythrophagocytosis D75.89
Erythrophobia F40.298
Erythroplakia, oral epithelium, and tongue
    K13.29
Erythroplasia (Queyrat) D07.4
  specified site —see Neoplasm, skin, in situ
  unspecified site D07.4
Escherichia coli (E. coli), as cause of disease
    classified elsewhere B96.20
  non-O157 Shiga toxin-producing (with
    known O group) B96.22
  non-Shiga toxin-producing B96.29
  O157 with confirmation of Shiga toxin when
    H antigen is unknown, or is not H7
    B96.21
  O157:H- (nonmotile) with confirmation of
    Shiga toxin B96.21
  O157:H7 with or without confirmation of
    Shiga toxin-production B96.21
  Shiga toxin-producing (with unspecified O
    group) (STEC) B96.23
  O157 B96.21
  O157:H7 with or without confirmation of
    Shiga toxin-production B96.21
  specified NEC B96.22
  specified NEC B96.29
Esophagismus K22.4
Esophagitis (acute) (alkaline) (chemical)
    (chronic) (infectional) (necrotic) (peptic)
    (postoperative) K20.9
  candidal B37.81
  due to gastrointestinal reflux disease K21.0
  eosinophilic K20.0
  reflux K21.0
  specified NEC K20.8
  tuberculous A18.83
  ulcerative K22.10
    with bleeding K22.11

Esophagocele K22.5
Esophagomalacia K22.8
Esophagospasm K22.4
Esophagostenosis K22.2
Esophagostomiasis B81.8
Esophagotracheal —see condition
Esophagus —see condition
Esophoria H50.51
  convergence, excess H51.12
  divergence, insufficiency H51.8
Esotropia —see Strabismus, convergent
    concomitant
Espundia B55.2
Essential —see condition
Esthesioneuroblastoma C30.0
Esthesioneurocytoma C30.0
Esthesioneuroepithelioma C30.0
Esthiomene A55
Estivo-autumnal malaria (fever) B50.9
Estrangement (marital) Z63.5
  parent-child NEC Z62.890
Estriasis —see Myiasis
Ethanolism —see Alcoholism
Etherism —see Dependence, drug, inhalant
Ethmoid, ethmoidal —see condition
Ethmoiditis (chronic) (nonpurulent)
    (purulent) —see also Sinusitis, ethmoidal
  influenzal —see Influenza, with, respiratory
    manifestations NEC
  Woakes' J33.1
Ethylism —see Alcoholism
Eulenburg's disease (congenital paramyotonia)
    G71.19
Eumycetoma B47.0
Eunuchoidism E29.1
  hypogonadotropic E23.0
European blastomycosis —see Cryptococcosis
Eustachian —see condition
Evaluation (for) (of)
  development state
    adolescent Z00.3
    period of
      delayed growth in childhood Z00.70
        with abnormal findings Z00.71
      rapid growth in childhood Z00.2
      puberty Z00.3
  growth and developmental state (period of
    rapid growth) Z00.2
  delayed growth Z00.70
    with abnormal findings Z00.71
  mental health (status) Z00.8
    requested by authority Z04.6
  period of
    delayed growth in childhood Z00.70
      with abnormal findings Z00.71
    rapid growth in childhood Z00.2
  suspected condition —see Observation
Evans syndrome D69.41
~~Event, apparent life threatening in newborn and
    infant (ALTE) R68.13~~
►**Event**
  ►apparent life threatening in newborn and
    infant (ALTE) R68.13
  ►brief resolved unexplained event (BRUE)
    R68.13
Eventration —see also Hernia, ventral
  colon into chest —see Hernia, diaphragm
  diaphragm (congenital) Q79.1
Eversion
  bladder N32.89
  cervix (uteri) N86
    with cervicitis N72
  foot NEC —see also Deformity, valgus, ankle
    congenital Q66.6
  punctum lacrimale (postinfectional) (senile)
    H04.52-●
  ureter (meatus) N28.89
  urethra (meatus) N36.8
  uterus N81.4
Evidence
  cytologic
    of malignancy on anal smear R85.614

Evidence *(Continued)*
  cytologic *(Continued)*
    of malignancy on cervical smear R87.614
    of malignancy on vaginal smear R87.624
Evisceration
  birth injury P15.8
  traumatic NEC
    eye —*see* Enucleated eye
Evulsion —*see* Avulsion
Ewing's sarcoma or tumor —*see* Neoplasm, bone, malignant
Examination (for) (following) (general) (of) (routine) Z00.00
  with abnormal findings Z00.01
  abuse, physical (alleged), ruled out
    adult Z04.71
    child Z04.72
  adolescent (development state) Z00.3
  alleged rape or sexual assault (victim), ruled out
    adult Z04.41
    child Z04.42
  allergy Z01.82
  annual (adult) (periodic) (physical) Z00.00
    with abnormal findings Z00.01
    gynecological Z01.419
      with abnormal findings Z01.411
  antibody response Z01.84
  blood —*see* Examination, laboratory
  blood pressure Z01.30
    with abnormal findings Z01.31
  cancer staging —*see* Neoplasm, malignant, by site
  cervical Papanicolaou smear Z12.4
    as part of routine gynecological examination Z01.419
      with abnormal findings Z01.411
  child (over 28 days old) Z00.129
    with abnormal findings Z00.121
    under 28 days old —*see* Newborn, examination
  clinical research control or normal comparison (control) (participant) Z00.6
  contraceptive (drug) maintenance (routine) Z30.8
    device (intrauterine) Z30.431
  dental Z01.20
    with abnormal findings Z01.21
  developmental —*see* Examination, child
  donor (potential) Z00.5
  ear Z01.10
    with abnormal findings NEC Z01.118
  eye Z01.00
    with abnormal findings Z01.01
  following
    accident NEC Z04.3
      transport Z04.1
      work Z04.2
    assault, alleged, ruled out
      adult Z04.71
      child Z04.72
    motor vehicle accident Z04.1
    treatment (for) Z09
      combined NEC Z09
        fracture Z09
        malignant neoplasm Z08
      malignant neoplasm Z08
      mental disorder Z09
      specified condition NEC Z09
  follow-up (routine) (following) Z09
    chemotherapy NEC Z09
      malignant neoplasm Z08
    fracture Z09
    malignant neoplasm Z08
    postpartum Z39.2
    psychotherapy Z09
    radiotherapy NEC Z09
      malignant neoplasm Z08
    surgery NEC Z09
      malignant neoplasm Z08

Examination *(Continued)*
  gynecological Z01.419
    with abnormal findings Z01.411
    for contraceptive maintenance Z30.8
  health —*see* Examination, medical
  hearing Z01.10
    with abnormal findings NEC Z01.118
    following failed hearing screening Z01.110
  immunity status testing Z01.84
  laboratory (as part of a general medical examination) Z00.00
    with abnormal findings Z00.01
    preprocedural Z01.812
  lactating mother Z39.1
  medical (adult) (for) (of) Z00.00
    with abnormal findings Z00.01
    administrative purpose only Z02.9
      specified NEC Z02.89
    admission to
      armed forces Z02.3
      old age home Z02.2
      prison Z02.89
      residential institution Z02.2
      school Z02.0
        following illness or medical treatment Z02.0
      summer camp Z02.89
    adoption Z02.82
    blood alcohol or drug level Z02.83
    camp (summer) Z02.89
    clinical research, normal subject (control) (participant) Z00.6
    control subject in clinical research (normal comparison) (participant) Z00.6
    donor (potential) Z00.5
    driving license Z02.4
    general (adult) Z00.00
      with abnormal findings Z00.01
    immigration Z02.89
    insurance purposes Z02.6
    marriage Z02.89
    medicolegal reasons NEC Z04.8
    naturalization Z02.89
    participation in sport Z02.5
    paternity testing Z02.81
    population survey Z00.8
    pre-employment Z02.1
    pre-operative —*see* Examination, pre-procedural
    pre-procedural
      cardiovascular Z01.810
      respiratory Z01.811
      specified NEC Z01.818
    preschool children
      for admission to school Z02.0
    prisoners
      for entrance into prison Z02.89
    recruitment for armed forces Z02.3
    specified NEC Z00.8
    sport competition Z02.5
  medicolegal reason NEC Z04.8
  newborn —*see* Newborn, examination
  pelvic (annual) (periodic) Z01.419
    with abnormal findings Z01.411
  period of rapid growth in childhood Z00.2
  periodic (adult) (annual) (routine) Z00.00
    with abnormal findings Z00.01
  physical (adult) —*see also* Examination, medical Z00.00
    sports Z02.5
  postpartum
    immediately after delivery Z39.0
    routine follow-up Z39.2
  pre-chemotherapy (antineoplastic) Z01.818
  prenatal (normal pregnancy) —*see also* Pregnancy, normal Z34.9-•
  pre-procedural (pre-operative)
    cardiovascular Z01.810
    laboratory Z01.812
    respiratory Z01.811
    specified NEC Z01.818

Examination *(Continued)*
  prior to chemotherapy (antineoplastic) Z01.818
  psychiatric NEC Z00.8
    follow-up not needing further care Z09
    requested by authority Z04.6
  radiological (as part of a general medical examination) Z00.00
    with abnormal findings Z00.01
  repeat cervical smear to confirm findings of recent normal smear following initial abnormal smear Z01.42
  skin (hypersensitivity) Z01.82
  special —*see also* Examination, by type Z01.89
    specified type NEC Z01.89
  specified type or reason NEC Z04.8
  teeth Z01.20
    with abnormal findings Z01.21
  urine —*see* Examination, laboratory
  vision Z01.00
    with abnormal findings Z01.01
Exanthem, exanthema —*see also* Rash
  with enteroviral vesicular stomatitis B08.4
  Boston A88.0
  epidemic with meningitis A88.0 *[G02]*
  subitum B08.20
    due to human herpesvirus 6 B08.21
    due to human herpesvirus 7 B08.22
  viral, virus B09
    specified type NEC B08.8
Excess, excessive, excessively
  alcohol level in blood R78.0
  androgen (ovarian) E28.1
  attrition, tooth, teeth K03.0
  carotene, carotin (dietary) E67.1
  cold, effects of T69.9
    specified effect NEC T69.8
  convergence H51.12
  crying
    in child, adolescent, or adult R45.83
    in infant R68.11
  development, breast N62
  divergence H51.8
  drinking (alcohol) NEC (without dependence) F10.10
    habitual (continual) (without remission) F10.20
  eating R63.2
  estrogen E28.0
  fat —*see also* Obesity
    in heart —*see* Degeneration, myocardial
    localized E65
  foreskin N47.8
  gas R14.0
  glucagon E16.3
  heat —*see* Heat
  intermaxillary vertical dimension of fully erupted teeth M26.37
  interocclusal distance of fully erupted teeth M26.37
  kalium E87.5
  large
    colon K59.39
      congenital Q43.8
    infant P08.0
    organ or site, congenital NEC —*see* Anomaly, by site
  long
    organ or site, congenital NEC —*see* Anomaly, by site
  menstruation (with regular cycle) N92.0
    with irregular cycle N92.1
  napping Z72.821
  natrium E87.0
  number of teeth K00.1
  nutrient (dietary) NEC R63.2
  potassium (K) E87.5
  salivation K11.7
  secretion —*see also* Hypersecretion
    milk O92.6
    sputum R09.3
    sweat R61

Excess, excessive, excessively *(Continued)*
  sexual drive F52.8
  short
    organ or site, congenital NEC —*see*
      Anomaly, by site
    umbilical cord in labor or delivery O69.3
  skin L98.7
    and subcutaneous tissue L98.7
      eyelid (acquired) —*see* Blepharochalasis
        congenital Q10.3
  sodium (Na) E87.0
  spacing of fully erupted teeth M26.32
  sputum R09.3
  sweating R61
  thirst R63.1
    due to deprivation of water T73.1
  tuberosity of jaw M26.07
  vitamin
    A (dietary) E67.0
      administered as drug (prolonged
        intake) —*see* Table of Drugs and
        Chemicals, vitamins, adverse
        effect
      overdose or wrong substance given
        or taken —*see* Table of Drugs and
        Chemicals, vitamins, poisoning
    D (dietary) E67.3
      administered as drug (prolonged
        intake) —*see* Table of Drugs and
        Chemicals, vitamins, adverse
        effect
      overdose or wrong substance given
        or taken —*see* Table of Drugs and
        Chemicals, vitamins, poisoning
  weight
    gain R63.5
    loss R63.4
Excitability, abnormal, under minor stress
  (personality disorder) F60.3
Excitation
  anomalous atrioventricular I45.6
  psychogenic F30.8
  reactive (from emotional stress, psychological
    trauma) F30.8
Excitement
  hypomanic F30.8
  manic F30.9
  mental, reactive (from emotional stress,
    psychological trauma) F30.8
  state, reactive (from emotional stress,
    psychological trauma) F30.8
Excoriation (traumatic) —*see also* Abrasion
  neurotic L98.1
  skin picking disorder F42.4
Exfoliation
  due to erythematous conditions according
    to extent of body surface involved
    L49.0
    10-19 percent of body surface L49.1
    20-29 percent of body surface L49.2
    30-39 percent of body surface L49.3
    40-49 percent of body surface L49.4
    50-59 percent of body surface L49.5
    60-69 percent of body surface L49.6
    70-79 percent of body surface L49.7
    80-89 percent of body surface L49.8
    90-99 percent of body surface L49.9
    less than 10 percent of body surface L49.0
  teeth, due to systemic causes K08.0
Exfoliative —*see* condition
Exhaustion, exhaustive (physical NEC) R53.83
  battle F43.0
  cardiac —*see* Failure, heart
  delirium F43.0
  due to
    cold T69.8
    excessive exertion T73.3
    exposure T73.2
    neurasthenia F48.8
  heart —*see* Failure, heart
  heat —*see also* Heat, exhaustion T67.5

Exhaustion, exhaustive *(Continued)*
  heat *(Continued)*
    due to
      salt depletion T67.4
      water depletion T67.3
  maternal, complicating delivery O75.81
  mental F48.8
  myocardium, myocardial —*see* Failure, heart
  nervous F48.8
  old age R54
  psychogenic F48.8
  psychosis F43.0
  senile R54
  vital NEC Z73.0
Exhibitionism F65.2
Exocervicitis —*see* Cervicitis
Exomphalos Q79.2
  meaning hernia —*see* Hernia, umbilicus
Exophoria H50.52
  convergence, insufficiency H51.11
  divergence, excess H51.8
Exophthalmos H05.2-●
  congenital Q15.8
  constant NEC H05.24-●
  displacement, globe —*see* Displacement,
    globe
  due to thyrotoxicosis (hyperthyroidism) —*see*
    Hyperthyroidism, with, goiter (diffuse)
  dysthyroid —*see* Hyperthyroidism, with,
    goiter (diffuse)
  goiter —*see* Hyperthyroidism, with, goiter
    (diffuse)
  intermittent NEC H05.25-●
  malignant —*see* Hyperthyroidism, with,
    goiter (diffuse)
  orbital
    edema —*see* Edema, orbit
    hemorrhage —*see* Hemorrhage, orbit
  pulsating NEC H05.26-●
  thyrotoxic, thyrotropic —*see*
    Hyperthyroidism, with, goiter (diffuse)
Exostosis —*see also* Disorder, bone
  cartilaginous —*see* Neoplasm, bone, benign
  congenital (multiple) Q78.6
  external ear canal H61.81-●
  gonococcal A54.49
  jaw (bone) M27.8
  multiple, congenital Q78.6
  orbit H05.35-●
  osteocartilaginous —*see* Neoplasm, bone,
    benign
  syphilitic A52.77
Exotropia —*see* Strabismus, divergent
  concomitant
Explanation of
  investigation finding Z71.2
  medication Z71.89
Exposure (to) —*see also* Contact, with T75.89
  acariasis Z20.7
  AIDS virus Z20.6
  air pollution Z77.110
  algae and algae toxins Z77.121
  algae bloom Z77.121
  anthrax Z20.810
  aromatic amines Z77.020
  aromatic (hazardous) compounds NEC
    Z77.028
  aromatic dyes NOS Z77.028
  arsenic Z77.010
  asbestos Z77.090
  bacterial disease NEC Z20.818
  benzene Z77.021
  blue-green algae bloom Z77.121
  body fluids (potentially hazardous) Z77.21
  brown tide Z77.121
  chemicals (chiefly nonmedicinal) (hazardous)
    NEC Z77.098
  cholera Z20.09
  chromium compounds Z77.018
  cold, effects of T69.9
    specified effect NEC T69.8

Exposure *(Continued)*
  communicable disease Z20.9
    bacterial NEC Z20.818
    specified NEC Z20.89
    viral NEC Z20.828
  cyanobacteria bloom Z77.121
  disaster Z65.5
  discrimination Z60.5
  dyes Z77.098
  effects of T73.9
  environmental tobacco smoke (acute)
    (chronic) Z77.22
  Escherichia coli (E. coli) Z20.01
  exhaustion due to T73.2
  fiberglass —*see* Table of Drugs and
    Chemicals, fiberglass
  German measles Z20.4
  gonorrhea Z20.2
  hazardous metals NEC Z77.018
  hazardous substances NEC Z77.29
  hazards in the physical environment NEC
    Z77.128
  hazards to health NEC Z77.9
  human immunodeficiency virus (HIV) Z20.6
  human T-lymphotropic virus type-1 (HTLV-1)
    Z20.89
  implanted
    mesh —*see* Complications, mesh
    prosthetic materials NEC —*see*
      Complications, prosthetic materials
      NEC
  infestation (parasitic) NEC Z20.7
  intestinal infectious disease NEC Z20.09
    Escherichia coli (E. coli) Z20.01
  lead Z77.011
  meningococcus Z20.811
  mold (toxic) Z77.120
  nickel dust Z77.018
  noise Z77.122
  occupational
    air contaminants NEC Z57.39
    dust Z57.2
    environmental tobacco smoke Z57.31
    extreme temperature Z57.6
    noise Z57.0
    radiation Z57.1
    risk factors Z57.9
      specified NEC Z57.8
    toxic agents (gases) (liquids) (solids)
      (vapors) in agriculture Z57.4
    toxic agents (gases) (liquids) (solids)
      (vapors) in industry NEC Z57.5
    vibration Z57.7
  parasitic disease NEC Z20.7
  pediculosis Z20.7
  persecution Z60.5
  pfiesteria piscicida Z77.121
  poliomyelitis Z20.89
  pollution
    air Z77.110
    environmental NEC Z77.118
    soil Z77.112
    water Z77.111
  polycyclic aromatic hydrocarbons
    Z77.028
  prenatal (drugs) (toxic chemicals) —*see*
    Newborn, affected by, noxious
    substances transmitted via placenta or
    breast milk
  rabies Z20.3
  radiation, naturally occurring NEC Z77.123
  radon Z77.123
  red tide (Florida) Z77.121
  rubella Z20.4
  second hand tobacco smoke (acute) (chronic)
    Z77.22
    in the perinatal period P96.81
  sexually-transmitted disease Z20.2
  smallpox (laboratory) Z20.89
  syphilis Z20.2
  terrorism Z65.4

Exposure *(Continued)*
  torture Z65.4
  tuberculosis Z20.1
  uranium Z77.012
  varicella Z20.820
  venereal disease Z20.2
  viral disease NEC Z20.828
  war Z65.5
  water pollution Z77.111
Exsanguination *—see* Hemorrhage
Exstrophy
  abdominal contents Q45.8
  bladder Q64.10
    cloacal Q64.12
    specified type NEC Q64.19
    supravesical fissure Q64.11
Extensive *—see* condition
Extra *—see also* Accessory
  marker chromosomes (normal individual)
    Q92.61
    in abnormal individual Q92.62

Extra *(Continued)*
  rib Q76.6
    cervical Q76.5
Extrasystoles (supraventricular) I49.49
  atrial I49.1
  auricular I49.1
  junctional I49.2
  ventricular I49.3
Extrauterine gestation or pregnancy *—see*
    Pregnancy, by site
Extravasation
  blood R58
  chyle into mesentery I89.8
  pelvicalyceal N13.8
  pyelosinus N13.8
  urine (from ureter) R39.0
  vesicant agent
    antineoplastic chemotherapy T80.810
    other agent NEC T80.818
Extremity *—see* condition, limb
Extrophy *—see* Exstrophy

Extroversion
  bladder Q64.19
  uterus N81.4
    complicating delivery O71.2
    postpartal (old) N81.4
Extruded tooth (teeth) M26.34
Extrusion
  breast implant (prosthetic) T85.42
  eye implant (globe) (ball) T85.328
  intervertebral disc *—see* Displacement,
    intervertebral disc
  ocular lens implant (prosthetic) *—see*
    Complications, intraocular lens
  vitreous *—see* Prolapse, vitreous
Exudate
  pleural *—see* Effusion, pleura
  retina H35.89
Exudative *—see* condition
Eye, eyeball, eyelid *—see* condition
Eyestrain *—see* Disturbance, vision, subjective
Eyeworm disease of Africa B74.3

F

Faber's syndrome (achlorhydric anemia) D50.9
Fabry (-Anderson) disease E75.21
Faciocephalalgia, autonomic —see also
    Neuropathy, peripheral, autonomic G90.09
Factor(s)
    psychic, associated with diseases classified
        elsewhere F54
    psychological
        affecting physical conditions F54
        or behavioral
            affecting general medical condition F54
            associated with disorders or diseases
                classified elsewhere F54
Fahr disease (of brain) G23.8
Fahr Volhard disease (of kidney) I12.-●
Failure, failed
    abortion —see Abortion, attempted
    aortic (valve) I35.8
        rheumatic I06.8
    attempted abortion —see Abortion, attempted
    biventricular I50.82
        due to left heart failure I50.814
    bone marrow —see Anemia, aplastic
    cardiac —see Failure, heart
    cardiorenal (chronic) —see also Failure, renal,
        and Failure, heart I50.9
        hypertensive I13.2
    cardiorespiratory (see also Failure, heart) R09.2
    cardiovascular (chronic) —see Failure, heart
    cerebrovascular I67.9
    cervical dilatation in labor O62.0
    circulation, circulatory (peripheral) R57.9
        newborn P29.89
    compensation —see Disease, heart
    compliance with medical treatment or
        regimen —see Noncompliance
    congestive —see Failure, heart, congestive
    dental implant (endosseous) M27.69
        due to
            failure of dental prosthesis M27.63
            lack of attached gingiva M27.62
            occlusal trauma (poor prosthetic design)
                M27.62
            parafunctional habits M27.62
            periodontal infection (peri-implantitis)
                M27.62
            poor oral hygiene M27.62
        osseointegration M27.61
            due to
                complications of systemic disease
                    M27.61
                poor bone quality M27.61
            iatrogenic M27.61
        post-osseointegration
            biological M27.62
            due to complications of systemic disease
                M27.62
            iatrogenic M27.62
            mechanical M27.63
        pre-integration M27.61
        pre-osseointegration M27.61
        specified NEC M27.69
    descent of head (at term) of pregnancy
        (mother) O32.4
    endosseous dental implant —see Failure,
        dental implant
    engagement of head (term of pregnancy)
        (mother) O32.4
    erection (penile) —see also Dysfunction,
        sexual, male, erectile N52.9
        nonorganic F52.21
    examination(s), anxiety concerning Z55.2
    expansion terminal respiratory units
        (newborn) (primary) P28.0
    forceps NOS (with subsequent cesarean
        delivery) O66.5
    gain weight (child over 28 days old) R62.51
        adult R62.7
        newborn P92.6

Failure, failed (Continued)
    genital response (male) F52.21
        female F52.22
    heart (acute) (senile) (sudden) I50.9
        with
            acute pulmonary edema —see Failure,
                ventricular, left
            decompensation —see also Failure, heart,
                by type as diastolic or systolic,
                acute and chronic I50.9
            dilatation —see Disease, heart
            normal ejection fraction —see Failure,
                heart, diastolic
            preserved ejection fraction —see Failure,
                heart, diastolic
            reduced ejection fraction —see Failure,
                heart, systolic
        arteriosclerotic I70.90
        biventricular I50.82
            due to left heart failure I50.814
        combined left-right sided I50.82
            due to left heart failure I50.814
        compensated —see also Failure, heart, by
            type as diastolic or systolic, chronic
            I50.9
        complicating
            anesthesia (general) (local) or other
                sedation
                in labor and delivery O74.2
                in pregnancy O29.12-●
                postpartum, puerperal O89.1
            delivery (cesarean) (instrumental) O75.4
        congestive I50.9
            with rheumatic fever (conditions in I00)
                active I01.8
                inactive or quiescent (with chorea)
                    I09.81
            newborn P29.0
            rheumatic (chronic) (inactive) (with
                chorea) I09.81
                active or acute I01.8
                    with chorea I02.0
        decompensated —see also Failure, heart, by
            type as diastolic or systolic, acute and
            chronic I50.9
        degenerative —see Degeneration,
            myocardial
        diastolic (congestive) (left ventricular)
            I50.30
            acute (congestive) I50.31
                and (on) chronic (congestive) I50.33
            chronic (congestive) I50.32
                and (on) acute (congestive) I50.33
            combined with systolic (congestive)
                I50.40
                acute (congestive) I50.41
                    and (on) chronic (congestive) I50.43
                chronic (congestive) I50.42
                  and (on) acute (congestive) I50.43
            due to presence of cardiac prosthesis I97.13-●
        end stage —see also Failure, heart, by type
            as diastolic or systolic, chronic I50.84
        following cardiac surgery I97.13-●
        high output NOS I50.83
        hypertensive —see Hypertension, heart
        left (ventricular) —see also Failure,
            ventricular, left
            combined diastolic and systolic —see
                Failure, heart, diastolic, combined
                with systolic
            diastolic —see Failure, heart, diastolic
            systolic —see Failure, heart, systolic
        low output (syndrome) NOS I50.9
        newborn P29.0
        organic —see Disease, heart
        peripartum O90.3
        postprocedural I97.13-●
        rheumatic (chronic) (inactive) I09.9
        right (isolated) (ventricular) I50.810
            acute I50.811
                and (on) chronic I50.813

Failure, failed (Continued)
    heart (Continued)
        right (Continued)
            chronic I50.812
                and acute I50.813
            secondary to left heart failure I50.814
            ~~systolic (congestive) I50.20~~
            ~~acute (congestive) I50.21~~
                ~~and (on) chronic (congestive)~~
                    ~~I50.23~~
            ~~chronic (congestive) I50.22~~
                ~~and (on) acute (congestive) I50.23~~
            ~~combined with diastolic (congestive)~~
                ~~I50.40~~
                ~~acute (congestive) I50.41~~
                    ~~and (on) chronic (congestive)~~
                    ~~I50.43~~
                ~~chronic (congestive) I50.42~~
                  ~~and (on) acute (congestive)~~
                    ~~I50.43~~
            ~~thyrotoxic —see also Thyrotoxicosis~~
                ~~E05.90 [I43]~~
                ~~with thyroid storm E05.91 [I43]~~
            ~~valvular —see Endocarditis~~
            specified NEC I50.89

> Note: heart failure stages A, B, C, and
> D are based on the American College of
> Cardiology and American Heart Association
> stages of heart failure, which complement
> and should not be confused with the New
> York Heart Association Classification of
> Heart Failure, into Class I, Class II, Class III,
> and Class IV

            stage A Z91.89
            stage B (see also Failure, heart, by type as
                diastolic or systolic) I50.9
            stage C (see also Failure, heart, by type as
                diastolic or systolic) I50.9
            stage D (see also Failure, heart, by type as
                diastolic or systolic, chronic) I50.84
            systolic (congestive) (left ventricular) I50.20
                acute (congestive) I50.21
                  and (on) chronic (congestive) I50.23
                chronic (congestive) I50.22
                  and (on) acute (congestive) I50.23
                combined with diastolic (congestive)
                  I50.40
                  acute (congestive) I50.41
                    and (on) chronic (congestive) I50.43
                  chronic (congestive) I50.42
                    and (on) acute (congestive) I50.43
            thyrotoxic (see also Thyrotoxicosis) E05.90
                [I43]
            with
                high output (see also Thyrotoxicosis)
                  I50.83
                thyroid storm E05.91 [I43]
                  high output (see also
                    Thyrotoxicosis) I50.83
            valvular —see Endocarditis
    hepatic K72.90
        with coma K72.91
        acute or subacute K72.00
            with coma K72.01
            due to drugs K71.10
                with coma K71.11
        alcoholic (acute) (chronic) (subacute)
            K70.40
            with coma K70.41
        chronic K72.10
            with coma K72.11
            due to drugs (acute) (subacute) (chronic)
                K71.10
                with coma K71.11
        due to drugs (acute) (subacute) (chronic)
            K71.10
            with coma K71.11
         postprocedural K91.82

Failure, failed *(Continued)*
  hepatorenal K76.7
  induction (of labor) O61.9
    abortion —*see* Abortion, attempted
    by
      oxytocic drugs O61.0
      prostaglandins O61.0
    instrumental O61.1
    mechanical O61.1
    medical O61.0
    specified NEC O61.8
    surgical O61.1
  intubation during anesthesia T88.4
    in pregnancy O29.6- •
    labor and delivery O74.7
    postpartum, puerperal O89.6
  involution, thymus (gland) E32.0
  kidney —*see also* Disease, kidney, chronic N19
    acute —*see also* Failure, renal, acute
      N17.9- •
    diabetic —*see* E08-E13 with .22
  lactation (complete) O92.3
    partial O92.4
  Leydig's cell, adult E29.1
  liver —*see* Failure, hepatic
  menstruation at puberty N91.0
  mitral I05.8
  myocardial, myocardium —*see also* Failure,
    heart I50.9
    chronic —*see also* Failure, heart, congestive
      I50.9
    congestive —*see also* Failure, heart,
      congestive I50.9
  orgasm (female) (psychogenic) F52.31
    male F52.32
  ovarian (primary) E28.39
    iatrogenic E89.40
      asymptomatic E89.40
      symptomatic E89.41
    postprocedural (postablative)
      (postirradiation) (postsurgical) E89.40
      asymptomatic E89.40
      symptomatic E89.41
  ovulation causing infertility N97.0
  polyglandular, autoimmune E31.0
  prosthetic joint implant —*see* Complications,
    joint prosthesis, mechanical, breakdown,
    by site
  renal N19
    with
      tubular necrosis (acute) N17.0
    acute N17.9
      with
        cortical necrosis N17.1
        medullary necrosis N17.2
        tubular necrosis N17.0
      specified NEC N17.8
    chronic N18.9
      hypertensive —*see* Hypertension, kidney
    congenital P96.0
    end stage (chronic) N18.6
      due to hypertension I12.0
    following
      abortion —*see* Abortion by type
        complicated by specified
          condition NEC
      crushing T79.5
      ectopic or molar pregnancy O08.4
      labor and delivery (acute) O90.4
    hypertensive —*see* Hypertension, kidney
    postprocedural N99.0
  respiration, respiratory J96.9
    with
      hypercapnia J96.92
      ►hypercarbia J96.02
      hypoxia J96.91
    acute J96.00
      with
        hypercapnia J96.02
        ►hypercarbia J96.02
        hypoxia J96.01

Failure, failed *(Continued)*
  respiration, respiratory *(Continued)*
    acute and (on) chronic J96.20
      with
        hypercapnia J96.22
        ►hypercarbia J96.22
        hypoxia J96.21
    center G93.89
    chronic J96.10
      with
        hypercapnia J96.12
        ►hypercarbia J96.12
        hypoxia J96.11
    newborn P28.5
    postprocedural (acute) J95.821
      acute and chronic J95.822
  rotation
    cecum Q43.3
    colon Q43.3
    intestine Q43.3
    kidney Q63.2
  sedation (conscious) (moderate) during
    procedure T88.52
    history of Z92.83
  segmentation —*see also* Fusion
    fingers —*see* Syndactylism, complex,
      fingers
    vertebra Q76.49
      with scoliosis Q76.3
  seminiferous tubule, adult E29.1
  senile (general) R54
  sexual arousal (male) F52.21
    female F52.22
  testicular endocrine function E29.1
  to thrive (child over 28 days old) R62.51
    adult R62.7
    newborn P92.6
  transplant T86.92
    bone T86.831
      marrow T86.02
    cornea T86.841
    heart T86.22
      with lung(s) T86.32
    intestine T86.851
    kidney T86.12
    liver T86.42
    lung(s) T86.811
      with heart T86.32
    pancreas T86.891
    skin (allograft) (autograft) T86.821
    specified organ or tissue NEC T86.891
    stem cell (peripheral blood) (umbilical
      cord) T86.5
  trial of labor (with subsequent cesarean
    delivery) O66.40
    following previous cesarean delivery
      O66.41
  tubal ligation N99.89
  urinary —*see* Disease, kidney, chronic
  vacuum extraction NOS (with subsequent
    cesarean delivery) O66.5
  vasectomy N99.89
  ventouse NOS (with subsequent cesarean
    delivery) O66.5
  ventricular —*see also* Failure, heart I50.9
  ➡left —*see also* Failure, heart, left I50.1
    with rheumatic fever (conditions in I00)
      active I01.8
        with chorea I02.0
      inactive or quiescent (with chorea)
        I09.81
      rheumatic (chronic) (inactive) (with
        chorea) I09.81
        active or acute I01.8
          with chorea I02.0
  ➡right —*see* Failure, heart, right
  ➡vital centers, newborn P91.88
Fainting (fit) R55
Fallen arches —*see* Deformity, limb, flat foot
Falling, falls (repeated) R29.6
  any organ or part —*see* Prolapse

Fallopian
  insufflation Z31.41
  tube —*see* condition
Fallot's
  pentalogy Q21.8
  tetrad or tetralogy Q21.3
  triad or trilogy Q22.3
False —*see also* condition
  croup J38.5
  joint —*see* Nonunion, fracture
  labor (pains) O47.9
    at or after 37 completed weeks of gestation
      O47.1
    before 37 completed weeks of gestation
      O47.0- •
  passage, urethra (prostatic) N36.5
  pregnancy F45.8
Family, familial —*see also* condition
  disruption Z63.8
    involving divorce or separation Z63.5
  Li-Fraumeni (syndrome) Z15.01
  planning advice Z30.09
  problem Z63.9
    specified NEC Z63.8
  retinoblastoma C69.2- •
Famine (effects of) T73.0
  edema —*see* Malnutrition, severe
Fanconi (-de Toni)(-Debré) syndrome E72.09
  with cystinosis E72.04
Fanconi's anemia (congenital pancytopenia)
  D61.09
Farber's disease or syndrome E75.29
Farcy A24.0
Farmer's
  lung J67.0
  skin L57.8
Farsightedness —*see* Hypermetropia
Fascia —*see* condition
Fasciculation R25.3
Fasciitis M72.9
  diffuse (eosinophilic) M35.4
  infective M72.8
    necrotizing M72.6
  necrotizing M72.6
  nodular M72.4
  perirenal (with ureteral obstruction) N13.5
    with infection N13.6
  plantar M72.2
  specified NEC M72.8
  traumatic (old) M72.8
    current - code by site under Sprain
Fascioliasis B66.3
Fasciolopsis, fasciolopsiasis (intestinal) B66.5
Fascioscapulohumeral myopathy G71.0
Fast pulse R00.0
Fat
  embolism —*see* Embolism, fat
  excessive —*see also* Obesity
    in heart —*see* Degeneration, myocardial
  in stool R19.5
  localized (pad) E65
    heart —*see* Degeneration, myocardial
    knee M79.4
    retropatellar M79.4
  necrosis
    breast N64.1
    mesentery K65.4
    omentum K65.4
  pad E65
    knee M79.4
Fatigue R53.83
  auditory deafness —*see* Deafness
  chronic R53.82
  combat F43.0
  general R53.83
    psychogenic F48.8
  heat (transient) T67.6
  muscle M62.89
  myocardium —*see* Failure, heart
  neoplasm-related R53.0
  nervous, neurosis F48.8

► New   ➡ Revised   ~~deleted~~ Deleted   • Use Additional Character(s)

Fever (Continued)
  Machupo (virus) hemorrhagic A96.1
  malaria, malarial —see Malaria
  Malta A23.9
  Marseilles A77.1
  marsh —see Malaria
  Mayaro (viral) A92.8
  Mediterranean —see also Brucellosis A23.9
    familial M04.1
    tick A77.1
  meningeal —see Meningitis
  Meuse A79.0
  Mexican A75.2
  mianeh A68.1
  miasmatic —see Malaria
  mosquito-borne (viral) A92.9
    hemorrhagic A92.8
  mountain —see also Brucellosis
    meaning Rocky Mountain spotted fever
      A77.0
    tick (American) (Colorado) (viral) A93.2
  Mucambo (viral) A92.8
  mud A27.9
  Neapolitan —see Brucellosis
  neutropenic D70.9
  newborn P81.9
    environmental P81.0
  Nine-Mile A78
  non-exanthematous tick A93.2
  North Asian tick-borne A77.2
  Omsk hemorrhagic A98.1
  O'nyong-nyong (viral) A92.1
  Oropouche (viral) A93.0
  Oroya A44.0
  paludal —see Malaria
  Panama (malarial) B50.9
  Pappataci A93.1
  paratyphoid A01.4
    A A01.1
    B A01.2
    C A01.3
  parrot A70
  periodic (Mediterranean) M04.1
  persistent (of unknown origin) R50.9
  petechial A39.0
  pharyngoconjunctival B30.2
  Philippine hemorrhagic A91
  phlebotomus A93.1
  Piry (virus) A93.8
  Pixuna (viral) A92.8
  Plasmodium ovale B53.0
  polioviral (nonparalytic) A80.4
  Pontiac A48.2
  postimmunization R50.83
  postoperative R50.82
  ➡due to infection T81.4
  posttransfusion R50.84
  postvaccination R50.83
  presenting with conditions classified
    elsewhere R50.81
  pretibial A27.89
  puerperal O86.4
  Q A78
  quadrilateral A78
  quartan (malaria) B52.9
  Queensland (coastal) (tick) A77.3
  quintan A79.0
  rabbit —see Tularemia
  rat-bite A25.9
    due to
      Spirillum A25.0
      Streptobacillus moniliformis A25.1
  recurrent —see Fever, relapsing
  relapsing (Borrelia) A68.9
    Carter's (Asiatic) A68.1
    Dutton's (West African) A68.1
    Koch's A68.9
    louse-borne A68.0
    Novy's
      louse-borne A68.0
      tick-borne A68.1

Fever (Continued)
  relapsing (Borrelia) (Continued)
    Obermeyer's (European) A68.0
    tick-borne A68.1
  remittent (bilious) (congestive) (gastric) —see
    Malaria
  rheumatic (active) (acute) (chronic) (subacute)
    I00
    with central nervous system involvement
      I02.9
    active with heart involvement —see
      category I01
    inactive or quiescent with
      cardiac hypertrophy I09.89
      carditis I09.9
      endocarditis I09.1
        aortic (valve) I06.9
          with mitral (valve) disease I08.0
        mitral (valve) I05.9
          with aortic (valve) disease I08.0
        pulmonary (valve) I09.89
        tricuspid (valve) I07.8
      heart disease NEC I09.89
      ➡heart failure (congestive) (conditions in
        I50.) I09.81
      ➡left ventricular failure (conditions in
        I50.- I50.4-) I09.81
      myocarditis, myocardial degeneration
        (conditions in I51.4) I09.0
      pancarditis I09.9
      pericarditis I09.2
  Rift Valley (viral) A92.4
  Rocky Mountain spotted A77.0
  rose J30.1
  Ross River B33.1
  Russian hemorrhagic A98.5
  San Joaquin (Valley) B38.0
  sandfly A93.1
  Sao Paulo A77.0
  scarlet A38.9
  seven day (leptospirosis) (autumnal)
    (Japanese) A27.89
    dengue A90
  shin-bone A79.0
  Singapore hemorrhagic A91
  solar A90
  Songo A98.5
  sore B00.1
  South African tick-bite A68.1
  Southeast Asia hemorrhagic A91
  spinal —see Meningitis
  spirillary A25.0
  splenic —see Anthrax
  spotted A77.9
    American A77.0
    Brazilian A77.0
    cerebrospinal meningitis A39.0
    Colombian A77.0
    due to Rickettsia
      australis A77.3
      conorii A77.1
      rickettsii A77.0
      sibirica A77.2
      specified type NEC A77.8
    Ehrlichiosis A77.40
      due to
        E. chafeensis A77.41
        specified organism NEC A77.49
    Rocky Mountain A77.0
  steroid R50.2
  streptobacillary A25.1
  subtertian B50.9
  Sumatran mite A75.3
  sun A90
  swamp A27.9
  swine A02.8
  sylvatic, yellow A95.0
  Tahyna B33.8
  tertian —see Malaria, tertian
  Thailand hemorrhagic A91
  thermic T67.0

Fever (Continued)
  three-day A93.1
  tick
    American mountain A93.2
    Colorado A93.2
    Kemerovo A93.8
    Mediterranean A77.1
    mountain A93.2
    nonexanthematous A93.2
    Quaranfil A93.8
  tick-bite NEC A93.8
  tick-borne (hemorrhagic) NEC A93.8
  trench A79.0
  tsutsugamushi A75.3
  typhogastric A01.00
  typhoid (abortive) (hemorrhagic)
    (intermittent) (malignant) A01.00
    complicated by
      arthritis A01.04
      heart involvement A01.02
      meningitis A01.01
      osteomyelitis A01.05
      pneumonia A01.03
      specified NEC A01.09
  typhomalarial —see Malaria
  typhus —see Typhus (fever)
  undulant —see Brucellosis
  unknown origin R50.9
  uveoparotid D86.89
  valley B38.0
  Venezuelan equine A92.2
  vesicular stomatitis A93.8
  viral hemorrhagic —see Fever, hemorrhagic,
    by type of virus
  Volhynian A79.0
  Wesselsbron (viral) A92.8
  West
    African B50.8
    Nile (viral) A92.30
      with
        complications NEC A92.39
        cranial nerve disorders A92.32
        encephalitis A92.31
        encephalomyelitis A92.31
        neurologic manifestation NEC
          A92.32
        optic neuritis A92.32
        polyradiculitis A92.32
  Whitmore's —see Melioidosis
  Wolhynian A79.0
  worm B83.9
  yellow A95.9
    jungle A95.0
    sylvatic A95.0
    urban A95.1
  Zika virus A92.5
Fibrillation
  atrial or auricular (established) I48.91
    chronic I48.2
    paroxysmal I48.0
    permanent I48.2
    persistent I48.1
  cardiac I49.8
  heart I49.8
  muscular M62.89
  ventricular I49.01
Fibrin
  ball or bodies, pleural (sac) J94.1
  chamber, anterior (eye) (gelatinous
    exudate) —see Iridocyclitis, acute
Fibrinogenolysis —see Fibrinolysis
Fibrinogenopenia D68.8
  acquired D65
  congenital D68.2
Fibrinolysis (hemorrhagic) (acquired) D65
  antepartum hemorrhage —see Hemorrhage,
    antepartum, with coagulation defect
  following
    abortion —see Abortion by type
      complicated by hemorrhage
    ectopic or molar pregnancy O08.1

▶ New   ⟹ Revised   ~~deleted~~ Deleted   ● Use Additional Character(s)

Fibrinolysis *(Continued)*
  intrapartum O67.0
  newborn, transient P60
  postpartum O72.3
Fibrinopenia (hereditary) D68.2
  acquired D68.4
Fibrinopurulent —*see* condition
Fibrinous —*see* condition
Fibroadenoma
  cellular intracanalicular D24-●
  giant D24-●
  intracanalicular
    cellular D24-●
    giant D24-●
    specified site —*see* Neoplasm, benign, by
      site
    unspecified site D24-●
  juvenile D24-●
  pericanalicular
    specified site —*see* Neoplasm, benign, by
      site
    unspecified site D24-●
  phyllodes D24-●
  prostate D29.1
  specified site NEC —*see* Neoplasm, benign,
    by site
  unspecified site D24-●
Fibroadenosis, breast (chronic) (cystic) (diffuse)
    (periodic) (segmental) N60.2-●
Fibroangioma —*see also* Neoplasm, benign, by
    site
  juvenile
    specified site —*see* Neoplasm, benign, by
      site
    unspecified site D10.6
Fibrochondrosarcoma —*see* Neoplasm,
    cartilage, malignant
Fibrocystic
  disease —*see also* Fibrosis, cystic
    breast —*see* Mastopathy, cystic
    jaw M27.49
    kidney (congenital) Q61.8
    liver Q44.6
    pancreas E84.9
  kidney (congenital) Q61.8
Fibrodysplasia ossificans progressiva —*see*
    Myositis, ossificans, progressiva
Fibroelastosis (cordis) (endocardial)
    (endomyocardial) I42.4
Fibroid (tumor) —*see also* Neoplasm, connective
    tissue, benign
  disease, lung (chronic) —*see* Fibrosis, lung
  heart (disease) —*see* Myocarditis
  in pregnancy or childbirth O34.1-●
    causing obstructed labor O65.5
  induration, lung (chronic) —*see* Fibrosis, lung
  lung —*see* Fibrosis, lung
  pneumonia (chronic) —*see* Fibrosis, lung
  uterus —*see also* Leiomyoma, uterus D25.9
Fibrolipoma —*see* Lipoma
Fibroliposarcoma —*see* Neoplasm, connective
    tissue, malignant
Fibroma —*see also* Neoplasm, connective tissue,
    benign
  ameloblastic —*see* Cyst, calcifying
    odontogenic
  bone (nonossifying) —*see* Disorder, bone,
    specified type NEC
    ossifying —*see* Neoplasm, bone, benign
  cementifying —*see* Neoplasm, bone, benign
  chondromyxoid —*see* Neoplasm, bone,
    benign
  desmoplastic —*see* Neoplasm, connective
    tissue, uncertain behavior
  durum —*see* Neoplasm, connective tissue,
    benign
  fascial —*see* Neoplasm, connective tissue,
    benign
  invasive —*see* Neoplasm, connective tissue,
    uncertain behavior
  molle —*see* Lipoma

Fibroma *(Continued)*
  myxoid —*see* Neoplasm, connective tissue,
    benign
  nasopharynx, nasopharyngeal (juvenile)
    D10.6
  nonosteogenic (nonossifying) —*see* Dysplasia,
    fibrous
  odontogenic (central) —*see* Cyst, calcifying
    odontogenic
  ossifying —*see* Neoplasm, bone, benign
  periosteal —*see* Neoplasm, bone, benign
  soft —*see* Lipoma
Fibromatosis M72.9
  abdominal —*see* Neoplasm, connective tissue,
    uncertain behavior
  aggressive —*see* Neoplasm, connective tissue,
    uncertain behavior
  congenital generalized —*see* Neoplasm,
    connective tissue, uncertain behavior
  Dupuytren's M72.0
  gingival K06.1
  palmar (fascial) M72.0
  plantar (fascial) M72.2
  pseudosarcomatous (proliferative)
    (subcutaneous) M72.4
  retroperitoneal D48.3
  specified NEC M72.8
Fibromyalgia M79.7
Fibromyoma —*see also* Neoplasm, connective
    tissue, benign
  uterus (corpus) —*see also* Leiomyoma, uterus
    in pregnancy or childbirth —*see* Fibroid, in
      pregnancy or childbirth
    causing obstructed labor O65.5
Fibromyositis M79.7
Fibromyxolipoma D17.9
Fibromyxoma —*see* Neoplasm, connective
    tissue, benign
Fibromyxosarcoma —*see* Neoplasm, connective
    tissue, malignant
Fibro-odontoma, ameloblastic —*see* Cyst,
    calcifying odontogenic
Fibro-osteoma —*see* Neoplasm, bone, benign
Fibroplasia, retrolental H35.17
Fibropurulent —*see* condition
Fibrosarcoma —*see also* Neoplasm, connective
    tissue, malignant
  ameloblastic C41.1
    upper jaw (bone) C41.0
  congenital —*see* Neoplasm, connective tissue,
    malignant
  fascial —*see* Neoplasm, connective tissue,
    malignant
  infantile —*see* Neoplasm, connective tissue,
    malignant
  odontogenic C41.1
    upper jaw (bone) C41.0
  periosteal —*see* Neoplasm, bone, malignant
Fibrosclerosis
  breast N60.3-●
  multifocal M35.5
  penis (corpora cavernosa) N48.6
Fibrosis, fibrotic
  adrenal (gland) E27.8
  amnion O41.8X-●
  anal papillae K62.89
  arteriocapillary —*see* Arteriosclerosis
  bladder N32.89
    interstitial —*see* Cystitis, chronic,
      interstitial
    localized submucosal —*see* Cystitis,
      chronic, interstitial
    panmural —*see* Cystitis, chronic, interstitial
  breast —*see* Fibrosclerosis, breast
  capillary —*see also* Arteriosclerosis I70.90
    lung (chronic) —*see* Fibrosis, lung
  cardiac —*see* Myocarditis
  cervix N88.8
  chorion O41.8X-●
  corpus cavernosum (sclerosing) N48.6
  cystic (of pancreas) E84.9

Fibrosis, fibrotic *(Continued)*
  cystic *(Continued)*
    with
      distal intestinal obstruction syndrome
        E84.19
      fecal impaction E84.19
      intestinal manifestations NEC E84.19
      pulmonary manifestations E84.0
      specified manifestations NEC E84.8
  due to device, implant or graft —*see also*
    Complications, by site and type,
      specified NEC T85.828
    arterial graft NEC T82.828
    breast (implant) T85.828
    catheter NEC T85.828
      dialysis (renal) T82.828
        intraperitoneal T85.828
      infusion NEC T82.828
        spinal (epidural) (subdural)
          T85.820
      urinary (indwelling) T83.82
    electronic (electrode) (pulse generator)
      (stimulator)
        bone T84.82
        cardiac T82.827
        nervous system (brain) (peripheral
          nerve) (spinal) T85.820
        urinary T83.82
    fixation, internal (orthopedic) NEC T84.82
    gastrointestinal (bile duct) (esophagus)
      T85.828
    genital NEC T83.82
    heart NEC T82.827
    joint prosthesis T84.82
    ocular (corneal graft) (orbital implant)
      NEC T85.828
    orthopedic NEC T84.82
    specified NEC T85.828
    urinary NEC T83.82
    vascular NEC T82.828
    ventricular intracranial shunt T85.820
  ejaculatory duct N50.89
  endocardium —*see* Endocarditis
  endomyocardial (tropical) I42.3
  epididymis N50.89
  eye muscle —*see* Strabismus, mechanical
  heart —*see* Myocarditis
  hepatic —*see* Fibrosis, liver
  hepatolienal (portal hypertension) K76.6
  hepatosplenic (portal hypertension) K76.6
  infrapatellar fat pad M79.4
  intrascrotal N50.89
  kidney N26.9
  liver K74.0
    with sclerosis K74.2
    alcoholic K70.2
  lung (atrophic) (chronic) (confluent)
    (massive) (perialveolar) (peribronchial)
    J84.10
    with
      anthracosilicosis J60
      anthracosis J60
      asbestosis J61
      bagassosis J67.1
      bauxite J63.1
      berylliosis J63.2
      byssinosis J66.0
      calcicosis J62.8
      chalicosis J62.8
      dust reticulation J64
      farmer's lung J67.0
      ganister disease J62.8
      graphite J63.3
      pneumoconiosis NOS J64
      siderosis J63.4
      silicosis J62.8
    capillary J84.10
    congenital P27.8
    diffuse (idiopathic) J84.10
      chemicals, gases, fumes or vapors
        (inhalation) J68.4

Fibrosis, fibrotic *(Continued)*
  lung *(Continued)*
    diffuse *(Continued)*
      interstitial J84.10
        acute J84.114
        talc J62.0
      following radiation J70.1
      idiopathic J84.112
      postinflammatory J84.10
      silicotic J62.8
      tuberculous —*see* Tuberculosis, pulmonary
  lymphatic gland I89.8
  median bar —*see* Hyperplasia, prostate
  mediastinum (idiopathic) J98.59
  meninges G96.19
  myocardium, myocardial —*see* Myocarditis
  ovary N83.8
  oviduct N83.8
  pancreas K86.89
  penis NEC N48.6
  pericardium I31.0
  perineum, in pregnancy or childbirth O34.7-●
    causing obstructed labor O65.5
  pleura J94.1
  popliteal fat pad M79.4
  prostate (chronic) —*see* Hyperplasia,
    prostate
  pulmonary —*see also* Fibrosis, lung J84.10
    congenital P27.8
    idiopathic J84.112
  rectal sphincter K62.89
  retroperitoneal, idiopathic (with ureteral
    obstruction) N13.5
    with infection N13.6
  sclerosing mesenteric (idiopathic) K65.4
  scrotum N50.89
  seminal vesicle N50.89
  senile R54
  skin L90.5
  spermatic cord N50.89
  spleen D73.89
    in schistosomiasis (bilharziasis) B65.9
      [D77]
  subepidermal nodular —*see* Neoplasm, skin,
    benign
  submucous (oral) (tongue) K13.5
  testis N44.8
    chronic, due to syphilis A52.76
  thymus (gland) E32.8
  tongue, submucous K13.5
  tunica vaginalis N50.89
  uterus (non-neoplastic) N85.8
  vagina N89.8
  valve, heart —*see* Endocarditis
  vas deferens N50.89
  vein I87.8
Fibrositis (periarticular) M79.7
  nodular, chronic (Jaccoud's) (rheumatoid) —
    see Arthropathy, postrheumatic, chronic
Fibrothorax J94.1
Fibrotic —*see* Fibrosis
Fibrous —*see* condition
Fibroxanthoma —*see also* Neoplasm, connective
  tissue, benign
  atypical —*see* Neoplasm, connective tissue,
    uncertain behavior
  malignant —*see* Neoplasm, connective tissue,
    malignant
Fibroxanthosarcoma —*see* Neoplasm,
  connective tissue, malignant
Fiedler's
  disease (icterohemorrhagic leptospirosis)
    A27.0
  myocarditis (acute) I40.1
Fifth disease B08.3
  venereal A55
Filaria, filarial, filariasis —*see* Infestation,
  filarial
Filatov's disease —*see* Mononucleosis,
  infectious
File-cutter's disease —*see* Poisoning, lead

Filling defect
  biliary tract R93.2
  bladder R93.41
  duodenum R93.3
  gallbladder R93.2
  gastrointestinal tract R93.3
  intestine R93.3
  kidney R93.42-●
  stomach R93.3
  ureter R93.41
  urinary organs, specified NEC R93.49
Fimbrial cyst Q50.4
Financial problem affecting care NOS Z59.9
  bankruptcy Z59.8
  foreclosure on loan Z59.8
Findings, abnormal, inconclusive, without
  diagnosis —*see also* Abnormal
  17-ketosteroids, elevated R82.5
  acetonuria R82.4
  alcohol in blood R78.0
  anisocytosis R71.8
  antenatal screening of mother O28.9
    biochemical O28.1
    chromosomal O28.5
    cytological O28.2
    genetic O28.5
    hematological O28.0
    radiological O28.4
    specified NEC O28.8
    ultrasonic O28.3
  antibody titer, elevated R76.0
  anticardiolipin antibody R76.0
  antiphosphatidylglycerol antibody R76.0
  antiphosphatidylinositol antibody R76.0
  antiphosphatidylserine antibody R76.0
  antiphospholipid antibody R76.0
  bacteriuria R82.71
  bicarbonate E87.8
  bile in urine R82.2
  blood sugar R73.09
    high R73.9
    low (transient) E16.2
  body fluid or substance, specified NEC R88.8
  casts, urine R82.99
  catecholamines R82.5
  cells, urine R82.99
  chloride E87.8
  cholesterol E78.9
    high E78.00
      with high triglycerides E78.2
  chyluria R82.0
  cloudy
    dialysis effluent R88.0
    urine R82.90
  creatinine clearance R94.4
  crystals, urine R82.99
  culture
    blood R78.81
    positive —*see* Positive, culture
  echocardiogram R93.1
  electrolyte level, urinary R82.99
  function study NEC R94.8
    bladder R94.8
    endocrine NEC R94.7
      thyroid R94.6
    kidney R94.4
    liver R94.5
    pancreas R94.8
    placenta R94.8
    pulmonary R94.2
    spleen R94.8
  gallbladder, nonvisualization R93.2
  glucose (tolerance test) (non-fasting)
    R73.09
  glycosuria R81
  heart
    shadow R93.1
    sounds R01.2
  hematinuria R82.3
  hematocrit drop (precipitous) R71.0
  hemoglobinuria R82.3

Findings, abnormal, inconclusive, without
  diagnosis *(Continued)*
  human papillomavirus (HPV) DNA test
    positive
    cervix
      high risk R87.810
      low risk R87.820
    vagina
      high risk R87.811
      low risk R87.821
  in blood (of substance not normally found in
    blood) R78.9
    addictive drug NEC R78.4
    alcohol (excessive level) R78.0
    cocaine R78.2
    hallucinogen R78.3
    heavy metals (abnormal level) R78.79
    lead R78.71
    lithium (abnormal level) R78.89
    opiate drug R78.1
    psychotropic drug R78.5
    specified substance NEC R78.89
    steroid agent R78.6
  indoleacetic acid, elevated R82.5
  ketonuria R82.4
  lactic acid dehydrogenase (LDH) R74.0
  liver function test R79.89
  mammogram NEC R92.8
    calcification (calculus) R92.1
    inconclusive result (due to dense breasts)
      R92.2
    microcalcification R92.0
  mediastinal shift R93.8
  melanin, urine R82.99
  myoglobinuria R82.1
  neonatal screening P09
  nonvisualization of gallbladder R93.2
  odor of urine NOS R82.90
  Papanicolaou cervix R87.619
    non-atypical endometrial cells R87.618
  pneumoencephalogram R93.0
  poikilocytosis R71.8
  potassium (deficiency) E87.6
    excess E87.5
  PPD R76.11
  radiologic (X-ray) R93.8
    abdomen R93.5
    biliary tract R93.2
    breast R92.8
    gastrointestinal tract R93.3
    genitourinary organs R93.8
    head R93.0
    inconclusive due to excess body fat of
      patient R93.9
    intrathoracic organs NEC R93.1
    placenta R93.8
    retroperitoneum R93.5
    skin R93.8
    skull R93.0
    subcutaneous tissue R93.8
  red blood cell (count) (morphology) (sickling)
    (volume) R71.8
  scan NEC R94.8
    bladder R94.8
    bone R94.8
    kidney R94.4
    liver R93.2
    lung R94.2
    pancreas R94.8
    placental R94.8
    spleen R94.8
    thyroid R94.6
  sedimentation rate, elevated R70.0
  SGOT R74.0
  SGPT R74.0
  sodium (deficiency) E87.1
    excess E87.0
  specified body fluid NEC R88.8
  stress test R94.39
  thyroid (function) (metabolic rate) (scan)
    (uptake) R94.6

Findings, abnormal, inconclusive, without diagnosis *(Continued)*
transaminase (level) R74.0
triglycerides E78.9
high E78.1
with high cholesterol E78.2
tuberculin skin test (without active tuberculosis) R76.11
urine R82.90
acetone R82.4
bacteria R82.71
bile R82.2
casts or cells R82.99
chyle R82.0
culture positive R82.79
glucose R81
hemoglobin R82.3
ketone R82.4
sugar R81
vanillylmandelic acid (VMA), elevated R82.5
vectorcardiogram (VCG) R94.39
ventriculogram R93.0
white blood cell (count) (differential) (morphology) D72.9
xerography R92.8
Finger —*see* condition
Fire, Saint Anthony's —*see* Erysipelas
Fire-setting
pathological (compulsive) F63.1
Fish hook stomach K31.89
Fishmeal-worker's lung J67.8
Fissure, fissured
anus, anal K60.2
acute K60.0
chronic K60.1
congenital Q43.8
ear, lobule, congenital Q17.8
epiglottis (congenital) Q31.8
larynx J38.7
congenital Q31.8
lip K13.0
congenital —*see* Cleft, lip
nipple N64.0
associated with
lactation O92.13
pregnancy O92.11-●
puerperium O92.12
nose Q30.2
palate (congenital) —*see* Cleft, palate
skin R23.4
spine (congenital) —*see also* Spina bifida
with hydrocephalus —*see* Spina bifida, by site, with hydrocephalus
tongue (acquired) K14.5
congenital Q38.3
Fistula (cutaneous) L98.8
abdomen (wall) K63.2
bladder N32.2
intestine NEC K63.2
ureter N28.89
uterus N82.5
abdominorectal K63.2
abdominosigmoidal K63.2
abdominothoracic J86.0
abdominouterine N82.5
congenital Q51.7
abdominovesical N32.2
accessory sinuses —*see* Sinusitis
actinomycotic —*see* Actinomycosis
alveolar antrum —*see* Sinusitis, maxillary
alveolar process K04.6
anorectal K60.5
antrobuccal —*see* Sinusitis, maxillary
antrum —*see* Sinusitis, maxillary
anus, anal (recurrent) (infectional) K60.3
congenital Q43.6
with absence, atresia and stenosis Q42.2
tuberculous A18.32
aorta-duodenal I77.2
appendix, appendicular K38.3

Fistula *(Continued)*
arteriovenous (acquired) (nonruptured) I77.0
brain I67.1
congenital Q28.2
ruptured I60.8
ruptured I60.8
cerebral —*see* Fistula, arteriovenous, brain
congenital (peripheral) —*see also* Malformation, arteriovenous
brain Q28.2
ruptured I60.8
coronary Q24.5
pulmonary Q25.72
coronary I25.41
congenital Q24.5
pulmonary I28.0
congenital Q25.72
surgically created (for dialysis) Z99.2
complication —*see* Complication, arteriovenous, fistula, surgically created
traumatic —*see* Injury, blood vessel
artery I77.2
aural (mastoid) —*see* Mastoiditis, chronic
auricle —*see also* Disorder, pinna, specified type NEC
congenital Q18.1
Bartholin's gland N82.8
bile duct (common) (hepatic) K83.3
with calculus, stones —*see* Calculus, bile duct
biliary (tract) —*see* Fistula, bile duct
bladder (sphincter) NEC —*see also* Fistula, vesico- N32.2
into seminal vesicle N32.2
bone —*see also* Disorder, bone, specified type NEC
with osteomyelitis, chronic —*see* Osteomyelitis, chronic, with draining sinus
brain G93.89
arteriovenous (acquired) I67.1
congenital Q28.2
branchial (cleft) Q18.0
branchiogenous Q18.0
breast N61.0
puerperal, postpartum or gestational, due to mastitis (purulent) —*see* Mastitis, obstetric, purulent
bronchial J86.0
bronchocutaneous, bronchomediastinal, bronchopleural, bronchopleuromediastinal (infective) J86.0
tuberculous NEC A15.5
bronchoesophageal J86.0
congenital Q39.2
with atresia of esophagus Q39.1
bronchovisceral J86.0
buccal cavity (infective) K12.2
cecosigmoidal K63.2
cecum K63.2
cerebrospinal (fluid) G96.0
cervical, lateral Q18.1
cervicoaural Q18.1
cervicosigmoidal N82.4
cervicovesical N82.1
cervix N82.8
chest (wall) J86.0
cholecystenteric —*see* Fistula, gallbladder
cholecystocolic —*see* Fistula, gallbladder
cholecystocolonic —*see* Fistula, gallbladder
cholecystoduodenal —*see* Fistula, gallbladder
cholecystogastric —*see* Fistula, gallbladder
cholecystointestinal —*see* Fistula, gallbladder
choledochoduodenal —*see* Fistula, bile duct
cholocolic K82.3
coccyx —*see* Sinus, pilonidal
colon K63.2
colostomy K94.09
common duct —*see* Fistula, bile duct

Fistula *(Continued)*
congenital, site not listed —*see* Anomaly, by site
coronary, arteriovenous I25.41
congenital Q24.5
costal region J86.0
cul-de-sac, Douglas' N82.8
cystic duct —*see also* Fistula, gallbladder
congenital Q44.5
dental K04.6
diaphragm J86.0
duodenum K31.6
ear (external) (canal) —*see* Disorder, ear, external, specified type NEC
enterocolic K63.2
enterocutaneous K63.2
enterouterine N82.4
congenital Q51.7
enterovaginal N82.4
congenital Q52.2
large intestine N82.3
small intestine N82.2
enterovesical N32.1
epididymis N50.89
tuberculous A18.15
esophagobronchial J86.0
congenital Q39.2
with atresia of esophagus Q39.1
esophagocutaneous K22.8
esophagopleural-cutaneous J86.0
esophagotracheal J86.0
congenital Q39.2
with atresia of esophagus Q39.1
esophagus K22.8
congenital Q39.2
with atresia of esophagus Q39.1
ethmoid —*see* Sinusitis, ethmoidal
eyeball (cornea) (sclera) —*see* Disorder, globe, hypotony
eyelid H01.8
fallopian tube, external N82.5
fecal K63.2
congenital Q43.6
from periapical abscess K04.6
frontal sinus —*see* Sinusitis, frontal
gallbladder K82.3
with calculus, cholelithiasis, stones —*see* Calculus, gallbladder
gastric K31.6
gastrocolic K31.6
congenital Q40.2
tuberculous A18.32
gastroenterocolic K31.6
gastroesophageal K31.6
gastrojejunal K31.6
gastrojejunocolic K31.6
genital tract (female) N82.9
specified NEC N82.8
to intestine NEC N82.4
to skin N82.5
hepatic artery-portal vein, congenital Q26.6
hepatopleural J86.0
hepatopulmonary J86.0
ileorectal or ileosigmoidal K63.2
ileovaginal N82.2
ileovesical N32.1
ileum K63.2
in ano K60.3
tuberculous A18.32
inner ear (labyrinth) —*see* subcategory H83.1
intestine NEC K63.2
intestinocolonic (abdominal) K63.2
intestinoureteral N28.89
intestinouterine N82.4
intestinovaginal N82.4
large intestine N82.3
small intestine N82.2
intestinovesical N32.1
ischiorectal (fossa) K61.3
jejunum K63.2

Fistula *(Continued)*
  joint M25.1Ø
    ankle M25.17-●
    elbow M25.12-●
    foot joint M25.17-●
    hand joint M25.14-●
    hip M25.15-●
    knee M25.16-●
    shoulder M25.11-●
    specified joint NEC M25.18
    tuberculous —*see* Tuberculosis, joint
    vertebrae M25.18
    wrist M25.13-●
  kidney N28.89
  labium (majus) (minus) N82.8
  labyrinth —*see* subcategory H83.1
  lacrimal (gland) (sac) H04.61-●
  lacrimonasal duct —*see* Fistula, lacrimal
  laryngotracheal, congenital Q34.8
  larynx J38.7
  lip K13.Ø
    congenital Q38.Ø
  lumbar, tuberculous A18.Ø1
  lung J86.Ø
  lymphatic I89.8
  mammary (gland) N61.Ø
  mastoid (process) (region) —*see* Mastoiditis,
    chronic
  maxillary J32.Ø
  medial, face and neck Q18.8
  mediastinal J86.Ø
  mediastinobronchial J86.Ø
  mediastinocutaneous J86.Ø
  middle ear —*see* subcategory H74.8
  mouth K12.2
  nasal J34.89
    sinus —*see* Sinusitis
  nasopharynx J39.2
  nipple N64.Ø
  nose J34.89
  oral (cutaneous) K12.2
    maxillary J32.Ø
    nasal (with cleft palate) —*see* Cleft, palate
  orbit, orbital —*see* Disorder, orbit, specified
    type NEC
  oroantral J32.Ø
  oviduct, external N82.5
  palate (hard) M27.8
  pancreatic K86.89
  pancreaticoduodenal K86.89
  parotid (gland) K11.4
    region K12.2
  penis N48.89
  perianal K60.3
  pericardium (pleura) (sac) —*see* Pericarditis
  pericecal K63.2
  perineorectal K6Ø.4 perineosigmoidal K63.2
  perineosigmoidal K63.2
  perineum, perineal (with urethral
    involvement) NEC N36.Ø
    tuberculous A18.13
    ureter N28.89
  perirectal K6Ø.4
    tuberculous A18.32
  peritoneum K65.9
  pharyngoesophageal J39.2
  pharynx J39.2
    branchial cleft (congenital) Q18.Ø
  pilonidal (infected) (rectum) —*see* Sinus,
    pilonidal
  pleura, pleural, pleurocutaneous,
    pleuroperitoneal J86.Ø
    tuberculous NEC A15.6
  pleuropericardial I31.8
  portal vein-hepatic artery, congenital
    Q26.6
  postauricular H7Ø.81-●
  postoperative, persistent T81.83
    specified site —*see* Fistula, by site
  preauricular (congenital) Q18.1
  prostate N42.89

Fistula *(Continued)*
  pulmonary J86.Ø
    arteriovenous I28.Ø
      congenital Q25.72
    tuberculous —*see* Tuberculosis, pulmonary
  pulmonoperitoneal J86.Ø
  rectolabial N82.4
  rectosigmoid (intercommunicating) K63.2
  rectoureteral N28.89
  rectourethral N36.Ø
    congenital Q64.73
  rectouterine N82.4
    congenital Q51.7
  rectovaginal N82.3
    congenital Q52.2
    tuberculous A18.18
  rectovesical N32.1
    congenital Q64.79
  rectovesicovaginal N82.3
  rectovulval N82.4
    congenital Q52.79
  rectum (to skin) K6Ø.4
    congenital Q43.6
      with absence, atresia and stenosis Q42.Ø
    tuberculous A18.32
  renal N28.89
  retroauricular —*see* Fistula, postauricular
  salivary duct or gland (any) K11.4
    congenital Q38.4
  scrotum (urinary) N5Ø.89
    tuberculous A18.15
  semicircular canals —*see* subcategory H83.1
  sigmoid K63.2
    to bladder N32.1
  sinus —*see* Sinusitis
  skin L98.8
    to genital tract (female) N82.5
  splenocolic D73.89
  stercoral K63.2
  stomach K31.6
  sublingual gland K11.4
  submandibular gland K11.4
  submaxillary (gland) K11.4
    region K12.2
  thoracic J86.Ø
    duct I89.8
  thoracoabdominal J86.Ø
  thoracogastric J86.Ø
  thoracointestinal J86.Ø
  thorax J86.Ø
  thyroglossal duct Q89.2
  thyroid EØ7.89
  trachea, congenital (external) (internal) Q32.1
  tracheoesophageal J86.Ø
    congenital Q39.2
      with atresia of esophagus Q39.1
    following tracheostomy J95.04
  traumatic arteriovenous —*see* Injury, blood
    vessel, by site
  tuberculous - code by site under Tuberculosis
  typhoid AØ1.Ø9
  umbilicourinary Q64.8
  urachus, congenital Q64.4
  ureter (persistent) N28.89
  ureteroabdominal N28.89
  ureterorectal N28.89
  ureterosigmoido-abdominal N28.89
  ureterovaginal N82.1
  ureterovesical N32.2
  urethra N36.Ø
    congenital Q64.79
    tuberculous A18.13
  urethroperineal N36.Ø
  urethroperineovesical N32.2
  urethrorectal N36.Ø
    congenital Q64.73
  urethroscrotal N5Ø.89
  urethrovaginal N82.1
  urethrovesical N32.2
  urinary (tract) (persistent) (recurrent)
    N36.Ø

Fistula *(Continued)*
  uteroabdominal N82.5
    congenital Q51.7
  uteroenteric, uterointestinal N82.4
    congenital Q51.7
  uterorectal N82.4
    congenital Q51.7
  uteroureteric N82.1
  uterourethral Q51.7
  uterovaginal N82.8
  uterovesical N82.1
    congenital Q51.7
  uterus N82.8
  vagina (postpartal) (wall) N82.8
  vaginocutaneous (postpartal) N82.5
  vaginointestinal NEC N82.4
    large intestine N82.3
    small intestine N82.2
  vaginoperineal N82.5
  vasocutaneous, congenital Q55.7
  vesical NEC N32.2
  vesicoabdominal N32.2
  vesicocervicovaginal N82.1
  vesicocolic N32.1
  vesicocutaneous N32.2
  vesicoenteric N32.1
  vesicointestinal N32.1
  vesicometrorectal N82.4
  vesicoperineal N32.2
  vesicorectal N32.1
    congenital Q64.79
  vesicosigmoidal N32.1
  vesicosigmoidovaginal N82.3
  vesicoureteral N32.2
  vesicoureterovaginal N82.1
  vesicourethral N32.2
  vesicourethrorectal N32.1
  vesicouterine N82.1
    congenital Q51.7
  vesicovaginal N82.Ø
  vulvorectal N82.4
    congenital Q52.79
Fit R56.9
  epileptic —*see* Epilepsy
  fainting R55
  hysterical F44.5
  newborn P9Ø
Fitting (and adjustment) (of)
  artificial
    arm —*see* Admission, adjustment, artificial,
      arm
    breast Z44.3
    eye Z44.2
    leg —*see* Admission, adjustment, artificial,
      leg
  automatic implantable cardiac defibrillator
    (with synchronous cardiac pacemaker)
    Z45.Ø2
  brain neuropacemaker Z46.2
    implanted Z45.42
  cardiac defibrillator —*see* Fitting (and
    adjustment) (of), automatic implantable
    cardiac defibrillator
  catheter, non-vascular Z46.82
  colostomy belt Z46.89
  contact lenses Z46.Ø
  CRT-D (resynchronization therapy
    defibrillator) Z45.Ø2
  CRT-P (cardiac resynchronization therapy
    pacemaker) Z45.Ø18
    pulse generator Z45.Ø1Ø
  cystostomy device Z46.6
  defibrillator, cardiac —*see* Fitting (and
    adjustment) (of), automatic implantable
    cardiac defibrillator
  dentures Z46.3
  device NOS Z46.9
    abdominal Z46.89
    gastrointestinal NEC Z46.59
    implanted NEC Z45.89
    nervous system Z46.2
      implanted —*see* Admission, adjustment,
        device, implanted, nervous system

Fitting *(Continued)*
  device NOS *(Continued)*
    orthodontic Z46.4
    orthoptic Z46.0
    orthotic Z46.89
    prosthetic (external) Z44.9
      breast Z44.3
      dental Z46.3
      eye Z44.2
      specified NEC Z44.8
    specified NEC Z46.89
    substitution
      auditory Z46.2
        implanted —*see* Admission,
          adjustment, device, implanted,
          hearing device
      nervous system Z46.2
        implanted —*see* Admission,
          adjustment, device, implanted,
          nervous system
      visual Z46.2
        implanted Z45.31
    urinary Z46.6
  gastric lap band Z46.51
  gastrointestinal appliance NEC Z46.59
  glasses (reading) Z46.0
  hearing aid Z46.1
  ileostomy device Z46.89
  insulin pump Z46.81
  intestinal appliance NEC Z46.89
  myringotomy device (stent) (tube) Z45.82
  neuropacemaker Z46.2
    implanted Z45.42
  non-vascular catheter Z46.82
  orthodontic device Z46.4
  orthopedic device (brace) (cast) (corset)
    (shoes) Z46.89
  pacemaker (cardiac) (cardiac
    resynchronization therapy (CRT-P))
    Z45.018
    nervous system (brain) (peripheral nerve)
      (spinal cord) Z46.2
      implanted Z45.42
    pulse generator Z45.010
  portacath (port-a-cath) Z45.2
  prosthesis (external) Z44.9
    arm —*see* Admission, adjustment, artificial,
      arm
    breast Z44.3
    dental Z46.3
    eye Z44.2
    leg —*see* Admission, adjustment, artificial,
      leg
    specified NEC Z44.8
  spectacles Z46.0
  wheelchair Z46.89
Fitzhugh-Curtis syndrome
  due to
    Chlamydia trachomatis A74.81
    Neisseria gonorrhorea (gonococcal
      peritonitis) A54.85
Fitz's syndrome (acute hemorrhagic
  pancreatitis) —*see also* Pancreatitis,
  acute K85.80
Fixation
  joint —*see* Ankylosis
  larynx J38.7
  stapes —*see* Ankylosis, ear ossicles
    deafness —*see* Deafness, conductive
  uterus (acquired) —*see* Malposition, uterus
  vocal cord J38.3
Flabby ridge K06.8
Flaccid —*see also* condition
  palate, congenital Q38.5
Flail
  chest S22.5-●
    newborn (birth injury) P13.8
  joint (paralytic) M25.20
    ankle M25.27-●
    elbow M25.22-●
    foot joint M25.27-●

Flail *(Continued)*
  joint *(Continued)*
    hand joint M25.24-●
    hip M25.25-●
    knee M25.26-●
    shoulder M25.21-●
    specified joint NEC M25.28
    wrist M25.23-●
Flajani's disease —*see* Hyperthyroidism, with,
  goiter (diffuse)
Flap, liver K71.3
Flashbacks (residual to hallucinogen use) F16.283
Flat
  chamber (eye) —*see* Disorder, globe,
    hypotony, flat anterior chamber
  chest, congenital Q67.8
  foot (acquired) (fixed type) (painful)
    (postural) —*see also* Deformity, limb,
    flat foot
    congenital (rigid) (spastic (everted)) Q66.5-●
    rachitic sequelae (late effect) E64.3
  organ or site, congenital NEC —*see* Anomaly,
    by site
  pelvis M95.5
    with disproportion (fetopelvic) O33.0
      causing obstructed labor O65.0
    congenital Q74.2
Flatau-Schilder disease G37.0
Flatback syndrome M40.30
  lumbar region M40.36
  lumbosacral region M40.37
  thoracolumbar region M40.35
Flattening
  head, femur M89.8X5
  hip —*see* Coxa, plana
  lip (congenital) Q18.8
  nose (congenital) Q67.4
    acquired M95.0
Flatulence R14.3
  psychogenic F45.8
Flatus R14.3
  vaginalis N89.8
Flax-dresser's disease J66.1
Flea bite —*see* Injury, bite, by site, superficial,
  insect
Flecks, glaucomatous (subcapsular) —*see*
  Cataract, complicated
Fleischer (-Kayser) ring (cornea) H18.04-●
Fleshy mole O02.0
Flexibilitas cerea —*see* Catalepsy
Flexion
  amputation stump (surgical) T87.89
  cervix —*see* Malposition, uterus
  contracture, joint —*see* Contraction, joint
  deformity, joint —*see also* Deformity, limb,
    flexion M21.20
    hip, congenital Q65.89
  uterus —*see also* Malposition, uterus
    lateral —*see* Lateroversion, uterus
Flexner-Boyd dysentery A03.2
Flexner's dysentery A03.1
Flexure —*see* Flexion
Flint murmur (aortic insufficiency) I35.1
Floater, vitreous —*see* Opacity, vitreous
Floating
  cartilage (joint) —*see also* Loose, body, joint
    knee —*see* Derangement, knee, loose body
  gallbladder, congenital Q44.1
  kidney N28.89
    congenital Q63.8
  spleen D73.89
Flooding N92.0
Floor —*see* condition
Floppy
  baby syndrome (nonspecific) P94.2
  iris syndrome (intraoperative) (IFIS) H21.81
  nonrheumatic mitral valve syndrome I34.1
Flu —*see also* Influenza
  avian —*see also* Influenza, due to, identified
    novel influenza A virus J09.X2
  bird —*see also* Influenza, due to, identified
    novel influenza A virus J09.X2

Flu *(Continued)*
  intestinal NEC A08.4
  swine (viruses that normally cause infections
    in pigs) —*see also* Influenza, due to,
    identified novel influenza A virus J09.X2
Fluctuating blood pressure I99.8
Fluid
  abdomen R18.8
  chest J94.8
  heart —*see* Failure, heart, congestive
  joint —*see* Effusion, joint
  loss (acute) E86.9
  lung —*see* Edema, lung
  overload E87.70
    specified NEC E87.79
  peritoneal cavity R18.8
  pleural cavity J94.8
  retention R60.9
Flukes NEC —*see also* Infestation, fluke
  blood NEC —*see* Schistosomiasis
  liver B66.3
Fluor (vaginalis) N89.8
  trichomonal or due to Trichomonas
    (vaginalis) A59.00
Fluorosis
  dental K00.3
  skeletal M85.10
    ankle M85.17-●
    foot M85.17-●
    forearm M85.13-●
    hand M85.14-●
    lower leg M85.16-●
    multiple site M85.19
    neck M85.18
    rib M85.18
    shoulder M85.11-●
    skull M85.18
    specified site NEC M85.18
    thigh M85.15-●
    toe M85.17-●
    upper arm M85.12-●
    vertebra M85.18
Flush syndrome E34.0
Flushing R23.2
  menopausal N95.1
Flutter
  atrial or auricular I48.92
    atypical I48.4
    type I I48.3
    type II I48.4
    typical I48.3
  heart I49.8
    atrial or auricular I48.92
      atypical I48.4
      type I I48.3
      type II I48.4
      typical I48.3
    ventricular I49.02
  ventricular I49.02
FNHTR (febrile nonhemolytic transfusion
  reaction) R50.84
Fochier's abscess - code by site under Abscess
Focus, Assmann's —*see* Tuberculosis,
  pulmonary
Fogo selvagem L10.3
Foix-Alajouanine syndrome G95.19
Fold, folds (anomalous) —*see also* Anomaly,
  by site
  Descemet's membrane —*see* Change, corneal
    membrane, Descemet's, fold
  epicanthic Q10.3
  heart Q24.8
Folie à deux F24
Follicle
  cervix (nabothian) (ruptured) N88.8
  graafian, ruptured, with hemorrhage N83.0-●
  nabothian N88.8
Follicular —*see* condition
Folliculitis (superficial) L73.9
  abscedens et suffodiens L66.3
  cyst N83.0-●

Folliculitis *(Continued)*
decalvans L66.2
deep —*see* Furuncle, by site
gonococcal (acute) (chronic) A54.01
keloid, keloidalis L73.0
pustular L01.02
ulerythematosa reticulata L66.4
Folliculome lipidique
specified site —*see* Neoplasm, benign, by site
unspecified site
female D27.9
male D29.20
Følling's disease E70.0
Follow-up —*see* Examination, follow-up
Fong's syndrome (hereditary osteo-onychodysplasia) Q87.2
Food
allergy L27.2
asphyxia (from aspiration or inhalation) —*see* Foreign body, by site
choked on —*see* Foreign body, by site
deprivation T73.0
specified kind of food NEC E63.8
intoxication —*see* Poisoning, food
lack of T73.0
poisoning —*see* Poisoning, food
rejection NEC —*see* Disorder, eating
strangulation or suffocation —*see* Foreign body, by site
toxemia —*see* Poisoning, food
Foot —*see* condition
Foramen ovale (nonclosure) (patent) (persistent) Q21.1
Forbes' glycogen storage disease E74.03
Fordyce-Fox disease L75.2
Fordyce's disease (mouth) Q38.6
Forearm —*see* condition
Foreign body
with
laceration —*see* Laceration, by site, with foreign body
puncture wound —*see* Puncture, by site, with foreign body
accidentally left following a procedure T81.509
aspiration T81.506
resulting in
adhesions T81.516
obstruction T81.526
perforation T81.536
specified complication NEC T81.596
cardiac catheterization T81.505
resulting in
acute reaction T81.60
aseptic peritonitis T81.61
specified NEC T81.69
adhesions T81.515
obstruction T81.525
perforation T81.535
specified complication NEC T81.595
causing
acute reaction T81.60
aseptic peritonitis T81.61
specified complication NEC T81.69
adhesions T81.519
aseptic peritonitis T81.61
obstruction T81.529
perforation T81.539
specified complication NEC T81.599
endoscopy T81.504
resulting in
adhesions T81.514
obstruction T81.524
perforation T81.534
specified complication NEC T81.594
immunization T81.503
resulting in
adhesions T81.513
obstruction T81.523
perforation T81.533
specified complication NEC T81.593

Foreign body *(Continued)*
accidentally left following a procedure *(Continued)*
infusion T81.501
resulting in
adhesions T81.511
obstruction T81.521
perforation T81.531
specified complication NEC T81.591
injection T81.503
resulting in
adhesions T81.513
obstruction T81.523
perforation T81.533
specified complication NEC T81.593
kidney dialysis T81.502
resulting in
adhesions T81.512
obstruction T81.522
perforation T81.532
specified complication NEC T81.592
packing removal T81.507
resulting in
acute reaction T81.60
aseptic peritonitis T81.61
specified NEC T81.69
adhesions T81.517
obstruction T81.527
perforation T81.537
specified complication NEC T81.597
puncture T81.506
resulting in
adhesions T81.516
obstruction T81.526
perforation T81.536
specified complication NEC T81.596
specified procedure NEC T81.508
resulting in
acute reaction T81.60
aseptic peritonitis T81.61
specified NEC T81.69
adhesions T81.518
obstruction T81.528
perforation T81.538
specified complication NEC T81.598
surgical operation T81.500
resulting in
acute reaction T81.60
aseptic peritonitis T81.61
specified NEC T81.69
adhesions T81.510
obstruction T81.520
perforation T81.530
specified complication NEC T81.590
transfusion T81.501
resulting in
adhesions T81.511
obstruction T81.521
perforation T81.531
specified complication NEC T81.591
alimentary tract T18.9
anus T18.5
colon T18.4
esophagus —*see* Foreign body, esophagus
mouth T18.0
multiple sites T18.8
rectosigmoid (junction) T18.5
rectum T18.5
small intestine T18.3
specified site NEC T18.8
stomach T18.2
anterior chamber (eye) S05.5-●
auditory canal —*see* Foreign body, entering through orifice, ear
bronchus T17.508
causing
asphyxiation T17.500
food (bone) (seed) T17.520
gastric contents (vomitus) T17.510
specified type NEC T17.590

Foreign body *(Continued)*
bronchus *(Continued)*
causing *(Continued)*
injury NEC T17.508
food (bone) (seed) T17.528
gastric contents (vomitus) T17.518
specified type NEC T17.598
canthus —*see* Foreign body, conjunctival sac
ciliary body (eye) S05.5-●
conjunctival sac T15.1-●
cornea T15.0-●
entering through orifice
accessory sinus T17.0
alimentary canal T18.9
multiple parts T18.8
specified part NEC T18.8
alveolar process T18.0
antrum (Highmore's) T17.0
anus T18.5
appendix T18.4
auditory canal —*see* Foreign body, entering through orifice, ear
auricle —*see* Foreign body, entering through orifice, ear
bladder T19.1
bronchioles —*see* Foreign body, respiratory tract, specified site NEC
bronchus (main) —*see* Foreign body, bronchus
buccal cavity T18.0
canthus (inner) —*see* Foreign body, conjunctival sac
cecum T18.4
cervix (canal) (uteri) T19.3
colon T18.4
conjunctival sac —*see* Foreign body, conjunctival sac
cornea —*see* Foreign body, cornea
digestive organ or tract NOS T18.9
multiple parts T18.8
specified part NEC T18.8
duodenum T18.3
ear (external) T16.-●
esophagus —*see* Foreign body, esophagus
eye (external) NOS T15.9-●
conjunctival sac —*see* Foreign body, conjunctival sac
cornea —*see* Foreign body, cornea
specified part NEC T15.8-●
eyeball —*see also* Foreign body, entering through orifice, eye, specified part NEC
with penetrating wound —*see* Puncture, eyeball
eyelid —*see also* Foreign body, conjunctival sac
with
laceration —*see* Laceration, eyelid, with foreign body
puncture —*see* Puncture, eyelid, with foreign body
superficial injury —*see* Foreign body, superficial, eyelid
gastrointestinal tract T18.9
multiple parts T18.8
specified part NEC T18.8
genitourinary tract T19.9
multiple parts T19.8
specified part NEC T19.8
globe —*see* Foreign body, entering through orifice, eyeball
gum T18.0
Highmore's antrum T17.0
hypopharynx —*see* Foreign body, pharynx
ileum T18.3
intestine (small) T18.3
large T18.4
lacrimal apparatus (punctum) —*see* Foreign body, entering through orifice, eye, specified part NEC
large intestine T18.4

▶ New   ⇒ Revised   ~~deleted~~ Deleted   ● Use Additional Character(s)

Foreign body *(Continued)*
  entering through orifice *(Continued)*
    larynx —*see* Foreign body, larynx
    lung —*see* Foreign body, respiratory tract,
        specified site NEC
    maxillary sinus T17.0
    mouth T18.0
    nasal sinus T17.0
    nasopharynx —*see* Foreign body, pharynx
    nose (passage) T17.1
    nostril T17.1
    oral cavity T18.0
    palate T18.0
    penis T19.4
    pharynx —*see* Foreign body, pharynx
    piriform sinus —*see* Foreign body, pharynx
    rectosigmoid (junction) T18.5
    rectum T18.5
    respiratory tract —*see* Foreign body,
        respiratory tract
    sinus (accessory) (frontal) (maxillary)
        (nasal) T17.0
      piriform —*see* Foreign body, pharynx
    small intestine T18.3
    stomach T18.2
    suffocation by —*see* Foreign body, by site
    tear ducts or glands —*see* Foreign body,
        entering through orifice, eye, specified
        part NEC
    throat —*see* Foreign body, pharynx
    tongue T18.0
    tonsil, tonsillar (fossa) —*see* Foreign body,
        pharynx
    trachea —*see* Foreign body, trachea
    ureter T19.8
    urethra T19.0
    uterus (any part) T19.3
    vagina T19.2
    vulva T19.2
  esophagus T18.108
    causing
      injury NEC T18.108
        food (bone) (seed) T18.128
        gastric contents (vomitus) T18.118
        specified type NEC T18.198
      tracheal compression T18.100
        food (bone) (seed) T18.120
        gastric contents (vomitus) T18.110
        specified type NEC T18.190
  ~~feeling of, in throat R09.89~~
▶ feeling of, in throat R09.89
  fragment —*see* Retained, foreign body
      fragments (type of)
  genitourinary tract T19.9
    bladder T19.1
    multiple parts T19.8
    penis T19.4
    specified site NEC T19.8
    urethra T19.0
    uterus T19.3
      IUD Z97.5
    vagina T19.2
      contraceptive device Z97.5
    vulva T19.2
  granuloma (old) (soft tissue) —*see also*
      Granuloma, foreign body
    skin L92.3
  in
    laceration —*see* Laceration, by site, with
        foreign body
    puncture wound —*see* Puncture, by site,
        with foreign body
    soft tissue (residual) M79.5
  inadvertently left in operation wound —*see*
      Foreign body, accidentally left during a
      procedure
  ingestion, ingested NOS T18.9
  inhalation or inspiration —*see* Foreign body,
      by site
  internal organ, not entering through a natural
      orifice - code as specific injury with
      foreign body

Foreign body *(Continued)*
  intraocular S05.5-●
    old, retained (nonmagnetic) H44.70-●
      anterior chamber H44.71-●
      ciliary body H44.72-●
      iris H44.72-●
      lens H44.73-●
      magnetic H44.60-●
        anterior chamber H44.61-●
        ciliary body H44.62-●
        iris H44.62-●
        lens H44.63-●
        posterior wall H44.64-●
        specified site NEC H44.69-●
        vitreous body H44.65-●
      posterior wall H44.74-●
      specified site NEC H44.79-●
      vitreous body H44.75-●
    iris —*see* Foreign body, intraocular
  lacrimal punctum —*see* Foreign body,
      entering through orifice, eye, specified
      part NEC
  larynx T17.308
    causing
      asphyxiation T17.300
        food (bone) (seed) T17.320
        gastric contents (vomitus) T17.310
        specified type NEC T17.390
      injury NEC T17.308
        food (bone) (seed) T17.328
        gastric contents (vomitus) T17.318
        specified type NEC T17.398
  lens —*see* Foreign body, intraocular
  ocular muscle S05.4-●
    old, retained —*see* Foreign body, orbit, old
  old or residual
    soft tissue (residual) M79.5
  operation wound, left accidentally —*see*
      Foreign body, accidentally left during a
      procedure
  orbit S05.4-●
    old, retained H05.5-●
  pharynx T17.208
    causing
      asphyxiation T17.200
        food (bone) (seed) T17.220
        gastric contents (vomitus)
            T17.210
        specified type NEC T17.290
      injury NEC T17.208
        food (bone) (seed) T17.228
        gastric contents (vomitus) T17.218
        specified type NEC T17.298
  respiratory tract T17.908
    bronchioles —*see* Foreign body, respiratory
        tract, specified site NEC
    bronchus —*see* Foreign body, bronchus
    causing
      asphyxiation T17.900
        food (bone) (seed) T17.920
        gastric contents (vomitus) T17.910
        specified type NEC T17.990
      injury NEC T17.908
        food (bone) (seed) T17.928
        gastric contents (vomitus) T17.918
        specified type NEC T17.998
    larynx —*see* Foreign body, larynx
    lung —*see* Foreign body, respiratory tract,
        specified site NEC
    multiple parts —*see* Foreign body,
        respiratory tract, specified site NEC
    nasal sinus T17.0
    nasopharynx —*see* Foreign body, pharynx
    nose T17.1
    nostril T17.1
    pharynx —*see* Foreign body, pharynx
    specified site NEC T17.808
      causing
        asphyxiation T17.800
          food (bone) (seed) T17.820
          gastric contents (vomitus) T17.810
          specified type NEC T17.890

Foreign body *(Continued)*
  respiratory tract *(Continued)*
    specified site NEC *(Continued)*
      causing *(Continued)*
        injury NEC T17.808
          food (bone) (seed) T17.828
          gastric contents (vomitus) T17.818
          specified type NEC T17.898
    throat —*see* Foreign body, pharynx
    trachea —*see* Foreign body, trachea
  retained (old) (nonmagnetic) (in)
    anterior chamber (eye) —*see* Foreign body,
        intraocular, old, retained, anterior
        chamber
      magnetic —*see* Foreign body, intraocular,
          old, retained, magnetic, anterior
          chamber
    ciliary body —*see* Foreign body,
        intraocular, old, retained, ciliary body
      magnetic —*see* Foreign body, intraocular,
          old, retained, magnetic, ciliary
          body
    eyelid H02.819
      left H02.816
        lower H02.815
        upper H02.814
      right H02.813
        lower H02.812
        upper H02.811
    fragments —*see* Retained, foreign body
        fragments (type of)
    globe —*see* Foreign body, intraocular, old,
        retained
      magnetic —*see* Foreign body, intraocular,
          old, retained, magnetic
    intraocular —*see* Foreign body, intraocular,
        old, retained
      magnetic —*see* Foreign body, intraocular,
          old, retained, magnetic
    iris —*see* Foreign body, intraocular, old,
        retained, iris
      magnetic —*see* Foreign body, intraocular,
          old, retained, magnetic, iris
    lens —*see* Foreign body, intraocular, old,
        retained, lens
      magnetic —*see* Foreign body, intraocular,
          old, retained, magnetic, lens
    muscle —*see* Foreign body, retained, soft
        tissue
    orbit —*see* Foreign body, orbit, old
    posterior wall of globe —*see* Foreign body,
        intraocular, old, retained, posterior
        wall
      magnetic —*see* Foreign body, intraocular,
          old, retained, magnetic, posterior
          wall
    retrobulbar —*see* Foreign body, orbit, old,
        retrobulbar
    soft tissue M79.5
    vitreous —*see* Foreign body, intraocular,
        old, retained, vitreous body
      magnetic —*see* Foreign body, intraocular,
          old, retained, magnetic, vitreous
          body
  retina S05.5-●
  superficial, without open wound
    abdomen, abdominal (wall) S30.851
    alveolar process S00.552
    ankle S90.55-●
    antecubital space —*see* Foreign body,
        superficial, forearm
    anus S30.857
    arm (upper) S40.85-●
    auditory canal —*see* Foreign body,
        superficial, ear
    auricle —*see* Foreign body, superficial, ear
    axilla —*see* Foreign body, superficial, arm
    back, lower S30.850
    breast S20.15-●
    brow S00.85
    buttock S30.850

Foreign body *(Continued)*
  superficial, without open wound *(Continued)*
    calf —*see* Foreign body, superficial, leg
    canthus —*see* Foreign body, superficial,
        eyelid
    cheek S00.85
      internal S00.552
    chest wall —*see* Foreign body, superficial,
        thorax
    chin S00.85
    clitoris S30.854
    costal region —*see* Foreign body,
        superficial, thorax
    digit(s)
      foot —*see* Foreign body, superficial, toe
      hand —*see* Foreign body, superficial,
          finger
    ear S00.45-•
    elbow S50.35-•
    epididymis S30.853
    epigastric region S30.851
    epiglottis S10.15
    esophagus, cervical S10.15
    eyebrow —*see* Foreign body, superficial,
        eyelid
    eyelid S00.25-•
    face S00.85
    finger(s) S60.459
      index S60.45-•
      little S60.45-•
      middle S60.45-•
      ring S60.45-•
    flank S30.851
    foot (except toe(s) alone) S90.85-•
      toe —*see* Foreign body, superficial, toe
    forearm S50.85-•
      elbow only —*see* Foreign body,
          superficial, elbow
    forehead S00.85
    genital organs, external
      female S30.856
      male S30.855
    groin S30.851
    gum S00.552
    hand S60.55-•
    head S00.95
      ear —*see* Foreign body, superficial, ear
      eyelid —*see* Foreign body, superficial,
          eyelid
      lip S00.551
      nose S00.35
      oral cavity S00.552
      scalp S00.05
      specified site NEC S00.85
    heel —*see* Foreign body, superficial, foot
    hip S70.25-•
    inguinal region S30.851
    interscapular region S20.459
    jaw S00.85
    knee S80.25-•
    labium (majus) (minus) S30.854
    larynx S10.15
    leg (lower) S80.85-•
      knee —*see* Foreign body, superficial,
          knee
      upper —*see* Foreign body, superficial,
          thigh
    lip S00.551
    lower back S30.850
    lumbar region S30.850
    malar region S00.85
    mammary —*see* Foreign body, superficial,
        breast
    mastoid region S00.85
    mouth S00.552
    nail
      finger —*see* Foreign body, superficial,
          finger
      toe —*see* Foreign body, superficial, toe
    nape S10.85
    nasal S00.35

Foreign body *(Continued)*
  superficial, without open wound *(Continued)*
    neck S10.95
      specified site NEC S10.85
      throat S10.15
    nose S00.35
    occipital region S00.05
    oral cavity S00.552
    orbital region —*see* Foreign body,
        superficial, eyelid
    palate S00.552
    palm —*see* Foreign body, superficial, hand
    parietal region S00.05
    pelvis S30.850
    penis S30.852
    perineum
      female S30.854
      male S30.850
    periocular area —*see* Foreign body,
        superficial, eyelid
    phalanges
      finger —*see* Foreign body, superficial,
          finger
      toe —*see* Foreign body, superficial, toe
    pharynx S10.15
    pinna —*see* Foreign body, superficial, ear
    popliteal space —*see* Foreign body,
        superficial, knee
    prepuce S30.852
    pubic region S30.850
    pudendum
      female S30.856
      male S30.855
    sacral region S30.850
    scalp S00.05
    scapular region —*see* Foreign body,
        superficial, shoulder
    scrotum S30.853
    shin —*see* Foreign body, superficial, leg
    shoulder S40.25-•
    sternal region S20.359
    submaxillary region S00.85
    submental region S00.85
    subungual
      finger(s) —*see* Foreign body, superficial,
          finger
      toe(s) —*see* Foreign body, superficial, toe
    supraclavicular fossa S10.85
    supraorbital S00.85
    temple S00.85
    temporal region S00.85
    testis S30.853
    thigh S70.35-•
    thorax, thoracic (wall) S20.95
      back S20.45-•
      front S20.35-•
    throat S10.15
    thumb S60.35-•
    toe(s) (lesser) S90.456
      great S90.45-•
    tongue S00.552
    trachea S10.15
    tunica vaginalis S30.853
    tympanum, tympanic membrane —*see*
        Foreign body, superficial, ear
    uvula S00.552
    vagina S30.854
    vocal cords S10.15
    vulva S30.854
    wrist S60.85-•
  swallowed T18.9
  trachea T17.408
    causing
      asphyxiation T17.400
        food (bone) (seed) T17.420
        gastric contents (vomitus) T17.410
        specified type NEC T17.490
      injury NEC T17.408
        food (bone) (seed) T17.428
        gastric contents (vomitus) T17.418
        specified type NEC T17.498

Foreign body *(Continued)*
  type of fragment —*see* Retained, foreign body
      fragments (type of)
  vitreous (humor) S05.5-•
Forestier's disease (rhizomelic
      pseudopolyarthritis) M35.3-•
  meaning ankylosing hyperostosis —*see*
      Hyperostosis, ankylosing
Formation
  hyalin in cornea —*see* Degeneration, cornea
  sequestrum in bone (due to infection) —*see*
      Osteomyelitis, chronic
  valve
    colon, congenital Q43.8
    ureter (congenital) Q62.39
Formication R20.2
Fort Bragg fever A27.89
Fossa —*see also* condition
  pyriform —*see* condition
Foster-Kennedy syndrome H47.14-•
Fothergill's
  disease (trigeminal neuralgia) —*see also*
      Neuralgia, trigeminal
  scarlatina anginosa A38.9
Foul breath R19.6
Foundling Z76.1
Fournier disease or gangrene N49.3
  female N76.89
Fourth
  cranial nerve —*see* condition
  molar K00.1
Foville's (peduncular) disease or syndrome
      G46.3
Fox (-Fordyce) disease (apocrine miliaria) L75.2
Fracture, burst —*see* Fracture, traumatic, by site
➡ **Fracture, chronic** —*see* Fracture, pathological,
      by site
➡ **Fracture, insufficiency** —*see* Fracture,
      pathological, by site
Fracture, nontraumatic, NEC
  atypical
    femur M84.750-•
      complete
        oblique M84.759
          left side M84.758
          right side M84.757
        transverse M84.756
          left side M84.755
          right side M84.754
      incomplete M84.753
        left side M84.752
        right side M84.751
Fracture, pathological (pathologic) —*see also*
      Fracture, traumatic M84.40
  ankle M84.47-•
  carpus M84.44-•
  clavicle M84.41-•
  compression (not due to trauma) —*see also*
      Collapse, vertebra M48.50-•
  dental implant M27.63
  dental restorative material K08.539
    with loss of material K08.531
    without loss of material K08.530
  due to
    neoplastic disease NEC —*see also*
        Neoplasm M84.50
      ankle M84.57-•
      carpus M84.54-•
      clavicle M84.51-•
      femur M84.55-•
      fibula M84.56-•
      finger M84.54-•
      hip M84.559
      humerus M84.52-•
      ilium M84.550
      ischium M84.550
      metacarpus M84.54-•
      metatarsus M84.57-•
      neck M84.58
      pelvis M84.550
      radius M84.53-•

▶ New   ⇨ Revised   ~~deleted~~ Deleted   • Use Additional Character(s)

Fracture, pathological *(Continued)*
  due to *(Continued)*
    neoplastic disease NEC *(Continued)*
      rib M84.58
      scapula M84.51-●
      skull M84.58
      specified site NEC M84.58
      tarsus M84.57-●
      tibia M84.56-●
      toe M84.57-●
      ulna M84.53-●
      vertebra M84.58
    osteoporosis M80.00
      disuse —*see* Osteoporosis, specified type
        NEC, with pathological fracture
      drug-induced —*see* Osteoporosis, drug
        induced, with pathological fracture
      idiopathic —*see* Osteoporosis, specified
        type NEC, with pathological
        fracture
      postmenopausal —*see* Osteoporosis,
        postmenopausal, with pathological
        fracture
      postoophorectomy —*see* Osteo-
        porosis, postoophorectomy, with
        pathological fracture
      postsurgical malabsorption —*see*
        Osteoporosis, specified type NEC,
        with pathological fracture
      specified cause NEC —*see* Osteoporosis,
        specified type NEC, with
        pathological fracture
    specified disease NEC M84.60
      ankle M84.67-●
      carpus M84.64-●
      clavicle M84.61-●
      femur M84.65-●
      fibula M84.66-●
      finger M84.64-●
      hip M84.65-●
      humerus M84.62-●
      ilium M84.650
      ischium M84.650
      metacarpus M84.64-●
      metatarsus M84.67-●
      neck M84.68
      radius M84.63-●
      rib M84.68
      scapula M84.61-●
      skull M84.68
      tarsus M84.67-●
      tibia M84.66-●
      toe M84.67-●
      ulna M84.63-●
      vertebra M84.68
    femur M84.45-●
    fibula M84.46-●
    finger M84.44-●
    hip M84.459
    humerus M84.42-●
    ilium M84.454
    ischium M84.454
    joint prosthesis —*see* Complications, joint
      prosthesis, mechanical, breakdown, by
      site
    periprosthetic —*see* Fracture, pathological,
      periprosthetic
    metacarpus M84.44-●
    metatarsus M84.47-●
    neck M84.48
    pelvis M84.454
    periprosthetic M97.9
      ankle M97.2-●
      elbow M97.4-●
      finger M97.8
      hip M97.0-●
      knee M97.1-●
      other specified joint M97.8
      shoulder M97.3-●
      spinal joint M97.8
      toe joint M97.8
      wrist joint M97.8

Fracture, pathological *(Continued)*
  radius M84.43-●
  restorative material (dental) K08.539
    with loss of material K08.531
    without loss of material K08.530
  rib M84.48
  scapula M84.41-●
  skull M84.48
  tarsus M84.47-●
  tibia M84.46-●
  toe M84.47-●
  ulna M84.43-●
  vertebra M84.48
Fracture, traumatic (abduction) (adduction)
    (separation) —*see also* Fracture,
    pathological T14.8
  acetabulum S32.40-●
    column
      anterior (displaced) (iliopubic) S32.43-●
        nondisplaced S32.436
      posterior (displaced) (ilioischial)
        S32.443
        nondisplaced S32.44-●
    dome (displaced) S32.48-●
      nondisplaced S32.48
    specified NEC S32.49-●
    transverse (displaced) S32.45-●
      with associated posterior wall fracture
        (displaced) S32.46-●
        nondisplaced S32.46-●
      nondisplaced S32.45-●
    wall
      anterior (displaced) S32.41-●
        nondisplaced S32.41-●
      medial (displaced) S32.47-●
        nondisplaced S32.47-●
      posterior (displaced) S32.42-●
        with associated transverse fracture
          (displaced) S32.46-●
          nondisplaced S32.46-●
        nondisplaced S32.42-●
  acromion —*see* Fracture, scapula, acromial
    process
  ankle S82.899
    bimalleolar (displaced) S82.84-●
      nondisplaced S82.84-●
    lateral malleolus only (displaced) S82.6-●
      nondisplaced S82.6-●
    medial malleolus (displaced) S82.5-●
      associated with Maisonneuve's
        fracture —*see* Fracture,
        Maisonneuve's
      nondisplaced S82.5-●
    talus —*see* Fracture, tarsal, talus
    trimalleolar (displaced) S82.85-●
      nondisplaced S82.85-●
  arm (upper) —*see also* Fracture, humerus,
    shaft
    humerus —*see* Fracture, humerus
    radius —*see* Fracture, radius
    ulna —*see* Fracture, ulna
  astragalus —*see* Fracture, tarsal, talus
  atlas —*see* Fracture, neck, cervical vertebra,
    first
  axis —*see* Fracture, neck, cervical vertebra,
    second
  back —*see* Fracture, vertebra
  Barton's —*see* Barton's fracture
  base of skull —*see* Fracture, skull, base
  basicervical (basal) (femoral) S72.0
  Bennett's —*see* Bennett's fracture
  bimalleolar —*see* Fracture, ankle,
    bimalleolar
  blow-out S02.3-●
  bone NEC T14.8
    birth injury P13.9
    following insertion of orthopedic implant,
      joint prosthesis or bone plate —*see*
      Fracture, following insertion of
      orthopedic implant, joint prosthesis or
      bone plate

Fracture, traumatic *(Continued)*
  bone NEC *(Continued)*
    in (due to) neoplastic disease NEC —
      see Fracture, pathological, due to,
      neoplastic disease
    pathological (cause unknown) —*see*
      Fracture, pathological
  breast bone —*see* Fracture, sternum
  bucket handle (semilunar cartilage) —*see*
    Tear, meniscus
  burst —*see* Fracture, traumatic, by site
  calcaneus —*see* Fracture, tarsal, calcaneus
  carpal bone(s) S62.10-●
    capitate (displaced) S62.13-●
      nondisplaced S62.13-●
    cuneiform —*see* Fracture, carpal bone,
      triquetrum
    hamate (body) (displaced) S62.143
      hook process (displaced) S62.15-●
        nondisplaced S62.15-●
      nondisplaced S62.14-●
    larger multangular —*see* Fracture, carpal
      bones, trapezium
    lunate (displaced) S62.12-●
      nondisplaced S62.12-●
    navicular S62.00-●
      distal pole (displaced) S62.01-●
        nondisplaced S62.01-●
      middle third (displaced) S62.02-●
        nondisplaced S62.02-●
      proximal third (displaced) S62.03-●
        nondisplaced S62.03-●
      volar tuberosity —*see* Fracture, carpal
        bones, navicular, distal pole
    os magnum —*see* Fracture, carpal bones,
      capitate
    pisiform (displaced) S62.16-●
      nondisplaced S62.16-●
    semilunar —*see* Fracture, carpal bones,
      lunate
    smaller multangular —*see* Fracture, carpal
      bones, trapezoid
    trapezium (displaced) S62.17-●
      nondisplaced S62.17-●
    trapezoid (displaced) S62.18-●
      nondisplaced S62.18-●
    triquetrum (displaced) S62.11-●
      nondisplaced S62.11-●
    unciform —*see* Fracture, carpal bones,
      hamate
  cervical —*see* Fracture, vertebra, cervical
  clavicle S42.00-●
    acromial end (displaced) S42.03-●
      nondisplaced S42.03-●
    birth injury P13.4
    lateral end —*see* Fracture, clavicle, acromial
      end
    shaft (displaced) S42.02-●
      nondisplaced S42.02-●
    sternal end (anterior) (displaced) S42.01-●
      nondisplaced S42.01-●
      posterior S42.01-●
  coccyx S32.2
  collapsed —*see* Collapse, vertebra
  collar bone —*see* Fracture, clavicle
  Colles' —*see* Colles' fracture
  coronoid process —*see* Fracture, ulna, upper
    end, coronoid process
  corpus cavernosum penis S39.840
  costochondral cartilage S23.41
  costochondral, costosternal junction —*see*
    Fracture, rib
  cranium —*see* Fracture, skull
  cricoid cartilage S12.8
  cuboid (ankle) —*see* Fracture, tarsal, cuboid
  cuneiform
    foot —*see* Fracture, tarsal, cuneiform
    wrist —*see* Fracture, carpal, triquetrum
  delayed union —*see* Delay, union, fracture
  dental restorative material K08.539
    with loss of material K08.531
    without loss of material K08.530

▶ New   ⇒ Revised   ~~deleted~~ Deleted   ● Use Additional Character(s)

Fracture, traumatic *(Continued)*
  due to
    birth injury —*see* Birth, injury, fracture
    osteoporosis —*see* Osteoporosis, with
      fracture
  Dupuytren's —*see* Fracture, ankle, lateral
    malleolus
  elbow S42.40-●
  ethmoid (bone) (sinus) —*see* Fracture, skull,
    base
  face bone S02.92
  fatigue —*see also* Fracture, stress
    vertebra M48.40
      cervical region M48.42
      cervicothoracic region M48.43
      lumbar region M48.46
      lumbosacral region M48.47
      occipito-atlanto-axial region M48.41
      sacrococcygeal region M48.48
      thoracic region M48.44
      thoracolumbar region M48.45
  femur, femoral S72.9-●
    basicervical (basal) S72.0
    birth injury P13.2
    capital epiphyseal S79.01-●
    condyles, epicondyles —*see* Fracture,
      femur, lower end
    distal end —*see* Fracture, femur, lower end
    epiphysis
      head —*see* Fracture, femur, upper end,
        epiphysis
      lower —*see* Fracture, femur, lower end,
        epiphysis
      upper —*see* Fracture, femur, upper end,
        epiphysis
    following insertion of implant, prosthesis
      or plate M96.66-●
    head —*see* Fracture, femur, upper end,
      head
    intertrochanteric —*see* Fracture, femur,
      trochanteric
    intratrochanteric —*see* Fracture, femur,
      trochanteric
    lower end S72.40-●
      condyle (displaced) S72.41-●
        lateral (displaced) S72.42-●
          nondisplaced S72.42-●
        medial (displaced) S72.43-●
          nondisplaced S72.43-●
        nondisplaced S72.41-●
      epiphysis (displaced) S72.44-●
        nondisplaced S72.44-●
      physeal S79.10-●
        Salter-Harris
          Type I S79.11-●
          Type II S79.12-●
          Type III S79.13-●
          Type IV S79.14-●
        specified NEC S79.19-●
      specified NEC S72.49-●
      supracondylar (displaced) S72.45-●
        with intracondylar extension
          (displaced) S72.46-●
          nondisplaced S72.46-●
        nondisplaced S72.45-●
      torus S72.47-●
    neck —*see* Fracture, femur, upper end, neck
    pertrochanteric —*see* Fracture, femur,
      trochanteric
    shaft (lower third) (middle third) (upper
      third) S72.30-●
      comminuted (displaced) S72.35-●
        nondisplaced S72.35-●
      oblique (displaced) S72.33-●
        nondisplaced S72.33-●
      segmental (displaced) S72.36-●
        nondisplaced S72.36-●
      specified NEC S72.39-●
      spiral (displaced) S72.34-●
        nondisplaced S72.34-●
      transverse (displaced) S72.32-●
        nondisplaced S72.32-●

Fracture, traumatic *(Continued)*
  femur, femoral *(Continued)*
    specified site NEC —*see* subcategory S72.8
    subcapital (displaced) S72.01-●
    subtrochanteric (region) (section)
      (displaced) S72.2-●
      nondisplaced S72.2-●
    transcervical —*see* Fracture, femur, upper
      end, neck
    transtrochanteric —*see* Fracture, femur,
      trochanteric
    trochanteric S72.10-●
      apophyseal (displaced) S72.13-●
        nondisplaced S72.13-●
      greater trochanter (displaced) S72.11-●
        nondisplaced S72.11-●
      intertrochanteric (displaced) S72.14-●
        nondisplaced S72.14-●
      lesser trochanter (displaced) S72.12-●
        nondisplaced S72.12-●
    upper end S72.00-●
      apophyseal (displaced) S72.13-●
        nondisplaced S72.13-●
      cervicotrochanteric —*see* Fracture,
        femur, upper end, neck, base
      epiphysis (displaced) S72.02-●
        nondisplaced S72.02-●
      head S72.05-●
        articular (displaced) S72.06-●
          nondisplaced S72.06-●
        specified NEC S72.09-●
      intertrochanteric (displaced) S72.14-●
        nondisplaced S72.14-●
      intracapsular S72.01-●
      midcervical (displaced) S72.03-●
        nondisplaced S72.03-●
      neck S72.00-●
        base (displaced) S72.04-●
          nondisplaced S72.04-●
        specified NEC S72.09-●
      pertrochanteric —*see* Fracture, femur,
        upper end, trochanteric
      physeal S79.00-●
        Salter-Harris type I S79.01-●
        specified NEC S79.09-●
      subcapital (displaced) S72.01-●
      subtrochanteric (displaced) S72.2-●
        nondisplaced S72.2-●
      transcervical —*see* Fracture, femur,
        upper end, midcervical
      trochanteric S72.10-●
        greater (displaced) S72.11-●
          nondisplaced S72.11-●
        lesser (displaced) S72.12-●
          nondisplaced S72.12-●
  fibula (shaft) (styloid) S82.40-●
    comminuted (displaced) S82.45-●
      nondisplaced S82.45-●
    following insertion of implant, prosthesis
      or plate M96.67-●
    involving ankle or malleolus —*see*
      Fracture, fibula, lateral malleolus
    lateral malleolus (displaced) S82.6-●
      nondisplaced S82.6-●
    lower end
      physeal S89.30-●
        Salter-Harris
          Type I S89.31-●
          Type II S89.32-●
        specified NEC S89.39-●
      specified NEC S82.83-●
      torus S82.82-●
    oblique (displaced) S82.43-●
      nondisplaced S82.43-●
    segmental (displaced) S82.46-●
      nondisplaced S82.46-●
    specified NEC S82.49-●
    spiral (displaced) S82.44-●
      nondisplaced S82.44-●
    transverse (displaced) S82.42-●
      nondisplaced S82.42-●

Fracture, traumatic *(Continued)*
  fibula (shaft) (styloid) *(Continued)*
    upper end
      physeal S89.20-●
        Salter-Harris
          Type I S89.21-●
          Type II S89.22-●
        specified NEC S89.29-●
      specified NEC S82.83-●
      torus S82.81-●
  finger (except thumb) S62.60-●
    distal phalanx (displaced) S62.63-●
      nondisplaced S62.66-●
    index S62.60-●
      distal phalanx (displaced) S62.63-●
        nondisplaced S62.66-●
      medial phalanx (displaced) S62.62-●
        nondisplaced S62.65-●
      proximal phalanx (displaced) S62.61-●
        nondisplaced S62.64-●
    little S62.60-●
      distal phalanx (displaced) S62.63-●
        nondisplaced S62.66-●
      medial phalanx (displaced) S62.62-●
        nondisplaced S62.65-●
      proximal phalanx (displaced) S62.61-●
        nondisplaced S62.64-●
    medial phalanx (displaced) S62.62-●
      nondisplaced S62.65-●
    middle S62.60-●
      distal phalanx (displaced) S62.63-●
        nondisplaced S62.66-●
      medial phalanx (displaced) S62.62-●
        nondisplaced S62.65-●
      proximal phalanx (displaced) S62.61-●
        nondisplaced S62.64-●
    proximal phalanx (displaced) S62.61-●
      nondisplaced S62.64-●
    ring S62.60-●
      distal phalanx (displaced) S62.63-●
        nondisplaced S62.66-●
      medial phalanx (displaced) S62.62-●
        nondisplaced S62.65-●
      proximal phalanx (displaced) S62.61-●
        nondisplaced S62.64-●
    thumb —*see* Fracture, thumb
  following insertion (intraoperative)
    (postoperative) of orthopedic implant,
    joint prosthesis or bone plate M96.69
    femur M96.66-●
    fibula M96.67-●
    humerus M96.62-●
    pelvis M96.65
    radius M96.63-●
    specified bone NEC M96.69
    tibia M96.67-●
    ulna M96.63-●
  foot S92.90-●
    astragalus —*see* Fracture, tarsal, talus
    calcaneus —*see* Fracture, tarsal, calcaneus
    cuboid —*see* Fracture, tarsal, cuboid
    cuneiform —*see* Fracture, tarsal, cuneiform
    metatarsal —*see* Fracture, metatarsal
    navicular —*see* Fracture, tarsal, navicular
    sesamoid S92.81-●
    specified NEC S92.81-●
    talus —*see* Fracture, tarsal, talus
    tarsal —*see* Fracture, tarsal
    toe —*see* Fracture, toe
  forearm S52.9-●
    radius —*see* Fracture, radius
    ulna —*see* Fracture, ulna
  fossa (anterior) (middle) (posterior) S02.19
  frontal (bone) (skull) S02.0
    sinus S02.19
  glenoid (cavity) (scapula) —*see* Fracture,
    scapula, glenoid cavity
  greenstick —*see* Fracture, by site
  hallux —*see* Fracture, toe, great
  hand S62.9-●
    carpal —*see* Fracture, carpal bone

▶ New   ⇒ Revised   ~~deleted~~ Deleted   ● Use Additional Character(s)

Fracture, traumatic *(Continued)*
  hand *(Continued)*
    finger (except thumb) —*see* Fracture, finger
    metacarpal —*see* Fracture, metacarpal
    navicular (scaphoid) (hand) —*see* Fracture, carpal bone, navicular
    thumb —*see* Fracture, thumb
  healed or old
    with complications - code by Nature of the complication
  heel bone —*see* Fracture, tarsal, calcaneus
  Hill-Sachs S42.29-●
  hip —*see* Fracture, femur, neck
  humerus S42.30-●
    anatomical neck —*see* Fracture, humerus, upper end
    articular process —*see* Fracture, humerus, lower end
    capitellum —*see* Fracture, humerus, lower end, condyle, lateral
    distal end —*see* Fracture, humerus, lower end
    epiphysis
      lower —*see* Fracture, humerus, lower end, physeal
      upper —*see* Fracture, humerus, upper end, physeal
    external condyle —*see* Fracture, humerus, lower end, condyle, lateral
    following insertion of implant, prosthesis or plate M96.62-●
    great tuberosity —*see* Fracture, humerus, upper end, greater tuberosity
    intercondylar —*see* Fracture, humerus, lower end
    internal epicondyle —*see* Fracture, humerus, lower end, epicondyle, medial
    lesser tuberosity —*see* Fracture, humerus, upper end, lesser tuberosity
    lower end S42.40-●
      condyle
        lateral (displaced) S42.45-●
          nondisplaced S42.45-●
        medial (displaced) S42.46-●
          nondisplaced S42.46-●
      epicondyle
        lateral (displaced) S42.43-●
          nondisplaced S42.43-●
        medial (displaced) S42.44-●
          incarcerated S42.44-●
          nondisplaced S42.44-●
      physeal S49.10-●
      Salter-Harris
        Type I S49.11-●
        Type II S49.12-●
        Type III S49.13-●
        Type IV S49.14-●
        specified NEC S49.19-●
      specified NEC (displaced) S42.49-●
        nondisplaced S42.49-●
      supracondylar (simple) (displaced) S42.41-●
        with intercondylar fracture —*see* Fracture, humerus, lower end
        comminuted (displaced) S42.42-●
          nondisplaced S42.42-●
        nondisplaced S42.41-●
      torus S42.48-●
      transcondylar (displaced) S42.47-●
        nondisplaced S42.47-●
    proximal end —*see* Fracture, humerus, upper end
    shaft S42.30-●
      comminuted (displaced) S42.35-●
        nondisplaced S42.35-●
      greenstick S42.31-●
      oblique (displaced) S42.33-●
        nondisplaced S42.33-●
      segmental (displaced) S42.36-●
        nondisplaced S42.36-●
      specified NEC S42.39-●

Fracture, traumatic *(Continued)*
  humerus *(Continued)*
    shaft *(Continued)*
      spiral (displaced) S42.34-●
        nondisplaced S42.34-●
      transverse (displaced) S42.32-●
        nondisplaced S42.32-●
    supracondylar —*see* Fracture, humerus, lower end
    surgical neck —*see* Fracture, humerus, upper end, surgical neck
    trochlea —*see* Fracture, humerus, lower end, condyle, medial
    tuberosity —*see* Fracture, humerus, upper end
    upper end S42.20-●
      anatomical neck —*see* Fracture, humerus, upper end, specified NEC
      articular head —*see* Fracture, humerus, upper end, specified NEC
      epiphysis —*see* Fracture, humerus, upper end, physeal
      greater tuberosity (displaced) S42.25-●
        nondisplaced S42.25-●
      lesser tuberosity (displaced) S42.26-●
        nondisplaced S42.26-●
      physeal S49.00-●
      Salter-Harris
        Type I S49.01-●
        Type II S49.02-●
        Type III S49.03-●
        Type IV S49.04-●
        specified NEC S49.09-●
      specified NEC (displaced) S42.29-●
        nondisplaced S42.29-●
      surgical neck (displaced) S42.21-●
        four-part S42.24-●
        nondisplaced S42.21-●
        three-part S42.23-●
        two-part (displaced) S42.22-●
          nondisplaced S42.22-●
      torus S42.27-●
      transepiphyseal —*see* Fracture, humerus, upper end, physeal
  hyoid bone S12.8
  ilium S32.30-●
    with disruption of pelvic ring —*see* Disruption, pelvic ring
    avulsion (displaced) S32.31-●
      nondisplaced S32.31-●
    specified NEC S32.39-●
  impaction, impacted - code as Fracture, by site
  innominate bone —*see* Fracture, ilium
  instep —*see* Fracture, foot
  ischium S32.60-●
    with disruption of pelvic ring —*see* Disruption, pelvic ring
    avulsion (displaced) S32.61-●
      nondisplaced S32.61-●
    specified NEC S32.69-●
  jaw (bone) (lower) —*see* Fracture, mandible
    upper —*see* Fracture, maxilla
  joint prosthesis —*see* Complications, joint prosthesis, mechanical, breakdown, by site
    periprosthetic —*see* Fracture, traumatic, periprosthetic
  knee cap —*see* Fracture, patella
  larynx S12.8
  late effects —*see* Sequelae, fracture
  leg (lower) S82.9-●
    ankle —*see* Fracture, ankle
    femur —*see* Fracture, femur
    fibula —*see* Fracture, fibula
    malleolus —*see* Fracture, ankle
    patella —*see* Fracture, patella
    specified site NEC S82.89-●
    tibia —*see* Fracture, tibia
  lumbar spine —*see* Fracture, vertebra, lumbar
  lumbosacral spine S32.9

Fracture, traumatic *(Continued)*
  Maisonneuve's (displaced) S82.86-●
    nondisplaced S82.86-●
  malar bone —*see also* Fracture, maxilla S02.400
    left side S02.40B
    right side S02.40A
  malleolus —*see* Fracture, ankle
  malunion —*see* Fracture, by site
  mandible (lower jawbone) S02.609
    alveolus S02.67-●
    angle (of jaw) S02.65-●
    body, unspecified S02.600-●
      left side S02.602
      right side S02.601
    condylar process S02.61-●
    coronoid process S02.63-●
    ramus, unspecified S02.64-●
    specified site NEC S02.69
    subcondylar process S02.62-●
    symphysis S02.66
  manubrium (sterni) S22.21
    dissociation from sternum S22.23
  march —*see* Fracture, traumatic, stress, by site
  maxilla, maxillary (bone) (sinus) (superior) (upper jaw) S02.401
    alveolus S02.42
    inferior —*see* Fracture, mandible
    LeFort I S02.411
    LeFort II S02.412
    LeFort III S02.413
    left side S02.40D
    right side S02.40C
  metacarpal S62.309
    base (displaced) S62.319
      nondisplaced S62.349
    fifth S62.30-●
      base (displaced) S62.31-●
        nondisplaced S62.34-●
      neck (displaced) S62.33-●
        nondisplaced S62.36-●
      shaft (displaced) S62.32-●
        nondisplaced S62.35-●
      specified NEC S62.398
    first S62.20-●
      base NEC (displaced) S62.23-●
        nondisplaced S62.23-●
      Bennett's —*see* Bennett's fracture
      neck (displaced) S62.25-●
        nondisplaced S62.25-●
      shaft (displaced) S62.24-●
        nondisplaced S62.24-●
      specified NEC S62.29-●
    fourth S62.30-●
      base (displaced) S62.31-●
        nondisplaced S62.34-●
      neck (displaced) S62.33-●
        nondisplaced S62.36-●
      shaft (displaced) S62.32-●
        nondisplaced S62.35-●
      specified NEC S62.39-●
    neck (displaced) S62.33-●
      nondisplaced S62.36-●
    Rolando's —*see* Rolando's fracture
    second S62.30-●
      base (displaced) S62.31-●
        nondisplaced S62.34-●
      neck (displaced) S62.33-●
        nondisplaced S62.36-●
      shaft (displaced) S62.32-●
        nondisplaced S62.35-●
      specified NEC S62.39-●
    shaft (displaced) S62.32-●
      nondisplaced S62.35-●
    specified NEC S62.399
    third S62.30-●
      base (displaced) S62.31-●
        nondisplaced S62.34-●
      neck (displaced) S62.33-●
        nondisplaced S62.36-●
      shaft (displaced) S62.32-●
        nondisplaced S62.35-●
      specified NEC S62.39-●

Fracture, traumatic *(Continued)*
  metastatic —*see* Fracture, pathological,
      due to, neoplastic disease —*see also*
      Neoplasm
  metatarsal bone S92.30-●
    fifth (displaced) S92.35-●
      nondisplaced S92.35-●
    first (displaced) S92.31-●
      nondisplaced S92.31-●
    fourth (displaced) S92.34-●
      nondisplaced S92.34-●
    physeal S99.10-●
      Salter-Harris
        Type I S99.11-●
        Type II S99.12-●
        Type III S99.13-●
        Type IV S99.14-●
      specified NEC S99.19-●
    second (displaced) S92.32-●
      nondisplaced S92.32-●
    third (displaced) S92.33-●
      nondisplaced S92.33-●
  Monteggia's —*see* Monteggia's
      fracture
  multiple
    hand (and wrist) NEC —*see* Fracture, by
        site
    ribs —*see* Fracture, rib, multiple
  nasal (bone(s)) S02.2
  navicular (scaphoid) (foot) —*see also* Fracture,
      tarsal, navicular
    hand —*see* Fracture, carpal, navicular
  neck S12.9
    cervical vertebra S12.9
      fifth (displaced) S12.400
        nondisplaced S12.401
        specified type NEC (displaced)
            S12.490
          nondisplaced S12.491
      first (displaced) S12.000
        burst (stable) S12.01
          unstable S12.02
        lateral mass (displaced) S12.040
          nondisplaced S12.041
        nondisplaced S12.001
        posterior arch (displaced) S12.030
          nondisplaced S12.031
        specified type NEC (displaced)
            S12.090
          nondisplaced S12.091
      fourth (displaced) S12.300
        nondisplaced S12.301
        specified type NEC (displaced)
            S12.390
          nondisplaced S12.391
      second (displaced) S12.100
        dens (anterior) (displaced) (type II)
            S12.110
          nondisplaced S12.112
          posterior S12.111
        specified type NEC (displaced)
            S12.120
          nondisplaced S12.121
        nondisplaced S12.101
        specified type NEC (displaced)
            S12.190
          nondisplaced S12.191
      seventh (displaced) S12.600
        nondisplaced S12.601
        specified type NEC (displaced) S12.690
          nondisplaced S12.691
      sixth (displaced) S12.500
        nondisplaced S12.501
        specified type NEC (displaced)
            S12.590
          nondisplaced S12.591
      third (displaced) S12.200
        nondisplaced S12.201
        specified type NEC (displaced)
            S12.290
          nondisplaced S12.291

Fracture, traumatic *(Continued)*
  neck *(Continued)*
    hyoid bone S12.8
    larynx S12.8
    specified site NEC S12.8
    thyroid cartilage S12.8
    trachea S12.8
  neoplastic NEC —*see* Fracture, pathological,
      due to, neoplastic disease
  neural arch —*see* Fracture, vertebra
  newborn —*see* Birth, injury, fracture
  nontraumatic —*see* Fracture, pathological
  nonunion —*see* Nonunion, fracture
  nose, nasal (bone) (septum) S02.2
  occiput —*see* Fracture, skull, base, occiput
  odontoid process —*see* Fracture, neck,
      cervical vertebra, second
  olecranon (process) (ulna) —*see* Fracture,
      ulna, upper end, olecranon process
  orbit, orbital (bone) (region) S02.8-●
    floor (blow-out) S02.3-●
    roof S02.19
  os
    calcis —*see* Fracture, tarsal, calcaneus
    magnum —*see* Fracture, carpal, capitate
    pubis —*see* Fracture, pubis
  palate S02.8-●
  parietal bone (skull) S02.0
  patella S82.00-●
    comminuted (displaced) S82.04-●
      nondisplaced S82.04-●
    longitudinal (displaced) S82.02-●
      nondisplaced S82.02-●
    osteochondral (displaced) S82.01-●
      nondisplaced S82.01-●
    specified NEC S82.09-●
    transverse (displaced) S82.03-●
      nondisplaced S82.03-●
  pedicle (of vertebral arch) —*see* Fracture,
      vertebra
  pelvis, pelvic (bone) S32.9
    acetabulum —*see* Fracture, acetabulum
    circle —*see* Disruption, pelvic ring
    following insertion of implant, prosthesis
        or plate M96.65
    ilium —*see* Fracture, ilium
    ischium —*see* Fracture, ischium
    multiple
      with disruption of pelvic ring (circle) —
          see Disruption, pelvic ring
      without disruption of pelvic ring (circle)
          S32.82
    pubis —*see* Fracture, pubis
    sacrum —*see* Fracture, sacrum
    specified site NEC S32.89
  periprosthetic, around internal prosthetic
      joint M97.9
    ankle M97.2-●
    elbow M97.4-●
    finger M97.8
    hip M97.0-●
    knee M97.1-●
    shoulder M97.3-●
    specified joint NEC M97.8
    spine M97.8
    toe M97.8
    wrist M97.8
  phalanx
    foot —*see* Fracture, toe
    hand —*see* Fracture, finger
  pisiform —*see* Fracture, carpal, pisiform
  pond —*see* Fracture, skull
  prosthetic device, internal —*see*
      Complications, prosthetic device, by site,
      mechanical
  pubis S32.50-●
    with disruption of pelvic ring —*see*
        Disruption, pelvic ring
    specified site NEC S32.59-●
    superior rim S32.59-●

Fracture, traumatic *(Continued)*
  radius S52.9-●
    distal end —*see* Fracture, radius,
        lower end
    following insertion of implant, prosthesis
        or plate M96.63-●
    head —*see* Fracture, radius, upper end,
        head
    lower end S52.50-●
      Barton's —*see* Barton's fracture
      Colles' —*see* Colles' fracture
      extraarticular NEC S52.55-●
      intraarticular NEC S52.57-●
      physeal S59.20-●
        Salter-Harris
          Type I S59.21-●
          Type II S59.22-●
          Type III S59.23-●
          Type IV S59.24-●
        specified NEC S59.29-●
      Smith's —*see* Smith's fracture
      specified NEC S52.59-●
      styloid process (displaced) S52.51-●
        nondisplaced S52.51-●
      torus S52.52-●
    neck —*see* Fracture, radius, upper end
    proximal end —*see* Fracture, radius, upper
        end
    shaft S52.30-●
      bent bone S52.38-●
      comminuted (displaced) S52.35-●
        nondisplaced S52.35-●
      Galeazzi's —*see* Galeazzi's fracture
      greenstick S52.31-●
      oblique (displaced) S52.33-●
        nondisplaced S52.33-●
      segmental (displaced) S52.36-●
        nondisplaced S52.36-●
      specified NEC S52.39-●
      spiral (displaced) S52.34-●
        nondisplaced S52.34-●
      transverse (displaced) S52.32-●
        nondisplaced S52.32-●
    upper end S52.10-●
      head (displaced) S52.12-●
        nondisplaced S52.12-●
      neck (displaced) S52.13-●
        nondisplaced S52.13-●
      physeal S59.10-●
        Salter-Harris
          Type I S59.11-●
          Type II S59.12-●
          Type III S59.13-●
          Type IV S59.14-●
        specified NEC S59.19-●
      specified NEC S52.18-●
      torus S52.11-●
  ramus
    inferior or superior, pubis —*see* Fracture,
        pubis
    mandible —*see* Fracture, mandible
  restorative material (dental) K08.539
    with loss of material K08.531
    without loss of material K08.530
  rib S22.3-●
    with flail chest —*see* Flail, chest
    multiple S22.4-●
      with flail chest —*see* Flail, chest
  root, tooth —*see* Fracture, tooth
  sacrum S32.10
    specified NEC S32.19
    Type
      1 S32.14
      2 S32.15
      3 S32.16
      4 S32.17
    Zone
      I S32.119
        displaced (minimally) S32.111
          severely S32.112
        nondisplaced S32.110

▶ New   ⇒ Revised   ~~deleted~~ Deleted   ● Use Additional Character(s)

Fracture, traumatic *(Continued)*
  sacrum *(Continued)*
    Zone *(Continued)*
      II S32.129
        displaced (minimally) S32.121
          severely S32.122
        nondisplaced S32.120
      III S32.139
        displaced (minimally) S32.131
          severely S32.132
        nondisplaced S32.130
  scaphoid (hand) —*see also* Fracture, carpal, navicular
    foot —*see* Fracture, tarsal, navicular
  scapula S42.10-•
    acromial process (displaced) S42.12-•
      nondisplaced S42.12-•
    body (displaced) S42.11-•
      nondisplaced S42.11-•
    coracoid process (displaced) S42.13-•
      nondisplaced S42.13-•
    glenoid cavity (displaced) S42.14-•
      nondisplaced S42.14-•
    neck (displaced) S42.15-•
      nondisplaced S42.15-•
    specified NEC S42.19-•
  semilunar bone, wrist —*see* Fracture, carpal, lunate
  sequelae —*see* Sequelae, fracture
  sesamoid bone
    foot S92.81-•
    hand —*see* Fracture, carpal
    other —*see* Fracture, traumatic, by site
  shepherd's —*see* Fracture, tarsal, talus
  shoulder (girdle) S42.9-•
    blade —*see* Fracture, scapula
  sinus (ethmoid) (frontal) S02.19
  skull S02.91
    base S02.10-•
      occiput S02.119
        condyle S02.113
          type I S02.110
            left side S02.11B
            right side S02.11A
          type II S02.111
            left side S02.11D
            right side S02.11C
          type III S02.112
            left side S02.11F
            right side S02.11E
          specified NEC S02.118
            left side S02.11H
            right side S02.11G
      specified NEC S02.19-•
    birth injury P13.0
    frontal bone S02.0
    parietal bone S02.0
    specified site NEC S02.8
    temporal bone S02.19
    vault S02.0
  Smith's —*see* Smith's fracture
  sphenoid (bone) (sinus) S02.19
  spine —*see* Fracture, vertebra
  spinous process —*see* Fracture, vertebra
  spontaneous (cause unknown) —*see* Fracture, pathological
  stave (of thumb) —*see* Fracture, metacarpal, first
  sternum S22.20
    with flail chest —*see* Flail, chest
    body S22.22
    manubrium S22.21
    xiphoid (process) S22.24
  stress M84.30
    ankle M84.37-•
    carpus M84.34-•
    clavicle M84.31-•
    femoral neck M84.359
    femur M84.35-•
    fibula M84.36-•
    finger M84.34-•

Fracture, traumatic *(Continued)*
  stress *(Continued)*
    hip M84.359
    humerus M84.32-•
    ilium M84.350
    ischium M84.350
    metacarpus M84.34-•
    metatarsus M84.37-•
    neck —*see* Fracture, fatigue, vertebra
    pelvis M84.350
    radius M84.33-•
    rib M84.38
    scapula M84.31-•
    skull M84.38
    tarsus M84.37-•
    tibia M84.36-•
    toe M84.37-•
    ulna M84.33-•
    vertebra —*see* Fracture, fatigue, vertebra
  supracondylar, elbow —*see* Fracture, humerus, lower end, supracondylar
  symphysis pubis —*see* Fracture, pubis
  talus (ankle bone) —*see* Fracture, tarsal, talus
  tarsal bone(s) S92.20-•
    astragalus —*see* Fracture, tarsal, talus
    calcaneus S92.00-•
      anterior process (displaced) S92.02-•
        nondisplaced S92.02-•
      body (displaced) S92.01-•
        nondisplaced S92.01-•
      extraarticular NEC (displaced) S92.05-•
        nondisplaced S92.05-•
      intraarticular (displaced) S92.06-•
        nondisplaced S92.06-•
      physeal S99.00-•
        Salter-Harris
          Type I S99.01-•
          Type II S99.02-•
          Type III S99.03-•
          Type IV S99.04-•
        specified NEC S99.09-•
      tuberosity (displaced) S92.04-•
        avulsion (displaced) S92.03-•
          nondisplaced S92.03-•
        nondisplaced S92.04-•
    cuboid (displaced) S92.21-•
      nondisplaced S92.21-•
    cuneiform
      intermediate (displaced) S92.23-•
        nondisplaced S92.23-•
      lateral (displaced) S92.22-•
        nondisplaced S92.22-•
      medial (displaced) S92.24-•
        nondisplaced S92.24-•
    navicular (displaced) S92.25-•
      nondisplaced S92.25-•
    scaphoid —*see* Fracture, tarsal, navicular
    talus S92.10-•
      avulsion (displaced) S92.15-•
        nondisplaced S92.15-•
      body (displaced) S92.12-•
        nondisplaced S92.12-•
      dome (displaced) S92.14-•
        nondisplaced S92.14-•
      head (displaced) S92.12-•
        nondisplaced S92.12-•
      lateral process (displaced) S92.14-•
        nondisplaced S92.14-•
      neck (displaced) S92.11-•
        nondisplaced S92.11-•
      posterior process (displaced) S92.13-•
        nondisplaced S92.13-•
      specified NEC S92.19-•
  temporal bone (styloid) S02.19
  thorax (bony) S22.9
    with flail chest —*see* Flail, chest
    rib S22.3-•
      multiple S22.4-•
        with flail chest —*see* Flail, chest

Fracture, traumatic *(Continued)*
  thorax *(Continued)*
    sternum S22.20
      body S22.22
      manubrium S22.21
      xiphoid process S22.24
    vertebra (displaced) S22.009
      burst (stable) S22.001
        unstable S22.002
      eighth S22.069
        burst (stable) S22.061
          unstable S22.062
        specified type NEC S22.068
        wedge compression S22.060
      eleventh S22.089
        burst (stable) S22.081
          unstable S22.082
        specified type NEC S22.088
        wedge compression S22.080
      fifth S22.059
        burst (stable) S22.051
          unstable S22.052
        specified type NEC S22.058
        wedge compression S22.050
      first S22.019
        burst (stable) S22.011
          unstable S22.012
        specified type NEC S22.018
        wedge compression S22.010
      fourth S22.049
        burst (stable) S22.041
          unstable S22.042
        specified type NEC S22.048
        wedge compression S22.040
      ninth S22.079
        burst (stable) S22.071
          unstable S22.072
        specified type NEC S22.078
        wedge compression S22.070
      nondisplaced S22.001
      second S22.029
        burst (stable) S22.021
          unstable S22.022
        specified type NEC S22.028
        wedge compression S22.020
      seventh S22.069
        burst (stable) S22.061
          unstable S22.062
        specified type NEC S22.068
        wedge compression S22.060
      sixth S22.059
        burst (stable) S22.051
          unstable S22.052
        specified type NEC S22.058
        wedge compression S22.050
      specified type NEC S22.008
      tenth S22.079
        burst (stable) S22.071
          unstable S22.072
        specified type NEC S22.078
        wedge compression S22.070
      third S22.039
        burst (stable) S22.031
          unstable S22.032
        specified type NEC S22.038
        wedge compression S22.030
      twelfth S22.089
        burst (stable) S22.081
          unstable S22.082
        specified type NEC S22.088
        wedge compression S22.080
      wedge compression S22.000
  thumb S62.50-•
    distal phalanx (displaced) S62.52-•
      nondisplaced S62.52-•
    proximal phalanx (displaced) S62.51-•
      nondisplaced S62.51-•
  thyroid cartilage S12.8
  tibia (shaft) S82.20-•
    comminuted (displaced) S82.25-•
      nondisplaced S82.25-•

Fracture, traumatic *(Continued)*
  tibia *(Continued)*
    condyles —*see* Fracture, tibia, upper end
    distal end —*see* Fracture, tibia, lower end
    epiphysis
      lower —*see* Fracture, tibia, lower end
      upper —*see* Fracture, tibia, upper end
    following insertion of implant, prosthesis
      or plate M96.67-●
    head (involving knee joint) —*see* Fracture,
      tibia, upper end
    intercondyloid eminence —*see* Fracture,
      tibia, upper end
    involving ankle or malleolus —*see*
      Fracture, ankle, medial malleolus
    lower end S82.30-●
      physeal S89.10-●
        Salter-Harris
          Type I S89.11-●
          Type II S89.12-●
          Type III S89.13-●
          Type IV S89.14-●
        specified NEC S89.19-●
      pilon (displaced) S82.87-●
        nondisplaced S82.87-●
      specified NEC S82.39-●
      torus S82.31-●
    malleolus —*see* Fracture, ankle, medial
      malleolus
    oblique (displaced) S82.23-●
      nondisplaced S82.23-●
    pilon —*see* Fracture, tibia, lower end, pilon
    proximal end —*see* Fracture, tibia, upper
      end
    segmental (displaced) S82.26-●
      nondisplaced S82.26-●
    specified NEC S82.29-●
➡spine —*see* Fracture, tibia, upper end, spine
    spiral (displaced) S82.24-●
      nondisplaced S82.24-●
    transverse (displaced) S82.22-●
      nondisplaced S82.22-●
    tuberosity —*see* Fracture, tibia, upper end,
      tuberosity
    upper end S82.10-●
      bicondylar (displaced) S82.14-●
        nondisplaced S82.14-●
      lateral condyle (displaced) S82.12-●
        nondisplaced S82.12-●
      medial condyle (displaced) S82.13-●
        nondisplaced S82.13-●
      physeal S89.00-●
        Salter-Harris
          Type I S89.01-●
          Type II S89.02-●
          Type III S89.03-●
          Type IV S89.04-●
        specified NEC S89.09-●
      plateau —*see* Fracture, tibia, upper end,
        bicondylar
      specified NEC S82.19-●
      spine (displaced) S82.11-●
        nondisplaced S82.11-●
      torus S82.16-●
      tuberosity (displaced) S82.15-●
        nondisplaced S82.15-●
  toe S92.91-●
    great (displaced) S92.40-●
      distal phalanx (displaced) S92.42-●
        nondisplaced S92.42-●
      nondisplaced S92.40-●
      proximal phalanx (displaced)
        S92.41-●
        nondisplaced S92.41-●
      specified NEC S92.49-●
    lesser (displaced) S92.50-●
      distal phalanx (displaced) S92.53-●
        nondisplaced S92.53-●
      medial phalanx (displaced) S92.52-●
        nondisplaced S92.52-●
      nondisplaced S92.50-●

Fracture, traumatic *(Continued)*
  toe *(Continued)*
    lesser *(Continued)*
      proximal phalanx (displaced) S92.51-●
        nondisplaced S92.51-●
      specified NEC S92.59-●
    physeal
      phalanx S99.20-●
        Salter-Harris
          Type I S99.21-●
          Type II S99.22-●
          Type III S99.23-●
          Type IV S99.24-●
        specified NEC S99.29-●
  tooth (root) S02.5
  trachea (cartilage) S12.8
  transverse process —*see* Fracture, vertebra
  trapezium or trapezoid bone —*see* Fracture,
    carpal
  trimalleolar —*see* Fracture, ankle, trimalleolar
  triquetrum (cuneiform of carpus) —*see*
    Fracture, carpal, triquetrum
  trochanter —*see* Fracture, femur, trochanteric
  tuberosity (external) —*see* Fracture,
    traumatic, by site
  ulna (shaft) S52.20-●
    bent bone S52.28-●
    coronoid process —*see* Fracture, ulna,
      upper end, coronoid process
    distal end —*see* Fracture, ulna, lower end
    following insertion of implant, prosthesis
      or plate M96.63-●
➡ head S52.60-●
    lower end S52.60-●
      physeal S59.00-●
        Salter-Harris
          Type I S59.01-●
          Type II S59.02-●
          Type III S59.03-●
          Type IV S59.04-●
        specified NEC S59.09-●
      specified NEC S52.69-●
      styloid process (displaced) S52.61-●
        nondisplaced S52.61-●
      torus S52.62-●
    proximal end —*see* Fracture, ulna, upper
      end
    shaft S52.20-●
      comminuted (displaced) S52.25-●
        nondisplaced S52.25-●
      greenstick S52.21-●
      Monteggia's —*see* Monteggia's fracture
      oblique (displaced) S52.23-●
        nondisplaced S52.23-●
      segmental (displaced) S52.26-●
        nondisplaced S52.26-●
      specified NEC S52.29-●
      spiral (displaced) S52.24-●
        nondisplaced S52.24-●
      transverse (displaced) S52.22-●
        nondisplaced S52.22-●
    upper end S52.00-●
      coronoid process (displaced) S52.04-●
        nondisplaced S52.04-●
      olecranon process (displaced) S52.02-●
        with intraarticular extension S52.03-●
        nondisplaced S52.02-●
          with intraarticular extension S52.03-●
      specified NEC S52.09-●
      torus S52.01-●
  unciform —*see* Fracture, carpal, hamate
  vault of skull S02.0
  vertebra, vertebral (arch) (body) (column)
    (neural arch) (pedicle) (spinous process)
    (transverse process)
    atlas —*see* Fracture, neck, cervical vertebra,
      first
    axis —*see* Fracture, neck, cervical vertebra,
      second
    cervical (teardrop) S12.9
      axis —*see* Fracture, neck, cervical
        vertebra, second

Fracture, traumatic *(Continued)*
  vertebra, vertebral *(Continued)*
    cervical *(Continued)*
      first (atlas) —*see* Fracture, neck, cervical
        vertebra, first
      second (axis) —*see* Fracture, neck,
        cervical vertebra, second
    chronic M84.48
    coccyx S32.2
    dorsal —*see* Fracture, thorax, vertebra
    lumbar S32.009
      burst (stable) S32.001
        unstable S32.002
      fifth S32.059
        burst (stable) S32.051
          unstable S32.052
        specified type NEC S32.058
        wedge compression S32.050
      first S32.019
        burst (stable) S32.011
          unstable S32.012
        specified type NEC S32.018
        wedge compression S32.010
      fourth S32.049
        burst (stable) S32.041
          unstable S32.042
        specified type NEC S32.048
        wedge compression S32.040
      second S32.029
        burst (stable) S32.021
          unstable S32.022
        specified type NEC S32.028
        wedge compression S32.020
      specified type NEC S32.008
      third S32.039
        burst (stable) S32.031
          unstable S32.032
        specified type NEC S32.038
        wedge compression S32.030
      wedge compression S32.000
    metastatic —*see* Collapse, vertebra, in,
      specified disease NEC —*see also*
      Neoplasm
    newborn (birth injury) P11.5
    sacrum S32.10
      specified NEC S32.19
      Type
        1 S32.14
        2 S32.15
        3 S32.16
        4 S32.17
      Zone
        I S32.119
          displaced (minimally) S32.111
            severely S32.112
          nondisplaced S32.110
        II S32.129
          displaced (minimally) S32.121
            severely S32.122
          nondisplaced S32.120
        III S32.139
          displaced (minimally) S32.131
            severely S32.132
          nondisplaced S32.130
    thoracic —*see* Fracture, thorax, vertebra
  vertex S02.0
  vomer (bone) S02.2
  wrist S62.10-●
    carpal —*see* Fracture, carpal bone
    navicular (scaphoid) (hand) —*see* Fracture,
      carpal, navicular
  xiphisternum, xiphoid (process) S22.24
  zygoma S02.442
    left side S02.40F
    right side S02.40E
Fragile, fragility
  autosomal site Q95.5
  bone, congenital (with blue sclera) Q78.0
  capillary (hereditary) D69.8
  hair L67.8
  nails L60.3
  non-sex chromosome site Q95.5
  X chromosome Q99.2

▶ New   ➡ Revised   ~~deleted~~ Deleted   ● Use Additional Character(s)

Fragilitas
  crinium L67.8
  ossium (with blue sclerae) (hereditary) Q78.0
  unguium L60.3
    congenital Q84.6
Fragments, cataract (lens), following cataract
    surgery H59.02-●
  retained foreign body —see Retained, foreign
      body fragments (type of)
Frailty (frail) R54
  mental R41.81
Frambesia, frambesial (tropica) —see also Yaws
  initial lesion or ulcer A66.0
  primary A66.0
Frambeside
  gummatous A66.4
  of early yaws A66.2
Frambesioma A66.1
Franceschetti-Klein (-Wildervanck) disease or
    syndrome Q75.4
Francis' disease —see Tularemia
Franklin disease C88.2
Frank's essential thrombocytopenia D69.3
Fraser's syndrome Q87.0
Freckle(s) L81.2
  malignant melanoma in —see Melanoma
  melanotic (Hutchinson's) —see Melanoma,
      in situ
  retinal D49.81
Frederickson's hyperlipoproteinemia, type
    I and V E78.3
  IIA E78.00
  IIB and III E78.2
  IV E78.1
Freeman Sheldon syndrome Q87.0
Freezing —see also Effect, adverse, cold T69.9
Freiberg's disease (infraction of metatarsal head
    or osteochondrosis) —see Osteochondrosis,
    juvenile, metatarsus
Frei's disease A55
Fremitus, friction, cardiac R01.2
Frenum, frenulum
  external os Q51.828
  tongue (shortening) (congenital) Q38.1
Frequency micturition (nocturnal) R35.0
  psychogenic F45.8
Frey's syndrome
  auriculotemporal G50.8
  hyperhidrosis L74.52
Friction
  burn —see Burn, by site
  fremitus, cardiac R01.2
  precordial R01.2
  sounds, chest R09.89
Friderichsen-Waterhouse syndrome or disease
    A39.1
Friedländer's B (bacillus) NEC —see also
    condition A49.8
Friedreich's
  ataxia G11.1
  combined systemic disease G11.1
  facial hemihypertrophy Q67.4
  sclerosis (cerebellum) (spinal cord) G11.1
Frigidity F52.22
Fröhlich's syndrome E23.6
Frontal —see also condition
  lobe syndrome F07.0
Frostbite (superficial) T33.90
  with
    partial thickness skin loss —see Frostbite
        (superficial), by site
    tissue necrosis T34.90
  abdominal wall T33.3
    with tissue necrosis T34.3
  ankle T33.81-●
    with tissue necrosis T34.81-●
  arm T33.4-●
  with tissue necrosis T34.4-●
    finger(s) —see Frostbite, finger
    hand —see Frostbite, hand
    wrist —see Frostbite, wrist

Frostbite (Continued)
  ear T33.01-●
    with tissue necrosis T34.01-●
  face T33.09
    with tissue necrosis T34.09
  finger T33.53-●
    with tissue necrosis T34.53-●
  foot T33.82-●
    with tissue necrosis T34.82-●
  hand T33.52-●
    with tissue necrosis T34.52-●
  head T33.09
    with tissue necrosis T34.09
    ear —see Frostbite, ear
    nose —see Frostbite, nose
  hip (and thigh) T33.6-●
    with tissue necrosis T34.6-●
  knee T33.7-●
    with tissue necrosis T34.7-●
  leg T33.9-●
    with tissue necrosis T34.9-●
    ankle —see Frostbite, ankle
    foot —see Frostbite, foot
    knee —see Frostbite, knee
    lower T33.7-●
      with tissue necrosis T34.7-●
    thigh —see Frostbite, hip
    toe —see Frostbite, toe
  limb
    lower T33.99
      with tissue necrosis T34.99
    upper —see Frostbite, arm
  neck T33.1
    with tissue necrosis T34.1
  nose T33.02
    with tissue necrosis T34.02
  pelvis T33.3
    with tissue necrosis T34.3
  specified site NEC T33.99
    with tissue necrosis T34.99
  thigh —see Frostbite, hip
  thorax T33.2
    with tissue necrosis T34.2
  toes T33.83-●
    with tissue necrosis T34.83-●
  trunk T33.99
    with tissue necrosis T34.99
  wrist T33.51-●
    with tissue necrosis T34.51-●
Frotteurism F65.81
Frozen —see also Effect, adverse, cold T69.9
  pelvis (female) N94.89
    male K66.8
  shoulder —see Capsulitis, adhesive
Fructokinase deficiency E74.11
Fructose 1,6 diphosphatase deficiency E74.19
Fructosemia (benign) (essential) E74.12
Fructosuria (benign) (essential) E74.11
Fuchs'
➡black spot (myopic) —see also Myopia,
    degenerative H44.2-●
  dystrophy (corneal endothelium) H18.51
  heterochromic cyclitis —see Cyclitis, Fuchs'
      heterochromic
Fucosidosis E77.1
Fugue R68.89
  dissociative F44.1
  hysterical (dissociative) F44.1
  postictal in epilepsy —see Epilepsy
  reaction to exceptional stress (transient)
      F43.0
Fulminant, fulminating —see condition
Functional —see also condition
  bleeding (uterus) N93.8
Functioning, intellectual, borderline R41.83
Fundus —see condition
Fungemia NOS B49
Fungus, fungous
  cerebral G93.89
  disease NOS B49
  infection —see Infection, fungus

Funiculitis (acute) (chronic) (endemic)
    N49.1
  gonococcal (acute) (chronic) A54.23
  tuberculous A18.15
Funnel
  breast (acquired) M95.4
    congenital Q67.6
    sequelae (late effect) of rickets E64.3
  chest (acquired) M95.4
    congenital Q67.6
    sequelae (late effect) of rickets E64.3
  pelvis (acquired) M95.5
    with disproportion (fetopelvic) O33.3
      causing obstructed labor O65.3
    congenital Q74.2
FUO (fever of unknown origin) R50.9
Furfur L21.0
  microsporon B36.0
Furrier's lung J67.8
Furrowed K14.5
  nail(s) (transverse) L60.4
    congenital Q84.6
  tongue K14.5
    congenital Q38.3
Furuncle L02.92
  abdominal wall L02.221
  ankle —see Furuncle, lower limb
  antecubital space —see Furuncle, upper
      limb
  anus K61.0
  arm —see Furuncle, upper limb
  auditory canal, external —see Abscess, ear,
      external
  auricle (ear) —see Abscess, ear, external
  axilla (region) L02.42-●
  back (any part) L02.222
  breast N61.1
  buttock L02.32
  cheek (external) L02.02
  chest wall L02.223
  chin L02.02
  corpus cavernosum N48.21
  ear, external —see Abscess, ear, external
  external auditory canal —see Abscess, ear,
      external
  eyelid —see Abscess, eyelid
  face L02.02
  femoral (region) —see Furuncle, lower
      limb
  finger —see Furuncle, hand
  flank L02.221
  foot L02.62-●
  forehead L02.02
  gluteal (region) L02.32
  groin L02.224
  hand L02.52-●
  head L02.821
    face L02.02
  hip —see Furuncle, lower limb
  kidney —see Abscess, kidney
  knee —see Furuncle, lower limb
  labium (majus) (minus) N76.4
  lacrimal
    gland —see Dacryoadenitis
    passages (duct) (sac) —see Inflammation,
        lacrimal, passages, acute
  leg (any part) —see Furuncle, lower limb
  lower limb L02.42-●
  malignant A22.0
  mouth K12.2
  navel L02.226
  neck L02.12
  nose J34.0
  orbit, orbital —see Abscess, orbit
  palmar (space) —see Furuncle, hand
  partes posteriores L02.32
  pectoral region L02.223
  penis N48.21
  perineum L02.225
  pinna —see Abscess, ear, external
  popliteal —see Furuncle, lower limb

Furuncle *(Continued)*
  prepatellar —*see* Furuncle, lower limb
  scalp L02.821
  seminal vesicle N49.0
  shoulder —*see* Furuncle, upper limb
  specified site NEC L02.828
  submandibular K12.2
  temple (region) L02.02
  thumb —*see* Furuncle, hand
  toe —*see* Furuncle, foot
  trunk L02.229
    abdominal wall L02.221
    back L02.222
    chest wall L02.223
    groin L02.224
    perineum L02.225
    umbilicus L02.226
  umbilicus L02.226
  upper limb L02.42-●
  vulva N76.4
Furunculosis —*see* Furuncle
Fused —*see* Fusion, fused
Fusion, fused (congenital)
  astragaloscaphoid Q74.2
  atria Q21.1
  auditory canal Q16.1
  auricles, heart Q21.1
  binocular with defective stereopsis H53.32
  bone Q79.8
  cervical spine M43.22

Fusion, fused *(Continued)*
  choanal Q30.0
  commissure, mitral valve Q23.2
  cusps, heart valve NEC Q24.8
    mitral Q23.2
    pulmonary Q22.1
    tricuspid Q22.4
  ear ossicles Q16.3
  fingers Q70.0-●
  hymen Q52.3
  joint (acquired) —*see also* Ankylosis
    congenital Q74.8
  kidneys (incomplete) Q63.1
  labium (majus) (minus) Q52.5
  larynx and trachea Q34.8
  limb, congenital Q74.8
    lower Q74.2
    upper Q74.0
  lobes, lung Q33.8
  lumbosacral (acquired) M43.27
    arthrodesis status Z98.1
    congenital Q76.49
    postprocedural status Z98.1
  nares, nose, nasal, nostril(s) Q30.0
  organ or site not listed —*see* Anomaly,
    by site
  ossicles Q79.9
    auditory Q16.3
  pulmonic cusps Q22.1
  ribs Q76.6

Fusion, fused *(Continued)*
  sacroiliac (joint) (acquired) M43.28
    arthrodesis status Z98.1
    congenital Q74.2
    postprocedural status Z98.1
  spine (acquired) NEC M43.20
    arthrodesis status Z98.1
    cervical region M43.22
    cervicothoracic region M43.23
    congenital Q76.49
    lumbar M43.26
    lumbosacral region M43.27
    occipito-atlanto-axial region M43.21
    postoperative status Z98.1
    sacrococcygeal region M43.28
    thoracic region M43.24
    thoracolumbar region M43.25
  sublingual duct with submaxillary duct at
    opening in mouth Q38.4
  testes Q55.1
  toes Q70.2
  tooth, teeth K00.2
  trachea and esophagus Q39.8
  twins Q89.4
  vagina Q52.4
  ventricles, heart Q21.0
  vertebra (arch) —*see* Fusion, spine
  vulva Q52.5
Fusospirillosis (mouth) (tongue) (tonsil) A69.1
Fussy baby R68.12

G

Gain in weight (abnormal) (excessive) —*see also* Weight, gain
Gaisböck's disease (polycythemia hypertonica) D75.1
Gait abnormality R26.9
  ataxic R26.0
  falling R29.6
  hysterical (ataxic) (staggering) F44.4
  paralytic R26.1
  spastic R26.1
  specified type NEC R26.89
  staggering R26.0
  unsteadiness R26.81
  walking difficulty NEC R26.2
Galactocele (breast) N64.89
  puerperal, postpartum O92.79
Galactokinase deficiency E74.29
Galactophoritis N61.0
  gestational, puerperal, postpartum O91.2-•
Galactorrhea O92.6
  not associated with childbirth N64.3
Galactosemia (classic) (congenital) E74.21
Galactosuria E74.29
Galacturia R82.0
  schistosomiasis (bilharziasis) B65.0
▶GALD (gestational alloimmune liver disease) P78.84
Galeazzi's fracture S52.37-•
Galen's vein —*see* condition
Galeophobia F40.218
Gall duct —*see* condition
Gallbladder —*see also* condition
  acute K81.0
Gallop rhythm R00.8
Gallstone (colic) (cystic duct) (gallbladder) (impacted) (multiple) —*see also* Calculus, gallbladder
  with
    cholecystitis —*see* Calculus, gallbladder, with cholecystitis
  bile duct (common) (hepatic) —*see* Calculus, bile duct
  causing intestinal obstruction K56.3
  specified NEC K80.80
    with obstruction K80.81
Gambling Z72.6
  pathological (compulsive) F63.0
Gammopathy (of undetermined significance [MGUS]) D47.2
  associated with lymphoplasmacytic dyscrasia D47.2
  monoclonal D47.2
  polyclonal D89.0
Gamna's disease (siderotic splenomegaly) D73.1
Gamophobia F40.298
Gampsodactylia (congenital) Q66.7
Gamstorp's disease (adynamia episodica hereditaria) G72.3
Gandy-Nanta disease (siderotic splenomegaly) D73.1
Gang
  membership offenses Z72.810
Gangliocytoma D36.10
Ganglioglioma —*see* Neoplasm, uncertain behavior, by site
Ganglion (compound) (diffuse) (joint) (tendon (sheath)) M67.40
  ankle M67.47-•
  foot M67.47-•
  forearm M67.43-•
  hand M67.44-•
  lower leg M67.46-•
  multiple sites M67.49
  of yaws (early) (late) A66.6
  pelvic region M67.45-•
  periosteal —*see* Periostitis
  shoulder region M67.41-•
  specified site NEC M67.48
  thigh region M67.45-•

Ganglion *(Continued)*
  tuberculous A18.09
  upper arm M67.42-•
  wrist M67.43-•
Ganglioneuroblastoma —*see* Neoplasm, nerve, malignant
Ganglioneuroma D36.10
  malignant —*see* Neoplasm, nerve, malignant
Ganglioneuromatosis D36.10
Ganglionitis
  fifth nerve —*see* Neuralgia, trigeminal
  gasserian (postherpetic) (postzoster) B02.21
  geniculate G51.1
    newborn (birth injury) P11.3
    postherpetic, postzoster B02.21
  herpes zoster B02.21
  postherpetic geniculate B02.21
Gangliosidosis E75.10
  GM1 E75.19
  GM2 E75.00
    other specified E75.09
    Sandhoff disease E75.01
    Tay-Sachs disease E75.02
  GM3 E75.19
  mucolipidosis IV E75.11
Gangosa A66.5
Gangrene, gangrenous (connective tissue) (dropsical) (dry) (moist) (skin) (ulcer) —*see also* Necrosis I96
  with diabetes (mellitus) —*see* Diabetes, gangrene
  abdomen (wall) I96
  alveolar M27.3
  appendix K35.80
    with
      perforation or rupture K35.2
      peritoneal abscess K35.3
      peritonitis NEC K35.3
        generalized (with perforation or rupture) K35.2
        localized (with perforation or rupture) K35.3
  arteriosclerotic (general) (senile) —*see* Arteriosclerosis, extremities, with, gangrene
  auricle I96
  Bacillus welchii A48.0
  bladder (infectious) —*see* Cystitis, specified type NEC
  bowel, cecum, or colon —*see* Gangrene, intestine
  Clostridium perfringens or welchii A48.0
  cornea H18.89-•
  corpora cavernosa N48.29
    noninfective N48.89
  cutaneous, spreading I96
  decubital —*see* Ulcer, pressure, by site
  diabetic (any site) —*see* Diabetes, gangrene
  emphysematous —*see* Gangrene, gas
  epidemic —*see* Poisoning, food, noxious, plant
  epididymis (infectional) N45.1
  erysipelas —*see* Erysipelas
  extremity (lower) (upper) I96
  Fournier N49.3
    female N76.89
  fusospirochetal A69.0
  gallbladder —*see* Cholecystitis, acute
  gas (bacillus) A48.0
    following
      abortion —*see* Abortion by type complicated by infection
      ectopic or molar pregnancy O08.0
  glossitis K14.0
  hernia —*see* Hernia, by site, with gangrene
  intestine, intestinal (hemorrhagic) (massive) — *see also* Infarct, intestine K55.069
    with
      mesenteric embolism —*see also* Infarct, intestine K55.069
      obstruction —*see* Obstruction, intestine

Gangrene, gangrenous *(Continued)*
  laryngitis J04.0
  limb (lower) (upper) I96
  lung J85.0
    spirochetal A69.8
  lymphangitis I89.1
  Meleney's (synergistic) —*see* Ulcer, skin
  mesentery —*see also* Infarct, intestine K55.069
    with
      embolism —*see also* Infarct, intestine K55.069
      intestinal obstruction —*see* Obstruction, intestine
  mouth A69.0
  ovary —*see* Oophoritis
  pancreas —*see* Pancreatitis, acute
  penis N48.29
    noninfective N48.89
  perineum I96
  pharynx —*see also* Pharyngitis
    Vincent's A69.1
  presenile I73.1
  progressive synergistic —*see* Ulcer, skin
  pulmonary J85.0
  pulpal (dental) K04.1
  quinsy J36
  Raynaud's (symmetric gangrene) I73.01
  retropharyngeal J39.2
  scrotum N49.3
    noninfective N50.89
  senile (atherosclerotic) —*see* Arteriosclerosis, extremities, with, gangrene
  spermatic cord N49.1
    noninfective N50.89
  spine I96
  spirochetal NEC A69.8
  spreading cutaneous I96
  stomatitis A69.0
  symmetrical I73.01
  testis (infectional) N45.2
    noninfective N44.8
  throat —*see also* Pharyngitis
    diphtheritic A36.0
    Vincent's A69.1
  thyroid (gland) E07.89
  tooth (pulp) K04.1
  tuberculous NEC —*see* Tuberculosis
  tunica vaginalis N49.1
    noninfective N50.89
  umbilicus I96
  uterus —*see* Endometritis
  uvulitis K12.2
  vas deferens N49.1
    noninfective N50.89
  vulva N76.89
Ganister disease J62.8
Ganser's syndrome (hysterical) F44.89
Gardner-Diamond syndrome (autoerythrocyte sensitization) D69.2
Gargoylism E76.01
Garré's disease, osteitis (sclerosing), osteomyelitis —*see* Osteomyelitis, specified type NEC
Garrod's pad, knuckle M72.1
Gartner's duct
  cyst Q52.4
  persistent Q50.6
Gas R14.3
  asphyxiation, inhalation, poisoning, suffocation NEC —*see* Table of Drugs and Chemicals
  excessive R14.0
  gangrene A48.0
    following
      abortion —*see* Abortion by type complicated by infection
      ectopic or molar pregnancy O08.0
  on stomach R14.0
  pains R14.1
Gastralgia —*see also* Pain, abdominal
Gastrectasis K31.0
  psychogenic F45.8

Gastric —see condition
Gastrinoma
  malignant
    pancreas C25.4
    specified site NEC —see Neoplasm,
      malignant, by site
    unspecified site C25.4
  specified site —see Neoplasm, uncertain
    behavior
  unspecified site D37.9
Gastritis (simple) K29.70
  with bleeding K29.71
  acute (erosive) K29.00
    with bleeding K29.01
  alcoholic K29.20
    with bleeding K29.21
  allergic K29.60
    with bleeding K29.61
  atrophic (chronic) K29.40
    with bleeding K29.41
  chronic (antral) (fundal) K29.50
    with bleeding K29.51
    atrophic K29.40
      with bleeding K29.41
    superficial K29.30
      with bleeding K29.31
  dietary counseling and surveillance Z71.3
  due to diet deficiency E63.9
  eosinophilic K52.81
  giant hypertrophic K29.60
    with bleeding K29.61
  granulomatous K29.60
    with bleeding K29.61
  hypertrophic (mucosa) K29.60
    with bleeding K29.61
  nervous F54
  spastic K29.60
    with bleeding K29.61
  specified NEC K29.60
    with bleeding K29.61
  superficial chronic K29.30
    with bleeding K29.31
  tuberculous A18.83
  viral NEC A08.4
Gastrocarcinoma —see Neoplasm, malignant,
  stomach
Gastrocolic —see condition
Gastrodisciasis, gastrodiscoidiasis B66.8
Gastroduodenitis K29.90
  with bleeding K29.91
  virus, viral A08.4
    specified type NEC A08.39
Gastrodynia —see Pain, abdominal
Gastroenteritis (acute) (chronic) (noninfectious)
    (see also Enteritis) K52.9
  allergic K52.29
  with
    eosinophilic gastritis or gastroenteritis
      K52.81
    food protein-induced enterocolitis
      syndrome K52.21
    food protein-induced enteropathy K52.22
  dietetic —see also Gastroenteritis, allergic
    K52.29
  drug-induced K52.1
  due to
    Cryptosporidium A07.2
    drugs K52.1
    food poisoning —see Intoxication,
      foodborne
    radiation K52.0
  eosinophilic K52.81
  epidemic (infectious) A09
  food hypersensitivity —see also
    Gastroenteritis, allergic K52.29
  infectious —see Enteritis, infectious
  influenzal —see Influenza, with
    gastroenteritis
  noninfectious K52.9
    specified NEC K52.89
  rotaviral A08.0

Gastroenteritis (Continued)
  Salmonella A02.0
  toxic K52.1
  viral NEC A08.4
    acute infectious A08.39
      type Norwalk A08.11
    infantile (acute) A08.39
    Norwalk agent A08.11
    rotaviral A08.0
    severe of infants A08.39
    specified type NEC A08.39
Gastroenteropathy —see also Gastroenteritis
  K52.9
  acute, due to Norovirus A08.11
  acute, due to Norwalk agent A08.11
  infectious A09
Gastroenteroptosis K63.4
Gastroesophageal laceration-hemorrhage
  syndrome K22.6
Gastrointestinal —see condition
Gastrojejunal —see condition
Gastrojejunitis —see also Enteritis K52.9
Gastrojejunocolic —see condition
Gastroliths K31.89
Gastromalacia K31.89
Gastroparalysis K31.84
  diabetic —see Diabetes, gastroparalysis
Gastroparesis K31.84
  diabetic —see Diabetes, by type, with
    gastroparesis
Gastropathy K31.9
  congestive portal K31.89
  erythematous K29.70
  exudative K90.89
  portal hypertensive K31.89
Gastroptosis K31.89
Gastrorrhagia K92.2
  psychogenic F45.8
Gastroschisis (congenital) Q79.3
Gastrospasm (neurogenic) (reflex) K31.89
  neurotic F45.8
  psychogenic F45.8
Gastrostaxis —see Gastritis, with bleeding
Gastrostenosis K31.89
Gastrostomy
  attention to Z43.1
  status Z93.1
Gastrosuccorrhea (continuous) (intermittent)
  K31.89
  neurotic F45.8
  psychogenic F45.8
Gatophobia F40.218
Gaucher's disease or splenomegaly (adult)
    (infantile) E75.22
Gee (-Herter)(-Thaysen) disease (nontropical
    sprue) K90.0
Gélineau's syndrome G47.419
  with cataplexy G47.411
Gemination, tooth, teeth K00.2
Gemistocytoma
  specified site —see Neoplasm, malignant, by
    site
  unspecified site C71.9
General, generalized —see condition
Genetic
  carrier (status)
    cystic fibrosis Z14.1
    hemophilia A (asymptomatic) Z14.01
      symptomatic Z14.02
    specified NEC Z14.8
  susceptibility to disease NEC Z15.89
    malignant neoplasm Z15.09
      breast Z15.01
      endometrium Z15.04
      ovary Z15.02
      prostate Z15.03
      specified NEC Z15.09
    multiple endocrine neoplasia Z15.81
Genital —see condition
Genito-anorectal syndrome A55
Genitourinary system —see condition

Genu
  congenital Q74.1
  extrorsum (acquired) —see also Deformity,
    varus, knee
    congenital Q74.1
    sequelae (late effect) of rickets E64.3
  introrsum (acquired) —see also Deformity,
    valgus, knee
    congenital Q74.1
    sequelae (late effect) of rickets E64.3
  rachitic (old) E64.3
  recurvatum (acquired) —see also Deformity,
    limb, specified type NEC, lower leg
    congenital Q68.2
    sequelae (late effect) of rickets E64.3
  valgum (acquired) (knock-knee) M21.06-●
    congenital Q74.1
    sequelae (late effect) of rickets E64.3
  varum (acquired) (bowleg) M21.16-●
    congenital Q74.1
    sequelae (late effect) of rickets E64.3
Geographic tongue K14.1
Geophagia —see Pica
Geotrichosis B48.3
  stomatitis B48.3
Gephyrophobia F40.242
Gerbode defect Q21.0
GERD (gastroesophageal reflux disease) K21.9
Gerhardt's
  disease (erythromelalgia) I73.81
  syndrome (vocal cord paralysis)
    J38.00
    bilateral J38.02
    unilateral J38.01
German measles —see also Rubella
  exposure to Z20.4
Germinoblastoma (diffuse) C85.9-●
  follicular C82.9-●
Germinoma —see Neoplasm, malignant, by site
Gerontoxon —see Degeneration, cornea, senile
Gerstmann-Sträussler-Scheinker syndrome
  (GSS) A81.82
Gerstmann's syndrome R48.8
  developmental F81.2
Gestation (period) —see also Pregnancy
  ectopic —see Pregnancy, by site
  multiple O30.9-●
    greater than quadruplets —see Pregnancy,
      multiple (gestation), specified NEC
    specified NEC —see Pregnancy, multiple
      (gestation), specified NEC
Gestational
  mammary abscess O91.11-●
  purulent mastitis O91.11-●
  subareolar abscess O91.11-●
Ghon tubercle, primary infection A15.7
Ghost
  teeth K00.4
  vessels (cornea) H16.41-●
Ghoul hand A66.3
Gianotti-Crosti disease L44.4
Giant
  cell
    epulis K06.8
    peripheral granuloma K06.8
  esophagus, congenital Q39.5
  kidney, congenital Q63.3
  urticaria T78.3
    hereditary D84.1
Giardiasis A07.1
Gibert's disease or pityriasis L42
Giddiness R42
  hysterical F44.89
  psychogenic F45.8
Gierke's disease (glycogenosis I) E74.01
Gigantism (cerebral) (hypophyseal) (pituitary)
  E22.0
  constitutional E34.4
Gilbert's disease or syndrome E80.4
Gilchrist's disease B40.9
Gilford-Hutchinson disease E34.8

▶ New   ⇒ Revised   ~~deleted~~ Deleted   ● Use Additional Character(s)

Gilles de la Tourette's disease or syndrome (motor-verbal tic) F95.2
Gingivitis K05.10
  acute (catarrhal) K05.00
    necrotizing A69.1
    nonplaque induced K05.01
    plaque induced K05.00
  chronic (desquamative) (hyperplastic) (simple marginal) (pregnancy associated) (ulcerative) K05.10
    nonplaque induced K05.11
    plaque induced K05.10
  expulsiva —see Periodontitis
  necrotizing ulcerative (acute) A69.1
  pellagrous E52
    acute necrotizing A69.1
  Vincent's A69.1
Gingivoglossitis K14.0
Gingivopericementitis —see Periodontitis
Gingivosis —see Gingivitis, chronic
Gingivostomatitis K05.10
  herpesviral B00.2
  necrotizing ulcerative (acute) A69.1
Gland, glandular —see condition
Glanders A24.0
Glanzmann (-Naegeli) disease or thrombasthenia D69.1
Glasgow coma scale
  total score
    3-8 R40.243
    9-12 R40.242
    13-15 R40.241
Glass-blower's disease (cataract) —see Cataract, specified NEC
Glaucoma H40.9
  with
    increased episcleral venous pressure H40.81-●
    pseudoexfoliation of lens —see Glaucoma, open angle, primary, capsular
  absolute H44.51-●
  angle-closure (primary) H40.20-●
    acute (attack) (crisis) H40.21-●
    chronic H40.22-●
    intermittent H40.23-●
    residual stage H40.24-●
  borderline H40.00-●
  capsular (with pseudoexfoliation of lens) —see Glaucoma, open angle, primary, capsular
  childhood Q15.0
  closed angle —see Glaucoma, angle-closure
  congenital Q15.0
  corticosteroid-induced —see Glaucoma, secondary, drugs
  hypersecretion H40.82-●
  in (due to)
    amyloidosis E85.4 [H42]
    aniridia Q13.1 [H42]
    concussion of globe —see Glaucoma, secondary, trauma
    dislocation of lens —see Glaucoma, secondary
    disorder of lens NEC —see Glaucoma, secondary
    drugs —see Glaucoma, secondary, drugs
    endocrine disease NOS E34.9 [H42]
    eye
      inflammation —see Glaucoma, secondary, inflammation
      trauma —see Glaucoma, secondary, trauma
    hypermature cataract —see Glaucoma, secondary
    iridocyclitis —see Glaucoma, secondary, inflammation
    lens disorder —see Glaucoma, secondary, Lowe's syndrome E72.03 [H42]
    metabolic disease NOS E88.9 [H42]
    ocular disorders NEC —see Glaucoma, secondary

Glaucoma (Continued)
  in (due to) (Continued)
    onchocerciasis B73.02
    pupillary block —see Glaucoma, secondary
    retinal vein occlusion —see Glaucoma, secondary
    Rieger's anomaly Q13.81 [H42]
    rubeosis of iris —see Glaucoma, secondary
    tumor of globe —see Glaucoma, secondary
  infantile Q15.0
  low tension —see Glaucoma, open angle, primary, low-tension
  malignant H40.83-●
  narrow angle —see Glaucoma, angle-closure
  newborn Q15.0
  noncongestive (chronic) —see Glaucoma, open angle
  nonobstructive —see Glaucoma, open angle
  obstructive —see also Glaucoma, angle-closure
    due to lens changes —see Glaucoma, secondary
  open angle H40.10-●
    primary H40.11-●
      capsular (with pseudoexfoliation of lens) H40.14-●
      low-tension H40.12-●
      pigmentary H40.13-●
      residual stage H40.15-●
  phacolytic —see Glaucoma, secondary
  pigmentary —see Glaucoma, open angle, primary, pigmentary
  postinfectious —see Glaucoma, secondary, inflammation
  secondary (to) H40.5-●
    drugs H40.6-●
    inflammation H40.4-●
    trauma H40.3-●
  simple (chronic) H40.11-●
  simplex H40.11-●
  specified type NEC H40.89
  suspect H40.00-●
  syphilitic A52.71
  traumatic —see also Glaucoma, secondary, trauma
    newborn (birth injury) P15.3
  tuberculous A18.59
Glaucomatous flecks (subcapsular) —see Cataract, complicated
Glazed tongue K14.4
Gleet (gonococcal) A54.01
Glénard's disease K63.4
Glioblastoma (multiforme)
  with sarcomatous component
    specified site —see Neoplasm, malignant, by site
    unspecified site C71.9
  giant cell
    specified site —see Neoplasm, malignant, tumor by site
    unspecified site C71.9
  specified site —see Neoplasm, malignant, by site
  unspecified site C71.9
Glioma (malignant)
  astrocytic
    specified site —see Neoplasm, malignant, by site
    unspecified site C71.9
  mixed
    specified site —see Neoplasm, malignant, by site
    unspecified site C71.9
  nose Q30.8
  specified site NEC —see Neoplasm, malignant, by site
  subependymal D43.2
    specified site —see Neoplasm, uncertain behavior, by site
    unspecified site D43.2
  unspecified site C71.9

Gliomatosis cerebri C71.0
Glioneuroma —see Neoplasm, uncertain behavior, by site
Gliosarcoma
  specified site —see Neoplasm, malignant, by site
  unspecified site C71.9
Gliosis (cerebral) G93.89
  spinal G95.89
Glisson's disease —see Rickets
Globinuria R82.3
Globus (hystericus) F45.8
Glomangioma D18.00
  intra-abdominal D18.03
  intracranial D18.02
  skin D18.01
  specified site NEC D18.09
Glomangiomyoma D18.00
  intra-abdominal D18.03
  intracranial D18.02
  skin D18.01
  specified site NEC D18.09
Glomangiosarcoma —see Neoplasm, connective tissue, malignant
Glomerular
  disease in syphilis A52.75
  nephritis —see Glomerulonephritis
Glomerulitis —see Glomerulonephritis
Glomerulonephritis —see also Nephritis N05.9
  with
    edema —see Nephrosis
    minimal change N05.0
    minor glomerular abnormality N05.0
  acute N00.9
  chronic N03.9
  crescentic (diffuse) NEC —see also N00-N07 with fourth character .7 N05.7
  dense deposit —see also N00-N07 with fourth character .6 N05.6
  diffuse
    crescentic —see also N00-N07 with fourth character .7 N05.7
    endocapillary proliferative —see also N00N07 with fourth character .4 N05.4
    membranous —see also N00-N07 with fourth character .2 N05.2
    mesangial proliferative —see also N00-N07 with fourth character .3 N05.3
    mesangiocapillary —see also N00-N07 with fourth character .5 N05.5
  sclerosing N18.9
  endocapillary proliferative (diffuse) NEC —see also N00-N07 with fourth character .4 N05.4
  extracapillary NEC —see also N00-N07 with fourth character .7 N05.7
  focal (and segmental) —see also N00-N07 with fourth character .1 N05.1
  hypocomplementemic —see Glomerulonephritis, membranoproliferative
  IgA —see Nephropathy, IgA
  immune complex (circulating) NEC N05.8
  in (due to)
    amyloidosis E85.4 [N08]
    bilharziasis B65.9 [N08]
    cryoglobulinemia D89.1 [N08]
    defibrination syndrome D65 [N08]
    diabetes mellitus —see Diabetes, glomerulosclerosis
    disseminated intravascular coagulation D65 [N08]
    Fabry (-Anderson) disease E75.21 [N08]
    Goodpasture's syndrome M31.0
    hemolytic-uremic syndrome D59.3
    Henoch (-Schönlein) purpura D69.0 [N08]
    lecithin cholesterol acyltransferase deficiency E78.6 [N08]

Glomerulonephritis *(Continued)*
  in *(Continued)*
    microscopic polyangiitis M31.7 *[N08]*
    multiple myeloma C90.0-● *[N08]*
    Plasmodium malariae B52.0
    schistosomiasis B65.9 *[N08]*
    sepsis A41.9-● *[N08]*
      streptococcal A40-● *[N08]*
    sickle-cell disorders D57.-● *[N08]*
    strongyloidiasis B78.9 *[N08]*
    subacute bacterial endocarditis I33.0
      [N08]
    syphilis (late) congenital A50.59 *[N08]*
    systemic lupus erythematosus M32.14
    thrombotic thrombocytopenic purpura
      M31.1 *[N08]*
    typhoid fever A01.09
    Waldenström macroglobulinemia C88.0
      [N08]
    Wegener's granulomatosis M31.31
  latent or quiescent N03.9
  lobular, lobulonodular —
    see Glomerulonephritis,
    membranoproliferative
  membranoproliferative (diffuse) (type 1
    or 3) —*see also* N00-N07 with fourth
    character .5 N05.5
    dense deposit (type 2) NEC —*see also*
      N00-N07 with fourth character .6
      N05.6
  membranous (diffuse) NEC —*see also*
    N00-N07 with fourth character .2 N05.2
  mesangial
    IgA/IgG —*see* Nephropathy, IgA
    proliferative (diffuse) NEC —*see also*
      N00-N07 with fourth character .3
      N05.3
  mesangiocapillary (diffuse) NEC —*see also*
    N00-N07 with fourth character .5 N05.5
  necrotic, necrotizing NEC —*see also* N00-N07
    with fourth character .8 N05.8
  nodular —*see* Glomerulonephritis,
    membranoproliferative
  poststreptococcal NEC N05.9
    acute N00.9
    chronic N03.9
    rapidly progressive N01.9
  proliferative NEC —*see also* N00-N07 with
    fourth character .8 N05.8
    diffuse (lupus) M32.14
  rapidly progressive N01.9
  sclerosing, diffuse N18.9
  specified pathology NEC —*see also* N00-N07
    with fourth character .8 N05.8
  subacute N01.9
Glomerulopathy —*see* Glomerulonephritis
Glomerulosclerosis —*see also* Sclerosis, renal
  intercapillary (nodular) (with diabetes) —*see*
    Diabetes, glomerulosclerosis
  intracapillary —*see* Diabetes,
    glomerulosclerosis
Glossagra K14.6
Glossalgia K14.6
Glossitis (chronic superficial) (gangrenous)
  (Moeller's) K14.0
  areata exfoliativa K14.1
  atrophic K14.4
  benign migratory K14.1
  cortical superficial, sclerotic K14.0
  Hunter's D51.0
  interstitial, sclerous K14.0
  median rhomboid K14.2
  pellagrous E52
  superficial, chronic K14.0
Glossocele K14.8
Glossodynia K14.6
  exfoliativa K14.4
Glossoncus K14.8
Glossopathy K14.9
Glossophytia K14.3
Glossoplegia K14.8

Glossoptosis K14.8
Glossopyrosis K14.6
Glossotrichia K14.3
Glossy skin L90.8
Glottis —*see* condition
Glottitis —*see also* Laryngitis J04.0
Glucagonoma
  pancreas
    benign D13.7
    malignant C25.4
    uncertain behavior D37.8
  specified site NEC
    benign —*see* Neoplasm, benign, by site
    malignant —*see* Neoplasm, malignant, by
      site
    uncertain behavior —*see* Neoplasm,
      uncertain behavior, by site
  unspecified site
    benign D13.7
    malignant C25.4
    uncertain behavior D37.8
Glucoglycinuria E72.51
Glucose-galactose malabsorption E74.39
Glue
  ear —*see* Otitis, media, nonsuppurative,
    chronic, mucoid
  sniffing (airplane) —*see* Abuse, drug,
    inhalant
    dependence —*see* Dependence, drug,
      inhalant
Glutaric aciduria E72.3
Glycinemia E72.51
Glycinuria (renal) (with ketosis) E72.09
Glycogen
  infiltration —*see* Disease, glycogen storage
  storage disease —*see* Disease, glycogen
    storage
Glycogenosis (diffuse) (generalized) —*see also*
  Disease, glycogen storage
  cardiac E74.02 *[I43]*
  diabetic, secondary —*see* Diabetes,
    glycogenosis, secondary
  pulmonary interstitial J84.842
Glycopenia E16.2
Glycosuria R81
  renal E74.8
Gnathostoma spinigerum (infection)
  (infestation), **gnathostomiasis** (wandering
  swelling) B83.1
Goiter (plunging) (substernal) E04.9
  with
    hyperthyroidism (recurrent) —*see*
      Hyperthyroidism, with, goiter
    thyrotoxicosis —*see* Hyperthyroidism,
      with, goiter
  adenomatous —*see* Goiter, nodular
  cancerous C73
  congenital (nontoxic) E03.0
    diffuse E03.0
    parenchymatous E03.0
    transitory, with normal functioning
      P72.0
  cystic E04.2
    due to iodine-deficiency E01.1
  due to
    enzyme defect in synthesis of thyroid
      hormone E07.1
    iodine-deficiency (endemic) E01.2
  dyshormonogenetic (familial) E07.1
  endemic (iodine-deficiency) E01.2
    diffuse E01.0
    multinodular E01.1
  exophthalmic —*see* Hyperthyroidism, with,
    goiter
  iodine-deficiency (endemic) E01.2
    diffuse E01.0
    multinodular E01.1
    nodular E01.1
  lingual Q89.2
  lymphadenoid E06.3
  malignant C73

Goiter *(Continued)*
  multinodular (cystic) (nontoxic) E04.2
    toxic or with hyperthyroidism E05.20
      with thyroid storm E05.21
  neonatal NEC P72.0
  nodular (nontoxic) (due to) E04.9
    with
      hyperthyroidism E05.20
        with thyroid storm E05.21
      thyrotoxicosis E05.20
        with thyroid storm E05.21
    endemic E01.1
    iodine-deficiency E01.1
    sporadic E04.9
    toxic E05.20
      with thyroid storm E05.21
  nontoxic E04.9
    diffuse (colloid) E04.0
    multinodular E04.2
    simple E04.0
    specified NEC E04.8
    uninodular E04.1
  simple E04.0
  toxic —*see* Hyperthyroidism, with, goiter
  uninodular (nontoxic) E04.1
    toxic or with hyperthyroidism E05.10
      with thyroid storm E05.11
Goiter-deafness syndrome E07.1
Goldberg syndrome Q89.8
Goldberg-Maxwell syndrome E34.51
Goldblatt's hypertension or kidney I70.1
Goldenhar (-Gorlin) syndrome Q87.0
Goldflam-Erb disease or syndrome G70.00
  with exacerbation (acute) G70.01
  in crisis G70.01
Goldscheider's disease Q81.8
Goldstein's disease (familial hemorrhagic
  telangiectasia) I78.0
Golfer's elbow —*see* Epicondylitis, medial
Gonadoblastoma
  specified site —*see* Neoplasm, uncertain
    behavior, by site
  unspecified site
    female D39.10
    male D40.10
Gonecystitis —*see* Vesiculitis
Gongylonemiasis B83.8
Goniosynechiae —*see* Adhesions, iris,
  goniosynechiae
Gonococcemia A54.86
Gonococcus, gonococcal (disease) (infection)
  —*see also* condition A54.9
  anus A54.6
  bursa, bursitis A54.49
  conjunctiva, conjunctivitis (neonatorum)
    A54.31
  endocardium A54.83
  eye A54.30
    conjunctivitis A54.31
    iridocyclitis A54.32
    keratitis A54.33
    newborn A54.31
    other specified A54.39
  fallopian tubes (acute) (chronic) A54.24
  genitourinary (organ) (system) (tract) (acute)
    lower A54.00
      with abscess (accessory gland)
        (periurethral) A54.1
    upper —*see also* condition A54.29
  heart A54.83
  iridocyclitis A54.32
  joint A54.42
  lymphatic (gland) (node) A54.89
  meninges, meningitis A54.81
  musculoskeletal A54.40
    arthritis A54.42
    osteomyelitis A54.43
    other specified A54.49
    spondylopathy A54.41
  pelviperitonitis A54.24
  pelvis (acute) (chronic) A54.24

Gonococcus, gonococcal (Continued)
  pharynx A54.5
  proctitis A54.6
  pyosalpinx (acute) (chronic) A54.24
  rectum A54.6
  skin A54.89
  specified site NEC A54.89
  tendon sheath A54.49
  throat A54.5
  urethra (acute) (chronic) A54.01
    with abscess (accessory gland)
      (periurethral) A54.1
  vulva (acute) (chronic) A54.02
Gonocytoma
  specified site —see Neoplasm, uncertain
    behavior, by site
  unspecified site
    female D39.10
    male D40.10
Gonorrhea (acute) (chronic) A54.9
  Bartholin's gland (acute) (chronic) (purulent)
    A54.02
    with abscess (accessory gland)
      (periurethral) A54.1
  bladder A54.01
  cervix A54.03
  conjunctiva, conjunctivitis (neonatorum)
    A54.31
  contact Z20.2
  Cowper's gland (with abscess) A54.1
  exposure to Z20.2
  fallopian tube (acute) (chronic) A54.24
  kidney (acute) (chronic) A54.21
  lower genitourinary tract A54.00
    with abscess (accessory gland)
      (periurethral) A54.1
  ovary (acute) (chronic) A54.24
  pelvis (acute) (chronic) A54.24
    female pelvic inflammatory disease A54.24
  penis A54.09
  prostate (acute) (chronic) A54.22
  seminal vesicle (acute) (chronic) A54.23
  specified site not listed —see also Gonococcus
    A54.89
  spermatic cord (acute) (chronic) A54.23
  urethra A54.01
    with abscess (accessory gland)
      (periurethral) A54.1
  vagina A54.02
  vas deferens (acute) (chronic) A54.23
  vulva A54.02
Goodall's disease A08.19
Goodpasture's syndrome M31.0
Gopalan's syndrome (burning feet) E53.0
Gorlin-Chaudry-Moss syndrome Q87.0
Gottron's papules L94.4
Gougerot's syndrome (trisymptomatic) L81.7
Gougerot-Blum syndrome (pigmented
  purpuric lichenoid dermatitis) L81.7
Gougerot-Carteaud disease or syndrome
  (confluent reticulate papillomatosis) L83
Gouley's syndrome (constrictive pericarditis)
  I31.1
Goundou A66.6
Gout, chronic (see also Gout, gouty) M1A.9-●
  drug-induced M1A.20
    ankle M1A.27-●
    elbow M1A.22-●
    foot joint M1A.27-●
    hand joint M1A.24-●
    hip M1A.25-●
    knee M1A.26-●
    multiple site M1A.29-●
    shoulder M1A.21-●
    vertebrae M1A.28
    wrist M1A.23-●
  idiopathic M1A.00
    ankle M1A.07-●
    elbow M1A.02-●
    foot joint M1A.07-●
    hand joint M1A.04-●

Gout, chronic (Continued)
  idiopathic (Continued)
    hip M1A.05-●
    knee M1A.06-●
    multiple site M1A.09
    shoulder M1A.01-●
    vertebrae M1A.08
    wrist M1A.03-●
  in (due to) renal impairment M1A.30
    ankle M1A.37-●
    elbow M1A.32-●
    foot joint M1A.37-●
    hand joint M1A.34-●
    hip M1A.35-●
    knee M1A.36-●
    multiple site M1A.39
    shoulder M1A.31-●
    vertebrae M1A.38
    wrist M1A.33-●
  lead-induced M1A.10
    ankle M1A.17-●
    elbow M1A.12-●
    foot joint M1A.17-●
    hand joint M1A.14-●
    hip M1A.15-●
    knee M1A.16-●
    multiple site M1A.19
    shoulder M1A.11-●
    vertebrae M1A.18
    wrist M1A.13-●
  primary —see Gout, chronic, idiopathic
  saturnine —see Gout, chronic, lead-induced
  secondary NEC M1A.40
    ankle M1A.47-●
    elbow M1A.42-●
    foot joint M1A.47-●
    hand joint M1A.44-●
    hip M1A.45-●
    knee M1A.46-●
    multiple site M1A.49
    shoulder M1A.41-●
    vertebrae M1A.48
    wrist M1A.43-●
  syphilitic —see also subcategory M14.8-●
    A52.77
  tophi M1A.9
Gout, gouty (acute) (attack) (flare) —see also
  Gout, chronic M10.9-●
  drug-induced M10.20
    ankle M10.27-●
    elbow M10.22-●
    foot joint M10.27-●
    hand joint M10.24-●
    hip M10.25-●
    knee M10.26-●
    multiple site M10.29
    shoulder M10.21-●
    vertebrae M10.28
    wrist M10.23-●
  idiopathic M10.00
    ankle M10.07-●
    elbow M10.02-●
    foot joint M10.07-●
    hand joint M10.04-●
    hip M10.05-●
    knee M10.06-●
    multiple site M10.09
    shoulder M10.01-●
    vertebrae M10.08
    wrist M10.03-●
  in (due to) renal impairment M10.30
    ankle M10.37-●
    elbow M10.32-●
    foot joint M10.37-●
    hand joint M10.34-●
    hip M10.35-●
    knee M10.36-●
    multiple site M10.39
    shoulder M10.31-●
    vertebrae M10.38
    wrist M10.33-●

Gout, gouty (Continued)
  lead-induced M10.10
    ankle M10.17-●
    elbow M10.12-●
    foot joint M10.17-●
    hand joint M10.14-●
    hip M10.15-●
    knee M10.16-●
    multiple site M10.19
    shoulder M10.11-●
    vertebrae M10.18
    wrist M10.13-●
  primary —see Gout, idiopathic
  saturnine —see Gout, lead-induced
  secondary NEC M10.40
    ankle M10.47-●
    elbow M10.42-●
    foot joint M10.47-●
    hand joint M10.44-●
    hip M10.45-●
    knee M10.46-●
    multiple site M10.49
    shoulder M10.41-●
    vertebrae M10.48
    wrist M10.43-●
  syphilitic —see also subcategory M14.8-●
    A52.77
  tophi NEC —see Gout, chronic
Gower's
  muscular dystrophy G71.0
  syndrome (vasovagal attack) R55
Gradenigo's syndrome —see Otitis, media,
  suppurative, acute
Graefe's disease —see Strabismus, paralytic,
  ophthalmoplegia, progressive
Graft-versus-host disease D89.813
  acute D89.810
  acute on chronic D89.812
  chronic D89.811
Grain mite (itch) B88.0
Grainhandler's disease or lung J67.8
Grand mal —see Epilepsy, generalized,
  specified NEC
Grand multipara status only (not pregnant)
  Z64.1
  pregnant —see Pregnancy, complicated by,
    grand multiparity
Granite worker's lung J62.8
Granular —see also condition
  inflammation, pharynx J31.2
  kidney (contracting) —see Sclerosis, renal
  liver K74.69
Granulation tissue (abnormal) (excessive) L92.9
  postmastoidectomy cavity —see
    Complications, postmastoidectomy,
    granulation
Granulocytopenia (primary) (malignant) —see
  Agranulocytosis
Granuloma L92.9
  abdomen K66.8
    from residual foreign body L92.3
    pyogenicum L98.0
  actinic L57.5
  annulare (perforating) L92.0
  apical K04.5
  aural —see Otitis, externa, specified NEC
  beryllium (skin) L92.3
  bone
    eosinophilic C96.6
    from residual foreign body —see
      Osteomyelitis, specified type NEC
    lung C96.6
  brain (any site) G06.0
    schistosomiasis B65.9 [G07]
  canaliculus lacrimalis —see Granuloma,
    lacrimal
  candidal (cutaneous) B37.2
  cerebral (any site) G06.0
  coccidioidal (primary) (progressive) B38.7
    lung B38.1
    meninges B38.4

Granuloma (*Continued*)
  colon K63.89
  conjunctiva H11.22-●
  dental K04.5
  ear, middle —*see* Cholesteatoma
  eosinophilic C96.6
    bone C96.6
    lung C96.6
    oral mucosa K13.4
    skin L92.2
  eyelid H01.8
  facial (e) L92.2
  foreign body (in soft tissue) NEC M60.20
    ankle M60.27-●
    foot M60.27-●
    forearm M60.23-●
    hand M60.24-●
    in operation wound —*see* Foreign body,
      accidentally left during a procedure
    lower leg M60.26-●
    pelvic region M60.25-●
    shoulder region M60.21-●
    skin L92.3
    specified site NEC M60.28
    subcutaneous tissue L92.3
    thigh M60.25-●
    upper arm M60.22-●
  gangraenescens M31.2
  genito-inguinale A58
  giant cell (central) (reparative) (jaw) M27.1
    gingiva (peripheral) K06.8
  gland (lymph) I88.8
  hepatic NEC K75.3
    in (due to)
      berylliosis J63.2 [K77]
      sarcoidosis D86.89
  Hodgkin C81.9
  ileum K63.89
  infectious B99.9
    specified NEC B99.8
  inguinale (Donovan) (venereal) A58
  intestine NEC K63.89
  intracranial (any site) G06.0
  intraspinal (any part) G06.1
  iridocyclitis —*see* Iridocyclitis, chronic
  jaw (bone) (central) M27.1
    reparative giant cell M27.1
  kidney —*see also* Infection, kidney N15.8
  lacrimal H04.81-●
  larynx J38.7
  lethal midline (faciale (e)) M31.2
  liver NEC —*see* Granuloma, hepatic
  lung (infectious) —*see also* Fibrosis, lung
    coccidioidal B38.1
    eosinophilic C96.6
  Majocchi's B35.8
  malignant (facial (e)) M31.2
  mandible (central) M27.1
  midline (lethal) M31.2
  monilial (cutaneous) B37.2
  nasal sinus —*see* Sinusitis
  operation wound T81.89
    foreign body —*see* Foreign body,
      accidentally left during a procedure
    stitch T81.89
    talc —*see* Foreign body, accidentally left
      during a procedure
  oral mucosa K13.4
  orbit, orbital H05.11-●
  paracoccidioidal B41.8
  penis, venereal A58
  periapical K04.5
  peritoneum K66.8
    due to ova of helminths NOS —*see also*
      Helminthiasis B83.9 [K67]
  postmastoidectomy cavity —*see*
      Complications, postmastoidectomy,
      recurrent cholesteatoma
  prostate N42.89
  pudendi (ulcerating) A58
  pulp, internal (tooth) K03.3

Granuloma (*Continued*)
  pyogenic, pyogenicum (of) (skin) L98.0
    gingiva K06.8
    maxillary alveolar ridge K04.5
    oral mucosa K13.4
  rectum K62.89
  reticulohistiocytic D76.3
  rubrum nasi L74.8
  Schistosoma —*see* Schistosomiasis
  septic (skin) L98.0
  silica (skin) L92.3
  sinus (accessory) (infective) (nasal) —*see*
      Sinusitis
  skin L92.9
    from residual foreign body L92.3
    pyogenicum L98.0
  spine
    syphilitic (epidural) A52.19
    tuberculous A18.01
  stitch (postoperative) T81.89
  suppurative (skin) L98.0
  swimming pool A31.1
  talc —*see also* Granuloma, foreign body
    in operation wound —*see* Foreign body,
      accidentally left during a procedure
  telangiectaticum (skin) L98.0
  tracheostomy J95.09
  trichophyticum B35.8
  tropicum A66.4
▶ umbilical P83.81
⇒ umbilicus P83.81
  urethra N36.8
  uveitis —*see* Iridocyclitis, chronic
  vagina A58
  venereum A58
  vocal cord J38.3
Granulomatosis L92.9
  lymphoid C83.8-●
  miliary (listerial) A32.89
  necrotizing, respiratory M31.30
  progressive septic D71
  specified NEC L92.8
  Wegener's M31.30
    with renal involvement M31.31
Granulomatous tissue (abnormal) (excessive)
    L92.9
Granulosis rubra nasi L74.8
Graphite fibrosis (of lung) J63.3
Graphospasm F48.8
  organic G25.89
Grating scapula M89.8X1
Gravel (urinary) —*see* Calculus, urinary
Graves' disease —*see* Hyperthyroidism, with,
    goiter
Gravis —*see* condition
Grawitz tumor C64.-●
Gray syndrome (newborn) P93.0
Grayness, hair (premature) L67.1
  congenital Q84.2
Green sickness D50.8
Greenfield's disease
  meaning
    concentric sclerosis (encephalitis periaxialis
      concentrica) G37.5
    metachromatic leukodystrophy E75.25
Greenstick fracture - code as Fracture, by site
Grey syndrome (newborn) P93.0
Grief F43.21
  prolonged F43.29
  reaction —*see also* Disorder, adjustment F43.20
Griesinger's disease B76.9
Grinder's lung or pneumoconiosis J62.8
Grinding, teeth
  psychogenic F45.8
  sleep related G47.63
Grip
  Dabney's B33.0
  devil's B33.0
Grippe, grippal —*see also* Influenza
  Balkan A78
  summer, of Italy A93.1
Grisel's disease M43.6

Groin —*see* condition
Grooved tongue K14.5
Ground itch B76.9
Grover's disease or syndrome L11.1
Growing pains, children R29.898
Growth (fungoid) (neoplastic) (new) —*see also*
    Neoplasm
  adenoid (vegetative) J35.8
  benign —*see* Neoplasm, benign, by site
  malignant —*see* Neoplasm, malignant, by site
  rapid, childhood Z00.2
  secondary —*see* Neoplasm, secondary, by site
Gruby's disease B35.0
Gubler-Millard paralysis or syndrome G46.3
Guerin-Stern syndrome Q74.3
Guidance, insufficient anterior (occlusal) M26.54
Guillain-Barré disease or syndrome G61.0
  sequelae G65.0
Guinea worms (infection) (infestation) B72
Guinon's disease (motor-verbal tic) F95.2
Gull's disease E03.4
Gum —*see* condition
Gumboil K04.7
  with sinus K04.6
Gumma (syphilitic) A52.79
  artery A52.09
    cerebral A52.04
  bone A52.77
    of yaws (late) A66.6
  brain A52.19
  cauda equina A52.19
  central nervous system A52.3
  ciliary body A52.71
  congenital A50.59
  eyelid A52.71
  heart A52.06
  intracranial A52.19
  iris A52.71
  kidney A52.75
  larynx A52.73
  leptomeninges A52.19
  liver A52.74
  meninges A52.19
  myocardium A52.06
  nasopharynx A52.73
  neurosyphilitic A52.3
  nose A52.73
  orbit A52.71
  palate (soft) A52.79
  penis A52.76
  pericardium A52.06
  pharynx A52.73
  pituitary A52.79
  scrofulous (tuberculous) A18.4
  skin A52.79
  specified site NEC A52.79
  spinal cord A52.19
  tongue A52.79
  tonsil A52.73
  trachea A52.73
  tuberculous A18.4
  ulcerative due to yaws A66.4
  ureter A52.75
  yaws A66.4
    bone A66.6
Gunn's syndrome Q07.8
Gunshot wound —*see also* Wound, open
  fracture - code as Fracture, by site
  internal organs —*see* Injury, by site
Gynandrism Q56.0
Gynandroblastoma
  specified site —*see* Neoplasm, uncertain
      behavior, by site
  unspecified site
    female D39.10
    male D40.10
Gynecological examination (periodic) (routine)
    Z01.419
  with abnormal findings Z01.411
Gynecomastia N62
Gynephobia F40.291
Gyrate scalp Q82.8

▶ New ⇒ Revised ~~deleted~~ Deleted ● Use Additional Character(s)

H

H (Hartnup's) disease E72.02
Haas' disease or osteochondrosis (juvenile)
(head of humerus) —*see* Osteochondrosis,
juvenile, humerus
Habit, habituation
bad sleep Z72.821
chorea F95.8
disturbance, child F98.9
drug —*see* Dependence, drug
irregular sleep Z72.821
laxative F55.2
spasm —*see* Tic
tic —*see* Tic
Haemophilus (H.) influenzae, as cause of
disease classified elsewhere B96.3
Haff disease —*see* Poisoning, mercury
Hageman's factor defect, deficiency or disease
D68.2
Haglund's disease or osteochondrosis
(juvenile) (os tibiale externum) —*see*
Osteochondrosis, juvenile, tarsus
Hailey-Hailey disease Q82.8
Hair —*see also* condition
plucking F63.3
in stereotyped movement disorder F98.4
tourniquet syndrome —*see also* Constriction,
external, by site
finger S60.44-●
penis S30.842
thumb S60.34-●
toe S90.44-●
Hairball in stomach T18.2
Hair-pulling, pathological (compulsive) F63.3
Hairy black tongue K14.3
Half vertebra Q76.49
Halitosis R19.6
Hallerman-Streiff syndrome Q87.0
Hallervorden-Spatz disease G23.0
Hallopeau's acrodermatitis or disease L40.2
Hallucination R44.3
auditory R44.0
gustatory R44.2
olfactory R44.2
specified NEC R44.2
tactile R44.2
visual R44.1
Hallucinosis (chronic) F28
alcoholic (acute) F10.951
in
abuse F10.151
dependence F10.251
drug-induced F19.951
cannabis F12.951
cocaine F14.951
hallucinogen F16.151
in
abuse F19.151
cannabis F12.151
cocaine F14.151
hallucinogen F16.151
inhalant F18.151
opioid F11.151
sedative, anxiolytic or hypnotic
F13.151
stimulant NEC F15.151
dependence F19.251
cannabis F12.251
cocaine F14.251
hallucinogen F16.251
inhalant F18.251
opioid F11.251
sedative, anxiolytic or hypnotic
F13.251
stimulant NEC F15.251
inhalant F18.951
opioid F11.951
sedative, anxiolytic or hypnotic F13.951
stimulant NEC F15.951
organic F06.0

Hallux
deformity (acquired) NEC M20.5X-●
limitus M20.5X-●
malleus (acquired) NEC M20.3-●
rigidus (acquired) M20.2-●
congenital Q74.2
sequelae (late effect) of rickets E64.3
valgus (acquired) M20.1-●
congenital Q66.6
varus (acquired) M20.3-●
congenital Q66.3
Halo, visual H53.19
Hamartoma, hamartoblastoma Q85.9
epithelial (gingival), odontogenic, central
or peripheral —*see* Cyst, calcifying
odontogenic
Hamartosis Q85.9
Hamman-Rich syndrome J84.114
Hammer toe (acquired) NEC —*see also*
Deformity, toe, hammer toe
congenital Q66.89
sequelae (late effect) of rickets E64.3
Hand —*see* condition
Hand-foot syndrome L27.1
Handicap, handicapped
educational Z55.9
specified NEC Z55.8
Hand-Schüller-Christian disease or syndrome
C96.5
Hanging (asphyxia) (strangulation)
(suffocation) —*see* Asphyxia, traumatic,
due to mechanical threat
Hangnail —*see also* Cellulitis, digit
with lymphangitis —*see* Lymphangitis, acute,
digit
Hangover (alcohol) F10.129
Hanhart's syndrome Q87.0
Hanot-Chauffard (-Troisier) syndrome E83.19
Hanot's cirrhosis or disease K74.3
Hansen's disease —*see* Leprosy
Hantaan virus disease (Korean hemorrhagic
fever) A98.5
Hantavirus disease (with renal manifestations)
(Dobrava) (Puumala) (Seoul) A98.5
with pulmonary manifestations (Andes)
(Bayou) (Bermejo) (Black Creek Canal)
(Choclo) (Juquitiba) (Laguna negra)
(Lechiguanas) (New York) (Oran) (Sin
nombre) B33.4
Happy puppet syndrome Q93.5
Harada's disease or syndrome H30.81-●
Hardening
artery —*see* Arteriosclerosis
brain G93.89
Harelip (complete) (incomplete) —*see* Cleft, lip
Harlequin (newborn) Q80.4
Harley's disease D59.6
Harmful use (of)
alcohol F10.10
anxiolytics —*see* Abuse, drug, sedative
cannabinoids —*see* Abuse, drug, cannabis
cocaine —*see* Abuse, drug, cocaine
drug —*see* Abuse, drug
hallucinogens —*see* Abuse, drug,
hallucinogen
hypnotics —*see* Abuse, drug, sedative -
opioids —*see* Abuse, drug, opioid
PCP (phencyclidine) —*see* Abuse, drug,
hallucinogen
sedatives —*see* Abuse, drug, sedative
stimulants NEC —*see* Abuse, drug, stimulant
Harris' lines —*see* Arrest, epiphyseal
Hartnup's disease E72.02
Harvester's lung J67.0
Harvesting ovum for in vitro fertilization
Z31.83
Hashimoto's disease or thyroiditis E06.3
Hashitoxicosis (transient) E06.3
Hassal-Henle bodies or warts (cornea) H18.49
Haut mal —*see* Epilepsy, generalized, specified
NEC

Haverhill fever A25.1
Hay fever —*see also* Fever, hay J30.1
Hayem-Widal syndrome D59.8
Haygarth's nodes M15.8
Haymaker's lung J67.0
Hb (abnormal)
Bart's disease D56.0
disease —*see* Disease, hemoglobin
trait —*see* Trait
Head —*see* condition
Headache R51
allergic NEC G44.89
associated with sexual activity
G44.82
chronic daily R51
cluster G44.009
chronic G44.029
intractable G44.021
not intractable G44.029
episodic G44.019
intractable G44.011
not intractable G44.019
intractable G44.001
not intractable G44.009
cough (primary) G44.83
daily chronic R51
drug-induced NEC G44.40
intractable G44.41
not intractable G44.40
exertional (primary) G44.84
histamine G44.009
intractable G44.001
not intractable G44.009
hypnic G44.81
lumbar puncture G97.1
medication overuse G44.40
intractable G44.41
not intractable G44.40
menstrual —*see* Migraine, menstrual
migraine (type) —*see also* Migraine
G43.909
nasal septum R51
neuralgiform, short lasting unilateral, with
conjunctival injection and tearing
(SUNCT) G44.059
intractable G44.051
not intractable G44.059
new daily persistent (NDPH) G44.52
orgasmic G44.82
periodic syndromes in adults and children
G43.C0
with refractory migraine G43.C1
intractable G43.C1
not intractable G43.C0
without refractory migraine G43.C0
postspinal puncture G97.1
post-traumatic G44.309
acute G44.319
intractable G44.311
not intractable G44.319
chronic G44.329
intractable G44.321
not intractable G44.329
intractable G44.301
not intractable G44.309
pre-menstrual —*see* Migraine, menstrual
preorgasmic G44.82
primary
cough G44.83
exertional G44.84
stabbing G44.85
thunderclap G44.53
rebound G44.40
intractable G44.41
not intractable G44.40
short lasting unilateral neuralgiform, with
conjunctival injection and tearing
(SUNCT) G44.059
intractable G44.051
not intractable G44.059
specified syndrome NEC G44.89

Headache *(Continued)*
  spinal and epidural anesthesia - induced
      T88.59
    in labor and delivery O74.5
    in pregnancy O29.4- ●
    postpartum, puerperal O89.4
  spinal fluid loss (from puncture) G97.1
  stabbing (primary) G44.85
  tension (-type) G44.209
    chronic G44.229
      intractable G44.221
      not intractable G44.229
    episodic G44.219
      intractable G44.211
      not intractable G44.219
    intractable G44.201
    not intractable G44.209
  thunderclap (primary) G44.53
  vascular NEC G44.1
Healthy
  infant
    accompanying sick mother Z76.3
    receiving care Z76.2
  person accompanying sick person Z76.3
Hearing examination Z01.10
  with abnormal findings NEC Z01.118
  following failed hearing screening Z01.110
  for hearing conservation and treatment
    Z01.12
Heart —*see* condition
Heart beat
  abnormality R00.9
    specified NEC R00.8
  awareness R00.2
  rapid R00.0
  slow R00.1
Heartburn R12
  psychogenic F45.8
▶Heartland virus disease A93.8
Heat (effects) T67.9
  apoplexy T67.0
  burn —*see also* Burn L55.9
  collapse T67.1
  cramps T67.2
  dermatitis or eczema L59.0
  edema T67.7
  erythema - code by site under Burn, first
    degree
  excessive T67.9
    specified effect NEC T67.8
  exhaustion T67.5
    anhydrotic T67.3
    due to
      salt (and water) depletion T67.4
      water depletion T67.3
        with salt depletion T67.4
  fatigue (transient) T67.6
  fever T67.0
  hyperpyrexia T67.0
  prickly L74.0
  prostration —*see* Heat, exhaustion
  pyrexia T67.0
  rash L74.0
  specified effect NEC T67.8
  stroke T67.0
  sunburn —*see* Sunburn
  syncope T67.1
Heavy-for-dates NEC (infant) (4000g to 4499g)
  P08.1
  exceptionally (4500g or more) P08.0
Hebephrenia, hebephrenic (schizophrenia) F20.1
Heberden's disease or nodes (with
  arthropathy) M15.1
Hebra's
  pityriasis L26
  prurigo L28.2
Heel —*see* condition
Heerfordt's disease D86.89
Hegglin's anomaly or syndrome D72.0
Heilmeyer-Schoner disease D45
Heine-Medin disease A80.9

Heinz body anemia, congenital D58.2
Heliophobia F40.228
Heller's disease or syndrome F84.3
HELLP syndrome (hemolysis, elevated liver
  enzymes and low platelet count) O14.2- ●
  complicating
    childbirth O14.24
    puerperium O14.25
Helminthiasis —*see also* Infestation, helminth
  Ancylostoma B76.0
  intestinal B82.0
    mixed types (types classifiable to more
      than one of the titles B65.0-B81.3 and
      B81.8) B81.4
    specified type NEC B81.8
  mixed types (intestinal) (types classifiable to
    more than one of the titles B65.0-B81.3
    and B81.8) B81.4
  Necator (americanus) B76.1
  specified type NEC B83.8
Heloma L84
Hemangioblastoma —*see* Neoplasm,
  connective tissue, uncertain behavior
  malignant —*see* Neoplasm, connective tissue,
    malignant
Hemangioendothelioma —*see also* Neoplasm,
  uncertain behavior, by site
  benign D18.00
    intra-abdominal D18.03
    intracranial D18.02
    skin D18.01
    specified site NEC D18.09
  bone (diffuse) —*see* Neoplasm, bone,
    malignant
  epithelioid —*see also* Neoplasm, uncertain
    behavior, by site
    malignant —*see* Neoplasm, malignant, by
      site
  malignant —*see* Neoplasm, connective tissue,
    malignant
Hemangiofibroma —*see* Neoplasm, benign,
  by site
Hemangiolipoma —*see* Lipoma
Hemangioma D18.00
  arteriovenous D18.00
    intra-abdominal D18.03
    intracranial D18.02
    skin D18.01
    specified site NEC D18.09
  capillary D18.00
    intra-abdominal D18.03
    intracranial D18.02
    skin D18.01
    specified site NEC D18.09
  cavernous D18.00
    intra-abdominal D18.03
    intracranial D18.02
    skin D18.01
    specified site NEC D18.09
  epithelioid D18.00
    intra-abdominal D18.03
    intracranial D18.02
    skin D18.01
    specified site NEC D18.09
  histiocytoid D18.00
    intra-abdominal D18.03
    intracranial D18.02
    skin D18.01
    specified site NEC D18.09
  infantile D18.00
    intra-abdominal D18.03
    intracranial D18.02
    skin D18.01
    specified site NEC D18.09
  intra-abdominal D18.03
  intracranial D18.02
  intramuscular D18.00
    intra-abdominal D18.03
    intracranial D18.02
    skin D18.01
    specified site NEC D18.09

Hemangioma *(Continued)*
  intrathoracic structures D18.09
  juvenile D18.00
  malignant —*see* Neoplasm, connective tissue,
    malignant
  plexiform D18.00
    intra-abdominal D18.03
    intracranial D18.02
    skin D18.01
    specified site NEC D18.09
  racemose D18.00
    intra-abdominal D18.03
    intracranial D18.02
    skin D18.01
    specified site NEC D18.09
  sclerosing —*see* Neoplasm, skin, benign
  simplex D18.00
    intra-abdominal D18.03
    intracranial D18.02
    skin D18.01
    specified site NEC D18.09
  skin D18.01
  specified site NEC D18.09
  venous D18.00
    intra-abdominal D18.03
    intracranial D18.02
    skin D18.01
    specified site NEC D18.09
  verrucous keratotic D18.00
    intra-abdominal D18.03
    intracranial D18.02
    skin D18.01
    specified site NEC D18.09
Hemangiomatosis (systemic) I78.8
  involving single site —*see* Hemangioma
Hemangiopericytoma —*see also* Neoplasm,
  connective tissue, uncertain behavior
  benign —*see* Neoplasm, connective tissue,
    benign
  malignant —*see* Neoplasm, connective tissue,
    malignant
Hemangiosarcoma —*see* Neoplasm, connective
  tissue, malignant
Hemarthrosis (nontraumatic) M25.00
  ankle M25.07- ●
  elbow M25.02- ●
  foot joint M25.07- ●
  hand joint M25.04- ●
  hip M25.05- ●
  in hemophilic arthropathy —*see* Arthropathy,
    hemophilic
  knee M25.06- ●
  shoulder M25.01- ●
  specified joint NEC M25.08
  traumatic —*see* Sprain, by site
  vertebrae M25.08
  wrist M25.03- ●
Hematemesis K92.0
  with ulcer - code by site under Ulcer, with
    hemorrhage K27.4
  newborn, neonatal P54.0
    due to swallowed maternal blood
      P78.2
Hematidrosis L74.8
Hematinuria —*see also* Hemoglobinuria
  malarial B50.8
Hematobilia K83.8
Hematocele
  female NEC N94.89
    with ectopic pregnancy O00.90
      with intrauterine pregnancy O00.91
    ovary N83.8
  male N50.1
Hematochezia —*see also* Melena K92.1
Hematochyluria —*see also* Infestation, filarial
  schistosomiasis (bilharziasis) B65.0
Hematocolpos (with hematometra or
  hematosalpinx) N89.7
Hematocornea —*see* Pigmentation, cornea,
  stromal
Hematogenous —*see* condition

Hematoma (traumatic) (skin surface intact) —
    see also Contusion
with
    injury of internal organs —see Injury, by site
    open wound —see Wound, open
amputation stump (surgical) (late) T87.89
aorta, dissecting I71.00
    abdominal I71.02
    thoracic I71.01
    thoracoabdominal I71.03
aortic intramural —see Dissection, aorta
arterial (complicating trauma) —see Injury,
    blood vessel, by site
auricle —see Contusion, ear
    nontraumatic —see Disorder, pinna,
        hematoma
birth injury NEC P15.8
brain (traumatic)
    with
        cerebral laceration or contusion
            (diffuse) —see Injury, intracranial,
                diffuse
            focal —see Injury, intracranial, focal
        cerebellar, traumatic S06.37-●
        intracerebral, traumatic —see Injury,
            intracranial, intracerebral hemorrhage
        newborn NEC P52.4
            birth injury P10.1
        nontraumatic —see Hemorrhage,
            intracranial
        subarachnoid, arachnoid, traumatic —see
            Injury, intracranial, subarachnoid
            hemorrhage
        subdural, traumatic —see Injury,
            intracranial, subdural hemorrhage
breast (nontraumatic) N64.89
broad ligament (nontraumatic) N83.7
    traumatic S37.892
cerebellar, traumatic S06.37-●
cerebral —see Hematoma, brain
cerebrum S06.36-●
    left S06.35-●
    right S06.34-●
cesarean delivery wound O90.2
complicating delivery (perineal) (pelvic)
    (vagina) (vulva) O71.7
corpus cavernosum (nontraumatic) N48.89
epididymis (nontraumatic) N50.1
epidural (traumatic) —see Injury, intracranial,
    epidural hemorrhage
    spinal —see Injury, spinal cord, by region
episiotomy O90.2
face, birth injury P15.4
genital organ NEC (nontraumatic)
    female (nonobstetric) N94.89
        traumatic S30.202
    male N50.1
        traumatic S30.201
internal organs —see Injury, by site
intracerebral, traumatic —see Injury,
    intracranial, intracerebral hemorrhage
intraoperative —see Complications,
    intraoperative, hemorrhage
labia (nontraumatic) (nonobstetric) N90.8
liver (subcapsular) (nontraumatic) K76.89
    birth injury P15.0
mediastinum —see Injury, intrathoracic
mesosalpinx (nontraumatic) N83.7
    traumatic S37.898
muscle - code by site under Contusion
nontraumatic
    muscle M79.81
    soft tissue M79.81
obstetrical surgical wound O90.2
orbit, orbital (nontraumatic) —see also
        Hemorrhage, orbit
    traumatic —see Contusion, orbit
pelvis (female) (nontraumatic) (nonobstetric)
    N94.89
    obstetric O71.7
    traumatic —see Injury, by site

Hematoma (Continued)
    penis (nontraumatic) N48.89
        birth injury P15.5
    perianal (nontraumatic) K64.5
    perineal S30.23
        complicating delivery O71.7
    perirenal —see Injury, kidney
    pinna —see Contusion, ear
        nontraumatic —see Disorder, pinna,
            hematoma
    placenta O43.89-●
    postoperative (postprocedural) —see
        Complication, postprocedural,
            hematoma
    retroperitoneal (nontraumatic) K66.1
        traumatic S36.892
    scrotum, superficial S30.22
        birth injury P15.5
    seminal vesicle (nontraumatic) N50.1
        traumatic S37.892
    spermatic cord (traumatic) S37.892
        nontraumatic N50.1
    spinal (cord) (meninges) —see also Injury,
        spinal cord, by region
        newborn (birth injury) P11.5
    spleen D73.5
        intraoperative —see Complications,
            intraoperative, hemorrhage, spleen
        postprocedural (postoperative) —see
            Complications, postprocedural,
                hemorrhage, spleen
    sternocleidomastoid, birth injury P15.2
    sternomastoid, birth injury P15.2
    subarachnoid (traumatic) —see Injury,
        intracranial, subarachnoid hemorrhage
        newborn (nontraumatic) P52.5
            due to birth injury P10.3
        nontraumatic —see Hemorrhage,
            intracranial, subarachnoid
    subdural (traumatic) —see Injury, intracranial,
        subdural hemorrhage
        newborn (localized) P52.8
            birth injury P10.0
        nontraumatic —see Hemorrhage,
            intracranial, subdural
    superficial, newborn P54.5
    testis (nontraumatic) N50.1
        birth injury P15.5
    tunica vaginalis (nontraumatic) N50.1
    umbilical cord, complicating delivery O69.5
    uterine ligament (broad) (nontraumatic)
        N83.7
        traumatic S37.892
    vagina (ruptured) (nontraumatic) N89.8
        complicating delivery O71.7
    vas deferens (nontraumatic) N50.1
        traumatic S37.892
    vitreous —see Hemorrhage, vitreous
    vulva (nontraumatic) (nonobstetric) N90.89
        complicating delivery O71.7
        newborn (birth injury) P15.5
Hematometra N85.7
    with hematocolpos N89.7
Hematomyelia (central) G95.19
    newborn (birth injury) P11.5
    traumatic T14.8
Hematomyelitis G04.90
Hematoperitoneum —see Hemoperitoneum
Hematopneumothorax (see Hemothorax)
Hematopoiesis, cyclic D70.4
Hematoporphyria —see Porphyria
Hematorachis, hematorrhachis G95.19
    newborn (birth injury) P11.5
Hematosalpinx N83.6
    with
        hematocolpos N89.7
        hematometra N85.7
            with hematocolpos N89.7
    infectional —see Salpingitis
Hematospermia R36.1

Hematothorax (see Hemothorax)
Hematuria R31.9
    benign (familial) (of childhood) —see also
        Hematuria, idiopathic
        essential microscopic R31.1
    due to sulphonamide, sulfonamide —see Table
        of Drugs and Chemicals, by drug
    endemic —see also Schistosomiasis B65.0
    gross R31.0
    idiopathic N02.9
        with glomerular lesion
            crescentic (diffuse) glomerulonephritis
                N02.7
            dense deposit disease N02.6
            endocapillary proliferative
                glomerulonephritis N02.4
            focal and segmental hyalinosis or
                sclerosis N02.1
            membranoproliferative (diffuse) N02.5
            membranous (diffuse) N02.2
            mesangial proliferative (diffuse) N02.3
            mesangiocapillary (diffuse) N02.5
            minor abnormality N02.0
            proliferative NEC N02.8
            specified pathology NEC N02.8
    intermittent —see Hematuria, idiopathic
    malarial B50.8
    microscopic NEC (with symptoms) R31.29
        asymptomatic R31.21
        benign essential R31.1
    paroxysmal —see also Hematuria, idiopathic
        nocturnal D59.5
    persistent —see Hematuria, idiopathic
    recurrent —see Hematuria, idiopathic
    tropical —see also Schistosomiasis B65.0
    tuberculous A18.13
Hemeralopia (day blindness) H53.11
    vitamin A deficiency E50.5
Hemi-akinesia R41.4
Hemianalgesia R20.0
Hemianencephaly Q00.0
Hemianesthesia R20.0
Hemianopia, hemianopsia (heteronymous)
    H53.47
    homonymous H53.46-●
    syphilitic A52.71
Hemiathetosis R25.8
Hemiatrophy R68.89
    cerebellar G31.9
    face, facial, progressive (Romberg) G51.8
    tongue K14.8
Hemiballism (us) G25.5
Hemicardia Q24.8
Hemicephalus, hemicephaly Q00.0
Hemichorea G25.5
Hemicolitis, left —see Colitis, left sided
Hemicrania
    congenital malformation Q00.0
    continua G44.51
    meaning migraine —see also Migraine G43.909
    paroxysmal G44.039
        chronic G44.049
            intractable G44.041
            not intractable G44.049
        episodic G44.039
            intractable G44.031
            not intractable G44.039
        intractable G44.031
        not intractable G44.039
Hemidystrophy —see Hemiatrophy
Hemiectromelia Q73.8
Hemihypalgesia R20.8
Hemihypesthesia R20.1
Hemi-inattention R41.4
Hemimelia Q73.8
    lower limb —see Defect, reduction, lower
        limb, specified type NEC
    upper limb —see Defect, reduction, upper
        limb, specified type NEC
Hemiparalysis —see Hemiplegia
Hemiparesis —see Hemiplegia

Hemiparesthesia R20.2
Hemiparkinsonism G20
Hemiplegia G81.9- ●
  alternans facialis G83.89
  ascending NEC G81.90
    spinal G95.89
  congenital (cerebral) G80.8
    spastic G80.2
  embolic (current episode) I63.4- ●
  flaccid G81.0- ●
  following
    cerebrovascular disease I69.959
      cerebral infarction I69.35- ●
      intracerebral hemorrhage I69.15- ●
      nontraumatic intracranial hemorrhage
        NEC I69.25- ●
      specified disease NEC I69.85- ●
      stroke NOS I69.35- ●
      subarachnoid hemorrhage I69.05- ●
  hysterical F44.4
  newborn NEC P91.88
    birth injury P11.9
  spastic G81.1- ●
    congenital G80.2
  thrombotic (current episode) I63.3- ●
Hemisection, spinal cord —see Injury, spinal
    cord, by region
Hemispasm (facial) R25.2
Hemisporosis B48.8
Hemitremor R25.1
Hemivertebra Q76.49
  failure of segmentation with scoliosis Q76.3
  fusion with scoliosis Q76.3
Hemochromatosis E83.119
  with refractory anemia D46.1
  due to repeated red blood cell transfusion
    E83.111
  hereditary (primary) E83.110
  neonatal P78.84
  primary E83.110
  specified NEC E83.118
Hemoglobin —see also condition
  abnormal (disease) —see Disease, hemoglobin
  AS genotype D57.3
  Constant Spring D58.2
  E-beta thalassemia D56.5
  fetal, hereditary persistence (HPFH) D56.4
  H Constant Spring D56.0
  low NOS D64.9
  S (Hb S), heterozygous D57.3
Hemoglobinemia D59.9
  due to blood transfusion T80.89
  paroxysmal D59.6
    nocturnal D59.5
Hemoglobinopathy (mixed) D58.2
  with thalassemia D56.8
  sickle-cell D57.1
    with thalassemia D57.40
      with crisis (vasoocclusive pain) D57.419
        with
          acute chest syndrome D57.411
          splenic sequestration D57.412
      without crisis D57.40
Hemoglobinuria R82.3
  with anemia, hemolytic, acquired (chronic)
    NEC D59.6
  cold (agglutinin) (paroxysmal) (with
    Raynaud's syndrome) D59.6
  due to exertion or hemolysis NEC D59.6
  intermittent D59.6
  malarial B50.8
  march D59.6
  nocturnal (paroxysmal) D59.5
  paroxysmal (cold) D59.6
    nocturnal D59.5
Hemolymphangioma D18.1
Hemolysis
  intravascular
    with
      abortion —see Abortion, by type,
        complicated by, hemorrhage
      ectopic or molar pregnancy O08.1

Hemolysis (Continued)
  intravascular (Continued)
    with (Continued)
      hemorrhage
        antepartum —see Hemorrhage,
          antepartum, with coagulation
          defect
        intrapartum —see also Hemorrhage,
          complicating, delivery O67.0
    postpartum O72.3
  neonatal (excessive) P58.9
    specified NEC P58.8
Hemolytic —see condition
Hemopericardium I31.2
  following acute myocardial infarction
    (current complication) I23.0
  newborn P54.8
  traumatic —see Injury, heart, with
    hemopericardium
Hemoperitoneum K66.1
  infectional K65.9
  traumatic S36.899
    with open wound —see Wound, open, with
      penetration into peritoneal cavity
Hemophilia (classical) (familial) (hereditary)
    D66
  A D66
  B D67
  C D68.1
  acquired D68.311
  autoimmune D68.311
  calcipriva —see also Defect, coagulation D68.4
  nonfamilial —see also Defect, coagulation
    D68.4
  secondary D68.311
  vascular D68.0
Hemophthalmos H44.81- ●
Hemopneumothorax —see also Hemothorax
  traumatic S27.2
Hemoptysis R04.2
  newborn P26.9
  tuberculous —see Tuberculosis, pulmonary
Hemorrhage, hemorrhagic (concealed) R58
  abdomen R58
  accidental antepartum —see Hemorrhage,
    antepartum
  acute idiopathic pulmonary, in infants
    R04.81
  adenoid J35.8
  adrenal (capsule) (gland) E27.49
    medulla E27.8
    newborn P54.4
  after delivery —see Hemorrhage, postpartum
  alveolar
    lung, newborn P26.8
    process K08.89
  alveolus K08.89
  amputation stump (surgical) T87.89
  anemia (chronic) D50.0
    acute D62
  antepartum (with) O46.90
    with coagulation defect O46.00- ●
      afibrinogenemia O46.01- ●
      disseminated intravascular coagulation
        O46.02- ●
      hypofibrinogenemia O46.01- ●
      specified defect NEC O46.09- ●
    before 20 weeks gestation O20.9
      specified type NEC O20.8
      threatened abortion O20.0
    due to
      abruptio placenta —see also Abruptio
        placentae O45.9- ●
      leiomyoma, uterus —see Hemorrhage,
        antepartum, specified cause NEC
      placenta previa O44.1- ●
    specified cause NEC —see subcategory
      O46.8X- ●
  anus (sphincter) K62.5
  apoplexy (stroke) —see Hemorrhage,
    intracranial, intracerebral

Hemorrhage, hemorrhagic (Continued)
  arachnoid —see Hemorrhage, intracranial,
    subarachnoid
  artery R58
    brain —see Hemorrhage, intracranial,
      intracerebral
  basilar (ganglion) I61.0
  bladder N32.89
  bowel K92.2
    newborn P54.3
  brain (miliary) (nontraumatic) —see
    Hemorrhage, intracranial, intracerebral
    due to
      birth injury P10.1
      syphilis A52.05
    epidural or extradural (traumatic) —
      see Injury, intracranial, epidural
      hemorrhage
    newborn P52.4
      birth injury P10.1
    subarachnoid —see Hemorrhage,
      intracranial, subarachnoid
    subdural —see Hemorrhage, intracranial,
      subdural
  brainstem (nontraumatic) I61.3
    traumatic S06.38- ●
  breast N64.59
  bronchial tube —see Hemorrhage, lung
  bronchopulmonary —see Hemorrhage, lung
  bronchus —see Hemorrhage, lung
  bulbar I61.5
  capillary I78.8
    primary D69.8
  cecum K92.2
  cerebellar, cerebellum (nontraumatic) I61.4
    newborn P52.6
    traumatic S06.37- ●
  cerebral, cerebrum —see also Hemorrhage,
    intracranial, intracerebral
    lobe I61.1
    newborn (anoxic) P52.4
      birth injury P10.1
  cerebromeningeal I61.8
  cerebrospinal —see Hemorrhage, intracranial,
    intracerebral
  cervix (uteri) (stump) NEC N88.8
  chamber, anterior (eye) —see Hyphema
  childbirth —see Hemorrhage, complicating,
    delivery
  choroid H31.30- ●
    expulsive H31.31- ●
  ciliary body —see Hyphema
  cochlea —see subcategory H83.8
  colon K92.2
  complicating
    abortion —see Abortion, by type,
      complicated by, hemorrhage
    delivery O67.9
      associated with coagulation defect
        (afibrinogenemia) (DIC)
        (hyperfibrinolysis) O67.0
      specified cause NEC O67.8
    surgical procedure —see Hemorrhage,
      intraoperative
  conjunctiva H11.3- ●
    newborn P54.8
  cord, newborn (stump) P51.9
  corpus luteum (ruptured) cyst N83.1- ●
  cortical (brain) I61.1
  cranial —see Hemorrhage, intracranial
  cutaneous R23.3
    due to autosensitivity, erythrocyte D69.2
    newborn P54.5
  delayed
    following ectopic or molar pregnancy
      O08.1
    postpartum O72.2
  diathesis (familial) D69.9
  disease D69.9
    newborn P53
    specified type NEC D69.8

Hemorrhage, hemorrhagic (Continued)
due to or associated with
afibrinogenemia or other coagulation defect
(conditions in categories D65-D69)
antepartum —see Hemorrhage,
antepartum, with coagulation
defect
intrapartum O67.0
dental implant M27.61
device, implant or graft —see also
Complications, by site and type,
specified NEC T85.838
arterial graft NEC T82.838
breast T85.838
catheter NEC T85.838
dialysis (renal) T82.838
intraperitoneal T85.838
infusion NEC T82.838
spinal (epidural) (subdural)
T85.830
urinary (indwelling) T83.83
electronic (electrode) (pulse generator)
(stimulator)
bone T84.83
cardiac T82.837
nervous system (brain) (peripheral
nerve) (spinal) T85.830
urinary T83.83
fixation, internal (orthopedic) NEC T84.83
gastrointestinal (bile duct) (esophagus)
T85.838
genital NEC T83.83
heart NEC T82.837
joint prosthesis T84.83
ocular (corneal graft) (orbital implant)
NEC T85.838
orthopedic NEC T84.83
bone graft T86.838
specified NEC T85.838
urinary NEC T83.83
vascular NEC T82.838
ventricular intracranial shunt T85.838
duodenum, duodenal K92.2
ulcer —see Ulcer, duodenum, with
hemorrhage
dura mater —see Hemorrhage, intracranial,
subdural
endotracheal —see Hemorrhage, lung
epicranial subaponeurotic (massive), birth
injury P12.2
epidural (traumatic) —see also Injury,
intracranial, epidural hemorrhage
nontraumatic I62.1
esophagus K22.8
varix I85.01
secondary I85.11
excessive, following ectopic gestation
(subsequent episode) O08.1
extradural (traumatic) —see Injury,
intracranial, epidural hemorrhage
birth injury P10.8
newborn (anoxic) (nontraumatic) P52.8
nontraumatic I62.1
eye NEC H57.8
fundus —see Hemorrhage, retina
lid —see Disorder, eyelid, specified type
NEC
fallopian tube N83.6
fibrinogenolysis —see Fibrinolysis
fibrinolytic (acquired) —see Fibrinolysis
from
ear (nontraumatic) —see Otorrhagia
tracheostomy stoma J95.01
fundus, eye —see Hemorrhage, retina
funis —see Hemorrhage, umbilicus, cord
gastric —see Hemorrhage, stomach
gastroenteric K92.2
newborn P54.3
gastrointestinal (tract) K92.2
newborn P54.3
genital organ, male N50.1

Hemorrhage, hemorrhagic (Continued)
genitourinary (tract) NOS R31.9
gingiva K06.8
globe (eye) —see Hemophthalmos
graafian follicle cyst (ruptured) N83.0-●
gum K06.8
heart I51.89
hypopharyngeal (throat) R04.1
intermenstrual (regular) N92.3
irregular N92.1
internal (organs) NEC R58
capsule I61.0
ear —see subcategory H83.8
newborn P54.8
intestine K92.2
newborn P54.3
intra-abdominal R58
intra-alveolar (lung), newborn P26.8
intracerebral (nontraumatic) —see
Hemorrhage, intracranial,
intracerebral
intracranial (nontraumatic) I62.9
birth injury P10.9
epidural, nontraumatic I62.1
extradural, nontraumatic I62.1
intracerebral (nontraumatic) (in) I61.9
brain stem I61.3
cerebellum I61.4
hemisphere I61.2
cortical (superficial) I61.1
subcortical (deep) I61.0
intraoperative
during a nervous system procedure
G97.31
during other procedure G97.32
intraventricular I61.5
multiple localized I61.6
newborn P52.4
birth injury P10.1
postprocedural
following a nervous system procedure
G97.51
following other procedure
G97.52
specified NEC I61.8
superficial I61.1
traumatic (diffuse) —see Injury,
intracranial, diffuse
focal —see Injury, intracranial, focal
newborn P52.9
specified NEC P52.8
subarachnoid (nontraumatic) (from) I60.9
intracranial (cerebral) artery I60.7
anterior communicating I60.2
basilar I60.4
carotid siphon and bifurcation
I60.0-●
communicating I60.7
anterior I60.2
posterior I60.3-●
middle cerebral I60.1-●
posterior communicating I60.3-●
specified artery NEC I60.6
vertebral I60.5-●
newborn P52.5
birth injury P10.3
specified NEC I60.8
traumatic S06.6X-●
subdural (nontraumatic) I62.00
acute I62.01
birth injury P10.0
chronic I62.03
newborn (anoxic) (hypoxic) P52.8
birth injury P10.0
spinal G95.19
subacute I62.02
traumatic —see Injury, intracranial,
subdural hemorrhage
traumatic —see Injury, intracranial, focal
brain injury
intramedullary NEC G95.19

Hemorrhage, hemorrhagic (Continued)
intraocular —see Hemophthalmos
intraoperative, intraprocedural —see
Complication, hemorrhage (hematoma),
intraoperative (intraprocedural), by site
intrapartum —see Hemorrhage, complicating,
delivery
intrapelvic
female N94.89
male K66.1
intraperitoneal K66.1
intrapontine I61.3
intraprocedural —see Complication,
hemorrhage (hematoma), intraoperative
(intraprocedural), by site
intrauterine N85.7
complicating delivery —see also Hemorrhage,
complicating, delivery O67.9
postpartum —see Hemorrhage, postpartum
intraventricular I61.5
newborn (nontraumatic) —see also Newborn,
affected by, hemorrhage P52.3
due to birth injury P10.2
grade
1 P52.0
2 P52.1
3 P52.21
4 P52.22
intravesical N32.89
iris (postinfectional) (postinflammatory)
(toxic) —see Hyphema
joint (nontraumatic) —see Hemarthrosis
kidney N28.89
knee (joint) (nontraumatic) —see
Hemarthrosis, knee
labyrinth —see subcategory H83.8
lenticular striate artery I61.0
ligature, vessel —see Hemorrhage,
postoperative
liver K76.89
lung R04.89
newborn P26.9
massive P26.1
specified NEC P26.8
tuberculous —see Tuberculosis, pulmonary
massive umbilical, newborn P51.0
mediastinum —see Hemorrhage, lung
medulla I61.3
membrane (brain) I60.8
spinal cord —see Hemorrhage, spinal cord
meninges, meningeal (brain) (middle) I60.8
spinal cord —see Hemorrhage, spinal cord
mesentery K66.1
metritis —see Endometritis
mouth K13.79
mucous membrane NEC R58
newborn P54.8
muscle M62.89
nail (subungual) L60.8
nasal turbinate R04.0
newborn P54.8
navel, newborn P51.9
newborn P54.9
specified NEC P54.8
nipple N64.59
nose R04.0
newborn P54.8
omentum K66.1
optic nerve (sheath) H47.02-●
orbit, orbital H05.23-●
ovary NEC N83.8
oviduct N83.6
pancreas K86.89
parathyroid (gland) (spontaneous) E21.4
parturition —see Hemorrhage, complicating,
delivery
penis N48.89
pericardium, pericarditis I31.2
peritoneum, peritoneal K66.1
peritonsillar tissue J35.8
due to infection J36

Hemorrhage, hemorrhagic *(Continued)*
petechial R23.3
    due to autosensitivity, erythrocyte D69.2
pituitary (gland) E23.6
pleura —*see* Hemorrhage, lung
polioencephalitis, superior E51.2
polymyositis —*see* Polymyositis
pons, pontine I61.3
posterior fossa (nontraumatic) I61.8
    newborn P52.6
postmenopausal N95.0
postnasal R04.0
postoperative —*see* Complications,
    postprocedural, hemorrhage, by site
postpartum NEC (following delivery of
    placenta) O72.1
    delayed or secondary O72.2
    retained placenta O72.0
    third stage O72.0
pregnancy —*see* Hemorrhage, antepartum
preretinal —*see* Hemorrhage, retina
prostate N42.1
puerperal —*see* Hemorrhage, postpartum
    delayed or secondary O72.2
pulmonary R04.89
    newborn P26.9
        massive P26.1
        specified NEC P26.8
    tuberculous —*see* Tuberculosis, pulmonary
purpura (primary) D69.3
rectum (sphincter) K62.5
    newborn P54.2
recurring, following initial hemorrhage at
    time of injury T79.2
renal N28.89
respiratory passage or tract R04.9
    specified NEC R04.89
retina, retinal (vessels) H35.6-●
    diabetic —*see* Diabetes, retinal, hemorrhage
retroperitoneal R58
scalp R58
scrotum N50.1
secondary (nontraumatic) R58
    following initial hemorrhage at time of
        injury T79.2
seminal vesicle N50.1
skin R23.3
    newborn P54.5
slipped umbilical ligature P51.8
spermatic cord N50.1
spinal (cord) G95.19
    newborn (birth injury) P11.5
spleen D73.5
    intraoperative —*see* Complications,
        intraoperative, hemorrhage, spleen
    postprocedural —*see* Complications,
        postprocedural, hemorrhage, spleen
stomach K92.2
    newborn P54.3
    ulcer —*see* Ulcer, stomach, with
        hemorrhage
subarachnoid (nontraumatic) —*see*
    Hemorrhage, intracranial, subarachnoid
subconjunctival —*see also* Hemorrhage,
    conjunctiva
    birth injury P15.3
subcortical (brain) I61.0
subcutaneous R23.3
subdiaphragmatic R58
subdural (acute) (nontraumatic) —*see*
    Hemorrhage, intracranial, subdural
subependymal
    newborn P52.0
        with intraventricular extension P52.1
        and intracerebral extension P52.22
subgaleal P12.2
subhyaloid —*see* Hemorrhage, retina
subperiosteal —*see* Disorder, bone, specified
    type NEC
subretinal —*see* Hemorrhage, retina
subtentorial —*see* Hemorrhage, intracranial,
    subdural

Hemorrhage, hemorrhagic *(Continued)*
subungual L60.8
suprarenal (capsule) (gland) E27.49
    newborn P54.4
tentorium (traumatic) NEC —*see*
    Hemorrhage, brain
    newborn (birth injury) P10.4
testis N50.1
third stage (postpartum) O72.0
thorax —*see* Hemorrhage, lung
throat R04.1
thymus (gland) E32.8
thyroid (cyst) (gland) E07.89
tongue K14.8
tonsil J35.8
trachea —*see* Hemorrhage, lung
tracheobronchial R04.89
    newborn P26.0
traumatic — code to specific injury
    cerebellar —*see* Hemorrhage, brain
    intracranial —*see* Hemorrhage, brain
    recurring or secondary (following initial
        hemorrhage at time of injury)
        T79.2
tuberculous NEC —*see also* Tuberculosis,
    pulmonary A15.0
tunica vaginalis N50.1
ulcer - code by site under Ulcer, with
    hemorrhage K27.4
umbilicus, umbilical
    cord
        after birth, newborn P51.9
        complicating delivery O69.5
    newborn P51.9
        massive P51.0
        slipped ligature P51.8
    stump P51.9
urethra (idiopathic) N36.8
uterus, uterine (abnormal) N93.9
    climacteric N92.4
    complicating delivery —*see* Hemorrhage,
        complicating, delivery
    dysfunctional or functional N93.8
    intermenstrual (regular) N92.3
        irregular N92.1
    postmenopausal N95.0
    postpartum —*see* Hemorrhage,
        postpartum
    preclimacteric or premenopausal N92.4
    prepubertal N93.8
    pubertal N92.2
vagina (abnormal) N93.9
    newborn P54.6
vas deferens N50.1
vasa previa O69.4
ventricular I61.5
vesical N32.89
viscera NEC R58
    newborn P54.8
vitreous (humor) (intraocular) H43.1-●
vulva N90.89

Hemorrhoids (bleeding) (without mention of
    degree) K64.9
1st degree (grade/stage I) (without prolapse
    outside of anal canal) K64.0
2nd degree (grade/stage II) (that prolapse
    with straining but retract spontaneously)
    K64.1
3rd degree (grade/stage III) (that prolapse
    with straining and require manual
    replacement back inside anal canal)
    K64.2
4th degree (grade/stage IV) (with prolapsed
    tissue that cannot be manually replaced)
    K64.3
complicating
    pregnancy O22.4
    puerperium O87.2
external K64.4
    with
        thrombosis K64.5

Hemorrhoids *(Continued)*
internal (without mention of degree) K64.8
prolapsed K64.8
skin tags
    anus K64.4
    residual K64.4
specified NEC K64.8
strangulated —*see also* Hemorrhoids, by
    degree K64.8
thrombosed —*see also* Hemorrhoids, by
    degree K64.5
ulcerated —*see also* Hemorrhoids, by degree
    K64.8
Hemosalpinx N83.6
with
    hematocolpos N89.7
    hematometra N85.7
        with hematocolpos N89.7
Hemosiderosis (dietary) E83.19
pulmonary, idiopathic E83.1 *[J84.03]*
transfusion T80.89
Hemothorax (bacterial) (nontuberculous) J94.2
newborn P54.8
traumatic S27.1
    with pneumothorax S27.2
tuberculous NEC A15.6
Henoch (-Schönlein) disease or syndrome
    (purpura) D69.0
Henpue, henpuye A66.6
Hepar lobatum (syphilitic) A52.74
Hepatalgia K76.89
Hepatitis K75.9
acute B17.9
    with coma K72.01
    with hepatic failure —*see* Failure, hepatic
    alcoholic —*see* Hepatitis, alcoholic
    infectious B15.9
    non-viral K72.0
    viral B17.9
alcoholic (acute) (chronic) K70.10
    with ascites K70.11
amebic —*see* Abscess, liver, amebic
anicteric (viral) —*see* Hepatitis, viral
antigen-associated (HAA) —*see* Hepatitis, B
Australia-antigen (positive) —*see* Hepatitis, B
autoimmune K75.4
B B19.10
    with hepatic coma B19.11
    acute B16.9
        with
            delta-agent (coinfection) (without
                hepatic coma) B16.1
                with hepatic coma B16.0
            hepatic coma (without delta-agent
                coinfection) B16.2
    chronic B18.1
        with delta-agent B18.0
    bacterial NEC K75.89
C (viral) B19.20
    with hepatic coma B19.21
    acute B17.10
        with hepatic coma B17.11
    chronic B18.2
catarrhal (acute) B15.9
    with hepatic coma B15.0
cholangiolitic K75.89
cholestatic K75.89
chronic K73.9
    active NEC K73.2
    lobular NEC K73.1
    persistent NEC K73.0
    specified NEC K73.8
cytomegaloviral B25.1
due to ethanol (acute) (chronic) —*see*
    Hepatitis, alcoholic
epidemic B15.9
    with hepatic coma B15.0
fulminant NEC (viral) —*see* Hepatitis,
    viral
granulomatous NEC K75.3
herpesviral B00.81

▶ New   ⇒ Revised   ~~deleted~~ Deleted   ● Use Additional Character(s)

Hepatitis (Continued)
  history of
    B Z86.19
    C Z86.19
  homologous serum —see Hepatitis, viral,
    type B
  in (due to)
    mumps B26.81
    toxoplasmosis (acquired) B58.1
      congenital (active) P37.1 [K77]
  infectious, infective B15.9
    acute (subacute) B17.9
    chronic B18.9
  inoculation —see Hepatitis, viral, type B
  interstitial (chronic) K74.69
  lupoid NEC K75.2
  malignant NEC (with hepatic failure)
    K72.90
    with coma K72.91
  neonatal giant cell P59.29
  neonatal (idiopathic) (toxic) P59.29
  newborn P59.29
  postimmunization —see Hepatitis, viral,
    type B
  post-transfusion —see Hepatitis, viral, type B
  reactive, nonspecific K75.2
  serum —see Hepatitis, viral, type B
  specified type NEC
    with hepatic failure —see Failure, hepatic
  syphilitic (late) A52.74
    congenital (early) A50.08 [K77]
      late A50.59 [K77]
    secondary A51.45
  toxic —see also Disease, liver, toxic K71.6
  tuberculous A18.83
  viral, virus B19.9
    with hepatic coma B19.0
    acute B17.9
    chronic B18.9
      specified NEC B18.8
      type
        B B18.1
          with delta-agent B18.0
        C B18.2
    congenital P35.3
    coxsackie B33.8 [K77]
    cytomegalic inclusion B25.1
    in remission, any type — code to Hepatitis,
      chronic, by type
    non-A, non-B B17.8
    specified type NEC (with or without coma)
      B17.8
    type
      A B15.9
        with hepatic coma B15.0
      B B19.10
        with hepatic coma B19.11
        acute B16.9
          with
            delta-agent (coinfection) (without
              hepatic coma) B16.1
              with hepatic coma B16.0
            hepatic coma (without delta-
              agent coinfection) B16.2
        chronic B18.1
          with delta-agent B18.0
      C B19.20
        with hepatic coma B19.21
        acute B17.10
          with hepatic coma B17.11
        chronic B18.2
      E B17.2
      non-A, non-B B17.8
Hepatization lung (acute) —see Pneumonia,
  lobar
Hepatoblastoma C22.2
Hepatocarcinoma C22.0
Hepatocholangiocarcinoma C22.0
Hepatocholangioma, benign D13.4
Hepatocholangitis K75.89
Hepatolenticular degeneration E83.01

Hepatoma (malignant) C22.0
  benign D13.4
  embryonal C22.0
Hepatomegaly —see also Hypertrophy, liver
  with splenomegaly R16.2
  congenital Q44.7
  in mononucleosis
    gammaherpesviral B27.09
    infectious specified NEC B27.89
Hepatoptosis K76.89
Hepatorenal syndrome following labor and
  delivery O90.4
Hepatosis K76.89
Hepatosplenomegaly R16.2
  hyperlipemic (Bürger-Grütz type) E78.3 [K77]
Hereditary —see condition
Heredodegeneration, macular —see Dystrophy,
  retina
Heredopathia atactica polyneuritiformis G60.1
Heredosyphilis —see Syphilis, congenital
Herlitz' syndrome Q81.1
Hermansky-Pudlak syndrome E70.331
Hermaphrodite, hermaphroditism (true)
  Q56.0
  46,XX with streak gonads Q99.1
  46,XX/46,XY Q99.0
  46,XY with streak gonads Q99.1
  chimera 46,XX/46,XY Q99.0
Hernia, hernial (acquired) (recurrent) K46.9
  with
    gangrene —see Hernia, by site, with,
      gangrene
    incarceration —see Hernia, by site, with,
      obstruction
    irreducible —see Hernia, by site, with,
      obstruction
    obstruction —see Hernia, by site, with,
      obstruction
    strangulation —see Hernia, by site, with,
      obstruction
  abdomen, abdominal K46.9
    with
      gangrene (and obstruction) K46.1
      obstruction K46.0
    femoral —see Hernia, femoral
    incisional —see Hernia, incisional
    inguinal —see Hernia, inguinal
    specified site NEC K45.8
      with
        gangrene (and obstruction) K45.1
        obstruction K45.0
    umbilical —see Hernia, umbilical
    wall —see Hernia, ventral
  appendix —see Hernia, abdomen
  bladder (mucosa) (sphincter)
    congenital (female) (male) Q79.51
    female —see Cystocele
    male N32.89
  brain, congenital —see Encephalocele
  cartilage, vertebra —see Displacement,
    intervertebral disc
  cerebral, congenital —see also Encephalocele
    endaural Q01.8
  ciliary body (traumatic) S05.2-●
  colon —see Hernia, abdomen
  Cooper's —see Hernia, abdomen, specified
    site NEC
  crural —see Hernia, femoral
  diaphragm, diaphragmatic K44.9
    with
      gangrene (and obstruction) K44.1
      obstruction K44.0
    congenital Q79.0
  direct (inguinal) —see Hernia, inguinal
  diverticulum, intestine —see Hernia,
    abdomen
  double (inguinal) —see Hernia, inguinal,
    bilateral
  ⮞due to adhesions (with obstruction) K56.50
  epigastric —see also Hernia, ventral K43.9
  esophageal hiatus —see Hernia, hiatal

Hernia, hernial (Continued)
  external (inguinal) —see Hernia, inguinal
  fallopian tube N83.4-●
  fascia M62.89
  femoral K41.90
    with
      gangrene (and obstruction) K41.40
        not specified as recurrent K41.40
        recurrent K41.41
      obstruction K41.30
        not specified as recurrent K41.30
        recurrent K41.31
    bilateral K41.20
      with
        gangrene (and obstruction) K41.10
          not specified as recurrent K41.10
          recurrent K41.11
        obstruction K41.00
          not specified as recurrent K41.00
          recurrent K41.01
      not specified as recurrent K41.20
      recurrent K41.21
    not specified as recurrent K41.90
    recurrent K41.91
    unilateral K41.90
      with
        gangrene (and obstruction) K41.40
          not specified as recurrent K41.40
          recurrent K41.41
        obstruction K41.30
          not specified as recurrent K41.30
          recurrent K41.31
      not specified as recurrent K41.90
      recurrent K41.91
  foramen magnum G93.5
    congenital Q01.8
  funicular (umbilical) —see also Hernia,
    umbilicus
    spermatic (cord) —see Hernia, inguinal
  gastrointestinal tract —see Hernia, abdomen
  Hesselbach's —see Hernia, femoral, specified
    site NEC
  hiatal (esophageal) (sliding) K44.9
    with
      gangrene (and obstruction) K44.1
      obstruction K44.0
    congenital Q40.1
  hypogastric —see Hernia, ventral
  incarcerated —see also Hernia, by site, with
    obstruction
    with gangrene —see Hernia, by site, with
      gangrene
  incisional K43.92
    with
      gangrene (and obstruction) K43.1
      obstruction K43.0
  indirect (inguinal) —see Hernia, inguinal
  inguinal (direct) (external) (funicular)
    (indirect) (internal) (oblique) (scrotal)
    (sliding) K40.90
    with
      gangrene (and obstruction) K40.40
        not specified as recurrent K40.40
        recurrent K40.41
      obstruction K40.30
        not specified as recurrent K40.30
        recurrent K40.31
    bilateral K40.20
      with
        gangrene (and obstruction)
          K40.10
          not specified as recurrent
            K40.10
          recurrent K40.11
        obstruction K40.00
          not specified as recurrent K40.00
          recurrent K40.01
      not specified as recurrent K40.20
      recurrent K40.21
    not specified as recurrent K40.90
    recurrent K40.91

Hernia, hernial (Continued)
  inguinal (Continued)
    unilateral K40.90
      with
        gangrene (and obstruction) K40.40
          not specified as recurrent K40.40
          recurrent K40.41
        obstruction K40.30
          not specified as recurrent K40.30
          recurrent K40.31
      not specified as recurrent K40.90
      recurrent K40.91
  internal —see also Hernia, abdomen
    inguinal —see Hernia, inguinal
  interstitial —see Hernia, abdomen
  intervertebral cartilage or disc —see
    Displacement, intervertebral disc
  intestine, intestinal —see Hernia, by site
  intra-abdominal —see Hernia, abdomen
  iris (traumatic) S05.2-●
  irreducible —see also Hernia, by site, with
    obstruction
    with gangrene —see Hernia, by site, with
      gangrene
  ischiatic —see Hernia, abdomen, specified
    site NEC
  ischiorectal —see Hernia, abdomen, specified
    site NEC
  lens (traumatic) S05.2-●
  linea (alba) (semilunaris) —see Hernia,
    ventral
  Littre's —see Hernia, abdomen
  lumbar —see Hernia, abdomen, specified site
    NEC
  lung (subcutaneous) J98.4
  mediastinum J98.59
  mesenteric (internal) —see Hernia, abdomen
  midline —see Hernia, ventral
  muscle (sheath) M62.89
  nucleus pulposus —see Displacement,
    intervertebral disc
  oblique (inguinal) —see Hernia, inguinal
  obstructive —see also Hernia, by site, with
    obstruction
    with gangrene —see Hernia, by site, with
      gangrene
  obturator —see Hernia, abdomen, specified
    site NEC
  omental —see Hernia, abdomen
  ovary N83.4-●
  oviduct N83.4-●
  paraesophageal —see also Hernia, diaphragm
    congenital Q40.1
  parastomal K43.5
    with
      gangrene (and obstruction) K43.4
      obstruction K43.3
  paraumbilical —see Hernia, umbilicus
  perineal —see Hernia, abdomen, specified
    site NEC
  Petit's —see Hernia, abdomen, specified site
    NEC
  postoperative —see Hernia, incisional
  pregnant uterus —see Abnormal, uterus in
    pregnancy or childbirth
  prevesical N32.89
  properitoneal —see Hernia, abdomen,
    specified site NEC
  pudendal —see Hernia, abdomen, specified
    site NEC
  rectovaginal N81.6
  retroperitoneal —see Hernia, abdomen,
    specified site NEC
  Richter's —see Hernia, abdomen, with
    obstruction
  Rieux's, Riex's —see Hernia, abdomen,
    specified site NEC
  sac condition (adhesion) (dropsy)
    (inflammation) (laceration)
    (suppuration) - code by site under
    Hernia

Hernia, hernial (Continued)
  sciatic —see Hernia, abdomen, specified site
    NEC
  scrotum, scrotal —see Hernia, inguinal
  sliding (inguinal) —see also Hernia,
    inguinal
    hiatus —see Hernia, hiatal
  spigelian —see Hernia, ventral
  spinal —see Spina bifida
  strangulated —see also Hernia, by site, with
    obstruction
    with gangrene —see Hernia, by site, with
      gangrene
  subxiphoid —see Hernia, ventral
  supra-umbilicus —see Hernia, ventral
  tendon —see Disorder, tendon, specified type
    NEC
  Treitz's (fossa) —see Hernia, abdomen,
    specified site NEC
  tunica vaginalis Q55.29
  umbilicus, umbilical K42.9
    with
      gangrene (and obstruction) K42.1
      obstruction K42.0
  ureter N28.89
  urethra, congenital Q64.79
  urinary meatus, congenital Q64.79
  uterus N81.4
    pregnant —see Abnormal, uterus in
      pregnancy or childbirth
  vaginal (anterior) (wall) —see Cystocele
  Velpeau's —see Hernia, femoral
  ventral K43.9
    with
      gangrene (and obstruction) K43.7
      obstruction K43.6
    incisional K43.2
      with
        gangrene (and obstruction) K43.1
        obstruction K43.0
      recurrent —see Hernia, incisional
    specified NEC K43.9
      with
        gangrene (and obstruction) K43.7
        obstruction K43.6
  vesical
    congenital (female) (male) Q79.51
    female —see Cystocele
    male N32.89
  vitreous (into wound) S05.2-●
    into anterior chamber —see Prolapse,
      vitreous
Herniation —see also Hernia
  brain (stem) G93.5
  cerebral G93.5
  mediastinum J98.59
  nucleus pulposus —see Displacement,
    intervertebral disc
Herpangina B08.5
Herpes, herpesvirus, herpetic B00.9
  anogenital A60.9
    perianal skin A60.1
    rectum A60.1
    urogenital tract A60.00
      cervix A60.03
      male genital organ NEC A60.02
      penis A60.01
      specified site NEC A60.09
      vagina A60.04
      vulva A60.04
  blepharitis (zoster) B02.39
    simplex B00.59
  circinatus B35.4
    bullosus L12.0
  conjunctivitis (simplex) B00.53
    zoster B02.31
  cornea B02.33
  encephalitis B00.4
    due to herpesvirus 6 B10.01
    due to herpesvirus 7 B10.09
    specified NEC B10.09

Herpes, herpesvirus, herpetic (Continued)
  eye (zoster) B02.30
    simplex B00.50
  eyelid (zoster) B02.39
    simplex B00.59
  facialis B00.1
  febrilis B00.1
  geniculate ganglionitis B02.21
  genital, genitalis A60.00
    female A60.09
    male A60.02
  gestational, gestationis O26.4-●
  gingivostomatitis B00.2
  human B00.9
    1 —see Herpes, simplex
    2 —see Herpes, simplex
    3 —see Varicella
    4 —see Mononucleosis, Epstein-Barr (virus)
    5 —see Disease, cytomegalic inclusion
      (generalized)
    6
      encephalitis B10.01
      specified NEC B10.81
    7
      encephalitis B10.09
      specified NEC B10.82
    8 B10.89
  infection NEC B10.89
    Kaposi's sarcoma associated B10.89
  iridocyclitis (simplex) B00.51
    zoster B02.32
  iris (vesicular erythema multiforme) L51.9
  iritis (simplex) B00.51
  Kaposi's sarcoma associated B10.89
  keratitis (simplex) (dendritic) (disciform)
    (interstitial) B00.52
    zoster (interstitial) B02.33
  keratoconjunctivitis (simplex) B00.52
    zoster B02.33
  labialis B00.1
  lip B00.1
  meningitis (simplex) B00.3
    zoster B02.1
  ophthalmicus (zoster) NEC B02.30
    simplex B00.50
  penis A60.01
  perianal skin A60.1
  pharyngitis, pharyngotonsillitis B00.2
  rectum A60.1
  scrotum A60.02
  sepsis B00.7
  simplex B00.9
    complicated NEC B00.89
    congenital P35.2
    conjunctivitis B00.53
    external ear B00.1
    eyelid B00.59
    hepatitis B00.81
    keratitis (interstitial) B00.52
    myleitis B00.82
    specified complication NEC B00.89
    visceral B00.89
  stomatitis B00.2
  tonsurans B35.0
  visceral B00.89
  vulva A60.04
  whitlow B00.89
  zoster —see also condition B02.9
    auricularis B02.21
    complicated NEC B02.8
    conjunctivitis B02.31
    disseminated B02.7
    encephalitis B02.0
    eye(lid) B02.39
    geniculate ganglionitis B02.21
    keratitis (interstitial) B02.33
    meningitis B02.1
    myelitis B02.24
    neuritis, neuralgia B02.29
    ophthalmicus NEC B02.30
    oticus B02.21

► New   ⮕ Revised   ~~deleted~~ Deleted   ● Use Additional Character(s)

Herpes, herpesvirus, herpetic *(Continued)*
zoster *(Continued)*
polyneuropathy B02.23
specified complication NEC B02.8
trigeminal neuralgia B02.22
Herpesvirus (human) —*see* Herpes
Herpetophobia F40.218
Herrick's anemia —*see* Disease, sickle-cell
Hers' disease E74.09
Herter-Gee syndrome K90.0
Herxheimer's reaction R68.89
Hesitancy
of micturition R39.11
urinary R39.11
Hesselbach's hernia —*see* Hernia, femoral, specified site NEC
Heterochromia (congenital) Q13.2
cataract —*see* Cataract, complicated
cyclitis (Fuchs) —*see* Cyclitis, Fuchs' heterochromic
hair L67.1
iritis —*see* Cyclitis, Fuchs' heterochromic
retained metallic foreign body (nonmagnetic) —*see* Foreign body, intraocular, old, retained
magnetic —*see* Foreign body, intraocular, old, retained, magnetic
uveitis —*see* Cyclitis, Fuchs' heterochromic
Heterophoria —*see* Strabismus, heterophoria
Heterophyes, heterophyiasis (small intestine) B66.8
Heterotopia, heterotopic —*see also* Malposition, congenital
cerebralis Q04.8
Heterotropia —*see* Strabismus
Heubner-Herter disease K90.0
Hexadactylism Q69.9
HGSIL (cytology finding) (high grade squamous intraepithelial lesion on cytologic smear) (Pap smear finding)
anus R85.613
cervix R87.613
biopsy (histology) finding — *see* Neoplasia, intraepithelial, cervix, grade II or grade III
vagina R87.623
biopsy (histology) finding — *see* Neoplasia, intraepithelial, vagina, grade II or grade III
Hibernoma —*see* Lipoma
Hiccup, hiccough R06.6
epidemic B33.0
psychogenic F45.8
Hidden penis (congenital) Q55.64
acquired N48.83
Hidradenitis (axillaris) (suppurative) L73.2
Hidradenoma (nodular) —*see also* Neoplasm, skin, benign
clear cell —*see* Neoplasm, skin, benign
papillary —*see* Neoplasm, skin, benign
Hidrocystoma —*see* Neoplasm, skin, benign
High
altitude effects T70.20
anoxia T70.29
on
ears T70.0
sinuses T70.1
polycythemia D75.1
arch
foot Q66.7
palate, congenital Q38.5
arterial tension —*see* Hypertension
basal metabolic rate R94.8
blood pressure —*see also* Hypertension
borderline R03.0
reading (incidental) (isolated) (nonspecific), without diagnosis of hypertension R03.0
cholesterol E78.00
with high triglycerides E78.2
diaphragm (congenital) Q79.1

High *(Continued)*
expressed emotional level within family Z63.8
head at term O32.4
palate, congenital Q38.5
risk
infant NEC Z76.2
sexual behavior (heterosexual) Z72.51
bisexual Z72.53
homosexual Z72.52
▶scrotal testis, testes
▶bilateral Q53.23
▶unilateral Q53.13
temperature (of unknown origin) R50.9
thoracic rib Q76.6
triglycerides E78.1
with high cholesterol E78.2
Hildenbrand's disease A75.0
Hilum —*see* condition
Hip —*see* condition
Hippel's disease Q85.8
Hippophobia F40.218
Hippus H57.09
Hirschsprung's disease or megacolon Q43.1
Hirsutism, hirsuties L68.0
Hirudiniasis
external B88.3
internal B83.4
Hiss-Russell dysentery A03.1
Histidinemia, histidinuria E70.41
Histiocytoma —*see also* Neoplasm, skin, benign
fibrous —*see also* Neoplasm, skin, benign
atypical —*see* Neoplasm, connective tissue, uncertain behavior
malignant —*see* Neoplasm, connective tissue, malignant
Histiocytosis D76.3
acute differentiated progressive C96.0
Langerhans' cell NEC C96.6
multifocal X
multisystemic (disseminated) C96.0
unisystemic C96.5
pulmonary, adult (adult PLCH) J84.82
unifocal (X) C96.6
lipid, lipoid D76.3
essential E75.29
malignant C96.A
mononuclear phagocytes NEC D76.1
Langerhans' cells C96.6
non-Langerhans cell D76.3
polyostotic sclerosing D76.3
sinus, with massive lymphadenopathy D76.3
syndrome NEC D76.3
X NEC C96.6
acute (progressive) C96.0
chronic C96.6
multifocal C96.5
multisystemic C96.0
unifocal C96.6
Histoplasmosis B39.9
with pneumonia NEC B39.2
African B39.5
American —*see* Histoplasmosis, capsulati
capsulati B39.4
disseminated B39.3
generalized B39.3
pulmonary B39.2
acute B39.0
chronic B39.1
Darling's B39.4
duboisii B39.5
lung NEC B39.2
History
family (of) —*see also* History, personal (of)
alcohol abuse Z81.1
allergy NEC Z84.89
anemia Z83.2
arthritis Z82.61
asthma Z82.5
blindness Z82.1
cardiac death (sudden) Z82.41
carrier of genetic disease Z84.81
chromosomal anomaly Z82.79

History *(Continued)*
family *(Continued)*
chronic
disabling disease NEC Z82.8
lower respiratory disease Z82.5
colonic polyps Z83.71
congenital malformations and deformations Z82.79
polycystic kidney Z82.71
consanguinity Z84.3
deafness Z82.2
diabetes mellitus Z83.3
disability NEC Z82.8
disease or disorder (of)
allergic NEC Z84.89
behavioral NEC Z81.8
blood and blood-forming organs Z83.2
cardiovascular NEC Z82.49
chronic disabling NEC Z82.8
digestive Z83.79
ear NEC Z83.52
endocrine NEC Z83.49
eye NEC Z83.518
glaucoma Z83.511
familial hypercholesterolemia Z83.42
genitourinary NEC Z84.2
glaucoma Z83.511
hematological Z83.2
immune mechanism Z83.2
infectious NEC Z83.1
ischemic heart Z82.49
kidney Z84.1
mental NEC Z81.8
metabolic Z83.49
musculoskeletal NEC Z82.69
neurological NEC Z82.0
nutritional Z83.49
parasitic NEC Z83.1
psychiatric NEC Z81.8
respiratory NEC Z83.6
skin and subcutaneous tissue NEC Z84.0
specified NEC Z84.89
drug abuse NEC Z81.3
epilepsy Z82.0
familial hypercholesterolemia Z83.42
genetic disease carrier Z84.81
glaucoma Z83.511
hearing loss Z82.2
human immunodeficiency virus (HIV) infection Z83.0
Huntington's chorea Z82.0
intellectual disability Z81.0
leukemia Z80.6
malignant neoplasm (of) NOS Z80.9
bladder Z80.52
breast Z80.3
bronchus Z80.1
digestive organ Z80.0
gastrointestinal tract Z80.0
genital organ Z80.49
ovary Z80.41
prostate Z80.42
specified organ NEC Z80.49
testis Z80.43
hematopoietic NEC Z80.7
intrathoracic organ NEC Z80.2
kidney Z80.51
lung Z80.1
lymphatic NEC Z80.7
ovary Z80.41
prostate Z80.42
respiratory organ NEC Z80.2
specified site NEC Z80.8
testis Z80.43
trachea Z80.1
urinary organ or tract Z80.59
bladder Z80.52
kidney Z80.51
mental
disorder NEC Z81.8
multiple endocrine neoplasia (MEN) syndrome Z83.41

▶ New   ⇒ Revised   ~~deleted~~ Deleted   ● Use Additional Character(s)

History *(Continued)*
　personal *(Continued)*
　　malignant neoplasm *(Continued)*
　　　digestive organ Z85.00
　　　　specified NEC Z85.09
　　　endocrine gland NEC Z85.858
　　　epididymis Z85.48
　　　esophagus Z85.01
　　　eye Z85.840
　　　gastrointestinal tract —*see* History,
　　　　　malignant neoplasm, digestive
　　　　　organ
　　　genital organ
　　　　female Z85.40
　　　　　specified NEC Z85.44
　　　　male Z85.45
　　　　　specified NEC Z85.49
　　　hematopoietic NEC Z85.79
　　　intrathoracic organ Z85.20-●
　　　kidney NEC Z85.528
　　　　carcinoid Z85.520
　　　large intestine NEC Z85.038
　　　　carcinoid Z85.030
　　　larynx Z85.21
　　　liver Z85.05
　　　lung NEC Z85.118
　　　　carcinoid Z85.110
　　　mediastinum Z85.29
　　　Merkel cell Z85.821
　　　middle ear Z85.22
　　　nasal cavities Z85.22
　　　nervous system NEC Z85.848
　　　oral cavity Z85.819
　　　　specified site NEC Z85.818
　　　ovary Z85.43
　　　pancreas Z85.07
　　　pelvis Z85.53
　　　pharynx Z85.819
　　　　specified site NEC Z85.818
　　　pleura Z85.29
　　　prostate Z85.46
　　　rectosigmoid junction NEC Z85.048
　　　　carcinoid Z85.040
　　　rectum NEC Z85.048
　　　　carcinoid Z85.040
　　　respiratory organ Z85.20
　　　sinuses, accessory Z85.22
　　　skin NEC Z85.828
　　　　melanoma Z85.820
　　　　Merkel cell Z85.821
　　　small intestine NEC Z85.068
　　　　carcinoid Z85.060
　　　soft tissue Z85.831
　　　specified site NEC Z85.89
　　　stomach NEC Z85.028
　　　　carcinoid Z85.020
　　　testis Z85.47
　　　thymus NEC Z85.238
　　　　carcinoid Z85.230
　　　thyroid Z85.850
　　　tongue Z85.810
　　　trachea Z85.12
　　　ureter Z85.54
　　　urinary organ or tract Z85.50
　　　　specified NEC Z85.59
　　　uterus Z85.42
　　maltreatment Z91.89
　　medical treatment NEC Z92.89
　　melanoma (malignant) (skin) Z85.820
　　meningitis Z86.61
　　mental disorder Z86.59
　　Merkel cell carcinoma (skin) Z85.821
　　Methicillin resistant Staphylococcus aureus
　　　(MRSA) Z86.14
　　military deployment Z91.82
　　military war, peacekeeping and
　　　humanitarian deployment (current or
　　　past conflict) Z91.82
　　myocardial infarction (old) I25.2
　　neglect (in)
　　　adult Z91.412
　　　childhood Z62.812

History *(Continued)*
　personal *(Continued)*
　　neoplasm
　　　benign Z86.018
　　　　brain Z86.011
　　　　colon polyp Z86.010
　　　in situ
　　　　breast Z86.000
　　　　cervix uteri Z86.001
　　　　specified NEC Z86.008
　　　malignant —*see* History of, malignant
　　　　　neoplasm
　　　uncertain behavior Z86.03
　　nephrotic syndrome Z87.441
　　nicotine dependence Z87.891
　　noncompliance with medical treatment or
　　　regimen —*see* Noncompliance
　　nutritional deficiency Z86.39
　　obstetric complications Z87.59
　　　childbirth Z87.59
　　　pregnancy Z87.59
　　　pre-term labor Z87.51
　　　puerperium Z87.59
　　osteoporosis fractures Z87.31
　　parasuicide (attempt) Z91.5
　　physical trauma NEC Z87.828
　　　self-harm or suicide attempt Z91.5
　　pneumonia (recurrent) Z87.01
　　poisoning NEC Z91.89
　　　self-harm or suicide attempt Z91.5
　　poor personal hygiene Z91.89
　　preterm labor Z87.51
　　procedure during pregnancy Z98.870
　　procedure while a fetus Z98.871
　　prolonged reversible ischemic neurologic
　　　deficit (PRINO) Z86.73
　　prostatic dysplasia Z87.430
　　psychiatric disorder NEC Z87.89
　　psychological
　　　abuse
　　　　adult Z91.411
　　　　child Z62.811
　　　trauma, specified NEC Z91.49
　　radiation therapy Z92.3
　　removal
　　　implant
　　　　breast Z98.86
　　　renal calculi Z87.442
　　respiratory condition NEC Z87.09
　　retained foreign body fully removed
　　　Z87.821
　　risk factors NEC Z91.89
　　self-harm Z91.5
　　self-poisoning attempt Z91.5
　　sex reassignment Z87.890
　　sleep-wake cycle problem Z72.821
　　specified NEC Z87.898
　　steroid therapy (systemic) Z92.241
　　　inhaled Z92.240
　　stroke without residual deficits Z86.73
　　~~substance abuse NEC F10-F19 with~~
　　　~~fifth character 1~~
　▶substance abuse NEC F10-F19
　　sudden cardiac arrest Z86.74
　　sudden cardiac death successfully
　　　resuscitated Z86.74
　　suicide attempt Z91.5
　　surgery NEC Z98.890
　　　with uterine scar Z98.891
　　　sex reassignment Z87.890
　　　transplant —*see* Transplant
　　thrombophlebitis Z86.72
　　thrombosis (venous) Z86.718
　　　pulmonary Z86.711
　　tobacco dependence Z87.891
　　transient ischemic attack (TIA) without
　　　residual deficits Z86.73
　　trauma (physical) NEC Z87.828
　　　psychological NEC Z91.49
　　　self-harm Z91.5
　　traumatic brain injury Z87.820
　　unhealthy sleep-wake cycle Z72.821

History *(Continued)*
　personal *(Continued)*
　　unintended awareness under general
　　　anesthesia Z92.84
　　urinary (recurrent) (tract) infection(s)
　　　Z87.440
　　urinary calculi Z87.42
　　uterine scar from previous surgery
　　　Z98.891
　　vaginal dysplasia Z87.411
　　venous thrombosis or embolism Z86.718
　　　pulmonary Z86.711
　　vulvar dysplasia Z87.412
His-Werner disease A79.0
HIV —*see also* Human, immunodeficiency virus
　B20
　laboratory evidence (nonconclusive) R75
　nonconclusive test (in infants) R75
　positive, seropositive Z21
Hives (bold) —*see* Urticaria
Hoarseness R49.0
Hobo Z59.0
Hodgkin disease —*see* Lymphoma,
　Hodgkin
Hodgson's disease I71.2
　ruptured I71.1
Hoffa-Kastert disease E88.89
Hoffa's disease E88.89
Hoffmann-Bouveret syndrome I47.9
Hoffmann's syndrome E03.9 *[G73.7]*
Hole (round)
　macula H35.34-●
　retina (without detachment) —*see* Break,
　　retina, round hole
　　with detachment —*see* Detachment, retina,
　　　with retinal, break
Holiday relief care Z75.5
Hollenhorst's plaque —*see* Occlusion, artery,
　retina
Hollow foot (congenital) Q66.7
　acquired —*see* Deformity, limb, foot, specified
　　NEC
Holoprosencephaly Q04.2
Holt-Oram syndrome Q87.2
Homelessness Z59.0
Homesickness —*see* Disorder, adjustment
Homocystinemia, homocystinuria E72.11
Homogentisate 1,2-dioxygenase deficiency
　E70.29
Homologous serum hepatitis (prophylactic)
　(therapeutic) —*see* Hepatitis, viral, type B
Honeycomb lung J98.4
　congenital Q33.0
Hooded
　clitoris Q52.6
　penis Q55.69
Hookworm (anemia) (disease) (infection)
　(infestation) B76.9
　specified NEC B76.8
Hordeolum (eyelid) (externum) (recurrent)
　H00.019
　internum H00.029
　　left H00.026
　　　lower H00.025
　　　upper H00.024
　　right H00.023
　　　lower H00.022
　　　upper H00.021
　left H00.016
　　lower H00.015
　　upper H00.014
　right H00.013
　　lower H00.012
　　upper H00.011
Horn
　cutaneous L85.8
　nail L60.2
　　congenital Q84.6
Horner (-Claude Bernard) syndrome G90.2
　traumatic —*see* Injury, nerve, cervical
　　sympathetic

Horseshoe kidney (congenital) Q63.1
Horton's headache or neuralgia G44.099
   intractable G44.091
   not intractable G44.099
Hospital hopper syndrome —see Disorder,
      factitious
Hospitalism in children —see Disorder,
      adjustment
Hostility R45.5
   towards child Z62.3
Hot flashes
   menopausal N95.1
Hourglass (contracture) —see also Contraction,
      hourglass
   stomach K31.89
      congenital Q40.2
      stricture K31.2
Household, housing circumstance affecting
      care Z59.9
   specified NEC Z59.8
Housemaid's knee —see Bursitis, prepatellar
Hudson (-Stähli) line (cornea) —see
      Pigmentation, cornea, anterior
Human
   bite (open wound) —see also Bite
      intact skin surface —see Bite, superficial
   herpesvirus —see Herpes
   immunodeficiency virus (HIV) disease
         (infection) B20
      asymptomatic status Z21
      contact Z20.6
      counseling Z71.7
      dementia B20 [F02.80]
         with behavioral disturbance B20 [F02.81]
      exposure to Z20.6
      laboratory evidence R75
      type-2 (HIV 2) as cause of disease classified
            elsewhere B97.35
   papillomavirus (HPV)
      DNA test positive
         high risk
            cervix R87.810
            vagina R87.811
         low risk
            cervix R87.820
            vagina R87.821
      screening for Z11.51
   T-cell lymphotropic virus
      type-1 (HTLV-I) infection B33.3
         as cause of disease classified elsewhere
               B97.33
         carrier Z22.6
      type-2 (HTLV-II) as cause of disease
            classified elsewhere B97.34
Humidifier lung or pneumonitis J67.7
Humiliation (experience) in childhood Z62.898
Humpback (acquired) —see Kyphosis
Hunchback (acquired) —see Kyphosis
Hunger T73.0
   air, psychogenic F45.8
Hungry bone syndrome E83.81
Hunner's ulcer —see Cystitis, chronic,
      interstitial
Hunter's
   glossitis D51.0
   syndrome E76.1
Huntington's disease or chorea G10
   with dementia G10 [F02.80]
      with behavioral disturbance G10 [F02.81]
Hunt's
   disease or syndrome (herpetic geniculate
         ganglionitis) B02.21
      dyssynergia cerebellaris myoclonica G11.1
   neuralgia B02.21
Hurler (-Scheie) disease or syndrome E76.02
Hurst's disease G36.1
Hurthle cell
   adenocarcinoma C73
   adenoma D34
   carcinoma C73
   tumor D34

Hutchinson-Boeck disease or syndrome —see
      Sarcoidosis
Hutchinson-Gilford disease or syndrome E34.8
Hutchinson's
   disease, meaning
      angioma serpiginosum L81.7
      pompholyx (cheiropompholyx) L30.1
      prurigo estivalis L56.4
      summer eruption or summer prurigo L56.4
   melanotic freckle —see Melanoma, in situ
      malignant melanoma in —see Melanoma
   teeth or incisors (congenital syphilis) A50.52
   triad (congenital syphilis) A50.53
Hyalin plaque, sclera, senile H15.89
Hyaline membrane (disease) (lung)
      (pulmonary) (newborn) P22.0
Hyalinosis
   cutis (et mucosae) E78.89
   focal and segmental (glomerular) —see also
         N00-N07 with fourth character .1 N05.1
Hyalitis, hyalosis, asteroid —see also Deposit,
      crystalline
   syphilitic (late) A52.71
Hydatid
   cyst or tumor —see Echinococcus
   mole —see Hydatidiform mole
   Morgagni
      female Q50.5
      male (epididymal) Q55.4
         testicular Q55.29
Hydatidiform mole (benign) (complicating
      pregnancy) (delivered) (undelivered) O01.9
   classical O01.0
   complete O01.0
   incomplete O01.1
   invasive D39.2
   malignant D39.2
   partial O01.1
Hydatidosis —see Echinococcus
Hydradenitis (axillaris) (suppurative) L73.2
Hydradenoma —see Hidradenoma
Hydramnios O40.-●
Hydrancephaly, hydranencephaly Q04.3
   with spina bifida —see Spina bifida, with
         hydrocephalus
Hydrargyrism NEC —see Poisoning, mercury
Hydrarthrosis —see also Effusion, joint
   gonococcal A54.42
   intermittent M12.40
      ankle M12.47-●
      elbow M12.42-●
      foot joint M12.47-●
      hand joint M12.44-●
      hip M12.45-●
      knee M12.46-●
      multiple site M12.49
      shoulder M12.41-●
      specified joint NEC M12.48
      wrist M12.43-●
   of yaws (early) (late) —see also subcategory
         M14.8-● A66.6
   syphilitic (late) A52.77
      congenital A50.55 [M12.80]
Hydremia D64.89
Hydrencephalocele (congenital) —see
      Encephalocele
Hydrencephalomeningocele (congenital) —see
      Encephalocele
Hydroa R23.8
   aestivale L56.4
   vacciniforme L56.4
Hydroadenitis (axillaris) (suppurative)
      L73.2
Hydrocalycosis —see Hydronephrosis
Hydrocele (spermatic cord) (testis) (tunica
      vaginalis) N43.3
   canal of Nuck N94.89
   communicating N43.2
      congenital P83.5
   congenital P83.5
   encysted N43.0

Hydrocele (Continued)
   female NEC N94.89
   infected N43.1
   newborn P83.5
   round ligament N94.89
   specified NEC N43.2
   spinalis —see Spina bifida
   vulva N90.89
Hydrocephalus (acquired) (external) (internal)
      (malignant) (recurrent) G91.9
   aqueduct Sylvius stricture Q03.0
   causing disproportion O33.6
      with obstructed labor O66.3
   communicating G91.0
   congenital (external) (internal) Q03.9
      with spina bifida Q05.4
         cervical Q05.0
         dorsal Q05.1
         lumbar Q05.2
         lumbosacral Q05.2
         sacral Q05.3
         thoracic Q05.1
         thoracolumbar Q05.1
      specified NEC Q03.8
   due to toxoplasmosis (congenital) P37.1
   foramen Magendie block (acquired) G91.1
      congenital —see also Hydrocephalus,
            congenital Q03.1
   in (due to)
      infectious disease NEC B89 [G91.4]
      neoplastic disease NEC (see also Neoplasm)
            G91.4
      parasitic disease B89 [G91.4]
   newborn Q03.9
      with spina bifida —see Spina bifida, with
            hydrocephalus
   noncommunicating G91.1
   normal pressure G91.2
      secondary G91.0
   obstructive G91.1
   otitic G93.2
   post-traumatic NEC G91.3
   secondary G91.4
      post-traumatic G91.3
   specified NEC G91.8
   syphilitic, congenital A50.49
Hydrocolpos (congenital) N89.8
Hydrocystoma —see Neoplasm, skin, benign
Hydroencephalocele (congenital) —see
      Encephalocele
Hydroencephalomeningocele (congenital) —
      see Encephalocele
Hydrohematopneumothorax —see Hemothorax
Hydromeningitis —see Meningitis
Hydromeningocele (spinal) —see also Spina
      bifida
   cranial —see Encephalocele
Hydrometra N85.8
Hydrometrocolpos N89.8
Hydromicrocephaly Q02
Hydromphalos (since birth) Q45.8
Hydromyelia Q06.4
Hydromyelocele —see Spina bifida
Hydronephrosis (atrophic) (early)
      (functionless) (intermittent) (primary)
      (secondary) NEC N13.30
   with
      infection N13.6
      obstruction (by) (of)
         renal calculus N13.2
            with infection N13.6
         ureteral NEC N13.1
            with infection N13.6
            calculus N13.2
               with infection N13.6
         ➡ureteropelvic junction (congenital)
               Q62.11
            acquired N13.0
               with infection N13.6
         ureteral stricture NEC N13.1
            with infection N13.6

▶ New   ➡ Revised   ~~deleted~~ Deleted   ● Use Additional Character(s)

Hydronephrosis NEC *(Continued)*
  congenital Q62.0
    due to acquired occlusion of ureteropelvic
      junction N13.0
    specified type NEC N13.39
    tuberculous A18.11
Hydropericarditis —*see* Pericarditis
Hydropericardium —*see* Pericarditis
Hydroperitoneum R18.8
Hydrophobia —*see* Rabies
Hydrophthalmos Q15.0
Hydropneumohemothorax —*see* Hemothorax
Hydropneumopericarditis —*see* Pericarditis
Hydropneumopericardium —*see* Pericarditis
Hydropneumothorax J94.8
  traumatic —*see* Injury, intrathoracic, lung
  tuberculous NEC A15.6
Hydrops R60.9
  abdominis R18.8
  articulorum intermittens —*see* Hydrarthrosis,
    intermittent
  cardiac —*see* Failure, heart, congestive
  causing obstructed labor (mother) O66.3
  endolymphatic H81.0-●
  fetal —*see* Pregnancy, complicated by,
    hydrops, fetalis
  fetalis P83.2
    due to
      ABO isoimmunization P56.0
      alpha thalassemia D56.0
      hemolytic disease P56.90
        specified NEC P56.99
      isoimmunization (ABO) (Rh) P56.0
      other specified nonhemolytic disease
        NEC P83.2
      Rh incompatibility P56.0
    during pregnancy —*see* Pregnancy,
      complicated by, hydrops, fetalis
  gallbladder K82.1
  joint —*see* Effusion, joint
  labyrinth H81.0
  newborn (idiopathic) P83.2
    due to
      ABO isoimmunization P56.0
      alpha thalassemia D56.0
      hemolytic disease P56.90
        specified NEC P56.99
      isoimmunization (ABO) (Rh) P56.0
      Rh incompatibility P56.0
  nutritional —*see* Malnutrition, severe
  pericardium —*see* Pericarditis
  pleura —*see* Hydrothorax
  spermatic cord —*see* Hydrocele
Hydropyonephrosis N13.6
Hydrorachis Q06.4
Hydrorrhea (nasal) J34.89
  pregnancy —*see* Rupture, membranes,
    premature
Hydrosadenitis (axillaris) (suppurative) L73.2
Hydrosalpinx (fallopian tube) (follicularis) N70.11
Hydrothorax (double) (pleura) J94.8
  chylous (nonfilarial) I89.8
    filarial —*see also* Infestation, filarial B74.9
      [J91.8]
  traumatic —*see* Injury, intrathoracic
  tuberculous NEC (non primary) A15.6
Hydroureter —*see also* Hydronephrosis N13.4
  with infection N13.6
  congenital Q62.39
Hydroureteronephrosis —*see* Hydronephrosis
Hydrourethra N36.8
Hydroxykynureninuria E70.8
Hydroxylysinemia E72.3
Hydroxyprolinemia E72.59
Hygiene, sleep
  abuse Z72.821
  inadequate Z72.821
  poor Z72.821
Hygroma (congenital) (cystic) D18.1
  praepatellare, prepatellar —*see* Bursitis,
    prepatellar

Hymen —*see* condition
Hymenolepis, hymenolepiasis (diminuta)
  (infection) (infestation) (nana) B71.0
Hypalgesia R20.8
Hyperacidity (gastric) K31.89
  psychogenic F45.8
Hyperactive, hyperactivity F90.9
  basal cell, uterine cervix —*see* Dysplasia,
    cervix
  bowel sounds R19.12
  cervix epithelial (basal) —*see* Dysplasia,
    cervix
  child F90.9
    attention deficit —*see* Disorder, attention-
      deficit hyperactivity
  detrusor muscle N32.81
  gastrointestinal K31.89
    psychogenic F45.8
  nasal mucous membrane J34.3
  stomach K31.89
  thyroid (gland) —*see* Hyperthyroidism
Hyperacusis H93.23-●
Hyperadrenalism E27.5
Hyperadrenocorticism E24.9
  congenital E25.0
  iatrogenic E24.2
    correct substance properly administered —
      see Table of Drugs and Chemicals, by
      drug, adverse effect
    overdose or wrong substance given
      or taken —*see* Table of Drugs and
      Chemicals, by drug, poisoning
  not associated with Cushing's syndrome E27.0
  pituitary-dependent E24.0
Hyperaldosteronism E26.9
  familial (type I) E26.02
  glucocorticoid-remediable E26.02
  primary (due to (bilateral) adrenal
    hyperplasia) E26.09
  primary NEC E26.09
  secondary E26.1
  specified NEC E26.89
Hyperalgesia R20.8
Hyperalimentation R63.2
  carotene, carotin E67.1
  specified NEC E67.8
  vitamin
    A E67.0
    D E67.3
Hyperaminoaciduria
  arginine E72.21
  cystine E72.01
  lysine E72.3
  ornithine E72.4
Hyperammonemia (congenital) E72.20
Hyperazotemia —*see* Uremia
Hyperbetalipoproteinemia (familial) E78.00
  with prebetalipoproteinemia E78.2
Hyperbilirubinemia
  constitutional E80.6
  familial conjugated E80.6
  neonatal (transient) —*see* Jaundice, newborn
Hypercalcemia, hypocalciuric, familial E83.52
Hypercalciuria, idiopathic E83.52
Hypercapnia R06.89
  newborn P84
Hypercarotenemia, hypercarotinemia (dietary)
  E67.1
Hypercementosis K03.4
Hyperchloremia E87.8
Hyperchlorhydria K31.89
  neurotic F45.8
  psychogenic F45.8
Hypercholesterinemia —*see*
  Hypercholesterolemia
Hypercholesterolemia (essential) (primary)
  (pure) E78.00
  with hyperglyceridemia, endogenous E78.2
  dietary counseling and surveillance Z71.3
  familial E78.01
  hereditary E78.01

Hyperchylia gastrica, psychogenic F45.8
Hyperchylomicronemia (familial) (primary)
  E78.3
  with hyperbetalipoproteinemia E78.3
Hypercoagulable (state) D68.59
  activated protein C resistance D68.51
  antithrombin (III) deficiency D68.59
  factor V Leiden mutation D68.51
  primary NEC D68.59
  protein C deficiency D68.59
  protein S deficiency D68.59
  prothrombin gene mutation D68.52
  secondary D68.69
  specified NEC D68.69
Hypercoagulation (state) D68.59
Hypercorticalism, pituitary-dependent E24.0
Hypercorticosolism —*see* Cushing's, syndrome
Hypercorticosteronism E24.2
  correct substance properly administered —*see*
    Table of Drugs and Chemicals, by drug,
    adverse effect
  overdose or wrong substance given
    or taken —*see* Table of Drugs and
    Chemicals, by drug, poisoning
Hypercortisonism E24.2
  correct substance properly administered —*see*
    Table of Drugs and Chemicals, by drug,
    adverse effect
  overdose or wrong substance given
    or taken —*see* Table of Drugs and
    Chemicals, by drug, poisoning
Hyperekplexia Q89.8
Hyperelectrolytemia E87.8
Hyperemesis R11.10
  with nausea R11.2
  gravidarum (mild) O21.0
    with
      carbohydrate depletion O21.1
      dehydration O21.1
      electrolyte imbalance O21.1
      metabolic disturbance O21.1
    severe (with metabolic disturbance) O21.1
  projectile R11.12
  psychogenic F45.8
Hyperemia (acute) (passive) R68.89
  anal mucosa K62.89
  bladder N32.89
  cerebral I67.89
  conjunctiva H11.43-●
  ear internal, acute —*see* subcategory H83.0
  enteric K59.8
  eye —*see* Hyperemia, conjunctiva
  eyelid (active) (passive) —*see* Disorder,
    eyelid, specified type NEC
  intestine K59.8
  iris —*see* Disorder, iris, vascular
  kidney N28.89
  labyrinth —*see* subcategory H83.0
  liver (active) K76.89
  lung (passive) —*see* Edema, lung
  pulmonary (passive) —*see* Edema, lung
  renal N28.89
  retina H35.89
  stomach K31.89
Hyperesthesia (body surface) R20.3
  larynx (reflex) J38.7
    hysterical F44.89
  pharynx (reflex) J39.2
    hysterical F44.89
Hyperestrogenism (drug-induced) (iatrogenic)
  E28.0
Hyperexplexia Q89.8
Hyperfibrinolysis —*see* Fibrinolysis
Hyperfructosemia E74.19
Hyperfunction
  adrenal cortex, not associated with Cushing's
    syndrome E27.0
    medulla E27.5
      adrenomedullary E27.5
    virilism E25.9
      congenital E25.0

Hyperfunction (*Continued*)
  ovarian E28.8
  pancreas K86.89
  parathyroid (gland) E21.3
  pituitary (gland) (anterior) E22.9
    specified NEC E22.8
  polyglandular E31.1
  testicular E29.0
Hypergammaglobulinemia D89.2
  polyclonal D89.0
  Waldenström D89.0
Hypergastrinemia E16.4
Hyperglobulinemia R77.1
Hyperglycemia, hyperglycemic (transient) R73.9
  coma —*see* Diabetes, by type, with coma
  postpancreatectomy E89.1
Hyperglyceridemia (endogenous) (essential)
    (familial) (hereditary) (pure) E78.1
  mixed E78.3
Hyperglycinemia (non-ketotic) E72.51
Hypergonadism
  ovarian E28.8
  testicular (primary) (infantile) E29.0
Hyperheparinemia D68.32
Hyperhidrosis, hyperidrosis R61
  focal
    primary L74.519
      axilla L74.510
      face L74.511
      palms L74.512
      soles L74.513
    secondary L74.52
  generalized R61
  localized
    primary L74.519
      axilla L74.510
      face L74.511
      palms L74.512
      soles L74.513
    secondary L74.52
  psychogenic F45.8
  secondary R61
    focal L74.52
Hyperhistidinemia E70.41
Hyperhomocysteinemia E72.11
Hyperhydroxyprolinemia E72.59
Hyperinsulinism (functional) E16.1
  with
    coma (hypoglycemic) E15
    encephalopathy E16.1 [G94]
  ectopic E16.1
  therapeutic misadventure (from
    administration of insulin) —*see*
    subcategory T38.3
Hyperkalemia E87.5
Hyperkeratosis —*see also* Keratosis L85.9
  cervix N88.0
  due to yaws (early) (late) (palmar or plantar)
    A66.3
  follicularis Q82.8
    penetrans (in cutem) L87.0
  palmoplantaris climacterica L85.1
  pinta A67.1
  senile (with pruritus) L57.0
  universalis congenita Q80.8
  vocal cord J38.3
  vulva N90.4
Hyperkinesia, hyperkinetic (disease) (reaction)
    (syndrome) (childhood) (adolescence) —*see*
    also Disorder, attention-deficit hyperactivity
  heart I51.89
Hyperleucine-isoleucinemia E71.19
Hyperlipemia, hyperlipidemia E78.5
  combined E78.2
    familial E78.4
  group
    A E78.00
    B E78.1
    C E78.2
    D E78.3
  mixed E78.2
  specified NEC E78.4

Hyperlipidosis E75.6
  hereditary NEC E75.5
Hyperlipoproteinemia E78.5
  Fredrickson's type
    I E78.3
    IIa E78.00
    IIb E78.2
    III E78.2
    IV E78.1
    V E78.3
  low-density-lipoprotein-type (LDL) E78.00
  very-low-density-lipoprotein-type (VLDL)
    E78.1
Hyperlucent lung, unilateral J43.0
Hyperlysinemia E72.3
Hypermagnesemia E83.41
  neonatal P71.8
Hypermenorrhea N92.0
Hypermethioninemia E72.19
Hypermetropia (congenital) H52.0-●
Hypermobility, hypermotility
  cecum —*see* Syndrome, irritable bowel
  coccyx —*see* subcategory M53.2
  colon —*see* Syndrome, irritable bowel
    psychogenic F45.8
  ileum K58.9
  intestine —*see also* Syndrome, irritable bowel
    K58.9
    psychogenic F45.8
  meniscus (knee) —*see* Derangement, knee,
    meniscus
  scapula —*see* Instability, joint, shoulder
  stomach K31.89
    psychogenic F45.8
  syndrome M35.7
  urethra N36.41
    with intrinsic sphincter deficiency N36.43
Hypernasality R49.21
Hypernatremia E87.0
Hypernephroma C64.-●
Hyperopia —*see* Hypermetropia
Hyperorexia nervosa F50.2
Hyperornithinemia E72.4
Hyperosmia R43.1
Hyperosmolality E87.0
Hyperostosis (monomelic) —*see also* Disorder,
    bone, density and structure, specified NEC
  ankylosing (spine) M48.10
    cervical region M48.12
    cervicothoracic region M48.13
    lumbar region M48.16
    lumbosacral region M48.17
    multiple sites M48.19
    occipito-atlanto-axial region M48.11
    sacrococcygeal region M48.18
    thoracic region M48.14
    thoracolumbar region M48.15
  cortical (skull) M85.2
    infantile M89.8X-●
  frontal, internal of skull M85.2
  interna frontalis M85.2
  skeletal, diffuse idiopathic —*see*
    Hyperostosis, ankylosing
  skull M85.2
    congenital Q75.8
  vertebral, ankylosing —*see* Hyperostosis,
    ankylosing
Hyperovarism E28.8
Hyperoxaluria (primary) E72.53
Hyperparathyroidism E21.3
  primary E21.0
  secondary (renal) N25.81
    non-renal E21.1
  specified NEC E21.2
  tertiary E21.2
Hyperpathia R20.8
Hyperperistalsis R19.2
  psychogenic F45.8
Hyperpermeability, capillary I78.8
Hyperphagia R63.2
Hyperphenylalaninemia NEC E70.1

Hyperphoria (alternating) H50.53
Hyperphosphatemia E83.39
Hyperpiesis, hyperpiesia —*see* Hypertension
Hyperpigmentation —*see also* Pigmentation
  melanin NEC L81.4
  postinflammatory L81.0
Hyperpinealism E34.8
Hyperpituitarism E22.9
Hyperplasia, hyperplastic
  adenoids J35.2
  adrenal (capsule) (cortex) (gland) E27.8
    with
      sexual precocity (male) E25.9
        congenital E25.0
      virilism, adrenal E25.9
        congenital E25.0
      virilization (female) E25.9
        congenital E25.0
    congenital E25.0
    salt-losing E25.0
  adrenomedullary E27.5
  angiolymphoid, eosinophilia (ALHE) D18.01
  appendix (lymphoid) K38.0
  artery, fibromuscular I77.3
  bone —*see also* Hypertrophy, bone
    marrow D75.89
  breast —*see also* Hypertrophy, breast
    ductal (atypical) N60.9-●
  C-cell, thyroid E07.0
  cementation (tooth) (teeth) K03.4
  cervical gland R59.0
  cervix (uteri) (basal cell) (endometrium)
    (polypoid) —*see also* Dysplasia, cervix
    congenital Q51.828
  clitoris, congenital Q52.6
  denture K06.2
  endocervicitis N72
  endometrium, endometrial (adenomatous)
    (benign) (cystic) (glandular) (glandular-
    cystic) (polypoid) N85.00
    with atypia N85.02
    cervix —*see* Dysplasia, cervix
    complex (without atypia) N85.01
    simple (without atypia) N85.01
  epithelial L85.9
    focal, oral, including tongue K13.29
    nipple N62
    skin L85.9
    tongue K13.29
    vaginal wall N89.3
  erythroid D75.89
  fibromuscular of artery (carotid) (renal)
    I77.3
  genital
    female NEC N94.89
    male N50.89
  gingiva K06.1
  glandularis cystica uteri (interstitialis) —*see*
    also Hyperplasia, endometrial N85.00-●
  gum K06.1
  hymen, congenital Q52.4
  irritative, edentulous (alveolar) K06.2
  jaw M26.09
    alveolar M26.79
    lower M26.03
      alveolar M26.72
    upper M26.01
      alveolar M26.71
  kidney (congenital) Q63.3
  labia N90.69
    epithelial N90.3
  liver (congenital) Q44.7
    nodular, focal K76.89
  lymph gland or node R59.9
  mandible, mandibular M26.03
    alveolar M26.72
    unilateral condylar M27.8
  maxilla, maxillary M26.01
    alveolar M26.71
  myometrium, myometrial N85.2
  neuroendocrine cell, of infancy J84.841

▶ New   ⇒ Revised   ~~deleted~~ Deleted   ● Use Additional Character(s)

Hyperplasia, hyperplastic *(Continued)*
  nose
    lymphoid J34.89
    polypoid J33.9
  oral mucosa (irritative) K13.6
  organ or site, congenital NEC —*see* Anomaly,
    by site
  ovary N83.8
  palate, papillary (irritative) K13.6
  pancreatic islet cells E16.9
    alpha E16.8
      with excess
        gastrin E16.4
        glucagon E16.3
    beta E16.1
  parathyroid (gland) E21.0
  pharynx (lymphoid) J39.2
  prostate (adenofibromatous) (nodular) N40.0
    with lower urinary tract symptoms (LUTS)
      N40.1
    without lower urinary tract symptoms
      (LUTS) N40.0
  renal artery I77.89
  reticulo-endothelial (cell) D75.89
  salivary gland (any) K11.1
  Schimmelbusch's —*see* Mastopathy, cystic
  suprarenal capsule (gland) E27.8
  thymus (gland) (persistent) E32.0
  thyroid (gland) —*see* Goiter
  tonsils (faucial) (infective) (lingual)
    (lymphoid) J35.1
    with adenoids J35.3
  unilateral condylar M27.8
  uterus, uterine N85.2
    endometrium (glandular) —*see also*
      Hyperplasia, endometrial N85.00-●
  vulva N90.69
    epithelial N90.3
Hyperpnea —*see* Hyperventilation
Hyperpotassemia E87.5
Hyperprebetalipoproteinemia (familial) E78.1
Hyperprolactinemia E22.1
Hyperprolinemia (type I) (type II) E72.59
Hyperproteinemia E88.09
Hyperprothrombinemia, causing coagulation
  factor deficiency D68.4
Hyperpyrexia R50.9
  heat (effects) T67.0
  malignant, due to anesthetic T88.3
  rheumatic —*see* Fever, rheumatic
  unknown origin R50.9
Hyper-reflexia R29.2
Hypersalivation K11.7
Hypersecretion
  ACTH (not associated with Cushing's
    syndrome) E27.0
    pituitary E24.0
  adrenaline E27.5
  adrenomedullary E27.5
  androgen (testicular) E29.0
    ovarian (drug-induced) (iatrogenic) E28.1
  calcitonin E07.0
  catecholamine E27.5
  corticoadrenal E24.9
  cortisol E24.9
  epinephrine E27.5
  estrogen E28.0
  gastric K31.89
    psychogenic F45.8
  gastrin E16.4
  glucagon E16.3
  hormone(s)
    ACTH (not associated with Cushing's
      syndrome) E27.0
      pituitary E24.0
    antidiuretic E22.2
    growth E22.0
    intestinal NEC E34.1
    ovarian androgen E28.1
    pituitary E22.9
    testicular E29.0

Hypersecretion *(Continued)*
  hormone *(Continued)*
    thyroid stimulating E05.80
      with thyroid storm E05.81
  insulin —*see* Hyperinsulinism
  lacrimal glands —*see* Epiphora
  medulloadrenal E27.5
  milk O92.6
  ovarian androgens E28.1
  salivary gland (any) K11.7
  thyrocalcitonin E07.0
  upper respiratory J39.8
Hypersegmentation, leukocytic, hereditary D72.0
Hypersensitiveness, hypersensitiveness,
  hypersensitivity —*see also* Allergy
  carotid sinus G90.01
  colon —*see* Irritable, colon
  drug T88.7
  gastrointestinal K52.29
    immediate K52.29
    psychogenic F45.8
  labyrinth —*see* subcategory H83.2
  pain R20.8
  pneumonitis —*see* Pneumonitis, allergic
  reaction T78.40
    upper respiratory tract NEC J39.3
Hypersomnia (organic) G47.10
  due to
    alcohol
      abuse F10.182
      dependence F10.282
      use F10.982
    amphetamines
      abuse F15.182
      dependence F15.282
      use F15.982
    caffeine
      abuse F15.182
      dependence F15.282
      use F15.982
    cocaine
      abuse F14.182
      dependence F14.282
      use F14.982
    drug NEC
      abuse F19.182
      dependence F19.282
      use F19.982
    medical condition G47.14
    mental disorder F51.13
    opioid
      abuse F11.182
      dependence F11.282
      use F11.982
    psychoactive substance NEC
      abuse F19.182
      dependence F19.282
      use F19.982
    sedative, hypnotic, or anxiolytic
      abuse F13.182
      dependence F13.282
      use F13.982
    stimulant NEC
      abuse F15.182
      dependence F15.282
      use F15.982
  idiopathic G47.11
    with long sleep time G47.11
    without long sleep time G47.12
  menstrual related G47.13
  nonorganic origin F51.11
    specified NEC F51.19
  not due to a substance or known
    physiological condition F51.11
    specified NEC F51.19
  primary F51.11
  recurrent G47.13
  specified NEC G47.19
Hypersplenia, hypersplenism D73.1
Hyperstimulation, ovaries (associated with
  induced ovulation) N98.1

Hypersusceptibility —*see* Allergy
Hypertelorism (ocular) (orbital) Q75.2
Hypertension, hypertensive (accelerated)
  (benign) (essential) (idiopathic)
  (malignant) (systemic) I10
  with
    ▶heart failure (congestive) I11.0
    ⇒heart involvement (conditions in I50.-,
      I51.4-I51.9 due to hypertension) —*see*
      Hypertension, heart
    kidney involvement —*see* Hypertension,
      kidney
  benign, intracranial G93.2
  borderline R03.0
  cardiorenal (disease) I13.10
    with heart failure I13.0
      with stage 1 through stage 4 chronic
        kidney disease I13.0
      with stage 5 or end stage renal disease
        I13.2
    without heart failure I13.10
      with stage 1 through stage 4 chronic
        kidney disease I13.10
      with stage 5 or end stage renal disease
        I13.11
  cardiovascular
    disease (arteriosclerotic) (sclerotic) —*see*
      Hypertension, heart
    renal (disease) —*see* Hypertension,
      cardiorenal
  chronic venous —*see* Hypertension, venous
    (chronic)
  complicating
    childbirth (labor) O16.4
    pre-existing O10.92
      with
        heart disease O10.12
          with renal disease O10.32
        pre-eclampsia O11.4
        renal disease O10.22
          with heart disease O10.32
      essential O10.02
      secondary O10.42
    pregnancy O16.-●
      with edema —*see also* Pre-eclampsia
        O14.9-●
      gestational (pregnancy induced)
        (without proteinuria) O13.-●
        with proteinuria O14.9-●
          mild pre-eclampsia O14.0-●
          moderate pre-eclampsia O14.0-●
          severe pre-eclampsia O14.1-●
            with hemolysis, elevated
              liver enzymes and low
              platelet count (HELLP)
              O14.2-●
      pre-existing O10.91-●
        with
          heart disease O10.11-●
            with renal disease O10.31-●
          pre-eclampsia —*see* category O11
          renal disease O10.21-●
            with heart disease O10.31-●
        essential O10.01-●
        secondary O10.41-●
      transient O13.-●
    puerperium pre-existing O16.5
    pre-existing
      with
        heart disease O10.13
          with renal disease O10.33
        pre-eclampsia O11.5
        renal disease O10.23
          with heart disease O10.33
        essential O10.03
    pregnancy-induced O13.9
    secondary O10.43
  crisis I16.9
  due to
    endocrine disorders I15.2
    pheochromocytoma I15.2

Hypertension, hypertensive *(Continued)*
  due to *(Continued)*
    renal disorders NEC I15.1
      arterial I15.0
    renovascular disorders I15.0
    specified disease NEC I15.8
  emergency I16.1
  encephalopathy I67.4
  gestational (without significant proteinuria)
    (pregnancy-induced) (transient) O13.-•
    with significant proteinuria —*see*
      Pre-eclampsia
    complicating
      delivery O13.4
      puerperium O13.5
  Goldblatt's I70.1
  heart (disease) (conditions in I51.4-I51.9 due
    to hypertension) I11.9
    with
      heart failure (congestive) I11.0
      kidney disease (chronic) —*see*
        Hypertension, cardiorenal
  intracranial (benign) G93.2
  kidney I12.9
    with
      heart disease —*see* Hypertension,
        cardiorenal
      stage 1 through stage 4 chronic kidney
        disease I12.9
      stage 5 chronic kidney disease (CKD) or
        end stage renal disease (ESRD) I12.0
  lesser circulation I27.0
  maternal O16.-•
  newborn P29.2
  pulmonary (persistent) P29.30
  ocular H40.05-•
  pancreatic duct — code to underlying condition
    with chronic pancreatitis K86.1
  portal (due to chronic liver disease)
    (idiopathic) K76.6
    gastropathy K31.89
    in (due to) schistosomiasis (bilharziasis)
      B65.9 *[K77]*
  postoperative I97.3
  psychogenic F45.8
  pulmonary NEC I27.20
    with
      cor pulmonale (chronic) I27.29
        acute I26.09
      right heart ventricular strain/failure
        I27.29
        acute I26.09
      right to left shunt related to congenital
        heart disease I27.83
      unclear multifactorial mechanisms I27.29
    arterial (associated) (drug-induced)
      (toxin-induced) I27.21
    chronic thromboembolic I27.24
    due to
      hematologic disorders I27.29
      left heart disease I27.22
      lung diseases and hypoxia I27.23
      metabolic disorders I27.29
      specified systemic disorders NEC I27.29
    group 1 (associated) (drug-induced)
      (toxin-induced) I27.21
    group 2 I27.22
    group 3 I27.23
    group 4 I27.24
    group 5 I27.29
    of newborn (persistent) P29.30
      secondary
        arterial I27.21
        specified NEC I27.29
    primary (idiopathic) I27.0
  renal —*see* Hypertension, kidney
  renovascular I15.0
  secondary NEC I15.9
    due to
      endocrine disorders I15.2
      pheochromocytoma I15.2

Hypertension, hypertensive *(Continued)*
  secondary NEC *(Continued)*
    due to *(Continued)*
      renal disorders NEC I15.1
        arterial I15.0
      renovascular disorders I15.0
    specified NEC I15.8
  transient, of pregnancy O13.-•
  urgency I16.0
  venous (chronic)
    due to
      deep vein thrombosis —*see* Syndrome,
        postthrombotic
    idiopathic I87.309
      with
        inflammation I87.32-•
          with ulcer I87.33-•
        specified complication NEC I87.39-•
        ulcer I87.31-•
          with inflammation I87.33-•
      asymptomatic I87.30-•
Hypertensive urgency —*see* Hypertension
Hyperthecosis ovary E28.8
Hyperthermia (of unknown origin) —*see also*
  Hyperpyrexia
  malignant, due to anesthesia T88.3
  newborn P81.9
    environmental P81.0
Hyperthyroid (recurrent) —*see*
  Hyperthyroidism
Hyperthyroidism (latent) (pre-adult)
  (recurrent) E05.90
  with
    goiter (diffuse) E05.00
      with thyroid storm E05.01
      nodular (multinodular) E05.20
        with thyroid storm E05.21
        uninodular E05.10
          with thyroid storm E05.11
    storm E05.91
  due to ectopic thyroid tissue E05.30
    with thyroid storm E05.31
  neonatal, transitory P72.1
  specified NEC E05.80
    with thyroid storm E05.81
Hypertony, hypertonia, hypertonicity
  bladder N31.8
  congenital P94.1
  stomach K31.89
    psychogenic F45.8
  uterus, uterine (contractions) (complicating
    delivery) O62.4
Hypertrichosis L68.9
  congenital Q84.2
  eyelid H02.869
    left H02.866
      lower H02.865
      upper H02.864
    right H02.863
      lower H02.862
      upper H02.861
  lanuginosa Q84.2
    acquired L68.1
  localized L68.2
  specified NEC L68.8
Hypertriglyceridemia, essential E78.1
Hypertrophy, hypertrophic
  adenofibromatous, prostate —*see*
    Enlargement, enlarged, prostate
  adenoids (infective) J35.2
    with tonsils J35.3
  adrenal cortex E27.8
  alveolar process or ridge —*see* Anomaly,
    alveolar
  anal papillae K62.89
  artery I77.89
    congenital NEC Q27.8
      digestive system Q27.8
      lower limb Q27.8
      specified site NEC Q27.8
      upper limb Q27.8

Hypertrophy, hypertrophic *(Continued)*
  auricular —*see* Hypertrophy, cardiac
  Bartholin's gland N75.8
  bile duct (common) (hepatic) K83.8
  bladder (sphincter) (trigone) N32.89
  bone M89.30
    carpus M89.34-•
    clavicle M89.31-•
    femur M89.35-•
    fibula M89.36-•
    finger M89.34-•
    humerus M89.32-•
    ilium M89.359
    ischium M89.359
    metacarpus M89.34-•
    metatarsus M89.37-•
    multiple sites M89.39
    neck M89.38
    radius M89.33-•
    rib M89.38
    scapula M89.31-•
    skull M89.38
    tarsus M89.37-•
    tibia M89.36-•
    toe M89.37-•
    ulna M89.33-•
    vertebra M89.38
  brain G93.89
  breast N62
    cystic —*see* Mastopathy, cystic
    newborn P83.4
    pubertal, massive N62
    puerperal, postpartum —*see* Disorder,
      breast, specified type NEC
    senile (parenchymatous) N62
  cardiac (chronic) (idiopathic) I51.7
    with rheumatic fever (conditions in I00)
      active I01.8
      inactive or quiescent (with chorea) I09.89
    congenital NEC Q24.8
    fatty —*see* Degeneration, myocardial
    hypertensive —*see* Hypertension, heart
    rheumatic (with chorea) I09.89
      active or acute I01.8
        with chorea I02.0
    valve —*see* Endocarditis
  cartilage —*see* Disorder, cartilage, specified
    type NEC
  cecum —*see* Megacolon
  cervix (uteri) N88.8
    congenital Q51.828
    elongation N88.4
  clitoris (cirrhotic) N90.89
    congenital Q52.6
  colon —*see also* Megacolon
    congenital Q43.2
  conjunctiva, lymphoid H11.89
  corpora cavernosa N48.89
  cystic duct K82.8
  duodenum K31.89
  endometrium (glandular) —*see also*
    Hyperplasia, endometrial N85.00-•
    cervix N88.8
  epididymis N50.89
  esophageal hiatus (congenital) Q79.1
    with hernia —*see* Hernia, hiatal
  eyelid —*see* Disorder, eyelid, specified type
    NEC
  fat pad E65
    knee (infrapatellar) (popliteal) (prepatellar)
      (retropatellar) M79.4
  foot (congenital) Q74.2
  frenulum, frenum (tongue) K14.8
    lip K13.0
  gallbladder K82.8
  gastric mucosa K29.60
    with bleeding K29.61
  gland, glandular R59.9
    generalized R59.1
    localized R59.0
  gum (mucous membrane) K06.1

Hypertrophy, hypertrophic (Continued)
heart (idiopathic) —see also Hypertrophy, cardiac
 valve —see also Endocarditis I38
hemifacial Q67.4
hepatic —see Hypertrophy, liver
hiatus (esophageal) Q79.1
hilus gland R59.0
hymen, congenital Q52.4
ileum K63.89
intestine NEC K63.89
jejunum K63.89
kidney (compensatory) N28.81
 congenital Q63.3
labium (majus) (minus) N90.60
ligament —see Disorder, ligament
lingual tonsil (infective) J35.1
 with adenoids J35.3
lip K13.0
 congenital Q18.6
liver R16.0
 acute K76.89
 cirrhotic —see Cirrhosis, liver
 congenital Q44.7
 fatty —see Fatty, liver
lymph, lymphatic gland R59.9
 generalized R59.1
 localized R59.0
 tuberculous —see Tuberculosis, lymph gland
mammary gland —see Hypertrophy, breast
Meckel's diverticulum (congenital) Q43.0
 malignant —see Table of Neoplasms, small intestine, malignant
median bar —see Hyperplasia, prostate
meibomian gland —see Chalazion
meniscus, knee, congenital Q74.1
metatarsal head —see Hypertrophy, bone, metatarsus
metatarsus —see Hypertrophy, bone, metatarsus
mucous membrane
 alveolar ridge K06.2
 gum K06.1
 nose (turbinate) J34.3
muscle M62.89
muscular coat, artery I77.89
myocardium —see also Hypertrophy, cardiac
 idiopathic I42.2
myometrium N85.2
nail L60.2
 congenital Q84.5
nasal J34.89
 alae J34.89
 bone J34.89
 cartilage J34.89
 mucous membrane (septum) J34.3
 sinus J34.89
 turbinate J34.3
nasopharynx, lymphoid (infectional) (tissue) (wall) J35.2
nipple N62
organ or site, congenital NEC —see Anomaly, by site - ovary N83.8
palate (hard) M27.8
 soft K13.79
pancreas, congenital Q45.3
parathyroid (gland) E21.0
parotid gland K11.1
penis N48.89
pharyngeal tonsil J35.2
pharynx J39.2
 lymphoid (infectional) (tissue) (wall) J35.2
pituitary (anterior) (fossa) (gland) E23.6
prepuce (congenital) N47.8
 female N90.89

Hypertrophy, hypertrophic (Continued)
prostate —see Enlargement, enlarged, prostate
 congenital Q55.4
pseudomuscular G71.0
pylorus (adult) (muscle) (sphincter) K31.1
 congenital or infantile Q40.0
rectal, rectum (sphincter) K62.89
rhinitis (turbinate) J31.0
salivary gland (any) K11.1
 congenital Q38.4
scaphoid (tarsal) —see Hypertrophy, bone, tarsus
scar L91.0
scrotum N50.89
seminal vesicle N50.89
sigmoid —see Megacolon
skin L91.9
 specified NEC L91.8
spermatic cord N50.89
spleen —see Splenomegaly
spondylitis —see Spondylosis
stomach K31.89
sublingual gland K11.1
submandibular gland K11.1
suprarenal cortex (gland) E27.8
synovial NEC M67.20
 acromioclavicular M67.21-●
 ankle M67.27-●
 elbow M67.22-●
 foot M67.27-●
 hand M67.24-●
 hip M67.25-●
 knee M67.26-●
 multiple sites M67.29
 specified site NEC M67.28
 wrist M67.23-●
tendon —see Disorder, tendon, specified type NEC
testis N44.8
 congenital Q55.29
thymic, thymus (gland) (congenital) E32.0
thyroid (gland) —see Goiter
toe (congenital) Q74.2
 acquired —see also Deformity, toe, specified NEC
tongue K14.8
 congenital Q38.2
 papillae (foliate) K14.3
tonsils (faucial) (infective) (lingual) (lymphoid) J35.1
 with adenoids J35.3
tunica vaginalis N50.89
ureter N28.89
urethra N36.8
uterus N85.2
 neck (with elongation) N88.4
 puerperal O90.89
uvula K13.79
vagina N89.8
vas deferens N50.89
vein I87.8
ventricle, ventricular (heart) —see also Hypertrophy, cardiac
 congenital Q24.8
 in tetralogy of Fallot Q21.3
verumontanum N36.8
vocal cord J38.3
vulva N90.60
 stasis (nonfilarial) N90.69
Hypertropia H50.2-●
Hypertyrosinemia E70.21
Hyperuricemia (asymptomatic) E79.0
Hypervalinemia E71.19
Hyperventilation (tetany) R06.4
 hysterical F45.8
 psychogenic F45.8
 syndrome F45.8

Hypervitaminosis (dietary) NEC E67.8
A E67.0
 administered as drug (prolonged intake) —see Table of Drugs and Chemicals, vitamins, adverse effect
 overdose or wrong substance given or taken —see Table of Drugs and Chemicals, vitamins, poisoning
B6 E67.2
D E67.3
 administered as drug (prolonged intake) —see Table of Drugs and Chemicals, vitamins, adverse effect
 overdose or wrong substance given or taken —see Table of Drugs and Chemicals, vitamins, poisoning
K E67.8
 administered as drug (prolonged intake) —see Table of Drugs and Chemicals, vitamins, adverse effect
 overdose or wrong substance given or taken —see Table of Drugs and Chemicals, vitamins, poisoning
Hypervolemia E87.70
 specified NEC E87.79
Hypesthesia R20.1
 cornea —see Anesthesia, cornea
Hyphema H21.0-●
 traumatic S05.1-●
Hypoacidity, gastric K31.89
 psychogenic F45.8
Hypoadrenalism, hypoadrenia E27.40
 primary E27.1
 tuberculous A18.7
Hypoadrenocorticism E27.40
 pituitary E23.0
 primary E27.1
Hypoalbuminemia E88.09
Hypoaldosteronism E27.40
Hypoalphalipoproteinemia E78.6
Hypobarism T70.29
Hypobaropathy T70.29
Hypobetalipoproteinemia (familial) E78.6
Hypocalcemia E83.51
 dietary E58
 neonatal P71.1
 due to cow's milk P71.0
 phosphate-loading (newborn) P71.1
Hypochloremia E87.8
Hypochlorhydria K31.89
 neurotic F45.8
 psychogenic F45.8
Hypochondria, hypochondriac, hypochondriasis (reaction) F45.21
 sleep F51.03
Hypochondrogenesis Q77.0
Hypochondroplasia Q77.4
Hypochromasia, blood cells D50.8
Hypodontia —see Anodontia
Hypoeosinophilia D72.89
Hypoesthesia R20.1
Hypofibrinogenemia D68.8
 acquired D65
 congenital (hereditary) D68.2
Hypofunction
 adrenocortical E27.40
 drug-induced E27.3
 postprocedural E89.6
 primary E27.1
 adrenomedullary, postprocedural E89.6
 cerebral R29.818
 corticoadrenal NEC E27.40
 intestinal K59.8
 labyrinth —see subcategory H83.2
 ovary E28.39
 pituitary (gland) (anterior) E23.0
 testicular E29.1
 postprocedural (postsurgical) (postirradiation) (iatrogenic) E89.5
Hypogalactia O92.4

Hypogammaglobulinemia —*see also*
    Agammaglobulinemia D80.1
    hereditary D80.0
    nonfamilial D80.1
    transient, of infancy D80.7
Hypogenitalism (congenital) —*see*
    Hypogonadism
Hypoglossia Q38.3
Hypoglycemia (spontaneous) E16.2
    coma E15
    ➠ diabetic —*see* Diabetes, by type, with
        hypoglycemia, with coma
    diabetic —*see* Diabetes, hypoglycemia
    dietary counseling and surveillance Z71.3
    drug-induced E16.0
      with coma (nondiabetic) E15
    due to insulin E16.0
      with coma (nondiabetic) E15
      therapeutic misadventure —*see*
        subcategory T38.3
    functional, nonhyperinsulinemic E16.1
    iatrogenic E16.0
      with coma (nondiabetic) E15
    in infant of diabetic mother P70.1
      gestational diabetes P70.0
    infantile E16.1
    leucine-induced E71.19
    neonatal (transitory) P70.4
      iatrogenic P70.3
    reactive (not drug-induced) E16.1
    transitory neonatal P70.4
Hypogonadism
    female E28.39
    hypogonadotropic E23.0
    male E29.1
    ovarian (primary) E28.39
    pituitary E23.0
    testicular (primary) E29.1
Hypohidrosis, hypoidrosis L74.4
Hypoinsulinemia, postprocedural E89.1
Hypokalemia E87.6
Hypoleukocytosis —*see* Agranulocytosis
Hypolipoproteinemia (alpha) (beta) E78.6
Hypomagnesemia E83.42
    neonatal P71.2
Hypomania, hypomanic reaction F30.8
Hypomenorrhea —*see* Oligomenorrhea
Hypometabolism R63.8
Hypomotility
    gastrointestinal (tract) K31.89
      psychogenic F45.8
    intestine K59.8
      psychogenic F45.8
    stomach K31.89
      psychogenic F45.8
Hyponasality R49.22
Hyponatremia E87.1
Hypo-osmolality E87.1
Hypo-ovarianism, hypo-ovarism E28.39
Hypoparathyroidism E20.9
    familial E20.8
    idiopathic E20.0
    neonatal, transitory P71.4
    postprocedural E89.2
    specified NEC E20.8
Hypoperfusion (in)
    newborn P96.89
Hypopharyngitis —*see* Laryngopharyngitis
Hypophoria H50.53
Hypophosphatemia, hypophosphatasia
    (acquired) (congenital) (renal) E83.39
    familial E83.31
Hypophyseal, hypophysis —*see also* condition
    dwarfism E23.0
    gigantism E22.0
Hypopiesis —*see* Hypotension
Hypopinealism E34.8
Hypopituitarism (juvenile) E23.0
    drug-induced E23.1
    due to
      hypophysectomy E89.3
      radiotherapy E89.3

Hypopituitarism *(Continued)*
    iatrogenic NEC E23.1
    postirradiation E89.3
    postpartum O99.285
    postprocedural E89.3
Hypoplasia, hypoplastic
    adrenal (gland), congenital Q89.1
    alimentary tract, congenital Q45.8
      upper Q40.8
    anus, anal (canal) Q42.3
      with fistula Q42.2
    aorta, aortic Q25.42
      ascending, in hypoplastic left heart
        syndrome Q23.4
      valve Q23.1
        in hypoplastic left heart syndrome
          Q23.4
    areola, congenital Q83.8
    arm (congenital) —*see* Defect, reduction,
      upper limb
    artery (peripheral) Q27.8
      brain (congenital) Q28.3
      coronary Q24.5
      digestive system Q27.8
      lower limb Q27.8
      pulmonary Q25.79
        functional, unilateral J43.0
      retinal (congenital) Q14.1
      specified site NEC Q27.8
      umbilical Q27.0
      upper limb Q27.8
    auditory canal Q17.8
      causing impairment of hearing Q16.9
    biliary duct or passage Q44.5
    bone NOS Q79.9
      face Q75.8
      marrow D61.9
        megakaryocytic D69.49
      skull —*see* Hypoplasia, skull
    brain Q02
      gyri Q04.3
      part of Q04.3
    breast (areola) N64.82
    bronchus Q32.4
    cardiac Q24.8
    carpus —*see* Defect, reduction, upper limb,
      specified type NEC
    cartilage hair Q78.8
    cecum Q42.8
    cementum K00.4
    cephalic Q02
    cerebellum Q04.3
    cervix (uteri), congenital Q51.821
    clavicle (congenital) Q74.0
    coccyx Q76.49
    colon Q42.9
      specified NEC Q42.8
    corpus callosum Q04.0
    cricoid cartilage Q31.2
    digestive organ(s) or tract NEC Q45.8
      upper (congenital) Q40.8
    ear (auricle) (lobe) Q17.2
      middle Q16.4
    enamel of teeth (neonatal) (postnatal)
      (prenatal) K00.4
    endocrine (gland) NEC Q89.2
    endometrium N85.8
    epididymis (congenital) Q55.4
    epiglottis Q31.2
    erythroid, congenital D61.01
    esophagus (congenital) Q39.8
    eustachian tube Q17.8
    eye Q11.2
    eyelid (congenital) Q10.3
    face Q18.8
      bone(s) Q75.8
    femur (congenital) —*see* Defect,
      reduction, lower limb, specified
      type NEC
    fibula (congenital) —*see* Defect, reduction,
      lower limb, specified type NEC

Hypoplasia, hypoplastic *(Continued)*
    finger (congenital) —*see* Defect, reduction,
      upper limb, specified type NEC
    focal dermal Q82.8
    foot —*see* Defect, reduction, lower limb,
      specified type NEC
    gallbladder Q44.0
    genitalia, genital organ(s)
      female, congenital Q52.8
        external Q52.79
        internal NEC Q52.8
      in adiposogenital dystrophy E23.6
    glottis Q31.2
    hair Q84.2
    hand (congenital) —*see* Defect, reduction,
      upper limb, specified type NEC
    heart Q24.8
    humerus (congenital) —*see* Defect, reduction,
      upper limb, specified type NEC
    intestine (small) Q41.9
      large Q42.9
        specified NEC Q42.8
    jaw M26.09
      alveolar M26.79
      lower M26.04
        alveolar M26.74
      upper M26.02
        alveolar M26.73
    kidney(s) Q60.5
      bilateral Q60.4
      unilateral Q60.3
    labium (majus) (minus), congenital Q52.79
    larynx Q31.2
    left heart syndrome Q23.4
    leg (congenital) —*see* Defect, reduction, lower
      limb
    limb Q73.8
      lower (congenital) —*see* Defect, reduction,
        lower limb
      upper (congenital) —*see* Defect, reduction,
        upper limb
    liver Q44.7
    lung (lobe) (not associated with short
      gestation) Q33.6
      associated with immaturity, low birth
        weight, prematurity, or short gestation
        P28.0
    mammary (areola), congenital Q83.8
    mandible, mandibular M26.04
      alveolar M26.74
      unilateral condylar M27.8
    maxillary M26.02
      alveolar M26.73
    medullary D61.9
    megakaryocytic D69.49
    metacarpus —*see* Defect, reduction, upper
      limb, specified type NEC
    metatarsus —*see* Defect, reduction, lower
      limb, specified type NEC
    muscle Q79.8
    nail(s) Q84.6
    nose, nasal Q30.1
    optic nerve H47.03-●
    osseous meatus (ear) Q17.8
    ovary, congenital Q50.39
    pancreas Q45.0
    parathyroid (gland) Q89.2
    parotid gland Q38.4
    patella Q74.1
    pelvis, pelvic girdle Q74.2
    penis (congenital) Q55.62
    peripheral vascular system Q27.8
      digestive system Q27.8
      lower limb Q27.8
      specified site NEC Q27.8
      upper limb Q27.8
    pituitary (gland) (congenital) Q89.2
    pulmonary (not associated with short
      gestation) Q33.6
      artery, functional J43.0
      associated with short gestation P28.0

▶ New   ➠ Revised   ~~deleted~~ Deleted   ● Use Additional Character(s)

Hypoplasia, hypoplastic (Continued)
  radioulnar —see Defect, reduction, upper limb, specified type NEC
  radius —see Defect, reduction, upper limb
  rectum Q42.1
    with fistula Q42.0
  respiratory system NEC Q34.8
  rib Q76.6
  right heart syndrome Q22.6
  sacrum Q76.49
  scapula Q74.0
  scrotum Q55.1
  shoulder girdle Q74.0
  skin Q82.8
  skull (bone) Q75.8
    with
      anencephaly Q00.0
      encephalocele —see Encephalocele
      hydrocephalus Q03.9
        with spina bifida —see Spina bifida, by site, with hydrocephalus
      microcephaly Q02
  spinal (cord) (ventral horn cell) Q06.1
  spine Q76.49
  sternum Q76.7
  tarsus —see Defect, reduction, lower limb, specified type NEC
  testis Q55.1
  thymic, with immunodeficiency D82.1
  thymus (gland) Q89.2
    with immunodeficiency D82.1
  thyroid (gland) E03.1
    cartilage Q31.2
  tibiofibular (congenital) —see Defect, reduction, lower limb, specified type NEC
  toe —see Defect, reduction, lower limb, specified type NEC
  tongue Q38.3
  Turner's K00.4
  ulna (congenital) —see Defect, reduction, upper limb
  umbilical artery Q27.0
  unilateral condylar M27.8
  ureter Q62.8
  uterus, congenital Q51.811
  vagina Q52.4
  vascular NEC peripheral Q27.8
    brain Q28.3
    digestive system Q27.8
    lower limb Q27.8
    specified site NEC Q27.8
    upper limb Q27.8
  vein(s) (peripheral) Q27.8
    brain Q28.3
    digestive system Q27.8
    great Q26.8
    lower limb Q27.8
    specified site NEC Q27.8
    upper limb Q27.8
  vena cava (inferior) (superior) Q26.8
  vertebra Q76.49
  vulva, congenital Q52.79
  zonule (ciliary) Q12.8
▶Hypopnea, obstructive sleep apnea G47.33

Hypopotassemia E87.6
Hypoproconvertinemia, congenital (hereditary) D68.2
Hypoproteinemia E77.8
Hypoprothrombinemia (congenital) (hereditary) (idiopathic) D68.2
  acquired D68.4
  newborn, transient P61.6
Hypoptyalism K11.7
Hypopyon (eye) (anterior chamber) —see Iridocyclitis, acute, hypopyon
Hypopyrexia R68.0
Hyporeflexia R29.2
Hyposecretion
  ACTH E23.0
  antidiuretic hormone E23.2
  ovary E28.39
  salivary gland (any) K11.7
  vasopressin E23.2
Hyposegmentation, leukocytic, hereditary D72.0
Hyposiderinemia D50.9
Hypospadias Q54.9
  balanic Q54.0
  coronal Q54.0
  glandular Q54.0
  penile Q54.1
  penoscrotal Q54.2
  perineal Q54.3
  specified NEC Q54.8
Hypospermatogenesis —see Oligospermia
Hyposplenism D73.0
Hypostasis pulmonary, passive —see Edema, lung
Hypostatic —see condition
Hyposthenuria N28.89
Hypotension (arterial) (constitutional) I95.9
  chronic I95.89
  drug-induced I95.2
  due to (of) hemodialysis I95.3
  iatrogenic I95.89
  idiopathic (permanent) I95.0
  intracranial, following ventricular shunting (ventriculostomy) G97.2
  intra-dialytic I95.3
  maternal, syndrome (following labor and delivery) O26.5-●
  neurogenic, orthostatic G90.3
  orthostatic (chronic) I95.1
    due to drugs I95.2
    neurogenic G90.3
  postoperative I95.81
  postural I95.1
  specified NEC I95.89
Hypothermia (accidental) T68
  due to anesthesia, anesthetic T88.51
  low environmental temperature T68
  neonatal P80.9
    environmental (mild) NEC P80.8
    mild P80.8
    severe (chronic) (cold injury syndrome) P80.0
    specified NEC P80.8
  not associated with low environmental temperature R68.0

Hypothyroidism (acquired) E03.9
▶autoimmune —see Thyroiditis, autoimmune
  congenital (without goiter) E03.1
    with goiter (diffuse) E03.0
  due to
    exogenous substance NEC E03.2
    iodine-deficiency, acquired E01.8
      subclinical E02
    irradiation therapy E89.0
    medicament NEC E03.2
    P-aminosalicylic acid (PAS) E03.2
    phenylbutazone E03.2
    resorcinol E03.2
    sulfonamide E03.2
    surgery E89.0
    thiourea group drugs E03.2
  iatrogenic NEC E03.2
  iodine-deficiency (acquired) E01.8
    congenital —see Syndrome, iodine-deficiency, congenital
    subclinical E02
  neonatal, transitory P72.2
  postinfectious E03.3
  postirradiation E89.0
  postprocedural E89.0
  postsurgical E89.0
  specified NEC E03.8
  subclinical, iodine-deficiency related E02
Hypotonia, hypotonicity, hypotony
  bladder N31.2
  congenital (benign) P94.2
  eye —see Disorder, globe, hypotony
Hypotrichosis —see Alopecia
Hypotropia H50.2-●
Hypoventilation R06.89
  congenital central alveolar G47.35
  sleep related
    idiopathic nonobstructive alveolar G47.34
    in conditions classified elsewhere G47.36
Hypovitaminosis —see Deficiency, vitamin
Hypovolemia E86.1
  surgical shock T81.19
  traumatic (shock) T79.4
Hypoxemia R09.02
  newborn P84
  sleep related, in conditions classified elsewhere G47.36
Hypoxia —see also Anoxia R09.02
  cerebral, during a procedure NEC G97.81
    postprocedural NEC G97.82
  intrauterine P84
  myocardial —see Insufficiency, coronary
  newborn P84
  sleep-related G47.34
Hypsarhythmia —see Epilepsy, generalized, specified NEC
Hysteralgia, pregnant uterus O26.89-●
Hysteria, hysterical (conversion) (dissociative state) F44.9
  anxiety F41.8
  convulsions F44.5
  psychosis, acute F44.9
Hysteroepilepsy F44.5

INDEX TO DISEASES AND INJURIES / IBDU

I

IBDU (colonic inflammatory bowel disease
   unclassified) K52.3
Ichthyoparasitism due to Vandellia cirrhosa
   B88.8
Ichthyosis (congenital) Q80.9
   acquired L85.0
   fetalis Q80.4
   hystrix Q80.8
   lamellar Q80.2
   lingual K13.29
   palmaris and plantaris Q82.8
   simplex Q80.0
   vera Q80.8
   vulgaris Q80.0
   X-linked Q80.1
Ichthyotoxism —see Poisoning, fish
   bacterial —see Intoxication, foodborne
Icteroanemia, hemolytic (acquired) D59.9
   congenital —see Spherocytosis
Icterus —see also Jaundice
   conjunctiva R17
   gravis, newborn P55.0
   hematogenous (acquired) D59.9
   hemolytic (acquired) D59.9
      congenital —see Spherocytosis
   hemorrhagic (acute) (leptospiral)
         (spirochetal) A27.0
      newborn P53
   infectious B15.9
      with hepatic coma B15.0
      leptospiral A27.0
      spirochetal A27.0
   neonatorum —see Jaundice, newborn
   newborn P59.9
   spirochetal A27.0
Ictus solaris, solis T67.0
Ideation
   homicidal R45.850
   suicidal R45.851
Identity disorder (child) F64.9
   gender role F64.2
   psychosexual F64.2
Idioglossia F80.0
Idiopathic —see condition
Idiot, idiocy (congenital) F73
   amaurotic (Bielschowsky(-Jansky)) (family)
         (infantile (late)) (juvenile (late)) (Vogt-
         Spielmeyer) E75.4
   microcephalic Q02
Id reaction (due to bacteria) L30.2
IgE asthma J45.909
IIAC (idiopathic infantile arterial calcification)
   Q28.8
Ileitis (chronic) (noninfectious) —see also
      Enteritis K52.9
   backwash —see Pancolitis, ulcerative
         (chronic)
   infectious A09
   regional (ulcerative) —see Enteritis, regional,
         small intestine
   segmental —see Enteritis, regional
   terminal (ulcerative) —see Enteritis, regional,
         small intestine
Ileocolitis —see also Enteritis K52.9
   infectious A09
   regional —see Enteritis, regional
▶ulcerative K51.0-●
Ileostomy
   attention to Z43.2
   malfunctioning K94.13
   status Z93.2
      with complication —see Complications,
            enterostomy
Ileotyphus —see Typhoid
Ileum —see condition
Ileus (bowel) (colon) (inhibitory) (intestine) K56.7
   adynamic K56.0
   due to gallstone (in intestine) K56.3
   duodenal (chronic) K31.5

Ileus (Continued)
   gallstone K56.3
➡mechanical NEC —see also Obstruction,
      intestine, specified K56.699
   meconium P76.0
      in cystic fibrosis E84.11
      meaning meconium plug (without cystic
            fibrosis) P76.0
   myxedema K59.8
   neurogenic K56.0
      Hirschsprung's disease or megacolon Q43.1
   newborn
      due to meconium P76.0
         in cystic fibrosis E84.11
         meaning meconium plug (without cystic
               fibrosis) P76.0
      transitory P76.1
➡obstructive —see also Obstruction, intestine,
      specified K56.699
   paralytic K56.0
▶postoperative K91.89
Iliac —see condition
Iliotibial band syndrome M76.3-●
Illiteracy Z55.0
Illness —see also Disease R69
   manic-depressive —see Disorder, bipolar
Imbalance R26.89
   autonomic G90.8
   constituents of food intake E63.1
   electrolyte E87.8
      with
         abortion —see Abortion by type,
               complicated by, electrolyte
               imbalance
         molar pregnancy O08.5
      due to hyperemesis gravidarum O21.1
      following ectopic or molar pregnancy
            O08.5
      neonatal, transitory NEC P74.4
         potassium P74.3
         sodium P74.2
   endocrine E34.9
   eye muscle NOS H50.9
   hormone E34.9
   hysterical F44.4
   labyrinth —see subcategory H83.2
   posture R29.3
   protein-energy —see Malnutrition
   sympathetic G90.8
Imbecile, imbecility (I.Q. 35-49) F71
Imbedding, intrauterine device T83.39
Imbibition, cholesterol (gallbladder) K82.4
Imbrication, teeth, fully erupted M26.30
Imerslund (-Gräsbeck) syndrome D51.1
Immature —see also Immaturity
   birth (less than 37 completed weeks) —see
         Preterm, newborn
      extremely (less than 28 completed
            weeks) —see Immaturity, extreme
   personality F60.89
Immaturity (less than 37 completed weeks) —
      see also Preterm, newborn
   extreme of newborn (less than 28
         completed weeks of gestation) (less
         than 196 completed days of gestation)
         (unspecified weeks of gestation) P07.20
      gestational age
         23 completed weeks (23 weeks, 0 days
               through 23 weeks, 6 days) P07.22
         24 completed weeks (24 weeks, 0 days
               through 24 weeks, 6 days) P07.23
         25 completed weeks (25 weeks, 0 days
               through 25 weeks, 6 days) P07.24
         26 completed weeks (26 weeks, 0 days
               through 26 weeks, 6 days) P07.25
         27 completed weeks (27 weeks, 0 days
               through 27 weeks, 6 days) P07.26
         less than 23 completed weeks P07.21
   fetus or infant light-for-dates —see
         Light-for-dates
   lung, newborn P28.0
   organ or site NEC —see Hypoplasia

Immaturity (Continued)
   pulmonary, newborn P28.0
   reaction F60.89
   sexual (female) (male), after puberty E30.0
Immersion T75.1
   foot T69.02-●
   hand T69.01-●
Immobile, immobility
   complete, due to severe physical disability or
         frailty R53.2
   intestine K59.8
   syndrome (paraplegic) M62.3
Immune reconstitution (inflammatory)
   syndrome [IRIS] D89.3
Immunization —see also Vaccination
   ABO —see Incompatibility, ABO
      in newborn P55.1
   complication —see Complications, vaccination
   encounter for Z23
   not done (not carried out) Z28.9
      because (of)
         acute illness of patient Z28.01
         allergy to vaccine (or component) Z28.04
         caregiver refusal Z28.82
         chronic illness of patient Z28.02
         contraindication NEC Z28.09
         group pressure Z28.1
         guardian refusal Z28.82
         immune compromised state of patient
               Z28.03
         parent refusal Z28.82
         patient's belief Z28.1
         patient had disease being vaccinated
               against Z28.81
         patient refusal Z28.21
         religious beliefs of patient Z28.1
         specified reason NEC Z28.89
            of patient Z28.29
         unspecified patient reason Z28.20
   Rh factor
      affecting management of pregnancy NEC
            O36.09-●
         anti-D antibody O36.01-●
      from transfusion —see Complication(s),
            transfusion, incompatibility reaction,
            Rh (factor)
Immunocytoma C83.0-●
Immunodeficiency D84.9
   with
      adenosine-deaminase deficiency D81.3
      antibody defects D80.9
         specified type NEC D80.8
      hyperimmunoglobulinemia D80.6
      increased immunoglobulin M (IgM) D80.5
      major defect D82.9
         specified type NEC D82.8
      partial albinism D82.8
      short-limbed stature D82.2
      thrombocytopenia and eczema D82.0
   antibody with
      hyperimmunoglobulinemia D80.6
      near-normal immunoglobulins D80.6
   autosomal recessive, Swiss type D80.0
   combined D81.9
      biotin-dependent carboxylase D81.819
         biotinidase D81.810
         holocarboxylase synthetase D81.818
         specified type NEC D81.818
      severe (SCID) D81.9
         with
            low or normal B-cell numbers D81.2
            low T- and B-cell numbers D81.1
            reticular dysgenesis D81.0
         specified type NEC D81.89
   common variable D83.9
      with
         abnormalities of B-cell numbers and
               function D83.0
         autoantibodies to B- or T-cells D83.2
         immunoregulatory T-cell disorders D83.1
         specified type NEC D83.8

Immunodeficiency *(Continued)*
  following hereditary defective response to
    Epstein-Barr virus (EBV) D82.3
  selective, immunoglobulin
    A (IgA) D80.2
    G (IgG) (subclasses) D80.3
    M (IgM) D80.4
  severe combined (SCID) D81.9
  specified type NEC D84.8
  X-linked, with increased IgM D80.5
Immunotherapy (encounter for)
  antineoplastic Z51.12
Impaction, impacted
  bowel, colon, rectum —*see also* Impaction,
    fecal K56.49
    by gallstone K56.3
  calculus —*see* Calculus
  cerumen (ear) (external) H61.2-●
  cuspid —*see* Impaction, tooth
  dental (same or adjacent tooth) K01.1
  fecal, feces K56.41
  fracture —*see* Fracture, by site
  gallbladder —*see* Calculus, gallbladder
  gallstone(s) —*see* Calculus, gallbladder
    bile duct (common) (hepatic) —*see*
      Calculus, bile duct
    cystic duct —*see* Calculus, gallbladder
    in intestine, with obstruction (any part) K56.3
  intestine (calculous) NEC —*see also*
    Impaction, fecal K56.49
    gallstone, with ileus K56.3
  intrauterine device (IUD) T83.39
  molar —*see* Impaction, tooth
  shoulder, causing obstructed labor O66.0
  tooth, teeth K01.1
  turbinate J34.89
Impaired, impairment (function)
  auditory discrimination —*see* Abnormal,
    auditory perception
  cognitive, mild, so stated G31.84
  dual sensory Z73.82
  fasting glucose R73.01
  glucose tolerance (oral) R73.02
  hearing —*see* Deafness
  heart —*see* Disease, heart
  kidney N28.9
    disorder resulting from N25.9
      specified NEC N25.89
  liver K72.90
    with coma K72.91
  mastication K08.89
  mild cognitive, so stated G31.84
  mobility
    ear ossicles —*see* Ankylosis, ear ossicles
    requiring care provider Z74.09
  myocardium, myocardial —*see* Insufficiency,
    myocardial
  rectal sphincter R19.8
  renal (acute) (chronic) N28.9
    disorder resulting from N25.9
      specified NEC N25.89
  vision NEC H54.7
    both eyes H54.3
Impediment, speech R47.9
  psychogenic (childhood) F98.8
  slurring R47.81
  specified NEC R47.89
Impending
  coronary syndrome I20.0
  delirium tremens F10.239
  myocardial infarction I20.0
Imperception auditory (acquired) —*see also*
    Deafness
  congenital H93.25
Imperfect
  aeration, lung (newborn) NEC —*see* Atelectasis
  closure (congenital)
    alimentary tract NEC Q45.8
      lower Q43.8
      upper Q40.8
    atrioventricular ostium Q21.2

Imperfect *(Continued)*
  closure *(Continued)*
    atrium (secundum) Q21.1
    branchial cleft or sinus Q18.0
    ►branchial cleft NOS Q18.2
      ►cyst Q18.0
      ►fistula Q18.0
      ►sinus Q18.0
    choroid Q14.3
    cricoid cartilage Q31.8
    cusps, heart valve NEC Q24.8
      pulmonary Q22.3
    ductus
      arteriosus Q25.0
      Botalli Q25.0
    ear drum (causing impairment of hearing)
      Q16.4
    esophagus with communication to
      bronchus or trachea Q39.1
    eyelid Q10.3
    foramen
      botalli Q21.1
      ovale Q21.1
    genitalia, genital organ(s) or system
      female Q52.8
        external Q52.79
        internal NEC Q52.8
      male Q55.8
    glottis Q31.8
    interatrial ostium or septum Q21.1
    interauricular ostium or septum Q21.1
    interventricular ostium or septum Q21.0
    larynx Q31.8
    lip —*see* Cleft, lip
    nasal septum Q30.3
    nose Q30.2
    omphalomesenteric duct Q43.0
    optic nerve entry Q14.2
    organ or site not listed —*see* Anomaly, by
      site
    ostium
      interatrial Q21.1
      interauricular Q21.1
      interventricular Q21.0
    palate —*see* Cleft, palate
    preauricular sinus Q18.1
    retina Q14.1
    roof of orbit Q75.8
    sclera Q13.5
    septum
      aorticopulmonary Q21.4
      atrial (secundum) Q21.1
      between aorta and pulmonary artery
        Q21.4
      heart Q21.9
      interatrial (secundum) Q21.1
      interauricular (secundum) Q21.1
      interventricular Q21.0
        in tetralogy of Fallot Q21.3
      nasal Q30.3
      ventricular Q21.0
        with pulmonary stenosis or atresia,
          dextraposition of aorta, and
          hypertrophy of right ventricle
          Q21.3
        in tetralogy of Fallot Q21.3
    skull Q75.0
      with
        anencephaly Q00.0
        encephalocele —*see* Encephalocele
        hydrocephalus Q03.9
          with spina bifida —*see* Spina bifida,
            by site, with hydrocephalus
        microcephaly Q02
    spine (with meningocele) —*see* Spina bifida
    trachea Q32.1
    tympanic membrane (causing impairment
      of hearing) Q16.4
    uterus Q51.818
    vitelline duct Q43.0
  erection —*see* Dysfunction, sexual, male,
    erectile

Imperfect *(Continued)*
  fusion —*see* Imperfect, closure
  inflation, lung (newborn) —*see* Atelectasis
  posture R29.3
  rotation, intestine Q43.3
  septum, ventricular Q21.0
Imperfectly descended testis —*see* Cryptorchid
Imperforate (congenital) —*see also* Atresia
  anus Q42.3
    with fistula Q42.2
  cervix (uteri) Q51.828
  esophagus Q39.0
    with tracheoesophageal fistula Q39.1
  hymen Q52.3
  jejunum Q41.1
  pharynx Q38.8
  rectum Q42.1
    with fistula Q42.0
  urethra Q64.39
  vagina Q52.4
Impervious (congenital) —*see also* Atresia
  anus Q42.3
    with fistula Q42.2
  bile duct Q44.2
  esophagus Q39.0
    with tracheoesophageal fistula Q39.1
  intestine (small) Q41.9
    large Q42.9
      specified NEC Q42.8
  rectum Q42.1
    with fistula Q42.0
  ureter —*see* Atresia, ureter
  urethra Q64.39
Impetiginization of dermatoses L01.1
Impetigo (any organism) (any site) (circinate)
    (contagiosa) (simplex) (vulgaris) L01.00
  Bockhart's L01.02
  bullous, bullosa L01.03
  external ear L01.00 *[H62.40]*
  follicularis L01.02
  furfuracea L30.5
  herpetiformis L40.1
    nonobstetrical L40.1
  neonatorum L01.03
  nonbullous L01.01
  specified type NEC L01.09
  ulcerative L01.09
Impingement (on teeth)
  soft tissue
    anterior M26.81
    posterior M26.82
Implant, endometrial N80.9
Implantation
  anomalous —*see* Anomaly, by site
    ureter Q62.63
  cyst
    external area or site (skin) NEC L72.0
    iris —*see* Cyst, iris, implantation
    vagina N89.8
    vulva N90.7
  dermoid (cyst) —*see* Implantation, cyst
Impotence (sexual) N52.9
  counseling Z70.1
  organic origin —*see also* Dysfunction, sexual,
    male, erectile N52.9
  psychogenic F52.21
Impression, basilar Q75.8
Imprisonment, anxiety concerning Z65.1
Improper care (child) (newborn) —*see*
    Maltreatment
Improperly tied umbilical cord (causing
    hemorrhage) P51.8
Impulsiveness (impulsive) R45.87
Inability to swallow —*see* Aphagia
Inaccessible, inaccessibility
  health care NEC Z75.3
    due to
      waiting period Z75.2
        for admission to facility elsewhere
          Z75.1
    other helping agencies Z75.4
Inactive —*see* condition

Inadequate, inadequacy
  aesthetics of dental restoration K08.56
  biologic, constitutional, functional, or social
    F60.7
  development
    child R62.50
    genitalia
      after puberty NEC E30.0
      congenital
        female Q52.8
          external Q52.79
          internal Q52.8
        male Q55.8
    lungs Q33.6
      associated with short gestation P28.0
    organ or site not listed —*see* Anomaly, by
      site
  diet (causing nutritional deficiency) E63.9
  eating habits Z72.4
  environment, household Z59.1
  family support Z63.8
  food (supply) NEC Z59.4
    hunger effects T73.0
  functional F60.7
  household care, due to
    family member
      handicapped or ill Z74.2
      on vacation Z75.5
      temporarily away from home Z74.2
    technical defects in home Z59.1
    temporary absence from home of person
      rendering care Z74.2
  housing (heating) (space) Z59.1
  income (financial) Z59.6
  intrafamilial communication Z63.8
  material resources Z59.9
  mental —*see* Disability, intellectual
  parental supervision or control of child
    Z62.0
  personality F60.7
  pulmonary
    function R06.89
      newborn P28.5
    ventilation, newborn P28.5
  sample of cytologic smear
    anus R85.615
    cervix R87.615
    vagina R87.625
  social F60.7
    insurance Z59.7
    skills NEC Z73.4
  supervision of child by parent Z62.0
  teaching affecting education Z55.8
  welfare support Z59.7
Inanition R64
  with edema —*see* Malnutrition, severe
  due to
    deprivation of food T73.0
    malnutrition —*see* Malnutrition
  fever R50.9
Inappropriate
  change in quantitative human chorionic
    gonadotropin (hCG) in early pregnancy
    O02.81
  diet or eating habits Z72.4
  level of quantitative human chorionic
    gonadotropin (hCG) for gestational age
    in early pregnancy O02.81
  secretion
    antidiuretic hormone (ADH) (excessive)
      E22.2
    deficiency E23.2
    pituitary (posterior) E22.2
Inattention at or after birth —*see* Neglect
Incarceration, incarcerated
  enterocele K46.0
    gangrenous K46.1
  epiplocele K46.0
    gangrenous K46.1
  exomphalos K42.0
    gangrenous K42.1

Incarceration, incarcerated *(Continued)*
  hernia —*see also* Hernia, by site, with
    obstruction
    with gangrene —*see* Hernia, by site, with
      gangrene
  iris, in wound —*see* Injury, eye, laceration,
    with prolapse
  lens, in wound —*see* Injury, eye, laceration,
    with prolapse
  omphalocele K42.0
  prison, anxiety concerning Z65.1
  rupture —*see* Hernia, by site
  sarcoepiplocele K46.0
    gangrenous K46.1
  sarcoepiplomphalocele K42.0
    with gangrene K42.1
  uterus N85.8
    gravid O34.51-●
      causing obstructed labor O65.5
Incised wound
  external —*see* Laceration
  internal organs —*see* Injury, by site
Incision, incisional
  hernia K43.2
    with
      gangrene (and obstruction) K43.1
      obstruction K43.0
  surgical, complication —*see* Complications,
    surgical procedure
  traumatic
    external —*see* Laceration
    internal organs —*see* Injury, by site
Inclusion
  azurophilic leukocytic D72.0
  blennorrhea (neonatal) (newborn) P39.1
  gallbladder in liver (congenital) Q44.1
Incompatibility
  ABO
    affecting management of pregnancy
      O36.11-●
      anti-A sensitization O36.11-●
      anti-B sensitization O36.19-●
      specified NEC O36.19-●
    infusion or transfusion reaction —*see*
      Complication(s), transfusion,
      incompatibility reaction, ABO
    newborn P55.1
  blood (group) (Duffy) (K(ell)) (Kidd) (Lewis)
    (M) (S) NEC
    affecting management of pregnancy
      O36.11-●
      anti-A sensitization O36.11-●
      anti-B sensitization O36.19-●
    infusion or transfusion reaction T80.89
    newborn P55.8
  divorce or estrangement Z63.5
  Rh (blood group) (factor) Z31.82
    affecting management of pregnancy NEC
      O36.09-●
      anti-D antibody O36.01-●
    infusion or transfusion reaction —*see*
      Complication(s), transfusion,
      incompatibility reaction, Rh (factor)
    newborn P55.0
  rhesus —*see* Incompatibility, Rh
Incompetency, incompetent, incompetence
  annular
    aortic (valve) —*see* Insufficiency, aortic
    mitral (valve) I34.0
    pulmonary valve (heart) I37.1
  aortic (valve) —*see* Insufficiency, aortic
  cardiac valve —*see* Endocarditis
  cervix, cervical (os) N88.3
    in pregnancy O34.3-●
  chronotropic I45.89
    with
      autonomic dysfunction G90.8
      ischemic heart disease I25.89
      left ventricular dysfunction I51.89
      sinus node dysfunction I49.8
  esophagogastric (junction) (sphincter) K22.0

Incompetency, incompetent, incompetence
    (Continued)
  mitral (valve) —*see* Insufficiency, mitral
  pelvic fundus N81.89
  pubocervical tissue N81.82
  pulmonary valve (heart) I37.1
    congenital Q22.3
  rectovaginal tissue N81.83
  tricuspid (annular) (valve) —*see* Insufficiency,
    tricuspid
  valvular —*see* Endocarditis
    congenital Q24.8
  vein, venous (saphenous) (varicose) —*see*
    Varix, leg
Incomplete —*see also* condition
  bladder, emptying R33.9
  defecation R15.0
  expansion lungs (newborn) NEC —*see*
    Atelectasis
  rotation, intestine Q43.3
Inconclusive
  diagnostic imaging due to excess body fat of
    patient R93.9
  findings on diagnostic imaging of breast NEC
    R92.8
  mammogram (due to dense breasts) R92.2
Incontinence R32
  anal sphincter R15.9
  coital N39.491
  feces R15.9
    nonorganic origin F98.1
  insensible (urinary) N39.42
  overflow N39.490
  postural (urinary) N39.492
  psychogenic F45.8
  rectal R15.9
  reflex N39.498
  stress (female) (male) N39.3
    and urge N39.46
  urethral sphincter R32
  urge N39.41
    and stress (female) (male) N39.46
  urine (urinary) R32
    continuous N39.45
    due to cognitive impairment, or severe
      physical disability or immobility R39.81
    functional R39.81
    insensible N39.42
    mixed (stress and urge) N39.46
    nocturnal N39.44
    nonorganic origin F98.0
    overflow N39.490
    post dribbling N39.43
    postural N39.492
    reflex N39.498
    specified NEC N39.498
    stress (female) (male) N39.3
      and urge N39.46
    total N39.498
    unaware N39.42
    urge N39.41
      and stress (female) (male) N39.46
Incontinentia pigmenti Q82.3
Incoordinate, incoordination
  esophageal-pharyngeal (newborn) —*see*
    Dysphagia
  muscular R27.8
  uterus (action) (contractions) (complicating
    delivery) O62.4
Increase, increased
  abnormal, in development R63.8
  androgens (ovarian) E28.1
  anticoagulants (antithrombin) (anti-VIIIa)
    (anti-IXa) (anti-Xa) (anti-XIa) —*see*
    Circulating anticoagulants
  cold sense R20.8
  estrogen E28.0
  function
    adrenal
      cortex —*see* Cushing's, syndrome
      medulla E27.5

▶ New   ⇒ Revised   ~~deleted~~ Deleted   ● Use Additional Character(s)

Increase, increased (Continued)
  function (Continued)
    pituitary (gland) (anterior) (lobe) E22.9
      posterior E22.2
  heat sense R20.8
  intracranial pressure (benign) G93.2
  permeability, capillaries I78.8
  pressure, intracranial G93.2
  secretion
    gastrin E16.4
    glucagon E16.3
    pancreas, endocrine E16.9
      growth hormone-releasing hormone E16.8
      pancreatic polypeptide E16.8
      somatostatin E16.8
      vasoactive-intestinal polypeptide E16.8
  sphericity, lens Q12.4
  splenic activity D73.1
  venous pressure I87.8
    portal K76.6
Increta placenta O43.22-•
Incrustation, cornea, foreign body (lead)
  (zinc) —see Foreign body, cornea
Incyclophoria H50.54
Incyclotropia —see Cyclotropia
Indeterminate sex Q56.4
India rubber skin Q82.8
Indigestion (acid) (bilious) (functional) K30
  catarrhal K31.89
  due to decomposed food NOS A05.9
  nervous F45.8
  psychogenic F45.8
Indirect —see condition
Induratio penis plastica N48.6
Induration, indurated
  brain G93.89
  breast (fibrous) N64.51
    puerperal, postpartum O92.29
  broad ligament N83.8
  chancre
    anus A51.1
    congenital A50.07
    extragenital NEC A51.2
  corpora cavernosa (penis) (plastic) N48.6
  liver (chronic) K76.89
  lung (black) (chronic) (fibroid) —see also
    Fibrosis, lung J84.10
    essential brown J84.03
  penile (plastic) N48.6
  phlebitic —see Phlebitis
  skin R23.4
Inebriety (without dependence) —see Alcohol,
  intoxication
Inefficiency, kidney N28.9
Inelasticity, skin R23.4
Inequality, leg (length) (acquired) —see also
  Deformity, limb, unequal length
  congenital —see Defect, reduction, lower limb
  lower leg —see Deformity, limb, unequal
    length
Inertia
  bladder (neurogenic) N31.2
  stomach K31.89
    psychogenic F45.8
  uterus, uterine during labor O62.2
    during latent phase of labor O62.0
    primary O62.0
    secondary O62.1
  vesical (neurogenic) N31.2
Infancy, infantile, infantilism —see also
  condition
  celiac K90.0
  genitalia, genitals (after puberty) E30.0
  Herter's (nontropical sprue) K90.0
  intestinal K90.0
  Lorain E23.0
  pancreatic K86.89
  pelvis M95.5
    with disproportion (fetopelvic) O33.1
      causing obstructed labor O65.1
  pituitary E23.0

Infancy, infantile, infantilism (Continued)
  renal N25.0
  uterus —see Infantile, genitalia
Infant(s) —see also Infancy
  excessive crying R68.11
  irritable child R68.12
  lack of care —see Neglect
  liveborn (singleton) Z38.2
    born in hospital Z38.00
      by cesarean Z38.01
    born outside hospital Z38.1
    multiple NEC Z38.8
      born in hospital Z38.68
        by cesarean Z38.69
      born outside hospital Z38.7
    quadruplet Z38.8
      born in hospital Z38.63
        by cesarean Z38.64
      born outside hospital Z38.7
    quintuplet Z38.8
      born in hospital Z38.65
        by cesarean Z38.66
      born outside hospital Z38.7
    triplet Z38.8
      born in hospital Z38.61
        by cesarean Z38.62
      born outside hospital Z38.7
    twin Z38.5
      born in hospital Z38.30
        by cesarean Z38.31
      born outside hospital Z38.4
  of diabetic mother (syndrome of) P70.1
    gestational diabetes P70.0
Infantile —see also condition
  genitalia, genitals E30.0
  os, uterine E30.0
  penis E30.0
  testis E29.1
  uterus E30.0
Infantilism —see Infancy
Infarct, infarction
  adrenal (capsule) (gland) E27.49
  appendices epiploicae —see also Infarct,
    intestine K55.069
  bowel —see also Infarct, intestine K55.069
  brain (stem) —see Infarct, cerebral
  breast N64.89
  brewer's (kidney) N28.0
  cardiac —see Infarct, myocardium
  cerebellar —see Infarct, cerebral
  cerebral —see also Occlusion, artery cerebral
    or precerebral, with infarction I63.9-•
    aborted I63.9
    cortical I63.9
    due to
      cerebral venous thrombosis,
        nonpyogenic I63.6
      embolism
        cerebral arteries I63.4-•
        precerebral arteries I63.1-•
      occlusion NEC
        cerebral arteries I63.5-•
        precerebral arteries I63.2-•
      stenosis NEC
        cerebral arteries I63.5-•
        precerebral arteries I63.2-•
      thrombosis
        cerebral artery I63.3-•
        precerebral artery I63.0-•
    intraoperative
      during cardiac surgery I97.810
      during other surgery I97.811
    postprocedural
      following cardiac surgery I97.820
      following other surgery I97.821
    specified NEC I63.8
  colon (acute) (agnogenic) (embolic)
    (hemorrhagic) (nonocclusive)
    (nonthrombotic) (occlusive) (segmental)
    (thrombotic) (with gangrene) —see also
    Infarct, intestine K55.049

Infarct, infarction (Continued)
  coronary artery —see Infarct, myocardium
  embolic —see Embolism
  fallopian tube N83.8
  gallbladder K82.8
  heart —see Infarct, myocardium
  hepatic K76.3
  hypophysis (anterior lobe) E23.6
  impending (myocardium) I20.0
  intestine (acute) (agnogenic) (embolic)
    (hemorrhagic) (nonocclusive)
    (nonthrombotic) (occlusive) (thrombotic)
    (with gangrene) K55.069
    diffuse K55.062
    focal K55.061
    large K55.049
      diffuse K55.042
      focal K55.041
    small K55.029
      diffuse K55.022
      focal K55.021
  kidney N28.0
  liver K76.3
  lung (embolic) (thrombotic) —see Embolism,
    pulmonary
  lymph node I89.8
  mesentery, mesenteric (embolic) (thrombotic)
    (with gangrene) —see also Infarct,
    intestine K55.069
  muscle (ischemic) M62.20
    ankle M62.27-•
    foot M62.27-•
    forearm M62.23-•
    hand M62.24-•
    lower leg M62.26-•
    pelvic region M62.25-•
    shoulder region M62.21-•
    specified site NEC M62.28
    thigh M62.25-•
    upper arm M62.22-•
⟹myocardium, myocardial (acute) (with stated
    duration of 4 weeks or less) I21.9
▶associated with revascularization
    procedure I21.A9
  diagnosed on ECG, but presenting no
    symptoms I25.2
▶due to
  ▶demand ischemia I21.A1
  ▶ischemic imbalance I21.A1
  healed or old I25.2
⟹intraoperative —see also Infarct,
    myocardium, associated with
    revascularization procedure
    during cardiac surgery I97.790
    during other surgery I97.791
  non-Q wave I21.4
  non-ST elevation (NSTEMI) I21.4
    subsequent I22.2
  nontransmural I21.4
  past (diagnosed on ECG or other
    investigation, but currently presenting
    no symptoms) I25.2
⟹postprocedural —see also Infarct,
    myocardium, associated with
    revascularization procedure
    ~~following cardiac surgery I97.190~~
  ▶following cardiac surgery —see also
    Infarct, myocardium, type 4 or
    type 5 I97.190
    following other surgery I97.191
  Q wave —see also Infarct, myocardium, by
    site I21.3
▶secondary to
  ▶demand ischemia I21.A1
  ▶ischemic imbalance I21.A1
  ST elevation (STEMI) I21.3
    anterior (anteroapical) (anterolateral)
      (anteroseptal) (Q wave) (wall) I21.09
      subsequent I22.0
    inferior (diaphragmatic) (inferolateral)
      (inferoposterior) (wall) NEC I21.19
      subsequent I22.1
    inferoposterior transmural (Q wave) I21.11

Infarct, infarction (Continued)
  myocardium, myocardial (Continued)
    ST elevation (Continued)
      involving
        coronary artery of anterior wall NEC
          I21.09
        coronary artery of inferior wall NEC
          I21.19
        diagonal coronary artery I21.02
        left anterior descending coronary
          artery I21.02
        left circumflex coronary artery I21.21
        left main coronary artery I21.01
        oblique marginal coronary artery
          I21.21
        right coronary artery I21.11
      lateral (apical-lateral) (basal-lateral)
        (high) I21.29
        subsequent I22.8
      posterior (posterobasal) (posterolateral)
        (posteroseptal) (true) I21.29
        subsequent I22.8
      septal I21.29
        subsequent I22.8
      specified NEC I21.29
        subsequent I22.8
      subsequent I22.9
    subsequent (recurrent) (reinfarction) I22.9
      anterior (anteroapical) (anterolateral)
        (anteroseptal) (wall) I22.0
      diaphragmatic (wall) I22.1
      inferior (diaphragmatic) (inferolateral)
        (inferoposterior) (wall) I22.1
      lateral (apical-lateral) (basal-lateral)
        (high) I22.8
      non-ST elevation (NSTEMI) I22.2
      posterior (posterobasal) (posterolateral)
        (posteroseptal) (true) I22.8
      septal I22.8
      specified NEC I22.8
      ST elevation I22.9
        anterior (anteroapical) (anterolateral)
          (anteroseptal) (wall) I22.0
        inferior (diaphragmatic) (inferolateral)
          (inferoposterior) (wall) I22.1
        specified NEC I22.8
      subendocardial I22.2
      transmural I22.9
        anterior (anteroapical) (anterolateral)
          (anteroseptal) (wall) I22.0
        diaphragmatic (wall) I22.1
        inferior (diaphragmatic) (inferolateral)
          (inferoposterior) (wall) I22.1
        lateral (apical-lateral) (basal-lateral)
          (high) I22.8
        posterior (posterobasal)
          (posterolateral) (posteroseptal)
          (true) I22.8
        specified NEC I22.8
    ▶type 1 —see also Infarction, myocardial,
        subsequent, by site, or by ST
        elevation or non-ST elevation I22.9
    ▶type 2 I21.A1
    ▶type 3 I21.A9
    ▶type 4 I21.A9
    ▶type 5 I21.A9
    syphilitic A52.06
  ⇒transmural I21.9
    anterior (anteroapical) (anterolateral)
      (anteroseptal) (Q wave) (wall) NEC
      I21.09
    inferior (diaphragmatic) (inferolateral)
      (inferoposterior) (Q wave) (wall)
      NEC I21.19
    inferoposterior (Q wave) I21.11
    lateral (apical-lateral) (basal-lateral)
      (high) NEC I21.29
    posterior (posterobasal) (posterolateral)
      (posteroseptal) (true) NEC I21.29
    septal NEC I21.29
    specified NEC I21.29

Infarct, infarction (Continued)
  myocardium, myocardial (Continued)
    ▶type 1 —see also Infarction, myocardial, by
        site, or by ST elevation or non-ST
        elevation I21.9
    ▶type 2 I21.A1
    ▶type 3 I21.A9
    ▶type 4 (a) (b) (c) I21.A9
    ▶type 5 I21.A9
    nontransmural I21.4
  omentum —see also Infarct, intestine K55.069
  ovary N83.8
  pancreas K86.89
  papillary muscle —see Infarct, myocardium
  parathyroid gland E21.4
  pituitary (gland) E23.6
  placenta O43.81-●
  prostate N42.89
  pulmonary (artery) (vein) (hemorrhagic) —
    see Embolism, pulmonary
  renal (embolic) (thrombotic) N28.0
  retina, retinal (artery) —see Occlusion, artery,
    retina
  spinal (cord) (acute) (embolic) (nonembolic)
    G95.11
  spleen D73.5
    embolic or thrombotic I74.8
  subendocardial (acute) (nontransmural) I21.4
  suprarenal (capsule) (gland) E27.49
  testis N50.1
  thrombotic —see also Thrombosis
    artery, arterial —see Embolism
  thyroid (gland) E07.89
  ventricle (heart) —see Infarct, myocardium
Infecting —see condition
Infection, infected, infective (opportunistic)
    B99.9
  with
    drug resistant organism —see Resistance
      (to), drug —see also specific organism
    lymphangitis —see Lymphangitis
    organ dysfunction (acute) R65.20
      with septic shock R65.21
  abscess (skin) - code by site under Abscess
  Absidia —see Mucormycosis
  Acanthamoeba —see Acanthamebiasis
  Acanthocheilonema (perstans) (streptocerca)
    B74.4
  accessory sinus (chronic) —see Sinusitis
  achorion —see Dermatophytosis
  Acremonium falciforme B47.0
  acromioclavicular M00.9
  Actinobacillus (actinomycetem-comitans)
    A28.8
    mallei A24.0
    muris A25.1
  Actinomadura B47.1
  Actinomyces (israelii) —see also
    Actinomycosis A42.9
  Actinomycetales —see Actinomycosis
  actinomycotic NOS —see Actinomycosis
  adenoid (and tonsil) J03.90
    chronic J35.02
  adenovirus NEC
    as cause of disease classified elsewhere
      B97.0
    unspecified nature or site B34.0
  aerogenes capsulatus A48.0
  aertrycke —see Infection, salmonella
  alimentary canal NOS —see Enteritis,
    infectious
  Allescheria boydii B48.2
  Alternaria B48.8
  alveolus, alveolar (process) K04.7
  Ameba, amebic (histolytica) —see Amebiasis
  amniotic fluid, sac or cavity O41.10-●
    chorioamnionitis O41.12-●
    placentitis O41.14-●
  amputation stump (surgical) —see
    Complication, amputation stump,
    infection

Infection, infected, infective (Continued)
  Ancylostoma (duodenalis) B76.0
  Anisakiasis, Anisakis larvae B81.0
  anthrax —see Anthrax
  antrum (chronic) —see Sinusitis, maxillary
  anus, anal (papillae) (sphincter) K62.89
  arbovirus (arbor virus) A94
    specified type NEC A93.8
  artificial insemination N98.0
  Ascaris lumbricoides —see Ascariasis
  Ascomycetes B47.0
  Aspergillus (flavus) (fumigatus) (terreus) —
    see Aspergillosis
  atypical
    acid-fast (bacilli) —see Mycobacterium,
      atypical
    mycobacteria —see Mycobacterium,
      atypical
    virus A81.9
      specified type NEC A81.89
  auditory meatus (external) —see Otitis,
    externa, infective
  auricle (ear) —see Otitis, externa, infective
  axillary gland (lymph) L04.2
  Bacillus A49.9
    abortus A23.1
    anthracis —see Anthrax
    Ducrey's (any location) A57
    Flexner's A03.1
    Friedländer's NEC A49.8
    gas (gangrene) A48.0
    mallei A24.0
    melitensis A23.0
    paratyphoid, paratyphosus A01.4
      A A01.1
      B A01.2
      C A01.3
    Shiga (-Kruse) A03.0
    suipestifer —see Infection, salmonella
    swimming pool A31.1
    typhosa A01.00
    welchii —see Gangrene, gas
  bacterial NOS A49.9
    as cause of disease classified elsewhere
      B96.89
      Bacteroides fragilis [B. fragilis] B96.6
      Clostridium perfringens [C. perfringens]
        B96.7
      Enterobacter sakazakii B96.89
      Enterococcus B95.2
      Escherichia coli [E. coli] (see also
        Escherichia coli) B96.20
      Helicobacter pylori [H.pylori] B96.81
      Hemophilus influenzae [H. influenzae]
        B96.3
      Klebsiella pneumoniae [K. pneumoniae]
        B96.1
      Mycoplasma pneumoniae [M.
        pneumoniae] B96.0
      Proteus (mirabilis) (morganii) B96.4
      Pseudomonas (aeruginosa) (mallei)
        (pseudomallei) B96.5
      Staphylococcus B95.8
        aureus (methicillin susceptible)
          (MSSA) B95.61
          methicillin resistant (MRSA)
            B95.62
        specified NEC B95.7
      Streptococcus B95.5
        group A B95.0
        group B B95.1
        pneumoniae B95.3
        specified NEC B95.4
      Vibrio vulnificus B96.82
    specified NEC A48.8
  Bacterium
    paratyphosum A01.4
      A A01.1
      B A01.2
      C A01.3
    typhosum A01.00

▶ New   ⇒ Revised   deleted Deleted   ● Use Additional Character(s)

Infection, infected, infective *(Continued)*
  Bacteroides NEC A49.8
    fragilis, as cause of disease classified
      elsewhere B96.6
  Balantidium coli A07.0
  Bartholin's gland N75.8
  Basidiobolus B46.8
  bile duct (common) (hepatic) —*see*
      Cholangitis
  bladder —*see* Cystitis
  Blastomyces, blastomycotic —*see also*
      Blastomycosis
    brasiliensis —*see* Paracoccidioidomycosis
    dermatitidis —*see* Blastomycosis
    European —*see* Cryptococcosis
    Loboi B48.0
    North American B40.9
    South American —*see*
      Paracoccidioidomycosis
  bleb, postprocedure —*see* Blebitis
  bone —*see* Osteomyelitis
  Bordetella —*see* Whooping cough
  Borrelia bergdorfi A69.20
  brain —*see also* Encephalitis G04.90
    membranes —*see* Meningitis
    septic G06.0
      meninges —*see* Meningitis, bacterial
  branchial cyst Q18.0
  breast —*see* Mastitis
  bronchus —*see* Bronchitis
  Brucella A23.9
    abortus A23.1
    canis A23.3
    melitensis A23.0
    mixed A23.8
    specified NEC A23.8
    suis A23.2
  Brugia (malayi) B74.1
    timori B74.2
  bursa —*see* Bursitis, infective
  buttocks (skin) L08.9
  Campylobacter, intestinal A04.5
    as cause of disease classified elsewhere
      B96.81
  Candida (albicans) (tropicalis) —*see*
      Candidiasis
  candiru B88.8
  Capillaria (intestinal) B81.1
    hepatica B83.8
    philippinensis B81.1
  cartilage —*see* Disorder, cartilage, specified
      type NEC
  catheter-related bloodstream (CRBSI) T80.211
  cat liver fluke B66.0
  cellulitis - code by site under Cellulitis
  central line-associated T80.219
    bloodstream (CLABSI) T80.211
    specified NEC T80.218
  Cephalosporium falciforme B47.0
  cerebrospinal —*see* Meningitis
  cervical gland (lymph) L04.0
  cervix —*see* Cervicitis
  cesarean delivery wound (puerperal) O86.0
  cestodes —*see* Infestation, cestodes
  chest J22
  Chilomastix (intestinal) A07.8
  Chlamydia, chlamydial A74.9
    anus A56.3
    genitourinary tract A56.2
      lower A56.00
      specified NEC A56.19
    lymphogranuloma A55
    pharynx A56.4
    psittaci A70
    rectum A56.3
    sexually transmitted NEC A56.8
  cholera —*see* Cholera
  Cladosporium
    bantianum (brain abscess) B43.1
    carrionii B43.0
    castellanii B36.1

Infection, infected, infective *(Continued)*
  Cladosporium *(Continued)*
    trichoides (brain abscess) B43.1
    werneckii B36.1
  Clonorchis (sinensis) (liver) B66.1
  Clostridium NEC
    bifermentans A48.0
    botulinum (food poisoning) A05.1
      infant A48.51
      wound A48.52
    difficile
      as cause of disease classified elsewhere
        B96.89
    ➠ foodborne (disease)
      ▶ not specified as recurrent
        A04.72
      ▶ recurrent A04.71
      gas gangrene A48.0
    ➠ necrotizing enterocolitis
      ▶ not specified as recurrent
        A04.72
      ▶ recurrent A04.71
      sepsis A41.4
    gas-forming NEC A48.0
    histolyticum A48.0
    novyi, causing gas gangrene A48.0
    oedematiens A48.0
    perfringens
      as cause of disease classified elsewhere
        B96.7
      due to food A05.2
      foodborne (disease) A05.2
      gas gangrene A48.0
      sepsis A41.4
    septicum, causing gas gangrene A48.0
    sordellii, causing gas gangrene A48.0
    welchii
      as cause of disease classified elsewhere
        B96.7
      foodborne (disease) A05.2
      gas gangrene A48.0
      necrotizing enteritis A05.2
      sepsis A41.4
  Coccidioides (immitis) —*see*
      Coccidioidomycosis
  colon —*see* Enteritis, infectious
  colostomy K94.02
  common duct —*see* Cholangitis
  congenital P39.9
    Candida (albicans) P37.5
    cytomegalovirus P35.1
    hepatitis, viral P35.3
    herpes simplex P35.2
    infectious or parasitic disease P37.9
      specified NEC P37.8
    listeriosis (disseminated) P37.2
    malaria NEC P37.4
      falciparum P37.3
    Plasmodium falciparum P37.3
    poliomyelitis P35.8
    rubella P35.0
    skin P39.4
    toxoplasmosis (acute) (subacute) (chronic)
      P37.1
    tuberculosis P37.0
    urinary (tract) P39.3
    vaccinia P35.8
    virus P35.9
      specified type NEC P35.8
  Conidiobolus B46.8
  coronavirus NEC B34.2
    as cause of disease classified elsewhere
      B97.29
    severe acute respiratory syndrome (SARS
      associated) B97.21
  corpus luteum —*see* Salpingo-oophoritis
  Corynebacterium diphtheriae —*see*
      Diphtheria
  cotia virus B08.8
  Coxiella burnetii A78
  coxsackie —*see* Coxsackie

Infection, infected, infective *(Continued)*
  Cryptococcus neoformans —*see*
      Cryptococcosis
  Cryptosporidium A07.2
  Cunninghamella —*see* Mucormycosis
  cyst —*see* Cyst
  cystic duct —*see also* Cholecystitis K81.9
  Cysticercus cellulosae —*see* Cysticercosis
  cytomegalovirus, cytomegaloviral B25.9
    congenital P35.1
    maternal, maternal care for (suspected)
      damage to fetus O35.3
    mononucleosis B27.10
      with
        complication NEC B27.19
        meningitis B27.12
        polyneuropathy B27.11
  delta-agent (acute), in hepatitis B carrier
      B17.0
  dental (pulpal origin) K04.7
  Deuteromycetes B47.0
  Dicrocoelium dendriticum B66.2
  Dipetalonema (perstans) (streptocerca) B74.4
  diphtherial —*see* Diphtheria
  Diphyllobothrium (adult) (latum) (pacificum)
      B70.0
    larval B70.1
  Diplogonoporus (grandis) B71.8
  Dipylidium caninum B67.4
  Dirofilaria B74.8
  Dracunculus medinensis B72
  Drechslera (hawaiiensis) B43.8
  Ducrey Haemophilus (any location) A57
  due to or resulting from
    artificial insemination N98.0
    central venous catheter T80.219
      bloodstream T80.211
      exit or insertion site T80.212
      localized T80.212
      port or reservoir T80.212
      specified NEC T80.218
      tunnel T80.212
    device, implant or graft —*see also*
      Complications, by site and type,
        infection or inflammation
        T85.79
    arterial graft NEC T82.7
    breast (implant) T85.79
    catheter NEC T85.79
      dialysis (renal) T82.7
        intraperitoneal T85.71
      infusion NEC T82.7
        cranial T85.735
        intrathecal T85.735
        spinal (epidural) (subdural)
          T85.735
        subarachnoid T85.735
      urinary T83.518
        cystostomy T83.510
        Hopkins T83.518
        ileostomy T83.518
        nephrostomy T83.512
        specified NEC T83.518
        urethral indwelling T83.511
        urostomy T83.518
    electronic (electrode) (pulse generator)
      (stimulator)
      bone T84.7
      cardiac T82.7
      nervous system T85.738
        brain T85.731
        cranial nerve T85.732
        gastric nerve T85.732
        generator pocket T85.734
        neurostimulator generator
          T85.734
        peripheral nerve T85.732
        sacral nerve T85.732
        spinal cord T85.733
        vagal nerve T85.732
      urinary T83.590

Infection, infected, infective *(Continued)*
  due to or resulting from *(Continued)*
    device, implant or graft *(Continued)*
      fixation, internal (orthopedic) NEC —
          see Complication, fixation device,
          infection
      gastrointestinal (bile duct) (esophagus)
          T85.79
        neurostimulator electrode (lead)
            T85.732
      genital NEC T83.69
      heart NEC T82.7
        valve (prosthesis) T82.6
          graft T82.7
      joint prosthesis —*see* Complication, joint
          prosthesis, infection
      ocular (corneal graft) (orbital implant)
          NEC T85.79
      orthopedic NEC T84.7
      penile (cylinder) (pump) (resevoir)
          T83.61
      specified NEC T85.79
      testicular T83.62
      urinary NEC T83.598
        ileal conduit stent T83.593
        implanted neurostimulation
            T83.590
        implanted sphincter T83.591
        indwelling ureteral stent T83.592
        nephroureteral stent T83.593
        specified stent NEC T83.593
      vascular NEC T82.7
      ventricular intracranial (communicating)
          shunt T85.730
    Hickman catheter T80.219
      bloodstream T80.211
      localized T80.212
      specified NEC T80.218
    immunization or vaccination T88.0
    infusion, injection or transfusion NEC
        T80.29
      acute T80.22
    injury NEC - code by site under Wound,
        open
    peripherally inserted central catheter
        (PICC) T80.219
      bloodstream T80.211
      localized T80.212
      specified NEC T80.218
    portacath (port-a-cath) T80.219
      bloodstream T80.211
      localized T80.212
      specified NEC T80.218
    pulmonary artery catheter —*see* Infection,
        due to or resulting from, central
        venous catheter
➡ surgery T81.4
    Swan Ganz catheter —*see* Infection, due to
        or resulting from, central venous
        catheter
    triple lumen catheter T80.219
      bloodstream T80.211
      localized T80.212
      specified NEC T80.218
    umbilical venous catheter T80.219
      bloodstream T80.211
      localized T80.212
      specified NEC T80.218
  during labor NEC O75.3
  ear (middle) —*see also* Otitis media
    external —*see* Otitis, externa, infective
    inner —*see* subcategory H83.0
  Eberthella typhosa A01.00
  Echinococcus —*see* Echinococcus
  echovirus
    as cause of disease classified elsewhere
        B97.12
    unspecified nature or site B34.1
  endocardium I33.0
  endocervix —*see* Cervicitis
  Entamoeba —*see* Amebiasis

  enteric —*see* Enteritis, infectious
  Enterobacter sakazakii B96.89
  Enterobius vermicularis B80
  enterostomy K94.12
  enterovirus B34.1
    as cause of disease classified elsewhere
        B97.10
      coxsackievirus B97.11
      echovirus B97.12
      specified NEC B97.19
  Entomophthora B46.8
  Epidermophyton —*see* Dermatophytosis
  epididymis —*see* Epididymitis
  episiotomy (puerperal) O86.0
  Erysipelothrix (insidiosa) (rhusiopathiae) —
      see Erysipeloid
  erythema infectiosum B08.3
  Escherichia (E.) coli NEC A49.8
    as cause of disease classified elsewhere —
        see also Escherichia coli B96.20
    congenital P39.8
      sepsis P36.4
    generalized A41.51
    intestinal —*see* Enteritis, infectious, due to,
        Escherichia coli
  ethmoidal (chronic) (sinus) —*see* Sinusitis,
      ethmoidal
  eustachian tube (ear) —*see* Salpingitis,
      eustachian
  external auditory canal (meatus) NEC —*see*
      Otitis, externa, infective
  eye (purulent) —*see* Endophthalmitis, purulent
  eyelid —*see* Inflammation, eyelid
  fallopian tube —*see* Salpingo-oophoritis
  Fasciola (gigantica) (hepatica) (indica) B66.3
  Fasciolopsis (buski) B66.5
  filarial —*see* Infestation, filarial
  finger (skin) L08.9
    nail L03.01-●
      fungus B35.1
  fish tapeworm B70.0
    larval B70.1
  flagellate, intestinal A07.9
  fluke —*see* Infestation, fluke
  focal
    teeth (pulpal origin) K04.7
    tonsils J35.01
  Fonsecaea (compactum) (pedrosoi) B43.0
  food —*see* Intoxication, foodborne
  foot (skin) L08.9
    dermatophytic fungus B35.3
  Francisella tularensis —*see* Tularemia
  frontal (sinus) (chronic) —*see* Sinusitis, frontal
  fungus NOS B49
    beard B35.0
    dermatophytic —*see* Dermatophytosis
    foot B35.3
    groin B35.6
    hand B35.2
    nail B35.1
    pathogenic to compromised host only B48.8
    perianal (area) B35.6
    scalp B35.0
    skin B36.9
      foot B35.3
      hand B35.2
      toenails B35.1
  Fusarium B48.8
  gallbladder —*see* Cholecystitis
  gas bacillus —*see* Gangrene, gas
  gastrointestinal —*see* Enteritis, infectious
  generalized NEC —*see* Sepsis
  generator pocket, implanted electronic
      neurostimulator T85.734
  genital organ or tract
    female —*see* Disease, pelvis, inflammatory
    male N49.9
      multiple sites N49.8
      specified NEC N49.8
  Ghon tubercle, primary A15.7

  Giardia lamblia A07.1
  gingiva (chronic) K05.10
    acute K05.00
      nonplaque induced K05.01
      plaque induced K05.00
    nonplaque induced K05.11
    plaque induced K05.10
  glanders A24.0
  glenosporopsis B48.0
  Gnathostoma (spinigerum) B83.1
  Gongylonema B83.8
  gonococcal —*see* Gonococcus
  gram-negative bacilli NOS A49.9
  guinea worm B72
  gum (chronic) K05.10
    acute K05.00
      nonplaque induced K05.01
      plaque induced K05.00
    nonplaque induced K05.11
    plaque induced K05.10
  Haemophilus —*see* Infection, Hemophilus
  heart —*see* Carditis
  Helicobacter pylori A04.8
    as cause of disease classified elsewhere
        B96.81
  helminths B83.9
    intestinal B82.0
      mixed (types classifiable to more than
          one of the titles B65.0-B81.3 and
          B81.8) B81.4
      specified type NEC B81.8
    specified type NEC B83.8
  Hemophilus
    aegyptius, systemic A48.4
    ducrey (any location) A57
    generalized A41.3
    influenzae NEC A49.2
      as cause of disease classified elsewhere
          B96.3
  herpes (simplex) —*see also* Herpes
    congenital P35.2
    disseminated B00.7
    zoster B02.9
  herpesvirus, herpesviral —*see* Herpes
  Heterophyes (heterophyes) B66.8
  hip (joint) NEC M00.9
    due to internal joint prosthesis
      left T84.52
      right T84.51
    skin NEC L08.9
  Histoplasma —*see* Histoplasmosis
    American B39.4
    capsulatum B39.4
  hookworm B76.9
  human
    papilloma virus A63.0
    T-cell lymphotropic virus type-1 (HTLV-1)
        B33.3
  hydrocele N43.0
  Hymenolepis B71.0
  hypopharynx —*see* Pharyngitis
  inguinal (lymph) glands L04.1
    due to soft chancre A57
  intervertebral disc, pyogenic M46.30
    cervical region M46.32
    cervicothoracic region M46.33
    lumbar region M46.36
    lumbosacral region M46.37
    multiple sites M46.39
    occipito-atlanto-axial region M46.31
    sacrococcygeal region M46.38
    thoracic region M46.34
    thoracolumbar region M46.35
  intestine, intestinal —*see* Enteritis, infectious
    specified NEC A08.8
  intra-amniotic affecting newborn NEC P39.2
  Isospora belli or hominis A07.3
  Japanese B encephalitis A83.0
  jaw (bone) (lower) (upper) M27.2
  joint NEC M00.9
    due to internal joint prosthesis T84.50

▶ New   ➡ Revised   ~~deleted~~ Deleted   ● Use Additional Character(s)

Infection, infected, infective *(Continued)*
  kidney (cortex) (hematogenous) N15.9
    with calculus N20.0
      with hydronephrosis N13.6
    following ectopic gestation O08.83
    pelvis and ureter (cystic) N28.85
    puerperal (postpartum) O86.21
    specified NEC N15.8
  Klebsiella (K.) pneumoniae NEC A49.8
    as cause of disease classified elsewhere B96.1
  knee (joint) NEC M00.9
    due to internal joint prosthesis
      left T84.54
      right T84.53
    joint M00.9
    skin L08.9
  Koch's —*see* Tuberculosis
  labia (majora) (minora) (acute) —*see* Vulvitis
  lacrimal
    gland —*see* Dacryoadenitis
    passages (duct) (sac) —*see* Inflammation, lacrimal, passages
  lancet fluke B66.2
  larynx NEC J38.7
  leg (skin) NOS L08.9
  Legionella pneumophila A48.1
    nonpneumonic A48.2
  Leishmania —*see also* Leishmaniasis
    aethiopica B55.1
    braziliensis B55.2
    chagasi B55.0
    donovani B55.0
    infantum B55.0
    major B55.1
    mexicana B55.1
    tropica B55.1
  lentivirus, as cause of disease classified elsewhere B97.31
  Leptosphaeria senegalensis B47.0
  Leptospira interrogans A27.9
    autumnalis A27.89
    canicola A27.89
    hebdomadis A27.89
    icterohaemorrhagiae A27.0
    pomona A27.89
    specified type NEC A27.89
  leptospirochetal NEC —*see* Leptospirosis
  Listeria monocytogenes —*see also* Listeriosis
    congenital P37.2
  Loa loa B74.3
    with conjunctival infestation B74.3
    eyelid B74.3
  Loboa loboi B48.0
  local, skin (staphylococcal) (streptococcal) L08.9
    abscess - code by site under Abscess
    cellulitis - code by site under Cellulitis
    specified NEC L08.89
    ulcer —*see* Ulcer, skin
  Loefflerella mallei A24.0
  lung —*see also* Pneumonia J18.9
    atypical Mycobacterium A31.0
    spirochetal A69.8
    tuberculous —*see* Tuberculosis, pulmonary
    virus —*see* Pneumonia, viral
  lymph gland —*see also* Lymphadenitis, acute
    mesenteric I88.0
  lymphoid tissue, base of tongue or posterior pharynx, NEC (chronic) J35.03
  Madurella (grisea) (mycetomii) B47.0
  major
    following ectopic or molar pregnancy O08.0
    puerperal, postpartum, childbirth O85
  Malassezia furfur B36.0
  Malleomyces
    mallei A24.0
    pseudomallei (whitmori) —*see* Melioidosis
  mammary gland N61.0
  Mansonella (ozzardi) (perstans) (streptocerca) B74.4
  mastoid —*see* Mastoiditis

Infection, infected, infective *(Continued)*
  maxilla, maxillary M27.2
    sinus (chronic) —*see* Sinusitis, maxillary
  mediastinum J98.51
  Medina (worm) B72
  meibomian cyst or gland —*see* Hordeolum
  meninges —*see* Meningitis, bacterial
  meningococcal —*see also* condition A39.9
    adrenals A39.1
    brain A39.81
    cerebrospinal A39.0
    conjunctiva A39.89
    endocardium A39.51
    heart A39.50
      endocardium A39.51
      myocardium A39.52
      pericardium A39.53
    joint A39.83
    meninges A39.0
    meningococcemia A39.4
      acute A39.2
      chronic A39.3
    myocardium A39.52
    pericardium A39.53
    retrobulbar neuritis A39.82
    specified site NEC A39.89
  mesenteric lymph nodes or glands NEC I88.0
  Metagonimus B66.8
  metatarsophalangeal M00.9
  methicillin
    resistant Staphylococcus aureus (MRSA) A49.02
    susceptible Staphylococcus aureus (MSSA) A49.01
  Microsporum, microsporic —*see* Dermatophytosis
  mixed flora (bacterial) NEC A49.8
  Monilia —*see* Candidiasis
  Monosporium apiospermum B48.2
  mouth, parasitic B37.0
  Mucor —*see* Mucormycosis
  muscle NEC —*see* Myositis, infective
  mycelium NOS B49
  mycetoma B47.9
    actinomycotic NEC B47.1
    mycotic NEC B47.0
  Mycobacterium, mycobacterial —*see* Mycobacterium
  Mycoplasma NEC A49.3
    pneumoniae, as cause of disease classified elsewhere B96.0
  mycotic NOS B49
    pathogenic to compromised host only B48.8
    skin NOS B36.9
  myocardium NEC I40.0
  nail (chronic)
    with lymphangitis —*see* Lymphangitis, acute, digit
    finger L03.01-●
      fungus B35.1
    ingrowing L60.0
    toe L03.03-●
      fungus B35.1
  nasal sinus (chronic) —*see* Sinusitis
  nasopharynx —*see* Nasopharyngitis
  navel L08.82
  Necator americanus B76.1
  Neisseria —*see* Gonococcus
  Neotestudina rosatii B47.0
  newborn P39.9
    intra-amniotic NEC P39.2
    skin P39.4
    specified type NEC P39.8
  nipple N61.0
    associated with
      lactation O91.03
      pregnancy O91.01-●
      puerperium O91.02
  Nocardia —*see* Nocardiosis
  obstetrical surgical wound (puerperal) O86.0
  Oesophagostomum (apiostomum) B81.8

Infection, infected, infective *(Continued)*
  Oestrus ovis —*see* Myiasis
  Oidium albicans B37.9
  Onchocerca (volvulus) —*see* Onchocerciasis - oncovirus, as cause of disease classified elsewhere B97.32
  ►operation wound T81.4
  Opisthorchis (felineus) (viverrini) B66.0
  orbit, orbital —*see* Inflammation, orbit
  orthopoxvirus NEC B08.09
  ovary —*see* Salpingo-oophoritis
  Oxyuris vermicularis B80
  pancreas (acute) —*see* Pancreatitis, acute
    abscess —*see* Pancreatitis, acute
    specified NEC —*see also* Pancreatitis, acute K85.80
  papillomavirus, as cause of disease classified elsewhere B97.7
  papovavirus NEC B34.4
  Paracoccidioides brasiliensis —*see* Paracoccidioidomycosis
  Paragonimus (westermani) B66.4
  parainfluenza virus B34.8
  parameningococcus NOS A39.9
  parapoxvirus B08.60
    specified NEC B08.69
  parasitic B89
  Parastrongylus
    cantonensis B83.2
    costaricensis B81.3
    paratyphoid A01.4
      Type A A01.1
      Type B A01.2
      Type C A01.3
  paraurethral ducts N34.2
  parotid gland —*see* Sialoadenitis
  parvovirus NEC B34.3
    as cause of disease classified elsewhere B97.6
  Pasteurella NEC A28.0
    multocida A28.0
    pestis —*see* Plague
    pseudotuberculosis A28.0
    septica (cat bite) (dog bite) A28.0
    tularensis —*see* Tularemia
  pelvic, female —*see* Disease, pelvis, inflammatory
  Penicillium (marneffei) B48.4
  penis (glans) (retention) NEC N48.29
  periapical K04.5
  peridental, periodontal K05.20
    generalized —*see* Peridontitis, aggressive, generalized
    localized —*see* Peridontitis, aggressive, localized
  perinatal period P39.9
    specified type NEC P39.8
  perineal repair (puerperal) O86.0
  periorbital —*see* Inflammation, orbit
  perirectal K62.89
  perirenal —*see* Infection, kidney
  peritoneal —*see* Peritonitis
  periureteral N28.89
  Petriellidium boydii B48.2
  pharynx —*see also* Pharyngitis
    coxsackievirus B08.5
    posterior, lymphoid (chronic) J35.03
  Phialophora
    gougerotii (subcutaneous abscess or cyst) B43.2
    jeanselmei (subcutaneous abscess or cyst) B43.2
    verrucosa (skin) B43.0
  Piedraia hortae B36.3
  pinta A67.9
    intermediate A67.1
    late A67.2
    mixed A67.3
    primary A67.0
  pinworm B80
  pityrosporum furfur B36.0
  pleuro-pneumonia-like organism (PPLO) NEC A49.3
    as cause of disease classified elsewhere B96.0

Infection, infected, infective *(Continued)*
  pneumococcus, pneumococcal NEC A49.1
    as cause of disease classified elsewhere B95.3
    generalized (purulent) A40.3
      with pneumonia J13
  Pneumocystis carinii (pneumonia) B59
  Pneumocystis jiroveci (pneumonia) B59
  port or reservoir T80.212
➠ postoperative T81.4
➠ postoperative wound T81.4
➠ postprocedural T81.4
    ~~deep incisional surgical site T81.42~~
    ~~organ and space surgical site T81.43~~
    ~~sepsis T81.49~~
    ~~specified surgical site NEC T81.48~~
    ~~superficial incisional surgical site T81.41~~
  postvaccinal T88.0
  prepuce NEC N47.7
    with penile inflammation N47.6
  prion —*see* Disease, prion, central nervous system
  prostate (capsule) —*see* Prostatitis
  Proteus (mirabilis) (morganii) (vulgaris) NEC A49.8
    as cause of disease classified elsewhere B96.4
  protozoal NEC B64
    intestinal A07.9
      specified NEC A07.8
    specified NEC B60.8
  Pseudoallescheria boydii B48.2
  Pseudomonas NEC A49.8
    as cause of disease classified elsewhere B96.5
    mallei A24.0
    pneumonia J15.1
    pseudomallei —*see* Melioidosis
  puerperal O86.4
    genitourinary tract NEC O86.89
    major or generalized O85
    minor O86.4
    specified NEC O86.89
  pulmonary —*see* Infection, lung
  purulent —*see* Abscess
  Pyrenochaeta romeroi B47.0
  Q fever A78
  rectum (sphincter) K62.89
  renal —*see also* Infection, kidney
    pelvis and ureter (cystic) N28.85
  reovirus, as cause of disease classified elsewhere B97.5
  respiratory (tract) NEC J98.8
    acute J22
    chronic J98.8
    influenzal (upper) (acute) —*see* Influenza, with, respiratory manifestations NEC
    lower (acute) J22
      chronic —*see* Bronchitis, chronic
    rhinovirus J00
    syncytial virus, as cause of disease classified elsewhere B97.4
    upper (acute) NOS J06.9
      chronic J39.8
      streptococcal J06.9
      viral NOS J06.9
  resulting from
    presence of internal prosthesis, implant, graft —*see* Complications, by site and type, infection
  retortamoniasis A07.8
  retroperitoneal NEC K68.9
  retrovirus B33.3
    as cause of disease classified elsewhere B97.30
    human
      immunodeficiency, type 2 (HIV 2) B97.35
      T-cell lymphotropic
        type I (HTLV-I) B97.33
        type II (HTLV-II) B97.34
    lentivirus B97.31
    oncovirus B97.32
    specified NEC B97.39
  Rhinosporidium (seeberi) B48.1

Infection, infected, infective *(Continued)*
  rhinovirus
    as cause of disease classified elsewhere B97.89
    unspecified nature or site B34.8
  Rhizopus —*see* Mucormycosis
  rickettsial NOS A79.9
  roundworm (large) NEC B82.0
    Ascariasis —*see also* Ascariasis B77.9
  rubella —*see* Rubella
  Saccharomyces —*see* Candidiasis
  salivary duct or gland (any) —*see* Sialoadenitis
  Salmonella (aertrycke) (arizonae) (callinarum) (cholerae-suis) (enteritidis) (suipestifer) (typhimurium) A02.9
    with
      (gastro) enteritis A02.0
      sepsis A02.1
      specified manifestation NEC A02.8
    due to food (poisoning) A02.9
    hirschfeldii A01.3
    localized A02.20
      arthritis A02.23
      meningitis A02.21
      osteomyelitis A02.24
      pneumonia A02.22
      pyelonephritis A02.25
      specified NEC A02.29
    paratyphi A01.4
      A A01.1
      B A01.2
      C A01.3
    schottmuelleri A01.2
    typhi, typhosa —*see* Typhoid
  Sarcocystis A07.8
  scabies B86
  Schistosoma —*see* Infestation, Schistosoma
  scrotum (acute) NEC N49.2
  seminal vesicle —*see* Vesiculitis
  septic
    localized, skin —*see* Abscess
  sheep liver fluke B66.3
  Shigella A03.9
    boydii A03.2
    dysenteriae A03.0
    flexneri A03.1
    group
      A A03.0
      B A03.1
      C A03.2
      D A03.3
    Schmitz (-Stutzer) A03.0
    schmitzii A03.0
    shigae A03.0
    sonnei A03.3
    specified NEC A03.8
  shoulder (joint) NEC M00.9
    due to internal joint prosthesis T84.59
    skin NEC L08.9
  sinus (accessory) (chronic) (nasal) —*see also* Sinusitis
    pilonidal —*see* Sinus, pilonidal
    skin NEC L08.89
  Skene's duct or gland —*see* Urethritis
  skin (local) (staphylococcal) (streptococcal) L08.9
    abscess - code by site under Abscess
    cellulitis - code by site under Cellulitis
    due to fungus B36.9
      specified type NEC B36.8
    mycotic B36.9
      specified type NEC B36.8
    newborn P39.4
    ulcer —*see* Ulcer, skin
  slow virus A81.9
    specified NEC A81.89
  Sparganum (mansoni) (proliferum) (baxteri) B70.1
  specific —*see also* Syphilis
    to perinatal period —*see* Infection, congenital

Infection, infected, infective *(Continued)*
  specified NEC B99.8
  spermatic cord NEC N49.1
  sphenoidal (sinus) —*see* Sinusitis, sphenoidal
  spinal cord NOS —*see also* Myelitis G04.91
    abscess G06.1
    meninges —*see* Meningitis
    streptococcal G04.89
  Spirillum A25.0
  spirochetal NOS A69.9
    lung A69.8
    specified NEC A69.8
  Spirometra larvae B70.1
  spleen D73.89
  Sporotrichum, Sporothrix (schenckii) —*see* Sporotrichosis
  staphylococcal, unspecified site
    aureus (methicillin susceptible) (MSSA) A49.01
      methicillin resistant (MRSA) A49.02
    as cause of disease classified elsewhere B95.8
      aureus (methicillin susceptible) (MSSA) B95.61
        methicillin resistant (MRSA) B95.62
      specified NEC B95.7
    food poisoning A05.0
    generalized (purulent) A41.2
    pneumonia —*see* Pneumonia, staphylococcal
  Stellantchasmus falcatus B66.8
  streptobacillus moniliformis A25.1
  streptococcal NEC A49.1
    as cause of disease classified elsewhere B95.5
    B genitourinary complicating
      childbirth O98.82
      pregnancy O98.81-●
      puerperium O98.83
    congenital
      sepsis P36.10
        group B P36.0
        specified NEC P36.19
    generalized (purulent) A40.9
  Streptomyces B47.1
  Strongyloides (stercoralis) —*see* Strongyloidiasis
  stump (amputation) (surgical) —*see* Complication, amputation stump, infection
  subcutaneous tissue, local L08.9
  suipestifer —*see* Infection, salmonella
  swimming pool bacillus A31.1
  Taenia —*see* Infestation, Taenia
  Taeniarhynchus saginatus B68.1
  tapeworm —*see* Infestation, tapeworm
  tendon (sheath) —*see* Tenosynovitis, infective NEC
  Ternidens diminutus B81.8
  testis —*see* Orchitis
  threadworm B80
  throat —*see* Pharyngitis
  thyroglossal duct K14.8
  toe (skin) L08.9
    cellulitis L03.03-●
      fungus B35.1
    nail L03.03-●
      fungus B35.1
  tongue NEC K14.0
    parasitic B37.0
  tonsil (and adenoid) (faucial) (lingual) (pharyngeal) —*see* Tonsillitis
  tooth, teeth K04.7
    irreversible K04.02
    periapical K04.7
    peridental, periodontal K05.20
      generalized —*see* Peridontitis, aggressive, generalized
      localized —*see* Peridontitis, aggressive, localized

▶ New   ➠ Revised   ~~deleted~~ Deleted   ● Use Additional Character(s)

Infection, infected, infective *(Continued)*
  tooth, teeth *(Continued)*
    pulp K04.01
    ▶irreversible K04.02
    ▶reversible K04.01
    ~~reversible K04.01~~
    ~~socket M27.3~~
  TORCH —*see* Infection, congenital without active infection P00.2
  Torula histolytica —*see* Cryptococcosis
  Toxocara (canis) (cati) (felis) B83.0
  Toxoplasma gondii —*see* Toxoplasma
  trachea, chronic J42
  trematode NEC —*see* Infestation, fluke
  trench fever A79.0
  Treponema pallidum —*see* Syphilis
  Trichinella (spiralis) B75
  Trichomonas A59.9
    cervix A59.09
    intestine A07.8
    prostate A59.02
    specified site NEC A59.8
    urethra A59.03
    urogenitalis A59.00
    vagina A59.01
    vulva A59.01
  Trichophyton, trichophytic —*see* Dermatophytosis
  Trichosporon (beigelii) cutaneum B36.2
  Trichostrongylus B81.2
  Trichuris (trichiura) B79
  Trombicula (irritans) B88.0
  Trypanosoma
    brucei
      gambiense B56.0
      rhodesiense B56.1
    cruzi —*see* Chagas' disease
  tubal —*see* Salpingo-oophoritis
  tuberculous NEC —*see* Tuberculosis
  tubo-ovarian —*see* Salpingo-oophoritis
  tunica vaginalis N49.1
  tunnel T80.212
  tympanic membrane NEC —*see* Myringitis
  typhoid (abortive) (ambulant) (bacillus) —*see* Typhoid
  typhus A75.9
    flea-borne A75.2
    mite-borne A75.3
    recrudescent A75.1
    tick-borne A77.9
      African A77.1
      North Asian A77.2
  umbilicus L08.82
  ureter N28.86
  urethra —*see* Urethritis
  urinary (tract) N39.0
    bladder —*see* Cystitis
    complicating
      pregnancy O23.4-●
        specified type NEC O23.3-●
    kidney —*see* Infection, kidney
    newborn P39.3
    puerperal (postpartum) O86.20
    tuberculous A18.13
    urethra —*see* Urethritis
  uterus, uterine —*see* Endometritis
  vaccination T88.0
  vaccinia not from vaccination B08.011
  vagina (acute) —*see* Vaginitis
  varicella B01.9
  varicose veins —*see* Varix
  vas deferens NEC N49.1
  vesical —*see* Cystitis
  Vibrio
    cholerae A00.0
      El Tor A00.1
    parahaemolyticus (food poisoning) A05.3
    vulnificus
      as cause of disease classified elsewhere B96.82
      foodborne intoxication A05.5
  Vincent's (gum) (mouth) (tonsil) A69.1

Infection, infected, infective *(Continued)*
  virus, viral NOS B34.9
    adenovirus
      as cause of disease classified elsewhere B97.0
      unspecified nature or site B34.0
    arborvirus, arbovirus arthropod-borne A94
    as cause of disease classified elsewhere B97.89
    adenovirus B97.0
    coronavirus B97.29
      SARS-associated B97.21
    coxsackievirus B97.11
    echovirus B97.12
    enterovirus B97.10
      coxsackievirus B97.11
      echovirus B97.12
      specified NEC B97.19
    human
      immunodeficiency, type 2 (HIV 2) B97.35
      metapneumovirus B97.81
      T-cell lymphotropic,
        type I (HTLV-I) B97.33
        type II (HTLV-II) B97.34
    papillomavirus B97.7
    parvovirus B97.6
    reovirus B97.5
    respiratory syncytial B97.4
    retrovirus B97.30
      human
        immunodeficiency, type 2 (HIV 2) B97.35
        T-cell lymphotropic,
          type I (HTLV-I) B97.33
          type II (HTLV-II) B97.34
      lentivirus B97.31
      oncovirus B97.32
      specified NEC B97.39
    specified NEC B97.89
  central nervous system A89
    atypical A81.9
      specified NEC A81.89
    enterovirus NEC A88.8
      meningitis A87.0
    slow virus A81.9
      specified NEC A81.89
    specified NEC A88.8
  chest J98.8
  cotia B08.8
  coxsackie —*see also* Infection, coxsackie B34.1
    as cause of disease classified elsewhere B97.11
  ECHO
    as cause of disease classified elsewhere B97.12
    unspecified nature or site B34.1
  encephalitis, tick-borne A84.9
  enterovirus, as cause of disease classified elsewhere B97.10
    coxsackievirus B97.11
    echovirus B97.12
    specified NEC B97.19
  exanthem NOS B09
  human metapneumovirus as cause of disease classified elsewhere B97.81
  human papilloma as cause of disease classified elsewhere B97.7
  intestine —*see* Enteritis, viral
  respiratory syncytial
    as cause of disease classified elsewhere B97.4
    bronchopneumonia J12.1
    common cold syndrome J00
    nasopharyngitis (acute) J00
  rhinovirus
    as cause of disease classified elsewhere B97.89
    unspecified nature or site B34.8
  slow A81.9
    specified NEC A81.89

Infection, infected, infective *(Continued)*
  virus, viral NOS *(Continued)*
    specified type NEC B33.8
      as cause of disease classified elsewhere B97.89
      unspecified nature or site B34.8
    unspecified nature or site B34.9
    West Nile —*see* Virus, West Nile
    vulva (acute) —*see* Vulvitis
  West Nile —*see* Virus, West Nile
  whipworm B79
  worms B83.9
    specified type NEC B83.8
  Wuchereria (bancrofti) B74.0
    malayi B74.1
    yatapoxvirus B08.70
      specified NEC B08.79
  yeast *(see also* Candidiasis) B37.9
  yellow fever —*see* Fever, yellow
  Yersinia
    enterocolitica (intestinal) A04.6
    pestis —*see* Plague
    pseudotuberculosis A28.2
  Zeis' gland —*see* Hordeolum
  Zika virus A92.5
  zoonotic bacterial NOS A28.9
  Zopfia senegalensis B47.0
Infective, infectious —*see* condition
Infertility
  female N97.9
    age-related N97.8
    associated with
      anovulation N97.0
      cervical (mucus) disease or anomaly N88.3
      congenital anomaly
        cervix N88.3
        fallopian tube N97.1
        uterus N97.2
        vagina N97.8
      dysmucorrhea N88.3
      fallopian tube disease or anomaly N97.1
      pituitary-hypothalamic origin E23.0
      specified origin NEC N97.8
      Stein-Leventhal syndrome E28.2
      uterine disease or anomaly N97.2
      vaginal disease or anomaly N97.8
    due to
      cervical anomaly N88.3
      fallopian tube anomaly N97.1
      ovarian failure E28.39
      Stein-Leventhal syndrome E28.2
      uterine anomaly N97.2
      vaginal anomaly N97.8
    nonimplantation N97.2
    origin
      cervical N88.3
      tubal (block) (occlusion) (stenosis) N97.1
      uterine N97.2
      vaginal N97.8
  male N46.9
    azoospermia N46.01
      extratesticular cause N46.029
        drug therapy N46.021
        efferent duct obstruction N46.023
        infection N46.022
        radiation N46.024
        specified cause NEC N46.029
        systemic disease N46.025
    oligospermia N46.11
      extratesticular cause N46.129
        drug therapy N46.121
        efferent duct obstruction N46.123
        infection N46.122
        radiation N46.124
        specified cause NEC N46.129
        systemic disease N46.125
    specified type NEC N46.8
Infestation B88.9
  Acanthocheilonema (perstans) (streptocerca) B74.4

Infestation *(Continued)*
  Acariasis B88.0
    demodex folliculorum B88.0
    sarcoptes scabiei B86
    trombiculae B88.0
  Agamofilaria streptocerca B74.4
  Ancylostoma, ankylostoma (braziliense)
      (caninum) (ceylanicum) (duodenale)
      B76.0
    americanum B76.1
    new world B76.1
  Anisakis larvae, anisakiasis B81.0
  arthropod NEC B88.2
  Ascaris lumbricoides —*see* Ascariasis
  Balantidium coli A07.0
  beef tapeworm B68.1
  Bothriocephalus (latus) B70.0
    larval B70.1
  broad tapeworm B70.0
    larval B70.1
  Brugia (malayi) B74.1
    timori B74.2
  candiru B88.8
  Capillaria
    hepatica B83.8
    philippinensis B81.1
  cat liver fluke B66.0
  cestodes B71.9
    diphyllobothrium —*see* Infestation,
        diphyllobothrium
    dipylidiasis B71.1
    hymenolepiasis B71.0
    specified type NEC B71.8
  chigger B88.0
  chigo, chigoe B88.1
  Clonorchis (sinensis) (liver) B66.1
  coccidial A07.3
  crab-lice B85.3
  Cysticercus cellulosae —*see* Cysticercosis
  Demodex (folliculorum) B88.0
  Dermanyssus gallinae B88.0
  Dermatobia (hominis) —*see* Myiasis
  Dibothriocephalus (latus) B70.0
    larval B70.1
  Dicrocoelium dendriticum B66.2
  Diphyllobothrium (adult) (latum) (intestinal)
      (pacificum) B70.0
    larval B70.1
  Diplogonoporus (grandis) B71.8
  Dipylidium caninum B67.4
  Distoma hepaticum B66.3
  dog tapeworm B67.4
  Dracunculus medinensis B72
  dragon worm B72
  dwarf tapeworm B71.0
  Echinococcus —*see* Echinococcus
  Echinostomum ilocanum B66.8
  Entamoeba (histolytica) —*see* Infection,
      Ameba
  Enterobius vermicularis B80
  eyelid
    in (due to)
      leishmaniasis B55.1
      loiasis B74.3
      onchocerciasis B73.09
      phthiriasis B85.3
      parasitic NOS B89
  eyeworm B74.3
  Fasciola (gigantica) (hepatica) (indica) B66.3
  Fasciolopsis (buski) (intestine) B66.5
  filarial B74.9
    bancroftian B74.0
    conjunctiva B74.9
    due to
      Acanthocheilonema (perstans)
          (streptocerca) B74.4
      Brugia (malayi) B74.1
        timori B74.2
      Dracunculus medinensis B72
      guinea worm B72
      loa loa B74.3

Infestation *(Continued)*
  filarial *(Continued)*
    due to *(Continued)*
      Mansonella (ozzardi) (perstans)
          (streptocerca) B74.4
      Onchocerca volvulus B73.00
        eye B73.00
        eyelid B73.09
      Wuchereria (bancrofti) B74.0
    Malayan B74.1
    ozzardi B74.4
    specified type NEC B74.8
  fish tapeworm B70.0
    larval B70.1
  fluke B66.9
    blood NOS —*see* Schistosomiasis
    cat liver B66.0
    intestinal B66.5
    lancet B66.2
    liver (sheep) B66.3
      cat B66.0
      Chinese B66.1
      due to clonorchiasis B66.1
      oriental B66.1
    lung (oriental) B66.4
    sheep liver B66.3
    specified type NEC B66.8
  fly larvae —*see* Myiasis
  Gasterophilus (intestinalis) —*see* Myiasis
  Gastrodiscoides hominis B66.8
  Giardia lamblia A07.1
  Gnathostoma (spinigerum) B83.1
  Gongylonema B83.8
  guinea worm B72
  helminth B83.9
    angiostrongyliasis B83.2
      intestinal B81.3
    gnathostomiasis B83.1
    hirudiniasis, internal B83.4
    intestinal B82.0
      angiostrongyliasis B81.3
      anisakiasis B81.0
      ascariasis —*see* Ascariasis
      capillariasis B81.1
      cysticercosis —*see* Cysticercosis
      diphyllobothriasis —*see* Infestation,
          diphyllobothriasis
      dracunculiasis B72
      echinococcus —*see* Echinococcosis
      enterobiasis B80
      filariasis —*see* Infestation, filarial
      fluke —*see* Infestation, fluke
      hookworm —*see* Infestation, hookworm
      mixed (types classifiable to more than
          one of the titles B65.0-B81.3 and
          B81.8) B81.4
      onchocerciasis —*see* Onchocerciasis
      schistosomiasis —*see* Infestation,
          schistosoma
      specified
        cestode NEC —*see* Infestation, cestode
        type NEC B81.8
      strongyloidiasis —*see* Strongyloidiasis
      taenia —*see* Infestation, taenia
      trichinellosis B75
      trichostrongyliasis B81.2
      trichuriasis B79
    specified type NEC B83.8
    syngamiasis B83.3
    visceral larva migrans B83.0
  Heterophyes (heterophyes) B66.8
  hookworm B76.9
    ancylostomiasis B76.0
    necatoriasis B76.1
    specified type NEC B76.8
  Hymenolepis (diminuta) (nana) B71.0
  intestinal NEC B82.9
  leeches (aquatic) (land) —*see* Hirudiniasis
  Leishmania —*see* Leishmaniasis
  lice, louse —*see* Infestation, Pediculus
  Linguatula B88.8

Infestation *(Continued)*
  Liponyssoides sanguineus B88.0
  Loa loa B74.3
    conjunctival B74.3
    eyelid B74.3
  louse —*see* Infestation, Pediculus
  maggots —*see* Myiasis
  Mansonella (ozzardi) (perstans) (streptocerca)
      B74.4
  Medina (worm) B72
  Metagonimus (yokogawai) B66.8
  microfilaria streptocerca —*see* Onchocerciasis
    eye B73.00
    eyelid B73.09
  mites B88.9
    scabic B86
  Monilia (albicans) —*see* Candidiasis
  mouth B37.0
  Necator americanus B76.1
  nematode NEC (intestinal) B82.0
    Ancylostoma B76.0
    conjunctiva NEC B83.9
    Enterobius vermicularis B80
    Gnathostoma spinigerum B83.1
    physaloptera B80
    specified NEC B81.8
    trichostrongylus B81.2
    trichuris (trichuria) B79
  Oesophagostomum (apiostomum) B81.8
  Oestrus ovis —*see also* Myiasis B87.9
  Onchocerca (volvulus) —*see* Onchocerciasis
  Opisthorchis (felineus) (viverrini) B66.0
  orbit, parasitic NOS B89
  Oxyuris vermicularis B80
  Paragonimus (westermani) B66.4
  parasite, parasitic B89
    eyelid B89
    intestinal NOS B82.9
    mouth B37.0
    skin B88.9
    tongue B37.0
  Parastrongylus
    cantonensis B83.2
    costaricensis B81.3
  Pediculus B85.2
    body B85.1
    capitis (humanus) (any site) B85.0
    corporis (humanus) (any site) B85.1
    head B85.0
    mixed (classifiable to more than one of the
        titles B85.0-B85.3) B85.4
    pubis (any site) B85.3
  Pentastoma B88.8
  Phthirus (pubis) (any site) B85.3
    with any infestation classifiable to
        B85.0-B85.2 B85.4
  pinworm B80
  pork tapeworm (adult) B68.0
  protozoal NEC B64
    intestinal A07.9
      specified NEC A07.8
    specified NEC B60.8
  pubic, louse B85.3
  rat tapeworm B71.0
  red bug B88.0
  roundworm (large) NEC B82.0
    Ascariasis —*see also* Ascariasis B77.9
  sandflea B88.1
  Sarcoptes scabiei B86
  scabies B86
  Schistosoma B65.9
    bovis B65.8
    cercariae B65.3
    haematobium B65.0
    intercalatum B65.8
    japonicum B65.2
    mansoni B65.1
    mattheei B65.8
    mekongi B65.8
    specified type NEC B65.8
    spindale B65.8

▶ New   ⇒ Revised   ~~deleted~~ Deleted   ● Use Additional Character(s)

Infestation *(Continued)*
    screw worms —*see* Myiasis
    skin NOS B88.9
    Sparganum (mansoni) (proliferum) (baxteri)
        B70.1
        larval B70.1
    specified type NEC B88.8
    Spirometra larvae B70.1
    Stellantchasmus falcatus B66.8
    Strongyloides stercoralis —*see*
        Strongyloidiasis
    Taenia B68.9
        diminuta B71.0
        echinococcus —*see* Echinococcus
        mediocanellata B68.1
        nana B71.0
        saginata B68.1
        solium (intestinal form) B68.0
            larval form —*see* Cysticercosis
    Taeniarhynchus saginatus B68.1
    tapeworm B71.9
        beef B68.1
        broad B70.0
            larval B70.1
        dog B67.4
        dwarf B71.0
        fish B70.0
            larval B70.1
        pork B68.0
        rat B71.0
    Ternidens diminutus B81.8
    Tetranychus molestissimus B88.0
    threadworm B80
    tongue B37.0
    Toxocara (canis) (cati) (felis) B83.0
    trematode(s) NEC —*see* Infestation, fluke
    Trichinella (spiralis) B75
    Trichocephalus B79
    Trichomonas —*see* Trichomoniasis
    Trichostrongylus B81.2
    Trichuris (trichiura) B79
    Trombicula (irritans) B88.0
    Tunga penetrans B88.1
    Uncinaria americana B76.1
    Vandellia cirrhosa B88.8
    whipworm B79
    worms B83.9
        intestinal B82.0
    Wuchereria (bancrofti) B74.0
Infiltrate, infiltration
    amyloid (generalized) (localized) —*see*
        Amyloidosis
    calcareous NEC R89.7
        localized —*see* Degeneration, by site
    calcium salt R89.7
    cardiac
        fatty —*see* Degeneration, myocardial
        glycogenic E74.02 *[I43]*
    corneal —*see* Edema, cornea
    eyelid —*see* Inflammation, eyelid
    glycogen, glycogenic —*see* Disease, glycogen
        storage
    heart, cardiac
        fatty —*see* Degeneration, myocardial
        glycogenic E74.02 *[I43]*
    inflammatory in vitreous H43.89
    kidney N28.89
    leukemic —*see* Leukemia
    liver K76.89
        fatty —*see* Fatty, liver NEC
        glycogen —*see also* Disease, glycogen
            storage E74.03 *[K77]*
    lung R91.8
        eosinophilic J82
    lymphatic —*see also* Leukemia, lymphatic
        C91.9-•
        gland I88.9
    muscle, fatty M62.89
    myocardium, myocardial
        fatty —*see* Degeneration, myocardial
        glycogenic E74.02 *[I43]*

Infiltrate, infiltration *(Continued)*
    on chest x-ray R91.8
    pulmonary R91.8
        with eosinophilia J82
    skin (lymphocytic) L98.6
    thymus (gland) (fatty) E32.8
    urine R39.0
    vesicant agent
        antineoplastic chemotherapy T80.810
        other agent NEC T80.818
    vitreous body H43.89
Infirmity R68.89
    senile R54
Inflammation, inflamed, inflammatory (with
        exudation)
    abducent (nerve) —*see* Strabismus, paralytic,
        sixth nerve
    accessory sinus (chronic) —*see* Sinusitis
    adrenal (gland) E27.8
    alveoli, teeth M27.3
        scorbutic E54
    anal canal, anus K62.89
    antrum (chronic) —*see* Sinusitis, maxillary
    appendix —*see* Appendicitis
    arachnoid —*see* Meningitis
    areola N61.1
        puerperal, postpartum or gestational —*see*
            Infection, nipple
    areolar tissue NOS L08.9
    artery —*see* Arteritis
    auditory meatus (external) —*see* Otitis,
        externa
    Bartholin's gland N75.8
    bile duct (common) (hepatic) or passage —*see*
        Cholangitis
    bladder —*see* Cystitis
    bone —*see* Osteomyelitis
    brain —*see also* Encephalitis
        membrane —*see* Meningitis
    breast N61.0
        puerperal, postpartum, gestational —*see*
            Mastitis, obstetric
    broad ligament —*see* Disease, pelvis,
        inflammatory
    bronchi —*see* Bronchitis
    catarrhal J00
    cecum —*see* Appendicitis
    cerebral —*see also* Encephalitis
        membrane —*see* Meningitis
    cerebrospinal
        meningococcal A39.0
    cervix (uteri) —*see* Cervicitis
    chest J98.8
    chorioretinal H30.9-•
        cyclitis —*see* Cyclitis
        disseminated H30.10-•
            generalized H30.13-•
            peripheral H30.12-•
            posterior pole H30.11-•
        epitheliopathy —*see* Epitheliopathy
        focal H30.00-•
            juxtapapillary H30.01-•
            macular H30.04-•
            paramacular —*see* Inflammation,
                chorioretinal, focal, macular
            peripheral H30.03-•
            posterior pole H30.02-•
        specified type NEC H30.89-•
    choroid —*see* Inflammation, chorioretinal
    chronic, postmastoidectomy cavity —*see*
        Complications, postmastoidectomy,
        inflammation
    colon —*see* Enteritis
    connective tissue (diffuse) NEC —*see*
        Disorder, soft tissue, specified type
        NEC
    cornea —*see* Keratitis
    corpora cavernosa N48.29
    cranial nerve —*see* Disorder, nerve, cranial
    Douglas' cul-de-sac or pouch (chronic)
        N73.0

Inflammation, inflamed, inflammatory
    (Continued)
    due to device, implant or graft —*see also*
        Complications, by site and type,
        infection or inflammation
        arterial graft T82.7
        breast (implant) T85.79
        catheter T85.79
            dialysis (renal) T82.7
                intraperitoneal T85.71
            infusion T82.7
                cranial T85.735
                intrathecal T85.735
                spinal (epidural) (subdural)
                    T85.735
                subarachnoid T85.735
            urinary T83.518
                cystostomy T83.510
                Hopkins T83.518
                ileostomy T83.518
                nephrostomy T83.512
                specified NEC T83.518
                urethral indwelling T83.511
                urostomy T83.518
        electronic (electrode) (pulse generator)
            (stimulator)
            bone T84.7
            cardiac T82.7
            nervous system T85.738
                brain T85.731
                cranial nerve T85.732
                gastric nerve T85.732
                neurostimulator generator T85.734
                peripheral nerve T85.732
                sacral nerve T85.732
                spinal cord T85.733
                vagal nerve T85.732
            urinary T83.590
        fixation, internal (orthopedic) NEC —
            see Complication, fixation device,
            infection
        gastrointestinal (bile duct) (esophagus)
            T85.79
            neurostimulator electrode (lead)
                T85.732
        genital NEC T83.69
        heart NEC T82.7
            valve (prosthesis) T82.6
                graft T82.7
        joint prosthesis —*see* Complication, joint
            prosthesis, infection
        ocular (corneal graft) (orbital implant)
            NEC T85.79
        orthopedic NEC T84.7
        penile (cylinder) (pump) (resevoir)
            T83.61
        specified NEC T85.79
        testicular T83.62
        urinary NEC T83.598
            ileal conduit stent T83.593
            implanted neurostimulation
                T83.590
            implanted sphincter T83.591
            indwelling ureteral stent T83.592
            nephroureteral stent T83.593
            specified stent NEC T83.593
        vascular NEC T82.7
        ventricular intracranial (communicating)
            shunt T85.730
    duodenum K29.80
        with bleeding K29.81
    dura mater —*see* Meningitis
    ear (middle) —*see also* Otitis, media
        external —*see* Otitis, externa
        inner —*see* subcategory H83.0
    epididymis —*see* Epididymitis
    esophagus K20.9
    ethmoidal (sinus) (chronic) —*see* Sinusitis,
        ethmoidal
    eustachian tube (catarrhal) —*see* Salpingitis,
        eustachian

Inflammation, inflamed, inflammatory
(*Continued*)
eyelid H01.9
    abscess —*see* Abscess, eyelid
    blepharitis —*see* Blepharitis
    chalazion —*see* Chalazion
    dermatosis (noninfectious) —*see*
        Dermatosis, eyelid
    hordeolum —*see* Hordeolum
    specified NEC H01.8
fallopian tube —*see* Salpingo-oophoritis
fascia —*see* Myositis
follicular, pharynx J31.2
frontal (sinus) (chronic) —*see* Sinusitis, frontal
gallbladder —*see* Cholecystitis
gastric —*see* Gastritis
gastrointestinal —*see* Enteritis
genital organ (internal) (diffuse)
    female —*see* Disease, pelvis, inflammatory
    male N49.9
        multiple sites N49.8
        specified NEC N49.8
gland (lymph) —*see* Lymphadenitis
glottis —*see* Laryngitis
granular, pharynx J31.2
gum K05.10
    nonplaque induced K05.11
    plaque induced K05.10
heart —*see* Carditis
hepatic duct —*see* Cholangitis
ileoanal (internal) pouch K91.850
ileum —*see also* Enteritis
    regional or terminal —*see* Enteritis, regional
intestinal pouch K91.850
intestine (any part) —*see* Enteritis
jaw (acute) (bone) (chronic) (lower)
    (suppurative) (upper) M27.2
joint NEC —*see* Arthritis
    sacroiliac M46.1
kidney —*see* Nephritis
knee (joint) M13.169
    tuberculous A18.02
labium (majus) (minus) —*see* Vulvitis
lacrimal
    gland —*see* Dacryoadenitis
    passages (duct) (sac) —*see also*
        Dacryocystitis
        canaliculitis —*see* Canaliculitis, lacrimal
larynx —*see* Laryngitis
leg NOS L08.9
lip K13.0
liver (capsule) —*see also* Hepatitis
    chronic K73.9
    suppurative K75.0
lung (acute) —*see also* Pneumonia
    chronic J98.4
lymphatic vessel —*see* Lymphangitis
lymph gland or node —*see* Lymphadenitis
maxilla, maxillary M27.2
    sinus (chronic) —*see* Sinusitis, maxillary
membranes of brain or spinal cord —*see*
    Meningitis
meninges —*see* Meningitis
mouth K12.1
muscle —*see* Myositis
myocardium —*see* Myocarditis
nasal sinus (chronic) —*see* Sinusitis
nasopharynx —*see* Nasopharyngitis
navel L08.82
nerve NEC —*see* Neuralgia
nipple N61.0
    puerperal, postpartum or gestational —*see*
        Infection, nipple
nose —*see* Rhinitis
oculomotor (nerve) —*see* Strabismus,
    paralytic, third nerve
optic nerve —*see* Neuritis, optic
orbit (chronic) H05.10
    acute H05.00
        abscess —*see* Abscess, orbit
        cellulitis —*see* Cellulitis, orbit

Inflammation, inflamed, inflammatory
(*Continued*)
orbit (chronic) (*Continued*)
    acute (*Continued*)
        osteomyelitis —*see* Osteomyelitis,
            orbit
        periostitis —*see* Periostitis, orbital
        tenonitis —*see* Tenonitis, eye
    granuloma —*see* Granuloma, orbit
    myositis —*see* Myositis, orbital
ovary —*see* Salpingo-oophoritis
oviduct —*see* Salpingo-oophoritis
pancreas (acute) —*see* Pancreatitis
parametrium N73.0
parotid region L08.9
pelvis, female —*see* Disease, pelvis,
    inflammatory
penis (corpora cavernosa) N48.29
perianal K62.89
pericardium —*see* Pericarditis
perineum (female) (male) L08.9
perirectal K62.89
peritoneum —*see* Peritonitis
periuterine —*see* Disease, pelvis,
    inflammatory
perivesical —*see* Cystitis
petrous bone (acute) (chronic) —*see* Petrositis
pharynx (acute) —*see* Pharyngitis
pia mater —*see* Meningitis
pleura —*see* Pleurisy
polyp, colon —*see also* Polyp, colon,
    inflammatory K51.40
prostate —*see also* Prostatitis
    specified type NEC N41.8
rectosigmoid —*see* Rectosigmoiditis
rectum —*see also* Proctitis K62.89
respiratory, upper —*see also* Infection,
    respiratory, upper J06.9
    acute, due to radiation J70.0
    chronic, due to external agent —*see*
        condition, respiratory, chronic, due to
    due to
        chemicals, gases, fumes or vapors
            (inhalation) J68.2
        radiation J70.1
retina —*see* Chorioretinitis
retrocecal —*see* Appendicitis
retroperitoneal —*see* Peritonitis
salivary duct or gland (any) (suppurative) —
    see Sialoadenitis
scorbutic, alveoli, teeth E54
scrotum N49.2
seminal vesicle —*see* Vesiculitis
sigmoid —*see* Enteritis
sinus —*see* Sinusitis
Skene's duct or gland —*see* Urethritis
skin L08.9
spermatic cord N49.1
sphenoidal (sinus) —*see* Sinusitis, sphenoidal
spinal
    cord —*see* Encephalitis
    membrane —*see* Meningitis
    nerve —*see* Disorder, nerve
spine —*see* Spondylopathy, inflammatory
spleen (capsule) D73.89
stomach —*see* Gastritis
subcutaneous tissue L08.9
suprarenal (gland) E27.8
synovial —*see* Tenosynovitis
tendon (sheath) NEC —*see* Tenosynovitis
testis —*see* Orchitis
throat (acute) —*see* Pharyngitis
thymus (gland) E32.8
thyroid (gland) —*see* Thyroiditis
tongue K14.0
tonsil —*see* Tonsillitis
trachea —*see* Tracheitis
trochlear (nerve) —*see* Strabismus, paralytic,
    fourth nerve
tubal —*see* Salpingo-oophoritis
tuberculous NEC —*see* Tuberculosis

Inflammation, inflamed, inflammatory
(*Continued*)
tubo-ovarian —*see* Salpingo-oophoritis
tunica vaginalis N49.1
tympanic membrane —*see* Tympanitis
umbilicus, umbilical L08.82
uterine ligament —*see* Disease, pelvis,
    inflammatory
uterus (catarrhal) —*see* Endometritis
uveal tract (anterior) NOS —*see also*
    Iridocyclitis
    posterior —*see* Chorioretinitis
vagina —*see* Vaginitis
vas deferens N49.1
vein —*see also* Phlebitis
    intracranial or intraspinal (septic) G08
    thrombotic I80.9
        leg —*see* Phlebitis, leg
        lower extremity —*see* Phlebitis, leg
vocal cord J38.3
vulva —*see* Vulvitis
Wharton's duct (suppurative) —*see*
    Sialoadenitis
Inflation, lung, imperfect (newborn) —*see*
    Atelectasis
Influenza (bronchial) (epidemic) (respiratory
    (upper)) (unidentified influenza virus)
    J11.1
with
    digestive manifestations J11.2
    encephalopathy J11.81
    enteritis J11.2
    gastroenteritis J11.2
    gastrointestinal manifestations J11.2
    laryngitis J11.1
    myocarditis J11.82
    otitis media J11.83
    pharyngitis J11.1
    pneumonia J11.00
        specified type J11.08
    respiratory manifestations NEC J11.1
    specified manifestation NEC J11.89
A/H5N1 —*see also* Influenza, due to,
    identified novel influenza A virus J09.X2
avian —*see also* Influenza, due to, identified
    novel influenza A virus J09.X2
bird —*see also* Influenza, due to, identified
    novel influenza A virus J09.X2
novel (2009) H1N1 influenza —*see also*
    Influenza, due to, identified influenza
    virus NEC J10.1
novel influenza A/H1N1 —*see also* Influenza,
    due to, identified influenza virus NEC
    J10.1
due to
    avian (*see also* Influenza, due to, identified
        novel influenza A virus) J09.X2
    identified influenza virus NEC J10.1
        with
            digestive manifestations J10.2
            encephalopathy J10.81
            enteritis J10.2
            gastroenteritis J10.2
            gastrointestinal manifestations J10.2
            laryngitis J10.1
            myocarditis J10.82
            otitis media J10.83
            pharyngitis J10.1
            pneumonia (unspecified type) J10.00
                with same identified influenza virus
                    J10.01
                specified type NEC J10.08
            respiratory manifestations NEC J10.1
            specified manifestation NEC J10.89
    identified novel influenza A virus J09.X2
        with
            digestive manifestations J09.X3
            encephalopathy J09.X9
            enteritis J09.X3
            gastroenteritis J09.X3
            gastrointestinal manifestations J09.X3

▶ New   ⇒ Revised   ~~deleted~~ Deleted   ● Use Additional Character(s)

Influenza *(Continued)*
 due to *(Continued)*
  identified novel influenza A virus
    (Continued)
   with *(Continued)*
    laryngitis J09.X2
    myocarditis J09.X9
    otitis media J09.X9
    pharyngitis J09.X2
    pneumonia J09.X1
    respiratory manifestations NEC J09.X2
    specified manifestation NEC J09.X9
    upper respiratory symptoms J09.X2
  of other animal origin, not bird or swine *(see
    also* Influenza, due to, identified novel
    influenza A virus) J09.X2
  swine (viruses that normally cause infections
    in pigs) —*see also* Influenza, due to,
    identified novel influenza A virus J09.X2
Influenza-like disease —*see* Influenza
Influenzal —*see* Influenza
Infraction, Freiberg's (metatarsal head) —*see*
  Osteochondrosis, juvenile, metatarsus
Infraeruption of tooth (teeth) M26.34
Infusion complication, misadventure, or
  reaction —*see* Complications, infusion
Ingestion
 chemical —*see* Table of Drugs and Chemicals,
  by substance, poisoning
 drug or medicament
  correct substance properly administered —
    see Table of Drugs and Chemicals, by
    drug, adverse effect
  overdose or wrong substance given
    or taken —*see* Table of Drugs and
    Chemicals, by drug, poisoning
 foreign body —*see* Foreign body, alimentary
  tract
 tularemia A21.3
Ingrowing
 hair (beard) L73.1
 nail (finger) (toe) L60.0
Inguinal —*see also* condition
 testicle Q53.9
  ⇒bilateral Q53.212
  ⇒unilateral Q53.112
Inhalant-induced
 anxiety disorder F18.980
 depressive disorder F18.94
 major neurocognitive disorder
  F18.97
 mild neurocognitive disorder
  F18.988
 psychotic disorder F18.959
Inhalation
 anthrax A22.1
 flame T27.3
 food or foreign body —*see* Foreign body, by
  site
 gases, fumes, or vapors NEC T59.9-●
  specified agent —*see* Table of Drugs and
    Chemicals, by substance
 liquid or vomitus —*see* Asphyxia
 meconium (newborn) P24.00
  with
   with respiratory symptoms P24.01
   pneumonia (pneumonitis) P24.01
 mucus —*see* Asphyxia, mucus
 oil or gasoline (causing suffocation) —*see*
  Foreign body, by site
 smoke J70.5
  due to chemicals, gases, fumes and vapors
    J68.9
 steam —*see* Toxicity, vapors
 stomach contents or secretions —*see* Foreign
  body, by site
  due to anesthesia (general) (local) or other
    sedation T88.59
   in labor and delivery O74.0
   in pregnancy O29.01-●
   postpartum, puerperal O89.01

Inhibition, orgasm
 female F52.31
 male F52.32
Inhibitor, systemic lupus erythematosus
  (presence of) D68.62
Iniencephalus, iniencephaly Q00.2
Injection, traumatic jet (air) (industrial) (water)
  (paint or dye) T70.4
Injury —*see also* specified injury type
  T14.90
 abdomen, abdominal S39.91
  blood vessel —*see* Injury, blood vessel,
    abdomen
  cavity —*see* Injury, intra-abdominal
  contusion S30.1
  internal —*see* Injury, intra-abdominal
  intra-abdominal organ —*see* Injury,
    intra-abdominal
  nerve —*see* Injury, nerve, abdomen
  open —*see* Wound, open, abdomen
  specified NEC S39.81
  superficial —*see* Injury, superficial,
    abdomen
 Achilles tendon S86.00-●
  laceration S86.02-●
  specified type NEC S86.09-●
  strain S86.01-●
 acoustic, resulting in deafness —*see* Injury,
  nerve, acoustic
 adrenal (gland) S37.819
  contusion S37.812
  laceration S37.813
  specified type NEC S37.818
 alveolar (process) S09.93
 ankle S99.91-●
  contusion —*see* Contusion, ankle
  dislocation —*see* Dislocation, ankle
  fracture —*see* Fracture, ankle
  nerve —*see* Injury, nerve, ankle
  open —*see* Wound, open, ankle
  specified type NEC S99.81-●
  sprain —*see* Sprain, ankle
  superficial —*see* Injury, superficial,
    ankle
 anterior chamber, eye —*see* Injury, eye,
  specified site NEC
 anus —*see* Injury, abdomen
 aorta (thoracic) S25.00
  abdominal S35.00
   laceration (minor) (superficial) S35.01
    major S35.02
   specified type NEC S35.09
  laceration (minor) (superficial) S25.01
   major S25.02
  specified type NEC S25.09
 arm (upper) S49.9-●
  blood vessel —*see* Injury, blood vessel, arm
  contusion —*see* Contusion, arm, upper
  fracture —*see* Fracture, humerus
  lower —*see* Injury, forearm
  muscle —*see* Injury, muscle, shoulder
  nerve —*see* Injury, nerve, arm
  open —*see* Wound, open, arm
  specified type NEC S49.8-●
  superficial —*see* Injury, superficial, arm
 artery (complicating trauma) —*see also* Injury,
  blood vessel, by site
  cerebral or meningeal —*see* Injury,
    intracranial
 auditory canal (external) (meatus) S09.91
 auricle, auris, ear S09.91
 axilla —*see* Injury, shoulder
 back —*see* Injury, back, lower
 bile duct S36.13
 birth —*see also* Birth, injury P15.9
 bladder (sphincter) S37.20
  at delivery O71.5
  contusion S37.22
  laceration S37.23
  obstetrical trauma O71.5
  specified type NEC S37.29

Injury *(Continued)*
 blast (air) (hydraulic) (immersion)
   (underwater) NEC T14.8
  acoustic nerve trauma —*see* Injury, nerve,
    acoustic
  bladder —*see* Injury, bladder
  brain —*see* Concussion
  colon —*see* Injury, intestine, large, blast
    injury
  ear (primary) S09.31-●
   secondary S09.39-●
  generalized T70.8
  lung —*see* Injury, intrathoracic, lung, blast
    injury
  multiple body organs T70.8
  peritoneum S36.81
  rectum S36.61
  retroperitoneum S36.898
  small intestine S36.419
   duodenum S36.410
   specified site NEC S36.418
  specified
   intra-abdominal organ NEC S36.898
   pelvic organ NEC S37.899
 blood vessel NEC T14.8
  abdomen S35.9-●
   aorta —*see* Injury, aorta, abdominal
   celiac artery —*see* Injury, blood vessel,
     celiac artery
   iliac vessel —*see* Injury, blood vessel,
     iliac
   laceration S35.91
   mesenteric vessel —*see* Injury,
     mesenteric
   portal vein —*see* Injury, blood vessel,
     portal vein
   renal vessel —*see* Injury, blood vessel,
     renal
   specified vessel NEC S35.8X-●
   splenic vessel —*see* Injury, blood vessel,
     splenic
   vena cava —*see* Injury, vena cava,
     inferior
  ankle —*see* Injury, blood vessel, foot
  aorta (abdominal) (thoracic) —*see* Injury,
    aorta
  arm (upper) NEC S45.90-●
   forearm —*see* Injury, blood vessel,
     forearm
   laceration S45.91-●
   specified
    site NEC S45.80-●
     laceration S45.81-●
     specified type NEC S45.89-●
    type NEC S45.99-●
   superficial vein S45.30-●
    laceration S45.31-●
    specified type NEC S45.39-●
  axillary
   artery S45.00-●
    laceration S45.01-●
    specified type NEC S45.09-●
   vein S45.20-●
    laceration S45.21-●
    specified type NEC S45.29-●
  azygos vein —*see* Injury, blood vessel,
    thoracic, specified site NEC
  brachial
   artery S45.10-●
    laceration S45.11-●
    specified type NEC S45.19-●
   vein S45.20-●
    laceration S45.219
    specified type NEC S45.29-●
  carotid artery (common) (external)
    (internal, extracranial) S15.00-●
   internal, intracranial S06.8-●
   laceration (minor) (superficial)
     S15.01-●
    major S15.02-●
   specified type NEC S15.09-●

Injury *(Continued)*
  blood vessel NEC *(Continued)*
    celiac artery S35.219
      branch S35.299
        laceration (minor) (superficial) S35.291
          major S35.292
          specified NEC S35.298
      laceration (minor) (superficial) S35.211
        major S35.212
        specified type NEC S35.218
    cerebral —*see* Injury, intracranial
    deep plantar —*see* Injury, blood vessel, plantar artery
    digital (hand) —*see* Injury, blood vessel, finger
    dorsal
      artery (foot) S95.00-●
        laceration S95.01-●
        specified type NEC S95.09-●
      vein (foot) S95.20-●
        laceration S95.21-●
        specified type NEC S95.29-●
    due to accidental laceration during procedure —*see* Laceration, accidental complicating surgery
    extremity —*see* Injury, blood vessel, limb
    femoral
      artery (common) (superficial) S75.00-●
        laceration (minor) (superficial) S75.01-●
          major S75.02-●
          specified type NEC S75.09-●
      vein (hip level) (thigh level) S75.10-●
        laceration (minor) (superficial) S75.11-●
          major S75.12-●
          specified type NEC S75.19-●
    finger S65.50-●
      index S65.50-●
        laceration S65.51-●
        specified type NEC S65.59-●
      laceration S65.51-●
      little S65.50-●
        laceration S65.51-●
        specified type NEC S65.59-●
      middle S65.50-●
        laceration S65.51-●
        specified type NEC S65.59-●
      specified type NEC S65.59-●
    thumb —*see* Injury, blood vessel, thumb
    foot S95.90-●
      dorsal
        artery —*see* Injury, blood vessel, dorsal, artery
        vein —*see* Injury, blood vessel, dorsal, vein
      laceration S95.91-●
      plantar artery —*see* Injury, blood vessel, plantar artery
      specified
        site NEC S95.80-●
          laceration S95.81-●
          specified type NEC S95.89-●
        specified type NEC S95.99-●
    forearm S55.90-●
      laceration S55.91-●
      radial artery —*see* Injury, blood vessel, radial artery
      specified
        site NEC S55.80-●
          laceration S55.81-●
          specified type NEC S55.89-●
        type NEC S55.99-●
      ulnar artery —*see* Injury, blood vessel, ulnar artery
      vein S55.20-●
        laceration S55.21-●
        specified type NEC S55.29-●
    gastric
      artery —*see* Injury, mesenteric, artery, branch
      vein —*see* Injury, blood vessel, abdomen

  blood vessel NEC *(Continued)*
    gastroduodenal artery —*see* Injury, mesenteric, artery, branch
    greater saphenous vein (lower leg level) S85.30-●
      hip (and thigh) level S75.20-●
        laceration (minor) (superficial) S75.21-●
          major S75.22-●
          specified type NEC S75.29-●
      laceration S85.31-●
      specified type NEC S85.39-●
    hand (level) S65.90-●
      finger —*see* Injury, blood vessel, finger
      laceration S65.91-●
      palmar arch —*see* Injury, blood vessel, palmar arch
      radial artery —*see* Injury, blood vessel, radial artery, hand
      specified
        site NEC S65.80-●
          laceration S65.81-●
          specified type NEC S65.89-●
        type NEC S65.99-●
      thumb —*see* Injury, blood vessel, thumb
      ulnar artery —*see* Injury, blood vessel, ulnar artery, hand
    head S09.0
      intracranial —*see* Injury, intracranial
      multiple S09.0
    hepatic
      artery —*see* Injury, mesenteric, artery
      vein —*see* Injury, vena cava, inferior
    hip S75.90-●
      femoral artery —*see* Injury, blood vessel, femoral, artery
      femoral vein —*see* Injury, blood vessel, femoral, vein
      greater saphenous vein —*see* Injury, blood vessel, greater saphenous, hip level
      laceration S75.91-●
      specified
        site NEC S75.80-●
          laceration S75.81-●
          specified type NEC S75.89-●
        type NEC S75.99-●
    hypogastric (artery) (vein) —*see* Injury, blood vessel, iliac
    iliac S35.5-●
      artery S35.51-●
      specified vessel NEC S35.5-●
      uterine vessel —*see* Injury, blood vessel, uterine
      vein S35.51-●
    innominate —*see* Injury, blood vessel, thoracic, innominate
    intercostal (artery) (vein) —*see* Injury, blood vessel, thoracic, intercostal
    jugular vein (external) S15.20-●
      internal S15.30-●
        laceration (minor) (superficial) S15.31-●
          major S15.32-●
          specified type NEC S15.39-●
      laceration (minor) (superficial) S15.21-●
        major S15.22-●
        specified type NEC S15.29-●
    leg (level) (lower) S85.90-●
      greater saphenous —*see* Injury, blood vessel, greater saphenous
      laceration S85.91-●
      lesser saphenous —*see* Injury, blood vessel, lesser saphenous
      peroneal artery —*see* Injury, blood vessel, peroneal artery
      popliteal
        artery —*see* Injury, blood vessel, popliteal, artery
        vein —*see* Injury, blood vessel, popliteal, vein

  blood vessel NEC *(Continued)*
    leg (level) (lower) *(Continued)*
      specified
        site NEC S85.80-●
          laceration S85.81-●
          specified type NEC S85.89-●
        type NEC S85.99-●
      thigh —*see* Injury, blood vessel, hip
      tibial artery —*see* Injury, blood vessel, tibial artery
      lesser saphenous vein (lower leg level) S85.40-●
        laceration S85.41-●
        specified type NEC S85.49-●
    limb
      lower —*see* Injury, blood vessel, leg
      upper —*see* Injury, blood vessel, arm
    lower back —*see* Injury, blood vessel, abdomen
    specified NEC —*see* Injury, blood vessel, abdomen, specified, site NEC
    mammary (artery) (vein) —*see* Injury, blood vessel, thoracic, specified site NEC
    mesenteric (inferior) (superior)
      artery —*see* Injury, mesenteric, artery
      vein —*see* Injury, mesenteric, vein
    neck S15.9
      specified site NEC S15.8
    ovarian (artery) (vein) —*see* subcategory S35.8
    palmar arch (superficial) S65.20-●
      deep S65.30-●
        laceration S65.31-●
        specified type NEC S65.39-●
      laceration S65.21-●
      specified type NEC S65.29-●
    pelvis —*see* Injury, blood vessel, abdomen
      specified NEC —*see* Injury, blood vessel, abdomen, specified, site NEC
    peroneal artery S85.20-●
      laceration S85.21-●
      specified type NEC S85.29-●
    plantar artery (deep) (foot) S95.10-●
      laceration S95.11-●
      specified type NEC S95.19-●
    popliteal
      artery S85.00-●
        laceration S85.01-●
        specified type NEC S85.09-●
      vein S85.50-●
        laceration S85.51-●
        specified type NEC S85.59-●
    portal vein S35.319
      laceration S35.311
      specified type NEC S35.318
    precerebral —*see* Injury, blood vessel, neck
    pulmonary (artery) (vein) —*see* Injury, blood vessel, thoracic, pulmonary
    radial artery (forearm level) S55.10-●
      hand and wrist (level) S65.10-●
        laceration S65.11-●
        specified type NEC S65.19-●
      laceration S55.11-●
      specified type NEC S55.19-●
    renal
      artery S35.40-●
        laceration S35.41-●
        specified NEC S35.49-●
      vein S35.40-●
        laceration S35.41-●
        specified NEC S35.49-●
    saphenous vein (greater) (lower leg level) —*see* Injury, blood vessel, greater saphenous
      hip and thigh level —*see* Injury, blood vessel, greater saphenous, hip level
      lesser —*see* Injury, blood vessel, lesser saphenous

▶ New ➡ Revised ~~deleted~~ Deleted ● Use Additional Character(s)

Injury *(Continued)*
  blood vessel NEC *(Continued)*
    shoulder
      specified NEC —*see* Injury, blood vessel, arm, specified site NEC
      superficial vein —*see* Injury, blood vessel, arm, superficial vein
    specified NEC T14.8
    splenic
      artery —*see* Injury, blood vessel, celiac artery, branch
      vein S35.329
        laceration S35.321
        specified NEC S35.328
    subclavian —*see* Injury, blood vessel, thoracic, innominate
    thigh —*see* Injury, blood vessel, hip
    thoracic S25.90
      aorta S25.00
        laceration (minor) (superficial) S25.01
          major S25.02
        specified type NEC S25.09
      azygos vein —*see* Injury, blood vessel, thoracic, specified, site NEC
      innominate
        artery S25.10-●
          laceration (minor) (superficial) S25.11-●
            major S25.12-●
          specified type NEC S25.19-●
        vein S25.30-●
          laceration (minor) (superficial) S25.31-●
            major S25.32-●
          specified type NEC S25.39-●
      intercostal S25.50-●
        laceration S25.51-●
        specified type NEC S25.59-●
      laceration S25.91
      mammary vessel —*see* Injury, blood vessel, thoracic, specified, site NEC
      pulmonary S25.40-●
        laceration (minor) (superficial) S25.41-●
          major S25.42-●
        specified type NEC S25.49-●
      specified
        site NEC S25.80-●
          laceration S25.81-●
          specified type NEC S25.89-●
        type NEC S25.99
      subclavian —*see* Injury, blood vessel, thoracic, innominate
      vena cava (superior) S25.20
        laceration (minor) (superficial) S25.21
          major S25.22
        specified type NEC S25.29
    thumb S65.40-●
      laceration S65.41-●
      specified type NEC S65.49-●
    tibial artery S85.10-●
      anterior S85.13-●
        laceration S85.14-●
        specified injury NEC S85.15-●
      laceration S85.11-●
      posterior S85.16-●
        laceration S85.17-●
        specified injury NEC S85.18-●
      specified injury NEC S85.12-●
    ulnar artery (forearm level) S55.00-●
      hand and wrist (level) S65.00-●
        laceration S65.01-●
        specified type NEC S65.09-●
      laceration S55.01-●
      specified type NEC S55.09-●
    upper arm (level) —*see* Injury, blood vessel, arm
      superficial vein —*see* Injury, blood vessel, arm, superficial vein
    uterine S35.5-●
      artery S35.53-●
      vein S35.53-●

Injury *(Continued)*
  blood vessel NEC *(Continued)*
    vena cava —*see* Injury, vena cava
    vertebral artery S15.10-●
      laceration (minor) (superficial) S15.11-●
        major S15.12-●
      specified type NEC S15.19-●
    wrist (level) —*see* Injury, blood vessel, hand
  brachial plexus S14.3
    newborn P14.3
  brain (traumatic) S06.9-●
    diffuse (axonal) S06.2X-●
    focal S06.30-●
  brainstem S06.38-●
  breast NOS S29.9
  broad ligament —*see* Injury, pelvic organ, specified site NEC
  bronchus, bronchi —*see* Injury, intrathoracic, bronchus
  brow S09.90
  buttock S39.92
  canthus, eye S05.90
  cardiac plexus —*see* Injury, nerve, thorax, sympathetic
  cauda equina S34.3
  cavernous sinus —*see* Injury, intracranial
  cecum —*see* Injury, colon
  celiac ganglion or plexus —*see* Injury, nerve, lumbosacral, sympathetic
  cerebellum —*see* Injury, intracranial
  cerebral —*see* Injury, intracranial
  cervix (uteri) —*see* Injury, uterus
  cheek (wall) S09.93
  chest —*see* Injury, thorax
  childbirth (newborn) —*see also* Birth, injury
    maternal NEC O71.9
  chin S09.93
  choroid (eye) —*see* Injury, eye, specified site NEC
  clitoris S39.94
  coccyx —*see also* Injury, back, lower
    complicating delivery O71.6
  colon —*see* Injury, intestine, large
  common bile duct —*see* Injury, liver
  conjunctiva (superficial) —*see* Injury, eye, conjunctiva
  conus medullaris —*see* Injury, spinal, sacral cord
    spermatic (pelvic region) S37.898
      scrotal region S39.848
    spinal —*see* Injury, spinal cord, by region
  cornea —*see* Injury, eye, specified site NEC
    abrasion —*see* Injury, eye, cornea, abrasion
  cortex (cerebral) —*see also* Injury, intracranial
    visual —*see* Injury, nerve, optic
  costal region NEC S29.9
  costochondral NEC S29.9
  cranial
    cavity —*see* Injury, intracranial
    nerve —*see* Injury, nerve, cranial
  crushing —*see* Crush
  cutaneous sensory nerve
  cystic duct —*see* Injury, liver
  deep tissue —*see* Contusion, by site
    meaning pressure ulcer —*see* Ulcer, pressure, unstageable, by site
  delivery (newborn) P15.9
    maternal NEC O71.9
  Descemet's membrane —*see* Injury, eyeball, penetrating
  diaphragm —*see* Injury, intrathoracic, diaphragm
  duodenum —*see* Injury, intestine, small, duodenum
  ear (auricle) (external) (canal) S09.91
    abrasion —*see* Abrasion, ear
    bite —*see* Bite, ear
    blister —*see* Blister, ear
    bruise —*see* Contusion, ear

Injury *(Continued)*
  ear *(Continued)*
    contusion —*see* Contusion, ear
    external constriction —*see* Constriction, external, ear
    hematoma —*see* Hematoma, ear
    inner —*see* Injury, ear, middle
    laceration —*see* Laceration, ear
    middle S09.30-●
      blast —*see* Injury, blast, ear
      specified NEC S09.39-●
    puncture —*see* Puncture, ear
    superficial —*see* Injury, superficial, ear
  eighth cranial nerve (acoustic or auditory) — *see* Injury, nerve, acoustic
  elbow S59.90-●
    contusion —*see* Contusion, elbow
    dislocation —*see* Dislocation, elbow
    fracture —*see* Fracture, ulna, upper end
    open —*see* Wound, open, elbow
    specified NEC S59.80-●
    sprain —*see* Sprain, elbow
    superficial —*see* Injury, superficial, elbow
  eleventh cranial nerve (accessory) —*see* Injury, nerve, accessory
  epididymis S39.94
  epigastric region S39.91
  epiglottis NEC S19.89
  esophageal plexus —*see* Injury, nerve, thorax, sympathetic
  esophagus (thoracic part) —*see also* Injury, intrathoracic, esophagus
    cervical NEC S19.85
  eustachian tube S09.30-●
  eye S05.9-●
    avulsion S05.7-●
    ball —*see* Injury, eyeball
    conjunctiva S05.0-●
    cornea
      abrasion S05.0-●
      laceration S05.3-●
        with prolapse S05.2-●
    lacrimal apparatus S05.8X-●
    orbit penetration S05.4-●
    specified site NEC S05.8X-●
  eyeball S05.8X-●
    contusion S05.1-●
    penetrating S05.6-●
      with
        foreign body S05.5-●
        prolapse or loss of intraocular tissue S05.2-●
        without prolapse or loss of intraocular tissue S05.3-●
    specified type NEC S05.8-●
  eyebrow S09.93
  eyelid S09.93
    abrasion —*see* Abrasion, eyelid
    contusion —*see* Contusion, eyelid
    open —*see* Wound, open, eyelid
  face S09.93
  fallopian tube S37.509
    bilateral S37.502
      blast injury S37.512
      contusion S37.522
      laceration S37.532
      specified type NEC S37.592
    blast injury (primary) S37.519
      bilateral S37.512
      secondary —*see* Injury, fallopian tube, specified type NEC
      unilateral S37.511
    contusion S37.529
      bilateral S37.522
      unilateral S37.521
    laceration S37.539
      bilateral S37.532
      unilateral S37.531
    specified type NEC S37.599
      bilateral S37.592
      unilateral S37.591

Injury *(Continued)*
  fallopian tube *(Continued)*
    unilateral S37.501
      blast injury S37.511
      contusion S37.521
      laceration S37.531
      specified type NEC S37.591
  fascia —*see* Injury, muscle
  fifth cranial nerve (trigeminal) —*see* Injury,
      nerve, trigeminal
  finger (nail) S69.9-●
    blood vessel —*see* Injury, blood vessel,
        finger
    contusion —*see* Contusion, finger
    dislocation —*see* Dislocation, finger
    fracture —*see* Fracture, finger
    muscle —*see* Injury, muscle, finger
    nerve —*see* Injury, nerve, digital, finger
    open —*see* Wound, open, finger
    specified NEC S69.8-●
    sprain —*see* Sprain, finger
    superficial —*see* Injury, superficial, finger
  first cranial nerve (olfactory) —*see* Injury,
      nerve, olfactory
  flank —*see* Injury, abdomen
  foot S99.92-●
    blood vessel —*see* Injury, blood vessel, foot
    contusion —*see* Contusion, foot
    dislocation —*see* Dislocation, foot
    fracture —*see* Fracture, foot
    muscle —*see* Injury, muscle, foot
    open —*see* Wound, open, foot
    specified type NEC S99.82-●
    sprain —*see* Sprain, foot
    superficial —*see* Injury, superficial, foot
  forceps NOS P15.9
  forearm S59.91-●
    blood vessel —*see* Injury, blood vessel,
        forearm
    contusion —*see* Contusion, forearm
    fracture —*see* Fracture, forearm
    muscle —*see* Injury, muscle, forearm
    nerve —*see* Injury, nerve, forearm
    open —*see* Wound, open, forearm
    specified NEC S59.81-●
    superficial —*see* Injury, superficial,
        forearm
  forehead S09.90
  fourth cranial nerve (trochlear) —*see* Injury,
      nerve, trochlear
  gallbladder S36.129
    contusion S36.122
    laceration S36.123
    specified NEC S36.128
  ganglion
    celiac, coeliac —*see* Injury, nerve,
        lumbosacral, sympathetic
    gasserian —*see* Injury, nerve, trigeminal
    stellate —*see* Injury, nerve, thorax,
        sympathetic
    thoracic sympathetic —*see* Injury, nerve,
        thorax, sympathetic
  gasserian ganglion —*see* Injury, nerve,
      trigeminal
  gastric artery —*see* Injury, blood vessel, celiac
      artery, branch
  gastroduodenal artery —*see* Injury, blood
      vessel, celiac artery, branch
  gastrointestinal tract —*see* Injury,
      intra-abdominal
    with open wound into abdominal cavity —
        see Wound, open, with penetration
        into peritoneal cavity
    colon —*see* Injury, intestine, large
    rectum —*see* Injury, intestine, large, rectum
      with open wound into abdominal cavity
          S36.61
    small intestine —*see* Injury, intestine, small
    specified site NEC —*see* Injury, intra-
        abdominal, specified, site NEC
    stomach —*see* Injury, stomach

Injury *(Continued)*
  genital organ(s)
    external S39.94
      specified NEC S39.848
    internal S37.90
      fallopian tube —*see* Injury, fallopian tube
      ovary —*see* Injury, ovary
      prostate —*see* Injury, prostate
      seminal vesicle —*see* Injury, pelvis,
          organ, specified site NEC
      uterus —*see* Injury, uterus
      vas deferens —*see* Injury, pelvis, organ,
          specified site NEC
    obstetrical trauma O71.9
  gland
    lacrimal laceration —*see* Injury, eye,
        specified site NEC
    salivary S09.93
    thyroid NEC S19.84
  globe (eye) S05.90
    specified NEC S05.8X-●
  groin —*see* Injury, abdomen
  gum S09.90
  hand S69.9-●
    blood vessel —*see* Injury, blood vessel,
        hand
    contusion —*see* Contusion, hand
    fracture —*see* Fracture, hand
    muscle —*see* Injury, muscle, hand
    nerve —*see* Injury, nerve, hand
    open —*see* Wound, open, hand
    specified NEC S69.8-●
    sprain —*see* Sprain, hand
    superficial —*see* Injury, superficial, hand
  head S09.90
    with loss of consciousness S06.9-●
    specified NEC S09.8-●
  heart S26.90
    with hemopericardium S26.00
      contusion S26.01
      laceration (mild) S26.020
        major S26.022
        moderate S26.021
      specified type NEC S26.09
    without hemopericardium S26.10
      contusion S26.11
      laceration S26.12
      specified type NEC S26.19
    contusion S26.91
    laceration S26.92
    specified type NEC S26.99
  heel —*see* Injury, foot
  hepatic
    artery —*see* Injury, blood vessel, celiac
        artery, branch
    duct —*see* Injury, liver
    vein —*see* Injury, vena cava, inferior
  hip S79.91-●
    blood vessel —*see* Injury, blood vessel,
        hip
    contusion —*see* Contusion, hip
    dislocation —*see* Dislocation, hip
    fracture —*see* Fracture, femur, neck
    muscle —*see* Injury, muscle, hip
    nerve —*see* Injury, nerve, hip
    open —*see* Wound, open, hip
    specified NEC S79.81-●
    sprain —*see* Sprain, hip
    superficial —*see* Injury, superficial, hip
  hymen S39.94
  hypogastric
    blood vessel —*see* Injury, blood vessel, iliac
    plexus —*see* Injury, nerve, lumbosacral,
        sympathetic
  ileum —*see* Injury, intestine, small
  iliac region S39.91
  instrumental (during surgery) —*see*
      Laceration, accidental complicating
      surgery
    birth injury —*see* Birth, injury
    nonsurgical —*see* Injury, by site

Injury *(Continued)*
  instrumental *(Continued)*
    obstetrical O71.9
      bladder O71.5
      cervix O71.3
      high vaginal O71.4
      perineal NOS O70.9
      urethra O71.5
      uterus O71.5
        with rupture or perforation O71.1
  internal T14.8
    aorta —*see* Injury, aorta
    bladder (sphincter) —*see* Injury, bladder
      with
        ectopic or molar pregnancy O08.6
        following ectopic or molar pregnancy
            O08.6
      obstetrical trauma O71.5
    bronchus, bronchi —*see* Injury,
        intrathoracic, bronchus
    cecum —*see* Injury, intestine, large
    cervix (uteri) —*see also* Injury, uterus
      with ectopic or molar pregnancy O08.6
      following ectopic or molar pregnancy
          O08.6
      obstetrical trauma O71.3
    chest —*see* Injury, intrathoracic
    gastrointestinal tract —*see* Injury,
        intra-abdominal
    heart —*see* Injury, heart
    intestine NEC —*see* Injury, intestine
    intrauterine —*see* Injury, uterus
    mesentery —*see* Injury, intra-abdominal,
        specified, site NEC
    pelvis, pelvic (organ) S37.90
      following ectopic or molar pregnancy
          (subsequent episode) O08.6
      obstetrical trauma NEC O71.5
        rupture or perforation O71.1
      specified NEC S39.83
    rectum —*see* Injury, intestine, large,
        rectum
    stomach —*see* Injury, stomach
    ureter —*see* Injury, ureter
    urethra (sphincter) following ectopic or
        molar pregnancy O08.6
    uterus —*see* Injury, uterus
  interscapular area —*see* Injury, thorax
  intestine
    large S36.509
      ascending (right) S36.500
        blast injury (primary) S36.510
          secondary S36.590
        contusion S36.520
        laceration S36.530
        specified type NEC S36.590
      blast injury (primary) S36.519
        ascending (right) S36.510
        descending (left) S36.512
        rectum S36.61
        sigmoid S36.513
        specified site NEC S36.518
        transverse S36.511
      contusion S36.529
        ascending (right) S36.520
        descending (left) S36.522
        rectum S36.62
        sigmoid S36.523
        specified site NEC S36.528
        transverse S36.521
      descending (left) S36.502
        blast injury (primary) S36.512
          secondary S36.592
        contusion S36.522
        laceration S36.532
        specified type NEC S36.592
      laceration S36.539
        ascending (right) S36.530
        descending (left) S36.532
        rectum S36.63
        sigmoid S36.533

▶ New ⇒ Revised ~~deleted~~ Deleted ● Use Additional Character(s)

Injury *(Continued)*
  intestine *(Continued)*
    large *(Continued)*
      laceration *(Continued)*
        specified site NEC S36.538
        transverse S36.531
      rectum S36.60
        blast injury (primary) S36.61
          secondary S36.69
        contusion S36.62
        laceration S36.63
        specified type NEC S36.69
      sigmoid S36.503
        blast injury (primary) S36.513
          secondary S36.593
        contusion S36.523
        laceration S36.533
        specified type NEC S36.593
      specified
        site NEC S36.508
          blast injury (primary) S36.518
            secondary S36.598
          contusion S36.528
          laceration S36.538
          specified type NEC S36.598
        type NEC S36.599
          ascending (right) S36.590
          descending (left) S36.592
          rectum S36.69
          sigmoid S36.593
          specified site NEC S36.598
          transverse S36.591
      transverse S36.501
        blast injury (primary) S36.511
          secondary S36.591
        contusion S36.521
        laceration S36.531
        specified type NEC S36.591
    small S36.409
      blast injury (primary) S36.419
        duodenum S36.410
        secondary S36.499
          duodenum S36.490
          specified site NEC S36.498
        specified site NEC S36.418
      contusion S36.429
        duodenum S36.420
        specified site NEC S36.428
      duodenum S36.400
        blast injury (primary) S36.410
          secondary S36.490
        contusion S36.420
        laceration S36.430
        specified NEC S36.490
      laceration S36.439
        duodenum S36.430
        specified site NEC S36.438
      specified
        site NEC S36.408
        type NEC S36.499
          duodenum S36.490
          specified site NEC S36.498
  intra-abdominal S36.90
    adrenal gland —*see* Injury, adrenal gland
    bladder —*see* Injury, bladder
    colon —*see* Injury, intestine, large
    contusion S36.92
    fallopian tube —*see* Injury, fallopian tube
    gallbladder —*see* Injury, gallbladder
    intestine —*see* Injury, intestine
    kidney —*see* Injury, kidney
    laceration S36.93
    liver —*see* Injury, liver
    ovary —*see* Injury, ovary
    pancreas —*see* Injury, pancreas
    pelvic NOS S37.90
    peritoneum —*see* Injury, intra-abdominal, specified, site NEC
    prostate —*see* Injury, prostate
    rectum —*see* Injury, intestine, large, rectum

Injury *(Continued)*
  intra-abdominal *(Continued)*
    retroperitoneum —*see* Injury, intra-abdominal, specified, site NEC
    seminal vesicle —*see* Injury, pelvis, organ, specified site NEC
    small intestine —*see* Injury, intestine, small
    specified
      pelvic S37.90
        specified
          site NEC S37.899
            specified type NEC S37.898
          type NEC S37.99
      site NEC S36.899
        contusion S36.892
        laceration S36.893
        specified type NEC S36.898
      type NEC S36.99
    spleen —*see* Injury, spleen
    stomach —*see* Injury, stomach
    ureter —*see* Injury, ureter
    urethra —*see* Injury, urethra
    uterus —*see* Injury, uterus
    vas deferens —*see* Injury, pelvis, organ, specified site NEC
  intracranial (traumatic) S06.9-●
    cerebellar hemorrhage, traumatic —*see* Injury, intracranial, focal
    cerebral edema, traumatic S06.1X-●
      diffuse S06.1X-●
      focal S06.1X-●
    diffuse (axonal) S06.2X-●
    epidural hemorrhage (traumatic) S06.4X-●
    focal brain injury S06.30-●
      contusion —*see* Contusion, cerebral
      laceration —*see* Laceration, cerebral
      intracerebral hemorrhage, traumatic S06.36-●
        left side S06.35-●
        right side S06.34-●
    subarachnoid hemorrhage, traumatic S06.6X-●
    subdural hemorrhage, traumatic S06.5X-●
  intraocular —*see* Injury, eyeball, penetrating
  intrathoracic S27.9
    bronchus S27.409
      bilateral S27.402
      blast injury (primary) S27.419
        bilateral S27.412
        secondary —*see* Injury, intrathoracic, bronchus, specified type NEC
        unilateral S27.411
      contusion S27.429
        bilateral S27.422
        unilateral S27.421
      laceration S27.439
        bilateral S27.432
        unilateral S27.431
      specified type NEC S27.499
        bilateral S27.492
        unilateral S27.491
      unilateral S27.401
    diaphragm S27.809
      contusion S27.802
      laceration S27.803
      specified type NEC S27.808
    esophagus (thoracic) S27.819
      contusion S27.812
      laceration S27.813
      specified type NEC S27.818
    heart —*see* Injury, heart
    hemopneumothorax S27.2
    hemothorax S27.1
    lung S27.309
      aspiration J69.0
      bilateral S27.302
      blast injury (primary) S27.319
        bilateral S27.312
        secondary —*see* Injury, intrathoracic, lung, specified type NEC
        unilateral S27.311

Injury *(Continued)*
  intrathoracic *(Continued)*
    bronchus *(Continued)*
      contusion S27.329
        bilateral S27.322
        unilateral S27.321
      laceration S27.339
        bilateral S27.332
        unilateral S27.331
      specified type NEC S27.399
        bilateral S27.392
        unilateral S27.391
      unilateral S27.301
    pleura S27.60
      laceration S27.63
      specified type NEC S27.69
    pneumothorax S27.0
    specified organ NEC S27.899
      contusion S27.892
      laceration S27.893
      specified type NEC S27.898
    thoracic duct —*see* Injury, intrathoracic, specified organ NEC
    thymus gland —*see* Injury, intrathoracic, specified organ NEC
    trachea, thoracic S27.50
      blast (primary) S27.51
      contusion S27.52
      laceration S27.53
      specified type NEC S27.59
  iris —*see* Injury, eye, specified site NEC
    penetrating —*see* Injury, eyeball, penetrating
  jaw S09.93
  jejunum —*see* Injury, intestine, small
  joint NOS T14.8
    old or residual —*see* Disorder, joint, specified type NEC
  kidney S37.00-●
    acute (nontraumatic) N17.9
    contusion —*see* Contusion, kidney
    laceration —*see* Laceration, kidney
    specified NEC S37.09-●
  knee S89.9-●
    contusion —*see* Contusion, knee
    dislocation —*see* Dislocation, knee
    meniscus (lateral) (medial) —*see* Sprain, knee, specified site NEC
      old injury or tear —*see* Derangement, knee, meniscus, due to old injury
    open —*see* Wound, open, knee
    specified NEC S89.8-●
    sprain —*see* Sprain, knee
    superficial —*see* Injury, superficial, knee
  labium (majus) (minus) S39.94
  labyrinth, ear S09.30-●
  lacrimal apparatus, duct, gland, or sac —*see* Injury, eye, specified site NEC
  larynx NEC S19.81
  leg (lower) S89.9-●
    blood vessel —*see* Injury, blood vessel, leg
    contusion —*see* Contusion, leg
    fracture —*see* Fracture, leg
    muscle —*see* Injury, muscle, leg
    nerve —*see* Injury, nerve, leg
    open —*see* Wound, open, leg
    specified NEC S89.8-●
    superficial —*see* Injury, superficial, leg
  lens, eye —*see* Injury, eye, specified site NEC
    penetrating —*see* Injury, eyeball, penetrating
  limb NEC T14.8
  lip S09.93
  liver S36.119
    contusion S36.112
    laceration S36.113
      major (stellate) S36.116
      minor S36.114
      moderate S36.115
    specified NEC S36.118
  lower back S39.92
    specified NEC S39.82

Injury *(Continued)*
  lumbar, lumbosacral (region) S39.92
    plexus —*see* Injury, lumbosacral plexus
  lumbosacral plexus S34.4
  lung —*see also* Injury, intrathoracic, lung
    aspiration J69.0
    transfusion-related (TRALI) J95.84
  lymphatic thoracic duct —*see* Injury,
    intrathoracic, specified organ NEC
  malar region S09.93
  mastoid region S09.90
  maxilla S09.93
  mediastinum —*see* Injury, intrathoracic,
    specified organ NEC
  membrane, brain —*see* Injury, intracranial
  meningeal artery —*see* Injury, intracranial,
    subdural hemorrhage
  meninges (cerebral) —*see* Injury, intracranial
  mesenteric
    artery
      branch S35.299
        laceration (minor) (superficial) S35.291
          major S35.292
        specified NEC S35.298
      inferior S35.239
        laceration (minor) (superficial) S35.231
          major S35.232
        specified NEC S35.238
      superior S35.229
        laceration (minor) (superficial) S35.221
          major S35.222
        specified NEC S35.228
      plexus (inferior) (superior) —*see* Injury,
        nerve, lumbosacral, sympathetic
    vein
      inferior S35.349
        laceration S35.341
        specified NEC S35.348
      superior S35.339
        laceration S35.331
        specified NEC S35.338
  mesentery —*see* Injury, intra-abdominal,
    specified site NEC
  mesosalpinx —*see* Injury, pelvic organ,
    specified site NEC
  middle ear S09.30-●
  midthoracic region NOS S29.9
  mouth S09.93
  multiple NOS T07
  muscle (and fascia) (and tendon)
    abdomen S39.001
      laceration S39.021
      specified type NEC S39.091
      strain S39.011
    abductor
      thumb, forearm level —*see* Injury,
        muscle, thumb, abductor
    adductor
      thigh S76.20-●
        laceration S76.22-●
        specified type NEC S76.29-●
        strain S76.21-●
    ankle —*see* Injury, muscle, foot
    anterior muscle group, at leg level (lower)
      S86.20-●
      laceration S86.22-●
      specified type NEC S86.29-●
      strain S86.21-●
    arm (upper) —*see* Injury, muscle,
      shoulder
    biceps (parts NEC) S46.20-●
      laceration S46.22-●
      long head S46.10-●
        laceration S46.12-●
        specified type NEC S46.19-●
        strain S46.11-●
      specified type NEC S46.29-●
      strain S46.21-●
    extensor
      finger(s) (other than thumb) —*see* Injury,
        muscle, finger by site, extensor

Injury *(Continued)*
  muscle *(Continued)*
    extensor *(Continued)*
      forearm level, specified NEC —*see*
        Injury, muscle, forearm, extensor
      thumb —*see* Injury, muscle, thumb,
        extensor
      toe (large) (ankle level) (foot level) —*see*
        Injury, muscle, toe, extensor
    finger
      extensor (forearm level) S56.40-●
        hand level S66.309
          laceration S66.329
          specified type NEC S66.399
          strain S66.319
        laceration S56.429
        specified type NEC S56.499
        strain S56.419
      flexor (forearm level) S56.10-●
        hand level S66.109
          laceration S66.129
          specified type NEC S66.199
          strain S66.119
        laceration S56.129
        specified type NEC S56.199
        strain S56.119
      index
        extensor (forearm level)
          hand level S66.308
            laceration S66.32-●
            specified type NEC S66.39-●
            strain S66.31-●
          specified type NEC S56.492-●
        flexor (forearm level)
          hand level S66.108
            laceration S66.12-●
            specified type NEC
              S66.19-●
            strain S66.11-●
          specified type NEC S56.19-●
          strain S56.11-●
        intrinsic S66.50-●
          laceration S66.52-●
          specified type NEC S66.59-●
          strain S66.51-●
      intrinsic S66.509
        laceration S66.529
        specified type NEC S66.599
        strain S66.519
      little
        extensor (forearm level)
          hand level S66.30-●
            laceration S66.32-●
            specified type NEC S66.39-●
            strain S66.31-●
          laceration S56.42-●
          specified type NEC S56.49-●
          strain S56.41-●
        flexor (forearm level)
          hand level S66.10-●
            laceration S66.12-●
            specified type NEC S66.19-●
            strain S66.11-●
          laceration S56.12-●
          specified type NEC S56.19-●
          strain S56.11-●
        intrinsic S66.50-●
          laceration S66.52-●
          specified type NEC S66.59-●
          strain S66.51-●
      middle
        extensor (forearm level)
          hand level S66.30-●
            laceration S66.32-●
            specified type NEC
              S66.39-●
            strain S66.31-●
          laceration S56.42-●
          specified type NEC
            S56.49-●
          strain S56.41-●

Injury *(Continued)*
  muscle *(Continued)*
    finger *(Continued)*
      middle *(Continued)*
        flexor (forearm level)
          hand level S66.10-●
            laceration S66.12-●
            specified type NEC
              S66.19-●
            strain S66.11-●
          laceration S56.12-●
          specified type NEC S56.19-●
          strain S56.11-●
        intrinsic S66.50-●
          laceration S66.52-●
          specified type NEC S66.59-●
          strain S66.51-●
      ring
        extensor (forearm level)
          hand level S66.30-●
            laceration S66.32-●
            specified type NEC S66.39-●
            strain S66.31-●
          laceration S56.42-●
          specified type NEC S56.49-●
          strain S56.41-●
        flexor (forearm level)
          hand level S66.10-●
            laceration S66.12-●
            specified type NEC S66.19-●
            strain S66.11-●
          laceration S56.12-●
          specified type NEC S56.19-●
          strain S56.11-●
        intrinsic S66.50-●
          laceration S66.52-●
          specified type NEC S66.59-●
          strain S66.51-●
    flexor
      finger(s) (other than thumb) — *see* Injury,
        muscle, finger
      forearm level, specified NEC — *see*
        Injury, muscle, forearm, flexor
      thumb —*see* Injury, muscle, thumb,
        flexor
      toe (long) (ankle level) (foot level) —*see*
        Injury, muscle, toe, flexor
    foot S96.90-●
      intrinsic S96.20-●
        laceration S96.22-●
        specified type NEC S96.29-●
        strain S96.21-●
      laceration S96.92-●
      long extensor, toe —*see* Injury, muscle,
        toe, extensor
      long flexor, toe —*see* Injury, muscle, toe,
        flexor
      specified
        site NEC S96.80-●
          laceration S96.82-●
          specified type NEC
            S96.89-●
          strain S96.81-●
        type NEC S96.99-●
      strain S96.91-●
    forearm (level) S56.90-●
      extensor S56.50-●
        laceration S56.52-●
        specified type NEC S56.59-●
        strain S56.51-●
      flexor S56.20-●
        laceration S56.22-●
        specified type NEC S56.29-●
        strain S56.21-●
      laceration S56.92-●
      specified S56.99-●
        site NEC S56.80-●
          laceration S56.82-●
          strain S56.81-●
        type NEC S56.89-●
      strain S56.91-●

Injury *(Continued)*
  muscle *(Continued)*
    hand (level) S66.90-●
      laceration S66.92-●
      specified
        site NEC S66.80-●
          laceration S66.82-●
          specified type NEC S66.89-●
          strain S66.81-●
        type NEC S66.99-●
      strain S66.91-●
    head S09.10
      laceration S09.12
      specified type NEC S09.19
      strain S09.11
    hip NEC S76.00-●
      laceration S76.02-●
      specified type NEC S76.09-●
      strain S76.01-●
    intrinsic
      ankle and foot level —*see* Injury, muscle, foot, intrinsic
      finger (other than thumb) —*see* Injury, muscle, finger by site, intrinsic
      foot (level) —*see* Injury, muscle, foot, intrinsic
      thumb —*see* Injury, muscle, thumb, intrinsic
    leg (level) (lower) S86.90-●
      Achilles tendon —*see* Injury, Achilles tendon
      anterior muscle group —*see* Injury, muscle, anterior muscle group
      laceration S86.92-●
      peroneal muscle group —*see* Injury, muscle, peroneal muscle group
      posterior muscle group —*see* Injury, muscle, posterior muscle group, leg level
      specified
        site NEC S86.80-●
          laceration S86.82-●
          specified type NEC S86.89-●
          strain S86.81-●
        type NEC S86.99-●
      strain S86.91-●
    long
      extensor toe, at ankle and foot level —*see* Injury, muscle, toe, extensor
      flexor, toe, at ankle and foot level —*see* Injury, muscle, toe, flexor
      head, biceps —*see* Injury, muscle, biceps, long head
    lower back S39.002
      laceration S39.022
      specified type NEC S39.092
      strain S39.012
    neck (level) S16.9
      laceration S16.2
      specified type NEC S16.8
      strain S16.1
    pelvis S39.003
      laceration S39.023
      specified type NEC S39.093
      strain S39.013
    peroneal muscle group, at leg level (lower) S86.30-●
      laceration S86.32-●
      specified type NEC S86.39-●
      strain S86.31-●
    posterior muscle (group)
      leg level (lower) S86.10-●
        laceration S86.12-●
        specified type NEC S86.19-●
        strain S86.11-●
      thigh level S76.30-●
        laceration S76.32-●
        specified type NEC S76.39-●
        strain S76.31-●

Injury *(Continued)*
  muscle *(Continued)*
    quadriceps (thigh) S76.10-●
      laceration S76.12-●
      specified type NEC S76.19-●
      strain S76.11-●
    shoulder S46.90-●
      laceration S46.92-●
      rotator cuff —*see* Injury, rotator cuff
      specified site NEC S46.80-●
        laceration S46.82-●
        specified type NEC S46.89-●
        strain S46.81-●
      specified type NEC S46.99-●
      strain S46.91-●
    thigh NEC (level) S76.90-●
      adductor —*see* Injury, muscle, adductor, thigh
      laceration S76.92-●
      posterior muscle (group) —*see* Injury, muscle, posterior muscle, thigh level
      quadriceps —*see* Injury, muscle, quadriceps
      specified
        site NEC S76.80-●
          laceration S76.82-●
          specified type NEC S76.89-●
          strain S76.81-●
        type NEC S76.99-●
      strain S76.91-●
    thorax (level) S29.009
      back wall S29.002
      front wall S29.001
      laceration S29.029
        back wall S29.022
        front wall S29.021
      specified type NEC S29.099
        back wall S29.092
        front wall S29.091
      strain S29.019
        back wall S29.012
        front wall S29.011
    thumb
      abductor (forearm level) S56.30-●
        laceration S56.32-●
        specified type NEC S56.39-●
        strain S56.31-●
      extensor (forearm level) S56.30-●
        hand level S66.20-●
          laceration S66.22-●
          specified type NEC S66.29-●
          strain S66.21-●
        laceration S56.32-●
        specified type NEC S56.39-●
        strain S56.31-●
      flexor (forearm level) S56.00-●
        hand level S66.00-●
          laceration S66.02-●
          specified type NEC S66.09-●
          strain S66.01-●
        laceration S56.02-●
        specified type NEC S56.09-●
        strain S56.01-●
        wrist level —*see* Injury, muscle, thumb, flexor, hand level
      intrinsic S66.40-●
        laceration S66.42-●
        specified type NEC S66.49-●
        strain S66.41-●
    toe —*see also* Injury, muscle, foot
      extensor, long S96.10-●
        laceration S96.12-●
        specified type NEC S96.19-●
        strain S96.11-●
      flexor, long S96.00-●
        laceration S96.02-●
        specified type NEC S96.09-●
        strain S96.01-●

Injury *(Continued)*
  muscle *(Continued)*
    triceps S46.30-●
      laceration S46.32-●
      specified type NEC S46.39-●
      strain S46.31-●
    wrist (and hand) level —*see* Injury, muscle, hand
  musculocutaneous nerve —*see* Injury, nerve, musculocutaneous
  myocardium —*see* Injury, heart
  nape —*see* Injury, neck
  nasal (septum) (sinus) S09.92
  nasopharynx S09.92
  neck S19.9
    specified NEC S19.80
      specified site NEC S19.89
  nerve NEC T14.8
    abdomen S34.9
      peripheral S34.6
      specified site NEC S34.8
    abducens S04.4-●
      contusion S04.4-●
      laceration S04.4-●
      specified type NEC S04.4-●
    abducent —*see* Injury, nerve, abducens
    accessory S04.7-●
      contusion S04.7-●
      laceration S04.7-●
      specified type NEC S04.7-●
    acoustic S04.6-●
      contusion S04.6-●
      laceration S04.6-●
      specified type NEC S04.6-●
    ankle S94.9-●
      cutaneous sensory S94.3-●
      specified site NEC —*see* subcategory S94.8
    anterior crural, femoral —*see* Injury, nerve, femoral
    arm (upper) S44.9-●
      axillary —*see* Injury, nerve, axillary
      cutaneous —*see* Injury, nerve, cutaneous, arm
      median —*see* Injury, nerve, median, upper arm
      musculocutaneous —*see* Injury, nerve, musculocutaneous
      radial —*see* Injury, nerve, radial, upper arm
      specified site NEC —*see* subcategory S44.8
      ulnar —*see* Injury, nerve, ulnar, arm
    auditory —*see* Injury, nerve, acoustic
    axillary S44.3-●
    brachial plexus —*see* Injury, brachial plexus
    cervical sympathetic S14.5
    cranial S04.9
      contusion S04.9
      eighth (acoustic or auditory) —*see* Injury, nerve, acoustic
      eleventh (accessory) —*see* Injury, nerve, accessory
      fifth (trigeminal) —*see* Injury, nerve, trigeminal
      first (olfactory) —*see* Injury, nerve, olfactory
      fourth (trochlear) —*see* Injury, nerve, trochlear
      laceration S04.9
      ninth (glossopharyngeal) —*see* Injury, nerve, glossopharyngeal
      second (optic) —*see* Injury, nerve, optic
      seventh (facial) —*see* Injury, nerve, facial
      sixth (abducent) —*see* Injury, nerve, abducens
      specified
        nerve NEC S04.89-●
          contusion S04.89-●
          laceration S04.89-●
          specified type NEC S04.89-●
        type NEC S04.9

Injury *(Continued)*
  nerve NEC *(Continued)*
    cranial *(Continued)*
      tenth (pneumogastric or vagus) —*see*
        Injury, nerve, vagus
      third (oculomotor) —*see* Injury, nerve,
        oculomotor
      twelfth (hypoglossal) —*see* Injury, nerve,
        hypoglossal
    cutaneous sensory
      ankle (level) S94.3- ●
      arm (upper) (level) S44.5- ●
      foot (level) —*see* Injury, nerve, cutaneous
        sensory, ankle
      forearm (level) S54.3- ●
      hip (level) S74.2- ●
      leg (lower level) S84.2- ●
      shoulder (level) —*see* Injury, nerve,
        cutaneous sensory, arm
      thigh (level) —*see* Injury, nerve,
        cutaneous sensory, hip
    deep peroneal —*see* Injury, nerve, peroneal,
      foot
    digital
      finger S64.4- ●
        index S64.49- ●
        little S64.49- ●
        middle S64.49- ●
        ring S64.49- ●
        thumb S64.3- ●
      toe —*see* Injury, nerve, ankle, specified
        site NEC
    eighth cranial (acoustic or auditory) —*see*
      Injury, nerve, acoustic
    eleventh cranial (accessory) —*see* Injury,
      nerve, accessory
    facial S04.5- ●
      contusion S04.5- ●
      laceration S04.5- ●
      newborn P11.3
      specified type NEC S04.5- ●
    femoral (hip level) (thigh level) S74.1- ●
    fifth cranial (trigeminal) —*see* Injury, nerve,
      trigeminal
    finger (digital) —*see* Injury, nerve, digital,
      finger
    first cranial (olfactory) —*see* Injury, nerve,
      olfactory
    foot S94.9- ●
      cutaneous sensory S94.3- ●
      deep peroneal S94.2- ●
      lateral plantar S94.0- ●
      medial plantar S94.1- ●
      specified site NEC —*see* subcategory
        S94.8
    forearm (level) S54.9- ●
      cutaneous sensory —*see* Injury, nerve,
        cutaneous sensory, forearm
      median —*see* Injury, nerve, median
      radial —*see* Injury, nerve, radial
      specified site NEC —*see* subcategory
        S54.8
      ulnar —*see* Injury, nerve, ulnar
    fourth cranial (trochlear) —*see* Injury,
      nerve, trochlear
    glossopharyngeal S04.89- ●
      specified type NEC S04.89- ●
    hand S64.9- ●
      median —*see* Injury, nerve, median,
        hand
      radial —*see* Injury, nerve, radial, hand
      specified NEC —*see* subcategory
        S64.8
      ulnar —*see* Injury, nerve, ulnar, hand
    hip (level) S74.9- ●
      cutaneous sensory —*see* Injury, nerve,
        cutaneous sensory, hip
      femoral —*see* Injury, nerve, femoral
      sciatic —*see* Injury, nerve, sciatic
      specified site NEC —*see* subcategory
        S74.8

Injury *(Continued)*
  nerve NEC *(Continued)*
    hypoglossal S04.89- ●
      specified type NEC S04.89- ●
    lateral plantar S94.0- ●
    leg (lower) S84.9- ●
      cutaneous sensory —*see* Injury, nerve,
        cutaneous sensory, leg
      peroneal —*see* Injury, nerve, peroneal
      specified site NEC —*see* subcategory
        S84.8
      tibial —*see* Injury, nerve, tibial
      upper —*see* Injury, nerve, thigh
    lower
      back —*see* Injury, nerve, abdomen,
        specified site NEC
        peripheral —*see* Injury, nerve,
          abdomen, peripheral
      limb —*see* Injury, nerve, leg
    lumbar plexus —*see* Injury, nerve,
      lumbosacral, sympathetic
    lumbar spinal —*see* Injury, nerve, spinal,
      lumbar
    lumbosacral
      plexus —*see* Injury, nerve, lumbosacral,
        sympathetic
      sympathetic S34.5
    medial plantar S94.1- ●
    median (forearm level) S54.1- ●
      hand (level) S64.1- ●
      upper arm (level) S44.1- ●
      wrist (level) —*see* Injury, nerve, median,
        hand
    musculocutaneous S44.4- ●
    musculospiral (upper arm level) —*see*
      Injury, nerve, radial, upper arm
    neck S14.9
      peripheral S14.4
      specified site NEC S14.8
      sympathetic S14.5
    ninth cranial (glossopharyngeal) —*see*
      Injury, nerve, glossopharyngeal
    oculomotor S04.1- ●
      contusion S04.1- ●
      laceration S04.1- ●
      specified type NEC S04.1- ●
    olfactory S04.81- ●
      specified type NEC S04.81- ●
    optic S04.01- ●
      contusion S04.01- ●
      laceration S04.01- ●
      specified type NEC S04.01- ●
    pelvic girdle —*see* Injury, nerve, hip
    pelvis —*see* Injury, nerve, abdomen,
      specified site NEC
      peripheral —*see* Injury, nerve, abdomen,
        peripheral
    peripheral NEC T14.8
      abdomen —*see* Injury, nerve, abdomen,
        peripheral
      lower back —*see* Injury, nerve, abdomen,
        peripheral
      neck —*see* Injury, nerve, neck, peripheral
      pelvis —*see* Injury, nerve, abdomen,
        peripheral
      specified NEC T14.8
    peroneal (lower leg level) S84.1- ●
      foot S94.2- ●
    plexus
      brachial —*see* Injury, brachial plexus
      celiac, coeliac —*see* Injury, nerve,
        lumbosacral, sympathetic
      mesenteric, inferior —*see* Injury, nerve,
        lumbosacral, sympathetic
      sacral —*see* Injury, lumbosacral
        plexus
      spinal
        brachial —*see* Injury, brachial
          plexus
        lumbosacral —*see* Injury, lumbosacral
          plexus

Injury *(Continued)*
  nerve NEC *(Continued)*
    pneumogastric —*see* Injury, nerve, vagus
    radial (forearm level) S54.2- ●
      hand (level) S64.2- ●
      upper arm (level) S44.2- ●
      wrist (level) —*see* Injury, nerve, radial,
        hand
    root —*see* Injury, nerve, spinal, root
    sacral plexus —*see* Injury, lumbosacral
      plexus
    sacral spinal —*see* Injury, nerve, spinal,
      sacral
    sciatic (hip level) (thigh level) S74.0- ●
    second cranial (optic) —*see* Injury, nerve,
      optic
    seventh cranial (facial) —*see* Injury, nerve,
      facial
    shoulder —*see* Injury, nerve, arm
    sixth cranial (abducent) —*see* Injury, nerve,
      abducens
    spinal
      plexus —*see* Injury, nerve, plexus, spinal
      root
        cervical S14.2
        dorsal S24.2
        lumbar S34.21
        sacral S34.22
        thoracic —*see* Injury, nerve, spinal,
          root, dorsal
    splanchnic —*see* Injury, nerve, lumbosacral,
      sympathetic
    sympathetic NEC —*see* Injury, nerve,
      lumbosacral, sympathetic
      cervical —*see* Injury, nerve, cervical
        sympathetic
    tenth cranial (pneumogastric or vagus) —
      see Injury, nerve, vagus
    thigh (level) —*see* Injury, nerve, hip
      cutaneous sensory —*see* Injury, nerve,
        cutaneous sensory, hip
      femoral —*see* Injury, nerve, femoral
      sciatic —*see* Injury, nerve, sciatic
      specified NEC —*see* Injury, nerve, hip
    third cranial (oculomotor) —*see* Injury,
      nerve, oculomotor
    thorax S24.9
      peripheral S24.3
      specified site NEC S24.8
      sympathetic S24.4
    thumb, digital —*see* Injury, nerve, digital,
      thumb
    tibial (lower leg level) (posterior) S84.0- ●
    toe —*see* Injury, nerve, ankle
    trigeminal S04.3- ●
      contusion S04.3- ●
      laceration S04.3- ●
      specified type NEC S04.3- ●
    trochlear S04.2- ●
      contusion S04.2- ●
      laceration S04.2- ●
      specified type NEC S04.2- ●
    twelfth cranial (hypoglossal) —*see* Injury,
      nerve, hypoglossal
    ulnar (forearm level) S54.0- ●
      arm (upper) (level) S44.0- ●
      hand (level) S64.0- ●
      wrist (level) —*see* Injury, nerve, ulnar,
        hand
    vagus S04.89- ●
      specified type NEC S04.89- ●
    wrist (level) —*see* Injury, nerve, hand
  ninth cranial nerve (glossopharyngeal) —*see*
    Injury, nerve, glossopharyngeal
  nose (septum) S09.92
  obstetrical O71.9
    specified NEC O71.89
  occipital (region) (scalp) S09.90
    lobe —*see* Injury, intracranial
  optic chiasm S04.02
  optic radiation S04.03- ●

Injury *(Continued)*
optic tract and pathways S04.03-●
orbit, orbital (region) —*see* Injury, eye
  penetrating (with foreign body) —*see*
    Injury, eye, orbit, penetrating
  specified NEC —*see* Injury, eye, specified
    site NEC
ovary, ovarian S37.409
  bilateral S37.402
    contusion S37.422
    laceration S37.432
    specified type NEC S37.492
  blood vessel —*see* Injury, blood vessel,
    ovarian
  contusion S37.429
    bilateral S37.422
    unilateral S37.421
  laceration S37.439
    bilateral S37.432
    unilateral S37.431
  specified type NEC S37.499
    bilateral S37.492
    unilateral S37.491
  unilateral S37.401
    contusion S37.421
    laceration S37.431
    specified type NEC S37.491
palate (hard) (soft) S09.93
pancreas S36.209
  body S36.201
    contusion S36.221
    laceration S36.231
      major S36.261
      minor S36.241
      moderate S36.251
    specified type NEC S36.291
  contusion S36.229
  head S36.200
    contusion S36.220
    laceration S36.230
      major S36.260
      minor S36.240
      moderate S36.250
    specified type NEC S36.290
  laceration S36.239
    major S36.269
    minor S36.249
    moderate S36.259
  specified type NEC S36.299
  tail S36.202
    contusion S36.222
    laceration S36.232
      major S36.262
      minor S36.242
      moderate S36.252
    specified type NEC S36.292
parietal (region) (scalp) S09.90
  lobe —*see* Injury, intracranial
patellar ligament (tendon) S76.10-●
  laceration S76.12-●
  specified NEC S76.19-●
  strain S76.11-●
pelvis, pelvic (floor) S39.93
  complicating delivery O70.1
  joint or ligament, complicating delivery
    O71.6
  organ S37.90
    with ectopic or molar pregnancy O08.6
    complication of abortion —*see* Abortion
    contusion S37.92
    following ectopic or molar pregnancy
      O08.6
    laceration S37.93
    obstetrical trauma NEC O71.5
    specified
      site NEC S37.899
        contusion S37.892
        laceration S37.893
        specified type NEC S37.898
      type NEC S37.99
  specified NEC S39.83

Injury *(Continued)*
penis S39.94
perineum S39.94
peritoneum S36.81
  laceration S36.893
periurethral tissue —*see* Injury, urethra
  complicating delivery O71.82
phalanges
  foot —*see* Injury, foot
  hand —*see* Injury, hand
pharynx NEC S19.85
pleura —*see* Injury, intrathoracic, pleura
plexus
  brachial —*see* Injury, brachial plexus
  cardiac —*see* Injury, nerve, thorax,
    sympathetic
  celiac, coeliac —*see* Injury, nerve,
    lumbosacral, sympathetic
  esophageal —*see* Injury, nerve, thorax,
    sympathetic
  hypogastric —*see* Injury, nerve,
    lumbosacral, sympathetic
  lumbar, lumbosacral —*see* Injury,
    lumbosacral plexus
  mesenteric —*see* Injury, nerve, lumbosacral,
    sympathetic
  pulmonary —*see* Injury, nerve, thorax,
    sympathetic
postcardiac surgery (syndrome) I97.0
prepuce S39.94
prostate S37.829
  contusion S37.822
  laceration S37.823
  specified type NEC S37.828
pubic region S39.94
pudendum S39.94
pulmonary plexus —*see* Injury, nerve, thorax,
  sympathetic
rectovaginal septum NEC S39.83
rectum —*see* Injury, intestine, large, rectum
retina —*see* Injury, eye, specified site NEC
  penetrating —*see* Injury, eyeball,
    penetrating
retroperitoneal —*see* Injury, intra-abdominal,
  specified site NEC
rotator cuff (muscle(s)) (tendon(s)) S46.00-●
  laceration S46.02-●
  specified type NEC S46.09-●
  strain S46.01-●
round ligament —*see* Injury, pelvic organ,
  specified site NEC
sacral plexus —*see* Injury, lumbosacral
  plexus
salivary duct or gland S09.93
scalp S09.90
  newborn (birth injury) P12.9
    due to monitoring (electrode) (sampling
      incision) P12.4
    specified NEC P12.89
      caput succedaneum P12.81
scapular region —*see* Injury, shoulder
sclera —*see* Injury, eye, specified site NEC
  penetrating —*see* Injury, eyeball,
    penetrating
scrotum S39.94
second cranial nerve (optic) —*see* Injury,
  nerve, optic
seminal vesicle —*see* Injury, pelvic organ,
  specified site NEC
seventh cranial nerve (facial) —*see* Injury,
  nerve, facial
shoulder S49.9-●
  blood vessel —*see* Injury, blood vessel,
    arm
  contusion —*see* Contusion, shoulder
  dislocation —*see* Dislocation, shoulder
  fracture —*see* Fracture, shoulder
  muscle —*see* Injury, muscle, shoulder
  nerve —*see* Injury, nerve, shoulder
  open —*see* Wound, open, shoulder
  specified type NEC S49.8-●

Injury *(Continued)*
shoulder *(Continued)*
  sprain —*see* Sprain, shoulder girdle
  superficial —*see* Injury, superficial,
    shoulder
sinus
  cavernous —*see* Injury, intracranial
  nasal S09.92
sixth cranial nerve (abducent) —*see* Injury,
  nerve, abducens
skeleton, birth injury P13.9
  specified part NEC P13.8
skin NEC T14.8
  surface intact —*see* Injury, superficial
skull NEC S09.90
specified NEC T14.8
spermatic cord (pelvic region) S37.898
  scrotal region S39.848
spinal (cord)
  cervical (neck) S14.109
    anterior cord syndrome S14.139
      C1 level S14.131
      C2 level S14.132
      C3 level S14.133
      C4 level S14.134
      C5 level S14.135
      C6 level S14.136
      C7 level S14.137
      C8 level S14.138
    Brown-Séquard syndrome S14.149
      C1 level S14.141
      C2 level S14.142
      C3 level S14.143
      C4 level S14.144
      C5 level S14.145
      C6 level S14.146
      C7 level S14.147
      C8 level S14.148
    C1 level S14.101
    C2 level S14.102
    C3 level S14.103
    C4 level S14.104
    C5 level S14.105
    C6 level S14.106
    C7 level S14.107
    C8 level S14.108
    central cord syndrome S14.129
      C1 level S14.121
      C2 level S14.122
      C3 level S14.123
      C4 level S14.124
      C5 level S14.125
      C6 level S14.126
      C7 level S14.127
      C8 level S14.128
    complete lesion S14.119
      C1 level S14.111
      C2 level S14.112
      C3 level S14.113
      C4 level S14.114
      C5 level S14.115
      C6 level S14.116
      C7 level S14.117
      C8 level S14.118
    concussion S14.0
    edema S14.0
    incomplete lesion specified NEC S14.159
      C1 level S14.151
      C2 level S14.152
      C3 level S14.153
      C4 level S14.154
      C5 level S14.155
      C6 level S14.156
      C7 level S14.157
      C8 level S14.158
    posterior cord syndrome S14.159
      C1 level S14.151
      C2 level S14.152
      C3 level S14.153
      C4 level S14.154
      C5 level S14.155

▶ New   ⇒ Revised   ~~deleted~~ Deleted   ● Use Additional Character(s)

Injury *(Continued)*
  superficial NEC *(Continued)*
    foot *(Continued)*
      blister —*see* Blister, foot
      contusion —*see* Contusion, foot
      external constriction —*see* Constriction, external, foot
      foreign body —*see* Foreign body, superficial, foot
    forearm S50.91-●
      abrasion —*see* Abrasion, forearm
      bite —*see* Bite, forearm, superficial
      blister —*see* Blister, forearm
      contusion —*see* Contusion, forearm
      elbow only —*see* Injury, superficial, elbow
      external constriction —*see* Constriction, external, forearm
      foreign body —*see* Foreign body, superficial, forearm
    forehead —*see* Injury, superficial, head NEC
    foreign body —*see* Foreign body, superficial
    genital organs, external
      female S30.97
      male S30.96
    globe (eye) —*see* Injury, eye, specified site NEC
    groin S30.92
    gum —*see* Injury, superficial, oral cavity
    hand S60.92-●
      abrasion —*see* Abrasion, hand
      bite —*see* Bite, superficial, hand
      contusion —*see* Contusion, hand
      external constriction —*see* Constriction, external, hand
      foreign body —*see* Foreign body, superficial, hand
    head S00.90
      ear —*see* Injury, superficial, ear
      eyelid —*see* Injury, superficial, eyelid
      nose S00.30
      oral cavity S00.502
      scalp S00.00
      specified site NEC S00.80
    heel —*see* Injury, superficial, foot
    hip S70.91-●
      abrasion —*see* Abrasion, hip
      bite —*see* Bite, superficial, hip
      blister —*see* Blister, hip
      contusion —*see* Contusion, hip
      external constriction —*see* Constriction, external, hip
      foreign body —*see* Foreign body, superficial, hip
    iliac region —*see* Injury, superficial, abdomen
    inguinal region —*see* Injury, superficial, abdomen
    insect bite —*see* Bite, by site, superficial, insect
    interscapular region —*see* Injury, superficial, thorax, back
    jaw —*see* Injury, superficial, head, specified NEC
    knee S80.91-●
      abrasion —*see* Abrasion, knee
      bite —*see* Bite, superficial, knee
      blister —*see* Blister, knee
      contusion —*see* Contusion, knee
      external constriction —*see* Constriction, external, knee
      foreign body —*see* Foreign body, superficial, knee
    labium (majus) (minus) S30.95
    lacrimal (apparatus) (gland) (sac) —*see* Injury, eye, specified site NEC
    larynx —*see* Injury, superficial, throat
    leg (lower) S80.92-●
      abrasion —*see* Abrasion, leg
      bite —*see* Bite, superficial, leg

Injury *(Continued)*
  superficial NEC *(Continued)*
    leg *(Continued)*
      contusion —*see* Contusion, leg
      external constriction —*see* Constriction, external, leg
      foreign body —*see* Foreign body, superficial, leg
      knee —*see* Injury, superficial, knee
    limb NEC T14.8
    lip S00.501
    lower back S30.91
    lumbar region S30.91
    malar region —*see* Injury, superficial, head, specified NEC
    mammary —*see* Injury, superficial, breast
    mastoid region —*see* Injury, superficial, head, specified NEC
    mouth —*see* Injury, superficial, oral cavity
    muscle NEC T14.8
    nail NEC T14.8
      finger —*see* Injury, superficial, finger
      toe —*see* Injury, superficial, toe
    nasal (septum) —*see* Injury, superficial, nose
    neck S10.90
      specified site NEC S10.80
    nose (septum) S00.30
    occipital region —*see* Injury, superficial, scalp
    oral cavity S00.502
    orbital region —*see* Injury, superficial, periocular area
    palate —*see* Injury, superficial, oral cavity
    palm —*see* Injury, superficial, hand
    parietal region —*see* Injury, superficial, scalp
    pelvis S30.91
      girdle —*see* Injury, superficial, hip
    penis S30.93
    perineum
      female S30.95
      male S30.91
    periocular area S00.20-●
      abrasion —*see* Abrasion, eyelid
      bite —*see* Bite, superficial, eyelid
      contusion —*see* Contusion, eyelid
      external constriction —*see* Constriction, external, eyelid
      foreign body —*see* Foreign body, superficial, eyelid
    phalanges
      finger —*see* Injury, superficial, finger
      toe —*see* Injury, superficial, toe
    pharynx —*see* Injury, superficial, throat
    pinna —*see* Injury, superficial, ear
    popliteal space —*see* Injury, superficial, knee
    prepuce S30.93
    pubic region S30.91
    pudendum
      female S30.97
      male S30.96
    sacral region S30.91
    scalp S00.00
    scapular region —*see* Injury, superficial, shoulder
    sclera —*see* Injury, eye, specified site NEC
    scrotum S30.94
    shin —*see* Injury, superficial, leg
    shoulder S40.91-●
      abrasion —*see* Abrasion, shoulder
      bite —*see* Bite, superficial, shoulder
      blister —*see* Blister, shoulder
      contusion —*see* Contusion, shoulder
      external constriction —*see* Constriction, external, shoulder
      foreign body —*see* Foreign body, superficial, shoulder

Injury *(Continued)*
  superficial NEC *(Continued)*
    skin NEC T14.8
    sternal region —*see* Injury, superficial, thorax, front
    subconjunctival —*see* Injury, eye, specified site NEC
    subcutaneous NEC T14.8
    submaxillary region —*see* Injury, superficial, head, specified NEC
    submental region —*see* Injury, superficial, head, specified NEC
    subungual
      finger(s) —*see* Injury, superficial, finger
      toe(s) —*see* Injury, superficial, toe
    supraclavicular fossa —*see* Injury, superficial, neck
    supraorbital —*see* Injury, superficial, head, specified NEC
    temple —*see* Injury, superficial, head, specified NEC
    temporal region —*see* Injury, superficial, head, specified NEC
    testis S30.94
    thigh S70.92-●
      abrasion —*see* Abrasion, thigh
      bite —*see* Bite, superficial, thigh
      blister —*see* Blister, thigh
      contusion —*see* Contusion, thigh
      external constriction —*see* Constriction, external, thigh
      foreign body —*see* Foreign body, superficial, thigh
    thorax, thoracic (wall) S20.90
      abrasion —*see* Abrasion, thorax
      back S20.40-●
      bite —*see* Bite, thorax, superficial
      blister —*see* Blister, thorax
      contusion —*see* Contusion, thorax
      external constriction —*see* Constriction, external, thorax
      foreign body —*see* Foreign body, superficial, thorax
      front S20.30-●
    throat S10.10
      abrasion S10.11
      bite S10.17
        insect S10.16
      blister S10.12
      contusion S10.0
      external constriction S10.14
      foreign body S10.15
    thumb S60.93-●
      abrasion —*see* Abrasion, thumb
      bite —*see* Bite, superficial, thumb
      blister —*see* Blister, thumb
      contusion —*see* Contusion, thumb
      external constriction —*see* Constriction, external, thumb
      foreign body —*see* Foreign body, superficial, thumb
      insect bite —*see* Bite, by site, superficial, insect
      specified type NEC S60.39-●
    toe(s) S90.93-●
      abrasion —*see* Abrasion, toe
      bite —*see* Bite, toe
      blister —*see* Blister, toe
      contusion —*see* Contusion, toe
      external constriction —*see* Constriction, external, toe
      foreign body —*see* Foreign body, superficial, toe
      great S90.93-●
    tongue —*see* Injury, superficial, oral cavity
    tooth, teeth —*see* Injury, superficial, oral cavity
    trachea S10.10
    tunica vaginalis S30.94
    tympanum, tympanic membrane —*see* Injury, superficial, ear

Injury *(Continued)*
  superficial NEC *(Continued)*
    uvula —*see* Injury, superficial, oral cavity
    vagina S30.95
    vocal cords —*see* Injury, superficial, throat
    vulva S30.95
    wrist S60.91-●
  supraclavicular region —*see* Injury, neck
  supraorbital S09.93
  suprarenal gland (multiple) —*see* Injury,
      adrenal
  surgical complication (external or internal
      site) —*see* Laceration, accidental
      complicating surgery
  temple S09.90
  temporal region S09.90
  tendon —*see also* Injury, muscle, by site
    abdomen —*see* Injury, muscle, abdomen
    Achilles —*see* Injury, Achilles tendon
    lower back —*see* Injury, muscle, lower back
    pelvic organs —*see* Injury, muscle, pelvis
  tenth cranial nerve (pneumogastric or
      vagus) —*see* Injury, nerve, vagus
  testis S39.94
  thigh S79.92-●
    blood vessel —*see* Injury, blood vessel, hip
    contusion —*see* Contusion, thigh
    fracture —*see* Fracture, femur
    muscle —*see* Injury, muscle, thigh
    nerve —*see* Injury, nerve, thigh
    open —*see* Wound, open, thigh
    specified NEC S79.82-●
    superficial —*see* Injury, superficial, thigh
  third cranial nerve (oculomotor) —*see* Injury,
      nerve, oculomotor
  thorax, thoracic S29.9
    blood vessel —*see* Injury, blood vessel,
        thorax
    cavity —*see* Injury, intrathoracic
    dislocation —*see* Dislocation, thorax
    external (wall) S29.9
      contusion —*see* Contusion, thorax
      nerve —*see* Injury, nerve, thorax
      open —*see* Wound, open, thorax
      specified NEC S29.8
      sprain —*see* Sprain, thorax
      superficial —*see* Injury, superficial,
          thorax
    fracture —*see* Fracture, thorax
    internal —*see* Injury, intrathoracic
    intrathoracic organ —*see* Injury,
        intrathoracic
    sympathetic ganglion —*see* Injury, nerve,
        thorax, sympathetic
  throat —*see also* Injury, neck S19.9
  thumb S69.9-●
    blood vessel —*see* Injury, blood vessel,
        thumb
    contusion —*see* Contusion, thumb
    dislocation —*see* Dislocation, thumb
    fracture —*see* Fracture, thumb
    muscle —*see* Injury, muscle, thumb
    nerve —*see* Injury, nerve, digital, thumb
    open —*see* Wound, open, thumb
    specified NEC S69.8-●
    sprain —*see* Sprain, thumb
    superficial —*see* Injury, superficial, thumb
  thymus (gland) —*see* Injury, intrathoracic,
      specified organ NEC
  thyroid (gland) NEC S19.84
  toe S99.92-●
    contusion —*see* Contusion, toe
    dislocation —*see* Dislocation, toe
    fracture —*see* Fracture, toe
    muscle —*see* Injury, muscle, toe
    open —*see* Wound, open, toe
    specified type NEC S99.82-●
    sprain —*see* Sprain, toe
    superficial —*see* Injury, superficial, toe
  tongue S09.93
  tonsil S09.93

Injury *(Continued)*
  tooth S09.93
  trachea (cervical) NEC S19.82
    thoracic —*see* Injury, intrathoracic, trachea,
        thoracic
  transfusion-related acute lung (TRALI) J95.84
  tunica vaginalis S39.94
  twelfth cranial nerve (hypoglossal) —*see*
      Injury, nerve, hypoglossal
  ureter S37.10
    contusion S37.12
    laceration S37.13
    specified type NEC S37.19
  urethra (sphincter) S37.30
    at delivery O71.5
    contusion S37.32
    laceration S37.33
    specified type NEC S37.38
  urinary organ S37.899
    contusion S37.92
    laceration S37.93
    specified
      site NEC S37.899
        contusion S37.892
        laceration S37.893
        specified type NEC S37.898
      type NEC S37.99
  uterus, uterine S37.60
    with ectopic or molar pregnancy O08.6
    blood vessel —*see* Injury, blood vessel, iliac
    contusion S37.62
    laceration S37.63
      cervix at delivery O71.3
    rupture associated with obstetrics —*see*
        Rupture, uterus
    specified type NEC S37.69
  uvula S09.93
  vagina S39.93
    abrasion S30.814
    bite S31.45
      insect S30.864
      superficial NEC S30.874
    contusion S30.23
    crush S38.03
    during delivery —*see* Laceration, vagina,
        during delivery
    external constriction S30.844
    insect bite S30.864
    laceration S31.41
      with foreign body S31.42
    open wound S31.40
    puncture S31.43
      with foreign body S31.44
    superficial S30.95
      foreign body S30.854
  vas deferens —*see* Injury, pelvic organ,
      specified site NEC
  vascular NEC T14.8
  vein —*see* Injury, blood vessel
  vena cava (superior) S25.20
    inferior S35.10
      laceration (minor) (superficial) S35.11
        major S35.12
      specified type NEC S35.19
    laceration (minor) (superficial) S25.21
      major S25.22
    specified type NEC S25.29
  vesical (sphincter) —*see* Injury, bladder
  visual cortex S04.04-●
  vitreous (humor) S05.90
    specified NEC S05.8X-●
  vocal cord NEC S19.83
  vulva S39.94
    abrasion S30.814
    bite S31.45
      insect S30.864
      superficial NEC S30.874
    contusion S30.23
    crush S38.03
    during delivery —*see* Laceration,
        perineum, female, during delivery

Injury *(Continued)*
  vulva *(Continued)*
    external constriction S30.844
    insect bite S30.864
    laceration S31.41
      with foreign body S31.42
    open wound S31.40
    puncture S31.43
      with foreign body S31.44
    superficial S30.95
      foreign body S30.854
  whiplash (cervical spine) S13.4
  wrist S69.9-●
    blood vessel —*see* Injury, blood vessel,
        hand
    contusion —*see* Contusion, wrist
    dislocation —*see* Dislocation, wrist
    fracture —*see* Fracture, wrist
    muscle —*see* Injury, muscle, hand
    nerve —*see* Injury, nerve, hand
    open —*see* Wound, open, wrist
    specified NEC S69.8-●
    sprain —*see* Sprain, wrist
    superficial —*see* Injury, superficial, wrist
Inoculation —*see also* Vaccination
  complication or reaction —*see* Complications,
      vaccination
Insanity, insane —*see also* Psychosis
  adolescent —*see* Schizophrenia
  confusional F28
    acute or subacute F05
  delusional F22
  senile F03
Insect
  bite —*see* Bite, by site, superficial, insect
  venomous, poisoning NEC (by) —*see* Venom,
      arthropod
Insensitivity
  adrenocorticotropin hormone (ACTH)
      E27.49
  androgen E34.50
    complete E34.51
    partial E34.52
Insertion
  cord (umbilical) lateral or velamentous
      O43.12-●
  intrauterine contraceptive device (encounter
      for) —*see* Intrauterine contraceptive
      device
Insolation (sunstroke) T67.0
Insomnia (organic) G47.00
  without objective findings F51.02
  adjustment F51.02
  adjustment disorder F51.02
  behavioral, of childhood Z73.819
    combined type Z73.812
    limit setting type Z73.811
    sleep-onset association type Z73.810
  childhood Z73.819
  chronic F51.04
    somatized tension F51.04
  conditioned F51.04
  due to
    alcohol
      abuse F10.182
      dependence F10.282
      use F10.982
    amphetamines
      abuse F15.182
      dependence F15.282
      use F15.982
    anxiety disorder F51.05
    caffeine
      abuse F15.182
      dependence F15.282
      use F15.982
    cocaine
      abuse F14.182
      dependence F14.282
      use F14.982
    depression F51.05

Insomnia (Continued)
  due to (Continued)
    drug NEC
      abuse F19.182
      dependence F19.282
      use F19.982
    medical condition G47.01
    mental disorder NEC F51.05
    opioid
      abuse F11.182
      dependence F11.282
      use F11.982
    psychoactive substance NEC
      abuse F19.182
      dependence F19.282
      use F19.982
    sedative, hypnotic, or anxiolytic
      abuse F13.182
      dependence F13.282
      use F13.982
    stimulant NEC
      abuse F15.182
      dependence F15.282
      use F15.982
  fatal familial (FFI) A81.83
  idiopathic F51.01
  learned F51.3
  nonorganic origin F51.01
  not due to a substance or known
      physiological condition F51.01
    specified NEC F51.09
  paradoxical F51.03
  primary F51.01
  psychiatric F51.05
  psychophysiologic F51.04
  related to psychopathology F51.05
  short-term F51.02
  specified NEC G47.09
  stress-related F51.02
  transient F51.02
Inspiration
  food or foreign body —see Foreign body, by
      site
  mucus —see Asphyxia, mucus
Inspissated bile syndrome (newborn)
    P59.1
Instability
  emotional (excessive) F60.3
  joint (post-traumatic) M25.30
    ankle M25.37-●
    due to old ligament injury —see Disorder,
        ligament
    elbow M25.32-●
    flail —see Flail, joint
    foot M25.37-●
    hand M25.34-●
    hip M25.35-●
    knee M25.36-●
    lumbosacral —see subcategory M53.2
    prosthesis —see Complications, joint
        prosthesis, mechanical, displacement,
        by site
    sacroiliac —see subcategory M53.2
    secondary to
      old ligament injury —see Disorder,
          ligament
      removal of joint prosthesis M96.89
    shoulder (region) M25.31-●
    spine —see subcategory M53.2
    wrist M25.33-●
  knee (chronic) M23.5-●
  lumbosacral —see subcategory M53.2
  nervous F48.8
  personality (emotional) F60.3
  spine —see Instability, joint, spine
  vasomotor R55
Institutional syndrome (childhood)
    F94.2
Institutionalization, affecting child
    Z62.22
  disinhibited attachment F94.2

Insufficiency, insufficient
  accommodation, old age H52.4
  adrenal (gland) E27.40
    primary E27.1
  adrenocortical E27.40
    drug-induced E27.3
    iatrogenic E27.3
    primary E27.1
  anatomic crown height K08.89
  anterior (occlusal) guidance M26.54
  anus K62.89
  aortic (valve) I35.1
    with
      mitral (valve) disease I08.0
        with tricuspid (valve) disease I08.3
      stenosis I35.2
      tricuspid (valve) disease I08.2
        with mitral (valve) disease I08.3
    congenital Q23.1
    rheumatic I06.1
      with
        mitral (valve) disease I08.0
          with tricuspid (valve) disease
              I08.3
        stenosis I06.2
          with mitral (valve) disease I08.0
            with tricuspid (valve) disease
                I08.3
        tricuspid (valve) disease I08.2
          with mitral (valve) disease I08.3
    specified cause NEC I35.1
    syphilitic A52.03
  arterial I77.1
    basilar G45.0
    carotid (hemispheric) G45.1
    cerebral I67.81
    coronary (acute or subacute) I24.8
    mesenteric K55.1
    peripheral I73.9
    precerebral (multiple) (bilateral) G45.2
    vertebral G45.0
  arteriovenous I99.8
  biliary K83.8
  cardiac —see also Insufficiency, myocardial
    due to presence of (cardiac) prosthesis
        I97.11-●
    postprocedural I97.11-●
  cardiorenal, hypertensive I13.2
  cardiovascular —see Disease, cardiovascular
  cerebrovascular (acute) I67.81
    with transient focal neurological signs and
        symptoms G45.8
  circulatory NEC I99.8
    newborn P29.89
  clinical crown length K08.89
  convergence H51.11
  coronary (acute or subacute) I24.8
    chronic or with a stated duration of over 4
        weeks I25.89
  corticoadrenal E27.40
    primary E27.1
  dietary E63.9
  divergence H51.8
  food T73.0
  gastroesophageal K22.8
  gonadal
    ovary E28.39
    testis E29.1
  heart —see also Insufficiency, myocardial
    newborn P29.0
    valve —see Endocarditis
  hepatic —see Failure, hepatic
  idiopathic autonomic G90.09
  interocclusal distance of fully erupted teeth
      (ridge) M26.36
  kidney N28.9
    acute N28.9
    chronic N18.9
  lacrimal (secretion) H04.12-●
    passages —see Stenosis, lacrimal
  liver —see Failure, hepatic

Insufficiency, insufficient (Continued)
  lung —see Insufficiency, pulmonary
  mental (congenital) —see Disability,
      intellectual
  mesenteric K55.1
  mitral (valve) I34.0
    with
      aortic valve disease I08.0
        with tricuspid (valve) disease
            I08.3
      obstruction or stenosis I05.2
        with aortic valve disease I08.0
      tricuspid (valve) disease I08.1
        with aortic (valve) disease I08.3
    congenital Q23.3
    rheumatic I05.1
      with
        aortic valve disease I08.0
          with tricuspid (valve) disease I08.3
        obstruction or stenosis I05.2
          with aortic valve disease I08.0
            with tricuspid (valve) disease
                I08.3
        tricuspid (valve) disease I08.1
          with aortic (valve) disease I08.3
      active or acute I01.1
        with chorea, rheumatic (Sydenham's)
            I02.0
    specified cause, except rheumatic I34.0
  muscle —see also Disease, muscle
    heart —see Insufficiency, myocardial
  ocular NEC H50.9
  ➡myocardial, myocardium (with
      arteriosclerosis) —see also Failure, heart
      I50.9
    with
      rheumatic fever (conditions in I00)
          I09.0
        active, acute or subacute I01.2
          with chorea I02.0
        inactive or quiescent (with chorea)
            I09.0
    congenital Q24.8
    hypertensive —see Hypertension, heart
    newborn P29.0
    rheumatic I09.0
      active, acute, or subacute I01.2
    syphilitic A52.06
  nourishment T73.0
  pancreatic K86.89
    exocrine K86.81
  parathyroid (gland) E20.9
  peripheral vascular (arterial) I73.9
  pituitary E23.0
  placental (mother) O36.51-●
  platelets D69.6
  prenatal care affecting management of
      pregnancy O09.3-●
  progressive pluriglandular E31.0
  pulmonary J98.4
    acute, following surgery (nonthoracic)
        J95.2
      thoracic J95.1
    chronic, following surgery J95.3
    following
      shock J98.4
      trauma J98.4
    newborn P28.5
    valve I37.1
      with stenosis I37.2
      congenital Q22.2
      rheumatic I09.89
        with aortic, mitral or tricuspid (valve)
            disease I08.8
  pyloric K31.89
  renal (acute) N28.9
    chronic N18.9
  respiratory R06.89
    newborn P28.5
  rotation —see Malrotation
  sleep syndrome F51.12

Insufficiency, insufficient (Continued)
  social insurance Z59.7
  suprarenal E27.40
    primary E27.1
  tarso-orbital fascia, congenital Q10.3
  testis E29.1
  thyroid (gland) (acquired) E03.9
    congenital E03.1
  tricuspid (valve) (rheumatic) I07.1
    with
      aortic (valve) disease I08.2
        with mitral (valve) disease I08.3
      mitral (valve) disease I08.1
        with aortic (valve) disease I08.3
      obstruction or stenosis I07.2
        with aortic (valve) disease I08.2
          with mitral (valve) disease I08.3
    congenital Q22.8
    nonrheumatic I36.1
      with stenosis I36.2
  urethral sphincter R32
➡valve, valvular (heart) I38
  ▶aortic —see Insufficiency, aortic (valve)
  ▶mitral —see Insufficiency, mitral (valve)
  ▶pulmonary —see Insufficiency, pulmonary, valve
  ▶tricuspid —see Insufficiency, tricuspid (valve)
    congenital Q24.8
  vascular I99.8
    intestine K55.9
      acute —see also Ischemia, intestine, acute K55.059
    mesenteric K55.1
    peripheral I73.9
    renal —see Hypertension, kidney
  velopharyngeal
    acquired K13.79
    congenital Q38.8
  venous (chronic) (peripheral) I87.2
  ventricular —see Insufficiency, myocardial
  welfare support Z59.7
Insufflation, fallopian Z31.41
Insular —see condition
Insulinoma
  pancreas
    benign D13.7
    malignant C25.4
    uncertain behavior D37.8
  specified site
    benign —see Neoplasm, by site, benign
    malignant —see Neoplasm, by site, malignant
    uncertain behavior —see Neoplasm, by site, uncertain behavior
  unspecified site
    benign D13.7
    malignant C25.4
    uncertain behavior D37.8
Insuloma —see Insulinoma
Interference
  balancing side M26.56
  non-working side M26.56
Intermenstrual —see condition
Intermittent —see condition
Internal —see condition
Interrogation
  cardiac defibrillator (automatic) (implantable) Z45.02
  cardiac pacemaker Z45.018
  cardiac (event) (loop) recorder Z45.09
  infusion pump (implanted) (intrathecal) Z45.1
  neurostimulator Z46.2
Interruption
  aortic arch Q25.21
  phase-shift, sleep cycle —see Disorder, sleep, circadian rhythm
  sleep phase-shift, or 24 hour sleep-wake cycle —see Disorder, sleep, circadian rhythm

Interstitial —see condition
Intertrigo L30.4
  labialis K13.0
Intervertebral disc —see condition
Intestine, intestinal —see condition
Intolerance
  carbohydrate K90.49
  disaccharide, hereditary E73.0
  fat NEC K90.49
    pancreatic K90.3
  food K90.49
    dietary counseling and surveillance Z71.3
  fructose E74.10
    hereditary E74.12
  glucose(-galactose) E74.39
  gluten K90.01
  lactose E73.9
    specified NEC E73.8
  lysine E72.3
  milk NEC K90.49
    lactose E73.9
  protein K90.49
  starch NEC K90.49
  sucrose (-isomaltose) E74.31
Intoxicated NEC (without dependence) —see Alcohol, intoxication
Intoxication
  acid E87.2
  alcoholic (acute) (without dependence) —see Alcohol, intoxication
  alimentary canal K52.1
  amphetamine (without dependence) — see Abuse, drug, stimulant, with intoxication
    with dependence —see Dependence, drug, stimulant, with intoxication
  anxiolytic (acute) (without dependence) —see Abuse, drug, sedative, with intoxication
    with dependence —see Dependence, drug, sedative, with intoxication
  caffeine F15.929
    with dependence —see Dependence, drug, stimulant, with intoxication
  cannabinoids (acute) (without dependence) —see Use, cannabis, with intoxication
    with
      abuse —see Abuse, drug, cannabis, with intoxication
      dependence —see Dependence, drug, cannabis, with intoxication
  chemical —see Table of Drugs and Chemicals
    via placenta or breast milk —see - Absorption, chemical, through placenta
  cocaine (acute) (without dependence) —see Abuse, drug, cocaine, with intoxication
    with dependence —see Dependence, drug, cocaine, with intoxication
  drug
    acute (without dependence) —see Abuse, drug, by type with intoxication
      with dependence —see Dependence, drug, by type with intoxication
    addictive
      via placenta or breast milk —see Absorption, drug, addictive, through placenta
    newborn P93.8
      gray baby syndrome P93.0
    overdose or wrong substance given or taken —see Table of Drugs and Chemicals, by drug, poisoning
  enteric K52.1
  foodborne A05.9
    bacterial A05.9
    classical (Clostridium botulinum) A05.1
    due to
      Bacillus cereus A05.4
      bacterium A05.9
        specified NEC A05.8

Intoxication (Continued)
  foodborne (Continued)
    due to (Continued)
      Clostridium
        botulinum A05.1
        perfringens A05.2
        welchii A05.2
      Salmonella A02.9
        with
          (gastro) enteritis A02.0
          localized infection(s) A02.20
            arthritis A02.23
            meningitis A02.21
            osteomyelitis A02.24
            pneumonia A02.22
            pyelonephritis A02.25
            specified NEC A02.29
          sepsis A02.1
          specified manifestation NEC A02.8
      Staphylococcus A05.0
      Vibrio
        parahaemolyticus A05.3
        vulnificus A05.5
      enterotoxin, staphylococcal A05.0
    noxious —see Poisoning, food, noxious
  gastrointestinal K52.1
  hallucinogenic (without dependence) — see Abuse, drug, hallucinogen, with intoxication
    with dependence —see Dependence, drug, hallucinogen, with intoxication
  hypnotic (acute) (without dependence) —see Abuse, drug, sedative, with intoxication
    with dependence —see Dependence, drug, sedative, with intoxication
  inhalant (acute) (without dependence) —see Abuse, drug, inhalant, with intoxication
    with dependence —see Dependence, drug, inhalant, with intoxication
  meaning
    inebriation —see category F10
    poisoning —see Table of Drugs and Chemicals
  methyl alcohol (acute) (without dependence) —see Alcohol, intoxication
  opioid (acute) (without dependence) —see Abuse, drug, opioid, with intoxication
    with dependence —see Dependence, drug, opioid, with intoxication
  pathologic NEC (without dependence) —see Alcohol, intoxication
  phencyclidine (without dependence) —see Abuse, drug, hallucinogen, with intoxication
    with dependence —see Dependence, drug, hallucinogen, with intoxication
  potassium (K) E87.5
  psychoactive substance NEC (without dependence) —see Abuse, drug, psychoactive NEC, with intoxication
    with dependence —see Dependence, drug, psychoactive NEC, with intoxication
  sedative (acute) (without dependence) —see Abuse, drug, sedative, with intoxication
    with dependence —see Dependence, drug, sedative, with intoxication
  serum —see also Reaction, serum T80.69
  uremic —see Uremia
  volatile solvents (acute) (without dependence) —see Abuse, drug, inhalant, with intoxication
    with dependence —see Dependence, drug, inhalant, with intoxication
  water E87.79
▶**Intraabdominal testis, testes**
  ▶bilateral Q53.211
  ▶unilateral Q53.111
Intracranial —see condition
Intrahepatic gallbladder Q44.1
Intraligamentous —see condition

▶ New   ➡ Revised   ~~deleted~~ Deleted   ● Use Additional Character(s)

Intrathoracic —see also condition
  kidney Q63.2
Intrauterine contraceptive device
  checking Z30.431
  in situ Z97.5
  insertion Z30.430
    immediately following removal Z30.433
  management Z30.431
  reinsertion Z30.433
  removal Z30.432
  replacement Z30.433
  retention in pregnancy O26.3-•
Intraventricular —see condition
Intrinsic deformity —see Deformity
Intubation, difficult or failed T88.4
Intumescence, lens (eye) (cataract) —see
  Cataract
Intussusception (bowel) (colon) (enteric)
    (ileocecal) (ileocolic) (intestine) (rectum)
    K56.1
  appendix K38.8
  congenital Q43.8
  ureter (with obstruction) N13.5
Invagination (bowel, colon, intestine or rectum)
    K56.1
Inversion
  albumin-globulin (A-G) ratio E88.09
  bladder N32.89
  cecum —see Intussusception
  cervix N88.8
  chromosome in normal individual Q95.1
  circadian rhythm —see Disorder, sleep,
    circadian rhythm
  nipple N64.59
    congenital Q83.8
    gestational —see Retraction, nipple
    puerperal, postpartum —see Retraction,
      nipple
  nyctohemeral rhythm —see Disorder, sleep,
    circadian rhythm
  optic papilla Q14.2
  organ or site, congenital NEC —see Anomaly,
    by site
  sleep rhythm —see Disorder, sleep, circadian
    rhythm
  testis (congenital) Q55.29
  uterus (chronic) (postinfectional) (postpartal,
    old) N85.5
    postpartum O71.2
  vagina (posthysterectomy) N99.3
  ventricular Q20.5
Investigation —see also Examination Z04.9
  clinical research subject (control) (normal
    comparison) (participant) Z00.6
Involuntary movement, abnormal R25.9
Involution, involutional —see also condition
  breast, cystic —see Dysplasia, mammary,
    specified type NEC
  depression (single episode) F32.89
    recurrent episode F33.9
  melancholia (single episode) F32.89
    recurrent episode F33.8
  ovary, senile —see Atrophy, ovary
  thymus failure E32.8
I.Q.
  under 20 F73
  20-34 F72
  35-49 F71
  50-69 F70
IRDS (type I) P22.0
  type II P22.1
Irideremia Q13.1
Iridis rubeosis —see Disorder, iris, vascular
Iridochoroiditis (panuveitis) —see Panuveitis
Iridocyclitis H20.9-•
  acute H20.0-•
    hypopyon H20.05-•
    primary H20.01-•
    recurrent H20.02-•
    secondary (noninfectious) H20.04-•
      infectious H20.03-•

Iridocyclitis (Continued)
  chronic H20.1-•
  due to allergy —see Iridocyclitis, acute,
    secondary
  endogenous —see Iridocyclitis, acute, primary
  Fuchs' —see Cyclitis, Fuchs' heterochromic
  gonococcal A54.32
  granulomatous —see Iridocyclitis, chronic
  herpes, herpetic (simplex) B00.51
    zoster B02.32
  hypopyon —see Iridocyclitis, acute,
    hypopyon
  in (due to)
    ankylosing spondylitis M45.9
    gonococcal infection A54.32
    herpes (simplex) virus B00.51
      zoster B02.32
    infectious disease NOS B99
    parasitic disease NOS B89 [H22]
    sarcoidosis D86.83
    syphilis A51.43
    tuberculosis A18.54
    zoster B02.32
  lens-induced H20.2-•
  nongranulomatous —see Iridocyclitis, acute
  recurrent —see Iridocyclitis, acute, recurrent
  rheumatic —see Iridocyclitis, chronic
  subacute —see Iridocyclitis, acute
  sympathetic —see Uveitis, sympathetic
  syphilitic (secondary) A51.43
  tuberculous (chronic) A18.54
  Vogt-Koyanagi H20.82-•
Iridocyclochoroiditis (panuveitis) —see
  Panuveitis
Iridodialysis H21.53-•
Iridodonesis H21.89
Iridoplegia (complete) (partial) (reflex) H57.09
Iridoschisis H21.25-•
Iris —see also condition
  bombé —see Membrane, pupillary
Iritis —see also Iridocyclitis
  chronic —see Iridocyclitis, chronic
  diabetic —see E08-E13 with .39
  due to
    herpes simplex B00.51
    leprosy A30.9 [H22]
  gonococcal A54.32
  gouty —see also Gout, by type M10.9 [H22]
  granulomatous —see Iridocyclitis, chronic
  lens induced —see Iridocyclitis, lens-induced
  papulosa (syphilitic) A52.71
  rheumatic —see Iridocyclitis, chronic
  syphilitic (secondary) A51.43
    congenital (early) A50.01
    late A52.71
  tuberculous A18.54
Iron —see condition
Iron-miner's lung J63.4
Irradiated enamel (tooth, teeth) K03.89
Irradiation effects, adverse T66
Irreducible, irreducibility —see condition
Irregular, irregularity
  action, heart I49.9
  alveolar process K08.89
  bleeding N92.6
  breathing R06.89
  contour of cornea (acquired) —see Deformity,
    cornea
    congenital Q13.4
  contour, reconstructed breast N65.0
  dentin (in pulp) K04.3
  eye movements H55.89
    nystagmus —see Nystagmus
    saccadic H55.81
  labor O62.2
  menstruation (cause unknown) N92.6
  periods N92.6
  prostate N42.9
  pupil —see Abnormality, pupillary
  reconstructed breast N65.0
  respiratory R06.89

Irregular, irregularity (Continued)
  septum (nasal) J34.2
  shape, organ or site, congenital NEC —see
    Distortion
  sleep-wake pattern (rhythm) G47.23
Irritable, irritability R45.4
  bladder N32.89
  bowel (syndrome) K58.9
    with
      constipation K58.1
      diarrhea K58.0
    mixed K58.2
    psychogenic F45.8
    specified NEC K58.8
  bronchial —see Bronchitis
  cerebral, in newborn P91.3
  colon —see also Irritable, bowel K58.9
    with diarrhea K58.0
    psychogenic F45.8
  duodenum K59.8
  heart (psychogenic) F45.8
  hip —see Derangement, joint, specified type
    NEC, hip
  ileum K59.8
  infant R68.12
  jejunum K59.8
  rectum K59.8
  stomach K31.89
    psychogenic F45.8
  sympathetic G90.8
  urethra N36.8
Irritation
  anus K62.89
  axillary nerve G54.0
  bladder N32.89
  brachial plexus G54.0
  bronchial —see Bronchitis
  cervical plexus G54.2
  cervix —see Cervicitis
  choroid, sympathetic —see Endophthalmitis
  cranial nerve —see Disorder, nerve, cranial
  gastric K31.89
    psychogenic F45.8
  globe, sympathetic —see Uveitis,
    sympathetic
  labyrinth —see subcategory H83.2
  lumbosacral plexus G54.1
  meninges (traumatic) —see Injury, intracranial
    nontraumatic —see Meningismus
  nerve —see Disorder, nerve
  nervous R45.0
  penis N48.89
  perineum NEC L29.3
  peripheral autonomic nervous system
    G90.8
  peritoneum —see Peritonitis
  pharynx J39.2
  plantar nerve —see Lesion, nerve, plantar
  spinal (cord) (traumatic) —see also Injury,
    spinal cord, by region
    nerve G58.9
      root NEC —see Radiculopathy
    nontraumatic —see Myelopathy
  stomach K31.89
    psychogenic F45.8
  sympathetic nerve NEC G90.8
  ulnar nerve —see Lesion, nerve, ulnar
  vagina N89.8
Ischemia, ischemic I99.8
  bowel (transient)
    acute —see also Ischemia, intestine, acute
      K55.059
    chronic K55.1
    due to mesenteric artery insufficiency
      K55.1
  brain —see Ischemia, cerebral
  cardiac (see Disease, heart, ischemic)
  cardiomyopathy I25.5
  cerebral (chronic) (generalized) I67.82
    arteriosclerotic I67.2
    intermittent G45.9

Ischemia, ischemic *(Continued)*
  cerebral (chronic) (generalized) *(Continued)*
    newborn P91.0
    recurrent focal G45.8
    transient G45.9
  colon chronic (due to mesenteric artery
    insufficiency) K55.1
  coronary —*see* Disease, heart, ischemic
  demand (coronary) —*see also* Angina I24.8
  ▶with myocardial infarction I21.A1
  ▶resulting in myocardial infarction I21.A1
  heart (chronic or with a stated duration of
    over 4 weeks) I25.9
    acute or with a stated duration of 4 weeks
      or less I24.9
    subacute I24.9
  infarction, muscle —*see* Infarct, muscle
  intestine (large) (small) (transient) K55.9
    acute K55.059
      diffuse K55.052
      focal K55.051
      large K55.039
        diffuse K55.032
        focal K55.031
      small K55.019
        diffuse K55.012
        focal K55.011
    chronic K55.1
    due to mesenteric artery insufficiency K55.1
  kidney N28.0
  mesenteric, acute —*see also* Ischemia,
    intestine, acute K55.059
  muscle, traumatic T79.6
  myocardium, myocardial (chronic or with a
    stated duration of over 4 weeks) I25.9
    acute, without myocardial infarction
      I51.3
    silent (asymptomatic) I25.6
    transient of newborn P29.4
  renal N28.0
  retina, retinal —*see* Occlusion, artery, retina
  small bowel
    acute K55.019
      diffuse K55.012
      focal K55.011
    chronic K55.1
    due to mesenteric artery insufficiency K55.1

Ischemia, ischemic *(Continued)*
  spinal cord G95.11
  subendocardial —*see* Insufficiency, coronary
  supply (coronary) —*see also* Angina I25.9
    due to vasospasm I20.1
Ischial spine —*see* condition
Ischialgia —*see* Sciatica
Ischiopagus Q89.4
Ischium, ischial —*see* condition
Ischuria R34
Iselin's disease or osteochondrosis —*see*
  Osteochondrosis, juvenile, metatarsus
Islands of
  parotid tissue in
    lymph nodes Q38.6
    neck structures Q38.6
  submaxillary glands in
    fascia Q38.6
    lymph nodes Q38.6
    neck muscles Q38.6
Islet cell tumor, pancreas D13.7
Isoimmunization NEC —*see also*
  Incompatibility
  affecting management of pregnancy (ABO)
    (with hydrops fetalis) O36.11-●
    anti-A sensitization O36.11-●
    anti-B sensitization O36.19-●
    anti-c sensitization O36.09-●
    anti-C sensitization O36.09-●
    anti-e sensitization O36.09-●
    anti-E sensitization O36.09-●
    Rh NEC O36.09-●
      anti-D antibody O36.01-●
    specified NEC O36.19-●
  newborn P55.9
    with
      hydrops fetalis P56.0
      kernicterus P57.0
    ABO (blood groups) P55.1
    Rhesus (Rh) factor P55.0
    specified type NEC P55.8
Isolation, isolated
  dwelling Z59.8
  family Z63.79
  social Z60.4
Isoleucinosis E71.19

Isomerism atrial appendages (with asplenia or
  polysplenia) Q20.6
Isosporiasis, isosporosis A07.3
Isovaleric acidemia E71.110
Issue of
  medical certificate Z02.79
    for disability determination Z02.71
  repeat prescription (appliance) (glasses)
    (medicinal substance, medicament,
    medicine) Z76.0
    contraception —*see* Contraception
Itch, itching —*see also* Pruritus
  baker's L23.6
  barber's B35.0
  bricklayer's L24.5
  cheese B88.0
  clam digger's B65.3
  coolie B76.9
  copra B88.0
  dew B76.9
  dhobi B35.6
  filarial —*see* Infestation, filarial
  grain B88.0
  grocer's B88.0
  ground B76.9
  harvest B88.0
  jock B35.6
  Malabar B35.5
    beard B35.0
    foot B35.3
    scalp B35.0
  meaning scabies B86
  Norwegian B86
  perianal L29.0
  poultrymen's B88.0
  sarcoptic B86
  scabies B86
  scrub B88.0
  straw B88.0
  swimmer's B65.3
  water B76.9
  winter L29.8
Ivemark's syndrome (asplenia with congenital
  heart disease) Q89.01
Ivory bones Q78.2
Ixodiasis NEC B88.8

▶ New   ⇒ Revised   ~~deleted~~ Deleted   ● Use Additional Character(s)

J

Jaccoud's syndrome —see Arthropathy, postrheumatic, chronic
Jackson's
  membrane Q43.3
  paralysis or syndrome G83.89
  veil Q43.3
Jacquet's dermatitis (diaper dermatitis) L22
Jadassohn-Pellizari's disease or anetoderma L90.2
Jadassohn's
  blue nevus —see Nevus
  intraepidermal epithelioma —see Neoplasm, skin, benign
Jaffe-Lichtenstein (-Uehlinger) syndrome —see Dysplasia, fibrous, bone NEC
Jakob-Creutzfeldt disease or syndrome —see Creutzfeldt-Jakob disease or syndrome
Jaksch-Luzet disease D64.89
Jamaican
  neuropathy G92
  paraplegic tropical ataxic-spastic syndrome G92
Janet's disease F48.8
Janiceps Q89.4
Jansky-Bielschowsky amaurotic idiocy E75.4
Japanese
  B-type encephalitis A83.0
  river fever A75.3
Jaundice (yellow) R17
  acholuric (familial) (splenomegalic) —see also Spherocytosis
    acquired D59.8
  breast-milk (inhibitor) P59.3
  catarrhal (acute) B15.9
    with hepatic coma B15.0
  cholestatic (benign) R17
  due to or associated with
    delayed conjugation P59.8
      associated with (due to) preterm delivery P59.0
    preterm delivery P59.0
  epidemic (catarrhal) B15.9
    with hepatic coma B15.0
    leptospiral A27.0
    spirochetal A27.0
  familial nonhemolytic (congenital) (Gilbert) E80.4
    Crigler-Najjar E80.5
  febrile (acute) B15.9
    with hepatic coma B15.0
    leptospiral A27.0
    spirochetal A27.0
  hematogenous D59.9
  hemolytic (acquired) D59.9
    congenital —see Spherocytosis

Jaundice (Continued)
  hemorrhagic (acute) (leptospiral) (spirochetal) A27.0
  infectious (acute) (subacute) B15.9
    with hepatic coma B15.0
    leptospiral A27.0
    spirochetal A27.0
  leptospiral (hemorrhagic) A27.0
  malignant (without coma) K72.90
    with coma K72.91
  neonatal —see Jaundice, newborn
  newborn P59.9
    due to or associated with
      ABO
        antibodies P55.1
        incompatibility, maternal/fetal P55.1
        isoimmunization P55.1
      absence or deficiency of enzyme system for bilirubin conjugation (congenital) P59.8
      bleeding P58.1
      breast milk inhibitors to conjugation P59.3
        associated with preterm delivery P59.0
      bruising P58.0
      Crigler-Najjar syndrome E80.5
      delayed conjugation P59.8
        associated with preterm delivery P59.0
      drugs or toxins
        given to newborn P58.42
        transmitted from mother P58.41
      excessive hemolysis P58.9
        due to
          bleeding P58.1
          bruising P58.0
          drugs or toxins
            given to newborn P58.42
            transmitted from mother P58.41
          infection P58.2
          polycythemia P58.3
          swallowed maternal blood P58.5
        specified type NEC P58.8
      galactosemia E74.21
      Gilbert syndrome E80.4
      hemolytic disease P55.9
        ABO isoimmunization P55.1
        Rh isoimmunization P55.0
        specified NEC P55.8
      hepatocellular damage P59.20
        specified NEC P59.29
      hereditary hemolytic anemia P58.8
      hypothyroidism, congenital E03.1
      incompatibility, maternal/fetal NOS P55.9
      infection P58.2

Jaundice (Continued)
  newborn (Continued)
    due to or associated with (Continued)
      inspissated bile syndrome P59.1
      isoimmunization NOS P55.9
      mucoviscidosis E84.9
      polycythemia P58.3
      preterm delivery P59.0
      Rh
        antibodies P55.0
        incompatibility, maternal/fetal P55.0
        isoimmunization P55.0
      specified cause NEC P59.8
      swallowed maternal blood P58.5
    spherocytosis (congenital) D58.0
    nonhemolytic congenital familial (Gilbert) E80.4
    nuclear, newborn —see also Kernicterus of newborn P57.9
    obstructive —see also Obstruction, bile duct K83.1
    post-immunization —see Hepatitis, viral, type, B
    post-transfusion —see Hepatitis, viral, type, B
    regurgitation —see also Obstruction, bile duct K83.1
    serum (homologous) (prophylactic) (therapeutic) —see Hepatitis, viral, type, B
    spirochetal (hemorrhagic) A27.0
    symptomatic R17
      newborn P59.9
Jaw —see condition
Jaw-winking phenomenon or syndrome Q07.8
Jealousy
  alcoholic F10.988
  childhood F93.8
  sibling F93.8
Jejunitis —see Enteritis
Jejunostomy status Z93.4
Jejunum, jejunal —see condition
Jensen's disease —see Inflammation, chorioretinal, focal, juxtapapillary
Jerks, myoclonic G25.3
Jervell-Lange-Nielsen syndrome I45.81
Jeune's disease Q77.2
Jigger disease B88.1
Job's syndrome (chronic granulomatous disease) D71
Joint —see also condition
  mice —see Loose, body, joint
    knee M23.4-●
Jordan's anomaly or syndrome D72.0
Joseph-Diamond-Blackfan anemia (congenital hypoplastic) D61.01
Jungle yellow fever A95.0
Jüngling's disease —see Sarcoidosis
Juvenile —see condition

K

Kahler's disease C90.0-●
Kakke E51.11
Kala-azar B55.0
Kallmann's syndrome E23.0
Kanner's syndrome (autism) —see Psychosis, childhood
Kaposi's
dermatosis (xeroderma pigmentosum) Q82.1
lichen ruber L44.0
acuminatus L44.0
sarcoma
colon C46.4
connective tissue C46.1
gastrointestinal organ C46.4
lung C46.5-●
lymph node (multiple) C46.3
palate (hard) (soft) C46.2
rectum C46.4
skin (multiple sites) C46.0
specified site NEC C46.7
stomach C46.4
unspecified site C46.9
varicelliform eruption B00.0
vaccinia T88.1
Kartagener's syndrome or triad (sinusitis, bronchiectasis, situs inversus) Q89.3
Karyotype
with abnormality except iso (Xq) Q96.2
45,X Q96.0
46,X
iso (Xq) Q96.1
46,XX Q98.3
with streak gonads Q50.32
hermaphrodite (true) Q99.1
male Q98.3
46,XY
with streak gonads Q56.1
female Q97.3
hermaphrodite (true) Q99.1
47,XXX Q97.0
47,XXY Q98.0
47,XYY Q98.5
Kaschin-Beck disease —see Disease, Kaschin-Beck
Katayama's disease or fever B65.2
Kawasaki's syndrome M30.3
Kayser-Fleischer ring (cornea) (pseudosclerosis) H18.04-●
Kaznelson's syndrome (congenital hypoplastic anemia) D61.01
Kearns-Sayre syndrome H49.81-●
Kedani fever A75.3
Kelis L91.0
Kelly (-Patterson) syndrome (sideropenic dysphagia) D50.1
Keloid, cheloid L91.0
acne L73.0
Addison's L94.0
cornea —see Opacity, cornea
Hawkin's L91.0
scar L91.0
Keloma L91.0
Kenya fever A77.1
Keratectasia —see also Ectasia, cornea
congenital Q13.4
Keratinization of alveolar ridge mucosa
excessive K13.23
minimal K13.22
Keratinized residual ridge mucosa
excessive K13.23
minimal K13.22
Keratitis (nodular) (nonulcerative) (simple) (zonular) H16.9
with ulceration (central) (marginal) (perforated) (ring) —see Ulcer, cornea
actinic —see Photokeratitis
arborescens (herpes simplex) B00.52
areolar H16.11-●
bullosa H16.8

Keratitis (Continued)
deep H16.309
specified type NEC H16.399
dendritic (a) (herpes simplex) B00.52
disciform (is) (herpes simplex) B00.52
varicella B01.81
filamentary H16.12-●
gonococcal (congenital or prenatal) A54.33
herpes, herpetic (simplex) B00.52
zoster B02.33
in (due to)
acanthamebiasis B60.13
adenovirus B30.0
exanthema —see also Exanthem B09
herpes (simplex) virus B00.52
measles B05.81
syphilis A50.31
tuberculosis A18.52
zoster B02.33
interstitial (nonsyphilitic) H16.30-●
diffuse H16.32-●
herpes, herpetic (simplex) B00.52
zoster B02.33
sclerosing H16.33-●
specified type NEC H16.39-●
syphilitic (congenital) (late) A50.31
tuberculous A18.52
macular H16.11-●
nummular H16.11-●
oyster shuckers' H16.8
parenchymatous —see Keratitis, interstitial
petrificans H16.8
postmeasles B05.81
punctata
leprosa A30.9 [H16.14-●]
syphilitic (profunda) A50.31
punctate H16.14-●
purulent H16.8
rosacea L71.8
sclerosing H16.33-●
specified type NEC H16.8
stellate H16.11-●
striate H16.11-●
superficial H16.10-●
with conjunctivitis —see Keratoconjunctivitis
due to light —see Photokeratitis
suppurative H16.8
syphilitic (congenital) (prenatal) A50.31
trachomatous A71.1
sequelae B94.0
tuberculous A18.52
vesicular H16.8
xerotic —see also Keratomalacia H16.8
vitamin A deficiency E50.4
Keratoacanthoma L85.8
Keratocele —see Descemetocele
Keratoconjunctivitis H16.20-●
Acanthamoeba B60.13
adenoviral B30.0
epidemic B30.0
exposure H16.21-●
herpes, herpetic (simplex) B00.52
zoster B02.33
in exanthema —see also Exanthem B09
infectious B30.0
lagophthalmic —see Keratoconjunctivitis, specified type NEC
neurotrophic H16.23-●
phlyctenular H16.25-●
postmeasles B05.81
shipyard B30.0
sicca (Sjogren's) M35.0-●
not Sjogren's H16.22-●
specified type NEC H16.29-●
tuberculous (phlyctenular) A18.52
vernal H16.26-●
Keratoconus H18.60-●
congenital Q13.4
stable H18.61-●
unstable H18.62-●

Keratocyst (dental) (odontogenic) —see Cyst, calcifying odontogenic
Keratoderma, keratodermia (congenital) (palmaris et plantaris) (symmetrical) Q82.8
acquired L85.1
in diseases classified elsewhere L86
climactericum L85.1
gonococcal A54.89
gonorrheal A54.89
punctata L85.2
Reiter's —see Reiter's disease
Keratodermatocele —see Descemetocele
Keratoglobus H18.79
congenital Q15.8
with glaucoma Q15.0
Keratohemia —see Pigmentation, cornea, stromal
Keratoiritis —see also Iridocyclitis
syphilitic A50.39
tuberculous A18.54
Keratoma L57.0
palmaris and plantaris hereditarium Q82.8
senile L57.0
Keratomalacia H18.44-●
vitamin A deficiency E50.4
Keratomegaly Q13.4
Keratomycosis B49
nigrans, nigricans (palmaris) B36.1
Keratopathy H18.9
band H18.42-●
bullous H18.1-●
bullous (aphakic), following cataract surgery H59.01-●
Keratoscleritis, tuberculous A18.52
Keratosis L57.0
actinic L57.0
arsenical L85.8
congenital, specified NEC Q80.8
female genital NEC N94.89
follicularis Q82.8
acquired L11.0
congenita Q82.8
et parafollicularis in cutem penetrans L87.0
spinulosa (decalvans) Q82.8
vitamin A deficiency E50.8
gonococcal A54.89
male genital (external) N50.89
nigricans L83
obturans, external ear (canal) —see Cholesteatoma, external ear
palmaris et plantaris (inherited) (symmetrical) Q82.8
acquired L85.1
penile N48.89
pharynx J39.2
pilaris, acquired L85.8
punctata (palmaris et plantaris) L85.2
scrotal N50.89
seborrheic L82.1
inflamed L82.0
senile L57.0
solar L57.0
tonsillaris J35.8
vagina N89.4
vegetans Q82.8
vitamin A deficiency E50.8
vocal cord J38.3
Kerato-uveitis —see Iridocyclitis
Kerion (celsi) B35.0
Kernicterus of newborn (not due to isoimmunization) P57.9
due to isoimmunization (conditions in P55.0-P55.9) P57.0
specified type NEC P57.8
Kerunoparalysis T75.09
Keshan disease E59
Ketoacidosis E87.2
diabetic —see Diabetes, by type, with ketoacidosis
Ketonuria R82.4

▶ New   ⇒ Revised   ~~deleted~~ Deleted   ● Use Additional Character(s)

Ketosis NEC E88.89
  diabetic —*see* Diabetes, by type, with
    ketoacidosis
Kew Garden fever A79.1
Kidney —*see* condition
Kienböck's disease —*see also* Osteochondrosis,
    juvenile, hand, carpal lunate
  adult M93.1
Kimmelstiel (-Wilson) disease —*see* Diabetes,
    Kimmelstiel (-Wilson) disease
Kimura disease D21.9
  specified site (*see* Neoplasm, connective
    tissue benign)
Kink, kinking
  artery I77.1
  hair (acquired) L67.8
  ileum or intestine —*see* Obstruction,
    intestine
  Lane's —*see* Obstruction, intestine
  organ or site, congenital NEC —*see* Anomaly,
    by site
  ureter (pelvic junction) N13.5
    with
      hydronephrosis N13.1
        with infection N13.6
      pyelonephritis (chronic) N11.1
    congenital Q62.39
  vein(s) I87.8
    caval I87.1
    peripheral I87.1
Kinnier Wilson's disease (hepatolenticular
    degeneration) E83.01
Kissing spine M48.20
  cervical region M48.22
  cervicothoracic region M48.23
  lumbar region M48.26
  lumbosacral region M48.27
  occipito-atlanto-axial region M48.21
  thoracic region M48.24
  thoracolumbar region M48.25
Klatskin's tumor C24.0
Klauder's disease A26.8
Klebs' disease —*see also* Glomerulonephritis
    N05.-•
Klebsiella (K.) pneumoniae, as cause of
    disease classified elsewhere B96.1
Klein (e)-Levin syndrome G47.13
Kleptomania F63.2
Klinefelter's syndrome Q98.4
  karyotype 47,XXY Q98.0
  male with more than two X chromosomes
    Q98.1
Klippel-Feil deficiency, disease, or syndrome
    (brevicollis) Q76.1
Klippel's disease I67.2
Klippel-Trenaunay (-Weber) syndrome
    Q87.2
Klumpke (-Déjerine) palsy, paralysis (birth)
    (newborn) P14.1
Knee —*see* condition
Knock knee (acquired) M21.06-•
  congenital Q74.1

Knot(s)
  intestinal, syndrome (volvulus) K56.2
    surfer S89.8-•
  umbilical cord (true) O69.2
Knotting (of)
  hair L67.8
  intestine K56.2
Knuckle pad (Garrod's) M72.1
Koch's
  infection —*see* Tuberculosis
  relapsing fever A68.9
Koch-Weeks' conjunctivitis —*see*
    Conjunctivitis, acute, mucopurulent
Köebner's syndrome Q81.8
Köenig's disease (osteochondritis dissecans) —
    see Osteochondritis, dissecans
Köhler-Pellegrini-Steida disease or syndrome
    (calcification, knee joint) —*see* Bursitis,
    tibial collateral
Köhler's disease
  patellar —*see* Osteochondrosis, juvenile,
    patella
  tarsal navicular —*see* Osteochondrosis,
    juvenile, tarsus
Koilonychia L60.3
  congenital Q84.6
Kojevnikov's, epilepsy —*see* Kozhevnikof's
    epilepsy
Koplik's spots B05.9
Kopp's asthma E32.8
Korsakoff's (Wernicke) disease, psychosis or
    syndrome (alcoholic) F10.96
  with dependence F10.26
  drug-induced
    due to drug abuse —*see* Abuse, drug, by
      type, with amnestic disorder
    due to drug dependence —*see* Dependence,
      drug, by type, with amnestic disorder
  nonalcoholic F04
Korsakov's disease, psychosis or syndrome —
    see Korsakoff's disease
Korsakow's disease, psychosis or syndrome —
    see Korsakoff's disease
Kostmann's disease or syndrome (infantile
    genetic agranulocytosis) —*see*
    Agranulocytosis
Kozhevnikof's epilepsy G40.109
  intractable G40.119
    with status epilepticus G40.111
    without status epilepticus G40.119
  not intractable G40.109
    with status epilepticus G40.101
    without status epilepticus G40.109
Krabbe's
  disease E75.23
  syndrome, congenital muscle hypoplasia
    Q79.8
Kraepelin-Morel disease —*see* Schizophrenia
Kraft-Weber-Dimitri disease Q85.8
Kraurosis
  ani K62.89
  penis N48.0

Kraurosis (*Continued*)
  vagina N89.8
  vulva N90.4
Kreotoxism A05.9
Krukenberg's
  spindle —*see* Pigmentation, cornea, posterior
    tumor C79.6-•
Kufs' disease E75.4
Kugelberg-Welander disease G12.1
Kuhnt-Junius degeneration —*see also*
    Degeneration, macula H35.32-•
Kümmell's disease or spondylitis —*see*
    Spondylopathy, traumatic
Kupffer cell sarcoma C22.3
Kuru A81.81
Kussmaul's
  disease M30.0
  respiration E87.2
    in diabetic acidosis —*see* Diabetes, by type,
      with ketoacidosis
Kwashiorkor E40
  marasmic, marasmus type E42
Kyasanur Forest disease A98.2
Kyphoscoliosis, kyphoscoliotic (acquired) —
    see also Scoliosis M41.9
  congenital Q67.5
  heart (disease) I27.1
  sequelae of rickets E64.3
  tuberculous A18.01
Kyphosis, kyphotic (acquired) M40.209
  cervical region M40.202
  cervicothoracic region M40.203
  congenital Q76.419
    cervical region Q76.412
    cervicothoracic region Q76.413
    occipito-atlanto-axial region Q76.411
    thoracic region Q76.414
    thoracolumbar region Q76.415
  Morquio-Brailsford type (spinal) —*see also*
    subcategory M49.8 E76.219
  postlaminectomy M96.3
  postradiation therapy M96.2
  postural (adolescent) M40.00
    cervicothoracic region M40.03
    thoracic region M40.04
    thoracolumbar region M40.05
  secondary NEC M40.10
    cervical region M40.12
    cervicothoracic region M40.13
    thoracic region M40.14
    thoracolumbar region M40.15
  sequelae of rickets E64.3
  specified type NEC M40.299
    cervical region M40.292
    cervicothoracic region M40.293
    thoracic region M40.294
    thoracolumbar region M40.295
  syphilitic, congenital A50.56
  thoracic region M40.204
  thoracolumbar region M40.205
  tuberculous A18.01
Kyrle disease L87.0

L

Labia, labium —*see* condition
Labile
  blood pressure R09.89
  vasomotor system I73.9
Labioglossal paralysis G12.29
Labium leporinum —*see* Cleft, lip
Labor —*see* Delivery
Labored breathing —*see* Hyperventilation
Labyrinthitis (circumscribed) (destructive)
    (diffuse) (inner ear) (latent) (purulent)
    (suppurative) (*see also* subcategory)
    H83.0
  syphilitic A52.79
Laceration
  with abortion —*see* Abortion, by type,
      complicated by laceration of pelvic
      organs
  abdomen, abdominal
    wall S31.119
      with
        foreign body S31.129
        penetration into peritoneal cavity
          S31.619
          with foreign body S31.629
      epigastric region S31.112
        with
          foreign body S31.122
          penetration into peritoneal cavity
            S31.612
            with foreign body S31.622
      left
        lower quadrant S31.114
          with
            foreign body S31.124
            penetration into peritoneal cavity
              S31.614
              with foreign body S31.624
        upper quadrant S31.111
          with
            foreign body S31.121
            penetration into peritoneal cavity
              S31.611
              with foreign body S31.621
      periumbilic region S31.115
        with
          foreign body S31.125
          penetration into peritoneal cavity
            S31.615
            with foreign body S31.625
      right
        lower quadrant S31.113
          with
            foreign body S31.123
            penetration into peritoneal cavity
              S31.613
              with foreign body S31.623
        upper quadrant S31.110
          with
            foreign body S31.120
            penetration into peritoneal cavity
              S31.610
              with foreign body S31.620
  accidental, complicating surgery —*see*
      Complications, surgical, accidental
      puncture or laceration
  Achilles tendon S86.02-●
  adrenal gland S37.813
  alveolar (process) —*see* Laceration, oral cavity
  ankle S91.01-●
    with
      foreign body S91.02-●
  antecubital space —*see* Laceration, elbow
  anus (sphincter) S31.831
    with
      ectopic or molar pregnancy O08.6
      foreign body S31.832
    complicating delivery —*see* Delivery,
        complicated, by, laceration, anus
        (sphincter)

Laceration (*Continued*)
  anus (*Continued*)
    following ectopic or molar pregnancy
      O08.6
    nontraumatic, nonpuerperal —*see* Fissure,
      anus
  arm (upper) S41.11-●
    with foreign body S41.12-●
    lower —*see* Laceration, forearm
  auditory canal (external) (meatus) —*see*
      Laceration, ear
  auricle, ear —*see* Laceration, ear
  axilla —*see* Laceration, arm
  back —*see also* Laceration, thorax, back
    lower S31.010
      with
        foreign body S31.020
          with penetration into
            retroperitoneal space S31.021
          penetration into retroperitoneal space
            S31.011
  bile duct S36.13
  bladder S37.23
    with ectopic or molar pregnancy O08.6
    following ectopic or molar pregnancy
      O08.6
    obstetrical trauma O71.5
  blood vessel —*see* Injury, blood vessel
  bowel —*see also* Laceration, intestine
    with ectopic or molar pregnancy O08.6
    complicating abortion —*see* Abortion,
        by type, complicated by, specified
        condition NEC
    following ectopic or molar pregnancy
      O08.6
    obstetrical trauma O71.5
  brain (any part) (cortex) (diffuse)
      (membrane) —*see also* Injury,
      intracranial, diffuse
    during birth P10.8
      with hemorrhage P10.1
    focal —*see* Injury, intracranial, focal brain
      injury
  brainstem S06.38-●
  breast S21.01-●
    with foreign body S21.02-●
  broad ligament S37.893
    with ectopic or molar pregnancy O08.6
    following ectopic or molar pregnancy
      O08.6
    laceration syndrome N83.8
    obstetrical trauma O71.6
    syndrome (laceration) N83.8
  buttock S31.801
    with foreign body S31.802
    left S31.821
      with foreign body S31.822
    right S31.811
      with foreign body S31.812
  calf —*see* Laceration, leg
  canaliculus lacrimalis —*see* Laceration,
      eyelid
  canthus, eye —*see* Laceration, eyelid
  capsule, joint —*see* Sprain
  causing eversion of cervix uteri (old) N86
  central (perineal), complicating delivery
    O70.9
  cerebellum, traumatic S06.37-●
  cerebral S06.33-●
    during birth P10.8
      with hemorrhage P10.1
    left side S06.32-●
    right side S06.31-●
  cervix (uteri)
    with ectopic or molar pregnancy O08.6
    following ectopic or molar pregnancy
      O08.6
    nonpuerperal, nontraumatic N88.1
    obstetrical trauma (current) O71.3
    old (postpartal) N88.1
    traumatic S37.63

Laceration (*Continued*)
  cheek (external) S01.41-●
    with foreign body S01.42-●
    internal —*see* Laceration, oral cavity
  chest wall —*see* Laceration, thorax
  chin —*see* Laceration, head, specified site
    NEC
  chordae tendinae NEC I51.1
    concurrent with acute myocardial
      infarction —*see* Infarct, myocardium
    following acute myocardial infarction
      (current complication) I23.4
  clitoris —*see* Laceration, vulva
  colon —*see* Laceration, intestine, large,
    colon
  common bile duct S36.13
  cortex (cerebral) —*see* Injury, intracranial,
    diffuse
  costal region —*see* Laceration, thorax
  cystic duct S36.13
  diaphragm S27.803
  digit(s)
    foot —*see* Laceration, toe
    hand —*see* Laceration, finger
  duodenum S36.430
  ear (canal) (external) S01.31-●
    with foreign body S01.32-●
    drum S09.2-●
  elbow S51.01-●
    with
      foreign body S51.02-●
  epididymis —*see* Laceration, testis
  epigastric region —*see* Laceration, abdomen,
    wall, epigastric region
  esophagus K22.8
    traumatic
      cervical S11.21
        with foreign body S11.22
      thoracic S27.813
  eye (ball) S05.3-●
    with prolapse or loss of intraocular tissue
      S05.2-●
    penetrating S05.6-●
  eyebrow —*see* Laceration, eyelid
  eyelid S01.11-●
    with foreign body S01.12-●
  face NEC —*see* Laceration, head, specified
    site NEC
  fallopian tube S37.539
    bilateral S37.532
    unilateral S37.531
  finger(s) S61.219
    with
      damage to nail S61.319
        with
          foreign body S61.329
      foreign body S61.229
    index S61.218
      with
        damage to nail S61.318
          with
            foreign body S61.328
        foreign body S61.228
      left S61.211
        with
          damage to nail S61.311
            with
              foreign body S61.321
          foreign body S61.221
      right S61.210
        with
          damage to nail S61.310
            with
              foreign body S61.320
          foreign body S61.220
    little S61.218
      with
        damage to nail S61.318
          with
            foreign body S61.328
        foreign body S61.228

▶ New   ⇒ Revised   ~~deleted~~ Deleted   ● Use Additional Character(s)

Laceration *(Continued)*
  finger *(Continued)*
    little *(Continued)*
      left S61.217
        with
          damage to nail S61.317
            with
              foreign body S61.327
          foreign body S61.227
      right S61.216
        with
          damage to nail S61.316
            with
              foreign body S61.326
          foreign body S61.226
    middle S61.218
      with
        damage to nail S61.318
          with
            foreign body S61.328
        foreign body S61.228
      left S61.213
        with
          damage to nail S61.313
            with
              foreign body S61.323
          foreign body S61.223
      right S61.212
        with
          damage to nail S61.312
            with
              foreign body S61.322
          foreign body S61.222
    ring S61.218
      with
        damage to nail S61.318
          with
            foreign body S61.328
        foreign body S61.228
      left S61.215
        with
          damage to nail S61.315
            with
              foreign body S61.325
          foreign body S61.225
      right S61.214
        with
          damage to nail S61.314
            with
              foreign body S61.324
          foreign body S61.224
  flank S31.119
    with foreign body S31.129
  foot (except toe(s) alone) S91.319
    with foreign body S91.329
    left S91.312
      with foreign body S91.322
    right S91.311
      with foreign body S91.321
    toe —*see* Laceration, toe
  forearm S51.819
    with
      foreign body S51.829
    elbow only —*see* Laceration,
      elbow
    left S51.812
      with
        foreign body S51.822
    right S51.811
      with
        foreign body S51.821
  forehead S01.81
    with foreign body S01.82
  fourchette O70.0
    with ectopic or molar pregnancy
      O08.6
    complicating delivery O70.0
    following ectopic or molar pregnancy
      O08.6
  gallbladder S36.123

Laceration *(Continued)*
  genital organs, external
    female S31.512
      with foreign body S31.522
      vagina —*see* Laceration, vagina
      vulva —*see* Laceration, vulva
    male S31.511
      with foreign body S31.521
      penis —*see* Laceration, penis
      scrotum —*see* Laceration, scrotum
      testis —*see* Laceration, testis
  groin —*see* Laceration, abdomen, wall
  gum —*see* Laceration, oral cavity
  hand S61.419
    with
      foreign body S61.429
    finger —*see* Laceration, finger
    left S61.412
      with
        foreign body S61.422
    right S61.411
      with
        foreign body S61.421
    thumb —*see* Laceration, thumb
  head S01.91
    with foreign body S01.92
    cheek —*see* Laceration, cheek
    ear —*see* Laceration, ear
    eyelid —*see* Laceration, eyelid
    lip —*see* Laceration, lip
    nose —*see* Laceration, nose
    oral cavity —*see* Laceration, oral
      cavity
    scalp S01.01
      with foreign body S01.02
    specified site NEC S01.81
      with foreign body S01.82
    temporomandibular area —*see* Laceration,
      cheek
  heart —*see* Injury, heart, laceration
  heel —*see* Laceration, foot
  hepatic duct S36.13
  hip S71.019
    with foreign body S71.029
    left S71.012
      with foreign body S71.022
    right S71.011
      with foreign body S71.021
  hymen —*see* Laceration, vagina
  hypochondrium —*see* Laceration, abdomen,
    wall
  hypogastric region —*see* Laceration,
    abdomen, wall
  ileum S36.438
  inguinal region —*see* Laceration, abdomen,
    wall
  instep —*see* Laceration, foot
  internal organ —*see* Injury, by site
  interscapular region —*see* Laceration, thorax,
    back
  intestine
    large
      colon S36.539
        ascending S36.530
        descending S36.532
        sigmoid S36.533
        specified site NEC S36.538
      rectum S36.63
        transverse S36.531
    small S36.439
      duodenum S36.430
      specified site NEC S36.438
  intra-abdominal organ S36.93
    intestine —*see* Laceration, intestine
    liver —*see* Laceration, liver
    pancreas —*see* Laceration, pancreas
    peritoneum S36.81
    specified site NEC S36.893
    spleen —*see* Laceration, spleen
    stomach —*see* Laceration, stomach

Laceration *(Continued)*
  intracranial NEC —*see also* Injury,
    intracranial, diffuse
    birth injury P10.9
  jaw —*see* Laceration, head, specified site NEC
  jejunum S36.438
  joint capsule —*see* Sprain, by site
  kidney S37.03-●
    major (greater than 3 cm) (massive)
      (stellate) S37.06-●
    minor (less than 1 cm) S37.04-●
    moderate (1 to 3 cm) S37.05-●
    multiple S37.06-●
  knee S81.01-●
    with foreign body S81.02-●
  labium (majus) (minus) —*see* Laceration,
    vulva
  lacrimal duct —*see* Laceration, eyelid
  large intestine —*see* Laceration, intestine,
    large
  larynx S11.011
    with foreign body S11.012
  leg (lower) S81.819
    with foreign body S81.829
    foot —*see* Laceration, foot
    knee —*see* Laceration, knee
    left S81.812
      with foreign body S81.822
    right S81.811
      with foreign body S81.821
    upper —*see* Laceration, thigh
  ligament —*see* Sprain
  lip S01.511
    with foreign body S01.521
  liver S36.113
    major (stellate) S36.116
    minor S36.114
    moderate S36.115
  loin —*see* Laceration, abdomen, wall
  lower back —*see* Laceration, back, lower
  lumbar region —*see* Laceration, back, lower
  lung S27.339
    bilateral S27.332
    unilateral S27.331
  malar region —*see* Laceration, head, specified
    site NEC
  mammary —*see* Laceration, breast
  mastoid region —*see* Laceration, head,
    specified site NEC
  meninges —*see* Injury, intracranial, diffuse
  meniscus —*see* Tear, meniscus
  mesentery S36.893
  mesosalpinx S37.893
  mouth —*see* Laceration, oral cavity
  muscle —*see* Injury, muscle, by site,
    laceration
  nail
    finger —*see* Laceration, finger, with
      damage to nail
    toe —*see* Laceration, toe, with damage to nail
  nasal (septum) (sinus) —*see* Laceration, nose
  nasopharynx —*see* Laceration, head, specified
    site NEC
  neck S11.91
    with foreign body S11.92
    involving
      cervical esophagus S11.21
        with foreign body S11.22
      larynx —*see* Laceration, larynx
      pharynx —*see* Laceration, pharynx
      thyroid gland —*see* Laceration, thyroid
        gland
      trachea —*see* Laceration, trachea
    specified site NEC S11.81
      with foreign body S11.82
  nerve —*see* Injury, nerve
  nose (septum) (sinus) S01.21
    with foreign body S01.22
  ocular NOS S05.3-●
    adnexa NOS S01.11-●

Laceration *(Continued)*
  oral cavity S01.512
    with foreign body S01.522
  orbit (eye) —*see* Wound, open, ocular, orbit
  ovary S37.439
    bilateral S37.432
    unilateral S37.431
  palate —*see* Laceration, oral cavity
  palm —*see* Laceration, hand
  pancreas S36.239
    body S36.231
      major S36.261
      minor S36.241
      moderate S36.251
    head S36.230
      major S36.260
      minor S36.240
      moderate S36.250
    major S36.269
    minor S36.249
    moderate S36.259
    tail S36.232
      major S36.262
      minor S36.242
      moderate S36.252
  pelvic S31.010
    with
      foreign body S31.020
        penetration into retroperitoneal cavity S31.021
      penetration into retroperitoneal cavity S31.011
    floor —*see also* Laceration, back, lower
      with ectopic or molar pregnancy O08.6
      complicating delivery O70.1
      following ectopic or molar pregnancy O08.6
      old (postpartal) N81.89
    organ S37.93
      with ectopic or molar pregnancy O08.6
      adrenal gland S37.813
      bladder S37.23
      fallopian tube —*see* Laceration, fallopian tube
      following ectopic or molar pregnancy O08.6
      kidney —*see* Laceration, kidney
      obstetrical trauma O71.5
      ovary —*see* Laceration, ovary
      prostate S37.823
      specified site NEC S37.893
      ureter S37.13
      urethra S37.33
      uterus S37.63
  penis S31.21
    with foreign body S31.22
  perineum
    female S31.41
      with
        ectopic or molar pregnancy O08.6
        foreign body S31.42
      during delivery O70.9
        first degree O70.0
        fourth degree O70.3
        second degree O70.1
        third degree —*see also* Delivery, complicated, by, laceration, perineum, third degree O70.20
      old (postpartal) N81.89
      postpartal N81.89
      secondary (postpartal) O90.1
    male S31.119
      with foreign body S31.129
  periocular area (with or without lacrimal passages) —*see* Laceration, eyelid
  peritoneum S36.893
  periumbilic region —*see* Laceration, abdomen, wall, periumbilic

Laceration *(Continued)*
  periurethral tissue —*see* Laceration, urethra
  phalanges
    finger —*see* Laceration, finger
    toe —*see* Laceration, toe
  pharynx S11.21
    with foreign body S11.22
  pinna —*see* Laceration, ear
  popliteal space —*see* Laceration, knee
  prepuce —*see* Laceration, penis
  prostate S37.823
  pubic region S31.119
    with foreign body S31.129
  pudendum —*see* Laceration, genital organs, external
  rectovaginal septum —*see* Laceration, vagina
  rectum S36.63
  retroperitoneum S36.893
  round ligament S37.893
  sacral region —*see* Laceration, back, lower
  sacroiliac region —*see* Laceration, back, lower
  salivary gland —*see* Laceration, oral cavity
  scalp S01.01
    with foreign body S01.02
  scapular region —*see* Laceration, shoulder
  scrotum S31.31
    with foreign body S31.32
  seminal vesicle S37.893
  shin —*see* Laceration, leg
  shoulder S41.019
    with foreign body S41.029
    left S41.012
      with foreign body S41.022
    right S41.011
      with foreign body S41.021
  small intestine —*see* Laceration, intestine, small
  spermatic cord —*see* Laceration, testis
  spinal cord (meninges) —*see also* Injury, spinal cord, by region
    due to injury at birth P11.5
    newborn (birth injury) P11.5
  spleen S36.039
    major (massive) (stellate) S36.032
    moderate S36.031
    superficial (minor) S36.030
  sternal region —*see* Laceration, thorax, front
  stomach S36.33
  submaxillary region —*see* Laceration, head, specified site NEC
  submental region —*see* Laceration, head, specified site NEC
  subungual
    finger(s) —*see* Laceration, finger, with damage to nail
    toe(s) —*see* Laceration, toe, with damage to nail
  suprarenal gland —*see* Laceration, adrenal gland
  temple, temporal region —*see* Laceration, head, specified site NEC
  temporomandibular area —*see* Laceration, cheek
  tendon —*see* Injury, muscle, by site, laceration
    Achilles S86.02-●
  tentorium cerebelli —*see* Injury, intracranial, diffuse
  testis S31.31
    with foreign body S31.32
  thigh S71.11-●
    with foreign body S71.12-●
  thorax, thoracic (wall) S21.91
    with foreign body S21.92
      back S21.22-●
        with penetration into thoracic cavity S21.42-●
      front S21.12-●
        with penetration into thoracic cavity S21.32-●

Laceration *(Continued)*
  thorax, thoracic *(Continued)*
    back S21.21-●
      with
        foreign body S21.22-●
          with penetration into thoracic cavity S21.42-●
        penetration into thoracic cavity S21.41-●
    breast —*see* Laceration, breast
    front S21.11-●
      with
        foreign body S21.12-●
          with penetration into thoracic cavity S21.32-●
        penetration into thoracic cavity S21.31-●
  thumb S61.019
    with
      damage to nail S61.119
        with foreign body S61.129
      foreign body S61.029
    left S61.012
      with
        damage to nail S61.112
          with foreign body S61.122
        foreign body S61.022
    right S61.011
      with
        damage to nail S61.111
          with foreign body S61.121
        foreign body S61.021
  thyroid gland S11.11
    with foreign body S11.12
  toe(s) S91.119
    with
      damage to nail S91.219
        with foreign body S91.229
      foreign body S91.129
    great S91.113
      with
        damage to nail S91.213
          with foreign body S91.223
        foreign body S91.123
      left S91.112
        with
          damage to nail S91.212
            with foreign body S91.222
          foreign body S91.122
      right S91.111
        with
          damage to nail S91.211
            with foreign body S91.221
          foreign body S91.121
    lesser S91.116
      with
        damage to nail S91.216
          with foreign body S91.226
        foreign body S91.126
      left S91.115
        with
          damage to nail S91.215
            with foreign body S91.225
          foreign body S91.125
      right S91.114
        with
          damage to nail S91.214
            with foreign body S91.224
          foreign body S91.124
  tongue —*see* Laceration, oral cavity

▶ New   ⟹ Revised   ~~deleted~~ Deleted   ● Use Additional Character(s)

Laceration *(Continued)*
  trachea S11.021
    with foreign body S11.022
  tunica vaginalis —*see* Laceration, testis
  tympanum, tympanic membrane —*see*
      Laceration, ear, drum
  umbilical region S31.115
    with foreign body S31.125
  ureter S37.13
  urethra S37.33
    with or following ectopic or molar
        pregnancy O08.6
    obstetrical trauma O71.5
  urinary organ NEC S37.893
  uterus S37.63
    with ectopic or molar pregnancy O08.6
    following ectopic or molar pregnancy O08.6
    nonpuerperal, nontraumatic N85.8
    obstetrical trauma NEC O71.81
    old (postpartal) N85.8
  uvula —*see* Laceration, oral cavity
  vagina S31.41
    with
        ectopic or molar pregnancy O08.6
        foreign body S31.42
    during delivery O71.4
        with perineal laceration —*see* Laceration,
            perineum, female, during delivery
    following ectopic or molar pregnancy
        O08.6
    nonpuerperal, nontraumatic N89.8
    old (postpartal) N89.8
  vas deferens S37.893
  vesical —*see* Laceration, bladder
  vocal cords S11.031
    with foreign body S11.032
  vulva S31.41
    with
        ectopic or molar pregnancy O08.6
        foreign body S31.42
    complicating delivery O70.0
    following ectopic or molar pregnancy
        O08.6
    nonpuerperal, nontraumatic N90.89
    old (postpartal) N90.89
  wrist S61.519
    with
        foreign body S61.529
    left S61.512
        with
            foreign body S61.522
    right S61.511
        with
            foreign body S61.521
Lack of
  achievement in school Z55.3
  adequate
    food Z59.4
    intermaxillary vertical dimension of fully
        erupted teeth M26.36
    sleep Z72.820
  appetite *(see* Anorexia) R63.0
  awareness R41.9
  care
    in home Z74.2
    of infant (at or after birth) T76.02
        confirmed T74.02
  cognitive functions R41.9
  coordination R27.9
    ataxia R27.0
    specified type NEC R27.8
  development (physiological) R62.50
    failure to thrive (child over 28 days old)
        R62.51
        adult R62.7
        newborn P92.6
    short stature R62.52
    specified type NEC R62.59
  energy R53.83
  financial resources Z59.6

Lack of *(Continued)*
  food T73.0
  growth R62.52
  heating Z59.1
  housing (permanent) (temporary) Z59.0
    adequate Z59.1
  learning experiences in childhood Z62.898
  leisure time (affecting life-style) Z73.2
  material resources Z59.9
  memory —*see also* Amnesia
    mild, following organic brain damage
        F06.8
  ovulation N97.0
  parental supervision or control of child Z62.0
  person able to render necessary care Z74.2
  physical exercise Z72.3
  play experience in childhood Z62.898
  posterior occlusal support M26.57
  relaxation (affecting life-style) Z73.2
  sexual
    desire F52.0
    enjoyment F52.1
  shelter Z59.0
  sleep (adequate) Z72.820
  supervision of child by parent Z62.0
  support, posterior occlusal M26.57
  water T73.1
Lacrimal —*see* condition
Lacrimation, abnormal —*see* Epiphora
Lacrimonasal duct —*see* condition
Lactation, lactating (breast) (puerperal,
    postpartum)
  associated
    cracked nipple O92.13
    retracted nipple O92.03
  defective O92.4
  disorder NEC O92.79
  excessive O92.6
  failed (complete) O92.3
    partial O92.4
  mastitis NEC —*see* Mastitis, obstetric
  mother (care and/or examination) Z39.1
  nonpuerperal N64.3
Lacticemia, excessive E87.2
Lacunar skull Q75.8
Laennec's cirrhosis K70.30
  with ascites K70.31
  nonalcoholic K74.69
Lafora's disease —*see* Epilepsy, generalized,
    idiopathic
Lag, lid (nervous) —*see* Retraction, lid
Lagophthalmos (eyelid) (nervous) H02.209
  cicatricial H02.219
    left H02.216
        lower H02.215
        upper H02.214
    right H02.213
        lower H02.212
        upper H02.211
  keratoconjunctivitis —*see* Keratoconjunctivitis
  left H02.206
    lower H02.205
    upper H02.204
  mechanical H02.229
    left H02.226
        lower H02.225
        upper H02.224
    right H02.223
        lower H02.222
        upper H02.221
  paralytic H02.239
    left H02.236
        lower H02.235
        upper H02.234
    right H02.233
        lower H02.232
        upper H02.231
  right H02.203
    lower H02.202
    upper H02.201

Laki-Lorand factor deficiency —*see* Defect,
    coagulation, specified type NEC
Lalling F80.0
Lambert-Eaton syndrome —*see* Syndrome,
    Lambert-Eaton
Lambliasis, lambliosis A07.1
Landau-Kleffner syndrome —*see* Epilepsy,
    specified NEC
Landouzy-Déjérine dystrophy or
    facioscapulohumeral atrophy G71.0
Landouzy's disease (icterohemorrhagic
    leptospirosis) A27.0
Landry-Guillain-Barré, syndrome or paralysis
    G61.0
Landry's disease or paralysis G61.0
Lane's
  band Q43.3
  kink —*see* Obstruction, intestine
  syndrome K90.2
Langdon Down's syndrome —*see* Trisomy, 21
Lapsed immunization schedule status Z28.3
Large
  baby (regardless of gestational age) (4000g to
      4499g) P08.1
  ear, congenital Q17.1
  physiological cup Q14.2
  stature R68.89
Large-for-dates NEC (infant) (4000g to 4499g)
    P08.1
  affecting management of pregnancy O36.6- ●
  exceptionally (4500g or more) P08.0
Larsen-Johansson disease
    orosteochondrosis —*see* Osteochondrosis,
    juvenile, patella
Larsen's syndrome (flattened facies and
    multiple congenital dislocations) Q74.8
Larva migrans
  cutaneous B76.9
    Ancylostoma B76.0
  visceral B83.0
Laryngeal —*see* condition
Laryngismus (stridulus) J38.5
  congenital P28.89
  diphtheritic A36.2
Laryngitis (acute) (edematous) (fibrinous)
    (infective) (infiltrative) (malignant)
    (membranous) (phlegmonous)
    (pneumococcal) (pseudomembranous)
    (septic) (subglottic) (suppurative)
    (ulcerative) J04.0
  with
    influenza, flu, or grippe —*see* Influenza,
        with, laryngitis
    tracheitis (acute) —*see* Laryngotracheitis
  atrophic J37.0
  catarrhal J37.0
  chronic J37.0
    with tracheitis (chronic) J37.1
  diphtheritic A36.2
  due to external agent —*see* Inflammation,
      respiratory, upper, due to
  Hemophilus influenzae J04.0
  H. influenzae J04.0
  hypertrophic J37.0
  influenzal —*see* Influenza, with, respiratory
      manifestations NEC
  obstructive J05.0
  sicca J37.0
  spasmodic J05.0
    acute J04.0
  streptococcal J04.0
  stridulous J05.0
  syphilitic (late) A52.73
    congenital A50.59 *[J99]*
        early A50.03 *[J99]*
  tuberculous A15.5
  Vincent's A69.1
Laryngocele (congenital) (ventricular) Q31.3
Laryngofissure J38.7
  congenital Q31.8
Laryngomalacia (congenital) Q31.5

Laryngopharyngitis (acute) J06.0
  chronic J37.0
  due to external agent —see Inflammation,
    respiratory, upper, due to
Laryngoplegia J38.00
  bilateral J38.02
  unilateral J38.01
Laryngoptosis J38.7
Laryngospasm J38.5
Laryngostenosis J38.6
Laryngotracheitis (acute) (Infectional)
    (infective) (viral) J04.2
  atrophic J37.1
  catarrhal J37.1
  chronic J37.1
  diphtheritic A36.2
  due to external agent —see Inflammation,
    respiratory, upper, due to
  Hemophilus influenzae J04.2
  hypertrophic J37.1
  influenzal —see Influenza, with, respiratory
    manifestations NEC
  pachydermic J38.7
  sicca J37.1
  spasmodic J38.5
    acute J05.0
  streptococcal J04.2
  stridulous J38.5
  syphilitic (late) A52.73
    congenital A50.59 [J99]
    early A50.03 [J99]
  tuberculous A15.5
  Vincent's A69.1
Laryngotracheobronchitis —see Bronchitis
Larynx, laryngeal —see condition
Lassa fever A96.2
Lassitude —see Weakness
Late
  talker R62.0
  walker R62.0
Late effect(s) —see Sequelae
Latent —see condition
Laterocession —see Lateroversion
Lateroflexion —see Lateroversion
Lateroversion
  cervix —see Lateroversion, uterus
  uterus, uterine (cervix) (postinfectional)
    (postpartal, old) N85.4
    congenital Q51.818
    in pregnancy or childbirth O34.59-●
Lathyrism —see Poisoning, food, noxious, plant
Launois' syndrome (pituitary gigantism) E22.0
Launois-Bensaude adenolipomatosis E88.89
Laurence-Moon (-Bardet)-Biedl syndrome
    Q87.89
Lax, laxity —see also Relaxation
  ligament (ous) —see also Disorder, ligament
    familial M35.7
    knee —see Derangement, knee
  skin (acquired) L57.4
    congenital Q82.8
Laxative habit F55.2
Lazy leukocyte syndrome D70.8
Lead miner's lung J63.6
Leak, leakage
  air NEC J93.82
    postprocedural J95.812
  amniotic fluid —see Rupture, membranes,
    premature
  blood (microscopic), fetal, into maternal
    circulation affecting management of
    pregnancy —see Pregnancy, complicated
    by
  cerebrospinal fluid G96.0
    from spinal (lumbar) puncture G97.0
  device, implant or graft —see also
    Complications, by site and type,
    mechanical
    arterial graft NEC —see Complication,
      cardiovascular device, mechanical,
      vascular

Leak, leakage (Continued)
  device, implant or graft (Continued)
    breast (implant) T85.43
    catheter NEC T85.638
      dialysis (renal) T82.43
        intraperitoneal T85.631
      infusion NEC T82.534
        spinal (epidural) (subdural)
          T85.630
      urinary T83.038
        cystostomy T83.030
        Hopkins T83.038
        ileostomy T83.038
        indwelling T83.031
        nephrostomy T83.032
        specified NEC T83.038
        urostomy T83.038
    gastrointestinal —see Complications,
      prosthetic device, mechanical,
      gastrointestinal device
    genital NEC T83.498
      penile prosthesis (cylinder) (implanted)
        (pump) (resevoir) T83.490
      testicular prosthesis T83.491
    heart NEC —see Complication,
      cardiovascular device, mechanical
    joint prosthesis —see Complications, joint
      prosthesis, mechanical, specified NEC,
      by site
    ocular NEC —see Complications,
      prosthetic device, mechanical,
      ocular device
    orthopedic NEC —see Complication,
      orthopedic, device, mechanical
    persistent air J93.82
    specified NEC T85.638
    urinary NEC —see also Complication,
      genitourinary, device, urinary,
      mechanical
      graft T83.23
    vascular NEC —see Complication,
      cardiovascular device, mechanical
    ventricular intracranial shunt T85.03
  urine —see Incontinence
Leaky heart —see Endocarditis
Learning defect (specific) F81.9
Leather bottle stomach C16.9
Leber's
  congenital amaurosis H35.50
  optic atrophy (hereditary) H47.22
Lederer's anemia D59.1
Leeches (external) —see Hirudiniasis
Leg —see condition
Legg (-Calvé)-Perthes disease, syndrome or
    osteochondrosis M91.1-●
Legionellosis A48.1
  nonpneumonic A48.2
Legionnaires'
  disease A48.1
    nonpneumonic A48.2
    pneumonia A48.1
Leigh's disease G31.82
Leiner's disease L21.1
Leiofibromyoma —see Leiomyoma
Leiomyoblastoma —see Neoplasm, connective
    tissue, benign
Leiomyofibroma —see also Neoplasm,
    connective tissue, benign
  uterus (cervix) (corpus) D25.9
Leiomyoma —see also Neoplasm, connective
    tissue, benign
  bizarre —see Neoplasm, connective tissue,
    benign
  cellular —see Neoplasm, connective tissue,
    benign
  epithelioid —see Neoplasm, connective
    tissue, benign
  uterus (cervix) (corpus) D25.9
    intramural D25.1
    submucous D25.0
    subserosal D25.2

Leiomyoma (Continued)
  vascular —see Neoplasm, connective tissue,
    benign
Leiomyoma, leiomyomatosis (intravascular) —
    see Neoplasm, connective tissue, uncertain
    behavior
Leiomyosarcoma —see also Neoplasm,
    connective tissue, malignant
  epithelioid —see Neoplasm, connective
    tissue, malignant
  myxoid —see Neoplasm, connective tissue,
    malignant
Leishmaniasis B55.9
  American (mucocutaneous) B55.2
    cutaneous B55.1
  Asian Desert B55.1
  Brazilian B55.2
  cutaneous (any type) B55.1
  dermal —see also Leishmaniasis, cutaneous
    post-kala-azar B55.0
  eyelid B55.1
  infantile B55.0
  Mediterranean B55.0
  mucocutaneous (American) (New World)
    B55.2
  naso-oral B55.2
  nasopharyngeal B55.2
  old world B55.1
  tegumentaria diffusa B55.1
  visceral B55.0
Leishmanoid, dermal —see also Leishmaniasis,
    cutaneous
  post-kala-azar B55.0
Lenegre's disease I44.2
Lengthening, leg —see Deformity, limb,
    unequal length
Lennert's lymphoma —see Lymphoma,
    Lennert's
Lennox-Gastaut syndrome G40.812
  intractable G40.814
    with status epilepticus G40.813
    without status epilepticus G40.814
  not intractable G40.812
    with status epilepticus G40.811
    without status epilepticus G40.812
Lens —see condition
Lenticonus (anterior) (posterior) (congenital)
    Q12.8
Lenticular degeneration, progressive E83.01
Lentiglobus (posterior) (congenital) Q12.8
Lentigo (congenital) L81.4
  maligna —see also Melanoma, in situ
    melanoma —see Melanoma
Lentivirus, as cause of disease classified
    elsewhere B97.31
Leontiasis
  ossium M85.2
  syphilitic (late) A52.78
    congenital A50.59
Lepothrix A48.8
Lepra —see Leprosy
Leprechaunism E34.8
Leprosy A30.-●
  with muscle disorder A30.9 [M63.80]
    ankle A30.9 [M63.87-●]
    foot A30.9 [M63.87-●]
    forearm A30.9 [M63.83-●]
    hand A30.9 [M63.84-●]
    lower leg A30.9 [M63.86-●]
    multiple sites A30.9 [M63.89]
    pelvic region A30.9 [M63.85-●]
    shoulder region A30.9 [M63.81-●]
    specified site NEC A30.9 [M63.88]
    thigh A30.9 [M63.85-●]
    upper arm A30.9 [M63.82-●]
  anesthetic A30.9
  BB A30.3
  BL A30.4
  borderline (infiltrated) (neuritic) A30.3
    lepromatous A30.4
    tuberculoid A30.2

Lesion *(Continued)*
　ulcerated or ulcerative —*see* Ulcer, skin
　uterus N85.9
　vagus nerve G52.2
　valvular —*see* Endocarditis
　vascular I99.9
　　affecting central nervous system I67.9
　　following trauma NEC T14.8
　　umbilical cord, complicating delivery
　　　O69.5
　warty —*see* Verruca
　white spot (tooth)
　　chewing surface K02.51
　　pit and fissure surface K02.51
　　smooth surface K02.61
Lethargic —*see* condition
Lethargy R53.83
Letterer-Siwe's disease C96.0
Leukemia, leukemic C95.9-●
　acute basophilic C94.8-●
　acute bilineal C95.0-●
　acute erythroid C94.0-●
　acute lymphoblastic C91.0-●
　acute megakaryoblastic C94.2-●
　acute megakaryocytic C94.2-●
　acute mixed lineage C95.0-●
　acute monoblastic (monoblastic/monocytic)
　　C93.0-●
　acute monocytic (monoblastic/monocytic)
　　C93.0-●
　acute myeloblastic (minimal differentiation)
　　(with maturation) C92.0-●
　acute myeloid
　　with
　　　11q23-abnormality C92.6-●
　　　dysplasia of remaining hematopoesis
　　　　and/or myelodysplastic disease in
　　　　its history C92.A-●
　　　multilineage dysplasia C92.A-●
　　　variation of MLL-gene C92.6-●
　　M6 (a)(b) C94.0-●
　　M7 C94.2-●
　acute myelomonocytic C92.5-●
　acute promyelocytic C92.4-●
　adult T-cell (HTLV-1-associated) (acute
　　variant) (chronic variant)
　　(lymphomatoid variant) (smouldering
　　variant) C91.5-●
　aggressive NK-cell C94.8-●
　AML (1/ETO) (M0) (M1) (M2) (without a
　　FAB classification) C92.0-●
　AML M3 C92.4-●
　AML M4 (Eo with inv(16) or t(16;16))
　　C92.5-●
　AML M5 C93.0-●
　AML M5a C93.0-●
　AML M5b C93.0-●
　AML Me with t (15;17) and variants C92.4-●
　atypical chronic myeloid, BCR/ABL-negative
　　C92.2-●
　biphenotypic acute C95.0-●
　blast cell C95.0-●
　Burkitt-type, mature B-cell C91.A-●
　chronic lymphocytic, of B-cell type C91.1-●
　chronic monocytic C93.1-●
　chronic myelogenous (Philadelphia
　　chromosome (Ph1) positive) (t(9;22))
　　(q34;q11) (with crisis of blast cells)
　　C92.1-●
　chronic myeloid, BCR/ABL-positive C92.1-●
　　atypical, BCR/ABL-negative C92.2-●
　chronic myelomonocytic C93.1-●
　chronic neutrophilic D47.1
　CMML (-1) (-2) (with eosinophilia) C93.1-●
　granulocytic —*see also* Category C92 C92.9-●
　hairy-cell C91.4-●
　juvenile myelomonocytic C93.3-●
　lymphoid C91.9-●
　　specified NEC C91.Z-●
　mast cell C94.3-●
　mature B-cell, Burkitt-type C91.A-●

Leukemia, leukemic *(Continued)*
　monocytic (subacute) C93.9-●
　　specified NEC C93.Z-●
　myelogenous —*see also* Category C92 C92.9-●
　myeloid C92.9-●
　　specified NEC C92.Z-●
　plasma cell C90.1-●
　plasmacytic C90.1-●
　prolymphocytic
　　of B-cell type C91.3-●
　　of T-cell type C91.6-●
　specified NEC C94.8-●
　stem cell, of unclear lineage C95.0-●
　subacute lymphocytic C91.9-●
　T-cell large granular lymphocytic C91.Z-●
　unspecified cell type C95.9-●
　　acute C95.0-●
　　chronic C95.1-●
Leukemoid reaction —*see also* Reaction,
　leukemoid D72.823-●
Leukoaraiosis (hypertensive) I67.81
Leukoariosis —*see* Leukoaraiosis
Leukocoria —*see* Disorder, globe, degenerated
　condition, leucocoria
Leukocytopenia D72.819
Leukocytosis D72.829
　eosinophilic D72.1
Leukoderma, leukodermia NEC L81.5
　syphilitic A51.39
　　late A52.79
Leukodystrophy E75.29
Leukoedema, oral epithelium K13.29
Leukoencephalitis G04.81
　acute (subacute) hemorrhagic G36.1
　　postimmunization or postvaccinal G04.02
　postinfectious G04.01
　subacute sclerosing A81.1
　van Bogaert's (sclerosing) A81.1
Leukoencephalopathy —*see also*
　Encephalopathy G93.49
　Binswanger's I67.3
　heroin vapor G92
　metachromatic E75.25
　multifocal (progressive) A81.2
　postimmunization and postvaccinal G04.02
　progressive multifocal A81.2
　reversible, posterior G93.6
　van Bogaert's (sclerosing) A81.1
　vascular, progressive I67.3
Leukoerythroblastosis D75.9
Leukokeratosis —*see also* Leukoplakia
　mouth K13.21
　nicotina palati K13.24
　oral mucosa K13.21
　tongue K13.21
　vocal cord J38.3
Leukokraurosis vulva (e) N90.4
Leukoma (cornea) —*see also* Opacity, cornea
　adherent H17.0-●
　interfering with central vision —*see* Opacity,
　　cornea, central
Leukomalacia, cerebral, newborn P91.2
　periventricular P91.2
Leukomelanopathy, hereditary D72.0
Leukonychia (punctata) (striata) L60.8
　congenital Q84.4
Leukopathia unguium L60.8
　congenital Q84.4
Leukopenia D72.819
　basophilic D72.818
　chemotherapy (cancer) induced D70.1
　congenital D70.0
　cyclic D70.0
　drug induced NEC D70.2
　　due to cytoreductive cancer chemotherapy
　　　D70.1
　eosinophilic D72.818
　familial D70.0
　infantile genetic D70.0
　malignant D70.9
　periodic D70.0
　transitory neonatal P61.5

Leukopenic —*see* condition
Leukoplakia
　anus K62.89
　bladder (postinfectional) N32.89
　buccal K13.21
　cervix (uteri) N88.0
　esophagus K22.8
　gingiva K13.21
　hairy (oral mucosa) (tongue) K13.3
　kidney (pelvis) N28.89
　larynx J38.7
　lip K13.21
　mouth K13.21
　oral epithelium, including tongue (mucosa)
　　K13.21
　palate K13.21
　pelvis (kidney) N28.89
　penis (infectional) N48.0
　rectum K62.89
　syphilitic (late) A52.79
　tongue K13.21
　ureter (postinfectional) N28.89
　urethra (postinfectional) N36.8
　uterus N85.8
　vagina N89.4
　vocal cord J38.3
　vulva N90.4
Leukorrhea N89.8
　due to Trichomonas (vaginalis)
　　A59.00
　trichomonal A59.00
Leukosarcoma C85.9
Levocardia (isolated) Q24.1
　with situs inversus Q89.3
Levotransposition Q20.5
Lev's disease or syndrome (acquired complete
　heart block) I44.2
Levulosuria —*see* Fructosuria
Levurid L30.2
Lewy body (ies) (dementia) (disease)
　G31.83
Leyden-Moebius dystrophy G71.0
Leydig cell
　carcinoma
　　specified site —*see* Neoplasm, malignant,
　　　by site
　　unspecified site
　　　female C56.9-●
　　　male C62.9-●
　tumor
　　benign
　　　specified site —*see* Neoplasm, benign,
　　　　by site
　　　unspecified site
　　　　female D27.-●
　　　　male D29.2-●
　　malignant
　　　specified site —*see* Neoplasm,
　　　　malignant, by site
　　　unspecified site
　　　　female C56.-●
　　　　male C62.9-●
　　specified site —*see* Neoplasm, uncertain
　　　behavior, by site
　　unspecified site
　　　female D39.1-●
　　　male D40.1-●
Leydig-Sertoli cell tumor
　specified site —*see* Neoplasm, benign,
　　by site
　unspecified site
　　female D27.-●
　　male D29.2-●
LGSIL (Low grade squamous intraepithelial
　lesion on cytologic smear of)
　anus R85.612
　cervix R87.612
　vagina R87.622
Liar, pathologic F60.2
Libido
　decreased R68.82

　▶ New　⟹ Revised　~~deleted~~ Deleted　● Use Additional Character(s)

Libman-Sacks disease M32.11
Lice (infestation) B85.2
  body (Pediculus corporis) B85.1
  crab B85.3
  head (Pediculus capitis) B85.0
  mixed (classifiable to more than one of the
      titles B85.0-B85.3) B85.4
  pubic (Phthirus pubis) B85.3
Lichen L28.0
  albus L90.0
    penis N48.0
    vulva N90.4
  amyloidosis E85.4 [L99]
  atrophicus L90.0
    penis N48.0
    vulva N90.4
  congenital Q82.8
  myxedematosus L98.5
  nitidus L44.1
  pilaris Q82.8
    acquired L85.8
  planopilaris L66.1
  planus (chronicus) L43.9
    annularis L43.8
    bullous L43.1
    follicular L66.1
    hypertrophic L43.0
    moniliformis L44.3
    of Wilson L43.9
    specified NEC L43.8
    subacute (active) L43.3
    tropicus L43.3
  ruber
    acuminatus L44.0
    moniliformis L44.3
    planus L43.9
  sclerosus (et atrophicus) L90.0
    penis N48.0
    vulva N90.4
  scrofulosus (primary) (tuberculous) A18.4
  simplex (chronicus) (circumscriptus) L28.0
  striatus L44.2
  urticatus L28.2
Lichenification L28.0
Lichenoides tuberculosis (primary) A18.4
Lichtheim's disease or syndrome —see
    Degeneration, combined
Lien migrans D73.89
Ligament —see condition
Light
  for gestational age —see Light for dates
  headedness R42
Light-for-dates (infant) P05.00
  with weight of
    499 grams or less P05.01
    500-749 grams P05.02
    750-999 grams P05.03
    1000-1249 grams P05.04
    1250-1499 grams P05.05
    1500-1749 grams P05.06
    1750-1999 grams P05.07
    2000-2499 grams P05.08
    2500 grams and over P05.09
  affecting management of pregnancy O36.59-●
  and small-for-dates —see Small for dates
  specified NEC P05.09
Lightning (effects) (stroke) (struck by) T75.00
  burn —see Burn
  foot E53.8
  shock T75.01
  specified effect NEC T75.09
Lightwood-Albright syndrome N25.89
Lightwood's disease or syndrome (renal
    tubular acidosis) N25.89
Lignac (-de Toni) (-Fanconi) (-Debré) disease or
    syndrome E72.09
  with cystinosis E72.04
Ligneous thyroiditis E06.5
Likoff's syndrome I20.8
Limb —see condition
Limbic epilepsy personality syndrome F07.0

Limitation, limited
  activities due to disability Z73.6
  cardiac reserve —see Disease, heart
  eye muscle duction, traumatic —see
      Strabismus, mechanical
  mandibular range of motion M26.52
Lindau (-von Hippel) disease Q85.8
Line(s)
  Beau's L60.4
  Harris' —see Arrest, epiphyseal
  Hudson's (cornea) —see Pigmentation,
      cornea, anterior
  Stähli's (cornea) —see Pigmentation, cornea,
      anterior
Linea corneae senilis —see Change, cornea,
    senile
Lingua
  geographica K14.1
  nigra (villosa) K14.3
  plicata K14.5
  tylosis K13.29
Lingual —see condition
Linguatulosis B88.8
Linitis (gastric) plastica C16.9
Lip —see condition
Lipedema —see Edema
Lipemia —see also Hyperlipidemia
  retina, retinalis E78.3
Lipidosis E75.6
  cerebral (infantile) (juvenile) (late) E75.4
  cerebroretinal E75.4
  cerebroside E75.22
  cholesterol (cerebral) E75.5
  glycolipid E75.21
  hepatosplenomegalic E78.3
  sphingomyelin —see Niemann-Pick disease
      or syndrome
  sulfatide E75.29
Lipoadenoma —see Neoplasm, benign, by site
Lipoblastoma —see Lipoma
Lipoblastomatosis —see Lipoma
Lipochondrodystrophy E76.01
Lipochrome histiocytosis (familial) D71
Lipodermatosclerosis —see Varix, leg, with,
    inflammation
  ulcerated —see Varix, leg, with, ulcer, with
      inflammation by site
Lipodystrophia progressiva E88.1
Lipodystrophy (progressive) E88.1
  insulin E88.1
  intestinal K90.81
  mesenteric K65.4
Lipofibroma —see Lipoma
Lipofuscinosis, neuronal (with ceroidosis)
    E75.4
Lipogranuloma, sclerosing L92.8
Lipogranulomatosis E78.89
Lipoid —see also condition
  histiocytosis D76.3
    essential E75.29
  nephrosis N04.9
  proteinosis of Urbach E78.89
Lipoidemia —see Hyperlipidemia
Lipoidosis —see Lipidosis
Lipoma D17.9
  fetal D17.9
  fat cell D17.9
  infiltrating D17.9
  intramuscular D17.9
  pleomorphic D17.9
  site classification
    arms (skin) (subcutaneous) D17.2-●
    connective tissue D17.30
      intra-abdominal D17.5
      intrathoracic D17.4
      peritoneum D17.79
      retroperitoneum D17.79
      specified site NEC D17.39
      spermatic cord D17.6
    face (skin) (subcutaneous) D17.0
    genitourinary organ NEC D17.72

Lipoma (Continued)
  site classification (Continued)
    head (skin) (subcutaneous) D17.0
    intra-abdominal D17.5
    intrathoracic D17.4
    kidney D17.71
    legs (skin) (subcutaneous) D17.2-●
    neck (skin) (subcutaneous) D17.0
    peritoneum D17.79
    retroperitoneum D17.79
    skin D17.30
      specified site NEC D17.39
    specified site NEC D17.79
    spermatic cord D17.6
    subcutaneous D17.30
      specified site NEC D17.39
    trunk (skin) (subcutaneous) D17.1
    unspecified D17.9
  spindle cell D17.9
Lipomatosis E88.2
  dolorosa (Dercum) E88.2
  fetal —see Lipoma
  Launois-Bensaude E88.89
Lipomyoma —see Lipoma
Lipomyxoma —see Lipoma
Lipomyxosarcoma —see Neoplasm, connective
    tissue, malignant
Lipoprotein metabolism disorder E78.9
Lipoproteinemia E78.5
  broad-beta E78.2
  floating-beta E78.2
  hyper-pre-beta E78.1
Liposarcoma —see also Neoplasm, connective
    tissue, malignant
  dedifferentiated —see Neoplasm, connective
      tissue, malignant
  differentiated type —see Neoplasm,
      connective tissue, malignant
  embryonal —see Neoplasm, connective tissue,
      malignant
  mixed type —see Neoplasm, connective
      tissue, malignant
  myxoid —see Neoplasm, connective tissue,
      malignant
  pleomorphic —see Neoplasm, connective
      tissue, malignant
  round cell —see Neoplasm, connective tissue,
      malignant
  well differentiated type —see Neoplasm,
      connective tissue, malignant
Liposynovitis prepatellaris E88.89
Lipping, cervix N86
Lipschütz disease or ulcer N76.6
Lipuria R82.0
  schistosomiasis (bilharziasis) B65.0
Lisping F80.0
Lissauer's paralysis A52.17
Lissencephalia, lissencephaly Q04.3
Listeriosis, listerellosis A32.9
  congenital (disseminated) P37.2
  cutaneous A32.0
  neonatal, newborn (disseminated) P37.2
  oculoglandular A32.81
  specified NEC A32.89
Lithemia E79.0
Lithiasis —see Calculus
Lithosis J62.8
Lithuria R82.99
Litigation, anxiety concerning Z65.3
Little leaguer's elbow —see Epicondylitis,
    medial
Little's disease G80.9
Littre's
  gland —see condition
  hernia —see Hernia, abdomen
Littritis —see Urethritis
Livedo (annularis) (racemosa) (reticularis)
    R23.1
Liver —see condition
Living alone (problems with) Z60.2
  with handicapped person Z74.2

Lloyd's syndrome —*see* Adenomatosis,
    endocrine
Loa loa, loaiasis, loasis B74.3
Lobar —*see* condition
Lobomycosis B48.0
Lobo's disease B48.0
Lobotomy syndrome F07.0
Lobstein (-Ekman) disease or syndrome Q78.0
Lobster-claw hand Q71.6-●
Lobulation (congenital) —*see also* Anomaly,
    by site
  kidney, Q63.1
  liver, abnormal Q44.7
  spleen Q89.09
Lobule, lobular —*see* condition
Local, localized —*see* condition
Locked twins causing obstructed labor
    O66.1
Locked-in state G83.5
Locking
  joint —*see* Derangement, joint, specified type
    NEC
    knee —*see* Derangement, knee
Lockjaw —*see* Tetanus
Löffler's
  endocarditis I42.3
  eosinophilia J82
  pneumonia J82
  syndrome (eosinophilic pneumonitis) J82
Loiasis (with conjunctival infestation) (eyelid)
    B74.3
Lone Star fever A77.0
Long
  labor O63.9
    first stage O63.0
    second stage O63.1
  QT syndrome I45.81
Long-term (current) (prophylactic) drug
    therapy (use of)
  agents affecting estrogen receptors and
    estrogen levels NEC Z79.818
  anastrozole (Arimidex) Z79.811
  antibiotics Z79.2
    short-term use - omit code
  anticoagulants Z79.01
  anti-inflammatory, non-steroidal (NSAID)
    Z79.1
  antiplatelet Z79.02
  antithrombotics Z79.02
  aromatase inhibitors Z79.811
  aspirin Z79.82
  birth control pill or patch Z79.3
  bisphosphonates Z79.83
  contraceptive, oral Z79.3
  drug, specified NEC Z79.899
  estrogen receptor downregulators Z79.818
  Evista Z79.810
  exemestane (Aromasin) Z79.811
  Fareston Z79.810
  fulvestrant (Faslodex) Z79.818
  gonadotropin-releasing hormone (GnRH)
    agonist Z79.818
  goserelin acetate (Zoladex) Z79.818
➡ hormone replacement Z79.890
  insulin Z79.4
  letrozole (Femara) Z79.811
  leuprolide acetate (leuprorelin) (Lupron)
    Z79.818
  megestrol acetate (Megace) Z79.818
  methadone for pain management Z79.891
  Nolvadex Z79.810
  non-steroidal anti-inflammatories (NSAID)
    Z79.1
  opiate analgesic Z79.891
  oral
    antidiabetic Z79.84
    contraceptive Z79.3
    hypoglycemic Z79.84
  raloxifene (Evista) Z79.810
  selective estrogen receptor modulators
    (SERMs) Z79.810

Long-term (*Continued*)
  steroids
    inhaled Z79.51
    systemic Z79.52
  tamoxifen (Nolvadex) Z79.810
  toremifene (Fareston) Z79.810
Longitudinal stripes or grooves, nails L60.8
  congenital Q84.6
Loop
  intestine —*see* Volvulus
  vascular on papilla (optic) Q14.2
Loose —*see also* condition
  body
    joint M24.00
      ankle M24.07-●
      elbow M24.02-●
      hand M24.04-●
      hip M24.05-●
      knee M23.4-●
      shoulder (region) M24.01-●
      specified site NEC M24.08
      toe M24.07-●
      vertebra M24.08
      wrist M24.03-●
    knee M23.4-●
    sheath, tendon —*see* Disorder, tendon,
      specified type NEC
  cartilage —*see* Loose, body, joint
  skin and subcutaneous tissue (following
    bariatric surgery weight loss) (following
    dietary weight loss) L98.7
  tooth, teeth K08.89
Loosening
  aseptic
    joint prosthesis —*see* Complications, joint
      prosthesis, mechanical, loosening,
      by site
    epiphysis —*see* Osteochondropathy
  mechanical
    joint prosthesis —*see* Complications, joint
      prosthesis, mechanical, loosening,
      by site
Looser-Milkman (-Debray) **syndrome** M83.8
Lop ear (deformity) Q17.3
Lorain (-Levi) **short stature syndrome** E23.0
Lordosis M40.50
  acquired —*see* Lordosis, specified type NEC
  congenital Q76.429
    lumbar region Q76.426
    lumbosacral region Q76.427
    sacral region Q76.428
    sacrococcygeal region Q76.428
    thoracolumbar region Q76.425
  lumbar region M40.56
  lumbosacral region M40.57
  postsurgical M96.4
  postural —*see* Lordosis, specified type NEC
  rachitic (late effect) (sequelae) E64.3
  sequelae of rickets E64.3
  specified type NEC M40.40
    lumbar region M40.46
    lumbosacral region M40.47
    thoracolumbar region M40.45
  thoracolumbar region M40.55
  tuberculous A18.01
Loss (of)
  appetite (*see* Anorexia) R63.0
    hysterical F50.89
    nonorganic origin F50.89
    psychogenic F50.89
  blood —*see* Hemorrhage
  bone —*see* Loss, substance of, bone
  consciousness, transient R55
    traumatic —*see* Injury, intracranial
  control, sphincter, rectum R15.9
    nonorganic origin F98.1
  elasticity, skin R23.4
  family (member) in childhood Z62.898
  fluid (acute) E86.9
  function of labyrinth —*see* subcategory H83.2
  hair, nonscarring —*see* Alopecia

Loss (*Continued*)
  hearing —*see also* Deafness
    central NOS H90.5
    conductive H90.2
      bilateral H90.0
      unilateral
        with
          restricted hearing on the
            contralateral side H90.A1-●
          unrestricted hearing on the
            contralateral side H90.1-●
    mixed conductive and sensorineural
      hearing loss H90.8
      bilateral H90.6
      unilateral
        with
          restricted hearing on the
            contralateral side H90.A3-●
          unrestricted hearing on the
            contralateral side H90.7-●
    neural NOS H90.5
    perceptive NOS H90.5
    sensorineural NOS H90.5
      bilateral H90.3
      unilateral
        with
          restricted hearing on the
            contralateral side H90.A2-●
          unrestricted hearing on the
            contralateral side H90.4-●
    sensory NOS H90.5
  height R29.890
  limb or member, traumatic, current —*see*
    Amputation, traumatic
  love relationship in childhood Z62.898
  memory —*see also* Amnesia
    mild, following organic brain damage
      F06.8
  mind —*see* Psychosis
  occlusal vertical dimension of fully erupted
    teeth M26.37
  organ or part —*see* Absence, by site, acquired
  ossicles, ear (partial) H74.32-●
  parent in childhood Z63.4
  pregnancy, recurrent N96
    without current pregnancy N96
    care in current pregnancy O26.2-●
  recurrent pregnancy —*see* Loss, pregnancy,
    recurrent
  self-esteem, in childhood Z62.898
  sense of
    smell —*see* Disturbance, sensation, smell
    taste —*see* Disturbance, sensation, taste
    touch R20.8
  sensory R44.9
    dissociative F44.6
  sexual desire F52.0
  sight (acquired) (complete) (congenital) —*see*
    Blindness
  substance of
    bone —*see* Disorder, bone, density and
      structure, specified NEC
      horizontal alveolar K06.3
    cartilage —*see* Disorder, cartilage, specified
      type NEC
      auricle (ear) —*see* Disorder, pinna,
        specified type NEC
    vitreous (humor) H15.89
  tooth, teeth —*see* Absence, teeth, acquired
  vision, visual H54.7
    both eyes H54.3
    one eye H54.60
      left (normal vision on right) H54.62
      right (normal vision on left) H54.61
    specified as blindness —*see* Blindness
    subjective
      sudden H53.13-●
      transient H53.12-●
  vitreous —*see* Prolapse, vitreous
  voice —*see* Aphonia
  weight (abnormal) (cause unknown) R63.4

Louis-Bar syndrome (ataxia-telangiectasia) G11.3
Louping ill (encephalitis) A84.8
Louse, lousiness —see Lice
Low
  achiever, school Z55.3
  back syndrome M54.5
  basal metabolic rate R94.8
  birthweight (2499 grams or less) P07.10
    with weight of
      1000-1249 grams P07.14
      1250-1499 grams P07.15
      1500-1749 grams P07.16
      1750-1999 grams P07.17
      2000-2499 grams P07.18
    extreme (999 grams or less) P07.00
      with weight of
        499 grams or less P07.01
        500-749 grams P07.02
        750-999 grams P07.03
    for gestational age —see Light for dates
  blood pressure —see also Hypotension
    reading (incidental) (isolated) (nonspecific) R03.1
  cardiac reserve —see Disease, heart
  function —see also Hypofunction
    kidney N28.9
  hematocrit D64.9
  hemoglobin D64.9
  income Z59.6
  level of literacy Z55.0
  lying
    kidney N28.89
    organ or site, congenital —see Malposition, congenital
  output syndrome (cardiac) —see Failure, heart
  platelets (blood) —see Thrombocytopenia
  reserve, kidney N28.89
  salt syndrome E87.1
  self esteem R45.81
  set ears Q17.4
  vision H54.2X-
    one eye (other eye normal) H54.50
      left (normal vision on right) H54.52A-
      other eye blind —see Blindness
      right (normal vision on left) H54.511-
Low-density-lipoprotein-type (LDL) hyperlipoproteinemia E78.00
Lowe's syndrome E72.03
Lown-Ganong-Levine syndrome I45.6
LSD reaction (acute) (without dependence) F16.90
  with dependence F16.20
L-shaped kidney Q63.8
Ludwig's angina or disease K12.2
Lues (venerea), luetic —see Syphilis
Luetscher's syndrome (dehydration) E86.0
Lumbago, lumbalgia M54.5
  with sciatica M54.4-●
    due to intervertebral disc disorder M51.17
  due to displacement, intervertebral disc M51.27
    with sciatica M51.17
Lumbar —see condition
Lumbarization, vertebra, congenital Q76.49
Lumbermen's itch B88.0
Lump —see also Mass
  breast N63.0
    axillary tail
      left N63.32
      right N63.31
    left
      lower inner quadrant N63.24
      lower outer quadrant N63.23
      unspecified quadrant N63.20
      upper inner quadrant N63.22
      upper outer quadrant N63.21
    right
      lower inner quadrant N63.14
      lower outer quadrant N63.13

Lump (Continued)
  breast (Continued)
    right (Continued)
      unspecified quadrant N63.10
      upper inner quadrant N63.12
      upper outer quadrant N63.11
    subareolar
      left N63.42
      right N63.41
Lunacy —see Psychosis
Lung —see condition
Lupoid (miliary) of Boeck D86.3
Lupus
  anticoagulant D68.62
    with
      hemorrhagic disorder D68.312
      hypercoagulable state D68.62
    finding without diagnosis R76.0
  discoid (local) L93.0
  erythematosus (discoid) (local) L93.0
    disseminated —see Lupus, erythematosus, systemic
    eyelid H01.129
      left H01.126
        lower H01.125
        upper H01.124
      right H01.123
        lower H01.122
        upper H01.121
    profundus L93.2
    specified NEC L93.2
    subacute cutaneous L93.1
    systemic M32.9
      with organ or system involvement M32.10
        endocarditis M32.11
        lung M32.13
        pericarditis M32.12
        renal (glomerular) M32.14
          tubulo-interstitial M32.15
        specified organ or system NEC M32.19
      drug-induced M32.0
      inhibitor (presence of) D68.62
        with
          hemorrhagic disorder D68.312
          hypercoagulable state D68.62
        finding without diagnosis R76.0
      specified NEC M32.8
  exedens A18.4
  hydralazine M32.0
    correct substance properly administered —see Table of Drugs and Chemicals, by drug, adverse effect
    overdose or wrong substance given or taken —see Table of Drugs and Chemicals, by drug, poisoning
  nephritis (chronic) M32.14
  nontuberculous, not disseminated L93.0
  panniculitis L93.2
  pernio (Besnier) D86.3
  systemic —see Lupus, erythematosus, systemic
  tuberculous A18.4
    eyelid A18.4
  vulgaris A18.4
    eyelid A18.4
Luteinoma D27.-●
Lutembacher's disease or syndrome (atrial septal defect with mitral stenosis) Q21.1
Luteoma D27.-●
Lutz (-Splendore-de Almeida) disease —see Paracoccidioidomycosis
Luxation —see also Dislocation
  eyeball (nontraumatic) —see Luxation, globe
    birth injury P15.3
  globe, nontraumatic H44.82-●
  lacrimal gland —see Dislocation, lacrimal gland
  lens (old) (partial) (spontaneous)
    congenital Q12.1
      syphilitic A50.39

Lycanthropy F22
Lyell's syndrome L51.2
  due to drug L51.2
    correct substance properly administered —see Table of Drugs and Chemicals, by drug, adverse effect
    overdose or wrong substance given or taken —see Table of Drugs and Chemicals, by drug, poisoning
Lyme disease A69.20
Lymph
  gland or node —see condition
  scrotum —see Infestation, filarial
Lymphadenitis I88.9
  with ectopic or molar pregnancy O08.0
  acute L04.9
    axilla L04.2
    face L04.0
    head L04.0
    hip L04.3
    limb
      lower L04.3
      upper L04.2
    neck L04.0
    shoulder L04.2
    specified site NEC L04.8
    trunk L04.1
  anthracosis (occupational) J60
  any site, except mesenteric I88.9
    chronic I88.1
    subacute I88.1
  breast
    gestational —see Mastitis, obstetric
    puerperal, postpartum (nonpurulent) O91.22
  chancroidal (congenital) A57
  chronic I88.1
    mesenteric I88.0
  due to
    Brugia (malayi) B74.1
      timori B74.2
    chlamydial lymphogranuloma A55
    diphtheria (toxin) A36.89
    lymphogranuloma venereum A55
    Wuchereria bancrofti B74.0
  following ectopic or molar pregnancy O08.0
  gonorrheal A54.89
  infective —see Lymphadenitis, acute
  mesenteric (acute) (chronic) (nonspecific) (subacute) I88.0
    due to Salmonella typhi A01.09
    tuberculous A18.39
  mycobacterial A31.8
  purulent —see Lymphadenitis, acute
  pyogenic —see Lymphadenitis, acute
  regional, nonbacterial I88.8
  septic —see Lymphadenitis, acute
  subacute, unspecified site I88.1
  suppurative —see Lymphadenitis, acute
  syphilitic (early) (secondary) A51.49
    late A52.79
  tuberculous —see Tuberculosis, lymph gland
  venereal (chlamydial) A55
Lymphadenoid goiter E06.3
Lymphadenopathy (generalized) R59.1
  angioimmunoblastic, with dysproteinemia (AILD) C86.5
  due to toxoplasmosis (acquired) B58.89
    congenital (acute) (subacute) (chronic) P37.1
  localized R59.0
  syphilitic (early) (secondary) A51.49
Lymphadenosis R59.1
Lymphangiectasis I89.0
  conjunctiva H11.89
  postinfectional I89.0
  scrotum I89.0
Lymphangiectatic elephantiasis, nonfilarial I89.0
Lymphangioendothelioma D18.1
  malignant —see Neoplasm, connective tissue, malignant
Lymphangioleiomyomatosis J84.81

Lymphoma *(Continued)*
    SALT C88.4
    skin-associated lymphoid tissue
            [SALT-lymphoma] C88.4
    small cell B-cell C83.Ø-•
    splenic marginal zone C83.Ø-•
    subcutaneous panniculitis-like T-cell C86.3
    T-precursor C83.5-•
    true histiocytic C96.A

Lymphomatosis —*see* Lymphoma
Lymphopathia venereum, veneris A55
Lymphopenia D72.81Ø
Lymphoplasmacytic leukemia —*see* Leukemia,
        chronic lymphocytic, B-cell type
Lymphoproliferation, X-linked disease D82.3
Lymphoreticulosis, benign (of inoculation)
        A28.1

Lymphorrhea I89.8
Lymphosarcoma (diffuse) —*see also* Lymphoma
        C85.9-•
Lymphostasis I89.8
Lypemania —*see* Melancholia
Lysine and hydroxylysine metabolism
        disorder E72.3
Lyssa —*see* Rabies

M

Macacus ear Q17.3
Maceration, wet feet, tropical (syndrome)
T69.02-•
MacLeod's syndrome J43.0
Macrocephalia, macrocephaly Q75.3
Macrocheilia, macrochilia (congenital)Q18.6
Macrocolon —see also Megacolon Q43.1
Macrocornea Q15.8
  with glaucoma Q15.0
Macrocytic —see condition
Macrocytosis D75.89
Macrodactylia, macrodactylism (fingers)
    (thumbs) Q74.0
  toes Q74.2
Macrodontia K00.2
Macrogenia M26.05
Macrogenitosomia (adrenal) (male) (praecox)
    E25.9
  congenital E25.0
Macroglobulinemia (idiopathic) (primary)
    C88.0
  monoclonal (essential) D47.2
  Waldenström C88.0
Macroglossia (congenital) Q38.2
  acquired K14.8
Macrognathia, macrognathism (congenital)
    (mandibular) (maxillary) M26.09
Macrogyria (congenital) Q04.8
Macrohydrocephalus —see Hydrocephalus
Macromastia —see Hypertrophy, breast
Macrophthalmos Q11.3
  in congenital glaucoma Q15.0
Macropsia H53.15
Macrosigmoid K59.39
  congenital Q43.2
Macrospondylitis, acromegalic E22.0
Macrostomia (congenital) Q18.4
Macrotia (external ear) (congenital) Q17.1
Macula
  cornea, corneal —see Opacity, cornea
  degeneration (atrophic) (exudative)
      (senile) —see also Degeneration, macula
    hereditary —see Dystrophy, retina
Maculae ceruleae — B85.1
Maculopathy, toxic —see Degeneration, macula,
    toxic
Madarosis (eyelid) H02.729
  left H02.726
    lower H02.725
    upper H02.724
  right H02.723
    lower H02.722
    upper H02.721
Madelung's
  deformity (radius) Q74.0
  disease
    radial deformity Q74.0
    symmetrical lipomas, neck E88.89
Madness —see Psychosis
Madura
  foot B47.9
    actinomycotic B47.1
    mycotic B47.0
Maduromycosis B47.0
Maffucci's syndrome Q78.4
Magnesium metabolism disorder —see
    Disorder, metabolism, magnesium
Main en griffe (acquired) —see also Deformity,
    limb, clawhand
  congenital Q74.0
Maintenance (encounter for)
  antineoplastic chemotherapy Z51.11
  antineoplastic radiation therapy Z51.0
  methadone F11.20
Majocchi's
  disease L81.7
  granuloma B35.8
Major —see condition
Malabar itch (any site) B35.5

Malabsorption K90.9
  calcium K90.89
  carbohydrate K90.49
  disaccharide E73.9
  fat K90.49
  galactose E74.20
  glucose(-galactose) E74.39
  intestinal K90.9
    specified NEC K90.89
  isomaltose E74.31
  lactose E73.9
  methionine E72.19
  monosaccharide E74.39
  postgastrectomy K91.2
  postsurgical K91.2
  protein K90.49
  starch K90.49
  sucrose E74.39
  syndrome K90.9
    postsurgical K91.2
Malacia, bone (adult) M83.9
  juvenile —see Rickets
Malacoplakia
  bladder N32.89
  pelvis (kidney) N28.89
  ureter N28.89
  urethra N36.8
Malacosteon, juvenile —see Rickets
Maladaptation —see Maladjustment
Maladie de Roger Q21.0
Maladjustment
  conjugal Z63.0
    involving divorce or estrangement Z63.5
  educational Z55.4
  family Z63.9
  marital Z63.0
    involving divorce or estrangement Z63.5
  occupational NEC Z56.89
  simple, adult —see Disorder, adjustment
  situational —see Disorder, adjustment
  social Z60.9
    due to
      acculturation difficulty Z60.3
      discrimination and persecution
          (perceived) Z60.5
      exclusion and isolation Z60.4
      life-cycle (phase of life) transition Z60.0
      rejection Z60.4
      specified reason NEC Z60.8
Malaise R53.81
Malakoplakia —see Malacoplakia
Malaria, malarial (fever) B54
  with
    blackwater fever B50.8
      hemoglobinuric (bilious) B50.8
      hemoglobinuria B50.8
    accidentally induced (therapeutically) - code
        by type under Malaria
  algid B50.9
  cerebral B50.0 [G94]
  clinically diagnosed (without parasitological
      confirmation) B54
  congenital NEC P37.4
    falciparum P37.3
  congestion, congestive B54
  continued (fever) B50.9
  estivo-autumnal B50.9
  falciparum B50.9
    with complications NEC B50.8
      cerebral B50.0 [G94]
      severe B50.8
  hemorrhagic B54
  malariae B52.9
    with
      complications NEC B52.8
      glomerular disorder B52.0
  malignant (tertian) —see Malaria, falciparum
  mixed infections — code to first listed type
      in B50-B53
  ovale B53.0
  parasitologically confirmed NEC B53.8

Malaria, malarial (Continued)
  pernicious, acute —see Malaria, falciparum
  Plasmodium (P.)
    falciparum NEC —see Malaria, falciparum
    malariae NEC B52.9
      with Plasmodium
        falciparum (and or vivax) —see
            Malaria, falciparum
        vivax —see also Malaria, vivax
            and falciparum —see Malaria,
            falciparum
    ovale B53.0
      with Plasmodium malariae —see also
          Malaria, malariae
        and vivax —see also Malaria, vivax
            and falciparum —see Malaria,
            falciparum
    simian B53.1
      with Plasmodium malariae —see also
          Malaria, malariae
        and vivax —see also Malaria, vivax
            and falciparum —see Malaria,
            falciparum
    vivax NEC B51.9
      with Plasmodium falciparum —see
          Malaria, falciparum
  quartan —see Malaria, malariae
  quotidian —see Malaria, falciparum
  recurrent B54
  remittent B54
  specified type NEC (parasitologically
      confirmed) B53.8
  spleen B54
  subtertian (fever) —see Malaria, falciparum
  tertian (benign) —see also Malaria, vivax
    malignant B50.9
  tropical B50.9
  typhoid B54
  vivax B51.9
    with
      complications NEC B51.8
      ruptured spleen B51.0
Malassez's disease (cystic) N50.89
Malassimilation K90.9
Mal de los pintos —see Pinta
Mal de mer T75.3
Maldescent, testis Q53.9
  bilateral Q53.20
    ➡abdominal Q53.211
    perineal Q53.22
  unilateral Q53.10
    ➡abdominal Q53.111
    perineal Q53.12
Maldevelopment —see also Anomaly
  brain Q07.9
  colon Q43.9
  hip Q74.2
    congenital dislocation Q65.2
      bilateral Q65.1
      unilateral Q65.0-•
  mastoid process Q75.8
  middle ear Q16.4
    except ossicles Q16.4
    ossicles Q16.3
  ossicles Q16.3
  spine Q76.49
  toe Q74.2
Male type pelvis Q74.2
  with disproportion (fetopelvic) O33.3
    causing obstructed labor O65.3
Malformation (congenital) —see also Anomaly
  adrenal gland Q89.1
  affecting multiple systems with skeletal
      changes NEC Q87.5
  alimentary tract Q45.9
    specified type NEC Q45.8
    upper Q40.9
      specified type NEC Q40.8
  aorta Q25.40
    absence Q25.41
    aneurysm, congenital Q25.43

▶ New   ➡ Revised   ~~deleted~~ Deleted   • Use Additional Character(s)

Malformation *(Continued)*
  aorta *(Continued)*
    aplasia Q25.41
    atresia Q25.29
      aortic arch Q25.21
    coarctation (preductal) (postductal) Q25.1
    dilatation, congenital Q25.44
    hypoplasia Q25.42
    patent ductus arteriosus Q25.0
    specified type NEC Q25.49
    stenosis Q25.1
      supravalvular Q25.3
  aortic valve Q23.9
    specified NEC Q23.8
  arteriovenous, aneurysmatic (congenital) Q27.30
    brain Q28.2
    cerebral Q28.2
    peripheral Q27.30
      digestive system Q27.33
      lower limb Q27.32
      other specified site Q27.39
      renal vessel Q27.34
      upper limb Q27.31
    precerebral vessels (nonruptured) Q28.0
  auricle
    ear (congenital) Q17.3
      acquired H61.119
        left H61.112
          with right H61.113
        right H61.111
          with left H61.113
  bile duct Q44.5
  bladder Q64.79
    aplasia Q64.5
    diverticulum Q64.6
    exstrophy —*see* Exstrophy, bladder
    neck obstruction Q64.31
  bone Q79.9
    face Q75.9
      specified type NEC Q75.8
    skull Q75.9
      specified type NEC Q75.8
  brain (multiple) Q04.9
    arteriovenous Q28.2
    specified type NEC Q04.8
  branchial cleft Q18.2
  breast Q83.9
    specified type NEC Q83.8
  broad ligament Q50.6
  bronchus Q32.4
  bursa Q79.9
  cardiac
    chambers Q20.9
      specified type NEC Q20.8
    septum Q21.9
      specified type NEC Q21.8
  cerebral Q04.9
    vessels Q28.3
  cervix uteri Q51.9
    specified type NEC Q51.828
  Chiari
    Type I G93.5
    Type II Q07.01
  choroid (congenital) Q14.3
    plexus Q07.8
  circulatory system Q28.9
  cochlea Q16.5
  cornea Q13.4
  coronary vessels Q24.5
  corpus callosum (congenital) Q04.0
  diaphragm Q79.1
  digestive system NEC, specified type NEC Q45.8
  dura Q07.9
    brain Q04.9
    spinal Q06.9
  ear Q17.9
    causing impairment of hearing Q16.9

Malformation *(Continued)*
  ear *(Continued)*
    external Q17.9
      accessory auricle Q17.0
      causing impairment of hearing Q16.9
        absence of
          auditory canal Q16.1
          auricle Q16.0
      macrotia Q17.1
      microtia Q17.2
      misplacement Q17.4
      misshapen NEC Q17.3
      prominence Q17.5
      specified type NEC Q17.8
    inner Q16.5
    middle Q16.4
      absence of eustachian tube Q16.2
      ossicles (fusion) Q16.3
    ossicles Q16.3
    specified type NEC Q17.8
  epididymis Q55.4
  esophagus Q39.9
    specified type NEC Q39.8
  eye Q15.9
    lid Q10.3
    specified NEC Q15.8
  fallopian tube Q50.6
  genital organ —*see* Anomaly, genitalia
  great
    artery Q25.9
      aorta —*see* Malformation, aorta
      pulmonary artery —*see* Malformation, pulmonary, artery
      specified type NEC Q25.8
    vein Q26.9
      anomalous
        portal venous connection Q26.5
        pulmonary venous connection Q26.4
          partial Q26.3
          total Q26.2
      persistent left superior vena cava Q26.1
      portal vein-hepatic artery fistula Q26.6
      specified type NEC Q26.8
      vena cava stenosis, congenital Q26.0
  gum Q38.6
  hair Q84.2
  heart Q24.9
    specified type NEC Q24.8
  integument Q84.9
    specified type NEC Q84.8
  internal ear Q16.5
  intestine Q43.9
    specified type NEC Q43.8
  iris Q13.2
  joint Q74.9
    ankle Q74.2
    lumbosacral Q76.49
    sacroiliac Q74.2
    specified type NEC Q74.8
  kidney Q63.9
    accessory Q63.0
    giant Q63.3
    horseshoe Q63.1
    hydronephrosis Q62.0
    malposition Q63.2
    specified type NEC Q63.8
  lacrimal apparatus Q10.6
  lingual Q38.3
  lip Q38.0
  liver Q44.7
  lung Q33.9
  meninges or membrane (congenital) Q07.9
    cerebral Q04.8
    spinal (cord) Q06.9
  middle ear Q16.4
    ossicles Q16.3
  mitral valve Q23.9
    specified NEC Q23.8
  Mondini's (congenital) (malformation, cochlea) Q16.5

Malformation *(Continued)*
  mouth (congenital) Q38.6
  multiple types NEC Q89.7
  musculoskeletal system Q79.9
  myocardium Q24.8
  nail Q84.6
  nervous system (central) Q07.9
  nose Q30.9
    specified type NEC Q30.8
  optic disc Q14.2
  orbit Q10.7
  ovary Q50.39
  palate Q38.5
  parathyroid gland Q89.2
  pelvic organs or tissues NEC
    in pregnancy or childbirth O34.8-●
      causing obstructed labor O65.5
  penis Q55.69
    aplasia Q55.5
    curvature (lateral) Q55.61
    hypoplasia Q55.62
  pericardium Q24.8
  peripheral vascular system Q27.9
    specified type NEC Q27.8
  pharynx Q38.8
  precerebral vessels Q28.1
  prostate Q55.4
  pulmonary
    arteriovenous Q25.72
    artery Q25.9
      atresia Q25.5
      specified type NEC Q25.79
      stenosis Q25.6
    valve Q22.3
  renal artery Q27.2
  respiratory system Q34.9
  retina Q14.1
  scrotum —*see* Malformation, testis and scrotum
  seminal vesicles Q55.4
  sense organs NEC Q07.9
  skin Q82.9
  specified NEC Q89.8
  spinal
    cord Q06.9
    nerve root Q07.8
  spine Q76.49
    kyphosis —*see* Kyphosis, congenital
    lordosis —*see* Lordosis, congenital
  spleen Q89.09
  stomach Q40.3
    specified type NEC Q40.2
  teeth, tooth K00.9
  tendon Q79.9
  testis and scrotum Q55.20
    aplasia Q55.0
    hypoplasia Q55.1
    polyorchism Q55.21
    retractile testis Q55.22
    scrotal transposition Q55.23
    specified NEC Q55.29
  thorax, bony Q76.9
  throat Q38.8
  thyroid gland Q89.2
  tongue (congenital) Q38.3
    hypertrophy Q38.2
    tie Q38.1
  trachea Q32.1
  tricuspid valve Q22.9
    specified type NEC Q22.8
  umbilical cord NEC (complicating delivery) O69.89
  umbilicus Q89.9
  ureter Q62.8
    agenesis Q62.4
    duplication Q62.5
    malposition —*see* Malposition, congenital, ureter
    obstructive defect —*see* Defect, obstructive, ureter
    vesico-uretero-renal reflux Q62.7

Malformation (Continued)
  urethra Q64.79
    aplasia Q64.5
    duplication Q64.74
    posterior valves Q64.2
    prolapse Q64.71
    stricture Q64.32
  urinary system Q64.9
  uterus Q51.9
    specified type NEC Q51.818
  vagina Q52.4
  vascular system, peripheral Q27.9
  vas deferens Q55.4
    atresia Q55.3
  venous —see Anomaly, vein(s)
  vulva Q52.70
Malfunction —see also Dysfunction
  cardiac electronic device T82.119
    electrode T82.110
    pulse generator T82.111
    specified type NEC T82.118
  catheter device NEC T85.618
    cystostomy T83.010
    dialysis (renal) (vascular) T82.41
      intraperitoneal T85.611
    infusion NEC T82.514
      cranial T85.610
      epidural T85.610
      intrathecal T85.610
      spinal T85.610
      subarachnoid T85.610
      subdural T85.610
    urinary —see also Breakdown, device,
        catheter T83.018
  colostomy K94.03
    valve K94.03
  cystostomy (stoma) N99.512
    catheter T83.010
  enteric stoma K94.13
  enterostomy K94.13
  esophagostomy K94.33
  gastroenteric K31.89
  gastrostomy K94.23
  ileostomy K94.13
    valve K94.13
  intrathecal infusion pump T85.615
  jejunostomy K94.13
  nervous system device, implant or graft,
      specified NEC T85.615
  pacemaker —see Malfunction, cardiac
      electronic device
  prosthetic device, internal —see
      Complications, prosthetic device, by site,
      mechanical
  tracheostomy J95.03
  urinary device NEC —see Complication,
      genitourinary, device, urinary,
      mechanical
  valve
    colostomy K94.03
    heart T82.09
    ileostomy K94.13
  vascular graft or shunt NEC —see
      Complication, cardiovascular device,
      mechanical, vascular
  ventricular (communicating shunt) T85.01
Malherbe's tumor —see Neoplasm, skin,
    benign
Malibu disease L98.8-●
Malignancy —see also Neoplasm, malignant,
    by site
  unspecified site (primary) C80.1
Malignant —see condition
Malingerer, malingering Z76.5
Mallet finger (acquired) —see Deformity, finger,
    mallet finger
  congenital Q74.0
  sequelae of rickets E64.3
Malleus A24.0
Mallory's bodies R89.7
Mallory-Weiss syndrome K22.6

Malnutrition E46
  degree
    first E44.1
    mild (protein) E44.1
    moderate (protein) E44.0
    second E44.0
    severe (protein-energy) E43
      intermediate form E42
        with
          kwashiorkor (and marasmus) E42
          marasmus E41
    third E43
  following gastrointestinal surgery K91.2
  intrauterine
    light-for-dates —see Light for dates
    small-for-dates —see Small for dates
  lack of care, or neglect (child) (infant) T76.02
    confirmed T74.02
  malignant E40
  protein E46
    calorie E46
      mild E44.1
      moderate E44.0
      severe E43
        intermediate form E42
          with
            kwashiorkor (and marasmus)
                E42
            marasmus E41
    energy E46
      mild E44.1
      moderate E44.0
      severe E43
        intermediate form E42
          with
            kwashiorkor (and marasmus)
                E42
            marasmus E41
  severe (protein-energy) E43
    with
      kwashiorkor (and marasmus) E42
      marasmus E41
Malocclusion (teeth) M26.4
  Angle's M26.219
    class I M26.211
    class II M26.212
    class III M26.213
  due to
    abnormal swallowing M26.59
    mouth breathing M26.59
    tongue, lip or finger habits M26.59
  temporomandibular (joint) M26.69
Malposition
  cervix —see Malposition, uterus
  congenital
    adrenal (gland) Q89.1
    alimentary tract Q45.8
      lower Q43.8
      upper Q40.8
    aorta Q25.49
    appendix Q43.8
    arterial trunk Q20.0
    artery (peripheral) Q27.8
      coronary Q24.5
      digestive system Q27.8
      lower limb Q27.8
      pulmonary Q25.79
      specified site NEC Q27.8
      upper limb Q27.8
    auditory canal Q17.8
      causing impairment of hearing Q16.9
    auricle (ear) Q17.4
      causing impairment of hearing Q16.9
    cervical Q18.2
    biliary duct or passage Q44.5
    bladder (mucosa) —see Exstrophy,
        bladder
    brachial plexus Q07.8
    brain tissue Q04.8
    breast Q83.8
    bronchus Q32.4

Malposition (Continued)
  congenital (Continued)
    cecum Q43.8
    clavicle Q74.0
    colon Q43.8
    digestive organ or tract NEC Q45.8
      lower Q43.8
      upper Q40.8
    ear (auricle) (external) Q17.4
      ossicles Q16.3
    endocrine (gland) NEC Q89.2
    epiglottis Q31.8
    eustachian tube Q17.8
    eye Q15.8
    facial features Q18.8
    fallopian tube Q50.6
    finger(s) Q68.1
      supernumerary Q69.0
    foot Q66.9
    gallbladder Q44.1
    gastrointestinal tract Q45.8
    genitalia, genital organ(s) or tract
      female Q52.8
        external Q52.79
        internal NEC Q52.8
      male Q55.8
    glottis Q31.8
    hand Q68.1
    heart Q24.8
      dextrocardia Q24.0
        with complete transposition of viscera
            Q89.3
    hepatic duct Q44.5
    hip (joint) Q65.89
    intestine (large) (small) Q43.8
      with anomalous adhesions, fixation or
          malrotation Q43.3
    joint NEC Q68.8
    kidney Q63.2
    larynx Q31.8
    limb Q68.8
      lower Q68.8
      upper Q68.8
    liver Q44.7
    lung (lobe) Q33.8
    nail(s) Q84.6
    nerve Q07.8
    nervous system NEC Q07.8
    nose, nasal (septum) Q30.8
    organ or site not listed —see Anomaly,
        by site
    ovary Q50.39
    pancreas Q45.3
    parathyroid (gland) Q89.2
    patella Q74.1
    peripheral vascular system Q27.8
    pituitary (gland) Q89.2
    respiratory organ or system NEC
        Q34.8
    rib (cage) Q76.6
      supernumerary in cervical region
          Q76.5
    scapula Q74.0
    shoulder Q74.0
    spinal cord Q06.8
    spleen Q89.09
    sternum NEC Q76.7
    stomach Q40.2
    symphysis pubis Q74.2
    thymus (gland) Q89.2
    thyroid (gland) (tissue) Q89.2
      cartilage Q31.8
    toe(s) Q66.9
      supernumerary Q69.2
    tongue Q38.3
    trachea Q32.1
    ureter Q62.60
      deviation Q62.61
      displacement Q62.62
      ectopia Q62.63
      specified type NEC Q62.69

M

Malposition *(Continued)*
  congenital *(Continued)*
    uterus Q51.818
    vein(s) (peripheral) Q27.8
      great Q26.8
    vena cava (inferior) (superior) Q26.8
  device, implant or graft —*see also*
      Complications, by site and type,
      mechanical T85.628
    arterial graft NEC —*see* Complication,
        cardiovascular device, mechanical,
        vascular
    breast (implant) T85.42
    catheter NEC T85.628
      cystostomy T83.020
      dialysis (renal) T82.42
        intraperitoneal T85.621
      infusion NEC T82.524
        spinal (epidural) (subdural) T85.620
      urinary —*see also* Displacement, device,
        catheter, urinary T83.028
    electronic (electrode) (pulse generator)
        (stimulator)
      bone T84.320
      cardiac T82.129
        electrode T82.120
        pulse generator T82.121
        specified type NEC T82.128
      nervous system —*see* Complication,
        prosthetic device, mechanical,
        electronic nervous system
        stimulator
      urinary —*see* Complication,
        genitourinary, device, urinary,
        mechanical
    fixation, internal (orthopedic) NEC —
        see Complication, fixation device,
        mechanical
    gastrointestinal —*see* Complications,
        prosthetic device, mechanical,
        gastrointestinal device
    genital NEC T83.428
      intrauterine contraceptive device (string)
        T83.32
      penile prosthesis (cylinder) (implanted)
        (pump) (resevoir) T83.420
      testicular prosthesis T83.421
    heart NEC —*see* Complication,
        cardiovascular device, mechanical
    joint prosthesis —*see* Complication, joint
        prosthesis, mechanical
    ocular NEC —*see* Complications,
        prosthetic device, mechanical,
        ocular device
    orthopedic NEC —*see* Complication,
        orthopedic, device, mechanical
    specified NEC T85.628
    urinary NEC —*see also* Complication,
        genitourinary, device, urinary,
        mechanical
      graft T83.22
    vascular NEC —*see* Complication,
        cardiovascular device, mechanical
    ventricular intracranial shunt T85.02
  fetus —*see* Pregnancy, complicated by
      (management affected by), presentation,
      fetal
  gallbladder K82.8
  gastrointestinal tract, congenital Q45.8
  heart, congenital NEC Q24.8
  joint prosthesis —*see* Complications, joint
      prosthesis, mechanical, displacement,
      by site
  stomach K31.89
    congenital Q40.2
  tooth, teeth, fully erupted M26.30
  uterus (acute) (acquired) (adherent)
      (asymptomatic) (postinfectional)
      (postpartal, old) N85.4
    anteflexion or anteversion N85.4
      congenital Q51.818

Malposition *(Continued)*
  uterus *(Continued)*
    flexion N85.4
      lateral —*see* Lateroversion, uterus
    inversion N85.5
    lateral (flexion) (version) —*see*
        Lateroversion, uterus
      in pregnancy or childbirth —*see*
        subcategory O34.5
    retroflexion or retroversion —*see*
        Retroversion, uterus
Malposture R29.3
Malrotation
  cecum Q43.3
  colon Q43.3
  intestine Q43.3
  kidney Q63.2
Malta fever —*see* Brucellosis
Maltreatment
  adult
    abandonment
      confirmed T74.01
      suspected T76.01
    confirmed T74.91
    history of Z91.419
    neglect
      confirmed T74.01
      suspected T76.01
    physical abuse
      confirmed T74.11
      suspected T76.11
    psychological abuse
      confirmed T74.31
      history of Z91.411
      suspected T76.31
    sexual abuse
      confirmed T74.21
      suspected T76.21
    suspected T76.91
  child
    abandonment
      confirmed T74.02
      suspected T76.02
    confirmed T74.92
    history of —*see* History, personal (of),
        abuse
    neglect
      confirmed T74.02
      history of —*see* History, personal (of),
          abuse
      suspected T76.02
    physical abuse
      confirmed T74.12
      history of —*see* History, personal (of),
          abuse
      suspected T76.12
    psychological abuse
      confirmed T74.32
      history of —*see* History, personal (of),
          abuse
      suspected T76.32
    sexual abuse
      confirmed T74.22
      history of —*see* History, personal (of),
          abuse
      suspected T76.22
    suspected T76.92
    personal history of Z91.89
Maltworker's lung J67.4
Malunion, fracture —*see* Fracture, by site
Mammillitis N61.0
  puerperal, postpartum O91.02
Mammitis —*see* Mastitis
Mammogram (examination) Z12.39
  routine Z12.31
Mammoplasia N62
Management (of)
  bone conduction hearing device (implanted)
      Z45.320
  cardiac pacemaker NEC Z45.018
  cerebrospinal fluid drainage device Z45.41

Management *(Continued)*
  cochlear device (implanted) Z45.321
  contraceptive Z30.9
    specified NEC Z30.8
  implanted device Z45.9
    specified NEC Z45.89
  infusion pump Z45.1
  procreative Z31.9
    male factor infertility in female Z31.81
    specified NEC Z31.89
  prosthesis (external) —*see also* Fitting Z44.9
    implanted Z45.9
      specified NEC Z45.89
  renal dialysis catheter Z49.01
  vascular access device Z45.2
Mangled —*see* specified injury by site
Mania (monopolar) —*see also* Disorder, mood,
    manic episode
  with psychotic symptoms F30.2
  without psychotic symptoms F30.10
    mild F30.11
    moderate F30.12
    severe F30.13
  Bell's F30.8
  chronic (recurrent) F31.89
  hysterical F44.89
  puerperal F30.8
  recurrent F31.89
► Manic depression F31.9
Manic-depressive insanity, psychosis, or
    syndrome —*see* Disorder, bipolar
Mannosidosis E77.1
Mansonelliasis, mansonellosis B74.4
Manson's
  disease B65.1
  schistosomiasis B65.1
Manual —*see* condition
Maple-bark-stripper's lung (disease) J67.6
Maple-syrup-urine disease E71.0
Marable's syndrome (celiac artery
    compression) I77.4
Marasmus E41
  due to malnutrition E41
  intestinal E41
  nutritional E41
  senile R54
  tuberculous NEC —*see* Tuberculosis
Marble
  bones Q78.2
  skin R23.8
Marburg virus disease A98.3
March
  fracture —*see* Fracture, traumatic, stress, by
      site
  hemoglobinuria D59.6
Marchesani (-Weill) syndrome Q87.0
Marchiafava (-Bignami) syndrome or disease
    G37.1
Marchiafava-Micheli syndrome D59.5
Marcus Gunn's syndrome Q07.8
Marfan's syndrome —*see* Syndrome, Marfan's
Marie-Bamberger disease —*see*
    Osteoarthropathy, hypertrophic, specified
    NEC
Marie-Charcot-Tooth neuropathic muscular
    atrophy G60.0
Marie's
  cerebellar ataxia (late-onset) G11.2
  disease or syndrome (acromegaly) E22.0
Marie-Strümpell arthritis, disease or
    spondylitis —*see* Spondylitis, ankylosing
Marion's disease (bladder neck obstruction)
    N32.0
Marital conflict Z63.0
Mark
  port wine Q82.5
  raspberry Q82.5
  strawberry Q82.5
  stretch L90.6
  tattoo L81.8
Marker heterochromatin —*see* Extra, marker
  chromosomes

M

Maroteaux-Lamy syndrome (mild) (severe)
    E76.29
Marrow (bone)
    arrest D61.9
    poor function D75.89
Marseilles fever A77.1
Marsh fever —*see* Malaria
Marshall's (hidrotic) **ectodermal dysplasia**
    Q82.4
Marsh's disease (exophthalmic goiter) E05.00
    with storm E05.01
Masculinization (female) **with adrenal**
    hyperplasia E25.9
    congenital E25.0
Masculinovoblastoma D27.-●
Masochism (sexual) F65.51
Mason's lung J62.8
Mass
    abdominal R19.00
        epigastric R19.06
        generalized R19.07
        left lower quadrant R19.04
        left upper quadrant R19.02
        periumbilic R19.05
        right lower quadrant R19.03
        right upper quadrant R19.01
        specified site NEC R19.09
    ⇒breast —*see also* Lump, breast N63.0
    chest R22.2
    cystic —*see* Cyst
    ear H93.8-●
    head R22.0
    intra-abdominal (diffuse) (generalized) —*see*
        Mass, abdominal
    kidney N28.89
    liver R16.0
    localized (skin) R22.9
        chest R22.2
        head R22.0
        limb
            lower R22.4-●
            upper R22.3-●
        neck R22.1
        trunk R22.2
    lung R91.8
    malignant —*see* Neoplasm, malignant,
        by site
    neck R22.1
    pelvic (diffuse) (generalized) —*see* Mass,
        abdominal
    specified organ NEC —*see* Disease, by site
    splenic R16.1
    substernal thyroid —*see* Goiter
    superficial (localized) R22.9
    umbilical (diffuse) (generalized) R19.09
Massive —*see* condition
Mast cell
    ⇒disease, systemic tissue D47.02
    leukemia C94.3-●
    ▶neoplasm
        ▶malignant C96.20
            ▶specified type NEC C96.29
        ▶of uncertain behavior NEC D47.09
    ⇒sarcoma C96.22
    ⇒tumor D47.09
        ~~malignant C96.2~~
Mastalgia N64.4
Masters-Allen syndrome N83.8
Mastitis (acute) (diffuse) (nonpuerperal)
        (subacute) N61.0
    with abscess N61.1
    chronic (cystic) —*see* Mastopathy, cystic
    cystic (Schimmelbusch's type) —*see*
        Mastopathy, cystic
    fibrocystic —*see* Mastopathy, cystic
    infective N61.0
        newborn P39.0
    interstitial, gestational or puerperal —*see*
        Mastitis, obstetric
    neonatal (noninfective) P83.4
        infective P39.0

Mastitis (*Continued*)
    obstetric (interstitial) (nonpurulent)
        associated with
            lactation O91.23
            pregnancy O91.21-●
            puerperium O91.22
        purulent
            associated with
                lactation O91.13
                pregnancy O91.11-●
                puerperium O91.12
    periductal —*see* Ectasia, mammary duct
    phlegmonous —*see* Mastopathy, cystic
    plasma cell —*see* Ectasia, mammary duct
    without abscess N61.0
⇒Mastocytoma (extracutaneous) D47.09
    ⇒malignant C96.29
    ▶solitary D47.01
⇒Mastocytosis D47.09
    ⇒aggressive systemic C96.21
    ▶cutaneous (diffuse) (maculopapular) D47.01
        ▶congenital Q82.2
        ▶of neonatal onset Q82.2
        ▶of newborn onset Q82.2
    ▶indolent systemic D47.02
    ▶isolated bone marrow D47.02
    ⇒malignant C96.29
        ~~systemic, associated with clonal hematopoetic~~
        ~~non-mast-cell disease (SM-AHNMD)~~
        ~~D47.0~~
    ▶systemic (indolent) (smoldering)
        ▶with an associated hematological non-mast
            cell lineage disease (SM-AHNMD)
            D47.02
Mastodynia N64.4
Mastoid —*see* condition
Mastoidalgia —*see* subcategory H92.0
Mastoiditis (coalescent) (hemorrhagic)
        (suppurative) H70.9-●
    acute, subacute H70.00-●
        complicated NEC H70.09-●
        subperiosteal H70.01-●
    chronic (necrotic) (recurrent) H70.1-●
    in (due to)
        infectious disease NEC B99 [H75.0-●]
        parasitic disease NEC B89 [H75.0-●]
        tuberculosis A18.03
    petrositis —*see* Petrositis
    postauricular fistula —*see* Fistula, postauricular
    specified NEC H70.89-●
    tuberculous A18.03
Mastopathy, mastopathia N64.9
    chronica cystica —*see* Mastopathy, cystic
    cystic (chronic) (diffuse) N60.1
        with epithelial proliferation N60.3-●
    diffuse cystic —*see* Mastopathy, cystic
    estrogenic, oestrogenica N64.89
    ovarian origin N64.89
Mastoplasia, mastoplastia N62
Masturbation (excessive) F98.8
Maternal care (for) —*see* Pregnancy
        (complicated by) (management affected by)
Matheiu's disease (leptospiral jaundice) A27.0
Mauclaire's disease or osteochondrosis —
    see Osteochondrosis, juvenile, hand,
    metacarpal
Maxcy's disease A75.2
Maxilla, maxillary —*see* condition
May (-Hegglin) **anomaly or syndrome** D72.0
McArdle (-Schmid)(-Pearson) **disease**
    (glycogen storage) E74.04
McCune-Albright syndrome Q78.1
McQuarrie's syndrome (idiopathic familial
    hypoglycemia) E16.2
Meadow's syndrome Q86.1
Measles (black) (hemorrhagic) (suppressed)
        B05.9
    with
        complications NEC B05.89
        encephalitis B05.0
        intestinal complications B05.4

Measles (*Continued*)
    with (*Continued*)
        keratitis (keratoconjunctivitis) B05.81
        meningitis B05.1
        otitis media B05.3
        pneumonia B05.2
    French —*see* Rubella
    German —*see* Rubella
    Liberty —*see* Rubella
Meatitis, urethral —*see* Urethritis
Meatus, meatal —*see* condition
Meat-wrappers' asthma J68.9
Meckel-Gruber syndrome Q61.9
Meckel's diverticulitis, diverticulum
    (displaced) (hypertrophic) Q43.0
Meconium
    ileus, newborn P76.0
        in cystic fibrosis E84.11
        meaning meconium plug (without cystic
            fibrosis) P76.0
    obstruction, newborn P76.0
        due to fecaliths P76.0
        in mucoviscidosis E84.11
    peritonitis P78.0
    plug syndrome (newborn) NEC P76.0
Median —*see also* condition
    arcuate ligament syndrome I77.4
    bar (prostate) (vesical orifice) —*see*
        Hyperplasia, prostate
    rhomboid glossitis K14.2
Mediastinal shift R93.8
Mediastinitis (acute) (chronic) J98.51
    syphilitic A52.73
    tuberculous A15.8
Mediastinopericarditis —*see also* Pericarditis
    acute I30.9
    adhesive I31.0
    chronic I31.8
        rheumatic I09.2
Mediastinum, mediastinal —*see* condition
Medicine poisoning —*see* Table of Drugs and
    Chemicals, by drug, poisoning
Mediterranean
    fever —*see* Brucellosis
        familial M04.1
        tick A77.1
    kala-azar B55.0
    leishmaniasis B55.0
    tick fever A77.1
Medulla —*see* condition
Medullary cystic kidney Q61.5
Medullated fibers
    optic (nerve) Q14.8
    retina Q14.1
Medulloblastoma
    desmoplastic C71.6
    specified site —*see* Neoplasm, malignant, by
        site
    unspecified site C71.6
Medulloepithelioma —*see also* Neoplasm,
    malignant, by site
    teratoid —*see* Neoplasm, malignant, by site
Medullomyoblastoma
    specified site —*see* Neoplasm, malignant, by
        site
    unspecified site C71.6
Meekeren-Ehlers-Danlos syndrome Q79.6
Megacolon (acquired) (functional) (not
    Hirschsprung's disease) (in) K59.39
    Chagas' disease B57.32
    congenital, congenitum (aganglionic) Q43.1
    Hirschsprung's (disease) Q43.1
    toxic NEC K59.31
    ⇒due to Clostridium difficile
        ▶not specified as recurrent A04.72
        ▶recurrent A04.71
Megaesophagus (functional) K22.0
    congenital Q39.5
    in (due to) Chagas' disease B57.31
Megalencephaly Q04.5
Megalerythema (epidemic) B08.3

▶ New   ⇒ Revised   ~~deleted~~ Deleted   ● Use Additional Character(s)

Megaloappendix Q43.8
Megalocephalus, megalocephaly NEC Q75.3
Megalocornea Q15.8
   with glaucoma Q15.0
Megalocytic anemia D53.1
Megalodactylia (fingers) (thumbs) (congenital)
   Q74.0
   toes Q74.2
Megaloduodenum Q43.8
Megaloesophagus (functional) K22.0
   congenital Q39.5
Megalogastria (acquired) K31.89
   congenital Q40.2
Megalophthalmos Q11.3
Megalopsia H53.15
Megalosplenia —see Splenomegaly
Megaloureter N28.82
   congenital Q62.2
Megarectum K62.89
Megasigmoid K59.39
   congenital Q43.2
Megaureter N28.82
   congenital Q62.2
Megavitamin-B6 syndrome E67.2
Megrim —see Migraine
Meibomian
   cyst, infected —see Hordeolum
   gland —see condition
   sty, stye —see Hordeolum
Meibomitis —see Hordeolum
Meige-Milroy disease (chronic hereditary
   edema) Q82.0
Meige's syndrome Q82.0
Melalgia, nutritional E53.8
Melancholia F32.9
   climacteric (single episode) F32.89
     recurrent episode F33.8
   hypochondriac F45.29
   intermittent (single episode) F32.89
     recurrent episode F33.8
   involutional (single episode) F32.89
     recurrent episode F33.8
   menopausal (single episode) F32.89
     recurrent episode F33.8
   puerperal F32.89
   reactive (emotional stress or trauma) F32.3
   recurrent F33.9
   senile F03
   stuporous (single episode) F32.89
     recurrent episode F33.8
Melanemia R79.89
Melanoameloblastoma —see Neoplasm, bone,
   benign
Melanoblastoma —see Melanoma
Melanocarcinoma —see Melanoma
Melanocytoma, eyeball D31.9-●
Melanocytosis, neurocutaneous Q82.8
Melanoderma, melanodermia L81.4
Melanodontia, infantile K03.89
Melanodontoclasia K03.89
Melanoepithelioma —see Melanoma
Melanoma (malignant) C43.9
   acral lentiginous, malignant —see Melanoma,
     skin, by site
   amelanotic —see Melanoma, skin, by site
   balloon cell —see Melanoma, skin, by site
   benign —see Nevus
   desmoplastic, malignant —see Melanoma,
     skin, by site
   epithelioid cell —see Melanoma, skin, by site
     with spindle cell, mixed —see Melanoma,
       skin, by site
   in
     giant pigmented nevus —see Melanoma,
       skin, by site
     Hutchinson's melanotic freckle —see
       Melanoma, skin, by site
     junctional nevus —see Melanoma, skin,
       by site
     precancerous melanosis —see Melanoma,
       skin, by site

Melanoma (Continued)
   in situ D03.9
     abdominal wall D03.59
     ala nasi D03.39
     ankle D03.7-●
     anus, anal (margin) (skin) D03.51
     arm D03.6-●
     auditory canal D03.2-●
     auricle (ear) D03.2-●
     auricular canal (external) D03.2-●
     axilla, axillary fold D03.59
     back D03.59
     breast D03.52
     brow D03.39
     buttock D03.59
     canthus (eye) D03.1-●
     cheek (external) D03.39
     chest wall D03.59
     chin D03.39
     choroid D03.8
     conjunctiva D03.8
     ear (external) D03.2-●
     external meatus (ear) D03.2-●
     eye D03.8
     eyebrow D03.39
     eyelid (lower) (upper) D03.1-●
     face D03.30
       specified NEC D03.39
     female genital organ (external) NEC D03.8
     finger D03.6-●
     flank D03.59
     foot D03.7-●
     forearm D03.6-●
     forehead D03.39
     foreskin D03.8
     gluteal region D03.59
     groin D03.59
     hand D03.6-●
     heel D03.7-●
     helix D03.2-●
     hip D03.7-●
     interscapular region D03.59
     iris D03.8
     jaw D03.39
     knee D03.7-●
     labium (majus) (minus) D03.8
     lacrimal gland D03.8
     leg D03.7-●
     lip (lower) (upper) D03.0
     lower limb NEC D03.7-●
     male genital organ (external) NEC D03.8
     nail D03.9
       finger D03.6-●
       toe D03.7-●
     neck D03.4
     nose (external) D03.39
     orbit D03.8
     penis D03.8
     perianal skin D03.51
     perineum D03.51
     pinna D03.2-●
     popliteal fossa or space D03.7-●
     prepuce D03.8
     pudendum D03.8
     retina D03.8
     retrobulbar D03.8
     scalp D03.4
     scrotum D03.8
     shoulder D03.6-●
     specified site NEC D03.8
     submammary fold D03.52
     temple D03.39
     thigh D03.7-●
     toe D03.7-●
     trunk NEC D03.59
     umbilicus D03.59
     upper limb NEC D03.6-●
     vulva D03.8
   juvenile —see Nevus
   malignant, of soft parts except skin —see
     Neoplasm, connective tissue, malignant

Melanoma (Continued)
   metastatic
     breast C79.81
     genital organ C79.82
     specified site NEC C79.89
   neurotropic, malignant —see Melanoma, skin,
     by site
   nodular —see Melanoma, skin, by site
   regressing, malignant —see Melanoma, skin,
     by site
   skin C43.9
     abdominal wall C43.59
     ala nasi C43.31
     ankle C43.7-●
     anus, anal (skin) C43.51
     arm C43.6-●
     auditory canal (external) C43.2-●
     auricle (ear) C43.2-●
     auricular canal (external) C43.2-●
     axilla, axillary fold C43.59
     back C43.59
     breast (female) (male) C43.52
     brow C43.39
     buttock C43.59
     canthus (eye) C43.1-●
     cheek (external) C43.39
     chest wall C43.59
     chin C43.39
     ear (external) C43.2-●
     elbow C43.6-●
     external meatus (ear) C43.2-●
     eyebrow C43.39
     eyelid (lower) (upper) C43.1-●
     face C43.30
       specified NEC C43.39
     female genital organ (external) NEC C51.9
     finger C43.6-●
     flank C43.59
     foot C43.7-●
     forearm C43.6-●
     forehead C43.39
     foreskin C60.0
     glabella C43.39
     gluteal region C43.59
     groin C43.59
     hand C43.6-●
     heel C43.7-●
     helix C43.2-●
     hip C43.7-●
     interscapular region C43.59
     jaw (external) C43.39
     knee C43.7-●
     labium C51.9
       majus C51.0
       minus C51.1
     leg C43.7-●
     lip (lower) (upper) C43.0
     lower limb NEC C43.7-●
     male genital organ (external) NEC C63.9
     nail
       finger C43.6-●
       toe C43.7-●
     nasolabial groove C43.39
     nates C43.59
     neck C43.4
     nose (external) C43.31
     overlapping site C43.8
     palpebra C43.1-●
     penis C60.9
     perianal skin C43.51
     perineum C43.51
     pinna C43.2-●
     popliteal fossa or space C43.7-●
     prepuce C60.0
     pudendum C51.9
     scalp C43.4
     scrotum C63.2
     shoulder C43.6-●
     skin NEC C43.9
     submammary fold C43.52
     temple C43.39

M

Melanoma *(Continued)*
  skin *(Continued)*
    thigh C43.7-●
    toe C43.7-●
    trunk NEC C43.59
    umbilicus C43.59
    upper limb NEC C43.6-●
    vulva C51.9
      overlapping sites C51.8
  spindle cell
    with epithelioid, mixed —*see* Melanoma, skin, by site
    type A C69.4-●
    type B C69.4-●
  superficial spreading —*see* Melanoma, skin, by site
Melanosarcoma —*see also* Melanoma
  epithelioid cell —*see* Melanoma
Melanosis L81.4
  addisonian E27.1
    tuberculous A18.7
  adrenal E27.1
  colon K63.89
  conjunctiva —*see* Pigmentation, conjunctiva
    congenital Q13.89
  cornea (presenile) (senile) —*see also* Pigmentation, cornea
    congenital Q13.4
  eye NEC H57.8
    congenital Q15.8
  lenticularis progressiva Q82.1
  liver K76.89
  precancerous —*see also* Melanoma, in situ
    malignant melanoma in —*see* Melanoma
  Riehl's L81.4
  sclera H15.89
    congenital Q13.89
  suprarenal E27.1
  tar L81.4
  toxic L81.4
Melanuria R82.99
MELAS syndrome E88.41
Melasma L81.1
  adrenal (gland) E27.1
  suprarenal (gland) E27.1
Melena K92.1
  with ulcer - code by site under Ulcer, with hemorrhage K27.4
  due to swallowed maternal blood P78.2
  newborn, neonatal P54.1
    due to swallowed maternal blood P78.2
Meleney's
  gangrene (cutaneous) —*see* Ulcer, skin
  ulcer (chronic undermining) —*see* Ulcer, skin
Melioidosis A24.9
  acute A24.1
  chronic A24.2
  fulminating A24.1
  pneumonia A24.1
  pulmonary (chronic) A24.2
    acute A24.1
    subacute A24.2
  sepsis A24.1
  specified NEC A24.3
  subacute A24.2
Melitensis, febris A23.0
Melkersson (-Rosenthal) syndrome G51.2
Mellitus, diabetes —*see* Diabetes
Melorheostosis (bone) —*see* Disorder, bone, density and structure, specified NEC
Meloschisis Q18.4
Melotia Q17.4
Membrana
  capsularis lentis posterior Q13.89
  epipapillaris Q14.2
Membranacea placenta O43.19-●
Membranaceous uterus N85.8
Membrane(s), membranous —*see also* condition
  cyclitic —*see* Membrane, pupillary
  folds, congenital —*see* Web
  Jackson's Q43.3

Membrane(s), membranous *(Continued)*
  over face of newborn P28.9
  premature rupture —*see* Rupture, membranes, premature
  pupillary H21.4-●
    persistent Q13.89
  retained (with hemorrhage) (complicating delivery) O72.2
    without hemorrhage O73.1
  secondary cataract —*see* Cataract, secondary
  unruptured (causing asphyxia) —*see* Asphyxia, newborn
  vitreous —*see* Opacity, vitreous, membranes and strands
Membranitis —*see* Chorioamnionitis
Memory disturbance, lack or loss —*see also* Amnesia
  mild, following organic brain damage F06.8
Menadione deficiency E56.1
Menarche
  delayed E30.0
  precocious E30.1
Mendacity, pathologic F60.2
Mendelson's syndrome (due to anesthesia) J95.4
  in labor and delivery O74.0
  in pregnancy O29.01-●
  obstetric O74.0
  postpartum, puerperal O89.01
Ménétrier's disease or syndrome K29.60
  with bleeding K29.61
Ménière's disease, syndrome or vertigo H81.0-●
Meninges, meningeal —*see* condition
Meningioma —*see also* Neoplasm, meninges, benign
  angioblastic —*see* Neoplasm, meninges, benign
  angiomatous —*see* Neoplasm, meninges, benign
  endotheliomatous —*see* Neoplasm, meninges, benign
  fibroblastic —*see* Neoplasm, meninges, benign
  fibrous —*see* Neoplasm, meninges, benign
  hemangioblastic —*see* Neoplasm, meninges, benign
  hemangiopericytic —*see* Neoplasm, meninges, benign
  malignant —*see* Neoplasm, meninges, malignant
  meningiothelial —*see* Neoplasm, meninges, benign
  meningotheliomatous —*see* Neoplasm, meninges, benign
  mixed —*see* Neoplasm, meninges, benign
  multiple —*see* Neoplasm, meninges, uncertain behavior
  papillary —*see* Neoplasm, meninges, uncertain behavior
  psammomatous —*see* Neoplasm, meninges, benign
  syncytial —*see* Neoplasm, meninges, benign
  transitional —*see* Neoplasm, meninges, benign
Meningiomatosis (diffuse) —*see* Neoplasm, meninges, uncertain behavior
Meningism —*see* Meningismus
Meningismus (infectional) (pneumococcal) R29.1
  due to serum or vaccine R29.1
  influenzal —*see* Influenza, with, manifestations NEC
Meningitis (basal) (basic) (brain) (cerebral) (cervical) (congestive) (diffuse) (hemorrhagic) infantile) (membranous) (metastatic) (nonspecific) (pontine) (progressive) (simple) (spinal) (subacute) (sympathetic) (toxic) G03.9
  abacterial G03.0
  actinomycotic A42.81
  adenoviral A87.1
  arbovirus A87.8
  aseptic (acute) G03.0

Meningitis *(Continued)*
  bacterial G00.9
    Escherichia coli (E. coli) G00.8
    Friedländer (bacillus) G00.8
    gram-negative G00.9
    H. influenzae G00.0
    Klebsiella G00.8
    pneumococcal G00.1
    specified organism NEC G00.8
    staphylococcal G00.3
    streptococcal (acute) G00.2
  benign recurrent (Mollaret) G03.2
  candidal B37.5
  caseous (tuberculous) A17.0
  cerebrospinal A39.0
  chronic NEC G03.1
  clear cerebrospinal fluid NEC G03.0
  coxsackievirus A87.0
  cryptococcal B45.1
  diplococcal (gram positive) A39.0
  echovirus A87.0
  enteroviral A87.0
  eosinophilic B83.2
  epidemic NEC A39.0
  Escherichia coli (E. coli) G00.8
  fibrinopurulent G00.9
    specified organism NEC G00.8
  Friedländer (bacillus) G00.8
  gonococcal A54.81
  gram-negative cocci G00.9
  gram-positive cocci G00.9
  Haemophilus (influenzae) G00.0
  H. influenzae G00.0
  in (due to)
    adenovirus A87.1
    African trypanosomiasis B56.9 *[G02]*
    anthrax A22.8
    bacterial disease NEC A48.8 *[G01]*
    Chagas' disease (chronic) B57.41
    chickenpox B01.0
    coccidioidomycosis B38.4
    Diplococcus pneumoniae G00.1
    enterovirus A87.0
    herpes (simplex) virus B00.3
      zoster B02.1
    infectious mononucleosis B27.92
    leptospirosis A27.81
    Listeria monocytogenes A32.11
    Lyme disease A69.21
    measles B05.1
    mumps (virus) B26.1
    neurosyphilis (late) A52.13
    parasitic disease NEC B89 *[G02]*
    poliovirus A80.9 *[G02]*
    preventive immunization, inoculation or vaccination G03.8
    rubella B06.02
    Salmonella infection A02.21
    specified cause NEC G03.8
    Streptococcal pneumoniae G00.1
    typhoid fever A01.01
    varicella B01.0
    viral disease NEC A87.8
    whooping cough A37.90
    zoster B02.1
  infectious G00.9
  influenzal (H. influenzae) G00.0
  Klebsiella G00.8
  leptospiral (aseptic) A27.81
  lymphocytic (acute) (benign) (serous) A87.2
  meningococcal A39.0
  Mima polymorpha G00.8
  Mollaret (benign recurrent) G03.2
  monilial B37.5
  mycotic NEC B49 *[G02]*
  Neisseria A39.0
  nonbacterial G03.0
  nonpyogenic NEC G03.0
  ossificans G96.19
  pneumococcal streptococcus pneumoniae G00.1

Meningitis *(Continued)*
  poliovirus A80.9 [G02]
  postmeasles B05.1
  purulent G00.9
    specified organism NEC G00.8
  pyogenic G00.9
    specified organism NEC G00.8
  Salmonella (arizonae) (Cholerae-Suis)
    (enteritidis) (typhimurium) A02.21
  septic G00.9
    specified organism NEC G00.8
  serosa circumscripta NEC G03.0
  serous NEC G93.2
  specified organism NEC G00.8
  sporotrichosis B42.81
  staphylococcal G00.3
  sterile G03.0
  Streptococcal (acute) G00.2
    pneumoniae G00.1
  suppurative G00.9
    specified organism NEC G00.8
  syphilitic (late) (tertiary) A52.13
    acute A51.41
    congenital A50.41
    secondary A51.41
  Torula histolytica (cryptococcal) B45.1
  traumatic (complication of injury) T79.8
  tuberculous A17.0
  typhoid A01.01
  viral NEC A87.9
  Yersinia pestis A20.3
Meningocele (spinal) —*see also* Spina bifida
  with hydrocephalus —*see* Spina bifida, by
    site, with hydrocephalus
  acquired (traumatic) G96.19
  cerebral —*see* Encephalocele
Meningocerebritis —*see* Meningoencephalitis
Meningococcemia A39.4
  acute A39.2
  chronic A39.3
Meningococcus, meningococcal —*see also*
    condition A39.9
  adrenalitis, hemorrhagic A39.1
  carrier (suspected) of Z22.31
  meningitis (cerebrospinal) A39.0
Meningoencephalitis —*see also* Encephalitis
    G04.90
  acute NEC —*see also* Encephalitis, viral A86
  bacterial NEC G04.2
  California A83.5
  diphasic A84.1
  eosinophilic B83.2
  epidemic A39.81
  herpesviral, herpetic B00.4
    due to herpesvirus 6 B10.01
    due to herpesvirus 7 B10.09
    specified NEC B10.09
  in (due to)
    blastomycosis NEC B40.81
    diseases classified elsewhere G05.3
    free-living ameba B60.2
    Hemophilus influenzae (H. influenzae)
      G00.0
    herpes B00.4
      due to herpesvirus 6 B10.01
      due to herpesvirus 7 B10.09
      specified NEC B10.09
    H. influenzae G00.0
    Lyme disease A69.22
    mercury —*see* subcategory T56.1
    mumps B26.2
    Naegleria (amebae) (organisms) (fowleri)
      B60.2
    Parastrongylus cantonensis B83.2
    toxoplasmosis (acquired) B58.2
      congenital P37.1
  infectious (acute) (viral) A86
  influenzal (H. influenzae) G00.0
  Listeria monocytogenes A32.12
  lymphocytic (serous) A87.2
  mumps B26.2

Meningoencephalitis *(Continued)*
  parasitic NEC B89 [G05.3]
  pneumococcal G04.2
  primary amebic B60.2
  specific (syphilitic) A52.14
  specified organism NEC G04.81
  staphylococcal G04.2
  streptococcal G04.2
  syphilitic A52.14
  toxic NEC G92
    due to mercury —*see* subcategory T56.1
  tuberculous A17.82
  virus NEC A86
Meningoencephalocele —*see also*
    Encephalocele
  syphilitic A52.19
    congenital A50.49
Meningoencephalomyelitis —*see also*
    Meningoencephalitis
  acute NEC (viral) A86
    disseminated G04.00
      postimmunization or postvaccination
        G04.02
      postinfectious G04.01
  due to
    actinomycosis A42.82
    Torula B45.1
    Toxoplasma or toxoplasmosis (acquired)
      B58.2
    congenital P37.1
  postimmunization or postvaccination G04.02
Meningoencephalomyelopathy G96.9
Meningoencephalopathy G96.9
Meningomyelitis —*see also*
    Meningoencephalitis
  bacterial NEC G04.2
  blastomycotic NEC B40.81
  cryptococcal B45.1
  in diseases classified elsewhere G05.4
  meningococcal A39.81
  syphilitic A52.14
  tuberculous A17.82
Meningomyelocele —*see also* Spina bifida
  syphilitic A52.19
Meningomyeloneuritis —*see*
    Meningoencephalitis
Meningoradiculitis —*see* Meningitis
Meningovascular —*see* condition
Menkes' disease or syndrome E83.09
  meaning maple-syrup-urine disease E71.0
Menometrorrhagia N92.1
Menopause, menopausal (asymptomatic)
    (state) Z78.0
  arthritis (any site) NEC —*see* Arthritis,
    specified form NEC
  bleeding N92.4
  depression (single episode) F32.89
    agitated (single episode) F32.2
      recurrent episode F33.9
    psychotic (single episode) F32.89
      recurrent episode F33.8
    recurrent episode F33.9
  melancholia (single episode) F32.89
    recurrent episode F33.8
  paranoid state F22
  premature E28.319
    asymptomatic E28.319
      postirradiation E89.40
      postsurgical E89.40
    symptomatic E28.310
      postirradiation E89.41
      postsurgical E89.41
  psychosis NEC F28
  symptomatic N95.1
  toxic polyarthritis NEC —*see* Arthritis,
    specified form NEC
Menorrhagia (primary) N92.0
  climacteric N92.4
    menopausal N92.4
  menopausal N92.4
  postclimacteric N95.0

Menorrhagia *(Continued)*
  postmenopausal N95.0
  preclimacteric or premenopausal N92.4
  pubertal (menses retained) N92.2
Menostaxis N92.0
Menses, retention N94.89
Menstrual —*see* Menstruation
Menstruation
  absent —*see* Amenorrhea
  anovulatory N97.0
  cycle, irregular N92.6
  delayed N91.0
  disorder N93.9
    psychogenic F45.8
  during pregnancy O20.8
  excessive (with regular cycle) N92.0
    with irregular cycle N92.1
    at puberty N92.2
  frequent N92.0
  infrequent —*see* Oligomenorrhea
  irregular N92.6
    specified NEC N92.5
  latent N92.5
  membranous N92.5
  painful —*see also* Dysmenorrhea N94.6
    primary N94.4
    psychogenic F45.8
    secondary N94.5
  passage of clots N92.0
  precocious E30.1
  protracted N92.5
  rare —*see* Oligomenorrhea
  retained N94.89
  retrograde N92.5
  scanty —*see* Oligomenorrhea
  suppression N94.89
  vicarious (nasal) N94.89
Mental —*see also* condition
  deficiency —*see* Disability, intellectual
  deterioration —*see* Psychosis
  disorder —*see* Disorder, mental
  exhaustion F48.8
  insufficiency (congenital) —*see* Disability,
    intellectual
  observation without need for further medical
    care Z03.89
  retardation —*see* Disability, intellectual
  subnormality —*see* Disability, intellectual
  upset —*see* Disorder, mental
Meralgia paresthetica G57.1-●
Mercurial —*see* condition
Mercurialism —*see* subcategory T56.1
MERRF syndrome (myoclonic epilepsy
    associated with ragged-red fiber) E88.42
Merkel cell tumor —*see* Carcinoma, Merkel cell
Merocele —*see* Hernia, femoral
Meromelia
  lower limb —*see* Defect, reduction, lower limb
    intercalary
      femur —*see* Defect, reduction, lower
        limb, specified type NEC
        tibiofibular (complete) (incomplete) —
          see Defect, reduction, lower limb
  upper limb —*see* Defect, reduction, upper
    limb
    intercalary, humeral, radioulnar —*see*
      Agenesis, arm, with hand present
Merzbacher-Pelizaeus disease E75.29
Mesaortitis —*see* Aortitis
Mesarteritis —*see* Arteritis
Mesencephalitis —*see* Encephalitis
Mesenchymoma —*see also* Neoplasm,
    connective tissue, uncertain behavior
  benign —*see* Neoplasm, connective tissue,
    benign
  malignant —*see* Neoplasm, connective tissue,
    malignant
Mesenteritis
  retractile K65.4
  sclerosing K65.4
Mesentery, mesenteric —*see* condition

Mesiodens, mesiodentes K00.1
Mesio-occlusion M26.213
Mesocolon —see condition
Mesonephroma (malignant) —see Neoplasm,
 malignant, by site
 benign —see Neoplasm, benign, by site
Mesophlebitis —see Phlebitis
Mesostromal dysgenesis Q13.89
Mesothelioma (malignant) C45.9
 benign
  mesentery D19.1
  mesocolon D19.1
  omentum D19.1
  peritoneum D19.1
  pleura D19.0
  specified site NEC D19.7
  unspecified site D19.9
 biphasic C45.9
  benign
   mesentery D19.1
   mesocolon D19.1
   omentum D19.1
   peritoneum D19.1
   pleura D19.0
   specified site NEC D19.7
   unspecified site D19.9
 cystic D48.4
 epithelioid C45.9
  benign
   mesentery D19.1
   mesocolon D19.1
   omentum D19.1
   peritoneum D19.1
   pleura D19.0
   specified site NEC D19.7
   unspecified site D19.9
 fibrous C45.9
  benign
   mesentery D19.1
   mesocolon D19.1
   omentum D19.1
   peritoneum D19.1
   pleura D19.0
   specified site NEC D19.7
   unspecified site D19.9
 site classification
  liver C45.7
  lung C45.7
  mediastinum C45.7
  mesentery C45.1
  mesocolon C45.1
  omentum C45.1
  pericardium C45.2
  peritoneum C45.1
  pleura C45.0
   parietal C45.0
  retroperitoneum C45.7
  specified site NEC C45.7
  unspecified C45.9
Metabolic syndrome E88.81
Metagonimiasis B66.8
Metagonimus infestation (intestine) B66.8
Metal
 pigmentation L81.8
 polisher's disease J62.8
Metamorphopsia H53.15
Metaplasia
 apocrine (breast) —see Dysplasia, mammary,
  specified type NEC
 cervix (squamous) —see Dysplasia, cervix
 endometrium (squamous) (uterus) N85.8
 esophagus K22.7-•
 kidney (pelvis) (squamous) N28.89
 myelogenous D73.1
 myeloid (agnogenic) (megakaryocytic)
  D73.1
 spleen D73.1
 squamous cell, bladder N32.89
Metastasis, metastatic
 abscess —see Abscess
 calcification E83.59

Metastasis, metastatic (Continued)
 cancer
  from specified site —see Neoplasm,
   malignant, by site
  to specified site —see Neoplasm, secondary,
   by site
  deposits (in) —see Neoplasm, secondary, by
   site
  disease (see also Neoplasm, secondary, by site)
   C79.9
  spread (to) —see Neoplasm, secondary, by site
Metastrongyliasis B83.8
Metatarsalgia M77.4-•
 anterior G57.6-•
 Morton's G57.6-•
Metatarsus, metatarsal —see also condition
 adductus, congenital Q66.22
 valgus (abductus), congenital Q66.6
 varus (congenital) Q66.22
  primus Q66.21
Methadone use —see Use, opioid
Methemoglobinemia D74.9
 acquired (with sulfhemoglobinemia) D74.8
 congenital D74.0
 enzymatic (congenital) D74.0
 Hb M disease D74.0
 hereditary D74.0
 toxic D74.8
Methemoglobinuria —see Hemoglobinuria
Methioninemia E72.19
Methylmalonic acidemia E71.120
Metritis (catarrhal) (hemorrhagic) (septic)
  (suppurative) —see also Endometritis
 cervical —see Cervicitis
Metropathia hemorrhagica N93.8
Metroperitonitis —see Peritonitis, pelvic, female
Metrorrhagia N92.1
 climacteric N92.4
 menopausal N92.4
 postpartum NEC (atonic) (following delivery
  of placenta) O72.1
  delayed or secondary O72.2
 preclimacteric or premenopausal N92.4
 psychogenic F45.8
Metrorrhexis —see Rupture, uterus
Metrosalpingitis N70.91
Metrostaxis N93.8
Metrovaginitis —see Endometritis
Meyer-Schwickerath and Weyers syndrome
 Q87.0
Meynert's amentia (nonalcoholic) F04
 alcoholic F10.96
  with dependence F10.26
Mibelli's disease (porokeratosis) Q82.8
Mice, joint —see Loose, body, joint
 knee M23.4
Micrencephalon, micrencephaly Q02
Microalbuminuria R80.9
Microaneurysm, retinal —see also Disorder,
  retina, microaneurysms
 diabetic —see E08-E13 with .31
Microangiopathy (peripheral) I73.9
 thrombotic M31.1
Microcalcifications, breast R92.0
Microcephalus, microcephalic, microcephaly
 Q02
 due to toxoplasmosis (congenital) P37.1
Microcheilia Q18.7
Microcolon (congenital) Q43.8
Microcornea (congenital) Q13.4
Microcytic —see condition D57.40
Microdeletions NEC Q93.88
Microdontia K00.2
Microdrepanocytosis D57.40
 with crisis (vasoocclusive pain) D57.419
  with
   acute chest syndrome D57.411
   splenic sequestration D57.412
Microembolism
 atherothrombotic —see Atheroembolism
 retinal —see Occlusion, artery, retina

Microencephalon Q02
Microfilaria streptocerca infestation —see
 Onchocerciasis
Microgastria (congenital) Q40.2
Microgenia M26.06
Microgenitalia, congenital
 female Q52.8
 male Q55.8
Microglioma —see Lymphoma, non-Hodgkin,
 specified NEC
Microglossia (congenital) Q38.3
Micrognathia, micrognathism (congenital)
 (mandibular) (maxillary) M26.09
Microgyria (congenital) Q04.3
Microinfarct of heart —see Insufficiency,
 coronary
Microlentia (congenital) Q12.8
Microlithiasis, alveolar, pulmonary J84.02
Micromastia N64.82
Micromyelia (congenital) Q06.8
Micropenis Q55.62
Microphakia (congenital) Q12.8
Microphthalmos, microphthalmia (congenital)
 Q11.2
 due to toxoplasmosis P37.1
Micropsia H53.15
Microscopic polyangiitis (polyarteritis) M31.7
Microsporidiosis B60.8
 intestinal A07.8
Microsporon furfur infestation B36.0
Microsporosis —see also Dermatophytosis
 nigra B36.1
Microstomia (congenital) Q18.5
Microtia (congenital) (external ear) Q17.2
Microtropia H50.40
Microvillus inclusion disease (MVD) (MVID)
 Q43.8
Micturition
 disorder NEC —see also Difficulty, micturition
  R39.198
  psychogenic F45.8
 frequency R35.0
  psychogenic F45.8
 hesitancy R39.11
 incomplete emptying R39.14
 nocturnal R35.1
 painful R30.9
  dysuria R30.0
  psychogenic F45.8
  tenesmus R30.1
 poor stream R39.12
 position dependent R39.192
 split stream R39.13
 straining R39.16
 urgency R39.15
Mid plane —see condition
Middle
 ear —see condition
 lobe (right) syndrome J98.19
Miescher's elastoma L87.2
Mietens' syndrome Q87.2
Migraine (idiopathic) G43.909
 with refractory migraine G43.919
  with status migrainosus G43.911
  without status migrainosus G43.919
 with aura (acute-onset) (prolonged) (typical)
  (without headache) G43.109
  with refractory migraine G43.119
   with status migrainosus G43.111
   without status migrainosus G43.119
  intractable G43.119
   with status migrainosus G43.111
   without status migrainosus G43.119
  not intractable G43.109
   with status migrainosus G43.101
   without status migrainosus G43.109
  persistent G43.509
   with cerebral infarction G43.609
    with refractory migraine G43.619
     with status migrainosus G43.611
     without status migrainosus G43.619

▶ New   ⇒ Revised   ~~deleted~~ Deleted   • Use Additional Character(s)

Migraine *(Continued)*
  with aura *(Continued)*
    persistent *(Continued)*
      with cerebral infarction *(Continued)*
        intractable G43.619
          with status migrainosus G43.611
          without status migrainosus G43.619
        not intractable G43.609
          with status migrainosus G43.601
          without status migrainosus G43.609
        without refractory migraine G43.609
          with status migrainosus G43.601
          without status migrainosus G43.609
      without cerebral infarction G43.509
        with refractory migraine G43.519
          with status migrainosus G43.511
          without status migrainosus G43.519
        intractable G43.519
          with status migrainosus G43.511
          without status migrainosus G43.519
        not intractable G43.509
          with status migrainosus G43.501
          without status migrainosus G43.509
        without refractory migraine G43.509
          with status migrainosus G43.501
          without status migrainosus G43.509
      without mention of refractory migraine G43.109
        with status migrainosus G43.101
        without status migrainosus G43.109
  abdominal G43.D0
    with refractory migraine G43.D1
    intractable G43.D1
    not intractable G43.D0
    without refractory migraine G43.D0
  basilar —*see* Migraine, with aura
  classical —*see* Migraine, with aura
  common —*see* Migraine, without aura
  complicated G43.109
  equivalents —*see* Migraine, with aura
  familiar —*see* Migraine, hemiplegic
  hemiplegic G43.409
    with refractory migraine G43.419
      with status migrainosus G43.411
      without status migrainosus G43.419
    intractable G43.419
      with status migrainosus G43.411
      without status migrainosus G43.419
    not intractable G43.409
      with status migrainosus G43.401
      without status migrainosus G43.409
    without refractory migraine G43.409
      with status migrainosus G43.401
      without status migrainosus G43.409
  intractable G43.919
    with status migrainosus G43.911
    without status migrainosus G43.919
  menstrual G43.829
    with refractory migraine G43.839
      with status migrainosus G43.831
      without status migrainosus G43.839
    intractable G43.839
      with status migrainosus G43.831
      without status migrainosus G43.839
    not intractable G43.829
      with status migrainosus G43.821
      without status migrainosus G43.829
    without refractory migraine G43.829
      with status migrainosus G43.821
      without status migrainosus G43.829
  menstrually related —*see* Migraine, menstrual
  not intractable G43.909
    with status migrainosus G43.901
    without status migrainosus G43.919
  ophthalmoplegic G43.B0
    with refractory migraine G43.B1
    intractable G43.B1
    not intractable G43.B0
    without refractory migraine G43.B0

Migraine *(Continued)*
  persistent aura (with, without) cerebral infarction —*see* Migraine, with aura, persistent
  preceded or accompanied by transient focal neurological phenomena —*see* Migraine, with aura
  pre-menstrual —*see* Migraine, menstrual
  pure menstrual —*see* Migraine, menstrual
  retinal —*see* Migraine, with aura
  specified NEC G43.809
    intractable G43.819
      with status migrainosus G43.811
      without status migrainosus G43.819
    not intractable G43.809
      with status migrainosus G43.801
      without status migrainosus G43.809
  sporadic —*see* Migraine, hemiplegic
  transformed —*see* Migraine, without aura, chronic
  triggered seizures —*see* Migraine, with aura
  without aura G43.009
    with refractory migraine G43.019
      with status migrainosus G43.011
      without status migrainosus G43.019
    chronic G43.709
      with refractory migraine G43.719
        with status migrainosus G43.711
        without status migrainosus G43.719
      intractable
        with status migrainosus G43.711
        without status migrainosus G43.719
      not intractable
        with status migrainosus G43.701
        without status migrainosus G43.709
      without refractory migraine G43.709
        with status migrainosus G43.701
        without status migrainosus G43.709
    intractable
      with status migrainosus G43.011
      without status migrainosus G43.019
    not intractable
      with status migrainosus G43.001
      without status migrainosus G43.009
    without mention of refractory migraine G43.009
      with status migrainosus G43.001
      without status migrainosus G43.009
  without refractory migraine G43.909
    with status migrainosus G43.901
    without status migrainosus G43.919
Migrant, social Z59.0
Migration, anxiety concerning Z60.3
Migratory, migrating —*see also* condition
  person Z59.0
  testis Q55.29
Mikity-Wilson disease or syndrome P27.0
Mikulicz' disease or syndrome K11.8
Miliaria L74.3
  alba L74.1
  apocrine L75.2
  crystallina L74.1
  profunda L74.2
  rubra L74.0
  tropicalis L74.2
Miliary —*see* condition
Milium L72.0
  colloid L57.8
Milk
  crust L21.0
  excessive secretion O92.6
  poisoning —*see* Poisoning, food, noxious
  retention O92.79
  sickness —*see* Poisoning, food, noxious
  spots I31.0
Milk-alkali disease or syndrome E83.52
Milk-leg (deep vessels) (nonpuerperal) —*see* Embolism, vein, lower extremity
  complicating pregnancy O22.3-●
  puerperal, postpartum, childbirth O87.1

Milkman's disease or syndrome M83.8
Milky urine —*see* Chyluria
Millard-Gubler (-Foville) paralysis or syndrome G46.3
Millar's asthma J38.5
Miller-Fisher syndrome G61.0
Mills' disease —*see* Hemiplegia
Millstone maker's pneumoconiosis J62.8
Milroy's disease (chronic hereditary edema) Q82.0
Minamata disease T56.1-●
Miners' asthma or lung J60
Minkowski-Chauffard syndrome —*see* Spherocytosis
Minor —*see* condition
Minor's disease (hematomyelia) G95.19
Minot's disease (hemorrhagic disease), newborn P53
Minot-von Willebrand-Jurgens disease or syndrome (angiohemophilia) D68.0
Minus (and plus) hand (intrinsic) —*see* Deformity, limb, specified type NEC, forearm
Miosis (pupil) H57.03
Mirizzi's syndrome (hepatic duct stenosis) K83.1
Mirror writing F81.0
Misadventure (of) (prophylactic) (therapeutic) — *see also* Complications T88.9
  administration of insulin (by accident) —*see* subcategory T38.3
  infusion —*see* Complications, infusion
  local applications (of fomentations, plasters, etc.) T88.9
    burn or scald —*see* Burn
    specified NEC T88.8
  medical care (early) (late) T88.9
    adverse effect of drugs or chemicals —*see* Table of Drugs and Chemicals
  medical care (early) (late)
    burn or scald —*see* Burn
    specified NEC T88.8
  specified NEC T88.8
  surgical procedure (early) (late) —*see* Complications, surgical procedure
  transfusion —*see* Complications, transfusion
  vaccination or other immunological procedure —*see* Complications, vaccination
Miscarriage O03.9
Misdirection, aqueous H40.83-●
Misperception, sleep state F51.02
Misplaced, misplacement
  ear Q17.4
  kidney (acquired) N28.89
    congenital Q63.2
  organ or site, congenital NEC —*see* Malposition, congenital
Missed
  abortion O02.1
  delivery O36.4
Missing —*see also* Absence
  string of intrauterine contraceptive device T83.32
Misuse of drugs F19.99
Mitchell's disease (erythromelalgia) I73.81
Mite(s) (infestation) B88.9
  diarrhea B88.0
  grain (itch) B88.0
  hair follicle (itch) B88.0
  in sputum B88.0
Mitral —*see* condition
Mittelschmerz N94.0
Mixed —*see* condition
MMN (multifocal motor neuropathy) G61.82
MNGIE (Mitochondrial Neurogastrointestinal Encephalopathy) syndrome E88.49
Mobile, mobility
  cecum Q43.3
  excessive —*see* Hypermobility
  gallbladder, congenital Q44.1

Mobile, mobility *(Continued)*
  kidney N28.89
  organ or site, congenital NEC —*see*
      Malposition, congenital
Mobitz heart block (atrioventricular) I44.1
Moebius, Möbius
  disease (ophthalmoplegic migraine) —*see*
      Migraine, ophthalmoplegic
  syndrome Q87.0
      congenital oculofacial paralysis (with other
          anomalies) Q87.0
      ophthalmoplegic migraine —*see* Migraine,
          ophthalmoplegic
Moeller's glossitis K14.0
Mohr's syndrome (Types I and II) Q87.0
Mola destruens D39.2
Molar pregnancy O02.0
Molarization of premolars K00.2
Molding, head (during birth) - omit code
Mole (pigmented) —*see also* Nevus
  blood O02.0
  Breus' O02.0
  cancerous —*see* Melanoma
  carneous O02.0
  destructive D39.2
  fleshy O02.0
  hydatid, hydatidiform (benign) (complicating
      pregnancy) (delivered) (undelivered)
      O01.9
      classical O01.0
      complete O01.0
      incomplete O01.1
      invasive D39.2
      malignant D39.2
      partial O01.1
  intrauterine O02.0
  invasive (hydatidiform) D39.2
  malignant
      meaning
          malignant hydatidiform mole D39.2
          melanoma —*see* Melanoma
  nonhydatidiform O02.0
  nonpigmented —*see* Nevus
  pregnancy NEC O02.0
  skin —*see* Nevus
  ▸tubal O00.10-
      ▸with intrauterine pregnancy O00.11-
  vesicular —*see* Mole, hydatidiform
Molimen, molimina (menstrual) N94.3
Molluscum contagiosum (epitheliale) B08.1
Mönckeberg's arteriosclerosis, disease, or
    sclerosis —*see* Arteriosclerosis, extremities
Mondini's malformation (cochlea) Q16.5
Mondor's disease I80.8
Monge's disease T70.29
Monilethrix (congenital) Q84.1
Moniliasis —*see also* Candidiasis B37.9
  neonatal P37.5
Monitoring (encounter for)
  therapeutic drug level Z51.81
Monkey malaria B53.1
Monkeypox B04
Monoarthritis M13.10
  ankle M13.17-•
  elbow M13.12-•
  foot joint M13.17-•
  hand joint M13.14-•
  hip M13.15-•
  knee M13.16-•
  shoulder M13.11-•
  wrist M13.13-•
Monoblastic —*see* condition
Monochromat (ism), monochromatopsia
    (acquired) (congenital) H53.51
Monocytic —*see* condition
Monocytopenia D72.818
Monocytosis (symptomatic) D72.821
Monomania —*see* Psychosis
Mononeuritis G58.9
  cranial nerve —*see* Disorder, nerve,
      cranial

Mononeuritis *(Continued)*
  femoral nerve G57.2-•
  lateral
      cutaneous nerve of thigh G57.1-•
      popliteal nerve G57.3-•
  lower limb G57.9-•
      specified nerve NEC G57.8-•
  medial popliteal nerve G57.4-•
  median nerve G56.1-•
  multiplex G58.7
  plantar nerve G57.6-•
  posterior tibial nerve G57.5-•
  radial nerve G56.3-•
  sciatic nerve G57.0-•
  specified NEC G58.8
  tibial nerve G57.4-•
  ulnar nerve G56.2-•
  upper limb G56.9-•
      specified nerve NEC G56.8-•
  vestibular —*see* subcategory H93.3
Mononeuropathy G58.9
  carpal tunnel syndrome —*see* Syndrome,
      carpal tunnel
  diabetic NEC —*see* E08-E13 with .41
  femoral nerve —*see* Lesion, nerve, femoral
  ilioinguinal nerve G57.8-•
  in diseases classified elsewhere —*see* category
      G59
  intercostal G58.0
  lower limb G57.9-•
      causalgia —*see* Causalgia, lower limb
      femoral nerve —*see* Lesion, nerve,
          femoral
      meralgia paresthetica G57.1-•
      plantar nerve —*see* Lesion, nerve, plantar
      popliteal nerve —*see* Lesion, nerve,
          popliteal
      sciatic nerve —*see* Lesion, nerve, sciatic
      specified NEC G57.8-•
      tarsal tunnel syndrome —*see* Syndrome,
          tarsal tunnel
  median nerve —*see* Lesion, nerve, median
  multiplex G58.7
  obturator nerve G57.8-•
  popliteal nerve —*see* Lesion, nerve,
      popliteal
  radial nerve —*see* Lesion, nerve, radial
  saphenous nerve G57.8-•
  specified NEC G58.8
  tarsal tunnel syndrome —*see* Syndrome,
      tarsal tunnel
  tuberculous A17.83
  ulnar nerve —*see* Lesion, nerve, ulnar
  upper limb G56.9-•
      carpal tunnel syndrome —*see* Syndrome,
          carpal tunnel
      causalgia —*see* Causalgia
      median nerve —*see* Lesion, nerve, median
      radial nerve —*see* Lesion, nerve, radial
      specified site NEC G56.8-•
      ulnar nerve —*see* Lesion, nerve, ulnar
Mononucleosis, infectious B27.90
  with
      complication NEC B27.99
      meningitis B27.92
      polyneuropathy B27.91
  cytomegaloviral B27.10
      with
          complication NEC B27.19
          meningitis B27.12
          polyneuropathy B27.11
  Epstein-Barr (virus) B27.00
      with
          complication NEC B27.09
          meningitis B27.02
          polyneuropathy B27.01
  gammaherpesviral B27.00
      with
          complication NEC B27.09
          meningitis B27.02
          polyneuropathy B27.01

Mononucleosis, infectious *(Continued)*
  specified NEC B27.80
      with
          complication NEC B27.89
          meningitis B27.82
          polyneuropathy B27.81
Monoplegia G83.3-•
  congenital (cerebral) G80.8
      spastic G80.1
  embolic (current episode) I63.4-•
  following
      cerebrovascular disease
          cerebral infarction
              lower limb I69.34-•
              upper limb I69.33-•
          intracerebral hemorrhage
              lower limb I69.14-•
              upper limb I69.13-•
          lower limb I69.94-•
          nontraumatic intracranial hemorrhage
              NEC
              lower limb I69.24-•
              upper limb I69.23-•
          specified disease NEC
              lower limb I69.84-•
              upper limb I69.83-•
          stroke NOS
              lower limb I69.34-•
              upper limb I69.33-•
          subarachnoid hemorrhage
              lower limb I69.04-•
              upper limb I69.03-•
          upper limb I69.93-•
  hysterical (transient) F44.4
  lower limb G83.1-•
  psychogenic (conversion reaction) F44.4
  thrombotic (current episode) I63.3-•
  transient R29.818
  upper limb G83.2-•
Monorchism, monorchidism Q55.0
Monosomy —*see also* Deletion, chromosome
    Q93.9
  specified NEC Q93.89
  whole chromosome
      meiotic nondisjunction Q93.0
      mitotic nondisjunction Q93.1
      mosaicism Q93.1
  X Q96.9
Monster, monstrosity (single) Q89.7
  acephalic Q00.0
  twin Q89.4
Monteggia's fracture (-dislocation) S52.27-•
Mooren's ulcer (cornea) —*see* Ulcer, cornea,
    Mooren's
Moore's syndrome —*see* Epilepsy, specified NEC
Mooser-Neill reaction A75.2
Mooser's bodies A75.2
Morbidity not stated or unknown R69
Morbilli —*see* Measles
Morbus —*see also* Disease
  angelicus, anglorum E55.0
  Beigel B36.2
  caducus —*see* Epilepsy
  celiacus K90.0
  comitialis —*see* Epilepsy
  cordis —*see also* Disease, heart I51.9
      valvulorum —*see* Endocarditis
  coxae senilis M16.9
      tuberculous A18.02
  hemorrhagicus neonatorum P53
  maculosus neonatorum P54.5
Morel (-Stewart)(-Morgagni) syndrome M85.2
Morel-Kraepelin disease —*see* Schizophrenia
Morel-Moore syndrome M85.2
Morgagni's
  cyst, organ, hydatid, or appendage
      female Q50.5
      male (epididymal) Q55.4
          testicular Q55.29
  syndrome M85.2
Morgagni-Stewart-Morel syndrome M85.2

▶ New   ⇒ Revised   ~~deleted~~ Deleted   • Use Additional Character(s)

Morgagni-Stokes-Adams syndrome I45.9
Morgagni-Turner (-Albright) syndrome Q96.9
Moria F07.0
Moron (I.Q. 50-69) F70
Morphea L94.0
Morphinism (without remission) F11.20
  with remission F11.21
Morphinomania (without remission) F11.20
  with remission F11.21
Morquio (-Ullrich)(-Brailsford) disease or
  syndrome —see Mucopolysaccharidosis
Mortification (dry) (moist) —see Gangrene
Morton's metatarsalgia (neuralgia)(neuroma)
  (syndrome) G57.6
Morvan's disease or syndrome G60.8
Mosaicism, mosaic (autosomal) (chromosomal)
  45,X/46,XX Q96.3
  45,X/other cell lines NEC with abnormal sex
    chromosome Q96.4
  sex chromosome
    female Q97.8
    lines with various numbers of
      X chromosomes Q97.2
    male Q98.7
  XY Q96.3
Moschowitz' disease M31.1
Mother yaw A66.0
Motion sickness (from travel, any vehicle)
  (from roundabouts or swings) T75.3
Mottled, mottling, teeth (enamel) (endemic)
  (nonendemic) K00.3
Mounier-Kuhn syndrome Q32.4
  with bronchiectasis J47.9
    exacerbation (acute) J47.1
    lower respiratory infection J47.0
  acquired J98.09
    with bronchiectasis J47.9
      with
        exacerbation (acute) J47.1
        lower respiratory infection J47.0
Mountain
  sickness T70.29
    with polycythemia , acquired (acute) D75.1
  tick fever A93.2
Mouse, joint —see Loose, body, joint
  knee M23.4-●
Mouth —see condition
Movable
  coccyx —see subcategory M53.2
  kidney N28.89
    congenital Q63.8
  spleen D73.89
Movements, dystonic R25.8
Moyamoya disease I67.5
MRSA (Methicillin resistant Staphylococcus
  aureus)
  infection A49.02
    as the cause of diseases classified
      elsewhere B95.62
  sepsis A41.02
MSSA (Methicillin susceptible Staphylococcus
  aureus)
  infection A49.01
    as the cause of diseases classified
      elsewhere B95.61
  sepsis A41.01
Mucha-Habermann disease L41.0
Mucinosis (cutaneous) (focal) (papular)
  (reticular erythematous) (skin) L98.5
  oral K13.79
Mucocele
  appendix K38.8
  buccal cavity K13.79
  gallbladder K82.1
  lacrimal sac, chronic H04.43-●
  nasal sinus J34.1
  nose J34.1
  salivary gland (any) K11.6
  sinus (accessory) (nasal) J34.1
  turbinate (bone) (middle) (nasal) J34.1
  uterus N85.8

Mucolipidosis
  I E77.1
  II, III E77.0
  IV E75.11
Mucopolysaccharidosis E76.3
  beta-gluduronidase deficiency E76.29
  cardiopathy E76.3 [I52]
  Hunter's syndrome E76.1
  Hurler's syndrome E76.01
  Hurler-Scheie syndrome E76.02
  Maroteaux-Lamy syndrome E76.29
  Morquio syndrome E76.219
    A E76.210
    B E76.211
    classic E76.210
  Sanfilippo syndrome E76.22
  Scheie's syndrome E76.03
  specified NEC E76.29
  type
    I
      Hurler's syndrome E76.01
      Hurler-Scheie syndrome E76.02
      Scheie's syndrome E76.03
    II E76.1
    III E76.22
    IV E76.219
    IVA E76.210
    IVB E76.211
    VI E76.29
    VII E76.29
Mucormycosis B46.5
  cutaneous B46.3
  disseminated B46.4
  gastrointestinal B46.2
  generalized B46.4
  pulmonary B46.0
  rhinocerebral B46.1
  skin B46.3
  subcutaneous B46.3
Mucositis (ulcerative) K12.30
  due to drugs NEC K12.32
  gastrointestinal K92.81
  mouth (oral) (oropharyngeal) K12.30
    due to antineoplastic therapy K12.31
    due to drugs NEC K12.32
    due to radiation K12.33
    specified NEC K12.39
    viral K12.39
  nasal J34.81
  oral cavity —see Mucositis, mouth
  oral soft tissues —see Mucositis, mouth
  vagina and vulva N76.81
Mucositis necroticans agranulocytica —see
  Agranulocytosis
Mucous —see also condition
  patches (syphilitic) A51.39
    congenital A50.07
Mucoviscidosis E84.9
  with meconium obstruction E84.11
Mucus
  asphyxia or suffocation —see Asphyxia,
    mucus
  in stool R19.5
  plug —see Asphyxia, mucus
Muguet B37.0
Mulberry molars (congenital syphilis)
  A50.52
Müllerian mixed tumor
  specified site —see Neoplasm, malignant, by
    site
  unspecified site C54.9
Multicystic kidney (development) Q61.4
Multiparity (grand) Z64.1
  affecting management of pregnancy, labor
    and delivery (supervision only)
    O09.4-●
  requiring contraceptive management —see
    Contraception
Multipartita placenta O43.19-●
Multiple, multiplex —see also condition
  digits (congenital) Q69.9

Multiple, multiplex (Continued)
  endocrine neoplasia —see Neoplasia,
    endocrine, multiple [MEN]
  personality F44.81
Mumps B26.9
  arthritis B26.85
  complication NEC B26.89
  encephalitis B26.2
  hepatitis B26.81
  meningitis (aseptic) B26.1
  meningoencephalitis B26.2
  myocarditis B26.82
  oophoritis B26.89
  orchitis B26.0
  pancreatitis B26.3
  polyneuropathy B26.84
Mumu —see also Infestation, filarial B74.9
  [N51]
Münchhausen's syndrome —see Disorder,
  factitious
Münchmeyer's syndrome —see Myositis,
  ossificans, progressiva
Mural —see condition
Murmur (cardiac) (heart) (organic) R01.1
  abdominal R19.15
  aortic (valve) —see Endocarditis, aortic
  benign R01.0
  diastolic —see Endocarditis
  Flint I35.1
  functional R01.0
  Graham Steell I37.1
  innocent R01.0
  mitral (valve) —see Insufficiency, mitral
  nonorganic R01.0
  presystolic, mitral —see Insufficiency, mitral
  pulmonic (valve) I37.8
  systolic R01.1
  tricuspid (valve) I07.9
  valvular —see Endocarditis
Murri's disease (intermittent hemoglobinuria)
  D59.6
Muscle, muscular —see also condition
  carnitine (palmityltransferase) deficiency
    E71.314
Musculoneuralgia —see Neuralgia
Mushroom-workers' (pickers') disease or lung
  J67.5
Mushrooming hip —see Derangement, joint,
  specified NEC, hip
Mutation(s)
  factor V Leiden D68.51
  surfactant, of lung J84.83
  prothrombin gene D68.52
Mutism —see also Aphasia
  deaf (acquired) (congenital) NEC H91.3
  elective (adjustment reaction) (childhood)
    F94.0
  hysterical F44.4
  selective (childhood) F94.0
MVD (microvillus inclusion disease) Q43.8
MVID (microvillus inclusion disease) Q43.8
Myalgia M79.1
  epidemic (cervical) B33.0
  traumatic NEC T14.8
Myasthenia G70.9
  congenital G70.2
  cordis —see Failure, heart
  developmental G70.2
  gravis G70.00
    with exacerbation (acute) G70.01
    in crisis G70.01
    neonatal, transient P94.0
    pseudoparalytica G70.00
      with exacerbation (acute) G70.01
      in crisis G70.01
  stomach, psychogenic F45.8
  syndrome
    in
      diabetes mellitus —see E08-E13 with .44
      neoplastic disease —see also Neoplasm
        D49.9 [G73.3]

Myasthenia (Continued)
  syndrome (Continued)
    in (Continued)
      pernicious anemia D51.0 [G73.3]
      thyrotoxicosis E05.90 [G73.3]
        with thyroid storm E05.91 [G73.3]
Myasthenic M62.81
Mycelium infection B49
Mycetismus —see Poisoning, food, noxious, mushroom
Mycetoma B47.9
  actinomycotic B47.1
  bone (mycotic) B47.9 [M90.80]
  eumycotic B47.0
  foot B47.9
    actinomycotic B47.1
    mycotic B47.0
  madurae NEC B47.9
    mycotic B47.0
  maduromycotic B47.0
  mycotic B47.0
  nocardial B47.1
Mycobacteriosis —see Mycobacterium
Mycobacterium, mycobacterial (infection) A31.9
  anonymous A31.9
  atypical A31.9
    cutaneous A31.1
    pulmonary A31.0
      tuberculous —see Tuberculosis, pulmonary
    specified site NEC A31.8
  avium (intracellulare complex) A31.0
  balnei A31.1
  Battey A31.0
  chelonei A31.8
  cutaneous A31.1
  extrapulmonary systemic A31.8
  fortuitum A31.8
  intracellulare (Battey bacillus) A31.0
  kakaferifu A31.8
  kansasii (yellow bacillus) A31.0
  kasongo A31.8
  leprae —see also Leprosy A30.9
  luciflavum A31.1
  marinum (M. balnei) A31.1
  nonspecific —see Mycobacterium, atypical
  pulmonary (atypical) A31.0
    tuberculous —see Tuberculosis, pulmonary
  scrofulaceum A31.8
  simiae A31.8
  systemic, extrapulmonary A31.8
  szulgai A31.8
  terrae A31.8
  triviale A31.8
  tuberculosis (human, bovine) —see Tuberculosis
  ulcerans A31.1
  xenopi A31.8
Mycoplasma (M.) **pneumoniae, as cause of disease classified elsewhere** B96.0
Mycosis, mycotic B49
  cutaneous NEC B36.9
  ear B36.9
    in
      aspergillosis B44.89
      candidiasis B37.84
      moniliasis B37.84
  fungoides (extranodal) (solid organ) C84.0-●
  mouth B37.0
  nails B35.1
  opportunistic B48.8
  skin NEC B36.9
  specified NEC B48.8
  stomatitis B37.0
  vagina, vaginitis (candidal) B37.3
Mydriasis (pupil) H57.04
Myelatelia Q06.1
Myelinolysis, pontine, central G37.2

Myelitis (acute) (ascending) (childhood) (chronic) (descending) (diffuse) (disseminated) (idiopathic) (pressure) (progressive) (spinal cord) (subacute) —see also Encephalitis G04.91
  herpes simplex B00.82
  herpes zoster B02.24
  in diseases classified elsewhere G05.4
  necrotizing, subacute G37.4
  optic neuritis in G36.0
  postchickenpox B01.12
  postherpetic B02.24
  postimmunization G04.02
  postinfectious NEC G04.89
  postvaccinal G04.02
  specified NEC G04.89
  syphilitic (transverse) A52.14
  toxic G92
  transverse (in demyelinating diseases of central nervous system) G37.3
  tuberculous A17.82
  varicella B01.12
Myeloblastic —see condition
Myeloblastoma
  granular cell —see also Neoplasm, connective tissue
    malignant —see Neoplasm, connective tissue, malignant
    tongue D10.1
Myelocele —see Spina bifida
Myelocystocele —see Spina bifida
Myelocytic —see condition
Myelodysplasia D46.9
  specified NEC D46.Z
  spinal cord (congenital) Q06.1
Myelodysplastic syndrome D46.9
  with
    5q deletion D46.C
    isolated del (5q) chromosomal abnormality C46.C
  specified NEC D46.Z
Myeloencephalitis —see Encephalitis
Myelofibrosis D75.81
  with myeloid metaplasia D47.4
  acute C94.4-●
  idiopathic (chronic) D47.4
  primary D47.1
  secondary D75.81
    in myeloproliferative disease D47.4
Myelogenous —see condition
Myeloid —see condition
Myelokathexis D70.9
Myeloleukodystrophy E75.29
Myelolipoma —see Lipoma
Myeloma (multiple) C90.0-●
  monostotic C90.3
    plasma cell C90.0-●
  plasma cell C90.0-●
  solitary —see also Plasmacytoma, solitary C90.3-●
Myelomalacia G95.89
Myelomatosis C90.0-●
Myelomeningitis —see Meningoencephalitis
Myelomeningocele (spinal cord) —see Spina bifida
Myelo-osteo-musculodysplasia hereditaria Q79.8
Myelopathic
  anemia D64.89
  muscle atrophy —see Atrophy, muscle, spinal
  pain syndrome G89.0
Myelopathy (spinal cord) G95.9
  drug-induced G95.89
  in (due to)
    degeneration or displacement, intervertebral disc NEC —see Disorder, disc, with, myelopathy
    infection —see Encephalitis
    intervertebral disc disorder —see also Disorder, disc, with, myelopathy
    mercury —see subcategory T56.1

Myelopathy (Continued)
  in (due to) (Continued)
    neoplastic disease —see also Neoplasm D49.9 [G99.2]
    pernicious anemia D51.0 [G99.2]
    spondylosis —see Spondylosis, with myelopathy NEC
  necrotic (subacute) (vascular) G95.19
  radiation-induced G95.89
  spondylogenic NEC —see Spondylosis, with myelopathy NEC
  toxic G95.89
  transverse, acute G37.3
  vascular G95.19
  vitamin B12 E53.8 [G32.0]
Myelophthisis D61.82
Myeloradiculitis G04.91
Myeloradiculodysplasia (spinal) Q06.1
Myelosarcoma C92.3-●
Myelosclerosis D75.89
  with myeloid metaplasia D47.4
  disseminated, of nervous system G35
  megakaryocytic D47.4
    with myeloid metaplasia D47.4
Myelosis
  acute C92.0-●
  aleukemic C92.9-●
  chronic D47.1
  erythremic (acute) C94.0-●
  megakaryocytic C94.2-●
  nonleukemic D72.828
  subacute C92.9-●
Myiasis (cavernous) B87.9
  aural B87.4
  creeping B87.0
  cutaneous B87.0
  dermal B87.0
  ear (external) (middle) B87.4
  eye B87.2
  genitourinary B87.81
  intestinal B87.82
  laryngeal B87.3
  nasopharyngeal B87.3
  ocular B87.2
  orbit B87.2
  skin B87.0
  specified site NEC B87.89
  traumatic B87.1
  wound B87.1
Myoadenoma, prostate —see Hyperplasia, prostate
Myoblastoma
  granular cell —see also Neoplasm, connective tissue, benign
    malignant —see Neoplasm, connective tissue, malignant
  tongue D10.1
Myocardial —see condition
Myocardiopathy (congestive) (constrictive) (familial) (hypertrophic nonobstructive) (idiopathic) (infiltrative) (obstructive) (primary) (restrictive) (sporadic) —see also Cardiomyopathy I42.9
  alcoholic I42.6
  cobalt-beer I42.6
  glycogen storage E74.02 [I43]
  hypertrophic obstructive I42.1
  in (due to)
    beriberi E51.12
    cardiac glycogenosis E74.02 [I43]
    Friedreich's ataxia G11.1 [I43]
    myotonia atrophica G71.11 [I43]
    progressive muscular dystrophy G71.0 [I43]
  obscure (African) I42.8
  secondary I42.9
  thyrotoxic E05.90 [I43]
    with storm E05.91 [I43]
  toxic NEC I42.7

▶ New   ▸ Revised   ~~deleted~~ Deleted   ● Use Additional Character(s)

Myocarditis (with arteriosclerosis) (chronic) (fibroid) (interstitial) (old) (progressive) (senile) I51.4
with
  rheumatic fever (conditions in I00) I09.0
    active —see Myocarditis, acute, rheumatic
    inactive or quiescent (with chorea) I09.0
active I40.9
  rheumatic I01.2
    with chorea (acute) (rheumatic) (Sydenham's) I02.0
acute or subacute (interstitial) I40.9
  due to
    streptococcus (beta-hemolytic) I01.2
  idiopathic I40.1
  rheumatic I01.2
    with chorea (acute) (rheumatic) (Sydenham's) I02.0
  specified NEC I40.8
aseptic of newborn B33.22
bacterial (acute) I40.0
Coxsackie (virus) B33.22
diphtheritic A36.81
eosinophilic I40.1
epidemic of newborn (Coxsackie) B33.22
Fiedler's (acute) (isolated) I40.1
giant cell (acute) (subacute) I40.1
gonococcal A54.83
granulomatous (idiopathic) (isolated) (nonspecific) I40.1
hypertensive —see Hypertension, heart
idiopathic (granulomatous) I40.1
in (due to)
  diphtheria A36.81
  epidemic louse-borne typhus A75.0 [I41]
  Lyme disease A69.29
  sarcoidosis D86.85
  scarlet fever A38.1
  toxoplasmosis (acquired) B58.81
  typhoid A01.02
  typhus NEC A75.9 [I41]
infective I40.0
influenzal —see Influenza, with, myocarditis
isolated (acute) I40.1
meningococcal A39.52
mumps B26.82
nonrheumatic, active I40.9
parenchymatous I40.9
pneumococcal I40.0
rheumatic (chronic) (inactive) (with chorea) I09.0
  active or acute I01.2
    with chorea (acute) (rheumatic) (Sydenham's) I02.0
rheumatoid —see Rheumatoid, carditis
septic I40.0
staphylococcal I40.0
suppurative I40.0
syphilitic (chronic) A52.06
toxic I40.8
  rheumatic —see Myocarditis, acute, rheumatic
tuberculous A18.84
typhoid A01.02
valvular —see Endocarditis
virus, viral I40.0
  of newborn (Coxsackie) B33.22
Myocardium, myocardial —see condition
Myocardosis —see Cardiomyopathy
Myoclonus, myoclonic, myoclonia (familial) (essential) (multifocal) (simplex) G25.3
drug-induced G25.3
epilepsy —see also Epilepsy, generalized, specified NEC G40.4-●
  familial (progressive) G25.3
epileptica G40.409
  with status epilepticus G40.401
facial G51.3
familial progressive G25.3
Friedreich's G25.3

Myoclonus, myoclonic, myoclonia (Continued)
jerks G25.3
massive G25.3
palatal G25.3
pharyngeal G25.3
Myocytolysis I51.5
Myodiastasis —see Diastasis, muscle
Myoendocarditis —see Endocarditis
Myoepithelioma —see Neoplasm, benign, by site
Myofasciitis (acute) —see Myositis
Myofibroma —see also Neoplasm, connective tissue, benign
uterus (cervix) (corpus) —see Leiomyoma
Myofibromatosis D48.1
infantile Q89.8
Myofibrosis M62.89
heart —see Myocarditis
scapulohumeral —see Lesion, shoulder, specified NEC
Myofibrositis M79.7
scapulohumeral —see Lesion, shoulder, specified NEC
Myoglobulinuria, myoglobinuria (primary) R82.1
Myokymia, facial G51.4
Myolipoma —see Lipoma
Myoma —see also Neoplasm, connective tissue, benign
malignant —see Neoplasm, connective tissue, malignant
prostate D29.1
uterus (cervix) (corpus) —see Leiomyoma
Myomalacia M62.89
Myometritis —see Endometritis
Myometrium —see condition
Myonecrosis, clostridial A48.0
Myopathy G72.9
acute
  necrotizing G72.81
  quadriplegic G72.81
alcoholic G72.1
benign congenital G71.2
central core G71.2
centronuclear G71.2
congenital (benign) G71.2
critical illness G72.81
distal G71.0
drug-induced G72.0
endocrine NEC E34.9 [G73.7]
extraocular muscles H05.82-●
facioscapulohumeral G71.0
hereditary G71.9
  specified NEC G71.8
immune NEC G72.49
in (due to)
  Addison's disease E27.1 [G73.7]
  alcohol G72.1
  amyloidosis E85.0 [G73.7]
  cretinism E00.9 [G73.7]
  Cushing's syndrome E24.9 [G73.7]
  drugs G72.0
  endocrine disease NEC E34.9 [G73.7]
  giant cell arteritis M31.6 [G73.7]
  glycogen storage disease E74.00 [G73.7]
  hyperadrenocorticism E24.9 [G73.7]
  hyperparathyroidism NEC E21.3 [G73.7]
  hypoparathyroidism E20.9 [G73.7]
  hypopituitarism E23.0 [G73.7]
  hypothyroidism E03.9 [G73.7]
  infectious disease NEC B99 [G73.7]
  lipid storage disease E75.6 [G73.7]
  metabolic disease NEC E88.9 [G73.7]
  myxedema E03.9 [G73.7]
  parasitic disease NEC B89 [G73.7]
  polyarteritis nodosa M30.0 [G73.7]
  rheumatoid arthritis —see Rheumatoid, myopathy
  sarcoidosis D86.87
  scleroderma M34.82
  sicca syndrome M35.03

Myopathy (Continued)
in (due to) (Continued)
  Sjögren's syndrome M35.03
  systemic lupus erythematosus M32.19
  thyrotoxicosis (hyperthyroidism) E05.90 [G73.7]
    with thyroid storm E05.91 [G73.7]
  toxic agent NEC G72.2
inflammatory NEC G72.49
intensive care (ICU) G72.81
limb-girdle G71.0
mitochondrial NEC G71.3
myotubular G71.2
mytonic, proximal (PROMM) G71.11
nemaline G71.2
ocular G71.0
oculopharyngeal G71.0
of critical illness G72.81
primary G71.9
  specified NEC G71.8
progressive NEC G72.89
proximal myotonic (PROMM) G71.11
rod G71.2
scapulohumeral G71.0
specified NEC G72.89
toxic G72.2
Myopericarditis —see also Pericarditis
chronic rheumatic I09.2
Myopia (axial) (congenital) H52.1-●
➥degenerative (malignant) H44.20
  ▶with
    ▶choroidal neovascularization H44.2A-●
    ▶foveoschisis H44.2D-●
    ▶macular hole H44.2B-●
    ▶retinal detachment H44.2C-●
    ▶specified maculopathy NEC H44.2E-●
  ▶bilateral H44.23
  ▶left eye H44.22
  ▶right eye H44.21
➥malignant —see also Myopia, degenerative H44.2-●
➥pernicious —see also Myopia, degenerative H44.2-●
➥progressive high (degenerative) —see also Myopia, degenerative H44.2-●
Myosarcoma —see Neoplasm, connective tissue, malignant
Myosis (pupil) H57.03
stromal (endolymphatic) D39.0
Myositis M60.9
clostridial A48.0
due to posture —see Myositis, specified type NEC
epidemic B33.0
fibrosa or fibrous (chronic), Volkmann's T79.6
foreign body granuloma —see Granuloma, foreign body
in (due to)
  bilharziasis B65.9 [M63.8-●]
  cysticercosis B69.81
  leprosy A30.9 [M63.8-●]
  mycosis B49 [M63.8-●]
  sarcoidosis D86.87
  schistosomiasis B65.9 [M63.8-●]
  syphilis
    late A52.78
    secondary A51.49
  toxoplasmosis (acquired) B58.82
  trichinellosis B75 [M63.8-●]
  tuberculosis A18.09
inclusion body [IBM] G72.41
infective M60.009
  arm M60.002
    left M60.001
    right M60.000
  leg M60.005
    left M60.004
    right M60.003
  lower limb M60.005
    ankle M60.07-●
    foot M60.07-●
    lower leg M60.06-●

Myositis *(Continued)*
  infective *(Continued)*
    lower limb *(Continued)*
      thigh M60.05-●
      toe M60.07-●
    multiple sites M60.09
    specified site NEC M60.08
    upper limb M60.002
      finger M60.04-●
      forearm M60.03-●
      hand M60.04-●
      shoulder region M60.01-●
      upper arm M60.02-●
  interstitial M60.10
    ankle M60.17-●
    foot M60.17-●
    forearm M60.13-●
    hand M60.14-●
    lower leg M60.16-●
    multiple sites M60.19
    shoulder region M60.11-●
    specified site NEC M60.18
    thigh M60.15-●
    upper arm M60.12-●
  mycotic B49 [M63.8-●]
  ossificans or ossifying (circumscripta) —see
    also Ossification, muscle, specified NEC
    in (due to)
      burns M61.30
        ankle M61.37-●
        foot M61.37-●
        forearm M61.33-●
        hand M61.34-●
        lower leg M61.36-●
        multiple sites M61.39
        pelvic region M61.35-●
        shoulder region M61.31-●
        specified site NEC M61.38
        thigh M61.35-●
        upper arm M61.32-●
      quadriplegia or paraplegia M61.20
        ankle M61.27-●
        foot M61.27-●
        forearm M61.23-●
        hand M61.24-●
        lower leg M61.26-●
        multiple sites M61.29
        pelvic region M61.25-●
        shoulder region M61.21-●
        specified site NEC M61.28
        thigh M61.25-●
        upper arm M61.22-●

Myositis *(Continued)*
  ossificans or ossifying *(Continued)*
    progressiva M61.10
      ankle M61.17-●
      finger M61.14-●
      foot M61.17-●
      forearm M61.13-●
      hand M61.14-●
      lower leg M61.16-●
      multiple sites M61.19
      pelvic region M61.15-●
      shoulder region M61.11-●
      specified site NEC M61.18
      thigh M61.15-●
      toe M61.17-●
      upper arm M61.12-●
    traumatica M61.00
      ankle M61.07-●
      foot M61.07-●
      forearm M61.03-●
      hand M61.04-●
      lower leg M61.06-●
      multiple sites M61.09
      pelvic region M61.05-●
      shoulder region M61.01-●
      specified site NEC M61.08
      thigh M61.05-●
      upper arm M61.02-●
  purulent —see Myositis, infective
  specified type NEC M60.80
    ankle M60.87-●
    foot M60.87-●
    forearm M60.83-●
    hand M60.84-●
    lower leg M60.86-●
    multiple sites M60.89
    pelvic region M60.85-●
    shoulder region M60.81-●
    specified site NEC M60.88
    thigh M60.85-●
    upper arm M60.82-●
  suppurative —see Myositis, infective
  traumatic (old) —see Myositis, specified type
    NEC
Myospasia impulsiva F95.2
Myotonia (acquisita) (intermittens) M62.89
  atrophica G71.11
  chondrodystrophic G71.13
  congenita (acetazolamide responsive)
    (dominant) (recessive) G71.12

Myotonia *(Continued)*
  drug-induced G71.14
  dystrophica G71.11
  fluctuans G71.19
  levior G71.12
  permanens G71.19
  symptomatic G71.19
Myotonic pupil —see Anomaly, pupil, function,
  tonic pupil
Myriapodiasis B88.2
Myringitis H73.2-●
  with otitis media —see Otitis, media
  acute H73.00-●
    bullous H73.01-●
    specified NEC H73.09-●
  bullous —see Myringitis, acute, bullous
  chronic H73.1-●
Mysophobia F40.228
Mytilotoxism —see Poisoning, fish
Myxadenitis labialis K13.0
Myxedema (adult) (idiocy) (infantile)
  (juvenile) —see also Hypothyroidism
  E03.9
  circumscribed E05.90
    with storm E05.91
  coma E03.5
  congenital E00.1
  cutis L98.5
  localized (pretibial) E05.90
    with storm E05.91
  papular L98.5
Myxochondrosarcoma —see Neoplasm,
  cartilage, malignant
Myxofibroma —see Neoplasm, connective
  tissue, benign
  odontogenic —see Cyst, calcifying
    odontogenic
Myxofibrosarcoma —see Neoplasm, connective
  tissue, malignant
Myxolipoma D17.9
Myxoliposarcoma —see Neoplasm, connective
  tissue, malignant
Myxoma —see also Neoplasm, connective tissue,
  benign
  nerve sheath —see Neoplasm, nerve,
    benign
  odontogenic —see Cyst, calcifying
    odontogenic
Myxosarcoma —see Neoplasm, connective
  tissue, malignant

M

▶ New   ⇒ Revised   ~~deleted~~ Deleted   ● Use Additional Character(s)

N

Naegeli's
   disease Q82.8
   leukemia, monocytic C93.1-•
Naegleriasis (with meningoencephalitis)
      B60.2
Naffziger's syndrome G54.0
Naga sore —see Ulcer, skin
Nägele's pelvis M95.5
   with disproportion (fetopelvic) O33.0
      causing obstructed labor O65.0
Nail —see also condition
   biting F98.8
   patella syndrome Q87.2
Nanism, nanosomia —see Dwarfism
Nanophyetiasis B66.8
Nanukayami A27.89
Napkin rash L22
Narcolepsy G47.419
   with cataplexy G47.411
   in conditions classified elsewhere
         G47.429
      with cataplexy G47.421
Narcosis R06.89
Narcotism —see Dependence
NARP (Neuropathy, Ataxia and Retinitis
      pigmentosa) syndrome E88.49
Narrow
   anterior chamber angle H40.03-•
   gingival width (of periodontal soft tissue)
         K05.5
   pelvis —see Contraction, pelvis
Narrowing —see also Stenosis
   artery I77.1
      auditory, internal I65.8
      basilar —see Occlusion, artery, basilar
      carotid —see Occlusion, artery, carotid
      cerebellar —see Occlusion, artery, cerebellar
      cerebral —see Occlusion artery, cerebral
      choroidal —see Occlusion, artery, cerebral,
            specified NEC
      communicating posterior —see Occlusion,
            artery, cerebral, specified NEC
      coronary —see also Disease, heart, ischemic,
            atherosclerotic
         congenital Q24.5
            syphilitic A50.54 [I52]
         due to syphilis NEC A52.06
      hypophyseal —see Occlusion, artery,
            cerebral, specified NEC
      pontine —see Occlusion, artery, cerebral,
            specified NEC
      precerebral —see Occlusion, artery,
            precerebral
      vertebral —see Occlusion, artery, vertebral
   auditory canal (external) —see Stenosis,
         external ear canal
   eustachian tube —see Obstruction, eustachian
         tube
   eyelid —see Disorder, eyelid function
   larynx J38.6
   mesenteric artery —see also Ischemia,
         intestine, acute K55.059
   palate M26.89
   palpebral fissure —see Disorder, eyelid
         function
   ureter N13.5
      with infection N13.6
   urethra —see Stricture, urethra
Narrowness, abnormal, eyelid Q10.3
Nasal —see condition
Nasolachrymal, nasolacrimal —see condition
Nasopharyngeal —see also condition
   pituitary gland Q89.2
   torticollis M43.6
Nasopharyngitis (acute) (infective)
      (streptococcal) (subacute) J00
   chronic (suppurative) (ulcerative) J31.1
Nasopharynx, nasopharyngeal —see condition
Natal tooth, teeth K00.6

Nausea (without vomiting) R11.0
   with vomiting R11.2
      gravidarum —see Hyperemesis, gravidarum
   marina T75.3
   navalis T75.3
Navel —see condition
Neapolitan fever —see Brucellosis
Near drowning T75.1
Nearsightedness —see Myopia
Near-syncope R55
Nebula, cornea —see Opacity, cornea
Necator americanus infestation B76.1
Necatoriasis B76.1
Neck —see condition
Necrobiosis R68.89
   lipoidica NEC L92.1
      with diabetes —see E08-E13 with .620
Necrolysis, toxic epidermal L51.2
   due to drug
      correct substance properly administered —
            see Table of Drugs and Chemicals, by
            drug, adverse effect
      overdose or wrong substance given
            or taken —see Table of Drugs and
            Chemicals, by drug, poisoning
Necrophilia F65.89
Necrosis, necrotic (ischemic) —see also
      Gangrene
   adrenal (capsule) (gland) E27.49
   amputation stump (surgical) (late) T87.50
      arm T87.5-•
      leg T87.5-•
   antrum J32.0
   aorta (hyaline) —see also Aneurysm, aorta
      cystic medial —see Dissection, aorta
   artery I77.5
   bladder (aseptic) (sphincter) N32.89
   bone —see also Osteonecrosis M87.9
      aseptic or avascular —see Osteonecrosis
         idiopathic M87.00
      ethmoid J32.2
      jaw M27.2
      tuberculous —see Tuberculosis, bone
   brain I67.89
   breast (aseptic) (fat) (segmental) N64.1
   bronchus J98.09
   central nervous system NEC I67.89
   cerebellar I67.89
   cerebral I67.89
   colon —see also Infarct, intestine K55.049
   cornea H18.89-•
   cortical (acute) (renal) N17.1
   cystic medial (aorta) —see Dissection, aorta
   dental pulp K04.1
   esophagus K22.8
   ethmoid (bone) J32.2
   eyelid —see Disorder, eyelid, degenerative
   fat, fatty (generalized) —see also Disorder, soft
         tissue, specified type NEC
      abdominal wall K65.4
      breast (aseptic) (segmental) N64.1
      localized —see Degeneration, by site, fatty
      mesentery K65.4
      omentum K65.4
      pancreas K86.89
      peritoneum K65.4
      skin (subcutaneous), newborn P83.0
      subcutaneous, due to birth injury P15.6
   gallbladder —see Cholecystitis, acute
   heart —see Infarct, myocardium
   hip, aseptic or avascular —see Osteonecrosis,
         by type, femur
   intestine (acute) (hemorrhagic) (massive) —
         see also Infarct, intestine K55.069
   jaw M27.2
   kidney (bilateral) N28.0
      acute N17.9
      cortical (acute) (bilateral) N17.1
         with ectopic or molar pregnancy O08.4
      medullary (bilateral) (in acute renal failure)
            (papillary) N17.2

Necrosis, necrotic (Continued)
   kidney (Continued)
      papillary (bilateral) (in acute renal
            failure) N17.2
      tubular N17.0
         with ectopic or molar pregnancy
               O08.4
         complicating
            abortion —see Abortion, by type,
                  complicated by, tubular necrosis
            ectopic or molar pregnancy O08.4
            pregnancy —see Pregnancy,
                  complicated by, diseases of,
                  specified type or system NEC
         following ectopic or molar pregnancy
               O08.4
      traumatic T79.5
   larynx J38.7
   liver (with hepatic failure) (cell) —see Failure,
         hepatic
      hemorrhagic, central K76.2
   lung J85.0
   lymphatic gland —see Lymphadenitis, acute
   mammary gland (fat) (segmental) N64.1
   mastoid (chronic) —see Mastoiditis, chronic
   medullary (acute) (renal) N17.2
   mesentery —see also Infarct, intestine
         K55.069
      fat K65.4
   mitral valve —see Insufficiency, mitral
   myocardium, myocardial —see Infarct,
         myocardium
   nose J34.0
   omentum (with mesenteric infarction) —see
         also Infarct, intestine K55.069
      fat K65.4
   orbit, orbital —see Osteomyelitis, orbit
   ossicles, ear —see Abnormal, ear ossicles
   ovary N70.92
   pancreas (aseptic) (duct) (fat) K86.89
      acute (infective) —see Pancreatitis, acute
      infective —see Pancreatitis, acute
   papillary (acute) (renal) N17.2
   perineum N90.89
   peritoneum (with mesenteric infarction) —see
         also Infarct, intestine K55.069
      fat K65.4
   pharynx J02.9
      in granulocytopenia —see Neutropenia
      Vincent's A69.1
   phosphorus —see subcategory T54.2
   pituitary (gland) E23.0
      postpartum O99.285
      Sheehan O99.285
   pressure —see Ulcer, pressure, by site
   pulmonary J85.0
   pulp (dental) K04.1
   radiation —see Necrosis, by site
   radium —see Necrosis, by site
   renal —see Necrosis, kidney
   sclera H15.89
   scrotum N50.89
   skin or subcutaneous tissue NEC I96
   spine, spinal (column) —see also
         Osteonecrosis, by type, vertebra
      cord G95.19
   spleen D73.5
   stomach K31.89
   stomatitis (ulcerative) A69.0
➡ subcutaneous fat, newborn P83.88
   subendocardial (acute) I21.4
      chronic I25.89
   suprarenal (capsule) (gland) E27.49
   testis N50.89
   thymus (gland) E32.8
   tonsil J35.8
   trachea J39.8
   tuberculous NEC —see Tuberculosis
   tubular (acute) (anoxic) (renal) (toxic)
         N17.0
      postprocedural N99.0

Necrosis, necrotic *(Continued)*
  vagina N89.8
  vertebra —*see also* Osteonecrosis, by type,
    vertebra
    tuberculous A18.01
  vulva N90.89
  X-ray —*see* Necrosis, by site
Necrospermia —*see* Infertility, male
Need (for)
  care provider because (of)
    assistance with personal care Z74.1
    continuous supervision required Z74.3
    impaired mobility Z74.09
    no other household member able to render
      care Z74.2
    specified reason NEC Z74.8
  immunization —*see* Vaccination
  vaccination —*see* Vaccination
Neglect
  adult
    confirmed T74.01
    history of Z91.412
    suspected T76.01
  child (childhood)
    confirmed T74.02
    history of Z62.812
    suspected T76.02
  emotional, in childhood Z62.898
  hemispatial R41.4
  left-sided R41.4
  sensory R41.4
  visuospatial R41.4
Neisserian infection NEC —*see* Gonococcus
Nelaton's syndrome G60.8
Nelson's syndrome E24.1
Nematodiasis (intestinal) B82.0
  Ancylostoma B76.0
Neonatal —*see also* Newborn
  acne L70.4
  bradycardia P29.12
  screening, abnormal findings on P09
  tachycardia P29.11
  tooth, teeth K00.6
Neonatorum —*see* condition
Neoplasia
  endocrine, multiple (MEN) E31.20
    type I E31.21
    type IIA E31.22
    type IIB E31.23
  intraepithelial (histologically confirmed)
    anal (AIN) (histologically confirmed)
      K62.82
      grade I K62.82
      grade II K62.82
      severe D01.3
    cervical glandular (histologically
      confirmed) D06.9
    cervix (uteri) (CIN) (histologically
      confirmed) N87.9
      glandular D06.9
      grade I N87.0
      grade II N87.1
      grade III (severe dysplasia) —*see also*
        Carcinoma, cervix uteri, in situ
        D06.9
    prostate (histologically confirmed) (PIN)
      N42.31
      grade I N42.31
      grade II N42.31
      grade III (severe dysplasia) D07.5
    vagina (histologically confirmed) (VAIN)
      N89.3
      grade I N89.0
      grade II N89.1
      grade III (severe dysplasia) D07.2
    vulva (histologically confirmed) (VIN)
      N90.3
      grade I N90.0
      grade II N90.1
      grade III (severe dysplasia)
        D07.1

Neoplasm, neoplastic —*see also* Table of
  Neoplasms
  lipomatous, benign —*see* Lipoma
▶malignant mast cell C96.20
  ▶specified type NEC C96.29
▶mast cell, of uncertain behavior NEC D47.09
Neovascularization
  ciliary body —*see* Disorder, iris, vascular
  cornea H16.40-●
    deep H16.44-●
    ghost vessels —*see* Ghost, vessels
    localized H16.43-●
    pannus —*see* Pannus
  iris —*see* Disorder, iris, vascular
  retina H35.05-●
Nephralgia N23
Nephritis, nephritic (albuminuric) (azotemic)
  (congenital) (disseminated) (epithelial)
  (familial) (focal) (granulomatous)
  (hemorrhagic) (infantile) (nonsuppurative,
  excretory) (uremic) N05.9
  with
    dense deposit disease N05.6
    diffuse
      crescentic glomerulonephritis N05.7
      endocapillary proliferative
        glomerulonephritis N05.4
      membranous glomerulonephritis N05.2
      mesangial proliferative
        glomerulonephritis N05.3
      mesangiocapillary glomerulonephritis
        N05.5
    edema —*see* Nephrosis
    focal and segmental glomerular lesions
      N05.1
    foot process disease N04.9
    glomerular lesion
      diffuse sclerosing N05.8
      hypocomplementemic —*see* Nephritis,
        membranoproliferative
      IgA —*see* Nephropathy, IgA
      lobular, lobulonodular —*see* Nephritis,
        membranoproliferative
      nodular —*see* Nephritis,
        membranoproliferative
    lesion of
      glomerulonephritis, proliferative N05.8
      renal necrosis N05.9
    minor glomerular abnormality N05.0
    specified morphological changes NEC
      N05.8
  acute N00.9
    with
      dense deposit disease N00.6
      diffuse
        crescentic glomerulonephritis
          N00.7
        endocapillary proliferative
          glomerulonephritis N00.4
        membranous glomerulonephritis
          N00.2
        mesangial proliferative
          glomerulonephritis N00.3
        mesangiocapillary glomerulonephritis
          N00.5
      focal and segmental glomerular lesions
        N00.1
      minor glomerular abnormality N00.0
      specified morphological changes NEC
        N00.8
  amyloid E85.4 *[N08]*
  antiglomerular basement membrane (anti-
    GBM) antibody NEC
    in Goodpasture's syndrome M31.0
  antitubular basement membrane (tubulo-
    interstitial) NEC N12
    toxic —*see* Nephropathy, toxic
  arteriolar —*see* Hypertension, kidney
  arteriosclerotic —*see* Hypertension, kidney
  ascending —*see* Nephritis, tubulo-interstitial
  atrophic N03.9

Nephritis, nephritic *(Continued)*
  Balkan (endemic) N15.0
  calculous, calculus —*see* Calculus,
    kidney
  cardiac —*see* Hypertension, kidney
  cardiovascular —*see* Hypertension,
    kidney
  chronic N03.9
    with
      dense deposit disease N03.6
      diffuse
        crescentic glomerulonephritis
          N03.7
        endocapillary proliferative
          glomerulonephritis N03.4
        membranous glomerulonephritis
          N03.2
        mesangial proliferative
          glomerulonephritis N03.3
        mesangiocapillary glomerulonephritis
          N03.5
      focal and segmental glomerular lesions
        N03.1
      minor glomerular abnormality
        N03.0
      specified morphological changes
        NEC N03.8
    arteriosclerotic —*see* Hypertension,
      kidney
  cirrhotic N26.9
  complicating pregnancy O26.83-●
  croupous N00.9
  degenerative —*see* Nephrosis
  diffuse sclerosing N05.8
  due to
    diabetes mellitus —*see* E08-E13 with .21
    subacute bacterial endocarditis I33.0
    systemic lupus erythematosus (chronic)
      M32.14
    typhoid fever A01.09
  gonococcal (acute) (chronic) A54.21
  hypocomplementemic —*see* Nephritis,
    membranoproliferative
  IgA —*see* Nephropathy, IgA
  immune complex (circulating) NEC N05.8
  infective —*see* Nephritis, tubulo-interstitial
  interstitial —*see* Nephritis, tubulo-interstitial
  lead N14.3
  membranoproliferative (diffuse) (type 1
    or 3) —*see also* N00-N07 with fourth
    character .5 N05.5
    type 2 —*see also* N00-N07 with fourth
      character .6 N05.6
  minimal change N05.0
  necrotic, necrotizing NEC —*see also*
    N00-N07 with fourth character .8
    N05.8
  nephrotic —*see* Nephrosis
  nodular —*see* Nephritis,
    membranoproliferative
  polycystic Q61.3
    adult type Q61.2
    autosomal
      dominant Q61.2
      recessive NEC Q61.19
    childhood type NEC Q61.19
    infantile type NEC Q61.19
  poststreptococcal N05.9
    acute N00.9
    chronic N03.9
    rapidly progressive N01.9
  proliferative NEC —*see also* N00-N07 with
    fourth character .8 N05.8
  purulent —*see* Nephritis, tubulo-interstitial
  rapidly progressive N01.9
    with
      dense deposit disease N01.6
      diffuse
        crescentic glomerulonephritis N01.7
        endocapillary proliferative
          glomerulonephritis N01.4

▶ New   ⇒ Revised   ~~deleted~~ Deleted   ● Use Additional Character(s)

Nephritis, nephritic *(Continued)*
  rapidly progressive *(Continued)*
    with *(Continued)*
      diffuse *(Continued)*
        membranous glomerulonephritis
          N01.2
        mesangial proliferative
          glomerulonephritis N01.3
        mesangiocapillary glomerulonephritis
          N01.5
        focal and segmental glomerular lesions
          N01.1
        minor glomerular abnormality N01.0
        specified morphological changes NEC
          N01.8
  salt losing or wasting NEC N28.89
  saturnine N14.3
  sclerosing, diffuse N05.8
  septic —*see* Nephritis, tubulo-interstitial
  specified pathology NEC —*see also* N00-N07
    with fourth character .8 N05.8
  subacute N01.9
  suppurative —*see* Nephritis,
    tubulo-interstitial
  syphilitic (late) A52.75
    congenital A50.59 *[N08]*
    early (secondary) A51.44
  toxic —*see* Nephropathy, toxic
  tubal, tubular —*see* Nephritis,
    tubulo-interstitial
  tuberculous A18.11
  tubulo-interstitial (in) N12
    acute (infectious) N10
    chronic (infectious) N11.9
      nonobstructive N11.8
        reflux-associated N11.0
      obstructive N11.1
      specified NEC N11.8
    due to
      brucellosis A23.9 *[N16]*
      cryoglobulinemia D89.1 *[N16]*
      glycogen storage disease E74.00
        [N16]
      Sjögren's syndrome M35.04
  vascular —*see* Hypertension, kidney
  war N00.9
Nephroblastoma (epithelial) (mesenchymal)
  C64-•
Nephrocalcinosis E83.59 *[N29]*
Nephrocystitis, pustular —*see* Nephritis,
  tubulo-interstitial
Nephrolithiasis (congenital) (pelvis)
  (recurrent) —*see also* Calculus, kidney
Nephroma C64-•
  mesoblastic D41.0-•
Nephronephritis —*see* Nephrosis
Nephronophthisis Q61.5
Nephropathia epidemica A98.5
Nephropathy —*see also* Nephritis N28.9
  with
    edema —*see* Nephrosis
    glomerular lesion —*see*
      Glomerulonephritis
  amyloid, hereditary E85.0
  analgesic N14.0
    with medullary necrosis, acute N17.2
  Balkan (endemic) N15.0
  chemical —*see* Nephropathy, toxic
  diabetic —*see* E08-E13 with .21
  drug-induced N14.2
    specified NEC N14.1
  focal and segmental hyalinosis or sclerosis
    N02.1
  heavy metal-induced N14.3
  hereditary NEC N07.9
    with
      dense deposit disease N07.6
      diffuse
        crescentic glomerulonephritis N07.7
        endocapillary proliferative
          glomerulonephritis N07.4

Nephropathy *(Continued)*
  hereditary NEC *(Continued)*
    with *(Continued)*
      diffuse *(Continued)*
        membranous glomerulonephritis
          N07.2
        mesangial proliferative
          glomerulonephritis N07.3
        mesangiocapillary glomerulonephritis
          N07.5
        focal and segmental glomerular lesions
          N07.1
        minor glomerular abnormality N07.0
        specified morphological changes NEC
          N07.8
  hypercalcemic N25.89
  hypertensive —*see* Hypertension, kidney
  hypokalemic (vacuolar) N25.89
  IgA N02.8
    with glomerular lesion N02.9
      focal and segmental hyalinosis or
        sclerosis N02.1
      membranoproliferative (diffuse) N02.5
      membranous (diffuse) N02.2
      mesangial proliferative (diffuse) N02.3
      mesangiocapillary (diffuse) N02.5
      proliferative NEC N02.8
      specified pathology NEC N02.8
  lead N14.3
  membranoproliferative (diffuse) N02.5
  membranous (diffuse) N02.2
  mesangial (IgA/IgG) —*see* Nephropathy, IgA
    proliferative (diffuse) N02.3
  mesangiocapillary (diffuse) N02.5
  obstructive N13.8
  phenacetin N17.2
  phosphate-losing N25.0
  potassium depletion N25.89
  pregnancy-related O26.83-•
  proliferative NEC (*see also* N00-N07 with
    fourth character .8) N05.8
  protein-losing N25.89
  saturnine N14.3
  sickle-cell D57.-• *[N08]*
  toxic NEC N14.4
    due to
      drugs N14.2
        analgesic N14.0
        specified NEC N14.1
      heavy metals N14.3
  vasomotor N17.0
  water-losing N25.89
Nephroptosis N28.83
Nephropyosis —*see* Abscess, kidney
Nephrorrhagia N28.89
Nephrosclerosis (arteriolar) (arteriosclerotic)
  (chronic) (hyaline) —*see also* Hypertension,
  kidney
  hyperplastic —*see* Hypertension, kidney
  senile N26.9
Nephrosis, nephrotic (Epstein's) (syndrome)
  (congenital) N04.9
  with
    foot process disease N04.9
    glomerular lesion N04.1
    hypocomplementemic N04.5
  acute N04.9
  anoxic —*see* Nephrosis, tubular
  chemical —*see* Nephrosis, tubular
  cholemic K76.7
  diabetic —*see* E08-E13 with .21
  Finnish type (congenital) Q89.8
  hemoglobin N10
  hemoglobinuric —*see* Nephrosis, tubular
  in
    amyloidosis E85.4 *[N08]*
    diabetes mellitus —*see* E08-E13 with .21
    epidemic hemorrhagic fever A98.5
    malaria (malariae) B52.0
  ischemic —*see* Nephrosis, tubular
  lipoid N04.9

Nephrosis, nephrotic *(Continued)*
  lower nephron —*see* Nephrosis, tubular
  malarial (malariae) B52.0
  minimal change N04.0
  myoglobin N10
  necrotizing —*see* Nephrosis, tubular
  osmotic (sucrose) N25.89
  radiation N04.9
  syphilitic (late) A52.75
  toxic —*see* Nephrosis, tubular
  tubular (acute) N17.0
    postprocedural N99.0
    radiation N04.9
Nephrosonephritis, hemorrhagic (endemic)
  A98.5
Nephrostomy
  attention to Z43.6
  status Z93.6
Nerve —*see also* condition
  injury —*see* Injury, nerve, by body site
Nerves R45.0
Nervous —*see also* condition R45.0
  heart F45.8
  stomach F45.8
  tension R45.0
Nervousness R45.0
Nesidioblastoma
  pancreas D13.7
  specified site NEC —*see* Neoplasm, benign,
    by site
  unspecified site D13.7
➡ **Nettleship's syndrome** —*see* Urticaria
  pigmentosa
Neumann's disease or syndrome L10.1
Neuralgia, neuralgic (acute) M79.2
  accessory (nerve) G52.8
  acoustic (nerve) —*see* subcategory H93.3
  auditory (nerve) —*see* subcategory H93.3
  ciliary G44.009
    intractable G44.001
    not intractable G44.009
  cranial
    nerve —*see also* Disorder, nerve, cranial
      fifth or trigeminal —*see* Neuralgia,
        trigeminal
      postherpetic, postzoster B02.29
  ear —*see* subcategory H92.0
  facialis vera G51.1
  Fothergill's —*see* Neuralgia, trigeminal
  glossopharyngeal (nerve) G52.1
  Horton's G44.009
    intractable G44.091
    not intractable G44.009
  Hunt's B02.21
  hypoglossal (nerve) G52.3
  infraorbital —*see* Neuralgia, trigeminal
  malarial —*see* Malaria
  migrainous G44.009
    intractable G44.001
    not intractable G44.009
  Morton's G57.6-•
  nerve, cranial —*see* Disorder, nerve, cranial
  nose G52.0
  occipital M54.81
  olfactory G52.0
  penis N48.9
  perineum R10.2
  postherpetic NEC B02.29
    trigeminal B02.22
  pubic region R10.2
  scrotum R10.2
  Sluder's G44.89
  specified nerve NEC G58.8
  spermatic cord R10.2
  sphenopalatine (ganglion) G90.09
  trifacial —*see* Neuralgia, trigeminal
  trigeminal G50.0
    postherpetic, postzoster B02.22
  vagus (nerve) G52.2
  writer's F48.8
    organic G25.89

Neurapraxia —*see* Injury, nerve
Neurasthenia F48.8
  cardiac F45.8
  gastric F45.8
  heart F45.8
Neurilemmoma —*see also* Neoplasm, nerve,
  benign
  acoustic (nerve) D33.3
  malignant —*see also* Neoplasm, nerve,
    malignant
    acoustic (nerve) C72.4
Neurilemmosarcoma —*see* Neoplasm, nerve,
  malignant
Neurinoma —*see* Neoplasm, nerve, benign
Neurinomatosis —*see* Neoplasm, nerve,
  uncertain behavior
Neuritis (rheumatoid) M79.2
  abducens (nerve) —*see* Strabismus, paralytic,
    sixth nerve
  accessory (nerve) G52.8
  acoustic (nerve) —*see also* subcategory H93.3
    in (due to)
      infectious disease NEC B99 [H94.0-●]
      parasitic disease NEC B89 [H94.0-●]
      syphilitic A52.15
  alcoholic G62.1
    with psychosis —*see* Psychosis, alcoholic
  amyloid, any site E85.4 [G63]
  auditory (nerve) —*see* subcategory H93.3
  brachial —*see* Radiculopathy
    due to displacement, intervertebral
      disc —*see* Disorder, disc, cervical, with
      neuritis
  cranial nerve
    due to Lyme disease A69.22
    eighth or acoustic or auditory —*see*
      subcategory H93.3
    eleventh or accessory G52.8
    fifth or trigeminal G51.0
    first or olfactory G52.0
    fourth or trochlear —*see* Strabismus,
      paralytic, fourth nerve
    second or optic —*see* Neuritis, optic
    seventh or facial G51.8
      newborn (birth injury) P11.3
    sixth or abducent —*see* Strabismus,
      paralytic, sixth nerve
    tenth or vagus G52.2
    third or oculomotor —*see* Strabismus,
      paralytic, third nerve
    twelfth or hypoglossal G52.3
  Déjérine-Sottas G60.0
  diabetic (mononeuropathy) —*see* E08-E13
    with .41
    polyneuropathy —*see* E08-E13 with .42
  due to
    beriberi E51.11
    displacement, prolapse or rupture,
      intervertebral disc —*see* Disorder, disc,
      with, radiculopathy
    herniation, nucleus pulposus M51.9 [G55]
  endemic E51.11
  facial G51.8
    newborn (birth injury) P11.3
  general —*see* Polyneuropathy
  geniculate ganglion G51.1
    due to herpes (zoster) B02.21
  gouty —*see also* Gout, by type M10.9 [G63]
  hypoglossal (nerve) G52.3
  ilioinguinal (nerve) G57.9-●
  infectious (multiple) NEC G61.0
  interstitial hypertrophic progressive G60.0
  lumbar M54.16
  lumbosacral M54.17
  multiple —*see also* Polyneuropathy
    endemic E51.11
    infective, acute G61.0
  multiplex endemica E51.11
  nerve root —*see* Radiculopathy
  oculomotor (nerve) —*see* Strabismus,
    paralytic, third nerve

Neuritis (*Continued*)
  olfactory nerve G52.0
  optic (nerve) (hereditary) (sympathetic) H46.9
    with demyelination G36.0
    in myelitis G36.0
    nutritional H46.2
    papillitis —*see* Papillitis, optic
    retrobulbar H46.1-●
    specified type NEC H46.8
    toxic H46.3
  peripheral (nerve) G62.9
    multiple —*see* Polyneuropathy
    single —*see* Mononeuritis
  pneumogastric (nerve) G52.2
  postherpetic, postzoster B02.29
  progressive hypertrophic interstitial G60.0
  retrobulbar —*see also* Neuritis, optic,
    retrobulbar
    in (due to)
      late syphilis A52.15
      meningococcal infection A39.82
      meningococcal A39.82
      syphilitic A52.15
  sciatic (nerve) —*see also* Sciatica
    due to displacement of intervertebral
      disc —*see* Disorder, disc, with,
      radiculopathy
  serum —*see also* Reaction, serum T80.69
  shoulder-girdle G54.5
  specified nerve NEC G58.8
  spinal (nerve) root —*see* Radiculopathy
  syphilitic A52.15
  thenar (median) G56.1-●
  thoracic M54.14
  toxic NEC G62.2
  trochlear (nerve) —*see* Strabismus, paralytic,
    fourth nerve
  vagus (nerve) G52.2
Neuroastrocytoma —*see* Neoplasm, uncertain
  behavior, by site
Neuroavitaminosis E56.9 [G99.8]
Neuroblastoma
  olfactory C30.0
  specified site —*see* Neoplasm, malignant, by
    site
  unspecified site C74.90
Neurochorioretinitis —*see* Chorioretinitis
Neurocirculatory asthenia F45.8
Neurocysticercosis B69.0
Neurocytoma —*see* Neoplasm, benign, by site
Neurodermatitis (circumscribed)
  (circumscripta) (local) L28.0
  atopic L20.81
  diffuse (Brocq) L20.81
  disseminated L20.81
Neuroencephalomyelopathy, optic G36.0
Neuroepithelioma —*see also* Neoplasm,
  malignant, by site
  olfactory C30.0
Neurofibroma —*see also* Neoplasm, nerve,
  benign
  melanotic —*see* Neoplasm, nerve, benign
  multiple —*see* Neurofibromatosis
  plexiform —*see* Neoplasm, nerve, benign
Neurofibromatosis (multiple) (nonmalignant)
  Q85.00
  acoustic Q85.02
  malignant —*see* Neoplasm, nerve, malignant
  specified NEC Q85.09
  type 1 (von Recklinghausen) Q85.01
  type 2 Q85.02
Neurofibrosarcoma —*see* Neoplasm, nerve,
  malignant
Neurogenic —*see also* condition
  bladder (see also Dysfunction, bladder,
    neuromuscular) N31.9
    cauda equina syndrome G83.4
  bowel NEC K59.2
  heart F45.8
Neuroglioma —*see* Neoplasm, uncertain
  behavior, by site

Neurolabyrinthitis (of Dix and Hallpike) —*see*
  Neuronitis, vestibular
Neurolathyrism —*see* Poisoning, food, noxious,
  plant
Neuroleprosy A30.9
Neuroma —*see also* Neoplasm, nerve, benign
  acoustic (nerve) D33.3
  amputation (stump) (traumatic) (surgical
    complication) (late) T87.3-●
    arm T87.3-●
    leg T87.3-●
  digital (toe) G57.6-●
  interdigital G58.8
    lower limb toe G57.8-●
    upper limb G56.8-●
  intermetatarsal G57.8-●
  Morton's G57.6-●
  nonneoplastic
    arm G56.9-●
    leg G57.9-●
    lower extremity G57.9-●
    upper extremity G56.9-●
  optic (nerve) D33.3
  plantar G57.6-●
  plexiform —*see* Neoplasm, nerve,
    benign
  surgical (nonneoplastic)
    arm G56.9-●
    leg G57.9-●
    lower extremity G57.9-●
    upper extremity G56.9-●
Neuromyalgia —*see* Neuralgia
Neuromyasthenia (epidemic) (postinfectious)
  G93.3
Neuromyelitis G36.9
  ascending G61.0
  optica G36.0
Neuromyopathy G70.9
  paraneoplastic D49.9 [G13.0]
Neuromyotonia (Isaacs) G71.19
Neuronevus —*see* Nevus
Neuronitis G58.9
  ascending (acute) G57.2-●
  vestibular H81.2-●
Neuroparalytic —*see* condition
Neuropathy, neuropathic G62.9
  acute motor G62.81
  alcoholic G62.1
    with psychosis —*see* Psychosis, alcoholic
  arm G56.9-●
  autonomic, peripheral —*see* Neuropathy,
    peripheral, autonomic
  axillary G56.9-●
  bladder N31.9
    atonic (motor) (sensory) N31.2
    autonomous N31.2
    flaccid N31.2
    nonreflex N31.2
    reflex N31.1
    uninhibited N31.0
  brachial plexus G54.0
  cervical plexus G54.2
  chronic
    progressive segmentally demyelinating
      G62.89
    relapsing demyelinating G62.89
  Déjérine-Sottas G60.0
  diabetic —*see* E08-E13 with .40
    mononeuropathy —*see* E08-E13 with .41
    polyneuropathy —*see* E08-E13 with .42
  entrapment G58.9
    iliohypogastric nerve G57.8-●
    ilioinguinal nerve G57.8-●
    lateral cutaneous nerve of thigh
      G57.1-●
    median nerve G56.0-●
    obturator nerve G57.8-●
    peroneal nerve G57.3-●
    posterior tibial nerve G57.5-●
    saphenous nerve G57.8-●
    ulnar nerve G56.2-●

Neuropathy, neuropathic (Continued)
facial nerve G51.9
hereditary G60.9
motor and sensory (types I-IV) G60.0
sensory G60.8
specified NEC G60.8
hypertrophic G60.0
Charcot-Marie-Tooth G60.0
Déjérine-Sottas G60.0
interstitial progressive G60.0
of infancy G60.0
Refsum G60.1
idiopathic G60.9
progressive G60.3
specified NEC G60.8
in association with hereditary ataxia G60.2
intercostal G58.0
ischemic —see Disorder, nerve
Jamaica (ginger) G62.2
leg NEC G57.9-●
lower extremity G57.9-●
lumbar plexus G54.1
median nerve G56.1-●
motor and sensory —see also Polyneuropathy
hereditary (types I-IV) G60.0
multifocal motor (MMN) G61.82
multiple (acute) (chronic) —see
Polyneuropathy
optic (nerve) —see also Neuritis, optic
ischemic H47.01-●
paraneoplastic (sensorial) (Denny Brown)
D49.9 [G13.0]
peripheral (nerve) —see also Polyneuropathy
G62.9
autonomic G90.9
idiopathic G90.09
in (due to)
amyloidosis E85.4 [G99.0]
diabetes mellitus —see E08-E13 with
.43
endocrine disease NEC E34.9 [G99.0]
gout M10.00 [G99.0]
hyperthyroidism E05.90 [G99.0]
with thyroid storm E05.91 [G99.0]
metabolic disease NEC E88.9 [G99.0]
idiopathic G60.9
progressive G60.3
in (due to)
antitetanus serum G62.0
arsenic G62.2
drugs NEC G62.0
lead G62.2
organophosphate compounds G62.2
toxic agent NEC G62.2
plantar nerves G57.6-●
progressive
hypertrophic interstitial G60.0
inflammatory G62.81
radicular NEC —see Radiculopathy
sacral plexus G54.1
sciatic G57.0-●
serum G61.1
toxic NEC G62.2
trigeminal sensory G50.8
ulnar nerve G56.2-●
uremic N18.9 [G63]
vitamin B12 E53.8 [G63]
with anemia (pernicious) D51.0 [G63]
due to dietary deficiency D51.3 [G63]
Neurophthisis —see also Disorder, nerve
peripheral, diabetic —see E08-E13 with .42
Neuroretinitis —see Chorioretinitis
Neuroretinopathy, hereditary optic H47.22
Neurosarcoma —see Neoplasm, nerve, malignant
Neurosclerosis —see Disorder, nerve
Neurosis, neurotic F48.9
anankastic F42.8
anxiety (state) F41.1
panic type F41.0
asthenic F48.8
bladder F45.8

Neurosis, neurotic (Continued)
cardiac (reflex) F45.8
cardiovascular F45.8
character F60.9
colon F45.8
compensation F68.1
compulsive, compulsion F42.8
conversion F44.9
craft F48.8
cutaneous F45.8
depersonalization F48.1
depressive (reaction) (type) F34.1
environmental F48.8
excoriation L98.1
fatigue F48.8
functional —see Disorder, somatoform
gastric F45.8
gastrointestinal F45.8
heart F45.8
hypochondriacal F45.21
hysterical F44.9
incoordination F45.8
larynx F45.8
vocal cord F45.8
intestine F45.8
larynx (sensory) F45.8
hysterical F44.4
mixed NEC F48.8
musculoskeletal F45.8
obsessional F42.8
obsessive-compulsive F42.8
occupational F48.8
ocular NEC F45.8
organ —see Disorder, somatoform
pharynx F45.8
phobic F40.9
posttraumatic (situational) F43.10
acute F43.11
chronic F43.12
psychasthenic (type) F48.8
railroad F48.8
rectum F45.8
respiratory F45.8
rumination F45.8
sexual F65.9
situational F48.8
social F40.10
generalized F40.11
specified type NEC F48.8
state F48.9
with depersonalization episode F48.1
stomach F45.8
traumatic F43.10
acute F43.11
chronic F43.12
vasomotor F45.8
visceral F45.8
war F48.8
Neurospongioblastosis diffusa Q85.1
Neurosyphilis (arrested) (early) (gumma) (late)
(latent) (recurrent) (relapse) A52.3
with ataxia (cerebellar) (locomotor) (spastic)
(spinal) A52.19
aneurysm (cerebral) A52.05
arachnoid (adhesive) A52.13
arteritis (any artery) (cerebral) A52.04
asymptomatic A52.2
congenital A50.40
dura (mater) A52.13
general paresis A52.17
hemorrhagic A52.05
juvenile (asymptomatic) (meningeal)
A50.40
leptomeninges (aseptic) A52.13
meningeal, meninges (adhesive) A52.13
meningitis A52.13
meningovascular (diffuse) A52.13
optic atrophy A52.15
parenchymatous (degenerative) A52.19
paresis, paretic A52.17
juvenile A50.45

Neurosyphilis (Continued)
remission in (sustained) A52.3
serological (without symptoms) A52.2
specified nature or site NEC A52.19
tabes, tabetic (dorsalis) A52.11
juvenile A50.45
taboparesis A52.17
juvenile A50.45
thrombosis (cerebral) A52.05
vascular (cerebral) NEC A52.05
Neurothekeoma —see Neoplasm, nerve, benign
Neurotic —see Neurosis
Neurotoxemia —see Toxemia
Neutroclusion M26.211
Neutropenia, neutropenic (chronic) (genetic)
(idiopathic) (immune) (infantile)
(malignant) (pernicious) (splenic) D70.9
congenital (primary) D70.0
cyclic D70.4
cytoreductive cancer chemotherapy sequela
D70.1
drug-induced D70.2
due to cytoreductive cancer chemotherapy
D70.1
due to infection D70.3
fever D70.9
neonatal, transitory (isoimmune) (maternal
transfer) P61.5
periodic D70.4
secondary (cyclic) (periodic) (splenic) D70.4
drug-induced D70.2
due to cytoreductive cancer
chemotherapy D70.1
toxic D70.8
Neutrophilia, hereditary giant D72.0
Nevocarcinoma —see Melanoma
Nevus D22.9
achromic —see Neoplasm, skin, benign
amelanotic —see Neoplasm, skin, benign
angiomatous D18.00
intra-abdominal D18.03
intracranial D18.02
skin D18.01
specified site NEC D18.09
araneus I78.1
balloon cell —see Neoplasm, skin, benign
bathing trunk D48.5
blue —see Neoplasm, skin, benign
cellular —see Neoplasm, skin, benign
giant —see Neoplasm, skin, benign
Jadassohn's —see Neoplasm, skin, benign
malignant —see Melanoma
capillary D18.00
intra-abdominal D18.03
intracranial D18.02
skin D18.01
specified site NEC D18.09
cavernous D18.00
intra-abdominal D18.03
intracranial D18.02
skin D18.01
specified site NEC D18.09
cellular —see Neoplasm, skin, benign
blue —see Neoplasm, skin, benign
choroid D31.3-●
comedonicus Q82.5
conjunctiva D31.0-●
dermal —see Neoplasm, skin, benign
with epidermal nevus —see Neoplasm,
skin, benign
dysplastic —see Neoplasm, skin, benign
eye D31.9-●
flammeus Q82.5
hemangiomatous D18.00
intra-abdominal D18.03
intracranial D18.02
skin D18.01
specified site NEC D18.09
iris D31.4-●
lacrimal gland D31.5-●
lymphatic D18.1

Nevus *(Continued)*
  magnocellular
    specified site —*see* Neoplasm, benign, by
        site
    unspecified site D31.40
  malignant —*see* Melanoma
  meaning hemangioma D18.00
    intra-abdominal D18.03
    intracranial D18.02
    skin D18.01
    specified site NEC D18.09
  mouth (mucosa) D10.30
    specified site NEC D10.39
    white sponge Q38.6
  multiplex Q85.1
  non-neoplastic I78.1
  oral mucosa D10.30
    specified site NEC D10.39
    white sponge Q38.6
  orbit D31.6-●
  pigmented
    giant —*see also* Neoplasm, skin, uncertain
        behavior D48.5
      malignant melanoma in —*see* Melanoma
  portwine Q82.5
  retina D31.2-●
  retrobulbar D31.6-●
  sanguineous Q82.5
  senile I78.1
  skin D22.9
    abdominal wall D22.5
    ala nasi D22.39
    ankle D22.7-●
    anus, anal D22.5
    arm D22.6-●
    auditory canal (external) D22.2-●
    auricle (ear) D22.2-●
    auricular canal (external) D22.2-●
    axilla, axillary fold D22.5
    back D22.5
    breast D22.5
    brow D22.39
    buttock D22.5
    canthus (eye) D22.1-●
    cheek (external) D22.39
    chest wall D22.5
    chin D22.39
    ear (external) D22.2-●
    external meatus (ear) D22.2-●
    eyebrow D22.39
    eyelid (lower) (upper) D22.1-●
    face D22.30
      specified NEC D22.39
    female genital organ (external) NEC D28.0
    finger D22.6-●
    flank D22.5
    foot D22.7-●
    forearm D22.6-●
    forehead D22.39
    foreskin D29.0
    genital organ (external) NEC
      female D28.0
      male D29.9
    gluteal region D22.5
    groin D22.5
    hand D22.6-●
    heel D22.7-●
    helix D22.2-●
    hip D22.7-●
    interscapular region D22.5
    jaw D22.39
    knee D22.7-●
    labium (majus) (minus) D28.0
    leg D22.7-●
    lip (lower) (upper) D22.0
    lower limb D22.7-●
    male genital organ (external) D29.9
    nail D22.9
      finger D22.6-●
      toe D22.7-●
    nasolabial groove D22.39
    nates D22.5

Nevus *(Continued)*
  skin *(Continued)*
    neck D22.4
    nose (external) D22.39
    palpebra D22.1-●
    penis D29.0
    perianal skin D22.5
    perineum D22.5
    pinna D22.2-●
    popliteal fossa or space D22.7-●
    prepuce D29.0
    pudendum D28.0
    scalp D22.4
    scrotum D29.4
    shoulder D22.6-●
    submammary fold D22.5
    temple D22.39
    thigh D22.7-●
    toe D22.7-●
    trunk NEC D22.5
    umbilicus D22.5
    upper limb D22.6-●
    vulva D28.0
  specified site NEC —*see* Neoplasm, benign,
      by site
  spider I78.1
  stellar I78.1
  strawberry Q82.5
  ~~Sutton's —see Neoplasm, skin, benign~~
  ▶ Sutton's benign D22.9
  unius lateris Q82.5
  Unna's Q82.5
  vascular Q82.5
  verrucous Q82.5
Newborn (infant) (liveborn) (singleton) Z38.2
  abstinence syndrome P96.1
  acne L70.4
  affected by
    abnormalities of membranes P02.9
      specified NEC P02.8
    abruptio placenta P02.1
    amino-acid metabolic disorder, transitory
        P74.8
    amniocentesis (while in utero) P00.6
    amnionitis P02.7
    apparent life threatening event (ALTE)
        R68.13
    bleeding (into)
      cerebral cortex P52.22
      germinal matrix P52.0
      ventricles P52.1
    breech delivery P03.0
    cardiac arrest P29.81
    cardiomyopathy I42.8
      congenital I42.4
    cerebral ischemia P91.0
    Cesarean delivery P03.4
    chemotherapy agents P04.1
    chorioamnionitis P02.7
    cocaine (crack) P04.41
    complications of labor and delivery P03.9
      specified NEC P03.89
    compression of umbilical cord NEC P02.5
    contracted pelvis P03.1
    delivery P03.9
      Cesarean P03.4
      forceps P03.2
      vacuum extractor P03.3
    entanglement (knot) in umbilical cord P02.5
    environmental chemicals P04.6
    fetal (intrauterine)
      growth retardation P05.9
      malnutrition not light or small for
          gestational age P05.2
    forceps delivery P03.2
    heart rate abnormalities
      bradycardia P29.12
      intrauterine P03.819
        before onset of labor P03.810
        during labor P03.811
      tachycardia P29.11

Newborn *(Continued)*
  affected by *(Continued)*
    hemorrhage (antepartum) P02.1
      cerebellar (nontraumatic) P52.6
      intracerebral (nontraumatic) P52.4
      intracranial (nontraumatic) P52.9
        specified NEC P52.8
      intraventricular (nontraumatic) P52.3
        grade 1 P52.0
        grade 2 P52.1
        grade 3 P52.21
        grade 4 P52.22
      posterior fossa (nontraumatic) P52.6
      subarachnoid (nontraumatic) P52.5
      subependymal P52.0
        with intracerebral extension P52.22
        with intraventricular extension P52.1
          with enlargment of ventricles
              P52.21
        without intraventricular extension
            P52.0
    hypoxic ischemic encephalopathy [HIE]
        P91.60
      mild P91.61
      moderate P91.62
      severe P91.63
    induction of labor P03.89
    intestinal perforation P78.0
    intrauterine (fetal) blood loss P50.9
      due to (from)
        cut end of co-twin cord P50.5
        hemorrhage into
          co-twin P50.3
          maternal circulation P50.4
        placenta P50.2
        ruptured cord blood P50.1
        vasa previa P50.0
      specified NEC P50.8
    intrauterine (fetal) hemorrhage P50.9
    intrauterine (in utero) procedure P96.5
    malpresentation (malposition) NEC P03.1
    maternal (complication of) (use of)
      alcohol P04.3
      analgesia (maternal) P04.0
      anesthesia (maternal) P04.0
      blood loss P02.1
      circulatory disease P00.3
      condition P00.9
        specified NEC P00.89
      delivery P03.9
        Cesarean P03.4
        forceps P03.2
        vacuum extractor P03.3
      diabetes mellitus (pre-existing) P70.1
      disorder P00.9
        specified NEC P00.89
      drugs (addictive) (illegal) NEC P04.49
      ectopic pregnancy P01.4
      gestational diabetes P70.0
      hemorrhage P02.1
      hypertensive disorder P00.0
      incompetent cervix P01.0
      infectious disease P00.2
      injury P00.5
      labor and delivery P03.9
      malpresentation before labor P01.7
      maternal death P01.6
      medical procedure P00.7
      medication P04.1
      multiple pregnancy P01.5
      nutritional disorder P00.4
      oligohydramnios P01.2
      parasitic disease P00.2
      periodontal disease P00.81
      placenta previa P02.0
      polyhydramnios P01.3
      precipitate delivery P03.5
      pregnancy P01.9
        specified P01.8
      premature rupture of membranes P01.1
      renal disease P00.1

Newborn *(Continued)*
  affected by *(Continued)*
    maternal *(Continued)*
      respiratory disease P00.3
      surgical procedure P00.6
      urinary tract disease P00.1
      uterine contraction (abnormal) P03.6
    meconium peritonitis P78.0
    medication (legal) (maternal use)
        (prescribed) P04.1
    membrane abnormalities P02.9
      specified NEC P02.8
    membranitis P02.7
    methamphetamine(s) P04.49
    mixed metabolic and respiratory acidosis
        P84
    neonatal abstinence syndrome P96.1
    noxious substances transmitted via
        placenta or breast milk P04.9
      specified NEC P04.8
    nutritional supplements P04.5
    placenta previa P02.0
    placental
      abnormality (functional)
          (morphological) P02.20
        specified NEC P02.29
      dysfunction P02.29
      infarction P02.29
      insufficiency P02.29
      separation NEC P02.1
      transfusion syndromes P02.3
    placentitis P02.7
    precipitate delivery P03.5
    prolapsed cord P02.4
    respiratory arrest P28.81
    slow intrauterine growth P05.9
    tobacco P04.2
    twin to twin transplacental transfusion
        P02.3
    umbilical cord (tightly) around neck
        P02.5
    umbilical cord condition P02.60
      short cord P02.69
      specified NEC P02.69
    uterine contractions (abnormal) P03.6
    vasa previa P02.69
      from intrauterine blood loss P50.0
  apnea P28.4
    obstructive P28.4
    primary P28.3
    sleep (central) (obstructive) (primary)
        P28.3
  born in hospital Z38.00
    by cesarean Z38.01
  born outside hospital Z38.1
  breast buds P96.89
  breast engorgement P83.4
  check-up —*see* Newborn, examination
  convulsion P90
  dehydration P74.1
  examination
    8 to 28 days old Z00.111
    under 8 days old Z00.110
  fever P81.9
    environmentally-induced P81.0
  hyperbilirubinemia P59.9
    of prematurity P59.0
  hypernatremia P74.2
  hyponatremia P74.2
  infection P39.9
    candidal P37.5
    specified NEC P39.8
    urinary tract P39.3
  jaundice P59.9
    due to
      breast milk inhibitor P59.3
      hepatocellular damage P59.20
        specified NEC P59.29
      preterm delivery P59.0
    of prematurity P59.0
    specified NEC P59.8

Newborn *(Continued)*
  late metabolic acidosis P74.0
  mastitis P39.0
    infective P39.0
    noninfective P83.4
  multiple born NEC Z38.8
    born in hospital Z38.68
      by cesarean Z38.69
    born outside hospital Z38.7
  omphalitis P38.9
    with mild hemorrhage P38.1
    without hemorrhage P38.9
  post-term P08.21
  prolonged gestation (over 42 completed
      weeks) P08.22
  quadruplet Z38.8
    born in hospital Z38.63
      by cesarean Z38.64
    born outside hospital Z38.7
  quintuplet Z38.8
    born in hospital Z38.65
      by cesarean Z38.66
    born outside hospital Z38.7
  seizure P90
  sepsis (congenital) P36.9
    due to
      anaerobes NEC P36.5
      Escherichia coli P36.4
      Staphylococcus P36.30
        aureus P36.2
        specified NEC P36.39
      Streptococcus P36.10
        group B P36.0
        specified NEC P36.19
      specified NEC P36.8
  triplet Z38.8
    born in hospital Z38.61
      by cesarean Z38.62
    born outside hospital Z38.7
  twin Z38.5
    born in hospital Z38.30
      by cesarean Z38.31
    born outside hospital Z38.4
  vomiting P92.09
    bilious P92.01
  weight check Z00.111
Newcastle conjunctivitis or disease B30.8
Nezelof's syndrome (pure alymphocytosis)
    D81.4
Niacin (amide) deficiency E52
Nicolas (-Durand)-Favre disease A55
Nicotine —*see* Tobacco
Nicotinic acid deficiency E52
Niemann-Pick disease or syndrome E75.249
  specified NEC E75.248
  type
    A E75.240
    B E75.241
    C E75.242
    D E75.243
Night
  blindness —*see* Blindness, night
  sweats R61
  terrors (child) F51.4
Nightmares (REM sleep type) F51.5
NIHSS (National Institutes of Health Stroke
    Scale) score R29.7-●
Nipple —*see* condition
Nisbet's chancre A57
Nishimoto (-Takeuchi) disease I67.5
Nitritoid crisis or reaction —*see* Crisis, nitritoid
Nitrosohemoglobinemia D74.8
Njovera A65
Nocardiosis, nocardiasis A43.9
  cutaneous A43.1
  lung A43.0
  pneumonia A43.0
  pulmonary A43.0
  specified site NEC A43.8
Nocturia R35.1
  psychogenic F45.8

Nocturnal —*see* condition
Nodal rhythm I49.8
Node(s) —*see also* Nodule
  Bouchard's (with arthropathy) M15.2
  Haygarth's M15.8
  Heberden's (with arthropathy) M15.1
  larynx J38.7
  lymph —*see* condition
  milker's B08.03
  Osler's I33.0
  Schmorl's —*see* Schmorl's disease
  singer's J38.2
  teacher's J38.2
  tuberculous —*see* Tuberculosis, lymph
      gland
  vocal cord J38.2
Nodule(s), nodular
  actinomycotic —*see* Actinomycosis
  ⇒breast NEC —*see also* Lump, breast N63.0
  colloid (cystic), thyroid E04.1
  cutaneous —*see* Swelling, localized
  endometrial (stromal) D26.1
  Haygarth's M15.8
  inflammatory —*see* Inflammation
  juxta-articular
    syphilitic A52.77
    yaws A66.7
  larynx J38.7
  lung, solitary (subsegmental branch of the
      bronchial tree) R91.1
    multiple R91.8
  milker's B08.03
  prostate N40.2
    with lower urinary tract symptoms (LUTS)
        N40.3
    without lower urinary tract symptoms
        (LUTS) N40.2
  pulmonary, solitary (subsegmental branch of
      the bronchial tree) R91.1
  retrocardiac R09.89
  rheumatoid M06.30
    ankle M06.37-●
    elbow M06.32-●
    foot joint M06.37-●
    hand joint M06.34-●
    hip M06.35-●
    knee M06.36-●
    multiple site M06.39
    shoulder M06.31-●
    vertebra M06.38
    wrist M06.33-●
  scrotum (inflammatory) N49.2
  singer's J38.2
  solitary, lung (subsegmental branch of the
      bronchial tree) R91.1
    multiple R91.8
  subcutaneous —*see* Swelling, localized
  teacher's J38.2
  thyroid (cold) (gland) (nontoxic) E04.1
    with thyrotoxicosis E05.20
      with thyroid storm E05.21
    toxic or with hyperthyroidism E05.20
      with thyroid storm E05.21
  vocal cord J38.2
Noma (gangrenous) (hospital) (infective)
    A69.0
  auricle I96
  mouth A69.0
  pudendi N76.89
  vulvae N76.89
Nomad, nomadism Z59.0
NOMID (neonatal onset multisystemic
    inflammatory disorder) M04.2
▶Nonadherence to medical treatment Z91.19
Nonautoimmune hemolytic anemia D59.4
  drug-induced D59.2
Nonclosure —*see also* Imperfect, closure
  ductus arteriosus (Botallo's) Q25.0
  foramen
    botalli Q21.1
    ovale Q21.1

Noncompliance Z91.19
  with
    dialysis Z91.15
    dietary regimen Z91.11
    medical treatment Z91.19
    medication regimen NEC Z91.14
      underdosing —*see also* Table of Drugs
        and Chemicals, categories T36-T50,
        with final character 6 Z91.14
      intentional NEC Z91.128
        due to financial hardship of patient
          Z91.120
      unintentional NEC Z91.138
        due to patient's age related debility
          Z91.130
    renal dialysis Z91.15
Nondescent (congenital) —*see also* Malposition,
    congenital
  cecum Q43.3
  colon Q43.3
  testicle Q53.9
    bilateral Q53.20
      abdominal Q53.211
      perineal Q53.22
    unilateral Q53.10
      abdominal Q53.111
      perineal Q53.12
Nondevelopment
  brain Q02
    part of Q04.3
  heart Q24.8
  organ or site, congenital NEC —*see*
    Hypoplasia
Nonengagement
  head NEC O32.4
    in labor, causing obstructed labor O64.8
Nonexanthematous tick fever A93.2
Nonexpansion, lung (newborn) P28.0
Nonfunctioning
  cystic duct —*see also* Disease, gallbladder
    K82.8
  gallbladder —*see also* Disease, gallbladder
    K82.8
  kidney N28.9
  labyrinth —*see* subcategory H83.2

Non-Hodgkin lymphoma NEC —*see*
    Lymphoma, non-Hodgkin
Nonimplantation, ovum N97.2
Noninsufflation, fallopian tube N97.1
Non-ketotic hyperglycinemia E72.51
Nonne-Milroy syndrome Q82.0
Nonovulation N97.0
▶Non-palpable testicle(s)
  ▶bilateral R39.84
  ▶unilateral R39.83
Nonpatent fallopian tube N97.1
Nonpneumatization, lung NEC P28.0
Nonrotation —*see* Malrotation
Nonsecretion, urine —*see* Anuria
Nonunion
  fracture —*see* Fracture, by site
  joint, following fusion or arthrodesis
    M96.0
  organ or site, congenital NEC —*see* Imperfect,
    closure
  symphysis pubis, congenital Q74.2
Nonvisualization, gallbladder R93.2
Nonvital, nonvitalized tooth K04.99
Non-working side interference
    M26.56
Noonan's syndrome Q87.1
Normocytic anemia (infectional) due to blood
    loss (chronic) D50.0
  acute D62
Norrie's disease (congenital) Q15.8
North American blastomycosis B40.9
Norwegian itch B86
Nose, nasal —*see* condition
Nosebleed R04.0
Nose-picking F98.8
Nosomania F45.21
Nosophobia F45.22
Nostalgia F43.20
Notch of iris Q13.2
Notching nose, congenital (tip)
    Q30.2
Nothnagel's
  syndrome —*see* Strabismus, paralytic, third
    nerve
  vasomotor acroparesthesia I73.89

Novy's relapsing fever A68.9
  louse-borne A68.0
  tick-borne A68.1
Noxious
  foodstuffs, poisoning by —*see* Poisoning,
    food, noxious, plant
  substances transmitted through placenta or
    breast milk P04.9
Nucleus pulposus —*see* condition
Numbness R20.0
Nuns' knee —*see* Bursitis, prepatellar
Nursemaid's elbow S53.03- •
Nutcracker esophagus K22.4
Nutmeg liver K76.1
Nutrient element deficiency E61.9
  specified NEC E61.8
Nutrition deficient or insufficient —*see also*
    Malnutrition E46
  due to
    insufficient food T73.0
    lack of
      care (child) T76.02
        adult T76.01
      food T73.0
Nutritional stunting E45
Nyctalopia (night blindness) —*see* Blindness,
    night
Nycturia R35.1
  psychogenic F45.8
Nymphomania F52.8
Nystagmus H55.00
  benign paroxysmal —*see* Vertigo, benign
    paroxysmal
  central positional H81.4- •
  congenital H55.01
  dissociated H55.04
  latent H55.02
  miners' H55.09
  positional
    benign paroxysmal H81.4- •
    central H81.4- •
  specified form NEC H55.09
  visual deprivation H55.03

▶ New   ⇒ Revised   ~~deleted~~ Deleted   • Use Additional Character(s)

O

Obermeyer's relapsing fever (European) A68.0
Obesity E66.9
  with alveolar hypoventilation E66.2
  adrenal E27.8
  complicating
    childbirth O99.214
    pregnancy O99.21-●
    puerperium O99.215
  constitutional E66.8
  dietary counseling and surveillance Z71.3
  drug-induced E66.1
  due to
    drug E66.1
    excess calories E66.09
      morbid E66.01
      severe E66.01
  endocrine E66.8
  endogenous E66.8
  exogenous E66.09
  familial E66.8
  glandular E66.8
  hypothyroid —see Hypothyroidism
  hypoventilation syndrome (OHS) E66.2
  morbid E66.01
    with
      alveolar hypoventilation E66.2
      obesity hypoventilation syndrome (OHS) E66.2
    due to excess calories E66.01
  nutritional E66.09
  pituitary E23.6
  severe E66.01
  specified type NEC E66.8
Oblique —see condition
Obliteration
  appendix (lumen) K38.8
  artery I77.1
  bile duct (noncalculous) K83.1
  common duct (noncalculous) K83.1
  cystic duct —see Obstruction, gallbladder
  disease, arteriolar I77.1
  endometrium N85.8
  eye, anterior chamber —see Disorder, globe, hypotony
  fallopian tube N97.1
  lymphatic vessel I89.0
    due to mastectomy I97.2
  organ or site, congenital NEC —see Atresia, by site
  ureter N13.5
    with infection N13.6
  urethra —see Stricture, urethra
  vein I87.8
  vestibule (oral) K08.89
Observation (following) (for) (without need for further medical care) Z04.9
  accident NEC Z04.3
    at work Z04.2
    transport Z04.1
  adverse effect of drug Z03.6
  alleged rape or sexual assault (victim), ruled out
    adult Z04.41
    child Z04.42
  criminal assault Z04.8
  development state
    adolescent Z00.3
    period of rapid growth in childhood Z00.2
    puberty Z00.3
  disease, specified NEC Z03.89
  following work accident Z04.2
  growth and development state —see Observation, development state
  injuries (accidental) NEC —see also Observation, accident

Observation (Continued)
  newborn (for)
    suspected condition, related to exposure from the mother or birth process — see Newborn, affected by, maternal
      ruled out Z05.9
        cardiac Z05.0
        connective tissue Z05.73
        gastrointestinal Z05.5
        genetic Z05.41
        genitourinary Z05.6
        immunologic Z05.43
        infectious Z05.1
        metabolic Z05.42
        musculoskeletal Z05.72
        neurological Z05.2
        respiratory Z05.3
        skin and subcutaneous tissue Z05.71
        specified condition NEC Z05.8
  postpartum
    immediately after delivery Z39.0
    routine follow-up Z39.2
  pregnancy (normal) (without complication) Z34.9-●
    high risk O09.9-●
  suicide attempt, alleged NEC Z03.89
    self-poisoning Z03.6
  suspected, ruled out —see also Suspected condition, ruled out
    abuse, physical
      adult Z04.71
      child Z04.72
    accident at work Z04.2
    adult battering victim Z04.71
    child battering victim Z04.72
    condition NEC Z03.89
      newborn —see also Observation, newborn (for), suspected condition, ruled out Z05.9
    drug poisoning or adverse effect Z03.6
    exposure (to)
      anthrax Z03.810
      biological agent NEC Z03.818
    inflicted injury NEC Z04.8
    suicide attempt, alleged Z03.89
      self-poisoning Z03.6
    toxic effects from ingested substance (drug) (poison) Z03.6
  toxic effects from ingested substance (drug) (poison) Z03.6
Obsession, obsessional state F42.8
  mixed thoughts and acts F42.2
Obsessive-compulsive neurosis or reaction F42.8
Obstetric embolism, septic —see Embolism, obstetric, septic
Obstetrical trauma (complicating delivery) O71.9
  with or following ectopic or molar pregnancy O08.6
  specified type NEC O71.89
Obstipation —see Constipation
Obstruction, obstructed, obstructive
  airway J98.8
    with
      allergic alveolitis J67.9
      asthma J45.909
        with
          exacerbation (acute) J45.901
          status asthmaticus J45.902
      bronchiectasis J47.9
        with
          exacerbation (acute) J47.1
          lower respiratory infection J47.0
      bronchitis (chronic) J44.9
      emphysema J43.9

Obstruction, obstructed, obstructive (Continued)
  airway (Continued)
    chronic J44.9
      with
        allergic alveolitis —see Pneumonitis, hypersensitivity
        bronchiectasis J47.9
          with
            exacerbation (acute) J47.1
            lower respiratory infection J47.0
    due to
      foreign body —see Foreign body, by site, causing asphyxia
      inhalation of fumes or vapors J68.9
      laryngospasm J38.5
  ampulla of Vater K83.1
  aortic (heart) (valve) —see Stenosis, aortic
  aortoiliac I74.09
  aqueduct of Sylvius G91.1
    congenital Q03.0
      with spina bifida —see Spina bifida, by site, with hydrocephalus
  Arnold-Chiari —see Arnold-Chiari disease
  artery (see also Atherosclerosis, artery) I70.9
    basilar (complete) (partial) —see Occlusion, artery, basilar
    carotid (complete) (partial) —see Occlusion, artery, carotid
    cerebellar —see Occlusion, artery, cerebellar
    cerebral (anterior) (middle) (posterior) — see Occlusion, artery, cerebral
    precerebral —see Occlusion, artery, precerebral
    renal N28.0
    retinal NEC —see Occlusion, artery, retina
    stent —see Restenosis, stent
    vertebral (complete) (partial) —see Occlusion, artery, vertebral
  band (intestinal) —see also Obstruction, intestine, specified NEC K56.699
  bile duct or passage (common) (hepatic) (noncalculous) K83.1
    with calculus K80.51
    congenital (causing jaundice) Q44.3
  biliary (duct) (tract) K83.1
    gallbladder K82.0
  bladder-neck (acquired) N32.0
    congenital Q64.31
    due to hyperplasia (hypertrophy) of prostate —see Hyperplasia, prostate
  bowel —see Obstruction, intestine
  bronchus J98.09
  canal, ear —see Stenosis, external ear canal
  cardia K22.2
  caval veins (inferior) (superior) I87.1
  cecum —see Obstruction, intestine
  circulatory I99.8
  colon —see Obstruction, intestine
  common duct (noncalculous) K83.1
  coronary (artery) —see Occlusion, coronary
  cystic duct —see also Obstruction, gallbladder
    with calculus K80.21
  device, implant or graft —see also Complications, by site and type, mechanical T85.698
    arterial graft NEC —see Complication, cardiovascular device, mechanical, vascular
    catheter NEC T85.628
      cystostomy T83.090
      dialysis (renal) T82.49
        intraperitoneal T85.691
      Hopkins T83.098
      ileostomy T83.098
      infusion NEC T82.594
        spinal (epidural) (subdural) T85.690
      nephrostomy T83.092
      urethral indwelling T83.091
      urinary T83.098
      urostomy T83.098

Obstruction, obstructed, obstructive
(Continued)
　device, implant or graft (Continued)
　　due to infection T85.79
　　gastrointestinal —see Complications,
　　　　prosthetic device, mechanical,
　　　　gastrointestinal device
　　genital NEC T83.498
　　　intrauterine contraceptive device T83.39
　　　penile prosthesis (cylinder) (implanted)
　　　　(pump) (resevoir) T83.490
　　　testicular prosthesis T83.491
　　heart NEC —see Complication,
　　　　cardiovascular device, mechanical
　　joint prosthesis —see Complications, joint
　　　　prosthesis, mechanical, specified NEC,
　　　　by site
　　orthopedic NEC —see Complication,
　　　　orthopedic, device, mechanical
　　specified NEC T85.628
　　urinary NEC —see also Complication,
　　　　genitourinary, device, urinary,
　　　　mechanical
　　　graft T83.29
　　vascular NEC —see Complication,
　　　　cardiovascular device, mechanical
　　ventricular intracranial shunt T85.09
　due to foreign body accidentally left in
　　　operative wound T81.529
　duodenum K31.5
　ejaculatory duct N50.89
　esophagus K22.2
　eustachian tube (complete) (partial) H68.10-●
　　cartilagenous (extrinsic) H68.13-●
　　　intrinsic H68.12-●
　　　osseous H68.11-●
　fallopian tube (bilateral) N97.1
　fecal K56.41
　　with hernia —see Hernia, by site, with
　　　obstruction
　foramen of Monro (congenital) Q03.8
　　with spina bifida —see Spina bifida,
　　　by site, with hydrocephalus
　foreign body —see Foreign body
　gallbladder K82.0
　　with calculus, stones K80.21
　　congenital Q44.1
　gastric outlet K31.1
　gastrointestinal —see Obstruction, intestine
　hepatic K76.89
　　duct (noncalculous) K83.1
　hepatobiliary K83.1
　ileum —see Obstruction, intestine
　iliofemoral (artery) I74.5
⇒intestine K56.609
　▶complete K56.601
　▶incomplete K56.600
　▶partial K56.600
　　with
　　⇒adhesions (intestinal) (peritoneal) K56.50
　　　▶complete K56.52
　　　▶incomplete K56.51
　　　▶partial K56.51
　　adynamic K56.0
　　by gallstone K56.3
　　congenital (small) Q41.9
　　　large Q42.9
　　　　specified part NEC Q42.8
　　neurogenic K56.0
　　　Hirschsprung's disease or megacolon
　　　　Q43.1
　　newborn P76.9
　　　due to
　　　　fecaliths P76.8
　　　　inspissated milk P76.2
　　　　meconium (plug) P76.0
　　　　　in mucoviscidosis E84.11
　　　specified NEC P76.8
⇒postoperative K91.30
　▶complete K91.32
　▶incomplete K91.31
　▶partial K91.31

Obstruction, obstructed, obstructive
(Continued)
　intestine (Continued)
　　reflex K56.0
⇒　specified NEC K56.699
　　　▶complete K56.691
　　　▶incomplete K56.690
　　　▶partial K56.690
　　volvulus K56.2
　intracardiac ball valve prosthesis T82.09
　jejunum —see Obstruction, intestine
　joint prosthesis —see Complications, joint
　　　prosthesis, mechanical, specified NEC,
　　　by site
　kidney (calices) N28.89
　labor —see Delivery
　lacrimal (passages) (duct)
　　by
　　　dacryolith —see Dacryolith
　　　stenosis —see Stenosis, lacrimal
　　congenital Q10.5
　　neonatal H04.53-●
　lacrimonasal duct —see Obstruction, lacrimal
　lacteal, with steatorrhea K90.2
　laryngitis —see Laryngitis
　larynx NEC J38.6
　　congenital Q31.8
　lung J98.4
　　disease, chronic J44.9
　lymphatic I89.0
　meconium (plug)
　　newborn P76.0
　　　due to fecaliths P76.0
　　　in mucoviscidosis E84.11
　mitral —see Stenosis, mitral
　nasal J34.89
　nasolacrimal duct —see also Obstruction,
　　　lacrimal
　　congenital Q10.5
　nasopharynx J39.2
　nose J34.89
　organ or site, congenital NEC —see Atresia,
　　　by site
　pancreatic duct K86.89
　parotid duct or gland K11.8
　pelviureteral junction N13.5
　　with hydronephrosis N13.0
　　congenital Q62.39
　pharynx J39.2
　portal (circulation) (vein) I81
　prostate —see also Hyperplasia, prostate
　　valve (urinary) N32.0
　pulmonary valve (heart) I37.0
　pyelonephritis (chronic) N11.1
　pylorus
　　adult K31.1
　　congenital or infantile Q40.0
　rectosigmoid —see Obstruction,
　　　intestine
　rectum K62.4
　renal N28.89
　　outflow N13.8
　　pelvis, congenital Q62.39
　respiratory J98.8
　　chronic J44.9
　retinal (vessels) H34.9
　salivary duct (any) K11.8
　　with calculus K11.5
　sigmoid —see Obstruction, intestine
　sinus (accessory) (nasal) J34.89
　Stensen's duct K11.8
　stomach NEC K31.89
　　acute K31.0
　　congenital Q40.2
　　due to pylorospasm K31.3
　submandibular duct K11.8
　submaxillary gland K11.8
　　with calculus K11.5
　thoracic duct I89.0
　thrombotic —see Thrombosis
　trachea J39.8

Obstruction, obstructed, obstructive
(Continued)
　tracheostomy airway J95.03
　tricuspid (valve) —see Stenosis, tricuspid
　upper respiratory, congenital Q34.8
　ureter (functional) (pelvic junction) NEC N13.5
　　with
　　　hydronephrosis N13.1
　　　　with infection N13.6
　　　pyelonephritis (chronic) N11.1
　　congenital Q62.39
　　due to calculus —see Calculus, ureter
　urethra NEC N36.8
　　congenital Q64.39
　urinary (moderate) N13.9
　　due to hyperplasia (hypertrophy) of
　　　prostate —see Hyperplasia, prostate
　　organ or tract (lower) N13.9
　　prostatic valve N32.0
　　specified NEC N13.8
　uropathy N13.9
　uterus N85.8
　vagina N89.5
　valvular —see Endocarditis
　vein, venous I87.1
　　caval (inferior) (superior) I87.1
　　thrombotic —see Thrombosis
　vena cava (inferior) (superior) I87.1
　vesical NEC N32.0
　vesicourethral orifice N32.0
　　congenital Q64.31
　vessel NEC I99.8
　　stent —see Restenosis, stent
Obturator —see condition
Occlusal wear, teeth K03.0
Occlusio pupillae —see Membrane, pupillary
Occlusion, occluded
　anus K62.4
　　congenital Q42.3
　　　with fistula Q42.2
　aortoiliac (chronic) I74.09
　aqueduct of Sylvius G91.1
　　congenital Q03.0
　　　with spina bifida —see Spina bifida, by
　　　　site, with hydrocephalus
⇒artery —see also Atherosclerosis, artery I70.9
　　auditory, internal I65.8
　　basilar I65.1
　　　with
　　　　infarction I63.22
　　　　　due to
　　　　　　embolism I63.12
　　　　　　thrombosis I63.02
　　brain or cerebral I66.9
　　　with infarction (due to) I63.5-●
　　　　embolism I63.4-●
　　　　thrombosis I63.3-●
　　carotid I65.2-●
　　　with
　　　　infarction I63.23-●
　　　　　due to
　　　　　　embolism I63.13-●
　　　　　　thrombosis I63.03-●
　　cerebellar (anterior inferior) (posterior
　　　inferior) (superior) I66.3
　　　with infarction I63.54-●
　　　　due to
　　　　　embolism I63.44-●
　　　　　thrombosis I63.34-●
　　cerebral I66.9
　　　with infarction I63.50
　　　　due to
　　　　　embolism I63.40
　　　　　　specified NEC I63.49
　　　　　thrombosis I63.30
　　　　　　specified NEC I63.39
　　　anterior I66.1-●
　　　　with infarction I63.52-●
　　　　　due to
　　　　　　embolism I63.42-●
　　　　　　thrombosis I63.32-●

▶ New　　⇒ Revised　　d̶e̶l̶e̶t̶e̶d̶ Deleted　　● Use Additional Character(s)

Occlusion, occluded (Continued)
  artery (Continued)
    cerebral (Continued)
      middle I66.0-●
        with infarction I63.51-●
          due to
            embolism I63.41-●
            thrombosis I63.31-●
      posterior I66.2-●
        with infarction I63.53-●
          due to
            embolism I63.43-●
            thrombosis I63.33-●
      specified NEC I66.8
        with infarction I63.59
          due to
            embolism I63.4-●
            thrombosis I63.3-●
    choroidal (anterior) —see Occlusion,
      artery, cerebral, specified NEC
    ⇒ communicating posterior —see Occlusion,
      artery, precerebral, specified NEC
    complete
      coronary I25.82
      extremities I70.92
    coronary (acute) (thrombotic) (without
      myocardial infarction) I24.0
      with myocardial infarction —see
        Infarction, myocardium
      chronic total I25.82
      complete I25.82
      healed or old I25.2
      total (chronic) I25.82
    hypophyseal —see Occlusion, artery,
      precerebral, specified NEC
    iliac I74.5
    lower extremities due to stenosis or
      stricture I77.1
    mesenteric (embolic) (thrombotic) —see also
      Infarct, intestine K55.069
    perforating —see Occlusion, artery,
      cerebral, specified NEC
    peripheral I77.9
      thrombotic or embolic I74.4
    ⇒ pontine —see Occlusion, artery, precerebral,
      specified NEC
    precerebral I65.9
      with infarction I63.20
        due to
          embolism I63.10
            specified NEC I63.19
          thrombosis I63.00
            specified NEC I63.09
        specified NEC I63.29
      basilar —see Occlusion, artery, basilar
      carotid —see Occlusion, artery, carotid
      puerperal O88.23
      specified NEC I65.8
        with infarction I63.29
          due to
            embolism I63.19
           ⇒ thrombosis I63.09
      vertebral —see Occlusion, artery,
        vertebral
    renal N28.0
    retinal
      branch H34.23-●
      central H34.1-●
      partial H34.21-●
      transient H34.0-●
    spinal —see Occlusion, artery, precerebral,
      vertebral
    total (chronic)
      coronary I25.82
      extremities I70.92
    vertebral I65.0-●
      with
        infarction I63.21-●
          due to
            embolism I63.11-●
            thrombosis I63.01-●

Occlusion, occluded (Continued)
  basilar artery —see Occlusion, artery, basilar
  bile duct (common) (hepatic) (noncalculous)
    K83.1
  bowel —see Obstruction, intestine
  carotid (artery) (common) (internal) —see
    Occlusion, artery, carotid
  centric (of teeth) M26.59
    maximum intercuspation discrepancy
      M26.55
  cerebellar (artery) —see Occlusion, artery,
    cerebellar
  cerebral (artery) —see Occlusion, artery,
    cerebral
  cerebrovascular —see also Occlusion, artery,
    cerebral
    with infarction I63.5-●
  cervical canal —see Stricture, cervix
  cervix (uteri) —see Stricture, cervix
  choanal Q30.0
  choroidal (artery) —see Occlusion, artery,
    precerebral, specified NEC
  colon —see Obstruction, intestine
  communicating posterior artery —see
    Occlusion, artery, precerebral, specified
    NEC
  coronary (artery) (vein) (thrombotic) —see
    also Infarct, myocardium
    chronic total I25.82
    healed or old I25.2
    not resulting in infarction I24.0
    total (chronic) I25.82
  cystic duct —see Obstruction, gallbladder
  embolic —see Embolism
  fallopian tube N97.1
    congenital Q50.6
  gallbladder —see also Obstruction,
    gallbladder
    congenital (causing jaundice) Q44.1
  gingiva, traumatic K06.2
  hymen N89.6
    congenital Q52.3
  hypophyseal (artery) —see Occlusion, artery,
    precerebral, specified NEC
  iliac artery I74.5
  intestine —see Obstruction, intestine
  lacrimal passages —see Obstruction, lacrimal
  lung J98.4
  lymph or lymphatic channel I89.0
  mammary duct N64.89
  mesenteric artery (embolic) (thrombotic) —
    see also Infarct, intestine K55.069
  nose J34.89
    congenital Q30.0
  organ or site, congenital NEC —see Atresia,
    by site
  oviduct N97.1
    congenital Q50.6
  peripheral arteries
    due to stricture or stenosis I77.1
    upper extremity I74.2
  pontine (artery) —see Occlusion, artery,
    precerebral, specified NEC
  posterior lingual, of mandibular teeth M26.29
  precerebral artery —see Occlusion, artery,
    precerebral
  punctum lacrimale —see Obstruction,
    lacrimal
  pupil —see Membrane, pupillary
  pylorus, adult —see also Stricture, pylorus
    K31.1
  renal artery N28.0
  retina, retinal
    artery —see Occlusion, artery, retinal
    vein (central) H34.81-●
      engorgement H34.82-●
      tributary H34.83-●
    vessels H34.9
  spinal artery —see Occlusion, artery,
    precerebral, vertebral
  teeth (mandibular) (posterior lingual) M26.29

Occlusion, occluded (Continued)
  thoracic duct I89.0
  thrombotic —see Thrombosis, artery
  traumatic
    edentulous (alveolar) ridge K06.2
    gingiva K06.2
    periodontal K05.5
  tubal N97.1
  ureter (complete) (partial) N13.5
    congenital Q62.10
  ureteropelvic junction N13.5
    congenital Q62.11
  ureterovesical orifice N13.5
    congenital Q62.12
  urethra —see Stricture, urethra
  uterus N85.8
  vagina N89.5
  vascular NEC I99.8
  vein —see Thrombosis
    retinal —see Occlusion, retinal, vein
  vena cava (inferior) (superior) —see
    Embolism, vena cava
  ventricle (brain) NEC G91.1
  vertebral (artery) —see Occlusion, artery,
    vertebral
  vessel (blood) I99.8
  vulva N90.5
Occult
  blood in feces (stools) R19.5
Occupational
  problems NEC Z56.89
Ochlophobia —see Agoraphobia
Ochronosis (endogenous) E70.29
Ocular muscle —see condition
Oculogyric crisis or disturbance H51.8
  psychogenic F45.8
Oculomotor syndrome H51.9
Oculopathy
  syphilitic NEC A52.71
    congenital
      early A50.01
      late A50.30
    early (secondary) A51.43
    late A52.71
Oddi's sphincter spasm K83.4
Odontalgia K08.89
Odontoameloblastoma —see Cyst, calcifying
  odontogenic
Odontoclasia K03.89
Odontodysplasia, regional K00.4
Odontogenesis imperfecta K00.5
Odontoma (ameloblastic) (complex)
  (compound) (fibroameloblastic) —see Cyst,
  calcifying odontogenic
Odontomyelitis (closed) (open) K04.01
  irreversible K04.02
  reversible K04.01
Odontorrhagia K08.89
Odontosarcoma, ameloblastic C41.1
  upper jaw (bone) C41.0
Oestriasis —see Myiasis
Oguchi's disease H53.63
Ohara's disease —see Tularemia
OHS (obesity hypoventilation syndrome) E66.2

Oidiomycosis —see Candidiasis
Oidium albicans infection —see Candidiasis
Old (previous) myocardial infarction
  I25.2
Old age (without mention of debility) R54-●
  dementia F03
Olfactory —see condition
Oligemia —see Anemia
Oligoastrocytoma
  specified site —see Neoplasm, malignant,
    by site
  unspecified site C71.9
Oligocythemia D64.9
Oligodendroblastoma
  specified site —see Neoplasm, malignant
  unspecified site C71.9

Oligodendroglioma
  anaplastic type
    specified site —see Neoplasm, malignant,
      by site
    unspecified site C71.9
  specified site —see Neoplasm, malignant,
    by site
  unspecified site C71.9
Oligodontia —see Anodontia
Oligoencephalon Q02
Oligohidrosis L74.4
Oligohydramnios O41.0-●
Oligohydrosis L74.4
Oligomenorrhea N91.5
  primary N91.3
  secondary N91.4
Oligophrenia —see also Disability, intellectual
  phenylpyruvic E70.0
Oligospermia N46.11
  due to
    drug therapy N46.121
    efferent duct obstruction N46.123
    infection N46.122
    radiation N46.124
    specified cause NEC N46.129
    systemic disease N46.125
Oligotrichia —see Alopecia
Oliguria R34
  with, complicating or following ectopic or
    molar pregnancy O08.4
  postprocedural N99.0
Ollier's disease Q78.4
Omenotocele —see Hernia, abdomen, specified
  site NEC
Omentitis —see Peritonitis
Omentum, omental —see condition
Omphalitis (congenital) (newborn) P38.9
  with mild hemorrhage P38.1
  without hemorrhage P38.9
  not of newborn L08.82
  tetanus A33
Omphalocele Q79.2
Omphalomesenteric duct, persistent Q43.0
Omphalorrhagia, newborn P51.9
Omsk hemorrhagic fever A98.1
Onanism (excessive) F98.8
Onchocerciasis, onchocercosis B73.1
  with
    eye disease B73.00
      endophthalmitis B73.01
      eyelid B73.09
      glaucoma B73.02
      specified NEC B73.09
  eye NEC B73.00
  eyelid B73.09
Oncocytoma —see Neoplasm, benign, by site
Oncovirus, as cause of disease classified
  elsewhere B97.32
Ondine's curse —see Apnea, sleep
Oneirophrenia F23
Onychauxis L60.2
  congenital Q84.5
Onychia —see also Cellulitis, digit
  with lymphangitis —see Lymphangitis, acute,
    digit
  candidal B37.2
  dermatophytic B35.1
Onychitis —see also Cellulitis, digit
  with lymphangitis —see Lymphangitis, acute,
    digit
Onychocryptosis L60.0
Onychodystrophy L60.3
  congenital Q84.6
Onychogryphosis, onychogryposis L60.2
Onycholysis L60.1
Onychomadesis L60.8
Onychomalacia L60.3
Onychomycosis (finger) (toe) B35.1
Onycho-osteodysplasia Q87.2
Onychophagia F98.8
Onychophosis L60.8

Onychoptosis L60.8
Onychorrhexis L60.3
  congenital Q84.6
Onychoschizia L60.3
Onyxis (finger) (toe) L60.0
Onyxitis —see also Cellulitis, digit
  with lymphangitis —see Lymphangitis, acute,
    digit
Oophoritis (cystic) (infectional) (interstitial)
  N70.92
  with salpingitis N70.93
  acute N70.02
    with salpingitis N70.03
  chronic N70.12
    with salpingitis N70.13
  complicating abortion —see Abortion, by
    type, complicated by, oophoritis
Oophorocele N83.4-●
Opacity, opacities
  cornea H17.-●
    central H17.1-●
    congenital Q13.3
    degenerative —see Degeneration, cornea
    hereditary —see Dystrophy, cornea
    inflammatory —see Keratitis
    minor H17.81-●
    peripheral H17.82-●
    sequelae of trachoma (healed) B94.0
    specified NEC H17.89
  enamel (teeth) (fluoride) (nonfluoride) K00.3
  lens —see Cataract
  snowball —see Deposit, crystalline
  vitreous (humor) NEC H43.39-●
    congenital Q14.0
    membranes and strands H43.31-●
Opalescent dentin (hereditary) K00.5
Open, opening
  abnormal, organ or site, congenital —see
    Imperfect, closure
  angle with
    borderline
      findings
        high risk H40.02-●
        low risk H40.01-●
      intraocular pressure H40.00-●
    cupping of discs H40.01-●
    glaucoma (primary) —see Glaucoma, open
      angle
  bite
    anterior M26.220
    posterior M26.221
  false —see Imperfect, closure
  margin on tooth restoration K08.51
  restoration margins of tooth K08.51
  wound —see Wound, open
Operational fatigue F48.8
Operative —see condition
Operculitis —see Periodontitis
Operculum —see Break, retina
Ophiasis L63.2
Ophthalmia —see also Conjunctivitis H10.9
  actinic rays —see Photokeratitis
  allergic (acute) —see Conjunctivitis, acute,
    atopic
  blennorrhagic (gonococcal) (neonatorum)
    A54.31
  diphtheritic A36.86
  Egyptian A71.1
  electrica —see Photokeratitis
  gonococcal (neonatorum) A54.31
  metastatic —see Endophthalmitis, purulent
  migraine —see Migraine, ophthalmoplegic
  neonatorum, newborn P39.1
    gonococcal A54.31
  nodosa H16.24-●
  purulent —see Conjunctivitis, acute,
    mucopurulent
  spring —see Conjunctivitis, acute, atopic
  sympathetic —see Uveitis, sympathetic
Ophthalmitis —see Ophthalmia
Ophthalmocele (congenital) Q15.8

Ophthalmoneuromyelitis G36.0
Ophthalmoplegia —see also Strabismus,
  paralytic
  anterior internuclear —see Ophthalmoplegia,
    internuclear
  ataxia-areflexia G61.0
  diabetic —see E08-E13 with .39
  exophthalmic E05.00
    with thyroid storm E05.01
  external H49.88-●
    progressive H49.4-●
      with pigmentary retinopathy —see
        Kearns-Sayre syndrome
    total H49.3-●
  internal (complete) (total) H52.51-●
  internuclear H51.2-●
  migraine —see Migraine, ophthalmoplegic
  Parinaud's H49.88-●
  progressive external —see Ophthalmoplegia,
    external, progressive
  supranuclear, progressive G23.1
  total (external) —see Ophthalmoplegia,
    external, total
Opioid(s)
  abuse —see Abuse, drug, opioids
  dependence —see Dependence, drug, opioids
  induced, without use disorder
    anxiety disorder F11.988
    delirium F11.921
    depressive disorder F11.94
    sexual dysfunction F11.981
    sleep disorder F11.982
Opisthognathism M26.09
Opisthorchiasis (felineus) (viverrini) B66.0
Opitz' disease D73.2
Opiumism —see Dependence, drug, opioid
Oppenheim's disease G70.2
Oppenheim-Urbach disease (necrobiosis
  lipoidica diabeticorum) —see E08-E13 with
  .620
Optic nerve —see condition
Orbit —see condition
Orchioblastoma C62.9-●
Orchitis (gangrenous) (nonspecific) (septic)
  (suppurative) N45.2
  blennorrhagic (gonococcal) (acute) (chronic)
    A54.23
  chlamydial A56.19
  filarial —see also Infestation, filarial B74.9
    [N51]
  gonococcal (acute) (chronic) A54.23
  mumps B26.0
  syphilitic A52.76
  tuberculous A18.15
Orf (virus disease) B08.02
Organic —see also condition
  brain syndrome F09
  heart —see Disease, heart
  mental disorder F09
  psychosis F09
Orgasm
  anejaculatory N53.13
Oriental
  bilharziasis B65.2
  schistosomiasis B65.2
Orifice —see condition
Origin of both great vessels from right
  ventricle Q20.1
Ormond's disease (with ureteral obstruction)
  N13.5
  with infection N13.6
Ornithine metabolism disorder E72.4
Ornithinemia (Type I) (Type II) E72.4
Ornithosis A70
Orotaciduria, oroticaciduria (congenital)
  (hereditary) (pyrimidine deficiency) E79.8
  anemia D53.0
Orthodontics
  adjustment Z46.4
  fitting Z46.4
Orthopnea R06.01

▶ New   ➡ Revised   ~~deleted~~ Deleted   ● Use Additional Character(s)

Orthopoxvirus B08.09
  specified NEC B08.09
Os, uterus —see condition
Osgood-Schlatter disease or
    osteochondrosis —see Osteochondrosis,
    juvenile, tibia
Osler (-Weber)-Rendu disease I78.0
Osler's nodes I33.0
Osmidrosis L75.0
Osseous —see condition
Ossification
  artery —see Arteriosclerosis
  auricle (ear) —see Disorder, pinna, specified
    type NEC
  bronchial J98.09
  cardiac —see Degeneration, myocardial
  cartilage (senile) —see Disorder, cartilage,
    specified type NEC
  coronary (artery) —see Disease, heart,
    ischemic, atherosclerotic
  diaphragm J98.6
  ear, middle —see Otosclerosis
  falx cerebri G96.19
  fontanel, premature Q75.0
  heart —see also Degeneration, myocardial
    valve —see Endocarditis
  larynx J38.7
  ligament —see Disorder, tendon, specified
    type NEC
    posterior longitudinal —see
      Spondylopathy, specified NEC
  meninges (cerebral) (spinal) G96.19
  multiple, eccentric centers —see Disorder,
    bone, development or growth
  muscle —see also Calcification, muscle
    due to burns —see Myositis, ossificans, in,
      burns
    paralytic —see Myositis, ossificans, in,
      quadriplegia
    progressive —see Myositis, ossificans,
      progressiva
    specified NEC M61.50
      ankle M61.57-●
      foot M61.57-●
      forearm M61.53-●
      hand M61.54-●
      lower leg M61.56-●
      multiple sites M61.59
      pelvic region M61.55-●
      shoulder region M61.51-●
      specified site NEC M61.58
      thigh M61.55-●
      upper arm M61.52-●
    traumatic —see Myositis, ossificans,
      traumatica
  myocardium, myocardial —see Degeneration,
    myocardial
  penis N48.89
  periarticular —see Disorder, joint, specified
    type NEC
  pinna —see Disorder, pinna, specified type
    NEC
  rider's bone —see Ossification, muscle,
    specified NEC
  sclera H15.89
  subperiosteal, post-traumatic M89.8X-●
  tendon —see Disorder, tendon, specified
    type NEC
  trachea J39.8
  tympanic membrane —see Disorder,
    tympanic membrane, specified NEC
  vitreous (humor) —see Deposit, crystalline
Osteitis —see also Osteomyelitis
  alveolar M27.3
  condensans M85.30
    ankle M85.37-●
    foot M85.37-●
    forearm M85.33-●
    hand M85.34-●
    lower leg M85.36-●
    multiple site M85.39

Osteitis (Continued)
  condensans (Continued)
    neck M85.38
    rib M85.38
    shoulder M85.31-●
    skull M85.38
    specified site NEC M85.38
    thigh M85.35-●
    toe M85.37-●
    upper arm M85.32-●
    vertebra M85.38
  deformans M88.9
    in (due to)
      malignant neoplasm of bone
        C41.9 [M90.60]
      neoplastic disease —see also Neoplasm
        D49.9 [M90.60]
        carpus D49.9 [M90.64-●]
        clavicle D49.9 [M90.61-●]
        femur D49.9 [M90.65-●]
        fibula D49.9 [M90.66-●]
        finger D49.9 [M90.64-●]
        humerus D49.9 [M90.62-●]
        ilium D49.9 [M90.65-●]
        ischium D49.9 [M90.65-●]
        metacarpus D49.9 [M90.64-●]
        metatarsus D49.9 [M90.67-●]
        multiple sites D49.9 [M90.69]
        neck D49.9 [M90.68]
        radius D49.9 [M90.63-●]
        rib D49.9 [M90.68]
        scapula D49.9 [M90.61-●]
        skull D49.9 [M90.68]
        tarsus D49.9 [M90.67-●]
        tibia D49.9 [M90.66-●]
        toe D49.9 [M90.67-●]
        ulna D49.9 [M90.63-●]
        vertebra D49.9 [M90.68]
    skull M88.0
    specified NEC —see Paget's disease, bone,
      by site
    vertebra M88.1
  due to yaws A66.6
  fibrosa NEC —see Cyst, bone, by site
    circumscripta —see Dysplasia, fibrous,
      bone NEC
    cystica (generalisata) E21.0
    disseminata Q78.1
    osteoplastica E21.0
  fragilitans Q78.0
  Garré's (sclerosing) —see Osteomyelitis,
    specified type NEC
  jaw (acute) (chronic) (lower) (suppurative)
    (upper) M27.2
  parathyroid E21.0
  petrous bone (acute) (chronic) —see Petrositis
  sclerotic, nonsuppurative —see Osteomyelitis,
    specified type NEC
  tuberculosa A18.09
    cystica D86.89
    multiplex cystoides D86.89
Osteoarthritis M19.90
  ankle M19.07-●
  elbow M19.02-●
  foot joint M19.07-●
  generalized M15.9
    erosive M15.4
    primary M15.0
    specified NEC M15.8
  hand joint M19.04-●
    first carpometacarpal joint M18.9-●
  hip M16.1-●
    bilateral M16.0
    due to hip dysplasia (unilateral)
      M16.3-●
      bilateral M16.2
  interphalangeal
    distal (Heberden) M15.1
    proximal (Bouchard) M15.2
⏩knee M17.1-●
    bilateral M17.0

Osteoarthritis (Continued)
  post-traumatic NEC M19.92
    ankle M19.17-●
    elbow M19.12-●
    foot joint M19.17-●
    hand joint M19.14-●
      first carpometacarpal joint M18.3-●
        bilateral M18.2
    hip M16.5-●
      bilateral M16.4
    knee M17.3-●
      bilateral M17.2
    shoulder M19.11-●
    wrist M19.13-●
  primary M19.91
    ankle M19.07-●
    elbow M19.02-●
    foot joint M19.07-●
    hand joint M19.04-●
      first carpometacarpal joint M18.1-●
        bilateral M18.0
    hip M16.1-●
      bilateral M16.0
    knee M17.1-●
      bilateral M17.0
    shoulder M19.01-●
    spine —see Spondylosis
    wrist M19.03-●
  secondary M19.93
    ankle M19.27-●
    elbow M19.22-●
    foot joint M19.27-●
    hand joint M19.24-●
      first carpometacarpal joint M18.5-●
        bilateral M18.4
    hip M16.7
      bilateral M16.6
    knee M17.5
      bilateral M17.4
    multiple M15.3
    shoulder M19.21-●
    spine —see Spondylosis
    wrist M19.23-●
  shoulder M19.01-●
  spine —see Spondylosis
  wrist M19.03-●
Osteoarthropathy (hypertrophic) M19.90
  ankle —see Osteoarthritis, primary, ankle
  elbow —see Osteoarthritis, primary, elbow
  foot joint —see Osteoarthritis, primary, foot
  hand joint —see Osteoarthritis, primary, hand
    joint
  knee joint —see Osteoarthritis, primary, knee
  multiple site —see Osteoarthritis, primary,
    multiple joint
  pulmonary —see also Osteoarthropathy,
    specified type NEC
    hypertrophic —see Osteoarthropathy,
      hypertrophic, specified type NEC
  secondary —see Osteoarthropathy, specified
    type NEC
  secondary hypertrophic —see
    Osteoarthropathy, specified type NEC
  shoulder —see Osteoarthritis, primary,
    shoulder
  specified joint NEC —see Osteoarthritis,
    primary, specified joint NEC
  specified type NEC M89.40
    carpus M89.44-●
    clavicle M89.41-●
    femur M89.45-●
    fibula M89.46-●
    finger M89.44-●
    humerus M89.42-●
    ilium M89.459
    ischium M89.459
    metacarpus M89.44-●
    metatarsus M89.47-●
    multiple sites M89.49
    neck M89.48
    radius M89.43-●

Osteoarthropathy (Continued)
  specified type NEC (Continued)
    rib M89.48
    scapula M89.41-●
    skull M89.48
    tarsus M89.47-●
    tibia M89.46-●
    toe M89.47-●
    ulna M89.43-●
    vertebra M89.48
  spine —see Spondylosis
  wrist —see Osteoarthritis, primary, wrist
Osteoarthrosis (degenerative) (hypertrophic)
    (joint) —see also Osteoarthritis
  deformans alkaptonurica E70.29 [M36.8]
  erosive M15.4
  generalized M15.9
    primary M15.0
  polyarticular M15.9
  spine —see Spondylosis
Osteoblastoma —see Neoplasm, bone, benign
  aggressive —see Neoplasm, bone, uncertain
    behavior
Osteochondroarthrosis deformans
    endemica —see Disease, Kaschin-Beck
Osteochondritis —see also Osteochondropathy,
    by site
  Brailsford's —see Osteochondrosis, juvenile,
    radius
  dissecans M93.20
    ankle M93.27-●
    elbow M93.22-●
    foot M93.27-●
    hand M93.24-●
    hip M93.25-●
    knee M93.26-●
    multiple sites M93.29
    shoulder joint M93.21-●
    specified site NEC M93.28
    wrist M93.23-●
  juvenile M92.9
    patellar —see Osteochondrosis, juvenile,
      patella
  syphilitic (congenital) (early) A50.02
    [M90.80]
    ankle A50.02 [M90.87-●]
    elbow A50.02 [M90.82-●]
    foot A50.02 [M90.87-●]
    forearm A50.02 [M90.83-●]
    hand A50.02 [M90.84-●]
    hip A50.02 [M90.85-●]
    knee A50.02 [M90.86●-]
    multiple sites A50.02 [M90.89]
    shoulder joint A50.02 [M90.81-●]
    specified site NEC A50.02 [M90.88]
Osteochondrodysplasia Q78.9
  with defects of growth of tubular bones and
    spine Q77.9
    specified NEC Q77.8
  specified NEC Q78.8
Osteochondrodystrophy E78.9
Osteochondrolysis —see Osteochondritis,
    dissecans
Osteochondroma —see Neoplasm, bone, benign
Osteochondromatosis D48.0
  syndrome Q78.4
Osteochondromyxosarcoma —see Neoplasm,
    bone, malignant
Osteochondropathy M93.90
  ankle M93.97-●
  elbow M93.92-●
  foot M93.97-●
  hand M93.94-●
  hip M93.95-●
  Kienböck's disease of adults M93.1
  knee M93.96-●
  multiple joints M93.99
  osteochondritis dissecans —see
    Osteochondritis, dissecans
  osteochondrosis —see Osteochondrosis
  shoulder region M93.91-●

Osteochondropathy (Continued)
  slipped upper femoral epiphysis —see
    Slipped, epiphysis, upper femoral
  specified joint NEC M93.98
  specified type NEC M93.80
    ankle M93.87-●
    elbow M93.82-●
    foot M93.87-●
    hand M93.84-●
    hip M93.85-●
    knee M93.86-●
    multiple joints M93.89
    shoulder region M93.81-●
    specified joint NEC M93.88
    wrist M93.83-●
  syphilitic, congenital
    early A50.02 [M90.80]
    late A50.56 [M90.80]
  wrist M93.93-●
Osteochondrosarcoma —see Neoplasm, bone,
    malignant
Osteochondrosis —see also Osteochondropathy,
    by site
  acetabulum (juvenile) M91.0
  adult —see Osteochondropathy, specified
    type NEC, by site
  astragalus (juvenile) —see Osteochondrosis,
    juvenile, tarsus
  Blount's —see Osteochondrosis, juvenile, tibia
  Buchanan's M91.0
  Burns' —see Osteochondrosis, juvenile, ulna
  calcaneus (juvenile) —see Osteochondrosis,
    juvenile, tarsus
  capitular epiphysis (femur) (juvenile) —see
    Legg-Calvé-Perthes disease
  carpal (juvenile) (lunate) (scaphoid) —see
    Osteochondrosis, juvenile, hand, carpal
    lunate
    adult M93.1
  coxae juvenilis —see Legg-Calvé-Perthes
    disease
  deformans juvenilis, coxae —see Legg-Calvé-
    Perthes disease
  Diaz's —see Osteochondrosis, juvenile, tarsus
  dissecans (knee) (shoulder) —see
    Osteochondritis, dissecans
  femoral capital epiphysis (juvenile) —see
    Legg-Calvé-Perthes disease
  femur (head), juvenile —see Legg-Calvé-
    Perthes disease
  fibula (juvenile) —see Osteochondrosis,
    juvenile, fibula
  foot NEC (juvenile) M92.8
  Freiberg's —see Osteochondrosis, juvenile,
    metatarsus
  Haas' (juvenile) —see Osteochondrosis,
    juvenile, humerus
  Haglund's —see Osteochondrosis, juvenile,
    tarsus
  hip (juvenile) —see Legg-Calvé-Perthes disease
  humerus (capitulum) (head) (juvenile) —see
    Osteochondrosis, juvenile, humerus
  ilium, iliac crest (juvenile) M91.0
  ischiopubic synchondrosis M91.0
  Iselin's —see Osteochondrosis, juvenile,
    metatarsus
  juvenile, juvenilis M92.9
    after congenital dislocation of hip
      reduction —see Osteochondrosis,
      juvenile, hip, specified NEC
    arm —see Osteochondrosis, juvenile, upper
      limb NEC
    capitular epiphysis (femur) —see Legg-
      Calvé-Perthes disease
    clavicle, sternal epiphysis —see
      Osteochondrosis, juvenile, upper limb
      NEC
    coxae —see Legg-Calvé-Perthes disease
    deformans M92.9
    fibula M92.5-●
    foot NEC M92.8

Osteochondrosis (Continued)
  juvenile, juvenilis (Continued)
    hand M92.20-●
      carpal lunate M92.21-●
      metacarpal head M92.22-●
      specified site NEC M92.29-●
    head of femur —see Legg-Calvé-Perthes
      disease
    hip and pelvis M91.9-●
      coxa plana —see Coxa, plana
      femoral head —see Legg-Calvé-Perthes
        disease
      pelvis M91.0
      pseudocoxalgia —see Pseudocoxalgia
      specified NEC M91.8-●
    humerus M92.0-●
    limb
      lower NEC M92.8
      upper NEC —see Osteochondrosis,
        juvenile, upper limb NEC
    medial cuneiform bone —see
      Osteochondrosis, juvenile, tarsus
    metatarsus M92.7-●
    patella M92.4-●
    radius M92.1-●
    specified site NEC M92.8
    spine M42.00
      cervical region M42.02
      cervicothoracic region M42.03
      lumbar region M42.06
      lumbosacral region M42.07
      multiple sites M42.09
      occipito-atlanto-axial region M42.01
      sacrococcygeal region M42.08
      thoracic region M42.04
      thoracolumbar region M42.05
    tarsus M92.6-●
    tibia M92.5-●
    ulna M92.1-●
    upper limb NEC M92.3-●
    vertebra (body) (epiphyseal plates)
      (Calvé's) (Scheuermann's) —see
      Osteochondrosis, juvenile, spine
  Kienböck's —see Osteochondrosis, juvenile,
    hand, carpal lunate
    adult M93.1
  Köhler's
    patellar —see Osteochondrosis, juvenile,
      patella
    tarsal navicular —see Osteochondrosis,
      juvenile, tarsus
  Legg-Perthes (-Calvé's) (-Waldenström) —see
    Legg-Calvé-Perthes disease
  limb
    lower NEC (juvenile) M92.8
    upper NEC (juvenile) —see
      Osteochondrosis, juvenile, upper limb
      NEC
  lunate bone (carpal) (juvenile) —see also
    Osteochondrosis, juvenile, hand, carpal
    lunate
    adult M93.1
  Mauclaire's —see Osteochondrosis, juvenile,
    hand, metacarpal
  metacarpal (head) (juvenile) —see
    Osteochondrosis, juvenile, hand,
    metacarpal
  metatarsus (fifth) (head) (juvenile)
    (second) —see Osteochondrosis, juvenile,
    metatarsus
  navicular (juvenile) —see Osteochondrosis,
    juvenile, tarsus
  os
    calcis (juvenile) —see Osteochondrosis,
      juvenile, tarsus
    tibiale externum (juvenile) —see
      Osteochondrosis, juvenile, tarsus
  Osgood-Schlatter —see Osteochondrosis,
    juvenile, tibia
  Panner's —see Osteochondrosis, juvenile,
    humerus

▶ New   ⇒ Revised   ~~deleted~~ Deleted   ● Use Additional Character(s)

Osteochondrosis *(Continued)*
  patellar center (juvenile) (primary)
    (secondary) —*see* Osteochondrosis,
    juvenile, patella
  pelvis (juvenile) M91.0
  Pierson's M91.0
  radius (head) (juvenile) —*see*
    Osteochondrosis, juvenile, radius
  Scheuermann's —*see* Osteochondrosis,
    juvenile, spine
  Sever's —*see* Osteochondrosis, juvenile,
    tarsus
  Sinding-Larsen —*see* Osteochondrosis,
    juvenile, patella
  spine M42.9
    adult M42.10
      cervical region M42.12
      cervicothoracic region M42.13
      lumbar region M42.16
      lumbosacral region M42.17
      multiple sites M42.19
      occipito-atlanto-axial region M42.11
      sacrococcygeal region M42.18
      thoracic region M42.14
      thoracolumbar region M42.15
    juvenile —*see* Osteochondrosis, juvenile,
      spine
  symphysis pubis (juvenile) M91.0
  syphilitic (congenital) A50.02
  talus (juvenile) —*see* Osteochondrosis,
    juvenile, tarsus
  tarsus (navicular) (juvenile) —*see*
    Osteochondrosis, juvenile, tarsus
  tibia (proximal) (tubercle) (juvenile) —*see*
    Osteochondrosis, juvenile, tibia
  tuberculous —*see* Tuberculosis, bone
  ulna (lower) (juvenile) —*see* Osteochondrosis,
    juvenile, ulna
  van Neck's M91.0
  vertebral —*see* Osteochondrosis,
    spine
Osteoclastoma D48.0
  malignant —*see* Neoplasm, bone,
    malignant
Osteodynia —*see* Disorder, bone,
  specified type NEC
Osteodystrophy Q78.9
  azotemic N25.0
  congenital Q78.9
  parathyroid, secondary E21.1
  renal N25.0
Osteofibroma —*see* Neoplasm, bone,
  benign
Osteofibrosarcoma —*see* Neoplasm,
  bone, malignant
Osteogenesis imperfecta Q78.0
Osteogenic —*see* condition
Osteolysis M89.50
  carpus M89.54-●
  clavicle M89.51-●
  femur M89.55-●
  fibula M89.56-●
  finger M89.54-●
  humerus M89.52-●
  ilium M89.559
  ischium M89.559
  joint prosthesis (periprosthetic) —*see*
    Complications, joint prosthesis,
    mechanical, periprosthetic, osteolysis,
    by site
  metacarpus M89.54-●
  metatarsus M89.57-●
  multiple sites M89.59
  neck M89.58
  periprosthetic —*see* Complications, joint
    prosthesis, mechanical, periprosthetic,
    osteolysis, by site
  radius M89.53-●
  rib M89.58
  scapula M89.51-●
  skull M89.58

Osteolysis *(Continued)*
  tarsus M89.57-●
  tibia M89.56-●
  toe M89.57-●
  ulna M89.53-●
  vertebra M89.58
Osteoma —*see also* Neoplasm, bone, benign
  osteoid —*see also* Neoplasm, bone, benign
    giant —*see* Neoplasm, bone, benign
Osteomalacia M83.9
  adult M83.9
    drug-induced NEC M83.5
    due to
      malabsorption (postsurgical) M83.2
      malnutrition M83.3
    specified NEC M83.8
  aluminium-induced M83.4
  infantile —*see* Rickets
  juvenile —*see* Rickets
  oncogenic E83.89
  pelvis M83.8
  puerperal M83.0
  senile M83.1
  vitamin-D-resistant in adults E83.31
    [M90.8-●]
    carpus E83.31 *[M90.84-●]*
    clavicle E83.31 *[M90.81-●]*
    femur E83.31 *[M90.85-●]*
    fibula E83.31 *[M90.86-●]*
    finger E83.31 *[M90.84-●]*
    humerus E83.31 *[M90.82-●]*
    ilium E83.31 *[M90.859]*
    ischium E83.31 *[M90.859]*
    metacarpus E83.31 *[M90.84-●]*
    metatarsus E83.31 *[M90.87-●]*
    multiple sites E83.31 *[M90.89]*
    neck E83.31 *[M90.88]*
    radius E83.31 *[M90.83-●]*
    rib E83.31 *[M90.88]*
    scapula E83.31 *[M90.819]*
    skull E83.31 *[M90.88]*
    tarsus E83.31 *[M90.879]*
    tibia E83.31 *[M90.869]*
    toe E83.31 *[M90.879]*
    ulna E83.31 *[M90.839]*
    vertebra E83.31 *[M90.88]*
Osteomyelitis (general) (infective)
  (localized) (neonatal) (purulent)
  (septic) (staphylococcal) (streptococcal)
  (suppurative) (with periostitis) M86.9
  acute M86.10
    carpus M86.14-●
    clavicle M86.11-●
    femur M86.15-●
    fibula M86.16-●
    finger M86.14-●
    hematogenous M86.00
      carpus M86.04-●
      clavicle M86.01-●
      femur M86.05-●
      fibula M86.06-●
      finger M86.04-●
      humerus M86.02-●
      ilium M86.059
      ischium M86.059
      mandible M27.2
      metacarpus M86.04-●
      metatarsus M86.07-●
      multiple sites M86.09
      neck M86.08
      orbit H05.02-●
      petrous bone —*see* Petrositis
      radius M86.03-●
      rib M86.08
      scapula M86.01-●
      skull M86.08
      tarsus M86.07-●
      tibia M86.06-●
      toe M86.07-●
      ulna M86.03-●
      vertebra —*see* Osteomyelitis, vertebra

Osteomyelitis *(Continued)*
  acute *(Continued)*
    humerus M86.12-●
    ilium M86.159
    ischium M86.159
    mandible M27.2
    metacarpus M86.14-●
    metatarsus M86.17-●
    multiple sites M86.19
    neck M86.18
    orbit H05.02-●
    petrous bone —*see* Petrositis
    radius M86.13-●
    rib M86.18
    scapula M86.11-●
    skull M86.18
    tarsus M86.17-●
    tibia M86.16-●
    toe M86.17-●
    ulna M86.13-●
    vertebra —*see* Osteomyelitis, vertebra
  chronic (or old) M86.60
    with draining sinus M86.40
      carpus M86.44-●
      clavicle M86.41-●
      femur M86.45-●
      fibula M86.46-●
      finger M86.44-●
      humerus M86.42-●
      ilium M86.459
      ischium M86.459
      mandible M27.2
      metacarpus M86.44-●
      metatarsus M86.47-●
      multiple sites M86.49
      neck M86.48
      orbit H05.02-●
      petrous bone —*see* Petrositis
      radius M86.43-●
      rib M86.48
      scapula M86.41-●
      skull M86.48
      tarsus M86.47-●
      tibia M86.46-●
      toe M86.47-●
      ulna M86.43-●
      vertebra —*see* Osteomyelitis,
        vertebra
    carpus M86.64-●
    clavicle M86.61-●
    femur M86.65-●
    fibula M86.66-●
    finger M86.64-●
    hematogenous NEC M86.50
      carpus M86.54-●
      clavicle M86.51-●
      femur M86.55-●
      fibula M86.56-●
      finger M86.54-●
      humerus M86.52-●
      ilium M86.559
      ischium M86.559
      mandible M27.2
      metacarpus M86.54-●
      metatarsus M86.57-●
      multifocal M86.30
        carpus M86.34-●
        clavicle M86.31-●
        femur M86.35-●
        fibula M86.36-●
        finger M86.34-●
        humerus M86.32-●
        ilium M86.359
        ischium M86.359
        metacarpus M86.34-●
        metatarsus M86.37-●
        multiple sites M86.39
        neck M86.38
        radius M86.33-●
        rib M86.38
        scapula M86.31-●

Osteomyelitis *(Continued)*
  chronic *(Continued)*
    hematogenous NEC *(Continued)*
      multifocal *(Continued)*
        skull M86.38
        tarsus M86.37-●
        tibia M86.36-●
        toe M86.37-●
        ulna M86.33-●
        vertebra —*see* Osteomyelitis, vertebra
      multiple sites M86.59
      neck M86.58
      orbit H05.02-●
      petrous bone —*see* Petrositis
      radius M86.53-●
      rib M86.58
      scapula M86.51-●
      skull M86.58
      tarsus M86.57-●
      tibia M86.56-●
      toe M86.57-●
      ulna M86.53-●
      vertebra —*see* Osteomyelitis, vertebra
    humerus M86.62-●
    ilium M86.659
    ischium M86.659
    mandible M27.2
    metacarpus M86.64-●
    metatarsus M86.67-●
    multifocal —*see* Osteomyelitis, chronic,
      hematogenous, multifocal
    multiple sites M86.69
    neck M86.68
    orbit H05.02-●
    petrous bone —*see* Petrositis
    radius M86.63-●
    rib M86.68
    scapula M86.61-●
    skull M86.68
    tarsus M86.67-●
    tibia M86.66-●
    toe M86.67-●
    ulna M86.63-●
    vertebra —*see* Osteomyelitis, vertebra
  echinococcal B67.2
  Garr's —*see* Osteomyelitis, specified type
    NEC
  in diabetes mellitus —*see* E08-E13 with .69
  jaw (acute) (chronic) (lower) (neonatal)
    (suppurative) (upper) M27.2
  nonsuppurating —*see* Osteomyelitis,
    specified type NEC
  orbit H05.02-●
  petrous bone —*see* Petrositis
  Salmonella (arizonae) (cholerae-suis)
    (enteritidis) (typhimurium) A02.24
  sclerosing, nonsuppurative —*see*
    Osteomyelitis, specified type NEC
  specified type NEC —*see also* subcategory
    M86.8X-●
    mandible M27.2
    orbit H05.02-●
    petrous bone —*see* Petrositis
    vertebra —*see* Osteomyelitis, vertebra
  subacute M86.20
    carpus M86.24-●
    clavicle M86.21-●
    femur M86.25-●
    fibula M86.26-●
    finger M86.24-●
    humerus M86.22-●
    mandible M27.2
    metacarpus M86.24-●
    metatarsus M86.27-●
    multiple sites M86.29
    neck M86.28
    orbit H05.02-●
    petrous bone —*see* Petrositis
    radius M86.23-●
    rib M86.28
    scapula M86.21-●

Osteomyelitis *(Continued)*
  subacute *(Continued)*
    skull M86.28
    tarsus M86.27-●
    tibia M86.26-●
    toe M86.27-●
    ulna M86.23-●
    vertebra —*see* Osteomyelitis, vertebra
  syphilitic A52.77
    congenital (early) A50.02 [M90.80]
  tuberculous —*see* Tuberculosis, bone
  typhoid A01.05
  vertebra M46.20
    cervical region M46.22
    cervicothoracic region M46.23
    lumbar region M46.26
    lumbosacral region M46.27
    occipito-atlanto-axial region
      M46.21
    sacrococcygeal region M46.28
    thoracic region M46.24
    thoracolumbar region M46.25
Osteomyelofibrosis D47.4
Osteomyeloscerosis D75.89
Osteonecrosis M87.9
  due to
    drugs —*see* Osteonecrosis, secondary, due
      to, drugs
    trauma —*see* Osteonecrosis, secondary, due
      to, trauma
  idiopathic aseptic M87.00
    ankle M87.07-●
    carpus M87.03-●
    clavicle M87.01-●
    femur M87.05-●
    fibula M87.06-●
    finger M87.04-●
    humerus M87.02-●
    ilium M87.050
    ischium M87.050
    metacarpus M87.04-●
    metatarsus M87.07-●
    multiple sites M87.09
    neck M87.08
    pelvis M87.050
    radius M87.03-●
    rib M87.08
    scapula M87.01-●
    skull M87.08
    tarsus M87.07-●
    tibia M87.06-●
    toe M87.07-●
    ulna M87.03-●
    vertebra M87.08
  secondary NEC M87.30
    carpus M87.33-●
    clavicle M87.31-●
    due to
      drugs M87.10
        carpus M87.13-●
        clavicle M87.11-●
        femur M87.15-●
        fibula M87.16-●
        finger M87.14-●
        humerus M87.12-●
        ilium M87.159
        ischium M87.159
        jaw M87.180
        metacarpus M87.14-●
        metatarsus M87.17-●
        multiple sites M87.19
        neck M87.18
        radius M87.13-●
        rib M87.18
        scapula M87.11-●
        skull M87.18
        tarsus M87.17-●
        tibia M87.16-●
        toe M87.17-●
        ulna M87.13-●
        vertebra M87.18

Osteonecrosis *(Continued)*
  secondary NEC *(Continued)*
    due to *(Continued)*
      hemoglobinopathy NEC D58.2
        [M90.50]
        carpus D58.2 [M90.54-●]
        clavicle D58.2 [M90.51-●]
        femur D58.2 [M90.55-●]
        fibula D58.2 [M90.56-●]
        finger D58.2 [M90.54-●]
        humerus D58.2 [M90.52-●]
        ilium D58.2 [M90.55-●]
        ischium D58.2 [M90.55-●]
        metacarpus D58.2 [M90.54-●]
        metatarsus D58.2 [M90.57-●]
        multiple sites D58.2 [M90.58]
        neck D58.2 [M90.58]
        radius D58.2 [M90.53-●]
        rib D58.2 [M90.58]
        scapula D58.2 [M90.51-●]
        skull D58.2 [M90.58]
        tarsus D58.2 [M90.57-●]
        tibia D58.2 [M90.56-●]
        toe D58.2 [M90.57-●]
        ulna D58.2 [M90.53-●]
        vertebra D58.2 [M90.58]
      trauma (previous) M87.20
        carpus M87.23-●
        clavicle M87.21-●
        femur M87.25-●
        fibula M87.26-●
        finger M87.24-●
        humerus M87.22-●
        ilium M87.25-●
        ischium M87.25-●
        metacarpus M87.24-●
        metatarsus M87.27-●
        multiple sites M87.29
        neck M87.28
        radius M87.23-●
        rib M87.28
        scapula M87.21-●
        skull M87.28
        tarsus M87.27-●
        tibia M87.26-●
        toe M87.27-●
        ulna M87.23-●
        vertebra M87.28
    femur M87.35-●
    fibula M87.36-●
    finger M87.34-●
    humerus M87.32
    ilium M87.350
    in
      caisson disease T70.3 [M90.50]
        carpus T70.3 [M90.54-●]
        clavicle T70.3 [M90.51-●]
        femur T70.3 [M90.55-●]
        fibula T70.3 [M90.56-●]
        finger T70.3 [M90.54-●]
        humerus T70.3 [M90.52-●]
        ilium T70.3 [M90.55-●]
        ischium T70.3 [M90.55-●]
        metacarpus T70.3 [M90.54-●]
        metatarsus T70.3 [M90.57-●]
        multiple sites T70.3 [M90.59]
        neck T70.3 [M90.58]
        radius T70.3 [M90.53-●]
        rib T70.3 [M90.58]
        scapula T70.3 [M90.51-●]
        skull T70.3 [M90.58]
        tarsus T70.3 [M90.57-●]
        tibia T70.3 [M90.56-●]
        toe T70.3 [M90.57-●]
        ulna T70.3 [M90.53-●]
        vertebra T70.3 [M90.58]
    ischium M87.350
    metacarpus M87.34-●
    metatarsus M87.37-●
    multiple site M87.39
    neck M87.38

▶ New   ⇒ Revised   ~~deleted~~ Deleted   ● Use Additional Character(s)

Osteonecrosis *(Continued)*
  secondary NEC *(Continued)*
    radius M87.33-●
    rib M87.38
    scapula M87.319
    skull M87.38
    tarsus M87.379
    tibia M87.366
    toe M87.379
    ulna M87.33-●
    vertebra M87.38
  specified type NEC M87.80
    carpus M87.83-●
    clavicle M87.81-●
    femur M87.85-●
    fibula M87.86-●
    finger M87.84-●
    humerus M87.82-●
    ilium M87.85-●
    ischium M87.85-●
    metacarpus M87.84-●
    metatarsus M87.87-●
    multiple sites M87.89
    neck M87.88
    radius M87.83-●
    rib M87.88-●
    scapula M87.81-●
    skull M87.88
    tarsus M87.87-●
    tibia M87.86-●
    toe M87.87-●
    ulna M87.83-●
    vertebra M87.88
Osteo-onycho-arthro-dysplasia Q87.2
Osteo-onychodysplasia, hereditary Q87.2
Osteopathia condensans disseminata Q78.8
Osteopathy —*see also* Osteomyelitis,
  Osteonecrosis, Osteoporosis
  after poliomyelitis M89.60
    carpus M89.64-●
    clavicle M89.61-●
    femur M89.65-●
    fibula M89.66-●
    finger M89.64-●
    humerus M89.62-●
    ilium M89.659
    ischium M89.659
    metacarpus M89.64-●
    metatarsus M89.67-●
    multiple sites M89.69
    neck M89.68
    radius M89.63-●
    rib M89.68
    scapula M89.61-●
    skull M89.68
    tarsus M89.67-●
    tibia M89.66-●
    toe M89.67-●
    ulna M89.63-●
    vertebra M89.68
  in (due to)
    renal osteodystrophy N25.0
    specified diseases classified elsewhere —
      see subcategory M90.8
Osteopenia M85.8-●
  borderline M85.8-●
Osteoperiostitis —*see* Osteomyelitis, specified
  type NEC
Osteopetrosis (familial) Q78.2
Osteophyte M25.70
  ankle M25.77-●
  elbow M25.72-●
  foot joint M25.77-●
  hand joint M25.74-●
  hip M25.75-●
  knee M25.76-●
  shoulder M25.71-●
  spine M25.78
  vertebrae M25.78
  wrist M25.73-●
Osteopoikilosis Q78.8

Osteoporosis (female) (male) M81.0
  with current pathological fracture M80.00
  age-related M81.0
    with current pathologic fracture M80.00
      carpus M80.04-●
      clavicle M80.01-●
      fibula M80.06-●
      finger M80.04-●
      humerus M80.02-●
      ilium M80.05-●
      ischium M80.05-●
      metacarpus M80.04-●
      metatarsus M80.07-●
      pelvis M80.05-●
      radius M80.03-●
      scapula M80.01-●
      tarsus M80.07-●
      tibia M80.06-●
      toe M80.07-●
      ulna M80.03-●
      vertebra M80.08
  disuse M81.8
    with current pathological fracture M80.80
      carpus M80.84-●
      clavicle M80.81-●
      fibula M80.86-●
      finger M80.84-●
      humerus M80.82-●
      ilium M80.85-●
      ischium M80.85-●
      metacarpus M80.84-●
      metatarsus M80.87-●
      pelvis M80.85-●
      radius M80.83-●
      scapula M80.81-●
      tarsus M80.87-●
      tibia M80.86-●
      toe M80.87-●
      ulna M80.83-●
      vertebra M80.88
  drug-induced —*see* Osteoporosis, specified
    type NEC
  idiopathic —*see* Osteoporosis, specified type
    NEC
  involutional —*see* Osteoporosis, age-related
  Lequesne M81.6
  localized M81.6
  postmenopausal M81.0
    with pathological fracture M80.00
      carpus M80.04-●
      clavicle M80.01-●
      fibula M80.06-●
      finger M80.04-●
      humerus M80.02-●
      ilium M80.05-●
      ischium M80.05-●
      metacarpus M80.04-●
      metatarsus M80.07-●
      pelvis M80.05-●
      radius M80.03-●
      scapula M80.01-●
      tarsus M80.07-●
      tibia M80.06-●
      toe M80.07-●
      ulna M80.03-●
      vertebra M80.08
  postoophorectomy —*see* Osteoporosis,
    specified type NEC
  postsurgical malabsorption —*see*
    Osteoporosis, specified type NEC
  post-traumatic —*see* Osteoporosis, specified
    type NEC
  senile —*see* Osteoporosis, age-related
  specified type NEC M81.8
    with pathological fracture M80.80
      carpus M80.84-●
      clavicle M80.81-●
      fibula M80.86-●
      finger M80.84-●
      humerus M80.82-●
      ilium M80.85-●

Osteoporosis *(Continued)*
  specified type NEC *(Continued)*
    with pathological fracture *(Continued)*
      ischium M80.85-●
      metacarpus M80.84-●
      metatarsus M80.87-●
      pelvis M80.85-●
      radius M80.83-●
      scapula M80.81-●
      tarsus M80.87-●
      tibia M80.86-●
      toe M80.87-●
      ulna M80.83-●
      vertebra M80.88
Osteopsathyrosis (idiopathica) Q78.0
Osteoradionecrosis, jaw (acute) (chronic)
  (lower) (suppurative) (upper)
  M27.2
Osteosarcoma (any form) —*see* Neoplasm,
  bone, malignant
Osteosclerosis Q78.2
  acquired M85.8-●
  congenita Q77.4
  fragilitas (generalisata) Q78.2
  myelofibrosis D75.81
Osteosclerotic anemia D64.89
Osteosis
  cutis L94.2
  renal fibrocystic N25.0
Österreicher-Turner syndrome Q87.2
Ostium
  atrioventriculare commune Q21.2
  primum (arteriosum) (defect) (persistent)
    Q21.2
  secundum (arteriosum) (defect) (patent)
    (persistent) Q21.1
Ostrum-Furst syndrome Q75.8
Otalgia —*see* subcategory H92.0
Otitis (acute) H66.90
  with effusion —*see also* Otitis, media,
    nonsuppurative
    purulent —*see* Otitis, media, suppurative
  adhesive —*see* subcategory H74.1
  chronic —*see also* Otitis, media, chronic
    with effusion —*see also* Otitis, media,
      nonsuppurative, chronic
  externa H60.9-●
    abscess —*see* Abscess, ear, external
    acute (noninfective) H60.50-●
      actinic H60.51-●
      chemical H60.52-●
      contact H60.53-●
      eczematoid H60.54-●
      infective —*see* Otitis, externa, infective
      reactive H60.55-●
      specified NEC H60.59-●
    cellulitis —*see* Cellulitis, ear
    chronic H60.6-●
    diffuse —*see* Otitis, externa, infective,
      diffuse
    hemorrhagic —*see* Otitis, externa, infective,
      hemorrhagic
    in (due to)
      aspergillosis B44.89
      candidiasis B37.84
      erysipelas A46 *[H62.40]*
      herpes (simplex) virus infection B00.1
        zoster B02.8
      impetigo L01.00 *[H62.40]*
      infectious disease NEC B99 *[H62.4-●]*
      mycosis NEC B36.9 *[H62.40]*
      parasitic disease NEC B89 *[H62.40]*
      viral disease NEC B34.9 *[H62.40]*
      zoster B02.8
    infective NEC H60.39-●
      abscess —*see* Abscess, ear, external
      cellulitis —*see* Cellulitis, ear
      diffuse H60.31-●
      hemorrhagic H60.32-●
      swimmer's ear —*see* Swimmer's, ear
    malignant H60.2-●

Otitis *(Continued)*
  externa *(Continued)*
    mycotic NEC B36.9 *[H62.40]*
      in
        aspergillosis B44.89
        candidiasis B37.84
        moniliasis B37.84
    necrotizing —*see* Otitis, externa, malignant
    Pseudomonas aeruginosa —*see* Otitis, externa, malignant
    reactive —*see* Otitis, externa, acute, reactive
    specified NEC —*see* subcategory H60.8
    tropical NEC B36.9 *[H62.40]*
      in
        aspergillosis B44.89
        candidiasis B37.84
        moniliasis B37.84
  insidiosa —*see* Otosclerosis
  interna —*see* subcategory H83.0
  media (hemorrhagic) (staphylococcal) (streptococcal) H66.9-●
    with effusion (nonpurulent) —*see* Otitis, media, nonsuppurative
    acute, subacute H66.90
      allergic —*see* Otitis, media, nonsuppurative, acute, allergic
      exudative —*see* Otitis, media, suppurative, acute
      mucoid —*see* Otitis, media, nonsuppurative, acute
      necrotizing —*see also* Otitis, media, suppurative, acute
        in
          measles B05.3
          scarlet fever A38.0
      nonsuppurative NEC —*see* Otitis, media, nonsuppurative, acute
      purulent —*see* Otitis, media, suppurative, acute
      sanguinous —*see* Otitis, media, nonsuppurative, acute
      secretory —*see* Otitis, media, nonsuppurative, acute, serous
      seromucinous —*see* Otitis, media, nonsuppurative, acute
      serous —*see* Otitis, media, nonsuppurative, acute, serous
      suppurative —*see* Otitis, media, suppurative, acute
    allergic —*see* Otitis, media, nonsuppurative
    catarrhal —*see* Otitis, media, nonsuppurative
    chronic H66.90
      with effusion (nonpurulent) —*see* Otitis, media, nonsuppurative, chronic
      allergic —*see* Otitis, media, nonsuppurative, chronic, allergic
      benign suppurative —*see* Otitis, media, suppurative, chronic, tubotympanic
      catarrhal —*see* Otitis, media, nonsuppurative, chronic, serous
      exudative —*see* Otitis, media, suppurative, chronic
      mucinous —*see* Otitis, media, nonsuppurative, chronic, mucoid
      mucoid —*see* Otitis, media, nonsuppurative, chronic, mucoid
      nonsuppurative NEC —*see* Otitis, media, nonsuppurative, chronic
      purulent —*see* Otitis, media, suppurative, chronic
      secretory —*see* Otitis, media, nonsuppurative, chronic, mucoid
      seromucinous —*see* Otitis, media, nonsuppurative, chronic
      serous —*see* Otitis, media, nonsuppurative, chronic, serous
      suppurative —*see* Otitis, media, suppurative, chronic

Otitis *(Continued)*
  media *(Continued)*
    chronic *(Continued)*
      transudative —*see* Otitis, media, nonsuppurative, chronic, mucoid
    exudative —*see* Otitis, media, nonsuppurative
    in (due to) (with)
      influenza —*see* Influenza, with, otitis media
      measles B05.3
      scarlet fever A38.0
      tuberculosis A18.6
      viral disease NEC B34.- ● *[H67.-●]*
    mucoid —*see* Otitis, media, nonsuppurative
    nonsuppurative H65.9-●
      acute or subacute NEC H65.19-●
        allergic H65.11-●
          recurrent H65.11-●
        recurrent H65.19-●
        secretory —*see* Otitis, media, nonsuppurative, serous
        serous H65.0-●
          recurrent H65.0-●
      chronic H65.49-●
        allergic H65.41-●
        mucoid H65.3-●
        serous H65.2-●
    postmeasles B05.3
    purulent —*see* Otitis, media, suppurative
    secretory —*see* Otitis, media, nonsuppurative
    seromucinous —*see* Otitis, media, nonsuppurative
    serous —*see* Otitis, media, nonsuppurative
    suppurative H66.4-●
      acute H66.00-●
        with rupture of ear drum H66.01-●
        recurrent H66.00-●
          with rupture of ear drum H66.01-●
      chronic —*see also* subcategory H66.3
        atticoantral H66.2-●
        benign —*see* Otitis, media, suppurative, chronic, tubotympanic
        tubotympanic H66.1-●
    transudative —*see* Otitis, media, nonsuppurative
    tuberculous A18.6
Otocephaly Q18.2
Otolith syndrome —*see* subcategory H81.8
Otomycosis (diffuse) NEC B36.9 *[H62.40]*
  in
    aspergillosis B44.89
    candidiasis B37.84
    moniliasis B37.84
Otoporosis —*see* Otosclerosis
Otorrhagia (nontraumatic) H92.2-●
  traumatic - code by Type of injury
Otorrhea H92.1-●
  cerebrospinal G96.0
Otosclerosis (general) H80.9-●
  cochlear (endosteal) H80.2-●
  involving
    otic capsule —*see* Otosclerosis, cochlear
    oval window
      nonobliterative H80.0-●
      obliterative H80.1-●
    round window —*see* Otosclerosis, cochlear
  nonobliterative —*see* Otosclerosis, involving, oval window, nonobliterative
  obliterative —*see* Otosclerosis, involving, oval window, obliterative
  specified NEC H80.8-●
Otospongiosis —*see* Otosclerosis
Otto's disease or pelvis M24.7
Outcome of delivery Z37.9
  multiple births Z37.9
    all liveborn Z37.50
      quadruplets Z37.52
      quintuplets Z37.53

Outcome of delivery *(Continued)*
  multiple births *(Continued)*
    all liveborn *(Continued)*
      sextuplets Z37.54
      specified number NEC Z37.59
      triplets Z37.51
    all stillborn Z37.7
    some liveborn Z37.60
      quadruplets Z37.62
      quintuplets Z37.63
      sextuplets Z37.64
      specified number NEC Z37.69
      triplets Z37.61
  single NEC Z37.9
    liveborn Z37.0
    stillborn Z37.1
  twins NEC Z37.9
    both liveborn Z37.2
    both stillborn Z37.4
    one liveborn, one stillborn Z37.3
Outlet —*see* condition
Ovalocytosis (congenital) (hereditary) —*see* Elliptocytosis
Ovarian —*see* Condition
Ovariocele N83.4-●
Ovaritis (cystic) —*see* Oophoritis
Ovary, ovarian —*see also* condition
  resistant syndrome E28.39
  vein syndrome N13.8
Overactive —*see also* Hyperfunction
  adrenal cortex NEC E27.0
  bladder N32.81
  hypothalamus E23.3
  thyroid —*see* Hyperthyroidism
Overactivity R46.3
  child —*see* Disorder, attention-deficit hyperactivity
Overbite (deep) (excessive) (horizontal) (vertical) M26.29
Overbreathing —*see* Hyperventilation
Overconscientious personality F60.5
Overdevelopment —*see* Hypertrophy
Overdistension —*see* Distension
Overdose, overdosage (drug) —*see* Table of Drugs and Chemicals, by drug, poisoning
Overeating R63.2
  nonorganic origin F50.89
  psychogenic F50.89
Overexertion (effects) (exhaustion) T73.3
Overexposure (effects) T73.9
  exhaustion T73.2
Overfeeding —*see* Overeating
  newborn P92.4
Overfill, endodontic M27.52
Overgrowth, bone —*see* Hypertrophy, bone
Overhanging of dental restorative material (unrepairable) K08.52
Overheated (places) (effects) —*see* Heat
Overjet (excessive horizontal) M26.23
Overlaid, overlying (suffocation) —*see* Asphyxia, traumatic, due to mechanical threat
Overlap, excessive horizontal (teeth) M26.23
Overlapping toe (acquired) —*see also* Deformity, toe, specified NEC
  congenital (fifth toe) Q66.89
Overload
  circulatory, due to transfusion (blood) (blood components) (TACO) E87.71
  fluid E87.70
    due to transfusion (blood) (blood components) E87.71
    specified NEC E87.79
  iron, due to repeated red blood cell transfusions E83.111
  potassium (K) E87.5
  sodium (Na) E87.0
Overnutrition —*see* Hyperalimentation
Overproduction —*see also* Hypersecretion
  ACTH E27.0
  catecholamine E27.5
  growth hormone E22.0

▶ New   ⇒ Revised   ~~deleted~~ Deleted   ● Use Additional Character(s)

Overprotection, child by parent Z62.1
Overriding
    aorta Q25.49
    finger (acquired) —*see* Deformity, finger
        congenital Q68.1
    toe (acquired) —*see also* Deformity, toe,
        specified NEC
        congenital Q66.89
Overstrained R53.83
    heart —*see* Hypertrophy, cardiac

Overuse, muscle NEC
    M70.8-●
Overweight E66.3
Overworked R53.83
Oviduct —*see* condition
Ovotestis Q56.0
Ovulation (cycle)
    failure or lack of N97.0
    pain N94.0
Ovum —*see* condition

Owren's disease or syndrome (parahemophilia)
    D68.2
Ox heart —*see* Hypertrophy, cardiac
Oxalosis E72.53
Oxaluria E72.53
Oxycephaly, oxycephalic Q75.0
    syphilitic, congenital A50.02
Oxyuriasis B80
Oxyuris vermicularis (infestation) B80
Ozena J31.0

P

Pachyderma, pachydermia L85.9
  larynx (verrucosa) J38.7
Pachydermatocele (congenital) Q82.8
Pachydermoperiostosis —see also
    Osteoarthropathy, hypertrophic, specified
    type NEC
  clubbed nail M89.40 [L62]
Pachygyria Q04.3
Pachymeningitis (adhesive) (basal) (brain)
    (cervical) (chronic) (circumscribed)
    (external) (fibrous) (hemorrhagic)
    (hypertrophic) (internal) (purulent) (spinal)
    (suppurative) —see Meningitis
Pachyonychia (congenital) Q84.5
Pacinian tumor —see Neoplasm, skin, benign
Pad, knuckle or Garrod's M72.1
Paget-Schroetter syndrome I82.890
Paget's disease
  with infiltrating duct carcinoma —see
      Neoplasm, breast, malignant
  bone M88.9
    carpus M88.84-●
    clavicle M88.81-●
    femur M88.85-●
    fibula M88.86-●
    finger M88.84-●
    humerus M88.82-●
    ilium M88.85-●
    in neoplastic disease —see Osteitis,
        deformans, in neoplastic disease
    ischium M88.85-●
    metacarpus M88.84-●
    metatarsus M88.87-●
    multiple sites M88.89
    neck M88.88
    radius M88.83-●
    rib M88.88
    scapula M88.81-●
    skull M88.0
    tarsus M88.87-●
    tibia M88.86-●
    toe M88.87-●
    ulna M88.83-●
    vertebra M88.88
  breast (female) C50.01-●
    male C50.02-●
  extramammary —see also Neoplasm, skin,
      malignant
    anus C21.0
      margin C44.590
      skin C44.590
  intraductal carcinoma —see Neoplasm,
      breast, malignant
  malignant —see Neoplasm, skin, malignant
    breast (female) C50.01-●
      male C50.02-●
    unspecified site (female) C50.01-●
      male C50.02-●
  mammary —see Paget's disease, breast
  nipple —see Paget's disease, breast
  osteitis deformans —see Paget's disease, bone
Pain(s) —see also Painful R52
  abdominal R10.9
    colic R10.83
    generalized R10.84
      with acute abdomen R10.0
    lower R10.30
      left quadrant R10.32
      pelvic or perineal R10.2
      periumbilical R10.33
      right quadrant R10.31
    rebound —see Tenderness, abdominal,
        rebound
    severe with abdominal rigidity R10.0
    tenderness —see Tenderness, abdominal
    upper R10.10
      epigastric R10.13
      left quadrant R10.12
      right quadrant R10.11

Pain (Continued)
  acute R52
    due to trauma G89.11
    neoplasm related G89.3
    postprocedural NEC G89.18
    post-thoracotomy G89.12
    specified by site — code to Pain, by site
  adnexa (uteri) R10.2
  anginoid —see Pain, precordial
  anus K62.89
  arm —see Pain, limb, upper
  axillary (axilla) M79.62-●
  back (postural) M54.9
  bladder R39.89
    associated with micturition —see
        Micturition, painful
    chronic R39.82
  bone —see Disorder, bone, specified type
      NEC
  breast N64.4
  broad ligament R10.2
  cancer associated (acute) (chronic) G89.3
  cecum —see Pain, abdominal
  cervicobrachial M53.1
  chest (central) R07.9
    anterior wall R07.89
    atypical R07.89
    ischemic I20.9
    musculoskeletal R07.89
    non-cardiac R07.89
    on breathing R07.1
    pleurodynia R07.81
    precordial R07.2
    wall (anterior) R07.89
  chronic G89.29
    associated with significant psychosocial
        dysfunction G89.4
    due to trauma G89.21
    neoplasm related G89.3
    postoperative NEC G89.28
    postprocedural NEC G89.28
    post-thoracotomy G89.22
    specified NEC G89.29
  coccyx M53.3
  colon —see Pain, abdominal
  coronary —see Angina
  costochondral R07.1
  diaphragm R07.1
  due to cancer G89.3
  due to device, implant or graft —see also
      Complications, by site and type,
      specified NEC T85.848
    arterial graft NEC T82.848
    breast (implant) T85.848
    catheter NEC T85.848
      dialysis (renal) T82.848
        intraperitoneal T85.848
      infusion NEC T82.848
        spinal (epidural) (subdural) T85.840
      urinary (indwelling) T83.84
    electronic (electrode) (pulse generator)
        (stimulator)
      bone T84.84
      cardiac T82.847
      nervous system (brain) (peripheral
          nerve) (spinal) T85.840
      urinary T83.84
    fixation, internal (orthopedic) NEC T84.84
    gastrointestinal (bile duct) (esophagus)
        T85.848
    genital NEC T83.84
    heart NEC T82.847
    infusion NEC T85.848
    joint prosthesis T84.84
    ocular (corneal graft) (orbital implant)
        NEC T85.848
    orthopedic NEC T84.84
    specified NEC T85.848
    urinary NEC T83.84
    vascular NEC T82.848
    ventricular intracranial shunt T85.840

Pain (Continued)
  due to malignancy (primary) (secondary)
      G89.3
  ear —see subcategory H92.0
  epigastric, epigastrium R10.13
  eye —see Pain, ocular
  face, facial R51
    atypical G50.1
  female genital organs NEC N94.89
  finger —see Pain, limb, upper
  flank —see Pain, abdominal
  foot —see Pain, limb, lower
  gallbladder K82.9
  gas (intestinal) R14.1
  gastric —see Pain, abdominal
  generalized NOS R52
  genital organ
    female N94.89
    male N50.89
  groin —see Pain, abdominal, lower
  hand —see Pain, limb, upper
  head —see Headache
  heart —see Pain, precordial
  infra-orbital —see Neuralgia, trigeminal
  intercostal R07.82
  intermenstrual N94.0
  jaw R68.84
  joint M25.50
    ankle M25.57-●
    elbow M25.52-●
    finger M25.54-●
    foot M25.57-●
    hand M25.54-●
    hip M25.55-●
    knee M25.56-●
    shoulder M25.51-●
    toe M25.57-●
    wrist M25.53-●
  kidney N23
  laryngeal R07.0
  leg —see Pain, limb, lower
  limb M79.609
    lower M79.60-●
      foot M79.67-●
      lower leg M79.66-●
      thigh M79.65-●
      toe M79.67-●
    upper M79.60-●
      axilla M79.62-●
      finger M79.64-●
      forearm M79.63-●
      hand M79.64-●
      upper arm M79.62-●
  loin M54.5
  low back M54.5
  lumbar region M54.5
  mandibular R68.84
  mastoid —see subcategory H92.0
  maxilla R68.84
  menstrual —see also Dysmenorrhea N94.6
  metacarpophalangeal (joint) —see Pain, joint,
      hand
  metatarsophalangeal (joint) —see Pain, joint,
      foot
  mouth K13.79
  muscle —see Myalgia
  musculoskeletal —see also Pain, by site M79.1
  myofascial M79.1
  nasal J34.89
  nasopharynx J39.2
  neck NEC M54.2
  nerve NEC —see Neuralgia
  neuromuscular —see Neuralgia
  nose J34.89
  ocular H57.1-●
  ophthalmic —see Pain, ocular
  orbital region —see Pain, ocular
  ovary N94.89
  over heart —see Pain, precordial
  ovulation N94.0
  pelvic (female) R10.2

▶ New   ⇒ Revised   ~~deleted~~ Deleted   ● Use Additional Character(s)

Pain *(Continued)*
  penis N48.89
  pericardial —*see* Pain, precordial
  perineal, perineum R10.2
  pharynx J39.2
  pleura, pleural, pleuritic R07.81
  postoperative NOS G89.18
  postprocedural NOS G89.18
  post-thoracotomy G89.12
  precordial (region) R07.2
  premenstrual N94.3
  psychogenic (persistent) (any site) F45.41
  radicular (spinal) —*see* Radiculopathy
  rectum K62.89
  respiration R07.1
  retrosternal R07.2
  rheumatoid, muscular —*see* Myalgia
  rib R07.81
  root (spinal) —*see* Radiculopathy
  round ligament (stretch) R10.2
  sacroiliac M53.3
  sciatic —*see* Sciatica
  scrotum N50.82
  seminal vesicle N50.89
  shoulder M25.51-●
  spermatic cord N50.89
  spinal root —*see* Radiculopathy
  spine M54.9
    cervical M54.2
    low back M54.5
      with sciatica M54.4-●
    thoracic M54.6
  stomach —*see* Pain, abdominal
  substernal R07.2
  temporomandibular (joint) M26.62-●
  testis N50.81-●
  thoracic spine M54.6
    with radicular and visceral pain M54.14
  throat R07.0
  tibia —*see* Pain, limb, lower
  toe —*see* Pain, limb, lower
  tongue K14.6
  tooth K08.89
  trigeminal —*see* Neuralgia, trigeminal
  tumor associated G89.3
  ureter N23
  urinary (organ) (system) N23
  uterus NEC N94.89
  vagina R10.2
  vertebrogenic (syndrome) M54.89
  vesical R39.89
    associated with micturition —*see* Micturition, painful
  vulva R10.2
Painful —*see also* Pain
  coitus
    female N94.10
    male N53.12
    psychogenic F52.6
  ejaculation (semen) N53.12
    psychogenic F52.6
  erection —*see* Priapism
  feet syndrome E53.8
  joint replacement (hip) (knee) T84.84
  menstruation —*see* Dysmenorrhea
    psychogenic F45.8
  micturition —*see* Micturition, painful
  respiration R07.1
  scar NEC L90.5
  wire sutures T81.89
Painter's colic —*see* subcategory T56.0
Palate —*see* condition
Palatoplegia K13.79
Palatoschisis —*see* Cleft, palate
Palilalia R48.8
Palliative care Z51.5
Pallor R23.1
  optic disc, temporal —*see* Atrophy, optic
Palmar —*see also* condition
  fascia —*see* condition

Palpable
  cecum K63.89
  kidney N28.89
  ovary N83.8
  prostate N42.9
  spleen —*see* Splenomegaly
Palpitations (heart) R00.2
  psychogenic F45.8
Palsy —*see also* Paralysis G83.9
  atrophic diffuse (progressive) G12.22
  Bell's —*see also* Palsy, facial
    newborn P11.3
  brachial plexus NEC G54.0
    newborn (birth injury) P14.3
  brain —*see* Palsy, cerebral
  bulbar (progressive) (chronic) G12.22
    of childhood (Fazio-Londe) G12.1
    pseudo NEC G12.29
    supranuclear (progressive) G23.1
  cerebral (congenital) G80.9
    ataxic G80.4
    athetoid G80.3
    choreathetoid G80.3
    diplegic G80.8
      spastic G80.1
    dyskinetic G80.3
      athetoid G80.3
      choreathetoid G80.3
      distonic G80.3
    dystonic G80.3
    hemiplegic G80.8
      spastic G80.2
    mixed G80.8
    monoplegic G80.8
      spastic G80.1
    paraplegic G80.8
      spastic G80.1
    quadriplegic G80.8
      spastic G80.0
    spastic G80.1
      diplegic G80.1
      hemiplegic G80.2
      monoplegic G80.1
      quadriplegic G80.0
      specified NEC G80.1
      tetrapelgic G80.0
    specified NEC G80.8
    syphilitic A52.12
      congenital A50.49
    tetraplegic G80.8
      spastic G80.0
  cranial nerve —*see also* Disorder, nerve, cranial
    multiple G52.7
      in
        infectious disease B99 *[G53]*
        neoplastic disease —*see also* Neoplasm D49.9 *[G53]*
        parasitic disease B89 *[G53]*
        sarcoidosis D86.82
  creeping G12.22
  diver's T70.3
  Erb's P14.0
  facial G51.0
    newborn (birth injury) P11.3
  glossopharyngeal G52.1
  Klumpke (-Déjérine) P14.1
  lead —*see* subcategory T56.0
  median nerve (tardy) G56.1-●
  nerve G58.9
    specified NEC G58.8
  peroneal nerve (acute) (tardy) G57.3-●
  progressive supranuclear G23.1
  pseudobulbar NEC G12.29
  radial nerve (acute) G56.3-●
  seventh nerve —*see also* Palsy, facial
    newborn P11.3
  shaking —*see* Parkinsonism
  spastic (cerebral) (spinal) G80.1
  ulnar nerve (tardy) G56.2-●
  wasting G12.29

Paludism —*see* Malaria
Panangiitis M30.0
Panaris, panaritium —*see also* Cellulitis, digit
  with lymphangitis —*see* Lymphangitis, acute, digit
Panarteritis nodosa M30.0
  brain or cerebral I67.7
Pancake heart R93.1
  with cor pulmonale (chronic) I27.81
Pancarditis (acute) (chronic) I51.89
  rheumatic I09.89
    active or acute I01.8
Pancoast's syndrome or tumor C34.1-●
Pancolitis, ulcerative (chronic) K51.00
  with
    abscess K51.014
    complication K51.019
    fistula K51.013
    obstruction K51.012
    rectal bleeding K51.011
    specified complication NEC K51.018
Pancreas, pancreatic —*see* condition
Pancreatitis (annular) (apoplectic) (calcareous) (edematous) (hemorrhagic) (malignant) (recurrent) (subacute) (suppurative) K85.90

  with necrosis (uninfected) K85.91
    infected K85.92
  acute (without necrosis or infection) K85.90
    with necrosis (uninfected) K85.91
      infected K85.92
    alcohol induced (without necrosis or infection) K85.20
      with necrosis (uninfected) K85.21
        infected K85.22
    biliary (without necrosis or infection) K85.10
      with necrosis (uninfected) K85.11
        infected K85.12
    drug induced (without necrosis or infection) K85.30
      with necrosis (uninfected) K85.31
        infected K85.32
    gallstone (without necrosis or infection) K85.10
      with necrosis (uninfected) K85.11
        infected K85.12
    idiopathic (without necrosis or infection) K85.00
      with necrosis (uninfected) K85.01
        infected K85.02
    specified NEC (without necrosis or infection) K85.80
      with necrosis (uninfected) K85.81
        infected K85.82
  chronic (infectious) K86.1
    alcohol-induced K86.0
    recurrent K86.1
    relapsing K86.1
  cystic (chronic) K86.1
  cytomegaloviral B25.2
  fibrous (chronic) K86.1
  gallstone (without necrosis or infection) K85.10
    with necrosis (uninfected) K85.11
      infected K85.12
  gangrenous —*see* Pancreatitis, acute
  interstitial (chronic) K86.1
    acute —*see also* Pancreatitis, acute K85.80
  mumps B26.3
  recurrent (chronic) K86.1
  relapsing, chronic K86.1
  syphilitic A52.74
Pancreatoblastoma —*see* Neoplasm, pancreas, malignant
Pancreolithiasis K86.89
Pancytolysis D75.89

Pancytopenia (acquired) D61.818
  with
    malformations D61.09
    myelodysplastic syndrome —see
      Syndrome, myelodysplastic
  antineoplastic chemotherapy induced
    D61.810
  congenital D61.09
  drug-induced NEC D61.811
▶PANDAS (pediatric autoimmune
    neuropsychiatric disorders associated with
    streptococcal infections syndrome) D89.89
Panencephalitis, subacute, sclerosing
  A81.1
Panhematopenia D61.9
  congenital D61.09
  constitutional D61.09
  splenic, primary D73.1
Panhemocytopenia D61.9
  congenital D61.09
  constitutional D61.09
Panhypogonadism E29.1
Panhypopituitarism E23.0
  prepubertal E23.0
Panic (attack) (state) F41.0
  reaction to exceptional stress (transient) F43.0
Panmyelopathy, familial, constitutional D61.09
Panmyelophthisis D61.82
  congenital D61.09
Panmyelosis (acute) (with myelofibrosis)
  C94.4-●
Panner's disease —see Osteochondrosis,
  juvenile, humerus
Panneuritis endemica E51.11
Panniculitis (nodular) (nonsuppurative) M79.3
  back M54.00
    cervical region M54.02
    cervicothoracic region M54.03
    lumbar region M54.06
    lumbosacral region M54.07
    multiple sites M54.09
    occipito-atlanto-axial region M54.01
    sacrococcygeal region M54.08
    thoracic region M54.04
    thoracolumbar region M54.05
  lupus L93.2
  mesenteric K65.4
  neck M54.02
    cervicothoracic region M54.03
    occipito-atlanto-axial region M54.01
  relapsing M35.6
Panniculus adiposus (abdominal) E65
Pannus (allergic) (cornea) (degenerativus)
  (keratic) H16.42-●
  abdominal (symptomatic) E65
  trachomatosus, trachomatous (active) A71.1
Panophthalmitis H44.01-●
Pansinusitis (chronic) (hyperplastic)
  (nonpurulent) (purulent) J32.4
  acute J01.40
    recurrent J01.41
  tuberculous A15.8
Panuveitis (sympathetic) H44.11-●
Panvalvular disease I08.9
  specified NEC I08.8
PAPA (pyogenic arthritis, pyoderma
  gangrenosum, and acne syndrome) M04.8
Papanicolaou smear, cervix Z12.4
  as part of routine gynecological examination
    Z01.419
    with abnormal findings Z01.411
  for suspected neoplasm Z12.4
  nonspecific abnormal finding R87.619
  routine Z01.419
    with abnormal findings Z01.411
Papilledema (choked disc) H47.10
  associated with
    decreased ocular pressure H47.12
    increased intracranial pressure H47.11
    retinal disorder H47.13
  Foster-Kennedy syndrome H47.14-●

Papillitis H46.00
  anus K62.89
  chronic lingual K14.4
  necrotizing, kidney N17.2
  optic H46.0-●
  rectum K62.89
  renal, necrotizing N17.2
  tongue K14.0
Papilloma —see also Neoplasm, benign,
  by site
  acuminatum (female) (male) (anogenital)
    A63.0
  basal cell L82.1
    inflamed L82.0
  benign pinta (primary) A67.0
  bladder (urinary) (transitional cell) D41.4
  choroid plexus (lateral ventricle) (third
    ventricle) D33.0
    anaplastic C71.5
    fourth ventricle D33.1
    malignant C71.5
  renal pelvis (transitional cell) D41.1-●
    benign D30.1-●
  Schneiderian
    specified site —see Neoplasm, benign, by
      site
    unspecified site D14.0
  serous surface
    borderline malignancy
      specified site —see Neoplasm, uncertain
        behavior, by site
      unspecified site D39.10
    specified site —see Neoplasm, benign, by
      site
    unspecified site D27.9
  transitional (cell)
    bladder (urinary) D41.4
    inverted type —see Neoplasm, uncertain
      behavior, by site
    renal pelvis D41.1-●
    ureter D41.2-●
  ureter (transitional cell) D41.2-●
    benign D30.2-●
  urothelial —see Neoplasm, uncertain
    behavior, by site
  villous —see Neoplasm, uncertain behavior,
    by site
    adenocarcinoma in —see Neoplasm,
      malignant, by site
    in situ —see Neoplasm, in situ
  yaws, plantar or palmar A66.1
Papillomata, multiple, of yaws A66.1
Papillomatosis —see also Neoplasm, benign,
  by site
  confluent and reticulated L83
  cystic, breast —see Mastopathy, cystic
  ductal, breast —see Mastopathy, cystic
  intraductal (diffuse) —see Neoplasm, benign,
    by site
  subareolar duct D24-●
Papillomavirus, as cause of disease classified
  elsewhere B97.7
Papillon-Léage and Psaume syndrome
  Q87.0
Papule(s) R23.8
  carate (primary) A67.0
  fibrous, of nose D22.39
  Gottron's L94.4
  pinta (primary) A67.0
Papulosis
  lymphomatoid C86.6
  malignant I77.89
Papyraceous fetus O31.0-●
Para-albuminemia E88.09
Paracephalus Q89.7
Parachute mitral valve Q23.2
Paracoccidioidomycosis B41.9
  disseminated B41.7
  generalized B41.7
  mucocutaneous-lymphangitic B41.8
  pulmonary B41.0

Paracoccidioidomycosis (Continued)
  specified NEC B41.8
  visceral B41.8
Paradentosis K05.4
Paraffinoma T88.8
Paraganglioma D44.7
  adrenal D35.0-●
    malignant C74.1-●
  aortic body D44.7
    malignant C75.5
  carotid body D44.6
    malignant C75.4
  chromaffin —see also Neoplasm, benign, by
    site
    malignant —see Neoplasm, malignant, by
      site
  extra-adrenal D44.7
    malignant C75.5
      specified site —see Neoplasm,
        malignant, by site
      unspecified site C75.5
    specified site —see Neoplasm, uncertain
      behavior, by site
    unspecified site D44.7
  gangliocytic D13.2
    specified site —see Neoplasm, benign, by
      site
    unspecified site D13.2
  glomus jugulare D44.7
    malignant C75.5
  jugular D44.7
  malignant C75.5
    specified site —see Neoplasm, malignant,
      by site
    unspecified site C75.5
  nonchromaffin D44.7
    malignant C75.5
      specified site —see Neoplasm,
        malignant, by site
      unspecified site C75.5
    specified site —see Neoplasm, uncertain
      behavior, by site
    unspecified site D44.7
  parasympathetic D44.7
    specified site —see Neoplasm, uncertain
      behavior, by site
    unspecified site D44.7
  specified site —see Neoplasm, uncertain
    behavior, by site
  sympathetic D44.7
    specified site —see Neoplasm, uncertain
      behavior, by site
    unspecified site D44.7
  unspecified site D44.7
Parageusia R43.2
  psychogenic F45.8
Paragonimiasis B66.4
▶Paragranuloma, Hodgkin —see Lymphoma,
  Hodgkin, specified NEC
Parahemophilia —see also Defect, coagulation
  D68.2
Parakeratosis R23.4
  variegata L41.0
Paralysis, paralytic (complete) (incomplete)
  G83.9
  with
    syphilis A52.17
  abducens, abducent (nerve) —see Strabismus,
    paralytic, sixth nerve
  abductor, lower extremity G57.9-●
  accessory nerve G52.8
  accommodation —see also Paresis, of
    accommodation
    hysterical F44.89
  acoustic nerve (except Deafness) —see
    subcategory H93.3
  agitans —see also Parkinsonism G20
    arteriosclerotic G21.4
  alternating (oculomotor) G83.89
  amyotrophic G12.21

▶ New   ⟹ Revised   ~~deleted~~ Deleted   ● Use Additional Character(s)

Paralysis, paralytic *(Continued)*
ankle G57.9-●
anus (sphincter) K62.89
arm —*see* Monoplegia, upper limb
ascending (spinal), acute G61.0
association G12.29
asthenic bulbar G70.00
   with exacerbation (acute) G70.01
   in crisis G70.01
ataxic (hereditary) G11.9
   general (syphilitic) A52.17
atrophic G58.9
   infantile, acute —*see* Poliomyelitis, paralytic
   progressive G12.22
   spinal (acute) —*see* Poliomyelitis, paralytic
axillary G54.0
Babinski-Nageotte's G83.89
Bell's G51.0
   newborn P11.3
Benedikt's G46.3
birth injury P14.9
   spinal cord P11.5
bladder (neurogenic) (sphincter)
   N31.2
bowel, colon or intestine K56.0
brachial plexus G54.0
   birth injury P14.3
   newborn (birth injury) P14.3
brain G83.9
   diplegia G83.0
   triplegia G83.89
bronchial J98.09
Brown-Séquard G83.81
bulbar (chronic) (progressive) G12.22
   infantile —*see* Poliomyelitis, paralytic
   poliomyelitic —*see* Poliomyelitis, paralytic
   pseudo G12.29
bulbospinal G70.00
   with exacerbation (acute) G70.01
   in crisis G70.01
cardiac —*see also* Failure, heart I50.9
cerebrocerebellar, diplegic G80.1
cervical
   plexus G54.2
   sympathetic G90.09
Céstan-Chenais G46.3
Charcot-Marie-Tooth type G60.0
Clark's G80.9
colon K56.0
compressed air T70.3
compression
   arm G56.9-●
   leg G57.9-●
   lower extremity G57.9-●
   upper extremity G56.9-●
congenital (cerebral) —*see* Palsy, cerebral
conjugate movement (gaze) (of eye) H51.0
   cortical (nuclear) (supranuclear) H51.0
cordis —*see* Failure, heart
cranial or cerebral nerve G52.9
creeping G12.22
crossed leg G83.89
crutch —*see* Injury, brachial plexus
deglutition R13.0
   hysterical F44.4
dementia A52.17
descending (spinal) NEC G12.29
diaphragm (flaccid) J98.6
   due to accidental dissection of phrenic
     nerve during procedure —*see*
     Puncture, accidental complicating
     surgery
digestive organs NEC K59.8
diplegic —*see* Diplegia
divergence (nuclear) H51.8
diver's T70.3
Duchenne's
   birth injury P14.0
   due to or associated with
     motor neuron disease G12.22
     muscular dystrophy G71.0

Paralysis, paralytic *(Continued)*
due to intracranial or spinal birth injury —*see*
   Palsy, cerebral
embolic (current episode) I63.4-●
Erb (-Duchenne) (birth) (newborn) P14.0
Erb's syphilitic spastic spinal A52.17
esophagus K22.8
eye muscle (extrinsic) H49.9
   intrinsic —*see also* Paresis, of
     accommodation
facial (nerve) G51.0
   birth injury P11.3
   congenital P11.3
   following operation NEC —*see* Puncture,
     accidental complicating surgery
   newborn (birth injury) P11.3
familial (recurrent) (periodic) G72.3
   spastic G11.4
fauces J39.2
finger G56.9-●
gait R26.1
gastric nerve (nondiabetic) G52.2
gaze, conjugate H51.0
general (progressive) (syphilitic) A52.17
   juvenile A50.45
glottis J38.00
   bilateral J38.02
   unilateral J38.01
gluteal G54.1
Gubler (-Millard) G46.3
hand —*see* Monoplegia, upper limb
heart —*see* Arrest, cardiac
hemiplegic —*see* Hemiplegia
hyperkalemic periodic (familial) G72.3
hypoglossal (nerve) G52.3
hypokalemic periodic G72.3
hysterical F44.4
ileus K56.0
infantile —*see also* Poliomyelitis, paralytic
   A80.30
   bulbar —*see* Poliomyelitis, paralytic
   cerebral —*see* Palsy, cerebral
   spastic —*see* Palsy, cerebral, spastic
infective —*see* Poliomyelitis, paralytic
inferior nuclear G83.9
internuclear —*see* Ophthalmoplegia,
   internuclear
intestine K56.0
iris H57.09
   due to diphtheria (toxin) A36.89
ischemic, Volkmann's (complicating trauma)
   T79.6
Jackson's G83.89
jake —*see* Poisoning, food, noxious, plant
Jamaica ginger (jake) G62.2
juvenile general A50.45
Klumpke (-Déjérine) (birth) (newborn) P14.1
labioglossal (laryngeal) (pharyngeal) G12.29
Landry's G61.0
laryngeal nerve (recurrent) (superior)
   (unilateral) J38.00
   bilateral J38.02
   unilateral J38.01
larynx J38.00
   bilateral J38.02
   due to diphtheria (toxin) A36.2
   unilateral J38.01
⇒lateral G12.23
lead —*see* subcategory T56.0
left side —*see* Hemiplegia
leg G83.1-●
   both —*see* Paraplegia
   crossed G83.89
   hysterical F44.4
   psychogenic F44.4
   transient or transitory R29.818
     traumatic NEC —*see* Injury, nerve, leg
levator palpebrae superioris —*see*
   Blepharoptosis, paralytic
limb —*see* Monoplegia
lip K13.0

Paralysis, paralytic *(Continued)*
Lissauer's A52.17
lower limb —*see* Monoplegia, lower
   limb
   both —*see* Paraplegia
lung J98.4
median nerve G56.1-●
medullary (tegmental) G83.89
mesencephalic NEC G83.89
   tegmental G83.89
middle alternating G83.89
Millard-Gubler-Foville G46.3
monoplegic —*see* Monoplegia
motor G83.9
muscle, muscular NEC G72.89
   due to nerve lesion G58.9
   eye (extrinsic) H49.9
     intrinsic —*see* Paresis, of
     accommodation
     oblique —*see* Strabismus, paralytic,
      fourth nerve
   iris sphincter H21.9
   ischemic (Volkmann's) (complicating
     trauma) T79.6
   progressive G12.21
   pseudohypertrophic G71.0
musculocutaneous nerve G56.9-●
musculospiral G56.9-●
nerve —*see also* Disorder, nerve
   abducent —*see* Strabismus, paralytic, sixth
     nerve
   accessory G52.8
   auditory (except Deafness) —*see*
     subcategory H93.3
   birth injury P14.9
   cranial or cerebral G52.9
   facial G51.0
     birth injury P11.3
     congenital P11.3
     newborn (birth injury) P11.3
   fourth or trochlear —*see* Strabismus,
     paralytic, fourth nerve
   newborn (birth injury) P14.9
   oculomotor —*see* Strabismus, paralytic,
     third nerve
   phrenic (birth injury) P14.2
   radial G56.3-●
   seventh or facial G51.0
     newborn (birth injury) P11.3
   sixth or abducent —*see* Strabismus,
     paralytic, sixth nerve
   syphilitic A52.15
   third or oculomotor —*see* Strabismus,
     paralytic, third nerve
   trigeminal G50.9
   trochlear —*see* Strabismus, paralytic,
     fourth nerve
   ulnar G56.2-●
normokalemic periodic G72.3
ocular H49.9
   alternating G83.89
oculofacial, congenital (Moebius) Q87.0
oculomotor (external bilateral) (nerve) —*see*
   Strabismus, paralytic, third nerve
palate (soft) K13.79
paratrigeminal G50.9
periodic (familial) (hyperkalemic)
   (hypokalemic) (myotonic)
   (normokalemic) (potassium sensitive)
   (secondary) G72.3
peripheral autonomic nervous system —*see*
   Neuropathy, peripheral, autonomic
peroneal (nerve) G57.3-●
pharynx J39.2
phrenic nerve G56.8-●
plantar nerve(s) G57.6-●
pneumogastric nerve G52.2
poliomyelitis (current) —*see* Poliomyelitis,
   paralytic
popliteal nerve G57.3-●
postepileptic transitory G83.84

Paralysis, paralytic *(Continued)*
  progressive (atrophic) (bulbar) (spinal) G12.22
    general A52.17
    infantile acute —*see* Poliomyelitis, paralytic
    supranuclear G23.1
  pseudobulbar G12.29
  pseudohypertrophic (muscle) G71.0
  psychogenic F44.4
  quadriceps G57.9-●
  quadriplegic —*see* Tetraplegia
  radial nerve G56.3-●
  rectus muscle (eye) H49.9
  recurrent isolated sleep G47.53
  respiratory (muscle) (system) (tract) R06.81
    center NEC G93.89
    congenital P28.89
    newborn P28.89
  right side —*see* Hemiplegia
  saturnine —*see* subcategory T56.0
  sciatic nerve G57.0-●
  senile G83.9
  shaking —*see* Parkinsonism
  shoulder G56.9-●
  sleep, recurrent isolated G47.53
  spastic G83.9
    cerebral —*see* Palsy, cerebral, spastic
    congenital (cerebral) —*see* Palsy, cerebral, spastic
    familial G11.4
    hereditary G11.4
    quadriplegic G80.0
    syphilitic (spinal) A52.17
  sphincter, bladder —*see* Paralysis, bladder
  spinal (cord) G83.9
    accessory nerve G52.8
    acute —*see* Poliomyelitis, paralytic
    ascending acute G61.0
    atrophic (acute) —*see also* Poliomyelitis, paralytic
      spastic, syphilitic A52.17
    congenital NEC —*see* Palsy, cerebral
    hereditary G95.89
    infantile —*see* Poliomyelitis, paralytic
    progressive G12.21
    sequelae NEC G83.89
  sternomastoid G52.8
  stomach K31.84
    diabetic —*see* Diabetes, by type, with gastroparesis
    nerve G52.2
      diabetic —*see* Diabetes, by type, with gastroparesis
  stroke —*see* Infarct, brain
  subcapsularis G56.8-●
  supranuclear (progressive) G23.1
  sympathetic G90.8
    cervical G90.09
    nervous system —*see* Neuropathy, peripheral, autonomic
  syndrome G83.9
    specified NEC G83.89
  syphilitic spastic spinal (Erb's) A52.17
  thigh G57.9-●
  throat J39.2
    diphtheritic A36.0
    muscle J39.2
  thrombotic (current episode) I63.3-●
  thumb G56.9-●
  tick —*see* Toxicity, venom, arthropod, specified NEC
  Todd's (postepileptic transitory paralysis) G83.84
  toe G57.6-●
  tongue K14.8
  transient R29.5
    arm or leg NEC R29.818
    traumatic NEC —*see* Injury, nerve
  trapezius G52.8
  traumatic, transient NEC —*see* Injury, nerve

Paralysis, paralytic *(Continued)*
  trembling —*see* Parkinsonism
  triceps brachii G56.9-●
  trigeminal nerve G50.9
  trochlear (nerve) —*see* Strabismus, paralytic, fourth nerve
  ulnar nerve G56.2-●
  upper limb —*see* Monoplegia, upper limb
  uremic N18.9 *[G99.8]*
  uveoparotitic D86.89
  uvula K13.79
    postdiphtheritic A36.0
  vagus nerve G52.2
  vasomotor NEC G90.8
  velum palati K13.79
  vesical —*see* Paralysis, bladder
  vestibular nerve (except Vertigo) —*see* subcategory H93.3
  vocal cords J38.00
    bilateral J38.02
    unilateral J38.01
  Volkmann's (complicating trauma) T79.6
  wasting G12.29
  Weber's G46.3
  wrist G56.9-●
Paramedial urethrovesical orifice Q64.79
Paramenia N92.6
Parametritis —*see also* Disease, pelvis, inflammatory N73.2
  acute N73.0
  complicating abortion —*see* Abortion, by type, complicated by, parametritis
Parametrium, parametric —*see* condition
Paramnesia —*see* Amnesia
Paramolar K00.1
▶Paramyloidosis E85.89
Paramyoclonus multiplex G25.3
Paramyotonia (congenita) G71.19
Parangi —*see* Yaws
Paranoia (querulans) F22
  senile F03
Paranoid
  dementia (senile) F03
    praecox —*see* Schizophrenia
  personality F60.0
  psychosis (climacteric) (involutional) (menopausal) F22
    psychogenic (acute) F23
    senile F03
  reaction (acute) F23
    chronic F22
  schizophrenia F20.0
  state (climacteric) (involutional) (menopausal) (simple) F22
    senile F03
  tendencies F60.0
  traits F60.0
  trends F60.0
  type, psychopathic personality F60.0
Paraparesis —*see* Paraplegia
Paraphasia R47.02
Paraphilia F65.9
Paraphimosis (congenital) N47.2
  chancroidal A57
Paraphrenia, paraphrenic (late) F22
  schizophrenia F20.0
Paraplegia (lower) G82.20
  ataxic —*see* Degeneration, combined, spinal cord
  complete G82.21
  congenital (cerebral) G80.8
    spastic G80.1
  familial spastic G11.4
  functional (hysterical) F44.4
  hereditary, spastic G11.4
  hysterical F44.4
  incomplete G82.22
  Pott's A18.01
  psychogenic F44.4

Paraplegia *(Continued)*
  spastic
    Erb's spinal, syphilitic A52.17
    hereditary G11.4
    tropical G04.1
  syphilitic (spastic) A52.17
  tropical spastic G04.1
Parapoxvirus B08.60
  specified NEC B08.69
Paraproteinemia D89.2
  benign (familial) D89.2
  monoclonal D47.2
  secondary to malignant disease D47.2
Parapsoriasis L41.9
  en plaques L41.4
  guttata L41.1
  large plaque L41.4
  retiform, retiformis L41.5
  small plaque L41.3
  specified NEC L41.8
  varioliformis (acuta) L41.0
Parasitic —*see also* condition
  disease NEC B89
  stomatitis B37.0
  sycosis (beard) (scalp) B35.0
  twin Q89.4
Parasitism B89
  intestinal B82.9
  skin B88.9
  specified —*see* Infestation
Parasitophobia F40.218
Parasomnia G47.50
  due to
    alcohol
      abuse F10.182
      dependence F10.282
      use F10.982
    amphetamines
      abuse F15.182
      dependence F15.282
      use F15.982
    caffeine
      abuse F15.182
      dependence F15.282
      use F15.982
    cocaine
      abuse F14.182
      dependence F14.282
      use F14.982
    drug NEC
      abuse F19.182
      dependence F19.282
      use F19.982
    opioid
      abuse F11.182
      dependence F11.282
      use F11.982
    psychoactive substance NEC
      abuse F19.182
      dependence F19.282
      use F19.982
    sedative, hypnotic, or anxiolytic
      abuse F13.182
      dependence F13.282
      use F13.982
    stimulant NEC
      abuse F15.182
      dependence F15.282
      use F15.982
  in conditions classified elsewhere G47.54
  nonorganic origin F51.8
  organic G47.50
  specified NEC G47.59
Paraspadias Q54.9
Paraspasmus facialis G51.8
Parasuicide (attempt)
  history of (personal) Z91.5
    in family Z81.8
Parathyroid gland —*see* condition
Parathyroid tetany E20.9
Paratrachoma A74.0

▶ New   ⇒ Revised   ~~deleted~~ Deleted   ● Use Additional Character(s)

Penicillosis B48.4

Penis —see condition

Penitis N48.29

Pentalogy of Fallot Q21.8

Pentasomy X syndrome Q97.1

Pentosuria (essential) E74.8

Percreta placenta O43.23- ●

Peregrinating patient —see Disorder, factitious

Perforation, perforated (nontraumatic) (of)
  accidental during procedure (blood vessel)
    (nerve) (organ) —see Complication,
    accidental puncture or laceration
  antrum —see Sinusitis, maxillary
  appendix K35.2
    with localized peritonitis K35.3
  atrial septum, multiple Q21.1
  attic, ear —see Perforation, tympanum, attic
  bile duct (common) (hepatic) K83.2
    cystic K82.2
  bladder (urinary)
    with or following ectopic or molar
      pregnancy O08.6
    obstetrical trauma O71.5
    traumatic S37.29
      at delivery O71.5
  bowel K63.1
    with or following ectopic or molar
      pregnancy O08.6
    newborn P78.0
    obstetrical trauma O71.5
    traumatic —see Laceration, intestine
  broad ligament N83.8
    with or following ectopic or molar
      pregnancy O08.6
    obstetrical trauma O71.6
  by
    device, implant or graft —see also
      Complications, by site and type,
      mechanical T85.628
      arterial graft NEC —see Complication,
        cardiovascular device, mechanical,
        vascular
      breast (implant) T85.49
      catheter NEC T85.698
        cystostomy T83.090
        dialysis (renal) T82.49
          intraperitoneal T85.691
        infusion NEC T82.594
          spinal (epidural) (subdural) T85.690
        urinary —see also Complications,
          catheter, urinary T83.098
      electronic (electrode) (pulse generator)
        (stimulator)
        bone T84.390
        cardiac T82.199
          electrode T82.190
          pulse generator T82.191
          specified type NEC T82.198
        nervous system —see Complication,
          prosthetic device, mechanical,
          electronic nervous system
          stimulator
        urinary —see Complication,
          genitourinary, device, urinary,
          mechanical
      fixation, internal (orthopedic) NEC —
        see Complication, fixation device,
        mechanical
      gastrointestinal —see Complications,
        prosthetic device, mechanical,
        gastrointestinal device
      genital NEC T83.498
        intrauterine contraceptive device
          T83.39
        penile prosthesis T83.490
      heart NEC —see Complication,
        cardiovascular device,
        mechanical
      joint prosthesis —see Complications,
        joint prosthesis, mechanical,
        specified NEC, by site

Perforation, perforated (Continued)
  by (Continued)
    urinary (Continued)
      ocular NEC —see Complications,
        prosthetic device, mechanical,
        ocular device
      orthopedic NEC —see Complication,
        orthopedic, device, mechanical
      specified NEC T85.628
      urinary NEC —see also Complication,
        genitourinary, device, urinary,
        mechanical
        graft T83.29
      vascular NEC —see Complication,
        cardiovascular device, mechanical
      ventricular intracranial shunt T85.09
    foreign body left accidentally in
      operative wound T81.539
    instrument (any) during a procedure,
      accidental —see Puncture, accidental
      complicating surgery
  cecum K35.2
    with localized peritonitis K35.3
  cervix (uteri) N88.8
    with or following ectopic or molar
      pregnancy O08.6
    obstetrical trauma O71.3
  colon K63.1
    newborn P78.0
    obstetrical trauma O71.5
    traumatic —see Laceration, intestine, large
  common duct (bile) K83.2
  cornea (due to ulceration) —see Ulcer,
    cornea, perforated
  cystic duct K82.2
  diverticulum (intestine) K57.80
    with bleeding K57.81
    large intestine K57.20
      with
        bleeding K57.21
        small intestine K57.40
          with bleeding K57.41
    small intestine K57.00
      with
        bleeding K57.01
        large intestine K57.40
          with bleeding K57.41
  ear drum —see Perforation, tympanum
  esophagus K22.3
  ethmoidal sinus —see Sinusitis, ethmoidal
  frontal sinus —see Sinusitis, frontal
  gallbladder K82.2
  heart valve —see Endocarditis
  ileum K63.1
    newborn P78.0
    obstetrical trauma O71.5
    traumatic —see Laceration, intestine, small
  instrumental, surgical (accidental) (blood
    vessel) (nerve) (organ) —see Puncture,
    accidental complicating surgery
  intestine NEC K63.1
    with ectopic or molar pregnancy O08.6
    newborn P78.0
    obstetrical trauma O71.5
    traumatic —see Laceration, intestine
    ulcerative NEC K63.1
      newborn P78.0
  jejunum, jejunal K63.1
    obstetrical trauma O71.5
    traumatic —see Laceration, intestine,
      small
    ulcer —see Ulcer, gastrojejunal, with
      perforation
  joint prosthesis —see Complications, joint
    prosthesis, mechanical, specified NEC,
    by site
  mastoid (antrum) (cell) —see Disorder,
    mastoid, specified NEC
  maxillary sinus —see Sinusitis, maxillary
  membrana tympani —see Perforation,
    tympanum

Perforation, perforated (Continued)
  nasal
    septum J34.89
      congenital Q30.3
      syphilitic A52.73
    sinus J34.89
      congenital Q30.8
      due to sinusitis —see Sinusitis
  palate —see also Cleft, palate Q35.9
    syphilitic A52.79
  palatine vault —see also Cleft, palate, hard Q35.1
    syphilitic A52.79
    congenital A50.59
  pars flaccida (ear drum) —see Perforation,
    tympanum, attic
  pelvic
    floor S31.030
      with
        ectopic or molar pregnancy O08.6
        penetration into retroperitoneal space
          S31.031
        retained foreign body S31.040
          with penetration into
            retroperitoneal space S31.041
      following ectopic or molar pregnancy
        O08.6
      obstetrical trauma O70.1
    organ S37.99
      adrenal gland S37.818
      bladder —see Perforation, bladder
      fallopian tube S37.599
        bilateral S37.592
        unilateral S37.591
      kidney S37.09- ●
      obstetrical trauma O71.5
      ovary S37.499
        bilateral S37.492
        unilateral S37.491
      prostate S37.828
      specified organ NEC S37.898
      ureter —see Perforation, ureter
      urethra —see Perforation, urethra
      uterus —see Perforation, uterus
  perineum —see Laceration, perineum
  pharynx J39.2
  rectum K63.1
    newborn P78.0
    obstetrical trauma O71.5
    traumatic S36.63
  root canal space due to endodontic treatment
    M27.51
  sigmoid K63.1
    newborn P78.0
    obstetrical trauma O71.5
    traumatic S36.533
  sinus (accessory) (chronic) (nasal) J34.89
  sphenoidal sinus —see Sinusitis, sphenoidal
  surgical (accidental) (by instrument) (blood
    vessel) (nerve) (organ) —see Puncture,
    accidental complicating surgery
  traumatic
    external —see Puncture
    eye —see Puncture, eyeball
    internal organ —see Injury, by site
  tympanum, tympanic (membrane) (persistent
    post-traumatic) (postinflammatory)
    H72.9- ●
    attic H72.1- ●
      multiple —see Perforation, tympanum,
        multiple
      total —see Perforation, tympanum, total
    central H72.0- ●
      multiple —see Perforation, tympanum,
        multiple
      total —see Perforation, tympanum, total
    marginal NEC —see subcategory H72.2
    multiple H72.81- ●
    pars flaccida —see Perforation, tympanum,
      attic
    total H72.82- ●
    traumatic, current episode S09.2- ●

  ▶ New   ⇛ Revised   ~~deleted~~ Deleted   ● Use Additional Character(s)

Perforation, perforated (Continued)
  typhoid, gastrointestinal —see Typhoid
  ulcer —see Ulcer, by site, with perforation
  ureter N28.89
    traumatic S37.19
  urethra N36.8
    with ectopic or molar pregnancy O08.6
    following ectopic or molar pregnancy
        O08.6
    obstetrical trauma O71.5
    traumatic S37.39
      at delivery O71.5
  uterus
    with ectopic or molar pregnancy O08.6
    by intrauterine contraceptive device T83.39
    following ectopic or molar pregnancy
        O08.6
    obstetrical trauma O71.1
    traumatic S37.69
      obstetric O71.1
  uvula K13.79
    syphilitic A52.79
  vagina
    obstetrical trauma O71.4
    other trauma - see Puncture, vagina
Periadenitis mucosa necrotica recurrens K12.0
Periappendicitis (acute) —see Appendicitis
Periarteritis nodosa (disseminated) (infectious)
    (necrotizing) M30.0
Periarthritis (joint) —see also Enthesopathy
  Duplay's M75.0-●
  gonococcal A54.42
  humeroscapularis —see Capsulitis, adhesive
  scapulohumeral —see Capsulitis, adhesive
  shoulder —see Capsulitis, adhesive
  wrist M77.2-●
Periarthrosis (angioneural) —see
    Enthesopathy
Pericapsulitis, adhesive (shoulder) —see
    Capsulitis, adhesive
Pericarditis (with decompensation) (with
    effusion) I31.9
  with rheumatic fever (conditions in I00)
    active —see Pericarditis, rheumatic
    inactive or quiescent I09.2
  acute (hemorrhagic) (nonrheumatic) (Sicca)
      I30.9
    with chorea (acute) (rheumatic)
        (Sydenham's) I02.0
    benign I30.8
    nonspecific I30.0
    rheumatic I01.0
      with chorea (acute) (Sydenham's)
          I02.0
  adhesive or adherent (chronic) (external)
      (internal) I31.0
    acute —see Pericarditis, acute
    rheumatic I09.2
  bacterial (acute) (subacute) (with serous or
      seropurulent effusion) I30.1
  calcareous I31.1
  cholesterol (chronic) I31.8
    acute I30.9
  chronic (nonrheumatic) I31.9
    rheumatic I09.2
  constrictive (chronic) I31.1
  coxsackie B33.23
  fibrinocaseous (tuberculous) A18.84
  fibrinopurulent I30.1
  fibrinous I30.8
  fibrous I31.0
  gonococcal A54.83
  idiopathic I30.0
  in systemic lupus erythematosus M32.12
  infective I30.1
  meningococcal A39.53
  neoplastic (chronic) I31.8
    acute I30.9
  obliterans, obliterating I31.0
  plastic I31.0
  pneumococcal I30.1

Pericarditis (Continued)
  postinfarction I24.1
  purulent I30.1
  rheumatic (active) (acute) (with effusion)
      (with pneumonia) I01.0
    with chorea (acute) (rheumatic)
        (Sydenham's) I02.0
    chronic or inactive (with chorea) I09.2
  rheumatoid —see Rheumatoid, carditis
  septic I30.1
  serofibrinous I30.8
  staphylococcal I30.1
  streptococcal I30.1
  suppurative I30.1
  syphilitic A52.06
  tuberculous A18.84
  uremic N18.9 [I32]
  viral I30.1
Pericardium, pericardial —see condition
Pericellulitis —see Cellulitis
Pericementitis (chronic) (suppurative) —see also
    Periodontitis
  acute K05.20
    generalized —see Peridontitis, aggressive,
        generalized
    localized —see Peridontitis, aggressive,
        localized
Perichondritis
  auricle —see Perichondritis, ear
  bronchus J98.09
  ear (external) H61.00-●
    acute H61.01-●
    chronic H61.02-●
  external auditory canal —see Perichondritis,
      ear
  larynx J38.7
    syphilitic A52.73
    typhoid A01.09
  nose J34.89
  pinna —see Perichondritis, ear
  trachea J39.8
Periclasia K05.4
Pericoronitis —see Periodontitis
Pericystitis N30.90
  with hematuria N30.91
Peridiverticulitis (intestine) K57.92
  cecum —see Diverticulitis, intestine, large
  colon —see Diverticulitis, intestine, large
  duodenum —see Diverticulitis, intestine,
      small
  intestine —see Diverticulitis, intestine
  jejunum —see Diverticulitis, intestine, small
  rectosigmoid —see Diverticulitis, intestine,
      large
  rectum —see Diverticulitis, intestine, large
  sigmoid —see Diverticulitis, intestine, large
Periendocarditis —see Endocarditis
Periepididymitis N45.1
Perifolliculitis L01.02
  abscedens, caput, scalp L66.3
  capitis, abscedens (et suffodiens) L66.3
  superficial pustular L01.02
Perihepatitis K65.8
Perilabyrinthitis (acute) —see subcategory H83.0
Perimeningitis —see Meningitis
Perimetritis —see Endometritis
Perimetrosalpingitis —see Salpingo-oophoritis
Perineocele N81.81
Perinephric, perinephritic —see condition
Perinephritis —see also Infection, kidney
  purulent —see Abscess, kidney
Perineum, perineal —see condition
Perineuritis NEC —see Neuralgia
Periodic —see condition
Periodontitis (chronic) (complex) (compound)
    (local) (simplex) K05.30
  acute K05.20
    generalized K05.229
      moderate K05.222
      severe K05.223
      slight K05.221

Periodontitis (Continued)
  acute (Continued)
    localized K05.219
      moderate K05.212
      severe K05.213
      slight K05.211
  apical K04.5
    acute (pulpal origin) K04.4
  generalized K05.329
    moderate K05.322
    severe K05.323
    slight K05.321
  localized K05.319
    moderate K05.312
    severe K05.313
    slight K05.311
Periodontoclasia K05.4
Periodontosis (juvenile) K05.4
Periods —see also Menstruation
  heavy N92.0
  irregular N92.6
  shortened intervals (irregular) N92.1
Perionychia —see also Cellulitis, digit
  with lymphangitis —see Lymphangitis, acute,
      digit
Perioophoritis —see Salpingo-oophoritis
Periorchitis N45.2
Periosteum, periosteal —see condition
Periostitis (albuminosa) (circumscribed)
    (diffuse) (infective) (monomelic) —see also
    Osteomyelitis
  alveolar M27.3
  alveolodental M27.3
  dental M27.3
  gonorrheal A54.43
  jaw (lower) (upper) M27.2
  orbit H05.03-●
  syphilitic A52.77
    congenital (early) A50.02 [M90.80]
    secondary A51.46
  tuberculous —see Tuberculosis, bone
  yaws (hypertrophic) (early) (late) A66.6
      [M90.80]
Periostosis (hyperplastic) —see also Disorder,
    bone, specified type NEC
  with osteomyelitis —see Osteomyelitis,
      specified type NEC
Peripartum
  cardiomyopathy O90.3
Periphlebitis —see Phlebitis
Periproctitis K62.89
Periprostatitis —see Prostatitis
Perirectal —see condition
Perirenal —see condition
Perisalpingitis —see Salpingo-oophoritis
Perisplenitis (infectional) D73.89
Peristalsis, visible or reversed R19.2
Peritendinitis —see Enthesopathy
Peritoneum, peritoneal —see condition
Peritonitis (adhesive) (bacterial) (fibrinous)
    (hemorrhagic) (idiopathic) (localized)
    (perforative) (primary) (with adhesions)
    (with effusion) K65.9
  with or following
    abscess K65.1
    appendicitis K35.3
      with perforation or rupture K35.2
      generalized K35.2
      localized K35.3
    diverticular disease (intestine) K57.80
      with bleeding K57.81
      ectopic or molar pregnancy O08.0
      large intestine K57.20
        with
          bleeding K57.21
          small intestine K57.40
            with bleeding K57.41
      small intestine K57.00
        with
          bleeding K57.01
          large intestine K57.40
            with bleeding K57.41

Peritonitis *(Continued)*
  acute (generalized) K65.0
  aseptic T81.61
  bile, biliary K65.3
  chemical T81.61
  chlamydial A74.81
  chronic proliferative K65.8
  complicating abortion —*see* Abortion, by
      type, complicated by, pelvic peritonitis
  congenital P78.1
  diaphragmatic K65.0
  diffuse K65.0
  diphtheritic A36.89
  disseminated K65.0
  due to
    bile K65.3
    foreign
      body or object accidentally left during
          a procedure (instrument) (sponge)
          (swab) T81.599
      substance accidentally left during a
          procedure (chemical) (powder)
          (talc) T81.61
    talc T81.61
    urine K65.8
  eosinophilic K65.8
    acute K65.0
  fibrocaseous (tuberculous) A18.31
  fibropurulent K65.0
  following ectopic or molar pregnancy
      O08.0
  general (ized) K65.0
  gonococcal A54.85
  meconium (newborn) P78.0
  neonatal P78.1
    meconium P78.0
  pancreatic K65.0
  paroxysmal, familial E85.0
    benign E85.0
  pelvic
    female N73.5
      acute N73.3
      chronic N73.4
        with adhesions N73.6
    male K65.0
  periodic, familial E85.0
  proliferative, chronic K65.8
  puerperal, postpartum, childbirth O85
  purulent K65.0
  septic K65.0
  specified NEC K65.8
  spontaneous bacterial K65.2
  subdiaphragmatic K65.0
  subphrenic K65.0
  suppurative K65.0
  syphilitic A52.74
    congenital (early) A50.08 *[K67]*
  talc T81.61
  tuberculous A18.31
  urine K65.8
Peritonsillar —*see* condition
Peritonsillitis J36
Perityphlitis K37
Periureteritis N28.89
Periurethral —*see* condition
Periurethritis (gangrenous) —*see* Urethritis
Periuterine —*see* condition
Perivaginitis —*see* Vaginitis
Perivasculitis, retinal H35.06-●
Perivasitis (chronic) N49.1
Perivesiculitis (seminal) —*see* Vesiculitis
Perlèche NEC K13.0
  due to
    candidiasis B37.83
    moniliasis B37.83
    riboflavin deficiency E53.0
    vitamin B2 (riboflavin) deficiency E53.0
Pernicious —*see* condition
Pernio, perniosis T69.1
Perpetrator (of abuse) —*see* Index to External
    Causes of Injury, Perpetrator

Persecution
  delusion F22
  social Z60.5
Perseveration (tonic) R48.8
Persistence, persistent (congenital)
  anal membrane Q42.3
    with fistula Q42.2
  arteria stapedia Q16.3
  atrioventricular canal Q21.2
  branchial cleft Q18.0
  ▶branchial cleft NOS Q18.2
    ▶cyst Q18.0
    ▶fistula Q18.0
    ▶sinus Q18.0
  bulbus cordis in left ventricle Q21.8
  canal of Cloquet Q14.0
  capsule (opaque) Q12.8
  cilioretinal artery or vein Q14.8
  cloaca Q43.7
  communication —*see* Fistula, congenital
  convolutions
    aortic arch Q25.46
    fallopian tube Q50.6
    oviduct Q50.6
    uterine tube Q50.6
  double aortic arch Q25.45
  ductus arteriosus (Botalli) Q25.0
  fetal
    ⇒circulation P29.38
    form of cervix (uteri) Q51.828
    hemoglobin, hereditary (HPFH) D56.4
  foramen
    Botalli Q21.1
    ovale Q21.1
  Gartner's duct Q52.4
  hemoglobin, fetal (hereditary) (HPFH) D56.4
  hyaloid
    artery (generally incomplete) Q14.0
    system Q14.8
  hymen, in pregnancy or childbirth —*see*
      Pregnancy, complicated by, abnormal,
      vulva
  lanugo Q84.2
  left
    posterior cardinal vein Q26.8
    root with right arch of aorta Q25.49
    superior vena cava Q26.1
  Meckel's diverticulum Q43.0
    malignant —*see* Table of Neoplasms, small
        intestine, malignant
  mucosal disease (middle ear) —*see*
      Otitis, media, suppurative, chronic,
      tubotympanic
  nail(s), anomalous Q84.6
  omphalomesenteric duct Q43.0
  organ or site not listed —*see* Anomaly, by site
  ostium
    atrioventriculare commune Q21.2
    primum Q21.2
    secundum Q21.1
  ovarian rests in fallopian tube Q50.6
  pancreatic tissue in intestinal tract Q43.8
  primary (deciduous)
    teeth K00.6
    vitreous hyperplasia Q14.0
  pupillary membrane Q13.89
  rhesus (Rh)titer —*see* Complication(s),
      transfusion, incompatibility reaction, Rh
      (factor)
  right aortic arch Q25.47
  sinus
    urogenitalis
      female Q52.8
      male Q55.8
    venosus with imperfect incorporation in
        right auricle Q26.8
  thymus (gland) (hyperplasia) E32.0
  thyroglossal duct Q89.2
  thyrolingual duct Q89.2
  truncus arteriosus or communis Q20.0
  tunica vasculosa lentis Q12.2

Persistence, persistent *(Continued)*
  umbilical sinus Q64.4
  urachus Q64.4
  vitelline duct Q43.0
Person (with)
  admitted for clinical research, as a
      control subject (normal comparison)
      (participant) Z00.6
  awaiting admission to adequate facility
      elsewhere Z75.1
  concern (normal) about sick person in family
      Z63.6
  consulting on behalf of another Z71.0
  feigning illness Z76.5
  living (in)
    without
      adequate housing (heating) (space) Z59.1
      housing (permanent) (temporary) Z59.0
      person able to render necessary care
          Z74.2
      shelter Z59.0
    alone Z60.2
    boarding school Z59.3
    residential institution Z59.3
  on waiting list Z75.1
  sick or handicapped in family Z63.6
Personality (disorder) F60.9
  accentuation of traits (type A pattern) Z73.1
  affective F34.0
  aggressive F60.3
  amoral F60.2
  anacastic, anankastic F60.5
  antisocial F60.2
  anxious F60.6
  asocial F60.2
  asthenic F60.7
  avoidant F60.6
  borderline F60.3
  change due to organic condition (enduring)
      F07.0
  compulsive F60.5
  cycloid F34.0
  cyclothymic F34.0
  dependent F60.7
  depressive F34.1
  dissocial F60.2
  dual F44.81
  eccentric F60.89
  emotionally unstable F60.3
  expansive paranoid F60.0
  explosive F60.3
  fanatic F60.0
  haltlose type F60.89
  histrionic F60.4
  hyperthymic F34.0
  hypothymic F34.1
  hysterical F60.4
  immature F60.89
  inadequate F60.7
  labile (emotional) F60.3
  mixed (nonspecific) F60.89
  morally defective F60.2
  multiple F44.81
  narcissistic F60.81
  obsessional F60.5
  obsessive (-compulsive) F60.5
  organic F07.0
  overconscientious F60.5
  paranoid F60.0
  passive (-dependent) F60.7
  passive-aggressive F60.89
  pathologic F60.9
  pattern defect or disturbance F60.9
  pseudopsychopathic (organic) F07.0
  pseudoretarded (organic) F07.0
  psychoinfantile F60.4
  psychoneurotic NEC F60.89
  psychopathic F60.2
  querulant F60.0
  sadistic F60.89
  schizoid F60.1

▶ New   ⇒ Revised   ~~deleted~~ Deleted   ● Use Additional Character(s)

Personality (Continued)
  self-defeating F60.7
  sensitive paranoid F60.0
  sociopathic (amoral) (antisocial) (asocial)
      (dissocial) F60.2
  specified NEC F60.89
  type A Z73.1
  unstable (emotional) F60.3
Perthes' disease —see Legg-Calvé-Perthes
    disease
Pertussis (see also Whooping cough) A37.90
Perversion, perverted
  appetite F50.89
    psychogenic F50.89
  function
    pituitary gland E23.2
      posterior lobe E22.2
  sense of smell and taste R43.8
    psychogenic F45.8
  sexual —see Deviation, sexual
Pervious, congenital —see also Imperfect, closure
  ductus arteriosus Q25.0
Pes (congenital) —see also Talipes
  acquired —see also Deformity, limb, foot,
      specified NEC
    planus —see Deformity, limb, flat foot
  adductus Q66.89
  cavus Q66.7
  deformity NEC, acquired —see Deformity,
      limb, foot, specified NEC
  planus (acquired) (any degree) —see also
      Deformity, limb, flat foot
    rachitic sequelae (late effect) E64.3
  valgus Q66.6
Pest, pestis —see Plague
Petechia, petechiae R23.3
  newborn P54.5
Petechial typhus A75.9
Peter's anomaly Q13.4
Petit mal seizure —see Epilepsy, generalized,
    specified NEC
Petit's hernia —see Hernia, abdomen, specified
    site NEC
Petrellidosis B48.2
Petrositis H70.20-●
  acute H70.21-●
  chronic H70.22-●
Peutz-Jeghers disease or syndrome Q85.8
Peyronie's disease N48.6
PFAPA (periodic fever, aphthous stomatitis,
    pharyngitis, and adenopathy syndrome)
    M04.8
Pfeiffer's disease —see Mononucleosis,
    infectious
Phagedena (dry) (moist) (sloughing) —see also
    Gangrene
  geometric L88
  penis N48.29
  tropical —see Ulcer, skin
  vulva N76.6
Phagedenic —see condition
Phakoma H35.89
Phakomatosis —see also specific eponymous
    syndromes Q85.9
  Bourneville's Q85.1
  specified NEC Q85.8
Phantom limb syndrome (without pain) G54.7
  with pain G54.6
Pharyngeal pouch syndrome D82.1
Pharyngitis (acute) (catarrhal) (gangrenous)
    (infective) (malignant) (membranous)
    (phlegmonous) (pseudomembranous)
    (simple) (subacute) (suppurative)
    (ulcerative) (viral) J02.9
  with influenza, flu, or grippe —see Influenza,
      with, pharyngitis
  aphthous B08.5
  atrophic J31.2
  chlamydial A56.4
  chronic (atrophic) (granular) (hypertrophic)
      J31.2

Pharyngitis (Continued)
  coxsackievirus B08.5
  diphtheritic A36.0
  enteroviral vesicular B08.5
  follicular (chronic) J31.2
  fusospirochetal A69.1
  gonococcal A54.5
  granular (chronic) J31.2
  herpesviral B00.2
  hypertrophic J31.2
  infectional, chronic J31.2
  influenzal —see Influenza, with, respiratory
      manifestations NEC
  lymphonodular, acute (enteroviral) B08.8
  pneumococcal J02.8
  purulent J02.9
  putrid J02.9
  septic J02.0
  sicca J31.2
  specified organism NEC J02.8
  staphylococcal J02.8
  streptococcal J02.0
  syphilitic, congenital (early) A50.03
  tuberculous A15.8
  vesicular, enteroviral B08.5
  viral NEC J02.8
Pharyngoconjunctivitis, viral B30.2
Pharyngolaryngitis (acute) J06.0
  chronic J37.0
Pharyngoplegia J39.2
Pharyngotonsillitis, herpesviral B00.2
Pharyngotracheitis, chronic J42
Pharynx, pharyngeal —see condition
Phencyclidine-induced
  anxiety disorder F16.980
  bipolar and related disorder F16.94
  depressive disorder F16.94
  psychotic disorder F16.959
Phenomenon
  Arthus' —see Arthus' phenomenon
  jaw-winking Q07.8
  lupus erythematosus (LE) cell M32.9
  Raynaud's (secondary) I73.00
    with gangrene I73.01
  vasomotor R55
  vasospastic I73.9
  vasovagal R55
  Wenckebach's I44.1
Phenylketonuria E70.1
  classical E70.0
  maternal E70.1
Pheochromoblastoma
  specified site —see Neoplasm, malignant, by
      site
  unspecified site C74.10
Pheochromocytoma
  malignant
    specified site —see Neoplasm, malignant,
        by site
    unspecified site C74.10
  specified site —see Neoplasm, benign, by site
  unspecified site D35.00
Pheohyphomycosis —see Chromomycosis
Pheomycosis —see Chromomycosis
Phimosis (congenital) (due to infection) N47.1
  chancroidal A57
Phlebectasia —see also Varix
  congenital Q27.4
Phlebitis (infective) (pyemic) (septic)
    (suppurative) I80.9
  antepartum —see Thrombophlebitis,
      antepartum
  blue —see Phlebitis, leg, deep
  breast, superficial I80.8
  cavernous (venous) sinus —see Phlebitis,
      vesicular (venous) sinus
  cerebral (venous) sinus —see Phlebitis,
      intracranial (venous) sinus
  chest wall, superficial I80.8
  cranial (venous) sinus —see Phlebitis,
      intracranial (venous) sinus

Phlebitis (Continued)
  deep (vessels) —see Phlebitis, leg, deep
  due to implanted device —see Complications,
      by site and type, specified NEC
  during or resulting from a procedure
      T81.72
  femoral vein (superficial) I80.1-●
  femoropopliteal vein I80.0-●
  gestational —see Phlebopathy, gestational
  hepatic veins I80.8
  iliofemoral —see Phlebitis, femoral vein
  intracranial (venous) sinus (any) G08
    nonpyogenic I67.6
  intraspinal venous sinuses and veins G08
    nonpyogenic G95.19
  lateral (venous) sinus —see Phlebitis,
      intracranial (venous) sinus
  leg I80.3
    antepartum —see Thrombophlebitis,
        antepartum
    deep (vessels) NEC I80.20-●
      iliac I80.21-●
      popliteal vein I80.22-●
      specified vessel NEC I80.29-●
      tibial vein I80.23-●
    femoral vein (superficial) I80.1-●
    superficial (vessels) I80.0-●
  longitudinal sinus —see Phlebitis, intracranial
      (venous) sinus
  lower limb —see Phlebitis, leg
  migrans, migrating (superficial) I82.1
  pelvic
    with ectopic or molar pregnancy O08.0
    following ectopic or molar pregnancy
        O08.0
    puerperal, postpartum O87.1
  popliteal vein —see Phlebitis, leg, deep,
      popliteal
  portal (vein) K75.1
  postoperative T81.72
  pregnancy —see Thrombophlebitis,
      antepartum
  puerperal, postpartum, childbirth O87.0
    deep O87.1
    pelvic O87.1
    superficial O87.0
  retina —see Vasculitis, retina
  saphenous (accessory) (great) (long)
      (small) —see Phlebitis, leg, superficial
  sinus (meninges) —see Phlebitis, intracranial
      (venous) sinus
  specified site NEC I80.8
  syphilitic A52.09
  tibial vein —see Phlebitis, leg, deep, tibial
  ulcerative I80.9
    leg —see Phlebitis, leg
  umbilicus I80.8
  uterus (septic) —see Endometritis
  varicose (leg) (lower limb) —see Varix, leg,
      with, inflammation
Phlebofibrosis I87.8
Phleboliths I87.8
Phlebopathy
  gestational O22.9-●
  puerperal O87.9
Phlebosclerosis I87.8
Phlebothrombosis —see also Thrombosis
  antepartum —see Thrombophlebitis,
      antepartum
  pregnancy —see Thrombophlebitis,
      antepartum
  puerperal —see Thrombophlebitis,
      puerperal
Phlebotomus fever A93.1
Phlegmasia
  alba dolens O87.1
    nonpuerperal —see Phlebitis, femoral
        vein
  cerulea dolens —see Phlebitis, leg, deep
Phlegmon —see Abscess
Phlegmonous —see condition

Phlyctenulosis (allergic) (keratoconjunctivitis) (nontuberculous) —*see also* Keratoconjunctivitis
  cornea —*see* Keratoconjunctivitis
  tuberculous A18.52
Phobia, phobic F40.9
  animal F40.218
    spiders F40.210
  examination F40.298
  reaction F40.9
  simple F40.298
  social F40.10
    generalized F40.11
  specific (isolated) F40.298
    animal F40.218
      spiders F40.210
    blood F40.230
    injection F40.231
    injury F40.233
    men F40.290
    natural environment F40.228
      thunderstorms F40.220
    situational F40.248
      bridges F40.242
      closed in spaces F40.240
      flying F40.243
      heights F40.241
    specified focus NEC F40.298
    transfusion F40.231
    women F40.291
  specified NEC F40.8
    medical care NEC F40.232
  state F40.9
Phocas' disease —*see* Mastopathy, cystic
Phocomelia Q73.1
  lower limb —*see* Agenesis, leg, with foot present
  upper limb —*see* Agenesis, arm, with hand present
Phoria H50.50
Phosphate-losing tubular disorder N25.0
Phosphatemia E83.39
Phosphaturia E83.39
Photodermatitis (sun) L56.8
  chronic L57.8
  due to drug L56.8
  light other than sun L59.8
Photokeratitis H16.13-●
Photophobia H53.14-●
Photophthalmia —*see* Photokeratitis
Photopsia H53.19
Photoretinitis —*see* Retinopathy, solar
Photosensitivity, photosensitization (sun) skin L56.8
  light other than sun L59.8
Phrenitis —*see* Encephalitis
Phrynoderma (vitamin A deficiency) E50.8
Phthiriasis (pubis) B85.3
  with any infestation classifiable to B85.0-B85.2 B85.4
Phthirus infestation —*see* Phthiriasis
Phthisis —*see also* Tuberculosis
  bulbi (infectional) —*see* Disorder, globe, degenerated condition, atrophy
  eyeball (due to infection) —*see* Disorder, globe, degenerated condition, atrophy
Phycomycosis —*see* Zygomycosis
Physalopteriasis B81.8
Physical restraint status Z78.1
Phytobezoar T18.9
  intestine T18.3
  stomach T18.2
Pian —*see* Yaws
Pianoma A66.1
Pica F50.89
  in adults F50.89
  infant or child F98.3
Picking, nose F98.8
Pick-Niemann disease —*see* Niemann-Pick disease or syndrome

Pick's
  cerebral atrophy G31.01 [F02.80]
    with behavioral disturbance G31.01 [F02.81]
  disease or syndrome (brain) G31.01 [F02.80]
    with behavioral disturbance G31.01 [F02.81]
    brain G31.01 [F02.80]
      with behavioral disturbance G31.01 [F02.81]
    pericardium (pericardial pseudocirrhosis of liver) I31.1
  syndrome
    brain G31.01 [F02.80]
      with behavioral disturbance G31.01 [F02.81]
    of heart (pericardial pseudocirrhosis of liver) I31.1
Pickwickian syndrome E66.2
Piebaldism E70.39
Piedra (beard) (scalp) B36.8
  black B36.3
  white B36.2
Pierre Robin deformity or syndrome Q87.0
Pierson's disease or osteochondrosis M91.0
Pig-bel A05.2
Pigeon
  breast or chest (acquired) M95.4
    congenital Q67.7
    rachitic sequelae (late effect) E64.3
  breeder's disease or lung J67.2
  fancier's disease or lung J67.2
  toe —*see* Deformity, toe, specified NEC
Pigmentation (abnormal) (anomaly) L81.9
  conjunctiva H11.13-●
  cornea (anterior) H18.01-●
    posterior H18.05-●
    stromal H18.06-●
  diminished melanin formation NEC L81.6
  iron L81.8
  lids, congenital Q82.8
  limbus corneae —*see* Pigmentation, cornea
  metals L81.8
  optic papilla, congenital Q14.2
  retina, congenital (grouped) (nevoid) Q14.1
  scrotum, congenital Q82.8
  tattoo L81.8
Piles —*see also* Hemorrhoids K64.9
Pili
  annulati or torti (congenital) Q84.1
  incarnati L73.1
Pill roller hand (intrinsic) —*see* Parkinsonism
Pilomatrixoma —*see* Neoplasm, skin, benign
  malignant —*see* Neoplasm, skin, malignant
Pilonidal —*see* condition
Pimple R23.8
PIN —*see* Neoplasia, intraepithelial, prostate
Pinched nerve —*see* Neuropathy, entrapment
Pindborg tumor —*see* Cyst, calcifying odontogenic
Pineal body or gland —*see* condition
Pinealoblastoma C75.3
Pinealoma D44.5
  malignant C75.3
Pineoblastoma C75.3
Pineocytoma D44.5
Pinguecula H11.15-●
Pingueculitis H10.81-●
Pinhole meatus —*see also* Stricture, urethra N35.9
Pink
  disease —*see* subcategory T56.1
  eye —*see* Conjunctivitis, acute, mucopurulent
Pinkus' disease (lichen nitidus) L44.1
Pinpoint
  meatus —*see* Stricture, urethra
  os (uteri) —*see* Stricture, cervix
Pins and needles R20.2
Pinta A67.9
  cardiovascular lesions A67.2
  chancre (primary) A67.0

Pinta (Continued)
  erythematous plaques A67.1
  hyperchromic lesions A67.1
  hyperkeratosis A67.1
  lesions A67.9
    cardiovascular A67.2
    hyperchromic A67.1
    intermediate A67.1
    late A67.2
    mixed A67.3
    primary A67.0
    skin (achromic) (cicatricial) (dyschromic) A67.2
      hyperchromic A67.1
      mixed (achromic and hyperchromic) A67.3
  papule (primary) A67.0
  skin lesions (achromic) (cicatricial) (dyschromic) A67.2
    hyperchromic A67.1
    mixed (achromic and hyperchromic) A67.3
  vitiligo A67.2
Pintids A67.1
Pinworm (disease) (infection) (infestation) B80
Piroplasmosis B60.0
Pistol wound —*see* Gunshot wound
Pitchers' elbow —*see* Derangement, joint, specified type NEC, elbow
Pithecoid pelvis Q74.2
  with disproportion (fetopelvic) O33.0
    causing obstructed labor O65.0
Pithiatism F48.8
Pitted —*see* Pitting
Pitting —*see also* Edema R60.9
  lip R60.0
  nail L60.8
  teeth K00.4
Pituitary gland —*see* condition
Pituitary-snuff-taker's disease J67.8
Pityriasis (capitis) L21.0
  alba L30.5
  circinata (et maculata) L42
  furfuracea L21.0
  Hebra's L26
  lichenoides L41.0
    chronica L41.1
    et varioliformis (acuta) L41.0
  maculata (et circinata) L30.5
  nigra B36.1
  pilaris, Hebra's L44.0
  rosea L42
  rotunda L44.8
  rubra (Hebra) pilaris L44.0
  simplex L30.5
  specified type NEC L30.5
  streptogenes L30.5
  versicolor (scrotal) B36.0
Placenta, placental —*see* Pregnancy, complicated by (care of) (management affected by), specified condition
Placentitis O41.14-●
Plagiocephaly Q67.3
Plague A20.9
  abortive A20.8
  ambulatory A20.8
  asymptomatic A20.8
  bubonic A20.0
  cellulocutaneous A20.1
  cutaneobubonic A20.1
  lymphatic gland A20.0
  meningitis A20.3
  pharyngeal A20.8
  pneumonic (primary) (secondary) A20.2
  pulmonary, pulmonic A20.2
  septicemic A20.7
  tonsillar A20.8
    septicemic A20.7
Planning, family
  contraception Z30.9
  procreation Z31.69

► New   ⇒ Revised   ~~deleted~~ Deleted   ● Use Additional Character(s)

Plaque(s)
  artery, arterial —*see* Arteriosclerosis
  calcareous —*see* Calcification
  coronary, lipid rich I25.83
  epicardial I31.8
  erythematous, of pinta A67.1
  Hollenhorst's —*see* Occlusion, artery,
      retina
  lipid rich, coronary I25.83
  pleural (without asbestos) J92.9
    with asbestos J92.0
  tongue K13.29
Plasmacytoma C90.3-●
  extramedullary C90.2-●
  medullary C90.0-●
  solitary C90.3-●
Plasmacytopenia D72.818
Plasmacytosis D72.822
Plaster ulcer —*see* Ulcer, pressure, by site
Plateau iris syndrome (post-iridectomy)
    (postprocedural) (without glaucoma)
    H21.82
  with glaucoma H40.22-●
Platybasia Q75.8
Platyonychia (congenital) Q84.6
  acquired L60.8
Platypelloid pelvis M95.5
  with disproportion (fetopelvic) O33.0
    causing obstructed labor O65.0
  congenital Q74.2
Platyspondylisis Q76.49
Plaut (-Vincent) disease —*see also* Vincent's
    A69.1
Plethora R23.2
  newborn P61.1
Pleura, pleural —*see* condition
Pleuralgia R07.81
Pleurisy (acute) (adhesive) (chronic) (costal)
    (diaphragmatic) (double) (dry) (fibrinous)
    (fibrous) (interlobar) (latent) (plastic)
    (primary) (residual) (sicca) (sterile)
    (subacute) (unresolved) R09.1
  with
    adherent pleura J86.0
    effusion J90
      chylous, chyliform J94.0
      tuberculous (non primary)
          A15.6
        primary (progressive) A15.7
      tuberculosis —*see* Pleurisy, tuberculous
          (non primary)
  encysted —*see* Pleurisy, with effusion
  exudative —*see* Pleurisy, with effusion
  fibrinopurulent, fibropurulent —*see*
      Pyothorax
  hemorrhagic —*see* Hemothorax
  pneumococcal J90
  purulent —*see* Pyothorax
  septic —*see* Pyothorax
  serofibrinous —*see* Pleurisy, with effusion
  seropurulent —*see* Pyothorax
  serous —*see* Pleurisy, with effusion
  staphylococcal J86.9
  streptococcal J90
  suppurative —*see* Pyothorax
  traumatic (post) (current) —*see* Injury,
      intrathoracic, pleura
  tuberculous (with effusion) (non primary)
      A15.6
    primary (progressive) A15.7
Pleuritis sicca —*see* Pleurisy
Pleurobronchopneumonia —*see* Pneumonia,
    broncho
Pleurodynia R07.81
  epidemic B33.0
  viral B33.0
Pleuropericarditis —*see also* Pericarditis
  acute I30.9
Pleuropneumonia (acute) (bilateral) (double)
    (septic) —*see also* Pneumonia J18.8
  chronic —*see* Fibrosis, lung

Pleuro-pneumonia-like-organism (PPLO),
    as cause of disease classified elsewhere
    B96.0
Pleurorrhea —*see* Pleurisy, with effusion
Plexitis, brachial G54.0
Plica
  polonica B85.0
  syndrome, knee M67.5
  tonsil J35.8
Plicated tongue K14.5
Plug
  bronchus NEC J98.09
  meconium (newborn) NEC syndrome P76.0
  mucus —*see* Asphyxia, mucus
Plumbism —*see* subcategory T56.0
Plummer's disease E05.20
  with thyroid storm E05.21
Plummer-Vinson syndrome D50.1
Pluricarential syndrome of infancy E40
Plus (and minus) hand (intrinsic) —*see*
    Deformity, limb, specified type NEC,
    forearm
Pneumathemia —*see* Air, embolism
Pneumatic hammer (drill) syndrome T75.21
Pneumatocele (lung) J98.4
  intracranial G93.89
  tension J44.9
Pneumatosis
  cystoides intestinalis K63.89
  intestinalis K63.89
  peritonei K66.8
Pneumaturia R39.89
Pneumoblastoma —*see* Neoplasm, lung,
    malignant
Pneumocephalus G93.89
Pneumococcemia A40.3
Pneumococcus, pneumococcal —*see* condition
Pneumoconiosis (due to) (inhalation of) J64
  with tuberculosis (any type in A15) J65
  aluminum J63.0
  asbestos J61
  bagasse, bagassosis J67.1
  bauxite J63.1
  beryllium J63.2
  coal miners' (simple) J60
  coalworkers' (simple) J60
  collier's J60
  cotton dust J66.0
  diatomite (diatomaceous earth) J62.8
  dust
    inorganic NEC J63.6
    lime J62.8
    marble J62.8
    organic NEC J66.8
  fumes or vapors (from silo) J68.9
  graphite J63.3
  grinder's J62.8
  kaolin J62.8
  mica J62.8
  millstone maker's J62.8
  mineral fibers NEC J61
  miner's J60
  moldy hay J67.0
  potter's J62.8
  rheumatoid —*see* Rheumatoid, lung
  sandblaster's J62.8
  silica, silicate NEC J62.8
    with carbon J60
  stonemason's J62.8
  talc (dust) J62.0
Pneumocystis carinii pneumonia B59
Pneumocystis jiroveci (pneumonia) B59
Pneumocystosis (with pneumonia) B59
Pneumohemopericardium I31.2
Pneumohemothorax J94.2
  traumatic S27.2
Pneumohydropericardium —*see* Pericarditis
Pneumohydrothorax —*see* Hydrothorax
Pneumomediastinum J98.2
  congenital or perinatal P25.2
Pneumomycosis B49 [J99]

Pneumonia (acute) (double) (migratory)
    (purulent) (septic) (unresolved) J18.9
with
  influenza —*see* Influenza, with, pneumonia
  lung abscess J85.1
    due to specified organism —*see*
        Pneumonia, in (due to)
adenoviral J12.0
adynamic J18.2
alba A50.04
allergic (eosinophilic) J82
alveolar —*see* Pneumonia, lobar
anaerobes J15.8
anthrax A22.1
apex, apical —*see* Pneumonia, lobar
Ascaris B77.81
aspiration J69.0
  due to
    aspiration of microorganisms
        bacterial J15.9
        viral J12.9
    food (regurgitated) J69.0
    gastric secretions J69.0
    milk (regurgitated) J69.0
    oils, essences J69.1
    solids, liquids NEC J69.8
    vomitus J69.0
  newborn P24.81
    amniotic fluid (clear) P24.11
    blood P24.21
    food (regurgitated) P24.31
    liquor (amnii) P24.11
    meconium P24.01
    milk P24.31
    mucus P24.11
    specified NEC P24.81
    stomach contents P24.31
  postprocedural J95.4
atypical NEC J18.9
bacillus J15.9
  specified NEC J15.8
bacterial J15.9
  specified NEC J15.8
Bacteroides (fragilis) (oralis)
    (melaninogenicus) J15.8
basal, basic, basilar —*see* Pneumonia, by type
bronchiolitis obliterans organized (BOOP)
    J84.89
broncho-, bronchial (confluent) (croupous)
    (diffuse) (disseminated) (hemorrhagic)
    (involving lobes) (lobar) (terminal) J18.0
  allergic (eosinophilic) J82
  aspiration —*see* Pneumonia, aspiration
  bacterial J15.9
    specified NEC J15.8
  chronic —*see* Fibrosis, lung
  diplococcal J13
  Eaton's agent J15.7
  Escherichia coli (E. coli) J15.5
  Friedländer's bacillus J15.0
  Hemophilus influenzae J14
  hypostatic J18.2
  inhalation —*see also* Pneumonia, aspiration
    due to fumes or vapors (chemical) J68.0
    of oils or essences J69.1
  Klebsiella (pneumoniae) J15.0
  lipid, lipoid J69.1
    endogenous J84.89
  Mycoplasma (pneumoniae) J15.7
  pleuro-pneumonia-like-organisms (PPLO)
      J15.7
  pneumococcal J13
  Proteus J15.6
  Pseudomonas J15.1
  Serratia marcescens J15.6
  specified organism NEC J16.8
  staphylococcal —*see* Pneumonia,
      staphylococcal
  streptococcal NEC J15.4
    group B J15.3
    pneumoniae J13
  viral, virus —*see* Pneumonia, viral

Pneumonia (Continued)
Butyrivibrio (fibriosolvens) J15.8
Candida B37.1
caseous —see Tuberculosis, pulmonary
catarrhal —see Pneumonia, broncho
chlamydial J16.0
   congenital P23.1
cholesterol J84.89
cirrhotic (chronic) —see Fibrosis, lung
Clostridium (haemolyticum) (novyi) J15.8
confluent —see Pneumonia, broncho
congenital (infective) P23.9
   due to
      bacterium NEC P23.6
      Chlamydia P23.1
      Escherichia coli P23.4
      Haemophilus influenzae P23.6
      infective organism NEC P23.8
      Klebsiella pneumoniae P23.6
      Mycoplasma P23.6
      Pseudomonas P23.5
      Staphylococcus P23.2
      Streptococcus (except group B) P23.6
         group B P23.3
      viral agent P23.0
   specified NEC P23.8
croupous —see Pneumonia, lobar
cryptogenic organizing J84.116
cytomegalic inclusion B25.0
cytomegaloviral B25.0
deglutition —see Pneumonia, aspiration
desquamative interstitial J84.117
diffuse —see Pneumonia, broncho
diplococcal, diplococcus (broncho-) (lobar) J13
disseminated (focal) —see Pneumonia, broncho
Eaton's agent J15.7
embolic, embolism —see Embolism, pulmonary
Enterobacter J15.6
eosinophilic J82
Escherichia coli (E. coli) J15.5
Eubacterium J15.8
fibrinous —see Pneumonia, lobar
fibroid, fibrous (chronic) —see Fibrosis, lung
Friedländer's bacillus J15.0
Fusobacterium (nucleatum) J15.8
gangrenous J85.0
giant cell (measles) B05.2
gonococcal A54.84
gram-negative bacteria NEC J15.6
   anaerobic J15.8
Hemophilus influenzae (broncho) (lobar) J14
human metapneumovirus J12.3
hypostatic (broncho) (lobar) J18.2
in (due to)
   actinomycosis A42.0
   adenovirus J12.0
   anthrax A22.1
   ascariasis B77.81
   aspergillosis B44.9
   Bacillus anthracis A22.1
   Bacterium anitratum J15.6
   candidiasis B37.1
   chickenpox B01.2
   Chlamydia J16.0
      neonatal P23.1
   coccidioidomycosis B38.2
      acute B38.0
      chronic B38.1
   cytomegalovirus disease B25.0
   Diplococcus (pneumoniae) J13
   Eaton's agent J15.7
   Enterobacter J15.6
   Escherichia coli (E. coli) J15.5
   Friedländer's bacillus J15.0
   fumes and vapors (chemical) (inhalation) J68.0
   gonorrhea A54.84
   Hemophilus influenzae (H. influenzae) J14

Pneumonia (Continued)
in (Continued)
   Herellea J15.6
   histoplasmosis B39.2
      acute B39.0
      chronic B39.1
   human metapneumovirus J12.3
   Klebsiella (pneumoniae) J15.0
   measles B05.2
   Mycoplasma (pneumoniae) J15.7
   nocardiosis, nocardiasis A43.0
   ornithosis A70
   parainfluenza virus J12.2
   pleuro-pneumonia-like-organism (PPLO) J15.7
   pneumococcus J13
   pneumocystosis (Pneumocystis carinii) (Pneumocystis jiroveci) B59
   Proteus J15.6
   Pseudomonas NEC J15.1
      pseudomallei A24.1
   psittacosis A70
   Q fever A78
   respiratory syncytial virus J12.1
   rheumatic fever I00 [J17]
   rubella B06.81
   Salmonella (infection) A02.22
      typhi A01.03
   schistosomiasis B65.9 [J17]
   Serratia marcescens J15.6
   specified
      bacterium NEC J15.8
      organism NEC J16.8
   spirochetal NEC A69.8
   Staphylococcus J15.20
      aureus (methicillin susceptible) (MSSA) J15.211
         methicillin resistant (MRSA) J15.212
      specified NEC J15.29
   Streptococcus J15.4
      group B J15.3
      pneumoniae J13
      specified NEC J15.4
   toxoplasmosis B58.3
   tularemia A21.2
   typhoid (fever) A01.03
   varicella B01.2
   virus —see Pneumonia, viral
   whooping cough A37.91
      due to
         Bordetella parapertussis A37.11
         Bordetella pertussis A37.01
         specified NEC A37.81
   Yersinia pestis A20.2
inhalation of food or vomit —see Pneumonia, aspiration
interstitial J84.9
   chronic J84.111
   desquamative J84.117
   due to
      collagen vascular disease J84.17
      known underlying cause J84.17
   idiopathic NOS J84.111
   in disease classified elsewhere J84.17
   lymphocytic (due to collagen vascular disease) (in diseases classified elsewhere) J84.17
   lymphoid J84.2
   non-specific J84.89
      due to
         collagen vascular disease J84.17
         known underlying cause J84.17
      idiopathic J84.113
      in diseases classified elsewhere J84.17
   plasma cell B59
   pseudomonas J15.1
   usual J84.112
      due to collagen vascular disease J84.17
      idiopathic J84.112
      in diseases classified elsewhere J84.17

Pneumonia (Continued)
Klebsiella (pneumoniae) J15.0
lipid, lipoid (exogenous) J69.1
   endogenous J84.89
lobar (disseminated) (double) (interstitial) J18.1
   bacterial J15.9
      specified NEC J15.8
   chronic —see Fibrosis, lung
   Escherichia coli (E. coli) J15.5
   Friedländer's bacillus J15.0
   Hemophilus influenzae J14
   hypostatic J18.2
   Klebsiella (pneumoniae) J15.0
   pneumococcal J13
   Proteus J15.6
   Pseudomonas J15.1
   specified organism NEC J16.8
   staphylococcal —see Pneumonia, staphylococcal
   streptococcal NEC J15.4
   Streptococcus pneumoniae J13
   viral, virus —see Pneumonia, viral
lobular —see Pneumonia, broncho
Löffler's J82
lymphoid interstitial J84.2
massive —see Pneumonia, lobar
meconium P24.01
MRSA (Methicillin resistant Staphylococcus aureus) J15.212
MSSA (methicillin susceptible Staphylococcus aureus) J15.211
multilobar —see Pneumonia, by type
Mycoplasma (pneumoniae) J15.7
necrotic J85.0
neonatal P23.9
   aspiration —see Aspiration, by substance, with pneumonia
nitrogen dioxide J68.0
organizing J84.89
   due to
      collagen vascular disease J84.17
      known underlying cause J84.17
   in diseases classified elsewhere J84.17
orthostatic J18.2
parainfluenza virus J12.2
parenchymatous —see Fibrosis, lung
passive J18.2
patchy —see Pneumonia, broncho
Peptococcus J15.8
Peptostreptococcus J15.8
plasma cell (of infants) B59
pleurolobar —see Pneumonia, lobar
pleuro-pneumonia-like organism (PPLO) J15.7
pneumococcal (broncho) (lobar) J13
Pneumocystis (carinii) (jiroveci) B59
postinfectional NEC B99 [J17]
postmeasles B05.2
Proteus J15.6
Pseudomonas J15.1
psittacosis A70
radiation J70.0
respiratory syncytial virus J12.1
resulting from a procedure J95.89
rheumatic I00 [J17]
Salmonella (arizonae) (cholerae-suis) (enteritidis) (typhimurium) A02.22
   typhi A01.03
   typhoid fever A01.03
SARS-associated coronavirus J12.81
segmented, segmental —see Pneumonia, broncho-●
Serratia marcescens J15.6
specified NEC J18.8
   bacterium NEC J15.8
   organism NEC J16.8
   virus NEC J12.89
spirochetal NEC A69.8

Pneumonia (Continued)
staphylococcal (broncho) (lobar) J15.20
  aureus (methicillin susceptible) (MSSA)
    J15.211
    methicillin resistant (MRSA) J15.212
  specified NEC J15.29
static, stasis J18.2
streptococcal NEC (broncho) (lobar) J15.4
  group
    A J15.4
    B J15.3
  specified NEC J15.4
Streptococcus pneumoniae J13
syphilitic, congenital (early) A50.04
traumatic (complication) (early) (secondary)
  T79.8
tuberculous (any) —see Tuberculosis,
  pulmonary
tularemic A21.2
varicella B01.2
Veillonella J15.8
ventilator associated J95.851
viral, virus (broncho) (interstitial) (lobar) J12.9
  adenoviral J12.0
  congenital P23.0
  human metapneumovirus J12.3
  parainfluenza J12.2
  respiratory syncytial J12.1
  SARS-associated coronavirus J12.81
  specified NEC J12.89
white (congenital) A50.04
Pneumonic —see condition
Pneumonitis (acute) (primary) —see also
  Pneumonia
air-conditioner J67.7
allergic (due to) J67.9
  organic dust NEC J67.8
  red cedar dust J67.8
  sequoiosis J67.8
  wood dust J67.8
aspiration J69.0
  due to
    anesthesia J95.4
      during
        labor and delivery O74.0
        pregnancy O29.01-●
        puerperium O89.01
    fumes or gases J68.0
  obstetric O74.0
chemical (due to gases, fumes or vapors)
  (inhalation) J68.0
  due to anesthesia J95.4
cholesterol J84.89
chronic —see Fibrosis, lung
congenital rubella P35.0
crack (cocaine) J68.0
due to
  beryllium J68.0
  cadmium J68.0
  crack (cocaine) J68.0
  detergent J69.8
  fluorocarbon-polymer J68.0
  food, vomit (aspiration) J69.0
  fumes or vapors J68.0
  gases, fumes or vapors (inhalation) J68.0
  inhalation
    blood J69.8
    essences J69.1
    food (regurgitated), milk, vomit
      J69.0
    oils, essences J69.1
    saliva J69.0
    solids, liquids NEC J69.8
  manganese J68.0
  nitrogen dioxide J68.0
  oils, essences J69.1
  solids, liquids NEC J69.8
  toxoplasmosis (acquired) B58.3
    congenital P37.1
  vanadium J68.0
  ventilator J95.851

Pneumonitis (Continued)
eosinophilic J82
hypersensitivity J67.9
  air conditioner lung J67.7
  bagassosis J67.1
  bird fancier's lung J67.2
  farmer's lung J67.0
  maltworker's lung J67.4
  maple bark-stripper's lung J67.6
  mushroom worker's lung J67.5
  specified organic dust NEC J67.8
  suberosis J67.3
interstitial (chronic) J84.89
  acute J84.114
  lymphoid J84.2
  non-specific J84.89
    idiopathic J84.113
lymphoid, interstitial J84.2
meconium P24.01
postanesthetic J95.4
  correct substance properly administered —
    see Table of Drugs and Chemcials, by
    drug, adverse effect
  in labor and delivery O74.0
  in pregnancy O29.01-●
  obstetric O74.0
  overdose or wrong substance given or taken
    (by accident) —see Table of Drugs and
    Chemicals, by drug, poisoning
  postpartum, puerperal O89.01
postoperative J95.4
  obstetric O74.0
radiation J70.0
rubella, congenital P35.0
ventilation (air-conditioning) J67.7
ventilator associated J95.851
wood-dust J67.8
Pneumonoconiosis —see Pneumoconiosis
Pneumoparotid K11.8
Pneumopathy NEC J98.4
alveolar J84.09
due to organic dust NEC J66.8
parietoalveolar J84.09
Pneumopericarditis —see also Pericarditis
acute I30.9
Pneumopericardium —see also Pericarditis
congenital P25.3
newborn P25.3
traumatic (post) —see Injury, heart
Pneumophagia (psychogenic) F45.8
Pneumopleurisy, pneumopleuritis —see also
  Pneumonia J18.8
Pneumopyopericardium I30.1
Pneumopyothorax —see Pyopneumothorax
  with fistula J86.0
Pneumorrhagia —see also Hemorrhage, lung
tuberculous —see Tuberculosis, pulmonary
Pneumothorax NOS J93.9
acute J93.83
chronic J93.81
congenital P25.1
perinatal period P25.1
postprocedural J95.811
specified NEC J93.83
spontaneous NOS J93.83
  newborn P25.1
  primary J93.11
  secondary J93.12
  tension J93.0
tense valvular, infectional J93.0
tension (spontaneous) J93.0
traumatic S27.0
  with hemothorax S27.2
tuberculous —see Tuberculosis, pulmonary
Podagra —see also Gout M10.9
Podencephalus Q01.9
Poikilocytosis R71.8
Poikiloderma L81.6
Civatte's L57.3
congenital Q82.8
vasculare atrophicans L94.5

Poikilodermatomyositis M33.10
with
  myopathy M33.12
  respiratory involvement M33.11
  specified organ involvement NEC M33.19
Pointed ear (congenital) Q17.3
Poison ivy, oak, sumac or other plant
  dermatitis (allergic) (contact) L23.7
Poisoning (acute) —see also Table of Drugs and
  Chemicals
algae and toxins T65.82-●
Bacillus B (aertrycke) (cholerae (suis))
  (paratyphosus) (suipestifer) A02.9
  botulinus A05.1
bacterial toxins A05.9
berries, noxious —see Poisoning, food,
  noxious, berries
botulism A05.1
ciguatera fish T61.0-●
Clostridium botulinum A05.1
death-cap (Amanita phalloides) (Amanita
  verna) —see Poisoning, food, noxious,
  mushrooms
drug —see Table of Drugs and Chemicals, by
  drug, poisoning
epidemic, fish (noxious) —see Poisoning,
  seafood
  bacterial A05.9
fava bean D55.0
fish (noxious) T61.9-●
  bacterial —see Intoxication, foodborne, by
    agent
  ciguatera fish —see Poisoning, ciguatera
    fish
  scombroid fish —see Poisoning, scombroid
    fish
  specified type NEC T61.77-●
food (acute) (diseased) (infected) (noxious)
  NEC T62.9-●
  bacterial —see Intoxication, foodborne, by
    agent
  due to
    Bacillus (aertrycke) (choleraesuis)
      (paratyphosus) (suipestifer) A02.9
      botulinus A05.1
    Clostridium (perfringens) (Welchii)
      A05.2
    salmonella (aertrycke) (callinarum)
      (choleraesuis) (enteritidis)
      (paratyphi) (suipestifer) A02.9
      with
        gastroenteritis A02.0
        sepsis A02.1
    staphylococcus A05.0
    Vibrio
      parahaemolyticus A05.3
      vulnificus A05.5
  noxious or naturally toxic T62.9-●
    berries —see subcategory T62.1-●
    fish —see Poisoning, seafood
    mushrooms —see subcategory T62.0X-●
    plants NEC —see subcategory T62.2X-●
    seafood —see Poisoning, seafood
    specified NEC —see subcategory
      T62.8X-●
ichthyotoxism —see Poisoning, seafood
kreotoxism, food A05.9
latex T65.81-●
lead T56.0-●
mushroom —see Poisoning, food, noxious,
  mushroom
mussels —see also Poisoning, shellfish
  bacterial —see Intoxication, foodborne, by
    agent
nicotine (tobacco) T65.2-●
noxious foodstuffs —see Poisoning, food,
  noxious
plants, noxious —see Poisoning, food,
  noxious, plants NEC
ptomaine —see Poisoning, food
radiation J70.0

Poisoning *(Continued)*
  Salmonella (arizonae) (cholerae-suis) (enteritidis) (typhimurium) A02.9
  scombroid fish T61.1-●
  seafood (noxious) T61.9-●
    bacterial —*see* Intoxication, foodborne, by agent
    fish —*see* Poisoning, fish
    shellfish —*see* Poisoning, shellfish
    specified NEC —*see* subcategory T61.8X-●
  shellfish (amnesic) (azaspiracid) (diarrheic) (neurotoxic) (noxious) (paralytic) T61.78-●
    bacterial —*see* Intoxication, foodborne, by agent
    ciguatera mollusk —*see* Poisoning, ciguatera fish
  specified substance NEC T65.891
  Staphylococcus, food A05.0
  tobacco (nicotine) T65.2-●
  water E87.79
Poker spine —*see* Spondylitis, ankylosing
Poland syndrome Q79.8
Polioencephalitis (acute) (bulbar) A80.9
  inferior G12.22
  influenzal —*see* Influenza, with, encephalopathy
  superior hemorrhagic (acute) (Wernicke's) E51.2
  Wernicke's E51.2
Polioencephalomyelitis (acute) (anterior) A80.9
  with beriberi E51.2
Polioencephalopathy, superior hemorrhagic E51.2
  with
    beriberi E51.11
    pellagra E52
Poliomeningoencephalitis —*see* Meningoencephalitis
Poliomyelitis (acute) (anterior) (epidemic) A80.9
  with paralysis (bulbar) —*see* Poliomyelitis, paralytic
  abortive A80.4
  ascending (progressive) —*see* Poliomyelitis, paralytic
  bulbar (paralytic) —*see* Poliomyelitis, paralytic
  congenital P35.8
  nonepidemic A80.9
  nonparalytic A80.4
  paralytic A80.30
    specified NEC A80.39
    vaccine-associated A80.0
    wild virus
      imported A80.1
      indigenous A80.2
  spinal, acute A80.9
Poliosis (eyebrow) (eyelashes) L67.1
  circumscripta, acquired L67.1
Pollakiuria R35.0
  psychogenic F45.8
Pollinosis J30.1
Pollitzer's disease L73.2
Polyadenitis —*see also* Lymphadenitis
  malignant A20.0
Polyalgia M79.89
Polyangiitis M30.0
  microscopic M31.7
  overlap syndrome M30.8
Polyarteritis
  microscopic M31.7
  nodosa M30.0
    with lung involvement M30.1
    juvenile M30.2
    related condition NEC M30.8
Polyarthralgia —*see* Pain, joint
Polyarthritis, polyarthropathy —*see also* Arthritis M13.0
  due to or associated with other specified conditions —*see* Arthritis

Polyarthritis, polyarthropathy *(Continued)*
  epidemic (Australian) (with exanthema) B33.1
  infective —*see* Arthritis, pyogenic or pyemic
  inflammatory M06.4
  juvenile (chronic) (seronegative) M08.3
  migratory —*see* Fever, rheumatic
  rheumatic, acute —*see* Fever, rheumatic
Polyarthrosis M15.9
  post-traumatic M15.3
  primary M15.0
  specified NEC M15.8
Polycarential syndrome of infancy E40
Polychondritis (atrophic) (chronic) —*see also* Disorder, cartilage, specified type NEC
  relapsing M94.1
Polycoria Q13.2
Polycystic (disease)
  degeneration, kidney Q61.3
    autosomal dominant (adult type) Q61.2
    autosomal recessive (infantile type) NEC Q61.19
  kidney Q61.3
    autosomal
      dominant Q61.2
      recessive NEC Q61.19
    autosomal dominant (adult type) Q61.2
    autosomal recessive (childhood type) NEC Q61.19
    infantile type NEC Q61.19
  liver Q44.6
  lung J98.4
    congenital Q33.0
  ovary, ovaries E28.2
  spleen Q89.09
Polycythemia (secondary) D75.1
  acquired D75.1
  benign (familial) D75.0
  due to
    donor twin P61.1
    erythropoietin D75.1
    fall in plasma volume D75.1
    high altitude D75.1
    maternal-fetal transfusion P61.1
    stress D75.1
  emotional D75.1
  erythropoietin D75.1
  familial (benign) D75.0
  Gaisböck's (hypertonica) D75.1
  high altitude D75.1
  hypertonica D75.1
  hypoxemic D75.1
  neonatorum P61.1
  nephrogenic D75.1
  relative D75.1
  secondary D75.1
  spurious D75.1
  stress D75.1
  vera D45
Polycytosis cryptogenica D75.1
Polydactylism, polydactyly Q69.9
  toes Q69.2
Polydipsia R63.1
Polydystrophy, pseudo-Hurler E77.0
Polyembryoma —*see* Neoplasm, malignant, by site
Polyglandular
  deficiency E31.0
  dyscrasia E31.9
  dysfunction E31.9
  syndrome E31.8
Polyhydramnios O40.-●
Polymastia Q83.1
Polymenorrhea N92.0
Polymyalgia M35.3
  arteritica, giant cell M31.5
  rheumatica M35.3
    with giant cell arteritis M31.5

Polymyositis (acute) (chronic) (hemorrhagic) M33.20
  with
    myopathy M33.22
    respiratory involvement M33.21
    skin involvement —*see* Dermatopolymyositis
    specified organ involvement NEC M33.29
  ossificans (generalisata) (progressiva) —*see* Myositis, ossificans, progressiva
Polyneuritis, polyneuritic —*see also* Polyneuropathy
  acute (post-)infective G61.0
  alcoholic G62.1
  cranialis G52.7
  demyelinating, chronic inflammatory (CIDP) G61.81
  diabetic —*see* Diabetes, polyneuropathy
  diphtheritic A36.83
  due to lack of vitamin NEC E56.9 *[G63]*
  endemic E51.11
  erythredema —*see* subcategory T56.1
  febrile, acute G61.0
  hereditary ataxic G60.1
  idiopathic, acute G61.0
  infective (acute) G61.0
  inflammatory, chronic demyelinating (CIDP) G61.81
  nutritional E63.9 *[G63]*
  postinfective (acute) G61.0
  specified NEC G62.89
Polyneuropathy (peripheral) G62.9
  alcoholic G62.1
  amyloid (Portuguese) E85.1 *[G63]*
    ▶transthyretin-related (ATTR) familial E85.1
  arsenical G62.2
  critical illness G62.81
  demyelinating, chronic inflammatory (CIDP) G61.81
  diabetic —*see* Diabetes, polyneuropathy
  drug-induced G62.0
  hereditary G60.9
    specified NEC G60.8
  idiopathic G60.9
    progressive G60.3
  in (due to)
    alcohol G62.1
      sequelae G65.2
    amyloidosis, familial (Portuguese) E85.1 *[G63]*
    antitetanus serum G61.1
    arsenic G62.2
      sequelae G65.2
    avitaminosis NEC E56.9 *[G63]*
    beriberi E51.11
    collagen vascular disease NEC M35.9 *[G63]*
    deficiency (of)
      B (-complex) vitamins E53.9 *[G63]*
      vitamin B6 E53.1 *[G63]*
    diabetes —*see* Diabetes, polyneuropathy
    diphtheria A36.83
    drug or medicament G62.0
      correct substance properly administered —*see* Table of Drugs and Chemicals, by drug, adverse effect
      overdose or wrong substance given or taken —*see* Table of Drugs and Chemicals, by drug, poisoning
    endocrine disease NEC E34.9 *[G63]*
    herpes zoster B02.23
    hypoglycemia E16.2 *[G63]*
    infectious
      disease NEC B99 *[G63]*
      mononucleosis B27.91
    lack of vitamin NEC E56.9 *[G63]*
    lead G62.2
      sequelae G65.2
    leprosy A30.9 *[G63]*
    Lyme disease A69.22
    metabolic disease NEC E88.9 *[G63]*

Polyneuropathy *(Continued)*
in *(Continued)*
microscopic polyangiitis M31.7 *[G63]*
mumps B26.84
neoplastic disease —*see also* Neoplasm
D49.9 *[G63]*
nutritional deficiency NEC E63.9 *[G63]*
organophosphate compounds G62.2
sequelae G65.2
parasitic disease NEC B89 *[G63]*
pellagra E52 *[G63]*
polyarteritis nodosa M30.0
porphyria E80.20 *[G63]*
radiation G62.82
rheumatoid arthritis —*see* Rheumatoid,
polyneuropathy
sarcoidosis D86.89
serum G61.1
syphilis (late) A52.15
congenital A50.43
systemic
connective tissue disorder M35.9 *[G63]*
lupus erythematosus M32.19
toxic agent NEC G62.2
sequelae G65.2
~~triorthocresyl phosphate G62.2~~
~~sequelae G65.2~~
~~tuberculosis A17.89~~
~~uremia N18.9 [G63]~~
~~vitamin B12 deficiency E53.8 [G63]~~
~~with anemia (pernicious) D51.0 [G63]~~
~~due to dietary deficiency D51.3 [G63]~~
~~zoster B02.23~~
▶transthyretin-related (ATTR) familial
amyloid E85.1
▶triorthocresyl phosphate G62.2
▶sequelae G65.2
▶tuberculosis A17.89
▶uremia N18.9 *[G63]*
▶vitamin B12 deficiency E53.8 *[G63]*
▶with anemia (pernicious) D51.0 *[G63]*
▶due to dietary deficiency D51.3 *[G63]*
▶zoster B02.23
inflammatory G61.9
chronic demyelinating (CIDP) G61.81
sequelae G65.1
specified NEC G61.89
lead G62.2
sequelae G65.2
nutritional NEC E63.9 *[G63]*
postherpetic (zoster) B02.23
progressive G60.3
radiation-induced G62.82
sensory (hereditary) (idiopathic) G60.8
specified NEC G62.89
syphilitic (late) A52.15
congenital A50.43
Polyopia H53.8
Polyorchism, polyorchidism Q55.21
Polyosteoarthritis —*see also* Osteoarthritis,
generalized M15.9-●
post-traumatic M15.3
specified NEC M15.8
Polyostotic fibrous dysplasia Q78.1
Polyotia Q17.0
Polyp, polypus
accessory sinus J33.8
adenocarcinoma in —*see* Neoplasm,
malignant, by site
adenocarcinoma in situ in —*see* Neoplasm, in
situ, by site
adenoid tissue J33.0
adenomatous —*see also* Neoplasm, benign,
by site
adenocarcinoma in —*see* Neoplasm,
malignant, by site
adenocarcinoma in situ in —*see* Neoplasm,
in situ, by site
carcinoma in —*see* Neoplasm, malignant,
by site
carcinoma in situ in —*see* Neoplasm, in
situ, by site

Polyp, polypus *(Continued)*
adenomatous *(Continued)*
multiple —*see* Neoplasm, benign
adenocarcinoma in —*see* Neoplasm,
malignant, by site
adenocarcinoma in situ in —*see*
Neoplasm, in situ, by site
antrum J33.8
anus, anal (canal) K62.0
Bartholin's gland N84.3
bladder D41.4
carcinoma in —*see* Neoplasm, malignant, by
site
carcinoma in situ in —*see* Neoplasm, in situ,
by site
cecum D12.0
cervix (uteri) N84.1
in pregnancy or childbirth —*see* Pregnancy,
complicated by, abnormal, cervix
mucous N84.1
nonneoplastic N84.1
choanal J33.0
cholesterol K82.4
clitoris N84.3
colon K63.5
adenomatous D12.6
ascending D12.2
cecum D12.0
descending D12.4
inflammatory K51.40
with
abscess K51.414
complication K51.419
specified NEC K51.418
fistula K51.413
intestinal obstruction K51.412
rectal bleeding K51.411
sigmoid D12.5
transverse D12.3
corpus uteri N84.0
dental K04.01
irreversible K04.02
reversible K04.01
duodenum K31.7
ear (middle) H74.4-●
endometrium N84.0
ethmoidal (sinus) J33.8
fallopian tube N84.8
female genital tract N84.9
specified NEC N84.8
frontal (sinus) J33.8
gallbladder K82.4
gingiva, gum K06.8
labia, labium (majus) (minus) N84.3
larynx (mucous) J38.1
adenomatous D14.1
malignant —*see* Neoplasm, malignant, by site
maxillary (sinus) J33.8
middle ear —*see* Polyp, ear (middle)
myometrium N84.0
nares
anterior J33.9
posterior J33.0
nasal (mucous) J33.9
cavity J33.0
septum J33.0
nasopharyngeal J33.0
nose (mucous) J33.9
oviduct N84.8
pharynx J39.2
placenta O90.89
prostate —*see* Enlargement, enlarged,
prostate
pudenda, pudendum N84.3
pulpal (dental) K04.01
irreversible K04.02
reversible K04.01
rectum (nonadenomatous) K62.1
adenomatous —*see* Polyp, adenomatous
septum (nasal) J33.0
sinus (accessory) (ethmoidal) (frontal)
(maxillary) (sphenoidal) J33.8

Polyp, polypus *(Continued)*
sphenoidal (sinus) J33.8
stomach K31.7
adenomatous D13.1
tube, fallopian N84.8
turbinate, mucous membrane J33.8
umbilical, newborn P83.6
ureter N28.89
urethra N36.2
uterus (body) (corpus) (mucous) N84.0
cervix N84.1
in pregnancy or childbirth —*see* Pregnancy,
complicated by, tumor, uterus
vagina N84.2
vocal cord (mucous) J38.1
vulva N84.3
Polyphagia R63.2
Polyploidy Q92.7
Polypoid —*see* condition
Polyposis —*see also* Polyp
coli (adenomatous) D12.6
adenocarcinoma in C18.9
adenocarcinoma in situ in —*see* Neoplasm,
in situ, by site
carcinoma in C18.9
colon (adenomatous) D12.6
familial D12.6
adenocarcinoma in situ in —*see* Neoplasm,
in situ, by site
intestinal (adenomatous) D12.6
malignant lymphomatous C83.1
multiple, adenomatous —*see also* Neoplasm,
benign D36.9
Polyradiculitis —*see* Polyneuropathy
Polyradiculoneuropathy (acute) (postinfective)
(segmentally demyelinating) G61.0
Polyserositis
due to pericarditis I31.1
pericardial I31.1
periodic, familial E85.0
tuberculous A19.9
acute A19.1
chronic A19.8
Polysplenia syndrome Q89.09
Polysyndactyly —*see also* Syndactylism,
syndactyly Q70.4
Polytrichia L68.3
Polyunguia Q84.6
Polyuria R35.8
nocturnal R35.1
psychogenic F45.8
Pompe's disease (glycogen storage) E74.02
Pompholyx L30.1
Poncet's disease (tuberculous rheumatism)
A18.09
Pond fracture —*see* Fracture, skull
Ponos B55.0
Pons, pontine —*see* condition
Poor
aesthetic of existing restoration of tooth
K08.56
contractions, labor O62.2
gingival margin to tooth restoration K08.51
personal hygiene R46.0
prenatal care, affecting management of
pregnancy —*see* Pregnancy, complicated
by, insufficient, prenatal care
sucking reflex (newborn) R29.2
urinary stream R39.12
vision NEC H54.7
Poradenitis, nostras inguinalis or venerea A55
Porencephaly (congenital) (developmental)
(true) Q04.6
acquired G93.0
nondevelopmental G93.0
traumatic (post) F07.89
Porocephaliasis B88.8
Porokeratosis Q82.8
Poroma, eccrine —*see* Neoplasm, skin, benign
Porphyria (South African) E80.20
acquired E80.20
acute intermittent (hepatic) (Swedish) E80.21

Porphyria *(Continued)*
  cutanea tarda (hereditary) (symptomatic) E80.1
  due to drugs E80.20
    correct substance properly administered —
      see Table of Drugs and Chemicals, by
      drug, adverse effect
    overdose or wrong substance given
      or taken —*see* Table of Drugs and
      Chemicals, by drug, poisoning
  erythropoietic (congenital) (hereditary) E80.0
  hepatocutaneous type E80.1
  secondary E80.20
  toxic NEC E80.20
  variegata E80.20
Porphyrinuria —*see* Porphyria
Porphyruria —*see* Porphyria
Portal —*see* condition
Port wine nevus, mark, or stain Q82.5
Posadas-Wernicke disease B38.9
Positive
  culture (nonspecific)
    blood R78.81
    bronchial washings R84.5
    cerebrospinal fluid R83.5
    cervix uteri R87.5
    nasal secretions R84.5
    nipple discharge R89.5
    nose R84.5
      staphylococcus (Methicillin susceptible)
        Z22.321
        Methicillin resistant Z22.322
    peritoneal fluid R85.5
    pleural fluid R84.5
    prostatic secretions R86.5
    saliva R85.5
    seminal fluid R86.5
    sputum R84.5
    synovial fluid R89.5
    throat scrapings R84.5
    urine R82.79
    vagina R87.5
    vulva R87.5
    wound secretions R89.5
  PPD (skin test) R76.11
  serology for syphilis A53.0
    with signs or symptoms - code as Syphilis,
      by site and stage
    false R76.8
  skin test, tuberculin (without active
    tuberculosis) R76.11
  test, human immunodeficiency virus (HIV)
    R75
  VDRL A53.0
    with signs or symptoms - code by site and
      stage under Syphilis A53.9
  Wassermann reaction A53.0
Postcardiotomy syndrome I97.0
Postcaval ureter Q62.62
Postcholecystectomy syndrome K91.5
Postclimacteric bleeding N95.0
Postcommissurotomy syndrome I97.0
Postconcussional syndrome F07.81
Postcontusional syndrome F07.81
Postcricoid region —*see* condition
Post-dates (40-42 weeks) (pregnancy) (mother)
  O48.0
  more than 42 weeks gestation O48.1
Postencephalitic syndrome F07.89
Posterior —*see* condition
Posterolateral sclerosis (spinal cord) —*see*
  Degeneration, combined
Postexanthematous —*see* condition
Postfebrile —*see* condition
Postgastrectomy dumping syndrome K91.1
Posthemiplegic chorea —*see* Monoplegia
Posthemorrhagic anemia (chronic) D50.0
  acute D62
  newborn P61.3
Postherpetic neuralgia (zoster) B02.29
  trigeminal B02.22
Posthitis N47.7

Postimmunization complication or reaction —
  see Complications, vaccination
Postinfectious —*see* condition
Postlaminectomy syndrome NEC M96.1
Postleukotomy syndrome F07.0
Postmastectomy lymphedema (syndrome) I97.2
Postmaturity, postmature (over 42 weeks)
  maternal (over 42 weeks gestation) O48.1
  newborn P08.22
Postmeasles complication NEC —*see also*
  condition B05.89
Postmenopausal
  endometrium (atrophic) N95.8
    suppurative —*see also* Endometritis N71.9
  osteoporosis —*see* Osteoporosis,
    postmenopausal
Postnasal drip R09.82
  due to
    allergic rhinitis —*see* Rhinitis, allergic
    common cold J00
    gastroesophageal reflux —*see* Reflux,
      gastroesophageal
    nasopharyngitis —*see* Nasopharyngitis
    other know condition — code to condition
    sinusitis —*see* Sinusitis
Postnatal —*see* condition
Postoperative (postprocedural) —*see*
  Complication, postoperative
  pneumothorax, therapeutic Z98.3
  state NEC Z98.890
Postpancreatectomy hyperglycemia E89.1
Postpartum —*see* Puerperal
Postphlebitic syndrome —*see* Syndrome,
  postthrombotic
Postpolio (myelitic) syndrome G14
Postpoliomyelitic —*see also* condition
  osteopathy —*see* Osteopathy, after
    poliomyelitis
Postprocedural —*see also* Postoperative
  hypoinsulinemia E89.1
Postschizophrenic depression F32.89
Postsurgery status —*see also* Status (post)
  pneumothorax, therapeutic Z98.3
Post-term (40-42 weeks) (pregnancy) (mother)
  O48.0
  infant P08.21
  more than 42 weeks gestation (mother) O48.1
Post-traumatic brain syndrome, nonpsychotic
  F07.81
Post-typhoid abscess A01.09
Postures, hysterical F44.2
Postvaccinal reaction or complication —*see*
  Complications, vaccination
Postvalvulotomy syndrome I97.0
Potain's
  disease (pulmonary edema) —*see* Edema, lung
  syndrome (gastrectasis with dyspepsia) K31.0
Potter's
  asthma J62.8
  facies Q60.6
  lung J62.8
  syndrome (with renal agenesis) Q60.6
Pott's
  curvature (spinal) A18.01
  disease or paraplegia A18.01
  spinal curvature A18.01
  tumor, puffy —*see* Osteomyelitis, specified
    type NEC
Pouch
  bronchus Q32.4
  Douglas' —*see* condition
  esophagus, esophageal, congenital Q39.6
    acquired K22.5
  gastric K31.4
  Hartmann's K82.8
  pharynx, pharyngeal (congenital) Q38.7
Pouchitis K91.850
Poultrymen's itch B88.0
Poverty NEC Z59.6
  extreme Z59.5
Poxvirus NEC B08.8

Prader-Willi syndrome Q87.1
Preauricular appendage or tag Q17.0
Prebetalipoproteinemia (acquired) (essential)
  (familial) (hereditary) (primary)
  (secondary) E78.1
  with chylomicronemia E78.3
Precipitate labor or delivery O62.3
Preclimacteric bleeding (menorrhagia) N92.4
Precocious
  adrenarche E30.1
  menarche E30.1
  menstruation E30.1
  pubarche E30.1
  puberty E30.1
    central E22.8
  sexual development NEC E30.1
  thelarche E30.8
Precocity, sexual (constitutional) (cryptogenic)
  (female) (idiopathic) (male) E30.1
  with adrenal hyperplasia E25.9
    congenital E25.0
Precordial pain R07.2
Predeciduous teeth K00.2
Prediabetes, prediabetic R73.03
  complicating
    pregnancy —*see* Pregnancy, complicated
      by, diseases of, specified type or
      system NEC
    puerperium O99.89
Predislocation status of hip at birth Q65.6
Pre-eclampsia O14.9-●
  with pre-existing hypertension —*see*
    Hypertension, complicating pregnancy,
    pre-existing, with, pre-eclampsia
  complicating
    childbirth O14.94
    puerperium O14.95
  mild O14.0-●
    complicating
      childbirth O14.04
      puerperium O14.05
  moderate O14.0-●
    complicating
      childbirth O14.04
      puerperium O14.05
  severe O14.1-●
    with hemolysis, elevated liver enzymes
      and low platelet count (HELLP)
      O14.2-●
    complicating
      childbirth O14.24
      puerperium O14.25
    complicating
      childbirth O14.14
      puerperium O14.15
Pre-eruptive color change, teeth, tooth
  K00.8
Pre-excitation atrioventricular conduction
  I45.6
Preglaucoma H40.00-●
Pregnancy (single) (uterine) —*see also* Delivery
  and Puerperal

> Note: The Tabular must be reviewed for assignment of the appropriate character indicating the trimester of the pregnancy
>
> Note: The Tabular must be reviewed for assignment of appropriate seventh character for multiple gestation codes in Chapter 15

  abdominal (ectopic) O00.00
    with intrauterine pregnancy O00.01
    with viable fetus O36.7-●
  ⇒ampullar O00.10-●
    ⇒with intrauterine pregnancy O00.11-●
    biochemical O02.81
    broad ligament O00.80
      with intrauterine pregnancy O00.81
    cervical O00.80
      with intrauterine pregnancy O00.81

Pregnancy *(Continued)*
  chemical O02.81
  complicated NOS O26.9-●
  complicated by (care of) (management affected by)
    abnormal, abnormality
      cervix O34.4-●
        causing obstructed labor O65.5
      cord (umbilical) O69.9
      ▶fetal heart rate or rhythm O36.83-●
      findings on antenatal screening of mother O28.9
        biochemical O28.1
        chromosomal O28.5
        cytological O28.2
        genetic O28.5
        hematological O28.0
        radiological O28.4
        specified NEC O28.8
        ultrasonic O28.3
      glucose (tolerance) NEC O99.810
      pelvic organs O34.9-●
        specified NEC O34.8-●
          causing obstructed labor O65.5
      pelvis (bony) (major) NEC O33.0
      perineum O34.7-●
      position
        placenta O44.0-●
          with hemorrhage O44.1-●
        uterus O34.59-●
      uterus O34.59-●
        causing obstructed labor O65.5
        congenital O34.0-●
      vagina O34.6-●
        causing obstructed labor O65.5
      vulva O34.7-●
        causing obstructed labor O65.5
    abruptio placentae —*see* Abruptio placentae
    abscess or cellulitis
      bladder O23.1-●
      breast O91.11-●
      genital organ or tract O23.9-●
    abuse
      physical O9A.31-●
      psychological O9A.51-●
      sexual O9A.41-●
    adverse effect anesthesia O29.9-●
      aspiration pneumonitis O29.01-●
      cardiac arrest O29.11-●
      cardiac complication NEC O29.19-●
      cardiac failure O29.12-●
      central nervous system complication NEC O29.29-●
      cerebral anoxia O29.21-●
      failed or difficult intubation O29.6-●
      inhalation of stomach contents or secretions NOS O29.01-●
      local, toxic reaction O29.3X
      Mendelson's syndrome O29.01-●
      pressure collapse of lung O29.02-●
      pulmonary complications NEC O29.09-●
      specified NEC O29.8X
      spinal and epidural type NEC O29.5X
        induced headache O29.4-●
    albuminuria —*see also* Proteinuria, gestational O12.1-●
    alcohol use O99.31-●
    amnionitis O41.12-●
    anaphylactoid syndrome of pregnancy O88.01-●
    anemia (conditions in D50-D64) (pre-existing) O99.01-●
      complicating the puerperium O99.03
    antepartum hemorrhage O46.9-●
      with coagulation defect —*see* Hemorrhage, antepartum, with coagulation defect
      specified NEC O46.8X-●
    appendicitis O99.61-●
    atrophy (yellow) (acute) liver (subacute) O26.61-●

Pregnancy *(Continued)*
  complicated by *(Continued)*
    bariatric surgery status O99.84-●
    bicornis or bicornuate uterus O34.0-●
    biliary tract problems O26.61-●
    breech presentation O32.1
    cardiovascular diseases (conditions in I00-I09, I20-I52, I70-I99) O99.41-●
    cerebrovascular disorders (conditions in I60-I69) O99.41-●
    cervical shortening O26.87-●
    cervicitis O23.51-●
    chloasma (gravidarum) O26.89-●
    cholecystitis O99.61-●
    cholestasis (intrahepatic) O26.61-●
    chorioamnionitis O41.12-●
    circulatory system disorder (conditions in I00-I09, I20-I99, O99.41-●)
    compound presentation O32.6
    conjoined twins O30.02-●
    connective system disorders (conditions in M00-M99) O99.89
    contracted pelvis (general) O33.1
      inlet O33.2
      outlet O33.3
    convulsions (eclamptic) (uremic) —*see also* Eclampsia O15.9-●
    cracked nipple O92.11-●
    cystitis O23.1-●
    cystocele O34.8-●
    death of fetus (near term) O36.4
      early pregnancy O02.1
      of one fetus or more in multiple gestation O31.2-●
    deciduitis O41.14-●
    decreased fetal movement O36.81-●
    dental problems O99.61-●
    diabetes (mellitus) O24.91-●
      gestational (pregnancy induced) —*see* Diabetes, gestational
      pre-existing O24.31-●
        specified NEC O24.81-●
        type 1 O24.01-●
        type 2 O24.11-●
    digestive system disorders (conditions in K00-K93) O99.61-●
    diseases of —*see* Pregnancy, complicated by, specified body system disease
      biliary tract O26.61-●
      blood NEC (conditions in D65-D77) O99.11-●
      liver O26.61-●
      specified NEC O99.89
    disorders of —*see* Pregnancy, complicated by, specified body system disorder
      amniotic fluid and membranes O41.9-●
        specified NEC O41.8X-●
      biliary tract O26.61-●
      ear and mastoid process (conditions in H60-H95) O99.89
      eye and adnexa (conditions in H00-H59) O99.89
      liver O26.61-●
      skin (conditions in L00-L99) O99.71-●
      specified NEC O99.89
    displacement, uterus NEC O34.59-●
      causing obstructed labor O65.5
    disproportion (due to) O33.9
      fetal (ascites) (hydrops) (meningomyelocele) (sacral teratoma) (tumor) deformities NEC O33.7
      generally contracted pelvis O33.1
      hydrocephalic fetus O33.6
      inlet contraction of pelvis O33.2
      mixed maternal and fetal origin O33.4
      specified NEC O33.8
    double uterus O34.0-●
      causing obstructed labor O65.5
    drug use (conditions in F11-F19) O99.32-●

Pregnancy *(Continued)*
  complicated by *(Continued)*
    eclampsia, eclamptic (coma) (convulsions) (delirium) (nephritis) (uremia) (*see also* Eclampsia) O15-●
    ectopic pregnancy —*see* Pregnancy, ectopic
    edema O12.0-●
      with
        gestational hypertension, mild —*see also* Pre-eclampsia O14.0-●
        proteinuria O12.2-●
    effusion, amniotic fluid —*see* Pregnancy, complicated by, premature rupture of membranes
    elderly
      multigravida O09.52-●
      primigravida O09.51-●
    embolism —*see also* Embolism, obstetric, pregnancy O88.-●
    endocrine diseases NEC O99.28-●
    endometritis O86.12
    excessive weight gain O26.0-●
    exhaustion O26.81-●
      during labor and delivery O75.81
    face presentation O32.3
    failed induction of labor O61.9
    failed or difficult intubation for anesthesia O29.6-●
      instrumental O61.1
      mechanical O61.1
      medical O61.0
      specified NEC O61.8
      surgical O61.1
    false labor (pains) O47.9
      at or after 37 completed weeks of pregnancy O47.1
      before 37 completed weeks of pregnancy O47.0-●
    fatigue O26.81-●
      during labor and delivery O75.81
    fatty metamorphosis of liver O26.61-●
    female genital mutilation O34.8-● *[N90.81-●]*
    fetal (maternal care for)
      abnormality or damage O35.9
        acid-base balance O68
        specified type NEC O35.8
      acidemia O68
      acidosis O68
      alkalosis O68
      anemia and thrombocytopenia O36.82-●
      anencephaly O35.0
      chromosomal abnormality (conditions in Q90-Q99) O35.1
      conjoined twins O30.02-●
      damage from
        amniocentesis O35.7
        biopsy procedures O35.7
        drug addiction O35.5
        hematological investigation O35.7
        intrauterine contraceptive device O35.7
        maternal
          alcohol addiction O35.4
          cytomegalovirus infection O35.3
          disease NEC O35.8
          drug addiction O35.5
          listeriosis O35.8
          rubella O35.3
          toxoplasmosis O35.8
          viral infection O35.3
        medical procedure NEC O35.7
        radiation O35.6
      death (near term) O36.4
        early pregnancy O02.1
      decreased movement O36.81-●
      disproportion due to deformity (fetal) O33.7
      excessive growth (large for dates) O36.6-●
      growth retardation O36.59-●
        light for dates O36.59-●
        small for dates O36.59-●

Pregnancy (Continued)
  complicated by (Continued)
    fetal (Continued)
      heart rate irregularity (bradycardia)
        (decelerations) (tachycardia) O76
      hereditary disease O35.2
      hydrocephalus O35.0
      intrauterine death O36.4
      poor growth O36.59-●
       light for dates O36.59-●
       small for dates O36.59-●
      problem O36.9-●
       specified NEC O36.89-●
      reduction (elective) O31.3-●
      selective termination O31.3-●
      spina bifida O35.0
      thrombocytopenia O36.82-●
    fibroid (tumor) (uterus) O34.1-●
    fissure of nipple O92.11-●
    gallstones O99.61-●
    gastric banding status O99.84-●
    gastric bypass status O99.84-●
➡   genital herpes (asymptomatic) (history of)
      (inactive) O98.3-●
    genital tract infection O23.9-●
    glomerular diseases (conditions in
      N00-N07) O26.83-●
      with hypertension, pre-existing —see
        Hypertension, complicating,
        pregnancy, pre-existing, with, renal
        disease
    gonorrhea O98.21-●
    grand multiparity O09.4
    habitual aborter —see Pregnancy,
      complicated by, recurrent pregnancy
      loss
    HELLP syndrome (hemolysis, elevated
      liver enzymes and low platelet count)
      O14.2-●
    hemorrhage
      antepartum —see Hemorrhage,
        antepartum
      before 20 completed weeks gestation
        O20.9
        specified NEC O20.8
      due to premature separation, placenta —
        see also Abruptio placentae O45.9-●
      early O20.9
        specified NEC O20.8
      threatened abortion O20.0
    hemorrhoids O22.4-●
    hepatitis (viral) O98.41-●
    herniation of uterus O34.59-●
    high
      head at term O32.4
      risk —see Supervision (of) (for), high-risk
    history of in utero procedure during
      previous pregnancy O09.82-●
    HIV O98.71-●
    human immunodeficiency virus (HIV)
      disease O98.71-●
    hydatidiform mole —see also Mole,
      hydatidiform O01.9-●
    hydramnios O40.-●
    hydrocephalic fetus (disproportion) O33.6
    hydrops
      amnii O40.-●
      fetalis O36.2-●
       associated with isoimmunization —see
        also Pregnancy, complicated by,
        isoimmunization O36.11-●
    hydrorrhea O42.90
    hyperemesis (gravidarum) (mild) —see also
      Hyperemesis, gravidarum O21.0-●
    hypertension —see Hypertension,
      complicating pregnancy
    hypertensive
      heart and renal disease, pre-existing —
        see Hypertension, complicating,
        pregnancy, pre-existing, with, heart
        disease, with renal disease

Pregnancy (Continued)
  complicated by (Continued)
    hypertensive (Continued)
      heart disease, pre-existing —see
        Hypertension, complicating,
        pregnancy, pre-existing, with, heart
        disease
      renal disease, pre-existing —see
        Hypertension, complicating,
        pregnancy, pre-existing, with, renal
        disease
    hypotension O26.5-●
    immune disorders NEC (conditions in
      D80-D89) O99.11-●
    incarceration, uterus O34.51-●
    incompetent cervix O34.3-●
    inconclusive fetal viability O36.80
    infection(s) O98.91-●
      amniotic fluid or sac O41.10-●
      bladder O23.1-●
      carrier state NEC O99.830
       streptococcus B O99.820
      genital organ or tract O23.9-●
       specified NEC O23.59-●
      genitourinary tract O23.9-●
      gonorrhea O98.21-●
      hepatitis (viral) O98.41-●
      HIV O98.71-●
      human immunodeficiency virus (HIV)
       O98.71-●
      kidney O23.0-●
      nipple O91.01-●
      parasitic disease O98.91-●
       specified NEC O98.81-●
      protozoal disease O98.61-●
      sexually transmitted NEC O98.31-●
      specified type NEC O98.81-●
      syphilis O98.11-●
      tuberculosis O98.01-●
      urethra O23.2-●
      urinary (tract) O23.4-●
       specified NEC O23.3-●
      viral disease O98.51-●
    injury or poisoning (conditions in S00-T88)
      O9A.21-●
      due to abuse
       physical O9A.31-●
       psychological O9A.51-●
       sexual O9A.41-●
    insufficient
      prenatal care O09.3-●
      weight gain O26.1-●
    insulin resistance O26.89
    intrauterine fetal death (near term) O36.4
      early pregnancy O02.1
      multiple gestation (one fetus or more)
       O31.2-●
    isoimmunization O36.11-●
      anti-A sensitization O36.11-●
      anti-B sensitization O36.19-●
      Rh O36.09-●
       anti-D antibody O36.01-●
      specified NEC O36.19-●
    laceration of uterus NEC O71.81
    malformation
      placenta, placental (vessel) O43.10-●
       specified NEC O43.19-●
      uterus (congenital) O34.0-●
    malnutrition (conditions in E40-E46)
      O25.1-●
    maternal hypotension syndrome O26.5-●
    mental disorders (conditions in F01-F09,
      F20-F99) O99.34-●
      alcohol use O99.31-●
      drug use O99.32-●
      smoking O99.33-●
    mentum presentation O32.3
    metabolic disorders O99.28-●
    missed
      abortion O02.1
      delivery O36.4

Pregnancy (Continued)
  complicated by (Continued)
    multiple gestations O30.9-●
      conjoined twins O30.02-●
      quadruplet —see Pregnancy, quadruplet
      specified complication NEC O31.8X-●
      specified number of multiples NEC —see
        Pregnancy, multiple (gestation),
        specified NEC
      triplet —see Pregnancy, triplet
      twin —see Pregnancy, twin
    musculoskeletal condition (conditions is
      M00-M99) O99.89
    necrosis, liver (conditions in K72)
      O26.61-●
    neoplasm
      benign
       cervix O34.4-●
       corpus uteri O34.1-●
       uterus O34.1-●
      malignant O9A.11-●
    nephropathy NEC O26.83-●
    nervous system condition (conditions in
      G00-G99) O99.35-●
    nutritional diseases NEC O99.28-●
    obesity (pre-existing) O99.21-●
    obesity surgery status O99.84-●
    oblique lie or presentation O32.2
    older mother —see Pregnancy, complicated
      by, elderly
    oligohydramnios O41.0-●
      with premature rupture of
        membranes —see also Pregnancy,
        complicated by, premature rupture
        of membranes O42-●
    onset (spontaneous) of labor after 37
      completed weeks of gestation but
      before 39 completed weeks gestation,
      with delivery by (planned) cesarean
      section O75.82
    oophoritis O23.52-●
    overdose, drug —see also Table of Drugs
      and Chemicals, by drug, poisoning
      O9A.21-●
    oversize fetus O33.5
    papyraceous fetus O31.0-●
    pelvic inflammatory disease O99.89
    periodontal disease O99.61-●
    peripheral neuritis O26.82-●
    peritoneal (pelvic) adhesions O99.89
    phlebitis O22.9-●
    phlebopathy O22.9-●
    phlebothrombosis (superficial) O22.2-●
      deep O22.3-●
    placenta accreta O43.21-●
    placenta increta O43.22-●
    placenta percreta O43.23-●
    placenta previa O44.0-●
      complete O44.0-●
       with hemorrhage O44.1-●
      marginal O44.2-●
       with hemorrhage O44.3-●
      partial O44.2-●
       with hemorrhage O44.3-●
    placental disorder O43.9-●
      specified NEC O43.89-●
    placental dysfunction O43.89-●
    placental infarction O43.81-●
    placental insufficiency O36.51-●
    placental transfusion syndromes
      fetomaternal O43.01-●
      fetus to fetus O43.02-●
      maternofetal O43.01-●
    placentitis O41.14-●
    pneumonia O99.51-●
    poisoning —see also Table of Drugs and
      Chemicals O9A.21-●
    polyhydramnios O40-●
    polymorphic eruption of pregnancy
      O26.86
    poor obstetric history NEC O09.29-●

▶ New   ➡ Revised   ~~deleted~~ Deleted   ● Use Additional Character(s)

Pregnancy *(Continued)*
  complicated by *(Continued)*
    postmaturity (post-term) (40 to 42 weeks) O48.0
      more than 42 completed weeks gestation (prolonged) O48.1
    pre-eclampsia O14.9-●
      mild O14.0-●
      moderate O14.0-●
      severe O14.1-●
        with hemolysis, elevated liver enzymes and low platelet count (HELLP) O14.2-●
    premature labor —*see* Pregnancy, complicated by, preterm labor
    premature rupture of membranes O42.90
      full-term, unspecified as to length of time between rupture and onset of labor O42.92
      with onset of labor
        within 24 hours O42.00
          at or after 37 weeks gestation, onset of labor within 24 hours of rupture O42.02
          pre-term (before 37 completed weeks of gestation) O42.01-●
        after 24 hours O42.10
          at or after 37 weeks gestation, onset of labor more than 24 hours following rupture O42.12
          pre-term (before 37 completed weeks of gestation) O42.11-●
      at or after 37 weeks gestation, unspecified as to length of time between rupture and onset of labor O42.92
      pre-term (before 37 completed weeks of gestation) O42.91-●
    premature separation of placenta —*see also* Abruptio placentae O45.9-●
    presentation, fetal —*see* Delivery, complicated by, malposition
    preterm delivery O60.10
    preterm labor
      with delivery O60.10
        preterm O60.10
        term O60.20
      second trimester
        with preterm delivery
          second trimester O60.12
          third trimester O60.13
        with term delivery O60.22
        without delivery O60.02
      third trimester
        with term delivery O60.23
        with third trimester preterm delivery O60.14
        without delivery O60.03
      without delivery O60.00
        second trimester O60.02
        third trimester O60.03
    previous history of —*see* Pregnancy, supervision of, high-risk
    prolapse, uterus O34.52-●
    proteinuria (gestational) —*see also* Proteinuria, gestational O12.1-●
      with edema O12.2-●
    pruritic urticarial papules and plaques of pregnancy (PUPPP) O26.86
    pruritus (neurogenic) O26.89-●
    psychosis or psychoneurosis (puerperal) F53
    ptyalism O26.89-●
    PUPPP (pruritic urticarial papules and plaques of pregnancy) O26.86
    pyelitis O23.0-●
    recurrent pregnancy loss O26.2-●

Pregnancy *(Continued)*
  complicated by *(Continued)*
    renal disease or failure NEC O26.83-●
      with secondary hypertension, pre-existing —*see* Hypertension, complicating, pregnancy, pre-existing, secondary
      hypertensive, pre-existing —*see* Hypertension, complicating, pregnancy, pre-existing, with, renal disease
    respiratory condition (conditions in J00-J99) O99.51-●
    retained, retention
      dead ovum O02.0
      intrauterine contraceptive device O26.3-●
    retroversion, uterus O34.53-●
    Rh immunization, incompatibility or sensitization NEC O36.09-●
      anti-D antibody O36.01-●
    rupture
      amnion (premature) —*see also* Pregnancy, complicated by, premature rupture of membranes O42-●
      membranes (premature) —*see also* Pregnancy, complicated by, premature rupture of membranes O42-●
      uterus (during labor) O71.1
        before onset of labor O71.0-●
    salivation (excessive) O26.89-●
    salpingitis O23.52-●
    salpingo-oophoritis O23.52-●
    sepsis (conditions in A40, A41) O98.81-●
    size date discrepancy (uterine) O26.84-●
    skin condition (conditions in L00-L99) O99.71-●
    smoking (tobacco) O99.33-●
    social problem O09.7-●
    specified condition NEC O26.89-●
    spotting O26.85-●
    streptococcus group B (GBS) carrier state O99.820
    subluxation of symphysis (pubis) O26.71-●
    syphilis (conditions in A50-A53) O98.11-●
    threatened
      abortion O20.0
      labor O47.9
        at or after 37 completed weeks of gestation O47.1
        before 37 completed weeks of gestation O47.0-●
    thrombophlebitis (superficial) O22.2-●
    thrombosis O22.9-●
      cerebral venous O22.5-●
      cerebrovenous sinus O22.5-●
      deep O22.3-●
    tobacco use disorder (smoking) O99.33-●
    torsion of uterus O34.59-●
    toxemia O14.9-●
    transverse lie or presentation O32.2
    tuberculosis (conditions in A15-A19) O98.01-●
    tumor (benign)
      cervix O34.4-●
      malignant O9A.11-●
      uterus O34.1-●
    unstable lie O32.0
    upper respiratory infection O99.51-●
    urethritis O23.2-●
    uterine size date discrepancy O26.84-●
    vaginitis or vulvitis O23.59-●
    varicose veins (lower extremities) O22.0-●
      genitals O22.1-●
      legs O22.0-●
      perineal O22.1-●
      vaginal or vulval O22.1-●
    venereal disease NEC (conditions in A63.8) O98.31-●

Pregnancy *(Continued)*
  complicated by *(Continued)*
    venous disorders O22.9-●
      specified NEC O22.8X-●
    very young mother —*see* Pregnancy, complicated by, young mother
    viral diseases (conditions in A80-B09, B25-B34) O98.51-●
    vomiting O21.9
      due to diseases classified elsewhere O21.8
      hyperemesis gravidarum (mild) —*see also* Hyperemesis, gravidarum O21.0-●
      late (occurring after 20 weeks of gestation) O21.2
    young mother
      multigravida O09.62-●
      primigravida O09.61-●
  concealed O09.3-●
  continuing following
    elective fetal reduction of one or more fetus O31.3-●
    intrauterine death of one or more fetus O31.2-●
    spontaneous abortion of one or more fetus O31.1-●
  cornual O00.80
    with intrauterine pregnancy O00.81
  ectopic (ruptured) O00.90
    with intrauterine pregnancy O00.91
    abdominal O00.00
      with
        intrauterine pregnancy O00.01
        viable fetus O36.7-●
    cervical O00.80
      with intrauterine pregnancy O00.81
    complicated (by) O08.9
      afibrinogenemia O08.1
      cardiac arrest O08.81
      chemical damage of pelvic organ(s) O08.6
      circulatory collapse O08.3
      defibrination syndrome O08.1
      electrolyte imbalance O08.5
      embolism (amniotic fluid) (blood clot) (pulmonary) (septic) O08.2
      endometritis O08.0
      genital tract and pelvic infection O08.0
      hemorrhage (delayed) (excessive) O08.1
      infection
        genital tract or pelvic O08.0
        kidney 008.83
        urinary tract O08.83
      intravascular coagulation O08.1
      laceration of pelvic organ(s) O08.6
      metabolic disorder O08.5
      oliguria O08.4
      oophoritis O08.0
      parametritis O08.0
      pelvic peritonitis O08.0
      perforation of pelvic organ(s) O08.6
      renal failure or shutdown O08.4
      salpingitis or salpingo-oophoritis O08.0
      sepsis O08.82
      shock O08.83
        septic O08.82
      specified condition NEC O08.89
      tubular necrosis (renal) O08.4
      uremia O08.4
      urinary infection O08.83
      venous complication NEC O08.7
        embolism O08.2
    cornual O00.80
      with intrauterine pregnancy O00.81
    intraligamentous O00.80
      with intrauterine pregnancy O00.81

Pregnancy (*Continued*)
  ectopic (*Continued*)
    mural O00.80
      with intrauterine pregnancy O00.81
    ➡ovarian O00.20-●
      ➡with intrauterine pregnancy O00.21-●
    specified site NEC O00.80
      with intrauterine pregnancy O00.81
    ➡tubal (ruptured) O00.10-●
      ➡with intrauterine pregnancy O00.11-●
  examination (normal) Z34.9-●
    first Z34.0-●
    high-risk —*see* Pregnancy, supervision of,
      high-risk
    specified Z34.8-●
  extrauterine —*see* Pregnancy, ectopic
  ➡fallopian O00.10-●
    ➡with intrauterine pregnancy O00.11-●
  false F45.8
  gestational carrier Z33.3
  hidden O09.3-●
  high-risk —*see* Pregnancy, supervision of,
    high-risk
  incidental finding Z33.1
  interstitial O00.80
    with intrauterine pregnancy O00.81
  intraligamentous O00.80
    with intrauterine pregnancy O00.81
  intramural O00.80
    with intrauterine pregnancy O00.81
  intraperitoneal O00.00
    with intrauterine pregnancy O00.01
  ➡isthmian O00.10-●
    ➡with intrauterine pregnancy O00.11-●
  mesometric (mural) O00.80
    with intrauterine pregnancy O00.81
  molar NEC O02.0
    complicated (by) O08.9
      afibrinogenemia O08.1
      cardiac arrest O08.81
      chemical damage of pelvic organ(s)
        O08.6
      circulatory collapse O08.3
      defibrination syndrome O08.1
      electrolyte imbalance O08.5
      embolism (amniotic fluid) (blood clot)
        (pulmonary) (septic) O08.2
      endometritis O08.0
      genital tract and pelvic infection
        O08.0
      hemorrhage (delayed) (excessive)
        O08.1
      infection
        genital tract or pelvic O08.0
        kidney O08.83
        urinary tract O08.83
      intravascular coagulation O08.1
      laceration of pelvic organ(s)
        O08.6
      metabolic disorder O08.5
      oliguria O08.4
      oophoritis O08.0
      parametritis O08.0
      pelvic peritonitis O08.0
      perforation of pelvic organ(s) O08.6
      renal failure or shutdown O08.4
      salpingitis or salpingo-oophoritis O08.0
      sepsis O08.82
      shock O08.3
        septic O08.82
      specified condition NEC O08.89
      tubular necrosis (renal) O08.4
      uremia O08.4
      urinary infection O08.83
      venous complication NEC O08.7
        embolism O08.2
    hydatidiform —*see also* Mole, hydatidiform
      O01.9-●
  multiple (gestation) O30.9-●
    greater than quadruplets —*see* Pregnancy,
      multiple (gestation), specified NEC

Pregnancy (*Continued*)
  multiple (gestation) (*Continued*)
    specified NEC O30.80-●
      with
        two or more monoamniotic fetuses
          O30.82-●
        two or more monochorionic fetuses
          O30.81-●
      two or more monoamniotic fetuses
        O30.82-●
      two or more monochorionic fetuses
        O30.81-●
      unable to determine number of placenta
        and number of amniotic sacs
        O30.89-●
      unspecified number of placenta and
        unspecified number of amniotic
        sacs O30.80-●
    mural O00.80
      with intrauterine pregnancy O00.81
    normal (supervision of) Z34.9-●
      first Z34.0-●
      high-risk —*see* Pregnancy, supervision of,
        high-risk
      specified Z34.8-●
    ➡ovarian O00.20-●
    ➡with intrauterine pregnancy O00.21-●
    postmature (40 to 42 weeks) O48.0
      more than 42 weeks gestation O48.1
    post-term (40 to 42 weeks) O48.0
    prenatal care only Z34.9-●
      first Z34.0-●
      high-risk —*see* Pregnancy, supervision of,
        high-risk
      specified Z34.8-●
    prolonged (more than 42 weeks gestation)
      O48.1
    quadruplet O30.20-●
      with
        two or more monoamniotic fetuses
          O30.22-●
        two or more monochorionic fetuses
          O30.21-●
      two or more monoamniotic fetuses O30.22-●
      two or more monochorionic fetuses
        O30.21-●
      unable to determine number of placenta
        and number of amniotic sacs O30.29-●
      unspecified number of placenta and
        unspecified number of amniotic sacs
        O30.20-●
    quintuplet —*see* Pregnancy, multiple
      (gestation), specified NEC
    sextuplet —*see* Pregnancy, multiple
      (gestation), specified NEC
    supervision of
      concealed pregnancy O09.3-●
      elderly mother
        multigravida O09.52-●
        primigravida O09.51-●
      hidden pregnancy O09.3-●
      high-risk O09.9-●
        due to (history of)
          ectopic pregnancy O09.1-●
          elderly —*see* Pregnancy, supervision,
            elderly mother
          grand multiparity O09.4
          infertility O09.0-●
          insufficient prenatal care O09.3-●
          in utero procedure during previous
            pregnancy O09.82-●
          in vitro fertilization O09.81-●
          molar pregnancy O09.A-●
          multiple previous pregnancies O09.4-●
          older mother —*see* Pregnancy,
            supervision of, elderly mother
          poor reproductive or obstetric history
            NEC O09.29-●
          pre-term labor O09.21-●
          previous
            neonatal death O09.29-●

Pregnancy (*Continued*)
  supervision of (*Continued*)
    high-risk (*Continued*)
      due to (*Continued*)
        social problems O09.7-●
        specified NEC O09.89-●
        very young mother —*see* Pregnancy,
          supervision, young mother
      resulting from in vitro fertilization
        O09.81-●
    normal Z34.9-●
      first Z34.0-●
      specified NEC Z34.8-●
    young mother
      multigravida O09.62-●
      primigravida O09.61-●
  triplet O30.10-●
    with
      two or more monoamniotic fetuses
        O30.12-●
      ~~two or more monochrorionic fetuses~~
        ~~O30.11-~~●
      ▶two or more monochorionic fetuses
        O30.11-●
    two or more monoamniotic fetuses O30.12-●
    ~~two or more monochrorionic fetuses~~
      ~~O30.11-~~●
    ▶two or more monochorionic fetuses O30.11-●
    unable to determine number of placenta
      and number of amniotic sacs O30.19-●
    unspecified number of placenta and
      unspecified number of amniotic sacs
      O30.10-●
  ➡tubal (with abortion) (with rupture) O00.10-●
    ➡with intrauterine pregnancy O00.11-●
  twin O30.00-●
    conjoined O30.02-●
    dichorionic/diamniotic (two placenta, two
      amniotic sacs) O30.04-●
    monochorionic/diamniotic (one placenta,
      two amniotic sacs) O30.03-●
    monochorionic/monoamniotic (one
      placenta, one amniotic sac) O30.01-●
    unable to determine number of placenta
      and number of amniotic sacs O30.09-●
    unspecified number of placenta and
      unspecified number of amniotic sacs
      O30.00-●
  unwanted Z64.0
  weeks of gestation
    8 weeks Z3A.08
    9 weeks Z3A.09
    10 weeks Z3A.10
    11 weeks Z3A.11
    12 weeks Z3A.12
    13 weeks Z3A.13
    14 weeks Z3A.14
    15 weeks Z3A.15
    16 weeks Z3A.16
    17 weeks Z3A.17
    18 weeks Z3A.18
    19 weeks Z3A.19
    20 weeks Z3A.20
    21 weeks Z3A.21
    22 weeks Z3A.22
    23 weeks Z3A.23
    24 weeks Z3A.24
    25 weeks Z3A.25
    26 weeks Z3A.26
    27 weeks Z3A.27
    28 weeks Z3A.28
    29 weeks Z3A.29
    30 weeks Z3A.30
    31 weeks Z3A.31
    32 weeks Z3A.32
    33 weeks Z3A.33
    34 weeks Z3A.34
    35 weeks Z3A.35
    36 weeks Z3A.36
    37 weeks Z3A.37
    38 weeks Z3A.38

    ▶ New   ➡ Revised   ~~deleted~~ Deleted   ● Use Additional Character(s)

Pregnancy *(Continued)*
  weeks of gestation *(Continued)*
    39 weeks Z3A.39
    40 weeks Z3A.40
    41 weeks Z3A.41
    42 weeks Z3A.42
    greater than 42 weeks Z3A.49
    less than 8 weeks Z3A.01
    not specified Z3A.00
Preiser's disease —*see* Osteonecrosis, secondary, due to, trauma, metacarpus
Pre-kwashiorkor —*see* Malnutrition, severe
Preleukemia (syndrome) D46.9
Preluxation, hip, congenital Q65.6
Premature —*see also* condition
  adrenarche E27.0
  aging E34.8
  beats I49.40
    atrial I49.1
    auricular I49.1
    supraventricular I49.1
  birth NEC —*see* Preterm, newborn
  closure, foramen ovale Q21.8
  contraction
    atrial I49.1
    atrioventricular I49.49
    auricular I49.1
    auriculoventricular I49.2
    heart (extrasystole) I49.49
    junctional I49.2
    ventricular I49.3
  delivery —*see also* Pregnancy, complicated by, preterm labor O60.10
  ejaculation F52.4
  infant NEC —*see* Preterm, newborn
    light-for-dates —*see* Light for dates
  labor —*see* Pregnancy, complicated by, preterm labor
  lungs P28.0
  menopause E28.319
    asymptomatic E28.319
    symptomatic E28.310
  newborn
    extreme (less than 28 completed weeks) — *see* Immaturity, extreme
    less than 37 completed weeks —*see* Preterm, newborn
  puberty E30.1
  rupture membranes or amnion —*see* Pregnancy, complicated by, premature rupture of membranes
  senility E34.8
  thelarche E30.8
  ventricular systole I49.3
Prematurity NEC (less than 37 completed weeks) —*see* Preterm, newborn
  extreme (less than 28 completed weeks) —*see* Immaturity, extreme
Premenstrual
  dysphoric disorder (PMDD) F32.81
  tension (syndrome) N94.3
Premolarization, cuspids K00.2
Prenatal
  care, normal pregnancy —*see* Pregnancy, normal
  screening of mother —*see also* Encounter, antenatal Z36.9
  teeth K00.6
Preparatory care for subsequent treatment NEC
  for dialysis Z49.01
    peritoneal Z49.02
Prepartum —*see* condition
Preponderance, left or right ventricular I51.7
Prepuce —*see* condition
PRES (posterior reversible encephalopathy syndrome) I67.83
Presbycardia R54
Presbycusis, presbyacusia H91.1-•
Presbyesophagus K22.8
Presbyophrenia F03
Presbyopia H52.4

Prescription of contraceptives (initial) Z30.019
  barrier Z30.018
  diaphragm Z30.018
  emergency (postcoital) Z30.012
  implantable subdermal Z30.017
  injectable Z30.013
  intrauterine contraceptive device Z30.014
  pills Z30.011
  postcoital (emergency) Z30.012
  repeat Z30.40
    barrier Z30.49
    diaphragm Z30.49
    implantable subdermal Z30.46
    injectable Z30.42
    pills Z30.41
    specified type NEC Z30.49
    transdermal patch hormonal Z30.45
    vaginal ring hormonal Z30.44
  specified type NEC Z30.018
    transdermal patch hormonal Z30.016
    vaginal ring hormonal Z30.015
Presence (of)
  ankle-joint implant (functional) (prosthesis) Z96.66-•
  aortocoronary (bypass) graft Z95.1
  arterial-venous shunt (dialysis) Z99.2
  artificial
    eye (globe) Z97.0
    heart (fully implantable) (mechanical) Z95.812
      valve Z95.2
    larynx Z96.3
    lens (intraocular) Z96.1
    limb (complete) (partial) Z97.1-•
      arm Z97.1-•
        bilateral Z97.15
      leg Z97.1-•
        bilateral Z97.16
  audiological implant (functional) Z96.29
  bladder implant (functional) Z96.0
  bone
    conduction hearing device Z96.29
    implant (functional) NEC Z96.7
    joint (prosthesis) —*see* Presence, joint implant
  cardiac
    defibrillator (functional) (with synchronous cardiac pacemaker)Z95.810
    implant or graft Z95.9
      specified type NEC Z95.818
    pacemaker Z95.0
    resynchronization therapy
      defibrillator Z95.810
      pacemaker Z95.0
  cerebrospinal fluid drainage device Z98.2
  cochlear implant (functional) Z96.21
  contact lens (es) Z97.3
  coronary artery graft or prosthesis Z95.5
  CRT-D (cardiac resynchronization therapy defibrillator) Z95.810
  CRT-P (cardiac resynchronization therapy pacemaker) Z95.0
  cardioverter-defibrillator (ICD) Z95.810
  CSF shunt Z98.2
  dental prosthesis device Z97.2
  dentures Z97.2
  device (external) NEC Z97.8
    cardiac NEC Z95.818
    heart assist Z95.811
    implanted (functional) Z96.9
      specified NEC Z96.89
    prosthetic Z97.8
  ear implant Z96.20
    cochlear implant Z96.21
    myringotomy tube Z96.22
    specified type NEC Z96.29
  elbow-joint implant (functional) (prosthesis) Z96.62-•
  endocrine implant (functional) NEC Z96.49
  eustachian tube stent or device (functional) Z96.29
  external hearing-aid or device Z97.4
  finger-joint implant (functional) (prosthetic) Z96.69-•

Presence *(Continued)*
  functional implant Z96.9
    specified NEC Z96.89
  graft
    cardiac NEC Z95.818
    vascular NEC Z95.828
  hearing-aid or device (external) Z97.4
    implant (bone) (cochlear) (functional) Z96.21
  heart assist device Z95.811
  heart valve implant (functional) Z95.2
    prosthetic Z95.2
    specified type NEC Z95.4
    xenogenic Z95.3
  hip-joint implant (functional) (prosthesis) Z96.64-•
  ICD (cardioverter-defibrillator) Z95.810
  implanted device (artificial) (functional) (prosthetic) Z96.9
    automatic cardiac defibrillator (with synchronous cardiac pacemaker) Z95.810
    cardiac pacemaker Z95.0
    cochlear Z96.21
    dental Z96.5
    heart Z95.812
    heart valve Z95.2
      prosthetic Z95.2
      specified NEC Z95.4
      xenogenic Z95.3
    insulin pump Z96.41
    intraocular lens Z96.1
    joint Z96.60
      ankle Z96.66-•
      elbow Z96.62-•
      finger Z96.69-•
      hip Z96.64-•
      knee Z96.65-•
      shoulder Z96.61-•
      specified NEC Z96.698
      wrist Z96.63-•
    larynx Z96.3
    myringotomy tube Z96.22
    otological Z96.20
      cochlear Z96.21
      eustachian stent Z96.29
      myringotomy Z96.22
      specified NEC Z96.29
      stapes Z96.29
    skin Z96.81
    skull plate Z96.7
    specified NEC Z96.89
    urogenital Z96.0
  insulin pump (functional) Z96.41
  intestinal bypass or anastomosis Z98.0
  intraocular lens (functional) Z96.1
  intrauterine contraceptive device (IUD) Z97.5
  intravascular implant (functional) (prosthetic) NEC Z95.9
    coronary artery Z95.5
    defibrillator (with synchronous cardiac pacemaker) Z95.810
    peripheral vessel (with angioplasty) Z95.820
  joint implant (prosthetic) (any) Z96.60
    ankle —*see* Presence, ankle joint implant
    elbow —*see* Presence, elbow joint implant
    finger —*see* Presence, finger joint implant
    hip —*see* Presence, hip joint implant
    knee —*see* Presence, knee joint implant
    shoulder —*see* Presence, shoulder joint implant
    specified joint NEC Z96.698
    wrist —*see* Presence, wrist joint implant
  knee-joint implant (functional) (prosthesis) Z96.65-•
  laryngeal implant (functional) Z96.3
  mandibular implant (dental) Z96.5
  myringotomy tube(s) Z96.22
  orthopedic-joint implant (prosthetic) (any) — *see* Presence, joint implant

Presence *(Continued)*
  otological implant (functional) Z96.29
  shoulder-joint implant (functional)
    (prosthesis) Z96.61-●
  skull-plate implant Z96.7
  spectacles Z97.3
  stapes implant (functional) Z96.29
  systemic lupus erythematosus [SLE] inhibitor
    D68.62
  tendon implant (functional) (graft) Z96.7
  tooth root(s) implant Z96.5
  ureteral stent Z96.0
  urethral stent Z96.0
  urogenital implant (functional) Z96.0
  vascular implant or device Z95.9
    access port device Z95.828
    specified type NEC Z95.828
  wrist-joint implant (functional) (prosthesis)
    Z96.63-●
Presenile —*see also* condition
  dementia F03
  premature aging E34.8
Presentation, fetal —*see* Delivery, complicated
  by, malposition
Prespondylolisthesis (congenital) Q76.2
Pressure
  area, skin —*see* Ulcer, pressure, by site
  brachial plexus G54.0
  brain G93.5
    injury at birth NEC P11.1
  cerebral —*see* Pressure, brain
  chest R07.89
  cone, tentorial G93.5
  hyposystolic —*see also* Hypotension
    incidental reading, without diagnosis of
      hypotension R03.1
  increased
    intracranial (benign) G93.2
      injury at birth P11.0
    intraocular H40.05-●
  lumbosacral plexus G54.1
  mediastinum J98.59
  necrosis (chronic) —*see* Ulcer, pressure,
    by site
  parental, inappropriate (excessive)
    Z62.6
  sore (chronic) —*see* Ulcer, pressure,
    by site
  spinal cord G95.20
  ulcer (chronic) —*see* Ulcer, pressure,
    by site
  venous, increased I87.8
Pre-syncope R55
Preterm
  delivery (*see also* Pregnancy, complicated by,
    preterm labor) O60.10
  labor —*see* Pregnancy, complicated by,
    preterm labor
  newborn (infant) P07.30
    gestational age
      28 completed weeks (28 weeks, 0 days
        through 28 weeks, 6 days) P07.31
      29 completed weeks (29 weeks, 0 days
        through 29 weeks, 6 days) P07.32
      30 completed weeks (30 weeks, 0 days
        through 30 weeks, 6 days) P07.33
      31 completed weeks (31 weeks, 0 days
        through 31 weeks, 6 days) P07.34
      32 completed weeks (32 weeks, 0 days
        through 32 weeks, 6 days) P07.35
      33 completed weeks (33 weeks, 0 days
        through 33 weeks, 6 days) P07.36
      34 completed weeks (34 weeks, 0 days
        through 34 weeks, 6 days) P07.37
      35 completed weeks (35 weeks, 0 days
        through 35 weeks, 6 days) P07.38
      36 completed weeks (36 weeks, 0 days
        through 36 weeks, 6 days) P07.39
Previa
  placenta (total) (without hemorrhage)
    O44.0-●

Previa *(Continued)*
  placenta *(Continued)*
    with hemorrhage O44.1-●
    complete O44.0-●
      with hemorrhage O44.1-●
    low —*see also* Delivery, complicated, by,
      placenta, low O44.4-●
      with hemorrhage O44.5-●
    marginal O44.2-●
      with hemorrhage O44.3-●
    partial O44.2-●
      with hemorrhage O44.3-●
  vasa O69.4
Priapism N48.30
  due to
    disease classified elsewhere N48.32
    drug N48.33
    specified cause NEC N48.39
    trauma N48.31
Prickling sensation (skin) R20.2
Prickly heat L74.0
Primary —*see* condition
Primigravida
  elderly, affecting management of pregnancy,
    labor and delivery (supervision only) —
    see Pregnancy, complicated by, elderly,
    primigravida
  older, affecting management of pregnancy,
    labor and delivery (supervision only) —
    see Pregnancy, complicated by, elderly,
    primigravida
  very young, affecting management of
    pregnancy, labor and delivery (supervision
    only) —*see* Pregnancy, complicated by,
    young mother, primigravida
Primipara
  elderly, affecting management of pregnancy,
    labor and delivery (supervision only) —
    see Pregnancy, complicated by, elderly,
    primigravida
  older, affecting management of pregnancy,
    labor and delivery (supervision only) —
    see Pregnancy, complicated by, elderly,
    primigravida
  very young, affecting management
    of pregnancy, labor and delivery
    (supervision only) —*see* Pregnancy,
    complicated by, young mother,
    primigravida
Primus varus (bilateral) Q66.2
PRIND (Prolonged reversible ischemic
  neurologic deficit) I63.9
Pringle's disease (tuberous sclerosis) Q85.1
Prinzmetal angina I20.1
Prizefighter ear —*see* Cauliflower ear
Problem (with) (related to)
  academic Z55.8
  acculturation Z60.3
  adjustment (to)
    change of job Z56.1
    life-cycle transition Z60.0
    pension Z60.0
    retirement Z60.0
  adopted child Z62.821
  alcoholism in family Z63.72
  atypical parenting situation Z62.9
  bankruptcy Z59.8
  behavioral (adult) F69
    drug seeking Z76.5
  birth of sibling affecting child Z62.898
  care (of)
    provider dependency Z74.9
      specified NEC Z74.8
    sick or handicapped person in family or
      household Z63.6
  child
    abuse (affecting the child) —*see*
      Maltreatment, child
    custody or support proceedings Z65.3
    in care of non-parental family member
      Z62.21

Problem *(Continued)*
  child *(Continued)*
    in foster care Z62.21
    in welfare custody Z62.21
    living in orphanage or group home Z62.22
  child-rearing Z62.9
    specified NEC Z62.898
  communication (developmental) F80.9
  conflict or discord (with)
    boss Z56.4
    classmates Z55.4
    counselor Z64.4
    employer Z56.4
    family Z63.9
      specified NEC Z63.8
    probation officer Z64.4
    social worker Z64.4
    teachers Z55.4
    workmates Z56.4
  conviction in legal proceedings Z65.0
    with imprisonment Z65.1
  counselor Z64.4
  creditors Z59.8
  digestive K92.9
  drug addict in family Z63.72
  ear —*see* Disorder, ear
  economic Z59.9
    affecting care Z59.9
    specified NEC Z59.8
  education Z55.9
    specified NEC Z55.8
  employment Z56.9
    change of job Z56.1
    discord Z56.4
    environment Z56.5
    sexual harassment Z56.81
    specified NEC Z56.89
    stress NEC Z56.6
    stressful schedule Z56.3
    threat of job loss Z56.2
    unemployment Z56.0
  enuresis, child F98.0
  eye H57.9
  failed examinations (school) Z55.2
  falling Z91.81
  family —*see also* Disruption, family Z63.9-●
    specified NEC Z63.8
  feeding (elderly) (infant) R63.3
    newborn P92.9
      breast P92.5
      overfeeding P92.4
      slow P92.2
      specified NEC P92.8
      underfeeding P92.3
    nonorganic F50.89
  finance Z59.9
    specified NEC Z59.8
  foreclosure on loan Z59.8
  foster child Z62.822
  frightening experience(s) in childhood
    Z62.898
  genital NEC
    female N94.9
    male N50.9
  health care Z75.9
    specified NEC Z75.8
  hearing —*see* Deafness
  homelessness Z59.0
  housing Z59.9
    inadequate Z59.1
    isolated Z59.8
    specified NEC Z59.8
  identity (of childhood) F93.8
  illegitimate pregnancy (unwanted) Z64.0
  illiteracy Z55.0
  impaired mobility Z74.09
  imprisonment or incarceration Z65.1
  inadequate teaching affecting education
    Z55.8
  inappropriate (excessive) parental pressure
    Z62.6

  ▶ New   ⇒ Revised   ~~deleted~~ Deleted   ● Use Additional Character(s)

Problem *(Continued)*
influencing health status NEC Z78.9
in-law Z63.1
institutionalization, affecting child
    Z62.22
intrafamilial communication Z63.8
jealousy, child F93.8
landlord Z59.2
language (developmental) F80.9
learning (developmental) F81.9
legal Z65.3
    conviction without imprisonment
        Z65.0
    imprisonment Z65.1
    release from prison Z65.2
life-management Z73.9
    specified NEC Z73.89
life-style Z72.9
    gambling Z72.6
    high-risk sexual behavior (heterosexual)
        Z72.51
        bisexual Z72.53
        homosexual Z72.52
    inappropriate eating habits Z72.4
    self-damaging behavior NEC Z72.89
    specified NEC Z72.89
    tobacco use Z72.0
literacy Z55.9
    low level Z55.0
    specified NEC Z55.8
living alone Z60.2
lodgers Z59.2
loss of love relationship in childhood
    Z62.898
marital Z63.0
    involving
        divorce Z63.5
        estrangement Z63.5
        gender identity F66
mastication K08.89
medical
    care, within family Z63.6
    facilities Z75.9
        specified NEC Z75.8
mental F48.9
multiparity Z64.1
negative life events in childhood Z62.9
    altered pattern of family relationships
        Z62.898
    frightening experience Z62.898
    loss of
        love relationship Z62.898
        self-esteem Z62.898
    physical abuse (alleged) —see
        Maltreatment, child
    removal from home Z62.29
    specified event NEC Z62.898
neighbor Z59.2
neurological NEC R29.818
new step-parent affecting child Z62.898
none (feared complaint unfounded) Z71.1
occupational NEC Z56.89
parent-child —see Conflict, parent-child
personal hygiene Z91.89
personality F69
phase-of-life transition, adjustment Z60.0
presence of sick or disabled person
    in family or household Z63.79
    needing care Z63.6
primary support group (family) Z63.9
    specified NEC Z63.8
probation officer Z64.4
psychiatric F99
psychosexual (development) F66
psychosocial Z65.9
▶religious or spiritual Z65.8
    specified NEC Z65.8
relationship Z63.9
    childhood F93.8
release from prison Z65.2
▶religious or spiritual Z65.8

Problem *(Continued)*
removal from home affecting child
    Z62.29
seeking and accepting known hazardous and
    harmful
    behavioral or psychological interventions
        Z65.8
    chemical, nutritional or physical
        interventions Z65.8
sexual function (nonorganic) F52.9
sight H54.7
sleep disorder, child F51.9
smell —see Disturbance, sensation, smell
social
    environment Z60.9
        specified NEC Z60.8
    exclusion and rejection Z60.4
    worker Z64.4
speech R47.9
    developmental F80.9
    specified NEC R47.89
swallowing —see Dysphagia
taste —see Disturbance, sensation, taste
tic, child F95.0
underachievement in school Z55.3
unemployment Z56.0
    threatened Z56.2
unwanted pregnancy Z64.0
upbringing Z62.9
    specified NEC Z62.898
urinary N39.9
voice production R47.89
work schedule (stressful) Z56.3
Procedure (surgical)
converted
    arthroscopic to open Z53.33
    laparoscopic to open Z53.31
    specified procedure NEC to open
        Z53.39
    thoracoscopic to open Z53.32
for purpose other than remedying health
    state Z41.9
    specified NEC Z41.8
not done Z53.9
    because of
        administrative reasons Z53.8
        contraindication Z53.09
            smoking Z53.01
        patient's decision Z53.20
            for reasons of belief or group pressure
                Z53.1
            left against medical advice (AMA)
                Z53.21
        specified reason NEC Z53.29
    specified reason NEC Z53.8
Procidentia (uteri) N81.3
Proctalgia K62.89
fugax K59.4
spasmodic K59.4
Proctitis K62.89
amebic (acute) A06.0
chlamydial A56.3
gonococcal A54.6
granulomatous —see Enteritis, regional, large
    intestine
herpetic A60.1
radiation K62.7
tuberculous A18.32
ulcerative (chronic) K51.20
    with
        complication K51.219
            abscess K51.214
            fistula K51.213
            obstruction K51.212
            rectal bleeding K51.211
            specified NEC K51.218
Proctocele
female (without uterine prolapse) N81.6
    with uterine prolapse N81.2
        complete N81.3
male K62.3

Proctocolitis
food-induced eosinophilic K52.82
food protein-induced K52.82
milk protein-induced K52.82
mucosal —see Rectosigmoiditis, ulcerative
Proctoptosis K62.3
Proctorrhagia K62.5
Proctosigmoiditis K63.89
ulcerative (chronic) —see Rectosigmoiditis,
    ulcerative
Proctospasm K59.4
psychogenic F45.8
Profichet's disease —see Disorder, soft tissue,
    specified type NEC
Progeria E34.8
Prognathism (mandibular) (maxillary) M26.19
Progonoma (melanotic) —see Neoplasm,
    benign, by site
Progressive —see condition
Prolactinoma
specified site —see Neoplasm, benign,
    by site
unspecified site D35.2
Prolapse, prolapsed
anus, anal (canal) (sphincter) K62.2
arm or hand O32.2
    causing obstructed labor O64.4
bladder (mucosa) (sphincter) (acquired)
    congenital Q79.4
    female —see Cystocele
    male N32.89
breast implant (prosthetic) T85.49
cecostomy K94.09
cecum K63.4
cervix, cervical (hypertrophied) N81.2
    anterior lip, obstructing labor O65.5
    congenital Q51.828
    postpartal, old N81.2
    stump N81.85
ciliary body (traumatic) —see Laceration,
    eye(ball), with prolapse or loss of
    interocular tissue
colon (pedunculated) K63.4
colostomy K94.09
disc (intervertebral) —see Displacement,
    intervertebral disc
eye implant (orbital) T85.398
    lens (ocular) —see Complications,
        intraocular lens
fallopian tube N83.4-●
gastric (mucosa) K31.89
genital, female N81.9
    specified NEC N81.89
globe, nontraumatic —see Luxation, globe
ileostomy bud K94.19
intervertebral disc —see Displacement,
    intervertebral disc
intestine (small) K63.4
iris (traumatic) —see Laceration, eye(ball),
    with prolapse or loss of interocular
    tissue
    nontraumatic H21.89
kidney N28.83
    congenital Q63.2
laryngeal muscles or ventricle J38.7
liver K76.89
meatus urinarius N36.8
mitral (valve) I34.1
ocular lens implant —see Complications,
    intraocular lens
organ or site, congenital NEC —see
    Malposition, congenital
ovary N83.4-●
pelvic floor, female N81.89
perineum, female N81.89
rectum (mucosa) (sphincter) K62.3
    due to trichuris trichuria B79
spleen D73.89
stomach K31.89
umbilical cord
    complicating delivery O69.0

Prolapse, prolapsed (Continued)
  urachus, congenital Q64.4
  ureter N28.89
    with obstruction N13.5
      with infection N13.6
  ureterovesical orifice N28.89
  urethra (acquired) (infected) (mucosa)
      N36.8
    congenital Q64.71
  urinary meatus N36.8
    congenital Q64.72
  uterovaginal N81.4
    complete N81.3
    incomplete N81.2
  uterus (with prolapse of vagina) N81.4
    complete N81.3
    congenital Q51.818
    first degree N81.2
    in pregnancy or childbirth —see
        Pregnancy, complicated by,
        abnormal, uterus
    incomplete N81.2
    postpartal (old) N81.4
    second degree N81.2
    third degree N81.3
  uveal (traumatic) —see Laceration, eye(ball),
      with prolapse or loss of interocular
      tissue
  vagina (anterior) (wall) —see Cystocele
    with prolapse of uterus N81.4
      complete N81.3
      incomplete N81.2
    posterior wall N81.6
    posthysterectomy N99.3
  vitreous (humor) H43.0-●
    in wound —see Laceration, eye(ball), with
        prolapse or loss of interocular tissue
  womb —see Prolapse, uterus
Prolapsus, female N81.9
  specified NEC N81.89
Proliferation(s)
  primary cutaneous CD30-positive large T-cell
      C86.6
  prostate, atypical small acinar N42.32
Proliferative —see condition
Prolonged, prolongation (of)
  bleeding (time) (idiopathic) R79.1
  coagulation (time) R79.1
  gestation (over 42 completed weeks)
    mother O48.1
    newborn P08.22
  interval I44.0
  labor O63.9
    first stage O63.0
    second stage O63.1
  partial thromboplastin time (PTT) R79.1
  pregnancy (more than 42 weeks gestation)
      O48.1
  prothrombin time R79.1
  QT interval I45.81
  uterine contractions in labor O62.4
Prominence, prominent
  with disproportion (fetopelvic) O33.0
    causing obstructed labor O65.0
  auricle (congenital) (ear) Q17.5
  ischial spine or sacral promontory
  nose (congenital) acquired M95.0
Promiscuity —see High, risk, sexual behavior
Pronation
  ankle —see Deformity, limb, foot, specified
      NEC
  foot —see also Deformity, limb, foot, specified
      NEC
    congenital Q74.2
Prophylactic
  administration of
    antibiotics, long-term Z79.2
      short-term use - omit code
    drug —see also Long-term (current) drug
        therapy (use of) Z79.899-●
  medication Z79.899

Prophylactic (Continued)
  organ removal (for neoplasia management)
      Z40.00
    breast Z40.01
    ▶fallopian tube(s) Z40.03
      ▶with ovary(s) Z40.02
    ⇒ovary(s) Z40.02
    specified site NEC Z40.09
  surgery Z40.9
    for risk factors related to malignant
        neoplasm —see Prophylactic, organ
        removal
    specified NEC Z40.8
  vaccination Z23
Propionic acidemia E71.121
Proptosis (ocular) —see also Exophthalmos
  thyroid —see Hyperthyroidism, with goiter
Prosecution, anxiety concerning Z65.3
Prosopagnosia R48.3
Prostadynia N42.81
Prostate, prostatic —see condition
Prostatism —see Hyperplasia, prostate
Prostatitis (congestive) (suppurative) (with
      cystitis) N41.9
  acute N41.0
  cavitary N41.8
  chronic N41.1
  diverticular N41.8
  due to Trichomonas (vaginalis) A59.02
  fibrous N41.1
  gonococcal (acute) (chronic) A54.22
  granulomatous N41.4
  hypertrophic N41.1
  subacute N41.1
  trichomonal A59.02
  tuberculous A18.14
Prostatocystitis N41.3
Prostatorrhea N42.89
Prostatosis N42.82
Prostration R53.83
  heat —see also Heat, exhaustion
    anhydrotic T67.3
    due to
      salt (and water) depletion T67.4
      water depletion T67.3
  nervous F48.8
  senile R54
Protanomaly (anomalous trichromat) H53.54
Protanopia (complete) (incomplete) H53.54
Protection (against) (from) —see Prophylactic
Protein
  deficiency NEC —see Malnutrition
  malnutrition —see Malnutrition
  sickness —see also Reaction, serum T80.69
Proteinemia R77.9
Proteinosis
  alveolar (pulmonary) J84.01
  lipid or lipoid (of Urbach) E78.89
Proteinuria R80.9
  Bence Jones R80.3
  complicating pregnancy —see Proteinuria,
      gestational
  gestational
    complicating
      childbirth O12.14
      pregnancy O12.1-●
        with edema O12.2-●
      puerperium O12.15
  idiopathic R80.0
  isolated R80.0
    with glomerular lesion N06.9
      dense deposit disease N06.6
      diffuse
        crescentic glomerulonephritis N06.7
        endocapillary proliferative
            glomerulonephritis N06.4
        mesangiocapillary glomerulonephritis
            N06.5
      focal and segmental hyalinosis or
          sclerosis N06.1
      membranous (diffuse) N06.2

Proteinuria (Continued)
  isolated (Continued)
    with glomerular lesion (Continued)
      mesangial proliferative (diffuse)
          N06.3
      minimal change N06.0
      specified pathology NEC N06.8
  orthostatic R80.2
    with glomerular lesion —see Proteinuria,
        isolated, with glomerular lesion
  persistent R80.1
    with glomerular lesion —see Proteinuria,
        isolated, with glomerular lesion
  postural R80.2
    with glomerular lesion —see Proteinuria,
        isolated, with glomerular lesion
  pre-eclamptic —see Pre-eclampsia
  puerperal O12.15
  specified type NEC R80.8
Proteolysis, pathologic D65
Proteus (mirabilis) (morganii), as cause of
      disease classified elsewhere B96.4
Prothrombin gene mutation D68.52
Protoporphyria, erythropoietic E80.0
Protozoal —see also condition
  disease B64
    specified NEC B60.8
Protrusion, protrusio
  acetabuli M24.7
  acetabulum (into pelvis) M24.7
  device, implant or graft —see also
      Complications, by site and type,
      mechanical T85.698
    arterial graft NEC —see Complication,
        cardiovascular device, mechanical,
        vascular
    breast (implant) T85.49
    catheter NEC T85.698
      cystostomy T83.090
      dialysis (renal) T82.49
        intraperitoneal T85.691
      infusion NEC T82.594
        spinal (epidural) (subdural)
            T85.690
      urinary —see also Complications,
          catheter, urinary T83.098
    electronic (electrode) (pulse generator)
        (stimulator)
      bone T84.390
      nervous system —see Complication,
          prosthetic device, mechanical,
          electronic nervous system
          stimulator
    fixation, internal (orthopedic) NEC —
        see Complication, fixation device,
        mechanical
    gastrointestinal —see Complications,
        prosthetic device, mechanical,
        gastrointestinal device
    genital NEC T83.498
      intrauterine contraceptive device
          T83.39
      penile prosthesis (cylinder) (implanted)
          (pump) (resevoir) T83.490
      testicular prosthesis T83.491
    heart NEC —see Complication,
        cardiovascular device, mechanical
    joint prosthesis —see Complications, joint
        prosthesis, mechanical, specified NEC,
        by site
    ocular NEC —see Complications, prosthetic
        device, mechanical, ocular device
    orthopedic NEC —see Complication,
        orthopedic, device, mechanical
    specified NEC T85.628
    urinary NEC —see also Complication,
        genitourinary, device, urinary,
        mechanical
      graft T83.29
    vascular NEC —see Complication,
        cardiovascular device, mechanical

Protrusion, protrusio *(Continued)*
device, implant or graft *(Continued)*
ventricular intracranial shunt T85.09
intervertebral disc —*see* Displacement, intervertebral disc
joint prosthesis —*see* Complications, joint prosthesis, mechanical, specified NEC, by site
nucleus pulposus —*see* Displacement, intervertebral disc
Prune belly (syndrome) Q79.4
Prurigo (ferox) (gravis) (Hebrae) (Hebra's) (mitis) (simplex) L28.2
Besnier's L20.0
estivalis L56.4
nodularis L28.1
psychogenic F45.8
Pruritus, pruritic (essential) L29.9
ani, anus L29.0
psychogenic F45.8
anogenital L29.3
psychogenic F45.8
due to onchocerca volvulus B73.1
gravidarum —*see* Pregnancy, complicated by, specified pregnancy-related condition NEC
hiemalis L29.8
neurogenic (any site) F45.8
perianal L29.0
psychogenic (any site) F45.8
scroti, scrotum L29.1
psychogenic F45.8
senile, senilis L29.8
specified NEC L29.8
psychogenic F45.8
Trichomonas A59.9
vulva, vulvae L29.2
psychogenic F45.8
Pseudarthrosis, pseudoarthrosis (bone) —*see* Nonunion, fracture
clavicle, congenital Q74.0
joint, following fusion or arthrodesis M96.0
Pseudoaneurysm —*see* Aneurysm
Pseudoangina (pectoris) —*see* Angina
Pseudoangioma I81
Pseudoarteriosus Q28.8
Pseudoarthrosis —*see* Pseudarthrosis
Pseudobulbar affect (PBA) F48.2
Pseudochromhidrosis L67.8
Pseudocirrhosis, liver, pericardial I31.1
Pseudocowpox B08.03
Pseudocoxalgia M91.3-•
Pseudocroup J38.5
Pseudo-Cushing's syndrome, alcohol-induced E24.4
Pseudocyesis F45.8
Pseudocyst
lung J98.4
pancreas K86.3
retina —*see* Cyst, retina
Pseudoelephantiasis neuroarthritica Q82.0
Pseudoexfoliation, capsule (lens) —*see* Cataract, specified NEC
Pseudofolliculitis barbae L73.1
Pseudoglioma H44.89
Pseudohemophilia (Bernuth's) (hereditary) (type B) D68.0
Type A D69.8
vascular D69.8
Pseudohermaphroditism Q56.3
adrenal E25.8
female Q56.2
with adrenocortical disorder E25.8
without adrenocortical disorder Q56.2
adrenal (congenital) E25.0
▶unspecified E25.9
male Q56.1
with
adrenocortical disorder E25.8
androgen resistance E34.51

Pseudohermaphroditism *(Continued)*
male *(Continued)*
with *(Continued)*
cleft scrotum Q56.1
feminizing testis E34.51
5-alpha-reductase deficiency E29.1
without gonadal disorder Q56.1
adrenal E25.8
▶unspecified E25.9
Pseudo-Hurler's polydystrophy E77.0
Pseudohydrocephalus G93.2
Pseudohypertrophic muscular dystrophy (Erb's) G71.0
Pseudohypertrophy, muscle G71.0
Pseudohypoparathyroidism E20.1
Pseudoinsomnia F51.03
Pseudoleukemia, infantile D64.89
Pseudomembranous —*see* condition
Pseudomeningocele (cerebral) (infective) (post-traumatic) G96.19
postprocedural (spinal) G97.82
Pseudomenses (newborn) P54.6
Pseudomenstruation (newborn) P54.6
Pseudomonas
aeruginosa, as cause of disease classified elsewhere B96.5
mallei infection A24.0
as cause of disease classified elsewhere B96.5
pseudomallei, as cause of disease classified elsewhere B96.5
Pseudomyotonia G71.19
Pseudomyxoma peritonei C78.6
Pseudoneuritis, optic (nerve) (disc) (papilla), congenital Q14.2
Pseudo-obstruction intestine (acute) (chronic) (idiopathic) (intermittent secondary) (primary) K59.8
Pseudopapilledema H47.33-•
congenital Q14.2
Pseudoparalysis
arm or leg R29.818
atonic, congenital P94.2
Pseudopelade L66.0
Pseudophakia Z96.1
Pseudopolyarthritis, rhizomelic M35.3
Pseudopolycythemia D75.1
Pseudopseudohypoparathyroidism E20.1
Pseudopterygium H11.81-•
Pseudoptosis (eyelid) —*see* Blepharochalasis
Pseudopuberty, precocious
female heterosexual E25.8
male isosexual E25.8
Pseudorickets (renal) N25.0
Pseudorubella B08.20
⟹**Pseudosclerema, newborn** P83.88
Pseudosclerosis (brain)
Jakob's —*see* Creutzfeldt-Jakob disease or syndrome
of Westphal (Strüümpell) E83.01
spastic —*see* Creutzfeldt-Jakob disease or syndrome
Pseudotetanus —*see* Convulsions
Pseudotetany R29.0
hysterical F44.5
Pseudotruncus arteriosus Q25.49
Pseudotuberculosis A28.2
enterocolitis A04.8
pasteurella (infection) A28.0
Pseudotumor
cerebri G93.2
orbital H05.11-•
Pseudoxanthoma elasticum Q82.8
Psilosis (sprue) (tropical) K90.1
nontropical K90.0
Psittacosis A70
Psoitis M60.88
Psoriasis L40.9
arthropathic L40.50
arthritis mutilans L40.52
distal interphalangeal L40.51

Psoriasis *(Continued)*
arthropathic *(Continued)*
juvenile L40.54
other specified L40.59
spondylitis L40.53
buccal K13.29
flexural L40.8
guttate L40.4
mouth K13.29
nummular L40.0
plaque L40.0
psychogenic F54
pustular (generalized) L40.1
palmaris et plantaris L40.3
specified NEC L40.8
vulgaris L40.0
Psychasthenia F48.8
Psychiatric disorder or problem F99
Psychogenic —*see also* condition
factors associated with physical conditions F54
Psychological and behavioral factors affecting medical condition F59
Psychoneurosis, psychoneurotic —*see also* Neurosis
anxiety (state) F41.1
depersonalization F48.1
hypochondriacal F45.21
hysteria F44.9
neurasthenic F48.8
personality NEC F60.89
Psychopathy, psychopathic
affectionless F94.2
autistic F84.5
constitution, post-traumatic F07.81
personality —*see* Disorder, personality
sexual —*see* Deviation, sexual
state F60.2
Psychosexual identity disorder of childhood F64.2
Psychosis, psychotic F29
acute (transient) F23
hysterical F44.9
affective —*see* Disorder, mood
alcoholic F10.959
with
abuse F10.159
anxiety disorder F10.980
with
abuse F10.180
dependence F10.280
delirium tremens F10.231
delusions F10.950
with
abuse F10.150
dependence F10.250
dementia F10.97
with dependence F10.27
dependence F10.259
hallucinosis F10.951
with
abuse F10.151
dependence F10.251
mood disorder F10.94
with
abuse F10.14
dependence F10.24
paranoia F10.950
with
abuse F10.150
dependence F10.250
persisting amnesia F10.96
with dependence F10.26
amnestic confabulatory F10.96
with dependence F10.26
delirium tremens F10.231
Korsakoff's, Korsakov's, Korsakow's F10.26
paranoid type F10.950
with
abuse F10.150
dependence F10.250

Psychosis, psychotic (Continued)
  anergastic —see Psychosis, organic
  arteriosclerotic (simple type) (uncomplicated)
      F01.50
    with behavioral disturbance F01.51
  childhood F84.0
    atypical F84.8
  climacteric —see Psychosis, involutional
  confusional F29
    acute or subacute F05
    reactive F23
  cycloid F23
  depressive —see Disorder, depressive
  disintegrative (childhood) F84.3
  drug-induced —see F11-F19 with .x59
    paranoid and hallucinatory states —see
        F11-F19 with .x50 or .x51
  due to or associated with
    addiction, drug —see F11-F19 with .X59
    dependence
      alcohol F10.259
      drug —see F11-F19 with .x59
    epilepsy F06.8
    Huntington's chorea F06.8
    ischemia, cerebrovascular (generalized)
        F06.8
    multiple sclerosis F06.8
    physical disease F06.8
    presenile dementia F03
    senile dementia F03
    vascular disease (arteriosclerotic) (cerebral)
        F01.50
      with behavioral disturbance F01.51
  epileptic F06.8
  episode F23
    due to or associated with physical
        condition F06.8
  exhaustive F43.0
  hallucinatory, chronic F28
  hypomanic F30.8
  hysterical (acute) F44.9
  induced F24
  infantile F84.0
    atypical F84.8
  infective (acute) (subacute) F05
  involutional F28
    depressive —see Disorder, depressive
    melancholic —see Disorder, depressive
    paranoid (state) F22
  Korsakoff's, Korsakov's, Korsakow's
      (nonalcoholic) F04
    alcoholic F10.96
      in dependence F10.26
    induced by other psychoactive
        substance —see categories F11-F19
        with .x5x
  mania, manic (single episode) F30.2
    recurrent type F31.89
  manic-depressive —see Disorder, bipolar
  menopausal —see Psychosis, involutional
  mixed schizophrenic and affective F25.8
  multi-infarct (cerebrovascular) F01.50
    with behavioral disturbance F01.51
  nonorganic F29
    specified NEC F28
  organic F09
    due to or associated with
      arteriosclerosis (cerebral) —see
          Psychosis, arteriosclerotic
      cerebrovascular disease,
          arteriosclerotic —see Psychosis,
          arteriosclerotic
      childbirth —see Psychosis, puerperal
      Creutzfeldt-Jakob disease or
          syndrome —see Creutzfeldt-Jakob
          disease or syndrome
      dependence, alcohol F10.259
      disease
        alcoholic liver F10.259
        brain, arteriosclerotic —see Psychosis,
            arteriosclerotic

Psychosis, psychotic (Continued)
  organic (Continued)
    due to or associated with (Continued)
      disease (Continued)
        cerebrovascular F01.50
          with behavioral disturbance
              F01.51
        Creutzfeldt-Jakob —see Creutzfeldt-
            Jakob disease or syndrome
        endocrine or metabolic F06.8
          acute or subacute F05
        liver, alcoholic F10.259
      epilepsy transient (acute) F05
      infection
        brain (intracranial) F06.8
          acute or subacute F05
      intoxication
        alcoholic (acute) F10.259
        drug F19 with .X59 F11-●
      ischemia, cerebrovascular (generalized) —
          see Psychosis, arteriosclerotic
      puerperium —see Psychosis, puerperal
      trauma, brain (birth) (from electric
          current) (surgical) F06.8
        acute or subacute F05
    infective F06.8
      acute or subacute F05
    post-traumatic F06.8
      acute or subacute F05
  paranoiac F22
  paranoid (climacteric) (involutional)
      (menopausal) F22
    psychogenic (acute) F23
    schizophrenic F20.0
    senile F03
  postpartum F53
  presbyophrenic (type) F03
  presenile F03
  psychogenic (paranoid) F23
    depressive F32.3
  puerperal F53
    specified type —see Psychosis, by type
  reactive (brief) (transient) (emotional stress)
      (psychological trauma) F23
    depressive F32.3
      recurrent F33.3
    excitative type F30.8
  schizoaffective F25.9
    depressive type F25.1
    manic type F25.0
  schizophrenia, schizophrenic —see
      Schizophrenia
  schizophrenia-like, in epilepsy F06.2
  schizophreniform F20.81
    affective type F25.9
    brief F23
    confusional type F23
    depressive type F25.1
    manic type F25.0
    mixed type F25.0
  senile NEC F03
    depressed or paranoid type F03
    simple deterioration F03
    specified type — code to condition
  shared F24
  situational (reactive) F23
  symbiotic (childhood) F84.3
  symptomatic F09
Psychosomatic —see Disorder, psychosomatic
Psychosyndrome, organic F07.9
Psychotic episode due to or associated with
    physical condition F06.8
Pterygium (eye) H11.00-●
  amyloid H11.01-●
  central H11.02-●
  colli Q18.3
  double H11.03-●
  peripheral
    progressive H11.05-●
    stationary H11.04-●
  recurrent H11.06-●

Ptilosis (eyelid) —see Madarosis
Ptomaine (poisoning) —see Poisoning, food
Ptosis —see also Blepharoptosis
  adiposa (false) —see Blepharoptosis
  breast N64.81
  cecum K63.4
  colon K63.4
  congenital (eyelid) Q10.0
    specified site NEC —see Anomaly, by site
  eyelid —see Blepharoptosis
    congenital Q10.0
  gastric K31.89
  intestine K63.4
  kidney N28.83
  liver K76.89
  renal N28.83
  splanchnic K63.4
  spleen D73.89
  stomach K31.89
  viscera K63.4
PTP D69.51
Ptyalism (periodic) K11.7
  hysterical F45.8
  pregnancy —see Pregnancy, complicated by,
      specified pregnancy-related condition
      NEC
  psychogenic F45.8
Ptyalolithiasis K11.5
Pubarche, precocious E30.1
Pubertas praecox E30.1
Puberty (development state) Z00.3
  bleeding (excessive) N92.2
  delayed E30.0
  precocious (constitutional) (cryptogenic)
      (idiopathic) E30.1
    central E22.8
    due to
      ovarian hyperfunction E28.1
        estrogen E28.0
      testicular hyperfunction E29.0
  premature E30.1
    due to
      adrenal cortical hyperfunction E25.8
      pineal tumor E34.8
      pituitary (anterior) hyperfunction E22.8
Puckering, macula —see Degeneration, macula,
    puckering
Pudenda, pudendum —see condition
Puente's disease (simple glandular cheilitis)
    K13.0
Puerperal, puerperium (complicated by,
    complications)
  abnormal glucose (tolerance test) O99.815
  abscess
    areola O91.02
      associated with lactation O91.03
    Bartholin's gland O86.19
    breast O91.12
      associated with lactation O91.13
    cervix (uteri) O86.11
    genital organ NEC O86.19
    kidney O86.21
    mammary O91.12
      associated with lactation O91.13
    nipple O91.02
      associated with lactation O91.03
    peritoneum O85
    subareolar O91.12
      associated with lactation O91.13
    urinary tract —see Puerperal, infection,
        urinary
    uterus O86.12
    vagina (wall) O86.13
    vaginorectal O86.13
    vulvovaginal gland O86.13
  adnexitis O86.19
  afibrinogenemia, or other coagulation defect
      O72.3
  albuminuria (acute) (subacute) —see
      Proteinuria, gestational
  alcohol use O99.315

▶ New   ➡ Revised   ~~deleted~~ Deleted   ● Use Additional Character(s)

Puerperal, puerperium *(Continued)*
anemia O90.81
  pre-existing (pre-pregnancy) O99.03
anesthetic death O89.8
apoplexy O99.43
bariatric surgery status O99.845
blood disorder NEC O99.13
blood dyscrasia O72.3
cardiomyopathy O90.3
cerebrovascular disorder (conditions in
    I60-I69) O99.43
cervicitis O86.11
circulatory system disorder O99.43
➠coagulopathy (any) O99.13
  ▶with hemorrhage O72.3
complications O90.9
  specified NEC O90.89
convulsions —*see* Eclampsia
cystitis O86.22
cystopyelitis O86.29
delirium NEC F05
diabetes O24.93
  gestational —*see* Puerperal, gestational
    diabetes
  pre-existing O24.33
    specified NEC O24.83
    type 1 O24.03
    type 2 O24.13
digestive system disorder O99.63
disease O90.9
  breast NEC O92.29
  cerebrovascular (acute) O99.43
  nonobstetric NEC O99.89
  tubo-ovarian O86.19
  Valsuani's O99.03
disorder O90.9
  biliary tract O26.63
  lactation O92.70
  liver O26.63
  nonobstetric NEC O99.89
disruption
  cesarean wound O90.0
  episiotomy wound O90.1
  perineal laceration wound O90.1
drug use O99.325
eclampsia (with pre-existing hypertension)
  O15.2
embolism (pulmonary) (blood clot) —*see*
  Embolism, obstetric, puerperal
endocrine, nutritional or metabolic disease
  NEC O99.285
endophlebitis —*see* Puerperal, phlebitis
endotrachelitis O86.11
failure
  lactation (complete) O92.3
    partial O92.4
  renal, acute O90.4
fever (of unknown origin) O86.4
  septic O85
fissure, nipple O92.12
  associated with lactation O92.13
fistula
  breast (due to mastitis) O91.12
    associated with lactation O91.13
  nipple O91.02
    associated with lactation O91.03
galactophoritis O91.22
  associated with lactation O91.23
galactorrhea O92.6
gastric banding status O99.845
gastric bypass status O99.845
gastrointestinal disease NEC O99.63
gestational
  diabetes O24.439
    diet controlled O24.430
    insulin (and diet) controlled O24.434
    oral drug controlled (antidiabetic)
      (hypoglycemic) O24.435
  edema O12.05
    with proteinuria O12.25
  proteinuria O12.15

Puerperal, puerperium *(Continued)*
gonorrhea O98.23
hematoma, subdural O99.43
hemiplegia, cerebral O99.355-●
  due to cerebrovascular disorder
    O99.43
hemorrhage O72.1
  brain O99.43
  bulbar O99.43
  cerebellar O99.43
  cerebral O99.43
  cortical O99.43
  delayed or secondary O72.2
  extradural O99.43
  internal capsule O99.43
  intracranial O99.43
  intrapontine O99.43
  meningeal O99.43
  pontine O99.43
  retained placenta O72.0
  subarachnoid O99.43
  subcortical O99.43
  subdural O99.43
  third stage O72.0
  uterine, delayed O72.2
  ventricular O99.43
hemorrhoids O87.2
hepatorenal syndrome O90.4
hypertension —*see* Hypertension,
  complicating, puerperium
hypertrophy, breast O92.29
induration breast (fibrous) O92.29
infection O86.4
  cervix O86.11
  generalized O85
  genital tract NEC O86.19
    obstetric surgical wound O86.0
  kidney (bacillus coli) O86.21
  maternal O98.93
    carrier state NEC O99.835
    gonorrhea O98.23
    human immunodeficiency virus (HIV)
      O98.73
    protozoal O98.63
    sexually transmitted NEC O98.33
    specified NEC O98.83
    streptococcus group B (GBS) carrier state
      O99.825
    syphilis O98.13
    tuberculosis O98.03
    viral hepatitis O98.43
    viral NEC O98.53
  nipple O91.02
    associated with lactation O91.03
  peritoneum O85
  renal O86.21
  specified NEC O86.89
  urinary (asymptomatic) (tract) NEC
    O86.20
    bladder O86.22
    kidney O86.21
    specified site NEC O86.29
    urethra O86.22
  vagina O86.13
  vein —*see* Puerperal, phlebitis
ischemia, cerebral O99.43
lymphangitis O86.89
  breast O91.22
    associated with lactation
      O91.23
malignancy O9A.13
malnutrition O25.3
mammillitis O91.02
  associated with lactation O91.03
mammitis O91.22
  associated with lactation O91.23
mania F30.8
mastitis O91.22
  associated with lactation O91.23
  purulent O91.12
    associated with lactation O91.13

Puerperal, puerperium *(Continued)*
melancholia —*see* Disorder, depressive
mental disorder NEC O99.345
metroperitonitis O85
metrorrhagia —*see* Hemorrhage,
  postpartum
metrosalpingitis O86.19
metrovaginitis O86.13
milk leg O87.1
monoplegia, cerebral O99.43
mood disturbance O90.6
necrosis, liver (acute) (subacute)
  (conditions in subcategory K72.0)
    O26.63
  with renal failure O90.4
nervous system disorder O99.355
neuritis O90.89
obesity (pre-existing prior to pregnancy)
  O99.215
obesity surgery status O99.845
occlusion, precerebral artery O99.43
paralysis
  bladder (sphincter) O90.89
  cerebral O99.43
paralytic stroke O99.43
parametritis O85
paravaginitis O86.13
pelviperitonitis O85
perimetritis O86.12
perimetrosalpingitis O86.19
perinephritis O86.21
periphlebitis —*see* Puerperal phlebitis
peritoneal infection O85
peritonitis (pelvic) O85
perivaginitis O86.13
phlebitis O87.0
  deep O87.1
  pelvic O87.1
  superficial O87.0
phlebothrombosis, deep O87.1
phlegmasia alba dolens O87.1
placental polyp O90.89
pneumonia, embolic —*see* Embolism,
  obstetric, puerperal
pre-eclampsia —*see* Pre-eclampsia
psychosis F53
pyelitis O86.21
pyelocystitis O86.29
pyelonephritis O86.21
pyelonephrosis O86.21
pyemia O85
pyocystitis O86.29
pyohemia O85
pyometra O86.12
pyonephritis O86.21
pyosalpingitis O86.19
pyrexia (of unknown origin) O86.4
renal
  disease NEC O90.89
  failure O90.4
respiratory disease NEC O99.53
retention
  decidua —*see* Retention, decidua
  placenta O72.0
  secundines —*see* Retention,
    secundines
retrated nipple O92.02
salpingo-ovaritis O86.19
salpingoperitonitis O85
secondary perineal tear O90.1
sepsis O85
sepsis (pelvic) O85
septic thrombophlebitis O86.81
skin disorder NEC O99.73
specified condition NEC O99.89
stroke O99.43
subinvolution (uterus) O90.89
subluxation of symphysis (pubis)
  O26.73
suppuration —*see* Puerperal, abscess
tetanus A34

Puerperal, puerperium *(Continued)*
thelitis O91.02
associated with lactation O91.03
thrombocytopenia O72.3
thrombophlebitis (superficial) O87.0
deep O87.1
pelvic O87.1
septic O86.81
thrombosis (venous) —*see* Thrombosis,
puerperal
thyroiditis O90.5
toxemia (eclamptic) (pre-eclamptic)
(with convulsions) O15.2
trauma, non-obstetric O9A.23
caused by abuse (physical) (suspected)
O9A.33
confirmed O9A.33
psychological (suspected)
O9A.53
confirmed O9A.53
sexual (suspected) O9A.43
confirmed O9A.43
uremia (due to renal failure)
O90.4
urethritis O86.22
vaginitis O86.13
varicose veins (legs) O87.4
vulva or perineum O87.8
venous O87.9
vulvitis O86.19
vulvovaginitis O86.13
white leg O87.1
Puerperium —*see* Puerperal
Pulmolithiasis J98.4
Pulmonary —*see* condition
Pulpitis (acute) (anachoretic) (chronic)
(hyperplastic) (putrescent) (suppurative)
(ulcerative) K04.01
irreversible K04.02
reversible K04.01
Pulpless tooth K04.99
Pulse
alternating R00.8
bigeminal R00.8
fast R00.0
feeble, rapid due to shock following injury
T79.4
rapid R00.0
weak R09.89
Pulsus alternans or trigeminus R00.8
Punch drunk F07.81
Punctum lacrimale occlusion —*see* Obstruction,
lacrimal
Puncture
abdomen, abdominal
wall S31.139
with
foreign body S31.149
penetration into peritoneal cavity
S31.639
with foreign body S31.649
epigastric region S31.132
with
foreign body S31.142
penetration into peritoneal cavity
S31.632
with foreign body S31.642
left
lower quadrant S31.134
with
foreign body S31.144
penetration into peritoneal cavity
S31.634
with foreign body S31.644
upper quadrant S31.131
with
foreign body S31.141
penetration into peritoneal cavity
S31.631
with foreign body S31.641

Puncture *(Continued)*
abdomen, abdominal *(Continued)*
wall *(Continued)*
periumbilic region S31.135
with
foreign body S31.145
penetration into peritoneal cavity
S31.635
with foreign body S31.645
right
lower quadrant S31.133
with
foreign body S31.143
penetration into peritoneal cavity
S31.633
with foreign body S31.643
upper quadrant S31.130
with
foreign body S31.140
penetration into peritoneal cavity
S31.630
with foreign body S31.640
accidental, complicating surgery —*see*
Complication, accidental puncture or
laceration
alveolar (process) —*see* Puncture, oral cavity
ankle S91.039
with
foreign body S91.049
left S91.032
with
foreign body S91.042
right S91.031
with
foreign body S91.041
anus S31.833
with foreign body S31.834
arm (upper) S41.139
with foreign body S41.149
left S41.132
with foreign body S41.142
lower —*see* Puncture, forearm
right S41.131
with foreign body S41.141
auditory canal (external) (meatus) —*see*
Puncture, ear
auricle, ear —*see* Puncture, ear
axilla —*see* Puncture, arm
back —*see also* Puncture, thorax, back
lower S31.030
with
foreign body S31.040
with penetration into
retroperitoneal space S31.041
penetration into retroperitoneal space
S31.031
bladder (traumatic) S37.29
nontraumatic N32.89
breast S21.039
with foreign body S21.049
left S21.032
with foreign body S21.042
right S21.031
with foreign body S21.041
buttock S31.803
with foreign body S31.804
left S31.823
with foreign body S31.824
right S31.813
with foreign body S31.814
by
device, implant or graft —*see*
Complications, by site and type,
mechanical
foreign body left accidentally in operative
wound T81.539
instrument (any) during a procedure,
accidental —*see* Puncture, accidental
complicating surgery
calf —*see* Puncture, leg
canaliculus lacrimalis —*see* Puncture, eyelid

Puncture *(Continued)*
canthus, eye —*see* Puncture, eyelid
cervical esophagus S11.23
with foreign body S11.24
cheek (external) S01.439
with foreign body S01.449
internal —*see* Puncture, oral cavity
left S01.432
with foreign body S01.442
right S01.431
with foreign body S01.441
chest wall —*see* Puncture, thorax
chin —*see* Puncture, head, specified site NEC
clitoris —*see* Puncture, vulva
costal region —*see* Puncture, thorax
digit(s)
foot —*see* Puncture, toe
hand —*see* Puncture, finger
ear (canal) (external) S01.339
with foreign body S01.349
drum S09.2-●
left S01.332
with foreign body S01.342
right S01.331
with foreign body S01.341
elbow S51.039
with
foreign body S51.049
left S51.032
with
foreign body S51.042
right S51.031
with
foreign body S51.041
epididymis —*see* Puncture, testis
epigastric region —*see* Puncture, abdomen,
wall, epigastric
epiglottis S11.83
with foreign body S11.84
esophagus
cervical S11.23
with foreign body S11.24
thoracic S27.818
eyeball S05.6-●
with foreign body S05.5-●
eyebrow —*see* Puncture, eyelid
eyelid S01.13-●
with foreign body S01.14-●
left S01.132
with foreign body S01.142
right S01.131
with foreign body S01.141
face NEC —*see* Puncture, head, specified site
NEC
finger(s) S61.239
with
damage to nail S61.339
with
foreign body S61.349
foreign body S61.249
index S61.238
with
damage to nail S61.338
with
foreign body S61.348
foreign body S61.248
left S61.231
with
damage to nail S61.331
with
foreign body S61.341
foreign body S61.241
right S61.230
with
damage to nail S61.330
with
foreign body S61.340
foreign body S61.240
little S61.238
with
damage to nail S61.338

Puncture *(Continued)*
  finger *(Continued)*
    with *(Continued)*
      with *(Continued)*
        damage to nail *(Continued)*
          with
            foreign body S61.348
          foreign body S61.248
        left S61.237
          with
            damage to nail S61.337
              with
                foreign body S61.347
            foreign body S61.247
        right S61.236
          with
            damage to nail S61.336
              with
                foreign body S61.346
            foreign body S61.246
    middle S61.238
      with
        damage to nail S61.338
          with
            foreign body S61.348
        foreign body S61.248
      left S61.233
        with
          damage to nail S61.333
            with
              foreign body S61.343
           foreign body S61.243
      right S61.232
        with
          damage to nail S61.332
            with
              foreign body S61.342
           foreign body S61.242
    ring S61.238
      with
        damage to nail S61.338
          with
            foreign body S61.348
        foreign body S61.248
      left S61.235
        with
          damage to nail S61.335
            with
              foreign body S61.345
           foreign body S61.245
      right S61.234
        with
          damage to nail S61.334
            with
              foreign body S61.344
           foreign body S61.244
  flank S31.139
    with foreign body S31.149
  foot (except toe(s) alone) S91.339
    with foreign body S91.349
    left S91.332
      with foreign body S91.342
    right S91.331
      with foreign body S91.341
    toe —*see* Puncture, toe
  forearm S51.839
    with
      foreign body S51.849
    elbow only —*see* Puncture, elbow
    left S51.832
      with
        foreign body S51.842
    right S51.831
      with
        foreign body S51.841
  forehead —*see* Puncture, head, specified site NEC
  genital organs, external
    female S31.532
      with foreign body S31.542
      vagina —*see* Puncture, vagina
      vulva —*see* Puncture, vulva

Puncture *(Continued)*
  genital organs, external *(Continued)*
    male S31.531
      with foreign body S31.541
      penis —*see* Puncture, penis
      scrotum —*see* Puncture, scrotum
      testis —*see* Puncture, testis
  groin —*see* Puncture, abdomen, wall
  gum —*see* Puncture, oral cavity
  hand S61.439
    with
      foreign body S61.449
    finger —*see* Puncture, finger
    left S61.432
      with
        foreign body S61.442
    right S61.431
      with
        foreign body S61.441
    thumb —*see* Puncture, thumb
  head S01.93
    with foreign body S01.94
    cheek —*see* Puncture, cheek
    ear —*see* Puncture, ear
    eyelid —*see* Puncture, eyelid
    lip —*see* Puncture, oral cavity
    nose —*see* Puncture, nose
    oral cavity —*see* Puncture, oral cavity
    scalp S01.03
      with foreign body S01.04
    specified site NEC S01.83
      with foreign body S01.84
    temporomandibular area —*see* Puncture, cheek
  heart S26.99
    with hemopericardium S26.09
    without hemopericardium S26.19
  heel —*see* Puncture, foot
  hip S71.039
    with foreign body S71.049
    left S71.032
      with foreign body S71.042
    right S71.031
      with foreign body S71.041
  hymen —*see* Puncture, vagina
  hypochondrium —*see* Puncture, abdomen, wall
  hypogastric region —*see* Puncture, abdomen, wall
  inguinal region —*see* Puncture, abdomen, wall
  instep —*see* Puncture, foot
  internal organs —*see* Injury, by site
  interscapular region —*see* Puncture, thorax, back
  intestine
    large
      colon S36.599
        ascending S36.590
        descending S36.592
        sigmoid S36.593
        specified site NEC S36.598
        transverse S36.591
      rectum S36.69
    small S36.499
      duodenum S36.490
      specified site NEC S36.498
  intra-abdominal organ S36.99
    gallbladder S36.128
    intestine —*see* Puncture, intestine
    liver S36.118
    pancreas —*see* Puncture, pancreas
    peritoneum S36.81
    specified site NEC S36.898
    spleen S36.09
    stomach S36.39
  jaw —*see* Puncture, head, specified site NEC
  knee S81.039
    with foreign body S81.049
    left S81.032
      with foreign body S81.042

Puncture *(Continued)*
  knee *(Continued)*
    right S81.031
      with foreign body S81.041
  labium (majus) (minus) —*see* Puncture, vulva
  lacrimal duct —*see* Puncture, eyelid
  larynx S11.013
    with foreign body S11.014
  leg (lower) S81.839
    with foreign body S81.849
    foot —*see* Puncture, foot
    knee —*see* Puncture, knee
    left S81.832
      with foreign body S81.842
    right S81.831
      with foreign body S81.841
    upper —*see* Puncture, thigh
  lip S01.531
    with foreign body S01.541
  loin —*see* Puncture, abdomen, wall
  lower back —*see* Puncture, back, lower
  lumbar region —*see* Puncture, back, lower
  malar region —*see* Puncture, head, specified site NEC
  mammary —*see* Puncture, breast
  mastoid region —*see* Puncture, head, specified site NEC
  mouth —*see* Puncture, oral cavity
  nail
    finger —*see* Puncture, finger, with damage to nail
    toe —*see* Puncture, toe, with damage to nail
  nasal (septum) (sinus) —*see* Puncture, nose
  nasopharynx —*see* Puncture, head, specified site NEC
  neck S11.93
    with foreign body S11.94
    involving
      cervical esophagus —*see* Puncture, cervical esophagus
      larynx —*see* Puncture, larynx
      pharynx —*see* Puncture, pharynx
      thyroid gland —*see* Puncture, thyroid gland
      trachea —*see* Puncture, trachea
    specified site NEC S11.83
      with foreign body S11.84
  nose (septum) (sinus) S01.23
    with foreign body S01.24
  ocular —*see* Puncture, eyeball - oral cavity S01.532
    with foreign body S01.542
  orbit S05.4-●
  palate —*see* Puncture, oral cavity
  palm —*see* Puncture, hand
  pancreas S36.299
    body S36.291
    head S36.290
    tail S36.292
  pelvis —*see* Puncture, back, lower
  penis S31.23
    with foreign body S31.24
  perineum
    female S31.43
      with foreign body S31.44
    male S31.139
      with foreign body S31.149
  periocular area (with or without lacrimal passages) —*see* Puncture, eyelid
  phalanges
    finger —*see* Puncture, finger
    toe —*see* Puncture, toe
  pharynx S11.23
    with foreign body S11.24
  pinna —*see* Puncture, ear
  popliteal space —*see* Puncture, knee
  prepuce —*see* Puncture, penis
  pubic region S31.139
    with foreign body S31.149

Puncture (Continued)

pudendum —see Puncture, genital organs, external

rectovaginal septum —see Puncture, vagina

sacral region —see Puncture, back, lower

sacroiliac region —see Puncture, back, lower

salivary gland —see Puncture, oral cavity

scalp S01.03

  with foreign body S01.04

scapular region —see Puncture, shoulder

scrotum S31.33

  with foreign body S31.34

shin —see Puncture, leg

shoulder S41.039

  with foreign body S41.049

  left S41.032

    with foreign body S41.042

  right S41.031

    with foreign body S41.041

spermatic cord —see Puncture, testis

sternal region —see Puncture, thorax, front

submaxillary region —see Puncture, head, specified site NEC

submental region —see Puncture, head, specified site NEC

subungual

  finger(s) —see Puncture, finger, with damage to nail

  toe —see Puncture, toe, with damage to nail

supraclavicular fossa —see Puncture, neck, specified site NEC

temple, temporal region —see Puncture, head, specified site NEC

temporomandibular area —see Puncture, cheek

testis S31.33

  with foreign body S31.34

thigh S71.139

  with foreign body S71.149

  left S71.132

    with foreign body S71.142

  right S71.131

    with foreign body S71.141

thorax, thoracic (wall) S21.93

  with foreign body S21.94

  back S21.23-●

    with

      foreign body S21.24-●

        with penetration S21.44

      penetration S21.43

  breast —see Puncture, breast

  front S21.13-●

    with

      foreign body S21.14-●

        with penetration S21.34

      penetration S21.33

throat —see Puncture, neck

thumb S61.039

  with

    damage to nail S61.139

      with

        foreign body S61.149

    foreign body S61.049

  left S61.032

    with

      damage to nail S61.132

        with

          foreign body S61.142

      foreign body S61.042

  right S61.031

    with

      damage to nail S61.131

        with

          foreign body S61.141

      foreign body S61.041

Puncture (Continued)

thyroid gland S11.13

  with foreign body S11.14

toe(s) S91.139

  with

    damage to nail S91.239

      with

        foreign body S91.249

    foreign body S91.149

  great S91.133

    with

      damage to nail S91.233

        with

          foreign body S91.243

      foreign body S91.143

    left S91.132

      with

        damage to nail S91.232

          with

            foreign body S91.242

        foreign body S91.142

    right S91.131

      with

        damage to nail S91.231

          with

            foreign body S91.241

        foreign body S91.141

  lesser S91.136

    with

      damage to nail S91.236

        with

          foreign body S91.246

      foreign body S91.146

    left S91.135

      with

        damage to nail S91.235

          with

            foreign body S91.245

        foreign body S91.145

    right S91.134

      with

        damage to nail S91.234

          with

            foreign body S91.244

        foreign body S91.144

tongue —see Puncture, oral cavity

trachea S11.023

  with foreign body S11.024

tunica vaginalis —see Puncture, testis

tympanum, tympanic membrane S09.2-●

umbilical region S31.135

  with foreign body S31.145

uvula —see Puncture, oral cavity

vagina S31.43

  with foreign body S31.44

vocal cords S11.033

  with foreign body S11.034

vulva S31.43

  with foreign body S31.44

wrist S61.539

  with

    foreign body S61.549

  left S61.532

    with

      foreign body S61.542

  right S61.531

    with

      foreign body S61.541

PUO (pyrexia of unknown origin) R50.9

Pupillary membrane (persistent) Q13.89

Pupillotonia —see Anomaly, pupil, function, tonic pupil

Purpura D69.2

abdominal D69.0

allergic D69.0

anaphylactoid D69.0

annularis telangiectodes L81.7

arthritic D69.0

autoerythrocyte sensitization D69.2

autoimmune D69.0

Purpura (Continued)

bacterial D69.0

Bateman's (senile) D69.2

capillary fragility (hereditary) (idiopathic) D69.8

cryoglobulinemic D89.1

Devil's pinches D69.2

fibrinolytic —see Fibrinolysis

fulminans, fulminous D65

gangrenous D65

hemorrhagic, hemorrhagica D69.3

  not due to thrombocytopenia D69.0

Henoch (-Schönlein) (allergic) D69.0

hypergammaglobulinemic (benign) (Waldenström's) D89.0

idiopathic (thrombocytopenic) D69.3

  nonthrombocytopenic D69.0

immune thrombocytopenic D69.3

infectious D69.0

malignant D69.0

neonatorum P54.5

nervosa D69.0

newborn P54.5

nonthrombocytopenic D69.2

  hemorrhagic D69.0

  idiopathic D69.0

nonthrombopenic D69.2

peliosis rheumatica D69.0

posttransfusion (post-transfusion) (from (fresh) whole blood or blood products) D69.51

primary D69.49

red cell membrane sensitivity D69.2

rheumatica D69.0

Schönlein (-Henoch) (allergic) D69.0

scorbutic E54 [D77]

senile D69.2

simplex D69.2

symptomatica D69.0

telangiectasia annularis L81.7

thrombocytopenic D69.49

  congenital D69.42

  hemorrhagic D69.3

  hereditary D69.42

  idiopathic D69.3

  immune D69.3

  neonatal, transitory P61.0

  thrombotic M31.1

thrombohemolytic —see Fibrinolysis

thrombolytic —see Fibrinolysis

thrombopenic D69.49

thrombotic, thrombocytopenic M31.1

toxic D69.0

vascular D69.0

visceral symptoms D69.0

Purpuric spots R23.3

Purulent —see condition

Pus

in

  stool R19.5

  urine N39.0

tube (rupture) —see Salpingo-oophoritis

Pustular rash L08.0

Pustule (nonmalignant) L08.9

malignant A22.0

Pustulosis palmaris et plantaris L40.3

Putnam (-Dana) disease or syndrome —see Degeneration, combined

Putrescent pulp (dental) K04.1

Pyarthritis, pyarthrosis —see Arthritis, pyogenic or pyemic

tuberculous —see Tuberculosis, joint

Pyelectasis —see Hydronephrosis

Pyelitis (congenital) (uremic) —see also Pyelonephritis

with

  calculus —see category N20

    with hydronephrosis N13.2

  contracted kidney N11.9

▶ New   ⮕ Revised   ~~deleted~~ Deleted   ● Use Additional Character(s)

Pyelitis *(Continued)*
 acute N1Ø
 chronic N11.9
  with calculus —*see* category N20
   with hydronephrosis N13.2
 cystica N28.84
 puerperal (postpartum) O86.21
 tuberculous A18.11
Pyelocystitis —*see* Pyelonephritis
Pyelonephritis —*see also* Nephritis,
  tubulo-interstitial
 with
  calculus —*see* category N20
   with hydronephrosis N13.2
  contracted kidney N11.9
 acute N1Ø
 calculus —*see* category N20
  with hydronephrosis N13.2
 chronic N11.9
  with calculus —*see* category N20
   with hydronephrosis N13.2
  associated with ureteral obstruction or
   stricture N11.1
  nonobstructive N11.8
   with reflux (vesicoureteral) N11.0
  obstructive N11.1
  specified NEC N11.8
 in (due to)
  brucellosis A23.9 *[N16]*
  cryoglobulinemia (mixed) D89.1 *[N16]*
  cystinosis E72.04
  diphtheria A36.84
  glycogen storage disease E74.09 *[N16]*
  leukemia NEC C95.9-• *[N16]*
  lymphoma NEC C85.90 *[N16]*
  multiple myeloma C90.0-• *[N16]*
  obstruction N11.1
  Salmonella infection A02.25
  sarcoidosis D86.84
  sepsis A41.9 *[N16]*
  Sjögren's disease M35.04
  toxoplasmosis B58.83
  transplant rejection T86.91 *[N16]*
  Wilson's disease E83.01 *[N16]*
 nonobstructive N12
  with reflux (vesicoureteral) N11.0
  chronic N11.8
 syphilitic A52.75

Pyelonephrosis (obstructive) N11.1
 chronic N11.9
Pyelophlebitis I80.8
Pyeloureteritis cystica N28.85
Pyemia, pyemic (fever) (infection) (purulent) —
   see also Sepsis
 joint —*see* Arthritis, pyogenic or pyemic
 liver K75.1
 pneumococcal A40.3
 portal K75.1
 postvaccinal T88.0
 puerperal, postpartum, childbirth O85
 specified organism NEC A41.89
 tuberculous —*see* Tuberculosis, miliary
Pygopagus Q89.4
Pyknoepilepsy (idiopathic) —*see* Pyknolepsy
Pyknolepsy G40.A09
 intractable G40.A19
  with status epilepticus G40.A11
  without status epilepticus G40.A19
 not intractable G40.A09
  with status epilepticus G40.A01
  without status epilepticus G40.A09
Pylephlebitis K75.1
Pyle's syndrome Q78.5
Pylethrombophlebitis K75.1
Pylethrombosis K75.1
Pyloritis K29.90
 with bleeding K29.91
Pylorospasm (reflex) NEC K31.3
 congenital or infantile Q40.0
 neurotic F45.8
 newborn Q40.0
 psychogenic F45.8
Pylorus, pyloric —*see* condition
Pyoarthrosis —*see* Arthritis, pyogenic or
  pyemic
Pyocele
 mastoid —*see* Mastoiditis, acute
 sinus (accessory) —*see* Sinusitis
 turbinate (bone) J32.9
 urethra —*see also* Urethritis N34.0
Pyocolpos —*see* Vaginitis
Pyocystitis N30.80
 with hematuria N30.81
Pyoderma, pyodermia L08.0
 gangrenosum L88
 newborn P39.4

Pyoderma, pyodermia *(Continued)*
 phagedenic L88
 vegetans L08.81
Pyodermatitis L08.0
 vegetans L08.81
Pyogenic —*see* condition
Pyohydronephrosis N13.6
Pyometra, pyometrium, pyometritis —*see*
  Endometritis
Pyomyositis (tropical) —*see* Myositis,
  infective
Pyonephritis N12
Pyonephrosis N13.6
 tuberculous A18.11
Pyo-oophoritis —*see* Salpingo-oophoritis
Pyo-ovarium —*see* Salpingo-oophoritis
Pyopericarditis, pyopericardium
  I30.1
Pyophlebitis —*see* Phlebitis
Pyopneumopericardium I30.1
Pyopneumothorax (infective) J86.9
 with fistula J86.0
 tuberculous NEC A15.6
Pyosalpinx, pyosalpingitis —*see also*
  Salpingo-oophoritis
Pyothorax J86.9
 with fistula J86.0
 tuberculous NEC A15.6
Pyoureter N28.89
 tuberculous A18.11
Pyramidopallidonigral syndrome
  G20
Pyrexia (of unknown origin) R50.9
 atmospheric T67.0
 during labor NEC O75.2
 heat T67.0
 newborn P81.9
  environmentally-induced P81.0
 persistent R50.9
 puerperal O86.4
Pyroglobulinemia NEC E88.09
Pyromania F63.1
Pyrosis R12
Pyuria (bacterial) N39.0

Q

Q fever A78
  with pneumonia A78
Quadricuspid aortic valve Q23.8
Quadrilateral fever A78
Quadriparesis —*see* Quadriplegia
  meaning muscle weakness M62.81
Quadriplegia G82.50-●
  complete
    C1-C4 level G82.51
    C5-C7 level G82.53
  congenital (cerebral) (spinal) G80.8
    spastic G80.0

Quadriplegia (*Continued*)
  embolic (current episode) I63.4-●
  functional R53.2
  incomplete
    C1-C4 level G82.52
    C5-C7 level G82.54
  thrombotic (current episode) I63.3-●
  traumatic — code to injury with seventh
      character S
    current episode —*see* Injury, spinal (cord),
        cervical
Quadruplet, pregnancy —*see* Pregnancy,
    quadruplet
Quarrelsomeness F60.3

Queensland fever A77.3
Quervain's disease M65.4
  thyroid E06.1
Queyrat's erythroplasia D07.4
  penis D07.4
  specified site —*see* Neoplasm, skin,
      in situ
  unspecified site D07.4
Quincke's disease or edema T78.3
  hereditary D84.1
Quinsy (gangrenous) J36
Quintan fever A79.0
Quintuplet, pregnancy —*see* Pregnancy,
    quintuplet

► New   ⇒ Revised   ~~deleted~~ Deleted   ● Use Additional Character(s)

R

Rabbit fever —*see* Tularemia
Rabies A82.9
    contact Z20.3
    exposure to Z20.3
    inoculation reaction —*see* Complications,
        vaccination
    sylvatic A82.0
    urban A82.1
Rachischisis —*see* Spina bifida
Rachitic —*see also* condition
    deformities of spine (late effect) (sequelae)
        E64.3
    pelvis (late effect) (sequelae) E64.3
        with disproportion (fetopelvic) O33.0
            causing obstructed labor O65.0
Rachitis, rachitism (acute) (tarda) —*see also*
        Rickets
    renalis N25.0
    sequelae E64.3
Radial nerve —*see* condition
Radiation
    burn —*see* Burn
    effects NOS T66
    sickness NOS T66
    therapy, encounter for Z51.0
Radiculitis (pressure) (vertebrogenic) —*see*
        Radiculopathy
Radiculomyelitis —*see also* Encephalitis
    toxic, due to
        Clostridium tetani A35
        Corynebacterium diphtheriae A36.82
Radiculopathy M54.10
    cervical region M54.12
    cervicothoracic region M54.13
    due to
        disc disorder
            C3 M50.11
            C4 M50.11
            C5 M50.121
            C6 M50.122
            C7 M50.123
            C8 M50.13
        displacement of intervertebral disc —*see*
            Disorder, disc, with, radiculopathy
    leg M54.1-●
    lumbar region M54.16
    lumbosacral region M54.17
    occipito-atlanto-axial region M54.11
    postherpetic B02.29
    sacrococcygeal region M54.18
    syphilitic A52.11
    thoracic region (with visceral pain)
        M54.14
    thoracolumbar region M54.15
Radiodermal burns (acute, chronic, or
        occupational) —*see* Burn
Radiodermatitis L58.9
    acute L58.0
    chronic L58.1
Radiotherapy session Z51.0
RAEB (refractory anemia with excess blasts)
        D46.2-●
Rage, meaning rabies —*see* Rabies
Ragpicker's disease A22.1
Ragsorter's disease A22.1
Raillietiniasis B71.8
Railroad neurosis F48.8
Railway spine F48.8
Raised —*see also* Elevated
    antibody titer R76.0
Rake teeth, tooth M26.39
Rales R09.89
Ramifying renal pelvis Q63.8
Ramsay-Hunt disease or syndrome —*see also*
        Hunt's disease B02.21
    meaning dyssynergia cerebellaris myoclonica
        G11.1
Ranula K11.6
    congenital Q38.4

Rape
    adult
        confirmed T74.21
        suspected T76.21
    alleged, observation or examination, ruled out
        adult Z04.41
        child Z04.42
    child
        confirmed T74.22
        suspected T76.22
Rapid
    feeble pulse, due to shock, following injury
        T79.4
    heart (beat) R00.0
        psychogenic F45.8
    second stage (delivery) O62.3
    time-zone change syndrome —*see* Disorder,
        sleep, circadian rhythm, psychogenic
Rarefaction, bone —*see* Disorder, bone, density
        and structure, specified NEC
Rash (toxic) R21
    canker A38.9
    diaper L22
    drug (internal use) L27.0
        contact —*see also* Dermatitis, due to, drugs,
            external L25.1
    following immunization T88.1
    food —*see* Dermatitis, due to, food
    heat L74.0
    napkin (psoriasiform) L22
    nettle —*see* Urticaria
    pustular L08.0
    rose R21
        epidemic B06.9
    scarlet A38.9
    serum —*see also* Reaction, serum T80.69
    wandering tongue K14.1
Rasmussen aneurysm —*see* Tuberculosis,
        pulmonary
Rasmussen encephalitis G04.81
Rat-bite fever A25.9
    due to Streptobacillus moniliformis A25.1
    spirochetal (morsus muris) A25.0
Rathke's pouch tumor D44.3
Raymond (-Céstan) syndrome I65.8
Raynaud's disease, phenomenon or syndrome
        (secondary) I73.00
    with gangrene (symmetric) I73.01
RDS (newborn) (type I) P22.0
    type II P22.1
Reaction —*see also* Disorder
    adaptation —*see* Disorder, adjustment
    adjustment (anxiety) (conduct disorder)
        (depressiveness) (distress) —*see*
        Disorder, adjustment
        with
            mutism, elective (child) (adolescent) F94.0
    adverse
        food (any) (ingested) NEC T78.1
            anaphylactic —*see* Shock, anaphylactic,
                due to food
    anaphylactoid —*see* Shock, anaphylactic
    affective —*see* Disorder, mood
    allergic —*see* Allergy
    anaphylactic —*see* Shock, anaphylactic
    anesthesia —*see* Anesthesia, complication
    antitoxin (prophylactic) (therapeutic) —*see*
        Complications, vaccination
    anxiety F41.1
    Arthus —*see* Arthus' phenomenon
    asthenic F48.8
    combat and operational stress F43.0
    compulsive F42.8
    conversion F44.9
    crisis, acute F43.0
    deoxyribonuclease (DNA) (DNase)
        hypersensitivity D69.2
    depressive (single episode) F32.9
        affective (single episode) F31.4
            recurrent episode F33.9
        neurotic F34.1
        psychoneurotic F34.1

Reaction *(Continued)*
    depressive *(Continued)*
        psychotic F32.3
        recurrent —*see* Disorder, depressive,
            recurrent
    dissociative F44.9
    drug NEC T88.7
        addictive —*see* Dependence, drug
            transmitted via placenta or breast
                milk —*see* Absorption, drug,
                addictive, through placenta
        allergic —*see* Allergy, drug
        lichenoid L43.2
        newborn P93.8
            gray baby syndrome P93.0
        overdose or poisoning (by accident) —*see*
            Table of Drugs and Chemicals, by
            drug, poisoning
        photoallergic L56.1
        phototoxic L56.0
        withdrawal —*see* Dependence, by drug,
            with, withdrawal
            infant of dependent mother P96.1
            newborn P96.1
        wrong substance given or taken (by
            accident) —*see* Table of Drugs and
            Chemicals, by drug, poisoning
    fear F40.9
        child (abnormal) F93.8
    febrile nonhemolytic transfusion (FNHTR)
        R50.84
    fluid loss, cerebrospinal G97.1
    foreign
        body NEC —*see* Granuloma, foreign body
            in operative wound (inadvertently
                left) —*see* Foreign body, accidentally
                left during a procedure
        substance accidentally left during a
            procedure (chemical) (powder) (talc)
            T81.60
            aseptic peritonitis T81.61
            body or object (instrument) (sponge)
                (swab) —*see* Foreign body,
                accidentally left during a
                procedure
            specified reaction NEC T81.69
    grief —*see* Disorder, adjustment
    Herxheimer's R68.89
    hyperkinetic —*see* Hyperkinesia
    hypochondriacal F45.20
    hypoglycemic, due to insulin E16.0
        with coma (diabetic) —*see* Diabetes, coma
            nondiabetic E15
        therapeutic misadventure —*see*
            subcategory T38.3
    hypomanic F30.8
    hysterical F44.9
    immunization —*see* Complications, vaccination
    incompatibility
        ABO blood group (infusion) (transfusion) —
            see Complication(s), transfusion,
            incompatibility reaction, ABO
        delayed serologic T80.39
        minor blood group (Duffy) (E) (K(ell))
            (Kidd) (Lewis) (M) (N) (P) (S)
            T80.89
        Rh (factor) (infusion) (transfusion) —
            see Complication(s), transfusion,
            incompatibility reaction, Rh (factor)
    inflammatory —*see* Infection
    infusion —*see* Complications, infusion
    inoculation (immune serum) —*see*
        Complications, vaccination
    insulin T38.3-●
    involutional psychotic —*see* Disorder,
        depressive
    leukemoid D72.823
        basophilic D72.823
        lymphocytic D72.823
        monocytic D72.823
        myelocytic D72.823
        neutrophilic D72.823

Reaction *(Continued)*
 LSD (acute)
  due to drug abuse —*see* Abuse, drug,
   hallucinogen
  due to drug dependence —*see* Dependence,
   drug, hallucinogen
 lumbar puncture G97.1
 manic-depressive —*see* Disorder, bipolar
 neurasthenic F48.8
 neurogenic —*see* Neurosis
 neurotic F48.9
 neurotic-depressive F34.1
 nitritoid —*see* Crisis, nitritoid - obsessive-
   compulsive F42
 nonspecific
  to
   cell mediated immunity measurement
    of gamma interferon antigen
    response without active
    tuberculosis R76.12
   QuantiFERON-TB test (QFT) without
    active tuberculosis R76.12
   tuberculin test —*see also* Reaction,
    tuberculin skin test R76.11
 obsessive-compulsive F42.8
 organic, acute or subacute —*see* Delirium
 paranoid (acute) F23
  chronic F22
  senile F03
 passive dependency F60.7
 phobic F40.9
 post-traumatic stress, uncomplicated
   Z73.3
 psychogenic F99
 psychoneurotic —*see also* Neurosis
  compulsive F42.8
  depersonalization F48.1
  depressive F34.1
  hypochondriacal F45.20
  neurasthenic F48.8
  obsessive F42.8
 psychophysiologic —*see* Disorder,
   somatoform
 psychosomatic —*see* Disorder, somatoform
 psychotic —*see* Psychosis
 scarlet fever toxin —*see* Complications,
   vaccination
 schizophrenic F23
  acute (brief) (undifferentiated) F23
  latent F21
  undifferentiated (acute) (brief) F23
 serological for syphilis —*see* Serology for
   syphilis
 serum T80.69
  anaphylactic (immediate) —*see also* Shock,
   anaphylactic T80.59
  specified reaction NEC
   due to
    administration of blood and blood
     products T80.61
    immunization T80.62
    serum specified NEC T80.69
    vaccination T80.62
 situational —*see* Disorder, adjustment
 somatization —*see* Disorder, somatoform
 spinal puncture G97.1
 stress (severe) F43.9
  acute (agitation) ("daze") (disorientation)
   (disturbance of consciousness) (flight
   reaction) (fugue) F43.0
  specified NEC F43.8
 surgical procedure —*see* Complications,
   surgical procedure
 tetanus antitoxin —*see* Complications,
   vaccination
 toxic, to local anesthesia T81.59
  in labor and delivery O74.4
  in pregnancy O29.3X- •
  postpartum, puerperal O89.3
 toxin-antitoxin —*see* Complications,
   vaccination

Reaction *(Continued)*
 transfusion (blood) (bone marrow)
   (lymphocytes) (allergic) —*see*
   Complications, transfusion
 tuberculin skin test, abnormal R76.11
 vaccination (any) —*see* Complications,
   vaccination
 withdrawing, child or adolescent F93.8
Reactive airway disease —*see* Asthma
Reactive depression —*see* Reaction, depressive
Rearrangement
 chromosomal
  balanced (in) Q95.9
   abnormal individual (autosomal) Q95.2
    non-sex (autosomal) chromosomes
     Q95.2
    sex/non-sex chromosomes Q95.3
   specified NEC Q95.8
Recalcitrant patient —*see* Noncompliance
Recanalization, thrombus —*see* Thrombosis
Recession, receding
 chamber angle (eye) H21.55- •
 chin M26.09
 ➡gingival (postinfective) (postoperative)
  ▶generalized K06.020
   ▶minimal K06.021
   ▶moderate K06.022
   ▶severe K06.023
  ▶localized K06.010
   ▶minimal K06.011
   ▶moderate K06.012
   ▶severe K06.013
  ~~Miller Class I K06.01~~
  ~~Miller Class II K06.02~~
  ~~Miller Class III K06.03~~
  ~~Miller Class IV K06.04~~
Recklinghausen's disease Q85.01
 bones E21.0
Reclus' disease (cystic) —*see* Mastopathy, cystic
Recrudescent typhus (fever) A75.1
Recruitment, auditory H93.21- •
Rectalgia K62.89
Rectitis K62.89
Rectocele
 female (without uterine prolapse) N81.6
  with uterine prolapse N81.4
   incomplete N81.2
 in pregnancy —*see* Pregnancy, complicated
   by, abnormal, pelvic organs or tissues
   NEC
 male K62.3
Rectosigmoid junction —*see* condition
Rectosigmoiditis K63.89
 ulcerative (chronic) K51.30
  with
   complication K51.319
    abscess K51.314
    fistula K51.313
    obstruction K51.312
    rectal bleeding K51.311
    specified NEC K51.318
Rectourethral —*see* condition
Rectovaginal —*see* condition
Rectovesical —*see* condition
Rectum, rectal —*see* condition
Recurrent —*see* condition
 pregnancy loss —*see* Loss (of), pregnancy,
   recurrent
Red bugs B88.0
Red-cedar lung or pneumonitis J67.8
Red tide —*see also* Table of Drugs and
   Chemicals T65.82- •
Reduced
 mobility Z74.09
 ventilatory or vital capacity R94.2
Redundant, redundancy
 anus (congenital) Q43.8
 clitoris N90.89
 colon (congenital) Q43.8
 foreskin (congenital) N47.8
 intestine (congenital) Q43.8

Redundant, redundancy *(Continued)*
 labia N90.69
 organ or site, congenital NEC —*see* Accessory
 panniculus (abdominal) E65
 prepuce (congenital) N47.8
 pylorus K31.89
 rectum (congenital) Q43.8
 scrotum N50.89
 sigmoid (congenital) Q43.8
 skin L98.7
  and subcutaneous tissue L98.7
  of face L57.4
   eyelids —*see* Blepharochalasis
 stomach K31.89
Reduplication —*see* Duplication
Reflex R29.2
 hyperactive gag J39.2
 pupillary, abnormal —*see* Anomaly, pupil,
   function
 vasoconstriction I73.9
 vasovagal R55
Reflux K21.9
 acid K21.9
 esophageal K21.9
  with esophagitis K21.0
  newborn P78.83
 gastroesophageal K21.9
  with esophagitis K21.0
 mitral —*see* Insufficiency, mitral
 ureteral —*see* Reflux, vesicoureteral
 vesicoureteral (with scarring) N13.70
  with
   nephropathy N13.729
    with hydroureter N13.739
     bilateral N13.732
     unilateral N13.731
    without hydroureter N13.729
     bilateral N13.722
     unilateral N13.721
    bilateral N13.722
    unilateral N13.721
   pyelonephritis (chronic) N11.0
  without nephropathy N13.71
  congenital Q62.7
Reforming, artificial openings —*see* Attention
   to, artificial, opening
Refractive error —*see* Disorder, refraction
Refsum's disease or syndrome G60.1
Refusal of
 food, psychogenic F50.89
 treatment (because of) Z53.20
  left against medical advice (AMA) Z53.21
  patient's decision NEC Z53.29
  reasons of belief or group pressure Z53.1
Regional —*see* condition
Regurgitation R11.10
 aortic (valve) —*see* Insufficiency, aortic
 food —*see also* Vomiting
  with reswallowing —*see* Rumination
  newborn P92.1
 gastric contents —*see* Vomiting
 heart —*see* Endocarditis
 mitral (valve) —*see* Insufficiency, mitral
  congenital Q23.3
 myocardial —*see* Endocarditis
 pulmonary (valve) (heart) I37.1
  congenital Q22.2
  syphilitic A52.03
 tricuspid —*see* Insufficiency, tricuspid
 valve, valvular —*see* Endocarditis
  congenital Q24.8
 vesicoureteral —*see* Reflux, vesicoureteral
Reichmann's disease or syndrome K31.89
Reifenstein syndrome E34.52
Reinsertion
 implantable subdermal contraceptive Z30.46
 intrauterine contraceptive device Z30.433
Reiter's disease, syndrome, or urethritis
   M02.30
 ankle M02.37- •
 elbow M02.32- •

▶ New   ➡ Revised   ~~deleted~~ Deleted   • Use Additional Character(s)

Reiter's disease, syndrome, or urethritis
(Continued)
  foot joint M02.37-●
  hand joint M02.34-●
  hip M02.35-●
  knee M02.36-●
  multiple site M02.39
  shoulder M02.31-●
  vertebra M02.38
  wrist M02.33-●
Rejection
  food, psychogenic F50.89
  transplant T86.91
    bone T86.830
      marrow T86.01
    cornea T86.840
    heart T86.21
      with lung(s) T86.31
    intestine T86.850
    kidney T86.11
    liver T86.41
    lung(s) T86.810
      with heart T86.31
    organ (immune or nonimmune cause) T86.91
    pancreas T86.890
    skin (allograft) (autograft) T86.820
    specified NEC T86.890
    stem cell (peripheral blood) (umbilical
      cord) T86.5
Relapsing fever A68.9
  Carter's (Asiatic) A68.1
  Dutton's (West African) A68.1
  Koch's A68.9
  louse-borne (epidemic) A68.0
  Novy's (American) A68.1
  Obermeyers's (European) A68.0
  Spirillum A68.9
  tick-borne (endemic) A68.1
Relationship
  occlusal
    open anterior M26.220
    open posterior M26.221
Relaxation
  anus (sphincter) K62.89
    psychogenic F45.8
  arch (foot) —see also Deformity, limb, flat foot
  back ligaments —see Instability, joint, spine
  bladder (sphincter) N31.2
  cardioesophageal K21.9
  cervix —see Incompetency, cervix
  diaphragm J98.6
  joint (capsule) (ligament) (paralytic) —see
    Flail, joint
    congenital NEC Q74.8
  lumbosacral (joint) —see subcategory M53.2
  pelvic floor N81.89
  perineum N81.89
  posture R29.3
  rectum (sphincter) K62.89
  sacroiliac (joint) —see subcategory M53.2
  scrotum N50.89
  urethra (sphincter) N36.44
  vesical N31.2
Release from prison, anxiety concerning Z65.2
Remains
  canal of Cloquet Q14.0
  capsule (opaque) Q14.8
Remittent fever (malarial) B54
Remnant
  canal of Cloquet Q14.0
  capsule (opaque) Q14.8
  cervix, cervical stump (acquired)
    (postoperative) N88.8
  cystic duct, postcholecystectomy K91.5
  fingernail L60.8
    congenital Q84.6
  meniscus, knee —see Derangement, knee,
    meniscus, specified NEC
  thyroglossal duct Q89.2
  tonsil J35.8
    infected (chronic) J35.01
  urachus Q64.4

Removal (from) (of)
  artificial
    arm Z44.00-●
      complete Z44.01-●
      partial Z44.02-●
    eye Z44.2-●
    leg Z44.10-●
      complete Z44.11-●
      partial Z44.12-●
  breast implant Z45.81
  cardiac pulse generator (battery) (end-of-life)
    Z45.010
  catheter (urinary) (indwelling) Z46.6
    from artificial opening —see Attention to,
      artificial, opening
    non-vascular Z46.82
    vascular NEC Z45.2
  device Z46.9
    contraceptive Z30.432
      implantable subdermal Z30.46
    implanted NEC Z45.89
    specified NEC Z46.89
  drains Z48.03
  dressing (nonsurgical) Z48.00
    surgical Z48.01
  external
    fixation device — code to fracture with
      seventh character D
    prosthesis, prosthetic device Z44.9
      breast Z44.3-●
      specified NEC Z44.8
  home in childhood (to foster home or
    institution) Z62.29
  ileostomy Z43.2
  insulin pump Z46.81
  myringotomy device (stent) (tube) Z45.82
  nervous system device NEC Z46.2
    brain neuropacemaker Z46.2
    visual substitution device Z46.2
      implanted Z45.31
  non-vascular catheter Z46.82
  organ, prophylactic (for neoplasia
    management) —see Prophylactic, organ
    removal
  orthodontic device Z46.4
  staples Z48.02
  stent
    ureteral Z46.6
  suture Z48.02
  urinary device Z46.6
  vascular access device or catheter Z45.2
Ren
  arcuatus Q63.1
  mobile, mobilis N28.89
    congenital Q63.8
  unguliformis Q63.1
Renal —see condition
Rendu-Osler-Weber disease or syndrome I78.0
Reninoma D41.0-●
Renon-Delille syndrome E23.3
Reovirus, as cause of disease classified
  elsewhere B97.5
Repeated falls NEC R29.6
Replaced chromosome by dicentric ring Q93.2
Replacement by artificial or mechanical device
  or prosthesis of
  bladder Z96.0
  blood vessel NEC Z95.828
  bone NEC Z96.7
  cochlea Z96.21
  coronary artery Z95.5
  eustachian tube Z96.29
  eye globe Z97.0
  heart Z95.812
    valve Z95.2
      prosthetic Z95.2
      specified NEC Z95.4
      xenogenic Z95.3
  intestine Z96.89
  joint Z96.60
    hip —see Presence, hip joint implant
    knee —see Presence, knee joint implant
    specified site NEC Z96.698

Replacement by artificial or mechanical device
  or prosthesis of (Continued)
  larynx Z96.3
  lens Z96.1
  limb(s) —see Presence, artificial, limb
  mandible NEC (for tooth root implant(s))
    Z96.5
  organ NEC Z96.89
  peripheral vessel NEC Z95.828
  stapes Z96.29
  teeth Z97.2
  tendon Z96.7
  tissue NEC Z96.89
  tooth root(s) Z96.5
  vessel NEC Z95.828
    coronary (artery) Z95.5
Request for expert evidence Z04.8
Reserve, decreased or low
  cardiac —see Disease, heart
  kidney N28.89
Residual —see also condition
  ovary syndrome N99.83
  state, schizophrenic F20.5
  urine R39.198
Resistance, resistant (to)
  activated protein C D68.51
  complicating pregnancy O26.89
  insulin E88.81
  organism(s)
    to
      drug Z16.30
        aminoglycosides Z16.29
        amoxicillin Z16.11
        ampicillin Z16.11
        antibiotic(s) Z16.20
          multiple Z16.24
          specified NEC Z16.29
        antifungal Z16.32
        antimicrobial (single) Z16.30
          multiple Z16.35
          specified NEC Z16.39
        antimycobacterial (single) Z16.341
          multiple Z16.342
        antiparasitic Z16.31
        antiviral Z16.33
        beta lactam antibiotics Z16.10
          specified NEC Z16.19
        cephalosporins Z16.19
        extended beta lactamase (ESBL) Z16.12
        fluoroquinolones Z16.23
        macrolides Z16.29
        methicillin —see MRSA
        multiple drugs (MDRO)
          antibiotics Z16.24
          antimicrobial Z16.35
          antimycobacterials Z16.342
        penicillins Z16.11
        quinine (and related compounds)
          Z16.31
        quinolones Z16.23
        sulfonamides Z16.29
        tetracyclines Z16.29
        tuberculostatics (single) Z16.341
          multiple Z16.342
        vancomycin Z16.21
          related antibiotics Z16.22
  thyroid hormone E07.89
Resorption
  dental (roots) K03.3
    alveoli M26.79
  teeth (external) (internal) (pathological)
    (roots) K03.3
Respiration
  Cheyne-Stokes R06.3
  decreased due to shock, following injury
    T79.4
  disorder of, psychogenic F45.8
  insufficient, or poor R06.89
    newborn P28.5
  painful R07.1
  sighing, psychogenic F45.8

Respiratory —*see also* condition
  distress syndrome (newborn) (type I)
      P22.0
    type II P22.1
  syncytial virus, as cause of disease classified
      elsewhere B97.4
Respite care Z75.5
Response (drug)
  photoallergic L56.1
  phototoxic L56.0
Restenosis
  stent
    vascular
      end stent
        adjacent to stent —*see*
            Arteriosclerosis
        within the stent
          coronary T82.855
          peripheral T82.856
      in stent
        coronary vessel T82.855
        peripheral vessel T82.856
Restless legs (syndrome) G25.81
Restlessness R45.1
Restoration (of)
  dental
    aesthetically inadequate or displeasing
        K08.56
    defective K08.50
      specified NEC K08.59
    failure of marginal integrity K08.51
    failure of periodontal anatomical intergrity
        K08.54
  organ continuity from previous sterilization
      (tuboplasty) (vasoplasty) Z31.0
    aftercare Z31.42
  tooth (existing)
    contours biologically incompatible with
        oral health K08.54
    open margins K08.51
    overhanging K08.52
    poor aesthetic K08.56
    poor gingival margins K08.51
  unsatisfactory, of tooth K08.50
    specified NEC K08.59
Restorative material (dental)
  allergy to K08.55
  fractured K08.539
    with loss of material K08.531
    without loss of material K08.530
  unrepairable overhanging of K08.52
Restriction of housing space Z59.1
Rests, ovarian, in fallopian tube Q50.6
Restzustand (schizophrenic) F20.5
Retained —*see also* Retention
  cholelithiasis following cholecystectomy
      K91.86
  foreign body fragments (type of) Z18.9
    acrylics Z18.2
    animal quill(s) or spines Z18.31
    cement Z18.83
    concrete Z18.83
    crystalline Z18.83
    depleted isotope Z18.09
    depleted uranium Z18.01
    diethylhexylphthalates Z18.2
    glass Z18.81
    isocyanate Z18.2
    magnetic metal Z18.11
    metal Z18.10
    nonmagnetic metal Z18.12
    nontherapeutic radioactive Z18.09
    organic NEC Z18.39
    plastic Z18.2
    quill(s) (animal) Z18.31
    radioactive (nontherapeutic) NEC Z18.09
    specified NEC Z18.89
    spine(s) (animal) Z18.31
    stone Z18.83
    tooth (teeth) Z18.32
    wood Z18.33

Retained (Continued)
    fragments (type of) Z18.9
      acrylics Z18.2
      animal quill(s) or spines Z18.31
      cement Z18.83
      concrete Z18.83
      crystalline Z18.83
      depleted isotope Z18.09
      depleted uranium Z18.01
      diethylhexylphthalates Z18.2
      glass Z18.81
      isocyanate Z18.2
      magnetic metal Z18.11
      metal Z18.10
      nonmagnectic metal Z18.12
      nontherapeutic radioactive Z18.09
      organic NEC Z18.39
      plastic Z18.2
      quill(s) (animal) Z18.31
      radioactive (nontherapeutic) NEC Z18.09
      specified NEC Z18.89
      spine(s) (animal) Z18.31
      stone Z18.83
      tooth (teeth) Z18.32
      wood Z18.33
  gallstones, following cholecystectomy K91.86
Retardation
  development, developmental, specific —*see*
      Disorder, developmental
  endochondral bone growth —*see* Disorder,
      bone, development or growth
  growth R62.50
    due to malnutrition E45
  mental —*see* Disability, intellectual
  motor function, specific F82
  physical (child) R62.52
    due to malnutrition E45
  reading (specific) F81.0
  spelling (specific) (without reading disorder)
      F81.81
Retching —*see* Vomiting
Retention —*see also* Retained
  bladder —*see* Retention, urine
  carbon dioxide E87.2
  cholelithiasis following cholecystectomy K91.86
  cyst —*see* Cyst
  dead
    fetus (at or near term) (mother) O36.4
      early fetal death O02.1
    ovum O02.0
  decidua (fragments) (following delivery)
      (with hemorrhage) O72.2
    without hemorrhage O73.1
  deciduous tooth K00.6
  dental root K08.3
  fecal —*see* Constipation
  fetus
    dead O36.4
      early O02.1
  fluid R60.9
  foreign body —*see also* Foreign body, retained
    current trauma - code as Foreign body, by
        site or type
  gallstones, following cholecystectomy K91.86
  gastric K31.89
  intrauterine contraceptive device, in
      pregnancy —*see* Pregnancy, complicated
      by, retention, intrauterine device
  membranes (complicating delivery) (with
      hemorrhage) O72.2
    with abortion —*see* Abortion, by type
    without hemorrhage O73.1
  meniscus —*see* Derangement, meniscus
  menses N94.89
  milk (puerperal, postpartum) O92.79
  nitrogen, extrarenal R39.2
  ovary syndrome N99.83
  placenta (total) (with hemorrhage) O72.0
    without hemorrhage O73.0
    portions or fragments (with hemorrhage)
        O72.2
      without hemorrhage O73.1

Retention (Continued)
  products of conception
    early pregnancy (dead fetus) O02.1
    following
      delivery (with hemorrhage) O72.2
        without hemorrhage O73.1
  secundines (following delivery) (with
      hemorrhage) O72.0
    without hemorrhage O73.0
  complicating puerperium (delayed
      hemorrhage) O72.2
  partial O72.2
    without hemorrhage O73.1
  smegma, clitoris N90.89
  urine R33.9
    drug-induced R33.0
    due to hyperplasia (hypertrophy) of
        prostate —*see* Hyperplasia, prostate
    organic R33.8
      drug-induced R33.0
    psychogenic F45.8
    specified NEC R33.8
  water (in tissues) —*see* Edema
Reticular erythematous mucinosis L98.5
Reticulation, dust —*see* Pneumoconiosis
Reticulocytosis R70.1
Reticuloendotheliosis
  acute infantile C96.0
  leukemic C91.4-●
  nonlipid C96.0
Reticulohistiocytoma (giant-cell) D76.3
Reticuloid, actinic L57.1
Reticulosis (skin)
  acute of infancy C96.0
  hemophagocytic, familial D76.1
  histiocytic medullary C96.A
  lipomelanotic I89.8
  malignant (midline) C86.0
  polymorphic C86.0
  Sézary —*see* Sézary disease
Retina, retinal —*see also* condition
  dark area D49.81
Retinitis —*see also* Inflammation,
    chorioretinal
  albuminurica N18.9 *[H32]*
  diabetic —*see* Diabetes, retinitis
  disciformis —*see* Degeneration, macula
  focal —*see* Inflammation, chorioretinal, focal
  gravidarum —*see* Pregnancy, complicated by,
      specified pregnancy-related condition
      NEC
  juxtapapillaris —*see* Inflammation,
      chorioretinal, focal, juxtapapillary
  luetic —*see* Retinitis, syphilitic
  pigmentosa H35.52
  proliferans —*see* Disorder, globe,
      degenerative, specified type NEC
  proliferating —*see* Disorder, globe,
      degenerative, specified type NEC
  renal N18.9 *[H32]*
  syphilitic (early) (secondary) A51.43
    central, recurrent A52.71
    congenital (early) A50.01 *[H32]*
    late A52.71
  tuberculous A18.53
Retinoblastoma C69.2-●
  differentiated C69.2-●
  undifferentiated C69.2-●
Retinochoroiditis —*see also* Inflammation,
    chorioretinal
  disseminated —*see* Inflammation,
      chorioretinal, disseminated
    syphilitic A52.71
  focal —*see* Inflammation, chorioretinal
  juxtapapillaris —*see* Inflammation,
      chorioretinal, focal, juxtapapillary
Retinopathy (background) H35.00
  arteriosclerotic I70.8 *[H35.0-●]*
  atherosclerotic I70.8 *[H35.0-●]*
  central serous —*see* Chorioretinopathy,
      central serous

▶ New   ⇒ Revised   ~~deleted~~ Deleted   ● Use Additional Character(s)

Retinopathy *(Continued)*
  Coats H35.02-●
  diabetic —*see* Diabetes, retinopathy
  exudative H35.02-●
  hypertensive H35.03-●
  in (due to)
    diabetes —*see* Diabetes, retinopathy
    sickle-cell disorders D57.-● *[H36]*
  of prematurity H35.10-●
    stage 0 H35.11-●
    stage 1 H35.12-●
    stage 2 H35.13-●
    stage 3 H35.14-●
    stage 4 H35.15-●
    stage 5 H35.16-●
  pigmentary, congenital —*see* Dystrophy,
    retina
  proliferative NEC H35.2-●
    diabetic —*see* Diabetes, retinopathy,
      proliferative
    sickle-cell D57.-● *[H36]*
  solar H31.02-●
Retinoschisis H33.10-●
  congenital Q14.1
  specified type NEC H33.19-●
Retortamoniasis A07.8
Retractile testis Q55.22
Retraction
  cervix —*see* Retroversion, uterus
  drum (membrane) —*see* Disorder, tympanic
    membrane, specified NEC
  finger —*see* Deformity, finger
  lid H02.539
    left H02.536
      lower H02.535
      upper H02.534
    right H02.533
      lower H02.532
      upper H02.531
  lung J98.4
  mediastinum J98.59
  nipple N64.53
    associated with
      lactation O92.03
      pregnancy O92.01-●
      puerperium O92.02
    congenital Q83.8
  palmar fascia M72.0
  pleura —*see* Pleurisy
  ring, uterus (Bandl's) (pathological)
    O62.4
  sternum (congenital) Q76.7
    acquired M95.4
  uterus —*see* Retroversion, uterus
  valve (heart) —*see* Endocarditis
Retrobulbar —*see* condition
Retrocecal —*see* condition
Retrocession —*see* Retroversion
Retrodisplacement —*see* Retroversion
Retroflection, retroflexion —*see* Retroversion
Retrognathia, retrognathism (mandibular)
    (maxillary) M26.19
Retrograde menstruation N92.5
Retroperineal —*see* condition
Retroperitoneal —*see* condition
Retroperitonitis K68.9
Retropharyngeal —*see* condition
Retroplacental —*see* condition
Retroposition —*see* Retroversion
Retroprosthetic membrane T85.398
Retrosternal thyroid (congenital) Q89.2
Retroversion, retroverted
  cervix —*see* Retroversion, uterus
  female NEC —*see* Retroversion, uterus
  iris H21.89
  testis (congenital) Q55.29
  uterus (acquired) (acute) (any degree)
      (asymptomatic) (cervix) (postinfectional)
      (postpartal, old) N85.4
    congenital Q51.818
    in pregnancy O34.53-●

Retrovirus, as cause of disease classified
    elsewhere B97.30
  human
    immunodeficiency, type 2 (HIV 2) B97.35
    T-cell lymphotropic
      type I (HTLV-I) B97.33
      type II (HTLV-II) B97.34
  lentivirus B97.31
  oncovirus B97.32
  specified NEC B97.39
Retrusion, premaxilla (developmental) M26.09
Rett's disease or syndrome F84.2
Reverse peristalsis R19.2
Reye's syndrome G93.7
Rh (factor)
  hemolytic disease (newborn) P55.0
  incompatibility, immunization or
      sensitization
    affecting management of pregnancy NEC
      O36.09-●
    anti-D antibody O36.01-●
    newborn P55.0
    transfusion reaction —*see* Complication(s),
      transfusion, incompatibility reaction,
      Rh (factor)
  negative mother affecting newborn P55.0
  titer elevated —*see* Complication(s),
    transfusion, incompatibility reaction, Rh
    (factor)
  transfusion reaction —*see* Complication(s),
    transfusion, incompatibility reaction, Rh
    (factor)
Rhabdomyolysis (idiopathic) NEC M62.82
  traumatic T79.6
Rhabdomyoma —*see also* Neoplasm, connective
    tissue, benign
  adult —*see* Neoplasm, connective tissue,
    benign
  fetal —*see* Neoplasm, connective tissue, benign
  glycogenic —*see* Neoplasm, connective tissue,
    benign
Rhabdomyosarcoma (any type) —*see*
    Neoplasm, connective tissue, malignant
Rhabdosarcoma —*see* Rhabdomyosarcoma
Rhesus (factor) incompatibility —*see* Rh,
    incompatibility
Rheumatic (acute) (subacute) (chronic)
  adherent pericardium I09.2
  coronary arteritis I01.9
  degeneration, myocardium I09.0
  fever (acute) —*see* Fever, rheumatic
  heart —*see* Disease, heart, rheumatic
  myocardial degeneration —*see* Degeneration,
    myocardium
  myocarditis (chronic) (inactive) (with chorea)
    I09.0
    with chorea (acute) (rheumatic)
      (Sydenham's) I02.0
    active or acute I01.2
  pancarditis, acute I01.8
    with chorea (acute) (rheumatic)
      Sydenham's) I02.0
  pericarditis (active) (acute) (with effusion)
      (with pneumonia) I01.0
    with chorea (acute) (rheumatic)
      (Sydenham's) I02.0
    chronic or inactive I09.2
  pneumonia I00 *[J17]*
  torticollis M43.6
  typhoid fever A01.09
Rheumatism (articular) (neuralgic)
    (nonarticular) M79.0
  gout —*see* Arthritis, rheumatoid
  intercostal, meaning Tietze's disease M94.0
  palindromic (any site) M12.30
    ankle M12.37-●
    elbow M12.32-●
    foot joint M12.37-●
    hand joint M12.34-●
    hip M12.35-●
    knee M12.36-●

Rheumatism *(Continued)*
  palindromic *(Continued)*
    multiple site M12.39
    shoulder M12.31-●
    specified joint NEC M12.38
    vertebrae M12.38
    wrist M12.33-●
  sciatic M54.4-●
Rheumatoid —*see also* condition
  arthritis —*see also* Arthritis, rheumatoid
    with involvement of organs NEC M05.60
      ankle M05.67-●
      elbow M05.62-●
      foot joint M05.67-●
      hand joint M05.64-●
      hip M05.65-●
      knee M05.66-●
      multiple site M05.69
      shoulder M05.61-●
      vertebra —*see* Spondylitis, ankylosing
      wrist M05.63-●
    seronegative —*see* Arthritis, rheumatoid,
      seronegative
    seropositive —*see* Arthritis, rheumatoid,
      seropositive
  carditis M05.30
    ankle M05.37-●
    elbow M05.32-●
    foot joint M05.37-●
    hand joint M05.34-●
    hip M05.35-●
    knee M05.36-●
    multiple site M05.39
    shoulder M05.31-●
    vertebra —*see* Spondylitis, ankylosing
    wrist M05.33-●
  endocarditis —*see* Rheumatoid, carditis
  lung (disease) M05.10
    ankle M05.17-●
    elbow M05.12-●
    foot joint M05.17-●
    hand joint M05.14-●
    hip M05.15-●
    knee M05.16-●
    multiple site M05.19
    shoulder M05.11-●
    vertebra —*see* Spondylitis, ankylosing
    wrist M05.13-●
  myocarditis —*see* Rheumatoid, carditis
  myopathy M05.40
    ankle M05.47-●
    elbow M05.42-●
    foot joint M05.47-●
    hand joint M05.44-●
    hip M05.45-●
    knee M05.46-●
    multiple site M05.49
    shoulder M05.41-●
    vertebra —*see* Spondylitis, ankylosing
    wrist M05.43-●
  pericarditis —*see* Rheumatoid, carditis
  polyarthritis —*see* Arthritis, rheumatoid
  polyneuropathy M05.50
    ankle M05.57-●
    elbow M05.52-●
    foot joint M05.57-●
    hand joint M05.54-●
    hip M05.55-●
    knee M05.56-●
    multiple site M05.59
    shoulder M05.51-●
    vertebra —*see* Spondylitis, ankylosing
    wrist M05.53-●
  vasculitis M05.20
    ankle M05.27-●
    elbow M05.22-●
    foot joint M05.27-●
    hand joint M05.24-●
    hip M05.25-●
    knee M05.26-●
    multiple site M05.29

Rheumatoid *(Continued)*
  vasculitis *(Continued)*
    shoulder M05.21-●
    vertebra —*see* Spondylitis, ankylosing
    wrist M05.23-●
Rhinitis (atrophic) (catarrhal) (chronic)
  (croupous) (fibrinous) (granulomatous)
  (hyperplastic) (hypertrophic)
  (membranous) (obstructive) (purulent)
  (suppurative) (ulcerative) J31.0
  with
    sore throat —*see* Nasopharyngitis
  acute J00
  allergic J30.9
    with asthma J45.909
      with
        exacerbation (acute) J45.901
        status asthmaticus J45.902
    due to
      food J30.5
      pollen J30.1
    nonseasonal J30.89
    perennial J30.89
    seasonal NEC J30.2
    specified NEC J30.89
  infective J00
  pneumococcal J00
  syphilitic A52.73
    congenital A50.05 [J99]
  tuberculous A15.8
  vasomotor J30.0
Rhinoantritis (chronic) —*see* Sinusitis,
  maxillary
Rhinodacryolith —*see* Dacryolith
Rhinolith (nasal sinus) J34.89
Rhinomegaly J34.89
Rhinopharyngitis (acute) (subacute) —*see also*
  Nasopharyngitis
  chronic J31.1
  destructive ulcerating A66.5
  mutilans A66.5
Rhinophyma L71.1
Rhinorrhea J34.89
  cerebrospinal (fluid) G96.0
  paroxysmal —*see* Rhinitis, allergic
  spasmodic —*see* Rhinitis, allergic
Rhinosalpingitis —*see* Salpingitis, eustachian
Rhinoscleroma A48.8
Rhinosporidiosis B48.1
Rhinovirus infection NEC B34.8
Rhizomelic chondrodysplasia punctata E71.540
Rhythm
  atrioventricular nodal I49.8
  disorder I49.9
    coronary sinus I49.8
    ectopic I49.8
    nodal I49.8
  escape I49.9
  heart, abnormal I49.9
  idioventricular I44.2
  nodal I49.8
  sleep, inversion G47.2-●
    nonorganic origin —*see* Disorder, sleep,
      circadian rhythm, psychogenic
Rhytidosis facialis L98.8
Rib —*see also* condition
  cervical Q76.5
Riboflavin deficiency E53.0
Rice bodies —*see also* Loose, body, joint
  knee M23.4-●
Richter syndrome —*see* Leukemia, chronic
  lymphocytic, B-cell type
Richter's hernia —*see* Hernia, abdomen, with
  obstruction
Ricinism —*see* Poisoning, food, noxious, plant
Rickets (active) (acute) (adolescent) (chest wall)
  (congenital) (current) (infantile) (intestinal)
  E55.0
  adult —*see* Osteomalacia
  celiac K90.0
  hypophosphatemic with nephrotic-glycosuric
    dwarfism E72.09
  inactive E64.3

Rickets *(Continued)*
  kidney N25.0
  renal N25.0
  sequelae, any E64.3
  vitamin-D-resistant E83.31 [M90.80]
Rickettsial disease A79.9
  specified type NEC A79.89
Rickettsialpox (Rickettsia akari) A79.1
Rickettsiosis A79.9
  due to
    Ehrlichia sennetsu A79.81
    Rickettsia akari (rickettsialpox) A79.1
  specified type NEC A79.89
  tick-borne A77.9
  vesicular A79.1
Rider's bone —*see* Ossification, muscle,
  specified NEC
Ridge, alveolus —*see also* condition
  flabby K06.8
Ridged ear, congenital Q17.3
Riedel's
  lobe, liver Q44.7
  struma, thyroiditis or disease E06.5
Rieger's anomaly or syndrome Q13.81
Riehl's melanosis L81.4
Rietti-Greppi-Micheli anemia D56.9
Rieux's hernia —*see* Hernia, abdomen, specified
  site NEC
Riga (-Fede) disease K14.0
Riggs' disease —*see* Periodontitis
Right aortic arch Q25.47
Right middle lobe syndrome J98.11
Rigid, rigidity —*see also* condition
  abdominal R19.30
    with severe abdominal pain R10.0
    epigastric R19.36
    generalized R19.37
    left lower quadrant R19.34
    left upper quadrant R19.32
    periumbilic R19.35
    right lower quadrant R19.33
    right upper quadrant R19.31
  articular, multiple, congenital Q68.8
  cervix (uteri) in pregnancy —*see* Pregnancy,
    complicated by, abnormal, cervix
  hymen (acquired) (congenital) N89.6
  nuchal R29.1
  pelvic floor in pregnancy —*see* Pregnancy,
    complicated by, abnormal, pelvic organs
    or tissues NEC
  perineum or vulva in pregnancy —*see*
    Pregnancy, complicated by, abnormal,
    vulva
  spine —*see* Dorsopathy, specified NEC
  vagina in pregnancy —*see* Pregnancy,
    complicated by, abnormal, vagina
Rigors R68.89
  with fever R50.9
Riley-Day syndrome G90.1
RIND (reversible ischemic neurologic deficit)
  I63.9
Ring(s)
  aorta (vascular) Q25.45
  Bandl's O62.4
  contraction, complicating delivery O62.4
  esophageal, lower (muscular) K22.2
  Fleischer's (cornea) H18.04-●
  hymenal, tight (acquired) (congenital) N89.6
  Kayser-Fleischer (cornea) H18.04-●
  retraction, uterus, pathological O62.4
  Schatzki's (esophagus) (lower) K22.2
    congenital Q39.3
  Soemmerring's —*see* Cataract, secondary
  vascular (congenital) Q25.8
    aorta Q25.45
Ringed hair (congenital) Q84.1
Ringworm B35.9
  beard B35.0
  black dot B35.0
  body B35.4
  Burmese B35.5
  corporeal B35.4
  foot B35.3

Ringworm *(Continued)*
  groin B35.6
  hand B35.2
  honeycomb B35.0
  nails B35.1
  perianal (area) B35.6
  scalp B35.0
  specified NEC B35.8
  Tokelau B35.5
Rise, venous pressure I87.8
Rising, PSA following treatment for malignant
  neoplasm of prostate R97.21
~~Risk, suicidal~~
  ~~meaning personal history of attempted~~
    ~~suicide Z91.5~~
  ~~meaning suicidal ideation — see Ideation,~~
    ~~suicidal~~
▶Risk
  ▶for
    ▶dental caries Z91.849
      ▶high Z91.843
      ▶low Z91.841
      ▶moderate Z91.842
  ▶suicidal
    ▶meaning personal history of attempted
      suicide Z91.5
    ▶meaning suicidal ideation —*see* Ideation,
      suicidal
Ritter's disease L00
Rivalry, sibling Z62.891
Rivalta's disease A42.2
River blindness B73.01
Robert's pelvis Q74.2
  with disproportion (fetopelvic) O33.0
    causing obstructed labor O65.0
Robin (-Pierre) syndrome Q87.0
Robinow-Silvermann-Smith syndrome Q87.1
Robinson's (hidrotic) ectodermal dysplasia or
  syndrome Q82.4
Robles' disease B73.01
Rocky Mountain (spotted) fever A77.0
Roetheln —*see* Rubella
Roger's disease Q21.0
Rokitansky-Aschoff sinuses (gallbladder) K82.8
Rolando's fracture (displaced) S62.22-●
  nondisplaced S62.22-●
Romano-Ward (prolonged QT interval)
  syndrome I45.81
Romberg's disease or syndrome G51.8
Roof, mouth —*see* condition
Rosacea L71.9
  acne L71.9
  keratitis L71.8
  specified NEC L71.8
Rosary, rachitic E55.0
Rose
  cold J30.1
  fever J30.1
  rash R21
    epidemic B06.9
Rosenbach's erysipeloid A26.0
Rosenthal's disease or syndrome D68.1
Roseola B09
  infantum B08.20
    due to human herpesvirus 6 B08.21
    due to human herpesvirus 7 B08.22
Ross River disease or fever B33.1
Rossbach's disease K31.89
  psychogenic F45.8
Rostan's asthma (cardiac) —*see* Failure,
  ventricular, left
Rotation
  anomalous, incomplete or insufficient,
    intestine Q43.3
  cecum (congenital) Q43.3
  colon (congenital) Q43.3
  spine, incomplete or insufficient —*see*
    Dorsopathy, deforming, specified NEC
  tooth, teeth, fully erupted M26.35
  vertebra, incomplete or insufficient —*see*
    Dorsopathy, deforming, specified NEC
Rotes Quérol disease or syndrome —*see*
  Hyperostosis, ankylosing

Roth (-Bernhardt) disease or syndrome —*see*
      Meralgia paraesthetica
Rothmund (-Thomson) syndrome Q82.8
Rotor's disease or syndrome E80.6
Round
   back (with wedging of vertebrae) —*see*
      Kyphosis
   sequelae (late effect) of rickets E64.3
   worms (large) (infestation) NEC B82.0
      Ascariasis —*see also* Ascariasis B77.9
Roussy-Lévy syndrome G60.0
Rubella (German measles) B06.9
   complication NEC B06.09
      neurological B06.00
   congenital P35.0
   contact Z20.4
   exposure to Z20.4
   maternal
      care for (suspected) damage to fetus O35.3
      manifest rubella in infant P35.0
      suspected damage to fetus affecting
         management of pregnancy O35.3
   specified complications NEC B06.89
Rubeola (meaning measles) —*see* Measles
   meaning rubella —*see* Rubella
Rubeosis, iris —*see* Disorder, iris, vascular
Rubinstein-Taybi syndrome Q87.2
Rudimentary (congenital) —*see also* Agenesis
   arm —*see* Defect, reduction, upper limb
   bone Q79.9
   cervix uteri Q51.828
   eye Q11.2
   lobule of ear Q17.3
   patella Q74.1
   respiratory organs in thoracopagus Q89.4
   tracheal bronchus Q32.4
   uterus Q51.818
      in male Q56.1
   vagina Q52.0
Ruled out condition —*see* Observation, suspected
Rumination R11.10
   with nausea R11.2
   disorder of infancy F98.21
   neurotic F42.8
   newborn P92.1
   obsessional F42.8
   psychogenic F42.8
Runeberg's disease D51.0
Runny nose R09.89
Rupia (syphilitic) A51.39
   congenital A50.06
   tertiary A52.79
Rupture, ruptured
   abscess (spontaneous) - code by site under
      Abscess
   aneurysm —*see* Aneurysm
   anus (sphincter) —*see* Laceration, anus
   aorta, aortic I71.8
      abdominal I71.3
      arch I71.1
      ascending I71.1
      descending I71.8
         abdominal I71.3
         thoracic I71.1
      syphilitic A52.01
      thoracoabdominal I71.5
      thorax, thoracic I71.1
      transverse I71.1
      traumatic —*see* Injury, aorta, laceration,
         major
      valve or cusp —*see also* Endocarditis, aortic
         I35.8
   appendix (with peritonitis) K35.2
      with localized peritonitis K35.3
   arteriovenous fistula, brain I60.8
   artery I77.2
      brain —*see* Hemorrhage, intracranial,
         intracerebral
      coronary —*see* Infarct, myocardium
      heart —*see* Infarct, myocardium
      pulmonary I28.8
      traumatic (complication) —*see* Injury,
         blood vessel

Rupture, ruptured (*Continued*)
   bile duct (common) (hepatic) K83.2
      cystic K82.2
   bladder (sphincter) (nontraumatic)
      (spontaneous) N32.89
      following ectopic or molar pregnancy O08.6
      obstetrical trauma O71.5
      traumatic S37.29
   blood vessel —*see also* Hemorrhage
      brain —*see* Hemorrhage, intracranial,
         intracerebral
      heart —*see* Infarct, myocardium
      traumatic (complication) —*see* Injury,
         blood vessel, laceration, major, by site
   bone —*see* Fracture
   bowel (nontraumatic) K63.1
   brain
      aneurysm (congenital) —*see also*
         Hemorrhage, intracranial,
         subarachnoid
         syphilitic A52.05
      hemorrhagic —*see* Hemorrhage,
         intracranial, intracerebral
   capillaries I78.8
   cardiac (auricle) (ventricle) (wall) I23.3
      with hemopericardium I23.0
      infectional I40.9
      traumatic —*see* Injury, heart
   cartilage (articular) (current) —*see also* Sprain
      knee S83.3-●
      semilunar —*see* Tear, meniscus
   cecum (with peritonitis) K65.0
      with peritoneal abscess K35.3
      traumatic S36.598
   celiac artery, traumatic —*see* Injury, blood
      vessel, celiac artery, laceration, major
   cerebral aneurysm (congenital) (*see*
      Hemorrhage, intracranial, subarachnoid)
   cervix (uteri)
      with ectopic or molar pregnancy O08.6
      following ectopic or molar pregnancy O08.6
      obstetrical trauma O71.3
      traumatic S37.69
   chordae tendineae NEC I51.1
      concurrent with acute myocardial
         infarction —*see* Infarct, myocardium
      following acute myocardial infarction
         (current complication) I23.4
   choroid (direct) (indirect) (traumatic) H31.32-●
   circle of Willis I60.6
   colon (nontraumatic) K63.1
      traumatic —*see* Injury, intestine, large
   cornea (traumatic) —*see* Injury, eye, laceration
   coronary (artery) (thrombotic) —*see* Infarct,
      myocardium
   corpus luteum (infected) (ovary) N83.1-●
   cyst —*see* Cyst
   cystic duct K82.2
   Descemet's membrane —*see* Change, corneal
      membrane, Descemet's, rupture
      traumatic —*see* Injury, eye, laceration
   diaphragm, traumatic —*see* Injury,
      intrathoracic, diaphragm
   disc —*see* Rupture, intervertebral disc
   diverticulum (intestine) K57.80
      with bleeding K57.81
      bladder N32.3
      large intestine K57.20
         with
            bleeding K57.21
            small intestine K57.40
               with bleeding K57.41
         small intestine K57.00
            with
               bleeding K57.01
               large intestine K57.40
                  with bleeding K57.41
   duodenal stump K31.89
   ear drum (nontraumatic) —*see also*
      Perforation, tympanum
      traumatic S09.2-●
      due to blast injury —*see* Injury, blast, ear
   esophagus K22.3

Rupture, ruptured (*Continued*)
   eye (without prolapse or loss of intraocular
      tissue) —*see* Injury, eye, laceration
   fallopian tube NEC (nonobstetric)
      (nontraumatic) N83.8
      ➠due to pregnancy O00.10-●
         ➠with intrauterine pregnancy O00.11-●
   fontanel P13.1
   gallbladder K82.2
      traumatic S36.128
   gastric —*see also* Rupture, stomach
      vessel K92.2
   globe (eye) (traumatic) —*see* Injury, eye,
      laceration
   graafian follicle (hematoma) N83.0-●
   heart —*see* Rupture, cardiac
   hymen (nontraumatic) (nonintentional) N89.8
   internal organ, traumatic —*see* Injury, by site
   intervertebral disc —*see* Displacement,
      intervertebral disc
      traumatic —*see* Rupture, traumatic,
         intervertebral disc
   intestine NEC (nontraumatic) K63.1
      traumatic —*see* Injury, intestine
   iris —*see also* Abnormality, pupillary
      traumatic —*see* Injury, eye, laceration
   joint capsule, traumatic —*see* Sprain
   kidney (traumatic) S37.06-●
      birth injury P15.8
      nontraumatic N28.89
   lacrimal duct (traumatic) —*see* Injury, eye,
      specified site NEC
   lens (cataract) (traumatic) —*see* Cataract,
      traumatic
   ligament, traumatic —*see* Rupture, traumatic,
      ligament, by site
   liver S36.116
      birth injury P15.0
   lymphatic vessel I89.8
   marginal sinus (placental) (with
      hemorrhage) —*see* Hemorrhage,
      antepartum, specified cause NEC
   membrana tympani (nontraumatic) —*see*
      Perforation, tympanum
   membranes (spontaneous)
      artificial
         delayed delivery following O75.5
      delayed delivery following —*see*
         Pregnancy, complicated by, premature
         rupture of membranes
   meningeal artery I60.8
   meniscus (knee) —*see also* Tear, meniscus
      old —*see* Derangement, meniscus
      site other than knee - code as Sprain
   mesenteric artery, traumatic —*see* Injury,
      mesenteric, artery, laceration, major
   mesentery (nontraumatic) K66.8
      traumatic —*see* Injury, intra-abdominal,
         specified, site NEC
   mitral (valve) I34.8
   muscle (traumatic) —*see also* Strain
      diastasis —*see* Diastasis, muscle
      nontraumatic M62.10
         ankle M62.17-●
         foot M62.17-●
         forearm M62.13-●
         hand M62.14-●
         lower leg M62.16-●
         pelvic region M62.15-●
         shoulder region M62.11-●
         specified site NEC M62.18
         thigh M62.15-●
         upper arm M62.12-●
      traumatic —*see* Strain, by site
   musculotendinous junction NEC,
      nontraumatic —*see* Rupture, tendon,
      spontaneous
   mycotic aneurysm causing cerebral
      hemorrhage —*see* Hemorrhage,
      intracranial, subarachnoid
   myocardium, myocardial —*see* Rupture,
      cardiac
      traumatic —*see* Injury, heart

Rupture, ruptured *(Continued)*
  nontraumatic, meaning hernia —*see* Hernia
  obstructed —*see* Hernia, by site, obstructed
  operation wound —*see* Disruption, wound,
      operation
  ovary, ovarian N83.8
    corpus luteum cyst N83.1-•
    follicle (graafian) N83.0-•
  oviduct (nonobstetric) (nontraumatic) N83.8
    ➡due to pregnancy O00.10-•
      ➡with intrauterine pregnancy O00.11-•
  pancreas (nontraumatic) K86.89
    traumatic S36.299
  papillary muscle NEC I51.2
    following acute myocardial infarction
        (current complication) I23.5
  pelvic
    floor, complicating delivery O70.1
    organ NEC, obstetrical trauma O71.5
  perineum (nonobstetric) (nontraumatic)
      N90.89
    complicating delivery —*see* Delivery,
        complicated, by, laceration, anus
        (sphincter)
  postoperative wound —*see* Disruption,
      wound, operation
  prostate (traumatic) S37.828
  pulmonary
    artery I28.8
    valve (heart) I37.8
    vein I28.8
    vessel I28.8
  pus tube —*see* Salpingitis
  pyosalpinx —*see* Salpingitis
  rectum (nontraumatic) K63.1
    traumatic S36.69
  retina, retinal (traumatic) (without
      detachment) —*see also* Break, retina
    with detachment —*see* Detachment, retina,
        with retinal, break
  rotator cuff (nontraumatic) M75.10-•
    complete M75.12-•
    incomplete M75.11-•
  sclera —*see* Injury, eye, laceration
  sigmoid (nontraumatic) K63.1
    traumatic S36.593
  spinal cord —*see also* Injury, spinal cord, by
      region
    due to injury at birth P11.5
    newborn (birth injury) P11.5
  spleen (traumatic) S36.09
    birth injury P15.1
    congenital (birth injury) P15.1
    due to P. vivax malaria B51.0
    nontraumatic D73.5
    spontaneous D73.5
  splenic vein R58
    traumatic —*see* Injury, blood vessel,
        splenic vein
  stomach (nontraumatic) (spontaneous) K31.89
    traumatic S36.39
  supraspinatus (complete) (incomplete)
      (nontraumatic) —*see* Tear, rotator cuff
  symphysis pubis
    obstetric O71.6
    traumatic S33.4
  synovium (cyst) M66.10
    ankle M66.17-•
    elbow M66.12-•
    finger M66.14-•
    foot M66.17-•
    forearm M66.13-•
    hand M66.14-•
    pelvic region M66.15-•
    shoulder region M66.11-•
    specified site NEC M66.18
    thigh M66.15-•
    toe M66.17-•
    upper arm M66.12-•
    wrist M66.13-•
  tendon (traumatic) —*see* Strain
    nontraumatic (spontaneous) M66.9
      ankle M66.87-•

Rupture, ruptured *(Continued)*
  tendon *(Continued)*
    nontraumatic *(Continued)*
      extensor M66.20
        ankle M66.27-•
        foot M66.27-•
        forearm M66.23-•
        hand M66.24-•
        lower leg M66.26-•
        multiple sites M66.29
        pelvic region M66.25-•
        shoulder region M66.21-•
        specified site NEC M66.28
        thigh M66.25-•
        upper arm M66.22-•
      flexor M66.30
        ankle M66.37-•
        foot M66.37-•
        forearm M66.33-•
        hand M66.34-•
        lower leg M66.36-•
        multiple sites M66.39
        pelvic region M66.35-•
        shoulder region M66.31-•
        specified site NEC M66.38
        thigh M66.35-•
        upper arm M66.32-•
      foot M66.87-•
      forearm M66.83-•
      hand M66.84-•
      lower leg M66.86-•
      multiple sites M66.89
      pelvic region M66.85-•
      shoulder region M66.81-•
      specified
        site NEC M66.88
        tendon M66.80
      thigh M66.85-•
      upper arm M66.82-•
  thoracic duct I89.8
  tonsil J35.8
  traumatic
    aorta —*see* Injury, aorta, laceration, major
    diaphragm —*see* Injury, intrathoracic,
        diaphragm
    external site —*see* Wound, open, by site
    eye —*see* Injury, eye, laceration
    internal organ —*see* Injury, by site
    intervertebral disc
      cervical S13.0
      lumbar S33.0
      thoracic S23.0
    kidney S37.06-•
    ligament —*see also* Sprain
      ankle —*see* Sprain, ankle
      carpus —*see* Rupture, traumatic,
          ligament, wrist
      collateral (hand) —*see* Rupture,
          traumatic, ligament, finger, collateral
      finger (metacarpophalangeal)
          (interphalangeal) S63.40-•
        collateral S63.41-•
          index S63.41-•
          little S63.41-•
          middle S63.41-•
          ring S63.41-•
        index S63.40-•
        little S63.40-•
        middle S63.40-•
        palmar S63.42-•
          index S63.42-•
          little S63.42-•
          middle S63.42-•
          ring S63.42-•
        ring S63.40-•
        specified site NEC S63.499
          index S63.49-•
          little S63.49-•
          middle S63.49-•
          ring S63.49-•
        volar plate S63.43-•
          index S63.43-•
          little S63.43-•

Rupture, ruptured *(Continued)*
  traumatic *(Continued)*
    ligament *(Continued)*
      finger *(Continued)*
        volar plate *(Continued)*
          middle S63.43-•
          ring S63.43-•
      foot —*see* Sprain, foot
      radial collateral S53.2-•
      radiocarpal —*see* Rupture, traumatic,
          ligament, wrist, radiocarpal
      ulnar collateral S53.3-•
      ulnocarpal —*see* Rupture, traumatic,
          ligament, wrist, ulnocarpal
      wrist S63.30-•
        collateral S63.31-•
        radiocarpal S63.32-•
        specified site NEC S63.39-•
        ulnocarpal (palmar) S63.33-•
    liver S36.116
    membrana tympani —*see* Rupture, ear
        drum, traumatic
    muscle or tendon —*see* Strain
    myocardium —*see* Injury, heart
    pancreas S36.299
    rectum S36.69
    sigmoid S36.593
    spleen S36.09
    stomach S36.39
    symphysis pubis S33.4
    tympanum, tympanic (membrane) —*see*
        Rupture, ear drum, traumatic
    ureter S37.19
    uterus S37.69
    vagina —*see* Injury, vagina
    vena cava —*see* Injury, vena cava,
        laceration, major
  tricuspid (heart) (valve) I07.8
  tube, tubal (nonobstetric) (nontraumatic)
      N83.8
    abscess —*see* Salpingitis
    ➡due to pregnancy O00.10-•
      ➡with intrauterine pregnancy O00.11-•
  tympanum, tympanic (membrane)
      (nontraumatic) —*see also* Perforation,
      tympanic membrane H72.9-•
    traumatic —*see* Rupture, ear drum, traumatic
  umbilical cord, complicating delivery O69.89
  ureter (traumatic) S37.19
    nontraumatic N28.89
  urethra (nontraumatic) N36.8
    with ectopic or molar pregnancy O08.6
    following ectopic or molar pregnancy
        O08.6
    obstetrical trauma O71.5
    traumatic S37.39
  uterosacral ligament (nonobstetric)
      (nontraumatic) N83.8
  uterus (traumatic) S37.69
    before labor O71.0-•
    during or after labor O71.1
    nonpuerperal, nontraumatic N85.8
    pregnant (during labor) O71.1
      before labor O71.0-•
  vagina —*see* Injury, vagina
  valve, valvular (heart) —*see* Endocarditis
  varicose vein —*see* Varix
  varix —*see* Varix
  vena cava R58
    traumatic —*see* Injury, vena cava,
        laceration, major
  vesical (urinary) N32.89
  vessel (blood) R58
    pulmonary I28.8
    traumatic —*see* Injury, blood vessel
  viscus R19.8
  vulva complicating delivery O70.0
Russell-Silver syndrome Q87.1
Russian spring-summer type encephalitis A84.0
Rust's disease (tuberculous cervical spondylitis)
    A18.01
Ruvalcaba-Myhre-Smith syndrome E71.440
Rytand-Lipsitch syndrome I44.2

▶ New   ➡ Revised   ~~deleted~~ Deleted   • Use Additional Character(s)

S

Saber, sabre shin or tibia (syphilitic) A50.56
[M90.8-●]
Sac lacrimal —see condition
Saccharomyces infection B37.9
Saccharopinuria E72.3
Saccular —see condition
Sacculation
  aorta (nonsyphilitic) —see Aneurysm, aorta
  bladder N32.3
  intralaryngeal (congenital) (ventricular)
    Q31.3
  larynx (congenital) (ventricular) Q31.3
  organ or site, congenital —see Distortion
  pregnant uterus —see Pregnancy, complicated
    by, abnormal, uterus
  ureter N28.89
  urethra N36.1
  vesical N32.3
Sachs' amaurotic familial idiocy or disease
  E75.02
Sachs-Tay disease E75.02
Sacks-Libman disease M32.11
Sacralgia M53.3
Sacralization Q76.49
Sacrodynia M53.3
Sacroiliac joint —see condition
Sacroiliitis NEC M46.1
Sacrum —see condition
Saddle
  back —see Lordosis
  embolus
    abdominal aorta I74.01
    pulmonary artery I26.92
      with acute cor pulmonale I26.02
  injury — code to condition
  nose M95.0
    due to syphilis A50.57
Sadism (sexual) F65.52
Sadness, postpartal O90.6
Sadomasochism F65.50
Saemisch's ulcer (cornea) —see Ulcer, cornea,
  central
Sagging
  skin and subcutaneous tissue (following
    bariatric surgery weight loss) (following
    dietary weight loss) L98.7
Sahib disease B55.0
Sailors' skin L57.8
Saint
  Anthony's fire —see Erysipelas
  triad —see Hernia, diaphragm
  Vitus' dance —see Chorea, Sydenham's
Salaam
  attack(s) —see Epilepsy, spasms
  tic R25.8
Salicylism
  abuse F55.8
  overdose or wrong substance given —see
    Table of Drugs and Chemicals, by drug,
    poisoning
Salivary duct or gland —see condition
Salivation, excessive K11.7
Salmonella —see Infection, Salmonella
Salmonellosis A02.0
Salpingitis (catarrhal) (fallopian tube) (nodular)
  (pseudofollicular) (purulent) (septic)
  N70.91
  with oophoritis N70.93
  acute N70.01
    with oophoritis N70.03
  chlamydial A56.11
  chronic N70.11
    with oophoritis N70.13
  complicating abortion —see Abortion, by
    type, complicated by, salpingitis
  ear —see Salpingitis, eustachian
  eustachian (tube) H68.00-●
    acute H68.01-●
    chronic H68.02-●

Salpingitis (Continued)
  follicularis N70.11
    with oophoritis N70.13
  gonococcal (acute) (chronic) A54.24
  interstitial, chronic N70.11
    with oophoritis N70.13
  isthmica nodosa N70.11
    with oophoritis N70.13
  specific (gonococcal) (acute) (chronic) A54.24
  tuberculous (acute) (chronic) A18.17
  venereal (gonococcal) (acute) (chronic) A54.24
Salpingocele N83.4-●
Salpingo-oophoritis (catarrhal) (purulent)
  (ruptured) (septic) (suppurative) N70.93
  acute N70.03
    with ectopic or molar pregnancy O08.0
    following ectopic or molar pregnancy
      O08.0
    gonococcal A54.24
  chronic N70.13
  following ectopic or molar pregnancy O08.0
  gonococcal (acute) (chronic) A54.24
  puerperal O86.19
  specific (gonococcal) (acute) (chronic) A54.24
  subacute N70.03
  tuberculous (acute) (chronic) A18.17
  venereal (gonococcal) (acute) (chronic) A54.24
Salpingo-ovaritis —see Salpingo-oophoritis
Salpingoperitonitis —see Salpingo-oophoritis
Salzmann's nodular dystrophy —see
  Degeneration, cornea, nodular
Sampson's cyst or tumor N80.1
San Joaquin (Valley) fever B38.0
Sandblaster's asthma, lung or pneumoconiosis
  J62.8
Sander's disease (paranoia) F22
Sandfly fever A93.1
Sandhoff's disease E75.01
Sanfilippo (Type B) (Type C) (Type D)
  syndrome E76.22
Sanger-Brown ataxia G11.2
Sao Paulo fever or typhus A77.0
Saponification, mesenteric K65.8
Sarcocele (benign)
  syphilitic A52.76
    congenital A50.59
Sarcocystosis A07.8
Sarcoepiplocele —see Hernia
Sarcoepiplomphalocele Q79.2
Sarcoid —see also Sarcoidosis
  arthropathy D86.86
  Boeck's D86.9
  Darier-Roussy D86.3
  iridocyclitis D86.83
  meningitis D86.81
  myocarditis D86.85
  myositis D86.87
  pyelonephritis D86.84
  Spiegler-Fendt L08.89
Sarcoidosis D86.9
  with
    cranial nerve palsies D86.82
    hepatic granuloma D86.89
    polyarthritis D86.86
    tubulo-interstitial nephropathy D86.84
  combined sites NEC D86.89
  lung D86.0
    and lymph nodes D86.2
  lymph nodes D86.1
    and lung D86.2
  meninges D86.81
  skin D86.3
  specified type NEC D86.89
Sarcoma (of) —see also Neoplasm, connective
  tissue, malignant
  alveolar soft part —see Neoplasm, connective
    tissue, malignant
  ameloblastic C41.1
    upper jaw (bone) C41.0
  botryoid —see Neoplasm, connective tissue,
    malignant

Sarcoma (Continued)
  botryoides —see Neoplasm, connective tissue,
    malignant
  cerebellar C71.6
    circumscribed (arachnoidal) C71.6
  circumscribed (arachnoidal) cerebellar
    C71.6
  clear cell —see also Neoplasm, connective
    tissue, malignant
    kidney C64.-●
  dendritic cells (accessory cells) C96.4
  embryonal —see Neoplasm, connective tissue,
    malignant
  endometrial (stromal) C54.1
    isthmus C54.0
  epithelioid (cell) —see Neoplasm, connective
    tissue, malignant
  Ewing's —see Neoplasm, bone, malignant
  follicular dendritic cell C96.4
  germinoblastic (diffuse) —see Lymphoma,
    diffuse, large cell
    follicular —see Lymphoma, follicular,
      specified NEC
  giant cell (except of bone) —see also Neoplasm,
    connective tissue, malignant
    bone —see Neoplasm, bone, malignant
  glomoid —see Neoplasm, connective tissue,
    malignant
  granulocytic C92.3-●
  hemangioendothelial —see Neoplasm,
    connective tissue, malignant
  hemorrhagic, multiple —see Sarcoma,
    Kaposi's
  histiocytic C96.A
  Hodgkin —see Lymphoma, Hodgkin
  immunoblastic (diffuse) —see Lymphoma,
    diffuse large cell
  interdigitating dendritic cell C96.4
  Kaposi's
    colon C46.4
    connective tissue C46.1
    gastrointestinal organ C46.4
    lung C46.5-●
    lymph node(s) C46.3
    palate (hard) (soft) C46.2
    rectum C46.4
    skin C46.0
    specified site NEC C46.7
    stomach C46.4
    unspecified site C46.9
  Kupffer cell C22.3
  Langerhans cell C96.4
  leptomeningeal —see Neoplasm, meninges,
    malignant
  liver NEC C22.4
  lymphangioendothelial —see Neoplasm,
    connective tissue, malignant
  lymphoblastic —see Lymphoma,
    lymphoblastic (diffuse)
  lymphocytic —see Lymphoma, small cell
    B-cell
  ⇒mast cell C96.22
  melanotic —see Melanoma
  meningeal —see Neoplasm, meninges,
    malignant
  meningothelial —see Neoplasm, meninges,
    malignant
  mesenchymal —see also Neoplasm,
    connective tissue, malignant
    mixed —see Neoplasm, connective tissue,
      malignant
  mesothelial —see Mesothelioma
  monstrocellular
    specified site —see Neoplasm, malignant,
      by site
    unspecified site C71.9
  myeloid C92.3-●
  neurogenic —see Neoplasm, nerve,
    malignant
  odontogenic C41.1
    upper jaw (bone) C41.0

Sarcoma (Continued)
- osteoblastic —see Neoplasm, bone, malignant
- osteogenic —see also Neoplasm, bone, malignant
  - juxtacortical —see Neoplasm, bone, malignant
  - periosteal —see Neoplasm, bone, malignant
- periosteal —see also Neoplasm, bone, malignant
  - osteogenic —see Neoplasm, bone, malignant
- pleomorphic cell —see Neoplasm, connective tissue, malignant
- reticulum cell (diffuse) —see Lymphoma, diffuse large cell
  - nodular —see Lymphoma, follicular
  - pleomorphic cell type —see Lymphoma, diffuse large cell
- rhabdoid —see Neoplasm, malignant, by site
- round cell —see Neoplasm, connective tissue, malignant
- small cell —see Neoplasm, connective tissue, malignant
- soft tissue —see Neoplasm, connective tissue, malignant
- spindle cell —see Neoplasm, connective tissue, malignant
- stromal (endometrial) C54.1
  - isthmus C54.0
- synovial —see also Neoplasm, connective tissue, malignant
  - biphasic —see Neoplasm, connective tissue, malignant
  - epithelioid cell —see Neoplasm, connective tissue, malignant
  - spindle cell —see Neoplasm, connective tissue, malignant

Sarcomatosis
- meningeal —see Neoplasm, meninges, malignant
- specified site NEC —see Neoplasm, connective tissue, malignant
- unspecified site C80.1

Sarcopenia (age-related) M62.84
Sarcosinemia E72.59
Sarcosporidiosis (intestinal) A07.8
Satiety, early R68.81
Saturnine —see condition
Saturnism
- overdose or wrong substance given or taken —see Table of Drugs and Chemicals, by drug, poisoning

Satyriasis F52.8
Sauriasis —see Ichthyosis
SBE (subacute bacterial endocarditis) I33.0
Scabies (any site) B86
Scabs R23.4
Scaglietti-Dagnini syndrome E22.0
Scald —see Burn
Scalenus anticus (anterior) **syndrome** G54.0
Scales R23.4
Scaling, skin R23.4
Scalp —see condition
Scapegoating affecting child Z62.3
Scaphocephaly Q75.0
Scapulalgia M89.8X1
Scapulohumeral myopathy G71.0
Scar, scarring —see also Cicatrix L90.5
- adherent L90.5
- atrophic L90.5
- cervix
  - in pregnancy or childbirth —see Pregnancy, complicated by, abnormal cervix
- cheloid L91.0
- chorioretinal H31.00-●
  - posterior pole macula H31.01-●
  - postsurgical H59.81-●
  - solar retinopathy H31.02-●
  - specified type NEC H31.09-●

Scar, scarring (Continued)
- choroid —see Scar, chorioretinal
- conjunctiva H11.24-●
- cornea H17.9
  - xerophthalmic —see also Opacity, cornea vitamin A deficiency E50.6
- duodenum, obstructive K31.5
- hypertrophic L91.0
- keloid L91.0
- labia N90.89
- lung (base) J98.4
- macula —see Scar, chorioretinal, posterior pole
- muscle M62.89
- myocardium, myocardial I25.2
- painful L90.5
- posterior pole (eye) —see Scar, chorioretinal, posterior pole
- retina —see Scar, chorioretinal
- trachea J39.8
- transmural uterine, in pregnancy O34.29
- uterus N85.8
  - in pregnancy O34.29
- vagina N89.8
  - postoperative N99.2
- vulva N90.89

Scarabiasis B88.2
⟹**Scarlatina** (anginosa) (maligna) A38.9
- myocarditis (acute) A38.1
  - old —see Myocarditis
- otitis media A38.0
▶ulcerosa A38.8
Scarlet fever (albuminuria) (angina) A38.9
Schamberg's disease (progressive pigmentary dermatosis) L81.7
Schatzki's ring (acquired) (esophagus) (lower) K22.2
- congenital Q39.3
Schaufenster krankheit I20.8
Schaumann's
- benign lymphogranulomatosis D86.1
- disease or syndrome —see Sarcoidosis
Scheie's syndrome E76.03
Schenck's disease B42.1
Scheuermann's disease or osteochondrosis — see Osteochondrosis, juvenile, spine
Schilder (-Flatau) **disease** G37.0
Schilling-type monocytic leukemia C93.0-●
Schimmelbusch's disease, cystic mastitis, or hyperplasia —see Mastopathy, cystic
Schistosoma infestation —see Infestation, Schistosoma
Schistosomiasis B65.9
- with muscle disorder B65.9 [M63.80]
  - ankle B65.9 [M63.87-●]
  - foot B65.9 [M63.87-●]
  - forearm B65.9 [M63.83-●]
  - hand B65.9 [M63.84-●]
  - lower leg B65.9 [M63.86-●]
  - multiple sites B65.9 [M63.89]
  - pelvic region B65.9 [M63.85-●]
  - shoulder region B65.9 [M63.81-●]
  - specified site NEC B65.9 [M63.88]
  - thigh B65.9 [M63.85-●]
  - upper arm B65.9 [M63.82-●]
- Asiatic B65.2
- bladder B65.0
- chestermani B65.8
- colon B65.1
- cutaneous B65.3
- due to
  - S. haematobium B65.0
  - S. japonicum B65.2
  - S. mansoni B65.1
  - S. mattheii B65.8
- Eastern B65.2
- genitourinary tract B65.0
- intestinal B65.1
- lung NEC B65.9 [J99]
  - pneumonia B65.9 [J17]
- Manson's (intestinal) B65.1

Schistosomiasis (Continued)
- oriental B65.2
- pulmonary NEC B65.9 [J99]
  - pneumonia B65.9
- Schistosoma
  - haematobium B65.0
  - japonicum B65.2
  - mansoni B65.1
- specified type NEC B65.8
- urinary B65.0
- vesical B65.0
Schizencephaly Q04.6
Schizoaffective psychosis F25.9
Schizodontia K00.2
Schizoid personality F60.1
Schizophrenia, schizophrenic F20.9
- acute (brief) (undifferentiated) F23
- atypical (form) F20.3
- borderline F21
- catalepsy F20.2
- catatonic (type) (excited) (withdrawn) F20.2
- cenesthopathic, cenesthesiopathic F20.89
- childhood type F84.5
- chronic undifferentiated F20.5
- cyclic F25.0
- disorganized (type) F20.1
- flexibilitas cerea F20.2
- hebephrenic (type) F20.1
- incipient F21
- latent F21
- negative type F20.5
- paranoid (type) F20.0
- paraphrenic F20.0
- post-psychotic depression F32.89
- prepsychotic F21
- prodromal F21
- pseudoneurotic F21
- pseudopsychopathic F21
- reaction F23
- residual (state) (type) F20.5
- restzustand F20.5
- schizoaffective (type) —see Psychosis, schizoaffective
- simple (type) F20.89
- simplex F20.89
- specified type NEC F20.89
▶spectrum and other psychotic disorder F29
  ▶specified NEC F28
- stupor F20.2
- syndrome of childhood F84.5
- undifferentiated (type) F20.3
  - chronic F20.5
Schizothymia (persistent) F60.1
Schlatter-Osgood disease or osteochondrosis —see Osteochondrosis, juvenile, tibia
Schlatter's tibia —see Osteochondrosis, juvenile, tibia
Schmidt's syndrome (polyglandular, autoimmune) E31.0
Schmincke's carcinoma or tumor —see Neoplasm, nasopharynx, malignant
Schmitz (-Stutzer) **dysentery** A03.0
Schmorl's disease or nodes
- lumbar region M51.46
- lumbosacral region M51.47
- sacrococcygeal region M53.3
- thoracic region M51.44
- thoracolumbar region M51.45
Schneiderian
- papilloma —see Neoplasm, nasopharynx benign
  - specified site —see Neoplasm, benign, by site
  - unspecified site D14.0
  - specified site —see Neoplasm, malignant, by site
  - unspecified site C30.0
Scholte's syndrome (malignant carcinoid) E34.0
Scholz (-Bielchowsky-Henneberg) **disease or syndrome** E75.25
Schönlein (-Henoch) **disease or purpura** (primary) (rheumatic) D69.0

▶ New   ⟹ Revised   ~~deleted~~ Deleted   ● Use Additional Character(s)

Schottmuller's disease A01.4
Schroeder's syndrome (endocrine hypertensive) E27.0
Schüller-Christian disease or syndrome C96.5
Schultze's type acroparesthesia, simple I73.89
Schultz's disease or syndrome —see Agranulocytosis
Schwalbe-Ziehen-Oppenheim disease G24.1
Schwannoma —see also Neoplasm, nerve, benign
  malignant —see also Neoplasm, nerve, malignant
    with rhabdomyoblastic differentiation — see Neoplasm, nerve, malignant
  melanocytic —see Neoplasm, nerve, benign
  pigmented —see Neoplasm, nerve, benign
Schwannomatosis Q85.03
Schwartz (-Jampel) syndrome G71.13
Schwartz-Bartter syndrome E22.2
Schweniger-Buzzi anetoderma L90.1
Sciatic —see condition
Sciatica (infective)
  with lumbago M54.4-●
    due to intervertebral disc disorder —see Disorder, disc, with, radiculopathy
  due to displacement of intervertebral disc (with lumbago) —see Disorder, disc, with, radiculopathy
  wallet M54.3-●
Scimitar syndrome Q26.8
Sclera —see condition
Sclerectasia H15.84-●
Scleredema
  adultorum —see Sclerosis, systemic
  Buschke's —see Sclerosis, systemic
  newborn P83.0
Sclerema (adiposum) (edematosum) (neonatorum) (newborn) P83.0
  adultorum —see Sclerosis, systemic
Scleriasis —see Scleroderma
Scleritis H15.00-●
  with corneal involvement H15.04-●
  anterior H15.01-●
  brawny H15.02-●
  in (due to) zoster B02.34
  posterior H15.03-●
  specified type NEC H15.09-●
  syphilitic A52.71
  tuberculous (nodular) A18.51
Sclerochoroiditis H31.8
Scleroconjunctivitis —see Scleritis
Sclerocystic ovary syndrome E28.2
Sclerodactyly, sclerodactylia L94.3
Scleroderma, sclerodermia (acrosclerotic) (diffuse) (generalized) (progressive) (pulmonary) —see also Sclerosis, systemic M34.9-●
  circumscribed L94.0
  linear L94.1
  localized L94.0
  ➡newborn P83.88
  systemic M34.9
Sclerokeratitis H16.8
  tuberculous A18.52
Scleroma nasi A48.8
Scleromalacia (perforans) H15.05-●
Scleromyxedema L98.5
Sclérose en plaques G35
Sclerosis, sclerotic
  adrenal (gland) E27.8
  Alzheimer's —see Disease, Alzheimer's
  amyotrophic (lateral) G12.21
  aorta, aortic I70.0
    valve —see Endocarditis, aortic
  artery, arterial, arteriolar, arteriovascular — see Arteriosclerosis
  ascending multiple G35
  brain (generalized) (lobular) G37.9
    artery, arterial I67.2
    diffuse G37.0
    disseminated G35

Sclerosis, sclerotic (Continued)
  brain (Continued)
    insular G35
    Krabbe's E75.23
    miliary G35
    multiple G35
    presenile (Alzheimer's) —see Disease, Alzheimer's, early onset
    senile (arteriosclerotic) I67.2
    stem, multiple G35
    tuberous Q85.1
  bulbar, multiple G35
  bundle of His I44.39
  cardiac —see Disease, heart, ischemic, atherosclerotic
  cardiorenal —see Hypertension, cardiorenal
  cardiovascular —see also Disease, cardiovascular
    renal —see Hypertension, cardiorenal
  cerebellar —see Sclerosis, brain
  cerebral —see Sclerosis, brain
  cerebrospinal (disseminated) (multiple) G35
  cerebrovascular I67.2
  choroid —see Degeneration, choroid
  combined (spinal cord) —see also Degeneration, combined
    multiple G35
  concentric (Balo) G37.5
  cornea —see Opacity, cornea
  coronary (artery) I25.10
    with angina pectoris —see Arteriosclerosis, coronary (artery),
  corpus cavernosum
    female N90.89
    male N48.6
  diffuse (brain) (spinal cord) G37.0
  disseminated G35
  dorsal G35
  dorsolateral (spinal cord) —see Degeneration, combined
  endometrium N85.5
  extrapyramidal G25.9
  eye, nuclear (senile) —see Cataract, senile, nuclear
  focal and segmental (glomerular) —see also N00-N07 with fourth character .1 N05.1
  Friedreich's (spinal cord) G11.1
  funicular (spermatic cord) N50.89
  general (vascular) —see Arteriosclerosis
  gland (lymphatic) I89.8
  hepatic K74.1
    alcoholic K70.2
  hereditary
    cerebellar G11.9
    spinal (Friedreich's ataxia) G11.1
  hippocampal G93.81
  insular G35
  kidney —see Sclerosis, renal
  larynx J38.7
  ➡lateral (amyotrophic) (descending) (spinal) G12.21
    ▶primary G12.23
  lens, senile nuclear —see Cataract, senile, nuclear
  liver K74.1
    with fibrosis K74.2
      alcoholic K70.2
    alcoholic K70.2
    cardiac K76.1
  lung —see Fibrosis, lung
  mastoid —see Mastoiditis, chronic
  mesial temporal G93.81
  mitral I05.8
  Mönckeberg's (medial) —see Arteriosclerosis, extremities
  multiple (brain stem) (cerebral) (generalized) (spinal cord) G35
  myocardium, myocardial —see Disease, heart, ischemic, atherosclerotic
  nuclear (senile), eye —see Cataract, senile, nuclear

Sclerosis, sclerotic (Continued)
  ovary N83.8
  pancreas K86.89
  penis N48.6
  peripheral arteries —see Arteriosclerosis, extremities
  plaques G35
  pluriglandular E31.8
  polyglandular E31.8
  posterolateral (spinal cord) —see Degeneration, combined
  presenile (Alzheimer's) —see Disease, Alzheimer's, early onset
  ➡primary, lateral G12.23
  progressive, systemic M34.0
  pulmonary —see Fibrosis, lung
    artery I27.0
    valve (heart) —see Endocarditis, pulmonary
  renal N26.9
    with
      cystine storage disease E72.09
      hypertensive heart disease (conditions in I11) —see Hypertension, cardiorenal
      arteriolar (hyaline) (hyperplastic) —see Hypertension, kidney
  retina (senile) (vascular) H35.00
  senile (vascular) —see Arteriosclerosis
  spinal (cord) (progressive) G95.89
    ascending G61.0
    combined —see also Degeneration, combined
      multiple G35
      syphilitic A52.11
    disseminated G35
    dorsolateral —see Degeneration, combined
    hereditary (Friedreich's) (mixed form) G11.1
    ➡lateral (amyotrophic) G12.23
    multiple G35
    posterior (syphilitic) A52.11
  stomach K31.89
  subendocardial, congenital I42.4
  systemic M34.9
    with
      lung involvement M34.81
      myopathy M34.82
      polyneuropathy M34.83
    drug-induced M34.2
    due to chemicals NEC M34.2
    progressive M34.0
    specified NEC M34.89
  temporal (mesial) G93.81
  tricuspid (heart) (valve) I07.8
  tuberous (brain) Q85.1
  tympanic membrane —see Disorder, tympanic membrane, specified NEC
  valve, valvular (heart) —see Endocarditis
  vascular —see Arteriosclerosis
  vein I87.8
Scoliosis (acquired) (postural) M41.9
  adolescent (idiopathic) —see Scoliosis, idiopathic, adolescent
  congenital Q67.5
    due to bony malformation Q76.3
    failure of segmentation (hemivertebra) Q76.3
    hemivertebra fusion Q76.3
    postural Q67.5
  idiopathic M41.20
    adolescent M41.129
      cervical region M41.122
      cervicothoracic region M41.123
      lumbar region M41.126
      lumbosacral region M41.127
      thoracic region M41.124
      thoracolumbar region M41.125
    cervical region M41.22
    cervicothoracic region M41.23

Scoliosis *(Continued)*
  idiopathic *(Continued)*
    infantile M41.00
      cervical region M41.02
      cervicothoracic region M41.03
      lumbar region M41.06
      lumbosacral region M41.07
      sacrococcygeal region M41.08
      thoracic region M41.04
      thoracolumbar region M41.05
    juvenile M41.119
      cervical region M41.112
      cervicothoracic region M41.113
      lumbar region M41.116
      lumbosacral region M41.117
      thoracic region M41.114
      thoracolumbar region M41.115
    lumbar region M41.26
    lumbosacral region M41.27
    thoracic region M41.24
    thoracolumbar region M41.25
  infantile —*see* Scoliosis, idiopathic,
    infantile
  neuromuscular M41.40
    cervical region M41.42
    cervicothoracic region M41.43
    lumbar region M41.46
    lumbosacral region M41.47
    occipito-atlanto-axial region M41.41
    thoracic region M41.44
    thoracolumbar region M41.45
  paralytic —*see* Scoliosis, neuromuscular
  postradiation therapy M96.5
  rachitic (late effect or sequelae) E64.3
    [M49.80]
    cervical region E64.3 *[M49.82]*
    cervicothoracic region E64.3 *[M49.83]*
    lumbar region E64.3 *[M49.86]*
    lumbosacral region E64.3 *[M49.87]*
    multiple sites E64.3 *[M49.89]*
    occipito-atlanto-axial region E64.3
      [M49.81]
    sacrococcygeal region E64.3 *[M49.88]*
    thoracic region E64.3 *[M49.84]*
    thoracolumbar region E64.3 *[M49.85]*
  sciatic M54.4-•
  secondary (to) NEC M41.50
    cerebral palsy, Friedreich's ataxia,
      poliomyelitis, neuromuscular
      disorders —*see* Scoliosis,
      neuromuscular
    cervical region M41.52
    cervicothoracic region M41.53
    lumbar region M41.56
    lumbosacral region M41.57
    thoracic region M41.54
    thoracolumbar region M41.55
  specified form NEC M41.80
    cervical region M41.82
    cervicothoracic region M41.83
    lumbar region M41.86
    lumbosacral region M41.87
    thoracic region M41.84
    thoracolumbar region M41.85
  thoracogenic M41.30
    thoracic region M41.34
    thoracolumbar region M41.35
  tuberculous A18.01
Scoliotic pelvis
  with disproportion (fetopelvic) O33.0
    causing obstructed labor O65.0
Scorbutus, scorbutic —*see also* Scurvy
  anemia D53.2
Score, NIHSS (National Institutes of Health
  Stroke Scale) R29.7-•
Scotoma (arcuate) (Bjerrum) (central) (ring) —
  see also Defect, visual field, localized,
  scotoma
  scintillating H53.19
Scratch —*see* Abrasion
Scratchy throat R09.89

Screening (for) Z13.9
  alcoholism Z13.89
  anemia Z13.0
  anomaly, congenital Z13.89
➔ antenatal, of mother —*see also* Encounter,
    antenatal Z36.9
  arterial hypertension Z13.6
  arthropod-borne viral disease NEC Z11.59
  bacteriuria, asymptomatic Z13.89
  behavioral disorder Z13.89
  brain injury, traumatic Z13.850
  bronchitis, chronic Z13.83
  brucellosis Z11.2
  cardiovascular disorder Z13.6
  cataract Z13.5
  chlamydial diseases Z11.8
  cholera Z11.0
  chromosomal abnormalities (nonprocreative)
    NEC Z13.79
  colonoscopy Z12.11
  congenital
    dislocation of hip Z13.89
    eye disorder Z13.5
    malformation or deformation Z13.89
  contamination NEC Z13.88
  cystic fibrosis Z13.228
  dengue fever Z11.59
  dental disorder Z13.84
  depression Z13.89
  developmental handicap Z13.42
    in early childhood Z13.42
    infant Z13.41
  diabetes mellitus Z13.1
  diphtheria Z11.2
  disability, intellectual Z13.42
    infant Z13.41
  disease or disorder Z13.9
    bacterial NEC Z11.2
      intestinal infectious Z11.0
      respiratory tuberculosis Z11.1
    blood or blood-forming organ Z13.0
    cardiovascular Z13.6
    Chagas' Z11.6
    chlamydial Z11.8
    dental Z13.89
    developmental Z13.42
      in child Z13.42
      infant Z13.41
    digestive tract NEC Z13.818
      lower GI Z13.811
      upper GI Z13.810
    ear Z13.5
    endocrine Z13.29
    eye Z13.5
    genitourinary Z13.89
    heart Z13.6
    human immunodeficiency virus (HIV)
      infection Z11.4
    immunity Z13.0
    infection
      intestinal Z11.0
      specified NEC Z11.6
    infectious Z11.9
    mental Z13.89
    metabolic Z13.228
    neurological Z13.89
    nutritional Z13.21
      metabolic Z13.228
      lipoid disorders Z13.220
    protozoal Z11.6
      intestinal Z11.0
    respiratory Z13.83
    rheumatic Z13.828
    rickettsial Z11.8
    sexually-transmitted NEC Z11.3
      human immunodeficiency virus (HIV)
        Z11.4
    sickle-cell (trait) Z13.0
    skin Z13.89
    specified NEC Z13.89
    spirochetal Z11.8

Screening *(Continued)*
  disease or disorder *(Continued)*
    thyroid Z13.29
    vascular Z13.6
    venereal Z11.3
    viral NEC Z11.59
      human immunodeficiency virus (HIV)
        Z11.4
      intestinal Z11.0
  elevated titer Z13.89
  emphysema Z13.83
  encephalitis, viral (mosquito- or tick-borne)
    Z11.59
  exposure to contaminants (toxic) Z13.88
  fever
    dengue Z11.59
    hemorrhagic Z11.59
    yellow Z11.59
  filariasis Z11.6
  galactosemia Z13.228
  gastrointestinal condition Z13.818
  genetic (nonprocreative)- for procreative
    management —*see* Testing, genetic, for
    procreative management
    disease carrier status (nonprocreative)
      Z13.71
    specified NEC (nonprocreative) Z13.79
  genitourinary condition Z13.89
  glaucoma Z13.5
  gonorrhea Z11.3
  gout Z13.89
  helminthiasis (intestinal) Z11.6
  hematopoietic malignancy Z12.89
  hemoglobinopathies NEC Z13.0
  hemorrhagic fever Z11.59
  Hodgkin disease Z12.89
  human immunodeficiency virus (HIV) Z11.4
  human papillomavirus Z11.51
  hypertension Z13.6
  immunity disorders Z13.0
  infection
    mycotic Z11.8
    parasitic Z11.8
  ingestion of radioactive substance Z13.88
  intellectual disability Z13.42
    infant Z13.41
  intestinal
    helminthiasis Z11.6
    infectious disease Z11.0
  leishmaniasis Z11.6
  leprosy Z11.2
  leptospirosis Z11.8
  leukemia Z12.89
  lymphoma Z12.89
  malaria Z11.6
  malnutrition Z13.29
    metabolic Z13.228
    nutritional Z13.21
  measles Z11.59
  mental disorder Z13.89
  metabolic errors, inborn Z13.228
  multiphasic Z13.89
  musculoskeletal disorder Z13.828
    osteoporosis Z13.820
  mycoses Z11.8
  myocardial infarction (acute) Z13.6
  neoplasm (malignant) (of) Z12.9
    bladder Z12.6
    blood Z12.89
    breast Z12.39
      routine mammogram Z12.31
    cervix Z12.4
    colon Z12.11
    genitourinary organs NEC Z12.79
      bladder Z12.6
      cervix Z12.4
      ovary Z12.73
      prostate Z12.5
      testis Z12.71
      vagina Z12.72
    hematopoietic system Z12.89

Screening *(Continued)*
 neoplasm *(Continued)*
  intestinal tract Z12.10
   colon Z12.11
   rectum Z12.12
   small intestine Z12.13
  lung Z12.2
  lymph (glands) Z12.89
  nervous system Z12.82
  oral cavity Z12.81
  prostate Z12.5
  rectum Z12.12
  respiratory organs Z12.2
  skin Z12.83
  small intestine Z12.13
  specified site NEC Z12.89
  stomach Z12.0
 nephropathy Z13.89
 nervous system disorders NEC Z13.858
 neurological condition Z13.89
 osteoporosis Z13.820
 parasitic infestation Z11.9
  specified NEC Z11.8
 phenylketonuria Z13.228
 plague Z11.2
 poisoning (chemical) (heavy metal) Z13.88
 poliomyelitis Z11.59
 postnatal, chromosomal abnormalities
  Z13.89
 ➡prenatal, of mother —*see also* Encounter,
  antenatal Z36.9
 protozoal disease Z11.6
  intestinal Z11.0
 pulmonary tuberculosis Z11.1
 radiation exposure Z13.88
 respiratory condition Z13.83
 respiratory tuberculosis Z11.1
 rheumatoid arthritis Z13.828
 rubella Z11.59
 schistosomiasis Z11.6
 sexually-transmitted disease NEC Z11.3
  human immunodeficiency virus (HIV)
   Z11.4
 sickle-cell disease or trait Z13.0
 skin condition Z13.89
 sleeping sickness Z11.6
 special Z13.9
  specified NEC Z13.89
 syphilis Z11.3
 tetanus Z11.2
 trachoma Z11.8
 traumatic brain injury Z13.850
 trypanosomiasis Z11.6
 tuberculosis, respiratory Z11.1
 venereal disease Z11.3
 viral encephalitis (mosquito- or tick-borne)
  Z11.59
 whooping cough Z11.2
 worms, intestinal Z11.6
 yaws Z11.8
 yellow fever Z11.59
Scrofula, scrofulosis (tuberculosis of cervical
 lymph glands) A18.2
Scrofulide (primary) (tuberculous) A18.4
Scrofuloderma, scrofulodermia (any site)
 (primary) A18.4
Scrofulosus lichen (primary) (tuberculous)
 A18.4
Scrofulous —*see* condition
Scrotal tongue K14.5
Scrotum —*see* condition
Scurvy, scorbutic E54
 anemia D53.2
 gum E54
 infantile E54
 rickets E55.0 [M90.80]
Sealpox B08.62
Seasickness T75.3
Seatworm (infection) (infestation) B80
Sebaceous —*see also* condition
 cyst —*see* Cyst, sebaceous

Seborrhea, seborrheic L21.9
 capillitii R23.8
 capitis L21.0
 dermatitis L21.9
  infantile L21.1
 eczema L21.9
  infantile L21.1
 sicca L21.0
Seckel's syndrome Q87.1
Seclusion, pupil —*see* Membrane, pupillary
Second hand tobacco smoke exposure (acute)
 (chronic) Z77.22
 in the perinatal period P96.81
Secondary
 dentin (in pulp) K04.3
 neoplasm, secondaries —*see* Table of
  Neoplasms, secondary
Secretion
 antidiuretic hormone, inappropriate E22.2
 catecholamine, by pheochromocytoma E27.5
 hormone
  antidiuretic, inappropriate (syndrome)
   E22.2
  by
   carcinoid tumor E34.0
   pheochromocytoma E27.5
  ectopic NEC E34.2
 urinary
  excessive R35.8
  suppression R34
Section
 nerve, traumatic —*see* Injury, nerve
Sedative, hypnotic, or anxiolytic-induced
 anxiety disorder F13.980
 bipolar and related disorder F13.94
 delirium F13.921
 depressive disorder F13.94
 major neurocognitive disorder F13.97
 mild neurocognitive disorder F13.988
 psychotic disorder F13.959
 sexual dysfunction F13.981
 sleep disorder F13.982
Segmentation, incomplete (congenital) —*see*
 also Fusion
 bone NEC Q78.8
 lumbosacral (joint) (vertebra) Q76.49
Seitelberger's syndrome (infantile neuraxonal
 dystrophy) G31.89
Seizure(s) —*see also* Convulsions R56.9
 akinetic —*see* Epilepsy, generalized, specified
  NEC
 atonic —*see* Epilepsy, generalized, specified
  NEC
 autonomic (hysterical) F44.5
 convulsive —*see* Convulsions
 cortical (focal) (motor) —*see* Epilepsy,
  localization-related, symptomatic, with
  simple partial seizures
 disorder —*see also* Epilepsy G40.909
 due to stroke —*see* Sequelae (of), disease,
  cerebrovascular, by type, specified NEC
 epileptic —*see* Epilepsy
 febrile (simple) R56.00
  with status epilepticus G40.901
  complex (atypical) (complicated) R56.01
   with status epilepticus G40.901
 grand mal G40.409
  intractable G40.419
   with status epilepticus G40.411
   without status epilepticus G40.419
  not intractable G40.409
   with status epilepticus G40.401
   without status epilepticus G40.409
 heart —*see* Disease, heart
 hysterical F44.5
 intractable G40.919
  with status epilepticus G40.911
 Jacksonian (focal) (motor type) (sensory
  type) —*see* Epilepsy, localization-related,
  symptomatic, with simple partial
  seizures

Seizure *(Continued)*
 newborn P90
 nonspecific epileptic
  atonic —*see* Epilepsy, generalized, specified
   NEC
  clonic —*see* Epilepsy, generalized, specified
   NEC
  myoclonic —*see* Epilepsy, generalized,
   specified NEC
  tonic —*see* Epilepsy, generalized, specified
   NEC
  tonic-clonic —*see* Epilepsy, generalized,
   specified NEC
 partial, developing into secondarily
  generalized seizures
  complex —*see* Epilepsy, localization-
   related, symptomatic, with complex
   partial seizures
  simple —*see* Epilepsy, localization-related,
   symptomatic, with simple partial
   seizures
 petit mal G40.409
  intractable G40.419
   with status epilepticus G40.411
   without status epilepticus G40.419
  not intractable G40.409
   with status epilepticus G40.401
   without status epilepticus G40.409
 post traumatic R56.1
 recurrent G40.909
 specified NEC G40.89
 uncinate —*see* Epilepsy, localization-related,
  symptomatic, with complex partial
  seizures
Selenium deficiency, dietary E59
Self-damaging behavior (life-style) Z72.89
Self-harm (attempted)
 history (personal) Z91.5
 in family Z81.8
Self-mutilation (attempted)
 history (personal) Z91.5
 in family Z81.8
Self-poisoning
 history (personal) Z91.5
 in family Z81.8
 observation following (alleged) attempt Z03.6
Semicoma R40.1
Seminal vesiculitis N49.0
Seminoma C62.9-●
 specified site —*see* Neoplasm, malignant, by
  site
Senear-Usher disease or syndrome L10.4
Senectus R54
Senescence (without mention of psychosis)
 R54
Senile, senility —*see also* condition R41.81
 with
  acute confusional state F05
  mental changes NOS F03
  psychosis NEC —*see* Psychosis, senile
 asthenia R54
 cervix (atrophic) N88.8
 debility R54
 endometrium (atrophic) N85.8
 fallopian tube (atrophic) —*see* Atrophy,
  fallopian tube
 heart (failure) R54
 ovary (atrophic) —*see* Atrophy, ovary
 premature E34.8
 vagina, vaginitis (atrophic) N95.2
 wart L82.1
Sensation
 burning (skin) R20.8
  tongue K14.6
 loss of R20.8
 prickling (skin) R20.2
 tingling (skin) R20.2
Sense loss
 smell —*see* Disturbance, sensation, smell
 taste —*see* Disturbance, sensation, taste
 touch R20.8

Sensibility disturbance (cortical) (deep)
  (vibratory) R20.9
Sensitive, sensitivity —see also Allergy
  carotid sinus G90.01
  child (excessive) F93.8
  cold, autoimmune D59.1
  dentin K03.89
  gluten (non-celiac) K90.41
  latex Z91.040
  methemoglobin D74.8
  tuberculin, without clinical or radiological
    symptoms R76.11
  visual
    glare H53.71
    impaired contrast H53.72
Sensitiver Beziehungswahn F22
Sensitization, auto-erythrocytic D69.2
Separation
  anxiety, abnormal (of childhood) F93.0
  apophysis, traumatic - code as Fracture, by
    site
  choroid —see Detachment, choroid
  epiphysis, epiphyseal
    nontraumatic —see also
      Osteochondropathy, specified type
      NEC
    upper femoral —see Slipped, epiphysis,
      upper femoral
    traumatic - code as Fracture, by site
  fracture —see Fracture
  infundibulum cardiac from right ventricle by
    a partition Q24.3
  joint (traumatic) (current) - code by site under
    Dislocation
  pubic bone, obstetrical trauma O71.6
  retina, retinal —see Detachment, retina
  symphysis pubis, obstetrical trauma O71.6
  tracheal ring, incomplete, congenital Q32.1
Sepsis (generalized) (unspecified organism)
    A41.9
  with
    organ dysfunction (acute) (multiple) R65.20
      with septic shock R65.21
  actinomycotic A42.7
  adrenal hemorrhage syndrome
    (meningococcal) A39.1
  anaerobic A41.4
  Bacillus anthracis A22.7
  Brucella —see also Brucellosis A23.9
  candidal B37.7
  cryptogenic A41.9
  due to device, implant or graft T85.79
    arterial graft NEC T82.7
    breast (implant) T85.79
    catheter NEC T85.79
      dialysis (renal) T82.7
        intraperitoneal T85.71
      infusion NEC T82.7
        spinal (cranial) (epidural) (intrathecal)
          (spinal) (subarachnoid)
          (subdural) T85.735
      urethral indwelling T83.511
      urinary T83.518
    ectopic or molar pregnancy O08.82
    electronic (electrode) (pulse generator)
      (stimulator)
      bone T84.7
      cardiac T82.7
      nervous system T85.738
        brain T85.731
        neurostimulator generator T85.734
        peripheral nerve T85.732
        spinal cord T85.733
      urinary T83.590
    fixation, internal (orthopedic) —see
      Complication, fixation device,
      infection
    gastrointestinal (bile duct) (esophagus)
      T85.79
    neurostimulator electrode (lead)
      T85.732

Sepsis (Continued)
  due to device, implant or graft (Continued)
    genital T83.69
    heart NEC T82.7
      valve (prosthesis) T82.6
        graft T82.7
    joint prosthesis —see Complication, joint
      prosthesis, infection
    ocular (corneal graft) (orbital implant)
      T85.79
    orthopedic NEC T84.7
      fixation device, internal —see
        Complication, fixation device,
        infection
    specified NEC T85.79
    vascular T82.7
    ventricular intracranial (communicating)
      shunt T85.730
  during labor O75.3
  Enterococcus A41.81
  Erysipelothrix (rhusiopathiae) (erysipeloid)
    A26.7
  Escherichia coli (E. coli) A41.5
  extraintestinal yersiniosis A28.2
  following
    abortion (subsequent episode) O08.0
      current episode —see Abortion
    ectopic or molar pregnancy O08.82
    immunization T88.0
    infusion, therapeutic injection or
      transfusion NEC T80.29
  gangrenous A41.9
  gonococcal A54.86
  Gram-negative (organism) A41.5
    anaerobic A41.4
  Haemophilus influenzae A41.3
  herpesviral B00.7
  intra-abdominal K65.1
  intraocular —see Endophthalmitis,
    purulent
  Listeria monocytogenes A32.7
  localized — code to specific localized
    infection
➠in operation wound T81.4
    skin —see Abscess
  malleus A24.0
  melioidosis A24.1
  meningeal —see Meningitis
  meningococcal A39.4
    acute A39.2
    chronic A39.3
  MSSA (Methicillin susceptible
    Staphylococcus aureus) A41.01
  newborn P36.9
    due to
      anaerobes NEC P36.5
      Escherichia coli P36.4
      Staphylococcus P36.30
        aureus P36.2
        specified NEC P36.39
      Streptococcus P36.10
        group B P36.0
        specified NEC P36.19
    specified NEC P36.8
  Pasteurella multocida A28.0
  pelvic, puerperal, postpartum, childbirth O85
  pneumococcal A40.3
➠postprocedural T81.4
  puerperal, postpartum, childbirth (pelvic)
    O85
  Salmonella (arizonae) (cholerae-suis)
    (enteritidis) (typhimurium) A02.1
  severe R65.20
    with septic shock R65.21
  Shigella (see also Dysentery, bacillary) A03.9
  skin, localized —see Abscess
  specified organism NEC A41.89
  Staphylococcus, staphylococcal A41.2
    aureus (methicillin susceptible) (MSSA)
      A41.01
      methicillin resistant (MRSA) A41.02

Sepsis (Continued)
  Staphylococcus, staphylococcal (Continued)
    coagulase-negative A41.1
    specified NEC A41.1
  Streptococcus, streptococcal A40.9
    agalactiae A40.1
    group
      A A40.0
      B A40.1
      D A41.81
    neonatal P36.10
      group B P36.0
      specified NEC P36.19
    pneumoniae A40.3
    pyogenes A40.0
    specified NEC A40.8
  tracheostomy stoma J95.02
  tularemic A21.7
  umbilical, umbilical cord (newborn) —see
    Sepsis, newborn
  Yersinia pestis A20.7
Septate —see Septum
Septic —see condition
  arm —see Cellulitis, upper limb
    with lymphangitis —see Lymphangitis,
      acute, upper limb
  embolus —see Embolism
  finger —see Cellulitis, digit
    with lymphangitis —see Lymphangitis,
      acute, digit
  foot —see Cellulitis, lower limb
    with lymphangitis —see Lymphangitis,
      acute, lower limb
  gallbladder (acute) K81.0
  hand —see Cellulitis, upper limb
    with lymphangitis —see Lymphangitis,
      acute, upper limb
  joint —see Arthritis, pyogenic or pyemic
  leg —see Cellulitis, lower limb
    with lymphangitis —see Lymphangitis,
      acute, lower limb
  nail —see also Cellulitis, digit
    with lymphangitis —see Lymphangitis,
      acute, digit
  sore —see also Abscess
    throat J02.0
      streptococcal J02.0
  spleen (acute) D73.89
  teeth, tooth (pulpal origin) K04.4
  throat —see Pharyngitis
  thrombus —see Thrombosis
  toe —see Cellulitis, digit
    with lymphangitis —see Lymphangitis,
      acute, digit
  tonsils, chronic J35.01
    with adenoiditis J35.03
  uterus —see Endometritis
Septicemia A41.9
  meaning sepsis —see Sepsis
Septum, septate (congenital) —see also
    Anomaly, by site
  anal Q42.3
    with fistula Q42.2
  aqueduct of Sylvius Q03.0
    with spina bifida —see Spina bifida, by site,
      with hydrocephalus
  uterus (complete) (partial) Q51.2
  vagina Q52.10
    in pregnancy —see Pregnancy,
      complicated by, abnormal
      vagina
    causing obstructed labor O65.5
    longitudinal Q52.129
      microperforate
        left side Q52.124
        right side Q52.123
      nonobstruction Q52.120
      obstructing Q52.129
        left side Q52.122
        right side Q52.121
    transverse Q52.11

Sequelae (of) —see also condition
  abscess, intracranial or intraspinal (conditions in G06) G09
  amputation — code to injury with seventh character S
  burn and corrosion — code to injury with seventh character S
  calcium deficiency E64.8
  cerebrovascular disease —see Sequelae, disease, cerebrovascular
  childbirth O94
  contusion — code to injury with seventh character S
  corrosion —see Sequelae, burn and corrosion
  crushing injury — code to injury with seventh character S
  disease
    cerebrovascular I69.90
      alteration of sensation I69.998
      aphasia I69.920
      apraxia I69.990
      ataxia I69.993
      cognitive deficits I69.91
      disturbance of vision I69.998
      dysarthria I69.922
      dysphagia I69.991
      dysphasia I69.921
      facial droop I69.992
      facial weakness I69.992
      fluency disorder I69.923
      hemiplegia I69.95-●
      hemorrhage
        intracerebral —see Sequelae, hemorrhage, intracerebral
        intracranial, nontraumatic NEC — see Sequelae, hemorrhage, intracranial, nontraumatic
        subarachnoid —see Sequelae, hemorrhage, subarachnoid
      language deficit I69.928
      monoplegia
        ⟱lower limb I69.94-●
        upper limb I69.93-●
      paralytic syndrome I69.96-●
      specified effect NEC I69.998
      specified type NEC I69.80
        alteration of sensation I69.898
        aphasia I69.820
        apraxia I69.890
        ataxia I69.893
        cognitive deficits I69.81
        disturbance of vision I69.898
        dysarthria I69.822
        dysphagia I69.891
        dysphasia I69.821
        facial droop I69.892
        facial weakness I69.892
        fluency disorder I69.823
        hemiplegia I69.85-●
        language deficit I69.828
        monoplegia
          lower limb I69.84-●
          upper limb I69.83-●
        paralytic syndrome I69.86-●
        specified effect NEC I69.898
      speech deficit I69.928
        speech deficit I69.828
      stroke NOS —see Sequelae, stroke NOS
  dislocation — code to injury with seventh character S
  encephalitis or encephalomyelitis (conditions in G04) G09
    in infectious disease NEC B94.8
    viral B94.1
  external cause — code to injury with seventh character S
  foreign body entering natural orifice — code to injury with seventh character S
  fracture — code to injury with seventh character S

Sequelae (Continued)
  frostbite — code to injury with seventh character S
  Hansen's disease B92
  hemorrhage
    intracerebral I69.10
      alteration of sensation I69.198
      aphasia I69.120
      apraxia I69.190
      ataxia I69.193
      cognitive deficits I69.11
      disturbance of vision I69.198
      dysarthria I69.122
      dysphagia I69.191
      dysphasia I69.121
      facial droop I69.192
      facial weakness I69.192
      fluency disorder I69.123
      hemiplegia I69.15-●
      language deficit NEC I69.128
      monoplegia
        lower limb I69.14-●
        upper limb I69.13-●
      paralytic syndrome I69.16-●
      specified effect NEC I69.198
      speech deficit NEC I69.128
    intracranial, nontraumatic NEC I69.20
      alteration of sensation I69.298
      aphasia I69.220
      apraxia I69.290
      ataxia I69.293
      cognitive deficits I69.21
      disturbance of vision I69.298
      dysarthria I69.222
      dysphagia I69.291
      dysphasia I69.221
      facial droop I69.292
      facial weakness I69.292
      fluency disorder I69.223
      hemiplegia I69.25-●
      language deficit NEC I69.228
      monoplegia
        lower limb I69.24-●
        upper limb I69.23-●
      paralytic syndrome I69.26-●
      specified effect NEC I69.298
      speech deficit NEC I69.228
    subarachnoid I69.00
      alteration of sensation I69.098
      aphasia I69.020
      apraxia I69.090
      ataxia I69.093
      cognitive deficits —see subcategory I69.01-●
      disturbance of vision I69.098
      dysarthria I69.022
      dysphagia I69.091
      dysphasia I69.021
      facial droop I69.092
      facial weakness I69.092
      fluency disorder I69.023
      hemiplegia I69.05-●
      language deficit NEC I69.028
      monoplegia
        lower limb I69.04-●
        upper limb I69.03-●
      paralytic syndrome I69.06-●
      specified effect NEC I69.098
      speech deficit NEC I69.028
  hepatitis, viral B94.2
  hyperalimentation E68
  infarction
    cerebral I69.30
      alteration of sensation I69.398
      aphasia I69.320
      apraxia I69.390
      ataxia I69.393
      cognitive deficits I69.31
      disturbance of vision I69.398
      dysarthria I69.322
      dysphagia I69.391

Sequelae (Continued)
  infarction (Continued)
    cerebral (Continued)
      dysphasia I69.321
      facial droop I69.392
      facial weakness I69.392
      fluency disorder I69.323
      hemiplegia I69.35-●
      language deficit NEC I69.328
      monoplegia
        lower limb I69.34-●
        upper limb I69.33-●
      paralytic syndrome I69.36-●
      specified effect NEC I69.398
      speech deficit NEC I69.328
  infection, pyogenic, intracranial or intraspinal G09
  infectious disease B94.9
    specified NEC B94.8
  injury — code to injury with seventh character S
  leprosy B92
  meningitis
    bacterial (conditions in G00) G09
    other or unspecified cause (conditions in G03) G09
  muscle (and tendon) injury — code to injury with seventh character S
  myelitis —see Sequelae, encephalitis
  niacin deficiency E64.8
  nutritional deficiency E64.9
    specified NEC E64.8
  obstetrical condition O94
  parasitic disease B94.9
  phlebitis or thrombophlebitis of intracranial or intraspinal venous sinuses and veins (conditions in G08) G09
  poisoning — code to poisoning with seventh character S
    nonmedicinal substance —see Sequelae, toxic effect, nonmedicinal substance
  poliomyelitis (acute) B91
  pregnancy O94
  protein-energy malnutrition E64.0
  puerperium O94
  rickets E64.3
  selenium deficiency E64.8
  sprain and strain — code to injury with seventh character S
  stroke NOS I69.30
    alteration in sensation I69.398
    aphasia I69.320
    apraxia I69.390
    ataxia I69.393
    cognitive deficits I69.31
    disturbance of vision I69.398
    dysarthria I69.322
    dysphagia I69.391
    dysphasia I69.321
    facial droop I69.392
    facial weakness I69.392
    hemiplegia I69.35-●
    language deficit NEC I69.328
    monoplegia
      lower limb I69.34-●
      upper limb I69.33-●
    paralytic syndrome I69.36-●
    specified effect NEC I69.398
    speech deficit NEC I69.328
  tendon and muscle injury — code to injury with seventh character S
  thiamine deficiency E64.8
  trachoma B94.0
  tuberculosis B90.9
    bones and joints B90.2
    central nervous system B90.0
    genitourinary B90.1
    pulmonary (respiratory) B90.9
    specified organs NEC B90.8

Sequelae (*Continued*)
   viral
     encephalitis B94.1
     hepatitis B94.2
   vitamin deficiency NEC E64.8
     A E64.1
     B E64.8
     C E64.2
   wound, open — code to injury with seventh
     character S
Sequestration —*see also* Sequestrum
   disk —*see* Displacement, intervertebral
     disk
   lung, congenital Q33.2
Sequestrum
   bone —*see* Osteomyelitis, chronic
   dental M27.2
   jaw bone M27.2
   orbit —*see* Osteomyelitis, orbit
   sinus (accessory) (nasal) —*see* Sinusitis
Sequoiosis lung or pneumonitis J67.8
Serology for syphilis
   doubtful
     with signs or symptoms - code by site and
       stage under Syphilis
     follow-up of latent syphilis —*see* Syphilis,
       latent
   negative, with signs or symptoms — code by
     site and stage under Syphilis
   positive A53.0
     with signs or symptoms - code by site and
       stage under Syphilis
   reactivated A53.0
Seroma —*see also* Hematoma
   postprocedural —*see* Complication,
     postprocedural, seroma
   traumatic, secondary and recurrent
     T79.2
Seropurulent —*see* condition
Serositis, multiple K65.8
   pericardial I31.1
   peritoneal K65.8
Serous —*see* condition
Sertoli cell
   adenoma
     specified site —*see* Neoplasm, benign, by
       site
     unspecified site
       female D27.9
       male D29.20
   carcinoma
     specified site —*see* Neoplasm, malignant,
       by site
     unspecified site (male) C62.9-●
       female C56.9
   tumor
     with lipid storage
       specified site —*see* Neoplasm, benign,
         by site
       unspecified site
         female D27.9
         male D29.20
     specified site —*see* Neoplasm, benign, by
       site
     unspecified site
       female D27.9
       male D29.20
Sertoli-Leydig cell tumor —*see* Neoplasm,
   benign, by site
   specified site —*see* Neoplasm, benign,
     by site
   unspecified site
     female D27.9
     male D29.20
Serum
   allergy, allergic reaction —*see also* Reaction,
     serum T80.69
     shock —*see also* Shock, anaphylactic T80.59
   arthritis —*see also* Reaction, serum T80.69
   complication or reaction NEC —*see also*
     Reaction, serum T80.69

Serum (*Continued*)
   disease NEC —*see also* Reaction, serum T80.69
   hepatitis —*see also* Hepatitis, viral, type B
     carrier (suspected) of B18.1
   intoxication —*see also* Reaction, serum T80.69
   neuritis —*see also* Reaction, serum T80.69
   neuropathy G61.1
   poisoning NEC —*see also* Reaction, serum
     T80.69
   rash NEC —*see also* Reaction, serum T80.69
   reaction NEC —*see also* Reaction, serum
     T80.69
   sickness NEC —*see also* Reaction, serum
     T80.69
   urticaria —*see also* Reaction, serum T80.69
Sesamoiditis M25.8-●
Sever's disease or osteochondrosis —*see*
   Osteochondrosis, juvenile, tarsus
Severe sepsis R65.20
   with septic shock R65.21
Sex
   chromosome mosaics Q97.8
     lines with various numbers of
       X chromosomes Q97.2
   education Z70.8
   reassignment surgery status Z87.890
Sextuplet pregnancy —*see* Pregnancy,
   sextuplet
Sexual
   function, disorder of (psychogenic) F52.9
   immaturity (female) (male) E30.0
   impotence (psychogenic) organic origin
     NEC —*see* Dysfunction, sexual, male
   precocity (constitutional) (cryptogenic)
     (female) (idiopathic) (male) E30.1
Sexuality, pathologic —*see* Deviation, sexual
Sézary disease C84.1-●
Shadow, lung R91.8
Shaking palsy or paralysis —*see* Parkinsonism
Shallowness, acetabulum —*see* Derangement,
   joint, specified type NEC, hip
Shaver's disease J63.1
Sheath (tendon) —*see* condition
Sheathing, retinal vessels H35.01-●
Shedding
   nail L60.8
   premature, primary (deciduous) teeth
     K00.6
Sheehan's disease or syndrome E23.0
Shelf, rectal K62.89
Shell teeth K00.5
Shellshock (current) F43.0
   lasting state —*see* Disorder, post-traumatic
     stress
Shield kidney Q63.1
Shift
   auditory threshold (temporary) H93.24-●
   mediastinal R93.8
Shifting sleep-work schedule (affecting sleep)
   G47.26
Shiga (-Kruse) dysentery A03.0
Shiga's bacillus A03.0
Shigella (dysentery) —*see* Dysentery,
   bacillary
Shigellosis A03.9
   Group A A03.0
   Group B A03.1
   Group C A03.2
   Group D A03.3
Shin splints S86.89
Shingles —*see* Herpes, zoster
Shipyard disease or eye B30.0
Shirodkar suture, in pregnancy —*see*
   Pregnancy, complicated by, incompetent
   cervix
Shock R57.9
   with ectopic or molar pregnancy O08.3
   adrenal (cortical) (Addisonian) E27.2
   adverse food reaction (anaphylactic) —*see*
     Shock, anaphylactic, due to food
   allergic —*see* Shock, anaphylactic

Shock (*Continued*)
   anaphylactic T78.2
     chemical —*see* Table of Drugs and
       Chemicals
     due to drug or medicinal substance
       correct substance properly administered
         T88.6
       overdose or wrong substance given or
         taken (by accident) —*see* Table of
         Drugs and Chemicals, by drug,
         poisoning
     due to food (nonpoisonous) T78.00
       additives T78.06
       dairy products T78.07
       eggs T78.08
       fish T78.03
         shellfish T78.02
       fruit T78.04
       milk T78.07
       nuts T78.05
         multiple types T78.05
         peanuts T78.01
       peanuts T78.01
       seeds T78.05
       specified type NEC T78.09
       vegetable T78.04
     following sting(s) —*see* Venom
     immunization T80.52
     serum T80.59
       blood and blood products T80.51
       immunization T80.52
       specified NEC T80.59
       vaccination T80.52
   anaphylactoid —*see* Shock, anaphylactic
   anesthetic
     correct substance properly administered
       T88.2
     overdose or wrong substance given
       or taken —*see* Table of Drugs and
       Chemicals, by drug, poisoning
     specified anesthetic —*see* Table of
       Drugs and Chemicals, by drug,
       poisoning
   cardiogenic R57.0
   chemical substance —*see* Table of Drugs and
     Chemicals
   complicating ectopic or molar pregnancy O08.3
   culture —*see* Disorder, adjustment
   drug
     due to correct substance properly
       administered T88.6
     overdose or wrong substance given or
       taken (by accident) —*see* Table of
       Drugs and Chemicals, by drug,
       poisoning
   during or after labor and delivery O75.1
   electric T75.4
     (taser) T75.4
   endotoxic R65.21
     postprocedural (resulting from a
       procedure, not elsewhere classified)
       T81.12
   following
     ectopic or molar pregnancy O08.3
     injury (immediate) (delayed) T79.4
     labor and delivery O75.1
   food (anaphylactic) —*see* Shock, anaphylactic,
     due to food
   from electroshock gun (taser) T75.4
   gram-negative R65.21
     postprocedural (resulting from a
       procedure, not elsewhere classified)
       T81.12
   hematologic R57.8
➡ hemorrhagic R57.8
     surgery (intraoperative) (postoperative)
       T81.19
     trauma T79.4
   hypovolemic R57.1
     surgical T81.19
     traumatic T79.4

► New   ➡ Revised   ~~deleted~~ Deleted   ● Use Additional Character(s)

Shock *(Continued)*
  insulin E15
    therapeutic misadventure —*see*
      subcategory T38.3
  kidney N17.0
    traumatic (following crushing) T79.5
  lightning T75.01
  liver K72.00
  lung J80
  obstetric O75.1
    with ectopic or molar pregnancy O08.3
    following ectopic or molar pregnancy
      O08.3
  pleural (surgical) T81.19
    due to trauma T79.4
  postprocedural (postoperative) T81.10
    with ectopic or molar pregnancy O08.3
    cardiogenic T81.11
    endotoxic T81.12
    following ectopic or molar pregnancy O08.3
    gram-negative T81.12
    hypovolemic T81.19
    septic T81.12
    specified type NEC T81.19
  psychic F43.0
  septic (due to severe sepsis) R65.21
  specified NEC R57.8
  surgical T81.10
  taser gun (taser) T75.4
  therapeutic misadventure NEC T81.10
  thyroxin
    overdose or wrong substance given
      or taken —*see* Table of Drugs and
      Chemicals, by drug, poisoning
  toxic, syndrome A48.3
  transfusion —*see* Complications, transfusion
  traumatic (immediate) (delayed) T79.4
Shoemaker's chest M95.4
Short, shortening, shortness
  arm (acquired) —*see also* Deformity, limb,
    unequal length
    congenital Q71.81-●
    forearm —*see* Deformity, limb, unequal
      length
  bowel syndrome K91.2
  breath R06.02
  cervical (complicating pregnancy) O26.87-●
    non-gravid uterus N88.3
  common bile duct, congenital Q44.5
  cord (umbilical), complicating delivery O69.3
  cystic duct, congenital Q44.5
  esophagus (congenital) Q39.8
  femur (acquired) —*see* Deformity, limb,
    unequal length, femur
    congenital —*see* Defect, reduction, lower
      limb, longitudinal, femur
  frenum, frenulum, linguae (congenital) Q38.1
  hip (acquired) —*see also* Deformity, limb,
    unequal length
    congenital Q65.89
  leg (acquired) —*see also* Deformity, limb,
    unequal length
    congenital Q72.81-●
    lower leg —*see also* Deformity, limb,
      unequal length
  limbed stature, with immunodeficiency D82.2
  lower limb (acquired) —*see also* Deformity,
    limb, unequal length
    congenital Q72.81-●
  organ or site, congenital NEC —*see* Distortion
  palate, congenital Q38.5
  radius (acquired) —*see also* Deformity, limb,
    unequal length
    congenital —*see* Defect, reduction, upper
      limb, longitudinal, radius
  rib syndrome Q77.2
  stature (child) (hereditary) (idiopathic) NEC
    R62.52
    constitutional E34.3
    due to endocrine disorder E34.3
    Laron-type E34.3

Short, shortening, shortness *(Continued)*
  tendon —*see also* Contraction, tendon
    with contracture of joint —*see* Contraction,
      joint
    Achilles (acquired) M67.0-●
      congenital Q66.89
    congenital Q79.8
  thigh (acquired) —*see also* Deformity, limb,
    unequal length, femur
    congenital —*see* Defect, reduction, lower
      limb, longitudinal, femur
  tibialis anterior (tendon) —*see* Contraction,
    tendon
  umbilical cord
    complicating delivery O69.3
  upper limb, congenital —*see* Defect,
    reduction, upper limb, specified type
    NEC
  urethra N36.8
  uvula, congenital Q38.5
  vagina (congenital) Q52.4
Shortsightedness —*see* Myopia
Shoshin (acute fulminating beriberi) E51.11
Shoulder —*see* condition
Shovel-shaped incisors K00.2
Shower, thromboembolic —*see* Embolism
Shunt
  arterial-venous (dialysis) Z99.2
  arteriovenous, pulmonary (acquired) I28.0
    congenital Q25.72
  cerebral ventricle (communicating) in situ
    Z98.2
  surgical, prosthetic, with complications —*see*
    Complications, cardiovascular, device or
    implant Shutdown, renal N28.9
Shutdown, renal N28.9
Shy-Drager syndrome G90.3
Sialadenitis, sialadenosis (any gland) (chronic)
  (periodic) (suppurative) —*see* Sialoadenitis
Sialectasia K11.8
Sialidosis E77.1
Sialitis, silitis (any gland) (chronic)
  (suppurative) —*see* Sialoadenitis
Sialoadenitis (any gland) (periodic)
  (suppurative) K11.20
  acute K11.21
    recurrent K11.22
  chronic K11.23
Sialoadenopathy K11.9
Sialoangitis —*see* Sialoadenitis
Sialodochitis (fibrinosa) —*see* Sialoadenitis
Sialodocholithiasis K11.5
Sialolithiasis K11.5
Sialometaplasia, necrotizing K11.8
Sialorrhea —*see also* Ptyalism
  periodic —*see* Sialoadenitis
Sialosis K11.7
Siamese twin Q89.4
Sibling rivalry Z62.891
Sicard's syndrome G52.7
Sicca syndrome M35.00
  with
    keratoconjunctivitis M35.01
    lung involvement M35.02
    myopathy M35.03
    renal tubulo-interstitial disorders M35.04
    specified organ involvement NEC M35.09
Sick R69
  or handicapped person in family Z63.79
    needing care at home Z63.6
  sinus (syndrome) I49.5
Sick-euthyroid syndrome E07.81
Sickle-cell
  anemia —*see* Disease, sickle-cell
  trait D57.3
Sicklemia —*see also* Disease, sickle-cell
  trait D57.3
Sickness
  air (travel) T75.3
  airplane T75.3
  alpine T70.29

Sickness *(Continued)*
  altitude T70.20
  Andes T70.29
  aviator's T70.29
  balloon T70.29
  car T75.3
  compressed air T70.3
  decompression T70.3
  green D50.8
  milk —*see* Poisoning, food, noxious
  motion T75.3
  mountain T70.29
    acute D75.1
  protein —*see also* Reaction, serum T80.69
  radiation T66
  roundabout (motion) T75.3
  sea T75.3
  serum NEC —*see also* Reaction, serum T80.69
  sleeping (African) B56.9
    by Trypanosoma B56.9
      brucei
        gambiense B56.0
        rhodesiense B56.1
    East African B56.1
    Gambian B56.0
    Rhodesian B56.1
    West African B56.0
  swing (motion) T75.3
  train (railway) (travel) T75.3
  travel (any vehicle) T75.3
Sideropenia —*see* Anemia, iron deficiency
Siderosilicosis J62.8
Siderosis (lung) J63.4
  eye (globe) —*see* Disorder, globe,
    degenerative, siderosis
Siemens' syndrome (ectodermal dysplasia) Q82.8
Sighing R06.89
  psychogenic F45.8
Sigmoid —*see also* condition
  flexure —*see* condition
  kidney Q63.1
Sigmoiditis —*see also* Enteritis K52.9
  infectious A09
  noninfectious K52.9
Silfversköld's syndrome Q78.9
Silicosiderosis J62.8
Silicosis, silicotic (simple) (complicated) J62.8
  with tuberculosis J65
Silicotuberculosis J65
Silo-fillers' disease J68.8
  bronchitis J68.0
  pneumonitis J68.0
  pulmonary edema J68.1
Silver's syndrome Q87.1
Simian malaria B53.1
Simmonds' cachexia or disease E23.0
Simons' disease or syndrome (progressive
  lipodystrophy) E88.1
Simple, simplex —*see* condition
Simulation, conscious (of illness) Z76.5
Simultanagnosia (asimultagnosia) R48.3
Sin Nombre virus disease (Hantavirus)
  (cardio)-pulmonary syndrome) B33.4
Sinding-Larsen disease or osteochondrosis —
  see Osteochondrosis, juvenile, patella
Singapore hemorrhagic fever A91
Singer's node or nodule J38.2
Single
  atrium Q21.2
  coronary artery Q24.5
  umbilical artery Q27.0
  ventricle Q20.4
Singultus R06.6
  epidemicus B33.0
Sinus —*see also* Fistula
  abdominal K63.89
  arrest I45.5
  arrhythmia I49.8
  bradycardia R00.1
  branchial cleft (internal) (external) Q18.0
  coccygeal —*see* Sinus, pilonidal

Sinus *(Continued)*
  dental K04.6
  dermal (congenital) Q06.8
    with abscess Q06.8
    coccygeal, pilonidal —*see* Sinus,
        coccygeal
  infected, skin NEC L08.89
  marginal, ruptured or bleeding —*see*
        Hemorrhage, antepartum, specified
        cause NEC
  medial, face and neck Q18.8
  pause I45.5
  pericranii Q01.9
  pilonidal (infected) (rectum) L05.92
    with abscess L05.02
  preauricular Q18.1
  rectovaginal N82.3
  Rokitansky-Aschoff (gallbladder) K82.8
  sacrococcygeal (dermoid) (infected) —*see*
        Sinus, pilonidal
  tachycardia R00.0
    paroxysmal I47.1
  tarsi syndrome M25.57-●
  testis N50.89
  tract (postinfective) —*see* Fistula
  urachus Q64.4
Sinusitis (accessory) (chronic) (hyperplastic)
      (nasal) (nonpurulent) (purulent) J32.9
  acute J01.90
    ethmoidal J01.20
      recurrent J01.21
    frontal J01.10
      recurrent J01.11
    involving more than one sinus, other than
        pansinusitis J01.80
      recurrent J01.81
    maxillary J01.00
      recurrent J01.01
    pansinusitis J01.40
      recurrent J01.41
    recurrent J01.91
    specified NEC J01.80
      recurrent J01.81
    sphenoidal J01.30
      recurrent J01.31
  allergic —*see* Rhinitis, allergic
  due to high altitude T70.1
  ethmoidal J32.2
    acute J01.20
      recurrent J01.21
  frontal J32.1
    acute J01.10
      recurrent J01.11
  influenzal —*see* Influenza, with, respiratory
        manifestations NEC
  involving more than one sinus but not
        pansinusitis J32.8
    acute J01.80
      recurrent J01.81
  maxillary J32.0
    acute J01.00
      recurrent J01.01
  sphenoidal J32.3
    acute J01.30
      recurrent J01.31
  tuberculous, any sinus A15.8
Sinusitis-bronchiectasis-situs inversus
      (syndrome) (triad) Q89.3
Sipple's syndrome E31.22
Sirenomelia (syndrome) Q87.2
Siriasis T67.0
Sirkari's disease B55.0
Siti A65
Situation, psychiatric F99
Situational
  disturbance (transient) —*see* Disorder,
        adjustment
    acute F43.0
  maladjustment —*see* Disorder, adjustment
  reaction —*see* Disorder, adjustment
    acute F43.0

Situs inversus or transversus (abdominalis)
      (thoracis) Q89.3
Sixth disease B08.20
  due to human herpesvirus 6 B08.21
  due to human herpesvirus 7 B08.22
Sjögren-Larsson syndrome Q87.1
Sjögren's syndrome or disease —*see* Sicca
      syndrome
Skeletal —*see* condition
Skene's gland —*see* condition
Skenitis —*see* Urethritis
Skerljevo A65
Skevas-Zerfus disease —*see* Toxicity, venom,
      marine animal, sea anemone
Skin —*see also* condition
  clammy R23.1
  donor —*see* Donor, skin
  hidebound M35.9
Slate-dressers' or slate-miners' lung J62.8
Sleep
  apnea —*see* Apnea, sleep
  deprivation Z72.820
  disorder or disturbance G47.9
    child F51.9
    nonorganic origin F51.9
    specified NEC G47.8
  disturbance G47.9
    nonorganic origin F51.9
  drunkenness F51.9
  rhythm inversion G47.2-●
  terrors F51.4
  walking F51.3
    hysterical F44.89
Sleep hygiene
  abuse Z72.821
  inadequate Z72.821
  poor Z72.821
Sleeping sickness —*see* Sickness, sleeping
Sleeplessness —*see* Insomnia
  menopausal N95.11
Sleep-wake schedule disorder G47.20
Slim disease (in HIV infection) B20
Slipped, slipping
  epiphysis (traumatic) —*see also*
        Osteochondropathy, specified type
        NEC
    capital femoral (traumatic)
      acute (on chronic) S79.01-●
    current traumatic - code as Fracture, by site
    upper femoral (nontraumatic) M93.00-●
      acute M93.01-●
        on chronic M93.03-●
      chronic M93.02-●
  intervertebral disc —*see* Displacement,
        intervertebral disc
  ligature, umbilical P51.8
  patella —*see* Disorder, patella, derangement
        NEC
  rib M89.8X8
  sacroiliac joint —*see* subcategory M53.2
  tendon —*see* Disorder, tendon
  ulnar nerve, nontraumatic —*see* Lesion,
        nerve, ulnar
  vertebra NEC —*see* Spondylolisthesis
Slocumb's syndrome E27.0
Sloughing (multiple) (phagedena) (skin) —*see*
      also Gangrene
  abscess —*see* Abscess
  appendix K38.8
  fascia —*see* Disorder, soft tissue, specified
        type NEC
  scrotum N50.89
  tendon —*see* Disorder, tendon
  transplanted organ —*see* Rejection, transplant
  ulcer —*see* Ulcer, skin
Slow
  feeding, newborn P92.2
  flow syndrome, coronary I20.8
  heart(beat) R00.1
Slowing, urinary stream R39.198
Sluder's neuralgia (syndrome) G44.89

Slurred, slurring speech R47.81
Small (ness)
  for gestational age —*see* Small for dates
  introitus, vagina N89.6
  kidney (unknown cause) N27.9
    bilateral N27.1
    unilateral N27.0
  ovary (congenital) Q50.39
  pelvis
    with disproportion (fetopelvic) O33.1
      causing obstructed labor O65.1
  uterus N85.8
  white kidney N03.9
Small-and-light-for-dates —*see* Small for
      dates
Small-for-dates (infant) P05.10
  with weight of
    499 grams or less P05.11
    500-749 grams P05.12
    750-999 grams P05.13
    1000-1249 grams P05.14
    1250-1499 grams P05.15
    1500-1749 grams P05.16
    1750-1999 grams P05.17
    2000-2499 grams P05.18
    2500 grams and over P05.19
  specified NEC P05.19
Smallpox B03
Smearing, fecal R15.1
Smith-Lemli-Opitz syndrome E78.72
Smith's fracture S52.54-●
Smoker —*see* Dependence, drug, nicotine
Smoker's
  bronchitis J41.0
  cough J41.0
  palate K13.24
  throat J31.2
  tongue K13.24
Smoking
  passive Z77.22
Smothering spells R06.81
Snaggle teeth, tooth M26.39
Snapping
  finger —*see* Trigger finger
  hip —*see* Derangement, joint, specified type
        NEC, hip
    involving the iliotiblial band M76.3-●
  knee —*see* Derangement, knee
    involving the iliotiblial band M76.3-●
Sneddon-Wilkinson disease or syndrome (sub-
      corneal pustular dermatosis) L13.1
Sneezing (intractable) R06.7
Sniffing
  cocaine
    abuse —*see* Abuse, drug, cocaine
    dependence —*see* Dependence, drug,
        cocaine
  gasoline
    abuse —*see* Abuse, drug, inhalant
    dependence —*see* Dependence, drug,
        inhalant
  glue (airplane)
    abuse —*see* Abuse, drug, inhalant
    drug dependence —*see* Dependence, drug,
        inhalant
Sniffles
  newborn P28.89
Snoring R06.83
Snow blindness —*see* Photokeratitis
Snuffles (non-syphilitic) R06.5
  newborn P28.89
  syphilitic (infant) A50.05 *[J99]*
Social
  exclusion Z60.4
    due to discrimination or persecution
        (perceived) Z60.5
  migrant Z59.0
    acculturation difficulty Z60.3
  rejection Z60.4
    due to discrimination or persecution
        Z60.5

▶ New   ⇒ Revised   ~~deleted~~ Deleted   ● Use Additional Character(s)

Social *(Continued)*
  role conflict NEC Z73.5
  skills inadequacy NEC Z73.4
  transplantation Z60.3
Sodoku A25.0
Soemmerring's ring —*see* Cataract, secondary
Soft —*see also* condition
  nails L60.3
Softening
  bone —*see* Osteomalacia
  brain (necrotic) (progressive) G93.89
    congenital Q04.8
    embolic I63.4-•
    hemorrhagic —*see* Hemorrhage,
      intracranial, intracerebral
    occlusive I63.5-•
    thrombotic I63.3-•
  cartilage M94.2-•
    patella M22.4-•
  cerebellar —*see* Softening, brain
  cerebral —*see* Softening, brain
  cerebrospinal —*see* Softening, brain
  myocardial, heart —*see* Degeneration,
    myocardial
  spinal cord G95.89
  stomach K31.89
Soldier's
  heart F45.8
  patches I31.0
Solitary
  cyst, kidney N28.1
  kidney, congenital Q60.0
Solvent abuse —*see* Abuse, drug, inhalant
  dependence —*see* Dependence, drug,
    inhalant
Somatization reaction, somatic reaction —*see*
    Disorder, somatoform
Somnambulism F51.3
  hysterical F44.89
Somnolence R40.0
  nonorganic origin F51.11
Sonne dysentery A03.3
Soor B37.0
Sore
  bed —*see* Ulcer, pressure, by site
  chiclero B55.1
  Delhi B55.1
  desert —*see* Ulcer, skin
  eye H57.1-•
  Lahore B55.1
  mouth K13.79
    canker K12.0
  muscle M79.1
  Naga —*see* Ulcer, skin
  of skin —*see* Ulcer, skin - oriental B55.1
  pressure —*see* Ulcer, pressure, by site
  skin L98.9
  soft A57
  throat (acute) —*see also* Pharyngitis
    with influenza, flu, or grippe —*see*
      Influenza, with, respiratory
      manifestations NEC
    chronic J31.2
    coxsackie (virus) B08.5
    diphtheritic A36.0
    herpesviral B00.2
    influenzal —*see* Influenza, with, respiratory
      manifestations NEC
    septic J02.0
    streptococcal (ulcerative) J02.0
    viral NEC J02.8
      coxsackie B08.5
  tropical —*see* Ulcer, skin
  veldt —*see* Ulcer, skin
Soto's syndrome (cerebral gigantism) Q87.3
South African cardiomyopathy syndrome I42.8
Southeast Asian hemorrhagic fever A91
Spacing
  abnormal, tooth, teeth, fully erupted M26.30
  excessive, tooth, fully erupted M26.32
Spade-like hand (congenital) Q68.1

Spading nail L60.8
  congenital Q84.6
Spanish collar N47.1
Sparganosis B70.1
Spasm(s), spastic, spasticity —*see also* condition
    R25.2
  accommodation —*see* Spasm, of
    accommodation
  ampulla of Vater K83.4
  anus, ani (sphincter) (reflex) K59.4
    psychogenic F45.8
  artery I73.9
    cerebral G45.9
  Bell's G51.3
  bladder (sphincter, external or internal) N32.89
    psychogenic F45.8
  bronchus, bronchiole J98.01
  cardia K22.0
  cardiac I20.1
  carpopedal —*see* Tetany
  cerebral (arteries) (vascular) G45.9
  cervix, complicating delivery O62.4
  ciliary body (of accommodation) —*see* Spasm,
    of accommodation
  colon —*see also* Irritable, bowel K58.9
    with diarrhea K58.0
    psychogenic F45.8
  common duct K83.8
  compulsive —*see* Tic
  conjugate H51.8
  coronary (artery) I20.1
  diaphragm (reflex) R06.6
    epidemic B33.0
    psychogenic F45.8
  duodenum K59.8
  epidemic diaphragmatic (transient) B33.0
  esophagus (diffuse) K22.4
    psychogenic F45.8
  facial G51.3
  fallopian tube N83.8
  gastrointestinal (tract) K31.89
    psychogenic F45.8
  glottis J38.5
    hysterical F44.4
    psychogenic F45.8
      conversion reaction F44.4
    reflex through recurrent laryngeal nerve
      J38.5
  habit —*see* Tic
  heart I20.1
  hemifacial (clonic) G51.3
  hourglass —*see* Contraction, hourglass
  hysterical F44.4
  infantile —*see* Epilepsy, spasms
  inferior oblique, eye H51.8
  intestinal —*see also* Syndrome, irritable bowel
    K58.9
    psychogenic F45.8
  larynx, laryngeal J38.5
    hysterical F44.4
    psychogenic F45.8
      conversion reaction F44.4
  levator palpebrae superioris —*see* Disorder,
    eyelid function
  muscle NEC M62.838
    back M62.830
  nerve, trigeminal G51.0
  nervous F45.8
  nodding F98.4
  occupational F48.8
  oculogyric H51.8
    psychogenic F45.8
  of accommodation H52.53-•
  ophthalmic artery —*see* Occlusion, artery,
    retina
  perineal, female N94.89
  peroneo-extensor —*see also* Deformity, limb,
    flat foot
  pharynx (reflex) J39.2
    hysterical F45.8
    psychogenic F45.8

Spasm(s), spastic, spasticity *(Continued)*
  psychogenic F45.8
  pylorus NEC K31.3
    adult hypertrophic K31.89
    congenital or infantile Q40.0
    psychogenic F45.8
  rectum (sphincter) K59.4
    psychogenic F45.8
  retinal (artery) —*see* Occlusion, artery, retina
  sigmoid —*see also* Syndrome, irritable bowel
    K58.9
    psychogenic F45.8
  sphincter of Oddi K83.4
  stomach K31.89
    neurotic F45.8
  throat J39.2
    hysterical F45.8
    psychogenic F45.8
  tic F95.9
    chronic F95.1
    transient of childhood F95.0
  tongue K14.8
  torsion (progressive) G24.1
  trigeminal nerve —*see* Neuralgia, trigeminal
  ureter N13.5
  urethra (sphincter) N35.9
  uterus N85.8
    complicating labor O62.4
  vagina N94.2
    psychogenic F52.5
  vascular I73.9
  vasomotor I73.9
  vein NEC I87.8
  viscera —*see* Pain, abdominal
Spasmodic —*see* condition
Spasmophilia —*see* Tetany
Spasmus nutans F98.4
Spastic, spasticity —*see also* Spasm
  child (cerebral) (congenital) (paralysis) G80.1
Speaker's throat R49.8
Specific, specified —*see* condition
Speech
  defect, disorder, disturbance, impediment
    R47.9
    psychogenic, in childhood and adolescence
      F98.8
    slurring R47.81
    specified NEC R47.89
Spencer's disease A08.19
Spens' syndrome (syncope with heart block)
    I45.9
Sperm counts (fertility testing) Z31.41
  postvasectomy Z30.8
  reversal Z31.42
Spermatic cord —*see* condition
Spermatocele N43.40
  congenital Q55.4
  multiple N43.42
  single N43.41
Spermatocystitis N49.0
Spermatocytoma C62.9-•
  specified site —*see* Neoplasm, malignant, by
    site
Spermatorrhea N50.89
Sphacelus —*see* Gangrene
Sphenoidal —*see* condition
Sphenoiditis (chronic) —*see* Sinusitis,
    sphenoidal
Sphenopalatine ganglion neuralgia G90.09
Sphericity, increased, lens (congenital)
    Q12.4
Spherocytosis (congenital) (familial)
    (hereditary) D58.0
  hemoglobin disease D58.0
  sickle-cell (disease) D57.8-•
Spherophakia Q12.4
Sphincter —*see* condition
Sphincteritis, sphincter of Oddi —*see*
    Cholangitis
Sphingolipidosis E75.3
  specified NEC E75.29

Sphingomyelinosis E75.3
Spicule tooth K00.2
Spider
  bite —see Toxicity, venom, spider
  fingers —see Syndrome, Marfan's
  nevus I78.1
  toes —see Syndrome, Marfan's
  vascular I78.1
Spiegler-Fendt
  benign lymphocytoma L98.8
  sarcoid L08.89
Spielmeyer-Vogt disease E75.4
Spina bifida (aperta) Q05.9
  with hydrocephalus NEC Q05.4
  cervical Q05.5
    with hydrocephalus Q05.0
  dorsal Q05.6
    with hydrocephalus Q05.1
  lumbar Q05.7
    with hydrocephalus Q05.2
  lumbosacral Q05.7
    with hydrocephalus Q05.2
  occulta Q76.0
  sacral Q05.8
    with hydrocephalus Q05.3
  thoracic Q05.6
    with hydrocephalus Q05.1
  thoracolumbar Q05.6
    with hydrocephalus Q05.1
Spindle, Krukenberg's —see Pigmentation,
  cornea, posterior
Spine, spinal —see condition
Spiradenoma (eccrine) —see Neoplasm, skin,
  benign
Spirillosis A25.0
Spirillum
  minus A25.0
  obermeieri infection A68.0
Spirochetal —see condition
Spirochetosis A69.9
  arthritic, arthritica A69.9
  bronchopulmonary A69.8
  icterohemorrhagic A27.0
  lung A69.8
Spirometrosis B70.1
Spitting blood —see Hemoptysis
Splanchnoptosis K63.4
Spleen, splenic —see condition
Splenectasis —see Splenomegaly
Splenitis (interstitial) (malignant) (nonspecific)
  D73.89
  malarial —see also Malaria B54 [D77]
  tuberculous A18.85
Splenocele D73.89
Splenomegaly, splenomegalia (Bengal)
  (cryptogenic) (idiopathic) (tropical) R16.1
  with hepatomegaly R16.2
  cirrhotic D73.2
  congenital Q89.09
  congestive, chronic D73.2
  Egyptian B65.1
  Gaucher's E75.22
  malarial —see also Malaria B54 [D77]
  neutropenic D73.81
  Niemann-Pick —see Niemann-Pick disease or
    syndrome
  siderotic D73.2
  syphilitic A52.79
    congenital (early) A50.08 [D77]
Splenopathy D73.9
Splenoptosis D73.89
Splenosis D73.89
Splinter —see Foreign body, superficial, by site
Split, splitting
  foot Q72.7-•
  hand Q71.6
  heart sounds R01.2
  lip, congenital —see Cleft, lip
  nails L60.3
  urinary stream R39.13
Spondylarthrosis —see Spondylosis

Spondylitis (chronic) —see also Spondylopathy,
  inflammatory
ankylopoietica —see Spondylitis, ankylosing
ankylosing (chronic) M45.9
  with lung involvement M45.9 [J99]
  cervical region M45.2
  cervicothoracic region M45.3
  juvenile M08.1
  lumbar region M45.6
  lumbosacral region M45.7
  multiple sites M45.0
  occipito-atlanto-axial region M45.1
  sacrococcygeal region M45.8
  thoracic region M45.4
  thoracolumbar region M45.5
atrophic (ligamentous) —see Spondylitis,
  ankylosing
deformans (chronic) —see Spondylosis
gonococcal A54.41
gouty —see also Gout, by type, vertebrae
  M10.08
in (due to)
  brucellosis A23.9 [M49.80]
    cervical region A23.9 [M49.82]
    cervicothoracic region A23.9 [M49.83]
    lumbar region A23.9 [M49.86]
    lumbosacral region A23.9 [M49.87]
    multiple sites A23.9 [M49.89]
    occipito-atlanto-axial region A23.9
      [M49.81]
    sacrococcygeal region A23.9 [M49.88]
    thoracic region A23.9 [M49.84]
    thoracolumbar region A23.9 [M49.85]
  enterobacteria —see also subcategory M49.8
    A04.9
  tuberculosis A18.01
infectious NEC —see Spondylopathy,
  infective
juvenile ankylosing (chronic) M08.1
Kümmell's —see Spondylopathy, traumatic
Marie-Strümpell —see Spondylitis,
  ankylosing
muscularis —see Spondylopathy, specified
  NEC
psoriatic L40.53
rheumatoid —see Spondylitis, ankylosing
rhizomelica —see Spondylitis, ankylosing
sacroiliac NEC M46.1
senescent, senile —see Spondylosis
traumatic (chronic) or post-traumatic —see
  Spondylopathy, traumatic
tuberculous A18.01
typhosa A01.05
Spondylolisthesis (acquired) (degenerative)
  M43.10
with disproportion (fetopelvic) O33.0
  causing obstructed labor O65.0
cervical region M43.12
cervicothoracic region M43.13
congenital Q76.2
lumbar region M43.16
lumbosacral region M43.17
multiple sites M43.19
occipito-atlanto-axial region M43.11
sacrococcygeal region M43.18
thoracic region M43.14
thoracolumbar region M43.15
traumatic (old) M43.10
  acute
    fifth cervical (displaced) S12.430
      nondisplaced S12.431
      specified type NEC (displaced)
        S12.450
        nondisplaced S12.451
      type III S12.44
    fourth cervical (displaced) S12.330
      nondisplaced S12.331
      specified type NEC (displaced)
        S12.350
        nondisplaced S12.351
      type III S12.34

Spondylolisthesis (Continued)
  traumatic (Continued)
    acute (Continued)
      second cervical (displaced) S12.130
        nondisplaced S12.131
        specified type NEC (displaced)
          S12.150
          nondisplaced S12.151
        type III S12.14
      seventh cervical (displaced) S12.630
        nondisplaced S12.631
        specified type NEC (displaced)
          S12.650
          nondisplaced S12.651
        type III S12.64
      sixth cervical (displaced) S12.530
        nondisplaced S12.531
        specified type NEC (displaced)
          S12.550
          nondisplaced S12.551
        type III S12.54
      third cervical (displaced) S12.230
        nondisplaced S12.231
        specified type NEC (displaced)
          S12.250
          nondisplaced S12.251
        type III S12.24
Spondylolysis (acquired) M43.00
  cervical region M43.02
  cervicothoracic region M43.03
  congenital Q76.2
  lumbar region M43.06
  lumbosacral region M43.07
    with disproportion (fetopelvic) O33.0
      causing obstructed labor O65.8
  multiple sites M43.09
  occipito-atlanto-axial region M43.01
  sacrococcygeal region M43.08
  thoracic region M43.04
  thoracolumbar region M43.05
Spondylopathy M48.9
  infective NEC M46.50
    cervical region M46.52
    cervicothoracic region M46.53
    lumbar region M46.56
    lumbosacral region M46.57
    multiple sites M46.59
    occipito-atlanto-axial region M46.51
    sacrococcygeal region M46.58
    thoracic region M46.54
    thoracolumbar region M46.55
  inflammatory M46.90
    cervical region M46.92
    cervicothoracic region M46.93
    lumbar region M46.96
    lumbosacral region M46.97
    multiple sites M46.99
    occipito-atlanto-axial region M46.91
    sacrococcygeal region M46.98
    specified type NEC M46.80
      cervical region M46.82
      cervicothoracic region M46.83
      lumbar region M46.86
      lumbosacral region M46.87
      multiple sites M46.89
      occipito-atlanto-axial region M46.81
      sacrococcygeal region M46.88
      thoracic region M46.84
      thoracolumbar region M46.85
    thoracic region M46.94
    thoracolumbar region M46.95
  neuropathic, in
    syringomyelia and syringobulbia G95.0
    tabes dorsalis A52.11
  specified NEC —see subcategory M48.8
  traumatic M48.30
    cervical region M48.32
    cervicothoracic region M48.33
    lumbar region M48.36
    lumbosacral region M48.37
    occipito-atlanto-axial region M48.31

▶ New   ⇒ Revised   ~~deleted~~ Deleted   • Use Additional Character(s)

Spondylopathy (Continued)
  traumatic (Continued)
    sacrococcygeal region M48.38
    thoracic region M48.34
    thoracolumbar region M48.35
Spondylosis M47.9
  with
    disproportion (fetopelvic) O33.0
      causing obstructed labor O65.0
    myelopathy NEC M47.10
      cervical region M47.12
      cervicothoracic region M47.13
      lumbar region M47.16
      occipito-atlanto-axial region M47.11
      thoracic region M47.14
      thoracolumbar region M47.15
    radiculopathy M47.20
      cervical region M47.22
      cervicothoracic region M47.23
      lumbar region M47.26
      lumbosacral region M47.27
      occipito-atlanto-axial region M47.21
      sacrococcygeal region M47.28
      thoracic region M47.24
      thoracolumbar region M47.25
  without myelopathy or radiculopathy M47.819
    cervical region M47.812
    cervicothoracic region M47.813
    lumbar region M47.816
    lumbosacral region M47.817
    occipito-atlanto-axial region M47.811
    sacrococcygeal region M47.818
    thoracic region M47.814
    thoracolumbar region M47.815
  specified NEC M47.899
    cervical region M47.892
    cervicothoracic region M47.893
    lumbar region M47.896
    lumbosacral region M47.897
    occipito-atlanto-axial region M47.891
    sacrococcygeal region M47.898
    thoracic region M47.894
    thoracolumbar region M47.895
  traumatic —see Spondylopathy, traumatic
Sponge
  inadvertently left in operation wound —see Foreign body, accidentally left during a procedure
  kidney (medullary) Q61.5
Sponge-diver's disease —see Toxicity, venom, marine animal, sea anemone
Spongioblastoma (any type) —see Neoplasm, malignant, by site
  specified site —see Neoplasm, malignant, by site
  unspecified site C71.9
Spongioneuroblastoma —see Neoplasm, malignant, by site
Spontaneous —see also condition
  fracture (cause unknown) —see Fracture, pathological
Spoon nail L60.3
  congenital Q84.6
Sporadic —see condition
Sporothrix schenckii infection —see Sporotrichosis
Sporotrichosis B42.9
  arthritis B42.82
  disseminated B42.7
  generalized B42.7
  lymphocutaneous (fixed) (progressive) B42.1
  pulmonary B42.0
  specified NEC B42.89
Spots, spotting (in) (of)
  Bitot's —see also Pigmentation, conjunctiva
    in the young child E50.1
      vitamin A deficiency E50.1

Spots, spotting (Continued)
  café, au lait L81.3
  Cayenne pepper I78.1
  cotton wool, retina —see Occlusion, artery, retina
  de Morgan's (senile angiomas) I78.1
  ➡Fuchs' black (myopic) —see also Myopia, degenerative H44.2-●
  intermenstrual (regular) N92.0
    irregular N92.1
  Koplik's B05.9
  liver L81.4
  pregnancy O26.85-●
  purpuric R23.3
  ruby I78.1
Spotted fever —see Fever, spotted N92.3
Sprain (joint) (ligament)
  acromioclavicular joint or ligament S43.5-●
  ankle S93.40-●
    calcaneofibular ligament S93.41-●
    deltoid ligament S93.42-●
    internal collateral ligament —see Sprain, ankle, specified ligament NEC
    specified ligament NEC S93.49-●
    talofibular ligament —see Sprain, ankle, specified ligament NEC
    tibiofibular ligament S93.43-●
  anterior longitudinal, cervical S13.4
  atlas, atlanto-axial, atlanto-occipital S13.4
  breast bone —see Sprain, sternum
  calcaneofibular —see Sprain, ankle
  carpal —see Sprain, wrist
  carpometacarpal —see Sprain, hand, specified site NEC
  cartilage
    costal S23.41
    semilunar (knee) —see Sprain, knee, specified site NEC
      with current tear —see Tear, meniscus
    thyroid region S13.5
    xiphoid —see Sprain, sternum
  cervical, cervicodorsal, cervicothoracic S13.4
  chondrosternal S23.421
  coracoclavicular S43.8-●
  coracohumeral S43.41-●
  coronary, knee —see Sprain, knee, specified site NEC
  costal cartilage S23.41
  cricoarytenoid articulation or ligament S13.5
  cricothyroid articulation S13.5
  cruciate, knee —see Sprain, knee, cruciate
  deltoid, ankle —see Sprain, ankle
  dorsal (spine) S23.3
  elbow S53.40-●
    radial collateral ligament S53.43-●
    radiohumeral S53.41-●
    rupture
      radial collateral ligament —see Rupture, traumatic, ligament, radial collateral
      ulnar collateral ligament —see Rupture, traumatic, ligament, ulnar collateral
    specified type NEC S53.49-●
    ulnar collateral ligament S53.44-●
    ulnohumeral S53.42-●
  femur, head —see Sprain, hip
  fibular collateral, knee —see Sprain, knee, collateral
  fibulocalcaneal —see Sprain, ankle
  finger(s) S63.61-●
    index S63.61-●
    interphalangeal (joint) S63.63-●
      index S63.63-●
      little S63.63-●
      middle S63.63-●
      ring S63.63-●
    little S63.61-●
    metacarpophalangeal (joint) S63.65-●
    middle S63.61-●
    ring S63.61-●

Sprain (Continued)
  finger(s) (Continued)
    specified site NEC S63.69-●
      index S63.69-●
      little S63.69-●
      middle S63.69-●
      ring S63.69-●
  foot S93.60-●
    specified ligament NEC S93.69-●
    tarsal ligament S93.61-●
    tarsometatarsal ligament S93.62-●
    toe —see Sprain, toe
  hand S63.9-●
    finger —see Sprain, finger
    specified site NEC —see subcategory S63.8
    thumb —see Sprain, thumb
  head S03.9
  hip S73.10-●
    iliofemoral ligament S73.11-●
    ischiocapsular (ligament) S73.12-●
    specified NEC S73.19-●
  iliofemoral —see Sprain, hip
  innominate
    acetabulum —see Sprain, hip
    sacral junction S33.6
  internal
    collateral, ankle —see Sprain, ankle
    semilunar cartilage —see Sprain, knee, specified site NEC
  interphalangeal
    finger —see Sprain, finger, interphalangeal (joint)
    toe —see Sprain, toe, interphalangeal joint
  ischiocapsular —see Sprain, hip
  ischiofemoral —see Sprain, hip
  jaw (articular disc) (cartilage) (meniscus) S03.4-●
    old M26.69
  knee S83.9-●
    collateral ligament S83.40-●
      lateral (fibular) S83.42-●
      medial (tibial) S83.41-●
    cruciate ligament S83.50-●
      anterior S83.51-●
      posterior S83.52-●
    lateral (fibular) collateral ligament S83.42-●
    medial (tibial) collateral ligament S83.41-●
    patellar ligament S76.11-●
    specified site NEC S83.8X-●
    superior tibiofibular joint (ligament) S83.6-●
  lateral collateral, knee —see Sprain, knee, collateral
  lumbar (spine) S33.5
  lumbosacral S33.9
  mandible (articular disc) S03.4-●
    old M26.69
  medial collateral, knee —see Sprain, knee, collateral
  meniscus
    jaw S03.4-●
      old M26.69
    knee —see Sprain, knee, specified site NEC
      with current tear —see Tear, meniscus
      old —see Derangement, knee, meniscus, due to old tear
    mandible S03.4-●
      old M26.69
  metacarpal (distal) (proximal) —see Sprain, hand, specified site NEC
  metacarpophalangeal —see Sprain, finger, metacarpophalangeal (joint)
  metatarsophalangeal —see Sprain, toe, metatarsophalangeal joint
  midcarpal —see Sprain, hand, specified site NEC
  midtarsal —see Sprain, foot, specified site NEC
  neck S13.9
    anterior longitudinal cervical ligament S13.4
    atlanto-axial joint S13.4

Sprain *(Continued)*
  neck *(Continued)*
    atlanto-occipital joint S13.4
    cervical spine S13.4
    cricoarytenoid ligament S13.5
    cricothyroid ligament S13.5
    specified site NEC S13.8
    thyroid region (cartilage) S13.5
  nose S03.8
  orbicular, hip —*see* Sprain, hip
  patella —*see* Sprain, knee, specified site NEC
  patellar ligament S76.11-●
  pelvis NEC S33.8
  phalanx
    finger —*see* Sprain, finger
    toe —*see* Sprain, toe
  pubofemoral —*see* Sprain, hip
  radiocarpal —*see* Sprain, wrist
  radiohumeral —*see* Sprain, elbow
  radius, collateral —*see* Rupture, traumatic,
    ligament, radial collateral
  rib (cage) S23.41
  rotator cuff (capsule) S43.42-●
  sacroiliac (region)
    chronic or old —*see* subcategory M53.2
    joint S33.6
  scaphoid (hand) —*see* Sprain, hand, specified
    site NEC
  scapula (r) —*see* Sprain, shoulder girdle,
    specified site NEC
  semilunar cartilage (knee) —*see* Sprain, knee,
    specified site NEC
    with current tear —*see* Tear, meniscus
      old —*see* Derangement, knee, meniscus,
        due to old tear
  shoulder joint S43.40-●
    acromioclavicular joint (ligament) —*see*
      Sprain, acromioclavicular joint
    blade —*see* Sprain, shoulder, girdle,
      specified site NEC
    coracoclavicular joint (ligament) —*see*
      Sprain, coracoclavicular joint
    coracohumeral ligament —*see* Sprain,
      coracohumeral joint
    girdle S43.9-●
      specified site NEC S43.8-●
    rotator cuff —*see* Sprain, rotator cuff
    specified site NEC S43.49-●
    sternoclavicular joint (ligament) —*see*
      Sprain, sternoclavicular joint
  spine
    cervical S13.4
    lumbar S33.5
    thoracic S23.3
  sternoclavicular joint S43.6-●
  sternum S23.429
    chondrosternal joint S23.421
    specified site NEC S23.428
    sternoclavicular (joint) (ligament)
      S23.420
  symphysis
    jaw S03.4-●
      old M26.69
    mandibular S03.4-●
      old M26.69
  talofibular —*see* Sprain, ankle
  tarsal —*see* Sprain, foot, specified site NEC
  tarsometatarsal —*see* Sprain, foot, specified
    site NEC
  temporomandibular S03.4-●
    old M26.69
  thorax S23.9
    ribs S23.41
    specified site NEC S23.8
    spine S23.3
    sternum —*see* Sprain, sternum
  thumb S63.60-●
    interphalangeal (joint) S63.62-●
    metacarpophalangeal (joint) S63.64-●
    specified site NEC S63.68-●
  thyroid cartilage or region S13.5

Sprain *(Continued)*
  tibia (proximal end) —*see* Sprain, knee,
    specified site NEC
  tibial collateral, knee —*see* Sprain, knee,
    collateral
  tibiofibular
    distal —*see* Sprain, ankle
    superior —*see* Sprain, knee, specified site
      NEC
  toe(s) S93.50-●
    great S93.50-●
    interphalangeal joint S93.51-●
      great S93.51-●
      lesser S93.51-●
    lesser S93.50-●
    metatarsophalangeal joint S93.52-●
      great S93.52-●
      lesser S93.52-●
  ulna, collateral —*see* Rupture, traumatic,
    ligament, ulnar collateral
  ulnohumeral —*see* Sprain, elbow
  wrist S63.50-●
    carpal S63.51-●
    radiocarpal S63.52-●
    specified site NEC S63.59-●
  xiphoid cartilage —*see* Sprain, sternum
Sprengel's deformity (congenital) Q74.0
Sprue (tropical) K90.1
  celiac K90.0
  idiopathic K90.49
  meaning thrush B37.0
  nontropical K90.0
Spur, bone —*see also* Enthesopathy
  calcaneal M77.3-●
  iliac crest M76.2-●
  nose (septum) J34.89
Spurway's syndrome Q78.0
Sputum
  abnormal (amount) (color) (odor) (purulent)
    R09.3
  blood-stained R04.2
  excessive (cause unknown) R09.3
Squamous —*see also* condition
  epithelium in
    cervical canal (congenital) Q51.828
    uterine mucosa (congenital) Q51.818
Squashed nose M95.0
  congenital Q67.4
Squeeze, diver's T70.3
Squint —*see also* Strabismus
  accommodative —*see* Strabismus, convergent
    concomitant
St. Hubert's disease A82.9
Stab —*see also* Laceration
  internal organs —*see* Injury, by site
Stafne's cyst or cavity M27.0
Staggering gait R26.0
  hysterical F44.4
Staghorn calculus —*see* Calculus, kidney
Stähli's line (cornea) (pigment) —*see*
  Pigmentation, cornea, anterior
Stain, staining
  meconium (newborn) P96.83
  port wine Q82.5
  tooth, teeth (hard tissues) (extrinsic) K03.6
    due to
      accretions K03.6
      deposits (betel) (black) (green) (materia
        alba) (orange) (soft) (tobacco) K03.6
      metals (copper) (silver) K03.7
      nicotine K03.6
      pulpal bleeding K03.7
      tobacco K03.6
    intrinsic K00.8
Stammering —*see also* Disorder, fluency F80.81
Standstill
  auricular I45.5
  cardiac —*see* Arrest, cardiac
  sinoatrial I45.5
  ventricular —*see* Arrest, cardiac
Stannosis J63.5

Stanton's disease —*see* Melioidosis
Staphylitis (acute) (catarrhal) (chronic)
  (gangrenous) (membranous) (suppurative)
  (ulcerative) K12.2
Staphylococcal scalded skin syndrome L00
Staphylococcemia A41.2
Staphylococcus, staphylococcal —*see also*
  condition
  as cause of disease classified elsewhere
    B95.8
    aureus (methicillin susceptible) (MSSA)
      B95.61
      methicillin resistant (MRSA) B95.62
    specified NEC, as cause of disease classified
      elsewhere B95.7
Staphyloma (sclera)
  cornea H18.72-●
  equatorial H15.81-●
  localized (anterior) H15.82-●
  posticum H15.83-●
  ring H15.85-●
Stargardt's disease —*see* Dystrophy, retina
Starvation (inanition) (due to lack of food)
  T73.0
  edema —*see* Malnutrition, severe
Stasis
  bile (noncalculous) K83.1
  bronchus J98.09
    with infection —*see* Bronchitis
  cardiac —*see* Failure, heart, congestive
  cecum K59.8
  colon K59.8
  dermatitis I87.2
    with
      varicose ulcer —*see* Varix, leg, with ulcer,
        with inflammation
      varicose veins —*see* Varix, leg, with,
        inflammation
    due to postthrombotic syndrome —*see*
      Syndrome, postthrombotic
  duodenal K31.5
  eczema —*see* Varix, leg, with, inflammation
  edema —*see* Hypertension, venous (chronic),
    idiopathic
  foot T69.0-●
  ileocecal coil K59.8
  ileum K59.8
  intestinal K59.8
  jejunum K59.8
  kidney N19
  liver (cirrhotic) K76.1
  lymphatic I89.8
  pneumonia J18.2
  pulmonary —*see* Edema, lung
  rectal K59.8
  renal N19
    tubular N17.0
  ulcer —*see* Varix, leg, with, ulcer
    without varicose veins I87.2
  urine —*see* Retention, urine
  venous I87.8
State (of)
  affective and paranoid, mixed, organic
    psychotic F06.8
  agitated R45.1
    acute reaction to stress F43.0
  anxiety (neurotic) F41.1
  apprehension F41.1
  burn-out Z73.0
  climacteric, female Z78.0
    symptomatic N95.1
  compulsive F42.8
    mixed with obsessional thoughts F42.2
  confusional (psychogenic) F44.89
    acute —*see also* Delirium
      with
        arteriosclerotic dementia F01.50
          with behavioral disturbance
            F01.51
        senility or dementia F05
      alcoholic F10.231

▶ New   ⇒ Revised   deleted Deleted   ● Use Additional Character(s)

State *(Continued)*
  confusional (psychogenic) *(Continued)*
    epileptic F05
    reactive (from emotional stress,
      psychological trauma) F44.89
    subacute —*see* Delirium
  convulsive —*see* Convulsions
  crisis F43.0
  depressive F32.9
    neurotic F34.1
  dissociative F44.9
  emotional shock (stress) R45.7
  hypercoagulation —*see* Hypercoagulable
  locked-in G83.5
  menopausal Z78.0
    symptomatic N95.1
  neurotic F48.9
    with depersonalization F48.1
  obsessional F42.8
  oneiroid (schizophrenia-like) F23
  organic
    hallucinatory (nonalcoholic) F06.0
    paranoid (-hallucinatory) F06.2
  panic F41.0
  paranoid F22
    climacteric F22
    involutional F22
    menopausal F22
    organic F06.2
    senile F03
    simple F22
  persistent vegetative R40.3
  phobic F40.9
  postleukotomy F07.0
  pregnant
    gestational carrier Z33.3
    incidental Z33.1
  psychogenic, twilight F44.89
  psychopathic (constitutional) F60.2
  psychotic, organic —*see also* Psychosis,
    organic
    mixed paranoid and affective F06.8
    senile or presenile F03
    transient NEC F06.8
      with
        depression F06.31
        hallucinations F06.0
  residual schizophrenic F20.5
  restlessness R45.1
  stress (emotional) R45.7
  tension (mental) F48.9
    specified NEC F48.8
  transient organic psychotic NEC F06.8
    depressive type F06.31
    hallucinatory type F06.0
  twilight
    epileptic F05
    psychogenic F44.89
  vegetative, persistent R40.3
  vital exhaustion Z73.0
  withdrawal —*see* Withdrawal, state
Status (post) —*see also* Presence (of)
  absence, epileptic —*see* Epilepsy, by type,
    with status epilepticus
  administration of tPA (rtPA) in a different
    facility within the last 24 hours prior to
    admission to the current facility
    Z92.82
  adrenalectomy (unilateral) (bilateral)
    E89.6
  anastomosis Z98.0
  anginosus I20.9
  angioplasty (peripheral) Z98.62
    with implant Z95.820
    coronary artery Z98.61
      with implant Z95.5
  aortocoronary bypass Z95.1
  arthrodesis Z98.1
  artificial opening (of) Z93.9
    gastrointestinal tract Z93.4
    specified NEC Z93.8

Status *(Continued)*
  artificial opening (of) *(Continued)*
    urinary tract Z93.6
    vagina Z93.8
  asthmaticus —*see* Asthma, by type, with
    status asthmaticus
  awaiting organ transplant Z76.82
  bariatric surgery Z98.84
  bed confinement Z74.01
  bleb, filtering (vitreous), after glaucoma
    surgery Z98.83
  breast implant Z98.82
    removal Z98.86
  cataract extraction Z98.4-●
  cholecystectomy Z90.49
  clitorectomy N90.811
    with excision of labia minora N90.812
  colectomy (complete) (partial) Z90.49
  colonization —*see* Carrier (suspected) of
  colostomy Z93.3
  convulsivus idiopathicus —*see* Epilepsy, by
    type, with status epilepticus
  coronary artery angioplasty —*see* Status,
    angioplasty, coronary artery
▶ coronary artery bypass graft Z95.1
  cystectomy (urinary bladder) Z90.6
  cystostomy Z93.50
    appendico-vesicostomy Z93.52
    cutaneous Z93.51
    specified NEC Z93.59
  delinquent immunization Z28.3
  dental Z98.818
    crown Z98.811
    fillings Z98.811
    restoration Z98.811
    sealant Z98.810
    specified NEC Z98.818
  deployment (current) (military) Z56.82
  dialysis (hemodialysis) (peritoneal) Z99.2
  do not resuscitate (DNR) Z66
  donor —*see* Donor
  embedded fragments —*see* Retained, foreign
    body fragments (type of)
  embedded splinter —*see* Retained, foreign
    body fragments (type of)
  enterostomy Z93.4
  epileptic, epilepticus —*see also* Epilepsy, by
    type, with status epilepticus G40.901
  estrogen receptor
    negative Z17.1
    positive Z17.0
  female genital cutting —*see* Female genital
    mutilation status
  female genital mutilation —*see* Female genital
    mutilation status
  filtering (vitreous) bleb after glaucoma
    surgery Z98.83
  gastrectomy (complete) (partial) Z90.3
  gastric banding Z98.84
  gastric bypass for obesity Z98.84
  gastrostomy Z93.1
  human immunodeficiency virus (HIV)
    infection, asymptomatic Z21
  hysterectomy (complete) (total) Z90.710
    partial (with remaining cervial stump)
      Z90.711
  ileostomy Z93.2
  implant
    breast Z98.82
  infibulation N90.813
  intestinal bypass Z98.0
  jejunostomy Z93.4
  lapsed immunization schedule Z28.3
  laryngectomy Z90.02
  lymphaticus E32.8
  malignancy
    castrate resistant prostate Z19.2
    hormone resistant Z19.2
    hormone sensitive Z19.1
  marmoratus G80.3
  mastectomy (unilateral) (bilateral)
    Z90.1-●

Status *(Continued)*
  military deployment status (current) Z56.82
    in theater or in support of military war,
      peacekeeping and humanitarian
      operations Z56.82
  nephrectomy (unilateral) (bilateral) Z90.5
  nephrostomy Z93.6
  obesity surgery Z98.84
  oophorectomy
    bilateral Z90.722
    unilateral Z90.721
  organ replacement
    by artificial or mechanical device or
      prosthesis of
      artery Z95.828
      bladder Z96.0
      blood vessel Z95.828
      breast Z97.8
      eye globe Z97.0
      heart Z95.812
        valve Z95.2
      intestine Z97.8
      joint Z96.60
        hip —*see* Presence, hip joint implant
        knee —*see* Presence, knee joint
          implant
        specified site NEC Z96.698
      kidney Z97.8
      larynx Z96.3
      lens Z96.1
      limbs —*see* Presence, artificial, limb
      liver Z97.8
      lung Z97.8
      pancreas Z97.8
    by organ transplant (heterologous)
      (homologous) —*see* Transplant
  pacemaker
    brain Z96.89
    cardiac Z95.0
    specified NEC Z96.89
  pancreatectomy Z90.410
    complete Z90.410
    partial Z90.411
    total Z90.410
  pneumonectomy (complete) (partial) Z90.2
  pneumothorax, therapeutic Z98.3
  postcommotio cerebri F07.81
  postoperative (postprocedural) NEC
    Z98.890
    breast implant Z98.82
    dental Z98.818
      crown Z98.811
      fillings Z98.811
      restoration Z98.811
      sealant Z98.810
      specified NEC Z98.818
    pneumothorax, therapeutic Z98.3
    uterine scar Z98.891
  postpartum (routine follow-up) Z39.2
    care immediately after delivery Z39.0
  postsurgical (postprocedural) NEC
    Z98.890
    pneumothorax, therapeutic Z98.3
  pregnancy, incidental Z33.1
  prosthesis coronary angioplasty Z95.5
  pseudophakia Z96.1
  renal dialysis (hemodialysis) (peritoneal)
    Z99.2
  retained foreign body —*see* Retained, foreign
    body fragments (type of)
  reversed jejunal transposition (for bypass
    Z98.0
  salpingo-oophorectomy
    bilateral Z90.722
    unilateral Z90.721
  sex reassignment surgery status Z87.890
  shunt
    arteriovenous (for dialysis) Z99.2
    cerebrospinal fluid Z98.2
    ventricular (communicating) (for
      drainage) Z98.2

Status (Continued)
  splenectomy Z90.81
  thymicolymphaticus E32.8
  thymicus E32.8
  thymolymphaticus E32.8
  thyroidectomy (hypothyroidism) E89.0
  tooth (teeth) extraction —see also Absence,
      teeth, acquired K08.409
  tPA (rtPA) administration in a different
      facility within the last 24 hours prior to
      admission to current facility Z92.82
  tracheostomy Z93.0
  transplant —see Transplant
      organ removed Z98.85
  tubal ligation Z98.51
  underimmunization Z28.3
  ureterostomy Z93.6
  urethrostomy Z93.6
  vagina, artificial Z93.8
  vasectomy Z98.52
  wheelchair confinement Z99.3
Stealing
  child problem F91.8
      in company with others Z72.810
  pathological (compulsive) F63.2
Steam burn —see Burn
Steatocystoma multiplex L72.2
Steatohepatitis (nonalcoholic) (NASH)
      K75.81
Steatoma L72.3
  eyelid (cystic) —see Dermatosis, eyelid
      infected —see Hordeolum
Steatorrhea (chronic) K90.9
  with lacteal obstruction K90.2
  idiopathic (adult) (infantile) K90.9
  pancreatic K90.3
  primary K90.0
  tropical K90.1
Steatosis E88.89
  heart —see Degeneration, myocardial
  kidney N28.89
  liver NEC K76.0
Steele-Richardson-Olszewski disease or
      syndrome G23.1
Steinbrocker's syndrome G90.8
Steinert's disease G71.11
Stein-Leventhal syndrome E28.2
Stein's syndrome E28.2
STEMI —see also Infarct, myocardium, ST
      elevation I21.3
Stenocardia I20.8
Stenocephaly Q75.8
Stenosis, stenotic (cicatricial) —see also
      Stricture
  ampulla of Vater K83.1
  anus, anal (canal) (sphincter) K62.4
      and rectum K62.4
      congenital Q42.3
          with fistula Q42.2
  aorta (ascending) (supraventricular)
      (congenital) Q25.1
      arteriosclerotic I70.0
      calcified I70.0
      supravalvular Q25.3
  aortic (valve) I35.0
      with insufficiency I35.2
      congenital Q23.0
      rheumatic I06.0
          with
              incompetency, insufficiency or
                  regurgitation I06.2
                  with mitral (valve) disease I08.0
                      with tricuspid (valve) disease
                          I08.3
                  mitral (valve) disease I08.0
                      with tricuspid (valve) disease
                          I08.3
                  tricuspid (valve) disease I08.2
                      with mitral (valve) disease I08.3
      specified cause NEC I35.0
      syphilitic A52.03

Stenosis, stenotic (Continued)
  aqueduct of Sylvius (congenital) Q03.0
      with spina bifida —see Spina bifida,
          by site, with hydrocephalus
      acquired G91.1
  artery NEC —see also Arteriosclerosis
      I77.1
      celiac I77.4
      cerebral —see Occlusion, artery, cerebral
      extremities —see Arteriosclerosis,
          extremities
      precerebral —see Occlusion, artery,
          precerebral
      pulmonary (congenital) Q25.6
          acquired I28.8
      renal I70.1
      stent
          coronary T82.855
          peripheral T82.856
  bile duct (common) (hepatic) K83.1
      congenital Q44.3
  bladder-neck (acquired) N32.0
      congenital Q64.31
  brain G93.89
  bronchus J98.09
      congenital Q32.3
      syphilitic A52.72
  cardia (stomach) K22.2
      congenital Q39.3
  cardiovascular —see Disease, cardiovascular
  caudal M48.08
  cervix, cervical (canal) N88.2
      congenital Q51.828
      in pregnancy or childbirth —see Pregnancy,
          complicated by, abnormal cervix
  colon —see also Obstruction, intestine
      congenital Q42.9
          specified NEC Q42.8
  colostomy K94.03
  common (bile) duct K83.1
      congenital Q44.3
  coronary (artery) —see Disease, heart,
      ischemic, atherosclerotic
  cystic duct —see Obstruction, gallbladder
  due to presence of device, implant or
      graft —see also Complications, by site
      and type, specified NEC T85.858
      arterial graft NEC T82.858
      breast (implant) T85.858
      catheter T85.858
          dialysis (renal) T82.858
              intraperitoneal T85.858
          infusion NEC T82.858
              spinal (epidural) (subdural)
                  T85.850
          urinary (indwelling) T83.85
      fixation, internal (orthopedic) NEC
          T84.85
      gastrointestinal (bile duct) (esophagus)
          T85.858
      genital NEC T83.85
      heart NEC T82.857
      joint prosthesis T84.85
      ocular (corneal graft) (orbital implant)
          NEC T85.858
      orthopedic NEC T84.85
      specified NEC T85.858
      urinary NEC T83.85
      vascular NEC T82.858
      ventricular intracranial shunt T85.850
  duodenum K31.5
      congenital Q41.0
  ejaculatory duct NEC N50.89
  endocervical os —see Stenosis, cervix
  enterostomy K94.13
  esophagus K22.2
      congenital Q39.3
      syphilitic A52.79
          congenital A50.59 [K23]
  eustachian tube —see Obstruction, eustachian
      tube

Stenosis, stenotic (Continued)
  external ear canal (acquired) H61.30-●
      congenital Q16.1
      due to
          inflammation H61.32-●
          trauma H61.31-●
      postprocedural H95.81-●
      specified cause NEC H61.39-●
  gallbladder —see Obstruction, gallbladder
  glottis J38.6
  heart valve (congenital) Q24.8
      aortic Q23.0
      mitral Q23.2
      pulmonary Q22.1
      tricuspid Q22.4
  hepatic duct K83.1
  hymen N89.6
  hypertrophic subaortic (idiopathic) I42.1
  ileum —see also Obstruction, intestine,
      specified NEC K56.699
      congenital Q41.2
  infundibulum cardia Q24.3
  intervertebral foramina —see also Lesion,
      biomechanical, specified NEC
      connective tissue M99.79
          abdomen M99.79
          cervical region M99.71
          cervicothoracic M99.71
          head region M99.70
          lumbar region M99.73
          lumbosacral M99.73
          occipitocervical M99.70
          sacral region M99.74
          sacrococcygeal M99.74
          sacroiliac M99.74
          specified NEC M99.79
          thoracic region M99.72
          thoracolumbar M99.72
      disc M99.79
          abdomen M99.79
          cervical region M99.71
          cervicothoracic M99.71
          head region M99.70
          lower extremity M99.76
          lumbar region M99.73
          lumbosacral M99.73
          occipitocervical M99.70
          pelvic M99.75
          rib cage M99.78
          sacral region M99.74
          sacrococcygeal M99.74
          sacroiliac M99.74
          specified NEC M99.79
          thoracic region M99.72
          thoracolumbar M99.72
          upper extremity M99.77
      osseous M99.69
          abdomen M99.69
          cervical region M99.61
          cervicothoracic M99.61
          head region M99.60
          lower extremity M99.66
          lumbar region M99.63
          lumbosacral M99.63
          occipitocervical M99.60
          pelvic M99.65
          rib cage M99.68
          sacral region M99.64
          sacrococcygeal M99.64
          sacroiliac M99.64
          specified NEC M99.69
          thoracic region M99.62
          thoracolumbar M99.62
          upper extremity M99.67
      subluxation —see Stenosis, intervertebral
          foramina, osseous
  intestine —see also Obstruction, intestine
      congenital (small) Q41.9
          large Q42.9
              specified NEC Q42.8
          specified NEC Q41.8

▶ New   ⟹ Revised   ~~deleted~~ Deleted   ● Use Additional Character(s)

Stenosis, stenotic *(Continued)*
⇒jejunum —*see also* Obstruction, intestine,
        specified NEC K56.699
    congenital Q41.1
  lacrimal (passage)
    canaliculi H04.54-•
      congenital Q10.5
    duct H04.55-•
    punctum H04.56-•
    sac H04.57-•
  lacrimonasal duct —*see* Stenosis, lacrimal, duct
    congenital Q10.5
  larynx J38.6
    congenital NEC Q31.8
      subglottic Q31.1
    syphilitic A52.73
      congenital A50.59 *[J99]*
  mitral (chronic) (inactive) (valve) I05.0
    with
      aortic valve disease I08.0
      incompetency, insufficiency or
          regurgitation I05.2
    active or acute I01.1
      with rheumatic or Sydenham's chorea
          I02.0
    congenital Q23.2
    specified cause, except rheumatic I34.2
    syphilitic A52.03
  myocardium, myocardial —*see also*
      Degeneration, myocardial
    hypertrophic subaortic (idiopathic) I42.1
  nares (anterior) (posterior) J34.89
    congenital Q30.0
  nasal duct —*see also* Stenosis, lacrimal, duct
    congenital Q10.5
  nasolacrimal duct —*see also* Stenosis, lacrimal,
      duct
    congenital Q10.5
  neural canal —*see also* Lesion, biomechanical,
      specified NEC
    connective tissue M99.49
      abdomen M99.49
      cervical region M99.41
      cervicothoracic M99.41
      head region M99.40
      lower extremity M99.46
      lumbar region M99.43
      lumbosacral M99.43
      occipitocervical M99.40
      pelvic M99.45
      rib cage M99.48
      sacral region M99.44
      sacrococcygeal M99.44
      sacroiliac M99.44
      specified NEC M99.49
      thoracic region M99.42
      thoracolumbar M99.42
      upper extremity M99.47
    intervertebral disc M99.59
      abdomen M99.59
      cervical region M99.51
      cervicothoracic M99.51
      head region M99.50
      lower extremity M99.56
      lumbar region M99.53
      lumbosacral M99.53
      occipitocervical M99.50
      pelvic M99.55
      rib cage M99.58
      sacral region M99.54
      sacrococcygeal M99.54
      sacroiliac M99.54
      specified NEC M99.59
      thoracic region M99.52
      thoracolumbar M99.52
      upper extremity M99.57
    osseous M99.39
      abdomen M99.39
      cervical region M99.31
      cervicothoracic M99.31
      head region M99.30

Stenosis, stenotic *(Continued)*
  neural canal *(Continued)*
    osseous *(Continued)*
      lower extremity M99.36
      lumbar region M99.33
      lumbosacral M99.33
      occipitocervical M99.30
      pelvic M99.35
      rib cage M99.38
      sacral region M99.34
      sacrococcygeal M99.34
      sacroiliac M99.34
      specified NEC M99.39
      thoracic region M99.32
      thoracolumbar M99.32
      upper extremity M99.37
    subluxation M99.29
      cervical region M99.21
      cervicothoracic M99.21
      head region M99.20
      lower extremity M99.26
      lumbar region M99.23
      lumbosacral M99.23
      occipitocervical M99.20
      pelvic M99.25
      rib cage M99.28
      sacral region M99.24
      sacrococcygeal M99.24
      sacroiliac M99.24
      specified NEC M99.29
      thoracic region M99.22
      thoracolumbar M99.22
      upper extremity M99.27
  organ or site, congenital NEC —*see* Atresia,
      by site
  papilla of Vater K83.1
  pulmonary (artery) (congenital) Q25.6
    with ventricular septal defect,
        transposition of aorta, and
        hypertrophy of right ventricle Q21.3
    acquired I28.8
    in tetralogy of Fallot Q21.3
    infundibular Q24.3
    subvalvular Q24.3
    supravalvular Q25.6
    valve I37.0
      with insufficiency I37.2
      congenital Q22.1
      rheumatic I09.89
        with aortic, mitral or tricuspid (valve)
            disease I08.8
    vein, acquired I28.8
    vessel NEC I28.8
  pulmonic (congenital) Q22.1
    infundibular Q24.3
    subvalvular Q24.3
  pylorus (hypertrophic) (acquired) K31.1
    adult K31.1
    congenital Q40.0
    infantile Q40.0
  rectum (sphincter) —*see* Stricture, rectum
  renal artery I70.1
    congenital Q27.1
  salivary duct (any) K11.8
  sphincter of Oddi K83.1
  spinal M48.00
    cervical region M48.02
    cervicothoracic region M48.03
⇒ lumbar region (NOS) (without neurogenic
      claudication) M48.061
    ▶with neurogenic claudication M48.062
    lumbosacral region M48.07
    occipito-atlanto-axial region M48.01
    sacrococcygeal region M48.08
    thoracic region M48.04
    thoracolumbar region M48.05
  stent
    vascular
      end stent
        adjacent to stent —*see*
            Arteriosclerosis

Stenosis, stenotic *(Continued)*
  stent *(Continued)*
    vascular *(Continued)*
      end stent *(Continued)*
        within the stent
          coronary T82.855
          peripheral T82.856
      in stent
        coronary vessel T82.855
        peripheral vessel T82.856
  stomach, hourglass K31.2
  subaortic (congenital) Q24.4
    hypertrophic (idiopathic) I42.1
  subglottic J38.6
    congenital Q31.1
    postprocedural J95.5
  trachea J39.8
    congenital Q32.1
    syphilitic A52.73
    tuberculous NEC A15.5
  tracheostomy J95.03
  tricuspid (valve) I07.0
    with
      aortic (valve) disease I08.2
      incompetency, insufficiency or
          regurgitation I07.2
        with aortic (valve) disease I08.2
          with mitral (valve) disease
              I08.3
      mitral (valve) disease I08.1
        with aortic (valve) disease I08.3
    congenital Q22.4
    nonrheumatic I36.0
      with insufficiency I36.2
  tubal N97.1
  ureter —*see* Atresia, ureter
  ureteropelvic junction, congenital
      Q62.11
  ureterovesical orifice, congenital Q62.12
  urethra (valve) —*see also* Stricture, urethra
    congenital Q64.32
  urinary meatus, congenital Q64.33
  vagina N89.5
    congenital Q52.4
    in pregnancy —*see* Pregnancy, complicated
        by, abnormal vagina
      causing obstructed labor O65.5
  valve (cardiac) (heart) —*see also* Endocarditis
      I38
    congenital Q24.8
      aortic Q23.0
      mitral Q23.2
      pulmonary Q22.1
      tricuspid Q22.4
  vena cava (inferior) (superior) I87.1
    congenital Q26.0
  vesicourethral orifice Q64.31
  vulva N90.5
Stent jail T82.897
Stercolith (impaction) K56.41
  appendix K38.1
Stercoraceous, stercoral ulcer K63.3
  anus or rectum K62.6
Stereotypies NEC F98.4
Sterility —*see* Infertility
Sterilization —*see* Encounter (for),
    sterilization
Sternalgia —*see* Angina
Sternopagus Q89.4
Sternum bifidum Q76.7
Steroid
  effects (adverse) (adrenocortical)
      (iatrogenic)
    cushingoid E24.2
      correct substance properly
          administered —*see* Table of Drugs
          and Chemicals, by drug, adverse
          effect
      overdose or wrong substance given
          or taken —*see* Table of Drugs and
          Chemicals, by drug, poisoning

Steroid *(Continued)*
 effects *(Continued)*
  diabetes —*see* category E09
   correct substance properly
    administered —*see* Table of Drugs
    and Chemicals, by drug, adverse
    effect
   overdose or wrong substance given
    or taken —*see* Table of Drugs and
    Chemicals, by drug, poisoning
  fever R50.2
  insufficiency E27.3
   correct substance properly
    administered —*see* Table of Drugs
    and Chemicals, by drug, adverse
    effect
   overdose or wrong substance given
    or taken —*see* Table of Drugs and
    Chemicals, by drug, poisoning
 responder H40.04-●
Stevens-Johnson disease or syndrome L51.1
 toxic epidermal necrolysis overlap L51.3
Stewart-Morel syndrome M85.2
Sticker's disease B08.3
Sticky eye —*see* Conjunctivitis, acute,
 mucopurulent
Stieda's disease —*see* Bursitis, tibial collateral
Stiff neck —*see* Torticollis
Stiff-man syndrome G25.82
Stiffness, joint NEC M25.60-●
 ankle M25.67-●
 ankylosis —*see* Ankylosis, joint
 contracture —*see* Contraction, joint
 elbow M25.62-●
 foot M25.67-●
 hand M25.64-●
 hip M25.65-●
 knee M25.66-●
 shoulder M25.61-●
 wrist M25.63-●
Stigmata congenital syphilis A50.59
Stillbirth P95
Still-Felty syndrome —*see* Felty's syndrome
Still's disease or syndrome (juvenile) M08.20
 adult-onset M06.1
 ankle M08.27-●
 elbow M08.22-●
 foot joint M08.27-●
 hand joint M08.24-●
 hip M08.25-●
 knee M08.26-●
 multiple site M08.29
 shoulder M08.21-●
 vertebra M08.28
 wrist M08.23-●
Stimulation, ovary E28.1
Sting (venomous) (with allergic or anaphylactic
 shock) —*see* Table of Drugs and Chemicals,
 by animal or substance, poisoning
Stippled epiphyses Q78.8
Stitch
➠abscess T81.4
 burst (in operation wound) —*see* Disruption,
  wound, operation
Stokes-Adams disease or syndrome I45.9
Stokes' disease E05.00
 with thyroid storm E05.01
Stokvis (-Talma) disease D74.8
Stoma malfunction
 colostomy K94.03
 enterostomy K94.13
 gastrostomy K94.23
 ileostomy K94.13
 tracheostomy J95.03
Stomach —*see* condition
Stomatitis (denture) (ulcerative) K12.1
 angular K13.0
  due to dietary or vitamin deficiency
   E53.0
 aphthous K12.0
 bovine B08.61

Stomatitis *(Continued)*
 candidal B37.0
 catarrhal K12.1
 diphtheritic A36.89
 due to
  dietary deficiency E53.0
  thrush B37.0
  vitamin deficiency
   B group NEC E53.9
   B2 (riboflavin) E53.0
 epidemic B08.8
 epizootic B08.8
 follicular K12.1
 gangrenous A69.0
 Geotrichum B48.3
 herpesviral, herpetic B00.2
 herpetiformis K12.0
 malignant K12.1
 membranous acute K12.1
 monilial B37.0
 mycotic B37.0
 necrotizing ulcerative A69.0
 parasitic B37.0
 septic K12.1
 spirochetal A69.1
 suppurative (acute) K12.2
 ulceromembranous A69.1
 vesicular K12.1
  with exanthem (enteroviral)
   B08.4
  virus disease A93.8
 Vincent's A69.1
Stomatocytosis D58.8
Stomatomycosis B37.0
Stomatorrhagia K13.79
Stone(s) —*see also* Calculus
 bladder (diverticulum) N21.0
 cystine E72.09
 heart syndrome I50.1
 kidney N20.0
 prostate N42.0
 pulpal (dental) K04.2
 renal N20.0
 salivary gland or duct (any) K11.5
 urethra (impacted) N21.1
 urinary (duct) (impacted) (passage)
  N20.9
  bladder (diverticulum) N21.0
  lower tract N21.9
  specified NEC N21.8
 xanthine E79.8 *[N22]*
Stonecutter's lung J62.8
**Stonemason's asthma, disease, lung or
 pneumoconiosis** J62.8
Stoppage
 heart —*see* Arrest, cardiac
 urine —*see* Retention, urine
Storm, thyroid —*see* Thyrotoxicosis
Strabismus (congenital) (nonparalytic)
 H50.9
 concomitant H50.40
  convergent —*see* Strabismus, convergent
   concomitant
  divergent —*see* Strabismus, divergent
   concomitant
 convergent concomitant H50.00
  accommodative component H50.43
  alternating H50.05
   with
    A pattern H50.06
    specified nonconcomitances NEC
     H50.08
    V pattern H50.07
  monocular H50.01-●
   with
    A pattern H50.02-●
    specified nonconcomitances NEC
     H50.04-●
    V pattern H50.03-●
  intermittent H50.31-●
   alternating H50.32

Strabismus *(Continued)*
 cyclotropia H50.41
 divergent concomitant H50.10
  alternating H50.15
   with
    A pattern H50.16
    specified noncomitances NEC
     H50.18
    V pattern H50.17
  monocular H50.11-●
   with
    A pattern H50.12-●
    specified noncomitances NEC
     H50.14-●
    V pattern H50.13-●
  intermittent H50.33-●
   alternating H50.34
 Duane's syndrome H50.81-●
 due to adhesions, scars H50.69
 heterophoria H50.50
  alternating H50.55
  cyclophoria H50.54
  esophoria H50.51
  exophoria H50.52
  vertical H50.53
 heterotropia H50.40
  intermittent H50.30
 hypertropia H50.2-●
 hypotropia —*see* Hypertropia
 latent H50.50
 mechanical H50.60
  Brown's sheath syndrome H50.61-●
  specified type NEC H50.69
 monofixation syndrome H50.42
 paralytic H49.9
  abducens nerve H49.2-●
  fourth nerve H49.1-●
  Kearns-Sayre syndrome H49.81-●
  ophthalmoplegia (external)
   progressive H49.4-●
    with pigmentary retinopathy H49.81-●
   total H49.3-●
  sixth nerve H49.2-●
  specified type NEC H49.88-●
  third nerve H49.0-●
  trochlear nerve H49.1-●
 specified type NEC H50.89
 vertical H50.2-●
Strain
 back S39.012
 cervical S16.1
 eye NEC —*see* Disturbance, vision, subjective
 heart —*see* Disease, heart
 low back S39.012
 mental NOS Z73.3
  work-related Z56.6
 muscle (tendon) —*see* Injury, muscle, by site,
  strain
 neck S16.1
 physical NOS Z73.3
  work-related Z56.6
 postural —*see also* Disorder, soft tissue, due
  to use
 psychological NEC Z73.3
 tendon —*see* Injury, muscle, by site, strain
Straining, on urination R39.16
Strand, vitreous —*see* Opacity, vitreous,
 membranes and strands
Strangulation, strangulated —*see also*
 Asphyxia, traumatic
 appendix K38.8
 bladder-neck N32.0
 bowel or colon K56.2
 food or foreign body —*see* Foreign body, by
  site
 hemorrhoids —*see* Hemorrhoids, with
  complication
 hernia —*see also* Hernia, by site, with
  obstruction
  with gangrene —*see* Hernia, by site, with
   gangrene

▶ New   ➠ Revised   ~~deleted~~ Deleted   ● Use Additional Character(s)

Strangulation, strangulated *(Continued)*
  intestine (large) (small) K56.2
    with hernia —*see also* Hernia, by site, with
      obstruction
      with gangrene —*see* Hernia, by site, with
        gangrene
  mesentery K56.2
  mucus —*see* Asphyxia, mucus
  omentum K56.2
  organ or site, congenital NEC —*see* Atresia,
    by site
  ovary —*see* Torsion, ovary
  penis N48.89
    foreign body T19.4
  rupture —*see* Hernia, by site, with obstruction
  stomach due to hernia —*see also* Hernia, by
    site, with obstruction
    with gangrene —*see* Hernia, by site, with
      gangrene
  vesicourethral orifice N32.0
Strangury R30.0
Straw itch B88.0
Strawberry
  gallbladder K82.4
  mark Q82.5
  tongue (red) (white) K14.3
Streak(s)
  macula, angioid H35.33
  ovarian Q50.32
Strephosymbolia F81.0
  secondary to organic lesion R48.8
Streptobacillary fever A25.1
Streptobacillosis A25.1
Streptobacillus moniliformis A25.1
Streptococcus, streptococcal —*see also*
  condition
  as cause of disease classified elsewhere B95.5
  group
    A, as cause of disease classified elsewhere
      B95.0
    B, as cause of disease classified elsewhere
      B95.1
    D, as cause of disease classified elsewhere
      B95.2
  pneumoniae, as cause of disease classified
    elsewhere B95.3
  specified NEC, as cause of disease classified
    elsewhere B95.4
Streptomycosis B47.1
Streptotrichosis A48.8
Stress F43.9
  family —*see* Disruption, family
  fetal P84
    complicating pregnancy O77.9
    due to drug administration O77.1
  mental NEC Z73.3
    work-related Z56.6
  physical NEC Z73.3
    work-related Z56.6
  polycythemia D75.1
  reaction —*see also* Reaction, stress F43.9
  work schedule Z56.3
Stretching, nerve —*see* Injury, nerve
Striae albicans, atrophicae or distensae
  (cutis) L90.6
Stricture —*see also* Stenosis
  ampulla of Vater K83.1
  anus (sphincter) K62.4
    congenital Q42.3
      with fistula Q42.2
    infantile Q42.3
      with fistula Q42.2
  aorta (ascending) (congenital) Q25.1
    arteriosclerotic I70.0
    calcified I70.0
    supravalvular, congenital Q25.3
  aortic (valve) —*see* Stenosis, aortic
  aqueduct of Sylvius (congenital) Q03.0
    with spina bifida —*see* Spina bifida, by site,
      with hydrocephalus
    acquired G91.1

Stricture *(Continued)*
  artery I77.1
    basilar —*see* Occlusion, artery, basilar
    carotid —*see* Occlusion, artery, carotid
    celiac I77.4
    congenital (peripheral) Q27.8
      cerebral Q28.3
      coronary Q24.5
      digestive system Q27.8
      lower limb Q27.8
      retinal Q14.1
      specified site NEC Q27.8
      umbilical Q27.0
      upper limb Q27.8
    coronary —*see* Disease, heart, ischemic,
      atherosclerotic
      congenital Q24.5
    precerebral —*see* Occlusion, artery,
      precerebral
    pulmonary (congenital) Q25.6
      acquired I28.8
    renal I70.1
    vertebral —*see* Occlusion, artery, vertebral
  auditory canal (external) (congenital)
    acquired —*see* Stenosis, external ear canal
  bile duct (common) (hepatic) K83.1
    congenital Q44.3
    postoperative K91.89
  bladder N32.89
    neck N32.0
  bowel —*see* Obstruction, intestine
  brain G93.89
  bronchus J98.09
    congenital Q32.3
    syphilitic A52.72
  cardia (stomach) K22.2
    congenital Q39.3
  cardiac —*see also* Disease, heart
    orifice (stomach) K22.2
  cecum —*see* Obstruction, intestine
  cervix, cervical (canal) N88.2
    congenital Q51.828
    in pregnancy —*see* Pregnancy, complicated
      by, abnormal cervix
      causing obstructed labor O65.5
  colon —*see also* Obstruction, intestine
    congenital Q42.9
      specified NEC Q42.8
  colostomy K94.03
  common (bile) duct K83.1
  coronary (artery) —*see* Disease, heart,
    ischemic, atherosclerotic
  cystic duct —*see* Obstruction, gallbladder
  digestive organs NEC, congenital Q45.8
  duodenum K31.5
    congenital Q41.0
  ear canal (external) (congenital) Q16.1
    acquired —*see* Stricture, auditory canal,
      acquired
  ejaculatory duct N50.89
  enterostomy K94.13
  esophagus K22.2
    congenital Q39.3
    syphilitic A52.79
      congenital A50.59 *[K23]*
  eustachian tube —*see also* Obstruction,
    eustachian tube
    congenital Q17.8
  fallopian tube N97.1
    gonococcal A54.24
    tuberculous A18.17
  gallbladder —*see* Obstruction, gallbladder
  glottis J38.6
  heart —*see also* Disease, heart
    valve (*see also* Endocarditis) I38
      aortic Q23.0
      mitral Q23.2
      pulmonary Q22.1
      tricuspid Q22.4
  hepatic duct K83.1
  hourglass, of stomach K31.2

Stricture *(Continued)*
  hymen N89.6
  hypopharynx J39.2
  ileum —*see also* Obstruction, intestine,
    specified NEC K56.699
    congenital Q41.2
  intestine —*see also* Obstruction, intestine
    congenital (small) Q41.9
      large Q42.9
        specified NEC Q42.8
      specified NEC Q41.8
    ischemic K55.1
  jejunum —*see also* Obstruction, intestine,
    specified NEC K56.699
    congenital Q41.1
  lacrimal passages —*see also* Stenosis, lacrimal
    congenital Q10.5
  larynx J38.6
    congenital NEC Q31.8
      subglottic Q31.1
    syphilitic A52.73
      congenital A50.59 *[J99]*
  meatus
    ear (congenital) Q16.1
      acquired —*see* Stricture, auditory canal,
        acquired
      osseous (ear) (congenital) Q16.1
        acquired —*see* Stricture, auditory canal,
          acquired
    urinarius —*see also* Stricture, urethra
      congenital Q64.33
  mitral (valve) —*see* Stenosis, mitral
  myocardium, myocardial I51.5
    hypertrophic subaortic (idiopathic) I42.1
  nares (anterior) (posterior) J34.89
    congenital Q30.0
  nasal duct —*see also* Stenosis, lacrimal, duct
    congenital Q10.5
  nasolacrimal duct —*see also* Stenosis, lacrimal,
    duct
    congenital Q10.5
  nasopharynx J39.2
    syphilitic A52.73
  nose J34.89
    congenital Q30.0
  nostril (anterior) (posterior) J34.89
    congenital Q30.0
    syphilitic A52.73
      congenital A50.59 *[J99]*
  organ or site, congenital NEC —*see* Atresia,
    by site
  os uteri —*see* Stricture, cervix
  osseous meatus (ear) (congenital) Q16.1
    acquired —*see* Stricture, auditory canal,
      acquired
  oviduct —*see* Stricture, fallopian tube
  pelviureteric junction (congenital) Q62.11
    acquired, with hydronephrosis N13.0
  penis, by foreign body T19.4
  pharynx J39.2
  prostate N42.89
  pulmonary, pulmonic
    artery (congenital) Q25.6
      acquired I28.8
      noncongenital I28.8
    infundibulum (congenital) Q24.3
    valve I37.0
      congenital Q22.1
    vein, acquired I28.8
    vessel NEC I28.8
  punctum lacrimale —*see also* Stenosis,
    lacrimal, punctum
    congenital Q10.5
  pylorus (hypertrophic) K31.1
    adult K31.1
    congenital Q40.0
    infantile Q40.0
  rectosigmoid —*see also* Obstruction, intestine,
    specified NEC K56.699
  rectum (sphincter) K62.4
    congenital Q42.1
      with fistula Q42.0

Stricture *(Continued)*
  rectum *(Continued)*
    due to
      chlamydial lymphogranuloma A55
      irradiation K91.89
      lymphogranuloma venereum A55
    gonococcal A54.6
    inflammatory (chlamydial) A55
    syphilitic A52.74
    tuberculous A18.32
  renal artery I70.1
    congenital Q27.1
  salivary duct or gland (any) K11.8
  sigmoid (flexure) —see Obstruction, intestine
  spermatic cord N50.89
  stoma (following) (of)
    colostomy K94.03
    enterostomy K94.13
    gastrostomy K94.23
    ileostomy K94.13
    tracheostomy J95.03
  stomach K31.89
    congenital Q40.2
    hourglass K31.2
  subaortic Q24.4
    hypertrophic (acquired) (idiopathic) I42.1
  subglottic J38.6
  syphilitic NEC A52.79
  trachea J39.8
    congenital Q32.1
    syphilitic A52.73
    tuberculous NEC A15.5
  tracheostomy J95.03
  tricuspid (valve) —see Stenosis, tricuspid
  tunica vaginalis N50.89
  ureter (postoperative) N13.5
    with
      hydronephrosis N13.1
        with infection N13.6
      pyelonephritis (chronic) N11.1
    congenital —see Atresia, ureter
    tuberculous A18.11
  ureteropelvic junction (congenital) Q62.11
    acquired, with hydronephrosis N13.0
  ureterovesical orifice N13.5
    with infection N13.6
  urethra (organic) (spasmodic) N35.9
    associated with schistosomiasis
      B65.0 [N37]
    congenital Q64.39
      valvular (posterior) Q64.2
    due to
      infection —see Stricture, urethra,
        postinfective
      trauma —see Stricture, urethra,
        post-traumatic
    gonococcal, gonorrheal A54.01
    infective NEC —see Stricture, urethra,
      postinfective
    late effect (sequelae) of injury —see
      Stricture, urethra, post-traumatic
    postcatheterization —see Stricture, urethra,
      postprocedural
    postinfective NEC
      female N35.12
      male N35.119
        anterior urethra N35.114
        bulbous urethra N35.112
        meatal N35.111
        membranous urethra N35.113
    postobstetric N35.021
    postoperative —see Stricture, urethra,
      postprocedural
    postprocedural
      female N99.12
      male N99.114
        anterior bulbous urethra N99.113
        bulbous urethra N99.111
        fossa navicularis N99.115
        meatal N99.110
        membranous urethra N99.112

Stricture *(Continued)*
  urethra (organic) (spasmodic) *(Continued)*
    post-traumatic
      female N35.028
        due to childbirth N35.021
      male N35.014
        anterior urethra N35.013
        bulbous urethra N35.011
        meatal N35.010
        membranous urethra N35.012
    sequela (late effect) of
      childbirth N35.021
      injury —see Stricture, urethra,
        post-traumatic
    specified cause NEC N35.8
    syphilitic A52.76
    traumatic —see Stricture, urethra,
      post-traumatic
    valvular (posterior), congenital Q64.2
  urinary meatus —see Stricture, urethra
  uterus, uterine (synechiae) N85.6
    os (external) (internal) —see Stricture, cervix
  vagina (outlet) —see Stenosis, vagina
  valve (cardiac) (heart) —see also Endocarditis
    congenital
      aortic Q23.0
      mitral Q23.2
      pulmonary Q22.1
      tricuspid Q22.4
  vas deferens N50.89
    congenital Q55.4
  vein I87.1
  vena cava (inferior) (superior) NEC I87.1
    congenital Q26.0
  vesicourethral orifice N32.0
    congenital Q64.31
  vulva (acquired) N90.5
Stridor R06.1
  congenital (larynx) P28.89
Stridulous —see condition
Stroke (apoplectic) (brain) (embolic) (ischemic)
  (paralytic) (thrombotic) I63.9
▶cryptogenic —see also infarction, cerebral
  I63.9
  epileptic —see Epilepsy
  heat T67.0
  in evolution I63.9
  intraoperative
    during cardiac surgery I97.810
    during other surgery I97.811
  lightning —see Lightning
  meaning
    cerebral hemorrhage — code to
      Hemorrhage, intracranial
    cerebral infarction — code to Infarction,
      cerebral
  postprocedural
    following cardiac surgery I97.820
    following other surgery I97.821
  unspecified (NOS) I63.9
Stromatosis, endometrial D39.0
Strongyloidiasis, strongyloidosis B78.9
  cutaneous B78.1
  disseminated B78.7
  intestinal B78.0
Strophulus pruriginosus L28.2
Struck by lightning —see Lightning
Struma —see also Goiter
  Hashimoto E06.3
  lymphomatosa E06.3
  nodosa (simplex) E04.9
    endemic E01.2
      multinodular E01.1
    multinodular E04.2
      iodine-deficiency related E01.1
    toxic or with hyperthyroidism E05.20
      with thyroid storm E05.21
      multinodular E05.20
        with thyroid storm E05.21
      uninodular E05.10
        with thyroid storm E05.11

Struma *(Continued)*
  nodosa (simplex) *(Continued)*
    toxicosa E05.20
      with thyroid storm E05.21
      multinodular E05.20
        with thyroid storm E05.21
      uninodular E05.10
        with thyroid storm E05.11
    uninodular E04.1
  ovarii D27.-•
  Riedel's E06.5
Strumipriva cachexia E03.4
Strümpell-Marie spine —see Spondylitis,
  ankylosing
Strümpell-Westphal pseudosclerosis E83.01
Stuart deficiency disease (factor X) D68.2
Stuart-Prower factor deficiency (factor X)
  D68.2
Student's elbow —see Bursitis, elbow,
  olecranon
Stump —see Amputation
Stunting, nutritional E45
Stupor (catatonic) R40.1
  depressive (single episode) F32.89
    recurrent episode F33.8
  dissociative F44.2
  manic F30.2
  manic-depressive F31.89
  psychogenic (anergic) F44.2
  reaction to exceptional stress (transient)
    F43.0
Sturge (-Weber) (-Dimitri) (-Kalischer) **disease**
  or syndrome Q85.8
Stuttering F80.81
  adult onset F98.5
  childhood onset F80.81
  following cerebrovascular disease —
    see Disorder, fluency, following
    cerebrovascular disease
  in conditions classified elsewhere R47.82
Sty, stye (external) (internal) (meibomian)
  (zeisian) —see Hordeolum
Subacidity, gastric K31.89
  psychogenic F45.8
Subacute —see condition
Subarachnoid —see condition
Subcortical —see condition
Subcostal syndrome, nerve compression —see
  Mononeuropathy, upper limb, specified
  site NEC
Subcutaneous, subcuticular —see condition
Subdural —see condition
Subendocardium —see condition
Subependymoma
  specified site —see Neoplasm, uncertain
    behavior, by site
  unspecified site D43.2
Suberosis J67.3
Subglossitis —see Glossitis
Subhemophilia D66
Subinvolution
  breast (postlactational) (postpuerperal)
    N64.89
  puerperal O90.89
  uterus (chronic) (nonpuerperal) N85.3
    puerperal O90.89
Sublingual —see condition
Sublinguitis —see Sialoadenitis
Subluxatable hip Q65.6
Subluxation —see also Dislocation
  acromioclavicular S43.11-•
  ankle S93.0-•
  atlantoaxial, recurrent M43.4
    with myelopathy M43.3
  carpometacarpal (joint) NEC S63.05-•
    thumb S63.04-•
  complex, vertebral —see Complex,
    subluxation
  congenital —see also Malposition, congenital
    hip —see Dislocation, hip, congenital,
      partial

▶ New   ⇒ Revised   ~~deleted~~ Deleted   • Use Additional Character(s)

Subluxation *(Continued)*
  congenital *(Continued)*
    joint (excluding hip)
      lower limb Q68.8
      shoulder Q68.8
      upper limb Q68.8
  elbow (traumatic) S53.10-●
    anterior S53.11-●
    lateral S53.14-●
    medial S53.13-●
    posterior S53.12-●
    specified type NEC S53.19-●
  finger S63.20-●
    index S63.20-●
    interphalangeal S63.22-●
      distal S63.24-●
        index S63.24-●
        little S63.24-●
        middle S63.24-●
        ring S63.24-●
      index S63.22-●
      little S63.22-●
      middle S63.22-●
      proximal S63.23-●
        index S63.23-●
        little S63.23-●
        middle S63.23-●
        ring S63.23-●
      ring S63.22-●
    little S63.20-●
    metacarpophalangeal S63.21-●
      index S63.21-●
      little S63.21-●
      middle S63.21-●
      ring S63.21-●
    middle S63.20-●
    ring S63.20-●
  foot S93.30-●
    specified site NEC S93.33-●
    tarsal joint S93.31-●
    tarsometatarsal joint S93.32-●
    toe —*see* Subluxation, toe
  hip S73.00-●
    anterior S73.03-●
      obturator S73.02-●
    central S73.04-●
    posterior S73.01-●
  interphalangeal (joint)
    finger S63.22-●
      distal joint S63.24-●
        index S63.24-●
        little S63.24-●
        middle S63.24-●
        ring S63.24-●
      index S63.22-●
      little S63.22-●
      middle S63.22-●
      proximal joint S63.23-●
        index S63.23-●
        little S63.23-●
        middle S63.23-●
        ring S63.23-●
      ring S63.22-●
    thumb S63.12-●
      distal joint S63.14-●
      proximal joint S63.13-●
    toe S93.13-●
      great S93.13-●
      lesser S93.13-●
  joint prosthesis —*see* Complications, joint
      prosthesis, mechanical, displacement,
      by site
  knee S83.10-●
    cap —*see* Subluxation, patella
    patella —*see* Subluxation, patella
    proximal tibia
      anteriorly S83.11-●
      laterally S83.14-●
      medially S83.13-●
      posteriorly S83.12-●
    specified type NEC S83.19-●

Subluxation *(Continued)*
  lens —*see* Dislocation, lens, partial
  ligament, traumatic —*see* Sprain, by site
  metacarpal (bone)
    proximal end S63.06-●
  metacarpophalangeal (joint)
    finger S63.21-●
      index S63.21-●
      little S63.21-●
      middle S63.21-●
      ring S63.21-●
    thumb S63.11-●
  metatarsophalangeal joint S93.14-●
    great toe S93.14-●
    lesser toe S93.14-●
  midcarpal (joint) S63.03-●
  patella S83.00-●
    lateral S83.01-●
    recurrent (nontraumatic) —*see* Dislocation,
      patella, recurrent, incomplete
    specified type NEC S83.09-●
  pathological —*see* Dislocation, pathological
  radial head S53.00-●
    anterior S53.01-●
    nursemaid's elbow S53.03-●
    posterior S53.02-●
    specified type NEC S53.09-●
  radiocarpal (joint) S63.02-●
  radioulnar (joint)
    distal S63.01-●
    proximal —*see* Subluxation, elbow
  shoulder
    congenital Q68.8
    girdle S43.30-●
      scapula S43.31-●
      specified site NEC S43.39-●
    traumatic S43.00-●
      anterior S43.01-●
      inferior S43.03-●
      posterior S43.02-●
      specified type NEC S43.08-●
  sternoclavicular (joint) S43.20-●
    anterior S43.21-●
    posterior S43.22-●
  symphysis (pubis)
  thumb S63.103
    interphalangeal joint —*see* Subluxation,
      interphalangeal (joint), thumb
    metacarpophalangeal joint —*see*
      Subluxation, metacarpophalangeal
      (joint), thumb
  toe(s) S93.10-●
    great S93.10-●
      interphalangeal joint S93.13-●
      metatarsophalangeal joint S93.14-●
    interphalangeal joint S93.13-●
    lesser S93.10-●
      interphalangeal joint S93.13-●
      metatarsophalangeal joint S93.14-●
    metatarsophalangeal joint S93.149
  ulnohumeral joint —*see* Subluxation,
    elbow
  vertebral
    recurrent NEC —*see* subcategory
      M43.5
    traumatic
      cervical S13.100
        atlantoaxial joint S13.120
        atlantooccipital joint S13.110
        atloidooccipital joint S13.110
        joint between
          C0 and C1 S13.110
          C1 and C2 S13.120
          C2 and C3 S13.130
          C3 and C4 S13.140
          C4 and C5 S13.150
          C5 and C6 S13.160
          C6 and C7 S13.170
          C7 and T1 S13.180
        occipitoatloid joint
          S13.110

Subluxation *(Continued)*
  vertebral *(Continued)*
    traumatic *(Continued)*
      lumbar S33.100
        joint between
          L1 and L2 S33.110
          L2 and L3 S33.120
          L3 and L4 S33.130
          L4 and L5 S33.140
      thoracic S23.100
        joint between
          T1 and T2 S23.110
          T2 and T3 S23.120
          T3 and T4 S23.122
          T4 and T5 S23.130
          T5 and T6 S23.132
          T6 and T7 S23.140
          T7 and T8 S23.142
          T8 and T9 S23.150
          T9 and T10 S23.152
          T10 and T11 S23.160
          T11 and T12 S23.162
          T12 and L1 S23.170
  ulna
    distal end S63.07-●
    proximal end —*see* Subluxation, elbow
  wrist (carpal bone) S63.00-●
    carpometacarpal joint —*see* Subluxation,
      carpometacarpal (joint)
    distal radioulnar joint —*see* Subluxation,
      radioulnar (joint), distal
    metacarpal bone, proximal —*see*
      Subluxation, metacarpal (bone),
      proximal end
    midcarpal —*see* Subluxation, midcarpal
      (joint)
    radiocarpal joint —*see* Subluxation,
      radiocarpal (joint)
    recurrent —*see* Dislocation, recurrent, wrist
    specified site NEC S63.09-●
    ulna —*see* Subluxation, ulna, distal end
Submaxillary —*see* condition
Submersion (fatal) (nonfatal) T75.1
Submucous —*see* condition
Subnormal, subnormality
  accommodation (old age) H52.4
  mental —*see* Disability, intellectual
  temperature (accidental) T68
Subphrenic —*see* condition
Subscapular nerve —*see* condition
Subseptus uterus Q51.2
Subsiding appendicitis K36
Substance (other psychoactive) -induced
  anxiety disorder F19.980
  bipolar and related disorder F19.94
  delirium F19.921
  depressive disorder F19.94
  major neurocognitive disorder F19.97
  mild neurocognitive disorder F19.988
  obsessive-compulsive and related disorder
    F19.988
  psychotic disorder F19.959
  sexual dysfunction F19.981
  sleep disorder F19.982
Substernal thyroid E04.9
  congenital Q89.2
Substitution disorder F44.9
Subtentorial —*see* condition
Subthyroidism (acquired) —*see also*
    Hypothyroidism
  congenital E03.1
Succenturiate placenta O43.19-●
Sucking thumb, child (excessive) F98.8
Sudamen, sudamina L74.1
Sudanese kala-azar B55.0
Sudden
  hearing loss —*see* Deafness, sudden
  heart failure —*see* Failure, heart
Sudeck's atrophy, disease, or syndrome —*see*
    Algoneurodystrophy
Suffocation —*see* Asphyxia, traumatic

Sugar
  blood
    high (transient) R73.9
    low (transient) E16.2
  in urine R81
Suicide, suicidal (attempted) T14.91
  by poisoning —see Table of Drugs and
      Chemicals
  history of (personal) Z91.5
    in family Z81.8
  ideation —see Ideation, suicidal
  risk
    meaning personal history of attempted
        suicide Z91.5
    meaning suicidal ideation —see Ideation,
        suicidal
  tendencies
    meaning personal history of attempted
        suicide Z91.5
    meaning suicidal ideation —see Ideation,
        suicidal
  trauma —see nature of injury by site
Suipestifer infection —see Infection, salmonella
Sulfhemoglobinemia, sulphemoglobinemia
    (acquired) (with methemoglobinemia)
    D74.8
Sumatran mite fever A75.3
Summer —see condition
Sunburn L55.9
  due to
    tanning bed (acute) L56.8
      chronic L57.8
    ultraviolet radiation (acute) L56.8
      chronic L57.8
  first degree L55.0
  second degree L55.1
  third degree L55.2
SUNCT (short lasting unilateral neuralgiform
    headache with conjunctival injection and
    tearing) G44.059
  intractable G44.051
  not intractable G44.059
▶Sundowning F05
Sunken acetabulum —see Derangement, joint,
    specified type NEC, hip
Sunstroke T67.0
Superfecundation —see Pregnancy, multiple
Superfetation —see Pregnancy, multiple
Superinvolution (uterus) N85.8
Supernumerary (congenital)
  aortic cusps Q23.8
  auditory ossicles Q16.3
  bone Q79.8
  breast Q83.1
  carpal bones Q74.0
  cusps, heart valve NEC Q24.8
    aortic Q23.8
    mitral Q23.2
    pulmonary Q22.3
  digit(s) Q69.9
  ear (lobule) Q17.0
  fallopian tube Q50.6
  finger Q69.0
  hymen Q52.4
  kidney Q63.0
  lacrimonasal duct Q10.6
  lobule (ear) Q17.0
  mitral cusps Q23.2
  muscle Q79.8
  nipple(s) Q83.3
  organ or site not listed —see Accessory
  ossicles, auditory Q16.3
  ovary Q50.31
  oviduct Q50.6
  pulmonary, pulmonic cusps Q22.3
  rib Q76.6
    cervical or first (syndrome) Q76.5
  roots (of teeth) K00.2
  spleen Q89.09
  tarsal bones Q74.2
  teeth K00.1

Supernumerary (Continued)
  testis Q55.29
  thumb Q69.1
  toe Q69.2
  uterus Q51.2
  vagina Q52.1
  vertebra Q76.49
Supervision (of)
  contraceptive —see Prescription,
      contraceptives
  dietary (for) Z71.3
    allergy (food) Z71.3
    colitis Z71.3
    diabetes mellitus Z71.3
    food allergy or intolerance Z71.3
    gastritis Z71.3
    hypercholesterolemia Z71.3
    hypoglycemia Z71.3
    intolerance (food) Z71.3
    obesity Z71.3
    specified NEC Z71.3
  healthy infant or child Z76.2
    foundling Z76.1
  high-risk pregnancy —see Pregnancy,
      complicated by, high, risk
  lactation Z39.1
  pregnancy —see Pregnancy, supervision of
Supplemental teeth K00.1
Suppression
  binocular vision H53.34
  lactation O92.5
  menstruation N94.89
  ovarian secretion E28.39
  renal N28.9
  urine, urinary secretion R34
Suppuration, suppurative —see also condition
  accessory sinus (chronic) —see Sinusitis
  adrenal gland
  antrum (chronic) —see Sinusitis, maxillary
  bladder —see Cystitis
  brain G06.0
    sequelae G09
  breast N61.1
    puerperal, postpartum or gestational —see
        Mastitis, obstetric, purulent
  dental periosteum M27.3
  ear (middle) —see also Otitis, media
    external NEC —see Otitis, externa,
        infective
    internal —see subcategory H83.0
  ethmoidal (chronic) (sinus) —see Sinusitis,
      ethmoidal
  fallopian tube —see Salpingo-oophoritis
  frontal (chronic) (sinus) —see Sinusitis,
      frontal
  gallbladder (acute) K81.0
  gum K05.20
    generalized —see Peridontitis, aggressive,
        generalized
    localized —see Peridontitis, aggressive,
        localized
  intracranial G06.0
  joint —see Arthritis, pyogenic or pyemic
  labyrinthine —see subcategory H83.0
  lung —see Abscess, lung
  mammary gland N61.1
    puerperal, postpartum O91.12
      associated with lactation O91.13
  maxilla, maxillary M27.2
    sinus (chronic) —see Sinusitis, maxillary
  muscle —see Myositis, infective
  nasal sinus (chronic) —see Sinusitis
  pancreas, acute —see also Pancreatitis, acute
      K85.80
  parotid gland —see Sialoadenitis
  pelvis, pelvic
    female —see Disease, pelvis, inflammatory
    male K65.0
  pericranial —see Osteomyelitis
  salivary duct or gland (any) —see
      Sialoadenitis

Suppuration, suppurative (Continued)
  sinus (accessory) (chronic) (nasal) —see
      Sinusitis
  sphenoidal sinus (chronic) —see Sinusitis,
      sphenoidal
  thymus (gland) E32.1
  thyroid (gland) E06.0
  tonsil —see Tonsillitis
  uterus —see Endometritis
Supraeruption of tooth (teeth) M26.34
Supraglottitis J04.30
  with obstruction J04.31
Suprarenal (gland) —see condition
Suprascapular nerve —see condition
Suprasellar —see condition
Surfer's knots or nodules S89.8-●
Surgical
  emphysema T81.82
  procedures, complication or misadventure —
      see Complications, surgical procedures
  shock T81.10
Surveillance (of) (for) —see also Observation
  alcohol abuse Z71.41
  contraceptive —see Prescription,
      contraceptives
  dietary Z71.3
  drug abuse Z71.51
Susceptibility to disease, genetic Z15.89
  malignant neoplasm Z15.09
    breast Z15.01
    endometrium Z15.04
    ovary Z15.02
    prostate Z15.03
    specified NEC Z15.09
  multiple endocrine neoplasia Z15.81
Suspected condition, ruled out —see also
    Observation, suspected
  amniotic cavity and membrane Z03.71
  cervical shortening Z03.75
  fetal anomaly Z03.73
  fetal growth Z03.74
  maternal and fetal conditions NEC Z03.79
  newborn —see also Observation, newborn,
      suspected condition ruled out Z05.9
  oligohydramnios Z03.71
  placental problem Z03.72
  polyhydramnios Z03.71
Suspended uterus
  in pregnancy or childbirth —see Pregnancy,
      complicated by, abnormal uterus
Sutton's nevus D22.9
Suture
  burst (in operation wound) T81.31
    external operation wound T81.31
    internal operation wound T81.32
  inadvertently left in operation wound —see
      Foreign body, accidentally left during a
      procedure
  removal Z48.02
Swab inadvertently left in operation wound —
    see Foreign body, accidentally left during a
    procedure
Swallowed, swallowing
  difficulty —see Dysphagia
  foreign body —see Foreign body, alimentary
      tract
Swan-neck deformity (finger) —see Deformity,
    finger, swan-neck
Swearing, compulsive F42.8
  in Gilles de la Tourette's syndrome F95.2
Sweat, sweats
  fetid L75.0
  night R61
Sweating, excessive R61
Sweeley-Klionsky disease E75.21
Sweet's disease or dermatosis L98.2
Swelling (of) R60.9
  abdomen, abdominal (not referable to any
      particular organ) —see Mass,
      abdominal
  ankle —see Effusion, joint, ankle

▶ New   ⇒ Revised   ~~deleted~~ Deleted   ● Use Additional Character(s)

Swelling *(Continued)*
  arm M79.89
    forearm M79.89
➡ breast —*see also* Lump, breast N63.0
  Calabar B74.3
  cervical gland R59.0
  chest, localized R22.2
  ear H93.8-•
  extremity (lower) (upper) —*see* Disorder, soft
    tissue, specified type NEC
  finger M79.89
  foot M79.89
  glands R59.9
    generalized R59.1
    localized R59.0
  hand M79.89
  head (localized) R22.0
  inflammatory —*see* Inflammation
  intra-abdominal —*see* Mass, abdominal
  joint —*see* Effusion, joint
  leg M79.89
    lower M79.89
  limb —*see* Disorder, soft tissue, specified type
    NEC
  localized (skin) R22.9
    chest R22.2
    head R22.0
    limb
      lower —*see* Mass, localized, limb, lower
      upper —*see* Mass, localized, limb, upper
    neck R22.1
    trunk R22.2
  neck (localized) R22.1
  pelvic —*see* Mass, abdominal
  scrotum N50.89
  splenic —*see* Splenomegaly
  testis N50.89
  toe M79.89
  umbilical R19.09
  wandering, due to Gnathostoma
    (spinigerum) B83.1
  white —*see* Tuberculosis, arthritis
Swift (-Feer) disease
  overdose or wrong substance given
    or taken —*see* Table of Drugs and
    Chemicals, by drug, poisoning
Swimmer's
  cramp T75.1
  ear H60.33-•
  itch B65.3
Swimming in the head R42
Swollen —*see* Swelling
Swyer syndrome Q99.1
Sycosis L73.8
  barbae (not parasitic) L73.8
  contagiosa (mycotic) B35.0
  lupoides L73.8
  mycotic B35.0
  parasitic B35.0
  vulgaris L73.8
Sydenham's chorea —*see* Chorea, Sydenham's
Sylvatic yellow fever A95.0
Sylvest's disease B33.0
Symblepharon H11.23-•
  congenital Q10.3
Symond's syndrome G93.2
Sympathetic —*see* condition
Sympatheticotonia G90.8
Sympathicoblastoma
  specified site —*see* Neoplasm, malignant, by
    site
  unspecified site C74.90
Sympathogonioma —*see* Sympathicoblastoma
Symphalangy (fingers) (toes) Q70.9
Symptoms NEC R68.89
  breast NEC N64.59
➤ cold J00
  development NEC R63.8
  factitious, self-induced —*see* Disorder,
    factitious
  genital organs, female R10.2

Symptoms NEC *(Continued)*
  involving
    abdomen NEC R19.8
    appearance NEC R46.89
    awareness R41.9
      altered mental status R41.82
      amnesia —*see* Amnesia
      borderline intellectual functioning
        R41.83
      coma —*see* Coma
      disorientation R41.0
      neurologic neglect syndrome R41.4
      senile cognitive decline R41.81
      specified symptom NEC R41.89
    behavior NEC R46.89
    cardiovascular system NEC R09.89
    chest NEC R09.89
    circulatory system NEC R09.89
    cognitive functions R41.9
      altered mental status R41.82
      amnesia —*see* Amnesia
      borderline intellectual functioning
        R41.83
      coma —*see* Coma
      disorientation R41.0
      neurologic neglect syndrome R41.4
      senile cognitive decline R41.81
      specified symptom NEC R41.89
    development NEC R62.50
    digestive system NEC R19.8
    emotional state NEC R45.89
      emotional lability R45.86
    food and fluid intake R63.8
    general perceptions and sensations
      R44.9
      specified NEC R44.8
    musculoskeletal system R29.91
      specified NEC R29.898
    nervous system R29.90
      specified NEC R29.818
    pelvis NEC R19.8
    respiratory system NEC R09.89
    skin and integument R23.9
    urinary system R39.9
  menopausal N95.1
  metabolism NEC R63.8
  neurotic F48.8
  of infancy R68.19
  pelvis NEC, female R10.2
  skin and integument NEC R23.9
  subcutaneous tissue NEC R23.9
➤ viral cold J00
Sympus Q74.2
Syncephalus Q89.4
Synchondrosis
  abnormal (congenital) Q78.8
  ischiopubic M91.0
Synchysis (scintillans) (senile) (vitreous body)
  H43.89
Syncope (near) (pre-) R55
  anginosa I20.9
  bradycardia R00.1
  cardiac R55
  carotid sinus G90.01
  due to spinal (lumbar) puncture G97.1
  heart R55
  heat T67.1
  laryngeal R05
  psychogenic F48.8
  tussive R05
  vasoconstriction R55
  vasodepressor R55
  vasomotor R55
  vasovagal R55
Syndactylism, syndactyly Q70.9
  complex (with synostosis)
    fingers Q70.0-•
    toes Q70.2-•
  simple (without synostosis)
    fingers Q70.1-•
    toes Q70.3-•

Syndrome —*see also* Disease
  5q minus NOS D46.C
  48,XXXX Q97.1
  49,XXXXX Q97.1
  abdominal
    acute R10.0
    muscle deficiency Q79.4
  abnormal innervation H02.519
    left H02.516
      lower H02.515
      upper H02.514
    right H02.513
      lower H02.512
      upper H02.511
  abstinence, neonatal P96.1
  acid pulmonary aspiration, obstetric O74.0
  acquired immunodeficiency —*see* Human,
    immunodeficiency virus (HIV) disease
  acute abdominal R10.0
  acute respiratory distress (adult) (child) J80
    idiopathic J84.114
  Adair-Dighton Q78.0
  Adams-Stokes (-Morgagni) I45.9
  adiposogenital E23.6
  adrenal
    hemorrhage (meningococcal) A39.1
    meningococcic A39.1
  adrenocortical —*see* Cushing's, syndrome
  adrenogenital E25.9
    congenital, associated with enzyme
      deficiency E25.0
  afferent loop NEC K91.89
  Alagille's Q44.7
  alcohol withdrawal (without convulsions) —
    see Dependence, alcohol, with,
    withdrawal
  Alder's D72.0
  Aldrich (-Wiskott) D82.0
  alien hand R41.4
  Alport Q87.81
  alveolar hypoventilation E66.2
  alveolocapillary block J84.10
  amnesic, amnestic (confabulatory) (due to) —
    see Disorder, amnesic
  amyostatic (Wilson's disease) E83.01
  androgen insensitivity E34.50
    complete E34.51
    partial E34.52
  androgen resistance (*see also* Syndrome,
    androgen insensitivity) E34.50
  Angelman Q93.5
  anginal —*see* Angina
  ankyloglossia superior Q38.1
  anterior
    chest wall R07.89
    cord G83.82
    spinal artery G95.19
      compression M47.019
        cervical region M47.012
        cervicothoracic region M47.013
        lumbar region M47.016
        occipito-atlanto-axial region M47.011
        thoracic region M47.014
        thoracolumbar region M47.015
    tibial M76.81-•
  antibody deficiency D80.9
    agammaglobulinemic D80.1
      hereditary D80.0
    congenital D80.0
    hypogammaglobulinemic D80.1
      hereditary D80.0
  anticardiolipin (-antibody) D68.61
➤ antidepressant discontinuation T43.205
  antiphospholipid (-antibody) D68.61
  aortic
    arch M31.4
    bifurcation I74.09
  aortomesenteric duodenum occlusion K31.5
  apical ballooning (transient left ventricular)
    I51.81
  arcuate ligament I77.4

Syndrome *(Continued)*
  argentaffin, argintaffinoma E34.0
  Arnold-Chiari —*see* Arnold-Chiari disease
  Arrillaga-Ayerza I27.0
  arterial tortuosity Q87.82
  arteriovenous steal T82.898-●
  Asherman's N85.6
  aspiration, of newborn —*see* Aspiration, by
    substance, with pneumonia
    meconium P24.01
  ataxia-telangiectasia G11.3
  auriculotemporal G50.8
  autoerythrocyte sensitization (Gardner-
    Diamond) D69.2
  autoimmune lymphoproliferative [ALPS]
    D89.82
  autoimmune polyglandular E31.0
  autoinflammatory M04.9
    specified type NEC M04.8
  autosomal —*see* Abnormal, autosomes
  Avellis' G46.8
  Ayerza (-Arrillaga) I27.0
  Babinski-Nageotte G83.89
  Bakwin-Krida Q78.5
  bare lymphocyte D81.6
  Barré-Guillain G61.0
  Barré-Liéou M53.0
  Barrett's —*see* Barrett's, esophagus
  Barsony-Polgar K22.4
  Barsony-Teschendorf K22.4
  Barth E78.71
  Bartter's E26.81
  basal cell nevus Q87.89
  Basedow's E05.00
    with thyroid storm E05.01
  basilar artery G45.0
  Batten-Steinert G71.11
  battered
    baby or child —*see* Maltreatment, child,
      physical abuse
    spouse —*see* Maltreatment, adult, physical
      abuse
  Beals Q87.40
  Beau's I51.5
  Beck's I65.8
  Benedikt's G46.3
  Béquez César (-Steinbrink-Chédiak-Higashi)
    D70.330
  Bernhardt-Roth —*see* Meralgia paresthetica
  ➡ Bernheim's —*see* Failure, heart, right
  big spleen D73.1
  bilateral polycystic ovarian E28.2
  Bing-Horton's —*see* Horton's headache
  Birt-Hogg-Dube syndrome Q87.89
  Björck (-Thorsen) E34.0
  black
    lung J60
    widow spider bite —*see* Toxicity, venom,
      spider, black widow
  Blackfan-Diamond D61.01
  Blau M04.8
  blind loop K90.2
    congenital Q43.8
    postsurgical K91.2
  blue sclera Q78.0
  blue toe I75.02-●
  Boder-Sedgewick G11.3
  Boerhaave's K22.3
  Borjeson Forssman Lehmann Q89.8
  Bouillaud's I01.9
  Bourneville (-Pringle) Q85.1
  Bouveret (-Hoffman) I47.9
  brachial plexus G54.0
  bradycardia-tachycardia I49.5
  brain (nonpsychotic) F09
    with psychosis, psychotic reaction F09
    acute or subacute —*see* Delirium
    congenital —*see* Disability, intellectual
    organic F09
      post-traumatic (nonpsychotic) F07.81
      psychotic F09

Syndrome *(Continued)*
  brain (nonpsychotic) *(Continued)*
    personality change F07.0
    postcontusional F07.81
    post-traumatic, nonpsychotic F07.81
    psycho-organic F09
    psychotic F06.8
  brain stem stroke G46.3
  Brandt's (acrodermatitis enteropathica) E83.2
  broad ligament laceration N83.8
  Brock's J98.11
  ➡ bronze baby P83.88
  Brown-Sequard G83.81
  ▶ Brugada I49.8
  bubbly lung P27.0
  Buchem's M85.2
  Budd-Chiari I82.0
  bulbar (progressive) G12.22
  Bürger-Grütz E78.3
  Burke's K86.89
  Burnett's (milk-alkali) E83.52
  burning feet E53.9
  Bywaters' T79.5
  Call-Fleming I67.841
  carbohydrate-deficient glycoprotein (CDGS)
    E77.8
  carcinogenic thrombophlebitis I82.1
  carcinoid E34.0
  cardiac asthma I50.1
  cardiacos negros I27.0
  cardiofaciocutaneous Q87.89
  cardiopulmonary-obesity E66.2
  cardiorenal —*see* Hypertension, cardiorenal
  cardiorespiratory distress (idiopathic),
    newborn P22.0
  cardiovascular renal —*see* Hypertension,
    cardiorenal
  carotid
    artery (hemispheric) (internal) G45.1
    body G90.01
    sinus G90.01
  carpal tunnel G56.0-●
  Cassidy (-Scholte) E34.0
  cat-cry Q93.4
  cat eye Q92.8
  cauda equina G83.4
  causalgia —*see* Causalgia
  celiac K90.0
    artery compression I77.4
    axis I77.4
  central pain G89.0
  cerebellar
    hereditary G11.9
    stroke G46.4
  cerebellomedullary malformation —*see* Spina
    bifida
  cerebral
    artery
      anterior G46.1
      middle G46.0
      posterior G46.2
    gigantism E22.0
  cervical (root) M53.1
    disc —*see* Disorder, disc, cervical, with
      neuritis
    fusion Q76.1
    posterior, sympathicus M53.0
    rib Q76.5
    sympathetic paralysis G90.2
  cervicobrachial (diffuse) M53.1
  cervicocranial M53.0
  cervicodorsal outlet G54.2
  cervicothoracic outlet G54.0
  Céstan (-Raymond) I65.8
  Charcot's (angina cruris) (intermittent
    claudication) I73.9
  Charcot-Weiss-Baker G90.09
  CHARGE Q89.8
  Chédiak-Higashi (-Steinbrink) E70.330
  chest wall R07.1
  Chiari's (hepatic vein thrombosis) I82.0

Syndrome *(Continued)*
  Chilaiditi's Q43.3
  child maltreatment —*see* Maltreatment, child
  chondrocostal junction M94.0
  chondroectodermal dysplasia Q77.6
  chromosome 4 short arm deletion Q93.3
  chromosome 5 short arm deletion Q93.4
  chronic
    infantile neurological, cutaneous and
      articular (CINCA) M04.2
    pain G89.4
      personality F68.8
  Clarke-Hadfield K86.89
  Clerambault's automatism G93.89
  Clouston's (hidrotic ectodermal dysplasia)
    Q82.4
  clumsiness, clumsy child F82
  cluster headache G44.009
    intractable G44.001
    not intractable G44.009
  Coffin-Lowry Q89.8
  cold injury (newborn) P80.0
  combined immunity deficiency D81.9
  compartment (deep) (posterior) (traumatic)
    T79.A0
    abdomen T79.A3
    lower extremity (hip, buttock, thigh, leg,
      foot, toes) T79.A2
    nontraumatic
      abdomen M79.A3
      lower extremity (hip, buttock, thigh, leg,
        foot, toes) M79.A2-●
      specified site NEC M79.A9
      upper extremity (shoulder, arm, forearm,
        wrist, hand, fingers) M79.A1-●
    postprocedural —*see* Syndrome
      compartment, nontraumatic
    specified site NEC T79.A9
    upper extremity (shoulder, arm, forearm,
      wrist, hand, fingers) T79.A1
  complex regional pain —*see* Syndrome, pain,
    complex regional
  compression T79.5
    anterior spinal —*see* Syndrome, anterior,
      spinal artery, compression
    cauda equina G83.4
    celiac artery I77.4
    vertebral artery M47.029
      cervical region M47.022
      occipito-atlanto-axial region M47.021
  concussion F07.81
  congenital
    affecting multiple systems NEC Q87.89
    central alveolar hypoventilation G47.35
    facial diplegia Q87.0
    muscular hypertrophy-cerebral Q87.89
    oculo-auriculovertebral Q87.0
    oculofacial diplegia (Moebius) Q87.0
    rubella (manifest) P35.0
  congestion-fibrosis (pelvic), female N94.89
  congestive dysmenorrhea N94.6
  Conn's E26.01
  connective tissue M35.9
    overlap NEC M35.1
  conus medullaris G95.81
  cord
    anterior G83.82
    posterior G83.83
  coronary
    acute NEC I24.9
    insufficiency or intermediate I20.0
    slow flow I20.8
  Costen's (complex) M26.69
  costochondral junction M94.0
  costoclavicular G54.0
  costovertebral E22.0
  Cowden Q85.8
  craniovertebral M53.0
  Creutzfeldt-Jakob —*see* Creutzfeldt-Jakob
    disease or syndrome
  cri-du-chat Q93.4

Syndrome *(Continued)*
  crib death R99
  cricopharyngeal —*see* Dysphagia
  croup J05.0
  CRPS I —*see* Syndrome, pain, complex
    regional I
  crush T79.5
  cubital tunnel —*see* Lesion, nerve, ulnar
  Curschmann (-Batten) (-Steinert) G71.11
  Cushing's E24.9
    alcohol-induced E24.4
    drug-induced E24.2
    due to
      alcohol
        drugs E24.2
      ectopic ACTH E24.3
      overproduction of pituitary ACTH E24.0
      overdose or wrong substance given
        or taken —*see* Table of Drugs and
        Chemicals, by drug, poisoning
    pituitary-dependent E24.0
    specified type NEC E24.8
  cryopyrin-associated periodic M04.2
  cryptophthalmos Q87.0
  cystic duct stump K91.5
  Dana-Putnam D51.0
  Danbolt (-Cross) (acrodermatitis
    enteropathica) E83.2
  Dandy-Walker Q03.1
    with spina bifida Q07.01
  Danlos' Q79.6
  defibrination —*see also* Fibrinolysis
    with
      antepartum hemorrhage —*see*
        Hemorrhage, antepartum, with
        coagulation defect
      intrapartum hemorrhage —*see*
        Hemorrhage, complicating,
        delivery
      newborn P60
      postpartum O72.3
  Degos' I77.8
  Déjérine-Roussy G89.0
  delayed sleep phase G47.21
  demyelinating G37.9
  dependence —*see* F10-F19 with fourth
    character .2
  depersonalization (-derealization) F48.1
  De Quervain E34.51
  de Toni-Fanconi (-Debré) E72.09
    with cystinosis E72.04
  diabetes mellitus-hypertension-nephrosis —
    see Diabetes, nephrosis
  diabetes mellitus in newborn infant P70.2
  diabetes-nephrosis —*see* Diabetes, nephrosis
  diabetic amyotrophy —*see* Diabetes,
    amyotrophy
  dialysis associated steal T82.898-●
  Diamond-Blackfan D61.01
  Diamond-Gardener D69.2
  DIC (diffuse or disseminated intravascular
    coagulopathy) D65
  di George's D82.1
  Dighton's Q78.0
  disequilibrium E87.8
  Döhle body-panmyelopathic D72.0
  dorsolateral medullary G46.4
  double athetosis G80.3
  Down (*see also* Down syndrome) Q90.9
  Dresbach's (elliptocytosis) D58.1
  Dressler's (postmyocardial infarction) I24.1
    postcardiotomy I97.0
  drug withdrawal, infant of dependent mother
    P96.1
  dry eye H04.12-●
  due to abnormality
    chromosomal Q99.9
      sex
        female phenotype Q97.9
        male phenotype Q98.9
      specified NEC Q99.8

Syndrome *(Continued)*
  dumping (postgastrectomy) K91.1
    nonsurgical K31.89
  Dupré's (meningism) R29.1
  dysmetabolic X E88.81
  dyspraxia, developmental F82
  Eagle-Barrett Q79.4
  Eaton-Lambert —*see* Syndrome,
    Lambert-Eaton
  Ebstein's Q22.5
  ectopic ACTH E24.3
  eczema-thrombocytopenia D82.0
  Eddowes' Q78.0
  effort (psychogenic) F45.8
  Ehlers-Danlos Q79.6
  ➡ Eisenmenger's I27.83
  Ekman's Q78.0
  electric feet E53.8
  Ellis-van Creveld Q77.6
  empty nest Z60.0
  endocrine-hypertensive E27.0
  entrapment —*see* Neuropathy,
    entrapment
  eosinophilia-myalgia M35.8
  epileptic —*see also* Epilepsy, by type
    absence G40.A09
      intractable G40.A19
        with status epilepticus G40.A11
        without status epilepticus G40.A19
      not intractable G40.A09
        with status epilepticus G40.A01
        without status epilepticus G40.A09
  Erdheim-Chester (ECD) E88.89
  Erdheim's E22.0
  erythrocyte fragmentation D59.4
  Evans D69.41
  exhaustion F48.8
  extrapyramidal G25.9
    specified NEC G25.89
  eye retraction —*see* Strabismus
  eyelid-malar-mandible Q87.0
  Faber's D50.9
  facial pain, paroxysmal G50.0
  Fallot's Q21.3
  familial cold autoinflammatory M04.2
  familial eczema-thrombocytopenia (Wiskott-
    Aldrich) D82.0
  Fanconi (-de Toni) (-Debré) E72.09
    with cystinosis E72.04
  Fanconi's (anemia) (congenital pancytopenia)
    D61.09
  fatigue
    chronic R53.82
    psychogenic F48.8
  faulty bowel habit K59.39
  Feil-Klippel (brevicollis) Q76.1
  Felty's —*see* Felty's syndrome
  fertile eunuch E23.0
  fetal
    alcohol (dysmorphic) Q86.0
    hydantoin Q86.1
  Fiedler's I40.1
  first arch Q87.0
  fish odor E72.8
  Fisher's G61.0
  Fitzhugh-Curtis
    due to
      Chlamydia trachomatis A74.81
      Neisseria gonorrhorea (gonococcal
        peritonitis) A54.85
  Fitz's —*see also* Pancreatitis, acute K85.80
  Flajani (-Basedow) E05.00
    with thyroid storm E05.01
  flatback —*see* Flatback syndrome
  floppy
    baby P94.2
    iris (intraoeprative) (IFIS) H21.81
    mitral valve I34.1
  flush E34.0
  Foix-Alajouanine G95.19
  Fong's Q87.2

Syndrome *(Continued)*
  food protein-induced enterocolitis K52.21
  foramen magnum G93.5
  Foster-Kennedy H47.14-●
  Foville's (peduncular) G46.3
  fragile X Q99.2
  Franceschetti Q75.4
  Frey's
    auriculotemporal G50.8
    hyperhidrosis L74.52
  Friderichsen-Waterhouse A39.1
  Froin's G95.89
  frontal lobe F07.0
  Fukuhara E88.49
  functional
    bowel K59.9
    prepubertal castrate E29.1
  Gaisböck's D75.1
  ganglion (basal ganglia brain) G25.9
    geniculi G51.1
  Gardner-Diamond D69.2
  gastroesophageal
    junction K22.0
    laceration-hemorrhage K22.6
  gastrojejunal loop obstruction K91.89
  Gee-Herter-Heubner K90.0
  Gelineau's G47.419
    with cataplexy G47.411
  genito-anorectal A55
  Gerstmann-Sträussler-Scheinker (GSS)
    A81.82
  Gianotti-Crosti L44.4
  giant platelet (Bernard-Soulier) D69.1
  Gilles de la Tourette's F95.2
  goiter-deafness E07.1
  Goldberg Q89.8
  Goldberg-Maxwell E34.51
  Good's D83.8
  Gopalan' (burning feet) E53.8
  Gorlin's Q87.89
  Gougerot-Blum L81.7
  Gouley's I31.1
  Gower's R55
  gray or grey (newborn) P93.0
    platelet D69.1
  Gubler-Millard G46.3
  Guillain-Barré (-Strohl) G61.0
  gustatory sweating G50.8
  Hadfield-Clarke K86.89
  hair tourniquet —*see* Constriction, external,
    by site
  Hamman's J98.19
  hand-foot L27.1
  hand-shoulder G90.8
  hantavirus (cardio)-pulmonary (HPS) (HCPS)
    B33.4
  happy puppet Q93.5
  Harada's H30.81-●
  Hayem-Faber D50.9
  headache NEC G44.89
    complicated NEC G44.59
  Heberden's I20.8
  Hedinger's E34.0
  Hegglin's D72.0
  HELLP (hemolysis, elevated liver enzymes
    and low platelet count) O14.2-●
    complicating
      childbirth O14.24
      puerperium O14.25
  hemolytic-uremic D59.3
  hemophagocytic, infection-associated
    D76.2
  Henoch-Schönlein D69.0
  hepatic flexure K59.8
  hepatopulmonary K76.81
  hepatorenal K76.7
    following delivery O90.4
    postoperative or postprocedural K91.83
    postpartum, puerperal O90.4
  hepatourologic K76.7
  Herter (-Gee) (nontropical sprue) K90.0

S

▶ New   ⟹ Revised   ~~deleted~~ Deleted   ● Use Additional Character(s)   **397**

Syndrome *(Continued)*
 Heubner-Herter K90.0
 Heyd's K76.7
 Hilger's G90.09
 histamine-like (fish poisoning) —*see* Poisoning, fish
 histiocytic D76.3
 histiocytosis NEC D76.3
 HIV infection, acute B20
 Hoffmann-Werdnig G12.0
 Hollander-Simons E88.1
 Hoppe-Goldflam G70.00
   with exacerbation (acute) G70.01
   in crisis G70.01
 Horner's G90.2
 hungry bone E83.81
 hunterian glossitis D51.0
 Hutchinson's triad A50.53
 hyperabduction G54.0
 hyperammonemia-hyperornithinemia-homocitrullinemia E72.4
 hypereosinophilic (idiopathic) D72.1
 hyperimmunoglobulin D M04.1
 hyperimmunoglobulin E (IgE) D82.4
 hyperkalemic E87.5
 hyperkinetic —*see* Hyperkinesia
 hypermobility M35.7
 hypernatremia E87.0
 hyperosmolarity E87.0
 hyperperfusion G97.82
 hypersplenic D73.1
 hypertransfusion, newborn P61.1
 hyperventilation F45.8
 hyperviscosity (of serum)
   polycythemic D75.1
   sclerothymic D58.8
 hypoglycemic (familial) (neonatal) E16.2
 hypokalemic E87.6
 hyponatremic E87.1
 hypopituitarism E23.0
 hypoplastic left-heart Q23.4
 hypopotassemia E87.6
 hyposmolality E87.1
 hypotension, maternal O26.5-●
 hypothenar hammer I73.89
 hypoventilation, obesity (OHS) E66.2
 ICF (intravascular coagulation-fibrinolysis) D65
 idiopathic
   cardiorespiratory distress, newborn P22.0
   nephrotic (infantile) N04.9
 iliotibial band M76.3-●
 immobility, immobilization (paraplegic) M62.3
 immune reconstitution D89.3
 immune reconstitution inflammatory [IRIS] D89.3
 immunity deficiency, combined D81.9
 immunodeficiency
   acquired —*see* Human, immunodeficiency virus (HIV) disease
   combined D81.9
 impending coronary I20.0
 impingement, shoulder M75.4-●
 inappropriate secretion of antidiuretic hormone E22.2
 infant
   gestational diabetes P70.0
   of diabetic mother P70.1
 infantilism (pituitary) E23.0
 inferior vena cava I87.1
 inspissated bile (newborn) P59.1
 institutional (childhood) F94.2
 insufficient sleep F51.12
 intermediate coronary (artery) I20.0
 interspinous ligament —*see* Spondylopathy, specified NEC
 intestinal
   carcinoid E34.0
   knot K56.2

Syndrome *(Continued)*
 intravascular coagulation-fibrinolysis (ICF) D65
 iodine-deficiency, congenital E00.9
   type
     mixed E00.2
     myxedematous E00.1
     neurological E00.0
 IRDS (idiopathic respiratory distress, newborn) P22.0
 irritable
   bowel K58.9
     with
       constipation K58.1
       diarrhea K58.0
     mixed K58.2
     psychogenic F45.8
     specified NEC K58.8
   heart (psychogenic) F45.8
   weakness F48.8
 ischemic
   bowel (transient) K55.9
     chronic K55.1
     due to mesenteric artery insufficiency K55.1
   steal T82.898
 IVC (intravascular coagulopathy) D65
 Ivemark's Q89.01
 Jaccoud's —*see* Arthropathy, postrheumatic, chronic
 Jackson's G83.89
 Jakob-Creutzfeldt —*see* Creutzfeldt-Jakob disease or syndrome
 jaw-winking Q07.8
 Jervell-Lange-Nielsen I45.81
 jet lag G47.25
 Job's D71
 Joseph-Diamond-Blackfan D61.01
 jugular foramen G52.7
 Kabuki Q89.8
 Kanner's (autism) F84.0
 Kartagener's Q89.3
 Kelly's D50.1
 Kimmelstiel-Wilson —*see* Diabetes, specified type, with Kimmelstiel-Wilson disease
 Klein (e)-Levine G47.13
 Klippel-Feil (brevicollis) Q76.1
 Köhler-Pellegrini-Steida —*see* Bursitis, tibial collateral
 König's K59.8
 Korsakoff (-Wernicke) (nonalcoholic) F04
   alcoholic F10.26
 Kostmann's D70.0
 Krabbe's congenital muscle hypoplasia Q79.8
 labyrinthine —*see* subcategory H83.2
 lacunar NEC G46.7
 Lambert-Eaton G70.80
   in
     neoplastic disease G73.1
     specified disease NEC G70.81
 Landau-Kleffner —*see* Epilepsy, specified NEC
 Larsen's Q74.8
 lateral
   cutaneous nerve of thigh G57.1-●
   medullary G46.4
 Launois' E22.0
 lazy
   leukocyte D70.8
   posture M62.3
 Lemiere I80.8
 Lennox-Gastaut G40.812
   intractable G40.814
     with status epilepticus G40.813
     without status epilepticus G40.814
   not intractable G40.812
     with status epilepticus G40.811
     without status epilepticus G40.812

Syndrome *(Continued)*
 lenticular, progressive E83.01
 Leopold-Levi's E05.90
 Lev's I44.2
 Li-Fraumeni Z15.01
 Lichtheim's D51.0
 Lightwood's N25.89
 Lignac (de Toni) (-Fanconi) (-Debré) E72.09
   with cystinosis E72.04
 Likoff's I20.8
 limbic epilepsy personality F07.0
 liver-kidney K76.7
 lobotomy F07.0
 Loffler's J82
 long arm 18 or 21 deletion Q93.89
 long QT I45.81
 Louis-Barré G11.3
 low
   atmospheric pressure T70.29
   back M54.5
   output (cardiac) I50.9
 lower radicular, newborn (birth injury) P14.8
 Luetscher's (dehydration) E86.0
 Lupus anticoagulant D68.62
 Lutembacher's Q21.1
 macrophage activation D76.1
   due to infection D76.2
 magnesium-deficiency R29.0
 Majeed M04.8
 Mal de Debarquement R42
 malabsorption K90.9
   postsurgical K91.2
 malformation, congenital, due to
   alcohol Q86.0
   exogenous cause NEC Q86.8
   hydantoin Q86.1
   warfarin Q86.2
 malignant
   carcinoid E34.0
   neuroleptic G21.0
 Mallory-Weiss K22.6
 mandibulofacial dysostosis Q75.4
 manic-depressive —*see* Disorder, bipolar
 maple-syrup-urine E71.0
 Marable's I77.4
 Marfan's Q87.40
   with
     cardiovascular manifestations Q87.418
       aortic dilation Q87.410
     ocular manifestations Q87.42
     skeletal manifestations Q87.43
 Marie's (acromegaly) E22.0
 mast cell activation —*see* Activation, mast cell
 maternal hypotension —*see* Syndrome, hypotension, maternal
 May (-Hegglin) D72.0
 McArdle (-Schmidt) (-Pearson) E74.04
 McQuarrie's E16.2
 meconium plug (newborn) P76.0
 median arcuate ligament I77.4
 Meekeren-Ehlers-Danlos Q79.6
 megavitamin-B6 E67.2
 Meige G24.4
 MELAS E88.41
 Mendelson's O74.0
 MERRF (myoclonic epilepsy associated with ragged-red fibers) E88.42
 mesenteric
   artery (superior) K55.1
   vascular insufficiency K55.1
 metabolic E88.81
 metastatic carcinoid E34.0
 micrognathia-glossoptosis Q87.0
 midbrain NEC G93.89
 middle lobe (lung) J98.19
 middle radicular G54.0
 migraine —*see also* Migraine G43.909-●
 Mikulicz' K11.8
 milk-alkali E83.52
 Millard-Gubler G46.3

▶ New   ⟹ Revised   ~~deleted~~ Deleted   ● Use Additional Character(s)

Syndrome *(Continued)*
  Miller-Dieker Q93.88
  Miller-Fisher G61.0
  Minkowski-Chauffard D58.0
  Mirizzi's K83.1
  MNGIE (Mitochondrial Neurogastrointestinal
    Encephalopathy) E88.49
  Möbius, ophthalmoplegic migraine *—see*
    Migraine, ophthalmoplegic
  monofixation H50.42
  Morel-Moore M85.2
  Morel-Morgagni M85.2
  Morgagni (-Morel) (-Stewart) M85.2
  Morgagni-Adams-Stokes I45.9
  Mounier-Kuhn Q32.4
    with bronchiectasis J47.9
      with
        exacerbation (acute) J47.1
        lower respiratory infection J47.0
    acquired J98.09
      with bronchiectasis J47.9
        with
          exacerbation (acute) J47.1
          lower respiratory infection J47.0
  Muckle-Wells M04.2
  mucocutaneous lymph node (acute febrile)
    (MCLS) M30.3
  multiple endocrine neoplasia (MEN) *—see*
    Neoplasia, endocrine, multiple (MEN}
  multiple operations *—see* Disorder, factitious
  myasthenic G70.9
    in
      diabetes mellitus *—see* Diabetes,
        amyotrophy
      endocrine disease NEC E34.9 *[G73.3]*
      neoplastic disease *—see also* Neoplasm
        D49.9 *[G73.3]*
      thyrotoxicosis (hyperthyroidism) E05.90
        [G73.3]
        with thyroid storm E05.91 *[G73.3]*
  myelodysplastic D46.9
    with
      5q deletion D46.C
      isolated del (5q) chromosomal
        abnormality D46.C
    lesions, low grade D46.20
    specified NEC D46.Z
  myelopathic pain G89.0
  myeloproliferative (chronic) D47.1
  myofascial pain M79.1
  Naffziger's G54.0
  nail patella Q87.2
  NARP (Neuropathy, Ataxia and Retinitis
    pigmentosa) E88.49
  neonatal abstinence P96.1
  nephritic *—see also* Nephritis
    with edema *—see* Nephrosis
    acute N00.9
    chronic N03.9
    rapidly progressive N01.9
  nephrotic (congenital) *—see also* Nephrosis
    N04.9
    with
      dense deposit disease N04.6
      diffuse
        crescentic glomerulonephritis
          N04.7
        endocapillary proliferative
          glomerulonephritis N04.4
        membranous glomerulonephritis
          N04.2
        mesangial proliferative
          glomerulonephritis N04.3
        mesangiocapillary glomerulonephritis
          N04.5
      focal and segmental glomerular lesions
        N04.1
      minor glomerular abnormality N04.0
      specified morphological changes NEC
        N04.8
    diabetic *—see* Diabetes, nephrosis

Syndrome *(Continued)*
  neurologic neglect R41.4
  Nezelof's D81.4
  Nonne-Milroy-Meige Q82.0
  Nothnagel's vasomotor acroparesthesia I73.89
  obesity hypoventilation (OHS) E66.2
  oculomotor H51.9
  ophthalmoplegia-cerebellar ataxia *—see*
    Strabismus, paralytic, third nerve
  oral allergy T78.1
  oral-facial-digital Q87.0
  organic
    affective F06.30
    amnesic (not alcohol- or drug-induced) F04
    brain F09
    depressive F06.31
    hallucinosis F06.0
    personality F07.0
  Ormond's N13.5
  oro-facial-digital Q87.0
  os trigonum Q68.8
  Osler-Weber-Rendu I78.0
  osteoporosis-osteomalacia M83.8
  Osterreicher-Turner Q87.2
  otolith *—see* subcategory H81.8
  oto-palatal-digital Q87.0
  outlet (thoracic) G54.0
  ovary
    polycystic E28.2
    resistant E28.39
    sclerocystic E28.2
  Owren's D68.2
  Paget-Schroetter I82.890
  pain *—see also* Pain
    complex regional I G90.50
      lower limb G90.52-•
      specified site NEC G90.59
      upper limb G90.51-•
    complex regional II *—see* Causalgia
  painful
    bruising D69.2
    feet E53.8
    prostate N42.81
  paralysis agitans *—see* Parkinsonism
  paralytic G83.9
    specified NEC G83.89
  Parinaud's H51.0
  parkinsonian *—see* Parkinsonism
  Parkinson's *—see* Parkinsonism
  paroxysmal facial pain G50.0
  Parry's E05.00
    with thyroid storm E05.01
  Parsonage (-Aldren)-Turner G54.5
  patella clunk M25.86-•
  Paterson (-Brown) (-Kelly) D50.1
  pectoral girdle I77.89
  pectoralis minor I77.89
▶ pediatric autoimmune neuropsychiatric
    disorders associated with streptococcal
    infections (PANDAS) D89.89
  Pelger-Huet D72.0
  pellagra-cerebellar ataxia-renal
    aminoaciduria E72.02
  pellagroid E52
  Pellegrini-Stieda *—see* Bursitis, tibial collateral
  pelvic congestion-fibrosis, female N94.89
  penta X Q97.1
  peptic ulcer *—see* Ulcer, peptic
  perabduction I77.89
  periodic fever M04.1
  periodic fever, aphthous stomatitis, pharyngitis,
    and adenopathy [PFAPA] M04.8
  periodic headache, in adults and children —
    see Headache, periodic syndromes in
    adults and children
  periurethral fibrosis N13.5
  phantom limb (without pain) G54.7
    with pain G54.6
  pharyngeal pouch D82.1
  Pick's *—see* Disease, Pick's
  Pickwickian E66.2

Syndrome *(Continued)*
  PIE (pulmonary infiltration with
    eosinophilia) J82
  pigmentary pallidal degeneration
    (progressive) G23.0
  pineal E34.8
  pituitary E22.0
  placental transfusion *—see* Pregnancy,
    complicated by, placental transfusion
    syndromes
  plantar fascia M72.2
  plateau iris (post-iridectomy)
    (postprocedural) H21.82
  Plummer-Vinson D50.1
  pluricarential of infancy E40
  plurideficiency E40
  pluriglandular (compensatory) E31.8
    autoimmune E31.0
  pneumatic hammer T75.21
  polyangiitis overlap M30.8
  polycarential of infancy E40
  polyglandular E31.8
    autoimmune E31.0
  polysplenia Q89.09
  pontine NEC G93.89
  popliteal
    artery entrapment I77.89
    web Q87.89
  postcardiac injury
    postcardiotomy I97.0
    postmyocardial infarction I24.1
  postcardiotomy I97.0
  post chemoembolization — code to
    associated conditions
  postcholecystectomy K91.5
  postcommissurotomy I97.0
  postconcussional F07.81
  postcontusional F07.81
  postencephalitic F07.89
  posterior
    cervical sympathetic M53.0
    cord G83.83
    fossa compression G93.5
    reversible encephalopathy (PRES) I67.83
  postgastrectomy (dumping) K91.1
  postgastric surgery K91.1
  postinfarction I24.1
  postlaminectomy NEC M96.1
  postleukotomy F07.0
  postmastectomy lymphedema I97.2
  postmyocardial infarction I24.1
  postoperative NEC T81.9
    blind loop K90.2
  postpartum panhypopituitary (Sheehan)
    E23.0
  postpolio (myelitic) G14
  postthrombotic I87.009
    with
      inflammation I87.02-•
        with ulcer I87.03-•
      specified complication NEC I87.09-•
      ulcer I87.01-•
        with inflammation I87.03-•
    asymptomatic I87.00-•
  postvagotomy K91.1
  postvalvulotomy I97.0
  postviral NEC G93.3
    fatigue G93.3
  Potain's K31.0
  potassium intoxication E87.5
  precerebral artery (multiple) (bilateral)
    G45.2
  preinfarction I20.0
  preleukemic D46.9
  premature senility E34.8
  premenstrual dysphoric F32.89
  premenstrual tension N94.3
  Prinzmetal-Massumi R07.1
  prune belly Q79.4
  pseudocarpal tunnel (sublimis) *—see*
    Syndrome, carpal tunnel

▶ New   ⟹ Revised   ~~deleted~~ Deleted   • Use Additional Character(s)

Syndrome (Continued)

pseudoparalytica G70.00
  with exacerbation (acute) G70.01
  in crisis G70.01
pseudo-Turner's Q87.1
psycho-organic (nonpsychotic severity) F07.9
  acute or subacute F05
  depressive type F06.31
  hallucinatory type F06.0
  nonpsychotic severity F07.0
  specified NEC F07.89
pulmonary
  arteriosclerosis I27.0
  dysmaturity (Wilson-Mikity) P27.0
  hypoperfusion (idiopathic) P22.0
  renal (hemorrhagic) (Goodpasture's) M31.0
pure
  motor lacunar G46.5
  sensory lacunar G46.6
Putnam-Dana D51.0
pyogenic arthritis, pyoderma gangrenosum, and acne [PAPA] M04.8
pyramidopallidonigral G20
pyriformis —see Lesion, nerve, sciatic
QT interval prolongation I45.81
radicular NEC —see Radiculopathy
  upper limbs, newborn (birth injury) P14.3
rapid time-zone change G47.25
Rasmussen G04.81
Raymond (-Céstan) I65.8
Raynaud's I73.00
  with gangrene I73.01
RDS (respiratory distress syndrome, newborn) P22.0
reactive airways dysfunction J68.3
Refsum's G60.1
Reifenstein E34.52
renal glomerulohyalinosis-diabetic —see Diabetes, nephrosis
Rendu-Osler-Weber I78.0
residual ovary N99.83
resistant ovary E28.39
respiratory
  distress
    acute J80
      adult J80
      child J80
      idiopathic J84.114
    newborn (idiopathic) (type I) P22.0
      type II P22.1
restless legs G25.81
retinoblastoma (familial) C69.2
retroperitoneal fibrosis N13.5
retroviral seroconversion (acute) Z21
Reye's G93.7
Richter —see Leukemia, chronic lymphocytic, B-cell type
Ridley's I50.1
right
  heart, hypoplastic Q22.6
  ventricular obstruction —see Failure, heart, congestive
Romano-Ward (prolonged QT interval) I45.81
rotator cuff, shoulder —see also Tear, rotator cuff M75.10-●
Rotes Quérol —see Hyperostosis, ankylosing
Roth —see Meralgia paresthetica
rubella (congenital) P35.0
Ruvalcaba-Myhre-Smith E71.440
Rytand-Lipsitch I44.2
salt
  depletion E87.1
    due to heat NEC T67.8
      causing heat exhaustion or prostration T67.4
  low E87.1
salt-losing N28.89
Scaglietti-Dagnini E22.0
scalenus anticus (anterior) G54.0
scapulocostal —see Mononeuropathy, upper limb, specified site NEC

Syndrome (Continued)

scapuloperoneal G71.0
schizophrenic, of childhood NEC F84.5
Schnitzler D47.2
Scholte's E34.0
Schroeder's E27.0
Schüller-Christian C96.5
Schwachman's —see Syndrome, Shwachman's
Schwartz (-Jampel) G71.13
Schwartz-Bartter E22.2
scimitar Q26.8
sclerocystic ovary E28.2
Seitelberger's G31.89
septicemic adrenal hemorrhage A39.1
seroconversion, retroviral (acute) Z21
serous meningitis G93.2
severe acute respiratory (SARS) J12.81
shaken infant T74.4
shock (traumatic) T79.4
  kidney N17.0
    following crush injury T79.5
  toxic A48.3
shock-lung J80
Shone's — code to specific anomalies
short
  bowel K91.2
  rib Q77.2
shoulder-hand —see Algoneurodystrophy
Shwachman's D70.4
sicca —see Sicca syndrome
sick
  cell E87.1
  sinus I49.5
sick-euthyroid E07.81
sideropenic D50.1
Siemens' ectodermal dysplasia Q82.4
Silfversköld's Q78.9
Simons' E88.1
sinus tarsi M25.57-●
sinusitis-bronchiectasis-situs inversus Q89.3
Sipple's E31.22
sirenomelia Q87.2
Slocumb's E27.0
slow flow, coronary I20.8
Sluder's G44.89
Smith-Magenis Q93.88
Sneddon-Wilkinson L13.1
Sotos' Q87.3
spasmodic
  upward movement, eyes H51.8
  winking F95.8
Spen's I45.9
splenic
  agenesis Q89.01
  flexure K59.8
  neutropenia D73.81
Spurway's Q78.0
staphylococcal scalded skin L00
steal
  arteriovenous T82.898-●
  ischemic T82.898-●
  subclavian G45.8
Stein-Leventhal E28.2
Stein's E28.2
Stevens-Johnson syndrome L51.1
  toxic epidermal necrolysis overlap L51.3
Stewart-Morel M85.2
Stickler Q89.8
stiff baby Q89.8
stiff man G25.82
Still-Felty —see Felty's syndrome
Stokes (-Adams) I45.9
stone heart I50.1
straight back, congenital Q76.49
subclavian steal G45.8
subcoracoid-pectoralis minor G54.0
subcostal nerve compression I77.89
subphrenic interposition Q43.3

Syndrome (Continued)

superior
  cerebellar artery I63.8
  mesenteric artery K55.1
  semi-circular canal dehiscence H83.8X-●
  vena cava I87.1
supine hypotensive (maternal) —see Syndrome, hypotension, maternal
suprarenal cortical E27.0
supraspinatus —see also Tear, rotator cuff M75.10-●
Susac G93.49
swallowed blood P78.2
sweat retention L74.0
Swyer Q99.1
Symond's G93.2
sympathetic
  cervical paralysis G90.2
  pelvic, female N94.89
systemic inflammatory response (SIRS), of non-infectious origin (without organ dysfunction) R65.10
  with acute organ dysfunction R65.11
tachycardia-bradycardia I49.5
takotsubo I51.81
TAR (thrombocytopenia with absent radius) Q87.2
tarsal tunnel G57.5-●
teething K00.7
tegmental G93.89
telangiectasic-pigmentation-cataract Q82.8
temporal pyramidal apex —see Otitis, media, suppurative, acute
temporomandibular joint-pain-dysfunction M26.62-●
➡ Terry's —see also Myopia, degenerative H44.2-●
testicular feminization —see also Syndrome, androgen insensitivity E34.51
thalamic pain (hyperesthetic) G89.0
thoracic outlet (compression) G54.0
Thorson-Björck E34.0
thrombocytopenia with absent radius (TAR) Q87.2
thyroid-adrenocortical insufficiency E31.0
tibial
  anterior M76.81-●
  posterior M76.82-●
Tietze's M94.0
time-zone (rapid) G47.25
Toni-Fanconi E72.09
  with cystinosis E72.04
Touraine's Q79.8
tourniquet —see Constriction, external, by site
toxic shock A48.3
transient left ventricular apical ballooning I51.81
traumatic vasospastic T75.22
Treacher Collins Q75.4
triple X, female Q97.0
trisomy Q92.9
  13 Q91.7
    meiotic nondisjunction Q91.4
    mitotic nondisjunction Q91.5
    mosaicism Q91.5
    translocation Q91.6
  18 Q91.3
    meiotic nondisjunction Q91.0
    mitotic nondisjunction Q91.1
    mosaicism Q91.1
    translocation Q91.2
  20 (q)(p) Q92.8
  21 Q90.9
    meiotic nondisjunction Q90.0
    mitotic nondisjunction Q90.1
    mosaicism Q90.1
    translocation Q90.2
  22 Q92.8
tropical wet feet T69.0-●
Trousseau's I82.1

▶ New   ➡ Revised   ~~deleted~~ Deleted   ● Use Additional Character(s)

Syndrome *(Continued)*
  tumor lysis (following antineoplastic chemotherapy) (spontaneous) NEC E88.3
  tumor necrosis factor receptor associated periodic (TRAPS) M04.1
  Twiddler's (due to)
    automatic implantable defibrillator T82.198
    cardiac pacemaker T82.198
  Unverricht (-Lundborg) —*see* Epilepsy, generalized, idiopathic
  upward gaze H51.8
  uremia, chronic —*see also* Disease, kidney, chronic N18.9
  urethral N34.3
  urethro-oculo-articular —*see* Reiter's disease
  urohepatic K76.7
  vago-hypoglossal G52.7
  van Buchem's M85.2
  van der Hoeve's Q78.0
  vascular NEC in cerebrovascular disease G46.8
  vasoconstriction, reversible cerebrovascular I67.841
  vasomotor I73.9
  vasospastic (traumatic) T75.22
  vasovagal R55
  VATER Q87.2
  velo-cardio-facial Q93.81
  vena cava (inferior) (superior) (obstruction) I87.1
  vertebral
    artery G45.0
      compression —*see* Syndrome, anterior, spinal artery, compression
    steal G45.0
  vertebro-basilar artery G45.0
  vertebrogenic (pain) M54.89
  vertiginous —*see* Disorder, vestibular function
  Vinson-Plummer D50.1
  virus B34.9
  visceral larva migrans B83.0
  visual disorientation H53.8
  vitamin B6 deficiency E53.1
  vitreal corneal H59.01-●
  vitreous (touch) H59.01-●
  Vogt-Koyanagi H20.82-●
  Volkmann's T79.6
  von Schroetter's I82.890
  von Willebrand (-Jürgen) D68.0
  Waldenström-Kjellberg D50.1
  Wallenberg's G46.3
  water retention E87.79
  Waterhouse (-Friderichsen) A39.1
  Weber-Gubler G46.3
  Weber-Leyden G46.3
  Weber's G46.3
  Wegener's M31.30
    with
      kidney involvement M31.31
      lung involvement M31.30
        with kidney involvement M31.31
  Weingarten's (tropical eosinophilia) J82
  Weiss-Baker G90.09
  Werdnig-Hoffman G12.0
  Werner's E31.21
  Werner's E34.8
  Wernicke-Korsakoff (nonalcoholic) F04
    alcoholic F10.26
  West's —*see* Epilepsy, spasms
  Westphal-Strümpell E83.01
  wet
    feet (maceration) (tropical) T69.0-●
    lung, newborn P22.1
  whiplash S13.4
  whistling face Q87.0
  Wilkie's K55.1
  Wilkinson-Sneddon L13.1
  Willebrand (-Jürgens) D68.0

Syndrome *(Continued)*
  Wilson's (hepatolenticular degeneration) E83.01
  Wiskott-Aldrich D82.0
  withdrawal —*see* Withdrawal, state
    drug
      infant of dependent mother P96.1
      therapeutic use, newborn P96.2
  Woakes' (ethmoiditis) J33.1
⇒ Wright's (hyperabduction) G54.0
  X I20.9
  XXXX Q97.1
  XXXXX Q97.1
  XXXXY Q98.1
  XXY Q98.0
  yellow nail L60.5
  Zahorsky's B08.5
  Zellweger syndrome E71.510
  Zellweger-like syndrome E71.541
Synechia (anterior) (iris) (posterior) (pupil) —*see also* Adhesions, iris
  intra-uterine (traumatic) N85.6
Synesthesia R20.8
Syngamiasis, syngamosis B83.3
Synodontia K00.2
Synorchidism, synorchism Q55.1
Synostosis (congenital) Q78.8
  astragalo-scaphoid Q74.2
  radioulnar Q74.0
Synovial sarcoma —*see* Neoplasm, connective tissue, malignant
Synovioma (malignant) —*see also* Neoplasm, connective tissue, malignant
  benign —*see* Neoplasm, connective tissue, benign
Synoviosarcoma —*see* Neoplasm, connective tissue, malignant
Synovitis —*see also* Tenosynovitis M65.9
  crepitant
    hand M70.0-●
    wrist M70.03-●
  gonococcal A54.49
  gouty —*see* Gout
  in (due to)
    crystals M65.8-●
    gonorrhea A54.49
    syphilis (late) A52.78
    use, overuse, pressure —*see* Disorder, soft tissue, due to use
  infective NEC —*see* Tenosynovitis, infective NEC
  specified NEC —*see* Tenosynovitis, specified type NEC
  syphilitic A52.78
    congenital (early) A50.02
  toxic —*see* Synovitis, transient
  transient M67.3-●
    ankle M67.37-●
    elbow M67.32-●
    foot joint M67.37-●
    hand joint M67.34-●
    hip M67.35-●
    knee M67.36-●
    multiple site M67.39
    pelvic region M67.35-●
    shoulder M67.31-●
    specified joint NEC M67.38
    wrist M67.33-●
  traumatic, current —*see* Sprain
  tuberculous —*see* Tuberculosis, synovitis
  villonodular (pigmented) M12.2-●
    ankle M12.27-●
    elbow M12.22-●
    foot joint M12.27-●
    hand joint M12.24-●
    hip M12.25-●
    knee M12.26-●
    multiple site M12.29
    pelvic region M12.25-●
    shoulder M12.21-●
    specified joint NEC M12.28

Synovitis *(Continued)*
  villonodular (pigmented) *(Continued)*
    vertebrae M12.28
    wrist M12.23-●
Syphilid A51.39
  congenital A50.06
  newborn A50.06
  tubercular (late) A52.79
Syphilis, syphilitic (acquired) A53.9
  abdomen (late) A52.79
  acoustic nerve A52.15
  adenopathy (secondary) A51.49
  adrenal (gland) (with cortical hypofunction) A52.79
  age under 2 years NOS —*see also* Syphilis, congenital, early
    acquired A51.9
  alopecia (secondary) A51.32
  anemia (late) A52.79 *[D63.8]*
  aneurysm (aorta) (ruptured) A52.01
    central nervous system A52.05
    congenital A50.54 *[I79.0]*
  anus (late) A52.74
    primary A51.1
    secondary A51.39
  aorta (arch) (abdominal) (thoracic) A52.02
    aneurysm A52.01
  aortic (insufficiency) (regurgitation) (stenosis)A52.03
    aneurysm A52.01
  arachnoid (adhesive) (cerebral) (spinal) A52.13
  asymptomatic —*see* Syphilis, latent
  ataxia (locomotor) A52.11
  atrophoderma maculatum A51.39
  auricular fibrillation A52.06
  bladder (late) A52.76
  bone A52.77
    secondary A51.46
  brain A52.17
  breast (late) A52.79
  bronchus (late) A52.72
  bubo (primary) A51.0
  bulbar palsy A52.19
  bursa (late) A52.78
  cardiac decompensation A52.06
  cardiovascular A52.00
  central nervous system (late) (recurrent) (relapse) (tertiary) A52.3
    with
      ataxia A52.11
      general paralysis A52.17
        juvenile A50.45
      paresis (general) A52.17
        juvenile A50.45
      tabes (dorsalis) A52.11
        juvenile A50.45
      taboparesis A52.17
        juvenile A50.45
    aneurysm A52.05
    congenital A50.40
    juvenile A50.40
    remission in (sustained) A52.3
    serology doubtful, negative, or positive A52.3
    specified nature or site NEC A52.19
    vascular A52.05
  cerebral A52.17
    meningovascular A52.13
    nerves (multiple palsies) A52.15
    sclerosis A52.17
    thrombosis A52.05
  cerebrospinal (tabetic type) A52.12
  cerebrovascular A52.05
  cervix (late) A52.76
  chancre (multiple) A51.0
    extragenital A51.2
    Rollet's A51.0
  Charcot's joint A52.16
  chorioretinitis A51.43
    congenital A50.01
    late A52.71
    prenatal A50.01

Syphilis, syphilitic *(Continued)*
   choroiditis —*see* Syphilitic chorioretinitis
   choroidoretinitis —*see* Syphilitic
      chorioretinitis
   ciliary body (secondary) A51.43
     late A52.71
   colon (late) A52.74
   combined spinal sclerosis A52.11
   condyloma (latum) A51.31
   congenital A50.9
     with
       paresis (general) A50.45
       tabes (dorsalis) A50.45
       taboparesis A50.45
     chorioretinitis, choroiditis A50.01 [H32]
     early, or less than 2 years after birth NEC
       A50.2
       with manifestations —*see* Syphilis,
         congenital, early, symptomatic
       latent (without manifestations) A50.1
         negative spinal fluid test A50.1
         serology positive A50.1
       symptomatic A50.09
         cutaneous A50.06
         mucocutaneous A50.07
         oculopathy A50.01
         osteochondropathy A50.02
         pharyngitis A50.03
         pneumonia A50.04
         rhinitis A50.05
         visceral A50.08
     interstitial keratitis A50.31
     juvenile neurosyphilis A50.45
     late, or 2 years or more after birth NEC
       A50.7
       chorioretinitis, choroiditis A50.32
       interstitial keratitis A50.31
       juvenile neurosyphilis A50.45
       latent (without manifestations) A50.6
         negative spinal fluid test A50.6
         serology positive A50.6
       symptomatic or with manifestations
         NEC A50.59
         arthropathy A50.55
         cardiovascular A50.54
         Clutton's joints A50.51
         Hutchinson's teeth A50.52
         Hutchinson's triad A50.53
         osteochondropathy A50.56
         saddle nose A50.57
   conjugal A53.9
     tabes A52.11
   conjunctiva (late) A52.71
   contact Z20.2
   cord bladder A52.19
   cornea, late A52.71
   coronary (artery) (sclerosis) A52.06
   coryza, congenital A50.05
   cranial nerve A52.15
     multiple palsies A52.15
   cutaneous —*see* Syphilis, skin
   dacryocystitis (late) A52.71
   degeneration, spinal cord A52.12
   dementia paralytica A52.17
     juvenilis A50.45
   destruction of bone A52.77
   dilatation, aorta A52.01
   due to blood transfusion A53.9
   dura mater A52.13
   ear A52.79
     inner A52.79
       nerve (eighth) A52.15
       neurorecurrence A52.15
   early A51.9
     cardiovascular A52.00
     central nervous system A52.3
     latent (without manifestations) (less than 2
       years after infection) A51.5
       negative spinal fluid test A51.5
       serological relapse after treatment A51.5
       serology positive A51.5

Syphilis, syphilitic *(Continued)*
   early *(Continued)*
     relapse (treated, untreated) A51.9
     skin A51.39
     symptomatic A51.9
       extragenital chancre A51.2
       primary, except extragenital chancre
         A51.0
       secondary —*see also* Syphilis, secondary
         A51.39
         relapse (treated, untreated) A51.49
     ulcer A51.39
   eighth nerve (neuritis) A52.15
   endemic A65
   endocarditis A52.03
     aortic A52.03
     pulmonary A52.03
   epididymis (late) A52.76
   epiglottis (late) A52.73
   epiphysitis (congenital) (early) A50.02
   episcleritis (late) A52.71
   esophagus A52.79
   eustachian tube A52.73
   exposure to Z20.2
   eye A52.71
   eyelid (late) (with gumma) A52.71
   fallopian tube (late) A52.76
   fracture A52.77
   gallbladder (late) A52.74
   gastric (polyposis) (late) A52.74
   general A53.9
     paralysis A52.17
       juvenile A50.45
   genital (primary) A51.0
   glaucoma A52.71
   gumma NEC A52.79
     cardiovascular system A52.00
     central nervous system A52.3
     congenital A50.59
   heart (block) (decompensation) (disease)
     (failure) A52.06 [I52]
     valve NEC A52.03
   hemianesthesia A52.19
   hemianopsia A52.71
   hemiparesis A52.17
   hemiplegia A52.17
   hepatic artery A52.09
   hepatis A52.74
   hepatomegaly, congenital A50.08
   hereditaria tarda —*see* Syphilis, congenital,
     late
   hereditary —*see* Syphilis, congenital
   Hutchinson's teeth A50.52
   hyalitis A52.71
   inactive —*see* Syphilis, latent
   infantum —*see* Syphilis, congenital
   inherited —*see* Syphilis, congenital
   internal ear A52.79
   intestine (late) A52.74
   iris, iritis (secondary) A51.43
     late A52.71
   joint (late) A52.77
   keratitis (congenital) (interstitial) (late) A50.31
   kidney (late) A52.75
   lacrimal passages (late) A52.71
   larynx (late) A52.73
   late A52.9
     cardiovascular A52.00
     central nervous system A52.3
     kidney A52.75
     latent or 2 years or more after infection
       (without manifestations) A52.8
       negative spinal fluid test A52.8
       serology positive A52.8
     paresis A52.17
     specified site NEC A52.79
     symptomatic or with manifestations A52.79
     tabes A52.11
   latent A53.0
     with signs or symptoms - code by site and
       stage under Syphilis

Syphilis, syphilitic *(Continued)*
   latent *(Continued)*
     central nervous system A52.2
     date of infection unspecified A53.0
     early, or less than 2 years after infection
       A51.5
     follow-up of latent syphilis A53.0
       date of infection unspecified A53.0
       late, or 2 years or more after infection
         A52.8
     late, or 2 years or more after infection
       A52.8
     positive serology (only finding) A53.0
       date of infection unspecified A53.0
       early, or less than 2 years after infection
         A51.5
       late, or 2 years or more after infection
         A52.8
   lens (late) A52.71
   leukoderma A51.39
     late A52.79
   lienitis A52.79
   lip A51.39
     chancre (primary) A51.2
     late A52.79
   Lissauer's paralysis A52.17
   liver A52.74
   locomotor ataxia A52.11
   lung A52.72
   lymph gland (early) (secondary) A51.49
     late A52.79
   lymphadenitis (secondary) A51.49
   macular atrophy of skin A51.39
     striated A52.79
   mediastinum (late) A52.73
   meninges (adhesive) (brain) (spinal cord)
     A52.13
   meningitis A52.13
     acute (secondary) A51.41
     congenital A50.41
   meningoencephalitis A52.14
   meningovascular A52.13
     congenital A50.41
   mesarteritis A52.09
     brain A52.04
   middle ear A52.77
   mitral stenosis A52.03
   monoplegia A52.17
   mouth (secondary) A51.39
     late A52.79
   mucocutaneous (secondary) A51.39
     late A52.79
   mucous
     membrane (secondary) A51.39
       late A52.79
     patches A51.39
       congenital A50.07
   mulberry molars A50.52
   muscle A52.78
   myocardium A52.06
   nasal sinus (late) A52.73
   neonatorum —*see* Syphilis, congenital
   nephrotic syndrome (secondary)
     A51.44
   nerve palsy (any cranial nerve) A52.15
     multiple A52.15
   nervous system, central A52.3
   neuritis A52.15
     acoustic A52.15
   neurorecidive of retina A52.19
   neuroretinitis A52.19
   newborn —*see* Syphilis, congenital
   nodular superficial (late) A52.79
   nonvenereal A65
   nose (late) A52.73
     saddle back deformity A50.57
   occlusive arterial disease A52.09
   oculopathy A52.71
   ophthalmic (late) A52.71
   optic nerve (atrophy) (neuritis) (papilla)
     A52.15

Syphilis, syphilitic *(Continued)*
orbit (late) A52.71
organic A53.9
osseous (late) A52.77
osteochondritis (congenital) (early) A50.02
[M90.80]
osteoporosis A52.77
ovary (late) A52.76
oviduct (late) A52.76
palate (late) A52.79
pancreas (late) A52.74
paralysis A52.17
general A52.17
juvenile A50.45
paresis (general) A52.17
juvenile A50.45
paresthesia A52.19
Parkinson's disease or syndrome A52.19
paroxysmal tachycardia A52.06
pemphigus (congenital) A50.06
penis (chancre) A51.0
late A52.76
pericardium A52.06
perichondritis, larynx (late) A52.73
periosteum (late) A52.77
congenital (early) A50.02 [M90.80]
early (secondary) A51.46
peripheral nerve A52.79
petrous bone (late) A52.77
pharynx (late) A52.73
secondary A51.39
pituitary (gland) A52.79
pleura (late) A52.73
pneumonia, white A50.04
pontine lesion A52.17
portal vein A52.09
primary A51.0
anal A51.1
and secondary —*see* Syphilis, secondary
central nervous system A52.3
extragenital chancre NEC A51.2
fingers A51.2
genital A51.0
lip A51.2
specified site NEC A51.2
tonsils A51.2
prostate (late) A52.76
ptosis (eyelid) A52.71
pulmonary (late) A52.72
artery A52.09
pyelonephritis (late) A52.75
recently acquired, symptomatic A51.9
rectum (late) A52.74
respiratory tract (late) A52.73
retina, late A52.71
retrobulbar neuritis A52.15
salpingitis A52.76
sclera (late) A52.71
sclerosis
cerebral A52.17
coronary A52.06
multiple A52.11
scotoma (central) A52.71
scrotum (late) A52.76

Syphilis, syphilitic *(Continued)*
secondary (and primary) A51.49
adenopathy A51.49
anus A51.39
bone A51.46
chorioretinitis, choroiditis A51.43
hepatitis A51.45
liver A51.45
lymphadenitis A51.49
meningitis (acute) A51.41
mouth A51.39
mucous membranes A51.39
periosteum, periostitis A51.46
pharynx A51.39
relapse (treated, untreated) A51.49
skin A51.39
specified form NEC A51.49
tonsil A51.39
ulcer A51.39
viscera NEC A51.49
vulva A51.39
seminal vesicle (late) A52.76
seronegative with signs or symptoms - code
by site and stage under Syphilis
seropositive
with signs or symptoms - code by site and
stage under Syphilis
follow-up of latent syphilis —*see* Syphilis,
latent
only finding —*see* Syphilis, latent
seventh nerve (paralysis) A52.15
sinus, sinusitis (late) A52.73
skeletal system A52.77
skin (with ulceration) (early) (secondary)
A51.39
late or tertiary A52.79
small intestine A52.74
spastic spinal paralysis A52.17
spermatic cord (late) A52.76
spinal (cord) A52.12
spleen A52.79
splenomegaly A52.79
spondylitis A52.77
staphyloma A52.71
stigmata (congenital) A50.59
stomach A52.74
synovium A52.78
tabes dorsalis (late) A52.11
juvenile A50.45
tabetic type A52.11
juvenile A50.45
taboparesis A52.17
juvenile A50.45
tachycardia A52.06
tendon (late) A52.78
tertiary A52.9
with symptoms NEC A52.79
cardiovascular A52.00
central nervous system A52.3
multiple NEC A52.79
specified site NEC A52.79
testis A52.76
thorax A52.73
throat A52.73

Syphilis, syphilitic *(Continued)*
thymus (gland) (late) A52.79
thyroid (late) A52.79
tongue (late) A52.79
tonsil (lingual) (late) A52.73
primary A51.2
secondary A51.39
trachea (late) A52.73
tunica vaginalis (late) A52.76
ulcer (any site) (early) (secondary)
A51.39
late A52.79
perforating A52.79
foot A52.11
urethra (late) A52.76
urogenital (late) A52.76
uterus (late) A52.76
uveal tract (secondary) A51.43
late A52.71
uveitis (secondary) A51.43
late A52.71
uvula (late) (perforated) A52.79
vagina A51.0
late A52.76
valvulitis NEC A52.03
vascular A52.00
brain (cerebral) A52.05
ventriculi A52.74
vesicae urinariae (late) A52.76
viscera (abdominal) (late) A52.74
secondary A51.49
vitreous (opacities) (late) A52.71
hemorrhage A52.71
vulva A51.0
late A52.76
secondary A51.39
Syphiloma A52.79
cardiovascular system A52.00
central nervous system A52.3
circulatory system A52.00
congenital A50.59
Syphilophobia F45.29
Syringadenoma —*see also* Neoplasm, skin,
benign
papillary —*see* Neoplasm, skin, benign
Syringobulbia G95.0
Syringocystadenoma —*see* Neoplasm, skin,
benign
papillary —*see* Neoplasm, skin, benign
Syringoma —*see also* Neoplasm, skin, benign
chondroid —*see* Neoplasm, skin, benign
Syringomyelia G95.0
Syringomyelitis —*see* Encephalitis
Syringomyelocele —*see* Spina bifida
Syringopontia G95.0
System, systemic —*see also* condition
disease, combined —*see* Degeneration,
combined
inflammatory response syndrome (SIRS) of
non-infectious origin (without organ
dysfunction) R65.10
with acute organ dysfunction R65.11
lupus erythematosus M32.9
inhibitor present D68.62

T

Tabacism, tabacosis, tabagism —*see also* Poisoning, tobacco
  meaning dependence (without remission) F17.200
    with
      disorder F17.299
      ~~remission F17.211~~
      ▶in remission F17.211
        specified disorder NEC F17.298
      withdrawal F17.203
Tabardillo A75.9
  flea-borne A75.2
  louse-borne A75.0
Tabes, tabetic A52.10
  with
    central nervous system syphilis A52.10
    Charcot's joint A52.16
    cord bladder A52.19
    crisis, viscera (any) A52.19
    paralysis, general A52.17
    paresis (general) A52.17
    perforating ulcer (foot) A52.19
  arthropathy (Charcot) A52.16
  bladder A52.19
  bone A52.11
  cerebrospinal A52.12
  congenital A50.45
  conjugal A52.10
  dorsalis A52.11
    juvenile A50.49
  juvenile A50.49
  latent A52.19
  mesenterica A18.39
  paralysis, insane, general A52.17
  spasmodic A52.17
  syphilis (cerebrospinal) A52.12
Taboparalysis A52.17
Taboparesis (remission) A52.17
  juvenile A50.45
TAC (trigeminal autonomic cephalgia) NEC G44.099
  intractable G44.091
  not intractable G44.099
Tache noir S60.22-●
Tachyalimentation K91.2
Tachyarrhythmia, tachyrhythmia —*see* Tachycardia
Tachycardia R00.0
  atrial (paroxysmal) I47.1
  auricular I47.1
  AV nodal re-entry (re-entrant) I47.1
  junctional (paroxysmal) I47.1
  newborn P29.11
  nodal (paroxysmal) I47.1
  non-paroxysmal AV nodal I45.89
  paroxysmal (sustained) (nonsustained) I47.9
    with sinus bradycardia I49.5
    atrial (PAT) I47.1
    atrioventricular (AV) (re-entrant) I47.1
      psychogenic F54
    junctional I47.1
      ectopic I47.1
    nodal I47.1
    psychogenic (atrial) (supraventricular) (ventricular) F54
    supraventricular (sustained) I47.1
      psychogenic F54
    ventricular I47.2
      psychogenic F54
  psychogenic F45.8
  sick sinus I49.5
  sinoauricular NOS R00.0
    paroxysmal I47.1
  sinus [sinusal] NOS R00.0
    paroxysmal I47.1
  supraventricular I47.1
  ventricular (paroxysmal) (sustained) I47.2
    psychogenic F54
Tachygastria K31.89

Tachypnea R06.82
  hysterical F45.8
  newborn (idiopathic) (transitory) P22.1
  psychogenic F45.8
  transitory, of newborn P22.1
TACO (transfusion associated circulatory overload) E87.71
Taenia (infection) (infestation) B68.9
  diminuta B71.0
  echinococcal infestation B67.90
  mediocanellata B68.1
  nana B71.0
  saginata B68.1
  solium (intestinal form) B68.0
    larval form —*see* Cysticercosis
Taeniasis (intestine) —*see* Taenia
Tag (hypertrophied skin) (infected) L91.8
  adenoid J35.8
  anus K64.4
  hemorrhoidal K64.4
  hymen N89.8
  perineal N90.89
  preauricular Q17.0
  sentinel K64.4
  skin L91.8
    accessory (congenital) Q82.8
    anus K64.4
    congenital Q82.8
    preauricular Q17.0
  tonsil J35.8
  urethra, urethral N36.8
  vulva N90.89
Tahyna fever B33.8
Takahara's disease E80.3
Takayasu's disease or syndrome M31.4
Talcosis (pulmonary) J62.0
Talipes (congenital) Q66.89
  acquired, planus —*see* Deformity, limb, flat foot
  asymmetric Q66.89
  calcaneovalgus Q66.4
  calcaneovarus Q66.1
  calcaneus Q66.89
  cavus Q66.7
  equinovalgus Q66.6
  equinovarus Q66.0
  equinus Q66.89
  percavus Q66.7
  planovalgus Q66.6
  planus (acquired) (any degree) —*see also* Deformity, limb, flat foot
    congenital Q66.5-●
    due to rickets (sequelae) E64.3
  valgus Q66.6
  varus Q66.3
Tall stature, constitutional E34.4
Talma's disease M62.89
Talon noir S90.3-●
  hand S60.22-●
  heel S90.3-●
  toe S90.1-●
Tamponade, heart I31.4
Tanapox (virus disease) B08.71
Tangier disease E78.6
Tantrum, child problem F91.8
Tapeworm (infection) (infestation) —*see* Infestation, tapeworm
Tapia's syndrome G52.7
TAR (thrombocytopenia with absent radius) syndrome Q87.2
Tarral-Besnier disease L44.0
Tarsal tunnel syndrome —*see* Syndrome, tarsal tunnel
Tarsalgia —*see* Pain, limb, lower
Tarsitis (eyelid) H01.8
  syphilitic A52.71
  tuberculous A18.4
Tartar (teeth) (dental calculus) K03.6
Tattoo (mark) L81.8
Tauri's disease E74.09
Taurodontism K00.2

Taussig-Bing syndrome Q20.1
Taybi's syndrome Q87.2
Tay-Sachs amaurotic familial idiocy or disease E75.02
TBI (traumatic brain injury) S06.9
Teacher's node or nodule J38.2
Tear, torn (traumatic) —*see also* Laceration
  with abortion —*see* Abortion
  annular fibrosis M51.35
  anus, anal (sphincter) S31.831
    complicating delivery
      with third degree perineal laceration — *see also* Delivery, complicated, by, laceration, perineum, third degree O70.20
        with mucosa O70.3
      without third degree perineal laceration O70.4
    nontraumatic (healed) (old) K62.81
  articular cartilage, old —*see* Derangement, joint, articular cartilage, by site
  bladder
    with ectopic or molar pregnancy O08.6
    following ectopic or molar pregnancy O08.6
    obstetrical O71.5
    traumatic —*see* Injury, bladder
  bowel
    with ectopic or molar pregnancy O08.6
    following ectopic or molar pregnancy O08.6
    obstetrical trauma O71.5
  broad ligament
    with ectopic or molar pregnancy O08.6
    following ectopic or molar pregnancy O08.6
    obstetrical trauma O71.6
  bucket handle (knee) (meniscus) —*see* Tear, meniscus
  capsule, joint —*see* Sprain
  cartilage —*see also* Sprain
    articular, old —*see* Derangement, joint, articular cartilage, by site
  cervix
    with ectopic or molar pregnancy O08.6
    following ectopic or molar pregnancy O08.6
    obstetrical trauma (current) O71.3
    old N88.1
    traumatic —*see* Injury, uterus
  dural G97.41
    nontraumatic G96.11
  internal organ —*see* Injury, by site
  knee cartilage
    articular (current) S83.3-●
    old —*see* Derangement, knee, meniscus, due to old tear
  ligament —*see* Sprain
  meniscus (knee) (current injury) S83.209
    bucket-handle S83.20-●
    lateral
      bucket-handle S83.25-●
      complex S83.27-●
      peripheral S83.26-●
      specified type NEC S83.28-●
    medial
      bucket-handle S83.21-●
      complex S83.23-●
      peripheral S83.22-●
      specified type NEC S83.24-●
    old —*see* Derangement, knee, meniscus, due to old tear
    site other than knee - code as Sprain
    specified type NEC S83.20-●
  muscle —*see* Strain
  pelvic
    floor, complicating delivery O70.1
    organ NEC, obstetrical trauma O71.5
      with ectopic or molar pregnancy O08.6
      following ectopic or molar pregnancy O08.6
  perineal, secondary O90.1

▶ New   ⇒ Revised   ~~deleted~~ Deleted   ● Use Additional Character(s)

Tear, torn *(Continued)*
  periurethral tissue, obstetrical trauma O71.82
    with ectopic or molar pregnancy O08.6
    following ectopic or molar pregnancy
        O08.6
  rectovaginal septum —*see* Laceration, vagina
  retina, retinal (without detachment)
        (horseshoe) —*see also* Break, retina,
        horseshoe
    with detachment —*see* Detachment, retina,
        with retinal, break
  rotator cuff (nontraumatic) M75.10-●
    complete M75.12-●
    incomplete M75.11-●
    traumatic S46.01-●
      capsule S43.42-●
  semilunar cartilage, knee —*see* Tear, meniscus
  supraspinatus (complete) (incomplete)
        (nontraumatic) —*see also* Tear, rotator
        cuff M75.10-●
  tendon —*see* Strain
  tentorial, at birth P10.4
  umbilical cord
    complicating delivery O69.89
  urethra
    with ectopic or molar pregnancy O08.6
    following ectopic or molar pregnancy
        O08.6
    obstetrical trauma O71.5
  uterus —*see* Injury, uterus
  vagina —*see* Laceration, vagina
  vessel, from catheter —*see* Puncture,
        accidental complicating surgery
  vulva, complicating delivery O70.0
Tear-stone —*see* Dacryolith
Teeth —*see also* condition
  grinding
    psychogenic F45.8
    sleep related G47.63
Teething (syndrome) K00.7
Telangiectasia, telangiectasis (verrucous) I78.1
  ataxic (cerebellar) (Louis-Bar) G11.3
  familial I78.0
  hemorrhagic, hereditary (congenital) (senile)
        I78.0
  hereditary, hemorrhagic (congenital) (senile)
        I78.0
  juxtafoveal H35.07-●
  macular H35.07-●
▶macularis eruptiva perstans D47.01
  parafoveal H35.07-●
  retinal (idiopathic) (juxtafoveal) (macular)
        (parafoveal) H35.07-●
  spider I78.1
Telephone scatologia F65.89
Telescoped bowel or intestine K56.1
  congenital Q43.8
Temperature
  body, high (of unknown origin) R50.9
  cold, trauma from T69.9
    newborn P80.0
    specified effect NEC T69.8
Temple —*see* condition
Temporal —*see* condition
Temporomandibular joint pain-dysfunction
      syndrome M26.62-●
Temporosphenoidal —*see* condition
Tendency
  bleeding —*see* Defect, coagulation
  suicide
    meaning personal history of attempted
        suicide Z91.5
    meaning suicidal ideation —*see* Ideation,
        suicidal
  to fall R29.6
Tenderness, abdominal R10.819
  epigastric R10.816
  generalized R10.817
  left lower quadrant R10.814
  left upper quadrant R10.812
  periumbilic R10.815

Tenderness, abdominal *(Continued)*
  rebound R10.829
    epigastric R10.826
    generalized R10.827
    left lower quadrant R10.824
    left upper quadrant R10.822
    periumbilic R10.825
    right lower quadrant R10.823
    right upper quadrant R10.821
  right lower quadrant R10.813
  right upper quadrant R10.811
Tendinitis, tendonitis —*see also* Enthesopathy
  Achilles M76.6-●
  adhesive —*see* Tenosynovitis, specified type
        NEC
    shoulder —*see* Capsulitis, adhesive
  bicipital M75.2-●
  calcific M65.2-●
    ankle M65.27-●
    foot M65.27-●
    forearm M65.23-●
    hand M65.24-●
    lower leg M65.26-●
    multiple sites M65.29
    pelvic region M65.25-●
    shoulder M75.3-●
    specified site NEC M65.28
    thigh M65.25-●
    upper arm M65.22-●
  due to use, overuse, pressure —*see also*
        Disorder, soft tissue, due to use
    specified NEC —*see* Disorder, soft tissue,
        due to use, specified NEC
  gluteal M76.0-●
  patellar M76.5-●
  peroneal M76.7-●
  psoas M76.1-●
  tibial (posterior) M76.82-●
    anterior M76.81-●
  trochanteric —*see* Bursitis, hip, trochanteric
Tendon —*see* condition
Tendosynovitis —*see* Tenosynovitis
Tenesmus (rectal) R19.8
  vesical R30.1
Tennis elbow —*see* Epicondylitis, lateral
Tenonitis —*see also* Tenosynovitis
  eye (capsule) H05.04-●
Tenontosynovitis —*see* Tenosynovitis
Tenontothecitis —*see* Tenosynovitis
Tenophyte —*see* Disorder, synovium, specified
      type NEC
Tenosynovitis —*see also* Synovitis M65.9
  adhesive —*see* Tenosynovitis, specified type
        NEC
    shoulder —*see* Capsulitis, adhesive
  bicipital (calcifying) —*see* Tendinitis,
        bicipital
  gonococcal A54.49
  in (due to)
    crystals M65.8-●
    gonorrhea A54.49
    syphilis (late) A52.78
    use, overuse, pressure —*see also* Disorder,
        soft tissue, due to use
      specified NEC —*see* Disorder, soft tissue,
        due to use, specified NEC
  infective NEC M65.1-●
    ankle M65.17-●
    foot M65.17-●
    forearm M65.13-●
    hand M65.14-●
    lower leg M65.16-●
    multiple sites M65.19
    pelvic region M65.15-●
    shoulder region M65.11-●
    specified site NEC M65.18
    thigh M65.15-●
    upper arm M65.12-●
  radial styloid M65.4
  shoulder region M65.81-●
    adhesive —*see* Capsulitis, adhesive

Tenosynovitis *(Continued)*
  specified type NEC M65.88-●
    ankle M65.87-●
    foot M65.87-●
    forearm M65.83-●
    hand M65.84-●
    lower leg M65.86-●
    multiple sites M65.89
    pelvic region M65.85-●
    shoulder region M65.81-●
    specified site NEC M65.88
    thigh M65.85-●
    upper arm M65.82-●
  tuberculous —*see* Tuberculosis, tenosynovitis
Tenovaginitis —*see* Tenosynovitis
Tension
  arterial, high —*see also* Hypertension
    without diagnosis of hypertension R03.0
  headache G44.209
    intractable G44.201
    not intractable G44.209
  nervous R45.0
  pneumothorax J93.0
  premenstrual N94.3
  state (mental) F48.9
Tentorium —*see* condition
Teratencephalus Q89.8
Teratism Q89.7
Teratoblastoma (malignant) —*see* Neoplasm,
      malignant, by site
Teratocarcinoma —*see also* Neoplasm,
      malignant, by site
  liver C22.7
Teratoma (solid) —*see also* Neoplasm, uncertain
      behavior, by site
  with embryonal carcinoma, mixed —*see*
        Neoplasm, malignant, by site
  with malignant transformation —*see*
        Neoplasm, malignant, by site
  adult (cystic) —*see* Neoplasm, benign, by site
  benign —*see* Neoplasm, benign, by site
  combined with choriocarcinoma —*see*
        Neoplasm, malignant, by site
  cystic (adult) —*see* Neoplasm, benign, by site
  differentiated —*see* Neoplasm, benign, by site
  embryonal —*see also* Neoplasm, malignant,
        by site
    liver C22.7
  immature —*see* Neoplasm, malignant, by site
  liver C22.7
    adult, benign, cystic, differentiated type or
        mature D13.4
  malignant —*see also* Neoplasm, malignant,
        by site
    anaplastic —*see* Neoplasm, malignant, by
        site
    intermediate —*see* Neoplasm, malignant,
        by site
    specified site —*see* Neoplasm,
        malignant, by site
    unspecified site C62.90
    undifferentiated —*see* Neoplasm,
        malignant, by site
  mature —*see* Neoplasm, uncertain behavior,
        by site
  malignant —*see* Neoplasm, by site,
        malignant, by site
  ovary D27.-●
    embryonal, immature or malignant C56.-●
  solid —*see* Neoplasm, uncertain behavior,
        by site
  testis C62.9-●
    adult, benign, cystic, differentiated type or
        mature D29.2-●
    scrotal C62.1-●
    undescended C62.0-●
Termination
  anomalous —*see also* Malposition,
        congenital
    right pulmonary vein Q26.3
  pregnancy, elective Z33.2

Ternidens diminutus infestation B81.8
Ternidensiasis B81.8
Terror(s) night (child) F51.4
Terrorism, victim of Z65.4
➡ Terry's syndrome —see also Myopia,
   degenerative H44.2-●
Tertiary —see condition
Test, tests, testing (for)
  adequacy (for dialysis)
    hemodialysis Z49.31
    peritoneal Z49.32
  blood pressure Z01.30
    abnormal reading —see Blood, pressure
  blood typing Z01.83
    Rh typing Z01.83
  blood-alcohol Z04.8
    positive —see Findings, abnormal, in
      blood
  blood-drug Z04.8
    positive —see Findings, abnormal, in
      blood
  cardiac pulse generator (battery) Z45.010
  fertility Z31.41
  genetic
    disease carrier status for procreative
      management
      female Z31.430
      male Z31.440
    male partner of patient with recurrent
      pregnancy loss Z31.441
    procreative management NEC
      female Z31.438
      male Z31.448
  hearing Z01.10
    with abnormal findings NEC Z01.118
  HIV (human immunodeficiency virus)
    nonconclusive (in infants) R75
    positive Z21
    seropositive Z21
  immunity status Z01.84
  intelligence NEC Z01.89
  laboratory (as part of a general medical
    examination) Z00.00
    with abnormal finding Z00.01
    for medicolegal reason NEC Z04.8
  male partner of patient with recurrent
    pregnancy loss Z31.441
  Mantoux (for tuberculosis) Z11.1
    abnormal result R76.11
  pregnancy, positive first pregnancy —see
    Pregnancy, normal, first
  procreative Z31.49
    fertility Z31.41
  skin, diagnostic
    allergy Z01.82
      special screening examination —see
        Screening, by name of disease
    Mantoux Z11.1
    tuberculin Z11.1
  specified NEC Z01.89
  tuberculin Z11.1
    abnormal result R76.11
  vision Z01.00
    with abnormal findings Z01.01
  Wassermann Z11.3
    positive —see Serology for syphilis,
      positive
Testicle, testicular, testis —see also condition
  feminization syndrome —see also Syndrome,
    androgen insensitivity E34.51
  migrans Q55.29
Tetanus, tetanic (cephalic) (convulsions) A35
  with
    abortion A34
    ectopic or molar pregnancy O08.0
  following ectopic or molar pregnancy O08.0
  inoculation reaction (due to serum) —see
    Complications, vaccination
  neonatorum A33
  obstetrical A34
  puerperal, postpartum, childbirth A34

Tetany (due to) R29.0
  alkalosis E87.3
  associated with rickets E55.0
  convulsions R29.0
    hysterical F44.5
  functional (hysterical) F44.5
  hyperkinetic R29.0
    hysterical F44.5
  hyperpnea R06.4
    hysterical F44.5
    psychogenic F45.8
  hyperventilation —see also Hyperventilation
    R06.4
    hysterical F44.5
  neonatal (without calcium or magnesium
    deficiency) P71.3
  parathyroid (gland) E20.9
  parathyroprival E89.2
  post- (para)thyroidectomy E89.2
  postoperative E89.2
  pseudotetany R29.0
  psychogenic (conversion reaction) F44.5
Tetralogy of Fallot Q21.3
Tetraplegia (chronic) —see also Quadriplegia
  G82.50-●
Thailand hemorrhagic fever A91
Thalassanemia —see Thalassemia
Thalassemia (anemia) (disease) D56.9
  with other hemoglobinopathy D56.8
  alpha (major) (severe) (triple gene defect)
    D56.0
    minor D56.3
    silent carrier D56.3
    trait D56.3
  beta (severe) D56.1
    homozygous D56.1
    major D56.1
    minor D56.3
    trait D56.3
  delta-beta (homozygous) D56.2
    minor D56.3
    trait D56.3
  dominant D56.8
  hemoglobin
    C D56.8
    E-beta D56.5
  intermedia D56.1
  major D56.1
  minor D56.3
  mixed D56.8
  sickle-cell —see Disease, sickle-cell,
    thalassemia
  specified type NEC D56.8
  trait D56.3
  variants D56.8
Thanatophoric dwarfism or short stature Q77.1
Thaysen-Gee disease (nontropical sprue) K90.0
Thaysen's disease K90.0
Thecoma D27-●
  luteinized D27-●
  malignant C56-●
Thelarche, premature E30.8
Thelaziasis B83.8
Thelitis N61.0
  puerperal, postpartum or gestational —see
    Infection, nipple
Therapeutic —see condition
Therapy
  drug, long-term (current) (prophylactic)
    agents affecting estrogen receptors and
      estrogen levels NEC Z79.818
    anastrozole (Arimidex) Z79.811
    antibiotics Z79.2
      short-term use - omit code
    anticoagulants Z79.01
    anti-inflammatory Z79.1
    antiplatelet Z79.02
    antithrombotics Z79.02
    aromatase inhibitors Z79.811
    aspirin Z79.82
    birth control pill or patch Z79.3

Therapy (Continued)
  drug, long-term (Continued)
    bisphosphonates Z79.83
    contraceptive, oral Z79.3
    drug, specified NEC Z79.899
    estrogen receptor downregulators
      Z79.818
    Evista Z79.810
    exemestane (Aromasin) Z79.811
    Fareston Z79.810
    fulvestrant (Faslodex) Z79.818
    gonadotropin-releasing hormone (GnRH)
      agonist Z79.818
    goserelin acetate (Zoladex) Z79.818
  ➡ hormone replacement Z79.890
    insulin Z79.4
    letrozole (Femara) Z79.811
    leuprolide acetate (leuprorelin) (Lupron)
      Z79.818
    megestrol acetate (Megace) Z79.818
    methadone
      for pain management Z79.891
      maintenance therapy F11.20
    Nolvadex Z79.810
    opiate analgesic Z79.891
    oral contraceptive Z79.3
    raloxifene (Evista) Z79.810
    selective estrogen receptor modulators
      (SERMs) Z79.810
    short term - omit code
    steroids
      inhaled Z79.51
      systemic Z79.52
    tamoxifen (Nolvadex) Z79.810
    toremifene (Fareston) Z79.810
Thermic —see condition
Thermography (abnormal) —see also Abnormal,
  diagnostic imaging R93.8
  breast R92.8
Thermoplegia T67.0
Thesaurismosis, glycogen —see Disease,
  glycogen storage
Thiamin deficiency E51.9
  specified NEC E51.8
Thiaminic deficiency with beriberi E51.11
Thibierge-Weissenbach syndrome —see
  Sclerosis, systemic
Thickening
  bone —see Hypertrophy, bone
  breast N64.59
  endometrium R93.8
  epidermal L85.9
    specified NEC L85.8
  hymen N89.6
  larynx J38.7
  nail L60.2
    congenital Q84.5
  periosteal —see Hypertrophy, bone
  pleura J92.9
    with asbestos J92.0
  skin R23.4
  subepiglottic J38.7
  tongue K14.8
  valve, heart —see Endocarditis
Thigh —see condition
Thinning vertebra —see Spondylopathy,
  specified NEC
Thirst, excessive R63.1
  due to deprivation of water T73.1
Thomsen disease G71.12
Thoracic —see also condition
  kidney Q63.2
  outlet syndrome G54.0
Thoracogastroschisis (congenital)
  Q79.8
Thoracopagus Q89.4
Thorax —see condition
Thorn's syndrome N28.89
Thorson-Björck syndrome E34.0
Threadworm (infection) (infestation)
  B80

▶ New   ➡ Revised   ~~deleted~~ Deleted   ● Use Additional Character(s)

Threatened
abortion O20.0
with subsequent abortion O03.9
job loss, anxiety concerning Z56.2
labor (without delivery) O47.9
at or after 37 completed weeks of gestation
O47.1
before 37 completed weeks of gestation
O47.0-●
loss of job, anxiety concerning Z56.2
miscarriage O20.0
unemployment, anxiety concerning Z56.2
Three-day fever A93.1
Threshers' lung J67.0
Thrix annulata (congenital) Q84.1
Throat —see condition
Thrombasthenia (Glanzmann) (hemorrhagic)
(hereditary) D69.1
Thromboangiitis I73.1
obliterans (general) I73.1
cerebral I67.89
vessels
brain I67.89
spinal cord I67.89
Thromboarteritis —see Arteritis
Thromboasthenia (Glanzmann) (hemorrhagic)
(hereditary) D69.1
Thrombocytasthenia (Glanzmann) D69.1
Thrombocythemia (essential) (hemorrhagic)
(idiopathic) (primary) D47.3
Thrombocytopathy (dystrophic) (granulopenic)
D69.1
Thrombocytopenia, thrombocytopenic
D69.6
with absent radius (TAR) Q87.2
congenital D69.42
dilutional D69.59
due to
drugs D69.59
extracorporeal circulation of blood
D69.59
(massive)blood transfusion D69.59
platelet alloimmunization D69.59
essential D69.3
heparin induced (HIT) D75.82
hereditary D69.42
idiopathic D69.3
neonatal, transitory P61.0
due to
exchange transfusion P61.0
idiopathic maternal thrombocytopenia
P61.0
isoimmunization P61.0
primary NEC D69.49
idiopathic D69.3
puerperal, postpartum O72.3
secondary D69.59
transient neonatal P61.0
Thrombocytosis, essential D47.3
primary D47.3
Thromboembolism —see Embolism
Thrombopathy (Bernard-Soulier) D69.1
constitutional D68.0
Willebrand-Jurgens D68.0
Thrombopenia —see Thrombocytopenia
Thrombophilia D68.59
primary NEC D68.59
secondary NEC D68.69
specified NEC D68.69
Thrombophlebitis I80.9
antepartum O22.2-●
deep O22.3-●
superficial O22.2-●
cavernous (venous) sinus G08
complicating pregnancy O22.5-●
nonpyogenic I67.6
cerebral (sinus) (vein) G08
nonpyogenic I67.6
sequelae G09
due to implanted device —see Complications,
by site and type, specified NEC

Thrombophlebitis (Continued)
during or resulting from a procedure NEC
T81.72
femoral vein (superficial) I80.1-●
femoropopliteal vein I80.0-●
hepatic (vein) I80.8
idiopathic, recurrent I82.1
iliofemoral I80.1-●
intracranial venous sinus (any) G08
nonpyogenic I67.6
sequelae G09
intraspinal venous sinuses and veins G08
nonpyogenic G95.19
lateral (venous) sinus G08
nonpyogenic I67.6
➡leg I80.3
superficial I80.0-●
longitudinal (venous) sinus G08
nonpyogenic I67.6
lower extremity I80.299
migrans, migrating I82.1
pelvic
with ectopic or molar pregnancy
O08.0
following ectopic or molar pregnancy
O08.0
puerperal O87.1
popliteal vein —see Phlebitis, leg, deep,
popliteal
portal (vein) K75.1
postoperative T81.72
pregnancy —see Thrombophlebitis,
antepartum
puerperal, postpartum, childbirth O87.0
deep O87.1
pelvic O87.1
septic O86.81
superficial O87.0
saphenous (greater) (lesser) I80.0-●
sinus (intracranial) G08
nonpyogenic I67.6
specified site NEC I80.8
tibial vein I80.23-●
Thrombosis, thrombotic (bland) (multiple)
(progressive) (silent) (vessel) I82.90
anal K64.5
antepartum —see Thrombophlebitis,
antepartum
aorta, aortic I74.10
abdominal I74.09
saddle I74.01
bifurcation I74.09
saddle I74.01
specified site NEC I74.19
terminal I74.09
thoracic I74.11
valve —see Endocarditis, aortic
apoplexy I63.3-●
artery, arteries (postinfectional) I74.9
auditory, internal —see Occlusion, artery,
precerebral, specified NEC
basilar —see Occlusion, artery, basilar
carotid (common) (internal) —see
Occlusion, artery, carotid
cerebellar (anterior inferior) (posterior
inferior) (superior) —see Occlusion,
artery, cerebellar
cerebral —see Occlusion, artery, cerebral
➡choroidal (anterior) —see Occlusion, artery,
precerebral, specified NEC
➡communicating, posterior —see Occlusion,
artery, precerebral, specified NEC
coronary —see also Infarct, myocardium
not resulting in infarction I24.0
hepatic I74.8
➡hypophyseal —see Occlusion, artery,
precerebral, specified NEC
iliac I74.5
limb I74.4
lower I74.3
upper I74.2

Thrombosis, thrombotic (Continued)
artery, arteries (Continued)
meningeal, anterior or posterior —see
Occlusion, artery, cerebral, specified
NEC
mesenteric (with gangrene) —see also
Infarct, intestine K55.069
ophthalmic —see Occlusion, artery, retina
➡pontine —see Occlusion, artery, precerebral,
specified NEC
precerebral —see Occlusion, artery,
precerebral
pulmonary (iatrogenic) —see Embolism,
pulmonary
renal N28.0
retinal —see Occlusion, artery, retina
spinal, anterior or posterior G95.11
traumatic NEC T14.8
vertebral —see Occlusion, artery, vertebral
atrium, auricular —see also Infarct, myocardium
following acute myocardial infarction
(current complication) I23.6
not resulting in infarction I51.3
▶old I51.3
basilar (artery) —see Occlusion, artery, basilar
brain (artery) (stem) —see also Occlusion,
artery, cerebral
due to syphilis A52.05
puerperal O99.43
sinus —see Thrombosis, intracranial
venous sinus
capillary I78.8
cardiac —see also Infarct, myocardium
not resulting in infarction I51.3
valve —see Endocarditis
▶old I51.3
carotid (artery) (common) (internal) —see
Occlusion, artery, carotid
cavernous (venous) sinus —see Thrombosis,
intracranial venous sinus
cerebellar artery (anterior inferior) (posterior
inferior) (superior) I66.3
cerebral (artery) —see Occlusion, artery,
cerebral
cerebrovenous sinus —see also Thrombosis,
intracranial venous sinus
puerperium O87.3
chronic I82.91
coronary (artery) (vein) —see also Infarct,
myocardium
not resulting in infarction I24.0
corpus cavernosum N48.89
cortical I66.9
deep —see Embolism, vein, lower extremity
due to device, implant or graft —see also
Complications, by site and type,
specified NEC T85.868
arterial graft NEC T82.868
breast (implant) T85.868
catheter NEC T85.868
dialysis (renal) T82.868
intraperitoneal T85.868
infusion NEC T82.868
spinal (epidural) (subdural) T85.860
urinary (indwelling) T83.86
electronic (electrode) (pulse generator)
(stimulator)
bone T84.86
cardiac T82.867
nervous system (brain) (peripheral
nerve) (spinal) T85.860
urinary T83.86
fixation, internal (orthopedic) NEC T84.86
gastrointestinal (bile duct) (esophagus)
T85.868
genital NEC T83.86
heart T82.867
joint prosthesis T84.86
ocular (corneal graft) (orbital implant)
NEC T85.868
orthopedic NEC T84.86

Thrombosis, thrombotic *(Continued)*
  due to device, implant or graft *(Continued)*
    specified NEC T85.868
    urinary NEC T83.86
    vascular NEC T82.868
    ventricular intracranial shunt T85.860
  during the puerperium —*see* Thrombosis, puerperal
  endocardial —*see also* Infarct, myocardium
    not resulting in infarction I51.3
  eye —*see* Occlusion, retina
  genital organ
    female NEC N94.89
      pregnancy —*see* Thrombophlebitis, antepartum
    male N50.1
  gestational —*see* Phlebopathy, gestational
  heart (chamber) —*see also* Infarct, myocardium
    not resulting in infarction I51.3
    ▶old I51.3
  hepatic (vein) I82.0
    artery I74.8
  history (of) Z86.718
  intestine (with gangrene) —*see also* Infarct, intestine K55.069
  intracardiac NEC (apical) (atrial) (auricular) (ventricular) (old) I51.3
  intracranial (arterial) I66.9
    venous sinus (any) G08
      nonpyogenic origin I67.6
      puerperium O87.3
  intramural —*see also* Infarct, myocardium
    not resulting in infarction I51.3
    ▶old I51.3
  intraspinal venous sinuses and veins G08
    nonpyogenic G95.19
  kidney (artery) N28.0
  lateral (venous) sinus —*see* Thrombosis, intracranial venous sinus
  leg —*see* Thrombosis, vein, lower extremity
    arterial I74.3
  liver (venous) I82.0
    artery I74.8
    portal vein I81
  longitudinal (venous) sinus —*see* Thrombosis, intracranial venous sinus
  lower limb —*see* Thrombosis, vein, lower extremity
  lung (iatrogenic) (postoperative) —*see* Embolism, pulmonary
  meninges (brain) (arterial) I66.8
  mesenteric (artery) (with gangrene) —*see also* Infarct, intestine K55.069
    vein (inferior) (superior) I81
  mitral I34.8
  mural —*see also* Infarct, myocardium
    due to syphilis A52.06
    not resulting in infarction I51.3
    ▶old I51.3
  omentum (with gangrene) —*see also* Infarct, intestine K55.069
  ophthalmic —*see* Occlusion, retina
  pampiniform plexus (male) N50.1
  parietal —*see also* Infarct, myocardium
    not resulting in infarction I24.0
  penis, superficial vein N48.81
  perianal venous K64.5
  peripheral arteries I74.4
    upper I74.2
  personal history (of) Z86.718
  portal I81
    due to syphilis A52.09
  precerebral artery —*see* Occlusion, artery, precerebral
  puerperal, postpartum O87.0
    brain (artery) O99.43
      venous (sinus) O87.3
    cardiac O99.43
    cerebral (artery) O99.43
      venous (sinus) O87.3
    superficial O87.0

Thrombosis, thrombotic *(Continued)*
  pulmonary (artery) (iatrogenic) (postoperative) (vein) —*see* Embolism, pulmonary
  renal (artery) N28.0
    vein I82.3
  resulting from presence of device, implant or graft —*see* Complications, by site and type, specified NEC
  retina, retinal —*see* Occlusion, retina
  scrotum N50.1
  seminal vesicle N50.1
  sigmoid (venous) sinus —*see* Thrombosis, intracranial venous sinus
  sinus, intracranial (any) —*see* Thrombosis, intracranial venous sinus
  specified site NEC I82.890
    chronic I82.891
  spermatic cord N50.1
  spinal cord (arterial) G95.11
    due to syphilis A52.09
    pyogenic origin G06.1
  spleen, splenic D73.5
    artery I74.8
  testis N50.1
  traumatic NEC T14.8
  tricuspid I07.8
  tumor —*see* Neoplasm, by site
  tunica vaginalis N50.1
  umbilical cord (vessels), complicating delivery O69.5
  vas deferens N50.1
  vein (acute) I82.90
    antecubital I82.61-●
      chronic I82.71-●
    axillary I82.A1-●
      chronic I82.A2-●
    basilic I82.61-●
      chronic I82.71-●
    brachial I82.62-●
      chronic I82.72-●
    brachiocephalic (innominate) I82.290
      chronic I82.291
    cerebral, nonpyogenic I67.6
    cephalic I82.61-●
      chronic I82.71-●
    chronic I82.91
    deep (DVT) I82.40-●
      calf I82.4Z-●
        chronic I82.5Z-●
      lower leg I82.4Z-●
        chronic I82.5Z-●
      thigh I82.4Y-●
        chronic I82.5Y-●
      upper leg I82.4Y
        chronic I82.5y-●
    femoral I82.41-●
      chronic I82.51-●
    iliac (iliofemoral) I82.42-●
      chronic I82.52-●
    innominate I82.290
      chronic I82.291
    internal jugular I82.C1-●
      chronic I82.C2-●
    lower extremity
      deep I82.40-●
        chronic I82.50-●
        specified NEC I82.49-●
          chronic NEC I82.59-●
      distal
        deep I82.4Z-●
      proximal
        deep I82.4Y-●
          chronic I82.5Y-●
      superficial I82.81-●
    perianal K64.5
    popliteal I82.43-●
      chronic I82.53-●
    radial I82.62-●
      chronic I82.72-●
    renal I82.3

Thrombosis, thrombotic *(Continued)*
  vein *(Continued)*
    saphenous (greater) (lesser) I82.81-●
    specified NEC I82.890
      chronic NEC I82.891
    subclavian I82.B1-●
      chronic I82.B2-●
    thoracic NEC I82.290
      chronic I82.291
    tibial I82.44-●
      chronic I82.54-●
    ulnar I82.62-●
      chronic I82.72-●
    upper extremity I82.60-●
      chronic I82.70-●
      deep I82.62-●
        chronic I82.72-●
      superficial I82.61-●
        chronic I82.71-●
  vena cava
    inferior I82.220
      chronic I82.221
    superior I82.210
      chronic I82.211
  venous, perianal K64.5
  ventricle —*see also* Infarct, myocardium
    following acute myocardial infarction (current complication) I23.6
    not resulting in infarction I24.0
    ▶old I51.3
Thrombus —*see* Thrombosis
Thrush —*see also* Candidiasis
  newborn P37.5
  oral B37.0
  vaginal B37.3
Thumb —*see also* condition
  sucking (child problem) F98.8
Thymitis E32.8
Thymoma (benign) D15.0
  malignant C37
Thymus, thymic (gland) —*see* condition
Thyrocele —*see* Goiter
Thyroglossal —*see also* condition
  cyst Q89.2
  duct, persistent Q89.2
Thyroid (gland) (body) —*see also* condition
  hormone resistance E07.89
  lingual Q89.2
  nodule (cystic) (nontoxic) (single) E04.1
Thyroiditis E06.9
  acute (nonsuppurative) (pyogenic) (suppurative) E06.0
  autoimmune E06.3
  chronic (nonspecific) (sclerosing) E06.5
    with thyrotoxicosis, transient E06.2
    fibrous E06.5
    lymphadenoid E06.3
    lymphocytic E06.3
    lymphoid E06.3
  de Quervain's E06.1
  drug-induced E06.4
  fibrous (chronic) E06.5
  giant-cell (follicular) E06.1
  granulomatous (de Quervain) (subacute) E06.1
  Hashimoto's (struma lymphomatosa) E06.3
  iatrogenic E06.4
  ligneous E06.5
  lymphocytic (chronic) E06.3
  lymphoid E06.3
  lymphomatous E06.3
  nonsuppurative E06.1
  postpartum, puerperal O90.5
  pseudotuberculous E06.1
  pyogenic E06.0
  radiation E06.4
  Riedel's E06.5
  subacute (granulomatous) E06.1
  suppurative E06.0
  tuberculous A18.81
  viral E06.1
  woody E06.5

▶ New   ⇒ Revised   ~~deleted~~ Deleted   ● Use Additional Character(s)

Thyrolingual duct, persistent Q89.2
Thyromegaly E01.0
Thyrotoxic
  crisis —see Thyrotoxicosis
  heart disease or failure —see also
      Thyrotoxicosis E05.90 [143]
    with thyroid storm E05.91 [143]
  storm —see Thyrotoxicosis
Thyrotoxicosis (recurrent) E05.90
  with
    goiter (diffuse) E05.00
      with thyroid storm E05.01
      adenomatous uninodular E05.10
        with thyroid storm E05.11
      multinodular E05.20
        with thyroid storm E05.21
      nodular E05.20
        with thyroid storm E05.21
      uninodular E05.10
        with thyroid storm E05.11
    infiltrative
      dermopathy E05.00
        with thyroid storm E05.01
      ophthalmopathy E05.00
        with thyroid storm E05.01
    single thyroid nodule E05.10
      with thyroid storm E05.11
    thyroid storm E05.91
  due to
    ectopic thyroid nodule or tissue E05.30
      with thyroid storm E05.31
    ingestion of (excessive) thyroid material
        E05.40
      with thyroid storm E05.41
    overproduction of thyroid-stimulating
        hormone E05.80
      with thyroid storm E05.81
    specified cause NEC E05.80
      with thyroid storm E05.81
  factitia E05.40
    with thyroid storm E05.41
  heart —see also Failure, heart, high-output
      E05.90 [143]
  with thyroid storm —see also Failure, heart,
      high-output E05.91 [143]
  failure —see also Failure, heart, high-output
      E05.90 [143]
  neonatal (transient) P72.1
  transient with chronic thyroiditis E06.2
Tibia vara —see Osteochondrosis, juvenile, tibia
Tic (disorder) F95.9
  breathing F95.8
  child problem F95.0
  compulsive F95.1
  de la Tourette F95.2
  degenerative (generalized) (localized) G25.69
    facial G25.69
  disorder
    chronic
      motor F95.1
      vocal F95.1
      combined vocal and multiple motor F95.2
      transient F95.0
  douloureux G50.0
    atypical G50.1
    postherpetic, postzoster B02.22
  drug-induced G25.61
  eyelid F95.8
  habit F95.9
    chronic F95.1
    transient of childhood F95.0
  lid, transient of childhood F95.0
  motor-verbal F95.2
  occupational F48.8
  orbicularis F95.8
    transient of childhood F95.0
  organic origin G25.69
  postchoreic G25.69
  provisional F95.0
  psychogenic, compulsive F95.1
  salaam R25.8

Tic (Continued)
  spasm (motor or vocal) F95.9
    chronic F95.1
    transient of childhood F95.0
  specified NEC F95.8
Tick-borne —see condition
Tietze's disease or syndrome M94.0
Tight, tightness
  anus K62.89
  chest R07.89
  fascia (lata) M62.89
  foreskin (congenital) N47.1
  hymen, hymenal ring N89.6
  introitus (acquired) (congenital) N89.6
  rectal sphincter K62.89
  tendon —see Short, tendon
  urethral sphincter N35.9
Tilting vertebra —see Dorsopathy, deforming,
    specified NEC
Timidity, child F93.8
Tin-miner's lung J63.5
Tinea (intersecta) (tarsi) B35.9
  amiantacea L44.8
  asbestina B35.0
  barbae B35.0
  beard B35.0
  black dot B35.0
  blanca B36.2
  capitis B35.0
  corporis B35.4
  cruris B35.6
  flava B36.0
  foot B35.3
  furfuracea B36.0
  imbricata (Tokelau) B35.5
  kerion B35.0
  manuum B35.2
  microsporic —see Dermatophytosis
  nigra B36.1
  nodosa —see Piedra
  pedis B35.3
  scalp B35.0
  specified site NEC B35.8
  ▶specified NEC B35.8
  sycosis B35.0
  tonsurans B35.0
  trichophytic —see Dermatophytosis
  unguium B35.1
  versicolor B36.0
Tingling sensation (skin) R20.2
Tinnitus NOS H93.1-●
  audible H93.1-●
  aurium H93.1-●
  pulsatile H93.A-●
  subjective H93.1-●
Tipped tooth (teeth) M26.33
Tipping
  pelvis M95.5
    with disproportion (fetopelvic) O33.0
      causing obstructed labor O65.0
  tooth (teeth), fully erupted M26.33
Tiredness R53.83
Tissue —see condition
Tobacco (nicotine)
  abuse —see Tobacco, use
  dependence —see Dependence, drug, nicotine
  harmful use Z72.0
  heart —see Tobacco, toxic effect
  maternal use, affecting newborn P04.2
  toxic effect —see Table of Drugs and
      Chemicals, by substance, poisoning
    chewing tobacco —see Table of Drugs
        and Chemicals, by substance, poisoning
    cigarettes —see Table of Drugs and
        Chemicals, by substance, poisoning
  use Z72.0
    complicating
      childbirth O99.334
      pregnancy O99.33-●
      puerperium O99.335
    counseling and surveillance Z71.6
    history Z87.891

Tobacco (Continued)
  withdrawal state —see also Dependence,
      drug, nicotine F17.203
Tocopherol deficiency E56.0
Todd's
  cirrhosis K74.3
  paralysis (postepileptic) (transitory) G83.84
Toe —see condition
Toilet, artificial opening —see Attention to,
    artificial, opening
Tokelau (ringworm) B35.5
Tollwut —see Rabies
Tommaselli's disease R31.9
  correct substance properly administered —see
      Table of Drugs and Chemicals, by drug,
      adverse effect
  overdose or wrong substance given
      or taken —see Table of Drugs and
      Chemicals, by drug, poisoning
Tongue —see also condition
  tie Q38.1
Tonic pupil —see Anomaly, pupil, function,
    tonic pupil
Toni-Fanconi syndrome (cystinosis) E72.09
  with cystinosis E72.04
Tonsil —see condition
Tonsillitis (acute) (catarrhal) (croupous)
    (follicular) (gangrenous) (infective)
    (lacunar) (lingual) (malignant)
    (membranous) (parenchymatous)
    (phlegmonous) (pseudomembranous)
    (purulent) (septic) (subacute) (suppurative)
    (toxic) (ulcerative) (vesicular) (viral) J03.90
  chronic J35.01
    with adenoiditis J35.03
  diphtheritic A36.0
  hypertrophic J35.01
    with adenoiditis J35.03
  recurrent J03.91
  specified organism NEC J03.80
    recurrent J03.81
  staphylococcal J03.80
    recurrent J03.81
  streptococcal J03.00
    recurrent J03.01
  tuberculous A15.8
  Vincent's A69.1
Tooth, teeth —see condition
Toothache K08.89
Topagnosis R20.8
Tophi —see Gout, chronic
TORCH infection —see Infection, congenital
  without active infection P00.2
Torn —see Tear
Tornwaldt's cyst or disease J39.2
Torsion
  accessory tube —see Torsion, fallopian tube
  adnexa (female) —see Torsion, fallopian tube
  aorta, acquired I77.1
  appendix epididymis N44.04
  appendix testis N44.03
  bile duct (common) (hepatic) K83.8
    congenital Q44.5
  bowel, colon or intestine K56.2
  cervix —see Malposition, uterus
  cystic duct K82.8
  dystonia —see Dystonia, torsion
  epididymis (appendix) N44.04
  fallopian tube N83.52-●
    with ovary N83.53
  gallbladder K82.8
    congenital Q44.1
  hydatid of Morgagni
    female N83.52-●
    male N44.03
  kidney (pedicle) (leading to infarction) N28.0
  Meckel's diverticulum (congenital) Q43.0
  malignant —see Table of Neoplasms, small
      intestine, malignant
  mesentery K56.2
  omentum K56.2

Torsion *(Continued)*
   organ or site, congenital NEC —*see* Anomaly,
      by site
   ovary (pedicle) N83.51-●
     with fallopian tube N83.53
     congenital Q50.2
   oviduct —*see* Torsion, fallopian tube
   penis (acquired) N48.82
     congenital Q55.63
   spasm —*see* Dystonia, torsion
   spermatic cord N44.02
     extravaginal N44.01
     intravaginal N44.02
   spleen D73.5
   testis, testicle N44.00
     appendix N44.03
   tibia —*see* Deformity, limb, specified type
     NEC, lower leg
   uterus —*see* Malposition, uterus
Torticollis (intermittent) (spastic) M43.6
   congenital (sternomastoid) Q68.0
   due to birth injury P15.8
   hysterical F44.4
   ocular R29.891
   psychogenic F45.8
     conversion reaction F44.4
   rheumatic M43.6
   rheumatoid M06.88
   spasmodic G24.3
   traumatic, current S13.4
Tortipelvis G24.1
Tortuous
   aortic arch Q25.46
   artery I77.1
   organ or site, congenital NEC —*see* Distortion
   retinal vessel, congenital Q14.1
   ureter N13.8
   urethra N36.8
   vein —*see* Varix
Torture, victim of Z65.4
Torula, torular (histolytica) (infection) —*see*
   Cryptococcosis
Torulosis —*see* Cryptococcosis
Torus (mandibularis) (palatinus) M27.0
   fracture —*see* Fracture, by site, torus
Touraine's syndrome Q79.8
Tourette's syndrome F95.2
Tourniquet syndrome —*see* Constriction,
   external, by site
Tower skull Q75.0
   with exophthalmos Q87.0
Toxemia R68.89
   bacterial —*see* Sepsis
   burn —*see* Burn
   eclamptic (with pre-existing hypertension) —
     see Eclampsia
   erysipelatous —*see* Erysipelas
   fatigue R68.89
   food —*see* Poisoning, food
   gastrointestinal K52.1
   intestinal K52.1
   kidney —*see* Uremia
   malarial —*see* Malaria
   myocardial —*see* Myocarditis, toxic
   of pregnancy —*see* Pre-eclampsia
   pre-eclamptic —*see* Pre-eclampsia
   small intestine K52.1
   staphylococcal, due to food A05.0
   stasis R68.89
   uremic —*see* Uremia
   urinary —*see* Uremia
Toxemica cerebropathia psychica
   (nonalcoholic) F04
   alcoholic —*see* Alcohol, amnestic disorder
Toxic (poisoning) —*see also* condition T65.91
   effect —*see* Table of Drugs and Chemicals, by
     substance, poisoning
   shock syndrome A48.3
   thyroid (gland) —*see* Thyrotoxicosis
Toxicemia —*see* Toxemia
Toxicity —*see* Table of Drugs and Chemicals, by
   substance, poisoning

Toxic *(Continued)*
   fava bean D55.0
   food, noxious —*see* Poisoning, food
   from drug or nonmedicinal substance —*see*
     Table of Drugs and Chemicals, by drug
Toxicosis —*see also* Toxemia
   capillary, hemorrhagic D69.0
Toxinfection, gastrointestinal K52.1
Toxocariasis B83.0
Toxoplasma, toxoplasmosis (acquired) B58.9
   with
     hepatitis B58.1
     meningoencephalitis B58.2
     ocular involvement B58.00
     other organ involvement B58.89
     pneumonia, pneumonitis B58.3
   congenital (acute) (subacute) (chronic) P37.1
   maternal, manifest toxoplasmosis in infant
     (acute) (subacute) (chronic) P37.1
tPA (rtPA) administration in a different facility
   within the last 24 hours prior to admission
   to current facility Z92.82
Trabeculation, bladder N32.89
Trachea —*see* condition
Tracheitis (catarrhal) (infantile) (membranous)
   (plastic) (septal) (suppurative) (viral) J04.10
   with
     bronchitis (15 years of age and above) J40
       acute or subacute —*see* Bronchitis, acute
       chronic J42
       tuberculous NEC A15.5
       under 15 years of age J20.9
     laryngitis (acute) J04.2
       chronic J37.1
       tuberculous NEC A15.5
   acute J04.10
     with obstruction J04.11
   chronic J42
     with
       bronchitis (chronic) J42
       laryngitis (chronic) J37.1
   diphtheritic (membranous) A36.89
   due to external agent —*see* Inflammation,
     respiratory, upper, due to
   syphilitic A52.73
   tuberculous A15.5
Trachelitis (nonvenereal) —*see* Cervicitis
Tracheobronchial —*see* condition
Tracheobronchitis (15 years of age and
   above) —*see also* Bronchitis
   due to
     Bordetella bronchiseptica A37.80
       with pneumonia A37.81
     Francisella tularensis A21.8
Tracheobronchomegaly Q32.4
   with bronchiectasis J47.9
     with
       exacerbation (acute) J47.1
       lower respiratory infection J47.0
   acquired J98.09
     with bronchiectasis J47.9
       with
         exacerbation (acute) J47.1
         lower respiratory infection J47.0
Tracheobronchopneumonitis —*see* Pneumonia,
   broncho-●
Tracheocele (external) (internal) J39.8
   congenital Q32.1
Tracheomalacia J39.8
   congenital Q32.0
Tracheopharyngitis (acute) J06.9
   chronic J42
   due to external agent —*see* Inflammation,
     respiratory, upper, due to
Tracheostenosis J39.8
Tracheostomy
   complication —*see* Complication,
     tracheostomy
   status Z93.0
     attention to Z43.0
     malfunctioning J95.03

Trachoma, trachomatous A71.9
   active (stage) A71.1
   contraction of conjunctiva A71.1
   dubium A71.0
   healed or sequelae B94.0
   initial (stage) A71.0
   pannus A71.1
   Türck's J37.0
Traction, vitreomacular H43.82-●
Train sickness T75.3
Trait(s)
   Hb-S D57.3
   hemoglobin
     abnormal NEC D58.2
       with thalassemia D56.3
     C —*see* Disease, hemoglobin C
     S (Hb-S) D57.3
   Lepore D56.3
   personality, accentuated Z73.1
   sickle-cell D57.3
     with elliptocytosis or spherocytosis D57.3
   type A personality Z73.1
Tramp Z59.0
Trance R41.89
   hysterical F44.89
Transaminasemia R74.0
Transection
   abdomen (partial) S38.3
   aorta (incomplete) —*see also* Injury, aorta
     complete —*see* Injury, aorta, laceration,
       major
   carotid artery (incomplete) —*see also* Injury,
     blood vessel, carotid, laceration
     complete —*see* Injury, blood vessel, carotid,
       laceration, major
   celiac artery (incomplete) S35.211
     branch (incomplete) S35.291
       complete S35.292
     complete S35.212
   innominate
     artery (incomplete) —*see also* Injury, blood
       vessel, thoracic, innominate, artery,
       laceration
       complete —*see* Injury, blood vessel,
         thoracic, innominate, artery,
         laceration, major
     vein (incomplete) —*see also* Injury, blood
       vessel, thoracic, innominate, vein,
       laceration
       complete —*see* Injury, blood vessel,
         thoracic, innominate, vein,
         laceration, major
   jugular vein (external) (incomplete) —*see*
     also Injury, blood vessel, jugular vein,
     laceration
     complete —*see* Injury, blood vessel, jugular
       vein, laceration, major
     internal (incomplete) —*see also* Injury,
       blood vessel, jugular vein, internal,
       laceration
       complete —*see* Injury, blood vessel,
         jugular vein, internal, laceration,
         major
   mesenteric artery (incomplete) —*see also*
     Injury, mesenteric, artery, laceration
     complete —*see* Injury, mesenteric artery,
       laceration, major
   pulmonary vessel (incomplete) —*see also*
     Injury, blood vessel, thoracic, pulmonary,
     laceration
     complete —*see* Injury, blood vessel,
       thoracic, pulmonary, laceration, major
   subclavian —*see* Transection, innominate
   vena cava (incomplete) —*see also* Injury, vena
     cava
     complete —*see* Injury, vena cava,
       laceration, major
   vertebral artery (incomplete) —*see also* Injury,
     blood vessel, vertebral, laceration
     complete —*see* Injury, blood vessel,
       vertebral, laceration, major

▶ New   ⇒ Revised   ~~deleted~~ Deleted   ● Use Additional Character(s)

Transfusion
  associated (red blood cell) hemochromatosis
    E83.111
  blood
    ABO incompatible —*see* Complication(s),
      transfusion, incompatibility reaction,
      ABO
    minor blood group (Duffy) (E) (K(ell))
      (Kidd) (Lewis) (M) (N) (P) (S)
      T80.89
    reaction or complication —*see*
      Complications, transfusion
  fetomaternal (mother) —*see* Pregnancy,
    complicated by, placenta, transfusion
    syndrome
  maternofetal (mother) —*see* Pregnancy,
    complicated by, placenta, transfusion
    syndrome
  placental (syndrome) (mother) —*see*
    Pregnancy, complicated by, placenta,
    transfusion syndrome
  reaction (adverse) —*see* Complications,
    transfusion
  related acute lung injury (TRALI) J95.84
  twin-to-twin —*see* Pregnancy, complicated
    by, placenta, transfusion syndrome, fetus
    to fetus
Transient (meaning homeless) —*see also*
  condition Z59.0
Translocation
  balanced autosomal Q95.9
    in normal individual Q95.0
  chromosomes NEC Q99.8
    balanced and insertion in normal
      individual Q95.0
  Down's syndrome Q90.2
  trisomy
    13 Q91.6
    18 Q91.2
    21 Q90.2
Translucency, iris —*see* Degeneration, iris
**Transmission of chemical substances through
  the placenta** —*see* Absorption, chemical,
  through placenta
Transparency, lung, unilateral J43.0
Transplant(ed) (status) Z94.9
  awaiting organ Z76.82
  bone Z94.6
    marrow Z94.81
  candidate Z76.82
  complication —*see* Complication, transplant
  cornea Z94.7
  heart Z94.1
    and lung(s) Z94.3
    valve Z95.2
      prosthetic Z95.2
      specified NEC Z95.4
      xenogenic Z95.3
  intestine Z94.82
  kidney Z94.0
  liver Z94.4
  lung(s) Z94.2
    and heart Z94.3
  organ (failure) (infection) (rejection)Z94.9
    removal status Z98.85
  pancreas Z94.83
  skin Z94.5
  social Z60.3
  specified organ or tissue NEC Z94.89
  stem cells Z94.84
  tissue Z94.9
Transplants, ovarian, endometrial N80.1
Transposed —*see* Transposition
Transposition (congenital) —*see also*
  Malposition, congenital
  abdominal viscera Q89.3
  aorta (dextra) Q20.3
  appendix Q43.8
  colon Q43.8
  corrected Q20.5
  great vessels (complete) (partial) Q20.3

Transposition *(Continued)*
  heart Q24.0
    with complete transposition of viscera
      Q89.3
  intestine (large) (small) Q43.8
  reversed jejunal (for bypass) (status) Z98.0
  scrotum Q55.23
  stomach Q40.2
    with general transposition of viscera
      Q89.3
  tooth, teeth, fully erupted M26.30
  vessels, great (complete) (partial) Q20.3
  viscera (abdominal) (thoracic) Q89.3
Transsexualism F64.0
Transverse —*see also* condition
  arrest (deep), in labor O64.0
  lie (mother) O32.2
    causing obstructed labor O64.8
Transvestism, transvestitism (dual-role)
  F64.1
  fetishistic F65.1
Trapped placenta (with hemorrhage) O72.0
  without hemorrhage O73.0
TRAPS (tumor necrosis factor receptor
  associated periodic syndrome) M04.1
Trauma, traumatism —*see also* Injury
  acoustic —*see* subcategory H83.3
  birth —*see* Birth, injury
  complicating ectopic or molar pregnancy
    O08.6
  during delivery O71.9
  following ectopic or molar pregnancy O08.6
  obstetric O71.9
    specified NEC O71.89
  occlusal
    primary K08.81
    secondary K08.82
Traumatic —*see also* condition
  brain injury S06.9
Treacher Collins syndrome Q75.4
Treitz's hernia —*see* Hernia, abdomen, specified
  site NEC
Trematode infestation —*see* Infestation, fluke
Trematodiasis —*see* Infestation, fluke
Trembling paralysis —*see* Parkinsonism
Tremor(s) R25.1
  drug induced G25.1
  essential (benign) G25.0
  familial G25.0
  hereditary G25.0
  hysterical F44.4
  intention G25.2
  medication induced postural G25.1
  mercurial —*see* subcategory T56.1
  Parkinson's —*see* Parkinsonism
  psychogenic (conversion reaction) F44.4
  senilis R54
  specified type NEC G25.2
Trench
  fever A79.0
  foot —*see* Immersion, foot
  mouth A69.1
Treponema pallidum infection —*see* Syphilis
Treponematosis
  due to
    T. pallidum —*see* Syphilis
    T. pertenue —*see* Yaws
Triad
  Hutchinson's (congenital syphilis) A50.53
  Kartagener's Q89.3
  Saint's —*see* Hernia, diaphragm
Trichiasis (eyelid) H02.059
  with entropion —*see* Entropion
  left H02.056
    lower H02.055
    upper H02.054
  right H02.053
    lower H02.052
    upper H02.051
Trichinella spiralis (infection) (infestation)
  B75

**Trichinellosis, trichiniasis, trichinelliasis,
  trichinosis** B75
  with muscle disorder B75 [M63.80]
    ankle B75 [M63.87-●]
    foot B75 [M63.87-●]
    forearm B75 [M63.83-●]
    hand B75 [M63.84-●]
    lower leg B75 [M63.86-●]
    multiple sites B75 [M63.89]
    pelvic region B75 [M63.85-●]
    shoulder region B75 [M63.81-●]
    specified site NEC B75 [M63.88]
    thigh B75 [M63.85-●]
    upper arm B75 [M63.82-●]
Trichobezoar T18.9
  intestine T18.3
  stomach T18.2
Trichocephaliasis, trichocephalosis B79
Trichocephalus infestation B79
Trichoclasis L67.8
Trichoepithelioma —*see also* Neoplasm, skin,
  benign
  malignant —*see* Neoplasm, skin, malignant
Trichofolliculoma —*see* Neoplasm, skin,
  benign
Tricholemmoma —*see* Neoplasm, skin,
  benign
Trichomoniasis A59.9
  bladder A59.03
  cervix A59.09
  intestinal A07.8
  prostate A59.02
  seminal vesicles A59.09
  specified site NEC A59.8
  urethra A59.03
  urogenitalis A59.00
  vagina A59.01
  vulva A59.01
Trichomycosis
  axillaris A48.8
  nodosa, nodularis B36.8
Trichonodosis L67.8
Trichophytid, trichophyton infection —*see*
  Dermatophytosis
Trichophytobezoar T18.9
  intestine T18.3
  stomach T18.2
Trichophytosis —*see* Dermatophytosis
Trichoptilosis L67.8
Trichorrhexis (nodosa) (invaginata) L67.0
Trichosis axillaris A48.8
Trichosporosis nodosa B36.2
Trichostasis spinulosa (congenital) Q84.1
Trichostrongyliasis, trichostrongylosis (small
  intestine) B81.2
Trichostrongylus infection B81.2
Trichotillomania F63.3
Trichromat, trichromatopsia, anomalous
  (congenital) H53.55
Trichuriasis B79
Trichuris trichiura (infection) (infestation) (any
  site) B79
Tricuspid (valve) —*see* condition
Trifid —*see also* Accessory
  kidney (pelvis) Q63.8
  tongue Q38.3
Trigeminal neuralgia —*see* Neuralgia,
  trigeminal
Trigeminy R00.8
Trigger finger (acquired) M65.30
  congenital Q74.0
  index finger M65.32-●
  little finger M65.35-●
  middle finger M65.33-●
  ring finger M65.34-●
  thumb M65.31-●
Trigonitis (bladder) (chronic)
  (pseudomembranous) N30.30
  with hematuria N30.31
Trigonocephaly Q75.0
Trilocular heart —*see* Cor triloculare

Trimethylaminuria E72.52
Tripartite placenta O43.19-●
Triphalangeal thumb Q74.0
Triple —see also Accessory
  kidneys Q63.0
  uteri Q51.818
  X, female Q97.0
Triplegia G83.89
  congenital G80.8
Triplet (newborn) —see also Newborn, triplet
  complicating pregnancy —see Pregnancy, triplet
Triplication —see Accessory
Triploidy Q92.7
Trismus R25.2
  neonatorum A33
  newborn A33
Trisomy (syndrome) Q92.9
  13 (partial) Q91.7
    meiotic nondisjunction Q91.4
    mitotic nondisjunction Q91.5
    mosaicism Q91.5
    translocation Q91.6
  18 (partial) Q91.3
    meiotic nondisjunction Q91.0
    mitotic nondisjunction Q91.1
    mosaicism Q91.1
    translocation Q91.2
  20 Q92.8
  21 (partial) Q90.9
    meiotic nondisjunction Q90.0
    mitotic nondisjunction Q90.1
    mosaicism Q90.1
    translocation Q90.2
  22 Q92.8
  autosomes Q92.9
  chromosome specified NEC Q92.8
    partial Q92.2
      due to unbalanced translocation Q92.5
    specified NEC Q92.8
    whole (nonsex chromosome)
      meiotic nondisjunction Q92.0
      mitotic nondisjunction Q92.1
      mosaicism Q92.1
  due to
    dicentrics —see Extra, marker chromosomes
    extra rings —see Extra, marker chromosomes
    isochromosomes —see Extra, marker chromosomes
  specified NEC Q92.8
  whole chromosome Q92.9
    meiotic nondisjunction Q92.0
    mitotic nondisjunction Q92.1
    mosaicism Q92.1
    partial Q92.9
    specified NEC Q92.8
Tritanomaly, tritanopia H53.55
Trombiculosis, trombiculiasis, trombidiosis B88.0
Trophedema (congenital) (hereditary) Q82.0
Trophoblastic disease —see also Mole, hydatidiform O01.9
Tropholymphedema Q82.0
Trophoneurosis NEC G96.8
  disseminated M34.9
Tropical —see condition
Trouble —see also Disease
  heart —see Disease, heart
  kidney —see Disease, renal
  nervous R45.0
  sinus —see Sinusitis
Trousseau's syndrome (thrombophlebitis migrans) I82.1
Truancy, childhood
  from school Z72.810
Truncus
  arteriosus (persistent) Q20.0
  communis Q20.0
Trunk —see condition

Trypanosomiasis
  African B56.9
    by Trypanosoma brucei
      gambiense B56.0
      rhodesiense B56.1
  American —see Chagas' disease
  Brazilian —see Chagas' disease
  by Trypanosoma
    brucei gambiense B56.0
    brucei rhodesiense B56.1
    cruzi —see Chagas' disease
  gambiensis, Gambian B56.0
  rhodesiensis, Rhodesian B56.1
  South American —see Chagas' disease
  where
    African trypanosomiasis is prevalent B56.9
    Chagas' disease is prevalent B57.2
T-shaped incisors K00.2
Tsutsugamushi (disease) (fever) A75.3
Tube, tubal, tubular —see condition
Tubercle —see also Tuberculosis
  brain, solitary A17.81
  Darwin's Q17.8
  Ghon, primary infection A15.7
Tuberculid, tuberculide (indurating, subcutaneous) (lichenoid) (miliary) (papulonecrotic) (primary) (skin) A18.4
Tuberculoma —see also Tuberculosis
  brain A17.81
  meninges (cerebral) (spinal) A17.1
  spinal cord A17.81
Tuberculosis, tubercular, tuberculous
  (calcification) (calcified) (caseous) (chromogenic acid-fast bacilli) (degeneration) (fibrocaseous) (fistula) (interstitial) (isolated circumscribed lesions) (necrosis) (parenchymatous) (ulcerative) A15.9
  with pneumoconiosis (any condition in J60-J64) J65
  abdomen (lymph gland) A18.39
  abscess (respiratory) A15.9
    bone A18.03
      hip A18.02
      knee A18.02
      sacrum A18.01
      specified site NEC A18.03
      spinal A18.01
      vertebra A18.01
    brain A17.81
    breast A18.89
    Cowper's gland A18.15
    dura (mater) (cerebral) (spinal) A17.81
    epidural (cerebral) (spinal) A17.81
    female pelvis A18.17
    frontal sinus A15.8
    genital organs NEC A18.10
    genitourinary A18.10
    gland (lymphatic) —see Tuberculosis, lymph gland
    hip A18.02
    intestine A18.32
    ischiorectal A18.32
    joint NEC A18.02
      hip A18.02
      knee A18.02
      specified NEC A18.02
      vertebral A18.01
    kidney A18.11
    knee A18.02
    latent R76.11
    lumbar (spine) A18.01
    lung —see Tuberculosis, pulmonary
    meninges (cerebral) (spinal) A17.0
    muscle A18.09
    perianal (fistula) A18.32
    perinephritic A18.11
    perirectal A18.32
    rectum A18.32
    retropharyngeal A15.8
    sacrum A18.01

Tuberculosis, tubercular, tuberculous
  (Continued)
  abscess (Continued)
    scrofulous A18.2
    scrotum A18.15
    skin (primary) A18.4
    spinal cord A17.81
    spine or vertebra (column) A18.01
    subdiaphragmatic A18.31
    testis A18.15
    urinary A18.13
    uterus A18.17
  accessory sinus —see Tuberculosis, sinus
  Addison's disease A18.7
  adenitis —see Tuberculosis, lymph gland
  adenoids A15.8
  adenopathy —see Tuberculosis, lymph gland
  adherent pericardium A18.84
  adnexa (uteri) A18.17
  adrenal (capsule) (gland) A18.7
  alimentary canal A18.32
  anemia A18.89
  ankle (joint) (bone) A18.02
  anus A18.32
  apex, apical —see Tuberculosis, pulmonary
  appendicitis, appendix A18.32
  arachnoid A17.0
  artery, arteritis A18.89
    cerebral A18.89
  arthritis (chronic) (synovial) A18.02
    spine or vertebra (column) A18.01
  articular —see Tuberculosis, joint
  ascites A18.31
  asthma —see Tuberculosis, pulmonary
  axilla, axillary (gland) A18.2
  bladder A18.12
  bone A18.03
    hip A18.02
    knee A18.02
    limb NEC A18.03
    sacrum A18.01
    spine or vertebral column A18.01
  bowel (miliary) A18.32
  brain A17.81
  breast A18.89
  broad ligament A18.17
  bronchi, bronchial, bronchus A15.5
    ectasia, ectasis (bronchiectasis) —see Tuberculosis, pulmonary
    fistula A15.5
      primary (progressive) A15.7
    gland or node A15.4
      primary (progressive) A15.7
    lymph gland or node A15.4
      primary (progressive) A15.7
  bronchiectasis —see Tuberculosis, pulmonary
  bronchitis A15.5
  bronchopleural A15.6
  bronchopneumonia, bronchopneumonic —see Tuberculosis, pulmonary
  bronchorrhagia A15.5
  bronchotracheal A15.5
  bronze disease A18.7
  buccal cavity A18.83
  bulbourethral gland A18.15
  bursa A18.09
  cachexia A15.9
  cardiomyopathy A18.84
  caries —see Tuberculosis, bone
  cartilage A18.02
    intervertebral A18.01
  catarrhal —see Tuberculosis, respiratory
  cecum A18.32
  cellulitis (primary) A18.4
  cerebellum A17.81
  cerebral, cerebrum A17.81
  cerebrospinal A17.81
    meninges A17.0
  cervical (lymph gland or node) A18.2
  cervicitis, cervix (uteri) A18.16
  chest —see Tuberculosis, respiratory

▶ New   ➡ Revised   ~~deleted~~ Deleted   ● Use Additional Character(s)

Tuberculosis, tubercular, tuberculous
  (Continued)
  chorioretinitis A18.53
  choroid, choroiditis A18.53
  ciliary body A18.54
  colitis A18.32
  collier's J65
  colliquativa (primary) A18.4
  colon A18.32
  complex, primary A15.7
  congenital P37.0
  conjunctiva A18.59
  connective tissue (systemic) A18.89
  contact Z20.1
  cornea (ulcer) A18.52
  Cowper's gland A18.15
  coxae A18.02
  coxalgia A18.02
  cul-de-sac of Douglas A18.17
  curvature, spine A18.01
  cutis (colliquativa) (primary) A18.4
  cyst, ovary A18.18
  cystitis A18.12
  dactylitis A18.03
  diarrhea A18.32
  diffuse —*see* Tuberculosis, miliary
  digestive tract A18.32
  disseminated —*see* Tuberculosis, miliary
  duodenum A18.32
  dura (mater) (cerebral) (spinal) A17.0
    abscess (cerebral) (spinal) A17.81
  dysentery A18.32
  ear (inner) (middle) A18.6
    bone A18.03
    external (primary) A18.4
    skin (primary) A18.4
  elbow A18.02
  emphysema —*see* Tuberculosis, pulmonary
  empyema A15.6
  encephalitis A17.82
  endarteritis A18.89
  endocarditis A18.84
    aortic A18.84
    mitral A18.84
    pulmonary A18.84
    tricuspid A18.84
  endocrine glands NEC A18.82
  endometrium A18.17
  enteric, enterica, enteritis A18.32
  enterocolitis A18.32
  epididymis, epididymitis A18.15
  epidural abscess (cerebral) (spinal) A17.81
  epiglottis A15.5
  episcleritis A18.51
  erythema (induratum) (nodosum) (primary)
    A18.4
  esophagus A18.83
  eustachian tube A18.6
  exposure (to) Z20.1
  exudative —*see* Tuberculosis, pulmonary
  eye A18.50
  eyelid (primary) (lupus) A18.4
  fallopian tube (acute) (chronic) A18.17
  fascia A18.09
  fauces A15.8
  female pelvic inflammatory disease A18.17
  finger A18.03
  first infection A15.7
  gallbladder A18.83
  ganglion A18.09
  gastritis A18.83
  gastrocolic fistula A18.32
  gastroenteritis A18.32
  gastrointestinal tract A18.32
  general, generalized —*see* Tuberculosis,
    miliary
  genital organs A18.10
  genitourinary A18.10
  genu A18.02
  glandula suprarenalis A18.7
  glandular, general A18.2

Tuberculosis, tubercular, tuberculous
  (Continued)
  glottis A15.5
  grinder's J65
  gum A18.83
  hand A18.03
  heart A18.84
  hematogenous —*see* Tuberculosis, miliary
  hemoptysis —*see* Tuberculosis, pulmonary
  hemorrhage NEC —*see* Tuberculosis,
    pulmonary
  hemothorax A15.6
  hepatitis A18.83
  hilar lymph nodes A15.4
    primary (progressive) A15.7
  hip (joint) (disease) (bone) A18.02
  hydropneumothorax A15.6
  hydrothorax A15.6
  hypoadrenalism A18.7
  hypopharynx A15.8
  ileocecal (hyperplastic) A18.32
  ileocolitis A18.32
  ileum A18.32
  iliac spine (superior) A18.03
  immunological findings only A15.7
  indurativa (primary) A18.4
  infantile A15.7
  infection A15.9
    without clinical manifestations A15.7
  infraclavicular gland A18.2
  inguinal gland A18.2
  inguinalis A18.2
  intestine (any part) A18.32
  iridocyclitis A18.54
  iris, iritis A18.54
  ischiorectal A18.32
  jaw A18.03
  jejunum A18.32
  joint A18.02
    vertebral A18.01
  keratitis (interstitial) A18.52
  keratoconjunctivitis A18.52
  kidney A18.11
  knee (joint) A18.02
  kyphosis, kyphoscoliosis A18.01
  laryngitis A15.5
  larynx A15.5
  latent R76.11
  leptomeninges, leptomeningitis (cerebral)
    (spinal) A17.0
  lichenoides (primary) A18.4
  linguae A18.83
  lip A18.83
  liver A18.83
  lordosis A18.01
  lung —*see* Tuberculosis, pulmonary
  lupus vulgaris A18.4
  lymph gland or node (peripheral) A18.2
    abdomen A18.39
    bronchial A15.4
      primary (progressive) A15.7
    cervical A18.2
    hilar A15.4
      primary (progressive) A15.7
    intrathoracic A15.4
      primary (progressive) A15.7
    mediastinal A15.4
      primary (progressive) A15.7
    mesenteric A18.39
    retroperitoneal A18.39
    tracheobronchial A15.4
      primary (progressive) A15.7
  lymphadenitis —*see* Tuberculosis, lymph
    gland
  lymphangitis —*see* Tuberculosis, lymph
    gland
  lymphatic (gland) (vessel) —*see* Tuberculosis,
    lymph gland
  mammary gland A18.89
  marasmus A15.9
  mastoiditis A18.03

Tuberculosis, tubercular, tuberculous
  (Continued)
  mediastinal lymph gland or node
    A15.4
    primary (progressive) A15.7
  mediastinitis A15.8
    primary (progressive) A15.7
  mediastinum A15.8
    primary (progressive) A15.7
  medulla A17.81
  melanosis, Addisonian A18.7
  meninges, meningitis (basilar) (cerebral)
    (cerebrospinal) (spinal) A17.0
  meningoencephalitis A17.82
  mesentery, mesenteric (gland or node)
    A18.39
  miliary A19.9
    acute A19.2
      multiple sites A19.1
      single specified site A19.0
    chronic A19.8
    specified NEC A19.8
  millstone makers' J65
  miner's J65
  molder's J65
  mouth A18.83
  multiple A19.9
    acute A19.1
    chronic A19.8
  muscle A18.09
  myelitis A17.82
  myocardium, myocarditis A18.84
  nasal (passage) (sinus) A15.8
  nasopharynx A15.8
  neck gland A18.2
  nephritis A18.11
  nerve (mononeuropathy) A17.83
  nervous system A17.9
  nose (septum) A15.8
  ocular A18.50
  omentum A18.31
  oophoritis (acute) (chronic) A18.17
  optic (nerve trunk) (papilla) A18.59
  orbit A18.59
  orchitis A18.15
  organ, specified NEC A18.89
  osseous —*see* Tuberculosis, bone
  osteitis —*see* Tuberculosis, bone
  osteomyelitis —*see* Tuberculosis, bone
  otitis media A18.6
  ovary, ovaritis (acute) (chronic) A18.17
  oviduct (acute) (chronic) A18.17
  pachymeningitis A17.0
  palate (soft) A18.83
  pancreas A18.83
  papulonecrotic (a) (primary) A18.4
  parathyroid glands A18.82
  paronychia (primary) A18.4
  parotid gland or region A18.83
  pelvis (bony) A18.03
  penis A18.15
  peribronchitis A15.5
  pericardium, pericarditis A18.84
  perichondritis, larynx A15.5
  periostitis —*see* Tuberculosis, bone
  perirectal fistula A18.32
  peritoneum NEC A18.31
  peritonitis A18.31
  pharynx, pharyngitis A15.8
  phlyctenulosis (keratoconjunctivitis) A18.52
  phthisis NEC —*see* Tuberculosis, pulmonary
  pituitary gland A18.82
  pleura, pleural, pleurisy, pleuritis (fibrinous)
    (obliterative) (purulent) (simple plastic)
    (with effusion) A15.6
    primary (progressive) A15.7
  pneumonia, pneumonic —*see* Tuberculosis,
    pulmonary
  pneumothorax (spontaneous) (tense
    valvular) —*see* Tuberculosis, pulmonary
  polyneuropathy A17.89

Tuberculosis, tubercular, tuberculous
  (Continued)
  polyserositis A19.9
    acute A19.1
    chronic A19.8
  potter's J65
  prepuce A18.15
  primary (complex) A15.7
  proctitis A18.32
  prostate, prostatitis A18.14
  pulmonalis —*see* Tuberculosis, pulmonary
  pulmonary (cavitated) (fibrotic) (infiltrative)
      (nodular) A15.0
    childhood type or first infection A15.7
    primary (complex) A15.7
  pyelitis A18.11
  pyelonephritis A18.11
  pyemia —*see* Tuberculosis, miliary
  pyonephrosis A18.11
  pyopneumothorax A15.6
  pyothorax A15.6
  rectum (fistula) (with abscess) A18.32
  reinfection stage —*see* Tuberculosis,
      pulmonary
  renal A18.11
  renis A18.11
  respiratory A15.9
    primary A15.7
    specified site NEC A15.8
  retina, retinitis A18.53
  retroperitoneal (lymph gland or node)
      A18.39
  rheumatism NEC A18.09
  rhinitis A15.8
  sacroiliac (joint) A18.01
  sacrum A18.01
  salivary gland A18.83
  salpingitis (acute) (chronic) A18.17
  sandblaster's J65
  sclera A18.51
  scoliosis A18.01
  scrofulous A18.2
  scrotum A18.15
  seminal tract or vesicle A18.15
  senile A15.9
  septic —*see* Tuberculosis, miliary
  shoulder (joint) A18.02
    blade A18.03
  sigmoid A18.32
  sinus (any nasal) A15.8
    bone A18.03
    epididymis A18.15
  skeletal NEC A18.03
  skin (any site) (primary) A18.4
  small intestine A18.32
  soft palate A18.83
  spermatic cord A18.15
  spine, spinal (column) A18.01
    cord A17.81
      medulla A17.81
      membrane A17.0
      meninges A17.0
  spleen, splenitis A18.85
  spondylitis A18.01
  sternoclavicular joint A18.02
  stomach A18.83
  stonemason's J65
  subcutaneous tissue (cellular) (primary)
      A18.4
  subcutis (primary) A18.4
  subdeltoid bursa A18.83
  submaxillary (region) A18.83
  supraclavicular gland A18.2
  suprarenal (capsule) (gland) A18.7
  swelling, joint —*see also* category M01 (*see also*
      Tuberculosis, joint) A18.02
  symphysis pubis A18.02
  synovitis A18.09
    articular A18.02
    spine or vertebra A18.01
  systemic —*see* Tuberculosis, miliary

Tuberculosis, tubercular, tuberculous
  (Continued)
  tarsitis A18.4
  tendon (sheath) —*see* Tuberculosis,
      tenosynovitis
  tenosynovitis A18.09
    spine or vertebra A18.01
  testis A18.15
  throat A15.8
  thymus gland A18.82
  thyroid gland A18.81
  tongue A18.83
  tonsil, tonsillitis A15.8
  trachea, tracheal A15.5
    lymph gland or node A15.4
      primary (progressive) A15.7
  tracheobronchial A15.5
    lymph gland or node A15.4
      primary (progressive) A15.7
  tubal (acute) (chronic) A18.17
  tubular (skin) (primary) A18.4
    bowel or intestine A18.32
    specified NEC - code under Tuberculosis,
        by site
  unspecified site A15.9
  ureter A18.11
  urethra, urethral (gland) A18.13
  urinary organ or tract A18.13
  uterus A18.17
  uveal tract A18.54
  uvula A18.83
  vagina A18.18
  vas deferens A18.15
  verruca, verrucosa (cutis) (primary) A18.4
  vertebra (column) A18.01
  vesiculitis A18.15
  vulva A18.18
  wrist (joint) A18.02
Tuberculum
  Carabelli —*see* Note at K00.2
  occlusal —*see* Note at K00.2
  paramolare K00.2
Tuberosity, enitre maxillary M26.07
Tuberous sclerosis (brain) Q85.1
Tubo-ovarian —*see* condition
Tuboplasty, after previous sterilization
      Z31.0
  aftercare Z31.42
Tubotympanitis, catarrhal (chronic) —*see* Otitis,
      media, nonsuppurative, chronic, serous
Tularemia A21.9
  with
    conjunctivitis A21.1
    pneumonia A21.2
  abdominal A21.3
  bronchopneumonic A21.2
  conjunctivitis A21.1
  cryptogenic A21.3
  enteric A21.3
  gastrointestinal A21.3
  generalized A21.7
  ingestion A21.3
  intestinal A21.3
  oculoglandular A21.1
  ophthalmic A21.1
  pneumonia (any), pneumonic A21.2
  pulmonary A21.2
  sepsis A21.7
  specified NEC A21.8
  typhoidal A21.7
  ulceroglandular A21.0
Tularensis conjunctivitis A21.1
Tumefaction —*see also* Swelling
  liver —*see* Hypertrophy, liver
Tumor —*see also* Neoplasm, unspecified
      behavior, by site
  acinar cell —*see* Neoplasm, uncertain
      behavior, by site
  acinic cell —*see* Neoplasm, uncertain
      behavior, by site

Tumor *(Continued)*
  adenocarcinoid —*see* Neoplasm, malignant,
      by site
  adenomatoid —*see also* Neoplasm, benign,
      by site
    odontogenic —*see* Cyst, calcifying
        odontogenic
  adnexal (skin) —*see* Neoplasm, skin, benign,
      by site
  adrenal
    cortical (benign) D35.0-●
      malignant C74.0-●
    rest —*see* Neoplasm, benign, by site
  alpha-cell
    malignant
      pancreas C25.4
      specified site NEC —*see* Neoplasm,
          malignant, by site
      unspecified site C25.4
    pancreas D13.7
    specified site NEC —*see* Neoplasm, benign,
        by site
    unspecified site D13.7
  aneurysmal —*see* Aneurysm
  aortic body D44.7
    malignant C75.5
  Askin's —*see* Neoplasm, connective tissue,
      malignant
  basal cell —*see also* Neoplasm, skin, uncertain
      behavior D48.5
  Bednar —*see* Neoplasm, skin, malignant
  benign (unclassified) —*see* Neoplasm, benign,
      by site
  beta-cell
    malignant
      pancreas C25.4
      specified site NEC —*see* Neoplasm,
          malignant, by site
      unspecified site C25.4
    pancreas D13.7
    specified site NEC —*see* Neoplasm, benign,
        by site
    unspecified site D13.7
  Brenner D27.9
    borderline malignancy D39.1-●
    malignant C56-●
    proliferating D39.1
  bronchial alveolar, intravascular D38.1
  Brooke's —*see* Neoplasm, skin, benign
  brown fat —*see* Lipoma
  Burkitt —*see* Lymphoma, Burkitt
  calcifying epithelial odontogenic —*see* Cyst,
      calcifying odontogenic
  carcinoid
    benign D3A.00
      appendix D3A.020
      ascending colon D3A.022
      bronchus (lung) D3A.090
      cecum D3A.021
      colon D3A.029
      descending colon D3A.024
      duodenum D3A.010
      foregut NOS D3A.094
      hindgut NOS D3A.096
      ileum D3A.012
      jejunum D3A.011
      kidney D3A.093
      large intestine D3A.029
      lung (bronchus) D3A.090
      midgut NOS D3A.095
      rectum D3A.026
      sigmoid colon D3A.025
      small intestine D3A.019
      specified NEC D3A.098
      stomach D3A.092
      thymus D3A.091
      transverse colon D3A.023
    malignant C7A.00
      appendix C7A.020
      ascending colon C7A.022
      bronchus (lung) C7A.090

▶ New ⇒ Revised ~~deleted~~ Deleted ● Use Additional Character(s)

Tumor *(Continued)*
  carcinoid *(Continued)*
    malignant *(Continued)*
      cecum C7A.021
      colon C7A.029
      descending colon C7A.024
      duodenum C7A.010
      foregut NOS C7A.094
      hindgut NOS C7A.096
      ileum C7A.012
      jejunum C7A.011
      kidney C7A.093
      large intestine C7A.029
      lung (bronchus) C7A.090
      midgut NOS C7A.095
      rectum C7A.026
      sigmoid colon C7A.025
      small intestine C7A.019
      specified NEC C7A.098
      stomach C7A.092
      thymus C7A.091
      transverse colon C7A.023
    mesentary metastasis C7B.04
    secondary C7B.00
      bone C7B.03
      distant lymph nodes C7B.01
      liver C7B.02
      peritoneum C7B.04
      specified NEC C7B.09
  carotid body D44.6
    malignant C75.4
  cells —*see also* Neoplasm, unspecified
    behavior, by site
    benign —*see* Neoplasm, benign,
      by site
    malignant —*see* Neoplasm, malignant,
      by site
    uncertain whether benign or malignant —
      see Neoplasm, uncertain behavior,
      by site
  cervix, in pregnancy or childbirth —*see*
    Pregnancy, complicated by, tumor,
    cervix
  chondromatous giant cell —*see* Neoplasm,
    bone, benign
  chromaffin —*see also* Neoplasm, benign, by
    site
    malignant —*see* Neoplasm, malignant, by
      site
  Cock's peculiar L72.3
  Codman's —*see* Neoplasm, bone, benign
  dentigerous, mixed —*see* Cyst, calcifying
    odontogenic
  dermoid —*see* Neoplasm, benign,
    by site
    with malignant transformation C56-●
  desmoid (extra-abdominal) —*see also*
    Neoplasm, connective tissue, uncertain
    behavior
    abdominal —*see* Neoplasm, connective
      tissue, uncertain behavior
  embolus —*see* Neoplasm, secondary,
    by site
  embryonal (mixed) —*see also* Neoplasm,
    uncertain behavior, by site
    liver C22.7
  endodermal sinus
    specified site —*see* Neoplasm, malignant,
      by site
    unspecified site
      female C56.-●
      male C62.90
  epithelial
    benign —*see* Neoplasm, benign,
      by site
    malignant —*see* Neoplasm, malignant, by
      site
  Ewing's —*see* Neoplasm, bone, malignant,
    by site
  fatty —*see* Lipoma
  fibroid —*see* Leiomyoma

Tumor *(Continued)*
  G cell
    malignant
      pancreas C25.4
      specified site NEC —*see* Neoplasm,
        malignant, by site
      unspecified site C25.4
    specified site —*see* Neoplasm, uncertain
      behavior, by site
    unspecified site D37.8
  germ cell —*see also* Neoplasm, malignant,
    by site
    mixed —*see* Neoplasm, malignant,
      by site
  ghost cell, odontogenic —*see* Cyst, calcifying
    odontogenic
  giant cell —*see also* Neoplasm, uncertain
    behavior, by site
    bone D48.0
      malignant —*see* Neoplasm, bone,
        malignant
    chondromatous —*see* Neoplasm, bone,
      benign
    malignant —*see* Neoplasm, malignant, by
      site
    soft parts —*see* Neoplasm, connective
      tissue, uncertain behavior
      malignant —*see* Neoplasm, connective
        tissue, malignant
  glomus D18.00
    intra-abdominal D18.03
    intracranial D18.02
    jugulare D44.7
      malignant C75.5
    skin D18.01
    specified site NEC D18.09
  gonadal stromal —*see* Neoplasm, uncertain
    behavior, by site
  granular cell —*see also* Neoplasm, connective
    tissue, benign
    malignant —*see* Neoplasm, connective
      tissue, malignant
  granulosa cell D39.1-●
    juvenile D39.1-●
    malignant C56-●
  granulosa cell-theca cell D39.1-●
    malignant C56-●
  Grawitz's C64-●
  hemorrhoidal —*see* Hemorrhoids
  hilar cell D27-●
  hilus cell D27-●
  Hurthle cell (benign) D34
    malignant C73
  hydatid —*see* Echinococcus
  hypernephroid —*see also* Neoplasm,
    uncertain behavior, by site
  interstitial cell —*see also* Neoplasm, uncertain
    behavior, by site
    benign —*see* Neoplasm, benign, by site
    malignant —*see* Neoplasm, malignant, by
      site
  intravascular bronchial alveolar D38.1
  islet cell —*see* Neoplasm, benign, by site
    malignant —*see* Neoplasm, malignant, by
      site
      pancreas C25.4
      specified site NEC —*see* Neoplasm,
        malignant, by site
      unspecified site C25.4
    pancreas D13.7
    specified site NEC —*see* Neoplasm, benign,
      by site
    unspecified site D13.7
  juxtaglomerular D41.0-●
  Klatskin's C24.0
  Krukenberg's C79.6-●
  Leydig cell —*see* Neoplasm, uncertain
    behavior, by site
    benign —*see* Neoplasm, benign, by site
      specified site —*see* Neoplasm, benign,
        by site

Tumor *(Continued)*
  Leydig cell *(Continued)*
    benign *(Continued)*
      unspecified site
        female D27.9
        male D29.20
    malignant —*see* Neoplasm, malignant, by
      site
      specified site —*see* Neoplasm,
        malignant, by site
      unspecified site
        female C56.9
        male C62.90
    specified site —*see* Neoplasm, uncertain
      behavior, by site
    unspecified site
      female D39.10
      male D40.10
  lipid cell, ovary D27-●
  lipoid cell, ovary D27-●
  malignant —*see also* Neoplasm, malignant, by
    site C80.1
    fusiform cell (type) C80.1
    giant cell (type) C80.1
    localized, plasma cell —*see* Plasmacytoma,
      solitary
    mixed NEC C80.1
    small cell (type) C80.1
    spindle cell (type) C80.1
    unclassified C80.1
  ➡ mast cell D47.09
    ~~malignant C96.2~~
  melanotic, neuroectodermal —*see* Neoplasm,
    benign, by site
  Merkel cell —*see* Carcinoma, Merkel cell
  mesenchymal
    malignant —*see* Neoplasm, connective
      tissue, malignant
    mixed —*see* Neoplasm, connective tissue,
      uncertain behavior
  mesodermal, mixed —*see also* Neoplasm,
    malignant, by site
    liver C22.4
  mesonephric —*see also* Neoplasm, uncertain
    behavior, by site
    malignant —*see* Neoplasm, malignant, by
      site
  metastatic
    from specified site —*see* Neoplasm,
      malignant, by site
    of specified site —*see* Neoplasm,
      malignant, by site
    to specified site —*see* Neoplasm, secondary,
      by site
  mixed NEC —*see also* Neoplasm, benign, by
    site
    malignant —*see* Neoplasm, malignant, by
      site
  mucinous of low malignant potential
    specified site —*see* Neoplasm, malignant,
      by site
    unspecified site C56.9
  mucocarcinoid
    specified site —*see* Neoplasm, malignant,
      by site
    unspecified site C18.1
  mucoepidermoid —*see* Neoplasm, uncertain
    behavior, by site
  Müllerian, mixed
    specified site —*see* Neoplasm, malignant,
      by site
    unspecified site C54.9
  myoepithelial —*see* Neoplasm, benign,
    by site
  neuroectodermal (peripheral) —*see*
    Neoplasm, malignant, by site
  primitive
    specified site —*see* Neoplasm,
      malignant,
      by site
    unspecified site C71.9

Tumor *(Continued)*
　neuroendocrine D3A.8
　　malignant poorly differentiated C7A.1
　　secondary NEC C7B.8
　　specified NEC C7A.8
　neurogenic olfactory C30.0
　nonencapsulated sclerosing C73
　odontogenic (adenomatoid) (benign)
　　　(calcifying epithelial) (keratocystic)
　　　(squamous) —*see* Cyst, calcifying
　　　odontogenic
　　malignant C41.1
　　　upper jaw (bone) C41.0
　ovarian stromal D39.1-●
　ovary, in pregnancy —*see* Pregnancy,
　　complicated by
　pacinian —*see* Neoplasm, skin, benign
　Pancoast's —*see* Pancoast's syndrome
　papillary —*see also* Papilloma
　　cystic D37.9
　　mucinous of low malignant potential C56-●
　　　specified site —*see* Neoplasm,
　　　　malignant, by site
　　　unspecified site C56.9
　　serous of low malignant potential
　　　specified site —*see* Neoplasm,
　　　　malignant, by site
　　　unspecified site C56.9
　pelvic, in pregnancy or childbirth —*see*
　　Pregnancy, complicated by
　phantom F45.8
　phyllodes D48.6-●
　　benign D24-●
　　malignant —*see* Neoplasm, breast,
　　　malignant
　Pindborg —*see* Cyst, calcifying odontogenic
　placental site trophoblastic D39.2
　plasma cell (malignant) (localized) —*see*
　　Plasmacytoma, solitary
　polyvesicular vitelline
　　specified site —*see* Neoplasm, malignant,
　　　by site
　　unspecified site
　　　female C56.9
　　　male C62.90
　Pott's puffy —*see* Osteomyelitis, specified NEC
　Rathke's pouch D44.3
　retinal anlage —*see* Neoplasm, benign, by site
　salivary gland type, mixed —*see* Neoplasm,
　　salivary gland, benign
　　malignant —*see* Neoplasm, salivary gland,
　　　malignant
　Sampson's N80.1
　Schmincke's —*see* Neoplasm, nasopharynx,
　　malignant
　sclerosing stromal D27-●
　sebaceous —*see* Cyst, sebaceous
　secondary —*see* Neoplasm, secondary, by site
　　carcinoid C7B.00
　　　bone C7B.03
　　　distant lymph nodes C7B.01
　　　liver C7B.02
　　　peritoneum C7B.04
　　　specified NEC C7B.09
　　neuroendocrine NEC C7B.8
　serous of low malignant potential
　　specified site —*see* Neoplasm, malignant,
　　　by site
　　unspecified site C56.9
　Sertoli cell —*see* Neoplasm, benign, by site
　　with lipid storage
　　　specified site —*see* Neoplasm, benign,
　　　　by site
　　　unspecified site
　　　　female D27.9
　　　　male D29.20
　　specified site —*see* Neoplasm, benign, by
　　　site
　　unspecified site
　　　female D27.9
　　　male D29.20

Tumor *(Continued)*
　Sertoli-Leydig cell —*see* Neoplasm, benign,
　　by site
　　specified site —*see* Neoplasm, benign, by
　　　site
　　unspecified site
　　　female D27.9
　　　male D29.20
　sex cord(-stromal) —*see* Neoplasm, uncertain
　　behavior, by site
　　with annular tubules D39.1-●
　skin appendage —*see* Neoplasm, skin,
　　benign
　smooth muscle —*see* Neoplasm, connective
　　tissue, uncertain behavior
　soft tissue
　　benign —*see* Neoplasm, connective tissue,
　　　benign
　　malignant —*see* Neoplasm, connective
　　　tissue, malignant
　sternomastoid (congenital) Q68.0
　stromal
　　endometrial D39.0
　　gastric D48.1
　　　benign D21.4
　　　malignant C16.9
　　　uncertain behavior D48.1
　　gastrointestinal C49.A-●
　　　benign D21.4
　　　esophagus C49.A1
　　　large intestine C49.A4
　　　malignant C49.A0
　　　　colon C49.A4
　　　　duodenum C49.A3
　　　　esophagus C49.A1
　　　　ileum C49.A3
　　　　jejunum C49.A3
　　　　Meckel diverticulum C49.A3
　　　　large intestine C49.A4
　　　　omentum C49.A9
　　　　peritoneum C49.A9
　　　　rectum C49.A5
　　　　small intestine C49.A3
　　　　specified site NEC C49.A9
　　　　stomach C49.A2
　　　large intestine C49.A4
　　　rectum C49.A5
　　　small intestine C49.A3
　　　specified site NEC C49.A9
　　　stomach C49.A2
　　　uncertain behavior D48.1
　　intestine
　　　benign D21.4
　　　malignant
　　　　large C49.A4
　　　　small C49.A3
　　　uncertain behavior D48.1
　　ovarian D39.1-●
　　stomach C49.A2
　　　benign D21.4
　　　malignant C49.A2
　　　uncertain behavior D48.1
　sweat gland —*see also* Neoplasm, skin,
　　uncertain behavior
　　benign —*see* Neoplasm, skin, benign
　　malignant —*see* Neoplasm, skin, malignant
　syphilitic, brain A52.17
　testicular D40.10
　testicular stromal D40.1-●
　theca cell D27.-●
　theca cell-granulosa cell D39.1-●
　Triton, malignant —*see* Neoplasm, nerve,
　　malignant
　trophoblastic, placental site D39.2
　turban D23.4
　uterus (body), in pregnancy or childbirth —
　　see Pregnancy, complicated by, tumor,
　　uterus
　vagina, in pregnancy or childbirth —*see*
　　Pregnancy, complicated by
　varicose —*see* Varix

Tumor *(Continued)*
　von Recklinghausen's —*see*
　　Neurofibromatosis
　vulva or perineum, in pregnancy or
　　childbirth —*see* Pregnancy, complicated
　　by
　　causing obstructed labor O65.5
　Warthin's —*see* Neoplasm, salivary gland,
　　benign
　Wilms' C64-●
　yolk sac —*see* Neoplasm, malignant, by site
　　specified site —*see* Neoplasm, malignant,
　　　by site
　　unspecified site
　　　female C56.9
　　　male C62.90
Tumor lysis syndrome (following
　antineoplastic chemotherapy)
　(spontaneous) NEC E88.3
Tumorlet —*see* Neoplasm, uncertain behavior,
　by site
Tungiasis B88.1
Tunica vasculosa lentis Q12.2
Turban tumor D23.4
Türck's trachoma J37.0
Turner-Kieser syndrome Q87.2
Turner-like syndrome Q87.1
Turner's
　hypoplasia (tooth) K00.4
　syndrome Q96.9
　　specified NEC Q96.8
　tooth K00.4
Turner-Ullrich syndrome Q96.9
Tussis convulsiva —*see* Whooping cough
Twiddler's syndrome (due to)
　automatic implantable defibrillator T82.198
　cardiac pacemaker T82.198
Twilight state
　epileptic F05
　psychogenic F44.89
Twin (newborn) —*see also* Newborn, twin
　conjoined Q89.4
▶pregnancy —*see* Pregnancy, twin
Twinning, teeth K00.2
Twist, twisted
　bowel, colon or intestine K56.2
　hair (congenital) Q84.1
　mesentery K56.2
　omentum K56.2
　organ or site, congenital NEC —*see* Anomaly,
　　by site
　ovarian pedicle —*see* Torsion, ovary
Twitching R25.3
Tylosis (acquired) L84
　buccalis K13.29
　linguae K13.29
　palmaris et plantaris (congenital) (inherited)
　　Q82.8
　　acquired L85.1
Tympanism R14.0
Tympanites (abdominal) (intestinal) R14.0
Tympanitis —*see* Myringitis
Tympanosclerosis —*see* subcategory H74.0
Tympanum —*see* condition
Tympany
　abdomen R14.0
　chest R09.89
Type A behavior pattern Z73.1
Typhlitis —*see* Appendicitis
Typhoenteritis —*see* Typhoid
Typhoid (abortive) (ambulant) (any site)
　　(clinical) (fever) (hemorrhagic) (infection)
　　(intermittent) (malignant) (rheumatic)
　　(Widal negative) A01.00
　with pneumonia A01.03
　abdominal A01.09
　arthritis A01.04
　carrier (suspected) of Z22.0
　cholecystitis (current) A01.09
　endocarditis A01.02
　heart involvement A01.02

▶ New　⇒ Revised　~~deleted~~ Deleted　● Use Additional Character(s)

Typhoid *(Continued)*
   inoculation reaction —*see* Complications,
      vaccination
   meningitis A01.01
   mesenteric lymph nodes A01.09
   myocarditis A01.02
   osteomyelitis A01.05
   perichondritis, larynx A01.09
   pneumonia A01.03
   specified NEC A01.09
   spine A01.05
   ulcer (perforating) A01.09
Typhomalaria (fever) —*see* Malaria
Typhomania A01.00
Typhoperitonitis A01.09
Typhus (fever) A75.9
   abdominal, abdominalis —*see* Typhoid
   African tick A77.1
   amarillic A95.9
   brain A75.9 *[G94]*

Typhus *(Continued)*
   cerebral A75.9 *[G94]*
   classical A75.0
   due to Rickettsia
      prowazekii A75.0
         recrudescent A75.1
      tsutsugamushi A75.3
      typhi A75.2
   endemic (flea-borne) A75.2
   epidemic (louse-borne) A75.0
   exanthematic NEC A75.0
   exanthematicus SAI A75.0
      brillii SAI A75.1
      mexicanus SAI A75.2
      typhus murinus A75.2
   flea-borne A75.2
   India tick A77.1
   Kenya (tick) A77.1
   louse-borne A75.0
   Mexican A75.2

Typhus *(Continued)*
   mite-borne A75.3
   murine A75.2
   North Asian tick-borne A77.2
   petechial A75.9
   Queensland tick A77.3
   rat A75.2
   recrudescent A75.1
   recurrens —*see* Fever, relapsing
   Sao Paulo A77.0
   scrub (China) (India) (Malaysia) (New
      Guinea) A75.3
   shop (of Malaysia) A75.2
   Siberian tick A77.2
   tick-borne A77.9
   tropical (mite-borne) A75.3
Tyrosinemia E70.21
   newborn, transitory P74.5
Tyrosinosis E70.21
Tyrosinuria E70.29

U

Uhl's anomaly or disease Q24.8
Ulcer, ulcerated, ulcerating, ulceration, ulcerative
  alveolar process M27.3
  amebic (intestine) A06.1
    skin A06.7
  anastomotic —see Ulcer, gastrojejunal
  anorectal K62.6
  antral —see Ulcer, stomach
  anus (sphincter) (solitary) K62.6
  aorta —see Aneurysm
  aphthous (oral) (recurrent) K12.0
    genital organ(s)
      female N76.6
      male N50.89
  artery I77.2
  atrophic —see Ulcer, skin
    decubitus —see Ulcer, pressure, by site
  back L98.429
    with
      ►bone involvement without evidence of
          necrosis L98.426
      bone necrosis L98.424
      exposed fat layer L98.422
      ►muscle involvement without evidence of
          necrosis L98.425
      muscle necrosis L98.423
      skin breakdown only L98.421
      ►specified severity NEC L98.428
  Barrett's (esophagus) K22.10
    with bleeding K22.11
  bile duct (common) (hepatic) K83.8
  bladder (solitary) (sphincter) NEC N32.89
    bilharzial B65.9 [N33]
    in schistosomiasis (bilharzial) B65.9 [N33]
    submucosal —see Cystitis, interstitial
    tuberculous A18.12
  bleeding K27.4
  bone —see Osteomyelitis, specified type NEC
  bowel —see Ulcer, intestine
  breast N61.1
  bronchus J98.09
  buccal (cavity) (traumatic) K12.1
  Buruli A31.1
  buttock L98.419
    with
      ►bone involvement without evidence of
          necrosis L98.416
      bone necrosis L98.414
      exposed fat layer L98.412
      ►muscle involvement without evidence of
          necrosis L98.415
      muscle necrosis L98.413
      skin breakdown only L98.411
      ►specified severity NEC L98.418
  cancerous —see Neoplasm, malignant, by site
  cardia K22.10
    with bleeding K22.11
  cardioesophageal (peptic) K22.10
    with bleeding K22.11
  cecum —see Ulcer, intestine
  cervix (uteri) (decubitus) (trophic) N86
    with cervicitis N72
  chancroidal A57
  chiclero B55.1
  chronic (cause unknown) —see Ulcer, skin
  Cochin-China B55.1
  colon —see Ulcer, intestine
  conjunctiva H10.89
  cornea H16.00-●
    with hypopyon H16.03-●
    central H16.01-●
    dendritic (herpes simplex) B00.52
    marginal H16.04-●
    Mooren's H16.05-●
    mycotic H16.06-●
    perforated H16.07-●
    ring H16.02-●
    tuberculous (phlyctenular) A18.52

Ulcer, ulcerated, ulcerating, ulceration, ulcerative (Continued)
  corpus cavernosum (chronic) N48.5
  crural —see Ulcer, lower limb
  Curling's —see Ulcer, peptic, acute
  Cushing's —see Ulcer, peptic, acute
  cystic duct K82.8
  cystitis (interstitial) —see Cystitis, interstitial
  decubitus —see Ulcer, pressure, by site
  dendritic, cornea (herpes simplex) B00.52
  diabetes, diabetic —see Diabetes, ulcer
  Dieulafoy's K25.0
  due to
    infection NEC —see Ulcer, skin
    radiation NEC L59.8
    trophic disturbance (any region) —see
        Ulcer, skin
    X-ray L58.1
  duodenum, duodenal (eroded) (peptic) K26.9
    with
      hemorrhage K26.4
        and perforation K26.6
      perforation K26.5
    acute K26.3
      with
        hemorrhage K26.0
          and perforation K26.2
        perforation K26.1
    chronic K26.7
      with
        hemorrhage K26.4
          and perforation K26.6
        perforation K26.5
  dysenteric A09
  elusive —see Cystitis, interstitial
  endocarditis (acute) (chronic) (subacute) I28.8
  epiglottis J38.7
  esophagus (peptic) K22.10
    with bleeding K22.11
    due to
      aspirin K22.10
        with bleeding K22.11
      gastrointestinal reflux disease K21.0
      ingestion of chemical or medicament
          K22.10
        with bleeding K22.11
      fungal K22.10
        with bleeding K22.11
      infective K22.10
        with bleeding K22.11
    varicose —see Varix, esophagus
  eyelid (region) H01.8
  fauces J39.2
  Fenwick (-Hunner) (solitary) —see Cystitis,
      interstitial
  fistulous —see Ulcer, skin
  foot (indolent) (trophic) —see Ulcer, lower
      limb
  frambesial, initial A66.0
  frenum (tongue) K14.0
  gallbladder or duct K82.8
  gangrenous —see Gangrene
  gastric —see Ulcer, stomach
  gastrocolic —see Ulcer, gastrojejunal
  gastroduodenal —see Ulcer, peptic
  gastroesophageal —see Ulcer, stomach
  gastrointestinal —see Ulcer, gastrojejunal
  gastrojejunal (peptic) K28.9
    with
      hemorrhage K28.4
        and perforation K28.6
      perforation K28.5
    acute K28.3
      with
        hemorrhage K28.0
          and perforation K28.2
        perforation K28.1
    chronic K28.7
      with
        hemorrhage K28.4
          and perforation K28.6
        perforation K28.5

Ulcer, ulcerated, ulcerating, ulceration, ulcerative (Continued)
  gastrojejunocolic —see Ulcer,
      gastrojejunal
  gingiva K06.8
  gingivitis K05.10
    nonplaque induced K05.11
    plaque induced K05.10
  glottis J38.7
  granuloma of pudenda A58
  gum K06.8
  gumma, due to yaws A66.4
  heel —see Ulcer, lower limb
  hemorrhoid —see also Hemorrhoids, by
      degree K64.8
  Hunner's —see Cystitis, interstitial
  hypopharynx J39.2
  hypopyon (chronic) (subacute) —see Ulcer,
      cornea, with hypopyon
  hypostaticum —see Ulcer, varicose
  ileum —see Ulcer, intestine
  intestine, intestinal K63.3
    with perforation K63.1
    amebic A06.1
    duodenal —see Ulcer, duodenum
    granulocytopenic (with hemorrhage) —see
        Neutropenia
    marginal —see Ulcer, gastrojejunal
    perforating K63.1
      newborn P78.0
    primary, small intestine K63.3
    rectum K62.6
    stercoraceous, stercoral K63.3
    tuberculous A18.32
    typhoid (fever) —see Typhoid
    varicose I86.8
  jejunum, jejunal —see Ulcer, gastrojejunal
  keratitis —see Ulcer, cornea
  knee —see Ulcer, lower limb
  labium (majus) (minus) N76.6
  laryngitis —see Laryngitis
  larynx (aphthous) (contact) J38.7
    diphtheritic A36.2
  leg —see Ulcer, lower limb
  lip K13.0
  Lipschütz's N76.6
  lower limb (atrophic) (chronic) (neurogenic)
      (perforating) (pyogenic) (trophic)
      (tropical) L97.909
    with
      ►bone involvement without evidence of
          necrosis L97.906
      bone necrosis L97.904
      exposed fat layer L97.902
      ►muscle involvement without evidence of
          necrosis L97.905
      muscle necrosis L97.903
      skin breakdown only L97.901
      ►specified severity NEC L97.908
    ankle L97.309
      with
        ►bone involvement without evidence of
            necrosis L97.306
        bone necrosis L97.304
        exposed fat layer L97.302
        ►muscle involvement without evidence
            of necrosis L97.305
        muscle necrosis L97.303
        skin breakdown only L97.301
        ►specified severity NEC L97.308
      left L97.329
        with
          ►bone involvement without evidence
              of necrosis L97.326
          bone necrosis L97.324
          exposed fat layer L97.322
          ►muscle involvement without
              evidence of necrosis L97.325
          muscle necrosis L97.323
          skin breakdown only L97.321
          ►specified severity NEC L97.328

► New   ➡ Revised   ~~deleted~~ Deleted   ● Use Additional Character(s)

Ulcer, ulcerated, ulcerating, ulceration, ulcerative *(Continued)*
  lower limb *(Continued)*
    ankle *(Continued)*
      right L97.319
        with
        ▶bone involvement without evidence
          of necrosis L97.316
        bone necrosis L97.314
        exposed fat layer L97.312
        ▶muscle involvement without
          evidence of necrosis L97.315
        muscle necrosis L97.313
        skin breakdown only L97.311
        ▶specified severity NEC L97.318
    calf L97.209
      with
      ▶bone involvement without evidence of
        necrosis L97.206
      bone necrosis L97.204
      exposed fat layer L97.202
      ▶muscle involvement without evidence
        of necrosis L97.205
      muscle necrosis L97.203
      skin breakdown only L97.201
      ▶specified severity NEC L97.208
      left L97.229
        with
        ▶bone involvement without evidence
          of necrosis L97.226
        bone necrosis L97.224
        exposed fat layer L97.222
        ▶muscle involvement without
          evidence of necrosis L97.225
        muscle necrosis L97.223
        skin breakdown only L97.221
        ▶specified severity NEC L97.228
      right L97.219
        with
        ▶bone involvement without evidence
          of necrosis L97.216
        bone necrosis L97.214
        exposed fat layer L97.212
        ▶muscle involvement without
          evidence of necrosis L97.215
        muscle necrosis L97.213
        skin breakdown only L97.211
        ▶specified severity NEC L97.218
    decubitus —*see* Ulcer, pressure, by site
    foot specified NEC L97.509
      with
      ▶bone involvement without evidence of
        necrosis L97.506
      bone necrosis L97.504
      exposed fat layer L97.502
      ▶muscle involvement without evidence
        of necrosis L97.505
      muscle necrosis L97.503
      skin breakdown only L97.501
      ▶specified severity NEC L97.508
      left L97.529
        with
        ▶bone involvement without evidence of
          necrosis L97.526
        bone necrosis L97.524
        exposed fat layer L97.522
        ▶muscle involvement without
          evidence of necrosis L97.525
        muscle necrosis L97.523
        skin breakdown only L97.521
        ▶specified severity NEC L97.528
      right L97.519
        with
        ▶bone involvement without evidence
          of necrosis L97.516
        bone necrosis L97.514
        exposed fat layer L97.512
        ▶muscle involvement without
          evidence of necrosis L97.515
        muscle necrosis L97.513
        skin breakdown only L97.511
        ▶specified severity NEC L97.518

Ulcer, ulcerated, ulcerating, ulceration, ulcerative *(Continued)*
  lower limb *(Continued)*
    heel L97.409
      with
      ▶bone involvement without evidence of
        necrosis L97.406
      bone necrosis L97.404
      exposed fat layer L97.402
      ▶muscle involvement without evidence
        of necrosis L97.405
      muscle necrosis L97.403
      skin breakdown only L97.401
      ▶specified severity NEC L97.408
      left L97.429
        with
        ▶bone involvement without evidence
          of necrosis L97.426
        bone necrosis L97.424
        exposed fat layer L97.422
        ▶muscle involvement without
          evidence of necrosis L97.425
        muscle necrosis L97.423
        skin breakdown only L97.421
        ▶specified severity NEC L97.428
      right L97.419
        with
        ▶bone involvement without evidence
          of necrosis L97.416
        bone necrosis L97.414
        exposed fat layer L97.412
        ▶muscle involvement without
          evidence of necrosis L97.415
        muscle necrosis L97.413
        skin breakdown only L97.411
        ▶specified severity NEC L97.418
    left L97.929
      with
      ▶bone involvement without evidence of
        necrosis L97.926
      bone necrosis L97.924
      exposed fat layer L97.922
      ▶muscle involvement without evidence
        of necrosis L97.925
      muscle necrosis L97.923
      skin breakdown only L97.921
      ▶specified severity NEC L97.928
    lower leg NOS L97.909
      with
      ▶bone involvement without evidence of
        necrosis L97.906
      bone necrosis L97.904
      exposed fat layer L97.902
      ▶muscle involvement without evidence
        of necrosis L97.905
      muscle necrosis L97.903
      skin breakdown only L97.901
      ▶specified severity NEC L97.908
      left L97.929
        with
        ▶bone involvement without evidence
          of necrosis L97.926
        bone necrosis L97.924
        exposed fat layer L97.922
        ▶muscle involvement without
          evidence of necrosis L97.925
        muscle necrosis L97.923
        skin breakdown only L97.921
        ▶specified severity NEC L97.928
      right L97.919
        with
        ▶bone involvement without evidence
          of necrosis L97.916
        bone necrosis L97.914
        exposed fat layer L97.912
        ▶muscle involvement without
          evidence of necrosis L97.915
        muscle necrosis L97.913
        skin breakdown only L97.911
        ▶specified severity NEC L97.918
    specified site NEC L97.809

Ulcer, ulcerated, ulcerating, ulceration, ulcerative *(Continued)*
  lower limb *(Continued)*
    lower leg NOS *(Continued)*
      specified site NEC *(Continued)*
        with
        ▶bone involvement without evidence
          of necrosis L97.806
        bone necrosis L97.804
        exposed fat layer L97.802
        ▶muscle involvement without
          evidence of necrosis L97.805
        muscle necrosis L97.803
        skin breakdown only L97.801
        ▶specified severity NEC L97.808
      left L97.829
        with
        ▶bone involvement without
          evidence of necrosis L97.826
        bone necrosis L97.824
        exposed fat layer L97.822
        ▶muscle involvement without
          evidence of necrosis L97.825
        muscle necrosis L97.823
        skin breakdown only L97.821
        ▶specified severity NEC L97.828
      right L97.819
        with
        ▶bone involvement without
          evidence of necrosis L97.816
        bone necrosis L97.814
        exposed fat layer L97.812
        ▶muscle involvement without
          evidence of necrosis L97.815
        muscle necrosis L97.813
        skin breakdown only L97.811
        ▶specified severity NEC L97.818
    midfoot L97.409
      with
      ▶bone involvement without evidence of
        necrosis L97.406
      bone necrosis L97.404
      exposed fat layer L97.402
      ▶muscle involvement without evidence
        of necrosis L97.405
      muscle necrosis L97.403
      skin breakdown only L97.401
      ▶specified severity NEC L97.408
      left L97.429
        with
        ▶bone involvement without evidence
          of necrosis L97.426
        bone necrosis L97.424
        exposed fat layer L97.422
        ▶muscle involvement without
          evidence of necrosis L97.425
        muscle necrosis L97.423
        skin breakdown only L97.421
        ▶specified severity NEC L97.428
      right L97.419
        with
        ▶bone involvement without evidence
          of necrosis L97.416
        bone necrosis L97.414
        exposed fat layer L97.412
        ▶muscle involvement without
          evidence of necrosis L97.415
        muscle necrosis L97.413
        skin breakdown only L97.411
        ▶specified severity NEC L97.418
      right L97.919
        with
        ▶bone involvement without evidence of
        necrosis L97.916
        bone necrosis L97.914
        exposed fat layer L97.912
        ▶muscle involvement without evidence
         of necrosis L97.915
        muscle necrosis L97.913
        skin breakdown only L97.911
        ▶specified severity NEC L97.918

▶ New   ➭ Revised   ~~deleted~~ Deleted   ● Use Additional Character(s)

Ulcer, ulcerated, ulcerating, ulceration, ulcerative *(Continued)*
  lower limb *(Continued)*
    thigh L97.109
      with
      ▶bone involvement without evidence of necrosis L97.106
        bone necrosis L97.104
        exposed fat layer L97.102
      ▶muscle involvement without evidence of necrosis L97.105
        muscle necrosis L97.103
        skin breakdown only L97.101
      ▶specified severity NEC L97.108
      left L97.129
        with
        ▶bone involvement without evidence of necrosis L97.126
          bone necrosis L97.124
          exposed fat layer L97.122
        ▶muscle involvement without evidence of necrosis L97.125
          muscle necrosis L97.123
          skin breakdown only L97.121
        ▶specified severity NEC L97.128
      right L97.119
        with
        ▶bone involvement without evidence of necrosis L97.116
          bone necrosis L97.114
          exposed fat layer L97.112
        ▶muscle involvement without evidence of necrosis L97.115
          muscle necrosis L97.113
          skin breakdown only L97.111
        ▶specified severity NEC L97.118
    toe L97.509
      with
      ▶bone involvement without evidence of necrosis L97.506
        bone necrosis L97.504
        exposed fat layer L97.502
      ▶muscle involvement without evidence of necrosis L97.505
        muscle necrosis L97.503
        skin breakdown only L97.501
      ▶specified severity NEC L97.508
      left L97.529
        with
        ▶bone involvement without evidence of necrosis L97.526
          bone necrosis L97.524
          exposed fat layer L97.522
        ▶muscle involvement without evidence of necrosis L97.525
          muscle necrosis L97.523
          skin breakdown only L97.521
        ▶specified severity NEC L97.528
      right L97.519
        with
        ▶bone involvement without evidence of necrosis L97.516
          bone necrosis L97.514
          exposed fat layer L97.512
        ▶muscle involvement without evidence of necrosis L97.515
          muscle necrosis L97.513
          skin breakdown only L97.511
        ▶specified severity NEC L97.518
  leprous A30.1
  syphilitic A52.19
  varicose —*see* Varix, leg, with, ulcer
  luetic —*see* Ulcer, syphilitic
  lung J98.4
    tuberculous —*see* Tuberculosis, pulmonary
  malignant —*see* Neoplasm, malignant, by site
  marginal NEC —*see* Ulcer, gastrojejunal
  meatus (urinarius) N34.2
  Meckel's diverticulum Q43.0
    malignant —*see* Table of Neoplasms, small intestine, malignant

Ulcer, ulcerated, ulcerating, ulceration, ulcerative *(Continued)*
  Meleney's (chronic undermining) —*see* Ulcer, skin
  Mooren's (cornea) —*see* Ulcer, cornea, Mooren's
  mycobacterial (skin) A31.1
  nasopharynx J39.2
  neck, uterus N86
  neurogenic NEC —*see* Ulcer, skin
  nose, nasal (passage) (infective) (septum) J34.0
    skin —*see* Ulcer, skin
    spirochetal A69.8
    varicose (bleeding) I86.8
  oral mucosa (traumatic) K12.1
  palate (soft) K12.1
  penis (chronic) N48.5
  peptic (site unspecified) K27.9
    with
      hemorrhage K27.4
        and perforation K27.6
      perforation K27.5
    acute K27.3
      with
        hemorrhage K27.0
          and perforation K27.2
        perforation K27.1
    chronic K27.7
      with
        hemorrhage K27.4
          and perforation K27.6
        perforation K27.5
    esophagus K22.10
      with bleeding K22.11
    newborn P78.82
  perforating K27.5
    skin —*see* Ulcer, skin
  peritonsillar J35.8
  phagedenic (tropical) —*see* Ulcer, skin
  pharynx J39.2
  phlebitis —*see* Phlebitis
  plaster —*see* Ulcer, pressure, by site
  popliteal space —*see* Ulcer, lower limb
  postpyloric —*see* Ulcer, duodenum
  prepuce N47.7
  prepyloric —*see* Ulcer, stomach
  pressure (pressure area) L89.9-●
    ankle L89.5-●
    back L89.1-●
    buttock L89.3-●
    coccyx L89.15-●
    contiguous site of back, buttock, hip L89.4-●
    elbow L89.0-●
    face L89.81-●
    head L89.81-●
    heel L89.6-●
    hip L89.2-●
    sacral region (tailbone) L89.15-●
    specified site NEC L89.89-●
    stage 1 (healing) (pre-ulcer skin changes limited to persistent focal edema)
      ankle L89.5-●
      back L89.1-●
      buttock L89.3-●
      coccyx L89.15-●
      contiguous site of back, buttock, hip L89.4-●
      elbow L89.0-●
      face L89.81-●
      head L89.81-●
      heel L89.6-●
      hip L89.2-●
      sacral region (tailbone) L89.15-●
      specified site NEC L89.89-●
    stage 2 (healing) (abrasion, blister, partial thickness skin loss involving epidermis and/or dermis)
      ankle L89.5-●
      back L89.1-●
      buttock L89.3-●

Ulcer, ulcerated, ulcerating, ulceration, ulcerative *(Continued)*
  pressure *(Continued)*
    stage 2 *(Continued)*
      coccyx L89.15-●
      contiguous site of back, buttock, hip L89.4-●
      elbow L89.0-●
      face L89.81-●
      head L89.81-●
      heel L89.6-●
      hip L89.2-●
      sacral region (tailbone) L89.15-●
      specified site NEC L89.89-●
    stage 3 (healing) (full thickness skin loss involving damage or necrosis of subcutaneous tissue)
      ankle L89.5-●
      back L89.1-●
      buttock L89.3-●
      coccyx L89.15-●
      contiguous site of back, buttock, hip L89.4-●
      elbow L89.0-●
      face L89.81-●
      head L89.81-●
      heel L89.6-●
      hip L89.2-●
      sacral region (tailbone) L89.15-●
      specified site NEC L89.89-●
    stage 4 (healing) (necrosis of soft tissues through to underlying muscle, tendon, or bone)
      ankle L89.5-●
      back L89.1-●
      buttock L89.3-●
      coccyx L89.15-●
      contiguous site of back, buttock, hip L89.4-●
      elbow L89.0-●
      face L89.81-●
      head L89.81-●
      heel L89.6-●
      hip L89.2-●
      sacral region (tailbone) L89.15-●
      specified site NEC L89.89-●
    unspecified stage
      ankle L89.5-●
      back L89.1-●
      buttock L89.3-●
      coccyx L89.15-●
      contiguous site of back, buttock, hip L89.4-●
      elbow L89.0-●
      face L89.81-●
      head L89.81-●
      heel L89.6-●
      hip L89.2-●
      sacral region (tailbone) L89.15-●
      specified site NEC L89.89-●
    unstageable
      ankle L89.5-●
      back L89.1-●
      buttock L89.3-●
      coccyx L89.15-●
      contiguous site of back, buttock, hip L89.4-●
      elbow L89.0-●
      face L89.81-●
      head L89.81-●
      heel L89.6-●
      hip L89.2-●
      sacral region (tailbone) L89.15-●
      specified site NEC L89.89-●
  primary of intestine K63.3
    with perforation K63.1
  prostate N41.9
  pyloric —*see* Ulcer, stomach
  rectosigmoid K63.3
    with perforation K63.1
  rectum (sphincter) (solitary) K62.6
    stercoraceous, stercoral K62.6

▶ New   ⇒ Revised   ~~deleted~~ Deleted   ● Use Additional Character(s)

Untruthfulness, child problem F91.8
Unverricht(-Lundborg) disease or epilepsy —
   see Epilepsy, generalized, idiopathic
Unwanted pregnancy Z64.0
Upbringing, institutional Z62.22
   away from parents NEC Z62.29
   in care of non-parental family member Z62.21
   in foster care Z62.21
   in orphanage or group home Z62.22
   in welfare custody Z62.21
Upper respiratory —see condition
Upset
   gastric K30
   gastrointestinal K30
      psychogenic F45.8
   intestinal (large) (small) K59.9
      psychogenic F45.8
   menstruation N93.9
   mental F48.9
   stomach K30
      psychogenic F45.8
Urachus —see also condition
   patent or persistent Q64.4
Urbach-Oppenheim disease (necrobiosis
   lipoidica diabeticorum) —see E08-E13 with
   .620
Urbach's lipoid proteinosis E78.89
Urbach-Wiethe disease E78.89
Urban yellow fever A95.1
Urea
   blood, high —see Uremia
   cycle metabolism disorder —see Disorder,
      urea cycle metabolism
Uremia, uremic N19
   with
      ectopic or molar pregnancy O08.4
      polyneuropathy N18.9 [G63]
   chronic — see also Disease, kidney, chronic
      N18.9
   due to hypertension — see Hypertensive,
      kidney
   ▶chronic NOS —see also Disease, kidney,
      chronic N18.9
      ▶due to hypertension —see Hypertensive,
         kidney
   complicating
      ectopic or molar pregnancy O08.4
   congenital P96.0
   extrarenal R39.2
   following ectopic or molar pregnancy O08.4
   newborn P96.0
   prerenal R39.2
Ureter, ureteral —see condition
Ureteralgia N23
Ureterectasis —see Hydroureter
Ureteritis N28.89
   cystica N28.86
   due to calculus N20.1
      with calculus, kidney N20.2
         with hydronephrosis N13.2
   gonococcal (acute) (chronic) A54.21
   nonspecific N28.89
Ureterocele N28.89
   congenital (orthotopic) Q62.31
      ectopic Q62.32
Ureterolith, ureterolithiasis —see Calculus,
   ureter
Ureterostomy
   attention to Z43.6
   status Z93.6
Urethra, urethral —see condition
Urethralgia R39.89
Urethritis (anterior) (posterior) N34.2
   calculous N21.1
   candidal B37.41
   chlamydial A56.01
   diplococcal (gonococcal) A54.01
      with abscess (accessory gland)
         (periurethral) A54.1
   gonococcal A54.01
      with abscess (accessory gland)
         (periurethral) A54.1

Urethritis (Continued)
   nongonococcal N34.1
      Reiter's —see Reiter's disease
   nonspecific N34.1
   nonvenereal N34.1
   postmenopausal N34.2
   puerperal O86.22
   Reiter's —see Reiter's disease
   specified NEC N34.2
   trichomonal or due to Trichomonas
      (vaginalis) A59.03
Urethrocele N81.0
   with
      cystocele —see Cystocele
      prolapse of uterus —see Prolapse, uterus
Urethrolithiasis (with colic or infection) N21.1
Urethrorectal —see condition
Urethrorrhagia N36.8
Urethrorrhea R36.9
Urethrostomy
   attention to Z43.6
   status Z93.6
Urethrotrigonitis —see Trigonitis
Urethrovaginal —see condition
Urgency
   fecal R15.2
   hypertensive —see Hypertension
   urinary N39.15
Urhidrosis, uridrosis L74.8
Uric acid in blood (increased) E79.0
Uricacidemia (asymptomatic) E79.0
Uricemia (asymptomatic) E79.0
Uricosuria R82.99
Urinary —see condition
Urination
   frequent R35.0
   painful R30.9
Urine
   blood in —see Hematuria
   discharge, excessive R35.8
   enuresis, nonorganic origin F98.0
   extravasation R39.0
   frequency R35.0
   incontinence R32
      nonorganic origin F98.0
   intermittent stream R39.198
   pus in N39.0
   retention or stasis R33.9
      organic R33.8
         drug-induced R33.0
      psychogenic F45.8
   secretion
      deficient R34
      excessive R35.8
      frequency R35.0
   stream
      intermittent R39.198
      slowing R39.198
      splitting R39.13
      weak R39.12
Urinemia —see Uremia
Urinoma, urethra N36.8
Uroarthritis, infectious (Reiter's) —see Reiter's
   disease
Urodialysis R34
Urolithiasis —see Calculus, urinary
Uronephrosis —see Hydronephrosis
Uropathy N39.9
   obstructive N13.9
      specified NEC N13.8
   reflux N13.9
      specified NEC N13.8
   vesicoureteral reflux-associated —see Reflux,
      vesicoureteral
Urosepsis — code to condition
Urticaria L50.9
   with angioneurotic edema T78.3
      hereditary D84.1
   allergic L50.0
   cholinergic L50.5
   chronic L50.8

Urticaria (Continued)
   cold, familial L50.2
   contact L50.6
   dermatographic L50.3
   due to
      cold or heat L50.2
      drugs L50.0
      food L50.0
      inhalants L50.0
      plants L50.6
      serum —see also Reaction, serum T80.69
   factitial L50.3
   familial cold M04.2
   giant T78.3
      hereditary D84.1
   gigantea T78.3
   idiopathic L50.1
   larynx T78.3
      hereditary D84.1
➡neonatorum P83.88
   nonallergic L50.1
   papulosa (Hebra) L28.2
➡pigmentosa D47.01
      ▶congenital Q82.2
      ▶of neonatal onset Q82.2
      ▶of newborn onset Q82.2
   recurrent periodic L50.8
   serum —see also Reaction, serum T80.69
   solar L56.3
   specified type NEC L50.8
   thermal (cold) (heat) L50.2
   vibratory L50.4
➡xanthelasmoidea —see Urticaria pigmentosa
Use (of)
   alcohol Z72.89
      with
         intoxication F10.929
         sleep disorder F10.982
      harmful —see Abuse, alcohol
   amphetamines —see Use, stimulant NEC
   caffeine —see Use, stimulant NEC
   cannabis F12.90
      with
         anxiety disorder F12.980
         intoxication F12.929
            with
               delirium F12.921
               perceptual disturbance F12.922
            uncomplicated F12.920
         other specified disorder F12.988
         psychosis F12.959
            delusions F12.950
            hallucinations F12.951
         unspecified disorder F12.99
   cocaine F14.90
      with
         anxiety disorder F14.980
         intoxication F14.929
            with
               delirium F14.921
               perceptual disturbance F14.922
            uncomplicated F14.920
         other specified disorder F14.988
         psychosis F14.959
            delusions F14.950
            hallucinations F14.951
         sexual dysfunction F14.981
         sleep disorder F14.982
         unspecified disorder F14.99
      harmful —see Abuse, drug, cocaine
   drug(s) NEC F19.90
      with sleep disorder F19.982
      harmful —see Abuse, drug, by type
   hallucinogen NEC F16.90
      with
         anxiety disorder F16.980
         intoxication F16.929
            with
               delirium F16.921
            uncomplicated F16.920
         mood disorder F16.94
         other specified disorder F16.988

▶ New   ➡ Revised   ~~deleted~~ Deleted   ● Use Additional Character(s)

Use *(Continued)*
  hallucinogen NEC *(Continued)*
    with *(Continued)*
      perception disorder (flashbacks) F16.983
      psychosis F16.959
        delusions F16.950
        hallucinations F16.951
      unspecified disorder F16.99
    harmful —*see* Abuse, drug, hallucinogen
      NEC
  inhalants F18.90
    with
      anxiety disorder F18.980
      intoxication F18.929
        with delirium F18.921
        uncomplicated F18.920
      mood disorder F18.94
      other specified disorder F18.988
      persisting dementia F18.97
      psychosis F18.959
        delusions F18.950
        hallucinations F18.951
      unspecified disorder F18.99
    harmful —*see* Abuse, drug, inhalant
  methadone —*see* Use, opioid
  nonprescribed drugs F19.90
    harmful —*see* Abuse, non-psychoactive
      substance
  opioid F11.90
    with
      disorder F11.99
        mood F11.94
        sleep F11.982
        specified type NEC F11.988
      intoxication F11.929
        with
          delirium F11.921
          perceptual disturbance F11.922
        uncomplicated F11.920
      withdrawal F11.93
    harmful —*see* Abuse, drug, opioid
  patent medicines F19.90
    harmful —*see* Abuse, non-psychoactive
      substance
  psychoactive drug NEC F19.90
    with
      anxiety disorder F19.980
      intoxication F19.929
        with
          delirium F19.921
          perceptual disturbance F19.922
        uncomplicated F19.920

Use *(Continued)*
  psychoactive drug NEC *(Continued)*
    with *(Continued)*
      mood disorder F19.94
      other specified disorder F19.988
      persisting
        amnestic disorder F19.96
        dementia F19.97
      psychosis F19.959
        delusions F19.950
        hallucinations F19.951
      sexual dysfunction F19.981
      sleep disorder F19.982
      unspecified disorder F19.99
      withdrawal F19.939
        with
          delirium F19.931
          perceptual disturbance F19.932
        uncomplicated F19.930
    harmful —*see* Abuse, drug NEC,
      psychoactive NEC
  sedative, hypnotic, or anxiolytic F13.90
    with
      anxiety disorder F13.980
      intoxication F13.929
        with
          delirium F13.921
        uncomplicated F13.920
      other specified disorder F13.988
      persisting
        amnestic disorder F13.96
        dementia F13.97
      psychosis F13.959
        delusions F13.950
        hallucinations F13.951
      sexual dysfunction F13.981
      sleep disorder F13.982
      unspecified disorder F13.99
    harmful —*see* Abuse, drug, sedative,
      hypnotic, or anxiolytic
  stimulant NEC F15.90
    with
      anxiety disorder F15.980
      intoxication F15.929
        with
          delirium F15.921
          perceptual disturbance F15.922
        uncomplicated F15.920
      mood disorder F15.94
      other specified disorder F15.988

Use *(Continued)*
  stimulant NEC *(Continued)*
    with *(Continued)*
      psychosis F15.959
        delusions F15.950
        hallucinations F15.951
      sexual dysfunction F15.981
      sleep disorder F15.982
      unspecified disorder F15.99
      withdrawal F15.93
    harmful —*see* Abuse, drug, stimulant
      NEC
  tobacco Z72.0
    with dependence —*see* Dependence,
      drug, nicotine
  volatile solvents —*see also* Use, inhalant
    F18.90
    harmful —*see* Abuse, drug, inhalant
Usher-Senear disease or syndrome L10.4
Uta B55.1
Uteromegaly N85.2
Uterovaginal —*see* condition
Uterovesical —*see* condition
Uveal —*see* condition
Uveitis (anterior) —*see also* Iridocyclitis
  acute —*see* Iridocyclitis, acute
  chronic —*see* Iridocyclitis, chronic
  due to toxoplasmosis (acquired) B58.09
    congenital P37.1
  granulomatous —*see* Iridocyclitis,
    chronic
  heterochromic —*see* Cyclitis, Fuchs'
    heterochromic
  lens-induced —*see* Iridocyclitis,
    lens-induced
  posterior —*see* Chorioretinitis
  sympathetic H44.13-●
  syphilitic (secondary) A51.43
    congenital (early) A50.01
    late A52.71
  tuberculous A18.54
Uveoencephalitis —*see* Inflammation,
  chorioretinal
Uveokeratitis —*see* Iridocyclitis
Uveoparotitis D86.89
Uvula —*see* condition
Uvulitis (acute) (catarrhal) (chronic)
  (membranous) (suppurative) (ulcerative)
  K12.2

V

Vaccination (prophylactic)
  complication or reaction —*see* Complications, vaccination
  delayed Z28.9
  encounter for Z23
  not done —*see* Immunization, not done, because (of)
Vaccinia (generalized) (localized) T88.1
  without vaccination B08.011
  congenital P35.8
Vacuum, in sinus (accessory) (nasal) J34.89
Vagabond, vagabondage Z59.0
Vagabond's disease B85.1
Vagina, vaginal —*see* condition
Vaginalitis (tunica) (testis) N49.1
Vaginismus (reflex) N94.2
  functional F52.5
  nonorganic F52.5
  psychogenic F52.5
  secondary N94.2
Vaginitis (acute) (circumscribed) (diffuse) (emphysematous) (nonvenereal) (ulcerative) N76.0
  with ectopic or molar pregnancy O08.0
  amebic A06.82
  atrophic, postmenopausal N95.2
  bacterial N76.0
  blennorrhagic (gonococcal) A54.02
  candidal B37.3
  chlamydial A56.02
  chronic N76.1
  due to Trichomonas (vaginalis) A59.01
  following ectopic or molar pregnancy O08.0
  gonococcal A54.02
    with abscess (accessory gland) (periurethral) A54.1
  granuloma A58
  in (due to)
    candidiasis B37.3
    herpesviral (herpes simplex) infection A60.04
    pinworm infection B80 [N77.1]
  monilial B37.3
  mycotic (candidal) B37.3
  postmenopausal atrophic N95.2
  puerperal (postpartum) O86.13
  senile (atrophic) N95.2
  subacute or chronic N76.1
  syphilitic (early) A51.0
    late A52.76
  trichomonal A59.01
  tuberculous A18.18
Vaginosis —*see* Vaginitis
Vagotonia G52.2
Vagrancy Z59.0
VAIN —*see* Neoplasia, intraepithelial, vagina
Vallecula —*see* condition
Valley fever B38.0
Valsuani's disease —*see* Anemia, obstetric
Valve, valvular (formation) —*see also* condition
  cerebral ventricle (communicating) in situ Z98.2
  cervix, internal os Q51.828
  congenital NEC —*see* Atresia, by site
  ureter (pelvic junction) (vesical orifice) Q62.39
  urethra (congenital) (posterior) Q64.2
Valvulitis (chronic) —*see* Endocarditis
Valvulopathy —*see* Endocarditis
Van Bogaert's leukoencephalopathy (sclerosing) (subacute) A81.1
Van Bogaert-Scherer-Epstein disease or syndrome E75.5
Van Buchem's syndrome M85.2
Van Creveld-von Gierke disease E74.01
Van der Hoeve (-de Kleyn) **syndrome** Q78.0
Van der Woude's syndrome Q38.0
Van Neck's disease or osteochondrosis M91.0
Vanishing lung J44.9

Vapor asphyxia or suffocation T59.9
  specified agent —*see* Table of Drugs and Chemicals
Variance, lethal ball, prosthetic heart valve T82.09
Variants, thalassemic D56.8
Variations in hair color L67.1
Varicella B01.9
  with
    complications NEC B01.89
    encephalitis B01.11
    encephalomyelitis B01.11
    meningitis B01.0
    myelitis B01.12
    pneumonia B01.2
  congenital P35.8
Varices —*see* Varix
Varicocele (scrotum) (thrombosed) I86.1
  ovary I86.2
  perineum I86.3
  spermatic cord (ulcerated) I86.1
Varicose
  aneurysm (ruptured) I77.0
  dermatitis —*see* Varix, leg, with, inflammation
  eczema —*see* Varix, leg, with, inflammation
  phlebitis —*see* Varix, with, inflammation
  tumor —*see* Varix
  ulcer (lower limb, any part) —*see also* Varix, leg, with, ulcer
    anus —*see also* Hemorrhoids K64.8
    esophagus —*see* Varix, esophagus
    inflamed or infected —*see* Varix, leg, with ulcer, with inflammation
    nasal septum I86.8
    perineum I86.3
    scrotum I86.1
    specified site NEC I86.8
  vein —*see* Varix
  vessel —*see* Varix, leg
Varicosis, varicosities, varicosity —*see* Varix
Variola (major) (minor) B03
Varioloid B03
Varix (lower limb) (ruptured) I83.90
  with
    edema I83.899
    inflammation I83.10
      with ulcer (venous) I83.209
    pain I83.819
    specified complication NEC I83.899
    stasis dermatitis I83.10
      with ulcer (venous) I83.209
    swelling I83.899
    ulcer I83.009
      with inflammation I83.209
  aneurysmal I77.0
  asymptomatic I83.9-●
  bladder I86.2
  broad ligament I86.2
  complicating
    childbirth (lower extremity) O87.4
      anus or rectum O87.2
      genital (vagina, vulva or perineum) O87.8
    pregnancy (lower extremity) O22.0-●
      anus or rectum O22.4-●
      genital (vagina, vulva or perineum) O22.1-●
    puerperium (lower extremity) O87.4
      anus or rectum O87.2
      genital (vagina, vulva, perineum) O87.8
  congenital (any site) Q27.8
  esophagus (idiopathic) (primary) (ulcerated) I85.00
    bleeding I85.01
    congenital Q27.8
    in (due to)
      alcoholic liver disease I85.10
        bleeding I85.11
      cirrhosis of liver I85.10
        bleeding I85.11

Varix (*Continued*)
  esophagus (*Continued*)
    in (*Continued*)
      portal hypertension I85.10
        bleeding I85.11
      schistosomiasis I85.10
        bleeding I85.11
      toxic liver disease I85.10
        bleeding I85.11
    secondary I85.10
      bleeding I85.11
  gastric I86.4
  inflamed or infected I83.10
    ulcerated I83.209
  labia (majora) I86.3
  leg (asymptomatic) I83.90
    with
      edema I83.899
      inflammation I83.10
        with ulcer —*see* Varix, leg, with, ulcer, with inflammation by site
      pain I83.819
      specified complication NEC I83.899
      swelling I83.899
      ulcer I83.009
        with inflammation I83.209
        ankle I83.003
          with inflammation I83.203
        calf I83.002
          with inflammation I83.202
        foot NEC I83.005
          with inflammation I83.205
        heel I83.004
          with inflammation I83.204
        lower leg NEC I83.008
          with inflammation I83.208
        midfoot I83.004
          with inflammation I83.204
        thigh I83.001
          with inflammation I83.201
    bilateral (asymptomatic) I83.93
      with
        edema I83.893
        pain I83.813
        specified complication NEC I83.893
        swelling I83.893
    ➡ ulcer I83.0-●
        with inflammation I83.209
    left (asymptomatic) I83.92
      with
        edema I83.892
        inflammation I83.12
          with ulcer —*see* Varix, leg, with, ulcer, with inflammation by site
        pain I83.812
        specified complication NEC I83.892
        swelling I83.892
        ulcer I83.029
          with inflammation I83.229
          ankle I83.023
            with inflammation I83.223
          calf I83.022
            with inflammation I83.222
          foot NEC I83.025
            with inflammation I83.225
          heel I83.024
            with inflammation I83.224
          lower leg NEC I83.028
            with inflammation I83.228
          midfoot I83.024
            with inflammation I83.224
          thigh I83.021
            with inflammation I83.221
    right (asymptomatic) I83.91
      with
        edema I83.891
        inflammation I83.11
          with ulcer —*see* Varix, leg, with, ulcer, with inflammation by site

▶ New   ⇒ Revised   ~~deleted~~ Deleted   ● Use Additional Character(s)

Varix *(Continued)*
  leg *(Continued)*
    right *(Continued)*
      with *(Continued)*
        pain I83.811
        specified complication NEC I83.891
        swelling I83.891
        ulcer I83.019
          with inflammation I83.219
          ankle I83.013
            with inflammation I83.213
          calf I83.012
            with inflammation I83.212
          foot NEC I83.015
            with inflammation I83.215
          heel I83.014
            with inflammation I83.214
          lower leg NEC I83.018
            with inflammation I83.218
          midfoot I83.014
            with inflammation I83.214
          thigh I83.011
            with inflammation I83.211
  nasal septum I86.8
  orbit I86.8
    congenital Q27.8
  ovary I86.2
  papillary I78.1
  pelvis I86.2
  perineum I86.3
  pharynx I86.8
  placenta O43.89-●
  renal papilla I86.8
  retina H35.09
  scrotum (ulcerated) I86.1
  sigmoid colon I86.8
  specified site NEC I86.8
  spinal (cord) (vessels) I86.8
  spleen, splenic (vein) (with phlebolith) I86.8
  stomach I86.4
  sublingual I86.0
  ulcerated I83.009
    inflamed or infected I83.209
  uterine ligament I86.2
  vagina I86.8
  vocal cord I86.8
  vulva I86.3
Vas deferens —*see* condition
Vas deferentitis N49.1
Vasa previa O69.4
  hemorrhage from, affecting newborn P50.0
Vascular —*see also* condition
  loop on optic papilla Q14.2
  spasm I73.9
  spider I78.1
Vascularization, cornea —*see* Neovascularization, cornea
Vasculitis I77.6
  allergic D69.0
  cryoglobulinemic D89.1
  disseminated I77.6
  hypocomplementemic M31.8
  kidney I77.89
  livedoid L95.0
  nodular L95.8
  retina H35.06-●
  rheumatic —*see* Fever, rheumatic
  rheumatoid —*see* Rheumatoid, vasculitis
  skin (limited to) L95.9
    specified NEC L95.8
  ▶systemic M31.8
Vasculopathy, necrotizing M31.9
  cardiac allograft T86.290
  specified NEC M31.8
Vasitis (nodosa) N49.1
  tuberculous A18.15
Vasodilation I73.9
Vasomotor —*see* condition
Vasoplasty, after previous sterilization Z31.0
  aftercare Z31.42

Vasospasm (vasoconstriction) I73.9
  cerebral (cerebrovascular) (artery) I67.848
    reversible I67.841
  coronary I20.1
  nerve
    arm —*see* Mononeuropathy, upper limb
    brachial plexus G54.0
    cervical plexus G54.2
    leg —*see* Mononeuropathy, lower limb
    peripheral NOS I73.9
  retina (artery) —*see* Occlusion, artery, retina
Vasospastic —*see* condition
Vasovagal attack (paroxysmal) R55
  psychogenic F45.8
VATER syndrome Q87.2
Vater's ampulla —*see* condition
Vegetation, vegetative
  adenoid (nasal fossa) J35.8
  endocarditis (acute) (any valve) (subacute) I33.0
  heart (mycotic) (valve) I33.0
Veil
  Jackson's Q43.3
Vein, venous —*see* condition
Veldt sore —*see* Ulcer, skin
Velpeau's hernia —*see* Hernia, femoral
Venereal
  bubo A55
  disease A64
  granuloma inguinale A58
  lymphogranuloma (Durand-Nicolas-Favre) A55
Venofibrosis I87.8
Venom, venomous —*see* Table of Drugs and Chemicals, by animal or substance, poisoning
Venous —*see* condition
Ventilator lung, newborn P27.8
Ventral —*see* condition
Ventricle, ventricular —*see also* condition
  escape I49.3
  inversion Q20.5
Ventriculitis (cerebral) —*see also* Encephalitis G04.90
Ventriculostomy status Z98.2
Vernet's syndrome G52.7
Verneuil's disease (syphilitic bursitis) A52.78
Verruca (due to HPV) (filiformis) (simplex) (viral) (vulgaris) B07.9
  acuminata A63.0
  necrogenica (primary) (tuberculosa) A18.4
  plana B07.8
  plantaris B07.0
  seborrheica L82.1
    inflamed L82.0
  senile (seborrheic) L82.1
    inflamed L82.0
  tuberculosa (primary) A18.4
  venereal A63.0
Verrucosities —*see* Verruca
Verruga peruana, peruviana A44.1
Version
  with extraction
  cervix —*see* Malposition, uterus
  uterus (postinfectional) (postpartal, old) -—*see* Malposition, uterus
Vertebra, vertebral —*see* condition
Vertical talus (congenital) Q66.80
  left foot Q66.82
  right foot Q66.81
Vertigo R42
  auditory —*see* Vertigo, aural
  aural H81.31-●
  benign paroxysmal (positional) H81.1-●
  central (origin) H81.4-●
  cerebral H81.4-●
  Dix and Hallpike (epidemic) —*see* Neuronitis, vestibular
  due to infrasound T75.23

Vertigo *(Continued)*
  epidemic A88.1
    Dix and Hallpike —*see* Neuronitis, vestibular
    Pedersen's —*see* Neuronitis, vestibular
    vestibular neuronitis —*see* Neuronitis, vestibular
  hysterical F44.89
  infrasound T75.23
  labyrinthine —*see* subcategory H81.0
  laryngeal R05
  malignant positional H81.4-●
  Ménière's —*see* subcategory H81.40
  menopausal N95.11
  otogenic —*see* Vertigo, aural
  paroxysmal positional, benign —*see* Vertigo, benign paroxysmal
  Pedersen's (epidemic) —*see* Neuronitis, vestibular
  peripheral NEC H81.39-●
  positional
    benign paroxysmal —*see* Vertigo, benign paroxysmal
    malignant H81.4-●
Very-low-density-lipoprotein-type (VLDL) hyperlipoproteinemia E78.1
Vesania —*see* Psychosis
Vesical —*see* condition
Vesicle
  cutaneous R23.8
  seminal —*see* condition
  skin R23.8
Vesicocolic —*see* condition
Vesicoperineal —*see* condition
Vesicorectal —*see* condition
Vesicourethrorectal —*see* condition
Vesicovaginal —*see* condition
Vesicular —*see* condition
Vesiculitis (seminal) N49.0
  amebic A06.82
  gonorrheal (acute) (chronic) A54.23
  trichomonal A59.09
  tuberculous A18.15
Vestibulitis (ear) —*see also* subcategory H83.0
  nose (external) J34.89
  vulvar N94.810
Vestibulopathy, acute peripheral (recurrent) — *see* Neuronitis, vestibular
Vestige, vestigial —*see also* Persistence
  branchial Q18.0
  structures in vitreous Q14.0
Vibration
  adverse effects T75.20
    pneumatic hammer syndrome T75.21
    specified effect NEC T75.29
    vasospastic syndrome T75.22
    vertigo from infrasound T75.23
  exposure (occupational) Z57.7
  vertigo T75.23
Vibriosis A28.9
Victim (of)
  crime Z65.4
  disaster Z65.5
  terrorism Z65.4
  torture Z65.4
  war Z65.5
Vidal's disease L28.0
Villaret's syndrome G52.7
Villous —*see* condition
VIN —*see* Neoplasia, intraepithelial, vulva
Vincent's infection (angina) (gingivitis) A69.1
  stomatitis NEC A69.1
Vinson-Plummer syndrome D50.1
Violence, physical R45.6
Viosterol deficiency —*see* Deficiency, calciferol
Vipoma —*see* Neoplasm, malignant, by site
Viremia B34.9
Virilism (adrenal) E25.9
  congenital E25.0
Virilization (female) (suprarenal) E25.9
  congenital E25.0
  isosexual E28.2

Virulent bubo A57
Virus, viral —*see also* condition
  as cause of disease classified elsewhere
    B97.89
  cytomegalovirus B25.9
  human immunodeficiency (HIV) —*see*
    Human, immunodeficiency virus (HIV)
    disease
  infection —*see* Infection, virus
  specified NEC B34.8
  swine influenza (viruses that normally cause
    infections in pigs) —*see also* Influenza,
    due to, identified novel influenza A virus
    J09.X2
  West Nile (fever) A92.30
    with
      complications NEC A92.39
      cranial nerve disorders A92.32
      encephalitis A92.31
      encephalomyelitis A92.31
      neurologic manifestation NEC A92.32
      optic neuritis A92.32
      polyradiculitis A92.32
Viscera, visceral —*see* condition
Visceroptosis K63.4
Visible peristalsis R19.2
Vision, visual
  binocular, suppression H53.34
  blurred, blurring H53.8
    hysterical F44.6
  defect, defective NEC H54.7
  disorientation (syndrome) H53.8
  disturbance H53.9
    hysterical F44.6
  double H53.2
  examination Z01.00
    with abnormal findings Z01.01
  field, limitation (defect) —*see* Defect, visual
    field
  hallucinations R44.1
  halos H53.19
  loss —*see* Loss, vision
    sudden —*see* Disturbance, vision,
      subjective, loss, sudden
  low (both eyes) —*see* Low, vision
  perception, simultaneous without fusion
    H53.33
Vitality, lack or want of R53.83
  newborn P96.89
Vitamin deficiency —*see* Deficiency, vitamin
Vitelline duct, persistent Q43.0
Vitiligo L80
  eyelid H02.739
    left H02.736
      lower H02.735
      upper H02.734
    right H02.733
      lower H02.732
      upper H02.731

Vitiligo *(Continued)*
  pinta A67.2
  vulva N90.89
Vitreal corneal syndrome H59.01-●
Vitreoretinopathy, proliferative —*see also*
    Retinopathy, proliferative
  with retinal detachment —*see* Detachment,
    retina, traction
Vitreous —*see also* condition
  touch syndrome —*see* Complication,
    postprocedural, following cataract
    surgery
Vocal cord —*see* condition
Vogt-Koyanagi syndrome H20.82-●
Vogt's disease or syndrome G80.3
Vogt-Spielmeyer amaurotic idiocy or disease
    E75.4
Voice
  change R49.9
    specified NEC R49.8
  loss —*see* Aphonia
Volhynian fever A79.0
Volkmann's ischemic contracture or paralysis
    (complicating trauma) T79.6
Volvulus (bowel) (colon) (intestine) K56.2
  with perforation K56.2
  congenital Q43.8
  duodenum K31.5
  fallopian tube —*see* Torsion, fallopian
    tube
  oviduct —*see* Torsion, fallopian tube
  stomach (due to absence of gastrocolic
    ligament) K31.89
Vomiting R11.10
  with nausea R11.2
  without nausea R11.11
  asphyxia —*see* Foreign body, by site, causing
    asphyxia, gastric contents
  bilious (cause unknown) R11.14
    following gastro-intestinal surgery
      K91.0
    in newborn P92.01
  blood —*see* Hematemesis
  causing asphyxia, choking, or suffocation —
    see Foreign body, by site
  cyclical G43.A0
    with refractory migraine G43.A1
    intractable G43.A1
    not intractable G43.A0
    psychogenic F50.89
    without refractory migraine G43.A0
  fecal mater R11.13
  following gastrointestinal surgery
    K91.0
    psychogenic F50.89
  functional K31.89
  hysterical F50.89

Vomiting *(Continued)*
  nervous F50.89
  neurotic F50.89
  newborn NEC P92.09
    bilious P92.01
  periodic R11.10
    psychogenic F50.89
  projectile R11.12
  psychogenic F50.89
  uremic —*see* Uremia
Vomito negro —*see* Fever, yellow
Von Bezold's abscess —*see* Mastoiditis,
    acute
Von Economo-Cruchet disease A85.8
Von Eulenburg's disease G71.19
Von Gierke's disease E74.01
Von Hippel (-Lindau) **disease or syndrome**
    Q85.8
Von Jaksch's anemia or disease D64.89
Von Recklinghausen
  disease (neurofibromatosis) Q85.01
    bones E21.0
Von Schroetter's syndrome I82.890
Von Willebrand (-Jurgens)(-Minot) **disease or**
    syndrome D68.0
Von Zumbusch's disease L40.1
Voyeurism F65.3
Vrolik's disease Q78.0
Vulva —*see* condition
Vulvismus N94.2
Vulvitis (acute) (allergic) (atrophic)
    (hypertrophic) (intertriginous) (senile)
    N76.2
  with ectopic or molar pregnancy O08.0
  adhesive, congenital Q52.79
  blennorrhagic (gonococcal) A54.02
  candidal B37.3
  chlamydial A56.02
  due to Haemophilus ducreyi A57
  following ectopic or molar pregnancy
    O08.0
  gonococcal A54.02
    with abscess (accessory gland)
      (periurethral) A54.1
  herpesviral A60.04
  leukoplakic N90.4
  monilial B37.3
  puerperal (postpartum) O86.19
  subacute or chronic N76.3
  syphilitic (early) A51.0
    late A52.76
  trichomonal A59.01
  tuberculous A18.18
Vulvodynia N94.819
  specified NEC N94.818
Vulvorectal —*see* condition
Vulvovaginitis (acute) —*see* Vaginitis

▶ New   ⇒ Revised   ~~deleted~~ Deleted   ● Use Additional Character(s)

W

Waiting list, person on Z75.1
  for organ transplant Z76.82
  undergoing social agency investigation
    Z75.2
Waldenström
  hypergammaglobulinemia D89.0
  syndrome or macroglobulinemia
    C88.0
Waldenström-Kjellberg syndrome
  D50.1
Walking
  difficulty R26.2
    psychogenic F44.4
  sleep F51.3
    hysterical F44.89
Wall, abdominal —see condition
Wallenberg's disease or syndrome G46.3
Wallgren's disease I87.8
Wandering
  gallbladder, congenital Q44.1
  in diseases classified elsewhere Z91.83
  kidney, congenital Q63.8
  organ or site, congenital NEC —see
    Malposition, congenital, by site
  pacemaker (heart) I49.8
  spleen D73.89
War neurosis F48.8
Wart (due to HPV) (filiform) (infectious)
  (viral) B07.9
  anogenital region (venereal) A63.0
  common B07.8
  external genital organs (venereal)
    A63.0
  flat B07.8
  Hassal-Henle's (of cornea) H18.49
  Peruvian A44.1
  plantar B07.0
  prosector (tuberculous) A18.4
  seborrheic L82.1
    inflamed L82.0
  senile (seborrheic) L82.1
    inflamed L82.0
  tuberculous A18.4
  venereal A63.0
Warthin's tumor —see Neoplasm, salivary
  gland, benign
Wassilieff's disease A27.0
Wasting
  disease R64
    due to malnutrition E41
  extreme (due to malnutrition) E41
  muscle NEC —see Atrophy, muscle
Water
  clefts (senile cataract) —see Cataract, senile,
    incipient
  deprivation of T73.1
  intoxication E87.79
  itch B76.9
  lack of T73.1
  loading E87.70
  on
    brain —see Hydrocephalus
    chest J94.8
  poisoning E87.79
Waterbrash R12
Waterhouse(-Friderichsen) syndrome or
  disease (meningococcal) A39.1
Water-losing nephritis N25.89
Watermelon stomach K31.819
  with hemorrhage K31.811
  without hemorrhage K31.819
Watsoniasis B66.8
Wax in ear —see Impaction, cerumen
Weak, weakening, weakness (generalized)
  R53.1
  arches (acquired) —see also Deformity, limb,
    flat foot
  bladder (sphincter) R32

Weak, weakening, weakness (Continued)
  facial R29.810
    following
      cerebrovascular disease I69.992
        cerebral infarction I69.392
        intracerebral hemorrhage I69.192
        nontraumatic intracranial hemorrhage
          NEC I69.292
        specified disease NEC I69.892
        stroke I69.392
        subarachnoid hemorrhage I69.092
  foot (double) —see Weak, arches
  heart, cardiac —see Failure, heart
  mind F70
  muscle M62.81
  myocardium —see Failure, heart
  newborn P96.89
  pelvic fundus N81.89
  pubocervical tissue N81.82
  rectovaginal tissue N81.83
  senile R54
  urinary stream R39.12
  valvular —see Endocarditis
Wear, worn (with normal or routine use)
  articular bearing surface of internal joint
    prosthesis —see Complications, joint
    prosthesis, mechanical, wear of articular
    bearing surfaces, by site
  device, implant or graft —see Complications,
    by site, mechanical complication
  tooth, teeth (approximal) (hard tissues)
    (interproximal) (occlusal) K03.0
Weather, weathered
  effects of
    cold T69.9
      specified effect NEC T69.8
    hot —see Heat
  skin L57.8
Weaver's syndrome Q87.3
Web, webbed (congenital)
  duodenal Q43.8
  esophagus Q39.4
  fingers Q70.1
  larynx (glottic) (subglottic) Q31.0
  neck (pterygium colli) Q18.3
  Paterson-Kelly D50.1
  popliteal syndrome Q87.89
  toes Q70.3
Weber-Christian disease M35.6
Weber-Cockayne syndrome (epidermolysis
  bullosa) Q81.8
Weber-Gubler syndrome G46.3
Weber-Leyden syndrome G46.3
Weber-Osler syndrome I78.0
Weber's paralysis or syndrome G46.3
Wedge-shaped or wedging vertebra —see
  Collapse, vertebra NEC
Wegener's granulomatosis or syndrome
  M31.30
  with
    kidney involvement M31.31
    lung involvement M31.30
      with kidney involvement M31.31
Wegner's disease A50.02
Weight
  1000-2499 grams at birth (low) —see Low,
    birthweight
  999 grams or less at birth (extremely low) —
    see Low, birthweight, extreme
  and length below 10th percentile for
    gestational age P05.1-●
  below but length above 10th percentile for
    gestational age P05.0-●
  gain (abnormal) (excessive) R63.5
    in pregnancy —see Pregnancy, complicated
      by, excessive weight gain
    low —see Pregnancy, complicated by,
      insufficient, weight gain
  loss (abnormal) (cause unknown) R63.4
Weightlessness (effect of) T75.82

Weil (l)-Marchesani syndrome Q87.1
Weil's disease A27.0
Weingarten's syndrome J82
Weir Mitchell's disease I73.81
Weiss-Baker syndrome G90.09
Wells' disease L98.3
Wen —see Cyst, sebaceous
Wenckebach's block or phenomenon I44.1
Werdnig-Hoffmann syndrome (muscular
  atrophy) G12.0
Werlhof's disease D69.3
Werner-His disease A79.0
Wermer's disease or syndrome E31.21
Werner's disease or syndrome E34.8
Wernicke-Korsakoff's syndrome or psychosis
  (alcoholic) F10.96
  with dependence F10.26
  drug-induced
    due to drug abuse —see Abuse, drug, by
      type, with amnestic disorder
    due to drug dependence —see
      Dependence, drug, by type, with
      amnestic disorder
  nonalcoholic F04
Wernicke-Posadas disease B38.9
Wernicke's
  developmental aphasia F80.2
  disease or syndrome E51.2
  encephalopathy E51.2
  polioencephalitis, superior E51.2
West African fever B50.8
Westphal-Strümpell syndrome E83.01
West's syndrome —see Epilepsy, spasms
Wet
  feet, tropical (maceration) (syndrome) —see
    Immersion, foot
  lung (syndrome), newborn P22.1
Wharton's duct —see condition
Wheal —see Urticaria
Wheezing R06.2
Whiplash injury S13.4
Whipple's disease —see also subcategory
  M14.8-● K90.81
Whipworm (disease) (infection) (infestation)
  B79
Whistling face Q87.0
White —see also condition
  kidney, small N03.9
  leg, puerperal, postpartum, childbirth O87.1
  mouth B37.0
  patches of mouth K13.29
  spot lesions, teeth
    chewing surface K02.51
    pit and fissure surface K02.51
    smooth surface K02.61
Whitehead L70.0
Whitlow —see also Cellulitis, digit
  with lymphangitis —see Lymphangitis, acute,
    digit
  herpesviral B00.89
Whitmore's disease or fever —see Melioidosis
Whooping cough A37.90
  with pneumonia A37.91
    due to Bordetella
      bronchiseptica A37.81
      parapertussis A37.11
      pertussis A37.01
      specified organism NEC A37.81
  due to
    Bordetella
      bronchiseptica A37.80
        with pneumonia A37.81
      parapertussis A37.10
        with pneumonia A37.11
      pertussis A37.00
        with pneumonia A37.01
    specified NEC A37.80
      with pneumonia A37.81
Wichman's asthma J38.5
Wide cranial sutures, newborn P96.3

▶ New   ➡ Revised   ~~deleted~~ Deleted   • Use Additional Character(s)

Wound, open (*Continued*)
  esophagus (thoracic) S27.819
    cervical —*see* Wound, open, cervical
      esophagus
    laceration S27.813
    specified type NEC S27.818
  eye —*see* Wound, open, ocular
  eyeball —*see* Wound, open, ocular
  eyebrow —*see* Wound, open, eyelid
  eyelid S01.10-●
    bite —*see* Bite, eyelid
    laceration —*see* Laceration, eyelid
    puncture —*see* Puncture, eyelid
  face NEC —*see* Wound, open, head, specified
    site NEC
  finger(s) S61.209
    with
      amputation —*see* Amputation,
        traumatic, finger
      damage to nail S61.309
    bite —*see* Bite, finger
    index S61.208
      with
        damage to nail S61.308
      left S61.201
        with
          damage to nail S61.301
      right S61.200
        with
          damage to nail S61.300
    laceration —*see* Laceration, finger
    little S61.208
      with
        damage to nail S61.308
      left S61.207
        with damage to nail S61.307
      right S61.206
        with damage to nail S61.306
    middle S61.208
      with
        damage to nail S61.308
      left S61.203
        with damage to nail S61.303
      right S61.202
        with damage to nail S61.302
    puncture —*see* Puncture, finger
    ring S61.208
      with
        damage to nail S61.308
      left S61.205
        with damage to nail S61.305
      right S61.204
        with damage to nail S61.304
  flank —*see* Wound, open, abdomen, wall
  foot (except toe(s) alone) S91.30-●
    with amputation —*see* Amputation,
      traumatic, foot
    bite —*see* Bite, foot
    laceration —*see* Laceration, foot
    puncture —*see* Puncture, foot
    toe —*see* Wound, open, toe
  forearm S51.80-●
    with
      amputation —*see* Amputation,
        traumatic, forearm
    bite —*see* Bite, forearm
    elbow only —*see* Wound, open, elbow
    laceration —*see* Laceration, forearm
    puncture —*see* Puncture, forearm
  forehead —*see* Wound, open, head, specified
    site NEC
  genital organs, external
    with amputation —*see* Amputation,
      traumatic, genital organs
    bite —*see* Bite, genital organ
    female S31.502
      vagina S31.40
      vulva S31.40
    laceration —*see* Laceration, genital
      organ

Wound, open (*Continued*)
  genital organs, external (*Continued*)
    male S31.501
      penis S31.20
      scrotum S31.30
      testes S31.30
    puncture —*see* Puncture, genital organ
  globe (eye) —*see* Wound, open, ocular
  groin —*see* Wound, open, abdomen, wall
  gum —*see* Wound, open, oral cavity
  hand S61.40-●
    with
      amputation —*see* Amputation,
        traumatic, hand
    bite —*see* Bite, hand
    finger(s) —*see* Wound, open, finger
    laceration —*see* Laceration, hand
    puncture —*see* Puncture, hand
    thumb —*see* Wound, open, thumb
  head S01.90
    bite —*see* Bite, head
    cheek —*see* Wound, open, cheek
    ear —*see* Wound, open, ear
    eyelid —*see* Wound, open, eyelid
    laceration —*see* Laceration, head
    lip —*see* Wound, open, lip
    nose S01.20
    oral cavity —*see* Wound, open, oral
      cavity
    puncture —*see* Puncture, head
    scalp —*see* Wound, open, scalp
    specified site NEC S01.80
    temporomandibular area —*see* Wound,
      open, cheek
  heel —*see* Wound, open, foot
  hip S71.00-●
    with amputation —*see* Amputation,
      traumatic, hip
    bite —*see* Bite, hip
    laceration —*see* Laceration, hip
    puncture —*see* Puncture, hip
  hymen S31.40
    bite —*see* Bite, vulva
    laceration —*see* Laceration, vagina
    puncture —*see* Puncture, vagina
  hypochondrium S31.109
    bite —*see* Bite, hypochondrium
    laceration —*see* Laceration,
      hypochondrium
    puncture —*see* Puncture, hypochondrium
  hypogastric region S31.109
    bite —*see* Bite, hypogastric region
    laceration —*see* Laceration, hypogastric
      region
    puncture —*see* Puncture, hypogastric
      region
  iliac (region) —*see* Wound, open, inguinal
    region
  inguinal region S31.109
    bite —*see* Bite, abdomen, wall, lower
      quadrant
    laceration —*see* Laceration, inguinal
      region
    puncture —*see* Puncture, inguinal
      region
  instep —*see* Wound, open, foot
  interscapular region —*see* Wound, open,
    thorax, back
  intraocular —*see* Wound, open, ocular
  iris —*see* Wound, open, ocular
  jaw —*see* Wound, open, head, specified site
    NEC
  knee S81.00-●
    bite —*see* Bite, knee
    laceration —*see* Laceration, knee
    puncture —*see* Puncture, knee
  labium (majus) (minus) —*see* Wound, open,
    vulva
  laceration —*see* Laceration, by site
  lacrimal duct —*see* Wound, open, eyelid

Wound, open (*Continued*)
  larynx S11.019
    bite —*see* Bite, larynx
    laceration —*see* Laceration, larynx
    puncture —*see* Puncture, larynx
  left
    lower quadrant S31.104
      with penetration into peritoneal cavity
        S31.604
      bite —*see* Bite, abdomen, wall, left, lower
        quadrant
      laceration —*see* Laceration, abdomen,
        wall, left, lower quadrant
      puncture —*see* Puncture, abdomen, wall,
        left, lower quadrant
    upper quadrant S31.101
      with penetration into peritoneal cavity
        S31.601
      bite —*see* Bite, abdomen, wall, left,
        upper quadrant
      laceration —*see* Laceration, abdomen,
        wall, left, upper quadrant
      puncture —*see* Puncture, abdomen, wall,
        left, upper quadrant
  leg (lower) S81.80-●
    with amputation —*see* Amputation,
      traumatic, leg
    ankle —*see* Wound, open, ankle
    bite —*see* Bite, leg
    foot —*see* Wound, open, foot
    knee —*see* Wound, open, knee
    laceration —*see* Laceration, leg
    puncture —*see* Puncture, leg
    toe —*see* Wound, open, toe
    upper —*see* Wound, open, thigh
  lip S01.501
    bite —*see* Bite, lip
    laceration —*see* Laceration, lip
    puncture —*see* Puncture, lip
  loin S31.109
    bite —*see* Bite, abdomen, wall
    laceration —*see* Laceration, loin
    puncture —*see* Puncture, loin
  lower back —*see* Wound, open, back,
    lower
  lumbar region —*see* Wound, open, back,
    lower
  malar region —*see* Wound, open, head,
    specified site NEC
  mammary —*see* Wound, open, breast
  mastoid region —*see* Wound, open, head,
    specified site NEC
  mouth —*see* Wound, open, oral cavity
  nail
    finger —*see* Wound, open, finger, with
      damage to nail
    toe —*see* Wound, open, toe, with damage
      to nail
  nape (neck) —*see* Wound, open, neck
  nasal (septum) (sinus) —*see* Wound, open,
    nose
  nasopharynx —*see* Wound, open, head,
    specified site NEC
  neck S11.90
    bite —*see* Bite, neck
    involving
      cervical esophagus S11.20
      larynx —*see* Wound, open, larynx
      pharynx S11.20
      thyroid S11.10
      trachea (cervical) S11.029
        bite —*see* Bite, trachea
        laceration S11.021
          with foreign body S11.022
        puncture S11.023
          with foreign body S11.024
    laceration —*see* Laceration, neck
    puncture —*see* Puncture, neck
    specified site NEC S11.80
      specified type NEC S11.89

W

Wound, open *(Continued)*
  nose (septum) (sinus) S01.20
    with amputation —*see* Amputation,
      traumatic, nose
    bite —*see* Bite, nose
    laceration —*see* Laceration, nose
    puncture —*see* Puncture, nose
  ocular S05.90
    avulsion (traumatic enucleation) S05.7-●
    eyeball S05.6-●
      with foreign body S05.5-●
    eyelid —*see* Wound, open, eyelid
    laceration and rupture S05.3-●
      with prolapse or loss of intraocular
        tissue S05.2-●
    orbit (penetrating) (with or without foreign
      body) S05.4-●
    periocular area —*see* Wound, open, eyelid
    specified NEC S05.8X-●
  oral cavity S01.502
    bite S01.552
    laceration —*see* Laceration, oral cavity
    puncture —*see* Puncture, oral cavity
  orbit —*see* Wound, open, ocular, orbit
  palate —*see* Wound, open, oral cavity
  palm —*see* Wound, open, hand
  pelvis, pelvic —*see also* Wound, open, back,
    lower
    girdle —*see* Wound, open, hip
  penetrating —*see* Puncture, by site
  penis S31.20
    with amputation —*see* Amputation,
      traumatic, penis
    bite S31.25
    laceration —*see* Laceration, penis
    puncture —*see* Puncture, penis
  perineum
    bite —*see* Bite, perineum
    female S31.502
    laceration —*see* Laceration, perineum
    male S31.501
    puncture —*see* Puncture, perineum
  periocular area (with or without lacrimal
    passages) —*see* Wound, open, eyelid
  periumbilic region S31.105
    with penetration into peritoneal cavity
      S31.605
    bite —*see* Bite, abdomen, wall, periumbilic
      region
    laceration —*see* Laceration, abdomen, wall,
      periumbilic region
    puncture —*see* Puncture, abdomen, wall,
      periumbilic region
  phalanges
    finger —*see* Wound, open, finger
    toe —*see* Wound, open, toe
  pharynx S11.20
  pinna —*see* Wound, open, ear
  popliteal space —*see* Wound, open, knee
  prepuce —*see* Wound, open, penis
  pubic region —*see* Wound, open, back, lower
  pudendum —*see* Wound, open, genital
    organs, external
  puncture wound —*see* Puncture
  rectovaginal septum —*see* Wound, open,
    vagina
  right
    lower quadrant S31.103
      with penetration into peritoneal cavity
        S31.603
      bite —*see* Bite, abdomen, wall, right,
        lower quadrant
      laceration —*see* Laceration, abdomen,
        wall, right, lower quadrant
      puncture —*see* Puncture, abdomen, wall,
        right, lower quadrant
    upper quadrant S31.100
      with penetration into peritoneal cavity
        S31.600

Wound, open *(Continued)*
  right *(Continued)*
    upper quadrant *(Continued)*
      bite —*see* Bite, abdomen, wall, right,
        upper quadrant
      laceration —*see* Laceration, abdomen,
        wall, right, upper quadrant
      puncture —*see* Puncture, abdomen, wall,
        right, upper quadrant
  sacral region —*see* Wound, open, back, lower
  sacroiliac region —*see* Wound, open, back,
    lower
  salivary gland —*see* Wound, open, oral cavity
  scalp S01.00
    bite S01.05
    laceration —*see* Laceration, scalp
    puncture —*see* Puncture, scalp
  scalpel, newborn (birth injury) P15.8
  scapular region —*see* Wound, open, shoulder
  sclera —*see* Wound, open, ocular
  scrotum S31.30
    with amputation —*see* Amputation,
      traumatic, scrotum
    bite S31.35
    laceration —*see* Laceration, scrotum
    puncture —*see* Puncture, scrotum
  shin —*see* Wound, open, leg
  shoulder S41.00-●
    with amputation —*see* Amputation,
      traumatic, arm
    bite —*see* Bite, shoulder
    laceration —*see* Laceration, shoulder
    puncture —*see* Puncture, shoulder
  skin NOS T14.8
  spermatic cord —*see* Wound, open, testis
  sternal region —*see* Wound, open, thorax,
    front wall
  submaxillary region —*see* Wound, open,
    head, specified site NEC
  submental region —*see* Wound, open, head,
    specified site NEC
  subungual
    finger(s) —*see* Wound, open, finger
    toe(s) —*see* Wound, open, toe
  supraclavicular region —*see* Wound, open,
    neck, specified site NEC
  temple, temporal region —*see* Wound, open,
    head, specified site NEC
  temporomandibular area —*see* Wound, open,
    cheek
  testis S31.30
    with amputation —*see* Amputation,
      traumatic, testes
    bite S31.35
    laceration —*see* Laceration, testis
    puncture —*see* Puncture, testis
  thigh S71.10-●
    with amputation —*see* Amputation,
      traumatic, hip
    bite —*see* Bite, thigh
    laceration —*see* Laceration, thigh
    puncture —*see* Puncture, thigh
  thorax, thoracic (wall) S21.90
    back S21.20-●
      with penetration S21.40
    bite —*see* Bite, thorax
    breast —*see* Wound, open, breast
    front S21.10-●
      with penetration S21.30
    laceration —*see* Laceration, thorax
    puncture —*see* Puncture, thorax
  throat —*see* Wound, open, neck
  thumb S61.009
    with
      amputation —*see* Amputation,
        traumatic, thumb
      damage to nail S61.109
    bite —*see* Bite, thumb
    laceration —*see* Laceration, thumb

Wound, open *(Continued)*
  thumb *(Continued)*
    left S61.002
      with
        damage to nail S61.102
      puncture —*see* Puncture, thumb
    right S61.001
      with
        damage to nail S61.101
  thyroid (gland) —*see* Wound, open, neck,
    thyroid
  toe(s) S91.109
    with
      amputation —*see* Amputation,
        traumatic, toe
      damage to nail S91.209
    bite —*see* Bite, toe
    great S91.103
      with
        damage to nail S91.203
      left S91.102
        with
          damage to nail S91.202
      right S91.101
        with
          damage to nail S91.201
    laceration —*see* Laceration, toe
    lesser S91.106
      with
        damage to nail S91.206
      left S91.105
        with
          damage to nail S91.205
      right S91.104
        with
          damage to nail S91.204
    puncture —*see* Puncture, toe
  tongue —*see* Wound, open, oral cavity
  trachea (cervical region) —*see* Wound, open,
    neck, trachea
  tunica vaginalis —*see* Wound, open, testis
  tympanum, tympanic membrane S09.2-●
    laceration —*see* Laceration, ear, drum
    puncture —*see* Puncture, tympanum
  umbilical region —*see* Wound, open,
    abdomen, wall, periumbilic region
  uvula —*see* Wound, open, oral cavity
  vagina S31.40
    bite S31.45
    laceration —*see* Laceration, vagina
    puncture —*see* Puncture, vagina
  vitreous (humor) —*see* Wound, open, ocular
  vocal cord S11.039
    bite —*see* Bite, vocal cord
    laceration S11.031
      with foreign body S11.032
    puncture S11.033
      with foreign body S11.034
  vulva S31.40
    with amputation —*see* Amputation,
      traumatic, vulva
    bite S31.45
    laceration —*see* Laceration, vulva
    puncture —*see* Puncture, vulva
  wrist S61.50-●
    bite —*see* Bite, wrist
    laceration —*see* Laceration, wrist
    puncture —*see* Puncture, wrist
Wound, superficial —*see* Injury (*see also*
  specified injury type)
Wright's syndrome G54.0
Wrist —*see* condition
Wrong drug (by accident) (given in error) —
  see Table of Drugs and Chemicals, by
  drug, poisoning
Wry neck —*see* Torticollis
Wuchereria (bancrofti) **infestation** B74.0
Wuchereriasis B74.0
Wuchernde Struma Langhans C73

W

X

Xanthelasma (eyelid) (palpebrarum) H02.60
  left H02.66
    lower H02.65
    upper H02.64
  right H02.63
    lower H02.62
    upper H02.61
Xanthelasmatosis (essential) E78.2
Xanthinuria, hereditary E79.8
Xanthoastrocytoma
  specified site —see Neoplasm, malignant, by
    site
  unspecified site C71.9
Xanthofibroma —see Neoplasm, connective
    tissue, benign
Xanthogranuloma D76.3
Xanthoma(s), xanthomatosis (primary)
    (familial) (hereditary) E75.5
  with
    hyperlipoproteinemia
      Type I E78.3
      Type III E78.2
      Type IV E78.1
      Type V E78.3
  bone (generalisata) C96.5
  cerebrotendinous E75.5
  cutaneotendinous E75.5

Xanthoma(s), xanthomatosis (Continued)
  disseminatum (skin) E78.2
  eruptive E78.2
  hypercholesterinemic E78.00
  hypercholesterolemic E78.00
  hyperlipidemic E78.5
  joint E75.5
  multiple (skin) E78.2
  tendon (sheath) E75.5
  tuberosum E78.2
  tuberous E78.2
  tubo-eruptive E78.2
  verrucous, oral mucosa K13.4
Xanthosis R23.8
Xenophobia F40.10
Xeroderma —see also Ichthyosis
  acquired L85.0
    eyelid H01.149
      left H01.146
        lower H01.145
        upper H01.144
      right H01.143
        lower H01.142
        upper H01.141
  pigmentosum Q82.1
  vitamin A deficiency E50.8
Xerophthalmia (vitamin A deficiency) E50.7
  unrelated to vitamin A deficiency —see
    Keratoconjunctivitis

Xerosis
  conjunctiva H11.14-●
    with Bitot's spots —see also Pigmentation,
      conjunctiva
      vitamin A deficiency E50.1
    vitamin A deficiency E50.0
  cornea H18.89-●
    with ulceration —see Ulcer, cornea
      vitamin A deficiency E50.3
    vitamin A deficiency E50.2
  cutis L85.3
  skin L85.3
Xerostomia K11.7
Xiphopagus Q89.4
XO syndrome Q96.9
X-ray (of)
  abnormal findings —see Abnormal,
    diagnostic imaging
  breast (mammogram) (routine) Z12.31
  chest
    routine (as part of a general medical
      examination) Z00.00
      with abnormal findings Z00.01
  routine (as part of a general medical
    examination) Z00.00
    with abnormal findings Z00.01
XXXXY syndrome Q98.1
XXY syndrome Q98.0

Y

Yaba pox virus disease B08.72
Yatapoxvirus B08.70
   specified NEC B08.79
Yawning R06.89
   psychogenic F45.8
Yaws A66.9
   bone lesions A66.6
   butter A66.1
   chancre A66.0
   cutaneous, less than five years after infection
         A66.2
   early (cutaneous) (macular) (maculopapular)
         (micropapular) (papular) A66.2
      frambeside A66.2
      skin lesions NEC A66.2
   eyelid A66.2
   ganglion A66.6
   gangosis, gangosa A66.5
   gumma, gummata A66.4
      bone A66.6
   gummatous
      frambeside A66.4
      osteitis A66.6
      periostitis A66.6
   hydrarthrosis —see also subcategory
         M14.8-● A66.6
   hyperkeratosis (early) (late) A66.3

Yaws *(Continued)*
   initial lesions A66.0
   joint lesions —see also subcategory
         M14.8-● A66.6
   juxta-articular nodules A66.7
   late nodular (ulcerated) A66.4
   latent (without clinical manifestations) (with
         positive serology) A66.8
   mother A66.0
   mucosal A66.7
   multiple papillomata A66.1
   nodular, late (ulcerated) A66.4
   osteitis A66.6
   papilloma, plantar or palmar A66.1
   periostitis (hypertrophic) A66.6
   specified NEC A66.7
   ulcers A66.4
   wet crab A66.1
Yeast infection —see also Candidiasis B37.9
Yellow
   atrophy (liver) —see Failure, hepatic
   fever —see Fever, yellow
   jack —see Fever, yellow
   jaundice —see Jaundice
   nail syndrome L60.5
Yersiniosis —see also Infection, Yersinia
   extraintestinal A28.2
   intestinal A04.6

Z

Zahorsky's syndrome (herpangina) B08.5
Zellweger's syndrome Q87.89
Zenker's diverticulum (esophagus) K22.5
Ziehen-Oppenheim disease G24.1
Zieve's syndrome K70.0
Zika NOS A92.5
Zinc
   deficiency, dietary E60
   metabolism disorder E83.2
Zollinger-Ellison syndrome E16.4
Zona —see Herpes, zoster
Zoophobia F40.218
Zoster (herpes) —see Herpes, zoster
Zygomycosis B46.9
   specified NEC B46.8
Zymotic —see condition

▶ New   ➡ Revised   ~~deleted~~ Deleted   ● Use Additional Character(s)

ICD-10-CM
Table of Neoplasms

The list below gives the code numbers for neoplasms by anatomical site. For each site there are six possible code numbers according to whether the neoplasm in question is malignant, benign, in situ, of uncertain behavior, or of unspecified nature. The description of the neoplasm will often indicate which of the six columns is appropriate; e.g., malignant melanoma of skin, benign fibroadenoma of breast, carcinoma in situ of cervix uteri.

Where such descriptors are not present, the remainder of the Index should be consulted where guidance is given to the appropriate column for each morphological (histological) variety listed; e.g., Mesonephroma — *see Neoplasm, malignant;* Embryoma — *see also Neoplasm, uncertain behavior;* Disease, Bowen's — *see Neoplasm, skin, in situ.* However, the guidance in the Index can be overridden if one of the descriptors mentioned above is present; e.g., malignant adenoma of colon is coded to C18.9 and not to D12.6 as the adjective "Malignant" overrides the Index entry 'Adenoma — *see also Neoplasm, benign.*'

Codes listed with a dash -, following the code have a required additional character for laterality. The Tablular must be reviewed for the complete code.

	Malignant Primary	Malignant Secondary	Ca in situ	Benign	Uncertain Behavior	Unspecified Behavior
Neoplasm, neoplastic	C80.1	C79.9	D09.9	D36.9	D48.9	D49.9
abdomen, abdominal	C76.2	C79.8-●	D09.8	D36.7	D48.7	D49.89
cavity	C76.2	C79.8-●	D09.8	D36.7	D48.7	D49.89
organ	C76.2	C79.8-●	D09.8	D36.7	D48.7	D49.89
viscera	C76.2	C79.8-●	D09.8	D36.7	D48.7	D49.89
wall — *see also Neoplasm, abdomen, wall, skin*	C44.509	C79.2-●	D04.5	D23.5	D48.5	D49.2
connective tissue	C49.4	C79.8-●	—	D21.4	D48.1	D49.2
skin	C44.509					
basal cell carcinoma	C44.519	—	—	—	—	—
specified type NEC	C44.599	—	—	—	—	—
squamous cell carcinoma	C44.529	—	—	—	—	—
abdominopelvic	C76.8	C79.8-●	—	D36.7	D48.7	D49.89
accessory sinus — *see Neoplasm, sinus*						
acoustic nerve	C72.4-●	C79.49	—	D33.3	D43.3	D49.7
adenoid (pharynx) (tissue)	C11.1	C79.89	D00.08	D10.6	D37.05	D49.0
adipose tissue — *see also Neoplasm, connective tissue*	C49.4	C79.89	—	D21.9	D48.1	D49.2
adnexa (uterine)	C57.4	C79.89	D07.39	D28.7	D39.8	D49.59
adrenal	C74.9-●	C79.7-●	D09.3	D35.0-●	D44.1-●	D49.7
capsule	C74.9-●	C79.7-●	D09.3	D35.0-●	D44.1-●	D49.7
cortex	C74.0-●	C79.7-●	D09.3	D35.0-●	D44.1-●	D49.7
gland	C74.9-●	C79.7-●	D09.3	D35.0-●	D44.1-●	D49.7
medulla	C74.1-●	C79.7-●	D09.3	D35.0-●	D44.1-●	D49.7
ala nasi (external) — *see also Neoplasm, skin, nose*	C44.301	C79.2	D04.39	D23.39	D48.5	D49.2
alimentary canal or tract NEC	C26.9	C78.80	D01.9	D13.9	D37.9	D49.0
alveolar	C03.9	C79.89	D00.03	D10.39	D37.09	D49.0
mucosa	C03.9	C79.89	D00.03	D10.39	D37.09	D49.0
lower	C03.1	C79.89	D00.03	D10.39	D37.09	D49.0
upper	C03.0	C79.89	D00.03	D10.39	D37.09	D49.0
ridge or process	C41.1	C79.51	—	D16.5-●	D48.0	D49.2
carcinoma	C03.9	C79.8-●	—	—	—	—
lower	C03.1	C79.8-●	—	—	—	—
upper	C03.0	C79.8-●	—	—	—	—
lower	C41.1	C79.51	—	D16.5-●	D48.0	D49.2
mucosa	C03.9	C79.89	D00.03	D10.39	D37.09	D49.0
lower	C03.1	C79.89	D00.03	D10.39	D37.09	D49.0
upper	C03.0	C79.89	D00.03	D10.39	D37.09	D49.0
upper	C41.0	C79.51	—	D16.4-●	D48.0	D49.2
sulcus	C06.1	C79.89	D00.02	D10.39	D37.09	D49.0
alveolus	C03.9	C79.89	D00.03	D10.39	D37.09	D49.0
lower	C03.1	C79.89	D00.03	D10.39	D37.09	D49.0
upper	C03.0	C79.89	D00.03	D10.39	D37.09	D49.0
ampulla of Vater	C24.1	C78.89	D01.5	D13.5	D37.6	D49.0
ankle NEC	C76.5-●	C79.89	D04.7-●	D36.7	D48.7	D49.89
anorectum, anorectal (junction)	C21.8	C78.5	D01.3	D12.9	D37.8	D49.0
antecubital fossa or space	C76.4-●	C79.89	D04.6-●	D36.7	D48.7	D49.89
antrum (Highmore) (maxillary)	C31.0	C78.39	D02.3	D14.0	D38.5	D49.1
pyloric	C16.3	C78.89	D00.2	D13.1	D37.1	D49.0
tympanicum	C30.1	C78.39	D02.3	D14.0	D38.5	D49.1
anus, anal	C21.0	C78.5	D01.3	D12.9	D37.8	D49.0
canal	C21.1	C78.5	D01.3	D12.9	D37.8	D49.0
cloacogenic zone	C21.2	C78.5	D01.3	D12.9	D37.8	D49.0
margin — *see also Neoplasm, anus, skin*	C44.500	C79.2	D04.5	D23.5	D48.5	D49.2
overlapping lesion with rectosigmoid junction or rectum	C21.8					
skin	C44.500	C79.2	D04.5	D23.5	D48.5	D49.2
basal cell carcinoma	C44.510	—	—	—	—	—
specified type NEC	C44.590	—	—	—	—	—
squamous cell carcinoma	C44.520	—	—	—	—	—
sphincter	C21.1	C78.5	D01.3	D12.9	D37.8	D49.0
aorta (thoracic)	C49.3	C79.89	—	D21.3	D48.1	D49.2
abdominal	C49.4	C79.89	—	D21.4	D48.1	D49.2
aortic body	C75.5	C79.89		D35.6	D44.7	D49.7
aponeurosis	C49.9	C79.89	—	D21.9	D48.1	D49.2
palmar	C49.1-●	C79.89	—	D21.1-●	D48.1	D49.2
plantar	C49.2-●	C79.89	—	D21.2-●	D48.1	D49.2

TABLE OF NEOPLASMS

	Malignant Primary	Malignant Secondary	Ca in situ	Benign	Uncertain Behavior	Unspecified Behavior
appendix	C18.1	C78.5	D01.0	D12.1	D37.3	D49.0
arachnoid	C70.9	C79.49	—	D32.9	D42.9	D49.7
cerebral	C70.0	C79.32	—	D32.0	D42.0	D49.7
spinal	C70.1	C79.49	—	D32.1	D42.1	D49.7
areola	C50.0-●	C79.81	D05.-●	D24.-●	D48.6-●	D49.3
arm NEC	C76.4-●	C79.89	D04.6-●	D36.7	D48.7	D49.89
artery — see Neoplasm, connective tissue						
aryepiglottic fold	C13.1	C79.89	D00.08	D10.7	D37.05	D49.0
hypopharyngeal aspect	C13.1	C79.89	D00.08	D10.7	D37.05	D49.0
laryngeal aspect	C32.1	C78.39	D02.0	D14.1	D38.0	D49.1
marginal zone	C13.1	C79.89	D00.08	D10.7	D37.05	D49.0
arytenoid (cartilage)	C32.3	C78.39	D02.0	D14.1	D38.0	D49.1
fold — see Neoplasm, aryepiglottic						
associated with transplanted organ	C80.2	—	—	—	—	—
atlas	C41.2	C79.51	—	D16.6	D48.0	D49.2
atrium, cardiac	C38.0	C79.89	—	D15.1	D48.7	D49.89
auditory						
canal (external) (skin)	C44.20-●	C79.2	D04.2-●	D23.2-●	D48.5	D49.2
internal	C30.1	C78.39	D02.3	D14.0	D38.5	D49.1
nerve	C72.4-●	C79.49	—	D33.3	D43.3	D49.7
tube	C30.1	C78.39	D02.3	D14.0	D38.5	D49.1
opening	C11.2	C79.89	D00.08	D10.6	D37.05	D49.0
auricle, ear — see also Neoplasm, skin, ear	C44.20-●	C79.2	D04.2-●	D23.2-●	D48.5	D49.2
auricular canal (external) — see also Neoplasm, skin, ear	C44.20-●	C79.2	D04.2-●	D23.2-●	D48.5	D49.2
internal	C30.1	C78.39	D02.3	D14.0	D38.5	D49.2
autonomic nerve or nervous system NEC (see Neoplasm, nerve, peripheral)						
axilla, axillary	C76.1	C79.89	D09.8	D36.7	D48.7	D49.89
fold — see also Neoplasm, skin, trunk	C44.509	C79.2	D04.5	D23.5	D48.5	D49.2
back NEC	C76.8	C79.89	D04.5	D36.7	D48.7	D49.89
Bartholin's gland	C51.0	C79.82	D07.1	D28.0	D39.8	D49.59
basal ganglia	C71.0	C79.31	—	D33.0	D43.0	D49.6
basis pedunculi	C71.7	C79.31	—	D33.1	D43.1	D49.6
bile or biliary (tract)	C24.9	C78.89	D01.5	D13.5	D37.6	D49.0
canaliculi (biliferi) (intrahepatic)	C22.1	C78.7	D01.5	D13.4	D37.6	D49.0
canals, interlobular	C22.1	C78.89	D01.5	D13.4	D37.6	D49.0

	Malignant Primary	Malignant Secondary	Ca in situ	Benign	Uncertain Behavior	Unspecified Behavior
bile or biliary (Continued)						
duct or passage (common) (cystic) (extrahepatic)	C24.0	C78.89	D01.5	D13.5	D37.6	D49.0
interlobular	C22.1	C78.89	D01.5	D13.4	D37.6	D49.0
intrahepatic	C22.1	C78.7	D01.5	D13.4	D37.6	D49.0
and extrahepatic	C24.8	C78.89	D01.5	D13.5	D37.6	D49.0
bladder (urinary)	C67.9	C79.11	D09.0	D30.3	D41.4	D49.4
dome	C67.1	C79.11	D09.0	D30.3	D41.4	D49.4
neck	C67.5	C79.11	D09.0	D30.3	D41.4	D49.4
orifice	C67.9	C79.11	D09.0	D30.3	D41.4	D49.4
ureteric	C67.6	C79.11	D09.0	D30.3	D41.4	D49.4
urethral	C67.5	C79.11	D09.0	D30.3	D41.4	D49.4
overlapping lesion	C67.8	—	—	—	—	—
sphincter	C67.8	C79.11	D09.0	D30.3	D41.4	D49.4
trigone	C67.0	C79.11	D09.0	D30.3	D41.4	D49.4
urachus	C67.7	C79.11	D09.0	D30.3	D41.4	D49.4
wall	C67.9	C79.11	D09.0	D30.3	D41.4	D49.4
anterior	C67.3	C79.11	D09.0	D30.3	D41.4	D49.4
lateral	C67.2	C79.11	D09.0	D30.3	D41.4	D49.4
posterior	C67.4	C79.11	D09.0	D30.3	D41.4	D49.4
blood vessel — see Neoplasm, connective tissue						
bone (periosteum)	C41.9	C79.51	—	D16.9-●	D48.0	D49.2
acetabulum	C41.4	C79.51	—	D16.8-●	D48.0	D49.2
ankle	C40.3-●	C79.51	—	D16.3-●	—	—
arm NEC	C40.0-●	C79.51	—	D16.0-●	—	—
astragalus	C40.3-●	C79.51	—	D16.3-●	—	—
atlas	C41.2	C79.51	—	D16.6-●	D48.0	D49.2
axis	C41.2	C79.51	—	D16.6-●	D48.0	D49.2
back NEC	C41.2	C79.51	—	D16.6-●	D48.0	D49.2
calcaneus	C40.3-●	C79.51	—	D16.3-●	—	—
calvarium	C41.0	C79.51	—	D16.4-●	D48.0	D49.2
carpus (any)	C40.1-●	C79.51	—	D16.1-●	—	—
cartilage NEC	C41.9	C79.51	—	D16.9-●	D48.0	D49.2
clavicle	C41.3	C79.51	—	D16.7-●	D48.0	D49.2
clivus	C41.0	C79.51	—	D16.4-●	D48.0	D49.2
coccygeal vertebra	C41.4	C79.51	—	D16.8-●	D48.0	D49.2
coccyx	C41.4	C79.51	—	D16.8-●	D48.0	D49.2
costal cartilage	C41.3	C79.51	—	D16.7-●	D48.0	D49.2
costovertebral joint	C41.3	C79.51	—	D16.7-●	D48.0	D49.2
cranial	C41.0	C79.51	—	D16.4-●	D48.0	D49.2
cuboid	C40.3-●	C79.51	—	D16.3-●	—	—
cuneiform	C41.9	C79.51	—	D16.9-●	D48.0	D49.2
elbow	C40.0-●	C79.51	—	D16.0-●	—	—

◀ New   ◀ Revised   ~~deleted~~ Deleted   ● Use Additional Character(s)

	Malignant Primary	Malignant Secondary	Ca in situ	Benign	Uncertain Behavior	Unspecified Behavior
bone *(Continued)*						
ethmoid (labyrinth)	C41.0	C79.51	—	D16.4-●	D48.0	D49.2
face	C41.0	C79.51	—	D16.4-●	D48.0	D49.2
femur (any part)	C40.2-●	C79.51	—	D16.2-●	—	—
fibula (any part)	C40.2-●	C79.51	—	D16.2-●	—	—
finger (any)	C40.1-●	C79.51	—	D16.1-●	—	—
foot	C40.3-●	C79.51	—	D16.3-●	—	—
forearm	C40.0-●	C79.51	—	D16.0-●	—	—
frontal	C41.0	C79.51	—	D16.4-●	D48.0	D49.2
hand	C40.1-●	C79.51	—	D16.1-●	—	—
heel	C40.3-●	C79.51	—	D16.3-●	—	—
hip	C41.4	C79.51	—	D16.8-●	D48.0	D49.2
humerus (any part)	C40.0-●	C79.51	—	D16.0-●	—	—
hyoid	C41.0	C79.51	—	D16.4-●	D48.0	D49.2
ilium	C41.4	C79.51	—	D16.8-●	D48.0	D49.2
innominate	C41.4	C79.51	—	D16.8-●	D48.0	D49.2
intervertebral cartilage or disc	C41.2	C79.51	—	D16.6-●	D48.0	D49.2
ischium	C41.4	C79.51	—	D16.8-●	D48.0	D49.2
jaw (lower)	C41.1	C79.51	—	D16.5-●	D48.0	D49.2
knee	C40.2-●	C79.51	—	D16.2-●	—	—
leg NEC	C40.2-●	C79.51	—	D16.2-●	—	—
limb NEC	C40.9-●	C79.51	—	D16.9-●	—	—
lower (long bones)	C40.2-●	C79.51	—	D16.2-●	—	—
short bones	C40.3-●	C79.51	—	D16.3-●	—	—
upper (long bones)	C40.0-●	C79.51	—	D16.0-●	—	—
short bones	C40.1-●	C79.51	—	D16.1-●	—	—
malar	C41.0	C79.51	—	D16.4-●	D48.0	D49.2
mandible	C41.1	C79.51	—	D16.5-●	D48.0	D49.2
marrow NEC (any bone)	C96.9	C79.52	—	—	D47.9	D49.89
mastoid	C41.0	C79.51	—	D16.4-●	D48.0	D49.2
maxilla, maxillary (superior)	C41.0	C79.51	—	D16.4-●	D48.0	D49.2
inferior	C41.1	C79.51	—	D16.5-●	D48.0	D49.2
metacarpus (any)	C40.1-●	C79.51	—	D16.1-●	—	—
metatarsus (any)	C40.3-●	C79.51	—	D16.3-●	—	—
overlapping sites	C40.8-●	—	—	—	—	—
navicular						
ankle	C40.3-●	C79.51	—	—	—	—
hand	C40.1-●	C79.51	—	—	—	—
nose, nasal	C41.0	C79.51	—	D16.4-●	D48.0	D49.2
occipital	C41.0	C79.51	—	D16.4-●	D48.0	D49.2
orbit	C41.0	C79.51	—	D16.4-●	D48.0	D49.2
parietal	C41.0	C79.51	—	D16.4-●	D48.0	D49.2
patella	C40.2-●	C79.51	—	—	—	—
pelvic	C41.4	C79.51	—	D16.8	D48.0	D49.2

	Malignant Primary	Malignant Secondary	Ca in situ	Benign	Uncertain Behavior	Unspecified Behavior
bone *(Continued)*						
phalanges						
foot	C40.3-●	C79.51	—	—	—	—
hand	C40.1-●	C79.51	—	—	—	—
pubic	C41.4	C79.51	—	D16.8	D48.0	D49.2
radius (any part)	C40.0-●	C79.51	—	D16.0-●	—	—
rib	C41.3	C79.51	—	D16.7	D48.0	D49.2
sacral vertebra	C41.4	C79.51	—	D16.8	D48.0	D49.2
sacrum	C41.4	C79.51	—	D16.8	D48.0	D49.2
scaphoid				—	—	—
of ankle	C40.3-●	C79.51	—	—	—	—
of hand	C40.1-●	C79.51	—	—	—	—
scapula (any part)	C40.0-●	C79.51	—	D16.0-●	—	—
sella turcica	C41.0	C79.51	—	D16.4-●	D48.0	D49.2
shoulder	C40.0-●	C79.51	—	D16.0-●	—	—
skull	C41.0	C79.51	—	D16.4-●	D48.0	D49.2
sphenoid	C41.0	C79.51	—	D16.4-●	D48.0	D49.2
spine, spinal (column)	C41.2	C79.51	—	D16.6	D48.0	D49.2
coccyx	C41.4	C79.51	—	D16.8	D48.0	D49.2
sacrum	C41.4	C79.51	—	D16.8	D48.0	D49.2
sternum	C41.3	C79.51	—	D16.7	D48.0	D49.2
tarsus (any)	C40.3-●	C79.51	—	—	—	—
temporal	C41.0	C79.51	—	D16.4-●	D48.0	D49.2
thumb	C40.1-●	C79.51	—	—	—	—
tibia (any part)	C40.2-●	C79.51	—	—	—	—
toe (any)	C40.3-●	C79.51	—	—	—	—
trapezium	C40.1-●	C79.51	—	—	—	—
trapezoid	C40.1-●	C79.51	—	—	—	—
turbinate	C41.0	C79.51	—	D16.4-●	D48.0	D49.2
ulna (any part)	C40.0-●	C79.51	—	D16.0-●	—	—
unciform	C40.1-●	C79.51	—	—	—	—
vertebra (column)	C41.2	C79.51	—	D16.6	D48.0	D49.2
coccyx	C41.4	C79.51	—	D16.8	D48.0	D49.2
sacrum	C41.4	C79.51	—	D16.8	D48.0	D49.2
vomer	C41.0	C79.51	—	D16.4-●	D48.0	D49.2
wrist	C40.1-●	C79.51	—	—	—	—
xiphoid process	C41.3	C79.51	—	D16.7	D48.0	D49.2
zygomatic	C41.0	C79.51	—	D16.4-●	D48.0	D49.2
book-leaf (mouth)	C06.89	C79.89	D00.00	D10.39	D37.09	D49.0
bowel — *see Neoplasm, intestine*						
brachial plexus	C47.1-●	C79.89	—	D36.12	D48.2	D49.2
brain NEC	C71.9	C79.31	—	D33.2	D43.2	D49.6
basal ganglia	C71.0	C79.31	—	D33.0	D43.0	D49.6
cerebellopontine angle	C71.6	C79.31	—	D33.1	D43.1	D49.6

TABLE OF NEOPLASMS

	Malignant Primary	Malignant Secondary	Ca in situ	Benign	Uncertain Behavior	Unspecified Behavior
brain NEC *(Continued)*						
cerebellum NOS	C71.6	C79.31	—	D33.1	D43.1	D49.6
cerebrum	C71.0	C79.31	—	D33.0	D43.0	D49.6
choroid plexus	C71.7	C79.31	—	D33.1	D43.1	D49.6
corpus callosum	C71.8	C79.31	—	D33.2	D43.2	D49.6
corpus striatum	C71.0	C79.31	—	D33.0	D43.0	D49.6
cortex (cerebral)	C71.0	C79.31	—	D33.0	D43.0	D49.6
frontal lobe	C71.1	C79.31	—	D33.0	D43.0	D49.6
globus pallidus	C71.0	C79.31	—	D33.0	D43.0	D49.6
hippocampus	C71.2	C79.31	—	D33.0	D43.0	D49.6
hypothalamus	C71.0	C79.31	—	D33.0	D43.0	D49.6
internal capsule	C71.0	C79.31	—	D33.0	D43.0	D49.6
medulla oblongata	C71.7	C79.31	—	D33.1	D43.1	D49.6
meninges	C70.0	C79.32	—	D32.0	D42.0	D49.7
midbrain	C71.7	C79.31	—	D33.1	D43.1	D49.6
occipital lobe	C71.4	C79.31	—	D33.0	D43.0	D49.6
overlapping lesion	C71.8	C79.31	—	—	—	—
parietal lobe	C71.3	C79.31	—	D33.0	D43.0	D49.6
peduncle	C71.7	C79.31	—	D33.1	D43.1	D49.6
pons	C71.7	C79.31	—	D33.1	D43.1	D49.6
stem	C71.7	C79.31	—	D33.1	D43.1	D49.6
tapetum	C71.8	C79.31	—	D33.2	D43.2	D49.6
temporal lobe	C71.2	C79.31	—	D33.0	D43.0	D49.6
thalamus	C71.0	C79.31	—	D33.0	D43.0	D49.6
uncus	C71.2	C79.31	—	D33.0	D43.0	D49.6
ventricle (floor)	C71.5	C79.31	—	D33.0	D43.0	D49.6
fourth	C71.7	C79.31	—	D33.1	D43.1	D49.6
branchial (cleft) (cyst) (vestiges)	C10.4	C79.89	D00.08	D10.5	D37.05	D49.0
breast (connective tissue) (glandular tissue) (soft parts)	C50.9-●	C79.81	D05.-●	D24.-●	D48.6-●	D49.3
areola	C50.0-●	C79.81	D05.-●	D24.-●	D48.6-●	D49.3
axillary tail	C50.6-●	C79.81	D05.-●	D24.-●	D48.6-●	D49.3
central portion	C50.1-●	C79.81	D05.-●	D24.-●	D48.6-●	D49.3
inner	C50.8-●	C79.81	D05.-●	D24.-●	D48.6-●	D49.3
lower	C50.8-●	C79.81	D05.-●	D24.-●	D48.6-●	D49.3
lower-inner quadrant	C50.3-●	C79.81	D05.-●	D24.-●	D48.6-●	D49.3
lower-outer quadrant	C50.5-●	C79.81	D05.-●	D24.-●	D48.6-●	D49.3
mastectomy site (skin) — *see also Neoplasm, breast, skin*	C44.501	C79.2	—	—	—	—
specified as breast tissue	C50.8-●	C79.81	—	—	—	—
midline	C50.8-●	C79.81	D05.-●	D24.-●	D48.6-●	D49.3
nipple	C50.0-●	C79.81	D05.-●	D24.-●	D48.6-●	D49.3
outer	C50.8-●	C79.81	D05.-●	D24.-●	D48.6-●	D49.3
overlapping lesion	C50.8-●	—	—	—	—	—

	Malignant Primary	Malignant Secondary	Ca in situ	Benign	Uncertain Behavior	Unspecified Behavior
breast *(Continued)*						
skin	C44.501	C79.2	D04.5	D23.5	D48.5	D49.2
basal cell carcinoma	C44.511	—	—	—	—	—
specified type NEC	C44.591	—	—	—	—	—
squamous cell carcinoma	C44.521	—	—	—	—	—
tail (axillary)	C50.6-●	C79.81	D05.-●	D24.-●	D48.6-●	D49.3
upper	C50.8-●	C79.81	D05.-●	D24.-●	D48.6-●	D49.3
upper-inner quadrant	C50.2-●	C79.81	D05.-●	D24.-●	D48.6-●	D49.3
upper-outer quadrant	C50.4-●	C79.81	D05.-●	D24.-●	D48.6-●	D49.3
broad ligament	C57.1	C79.82	D07.39	D28.2	D39.8	D49.59
bronchiogenic, bronchogenic (lung)	C34.9-●	C78.0-●	D02.2-●	D14.3-●	D38.1	D49.1
bronchiole	C34.9-●	C78.0-●	D02.2-●	D14.3-●	D38.1	D49.1
bronchus	C34.9-●	C78.0-●	D02.2-●	D14.3-●	D38.1	D49.1
carina	C34.0-●	C78.0-●	D02.2-●	D14.3-●	D38.1	D49.1
lower lobe of lung	C34.3-●	C78.0-●	D02.2-●	D14.3-●	D38.1	D49.1
main	C34.0-●	C78.0-●	D02.2-●	D14.3-●	D38.1	D49.1
middle lobe of lung	C34.2	C78.0-●	D02.21	D14.31	D38.1	D49.1
overlapping lesion	C34.8-●	—	—	—	—	—
upper lobe of lung	C34.1-●	C78.0-●	D02.2-●	D14.3-●	D38.1	D49.1
brow	C44.309	C79.2	D04.39	D23.39	D48.5	D49.2
basal cell carcinoma	C44.319	—	—	—	—	—
specified type NEC	C44.399	—	—	—	—	—
squamous cell carcinoma	C44.329	—	—	—	—	—
buccal (cavity)	C06.9	C79.89	D00.00	D10.39	D37.09	D49.0
commissure	C06.0	C79.89	D00.02	D10.39	D37.09	D49.0
groove (lower) (upper)	C06.1	C79.89	D00.02	D10.39	D37.09	D49.0
mucosa	C06.0	C79.89	D00.02	D10.39	D37.09	D49.0
sulcus (lower) (upper)	C06.1	C79.89	D00.02	D10.39	D37.09	D49.0
bulbourethral gland	C68.0	C79.19	D09.19	D30.4	D41.3	D49.59
bursa — *see Neoplasm, connective tissue*						
buttock NEC	C76.3	C79.89	D04.5	D36.7	D48.7	D49.89
calf	C76.5-●	C79.89	D04.7-●	D36.7	D48.7	D49.89
calvarium	C41.0	C79.51	—	D16.4-●	D48.0	D49.2
calyx, renal	C65.-●	C79.0-●	D09.19	D30.1-●	D41.1-●	D49.51-●
canal						
anal	C21.1	C78.5	D01.3	D12.9	D37.8	D49.0
auditory (external) — *see also Neoplasm, skin, ear*	C44.20-●	C79.2	D04.2-●	D23.2-●	D48.5	D49.2
auricular (external) — *see also Neoplasm, skin, ear*	C44.20-●	C79.2	D04.2-●	D23.2-●	D48.5	D49.2
canaliculi, biliary (biliferi) (intrahepatic)	C22.1	C78.7	D01.5	D13.4	D37.6	D49.0

◀ New   ◀◀ Revised   ~~deleted~~ Deleted   ● Use Additional Character(s)

	Malignant Primary	Malignant Secondary	Ca in situ	Benign	Uncertain Behavior	Unspecified Behavior
canthus (eye) (inner) (outer)	C44.10-•	C79.2	D04.1-•	D23.1-•	D48.5	D49.2
basal cell carcinoma	C44.11-•	—	—	—	—	—
specified type NEC	C44.19-•	—	—	—	—	—
squamous cell carcinoma	C44.12-•	—	—	—	—	—
capillary — *see Neoplasm, connective tissue*						
caput coli	C18.0	C78.5	D01.0	D12.0	D37.4	D49.0
carcinoid — *see Tumor, carcinoid*						
cardia (gastric)	C16.0	C78.89	D00.2	D13.1	D37.1	D49.0
cardiac orifice (stomach)	C16.0	C78.89	D00.2	D13.1	D37.1	D49.0
cardio-esophageal junction	C16.0	C78.89	D00.2	D13.1	D37.1	D49.0
cardio-esophagus	C16.0	C78.89	D00.2	D13.1	D37.1	D49.0
carina (bronchus)	C34.0-•	C78.0-•	D02.2-•	D14.3-•	D38.1	D49.1
carotid (artery)	C49.0	C79.89	—	D21.0	D48.1	D49.2
body	C75.4	C79.89	—	D35.5	D44.6	D49.7
carpus (any bone)	C40.1-•	C79.51	—	D16.1-•	—	—
cartilage (articular) (joint) NEC — *see also Neoplasm, bone*	C41.9	C79.51	—	D16.9-•	D48.0	D49.2
arytenoid	C32.3	C78.39	D02.0	D14.1	D38.0	D49.1
auricular	C49.0	C79.89	—	D21.0	D48.1	D49.2
bronchi	C34.0-•	C78.39	—	D14.3-•	D38.1	D49.1
costal	C41.3	C79.51	—	D16.7	D48.0	D49.2
cricoid	C32.3	C78.39	D02.0	D14.1	D38.0	D49.1
cuneiform	C32.3	C78.39	D02.0	D14.1	D38.0	D49.1
ear (external)	C49.0	C79.89	—	D21.0	D48.1	D49.2
ensiform	C41.3	C79.51	—	D16.7	D48.0	D49.2
epiglottis	C32.1	C78.39	D02.0	D14.1	D38.0	D49.1
anterior surface	C10.1	C79.89	D00.08	D10.5	D37.05	D49.0
eyelid	C49.0	C79.89	—	D21.0	D48.1	D49.2
intervertebral	C41.2	C79.51	—	D16.6	D48.0	D49.2
larynx, laryngeal	C32.3	C78.39	D02.0	D14.1	D38.0	D49.1
nose, nasal	C30.0	C78.39	D02.3	D14.0	D38.5	D49.1
pinna	C49.0	C79.89	—	D21.0	D48.1	D49.2
rib	C41.3	C79.51	—	D16.7	D48.0	D49.2
semilunar (knee)	C40.2-•	C79.51	—	D16.2-•	D48.0	D49.2
thyroid	C32.3	C78.39	D02.0	D14.1	D38.0	D49.1
trachea	C33	C78.39	D02.1	D14.2	D38.1	D49.1
cauda equina	C72.1	C79.49	—	D33.4	D43.4	D49.7
cavity						
buccal	C06.9	C79.89	D00.00	D10.30	D37.09	D49.0
nasal	C30.0	C78.39	D02.3	D14.0	D38.5	D49.1
oral	C06.9	C79.89	D00.00	D10.30	D37.09	D49.0
peritoneal	C48.2	C78.6	—	D20.1	D48.4	D49.0
tympanic	C30.1	C78.39	D02.3	D14.0	D38.5	D49.1

	Malignant Primary	Malignant Secondary	Ca in situ	Benign	Uncertain Behavior	Unspecified Behavior
cecum	C18.0	C78.5	D01.0	D12.0	D37.4	D49.0
central nervous system	C72.9	C79.40	—	—	—	—
cerebellopontine (angle)	C71.6	C79.31	—	D33.1	D43.1	D49.6
cerebellum, cerebellar	C71.6	C79.31	—	D33.1	D43.1	D49.6
cerebrum, cerebral (cortex) (hemisphere) (white matter)	C71.0	C79.31	—	D33.0	D43.0	D49.6
meninges	C70.0	C79.32	—	D32.0	D42.0	D49.7
peduncle	C71.7	C79.31	—	D33.1	D43.1	D49.6
ventricle	C71.5	C79.31	—	D33.0	D43.0	D49.6
fourth	C71.7	C79.31	—	D33.1	D43.1	D49.6
cervical region	C76.0	C79.89	D09.8	D36.7	D48.7	D49.89
cervix (cervical) (uteri) (uterus)	C53.9	C79.82	D06.9	D26.0	D39.0	D49.59
canal	C53.0	C79.82	D06.0	D26.0	D39.0	D49.59
endocervix (canal) (gland)	C53.0	C79.82	D06.0	D26.0	D39.0	D49.59
exocervix	C53.1	C79.82	D06.1	D26.0	D39.0	D49.59
external os	C53.1	C79.82	D06.1	D26.0	D39.0	D49.59
internal os	C53.0	C79.82	D06.0	D26.0	D39.0	D49.59
nabothian gland	C53.0	C79.82	D06.0	D26.0	D39.0	D49.59
overlapping lesion	C53.8	—	—	—	—	—
squamocolumnar junction	C53.8	C79.82	D06.7	D26.0	D39.0	D49.59
stump	C53.8	C79.82	D06.7	D26.0	D39.0	D49.59
cheek	C76.0	C79.89	D09.8	D36.7	D48.7	D49.89
external	C44.309	C79.2	D04.39	D23.39	D48.5	D49.2
basal cell carcinoma	C44.319	—	—	—	—	—
specified type NEC	C44.399	—	—	—	—	—
squamous cell carcinoma	C44.329	—	—	—	—	—
inner aspect	C06.0	C79.89	D00.02	D10.39	D37.09	D49.0
internal	C06.0	C79.89	D00.02	D10.39	D37.09	D49.0
mucosa	C06.0	C79.89	D00.02	D10.39	D37.09	D49.0
chest (wall) NEC	C76.1	C79.89	D09.8	D36.7	D48.7	D49.89
chiasma opticum	C72.3-•	C79.49	—	D33.3	D43.3	D49.7
chin	C44.309	C79.2	D04.39	D23.39	D48.5	D49.2
basal cell carcinoma	C44.319	—	—	—	—	—
specified type NEC	C44.399	—	—	—	—	—
squamous cell carcinoma	C44.329	—	—	—	—	—
choana	C11.3	C79.89	D00.08	D10.6	D37.05	D49.0
cholangiole	C22.1	C78.89	D01.5	D13.4	D37.6	D49.0
choledochal duct	C24.0	C78.89	D01.5	D13.5	D37.6	D49.0
choroid	C69.3-•	C79.49	D09.2-•	D31.3-•	D48.7	D49.81
plexus	C71.5	C79.31	—	D33.0	D43.0	D49.6
ciliary body	C69.4-•	C79.49	D09.2-•	D31.4-•	D48.7	D49.89
clavicle	C41.3	C79.51	—	D16.7	D48.0	D49.2
clitoris	C51.2	C79.82	D07.1	D28.0	D39.8	D49.59
clivus	C41.0	C79.51	—	D16.4-•	D48.0	D49.2

◀ New   ◀|||| Revised   ~~deleted~~ Deleted   • Use Additional Character(s)

TABLE OF NEOPLASMS

TABLE OF NEOPLASMS

	Malignant Primary	Malignant Secondary	Ca in situ	Benign	Uncertain Behavior	Unspecified Behavior
cloacogenic zone	C21.2	C78.5	D01.3	D12.9	D37.8	D49.0
coccygeal						
body or glomus	C49.5	C79.89	—	D21.5	D48.1	D49.2
vertebra	C41.4	C79.51	—	D16.8	D48.0	D49.2
coccyx	C41.4	C79.51	—	D16.8	D48.0	D49.2
colon — see also Neoplasm, intestine, large	C18.9	C78.5	—	—	—	—
with rectum	C19	C78.5	D01.1	D12.7	D37.5	D49.0
column, spinal — see Neoplasm, spine						
columnella — see also Neoplasm, skin, face	C44.390	C79.2	D04.39	D23.39	D48.5	D49.2
commissure						
labial, lip	C00.6	C79.89	D00.01	D10.39	D37.01	D49.0
laryngeal	C32.0	C78.39	D02.0	D14.1	D38.0	D49.1
common (bile) duct	C24.0	C78.89	D01.5	D13.5	D37.6	D49.0
concha — see also Neoplasm, skin, ear	C44.20-●	C79.2	D04.2-●	D23.2-●	D48.5	D49.2
nose	C30.0	C78.39	D02.3	D14.0	D38.5	D49.1
conjunctiva	C69.0-●	C79.49	D09.2-●	D31.0-●	D48.7	D49.89
connective tissue NEC	C49.9	C79.89	—	D21.9	D48.1	D49.2

Note: For neoplasms of connective tissue (blood vessel, bursa, fascia, ligament, muscle, peripheral nerves, sympathetic and parasympathetic nerves and ganglia, synovia, tendon, etc.) or of morphological types that indicate connective tissue, code according to the list under "Neoplasm, connective tissue". For sites that do not appear in this list, code to neoplasm of that site; e.g., fibrosarcoma, pancreas (C25.9)

Note: Morphological types that indicate connective tissue appear in their proper place in the alphabetic index with the instruction "see Neoplasm, connective tissue ...."

	Malignant Primary	Malignant Secondary	Ca in situ	Benign	Uncertain Behavior	Unspecified Behavior
abdomen	C49.4	C79.89	—	D21.4	D48.1	D49.2
abdominal wall	C49.4	C79.89	—	D21.4	D48.1	D49.2
ankle	C49.2-●	C79.89	—	D21.2-●	D48.1	D49.2
antecubital fossa or space	C49.1-●	C79.89	—	D21.1-●	D48.1	D49.2
arm	C49.1-●	C79.89	—	D21.1-●	D48.1	D49.2
auricle (ear)	C49.0	C79.89	—	D21.0	D48.1	D49.2
axilla	C49.3	C79.89	—	D21.3	D48.1	D49.2
back	C49.6	C79.89	—	D21.6	D48.1	D49.2
breast — see Neoplasm, breast						
buttock	C49.5	C79.89	—	D21.5	D48.1	D49.2
calf	C49.2-●	C79.89	—	D21.2-●	D48.1	D49.2
cervical region	C49.0	C79.89	—	D21.0	D48.1	D49.2
cheek	C49.0	C79.89	—	D21.0	D48.1	D49.2
chest (wall)	C49.3	C79.89	—	D21.3	D48.1	D49.2
chin	C49.0	C79.89	—	D21.0	D48.1	D49.2

connective tissue NEC *(Continued)*	Malignant Primary	Malignant Secondary	Ca in situ	Benign	Uncertain Behavior	Unspecified Behavior
diaphragm	C49.3	C79.89	—	D21.3	D48.1	D49.2
ear (external)	C49.0	C79.89	—	D21.0	D48.1	D49.2
elbow	C49.1-●	C79.89	—	D21.1-●	D48.1	D49.2
extrarectal	C49.5	C79.89	—	D21.5	D48.1	D49.2
extremity	C49.9	C79.89	—	D21.9	D48.1	D49.2
lower	C49.2-●	C79.89	—	D21.2-●	D48.1	D49.2
upper	C49.1-●	C79.89	—	D21.1-●	D48.1	D49.2
eyelid	C49.0	C79.89	—	D21.0	D48.1	D49.2
face	C49.0	C79.89	—	D21.0	D48.1	D49.2
finger	C49.1-●	C79.89	—	D21.1-●	D48.1	D49.2
flank	C49.6	C79.89	—	D21.6	D48.1	D49.2
foot	C49.2-●	C79.89	—	D21.2-●	D48.1	D49.2
forearm	C49.1-●	C79.89	—	D21.1-●	D48.1	D49.2
forehead	C49.0	C79.89	—	D21.0	D48.1	D49.2
gastric	C49.4	C79.89	—	D21.4	D48.1	D49.2
gastrointestinal	C49.4	C79.89	—	D21.4	D48.1	D49.2
gluteal region	C49.5	C79.89	—	D21.5	D48.1	D49.2
great vessels NEC	C49.3	C79.89	—	D21.3	D48.1	D49.2
groin	C49.5	C79.89	—	D21.5	D48.1	D49.2
hand	C49.1-●	C79.89	—	D21.1-●	D48.1	D49.2
head	C49.0	C79.89	—	D21.0	D48.1	D49.2
heel	C49.2-●	C79.89	—	D21.2-●	D48.1	D49.2
hip	C49.2-●	C79.89	—	D21.2-●	D48.1	D49.2
hypochondrium	C49.4	C79.89	—	D21.4	D48.1	D49.2
iliopsoas muscle	C49.5	C79.89	—	D21.5	D48.1	D49.2
infraclavicular region	C49.3	C79.89	—	D21.3	D48.1	D49.2
inguinal (canal) (region)	C49.5	C79.89	—	D21.5	D48.1	D49.2
intestinal	C49.4	C79.89	—	D21.4	D48.1	D49.2
intrathoracic	C49.3	C79.89	—	D21.3	D48.1	D49.2
ischiorectal fossa	C49.5	C79.89	—	D21.5	D48.1	D49.2
jaw	C03.9	C79.89	D00.03	D10.39	D48.1	D49.0
knee	C49.2-●	C79.89	—	D21.2-●	D48.1	D49.2
leg	C49.2-●	C79.89	—	D21.2-●	D48.1	D49.2
limb NEC	C49.9	C79.89	—	D21.9	D48.1	D49.2
lower	C49.2-●	C79.89	—	D21.2-●	D48.1	D49.2
upper	C49.1-●	C79.89	—	D21.1-●	D48.1	D49.2
nates	C49.5	C79.89	—	D21.5	D48.1	D49.2
neck	C49.0	C79.89	—	D21.0	D48.1	D49.2
orbit	C69.6-●	C79.49	D09.2-●	D31.6-●	D48.1	D49.89
overlapping lesion	C49.8	—	—	—	—	—
pararectal	C49.5	C79.89	—	D21.5	D48.1	D49.2
para-urethral	C49.5	C79.89	—	D21.5	D48.1	D49.2
paravaginal	C49.5	C79.89	—	D21.5	D48.1	D49.2

◀ New   ◀ Revised   ~~deleted~~ Deleted   ● Use Additional Character(s)

	Malignant Primary	Malignant Secondary	Ca in situ	Benign	Uncertain Behavior	Unspecified Behavior
connective tissue NEC *(Continued)*						
pelvis (floor)	C49.5	C79.89	—	D21.5	D48.1	D49.2
pelvo-abdominal	C49.8	C79.89	—	D21.6	D48.1	D49.2
perineum	C49.5	C79.89	—	D21.5	D48.1	D49.2
perirectal (tissue)	C49.5	C79.89	—	D21.5	D48.1	D49.2
periurethral (tissue)	C49.5	C79.89	—	D21.5	D48.1	D49.2
popliteal fossa or space	C49.2-●	C79.89	—	D21.2-●	D48.1	D49.2
presacral	C49.5	C79.89	—	D21.5	D48.1	D49.2
psoas muscle	C49.4	C79.89	—	D21.4	D48.1	D49.2
pterygoid fossa	C49.0	C79.89	—	D21.0	D48.1	D49.2
rectovaginal septum or wall	C49.5	C79.89	—	D21.5	D48.1	D49.2
rectovesical	C49.5	C79.89	—	D21.5	D48.1	D49.2
retroperitoneum	C48.0	C78.6	—	D20.0	D48.3	D49.0
sacrococcygeal region	C49.5	C79.89	—	D21.5	D48.1	D49.2
scalp	C49.0	C79.89	—	D21.0	D48.1	D49.2
scapular region	C49.3	C79.89	—	D21.3	D48.1	D49.2
shoulder	C49.1-●	C79.89	—	D21.1-●	D48.1	D49.2
skin (dermis) NEC — *see also Neoplasm, skin, by site*	C44.90	C79.2	D04.9	D23.9	D48.5	D49.2
stomach	C49.4	C79.89	—	D21.4	D48.1	D49.2
submental	C49.0	C79.89	—	D21.0	D48.1	D49.2
supraclavicular region	C49.0	C79.89	—	D21.0	D48.1	D49.2
temple	C49.0	C79.89	—	D21.0	D48.1	D49.2
temporal region	C49.0	C79.89	—	D21.0	D48.1	D49.2
thigh	C49.2-●	C79.89	—	D21.2-●	D48.1	D49.2
thoracic (duct) (wall)	C49.3	C79.89	—	D21.3	D48.1	D49.2
thorax	C49.3	C79.89	—	D21.3	D48.1	D49.2
thumb	C49.1-●	C79.89	—	D21.1-●	D48.1	D49.2
toe	C49.2-●	C79.89	—	D21.2-●	D48.1	D49.2
trunk	C49.6	C79.89	—	D21.6	D48.1	D49.2
umbilicus	C49.4	C79.89	—	D21.4	D48.1	D49.2
vesicorectal	C49.5	C79.89	—	D21.5	D48.1	D49.2
wrist	C49.1-●	C79.89	—	D21.1-●	D48.1	D49.2
conus medullaris	C72.0	C79.49	—	D33.4	D43.4	D49.7
cord (true) (vocal)	C32.0	C78.39	D02.0	D14.1	D38.0	D49.1
false	C32.1	C78.39	D02.0	D14.1	D38.0	D49.1
spermatic	C63.1-●	C79.82	D07.69	D29.8	D40.8	D49.59
spinal (cervical) (lumbar) (thoracic)	C72.0	C79.49	—	D33.4	D43.4	D49.7
cornea (limbus)	C69.1-●	C79.49	D09.2-●	D31.1-●	D48.7	D49.89
corpus						
albicans	C56.-●	C79.6-●	D07.39	D27.-●	D39.1-●	D49.59
callosum, brain	C71.0	C79.31	—	D33.2	D43.2	D49.6
cavernosum	C60.2	C79.82	D07.4	D29.0	D40.8	D49.59

	Malignant Primary	Malignant Secondary	Ca in situ	Benign	Uncertain Behavior	Unspecified Behavior
corpus *(Continued)*						
gastric	C16.2	C78.89	D00.2	D13.1	D37.1	D49.0
overlapping sites	C54.8	—	—	—	—	—
penis	C60.2	C79.82	D07.4	D29.0	D40.8	D49.59
striatum, cerebrum	C71.0	C79.31	—	D33.0	D43.0	D49.6
uteri	C54.9	C79.82	D07.0	D26.1	D39.0	D49.59
isthmus	C54.0	C79.82	D07.0	D26.1	D39.0	D49.59
cortex						
adrenal	C74.0-●	C79.7-●	D09.3	D35.0-●	D44.1-●	D49.7
cerebral	C71.0	C79.31	—	D33.0	D43.0	D49.6
costal cartilage	C41.3	C79.51	—	D16.7	D48.0	D49.2
costovertebral joint	C41.3	C79.51	—	D16.7	D48.0	D49.2
Cowper's gland	C68.0	C79.19	D09.19	D30.4	D41.3	D49.59
cranial (fossa, any)	C71.9	C79.31	—	D33.2	D43.2	D49.6
meninges	C70.0	C79.32	—	D32.0	D42.0	D49.7
nerve	C72.50	C79.49	—	D33.3	D43.3	D49.7
specified NEC	C72.59	C79.49	—	D33.3	D43.3	D49.7
craniobuccal pouch	C75.2	C79.89	D09.3	D35.2	D44.3	D49.7
craniopharyngeal (duct) (pouch)	C75.2	C79.89	D09.3	D35.3	D44.4	D49.7
cricoid	C13.0	C79.89	D00.08	D10.7	D37.05	D49.0
cartilage	C32.3	C78.39	D02.0	D14.1	D38.0	D49.1
cricopharynx	C13.0	C79.89	D00.08	D10.7	D37.05	D49.0
crypt of Morgagni	C21.8	C78.5	D01.3	D12.9	D37.8	D49.0
crystalline lens	C69.4-●	C79.49	D09.2-●	D31.4-●	D48.7	D49.89
cul-de-sac (Douglas')	C48.1	C78.6	—	D20.1	D48.4	D49.0
cuneiform cartilage	C32.3	C78.39	D02.0	D14.1	D38.0	D49.1
cutaneous — *see Neoplasm, skin*						
cutis — *see Neoplasm, skin*						
cystic (bile) duct (common)	C24.0	C78.89	D01.5	D13.5	D37.6	D49.0
dermis — *see Neoplasm, skin*						
diaphragm	C49.3	C79.89	—	D21.3	D48.1	D49.2
digestive organs, system, tube, or tract NEC	C26.9	C78.89	D01.9	D13.9	D37.9	D49.0
disc, intervertebral	C41.2	C79.51	—	D16.6	D48.0	D49.2
disease, generalized	C80.0	—	—	—	—	—
disseminated	C80.0	—	—	—	—	—
Douglas' cul-de-sac or pouch	C48.1	C78.6	—	D20.1	D48.4	D49.0
duodenojejunal junction	C17.8	C78.4	D01.49	D13.39	D37.2	D49.0
duodenum	C17.0	C78.4	D01.49	D13.2	D37.2	D49.0
dura (cranial) (mater)	C70.9	C79.49	—	D32.9	D42.9	D49.7
cerebral	C70.0	C79.32	—	D32.0	D42.0	D49.7
spinal	C70.1	C79.49	—	D32.1	D42.1	D49.7

TABLE OF NEOPLASMS

TABLE OF NEOPLASMS

	Malignant Primary	Malignant Secondary	Ca in situ	Benign	Uncertain Behavior	Unspecified Behavior
ear (external) — see also Neoplasm, skin, ear	C44.20-●	C79.2	D04.2-●	D23.2-●	D48.5	D49.2
auricle or auris — see also Neoplasm, skin, ear	C44.20-●	C79.2	D04.2-●	D23.2-●	D48.5	D49.2
canal, external — see also Neoplasm, skin, ear	C44.20-●	C79.2	D04.2-●	D23.2-●	D48.5	D49.2
cartilage	C49.0	C79.89	—	D21.0	D48.1	D49.2
external meatus — see also Neoplasm, skin, ear	C44.20-●	C79.2	D04.2-●	D23.2-●	D48.5	D49.2
inner	C30.1	C78.39	D02.3	D14.0	D38.5	D49.1
lobule — see also Neoplasm, skin, ear	C44.20-●	C79.2	D04.2-●	D23.2-●	D48.5	D49.2
middle	C30.1	C78.39	D02.3	D14.0	D38.5	D49.1
overlapping lesion with accessory sinuses	C31.8	—	—	—	—	—
skin	C44.20-●	C79.2	D04.2-●	D23.2-●	D48.5	D49.2
basal cell carcinoma	C44.21-●	—	—	—	—	—
specified type NEC	C44.29-●	—	—	—	—	—
squamous cell carcinoma	C44.22-●	—	—	—	—	—
earlobe	C44.20-●	C79.2	D04.2-●	D23.2-●	D48.5	D49.2
basal cell carcinoma	C44.21-●	—	—	—	—	—
specified type NEC	C44.29-●	—	—	—	—	—
squamous cell carcinoma	C44.22-●	—	—	—	—	—
ejaculatory duct	C63.7	C79.82	D07.69	D29.8	D40.8	D49.59
elbow NEC	C76.4-●	C79.89	D04.6-●	D36.7	D48.7	D49.89
endocardium	C38.0	C79.89	—	D15.1	D48.7	D49.89
endocervix (canal) (gland)	C53.0	C79.82	D06.0	D26.0	D39.0	D49.59
endocrine gland NEC	C75.9	C79.89	D09.3	D35.9	D44.9	D49.7
pluriglandular	C75.8	C79.89	D09.3	D35.7	D44.9	D49.7
endometrium (gland) (stroma)	C54.1	C79.82	D07.0	D26.1	D39.0	D49.59
ensiform cartilage	C41.3	C79.51	—	D16.7	D48.0	D49.2
enteric — see Neoplasm, intestine						
ependyma (brain)	C71.5	C79.31	—	D33.0	D43.0	D49.6
fourth ventricle	C71.7	C79.31	—	D33.1	D43.1	D49.6
epicardium	C38.0	C79.89	—	D15.1	D48.7	D49.89
epididymis	C63.0-●	C79.82	D07.69	D29.3-●	D40.8	D49.59
epidural	C72.9	C79.49	—	D33.9	D43.9	D49.7
epiglottis	C32.1	C78.39	D02.0	D14.1	D38.0	D49.1
anterior aspect or surface	C10.1	C79.89	D00.08	D10.5	D37.05	D49.0
cartilage	C32.3	C78.39	D02.0	D14.1	D38.0	D49.1
free border (margin)	C10.1	C79.89	D00.08	D10.5	D37.05	D49.0
junctional region	C10.8	C79.89	D00.08	D10.5	D37.05	D49.0
posterior (laryngeal) surface	C32.1	C78.39	D02.0	D14.1	D38.0	D49.1
suprahyoid portion	C32.1	C78.39	D02.0	D14.1	D38.0	D49.1

	Malignant Primary	Malignant Secondary	Ca in situ	Benign	Uncertain Behavior	Unspecified Behavior
esophagogastric junction	C16.0	C78.89	D00.2	D13.1	D37.1	D49.0
esophagus	C15.9	C78.89	D00.1	D13.0	D37.8	D49.0
abdominal	C15.5	C78.89	D00.1	D13.0	D37.8	D49.0
cervical	C15.3	C78.89	D00.1	D13.0	D37.8	D49.0
distal (third)	C15.5	C78.89	D00.1	D13.0	D37.8	D49.0
lower (third)	C15.5	C78.89	D00.1	D13.0	D37.8	D49.0
middle (third)	C15.4	C78.89	D00.1	D13.0	D37.8	D49.0
overlapping lesion	C15.8	—	—	—	—	—
proximal (third)	C15.3	C78.89	D00.1	D13.0	D37.8	D49.0
thoracic	C15.4	C78.89	D00.1	D13.0	D37.8	D49.0
upper (third)	C15.3	C78.89	D00.1	D13.0	D37.8	D49.0
ethmoid (sinus)	C31.1	C78.39	D02.3	D14.0	D38.5	D49.1
bone or labyrinth	C41.0	C79.51	—	D16.4-●	D48.0	D49.2
eustachian tube	C30.1	C78.39	D02.3	D14.0	D38.5	D49.1
exocervix	C53.1	C79.82	D06.1	D26.0	D39.0	D49.59
external						
meatus (ear) — see also Neoplasm, skin, ear	C44.20-●	C79.2	D04.2-●	D23.2-●	D48.5	D49.2
os, cervix uteri	C53.1	C79.82	D06.1	D26.0	D39.0	D49.59
extradural	C72.9	C79.49	—	D33.9	D43.9	D49.7
extrahepatic (bile) duct	C24.0	C78.89	D01.5	D13.5	D37.6	D49.0
overlapping lesion with gallbladder	C24.8	—	—	—	—	—
extraocular muscle	C69.6-●	C79.49	D09.2-●	D31.6-●	D48.7	D49.89
extrarectal	C76.3	C79.89	D09.8	D36.7	D48.7	D49.89
extremity	C76.8	C79.89	D04.8	D36.7	D48.7	D49.89
lower	C76.5-●	C79.89	D04.7-●	D36.7	D48.7	D49.89
upper	C76.4-●	C79.89	D04.6-●	D36.7	D48.7	D49.89
eye NEC	C69.9-●	C79.49	D09.2	D31.9	D48.7	D49.89
overlapping sites	C69.8	—	—	—	—	—
eyeball	C69.9-●	C79.49	D09.2-●	D31.9-●	D48.7	D49.89
eyebrow	C44.309	C79.2	D04.39	D23.39	D48.5	D49.2
basal cell carcinoma	C44.319	—	—	—	—	—
specified type NEC	C44.399	—	—	—	—	—
squamous cell carcinoma	C44.329	—	—	—	—	—
eyelid (lower) (skin) (upper)	C44.10-●	—	—	—	—	—
basal cell carcinoma	C44.11-●	—	—	—	—	—
cartilage	C49.0	C79.89	—	D21.0	D48.1	D49.2
specified type NEC	C44.19-●	—	—	—	—	—
squamous cell carcinoma	C44.12-●	—	—	—	—	—
face NEC	C76.0	C79.89	D04.39	D36.7	D48.7	D49.89
fallopian tube (accessory)	C57.0-●	C79.82	D07.39	D28.2	D39.8	D49.59
falx (cerebella) (cerebri)	C70.0	C79.32	—	D32.0	D42.0	D49.7

◀ New   ◀❚ Revised   ~~deleted~~ Deleted   ● Use Additional Character(s)

	Malignant Primary	Malignant Secondary	Ca in situ	Benign	Uncertain Behavior	Unspecified Behavior
fascia — *see also Neoplasm, connective tissue*						
palmar	C49.1-●	C79.89	—	D21.1-●	D48.1	D49.2
plantar	C49.2-●	C79.89	—	D21.2-●	D48.1	D49.2
fatty tissue — *see Neoplasm, connective tissue*						
fauces, faucial NEC	C10.9	C79.89	D00.08	D10.5	D37.05	D49.0
pillars	C09.1	C79.89	D00.08	D10.5	D37.05	D49.0
tonsil	C09.9	C79.89	D00.08	D10.4	D37.05	D49.0
femur (any part)	C40.2-●	—	—	D16.2-●	—	—
fetal membrane	C58	C79.82	D07.0	D26.7	D39.2	D49.59
fibrous tissue — *see Neoplasm, connective tissue*						
fibula (any part)	C40.2-●	C79.51	—	D16.2-●	—	—
filum terminale	C72.0	C79.49	—	D33.4	D43.4	D49.7
finger NEC	C76.4-●	C79.89	D04.6-●	D36.7	D48.7	D49.89
flank NEC	C76.8	C79.89	D04.5	D36.7	D48.7	D49.89
follicle, nabothian	C53.0	C79.82	D06.0	D26.0	D39.0	D49.59
foot NEC	C76.5-●	C79.89	D04.7-●	D36.7	D48.7	D49.89
forearm NEC	C76.4-●	C79.89	D04.6-●	D36.7	D48.7	D49.89
forehead (skin)	C44.309	C79.2	D04.39	D23.39	D48.5	D49.2
basal cell carcinoma	C44.319	—	—	—	—	—
specified type NEC	C44.399	—	—	—	—	—
squamous cell carcinoma	C44.329	—	—	—	—	—
foreskin	C60.0	C79.82	D07.4	D29.0	D40.8	D49.59
fornix						
pharyngeal	C11.3	C79.89	D00.08	D10.6	D37.05	D49.0
vagina	C52	C79.82	D07.2	D28.1	D39.8	D49.59
fossa (of)						
anterior (cranial)	C71.9	C79.31	—	D33.2	D43.2	D49.6
cranial	C71.9	C79.31	—	D33.2	D43.2	D49.6
ischiorectal	C76.3	C79.89	D09.8	D36.7	D48.7	D49.89
middle (cranial)	C71.9	C79.31	—	D33.2	D43.2	D49.6
piriform	C12	C79.89	D00.08	D10.7	D37.05	D49.0
pituitary	C75.1	C79.89	D09.3	D35.2	D44.3	D49.7
posterior (cranial)	C71.9	C79.31	—	D33.2	D43.2	D49.6
pterygoid	C49.0	C79.89	—	D21.0	D48.1	D49.2
pyriform	C12	C79.89	D00.08	D10.7	D37.05	D49.0
Rosenmuller	C11.2	C79.89	D00.08	D10.6	D37.05	D49.0
tonsillar	C09.0	C79.89	D00.08	D10.5	D37.05	D49.0
fourchette	C51.9	C79.82	D07.1	D28.0	D39.8	D49.59
frenulum						
labii — *see Neoplasm, lip, internal*						
linguae	C02.2	C79.89	D00.07	D10.1	D37.02	D49.0

	Malignant Primary	Malignant Secondary	Ca in situ	Benign	Uncertain Behavior	Unspecified Behavior
frontal						
bone	C41.0	C79.51	—	D16.4-●	D48.0	D49.2
lobe, brain	C71.1	C79.31	—	D33.0	D43.0	D49.6
pole	C71.1	C79.31	—	D33.0	D43.0	D49.6
sinus	C31.2	C78.39	D02.3	D14.0	D38.5	D49.1
fundus						
stomach	C16.1	C78.89	D00.2	D13.1	D37.1	D49.0
uterus	C54.3	C79.82	D07.0	D26.1	D39.0	D49.59
gall duct (extrahepatic)	C24.0	C78.89	D01.5	D13.5	D37.6	D49.0
intrahepatic	C22.1	C78.7	D01.5	D13.4	D37.6	D49.0
gallbladder	C23	C78.89	D01.5	D13.5	D37.6	D49.0
overlapping lesion with extrahepatic bile ducts	C24.8	—	—	—	—	—
ganglia — *see also Neoplasm, nerve, peripheral*	C47.9	C79.89	—	D36.10	D48.2	D49.2
basal	C71.0	C79.31	—	D33.0	D43.0	D49.6
cranial nerve	C72.50	C79.49	—	D33.3	D43.3	D49.7
Gartner's duct	C52	C79.82	D07.2	D28.1	D39.8	D49.59
gastric — *see Neoplasm, stomach*						
gastrocolic	C26.9	C78.89	D01.9	D13.9	D37.9	D49.0
gastroesophageal junction	C16.0	C78.89	D00.2	D13.1	D37.1	D49.0
gastrointestinal (tract) NEC	C26.9	C78.89	D01.9	D13.9	D37.9	D49.0
generalized	C80.0	—	—	—	—	—
genital organ or tract						
female NEC	C57.9	C79.82	D07.30	D28.9	D39.9	D49.59
overlapping lesion	C57.8	—	—	—	—	—
specified site NEC	C57.7	C79.82	D07.39	D28.7	D39.8	D49.59
male NEC	C63.9	C79.82	D07.60	D29.9	D40.9	D49.59
overlapping lesion	C63.8	—	—	—	—	—
specified site NEC	C63.7	C79.82	D07.69	D29.8	D40.8	D49.59
genitourinary tract						
female	C57.9	C79.82	D07.30	D28.9	D39.9	D49.59
male	C63.9	C79.82	D07.60	D29.9	D40.9	D49.59
gingiva (alveolar) (marginal)	C03.9	C79.89	D00.03	D10.39	D37.09	D49.0
lower	C03.1	C79.89	D00.03	D10.39	D37.09	D49.0
mandibular	C03.1	C79.89	D00.03	D10.39	D37.09	D49.0
maxillary	C03.0	C79.89	D00.03	D10.39	D37.09	D49.0
upper	C03.0	C79.89	D00.03	D10.39	D37.09	D49.0
gland, glandular (lymphatic) (system) — *see also Neoplasm, lymph gland*						
endocrine NEC	C75.9	C79.89	D09.3	D35.9	D44.9	D49.7
salivary — *see Neoplasm, salivary gland*						

TABLE OF NEOPLASMS

	Malignant Primary	Malignant Secondary	Ca in situ	Benign	Uncertain Behavior	Unspecified Behavior
glans penis	C60.1	C79.82	D07.4	D29.0	D40.8	D49.59
globus pallidus	C71.0	C79.31	—	D33.0	D43.0	D49.6
glomus						
coccygeal	C49.5	C79.89	—	D21.5	D48.1	D49.2
jugularis	C75.5	C79.89	—	D35.6	D44.7	D49.7
glosso-epiglottic fold(s)	C10.1	C79.89	D00.08	D10.5	D37.05	D49.0
glossopalatine fold	C09.1	C79.89	D00.08	D10.5	D37.05	D49.0
glossopharyngeal sulcus	C09.0	C79.89	D00.08	D10.5	D37.05	D49.0
glottis	C32.0	C78.39	D02.0	D14.1	D38.0	D49.1
gluteal region	C76.3	C79.89	D04.5	D36.7	D48.7	D49.89
great vessels NEC	C49.3	C79.89	—	D21.3	D48.1	D49.2
groin NEC	C76.3	C79.89	D04.5	D36.7	D48.7	D49.89
gum	C03.9	C79.89	D00.03	D10.39	D37.09	D49.0
lower	C03.1	C79.89	D00.03	D10.39	D37.09	D49.0
upper	C03.0	C79.89	D00.03	D10.39	D37.09	D49.0
hand NEC	C76.4-●	C79.89	D04.6-●	D36.7	D48.7	D49.89
head NEC	C76.0	C79.89	D04.4	D36.7	D48.7	D49.89
heart	C38.0	C79.89	—	D15.1	D48.7	D49.89
heel NEC	C76.5-●	C79.89	D04.7-●	D36.7	D48.7	D49.89
helix — *see also Neoplasm, skin, ear*	C44.20-●	C79.2	D04.2-●	D23.2-●	D48.5	D49.2
hematopoietic, hemopoietic tissue NEC	C96.9	—	—	—	—	—
specified NEC	C96.Z	—	—	—	—	—
hemisphere, cerebral	C71.0	C79.31	—	D33.0	D43.0	D49.6
hemorrhoidal zone	C21.1	C78.5	D01.3	D12.9	D37.8	D49.0
hepatic — *see also Index to disease, by histology*	C22.9	C78.7	D01.5	D13.4	D37.6	D49.0
duct (bile)	C24.0	C78.89	D01.5	D13.5	D37.6	D49.0
flexure (colon)	C18.3	C78.5	D01.0	D12.3	D37.4	D49.0
primary	C22.8	C78.7	D01.5	D13.4	D37.6	D49.0
hepatobiliary	C24.9	C79.89	D01.5	D13.5	D37.6	D49.0
hepatoblastoma	C22.2	C78.7	D01.5	D13.4	D37.6	D49.0
hepatoma	C22.0	C78.7	D01.5	D13.4	D37.6	D49.0
hilus of lung	C34.0-●	C78.0-●	D02.2-●	D14.3-●	D38.1	D49.1
hip NEC	C76.5-●	C79.89	D04.7-●	D36.7	D48.7	D49.89
hippocampus, brain	C71.2	C79.31	—	D33.0	D43.0	D49.6
humerus (any part)	C40.0-●	C79.51	—	D16.0-●	—	—
hymen	C52	C79.82	D07.2	D28.1	D39.8	D49.59
hypopharynx, hypopharyngeal NEC	C13.9	C79.89	D00.08	D10.7	D37.05	D49.0
overlapping lesion	C13.8	—	—	—	—	—
postcricoid region	C13.0	C79.89	D00.08	D10.7	D37.05	D49.0
posterior wall	C13.2	C79.89	D00.08	D10.7	D37.05	D49.0
pyriform fossa (sinus)	C12	C79.89	D00.08	D10.7	D37.05	D49.0
hypophysis	C75.1	C79.89	D09.3	D35.2	D44.3	D49.7

	Malignant Primary	Malignant Secondary	Ca in situ	Benign	Uncertain Behavior	Unspecified Behavior
hypothalamus	C71.0	C79.31	—	D33.0	D43.0	D49.6
ileocecum, ileocecal (coil) (junction) (valve)	C18.0	C78.5	D01.0	D12.0	D37.4	D49.0
ileum	C17.2	C78.4	D01.49	D13.39	D37.2	D49.0
ilium	C41.4	C79.51	—	D16.8	D48.0	D49.2
immunoproliferative NEC	C88.9	—	—	—	—	—
infraclavicular (region)	C76.1	C79.89	D04.5	D36.7	D48.7	D49.89
inguinal (region)	C76.3	C79.89	D04.5	D36.7	D48.7	D49.89
insula	C71.0	C79.31	—	D33.0	D43.0	D49.6
insular tissue (pancreas)	C25.4	C78.89	D01.7	D13.7	D37.8	D49.0
brain	C71.0	C79.31	—	D33.0	D43.0	D49.6
interarytenoid fold	C13.1	C79.89	D00.08	D10.7	D37.05	D49.0
hypopharyngeal aspect	C13.1	C79.89	D00.08	D10.7	D37.05	D49.0
laryngeal aspect	C32.1	C78.39	D02.0	D14.1	D38.0	D49.1
marginal zone	C13.1	C79.89	D00.08	D10.7	D37.05	D49.0
interdental papillae	C03.9	C79.89	D00.03	D10.39	D37.09	D49.0
lower	C03.1	C79.89	D00.03	D10.39	D37.09	D49.0
upper	C03.0	C79.89	D00.03	D10.39	D37.09	D49.0
internal						
capsule	C71.0	C79.31	—	D33.0	D43.0	D49.6
os (cervix)	C53.0	C79.82	D06.0	D26.0	D39.0	D49.59
intervertebral cartilage or disc	C41.2	C79.51	—	D16.6	D48.0	D49.2
intestine, intestinal	C26.0	C78.80	D01.40	D13.9	D37.8	D49.0
large	C18.9	C78.5	D01.0	D12.6	D37.4	D49.0
appendix	C18.1	C78.5	D01.0	D12.1	D37.3	D49.0
caput coli	C18.0	C78.5	D01.0	D12.0	D37.4	D49.0
cecum	C18.0	C78.5	D01.0	D12.0	D37.4	D49.0
colon	C18.9	C78.5	D01.0	D12.6	D37.4	D49.0
and rectum	C19	C78.5	D01.1	D12.7	D37.5	D49.0
ascending	C18.2	C78.5	D01.0	D12.2	D37.4	D49.0
caput	C18.0	C78.5	D01.0	D12.0	D37.4	D49.0
descending	C18.6	C78.5	D01.0	D12.4	D37.4	D49.0
distal	C18.6	C78.5	D01.0	D12.4	D37.4	D49.0
left	C18.6	C78.5	D01.0	D12.4	D37.4	D49.0
overlapping lesion	C18.8	—	—	—	—	—
pelvic	C18.7	C78.5	D01.0	D12.5	D37.4	D49.0
right	C18.2	C78.5	D01.0	D12.2	D37.4	D49.0
sigmoid (flexure)	C18.7	C78.5	D01.0	D12.5	D37.4	D49.0
transverse	C18.4	C78.5	D01.0	D12.3	D37.4	D49.0
hepatic flexure	C18.3	C78.5	D01.0	D12.3	D37.4	D49.0
ileocecum, ileocecal (coil) (valve)	C18.0	C78.5	D01.0	D12.0	D37.4	D49.0
overlapping lesion	C18.8	—	—	—	—	—

◀ New   ◀❚ Revised   ~~deleted~~ Deleted   ● Use Additional Character(s)

	Malignant Primary	Malignant Secondary	Ca in situ	Benign	Uncertain Behavior	Unspecified Behavior
intestine, intestinal *(Continued)*						
large *(Continued)*						
sigmoid flexure (lower) (upper)	C18.7	C78.5	D01.0	D12.5	D37.4	D49.0
splenic flexure	C18.5	C78.5	D01.0	D12.3	D37.4	D49.0
small	C17.9	C78.4	D01.40	D13.30	D37.2	D49.0
duodenum	C17.0	C78.4	D01.49	D13.2	D37.2	D49.0
ileum	C17.2	C78.4	D01.49	D13.39	D37.2	D49.0
jejunum	C17.1	C78.4	D01.49	D13.39	D37.2	D49.0
overlapping lesion	C17.8	—	—	—	—	—
tract NEC	C26.0	C78.89	D01.40	D13.9	D37.8	D49.0
intra-abdominal	C76.2	C79.89	D09.8	D36.7	D48.7	D49.89
intracranial NEC	C71.9	C79.31	—	D33.2	D43.2	D49.6
intrahepatic (bile) duct	C22.1	C78.7	D01.5	D13.4	D37.6	D49.0
intraocular	C69.9-●	C79.49	D09.2-●	D31.9-●	D48.7	D49.89
intraorbital	C69.6-●	C79.49	D09.2-●	D31.6-●	D48.7	D49.89
intrasellar	C75.1	C79.89	D09.3	D35.2	D44.3	D49.7
intrathoracic (cavity) (organs)	C76.1	C79.89	D09.8	D15.9	D48.7	D49.89
specified NEC	C76.1	C79.89	D09.8	D15.7	—	—
iris	C69.4-●	C79.49	D09.2-●	D31.4-●	D48.7	D49.89
ischiorectal (fossa)	C76.3	C79.89	D09.8	D36.7	D48.7	D49.89
ischium	C41.4	C79.51	—	D16.8	D48.0	D49.2
island of Reil	C71.0	C79.31	—	D33.0	D43.0	D49.6
islands or islets of Langerhans	C25.4	C78.89	D01.7	D13.7	D37.8	D49.0
isthmus uteri	C54.0	C79.82	D07.0	D26.1	D39.0	D49.59
jaw	C76.0	C79.89	D09.8	D36.7	D48.7	D49.89
bone	C41.1	C79.51	—	D16.5-●	D48.0	D49.2
lower	C41.1	C79.51	—	D16.5-●	—	—
upper	C41.0	C79.51	—	D16.4-●	—	—
carcinoma (any type) (lower) (upper)	C76.0	C79.89				
skin — *see also Neoplasm, skin, face*	C44.309	C79.2	D04.39	D23.39	D48.5	D49.2
soft tissues	C03.9	C79.89	D00.03	D10.39	D37.09	D49.0
lower	C03.1	C79.89	D00.03	D10.39	D37.09	D49.0
upper	C03.0	C79.89	D00.03	D10.39	D37.09	D49.0
jejunum	C17.1	C78.4	D01.49	D13.39	D37.2	D49.0
joint NEC — *see also Neoplasm, bone*	C41.9	C79.51	—	D16.9-●	D48.0	D49.2
acromioclavicular	C40.0-●	C79.51	—	D16.0-●	—	—
bursa or synovial membrane — *see Neoplasm, connective tissue*						
costovertebral	C41.3	C79.51	—	D16.7	D48.0	D49.2
sternocostal	C41.3	C79.51	—	D16.7	D48.0	D49.2
temporomandibular	C41.1	C79.51	—	D16.5-●	D48.0	D49.2

	Malignant Primary	Malignant Secondary	Ca in situ	Benign	Uncertain Behavior	Unspecified Behavior
junction						
anorectal	C21.8	C78.5	D01.3	D12.9	D37.8	D49.0
cardioesophageal	C16.0	C78.89	D00.2	D13.1	D37.1	D49.0
esophagogastric	C16.0	C78.89	D00.2	D13.1	D37.1	D49.0
gastroesophageal	C16.0	C78.89	D00.2	D13.1	D37.1	D49.0
hard and soft palate	C05.9	C79.89	D00.00	D10.39	D37.09	D49.0
ileocecal	C18.0	C78.5	D01.0	D12.0	D37.4	D49.0
pelvirectal	C19	C78.5	D01.1	D12.7	D37.5	D49.0
pelviureteric	C65.-●	C79.0-●	D09.19	D30.1-●	D41.1-●	D49.59
rectosigmoid	C19	C78.5	D01.1	D12.7	D37.5	D49.0
squamocolumnar, of cervix	C53.8	C79.82	D06.7	D26.0	D39.0	D49.59
Kaposi's sarcoma — *see Kaposi's, sarcoma*						
kidney (parenchymal)	C64.-●	C79.0-●	D09.19	D30.0-●	D41.0-●	D49.51-●
calyx	C65.-●	C79.0-●	D09.19	D30.1-●	D41.1-●	D49.51-●
hilus	C65.-●	C79.0-●	D09.19	D30.1-●	D41.1-●	D49.51-●
pelvis	C65.-●	C79.0-●	D09.19	D30.1-●	D41.1-●	D49.51-●
knee NEC	C76.5-●	C79.89	D04.7-●	D36.7	D48.7	D49.89
labia (skin)	C51.9	C79.82	D07.1	D28.0	D39.8	D49.59
majora	C51.0	C79.82	D07.1	D28.0	D39.8	D49.59
minora	C51.1	C79.82	D07.1	D28.0	D39.8	D49.59
labial — *see also Neoplasm, lip*	C00.9	C79.89	D00.01	D10.0	D37.01	D49.0
sulcus (lower) (upper)	C06.1	C79.89	D00.02	D10.39	D37.09	D49.0
labium (skin)	C51.9	C79.82	D07.1	D28.0	D39.8	D49.59
majus	C51.0	C79.82	D07.1	D28.0	D39.8	D49.59
minus	C51.1	C79.82	D07.1	D28.0	D39.8	D49.59
lacrimal						
canaliculi	C69.5-●	C79.49	D09.2-●	D31.5-●	D48.7	D49.89
duct (nasal)	C69.5-●	C79.49	D09.2-●	D31.5-●	D48.7	D49.89
gland	C69.5-●	C79.49	D09.2-●	D31.5-●	D48.7	D49.89
punctum	C69.5-●	C79.49	D09.2-●	D31.5-●	D48.7	D49.89
sac	C69.5-●	C79.49	D09.2-●	D31.5-●	D48.7	D49.89
Langerhans, islands or islets	C25.4	C78.89	D01.7	D13.7	D37.8	D49.0
laryngopharynx	C13.9	C79.89	D00.08	D10.7	D37.05	D49.0
larynx, laryngeal NEC	C32.9	C78.39	D02.0	D14.1	D38.0	D49.1
aryepiglottic fold	C32.1	C78.39	D02.0	D14.1	D38.0	D49.1
cartilage (arytenoid) (cricoid) (cuneiform) (thyroid)	C32.3	C78.39	D02.0	D14.1	D38.0	D49.1
commissure (anterior) (posterior)	C32.0	C78.39	D02.0	D14.1	D38.0	D49.1
extrinsic NEC	C32.1	C78.39	D02.0	D14.1	D38.0	D49.1
meaning hypopharynx	C13.9	C79.89	D00.08	D10.7	D37.05	D49.0
interarytenoid fold	C32.1	C78.39	D02.0	D14.1	D38.0	D49.1
intrinsic	C32.0	C78.39	D02.0	D14.1	D38.0	D49.1

◀ New   ◀▮ Revised   ~~deleted~~ Deleted   ● Use Additional Character(s)

	Malignant Primary	Malignant Secondary	Ca in situ	Benign	Uncertain Behavior	Unspecified Behavior
larynx, laryngeal NEC *(Continued)*						
overlapping lesion	C32.8	—	—	—	—	—
ventricular band	C32.1	C78.39	D02.0	D14.1	D38.0	D49.1
leg NEC	C76.5-●	C79.89	D04.7-●	D36.7	D48.7	D49.89
lens, crystalline	C69.4-●	C79.49	D09.2-●	D31.4-●	D48.7	D49.89
lid (lower) (upper)	C44.10-●	C79.2	D04.1-●	D23.1-●	D48.5	D49.2
basal cell carcinoma	C44.11-●	—	—	—	—	—
specified type NEC	C44.19-●	—	—	—	—	—
squamous cell carcinoma	C44.12-●	—	—	—	—	—
ligament — *see also Neoplasm, connective tissue*						
broad	C57.1	C79.82	D07.39	D28.2	D39.8	D49.59
Mackenrodt's	C57.7	C79.82	D07.39	D28.7	D39.8	D49.59
non-uterine — *see Neoplasm, connective tissue*						
round	C57.2	C79.82	—	D28.2	D39.8	D49.59
sacro-uterine	C57.3	C79.82	—	D28.2	D39.8	D49.59
uterine	C57.3	C79.82	—	D28.2	D39.8	D49.59
utero-ovarian	C57.7	C79.82	D07.39	D28.2	D39.8	D49.59
uterosacral	C57.3	C79.82	—	D28.2	D39.8	D49.59
limb	C76.8	C79.89	D04.8	D36.7	D48.7	D49.89
lower	C76.5-●	C79.89	D04.7-●	D36.7	D48.7	D49.89
upper	C76.4-●	C79.89	D04.6-●	D36.7	D48.7	D49.89
limbus of cornea	C69.1-●	C79.49	D09.2-●	D31.1-●	D48.7	D49.89
lingual NEC — *see also Neoplasm, tongue*	C02.9	C79.89	D00.07	D10.1	D37.02	D49.0
lingula, lung	C34.1-●	C78.0-●	D02.2-●	D14.3-●	D38.1	D49.1
lip	C00.9	C79.89	D00.01	D10.0	D37.01	D49.0
buccal aspect — *see Neoplasm, lip, internal*						
commissure	C00.6	C79.89	D00.01	D10.0	D37.01	D49.0
external	C00.2	C79.89	D00.01	D10.0	D37.01	D49.0
lower	C00.1	C79.89	D00.01	D10.0	D37.01	D49.0
upper	C00.0	C79.89	D00.01	D10.0	D37.01	D49.0
frenulum — *see Neoplasm, lip, internal*						
inner aspect — *see Neoplasm, lip, internal*						
internal	C00.5	C79.89	D00.01	D10.0	D37.01	D49.0
lower	C00.4	C79.89	D00.01	D10.0	D37.01	D49.0
upper	C00.3	C79.89	D00.01	D10.0	D37.01	D49.0
lipstick area	C00.2	C79.89	D00.01	D10.0	D37.01	D49.0
lower	C00.1	C79.89	D00.01	D10.0	D37.01	D49.0
upper	C00.0	C79.89	D00.01	D10.0	D37.01	D49.0
lip *(Continued)*						
lower	C00.1	C79.89	D00.01	D10.0	D37.01	D49.0
internal	C00.4	C79.89	D00.01	D10.0	D37.01	D49.0
mucosa — *see Neoplasm, lip, internal*						
oral aspect — *see Neoplasm, lip, internal*						
overlapping lesion	C00.8	—	—	—	—	—
with oral cavity or pharynx	C14.8	—	—	—	—	—
skin (commissure) (lower) (upper)	C44.00	C79.2	D04.0	D23.0	D48.5	D49.2
basal cell carcinoma	C44.01	—	—	—	—	—
specified type NEC	C44.09	—	—	—	—	—
squamous cell carcinoma	C44.02	—	—	—	—	—
upper	C00.0	C79.89	D00.01	D10.0	D37.01	D49.0
internal	C00.3	C79.89	D00.01	D10.0	D37.01	D49.0
vermilion border	C00.2	C79.89	D00.01	D10.0	D37.01	D49.0
lower	C00.1	C79.89	D00.01	D10.0	D37.01	D49.0
upper	C00.0	C79.89	D00.01	D10.0	D37.01	D49.0
lipomatous — *see Lipoma, by site*						
liver — *see also Index to disease, by histology*	C22.9	C78.7	D01.5	D13.4	D37.6	D49.0
primary	C22.8	C78.7	D01.5	D13.4	D37.6	D49.0
lumbosacral plexus	C47.5	C79.89	—	D36.16	D48.2	D49.2
lung	C34.9-●	C78.0-●	D02.2-●	D14.3-●	D38.1	D49.1
azygos lobe	C34.1-●	C78.0-●	D02.2-●	D14.3-●	D38.1	D49.1
carina	C34.0-●	C78.0-●	D02.2-●	D14.3-●	D38.1	D49.1
hilus	C34.0-●	C78.0-●	D02.2-●	D14.3-●	D38.1	D49.1
lingula	C34.1-●	C78.0-●	D02.2-●	D14.3-●	D38.1	D49.1
lobe NEC	C34.9-●	C78.0-●	D02.2-●	D14.3-●	D38.1	D49.1
lower lobe	C34.3-●	C78.0-●	D02.2-●	D14.3-●	D38.1	D49.1
main bronchus	C34.0-●	C78.0-●	D02.2-●	D14.3-●	D38.1	D49.1
mesothelioma — *see Mesothelioma*						
middle lobe	C34.2	C78.0-●	D02.21	D14.31	D38.1	D49.1
overlapping lesion	C34.8-●	—	—	—	—	—
upper lobe	C34.1-●	C78.0-●	D02.2-●	D14.3-●	D38.1	D49.1
lymph, lymphatic channel NEC	C49.9	C79.89	—	D21.9	D48.1	D49.2
gland (secondary)	—	C77.9	—	D36.0	D48.7	D49.89
abdominal	—	C77.2	—	D36.0	D48.7	D49.89
aortic	—	C77.2	—	D36.0	D48.7	D49.89
arm	—	C77.3	—	D36.0	D48.7	D49.89
auricular (anterior) (posterior)	—	C77.0	—	D36.0	D48.7	D49.89

◄ New   ◄█ Revised   ~~deleted~~ Deleted   ● Use Additional Character(s)

lymph, lymphatic channel NEC (Continued) gland (Continued)	Malignant Primary	Malignant Secondary	Ca in situ	Benign	Uncertain Behavior	Unspecified Behavior
axilla, axillary	—	C77.3	—	D36.0	D48.7	D49.89
brachial	—	C77.3	—	D36.0	D48.7	D49.89
bronchial	—	C77.1	—	D36.0	D48.7	D49.89
bronchopulmonary	—	C77.1	—	D36.0	D48.7	D49.89
celiac	—	C77.2	—	D36.0	D48.7	D49.89
cervical	—	C77.0	—	D36.0	D48.7	D49.89
cervicofacial	—	C77.0	—	D36.0	D48.7	D49.89
Cloquet	—	C77.4	—	D36.0	D48.7	D49.89
colic	—	C77.2	—	D36.0	D48.7	D49.89
common duct	—	C77.2	—	D36.0	D48.7	D49.89
cubital	—	C77.3	—	D36.0	D48.7	D49.89
diaphragmatic	—	C77.1	—	D36.0	D48.7	D49.89
epigastric, inferior	—	C77.1	—	D36.0	D48.7	D49.89
epitrochlear	—	C77.3	—	D36.0	D48.7	D49.89
esophageal	—	C77.1	—	D36.0	D48.7	D49.89
face	—	C77.0	—	D36.0	D48.7	D49.89
femoral	—	C77.4	—	D36.0	D48.7	D49.89
gastric	—	C77.2	—	D36.0	D48.7	D49.89
groin	—	C77.4	—	D36.0	D48.7	D49.89
head	—	C77.0	—	D36.0	D48.7	D49.89
hepatic	—	C77.2	—	D36.0	D48.7	D49.89
hilar (pulmonary)	—	C77.1	—	D36.0	D48.7	D49.89
splenic	—	C77.2	—	D36.0	D48.7	D49.89
hypogastric	—	C77.5	—	D36.0	D48.7	D49.89
ileocolic	—	C77.2	—	D36.0	D48.7	D49.89
iliac	—	C77.5	—	D36.0	D48.7	D49.89
infraclavicular	—	C77.3	—	D36.0	D48.7	D49.89
inguina, inguinal	—	C77.4	—	D36.0	D48.7	D49.89
innominate	—	C77.1	—	D36.0	D48.7	D49.89
intercostal	—	C77.1	—	D36.0	D48.7	D49.89
intestinal	—	C77.2	—	D36.0	D48.7	D49.89
intrabdominal	—	C77.2	—	D36.0	D48.7	D49.89
intrapelvic	—	C77.5	—	D36.0	D48.7	D49.89
intrathoracic	—	C77.1	—	D36.0	D48.7	D49.89
jugular	—	C77.0	—	D36.0	D48.7	D49.89
leg	—	C77.4	—	D36.0	D48.7	D49.89
limb						
lower	—	C77.4	—	D36.0	D48.7	D49.89
upper	—	C77.3	—	D36.0	D48.7	D49.89
lower limb	—	C77.4	—	D36.0	D48.7	D49.89
lumbar	—	C77.2	—	D36.0	D48.7	D49.89

lymph, lymphatic channel NEC (Continued) gland (Continued)	Malignant Primary	Malignant Secondary	Ca in situ	Benign	Uncertain Behavior	Unspecified Behavior
mandibular	—	C77.0	—	D36.0	D48.7	D49.89
mediastinal	—	C77.1	—	D36.0	D48.7	D49.89
mesenteric (inferior) (superior)	—	C77.2	—	D36.0	D48.7	D49.89
midcolic	—	C77.2	—	D36.0	D48.7	D49.89
multiple sites in categories C77.0 - C77.5	—	C77.8	—	D36.0	D48.7	D49.89
neck	—	C77.0	—	D36.0	D48.7	D49.89
obturator	—	C77.5	—	D36.0	D48.7	D49.89
occipital	—	C77.0	—	D36.0	D48.7	D49.89
pancreatic	—	C77.2	—	D36.0	D48.7	D49.89
para-aortic	—	C77.2	—	D36.0	D48.7	D49.89
paracervical	—	C77.5	—	D36.0	D48.7	D49.89
parametrial	—	C77.5	—	D36.0	D48.7	D49.89
parasternal	—	C77.1	—	D36.0	D48.7	D49.89
parotid	—	C77.0	—	D36.0	D48.7	D49.89
pectoral	—	C77.3	—	D36.0	D48.7	D49.89
pelvic	—	C77.5	—	D36.0	D48.7	D49.89
peri-aortic	—	C77.2	—	D36.0	D48.7	D49.89
peripancreatic	—	C77.2	—	D36.0	D48.7	D49.89
popliteal	—	C77.4	—	D36.0	D48.7	D49.89
porta hepatis	—	C77.2	—	D36.0	D48.7	D49.89
portal	—	C77.2	—	D36.0	D48.7	D49.89
preauricular	—	C77.0	—	D36.0	D48.7	D49.89
prelaryngeal	—	C77.0	—	D36.0	D48.7	D49.89
presymphysial	—	C77.5	—	D36.0	D48.7	D49.89
pretracheal	—	C77.0	—	D36.0	D48.7	D49.89
primary (any site) NEC	C96.9	—	—	—	—	—
pulmonary (hiler)	—	C77.1	—	D36.0	D48.7	D49.89
pyloric	—	C77.2	—	D36.0	D48.7	D49.89
retroperitoneal	—	C77.2	—	D36.0	D48.7	D49.89
retropharyngeal	—	C77.0	—	D36.0	D48.7	D49.89
Rosenmuller's	—	C77.4	—	D36.0	D48.7	D49.89
sacral	—	C77.5	—	D36.0	D48.7	D49.89
scalene	—	C77.0	—	D36.0	D48.7	D49.89
site NEC	—	C77.9	—	D36.0	D48.7	D49.89
splenic (hilar)	—	C77.2	—	D36.0	D48.7	D49.89
subclavicular	—	C77.3	—	D36.0	D48.7	D49.89
subinguinal	—	C77.4	—	D36.0	D48.7	D49.89
sublingual	—	C77.0	—	D36.0	D48.7	D49.89
submandibular	—	C77.0	—	D36.0	D48.7	D49.89

◀ New   ◀ Revised   ~~deleted~~ Deleted   ● Use Additional Character(s)

	Malignant Primary	Malignant Secondary	Ca in situ	Benign	Uncertain Behavior	Unspecified Behavior
lymph, lymphatic channel NEC *(Continued)*						
gland *(Continued)*						
submaxillary	—	C77.0	—	D36.0	D48.7	D49.89
submental	—	C77.0	—	D36.0	D48.7	D49.89
subscapular	—	C77.3	—	D36.0	D48.7	D49.89
supraclavicular	—	C77.0	—	D36.0	D48.7	D49.89
thoracic	—	C77.1	—	D36.0	D48.7	D49.89
tibial	—	C77.4	—	D36.0	D48.7	D49.89
tracheal	—	C77.1	—	D36.0	D48.7	D49.89
tracheobronchial	—	C77.1	—	D36.0	D48.7	D49.89
upper limb	—	C77.3	—	D36.0	D48.7	D49.89
Virchow's	—	C77.0	—	D36.0	D48.7	D49.89
node — *see also Neoplasm, lymph gland*						
primary NEC	C96.9	—	—	—	—	—
vessel — *see also Neoplasm, connective tissue*	C49.9	C79.89	—	D21.9	D48.1	D49.2
Mackenrodt's ligament	C57.7	C79.82	D07.39	D28.7	D39.8	D49.59
malar	C41.0	C79.51	—	D16.4-●	D48.0	D49.2
region — *see Neoplasm, cheek*						
mammary gland — *see Neoplasm, breast*						
mandible	C41.1	C79.51	—	D16.5-●	D48.0	D49.2
alveolar						
mucosa (carcinoma)	C03.1	C79.89	D00.03	D10.39	D37.09	D49.0
ridge or process	C41.1	C79.51	—	D16.5-●	D48.0	D49.2
marrow (bone) NEC	C96.9	C79.52	—	—	D47.9	D49.89
mastectomy site (skin) — *see also Neoplasm, breast, skin*	C44.501	C79.2	—	—	—	—
specified as breast tissue	C50.8-●	C79.81	—	—	—	—
mastoid (air cells) (antrum) (cavity)	C30.1	C78.39	D02.3	D14.0	D38.5	D49.1
bone or process	C41.0	C79.51	—	D16.4-●	D48.0	D49.2
maxilla, maxillary (superior)	C41.0	C79.51	—	D16.4-●	D48.0	D49.2
alveolar						
mucosa	C03.0	C79.89	D00.03	D10.39	D37.09	D49.0
ridge or process (carcinoma)	C41.0	C79.51	—	D16.4-●	D48.0	D49.2
antrum	C31.0	C78.39	D02.3	D14.0	D38.5	D49.1
carcinoma	C03.0	C79.51	—	—	—	—
inferior — *see Neoplasm, mandible*						
sinus	C31.0	C78.39	D02.3	D14.0	D38.5	D49.1
meatus external (ear) — *see also Neoplasm, skin, ear*	C44.20-●	C79.2	D04.2-●	D23.2-●	D48.5	D49.2
Meckel diverticulum, malignant	C17.3	C78.4	D01.49	D13.39	D37.2	D49.0

	Malignant Primary	Malignant Secondary	Ca in situ	Benign	Uncertain Behavior	Unspecified Behavior
mediastinum, mediastinal	C38.3	C78.1	—	D15.2	D38.3	D49.89
anterior	C38.1	C78.1	—	D15.2	D38.3	D49.89
posterior	C38.2	C78.1	—	D15.2	D38.3	D49.89
medulla						
adrenal	C74.1-●	C79.7-●	D09.3	D35.0-●	D44.1-●	D49.7
oblongata	C71.7	C79.31	—	D33.1	D43.1	D49.6
meibomian gland	C44.10-●	C79.2	D04.1-●	D23.1-●	D48.5	D49.2
basal cell carcinoma	C44.11-●	—	—	—	—	—
specified type NEC	C44.19-●	—	—	—	—	—
squamous cell carcinoma	C44.12-●	—	—	—	—	—
melanoma — *see Melanoma*						
meninges	C70.9	C79.49	—	D32.9	D42.9	D49.7
brain	C70.0	C79.32	—	D32.0	D42.0	D49.7
cerebral	C70.0	C79.32	—	D32.0	D42.0	D49.7
crainial	C70.0	C79.32	—	D32.0	D42.0	D49.7
intracranial	C70.0	C79.32	—	D32.0	D42.0	D49.7
spinal (cord)	C70.1	C79.49	—	D32.1	D42.1	D49.7
meniscus, knee joint (lateral) (medial)	C40.2-●	C79.51	—	D16.2-●	D48.0	D49.2
Merkel cell — *see Carcinoma, Merkel cell*						
mesentery, mesenteric	C48.1	C78.6	—	D20.1	D48.4	D49.0
mesoappendix	C48.1	C78.6	—	D20.1	D48.4	D49.0
mesocolon	C48.1	C78.6	—	D20.1	D48.4	D49.0
mesopharynx — *see Neoplasm, oropharynx*						
mesosalpinx	C57.1	C79.82	D07.39	D28.2	D39.8	D49.59
mesothelial tissue — *see Mesothelioma*						
mesothelioma — *see Mesothelioma*						
mesovarium	C57.1	C79.82	D07.39	D28.2	D39.8	D49.59
metacarpus (any bone)	C40.1-●	C79.51	—	D16.1-●	—	—
metastatic NEC — *see also Neoplasm, by site, secondary*	—	C79.9	—	—	—	—
metatarsus (any bone)	C40.3-●	C79.51	—	D16.3-●	—	—
midbrain	C71.7	C79.31	—	D33.1	D43.1	D49.6
milk duct — *see Neoplasm, breast*						
mons						
pubis	C51.9	C79.82	D07.1	D28.0	D39.8	D49.59
veneris	C51.9	C79.82	D07.1	D28.0	D39.8	D49.59
motor tract	C72.9	C79.49	—	D33.9	D43.9	D49.7
brain	C71.9	C79.31	—	D33.2	D43.2	D49.6
cauda equina	C72.1	C79.49	—	D33.4	D43.4	D49.7
spinal	C72.0	C79.49	—	D33.4	D43.4	D49.7

◀ New   ◀ Revised   ~~deleted~~ Deleted   ● Use Additional Character(s)

	Malignant Primary	Malignant Secondary	Ca in situ	Benign	Uncertain Behavior	Unspecified Behavior
mouth	C06.9	C79.89	D00.00	D10.30	D37.09	D49.0
book-leaf	C06.89	C79.89	—	—	—	—
floor	C04.9	C79.89	D00.06	D10.2	D37.09	D49.0
anterior portion	C04.0	C79.89	D00.06	D10.2	D37.09	D49.0
lateral portion	C04.1	C79.89	D00.06	D10.2	D37.09	D49.0
overlapping lesion	C04.8	—	—	—	—	—
overlapping NEC	C06.80	—	—	—	—	—
roof	C05.9	C79.89	D00.00	D10.39	D37.09	D49.0
specified part NEC	C06.89	C79.89	D00.00	D10.39	D37.09	D49.0
vestibule	C06.1	C79.89	D00.00	D10.39	D37.09	D49.0
mucosa						
alveolar (ridge or process)	C03.9	C79.89	D00.03	D10.39	D37.09	D49.0
lower	C03.1	C79.89	D00.03	D10.39	D37.09	D49.0
upper	C03.0	C79.89	D00.03	D10.39	D37.09	D49.0
buccal	C06.0	C79.89	D00.02	D10.39	D37.09	D49.0
cheek	C06.0	C79.89	D00.02	D10.39	D37.09	D49.0
lip — see Neoplasm, lip, internal						
nasal	C30.0	C78.39	D02.3	D14.0	D38.5	D49.1
oral	C06.0	C79.89	D00.02	D10.39	D37.09	D49.0
Mullerian duct						
female	C57.7	C79.82	D07.39	D28.7	D39.8	D49.59
male	C63.7	C79.82	D07.69	D29.8	D40.8	D49.59
muscle — see also Neoplasm, connective tissue						
extraocular	C69.6-●	C79.49	D09.2-●	D31.6-●	D48.7	D49.89
myocardium	C38.0	C79.89	—	D15.1	D48.7	D49.89
myometrium	C54.2	C79.82	D07.0	D26.1	D39.0	D49.59
myopericardium	C38.0	C79.89	—	D15.1	D48.7	D49.89
nabothian gland (follicle)	C53.0	C79.82	D06.0	D26.0	D39.0	D49.59
nail — see also Neoplasm, skin, limb	C44.90	C79.2	D04.9	D23.9	D48.5	D49.2
finger — see also Neoplasm, skin, limb, upper	C44.60-●	C79.2	D04.6-●	D23.6-●	D48.5	D49.2
toe — see also Neoplasm, skin, limb, lower	C44.70-●	C79.2	D04.7-●	D23.7-●	D48.5	D49.2
nares, naris (anterior) (posterior)	C30.0	C78.39	D02.3	D14.0	D38.5	D49.1
nasal — see Neoplasm, nose						
nasolabial groove — see also Neoplasm, skin, face	C44.309	C79.2	D04.39	D23.39	D48.5	D49.2
nasolacrimal duct	C69.5-●	C79.49	D09.2-●	D31.5-●	D48.7	D49.89
nasopharynx, nasopharyngeal	C11.9	C79.89	D00.08	D10.6	D37.05	D49.0
floor	C11.3	C79.89	D00.08	D10.6	D37.05	D49.0
overlapping lesion	C11.8	—	—	—	—	—
roof	C11.0	C79.89	D00.08	D10.6	D37.05	D49.0

	Malignant Primary	Malignant Secondary	Ca in situ	Benign	Uncertain Behavior	Unspecified Behavior
nasopharynx, nasopharyngeal (Continued)						
wall	C11.9	C79.89	D00.08	D10.6	D37.05	D49.0
anterior	C11.3	C79.89	D00.08	D10.6	D37.05	D49.0
lateral	C11.2	C79.89	D00.08	D10.6	D37.05	D49.0
posterior	C11.1	C79.89	D00.08	D10.6	D37.05	D49.0
superior	C11.0	C79.89	D00.08	D10.6	D37.05	D49.0
nates — see also Neoplasm, skin, trunk	C44.509	C79.2	D04.5	D23.5	D48.5	D49.2
neck NEC	C76.0	C79.89	D09.8	D36.7	D48.7	D49.89
skin	C44.40	—	—	—	—	—
basal cell carcinoma	C44.41	—	—	—	—	—
specified type NEC	C44.49	—	—	—	—	—
squamous cell carcinoma	C44.42	—	—	—	—	—
nerve (ganglion)	C47.9	C79.89	—	D36.10	D48.2	D49.2
abducens	C72.59	C79.49	—	D33.3	D43.3	D49.7
accessory (spinal)	C72.59	C79.49	—	D33.3	D43.3	D49.7
acoustic	C72.4-●	C79.49	—	D33.3	D43.3	D49.7
auditory	C72.4-●	C79.49	—	D33.3	D43.3	D49.7
autonomic NEC — see also Neoplasm, nerve, peripheral	C47.9	C79.89	—	D36.10	D48.2	D49.2
brachial	C47.1-●	C79.89	—	D36.12	D48.2	D49.2
cranial	C72.50	C79.49	—	D33.3	D43.3	D49.7
specified NEC	C72.59	C79.49	—	D33.3	D43.3	D49.7
facial	C72.59	C79.49	—	D33.3	D43.3	D49.7
femoral	C47.2-●	C79.89	—	D36.13	D48.2	D49.2
ganglion NEC — see also Neoplasm, nerve, peripheral	C47.9	C79.89	—	D36.10	D48.2	D49.2
glossopharyngeal	C72.59	C79.49	—	D33.3	D43.3	D49.7
hypoglossal	C72.59	C79.49	—	D33.3	D43.3	D49.7
intercostal	C47.3	C79.89	—	D36.14	D48.2	D49.2
lumbar	C47.6	C79.89	—	D36.17	D48.2	D49.2
median	C47.1-●	C79.89	—	D36.12	D48.2	D49.2
obturator	C47.2-●	C79.89	—	D36.13	D48.2	D49.2
oculomotor	C72.59	C79.49	—	D33.3	D43.3	D49.7
olfactory	C47.2-●	C79.49	—	D33.3	D43.3	D49.7
optic	C72.3-●	C79.49	—	D33.3	D43.3	D49.7
parasympathetic NEC	C47.9	C79.89	—	D36.10	D48.2	D49.2
peripheral NEC	C47.9	C79.89	—	D36.10	D48.2	D49.2
abdomen	C47.4	C79.89	—	D36.15	D48.2	D49.2
abdominal wall	C47.4	C79.89	—	D36.15	D48.2	D49.2
ankle	C47.2-●	C79.89	—	D36.13	D48.2	D49.2

TABLE OF NEOPLASMS

	Malignant Primary	Malignant Secondary	Ca in situ	Benign	Uncertain Behavior	Unspecified Behavior
nerve *(Continued)*						
peripheral NEC *(Continued)*						
antecubital fossa or space	C47.1-●	C79.89	—	D36.12	D48.2	D49.2
arm	C47.1-●	C79.89	—	D36.12	D48.2	D49.2
auricle (ear)	C47.0	C79.89	—	D36.11	D48.2	D49.2
axilla	C47.3	C79.89	—	D36.12	D48.2	D49.2
back	C47.6	C79.89	—	D36.17	D48.2	D49.2
buttock	C47.5	C79.89	—	D36.16	D48.2	D49.2
calf	C47.2-●	C79.89	—	D36.13	D48.2	D49.2
cervical region	C47.0	C79.89	—	D36.11	D48.2	D49.2
cheek	C47.0	C79.89	—	D36.11	D48.2	D49.2
chest (wall)	C47.3	C79.89	—	D36.14	D48.2	D49.2
chin	C47.0	C79.89	—	D36.11	D48.2	D49.2
ear (external)	C47.0	C79.89	—	D36.11	D48.2	D49.2
elbow	C47.1-●	C79.89	—	D36.12	D48.2	D49.2
extrarectal	C47.5	C79.89	—	D36.16	D48.2	D49.2
extremity	C47.9	C79.89	—	D36.10	D48.2	D49.2
lower	C47.2-●	C79.89	—	D36.13	D48.2	D49.2
upper	C47.1-●	C79.89	—	D36.12	D48.2	D49.2
eyelid	C47.0	C79.89	—	D36.11	D48.2	D49.2
face	C47.0	C79.89	—	D36.11	D48.2	D49.2
finger	C47.1-●	C79.89	—	D36.12	D48.2	D49.2
flank	C47.6	C79.89	—	D36.17	D48.2	D49.2
foot	C47.2-●	C79.89	—	D36.13	D48.2	D49.2
forearm	C47.1-●	C79.89	—	D36.12	D48.2	D49.2
forehead	C47.0	C79.89	—	D36.11	D48.2	D49.2
gluteal region	C47.5	C79.89	—	D36.16	D48.2	D49.2
groin	C47.5	C79.89	—	D36.16	D48.2	D49.2
hand	C47.1-●	C79.89	—	D36.12	D48.2	D49.2
head	C47.0	C79.89	—	D36.11	D48.2	D49.2
heel	C47.2-●	C79.89	—	D36.13	D48.2	D49.2
hip	C47.2-●	C79.89	—	D36.13	D48.2	D49.2
infraclavicular region	C47.3	C79.89	—	D36.14	D48.2	D49.2
inguinal (canal) (region)	C47.5	C79.89	—	D36.16	D48.2	D49.2
intrathoracic	C47.3	C79.89	—	D36.14	D48.2	D49.2
ischiorectal fossa	C47.5	C79.89	—	D36.16	D48.2	D49.2
knee	C47.2-●	C79.89	—	D36.13	D48.2	D49.2
leg	C47.2-●	C79.89	—	D36.13	D48.2	D49.2
limb NEC	C47.9	C79.89	—	D36.10	D48.2	D49.2
lower	C47.2-●	C79.89	—	D36.13	D48.2	D49.2
upper	C47.1-●	C79.89	—	D36.12	D48.2	D49.2
nates	C47.5	C79.89	—	D36.16	D48.2	D49.2
neck	C47.0	C79.89	—	D36.11	D48.2	D49.2
orbit	C69.6-●	C79.49	—	D31.6-●	D48.7	D49.2
pararectal	C47.5	C79.89	—	D36.16	D48.2	D49.2
paraurethral	C47.5	C79.89	—	D36.16	D48.2	D49.2
paravaginal	C47.5	C79.89	—	D36.16	D48.2	D49.2
pelvis (floor)	C47.5	C79.89	—	D36.16	D48.2	D49.2
pelvoabdominal	C47.8	C79.89	—	D36.17	D48.2	D49.2
perineum	C47.5	C79.89	—	D36.16	D48.2	D49.2
perirectal (tissue)	C47.5	C79.89	—	D36.16	D48.2	D49.2
periurethral (tissue)	C47.5	C79.89	—	D36.16	D48.2	D49.2
popliteal fossa or space	C47.2-●	C79.89	—	D36.13	D48.2	D49.2
presacral	C47.5	C79.89	—	D36.16	D48.2	D49.2
pterygoid fossa	C47.0	C79.89	—	D36.11	D48.2	D49.2
rectovaginal septum or wall	C47.5	C79.89	—	D36.16	D48.2	D49.2
rectovesical	C47.5	C79.89	—	D36.16	D48.2	D49.2
sacrococcygeal region	C47.5	C79.89	—	D36.16	D48.2	D49.2
scalp	C47.0	C79.89	—	D36.11	D48.2	D49.2
scapular region	C47.3	C79.89	—	D36.14	D48.2	D49.2
shoulder	C47.1-●	C79.89	—	D36.12	D48.2	D49.2
submental	C47.0	C79.89	—	D36.11	D48.2	D49.2
supraclavicular region	C47.0	C79.89	—	D36.11	D48.2	D49.2
temple	C47.0	C79.89	—	D36.11	D48.2	D49.2
temporal region	C47.0	C79.89	—	D36.11	D48.2	D49.2
thigh	C47.2-●	C79.89	—	D36.13	D48.2	D49.2
thoracic (duct) (wall)	C47.3	C79.89	—	D36.14	D48.2	D49.2
thorax	C47.3	C79.89	—	D36.14	D48.2	D49.2
thumb	C47.1-●	C79.89	—	D36.12	D48.2	D49.2
toe	C47.2-●	C79.89	—	D36.13	D48.2	D49.2
trunk	C47.6	C79.89	—	D36.17	D48.2	D49.2
umbilicus	C47.4	C79.89	—	D36.15	D48.2	D49.2
vesicorectal	C47.5	C79.89	—	D36.16	D48.2	D49.2
wrist	C47.1-●	C79.89	—	D36.12	D48.2	D49.2
radial	C47.1-●	C79.89	—	D36.12	D48.2	D49.2
sacral	C47.5	C79.89	—	D36.16	D48.2	D49.2
sciatic	C47.2-●	C79.89	—	D36.13	D48.2	D49.2
spinal NEC	C47.9	C79.89	—	D36.10	D48.2	D49.2
accessory	C72.59	C79.49	—	D33.3	D43.3	D49.7
sympathetic NEC — *see also Neoplasm, nerve, peripheral*	C47.9	C79.89	—	D36.10	D48.2	D49.2
trigeminal	C72.59	C79.49	—	D33.3	D43.3	D49.7
trochlear	C72.59	C79.49	—	D33.3	D43.3	D49.7
ulnar	C47.1-●	C79.89	—	D36.12	D48.2	D49.2
vagus	C72.59	C79.49	—	D33.3	D43.3	D49.7

◄ New ◀▌ Revised ~~deleted~~ Deleted ● Use Additional Character(s)

	Malignant Primary	Malignant Secondary	Ca in situ	Benign	Uncertain Behavior	Unspecified Behavior
nervous system (central)	C72.9	C79.40	—	D33.9	D43.9	D49.7
autonomic — *see Neoplasm, nerve, peripheral*						
parasympathetic — *see Neoplasm, nerve, peripheral*						
specified site NEC	—	C79.49	—	D33.7	D43.8	—
sympathetic — *see Neoplasm, nerve, peripheral*						
nevus — *see Nevus*						
nipple	C50.0-●	C79.81	D05.-●	D24.-●	—	—
nose, nasal	C76.0	C79.89	D09.8	D36.7	D48.7	D49.89
ala (external) (nasi) — *see also Neoplasm, nose, skin*	C44.301	C79.2	D04.39	D23.39	D48.5	D49.2
bone	C41.0	C79.51	—	D16.4-●	D48.0	D49.2
cartilage	C30.0	C78.39	D02.3	D14.0	D38.5	D49.1
cavity	C30.0	C78.39	D02.3	D14.0	D38.5	D49.1
choana	C11.3	C79.89	D00.08	D10.6	D37.05	D49.0
external (skin) — *see also Neoplasm, nose, skin*	C44.301	C79.2	D04.39	D23.39	D48.5	D49.2
fossa	C30.0	C78.39	D02.3	D14.0	D38.5	D49.1
internal	C30.0	C78.39	D02.3	D14.0	D38.5	D49.1
mucosa	C30.0	C78.39	D02.3	D14.0	D38.5	D49.1
septum	C30.0	C78.39	D02.3	D14.0	D38.5	D49.1
posterior margin	C11.3	C79.89	D00.08	D10.6	D37.05	D49.0
sinus — *see Neoplasm, sinus*						
skin	C44.301	C79.2	D04.39	D23.39	D48.5	D49.2
basal cell carcinoma	C44.311	—	—	—	—	—
specified type NEC	C44.391	—	—	—	—	—
squamous cell carcinoma	C44.321	—	—	—	—	—
turbinate (mucosa)	C30.0	C78.39	D02.3	D14.0	D38.5	D49.1
bone	C41.0	C79.51	—	D16.4-●	D48.0	D49.2
vestibule	C30.0	C78.39	D02.3	D14.0	D38.5	D49.1
nostril	C30.0	C78.39	D02.3	D14.0	D38.5	D49.1
nucleus pulposus	C41.2	C79.51	—	D16.6	D48.0	D49.2
occipital						
bone	C41.0	C79.51	—	D16.4-●	D48.0	D49.2
lobe or pole, brain	C71.4	C79.31	—	D33.0	D43.0	D49.6
odontogenic — *see Neoplasm, jaw bone*						
olfactory nerve or bulb	C72.2-●	C79.49	—	D33.3	D43.3	D49.7
olive (brain)	C71.7	C79.31	—	D33.1	D43.1	D49.6
omentum	C48.1	C78.6	—	D20.1	D48.4	D49.0
operculum (brain)	C71.0	C79.31	—	D33.0	D43.0	D49.6

	Malignant Primary	Malignant Secondary	Ca in situ	Benign	Uncertain Behavior	Unspecified Behavior
optic nerve, chiasm, or tract	C72.3-●	C79.49	—	D33.3	D43.3	D49.7
oral (cavity)	C06.9	C79.89	D00.00	D10.30	D37.09	D49.0
ill-defined	C14.8	C79.89	D00.00	D10.30	D37.09	D49.0
mucosa	C06.0	C79.89	D00.02	D10.39	D37.09	D49.0
orbit	C69.6-●	C79.49	D09.2-●	D31.6-●	D48.7	D49.89
autonomic nerve	C69.6-●	C79.49	—	D31.6-●	D48.7	D49.2
bone	C41.0	C79.51	—	D16.4-●	D48.0	D49.2
eye	C69.6-●	C79.49	D09.2-●	D31.6-●	D48.7	D49.89
peripheral nerves	C69.6-●	C79.49	—	D31.6-●	D48.7	D49.2
soft parts	C69.6-●	C79.49	D09.2-●	D31.6-●	D48.7	D49.89
organ of Zuckerkandl	C75.5	C79.89	—	D35.6	D44.7	D49.7
oropharynx	C10.9	C79.89	D00.08	D10.5	D37.05	D49.0
branchial cleft (vestige)	C10.4	C79.89	D00.08	D10.5	D37.05	D49.0
junctional region	C10.8	C79.89	D00.08	D10.5	D37.05	D49.0
lateral wall	C10.2	C79.89	D00.08	D10.5	D37.05	D49.0
overlapping lesion	C10.8	—	—	—	—	—
pillars or fauces	C09.1	C79.89	D00.08	D10.5	D37.05	D49.0
posterior wall	C10.3	C79.89	D00.08	D10.5	D37.05	D49.0
vallecula	C10.0	C79.89	D00.08	D10.5	D37.05	D49.0
os						
external	C53.1	C79.82	D06.1	D26.0	D39.0	D49.59
internal	C53.0	C79.82	D06.0	D26.0	D39.0	D49.59
ovary	C56.-●	C79.6-●	D07.39	D27.-●	D39.1-●	D49.59
oviduct	C57.0-●	C79.82	D07.39	D28.2	D39.8	D49.59
palate	C05.9	C79.89	D00.00	D10.39	D37.09	D49.0
hard	C05.0	C79.89	D00.05	D10.39	D37.09	D49.0
junction of hard and soft palate	C05.9	C79.89	D00.00	D10.39	D37.09	D49.0
overlapping lesions	C05.8	—	D00.00	—	—	—
soft	C05.1	C79.89	D00.04	D10.39	D37.09	D49.0
nasopharyngeal surface	C11.3	C79.89	D00.08	D10.6	D37.05	D49.0
posterior surface	C11.3	C79.89	D00.08	D10.6	D37.05	D49.0
superior surface	C11.3	C79.89	D00.08	D10.6	D37.05	D49.0
palatoglossal arch	C09.1	C79.89	D00.00	D10.5	D37.09	D49.0
palatopharyngeal arch	C09.1	C79.89	D00.00	D10.5	D37.09	D49.0
pallium	C71.0	C79.31	—	D33.0	D43.0	D49.6
palpebra	C44.10-●	C79.2	D04.1-●	D23.1-●	D48.5	D49.2
basal cell carcinoma	C44.11-●	—	—	—	—	—
specified type NEC	C44.19-●	—	—	—	—	—
squamous cell carcinoma	C44.12-●	—	—	—	—	—
pancreas	C25.9	C78.89	D01.7	D13.6	D37.8	D49.0
body	C25.1	C78.89	D01.7	D13.6	D37.8	D49.0
duct (of Santorini) (of Wirsung)	C25.3	C78.89	D01.7	D13.6	D37.8	D49.0
ectopic tissue	C25.7	C78.89	—	D13.6	D37.8	D49.0
head	C25.0	C78.89	D01.7	D13.6	D37.8	D49.0

◄ New   ◄| Revised   ~~deleted~~ Deleted   ● Use Additional Character(s)

TABLE OF NEOPLASMS

	Malignant Primary	Malignant Secondary	Ca in situ	Benign	Uncertain Behavior	Unspecified Behavior
pancreas (Continued)						
islet cells	C25.4	C78.89	D01.7	D13.7	D37.8	D49.0
neck	C25.7	C78.89	D01.7	D13.6	D37.8	D49.0
overlapping lesion	C25.8	—	—	—	—	—
tail	C25.2	C78.89	D01.7	D13.6	D37.8	D49.0
para-aortic body	C75.5	C79.89	—	D35.6	D44.7	D49.7
paraganglion NEC	C75.5	C79.89	—	D35.6	D44.7	D49.7
parametrium	C57.3	C79.82	—	D28.2	D39.8	D49.59
paranephric	C48.0	C78.6	—	D20.0	D48.3	D49.0
pararectal	C76.3	C79.89	—	D36.7	D48.7	D49.89
parasagittal (region)	C76.0	C79.89	D09.8	D36.7	D48.7	D49.89
parasellar	C72.9	C79.49	—	D33.9	D43.8	D49.7
parathyroid (gland)	C75.0	C79.89	D09.3	D35.1	D44.2	D49.7
paraurethral	C76.3	C79.89	—	D36.7	D48.7	D49.89
gland	C68.1	C79.19	D09.19	D30.8	D41.8	D49.59
paravaginal	C76.3	C79.89	—	D36.7	D48.7	D49.89
parenchyma, kidney	C64.-●	C79.0-●	D09.19	D30.0-●	D41.0-●	D49.51-●
parietal						
bone	C41.0	C79.51	—	D16.4-●	D48.0	D49.2
lobe, brain	C71.3	C79.31	—	D33.0	D43.0	D49.6
paroophoron	C57.1	C79.82	D07.39	D28.2	D39.8	D49.59
parotid (duct) (gland)	C07	C79.89	D00.00	D11.0	D37.030	D49.0
parovarium	C57.1	C79.82	D07.39	D28.2	D39.8	D49.59
patella	C40.20	C79.51	—	—	—	—
peduncle, cerebral	C71.7	C79.31	—	D33.1	D43.1	D49.6
pelvirectal junction	C19	C78.5	D01.1	D12.7	D37.5	D49.0
pelvis, pelvic	C76.3	C79.89	D09.8	D36.7	D48.7	D49.89
bone	C41.4	C79.51	—	D16.8	D48.0	D49.2
floor	C76.3	C79.89	D09.8	D36.7	D48.7	D49.89
renal	C65.-●	C79.0-●	D09.19	D30.1-●	D41.1-●	D49.51-●
viscera	C76.3	C79.89	D09.8	D36.7	D48.7	D49.89
wall	C76.3	C79.89	D09.8	D36.7	D48.7	D49.89
pelvo-abdominal	C76.8	C79.89	D09.8	D36.7	D48.7	D49.89
penis	C60.9	C79.82	D07.4	D29.0	D40.8	D49.59
body	C60.2	C79.82	D07.4	D29.0	D40.8	D49.59
corpus (cavernosum)	C60.2	C79.82	D07.4	D29.0	D40.8	D49.59
glans	C60.1	C79.82	D07.4	D29.0	D40.8	D49.59
overlapping sites	C60.8	—	—	—	—	—
skin NEC	C60.9	C79.82	D07.4	D29.0	D40.8	D49.59
periadrenal (tissue)	C48.0	C78.6	—	D20.0	D48.3	D49.0
perianal (skin) — see also Neoplasm, anus, skin	C44.500	C79.2	D04.5	D23.5	D48.5	D49.2
pericardium	C38.0	C79.89	—	D15.1	D48.7	D49.89
perinephric	C48.0	C78.6	—	D20.0	D48.3	D49.0
perineum	C76.3	C79.89	D09.8	D36.7	D48.7	D49.89
periodontal tissue NEC	C03.9	C79.89	D00.03	D10.39	D37.09	D49.0
periosteum — see Neoplasm, bone						
peripancreatic	C48.0	C78.6	—	D20.0	D48.3	D49.0
peripheral nerve NEC	C47.9	C79.89	—	D36.10	D48.2	D49.2
perirectal (tissue)	C76.3	C79.89	—	D36.7	D48.7	D49.89
perirenal (tissue)	C48.0	C78.6	—	D20.0	D48.3	D49.0
peritoneum, peritoneal (cavity)	C48.2	C78.6	—	D20.1	D48.4	D49.0
benign mesothelial tissue — see Mesothelioma, benign						
overlapping lesion	C48.8	—	—	—	—	—
with digestive organs	C26.9	—	—	—	—	—
parietal	C48.1	C78.6	—	D20.1	D48.4	D49.0
pelvic	C48.1	C78.6	—	D20.1	D48.4	D49.0
specified part NEC	C48.1	C78.6	—	D20.1	D48.4	D49.0
peritonsillar (tissue)	C76.0	C79.89	D09.8	D36.7	D48.7	D49.89
periurethral tissue	C76.3	C79.89	—	D36.7	D48.7	D49.89
phalanges						
foot	C40.3-●	C79.51	—	D16.3-●	—	—
hand	C40.1-●	C79.51	—	D16.1-●	—	—
pharynx, pharyngeal	C14.0	C79.89	D00.08	D10.9	D37.05	D49.0
bursa	C11.1	C79.89	D00.08	D10.6	D37.05	D49.0
fornix	C11.3	C79.89	D00.08	D10.6	D37.05	D49.0
recess	C11.2	C79.89	D00.08	D10.6	D37.05	D49.0
region	C14.0	C79.89	D00.08	D10.9	D37.05	D49.0
tonsil	C11.1	C79.89	D00.08	D10.6	D37.05	D49.0
wall (lateral) (posterior)	C14.0	C79.89	D00.08	D10.9	D37.05	D49.0
pia mater	C70.9	C79.40	—	D32.9	D42.9	D49.7
cerebral	C70.0	C79.32	—	D32.0	D42.0	D49.7
cranial	C70.0	C79.32	—	D32.0	D42.0	D49.7
spinal	C70.1	C79.49	—	D32.1	D42.1	D49.7
pillars of fauces	C09.1	C79.89	D00.08	D10.5	D37.05	D49.0
pineal (body) (gland)	C75.3	C79.89	D09.3	D35.4	D44.5	D49.7
pinna (ear) NEC — see also Neoplasm, skin, ear	C44.20-●	C79.2	D04.2-●	D23.2-●	D48.5	D49.2
piriform fossa or sinus	C12	C79.89	D00.08	D10.7	D37.05	D49.0
pituitary (body) (fossa) (gland) (lobe)	C75.1	C79.89	D09.3	D35.2	D44.3	D49.7
placenta	C58	C79.82	D07.0	D26.7	D39.2	D49.59
pleura, pleural (cavity)	C38.4	C78.2	—	D19.0	D38.2	D49.1
overlapping lesion with heart or mediastinum	C38.8	—	—	—	—	—
parietal	C38.4	C78.2	—	D19.0	D38.2	D49.1
visceral	C38.4	C78.2	—	D19.0	D38.2	D49.1

◀ New　◀◀ Revised　~~deleted~~ Deleted　● Use Additional Character(s)

	Malignant Primary	Malignant Secondary	Ca in situ	Benign	Uncertain Behavior	Unspecified Behavior
plexus						
brachial	C47.1-●	C79.89	—	D36.12	D48.2	D49.2
cervical	C47.0	C79.89	—	D36.11	D48.2	D49.2
choroid	C71.5	C79.31	—	D33.0	D43.0	D49.6
lumbosacral	C47.5	C79.89	—	D36.16	D48.2	D49.2
sacral	C47.5	C79.89	—	D36.16	D48.2	D49.2
pluriendocrine	C75.8	C79.89	D09.3	D35.7	D44.9	D49.7
pole						
frontal	C71.1	C79.31	—	D33.0	D43.0	D49.6
occipital	C71.4	C79.31	—	D33.0	D43.0	D49.6
pons (varolii)	C71.7	C79.31	—	D33.1	D43.1	D49.6
popliteal fossa or space	C76.5-●	C79.89	D04.7-●	D36.7	D48.7	D49.89
postcricoid (region)	C13.0	C79.89	D00.08	D10.7	D37.05	D49.0
posterior fossa (cranial)	C71.9	C79.31	—	D33.2	D43.2	D49.6
postnasal space	C11.9	C79.89	D00.08	D10.6	D37.05	D49.0
prepuce	C60.0	C79.82	D07.4	D29.0	D40.8	D49.59
prepylorus	C16.4	C78.89	D00.2	D13.1	D37.1	D49.0
presacral (region)	C76.3	C79.89	—	D36.7	D48.7	D49.89
prostate (gland)	C61	C79.82	D07.5	D29.1	D40.0	D49.59
utricle	C68.0	C79.19	D09.19	D30.4	D41.3	D49.59
pterygoid fossa	C49.0	C79.89	—	D21.0	D48.1	D49.2
pubic bone	C41.4	C79.51	—	D16.8	D48.0	D49.2
pudenda, pudendum (female)	C51.9	C79.82	D07.1	D28.0	D39.8	D49.59
pulmonary — *see also Neoplasm, lung*	C34.9-●	C78.0-●	D02.2-●	D14.3-●	D38.1	D49.1
putamen	C71.0	C79.31	—	D33.0	D43.0	D49.6
pyloric						
antrum	C16.3	C78.89	D00.2	D13.1	D37.1	D49.0
canal	C16.4	C78.89	D00.2	D13.1	D37.1	D49.0
pylorus	C16.4	C78.89	D00.2	D13.1	D37.1	D49.0
pyramid (brain)	C71.7	C79.31	—	D33.1	D43.1	D49.6
pyriform fossa or sinus	C12	C79.89	D00.08	D10.7	D37.05	D49.0
radius (any part)	C40.0-●	C79.51	—	D16.0-●	—	—
Rathke's pouch	C75.1	C79.89	D09.3	D35.2	D44.3	D49.7
rectosigmoid (junction)	C19	C78.5	D01.1	D12.7	D37.5	D49.0
overlapping lesion with anus or rectum	C21.8	—	—	—	—	—
rectouterine pouch	C48.1	C78.6	—	D20.1	D48.4	D49.0
rectovaginal septum or wall	C76.3	C79.89	D09.8	D36.7	D48.7	D49.89
rectovesical septum	C76.3	C79.89	D09.8	D36.7	D48.7	D49.89
rectum (ampulla)	C20	C78.5	D01.2	D12.8	D37.5	D49.0
and colon	C19	C78.5	D01.1	D12.7	D37.5	D49.0
overlapping lesion with anus or rectosigmoid junction	C21.8	—	—	—	—	—

	Malignant Primary	Malignant Secondary	Ca in situ	Benign	Uncertain Behavior	Unspecified Behavior
renal	C64.-●	C79.0-●	D09.19	D30.0-●	D41.0-●	D49.51-●
calyx	C65.-●	C79.0-●	D09.19	D30.1-●	D41.1-●	D49.51-●
hilus	C65.-●	C79.0-●	D09.19	D30.1-●	D41.1-●	D49.51-●
parenchyma	C64.-●	C79.0-●	D09.19	D30.0-●	D41.0-●	D49.51-●
pelvis	C65.-●	C79.0-●	D09.19	D30.1-●	D41.1-●	D49.51-●
respiratory						
organs or system NEC	C39.9	C78.30	D02.4	D14.4	D38.6	D49.1
tract NEC	C39.9	C78.30	D02.4	D14.4	D38.5	D49.1
upper	C39.0	C78.30	D02.4	D14.4	D38.5	D49.1
retina	C69.2-●	C79.49	D09.2-●	D31.2-●	D48.7	D49.81
retrobulbar	C69.6-●	C79.49	—	D31.6-●	D48.7	D49.89
retrocecal	C48.0	C78.6	—	D20.0	D48.3	D49.0
retromolar (area) (triangle) (trigone)	C06.2	C79.89	D00.00	D10.39	D37.09	D49.0
retro-orbital	C76.0	C79.89	D09.8	D36.7	D48.7	D49.89
retroperitoneal (space) (tissue)	C48.0	C78.6	—	D20.0	D48.3	D49.0
retroperitoneum	C48.0	C78.6	—	D20.0	D48.3	D49.0
retropharyngeal	C14.0	C79.89	D00.08	D10.9	D37.05	D49.0
retrovesical (septum)	C76.3	C79.89	D09.8	D36.7	D48.7	D49.89
rhinencephalon	C71.0	C79.31	—	D33.0	D43.0	D49.6
rib	C41.3	C79.51	—	D16.7	D48.0	D49.2
Rosenmuller's fossa	C11.2	C79.89	D00.08	D10.6	D37.05	D49.0
round ligament	C57.2	C79.82	—	D28.2	D39.8	D49.59
sacrococcyx, sacrococcygeal	C41.4	C79.51	—	D16.8	D48.0	D49.2
region	C76.3	C79.89	D09.8	D36.7	D48.7	D49.89
sacrouterine ligament	C57.3	C79.82	—	D28.2	D39.8	D49.59
sacrum, sacral (vertebra)	C41.4	C79.51	—	D16.8	D48.0	D49.2
salivary gland or duct (major)	C08.9	C79.89	D00.00	D11.9	D37.039	D49.0
minor NEC	C06.9	C79.89	D00.00	D10.39	D37.04	D49.0
overlapping lesion	C08.9	—	—	—	—	—
parotid	C07	C79.89	D00.00	D11.0	D37.030	D49.0
pluriglandular	C08.9	C79.89	D00.00	D11.9	D37.039	D49.0
sublingual	C08.1	C79.89	D00.00	D11.7	D37.031	D49.0
submandibular	C08.0	C79.89	D00.00	D11.7	D37.032	D49.0
submaxillary	C08.0	C79.89	D00.00	D11.7	D37.032	D49.0
salpinx (uterine)	C57.0-●	C79.82	D07.39	D28.2	D39.8	D49.59
Santorini's duct	C25.3	C78.89	D01.7	D13.6	D37.8	D49.0
scalp	C44.40	C79.2	D04.4	D23.4	D48.5	D49.2
basal cell carcinoma	C44.41	—	—	—	—	—
specified type NEC	C44.49	—	—	—	—	—
squamous cell carcinoma	C44.42	—	—	—	—	—
scapula (any part)	C40.0-●	C79.51	—	D16.0-●	—	—
scapular region	C76.1	C79.89	D09.8	D36.7	D48.7	D49.89

TABLE OF NEOPLASMS

	Malignant Primary	Malignant Secondary	Ca in situ	Benign	Uncertain Behavior	Unspecified Behavior
scar NEC — see also Neoplasm, skin, by site	C44.90	C79.2	D04.9	D23.9	D48.5	D49.2
sciatic nerve	C47.2-●	C79.89	—	D36.13	D48.2	D49.2
sclera	C69.4-●	C79.49	D09.2-●	D31.4-●	D48.7	D49.89
scrotum (skin)	C63.2	C79.82	D07.61	D29.4	D40.8	D49.59
sebaceous gland — see Neoplasm, skin						
sella turcica	C75.1	C79.89	D09.3	D35.2	D44.3	D49.7
bone	C41.0	C79.51	—	D16.4-●	D48.0	D49.2
semilunar cartilage (knee)	C40.2-●	C79.51	—	D16.2-●	D48.0	D49.2
seminal vesicle	C63.7	C79.82	D07.69	D29.8	D40.8	D49.59
septum						
nasal	C30.0	C78.39	D02.3	D14.0	D38.5	D49.1
posterior margin	C11.3	C79.89	D00.08	D10.6	D37.05	D49.0
rectovaginal	C76.3	C79.89	D09.8	D36.7	D48.7	D49.89
rectovesical	C76.3	C79.89	D09.8	D36.7	D48.7	D49.89
urethrovaginal	C57.9	C79.82	D07.30	D28.9	D39.9	D49.59
vesicovaginal	C57.9	C79.82	D07.30	D28.9	D39.9	D49.59
shoulder NEC	C76.4-●	C79.89	D04.6-●	D36.7	D48.7	D49.89
sigmoid flexure (lower) (upper)	C18.7	C78.5	D01.0	D12.5	D37.4	D49.0
sinus (accessory)	C31.9	C78.39	D02.3	D14.0	D38.5	D49.1
bone (any)	C41.0	C79.51	—	D16.4-●	D48.0	D49.2
ethmoidal	C31.1	C78.39	D02.3	D14.0	D38.5	D49.1
frontal	C31.2	C78.39	D02.3	D14.0	D38.5	D49.1
maxillary	C31.0	C78.39	D02.3	D14.0	D38.5	D49.1
nasal, paranasal NEC	C31.9	C78.39	D02.3	D14.0	D38.5	D49.1
overlapping lesion	C31.8	—	—	—	—	—
pyriform	C12	C79.89	D00.08	D10.7	D37.05	D49.0
sphenoid	C31.3	C78.39	D02.3	D14.0	D38.5	D49.1
skeleton, skeletal NEC	C41.9	C79.51	—	D16.9-●	D48.0	D49.2
Skene's gland	C68.1	C79.19	D09.19	D30.8	D41.8	D49.59
skin NOS	C44.90	C79.2	D04.9	D23.9	D48.5	D49.2
abdominal wall	C44.509	C79.2	D04.5	D23.5	D48.5	D49.2
basal cell carcinoma	C44.519	—	—	—	—	—
specified type NEC	C44.599	—	—	—	—	—
squamous cell carcinoma	C44.529	—	—	—	—	—
ala nasi — see also Neoplasm, nose, skin	C44.301	C79.2	D04.39	D23.39	D48.5	D49.2
ankle — see also Neoplasm, skin, limb, lower	C44.70-●	C79.2	D04.7-●	D23.7-●	D48.5	D49.2
antecubital space — see also Neoplasm, skin, limb, upper	C44.60-●	C79.2	D04.6-●	D23.6-●	D48.5	D49.2

	Malignant Primary	Malignant Secondary	Ca in situ	Benign	Uncertain Behavior	Unspecified Behavior
skin NOS (Continued)						
anus	C44.500	C79.2	D04.5	D23.5	D48.5	D49.2
basal cell carcinoma	C44.510	—	—	—	—	—
specified type NEC	C44.590	—	—	—	—	—
squamous cell carcinoma	C44.520	—	—	—	—	—
arm — see also Neoplasm, skin, limb, upper	C44.60-●	C79.2	D04.6-●	D23.6-●	D48.5	D49.2
auditory canal (external) — see also Neoplasm, skin, ear	C44.20-●	C79.2	D04.2-●	D23.2-●	D48.5	D49.2
auricle (ear) — see also Neoplasm, skin, ear	C44.20-●	C79.2	D04.2-●	D23.2-●	D48.5	D49.2
auricular canal (external) — see also Neoplasm, skin, ear	C44.20-●	C79.2	D04.2-●	D23.2-●	D48.5	D49.2
axilla, axillary fold — see also Neoplasm, skin, trunk	C44.509	C79.2	D04.5	D23.5	D48.5	D49.2
back — see also Neoplasm, skin, trunk	C44.509	C79.2	D04.5	D23.5	D48.5	D49.2
basal cell carcinoma	C44.91					
breast	C44.501	C79.2	D04.5	D23.5	D48.5	D49.2
basal cell carcinoma	C44.511	—	—	—	—	—
specified type NEC	C44.591	—	—	—	—	—
squamous cell carcinoma	C44.521	—	—	—	—	—
brow — see also Neoplasm, skin, face	C44.309	C79.2	D04.39	D23.39	D48.5	D49.2
buttock — see also Neoplasm, skin, trunk	C44.509	C79.2	D04.5	D23.5	D48.5	D49.2
calf — see also Neoplasm, skin, limb, lower	C44.70-●	C79.2	D04.7-●	D23.7-●	D48.5	D49.2
canthus (eye) (inner) (outer)	C44.10-●	C79.2	D04.1-●	D23.1-●	D48.5	D49.2
basal cell carcinoma	C44.11-●	—	—	—	—	—
specified type NEC	C44.19-●	—	—	—	—	—
squamous cell carcinoma	C44.12-●	—	—	—	—	—
cervical region — see also Neoplasm, skin, neck	C44.40	C79.2	D04.4	D23.4	D48.5	D49.2
cheek (external) — see also Neoplasm, skin, face	C44.309	C79.2	D04.39	D23.39	D48.5	D49.2
chest (wall) — see also Neoplasm, skin, trunk	C44.509	C79.2	D04.5	D23.5	D48.5	D49.2
chin — see also Neoplasm, skin, face	C44.309	C79.2	D04.39	D23.39	D48.5	D49.2
clavicular area — see also Neoplasm, skin, trunk	C44.509	C79.2	D04.5	D23.5	D48.5	D49.2
clitoris	C51.2	C79.82	D07.1	D28.0	D39.8	D49.59
columnella — see also Neoplasm, skin, face	C44.309	C79.2	D04.39	D23.39	D48.5	D49.2

◄ New   ◄█ Revised   ~~deleted~~ Deleted   ● Use Additional Character(s)

TABLE OF NEOPLASMS (side tab)

	Malignant Primary	Malignant Secondary	Ca in situ	Benign	Uncertain Behavior	Unspecified Behavior
skin NOS *(Continued)*						
concha — *see also Neoplasm, skin, ear*	C44.20-●	C79.2	D04.2-●	D23.2-●	D48.5	D49.2
ear (external)	C44.20-●	C79.2	D04.2-●	D23.2-●	D48.5	D49.2
basal cell carcinoma	C44.21-●	—	—	—	—	—
specified type NEC	C44.29-●	—	—	—	—	—
squamous cell carcinoma	C44.22-●	—	—	—	—	—
elbow — *see also Neoplasm, skin, limb, upper*	C44.60-●	C79.2	D04.6-●	D23.6-●	D48.5	D49.2
eyebrow — *see also Neoplasm, skin, face*	C44.309	C79.2	D04.39	D23.39	D48.5	D49.2
eyelid	C44.10-●	C79.2	D04.1-●	D23.1-●	D48.5	D49.2
basal cell carcinoma	C44.11-●	—	—	—	—	—
specified type NEC	C44.19-●	—	—	—	—	—
squamous cell carcinoma	C44.12-●	—	—	—	—	—
face NOS	C44.300	C79.2	D04.30	D23.30	D48.5	D49.2
basal cell carcinoma	C44.310	—	—	—	—	—
specified type NEC	C44.390	—	—	—	—	—
squamous cell carcinoma	C44.320	—	—	—	—	—
female genital organs (external)	C51.9	C79.82	D07.1	D28.0	D39.8	D49.59
clitoris	C51.2	C79.82	D07.1	D28.0	D39.8	D49.59
labium NEC	C51.9	C79.82	D07.1	D28.0	D39.8	D49.59
majus	C51.0	C79.82	D07.1	D28.0	D39.8	D49.59
minus	C51.1	C79.82	D07.1	D28.0	D39.8	D49.59
pudendum	C51.9	C79.82	D07.1	D28.0	D39.8	D49.59
vulva	C51.9	C79.82	D07.1	D28.0	D39.8	D49.59
finger — *see also Neoplasm, skin, limb, upper*	C44.60-●	C79.2	D04.6-●	D23.6-●	D48.5	D49.2
flank — *see also Neoplasm, skin, trunk*	C44.509	C79.2	D04.5	D23.5	D48.5	D49.2
foot — *see also Neoplasm, skin, limb, lower*	C44.70-●	C79.2	D04.7-●	D23.7-●	D48.5	D49.2
forearm — *see also Neoplasm, skin, limb, upper*	C44.60-●	C79.2	D04.6-●	D23.6-●	D48.5	D49.2
forehead — *see also Neoplasm, skin, face*	C44.309	C79.2	D04.39	D23.39	D48.5	D49.2
glabella — *see also Neoplasm, skin, face*	C44.309	C79.2	D04.39	D23.39	D48.5	D49.2
gluteal region — *see also Neoplasm, skin, trunk*	C44.509	C79.2	D04.5	D23.5	D48.5	D49.2
groin — *see also Neoplasm, skin, trunk*	C44.509	C79.2	D04.5	D23.5	D48.5	D49.2
hand — *see also Neoplasm, skin, limb, upper*	C44.60-●	C79.2	D04.6-●	D23.6-●	D48.5	D49.2
skin NOS *(Continued)*						
head NEC — *see also Neoplasm, skin, scalp*	C44.40	C79.2	D04.4	D23.4	D48.5	D49.2
heel — *see also Neoplasm, skin, limb, lower*	C44.70-●	C79.2	D04.7-●	D23.7-●	D48.5	D49.2
helix — *see also Neoplasm, skin, ear*	C44.20-●	C79.2	D04.2-●	D23.2-●	D48.5	D49.2
hip — *see also Neoplasm, skin, limb, lower*	C44.70-●	C79.2	D04.7-●	D23.7-●	D48.5	D49.2
infraclavicular region — *see also Neoplasm, skin, trunk*	C44.509	C79.2	D04.5	D23.5	D48.5	D49.2
inguinal region — *see also Neoplasm, skin, trunk*	C44.509	C79.2	D04.5	D23.5	D48.5	D49.2
jaw — *see also Neoplasm, skin, face*	C44.309	C79.2	D04.39	D23.39	D48.5	D49.2
Kaposi's sarcoma — *see Kaposi's, sarcoma, skin*						
knee — *see also Neoplasm, skin, limb, lower*	C44.70-●	C79.2	D04.7-●	D23.7-●	D48.5	D49.2
labia						
majora	C51.0	C79.82	D07.1	D28.0	D39.8	D49.59
minora	C51.1	C79.82	D07.1	D28.0	D39.8	D49.59
leg — *see also Neoplasm, skin, limb, lower*	C44.70-●	C79.2	D04.7-●	D23.7-●	D48.5	D49.2
lid (lower) (upper)	C44.10-●	C79.2	D04.1-●	D23.1-●	D48.5	D49.2
basal cell carcinoma	C44.11-●	—	—	—	—	—
specified type NEC	C44.19-●	—	—	—	—	—
squamous cell carcinoma	C44.12-●	—	—	—	—	—
limb NEC	C44.90	C79.2	D04.9	D23.9	D48.5	D49.2
basal cell carcinoma	C44.91					
lower	C44.70-●	C79.2	D04.7-●	D23.7-●	D48.5	D49.2
basal cell carcinoma	C44.71-●	—	—	—	—	—
specified type NEC	C44.79-●	—	—	—	—	—
squamous cell carcinoma	C44.72-●	—	—	—	—	—
upper	C44.60-●	C79.2	D04.6-●	D23.6-●	D48.5	D49.2
basal cell carcinoma	C44.61-●	—	—	—	—	—
specified type NEC	C44.69-●	—	—	—	—	—
squamous cell carcinoma	C44.62-●	—	—	—	—	—
lip (lower) (upper)	C44.00	C79.2	D04.0	D23.0	D48.5	D49.2
basal cell carcinoma	C44.01	—	—	—	—	—
specified type NEC	C44.09	—	—	—	—	—
squamous cell carcinoma	C44.02	—	—	—	—	—

TABLE OF NEOPLASMS

	Malignant Primary	Malignant Secondary	Ca in situ	Benign	Uncertain Behavior	Unspecified Behavior
skin NOS *(Continued)*						
male genital organs	C63.9	C79.82	D07.60	D29.9	D40.8	D49.59
penis	C60.9	C79.82	D07.4	D29.0	D40.8	D49.59
prepuce	C60.0	C79.82	D07.4	D29.0	D40.8	D49.59
scrotum	C63.2	C79.82	D07.61	D29.4	D40.8	D49.59
mastectomy site (skin) — *see also Neoplasm, skin, breast*	C44.501	C79.2	—	—	—	—
specified as breast tissue	C50.8-●	C79.81	—	—	—	—
meatus, acoustic (external) — *see also Neoplasm, skin, ear*	C44.20-●	C79.2	D04.2-●	D23.2-●	D48.5	D49.2
melanotic — *see Melanoma*						
Merkel cell — *see Carcinoma, Merkel cell*						
nates — *see also Neoplasm, skin, trunk*	C44.509	C79.2	D04.5	D23.5	D48.5	D49.2
neck	C44.40	C79.2	D04.4	D23.4	D48.5	D49.2
basal cell carcinoma	C44.41	—	—	—	—	—
specified type NEC	C44.49	—	—	—	—	—
squamous cell carcinoma	C44.42	—	—	—	—	—
nevus — *see Nevus, skin*						
nose (external) — *see also Neoplasm, nose, skin*	C44.301	C79.2	D04.39	D23.39	D48.5	D49.2
overlapping lesion	C44.80	—	—	—	—	—
basal cell carcinoma	C44.81	—	—	—	—	—
specified type NEC	C44.89	—	—	—	—	—
squamous cell carcinoma	C44.82	—	—	—	—	—
palm — *see also Neoplasm, skin, limb, upper*	C44.60-●	C79.2	D04.6-●	D23.6-●	D48.5	D49.2
palpebra	C44.10-●	C79.2	D04.1-●	D23.1-●	D48.5	D49.2
basal cell carcinoma	C44.11-●	—	—	—	—	—
specified type NEC	C44.19-●	—	—	—	—	—
squamous cell carcinoma	C44.12-●	—	—	—	—	—
penis NEC	C60.9	C79.82	D07.4	D29.0	D40.8	D49.59
perianal — *see also Neoplasm, skin, anus*	C44.500	C79.2	D04.5	D23.5	D48.5	D49.2
perineum — *see also Neoplasm, skin, anus*	C44.500	C79.2	D04.5	D23.5	D48.5	D49.2
pinna — *see also Neoplasm, skin, ear*	C44.20-●	C79.2	D04.2-●	D23.2-●	D48.5	D49.2
plantar — *see also Neoplasm, skin, limb, lower*	C44.70-●	C79.2	D04.7-●	D23.7-●	D48.5	D49.2
popliteal fossa or space — *see also Neoplasm, skin, limb, lower*	C44.70-●	C79.2	D04.7-●	D23.7-●	D48.5	D49.2
prepuce	C60.0	C79.82	D07.4	D29.0	D40.8	D49.59

	Malignant Primary	Malignant Secondary	Ca in situ	Benign	Uncertain Behavior	Unspecified Behavior
skin NOS *(Continued)*						
pubes — *see also Neoplasm, skin, trunk*	C44.509	C79.2	D04.5	D23.5	D48.5	D49.2
sacrococcygeal region — *see also Neoplasm, skin, trunk*	C44.509	C79.2	D04.5	D23.5	D48.5	D49.2
scalp	C44.40	C79.2	D04.4	D23.4	D48.5	D49.2
basal cell carcinoma	C44.41	—	—	—	—	—
specified type NEC	C44.49	—	—	—	—	—
squamous cell carcinoma	C44.42	—	—	—	—	—
scapular region — *see also Neoplasm, skin, trunk*	C44.509	C79.2	D04.5	D23.5	D48.5	D49.2
scrotum	C63.2	C79.82	D07.61	D29.4	D40.8	D49.59
shoulder — *see also Neoplasm, skin, limb, upper*	C44.60-●	C79.2	D04.6-●	D23.6-●	D48.5	D49.2
sole (foot) — *see also Neoplasm, skin, limb, lower*	C44.70-●	C79.2	D04.7-●	D23.7-●	D48.5	D49.2
specified sites NEC	C44.80	C79.2	D04.8	D23.9	D48.5	D49.2
basal cell carcinoma	C44.81	—	—	—	—	—
specified type NEC	C44.89	—	—	—	—	—
squamous cell carcinoma	C44.82	—	—	—	—	—
specified type NEC	C44.99	—	—	—	—	—
squamous cell carcinoma	C44.92	—	—	—	—	—
submammary fold — *see also Neoplasm, skin, trunk*	C44.509	C79.2	D04.5	D23.5	D48.5	D49.2
supraclavicular region — *see also Neoplasm, skin, neck*	C44.40	C79.2	D04.4	D23.4	D48.5	D49.2
temple — *see also Neoplasm, skin, face*	C44.309	C79.2	D04.39	D23.39	D48.5	D49.2
thigh — *see also Neoplasm, skin, limb, lower*	C44.70-●	C79.2	D04.7-●	D23.7-●	D48.5	D49.2
thoracic wall — *see also Neoplasm, skin, trunk*	C44.509	C79.2	D04.5	D23.5	D48.5	D49.2
thumb — *see also Neoplasm, skin, limb, upper*	C44.60-●	C79.2	D04.6-●	D23.6-●	D48.5	D49.2
toe — *see also Neoplasm, skin, limb, lower*	C44.70-●	C79.2	D04.7-●	D23.7-●	D48.5	D49.2
tragus — *see also Neoplasm, skin, ear*	C44.20-●	C79.2	D04.2-●	D23.2-●	D48.5	D49.2
trunk	C44.509	C79.2	D04.5	D23.5	D48.5	D49.2
basal cell carcinoma	C44.519	—	—	—	—	—
specified type NEC	C44.599	—	—	—	—	—
squamous cell carcinoma	C44.529	—	—	—	—	—
umbilicus — *see also Neoplasm, skin, trunk*	C44.509	C79.2	D04.5	D23.5	D48.5	D49.2

◀ New   ◀ Revised   ~~deleted~~ Deleted   ● Use Additional Character(s)

TABLE OF NEOPLASMS

	Malignant Primary	Malignant Secondary	Ca in situ	Benign	Uncertain Behavior	Unspecified Behavior
skin NOS *(Continued)*						
vulva	C51.9	C79.82	D07.1	D28.0	D39.8	D49.59
overlapping lesion	C51.8	—	—	—	—	—
wrist — *see also Neoplasm, skin, limb, upper*	C44.60-●	C79.2	D04.6-●	D23.6-●	D48.5	D49.2
skull	C41.0	C79.51	—	D16.4-●	D48.0	D49.2
soft parts or tissues — *see Neoplasm, connective tissue*						
specified site NEC	C76.8	C79.89	D09.8	D36.7	D48.7	D49.89
spermatic cord	C63.1-●	C79.82	D07.69	D29.8	D40.8	D49.59
sphenoid	C31.3	C78.39	D02.3	D14.0	D38.5	D49.1
bone	C41.0	C79.51	—	D16.4-●	D48.0	D49.2
sinus	C31.3	C78.39	D02.3	D14.0	D38.5	D49.1
sphincter						
anal	C21.1	C78.5	D01.3	D12.9	D37.8	D49.0
of Oddi	C24.0	C78.89	D01.5	D13.5	D37.6	D49.0
spine, spinal (column)	C41.2	C79.51	—	D16.6	D48.0	D49.2
bulb	C71.7	C79.31	—	D33.1	D43.1	D49.6
coccyx	C41.4	C79.51	—	D16.8	D48.0	D49.2
cord (cervical) (lumbar) (sacral) (thoracic)	C72.0	C79.49	—	D33.4	D43.4	D49.7
dura mater	C70.1	C79.49	—	D32.1	D42.1	D49.7
lumbosacral	C41.2	C79.51	—	D16.6	D48.0	D49.2
marrow NEC	C96.9	C79.52	—	—	D47.9	D49.89
membrane	C70.1	C79.49	—	D32.1	D42.1	D49.7
meninges	C70.1	C79.49	—	D32.1	D42.1	D49.7
nerve (root)	C47.9	C79.89	—	D36.10	D48.2	D49.2
pia mater	C70.1	C79.49	—	D32.1	D42.1	D49.7
root	C47.9	C79.89	—	D36.10	D48.2	D49.2
sacrum	C41.4	C79.51	—	D16.8	D48.0	D49.2
spleen, splenic NEC	C26.1	C78.89	D01.7	D13.9	D37.8	D49.0
flexure (colon)	C18.5	C78.5	D01.0	D12.3	D37.4	D49.0
stem, brain	C71.7	C79.31	—	D33.1	D43.1	D49.6
Stensen's duct	C07	C79.89	D00.00	D11.0	D37.030	D49.0
sternum	C41.3	C79.51	—	D16.7	D48.0	D49.2
stomach	C16.9	C78.89	D00.2	D13.1	D37.1	D49.0
antrum (pyloric)	C16.3	C78.89	D00.2	D13.1	D37.1	D49.0
body	C16.2	C78.89	D00.2	D13.1	D37.1	D49.0
cardia	C16.0	C78.89	D00.2	D13.1	D37.1	D49.0
cardiac orifice	C16.0	C78.89	D00.2	D13.1	D37.1	D49.0
corpus	C16.2	C78.89	D00.2	D13.1	D37.1	D49.0
fundus	C16.1	C78.89	D00.2	D13.1	D37.1	D49.0
greater curvature NEC	C16.6	C78.89	D00.2	D13.1	D37.1	D49.0
lesser curvature NEC	C16.5	C78.89	D00.2	D13.1	D37.1	D49.0
stomach *(Continued)*						
overlapping lesion	C16.8	—	—	—	—	—
prepylorus	C16.4	C78.89	D00.2	D13.1	D37.1	D49.0
pylorus	C16.4	C78.89	D00.2	D13.1	D37.1	D49.0
wall NEC	C16.9	C78.89	D00.2	D13.1	D37.1	D49.0
anterior NEC	C16.8	C78.89	D00.2	D13.1	D37.1	D49.0
posterior NEC	C16.8	C78.89	D00.2	D13.1	D37.1	D49.0
stroma, endometrial	C54.1	C79.82	D07.0	D26.1	D39.0	D49.59
stump, cervical	C53.8	C79.82	D06.7	D26.0	D39.0	D49.59
subcutaneous (nodule) (tissue) NEC — *see Neoplasm, connective tissue*						
subdural	C70.9	C79.32	—	D32.9	D42.9	D49.7
subglottis, subglottic	C32.2	C78.39	D02.0	D14.1	D38.0	D49.1
sublingual	C04.9	C79.89	D00.06	D10.2	D37.09	D49.0
gland or duct	C08.1	C79.89	D00.00	D11.7	D37.031	D49.0
submandibular gland	C08.0	C79.89	D00.00	D11.7	D37.032	D49.0
submaxillary gland or duct	C08.0	C79.89	D00.00	D11.7	D37.032	D49.0
submental	C76.0	C79.89	D09.8	D36.7	D48.7	D49.89
subpleural	C34.9-●	C78.0-●	D02.2-●	D14.3-●	D38.1	D49.1
substernal	C38.1	C78.1	—	D15.2	D38.3	D49.89
sudoriferous, sudoriparous gland, site unspecified	C44.90	C79.2	D04.9	D23.9	D48.5	D49.2
specified site — *see Neoplasm, skin*						
supraclavicular region	C76.0	C79.89	D09.8	D36.7	D48.7	D49.89
supraglottis	C32.1	C78.39	D02.0	D14.1	D38.0	D49.1
suprarenal	C74.9-●	C79.7-●	D09.3	D35.0-●	D44.1-●	D49.7
capsule	C74.9-●	C79.7-●	D09.3	D35.0-●	D44.1-●	D49.7
cortex	C74.0-●	C79.7-●	D09.3	D35.0-●	D44.1-●	D49.7
gland	C74.9-●	C79.7-●	D09.3	D35.0-●	D44.1-●	D49.7
medulla	C74.1-●	C79.7-●	D09.3	D35.0-●	D44.1-●	D49.7
suprasellar (region)	C71.9	C79.31	—	D33.2	D43.2	D49.6
supratentorial (brain) NEC	C71.0	C79.31	—	D33.0	D43.0	D49.6
sweat gland (apocrine) (eccrine), site unspecified	C44.90	C79.2	D04.9	D23.9	D48.5	D49.2
specified site — *see Neoplasm, skin*						
sympathetic nerve or nervous system NEC	C47.9	C79.89	—	D36.10	D48.2	D49.2
symphysis pubis	C41.4	C79.51	—	D16.8	D48.0	D49.2
synovial membrane — *see Neoplasm, connective tissue*						
tapetum, brain	C71.8	C79.31	—	D33.2	D43.2	D49.6

◀ New   ◀ Revised   ~~deleted~~ Deleted   ● Use Additional Character(s)

TABLE OF NEOPLASMS

TABLE OF NEOPLASMS

	Malignant Primary	Malignant Secondary	Ca in situ	Benign	Uncertain Behavior	Unspecified Behavior
tarsus (any bone)	C40.3-●	C79.51	—	D16.3-●	—	—
temple (skin) — see also Neoplasm, skin, face	C44.309	C79.2	D04.39	D23.39	D48.5	D49.2
temporal						
bone	C41.0	C79.51	—	D16.4-●	D48.0	D49.2
lobe or pole	C71.2	C79.31	—	D33.0	D43.0	D49.6
region	C76.0	C79.89	D09.8	D36.7	D48.7	D49.89
skin — see also Neoplasm, skin, face	C44.309	C79.2	D04.39	D23.39	D48.5	D49.2
tendon (sheath) — see Neoplasm, connective tissue						
tentorium (cerebelli)	C70.0	C79.32	—	D32.0	D42.0	D49.7
testis, testes	C62.9-●	C79.82	D07.69	D29.2-●	D40.1-●	D49.59
descended	C62.1-●	C79.82	D07.69	D29.2-●	D40.1-●	D49.59
ectopic	C62.0-●	C79.82	D07.69	D29.2-●	D40.1-●	D49.59
retained	C62.0-●	C79.82	D07.69	D29.2-●	D40.1-●	D49.59
scrotal	C62.1-●	C79.82	D07.69	D29.2-●	D40.1-●	D49.59
undescended	C62.0-●	C79.82	D07.69	D29.2-●	D40.1-●	D49.59
unspecified whether descended or undescended	C62.9-●	C79.82	D07.69	D29.2-●	D40.1-●	D49.59
thalamus	C71.0	C79.31	—	D33.0	D43.0	D49.6
thigh NEC	C76.5-●	C79.89	D04.7-●	D36.7	D48.7	D49.89
thorax, thoracic (cavity) (organs NEC)	C76.1	C79.89	D09.8	D36.7	D48.7	D49.89
duct	C49.3	C79.89	—	D21.3	D48.1	D49.2
wall NEC	C76.1	C79.89	D09.8	D36.7	D48.7	D49.89
throat	C14.0	C79.89	D00.08	D10.9	D37.05	D49.0
thumb NEC	C76.4-●	C79.89	D04.6-●	D36.7	D48.7	D49.89
thymus (gland)	C37	C79.89	D09.3	D15.0	D38.4	D49.89
thyroglossal duct	C73	C79.89	D09.3	D34	D44.0	D49.7
thyroid (gland)	C73	C79.89	D09.3	D34	D44.0	D49.7
cartilage	C32.3	C78.39	D02.0	D14.1	D38.0	D49.1
tibia (any part)	C40.2-●	C79.51	—	D16.2-●	—	—
toe NEC	C76.5-●	C79.89	D04.7-●	D36.7	D48.7	D49.89
tongue	C02.9	C79.89	D00.07	D10.1	D37.02	D49.0
anterior (two-thirds) NEC	C02.3	C79.89	D00.07	D10.1	D37.02	D49.0
dorsal surface	C02.0	C79.89	D00.07	D10.1	D37.02	D49.0
ventral surface	C02.2	C79.89	D00.07	D10.1	D37.02	D49.0
base (dorsal surface)	C01	C79.89	D00.07	D10.1	D37.02	D49.0
border (lateral)	C02.1	C79.89	D00.07	D10.1	D37.02	D49.0
dorsal surface NEC	C02.0	C79.89	D00.07	D10.1	D37.02	D49.0
fixed part NEC	C01	C79.89	D00.07	D10.1	D37.02	D49.0
foreamen cecum	C02.0	C79.89	D00.07	D10.1	D37.02	D49.0
frenulum linguae	C02.2	C79.89	D00.07	D10.1	D37.02	D49.0
tongue (Continued)						
junctional zone	C02.8	C79.89	D00.07	D10.1	D37.02	D49.0
margin (lateral)	C02.1	C79.89	D00.07	D10.1	D37.02	D49.0
midline NEC	C02.0	C79.89	D00.07	D10.1	D37.02	D49.0
mobile part NEC	C02.3	C79.89	D00.07	D10.1	D37.02	D49.0
overlapping lesion	C02.8	—	—	—	—	—
posterior (third)	C01	C79.89	D00.07	D10.1	D37.02	D49.0
root	C01	C79.89	D00.07	D10.1	D37.02	D49.0
surface (dorsal)	C02.0	C79.89	D00.07	D10.1	D37.02	D49.0
base	C01	C79.89	D00.07	D10.1	D37.02	D49.0
ventral	C02.2	C79.89	D00.07	D10.1	D37.02	D49.0
tip	C02.1	C79.89	D00.07	D10.1	D37.02	D49.0
tonsil	C02.4	C79.89	D00.07	D10.1	D37.02	D49.0
tonsil	C09.9	C79.89	D00.08	D10.4	D37.05	D49.0
fauces, faucial	C09.9	C79.89	D00.08	D10.4	D37.05	D49.0
lingual	C02.4	C79.89	D00.07	D10.1	D37.02	D49.0
overlapping sites	C09.8	—	—	—	—	—
palatine	C09.9	C79.89	D00.08	D10.4	D37.05	D49.0
pharyngeal	C11.1	C79.89	D00.08	D10.6	D37.05	D49.0
pillar (anterior) (posterior)	C09.1	C79.89	D00.08	D10.5	D37.05	D49.0
tonsillar fossa	C09.0	C79.89	D00.08	D10.5	D37.05	D49.0
tooth socket NEC	C03.9	C79.89	D00.03	D10.39	D37.09	D49.0
trachea (cartilage) (mucosa)	C33	C78.39	D02.1	D14.2	D38.1	D49.1
overlapping lesion with bronchus or lung	C34.8-●	—	—	—	—	—
tracheobronchial	C34.8-●	C78.39	D02.1	D14.2	D38.1	D49.1
overlapping lesion with lung	C34.8-●	—	—	—	—	—
tragus — see also Neoplasm, skin, ear	C44.20-●	C79.2	D04.2-●	D23.2-●	D48.5	D49.2
trunk NEC	C76.8	C79.89	D04.5	D36.7	D48.7	D49.89
tubo-ovarian	C57.8	C79.82	D07.39	D28.7	D39.8	D49.59
tunica vaginalis	C63.7	C79.82	D07.69	D29.8	D40.8	D49.59
turbinate (bone)	C41.0	C79.51	—	D16.4-●	D48.0	D49.2
nasal	C30.0	C78.39	D02.3	D14.0	D38.5	D49.1
tympanic cavity	C30.1	C78.39	D02.3	D14.0	D38.5	D49.1
ulna (any part)	C40.0-●	C79.51	—	D16.0-●	—	—
umbilicus, umbilical — see also Neoplasm, skin, trunk	C44.509	C79.2	D04.5	D23.5	D48.5	D49.2
uncus, brain	C71.2	C79.31	—	D33.0	D43.0	D49.6
unknown site or unspecified	C80.1	C79.9	D09.9	D36.9	D48.9	D49.9
urachus	C67.7	C79.11	D09.0	D30.3	D41.4	D49.4
ureter, ureteral	C66.-●	C79.19	D09.19	D30.2-●	D41.2-●	D49.59
orifice (bladder)	C67.6	C79.11	D09.0	D30.3	D41.4	D49.4
ureter-bladder (junction)	C67.6	C79.11	D09.0	D30.3	D41.4	D49.4

◀ New   ◀▮ Revised   ~~deleted~~ Deleted   ● Use Additional Character(s)

	Malignant Primary	Malignant Secondary	Ca in situ	Benign	Uncertain Behavior	Unspecified Behavior
urethra, urethral (gland)	C68.0	C79.19	D09.19	D30.4	D41.3	D49.59
orifice, internal	C67.5	C79.11	D09.0	D30.3	D41.4	D49.4
urethrovaginal (septum)	C57.9	C79.82	D07.30	D28.9	D39.8	D49.59
urinary organ or system	C68.9	C79.10	D09.10	D30.9	D41.9	D49.59
bladder — see Neoplasm, bladder						
overlapping lesion	C68.8	—	—	—	—	—
specified sites NEC	C68.8	C79.19	D09.19	D30.8	D41.8	D49.59
utero-ovarian	C57.8	C79.82	D07.39	D28.7	D39.8	D49.59
ligament	C57.1	C79.82	D07.39	D28.2	D39.8	D49.59
uterosacral ligament	C57.3	C79.82	—	D28.2	D39.8	D49.59
uterus, uteri, uterine	C55	C79.82	D07.0	D26.9	D39.0	D49.59
adnexa NEC	C57.4	C79.82	D07.39	D28.7	D39.8	D49.59
body	C54.9	C79.82	D07.0	D26.1	D39.0	D49.59
cervix	C53.9	C79.82	D06.9	D26.0	D39.0	D49.59
cornu	C54.9	C79.82	D07.0	D26.1	D39.0	D49.59
corpus	C54.9	C79.82	D07.0	D26.1	D39.0	D49.59
endocervix (canal) (gland)	C53.0	C79.82	D06.0	D26.0	D39.0	D49.59
endometrium	C54.1	C79.82	D07.0	D26.1	D39.0	D49.59
exocervix	C53.1	C79.82	D06.1	D26.0	D39.0	D49.59
external os	C53.1	C79.82	D06.1	D26.0	D39.0	D49.59
fundus	C54.3	C79.82	D07.0	D26.1	D39.0	D49.59
internal os	C53.0	C79.82	D06.0	D26.0	D39.0	D49.59
isthmus	C54.0	C79.82	D07.0	D26.1	D39.0	D49.59
ligament	C57.3	C79.82	—	D28.2	D39.8	D49.59
broad	C57.1	C79.82	D07.39	D28.2	D39.8	D49.59
round	C57.2	C79.82	—	D28.2	D39.8	D49.59
lower segment	C54.0	C79.82	D07.0	D26.1	D39.0	D49.59
myometrium	C54.2	C79.82	D07.0	D26.1	D39.0	D49.59
overlapping sites	C54.8	—	—	—	—	—
squamocolumnar junction	C53.8	C79.82	D06.7	D26.0	D39.0	D49.59
tube	C57.0-●	C79.82	D07.39	D28.2	D39.8	D49.59
utricle, prostatic	C68.0	C79.19	D09.19	D30.4	D41.3	D49.59
uveal tract	C69.4-●	C79.49	D09.2-●	D31.4-●	D48.7	D49.89
uvula	C05.2	C79.89	D00.04	D10.39	D37.09	D49.0
vagina, vaginal (fornix) (vault) (wall)	C52	C79.82	D07.2	D28.1	D39.8	D49.59
vaginovesical	C57.9	C79.82	D07.30	D28.9	D39.9	D49.59
septum	C57.9	C79.82	D07.30	D28.9	D39.9	D49.59
vallecula (epiglottis)	C10.0	C79.89	D00.08	D10.5	D37.05	D49.0
vas deferens	C63.1-●	C79.82	D07.69	D29.8	D40.8	D49.59
vascular — see Neoplasm, connective tissue						

	Malignant Primary	Malignant Secondary	Ca in situ	Benign	Uncertain Behavior	Unspecified Behavior
Vater's ampulla	C24.1	C78.89	D01.5	D13.5	D37.6	D49.0
vein, venous — see Neoplasm, connective tissue						
vena cava (abdominal) (inferior)	C49.4	C79.89	—	D21.4	D48.1	D49.2
superior	C49.3	C79.89	—	D21.3	D48.1	D49.2
ventricle (cerebral) (floor) (lateral) (third)	C71.5	C79.31	—	D33.0	D43.0	D49.6
cardiac (left) (right)	C38.0	C79.89	—	D15.1	D48.7	D49.89
fourth	C71.7	C79.31	—	D33.1	D43.1	D49.6
ventricular band of larynx	C32.1	C78.39	D02.0	D14.1	D38.0	D49.1
ventriculus — see Neoplasm, stomach						
vermillion border — see Neoplasm, lip						
vermis, cerebellum	C71.6	C79.31	—	D33.1	D43.1	D49.6
vertebra (column)	C41.2	C79.51	—	D16.6	D48.0	D49.2
coccyx	C41.4	C79.51	—	D16.8-●	D48.0	D49.2
marrow NEC	C96.9	C79.52	—	D47.9	D49.89	
sacrum	C41.4	C79.51	—	D16.8-●	D48.0	D49.2
vesical — see Neoplasm, bladder						
vesicle, seminal	C63.7	C79.82	D07.69	D29.8	D40.8	D49.59
vesicocervical tissue	C57.9	C79.82	D07.30	D28.9	D39.9	D49.59
vesicorectal	C76.3	C79.82	D09.8	D36.7	D48.7	D49.89
vesicovaginal	C57.9	C79.82	D07.30	D28.9	D39.9	D49.59
septum	C57.9	C79.82	D07.30	D28.9	D39.8	D49.59
vessel (blood) — see Neoplasm, connective tissue						
vestibular gland, greater	C51.0	C79.82	D07.1	D28.0	D39.8	D49.59
vestibule						
mouth	C06.1	C79.89	D00.00	D10.39	D37.09	D49.0
nose	C30.0	C78.39	D02.3	D14.0	D38.5	D49.1
Virchow's gland	C77.0	C77.0	—	D36.0	D48.7	D49.89
viscera NEC	C76.8	C79.89	D09.8	D36.7	D48.7	D49.89
vocal cords (true)	C32.0	C78.39	D02.0	D14.1	D38.0	D49.1
false	C32.1	C78.39	D02.0	D14.1	D38.0	D49.1
vomer	C41.0	C79.51	—	D16.4-●	D48.0	D49.2
vulva	C51.9	C79.82	D07.1	D28.0	D39.8	D49.59
vulvovaginal gland	C51.0	C79.82	D07.1	D28.0	D39.8	D49.59
Waldeyer's ring	C14.2	C79.89	D00.08	D10.9	D37.05	D49.0
Wharton's duct	C08.0	C79.89	D00.00	D11.7	D37.032	D49.0
white matter (central) (cerebral)	C71.0	C79.31	—	D33.0	D43.0	D49.6
windpipe	C33	C78.39	D02.1	D14.2	D38.1	D49.1

TABLE OF NEOPLASMS

	Malignant Primary	Malignant Secondary	Ca in situ	Benign	Uncertain Behavior	Unspecified Behavior
Wirsung's duct	C25.3	C78.89	D01.7	D13.6	D37.8	D49.0
wolffian (body) (duct)						
female	C57.7	C79.82	D07.39	D28.7	D39.8	D49.59
male	C63.7	C79.82	D07.69	D29.8	D40.8	D49.59

	Malignant Primary	Malignant Secondary	Ca in situ	Benign	Uncertain Behavior	Unspecified Behavior
womb — *see Neoplasm, uterus*						
wrist NEC	C76.4-●	C79.89	D04.6-●	D36.7	D48.7	D49.89
xiphoid process	C41.3	C79.51	—	D16.7	D48.0	D49.2
Zuckerkandl organ	C75.5	C79.89	—	D35.6	D44.7	D49.7

◀ New   ◀ Revised   ~~deleted~~ Deleted   ● Use Additional Character(s)

TABLE OF NEOPLASMS

ICD-10-CM
Table of Drugs and Chemicals

Substance	Poisoning, Accidental (Unintentional)	Poisoning, Intentional Self-Harm	Poisoning, Assault	Poisoning, Undetermined	Adverse Effect	Underdosing
#						
1-propanol	T51.3X1	T51.3X2	T51.3X3	T51.3X4	—	—
2-propanol	T51.2X1	T51.2X2	T51.2X3	T51.2X4	—	—
2,4-D (dichlorophen-oxyacetic acid)	T60.3X1	T60.3X2	T60.3X3	T60.3X4	—	—
2,4-toluene diisocyanate	T65.0X1	T65.0X2	T65.0X3	T65.0X4	—	—
2,4,5-T (trichloro-phenoxyacetic acid)	T60.1X1	T60.1X2	T60.1X3	T60.1X4	—	—
14-hydroxydihydro-morphinone	T40.2X1	T40.2X2	T40.2X3	T40.2X4	T40.2X5	T40.2X6
A						
ABOB	T37.5X1	T37.5X2	T37.5X3	T37.5X4	T37.5X5	T37.5X6
Abrine	T62.2X1	T62.2X2	T62.2X3	T62.2X4	—	—
Abrus (seed)	T62.2X1	T62.2X2	T62.2X3	T62.2X4	—	—
Absinthe	T51.0X1	T51.0X2	T51.0X3	T51.0X4	—	—
beverage	T51.0X1	T51.0X2	T51.0X3	T51.0X4	—	—
Acaricide	T60.8X1	T60.8X2	T60.8X3	T60.8X4	—	—
Acebutolol	T44.7X1	T44.7X2	T44.7X3	T44.7X4	T44.7X5	T44.7X6
Acecarbromal	T42.6X1	T42.6X2	T42.6X3	T42.6X4	T42.6X5	T42.6X6
Aceclidine	T44.1X1	T44.1X2	T44.1X3	T44.1X4	T44.1X5	T44.1X6
Acedapsone	T37.0X1	T37.0X2	T37.0X3	T37.0X4	T37.0X5	T37.0X6
Acefylline piperazine	T48.6X1	T48.6X2	T48.6X3	T48.6X4	T48.6X5	T48.6X6
Acemorphan	T40.2X1	T40.2X2	T40.2X3	T40.2X4	T40.2X5	T40.2X6
Acenocoumarin	T45.511	T45.512	T45.513	T45.514	T45.515	T45.516
Acenocoumarol	T45.511	T45.512	T45.513	T45.514	T45.515	T45.516
Acepifylline	T48.6X1	T48.6X2	T48.6X3	T48.6X4	T48.6X5	T48.6X6
Acepromazine	T43.3X1	T43.3X2	T43.3X3	T43.3X4	T43.3X5	T43.3X6
Acesulfamethoxypyridazine	T37.0X1	T37.0X2	T37.0X3	T37.0X4	T37.0X5	T37.0X6
Acetal	T52.8X1	T52.8X2	T52.8X3	T52.8X4	—	—
Acetaldehyde (vapor)	T52.8X1	T52.8X2	T52.8X3	T52.8X4	—	—
liquid	T65.891	T65.892	T65.893	T65.894	—	—
P-Acetamidophenol	T39.1X1	T39.1X2	T39.1X3	T39.1X4	T39.1X5	T39.1X6
Acetaminophen	T39.1X1	T39.1X2	T39.1X3	T39.1X4	T39.1X5	T39.1X6
Acetaminosalol	T39.1X1	T39.1X2	T39.1X3	T39.1X4	T39.1X5	T39.1X6
Acetanilide	T39.1X1	T39.1X2	T39.1X3	T39.1X4	T39.1X5	T39.1X6
Acetarsol	T37.3X1	T37.3X2	T37.3X3	T37.3X4	T37.3X5	T37.3X6
Acetazolamide	T50.2X1	T50.2X2	T50.2X3	T50.2X4	T50.2X5	T50.2X6
Acetiamine	T45.2X1	T45.2X2	T45.2X3	T45.2X4	T45.2X5	T45.2X6
Acetic						
acid	T54.2X1	T54.2X2	T54.2X3	T54.2X4	—	—
with sodium acetate (ointment)	T49.3X1	T49.3X2	T49.3X3	T49.3X4	T49.3X5	T49.3X6

Substance	Poisoning, Accidental (Unintentional)	Poisoning, Intentional Self-Harm	Poisoning, Assault	Poisoning, Undetermined	Adverse Effect	Underdosing
Acetic (Continued)						
acid (Continued)						
ester (solvent) (vapor)	T52.8X1	T52.8X2	T52.8X3	T52.8X4	—	—
irrigating solution	T50.3X1	T50.3X2	T50.3X3	T50.3X4	T50.3X5	T50.3X6
medicinal (lotion)	T49.2X1	T49.2X2	T49.2X3	T49.2X4	T49.2X5	T49.2X6
anhydride	T65.891	T65.892	T65.893	T65.894		
ether (vapor)	T52.8X1	T52.8X2	T52.8X3	T52.8X4	—	—
Acetohexamide	T38.3X1	T38.3X2	T38.3X3	T38.3X4	T38.3X5	T38.3X6
Acetohydroxamic acid	T50.991	T50.992	T50.993	T50.994	T50.995	T50.996
Acetomenaphthone	T45.7X1	T45.7X2	T45.7X3	T45.7X4	T45.7X5	T45.7X6
Acetomorphine	T40.1X1	T40.1X2	T40.1X3	T40.1X4	—	—
Acetone (oils)	T52.4X1	T52.4X2	T52.4X3	T52.4X4		
chlorinated	T52.4X1	T52.4X2	T52.4X3	T52.4X4		
vapor	T52.4X1	T52.4X2	T52.4X3	T52.4X4		
Acetonitrile	T52.8X1	T52.8X2	T52.8X3	T52.8X4		
Acetophenazine	T43.3X1	T43.3X2	T43.3X3	T43.3X4	T43.3X5	T43.3X6
Acetophenetedin	T39.1X1	T39.1X2	T39.1X3	T39.1X4	T39.1X5	T39.1X6
Acetophenone	T52.4X1	T52.4X2	T52.4X3	T52.4X4		
Acetorphine	T40.2X1	T40.2X2	T40.2X3	T40.2X4	—	—
Acetosulfone (sodium)	T37.1X1	T37.1X2	T37.1X3	T37.1X4	T37.1X5	T37.1X6
Acetrizoate (sodium)	T50.8X1	T50.8X2	T50.8X3	T50.8X4	T50.8X5	T50.8X6
Acetylcarbromal	T42.6X1	T42.6X2	T42.6X3	T42.6X4	T42.6X5	T42.6X6
Acetrizoic acid	T50.8X1	T50.8X2	T50.8X3	T50.8X4	T50.8X5	T50.8X6
Acetyl						
bromide	T53.6X1	T53.6X2	T53.6X3	T53.6X4		
chloride	T53.6X1	T53.6X2	T53.6X3	T53.6X4	—	—
Acetylcholine						
chloride	T44.1X1	T44.1X2	T44.1X3	T44.1X4	T44.1X5	T44.1X6
derivative	T44.1X1	T44.1X2	T44.1X3	T44.1X4	T44.1X5	T44.1X6
Acetylcysteine	T48.4X1	T48.4X2	T48.4X3	T48.4X4	T48.4X5	T48.4X6
Acetyldigitoxin	T46.0X1	T46.0X2	T46.0X3	T46.0X4	T46.0X5	T46.0X6
Acetyldigoxin	T46.0X1	T46.0X2	T46.0X3	T46.0X4	T46.0X5	T46.0X6
Acetyldihydrocodeine	T40.2X1	T40.2X2	T40.2X3	T40.2X4	—	—
Acetyldihydrocodeinone	T40.2X1	T40.2X2	T40.2X3	T40.2X4	—	—
Acetylene (gas)	T59.891	T59.892	T59.893	T59.894	—	—
dichloride	T53.6X1	T53.6X2	T53.6X3	T53.6X4		
incomplete combustion of	T58.11	T58.12	T58.13	T58.14		
industrial	T59.891	T59.892	T59.893	T59.894	—	—
tetrachloride	T53.6X1	T53.6X2	T53.6X3	T53.6X4		
vapor	T53.6X1	T53.6X2	T53.6X3	T53.6X4		
Acetylphenylhydrazine	T39.8X1	T39.8X2	T39.8X3	T39.8X4	T39.8X5	T39.8X6
Acetylpheneturide	T42.6X1	T42.6X2	T42.6X3	T42.6X4	T42.6X5	T42.6X6

◀ New   ◀| Revised   ~~deleted~~ Deleted

TABLE OF DRUGS AND CHEMICALS

Substance	Poisoning, Accidental (Unintentional)	Poisoning, Intentional Self-Harm	Poisoning, Assault	Poisoning, Undetermined	Adverse Effect	Underdosing
Acetylsalicylic acid (salts)	T39.011	T39.012	T39.013	T39.014	T39.015	T39.016
enteric coated	T39.011	T39.012	T39.013	T39.014	T39.015	T39.016
Acetylsulfamethoxypyridazine	T37.0X1	T37.0X2	T37.0X3	T37.0X4	T37.0X5	T37.0X6
Achromycin	T36.4X1	T36.4X2	T36.4X3	T36.4X4	T36.4X5	T36.4X6
ophthalmic preparation	T49.5X1	T49.5X2	T49.5X3	T49.5X4	T49.5X5	T49.5X6
topical NEC	T49.0X1	T49.0X2	T49.0X3	T49.0X4	T49.0X5	T49.0X6
Aciclovir	T37.5X1	T37.5X2	T37.5X3	T37.5X4	T37.5X5	T37.5X6
Acid (corrosive) NEC	T54.2X1	T54.2X2	T54.2X3	T54.2X4	—	—
Acidifying agent NEC	T50.901	T50.902	T50.903	T50.904	T50.905	T50.906
Acipimox	T46.6X1	T46.6X2	T46.6X3	T46.6X4	T46.6X5	T46.6X6
Acitretin	T50.991	T50.992	T50.993	T50.994	T50.995	T50.996
Aclarubicin	T45.1X1	T45.1X2	T45.1X3	T45.1X4	T45.1X5	T45.1X6
Aclatonium napadisilate	T48.1X1	T48.1X2	T48.1X3	T48.1X4	T48.1X5	T48.1X6
Aconite (wild)	T46.991	T46.992	T46.993	T46.994	T46.995	T46.996
Aconitine	T46.991	T46.992	T46.993	T46.994	T46.995	T46.996
Aconitum ferox	T46.991	T46.992	T46.993	T46.994	T46.995	T46.996
Acridine	T65.6X1	T65.6X2	T65.6X3	T65.6X4	—	—
vapor	T59.891	T59.892	T59.893	T59.894	—	—
Acriflavine	T37.91	T37.92	T37.93	T37.94	T37.95	T37.96
Acriflavinium chloride	T49.0X1	T49.0X2	T49.0X3	T49.0X4	T49.0X5	T49.0X6
Acrinol	T49.0X1	T49.0X2	T49.0X3	T49.0X4	T49.0X5	T49.0X6
Acrisorcin	T49.0X1	T49.0X2	T49.0X3	T49.0X4	T49.0X5	T49.0X6
Acrivastine	T45.0X1	T45.0X2	T45.0X3	T45.0X4	T45.0X5	T45.0X6
Acrolein (gas)	T59.891	T59.892	T59.893	T59.894	—	—
liquid	T54.1X1	T54.1X2	T54.1X3	T54.1X4	—	—
Acrylamide	T65.891	T65.892	T65.893	T65.894	—	—
Acrylic resin	T49.3X1	T49.3X2	T49.3X3	T49.3X4	T49.3X5	T49.3X6
Acrylonitrile	T65.891	T65.892	T65.893	T65.894	—	—
Actaea spicata	T62.2X1	T62.2X2	T62.2X3	T62.2X4	—	—
berry	T62.1X1	T62.1X2	T62.1X3	T62.1X4	—	—
Acterol	T37.3X1	T37.3X2	T37.3X3	T37.3X4	T37.3X5	T37.3X6
ACTH	T38.811	T38.812	T38.813	T38.814	T38.815	T38.816
Actinomycin C	T45.1X1	T45.1X2	T45.1X3	T45.1X4	T45.1X5	T45.1X6
Actinomycin D	T45.1X1	T45.1X2	T45.1X3	T45.1X4	T45.1X5	T45.1X6
Activated charcoal — see also Charcoal, medicinal	T47.6X1	T47.6X2	T47.6X3	T47.6X4	T47.6X5	T47.6X6
Acyclovir	T37.5X1	T37.5X2	T37.5X3	T37.5X4	T37.5X5	T37.5X6
Adenine	T45.2X1	T45.2X2	T45.2X3	T45.2X4	T45.2X5	T45.2X6
arabinoside	T37.5X1	T37.5X2	T37.5X3	T37.5X4	T37.5X5	T37.5X6
Adenosine (phosphate)	T46.2X1	T46.2X2	T46.2X3	T46.2X4	T46.2X5	T46.2X6
ADH	T38.891	T38.892	T38.893	T38.894	T38.895	T38.896
Adhesive NEC	T65.891	T65.892	T65.893	T65.894	—	—

Substance	Poisoning, Accidental (Unintentional)	Poisoning, Intentional Self-Harm	Poisoning, Assault	Poisoning, Undetermined	Adverse Effect	Underdosing
Adicillin	T36.0X1	T36.0X2	T36.0X3	T36.0X4	T36.0X5	T36.0X6
Adiphenine	T44.3X1	T44.3X2	T44.3X3	T44.3X4	T44.3X5	T44.3X6
Adipiodone	T50.8X1	T50.8X2	T50.8X3	T50.8X4	T50.8X5	T50.8X6
Adjunct, pharmaceutical	T50.901	T50.902	T50.903	T50.904	T50.905	T50.906
Adrenal (extract, cortex or medulla) (glucocorticoids) (hormones) (mineralo corticoids)	T38.0X1	T38.0X2	T38.0X3	T38.0X4	T38.0X5	T38.0X6
ENT agent	T49.6X1	T49.6X2	T49.6X3	T49.6X4	T49.6X5	T49.6X6
ophthalmic preparation	T49.5X1	T49.5X2	T49.5X3	T49.5X4	T49.5X5	T49.5X6
topical NEC	T49.0X1	T49.0X2	T49.0X3	T49.0X4	T49.0X5	T49.0X6
Adrenaline	T44.5X1	T44.5X2	T44.5X3	T44.5X4	T44.5X5	T44.5X6
Adrenalin — see Adrenaline						
Adrenergic NEC	T44.901	T44.902	T44.903	T44.904	T44.905	T44.906
blocking agent NEC	T44.8X1	T44.8X2	T44.8X3	T44.8X4	T44.8X5	T44.8X6
beta, heart	T44.7X1	T44.7X2	T44.7X3	T44.7X4	T44.7X5	T44.7X6
specified NEC	T44.991	T44.992	T44.993	T44.994	T44.995	T44.996
Adrenochrome						
(mono) semicarbazone	T46.991	T46.992	T46.993	T46.994	T46.995	T46.996
derivative	T46.991	T46.992	T46.993	T46.994	T46.995	T46.996
Adrenocorticotrophic hormone	T38.811	T38.812	T38.813	T38.814	T38.815	T38.816
Adrenocorticotrophin	T38.811	T38.812	T38.813	T38.814	T38.815	T38.816
Adriamycin	T45.1X1	T45.1X2	T45.1X3	T45.1X4	T45.1X5	T45.1X6
Aerosol spray NEC	T65.91	T65.92	T65.93	T65.94	—	—
Aerosporin	T36.8X1	T36.8X2	T36.8X3	T36.8X4	T36.8X5	T36.8X6
ENT agent	T49.6X1	T49.6X2	T49.6X3	T49.6X4	T49.6X5	T49.6X6
ophthalmic preparation	T49.5X1	T49.5X2	T49.5X3	T49.5X4	T49.5X5	T49.5X6
topical NEC	T49.0X1	T49.0X2	T49.0X3	T49.0X4	T49.0X5	T49.0X6
Aethusa cynapium	T62.2X1	T62.2X2	T62.2X3	T62.2X4	—	—
Afghanistan black	T40.7X1	T40.7X2	T40.7X3	T40.7X4	T40.7X5	T40.7X6
Aflatoxin	T64.01	T64.02	T64.03	T64.04	—	—
Afloqualone	T42.8X1	T42.8X2	T42.8X3	T42.8X4	T42.8X5	T42.8X6
African boxwood	T62.2X1	T62.2X2	T62.2X3	T62.2X4	—	—
Agar	T47.4X1	T47.4X2	T47.4X3	T47.4X4	T47.4X5	T47.4X6
Agonist						
predominantly						
alpha-adrenoreceptor	T44.4X1	T44.4X2	T44.4X3	T44.4X4	T44.4X5	T44.4X6
beta-adrenoreceptor	T44.5X1	T44.5X2	T44.5X3	T44.5X4	T44.5X5	T44.5X6
Agricultural agent NEC	T65.91	T65.92	T65.93	T65.94	—	—
Agrypnal	T42.3X1	T42.3X2	T42.3X3	T42.3X4	T42.3X5	T42.3X6
AHLG	T50.Z11	T50.Z12	T50.Z13	T50.Z14	T50.Z15	T50.Z16
Air contaminant(s), source/type NOS	T65.91	T65.92	T65.93	T65.94	—	—

◀ New ◀ Revised ~~deleted~~ Deleted

Substance	External Cause (T-Code)					
	Poisoning, Accidental (Unintentional)	Poisoning, Intentional Self-Harm	Poisoning, Assault	Poisoning, Undetermined	Adverse Effect	Underdosing
Ajmaline	T46.2X1	T46.2X2	T46.2X3	T46.2X4	T46.2X5	T46.2X6
Akritoin	T37.8X1	T37.8X2	T37.8X3	T37.8X4	T37.8X5	T37.8X6
Akee	T62.1X1	T62.1X2	T62.1X3	T62.1X4	—	—
Akrinol	T49.0X1	T49.0X2	T49.0X3	T49.0X4	T49.0X5	T49.0X6
Alacepril	T46.4X1	T46.4X2	T46.4X3	T46.4X4	T46.4X5	T46.4X6
Alantolactone	T37.4X1	T37.4X2	T37.4X3	T37.4X4	T37.4X5	T37.4X6
Albamycin	T36.8X1	T36.8X2	T36.8X3	T36.8X4	T36.8X5	T36.8X6
Albendazole	T37.4X1	T37.4X2	T37.4X3	T37.4X4	T37.4X5	T37.4X6
Albumin						
bovine	T45.8X1	T45.8X2	T45.8X3	T45.8X4	T45.8X5	T45.8X6
human serum	T45.8X1	T45.8X2	T45.8X3	T45.8X4	T45.8X5	T45.8X6
salt-poor	T45.8X1	T45.8X2	T45.8X3	T45.8X4	T45.8X5	T45.8X6
normal human serum	T45.8X1	T45.8X2	T45.8X3	T45.8X4	T45.8X5	T45.8X6
Albuterol	T48.6X1	T48.6X2	T48.6X3	T48.6X4	T48.6X5	T48.6X6
Albutoin	T42.0X1	T42.0X2	T42.0X3	T42.0X4	T42.0X5	T42.0X6
Alclometasone	T49.0X1	T49.0X2	T49.0X3	T49.0X4	T49.0X5	T49.0X6
Alcohol	T51.91	T51.92	T51.93	T51.94	—	—
absolute	T51.0X1	T51.0X2	T51.0X3	T51.0X4	—	—
beverage	T51.0X1	T51.0X2	T51.0X3	T51.0X4	—	—
allyl	T51.8X1	T51.8X2	T51.8X3	T51.8X4	—	—
amyl	T51.3X1	T51.3X2	T51.3X3	T51.3X4	—	—
antifreeze	T51.1X1	T51.1X2	T51.1X3	T51.1X4	—	—
beverage	T51.0X1	T51.0X2	T51.0X3	T51.0X4	—	—
butyl	T51.3X1	T51.3X2	T51.3X3	T51.3X4	—	—
dehydrated	T51.0X1	T51.0X2	T51.0X3	T51.0X4	—	—
beverage	T51.0X1	T51.0X2	T51.0X3	T51.0X4	—	—
denatured	T51.0X1	T51.0X2	T51.0X3	T51.0X4	—	—
deterrent NEC	T50.6X1	T50.6X2	T50.6X3	T50.6X4	T50.6X5	T50.6X6
diagnostic (gastric function)	T50.8X1	T50.8X2	T50.8X3	T50.8X4	T50.8X5	T50.8X6
ethyl	T51.0X1	T51.0X2	T51.0X3	T51.0X4	—	—
beverage	T51.0X1	T51.0X2	T51.0X3	T51.0X4	—	—
grain	T51.0X1	T51.0X2	T51.0X3	T51.0X4	—	—
beverage	T51.0X1	T51.0X2	T51.0X3	T51.0X4	—	—
industrial	T51.0X1	T51.0X2	T51.0X3	T51.0X4	—	—
isopropyl	T51.2X1	T51.2X2	T51.2X3	T51.2X4	—	—
methyl	T51.1X1	T51.1X2	T51.1X3	T51.1X4	—	—
preparation for consumption	T51.0X1	T51.0X2	T51.0X3	T51.0X4	—	—
propyl	T51.3X1	T51.3X2	T51.3X3	T51.3X4	—	—
secondary	T51.2X1	T51.2X2	T51.2X3	T51.2X4	—	—
radiator	T51.1X1	T51.1X2	T51.1X3	T51.1X4	—	—
rubbing	T51.2X1	T51.2X2	T51.2X3	T51.2X4	—	—
specified type NEC	T51.8X1	T51.8X2	T51.8X3	T51.8X4	—	—

Substance	External Cause (T-Code)					
	Poisoning, Accidental (Unintentional)	Poisoning, Intentional Self-Harm	Poisoning, Assault	Poisoning, Undetermined	Adverse Effect	Underdosing
Alcohol *(Continued)*						
surgical	T51.0X1	T51.0X2	T51.0X3	T51.0X4	—	—
vapor (from any type of Alcohol)	T59.891	T59.892	T59.893	T59.894	—	—
wood	T51.1X1	T51.1X2	T51.1X3	T51.1X4	—	—
Alcuronium (chloride)	T48.1X1	T48.1X2	T48.1X3	T48.1X4	T48.1X5	T48.1X6
Aldactone	T50.0X1	T50.0X2	T50.0X3	T50.0X4	T50.0X5	T50.0X6
Aldesulfone sodium	T37.1X1	T37.1X2	T37.1X3	T37.1X4	T37.1X5	T37.1X6
Aldicarb	T60.0X1	T60.0X2	T60.0X3	T60.0X4	—	—
Aldomet	T46.5X1	T46.5X2	T46.5X3	T46.5X4	T46.5X5	T46.5X6
Aldosterone	T50.0X1	T50.0X2	T50.0X3	T50.0X4	T50.0X5	T50.0X6
Aldrin (dust)	T60.1X1	T60.1X2	T60.1X3	T60.1X4	—	—
Aleve — *see* Naproxen						
Alexitol sodium	T47.1X1	T47.1X2	T47.1X3	T47.1X4	T47.1X5	T47.1X6
Alfacalcidol	T45.2X1	T45.2X2	T45.2X3	T45.2X4	T45.2X5	T45.2X6
Alfadolone	T41.1X1	T41.1X2	T41.1X3	T41.1X4	T41.1X5	T41.1X6
Alfaxalone	T41.1X1	T41.1X2	T41.1X3	T41.1X4	T41.1X5	T41.1X6
Alfentanil	T40.4X1	T40.4X2	T40.4X3	T40.4X4	T40.4X5	T40.4X6
Alfuzosin (hydrochloride)	T44.8X1	T44.8X2	T44.8X3	T44.8X4	T44.8X5	T44.8X6
Algae (harmful) (toxin)	T65.821	T65.822	T65.823	T65.824	—	—
Algeldrate	T47.1X1	T47.1X2	T47.1X3	T47.1X4	T47.1X5	T47.1X6
Algin	T47.8X1	T47.8X2	T47.8X3	T47.8X4	T47.8X5	T47.8X6
Alglucerase	T45.3X1	T45.3X2	T45.3X3	T45.3X4	T45.3X5	T45.3X6
Alidase	T45.3X1	T45.3X2	T45.3X3	T45.3X4	T45.3X5	T45.3X6
Alimemazine	T43.3X1	T43.3X2	T43.3X3	T43.3X4	T43.3X5	T43.3X6
Aliphatic thiocyanates	T65.0X1	T65.0X2	T65.0X3	T65.0X4	—	—
Alizapride	T45.0X1	T45.0X2	T45.0X3	T45.0X4	T45.0X5	T45.0X6
Alkali (caustic)	T54.3X1	T54.3X2	T54.3X3	T54.3X4	—	—
Alkalizing agent NEC	T50.901	T50.902	T50.903	T50.904	T50.905	T50.906
Alkaline antiseptic solution (aromatic)	T49.6X1	T49.6X2	T49.6X3	T49.6X4	T49.6X5	T49.6X6
Alkalinizing agents (medicinal)	T50.901	T50.902	T50.903	T50.904	T50.905	T50.906
Alka-seltzer	T39.011	T39.012	T39.013	T39.014	T39.015	T39.016
Alkavervir	T46.5X1	T46.5X2	T46.5X3	T46.5X4	T46.5X5	T46.5X6
Alkonium (bromide)	T49.0X1	T49.0X2	T49.0X3	T49.0X4	T49.0X5	T49.0X6
Alkylating drug NEC	T45.1X1	T45.1X2	T45.1X3	T45.1X4	T45.1X5	T45.1X6
antimyeloproliferative	T45.1X1	T45.1X2	T45.1X3	T45.1X4	T45.1X5	T45.1X6
lymphatic	T45.1X1	T45.1X2	T45.1X3	T45.1X4	T45.1X5	T45.1X6
Alkylisocyanate	T65.0X1	T65.0X2	T65.0X3	T65.0X4	—	—
Allantoin	T49.411	T49.412	T49.413	T49.414	T49.415	T49.416
Allegron	T43.0X1	T43.0X2	T43.0X3	T43.0X4	T43.0X5	T43.0X6
Allethrin	T49.0X1	T49.0X2	T49.0X3	T49.0X4	T49.0X5	T49.0X6
Allobarbital	T42.3X1	T42.3X2	T42.3X3	T42.3X4	T42.3X5	T42.3X6

◄ New   ◄ Revised   ~~deleted~~ Deleted

TABLE OF DRUGS AND CHEMICALS

Substance	Poisoning, Accidental (Unintentional)	Poisoning, Intentional Self-Harm	Poisoning, Assault	Poisoning, Undetermined	Adverse Effect	Underdosing
Allopurinol	T50.4X1	T50.4X2	T50.4X3	T50.4X4	T50.4X5	T50.4X6
Allyl						
alcohol	T51.8X1	T51.8X2	T51.8X3	T51.8X4	—	—
disulfide	T46.6X1	T46.6X2	T46.6X3	T46.6X4	T46.6X5	T46.6X6
Allylestrenol	T38.5X1	T38.5X2	T38.5X3	T38.5X4	T38.5X5	T38.5X6
Allylisopropylacetylurea	T42.6X1	T42.6X2	T42.6X3	T42.6X4	T42.6X5	T42.6X6
Allylisopropylmalonylurea	T42.3X1	T42.3X2	T42.3X3	T42.3X4	T42.3X5	T42.3X6
Allylthiourea	T49.3X1	T49.3X2	T49.3X3	T49.3X4	T49.3X5	T49.3X6
Allyltribromide	T42.6X1	T42.6X2	T42.6X3	T42.6X4	T42.6X5	T42.6X6
Allypropymal	T42.3X1	T42.3X2	T42.3X3	T42.3X4	T42.3X5	T42.3X6
Almagate	T47.1X1	T47.1X2	T47.1X3	T47.1X4	T47.1X5	T47.1X6
Almasilate	T47.1X1	T47.1X2	T47.1X3	T47.1X4	T47.1X5	T47.1X6
Almitrine	T50.7X1	T50.7X2	T50.7X3	T50.7X4	T50.7X5	T50.7X6
Aloes	T47.2X1	T47.2X2	T47.2X3	T47.2X4	T47.2X5	T47.2X6
Aloglutamol	T47.1X1	T47.1X2	T47.1X3	T47.1X4	T47.1X5	T47.1X6
Aloin	T47.2X1	T47.2X2	T47.2X3	T47.2X4	T47.2X5	T47.2X6
Aloxidone	T42.2X1	T42.2X2	T42.2X3	T42.2X4	T42.2X5	T42.2X6
Alpha						
acetyldigoxin	T46.0X1	T46.0X2	T46.0X3	T46.0X4	T46.0X5	T46.0X6
adrenergic blocking drug	T44.6X1	T44.6X2	T44.6X3	T44.6X4	T44.6X5	T44.6X6
amylase	T45.3X1	T45.3X2	T45.3X3	T45.3X4	T45.3X5	T45.3X6
tocoferol (acetate)	T45.2X1	T45.2X2	T45.2X3	T45.2X4	T45.2X5	T45.2X6
tocopherol	T45.2X1	T45.2X2	T45.2X3	T45.2X4	T45.2X5	T45.2X6
Alphadolone	T41.1X1	T41.1X2	T41.1X3	T41.1X4	T41.1X5	T41.1X6
Alphaprodine	T40.4X1	T40.4X2	T40.4X3	T40.4X4	T40.4X5	T40.4X6
Alphaxalone	T41.1X1	T41.1X2	T41.1X3	T41.1X4	T41.1X5	T41.1X6
Alprazolam	T42.4X1	T42.4X2	T42.4X3	T42.4X4	T42.4X5	T42.4X6
Alprenolol	T44.7X1	T44.7X2	T44.7X3	T44.7X4	T44.7X5	T44.7X6
Alprostadil	T46.7X1	T46.7X2	T46.7X3	T46.7X4	T46.7X5	T46.7X6
Alsactide	T38.811	T38.812	T38.813	T38.814	T38.815	T38.816
Alseroxylon	T46.5X1	T46.5X2	T46.5X3	T46.5X4	T46.5X5	T46.5X6
Alteplase	T45.611	T45.612	T45.613	T45.614	T45.615	T45.616
Altizide	T50.2X1	T50.2X2	T50.2X3	T50.2X4	T50.2X5	T50.2X6
Altretamine	T45.1X1	T45.1X2	T45.1X3	T45.1X4	T45.1X5	T45.1X6
Alum (medicinal)	T49.4X1	T49.4X2	T49.4X3	T49.4X4	T49.4X5	T49.4X6
nonmedicinal (ammonium) (potassium)	T56.891	T56.892	T56.893	T56.894	—	—
Aluminium, aluminum						
acetate	T49.2X1	T49.2X2	T49.2X3	T49.2X4	T49.2X5	T49.2X6
solution	T49.0X1	T49.0X2	T49.0X3	T49.0X4	T49.0X5	T49.0X6
aspirin	T39.011	T39.012	T39.013	T39.014	T39.015	T39.016
bis (acetylsalicylate)	T39.011	T39.012	T39.013	T39.014	T39.015	T39.016

Substance	Poisoning, Accidental (Unintentional)	Poisoning, Intentional Self-Harm	Poisoning, Assault	Poisoning, Undetermined	Adverse Effect	Underdosing
Aluminium, aluminum (Continued)						
carbonate (gel, basic)	T47.1X1	T47.1X2	T47.1X3	T47.1X4	T47.1X5	T47.1X6
chlorhydroxide-complex	T47.1X1	T47.1X2	T47.1X3	T47.1X4	T47.1X5	T47.1X6
chloride	T49.2X1	T49.2X2	T49.2X3	T49.2X4	T49.2X5	T49.2X6
clofibrate	T46.6X1	T46.6X2	T46.6X3	T46.6X4	T46.6X5	T46.6X6
diacetate	T49.2X1	T49.2X2	T49.2X3	T49.2X4	T49.2X5	T49.2X6
glycinate	T47.1X1	T47.1X2	T47.1X3	T47.1X4	T47.1X5	T47.1X6
hydroxide (gel)	T47.1X1	T47.1X2	T47.1X3	T47.1X4	T47.1X5	T47.1X6
hydroxide-magnesium carb. gel	T47.1X1	T47.1X2	T47.1X3	T47.1X4	T47.1X5	T47.1X6
magnesium silicate	T47.1X1	T47.1X2	T47.1X3	T47.1X4	T47.1X5	T47.1X6
nicotinate	T46.7X1	T46.7X2	T46.7X3	T46.7X4	T46.7X5	T46.7X6
ointment (surgical) (topical)	T49.3X1	T49.3X2	T49.3X3	T49.3X4	T49.3X5	T49.3X6
phosphate	T47.1X1	T47.1X2	T47.1X3	T47.1X4	T47.1X5	T47.1X6
salicylate	T39.091	T39.092	T39.093	T39.094	T39.095	T39.096
silicate	T47.1X1	T47.1X2	T47.1X3	T47.1X4	T47.1X5	T47.1X6
sodium silicate	T47.1X1	T47.1X2	T47.1X3	T47.1X4	T47.1X5	T47.1X6
subacetate	T49.2X1	T49.2X2	T49.2X3	T49.2X4	T49.2X5	T49.2X6
sulfate	T49.0X1	T49.0X2	T49.0X3	T49.0X4	T49.0X5	T49.0X6
tannate	T47.6X1	T47.6X2	T47.6X3	T47.6X4	T47.6X5	T47.6X6
topical NEC	T49.3X1	T49.3X2	T49.3X3	T49.3X4	T49.3X5	T49.3X6
Alurate	T42.3X1	T42.3X2	T42.3X3	T42.3X4	T42.3X5	T42.3X6
Alverine	T44.3X1	T44.3X2	T44.3X3	T44.3X4	T44.3X5	T44.3X6
Alvodine	T40.2X1	T40.2X2	T40.2X3	T40.2X4	T40.2X5	T40.2X6
Amanita phalloides	T62.0X1	T62.0X2	T62.0X3	T62.0X4	—	—
Amanitine	T62.0X1	T62.0X2	T62.0X3	T62.0X4	—	—
Amantadine	T42.8X1	T42.8X2	T42.8X3	T42.8X4	T42.8X5	T42.8X6
Ambazone	T49.6X1	T49.6X2	T49.6X3	T49.6X4	T49.6X5	T49.6X6
Ambenonium (chloride)	T44.0X1	T44.0X2	T44.0X3	T44.0X4	T44.0X5	T44.0X6
Ambroxol	T48.4X1	T48.4X2	T48.4X3	T48.4X4	T48.4X5	T48.4X6
Ambuphylline	T48.6X1	T48.6X2	T48.6X3	T48.6X4	T48.6X5	T48.6X6
Ambutonium bromide	T44.3X1	T44.3X2	T44.3X3	T44.3X4	T44.3X5	T44.3X6
Amcinonide	T49.0X1	T49.0X2	T49.0X3	T49.0X4	T49.0X5	T49.0X6
Amdinocilline	T36.0X1	T36.0X2	T36.0X3	T36.0X4	T36.0X5	T36.0X6
Ametazole	T50.8X1	T50.8X2	T50.8X3	T50.8X4	T50.8X5	T50.8X6
Amethocaine	T41.3X1	T41.3X2	T41.3X3	T41.3X4	T41.3X5	T41.3X6
regional	T41.3X1	T41.3X2	T41.3X3	T41.3X4	T41.3X5	T41.3X6
spinal	T41.3X1	T41.3X2	T41.3X3	T41.3X4	T41.3X5	T41.3X6
Amethopterin	T45.1X1	T45.1X2	T45.1X3	T45.1X4	T45.1X5	T45.1X6
Amezinium metilsulfate	T44.991	T44.992	T44.993	T44.994	T44.995	T44.996
Amfebutamone	T43.291	T43.292	T43.293	T43.294	T43.295	T43.296
Amfepramone	T50.5X1	T50.5X2	T50.5X3	T50.5X4	T50.5X5	T50.5X6

◀ New ◀ Revised ~~deleted~~ Deleted

Substance	Poisoning, Accidental (Unintentional)	Poisoning, Intentional Self-Harm	Poisoning, Assault	Poisoning, Undetermined	Adverse Effect	Underdosing
Amfetamine	T43.621	T43.622	T43.623	T43.624	T43.625	T43.626
Amfetaminil	T43.621	T43.622	T43.623	T43.624	T43.625	T43.626
Amfomycin	T36.8X1	T36.8X2	T36.8X3	T36.8X4	T36.8X5	T36.8X6
Amidefrine mesilate	T48.5X1	T48.5X2	T48.5X3	T48.5X4	T48.5X5	T48.5X6
Amidone	T40.3X1	T40.3X2	T40.3X3	T40.3X4	T40.3X5	T40.3X6
Amidopyrine	T39.2X1	T39.2X2	T39.2X3	T39.2X4	T39.2X5	T39.2X6
Amidotrizoate	T50.8X1	T50.8X2	T50.8X3	T50.8X4	T50.8X5	T50.8X6
Amiflamine	T43.1X1	T43.1X2	T43.1X3	T43.1X4	T43.1X5	T43.1X6
Amikacin	T36.5X1	T36.5X2	T36.5X3	T36.5X4	T36.5X5	T36.5X6
Amikhelline	T46.3X1	T46.3X2	T46.3X3	T46.3X4	T46.3X5	T46.3X6
Amiloride	T50.2X1	T50.2X2	T50.2X3	T50.2X4	T50.2X5	T50.2X6
Aminacrine	T49.0X1	T49.0X2	T49.0X3	T49.0X4	T49.0X5	T49.0X6
Amineptine	T43.011	T43.012	T43.013	T43.014	T43.015	T43.016
Aminitrozole	T37.3X1	T37.3X2	T37.3X3	T37.3X4	T37.3X5	T37.3X6
Aminoacetic acid (derivatives)	T50.3X1	T50.3X2	T50.3X3	T50.3X4	T50.3X5	T50.3X6
Amino acids	T50.3X1	T50.3X2	T50.3X3	T50.3X4	T50.3X5	T50.3X6
Aminoacridine	T49.0X1	T49.0X2	T49.0X3	T49.0X4	T49.0X5	T49.0X6
Aminobenzoic acid (-p)	T49.3X1	T49.3X2	T49.3X3	T49.3X4	T49.3X5	T49.3X6
4-Aminobutyric acid	T43.8X1	T43.8X2	T43.8X3	T43.8X4	T43.8X5	T43.8X6
Aminocaproic acid	T45.621	T45.622	T45.623	T45.624	T45.625	T45.626
Aminofenazone	T39.2X1	T39.2X2	T39.2X3	T39.2X4	T39.2X5	T39.2X6
Aminoethylisothiourium	T45.8X1	T45.8X2	T45.8X3	T45.8X4	T45.8X5	T45.8X6
Aminoglutethimide	T45.1X1	T45.1X2	T45.1X3	T45.1X4	T45.1X5	T45.1X6
Aminohippuric acid	T50.8X1	T50.8X2	T50.8X3	T50.8X4	T50.8X5	T50.8X6
Aminomethylbenzoic acid	T45.691	T45.692	T45.693	T45.694	T45.695	T45.696
Aminometradine	T50.2X1	T50.2X2	T50.2X3	T50.2X4	T50.2X5	T50.2X6
Aminopentamide	T44.3X1	T44.3X2	T44.3X3	T44.3X4	T44.3X5	T44.3X6
Aminophenazone	T39.2X1	T39.2X2	T39.2X3	T39.2X4	T39.2X5	T39.2X6
Aminophenol	T54.0X1	T54.0X2	T54.0X3	T54.0X4	—	—
4-Aminophenol derivatives	T39.1X1	T39.1X2	T39.1X3	T39.1X4	T39.1X5	T39.1X6
Aminophenylpyridone	T43.591	T43.592	T43.593	T43.594	T43.595	T43.596
Aminophylline	T48.6X1	T48.6X2	T48.6X3	T48.6X4	T48.6X5	T48.6X6
Aminopterin sodium	T45.1X1	T45.1X2	T45.1X3	T45.1X4	T45.1X5	T45.1X6
Aminopyrine	T39.2X1	T39.2X2	T39.2X3	T39.2X4	T39.2X5	T39.2X6
8-Aminoquinoline drugs	T37.2X1	T37.2X2	T37.2X3	T37.2X4	T37.2X5	T37.2X6
Aminorex	T50.5X1	T50.5X2	T50.5X3	T50.5X4	T50.5X5	T50.5X6
Aminosalicylic acid	T37.1X1	T37.1X2	T37.1X3	T37.1X4	T37.1X5	T37.1X6
Aminosalylum	T37.1X1	T37.1X2	T37.1X3	T37.1X4	T37.1X5	T37.1X6
Amiodarone	T46.2X1	T46.2X2	T46.2X3	T46.2X4	T46.2X5	T46.2X6
Amiphenazole	T50.7X1	T50.7X2	T50.7X3	T50.7X4	T50.7X5	T50.7X6
Amiquinsin	T46.5X1	T46.5X2	T46.5X3	T46.5X4	T46.5X5	T46.5X6
Amisometradine	T50.2X1	T50.2X2	T50.2X3	T50.2X4	T50.2X5	T50.2X6

Substance	Poisoning, Accidental (Unintentional)	Poisoning, Intentional Self-Harm	Poisoning, Assault	Poisoning, Undetermined	Adverse Effect	Underdosing
Amisulpride	T43.591	T43.592	T43.593	T43.594	T43.595	T43.596
Amitriptyline	T43.021	T43.022	T43.023	T43.024	T43.025	T43.026
Amitriptylinoxide	T43.021	T43.022	T43.023	T43.024	T43.025	T43.026
Amlexanox	T48.6X1	T48.6X2	T48.6X3	T48.6X4	T48.6X5	T48.6X6
Ammonia (fumes) (gas) (vapor)	T59.891	T59.892	T59.893	T59.894	—	—
aromatic spirit	T48.991	T48.992	T48.993	T48.994	T48.995	T48.996
liquid (household)	T54.3X1	T54.3X2	T54.3X3	T54.3X4	—	—
Ammoniated mercury	T49.0X1	T49.0X2	T49.0X3	T49.0X4	T49.0X5	T49.0X6
Ammonium						
acid tartrate	T49.5X1	T49.5X2	T49.5X3	T49.5X4	T49.5X5	T49.5X6
bromide	T42.6X1	T42.6X2	T42.6X3	T42.6X4	T42.6X5	T42.6X6
carbonate	T54.3X1	T54.3X2	T54.3X3	T54.3X4	—	—
chloride	T50.991	T50.992	T50.993	T50.994	T50.995	T50.996
expectorant	T48.4X1	T48.4X2	T48.4X3	T48.4X4	T48.4X5	T48.4X6
compounds (household) NEC	T54.3X1	T54.3X2	T54.3X3	T54.3X4	—	—
fumes (any usage)	T59.891	T59.892	T59.893	T59.894	—	—
industrial	T54.3X1	T54.3X2	T54.3X3	T54.3X4	—	—
ichthyosulronate	T49.4X1	T49.4X2	T49.4X3	T49.4X4	T49.4X5	T49.4X6
mandelate	T37.91	T37.92	T37.93	T37.94	T37.95	T37.96
sulfamate	T60.3X1	T60.3X2	T60.3X3	T60.3X4	—	—
sulfonate resin	T47.8X1	T47.8X2	T47.8X3	T47.8X4	T47.8X5	T47.8X6
Amobarbital (sodium)	T42.3X1	T42.3X2	T42.3X3	T42.3X4	T42.3X5	T42.3X6
Amodiaquine	T37.2X1	T37.2X2	T37.2X3	T37.2X4	T37.2X5	T37.2X6
Amopyroquin(e)	T37.2X1	T37.2X2	T37.2X3	T37.2X4	T37.2X5	T37.2X6
Amoxapine	T43.011	T43.012	T43.013	T43.014	T43.015	T43.016
Amoxicillin	T36.0X1	T36.0X2	T36.0X3	T36.0X4	T36.0X5	T36.0X6
Amperozide	T43.591	T43.592	T43.593	T43.594	T43.595	T43.596
Amphenidone	T43.591	T43.592	T43.593	T43.594	T43.595	T43.596
Amphetamine NEC	T43.621	T43.622	T43.623	T43.624	T43.625	T43.626
Amphomycin	T36.8X1	T36.8X2	T36.8X3	T36.8X4	T36.8X5	T36.8X6
Amphotalide	T37.4X1	T37.4X2	T37.4X3	T37.4X4	T37.4X5	T37.4X6
Amphotericin B	T36.7X1	T36.7X2	T36.7X3	T36.7X4	T36.7X5	T36.7X6
topical	T49.0X1	T49.0X2	T49.0X3	T49.0X4	T49.0X5	T49.0X6
Ampicillin	T36.0X1	T36.0X2	T36.0X3	T36.0X4	T36.0X5	T36.0X6
Amprotropine	T44.3X1	T44.3X2	T44.3X3	T44.3X4	T44.3X5	T44.3X6
Amsacrine	T45.1X1	T45.1X2	T45.1X3	T45.1X4	T45.1X5	T45.1X6
Amygdaline	T62.2X1	T62.2X2	T62.2X3	T62.2X4		
Amyl						
acetate	T52.8X1	T52.8X2	T52.8X3	T52.8X4	—	—
vapor	T59.891	T59.892	T59.893	T59.894	—	—
alcohol	T51.3X1	T51.3X2	T51.3X3	T51.3X4	—	—
chloride	T53.6X1	T53.6X2	T53.6X3	T53.6X4	—	—

◀ New   ◀ Revised   ~~deleted~~ Deleted

Substance	External Cause (T-Code) Poisoning, Accidental (Unintentional)	Poisoning, Intentional Self-Harm	Poisoning, Assault	Poisoning, Undetermined	Adverse Effect	Underdosing
Amyl *(Continued)*						
formate	T52.8X1	T52.8X2	T52.8X3	T52.8X4	—	—
nitrite	T46.3X1	T46.3X2	T46.3X3	T46.3X4	T46.3X5	T46.3X6
propionate	T65.891	T65.892	T65.893	T65.894	—	—
Amylase	T47.5X1	T47.5X2	T47.5X3	T47.5X4	T47.5X5	T47.5X6
Amyleine, regional	T41.3X1	T41.3X2	T41.3X3	T41.3X4	T41.3X5	T41.3X6
Amylene						
dichloride	T53.6X1	T53.6X2	T53.6X3	T53.6X4	—	—
hydrate	T51.3X1	T51.3X2	T51.3X3	T51.3X4	—	—
Amylmetacresol	T49.6X1	T49.6X2	T49.6X3	T49.6X4	T49.6X5	T49.6X6
Amylobarbitone	T42.3X1	T42.3X2	T42.3X3	T42.3X4	T42.3X5	T42.3X6
Amylocaine, regional	T41.3X1	T41.3X2	T41.3X3	T41.3X4	T41.3X5	T41.3X6
infiltration (subcutaneous)	T41.3X1	T41.3X2	T41.3X3	T41.3X4	T41.3X5	T41.3X6
nerve block (peripheral) (plexus)	T41.3X1	T41.3X2	T41.3X3	T41.3X4	T41.3X5	T41.3X6
spinal	T41.3X1	T41.3X2	T41.3X3	T41.3X4	T41.3X5	T41.3X6
topical (surface)	T41.3X1	T41.3X2	T41.3X3	T41.3X4	T41.3X5	T41.3X6
Amylopectin	T47.6X1	T47.6X2	T47.6X3	T47.6X4	T47.6X5	T47.6X6
Amytal (sodium)	T42.3X1	T42.3X2	T42.3X3	T42.3X4	T42.3X5	T42.3X6
Anabolic steroid	T38.7X1	T38.7X2	T38.7X3	T38.7X4	T38.7X5	T38.7X6
Analeptic NEC	T50.7X1	T50.7X2	T50.7X3	T50.7X4	T50.7X5	T50.7X6
Analgesic	T39.91	T39.92	T39.93	T39.94	T39.95	T39.96
anti-inflammatory NEC	T39.91	T39.92	T39.93	T39.94	T39.95	T39.96
propionic acid derivative	T39.311	T39.312	T39.313	T39.314	T39.315	T39.316
antirheumatic NEC	T39.4X1	T39.4X2	T39.4X3	T39.4X4	T39.4X5	T39.4X6
aromatic NEC	T39.1X1	T39.1X2	T39.1X3	T39.1X4	T39.1X5	T39.1X6
narcotic NEC	T40.601	T40.602	T40.603	T40.604	T40.605	T40.606
combination	T40.601	T40.602	T40.603	T40.604	T40.605	T40.606
obstetric	T40.601	T40.602	T40.603	T40.604	T40.605	T40.606
non-narcotic NEC	T39.91	T39.92	T39.93	T39.94	T39.95	T39.96
combination	T39.91	T39.92	T39.93	T39.94	T39.95	T39.96
pyrazole	T39.2X1	T39.2X2	T39.2X3	T39.2X4	T39.2X5	T39.2X6
specified NEC	T39.8X1	T39.8X2	T39.8X3	T39.8X4	T39.8X5	T39.8X6
Analgin	T39.2X1	T39.2X2	T39.2X3	T39.2X4	T39.2X5	T39.2X6
Anamirta cocculus	T62.1X1	T62.1X2	T62.1X3	T62.1X4	—	—
Ancillin	T36.0X1	T36.0X2	T36.0X3	T36.0X4	T36.0X5	T36.0X6
Ancrod	T45.691	T45.692	T45.693	T45.694	T45.695	T45.696
Androgen	T38.7X1	T38.7X2	T38.7X3	T38.7X4	T38.7X5	T38.7X6
Androgen-estrogen mixture	T38.7X1	T38.7X2	T38.7X3	T38.7X4	T38.7X5	T38.7X6
Androstalone	T38.7X1	T38.7X2	T38.7X3	T38.7X4	T38.7X5	T38.7X6
Androstanolone	T38.7X1	T38.7X2	T38.7X3	T38.7X4	T38.7X5	T38.7X6
Androsterone	T38.7X1	T38.7X2	T38.7X3	T38.7X4	T38.7X5	T38.7X6

Substance	External Cause (T-Code) Poisoning, Accidental (Unintentional)	Poisoning, Intentional Self-Harm	Poisoning, Assault	Poisoning, Undetermined	Adverse Effect	Underdosing
Anemone pulsatilla	T62.2X1	T62.2X2	T62.2X3	T62.2X4	—	—
Anesthesia						
caudal	T41.3X1	T41.3X2	T41.3X3	T41.3X4	T41.3X5	T41.3X6
endotracheal	T41.0X1	T41.0X2	T41.0X3	T41.0X4	T41.0X5	T41.0X6
epidural	T41.3X1	T41.3X2	T41.3X3	T41.3X4	T41.3X5	T41.3X6
inhalation	T41.0X1	T41.0X2	T41.0X3	T41.0X4	T41.0X5	T41.0X6
local	T41.3X1	T41.3X2	T41.3X3	T41.3X4	T41.3X5	T41.3X6
mucosal	T41.3X1	T41.3X2	T41.3X3	T41.3X4	T41.3X5	T41.3X6
muscle relaxation	T48.1X1	T48.1X2	T48.1X3	T48.1X4	T48.1X5	T48.1X6
nerve blocking	T41.3X1	T41.3X2	T41.3X3	T41.3X4	T41.3X5	T41.3X6
plexus blocking	T41.3X1	T41.3X2	T41.3X3	T41.3X4	T41.3X5	T41.3X6
potentiated	T41.201	T41.202	T41.203	T41.204	T41.205	T41.206
rectal	T41.201	T41.202	T41.203	T41.204	T41.205	T41.206
general	T41.201	T41.202	T41.203	T41.204	T41.205	T41.206
local	T41.3X1	T41.3X2	T41.3X3	T41.3X4	T41.3X5	T41.3X6
regional	T41.3X1	T41.3X2	T41.3X3	T41.3X4	T41.3X5	T41.3X6
surface	T41.3X1	T41.3X2	T41.3X3	T41.3X4	T41.3X5	T41.3X6
Anesthetic NEC — *see also Anesthesia*	T41.41	T41.42	T41.43	T41.44	T41.45	T41.46
with muscle relaxant	T41.201	T41.202	T41.203	T41.204	T41.205	T41.206
general	T41.201	T41.202	T41.203	T41.204	T41.205	T41.206
local	T41.3X1	T41.3X2	T41.3X3	T41.3X4	T41.3X5	T41.3X6
gaseous NEC	T41.0X1	T41.0X2	T41.0X3	T41.0X4	T41.0X5	T41.0X6
general NEC	T41.201	T41.202	T41.203	T41.204	T41.205	T41.206
halogenated hydrocarbon derivatives NEC	T41.0X1	T41.0X2	T41.0X3	T41.0X4	T41.0X5	T41.0X6
infiltration NEC	T41.3X1	T41.3X2	T41.3X3	T41.3X4	T41.3X5	T41.3X6
intravenous NEC	T41.1X1	T41.1X2	T41.1X3	T41.1X4	T41.1X5	T41.1X6
local NEC	T41.3X1	T41.3X2	T41.3X3	T41.3X4	T41.3X5	T41.3X6
rectal	T41.201	T41.202	T41.203	T41.204	T41.205	T41.206
general	T41.201	T41.202	T41.203	T41.204	T41.205	T41.206
local	T41.3X1	T41.3X2	T41.3X3	T41.3X4	T41.3X5	T41.3X6
regional NEC	T41.3X1	T41.3X2	T41.3X3	T41.3X4	T41.3X5	T41.3X6
spinal NEC	T41.3X1	T41.3X2	T41.3X3	T41.3X4	T41.3X5	T41.3X6
thiobarbiturate	T41.1X1	T41.1X2	T41.1X3	T41.1X4	T41.1X5	T41.1X6
topical	T41.3X1	T41.3X2	T41.3X3	T41.3X4	T41.3X5	T41.3X6
Aneurine	T45.2X1	T45.2X2	T45.2X3	T45.2X4	T45.2X5	T45.2X6
Angio-Conray	T50.8X1	T50.8X2	T50.8X3	T50.8X4	T50.8X5	T50.8X6
Angiotensin	T44.5X1	T44.5X2	T44.5X3	T44.5X4	T44.5X5	T44.5X6
Angiotensinamide	T44.991	T44.992	T44.993	T44.994	T44.995	T44.996
Anhydrohydroxy-progesterone	T38.5X1	T38.5X2	T38.5X3	T38.5X4	T38.5X5	T38.5X6
Anhydron	T50.2X1	T50.2X2	T50.2X3	T50.2X4	T50.2X5	T50.2X6
Anileridine	T40.4X1	T40.4X2	T40.4X3	T40.4X4	T40.4X5	T40.4X6

◀ New   ◀ Revised   ~~deleted~~ Deleted

	External Cause (T-Code)					
Substance	Poisoning, Accidental (Unintentional)	Poisoning, Intentional Self-Harm	Poisoning, Assault	Poisoning, Undetermined	Adverse Effect	Underdosing
Aniline (dye) (liquid)	T65.3X1	T65.3X2	T65.3X3	T65.3X4	—	—
analgesic	T39.1X1	T39.1X2	T39.1X4	T39.1X4	T39.1X5	T39.1X6
derivatives, therapeutic NEC	T39.1X1	T39.1X2	T39.1X3	T39.1X4	T39.1X5	T39.1X6
vapor	T65.3X1	T65.3X2	T65.3X3	T65.3X4	—	—
Anise oil	T47.5X1	T47.5X2	T47.5X3	T47.5X4	T47.5X5	T47.5X6
Aniscoropine	T44.3X1	T44.3X2	T44.3X3	T44.3X4	T44.3X5	T44.3X6
Anisidine	T65.3X1	T65.3X2	T65.3X3	T65.3X4	—	—
Anisindione	T45.511	T45.512	T45.513	T45.514	T45.515	T45.516
Anisotropine methyl-bromide	T44.3X1	T44.3X2	T44.3X3	T44.3X4	T44.3X5	T44.3X6
Anistreplase	T45.611	T45.612	T45.613	T45.614	T45.615	T45.616
Anorexiant (central)	T50.5X1	T50.5X2	T50.5X3	T50.5X4	T50.5X5	T50.5X6
Anorexic agents	T50.5X1	T50.5X2	T50.5X3	T50.5X4	T50.5X5	T50.5X6
Ansamycin	T36.6X1	T36.6X2	T36.6X3	T36.6X4	T36.6X5	T36.6X6
Ant (bite) (sting)	T63.421	T63.422	T63.423	T63.424	—	—
Antabuse	T50.6X1	T50.6X2	T50.6X3	T50.6X4	T50.6X5	T50.6X6
Ant poison — *see Insecticide*						
Antacid NEC	T47.1X1	T47.1X2	T47.1X3	T47.1X4	T47.1X5	T47.1X6
Antagonist						
Aldosterone	T50.0X1	T50.0X2	T50.0X3	T50.0X4	T50.0X5	T50.0X6
alpha-adrenoreceptor	T44.6X1	T44.6X2	T44.6X3	T44.6X4	T44.6X5	T44.6X6
anticoagulant	T45.7X1	T45.7X2	T45.7X3	T45.7X4	T45.7X5	T45.7X6
beta-adrenoreceptor	T44.7X1	T44.7X2	T44.7X3	T44.7X4	T44.7X5	T44.7X6
extrapyramidal NEC	T44.3X1	T44.3X2	T44.3X3	T44.3X4	T44.3X5	T44.3X6
folic acid	T45.1X1	T45.1X2	T45.1X3	T45.1X4	T45.1X5	T45.1X6
H2 receptor	T47.0X1	T47.0X2	T47.0X3	T47.0X4	T47.0X5	T47.0X6
heavy metal	T45.8X1	T45.8X2	T45.8X3	T45.8X4	T45.8X5	T45.8X6
narcotic analgesic	T50.7X1	T50.7X2	T50.7X3	T50.7X4	T50.7X5	T50.7X6
opiate	T50.7X1	T50.7X2	T50.7X3	T50.7X4	T50.7X5	T50.7X6
pyrimidine	T45.1X1	T45.1X2	T45.1X3	T45.1X4	T45.1X5	T45.1X6
serotonin	T46.5X1	T46.5X2	T46.5X3	T46.5X4	T46.5X5	T46.5X6
Antazolin(e)	T45.0X1	T45.0X2	T45.0X3	T45.0X4	T45.0X5	T45.0X6
Anterior pituitary hormone NEC	T38.811	T38.812	T38.813	T38.814	T38.815	T38.816
Anthelmintic NEC	T37.4X1	T37.4X2	T37.4X3	T37.4X4	T37.4X5	T37.4X6
Anthiolimine	T37.4X1	T37.4X2	T37.4X3	T37.4X4	T37.4X5	T37.4X6
Anthralin	T49.4X1	T49.4X2	T49.4X3	T49.4X4	T49.4X5	T49.4X6
Anthramycin	T45.1X1	T45.1X2	T45.1X3	T45.1X4	T45.1X5	T45.1X6
Antiadrenergic NEC	T44.8X1	T44.8X2	T44.8X3	T44.8X4	T44.8X5	T44.8X6
Antiallergic NEC	T45.0X1	T45.0X2	T45.0X3	T45.0X4	T45.0X5	T45.0X6
Anti-anemic (drug) (preparation)	T45.8X1	T45.8X2	T45.8X3	T45.8X4	T45.8X5	T45.8X6
Antiandrogen NEC	T38.6X1	T38.6X2	T38.6X3	T38.6X4	T38.6X5	T38.6X6
Antianxiety drug NEC	T43.501	T43.502	T43.503	T43.504	T43.505	T43.506
Antiaris toxicaria	T65.891	T65.892	T65.893	T65.894	—	—

	External Cause (T-Code)					
Substance	Poisoning, Accidental (Unintentional)	Poisoning, Intentional Self-Harm	Poisoning, Assault	Poisoning, Undetermined	Adverse Effect	Underdosing
Antiarteriosclerotic drug	T46.6X1	T46.6X2	T46.6X3	T46.6X4	T46.6X5	T46.6X6
Antiasthmatic drug NEC	T48.6X1	T48.6X2	T48.6X3	T48.6X4	T48.6X5	T48.6X6
Antibiotic NEC	T36.91	T36.92	T36.93	T36.94	T36.95	T36.96
aminoglycoside	T36.5X1	T36.5X2	T36.5X3	T36.5X4	T36.5X5	T36.5X6
anticancer	T45.1X1	T45.1X2	T45.1X3	T45.1X4	T45.1X5	T45.1X6
antifungal	T36.7X1	T36.7X2	T36.7X3	T36.7X4	T36.7X5	T36.7X6
antimycobacterial	T36.5X1	T36.5X2	T36.5X3	T36.5X4	T36.5X5	T36.5X6
antineoplastic	T45.1X1	T45.1X2	T45.1X3	T45.1X4	T45.1X5	T45.1X6
cephalosporin (group)	T36.1X1	T36.1X2	T36.1X3	T36.1X4	T36.1X5	T36.1X6
chloramphenicol (group)	T36.2X1	T36.2X2	T36.2X3	T36.2X4	T36.2X5	T36.2X6
ENT	T49.6X1	T49.6X2	T49.6X3	T49.6X4	T49.6X5	T49.6X6
eye	T49.5X1	T49.5X2	T49.5X3	T49.5X4	T49.5X5	T49.5X6
fungicidal (local)	T49.0X1	T49.0X2	T49.0X3	T49.0X4	T49.0X5	T49.0X6
intestinal	T36.8X1	T36.8X2	T36.8X3	T36.8X4	T36.8X5	T36.8X6
b-lactam NEC	T36.1X1	T36.1X2	T36.1X3	T36.1X4	T36.1X5	T36.1X6
local	T49.0X1	T49.0X2	T49.0X3	T49.0X4	T49.0X5	T49.0X6
macrolides	T36.3X1	T36.3X2	T36.3X3	T36.3X4	T36.3X5	T36.3X6
polypeptide	T36.8X1	T36.8X2	T36.8X3	T36.8X4	T36.8X5	T36.8X6
specified NEC	T36.8X1	T36.8X2	T36.8X3	T36.8X4	T36.8X5	T36.8X6
tetracycline (group)	T36.4X1	T36.4X2	T36.4X3	T36.4X4	T36.4X5	T36.4X6
throat	T49.6X1	T49.6X2	T49.6X3	T49.6X4	T49.6X5	T49.6X6
Anticancer agents NEC	T45.1X1	T45.1X2	T45.1X3	T45.1X4	T45.1X5	T45.1X6
Anticholesterolemic drug NEC	T46.6X1	T46.6X2	T46.6X3	T46.6X4	T46.6X5	T46.6X6
Anticholinergic NEC	T44.3X1	T44.3X2	T44.3X3	T44.3X4	T44.3X5	T44.3X6
Anticholinesterase	T44.0X1	T44.0X2	T44.0X3	T44.0X4	T44.0X5	T44.0X6
organophosphorus	T44.0X1	T44.0X2	T44.0X3	T44.0X4	T44.0X5	T44.0X6
insecticide	T60.0X1	T60.0X2	T60.0X3	T60.0X4	—	—
nerve gas	T59.891	T59.892	T59.893	T59.894	—	—
reversible	T44.0X1	T44.0X2	T44.0X3	T44.0X4	T44.0X5	T44.0X6
ophthalmological	T49.5X1	T49.5X2	T49.5X3	T49.5X4	T49.5X5	T49.5X6
Anticoagulant NEC	T45.511	T45.512	T45.513	T45.514	T45.515	T45.516
Antagonist	T45.7X1	T45.7X2	T45.7X3	T45.7X4	T45.7X5	T45.7X6
Anti-common-cold drug NEC	T48.5X1	T48.5X2	T48.5X3	T48.5X4	T48.5X5	T48.5X6
Anticonvulsant	T42.71	T42.72	T42.73	T42.74	T42.75	T42.76
barbiturate	T42.3X1	T42.3X2	T42.3X3	T42.3X4	T42.3X5	T42.3X6
combination (with barbiturate)	T42.3X1	T42.3X2	T42.3X3	T42.3X4	T42.3X5	T42.3X6
hydantoin	T42.0X1	T42.0X2	T42.0X3	T42.0X4	T42.0X5	T42.0X6
hypnotic NEC	T42.6X1	T42.6X2	T42.6X3	T42.6X4	T42.6X5	T42.6X6
oxazolidinedione	T42.2X1	T42.2X2	T42.2X3	T42.2X4	T42.2X5	T42.2X6
pyrimidinedione	T42.6X1	T42.6X2	T42.6X3	T42.6X4	T42.6X5	T42.6X6
specified NEC	T42.6X1	T42.6X2	T42.6X3	T42.6X4	T42.6X5	T42.6X6
succinimide	T42.2X1	T42.2X2	T42.2X3	T42.2X4	T42.2X5	T42.2X6

◀ New   ◀ Revised   ~~deleted~~ Deleted

TABLE OF DRUGS AND CHEMICALS

Substance	External Cause (T-Code)					
	Poisoning, Accidental (Unintentional)	Poisoning, Intentional Self-Harm	Poisoning, Assault	Poisoning, Undetermined	Adverse Effect	Underdosing
Anti-D immunoglobulin (human)	T50.Z11	T50.Z12	T50.Z13	T50.Z14	T50.Z15	T50.Z16
Antidepressant NEC	T43.201	T43.202	T43.203	T43.204	T43.205	T43.206
monoamine oxidase inhibitor	T43.1X1	T43.1X2	T43.1X3	T43.1X4	T43.1X5	T43.1X6
selective serotonin norepinephrine reuptake inhibitor	T43.211	T43.212	T43.213	T43.214	T43.215	T43.216
selective serotonin reuptake inhibitor	T43.221	T43.222	T43.223	T43.224	T43.225	T43.226
specified NEC	T43.291	T43.292	T43.293	T43.294	T43.295	T43.296
tetracyclic	T43.021	T43.022	T43.023	T43.024	T43.025	T43.026
triazolopyridine	T43.221	T43.222	T43.223	T43.224	T43.225	T43.226
tricyclic	T43.011	T43.012	T43.013	T43.014	T43.015	T43.016
Antidiabetic NEC	T38.3X1	T38.3X2	T38.3X3	T38.3X4	T38.3X5	T38.3X6
biguanide	T38.3X1	T38.3X2	T38.3X3	T38.3X4	T38.3X5	T38.3X6
and sulfonyl combined	T38.3X1	T38.3X2	T38.3X3	T38.3X4	T38.3X5	T38.3X6
combined	T38.3X1	T38.3X2	T38.3X3	T38.3X4	T38.3X5	T38.3X6
sulfonylurea	T38.3X1	T38.3X2	T38.3X3	T38.3X4	T38.3X5	T38.3X6
Antidiarrheal drug NEC	T47.6X1	T47.6X2	T47.6X3	T47.6X4	T47.6X5	T47.6X6
absorbent	T47.6X1	T47.6X2	T47.6X3	T47.6X4	T47.6X5	T47.6X6
Antidiphtheria serum	T50.Z11	T50.Z12	T50.Z13	T50.Z14	T50.Z15	T50.Z16
Antidiuretic hormone	T38.891	T38.892	T38.893	T38.894	T38.895	T38.896
Antidote NEC	T50.6X1	T50.6X2	T50.6X3	T50.6X4	T50.6X5	T50.6X6
heavy metal	T45.8X1	T45.8X2	T45.8X3	T45.8X4	T45.8X5	T45.8X6
Antidysrhythmic NEC	T46.2X1	T46.2X2	T46.2X3	T46.2X4	T46.2X5	T46.2X6
Antiemetic drug	T45.0X1	T45.0X2	T45.0X3	T45.0X4	T45.0X5	T45.0X6
Antiepilepsy agent	T42.71	T42.72	T42.73	T42.74	T42.75	T42.76
combination	T42.5X1	T42.5X2	T42.5X3	T42.5X4	T42.5X5	T42.5X6
mixed	T42.5X1	T42.5X2	T42.5X3	T42.5X4	T42.5X5	T42.5X6
specified, NEC	T42.6X1	T42.6X2	T42.6X3	T42.6X4	T42.6X5	T42.6X6
Antiestrogen NEC	T38.6X1	T38.6X2	T38.6X3	T38.6X4	T38.6X5	T38.6X6
Antifertility pill	T38.4X1	T38.4X2	T38.4X3	T38.4X4	T38.4X5	T38.4X6
Antifibrinolytic drug	T45.621	T45.622	T45.623	T45.624	T45.625	T45.626
Antifilarial drug	T37.4X1	T37.4X2	T37.4X3	T37.4X4	T37.4X5	T37.4X6
Antiflatulent	T47.5X1	T47.5X2	T47.5X3	T47.5X4	T47.5X5	T47.5X6
Antifreeze	T65.91	T65.92	T65.93	T65.94	—	—
alcohol	T51.1X1	T51.1X2	T51.1X3	T51.1X4	—	—
ethylene glycol	T51.8X1	T51.8X2	T51.8X3	T51.8X4	—	—
Antifungal						
antibiotic (systemic)	T36.7X1	T36.7X2	T36.7X3	T36.7X4	T36.7X5	T36.7X6
anti-infective NEC	T37.91	T37.92	T37.93	T37.94	T37.95	T37.96
disinfectant, local	T49.0X1	T49.0X2	T49.0X3	T49.0X4	T49.0X5	T49.0X6
nonmedicinal (spray)	T60.3X1	T60.3X2	T60.3X3	T60.3X4	—	—
topical	T49.0X1	T49.0X2	T49.0X3	T49.0X4	T49.0X5	T49.0X6

Substance	External Cause (T-Code)					
	Poisoning, Accidental (Unintentional)	Poisoning, Intentional Self-Harm	Poisoning, Assault	Poisoning, Undetermined	Adverse Effect	Underdosing
Anti-gastric-secretion drug NEC	T47.1X1	T47.1X2	T47.1X3	T47.1X4	T47.1X5	T47.1X6
Antigonadotrophin NEC	T38.6X1	T38.6X2	T38.6X3	T38.6X4	T38.6X5	T38.6X6
Antihallucinogen	T43.501	T43.502	T43.503	T43.504	T43.505	T43.506
Antihelmintics	T37.4X1	T37.4X2	T37.4X3	T37.4X4	T37.4X5	T37.4X6
Antihemophilic						
factor	T45.8X1	T45.8X2	T45.8X3	T45.8X4	T45.8X5	T45.8X6
fraction	T45.8X1	T45.8X2	T45.8X3	T45.8X4	T45.8X5	T45.8X6
globulin concentrate	T45.7X1	T45.7X2	T45.7X3	T45.7X4	T45.7X5	T45.7X6
human plasma	T45.8X1	T45.8X2	T45.8X3	T45.8X4	T45.8X5	T45.8X6
plasma, dried	T45.7X1	T45.7X2	T45.7X3	T45.7X4	T45.7X5	T45.7X6
Antihemorrhoidal preparation	T49.2X1	T49.2X2	T49.2X3	T49.2X4	T49.2X5	T49.2X6
Antiheparin drug	T45.7X1	T45.7X2	T45.7X3	T45.7X4	T45.7X5	T45.7X6
Antihistamine	T45.0X1	T45.0X2	T45.0X3	T45.0X4	T45.0X5	T45.0X6
Antihookworm drug	T37.4X1	T37.4X2	T37.4X3	T37.4X4	T37.4X5	T37.4X6
Anti-human lymphocytic globulin	T50.Z11	T50.Z12	T50.Z13	T50.Z14	T50.Z15	T50.Z16
Antihyperlipidemic drug	T46.6X1	T46.6X2	T46.6X3	T46.6X4	T46.6X5	T46.6X6
Antihypertensive drug NEC	T46.5X1	T46.5X2	T46.5X3	T46.5X4	T46.5X5	T46.5X6
Anti-infective NEC	T37.91	T37.92	T37.93	T37.94	T37.95	T37.96
anthelmintic	T37.4X1	T37.4X2	T37.4X3	T37.4X4	T37.4X5	T37.4X6
antibiotics	T36.91	T36.92	T36.93	T36.94	T36.95	T36.96
specified NEC	T36.8X1	T36.8X2	T36.8X3	T36.8X4	T36.8X5	T36.8X6
antimalarial	T37.2X1	T37.2X2	T37.2X3	T37.2X4	T37.2X5	T37.2X6
antimycobacterial NEC	T37.1X1	T37.1X2	T37.1X3	T37.1X4	T37.1X5	T37.1X6
antibiotics	T36.5X1	T36.5X2	T36.5X3	T36.5X4	T36.5X5	T36.5X6
antiprotozoal NEC	T37.3X1	T37.3X2	T37.3X3	T37.3X4	T37.3X5	T37.3X6
blood	T37.2X1	T37.2X2	T37.2X3	T37.2X4	T37.2X5	T37.2X6
antiviral	T37.5X1	T37.5X2	T37.5X3	T37.5X4	T37.5X5	T37.5X6
arsenical	T37.8X1	T37.8X2	T37.8X3	T37.8X4	T37.8X5	T37.8X6
bismuth, local	T49.0X1	T49.0X2	T49.0X3	T49.0X4	T49.0X5	T49.0X6
ENT	T49.6X1	T49.6X2	T49.6X3	T49.6X4	T49.6X5	T49.6X6
eye NEC	T49.5X1	T49.5X2	T49.5X3	T49.5X4	T49.5X5	T49.5X6
heavy metals NEC	T37.8X1	T37.8X2	T37.8X3	T37.8X4	T37.8X5	T37.8X6
local NEC	T49.0X1	T49.0X2	T49.0X3	T49.0X4	T49.0X5	T49.0X6
specified NEC	T49.0X1	T49.0X2	T49.0X3	T49.0X4	T49.0X5	T49.0X6
mixed	T37.91	T37.92	T37.93	T37.94	T37.95	T37.96
ophthalmic preparation	T49.5X1	T49.5X2	T49.5X3	T49.5X4	T49.5X5	T49.5X6
topical NEC	T49.0X1	T49.0X2	T49.0X3	T49.0X4	T49.0X5	T49.0X6
Anti-inflammatory drug NEC	T49.0X1	T49.0X2	T49.0X3	T49.0X4	T49.0X5	T49.0X6
local	T49.0X1	T49.0X2	T49.0X3	T49.0X4	T49.0X5	T49.0X6
nonsteroidal NEC	T39.391	T39.392	T39.393	T39.394	T39.395	T39.396
propionic acid derivative	T39.311	T39.312	T39.313	T39.314	T39.315	T39.316
specified NEC	T39.391	T39.392	T39.393	T39.394	T39.395	T39.396

◀ New   ◀ Revised   ~~deleted~~ Deleted

Substance	Poisoning, Accidental (Unintentional)	Poisoning, Intentional Self-Harm	Poisoning, Assault	Poisoning, Undetermined	Adverse Effect	Underdosing
Antikaluretic	T50.3X1	T50.3X2	T50.3X3	T50.3X4	T50.3X5	T50.3X6
Antiknock (tetraethyl lead)	T56.0X1	T56.0X2	T56.0X3	T56.0X4	—	—
Antilipemic drug NEC	T46.6X1	T46.6X2	T46.6X3	T46.6X4	T46.6X5	T46.6X6
Antimalarial	T37.2X1	T37.2X2	T37.2X3	T37.2X4	T37.2X5	T37.2X6
prophylactic NEC	T37.2X1	T37.2X2	T37.2X3	T37.2X4	T37.2X5	T37.2X6
pyrimidine derivative	T37.2X1	T37.2X2	T37.2X3	T37.2X4	T37.2X5	T37.2X6
Antimetabolite	T45.1X1	T45.1X2	T45.1X3	T45.1X4	T45.1X5	T45.1X6
Antimitotic agent	T45.1X1	T45.1X2	T45.1X3	T45.1X4	T45.1X5	T45.1X6
Antimony (compounds) (vapor) NEC	T56.891	T56.892	T56.893	T56.894	—	—
anti-infectives	T37.8X1	T37.8X2	T37.8X3	T37.8X4	T37.8X5	T37.8X6
dimercaptosuccinate	T37.3X1	T37.3X2	T37.3X3	T37.3X4	T37.3X5	T37.3X6
hydride	T56.891	T56.892	T56.893	T56.894	—	—
pesticide (vapor)	T60.8X1	T60.8X2	T60.8X3	T60.8X4	—	—
potassium (sodium) tartrate	T37.8X1	T37.8X2	T37.8X3	T37.8X4	T37.8X5	T37.8X6
sodium dimercaptosuccinate	T37.3X1	T37.3X2	T37.3X3	T37.3X4	T37.3X5	T37.3X6
tartrated	T37.8X1	T37.8X2	T37.8X3	T37.8X4	T37.8X5	T37.8X6
Antimuscarinic NEC	T44.3X1	T44.3X2	T44.3X3	T44.3X4	T44.3X5	T44.3X6
Antimycobacterial drug NEC	T37.1X1	T37.1X2	T37.1X3	T37.1X4	T37.1X5	T37.1X6
antibiotics	T36.5X1	T36.5X2	T36.5X3	T36.5X4	T36.5X5	T36.5X6
combination	T37.1X1	T37.1X2	T37.1X3	T37.1X4	T37.1X5	T37.1X6
Antinausea drug	T45.0X1	T45.0X2	T45.0X3	T45.0X4	T45.0X5	T45.0X6
Antinematode drug	T37.4X1	T37.4X2	T37.4X3	T37.4X4	T37.4X5	T37.4X6
Antineoplastic NEC	T45.1X1	T45.1X2	T45.1X3	T45.1X4	T45.1X5	T45.1X6
alkaloidal	T45.1X1	T45.1X2	T45.1X3	T45.1X4	T45.1X5	T45.1X6
antibiotics	T45.1X1	T45.1X2	T45.1X3	T45.1X4	T45.1X5	T45.1X6
combination	T45.1X1	T45.1X2	T45.1X3	T45.1X4	T45.1X5	T45.1X6
estrogen	T38.5X1	T38.5X2	T38.5X3	T38.5X4	T38.5X5	T38.5X6
steroid	T38.7X1	T38.7X2	T38.7X3	T38.7X4	T38.7X5	T38.7X6
Antiparasitic drug (systemic)	T37.91	T37.92	T37.93	T37.94	T37.95	T37.96
local	T49.0X1	T49.0X2	T49.0X3	T49.0X4	T49.0X5	T49.0X6
specified NEC	T37.8X1	T37.8X2	T37.8X3	T37.8X4	T37.8X5	T37.8X6
Antiparkinsonism drug NEC	T42.8X1	T42.8X2	T42.8X3	T42.8X4	T42.8X5	T42.8X6
Antiperspirant NEC	T49.2X1	T49.2X2	T49.2X3	T49.2X4	T49.2X5	T49.2X6
Antiphlogistic NEC	T39.4X1	T39.4X2	T39.4X3	T39.4X4	T39.4X5	T39.4X6
Antiplatyhelmintic drug	T37.4X1	T37.4X2	T37.4X3	T37.4X4	T37.4X5	T37.4X6
Antiprotozoal drug NEC	T37.3X1	T37.3X2	T37.3X3	T37.3X4	T37.3X5	T37.3X6
blood	T37.2X1	T37.2X2	T37.2X3	T37.2X4	T37.2X5	T37.2X6
local	T49.0X1	T49.0X2	T49.0X3	T49.0X4	T49.0X5	T49.0X6
Antipruritic drug NEC	T49.1X1	T49.1X2	T49.1X3	T49.1X4	T49.1X5	T49.1X6
Antipsychotic drug	T43.501	T43.502	T43.503	T43.504	T43.505	T43.506
specified NEC	T43.591	T43.592	T43.593	T43.594	T43.595	T43.596

Substance	Poisoning, Accidental (Unintentional)	Poisoning, Intentional Self-Harm	Poisoning, Assault	Poisoning, Undetermined	Adverse Effect	Underdosing
Antipyretic	T39.91	T39.92	T39.93	T39.94	T39.95	T39.96
specified NEC	T39.8X1	T39.8X2	T39.8X3	T39.8X4	T39.8X5	T39.8X6
Antipyrine	T39.2X1	T39.2X2	T39.2X3	T39.2X4	T39.2X5	T39.2X6
Antirabies hyperimmune serum	T50.Z11	T50.Z12	T50.Z13	T50.Z14	T50.Z15	T50.Z16
Antirheumatic NEC	T39.4X1	T39.4X2	T39.4X3	T39.4X4	T39.4X5	T39.4X6
Antirigidity drug NEC	T42.8X1	T42.8X2	T42.8X3	T42.8X4	T42.8X5	T42.8X6
Antischistosomal drug	T37.4X1	T37.4X2	T37.4X3	T37.4X4	T37.4X5	T37.4X6
Antiscorpion sera	T50.Z11	T50.Z12	T50.Z13	T50.Z14	T50.Z15	T50.Z16
Antiseborrheics	T49.4X1	T49.4X2	T49.4X3	T49.4X4	T49.4X5	T49.4X6
Antiseptics (external) (medicinal)	T49.0X1	T49.0X2	T49.0X3	T49.0X4	T49.0X5	T49.0X6
Antistine	T45.0X1	T45.0X2	T45.0X3	T45.0X4	T45.0X5	T45.0X6
Antitapeworm drug	T37.4X1	T37.4X2	T37.4X3	T37.4X4	T37.4X5	T37.4X6
Antitetanus immunoglobulin	T50.Z11	T50.Z12	T50.Z13	T50.Z14	T50.Z15	T50.Z16
Antithrombotic	T45.521	T45.522	T45.523	T45.524	T45.525	T45.526
Antithyroid drug NEC	T38.2X1	T38.2X2	T38.2X3	T38.2X4	T38.2X5	T38.2X6
Antitoxin	T50.Z11	T50.Z12	T50.Z13	T50.Z14	T50.Z15	T50.Z16
diphtheria	T50.Z11	T50.Z12	T50.Z13	T50.Z14	T50.Z15	T50.Z16
gas gangrene	T50.Z11	T50.Z12	T50.Z13	T50.Z14	T50.Z15	T50.Z16
tetanus	T50.Z11	T50.Z12	T50.Z13	T50.Z14	T50.Z15	T50.Z16
Antitoxin, any	T50.901	T50.902	T50.903	T50.904	T50.905	T50.906
Antitrichomonal drug	T37.3X1	T37.3X2	T37.3X3	T37.3X4	T37.3X5	T37.3X6
Antituberculars	T37.1X1	T37.1X2	T37.1X3	T37.1X4	T37.1X5	T37.1X6
antibiotics	T36.5X1	T36.5X2	T36.5X3	T36.5X4	T36.5X5	T36.5X6
Antitussive NEC	T48.3X1	T48.3X2	T48.3X3	T48.3X4	T48.3X5	T48.3X6
codeine mixture	T40.2X1	T40.2X2	T40.2X3	T40.2X4	T40.2X5	T40.2X6
opiate	T40.2X1	T40.2X2	T40.2X3	T40.2X4	T40.2X5	T40.2X6
Antivaricose drug	T46.8X1	T46.8X2	T46.8X3	T46.8X4	T46.8X5	T46.8X6
Antivenin, antivenom (sera)	T50.Z11	T50.Z12	T50.Z13	T50.Z14	T50.Z15	T50.Z16
crotaline	T50.Z11	T50.Z12	T50.Z13	T50.Z14	T50.Z15	T50.Z16
spider bite	T50.Z11	T50.Z12	T50.Z13	T50.Z14	T50.Z15	T50.Z16
Antivertigo drug	T45.0X1	T45.0X2	T45.0X3	T45.0X4	T45.0X5	T45.0X6
Antiviral drug NEC	T37.5X1	T37.5X2	T37.5X3	T37.5X4	T37.5X5	T37.5X6
eye	T49.5X1	T49.5X2	T49.5X3	T49.5X4	T49.5X5	T49.5X6
Antiwhipworm drug	T37.4X1	T37.4X2	T37.4X3	T37.4X4	T37.4X5	T37.4X6
Ant poisons — see Pesticides						
Antrol — see also by specific chemical substance	T60.91	T60.92	T60.93	T60.94	—	—
fungicide	T60.91	T60.92	T60.93	T60.94	—	—
ANTU (alpha naphthylthiourea)	T60.4X1	T60.4X2	T60.4X3	T60.4X4	—	—
Apalcillin	T36.0X1	T36.0X2	T36.0X3	T36.0X4	T36.0X5	T36.0X6
APC	T48.5X1	T48.5X2	T48.5X3	T48.5X4	T48.5X5	T48.5X6
Aplonidine	T44.4X1	T44.4X2	T44.4X3	T44.4X4	T44.4X5	T44.4X6
Apomorphine	T47.7X1	T47.7X2	T47.7X3	T47.7X4	T47.7X5	T47.7X6

TABLE OF DRUGS AND CHEMICALS

Substance	External Cause (T-Code)					
	Poisoning, Accidental (Unintentional)	Poisoning, Intentional Self-Harm	Poisoning, Assault	Poisoning, Undetermined	Adverse Effect	Underdosing
Appetite depressants, central	T50.5X1	T50.5X2	T50.5X3	T50.5X4	T50.5X5	T50.5X6
Apraclonidine (hydrochloride)	T44.4X1	T44.4X2	T44.4X3	T44.4X4	T44.4X5	T44.4X6
Apresoline	T46.5X1	T46.5X2	T46.5X3	T46.5X4	T46.5X5	T46.5X6
Aprindine	T46.2X1	T46.2X2	T46.2X3	T46.2X4	T46.2X5	T46.2X6
Aprobarbital	T42.3X1	T42.3X2	T42.3X3	T42.3X4	T42.3X5	T42.3X6
Apronalide	T42.6X1	T42.6X2	T42.6X3	T42.6X4	T42.6X5	T42.6X6
Aprotinin	T45.621	T45.622	T45.623	T45.624	T45.625	T45.626
Aptocaine	T41.3X1	T41.3X2	T41.3X3	T41.3X4	T41.3X5	T41.3X6
Aqua fortis	T54.2X1	T54.2X2	T54.2X3	T54.2X4	—	—
Ara-A	T37.5X1	T37.5X2	T37.5X3	T37.5X4	T37.5X5	T37.5X6
Ara-C	T45.1X1	T45.1X2	T45.1X3	T45.1X4	T45.1X5	T45.1X6
Arachis oil	T49.3X1	T49.3X2	T49.3X3	T49.3X4	T49.3X5	T49.3X6
cathartic	T47.4X1	T47.4X2	T47.4X3	T47.4X4	T47.4X5	T47.4X6
Aralen	T37.2X1	T37.2X2	T37.2X3	T37.2X4	T37.2X5	T37.2X6
Arecoline	T44.1X1	T44.1X2	T44.1X3	T44.1X4	T44.1X5	T44.1X6
Arginine	T50.991	T50.992	T50.993	T50.994	T50.995	T50.996
glutamate	T50.991	T50.992	T50.993	T50.994	T50.995	T50.996
Argyrol	T49.0X1	T49.0X2	T49.0X3	T49.0X4	T49.0X5	T49.0X6
ENT agent	T49.6X1	T49.6X2	T49.6X3	T49.6X4	T49.6X5	T49.6X6
ophthalmic preparation	T49.5X1	T49.5X2	T49.5X3	T49.5X4	T49.5X5	T49.5X6
Aristocort	T38.0X1	T38.0X2	T38.0X3	T38.0X4	T38.0X5	T38.0X6
ENT agent	T49.6X1	T49.6X2	T49.6X3	T49.6X4	T49.6X5	T49.6X6
ophthalmic preparation	T49.5X1	T49.5X2	T49.5X3	T49.5X4	T49.5X5	T49.5X6
topical NEC	T49.0X1	T49.0X2	T49.0X3	T49.0X4	T49.0X5	T49.0X6
Aromatics, corrosive	T54.1X1	T54.1X2	T54.1X3	T54.1X4	—	—
disinfectants	T54.1X1	T54.1X2	T54.1X3	T54.1X4	—	—
Arsenate of lead	T57.0X1	T57.0X2	T57.0X3	T57.0X4	—	—
herbicide	T57.0X1	T57.0X2	T57.0X3	T57.0X4	—	—
Arsenic, arsenicals (compounds) (dust) (vapor) NEC	T57.0X1	T57.0X2	T57.0X3	T57.0X4	—	—
anti-infectives	T37.8X1	T37.8X2	T37.8X3	T37.8X4	T37.8X5	T37.8X6
pesticide (dust) (fumes)	T57.0X1	T57.0X2	T57.0X3	T57.0X4	—	—
Arsine (gas)	T57.0X1	T57.0X2	T57.0X3	T57.0X4	—	—
Arsphenamine (silver)	T37.8X1	T37.8X2	T37.8X3	T37.8X4	T37.8X5	T37.8X6
Arsthinol	T37.3X1	T37.3X2	T37.3X3	T37.3X4	T37.3X5	T37.3X6
Artane	T44.3X1	T44.3X2	T44.3X3	T44.3X4	T44.3X5	T44.3X6
Arthropod (venomous) NEC	T63.481	T63.482	T63.483	T63.484	—	—
Articaine	T41.3X1	T41.3X2	T41.3X3	T41.3X4	T41.3X5	T41.3X6
Asbestos	T57.8X1	T57.8X2	T57.8X3	T57.8X4	—	—
Ascaridole	T37.4X1	T37.4X2	T37.4X3	T37.4X4	T37.4X5	T37.4X6
Ascorbic acid	T45.2X1	T45.2X2	T45.2X3	T45.2X4	T45.2X5	T45.2X6
Asiaticoside	T49.0X1	T49.0X2	T49.0X3	T49.0X4	T49.0X5	T49.0X6

Substance	External Cause (T-Code)					
	Poisoning, Accidental (Unintentional)	Poisoning, Intentional Self-Harm	Poisoning, Assault	Poisoning, Undetermined	Adverse Effect	Underdosing
Asparaginase	T45.1X1	T45.1X2	T45.1X3	T45.1X4	T45.1X5	T45.1X6
Aspidium (oleoresin)	T37.4X1	T37.4X2	T37.4X3	T37.4X4	T37.4X5	T37.4X6
Aspirin (aluminum) (soluble)	T39.011	T39.012	T39.013	T39.014	T39.015	T39.016
Aspoxicillin	T36.0X1	T36.0X2	T36.0X3	T36.0X4	T36.0X5	T36.0X6
Astemizole	T45.0X1	T45.0X2	T45.0X3	T45.0X4	T45.0X5	T45.0X6
Astringent (local)	T49.2X1	T49.2X2	T49.2X3	T49.2X4	T49.2X5	T49.2X6
specified NEC	T49.2X1	T49.2X2	T49.2X3	T49.2X4	T49.2X5	T49.2X6
Astromicin	T36.5X1	T36.5X2	T36.5X3	T36.5X4	T36.5X5	T36.5X6
Ataractic drug NEC	T43.501	T43.502	T43.503	T43.504	T43.505	T43.506
Atenolol	T44.7X1	T44.7X2	T44.7X3	T44.7X4	T44.7X5	T44.7X6
Atonia drug, intestinal	T47.4X1	T47.4X2	T47.4X3	T47.4X4	T47.4X5	T47.4X6
Atophan	T50.4X1	T50.4X2	T50.4X3	T50.4X4	T50.4X5	T50.4X6
Atracurium besilate	T48.1X1	T48.1X2	T48.1X3	T48.1X4	T48.1X5	T48.1X6
Atropine	T44.3X1	T44.3X2	T44.3X3	T44.3X4	T44.3X5	T44.3X6
derivative	T44.3X1	T44.3X2	T44.3X3	T44.3X4	T44.3X5	T44.3X6
methonitrate	T44.3X1	T44.3X2	T44.3X3	T44.3X4	T44.3X5	T44.3X6
Attapulgite	T47.6X1	T47.6X2	T47.6X3	T47.6X4	T47.6X5	T47.6X6
Attenuvax	T50.991	T50.992	T50.993	T50.994	T50.995	T50.996
Auramine	T65.891	T65.892	T65.893	T65.894	—	—
dye	T65.6X1	T65.6X2	T65.6X3	T65.6X4	—	—
fungicide	T60.3X1	T60.3X2	T60.3X3	T60.3X4	—	—
Auranofin	T39.4X1	T39.4X2	T39.4X3	T39.4X4	T39.4X5	T39.4X6
Aurantiin	T46.991	T46.992	T46.993	T46.994	T46.995	T46.996
Aureomycin	T36.4X1	T36.4X2	T36.4X3	T36.4X4	T36.4X5	T36.4X6
ophthalmic preparation	T49.5X1	T49.5X2	T49.5X3	T49.5X4	T49.5X5	T49.5X6
topical NEC	T49.0X1	T49.0X2	T49.0X3	T49.0X4	T49.0X5	T49.0X6
Aurothioglucose	T39.4X1	T39.4X2	T39.4X3	T39.4X4	T39.4X5	T39.4X6
Aurothioglycanide	T39.4X1	T39.4X2	T39.4X3	T39.4X4	T39.4X5	T39.4X6
Aurothiomalate sodium	T39.4X1	T39.4X2	T39.4X3	T39.4X4	T39.4X5	T39.4X6
Aurotioprol	T39.4X1	T39.4X2	T39.4X3	T39.4X4	T39.4X5	T39.4X6
Automobile fuel	T52.0X1	T52.0X2	T52.0X3	T52.0X4	—	—
Autonomic nervous system agent NEC	T44.901	T44.902	T44.903	T44.904	T44.905	T44.906
Avlosulfon	T37.1X1	T37.1X2	T37.1X3	T37.1X4	T37.1X5	T37.1X6
Avomine	T42.6X1	T42.6X2	T42.6X3	T42.6X4	T42.6X5	T42.6X6
Axerophthol	T45.2X1	T45.2X2	T45.2X3	T45.2X4	T45.2X5	T45.2X6
Azacitidine	T45.1X1	T45.1X2	T45.1X3	T45.1X4	T45.1X5	T45.1X6
Azacyclonol	T43.591	T43.592	T43.593	T43.594	T43.595	T43.596
Azadirachta	T60.2X1	T60.2X2	T60.2X3	T60.2X4	—	—
Azanidazole	T37.3X1	T37.3X2	T37.3X3	T37.3X4	T37.3X5	T37.3X6
Azapetine	T46.7X1	T46.7X2	T46.7X3	T46.7X4	T46.7X5	T46.7X6
Azapropazone	T39.2X1	T39.2X2	T39.2X3	T39.2X4	T39.2X5	T39.2X6

◀ New   ◀▮ Revised   ~~deleted~~ Deleted

Substance	External Cause (T-Code) Poisoning, Accidental (Unintentional)	Poisoning, Intentional Self-Harm	Poisoning, Assault	Poisoning, Undetermined	Adverse Effect	Underdosing
Azaribine	T45.1X1	T45.1X2	T45.1X3	T45.1X4	T45.1X5	T45.1X6
Azaserine	T45.1X1	T45.1X2	T45.1X3	T45.1X4	T45.1X5	T45.1X6
Azatadine	T45.0X1	T45.0X2	T45.0X3	T45.0X4	T45.0X5	T45.0X6
Azatepa	T45.1X1	T45.1X2	T45.1X3	T45.1X4	T45.1X5	T45.1X6
Azathioprine	T45.1X1	T45.1X2	T45.1X3	T45.1X4	T45.1X5	T45.1X6
Azelaic acid	T49.0X1	T49.0X2	T49.0X3	T49.0X4	T49.0X5	T49.0X6
Azelastine	T45.0X1	T45.0X2	T45.0X3	T45.0X4	T45.0X5	T45.0X6
Azidocillin	T36.0X1	T36.0X2	T36.0X3	T36.0X4	T36.0X5	T36.0X6
Azidothymidine	T37.5X1	T37.5X2	T37.5X3	T37.5X4	T37.5X5	T37.5X6
Azinphos (ethyl) (methyl)	T60.0X1	T60.0X2	T60.0X3	T60.0X4	—	—
Aziridine (chelating)	T54.1X1	T54.1X2	T54.1X3	T54.1X4	—	—
Azithromycin	T36.3X1	T36.3X2	T36.3X3	T36.3X4	T36.3X5	T36.3X6
Azlocillin	T36.01	T36.02	T36.03	T36.04	T36.05	T36.06
Azobenzene smoke	T65.3X1	T65.3X2	T65.3X3	T65.3X4	—	—
acaricide	T60.8X1	T60.8X2	T60.8X3	T60.8X4	—	—
Azosulfamide	T37.0X1	T37.0X2	T37.0X3	T37.0X4	T37.0X5	T37.0X6
AZT	T37.5X1	T37.5X2	T37.5X3	T37.5X4	T37.5X5	T37.5X6
Aztreonam	T36.1X1	T36.1X2	T36.1X3	T36.1X4	T36.1X5	T36.1X6
Azulfidine	T37.0X1	T37.0X2	T37.0X3	T37.0X4	T37.0X5	T37.0X6
Azuresin	T50.8X1	T50.8X2	T50.8X3	T50.8X4	T50.8X5	T50.8X6
B						
Bacampicillin	T36.0X1	T36.0X2	T36.0X3	T36.0X4	T36.0X5	T36.0X6
Bacillus						
lactobacillus	T47.8X1	T47.8X2	T47.8X3	T47.8X4	T47.8X5	T47.8X6
subtilis	T47.6X1	T47.6X2	T47.6X3	T47.6X4	T47.6X5	T47.6X6
Bacimycin	T49.0X1	T49.0X2	T49.0X3	T49.0X4	T49.0X5	T49.0X6
ophthalmic preparation	T49.5X1	T49.5X2	T49.5X3	T49.5X4	T49.5X5	T49.5X6
Bacitracin zinc	T49.0X1	T49.0X2	T49.0X3	T49.0X4	T49.0X5	T49.0X6
with neomycin	T49.0X1	T49.0X2	T49.0X3	T49.0X4	T49.0X5	T49.0X6
ENT agent	T49.6X1	T49.6X2	T49.6X3	T49.6X4	T49.6X5	T49.6X6
ophthalmic preparation	T49.5X1	T49.5X2	T49.5X3	T49.5X4	T49.5X5	T49.5X6
topical NEC	T49.0X1	T49.0X2	T49.0X3	T49.0X4	T49.0X5	T49.0X6
Baclofen	T42.8X1	T42.8X2	T42.8X3	T42.8X4	T42.8X5	T42.8X6
Baking soda	T50.991	T50.992	T50.993	T50.994	T50.995	T50.996
BAL	T45.8X1	T45.8X2	T45.8X3	T45.8X4	T45.8X5	T45.8X6
Bambuterol	T48.6X1	T48.6X2	T48.6X3	T48.6X4	T48.6X5	T48.6X6
Bamethan (sulfate)	T46.7X1	T46.7X2	T46.7X3	T46.7X4	T46.7X5	T46.7X6
Bamifylline	T48.6X1	T48.6X2	T48.6X3	T48.6X4	T48.6X5	T48.6X6
Bamipine	T45.0X1	T45.0X2		T45.0X4	T45.0X5	T45.0X6
Baneberry — see Actaea spicata						
Banewort — see Belladonna						

Substance	External Cause (T-Code) Poisoning, Accidental (Unintentional)	Poisoning, Intentional Self-Harm	Poisoning, Assault	Poisoning, Undetermined	Adverse Effect	Underdosing
Barbenyl	T42.3X1	T42.3X2	T42.3X3	T42.3X4	T42.3X5	T42.3X6
Barbexaclone	T42.6X1	T42.6X2	T42.6X3	T42.6X4	T42.6X5	T42.6X6
Barbital	T42.3X1	T42.3X2	T42.3X3	T42.3X4	T42.3X5	T42.3X6
sodium	T42.3X1	T42.3X2	T42.3X3	T42.3X4	T42.3X5	T42.3X6
Barbitone	T42.3X1	T42.3X2	T42.3X3	T42.3X4	T42.3X5	T42.3X6
Barbiturate NEC	T42.3X1	T42.3X2	T42.3X3	T42.3X4	T42.3X5	T42.3X6
with tranquilizer	T42.3X1	T42.3X2	T42.3X3	T42.3X4	T42.3X5	T42.3X6
anesthetic (intravenous)	T41.1X1	T41.1X2	T41.1X3	T41.1X4	T41.1X5	T41.1X6
Barium (carbonate) (chloride) (sulfite)	T57.8X1	T57.8X2	T57.8X3	T57.8X4	—	—
diagnostic agent	T50.8X1	T50.8X2	T50.8X3	T50.8X4	T50.8X5	T50.8X6
pesticide	T60.4X1	T60.4X2	T60.4X3	T60.4X4	—	—
rodenticide	T60.4X1	T60.4X2	T60.4X3	T60.4X4	—	—
sulfate (medicinal)	T50.8X1	T50.8X2	T50.8X3	T50.8X4	T50.8X5	T50.8X6
Barrier cream	T49.3X1	T49.3X2	T49.3X3	T49.3X4	T49.3X5	T49.3X6
Basic fuchsin	T49.0X1	T49.0X2	T49.0X3	T49.0X4	T49.0X5	T49.0X6
Battery acid or fluid	T54.2X1	T54.2X2	T54.2X3	T54.2X4	—	—
Bay rum	T51.8X1	T51.8X2	T51.8X3	T51.8X4	—	—
BCG (vaccine)	T50.A91	T50.A92	T50.A93	T50.A94	T50.A95	T50.A96
BCNU	T45.1X1	T45.1X2	T45.1X3	T45.1X4	T45.1X5	T45.1X6
Bearsfoot	T62.2X1	T62.2X2	T62.2X3	T62.2X4	—	—
Beclamide	T42.6X1	T42.6X2	T42.6X3	T42.6X4	T42.6X5	T42.6X6
Beclomethasone	T44.5X1	T44.5X2	T44.5X3	T44.5X4	T44.5X5	T44.5X6
Bee (sting) (venom)	T63.441	T63.442	T63.443	T63.444		
Befunolol	T49.5X1	T49.5X2	T49.5X3	T49.5X4	T49.5X5	T49.5X6
Bekanamycin	T36.5X1	T36.5X2	T36.5X3	T36.5X4	T36.5X5	T36.5X6
Belladonna — see also Nightshade						
alkaloids	T44.3X1	T44.3X2	T44.3X3	T44.3X4	T44.3X5	T44.3X6
extract	T44.3X1	T44.3X2	T44.3X3	T44.3X4	T44.3X5	T44.3X6
herb	T44.3X1	T44.3X2	T44.3X3	T44.3X4	T44.3X5	T44.3X6
Bemegride	T50.7X1	T50.7X2	T50.7X3	T50.7X4	T50.7X5	T50.7X6
Benactyzine	T44.3X1	T44.3X2	T44.3X3	T44.3X4	T44.3X5	T44.3X6
Benadryl	T45.0X1	T45.0X2	T45.0X3	T45.0X4	T45.0X5	T45.0X6
Benaprizine	T44.3X1	T44.3X2	T44.3X3	T44.3X4	T44.3X5	T44.3X6
Benazepril	T46.4X1	T46.4X2	T46.4X3	T46.4X4	T46.4X5	T46.4X6
Bencyclane	T46.7X1	T46.7X2	T46.7X3	T46.7X4	T46.7X5	T46.7X6
Bendazol	T46.3X1	T46.3X2	T46.3X3	T46.3X4	T46.3X5	T46.3X6
Bendrofluazide	T50.2X1	T50.2X2	T50.2X3	T50.2X4	T50.2X5	T50.2X6
Bendroflumethiazide	T50.2X1	T50.2X2	T50.2X3	T50.2X4	T50.2X5	T50.2X6
Benemid	T50.4X1	T50.4X2	T50.4X3	T50.4X4	T50.4X5	T50.4X6
Benethamine penicillin	T36.0X1	T36.0X2	T36.0X3	T36.0X4	T36.0X5	T36.0X6
Benisone	T49.0X1	T49.0X2	T49.0X3	T49.0X4	T49.0X5	T49.0X6

◀ New　◀‖‖ Revised　deleted Deleted

TABLE OF DRUGS AND CHEMICALS

Substance	External Cause (T-Code)					
	Poisoning, Accidental (Unintentional)	Poisoning, Intentional Self-Harm	Poisoning, Assault	Poisoning, Undetermined	Adverse Effect	Underdosing
Benexate	T47.1X1	T47.1X2	T47.1X3	T47.1X4	T47.1X5	T47.1X6
Benfluorex	T46.6X1	T46.6X2	T46.6X3	T46.6X4	T46.6X5	T46.6X6
Benfotiamine	T45.2X1	T45.2X2	T45.2X3	T45.2X4	T45.2X5	T45.2X6
Benomyl	T60.0X1	T60.0X2	T60.0X3	T60.0X4	—	—
Benoquin	T49.8X1	T49.8X2	T49.8X3	T49.8X4	T49.8X5	T49.8X6
Benoxinate	T41.3X1	T41.3X2	T41.3X3	T41.3X4	T41.3X5	T41.3X6
Benperidol	T43.4X1	T43.4X2	T43.4X3	T43.4X4	T43.4X5	T43.4X6
Benproperine	T48.3X1	T48.3X2	T48.3X3	T48.3X4	T48.3X5	T48.3X6
Benserazide	T42.8X1	T42.8X2	T42.8X3	T42.8X4	T42.8X5	T42.8X6
Bentazepam	T42.4X1	T42.4X2	T42.4X3	T42.4X4	T42.4X5	T42.4X6
Bentiromide	T50.8X1	T50.8X2	T50.8X3	T50.8X4	T50.8X5	T50.8X6
Bentonite	T49.3X1	T49.3X2	T49.3X3	T49.3X4	T49.3X5	T49.3X6
Benzalbutyramide	T46.6X1	T46.6X2	T46.6X3	T46.6X4	T46.6X5	T46.6X6
Benzalkonium (chloride)	T49.0X1	T49.0X2	T49.0X3	T49.0X4	T49.0X5	T49.0X6
ophthalmic preparation	T49.5X1	T49.5X2	T49.5X3	T49.5X4	T49.5X5	T49.5X6
Benzamine	T41.3X1	T41.3X2	T41.3X3	T41.3X4	T41.3X5	T41.3X6
lactate	T49.1X1	T49.1X2	T49.1X3	T49.1X4	T49.1X5	T49.1X6
Benzamidosalicylate (calcium)	T37.1X1	T37.1X2	T37.1X3	T37.1X4	T37.1X5	T37.1X6
Benzamphetamine	T50.5X1	T50.5X2	T50.5X3	T50.5X4	T50.5X5	T50.5X6
Benzapril hydrochloride	T46.5X1	T46.5X2	T46.5X3	T46.5X4	T46.5X5	T46.5X6
Benzathine benzylpenicillin	T36.0X1	T36.0X2	T36.0X3	T36.0X4	T36.0X5	T36.0X6
Benzathine penicillin	T36.0X1	T36.0X2	T36.0X3	T36.0X4	T36.0X5	T36.0X6
Benzatropine	T42.8X1	T42.8X2	T42.8X3	T42.8X4	T42.8X5	T42.8X6
Benzbromarone	T50.4X1	T50.4X2	T50.4X3	T50.4X4	T50.4X5	T50.4X6
Benzcarbimine	T45.1X1	T45.1X2	T45.1X3	T45.1X4	T45.1X5	T45.1X6
Benzedrex	T44.991	T44.992	T44.993	T44.994	T44.995	T44.996
Benzedrine (amphetamine)	T43.621	T43.622	T43.623	T43.624	T43.625	T43.626
Benzenamine	T65.3X1	T65.3X2	T65.3X3	T65.3X4	—	—
Benzene	T52.1X1	T52.1X2	T52.1X3	T52.1X4	—	—
homologues (acetyl) (dimethyl) (methyl) (solvent)	T52.2X1	T52.2X2	T52.2X3	T52.2X4	—	—
Benzethonium (chloride)	T49.0X1	T49.0X2	T49.0X3	T49.0X4	T49.0X5	T49.0X6
Benzfetamine	T50.5X1	T50.5X2	T50.5X3	T50.5X4	T50.5X5	T50.5X6
Benzhexol	T44.3X1	T44.3X2	T44.3X3	T44.3X4	T44.3X5	T44.3X6
Benzhydramine (chloride)	T45.0X1	T45.0X2	T45.0X3	T45.0X4	T45.0X5	T45.0X6
Benzidine	T65.891	T65.892	T65.893	T65.894	—	—
Benzilonium bromide	T44.3X1	T44.3X2	T44.3X3	T44.3X4	T44.3X5	T44.3X6
Benzimidazole	T60.3X1	T60.3X2	T60.3X3	T60.3X4	—	—
Benzin(e) — *see Ligroin*						
Benziodarone	T46.3X1	T46.3X2	T46.3X3	T46.3X4	T46.3X5	T46.3X6
Benznidazole	T37.3X1	T37.3X2	T37.3X3	T37.3X4	T37.3X5	T37.3X6
Benzocaine	T41.3X1	T41.3X2	T41.3X3	T41.3X4	T41.3X5	T41.3X6

Substance	External Cause (T-Code)					
	Poisoning, Accidental (Unintentional)	Poisoning, Intentional Self-Harm	Poisoning, Assault	Poisoning, Undetermined	Adverse Effect	Underdosing
Benzoctamine	T43.0X1	T43.0X2	T43.0X3	T43.0X4	T43.0X5	T43.0X6
Benzodiapin	T42.4X1	T42.4X2	T42.4X3	T42.4X4	T42.4X5	T42.4X6
Benzodiazepine NEC	T42.4X1	T42.4X2	T42.4X3	T42.4X4	T42.4X5	T42.4X6
Benzoic acid	T49.0X1	T49.0X2	T49.0X3	T49.0X4	T49.0X5	T49.0X6
with salicylic acid	T49.0X1	T49.0X2	T49.0X3	T49.0X4	T49.0X5	T49.0X6
Benzoin (tincture)	T48.5X1	T48.5X2	T48.5X3	T48.5X4	T48.5X5	T48.5X6
Benzol (benzene)	T52.1X1	T52.1X2	T52.1X3	T52.1X4	—	—
vapor	T52.0X1	T52.0X2	T52.0X3	T52.0X4	—	—
Benzomorphan	T40.2X1	T40.2X2	T40.2X3	T40.2X4	T40.2X5	T40.2X6
Benzonatate	T48.3X1	T48.3X2	T48.3X3	T48.3X4	T48.3X5	T48.3X6
Benzophenones	T49.3X1	T49.3X2	T49.3X3	T49.3X4	T49.3X5	T49.3X6
Benzopyrone	T46.991	T46.992	T46.993	T46.994	T46.995	T46.996
Benzothiadiazides	T50.2X1	T50.2X2	T50.2X3	T50.2X4	T50.2X5	T50.2X6
Benzoxonium chloride	T49.0X1	T49.0X2	T49.0X3	T49.0X4	T49.0X5	T49.0X6
Benzoyl peroxide	T49.0X1	T49.0X2	T49.0X3	T49.0X4	T49.0X5	T49.0X6
Benzoylpas calcium	T37.1X1	T37.1X2	T37.1X3	T37.1X4	T37.1X5	T37.1X6
Benzperidin	T43.591	T43.592	T43.593	T43.594	T43.595	T43.596
Benzperidol	T43.591	T43.592	T43.593	T43.594	T43.595	T43.596
Benzphetamine	T50.5X1	T50.5X2	T50.5X3	T50.5X4	T50.5X5	T50.5X6
Benzpyrinium bromide	T44.1X1	T44.1X2	T44.1X3	T44.1X4	T44.1X5	T44.1X6
Benzquinamide	T45.0X1	T45.0X2	T45.0X3	T45.0X4	T45.0X5	T45.0X6
Benzthiazide	T50.2X1	T50.2X2	T50.2X3	T50.2X4	T50.2X5	T50.2X6
Benztropine						
anticholinergic	T44.3X1	T44.3X2	T44.3X3	T44.3X4	T44.3X5	T44.3X6
antiparkinson	T42.8X1	T42.8X2	T42.8X3	T42.8X4	T42.8X5	T42.8X6
Benzydamine	T49.0X1	T49.0X2	T49.0X3	T49.0X4	T49.0X5	T49.0X6
Benzyl						
acetate	T52.8X1	T52.8X2	T52.8X3	T52.8X4	—	—
alcohol	T49.0X1	T49.0X2	T49.0X3	T49.0X4	T49.0X5	T49.0X6
benzoate	T49.0X1	T49.0X2	T49.0X3	T49.0X4	T49.0X5	T49.0X6
Benzoic acid	T49.0X1	T49.0X2	T49.0X3	T49.0X4	T49.0X5	T49.0X6
morphine	T40.2X1	T40.2X2	T40.2X3	T40.2X4	—	—
nicotinate	T46.6X1	T46.6X2	T46.6X3	T46.6X4	T46.6X5	T46.6X6
penicillin	T36.0X1	T36.0X2	T36.0X3	T36.0X4	T36.0X5	T36.0X6
Benzylhydrochlorthia-zide	T50.2X1	T50.2X2	T50.2X3	T50.2X4	T50.2X5	T50.2X6
Benzylpenicillin	T36.0X1	T36.0X2	T36.0X3	T36.0X4	T36.0X5	T36.0X6
Benzylthiouracil	T38.2X1	T38.2X2	T38.2X3	T38.2X4	T38.2X5	T38.2X6
Bephenium hydroxy-naphthoate	T37.4X1	T37.4X2	T37.4X3	T37.4X4	T37.4X5	T37.4X6
Bepridil	T46.1X1	T46.1X2	T46.1X3	T46.1X4	T46.1X5	T46.1X6
Bergamot oil	T65.891	T65.892	T65.893	T65.894	—	—
Bergapten	T50.991	T50.992	T50.993	T50.994	T50.995	T50.996
Berries, poisonous	T62.1X1	T62.1X2	T62.1X3	T62.1X4	—	—

◀ New   ◀ Revised   ~~deleted~~ Deleted

Substance	External Cause (T-Code) Poisoning, Accidental (Unintentional)	Poisoning, Intentional Self-Harm	Poisoning, Assault	Poisoning, Undetermined	Adverse Effect	Underdosing
Beryllium (compounds)	T56.7X1	T56.7X2	T56.7X3	T56.7X4	—	—
b-acetyldigoxin	T46.0X1	T46.0X2	T46.0X3	T46.0X4	T46.0X5	T46.0X6
beta adrenergic blocking agent, heart	T44.7X1	T44.7X2	T44.7X3	T44.7X4	T44.7X5	T44.7X6
b-benzalbutyramide	T46.6X1	T46.6X2	T46.6X3	T46.6X4	T46.6X5	T46.6X6
Betacarotene	T45.2X1	T45.2X2	T45.2X3	T45.2X4	T45.2X5	T45.2X6
b-eucaine	T49.1X1	T49.1X2	T49.1X3	T49.1X4	T49.1X5	T49.1X6
Beta-Chlor	T42.6X1	T42.6X2	T42.6X3	T42.6X4	T42.6X5	T42.6X6
b-galactosidase	T47.5X1	T47.5X2	T47.5X3	T47.5X4	T47.5X5	T47.5X6
Betahistine	T46.7X1	T46.7X2	T46.7X3	T46.7X4	T46.7X5	T46.7X6
Betaine	T47.5X1	T47.5X2	T47.5X3	T47.5X4	T47.5X5	T47.5X6
Betamethasone	T49.0X1	T49.0X2	T49.0X3	T49.0X4	T49.0X5	T49.0X6
topical	T49.0X1	T49.0X2	T49.0X3	T49.0X4	T49.0X5	T49.0X6
Betamicin	T36.8X1	T36.8X2	T36.8X3	T36.8X4	T36.8X5	T36.8X6
Betanidine	T46.5X1	T46.5X2	T46.5X3	T46.5X4	T46.5X5	T46.5X6
b-sitosterol(s)	T46.6X1	T46.6X2	T46.6X3	T46.6X4	T46.6X5	T46.6X6
Betaxolol	T44.7X1	T44.7X2	T44.7X3	T44.7X4	T44.7X5	T44.7X6
Betazole	T50.8X1	T50.8X2	T50.8X3	T50.8X4	T50.8X5	T50.8X6
Bethanechol	T44.1X1	T44.1X2	T44.1X3	T44.1X4	T44.1X5	T44.1X6
chloride	T44.1X1	T44.1X2	T44.1X3	T44.1X4	T44.1X5	T44.1X6
Bethanidine	T46.5X1	T46.5X2	T46.5X3	T46.5X4	T46.5X5	T46.5X6
Betoxycaine	T41.3X1	T41.3X2	T41.3X3	T41.3X4	T41.3X5	T41.3X6
Betula oil	T49.3X1	T49.3X2	T49.3X3	T49.3X4	T49.3X5	T49.3X6
Bevantolol	T44.7X1	T44.7X2	T44.7X3	T44.7X4	T44.7X5	T44.7X6
Bevonium metilsulfate	T44.3X1	T44.3X2	T44.3X3	T44.3X4	T44.3X5	T44.3X6
Bezafibrate	T46.6X1	T46.6X2	T46.6X3	T46.6X4	T46.6X5	T46.6X6
Bezitramide	T40.4X1	T40.4X2	T40.4X3	T40.4X4	T40.4X5	T40.4X6
BHA	T50.991	T50.992	T50.993	T50.994	T50.995	T50.996
Bhang	T40.7X1	T40.7X2	T40.7X3	T40.7X4	T40.7X5	T40.7X6
BHC (medicinal)	T49.0X1	T49.0X2	T49.0X3	T49.0X4	T49.0X5	T49.0X6
nonmedicinal (vapor)	T53.6X1	T53.6X2	T53.6X3	T53.6X4	—	—
Bialamicol	T37.3X1	T37.3X2	T37.3X3	T37.3X4	T37.3X5	T37.3X6
Bibenzonium bromide	T48.3X1	T48.3X2	T48.3X3	T48.3X4	T48.3X5	T48.3X6
Bibrocathol	T49.5X1	T49.5X2	T49.5X3	T49.5X4	T49.5X5	T49.5X6
Bichloride of mercury — see Mercury, chloride						
Bichromates (calcium) (potassium) (sodium) (crystals)	T57.8X1	T57.8X2	T57.8X3	T57.8X4	—	—
fumes	T56.2X1	T56.2X2	T56.2X3	T56.2X4	—	—
Biclotymol	T49.6X1	T49.6X2	T49.6X3	T49.6X4	T49.6X5	T49.6X6
Bicucculine	T50.7X1	T50.7X2	T50.7X3	T50.7X4	T50.7X5	T50.7X6
Bifemelane	T43.291	T43.292	T43.293	T43.294	T43.295	T43.296
Biguanide derivatives, oral	T38.3X1	T38.3X2	T38.3X3	T38.3X4	T38.3X5	T38.3X6

Substance	External Cause (T-Code) Poisoning, Accidental (Unintentional)	Poisoning, Intentional Self-Harm	Poisoning, Assault	Poisoning, Undetermined	Adverse Effect	Underdosing
Biligrafin	T50.8X1	T50.8X2	T50.8X3	T50.8X4	T50.8X5	T50.8X6
Bile salts	T47.5X1	T47.5X2	T47.5X3	T47.5X4	T47.5X5	T47.5X6
Bilopaque	T50.8X1	T50.8X2	T50.8X3	T50.8X4	T50.8X5	T50.8X6
Binifibrate	T46.6X1	T46.6X2	T46.6X3	T46.6X4	T46.6X5	T46.6X6
Binitrobenzol	T65.3X1	T65.3X2	T65.3X3	T65.3X4	—	—
Bioflavonoid(s)	T46.991	T46.992	T46.993	T46.994	T46.995	T46.996
Biological substance NEC	T50.901	T50.902	T50.903	T50.904	T50.905	T50.906
Biotin	T45.2X1	T45.2X2	T45.2X3	T45.2X4	T45.2X5	T45.2X6
Biperiden	T44.3X1	T44.3X2	T44.3X3	T44.3X4	T44.3X5	T44.3X6
Bisacodyl	T47.2X1	T47.2X2	T47.2X3	T47.2X4	T47.2X5	T47.2X6
Bisbentiamine	T45.2X1	T45.2X2	T45.2X3	T45.2X4	T45.2X5	T45.2X6
Bisbutiamine	T45.2X1	T45.2X2	T45.2X3	T45.2X4	T45.2X5	T45.2X6
Bisdequalinium (salts) (diacetate)	T49.6X1	T49.6X2	T49.6X3	T49.6X4	T49.6X5	T49.6X6
Bishydroxycoumarin	T45.511	T45.512	T45.513	T45.514	T45.515	T45.516
Bismarsen	T37.8X1	T37.8X2	T37.8X3	T37.8X4	T37.8X5	T37.8X6
Bismuth salts	T47.6X1	T47.6X2	T47.6X3	T47.6X4	T47.6X5	T47.6X6
aluminate	T47.1X1	T47.1X2	T47.1X3	T47.1X4	T47.1X5	T47.1X6
anti-infectives	T37.8X1	T37.8X2	T37.8X3	T37.8X4	T37.8X5	T37.8X6
formic iodide	T49.0X1	T49.0X2	T49.0X3	T49.0X4	T49.0X5	T49.0X6
glycolylarsenate	T49.0X1	T49.0X2	T49.0X3	T49.0X4	T49.0X5	T49.0X6
nonmedicinal (compounds) NEC	T65.91	T65.92	T65.93	T65.94	—	—
subcarbonate	T47.6X1	T47.6X2	T47.6X3	T47.6X4	T47.6X5	T47.6X6
subsalicylate	T37.8X1	T37.8X2	T37.8X3	T37.8X4	T37.8X5	T37.8X6
sulfarsphenamine	T37.8X1	T37.8X2	T37.8X3	T37.8X4	T37.8X5	T37.8X6
Bisoprolol	T44.7X1	T44.7X2	T44.7X3	T44.7X4	T44.7X5	T44.7X6
Bisoxatin	T47.2X1	T47.2X2	T47.2X3	T47.2X4	T47.2X5	T47.2X6
Bisulepin (hydrochloride)	T45.0X1	T45.0X2	T45.0X3	T45.0X4	T45.0X5	T45.0X6
Bithionol	T37.8X1	T37.8X2	T37.8X3	T37.8X4	T37.8X5	T37.8X6
anthelminthic	T37.4X1	T37.4X2	T37.4X3	T37.4X4	T37.4X5	T37.4X6
Bitolterol	T48.6X1	T48.6X2	T48.6X3	T48.6X4	T48.6X5	T48.6X6
Bitoscanate	T37.4X1	T37.4X2	T37.4X3	T37.4X4	T37.4X5	T37.4X6
Bitter almond oil	T62.8X1	T62.8X2	T62.8X3	T62.8X4	—	—
Bittersweet	T62.2X1	T62.2X2	T62.2X3	T62.2X4	—	—
Black						
flag	T60.91	T60.92	T60.93	T60.94	—	—
henbane	T62.2X1	T62.2X2	T62.2X3	T62.2X4	—	—
leaf (40)	T60.91	T60.92	T60.93	T60.94	—	—
widow spider (bite)	T63.311	T63.312	T63.313	T63.314	—	—
antivenin	T50.Z11	T50.Z12	T50.Z13	T50.Z14	T50.Z15	T50.Z16
Blast furnace gas (carbon monoxide from)	T58.8X1	T58.8X2	T58.8X3	T58.8X4	—	—
Bleach	T54.91	T54.92	T54.93	T54.94		

◀ New   ◀ Revised   ~~deleted~~ Deleted

Substance	External Cause (T-Code)					
	Poisoning, Accidental (Unintentional)	Poisoning, Intentional Self-Harm	Poisoning, Assault	Poisoning, Undetermined	Adverse Effect	Underdosing
Bleaching agent (medicinal)	T49.4X1	T49.4X2	T49.4X3	T49.4X4	T49.4X5	T49.4X6
Bleomycin	T45.1X1	T45.1X2	T45.1X3	T45.1X4	T45.1X5	T45.1X6
Blockain	T41.3X1	T41.3X2	T41.3X3	T41.3X4	T41.3X5	T41.3X6
infiltration (subcutaneous)	T41.3X1	T41.3X2	T41.3X3	T41.3X4	T41.3X5	T41.3X6
nerve block (peripheral) (plexus)	T41.3X1	T41.3X2	T41.3X3	T41.3X4	T41.3X5	T41.3X6
topical (surface)	T41.3X1	T41.3X2	T41.3X3	T41.3X4	T41.3X5	T41.3X6
Blockers, calcium channel	T46.1X1	T46.1X2	T46.1X3	T46.1X4	T46.1X5	T46.1X6
Blood (derivatives) (natural) (plasma) (whole)	T45.8X1	T45.8X2	T45.8X3	T45.8X4	T45.8X5	T45.8X6
dried	T45.8X1	T45.8X2	T45.8X3	T45.8X4	T45.8X5	T45.8X6
drug affecting NEC	T45.91	T45.92	T45.93	T45.94	T45.95	T45.96
expander NEC	T45.8X1	T45.8X2	T45.8X3	T45.8X4	T45.8X5	T45.8X6
fraction NEC	T45.8X1	T45.8X2	T45.8X3	T45.8X4	T45.8X5	T45.8X6
substitute (macromolecular)	T45.8X1	T45.8X2	T45.8X3	T45.8X4	T45.8X5	T45.8X6
Blue velvet	T40.2X1	T40.2X2	T40.2X3	T40.2X4	—	—
Bone meal	T62.8X1	T62.8X2	T62.8X3	T62.8X4	—	—
Bonine	T45.0X1	T45.0X2	T45.0X3	T45.0X4	T45.0X5	T45.0X6
Bopindolol	T44.7X1	T44.7X2	T44.7X3	T44.7X4	T44.7X5	T44.7X6
Boracic acid	T49.0X1	T49.0X2	T49.0X3	T49.0X4	T49.0X5	T49.0X6
ENT agent	T49.6X1	T49.6X2	T49.6X3	T49.6X4	T49.6X5	T49.6X6
ophthalmic preparation	T49.5X1	T49.5X2	T49.5X3	T49.5X4	T49.5X5	T49.5X6
Borane complex	T57.8X1	T57.8X2	T57.8X3	T57.8X4	—	—
Borate(s)	T57.8X1	T57.8X2	T57.8X3	T57.8X4	—	—
buffer	T50.991	T50.992	T50.993	T50.994	T50.995	T50.996
cleanser	T54.91	T54.92	T54.93	T54.94	—	—
sodium	T57.8X1	T57.8X2	T57.8X3	T57.8X4	—	—
Borax (cleanser)	T54.91	T54.92	T54.93	T54.94	—	—
Bordeaux mixture	T60.3X1	T60.3X2	T60.3X3	T60.3X4	—	—
Boric acid	T49.0X1	T49.0X2	T49.0X3	T49.0X4	T49.0X5	T49.0X6
ENT agent	T49.6X1	T49.6X2	T49.6X3	T49.6X4	T49.6X5	T49.6X6
ophthalmic preparation	T49.5X1	T49.5X2	T49.5X3	T49.5X4	T49.5X5	T49.5X6
Bornaprine	T44.3X1	T44.3X2	T44.3X3	T44.3X4	T44.3X5	T44.3X6
Boron	T57.8X1	T57.8X2	T57.8X3	T57.8X4	—	—
hydride NEC	T57.8X1	T57.8X2	T57.8X3	T57.8X4	—	—
fumes or gas	T57.8X1	T57.8X2	T57.8X3	T57.8X4	—	—
trifluoride	T59.891	T59.892	T59.893	T59.894	—	—
Botox	T48.291	T48.292	T48.293	T48.294	T48.295	T48.296
Botulinus anti-toxin (type A, B)	T50.Z11	T50.Z12	T50.Z13	T50.Z14	T50.Z15	T50.Z16
Brake fluid vapor	T59.891	T59.892	T59.893	T59.894	—	—
Brallobarbital	T42.3X1	T42.3X2	T42.3X3	T42.3X4	T42.3X5	T42.3X6
Bran (wheat)	T47.4X1	T47.4X2	T47.4X3	T47.4X4	T47.4X5	T47.4X6
Brass (fumes)	T56.891	T56.892	T56.893	T56.894	—	—

Substance	External Cause (T-Code)					
	Poisoning, Accidental (Unintentional)	Poisoning, Intentional Self-Harm	Poisoning, Assault	Poisoning, Undetermined	Adverse Effect	Underdosing
Brasso	T52.0X1	T52.0X2	T52.0X3	T52.0X4	—	—
Bretylium tosilate	T46.2X1	T46.2X2	T46.2X3	T46.2X4	T46.2X5	T46.2X6
Brevital (sodium)	T41.1X1	T41.1X2	T41.1X3	T41.1X4	T41.1X5	T41.1X6
Brinase	T45.3X1	T45.3X2	T45.3X3	T45.3X4	T45.3X5	T45.3X6
British antilewisite	T45.8X1	T45.8X2	T45.8X3	T45.8X4	T45.8X5	T45.8X6
Brodifacoum	T60.4X1	T60.4X2	T60.4X3	T60.4X4	—	—
Bromal (hydrate)	T42.6X1	T42.6X2	T42.6X3	T42.6X4	T42.6X5	T42.6X6
Bromazepam	T42.4X1	T42.4X2	T42.4X3	T42.4X4	T42.4X5	T42.4X6
Bromazine	T45.0X1	T45.0X2	T45.0X3	T45.0X4	T45.0X5	T45.0X6
Brombenzylcyanide	T59.3X1	T59.3X2	T59.3X3	T59.3X4	—	—
Bromelains	T45.3X1	T45.3X2	T45.3X3	T45.3X4	T45.3X5	T45.3X6
Bromethalin	T60.4X1	T60.4X2	T60.4X3	T60.4X4	—	—
Bromhexine	T48.4X1	T48.4X2	T48.4X3	T48.4X4	T48.4X5	T48.4X6
Bromide salts	T42.6X1	T42.6X2	T42.6X3	T42.6X4	T42.6X5	T42.6X6
Bromindione	T45.511	T45.512	T45.513	T45.514	T45.515	T45.516
Bromine						
compounds (medicinal)	T42.6X1	T42.6X2	T42.6X3	T42.6X4	T42.6X5	T42.6X6
sedative	T42.6X1	T42.6X2	T42.6X3	T42.6X4	T42.6X5	T42.6X6
vapor	T59.891	T59.892	T59.893	T59.894	—	—
Bromisovalum	T42.6X1	T42.6X2	T42.6X3	T42.6X4	T42.6X5	T42.6X6
Bromisoval	T42.6X1	T42.6X2	T42.6X3	T42.6X4	T42.6X5	T42.6X6
Bromobenzylcyanide	T59.3X1	T59.3X2	T59.3X3	T59.3X4	—	—
Bromochlorosalicylani-lide	T49.0X1	T49.0X2	T49.0X3	T49.0X4	T49.0X5	T49.0X6
Bromocriptine	T42.8X1	T42.8X2	T42.8X3	T42.8X4	T42.8X5	T42.8X6
Bromodiphenhydramine	T45.0X1	T45.0X2	T45.0X3	T45.0X4	T45.0X5	T45.0X6
Bromoform	T42.6X1	T42.6X2	T42.6X3	T42.6X4	T42.6X5	T42.6X6
Bromophenol blue reagent	T50.991	T50.992	T50.993	T50.994	T50.995	T50.996
Bromopride	T47.8X1	T47.8X2	T47.8X3	T47.8X4	T47.8X5	T47.8X6
Bromosalicylchloranitide	T49.0X1	T49.0X2	T49.0X3	T49.0X4	T49.0X5	T49.0X6
Bromosalicylhydroxamic acid	T37.1X1	T37.1X2	T37.1X3	T37.1X4	T37.1X5	T37.1X6
Bromo-seltzer	T39.1X1	T39.1X2	T39.1X3	T39.1X4	T39.1X5	T39.1X6
Bromoxynil	T60.3X1	T60.3X2	T60.3X3	T60.3X4	—	—
Bromperidol	T43.4X1	T43.4X2	T43.4X3	T43.4X4	T43.4X5	T43.4X6
Brompheniramine	T45.0X1	T45.0X2	T45.0X3	T45.0X4	T45.0X5	T45.0X6
Bromsulfophthalein	T50.8X1	T50.8X2	T50.8X3	T50.8X4	T50.8X5	T50.8X6
Bromural	T42.6X1	T42.6X2	T42.6X3	T42.6X4	T42.6X5	T42.6X6
Bromvaletone	T42.6X1	T42.6X2	T42.6X3	T42.6X4	T42.6X5	T42.6X6
Bronchodilator NEC	T48.6X1	T48.6X2	T48.6X3	T48.6X4	T48.6X5	T48.6X6
Brotizolam	T42.4X1	T42.4X2	T42.4X3	T42.4X4	T42.4X5	T42.4X6
Brovincamine	T46.7X1	T46.7X2	T46.7X3	T46.7X4	T46.7X5	T46.7X6
Brown spider (bite) (venom)	T63.391	T63.392	T63.393	T63.394	—	—

◀ New　　◀ Revised　　~~deleted~~ Deleted

Substance	Poisoning, Accidental (Unintentional)	Poisoning, Intentional Self-Harm	Poisoning, Assault	Poisoning, Undetermined	Adverse Effect	Underdosing
Brown recluse spider (bite) (venom)	T63.331	T63.332	T63.333	T63.334	—	—
Broxaterol	T48.6X1	T48.6X2	T48.6X3	T48.6X4	T48.6X5	T48.6X6
Broxuridine	T45.1X1	T45.1X2	T45.1X3	T45.1X4	T45.1X5	T45.1X6
Broxyquinoline	T37.8X1	T37.8X2	T37.8X3	T37.8X4	T37.8X5	T37.8X6
Bruceine	T48.291	T48.292	T48.293	T48.294	T48.295	T48.296
Brucia	T62.2X1	T62.2X2	T62.2X3	T62.2X4	—	—
Brucine	T65.1X1	T65.1X2	T65.1X3	T65.1X4	—	—
Brunswick green — *see Copper*						
Bruten — *see Ibuprofen*						
Bryonia	T47.2X1	T47.2X2	T47.2X3	T47.2X4	T47.2X5	T47.2X6
Buclizine	T45.0X1	T45.0X2	T45.0X3	T45.0X4	T45.0X5	T45.0X6
Buclosamide	T49.0X1	T49.0X2	T49.0X3	T49.0X4	T49.0X5	T49.0X6
Budesonide	T44.5X1	T44.5X2	T44.5X3	T44.5X4	T44.5X5	T44.5X6
Budralazine	T46.5X1	T46.5X2	T46.5X3	T46.5X4	T46.5X5	T46.5X6
Bufferin	T39.011	T39.012	T39.013	T39.014	T39.015	T39.016
Buflomedil	T46.7X1	T46.7X2	T46.7X3	T46.7X4	T46.7X5	T46.7X6
Buformin	T38.3X1	T38.3X2	T38.3X3	T38.3X4	T38.3X5	T38.3X6
Bufotenine	T40.991	T40.992	T40.993	T40.994	—	—
Bufrolin	T48.6X1	T48.6X2	T48.6X3	T48.6X4	T48.6X5	T48.6X6
Bufylline	T48.6X1	T48.6X2	T48.6X3	T48.6X4	T48.6X5	T48.6X6
Bulk filler	T50.5X1	T50.5X2	T50.5X3	T50.5X4	T50.5X5	T50.5X6
cathartic	T47.4X1	T47.4X2	T47.4X3	T47.4X4	T47.4X5	T47.4X6
Bumetanide	T50.1X1	T50.1X2	T50.1X3	T50.1X4	T50.1X5	T50.1X6
Bunaftine	T46.2X1	T46.2X2	T46.2X3	T46.2X4	T46.2X5	T46.2X6
Bunamiodyl	T50.8X1	T50.8X2	T50.8X3	T50.8X4	T50.8X5	T50.8X6
Bunazosin	T44.6X1	T44.6X2	T44.6X3	T44.6X4	T44.6X5	T44.6X6
Bunitrolol	T44.7X1	T44.7X2	T44.7X3	T44.7X4	T44.7X5	T44.7X6
Buphenine	T46.7X1	T46.7X2	T46.7X3	T46.7X4	T46.7X5	T46.7X6
Bupivacaine	T41.3X1	T41.3X2	T41.3X3	T41.3X4	T41.3X5	T41.3X6
infiltration (subcutaneous)	T41.3X1	T41.3X2	T41.3X3	T41.3X4	T41.3X5	T41.3X6
nerve block (peripheral) (plexus)	T41.3X1	T41.3X2	T41.3X3	T41.3X4	T41.3X5	T41.3X6
spinal	T41.3X1	T41.3X2	T41.3X3	T41.3X4	T41.3X5	T41.3X6
Bupranolol	T44.7X1	T44.7X2	T44.7X3	T44.7X4	T44.7X5	T44.7X6
Buprenorphine	T40.4X1	T40.4X2	T40.4X3	T40.4X4	T40.4X5	T40.4X6
Bupropion	T43.291	T43.292	T43.293	T43.294	T43.295	T43.296
Burimamide	T47.1X1	T47.1X2	T47.1X3	T47.1X4	T47.1X5	T47.1X6
Buserelin	T38.891	T38.892	T38.893	T38.894	T38.895	T38.896
Buspirone	T43.591	T43.592	T43.593	T43.594	T43.595	T43.596
Busulfan, busulphan	T45.1X1	T45.1X2	T45.1X3	T45.1X4	T45.1X5	T45.1X6
Butabarbital (sodium)	T42.3X1	T42.3X2	T42.3X3	T42.3X4	T42.3X5	T42.3X6
Butabarbitone	T42.3X1	T42.3X2	T42.3X3	T42.3X4	T42.3X5	T42.3X6

Substance	Poisoning, Accidental (Unintentional)	Poisoning, Intentional Self-Harm	Poisoning, Assault	Poisoning, Undetermined	Adverse Effect	Underdosing
Butabarpal	T42.3X1	T42.3X2	T42.3X3	T42.3X4	T42.3X5	T42.3X6
Butacaine	T41.3X1	T41.3X2	T41.3X3	T41.3X4	T41.3X5	T41.3X6
Butalamine	T46.7X1	T46.7X2	T46.7X3	T46.7X4	T46.7X5	T46.7X6
Butalbital	T42.3X1	T42.3X2	T42.3X3	T42.3X4	T42.3X5	T42.3X6
Butallylonal	T42.3X1	T42.3X2	T42.3X3	T42.3X4	T42.3X5	T42.3X6
Butamben	T41.3X1	T41.3X2	T41.3X3	T41.3X4	T41.3X5	T41.3X6
Butamirate	T48.3X1	T48.3X2	T48.3X3	T48.3X4	T48.3X5	T48.3X6
Butane (distributed in mobile container)	T59.891	T59.892	T59.893	T59.894	—	—
distributed through pipes	T59.891	T59.892	T59.893	T59.894	—	—
incomplete combustion	T58.11	T58.12	T58.13	T58.14		
Butanilicaine	T41.3X1	T41.3X2	T41.3X3	T41.3X4	T41.3X5	T41.3X6
Butanol	T51.3X1	T51.3X2	T51.3X3	T51.3X4	—	—
Butanone, 2-butanone	T52.4X1	T52.4X2	T52.4X3	T52.4X4	—	—
Butantrone	T49.4X1	T49.4X2	T49.4X3	T49.4X4	T49.4X5	T49.4X6
Butaperazine	T43.3X1	T43.3X2	T43.3X3	T43.3X4	T43.3X5	T43.3X6
Butazolidin	T39.2X1	T39.2X2	T39.2X3	T39.2X4	T39.2X5	T39.2X6
Butetamate	T48.6X1	T48.6X2	T48.6X3	T48.6X4	T48.6X5	T48.6X6
Butethal	T42.3X1	T42.3X2	T42.3X3	T42.3X4	T42.3X5	T42.3X6
Butethamate	T44.3X1	T44.3X2	T44.3X3	T44.3X4	T44.3X5	T44.3X6
Buthalitone (sodium)	T41.1X1	T41.1X2	T41.1X3	T41.1X4	T41.1X5	T41.1X6
Butisol (sodium)	T42.3X1	T42.3X2	T42.3X3	T42.3X4	T42.3X5	T42.3X6
Butizide	T50.2X1	T50.2X2	T50.2X3	T50.2X4	T50.2X5	T50.2X6
Butobarbital	T42.3X1	T42.3X2	T42.3X3	T42.3X4	T42.3X5	T42.3X6
sodium	T42.3X1	T42.3X2	T42.3X3	T42.3X4	T42.3X5	T42.3X6
Butobarbitone	T42.3X1	T42.3X2	T42.3X3	T42.3X4	T42.3X5	T42.3X6
Butoconazole (nitrate)	T49.0X1	T49.0X2	T49.0X3	T49.0X4	T49.0X5	T49.0X6
Butorphanol	T40.4X1	T40.4X2	T40.4X3	T40.4X4	T40.4X5	T40.4X6
Butriptyline	T43.011	T43.012	T43.013	T43.014	T43.015	T43.016
Butropium bromide	T44.3X1	T44.3X2	T44.3X3	T44.3X4	T44.3X5	T44.3X6
Buttercups	T62.2X1	T62.2X2	T62.2X3	T62.2X4	—	—
Butter of antimony — *see Antimony*						
Butyl						
acetate (secondary)	T52.8X1	T52.8X2	T52.8X3	T52.8X4	—	—
alcohol	T51.3X1	T51.3X2	T51.3X3	T51.3X4	—	—
aminobenzoate	T41.3X1	T41.3X2	T41.3X3	T41.3X4	T41.3X5	T41.3X6
butyrate	T52.8X1	T52.8X2	T52.8X3	T52.8X4	—	—
carbinol	T51.3X1	T51.3X2	T51.3X3	T51.3X4	—	—
carbitol	T52.3X1	T52.3X2	T52.3X3	T52.3X4	—	—
cellosolve	T52.3X1	T52.3X2	T52.3X3	T52.3X4	—	—
chloral (hydrate)	T42.6X1	T42.6X2	T42.6X3	T42.6X4	T42.6X5	T42.6X6
formate	T52.8X1	T52.8X2	T52.8X3	T52.8X4	—	—

TABLE OF DRUGS AND CHEMICALS

Substance	Poisoning, Accidental (Unintentional)	Poisoning, Intentional Self-Harm	Poisoning, Assault	Poisoning, Undetermined	Adverse Effect	Underdosing
Butyl *(Continued)*						
lactate	T52.8X1	T52.8X2	T52.8X3	T52.8X4	—	—
propionate	T52.8X1	T52.8X2	T52.8X3	T52.8X4	—	—
scopolamine bromide	T44.3X1	T44.3X2	T44.3X3	T44.3X4	T44.3X5	T44.3X6
thiobarbital sodium	T41.1X1	T41.1X2	T41.1X3	T41.1X4	T41.1X5	T41.1X6
Butylated hydroxy-anisole	T50.991	T50.992	T50.993	T50.994	T50.995	T50.996
Butylchloral hydrate	T42.6X1	T42.6X2	T42.6X3	T42.6X4	T42.6X5	T42.6X6
Butyltoluene	T52.2X1	T52.2X2	T52.2X3	T52.2X4	—	—
Butyn	T41.3X1	T41.3X2	T41.3X3	T41.3X4	T41.3X5	T41.3X6
Butyrophenone (-based tranquilizers)	T43.4X1	T43.4X2	T43.4X3	T43.4X4	T43.4X5	T43.4X6
C						
Cabergoline	T42.8X1	T42.8X2	T42.8X3	T42.8X4	T42.8X5	T42.8X6
Cacodyl, cacodylic acid	T57.0X1	T57.0X2	T57.0X3	T57.0X4	—	—
Cactinomycin	T45.1X1	T45.1X2	T45.1X3	T45.1X4	T45.1X5	T45.1X6
Cade oil	T49.4X1	T49.4X2	T49.4X3	T49.4X4	T49.4X5	T49.4X6
Cadexomer iodine	T49.0X1	T49.0X2	T49.0X3	T49.0X4	T49.0X5	T49.0X6
Cadmium (chloride) (fumes) (oxide)	T56.3X1	T56.3X2	T56.3X3	T56.3X4	—	—
sulfide (medicinal) NEC	T49.4X1	T49.4X2	T49.4X3	T49.4X4	T49.4X5	T49.4X6
Cadralazine	T46.5X1	T46.5X2	T46.5X3	T46.5X4	T46.5X5	T46.5X6
Caffeine	T43.611	T43.612	T43.613	T43.614	T43.615	T43.616
Calabar bean	T62.2X1	T62.2X2	T62.2X3	T62.2X4	—	—
Caladium seguinum	T62.2X1	T62.2X2	T62.2X3	T62.2X4	—	—
Calamine (lotion)	T49.3X1	T49.3X2	T49.3X3	T49.3X4	T49.3X5	T49.3X6
Calcifediol	T45.2X1	T45.2X2	T45.2X3	T45.2X4	T45.2X5	T45.2X6
Calciferol	T45.2X1	T45.2X2	T45.2X3	T45.2X4	T45.2X5	T45.2X6
Calcitonin	T50.991	T50.992	T50.993	T50.994	T50.995	T50.996
Calcitriol	T45.2X1	T45.2X2	T45.2X3	T45.2X4	T45.2X5	T45.2X6
Calcium	T50.3X1	T50.3X2	T50.3X3	T50.3X4	T50.3X5	T50.3X6
actylsalicylate	T39.011	T39.012	T39.013	T39.014	T39.015	T39.016
benzamidosalicylate	T37.1X1	T37.1X2	T37.1X3	T37.1X4	T37.1X5	T37.1X6
bromide	T42.6X1	T42.6X2	T42.6X3	T42.6X4	T42.6X5	T42.6X6
bromolactobionate	T42.6X1	T42.6X2	T42.6X3	T42.6X4	T42.6X5	T42.6X6
carbaspirin	T39.011	T39.012	T39.013	T39.014	T39.015	T39.016
carbimide	T50.6X1	T50.6X2	T50.6X3	T50.6X4	T50.6X5	T50.6X6
carbonate	T47.1X1	T47.1X2	T47.1X3	T47.1X4	T47.1X5	T47.1X6
chloride	T50.991	T50.992	T50.993	T50.994	T50.995	T50.996
anhydrous	T50.991	T50.992	T50.993	T50.994	T50.995	T50.996
cyanide	T57.8X1	T57.8X2	T57.8X3	T57.8X4	—	—
dioctyl sulfosuccinate	T47.4X1	T47.4X2	T47.4X3	T47.4X4	T47.4X5	T47.4X6
disodium edathamil	T45.8X1	T45.8X2	T45.8X3	T45.8X4	T45.8X5	T45.8X6

Substance	Poisoning, Accidental (Unintentional)	Poisoning, Intentional Self-Harm	Poisoning, Assault	Poisoning, Undetermined	Adverse Effect	Underdosing
Calcium *(Continued)*						
disodium edetate	T45.8X1	T45.8X2	T45.8X3	T45.8X4	T45.8X5	T45.8X6
dobesilate	T46.991	T46.992	T46.993	T46.994	T46.995	T46.996
EDTA	T45.8X1	T45.8X2	T45.8X3	T45.8X4	T45.8X5	T45.8X6
ferrous citrate	T45.4X1	T45.4X2	T45.4X3	T45.4X4	T45.4X5	T45.4X6
folinate	T45.8X1	T45.8X2	T45.8X3	T45.8X4	T45.8X5	T45.8X6
glubionate	T50.3X1	T50.3X2	T50.3X3	T50.3X4	T50.3X5	T50.3X6
gluconate	T50.3X1	T50.3X2	T50.3X3	T50.3X4	T50.3X5	T50.3X6
gluconogalactogluconate	T50.3X1	T50.3X2	T50.3X3	T50.3X4	T50.3X5	T50.3X6
hydrate, hydroxide	T54.3X1	T54.3X2	T54.3X3	T54.3X4	—	—
hypochlorite	T54.3X1	T54.3X2	T54.3X3	T54.3X4	—	—
iodide	T48.4X1	T48.4X2	T48.4X3	T48.4X4	T48.4X5	T48.4X6
ipodate	T50.8X1	T50.8X2	T50.8X3	T50.8X4	T50.8X5	T50.8X6
lactate	T50.3X1	T50.3X2	T50.3X3	T50.3X4	T50.3X5	T50.3X6
leucovorin	T45.8X1	T45.8X2	T45.8X3	T45.8X4	T45.8X5	T45.8X6
mandelate	T37.91	T37.92	T37.93	T37.94	T37.95	T37.96
oxide	T54.3X1	T54.3X2	T54.3X3	T54.3X4	—	—
pantothenate	T45.2X1	T45.2X2	T45.2X3	T45.2X4	T45.2X5	T45.2X6
phosphate	T50.3X1	T50.3X2	T50.3X3	T50.3X4	T50.3X5	T50.3X6
salicylate	T39.091	T39.092	T39.093	T39.094	T39.095	T39.096
salts	T50.3X1	T50.3X2	T50.3X3	T50.3X4	T50.3X5	T50.3X6
Calculus-dissolving drug	T50.991	T50.992	T50.993	T50.994	T50.995	T50.996
Calomel	T49.0X1	T49.0X2	T49.0X3	T49.0X4	T49.0X5	T49.0X6
Caloric agent	T50.3X1	T50.3X2	T50.3X3	T50.3X4	T50.3X5	T50.3X6
Calusterone	T38.7X1	T38.7X2	T38.7X3	T38.7X4	T38.7X5	T38.7X6
Camazepam	T42.4X1	T42.4X2	T42.4X3	T42.4X4	T42.4X5	T42.4X6
Camomile	T49.0X1	T49.0X2	T49.0X3	T49.0X4	T49.0X5	T49.0X6
Camoquin	T37.2X1	T37.2X2	T37.2X3	T37.2X4	T37.2X5	T37.2X6
Camphor						
insecticide	T60.2X1	T60.2X2	T60.2X3	T60.2X4	—	—
medicinal	T49.8X1	T49.8X2	T49.8X3	T49.8X4	T49.8X5	T49.8X6
Camylofin	T44.3X1	T44.3X2	T44.3X3	T44.3X4	T44.3X5	T44.3X6
Cancer chemotherapy drug regimen	T45.1X1	T45.1X2	T45.1X3	T45.1X4	T45.1X5	T45.1X6
Candeptin	T49.0X1	T49.0X2	T49.0X3	T49.0X4	T49.0X5	T49.0X6
Candicidin	T49.0X1	T49.0X2	T49.0X3	T49.0X4	T49.0X5	T49.0X6
Cannabinol	T40.7X1	T40.7X2	T40.7X3	T40.7X4	T40.7X5	T40.7X6
Cannabis (derivatives)	T40.7X1	T40.7X2	T40.7X3	T40.7X4	T40.7X5	T40.7X6
Canned heat	T51.1X1	T51.1X2	T51.1X3	T51.1X4	—	—
Canrenoic acid	T50.0X1	T50.0X2	T50.0X3	T50.0X4	T50.0X5	T50.0X6
Canrenone	T50.0X1	T50.0X2	T50.0X3	T50.0X4	T50.0X5	T50.0X6
Cantharides, cantharidin, cantharis	T49.8X1	T49.8X2	T49.8X3	T49.8X4	T49.8X5	T49.8X6

◀ New ◀ Revised ~~deleted~~ Deleted

Substance	External Cause (T-Code)					
	Poisoning, Accidental (Unintentional)	Poisoning, Intentional Self-Harm	Poisoning, Assault	Poisoning, Undetermined	Adverse Effect	Underdosing
Canthaxanthin	T50.991	T50.992	T50.993	T50.994	T50.995	T50.996
Capillary-active drug NEC	T46.901	T46.902	T46.903	T46.904	T46.905	T46.906
Capreomycin	T36.8X1	T36.8X2	T36.8X3	T36.8X4	T36.8X5	T36.8X6
Capsicum	T49.4X1	T49.4X2	T49.4X3	T49.4X4	T49.4X5	T49.4X6
Captafol	T60.3X1	T60.3X2	T60.3X3	T60.3X4	—	—
Captan	T60.3X1	T60.3X2	T60.3X3	T60.3X4	—	—
Captodiame, captodiamine	T43.591	T43.592	T43.593	T43.594	T43.595	T43.596
Captopril	T46.4X1	T46.4X2	T46.4X3	T46.4X4	T46.4X5	T46.4X6
Caramiphen	T44.3X1	T44.3X2	T44.3X3	T44.3X4	T44.3X5	T44.3X6
Carazolol	T44.7X1	T44.7X2	T44.7X3	T44.7X4	T44.7X5	T44.7X6
Carbachol	T44.1X1	T44.1X2	T44.1X3	T44.1X4	T44.1X5	T44.1X6
Carbacrylamine (resin)	T50.3X1	T50.3X2	T50.3X3	T50.3X4	T50.3X5	T50.3X6
Carbamate (insecticide)	T60.0X1	T60.0X2	T60.0X3	T60.0X4	—	—
Carbamate (sedative)	T42.6X1	T42.6X2	T42.6X3	T42.6X4	T42.6X5	T42.6X6
herbicide	T60.0X1	T60.0X2	T60.0X3	T60.0X4	—	—
insecticide	T60.0X1	T60.0X2	T60.0X3	T60.0X4	—	—
Carbamazepine	T42.1X1	T42.1X2	T42.1X3	T42.1X4	T42.1X5	T42.1X6
Carbamide	T47.3X1	T47.3X2	T47.3X3	T47.3X4	T47.3X5	T47.3X6
peroxide	T49.0X1	T49.0X2	T49.0X3	T49.0X4	T49.0X5	T49.0X6
topical	T49.8X1	T49.8X2	T49.8X3	T49.8X4	T49.8X5	T49.8X6
Carbamylcholine chloride	T44.1X1	T44.1X2	T44.1X3	T44.1X4	T44.1X5	T44.1X6
Carbaril	T60.0X1	T60.0X2	T60.0X3	T60.0X4	—	—
Carbarsone	T37.3X1	T37.3X2	T37.3X3	T37.3X4	T37.3X5	T37.3X6
Carbaryl	T60.0X1	T60.0X2	T60.0X3	T60.0X4	—	—
Carbaspirin	T39.011	T39.012	T39.013	T39.014	T39.015	T39.016
Carbazochrome (salicylate) (sodium sulfonate)	T49.4X1	T49.4X2	T49.4X3	T49.4X4	T49.4X5	T49.4X6
Carbenicillin	T36.0X1	T36.0X2	T36.0X3	T36.0X4	T36.0X5	T36.0X6
Carbenoxolone	T47.1X1	T47.1X2	T47.1X3	T47.1X4	T47.1X5	T47.1X6
Carbetapentane	T48.3X1	T48.3X2	T48.3X3	T48.3X4	T48.3X5	T48.3X6
Carbethyl salicylate	T39.091	T39.092	T39.093	T39.094	T39.095	T39.096
Carbidopa (with levodopa)	T42.8X1	T42.8X2	T42.8X3	T42.8X4	T42.8X5	T42.8X6
Carbimazole	T38.2X1	T38.2X2	T38.2X3	T38.2X4	T38.2X5	T38.2X6
Carbinol	T51.1X1	T51.1X2	T51.1X3	T51.1X4	—	—
Carbinoxamine	T45.0X1	T45.0X2	T45.0X3	T45.0X4	T45.0X5	T45.0X6
Carbiphene	T39.8X1	T39.8X2	T39.8X3	T39.8X4	T39.8X5	T39.8X6
Carbitol	T52.3X1	T52.3X2	T52.3X3	T52.3X4	—	—
Carbocaine	T41.3X1	T41.3X2	T41.3X3	T41.3X4	T41.3X5	T41.3X6
infiltration (subcutaneous)	T41.3X1	T41.3X2	T41.3X3	T41.3X4	T41.3X5	T41.3X6
nerve block (peripheral) (plexus)	T41.3X1	T41.3X2	T41.3X3	T41.3X4	T41.3X5	T41.3X6
topical (surface)	T41.3X1	T41.3X2	T41.3X3	T41.3X4	T41.3X5	T41.3X6
Carbo medicinalis	T47.6X1	T47.6X2	T47.6X4	T47.6X4	T47.6X5	T47.6X6

Substance	External Cause (T-Code)					
	Poisoning, Accidental (Unintentional)	Poisoning, Intentional Self-Harm	Poisoning, Assault	Poisoning, Undetermined	Adverse Effect	Underdosing
Carbomycin	T36.8X1	T36.8X2	T36.8X3	T36.8X4	T36.8X5	T36.8X6
Carbocisteine	T48.4X1	T48.4X2	T48.4X3	T48.4X4	T48.4X5	T48.4X6
Carbocromen	T46.3X1	T46.3X2	T46.3X3	T46.3X4	T46.3X5	T46.3X6
Carbol fuchsin	T49.0X1	T49.0X2	T49.0X3	T49.0X4	T49.0X5	T49.0X6
Carbolic acid — see also Phenol	T54.0X1	T54.0X2	T54.0X3	T54.0X4	—	—
Carbolonium (bromide)	T48.1X1	T48.1X2	T48.1X3	T48.1X4	T48.1X5	T48.1X6
Carbon						
bisulfide (liquid)	T65.4X1	T65.4X2	T65.4X3	T65.4X4		
vapor	T65.4X1	T65.4X2	T65.4X3	T65.4X4	—	—
dioxide (gas)	T59.7X1	T59.7X2	T59.7X3	T59.7X4		
medicinal	T41.5X1	T41.5X2	T41.5X3	T41.5X4	T41.5X5	T41.5X6
nonmedicinal	T59.7X1	T59.7X2	T59.7X3	T59.7X4	—	—
snow	T49.4X1	T49.4X2	T49.4X3	T49.4X4	T49.4X5	T49.4X6
disulfide (liquid)	T65.4X1	T65.4X2	T65.4X3	T65.4X4		
vapor	T65.4X1	T65.4X2	T65.4X3	T65.4X4	—	—
monoxide (from incomplete combustion)	T58.91	T58.92	T58.93	T58.94	—	—
blast furnace gas	T58.8X1	T58.8X2	T58.8X3	T58.8X4		
butane (distributed in mobile container)	T58.11	T58.12	T58.13	T58.14		
distributed through pipes	T58.11	T58.12	T58.13	T58.14		
charcoal fumes	T58.2X1	T58.2X2	T58.2X3	T58.2X4		
coal	T58.2X1	T58.2X2	T58.2X3	T58.2X4		
coke (in domestic stoves, fireplaces)	T58.2X1	T58.2X2	T58.2X3	T58.2X4		
gas (piped)	T58.11	T58.12	T58.13	T58.14		
solid (in domestic stoves, fireplaces)	T58.2X1	T58.2X2	T58.2X3	T58.2X4	—	—
exhaust gas (motor) not in transit	T58.01	T58.02	T58.03	T58.04	—	—
combustion engine, any not in watercraft	T58.01	T58.02	T58.03	T58.04		
farm tractor, not in transit	T58.01	T58.02	T58.03	T58.04		
gas engine	T58.01	T58.02	T58.03	T58.04	—	—
motor pump	T58.01	T58.02	T58.03	T58.04	—	—
motor vehicle, not in transit	T58.01	T58.02	T58.03	T58.04		
fuel (in domestic use)	T58.2X1	T58.2X2	T58.2X3	T58.2X4		
gas (piped)	T58.11	T58.12	T58.13	T58.14	—	—
in mobile container	T58.11	T58.12	T58.13	T58.14		
utility	T58.11	T58.12	T58.13	T58.14	—	—
in mobile container	T58.11	T58.12	T58.13	T58.14		
piped (natural)	T58.11	T58.12	T58.13	T58.14		

◀ New ◀ Revised ~~deleted~~ Deleted

	External Cause (T-Code)					
Substance	Poisoning, Accidental (Unintentional)	Poisoning, Intentional Self-Harm	Poisoning, Assault	Poisoning, Undetermined	Adverse Effect	Underdosing
Carbon *(Continued)*						
monoxide *(Continued)*						
illuminating gas	T58.11	T58.12	T58.13	T58.14	—	—
industrial fuels or gases, any	T58.8X1	T58.8X2	T58.8X3	T58.8X4	—	—
kerosene (in domestic stoves, fireplaces)	T58.2X1	T58.2X2	T58.2X3	T58.2X4	—	—
kiln gas or vapor	T58.8X1	T58.8X2	T58.8X3	T58.8X4	—	—
motor exhaust gas, not in transit	T58.01	T58.02	T58.03	T58.04	—	—
piped gas (manufactured) (natural)	T58.11	T58.12	T58.13	T58.14	—	—
producer gas	T58.8X1	T58.8X2	T58.8X3	T58.8X4	—	—
propane (distributed in mobile container)	T58.11	T58.12	T58.13	T58.14	—	—
distributed through pipes	T58.11	T58.12	T58.13	T58.14	—	—
specified source NEC	T58.8X1	T58.8X2	T58.8X3	T58.8X4	—	—
stove gas	T58.11	T58.12	T58.13	T58.14	—	—
piped	T58.11	T58.12	T58.13	T58.14	—	—
utility gas	T58.11	T58.12	T58.13	T58.14	—	—
piped	T58.11	T58.12	T58.13	T58.14	—	—
water gas	T58.11	T58.12	T58.13	T58.14	—	—
wood (in domestic stoves, fireplaces)	T58.2X1	T58.2X2	T58.2X3	T58.2X4	—	—
tetrachloride (vapor) NEC	T53.0X1	T53.0X2	T53.0X3	T53.0X4	—	—
liquid (cleansing agent) NEC	T53.0X1	T53.0X2	T53.0X3	T53.0X4	—	—
solvent	T53.0X1	T53.0X2	T53.0X3	T53.0X4	—	—
Carbonic acid gas	T59.7X1	T59.7X2	T59.7X3	T59.7X4	—	—
anhydrase inhibitor NEC	T50.2X1	T50.2X2	T50.2X3	T50.2X4	T50.2X5	T50.2X6
Carbophenothion	T60.0X1	T60.0X2	T60.0X3	T60.0X4	—	—
Carboplatin	T45.1X1	T45.1X2	T45.1X3	T45.1X4	T45.1X5	T45.1X6
Carboprost	T48.0X1	T48.0X2	T48.0X3	T48.0X4	T48.0X5	T48.0X6
Carboquone	T45.1X1	T45.1X2	T45.1X3	T45.1X4	T45.1X5	T45.1X6
Carbowax	T49.3X1	T49.3X2	T49.3X3	T49.3X4	T49.3X5	T49.3X6
Carboxymethyl-cellulose	T47.4X1	T47.4X2	T47.4X3	T47.4X4	T47.4X5	T47.4X6
S-Carboxymethyl-cysteine	T48.4X1	T48.4X2	T48.4X3	T48.4X4	T48.4X5	T48.4X6
Carbrital	T42.3X1	T42.3X2	T42.3X3	T42.3X4	T42.3X5	T42.3X6
Carbromal	T42.6X1	T42.6X2	T42.6X3	T42.6X4	T42.6X5	T42.6X6
Carbutamide	T38.3X1	T38.3X2	T38.3X3	T38.3X4	T38.3X5	T38.3X6
Carbuterol	T48.6X1	T48.6X2	T48.6X3	T48.6X4	T48.6X5	T48.6X6
Cardiac						
depressants	T46.2X1	T46.2X2	T46.2X3	T46.2X4	T46.2X5	T46.2X6
rhythm regulator	T46.2X1	T46.2X2	T46.2X3	T46.2X4	T46.2X5	T46.2X6
specified NEC	T46.2X1	T46.2X2	T46.2X3	T46.2X4	T46.2X5	T46.2X6

	External Cause (T-Code)					
Substance	Poisoning, Accidental (Unintentional)	Poisoning, Intentional Self-Harm	Poisoning, Assault	Poisoning, Undetermined	Adverse Effect	Underdosing
Cardiografin	T50.8X1	T50.8X2	T50.8X3	T50.8X4	T50.8X5	T50.8X6
Cardio-green	T50.8X1	T50.8X2	T50.8X3	T50.8X4	T50.8X5	T50.8X6
Cardiotonic (glycoside) NEC	T46.0X1	T46.0X2	T46.0X3	T46.0X4	T46.0X5	T46.0X6
Cardiovascular drug NEC	T46.901	T46.902	T46.903	T46.904	T46.905	T46.906
Cardrase	T50.2X1	T50.2X2	T50.2X3	T50.2X4	T50.2X5	T50.2X6
Carfusin	T49.0X1	T49.0X2	T49.0X3	T49.0X4	T49.0X5	T49.0X6
Carfecillin	T36.0X1	T36.0X2	T36.0X3	T36.0X4	T36.0X5	T36.0X6
Carfenazine	T43.3X1	T43.3X2	T43.3X3	T43.3X4	T43.3X5	T43.3X6
Carindacillin	T36.0X1	T36.0X2	T36.0X3	T36.0X4	T36.0X5	T36.0X6
Carisoprodol	T42.8X1	T42.8X2	T42.8X3	T42.8X4	T42.8X5	T42.8X6
Carmellose	T47.4X1	T47.4X2	T47.4X3	T47.4X4	T47.4X5	T47.4X6
Carminative	T47.5X1	T47.5X2	T47.5X3	T47.5X4	T47.5X5	T47.5X6
Carmofur	T45.1X1	T45.1X2	T45.1X3	T45.1X4	T45.1X5	T45.1X6
Carmustine	T45.1X1	T45.1X2	T45.1X3	T45.1X4	T45.1X5	T45.1X6
Carotene	T45.2X1	T45.2X2	T45.2X3	T45.2X4	T45.2X5	T45.2X6
Carphenazine	T43.3X1	T43.3X2	T43.3X3	T43.3X4	T43.3X5	T43.3X6
Carpipramine	T42.4X1	T42.4X2	T42.4X3	T42.4X4	T42.4X5	T42.4X6
Carprofen	T39.311	T39.312	T39.313	T39.314	T39.315	T39.316
Carpronium chloride	T44.3X1	T44.3X2	T44.3X3	T44.3X4	T44.3X5	T44.3X6
Carrageenan	T47.8X1	T47.8X2	T47.8X3	T47.8X4	T47.8X5	T47.8X6
Carteolol	T44.7X1	T44.7X2	T44.7X3	T44.7X4	T44.7X5	T44.7X6
Carter's Little Pills	T47.2X1	T47.2X2	T47.2X3	T47.2X4	T47.2X5	T47.2X6
Cascara (sagrada)	T47.2X1	T47.2X2	T47.2X3	T47.2X4	T47.2X5	T47.2X6
Cassava	T62.2X1	T62.2X2	T62.2X3	T62.2X4	—	—
Castellani's paint	T49.0X1	T49.0X2	T49.0X3	T49.0X4	T49.0X5	T49.0X6
Castor						
bean	T62.2X1	T62.2X2	T62.2X3	T62.2X4	—	—
oil	T47.2X1	T47.2X2	T47.2X3	T47.2X4	T47.2X5	T47.2X6
Catalase	T45.3X1	T45.3X2	T45.3X3	T45.3X4	T45.3X5	T45.3X6
Caterpillar (sting)	T63.431	T63.432	T63.433	T63.434	—	—
Catha (edulis) (tea)	T43.691	T43.692	T43.693	T43.694	—	—
Cathartic NEC	T47.4X1	T47.4X2	T47.4X3	T47.4X4	T47.4X5	T47.4X6
anthacene derivative	T47.2X1	T47.2X2	T47.2X3	T47.2X4	T47.2X5	T47.2X6
bulk	T47.4X1	T47.4X2	T47.4X3	T47.4X4	T47.4X5	T47.4X6
contact	T47.2X1	T47.2X2	T47.2X3	T47.2X4	T47.2X5	T47.2X6
emollient NEC	T47.4X1	T47.4X2	T47.4X3	T47.4X4	T47.4X5	T47.4X6
irritant NEC	T47.2X1	T47.2X2	T47.2X3	T47.2X4	T47.2X5	T47.2X6
mucilage	T47.4X1	T47.4X2	T47.4X3	T47.4X4	T47.4X5	T47.4X6
saline	T47.3X1	T47.3X2	T47.3X3	T47.3X4	T47.3X5	T47.3X6
vegetable	T47.2X1	T47.2X2	T47.2X3	T47.2X4	T47.2X5	T47.2X6
Cathine	T50.5X1	T50.5X2	T50.5X3	T50.5X4	T50.5X5	T50.5X6
Cathomycin	T36.8X1	T36.8X2	T36.8X3	T36.8X4	T36.8X5	T36.8X6

◀ New ◀ Revised ~~deleted~~ Deleted

Substance	External Cause (T-Code)					
	Poisoning, Accidental (Unintentional)	Poisoning, Intentional Self-Harm	Poisoning, Assault	Poisoning, Undetermined	Adverse Effect	Underdosing
Cation exchange resin	T50.3X1	T50.3X2	T50.3X3	T50.3X4	T50.3X5	T50.3X6
Caustic(s) NEC	T54.91	T54.92	T54.93	T54.94	—	—
alkali	T54.3X1	T54.3X2	T54.3X3	T54.3X4	—	—
hydroxide	T54.3X1	T54.3X2	T54.3X3	T54.3X4	—	—
potash	T54.3X1	T54.3X2	T54.3X3	T54.3X4	—	—
soda	T54.3X1	T54.3X2	T54.3X3	T54.3X4	—	—
specified NEC	T54.91	T54.92	T54.93	T54.94	—	—
Ceepryn	T49.0X1	T49.0X2	T49.0X3	T49.0X4	T49.0X5	T49.0X6
ENT agent	T49.6X1	T49.6X2	T49.6X3	T49.6X4	T49.6X5	T49.6X6
lozenges	T49.6X1	T49.6X2	T49.6X3	T49.6X4	T49.6X5	T49.6X6
Cefacetrile	T36.1X1	T36.1X2	T36.1X3	T36.1X4	T36.1X5	T36.1X6
Cefaclor	T36.1X1	T36.1X2	T36.1X3	T36.1X4	T36.1X5	T36.1X6
Cefadroxil	T36.1X1	T36.1X2	T36.1X3	T36.1X4	T36.1X5	T36.1X6
Cefalexin	T36.1X1	T36.1X2	T36.1X3	T36.1X4	T36.1X5	T36.1X6
Cefaloglycin	T36.1X1	T36.1X2	T36.1X3	T36.1X4	T36.1X5	T36.1X6
Cefaloridine	T36.1X1	T36.1X2	T36.1X3	T36.1X4	T36.1X5	T36.1X6
Cefalosporins	T36.1X1	T36.1X2	T36.1X3	T36.1X4	T36.1X5	T36.1X6
Cefalotin	T36.1X1	T36.1X2	T36.1X3	T36.1X4	T36.1X5	T36.1X6
Cefamandole	T36.1X1	T36.1X2	T36.1X3	T36.1X4	T36.1X5	T36.1X6
Cefamycin antibiotic	T36.1X1	T36.1X2	T36.1X3	T36.1X4	T36.1X5	T36.1X6
Cefapirin	T36.1X1	T36.1X2	T36.1X3	T36.1X4	T36.1X5	T36.1X6
Cefatrizine	T36.1X1	T36.1X2	T36.1X3	T36.1X4	T36.1X5	T36.1X6
Cefazedone	T36.1X1	T36.1X2	T36.1X3	T36.1X4	T36.1X5	T36.1X6
Cefazolin	T36.1X1	T36.1X2	T36.1X3	T36.1X4	T36.1X5	T36.1X6
Cefbuperazone	T36.1X1	T36.1X2	T36.1X3	T36.1X4	T36.1X5	T36.1X6
Cefetamet	T36.1X1	T36.1X2	T36.1X3	T36.1X4	T36.1X5	T36.1X6
Cefixime	T36.1X1	T36.1X2	T36.1X3	T36.1X4	T36.1X5	T36.1X6
Cefmenoxime	T36.1X1	T36.1X2	T36.1X3	T36.1X4	T36.1X5	T36.1X6
Cefmetazole	T36.1X1	T36.1X2	T36.1X3	T36.1X4	T36.1X5	T36.1X6
Cefminox	T36.1X1	T36.1X2	T36.1X3	T36.1X4	T36.1X5	T36.1X6
Cefonicid	T36.1X1	T36.1X2	T36.1X3	T36.1X4	T36.1X5	T36.1X6
Cefoperazone	T36.1X1	T36.1X2	T36.1X3	T36.1X4	T36.1X5	T36.1X6
Ceforanide	T36.1X1	T36.1X2	T36.1X3	T36.1X4	T36.1X5	T36.1X6
Cefotaxime	T36.1X1	T36.1X2	T36.1X3	T36.1X4	T36.1X5	T36.1X6
Cefotetan	T36.1X1	T36.1X2	T36.1X3	T36.1X4	T36.1X5	T36.1X6
Cefotiam	T36.1X1	T36.1X2	T36.1X3	T36.1X4	T36.1X5	T36.1X6
Cefoxitin	T36.1X1	T36.1X2	T36.1X3	T36.1X4	T36.1X5	T36.1X6
Cefpimizole	T36.1X1	T36.1X2	T36.1X3	T36.1X4	T36.1X5	T36.1X6
Cefpiramide	T36.1X1	T36.1X2	T36.1X3	T36.1X4	T36.1X5	T36.1X6
Cefradine	T36.1X1	T36.1X2	T36.1X3	T36.1X4	T36.1X5	T36.1X6
Cefroxadine	T36.1X1	T36.1X2	T36.1X3	T36.1X4	T36.1X5	T36.1X6
Cefsulodin	T36.1X1	T36.1X2	T36.1X3	T36.1X4	T36.1X5	T36.1X6

Substance	External Cause (T-Code)					
	Poisoning, Accidental (Unintentional)	Poisoning, Intentional Self-Harm	Poisoning, Assault	Poisoning, Undetermined	Adverse Effect	Underdosing
Ceftazidime	T36.1X1	T36.1X2	T36.1X3	T36.1X4	T36.1X5	T36.1X6
Cefteram	T36.1X1	T36.1X2	T36.1X3	T36.1X4	T36.1X5	T36.1X6
Ceftezole	T36.1X1	T36.1X2	T36.1X3	T36.1X4	T36.1X5	T36.1X6
Ceftizoxime	T36.1X1	T36.1X2	T36.1X3	T36.1X4	T36.1X5	T36.1X6
Ceftriaxone	T36.1X1	T36.1X2	T36.1X3	T36.1X4	T36.1X5	T36.1X6
Cefuroxime	T36.1X1	T36.1X2	T36.1X3	T36.1X4	T36.1X5	T36.1X6
Cefuzonam	T36.1X1	T36.1X2	T36.1X3	T36.1X4	T36.1X5	T36.1X6
Celestone	T38.0X1	T38.0X2	T38.0X3	T38.0X4	T38.0X5	T38.0X6
topical	T49.0X1	T49.0X2	T49.0X3	T49.0X4	T49.0X5	T49.0X6
Celiprolol	T44.7X1	T44.7X2	T44.7X3	T44.7X4	T44.7X5	T44.7X6
Cellosolve	T52.91	T52.92	T52.93	T52.94	—	—
Cell stimulants and proliferants	T49.8X1	T49.8X2	T49.8X3	T49.8X4	T49.8X5	T49.8X6
Cellulose						
cathartic	T47.4X1	T47.4X2	T47.4X3	T47.4X4	T47.4X5	T47.4X6
hydroxyethyl	T47.4X1	T47.4X2	T47.4X3	T47.4X4	T47.4X5	T47.4X6
nitrates (topical)	T49.3X1	T49.3X2	T49.3X3	T49.3X4	T49.3X5	T49.3X6
oxidized	T49.4X1	T49.4X2	T49.4X3	T49.4X4	T49.4X5	T49.4X6
Centipede (bite)	T63.411	T63.412	T63.413	T63.414	—	—
Central nervous system						
depressants	T42.71	T42.72	T42.73	T42.74	T42.75	T42.76
anesthetic (general) NEC	T41.201	T41.202	T41.203	T41.204	T41.205	T41.206
gases NEC	T41.0X1	T41.0X2	T41.0X3	T41.0X4	T41.0X5	T41.0X6
intravenous	T41.1X1	T41.1X2	T41.1X3	T41.1X4	T41.1X5	T41.1X6
barbiturates	T42.3X1	T42.3X2	T42.3X3	T42.3X4	T42.3X5	T42.3X6
benzodiazepines	T42.4X1	T42.4X2	T42.4X3	T42.4X4	T42.4X5	T42.4X6
bromides	T42.6X1	T42.6X2	T42.6X3	T42.6X4	T42.6X5	T42.6X6
cannabis sativa	T40.7X1	T40.7X2	T40.7X3	T40.7X4	T40.7X5	T40.7X6
chloral hydrate	T42.6X1	T42.6X2	T42.6X3	T42.6X4	T42.6X5	T42.6X6
ethanol	T51.0X1	T51.0X2	T51.0X3	T51.0X4	—	—
hallucinogenics	T40.901	T40.902	T40.903	T40.904	T40.905	T40.906
hypnotics	T42.71	T42.72	T42.73	T42.74	T42.75	T42.76
specified NEC	T42.6X1	T42.6X2	T42.6X3	T42.6X4	T42.6X5	T42.6X6
muscle relaxants	T42.8X1	T42.8X2	T42.8X3	T42.8X4	T42.8X5	T42.8X6
paraldehyde	T42.6X1	T42.6X2	T42.6X3	T42.6X4	T42.6X5	T42.6X6
sedatives; sedative-hypnotics	T42.71	T42.72	T42.73	T42.74	T42.75	T42.76
mixed NEC	T42.6X1	T42.6X2	T42.6X3	T42.6X4	T42.6X5	T42.6X6
specified NEC	T42.6X1	T42.6X2	T42.6X3	T42.6X4	T42.6X5	T42.6X6
muscle-tone depressants	T42.8X1	T42.8X2	T42.8X3	T42.8X4	T42.8X5	T42.8X6
stimulants	T43.601	T43.602	T43.603	T43.604	T43.605	T43.606
amphetamines	T43.621	T43.622	T43.623	T43.624	T43.625	T43.626
analeptics	T50.7X1	T50.7X2	T50.7X3	T50.7X4	T50.7X5	T50.7X6

◀ New ◀ Revised ~~deleted~~ Deleted

Substance	Poisoning, Accidental (Unintentional)	Poisoning, Intentional Self-Harm	Poisoning, Assault	Poisoning, Undetermined	Adverse Effect	Underdosing
External Cause (T-Code)						
Central nervous system *(Continued)*						
stimulants *(Continued)*						
antidepressants	T43.201	T43.202	T43.203	T43.204	T43.205	T43.206
opiate antagonists	T50.7X1	T50.7X2	T50.7X3	T50.7X4	T50.7X5	T50.7X6
specified NEC	T43.691	T43.692	T43.693	T43.694	T43.695	T43.696
Cephalexin	T36.1X1	T36.1X2	T36.1X3	T36.1X4	T36.1X5	T36.1X6
Cephaloglycin	T36.1X1	T36.1X2	T36.1X3	T36.1X4	T36.1X5	T36.1X6
Cephaloridine	T36.1X1	T36.1X2	T36.1X3	T36.1X4	T36.1X5	T36.1X6
Cephalosporins	T36.1X1	T36.1X2	T36.1X3	T36.1X4	T36.1X5	T36.1X6
N (adicillin)	T36.0X1	T36.0X2	T36.0X3	T36.0X4	T36.0X5	T36.0X6
Cephalothin	T36.1X1	T36.1X2	T36.1X3	T36.1X4	T36.1X5	T36.1X6
Cephalotin	T36.1X1	T36.1X2	T36.1X3	T36.1X4	T36.1X5	T36.1X6
Cephradine	T36.1X1	T36.1X2	T36.1X3	T36.1X4	T36.1X5	T36.1X6
Cerbera (odallam)	T62.2X1	T62.2X2	T62.2X3	T62.2X4	—	—
Cerberin	T46.0X1	T46.0X2	T46.0X3	T46.0X4	T46.0X5	T46.0X6
Cerebral stimulants	T43.601	T43.602	T43.603	T43.604	T43.605	T43.606
psychotherapeutic	T43.601	T43.602	T43.603	T43.604	T43.605	T43.606
specified NEC	T43.691	T43.692	T43.693	T43.694	T43.695	T43.696
Cerium oxalate	T45.0X1	T45.0X2	T45.0X3	T45.0X4	T45.0X5	T45.0X6
Cerous oxalate	T45.0X1	T45.0X2	T45.0X3	T45.0X4	T45.0X5	T45.0X6
Ceruletide	T50.8X1	T50.8X2	T50.8X3	T50.8X4	T50.8X5	T50.8X6
Cetalkonium (chloride)	T49.0X1	T49.0X2	T49.0X3	T49.0X4	T49.0X5	T49.0X6
Cethexonium chloride	T49.0X1	T49.0X2	T49.0X3	T49.0X4	T49.0X5	T49.0X6
Cetiedil	T46.7X1	T46.7X2	T46.7X3	T46.7X4	T46.7X5	T46.7X6
Cetirizine	T45.0X1	T45.0X2	T45.0X3	T45.0X4	T45.0X5	T45.0X6
Cetomacrogol	T50.991	T50.992	T50.993	T50.994	T50.995	T50.996
Cetotiamine	T45.2X1	T45.2X2	T45.2X3	T45.2X4	T45.2X5	T45.2X6
Cetoxime	T45.0X1	T45.0X2	T45.0X3	T45.0X4	T45.0X5	T45.0X6
Cetraxate	T47.1X1	T47.1X2	T47.1X3	T47.1X4	T47.1X5	T47.1X6
Cetrimide	T49.0X1	T49.0X2	T49.0X3	T49.0X4	T49.0X5	T49.0X6
Cetrimonium (bromide)	T49.0X1	T49.0X2	T49.0X3	T49.0X4	T49.0X5	T49.0X6
Cetylpyridinium chloride	T49.0X1	T49.0X2	T49.0X3	T49.0X4	T49.0X5	T49.0X6
ENT agent	T49.6X1	T49.6X2	T49.6X3	T49.6X4	T49.6X5	T49.6X6
lozenges	T49.6X1	T49.6X2	T49.6X3	T49.6X4	T49.6X5	T49.6X6
Cevadillasee Sabadilla						
Cevitamic acid	T45.2X1	T45.2X2	T45.2X3	T45.2X4	T45.2X5	T45.2X6
Chalk, precipitated	T47.1X1	T47.1X2	T47.1X3	T47.1X4	T47.1X5	T47.1X6
Chamomile	T49.0X1	T49.0X2	T49.0X3	T49.0X4	T49.0X5	T49.0X6
Ch'an su	T46.0X1	T46.0X2	T46.0X3	T46.0X4	T46.0X5	T46.0X6
Charcoal	T47.6X1	T47.6X2	T47.6X3	T47.6X4	T47.6X5	T47.6X6
activated — *see also* Charcoal, medicinal	T47.6X1	T47.6X2	T47.6X3	T47.6X4	T47.6X5	T47.6X6

Substance	Poisoning, Accidental (Unintentional)	Poisoning, Intentional Self-Harm	Poisoning, Assault	Poisoning, Undetermined	Adverse Effect	Underdosing
External Cause (T-Code)						
Charcoal *(Continued)*						
fumes (Carbon monoxide)	T58.2X1	T58.2X2	T58.2X3	T58.2X4	—	—
industrial	T58.8X1	T58.8X2	T58.8X3	T58.8X4	—	—
medicinal (activated)	T47.6X1	T47.6X2	T47.6X3	T47.6X4	T47.6X5	T47.6X6
antidiarrheal	T47.6X1	T47.6X2	T47.6X3	T47.6X4	T47.6X5	T47.6X6
poison control	T47.8X1	T47.8X2	T47.8X3	T47.8X4	T47.8X5	T47.8X6
specified use other than for diarrhea	T47.8X1	T47.8X2	T47.8X3	T47.8X4	T47.8X5	T47.8X6
topical	T49.8X1	T49.8X2	T49.8X3	T49.8X4	T49.8X5	T49.8X6
Chaulmosulfone	T37.1X1	T37.1X2	T37.1X3	T37.1X4	T37.1X5	T37.1X6
Chelating agent NEC	T50.6X1	T50.6X2	T50.6X3	T50.6X4	T50.6X5	T50.6X6
Chelidonium majus	T62.2X1	T62.2X2	T62.2X3	T62.2X4	—	—
Chemical substance NEC	T65.91	T65.92	T65.93	T65.94	—	—
Chenodeoxycholic acid	T47.5X1	T47.5X2	T47.5X3	T47.5X4	T47.5X5	T47.5X6
Chenodiol	T47.5X1	T47.5X2	T47.5X3	T47.5X4	T47.5X5	T47.5X6
Chenopodium	T37.4X1	T37.4X2	T37.4X3	T37.4X4	T37.4X5	T37.4X6
Cherry laurel	T62.2X1	T62.2X2	T62.2X3	T62.2X4	—	—
Chinidin(e)	T46.2X1	T46.2X2	T46.2X3	T46.2X4	T46.2X5	T46.2X6
Chiniofon	T37.8X1	T37.8X2	T37.8X3	T37.8X4	T37.8X5	T37.8X6
Chlophedianol	T48.3X1	T48.3X2	T48.3X3	T48.3X4	T48.3X5	T48.3X6
Chloral	T42.6X1	T42.6X2	T42.6X3	T42.6X4	T42.6X5	T42.6X6
derivative	T42.6X1	T42.6X2	T42.6X3	T42.6X4	T42.6X5	T42.6X6
hydrate	T42.6X1	T42.6X2	T42.6X3	T42.6X4	T42.6X5	T42.6X6
Chloralamide	T42.6X1	T42.6X2	T42.6X3	T42.6X4	T42.6X5	T42.6X6
Chloralodol	T42.6X1	T42.6X2	T42.6X3	T42.6X4	T42.6X5	T42.6X6
Chloralose	T60.4X1	T60.4X2	T60.4X3	T60.4X4	—	—
Chlorambucil	T45.1X1	T45.1X2	T45.1X3	T45.1X4	T45.1X5	T45.1X6
Chloramine	T57.8X1	T57.8X2	T57.8X3	T57.8X4	—	—
T	T49.0X1	T49.0X2	T49.0X3	T49.0X4	T49.0X5	T49.0X6
topical	T49.0X1	T49.0X2	T49.0X3	T49.0X4	T49.0X5	T49.0X6
Chloramphenicol	T36.2X1	T36.2X2	T36.2X3	T36.2X4	T36.2X5	T36.2X6
ENT agent	T49.6X1	T49.6X2	T49.6X3	T49.6X4	T49.6X5	T49.6X6
ophthalmic preparation	T49.5X1	T49.5X2	T49.5X3	T49.5X4	T49.5X5	T49.5X6
topical NEC	T49.0X1	T49.0X2	T49.0X3	T49.0X4	T49.0X5	T49.0X6
Chlorate (potassium) (sodium) NEC	T60.3X1	T60.3X2	T60.3X3	T60.3X4		
herbicide	T60.3X1	T60.3X2	T60.3X3	T60.3X4	—	—
Chlorazanil	T50.2X1	T50.2X2	T50.2X3	T50.2X4	T50.2X5	T50.2X6
Chlorbenzene, chlorbenzol	T53.7X1	T53.7X2	T53.7X3	T53.7X4		
Chlorbenzoxamine	T44.3X1	T44.3X2	T44.3X3	T44.3X4	T44.3X5	T44.3X6
Chlorbutol	T42.6X1	T42.6X2	T42.6X3	T42.6X4	T42.6X5	T42.6X6
Chlorcyclizine	T45.0X1	T45.0X2	T45.0X3	T45.0X4	T45.0X5	T45.0X6

◀ New ◀ Revised ~~deleted~~ Deleted

Substance	Poisoning, Accidental (Unintentional)	Poisoning, Intentional Self-Harm	Poisoning, Assault	Poisoning, Undetermined	Adverse Effect	Underdosing
Chlordan(e) (dust)	T60.1X1	T60.1X2	T60.1X3	T60.1X4	—	—
Chlordantoin	T49.0X1	T49.0X2	T49.0X3	T49.0X4	T49.0X5	T49.0X6
Chlordiazepoxide	T42.4X1	T42.4X2	T42.4X3	T42.4X4	T42.4X5	T42.4X6
Chlordiethyl benzamide	T49.3X1	T49.3X2	T49.3X3	T49.3X4	T49.3X5	T49.3X6
Chloresium	T49.8X1	T49.8X2	T49.8X3	T49.8X4	T49.8X5	T49.8X6
Chlorethiazol	T42.6X1	T42.6X2	T42.6X3	T42.6X4	T42.6X5	T42.6X6
Chlorethyl — see Ethyl chloride						
Chloretone	T42.6X1	T42.6X2	T42.6X3	T42.6X4	T42.6X5	T42.6X6
Chlorex	T53.6X1	T53.6X2	T53.6X3	T53.6X4	—	—
insecticide	T60.1X1	T60.1X2	T60.1X3	T60.1X4	—	—
Chlorfenvinphos	T60.0X1	T60.0X2	T60.0X3	T60.0X4	—	—
Chlorhexadol	T42.6X1	T42.6X2	T42.6X3	T42.6X4	T42.6X5	T42.6X6
Chlorhexamide	T45.1X1	T45.1X2	T45.1X3	T45.1X4	T45.1X5	T45.1X6
Chlorhexidine	T49.0X1	T49.0X2	T49.0X3	T49.0X4	T49.0X5	T49.0X6
Chlorhydroxyquinolin	T49.0X1	T49.0X2	T49.0X3	T49.0X4	T49.0X5	T49.0X6
Chloride of lime (bleach)	T54.3X1	T54.3X2	T54.3X3	T54.3X4	—	—
Chlorimipramine	T43.011	T43.012	T43.013	T43.014	T43.015	T43.016
Chlorinated						
camphene	T53.6X1	T53.6X2	T53.6X3	T53.6X4	—	—
diphenyl	T53.7X1	T53.7X2	T53.7X3	T53.7X4	—	—
hydrocarbons NEC	T53.91	T53.92	T53.93	T53.94	—	—
solvents	T53.91	T53.92	T53.93	T53.94	—	—
lime (bleach)	T54.3X1	T54.3X2	T54.3X3	T54.3X4	—	—
and boric acid solution	T49.0X1	T49.0X2	T49.0X3	T49.0X4	T49.0X5	T49.0X6
naphthalene (insecticide)	T60.1X1	T60.1X2	T60.1X3	T60.1X4	—	—
industrial (non-pesticide)	T53.7X1	T53.7X2	T53.7X3	T53.7X4	—	—
pesticide NEC	T60.8X1	T60.8X2	T60.8X3	T60.8X4	—	—
soda — see also sodium hypochlorite						
solution	T49.0X1	T49.0X2	T49.0X3	T49.0X4	T49.0X5	T49.0X6
Chlorine (fumes) (gas)	T59.4X1	T59.4X2	T59.4X3	T59.4X4	—	—
bleach	T54.3X1	T54.3X2	T54.3X3	T54.3X4	—	—
compound gas NEC	T59.4X1	T59.4X2	T59.4X3	T59.4X4	—	—
disinfectant	T59.4X1	T59.4X2	T59.4X3	T59.4X4	—	—
releasing agents NEC	T59.4X1	T59.4X2	T59.4X3	T59.4X4	—	—
Chlorisondamine chloride	T46.991	T46.992	T46.993	T46.994	T46.995	T46.996
Chlormadinone	T38.5X1	T38.5X2	T38.5X3	T38.5X4	T38.5X5	T38.5X6
Chlormephos	T60.0X1	T60.0X2	T60.0X3	T60.0X4	—	—
Chlormerodrin	T50.2X1	T50.2X2	T50.2X3	T50.2X4	T50.2X5	T50.2X6
Chlormethiazole	T42.6X1	T42.6X2	T42.6X3	T42.6X4	T42.6X5	T42.6X6
Chlormethine	T45.1X1	T45.1X2	T45.1X3	T45.1X4	T45.1X5	T45.1X6
Chlormethylenecycline	T36.4X1	T36.4X2	T36.4X3	T36.4X4	T36.4X5	T36.4X6

Substance	Poisoning, Accidental (Unintentional)	Poisoning, Intentional Self-Harm	Poisoning, Assault	Poisoning, Undetermined	Adverse Effect	Underdosing
Chlormezanone	T42.6X1	T42.6X2	T42.6X3	T42.6X4	T42.6X5	T42.6X6
Chloroacetic acid	T60.3X1	T60.3X2	T60.3X3	T60.3X4	—	—
Chloroacetone	T59.3X1	T59.3X2	T59.3X3	T59.3X4	—	—
Chloroacetophenone	T59.3X1	T59.3X2	T59.3X3	T59.3X4	—	—
Chloroaniline	T53.7X1	T53.7X2	T53.7X3	T53.7X4	—	—
Chlorobenzene, chlorobenzol	T53.7X1	T53.7X2	T53.7X3	T53.7X4	—	—
Chlorobromomethane (fire extinguisher)	T53.6X1	T53.6X2	T53.6X3	T53.6X4	—	—
Chlorobutanol	T49.0X1	T49.0X2	T49.0X3	T49.0X4	T49.0X5	T49.0X6
Chlorocresol	T49.0X1	T49.0X2	T49.0X3	T49.0X4	T49.0X5	T49.0X6
Chlorodehydro-methyltestosterone	T38.7X1	T38.7X2	T38.7X3	T38.7X4	T38.7X5	T38.7X6
Chlorodinitrobenzene	T53.7X1	T53.7X2	T53.7X3	T53.7X4	—	—
dust or vapor	T53.7X1	T53.7X2	T53.7X3	T53.7X4	—	—
Chlorodiphenyl	T53.7X1	T53.7X2	T53.7X3	T53.7X4	—	—
Chloroethane — see Ethyl chloride						
Chloroethylene	T53.6X1	T53.6X2	T53.6X3	T53.6X4	—	—
Chlorofluorocarbons	T53.5X1	T53.5X2	T53.5X3	T53.5X4	—	—
Chloroform (fumes) (vapor)	T53.1X1	T53.1X2	T53.1X3	T53.1X4	—	—
anesthetic	T41.0X1	T41.0X2	T41.0X3	T41.0X4	T41.0X5	T41.0X6
solvent	T53.1X1	T53.1X2	T53.1X3	T53.1X4	—	—
water, concentrated	T41.0X1	T41.0X2	T41.0X3	T41.0X4	T41.0X5	T41.0X6
Chloroguanide	T37.2X1	T37.2X2	T37.2X3	T37.2X4	T37.2X5	T37.2X6
Chloromycetin	T36.2X1	T36.2X2	T36.2X3	T36.2X4	T36.2X5	T36.2X6
ENT agent	T49.6X1	T49.6X2	T49.6X3	T49.6X4	T49.6X5	T49.6X6
ophthalmic preparation	T49.5X1	T49.5X2	T49.5X3	T49.5X4	T49.5X5	T49.5X6
otic solution	T49.6X1	T49.6X2	T49.6X3	T49.6X4	T49.6X5	T49.6X6
topical NEC	T49.0X1	T49.0X2	T49.0X3	T49.0X4	T49.0X5	T49.0X6
Chloronitrobenzene	T53.7X1	T53.7X2	T53.7X3	T53.7X4	—	—
dust or vapor	T53.7X1	T53.7X2	T53.7X3	T53.7X4	—	—
Chlorophacinone	T60.4X1	T60.4X2	T60.4X3	T60.4X4	—	—
Chlorophenol	T53.7X1	T53.7X2	T53.7X3	T53.7X4	—	—
Chlorophenothane	T60.1X1	T60.1X2	T60.1X3	T60.1X4	—	—
Chlorophyll	T50.991	T50.992	T50.993	T50.994	T50.995	T50.996
Chloropicrin (fumes)	T53.6X1	T53.6X2	T53.6X3	T53.6X4	—	—
fumigant	T60.8X1	T60.8X2	T60.8X3	T60.8X4	—	—
fungicide	T60.3X1	T60.3X2	T60.3X3	T60.3X4	—	—
pesticide	T60.8X1	T60.8X2	T60.8X3	T60.8X4	—	—
Chloroprocaine	T41.3X1	T41.3X2	T41.3X3	T41.3X4	T41.3X5	T41.3X6
infiltration (subcutaneous)	T41.3X1	T41.3X2	T41.3X3	T41.3X4	T41.3X5	T41.3X6
nerve block (peripheral) (plexus)	T41.3X1	T41.3X2	T41.3X3	T41.3X4	T41.3X5	T41.3X6
spinal	T41.3X1	T41.3X2	T41.3X3	T41.3X4	T41.3X5	T41.3X6

◀ New   ◀ Revised   ~~deleted~~ Deleted

	External Cause (T-Code)					
Substance	Poisoning, Accidental (Unintentional)	Poisoning, Intentional Self-Harm	Poisoning, Assault	Poisoning, Undetermined	Adverse Effect	Underdosing
Chloroptic	T49.5X1	T49.5X2	T49.5X3	T49.5X4	T49.5X5	T49.5X6
Chloropurine	T45.1X1	T45.1X2	T45.1X3	T45.1X4	T45.1X5	T45.1X6
Chloropyramine	T45.0X1	T45.0X2	T45.0X3	T45.0X4	T45.0X5	T45.0X6
Chloropyrifos	T60.0X1	T60.0X2	T60.0X3	T60.0X4	—	—
Chloropyrilene	T45.0X1	T45.0X2	T45.0X3	T45.0X4	T45.0X5	T45.0X6
Chloroquine	T37.2X1	T37.2X2	T37.2X3	T37.2X4	T37.2X5	T37.2X6
Chlorothalonil	T60.3X1	T60.3X2	T60.3X3	T60.3X4	—	—
Chlorothen	T45.0X1	T45.0X2	T45.0X3	T45.0X4	T45.0X5	T45.0X6
Chlorothiazide	T50.2X1	T50.2X2	T50.2X3	T50.2X4	T50.2X5	T50.2X6
Chlorothymol	T49.4X1	T49.4X2	T49.4X3	T49.4X4	T49.4X5	T49.4X6
Chlorotrianisene	T38.5X1	T38.5X2	T38.5X3	T38.5X4	T38.5X5	T38.5X6
Chlorovinyldichloro-arsine, not in war	T57.0X1	T57.0X2	T57.0X3	T57.0X4	—	—
Chloroxine	T49.4X1	T49.4X2	T49.4X3	T49.4X4	T49.4X5	T49.4X6
Chloroxylenol	T49.0X1	T49.0X2	T49.0X3	T49.0X4	T49.0X5	T49.0X6
Chlorphenamine	T45.0X1	T45.0X2	T45.0X3	T45.0X4	T45.0X5	T45.0X6
Chlorphenesin	T42.8X1	T42.8X2	T42.8X3	T42.8X4	T42.8X5	T42.8X6
topical (antifungal)	T49.0X1	T49.0X2	T49.0X3	T49.0X4	T49.0X5	T49.0X6
Chlorpheniramine	T45.0X1	T45.0X2	T45.0X3	T45.0X4	T45.0X5	T45.0X6
Chlorphenoxamine	T45.0X1	T45.0X2	T45.0X3	T45.0X4	T45.0X5	T45.0X6
Chlorphentermine	T50.5X1	T50.5X2	T50.5X3	T50.5X4	T50.5X5	T50.5X6
Chlorprocaine — see Chloroprocaine						
Chlorproguanil	T37.2X1	T37.2X2	T37.2X3	T37.2X4	T37.2X5	T37.2X6
Chlorpromazine	T43.3X1	T43.3X2	T43.3X3	T43.3X4	T43.3X5	T43.3X6
Chlorpropamide	T38.3X1	T38.3X2	T38.3X3	T38.3X4	T38.3X5	T38.3X6
Chlorprothixene	T43.4X1	T43.4X2	T43.4X3	T43.4X4	T43.4X5	T43.4X6
Chlorquinaldol	T49.0X1	T49.0X2	T49.0X3	T49.0X4	T49.0X5	T49.0X6
Chlorquinol	T49.0X1	T49.0X2	T49.0X3	T49.0X4	T49.0X5	T49.0X6
Chlortalidone	T50.2X1	T50.2X2	T50.2X3	T50.2X4	T50.2X5	T50.2X6
Chlortetracycline	T36.4X1	T36.4X2	T36.4X3	T36.4X4	T36.4X5	T36.4X6
Chlorthalidone	T50.2X1	T50.2X2	T50.2X3	T50.2X4	T50.2X5	T50.2X6
Chlorthiophos	T60.0X1	T60.0X2	T60.0X3	T60.0X4	—	—
Chlorotrianisene	T38.5X1	T38.5X2	T38.5X3	T38.5X4	T38.5X5	T38.5X6
Chlor-Trimeton	T45.0X1	T45.0X2	T45.0X3	T45.0X4	T45.0X5	T45.0X6
Chlorthion	T60.0X1	T60.0X2	T60.0X3	T60.0X4	—	—
Chlorzoxazone	T42.8X1	T42.8X2	T42.8X3	T42.8X4	T42.8X5	T42.8X6
Choke damp	T59.7X1	T59.7X2	T59.7X3	T59.7X4	—	—
Cholagogues	T47.5X1	T47.5X2	T47.5X3	T47.5X4	T47.5X5	T47.5X6
Cholebrine	T50.8X1	T50.8X2	T50.8X3	T50.8X4	T50.8X5	T50.8X6
Cholecalciferol	T45.2X1	T45.2X2	T45.2X3	T45.2X4	T45.2X5	T45.2X6
Cholecystokinin	T50.8X1	T50.8X2	T50.8X3	T50.8X4	T50.8X5	T50.8X6
Cholera vaccine	T50.A91	T50.A92	T50.A93	T50.A94	T50.A95	T50.A96

	External Cause (T-Code)					
Substance	Poisoning, Accidental (Unintentional)	Poisoning, Intentional Self-Harm	Poisoning, Assault	Poisoning, Undetermined	Adverse Effect	Underdosing
Choleretic	T47.5X1	T47.5X2	T47.5X3	T47.5X4	T47.5X5	T47.5X6
Cholesterol-lowering agents	T46.6X1	T46.6X2	T46.6X3	T46.6X4	T46.6X5	T46.6X6
Cholestyramine (resin)	T46.6X1	T46.6X2	T46.6X3	T46.6X4	T46.6X5	T46.6X6
Cholic acid	T47.5X1	T47.5X2	T47.5X3	T47.5X4	T47.5X5	T47.5X6
Choline	T48.6X1	T48.6X2	T48.6X3	T48.6X4	T48.6X5	T48.6X6
chloride	T50.991	T50.992	T50.993	T50.994	T50.995	T50.996
dihydrogen citrate	T50.991	T50.992	T50.993	T50.994	T50.995	T50.996
salicylate	T39.091	T39.092	T39.093	T39.094	T39.095	T39.096
theophyllinate	T48.6X1	T48.6X2	T48.6X3	T48.6X4	T48.6X5	T48.6X6
Cholinergic (drug) NEC	T44.1X1	T44.1X2	T44.1X3	T44.1X4	T44.1X5	T44.1X6
muscle tone enhancer	T44.1X1	T44.1X2	T44.1X3	T44.1X4	T44.1X5	T44.1X6
organophosphorus	T44.0X1	T44.0X2	T44.0X3	T44.0X4	T44.0X5	T44.0X6
insecticide	T60.0X1	T60.0X2	T60.0X3	T60.0X4	—	—
nerve gas	T59.891	T59.892	T59.893	T59.894	—	—
trimethyl ammonium propanediol	T44.1X1	T44.1X2	T44.1X3	T44.1X4	T44.1X5	T44.1X6
Cholinesterase reactivator	T50.6X1	T50.6X2	T50.6X3	T50.6X4	T50.6X5	T50.6X6
Cholografin	T50.8X1	T50.8X2	T50.8X3	T50.8X4	T50.8X5	T50.8X6
Chorionic gonadotropin	T38.891	T38.892	T38.893	T38.894	T38.895	T38.896
Chromate	T56.2X1	T56.2X2	T56.2X3	T56.2X4	—	—
dust or mist	T56.2X1	T56.2X2	T56.2X3	T56.2X4	—	—
lead — see also lead	T56.0X1	T56.0X2	T56.0X3	T56.0X4	—	—
paint	T56.0X1	T56.0X2	T56.0X3	T56.0X4	—	—
Chromic						
acid	T56.2X1	T56.2X2	T56.2X3	T56.2X4	—	—
dust or mist	T56.2X1	T56.2X2	T56.2X3	T56.2X4	—	—
phosphate 32P	T45.1X1	T45.1X2	T45.1X3	T45.1X4	T45.1X5	T45.1X6
Chromium	T56.2X1	T56.2X2	T56.2X3	T56.2X4	—	—
compounds — see Chromate						
sesquioxide	T50.8X1	T50.8X2	T50.8X3	T50.8X4	T50.8X5	T50.8X6
Chromomycin A3	T45.1X1	T45.1X2	T45.1X3	T45.1X4	T45.1X5	T45.1X6
Chromonar	T46.3X1	T46.3X2	T46.3X3	T46.3X4	T46.3X5	T46.3X6
Chromyl chloride	T56.2X1	T56.2X2	T56.2X3	T56.2X4	—	—
Chrysarobin	T49.4X1	T49.4X2	T49.4X3	T49.4X4	T49.4X5	T49.4X6
Chrysazin	T47.2X1	T47.2X2	T47.2X3	T47.2X4	T47.2X5	T47.2X6
Chymar	T45.3X1	T45.3X2	T45.3X3	T45.3X4	T45.3X5	T45.3X6
ophthalmic preparation	T49.5X1	T49.5X2	T49.5X3	T49.5X4	T49.5X5	T49.5X6
Chymopapain	T45.3X1	T45.3X2	T45.3X3	T45.3X4	T45.3X5	T45.3X6
Chymotrypsin	T45.3X1	T45.3X2	T45.3X3	T45.3X4	T45.3X5	T45.3X6
ophthalmic preparation	T49.5X1	T49.5X2	T49.5X3	T49.5X4	T49.5X5	T49.5X6
Cianidanol	T50.991	T50.992	T50.993	T50.994	T50.995	T50.996
Cianopramine	T43.011	T43.012	T43.013	T43.014	T43.015	T43.016
Cibenzoline	T46.2X1	T46.2X2	T46.2X3	T46.2X4	T46.2X5	T46.2X6

◀ New   ◀◀ Revised   ~~deleted~~ Deleted

Substance	Poisoning, Accidental (Unintentional)	Poisoning, Intentional Self-Harm	Poisoning, Assault	Poisoning, Undetermined	Adverse Effect	Underdosing
Ciclacillin	T36.0X1	T36.0X2	T36.0X3	T36.0X4	T36.0X5	T36.0X6
Ciclobarbital — see Hexobarbital						
Ciclonicate	T46.7X1	T46.7X2	T46.7X3	T46.7X4	T46.7X5	T46.7X6
Ciclopirox (olamine)	T49.0X1	T49.0X2	T49.0X3	T49.0X4	T49.0X5	T49.0X6
Ciclosporin	T45.1X1	T45.1X2	T45.1X3	T45.1X4	T45.1X5	T45.1X6
Cicuta maculata or virosa	T62.2X1	T62.2X2	T62.2X3	T62.2X4	—	—
Cicutoxin	T62.2X1	T62.2X2	T62.2X3	T62.2X4	—	—
Cigarette lighter fluid	T52.0X1	T52.0X2	T52.0X3	T52.0X4	—	—
Cigarettes (tobacco)	T65.221	T65.222	T65.223	T65.224		
Ciguatoxin	T61.01	T61.02	T61.03	T61.04	—	—
Cilazapril	T46.4X1	T46.4X2	T46.4X3	T46.4X4	T46.4X5	T46.4X6
Cimetidine	T47.0X1	T47.0X2	T47.0X3	T47.0X4	T47.0X5	T47.0X6
Cimetropium bromide	T44.3X1	T44.3X2	T44.3X3	T44.3X4	T44.3X5	T44.3X6
Cinchocaine	T41.3X1	T41.3X2	T41.3X3	T41.3X4	T41.3X5	T41.3X6
topical (surface)	T41.3X1	T41.3X2	T41.3X3	T41.3X4	T41.3X5	T41.3X6
Cinchona	T37.2X1	T37.2X2	T37.2X3	T37.2X4	T37.2X5	T37.2X6
Cinchonine alkaloids	T37.2X1	T37.2X2	T37.2X3	T37.2X4	T37.2X5	T37.2X6
Cinchophen	T50.4X1	T50.4X2	T50.4X3	T50.4X4	T50.4X5	T50.4X6
Cinepazide	T46.7X1	T46.7X2	T46.7X3	T46.7X4	T46.7X5	T46.7X6
Cinnamedrine	T48.5X1	T48.5X2	T48.5X3	T48.5X4	T48.5X5	T48.5X6
Cinnarizine	T45.0X1	T45.0X2	T45.0X3	T45.0X4	T45.0X5	T45.0X6
Cinoxacin	T37.8X1	T37.8X2	T37.8X3	T37.8X4	T37.8X5	T37.8X6
Ciprofibrate	T46.6X1	T46.6X2	T46.6X3	T46.6X4	T46.6X5	T46.6X6
Ciprofloxacin	T36.8X1	T36.8X2	T36.8X3	T36.8X4	T36.8X5	T36.8X6
Cisapride	T47.8X1	T47.8X2	T47.8X3	T47.8X4	T47.8X5	T47.8X6
Cisplatin	T45.1X1	T45.1X2	T45.1X3	T45.1X4	T45.1X5	T45.1X6
Citalopram	T43.221	T43.222	T43.223	T43.224	T43.225	T43.226
Citanest	T41.3X1	T41.3X2	T41.3X3	T41.3X4	T41.3X5	T41.3X6
infiltration (subcutaneous)	T41.3X1	T41.3X2	T41.3X3	T41.3X4	T41.3X5	T41.3X6
nerve block (peripheral) (plexus)	T41.3X1	T41.3X2	T41.3X3	T41.3X4	T41.3X5	T41.3X6
Citric acid	T47.5X1	T47.5X2	T47.5X3	T47.5X4	T47.5X5	T47.5X6
Citrovorum (factor)	T45.8X1	T45.8X2	T45.8X3	T45.8X4	T45.8X5	T45.8X6
Claviceps purpurea	T62.2X1	T62.2X2	T62.2X3	T62.2X4	—	—
Clavulanic acid	T36.1X1	T36.1X2	T36.1X3	T36.1X4	T36.1X5	T36.1X6
Cleaner, cleansing agent, type not specified	T65.891	T65.892	T65.893	T65.894	—	—
of paint or varnish	T52.91	T52.92	T52.93	T52.94	—	—
specified type NEC	T65.891	T65.892	T65.893	T65.894	—	—
Clebopride	T47.8X1	T47.8X2	T47.8X3	T47.8X4	T47.8X5	T47.8X6
Clefamide	T37.3X1	T37.3X2	T37.3X3	T37.3X4	T37.3X5	T37.3X6
Clemastine	T45.0X1	T45.0X2	T45.0X3	T45.0X4	T45.0X5	T45.0X6
Clematis vitalba	T62.2X1	T62.2X2	T62.2X3	T62.2X4	—	—

Substance	Poisoning, Accidental (Unintentional)	Poisoning, Intentional Self-Harm	Poisoning, Assault	Poisoning, Undetermined	Adverse Effect	Underdosing
Clemizole	T45.0X1	T45.0X2	T45.0X3	T45.0X4	T45.0X5	T45.0X6
penicillin	T36.0X1	T36.0X2	T36.0X3	T36.0X4	T36.0X5	T36.0X6
Clenbuterol	T48.6X1	T48.6X2	T48.6X3	T48.6X4	T48.6X5	T48.6X6
Clidinium bromide	T44.3X1	T44.3X2	T44.3X3	T44.3X4	T44.3X5	T44.3X6
Clindamycin	T36.8X1	T36.8X2	T36.8X3	T36.8X4	T36.8X5	T36.8X6
Clinofibrate	T46.6X1	T46.6X2	T46.6X3	T46.6X4	T46.6X5	T46.6X6
Clioquinol	T37.8X1	T37.8X2	T37.8X3	T37.8X4	T37.8X5	T37.8X6
Cliradon	T40.2X1	T40.2X2	T40.2X3	T40.2X4	—	—
Clobazam	T42.4X1	T42.4X2	T42.4X3	T42.4X4	T42.4X5	T42.4X6
Clobenzorex	T50.5X1	T50.5X2	T50.5X3	T50.5X4	T50.5X5	T50.5X6
Clobetasol	T49.0X1	T49.0X2	T49.0X3	T49.0X4	T49.0X5	T49.0X6
Clobetasone	T49.0X1	T49.0X2	T49.0X3	T49.0X4	T49.0X5	T49.0X6
Clobutinol	T48.3X1	T48.3X2	T48.3X3	T48.3X4	T48.3X5	T48.3X6
Clocapramine	T43.0X1	T43.0X2	T43.0X3	T43.0X4	T43.0X5	T43.0X6
Clocortolone	T38.0X1	T38.0X2	T38.0X3	T38.0X4	T38.0X5	T38.0X6
Clodantoin	T49.0X1	T49.0X2	T49.0X3	T49.0X4	T49.0X5	T49.0X6
Clodronic acid	T50.991	T50.992	T50.993	T50.994	T50.995	T50.996
Clofazimine	T37.1X1	T37.1X2	T37.1X3	T37.1X4	T37.1X5	T37.1X6
Clofedanol	T48.3X1	T48.3X2	T48.3X3	T48.3X4	T48.3X5	T48.3X6
Clofenamide	T50.2X1	T50.2X2	T50.2X3	T50.2X4	T50.2X5	T50.2X6
Clofenotane	T49.0X1	T49.0X2	T49.0X3	T49.0X4	T49.0X5	T49.0X6
Clofezone	T39.2X1	T39.2X2	T39.2X3	T39.2X4	T39.2X5	T39.2X6
Clofibrate	T46.6X1	T46.6X2	T46.6X3	T46.6X4	T46.6X5	T46.6X6
Clofibride	T46.6X1	T46.6X2	T46.6X3	T46.6X4	T46.6X5	T46.6X6
Cloforex	T50.5X1	T50.5X2	T50.5X3	T50.5X4	T50.5X5	T50.5X6
Clomacran	T43.0X1	T43.0X2	T43.0X3	T43.0X4	T43.0X5	T43.0X6
Clomethiazole	T42.6X1	T42.6X2	T42.6X3	T42.6X4	T42.6X5	T42.6X6
Clometocillin	T36.0X1	T36.0X2	T36.0X3	T36.0X4	T36.0X5	T36.0X6
Clomifene	T38.5X1	T38.5X2	T38.5X3	T38.5X4	T38.5X5	T38.5X6
Clomiphene	T38.5X1	T38.5X2	T38.5X3	T38.5X4	T38.5X5	T38.5X6
Clomipramine	T43.011	T43.012	T43.013	T43.014	T43.015	T43.016
Clomocycline	T36.4X1	T36.4X2	T36.4X3	T36.4X4	T36.4X5	T36.4X6
Clonazepam	T42.4X1	T42.4X2	T42.4X3	T42.4X4	T42.4X5	T42.4X6
Clonidine	T46.5X1	T46.5X2	T46.5X3	T46.5X4	T46.5X5	T46.5X6
Clonixin	T39.8X1	T39.8X2	T39.8X3	T39.8X4	T39.8X5	T39.8X6
Clopamide	T50.2X1	T50.2X2	T50.2X3	T50.2X4	T50.2X5	T50.2X6
Clopenthixol	T43.4X1	T43.4X2	T43.4X3	T43.4X4	T43.4X5	T43.4X6
Cloperastine	T48.3X1	T48.3X2	T48.3X3	T48.3X4	T48.3X5	T48.3X6
Clophedianol	T48.3X1	T48.3X2	T48.3X3	T48.3X4	T48.3X5	T48.3X6
Cloponone	T36.2X1	T36.2X2	T36.2X3	T36.2X4	T36.2X5	T36.2X6
Cloprednol	T38.0X1	T38.0X2	T38.0X3	T38.0X4	T38.0X5	T38.0X6
Cloral betaine	T42.6X1	T42.6X2	T42.6X3	T42.6X4	T42.6X5	T42.6X6

◀ New   ◀ Revised   ~~deleted~~ Deleted

TABLE OF DRUGS AND CHEMICALS

Substance	External Cause (T-Code)					
	Poisoning, Accidental (Unintentional)	Poisoning, Intentional Self-Harm	Poisoning, Assault	Poisoning, Undetermined	Adverse Effect	Underdosing
Cloramfenicol	T36.2X1	T36.2X2	T36.2X3	T36.2X4	T36.2X5	T36.2X6
Clorazepate (dipotassium)	T42.4X1	T42.4X2	T42.4X3	T42.4X4	T42.4X5	T42.4X6
Clorexolone	T50.2X1	T50.2X2	T50.2X3	T50.2X4	T50.2X5	T50.2X6
Clorox (bleach)	T54.91	T54.92	T54.93	T54.94	—	—
Clorfenamine	T45.0X1	T45.0X2	T45.0X3	T45.0X4	T45.0X5	T45.0X6
Clorgiline	T43.1X1	T43.1X2	T43.1X3	T43.1X4	T43.1X5	T43.1X6
Clorotepine	T44.3X1	T44.3X2	T44.3X3	T44.3X4	T44.3X5	T44.3X6
Clorprenaline	T48.6X1	T48.6X2	T48.6X3	T48.6X4	T48.6X5	T48.6X6
Clortermine	T50.5X1	T50.5X2	T50.5X3	T50.5X4	T50.5X5	T50.5X6
Clotiapine	T43.591	T43.592	T43.593	T43.594	T43.595	T43.596
Clotiazepam	T42.4X1	T42.4X2	T42.4X3	T42.4X4	T42.4X5	T42.4X6
Clotibric acid	T46.6X1	T46.6X2	T46.6X3	T46.6X4	T46.6X5	T46.6X6
Clotrimazole	T49.0X1	T49.0X2	T49.0X3	T49.0X4	T49.0X5	T49.0X6
Cloxacillin	T36.0X1	T36.0X2	T36.0X3	T36.0X4	T36.0X5	T36.0X6
Cloxazolam	T42.4X1	T42.4X2	T42.4X3	T42.4X4	T42.4X5	T42.4X6
Cloxiquine	T49.0X1	T49.0X2	T49.0X3	T49.0X4	T49.0X5	T49.0X6
Clozapine	T42.4X1	T42.4X2	T42.4X3	T42.4X4	T42.4X5	T42.4X6
Coagulant NEC	T45.7X1	T45.7X2	T45.7X3	T45.7X4	T45.7X5	T45.7X6
Coal (carbon monoxide from) — see also Carbon, monoxide, coal	T58.2X1	T58.2X2	T58.2X3	T58.2X4	—	—
oil — see Kerosene						
tar	T49.1X1	T49.1X2	T49.1X3	T49.1X4	T49.1X5	T49.1X6
fumes	T59.891	T59.892	T59.893	T59.894	—	—
medicinal (ointment)	T49.4X1	T49.4X2	T49.4X3	T49.4X4	T49.4X5	T49.4X6
analgesics NEC	T39.2X1	T39.2X2	T39.2X3	T39.2X4	T39.2X5	T39.2X6
naphtha (solvent)	T52.0X1	T52.0X2	T52.0X3	T52.0X4		
Cobalamine	T45.2X1	T45.2X2	T45.2X3	T45.2X4	T45.2X5	T45.2X6
Cobalt (nonmedicinal) (fumes) (industrial)	T56.891	T56.892	T56.893	T56.894		
medicinal (trace) (chloride)	T45.8X1	T45.8X2	T45.8X3	T45.8X4	T45.8X5	T45.8X6
Cobra (venom)	T63.041	T63.042	T63.043	T63.044		
Coca (leaf)	T40.5X1	T40.5X2	T40.5X3	T40.5X4	T40.5X5	T40.5X6
Cocaine	T40.5X1	T40.5X2	T40.5X3	T40.5X4	T40.5X5	T40.5X6
topical anesthetic	T41.3X1	T41.3X2	T41.3X3	T41.3X4	T41.3X5	T41.3X6
Cocarboxylase	T45.3X1	T45.3X2	T45.3X3	T45.3X4	T45.3X5	T45.3X6
Coccidioidin	T50.8X1	T50.8X2	T50.8X3	T50.8X4	T50.8X5	T50.8X6
Cocculus indicus	T62.1X1	T62.1X2	T62.1X3	T62.1X4		
Cochineal	T65.6X1	T65.6X2	T65.6X3	T65.6X4		
medicinal products	T50.991	T50.992	T50.993	T50.994	T50.995	T50.996
Codeine	T40.2X1	T40.2X2	T40.2X3	T40.2X4	T40.2X5	T40.2X6
Cod-liver oil	T45.2X1	T45.2X2	T45.2X3	T45.2X4	T45.2X5	T45.2X6

Substance	External Cause (T-Code)					
	Poisoning, Accidental (Unintentional)	Poisoning, Intentional Self-Harm	Poisoning, Assault	Poisoning, Undetermined	Adverse Effect	Underdosing
Coenzyme A	T50.991	T50.992	T50.993	T50.994	T50.995	T50.996
Coffee	T62.8X1	T62.8X2	T62.8X3	T62.8X4	—	—
Cogalactoisomerase	T50.991	T50.992	T50.993	T50.994	T50.995	T50.996
Cogentin	T44.3X1	T44.3X2	T44.3X3	T44.3X4	T44.3X5	T44.3X6
Coke fumes or gas (carbon monoxide)	T58.2X1	T58.2X2	T58.2X3	T58.2X4	—	—
industrial use	T58.8X1	T58.8X2	T58.8X3	T58.8X4	—	—
Colace	T47.4X1	T47.4X2	T47.4X3	T47.4X4	T47.4X5	T47.4X6
Colaspase	T45.1X1	T45.1X2	T45.1X3	T45.1X4	T45.1X5	T45.1X6
Colchicine	T50.4X1	T50.4X2	T50.4X3	T50.4X4	T50.4X5	T50.4X6
Colchicum	T62.2X1	T62.2X2	T62.2X3	T62.2X4	—	—
Cold cream	T49.3X1	T49.3X2	T49.3X3	T49.3X4	T49.3X5	T49.3X6
Colecalciferol	T45.2X1	T45.2X2	T45.2X3	T45.2X4	T45.2X5	T45.2X6
Colestipol	T46.6X1	T46.6X2	T46.6X3	T46.6X4	T46.6X5	T46.6X6
Colestyramine	T46.6X1	T46.6X2	T46.6X3	T46.6X4	T46.6X5	T46.6X6
Colimycin	T36.8X1	T36.8X2	T36.8X3	T36.8X4	T36.8X5	T36.8X6
Colistimethate	T36.8X1	T36.8X2	T36.8X3	T36.8X4	T36.8X5	T36.8X6
Colistin	T36.8X1	T36.8X2	T36.8X3	T36.8X4	T36.8X5	T36.8X6
sulfate (eye preparation)	T49.5X1	T49.5X2	T49.5X3	T49.5X4	T49.5X5	T49.5X6
Collagen	T50.991	T50.992	T50.993	T50.994	T50.995	T50.996
Collagenase	T49.4X1	T49.4X2	T49.4X3	T49.4X4	T49.4X5	T49.4X6
Collodion	T49.3X1	T49.3X2	T49.3X3	T49.3X4	T49.3X5	T49.3X6
Colocynth	T47.2X1	T47.2X2	T47.2X3	T47.2X4	T47.2X5	T47.2X6
Colophony adhesive	T49.3X1	T49.3X2	T49.3X3	T49.3X4	T49.3X5	T49.3X6
Colorant — see also Dye	T50.991	T50.992	T50.993	T50.994	T50.995	T50.996
Coloring matter — see Dye(s)						
Combustion gas (after combustion) — see Carbon, monoxide						
prior to combustion	T59.891	T59.892	T59.893	T59.894	—	—
Compazine	T43.3X1	T43.3X2	T43.3X3	T43.3X4	T43.3X5	T43.3X6
Compound						
42 (warfarin)	T60.4X1	T60.4X2	T60.4X3	T60.4X4	—	—
269 (endrin)	T60.1X1	T60.1X2	T60.1X3	T60.1X4	—	—
497 (dieldrin)	T60.1X1	T60.1X2	T60.1X3	T60.1X4	—	—
1080 (sodium fluoroacetate)	T60.4X1	T60.4X2	T60.4X3	T60.4X4	—	—
3422 (parathion)	T60.0X1	T60.0X2	T60.0X3	T60.0X4	—	—
3911 (phorate)	T60.0X1	T60.0X2	T60.0X3	T60.0X4	—	—
3956 (toxaphene)	T60.1X1	T60.1X2	T60.1X3	T60.1X4	—	—
4049 (malathion)	T60.0X1	T60.0X2	T60.0X3	T60.0X4	—	—
4069 (malathion)	T60.0X1	T60.0X2	T60.0X3	T60.0X4	—	—
4124 (dicapthon)	T60.0X1	T60.0X2	T60.0X3	T60.0X4	—	—

◀ New   ◀ Revised   ~~deleted~~ Deleted

	External Cause (T-Code)					
Substance	Poisoning, Accidental (Unintentional)	Poisoning, Intentional Self-Harm	Poisoning, Assault	Poisoning, Undetermined	Adverse Effect	Underdosing
Compound *(Continued)*						
E (cortisone)	T38.0X1	T38.0X2	T38.0X3	T38.0X4	T38.0X5	T38.0X6
F (hydrocortisone)	T38.0X1	T38.0X2	T38.0X3	T38.0X4	T38.0X5	T38.0X6
Congener, anabolic	T38.7X1	T38.7X2	T38.7X3	T38.7X4	T38.7X5	T38.7X6
Congo red	T50.8X1	T50.8X2	T50.8X3	T50.8X4	T50.8X5	T50.8X6
Coniine, conine	T62.2X1	T62.2X2	T62.2X3	T62.2X4	—	—
Conium (maculatum)	T62.2X1	T62.2X2	T62.2X3	T62.2X4	—	—
Conjugated estrogenic substances	T38.5X1	T38.5X2	T38.5X3	T38.5X4	T38.5X5	T38.5X6
Contac	T48.5X1	T48.5X2	T48.5X3	T48.5X4	T48.5X5	T48.5X6
Contact lens solution	T49.5X1	T49.5X2	T49.5X3	T49.5X4	T49.5X5	T49.5X6
Contraceptive (oral)	T38.4X1	T38.4X2	T38.4X3	T38.4X4	T38.4X5	T38.4X6
vaginal	T49.8X1	T49.8X2	T49.8X3	T49.8X4	T49.8X5	T49.8X6
Contrast medium, radiography	T50.8X1	T50.8X2	T50.8X3	T50.8X4	T50.8X5	T50.8X6
Convallaria glycosides	T46.0X1	T46.0X2	T46.0X3	T46.0X4	T46.0X5	T46.0X6
Convallaria majalis	T62.2X1	T62.2X2	T62.2X3	T62.2X4	—	—
berry	T62.1X1	T62.1X2	T62.1X3	T62.1X4	—	—
Copper (dust) (fumes) (nonmedicinal) NEC	T56.4X1	T56.4X2	T56.4X3	T56.4X4	—	—
arsenate, arsenite	T57.0X1	T57.0X2	T57.0X3	T57.0X4	—	—
insecticide	T60.2X1	T60.2X2	T60.2X3	T60.2X4	—	—
emetic	T47.7X1	T47.7X2	T47.7X3	T47.7X4	T47.7X5	T47.7X6
fungicide	T60.3X1	T60.3X2	T60.3X3	T60.3X4	—	—
gluconate	T49.0X1	T49.0X2	T49.0X3	T49.0X4	T49.0X5	T49.0X6
insecticide	T60.2X1	T60.2X2	T60.2X3	T60.2X4	—	—
medicinal (trace)	T45.8X1	T45.8X2	T45.8X3	T45.8X4	T45.8X5	T45.8X6
oleate	T49.0X1	T49.0X2	T49.0X3	T49.0X4	T49.0X5	T49.0X6
sulfate	T56.4X1	T56.4X2	T56.4X3	T56.4X4	—	—
cupric	T56.4X1	T56.4X2	T56.4X3	T56.4X4	—	—
fungicide	T60.3X1	T60.3X2	T60.3X3	T60.3X4	—	—
medicinal						
ear	T49.6X1	T49.6X2	T49.6X3	T49.6X4	T49.6X5	T49.6X6
emetic	T47.7X1	T47.7X2	T47.7X3	T47.7X4	T47.7X5	T47.7X6
eye	T49.5X1	T49.5X2	T49.5X3	T49.5X4	T49.5X5	T49.5X6
cuprous	T56.4X1	T56.4X2	T56.4X3	T56.4X4	—	—
fungicide	T60.3X1	T60.3X2	T60.3X3	T60.3X4	—	—
medicinal						
ear	T49.6X1	T49.6X2	T49.6X3	T49.6X4	T49.6X5	T49.6X6
emetic	T47.7X1	T47.7X2	T47.7X3	T47.7X4	T47.7X5	T47.7X6
eye	T49.5X1	T49.5X2	T49.5X3	T49.5X4	T49.5X5	T49.5X6
Copperhead snake (bite) (venom)	T63.061	T63.062	T63.063	T63.064	—	—
Coral (sting)	T63.691	T63.692	T63.693	T63.694	—	—
snake (bite) (venom)	T63.021	T63.022	T63.023	T63.024	—	—

	External Cause (T-Code)					
Substance	Poisoning, Accidental (Unintentional)	Poisoning, Intentional Self-Harm	Poisoning, Assault	Poisoning, Undetermined	Adverse Effect	Underdosing
Corbadrine	T49.6X1	T49.6X2	T49.6X3	T49.6X4	T49.6X5	T49.6X6
Cordran	T49.0X1	T49.0X2	T49.0X3	T49.0X4	T49.0X5	T49.0X6
Cordite	T65.891	T65.892	T65.893	T65.894	—	—
vapor	T59.891	T59.892	T59.893	T59.894	—	—
Corn cures	T49.4X1	T49.4X2	T49.4X3	T49.4X4	T49.4X5	T49.4X6
Cornhusker's lotion	T49.3X1	T49.3X2	T49.3X3	T49.3X4	T49.3X5	T49.3X6
Corn starch	T49.3X1	T49.3X2	T49.3X3	T49.3X4	T49.3X5	T49.3X6
Coronary vasodilator NEC	T46.3X1	T46.3X2	T46.3X3	T46.3X4	T46.3X5	T46.3X6
Corrosive NEC	T54.91	T54.92	T54.93	T54.94	—	—
acid NEC	T54.2X1	T54.2X2	T54.2X3	T54.2X4	—	—
aromatics	T54.1X1	T54.1X2	T54.1X3	T54.1X4	—	—
disinfectant	T54.1X1	T54.1X2	T54.1X3	T54.1X4	—	—
fumes NEC	T54.91	T54.92	T54.93	T54.94	—	—
specified NEC	T54.91	T54.92	T54.93	T54.94	—	—
sublimate	T56.1X1	T56.1X2	T56.1X3	T56.1X4	—	—
Cortate	T38.0X1	T38.0X2	T38.0X3	T38.0X4	T38.0X5	T38.0X6
Cort-Dome	T38.0X1	T38.0X2	T38.0X3	T38.0X4	T38.0X5	T38.0X6
ENT agent	T49.6X1	T49.6X2	T49.6X3	T49.6X4	T49.6X5	T49.6X6
ophthalmic preparation	T49.5X1	T49.5X2	T49.5X3	T49.5X4	T49.5X5	T49.5X6
topical NEC	T49.0X1	T49.0X2	T49.0X3	T49.0X4	T49.0X5	T49.0X6
Cortef	T38.0X1	T38.0X2	T38.0X3	T38.0X4	T38.0X5	T38.0X6
ENT agent	T49.6X1	T49.6X2	T49.6X3	T49.6X4	T49.6X5	T49.6X6
ophthalmic preparation	T49.5X1	T49.5X2	T49.5X3	T49.5X4	T49.5X5	T49.5X6
topical NEC	T49.0X1	T49.0X2	T49.0X3	T49.0X4	T49.0X5	T49.0X6
Corticosteroid	T38.0X1	T38.0X2	T38.0X3	T38.0X4	T38.0X5	T38.0X6
ENT agent	T49.6X1	T49.6X2	T49.6X3	T49.6X4	T49.6X5	T49.6X6
mineral	T50.0X1	T50.0X2	T50.0X3	T50.0X4	T50.0X5	T50.0X6
ophthalmic	T49.5X1	T49.5X2	T49.5X3	T49.5X4	T49.5X5	T49.5X6
topical NEC	T49.0X1	T49.0X2	T49.0X3	T49.0X4	T49.0X5	T49.0X6
Corticotropin	T38.811	T38.812	T38.813	T38.814	T38.815	T38.816
Cortisol	T49.0X1	T49.0X2	T49.0X3	T49.0X4	T49.0X5	T49.0X6
ENT agent	T49.6X1	T49.6X2	T49.6X3	T49.6X4	T49.6X5	T49.6X6
ophthalmic preparation	T49.5X1	T49.5X2	T49.5X3	T49.5X4	T49.5X5	T49.5X6
topical NEC	T49.0X1	T49.0X2	T49.0X3	T49.0X4	T49.0X5	T49.0X6
Cortisone (acetate)	T38.0X1	T38.0X2	T38.0X3	T38.0X4	T38.0X5	T38.0X6
ENT agent	T49.6X1	T49.6X2	T49.6X3	T49.6X4	T49.6X5	T49.6X6
ophthalmic preparation	T49.5X1	T49.5X2	T49.5X3	T49.5X4	T49.5X5	T49.5X6
topical NEC	T49.0X1	T49.0X2	T49.0X3	T49.0X4	T49.0X5	T49.0X6
Cortivazol	T38.0X1	T38.0X2	T38.0X3	T38.0X4	T38.0X5	T38.0X6
Cortogen	T38.0X1	T38.0X2	T38.0X3	T38.0X4	T38.0X5	T38.0X6
ENT agent	T49.6X1	T49.6X2	T49.6X3	T49.6X4	T49.6X5	T49.6X6
ophthalmic preparation	T49.5X1	T49.5X2	T49.5X3	T49.5X4	T49.5X5	T49.5X6

TABLE OF DRUGS AND CHEMICALS

Substance	External Cause (T-Code)					
	Poisoning, Accidental (Unintentional)	Poisoning, Intentional Self-Harm	Poisoning, Assault	Poisoning, Undetermined	Adverse Effect	Underdosing
Cortone	T38.0X1	T38.0X2	T38.0X3	T38.0X4	T38.0X5	T38.0X6
ENT agent	T49.6X1	T49.6X2	T49.6X3	T49.6X4	T49.6X5	T49.6X6
ophthalmic preparation	T49.5X1	T49.5X2	T49.5X3	T49.5X4	T49.5X5	T49.5X6
Cortril	T38.0X1	T38.0X2	T38.0X3	T38.0X4	T38.0X5	T38.0X6
ENT agent	T49.6X1	T49.6X2	T49.6X3	T49.6X4	T49.6X5	T49.6X6
ophthalmic preparation	T49.5X1	T49.5X2	T49.5X3	T49.5X4	T49.5X5	T49.5X6
topical NEC	T49.0X1	T49.0X2	T49.0X3	T49.0X4	T49.0X5	T49.0X6
Corynebacterium parvum	T45.1X1	T45.1X2	T45.1X3	T45.1X4	T45.1X5	T45.1X6
Cosmetic preparation	T49.8X1	T49.8X2	T49.8X3	T49.8X4	T49.8X5	T49.8X6
Cosmetics	T49.8X1	T49.8X2	T49.8X3	T49.8X4	T49.8X5	T49.8X6
Cosyntropin	T38.811	T38.812	T38.813	T38.814	T38.815	T38.816
Cotarnine	T45.7X1	T45.7X2	T45.7X3	T45.7X4	T45.7X5	T45.7X6
Co-trimoxazole	T36.8X1	T36.8X2	T36.8X3	T36.8X4	T36.8X5	T36.8X6
Cottonseed oil	T49.3X1	T49.3X2	T49.3X3	T49.3X4	T49.3X5	T49.3X6
Cough mixture (syrup)	T48.4X1	T48.4X2	T48.4X3	T48.4X4	T48.4X5	T48.4X6
containing opiates	T40.2X1	T40.2X2	T40.2X3	T40.2X4	T40.2X5	T40.2X6
expectorants	T48.4X1	T48.4X2	T48.4X3	T48.4X4	T48.4X5	T48.4X6
Coumadin	T45.511	T45.512	T45.513	T45.514	T45.515	T45.516
rodenticide	T60.4X1	T60.4X2	T60.4X3	T60.4X4	—	—
Coumaphos	T60.0X1	T60.0X2	T60.0X3	T60.0X4	—	—
Coumarin	T45.511	T45.512	T45.513	T45.514	T45.515	T45.516
Coumetarol	T45.511	T45.512	T45.513	T45.514	T45.515	T45.516
Cowbane	T62.2X1	T62.2X2	T62.2X3	T62.2X4	—	—
Cozyme	T45.2X1	T45.2X2	T45.2X3	T45.2X4	T45.2X5	T45.2X6
Crack	T40.5X1	T40.5X2	T40.5X3	T40.5X4	—	—
Crataegus extract	T46.0X1	T46.0X2	T46.0X3	T46.0X4	T46.0X5	T46.0X6
Creolin	T54.1X1	T54.1X2	T54.1X3	T54.1X4	—	—
disinfectant	T54.1X1	T54.1X2	T54.1X3	T54.1X4	—	—
Creosol (compound)	T49.0X1	T49.0X2	T49.0X3	T49.0X4	T49.0X5	T49.0X6
Creosote (coal tar) (beechwood)	T49.0X1	T49.0X2	T49.0X3	T49.0X4	T49.0X5	T49.0X6
medicinal (expectorant)	T48.4X1	T48.4X2	T48.4X3	T48.4X4	T48.4X5	T48.4X6
syrup	T48.4X1	T48.4X2	T48.4X3	T48.4X4	T48.4X5	T48.4X6
Cresol(s)	T49.0X1	T49.0X2	T49.0X3	T49.0X4	T49.0X5	T49.0X6
and soap solution	T49.0X1	T49.0X2	T49.0X3	T49.0X4	T49.0X5	T49.0X6
Cresyl acetate	T49.0X1	T49.0X2	T49.0X3	T49.0X4	T49.0X5	T49.0X6
Cresylic acid	T49.0X1	T49.0X2	T49.0X3	T49.0X4	T49.0X5	T49.0X6
Crimidine	T60.4X1	T60.4X2	T60.4X3	T60.4X4	—	—
Croconazole	T37.8X1	T37.8X2	T37.8X3	T37.8X4	T37.8X5	T37.8X6
Cromoglicic acid	T48.6X1	T48.6X2	T48.6X3	T48.6X4	T48.6X5	T48.6X6
Cromolyn	T48.6X1	T48.6X2	T48.6X3	T48.6X4	T48.6X5	T48.6X6
Cromonar	T46.3X1	T46.3X2	T46.3X3	T46.3X4	T46.3X5	T46.3X6

Substance	External Cause (T-Code)					
	Poisoning, Accidental (Unintentional)	Poisoning, Intentional Self-Harm	Poisoning, Assault	Poisoning, Undetermined	Adverse Effect	Underdosing
Cropropamide	T39.8X1	T39.8X2	T39.8X3	T39.8X4	T39.8X5	T39.8X6
with crotethamide	T50.7X1	T50.7X2	T50.7X3	T50.7X4	T50.7X5	T50.7X6
Crotamiton	T49.0X1	T49.0X2	T49.0X3	T49.0X4	T49.0X5	T49.0X6
Crotethamide	T39.8X1	T39.8X2	T39.8X3	T39.8X4	T39.8X5	T39.8X6
with cropropamide	T50.7X1	T50.7X2	T50.7X3	T50.7X4	T50.7X5	T50.7X6
Croton (oil)	T47.2X1	T47.2X2	T47.2X3	T47.2X4	T47.2X5	T47.2X6
chloral	T42.6X1	T42.6X2	T42.6X3	T42.6X4	T42.6X5	T42.6X6
Crude oil	T52.0X1	T52.0X2	T52.0X3	T52.0X4	—	—
Cryogenine	T39.8X1	T39.8X2	T39.8X3	T39.8X4	T39.8X5	T39.8X6
Cryolite (vapor)	T60.1X1	T60.1X2	T60.1X3	T60.1X4	—	—
insecticide	T60.1X1	T60.1X2	T60.1X3	T60.1X4	—	—
Cryptenamine (tannates)	T46.5X1	T46.5X2	T46.5X3	T46.5X4	T46.5X5	T46.5X6
Crystal violet	T49.0X1	T49.0X2	T49.0X3	T49.0X4	T49.0X5	T49.0X6
Cuckoopint	T62.2X1	T62.2X2	T62.2X3	T62.2X4	—	—
Cumetharol	T45.511	T45.512	T45.513	T45.514	T45.515	T45.516
Cupric						
acetate	T60.3X1	T60.3X2	T60.3X3	T60.3X4	—	—
acetoarsenite	T57.0X1	T57.0X2	T57.0X3	T57.0X4	—	—
arsenate	T57.0X1	T57.0X2	T57.0X3	T57.0X4	—	—
gluconate	T49.0X1	T49.0X2	T49.0X3	T49.0X4	T49.0X5	T49.0X6
oleate	T49.0X1	T49.0X2	T49.0X3	T49.0X4	T49.0X5	T49.0X6
sulfate	T56.4X1	T56.4X2	T56.4X3	T56.4X4		
Cuprous sulfate — see also Copper sulfate	T56.4X1	T56.4X2	T56.4X3	T56.4X4	—	—
Curare, curarine	T48.1X1	T48.1X2	T48.1X3	T48.1X4	T48.1X5	T48.1X6
Cyamemazine	T43.3X1	T43.3X2	T43.3X3	T43.3X4	T43.3X5	T43.3X6
Cyamopsis tetragono-loba	T46.6X1	T46.6X2	T46.6X3	T46.6X4	T46.6X5	T46.6X6
Cyanacetyl hydrazide	T37.1X1	T37.1X2	T37.1X3	T37.1X4	T37.1X5	T37.1X6
Cyanic acid (gas)	T59.891	T59.892	T59.893	T59.894		
Cyanide(s) (compounds) (potassium) (sodium) NEC	T65.0X1	T65.0X2	T65.0X3	T65.0X4		
dust or gas (inhalation) NEC	T57.3X1	T57.3X2	T57.3X3	T57.3X4		
fumigant	T65.0X1	T65.0X2	T65.0X3	T65.0X4	—	—
hydrogen	T57.3X1	T57.3X2	T57.3X3	T57.3X4		
mercuric — see Mercury						
pesticide (dust) (fumes)	T65.0X1	T65.0X2	T65.0X3	T65.0X4	—	—
Cyanoacrylate adhesive	T49.3X1	T49.3X2	T49.3X3	T49.3X4	T49.3X5	T49.3X6
Cyanocobalamin	T45.8X1	T45.8X2	T45.8X3	T45.8X4	T45.8X5	T45.8X6
Cyanogen (chloride) (gas) NEC	T59.891	T59.892	T59.893	T59.894	—	—
Cyclacillin	T36.0X1	T36.0X2	T36.0X3	T36.0X4	T36.0X5	T36.0X6
Cyclaine	T41.3X1	T41.3X2	T41.3X3	T41.3X4	T41.3X5	T41.3X6
Cyclamate	T50.991	T50.992	T50.993	T50.994	T50.995	T50.996

◀ New   ◀| Revised   ~~deleted~~ Deleted

	External Cause (T-Code)					
Substance	Poisoning, Accidental (Unintentional)	Poisoning, Intentional Self-Harm	Poisoning, Assault	Poisoning, Undetermined	Adverse Effect	Underdosing
Cyclamen europaeum	T62.2X1	T62.2X2	T62.2X3	T62.2X4	—	—
Cyclandelate	T46.7X1	T46.7X2	T46.7X3	T46.7X4	T46.7X5	T46.7X6
Cyclazocine	T50.7X1	T50.7X2	T50.7X3	T50.7X4	T50.7X5	T50.7X6
Cyclizine	T45.0X1	T45.0X2	T45.0X3	T45.0X4	T45.0X5	T45.0X6
Cyclobarbital	T42.3X1	T42.3X2	T42.3X3	T42.3X4	T42.3X5	T42.3X6
Cyclobarbitone	T42.3X1	T42.3X2	T42.3X3	T42.3X4	T42.3X5	T42.3X6
Cyclobenzaprine	T48.1X1	T48.1X2	T48.1X3	T48.1X4	T48.1X5	T48.1X6
Cyclodrine	T44.3X1	T44.3X2	T44.3X3	T44.3X4	T44.3X5	T44.3X6
Cycloguanil embonate	T37.2X1	T37.2X2	T37.2X3	T37.2X4	T37.2X5	T37.2X6
Cycloheptadiene	T43.291	T43.292	T43.293	T43.294	T43.295	T43.296
Cyclohexane	T52.8X1	T52.8X2	T52.8X3	T52.8X4	—	—
Cyclohexanol	T51.8X1	T51.8X2	T51.8X3	T51.8X4	—	—
Cyclohexanone	T52.4X1	T52.4X2	T52.4X3	T52.4X4	—	—
Cycloheximide	T60.3X1	T60.3X2	T60.3X3	T60.3X4	—	—
Cyclohexyl acetate	T52.8X1	T52.8X2	T52.8X3	T52.8X4	—	—
Cycloleucin	T45.1X1	T45.1X2	T45.1X3	T45.1X4	T45.1X5	T45.1X6
Cyclomethycaine	T41.3X1	T41.3X2	T41.3X3	T41.3X4	T41.3X5	T41.3X6
Cyclopentamine	T44.4X1	T44.4X2	T44.4X3	T44.4X4	T44.4X5	T44.4X6
Cyclopenthiazide	T50.2X1	T50.2X2	T50.2X3	T50.2X4	T50.2X5	T50.2X6
Cyclopentolate	T44.3X1	T44.3X2	T44.3X3	T44.3X4	T44.3X5	T44.3X6
Cyclophosphamide	T45.1X1	T45.1X2	T45.1X3	T45.1X4	T45.1X5	T45.1X6
Cycloplegic drug	T49.5X1	T49.5X2	T49.5X3	T49.5X4	T49.5X5	T49.5X6
Cyclopropane	T41.291	T41.292	T41.293	T41.294	T41.295	T41.296
Cyclopyrabital	T39.8X1	T39.8X2	T39.8X3	T39.8X4	T39.8X5	T39.8X6
Cycloserine	T37.1X1	T37.1X2	T37.1X3	T37.1X4	T37.1X5	T37.1X6
Cyclosporin	T45.1X1	T45.1X2	T45.1X3	T45.1X4	T45.1X5	T45.1X6
Cyclothiazide	T50.2X1	T50.2X2	T50.2X3	T50.2X4	T50.2X5	T50.2X6
Cycrimine	T44.3X1	T44.3X2	T44.3X3	T44.3X4	T44.3X5	T44.3X6
Cyhalothrin	T60.1X1	T60.1X2	T60.1X3	T60.1X4	—	—
Cymarin	T46.0X1	T46.0X2	T46.0X3	T46.0X4	T46.0X5	T46.0X6
Cypermethrin	T60.1X1	T60.1X2	T60.1X3	T60.1X4	—	—
Cyphenothrin	T60.2X1	T60.2X2	T60.2X3	T60.2X4	—	—
Cyproheptadine	T45.0X1	T45.0X2	T45.0X3	T45.0X4	T45.0X5	T45.0X6
Cyprolidol	T43.291	T43.292	T43.293	T43.294	T43.295	T43.296
Cyproterone	T38.6X1	T38.6X2	T38.6X3	T38.6X4	T38.6X5	T38.6X6
Cysteamine	T50.6X1	T50.6X2	T50.6X3	T50.6X4	T50.6X5	T50.6X6
Cytarabine	T45.1X1	T45.1X2	T45.1X3	T45.1X4	T45.1X5	T45.1X6
Cytisus						
laburnum	T62.2X1	T62.2X2	T62.2X3	T62.2X4	—	—
scoparius	T62.2X1	T62.2X2	T62.2X3	T62.2X4	—	—
Cytochrome C	T47.5X1	T47.5X2	T47.5X3	T47.5X4	T47.5X5	T47.5X6
Cytomel	T38.1X1	T38.1X2	T38.1X3	T38.1X4	T38.1X5	T38.1X6

	External Cause (T-Code)					
Substance	Poisoning, Accidental (Unintentional)	Poisoning, Intentional Self-Harm	Poisoning, Assault	Poisoning, Undetermined	Adverse Effect	Underdosing
Cytosine arabinoside	T45.1X1	T45.1X2	T45.1X3	T45.1X4	T45.1X5	T45.1X6
Cytoxan	T45.1X1	T45.1X2	T45.1X3	T45.1X4	T45.1X5	T45.1X6
Cytozyme	T45.7X1	T45.7X2	T45.7X3	T45.7X4	T45.7X5	T45.7X6
2,4-D	T60.3X1	T60.3X2	T60.3X3	T60.3X4	—	—
D						
Dacarbazine	T45.1X1	T45.1X2	T45.1X3	T45.1X4	T45.1X5	T45.1X6
Dactinomycin	T45.1X1	T45.1X2	T45.1X3	T45.1X4	T45.1X5	T45.1X6
DADPS	T37.1X1	T37.1X2	T37.1X3	T37.1X4	T37.1X5	T37.1X6
Dakin's solution	T49.0X1	T49.0X2	T49.0X3	T49.0X4	T49.0X5	T49.0X6
Dalapon (sodium)	T60.3X1	T60.3X2	T60.3X3	T60.3X4	—	—
Dalmane	T42.4X1	T42.4X2	T42.4X3	T42.4X4	T42.4X5	T42.4X6
Danazol	T38.6X1	T38.6X2	T38.6X3	T38.6X4	T38.6X5	T38.6X6
Danilone	T45.511	T45.512	T45.513	T45.514	T45.515	T45.516
Danthron	T47.2X1	T47.2X2	T47.2X3	T47.2X4	T47.2X5	T47.2X6
Dantrolene	T42.8X1	T42.8X2	T42.8X3	T42.8X4	T42.8X5	T42.8X6
Dantron	T47.2X1	T47.2X2	T47.2X3	T47.2X4	T47.2X5	T47.2X6
Daphne (gnidium) (mezereum)	T62.2X1	T62.2X2	T62.2X3	T62.2X4	—	—
berry	T62.1X1	T62.1X2	T62.1X3	T62.1X4		
Dapsone	T37.1X1	T37.1X2	T37.1X3	T37.1X4	T37.1X5	T37.1X6
Daraprim	T37.2X1	T37.2X2	T37.2X3	T37.2X4	T37.2X5	T37.2X6
Darnel	T62.2X1	T62.2X2	T62.2X3	T62.2X4	—	—
Darvon	T39.8X1	T39.8X2	T39.8X3	T39.8X4	T39.8X5	T39.8X6
Daunomycin	T45.1X1	T45.1X2	T45.1X3	T45.1X4	T45.1X5	T45.1X6
Daunorubicin	T45.1X1	T45.1X2	T45.1X3	T45.1X4	T45.1X5	T45.1X6
DBI	T38.3X1	T38.3X2	T38.3X3	T38.3X4	T38.3X5	T38.3X6
D-Con	T60.91	T60.92	T60.93	T60.94	—	—
insecticide	T60.2X1	T60.2X2	T60.2X3	T60.2X4	—	—
rodenticide	T60.4X1	T60.4X2	T60.4X3	T60.4X4	—	—
DDAVP	T38.891	T38.892	T38.893	T38.894	T38.895	T38.896
DDE (bis(chlorophenyl)-dichloroethylene)	T60.2X1	T60.2X2	T60.2X3	T60.2X4	—	—
DDS	T37.1X1	T37.1X2	T37.1X3	T37.1X4	T37.1X5	T37.1X6
DDT (dust)	T60.1X1	T60.1X2	T60.1X3	T60.1X4	—	—
Deadly nightshade — see also Belladonna	T62.2X1	T62.2X2	T62.2X3	T62.2X4	—	—
berry	T62.1X1	T62.1X2	T62.1X3	T62.1X4	—	—
Deamino-D-arginine vasopressin	T38.891	T38.892	T38.893	T38.894	T38.895	T38.896
Deanol (aceglumate)	T50.991	T50.992	T50.993	T50.994	T50.995	T50.996
Debrisoquine	T46.5X1	T46.5X2	T46.5X3	T46.5X4	T46.5X5	T46.5X6
Decaborane	T57.8X1	T57.8X2	T57.8X3	T57.8X4	—	—
fumes	T59.891	T59.892	T59.893	T59.894	—	—

◀ New   ◀ Revised   ~~deleted~~ Deleted

	External Cause (T-Code)					
Substance	Poisoning, Accidental (Unintentional)	Poisoning, Intentional Self-Harm	Poisoning, Assault	Poisoning, Undetermined	Adverse Effect	Underdosing
Decadron	T38.0X1	T38.0X2	T38.0X3	T38.0X4	T38.0X5	T38.0X6
ENT agent	T49.6X1	T49.6X2	T49.6X3	T49.6X4	T49.6X5	T49.6X6
ophthalmic preparation	T49.5X1	T49.5X2	T49.5X3	T49.5X4	T49.5X5	T49.5X6
topical NEC	T49.0X1	T49.0X2	T49.0X3	T49.0X4	T49.0X5	T49.0X6
Decahydronaphthalene	T52.8X1	T52.8X2	T52.8X3	T52.8X4	—	—
Decalin	T52.8X1	T52.8X2	T52.8X3	T52.8X4	—	—
Decamethonium (bromide)	T48.1X1	T48.1X2	T48.1X3	T48.1X4	T48.1X5	T48.1X6
Decholin	T47.5X1	T47.5X2	T47.5X3	T47.5X4	T47.5X5	T47.5X6
Declomycin	T36.4X1	T36.4X2	T36.4X3	T36.4X4	T36.4X5	T36.4X6
Decongestant, nasal (mucosa)	T48.5X1	T48.5X2	T48.5X3	T48.5X4	T48.5X5	T48.5X6
combination	T48.5X1	T48.5X2	T48.5X3	T48.5X4	T48.5X5	T48.5X6
Deet	T60.8X1	T60.8X2	T60.8X3	T60.8X4	—	—
Deferoxamine	T45.8X1	T45.8X2	T45.8X3	T45.8X4	T45.8X5	T45.8X6
Deflazacort	T38.0X1	T38.0X2	T38.0X3	T38.0X4	T38.0X5	T38.0X6
Deglycyrrhizinized extract of licorice	T48.4X1	T48.4X2	T48.4X3	T48.4X4	T48.4X5	T48.4X6
Dehydrocholic acid	T47.5X1	T47.5X2	T47.5X3	T47.5X4	T47.5X5	T47.5X6
Dehydroemetine	T37.3X1	T37.3X2	T37.3X3	T37.3X4	T37.3X5	T37.3X6
Dekalin	T52.8X1	T52.8X2	T52.8X3	T52.8X4	—	—
Delalutin	T38.5X1	T38.5X2	T38.5X3	T38.5X4	T38.5X5	T38.5X6
Delphinium	T62.2X1	T62.2X2	T62.2X3	T62.2X4	—	—
Deltasone	T38.0X1	T38.0X2	T38.0X3	T38.0X4	T38.0X5	T38.0X6
Deltra	T38.0X1	T38.0X2	T38.0X3	T38.0X4	T38.0X5	T38.0X6
Delvinal	T42.3X1	T42.3X2	T42.3X3	T42.3X4	T42.3X5	T42.3X6
Delorazepam	T42.4X1	T42.4X2	T42.4X3	T42.4X4	T42.4X5	T42.4X6
Deltamethrin	T60.1X1	T60.1X2	T60.1X3	T60.1X4	—	—
Demecarium (bromide)	T49.5X1	T49.5X2	T49.5X3	T49.5X4	T49.5X5	T49.5X6
Demeclocycline	T36.4X1	T36.4X2	T36.4X3	T36.4X4	T36.4X5	T36.4X6
Demecolcine	T45.1X1	T45.1X2	T45.1X3	T45.1X4	T45.1X5	T45.1X6
Demegestone	T38.5X1	T38.5X2	T38.5X3	T38.5X4	T38.5X5	T38.5X6
Demelanizing agents	T49.8X1	T49.8X2	T49.8X3	T49.8X4	T49.8X5	T49.8X6
Demephion -O and -S	T60.0X1	T60.0X2	T60.0X3	T60.0X4	—	—
Demerol	T40.2X1	T40.2X2	T40.2X3	T40.2X4	T40.2X5	T40.2X6
Demethylchlortetracycline	T36.4X1	T36.4X2	T36.4X3	T36.4X4	T36.4X5	T36.4X6
Demethyltetracycline	T36.4X1	T36.4X2	T36.4X3	T36.4X4	T36.4X5	T36.4X6
Demeton -O and -S	T60.0X1	T60.0X2	T60.0X3	T60.0X4	—	—
Demulcent (external)	T49.3X1	T49.3X2	T49.3X3	T49.3X4	T49.3X5	T49.3X6
specified NEC	T49.3X1	T49.3X2	T49.3X3	T49.3X4	T49.3X5	T49.3X6
Demulen	T38.4X1	T38.4X2	T38.4X3	T38.4X4	T38.4X5	T38.4X6
Denatured alcohol	T51.0X1	T51.0X2	T51.0X3	T51.0X4	—	—
Dendrid	T49.5X1	T49.5X2	T49.5X3	T49.5X4	T49.5X5	T49.5X6
Dental drug, topical application NEC	T49.7X1	T49.7X2	T49.7X3	T49.7X4	T49.7X5	T49.7X6

	External Cause (T-Code)					
Substance	Poisoning, Accidental (Unintentional)	Poisoning, Intentional Self-Harm	Poisoning, Assault	Poisoning, Undetermined	Adverse Effect	Underdosing
Dentifrice	T49.7X1	T49.7X2	T49.7X3	T49.7X4	T49.7X5	T49.7X6
Deodorant spray (feminine hygiene)	T49.8X1	T49.8X2	T49.8X3	T49.8X4	T49.8X5	T49.8X6
Deoxycortone	T50.0X1	T50.0X2	T50.0X3	T50.0X4	T50.0X5	T50.0X6
2-Deoxy-5-fluorouridine	T45.1X1	T45.1X2	T45.1X3	T45.1X4	T45.1X5	T45.1X6
5-Deoxy-5-fluorouridine	T45.1X1	T45.1X2	T45.1X3	T45.1X4	T45.1X5	T45.1X6
Deoxyribonuclease (pancreatic)	T45.3X1	T45.3X2	T45.3X3	T45.3X4	T45.3X5	T45.3X6
Depilatory	T49.4X1	T49.4X2	T49.4X3	T49.4X4	T49.4X5	T49.4X6
Deprenalin	T42.8X1	T42.8X2	T42.8X3	T42.8X4	T42.8X5	T42.8X6
Deprenyl	T42.8X1	T42.8X2	T42.8X3	T42.8X4	T42.8X5	T42.8X6
Depressant, appetite	T50.5X1	T50.5X2	T50.5X3	T50.5X4	T50.5X5	T50.5X6
Depressant						
appetite, central	T50.5X1	T50.5X2	T50.5X3	T50.5X4	T50.5X5	T50.5X6
cardiac	T46.2X1	T46.2X2	T46.2X3	T46.2X4	T46.2X5	T46.2X6
central nervous system (anesthetic) — see also Central nervous system, depressants	T42.71	T42.72	T42.73	T42.74	T42.75	T42.76
general anesthetic	T41.201	T41.202	T41.203	T41.204	T41.205	T41.206
muscle tone	T42.8X1	T42.8X2	T42.8X3	T42.8X4	T42.8X5	T42.8X6
muscle tone, central	T42.8X1	T42.8X2	T42.8X3	T42.8X4	T42.8X5	T42.8X6
psychotherapeutic	T43.501	T43.502	T43.503	T43.504	T43.505	T43.506
Deptropine	T45.0X1	T45.0X2	T45.0X3	T45.0X4	T45.0X5	T45.0X6
Dequalinium (chloride)	T49.0X1	T49.0X2	T49.0X3	T49.0X4	T49.0X5	T49.0X6
Derris root	T60.2X1	T60.2X2	T60.2X3	T60.2X4	—	—
Deserpidine	T43.011	T43.012	T43.013	T43.014	T43.015	T43.016
Desferrioxamine	T45.8X1	T45.8X2	T45.8X3	T45.8X4	T45.8X5	T45.8X6
Desipramine	T43.0X1	T43.0X2	T43.0X3	T43.0X4	T43.0X5	T43.0X6
Deslanoside	T46.0X1	T46.0X2	T46.0X3	T46.0X4	T46.0X5	T46.0X6
Desloughing agent	T49.4X1	T49.4X2	T49.4X3	T49.4X4	T49.4X5	T49.4X6
Desmethylimipramine	T43.011	T43.012	T43.013	T43.014	T43.015	T43.016
Desmopressin	T38.891	T38.892	T38.893	T38.894	T38.895	T38.896
Desocodeine	T40.2X1	T40.2X2	T40.2X3	T40.2X4	T40.2X5	T40.2X6
Desogestrel	T38.5X1	T38.5X2	T38.5X3	T38.5X4	T38.5X5	T38.5X6
Desomorphine	T40.2X1	T40.2X2	T40.2X3	T40.2X4	—	—
Desonide	T49.0X1	T49.0X2	T49.0X3	T49.0X4	T49.0X5	T49.0X6
Desoximetasone	T49.0X1	T49.0X2	T49.0X3	T49.0X4	T49.0X5	T49.0X6
Desoxycorticosteroid	T50.0X1	T50.0X2	T50.0X3	T50.0X4	T50.0X5	T50.0X6
Desoxycortone	T50.0X1	T50.0X2	T50.0X3	T50.0X4	T50.0X5	T50.0X6
Desoxyephedrine	T43.621	T43.622	T43.623	T43.624	T43.625	T43.626
Detaxtran	T46.6X1	T46.6X2	T46.6X3	T46.6X4	T46.6X5	T46.6X6
Detergent	T49.2X1	T49.2X2	T49.2X3	T49.2X4	T49.2X5	T49.2X6
external medication	T49.2X1	T49.2X2	T49.2X3	T49.2X4	T49.2X5	T49.2X6
local	T49.2X1	T49.2X2	T49.2X3	T49.2X4	T49.2X5	T49.2X6

◀ New   ◀◀ Revised   ~~deleted~~ Deleted

Substance	Poisoning, Accidental (Unintentional)	Poisoning, Intentional Self-Harm	Poisoning, Assault	Poisoning, Undetermined	Adverse Effect	Underdosing
Detergent *(Continued)*						
medicinal	T49.2X1	T49.2X2	T49.2X3	T49.2X4	T49.2X5	T49.2X6
nonmedicinal	T55.1X1	T55.1X2	T55.1X3	T55.1X4	—	—
specified NEC	T55.1X1	T55.1X2	T55.1X3	T55.1X4	T55.1X5	T55.1X6
Deterrent, alcohol	T50.6X1	T50.6X2	T50.6X3	T50.6X4	T50.6X5	T50.6X6
Detoxifying agent	T50.6X1	T50.6X2	T50.6X3	T50.6X4	T50.6X5	T50.6X6
Detrothyronine	T38.1X1	T38.1X2	T38.1X3	T38.1X4	T38.1X5	T38.1X6
Dettol (external medication)	T49.0X1	T49.0X2	T49.0X3	T49.0X4	T49.0X5	T49.0X6
Dexamethasone	T38.0X1	T38.0X2	T38.0X3	T38.0X4	T38.0X5	T38.0X6
ENT agent	T49.6X1	T49.6X2	T49.6X3	T49.6X4	T49.6X5	T49.6X6
ophthalmic preparation	T49.5X1	T49.5X2	T49.5X3	T49.5X4	T49.5X5	T49.5X6
topical NEC	T49.0X1	T49.0X2	T49.0X3	T49.0X4	T49.0X5	T49.0X6
Dexamfetamine	T43.621	T43.622	T43.623	T43.624	T43.625	T43.626
Dexamphetamine	T43.621	T43.622	T43.623	T43.624	T43.625	T43.626
Dexbrompheniramine	T45.0X1	T45.0X2	T45.0X3	T45.0X4	T45.0X5	T45.0X6
Dexchlorpheniramine	T45.0X1	T45.0X2	T45.0X3	T45.0X4	T45.0X5	T45.0X6
Dexedrine	T43.621	T43.622	T43.623	T43.624	T43.625	T43.626
Dexetimide	T44.3X1	T44.3X2	T44.3X3	T44.3X4	T44.3X5	T44.3X6
Dexfenfluramine	T50.5X1	T50.5X2	T50.5X3	T50.5X4	T50.5X5	T50.5X6
Dexpanthenol	T45.2X1	T45.2X2	T45.2X3	T45.2X4	T45.2X5	T45.2X6
Dextran (40) (70) (150)	T45.8X1	T45.8X2	T45.8X3	T45.8X4	T45.8X5	T45.8X6
Dextriferron	T45.4X1	T45.4X2	T45.4X3	T45.4X4	T45.4X5	T45.4X6
Dextroamphetamine	T43.621	T43.622	T43.623	T43.624	T43.625	T43.626
Dextro calcium pantothenate	T45.2X1	T45.2X2	T45.2X3	T45.2X4	T45.2X5	T45.2X6
Dextromethorphan	T48.3X1	T48.3X2	T48.3X3	T48.3X4	T48.3X5	T48.3X6
Dextromoramide	T40.4X1	T40.4X2	T40.4X3	T40.4X4	—	—
topical	T49.8X1	T49.8X2	T49.8X3	T49.8X4	T49.8X5	T49.8X6
Dextro pantothenyl alcohol	T45.2X1	T45.2X2	T45.2X3	T45.2X4	T45.2X5	T45.2X6
Dextropropoxyphene	T40.4X1	T40.4X2	T40.4X3	T40.4X4	T40.4X5	T40.4X6
Dextrorphan	T40.2X1	T40.2X2	T40.2X3	T40.2X4	T40.2X5	T40.2X6
Dextrose	T50.3X1	T50.3X2	T50.3X3	T50.3X4	T50.3X5	T50.3X6
concentrated solution, intravenous	T46.8X1	T46.8X2	T46.8X3	T46.8X4	T46.8X5	T46.8X6
Dextrothyroxin	T38.1X1	T38.1X2	T38.1X3	T38.1X4	T38.1X5	T38.1X6
Dextrothyroxine sodium	T38.1X1	T38.1X2	T38.1X3	T38.1X4	T38.1X5	T38.1X6
DFP	T44.0X1	T44.0X2	T44.0X3	T44.0X4	T44.0X5	T44.0X6
DHE	T37.3X1	T37.3X2	T37.3X3	T37.3X4	T37.3X5	T37.3X6
45	T46.5X1	T46.5X2	T46.5X3	T46.5X4	T46.5X5	T46.5X6
Diabinese	T38.3X1	T38.3X2	T38.3X3	T38.3X4	T38.3X5	T38.3X6
Diacetone alcohol	T52.4X1	T52.4X2	T52.4X3	T52.4X4	—	—
Diacetyl monoxime	T50.991	T50.992	T50.993	T50.994	—	—
Diacetylmorphine	T40.1X1	T40.1X2	T40.1X3	T40.1X4	—	—

Substance	Poisoning, Accidental (Unintentional)	Poisoning, Intentional Self-Harm	Poisoning, Assault	Poisoning, Undetermined	Adverse Effect	Underdosing
Diachylon plaster	T49.4X1	T49.4X2	T49.4X3	T49.4X4	T49.4X5	T49.4X6
Diaethylstilboestrolum	T38.5X1	T38.5X2	T38.5X3	T38.5X4	T38.5X5	T38.5X6
Diagnostic agent NEC	T50.8X1	T50.8X2	T50.8X3	T50.8X4	T50.8X5	T50.8X6
Dial (soap)	T49.2X1	T49.2X2	T49.2X3	T49.2X4	T49.2X5	T49.2X6
sedative	T42.3X1	T42.3X2	T42.3X3	T42.3X4	T42.3X5	T42.3X6
Dialkyl carbonate	T52.91	T52.92	T52.93	T52.94	—	—
Diallylbarbituric acid	T42.3X1	T42.3X2	T42.3X3	T42.3X4	T42.3X5	T42.3X6
Diallymal	T42.3X1	T42.3X2	T42.3X3	T42.3X4	T42.3X5	T42.3X6
Dialysis solution (intraperitoneal)	T50.3X1	T50.3X2	T50.3X3	T50.3X4	T50.3X5	T50.3X6
Diaminodiphenylsulfone	T37.1X1	T37.1X2	T37.1X3	T37.1X4	T37.1X5	T37.1X6
Diamorphine	T40.1X1	T40.1X2	T40.1X3	T40.1X4	—	—
Diamox	T50.2X1	T50.2X2	T50.2X3	T50.2X4	T50.2X5	T50.2X6
Diamthazole	T49.0X1	T49.0X2	T49.0X3	T49.0X4	T49.0X5	T49.0X6
Dianthone	T47.2X1	T47.2X2	T47.2X3	T47.2X4	T47.2X5	T47.2X6
Diaphenylsulfone	T37.0X1	T37.0X2	T37.0X3	T37.0X4	T37.0X5	T37.0X6
Diasone (sodium)	T37.1X1	T37.1X2	T37.1X3	T37.1X4	T37.1X5	T37.1X6
Diastase	T47.5X1	T47.5X2	T47.5X3	T47.5X4	T47.5X5	T47.5X6
Diatrizoate	T50.8X1	T50.8X2	T50.8X3	T50.8X4	T50.8X5	T50.8X6
Diazepam	T42.4X1	T42.4X2	T42.4X3	T42.4X4	T42.4X5	T42.4X6
Diazinon	T60.0X1	T60.0X2	T60.0X3	T60.0X4	—	—
Diazomethane (gas)	T59.891	T59.892	T59.893	T59.894	—	—
Diazoxide	T46.5X1	T46.5X2	T46.5X3	T46.5X4	T46.5X5	T46.5X6
Dibekacin	T36.5X1	T36.5X2	T36.5X3	T36.5X4	T36.5X5	T36.5X6
Dibenamine	T44.6X1	T44.6X2	T44.6X3	T44.6X4	T44.6X5	T44.6X6
Dibenzepin	T43.011	T43.012	T43.013	T43.014	T43.015	T43.016
Dibenzheptropine	T45.0X1	T45.0X2	T45.0X3	T45.0X4	T45.0X5	T45.0X6
Dibenzyline	T44.6X1	T44.6X2	T44.6X3	T44.6X4	T44.6X5	T44.6X6
Diborane (gas)	T59.891	T59.892	T59.893	T59.894	—	—
Dibromochloropropane	T60.8X1	T60.8X2	T60.8X3	T60.8X4	—	—
Dibromodulcitol	T45.1X1	T45.1X2	T45.1X3	T45.1X4	T45.1X5	T45.1X6
Dibromoethane	T53.6X1	T53.6X2	T53.6X3	T53.6X4	—	—
Dibromomannitol	T45.1X1	T45.1X2	T45.1X3	T45.1X4	T45.1X5	T45.1X6
Dibromopropamidine isethionate	T49.0X1	T49.0X2	T49.0X3	T49.0X4	T49.0X5	T49.0X6
Dibrompropamidine	T49.0X1	T49.0X2	T49.0X3	T49.0X4	T49.0X5	T49.0X6
Dibucaine	T41.3X1	T41.3X2	T41.3X3	T41.3X4	T41.3X5	T41.3X6
topical (surface)	T41.3X1	T41.3X2	T41.3X3	T41.3X4	T41.3X5	T41.3X6
Dibunate sodium	T48.3X1	T48.3X2	T48.3X3	T48.3X4	T48.3X5	T48.3X6
Dibutoline sulfate	T44.3X1	T44.3X2	T44.3X3	T44.3X4	T44.3X5	T44.3X6
Dicamba	T60.3X1	T60.3X2	T60.3X3	T60.3X4	—	—
Dicapthon	T60.0X1	T60.0X2	T60.0X3	T60.0X4	—	—
Dichlobenil	T60.3X1	T60.3X2	T60.3X3	T60.3X4	—	—
Dichlone	T60.3X1	T60.3X2	T60.3X3	T60.3X4	—	—

◀ New   ◀ Revised   ~~deleted~~ Deleted

Substance	Poisoning, Accidental (Unintentional)	Poisoning, Intentional Self-Harm	Poisoning, Assault	Poisoning, Undetermined	Adverse Effect	Underdosing
Dichloralphenozone	T42.6X1	T42.6X2	T42.6X3	T42.6X4	T42.6X5	T42.6X6
Dichlorbenzidine	T65.3X1	T65.3X2	T65.3X3	T65.3X4	—	—
Dichlorhydrin	T52.8X1	T52.8X2	T52.8X3	T52.8X4	—	—
Dichlorhydroxyquinoline	T37.8X1	T37.8X2	T37.8X3	T37.8X4	T37.8X5	T37.8X6
Dichlorobenzene	T53.7X1	T53.7X2	T53.7X3	T53.7X4	—	—
Dichlorobenzyl alcohol	T49.6X1	T49.6X2	T49.6X3	T49.6X4	T49.6X5	T49.6X6
Dichlorodifluoromethane	T53.5X1	T53.5X2	T53.5X3	T53.5X4	—	—
Dichloroethane	T52.8X1	T52.8X2	T52.8X3	T52.8X4	—	—
Sym-Dichloroethyl ether	T53.6X1	T53.6X2	T53.6X3	T53.6X4	—	—
Dichloroethyl sulfide, not in war	T59.891	T59.892	T59.893	T59.894	—	—
Dichloroethylene	T53.6X1	T53.6X2	T53.6X3	T53.6X4	—	—
Dichloroformoxine, not in war	T59.891	T59.892	T59.893	T59.894	—	—
Dichlorohydrin, alpha-dichlorohydrin	T52.8X1	T52.8X2	T52.8X3	T52.8X4	—	—
Dichloromethane (solvent)	T53.4X1	T53.4X2	T53.4X3	T53.4X4	—	—
vapor	T53.4X1	T53.4X2	T53.4X3	T53.4X4	—	—
Dichloronaphthoquinone	T60.3X1	T60.3X2	T60.3X3	T60.3X4	—	—
Dichlorophen	T37.4X1	T37.4X2	T37.4X3	T37.4X4	T37.4X5	T37.4X6
2,4-Dichlorophenoxy-acetic acid	T60.3X1	T60.3X2	T60.3X3	T60.3X4	—	—
Dichloropropene	T60.3X1	T60.3X2	T60.3X3	T60.3X4	—	—
Dichloropropionic acid	T60.3X1	T60.3X2	T60.3X3	T60.3X4	—	—
Dichlorphenamide	T50.2X1	T50.2X2	T50.2X3	T50.2X4	T50.2X5	T50.2X6
Dichlorvos	T60.0X1	T60.0X2	T60.0X3	T60.0X4	—	—
Diclofenac	T39.391	T39.392	T39.393	T39.394	T39.395	T39.396
Diclofenamide	T50.2X1	T50.2X2	T50.2X3	T50.2X4	T50.2X5	T50.2X6
Diclofensine	T43.291	T43.292	T43.293	T43.294	T43.295	T43.296
Diclonixine	T39.8X1	T39.8X2	T39.8X3	T39.8X4	T39.8X5	T39.8X6
Dicloxacillin	T36.0X1	T36.0X2	T36.0X3	T36.0X4	T36.0X5	T36.0X6
Dicophane	T49.0X1	T49.0X2	T49.0X3	T49.0X4	T49.0X5	T49.0X6
Dicoumarol, dicoumarin, dicumarol	T45.511	T45.512	T45.513	T45.514	T45.515	T45.516
Dicrotophos	T60.0X1	T60.0X2	T60.0X3	T60.0X4	—	—
Dicyanogen (gas)	T65.0X1	T65.0X2	T65.0X3	T65.0X4	—	—
Dicyclomine	T44.3X1	T44.3X2	T44.3X3	T44.3X4	T44.3X5	T44.3X6
Dicycloverine	T44.3X1	T44.3X2	T44.3X3	T44.3X4	T44.3X5	T44.3X6
Dideoxycytidine	T37.5X1	T37.5X2	T37.5X3	T37.5X4	T37.5X5	T37.5X6
Dideoxyinosine	T37.5X1	T37.5X2	T37.5X3	T37.5X4	T37.5X5	T37.5X6
Dieldrin (vapor)	T60.1X1	T60.1X2	T60.1X3	T60.1X4	—	—
Diemal	T42.3X1	T42.3X2	T42.3X3	T42.3X4	T42.3X5	T42.3X6
Dienestrol	T38.5X1	T38.5X2	T38.5X3	T38.5X4	T38.5X5	T38.5X6
Dienoestrol	T38.5X1	T38.5X2	T38.5X3	T38.5X4	T38.5X5	T38.5X6
Dietetic drug NEC	T50.901	T50.902	T50.903	T50.904	T50.905	T50.906
Diethazine	T42.8X1	T42.8X2	T42.8X3	T42.8X4	T42.8X5	T42.8X6

Substance	Poisoning, Accidental (Unintentional)	Poisoning, Intentional Self-Harm	Poisoning, Assault	Poisoning, Undetermined	Adverse Effect	Underdosing
Diethyl						
barbituric acid	T42.3X1	T42.3X2	T42.3X3	T42.3X4	T42.3X5	T42.3X6
carbamazine	T37.4X1	T37.4X2	T37.4X3	T37.4X4	T37.4X5	T37.4X6
carbinol	T51.3X1	T51.3X2	T51.3X3	T51.3X4	—	—
carbonate	T52.8X1	T52.8X2	T52.8X3	T52.8X4	—	—
ether (vapor) — see also ether	T41.0X1	T41.0X2	T41.0X3	T41.0X4	T41.0X5	T41.0X6
oxide	T52.8X1	T52.8X2	T52.8X3	T52.8X4	—	—
propion	T50.5X1	T50.5X2	T50.5X3	T50.5X4	T50.5X5	T50.5X6
stilbestrol	T38.5X1	T38.5X2	T38.5X3	T38.5X4	T38.5X5	T38.5X6
toluamide (nonmedicinal)	T60.8X1	T60.8X2	T60.8X3	T60.8X4	—	—
medicinal	T49.3X1	T49.3X2	T49.3X3	T49.3X4	T49.3X5	T49.3X6
Diethylcarbamazine	T37.4X1	T37.4X2	T37.4X3	T37.4X4	T37.4X5	T37.4X6
Diethylene						
dioxide	T52.8X1	T52.8X2	T52.8X3	T52.8X4	—	—
glycol (monoacetate) (monobutyl ether) (monoethyl ether)	T52.3X1	T52.3X2	T52.3X3	T52.3X4	—	—
Diethylhexylphthalate	T65.891	T65.892	T65.893	T65.894	—	—
Diethylpropion	T50.5X1	T50.5X2	T50.5X3	T50.5X4	T50.5X5	T50.5X6
Diethylstilbestrol	T38.5X1	T38.5X2	T38.5X3	T38.5X4	T38.5X5	T38.5X6
Diethylstilboestrol	T38.5X1	T38.5X2	T38.5X3	T38.5X4	T38.5X5	T38.5X6
Diethylsulfone-diethylmethane	T42.6X1	T42.6X2	T42.6X3	T42.6X4	T42.6X5	T42.6X6
Diethyltoluamide	T49.0X1	T49.0X2	T49.0X3	T49.0X4	T49.0X5	T49.0X6
Diethyltryptamine (DET)	T40.991	T40.992	T40.993	T40.994	—	—
Difebarbamate	T42.3X1	T42.3X2	T42.3X3	T42.3X4	T42.3X5	T42.3X6
Difencloxazine	T40.2X1	T40.2X2	T40.2X3	T40.2X4	T40.2X5	T40.2X6
Difenidol	T45.0X1	T45.0X2	T45.0X3	T45.0X4	T45.0X5	T45.0X6
Difenoxin	T47.6X1	T47.6X2	T47.6X3	T47.6X4	T47.6X5	T47.6X6
Difetarsone	T37.3X1	T37.3X2	T37.3X3	T37.3X4	T37.3X5	T37.3X6
Diffusin	T45.3X1	T45.3X2	T45.3X3	T45.3X4	T45.3X5	T45.3X6
Diflorasone	T49.0X1	T49.0X2	T49.0X3	T49.0X4	T49.0X5	T49.0X6
Diflubenzuron	T60.1X1	T60.1X2	T60.1X3	T60.1X4	—	—
Diflos	T44.0X1	T44.0X2	T44.0X3	T44.0X4	T44.0X5	T44.0X6
Diflucortolone	T49.0X1	T49.0X2	T49.0X3	T49.0X4	T49.0X5	T49.0X6
Diflunisal	T39.091	T39.092	T39.093	T39.094	T39.095	T39.096
Difluoromethyldopa	T42.8X1	T42.8X2	T42.8X3	T42.8X4	T42.8X5	T42.8X6
Difluorophate	T44.0X1	T44.0X2	T44.0X3	T44.0X4	T44.0X5	T44.0X6
Digestant NEC	T47.5X1	T47.5X2	T47.5X3	T47.5X4	T47.5X5	T47.5X6
Digitalin(e)	T46.0X1	T46.0X2	T46.0X3	T46.0X4	T46.0X5	T46.0X6
Digitalis (leaf) (glycoside)	T46.0X1	T46.0X2	T46.0X3	T46.0X4	T46.0X5	T46.0X6
lanata	T46.0X1	T46.0X2	T46.0X3	T46.0X4	T46.0X5	T46.0X6
purpurea	T46.0X1	T46.0X2	T46.0X3	T46.0X4	T46.0X5	T46.0X6
Digitoxin	T46.0X1	T46.0X2	T46.0X3	T46.0X4	T46.0X5	T46.0X6

◀ New   ◀ Revised   ~~deleted~~ Deleted

	External Cause (T-Code)					
Substance	Poisoning, Accidental (Unintentional)	Poisoning, Intentional Self-Harm	Poisoning, Assault	Poisoning, Undetermined	Adverse Effect	Underdosing
Digitoxose	T46.0X1	T46.0X2	T46.0X3	T46.0X4	T46.0X5	T46.0X6
Digoxin	T46.0X1	T46.0X2	T46.0X3	T46.0X4	T46.0X5	T46.0X6
Digoxine	T46.0X1	T46.0X2	T46.0X3	T46.0X4	T46.0X5	T46.0X6
Dihydralazine	T46.5X1	T46.5X2	T46.5X3	T46.5X4	T46.5X5	T46.5X6
Dihydrazine	T46.5X1	T46.5X2	T46.5X3	T46.5X4	T46.5X5	T46.5X6
Dihydrocodeinone	T40.2X1	T40.2X2	T40.2X3	T40.2X4	T40.2X5	T40.2X6
Dihydroergocornine	T46.7X1	T46.7X2	T46.7X3	T46.7X4	T46.7X5	T46.7X6
Dihydroergocristine (mesilate)	T46.7X1	T46.7X2	T46.7X3	T46.7X4	T46.7X5	T46.7X6
Dihydroergokryptine	T46.7X1	T46.7X2	T46.7X3	T46.7X4	T46.7X5	T46.7X6
Dihydroergotamine	T46.5X1	T46.5X2	T46.5X3	T46.5X4	T46.5X5	T46.5X6
Dihydroergotoxine	T46.7X1	T46.7X2	T46.7X3	T46.7X4	T46.7X5	T46.7X6
mesilate	T46.7X1	T46.7X2	T46.7X3	T46.7X4	T46.7X5	T46.7X6
Dihydrohydroxycodein-one	T40.2X1	T40.2X2	T40.2X3	T40.2X4	T40.2X5	T40.2X6
Dihydrohydroxymorphinone	T40.2X1	T40.2X2	T40.2X3	T40.2X4	T40.2X5	T40.2X6
Dihydroisocodeine	T40.2X1	T40.2X2	T40.2X3	T40.2X4	T40.2X5	T40.2X6
Dihydromorphine	T40.2X1	T40.2X2	T40.2X3	T40.2X4	—	—
Dihydromorphinone	T40.2X1	T40.2X2	T40.2X3	T40.2X4	T40.2X5	T40.2X6
Dihydrostreptomycin	T36.5X1	T36.5X2	T36.5X3	T36.5X4	T36.5X5	T36.5X6
Dihydrotachysterol	T45.2X1	T45.2X2	T45.2X3	T45.2X4	T45.2X5	T45.2X6
Dihydroxyaluminum aminoacetate	T47.1X1	T47.1X2	T47.1X3	T47.1X4	T47.1X5	T47.1X6
Dihydroxyaluminum sodium carbonate	T47.1X1	T47.1X2	T47.1X3	T47.1X4	T47.1X5	T47.1X6
Dihydroxyanthraquinone	T47.2X1	T47.2X2	T47.2X3	T47.2X4	T47.2X5	T47.2X6
Dihydroxycodeinone	T40.2X1	T40.2X2	T40.2X3	T40.2X4	T40.2X5	T40.2X6
Dihydroxypropyl theophylline	T50.2X1	T50.2X2	T50.2X3	T50.2X4	T50.2X5	T50.2X6
Diiodohydroxyquin	T37.8X1	T37.8X2	T37.8X3	T37.8X4	T37.8X5	T37.8X6
topical	T49.0X1	T49.0X2	T49.0X3	T49.0X4	T49.0X5	T49.0X6
Diiodohydroxyquinoline	T37.8X1	T37.8X2	T37.8X3	T37.8X4	T37.8X5	T37.8X6
Diiodotyrosine	T38.2X1	T38.2X2	T38.2X3	T38.2X4	T38.2X5	T38.2X6
Diisopromine	T44.3X1	T44.3X2	T44.3X3	T44.3X4	T44.3X5	T44.3X6
Diisopropylamine	T46.3X1	T46.3X2	T46.3X3	T46.3X4	T46.3X5	T46.3X6
Diisopropylfluorophosphonate	T44.0X1	T44.0X2	T44.0X3	T44.0X4	T44.0X5	T44.0X6
Dilantin	T42.0X1	T42.0X2	T42.0X3	T42.0X4	T42.0X5	T42.0X6
Dilaudid	T40.2X1	T40.2X2	T40.2X3	T40.2X4	T40.2X5	T40.2X6
Dilazep	T46.3X1	T46.3X2	T46.3X3	T46.3X4	T46.3X5	T46.3X6
Dill	T47.5X1	T47.5X2	T47.5X3	T47.5X4	T47.5X5	T47.5X6
Diloxanide	T37.3X1	T37.3X2	T37.3X3	T37.3X4	T37.3X5	T37.3X6
Diltiazem	T46.1X1	T46.1X2	T46.1X3	T46.1X4	T46.1X5	T46.1X6
Dimazole	T49.0X1	T49.0X2	T49.0X3	T49.0X4	T49.0X5	T49.0X6
Dimefline	T50.7X1	T50.7X2	T50.7X3	T50.7X4	T50.7X5	T50.7X6
Dimefox	T60.0X1	T60.0X2	T60.0X3	T60.0X4	—	—

	External Cause (T-Code)					
Substance	Poisoning, Accidental (Unintentional)	Poisoning, Intentional Self-Harm	Poisoning, Assault	Poisoning, Undetermined	Adverse Effect	Underdosing
Dimemorfan	T48.3X1	T48.3X2	T48.3X3	T48.3X4	T48.3X5	T48.3X6
Dimenhydrinate	T45.0X1	T45.0X2	T45.0X3	T45.0X4	T45.0X5	T45.0X6
Dimercaprol (British anti-lewisite)	T45.8X1	T45.8X2	T45.8X3	T45.8X4	T45.8X5	T45.8X6
Dimercaptopropanol	T45.8X1	T45.8X2	T45.8X3	T45.8X4	T45.8X5	T45.8X6
Dimestrol	T38.5X1	T38.5X2	T38.5X3	T38.5X4	T38.5X5	T38.5X6
Dimetane	T45.0X1	T45.0X2	T45.0X3	T45.0X4	T45.0X5	T45.0X6
Dimethicone	T47.1X1	T47.1X2	T47.1X3	T47.1X4	T47.1X5	T47.1X6
Dimethindene	T45.0X1	T45.0X2	T45.0X3	T45.0X4	T45.0X5	T45.0X6
Dimethisoquin	T49.1X1	T49.1X2	T49.1X3	T49.1X4	T49.1X5	T49.1X6
Dimethisterone	T38.5X1	T38.5X2	T38.5X3	T38.5X4	T38.5X5	T38.5X6
Dimethoate	T60.0X1	T60.0X2	T60.0X3	T60.0X4	—	—
Dimethocaine	T41.3X1	T41.3X2	T41.3X3	T41.3X4	T41.3X5	T41.3X6
Dimethoxanate	T48.3X1	T48.3X2	T48.3X3	T48.3X4	T48.3X5	T48.3X6
Dimethyl						
arsine, arsinic acid	T57.0X1	T57.0X2	T57.0X3	T57.0X4	—	—
carbinol	T51.2X1	T51.2X2	T51.2X3	T51.2X4	—	—
carbonate	T52.8X1	T52.8X2	T52.8X3	T52.8X4	—	—
diguanide	T38.3X1	T38.3X2	T38.3X3	T38.3X4	T38.3X5	T38.3X6
ketone	T52.4X1	T52.4X2	T52.4X3	T52.4X4	—	—
vapor	T52.4X1	T52.4X2	T52.4X3	T52.4X4	—	—
meperidine	T40.2X1	T40.2X2	T40.2X3	T40.2X4	T40.2X5	T40.2X6
parathion	T60.0X1	T60.0X2	T60.0X3	T60.0X4	—	—
phthlate	T49.3X1	T49.3X2	T49.3X3	T49.3X4	T49.3X5	T49.3X6
polysiloxane	T47.8X1	T47.8X2	T47.8X3	T47.8X4	T47.8X5	T47.8X6
sulfate (fumes)	T59.891	T59.892	T59.893	T59.894		
liquid	T65.891	T65.892	T65.893	T65.894	—	—
sulfoxide (nonmedicinal)	T52.8X1	T52.8X2	T52.8X3	T52.8X4	—	—
medicinal	T49.4X1	T49.4X2	T49.4X3	T49.4X4	T49.4X5	T49.4X6
tryptamine	T40.991	T40.992	T40.993	T40.994	—	—
tubocurarine	T48.1X1	T48.1X2	T48.1X3	T48.1X4	T48.1X5	T48.1X6
Dimethylamine sulfate	T49.4X1	T49.4X2	T49.4X3	T49.4X4	T49.4X5	T49.4X6
Dimethylformamide	T52.8X1	T52.8X2	T52.8X3	T52.8X4	—	—
Dimethyltubocurarinium chloride	T48.1X1	T48.1X2	T48.1X3	T48.1X4	T48.1X5	T48.1X6
Dimeticone	T47.1X1	T47.1X2	T47.1X3	T47.1X4	T47.1X5	T47.1X6
Dimetilan	T60.0X1	T60.0X2	T60.0X3	T60.0X4	—	—
Dimetindene	T45.0X1	T45.0X2	T45.0X3	T45.0X4	T45.0X5	T45.0X6
Dimetotiazine	T43.3X1	T43.3X2	T43.3X3	T43.3X4	T43.3X5	T43.3X6
Dimorpholamine	T50.7X1	T50.7X2	T50.7X3	T50.7X4	T50.7X5	T50.7X6
Dimoxyline	T46.3X1	T46.3X2	T46.3X3	T46.3X4	T46.3X5	T46.3X6
Dinitrobenzene	T65.3X1	T65.3X2	T65.3X3	T65.3X4	—	—
vapor	T59.891	T59.892	T59.893	T59.894		

TABLE OF DRUGS AND CHEMICALS

Substance	Poisoning, Accidental (Unintentional)	Poisoning, Intentional Self-Harm	Poisoning, Assault	Poisoning, Undetermined	Adverse Effect	Underdosing
Dinitrobenzol	T65.3X1	T65.3X2	T65.3X3	T65.3X4	—	—
vapor	T59.891	T59.892	T59.893	T59.894	—	—
Dinitrobutylphenol	T65.3X1	T65.3X2	T65.3X3	T65.3X4	—	—
Dinitro (-ortho-)cresol (pesticide) (spray)	T65.3X1	T65.3X2	T65.3X3	T65.3X4	—	—
Dinitrocyclohexylphenol	T65.3X1	T65.3X2	T65.3X3	T65.3X4	—	—
Dinitrophenol	T65.3X1	T65.3X2	T65.3X3	T65.3X4	—	—
Dinoprost	T48.0X1	T48.0X2	T48.0X3	T48.0X4	T48.0X5	T48.0X6
Dinoprostone	T48.0X1	T48.0X2	T48.0X3	T48.0X4	T48.0X5	T48.0X6
Dinoseb	T60.3X1	T60.3X2	T60.3X3	T60.3X4	—	—
Dioctyl sulfosuccinate (calcium) (sodium)	T47.4X1	T47.4X2	T47.4X3	T47.4X4	T47.4X5	T47.4X6
Diodone	T50.8X1	T50.8X2	T50.8X3	T50.8X4	T50.8X5	T50.8X6
Diodoquin	T37.8X1	T37.8X2	T37.8X3	T37.8X4	T37.8X5	T37.8X6
Dionin	T40.2X1	T40.2X2	T40.2X3	T40.2X4	T40.2X5	T40.2X6
Diosmin	T46.991	T46.992	T46.993	T46.994	T46.995	T46.996
Dioxane	T52.8X1	T52.8X2	T52.8X3	T52.8X4	—	—
Dioxathion	T60.0X1	T60.0X2	T60.0X3	T60.0X4	—	—
Dioxin	T53.7X1	T53.7X2	T53.7X3	T53.7X4	—	—
Dioxopromethazine	T43.3X1	T43.3X2	T43.3X3	T43.3X4	T43.3X5	T43.3X6
Dioxyline	T46.3X1	T46.3X2	T46.3X3	T46.3X4	T46.3X5	T46.3X6
Dipentene	T52.8X1	T52.8X2	T52.8X3	T52.8X4	—	—
Diperodon	T41.3X1	T41.3X2	T41.3X3	T41.3X4	T41.3X5	T41.3X6
Diphacinone	T60.4X1	T60.4X2	T60.4X3	T60.4X4	—	—
Diphemanil	T44.3X1	T44.3X2	T44.3X3	T44.3X4	T44.3X5	T44.3X6
metilsulfate	T44.3X1	T44.3X2	T44.3X3	T44.3X4	T44.3X5	T44.3X6
Diphenadione	T45.511	T45.512	T45.513	T45.514	T45.515	T45.516
rodenticide	T60.4X1	T60.4X2	T60.4X3	T60.4X4	—	—
Diphenhydramine	T45.0X1	T45.0X2	T45.0X3	T45.0X4	T45.0X5	T45.0X6
Diphenidol	T45.0X1	T45.0X2	T45.0X3	T45.0X4	T45.0X5	T45.0X6
Diphenoxylate	T47.6X1	T47.6X2	T47.6X3	T47.6X4	T47.6X5	T47.6X6
Diphenylamine	T65.3X1	T65.3X2	T65.3X3	T65.3X4	—	—
Diphenylbutazone	T39.2X1	T39.2X2	T39.2X3	T39.2X4	T39.2X5	T39.2X6
Diphenylchloroarsine, not in war	T57.0X1	T57.0X2	T57.0X3	T57.0X4	—	—
Diphenylhydantoin	T42.0X1	T42.0X2	T42.0X3	T42.0X4	T42.0X5	T42.0X6
Diphenylmethane dye	T52.1X1	T52.1X2	T52.1X3	T52.1X4	—	—
Diphenylpyraline	T45.0X1	T45.0X2	T45.0X3	T45.0X4	T45.0X5	T45.0X6
Diphtheria						
antitoxin	T50.Z11	T50.Z12	T50.Z13	T50.Z14	T50.Z15	T50.Z16
toxoid	T50.A91	T50.A92	T50.A93	T50.A94	T50.A95	T50.A96
with tetanus toxoid	T50.A21	T50.A22	T50.A23	T50.A24	T50.A25	T50.A26
with pertussis component	T50.A11	T50.A12	T50.A13	T50.A14	T50.A15	T50.A16

Substance	Poisoning, Accidental (Unintentional)	Poisoning, Intentional Self-Harm	Poisoning, Assault	Poisoning, Undetermined	Adverse Effect	Underdosing
Diphtheria (Continued)						
vaccine (combination)	T50.A91	T50.A92	T50.A93	T50.A94	T50.A95	T50.A96
combination						
including pertussis	T50.A11	T50.A12	T50.A13	T50.A14	T50.A15	T50.A16
without pertussis	T50.A21	T50.A22	T50.A23	T50.A24	T50.A25	T50.A26
Diphylline	T50.2X1	T50.2X2	T50.2X3	T50.2X4	T50.2X5	T50.2X6
Dipipanone	T40.4X1	T40.4X2	T40.4X3	T40.4X4	—	—
Dipivefrine	T49.5X1	T49.5X2	T49.5X3	T49.5X4	T49.5X5	T49.5X6
Diplovax	T50.B91	T50.B92	T50.B93	T50.B94	T50.B95	T50.B96
Diprophylline	T50.2X1	T50.2X2	T50.2X3	T50.2X4	T50.2X5	T50.2X6
Dipropyline	T48.291	T48.292	T48.293	T48.294	T48.295	T48.296
Dipyridamole	T46.3X1	T46.3X2	T46.3X3	T46.3X4	T46.3X5	T46.3X6
Dipyrone	T39.2X1	T39.2X2	T39.2X3	T39.2X4	T39.2X5	T39.2X6
Diquat (dibromide)	T60.3X1	T60.3X2	T60.3X3	T60.3X4	—	—
Disinfectant	T65.891	T65.892	T65.893	T65.894	—	—
alkaline	T54.3X1	T54.3X2	T54.3X3	T54.3X4	—	—
aromatic	T54.1X1	T54.1X2	T54.1X3	T54.1X4	—	—
intestinal	T37.8X1	T37.8X2	T37.8X3	T37.8X4	T37.8X5	T37.8X6
Disipal	T42.8X1	T42.8X2	T42.8X3	T42.8X4	T42.8X5	T42.8X6
Disodium edetate	T50.6X1	T50.6X2	T50.6X3	T50.6X4	T50.6X5	T50.6X6
Disoprofol	T41.291	T41.292	T41.293	T41.294	T41.295	T41.296
Disopyramide	T46.2X1	T46.2X2	T46.2X3	T46.2X4	T46.2X5	T46.2X6
Distigmine (bromide)	T44.0X1	T44.0X2	T44.0X3	T44.0X4	T44.0X5	T44.0X6
Disulfamide	T50.2X1	T50.2X2	T50.2X3	T50.2X4	T50.2X5	T50.2X6
Disulfanilamide	T37.0X1	T37.0X2	T37.0X3	T37.0X4	T37.0X5	T37.0X6
Disulfiram	T50.6X1	T50.6X2	T50.6X3	T50.6X4	T50.6X5	T50.6X6
Disulfoton	T60.0X1	T60.0X2	T60.0X3	T60.0X4	—	—
Dithiazanine iodide	T37.4X1	T37.4X2	T37.4X3	T37.4X4	T37.4X5	T37.4X6
Dithiocarbamate	T60.0X1	T60.0X2	T60.0X3	T60.0X4	—	—
Dithranol	T49.4X1	T49.4X2	T49.4X3	T49.4X4	T49.4X5	T49.4X6
Diucardin	T50.2X1	T50.2X2	T50.2X3	T50.2X4	T50.2X5	T50.2X6
Diupres	T50.2X1	T50.2X2	T50.2X3	T50.2X4	T50.2X5	T50.2X6
Diuretic NEC	T50.2X1	T50.2X2	T50.2X3	T50.2X4	T50.2X5	T50.2X6
benzothiadiazine	T50.2X1	T50.2X2	T50.2X3	T50.2X4	T50.2X5	T50.2X6
carbonic acid anhydrase inhibitors	T50.2X1	T50.2X2	T50.2X3	T50.2X4	T50.2X5	T50.2X6
furfuryl NEC	T50.2X1	T50.2X2	T50.2X3	T50.2X4	T50.2X5	T50.2X6
loop (high-ceiling)	T50.1X1	T50.1X2	T50.1X3	T50.1X4	T50.1X5	T50.1X6
mercurial NEC	T50.2X1	T50.2X2	T50.2X3	T50.2X4	T50.2X5	T50.2X6
osmotic	T50.2X1	T50.2X2	T50.2X3	T50.2X4	T50.2X5	T50.2X6
purine NEC	T50.2X1	T50.2X2	T50.2X3	T50.2X4	T50.2X5	T50.2X6
saluretic NEC	T50.2X1	T50.2X2	T50.2X3	T50.2X4	T50.2X5	T50.2X6

◄ New   ◄|| Revised   ~~deleted~~ Deleted

Substance	Poisoning, Accidental (Unintentional)	Poisoning, Intentional Self-Harm	Poisoning, Assault	Poisoning, Undetermined	Adverse Effect	Underdosing
Diuretic NEC *(Continued)*						
sulfonamide	T50.2X1	T50.2X2	T50.2X3	T50.2X4	T50.2X5	T50.2X6
thiazide NEC	T50.2X1	T50.2X2	T50.2X3	T50.2X4	T50.2X5	T50.2X6
xanthine	T50.2X1	T50.2X2	T50.2X3	T50.2X4	T50.2X5	T50.2X6
Diurgin	T50.2X1	T50.2X2	T50.2X3	T50.2X4	T50.2X5	T50.2X6
Diuril	T50.2X1	T50.2X2	T50.2X3	T50.2X4	T50.2X5	T50.2X6
Diuron	T60.3X1	T60.3X2	T60.3X3	T60.3X4	—	—
Divalproex	T42.6X1	T42.6X2	T42.6X3	T42.6X4	T42.6X5	T42.6X6
Divinyl ether	T41.0X1	T41.0X2	T41.0X3	T41.0X4	T41.0X5	T41.0X6
Dixanthogen	T49.0X1	T49.0X2	T49.0X3	T49.0X4	T49.0X5	T49.0X6
Dixyrazine	T43.3X1	T43.3X2	T43.3X3	T43.3X4	T43.3X5	T43.3X6
D-lysergic acid diethylamide	T40.8X1	T40.8X2	T40.8X3	T40.8X4	—	—
DMCT	T36.4X1	T36.4X2	T36.4X3	T36.4X4	T36.4X5	T36.4X6
DMSO — *see Dimethyl sulfoxide*						
DNBP	T60.3X1	T60.3X2	T60.3X3	T60.3X4	—	—
DNOC	T65.3X1	T65.3X2	T65.3X3	T65.3X4	—	—
DOCA	T38.0X1	T38.0X2	T38.0X3	T38.0X4	T38.0X5	T38.0X6
Dobutamine	T44.5X1	T44.5X2	T44.5X3	T44.5X4	T44.5X5	T44.5X6
Docusate sodium	T47.4X1	T47.4X2	T47.4X3	T47.4X4	T47.4X5	T47.4X6
Dodicin	T49.0X1	T49.0X2	T49.0X3	T49.0X4	T49.0X5	T49.0X6
Dofamium chloride	T49.0X1	T49.0X2	T49.0X3	T49.0X4	T49.0X5	T49.0X6
Dolophine	T40.3X1	T40.3X2	T40.3X3	T40.3X4	T40.3X5	T40.3X6
Doloxene	T39.8X1	T39.8X2	T39.8X3	T39.8X4	T39.8X5	T39.8X6
Domestic gas (after combustion) — *see Gas, utility*						
prior to combustion	T59.891	T59.892	T59.893	T59.894	—	—
Domiodol	T48.4X1	T48.4X2	T48.4X3	T48.4X4	T48.4X5	T48.4X6
Domiphen (bromide)	T49.0X1	T49.0X2	T49.0X3	T49.0X4	T49.0X5	T49.0X6
Domperidone	T45.0X1	T45.0X2	T45.0X3	T45.0X4	T45.0X5	T45.0X6
Dopa	T42.8X1	T42.8X2	T42.8X3	T42.8X4	T42.8X5	T42.8X6
Dopamine	T44.991	T44.992	T44.993	T44.994	T44.995	T44.996
Doriden	T42.6X1	T42.6X2	T42.6X3	T42.6X4	T42.6X5	T42.6X6
Dormiral	T42.3X1	T42.3X2	T42.3X3	T42.3X4	T42.3X5	T42.3X6
Dormison	T42.6X1	T42.6X2	T42.6X3	T42.6X4	T42.6X5	T42.6X6
Dornase	T48.4X1	T48.4X2	T48.4X3	T48.4X4	T48.4X5	T48.4X6
Dorsacaine	T41.3X1	T41.3X2	T41.3X3	T41.3X4	T41.3X5	T41.3X6
Dosulepin	T43.011	T43.012	T43.013	T43.014	T43.015	T43.016
Dothiepin	T43.011	T43.012	T43.013	T43.014	T43.015	T43.016
Doxantrazole	T48.6X1	T48.6X2	T48.6X3	T48.6X4	T48.6X5	T48.6X6
Doxapram	T50.7X1	T50.7X2	T50.7X3	T50.7X4	T50.7X5	T50.7X6
Doxazosin	T44.6X1	T44.6X2	T44.6X3	T44.6X4	T44.6X5	T44.6X6
Doxepin	T43.011	T43.012	T43.013	T43.014	T43.015	T43.016

Substance	Poisoning, Accidental (Unintentional)	Poisoning, Intentional Self-Harm	Poisoning, Assault	Poisoning, Undetermined	Adverse Effect	Underdosing
Doxifluridine	T45.1X1	T45.1X2	T45.1X3	T45.1X4	T45.1X5	T45.1X6
Doxorubicin	T45.1X1	T45.1X2	T45.1X3	T45.1X4	T45.1X5	T45.1X6
Doxycycline	T36.4X1	T36.4X2	T36.4X3	T36.4X4	T36.4X5	T36.4X6
Doxylamine	T45.0X1	T45.0X2	T45.0X3	T45.0X4	T45.0X5	T45.0X6
Dramamine	T45.0X1	T45.0X2	T45.0X3	T45.0X4	T45.0X5	T45.0X6
Drano (drain cleaner)	T54.3X1	T54.3X2	T54.3X3	T54.3X4	—	—
Dressing, live pulp	T49.7X1	T49.7X2	T49.7X3	T49.7X4	T49.7X5	T49.7X6
Drocode	T40.2X1	T40.2X2	T40.2X3	T40.2X4	T40.2X5	T40.2X6
Dromoran	T40.2X1	T40.2X2	T40.2X3	T40.2X4	T40.2X5	T40.2X6
Dromostanolone	T38.7X1	T38.7X2	T38.7X3	T38.7X4	T38.7X5	T38.7X6
Dronabinol	T40.7X1	T40.7X2	T40.7X3	T40.7X4	T40.7X5	T40.7X6
Droperidol	T43.591	T43.592	T43.593	T43.594	T43.595	T43.596
Dropropizine	T48.3X1	T48.3X2	T48.3X3	T48.3X4	T48.3X5	T48.3X6
Drostanolone	T38.7X1	T38.7X2	T38.7X3	T38.7X4	T38.7X5	T38.7X6
Drotaverine	T44.3X1	T44.3X2	T44.3X3	T44.3X4	T44.3X5	T44.3X6
Drotrecogin alfa	T45.511	T45.512	T45.513	T45.514	T45.515	T45.516
Drug NEC	T50.901	T50.902	T50.903	T50.904	T50.905	T50.906
specified NEC	T50.991	T50.992	T50.993	T50.994	T50.995	T50.996
DTIC	T45.1X1	T45.1X2	T45.1X3	T45.1X4	T45.1X5	T45.1X6
Duboisine	T44.3X1	T44.3X2	T44.3X3	T44.3X4	T44.3X5	T44.3X6
Dulcolax	T47.2X1	T47.2X2	T47.2X3	T47.2X4	T47.2X5	T47.2X6
Duponol (C) (EP)	T49.2X1	T49.2X2	T49.2X3	T49.2X4	T49.2X5	T49.2X6
Durabolin	T38.7X1	T38.7X2	T38.7X3	T38.7X4	T38.7X5	T38.7X6
Dyclone	T41.3X1	T41.3X2	T41.3X3	T41.3X4	T41.3X5	T41.3X6
Dyclonine	T41.3X1	T41.3X2	T41.3X3	T41.3X4	T41.3X5	T41.3X6
Dydrogesterone	T38.5X1	T38.5X2	T38.5X3	T38.5X4	T38.5X5	T38.5X6
Dye NEC	T65.6X1	T65.6X2	T65.6X3	T65.6X4	—	—
antiseptic	T49.0X1	T49.0X2	T49.0X3	T49.0X4	T49.0X5	T49.0X6
diagnostic agents	T50.8X1	T50.8X2	T50.8X3	T50.8X4	T50.8X5	T50.8X6
pharmaceutical NEC	T50.901	T50.902	T50.903	T50.904	T50.905	T50.906
Dyflos	T44.0X1	T44.0X2	T44.0X3	T44.0X4	T44.0X5	T44.0X6
Dymelor	T38.3X1	T38.3X2	T38.3X3	T38.3X4	T38.3X5	T38.3X6
Dynamite	T65.3X1	T65.3X2	T65.3X3	T65.3X4	—	—
fumes	T59.891	T59.892	T59.893	T59.894	—	—
Dyphylline	T44.3X1	T44.3X2	T44.3X3	T44.3X4	T44.3X5	T44.3X6
E						
Ear drug NEC	T49.6X1	T49.6X2	T49.6X3	T49.6X4	T49.6X5	T49.6X6
Ear preparations	T49.6X1	T49.6X2	T49.6X3	T49.6X4	T49.6X5	T49.6X6
Econazole	T49.0X1	T49.0X2	T49.0X3	T49.0X4	T49.0X5	T49.0X6
Ecothiopate iodide	T49.5X1	T49.5X2	T49.5X3	T49.5X4	T49.5X5	T49.5X6
Echothiophate, echothiopate, ecothiopate	T49.5X1	T49.5X2	T49.5X3	T49.5X4	T49.5X5	T49.5X6

TABLE OF DRUGS AND CHEMICALS

Substance	External Cause (T-Code)					
	Poisoning, Accidental (Unintentional)	Poisoning, Intentional Self-Harm	Poisoning, Assault	Poisoning, Undetermined	Adverse Effect	Underdosing
Ecstasy	T43.621	T43.622	T43.623	T43.624	T43.625	T43.626
Ectylurea	T42.6X1	T42.6X2	T42.6X3	T42.6X4	T42.6X5	T42.6X6
Edathamil disodium	T45.8X1	T45.8X2	T45.8X3	T45.8X4	T45.8X5	T45.8X6
Edecrin	T50.1X1	T50.1X2	T50.1X3	T50.1X4	T50.1X5	T50.1X6
Edetate, disodium (calcium)	T45.8X1	T45.8X2	T45.8X3	T45.8X4	T45.8X5	T45.8X6
Edoxudine	T49.5X1	T49.5X2	T49.5X3	T49.5X4	T49.5X5	T49.5X6
Edrophonium	T44.0X1	T44.0X2	T44.0X3	T44.0X4	T44.0X5	T44.0X6
chloride	T44.0X1	T44.0X2	T44.0X3	T44.0X4	T44.0X5	T44.0X6
EDTA	T50.6X1	T50.6X2	T50.6X3	T50.6X4	T50.6X5	T50.6X6
Eflornithine	T37.2X1	T37.2X2	T37.2X3	T37.2X4	T37.2X5	T37.2X6
Efloxate	T46.3X1	T46.3X2	T46.3X3	T46.3X4	T46.3X5	T46.3X6
Elase	T49.8X1	T49.8X2	T49.8X3	T49.8X4	T49.8X5	T49.8X6
Elastase	T47.5X1	T47.5X2	T47.5X3	T47.5X4	T47.5X5	T47.5X6
Elaterium	T47.2X1	T47.2X2	T47.2X3	T47.2X4	T47.2X5	T47.2X6
Elcatonin	T50.991	T50.992	T50.993	T50.994	T50.995	T50.996
Elder	T62.2X1	T62.2X2	T62.2X3	T62.2X4	—	—
berry (unripe)	T62.1X1	T62.1X2	T62.1X3	T62.1X4	—	—
Electrolyte balance drug	T50.3X1	T50.3X2	T50.3X3	T50.3X4	T50.3X5	T50.3X6
Electrolytes NEC	T50.3X1	T50.3X2	T50.3X3	T50.3X4	T50.3X5	T50.3X6
Electrolytic agent NEC	T50.3X1	T50.3X2	T50.3X3	T50.3X4	T50.3X5	T50.3X6
Elemental diet	T50.901	T50.902	T50.903	T50.904	T50.905	T50.906
Elliptinium acetate	T45.1X1	T45.1X2	T45.1X3	T45.1X4	T45.1X5	T45.1X6
Embramine	T45.0X1	T45.0X2	T45.0X3	T45.0X4	T45.0X5	T45.0X6
Emepronium (salts)	T44.3X1	T44.3X2	T44.3X3	T44.3X4	T44.3X5	T44.3X6
bromide	T44.3X1	T44.3X2	T44.3X3	T44.3X4	T44.3X5	T44.3X6
Emetic NEC	T47.7X1	T47.7X2	T47.7X3	T47.7X4	T47.7X5	T47.7X6
Emetine	T37.3X1	T37.3X2	T37.3X3	T37.3X4	T37.3X5	T37.3X6
Emollient NEC	T49.3X1	T49.3X2	T49.3X3	T49.3X4	T49.3X5	T49.3X6
Emorfazone	T39.8X1	T39.8X2	T39.8X3	T39.8X4	T39.8X5	T39.8X6
Emylcamate	T43.591	T43.592	T43.593	T43.594	T43.595	T43.596
Enalapril	T46.4X1	T46.4X2	T46.4X3	T46.4X4	T46.4X5	T46.4X6
Enalaprilat	T46.4X1	T46.4X2	T46.4X3	T46.4X4	T46.4X5	T46.4X6
Encainide	T46.2X1	T46.2X2	T46.2X3	T46.2X4	T46.2X5	T46.2X6
Endocaine	T41.3X1	T41.3X2	T41.3X3	T41.3X4	T41.3X5	T41.3X6
Endosulfan	T60.2X1	T60.2X2	T60.2X3	T60.2X4	—	—
Endothall	T60.3X1	T60.3X2	T60.3X3	T60.3X4	—	—
Endralazine	T46.5X1	T46.5X2	T46.5X3	T46.5X4	T46.5X5	T46.5X6
Endrin	T60.1X1	T60.1X2	T60.1X3	T60.1X4	—	—
Enflurane	T41.0X1	T41.0X2	T41.0X3	T41.0X4	T41.0X5	T41.0X6
Enhexymal	T42.3X1	T42.3X2	T42.3X3	T42.3X4	T42.3X5	T42.3X6
Enocitabine	T45.1X1	T45.1X2	T45.1X3	T45.1X4	T45.1X5	T45.1X6
Enovid	T38.4X1	T38.4X2	T38.4X3	T38.4X4	T38.4X5	T38.4X6

Substance	External Cause (T-Code)					
	Poisoning, Accidental (Unintentional)	Poisoning, Intentional Self-Harm	Poisoning, Assault	Poisoning, Undetermined	Adverse Effect	Underdosing
Enoxacin	T36.8X1	T36.8X2	T36.8X3	T36.8X4	T36.8X5	T36.8X6
Enoxaparin (sodium)	T45.511	T45.512	T45.513	T45.514	T45.515	T45.516
Enpiprazole	T43.591	T43.592	T43.593	T43.594	T43.595	T43.596
Enprofylline	T48.6X1	T48.6X2	T48.6X3	T48.6X4	T48.6X5	T48.6X6
Enprostil	T47.1X1	T47.1X2	T47.1X3	T47.1X4	T47.1X5	T47.1X6
ENT preparations (anti-infectives)	T49.6X1	T49.6X2	T49.6X3	T49.6X4	T49.6X5	T49.6X6
Enviomycin	T36.8X1	T36.8X2	T36.8X3	T36.8X4	T36.8X5	T36.8X6
Enzodase	T45.3X1	T45.3X2	T45.3X3	T45.3X4	T45.3X5	T45.3X6
Enzyme NEC	T45.3X1	T45.3X2	T45.3X3	T45.3X4	T45.3X5	T45.3X6
depolymerizing	T49.8X1	T49.8X2	T49.8X3	T49.8X4	T49.8X5	T49.8X6
fibrolytic	T45.3X1	T45.3X2	T45.3X3	T45.3X4	T45.3X5	T45.3X6
gastric	T47.5X1	T47.5X2	T47.5X3	T47.5X4	T47.5X5	T47.5X6
intestinal	T47.5X1	T47.5X2	T47.5X3	T47.5X4	T47.5X5	T47.5X6
local action	T49.4X1	T49.4X2	T49.4X3	T49.4X4	T49.4X5	T49.4X6
proteolytic	T49.4X1	T49.4X2	T49.4X3	T49.4X4	T49.4X5	T49.4X6
thrombolytic	T45.3X1	T45.3X2	T45.3X3	T45.3X4	T45.3X5	T45.3X6
EPAB	T41.3X1	T41.3X2	T41.3X3	T41.3X4	T41.3X5	T41.3X6
Epanutin	T42.0X1	T42.0X2	T42.0X3	T42.0X4	T42.0X5	T42.0X6
Ephedra	T44.991	T44.992	T44.993	T44.994	T44.995	T44.996
Ephedrine	T44.991	T44.992	T44.993	T44.994	T44.995	T44.996
Epichlorhydrin, epichlorohydrin	T52.8X1	T52.8X2	T52.8X3	T52.8X4	—	—
Epicillin	T36.0X1	T36.0X2	T36.0X3	T36.0X4	T36.0X5	T36.0X6
Epiestriol	T38.5X1	T38.5X2	T38.5X3	T38.5X4	T38.5X5	T38.5X6
Epilim — see Sodium valproate						
Epimestrol	T38.5X1	T38.5X2	T38.5X3	T38.5X4	T38.5X5	T38.5X6
Epinephrine	T44.5X1	T44.5X2	T44.5X3	T44.5X4	T44.5X5	T44.5X6
Epirubicin	T45.1X1	T45.1X2	T45.1X3	T45.1X4	T45.1X5	T45.1X6
Epitiostanol	T38.7X1	T38.7X2	T38.7X3	T38.7X4	T38.7X5	T38.7X6
Epitizide	T50.2X1	T50.2X2	T50.2X3	T50.2X4	T50.2X5	T50.2X6
EPN	T60.0X1	T60.0X2	T60.0X3	T60.0X4	—	—
EPO	T45.8X1	T45.8X2	T45.8X3	T45.8X4	T45.8X5	T45.8X6
Epoetin alpha	T45.8X1	T45.8X2	T45.8X3	T45.8X4	T45.8X5	T45.8X6
Epomediol	T50.991	T50.992	T50.993	T50.994	T50.995	T50.996
Epoprostenol	T45.521	T45.522	T45.523	T45.524	T45.525	T45.526
Epoxy resin	T65.891	T65.892	T65.893	T65.894	—	—
Eprazinone	T48.4X1	T48.4X2	T48.4X3	T48.4X4	T48.4X5	T48.4X6
Epsilon amino-caproic acid	T45.621	T45.622	T45.623	T45.624	T45.625	T45.626
Epsom salt	T47.3X1	T47.3X2	T47.3X3	T47.3X4	T47.3X5	T47.3X6
Eptazocine	T40.4X1	T40.4X2	T40.4X3	T40.4X4	T40.4X5	T40.4X6
Equanil	T43.591	T43.592	T43.593	T43.594	T43.595	T43.596
Equisetum	T62.2X1	T62.2X2	T62.2X3	T62.2X4	—	—
diuretic	T50.2X1	T50.2X2	T50.2X3	T50.2X4	T50.2X5	T50.2X6

◀ New   ◀ Revised   ~~deleted~~ Deleted

Substance	External Cause (T-Code)					
	Poisoning, Accidental (Unintentional)	Poisoning, Intentional Self-Harm	Poisoning, Assault	Poisoning, Undetermined	Adverse Effect	Underdosing
Ergobasine	T48.0X1	T48.0X2	T48.0X3	T48.0X4	T48.0X5	T48.0X6
Ergocalciferol	T45.2X1	T45.2X2	T45.2X3	T45.2X4	T45.2X5	T45.2X6
Ergoloid mesylates	T46.7X1	T46.7X2	T46.7X3	T46.7X4	T46.7X5	T46.7X6
Ergometrine	T48.0X1	T48.0X2	T48.0X3	T48.0X4	T48.0X5	T48.0X6
Ergonovine	T48.0X1	T48.0X2	T48.0X3	T48.0X4	T48.0X5	T48.0X6
Ergot NEC	T64.81	T64.82	T64.83	T64.84	—	—
derivative	T48.0X1	T48.0X2	T48.0X3	T48.0X4	T48.0X5	T48.0X6
medicinal (alkaloids)	T48.0X1	T48.0X2	T48.0X3	T48.0X4	T48.0X5	T48.0X6
prepared	T48.0X1	T48.0X2	T48.0X3	T48.0X4	T48.0X5	T48.0X6
Ergotamine	T46.5X1	T46.5X2	T46.5X3	T46.5X4	T46.5X5	T46.5X6
Ergotocine	T48.0X1	T48.0X2	T48.0X3	T48.0X4	T48.0X5	T48.0X6
Ergotrate	T48.0X1	T48.0X2	T48.0X3	T48.0X4	T48.0X5	T48.0X6
Eritrityl tetranitrate	T46.3X1	T46.3X2	T46.3X3	T46.3X4	T46.3X5	T46.3X6
Erythrityl tetranitrate	T46.3X1	T46.3X2	T46.3X3	T46.3X4	T46.3X5	T46.3X6
Erythrol tetranitrate	T46.3X1	T46.3X2	T46.3X3	T46.3X4	T46.3X5	T46.3X6
Erythromycin (salts)	T36.3X1	T36.3X2	T36.3X3	T36.3X4	T36.3X5	T36.3X6
ophthalmic preparation	T49.5X1	T49.5X2	T49.5X3	T49.5X4	T49.5X5	T49.5X6
topical NEC	T49.0X1	T49.0X2	T49.0X3	T49.0X4	T49.0X5	T49.0X6
Erythropoietin	T45.8X1	T45.8X2	T45.8X3	T45.8X4	T45.8X5	T45.8X6
human	T45.8X1	T45.8X2	T45.8X3	T45.8X4	T45.8X5	T45.8X6
Escin	T46.991	T46.992	T46.993	T46.994	T46.995	T46.996
Esculin	T45.2X1	T45.2X2	T45.2X3	T45.2X4	T45.2X5	T45.2X6
Esculoside	T45.2X1	T45.2X2	T45.2X3	T45.2X4	T45.2X5	T45.2X6
ESDT (ether-soluble tar distillate)	T49.1X1	T49.1X2	T49.1X3	T49.1X4	T49.1X5	T49.1X6
Eserine	T49.5X1	T49.5X2	T49.5X3	T49.5X4	T49.5X5	T49.5X6
Esflurbiprofen	T39.311	T39.312	T39.313	T39.314	T39.315	T39.316
Eskabarb	T42.3X1	T42.3X2	T42.3X3	T42.3X4	T42.3X5	T42.3X6
Eskalith	T43.8X1	T43.8X2	T43.8X3	T43.8X4	T43.8X5	T43.8X6
Esmolol	T44.7X1	T44.7X2	T44.7X3	T44.7X4	T44.7X5	T44.7X6
Estanozolol	T38.7X1	T38.7X2	T38.7X3	T38.7X4	T38.7X5	T38.7X6
Estazolam	T42.4X1	T42.4X2	T42.4X3	T42.4X4	T42.4X5	T42.4X6
Estradiol	T38.5X1	T38.5X2	T38.5X3	T38.5X4	T38.5X5	T38.5X6
with testosterone	T38.7X1	T38.7X2	T38.7X3	T38.7X4	T38.7X5	T38.7X6
benzoate	T38.5X1	T38.5X2	T38.5X3	T38.5X4	T38.5X5	T38.5X6
Estramustine	T45.1X1	T45.1X2	T45.1X3	T45.1X4	T45.1X5	T45.1X6
Estriol	T38.5X1	T38.5X2	T38.5X3	T38.5X4	T38.5X5	T38.5X6
Estrogen	T38.5X1	T38.5X2	T38.5X3	T38.5X4	T38.5X5	T38.5X6
with progesterone	T38.5X1	T38.5X2	T38.5X3	T38.5X4	T38.5X5	T38.5X6
conjugated	T38.5X1	T38.5X2	T38.5X3	T38.5X4	T38.5X5	T38.5X6
Estrone	T38.5X1	T38.5X2	T38.5X3	T38.5X4	T38.5X5	T38.5X6
Estropipate	T38.5X1	T38.5X2	T38.5X3	T38.5X4	T38.5X5	T38.5X6

Substance	External Cause (T-Code)					
	Poisoning, Accidental (Unintentional)	Poisoning, Intentional Self-Harm	Poisoning, Assault	Poisoning, Undetermined	Adverse Effect	Underdosing
Etacrynate sodium	T50.1X1	T50.1X2	T50.1X3	T50.1X4	T50.1X5	T50.1X6
Etacrynic acid	T50.1X1	T50.1X2	T50.1X3	T50.1X4	T50.1X5	T50.1X6
Etafedrine	T48.6X1	T48.6X2	T48.6X3	T48.6X4	T48.6X5	T48.6X6
Etafenone	T46.3X1	T46.3X2	T46.3X3	T46.3X4	T46.3X5	T46.3X6
Etambutol	T37.1X1	T37.1X2	T37.1X3	T37.1X4	T37.1X5	T37.1X6
Etamiphyllin	T48.6X1	T48.6X2	T48.6X3	T48.6X4	T48.6X5	T48.6X6
Etamivan	T50.7X1	T50.7X2	T50.7X3	T50.7X4	T50.7X5	T50.7X6
Etamsylate	T45.7X1	T45.7X2	T45.7X3	T45.7X4	T45.7X5	T45.7X6
Etebenecid	T50.4X1	T50.4X2	T50.4X3	T50.4X4	T50.4X5	T50.4X6
Ethacridine	T49.0X1	T49.0X2	T49.0X3	T49.0X4	T49.0X5	T49.0X6
Ethacrynic acid	T50.1X1	T50.1X2	T50.1X3	T50.1X4	T50.1X5	T50.1X6
Ethadione	T42.2X1	T42.2X2	T42.2X3	T42.2X4	T42.2X5	T42.2X6
Ethambutol	T37.1X1	T37.1X2	T37.1X3	T37.1X4	T37.1X5	T37.1X6
Ethamide	T50.2X1	T50.2X2	T50.2X3	T50.2X4	T50.2X5	T50.2X6
Ethamivan	T50.7X1	T50.7X2	T50.7X3	T50.7X4	T50.7X5	T50.7X6
Ethamsylate	T45.7X1	T45.7X2	T45.7X3	T45.7X4	T45.7X5	T45.7X6
Ethanol	T51.0X1	T51.0X2	T51.0X3	T51.0X4	—	—
beverage	T51.0X1	T51.0X2	T51.0X3	T51.0X4	—	—
Ethanolamine oleate	T46.8X1	T46.8X2	T46.8X3	T46.8X4	T46.8X5	T46.8X6
Ethaverine	T44.3X1	T44.3X2	T44.3X3	T44.3X4	T44.3X5	T44.3X6
Ethchlorvynol	T42.6X1	T42.6X2	T42.6X3	T42.6X4	T42.6X5	T42.6X6
Ethebenecid	T50.4X1	T50.4X2	T50.4X3	T50.4X4	T50.4X5	T50.4X6
Ether (vapor)	T41.0X1	T41.0X2	T41.0X3	T41.0X4	T41.0X5	T41.0X6
anesthetic	T41.0X1	T41.0X2	T41.0X3	T41.0X4	T41.0X5	T41.0X6
divinyl	T41.0X1	T41.0X2	T41.0X3	T41.0X4	T41.0X5	T41.0X6
ethyl (medicinal)	T41.0X1	T41.0X2	T41.0X3	T41.0X4	T41.0X5	T41.0X6
nonmedicinal	T52.8X1	T52.8X2	T52.8X3	T52.8X4	—	—
petroleum — *see* Ligroin						
solvent	T52.8X1	T52.8X2	T52.8X3	T52.8X4	—	—
Ethiazide	T50.2X1	T50.2X2	T50.2X3	T50.2X4	T50.2X5	T50.2X6
Ethidium chloride (vapor)	T59.891	T59.892	T59.893	T59.894	—	—
Ethinamate	T42.6X1	T42.6X2	T42.6X3	T42.6X4	T42.6X5	T42.6X6
Ethinylestradiol, ethinyloestradiol	T38.5X1	T38.5X2	T38.5X3	T38.5X4	T38.5X5	T38.5X6
with						
levonorgestrel	T38.4X1	T38.4X2	T38.4X3	T38.4X4	T38.4X5	T38.4X6
norethisterone	T38.4X1	T38.4X2	T38.4X3	T38.4X4	T38.4X5	T38.4X6
Ethiodized oil (131 I)	T50.8X1	T50.8X2	T50.8X3	T50.8X4	T50.8X5	T50.8X6
Ethion	T60.0X1	T60.0X2	T60.0X3	T60.0X4	—	—
Ethionamide	T37.1X1	T37.1X2	T37.1X3	T37.1X4	T37.1X5	T37.1X6
Ethioniamide	T37.1X1	T37.1X2	T37.1X3	T37.1X4	T37.1X5	T37.1X6
Ethisterone	T38.5X1	T38.5X2	T38.5X3	T38.5X4	T38.5X5	T38.5X6
Ethobral	T42.3X1	T42.3X2	T42.3X3	T42.3X4	T42.3X5	T42.3X6

TABLE OF DRUGS AND CHEMICALS

Substance	Poisoning, Accidental (Unintentional)	Poisoning, Intentional Self-Harm	Poisoning, Assault	Poisoning, Undetermined	Adverse Effect	Underdosing
Ethocaine (infiltration) (topical)	T41.3X1	T41.3X2	T41.3X3	T41.3X4	T41.3X5	T41.3X6
nerve block (peripheral) (plexus)	T41.3X1	T41.3X2	T41.3X3	T41.3X4	T41.3X5	T41.3X6
spinal	T41.3X1	T41.3X2	T41.3X3	T41.3X4	T41.3X5	T41.3X6
Ethoheptazine	T40.4X1	T40.4X2	T40.4X3	T40.4X4	T40.4X5	T40.4X6
Ethopropazine	T44.3X1	T44.3X2	T44.3X3	T44.3X4	T44.3X5	T44.3X6
Ethosuximide	T42.2X1	T42.2X2	T42.2X3	T42.2X4	T42.2X5	T42.2X6
Ethotoin	T42.0X1	T42.0X2	T42.0X3	T42.0X4	T42.0X5	T42.0X6
Ethoxazene	T37.91	T37.92	T37.93	T37.94	T37.95	T37.96
Ethoxazorutoside	T46.991	T46.992	T46.993	T46.994	T46.995	T46.996
2-Ethoxyethanol	T52.3X1	T52.3X2	T52.3X3	T52.3X4	—	—
Ethoxzolamide	T50.2X1	T50.2X2	T50.2X3	T50.2X4	T50.2X5	T50.2X6
Ethyl						
acetate	T52.8X1	T52.8X2	T52.8X3	T52.8X4	—	—
alcohol	T51.0X1	T51.0X2	T51.0X3	T51.0X4	—	—
beverage	T51.0X1	T51.0X2	T51.0X3	T51.0X4	—	—
aldehyde (vapor)	T59.891	T59.892	T59.893	T59.894	—	—
liquid	T52.8X1	T52.8X2	T52.8X3	T52.8X4	—	—
aminobenzoate	T41.3X1	T41.3X2	T41.3X3	T41.3X4	T41.3X5	T41.3X6
aminophenothiazine	T43.3X1	T43.3X2	T43.3X3	T43.3X4	T43.3X5	T43.3X6
benzoate	T52.8X1	T52.8X2	T52.8X3	T52.8X4	—	—
biscoumacetate	T45.511	T45.512	T45.513	T45.514	T45.515	T45.516
bromide (anesthetic)	T41.0X1	T41.0X2	T41.0X3	T41.0X4	T41.0X5	T41.0X6
carbamate	T45.1X1	T45.1X2	T45.1X3	T45.1X4	T45.1X5	T45.1X6
carbinol	T51.3X1	T51.3X2	T51.3X3	T51.3X4	—	—
carbonate	T52.8X1	T52.8X2	T52.8X3	T52.8X4	—	—
chaulmoograte	T37.1X1	T37.1X2	T37.1X3	T37.1X4	T37.1X5	T37.1X6
chloride (anesthetic)	T41.0X1	T41.0X2	T41.0X3	T41.0X4	T41.0X5	T41.0X6
anesthetic (local)	T41.3X1	T41.3X2	T41.3X3	T41.3X4	T41.3X5	T41.3X6
inhaled	T41.0X1	T41.0X2	T41.0X3	T41.0X4	T41.0X5	T41.0X6
local	T49.4X1	T49.4X2	T49.4X3	T49.4X4	T49.4X5	T49.4X6
solvent	T53.6X1	T53.6X2	T53.6X3	T53.6X4	—	—
dibunate	T48.3X1	T48.3X2	T48.3X3	T48.3X4	T48.3X5	T48.3X6
dichloroarsine (vapor)	T57.0X1	T57.0X2	T57.0X3	T57.0X4	—	—
estranol	T38.7X1	T38.7X2	T38.7X3	T38.7X4	T38.7X5	T38.7X6
ether — see also ether	T52.8X1	T52.8X2	T52.8X3	T52.8X4	—	—
formate NEC (solvent)	T52.0X1	T52.0X2	T52.0X3	T52.0X4	—	—
fumarate	T49.4X1	T49.4X2	T49.4X3	T49.4X4	T49.4X5	T49.4X6
hydroxyisobutyrate NEC (solvent)	T52.8X1	T52.8X2	T52.8X3	T52.8X4	—	—
iodoacetate	T59.3X1	T59.3X2	T59.3X3	T59.3X4	—	—
lactate NEC (solvent)	T52.8X1	T52.8X2	T52.8X3	T52.8X4	—	—
loflazepate	T42.4X1	T42.4X2	T42.4X3	T42.4X4	T42.4X5	T42.4X6

Substance	Poisoning, Accidental (Unintentional)	Poisoning, Intentional Self-Harm	Poisoning, Assault	Poisoning, Undetermined	Adverse Effect	Underdosing
Ethyl *(Continued)*						
mercuric chloride	T56.1X1	T56.1X2	T56.1X3	T56.1X4	—	—
methylcarbinol	T51.8X1	T51.8X2	T51.8X3	T51.8X4	—	—
morphine	T40.2X1	T40.2X2	T40.2X3	T40.2X4	T40.2X5	T40.2X6
noradrenaline	T48.6X1	T48.6X2	T48.6X3	T48.6X4	T48.6X5	T48.6X6
oxybutyrate NEC (solvent)	T52.8X1	T52.8X2	T52.8X3	T52.8X4	—	—
Ethylene (gas)	T59.891	T59.892	T59.893	T59.894	—	—
anesthetic (general)	T41.0X1	T41.0X2	T41.0X3	T41.0X4	T41.0X5	T41.0X6
chlorohydrin	T52.8X1	T52.8X2	T52.8X3	T52.8X4	—	—
vapor	T53.6X1	T53.6X2	T53.6X3	T53.6X4	—	—
dichloride	T52.8X1	T52.8X2	T52.8X3	T52.8X4	—	—
vapor	T53.6X1	T53.6X2	T53.6X3	T53.6X4	—	—
dinitrate	T52.3X1	T52.3X2	T52.3X3	T52.3X4	—	—
glycol(s)	T52.8X1	T52.8X2	T52.8X3	T52.8X4	—	—
dinitrate	T52.3X1	T52.3X2	T52.3X3	T52.3X4	—	—
monobutyl ether	T52.3X1	T52.3X2	T52.3X3	T52.3X4	—	—
imine	T54.1X1	T54.1X2	T54.1X3	T54.1X4	—	—
oxide (fumigant) (nonmedicinal)	T59.891	T59.892	T59.893	T59.894	—	—
medicinal	T49.0X1	T49.0X2	T49.0X3	T49.0X4	T49.0X5	T49.0X6
Ethylenediamine theophylline	T48.6X1	T48.6X2	T48.6X3	T48.6X4	T48.6X5	T48.6X6
Ethylenediaminetetra-acetic acid	T50.6X1	T50.6X2	T50.6X3	T50.6X4	T50.6X5	T50.6X6
Ethylenedinitrilotetra-acetate	T50.6X1	T50.6X2	T50.6X3	T50.6X4	T50.6X5	T50.6X6
Ethylestrenol	T38.7X1	T38.7X2	T38.7X3	T38.7X4	T38.7X5	T38.7X6
Ethylhydroxycellulose	T47.4X1	T47.4X2	T47.4X3	T47.4X4	T47.4X5	T47.4X6
Ethylidene						
chloride NEC	T53.6X1	T53.6X2	T53.6X3	T53.6X4	—	—
diacetate	T60.3X1	T60.3X2	T60.3X3	T60.3X4	—	—
dicoumarin	T45.511	T45.512	T45.513	T45.514	T45.515	T45.516
dicoumarol	T45.511	T45.512	T45.513	T45.514	T45.515	T45.516
diethyl ether	T52.0X1	T52.0X2	T52.0X3	T52.0X4	—	—
Ethylmorphine	T40.2X1	T40.2X2	T40.2X3	T40.2X4	T40.2X5	T40.2X6
Ethylnorepinephrine	T48.6X1	T48.6X2	T48.6X3	T48.6X4	T48.6X5	T48.6X6
Ethylparachlorophen-oxyisobutyrate	T46.6X1	T46.6X2	T46.6X3	T46.6X4	T46.6X5	T46.6X6
Ethynodiol	T38.4X1	T38.4X2	T38.4X3	T38.4X4	T38.4X5	T38.4X6
with mestranol diacetate	T38.4X1	T38.4X2	T38.4X3	T38.4X4	T38.4X5	T38.4X6
Etidocaine	T41.3X1	T41.3X2	T41.3X3	T41.3X4	T41.3X5	T41.3X6
infiltration (subcutaneous)	T41.3X1	T41.3X2	T41.3X3	T41.3X4	T41.3X5	T41.3X6
nerve (peripheral) (plexus)	T41.3X1	T41.3X2	T41.3X3	T41.3X4	T41.3X5	T41.3X6
Etidronate	T50.991	T50.992	T50.993	T50.994	T50.995	T50.996
Etidronic acid (disodium salt)	T50.991	T50.992	T50.993	T50.994	T50.995	T50.996
Etifoxine	T42.6X1	T42.6X2	T42.6X3	T42.6X4	T42.6X5	T42.6X6

◀ New   ◀| Revised   ~~deleted~~ Deleted

Substance	Poisoning, Accidental (Unintentional)	Poisoning, Intentional Self-Harm	Poisoning, Assault	Poisoning, Undetermined	Adverse Effect	Underdosing
Etilefrine	T44.4X1	T44.4X2	T44.4X3	T44.4X4	T44.4X5	T44.4X6
Etilfen	T42.3X1	T42.3X2	T42.3X3	T42.3X4	T42.3X5	T42.3X6
Etinodiol	T38.4X1	T38.4X2	T38.4X3	T38.4X4	T38.4X5	T38.4X6
Etiroxate	T46.6X1	T46.6X2	T46.6X3	T46.6X4	T46.6X5	T46.6X6
Etizolam	T42.4X1	T42.4X2	T42.4X3	T42.4X4	T42.4X5	T42.4X6
Etodolac	T39.391	T39.392	T39.393	T39.394	T39.395	T39.396
Etofamide	T37.3X1	T37.3X2	T37.3X3	T37.3X4	T37.3X5	T37.3X6
Etofibrate	T46.6X1	T46.6X2	T46.6X3	T46.6X4	T46.6X5	T46.6X6
Etofylline	T46.7X1	T46.7X2	T46.7X3	T46.7X4	T46.7X5	T46.7X6
clofibrate	T46.6X1	T46.6X2	T46.6X3	T46.6X4	T46.6X5	T46.6X6
Etoglucid	T45.1X1	T45.1X2	T45.1X3	T45.1X4	T45.1X5	T45.1X6
Etomidate	T41.1X1	T41.1X2	T41.1X3	T41.1X4	T41.1X5	T41.1X6
Etomide	T39.8X1	T39.8X2	T39.8X3	T39.8X4	T39.8X5	T39.8X6
Etomidoline	T44.3X1	T44.3X2	T44.3X3	T44.3X4	T44.3X5	T44.3X6
Etoposide	T45.1X1	T45.1X2	T45.1X3	T45.1X4	T45.1X5	T45.1X6
Etorphine	T40.2X1	T40.2X2	T40.2X3	T40.2X4	T40.2X5	T40.2X6
Etoval	T42.3X1	T42.3X2	T42.3X3	T42.3X4	T42.3X5	T42.3X6
Etozolin	T50.1X1	T50.1X2	T50.1X3	T50.1X4	T50.1X5	T50.1X6
Etretinate	T50.991	T50.992	T50.993	T50.994	T50.995	T50.996
Etryptamine	T43.691	T43.692	T43.693	T43.694	T43.695	T43.696
Etybenzatropine	T44.3X1	T44.3X2	T44.3X3	T44.3X4	T44.3X5	T44.3X6
Etynodiol	T38.4X1	T38.4X2	T38.4X3	T38.4X4	T38.4X5	T38.4X6
Eucaine	T41.3X1	T41.3X2	T41.3X3	T41.3X4	T41.3X5	T41.3X6
Eucalyptus oil	T49.7X1	T49.7X2	T49.7X3	T49.7X4	T49.7X5	T49.7X6
Eucatropine	T49.5X1	T49.5X2	T49.5X3	T49.5X4	T49.5X5	T49.5X6
Eucodal	T40.2X1	T40.2X2	T40.2X3	T40.2X4	T40.2X5	T40.2X6
Euneryl	T42.3X1	T42.3X2	T42.3X3	T42.3X4	T42.3X5	T42.3X6
Euphthalmine	T44.3X1	T44.3X2	T44.3X3	T44.3X4	T44.3X5	T44.3X6
Eurax	T49.0X1	T49.0X2	T49.0X3	T49.0X4	T49.0X5	T49.0X6
Euresol	T49.4X1	T49.4X2	T49.4X3	T49.4X4	T49.4X5	T49.4X6
Euthroid	T38.1X1	T38.1X2	T38.1X3	T38.1X4	T38.1X5	T38.1X6
Evans blue	T50.8X1	T50.8X2	T50.8X3	T50.8X4	T50.8X5	T50.8X6
Evipal	T42.3X1	T42.3X2	T42.3X3	T42.3X4	T42.3X5	T42.3X6
sodium	T41.1X1	T41.1X2	T41.1X3	T41.1X4	T41.1X5	T41.1X6
Evipan	T42.3X1	T42.3X2	T42.3X3	T42.3X4	T42.3X5	T42.3X6
sodium	T41.1X1	T41.1X2	T41.1X3	T41.1X4	T41.1X5	T41.1X6
Exalamide	T49.0X1	T49.0X2	T49.0X3	T49.0X4	T49.0X5	T49.0X6
Exalgin	T39.1X1	T39.1X2	T39.1X3	T39.1X4	T39.1X5	T39.1X6
Excipients, pharmaceutical	T50.901	T50.902	T50.903	T50.904	T50.905	T50.906
Exhaust gas (engine) (motor vehicle)	T58.01	T58.02	T58.03	T58.04	—	—
Ex-Lax (phenolphthalein)	T47.2X1	T47.2X2	T47.2X3	T47.2X4	T47.2X5	T47.2X6
Expectorant NEC	T48.4X1	T48.4X2	T48.4X3	T48.4X4	T48.4X5	T48.4X6

Substance	Poisoning, Accidental (Unintentional)	Poisoning, Intentional Self-Harm	Poisoning, Assault	Poisoning, Undetermined	Adverse Effect	Underdosing
Extended insulin zinc suspension	T38.3X1	T38.3X2	T38.3X3	T38.3X4	T38.3X5	T38.3X6
External medications (skin) (mucous membrane)	T49.91	T49.92	T49.93	T49.94	T49.95	T49.96
dental agent	T49.7X1	T49.7X2	T49.7X3	T49.7X4	T49.7X5	T49.7X6
ENT agent	T49.6X1	T49.6X2	T49.6X3	T49.6X4	T49.6X5	T49.6X6
ophthalmic preparation	T49.5X1	T49.5X2	T49.5X3	T49.5X4	T49.5X5	T49.5X6
specified NEC	T49.8X1	T49.8X2	T49.8X3	T49.8X4	T49.8X5	T49.8X6
Extrapyramidal antagonist NEC	T44.3X1	T44.3X2	T44.3X3	T44.3X4	T44.3X5	T44.3X6
Eye agents (anti-infective)	T49.5X1	T49.5X2	T49.5X3	T49.5X4	T49.5X5	T49.5X6
Eye drug NEC	T49.5X1	T49.5X2	T49.5X3	T49.5X4	T49.5X5	T49.5X6
F						
FAC (fluorouracil + doxorubicin + cyclophosphamide)	T45.1X1	T45.1X2	T45.1X3	T45.1X4	T45.1X5	T45.1X6
Factor						
I (fibrinogen)	T45.8X1	T45.8X2	T45.8X3	T45.8X4	T45.8X5	T45.8X6
III (thromboplastin)	T45.8X1	T45.8X2	T45.8X3	T45.8X4	T45.8X5	T45.8X6
VIII (antihemophilic Factor) (Concentrate)	T45.8X1	T45.8X2	T45.8X3	T45.8X4	T45.8X5	T45.8X6
IX complex	T45.7X1	T45.7X2	T45.7X3	T45.7X4	T45.7X5	T45.7X6
human	T45.8X1	T45.8X2	T45.8X3	T45.8X4	T45.8X5	T45.8X6
Famotidine	T47.0X1	T47.0X2	T47.0X3	T47.0X4	T47.0X5	T47.0X6
Fat suspension, intravenous	T50.991	T50.992	T50.993	T50.994	T50.995	T50.996
Fazadinium bromide	T48.1X1	T48.1X2	T48.1X3	T48.1X4	T48.1X5	T48.1X6
Febarbamate	T42.3X1	T42.3X2	T42.3X3	T42.3X4	T42.3X5	T42.3X6
Fecal softener	T47.4X1	T47.4X2	T47.4X3	T47.4X4	T47.4X5	T47.4X6
Fedrilate	T48.3X1	T48.3X2	T48.3X3	T48.3X4	T48.3X5	T48.3X6
Felodipine	T46.1X1	T46.1X2	T46.1X3	T46.1X4	T46.1X5	T46.1X6
Felypressin	T38.891	T38.892	T38.893	T38.894	T38.895	T38.896
Femoxetine	T43.221	T43.222	T43.223	T43.224	T43.225	T43.226
Fenalcomine	T46.3X1	T46.3X2	T46.3X3	T46.3X4	T46.3X5	T46.3X6
Fenamisal	T37.1X1	T37.1X2	T37.1X3	T97.1X4	T37.1X5	T37.1X6
Fenazone	T39.2X1	T39.2X2	T39.2X3	T39.2X4	T39.2X5	T39.2X6
Fenbendazole	T37.4X1	T37.4X2	T37.4X3	T37.4X4	T37.4X5	T37.4X6
Fenbutrazate	T50.5X1	T50.5X2	T50.5X3	T50.5X4	T50.5X5	T50.5X6
Fencamfamine	T43.691	T43.692	T43.693	T43.694	T43.695	T43.696
Fendiline	T46.1X1	T46.1X2	T46.1X3	T46.1X4	T46.1X5	T46.1X6
Fenetylline	T43.691	T43.692	T43.693	T43.694	T43.695	T43.696
Fenflumizole	T39.391	T39.392	T39.393	T39.394	T39.395	T39.396
Fenfluramine	T50.5X1	T50.5X2	T50.5X3	T50.5X4	T50.5X5	T50.5X6
Fenobarbital	T42.3X1	T42.3X2	T42.3X3	T42.3X4	T42.3X5	T42.3X6
Fenofibrate	T46.6X1	T46.6X2	T46.6X3	T46.6X4	T46.6X5	T46.6X6
Fenoprofen	T39.311	T39.312	T39.313	T39.314	T39.315	T39.316
Fenoterol	T48.6X1	T48.6X2	T48.6X3	T48.6X4	T48.6X5	T48.6X6

TABLE OF DRUGS AND CHEMICALS

Substance	Poisoning, Accidental (Unintentional)	Poisoning, Intentional Self-Harm	Poisoning, Assault	Poisoning, Undetermined	Adverse Effect	Underdosing
Fenoverine	T44.3X1	T44.3X2	T44.3X3	T44.3X4	T44.3X5	T44.3X6
Fenoxazoline	T48.5X1	T48.5X2	T48.5X3	T48.5X4	T48.5X5	T48.5X6
Fenproporex	T50.5X1	T50.5X2	T50.5X3	T50.5X4	T50.5X5	T50.5X6
Fenquizone	T50.2X1	T50.2X2	T50.2X3	T50.2X4	T50.2X5	T50.2X6
Fentanyl	T40.4X1	T40.4X2	T40.4X3	T40.4X4	T40.4X5	T40.4X6
Fentazin	T43.3X1	T43.3X2	T43.3X3	T43.3X4	T43.3X5	T43.3X6
Fenthion	T60.0X1	T60.0X2	T60.0X3	T60.0X4	—	—
Fenticlor	T49.0X1	T49.0X2	T49.0X3	T49.0X4	T49.0X5	T49.0X6
Fenylbutazone	T39.2X1	T39.2X2	T39.2X3	T39.2X4	T39.2X5	T39.2X6
Feprazone	T39.2X1	T39.2X2	T39.2X3	T39.2X4	T39.2X5	T39.2X6
Fer de lance (bite) (venom)	T63.061	T63.062	T63.063	T63.064	—	—
Ferric — see also Iron						
chloride	T45.4X1	T45.4X2	T45.4X3	T45.4X4	T45.4X5	T45.4X6
citrate	T45.4X1	T45.4X2	T45.4X3	T45.4X4	T45.4X5	T45.4X6
hydroxide						
colloidal	T45.4X1	T45.4X2	T45.4X3	T45.4X4	T45.4X5	T45.4X6
polymaltose	T45.4X1	T45.4X2	T45.4X3	T45.4X4	T45.4X5	T45.4X6
pyrophosphate	T45.4X1	T45.4X2	T45.4X3	T45.4X4	T45.4X5	T45.4X6
Ferritin	T45.4X1	T45.4X2	T45.4X3	T45.4X4	T45.4X5	T45.4X6
Ferrocholinate	T45.4X1	T45.4X2	T45.4X3	T45.4X4	T45.4X5	T45.4X6
Ferrodextrane	T45.4X1	T45.4X2	T45.4X3	T45.4X4	T45.4X5	T45.4X6
Ferropolimaler	T45.4X1	T45.4X2	T45.4X3	T45.4X4	T45.4X5	T45.4X6
Ferrous — see also Iron						
phosphate	T45.4X1	T45.4X2	T45.4X3	T45.4X4	T45.4X5	T45.4X6
salt	T45.4X1	T45.4X2	T45.4X3	T45.4X4	T45.4X5	T45.4X6
with folic acid	T45.4X1	T45.4X2	T45.4X3	T45.4X4	T45.4X5	T45.4X6
Ferrous fumarate, gluconate, lactate, salt NEC, sulfate (medicinal)	T45.4X1	T45.4X2	T45.4X3	T45.4X4	T45.4X5	T45.4X6
Ferrovanadium (fumes)	T59.891	T59.892	T59.893	T59.894	—	—
Ferrum — see Iron						
Fertilizers NEC	T65.891	T65.892	T65.893	T65.894	—	—
with herbicide mixture	T60.3X1	T60.3X2	T60.3X3	T60.3X4	—	—
Fetoxilate	T47.6X1	T47.6X2	T47.6X3	T47.6X4	T47.6X5	T47.6X6
Fiber, dietary	T47.4X1	T47.4X2	T47.4X3	T47.4X4	T47.4X5	T47.4X6
Fibrinogen (human)	T45.8X1	T45.8X2	T45.8X3	T45.8X4	T45.8X5	T45.8X6
Fibrinolysin (human)	T45.691	T45.692	T45.693	T45.694	T45.695	T45.696
Fibrinolysis						
affecting drug	T45.601	T45.602	T45.603	T45.604	T45.605	T45.606
inhibitor NEC	T45.621	T45.622	T45.623	T45.624	T45.625	T45.626
Fibrinolytic drug	T45.611	T45.612	T45.613	T45.614	T45.615	T45.616
Filix mas	T37.4X1	T37.4X2	T37.4X3	T37.4X4	T37.4X5	T37.4X6
Filtering cream	T49.3X1	T49.3X2	T49.3X3	T49.3X4	T49.3X5	T49.3X6

Substance	Poisoning, Accidental (Unintentional)	Poisoning, Intentional Self-Harm	Poisoning, Assault	Poisoning, Undetermined	Adverse Effect	Underdosing
Fiorinal	T39.011	T39.012	T39.013	T39.014	T39.015	T39.016
Firedamp	T59.891	T59.892	T59.893	T59.894	—	—
Fish, noxious, nonbacterial	T61.91	T61.92	T61.93	T61.94	—	—
ciguatera	T61.01	T61.02	T61.03	T61.04	—	—
scombroid	T61.11	T61.12	T61.13	T61.14	—	—
shell	T61.781	T61.782	T61.783	T61.784	—	—
specified NEC	T61.771	T61.772	T61.773	T61.774	—	—
Flagyl	T37.3X1	T37.3X2	T37.3X3	T37.3X4	T37.3X5	T37.3X6
Flavine adenine dinucleotide	T45.2X1	T45.2X2	T45.2X3	T45.2X4	T45.2X5	T45.2X6
Flavodic acid	T46.991	T46.992	T46.993	T46.994	T46.995	T46.996
Flavoxate	T44.3X1	T44.3X2	T44.3X3	T44.3X4	T44.3X5	T44.3X6
Flaxedil	T48.1X1	T48.1X2	T48.1X3	T48.1X4	T48.1X5	T48.1X6
Flaxseed (medicinal)	T49.3X1	T49.3X2	T49.3X3	T49.3X4	T49.3X5	T49.3X6
Flecainide	T46.2X1	T46.2X2	T46.2X3	T46.2X4	T46.2X5	T46.2X6
Fleroxacin	T36.8X1	T36.8X2	T36.8X3	T36.8X4	T36.8X5	T36.8X6
Floctafenine	T39.8X1	T39.8X2	T39.8X3	T39.8X4	T39.8X5	T39.8X6
Flomax	T44.6X1	T44.6X2	T44.6X3	T44.6X4	T44.6X5	T44.6X6
Flomoxef	T36.1X1	T36.1X2	T36.1X3	T36.1X4	T36.1X5	T36.1X6
Flopropione	T44.3X1	T44.3X2	T44.3X3	T44.3X4	T44.3X5	T44.3X6
Florantyrone	T47.5X1	T47.5X2	T47.5X3	T47.5X4	T47.5X5	T47.5X6
Floraquin	T37.8X1	T37.8X2	T37.8X3	T37.8X4	T37.8X5	T37.8X6
Florinef	T38.0X1	T38.0X2	T38.0X3	T38.0X4	T38.0X5	T38.0X6
ENT agent	T49.6X1	T49.6X2	T49.6X3	T49.6X4	T49.6X5	T49.6X6
ophthalmic preparation	T49.5X1	T49.5X2	T49.5X3	T49.5X4	T49.5X5	T49.5X6
topical NEC	T49.0X1	T49.0X2	T49.0X3	T49.0X4	T49.0X5	T49.0X6
Flowers of sulfur	T49.4X1	T49.4X2	T49.4X3	T49.4X4	T49.4X5	T49.4X6
Floxuridine	T45.1X1	T45.1X2	T45.1X3	T45.1X4	T45.1X5	T45.1X6
Fluanisone	T43.4X1	T43.4X2	T43.4X3	T43.4X4	T43.4X5	T43.4X6
Flubendazole	T37.4X1	T37.4X2	T37.4X3	T37.4X4	T37.4X5	T37.4X6
Fluclorolone acetonide	T49.0X1	T49.0X2	T49.0X3	T49.0X4	T49.0X5	T49.0X6
Flucloxacillin	T36.0X1	T36.0X2	T36.0X3	T36.0X4	T36.0X5	T36.0X6
Fluconazole	T37.8X1	T37.8X2	T37.8X3	T37.8X4	T37.8X5	T37.8X6
Flucytosine	T37.8X1	T37.8X2	T37.8X3	T37.8X4	T37.8X5	T37.8X6
Fludeoxyglucose (18F)	T50.8X1	T50.8X2	T50.8X3	T50.8X4	T50.8X5	T50.8X6
Fludiazepam	T42.4X1	T42.4X2	T42.4X3	T42.4X4	T42.4X5	T42.4X6
Fludrocortisone	T50.0X1	T50.0X2	T50.0X3	T50.0X4	T50.0X5	T50.0X6
ENT agent	T49.6X1	T49.6X2	T49.6X3	T49.6X4	T49.6X5	T49.6X6
ophthalmic preparation	T49.5X1	T49.5X2	T49.5X3	T49.5X4	T49.5X5	T49.5X6
topical NEC	T49.0X1	T49.0X2	T49.0X3	T49.0X4	T49.0X5	T49.0X6
Fludroxycortide	T49.0X1	T49.0X2	T49.0X3	T49.0X4	T49.0X5	T49.0X6
Flufenamic acid	T39.391	T39.392	T39.393	T39.394	T39.395	T39.396
Fluindione	T45.511	T45.512	T45.513	T45.514	T45.515	T45.516

◀ New   ◀ Revised   ~~deleted~~ Deleted

Substance	Poisoning, Accidental (Unintentional)	Poisoning, Intentional Self-Harm	Poisoning, Assault	Poisoning, Undetermined	Adverse Effect	Underdosing
Flumequine	T37.8X1	T37.8X2	T37.8X3	T37.8X4	T37.8X5	T37.8X6
Flumethasone	T49.0X1	T49.0X2	T49.0X3	T49.0X4	T49.0X5	T49.0X6
Flumethiazide	T50.2X1	T50.2X2	T50.2X3	T50.2X4	T50.2X5	T50.2X6
Flumidin	T37.5X1	T37.5X2	T37.5X3	T37.5X4	T37.5X5	T37.5X6
Flunarizine	T46.7X1	T46.7X2	T46.7X3	T46.7X4	T46.7X5	T46.7X6
Flunidazole	T37.8X1	T37.8X2	T37.8X3	T37.8X4	T37.8X5	T37.8X6
Flunisolide	T48.6X1	T48.6X2	T48.6X3	T48.6X4	T48.6X5	T48.6X6
Flunitrazepam	T42.4X1	T42.4X2	T42.4X3	T42.4X4	T42.4X5	T42.4X6
Fluocinolone (acetonide)	T49.0X1	T49.0X2	T49.0X3	T49.0X4	T49.0X5	T49.0X6
Fluocinonide	T49.0X1	T49.0X2	T49.0X3	T49.0X4	T49.0X5	T49.0X6
Fluocortin (butyl)	T49.0X1	T49.0X2	T49.0X3	T49.0X4	T49.0X5	T49.0X6
Fluocortolone	T49.0X1	T49.0X2	T49.0X3	T49.0X4	T49.0X5	T49.0X6
Fluohydrocortisone	T38.0X1	T38.0X2	T38.0X3	T38.0X4	T38.0X5	T38.0X6
ENT agent	T49.6X1	T49.6X2	T49.6X3	T49.6X4	T49.6X5	T49.6X6
ophthalmic preparation	T49.5X1	T49.5X2	T49.5X3	T49.5X4	T49.5X5	T49.5X6
topical NEC	T49.0X1	T49.0X2	T49.0X3	T49.0X4	T49.0X5	T49.0X6
Fluonid	T49.0X1	T49.0X2	T49.0X3	T49.0X4	T49.0X5	T49.0X6
Fluopromazine	T43.3X1	T43.3X2	T43.3X3	T43.3X4	T43.3X5	T43.3X6
Fluoroacetate	T60.8X1	T60.8X2	T60.8X3	T60.8X4	—	—
Fluorescein	T50.8X1	T50.8X2	T50.8X3	T50.8X4	T50.8X5	T50.8X6
Fluorhydrocortisone	T50.0X1	T50.0X2	T50.0X3	T50.0X4	T50.0X5	T50.0X6
Fluoride (nonmedicinal) (pesticide) (sodium) NEC	T60.8X1	T60.8X2	T60.8X3	T60.8X4	—	—
hydrogen — see Hydrofluoric acid						
medicinal NEC	T50.991	T50.992	T50.993	T50.994	T50.995	T50.996
dental use	T49.7X1	T49.7X2	T49.7X3	T49.7X4	T49.7X5	T49.7X6
not pesticide NEC	T54.91	T54.92	T54.93	T54.94	—	—
stannous	T49.7X1	T49.7X2	T49.7X3	T49.7X4	T49.7X5	T49.7X6
Fluorinated corticosteroids	T38.0X1	T38.0X2	T38.0X3	T38.0X4	T38.0X5	T38.0X6
Fluorine (gas)	T59.5X1	T59.5X2	T59.5X3	T59.5X4		
salt — see Fluoride(s)						
Fluoristan	T49.7X1	T49.7X2	T49.7X3	T49.7X4	T49.7X5	T49.7X6
Fluormetholone	T49.0X1	T49.0X2	T49.0X3	T49.0X4	T49.0X5	T49.0X6
Fluoroacetate	T60.8X1	T60.8X2	T60.8X3	T60.8X4	—	—
Fluorocarbon monomer	T53.6X1	T53.6X2	T53.6X3	T53.6X4	—	—
Fluorocytosine	T37.8X1	T37.8X2	T37.8X3	T37.8X4	T37.8X5	T37.8X6
Fluorodeoxyuridine	T45.1X1	T45.1X2	T45.1X3	T45.1X4	T45.1X5	T45.1X6
Fluorometholone	T49.0X1	T49.0X2	T49.0X3	T49.0X4	T49.0X5	T49.0X6
ophthalmic preparation	T49.5X1	T49.5X2	T49.5X3	T49.5X4	T49.5X5	T49.5X6
Fluorophosphate insecticide	T60.0X1	T60.0X2	T60.0X3	T60.0X4	—	—
Fluorosol	T46.3X1	T46.3X2	T46.3X3	T46.3X4	T46.3X5	T46.3X6
Fluorouracil	T45.1X1	T45.1X2	T45.1X3	T45.1X4	T45.1X5	T45.1X6

Substance	Poisoning, Accidental (Unintentional)	Poisoning, Intentional Self-Harm	Poisoning, Assault	Poisoning, Undetermined	Adverse Effect	Underdosing
Fluorphenylalanine	T49.5X1	T49.5X2	T49.5X3	T49.5X4	T49.5X5	T49.5X6
Fluothane	T41.0X1	T41.0X2	T41.0X3	T41.0X4	T41.0X5	T41.0X6
Fluoxetine	T43.221	T43.222	T43.223	T43.224	T43.225	T43.226
Fluoxymesterone	T38.7X1	T38.7X2	T38.7X3	T38.7X4	T38.7X5	T38.7X6
Flupenthixol	T43.4X1	T43.4X2	T43.4X3	T43.4X4	T43.4X5	T43.4X6
Flupentixol	T43.4X1	T43.4X2	T43.4X3	T43.4X4	T43.4X5	T43.4X6
Fluphenazine	T43.3X1	T43.3X2	T43.3X3	T43.3X4	T43.3X5	T43.3X6
Fluprednidene	T49.0X1	T49.0X2	T49.0X3	T49.0X4	T49.0X5	T49.0X6
Fluprednisolone	T38.0X1	T38.0X2	T38.0X3	T38.0X4	T38.0X5	T38.0X6
Fluradoline	T39.8X1	T39.8X2	T39.8X3	T39.8X4	T39.8X5	T39.8X6
Flurandrenolide	T49.0X1	T49.0X2	T49.0X3	T49.0X4	T49.0X5	T49.0X6
Flurandrenolone	T49.0X1	T49.0X2	T49.0X3	T49.0X4	T49.0X5	T49.0X6
Flurazepam	T42.4X1	T42.4X2	T42.4X3	T42.4X4	T42.4X5	T42.4X6
Flurbiprofen	T39.311	T39.312	T39.313	T39.314	T39.315	T39.316
Flurobate	T49.0X1	T49.0X2	T49.0X3	T49.0X4	T49.0X5	T49.0X6
Flurotyl	T43.291	T43.292	T43.293	T43.294	T43.295	T43.296
Fluroxene	T41.0X1	T41.0X2	T41.0X3	T41.0X4	T41.0X5	T41.0X6
Fluspirilene	T43.591	T43.592	T43.593	T43.594	T43.595	T43.596
Flutamide	T38.6X1	T38.6X2	T38.6X3	T38.6X4	T38.6X5	T38.6X6
Flutazolam	T42.4X1	T42.4X2	T42.4X3	T42.4X4	T42.4X5	T42.4X6
Fluticasone propionate	T38.0X1	T38.0X2	T38.0X3	T38.0X4	T38.0X5	T38.0X6
Flutoprazepam	T42.4X1	T42.4X2	T42.4X3	T42.4X4	T42.4X5	T42.4X6
Flutropium bromide	T48.6X1	T48.6X2	T48.6X3	T48.6X4	T48.6X5	T48.6X6
Fluvoxamine	T43.221	T43.222	T43.223	T43.224	T43.225	T43.226
Folacin	T45.8X1	T45.8X2	T45.8X3	T45.8X4	T45.8X5	T45.8X6
Folic acid	T45.8X1	T45.8X2	T45.8X3	T45.8X4	T45.8X5	T45.8X6
with ferrous salt	T45.2X1	T45.2X2	T45.2X3	T45.2X4	T45.2X5	T45.2X6
antagonist	T45.1X1	T45.1X2	T45.1X3	T45.1X4	T45.1X5	T45.1X6
Folinic acid	T45.8X1	T45.8X2	T45.8X3	T45.8X4	T45.8X5	T45.8X6
Folium stramoniae	T48.6X1	T48.6X2	T48.6X3	T48.6X4	T48.6X5	T48.6X6
Follicle-stimulating hormone, human	T38.811	T38.812	T38.813	T38.814	T38.815	T38.816
Folpet	T60.3X1	T60.3X2	T60.3X3	T60.3X4	—	—
Fominoben	T48.3X1	T48.3X2	T48.3X3	T48.3X4	T48.3X5	T48.3X6
Food, foodstuffs, noxious, nonbacterial, NEC	T62.91	T62.92	T62.93	T62.94	—	—
berries	T62.1X1	T62.1X2	T62.1X3	T62.1X4	—	—
fish — see also Fish	T61.91	T61.92	T61.93	T61.94	—	—
mushrooms	T62.0X1	T62.0X2	T62.0X3	T62.0X4	—	—
plants	T62.2X1	T62.2X2	T62.2X3	T62.2X4	—	—
seafood	T61.91	T61.92	T61.93	T61.94	—	—
specified NEC	T61.8X1	T61.8X2	T61.8X3	T61.8X4	—	—
seeds	T62.2X1	T62.2X2	T62.2X3	T62.2X4	—	—

◀ New ◀ Revised ~~deleted~~ Deleted

TABLE OF DRUGS AND CHEMICALS

Substance	External Cause (T-Code)					
	Poisoning, Accidental (Unintentional)	Poisoning, Intentional Self-Harm	Poisoning, Assault	Poisoning, Undetermined	Adverse Effect	Underdosing
Food, foodstuffs, noxious, nonbacterial, NEC (Continued)						
shellfish	T61.781	T61.782	T61.783	T61.784	—	—
specified NEC	T62.8X1	T62.8X2	T62.8X3	T62.8X4	—	—
Fool's parsley	T62.2X1	T62.2X2	T62.2X3	T62.2X4	—	—
Formaldehyde (solution), gas or vapor	T59.2X1	T59.2X2	T59.2X3	T59.2X4	—	—
fungicide	T60.3X1	T60.3X2	T60.3X3	T60.3X4	—	—
Formalin	T59.2X1	T59.2X2	T59.2X3	T59.2X4	—	—
fungicide	T60.3X1	T60.3X2	T60.3X3	T60.3X4	—	—
vapor	T59.2X1	T59.2X2	T59.2X3	T59.2X4	—	—
Formic acid	T54.2X1	T54.2X2	T54.2X3	T54.2X4	—	—
vapor	T59.891	T59.892	T59.893	T59.894	—	—
Foscarnet sodium	T37.5X1	T37.5X2	T37.5X3	T37.5X4	T37.5X5	T37.5X6
Fosfestrol	T38.5X1	T38.5X2	T38.5X3	T38.5X4	T38.5X5	T38.5X6
Fosfomycin	T36.8X1	T36.8X2	T36.8X3	T36.8X4	T36.8X5	T36.8X6
Fosfonet sodium	T37.5X1	T37.5X2	T37.5X3	T37.5X4	T37.5X5	T37.5X6
Fosinopril	T46.4X1	T46.4X2	T46.4X3	T46.4X4	T46.4X5	T46.4X6
sodium	T46.4X1	T46.4X2	T46.4X3	T46.4X4	T46.4X5	T46.4X6
Fowler's solution	T57.0X1	T57.0X2	T57.0X3	T57.0X4	—	—
Foxglove	T62.2X1	T62.2X2	T62.2X3	T62.2X4	—	—
Framycetin	T36.5X1	T36.5X2	T36.5X3	T36.5X4	T36.5X5	T36.5X6
Frangula	T47.2X1	T47.2X2	T47.2X3	T47.2X4	T47.2X5	T47.2X6
extract	T47.2X1	T47.2X2	T47.2X3	T47.2X4	T47.2X5	T47.2X6
Frei antigen	T50.8X1	T50.8X2	T50.8X3	T50.8X4	T50.8X5	T50.8X6
Freon	T53.5X1	T53.5X2	T53.5X3	T53.5X4	—	—
Fructose	T50.3X1	T50.3X2	T50.3X3	T50.3X4	T50.3X5	T50.3X6
Frusemide	T50.1X1	T50.1X2	T50.1X3	T50.1X4	T50.1X5	T50.1X6
FSH	T38.811	T38.812	T38.813	T38.814	T38.815	T38.816
Ftorafur	T45.1X1	T45.1X2	T45.1X3	T45.1X4	T45.1X5	T45.1X6
Fuel						
automobile	T52.0X1	T52.0X2	T52.0X3	T52.0X4	—	—
exhaust gas, not in transit	T58.01	T58.02	T58.03	T58.04	—	—
vapor NEC	T52.0X1	T52.0X2	T52.0X3	T52.0X4	—	—
gas (domestic use) — see also Carbon, monoxide, fuel, utility	T59.891	T59.892	T59.893	T59.894	—	—
utility	T59.891	T59.892	T59.893	T59.894	—	—
in mobile container	T59.891	T59.892	T59.893	T59.894	—	—
incomplete combustion of — see Carbon, monoxide, fuel, utility						
piped (natural)	T59.891	T59.892	T59.893	T59.894	—	—
industrial, incomplete combustion	T58.8X1	T58.8X2	T58.8X3	T58.8X4	—	—

Substance	External Cause (T-Code)					
	Poisoning, Accidental (Unintentional)	Poisoning, Intentional Self-Harm	Poisoning, Assault	Poisoning, Undetermined	Adverse Effect	Underdosing
Fugillin	T36.8X1	T36.8X2	T36.8X3	T36.8X4	T36.8X5	T36.8X6
Fulminate of mercury	T56.1X1	T56.1X2	T56.1X3	T56.1X4	—	—
Fulvicin	T36.7X1	T36.7X2	T36.7X3	T36.7X4	T36.7X5	T36.7X6
Fumadil	T36.8X1	T36.8X2	T36.8X3	T36.8X4	T36.8X5	T36.8X6
Fumagillin	T36.8X1	T36.8X2	T36.8X3	T36.8X4	T36.8X5	T36.8X6
Fumaric acid	T49.4X1	T49.4X2	T49.4X3	T49.4X4	T49.4X5	T49.4X6
Fumes (from)	T59.91	T59.92	T59.93	T59.94	—	—
carbon monoxide — see Carbon, monoxide						
charcoal (domestic use) — see Charcoal, fumes						
chloroform — see Chloroform						
coke (in domestic stoves, fireplaces) — see Coke, fumes						
corrosive NEC	T54.91	T54.92	T54.93	T54.94	—	—
ether — see ether						
freons	T53.5X1	T53.5X2	T53.5X3	T53.5X4	—	—
hydrocarbons	T59.891	T59.892	T59.893	T59.894	—	—
petroleum (liquefied)	T59.891	T59.892	T59.893	T59.894	—	—
distributed through pipes (pure or mixed with air)	T59.891	T59.892	T59.893	T59.894	—	—
lead — see lead						
metal — see Metals, or the specified metal						
nitrogen dioxide	T59.0X1	T59.0X2	T59.0X3	T59.0X4	—	—
pesticides — see Pesticides						
petroleum (liquefied)	T59.891	T59.892	T59.893	T59.894	—	—
distributed through pipes (pure or mixed with air)	T59.891	T59.892	T59.893	T59.894	—	—
polyester	T59.891	T59.892	T59.893	T59.894	—	—
specified source NEC — see also substance specified	T59.891	T59.892	T59.893	T59.894	—	—
sulfur dioxide	T59.1X1	T59.1X2	T59.1X3	T59.1X4	—	—
Fumigant NEC	T60.91	T60.92	T60.93	T60.94	—	—
Fungi, noxious, used as food	T62.0X1	T62.0X2	T62.0X3	T62.0X4	—	—
Fungicide NEC (nonmedicinal)	T60.3X1	T60.3X2	T60.3X3	T60.3X4	—	—
Fungizone	T36.7X1	T36.7X2	T36.7X3	T36.7X4	T36.7X5	T36.7X6
topical	T49.0X1	T49.0X2	T49.0X3	T49.0X4	T49.0X5	T49.0X6
Furacin	T49.0X1	T49.0X2	T49.0X3	T49.0X4	T49.0X5	T49.0X6
Furadantin	T37.91	T37.92	T37.93	T37.94	T37.95	T37.96
Furazolidone	T37.8X1	T37.8X2	T37.8X3	T37.8X4	T37.8X5	T37.8X6
Furazolium chloride	T49.0X1	T49.0X2	T49.0X3	T49.0X4	T49.0X5	T49.0X6
Furfural	T52.8X1	T52.8X2	T52.8X3	T52.8X4	—	—

TABLE OF DRUGS AND CHEMICALS

Substance	Poisoning, Accidental (Unintentional)	Poisoning, Intentional Self-Harm	Poisoning, Assault	Poisoning, Undetermined	Adverse Effect	Underdosing
Furnace (coal burning) (domestic), gas from industrial	T58.2X1	T58.2X2	T58.2X3	T58.2X4	—	—
industrial	T58.8X1	T58.8X2	T58.8X3	T58.8X4	—	—
Furniture polish	T65.891	T65.892	T65.893	T65.894	—	—
Furosemide	T50.1X1	T50.1X2	T50.1X3	T50.1X4	T50.1X5	T50.1X6
Furoxone	T37.91	T37.92	T37.93	T37.94	T37.95	T37.96
Fursultiamine	T45.2X1	T45.2X2	T45.2X3	T45.2X4	T45.2X5	T45.2X6
Fusafungine	T36.8X1	T36.8X2	T36.8X3	T36.8X4	T36.8X5	T36.8X6
Fusel oil (any) (amyl) (butyl) (propyl), vapor	T51.3X1	T51.3X2	T51.3X3	T51.3X4	—	—
Fusidate (ethanolamine) (sodium)	T36.8X1	T36.8X2	T36.8X3	T36.8X4	T36.8X5	T36.8X6
Fusidic acid	T36.8X1	T36.8X2	T36.8X3	T36.8X4	T36.8X5	T36.8X6
Fytic acid, nonasodium	T50.6X1	T50.6X2	T50.6X3	T50.6X4	T50.6X5	T50.6X6
G						
GABA	T43.8X1	T43.8X2	T43.8X3	T43.8X4	T43.8X5	T43.8X6
Gadopentetic acid	T50.8X1	T50.8X2	T50.8X3	T50.8X4	T50.8X5	T50.8X6
Galactose	T50.3X1	T50.3X2	T50.3X3	T50.3X4	T50.3X5	T50.3X6
b-Galactosidase	T47.5X1	T47.5X2	T47.5X3	T47.5X4	T47.5X5	T47.5X6
Galantamine	T44.0X1	T44.0X2	T44.0X3	T44.0X4	T44.0X5	T44.0X6
Gallamine (triethiodide)	T48.1X1	T48.1X2	T48.1X3	T48.1X4	T48.1X5	T48.1X6
Gallium citrate	T50.991	T50.992	T50.993	T50.994	T50.995	T50.996
Gallopamil	T46.1X1	T46.1X2	T46.1X3	T46.1X4	T46.1X5	T46.1X6
Gamboge	T47.2X1	T47.2X2	T47.2X3	T47.2X4	T47.2X5	T47.2X6
Gamimune	T50.Z11	T50.Z12	T50.Z13	T50.Z14	T50.Z15	T50.Z16
Gamma-aminobutyric acid	T43.8X1	T43.8X2	T43.8X3	T43.8X4	T43.8X5	T43.8X6
Gamma-benzene hexachloride (medicinal)	T49.0X1	T49.0X2	T49.0X3	T49.0X4	T49.0X5	T49.0X6
nonmedicinal, vapor	T53.6X1	T53.6X2	T53.6X3	T53.6X4	—	—
Gamma-BHC (medicinal) — see also Gamma-benzene hexachloride	T49.0X1	T49.0X2	T49.0X3	T49.0X4	T49.0X5	T49.0X6
Gamma globulin	T50.Z11	T50.Z12	T50.Z13	T50.Z14	T50.Z15	T50.Z16
Gamulin	T50.Z11	T50.Z12	T50.Z13	T50.Z14	T50.Z15	T50.Z16
Ganciclovir (sodium)	T37.5X1	T37.5X2	T37.5X3	T37.5X4	T37.5X5	T37.5X6
Ganglionic blocking drug NEC	T44.2X1	T44.2X2	T44.2X3	T44.2X4	T44.2X5	T44.2X6
specified NEC	T44.2X1	T44.2X2	T44.2X3	T44.2X4	T44.2X5	T44.2X6
Ganja	T40.7X1	T40.7X2	T40.7X3	T40.7X4	T40.7X5	T40.7X6
Garamycin	T36.5X1	T36.5X2	T36.5X3	T36.5X4	T36.5X5	T36.5X6
ophthalmic preparation	T49.5X1	T49.5X2	T49.5X3	T49.5X4	T49.5X5	T49.5X6
topical NEC	T49.0X1	T49.0X2	T49.0X3	T49.0X4	T49.0X5	T49.0X6
Gardenal	T42.3X1	T42.3X2	T42.3X3	T42.3X4	T42.3X5	T42.3X6
Gardepanyl	T42.3X1	T42.3X2	T42.3X3	T42.3X4	T42.3X5	T42.3X6

Substance	Poisoning, Accidental (Unintentional)	Poisoning, Intentional Self-Harm	Poisoning, Assault	Poisoning, Undetermined	Adverse Effect	Underdosing
~~Gas~~	~~T59.91~~	~~T59.92~~	~~T59.93~~	~~T59.94~~	—	—
~~acetylene~~	~~T59.891~~	~~T59.892~~	~~T59.893~~	~~T59.894~~	—	—
~~incomplete combustion of~~	~~T58.11~~	~~T58.12~~	~~T58.13~~	~~T58.14~~	—	—
~~air contaminants, source or type not specified~~	~~T59.91~~	~~T59.92~~	~~T59.93~~	~~T59.94~~	—	—
~~anesthetic~~	~~T41.0X1~~	~~T41.0X2~~	~~T41.0X3~~	~~T41.0X4~~	~~T41.0X5~~	~~T41.0X6~~
~~blast furnace~~	~~T58.8X1~~	~~T58.8X2~~	~~T58.8X3~~	~~T58.8X4~~	—	—
~~butane — see butane~~						
~~carbon monoxide — see Carbon, monoxide~~						
~~chlorine~~	~~T59.4X1~~	~~T59.4X2~~	~~T59.4X3~~	~~T59.4X4~~	—	—
~~coal~~	~~T58.2X1~~	~~T58.2X2~~	~~T58.2X3~~	~~T58.2X4~~	—	—
~~cyanide~~	~~T57.3X1~~	~~T57.3X2~~	~~T57.3X3~~	~~T57.3X4~~	—	—
~~dicyanogen~~	~~T65.0X1~~	~~T65.0X2~~	~~T65.0X3~~	~~T65.0X4~~	—	—
~~domestic — see Domestic gas~~	~~T57.91~~	~~T57.92~~	~~T57.93~~	~~T57.94~~	—	—
~~exhaust~~	~~T57.91~~	~~T57.92~~	~~T57.93~~	~~T57.94~~	—	—
~~from utility (for cooking, heating, or lighting) (after combustion) — see Carbon, monoxide, fuel, utility~~						
~~prior to combustion~~	~~T59.891~~	~~T59.892~~	~~T59.893~~	~~T59.894~~	—	—
~~from wood or coal-burning stove or fireplace~~	~~T57.91~~	~~T57.92~~	~~T57.93~~	~~T57.94~~	—	—
~~fuel (domestic use) (after combustion) — see also Carbon, monoxide, fuel~~	~~T57.91~~	~~T57.92~~	~~T57.93~~	~~T57.94~~	—	—
~~industrial use~~	~~T58.8X1~~	~~T58.8X2~~	~~T58.8X3~~	~~T58.8X4~~	—	—
~~prior to combustion~~	~~T59.891~~	~~T59.892~~	~~T59.893~~	~~T59.894~~	—	—
~~utility~~	~~T59.891~~	~~T59.892~~	~~T59.893~~	~~T59.894~~	—	—
~~in mobile container~~	~~T59.891~~	~~T59.892~~	~~T59.893~~	~~T59.894~~	—	—
~~incomplete combustion of — see Carbon, monoxide, fuel, utility~~						
~~piped (natural)~~	~~T59.891~~	~~T59.892~~	~~T59.893~~	~~T59.894~~	—	—
~~garage~~	~~T58.01~~	~~T58.02~~	~~T58.03~~	~~T58.04~~	—	—
~~hydrocarbon NEC~~	~~T59.891~~	~~T59.892~~	~~T59.893~~	~~T59.894~~	—	—
~~incomplete combustion of — see Carbon, monoxide, fuel, utility~~						
~~liquefied — see butane~~						
~~piped~~	~~T59.891~~	~~T59.892~~	~~T59.893~~	~~T59.894~~	—	—
~~hydrocyanic acid~~	~~T65.0X1~~	~~T65.0X2~~	~~T65.0X3~~	~~T65.0X4~~	—	—

◀ New　◀ Revised　~~deleted~~ Deleted

Substance	Poisoning, Accidental (Unintentional)	Poisoning, Intentional Self-Harm	Poisoning, Assault	Poisoning, Undetermined	Adverse Effect	Underdosing
Gas (Continued)						
~~illuminating (after combustion)~~	~~T58.11~~	~~T58.12~~	~~T58.13~~	~~T58.14~~	~~—~~	~~—~~
~~prior to combustion~~	~~T59.891~~	~~T59.892~~	~~T59.893~~	~~T59.894~~		
~~incomplete combustion, any — see Carbon, monoxide~~						
~~kiln~~	~~T58.8X1~~	~~T58.8X2~~	~~T58.8X3~~	~~T58.8X4~~	~~—~~	~~—~~
~~lacrimogenic~~	~~T59.3X1~~	~~T59.3X2~~	~~T59.3X3~~	~~T59.3X4~~	~~—~~	~~—~~
~~liquefied petroleum — see butane~~						
~~marsh~~	~~T59.891~~	~~T59.892~~	~~T59.893~~	~~T59.894~~		
~~motor exhaust, not in transit~~	~~T58.01~~	~~T58.02~~	~~T58.03~~	~~T58.04~~		
~~mustard, not in war~~	~~T59.891~~	~~T59.892~~	~~T59.893~~	~~T59.894~~		
~~natural~~	~~T59.891~~	~~T59.892~~	~~T59.893~~	~~T59.894~~		
~~nerve, not in war~~	~~T59.91~~	~~T59.92~~	~~T59.93~~	~~T59.94~~		
~~oil~~	~~T52.0X1~~	~~T52.0X2~~	~~T52.0X3~~	~~T52.0X4~~		
~~petroleum (liquefied) (distributed in mobile containers)~~	~~T59.891~~	~~T59.892~~	~~T59.893~~	~~T59.894~~		
~~piped (pure or mixed with air)~~	~~T59.891~~	~~T59.892~~	~~T59.893~~	~~T59.894~~		
~~piped (manufactured) (natural) NEC~~	~~T59.891~~	~~T59.892~~	~~T59.893~~	~~T59.894~~		
~~producer~~	~~T58.8X1~~	~~T58.8X2~~	~~T58.8X3~~	~~T58.8X4~~		
~~propane — see propane~~						
~~refrigerant (chlorofluoro-carbon)~~	~~T53.5X1~~	~~T53.5X2~~	~~T53.5X3~~	~~T53.5X4~~		
~~not chlorofluoro-carbon~~	~~T59.891~~	~~T59.892~~	~~T59.893~~	~~T59.894~~		
~~sewer~~	~~T59.91~~	~~T59.92~~	~~T59.93~~	~~T59.94~~		
~~specified source NEC~~	~~T59.91~~	~~T59.92~~	~~T59.93~~	~~T59.94~~		
~~stove (after combustion)~~	~~T58.11~~	~~T58.12~~	~~T58.13~~	~~T58.14~~		
~~tear~~	~~T59.3X1~~	~~T59.3X2~~	~~T59.3X3~~	~~T59.3X4~~		
~~therapeutic~~	~~T41.5X1~~	~~T41.5X2~~	~~T41.5X3~~	~~T41.5X4~~	~~T41.5X5~~	~~T41.5X6~~
~~utility (for cooking, heating, or lighting) (piped) NEC~~	~~T59.891~~	~~T59.892~~	~~T59.893~~	~~T59.894~~		
~~in mobile container~~	~~T59.891~~	~~T59.892~~	~~T59.893~~	~~T59.894~~		
~~incomplete combustion of — see Carbon, monoxide, fuel, utility~~						
~~piped (natural)~~	~~T59.891~~	~~T59.892~~	~~T59.893~~	~~T59.894~~		
~~water~~	~~T58.11~~	~~T58.12~~	~~T58.13~~	~~T58.14~~		
~~incomplete combustion of — see Carbon, monoxide, fuel, utility~~						

Substance	Poisoning, Accidental (Unintentional)	Poisoning, Intentional Self-Harm	Poisoning, Assault	Poisoning, Undetermined	Adverse Effect	Underdosing
Gas NEC	T59.91	T59.92	T59.93	T59.94	—	—
acetylene	T59.891	T59.892	T59.893	T59.894	—	—
incomplete combustion of	T58.11	T58.12	T58.13	T58.14		
air contaminants, source or type not specified	T59.91	T59.92	T59.93	T59.94	—	—
anesthetic	T41.0X1	T41.0X2	T41.0X3	T41.0X4	T41.0X5	T41.0X6
blast furnace	T58.8X1	T58.8X2	T58.8X3	T58.8X4		
butane — see butane						
carbon monoxide — see Carbon, monoxide						
chlorine	T59.4X1	T59.4X2	T59.4X3	T59.4X4		
coal	T58.2X1	T58.2X2	T58.2X3	T58.2X4		
cyanide	T57.3X1	T57.3X2	T57.3X3	T57.3X4		
dicyanogen	T65.0X1	T65.0X2	T65.0X3	T65.0X4		
domestic — see Domestic gas	T57.91	T57.92	T57.93	T57.94		
exhaust	T57.91	T57.92	T57.93	T57.94		
from utility (for cooking, heating, or lighting) (after combustion) — see Carbon, monoxide, fuel, utility						
prior to combustion	T59.891	T59.892	T59.893	T59.894		
from wood or coal-burning stove or fireplace	T57.91	T57.92	T57.93	T57.94		
fuel (domestic use) (after combustion) — see also Carbon, monoxide, fuel	T57.91	T57.92	T57.93	T57.94	—	—
industrial use	T58.8X1	T58.8X2	T58.8X3	T58.8X4		
prior to combustion	T59.891	T59.892	T59.893	T59.894		
utility	T59.891	T59.892	T59.893	T59.894		
in mobile container	T59.891	T59.892	T59.893	T59.894		
incomplete combustion of — see Carbon, monoxide, fuel, utility						
piped (natural)	T59.891	T59.892	T59.893	T59.894		
garage	T58.01	T58.02	T58.03	T58.04		
hydrocarbon NEC	T59.891	T59.892	T59.893	T59.894		
incomplete combustion of — see Carbon, monoxide, fuel, utility						
liquefied — see butane						
piped	T59.891	T59.892	T59.893	T59.894	—	—
hydrocyanic acid	T65.0X1	T65.0X2	T65.0X3	T65.0X4	—	—

TABLE OF DRUGS AND CHEMICALS

◀ New　◀ Revised　~~deleted~~ Deleted

Substance	External Cause (T-Code)					
	Poisoning, Accidental (Unintentional)	Poisoning, Intentional Self-Harm	Poisoning, Assault	Poisoning, Undetermined	Adverse Effect	Underdosing
Gas (Continued)						
illuminating (after combustion)	T58.11	T58.12	T58.13	T58.14	—	—
prior to combustion	T59.891	T59.892	T59.893	T59.894	—	—
incomplete combustion, any — see Carbon, monoxide						
kiln	T58.8X1	T58.8X2	T58.8X3	T58.8X4		
lacrimogenic	T59.3X1	T59.3X2	T59.3X3	T59.3X4		
liquefied petroleum — see butane						
marsh	T59.891	T59.892	T59.893	T59.894	—	—
motor exhaust, not in transit	T58.01	T58.02	T58.03	T58.04		
mustard, not in war	T59.891	T59.892	T59.893	T59.894		
natural	T59.891	T59.892	T59.893	T59.894		
nerve, not in war	T59.91	T59.92	T59.93	T59.94		
oil	T52.0X1	T52.0X2	T52.0X3	T52.0X4	—	
petroleum (liquefied) (distributed in mobile containers)	T59.891	T59.892	T59.893	T59.894	—	—
piped (pure or mixed with air)	T59.891	T59.892	T59.893	T59.894	—	—
piped (manufactured) (natural) NEC	T59.891	T59.892	T59.893	T59.894	—	—
producer	T58.8X1	T58.8X2	T58.8X3	T58.8X4		
propane — see propane						
refrigerant (chlorofluoro-carbon)	T53.5X1	T53.5X2	T53.5X3	T53.5X4	—	—
not chlorofluoro-carbon	T59.891	T59.892	T59.893	T59.894	—	—
sewer	T59.91	T59.92	T59.93	T59.94		
specified source NEC	T59.91	T59.92	T59.93	T59.94		
stove (after combustion)	T58.11	T58.12	T58.13	T58.14		
tear	T59.3X1	T59.3X2	T59.3X3	T59.3X4		
therapeutic	T41.5X1	T41.5X2	T41.5X3	T41.5X4	T41.5X5	T41.5X6
utility (for cooking, heating, or lighting) (piped) NEC	T59.891	T59.892	T59.893	T59.894	—	—
in mobile container	T59.891	T59.892	T59.893	T59.894	—	—
incomplete combustion of — see Carbon, monoxide, fuel, utilty						
piped (natural)	T59.891	T59.892	T59.893	T59.894	—	—
water	T58.11	T58.12	T58.13	T58.14	—	—
incomplete combustion of — see Carbon, monoxide, fuel, utility						

Substance	External Cause (T-Code)					
	Poisoning, Accidental (Unintentional)	Poisoning, Intentional Self-Harm	Poisoning, Assault	Poisoning, Undetermined	Adverse Effect	Underdosing
Gaseous substance — see Gas						
Gasoline	T52.0X1	T52.0X2	T52.0X3	T52.0X4	—	—
vapor	T52.0X1	T52.0X2	T52.0X3	T52.0X4	—	—
Gastric enzymes	T47.5X1	T47.5X2	T47.5X3	T47.5X4	T47.5X5	T47.5X6
Gastrografin	T50.8X1	T50.8X2	T50.8X3	T50.8X4	T50.8X5	T50.8X6
Gastrointestinal drug	T47.91	T47.92	T47.93	T47.94	T47.95	T47.96
biological	T47.8X1	T47.8X2	T47.8X3	T47.8X4	T47.8X5	T47.8X6
specified NEC	T47.8X1	T47.8X2	T47.8X3	T47.8X4	T47.8X5	T47.8X6
Gaultheria procumbens	T62.2X1	T62.2X2	T62.2X3	T62.2X4	—	—
Gelatin (intravenous)	T45.8X1	T45.8X2	T45.8X3	T45.8X4	T45.8X5	T45.8X6
absorbable (sponge)	T45.7X1	T45.7X2	T45.7X3	T45.7X4	T45.7X5	T45.7X6
Gefarnate	T44.3X1	T44.3X2	T44.3X3	T44.3X4	T44.3X5	T44.3X6
Gelfilm	T49.8X1	T49.8X2	T49.8X3	T49.8X4	T49.8X5	T49.8X6
Gelfoam	T45.7X1	T45.7X2	T45.7X3	T45.7X4	T45.7X5	T45.7X6
Gelsemine	T50.991	T50.992	T50.993	T50.994	T50.995	T50.996
Gelsemium (sempervirens)	T62.2X1	T62.2X2	T62.2X3	T62.2X4	—	—
Gemeprost	T48.0X1	T48.0X2	T48.0X3	T48.0X4	T48.0X5	T48.0X6
Gemfibrozil	T46.6X1	T46.6X2	T46.6X3	T46.6X4	T46.6X5	T46.6X6
Gemonil	T42.3X1	T42.3X2	T42.3X3	T42.3X4	T42.3X5	T42.3X6
Gentamicin	T36.5X1	T36.5X2	T36.5X3	T36.5X4	T36.5X5	T36.5X6
ophthalmic preparation	T49.5X1	T49.5X2	T49.5X3	T49.5X4	T49.5X5	T49.5X6
topical NEC	T49.0X1	T49.0X2	T49.0X3	T49.0X4	T49.0X5	T49.0X6
Gentian	T47.5X1	T47.5X2	T47.5X3	T47.5X4	T47.5X5	T47.5X6
violet	T49.0X1	T49.0X2	T49.0X3	T49.0X4	T49.0X5	T49.0X6
Gepefrine	T44.4X1	T44.4X2	T44.4X3	T44.4X4	T44.4X5	T44.4X6
Gestonorone caproate	T38.5X1	T38.5X2	T38.5X3	T38.5X4	T38.5X5	T38.5X6
Gexane	T49.0X1	T49.0X2	T49.0X3	T49.0X4	T49.0X5	T49.0X6
Gila monster (venom)	T63.111	T63.112	T63.113	T63.114	—	—
Ginger	T47.5X1	T47.5X2	T47.5X3	T47.5X4	T47.5X5	T47.5X6
Jamaica — see Jamaica, ginger						
Gitalin	T46.0X1	T46.0X2	T46.0X3	T46.0X4	T46.0X5	T46.0X6
amorphous	T46.0X1	T46.0X2	T46.0X3	T46.0X4	T46.0X5	T46.0X6
Gitaloxin	T46.0X1	T46.0X2	T46.0X3	T46.0X4	T46.0X5	T46.0X6
Gitoxin	T46.0X1	T46.0X2	T46.0X3	T46.0X4	T46.0X5	T46.0X6
Glafenine	T39.8X1	T39.8X2	T39.8X3	T39.8X4	T39.8X5	T39.8X6
Glandular extract (medicinal) NEC	T50.Z91	T50.Z92	T50.Z93	T50.Z94	T50.Z95	T50.Z96
Glaucarubin	T37.3X1	T37.3X2	T37.3X3	T37.3X4	T37.3X5	T37.3X6
Glibenclamide	T38.3X1	T38.3X2	T38.3X3	T38.3X4	T38.3X5	T38.3X6
Glibornuride	T38.3X1	T38.3X2	T38.3X3	T38.3X4	T38.3X5	T38.3X6
Gliclazide	T38.3X1	T38.3X2	T38.3X3	T38.3X4	T38.3X5	T38.3X6
Glimidine	T38.3X1	T38.3X2	T38.3X3	T38.3X4	T38.3X5	T38.3X6

◄ New   ◄|| Revised   ~~deleted~~ Deleted

TABLE OF DRUGS AND CHEMICALS

Substance	Poisoning, Accidental (Unintentional)	Poisoning, Intentional Self-Harm	Poisoning, Assault	Poisoning, Undetermined	Adverse Effect	Underdosing
Glipizide	T38.3X1	T38.3X2	T38.3X3	T38.3X4	T38.3X5	T38.3X6
Gliquidone	T38.3X1	T38.3X2	T38.3X3	T38.3X4	T38.3X5	T38.3X6
Glisolamide	T38.3X1	T38.3X2	T38.3X3	T38.3X4	T38.3X5	T38.3X6
Glisoxepide	T38.3X1	T38.3X2	T38.3X3	T38.3X4	T38.3X5	T38.3X6
Globin zinc insulin	T38.3X1	T38.3X2	T38.3X3	T38.3X4	T38.3X5	T38.3X6
Globulin						
antilymphocytic	T50.Z11	T50.Z12	T50.Z13	T50.Z14	T50.Z15	T50.Z16
antirhesus	T50.Z11	T50.Z12	T50.Z13	T50.Z14	T50.Z15	T50.Z16
antivenin	T50.Z11	T50.Z12	T50.Z13	T50.Z14	T50.Z15	T50.Z16
antiviral	T50.Z11	T50.Z12	T50.Z13	T50.Z14	T50.Z15	T50.Z16
Glucagon	T38.3X1	T38.3X2	T38.3X3	T38.3X4	T38.3X5	T38.3X6
Glucocorticoids	T38.0X1	T38.0X2	T38.0X3	T38.0X4	T38.0X5	T38.0X6
Glucocorticosteroid	T38.0X1	T38.0X2	T38.0X3	T38.0X4	T38.0X5	T38.0X6
Gluconic acid	T50.991	T50.992	T50.993	T50.994	T50.995	T50.996
Glucosamine sulfate	T39.4X1	T39.4X2	T39.4X3	T39.4X4	T39.4X5	T39.4X6
Glucose	T50.3X1	T50.3X2	T50.3X3	T50.3X4	T50.3X5	T50.3X6
with sodium chloride	T50.3X1	T50.3X2	T50.3X3	T50.3X4	T50.3X5	T50.3X6
Glucosulfone sodium	T37.1X1	T37.1X2	T37.1X3	T37.1X4	T37.1X5	T37.1X6
Glucurolactone	T47.8X1	T47.8X2	T47.8X3	T47.8X4	T47.8X5	T47.8X6
Glue NEC	T52.8X1	T52.8X2	T52.8X3	T52.8X4	—	—
Glutamic acid	T47.5X1	T47.5X2	T47.5X3	T47.5X4	T47.5X5	T47.5X6
Glutaral (medicinal)	T49.0X1	T49.0X2	T49.0X3	T49.0X4	T49.0X5	T49.0X6
nonmedicinal	T65.891	T65.892	T65.893	T65.894	—	—
Glutaraldehyde (nonmedicinal)	T65.891	T65.892	T65.893	T65.894	—	—
medicinal	T49.0X1	T49.0X2	T49.0X3	T49.0X4	T49.0X5	T49.0X6
Glutathione	T50.6X1	T50.6X2	T50.6X3	T50.6X4	T50.6X5	T50.6X6
Glutethimide	T42.6X1	T42.6X2	T42.6X3	T42.6X4	T42.6X5	T42.6X6
Glyburide	T38.3X1	T38.3X2	T38.3X3	T38.3X4	T38.3X5	T38.3X6
Glycerin	T47.4X1	T47.4X2	T47.4X3	T47.4X4	T47.4X5	T47.4X6
Glycerol	T47.4X1	T47.4X2	T47.4X3	T47.4X4	T47.4X5	T47.4X6
borax	T49.6X1	T49.6X2	T49.6X3	T49.6X4	T49.6X5	T49.6X6
intravenous	T50.3X1	T50.3X2	T50.3X3	T50.3X4	T50.3X5	T50.3X6
iodinated	T48.4X1	T48.4X2	T48.4X3	T48.4X4	T48.4X5	T48.4X6
Glycerophosphate	T50.991	T50.992	T50.993	T50.994	T50.995	T50.996
Glyceryl						
gualacolate	T48.4X1	T48.4X2	T48.4X3	T48.4X4	T48.4X5	T48.4X6
nitrate	T46.3X1	T46.3X2	T46.3X3	T46.3X4	T46.3X5	T46.3X6
triacetate (topical)	T49.0X1	T49.0X2	T49.0X3	T49.0X4	T49.0X5	T49.0X6
trinitrate	T46.3X1	T46.3X2	T46.3X3	T46.3X4	T46.3X5	T46.3X6
Glycine	T50.3X1	T50.3X2	T50.3X3	T50.3X4	T50.3X5	T50.3X6
Glyclopyramide	T38.3X1	T38.3X2	T38.3X3	T38.3X4	T38.3X5	T38.3X6
Glycobiarsol	T37.3X1	T37.3X2	T37.3X3	T37.3X4	T37.3X5	T37.3X6

Substance	Poisoning, Accidental (Unintentional)	Poisoning, Intentional Self-Harm	Poisoning, Assault	Poisoning, Undetermined	Adverse Effect	Underdosing
Glycols (ether)	T52.3X1	T52.3X2	T52.3X3	T52.3X4	—	—
Glyconiazide	T37.1X1	T37.1X2	T37.1X3	T37.1X4	T37.1X5	T37.1X6
Glycopyrrolate	T44.3X1	T44.3X2	T44.3X3	T44.3X4	T44.3X5	T44.3X6
Glycopyrronium	T44.3X1	T44.3X2	T44.3X3	T44.3X4	T44.3X5	T44.3X6
bromide	T44.3X1	T44.3X2	T44.3X3	T44.3X4	T44.3X5	T44.3X6
Glycoside, cardiac (stimulant)	T46.0X1	T46.0X2	T46.0X3	T46.0X4	T46.0X5	T46.0X6
Glycyclamide	T38.3X1	T38.3X2	T38.3X3	T38.3X4	T38.3X5	T38.3X6
Glycyrrhiza extract	T48.4X1	T48.4X2	T48.4X3	T48.4X4	T48.4X5	T48.4X6
Glycyrrhizic acid	T48.4X1	T48.4X2	T48.4X3	T48.4X4	T48.4X5	T48.4X6
Glycyrrhizinate potassium	T48.4X1	T48.4X2	T48.4X3	T48.4X4	T48.4X5	T48.4X6
Glymidine sodium	T38.3X1	T38.3X2	T38.3X3	T38.3X4	T38.3X5	T38.3X6
Glyphosate	T60.3X1	T60.3X2	T60.3X3	T60.3X4	—	—
Glyphylline	T48.6X1	T48.6X2	T48.6X3	T48.6X4	T48.6X5	T48.6X6
Gold						
colloidal (l98Au)	T45.1X1	T45.1X2	T45.1X3	T45.1X4	T45.1X5	T45.1X6
salts	T39.4X1	T39.4X2	T39.4X3	T39.4X4	T39.4X5	T39.4X6
Golden sulfide of antimony	T56.891	T56.892	T56.893	T56.894	—	—
Goldylocks	T62.2X1	T62.2X2	T62.2X3	T62.2X4	—	—
Gonadal tissue extract	T38.901	T38.902	T38.903	T38.904	T38.905	T38.906
female	T38.5X1	T38.5X2	T38.5X3	T38.5X4	T38.5X5	T38.5X6
male	T38.7X1	T38.7X2	T38.7X3	T38.7X4	T38.7X5	T38.7X6
Gonadorelin	T38.891	T38.892	T38.893	T38.894	T38.895	T38.896
Gonadotropin	T38.891	T38.892	T38.893	T38.894	T38.895	T38.896
chorionic	T38.891	T38.892	T38.893	T38.894	T38.895	T38.896
pituitary	T38.811	T38.812	T38.813	T38.814	T38.815	T38.816
Goserelin	T45.1X1	T45.1X2	T45.1X3	T45.1X4	T45.1X5	T45.1X6
Grain alcohol	T51.0X1	T51.0X2	T51.0X3	T51.0X4	—	—
Gramicidin	T49.0X1	T49.0X2	T49.0X3	T49.0X4	T49.0X5	T49.0X6
Granisetron	T45.0X1	T45.0X2	T45.0X3	T45.0X4	T45.0X5	T45.0X6
Gratiola officinalis	T62.2X1	T62.2X2	T62.2X3	T62.2X4	—	—
Grease	T65.891	T65.892		T65.893	T65.894	—	—
Green hellebore	T62.2X1	T62.2X2	T62.2X3	T62.2X4	—	—
Green soap	T49.2X1	T49.2X2	T49.2X3	T49.2X4	T49.2X5	T49.2X6
Grifulvin	T36.7X1	T36.7X2	T36.7X3	T36.7X4	T36.7X5	T36.7X6
Griseofulvin	T36.7X1	T36.7X2	T36.7X3	T36.7X4	T36.7X5	T36.7X6
Growth hormone	T38.811	T38.812	T38.813	T38.814	T38.815	T38.816
Guaiacol derivatives	T48.4X1	T48.4X2	T48.4X3	T48.4X4	T48.4X5	T48.4X6
Guaiac reagent	T50.991	T50.992	T50.993	T50.994	T50.995	T50.996
Guaifenesin	T48.4X1	T48.4X2	T48.4X3	T48.4X4	T48.4X5	T48.4X6
Guaimesal	T48.4X1	T48.4X2	T48.4X3	T48.4X4	T48.4X5	T48.4X6
Guaiphenesin	T48.4X1	T48.4X2	T48.4X3	T48.4X4	T48.4X5	T48.4X6
Guamecycline	T36.4X1	T36.4X2	T36.4X3	T36.4X4	T36.4X5	T36.4X6

◀ New   ◀ Revised   ~~deleted~~ Deleted

Substance	Poisoning, Accidental (Unintentional)	Poisoning, Intentional Self-Harm	Poisoning, Assault	Poisoning, Undetermined	Adverse Effect	Underdosing
Guanabenz	T46.5X1	T46.5X2	T46.5X3	T46.5X4	T46.5X5	T46.5X6
Guanacline	T46.5X1	T46.5X2	T46.5X3	T46.5X4	T46.5X5	T46.5X6
Guanadrel	T46.5X1	T46.5X2	T46.5X3	T46.5X4	T46.5X5	T46.5X6
Guanatol	T37.2X1	T37.2X2	T37.2X3	T37.2X4	T37.2X5	T37.2X6
Guanethidine	T46.5X1	T46.5X2	T46.5X3	T46.5X4	T46.5X5	T46.5X6
Guanfacine	T46.5X1	T46.5X2	T46.5X3	T46.5X4	T46.5X5	T46.5X6
Guano	T65.891	T65.892	T65.893	T65.894	—	—
Guanochlor	T46.5X1	T46.5X2	T46.5X3	T46.5X4	T46.5X5	T46.5X6
Guanoclor	T46.5X1	T46.5X2	T46.5X3	T46.5X4	T46.5X5	T46.5X6
Guanoctine	T46.5X1	T46.5X2	T46.5X3	T46.5X4	T46.5X5	T46.5X6
Guanoxabenz	T46.5X1	T46.5X2	T46.5X3	T46.5X4	T46.5X5	T46.5X6
Guanoxan	T46.5X1	T46.5X2	T46.5X3	T46.5X4	T46.5X5	T46.5X6
Guar gum (medicinal)	T46.6X1	T46.6X2	T46.6X3	T46.6X4	T46.6X5	T46.6X6
H						
Hachimycin	T36.7X1	T36.7X2	T36.7X3	T36.7X4	T36.7X5	T36.7X6
Hair						
dye	T49.4X1	T49.4X2	T49.4X3	T49.4X4	T49.4X5	T49.4X6
preparation NEC	T49.4X1	T49.4X2	T49.4X3	T49.4X4	T49.4X5	T49.4X6
Halazepam	T42.4X1	T42.4X2	T42.4X3	T42.4X4	T42.4X5	T42.4X6
Halcinolone	T49.0X1	T49.0X2	T49.0X3	T49.0X4	T49.0X5	T49.0X6
Halcinonide	T49.0X1	T49.0X2	T49.0X3	T49.0X4	T49.0X5	T49.0X6
Halethazole	T49.0X1	T49.0X2	T49.0X3	T49.0X4	T49.0X5	T49.0X6
Hallucinogen NEC	T40.901	T40.902	T40.903	T40.904	T40.905	T40.906
Halofantrine	T37.2X1	T37.2X2	T37.2X3	T37.2X4	T37.2X5	T37.2X6
Halofenate	T46.6X1	T46.6X2	T46.6X3	T46.6X4	T46.6X5	T46.6X6
Halometasone	T49.0X1	T49.0X2	T49.0X3	T49.0X4	T49.0X5	T49.0X6
Haloperidol	T43.4X1	T43.4X2	T43.4X3	T43.4X4	T43.4X5	T43.4X6
Haloprogin	T49.0X1	T49.0X2	T49.0X3	T49.0X4	T49.0X5	T49.0X6
Halotex	T49.0X1	T49.0X2	T49.0X3	T49.0X4	T49.0X5	T49.0X6
Halothane	T41.0X1	T41.0X2	T41.0X3	T41.0X4	T41.0X5	T41.0X6
Haloxazolam	T42.4X1	T42.4X2	T42.4X3	T42.4X4	T42.4X5	T42.4X6
Halquinols	T49.0X1	T49.0X2	T49.0X3	T49.0X4	T49.0X5	T49.0X6
Hamamelis	T49.2X1	T49.2X2	T49.2X3	T49.2X4	T49.2X5	T49.2X6
Haptendextran	T45.8X1	T45.8X2	T45.8X3	T45.8X4	T45.8X5	T45.8X6
Harmonyl	T46.5X1	T46.5X2	T46.5X3	T46.5X4	T46.5X5	T46.5X6
Hartmann's solution	T50.3X1	T50.3X2	T50.3X3	T50.3X4	T50.3X5	T50.3X6
Hashish	T40.7X1	T40.7X2	T40.7X3	T40.7X4	T40.7X5	T40.7X6
Hawaiian Woodrose seeds	T40.991	T40.992	T40.993	T40.994	—	—
HCB	T60.3X1	T60.3X2	T60.3X3	T60.3X4	—	—
HCH	T53.6X1	T53.6X2	T53.6X3	T53.6X4	—	—
medicinal	T49.0X1	T49.0X2	T49.0X3	T49.0X4	T49.0X5	T49.0X6
HCN	T57.3X1	T57.3X2	T57.3X3	T57.3X4	—	—
Headache cures, drugs, powders NEC	T50.901	T50.902	T50.903	T50.904	T50.905	T50.906
Heavenly Blue (morning glory)	T40.991	T40.992	T40.993	T40.994		
Heavy metal antidote	T45.8X1	T45.8X2	T45.8X3	T45.8X4	T45.8X5	T45.8X6
Hedaquinium	T49.0X1	T49.0X2	T49.0X3	T49.0X4	T49.0X5	T49.0X6
Hedge hyssop	T62.2X1	T62.2X2	T62.2X3	T62.2X4		
Heet	T49.8X1	T49.8X2	T49.8X3	T49.8X4	T49.8X5	T49.8X6
Helium	T48.991	T48.992	T48.993	T48.994	T48.995	T48.996
Helenin	T37.4X1	T37.4X2	T37.4X3	T37.4X4	T37.4X5	T37.4X6
Hellebore (black) (green) (white)	T62.2X1	T62.2X2	T62.2X3	T62.2X4		
Helium (nonmedicinal) NEC	T59.891	T59.892	T59.893	T59.894	—	—
medicinal	T48.991	T48.992	T48.993	T48.994	T48.995	T48.996
Hematin	T45.8X1	T45.8X2	T45.8X3	T45.8X4	T45.8X5	T45.8X6
Hematinic preparation	T45.8X1	T45.8X2	T45.8X3	T45.8X4	T45.8X5	T45.8X6
Hemlock	T62.2X1	T62.2X2	T62.2X3	T62.2X4	—	—
Hemostatic	T45.621	T45.622	T45.623	T45.624	T45.625	T45.626
drug, systemic	T45.621	T45.622	T45.623	T45.624	T45.625	T45.626
Hemostyptic	T49.4X1	T49.4X2	T49.4X3	T49.4X4	T49.4X5	T49.4X6
Henbane	T62.2X1	T62.2X2	T62.2X3	T62.2X4		
Heparin (sodium)	T45.511	T45.512	T45.513	T45.514	T45.515	T45.516
action reverser	T45.7X1	T45.7X2	T45.7X3	T45.7X4	T45.7X5	T45.7X6
Heparin-fraction	T45.511	T45.512	T45.513	T45.514	T45.515	T45.516
Heparinoid (systemic)	T45.511	T45.512	T45.513	T45.514	T45.515	T45.516
Hepatic secretion stimulant	T47.8X1	T47.8X2	T47.8X3	T47.8X4	T47.8X5	T47.8X6
Hepatitis B						
immune globulin	T50.Z11	T50.Z12	T50.Z13	T50.Z14	T50.Z15	T50.Z16
vaccine	T50.B91	T50.B92	T50.B93	T50.B94	T50.B95	T50.B96
Hepronicate	T46.7X1	T46.7X2	T46.7X3	T46.7X4	T46.7X5	T46.7X6
Heptabarb	T42.3X1	T42.3X2	T42.3X3	T42.3X4	T42.3X5	T42.3X6
Heptabarbitone	T42.3X1	T42.3X2	T42.3X3	T42.3X4	T42.3X5	T42.3X6
Heptabarbital	T42.3X1	T42.3X2	T42.3X3	T42.3X4	T42.3X5	T42.3X6
Heptachlor	T60.1X1	T60.1X2	T60.1X3	T60.1X4	—	—
Heptalgin	T40.2X1	T40.2X2	T40.2X3	T40.2X4	T40.2X5	T40.2X6
Heptaminol	T46.3X1	T46.3X2	T46.3X3	T46.3X4	T46.3X5	T46.3X6
Herbicide NEC	T60.3X1	T60.3X2	T60.3X3	T60.3X4	—	—
Heroin	T40.1X1	T40.1X2	T40.1X3	T40.1X4	—	—
Herplex	T49.5X1	T49.5X2	T49.5X3	T49.5X4	T49.5X5	T49.5X6
HES	T45.8X1	T45.8X2	T45.8X3	T45.8X4	T45.8X5	T45.8X6
Hesperidin	T46.991	T46.992	T46.993	T46.994	T46.995	T46.996
Hetacillin	T36.0X1	T36.0X2	T36.0X3	T36.0X4	T36.0X5	T36.0X6

◀ New ◀ Revised ~~deleted~~ Deleted

	External Cause (T-Code)					
Substance	Poisoning, Accidental (Unintentional)	Poisoning, Intentional Self-Harm	Poisoning, Assault	Poisoning, Undetermined	Adverse Effect	Underdosing
Hetastarch	T45.8X1	T45.8X2	T45.8X3	T45.8X4	T45.8X5	T45.8X6
HETP	T60.0X1	T60.0X2	T60.0X3	T60.0X4	—	—
Hexachlorobenzene (vapor)	T60.3X1	T60.3X2	T60.3X3	T60.3X4	—	—
Hexachlorocyclohexane	T53.6X1	T53.6X2	T53.6X3	T53.6X4	—	—
Hexachlorophene	T49.0X1	T49.0X2	T49.0X3	T49.0X4	T49.0X5	T49.0X6
Hexadiline	T46.3X1	T46.3X2	T46.3X3	T46.3X4	T46.3X5	T46.3X6
Hexadimethrine (bromide)	T45.7X1	T45.7X2	T45.7X3	T45.7X4	T45.7X5	T45.7X6
Hexadylamine	T46.3X1	T46.3X2	T46.3X3	T46.3X4	T46.3X5	T46.3X6
Hexaethyl tetraphosphate	T60.0X1	T60.0X2	T60.0X3	T60.0X4	—	—
Hexafluorenium bromide	T48.1X1	T48.1X2	T48.1X3	T48.1X4	T48.1X5	T48.1X6
Hexafluorodiethyl ether	T43.291	T43.292	T43.293	T43.294	T43.295	T43.296
Hexaflurium (bromide)	T48.1X1	T48.1X2	T48.1X3	T48.1X4	T48.1X5	T48.1X6
Hexahydrobenzol	T52.8X1	T52.8X2	T52.8X3	T52.8X4	—	—
Hexahydrocresol(s)	T51.8X1	T51.8X2	T51.8X3	T51.8X4	—	—
arsenide	T57.0X1	T57.0X2	T57.0X3	T57.0X4	—	—
arseniurated	T57.0X1	T57.0X2	T57.0X3	T57.0X4	—	—
cyanide	T57.3X1	T57.3X2	T57.3X3	T57.3X4	—	—
gas	T59.891	T59.892	T59.893	T59.894	—	—
Fluoride (liquid)	T57.8X1	T57.8X2	T57.8X3	T57.8X4	—	—
vapor	T59.891	T59.892	T59.893	T59.894	—	—
phophorated	T60.0X1	T60.0X2	T60.0X3	T60.0X4	—	—
sulfate	T57.8X1	T57.8X2	T57.8X3	T57.8X4	—	—
sulfide (gas)	T59.6X1	T59.6X2	T59.6X3	T59.6X4	—	—
arseniurated	T57.0X1	T57.0X2	T57.0X3	T57.0X4	—	—
sulfurated	T57.8X1	T57.8X2	T57.8X3	T57.8X4	—	—
Hexahydrophenol	T51.8X1	T51.8X2	T51.8X3	T51.8X4	—	—
Hexa-germ	T49.2X1	T49.2X2	T49.2X3	T49.2X4	T49.2X5	T49.2X6
Hexalen	T51.8X1	T51.8X2	T51.8X3	T51.8X4	—	—
Hexamethonium bromide	T44.2X1	T44.2X2	T44.2X3	T44.2X4	T44.2X5	T44.2X6
Hexamethylene	T52.8X1	T52.8X2	T52.8X3	T52.8X4	—	—
Hexamethylmelamine	T45.1X1	T45.1X2	T45.1X3	T45.1X4	T45.1X5	T45.1X6
Hexamidine	T49.0X1	T49.0X2	T49.0X3	T49.0X4	T49.0X5	T49.0X6
Hexamine (mandelate)	T37.8X1	T37.8X2	T37.8X3	T37.8X4	T37.8X5	T37.8X6
Hexanone, 2-hexanone	T52.4X1	T52.4X2	T52.4X3	T52.4X4	—	—
Hexanuorenium	T48.1X1	T48.1X2	T48.1X3	T48.1X4	T48.1X5	T48.1X6
Hexapropymate	T42.6X1	T42.6X2	T42.6X3	T42.6X4	T42.6X5	T42.6X6
Hexasonium iodide	T44.3X1	T44.3X2	T44.3X3	T44.3X4	T44.3X5	T44.3X6
Hexcarbacholine bromide	T48.1X1	T48.1X2	T48.1X3	T48.1X4	T48.1X5	T48.1X6
Hexemal	T42.3X1	T42.3X2	T42.3X3	T42.3X4	T42.3X5	T42.3X6
Hexestrol	T38.5X1	T38.5X2	T38.5X3	T38.5X4	T38.5X5	T38.5X6
Hexethal (sodium)	T42.3X1	T42.3X2	T42.3X3	T42.3X4	T42.3X5	T42.3X6
Hexetidine	T37.8X1	T37.8X2	T37.8X3	T37.8X4	T37.8X5	T37.8X6

	External Cause (T-Code)					
Substance	Poisoning, Accidental (Unintentional)	Poisoning, Intentional Self-Harm	Poisoning, Assault	Poisoning, Undetermined	Adverse Effect	Underdosing
Hexobarbital	T42.3X1	T42.3X2	T42.3X3	T42.3X4	T42.3X5	T42.3X6
rectal	T41.291	T41.292	T41.293	T41.294	T41.295	T41.296
sodium	T41.1X1	T41.1X2	T41.1X3	T41.1X4	T41.1X5	T41.1X6
Hexobendine	T46.3X1	T46.3X2	T46.3X3	T46.3X4	T46.3X5	T46.3X6
Hexocyclium	T44.3X1	T44.3X2	T44.3X3	T44.3X4	T44.3X5	T44.3X6
metilsulfate	T44.3X1	T44.3X2	T44.3X3	T44.3X4	T44.3X5	T44.3X6
Hexoestrol	T38.5X1	T38.5X2	T38.5X3	T38.5X4	T38.5X5	T38.5X6
Hexone	T52.4X1	T52.4X2	T52.4X3	T52.4X4	—	—
Hexoprenaline	T48.6X1	T48.6X2	T48.6X3	T48.6X4	T48.6X5	T48.6X6
Hexylcaine	T41.3X1	T41.3X2	T41.3X3	T41.3X4	T41.3X5	T41.3X6
Hexylresorcinol	T52.2X1	T52.2X2	T52.2X3	T52.2X4	—	—
HGH (human growth hormone)	T38.811	T38.812	T38.813	T38.814	T38.815	T38.816
Hinkle's pills	T47.2X1	T47.2X2	T47.2X3	T47.2X4	T47.2X5	T47.2X6
Histalog	T50.8X1	T50.8X2	T50.8X3	T50.8X4	T50.8X5	T50.8X6
Histamine (phosphate)	T50.8X1	T50.8X2	T50.8X3	T50.8X4	T50.8X5	T50.8X6
Histoplasmin	T50.8X1	T50.8X2	T50.8X3	T50.8X4	T50.8X5	T50.8X6
Holly berries	T62.2X1	T62.2X2	T62.2X3	T62.2X4	—	—
Homatropine	T44.3X1	T44.3X2	T44.3X3	T44.3X4	T44.3X5	T44.3X6
methylbromide	T44.3X1	T44.3X2	T44.3X3	T44.3X4	T44.3X5	T44.3X6
Homochlorcyclizine	T45.0X1	T45.0X2	T45.0X3	T45.0X4	T45.0X5	T45.0X6
Homosalate	T49.3X1	T49.3X2	T49.3X3	T49.3X4	T49.3X5	T49.3X6
Homo-tet	T50.Z11	T50.Z12	T50.Z13	T50.Z14	T50.Z15	T50.Z16
Hormone	T38.801	T38.802	T38.803	T38.804	T38.805	T38.806
adrenal cortical steroids	T38.0X1	T38.0X2	T38.0X3	T38.0X4	T38.0X5	T38.0X6
androgenic	T38.7X1	T38.7X2	T38.7X3	T38.7X4	T38.7X5	T38.7X6
anterior pituitary NEC	T38.811	T38.812	T38.813	T38.814	T38.815	T38.816
antidiabetic agents	T38.3X1	T38.3X2	T38.3X3	T38.3X4	T38.3X5	T38.3X6
antidiuretic	T38.891	T38.892	T38.893	T38.894	T38.895	T38.896
cancer therapy	T45.1X1	T45.1X2	T45.1X3	T45.1X4	T45.1X5	T45.1X6
follicle stimulating	T38.811	T38.812	T38.813	T38.814	T38.815	T38.816
gonadotropic	T38.891	T38.892	T38.893	T38.894	T38.895	T38.896
pituitary	T38.811	T38.812	T38.813	T38.814	T38.815	T38.816
growth	T38.811	T38.812	T38.813	T38.814	T38.815	T38.816
luteinizing	T38.811	T38.812	T38.813	T38.814	T38.815	T38.816
ovarian	T38.5X1	T38.5X2	T38.5X3	T38.5X4	T38.5X5	T38.5X6
oxytocic	T48.0X1	T48.0X2	T48.0X3	T48.0X4	T48.0X5	T48.0X6
parathyroid (derivatives)	T50.991	T50.992	T50.993	T50.994	T50.995	T50.996
pituitary (posterior) NEC	T38.891	T38.892	T38.893	T38.894	T38.895	T38.896
anterior	T38.811	T38.812	T38.813	T38.814	T38.815	T38.816
specified, NEC	T38.891	T38.892	T38.893	T38.894	T38.895	T38.896
thyroid	T38.1X1	T38.1X2	T38.1X3	T38.1X4	T38.1X5	T38.1X6
Hornet (sting)	T63.451	T63.452	T63.453	T63.454	—	—

◀ New ◀ Revised ~~deleted~~ Deleted

Substance	Poisoning, Accidental (Unintentional)	Poisoning, Intentional Self-Harm	Poisoning, Assault	Poisoning, Undetermined	Adverse Effect	Underdosing
Horse anti-human lymphocytic serum	T50.Z11	T50.Z12	T50.Z13	T50.Z14	T50.Z15	T50.Z16
Horticulture agent NEC	T65.91	T65.92	T65.93	T65.94	—	—
with pesticide	T60.91	T60.92	T60.93	T60.94	—	—
Human						
albumin	T45.8X1	T45.8X2	T45.8X3	T45.8X4	T45.8X5	T45.8X6
growth hormone (HGH)	T38.811	T38.812	T38.813	T38.814	T38.815	T38.816
immune serum	T50.Z11	T50.Z12	T50.Z13	T50.Z14	T50.Z15	T50.Z16
Hyaluronidase	T45.3X1	T45.3X2	T45.3X3	T45.3X4	T45.3X5	T45.3X6
Hyazyme	T45.3X1	T45.3X2	T45.3X3	T45.3X4	T45.3X5	T45.3X6
Hycodan	T40.2X1	T40.2X2	T40.2X3	T40.2X4	T40.2X5	T40.2X6
Hydantoin derivative NEC	T42.0X1	T42.0X2	T42.0X3	T42.0X4	T42.0X5	T42.0X6
Hydeltra	T38.0X1	T38.0X2	T38.0X3	T38.0X4	T38.0X5	T38.0X6
Hydergine	T44.6X1	T44.6X2	T44.6X3	T44.6X4	T44.6X5	T44.6X6
Hydrabamine penicillin	T36.0X1	T36.0X2	T36.0X3	T36.0X4	T36.0X5	T36.0X6
Hydralazine	T46.5X1	T46.5X2	T46.5X3	T46.5X4	T46.5X5	T46.5X6
Hydrargaphen	T49.0X1	T49.0X2	T49.0X3	T49.0X4	T49.0X5	T49.0X6
Hydrargyri amino-chloridum	T49.0X1	T49.0X2	T49.0X3	T49.0X4	T49.0X5	T49.0X6
Hydrastine	T48.291	T48.292	T48.293	T48.294	T48.295	T48.296
Hydrazine	T54.1X1	T54.1X2	T54.1X3	T54.1X4	—	—
monoamine oxidase inhibitors	T43.1X1	T43.1X2	T43.1X3	T43.1X4	T43.1X5	T43.1X6
Hydrazoic acid, azides	T54.2X1	T54.2X2	T54.2X3	T54.2X4	—	—
Hydriodic acid	T48.4X1	T48.4X2	T48.4X3	T48.4X4	T48.4X5	T48.4X6
Hydrocarbon gas	T59.891	T59.892	T59.893	T59.894	—	—
incomplete combustion of — see Carbon, monoxide, fuel, utility						
liquefied (mobile container)	T59.891	T59.892	T59.893	T59.894	—	—
piped (natural)	T59.891	T59.892	T59.893	T59.894	—	—
Hydrochloric acid (liquid)	T54.2X1	T54.2X2	T54.2X3	T54.2X4	—	—
medicinal (digestant)	T47.5X1	T47.5X2	T47.5X3	T47.5X4	T47.5X5	T47.5X6
vapor	T59.891	T59.892	T59.893	T59.894	—	—
Hydrochlorothiazide	T50.2X1	T50.2X2	T50.2X3	T50.2X4	T50.2X5	T50.2X6
Hydrocodone	T40.2X1	T40.2X2	T40.2X3	T40.2X4	T40.2X5	T40.2X6
Hydrocortisone (derivatives)	T38.0X1	T38.0X2	T38.0X3	T38.0X4	T38.0X5	T38.0X6
aceponate	T49.0X1	T49.0X2	T49.0X3	T49.0X4	T49.0X5	T49.0X6
ENT agent	T49.6X1	T49.6X2	T49.6X3	T49.6X4	T49.6X5	T49.6X6
ophthalmic preparation	T49.5X1	T49.5X2	T49.5X3	T49.5X4	T49.5X5	T49.5X6
topical NEC	T49.0X1	T49.0X2	T49.0X3	T49.0X4	T49.0X5	T49.0X6
Hydrocortone	T38.0X1	T38.0X2	T38.0X3	T38.0X4	T38.0X5	T38.0X6
ENT agent	T49.6X1	T49.6X2	T49.6X3	T49.6X4	T49.6X5	T49.6X6
ophthalmic preparation	T49.5X1	T49.5X2	T49.5X3	T49.5X4	T49.5X5	T49.5X6
topical NEC	T49.0X1	T49.0X2	T49.0X3	T49.0X4	T49.0X5	T49.0X6

Substance	Poisoning, Accidental (Unintentional)	Poisoning, Intentional Self-Harm	Poisoning, Assault	Poisoning, Undetermined	Adverse Effect	Underdosing
Hydrocyanic acid (liquid)	T57.3X1	T57.3X2	T57.3X3	T57.3X4	—	—
gas	T65.0X1	T65.0X2	T65.0X3	T65.0X4	—	—
Hydroflumethiazide	T50.2X1	T50.2X2	T50.2X3	T50.2X4	T50.2X5	T50.2X6
Hydrofluoric acid (liquid)	T54.2X1	T54.2X2	T54.2X3	T54.2X4	—	—
vapor	T59.891	T59.892	T59.893	T59.894	—	—
Hydrogen	T59.891	T59.892	T59.893	T59.894	—	—
arsenide	T57.0X1	T57.0X2	T57.0X3	T57.0X4	—	—
arseniureted	T57.0X1	T57.0X2	T57.0X3	T57.0X4	—	—
chloride	T57.8X1	T57.8X2	T57.8X3	T57.8X4	—	—
cyanide (salts)	T57.3X1	T57.3X2	T57.3X3	T57.3X4	—	—
gas	T57.3X1	T57.3X2	T57.3X3	T57.3X4	—	—
Fluoride	T59.5X1	T59.5X2	T59.5X3	T59.5X4	—	—
vapor	T59.5X1	T59.5X2	T59.5X3	T59.5X4	—	—
peroxide	T49.0X1	T49.0X2	T49.0X3	T49.0X4	T49.0X5	T49.0X6
phosphureted	T57.1X1	T57.1X2	T57.1X3	T57.1X4	—	—
sulfide	T59.6X1	T59.6X2	T59.6X3	T59.6X4	—	—
arseniureted	T57.0X1	T57.0X2	T57.0X3	T57.0X4	—	—
sulfureted	T59.6X1	T59.6X2	T59.6X3	T59.6X4	—	—
Hydromethylpyridine	T46.7X1	T46.7X2	T46.7X3	T46.7X4	T46.7X5	T46.7X6
Hydromorphinol	T40.2X1	T40.2X2	T40.2X3	T40.2X4	—	—
Hydromorphinone	T40.2X1	T40.2X2	T40.2X3	T40.2X4	T40.2X5	T40.2X6
Hydromorphone	T40.2X1	T40.2X2	T40.2X3	T40.2X4	T40.2X5	T40.2X6
Hydromox	T50.2X1	T50.2X2	T50.2X3	T50.2X4	T50.2X5	T50.2X6
Hydrophilic lotion	T49.3X1	T49.3X2	T49.3X3	T49.3X4	T49.3X5	T49.3X6
Hydroquinidine	T46.2X1	T46.2X2	T46.2X3	T46.2X4	T46.2X5	T46.2X6
Hydroquinone	T52.2X1	T52.2X2	T52.2X3	T52.2X4	—	—
vapor	T59.891	T59.892	T59.893	T59.894	—	—
Hydrosulfuric acid (gas)	T59.6X1	T59.6X2	T59.6X3	T59.6X4	—	—
Hydrotalcite	T47.1X1	T47.1X2	T47.1X3	T47.1X4	T47.1X5	T47.1X6
Hydrous wool fat	T49.3X1	T49.3X2	T49.3X3	T49.3X4	T49.3X5	T49.3X6
Hydroxide, caustic	T54.3X1	T54.3X2	T54.3X3	T54.3X4	—	—
Hydroxocobalamin	T45.8X1	T45.8X2	T45.8X3	T45.8X4	T45.8X5	T45.8X6
Hydroxyamphetamine	T49.5X1	T49.5X2	T49.5X3	T49.5X4	T49.5X5	T49.5X6
Hydroxycarbamide	T45.1X1	T45.1X2	T45.1X3	T45.1X4	T45.1X5	T45.1X6
Hydroxychloroquine	T37.8X1	T37.8X2	T37.8X3	T37.8X4	T37.8X5	T37.8X6
Hydroxydihydrocodeinone	T40.2X1	T40.2X2	T40.2X3	T40.2X4	T40.2X5	T40.2X6
Hydroxyestrone	T38.5X1	T38.5X2	T38.5X3	T38.5X4	T38.5X5	T38.5X6
Hydroxyethyl starch	T45.8X1	T45.8X2	T45.8X3	T45.8X4	T45.8X5	T45.8X6
Hydroxymethylpentanone	T52.4X1	T52.4X2	T52.4X3	T52.4X4	—	—
Hydroxyphenamate	T43.591	T43.592	T43.593	T43.594	T43.595	T43.596
Hydroxyphenylbutazone	T39.2X1	T39.2X2	T39.2X3	T39.2X4	T39.2X5	T39.2X6

TABLE OF DRUGS AND CHEMICALS

Substance	Poisoning, Accidental (Unintentional)	Poisoning, Intentional Self-Harm	Poisoning, Assault	Poisoning, Undetermined	Adverse Effect	Underdosing
Hydroxyprogesterone	T38.5X1	T38.5X2	T38.5X3	T38.5X4	T38.5X5	T38.5X6
caproate	T38.5X1	T38.5X2	T38.5X3	T38.5X4	T38.5X5	T38.5X6
Hydroxyquinoline (derivatives) NEC	T37.8X1	T37.8X2	T37.8X3	T37.8X4	T37.8X5	T37.8X6
Hydroxystilbamidine	T37.3X1	T37.3X2	T37.3X3	T37.3X4	T37.3X5	T37.3X6
Hydroxytoluene (nonmedicinal)	T54.0X1	T54.0X2	T54.0X3	T54.0X4	—	—
medicinal	T49.0X1	T49.0X2	T49.0X3	T49.0X4	T49.0X5	T49.0X6
Hydroxyurea	T45.1X1	T45.1X2	T45.1X3	T45.1X4	T45.1X5	T45.1X6
Hydroxyzine	T43.591	T43.592	T43.593	T43.594	T43.595	T43.596
Hyoscine	T44.3X1	T44.3X2	T44.3X3	T44.3X4	T44.3X5	T44.3X6
Hyoscyamine	T44.3X1	T44.3X2	T44.3X3	T44.3X4	T44.3X5	T44.3X6
Hyoscyamus	T44.3X1	T44.3X2	T44.3X3	T44.3X4	T44.3X5	T44.3X6
dry extract	T44.3X1	T44.3X2	T44.3X3	T44.3X4	T44.3X5	T44.3X6
Hypaque	T50.8X1	T50.8X2	T50.8X3	T50.8X4	T50.8X5	T50.8X6
Hypertussis	T50.Z11	T50.Z12	T50.Z13	T50.Z14	T50.Z15	T50.Z16
Hypnotic	T42.71	T42.72	T42.73	T42.74	T42.75	T42.76
anticonvulsant	T42.71	T42.72	T42.73	T42.74	T42.75	T42.76
specified NEC	T42.6X1	T42.6X2	T42.6X3	T42.6X4	T42.6X5	T42.6X6
Hypochlorite	T49.0X1	T49.0X2	T49.0X3	T49.0X4	T49.0X5	T49.0X6
Hypophysis, posterior	T38.891	T38.892	T38.893	T38.894	T38.895	T38.896
Hypotensive NEC	T46.5X1	T46.5X2	T46.5X3	T46.5X4	T46.5X5	T46.5X6
Hypromellose	T49.5X1	T49.5X2	T49.5X3	T49.5X4	T49.5X5	T49.5X6

I

Substance	Poisoning, Accidental (Unintentional)	Poisoning, Intentional Self-Harm	Poisoning, Assault	Poisoning, Undetermined	Adverse Effect	Underdosing
Ibacitabine	T37.5X1	T37.5X2	T37.5X4	T37.5X5	T37.5X6	
Ibopamine	T44.991	T44.992	T44.993	T44.994	T44.995	T44.996
Ibufenac	T39.311	T39.312	T39.313	T39.314	T39.315	T39.316
Ibuprofen	T39.311	T39.312	T39.313	T39.314	T39.315	T39.316
Ibuproxam	T39.311	T39.312	T39.313	T39.314	T39.315	T39.316
Ibuterol	T48.6X1	T48.6X2	T48.6X3	T48.6X4	T48.6X5	T48.6X6
Ichthammol	T49.0X1	T49.0X2	T49.0X3	T49.0X4	T49.0X5	T49.0X6
Ichthyol	T49.4X1	T49.4X2	T49.4X3	T49.4X4	T49.4X5	T49.4X6
Idarubicin	T45.1X1	T45.1X2	T45.1X3	T45.1X4	T45.1X5	T45.1X6
Idrocilamide	T42.8X1	T42.8X2	T42.8X3	T42.8X4	T42.8X5	T42.8X6
Ifenprodil	T46.7X1	T46.7X2	T46.7X3	T46.7X4	T46.7X5	T46.7X6
Ifosfamide	T45.1X1	T45.1X2	T45.1X3	T45.1X4	T45.1X5	T45.1X6
Iletin	T38.3X1	T38.3X2	T38.3X3	T38.3X4	T38.3X5	T38.3X6
Ilex	T62.2X1	T62.2X2	T62.2X3	T62.2X4	—	—
Illuminating gas (after combustion)	T58.11	T58.12	T58.13	T58.14	—	—
prior to combustion	T59.891	T59.892	T59.893	T59.894	—	—
Ilopan	T45.2X1	T45.2X2	T45.2X3	T45.2X4	T45.2X5	T45.2X6
Iloprost	T46.7X1	T46.7X2	T46.7X3	T46.7X4	T46.7X5	T46.7X6

Substance	Poisoning, Accidental (Unintentional)	Poisoning, Intentional Self-Harm	Poisoning, Assault	Poisoning, Undetermined	Adverse Effect	Underdosing
Ilotycin	T36.3X1	T36.3X2	T36.3X3	T36.3X4	T36.3X5	T36.3X6
ophthalmic preparation	T49.5X1	T49.5X2	T49.5X3	T49.5X4	T49.5X5	T49.5X6
topical NEC	T49.0X1	T49.0X2	T49.0X3	T49.0X4	T49.0X5	T49.0X6
Imidazole-4-carboxamide	T45.1X1	T45.1X2	T45.1X3	T45.1X4	T45.1X5	T45.1X6
Imipenem	T36.0X1	T36.0X2	T36.0X3	T36.0X4	T36.0X5	T36.0X6
Imipramine	T43.011	T43.012	T43.013	T43.014	T43.015	T43.016
Iminostilbene	T42.1X1	T42.1X2	T42.1X3	T42.1X4	T42.1X5	T42.1X6
Immu-G	T50.Z11	T50.Z12	T50.Z13	T50.Z14	T50.Z15	T50.Z16
Immuglobin	T50.Z11	T50.Z12	T50.Z13	T50.Z14	T50.Z15	T50.Z16
Immune						
globulin	T50.Z11	T50.Z12	T50.Z13	T50.Z14	T50.Z15	T50.Z16
serum globulin	T50.Z11	T50.Z12	T50.Z13	T50.Z14	T50.Z15	T50.Z16
Immunoglobin human (intravenous) (normal)	T50.Z11	T50.Z12	T50.Z13	T50.Z14	T50.Z15	T50.Z16
unmodified	T50.Z11	T50.Z12	T50.Z13	T50.Z14	T50.Z15	T50.Z16
Immunosuppressive drug	T45.1X1	T45.1X2	T45.1X3	T45.1X4	T45.1X5	T45.1X6
Immu-tetanus	T50.Z11	T50.Z12	T50.Z13	T50.Z14	T50.Z15	T50.Z16
Indalpine	T43.221	T43.222	T43.223	T43.224	T43.225	T43.226
Indanazoline	T48.5X1	T48.5X2	T48.5X3	T48.5X4	T48.5X5	T48.5X6
Indandione (derivatives)	T45.511	T45.512	T45.513	T45.514	T45.515	T45.516
Indapamide	T46.5X1	T46.5X2	T46.5X3	T46.5X4	T46.5X5	T46.5X6
Indendione (derivatives)	T45.511	T45.512	T45.513	T45.514	T45.515	T45.516
Indenolol	T44.7X1	T44.7X2	T44.7X3	T44.7X4	T44.7X5	T44.7X6
Inderal	T44.7X1	T44.7X2	T44.7X3	T44.7X4	T44.7X5	T44.7X6
Indian						
hemp	T40.7X1	T40.7X2	T40.7X3	T40.7X4	T40.7X5	T40.7X6
tobacco	T62.2X1	T62.2X2	T62.2X3	T62.2X4	—	—
Indigo carmine	T50.8X1	T50.8X2	T50.8X3	T50.8X4	T50.8X5	T50.8X6
Indobufen	T45.521	T45.522	T45.523	T45.524	T45.525	T45.526
Indocin	T39.2X1	T39.2X2	T39.2X3	T39.2X4	T39.2X5	T39.2X6
Indocyanine green	T50.8X1	T50.8X2	T50.8X3	T50.8X4	T50.8X5	T50.8X6
Indometacin	T39.391	T39.392	T39.393	T39.394	T39.395	T39.396
Indomethacin	T39.391	T39.392	T39.393	T39.394	T39.395	T39.396
farnesil	T39.4X1	T39.4X2	T39.4X3	T39.4X4	T39.4X5	T39.4X6
Indoramin	T44.6X1	T44.6X2	T44.6X3	T44.6X4	T44.6X5	T44.6X6
Industrial						
alcohol	T51.0X1	T51.0X2	T51.0X3	T51.0X4	—	—
fumes	T59.891	T59.892	T59.893	T59.894	—	—
solvents (fumes) (vapors)	T52.91	T52.92	T52.93	T52.94	—	—
Influenza vaccine	T50.B91	T50.B92	T50.B93	T50.B94	T50.B95	T50.B96
Ingested substance NEC	T65.91	T65.92	T65.93	T65.94	—	—
INH	T37.1X1	T37.1X2	T37.1X3	T37.1X4	T37.1X5	T37.1X6

◀ New   ◀ Revised   ~~deleted~~ Deleted

Substance	Poisoning, Accidental (Unintentional)	Poisoning, Intentional Self-Harm	Poisoning, Assault	Poisoning, Undetermined	Adverse Effect	Underdosing
Inhalation, gas (noxious) — see Gas						
Inhibitor						
angiotensin-converting enzyme	T46.4X1	T46.4X2	T46.4X3	T46.4X4	T46.4X5	T46.4X6
carbonic anhydrase	T50.2X1	T50.2X2	T50.2X3	T50.2X4	T50.2X5	T50.2X6
fibrinolysis	T45.621	T45.622	T45.623	T45.624	T45.625	T45.626
monoamine oxidase NEC	T43.1X1	T43.1X2	T43.1X3	T43.1X4	T43.1X5	T43.1X6
hydrazine	T43.1X1	T43.1X2	T43.1X3	T43.1X4	T43.1X5	T43.1X6
postsynaptic	T43.8X1	T43.8X2	T43.8X3	T43.8X4	T43.8X5	T43.8X6
prothrombin synthesis	T45.511	T45.512	T45.513	T45.514	T45.515	T45.516
Ink	T65.891	T65.892	T65.893	T65.894	—	—
Inorganic substance NEC	T57.91	T57.92	T57.93	T57.94	—	—
Inosine pranobex	T37.5X1	T37.5X2	T37.5X3	T37.5X4	T37.5X5	T37.5X6
Inositol	T50.991	T50.992	T50.993	T50.994	T50.995	T50.996
nicotinate	T46.7X1	T46.7X2	T46.7X3	T46.7X4	T46.7X5	T46.7X6
Inproquone	T45.1X1	T45.1X2	T45.1X3	T45.1X4	T45.1X5	T45.1X6
Insect (sting), venomous	T63.481	T63.482	T63.483	T63.484	—	—
ant	T63.421	T63.422	T63.423	T63.424	—	—
bee	T63.441	T63.442	T63.443	T63.444	—	—
caterpillar	T63.431	T63.432	T63.433	T63.434	—	—
hornet	T63.451	T63.452	T63.453	T63.454	—	—
wasp	T63.461	T63.462	T63.463	T63.464	—	—
Insecticide NEC	T60.91	T60.92	T60.93	T60.94	—	—
carbamate	T60.0X1	T60.0X2	T60.0X3	T60.0X4	—	—
chlorinated	T60.1X1	T60.1X2	T60.1X3	T60.1X4	—	—
mixed	T60.91	T60.92	T60.93	T60.94	—	—
organochlorine	T60.1X1	T60.1X2	T60.1X3	T60.1X4	—	—
organophosphorus	T60.0X1	T60.0X2	T60.0X3	T60.0X4	—	—
Insular tissue extract	T38.3X1	T38.3X2	T38.3X3	T38.3X4	T38.3X5	T38.3X6
Insulin (amorphous) (globin) (isophane) (Lente) (NPH) (Semilente) (Ultralente)	T38.3X1	T38.3X2	T38.3X3	T38.3X4	T38.3X5	T38.3X6
defalan	T38.3X1	T38.3X2	T38.3X3	T38.3X4	T38.3X5	T38.3X6
human	T38.3X1	T38.3X2	T38.3X3	T38.3X4	T38.3X5	T38.3X6
injection, soluble	T38.3X1	T38.3X2	T38.3X3	T38.3X4	T38.3X5	T38.3X6
biphasic	T38.3X1	T38.3X2	T38.3X3	T38.3X4	T38.3X5	T38.3X6
intermediate acting	T38.3X1	T38.3X2	T38.3X3	T38.3X4	T38.3X5	T38.3X6
protamine zinc	T38.3X1	T38.3X2	T38.3X3	T38.3X4	T38.3X5	T38.3X6
slow acting	T38.3X1	T38.3X2	T38.3X3	T38.3X4	T38.3X5	T38.3X6
zinc						
protamine injection	T38.3X1	T38.3X2	T38.3X3	T38.3X4	T38.3X5	T38.3X6
suspension (amorphous) (crystalline)	T38.3X1	T38.3X2	T38.3X3	T38.3X4	T38.3X5	T38.3X6

Substance	Poisoning, Accidental (Unintentional)	Poisoning, Intentional Self-Harm	Poisoning, Assault	Poisoning, Undetermined	Adverse Effect	Underdosing
Interferon (alpha) (beta) (gamma)	T37.5X1	T37.5X2	T37.5X3	T37.5X4	T37.5X5	T37.5X6
Intestinal motility control drug	T47.6X1	T47.6X2	T47.6X3	T47.6X4	T47.6X5	T47.6X6
biological	T47.8X1	T47.8X2	T47.8X3	T47.8X4	T47.8X5	T47.8X6
Intranarcon	T41.1X1	T41.1X2	T41.1X3	T41.1X4	T41.1X5	T41.1X6
Intravenous						
amino acids	T50.991	T50.992	T50.993	T50.994	T50.995	T50.996
fat suspension	T50.991	T50.992	T50.993	T50.994	T50.995	T50.996
Inulin	T50.8X1	T50.8X2	T50.8X3	T50.8X4	T50.8X5	T50.8X6
Invert sugar	T50.3X1	T50.3X2	T50.3X3	T50.3X4	T50.3X5	T50.3X6
Inza — see Naproxen						
Iobenzamic acid	T50.8X1	T50.8X2	T50.8X3	T50.8X4	T50.8X5	T50.8X6
Iocarmic acid	T50.8X1	T50.8X2	T50.8X3	T50.8X4	T50.8X5	T50.8X6
Iocetamic acid	T50.8X1	T50.8X2	T50.8X3	T50.8X4	T50.8X5	T50.8X6
Iodamide	T50.8X1	T50.8X2	T50.8X3	T50.8X4	T50.8X5	T50.8X6
Iodide NEC — see also Iodine	T49.0X1	T49.0X2	T49.0X3	T49.0X4	T49.0X5	T49.0X6
mercury (ointment)	T49.0X1	T49.0X2	T49.0X3	T49.0X4	T49.0X5	T49.0X6
methylate	T49.0X1	T49.0X2	T49.0X3	T49.0X4	T49.0X5	T49.0X6
potassium (expectorant) NEC	T48.4X1	T48.4X2	T48.4X3	T48.4X4	T48.4X5	T48.4X6
Iodinated						
contrast medium	T50.8X1	T50.8X2	T50.8X3	T50.8X4	T50.8X5	T50.8X6
glycerol	T48.4X1	T48.4X2	T48.4X3	T48.4X4	T48.4X5	T48.4X6
human serum albumin (131I)	T50.8X1	T50.8X2	T50.8X3	T50.8X4	T50.8X5	T50.8X6
Iodine (antiseptic, external) (tincture) NEC	T49.0X1	T49.0X2	T49.0X3	T49.0X4	T49.0X5	T49.0X6
125 — see also Radiation sickness, and Exposure to radioactivce isotopes	T50.8X1	T50.8X2	T50.8X3	T50.8X4	T50.8X5	T50.8X6
therapeutic	T50.991	T50.992	T50.993	T50.994	T50.995	T50.996
131 — see also Radiation sickness, and Exposure to radioactivce isotopes	T50.8X1	T50.8X2	T50.8X3	T50.8X4	T50.8X5	T50.8X6
therapeutic	T38.2X1	T38.2X2	T38.2X3	T38.2X4	T38.2X5	T38.2X6
diagnostic	T50.8X1	T50.8X2	T50.8X3	T50.8X4	T50.8X5	T50.8X6
for thyroid conditions (antithyroid)	T38.2X1	T38.2X2	T38.2X3	T38.2X4	T38.2X5	T38.2X6
solution	T49.0X1	T49.0X2	T49.0X3	T49.0X4	T49.0X5	T49.0X6
vapor	T59.891	T59.892	T59.893	T59.894	—	—
Iodipamide	T50.8X1	T50.8X2	T50.8X3	T50.8X4	T50.8X5	T50.8X6
Iodized (poppy seed) oil	T50.8X1	T50.8X2	T50.8X3	T50.8X4	T50.8X5	T50.8X6
Iodobismitol	T37.8X1	T37.8X2	T37.8X3	T37.8X4	T37.8X5	T37.8X6
Iodochlorhydroxyquin	T37.8X1	T37.8X2	T37.8X3	T37.8X4	T37.8X5	T37.8X6
topical	T49.0X1	T49.0X2	T49.0X3	T49.0X4	T49.0X5	T49.0X6
Iodochlorhydroxyquino-line	T37.8X1	T37.8X2	T37.8X3	T37.8X4	T37.8X5	T37.8X6
Iodocholesterol (131I)	T50.8X1	T50.8X2	T50.8X3	T50.8X4	T50.8X5	T50.8X6

◀ New ◀ Revised ~~deleted~~ Deleted

TABLE OF DRUGS AND CHEMICALS

Substance	External Cause (T-Code)					
	Poisoning, Accidental (Unintentional)	Poisoning, Intentional Self-Harm	Poisoning, Assault	Poisoning, Undetermined	Adverse Effect	Underdosing
Iodoform	T49.0X1	T49.0X2	T49.0X3	T49.0X4	T49.0X5	T49.0X6
Iodohippuric acid	T50.8X1	T50.8X2	T50.8X3	T50.8X4	T50.8X5	T50.8X6
Iodopanoic acid	T50.8X1	T50.8X2	T50.8X3	T50.8X4	T50.8X5	T50.8X6
Iodophthalein (sodium)	T50.8X1	T50.8X2	T50.8X3	T50.8X4	T50.8X5	T50.8X6
Iodopyracet	T50.8X1	T50.8X2	T50.8X3	T50.8X4	T50.8X5	T50.8X6
Iodoquinol	T37.8X1	T37.8X2	T37.8X3	T37.8X4	T37.8X5	T37.8X6
Iodoxamic acid	T50.8X1	T50.8X2	T50.8X3	T50.8X4	T50.8X5	T50.8X6
Iofendylate	T50.8X1	T50.8X2	T50.8X3	T50.8X4	T50.8X5	T50.8X6
Ioglycamic acid	T50.8X1	T50.8X2	T50.8X3	T50.8X4	T50.8X5	T50.8X6
Iohexol	T50.8X1	T50.8X2	T50.8X3	T50.8X4	T50.8X5	T50.8X6
Ion exchange resin						
anion	T47.8X1	T47.8X2	T47.8X3	T47.8X4	T47.8X5	T47.8X6
cation	T50.3X1	T50.3X2	T50.3X3	T50.3X4	T50.3X5	T50.3X6
cholestyramine	T46.6X1	T46.6X2	T46.6X3	T46.6X4	T46.6X5	T46.6X6
intestinal	T47.8X1	T47.8X2	T47.8X3	T47.8X4	T47.8X5	T47.8X6
Iopamidol	T50.8X1	T50.8X2	T50.8X3	T50.8X4	T50.8X5	T50.8X6
Iopanoic acid	T50.8X1	T50.8X2	T50.8X3	T50.8X4	T50.8X5	T50.8X6
Iophenoic acid	T50.8X1	T50.8X2	T50.8X3	T50.8X4	T50.8X5	T50.8X6
Iopodate, sodium	T50.8X1	T50.8X2	T50.8X3	T50.8X4	T50.8X5	T50.8X6
Iopodic acid	T50.8X1	T50.8X2	T50.8X3	T50.8X4	T50.8X5	T50.8X6
Iopromide	T50.8X1	T50.8X2	T50.8X3	T50.8X4	T50.8X5	T50.8X6
Iopydol	T50.8X1	T50.8X2	T50.8X3	T50.8X4	T50.8X5	T50.8X6
Iotalamic acid	T50.8X1	T50.8X2	T50.8X3	T50.8X4	T50.8X5	T50.8X6
Iothalamate	T50.8X1	T50.8X2	T50.8X3	T50.8X4	T50.8X5	T50.8X6
Iothiouracil	T38.2X1	T38.2X2	T38.2X3	T38.2X4	T38.2X5	T38.2X6
Iotrol	T50.8X1	T50.8X2	T50.8X3	T50.8X4	T50.8X5	T50.8X6
Iotrolan	T50.8X1	T50.8X2	T50.8X3	T50.8X4	T50.8X5	T50.8X6
Iotroxate	T50.8X1	T50.8X2	T50.8X3	T50.8X4	T50.8X5	T50.8X6
Iotroxic acid	T50.8X1	T50.8X2	T50.8X3	T50.8X4	T50.8X5	T50.8X6
Ioversol	T50.8X1	T50.8X2	T50.8X3	T50.8X4	T50.8X5	T50.8X6
Ioxaglate	T50.8X1	T50.8X2	T50.8X3	T50.8X4	T50.8X5	T50.8X6
Ioxaglic acid	T50.8X1	T50.8X2	T50.8X3	T50.8X4	T50.8X5	T50.8X6
Ioxitalamic acid	T50.8X1	T50.8X2	T50.8X3	T50.8X4	T50.8X5	T50.8X6
Ipecac	T47.7X1	T47.7X2	T47.7X3	T47.7X4	T47.7X5	T47.7X6
Ipecacuanha	T48.4X1	T48.4X2	T48.4X3	T48.4X4	T48.4X5	T48.4X6
Ipodate, calcium	T50.8X1	T50.8X2	T50.8X3	T50.8X4	T50.8X5	T50.8X6
Ipral	T42.3X1	T42.3X2	T42.3X3	T42.3X4	T42.3X5	T42.3X6
Ipratropium (bromide)	T48.6X1	T48.6X2	T48.6X3	T48.6X4	T48.6X5	T48.6X6
Ipriflavone	T46.3X1	T46.3X2	T46.3X3	T46.3X4	T46.3X5	T46.3X6
Iprindole	T43.011	T43.012	T43.013	T43.014	T43.015	T43.016
Iproclozide	T43.1X1	T43.1X2	T43.1X3	T43.1X4	T43.1X5	T43.1X6
Iprofenin	T50.8X1	T50.8X2	T50.8X3	T50.8X4	T50.8X5	T50.8X6

Substance	External Cause (T-Code)					
	Poisoning, Accidental (Unintentional)	Poisoning, Intentional Self-Harm	Poisoning, Assault	Poisoning, Undetermined	Adverse Effect	Underdosing
Iproheptine	T49.2X1	T49.2X2	T49.2X3	T49.2X4	T49.2X5	T49.2X6
Iproniazid	T43.1X1	T43.1X2	T43.1X3	T43.1X4	T43.1X5	T43.1X6
Iproplatin	T45.1X1	T45.1X2	T45.1X3	T45.1X4	T45.1X5	T45.1X6
Iproveratril	T46.1X1	T46.1X2	T46.1X3	T46.1X4	T46.1X5	T46.1X6
Iron (compounds) (medicinal) NEC	T45.4X1	T45.4X2	T45.4X3	T45.4X4	T45.4X5	T45.4X6
ammonium	T45.4X1	T45.4X2	T45.4X3	T45.4X4	T45.4X5	T45.4X6
dextran injection	T45.4X1	T45.4X2	T45.4X3	T45.4X4	T45.4X5	T45.4X6
nonmedicinal	T56.891	T56.892	T56.893	T56.894	—	—
salts	T45.4X1	T45.4X2	T45.4X3	T45.4X4	T45.4X5	T45.4X6
sorbitex	T45.4X1	T45.4X2	T45.4X3	T45.4X4	T45.4X5	T45.4X6
sorbitol citric acid complex	T45.4X1	T45.4X2	T45.4X3	T45.4X4	T45.4X5	T45.4X6
Irrigating fluid (vaginal)	T49.8X1	T49.8X2	T49.8X3	T49.8X4	T49.8X5	T49.8X6
eye	T49.5X1	T49.5X2	T49.5X3	T49.5X4	T49.5X5	T49.5X6
Isepamicin	T36.5X1	T36.5X2	T36.5X3	T36.5X4	T36.5X5	T36.5X6
Isoaminile (citrate)	T48.3X1	T48.3X2	T48.3X3	T48.3X4	T48.3X5	T48.3X6
Isoamyl nitrite	T46.3X1	T46.3X2	T46.3X3	T46.3X4	T46.3X5	T46.3X6
Isobenzan	T60.1X1	T60.1X2	T60.1X3	T60.1X4	—	—
Isobutyl acetate	T52.8X1	T52.8X2	T52.8X3	T52.8X4	—	—
Isocarboxazid	T43.1X1	T43.1X2	T43.1X3	T43.1X4	T43.1X5	T43.1X6
Isoconazole	T49.0X1	T49.0X2	T49.0X3	T49.0X4	T49.0X5	T49.0X6
Isocyanate	T65.0X1	T65.0X2	T65.0X3	T65.0X4	—	—
Isoephedrine	T44.991	T44.992	T44.993	T44.994	T44.995	T44.996
Isoetarine	T48.6X1	T48.6X2	T48.6X3	T48.6X4	T48.6X5	T48.6X6
Isoethadione	T42.2X1	T42.2X2	T42.2X3	T42.2X4	T42.2X5	T42.2X6
Isoetharine	T44.5X1	T44.5X2	T44.5X3	T44.5X4	T44.5X5	T44.5X6
Isoflurane	T41.0X1	T41.0X2	T41.0X3	T41.0X4	T41.0X5	T41.0X6
Isoflurophate	T44.0X1	T44.0X2	T44.0X3	T44.0X4	T44.0X5	T44.0X6
Isomaltose, ferric complex	T45.4X1	T45.4X2	T45.4X3	T45.4X4	T45.4X5	T45.4X6
Isometheptene	T44.3X1	T44.3X2	T44.3X3	T44.3X4	T44.3X5	T44.3X6
Isoniazid	T37.1X1	T37.1X2	T37.1X3	T37.1X4	T37.1X5	T37.1X6
with						
rifampicin	T36.6X1	T36.6X2	T36.6X3	T36.6X4	T36.6X5	T36.6X6
thioacetazone	T37.1X1	T37.1X2	T37.1X3	T37.1X4	T37.1X5	T37.1X6
Isonicotinic acid hydrazide	T37.1X1	T37.1X2	T37.1X3	T37.1X4	T37.1X5	T37.1X6
Isonipecaine	T40.4X1	T40.4X2	T40.4X3	T40.4X4	T40.4X5	T40.4X6
Isopentaquine	T37.2X1	T37.2X2	T37.2X3	T37.2X4	T37.2X5	T37.2X6
Isophane insulin	T38.3X1	T38.3X2	T38.3X3	T38.3X4	T38.3X5	T38.3X6
Isophorone	T65.891	T65.892	T65.893	T65.894	—	—
Isophosphamide	T45.1X1	T45.1X2	T45.1X3	T45.1X4	T45.1X5	T45.1X6
Isopregnenone	T38.5X1	T38.5X2	T38.5X3	T38.5X4	T38.5X5	T38.5X6
Isoprenaline	T48.6X1	T48.6X2	T48.6X3	T48.6X4	T48.6X5	T48.6X6
Isopromethazine	T43.3X1	T43.3X2	T43.3X3	T43.3X4	T43.3X5	T43.3X6

◀ New   ◀ Revised   ~~deleted~~ Deleted

TABLE OF DRUGS AND CHEMICALS

Substance	External Cause (T-Code)					
	Poisoning, Accidental (Unintentional)	Poisoning, Intentional Self-Harm	Poisoning, Assault	Poisoning, Undetermined	Adverse Effect	Underdosing
Isopropamide	T44.3X1	T44.3X2	T44.3X3	T44.3X4	T44.3X5	T44.3X6
iodide	T44.3X1	T44.3X2	T44.3X3	T44.3X4	T44.3X5	T44.3X6
Isopropanol	T51.2X1	T51.2X2	T51.2X3	T51.2X4	—	—
Isopropyl						
acetate	T52.8X1	T52.8X2	T52.8X3	T52.8X4	—	—
alcohol	T51.2X1	T51.2X2	T51.2X3	T51.2X4	—	—
medicinal	T49.4X1	T49.4X2	T49.4X3	T49.4X4	T49.4X5	T49.4X6
ether	T52.8X1	T52.8X2	T52.8X3	T52.8X4	—	—
Isopropylaminophena-zone	T39.2X1	T39.2X2	T39.2X3	T39.2X4	T39.2X5	T39.2X6
Isoproterenol	T48.6X1	T48.6X2	T48.6X3	T48.6X4	T48.6X5	T48.6X6
Isosorbide dinitrate	T46.3X1	T46.3X2	T46.3X3	T46.3X4	T46.3X5	T46.3X6
Isothipendyl	T45.0X1	T45.0X2	T45.0X4	T45.0X4	T45.0X5	T45.0X6
Isotretinoin	T50.991	T50.992	T50.993	T50.994	T50.995	T50.996
Isoxazolyl penicillin	T36.0X1	T36.0X2	T36.0X3	T36.0X4	T36.0X5	T36.0X6
Isoxicam	T39.391	T39.392	T39.393	T39.394	T39.395	T39.396
Isoxsuprine	T46.7X1	T46.7X2	T46.7X3	T46.7X4	T46.7X5	T46.7X6
Ispagula	T47.4X1	T47.4X2	T47.4X3	T47.4X4	T47.4X5	T47.4X6
husk	T47.4X1	T47.4X2	T47.4X3	T47.4X4	T47.4X5	T47.4X6
Isradipine	T46.1X1	T46.1X2	T46.1X3	T46.1X4	T46.1X5	T46.1X6
I-thyroxine sodium	T38.1X1	T38.1X2	T38.1X3	T38.1X4	T38.1X5	T38.1X6
Itraconazole	T37.8X1	T37.8X2	T37.8X3	T37.8X4	T37.8X5	T37.8X6
Itramin tosilate	T46.3X1	T46.3X2	T46.3X3	T46.3X4	T46.3X5	T46.3X6
Ivermectin	T37.4X1	T37.4X2	T37.4X3	T37.4X4	T37.4X5	T37.4X6
Izoniazid	T37.1X1	T37.1X2	T37.1X3	T37.1X4	T37.1X5	T37.1X6
with thioacetazone	T37.1X1	T37.1X2	T37.1X3	T37.1X4	T37.1X5	T37.1X6

J

Substance	Poisoning, Accidental (Unintentional)	Poisoning, Intentional Self-Harm	Poisoning, Assault	Poisoning, Undetermined	Adverse Effect	Underdosing
Jalap	T47.2X1	T47.2X2	T47.2X3	T47.2X4	T47.2X5	T47.2X6
Jamaica						
dogwood (bark)	T39.8X1	T39.8X2	T39.8X3	T39.8X4	T39.8X5	T39.8X6
ginger	T65.891	T65.892	T65.893	T65.894	—	—
root	T62.2X1	T62.2X2	T62.2X3	T62.2X4	—	—
Jatropha	T62.2X1	T62.2X2	T62.2X3	T62.2X4	—	—
curcas	T62.2X1	T62.2X2	T62.2X3	T62.2X4	—	—
Jectofer	T45.4X1	T45.4X2	T45.4X3	T45.4X4	T45.4X5	T45.4X6
Jellyfish (sting)	T63.621	T63.622	T63.623	T63.624	—	—
Jequirity (bean)	T62.2X1	T62.2X2	T62.2X3	T62.2X4	—	—
Jimson weed (stramonium)	T62.2X1	T62.2X2	T62.2X3	T62.2X4	—	—
seeds	T62.2X1	T62.2X2	T62.2X3	T62.2X4	—	—
Josamycin	T36.3X1	T36.3X2	T36.3X3	T36.3X4	T36.3X5	T36.3X6
Juniper tar	T49.1X1	T49.1X2	T49.1X3	T49.1X4	T49.1X5	T49.1X6

Substance	External Cause (T-Code)					
	Poisoning, Accidental (Unintentional)	Poisoning, Intentional Self-Harm	Poisoning, Assault	Poisoning, Undetermined	Adverse Effect	Underdosing

K

Substance	Poisoning, Accidental (Unintentional)	Poisoning, Intentional Self-Harm	Poisoning, Assault	Poisoning, Undetermined	Adverse Effect	Underdosing
Kallidinogenase	T46.7X1	T46.7X2	T46.7X3	T46.7X4	T46.7X5	T46.7X6
Kallikrein	T46.7X1	T46.7X2	T46.7X3	T46.7X4	T46.7X5	T46.7X6
Kanamycin	T36.5X1	T36.5X2	T36.5X3	T36.5X4	T36.5X5	T36.5X6
Kantrex	T36.5X1	T36.5X2	T36.5X3	T36.5X4	T36.5X5	T36.5X6
Kaolin	T47.6X1	T47.6X2	T47.6X3	T47.6X4	T47.6X5	T47.6X6
light	T47.6X1	T47.6X2	T47.6X3	T47.6X4	T47.6X5	T47.6X6
Karaya (gum)	T47.4X1	T47.4X2	T47.4X3	T47.4X4	T47.4X5	T47.4X6
Kebuzone	T39.2X1	T39.2X2	T39.2X3	T39.2X4	T39.2X5	T39.2X6
Kelevan	T60.1X1	T60.1X2	T60.1X3	T60.1X4	—	—
Kemithal	T41.1X1	T41.1X2	T41.1X3	T41.1X4	T41.1X5	T41.1X6
Kenacort	T38.0X1	T38.0X2	T38.0X3	T38.0X4	T38.0X5	T38.0X6
Keratolytic drug NEC	T49.4X1	T49.4X2	T49.4X3	T49.4X4	T49.4X5	T49.4X6
anthracene	T49.4X1	T49.4X2	T49.4X3	T49.4X4	T49.4X5	T49.4X6
Keratoplastic NEC	T49.4X1	T49.4X2	T49.4X3	T49.4X4	T49.4X5	T49.4X6
Kerosene, kerosine (fuel) (solvent) NEC	T52.0X1	T52.0X2	T52.0X3	T52.0X4	—	—
insecticide	T52.0X1	T52.0X2	T52.0X3	T52.0X4	—	—
vapor	T52.0X1	T52.0X2	T52.0X3	T52.0X4	—	—
Ketamine	T41.291	T41.292	T41.293	T41.294	T41.295	T41.296
Ketazolam	T42.4X1	T42.4X2	T42.4X3	T42.4X4	T42.4X5	T42.4X6
Ketazon	T39.2X1	T39.2X2	T39.2X3	T39.2X4	T39.2X5	T39.2X6
Ketobemidone	T40.4X1	T40.4X2	T40.4X3	T40.4X4	—	—
Ketoconazole	T49.0X1	T49.0X2	T49.0X3	T49.0X4	T49.0X5	T49.0X6
Ketols	T52.4X1	T52.4X2	T52.4X3	T52.4X4	—	—
Ketone oils	T52.4X1	T52.4X2	T52.4X3	T52.4X4	—	—
Ketoprofen	T39.311	T39.312	T39.313	T39.314	T39.315	T39.316
Ketorolac	T39.8X1	T39.8X2	T39.8X3	T39.8X4	T39.8X5	T39.8X6
Ketotifen	T45.0X1	T45.0X2	T45.0X3	T45.0X4	T45.0X5	T45.0X6
Khat	T43.691	T43.692	T43.693	T43.694	—	—
Khellin	T46.3X1	T46.3X2	T46.3X3	T46.3X4	T46.3X5	T46.3X6
Khelloside	T46.3X1	T46.3X2	T46.3X3	T46.3X4	T46.3X5	T46.3X6
Kiln gas or vapor (carbon monoxide)	T58.8X1	T58.8X2	T58.8X3	T58.8X4	—	—
Kitasamycin	T36.3X1	T36.3X2	T36.3X3	T36.3X4	T36.3X5	T36.3X6
Konsyl	T47.4X1	T47.4X2	T47.4X3	T47.4X4	T47.4X5	T47.4X6
Kosam seed	T62.2X1	T62.2X2	T62.2X3	T62.2X4	—	—
Krait (venom)	T63.091	T63.092	T63.093	T63.094	—	—
Kwell (insecticide)	T60.1X1	T60.1X2	T60.1X3	T60.1X4	—	—
anti-infective (topical)	T49.0X1	T49.0X2	T49.0X3	T49.0X4	T49.0X5	T49.0X6

◀ New ◀▮ Revised ~~deleted~~ Deleted

TABLE OF DRUGS AND CHEMICALS

Substance	External Cause (T-Code)					
	Poisoning, Accidental (Unintentional)	Poisoning, Intentional Self-Harm	Poisoning, Assault	Poisoning, Undetermined	Adverse Effect	Underdosing
L						
Labetalol	T44.8X1	T44.8X2	T44.8X3	T44.8X4	T44.8X5	T44.8X6
Laburnum (seeds)	T62.2X1	T62.2X2	T62.2X3	T62.2X4	—	—
leaves	T62.2X1	T62.2X2	T62.2X3	T62.2X4	—	—
Lachesine	T49.5X1	T49.5X2	T49.5X3	T49.5X4	T49.5X5	T49.5X6
Lacidipine	T46.5X1	T46.5X2	T46.5X3	T46.5X4	T46.5X5	T46.5X6
Lacquer	T65.6X1	T65.6X2	T65.6X3	T65.6X4	—	—
Lacrimogenic gas	T59.3X1	T59.3X2	T59.3X3	T59.3X4	—	—
Lactated potassic saline	T50.3X1	T50.3X2	T50.3X3	T50.3X4	T50.3X5	T50.3X6
Lactic acid	T49.8X1	T49.8X2	T49.8X3	T49.8X4	T49.8X5	T49.8X6
Lactobacillus						
acidophilus	T47.6X1	T47.6X2	T47.6X3	T47.6X4	T47.6X5	T47.6X6
compound	T47.6X1	T47.6X2	T47.6X3	T47.6X4	T47.6X5	T47.6X6
bifidus, lyophilized	T47.6X1	T47.6X2	T47.6X3	T47.6X4	T47.6X5	T47.6X6
bulgaricus	T47.6X1	T47.6X2	T47.6X3	T47.6X4	T47.6X5	T47.6X6
sporogenes	T47.6X1	T47.6X2	T47.6X3	T47.6X4	T47.6X5	T47.6X6
Lactoflavin	T45.2X1	T45.2X2	T45.2X3	T45.2X4	T45.2X5	T45.2X6
Lactose (as excipient)	T50.901	T50.902	T50.903	T50.904	T50.905	T50.906
Lactuca (virosa) (extract)	T42.6X1	T42.6X2	T42.6X3	T42.6X4	T42.6X5	T42.6X6
Lactucarium	T42.6X1	T42.6X2	T42.6X3	T42.6X4	T42.6X5	T42.6X6
Lactulose	T47.3X1	T47.3X2	T47.3X3	T47.3X4	T47.3X5	T47.3X6
Laevo — see Levo-						
Lanatosides	T46.0X1	T46.0X2	T46.0X3	T46.0X4	T46.0X5	T46.0X6
Lanolin	T49.3X1	T49.3X2	T49.3X3	T49.3X4	T49.3X5	T49.3X6
Largactil	T43.3X1	T43.3X2	T43.3X3	T43.3X4	T43.3X5	T43.3X6
Larkspur	T62.2X1	T62.2X2	T62.2X3	T62.2X4	—	—
Laroxyl	T43.011	T43.012	T43.013	T43.014	T43.015	T43.016
Lassar's paste	T49.4X1	T49.4X2	T49.4X3	T49.4X4	T49.4X5	T49.4X6
Lasix	T50.1X1	T50.1X2	T50.1X3	T50.1X4	T50.1X5	T50.1X6
Latamoxef	T36.1X1	T36.1X2	T36.1X3	T36.1X4	T36.1X5	T36.1X6
Latex	T65.811	T65.812	T65.813	T65.814	—	—
Lathyrus (seed)	T62.2X1	T62.2X2	T62.2X3	T62.2X4	—	—
Laudanum	T40.0X1	T40.0X2	T40.0X3	T40.0X4	T40.0X5	T40.0X6
Laudexium	T48.1X1	T48.1X2	T48.1X3	T48.1X4	T48.1X5	T48.1X6
Laughing gas	T41.0X1	T41.0X2	T41.0X3	T41.0X4	T41.0X5	T41.0X6
Laurel, black or cherry	T62.2X1	T62.2X2	T62.2X3	T62.2X4	—	—
Laurolinium	T49.0X1	T49.0X2	T49.0X3	T49.0X4	T49.0X5	T49.0X6
Lauryl sulfoacetate	T49.2X1	T49.2X2	T49.2X3	T49.2X4	T49.2X5	T49.2X6

Substance	External Cause (T-Code)					
	Poisoning, Accidental (Unintentional)	Poisoning, Intentional Self-Harm	Poisoning, Assault	Poisoning, Undetermined	Adverse Effect	Underdosing
Laxative NEC	T47.4X1	T47.4X2	T47.4X3	T47.4X4	T47.4X5	T47.4X6
osmotic	T47.3X1	T47.3X2	T47.3X3	T47.3X4	T47.3X5	T47.3X6
saline	T47.3X1	T47.3X2	T47.3X3	T47.3X4	T47.3X5	T47.3X6
stimulant	T47.2X1	T47.2X2	T47.2X3	T47.2X4	T47.2X5	T47.2X6
L-dopa	T42.8X1	T42.8X2	T42.8X3	T42.8X4	T42.8X5	T42.8X6
Lead (dust) (fumes) (vapor) NEC	T56.0X1	T56.0X2	T56.0X3	T56.0X4	—	—
acetate	T49.2X1	T49.2X2	T49.2X3	T49.2X4	T49.2X5	T49.2X6
alkyl (fuel additive)	T56.0X1	T56.0X2	T56.0X3	T56.0X4	—	—
anti-infectives	T37.8X1	T37.8X2	T37.8X3	T37.8X4	T37.8X5	T37.8X6
antiknock compound (tetraethyl)	T56.0X1	T56.0X2	T56.0X3	T56.0X4	—	—
arsenate, arsenite (dust) (herbicide) (insecticide) (vapor)	T57.0X1	T57.0X2	T57.0X3	T57.0X4	—	—
carbonate	T56.0X1	T56.0X2	T56.0X3	T56.0X4	—	—
paint	T56.0X1	T56.0X2	T56.0X3	T56.0X4	—	—
chromate	T56.0X1	T56.0X2	T56.0X3	T56.0X4	—	—
paint	T56.0X1	T56.0X2	T56.0X3	T56.0X4	—	—
dioxide	T56.0X1	T56.0X2	T56.0X3	T56.0X4	—	—
inorganic	T56.0X1	T56.0X2	T56.0X3	T56.0X4	—	—
iodide	T56.0X1	T56.0X2	T56.0X3	T56.0X4	—	—
pigment (paint)	T56.0X1	T56.0X2	T56.0X3	T56.0X4	—	—
monoxide (dust)	T56.0X1	T56.0X2	T56.0X3	T56.0X4	—	—
paint	T56.0X1	T56.0X2	T56.0X3	T56.0X4	—	—
organic	T56.0X1	T56.0X2	T56.0X3	T56.0X4	—	—
oxide	T56.0X1	T56.0X2	T56.0X3	T56.0X4	—	—
paint	T56.0X1	T56.0X2	T56.0X3	T56.0X4	—	—
paint	T56.0X1	T56.0X2	T56.0X3	T56.0X4	—	—
salts	T56.0X1	T56.0X2	T56.0X3	T56.0X4	—	—
specified compound NEC	T56.0X1	T56.0X2	T56.0X3	T56.0X4	—	—
tetra-ethyl	T56.0X1	T56.0X2	T56.0X3	T56.0X4	—	—
Lebanese red	T40.7X1	T40.7X2	T40.7X3	T40.7X4	T40.7X5	T40.7X6
Lefetamine	T39.8X1	T39.8X2	T39.8X3	T39.8X4	T39.8X5	T39.8X6
Lenperone	T43.4X1	T43.4X2	T43.4X3	T43.4X4	T43.4X5	T43.4X6
Lente lietin (insulin)	T38.3X1	T38.3X2	T38.3X3	T38.3X4	T38.3X5	T38.3X6
Leptazol	T50.7X1	T50.7X2	T50.7X3	T50.7X4	T50.7X5	T50.7X6
Leptophos	T60.0X1	T60.0X2	T60.0X3	T60.0X4	—	—
Leritine	T40.2X1	T40.2X2	T40.2X3	T40.2X4	T40.2X5	T40.2X6
Letosteine	T48.4X1	T48.4X2	T48.4X3	T48.4X4	T48.4X5	T48.4X6
Letter	T38.1X1	T38.1X2	T38.1X3	T38.1X4	T38.1X5	T38.1X6
Lettuce opium	T42.6X1	T42.6X2	T42.6X3	T42.6X4	T42.6X5	T42.6X6
Leucinocaine	T41.3X1	T41.3X2	T41.3X3	T41.3X4	T41.3X5	T41.3X6

◄ New   ◄◄ Revised   ~~deleted~~ Deleted

Substance	Poisoning, Accidental (Unintentional)	Poisoning, Intentional Self-Harm	Poisoning, Assault	Poisoning, Undetermined	Adverse Effect	Underdosing
Leucocianidol	T46.991	T46.992	T46.993	T46.994	T46.995	T46.996
Leucovorin (factor)	T45.8X1	T45.8X2	T45.8X3	T45.8X4	T45.8X5	T45.8X6
Leukeran	T45.1X1	T45.1X2	T45.1X3	T45.1X4	T45.1X5	T45.1X6
Leuprolide	T38.891	T38.892	T38.893	T38.894	T38.895	T38.896
Levalbuterol	T48.6X1	T48.6X2	T48.6X3	T48.6X4	T48.6X5	T48.6X6
Levallorphan	T50.7X1	T50.7X2	T50.7X3	T50.7X4	T50.7X5	T50.7X6
Levamisole	T37.4X1	T37.4X2	T37.4X3	T37.4X4	T37.4X5	T37.4X6
Levanil	T42.6X1	T42.6X2	T42.6X3	T42.6X4	T42.6X5	T42.6X6
Levarterenol	T44.4X1	T44.4X2	T44.4X3	T44.4X4	T44.4X5	T44.4X6
Levdropropizine	T48.3X1	T48.3X2	T48.3X3	T48.3X4	T48.3X5	T48.3X6
Levobunolol	T49.5X1	T49.5X2	T49.5X3	T49.5X4	T49.5X5	T49.5X6
Levocabastine (hydrochloride)	T45.0X1	T45.0X2	T45.0X3	T45.0X4	T45.0X5	T45.0X6
Levocarnitine	T50.991	T50.992	T50.993	T50.994	T50.995	T50.996
Levodopa	T42.8X1	T42.8X2	T42.8X3	T42.8X4	T42.8X5	T42.8X6
with carbidopa	T42.8X1	T42.8X2	T42.8X3	T42.8X4	T42.8X5	T42.8X6
Levo-dromoran	T40.2X1	T40.2X2	T40.2X3	T40.2X4	T40.2X5	T40.2X6
Levoglutamide	T50.991	T50.992	T50.993	T50.994	T50.995	T50.996
Levoid	T38.1X1	T38.1X2	T38.1X3	T38.1X4	T38.1X5	T38.1X6
Levo-iso-methadone	T40.3X1	T40.3X2	T40.3X3	T40.3X4	T40.3X5	T40.3X6
Levomepromazine	T43.3X1	T43.3X2	T43.3X3	T43.3X4	T43.3X5	T43.3X6
Levonordefrin	T49.6X1	T49.6X2	T49.6X3	T49.6X4	T49.6X5	T49.6X6
Levonorgestrel	T38.4X1	T38.4X2	T38.4X3	T38.4X4	T38.4X5	T38.4X6
with ethinylestradiol	T38.5X1	T38.5X2	T38.5X3	T38.5X4	T38.5X5	T38.5X6
Levopromazine	T43.3X1	T43.3X2	T43.3X3	T43.3X4	T43.3X5	T43.3X6
Levoprome	T42.6X1	T42.6X2	T42.6X3	T42.6X4	T42.6X5	T42.6X6
Levopropoxyphene	T40.4X1	T40.4X2	T40.4X3	T40.4X4	T40.4X5	T40.4X6
Levopropylhexedrine	T50.5X1	T50.5X2	T50.5X3	T50.5X4	T50.5X5	T50.5X6
Levoproxyphylline	T48.6X1	T48.6X2	T48.6X3	T48.6X4	T48.6X5	T48.6X6
Levorphanol	T40.4X1	T40.4X2	T40.4X3	T40.4X4	T40.4X5	T40.4X6
Levothyroxine	T38.1X1	T38.1X2	T38.1X3	T38.1X4	T38.1X5	T38.1X6
sodium	T38.1X1	T38.1X2	T38.1X3	T38.1X4	T38.1X5	T38.1X6
Levsin	T44.3X1	T44.3X2	T44.3X3	T44.3X4	T44.3X5	T44.3X6
Levulose	T50.3X1	T50.3X2	T50.3X3	T50.3X4	T50.3X5	T50.3X6
Lewisite (gas), not in war	T57.0X1	T57.0X2	T57.0X3	T57.0X4	—	—
Librium	T42.4X1	T42.4X2	T42.4X3	T42.4X4	T42.4X5	T42.4X6
Lidex	T49.0X1	T49.0X2	T49.0X3	T49.0X4	T49.0X5	T49.0X6
Lidocaine	T41.3X1	T41.3X2	T41.3X3	T41.3X4	T41.3X5	T41.3X6
regional	T41.3X1	T41.3X2	T41.3X3	T41.3X4	T41.3X5	T41.3X6
spinal	T41.3X1	T41.3X2	T41.3X3	T41.3X4	T41.3X5	T41.3X6
Lidofenin	T50.8X1	T50.8X2	T50.8X3	T50.8X4	T50.8X5	T50.8X6
Lidoflazine	T46.1X1	T46.1X2	T46.1X3	T46.1X4	T46.1X5	T46.1X6
Lighter fluid	T52.0X1	T52.0X2	T52.0X3	T52.0X4	—	—

Substance	Poisoning, Accidental (Unintentional)	Poisoning, Intentional Self-Harm	Poisoning, Assault	Poisoning, Undetermined	Adverse Effect	Underdosing
Lignin hemicellulose	T47.6X1	T47.6X2	T47.6X3	T47.6X4	T47.6X5	T47.6X6
Lignocaine	T41.3X1	T41.3X2	T41.3X3	T41.3X4	T41.3X5	T41.3X6
regional	T41.3X1	T41.3X2	T41.3X3	T41.3X4	T41.3X5	T41.3X6
spinal	T41.3X1	T41.3X2	T41.3X3	T41.3X4	T41.3X5	T41.3X6
Ligroin(e) (solvent)	T52.0X1	T52.0X2	T52.0X3	T52.0X4	—	—
vapor	T59.891	T59.892	T59.893	T59.894	—	—
Ligustrum vulgare	T62.2X1	T62.2X2	T62.2X3	T62.2X4	—	—
Lily of the valley	T62.2X1	T62.2X2	T62.2X3	T62.2X4	—	—
Lime (chloride)	T54.3X1	T54.3X2	T54.3X3	T54.3X4	—	—
Limonene	T52.8X1	T52.8X2	T52.8X3	T52.8X4	—	—
Lincomycin	T36.8X1	T36.8X2	T36.8X3	T36.8X4	T36.8X5	T36.8X6
Lindane (insecticide) (nonmedicinal) (vapor)	T53.6X1	T53.6X2	T53.6X3	T53.6X4	—	—
medicinal	T49.0X1	T49.0X2	T49.0X3	T49.0X4	T49.0X5	T49.0X6
Liniments NEC	T49.91	T49.92	T49.93	T49.94	T49.95	T49.96
Linoleic acid	T46.6X1	T46.6X2	T46.6X3	T46.6X4	T46.6X5	T46.6X6
Linolenic acid	T46.6X1	T46.6X2	T46.6X3	T46.6X4	T46.6X5	T46.6X6
Linseed	T47.4X1	T47.4X2	T47.4X3	T47.4X4	T47.4X5	T47.4X6
Liothyronine	T38.1X1	T38.1X2	T38.1X3	T38.1X4	T38.1X5	T38.1X6
Liotrix	T38.1X1	T38.1X2	T38.1X3	T38.1X4	T38.1X5	T38.1X6
Lipancreatin	T47.5X1	T47.5X2	T47.5X3	T47.5X4	T47.5X5	T47.5X6
Lipo-alprostadil	T46.7X1	T46.7X2	T46.7X3	T46.7X4	T46.7X5	T46.7X6
Lipo-Lutin	T38.5X1	T38.5X2	T38.5X3	T38.5X4	T38.5X5	T38.5X6
Lipotropic drug NEC	T50.901	T50.902	T50.903	T50.904	T50.905	T50.906
Liquefied petroleum gases	T59.891	T59.892	T59.893	T59.894	—	—
piped (pure or mixed with air)	T59.891	T59.892	T59.893	T59.894	—	—
Liquid						
paraffin	T47.4X1	T47.4X2	T47.4X3	T47.4X4	T47.4X5	T47.4X6
petrolatum	T47.4X1	T47.4X2	T47.4X3	T47.4X4	T47.4X5	T47.4X6
topical	T49.3X1	T49.3X2	T49.3X3	T49.3X4	T49.3X5	T49.3X6
specified NEC	T65.891	T65.892	T65.893	T65.894	—	—
substance	T65.91	T65.92	T65.93	T65.94	—	—
Liquor creosolis compositus	T65.891	T65.892	T65.893	T65.894	—	—
Liquorice	T48.4X1	T48.4X2	T48.4X3	T48.4X4	T48.4X5	T48.4X6
extract	T47.8X1	T47.8X2	T47.8X3	T47.8X4	T47.8X5	T47.8X6
Lirugen	T50.991	T50.992	T50.993	T50.994	T50.995	T50.996
Lisinopril	T46.4X1	T46.4X2	T46.4X3	T46.4X4	T46.4X5	T46.4X6
Lisuride	T42.8X1	T42.8X2	T42.8X3	T42.8X4	T42.8X5	T42.8X6
Lithane	T43.8X1	T43.8X2	T43.8X3	T43.8X4	T43.8X5	T43.8X6
Lithium	T56.891	T56.892	T56.893	T56.894		
gluconate	T43.591	T43.592	T43.593	T43.594	T43.595	T43.596
salts (carbonate)	T43.591	T43.592	T43.593	T43.594	T43.595	T43.596

◄ New ◄▌ Revised ~~deleted~~ Deleted

TABLE OF DRUGS AND CHEMICALS

TABLE OF DRUGS AND CHEMICALS

Substance	Poisoning, Accidental (Unintentional)	Poisoning, Intentional Self-Harm	Poisoning, Assault	Poisoning, Undetermined	Adverse Effect	Underdosing
Lithonate	T43.8X1	T43.8X2	T43.8X3	T43.8X4	T43.8X5	T43.8X6
Liver						
extract	T45.8X1	T45.8X2	T45.8X3	T45.8X4	T45.8X5	T45.8X6
for parenteral use	T45.8X1	T45.8X2	T45.8X3	T45.8X4	T45.8X5	T45.8X6
fraction 1	T45.8X1	T45.8X2	T45.8X3	T45.8X4	T45.8X5	T45.8X6
hydrolysate	T45.8X1	T45.8X2	T45.8X3	T45.8X4	T45.8X5	T45.8X6
Lizard (bite) (venom)	T63.121	T63.122	T63.123	T63.124	—	—
LMD	T45.8X1	T45.8X2	T45.8X3	T45.8X4	T45.8X5	T45.8X6
Lobelia	T62.2X1	T62.2X2	T62.2X3	T62.2X4		
Lobeline	T50.7X1	T50.7X2	T50.7X3	T50.7X4	T50.7X5	T50.7X6
Local action drug NEC	T49.8X1	T49.8X2	T49.8X3	T49.8X4	T49.8X5	T49.8X6
Locorten	T49.0X1	T49.0X2	T49.0X3	T49.0X4	T49.0X5	T49.0X6
Lofepramine	T43.011	T43.012	T43.013	T43.014	T43.015	T43.016
Lolium temulentum	T62.2X1	T62.2X2	T62.2X3	T62.2X4	—	—
Lomotil	T47.6X1	T47.6X2	T47.6X3	T47.6X4	T47.6X5	T47.6X6
Lomustine	T45.1X1	T45.1X2	T45.1X3	T45.1X4	T45.1X5	T45.1X6
Lonidamine	T45.1X1	T45.1X2	T45.1X3	T45.1X4	T45.1X5	T45.1X6
Loperamide	T47.6X1	T47.6X2	T47.6X3	T47.6X4	T47.6X5	T47.6X6
Loprazolam	T42.4X1	T42.4X2	T42.4X3	T42.4X4	T42.4X5	T42.4X6
Lorajmine	T46.2X1	T46.2X2	T46.2X3	T46.2X4	T46.2X5	T46.2X6
Loratidine	T45.0X1	T45.0X2	T45.0X3	T45.0X4	T45.0X5	T45.0X6
Lorazepam	T42.4X1	T42.4X2	T42.4X3	T42.4X4	T42.4X5	T42.4X6
Lorcainide	T46.2X1	T46.2X2	T46.2X3	T46.2X4	T46.2X5	T46.2X6
Lormetazepam	T42.4X1	T42.4X2	T42.4X3	T42.4X4	T42.4X5	T42.4X6
Lotions NEC	T49.91	T49.92	T49.93	T49.94	T49.95	T49.96
Lotusate	T42.3X1	T42.3X2	T42.3X3	T42.3X4	T42.3X5	T42.3X6
Lovastatin	T46.6X1	T46.6X2	T46.6X3	T46.6X4	T46.6X5	T46.6X6
Loxapine	T43.591	T43.592	T43.593	T43.594	T43.595	T43.596
Lowila	T49.2X1	T49.2X2	T49.2X3	T49.2X4	T49.2X5	T49.2X6
Lozenges (throat)	T49.6X1	T49.6X2	T49.6X3	T49.6X4	T49.6X5	T49.6X6
LSD	T40.8X1	T40.8X2	T40.8X3	T40.8X4	—	—
L-Tryptophan—see amino acid						
Lubricant, eye	T49.5X1	T49.5X2	T49.5X3	T49.5X4	T49.5X5	T49.5X6
Lubricating oil NEC	T52.0X1	T52.0X2	T52.0X3	T52.0X4	—	—
Lucanthone	T37.4X1	T37.4X2	T37.4X3	T37.4X4	T37.4X5	T37.4X6
Luminal	T42.3X1	T42.3X2	T42.3X3	T42.3X4	T42.3X5	T42.3X6
Lung irritant (gas) NEC	T59.91	T59.92	T59.93	T59.94	—	—
Luteinizing hormone	T38.811	T38.812	T38.813	T38.814	T38.815	T38.816
Lutocylol	T38.5X1	T38.5X2	T38.5X3	T38.5X4	T38.5X5	T38.5X6
Lutromone	T38.5X1	T38.5X2	T38.5X3	T38.5X4	T38.5X5	T38.5X6
Lututrin	T48.291	T48.292	T48.293	T48.294	T48.295	T48.296
Lye (Concentrated)	T54.3X1	T54.3X2	T54.3X3	T54.3X4	—	—

Substance	Poisoning, Accidental (Unintentional)	Poisoning, Intentional Self-Harm	Poisoning, Assault	Poisoning, Undetermined	Adverse Effect	Underdosing
Lygranum (skin test)	T50.8X1	T50.8X2	T50.8X3	T50.8X4	T50.8X5	T50.8X6
Lymecycline	T36.4X1	T36.4X2	T36.4X3	T36.4X4	T36.4X5	T36.4X6
Lymphogranuloma venereum antigen	T50.8X1	T50.8X2	T50.8X3	T50.8X4	T50.8X5	T50.8X6
Lynestrenol	T38.4X1	T38.4X2	T38.4X3	T38.4X4	T38.4X5	T38.4X6
Lypressin	T38.891	T38.892	T38.893	T38.894	T38.895	T38.896
Lyovac Sodium Edecrin	T50.1X1	T50.1X2	T50.1X4	T50.1X4	T50.1X5	T50.1X6
Lysergic acid diethylamide	T40.8X1	T40.8X2	T40.8X3	T40.8X4	—	—
Lysergide	T40.8X1	T40.8X2	T40.8X3	T40.8X4	—	—
Lysine vasopressin	T38.891	T38.892	T38.893	T38.894	T38.895	T38.896
Lysol	T54.1X1	T54.1X2	T54.1X3	T54.1X4	—	—
Lysozyme	T49.0X1	T49.0X2	T49.0X3	T49.0X4	T49.0X5	T49.0X6
Lytta (vitatta)	T49.8X1	T49.8X2	T49.8X3	T49.8X4	T49.8X5	T49.8X6
M						
Mace	T59.3X1	T59.3X2	T59.3X3	T59.3X4	—	—
Macrogol	T50.991	T50.992	T50.993	T50.994	T50.995	T50.996
Macrolide						
anabolic drug	T38.7X1	T38.7X2	T38.7X3	T38.7X4	T38.7X5	T38.7X6
antibiotic	T36.3X1	T36.3X2	T36.3X3	T36.3X4	T36.3X5	T36.3X6
Mafenide	T49.0X1	T49.0X2	T49.0X3	T49.0X4	T49.0X5	T49.0X6
Magaldrate	T47.1X1	T47.1X2	T47.1X3	T47.1X4	T47.1X5	T47.1X6
Magic mushroom	T40.991	T40.992	T40.993	T40.994	—	—
Magnamycin	T36.8X1	T36.8X2	T36.8X3	T36.8X4	T36.8X5	T36.8X6
Magnesia magma	T47.1X1	T47.1X2	T47.1X3	T47.1X4	T47.1X5	T47.1X6
Magnesium NEC	T56.891	T56.892	T56.893	T56.894		
carbonate	T47.1X1	T47.1X2	T47.1X3	T47.1X4	T47.1X5	T47.1X6
citrate	T47.4X1	T47.4X2	T47.4X3	T47.4X4	T47.4X5	T47.4X6
hydroxide	T47.1X1	T47.1X2	T47.1X3	T47.1X4	T47.1X5	T47.1X6
oxide	T47.1X1	T47.1X2	T47.1X3	T47.1X4	T47.1X5	T47.1X6
peroxide	T49.0X1	T49.0X2	T49.0X3	T49.0X4	T49.0X5	T49.0X6
salicylate	T39.091	T39.092	T39.093	T39.094	T39.095	T39.096
silicofluoride	T50.3X1	T50.3X2	T50.3X3	T50.3X4	T50.3X5	T50.3X6
sulfate	T47.4X1	T47.4X2	T47.4X3	T47.4X4	T47.4X5	T47.4X6
thiosulfate	T45.0X1	T45.0X2	T45.0X3	T45.0X4	T45.0X5	T45.0X6
trisilicate	T47.1X1	T47.1X2	T47.1X3	T47.1X4	T47.1X5	T47.1X6
Malathion (medicinal)	T49.0X1	T49.0X2	T49.0X3	T49.0X4	T49.0X5	T49.0X6
insecticide	T60.0X1	T60.0X2	T60.0X3	T60.0X4	—	—
Male fern extract	T37.4X1	T37.4X2	T37.4X3	T37.4X4	T37.4X5	T37.4X6
M-AMSA	T45.1X1	T45.1X2	T45.1X3	T45.1X4	T45.1X5	T45.1X6
Mandelic acid	T37.8X1	T37.8X2	T37.8X3	T37.8X4	T37.8X5	T37.8X6
Manganese (dioxide) (salts)	T57.2X1	T57.2X2	T57.2X3	T57.2X4	—	—
medicinal	T50.991	T50.992	T50.993	T50.994	T50.995	T50.996

◄ New   ◄ Revised   ~~deleted~~ Deleted

Substance	Poisoning, Accidental (Unintentional)	Poisoning, Intentional Self-Harm	Poisoning, Assault	Poisoning, Undetermined	Adverse Effect	Underdosing
Mannitol	T47.3X1	T47.3X2	T47.3X3	T47.3X4	T47.3X5	T47.3X6
hexanitrate	T46.3X1	T46.3X2	T46.3X3	T46.3X4	T46.3X5	T46.3X6
Mannomustine	T45.1X1	T45.1X2	T45.1X3	T45.1X4	T45.1X5	T45.1X6
MAO inhibitors	T43.1X1	T43.1X2	T43.1X3	T43.1X4	T43.1X5	T43.1X6
Mapharsen	T37.8X1	T37.8X2	T37.8X3	T37.8X4	T37.8X5	T37.8X6
Maphenide	T49.0X1	T49.0X2	T49.0X3	T49.0X4	T49.0X5	T49.0X6
Maprotiline	T43.021	T43.022	T43.023	T43.024	T43.025	T43.026
Marcaine	T41.3X1	T41.3X2	T41.3X3	T41.3X4	T41.3X5	T41.3X6
infiltration (subcutaneous)	T41.3X1	T41.3X2	T41.3X3	T41.3X4	T41.3X5	T41.3X6
nerve block (peripheral) (plexus)	T41.3X1	T41.3X2	T41.3X3	T41.3X4	T41.3X5	T41.3X6
Marezine	T45.0X1	T45.0X2	T45.0X3	T45.0X4	T45.0X5	T45.0X6
Marihuana	T40.7X1	T40.7X2	T40.7X3	T40.7X4	T40.7X5	T40.7X6
Marijuana	T40.7X1	T40.7X2	T40.7X3	T40.7X4	T40.7X5	T40.7X6
Marine (sting)	T63.691	T63.692	T63.693	T63.694	—	—
animals (sting)	T63.691	T63.692	T63.693	T63.694	—	—
plants (sting)	T63.711	T63.712	T63.713	T63.714	—	—
Marplan	T43.1X1	T43.1X2	T43.1X3	T43.1X4	T43.1X5	T43.1X6
Marsh gas	T59.891	T59.892	T59.893	T59.894	—	—
Marsilid	T43.1X1	T43.1X2	T43.1X3	T43.1X4	T43.1X5	T43.1X6
Matulane	T45.1X1	T45.1X2	T45.1X3	T45.1X4	T45.1X5	T45.1X6
Mazindol	T50.5X1	T50.5X2	T50.5X3	T50.5X4	T50.5X5	T50.5X6
MCPA	T60.3X1	T60.3X2	T60.3X3	T60.3X4	—	—
MDMA	T43.621	T43.622	T43.623	T43.624	T43.625	T43.626
Meadow saffron	T62.2X1	T62.2X2	T62.2X3	T62.2X4	—	—
Measles virus vaccine (attenuated)	T50.B91	T50.B92	T50.B93	T50.B94	T50.B95	T50.B96
Meat, noxious	T62.8X1	T62.8X2	T62.8X3	T62.8X4	—	—
Meballymal	T42.3X1	T42.3X2	T42.3X3	T42.3X4	T42.3X5	T42.3X6
Mebanazine	T43.1X1	T43.1X2	T43.1X3	T43.1X4	T43.1X5	T43.1X6
Mebaral	T42.3X1	T42.3X2	T42.3X3	T42.3X4	T42.3X5	T42.3X6
Mebendazole	T37.4X1	T37.4X2	T37.4X3	T37.4X4	T37.4X5	T37.4X6
Mebeverine	T44.3X1	T44.3X2	T44.3X3	T44.3X4	T44.3X5	T44.3X6
Mebhydrolin	T45.0X1	T45.0X2	T45.0X3	T45.0X4	T45.0X5	T45.0X6
Mebumal	T42.3X1	T42.3X2	T42.3X3	T42.3X4	T42.3X5	T42.3X6
Mebutamate	T43.591	T43.592	T43.593	T43.594	T43.595	T43.596
Mecamylamine	T44.2X1	T44.2X2	T44.2X3	T44.2X4	T44.2X5	T44.2X6
Mechlorethamine	T45.1X1	T45.1X2	T45.1X3	T45.1X4	T45.1X5	T45.1X6
Mecillinam	T36.0X1	T36.0X2	T36.0X3	T36.0X4	T36.0X5	T36.0X6
Meclizine (hydrochloride)	T45.0X1	T45.0X2	T45.0X3	T45.0X4	T45.0X5	T45.0X6
Meclocycline	T36.4X1	T36.4X2	T36.4X3	T36.4X4	T36.4X5	T36.4X6
Meclofenamate	T39.391	T39.392	T39.393	T39.394	T39.395	T39.396
Meclofenamic acid	T39.391	T39.392	T39.393	T39.394	T39.395	T39.396
Meclofenoxate	T43.691	T43.692	T43.693	T43.694	T43.695	T43.696
Meclozine	T45.0X1	T45.0X2	T45.0X3	T45.0X4	T45.0X5	T45.0X6
Mecobalamin	T45.8X1	T45.8X2	T45.8X3	T45.8X4	T45.8X5	T45.8X6
Mecoprop	T60.3X1	T60.3X2	T60.3X3	T60.3X4	—	—
Mecrilate	T49.3X1	T49.3X2	T49.3X3	T49.3X4	T49.3X5	T49.3X6
Mecysteine	T48.4X1	T48.4X2	T48.4X3	T48.4X4	T48.4X5	T48.4X6
Medazepam	T42.4X1	T42.4X2	T42.4X3	T42.4X4	T42.4X5	T42.4X6
Medicament NEC	T50.901	T50.902	T50.903	T50.904	T50.905	T50.906
Medinal	T42.3X1	T42.3X2	T42.3X3	T42.3X4	T42.3X5	T42.3X6
Medomin	T42.3X1	T42.3X2	T42.3X3	T42.3X4	T42.3X5	T42.3X6
Medrogestone	T38.5X1	T38.5X2	T38.5X3	T38.5X4	T38.5X5	T38.5X6
Medroxalol	T44.8X1	T44.8X2	T44.8X3	T44.8X4	T44.8X5	T44.8X6
Medroxyprogesterone acetate (depot)	T38.5X1	T38.5X2	T38.5X3	T38.5X4	T38.5X5	T38.5X6
Medrysone	T49.0X1	T49.0X2	T49.0X3	T49.0X4	T49.0X5	T49.0X6
Mefenamic acid	T39.391	T39.392	T39.393	T39.394	T39.395	T39.396
Mefenorex	T50.5X1	T50.5X2	T50.5X3	T50.5X4	T50.5X5	T50.5X6
Mefloquine	T37.2X1	T37.2X2	T37.2X3	T37.2X4	T37.2X5	T37.2X6
Mefruside	T50.2X1	T50.2X2	T50.2X3	T50.2X4	T50.2X5	T50.2X6
Megahallucinogen	T40.901	T40.902	T40.903	T40.904	T40.905	T40.906
Megestrol	T38.5X1	T38.5X2	T38.5X3	T38.5X4	T38.5X5	T38.5X6
Meglumine						
antimoniate	T37.8X1	T37.8X2	T37.8X3	T37.8X4	T37.8X5	T37.8X6
diatrizoate	T50.8X1	T50.8X2	T50.8X3	T50.8X4	T50.8X5	T50.8X6
iodipamide	T50.8X1	T50.8X2	T50.8X3	T50.8X4	T50.8X5	T50.8X6
iotroxate	T50.8X1	T50.8X2	T50.8X3	T50.8X4	T50.8X5	T50.8X6
MEK (methyl ethyl ketone)	T52.4X1	T52.4X2	T52.4X3	T52.4X4	—	—
Meladrazine	T44.3X1	T44.3X2	T44.3X3	T44.3X4	T44.3X5	T44.3X6
Meladinin	T49.3X1	T49.3X2	T49.3X3	T49.3X4	T49.3X5	T49.3X6
Melaleuca alternifolia oil	T49.0X1	T49.0X2	T49.0X3	T49.0X4	T49.0X5	T49.0X6
Melanizing agents	T49.3X1	T49.3X2	T49.3X3	T49.3X4	T49.3X5	T49.3X6
Melanocyte-stimulating hormone	T38.891	T38.892	T38.893	T38.894	T38.895	T38.896
Melarsonyl potassium	T37.3X1	T37.3X2	T37.3X3	T37.3X4	T37.3X5	T37.3X6
Melarsoprol	T37.3X1	T37.3X2	T37.3X3	T37.3X4	T37.3X5	T37.3X6
Melia azedarach	T62.2X1	T62.2X2	T62.2X3	T62.2X4	—	—
Melitracen	T43.011	T43.012	T43.013	T43.014	T43.015	T43.016
Mellaril	T43.3X1	T43.3X2	T43.3X3	T43.3X4	T43.3X5	T43.3X6
Meloxine	T49.3X1	T49.3X2	T49.3X3	T49.3X4	T49.3X5	T49.3X6
Melperone	T43.4X1	T43.4X2	T43.4X3	T43.4X4	T43.4X5	T43.4X6
Melphalan	T45.1X1	T45.1X2	T45.1X3	T45.1X4	T45.1X5	T45.1X6
Memantine	T43.8X1	T43.8X2	T43.8X3	T43.8X4	T43.8X5	T43.8X6

Substance	Poisoning, Accidental (Unintentional)	Poisoning, Intentional Self-Harm	Poisoning, Assault	Poisoning, Undetermined	Adverse Effect	Underdosing
Menadiol	T45.7X1	T45.7X2	T45.7X3	T45.7X4	T45.7X5	T45.7X6
sodium sulfate	T45.7X1	T45.7X2	T45.7X3	T45.7X4	T45.7X5	T45.7X6
Menadione	T45.7X1	T45.7X2	T45.7X3	T45.7X4	T45.7X5	T45.7X6
sodium bisulfite	T45.7X1	T45.7X2	T45.7X3	T45.7X4	T45.7X5	T45.7X6
Menaphthone	T45.7X1	T45.7X2	T45.7X3	T45.7X4	T45.7X5	T45.7X6
Menaquinone	T45.7X1	T45.7X2	T45.7X3	T45.7X4	T45.7X5	T45.7X6
Menatetrenone	T45.7X1	T45.7X2	T45.7X3	T45.7X4	T45.7X5	T45.7X6
Meningococcal vaccine	T50.A91	T50.A92	T50.A93	T50.A94	T50.A95	T50.A96
Menningovax (-AC) (-C)	T50.A91	T50.A92	T50.A93	T50.A94	T50.A95	T50.A96
Menotropins	T38.811	T38.812	T38.813	T38.814	T38.815	T38.816
Menthol	T48.5X1	T48.5X2	T48.5X3	T48.5X4	T48.5X5	T48.5X6
Mepacrine	T37.2X1	T37.2X2	T37.2X3	T37.2X4	T37.2X5	T37.2X6
Meparfynol	T42.6X1	T42.6X2	T42.6X3	T42.6X4	T42.6X5	T42.6X6
Mepartricin	T36.7X1	T36.7X2	T36.7X3	T36.7X4	T36.7X5	T36.7X6
Mepazine	T43.3X1	T43.3X2	T43.3X3	T43.3X4	T43.3X5	T43.3X6
Mepenzolate	T44.3X1	T44.3X2	T44.3X3	T44.3X4	T44.3X5	T44.3X6
bromide	T44.3X1	T44.3X2	T44.3X3	T44.3X4	T44.3X5	T44.3X6
Meperidine	T40.4X1	T40.4X2	T40.4X3	T40.4X4	T40.4X5	T40.4X6
Mephebarbital	T42.3X1	T42.3X2	T42.3X3	T42.3X4	T42.3X5	T42.3X6
Mephenamin(e)	T42.8X1	T42.8X2	T42.8X3	T42.8X4	T42.8X5	T42.8X6
Mephenesin	T42.8X1	T42.8X2	T42.8X3	T42.8X4	T42.8X5	T42.8X6
Mephenhydramine	T45.0X1	T45.0X2	T45.0X3	T45.0X4	T45.0X5	T45.0X6
Mephenoxalone	T42.8X1	T42.8X2	T42.8X3	T42.8X4	T42.8X5	T42.8X6
Mephentermine	T44.991	T44.992	T44.993	T44.994	T44.995	T44.996
Mephenytoin	T42.0X1	T42.0X2	T42.0X3	T42.0X4	T42.0X5	T42.0X6
with phenobarbital	T42.3X1	T42.3X2	T42.3X3	T42.3X4	T42.3X5	T42.3X6
Mephobarbital	T42.3X1	T42.3X2	T42.3X3	T42.3X4	T42.3X5	T42.3X6
Mephosfolan	T60.0X1	T60.0X2	T60.0X3	T60.0X4	—	—
Mepindolol	T44.7X1	T44.7X2	T44.7X3	T44.7X4	T44.7X5	T44.7X6
Mepiperphenidol	T44.3X1	T44.3X2	T44.3X3	T44.3X4	T44.3X5	T44.3X6
Mepitiostane	T38.7X1	T38.7X2	T38.7X3	T38.7X4	T38.7X5	T38.7X6
Mepivacaine	T41.3X1	T41.3X2	T41.3X3	T41.3X4	T41.3X5	T41.3X6
epidural	T41.3X1	T41.3X2	T41.3X3	T41.3X4	T41.3X5	T41.3X6
Meprednisone	T38.0X1	T38.0X2	T38.0X3	T38.0X4	T38.0X5	T38.0X6
Meprobam	T43.591	T43.592	T43.593	T43.594	T43.595	T43.596
Meprobamate	T43.591	T43.592	T43.593	T43.594	T43.595	T43.596
Meproscillarin	T46.0X1	T46.0X2	T46.0X3	T46.0X4	T46.0X5	T46.0X6
Meprylcaine	T41.3X1	T41.3X2	T41.3X3	T41.3X4	T41.3X5	T41.3X6
Meptazinol	T39.8X1	T39.8X2	T39.8X3	T39.8X4	T39.8X5	T39.8X6
Mepyramine	T45.0X1	T45.0X2	T45.0X3	T45.0X4	T45.0X5	T45.0X6
Mequitazine	T43.3X1	T43.3X2	T43.3X3	T43.3X4	T43.3X5	T43.3X6
Meralluride	T50.2X1	T50.2X2	T50.2X3	T50.2X4	T50.2X5	T50.2X6

Substance	Poisoning, Accidental (Unintentional)	Poisoning, Intentional Self-Harm	Poisoning, Assault	Poisoning, Undetermined	Adverse Effect	Underdosing
Merbaphen	T50.2X1	T50.2X2	T50.2X3	T50.2X4	T50.2X5	T50.2X6
Merbromin	T49.0X1	T49.0X2	T49.0X3	T49.0X4	T49.0X5	T49.0X6
Mercaptobenzothiazole salts	T49.0X1	T49.0X2	T49.0X3	T49.0X4	T49.0X5	T49.0X6
Mercaptomerin	T50.2X1	T50.2X2	T50.2X3	T50.2X4	T50.2X5	T50.2X6
Mercaptopurine	T45.1X1	T45.1X2	T45.1X3	T45.1X4	T45.1X5	T45.1X6
Mercumatilin	T50.2X1	T50.2X2	T50.2X3	T50.2X4	T50.2X5	T50.2X6
Mercuramide	T50.2X1	T50.2X2	T50.2X3	T50.2X4	T50.2X5	T50.2X6
Mercurochrome	T49.0X1	T49.0X2	T49.0X3	T49.0X4	T49.0X5	T49.0X6
Mercurophylline	T50.2X1	T50.2X2	T50.2X3	T50.2X4	T50.2X5	T50.2X6
Mercury, mercurial, mercuric, mercurous (compounds) (cyanide) (fumes) (nonmedicinal) (vapor) NEC	T56.1X1	T56.1X2	T56.1X3	T56.1X4	—	—
ammoniated	T49.0X1	T49.0X2	T49.0X3	T49.0X4	T49.0X5	T49.0X6
anti-infective						
local	T49.0X1	T49.0X2	T49.0X3	T49.0X4	T49.0X5	T49.0X6
systemic	T37.8X1	T37.8X2	T37.8X3	T37.8X4	T37.8X5	T37.8X6
topical	T49.0X1	T49.0X2	T49.0X3	T49.0X4	T49.0X5	T49.0X6
chloride (ammoniated)	T49.0X1	T49.0X2	T49.0X3	T49.0X4	T49.0X5	T49.0X6
fungicide	T56.1X1	T56.1X2	T56.1X3	T56.1X4	—	—
diuretic NEC	T50.2X1	T50.2X2	T50.2X3	T50.2X4	T50.2X5	T50.2X6
fungicide	T56.1X1	T56.1X2	T56.1X3	T56.1X4	—	—
organic (fungicide)	T56.1X1	T56.1X2	T56.1X3	T56.1X4	—	—
oxide, yellow	T49.0X1	T49.0X2	T49.0X3	T49.0X4	T49.0X5	T49.0X6
Mersalyl	T50.2X1	T50.2X2	T50.2X3	T50.2X4	T50.2X5	T50.2X6
Merthiolate	T49.0X1	T49.0X2	T49.0X3	T49.0X4	T49.0X5	T49.0X6
ophthalmic preparation	T49.5X1	T49.5X2	T49.5X3	T49.5X4	T49.5X5	T49.5X6
Meruvax	T50.B91	T50.B92	T50.B93	T50.B94	T50.B95	T50.B96
Mesalazine	T47.8X1	T47.8X2	T47.8X3	T47.8X4	T47.8X5	T47.8X6
Mescal buttons	T40.991	T40.992	T40.993	T40.994	—	—
Mescaline	T40.991	T40.992	T40.993	T40.994	—	—
Mesna	T48.4X1	T48.4X2	T48.4X3	T48.4X4	T48.4X5	T48.4X6
Mesoglycan	T46.6X1	T46.6X2	T46.6X3	T46.6X4	T46.6X5	T46.6X6
Mesoridazine	T43.3X1	T43.3X2	T43.3X3	T43.3X4	T43.3X5	T43.3X6
Mestanolone	T38.7X1	T38.7X2	T38.7X3	T38.7X4	T38.7X5	T38.7X6
Mesterolone	T38.7X1	T38.7X2	T38.7X3	T38.7X4	T38.7X5	T38.7X6
Mestranol	T38.5X1	T38.5X2	T38.5X3	T38.5X4	T38.5X5	T38.5X6
Mesulergine	T42.8X1	T42.8X2	T42.8X3	T42.8X4	T42.8X5	T42.8X6
Mesulfen	T49.0X1	T49.0X2	T49.0X3	T49.0X4	T49.0X5	T49.0X6
Mesuximide	T42.2X1	T42.2X2	T42.2X3	T42.2X4	T42.2X5	T42.2X6
Metabutethamine	T41.3X1	T41.3X2	T41.3X3	T41.3X4	T41.3X5	T41.3X6
Metactesylacetate	T49.0X1	T49.0X2	T49.0X3	T49.0X4	T49.0X5	T49.0X6

◀ New   ◀ Revised   ~~deleted~~ Deleted

Substance	Poisoning, Accidental (Unintentional)	Poisoning, Intentional Self-Harm	Poisoning, Assault	Poisoning, Undetermined	Adverse Effect	Underdosing
Metacycline	T36.4X1	T36.4X2	T36.4X3	T36.4X4	T36.4X5	T36.4X6
Metaldehyde (snail killer) NEC	T60.8X1	T60.8X2	T60.8X3	T60.8X4	—	—
Metals (heavy) (nonmedicinal)	T56.91	T56.92	T56.93	T56.94	—	—
dust, fumes, or vapor NEC	T56.91	T56.92	T56.93	T56.94	—	—
light NEC	T56.91	T56.92	T56.93	T56.94	—	—
dust, fumes, or vapor NEC	T56.91	T56.92	T56.93	T56.94	—	—
specified NEC	T56.891	T56.892	T56.893	T56.894	—	—
thallium	T56.811	T56.812	T56.813	T56.814	—	—
Metamfetamine	T43.621	T43.622	T43.623	T43.624	T43.625	T43.626
Metamizole sodium	T39.2X1	T39.2X2	T39.2X3	T39.2X4	T39.2X5	T39.2X6
Metampicillin	T36.0X1	T36.0X2	T36.0X3	T36.0X4	T36.0X5	T36.0X6
Metamucil	T47.4X1	T47.4X2	T47.4X3	T47.4X4	T47.4X5	T47.4X6
Metaphen	T49.0X1	T49.0X2	T49.0X3	T49.0X4	T49.0X5	T49.0X6
Metandienone	T38.7X1	T38.7X2	T38.7X3	T38.7X4	T38.7X5	T38.7X6
Metandrostenolone	T38.7X1	T38.7X2	T38.7X3	T38.7X4	T38.7X5	T38.7X6
Metaphos	T60.0X1	T60.0X2	T60.0X3	T60.0X4	—	—
Metapramine	T43.011	T43.012	T43.013	T43.014	T43.015	T43.016
Metaproterenol	T48.291	T48.292	T48.293	T48.294	T48.295	T48.296
Metaraminol	T44.4X1	T44.4X2	T44.4X3	T44.4X4	T44.4X5	T44.4X6
Metaxalone	T42.8X1	T42.8X2	T42.8X3	T42.8X4	T42.8X5	T42.8X6
Metenolone	T38.7X1	T38.7X2	T38.7X3	T38.7X4	T38.7X5	T38.7X6
Metergoline	T42.8X1	T42.8X2	T42.8X3	T42.8X4	T42.8X5	T42.8X6
Metescufylline	T46.991	T46.992	T46.993	T46.994	T46.995	T46.996
Metetoin	T42.0X1	T42.0X2	T42.0X3	T42.0X4	T42.0X5	T42.0X6
Metformin	T38.3X1	T38.3X2	T38.3X3	T38.3X4	T38.3X5	T38.3X6
Methacholine	T44.1X1	T44.1X2	T44.1X3	T44.1X4	T44.1X5	T44.1X6
Methacycline	T36.4X1	T36.4X2	T36.4X3	T36.4X4	T36.4X5	T36.4X6
Methadone	T40.3X1	T40.3X2	T40.3X3	T40.3X4	T40.3X5	T40.3X6
Methallenestril	T38.5X1	T38.5X2	T38.5X3	T38.5X4	T38.5X5	T38.5X6
Methallenoestril	T38.5X1	T38.5X2	T38.5X3	T38.5X4	T38.5X5	T38.5X6
Methamphetamine	T43.621	T43.622	T43.623	T43.624	T43.625	T43.626
Methampyrone	T39.2X1	T39.2X2	T39.2X3	T39.2X4	T39.2X5	T39.2X6
Methandienone	T38.7X1	T38.7X2	T38.7X3	T38.7X4	T38.7X5	T38.7X6
Methandriol	T38.7X1	T38.7X2	T38.7X3	T38.7X4	T38.7X5	T38.7X6
Methandrostenolone	T38.7X1	T38.7X2	T38.7X3	T38.7X4	T38.7X5	T38.7X6
Methane	T59.891	T59.892	T59.893	T59.894	—	—
Methanethiol	T59.891	T59.892	T59.893	T59.894	—	—
Methaniazide	T37.1X1	T37.1X2	T37.1X3	T37.1X4	T37.1X5	T37.1X6
Methanol (vapor)	T51.1X1	T51.1X2	T51.1X3	T51.1X4		
Methantheline	T44.3X1	T44.3X2	T44.3X3	T44.3X4	T44.3X5	T44.3X6
Methanthelinium bromide	T44.3X1	T44.3X2	T44.3X3	T44.3X4	T44.3X5	T44.3X6
Methaphenilene	T45.0X1	T45.0X2	T45.0X3	T45.0X4	T45.0X5	T45.0X6

Substance	Poisoning, Accidental (Unintentional)	Poisoning, Intentional Self-Harm	Poisoning, Assault	Poisoning, Undetermined	Adverse Effect	Underdosing
Methapyrilene	T45.0X1	T45.0X2	T45.0X3	T45.0X4	T45.0X5	T45.0X6
Methaqualone (compound)	T42.6X1	T42.6X2	T42.6X3	T42.6X4	T42.6X5	T42.6X6
Metharbital	T42.3X1	T42.3X2	T42.3X3	T42.3X4	T42.3X5	T42.3X6
Methazolamide	T50.2X1	T50.2X2	T50.2X3	T50.2X4	T50.2X5	T50.2X6
Methdilazine	T43.3X1	T43.3X2	T43.3X3	T43.3X4	T43.3X5	T43.3X6
Methedrine	T43.621	T43.622	T43.623	T43.624	T43.625	T43.626
Methenamine (mandelate)	T37.8X1	T37.8X2	T37.8X3	T37.8X4	T37.8X5	T37.8X6
Methenolone	T38.7X1	T38.7X2	T38.7X3	T38.7X4	T38.7X5	T38.7X6
Methergine	T48.0X1	T48.0X2	T48.0X3	T48.0X4	T48.0X5	T48.0X6
Methetoin	T42.0X1	T42.0X2	T42.0X3	T42.0X4	T42.0X5	T42.0X6
Methiacil	T38.2X1	T38.2X2	T38.2X3	T38.2X4	T38.2X5	T38.2X6
Methicillin	T36.0X1	T36.0X2	T36.0X3	T36.0X4	T36.0X5	T36.0X6
Methimazole	T38.2X1	T38.2X2	T38.2X3	T38.2X4	T38.2X5	T38.2X6
Methiodal sodium	T50.8X1	T50.8X2	T50.8X3	T50.8X4	T50.8X5	T50.8X6
Methionine	T50.991	T50.992	T50.993	T50.994	T50.995	T50.996
Methisazone	T37.5X1	T37.5X2	T37.5X3	T37.5X4	T37.5X5	T37.5X6
Methisoprinol	T37.5X1	T37.5X2	T37.5X3	T37.5X4	T37.5X5	T37.5X6
Methitural	T42.3X1	T42.3X2	T42.3X3	T42.3X4	T42.3X5	T42.3X6
Methixene	T44.3X1	T44.3X2	T44.3X3	T44.3X4	T44.3X5	T44.3X6
Methobarbital, methobarbitone	T42.3X1	T42.3X2	T42.3X3	T42.3X4	T42.3X5	T42.3X6
Methocarbamol	T42.8X1	T42.8X2	T42.8X3	T42.8X4	T42.8X5	T42.8X6
skeletal muscle relaxant	T48.1X1	T48.1X2	T48.1X3	T48.1X4	T48.1X5	T48.1X6
Methohexital	T41.1X1	T41.1X2	T41.1X3	T41.1X4	T41.1X5	T41.1X6
Methohexitone	T41.1X1	T41.1X2	T41.1X3	T41.1X4	T41.1X5	T41.1X6
Methoin	T42.0X1	T42.0X2	T42.0X3	T42.0X4	T42.0X5	T42.0X6
Methopholine	T39.8X1	T39.8X2	T39.8X3	T39.8X4	T39.8X5	T39.8X6
Methopromazine	T43.3X1	T43.3X2	T43.3X3	T43.3X4	T43.3X5	T43.3X6
Methorate	T48.3X1	T48.3X2	T48.3X3	T48.3X4	T48.3X5	T48.3X6
Methoserpidine	T46.5X1	T46.5X2	T46.5X3	T46.5X4	T46.5X5	T46.5X6
Methotrexate	T45.1X1	T45.1X2	T45.1X3	T45.1X4	T45.1X5	T45.1X6
Methotrimeprazine	T43.3X1	T43.3X2	T43.3X3	T43.3X4	T43.3X5	T43.3X6
Methoxa-Dome	T49.3X1	T49.3X2	T49.3X3	T49.3X4	T49.3X5	T49.3X6
Methoxamine	T44.4X1	T44.4X2	T44.4X3	T44.4X4	T44.4X5	T44.4X6
Methoxsalen	T50.991	T50.992	T50.993	T50.994	T50.995	T50.996
Methoxyaniline	T65.3X1	T65.3X2	T65.3X3	T65.3X4	—	—
Methoxybenzyl penicillin	T36.0X1	T36.0X2	T36.0X3	T36.0X4	T36.0X5	T36.0X6
Methoxychlor	T53.7X1	T53.7X2	T53.7X3	T53.7X4		
Methoxy-DDT	T53.7X1	T53.7X2	T53.7X3	T53.7X4	—	—
2-Methoxyethanol	T52.3X1	T52.3X2	T52.3X3	T52.3X4	—	—
Methoxyflurane	T41.0X1	T41.0X2	T41.0X3	T41.0X4	T41.0X5	T41.0X6
Methoxyphenamine	T48.6X1	T48.6X2	T48.6X3	T48.6X4	T48.6X5	T48.6X6
Methoxypromazine	T43.3X1	T43.3X2	T43.3X3	T43.3X4	T43.3X5	T43.3X6

◀ New ◀▏ Revised ~~deleted~~ Deleted

Substance	External Cause (T-Code)					
	Poisoning, Accidental (Unintentional)	Poisoning, Intentional Self-Harm	Poisoning, Assault	Poisoning, Undetermined	Adverse Effect	Underdosing
5-Methoxypsoralen (5-MOP)	T50.991	T50.992	T50.993	T50.994	T50.995	T50.996
8-Methoxypsoralen (8-MOP)	T50.991	T50.992	T50.993	T50.994	T50.995	T50.996
Methscopolamine bromide	T44.3X1	T44.3X2	T44.3X3	T44.3X4	T44.3X5	T44.3X6
Methsuximide	T42.2X1	T42.2X2	T42.2X3	T42.2X4	T42.2X5	T42.2X6
Methyclothiazide	T50.2X1	T50.2X2	T50.2X3	T50.2X4	T50.2X5	T50.2X6
Methyl						
acetate	T52.4X1	T52.4X2	T52.4X3	T52.4X4	—	—
acetone	T52.4X1	T52.4X2	T52.4X3	T52.4X4	—	—
acrylate	T65.891	T65.892	T65.893	T65.894		
alcohol	T51.1X1	T51.1X2	T51.1X3	T51.1X4	—	—
aminophenol	T65.3X1	T65.3X2	T65.3X3	T65.3X4	—	—
amphetamine	T43.621	T43.622	T43.623	T43.624	T43.625	T43.626
androstanolone	T38.7X1	T38.7X2	T38.7X3	T38.7X4	T38.7X5	T38.7X6
atropine	T44.3X1	T44.3X2	T44.3X3	T44.3X4	T44.3X5	T44.3X6
benzene	T52.2X1	T52.2X2	T52.2X3	T52.2X4	—	—
benzoate	T52.8X1	T52.8X2	T52.8X3	T52.8X4	—	—
benzol	T52.2X1	T52.2X2	T52.2X3	T52.2X4	—	—
bromide (gas)	T59.891	T59.892	T59.893	T59.894	—	—
fumigant	T60.8X1	T60.8X2	T60.8X3	T60.8X4	—	—
butanol	T51.3X1	T51.3X2	T51.3X3	T51.3X4	—	—
carbinol	T51.1X1	T51.1X2	T51.1X3	T51.1X4	—	—
carbonate	T52.8X1	T52.8X2	T52.8X3	T52.8X4	—	—
CCNU	T45.1X1	T45.1X2	T45.1X3	T45.1X4	T45.1X5	T45.1X6
cellosolve	T52.91	T52.92	T52.93	T52.94	—	—
cellulose	T47.4X1	T47.4X2	T47.4X3	T47.4X4	T47.4X5	T47.4X6
chloride (gas)	T59.891	T59.892	T59.893	T59.894	—	—
chloroformate	T59.3X1	T59.3X2	T59.3X3	T59.3X4	—	—
cyclohexane	T52.8X1	T52.8X2	T52.8X3	T52.8X4	—	—
cyclohexanol	T51.8X1	T51.8X2	T51.8X3	T51.8X4	—	—
cyclohexanone	T52.8X1	T52.8X2	T52.8X3	T52.8X4	—	—
cyclohexyl acetate	T52.8X1	T52.8X2	T52.8X3	T52.8X4	—	—
demeton	T60.0X1	T60.0X2	T60.0X3	T60.0X4	—	—
dihydromorphinone	T40.2X1	T40.2X2	T40.2X3	T40.2X4	T40.2X5	T40.2X6
ergometrine	T48.0X1	T48.0X2	T48.0X3	T48.0X4	T48.0X5	T48.0X6
ergonovine	T48.0X1	T48.0X2	T48.0X3	T48.0X4	T48.0X5	T48.0X6
ethyl ketone	T52.4X1	T52.4X2	T52.4X3	T52.4X4	—	—
glucamine antimonate	T37.8X1	T37.8X2	T37.8X3	T37.8X4	T37.8X5	T37.8X6
hydrazine	T65.891	T65.892	T65.893	T65.894	—	—
iodide	T65.891	T65.892	T65.893	T65.894	—	—
isobutyl ketone	T52.4X1	T52.4X2	T52.4X3	T52.4X4	—	—
isothiocyanate	T60.3X1	T60.3X2	T60.3X3	T60.3X4	—	—
mercaptan	T59.891	T59.892	T59.893	T59.894		

Substance	External Cause (T-Code)					
	Poisoning, Accidental (Unintentional)	Poisoning, Intentional Self-Harm	Poisoning, Assault	Poisoning, Undetermined	Adverse Effect	Underdosing
Methyl *(Continued)*						
morphine NEC	T40.2X1	T40.2X2	T40.2X3	T40.2X4	T40.2X5	T40.2X6
nicotinate	T49.4X1	T49.4X2	T49.4X3	T49.4X4	T49.4X5	T49.4X6
paraben	T49.0X1	T49.0X2	T49.0X3	T49.0X4	T49.0X5	T49.0X6
parafynol	T42.6X1	T42.6X2	T42.6X3	T42.6X4	T42.6X5	T42.6X6
parathion	T60.0X1	T60.0X2	T60.0X3	T60.0X4	—	—
peridol	T43.4X1	T43.4X2	T43.4X3	T43.4X4	T43.4X5	T43.4X6
phenidate	T43.631	T43.632	T43.633	T43.634	T43.635	T43.636
prednisolone	T38.0X1	T38.0X2	T38.0X3	T38.0X4	T38.0X5	T38.0X6
ENT agent	T49.6X1	T49.6X2	T49.6X3	T49.6X4	T49.6X5	T49.6X6
ophthalmic preparation	T49.5X1	T49.5X2	T49.5X3	T49.5X4	T49.5X5	T49.5X6
topical NEC	T49.0X1	T49.0X2	T49.0X3	T49.0X4	T49.0X5	T49.0X6
propylcarbinol	T51.3X1	T51.3X2	T51.3X3	T51.3X4	—	—
rosaniline NEC	T49.0X1	T49.0X2	T49.0X3	T49.0X4	T49.0X5	T49.0X6
salicylate	T49.2X1	T49.2X2	T49.2X3	T49.2X4	T49.2X5	T49.2X6
sulfate (fumes)	T59.891	T59.892	T59.893	T59.894	—	—
liquid	T52.8X1	T52.8X2	T52.8X3	T52.8X4	—	—
sulfonal	T42.6X1	T42.6X2	T42.6X3	T42.6X4	T42.6X5	T42.6X6
testosterone	T38.7X1	T38.7X2	T38.7X3	T38.7X4	T38.7X5	T38.7X6
thiouracil	T38.2X1	T38.2X2	T38.2X3	T38.2X4	T38.2X5	T38.2X6
Methylamphetamine	T43.621	T43.622	T43.623	T43.624	T43.625	T43.626
Methylated spirit	T51.1X1	T51.1X2	T51.1X3	T51.1X4	—	—
Methylatropine nitrate	T44.3X1	T44.3X2	T44.3X3	T44.3X4	T44.3X5	T44.3X6
Methylbenactyzium bromide	T44.3X1	T44.3X2	T44.3X3	T44.3X4	T44.3X5	T44.3X6
Methylbenzethonium chloride	T49.0X1	T49.0X2	T49.0X3	T49.0X4	T49.0X5	T49.0X6
Methylcellulose	T47.4X1	T47.4X2	T47.4X3	T47.4X4	T47.4X5	T47.4X6
laxative	T47.4X1	T47.4X2	T47.4X3	T47.4X4	T47.4X5	T47.4X6
Methylchlorophenoxy-acetic acid	T60.3X1	T60.3X2	T60.3X3	T60.3X4	—	—
Methyldopa	T46.5X1	T46.5X2	T46.5X3	T46.5X4	T46.5X5	T46.5X6
Methyldopate	T46.5X1	T46.5X2	T46.5X3	T46.5X4	T46.5X5	T46.5X6
Methylene						
blue	T50.6X1	T50.6X2	T50.6X3	T50.6X4	T50.6X5	T50.6X6
chloride or dichloride (solvent) NEC	T53.4X1	T53.4X2	T53.4X3	T53.4X4		
Methylenedioxyamphet-amine	T43.621	T43.622	T43.623	T43.624	T43.625	T43.626
Methylenedioxymethamphetamine	T43.621	T43.622	T43.623	T43.624	T43.625	T43.626
Methylergometrine	T48.0X1	T48.0X2	T48.0X3	T48.0X4	T48.0X5	T48.0X6
Methylergonovine	T48.0X1	T48.0X2	T48.0X3	T48.0X4	T48.0X5	T48.0X6
Methylestrenolone	T38.5X1	T38.5X2	T38.5X3	T38.5X4	T38.5X5	T38.5X6
Methylethyl cellulose	T50.991	T50.992	T50.993	T50.994	T50.995	T50.996
Methylhexabital	T42.3X1	T42.3X2	T42.3X3	T42.3X4	T42.3X5	T42.3X6
Methylmorphine	T40.2X1	T40.2X2	T40.2X3	T40.2X4	T40.2X5	T40.2X6

◀ New   ◀|| Revised   ~~deleted~~ Deleted

TABLE OF DRUGS AND CHEMICALS

Substance	Poisoning, Accidental (Unintentional)	Poisoning, Intentional Self-Harm	Poisoning, Assault	Poisoning, Undetermined	Adverse Effect	Underdosing
Methylparaben (ophthalmic)	T49.5X1	T49.5X2	T49.5X3	T49.5X4	T49.5X5	T49.5X6
Methylparafynol	T42.6X1	T42.6X2	T42.6X3	T42.6X4	T42.6X5	T42.6X6
Methylpentynol, methylpenthynol	T42.6X1	T42.6X2	T42.6X3	T42.6X4	T42.6X5	T42.6X6
Methylphenidate	T43.631	T43.632	T43.633	T43.634	T43.635	T43.636
Methylphenobarbital	T42.3X1	T42.3X2	T42.3X3	T42.3X4	T42.3X5	T42.3X6
Methylpolysiloxane	T47.1X1	T47.1X2	T47.1X3	T47.1X4	T47.1X5	T47.1X6
Methylprednisolone — see Methyl, prednisolone						
Methylrosaniline	T49.0X1	T49.0X2	T49.0X3	T49.0X4	T49.0X5	T49.0X6
Methylrosanilinium chloride	T49.0X1	T49.0X2	T49.0X3	T49.0X4	T49.0X5	T49.0X6
Methyltestosterone	T38.7X1	T38.7X2	T38.7X3	T38.7X4	T38.7X5	T38.7X6
Methylthionine chloride	T50.6X1	T50.6X2	T50.6X3	T50.6X4	T50.6X5	T50.6X6
Methylthioninium chloride	T50.6X1	T50.6X2	T50.6X3	T50.6X4	T50.6X5	T50.6X6
Methylthiouracil	T38.2X1	T38.2X2	T38.2X3	T38.2X4	T38.2X5	T38.2X6
Methyprylon	T42.6X1	T42.6X2	T42.6X3	T42.6X4	T42.6X5	T42.6X6
Methysergide	T46.5X1	T46.5X2	T46.5X3	T46.5X4	T46.5X5	T46.5X6
Metiamide	T47.1X1	T47.1X2	T47.1X3	T47.1X4	T47.1X5	T47.1X6
Meticillin	T36.0X1	T36.0X2	T36.0X3	T36.0X4	T36.0X5	T36.0X6
Meticrane	T50.2X1	T50.2X2	T50.2X3	T50.2X4	T50.2X5	T50.2X6
Metildigoxin	T46.0X1	T46.0X2	T46.0X3	T46.0X4	T46.0X5	T46.0X6
Metipranolol	T49.5X1	T49.5X2	T49.5X3	T49.5X4	T49.5X5	T49.5X6
Metirosine	T46.5X1	T46.5X2	T46.5X3	T46.5X4	T46.5X5	T46.5X6
Metisazone	T37.5X1	T37.5X2	T37.5X3	T37.5X4	T37.5X5	T37.5X6
Metixene	T44.3X1	T44.3X2	T44.3X3	T44.3X4	T44.3X5	T44.3X6
Metizoline	T48.5X1	T48.5X2	T48.5X3	T48.5X4	T48.5X5	T48.5X6
Metoclopramide	T45.0X1	T45.0X2	T45.0X3	T45.0X4	T45.0X5	T45.0X6
Metofenazate	T43.3X1	T43.3X2	T43.3X3	T43.3X4	T43.3X5	T43.3X6
Metofoline	T39.8X1	T39.8X2	T39.8X3	T39.8X4	T39.8X5	T39.8X6
Metolazone	T50.2X1	T50.2X2	T50.2X3	T50.2X4	T50.2X5	T50.2X6
Metopon	T40.2X1	T40.2X2	T40.2X3	T40.2X4	T40.2X5	T40.2X6
Metoprine	T45.1X1	T45.1X2	T45.1X3	T45.1X4	T45.1X5	T45.1X6
Metoprolol	T44.7X1	T44.7X2	T44.7X3	T44.7X4	T44.7X5	T44.7X6
Metrifonate	T60.0X1	T60.0X2	T60.0X3	T60.0X4	—	—
Metrizamide	T50.8X1	T50.8X2	T50.8X3	T50.8X4	T50.8X5	T50.8X6
Metrizoic acid	T50.8X1	T50.8X2	T50.8X3	T50.8X4	T50.8X5	T50.8X6
Metronidazole	T37.8X1	T37.8X2	T37.8X3	T37.8X4	T37.8X5	T37.8X6
Metycaine	T41.3X1	T41.3X2	T41.3X3	T41.3X4	T41.3X5	T41.3X6
infiltration (subcutaneous)	T41.3X1	T41.3X2	T41.3X3	T41.3X4	T41.3X5	T41.3X6
nerve block (peripheral) (plexus)	T41.3X1	T41.3X2	T41.3X3	T41.3X4	T41.3X5	T41.3X6
topical (surface)	T41.3X1	T41.3X2	T41.3X3	T41.3X4	T41.3X5	T41.3X6
Metyrapone	T50.8X1	T50.8X2	T50.8X3	T50.8X4	T50.8X5	T50.8X6
Mevinphos	T60.0X1	T60.0X2	T60.0X3	T60.0X4	—	—

Substance	Poisoning, Accidental (Unintentional)	Poisoning, Intentional Self-Harm	Poisoning, Assault	Poisoning, Undetermined	Adverse Effect	Underdosing
Mexazolam	T42.4X1	T42.4X2	T42.4X3	T42.4X4	T42.4X5	T42.4X6
Mexenone	T49.3X1	T49.3X2	T49.3X3	T49.3X4	T49.3X5	T49.3X6
Mexiletine	T46.2X1	T46.2X2	T46.2X3	T46.2X4	T46.2X5	T46.2X6
Mezereon	T62.2X1	T62.2X2	T62.2X3	T62.2X4	—	—
berries	T62.1X1	T62.1X2	T62.1X3	T62.1X4	—	—
Mezlocillin	T36.0X1	T36.0X2	T36.0X3	T36.0X4	T36.0X5	T36.0X6
Mianserin	T43.021	T43.022	T43.023	T43.024	T43.025	T43.026
Micatin	T49.0X1	T49.0X2	T49.0X3	T49.0X4	T49.0X5	T49.0X6
Miconazole	T49.0X1	T49.0X2	T49.0X3	T49.0X4	T49.0X5	T49.0X6
Micronomicin	T36.5X1	T36.5X2	T36.5X3	T36.5X4	T36.5X5	T36.5X6
Midazolam	T42.4X1	T42.4X2	T42.4X3	T42.4X4	T42.4X5	T42.4X6
Midecamycin	T36.3X1	T36.3X2	T36.3X3	T36.3X4	T36.3X5	T36.3X6
Mifepristone	T38.6X1	T38.6X2	T38.6X3	T38.6X4	T38.6X5	T38.6X6
Milk of magnesia	T47.1X1	T47.1X2	T47.1X3	T47.1X4	T47.1X5	T47.1X6
Millipede (tropical) (venomous)	T63.411	T63.412	T63.413	T63.414	—	—
Miltown	T43.591	T43.592	T43.593	T43.594	T43.595	T43.596
Milverine	T44.3X1	T44.3X2	T44.3X3	T44.3X4	T44.3X5	T44.3X6
Minaprine	T43.291	T43.292	T43.293	T43.294	T43.295	T43.296
Minaxolone	T41.291	T41.292	T41.293	T41.294	T41.295	T41.296
Mineral						
acids	T54.2X1	T54.2X2	T54.2X3	T54.2X4	—	—
oil (laxative) (medicinal)	T47.4X1	T47.4X2	T47.4X3	T47.4X4	T47.4X5	T47.4X6
emulsion	T47.2X1	T47.2X2	T47.2X3	T47.2X4	T47.2X5	T47.2X6
nonmedicinal	T52.0X1	T52.0X2	T52.0X3	T52.0X4	—	—
topical	T49.3X1	T49.3X2	T49.3X3	T49.3X4	T49.3X5	T49.3X6
salt NEC	T50.3X1	T50.3X2	T50.3X3	T50.3X4	T50.3X5	T50.3X6
spirits	T52.0X1	T52.0X2	T52.0X3	T52.0X4	—	—
Mineralocorticosteroid	T50.0X1	T50.0X2	T50.0X3	T50.0X4	T50.0X5	T50.0X6
Minocycline	T36.4X1	T36.4X2	T36.4X3	T36.4X4	T36.4X5	T36.4X6
Minoxidil	T46.7X1	T46.7X2	T46.7X3	T46.7X4	T46.7X5	T46.7X6
Miokamycin	T36.3X1	T36.3X2	T36.3X3	T36.3X4	T36.3X5	T36.3X6
Miotic drug	T49.5X1	T49.5X2	T49.5X3	T49.5X4	T49.5X5	T49.5X6
Mipafox	T60.0X1	T60.0X2	T60.0X3	T60.0X4	—	—
Mirex	T60.1X1	T60.1X2	T60.1X3	T60.1X4	—	—
Mirtazapine	T43.021	T43.022	T43.023	T43.024	T43.025	T43.026
Misonidazole	T37.3X1	T37.3X2	T37.3X3	T37.3X4	T37.3X5	T37.3X6
Misoprostol	T47.1X1	T47.1X2	T47.1X3	T47.1X4	T47.1X5	T47.1X6
Mithramycin	T45.1X1	T45.1X2	T45.1X3	T45.1X4	T45.1X5	T45.1X6
Mitobronitol	T45.1X1	T45.1X2	T45.1X3	T45.1X4	T45.1X5	T45.1X6
Mitoguazone	T45.1X1	T45.1X2	T45.1X3	T45.1X4	T45.1X5	T45.1X6
Mitolactol	T45.1X1	T45.1X2	T45.1X3	T45.1X4	T45.1X5	T45.1X6
Mitomycin	T45.1X1	T45.1X2	T45.1X3	T45.1X4	T45.1X5	T45.1X6

◀ New ◀ Revised ~~deleted~~ Deleted

Substance	External Cause (T-Code)					
	Poisoning, Accidental (Unintentional)	Poisoning, Intentional Self-Harm	Poisoning, Assault	Poisoning, Undetermined	Adverse Effect	Underdosing
Mitopodozide	T45.1X1	T45.1X2	T45.1X3	T45.1X4	T45.1X5	T45.1X6
Mitotane	T45.1X1	T45.1X2	T45.1X3	T45.1X4	T45.1X5	T45.1X6
Mitoxantrone	T45.1X1	T45.1X2	T45.1X3	T45.1X4	T45.1X5	T45.1X6
Mivacurium chloride	T48.1X1	T48.1X2	T48.1X3	T48.1X4	T48.1X5	T48.1X6
Miyari bacteria	T47.6X1	T47.6X2	T47.6X3	T47.6X4	T47.6X5	T47.6X6
Moclobemide	T43.1X1	T43.1X2	T43.1X3	T43.1X4	T43.1X5	T43.1X6
Moderil	T46.5X1	T46.5X2	T46.5X3	T46.5X4	T46.5X5	T46.5X6
Mofebutazone	T39.2X1	T39.2X2	T39.2X3	T39.2X4	T39.2X5	T39.2X6
Mogadon — see Nitrazepam						
Molindone	T43.591	T43.592	T43.593	T43.594	T43.595	T43.596
Molsidomine	T46.3X1	T46.3X2	T46.3X3	T46.3X4	T46.3X5	T46.3X6
Mometasone	T49.0X1	T49.0X2	T49.0X3	T49.0X4	T49.0X5	T49.0X6
Monistat	T49.0X1	T49.0X2	T49.0X3	T49.0X4	T49.0X5	T49.0X6
Monkshood	T62.2X1	T62.2X2	T62.2X3	T62.2X4	—	—
Monoamine oxidase inhibitor NEC	T43.1X1	T43.1X2	T43.1X3	T43.1X4	T43.1X5	T43.1X6
hydrazine	T43.1X1	T43.1X2	T43.1X3	T43.1X4	T43.1X5	T43.1X6
Monobenzone	T49.4X1	T49.4X2	T49.4X3	T49.4X4	T49.4X5	T49.4X6
Monochloroacetic acid	T60.3X1	T60.3X2	T60.3X3	T60.3X4	—	—
Monochlorobenzene	T53.7X1	T53.7X2	T53.7X3	T53.7X4	—	—
Monoethanolamine	T46.8X1	T46.8X2	T46.8X3	T46.8X4	T46.8X5	T46.8X6
oleate	T46.8X1	T46.8X2	T46.8X3	T46.8X4	T46.8X5	T46.8X6
Monooctanoin	T50.991	T50.992	T50.993	T50.994	T50.995	T50.996
Monophenylbutazone	T39.2X1	T39.2X2	T39.2X3	T39.2X4	T39.2X5	T39.2X6
Monosodium glutamate	T65.891	T65.892	T65.893	T65.894	—	—
Monosulfiram	T49.0X1	T49.0X2	T49.0X3	T49.0X4	T49.0X5	T49.0X6
Monoxide, carbon — see Carbon, monoxide	T57.91	T57.92	T57.93	T57.94	—	—
Monoxidine hydrochloride	T46.1X1	T46.1X2	T46.1X3	T46.1X4	T46.1X5	T46.1X6
Monuron	T60.3X1	T60.3X2	T60.3X3	T60.3X4	—	—
Moperone	T43.4X1	T43.4X2	T43.4X3	T43.4X4	T43.4X5	T43.4X6
Mopidamol	T45.1X1	T45.1X2	T45.1X3	T45.1X4	T45.1X5	T45.1X6
MOPP (mechlorethamine + vincristine + prednisone + procarbazine)	T45.1X1	T45.1X2	T45.1X3	T45.1X4	T45.1X5	T45.1X6
Morfin	T40.2X1	T40.2X2	T40.2X3	T40.2X4	T40.2X5	T40.2X6
Morinamide	T37.1X1	T37.1X2	T37.1X3	T37.1X4	T37.1X5	T37.1X6
Morning glory seeds	T40.991	T40.992	T40.993	T40.994	—	—
Moroxydine	T37.5X1	T37.5X2	T37.5X3	T37.5X4	T37.5X5	T37.5X6
Morphazinamide	T37.1X1	T37.1X2	T37.1X3	T37.1X4	T37.1X5	T37.1X6
Morphine	T40.2X1	T40.2X2	T40.2X3	T40.2X4	T40.2X5	T40.2X6
antagonist	T50.7X1	T50.7X2	T50.7X3	T50.7X4	T50.7X5	T50.7X6
Morpholinylethylmorphine	T40.2X1	T40.2X2	T40.2X3	T40.2X4	—	—
Morsuximide	T42.2X1	T42.2X2	T42.2X3	T42.2X4	T42.2X5	T42.2X6

Substance	External Cause (T-Code)					
	Poisoning, Accidental (Unintentional)	Poisoning, Intentional Self-Harm	Poisoning, Assault	Poisoning, Undetermined	Adverse Effect	Underdosing
Mosapramine	T43.591	T43.592	T43.593	T43.594	T43.595	T43.596
Moth balls — see also Pesticides	T60.2X1	T60.2X2	T60.2X3	T60.2X4	—	—
naphthalene	T60.2X1	T60.2X2	T60.2X3	T60.2X4	—	—
paradichlorobenzene	T60.1X1	T60.1X2	T60.1X3	T60.1X4	—	—
Motor exhaust gas	T58.01	T58.02	T58.03	T58.04		
Mouthwash (antiseptic) (zinc chloride)	T49.6X1	T49.6X2	T49.6X3	T49.6X4	T49.6X5	T49.6X6
Moxastine	T45.0X1	T45.0X2	T45.0X3	T45.0X4	T45.0X5	T45.0X6
Moxaverine	T44.3X1	T44.3X2	T44.3X3	T44.3X4	T44.3X5	T44.3X6
Moxifensine	T43.291	T43.292	T43.293	T43.294	T43.295	T43.296
Moxisylyte	T46.7X1	T46.7X2	T46.7X3	T46.7X4	T46.7X5	T46.7X6
Mucilage, plant	T47.4X1	T47.4X2	T47.4X3	T47.4X4	T47.4X5	T47.4X6
Mucolytic drug	T48.4X1	T48.4X2	T48.4X3	T48.4X4	T48.4X5	T48.4X6
Mucomyst	T48.4X1	T48.4X2	T48.4X3	T48.4X4	T48.4X5	T48.4X6
Mucous membrane agents (external)	T49.91	T49.92	T49.93	T49.94	T49.95	T49.96
specified NEC	T49.8X1	T49.8X2	T49.8X3	T49.8X4	T49.8X5	T49.8X6
Mumps						
immune globulin (human)	T50.Z11	T50.Z12	T50.Z13	T50.Z14	T50.Z15	T50.Z16
skin test antigen	T50.8X1	T50.8X2	T50.8X3	T50.8X4	T50.8X5	T50.8X6
vaccine	T50.B91	T50.B92	T50.B93	T50.B94	T50.B95	T50.B96
Mumpsvax	T50.B91	T50.B92	T50.B93	T50.B94	T50.B95	T50.B96
Mupirocin	T49.0X1	T49.0X2	T49.0X3	T49.0X4	T49.0X5	T49.0X6
Muriatic acid — see Hydrochloric acid						
Muromonab-CD3	T45.1X1	T45.1X2	T45.1X3	T45.1X4	T45.1X5	T45.1X6
Muscle relaxant — see Relaxant, muscle						
Muscle-action drug NEC	T48.201	T48.202	T48.203	T48.204	T48.205	T48.206
Muscle affecting agents NEC	T48.201	T48.202	T48.203	T48.204	T48.205	T48.206
oxytocic	T48.0X1	T48.0X2	T48.0X3	T48.0X4	T48.0X5	T48.0X6
relaxants	T48.201	T48.202	T48.203	T48.204	T48.205	T48.206
central nervous system	T42.8X1	T42.8X2	T42.8X3	T42.8X4	T42.8X5	T42.8X6
skeletal	T48.1X1	T48.1X2	T48.1X3	T48.1X4	T48.1X5	T48.1X6
smooth	T44.3X1	T44.3X2	T44.3X3	T44.3X4	T44.3X5	T44.3X6
Muscle-tone depressant, central NEC	T42.8X1	T42.8X2	T42.8X3	T42.8X4	T42.8X5	T42.8X6
specified NEC	T42.8X1	T42.8X2	T42.8X3	T42.8X4	T42.8X5	T42.8X6
Mushroom, noxious	T62.0X1	T62.0X2	T62.0X3	T62.0X4	—	—
Mussel, noxious	T61.781	T61.782	T61.783	T61.784	—	—
Mustard (emetic)	T47.7X1	T47.7X2	T47.7X3	T47.7X4	T47.7X5	T47.7X6
black	T47.7X1	T47.7X2	T47.7X3	T47.7X4	T47.7X5	T47.7X6
gas, not in war	T59.91	T59.92	T59.93	T59.94	—	—
nitrogen	T45.1X1	T45.1X2	T45.1X3	T45.1X4	T45.1X5	T45.1X6

◀ New   ◀ Revised   ~~deleted~~ Deleted

Substance	Poisoning, Accidental (Unintentional)	Poisoning, Intentional Self-Harm	Poisoning, Assault	Poisoning, Undetermined	Adverse Effect	Underdosing
Mustine	T45.1X1	T45.1X2	T45.1X3	T45.1X4	T45.1X5	T45.1X6
M-vac	T45.1X1	T45.1X2	T45.1X3	T45.1X4	T45.1X5	T45.1X6
Mycifradin	T36.5X1	T36.5X2	T36.5X3	T36.5X4	T36.5X5	T36.5X6
topical	T49.0X1	T49.0X2	T49.0X3	T49.0X4	T49.0X5	T49.0X6
Mycitracin	T36.8X1	T36.8X2	T36.8X3	T36.8X4	T36.8X5	T36.8X6
ophthalmic preparation	T49.5X1	T49.5X2	T49.5X3	T49.5X4	T49.5X5	T49.5X6
Mycostatin	T36.7X1	T36.7X2	T36.7X3	T36.7X4	T36.7X5	T36.7X6
topical	T49.0X1	T49.0X2	T49.0X3	T49.0X4	T49.0X5	T49.0X6
Mycotoxins	T64.81	T64.82	T64.83	T64.84	—	—
aflatoxin	T64.01	T64.02	T64.03	T64.04	—	—
specified NEC	T64.81	T64.82	T64.83	T64.84	—	—
Mydriacyl	T44.3X1	T44.3X2	T44.3X3	T44.3X4	T44.3X5	T44.3X6
Mydriatic drug	T49.5X1	T49.5X2	T49.5X3	T49.5X4	T49.5X5	T49.5X6
Myelobromal	T45.1X1	T45.1X2	T45.1X3	T45.1X4	T45.1X5	T45.1X6
Myleran	T45.1X1	T45.1X2	T45.1X3	T45.1X4	T45.1X5	T45.1X6
Myochrysin(e)	T39.2X1	T39.2X2	T39.2X3	T39.2X4	T39.2X5	T39.2X6
Myoneural blocking agents	T48.1X1	T48.1X2	T48.1X3	T48.1X4	T48.1X5	T48.1X6
Myralact	T49.0X1	T49.0X2	T49.0X3	T49.0X4	T49.0X5	T49.0X6
Myristica fragrans	T62.2X1	T62.2X2	T62.2X3	T62.2X4	—	—
Myristicin	T65.891	T65.892	T65.893	T65.894	—	—
Mysoline	T42.3X1	T42.3X2	T42.3X3	T42.3X4	T42.3X5	T42.3X6
N						
Nabilone	T40.7X1	T40.7X2	T40.7X3	T40.7X4	T40.7X5	T40.7X6
Nabumetone	T39.391	T39.392	T39.393	T39.394	T39.395	T39.396
Nadolol	T44.7X1	T44.7X2	T44.7X3	T44.7X4	T44.7X5	T44.7X6
Nafcillin	T36.0X1	T36.0X2	T36.0X3	T36.0X4	T36.0X5	T36.0X6
Nafoxidine	T38.6X1	T38.6X2	T38.6X3	T38.6X4	T38.6X5	T38.6X6
Naftazone	T46.991	T46.992	T46.993	T46.994	T46.995	T46.996
Naftidrofuryl (oxalate)	T46.7X1	T46.7X2	T46.7X3	T46.7X4	T46.7X5	T46.7X6
Naftifine	T49.0X1	T49.0X2	T49.0X3	T49.0X4	T49.0X5	T49.0X6
Nail polish remover	T52.91	T52.92	T52.93	T52.94	—	—
Nalbuphine	T40.4X1	T40.4X2	T40.4X3	T40.4X4	T40.4X5	T40.4X6
Naled	T60.0X1	T60.0X2	T60.0X3	T60.0X4	—	—
Nalidixic acid	T37.8X1	T37.8X2	T37.8X3	T37.8X4	T37.8X5	T37.8X6
Nalorphine	T50.7X1	T50.7X2	T50.7X3	T50.7X4	T50.7X5	T50.7X6
Naloxone	T50.7X1	T50.7X2	T50.7X3	T50.7X4	T50.7X5	T50.7X6
Naltrexone	T50.7X1	T50.7X2	T50.7X3	T50.7X4	T50.7X5	T50.7X6
Namenda	T43.8X1	T43.8X2	T43.8X3	T43.8X4	T43.8X5	T43.8X6
Nandrolone	T38.7X1	T38.7X2	T38.7X3	T38.7X4	T38.7X5	T38.7X6
Naphazoline	T48.5X1	T48.5X2	T48.5X3	T48.5X4	T48.5X5	T48.5X6

Substance	Poisoning, Accidental (Unintentional)	Poisoning, Intentional Self-Harm	Poisoning, Assault	Poisoning, Undetermined	Adverse Effect	Underdosing
Naphtha (painters') (petroleum)	T52.0X1	T52.0X2	T52.0X3	T52.0X4	—	—
solvent	T52.0X1	T52.0X2	T52.0X3	T52.0X4	—	—
vapor	T52.0X1	T52.0X2	T52.0X3	T52.0X4	—	—
Naphthalene (non-chlorinated)	T60.2X1	T60.2X2	T60.2X3	T60.2X4	—	—
chlorinated	T60.1X1	T60.1X2	T60.1X3	T60.1X4	—	—
vapor	T60.1X1	T60.1X2	T60.1X3	T60.1X4	—	—
insecticide or moth repellent	T60.2X1	T60.2X2	T60.2X3	T60.2X4	—	—
chlorinated	T60.1X1	T60.1X2	T60.1X3	T60.1X4	—	—
vapor	T60.2X1	T60.2X2	T60.2X3	T60.2X4	—	—
chlorinated	T60.1X1	T60.1X2	T60.1X3	T60.1X4	—	—
Naphthol	T65.891	T65.892	T65.893	T65.894	—	—
Naphthylamine	T65.891	T65.892	T65.893	T65.894	—	—
Naphthylthiourea (ANTU)	T60.4X1	T60.4X2	T60.4X3	T60.4X4	—	—
Naprosyn — see Naproxen						
Naproxen	T39.311	T39.312	T39.313	T39.314	T39.315	T39.316
Narcotic (drug)	T40.601	T40.602	T40.603	T40.604	T40.605	T40.606
analgesic NEC	T40.601	T40.602	T40.603	T40.604	T40.605	T40.606
antagonist	T50.7X1	T50.7X2	T50.7X3	T50.7X4	T50.7X5	T50.7X6
specified NEC	T40.691	T40.692	T40.693	T40.694	T40.695	T40.696
synthetic	T40.4X1	T40.4X2	T40.4X3	T40.4X4	T40.4X5	T40.4X6
Narcotine	T48.3X1	T48.3X2	T48.3X3	T48.3X4	T48.3X5	T48.3X6
Nardil	T43.1X1	T43.1X2	T43.1X3	T43.1X4	T43.1X5	T43.1X6
Nasal drug NEC	T49.6X1	T49.6X2	T49.6X3	T49.6X4	T49.6X5	T49.6X6
Natamycin	T49.0X1	T49.0X2	T49.0X3	T49.0X4	T49.0X5	T49.0X6
Natrium cyanide — see Cyanide(s)						
Natural gas	T59.891	T59.892	T59.893	T59.894	—	—
incomplete combustion	T57.91	T57.92	T57.93	T57.94	—	—
Natural						
blood (product)	T45.8X1	T45.8X2	T45.8X3	T45.8X4	T45.8X5	T45.8X6
gas (piped)	T59.891	T59.892	T59.893	T59.894	—	—
incomplete combustion	T58.11	T58.12	T58.13	T58.14	—	—
Nealbarbital	T42.3X1	T42.3X2	T42.3X3	T42.3X4	T42.3X5	T42.3X6
Nectadon	T48.3X1	T48.3X2	T48.3X3	T48.3X4	T48.3X5	T48.3X6
Nedocromil	T48.6X1	T48.6X2	T48.6X3	T48.6X4	T48.6X5	T48.6X6
Nefopam	T39.8X1	T39.8X2	T39.8X3	T39.8X4	T39.8X5	T39.8X6
Nematocyst (sting)	T63.691	T63.692	T63.693	T63.694	—	—
Nembutal	T42.3X1	T42.3X2	T42.3X3	T42.3X4	T42.3X5	T42.3X6
Nemonapride	T43.591	T43.592	T43.593	T43.594	T43.595	T43.596
Neoarsphenamine	T37.8X1	T37.8X2	T37.8X3	T37.8X4	T37.8X5	T37.8X6

TABLE OF DRUGS AND CHEMICALS

Substance	External Cause (T-Code)					
	Poisoning, Accidental (Unintentional)	Poisoning, Intentional Self-Harm	Poisoning, Assault	Poisoning, Undetermined	Adverse Effect	Underdosing
Neocinchophen	T50.4X1	T50.4X2	T50.4X3	T50.4X4	T50.4X5	T50.4X6
Neomycin (derivatives)	T36.5X1	T36.5X2	T36.5X3	T36.5X4	T36.5X5	T36.5X6
with						
bacitracin	T49.0X1	T49.0X2	T49.0X3	T49.0X4	T49.0X5	T49.0X6
neostigmine	T44.0X1	T44.0X2	T44.0X3	T44.0X4	T44.0X5	T44.0X6
ENT agent	T49.6X1	T49.6X2	T49.6X3	T49.6X4	T49.6X5	T49.6X6
ophthalmic preparation	T49.5X1	T49.5X2	T49.5X3	T49.5X4	T49.5X5	T49.5X6
topical NEC	T49.0X1	T49.0X2	T49.0X3	T49.0X4	T49.0X5	T49.0X6
Neonal	T42.3X1	T42.3X2	T42.3X3	T42.3X4	T42.3X5	T42.3X6
Neoprontosil	T37.0X1	T37.0X2	T37.0X3	T37.0X4	T37.0X5	T37.0X6
Neosalvarsan	T37.8X1	T37.8X2	T37.8X3	T37.8X4	T37.8X5	T37.8X6
Neosilversalvarsan	T37.8X1	T37.8X2	T37.8X3	T37.8X4	T37.8X5	T37.8X6
Neosporin	T36.8X1	T36.8X2	T36.8X3	T36.8X4	T36.8X5	T36.8X6
ENT agent	T49.6X1	T49.6X2	T49.6X3	T49.6X4	T49.6X5	T49.6X6
opthalmic preparation	T49.5X1	T49.5X2	T49.5X3	T49.5X4	T49.5X5	T49.5X6
topical NEC	T49.0X1	T49.0X2	T49.0X3	T49.0X4	T49.0X5	T49.0X6
Neostigmine bromide	T44.0X1	T44.0X2	T44.0X3	T44.0X4	T44.0X5	T44.0X6
Neraval	T42.3X1	T42.3X2	T42.3X3	T42.3X4	T42.3X5	T42.3X6
Neravan	T42.3X1	T42.3X2	T42.3X3	T42.3X4	T42.3X5	T42.3X6
Nerium oleander	T62.2X1	T62.2X2	T62.2X3	T62.2X4	—	—
Nerve gas, not in war	T59.91	T59.92	T59.93	T59.94	—	—
Nesacaine	T41.3X1	T41.3X2	T41.3X3	T41.3X4	T41.3X5	T41.3X6
infiltration (subcutaneous)	T41.3X1	T41.3X2	T41.3X3	T41.3X4	T41.3X5	T41.3X6
nerve block (peripheral) (plexus)	T41.3X1	T41.3X2	T41.3X3	T41.3X4	T41.3X5	T41.3X6
Netilmicin	T36.5X1	T36.5X2	T36.5X3	T36.5X4	T36.5X5	T36.5X6
Neurobarb	T42.3X1	T42.3X2	T42.3X3	T42.3X4	T42.3X5	T42.3X6
Neuroleptic drug NEC	T43.501	T43.502	T43.503	T43.504	T43.505	T43.506
Neuromuscular blocking drug	T48.1X1	T48.1X2	T48.1X3	T48.1X4	T48.1X5	T48.1X6
Neutral insulin injection	T38.3X1	T38.3X2	T38.3X3	T38.3X4	T38.3X5	T38.3X6
Neutral spirits	T51.0X1	T51.0X2	T51.0X3	T51.0X4	—	—
beverage	T51.0X1	T51.0X2	T51.0X3	T51.0X4	—	—
Niacin	T46.7X1	T46.7X2	T46.7X3	T46.7X4	T46.7X5	T46.7X6
Niacinamide	T45.2X1	T45.2X2	T45.2X3	T45.2X4	T45.2X5	T45.2X6
Nialamide	T43.1X1	T43.1X2	T43.1X3	T43.1X4	T43.1X5	T43.1X6
Niaprazine	T42.6X1	T42.6X2	T42.6X3	T42.6X4	T42.6X5	T42.6X6
Nicametate	T46.7X1	T46.7X2	T46.7X3	T46.7X4	T46.7X5	T46.7X6
Nicardipine	T46.1X1	T46.1X2	T46.1X3	T46.1X4	T46.1X5	T46.1X6
Nicergoline	T46.7X1	T46.7X2	T46.7X3	T46.7X4	T46.7X5	T46.7X6
Nickel (carbonyl) (tetra-carbonyl) (fumes) (vapor)	T56.891	T56.892	T56.893	T56.894	—	—

Substance	External Cause (T-Code)					
	Poisoning, Accidental (Unintentional)	Poisoning, Intentional Self-Harm	Poisoning, Assault	Poisoning, Undetermined	Adverse Effect	Underdosing
Nickelocene	T56.891	T56.892	T56.893	T56.894	—	—
Niclosamide	T37.4X1	T37.4X2	T37.4X3	T37.4X4	T37.4X5	T37.4X6
Nicofuranose	T46.7X1	T46.7X2	T46.7X3	T46.7X4	T46.7X5	T46.7X6
Nicomorphine	T40.2X1	T40.2X2	T40.2X3	T40.2X4	—	—
Nicorandil	T46.3X1	T46.3X2	T46.3X3	T46.3X4	T46.3X5	T46.3X6
Nicotiana (plant)	T62.2X1	T62.2X2	T62.2X3	T62.2X4	—	—
Nicotinamide	T45.2X1	T45.2X2	T45.2X3	T45.2X4	T45.2X5	T45.2X6
Nicotine (insecticide) (spray) (sulfate) NEC	T60.2X1	T60.2X2	T60.2X3	T60.2X4	—	—
from tobacco	T65.291	T65.292	T65.293	T65.294		
cigarettes	T65.221	T65.222	T65.223	T65.224		
not insecticide	T65.291	T65.292	T65.293	T65.294	—	—
Nicotinic acid	T46.7X1	T46.7X2	T46.7X3	T46.7X4	T46.7X5	T46.7X6
Nicotinyl alcohol	T46.7X1	T46.7X2	T46.7X3	T46.7X4	T46.7X5	T46.7X6
Nicoumalone	T45.511	T45.512	T45.513	T45.514	T45.515	T45.516
Nifedipine	T46.1X1	T46.1X2	T46.1X3	T46.1X4	T46.1X5	T46.1X6
Nifenazone	T39.2X1	T39.2X2	T39.2X3	T39.2X4	T39.2X5	T39.2X6
Nifuraldezone	T37.91	T37.92	T37.93	T37.94	T37.95	T37.96
Nifuratel	T37.8X1	T37.8X2	T37.8X3	T37.8X4	T37.8X5	T37.8X6
Nifurtimox	T37.3X1	T37.3X2	T37.3X3	T37.3X4	T37.3X5	T37.3X6
Nifurtoinol	T37.8X1	T37.8X2	T37.8X3	T37.8X4	T37.8X5	T37.8X6
Nightshade, deadly (solanum) — see also Belladonna	T62.2X1	T62.2X2	T62.2X3	T62.2X4	—	—
berry	T62.1X1	T62.1X2	T62.1X3	T62.1X4	—	—
Nikethamide	T50.7X1	T50.7X2	T50.7X3	T50.7X4	T50.7X5	T50.7X6
Nilstat	T36.7X1	T36.7X2	T36.7X3	T36.7X4	T36.7X5	T36.7X6
topical	T49.0X1	T49.0X2	T49.0X3	T49.0X4	T49.0X5	T49.0X6
Nilutamide	T38.6X1	T38.6X2	T38.6X3	T38.6X4	T38.6X5	T38.6X6
Nimesulide	T39.391	T39.392	T39.393	T39.394	T39.395	T39.396
Nimetazepam	T42.4X1	T42.4X2	T42.4X3	T42.4X4	T42.4X5	T42.4X6
Nimodipine	T46.1X1	T46.1X2	T46.1X3	T46.1X4	T46.1X5	T46.1X6
Nimorazole	T37.3X1	T37.3X2	T37.3X3	T37.3X4	T37.3X5	T37.3X6
Nimustine	T45.1X1	T45.1X2	T45.1X3	T45.1X4	T45.1X5	T45.1X6
Niridazole	T37.4X1	T37.4X2	T37.4X3	T37.4X4	T37.4X5	T37.4X6
Nisentil	T40.2X1	T40.2X2	T40.2X3	T40.2X4	T40.2X5	T40.2X6
Nisoldipine	T46.1X1	T46.1X2	T46.1X3	T46.1X4	T46.1X5	T46.1X6
Nitramine	T65.3X1	T65.3X2	T65.3X3	T65.3X4	—	—
Nitrate, organic	T46.3X1	T46.3X2	T46.3X3	T46.3X4	T46.3X5	T46.3X6
Nitrazepam	T42.4X1	T42.4X2	T42.4X3	T42.4X4	T42.4X5	T42.4X6
Nitrefazole	T50.6X1	T50.6X2	T50.6X3	T50.6X4	T50.6X5	T50.6X6
Nitrendipine	T46.1X1	T46.1X2	T46.1X3	T46.1X4	T46.1X5	T46.1X6

◀ New   ◀ Revised   ~~deleted~~ Deleted

Substance	Poisoning, Accidental (Unintentional)	Poisoning, Intentional Self-Harm	Poisoning, Assault	Poisoning, Undetermined	Adverse Effect	Underdosing
Nitric						
acid (liquid)	T54.2X1	T54.2X2	T54.2X3	T54.2X4	—	—
vapor	T59.891	T59.892	T59.893	T59.894	—	—
oxide (gas)	T59.0X1	T59.0X2	T59.0X3	T59.0X4	—	—
Nitrimidazine	T37.3X1	T37.3X2	T37.3X3	T37.3X4	T37.3X5	T37.3X6
Nitrite, amyl (medicinal) (vapor)	T46.3X1	T46.3X2	T46.3X3	T46.3X4	T46.3X5	T46.3X6
Nitroaniline	T65.3X1	T65.3X2	T65.3X3	T65.3X4	—	—
vapor	T59.891	T59.892	T59.893	T59.894	—	—
Nitrobenzene, nitrobenzol	T65.3X1	T65.3X2	T65.3X3	T65.3X4	—	—
vapor	T65.3X1	T65.3X2	T65.3X3	T65.3X4	—	—
Nitrocellulose	T65.891	T65.892	T65.893	T65.894	—	—
lacquer	T65.891	T65.892	T65.893	T65.894	—	—
Nitrodiphenyl	T65.3X1	T65.3X2	T65.3X3	T65.3X4	—	—
Nitrofural	T49.0X1	T49.0X2	T49.0X3	T49.0X4	T49.0X5	T49.0X6
Nitrofurantoin	T37.8X1	T37.8X2	T37.8X3	T37.8X4	T37.8X5	T37.8X6
Nitrofurazone	T49.0X1	T49.0X2	T49.0X3	T49.0X4	T49.0X5	T49.0X6
Nitrogen	T59.0X1	T59.0X2	T59.0X3	T59.0X4	—	—
mustard	T45.1X1	T45.1X2	T45.1X3	T45.1X4	T45.1X5	T45.1X6
Nitroglycerin, nitro-glycerol (medicinal)	T46.3X1	T46.3X2	T46.3X3	T46.3X4	T46.3X5	T46.3X6
nonmedicinal	T65.5X1	T65.5X2	T65.5X3	T65.5X4	—	—
fumes	T65.5X1	T65.5X2	T65.5X3	T65.5X4	—	—
Nitroglycol	T52.3X1	T52.3X2	T52.3X3	T52.3X4	—	—
Nitrohydrochloric acid	T54.2X1	T54.2X2	T54.2X3	T54.2X4	—	—
Nitromersol	T49.0X1	T49.0X2	T49.0X3	T49.0X4	T49.0X5	T49.0X6
Nitronaphthalene	T65.891	T65.892	T65.893	T65.894	—	—
Nitrophenol	T54.0X1	T54.0X2	T54.0X3	T54.0X4	—	—
Nitropropane	T52.8X1	T52.8X2	T52.8X3	T52.8X4	—	—
Nitroprusside	T46.5X1	T46.5X2	T46.5X3	T46.5X4	T46.5X5	T46.5X6
Nitrosodimethylamine	T65.3X1	T65.3X2	T65.3X3	T65.3X4	—	—
Nitrothiazol	T37.4X1	T37.4X2	T37.4X3	T37.4X4	T37.4X5	T37.4X6
Nitrotoluene, nitrotoluol	T65.3X1	T65.3X2	T65.3X3	T65.3X4	—	—
vapor	T65.3X1	T65.3X2	T65.3X3	T65.3X4	—	—
Nitrous						
acid (liquid)	T54.2X1	T54.2X2	T54.2X3	T54.2X4	—	—
fumes	T59.891	T59.892	T59.893	T59.894	—	—
ether spirit	T46.3X1	T46.3X2	T46.3X3	T46.3X4	T46.3X5	T46.3X6
oxide	T41.0X1	T41.0X2	T41.0X3	T41.0X4	T41.0X5	T41.0X6
Nitroxoline	T37.8X1	T37.8X2	T37.8X3	T37.8X4	T37.8X5	T37.8X6
Nitrozone	T49.0X1	T49.0X2	T49.0X3	T49.0X4	T49.0X5	T49.0X6
Nizatidine	T47.0X1	T47.0X2	T47.0X3	T47.0X4	T47.0X5	T47.0X6
Nizofenone	T43.8X1	T43.8X2	T43.8X3	T43.8X4	T43.8X5	T43.8X6
Noctec	T42.6X1	T42.6X2	T42.6X3	T42.6X4	T42.6X5	T42.6X6
Noludar	T42.6X1	T42.6X2	T42.6X3	T42.6X4	T42.6X5	T42.6X6
Noptil	T42.3X1	T42.3X2	T42.3X3	T42.3X4	T42.3X5	T42.3X6
Nomegestrol	T38.5X1	T38.5X2	T38.5X3	T38.5X4	T38.5X5	T38.5X6
Nomifensine	T43.291	T43.292	T43.293	T43.294	T43.295	T43.296
Nonoxinol	T49.8X1	T49.8X2	T49.8X3	T49.8X4	T49.8X5	T49.8X6
Nonylphenoxy (polyethoxy-ethanol)	T49.8X1	T49.8X2	T49.8X3	T49.8X4	T49.8X5	T49.8X6
Noptil	T42.3X1	T42.3X2	T42.3X3	T42.3X4	T42.3X5	T42.3X6
Noradrenaline	T44.4X1	T44.4X2	T44.4X3	T44.4X4	T44.4X5	T44.4X6
Noramidopyrine	T39.2X1	T39.2X2	T39.2X3	T39.2X4	T39.2X5	T39.2X6
methanesulfonate sodium	T39.2X1	T39.2X2	T39.2X3	T39.2X4	T39.2X5	T39.2X6
Norbormide	T60.4X1	T60.4X2	T60.4X3	T60.4X4	—	—
Nordazepam	T42.4X1	T42.4X2	T42.4X3	T42.4X4	T42.4X5	T42.4X6
Norepinephrine	T44.4X1	T44.4X2	T44.4X3	T44.4X4	T44.4X5	T44.4X6
Norethandrolone	T38.7X1	T38.7X2	T38.7X3	T38.7X4	T38.7X5	T38.7X6
Norethindrone	T38.4X1	T38.4X2	T38.4X3	T38.4X4	T38.4X5	T38.4X6
Norethisterone (acetate) (enantate)	T38.4X1	T38.4X2	T38.4X3	T38.4X4	T38.4X5	T38.4X6
with ethinylestradiol	T38.5X1	T38.5X2	T38.5X3	T38.5X4	T38.5X5	T38.5X6
Noretynodrel	T38.5X1	T38.5X2	T38.5X3	T38.5X4	T38.5X5	T38.5X6
Norfenefrine	T44.4X1	T44.4X2	T44.4X3	T44.4X4	T44.4X5	T44.4X6
Norfloxacin	T36.8X1	T36.8X2	T36.8X3	T36.8X4	T36.8X5	T36.8X6
Norgestrel	T38.4X1	T38.4X2	T38.4X3	T38.4X4	T38.4X5	T38.4X6
Norgestrienone	T38.4X1	T38.4X2	T38.4X3	T38.4X4	T38.4X5	T38.4X6
Norlestrin	T38.4X1	T38.4X2	T38.4X3	T38.4X4	T38.4X5	T38.4X6
Norlutin	T38.4X1	T38.4X2	T38.4X3	T38.4X4	T38.4X5	T38.4X6
Normal serum albumin (human), salt-poor	T45.8X1	T45.8X2	T45.8X3	T45.8X4	T45.8X5	T45.8X6
Normethandrone	T38.5X1	T38.5X2	T38.5X3	T38.5X4	T38.5X5	T38.5X6
Normison — see Benzodiazepines						
Normorphine	T40.2X1	T40.2X2	T40.2X3	T40.2X4	—	—
Norpseudoephedrine	T50.5X1	T50.5X2	T50.5X3	T50.5X4	T50.5X5	T50.5X6
Nortestosterone (furanpropionate)	T38.7X1	T38.7X2	T38.7X3	T38.7X4	T38.7X5	T38.7X6
Nortriptyline	T43.011	T43.012	T43.013	T43.014	T43.015	T43.016
Noscapine	T48.3X1	T48.3X2	T48.3X3	T48.3X4	T48.3X5	T48.3X6
Nose preparations	T49.6X1	T49.6X2	T49.6X3	T49.6X4	T49.6X5	T49.6X6
Novobiocin	T36.5X1	T36.5X2	T36.5X3	T36.5X4	T36.5X5	T36.5X6
Novocain (infiltration) (topical)	T41.3X1	T41.3X2	T41.3X3	T41.3X4	T41.3X5	T41.3X6
nerve block (peripheral) (plexus)	T41.3X1	T41.3X2	T41.3X3	T41.3X4	T41.3X5	T41.3X6
spinal	T41.3X1	T41.3X2	T41.3X3	T41.3X4	T41.3X5	T41.3X6

◀ New　◀ Revised　~~deleted~~ Deleted

TABLE OF DRUGS AND CHEMICALS

Substance	External Cause (T-Code)					
	Poisoning, Accidental (Unintentional)	Poisoning, Intentional Self-Harm	Poisoning, Assault	Poisoning, Undetermined	Adverse Effect	Underdosing
Noxious foodstuff	T62.91	T62.92	T62.93	T62.94	—	—
specified NEC	T62.8X1	T62.8X2	T62.8X3	T62.8X4	—	—
Noxiptiline	T43.011	T43.012	T43.013	T43.014	T43.015	T43.016
Noxytiolin	T49.0X1	T49.0X2	T49.0X3	T49.0X4	T49.0X5	T49.0X6
NPH Iletin (insulin)	T38.3X1	T38.3X2	T38.3X3	T38.3X4	T38.3X5	T38.3X6
Numorphan	T40.2X1	T40.2X2	T40.2X3	T40.2X4	T40.2X5	T40.2X6
Nunol	T42.3X1	T42.3X2	T42.3X3	T42.3X4	T42.3X5	T42.3X6
Nupercaine (spinal anesthetic)	T41.3X1	T41.3X2	T41.3X3	T41.3X4	T41.3X5	T41.3X6
topical (surface)	T41.3X1	T41.3X2	T41.3X3	T41.3X4	T41.3X5	T41.3X6
Nutmeg oil (liniment)	T49.3X1	T49.3X2	T49.3X3	T49.3X4	T49.3X5	T49.3X6
Nutritional supplement	T50.901	T50.902	T50.903	T50.904	T50.905	T50.906
Nux vomica	T65.1X1	T65.1X2	T65.1X3	T65.1X4	—	—
Nydrazid	T37.1X1	T37.1X2	T37.1X3	T37.1X4	T37.1X5	T37.1X6
Nylidrin	T46.7X1	T46.7X2	T46.7X3	T46.7X4	T46.7X5	T46.7X6
Nystatin	T36.7X1	T36.7X2	T36.7X3	T36.7X4	T36.7X5	T36.7X6
topical	T49.0X1	T49.0X2	T49.0X3	T49.0X4	T49.0X5	T49.0X6
Nytol	T45.0X1	T45.0X2	T45.0X3	T45.0X4	T45.0X5	T45.0X6
O						
Obidoxime chloride	T50.6X1	T50.6X2	T50.6X3	T50.6X4	T50.6X5	T50.6X6
Octafonium (chloride)	T49.3X1	T49.3X2	T49.3X3	T49.3X4	T49.3X5	T49.3X6
Octamethyl pyrophos-phoramide	T60.0X1	T60.0X2	T60.0X3	T60.0X4	—	—
Octanoin	T50.991	T50.992	T50.993	T50.994	T50.995	T50.996
Octatropine methyl-bromide	T44.3X1	T44.3X2	T44.3X3	T44.3X4	T44.3X5	T44.3X6
Octotiamine	T45.2X1	T45.2X2	T45.2X3	T45.2X4	T45.2X5	T45.2X6
Octoxinol (9)	T49.8X1	T49.8X2	T49.8X3	T49.8X4	T49.8X5	T49.8X6
Octreotide	T38.991	T38.992	T38.993	T38.994	T38.995	T38.996
Octyl nitrite	T46.3X1	T46.3X2	T46.3X3	T46.3X4	T46.3X5	T46.3X6
Oestradiol	T38.5X1	T38.5X2	T38.5X3	T38.5X4	T38.5X5	T38.5X6
Oestriol	T38.5X1	T38.5X2	T38.5X3	T38.5X4	T38.5X5	T38.5X6
Oestrogen	T38.5X1	T38.5X2	T38.5X3	T38.5X4	T38.5X5	T38.5X6
Oestrone	T38.5X1	T38.5X2	T38.5X3	T38.5X4	T38.5X5	T38.5X6
Ofloxacin	T36.8X1	T36.8X2	T36.8X3	T36.8X4	T36.8X5	T36.8X6
Oil (of)	T65.891	T65.892	T65.893	T65.894	—	—
bitter almond	T62.8X1	T62.8X2	T62.8X3	T62.8X4	—	—
cloves	T49.7X1	T49.7X2	T49.7X3	T49.7X4	T49.7X5	T49.7X6
colors	T65.6X1	T65.6X2	T65.6X3	T65.6X4	—	—
fumes	T59.891	T59.892	T59.893	T59.894	—	—
lubricating	T52.0X1	T52.0X2	T52.0X3	T52.0X4	—	—
Niobe	T52.8X1	T52.8X2	T52.8X3	T52.8X4	—	—

Substance	External Cause (T-Code)					
	Poisoning, Accidental (Unintentional)	Poisoning, Intentional Self-Harm	Poisoning, Assault	Poisoning, Undetermined	Adverse Effect	Underdosing
Oil (of) *(Continued)*						
vitriol (liquid)	T54.2X1	T54.2X2	T54.2X3	T54.2X4	—	—
fumes	T54.2X1	T54.2X2	T54.2X3	T54.2X4	—	—
wintergreen (bitter) NEC	T49.3X1	T49.3X2	T49.3X3	T49.3X4	T49.3X5	T49.3X6
Oily preparation (for skin)	T49.3X1	T49.3X2	T49.3X3	T49.3X4	T49.3X5	T49.3X6
Ointment NEC	T49.3X1	T49.3X2	T49.3X3	T49.3X4	T49.3X5	T49.3X6
Olanzapine	T43.591	T43.592	T43.593	T43.594	T43.595	T43.596
Oleander	T62.2X1	T62.2X2	T62.2X3	T62.2X4	—	—
Oleandomycin	T36.3X1	T36.3X2	T36.3X3	T36.3X4	T36.3X5	T36.3X6
Oleandrin	T46.0X1	T46.0X2	T46.0X3	T46.0X4	T46.0X5	T46.0X6
Oleic acid	T46.6X1	T46.6X2	T46.6X3	T46.6X4	T46.6X5	T46.6X6
Oleovitamin A	T45.2X1	T45.2X2	T45.2X3	T45.2X4	T45.2X5	T45.2X6
Oleum ricini	T47.2X1	T47.2X2	T47.2X3	T47.2X4	T47.2X5	T47.2X6
Olive oil (medicinal) NEC	T47.4X1	T47.4X2	T47.4X3	T47.4X4	T47.4X5	T47.4X6
Olivomycin	T45.1X1	T45.1X2	T45.1X3	T45.1X4	T45.1X5	T45.1X6
Olsalazine	T47.8X1	T47.8X2	T47.8X3	T47.8X4	T47.8X5	T47.8X6
Omeprazole	T47.1X1	T47.1X2	T47.1X3	T47.1X4	T47.1X5	T47.1X6
OMPA	T60.0X1	T60.0X2	T60.0X3	T60.0X4	—	—
Ondansetron	T45.0X1	T45.0X2	T45.0X3	T45.0X4	T45.0X5	T45.0X6
Oncovin	T45.1X1	T45.1X2	T45.1X3	T45.1X4	T45.1X5	T45.1X6
Ophthaine	T41.3X1	T41.3X2	T41.3X3	T41.3X4	T41.3X5	T41.3X6
Ophthetic	T41.3X1	T41.3X2	T41.3X3	T41.3X4	T41.3X5	T41.3X6
Opiate NEC	T40.601	T40.602	T40.603	T40.604	T40.605	T40.606
antagonists	T50.7X1	T50.7X2	T50.7X3	T50.7X4	T50.7X5	T50.7X6
Opioid NEC	T40.2X1	T40.2X2	T40.2X3	T40.2X4	T40.2X5	T40.2X6
Opipramol	T43.011	T43.012	T43.013	T43.014	T43.015	T43.016
Opium alkaloids (total)	T40.0X1	T40.0X2	T40.0X3	T40.0X4	T40.0X5	T40.0X6
standardized powdered	T40.0X1	T40.0X2	T40.0X3	T40.0X4	T40.0X5	T40.0X6
tincture (camphorated)	T40.0X1	T40.0X2	T40.0X3	T40.0X4	T40.0X5	T40.0X6
Oracon	T38.4X1	T38.4X2	T38.4X3	T38.4X4	T38.4X5	T38.4X6
Oragrafin	T50.8X1	T50.8X2	T50.8X3	T50.8X4	T50.8X5	T50.8X6
Oral contraceptives	T38.4X1	T38.4X2	T38.4X3	T38.4X4	T38.4X5	T38.4X6
Oral rehydration salts	T50.3X1	T50.3X2	T50.3X3	T50.3X4	T50.3X5	T50.3X6
Orazamide	T50.991	T50.992	T50.993	T50.994	T50.995	T50.996
Orciprenaline	T48.291	T48.292	T48.293	T48.294	T48.295	T48.296
Organidin	T48.4X1	T48.4X2	T48.4X3	T48.4X4	T48.4X5	T48.4X6
Organonitrate NEC	T46.3X1	T46.3X2	T46.3X3	T46.3X4	T46.3X5	T46.3X6
Organophosphates	T60.0X1	T60.0X2	T60.0X3	T60.0X4	—	—
Orimune	T50.B91	T50.B92	T50.B93	T50.B94	T50.B95	T50.B96
Orinase	T38.3X1	T38.3X2	T38.3X3	T38.3X4	T38.3X5	T38.3X6
Ormeloxifene	T38.6X1	T38.6X2	T38.6X3	T38.6X4	T38.6X5	T38.6X6

Substance	Poisoning, Accidental (Unintentional)	Poisoning, Intentional Self-Harm	Poisoning, Assault	Poisoning, Undetermined	Adverse Effect	Underdosing
Ornidazole	T37.3X1	T37.3X2	T37.3X3	T37.3X4	T37.3X5	T37.3X6
Ornithine aspartate	T50.991	T50.992	T50.993	T50.994	T50.995	T50.996
Ornoprostil	T47.1X1	T47.1X2	T47.1X3	T47.1X4	T47.1X5	T47.1X6
Orphenadrine (hydrochloride)	T42.8X1	T42.8X2	T42.8X3	T42.8X4	T42.8X5	T42.8X6
Ortal (sodium)	T42.3X1	T42.3X2	T42.3X3	T42.3X4	T42.3X5	T42.3X6
Orthoboric acid	T49.0X1	T49.0X2	T49.0X3	T49.0X4	T49.0X5	T49.0X6
ENT agent	T49.6X1	T49.6X2	T49.6X3	T49.6X4	T49.6X5	T49.6X6
ophthalmic preparation	T49.5X1	T49.5X2	T49.5X3	T49.5X4	T49.5X5	T49.5X6
Orthocaine	T41.3X1	T41.3X2	T41.3X3	T41.3X4	T41.3X5	T41.3X6
Orthodichlorobenzene	T53.7X1	T53.7X2	T53.7X3	T53.7X4	—	—
Ortho-Novum	T38.4X1	T38.4X2	T38.4X3	T38.4X4	T38.4X5	T38.4X6
Orthotolidine (reagent)	T54.2X1	T54.2X2	T54.2X3	T54.2X4	—	—
Osmic acid (liquid)	T54.2X1	T54.2X2	T54.2X3	T54.2X4	—	—
fumes	T54.2X1	T54.2X2	T54.2X3	T54.2X4	—	—
Osmotic diuretics	T50.2X1	T50.2X2	T50.2X3	T50.2X4	T50.2X5	T50.2X6
Otilonium bromide	T44.3X1	T44.3X2	T44.3X3	T44.3X4	T44.3X5	T44.3X6
Otorhinolaryngological drug NEC	T49.6X1	T49.6X2	T49.6X3	T49.6X4	T49.6X5	T49.6X6
Ouabain(e)	T46.0X1	T46.0X2	T46.0X3	T46.0X4	T46.0X5	T46.0X6
Ovarian						
hormone	T38.5X1	T38.5X2	T38.5X3	T38.5X4	T38.5X5	T38.5X6
stimulant	T38.5X1	T38.5X2	T38.5X3	T38.5X4	T38.5X5	T38.5X6
Ovral	T38.4X1	T38.4X2	T38.4X3	T38.4X4	T38.4X5	T38.4X6
Ovulen	T38.4X1	T38.4X2	T38.4X3	T38.4X4	T38.4X5	T38.4X6
Oxacillin	T36.0X1	T36.0X2	T36.0X3	T36.0X4	T36.0X5	T36.0X6
Oxalic acid	T54.2X1	T54.2X2	T54.2X3	T54.2X4	—	—
ammonium salt	T50.991	T50.992	T50.993	T50.994	T50.995	T50.996
Oxamniquine	T37.4X1	T37.4X2	T37.4X3	T37.4X4	T37.4X5	T37.4X6
Oxanamide	T43.591	T43.592	T43.593	T43.594	T43.595	T43.596
Oxandrolone	T38.7X1	T38.7X2	T38.7X3	T38.7X4	T38.7X5	T38.7X6
Oxantel	T37.4X1	T37.4X2	T37.4X3	T37.4X4	T37.4X5	T37.4X6
Oxapium iodide	T44.3X1	T44.3X2	T44.3X3	T44.3X4	T44.3X5	T44.3X6
Oxaprotiline	T43.021	T43.022	T43.023	T43.024	T43.025	T43.026
Oxaprozin	T39.311	T39.312	T39.313	T39.314	T39.315	T39.316
Oxatomide	T45.0X1	T45.0X2	T45.0X3	T45.0X4	T45.0X5	T45.0X6
Oxazepam	T42.4X1	T42.4X2	T42.4X3	T42.4X4	T42.4X5	T42.4X6
Oxazimedrine	T50.5X1	T50.5X2	T50.5X3	T50.5X4	T50.5X5	T50.5X6
Oxazolam	T42.4X1	T42.4X2	T42.4X3	T42.4X4	T42.4X5	T42.4X6
Oxazolidine derivatives	T42.2X1	T42.2X2	T42.2X3	T42.2X4	T42.2X5	T42.2X6
Oxazolidinedione (derivative)	T42.2X1	T42.2X2	T42.2X3	T42.2X4	T42.2X5	T42.2X6
Ox bile extract	T47.5X1	T47.5X2	T47.5X3	T47.5X4	T47.5X5	T47.5X6
Oxcarbazepine	T42.1X1	T42.1X2	T42.1X3	T42.1X4	T42.1X5	T42.1X6
Oxedrine	T44.4X1	T44.4X2	T44.4X3	T44.4X4	T44.4X5	T44.4X6
Oxeladin (citrate)	T48.3X1	T48.3X2	T48.3X3	T48.3X4	T48.3X5	T48.3X6
Oxendolone	T38.5X1	T38.5X2	T38.5X3	T38.5X4	T38.5X5	T38.5X6
Oxetacaine	T41.3X1	T41.3X2	T41.3X3	T41.3X4	T41.3X5	T41.3X6
Oxethazine	T41.3X1	T41.3X2	T41.3X3	T41.3X4	T41.3X5	T41.3X6
Oxetorone	T39.8X1	T39.8X2	T39.8X3	T39.8X4	T39.8X5	T39.8X6
Oxiconazole	T49.0X1	T49.0X2	T49.0X3	T49.0X4	T49.0X5	T49.0X6
Oxidizing agent NEC	T54.91	T54.92	T54.93	T54.94	—	—
Oxipurinol	T50.4X1	T50.4X2	T50.4X3	T50.4X4	T50.4X5	T50.4X6
Oxitriptan	T43.291	T43.292	T43.293	T43.294	T43.295	T43.296
Oxitropium bromide	T48.6X1	T48.6X2	T48.6X3	T48.6X4	T48.6X5	T48.6X6
Oxodipine	T46.1X1	T46.1X2	T46.1X3	T46.1X4	T46.1X5	T46.1X6
Oxolamine	T48.3X1	T48.3X2	T48.3X3	T48.3X4	T48.3X5	T48.3X6
Oxolinic acid	T37.8X1	T37.8X2	T37.8X3	T37.8X4	T37.8X5	T37.8X6
Oxomemazine	T43.3X1	T43.3X2	T43.3X3	T43.3X4	T43.3X5	T43.3X6
Oxophenarsine	T37.3X1	T37.3X2	T37.3X3	T37.3X4	T37.3X5	T37.3X6
Oxprenolol	T44.7X1	T44.7X2	T44.7X3	T44.7X4	T44.7X5	T44.7X6
Oxsoralen	T49.3X1	T49.3X2	T49.3X3	T49.3X4	T49.3X5	T49.3X6
Oxtriphylline	T48.6X1	T48.6X2	T48.6X3	T48.6X4	T48.6X5	T48.6X6
Oxybate sodium	T41.291	T41.292	T41.293	T41.294	T41.295	T41.296
Oxybuprocaine	T41.3X1	T41.3X2	T41.3X3	T41.3X4	T41.3X5	T41.3X6
Oxybutynin	T44.3X1	T44.3X2	T44.3X3	T44.3X4	T44.3X5	T44.3X6
Oxychlorosene	T49.0X1	T49.0X2	T49.0X3	T49.0X4	T49.0X5	T49.0X6
Oxycodone	T40.2X1	T40.2X2	T40.2X3	T40.2X4	T40.2X5	T40.2X6
Oxyfedrine	T46.3X1	T46.3X2	T46.3X3	T46.3X4	T46.3X5	T46.3X6
Oxygen	T41.5X1	T41.5X2	T41.5X3	T41.5X4	T41.5X5	T41.5X6
Oxylone	T49.0X1	T49.0X2	T49.0X3	T49.0X4	T49.0X5	T49.0X6
ophthalmic preparation	T49.5X1	T49.5X2	T49.5X3	T49.5X4	T49.5X5	T49.5X6
Oxymesterone	T38.7X1	T38.7X2	T38.7X3	T38.7X4	T38.7X5	T38.7X6
Oxymetazoline	T48.5X1	T48.5X2	T48.5X3	T48.5X4	T48.5X5	T48.5X6
Oxymetholone	T38.7X1	T38.7X2	T38.7X3	T38.7X4	T38.7X5	T38.7X6
Oxymorphone	T40.2X1	T40.2X2	T40.2X3	T40.2X4	T40.2X5	T40.2X6
Oxypertine	T43.591	T43.592	T43.593	T43.594	T43.595	T43.596
Oxyphenbutazone	T39.2X1	T39.2X2	T39.2X3	T39.2X4	T39.2X5	T39.2X6
Oxyphencyclimine	T44.3X1	T44.3X2	T44.3X3	T44.3X4	T44.3X5	T44.3X6
Oxyphenisatine	T47.2X1	T47.2X2	T47.2X3	T47.2X4	T47.2X5	T47.2X6
Oxyphenonium bromide	T44.3X1	T44.3X2	T44.3X3	T44.3X4	T44.3X5	T44.3X6
Oxypolygelatin	T45.8X1	T45.8X2	T45.8X3	T45.8X4	T45.8X5	T45.8X6
Oxyquinoline (derivatives)	T37.8X1	T37.8X2	T37.8X3	T37.8X4	T37.8X5	T37.8X6
Oxytetracycline	T36.4X1	T36.4X2	T36.4X3	T36.4X4	T36.4X5	T36.4X6
Oxytocic drug NEC	T48.0X1	T48.0X2	T48.0X3	T48.0X4	T48.0X5	T48.0X6
Oxytocin (synthetic)	T48.0X1	T48.0X2	T48.0X3	T48.0X4	T48.0X5	T48.0X6
Ozone	T59.891	T59.892	T59.893	T59.894	—	—

◀ New   ◀ Revised   ~~deleted~~ Deleted

TABLE OF DRUGS AND CHEMICALS

Substance	External Cause (T-Code) Poisoning, Accidental (Unintentional)	Poisoning, Intentional Self-Harm	Poisoning, Assault	Poisoning, Undetermined	Adverse Effect	Underdosing
P						
PABA	T49.3X1	T49.3X2	T49.3X3	T49.3X4	T49.3X5	T49.3X6
Packed red cells	T45.8X1	T45.8X2	T45.8X3	T45.8X4	T45.8X5	T45.8X6
Padimate	T49.3X1	T49.3X2	T49.3X3	T49.3X4	T49.3X5	T49.3X6
Paint NEC	T65.6X1	T65.6X2	T65.6X3	T65.6X4	—	—
cleaner	T52.91	T52.92	T52.93	T52.94	—	—
fumes NEC	T59.891	T59.892	T59.893	T59.894	—	—
lead (fumes)	T56.0X1	T56.0X2	T56.0X3	T56.0X4	—	—
solvent NEC	T52.8X1	T52.8X2	T52.8X3	T52.8X4	—	—
stripper	T52.8X1	T52.8X2	T52.8X3	T52.8X4	—	—
Palfium	T40.2X1	T40.2X2	T40.2X3	T40.2X4	—	—
Palm kernel oil	T50.991	T50.992	T50.993	T50.994	T50.995	T50.996
Paludrine	T37.2X1	T37.2X2	T37.2X3	T37.2X4	T37.2X5	T37.2X6
PAM (pralidoxime)	T50.6X1	T50.6X2	T50.6X3	T50.6X4	T50.6X5	T50.6X6
Pamaquine (naphthoute)	T37.2X1	T37.2X2	T37.2X3	T37.2X4	T37.2X5	T37.2X6
Panadol	T39.1X1	T39.1X2	T39.1X3	T39.1X4	T39.1X5	T39.1X6
Pancreatic						
digestive secretion stimulant	T47.8X1	T47.8X2	T47.8X3	T47.8X4	T47.8X5	T47.8X6
dornase	T45.3X1	T45.3X2	T45.3X3	T45.3X4	T45.3X5	T45.3X6
Pancreatin	T47.5X1	T47.5X2	T47.5X3	T47.5X4	T47.5X5	T47.5X6
Pancrelipase	T47.5X1	T47.5X2	T47.5X3	T47.5X4	T47.5X5	T47.5X6
Pancuronium (bromide)	T48.1X1	T48.1X2	T48.1X3	T48.1X4	T48.1X5	T48.1X6
Pangamic acid	T45.2X1	T45.2X2	T45.2X3	T45.2X4	T45.2X5	T45.2X6
Panthenol	T45.2X1	T45.2X2	T45.2X3	T45.2X4	T45.2X5	T45.2X6
topical	T49.8X1	T49.8X2	T49.8X3	T49.8X4	T49.8X5	T49.8X6
Pantopon	T40.0X1	T40.0X2	T40.0X3	T40.0X4	T40.0X5	T40.0X6
Pantothenic acid	T45.2X1	T45.2X2	T45.2X3	T45.2X4	T45.2X5	T45.2X6
Panwarfin	T45.511	T45.512	T45.513	T45.514	T45.515	T45.516
Papain	T47.5X1	T47.5X2	T47.5X3	T47.5X4	T47.5X5	T47.5X6
digestant	T47.5X1	T47.5X2	T47.5X3	T47.5X4	T47.5X5	T47.5X6
Papaveretum	T40.0X1	T40.0X2	T40.0X3	T40.0X4	T40.0X5	T40.0X6
Papaverine	T44.3X1	T44.3X2	T44.3X3	T44.3X4	T44.3X5	T44.3X6
Para-acetamidophenol	T39.1X1	T39.1X2	T39.1X3	T39.1X4	T39.1X5	T39.1X6
Para-aminobenzoic acid	T49.3X1	T49.3X2	T49.3X3	T49.3X4	T49.3X5	T49.3X6
Para-aminophenol derivatives	T39.1X1	T39.1X2	T39.1X3	T39.1X4	T39.1X5	T39.1X6
Para-aminosalicylic acid	T37.1X1	T37.1X2	T37.1X3	T37.1X4	T37.1X5	T37.1X6
Paracetaldehyde	T42.6X1	T42.6X2	T42.6X3	T42.6X4	T42.6X5	T42.6X6
Paracetamol	T39.1X1	T39.1X2	T39.1X3	T39.1X4	T39.1X5	T39.1X6
Parachlorophenol (camphorated)	T49.0X1	T49.0X2	T49.0X3	T49.0X4	T49.0X5	T49.0X6
Paracodin	T40.2X1	T40.2X2	T40.2X3	T40.2X4	T40.2X5	T40.2X6
Paradione	T42.2X1	T42.2X2	T42.2X3	T42.2X4	T42.2X5	T42.2X6

Substance	External Cause (T-Code) Poisoning, Accidental (Unintentional)	Poisoning, Intentional Self-Harm	Poisoning, Assault	Poisoning, Undetermined	Adverse Effect	Underdosing
Paraffin(s) (wax)	T52.0X1	T52.0X2	T52.0X3	T52.0X4	—	—
liquid (medicinal)	T47.4X1	T47.4X2	T47.4X3	T47.4X4	T47.4X5	T47.4X6
nonmedicinal	T52.0X1	T52.0X2	T52.0X3	T52.0X4	—	—
Paraformaldehyde	T60.3X1	T60.3X2	T60.3X3	T60.3X4	—	—
Paraldehyde	T42.6X1	T42.6X2	T42.6X3	T42.6X4	T42.6X5	T42.6X6
Paramethadione	T42.2X1	T42.2X2	T42.2X3	T42.2X4	T42.2X5	T42.2X6
Paramethasone	T38.0X1	T38.0X2	T38.0X3	T38.0X4	T38.0X5	T38.0X6
acetate	T49.0X1	T49.0X2	T49.0X3	T49.0X4	T49.0X5	T49.0X6
Paraoxon	T60.0X1	T60.0X2	T60.0X3	T60.0X4	—	—
Paraquat	T60.3X1	T60.3X2	T60.3X3	T60.3X4	—	—
Parasympatholytic NEC	T44.3X1	T44.3X2	T44.3X3	T44.3X4	T44.3X5	T44.3X6
Parasympathomimetic drug NEC	T44.1X1	T44.1X2	T44.1X3	T44.1X4	T44.1X5	T44.1X6
Parathion	T60.0X1	T60.0X2	T60.0X3	T60.0X4	—	—
Parathormone	T50.991	T50.992	T50.993	T50.994	T50.995	T50.996
Parathyroid extract	T50.991	T50.992	T50.993	T50.994	T50.995	T50.996
Paratyphoid vaccine	T50.A91	T50.A92	T50.A93	T50.A94	T50.A95	T50.A96
Paredrine	T44.4X1	T44.4X2	T44.4X3	T44.4X4	T44.4X5	T44.4X6
Paregoric	T40.0X1	T40.0X2	T40.0X3	T40.0X4	T40.0X5	T40.0X6
Pargyline	T46.5X1	T46.5X2	T46.5X3	T46.5X4	T46.5X5	T46.5X6
Paris green	T57.0X1	T57.0X2	T57.0X3	T57.0X4	—	—
insecticide	T57.0X1	T57.0X2	T57.0X3	T57.0X4	—	—
Parnate	T43.1X1	T43.1X2	T43.1X3	T43.1X4	T43.1X5	T43.1X6
Paromomycin	T36.5X1	T36.5X2	T36.5X3	T36.5X4	T36.5X5	T36.5X6
Paroxypropione	T45.1X1	T45.1X2	T45.1X3	T45.1X4	T45.1X5	T45.1X6
Parzone	T40.2X1	T40.2X2	T40.2X3	T40.2X4	T40.2X5	T40.2X6
PAS	T37.1X1	T37.1X2	T37.1X3	T37.1X4	T37.1X5	T37.1X6
Pasiniazid	T37.1X1	T37.1X2	T37.1X3	T37.1X4	T37.1X5	T37.1X6
PBB (polybrominated biphenyls)	T65.891	T65.892	T65.893	T65.894	—	—
PCB	T65.891	T65.892	T65.893	T65.894	—	—
PCP						
meaning pentachlorophenol	T60.1X1	T60.1X2	T60.1X3	T60.1X4	—	—
fungicide	T60.3X1	T60.3X2	T60.3X3	T60.3X4	—	—
herbicide	T60.3X1	T60.3X2	T60.3X3	T60.3X4	—	—
insecticide	T60.1X1	T60.1X2	T60.1X3	T60.1X4	—	—
meaning phencyclidine	T40.991	T40.992	T40.993	T40.994	—	—
Peach kernel oil (emulsion)	T47.4X1	T47.4X2	T47.4X3	T47.4X4	T47.4X5	T47.4X6
Peanut oil (emulsion) NEC	T47.4X1	T47.4X2	T47.4X3	T47.4X4	T47.4X5	T47.4X6
topical	T49.3X1	T49.3X2	T49.3X3	T49.3X4	T49.3X5	T49.3X6
Pearly Gates (morning glory seeds)	T40.991	T40.992	T40.993	T40.994	—	—
Pecazine	T43.3X1	T43.3X2	T43.3X3	T43.3X4	T43.3X5	T43.3X6
Pectin	T47.6X1	T47.6X2	T47.6X3	T47.6X4	T47.6X5	T47.6X6

◀ New ◀ Revised ~~deleted~~ Deleted

Substance	Poisoning, Accidental (Unintentional)	Poisoning, Intentional Self-Harm	Poisoning, Assault	Poisoning, Undetermined	Adverse Effect	Underdosing
Pefloxacin	T37.8X1	T37.8X2	T37.8X3	T37.8X4	T37.8X5	T37.8X6
Pegademase, bovine	T50.Z91	T50.Z92	T50.Z93	T50.Z94	T50.Z95	T50.Z96
Pelletierine tannate	T37.4X1	T37.4X2	T37.4X3	T37.4X4	T37.4X5	T37.4X6
Pemirolast (potassium)	T48.6X1	T48.6X2	T48.6X3	T48.6X4	T48.6X5	T48.6X6
Pemoline	T50.7X1	T50.7X2	T50.7X3	T50.7X4	T50.7X5	T50.7X6
Pempidine	T44.2X1	T44.2X2	T44.2X3	T44.2X4	T44.2X5	T44.2X6
Penamecillin	T36.0X1	T36.0X2	T36.0X3	T36.0X4	T36.0X5	T36.0X6
Penbutolol	T44.7X1	T44.7X2	T44.7X3	T44.7X4	T44.7X5	T44.7X6
Penethamate	T36.0X1	T36.0X2	T36.0X3	T36.0X4	T36.0X5	T36.0X6
Penfluridol	T43.591	T43.592	T43.593	T43.594	T43.595	T43.596
Penflutizide	T50.2X1	T50.2X2	T50.2X3	T50.2X4	T50.2X5	T50.2X6
Pengitoxin	T46.0X1	T46.0X2	T46.0X3	T46.0X4	T46.0X5	T46.0X6
Penicillamine	T50.6X1	T50.6X2	T50.6X3	T50.6X4	T50.6X5	T50.6X6
Penicillin (any)	T36.0X1	T36.0X2	T36.0X3	T36.0X4	T36.0X5	T36.0X6
Penicillinase	T45.3X1	T45.3X2	T45.3X3	T45.3X4	T45.3X5	T45.3X6
Penicilloyl polylysine	T50.8X1	T50.8X2	T50.8X3	T50.8X4	T50.8X5	T50.8X6
Penimepicycline	T36.4X1	T36.4X2	T36.4X3	T36.4X4	T36.4X5	T36.4X6
Pentachloroethane	T53.6X1	T53.6X2	T53.6X3	T53.6X4	—	—
Pentachloronaphthalene	T53.7X1	T53.7X2	T53.7X3	T53.7X4	—	—
Pentachlorophenol (pesticide)	T60.1X1	T60.1X2	T60.1X3	T60.1X4	—	—
fungicide	T60.3X1	T60.3X2	T60.3X3	T60.3X4	—	—
herbicide	T60.3X1	T60.3X2	T60.3X3	T60.3X4	—	—
insecticide	T60.1X1	T60.1X2	T60.1X3	T60.1X4	—	—
Pentaerythritol tetranitrate	T46.3X1	T46.3X2	T46.3X3	T46.3X4	T46.3X5	T46.3X6
Pentaerythritol	T46.3X1	T46.3X2	T46.3X3	T46.3X4	T46.3X5	T46.3X6
chloral	T42.6X1	T42.6X2	T42.6X3	T42.6X4	T42.6X5	T42.6X6
tetranitrate NEC	T46.3X1	T46.3X2	T46.3X3	T46.3X4	T46.3X5	T46.3X6
Pentagastrin	T50.8X1	T50.8X2	T50.8X3	T50.8X4	T50.8X5	T50.8X6
Pentalin	T53.6X1	T53.6X2	T53.6X3	T53.6X4	—	—
Pentamethonium bromide	T44.2X1	T44.2X2	T44.2X3	T44.2X4	T44.2X5	T44.2X6
Pentamidine	T37.3X1	T37.3X2	T37.3X3	T37.3X4	T37.3X5	T37.3X6
Pentanol	T51.3X1	T51.3X2	T51.3X3	T51.3X4	—	—
Pentapyrrolinium (bitartrate)	T44.2X1	T44.2X2	T44.2X3	T44.2X4	T44.2X5	T44.2X6
Pentaquine	T37.2X1	T37.2X2	T37.2X3	T37.2X4	T37.2X5	T37.2X6
Pentazocine	T40.4X1	T40.4X2	T40.4X3	T40.4X4	T40.4X5	T40.4X6
Pentetrazole	T50.7X1	T50.7X2	T50.7X3	T50.7X4	T50.7X5	T50.7X6
Penthienate bromide	T44.3X1	T44.3X2	T44.3X3	T44.3X4	T44.3X5	T44.3X6
Pentifylline	T46.7X1	T46.7X2	T46.7X3	T46.7X4	T46.7X5	T46.7X6
Pentobarbital	T42.3X1	T42.3X2	T42.3X3	T42.3X4	T42.3X5	T42.3X6
sodium	T42.3X1	T42.3X2	T42.3X3	T42.3X4	T42.3X5	T42.3X6
Pentobarbitone	T42.3X1	T42.3X2	T42.3X3	T42.3X4	T42.3X5	T42.3X6
Pentolonium tartrate	T44.2X1	T44.2X2	T44.2X3	T44.2X4	T44.2X5	T44.2X6

Substance	Poisoning, Accidental (Unintentional)	Poisoning, Intentional Self-Harm	Poisoning, Assault	Poisoning, Undetermined	Adverse Effect	Underdosing
Pentosan polysulfate (sodium)	T39.8X1	T39.8X2	T39.8X3	T39.8X4	T39.8X5	T39.8X6
Pentostatin	T45.1X1	T45.1X2	T45.1X3	T45.1X4	T45.1X5	T45.1X6
Pentothal	T41.1X1	T41.1X2	T41.1X3	T41.1X4	T41.1X5	T41.1X6
Pentoxifylline	T46.7X1	T46.7X2	T46.7X3	T46.7X4	T46.7X5	T46.7X6
Pentoxyverine	T48.3X1	T48.3X2	T48.3X3	T48.3X4	T48.3X5	T48.3X6
Pentrinat	T46.3X1	T46.3X2	T46.3X3	T46.3X4	T46.3X5	T46.3X6
Pentylenetetrazole	T50.7X1	T50.7X2	T50.7X3	T50.7X4	T50.7X5	T50.7X6
Pentylsalicylamide	T37.1X1	T37.1X2	T37.1X3	T37.1X4	T37.1X5	T37.1X6
Pentymal	T42.3X1	T42.3X2	T42.3X3	T42.3X4	T42.3X5	T42.3X6
Peplomycin	T45.1X1	T45.1X2	T45.1X3	T45.1X4	T45.1X5	T45.1X6
Peppermint (oil)	T47.5X1	T47.5X2	T47.5X3	T47.5X4	T47.5X5	T47.5X6
Pepsin	T47.5X1	T47.5X2	T47.5X3	T47.5X4	T47.5X5	T47.5X6
digestant	T47.5X1	T47.5X2	T47.5X3	T47.5X4	T47.5X5	T47.5X6
Pepstatin	T47.1X1	T47.1X2	T47.1X3	T47.1X4	T47.1X5	T47.1X6
Peptavlon	T50.8X1	T50.8X2	T50.8X3	T50.8X4	T50.8X5	T50.8X6
Perazine	T43.3X1	T43.3X2	T43.3X3	T43.3X4	T43.3X5	T43.3X6
Percaine (spinal)	T41.3X1	T41.3X2	T41.3X3	T41.3X4	T41.3X5	T41.3X6
topical (surface)	T41.3X1	T41.3X2	T41.3X3	T41.3X4	T41.3X5	T41.3X6
Perchloroethylene	T53.3X1	T53.3X2	T53.3X3	T53.3X4	—	—
medicinal	T37.4X1	T37.4X2	T37.4X3	T37.4X4	T37.4X5	T37.4X6
vapor	T53.3X1	T53.3X2	T53.3X3	T53.3X4	—	—
Percodan	T40.2X1	T40.2X2	T40.2X3	T40.2X4	T40.2X5	T40.2X6
Percogesic — *see also acetaminophen*	T45.0X1	T45.0X2	T45.0X3	T45.0X4	T45.0X5	T45.0X6
Percorten	T38.0X1	T38.0X2	T38.0X3	T38.0X4	T38.0X5	T38.0X6
Pergolide	T42.8X1	T42.8X2	T42.8X3	T42.8X4	T42.8X5	T42.8X6
Pergonal	T38.811	T38.812	T38.813	T38.814	T38.815	T38.816
Perhexilene	T46.3X1	T46.3X2	T46.3X3	T46.3X4	T46.3X5	T46.3X6
Perhexiline (maleate)	T46.3X1	T46.3X2	T46.3X3	T46.3X4	T46.3X5	T46.3X6
Periactin	T45.0X1	T45.0X2	T45.0X3	T45.0X4	T45.0X5	T45.0X6
Periciazine	T43.3X1	T43.3X2	T43.3X3	T43.3X4	T43.3X5	T43.3X6
Periclor	T42.6X1	T42.6X2	T42.6X3	T42.6X4	T42.6X5	T42.6X6
Perindopril	T46.4X1	T46.4X2	T46.4X3	T46.4X4	T46.4X5	T46.4X6
Perisoxal	T39.8X1	T39.8X2	T39.8X3	T39.8X4	T39.8X5	T39.8X6
Peritrate	T46.3X1	T46.3X2	T46.3X3	T46.3X4	T46.3X5	T46.3X6
Peritoneal dialysis solution	T50.3X1	T50.3X2	T50.3X3	T50.3X4	T50.3X5	T50.3X6
Perlapine	T42.4X1	T42.4X2	T42.4X3	T42.4X4	T42.4X5	T42.4X6
Permanganate	T65.891	T65.892	T65.893	T65.894	—	—
Permethrin	T60.1X1	T60.1X2	T60.1X3	T60.1X4	—	—
Pernocton	T42.3X1	T42.3X2	T42.3X3	T42.3X4	T42.3X5	T42.3X6
Pernoston	T42.3X1	T42.3X2	T42.3X3	T42.3X4	T42.3X5	T42.3X6
Peronine	T40.2X1	T40.2X2	T40.2X3	T40.2X4	—	—
Perphenazine	T43.3X1	T43.3X2	T43.3X3	T43.3X4	T43.3X5	T43.3X6

◀ New   ◀ Revised   ~~deleted~~ Deleted

TABLE OF DRUGS AND CHEMICALS

Substance	External Cause (T-Code)					
	Poisoning, Accidental (Unintentional)	Poisoning, Intentional Self-Harm	Poisoning, Assault	Poisoning, Undetermined	Adverse Effect	Underdosing
Pertofrane	T43.011	T43.012	T43.013	T43.014	T43.015	T43.016
Pertussis						
immune serum (human)	T50.Z11	T50.Z12	T50.Z13	T50.Z14	T50.Z15	T50.Z16
vaccine (with diphtheria toxoid) (with tetanus toxoid)	T50.A11	T50.A12	T50.A13	T50.A14	T50.A15	T50.A16
Peruvian balsam	T49.0X1	T49.0X2	T49.0X3	T49.0X4	T49.0X5	T49.0X6
Peruvoside	T46.0X1	T46.0X2	T46.0X3	T46.0X4	T46.0X5	T46.0X6
Pesticide (dust) (fumes) (vapor) NEC	T60.91	T60.92	T60.93	T60.94	—	—
arsenic	T57.0X1	T57.0X2	T57.0X3	T57.0X4	—	—
chlorinated	T60.1X1	T60.1X2	T60.1X3	T60.1X4	—	—
cyanide	T65.0X1	T65.0X2	T65.0X3	T65.0X4	—	—
kerosene	T52.0X1	T52.0X2	T52.0X3	T52.0X4	—	—
mixture (of compounds)	T60.91	T60.92	T60.93	T60.94	—	—
naphthalene	T60.2X1	T60.2X2	T60.2X3	T60.2X4	—	—
organochlorine (compounds)	T60.1X1	T60.1X2	T60.1X3	T60.1X4	—	—
petroleum (distillate) (products) NEC	T60.8X1	T60.8X2	T60.8X3	T60.8X4	—	—
specified ingredient NEC	T60.8X1	T60.8X2	T60.8X3	T60.8X4	—	—
strychnine	T65.1X1	T65.1X2	T65.1X3	T65.1X4	—	—
thallium	T60.4X1	T60.4X2	T60.4X3	T60.4X4	—	—
Pethidine	T40.4X1	T40.4X2	T40.4X3	T40.4X4	T40.4X5	T40.4X6
Petrichloral	T42.6X1	T42.6X2	T42.6X3	T42.6X4	T42.6X5	T42.6X6
Petrol	T52.0X1	T52.0X2	T52.0X3	T52.0X4	—	—
vapor	T52.0X1	T52.0X2	T52.0X3	T52.0X4	—	—
Petrolatum	T49.3X1	T49.3X2	T49.3X3	T49.3X4	T49.3X5	T49.3X6
hydrophilic	T49.3X1	T49.3X2	T49.3X3	T49.3X4	T49.3X5	T49.3X6
liquid	T47.4X1	T47.4X2	T47.4X3	T47.4X4	T47.4X5	T47.4X6
topical	T49.3X1	T49.3X2	T49.3X3	T49.3X4	T49.3X5	T49.3X6
nonmedicinal	T52.0X1	T52.0X2	T52.0X3	T52.0X4	—	—
red veterinary	T49.3X1	T49.3X2	T49.3X3	T49.3X4	T49.3X5	T49.3X6
white	T49.3X1	T49.3X2	T49.3X3	T49.3X4	T49.3X5	T49.3X6
Petroleum (products) NEC	T52.0X1	T52.0X2	T52.0X3	T52.0X4	—	—
benzine(s) — see Ligroin						
ether — see Ligroin						
jelly — see Petrolatum						
naphtha — see Ligroin						
pesticide	T60.8X1	T60.8X2	T60.8X3	T60.8X4		
solids	T52.0X1	T52.0X2	T52.0X3	T52.0X4	—	—
solvents	T52.0X1	T52.0X2	T52.0X3	T52.0X4	—	—
vapor	T52.0X1	T52.0X2	T52.0X3	T52.0X4	—	—
Peyote	T40.991	T40.992	T40.993	T40.994		—
Phanodorm, phanodorn	T42.3X1	T42.3X2	T42.3X3	T42.3X4	T42.3X5	T42.3X6

Substance	External Cause (T-Code)					
	Poisoning, Accidental (Unintentional)	Poisoning, Intentional Self-Harm	Poisoning, Assault	Poisoning, Undetermined	Adverse Effect	Underdosing
Phanquinone	T37.3X1	T37.3X2	T37.3X3	T37.3X4	T37.3X5	T37.3X6
Phanquone	T37.3X1	T37.3X2	T37.3X3	T37.3X4	T37.3X5	T37.3X6
Pharmaceutical						
adjunct NEC	T50.901	T50.902	T50.903	T50.904	T50.905	T50.906
excipient NEC	T50.901	T50.902	T50.903	T50.904	T50.905	T50.906
sweetener	T50.901	T50.902	T50.903	T50.904	T50.905	T50.906
viscous agent	T50.901	T50.902	T50.903	T50.904	T50.905	T50.906
Phemitone	T42.3X1	T42.3X2	T42.3X3	T42.3X4	T42.3X5	T42.3X6
Phenacaine	T41.3X1	T41.3X2	T41.3X3	T41.3X4	T41.3X5	T41.3X6
Phenacemide	T42.6X1	T42.6X2	T42.6X3	T42.6X4	T42.6X5	T42.6X6
Phenacetin	T39.1X1	T39.1X2	T39.1X3	T39.1X4	T39.1X5	T39.1X6
Phenadoxone	T40.2X1	T40.2X2	T40.2X3	T40.2X4	—	—
Phenaglycodol	T43.591	T43.592	T43.593	T43.594	T43.595	T43.596
Phenantoin	T42.0X1	T42.0X2	T42.0X3	T42.0X4	T42.0X5	T42.0X6
Phenaphthazine reagent	T50.991	T50.992	T50.993	T50.994	T50.995	T50.996
Phenazocine	T40.4X1	T40.4X2	T40.4X3	T40.4X4	T40.4X5	T40.4X6
Phenazone	T39.2X1	T39.2X2	T39.2X3	T39.2X4	T39.2X5	T39.2X6
Phenazopyridine	T39.8X1	T39.8X2	T39.8X3	T39.8X4	T39.8X5	T39.8X6
Phenbenicillin	T36.0X1	T36.0X2	T36.0X3	T36.0X4	T36.0X5	T36.0X6
Phenbutrazate	T50.5X1	T50.5X2	T50.5X3	T50.5X4	T50.5X5	T50.5X6
Phencyclidine	T40.991	T40.992	T40.993	T40.994	T40.995	T40.996
Phendimetrazine	T50.5X1	T50.5X2	T50.5X3	T50.5X4	T50.5X5	T50.5X6
Phenelzine	T43.1X1	T43.1X2	T43.1X3	T43.1X4	T43.1X5	T43.1X6
Phenemal	T42.3X1	T42.3X2	T42.3X3	T42.3X4	T42.3X5	T42.3X6
Phenergan	T42.6X1	T42.6X2	T42.6X3	T42.6X4	T42.6X5	T42.6X6
Pheneticillin	T36.0X1	T36.0X2	T36.0X3	T36.0X4	T36.0X5	T36.0X6
Pheneturide	T42.6X1	T42.6X2	T42.6X3	T42.6X4	T42.6X5	T42.6X6
Phenformin	T38.3X1	T38.3X2	T38.3X3	T38.3X4	T38.3X5	T38.3X6
Phenglutarimide	T44.3X1	T44.3X2	T44.3X3	T44.3X4	T44.3X5	T44.3X6
Phenicarbazide	T39.8X1	T39.8X2	T39.8X3	T39.8X4	T39.8X5	T39.8X6
Phenindamine	T45.0X1	T45.0X2	T45.0X3	T45.0X4	T45.0X5	T45.0X6
Phenindione	T45.511	T45.512	T45.513	T45.514	T45.515	T45.516
Pheniprazine	T43.1X1	T43.1X2	T43.1X3	T43.1X4	T43.1X5	T43.1X6
Pheniramine	T45.0X1	T45.0X2	T45.0X3	T45.0X4	T45.0X5	T45.0X6
Phenisatin	T47.2X1	T47.2X2	T47.2X3	T47.2X4	T47.2X5	T47.2X6
Phenmetrazine	T50.5X1	T50.5X2	T50.5X3	T50.5X4	T50.5X5	T50.5X6
Phenobal	T42.3X1	T42.3X2	T42.3X3	T42.3X4	T42.3X5	T42.3X6
Phenobarbital	T42.3X1	T42.3X2	T42.3X3	T42.3X4	T42.3X5	T42.3X6
with						
mephenytoin	T42.3X1	T42.3X2	T42.3X3	T42.3X4	T42.3X5	T42.3X6
phenytoin	T42.3X1	T42.3X2	T42.3X3	T42.3X4	T42.3X5	T42.3X6
sodium	T42.3X1	T42.3X2	T42.3X3	T42.3X4	T42.3X5	T42.3X6

◀ New ◀ Revised ~~deleted~~ Deleted

Substance	External Cause (T-Code)					
	Poisoning, Accidental (Unintentional)	Poisoning, Intentional Self-Harm	Poisoning, Assault	Poisoning, Undetermined	Adverse Effect	Underdosing
Phenobarbitone	T42.3X1	T42.3X2	T42.3X3	T42.3X4	T42.3X5	T42.3X6
Phenobutiodil	T50.8X1	T50.8X2	T50.8X3	T50.8X4	T50.8X5	T50.8X6
Phenoctide	T49.0X1	T49.0X2	T49.0X3	T49.0X4	T49.0X5	T49.0X6
Phenol	T49.0X1	T49.0X2	T49.0X3	T49.0X4	T49.0X5	T49.0X6
disinfectant	T54.0X1	T54.0X2	T54.0X3	T54.0X4	—	—
in oil injection	T46.8X1	T46.8X2	T46.8X3	T46.8X4	T46.8X5	T46.8X6
medicinal	T49.1X1	T49.1X2	T49.1X3	T49.1X4	T49.1X5	T49.1X6
nonmedicinal NEC	T54.0X1	T54.0X2	T54.0X3	T54.0X4	—	—
pesticide	T60.8X1	T60.8X2	T60.8X3	T60.8X4	—	—
red	T50.8X1	T50.8X2	T50.8X3	T50.8X4	T50.8X5	T50.8X6
Phenolic preparation	T49.1X1	T49.1X2	T49.1X3	T49.1X4	T49.1X5	T49.1X6
Phenolphthalein	T47.2X1	T47.2X2	T47.2X3	T47.2X4	T47.2X5	T47.2X6
Phenolsulfonphthalein	T50.8X1	T50.8X2	T50.8X3	T50.8X4	T50.8X5	T50.8X6
Phenomorphan	T40.2X1	T40.2X2	T40.2X3	T40.2X4	—	—
Phenonyl	T42.3X1	T42.3X2	T42.3X3	T42.3X4	T42.3X5	T42.3X6
Phenoperidine	T40.4X1	T40.4X2	T40.4X3	T40.4X4	—	—
Phenopyrazone	T46.991	T46.992	T46.993	T46.994	T46.995	T46.996
Phenoquin	T50.4X1	T50.4X2	T50.4X3	T50.4X4	T50.4X5	T50.4X6
Phenothiazine (psychotropic) NEC	T43.3X1	T43.3X2	T43.3X3	T43.3X4	T43.3X5	T43.3X6
insecticide	T60.2X1	T60.2X2	T60.2X3	T60.2X4	—	—
Phenothrin	T49.0X1	T49.0X2	T49.0X3	T49.0X4	T49.0X5	T49.0X6
Phenoxybenzamine	T46.7X1	T46.7X2	T46.7X3	T46.7X4	T46.7X5	T46.7X6
Phenoxyethanol	T49.0X1	T49.0X2	T49.0X3	T49.0X4	T49.0X5	T49.0X6
Phenoxymethyl penicillin	T36.0X1	T36.0X2	T36.0X3	T36.0X4	T36.0X5	T36.0X6
Phenprobamate	T42.8X1	T42.8X2	T42.8X3	T42.8X4	T42.8X5	T42.8X6
Phenprocoumon	T45.511	T45.512	T45.513	T45.514	T45.515	T45.516
Phensuximide	T42.2X1	T42.2X2	T42.2X3	T42.2X4	T42.2X5	T42.2X6
Phentermine	T50.5X1	T50.5X2	T50.5X3	T50.5X4	T50.5X5	T50.5X6
Phenthicillin	T36.0X1	T36.0X2	T36.0X3	T36.0X4	T36.0X5	T36.0X6
Phentolamine	T46.7X1	T46.7X2	T46.7X3	T46.7X4	T46.7X5	T46.7X6
Phenyl						
butazone	T39.2X1	T39.2X2	T39.2X3	T39.2X4	T39.2X5	T39.2X6
enediamine	T65.3X1	T65.3X2	T65.3X3	T65.3X4	—	—
hydrazine	T65.3X1	T65.3X2	T65.3X3	T65.3X4	—	—
antineoplastic	T45.1X1	T45.1X2	T45.1X3	T45.1X4	T45.1X5	T45.1X6
mercuric compounds — see Mercury						
salicylate	T49.3X1	T49.3X2	T49.3X3	T49.3X4	T49.3X5	T49.3X6
Phenylalanine mustard	T45.1X1	T45.1X2	T45.1X3	T45.1X4	T45.1X5	T45.1X6
Phenylbutazone	T39.2X1	T39.2X2	T39.2X3	T39.2X4	T39.2X5	T39.2X6
Phenylenediamine	T65.3X1	T65.3X2	T65.3X3	T65.3X4	—	—
Phenylephrine	T44.4X1	T44.4X2	T44.4X3	T44.4X4	T44.4X5	T44.4X6

Substance	External Cause (T-Code)					
	Poisoning, Accidental (Unintentional)	Poisoning, Intentional Self-Harm	Poisoning, Assault	Poisoning, Undetermined	Adverse Effect	Underdosing
Phenylethylbiguanide	T38.3X1	T38.3X2	T38.3X3	T38.3X4	T38.3X5	T38.3X6
Phenylmercuric						
acetate	T49.0X1	T49.0X2	T49.0X3	T49.0X4	T49.0X5	T49.0X6
borate	T49.0X1	T49.0X2	T49.0X3	T49.0X4	T49.0X5	T49.0X6
nitrate	T49.0X1	T49.0X2	T49.0X3	T49.0X4	T49.0X5	T49.0X6
Phenylmethylbarbitone	T42.3X1	T42.3X2	T42.3X3	T42.3X4	T42.3X5	T42.3X6
Phenylpropanol	T47.5X1	T47.5X2	T47.5X3	T47.5X4	T47.5X5	T47.5X6
Phenylpropanolamine	T44.991	T44.992	T44.993	T44.994	T44.995	T44.996
Phenylsulfthion	T60.0X1	T60.0X2	T60.0X3	T60.0X4	—	—
Phenyltoloxamine	T45.0X1	T45.0X2	T45.0X3	T45.0X4	T45.0X5	T45.0X6
Phenyramidol, phenyramidon	T39.8X1	T39.8X2	T39.8X3	T39.8X4	T39.8X5	T39.8X6
Phenytoin	T42.0X1	T42.0X2	T42.0X3	T42.0X4	T42.0X5	T42.0X6
with Phenobarbital	T42.3X1	T42.3X2	T42.3X3	T42.3X4	T42.3X5	T42.3X6
pHisoHex	T49.2X1	T49.2X2	T49.2X3	T49.2X4	T49.2X5	T49.2X6
Pholcodine	T48.3X1	T48.3X2	T48.3X3	T48.3X4	T48.3X5	T48.3X6
Pholedrine	T46.991	T46.992	T46.993	T46.994	T46.995	T46.996
Phorate	T60.0X1	T60.0X2	T60.0X3	T60.0X4	—	—
Phosdrin	T60.0X1	T60.0X2	T60.0X3	T60.0X4	—	—
Phosfolan	T60.0X1	T60.0X2	T60.0X3	T60.0X4	—	—
Phosgene (gas)	T59.891	T59.892	T59.893	T59.894	—	—
Phosphamidon	T60.0X1	T60.0X2	T60.0X3	T60.0X4	—	—
Phosphate	T65.891	T65.892	T65.893	T65.894	—	—
laxative	T47.4X1	T47.4X2	T47.4X3	T47.4X4	T47.4X5	T47.4X6
organic	T60.0X1	T60.0X2	T60.0X3	T60.0X4	—	—
solvent	T52.91	T52.92	T52.93	T52.94	—	—
tricresyl	T65.891	T65.892	T65.893	T65.894	—	—
Phosphine	T57.1X1	T57.1X2	T57.1X3	T57.1X4	—	—
fumigant	T57.1X1	T57.1X2	T57.1X3	T57.1X4	—	—
Pholpholine	T49.5X1	T49.5X2	T49.5X3	T49.5X4	T49.5X5	T49.5X6
Phosphoric acid	T54.2X1	T54.2X2	T54.2X3	T54.2X4	—	—
Phosphorus (compound) NEC	T57.1X1	T57.1X2	T57.1X3	T57.1X4	—	—
pesticide	T60.0X1	T60.0X2	T60.0X3	T60.0X4	—	—
Phthalates	T65.891	T65.892	T65.893	T65.894	—	—
Phthalic anhydride	T65.891	T65.892	T65.893	T65.894	—	—
Phthalimidoglutarimide	T42.6X1	T42.6X2	T42.6X3	T42.6X4	T42.6X5	T42.6X6
Phthalylsulfathiazole	T37.0X1	T37.0X2	T37.0X3	T37.0X4	T37.0X5	T37.0X6
Phylloquinone	T45.7X1	T45.7X2	T45.7X3	T45.7X4	T45.7X5	T45.7X6
Physeptone	T40.3X1	T40.3X2	T40.3X3	T40.3X4	T40.3X5	T40.3X6
Physostigma venenosum	T62.2X1	T62.2X2	T62.2X3	T62.2X4	—	—
Physostigmine	T49.5X1	T49.5X2	T49.5X3	T49.5X4	T49.5X5	T49.5X6
Phytolacca decandra	T62.2X1	T62.2X2	T62.2X3	T62.2X4	—	—
berries	T62.1X1	T62.1X2	T62.1X3	T62.1X4	—	—

TABLE OF DRUGS AND CHEMICALS

Substance	Poisoning, Accidental (Unintentional)	Poisoning, Intentional Self-Harm	Poisoning, Assault	Poisoning, Undetermined	Adverse Effect	Underdosing
Phytomenadione	T45.7X1	T45.7X2	T45.7X3	T45.7X4	T45.7X5	T45.7X6
Phytonadione	T45.7X1	T45.7X2	T45.7X3	T45.7X4	T45.7X5	T45.7X6
Picoperine	T48.3X1	T48.3X2	T48.3X3	T48.3X4	T48.3X5	T48.3X6
Picosulfate (sodium)	T47.2X1	T47.2X2	T47.2X3	T47.2X4	T47.2X5	T47.2X6
Picric (acid)	T54.2X1	T54.2X2	T54.2X3	T54.2X4	—	—
Picrotoxin	T50.7X1	T50.7X2	T50.7X3	T50.7X4	T50.7X5	T50.7X6
Piketoprofen	T49.0X1	T49.0X2	T49.0X3	T49.0X4	T49.0X5	T49.0X6
Pilocarpine	T44.1X1	T44.1X2	T44.1X3	T44.1X4	T44.1X5	T44.1X6
Pilocarpus (jaborandi) extract	T44.1X1	T44.1X2	T44.1X3	T44.1X4	T44.1X5	T44.1X6
Pilsicainide (hydrochloride)	T46.2X1	T46.2X2	T46.2X3	T46.2X4	T46.2X5	T46.2X6
Pimaricin	T36.7X1	T36.7X2	T36.7X3	T36.7X4	T36.7X5	T36.7X6
Pimeclone	T50.7X1	T50.7X2	T50.7X3	T50.7X4	T50.7X5	T50.7X6
Pimelic ketone	T52.8X1	T52.8X2	T52.8X3	T52.8X4	—	—
Pimethixene	T45.0X1	T45.0X2	T45.0X3	T45.0X4	T45.0X5	T45.0X6
Piminodine	T40.2X1	T40.2X2	T40.2X3	T40.2X4	T40.2X5	T40.2X6
Pimozide	T43.591	T43.592	T43.593	T43.594	T43.595	T43.596
Pinacidil	T46.5X1	T46.5X2	T46.5X3	T46.5X4	T46.5X5	T46.5X6
Pinaverium bromide	T44.3X1	T44.3X2	T44.3X3	T44.3X4	T44.3X5	T44.3X6
Pinazepam	T42.4X1	T42.4X2	T42.4X3	T42.4X4	T42.4X5	T42.4X6
Pindolol	T44.7X1	T44.7X2	T44.7X3	T44.7X4	T44.7X5	T44.7X6
Pindone	T60.4X1	T60.4X2	T60.4X3	T60.4X4	—	—
Pine oil (disinfectant)	T65.891	T65.892	T65.893	T65.894	—	—
Pinkroot	T37.4X1	T37.4X2	T37.4X3	T37.4X4	T37.4X5	T37.4X6
Pipadone	T40.2X1	T40.2X2	T40.2X3	T40.2X4	—	—
Pipamazine	T45.0X1	T45.0X2	T45.0X3	T45.0X4	T45.0X5	T45.0X6
Pipamperone	T43.4X1	T43.4X2	T43.4X3	T43.4X4	T43.4X5	T43.4X6
Pipazetate	T48.3X1	T48.3X2	T48.3X3	T48.3X4	T48.3X5	T48.3X6
Pipemidic acid	T37.8X1	T37.8X2	T37.8X3	T37.8X4	T37.8X5	T37.8X6
Pipenzolate bromide	T44.3X1	T44.3X2	T44.3X3	T44.3X4	T44.3X5	T44.3X6
Piperacetazine	T43.3X1	T43.3X2	T43.3X3	T43.3X4	T43.3X5	T43.3X6
Piperacillin	T36.0X1	T36.0X2	T36.0X3	T36.0X4	T36.0X5	T36.0X6
Piperazine	T37.4X1	T37.4X2	T37.4X3	T37.4X4	T37.4X5	T37.4X6
estrone sulfate	T38.5X1	T38.5X2	T38.5X3	T38.5X4	T38.5X5	T38.5X6
Piper cubeba	T62.2X1	T62.2X2	T62.2X3	T62.2X4	—	—
Piperidione	T48.3X1	T48.3X2	T48.3X3	T48.3X4	—	—
Piperidolate	T44.3X1	T44.3X2	T44.3X3	T44.3X4	T44.3X5	T44.3X6
Piperocaine	T41.3X1	T41.3X2	T41.3X3	T41.3X4	T41.3X5	T41.3X6
infiltration (subcutaneous)	T41.3X1	T41.3X2	T41.3X3	T41.3X4	T41.3X5	T41.3X6
nerve block (peripheral) (plexus)	T41.3X1	T41.3X2	T41.3X3	T41.3X4	T41.3X5	T41.3X6
topical (surface)	T41.3X1	T41.3X2	T41.3X3	T41.3X4	T41.3X5	T41.3X6
Piperonyl butoxide	T60.8X1	T60.8X2	T60.8X3	T60.8X4	—	—
Pipethanate	T44.3X1	T44.3X2	T44.3X3	T44.3X4	T44.3X5	T44.3X6

Substance	Poisoning, Accidental (Unintentional)	Poisoning, Intentional Self-Harm	Poisoning, Assault	Poisoning, Undetermined	Adverse Effect	Underdosing
Pipobroman	T45.1X1	T45.1X2	T45.1X3	T45.1X4	T45.1X5	T45.1X6
Pipofezine	T43.0X1	T43.0X2	T43.0X3	T43.0X4	T43.0X5	T43.0X6
Pipotiazine	T43.3X1	T43.3X2	T43.3X3	T43.3X4	T43.3X5	T43.3X6
Pipoxizine	T45.0X1	T45.0X2	T45.0X3	T45.0X4	T45.0X5	T45.0X6
Pipradrol	T43.691	T43.692	T43.693	T43.694	T43.695	T43.696
Piprinhydrinate	T45.0X1	T45.0X2	T45.0X3	T45.0X4	T45.0X5	T45.0X6
Pirarubicin	T45.1X1	T45.1X2	T45.1X3	T45.1X4	T45.1X5	T45.1X6
Pirazinamide	T37.1X1	T37.1X2	T37.1X3	T37.1X4	T37.1X5	T37.1X6
Pirbuterol	T48.6X1	T48.6X2	T48.6X3	T48.6X4	T48.6X5	T48.6X6
Pirenzepine	T47.1X1	T47.1X2	T47.1X3	T47.1X4	T47.1X5	T47.1X6
Piretanide	T50.1X1	T50.1X2	T50.1X3	T50.1X4	T50.1X5	T50.1X6
Piribedil	T42.8X1	T42.8X2	T42.8X3	T42.8X4	T42.8X5	T42.8X6
Piridoxilate	T46.3X1	T46.3X2	T46.3X3	T46.3X4	T46.3X5	T46.3X6
Piritramide	T40.4X1	T40.4X2	T40.4X3	T40.4X4	—	—
Pirlindole	T43.0X1	T43.0X2	T43.0X3	T43.0X4	T43.0X5	T43.0X6
Piromidic acid	T37.8X1	T37.8X2	T37.8X3	T37.8X4	T37.8X5	T37.8X6
Piroxicam	T39.391	T39.392	T39.393	T39.394	T39.395	T39.396
beta-cyclodextrin complex	T39.8X1	T39.8X2	T39.8X3	T39.8X4	T39.8X5	T39.8X6
Pirozadil	T46.6X1	T46.6X2	T46.6X3	T46.6X4	T46.6X5	T46.6X6
Piscidia (bark) (erythrina)	T39.8X1	T39.8X2	T39.8X3	T39.8X4	T39.8X5	T39.8X6
Pitch	T65.891	T65.892	T65.893	T65.894	—	—
Pitkin's solution	T41.3X1	T41.3X2	T41.3X3	T41.3X4	T41.3X5	T41.3X6
Pitocin	T48.0X1	T48.0X2	T48.0X3	T48.0X4	T48.0X5	T48.0X6
Pitressin (tannate)	T38.891	T38.892	T38.893	T38.894	T38.895	T38.896
Pituitary extracts (posterior)	T38.891	T38.892	T38.893	T38.894	T38.895	T38.896
anterior	T38.811	T38.812	T38.813	T38.814	T38.815	T38.816
Pituitrin	T38.891	T38.892	T38.893	T38.894	T38.895	T38.896
Pivampicillin	T36.0X1	T36.0X2	T36.0X3	T36.0X4	T36.0X5	T36.0X6
Pivmecillinam	T36.0X1	T36.0X2	T36.0X3	T36.0X4	T36.0X5	T36.0X6
Placental hormone	T38.891	T38.892	T38.893	T38.894	T38.895	T38.896
Placidyl	T42.6X1	T42.6X2	T42.6X3	T42.6X4	T42.6X5	T42.6X6
Plague vaccine	T50.A91	T50.A92	T50.A93	T50.A94	T50.A95	T50.A96
Plant						
food or fertilizer NEC	T65.891	T65.892	T65.893	T65.894	—	—
containing herbicide	T60.3X1	T60.3X2	T60.3X3	T60.3X4	—	—
noxious, used as food	T62.2X1	T62.2X2	T62.2X3	T62.2X4	—	—
berries	T62.1X1	T62.1X2	T62.1X3	T62.1X4	—	—
seeds	T62.2X1	T62.2X2	T62.2X3	T62.2X4	—	—
specified type NEC	T62.2X1	T62.2X2	T62.2X3	T62.2X4	—	—
Plasma	T45.8X1	T45.8X2	T45.8X3	T45.8X4	T45.8X5	T45.8X6
expander NEC	T45.8X1	T45.8X2	T45.8X3	T45.8X4	T45.8X5	T45.8X6
protein fraction (human)	T45.8X1	T45.8X2	T45.8X3	T45.8X4	T45.8X5	T45.8X6

◀ New ◀ Revised ~~deleted~~ Deleted

Substance	External Cause (T-Code)					
	Poisoning, Accidental (Unintentional)	Poisoning, Intentional Self-Harm	Poisoning, Assault	Poisoning, Undetermined	Adverse Effect	Underdosing
Plasmanate	T45.8X1	T45.8X2	T45.8X3	T45.8X4	T45.8X5	T45.8X6
Plasminogen (tissue) activator	T45.611	T45.612	T45.613	T45.614	T45.615	T45.616
Plaster dressing	T49.3X1	T49.3X2	T49.3X3	T49.3X4	T49.3X5	T49.3X6
Plastic dressing	T49.3X1	T49.3X2	T49.3X3	T49.3X4	T49.3X5	T49.3X6
Plegicil	T43.3X1	T43.3X2	T43.3X3	T43.3X4	T43.3X5	T43.3X6
Plicamycin	T45.1X1	T45.1X2	T45.1X3	T45.1X4	T45.1X5	T45.1X6
Podophyllotoxin	T49.8X1	T49.8X2	T49.8X3	T49.8X4	T49.8X5	T49.8X6
Podophyllum (resin)	T49.4X1	T49.4X2	T49.4X3	T49.4X4	T49.4X5	T49.4X6
Poison NEC	T65.91	T65.92	T65.93	T65.94	—	—
Poisonous berries	T62.1X1	T62.1X2	T62.1X3	T62.1X4	—	—
Pokeweed (any part)	T62.2X1	T62.2X2	T62.2X3	T62.2X4	—	—
Poldine metilsulfate	T44.3X1	T44.3X2	T44.3X3	T44.3X4	T44.3X5	T44.3X6
Polidexide (sulfate)	T46.6X1	T46.6X2	T46.6X3	T46.6X4	T46.6X5	T46.6X6
Polidocanol	T46.8X1	T46.8X2	T46.8X3	T46.8X4	T46.8X5	T46.8X6
Poliomyelitis vaccine	T50.B91	T50.B92	T50.B93	T50.B94	T50.B95	T50.B96
Polish (car) (floor) (furniture) (metal) (porcelain) (silver)	T65.891	T65.892	T65.893	T65.894	—	—
abrasive	T65.891	T65.892	T65.893	T65.894	—	—
porcelain	T65.891	T65.892	T65.893	T65.894	—	—
Poloxalkol	T47.4X1	T47.4X2	T47.4X3	T47.4X4	T47.4X5	T47.4X6
Poloxamer	T47.4X1	T47.4X2	T47.4X3	T47.4X4	T47.4X5	T47.4X6
Polyaminostyrene resins	T50.3X1	T50.3X2	T50.3X3	T50.3X4	T50.3X5	T50.3X6
Polycarbophil	T47.4X1	T47.4X2	T47.4X3	T47.4X4	T47.4X5	T47.4X6
Polychlorinated biphenyl	T65.891	T65.892	T65.893	T65.894	—	—
Polycycline	T36.4X1	T36.4X2	T36.4X3	T36.4X4	T36.4X5	T36.4X6
Polyester fumes	T59.891	T59.892	T59.893	T59.894	—	—
Polyester resin hardener	T52.91	T52.92	T52.93	T52.94	—	—
fumes	T59.891	T59.892	T59.893	T59.894	—	—
Polyestradiol phosphate	T38.5X1	T38.5X2	T38.5X3	T38.5X4	T38.5X5	T38.5X6
Polyethanolamine alkyl sulfate	T49.2X1	T49.2X2	T49.2X3	T49.2X4	T49.2X5	T49.2X6
Polyethylene adhesive	T49.3X1	T49.3X2	T49.3X3	T49.3X4	T49.3X5	T49.3X6
Polyferose	T45.4X1	T45.4X2	T45.4X3	T45.4X4	T45.4X5	T45.4X6
Polygeline	T45.8X1	T45.8X2	T45.8X3	T45.8X4	T45.8X5	T45.8X6
Polymyxin	T36.8X1	T36.8X2	T36.8X3	T36.8X4	T36.8X5	T36.8X6
B	T36.8X1	T36.8X2	T36.8X3	T36.8X4	T36.8X5	T36.8X6
ENT agent	T49.6X1	T49.6X2	T49.6X3	T49.6X4	T49.6X5	T49.6X6
ophthalmic preparation	T49.5X1	T49.5X2	T49.5X3	T49.5X4	T49.5X5	T49.5X6
topical NEC	T49.0X1	T49.0X2	T49.0X3	T49.0X4	T49.0X5	T49.0X6
E sulfate (eye preparation)	T49.5X1	T49.5X2	T49.5X3	T49.5X4	T49.5X5	T49.5X6
Polynoxylin	T49.0X1	T49.0X2	T49.0X3	T49.0X4	T49.0X5	T49.0X6
Polyoestradiol phosphate	T38.5X1	T38.5X2	T38.5X3	T38.5X4	T38.5X5	T38.5X6
Polyoxymethyleneurea	T49.0X1	T49.0X2	T49.0X3	T49.0X4	T49.0X5	T49.0X6

Substance	External Cause (T-Code)					
	Poisoning, Accidental (Unintentional)	Poisoning, Intentional Self-Harm	Poisoning, Assault	Poisoning, Undetermined	Adverse Effect	Underdosing
Polysilane	T47.8X1	T47.8X2	T47.8X3	T47.8X4	T47.8X5	T47.8X6
Polytetrafluoroethylene (inhaled)	T59.891	T59.892	T59.893	T59.894	—	—
Polythiazide	T50.2X1	T50.2X2	T50.2X3	T50.2X4	T50.2X5	T50.2X6
Polyvidone	T45.8X1	T45.8X2	T45.8X3	T45.8X4	T45.8X5	T45.8X6
Polyvinylpyrrolidone	T45.8X1	T45.8X2	T45.8X3	T45.8X4	T45.8X5	T45.8X6
Pontocaine (hydrochloride) (infiltration) (topical)	T41.3X1	T41.3X2	T41.3X3	T41.3X4	T41.3X5	T41.3X6
nerve block (peripheral) (plexus)	T41.3X1	T41.3X2	T41.3X3	T41.3X4	T41.3X5	T41.3X6
spinal	T41.3X1	T41.3X2	T41.3X3	T41.3X4	T41.3X5	T41.3X6
Porfiromycin	T45.1X1	T45.1X2	T45.1X3	T45.1X4	T45.1X5	T45.1X6
Posterior pituitary hormone NEC	T38.891	T38.892	T38.893	T38.894	T38.895	T38.896
Pot	T40.7X1	T40.7X2	T40.7X3	T40.7X4	T40.7X5	T40.7X6
Potash (caustic)	T54.3X1	T54.3X2	T54.3X3	T54.3X4	—	—
Potassic saline injection (lactated)	T50.3X1	T50.3X2	T50.3X3	T50.3X4	T50.3X5	T50.3X6
Potassium (salts) NEC	T50.3X1	T50.3X2	T50.3X3	T50.3X4	T50.3X5	T50.3X6
aminobenzoate	T45.8X1	T45.8X2	T45.8X3	T45.8X4	T45.8X5	T45.8X6
aminosalicylate	T37.1X1	T37.1X2	T37.1X3	T37.1X4	T37.1X5	T37.1X6
antimony 'tartrate'	T37.8X1	T37.8X2	T37.8X3	T37.8X4	T37.8X5	T37.8X6
arsenite (solution)	T57.0X1	T57.0X2	T57.0X3	T57.0X4	—	—
bichromate	T56.2X1	T56.2X2	T56.2X3	T56.2X4	—	—
bisulfate	T47.3X1	T47.3X2	T47.3X3	T47.3X4	T47.3X5	T47.3X6
bromide	T42.6X1	T42.6X2	T42.6X3	T42.6X4	T42.6X5	T42.6X6
canrenoate	T50.0X1	T50.0X2	T50.0X3	T50.0X4	T50.0X5	T50.0X6
carbonate	T54.3X1	T54.3X2	T54.3X3	T54.3X4	—	—
chlorate NEC	T65.891	T65.892	T65.893	T65.894	—	—
chloride	T50.3X1	T50.3X2	T50.3X3	T50.3X4	T50.3X5	T50.3X6
citrate	T50.991	T50.992	T50.993	T50.994	T50.995	T50.996
cyanide	T65.0X1	T65.0X2	T65.0X3	T65.0X4	—	—
ferric hexacyanoferrate (medicinal)	T50.6X1	T50.6X2	T50.6X3	T50.6X4	T50.6X5	T50.6X6
nonmedicinal	T65.891	T65.892	T65.893	T65.894	—	—
Fluoride	T57.8X1	T57.8X2	T57.8X3	T57.8X4	—	—
glucaldrate	T47.1X1	T47.1X2	T47.1X3	T47.1X4	T47.1X5	T47.1X6
hydroxide	T54.3X1	T54.3X2	T54.3X3	T54.3X4	—	—
iodate	T49.0X1	T49.0X2	T49.0X3	T49.0X4	T49.0X5	T49.0X6
iodide	T48.4X1	T48.4X2	T48.4X3	T48.4X4	T48.4X5	T48.4X6
nitrate	T57.8X1	T57.8X2	T57.8X3	T57.8X4	—	—
oxalate	T65.891	T65.892	T65.893	T65.894	—	—
perchlorate (nonmedicinal) NEC	T65.891	T65.892	T65.893	T65.894	—	—
antithyroid	T38.2X1	T38.2X2	T38.2X3	T38.2X4	T38.2X5	T38.2X6
medicinal	T38.2X1	T38.2X2	T38.2X3	T38.2X4	T38.2X5	T38.2X6

◀ New ◀ Revised ~~deleted~~ Deleted

TABLE OF DRUGS AND CHEMICALS

Substance	External Cause (T-Code)					
	Poisoning, Accidental (Unintentional)	Poisoning, Intentional Self-Harm	Poisoning, Assault	Poisoning, Undetermined	Adverse Effect	Underdosing
Permanganate (nonmedicinal)	T65.891	T65.892	T65.893	T65.894	—	—
medicinal	T49.0X1	T49.0X2	T49.0X3	T49.0X4	T49.0X5	T49.0X6
sulfate	T47.2X1	T47.2X2	T47.2X3	T47.2X4	T47.2X5	T47.2X6
Potassium-removing resin	T50.3X1	T50.3X2	T50.3X3	T50.3X4	T50.3X5	T50.3X6
Potassium-retaining drug	T50.3X1	T50.3X2	T50.3X3	T50.3X4	T50.3X5	T50.3X6
Povidone	T45.8X1	T45.8X2	T45.8X3	T45.8X4	T45.8X5	T45.8X6
iodine	T49.0X1	T49.0X2	T49.0X3	T49.0X4	T49.0X5	T49.0X6
Practolol	T44.7X1	T44.7X2	T44.7X3	T44.7X4	T44.7X5	T44.7X6
Prajmalium bitartrate	T46.2X1	T46.2X2	T46.2X3	T46.2X4	T46.2X5	T46.2X6
Pralidoxime (iodide)	T50.6X1	T50.6X2	T50.6X3	T50.6X4	T50.6X5	T50.6X6
chloride	T50.6X1	T50.6X2	T50.6X3	T50.6X4	T50.6X5	T50.6X6
Pramiverine	T44.3X1	T44.3X2	T44.3X3	T44.3X4	T44.3X5	T44.3X6
Pramocaine	T49.1X1	T49.1X2	T49.1X3	T49.1X4	T49.1X5	T49.1X6
Pramoxine	T49.1X1	T49.1X2	T49.1X3	T49.1X4	T49.1X5	T49.1X6
Prasterone	T38.7X1	T38.7X2	T38.7X3	T38.7X4	T38.7X5	T38.7X6
Pravastatin	T46.6X1	T46.6X2	T46.6X3	T46.6X4	T46.6X5	T46.6X6
Prazepam	T42.4X1	T42.4X2	T42.4X3	T42.4X4	T42.4X5	T42.4X6
Praziquantel	T37.4X1	T37.4X2	T37.4X3	T37.4X4	T37.4X5	T37.4X6
Prazitone	T43.291	T43.292	T43.293	T43.294	T43.295	T43.296
Prazosin	T44.6X1	T44.6X2	T44.6X3	T44.6X4	T44.6X5	T44.6X6
Prednicarbate	T49.0X1	T49.0X2	T49.0X3	T49.0X4	T49.0X5	T49.0X6
Prednimustine	T45.1X1	T45.1X2	T45.1X3	T45.1X4	T45.1X5	T45.1X6
Prednisolone	T38.0X1	T38.0X2	T38.0X3	T38.0X4	T38.0X5	T38.0X6
ENT agent	T49.6X1	T49.6X2	T49.6X3	T49.6X4	T49.6X5	T49.6X6
ophthalmic preparation	T49.5X1	T49.5X2	T49.5X3	T49.5X4	T49.5X5	T49.5X6
steaglate	T49.0X1	T49.0X2	T49.0X3	T49.0X4	T49.0X5	T49.0X6
topical NEC	T49.0X1	T49.0X2	T49.0X3	T49.0X4	T49.0X5	T49.0X6
Prednisone	T38.0X1	T38.0X2	T38.0X3	T38.0X4	T38.0X5	T38.0X6
Prednylidene	T38.0X1	T38.0X2	T38.0X3	T38.0X4	T38.0X5	T38.0X6
Pregnandiol	T38.5X1	T38.5X2	T38.5X3	T38.5X4	T38.5X5	T38.5X6
Pregneninolone	T38.5X1	T38.5X2	T38.5X3	T38.5X4	T38.5X5	T38.5X6
Preludin	T43.691	T43.692	T43.693	T43.694	T43.695	T43.696
Premarin	T38.5X1	T38.5X2	T38.5X3	T38.5X4	T38.5X5	T38.5X6
Premedication anesthetic	T41.201	T41.202	T41.203	T41.204	T41.205	T41.206
Prenalterol	T44.5X1	T44.5X2	T44.5X3	T44.5X4	T44.5X5	T44.5X6
Prenoxdiazine	T48.3X1	T48.3X2	T48.3X3	T48.3X4	T48.3X5	T48.3X6
Prenylamine	T46.3X1	T46.3X2	T46.3X3	T46.3X4	T46.3X5	T46.3X6
Preparation, local	T49.4X1	T49.4X2	T49.4X3	T49.4X4	T49.4X5	T49.4X6
Preparation H	T49.8X1	T49.8X2	T49.8X3	T49.8X4	T49.8X5	T49.8X6
Preservative (nonmedicinal)	T65.891	T65.892	T65.893	T65.894	—	—
medicinal	T50.901	T50.902	T50.903	T50.904	T50.905	T50.906
wood	T60.91	T60.92	T60.93	T60.94		—

Substance	External Cause (T-Code)					
	Poisoning, Accidental (Unintentional)	Poisoning, Intentional Self-Harm	Poisoning, Assault	Poisoning, Undetermined	Adverse Effect	Underdosing
Prethcamide	T50.7X1	T50.7X2	T50.7X3	T50.7X4	T50.7X5	T50.7X6
Pride of China	T62.2X1	T62.2X2	T62.2X3	T62.2X4	—	—
Pridinol	T44.3X1	T44.3X2	T44.3X3	T44.3X4	T44.3X5	T44.3X6
Prifinium bromide	T44.3X1	T44.3X2	T44.3X3	T44.3X4	T44.3X5	T44.3X6
Prilocaine	T41.3X1	T41.3X2	T41.3X3	T41.3X4	T41.3X5	T41.3X6
infiltration (subcutaneous)	T41.3X1	T41.3X2	T41.3X3	T41.3X4	T41.3X5	T41.3X6
nerve block (peripheral) (plexus)	T41.3X1	T41.3X2	T41.3X3	T41.3X4	T41.3X5	T41.3X6
regional	T41.3X1	T41.3X2	T41.3X3	T41.3X4	T41.3X5	T41.3X6
Primaquine	T37.2X1	T37.2X2	T37.2X3	T37.2X4	T37.2X5	T37.2X6
Primidone	T42.6X1	T42.6X2	T42.6X3	T42.6X4	T42.6X5	T42.6X6
Primula (veris)	T62.2X1	T62.2X2	T62.2X3	T62.2X4	—	—
Prinadol	T40.2X1	T40.2X2	T40.2X3	T40.2X4	T40.2X5	T40.2X6
Priscol, Priscoline	T44.6X1	T44.6X2	T44.6X3	T44.6X4	T44.6X5	T44.6X6
Pristinamycin	T36.3X1	T36.3X2	T36.3X3	T36.3X4	T36.3X5	T36.3X6
Privet	T62.2X1	T62.2X2	T62.2X3	T62.2X4	—	—
berries	T62.1X1	T62.1X2	T62.1X3	T62.1X4	—	—
Privine	T44.4X1	T44.4X2	T44.4X3	T44.4X4	T44.4X5	T44.4X6
Pro-Banthine	T44.3X1	T44.3X2	T44.3X3	T44.3X4	T44.3X5	T44.3X6
Probarbital	T42.3X1	T42.3X2	T42.3X3	T42.3X4	T42.3X5	T42.3X6
Probenecid	T50.4X1	T50.4X2	T50.4X3	T50.4X4	T50.4X5	T50.4X6
Probucol	T46.6X1	T46.6X2	T46.6X3	T46.6X4	T46.6X5	T46.6X6
Procainamide	T46.2X1	T46.2X2	T46.2X3	T46.2X4	T46.2X5	T46.2X6
Procaine	T41.3X1	T41.3X2	T41.3X3	T41.3X4	T41.3X5	T41.3X6
benzylpenicillin	T36.0X1	T36.0X2	T36.0X3	T36.0X4	T36.0X5	T36.0X6
nerve block (periphreal) (plexus)	T41.3X1	T41.3X2	T41.3X3	T41.3X4	T41.3X5	T41.3X6
penicillin G	T36.0X1	T36.0X2	T36.0X3	T36.0X4	T36.0X5	T36.0X6
regional	T41.3X1	T41.3X2	T41.3X3	T41.3X4	T41.3X5	T41.3X6
spinal	T41.3X1	T41.3X2	T41.3X3	T41.3X4	T41.3X5	T41.3X6
Procalmidol	T43.591	T43.592	T43.593	T43.594	T43.595	T43.596
Procarbazine	T45.1X1	T45.1X2	T45.1X3	T45.1X4	T45.1X5	T45.1X6
Procaterol	T44.5X1	T44.5X2	T44.5X3	T44.5X4	T44.5X5	T44.5X6
Prochlorperazine	T43.3X1	T43.3X2	T43.3X3	T43.3X4	T43.3X5	T43.3X6
Procyclidine	T44.3X1	T44.3X2	T44.3X3	T44.3X4	T44.3X5	T44.3X6
Producer gas	T58.8X1	T58.8X2	T58.8X3	T58.8X4	—	—
Profadol	T40.4X1	T40.4X2	T40.4X3	T40.4X4	T40.4X5	T40.4X6
Profenamine	T44.3X1	T44.3X2	T44.3X3	T44.3X4	T44.3X5	T44.3X6
Profenil	T44.3X1	T44.3X2	T44.3X3	T44.3X4	T44.3X5	T44.3X6
Proflavine	T49.0X1	T49.0X2	T49.0X3	T49.0X4	T49.0X5	T49.0X6
Progabide	T42.6X1	T42.6X2	T42.6X3	T42.6X4	T42.6X5	T42.6X6
Progestin	T38.5X1	T38.5X2	T38.5X3	T38.5X4	T38.5X5	T38.5X6
oral contraceptive	T38.4X1	T38.4X2	T38.4X3	T38.4X4	T38.4X5	T38.4X6

◀ New ◀ Revised ~~deleted~~ Deleted

Substance	Poisoning, Accidental (Unintentional)	Poisoning, Intentional Self-Harm	Poisoning, Assault	Poisoning, Undetermined	Adverse Effect	Underdosing
Progesterone	T38.5X1	T38.5X2	T38.5X3	T38.5X4	T38.5X5	T38.5X6
Progestogen NEC	T38.5X1	T38.5X2	T38.5X3	T38.5X4	T38.5X5	T38.5X6
Progestone	T38.5X1	T38.5X2	T38.5X3	T38.5X4	T38.5X5	T38.5X6
Proglumide	T47.1X1	T47.1X2	T47.1X3	T47.1X4	T47.1X5	T47.1X6
Proguanil	T37.2X1	T37.2X2	T37.2X3	T37.2X4	T37.2X5	T37.2X6
Prolactin	T38.811	T38.812	T38.813	T38.814	T38.815	T38.816
Prolintane	T43.691	T43.692	T43.693	T43.694	T43.695	T43.696
Proloid	T38.1X1	T38.1X2	T38.1X3	T38.1X4	T38.1X5	T38.1X6
Proluton	T38.5X1	T38.5X2	T38.5X3	T38.5X4	T38.5X5	T38.5X6
Promacetin	T37.1X1	T37.1X2	T37.1X3	T37.1X4	T37.1X5	T37.1X6
Promazine	T43.3X1	T43.3X2	T43.3X3	T43.3X4	T43.3X5	T43.3X6
Promedol	T40.2X1	T40.2X2	T40.2X3	T40.2X4	—	—
Promegestone	T38.5X1	T38.5X2	T38.5X3	T38.5X4	T38.5X5	T38.5X6
Promethazine (teoclate)	T43.3X1	T43.3X2	T43.3X3	T43.3X4	T43.3X5	T43.3X6
Promin	T37.1X1	T37.1X2	T37.1X3	T37.1X4	T37.1X5	T37.1X6
Pronase	T45.3X1	T45.3X2	T45.3X3	T45.3X4	T45.3X5	T45.3X6
Pronestyl (hydrochloride)	T46.2X1	T46.2X2	T46.2X3	T46.2X4	T46.2X5	T46.2X6
Pronetalol	T44.7X1	T44.7X2	T44.7X3	T44.7X4	T44.7X5	T44.7X6
Prontosil	T37.0X1	T37.0X2	T37.0X3	T37.0X4	T37.0X5	T37.0X6
Propachlor	T60.3X1	T60.3X2	T60.3X3	T60.3X4	—	—
Propafenone	T46.2X1	T46.2X2	T46.2X3	T46.2X4	T46.2X5	T46.2X6
Propallylonal	T42.3X1	T42.3X2	T42.3X3	T42.3X4	T42.3X5	T42.3X6
Propamidine	T49.0X1	T49.0X2	T49.0X3	T49.0X4	T49.0X5	T49.0X6
Propane (distributed in mobile container)	T59.891	T59.892	T59.893	T59.894	—	—
distributed through pipes	T59.891	T59.892	T59.893	T59.894	—	—
incomplete combustion	T57.11	T57.12	T57.13	T57.14	—	—
Propanidid	T41.291	T41.292	T41.293	T41.294	T41.295	T41.296
Propanil	T60.3X1	T60.3X2	T60.3X3	T60.3X4	—	—
1-Propanol	T51.3X1	T51.3X2	T51.3X3	T51.3X4	—	—
2-Propanol	T51.2X1	T51.2X2	T51.2X3	T51.2X4	—	—
Propantheline	T44.3X1	T44.3X2	T44.3X3	T44.3X4	T44.3X5	T44.3X6
bromide	T44.3X1	T44.3X2	T44.3X3	T44.3X4	T44.3X5	T44.3X6
Proparacaine	T41.3X1	T41.3X2	T41.3X3	T41.3X4	T41.3X5	T41.3X6
Propatylnitrate	T46.3X1	T46.3X2	T46.3X3	T46.3X4	T46.3X5	T46.3X6
Propicillin	T36.0X1	T36.0X2	T36.0X3	T36.0X4	T36.0X5	T36.0X6
Propiolactone	T49.0X1	T49.0X2	T49.0X3	T49.0X4	T49.0X5	T49.0X6
Propiomazine	T45.0X1	T45.0X2	T45.0X3	T45.0X4	T45.0X5	T45.0X6
Propionaldehyde (medicinal)	T42.6X1	T42.6X2	T42.6X3	T42.6X4	T42.6X5	T42.6X6
Propionate (calcium) (sodium)	T49.0X1	T49.0X2	T49.0X3	T49.0X4	T49.0X5	T49.0X6
Propion gel	T49.0X1	T49.0X2	T49.0X3	T49.0X4	T49.0X5	T49.0X6
Propitocaine	T41.3X1	T41.3X2	T41.3X3	T41.3X4	T41.3X5	T41.3X6
infiltration (subcutaneous)	T41.3X1	T41.3X2	T41.3X3	T41.3X4	T41.3X5	T41.3X6
nerve block (peripheral) (plexus)	T41.3X1	T41.3X2	T41.3X3	T41.3X4	T41.3X5	T41.3X6
Propofol	T41.291	T41.292	T41.293	T41.294	T41.295	T41.296
Propoxur	T60.0X1	T60.0X2	T60.0X3	T60.0X4	—	—
Propoxycaine	T41.3X1	T41.3X2	T41.3X3	T41.3X4	T41.3X5	T41.3X6
infiltration (subcutaneous)	T41.3X1	T41.3X2	T41.3X3	T41.3X4	T41.3X5	T41.3X6
nerve block (peripheral) (plexus)	T41.3X1	T41.3X2	T41.3X3	T41.3X4	T41.3X5	T41.3X6
topical (surface)	T41.3X1	T41.3X2	T41.3X3	T41.3X4	T41.3X5	T41.3X6
Propoxyphene	T40.4X1	T40.4X2	T40.4X3	T40.4X4	T40.4X5	T40.4X6
Propranolol	T44.7X1	T44.7X2	T44.7X3	T44.7X4	T44.7X5	T44.7X6
Propyl						
alcohol	T51.3X1	T51.3X2	T51.3X3	T51.3X4	—	—
carbinol	T51.3X1	T51.3X2	T51.3X3	T51.3X4	—	—
hexadrine	T44.4X1	T44.4X2	T44.4X3	T44.4X4	T44.4X5	T44.4X6
iodone	T50.8X1	T50.8X2	T50.8X3	T50.8X4	T50.8X5	T50.8X6
thiouracil	T38.2X1	T38.2X2	T38.2X3	T38.2X4	T38.2X5	T38.2X6
Propylaminophenothiazine	T43.3X1	T43.3X2	T43.3X3	T43.3X4	T43.3X5	T43.3X6
Propylene	T59.891	T59.892	T59.893	T59.894	—	—
Propylhexedrine	T48.5X1	T48.5X2	T48.5X3	T48.5X4	T48.5X5	T48.5X6
Propyliodone	T50.8X1	T50.8X2	T50.8X3	T50.8X4	T50.8X5	T50.8X6
Propylthiouracil	T38.2X1	T38.2X2	T38.2X3	T38.2X4	T38.2X5	T38.2X6
Propylparaben (ophthalmic)	T49.5X1	T49.5X2	T49.5X3	T49.5X4	T49.5X5	T49.5X6
Propyphenazone	T39.2X1	T39.2X2	T39.2X3	T39.2X4	T39.2X5	T39.2X6
Proquazone	T39.391	T39.392	T39.393	T39.394	T39.395	T39.396
Proscillaridin	T46.0X1	T46.0X2	T46.0X3	T46.0X4	T46.0X5	T46.0X6
Prostacyclin	T45.521	T45.522	T45.523	T45.524	T45.525	T45.526
Prostaglandin (I2)	T45.521	T45.522	T45.523	T45.524	T45.525	T45.526
E1	T46.7X1	T46.7X2	T46.7X3	T46.7X4	T46.7X5	T46.7X6
E2	T48.0X1	T48.0X2	T48.0X3	T48.0X4	T48.0X5	T48.0X6
F2 alpha	T48.0X1	T48.0X2	T48.0X3	T48.0X4	T48.0X5	T48.0X6
Prostigmin	T44.0X1	T44.0X2	T44.0X3	T44.0X4	T44.0X5	T44.0X6
Prosultiamine	T45.2X1	T45.2X2	T45.2X3	T45.2X4	T45.2X5	T45.2X6
Protamine sulfate	T45.7X1	T45.7X2	T45.7X3	T45.7X4	T45.7X5	T45.7X6
zinc insulin	T38.3X1	T38.3X2	T38.3X3	T38.3X4	T38.3X5	T38.3X6
Protease	T47.5X1	T47.5X2	T47.5X3	T47.5X4	T47.5X5	T47.5X6
Protectant, skin NEC	T49.3X1	T49.3X2	T49.3X3	T49.3X4	T49.3X5	T49.3X6
Protein hydrolysate	T50.991	T50.992	T50.993	T50.994	T50.995	T50.996
Prothiaden—see Dothiepin hydrochloride						
Prothionamide	T37.1X1	T37.1X2	T37.1X3	T37.1X4	T37.1X5	T37.1X6

Substance	External Cause (T-Code)					
	Poisoning, Accidental (Unintentional)	Poisoning, Intentional Self-Harm	Poisoning, Assault	Poisoning, Undetermined	Adverse Effect	Underdosing
Prothipendyl	T43.591	T43.592	T43.593	T43.594	T43.595	T43.596
Prothoate	T60.0X1	T60.0X2	T60.0X3	T60.0X4	—	—
Prothrombin						
activator	T45.7X1	T45.7X2	T45.7X3	T45.7X4	T45.7X5	T45.7X6
synthesis inhibitor	T45.511	T45.512	T45.513	T45.514	T45.515	T45.516
Protionamide	T37.1X1	T37.1X2	T37.1X3	T37.1X4	T37.1X5	T37.1X6
Protirelin	T38.891	T38.892	T38.893	T38.894	T38.895	T38.896
Protokylol	T48.6X1	T48.6X2	T48.6X3	T48.6X4	T48.6X5	T48.6X6
Protopam	T50.6X1	T50.6X2	T50.6X3	T50.6X4	T50.6X5	T50.6X6
Protoveratrine(s) (A) (B)	T46.5X1	T46.5X2	T46.5X3	T46.5X4	T46.5X5	T46.5X6
Protriptyline	T43.011	T43.012	T43.013	T43.014	T43.015	T43.016
Provera	T38.5X1	T38.5X2	T38.5X3	T38.5X4	T38.5X5	T38.5X6
Provitamin A	T45.2X1	T45.2X2	T45.2X3	T45.2X4	T45.2X5	T45.2X6
Proxibarbal	T42.3X1	T42.3X2	T42.3X3	T42.3X4	T42.3X5	T42.3X6
Proxymetacaine	T41.3X1	T41.3X2	T41.3X3	T41.3X4	T41.3X5	T41.3X6
Proxyphylline	T48.6X1	T48.6X2	T48.6X3	T48.6X4	T48.6X5	T48.6X6
Prozac — see Fluoxetine hydrochloride						
Prunus						
laurocerasus	T62.2X1	T62.2X2	T62.2X3	T62.2X4	—	—
virginiana	T62.2X1	T62.2X2	T62.2X3	T62.2X4	—	—
Prussian blue						
commercial	T65.891	T65.892	T65.893	T65.894	—	—
therapeutic	T50.6X1	T50.6X2	T50.6X3	T50.6X4	T50.6X5	T50.6X6
Prussic acid	T65.0X1	T65.0X2	T65.0X3	T65.0X4	—	—
vapor	T57.3X1	T57.3X2	T57.3X3	T57.3X4	—	—
Pseudoephedrine	T44.991	T44.992	T44.993	T44.994	T44.995	T44.996
Psilocin	T40.991	T40.992	T40.993	T40.994	—	—
Psilocybin	T40.991	T40.992	T40.993	T40.994	—	—
Psilocybine	T40.991	T40.992	T40.993	T40.994	—	—
Psoralene (nonmedicinal)	T65.891	T65.892	T65.893	T65.894	—	—
Psoralens (medicinal)	T50.991	T50.992	T50.993	T50.994	T50.995	T50.996
PSP (phenolsulfonphthalein)	T50.8X1	T50.8X2	T50.8X3	T50.8X4	T50.8X5	T50.8X6
Psychodysleptic drug NEC	T40.901	T40.902	T40.903	T40.904	T40.905	T40.906
Psychostimulant	T43.601	T43.602	T43.603	T43.604	T43.605	T43.606
amphetamine	T43.621	T43.622	T43.623	T43.624	T43.625	T43.626
caffeine	T43.611	T43.612	T43.613	T43.614	T43.615	T43.616
methylphenidate	T43.631	T43.632	T43.633	T43.634	T43.635	T43.636
specified NEC	T43.691	T43.692	T43.693	T43.694	T43.695	T43.696
Psychotherapeutic drug NEC	T43.91	T43.92	T43.93	T43.94	T43.95	T43.96
antidepressants — see also Antidepressant	T43.201	T43.202	T43.203	T43.204	T43.205	T43.206

Substance	External Cause (T-Code)					
	Poisoning, Accidental (Unintentional)	Poisoning, Intentional Self-Harm	Poisoning, Assault	Poisoning, Undetermined	Adverse Effect	Underdosing
Psychotherapeutic drug NEC (Continued)						
specified NEC	T43.8X1	T43.8X2	T43.8X3	T43.8X4	T43.8X5	T43.8X6
tranquilizers NEC	T43.501	T43.502	T43.503	T43.504	T43.505	T43.506
Psychotomimetic agents	T40.901	T40.902	T40.903	T40.904	T40.905	T40.906
Psychotropic drug NEC	T43.91	T43.92	T43.93	T43.94	T43.95	T43.96
specified NEC	T43.8X1	T43.8X2	T43.8X3	T43.8X4	T43.8X5	T43.8X6
Psyllium hydrophilic mucilloid	T47.4X1	T47.4X2	T47.4X3	T47.4X4	T47.4X5	T47.4X6
Pteroylglutamic acid	T45.8X1	T45.8X2	T45.8X3	T45.8X4	T45.8X5	T45.8X6
Pteroyltriglutamate	T45.1X1	T45.1X2	T45.1X3	T45.1X4	T45.1X5	T45.1X6
PTFE — see Polytetrafluoroethylene						
Pulp						
devitalizing paste	T49.7X1	T49.7X2	T49.7X3	T49.7X4	T49.7X5	T49.7X6
dressing	T49.7X1	T49.7X2	T49.7X3	T49.7X4	T49.7X5	T49.7X6
Pulsatilla	T62.2X1	T62.2X2	T62.2X3	T62.2X4	—	—
Pumpkin seed extract	T37.4X1	T37.4X2	T37.4X3	T37.4X4	T37.4X5	T37.4X6
Purex (bleach)	T54.91	T54.92	T54.93	T54.94		
Purgative NEC — see also Cathartic	T47.4X1	T47.4X2	T47.4X3	T47.4X4	T47.4X5	T47.4X6
Purine analogue (antineoplastic)	T45.1X1	T45.1X2	T45.1X3	T45.1X4	T45.1X5	T45.1X6
Purine diuretics	T50.2X1	T50.2X2	T50.2X3	T50.2X4	T50.2X5	T50.2X6
Purinethol	T45.1X1	T45.1X2	T45.1X3	T45.1X4	T45.1X5	T45.1X6
PVP	T45.8X1	T45.8X2	T45.8X3	T45.8X4	T45.8X5	T45.8X6
Pyrabital	T39.8X1	T39.8X2	T39.8X3	T39.8X4	T39.8X5	T39.8X6
Pyramidon	T39.2X1	T39.2X2	T39.2X3	T39.2X4	T39.2X5	T39.2X6
Pyrantel	T37.4X1	T37.4X2	T37.4X3	T37.4X4	T37.4X5	T37.4X6
Pyrathiazine	T45.0X1	T45.0X2	T45.0X3	T45.0X4	T45.0X5	T45.0X6
Pyrazinamide	T37.1X1	T37.1X2	T37.1X3	T37.1X4	T37.1X5	T37.1X6
Pyrazinoic acid (amide)	T37.1X1	T37.1X2	T37.1X3	T37.1X4	T37.1X5	T37.1X6
Pyrazole (derivatives)	T39.2X1	T39.2X2	T39.2X3	T39.2X4	T39.2X5	T39.2X6
Pyrazolone analgesic NEC	T39.2X1	T39.2X2	T39.2X3	T39.2X4	T39.2X5	T39.2X6
Pyrethrin, pyrethrum (nonmedicinal)	T60.2X1	T60.2X2	T60.2X3	T60.2X4	—	—
Pyrethrum extract	T49.0X1	T49.0X2	T49.0X3	T49.0X4	T49.0X5	T49.0X6
Pyribenzamine	T45.0X1	T45.0X2	T45.0X3	T45.0X4	T45.0X5	T45.0X6
Pyridine	T52.8X1	T52.8X2	T52.8X3	T52.8X4	—	—
aldoxime methiodide	T50.6X1	T50.6X2	T50.6X3	T50.6X4	T50.6X5	T50.6X6
aldoxime methyl chloride	T50.6X1	T50.6X2	T50.6X3	T50.6X4	T50.6X5	T50.6X6
vapor	T59.891	T59.892	T59.893	T59.894	—	—
Pyridium	T39.8X1	T39.8X2	T39.8X3	T39.8X4	T39.8X5	T39.8X6
Pyridostigmine bromide	T44.0X1	T44.0X2	T44.0X3	T44.0X4	T44.0X5	T44.0X6
Pyridoxal phosphate	T45.2X1	T45.2X2	T45.2X3	T45.2X4	T45.2X5	T45.2X6

◀ New　⫸ Revised　deleted Deleted

Substance	Poisoning, Accidental (Unintentional)	Poisoning, Intentional Self-Harm	Poisoning, Assault	Poisoning, Undetermined	Adverse Effect	Underdosing
Pyridoxine	T45.2X1	T45.2X2	T45.2X3	T45.2X4	T45.2X5	T45.2X6
Pyrilamine	T45.0X1	T45.0X2	T45.0X3	T45.0X4	T45.0X5	T45.0X6
Pyrimethamine	T37.2X1	T37.2X2	T37.2X3	T37.2X4	T37.2X5	T37.2X6
with sulfadoxine	T37.2X1	T37.2X2	T37.2X3	T37.2X4	T37.2X5	T37.2X6
Pyrimidine antagonist	T45.1X1	T45.1X2	T45.1X3	T45.1X4	T45.1X5	T45.1X6
Pyriminil	T60.4X1	T60.4X2	T60.4X3	T60.4X4	—	—
Pyrithione zinc	T49.4X1	T49.4X2	T49.4X3	T49.4X4	T49.4X5	T49.4X6
Pyrithyldione	T42.6X1	T42.6X2	T42.6X3	T42.6X4	T42.6X5	T42.6X6
Pyrogallic acid	T49.0X1	T49.0X2	T49.0X3	T49.0X4	T49.0X5	T49.0X6
Pyrogallol	T49.0X1	T49.0X2	T49.0X3	T49.0X4	T49.0X5	T49.0X6
Pyroxylin	T49.3X1	T49.3X2	T49.3X3	T49.3X4	T49.3X5	T49.3X6
Pyrrobutamine	T45.0X1	T45.0X2	T45.0X3	T45.0X4	T45.0X5	T45.0X6
Pyrrolizidine alkaloids	T62.8X1	T62.8X2	T62.8X3	T62.8X4	—	—
Pyrvinium chloride	T37.4X1	T37.4X2	T37.4X3	T37.4X4	T37.4X5	T37.4X6
PZI	T38.3X1	T38.3X2	T38.3X3	T38.3X4	T38.3X5	T38.3X6

Q

Substance	Poisoning, Accidental (Unintentional)	Poisoning, Intentional Self-Harm	Poisoning, Assault	Poisoning, Undetermined	Adverse Effect	Underdosing
Quaalude	T42.6X1	T42.6X2	T42.6X3	T42.6X4	T42.6X5	T42.6X6
Quarternary ammonium						
anti-infective	T49.0X1	T49.0X2	T49.0X3	T49.0X4	T49.0X5	T49.0X6
ganglion blocking	T44.2X1	T44.2X2	T44.2X3	T44.2X4	T44.2X5	T44.2X6
parasympatholytic	T44.3X1	T44.3X2	T44.3X3	T44.3X4	T44.3X5	T44.3X6
Quazepam	T42.4X1	T42.4X2	T42.4X3	T42.4X4	T42.4X5	T42.4X6
Quicklime	T54.3X1	T54.3X2	T54.3X3	T54.3X4	—	—
Quillaja extract	T48.4X1	T48.4X2	T48.4X3	T48.4X4	T48.4X5	T48.4X6
Quinacrine	T37.2X1	T37.2X2	T37.2X3	T37.2X4	T37.2X5	T37.2X6
Quinaglute	T46.2X1	T46.2X2	T46.2X3	T46.2X4	T46.2X5	T46.2X6
Quinalbarbital	T42.3X1	T42.3X2	T42.3X3	T42.3X4	T42.3X5	T42.3X6
Quinalbarbitone sodium	T42.3X1	T42.3X2	T42.3X3	T42.3X4	T42.3X5	T42.3X6
Quinalphos	T60.0X1	T60.0X2	T60.0X3	T60.0X4	—	—
Quinapril	T46.4X1	T46.4X2	T46.4X3	T46.4X4	T46.4X5	T46.4X6
Quinestradiol	T38.5X1	T38.5X2	T38.5X3	T38.5X4	T38.5X5	T38.5X6
Quinestradol	T38.5X1	T38.5X2	T38.5X3	T38.5X4	T38.5X5	T38.5X6
Quinestrol	T38.5X1	T38.5X2	T38.5X3	T38.5X4	T38.5X5	T38.5X6
Quinethazone	T50.2X1	T50.2X2	T50.2X3	T50.2X4	T50.2X5	T50.2X6
Quingestanol	T38.4X1	T38.4X2	T38.4X3	T38.4X4	T38.4X5	T38.4X6
Quinidine	T46.2X1	T46.2X2	T46.2X3	T46.2X4	T46.2X5	T46.2X6
Quinine	T37.2X1	T37.2X2	T37.2X3	T37.2X4	T37.2X5	T37.2X6
Quiniobine	T37.8X1	T37.8X2	T37.8X3	T37.8X4	T37.8X5	T37.8X6
Quinisocaine	T49.1X1	T49.1X2	T49.1X3	T49.1X4	T49.1X5	T49.1X6
Quinocide	T37.2X1	T37.2X2	T37.2X3	T37.2X4	T37.2X5	T37.2X6
Quinoline (derivatives) NEC	T37.8X1	T37.8X2	T37.8X3	T37.8X4	T37.8X5	T37.8X6

Substance	Poisoning, Accidental (Unintentional)	Poisoning, Intentional Self-Harm	Poisoning, Assault	Poisoning, Undetermined	Adverse Effect	Underdosing
Quinupramine	T43.011	T43.012	T43.013	T43.014	T43.015	T43.016
Quotane	T41.3X1	T41.3X2	T41.3X3	T41.3X4	T41.3X5	T41.3X6

R

Substance	Poisoning, Accidental (Unintentional)	Poisoning, Intentional Self-Harm	Poisoning, Assault	Poisoning, Undetermined	Adverse Effect	Underdosing
Rabies						
immune globulin (human)	T50.Z11	T50.Z12	T50.Z13	T50.Z14	T50.Z15	T50.Z16
vaccine	T50.B91	T50.B92	T50.B93	T50.B94	T50.B95	T50.B96
Racemoramide	T40.2X1	T40.2X2	T40.2X3	T40.2X4	—	—
Racemorphan	T40.2X1	T40.2X2	T40.2X3	T40.2X4	T40.2X5	T40.2X6
Racepinefrin	T44.5X1	T44.5X2	T44.5X3	T44.5X4	T44.5X5	T44.5X6
Raclopride	T43.591	T43.592	T43.593	T43.594	T43.595	T43.596
Radiator alcohol	T51.1X1	T51.1X2	T51.1X3	T51.1X4	—	—
Radioactive drug NEC	T50.8X1	T50.8X2	T50.8X3	T50.8X4	T50.8X5	T50.8X6
Radio-opaque (drugs) (materials)	T50.8X1	T50.8X2	T50.8X3	T50.8X4	T50.8X5	T50.8X6
Ramifenazone	T39.2X1	T39.2X2	T39.2X3	T39.2X4	T39.2X5	T39.2X6
Ramipril	T46.4X1	T46.4X2	T46.4X3	T46.4X4	T46.4X5	T46.4X6
Ranitidine	T47.0X1	T47.0X2	T47.0X3	T47.0X4	T47.0X5	T47.0X6
Ranunculus	T62.2X1	T62.2X2	T62.2X3	T62.2X4	—	—
Rat poison NEC	T60.4X1	T60.4X2	T60.4X3	T60.4X4	—	—
Rattlesnake (venom)	T63.011	T63.012	T63.013	T63.014	—	—
Raubasine	T46.7X1	T46.7X2	T46.7X3	T46.7X4	T46.7X5	T46.7X6
Raudixin	T46.5X1	T46.5X2	T46.5X3	T46.5X4	T46.5X5	T46.5X6
Rautensin	T46.5X1	T46.5X2	T46.5X3	T46.5X4	T46.5X5	T46.5X6
Rautina	T46.5X1	T46.5X2	T46.5X3	T46.5X4	T46.5X5	T46.5X6
Rautotal	T46.5X1	T46.5X2	T46.5X3	T46.5X4	T46.5X5	T46.5X6
Rauwiloid	T46.5X1	T46.5X2	T46.5X3	T46.5X4	T46.5X5	T46.5X6
Rauwoldin	T46.5X1	T46.5X2	T46.5X3	T46.5X4	T46.5X5	T46.5X6
Rauwolfia (alkaloids)	T46.5X1	T46.5X2	T46.5X3	T46.5X4	T46.5X5	T46.5X6
Razoxane	T45.1X1	T45.1X2	T45.1X3	T45.1X4	T45.1X5	T45.1X6
Realgar	T57.0X1	T57.0X2	T57.0X3	T57.0X4	—	—
Recombinant (R) — see specific protein						
Red blood cells, packed	T45.8X1	T45.8X2	T45.8X3	T45.8X4	T45.8X5	T45.8X6
Red squill (scilliroside)	T60.4X1	T60.4X2	T60.4X3	T60.4X4	—	—
Reducing agent, industrial NEC	T65.891	T65.892	T65.893	T65.894	—	—
Refrigerant gas (chlorofluoro-carbon)	T53.5X1	T53.5X2	T53.5X3	T53.5X4	—	—
not chlorofluoro-carbon	T59.891	T59.892	T59.893	T59.894	—	—
Regroton	T50.2X1	T50.2X2	T50.2X3	T50.2X4	T50.2X5	T50.2X6
Rehydration salts (oral)	T50.3X1	T50.3X2	T50.3X3	T50.3X4	T50.3X5	T50.3X6
Rela	T42.8X1	T42.8X2	T42.8X3	T42.8X4	T42.8X5	T42.8X6

◀ New ◀ Revised ~~deleted~~ Deleted

TABLE OF DRUGS AND CHEMICALS

Substance	Poisoning, Accidental (Unintentional)	Poisoning, Intentional Self-Harm	Poisoning, Assault	Poisoning, Undetermined	Adverse Effect	Underdosing
Relaxant, muscle						
anesthetic	T48.1X1	T48.1X2	T48.1X3	T48.1X4	T48.1X5	T48.1X6
central nervous system	T42.8X1	T42.8X2	T42.8X3	T42.8X4	T42.8X5	T42.8X6
skeletal NEC	T48.1X1	T48.1X2	T48.1X3	T48.1X4	T48.1X5	T48.1X6
smooth NEC	T44.3X1	T44.3X2	T44.3X3	T44.3X4	T44.3X5	T44.3X6
Remoxipride	T43.591	T43.592	T43.593	T43.594	T43.595	T43.596
Renese	T50.2X1	T50.2X2	T50.2X3	T50.2X4	T50.2X5	T50.2X6
Renografin	T50.8X1	T50.8X2	T50.8X3	T50.8X4	T50.8X5	T50.8X6
Replacement solution	T50.3X1	T50.3X2	T50.3X3	T50.3X4	T50.3X5	T50.3X6
Reproterol	T48.6X1	T48.6X2	T48.6X3	T48.6X4	T48.6X5	T48.6X6
Rescinnamine	T46.5X1	T46.5X2	T46.5X3	T46.5X4	T46.5X5	T46.5X6
Reserpin(e)	T46.5X1	T46.5X2	T46.5X3	T46.5X4	T46.5X5	T46.5X6
Resorcin, resorcinol (nonmedicinal)	T65.891	T65.892	T65.893	T65.894	—	—
medicinal	T49.4X1	T49.4X2	T49.4X3	T49.4X4	T49.4X5	T49.4X6
Respaire	T48.4X1	T48.4X2	T48.4X3	T48.4X4	T48.4X5	T48.4X6
Respiratory drug NEC	T48.901	T48.902	T48.903	T48.904	T48.905	T48.906
antiasthmatic NEC	T48.6X1	T48.6X2	T48.6X3	T48.6X4	T48.6X5	T48.6X6
anti-common-cold NEC	T48.5X1	T48.5X2	T48.5X3	T48.5X4	T48.5X5	T48.5X6
expectorant NEC	T48.4X1	T48.4X2	T48.4X3	T48.4X4	T48.4X5	T48.4X6
stimulant	T48.901	T48.902	T48.903	T48.904	T48.905	T48.906
Retinoic acid	T49.0X1	T49.0X2	T49.0X3	T49.0X4	T49.0X5	T49.0X6
Retinol	T45.2X1	T45.2X2	T45.2X3	T45.2X4	T45.2X5	T45.2X6
Rh (D) immune globulin (human)	T50.Z11	T50.Z12	T50.Z13	T50.Z14	T50.Z15	T50.Z16
Rhodine	T39.011	T39.012	T39.013	T39.014	T39.015	T39.016
RhoGAM	T50.Z11	T50.Z12	T50.Z13	T50.Z14	T50.Z15	T50.Z16
Rhubarb						
dry extract	T47.2X1	T47.2X2	T47.2X3	T47.2X4	T47.2X5	T47.2X6
tincture, compound	T47.2X1	T47.2X2	T47.2X3	T47.2X4	T47.2X5	T47.2X6
Ribavirin	T37.5X1	T37.5X2	T37.5X3	T37.5X4	T37.5X5	T37.5X6
Riboflavin	T45.2X1	T45.2X2	T45.2X3	T45.2X4	T45.2X5	T45.2X6
Ribostamycin	T36.5X1	T36.5X2	T36.5X3	T36.5X4	T36.5X5	T36.5X6
Ricin	T62.2X1	T62.2X2	T62.2X3	T62.2X4	—	—
Ricinus communis	T62.2X1	T62.2X2	T62.2X3	T62.2X4	—	—
Rickettsial vaccine NEC	T50.A91	T50.A92	T50.A93	T50.A94	T50.A95	T50.A96
Rifabutin	T36.6X1	T36.6X2	T36.6X3	T36.6X4	T36.6X5	T36.6X6
Rifamide	T36.6X1	T36.6X2	T36.6X3	T36.6X4	T36.6X5	T36.6X6
Rifampicin	T36.6X1	T36.6X2	T36.6X3	T36.6X4	T36.6X5	T36.6X6
with isoniazid	T37.1X1	T37.1X2	T37.1X3	T37.1X4	T37.1X5	T37.1X6
Rifampin	T36.6X1	T36.6X2	T36.6X3	T36.6X4	T36.6X5	T36.6X6
Rifamycin	T36.6X1	T36.6X2	T36.6X3	T36.6X4	T36.6X5	T36.6X6
Rifaximin	T36.6X1	T36.6X2	T36.6X3	T36.6X4	T36.6X5	T36.6X6

Substance	Poisoning, Accidental (Unintentional)	Poisoning, Intentional Self-Harm	Poisoning, Assault	Poisoning, Undetermined	Adverse Effect	Underdosing
Rimantadine	T37.5X1	T37.5X2	T37.5X3	T37.5X4	T37.5X5	T37.5X6
Rimazolium metilsulfate	T39.8X1	T39.8X2	T39.8X3	T39.8X4	T39.8X5	T39.8X6
Rimifon	T37.1X1	T37.1X2	T37.1X3	T37.1X4	T37.1X5	T37.1X6
Rimiterol	T48.6X1	T48.6X2	T48.6X3	T48.6X4	T48.6X5	T48.6X6
Ringer (lactate) solution	T50.3X1	T50.3X2	T50.3X3	T50.3X4	T50.3X5	T50.3X6
Ristocetin	T36.8X1	T36.8X2	T36.8X3	T36.8X4	T36.8X5	T36.8X6
Ritalin	T43.631	T43.632	T43.633	T43.634	T43.635	T43.636
Ritodrine	T44.5X1	T44.5X2	T44.5X3	T44.5X4	T44.5X5	T44.5X6
Roach killer — *see Insecticide*						
Rociverine	T44.3X1	T44.3X2	T44.3X3	T44.3X4	T44.3X5	T44.3X6
Rocky Mountain spotted fever vaccine	T50.A91	T50.A92	T50.A93	T50.A94	T50.A95	T50.A96
Rodenticide NEC	T60.4X1	T60.4X2	T60.4X3	T60.4X4	—	—
Rohypnol	T42.4X1	T42.4X2	T42.4X3	T42.4X4	T42.4X5	T42.4X6
Rokitamycin	T36.3X1	T36.3X2	T36.3X3	T36.3X4	T36.3X5	T36.3X6
Rolaids	T47.1X1	T47.1X2	T47.1X3	T47.1X4	T47.1X5	T47.1X6
Rolitetracycline	T36.4X1	T36.4X2	T36.4X3	T36.4X4	T36.4X5	T36.4X6
Romilar	T48.3X1	T48.3X2	T48.3X3	T48.3X4	T48.3X5	T48.3X6
Ronifibrate	T46.6X1	T46.6X2	T46.6X3	T46.6X4	T46.6X5	T46.6X6
Rosaprostol	T47.1X1	T47.1X2	T47.1X3	T47.1X4	T47.1X5	T47.1X6
Rose bengal sodium (131I)	T50.8X1	T50.8X2	T50.8X3	T50.8X4	T50.8X5	T50.8X6
Rose water ointment	T49.3X1	T49.3X2	T49.3X3	T49.3X4	T49.3X5	T49.3X6
Rosoxacin	T37.8X1	T37.8X2	T37.8X3	T37.8X4	T37.8X5	T37.8X6
Rotenone	T60.2X1	T60.2X2	T60.2X3	T60.2X4	—	—
Rotoxamine	T45.0X1	T45.0X2	T45.0X3	T45.0X4	T45.0X5	T45.0X6
Rough-on-rats	T60.4X1	T60.4X2	T60.4X3	T60.4X4	—	—
Roxatidine	T47.0X1	T47.0X2	T47.0X3	T47.0X4	T47.0X5	T47.0X6
Roxithromycin	T36.3X1	T36.3X2	T36.3X3	T36.3X4	T36.3X5	T36.3X6
Rt-PA	T45.611	T45.612	T45.613	T45.614	T45.615	T45.616
Rubbing alcohol	T51.2X1	T51.2X2	T51.2X3	T51.2X4	—	—
Rubefacient	T49.4X1	T49.4X2	T49.4X3	T49.4X4	T49.4X5	T49.4X6
Rubella vaccine	T50.B91	T50.B92	T50.B93	T50.B94	T50.B95	T50.B96
Rubelogen	T50.B91	T50.B92	T50.B93	T50.B94	T50.B95	T50.B96
Rubeovax	T50.991	T50.992	T50.993	T50.994	T50.995	T50.996
Rubidium chloride Rb82	T50.8X1	T50.8X2	T50.8X3	T50.8X4	T50.8X5	T50.8X6
Rubidomycin	T45.1X1	T45.1X2	T45.1X3	T45.1X4	T45.1X5	T45.1X6
Rue	T62.2X1	T62.2X2	T62.2X3	T62.2X4	—	—
Rufocromomycin	T45.1X1	T45.1X2	T45.1X3	T45.1X4	T45.1X5	T45.1X6
Russel's viper venin	T45.7X1	T45.7X2	T45.7X3	T45.7X4	T45.7X5	T45.7X6
Ruta (graveolens)	T62.2X1	T62.2X2	T62.2X3	T62.2X4	—	—
Rutinum	T46.991	T46.992	T46.993	T46.994	T46.995	T46.996
Rutoside	T46.991	T46.992	T46.993	T46.994	T46.995	T46.996

◀ New   ◀ Revised   ~~deleted~~ Deleted

	External Cause (T-Code)					
Substance	Poisoning, Accidental (Unintentional)	Poisoning, Intentional Self-Harm	Poisoning, Assault	Poisoning, Undetermined	Adverse Effect	Underdosing
S						
Sabadilla (plant)	T62.2X1	T62.2X2	T62.2X3	T62.2X4	—	—
pesticide	T60.2X1	T60.2X2	T60.2X3	T60.2X4	—	—
Saccharated iron oxide	T45.8X1	T45.8X2	T45.8X3	T45.8X4	T45.8X5	T45.8X6
Saccharin	T50.901	T50.902	T50.903	T50.904	T50.905	T50.906
Saccharomyces boulardii	T47.6X1	T47.6X2	T47.6X3	T47.6X4	T47.6X5	T47.6X6
Safflower oil	T46.6X1	T46.6X2	T46.6X3	T46.6X4	T46.6X5	T46.6X6
Safrazine	T43.1X1	T43.1X2	T43.1X3	T43.1X4	T43.1X5	T43.1X6
Salazosulfapyridine	T37.0X1	T37.0X2	T37.0X3	T37.0X4	T37.0X5	T37.0X6
Salbutamol	T48.6X1	T48.6X2	T48.6X3	T48.6X4	T48.6X5	T48.6X6
Salicylamide	T39.091	T39.092	T39.093	T39.094	T39.095	T39.096
Salicylate NEC	T39.091	T39.092	T39.093	T39.094	T39.095	T39.096
methyl	T49.3X1	T49.3X2	T49.3X3	T49.3X4	T49.3X5	T49.3X6
theobromine calcium	T50.2X1	T50.2X2	T50.2X3	T50.2X4	T50.2X5	T50.2X6
Salicylazosulfapyridine	T37.0X1	T37.0X2	T37.0X3	T37.0X4	T37.0X5	T37.0X6
Salicylhydroxamic acid	T49.0X1	T49.0X2	T49.0X3	T49.0X4	T49.0X5	T49.0X6
Salicylic acid	T49.4X1	T49.4X2	T49.4X3	T49.4X4	T49.4X5	T49.4X6
with benzoic acid	T49.4X1	T49.4X2	T49.4X3	T49.4X4	T49.4X5	T49.4X6
congeners	T39.091	T39.092	T39.093	T39.094	T39.095	T39.096
derivative	T39.091	T39.092	T39.093	T39.094	T39.095	T39.096
salts	T39.091	T39.092	T39.093	T39.094	T39.095	T39.096
Salinazid	T37.1X1	T37.1X2	T37.1X3	T37.1X4	T37.1X5	T37.1X6
Salmeterol	T48.6X1	T48.6X2	T48.6X3	T48.6X4	T48.6X5	T48.6X6
Salol	T49.3X1	T49.3X2	T49.3X3	T49.3X4	T49.3X5	T49.3X6
Salsalate	T39.091	T39.092	T39.093	T39.094	T39.095	T39.096
Salt substitute	T50.901	T50.902	T50.903	T50.904	T50.905	T50.906
Salt-replacing drug	T50.901	T50.902	T50.903	T50.904	T50.905	T50.906
Salt-retaining mineralocorticoid	T50.0X1	T50.0X2	T50.0X3	T50.0X4	T50.0X5	T50.0X6
Saluretic NEC	T50.2X1	T50.2X2	T50.2X3	T50.2X4	T50.2X5	T50.2X6
Saluron	T50.2X1	T50.2X2	T50.2X3	T50.2X4	T50.2X5	T50.2X6
Salvarsan 606 (neosilver) (silver)	T37.8X1	T37.8X2	T37.8X3	T37.8X4	T37.8X5	T37.8X6
Sambucus canadensis	T62.2X1	T62.2X2	T62.2X3	T62.2X4	—	—
berry	T62.1X1	T62.1X2	T62.1X3	T62.1X4	—	—
Sandril	T46.5X1	T46.5X2	T46.5X3	T46.5X4	T46.5X5	T46.5X6
Sanguinaria canadensis	T62.2X1	T62.2X2	T62.2X3	T62.2X4	—	—
Saniflush (cleaner)	T54.2X1	T54.2X2	T54.2X3	T54.2X4	—	—
Santonin	T37.4X1	T37.4X2	T37.4X3	T37.4X4	T37.4X5	T37.4X6
Santyl	T49.8X1	T49.8X2	T49.8X3	T49.8X4	T49.8X5	T49.8X6
Saralasin	T46.5X1	T46.5X2	T46.5X3	T46.5X4	T46.5X5	T46.5X6
Sarcolysin	T45.1X1	T45.1X2	T45.1X3	T45.1X4	T45.1X5	T45.1X6
Sarkomycin	T45.1X1	T45.1X2	T45.1X3	T45.1X4	T45.1X5	T45.1X6
Saroten	T43.011	T43.012	T43.013	T43.014	T43.015	T43.016

	External Cause (T-Code)					
Substance	Poisoning, Accidental (Unintentional)	Poisoning, Intentional Self-Harm	Poisoning, Assault	Poisoning, Undetermined	Adverse Effect	Underdosing
Saturnine—see Lead						
Savin (oil)	T49.4X1	T49.4X2	T49.4X3	T49.4X4	T49.4X5	T49.4X6
Scammony	T47.2X1	T47.2X2	T47.2X3	T47.2X4	T47.2X5	T47.2X6
Scarlet red	T49.8X1	T49.8X2	T49.8X3	T49.8X4	T49.8X5	T49.8X6
Scheele's green	T57.0X1	T57.0X2	T57.0X3	T57.0X4	—	—
insecticide	T57.0X1	T57.0X2	T57.0X3	T57.0X4	—	—
Schizontozide (blood) (tissue)	T37.2X1	T37.2X2	T37.2X3	T37.2X4	T37.2X5	T37.2X6
Schradan	T60.0X1	T60.0X2	T60.0X3	T60.0X4	—	—
Schweinfurth green	T57.0X1	T57.0X2	T57.0X3	T57.0X4	—	—
insecticide	T57.0X1	T57.0X2	T57.0X3	T57.0X4	—	—
Scilla, rat poison	T60.4X1	T60.4X2	T60.4X3	T60.4X4	—	—
Scillaren	T60.4X1	T60.4X2	T60.4X3	T60.4X4	—	—
Sclerosing agent	T46.8X1	T46.8X2	T46.8X3	T46.8X4	T46.8X5	T46.8X6
Scombrotoxin	T61.11	T61.12	T61.13	T61.14	—	—
Scopolamine	T44.3X1	T44.3X2	T44.3X3	T44.3X4	T44.3X5	T44.3X6
Scopolia extract	T44.3X1	T44.3X2	T44.3X3	T44.3X4	T44.3X5	T44.3X6
Scouring powder	T65.891	T65.892	T65.893	T65.894	—	—
Sea						
anemone (sting)	T63.631	T63.632	T63.633	T63.634	—	—
cucumber (sting)	T63.691	T63.692	T63.693	T63.694	—	—
snake (bite) (venom)	T63.091	T63.092	T63.093	T63.094	—	—
urchin spine (puncture)	T63.691	T63.692	T63.693	T63.694	—	—
Seafood	T61.91	T61.92	T61.93	T61.94	—	—
specified NEC	T61.8X1	T61.8X2	T61.8X3	T61.8X4	—	—
Secbutabarbital	T42.3X1	T42.3X2	T42.3X3	T42.3X4	T42.3X5	T42.3X6
Secbutabarbitone	T42.3X1	T42.3X2	T42.3X3	T42.3X4	T42.3X5	T42.3X6
Secnidazole	T37.3X1	T37.3X2	T37.3X3	T37.3X4	T37.3X5	T37.3X6
Secobarbital	T42.3X1	T42.3X2	T42.3X3	T42.3X4	T42.3X5	T42.3X6
Seconal	T42.3X1	T42.3X2	T42.3X3	T42.3X4	T42.3X5	T42.3X6
Secretin	T50.8X1	T50.8X2	T50.8X3	T50.8X4	T50.8X5	T50.8X6
Sedative NEC	T42.71	T42.72	T42.73	T42.74	T42.75	T42.76
mixed NEC	T42.6X1	T42.6X2	T42.6X3	T42.6X4	T42.6X5	T42.6X6
Sedormid	T42.6X1	T42.6X2	T42.6X3	T42.6X4	T42.6X5	T42.6X6
Seed disinfectant or dressing	T60.8X1	T60.8X2	T60.8X3	T60.8X4	—	—
Seeds (poisonous)	T62.2X1	T62.2X2	T62.2X3	T62.2X4	—	—
Selegiline	T42.8X1	T42.8X2	T42.8X3	T42.8X4	T42.8X5	T42.8X6
Selenium NEC	T56.891	T56.892	T56.893	T56.894	—	—
disulfide or sulfide	T49.4X1	T49.4X2	T49.4X3	T49.4X4	T49.4X5	T49.4X6
fumes	T59.891	T59.892	T59.893	T59.894	—	—
sulfide	T49.4X1	T49.4X2	T49.4X3	T49.4X4	T49.4X5	T49.4X6
Selenomethionine (75Se)	T50.8X1	T50.8X2	T50.8X3	T50.8X4	T50.8X5	T50.8X6
Selsun	T49.4X1	T49.4X2	T49.4X3	T49.4X4	T49.4X5	T49.4X6

Substance	Poisoning, Accidental (Unintentional)	Poisoning, Intentional Self-Harm	Poisoning, Assault	Poisoning, Undetermined	Adverse Effect	Underdosing
Semustine	T45.1X1	T45.1X2	T45.1X4	T45.1X4	T45.1X5	T45.1X6
Senega syrup	T48.4X1	T48.4X2	T48.4X3	T48.4X4	T48.4X5	T48.4X6
Senna	T47.2X1	T47.2X2	T47.2X3	T47.2X4	T47.2X5	T47.2X6
Sennoside A+B	T47.2X1	T47.2X2	T47.2X3	T47.2X4	T47.2X5	T47.2X6
Septisol	T49.2X1	T49.2X2	T49.2X3	T49.2X4	T49.2X5	T49.2X6
Seractide	T38.811	T38.812	T38.813	T38.814	T38.815	T38.816
Serax	T42.4X1	T42.4X2	T42.4X3	T42.4X4	T42.4X5	T42.4X6
Serenesil	T42.6X1	T42.6X2	T42.6X3	T42.6X4	T42.6X5	T42.6X6
Serenium (hydrochloride)	T37.91	T37.92	T37.93	T37.94	T37.95	T37.96
Serepax — see Oxazepam						
Sermorelin	T38.891	T38.892	T38.893	T38.894	T38.895	T38.896
Sernyl	T41.1X1	T41.1X2	T41.1X3	T41.1X4	T41.1X5	T41.1X6
Serotonin	T50.991	T50.992	T50.993	T50.994	T50.995	T50.996
Serpasil	T46.5X1	T46.5X2	T46.5X3	T46.5X4	T46.5X5	T46.5X6
Serrapeptase	T45.3X1	T45.3X2	T45.3X3	T45.3X4	T45.3X5	T45.3X6
Serum						
antibotulinus	T50.Z11	T50.Z12	T50.Z13	T50.Z14	T50.Z15	T50.Z16
anticytotoxic	T50.Z11	T50.Z12	T50.Z13	T50.Z14	T50.Z15	T50.Z16
antidiphtheria	T50.Z11	T50.Z12	T50.Z13	T50.Z14	T50.Z15	T50.Z16
antimeningococcus	T50.Z11	T50.Z12	T50.Z13	T50.Z14	T50.Z15	T50.Z16
anti-Rh	T50.Z11	T50.Z12	T50.Z13	T50.Z14	T50.Z15	T50.Z16
anti-snake-bite	T50.Z11	T50.Z12	T50.Z13	T50.Z14	T50.Z15	T50.Z16
antitetanic	T50.Z11	T50.Z12	T50.Z13	T50.Z14	T50.Z15	T50.Z16
antitoxic	T50.Z11	T50.Z12	T50.Z13	T50.Z14	T50.Z15	T50.Z16
complement (inhibitor)	T45.8X1	T45.8X2	T45.8X3	T45.8X4	T45.8X5	T45.8X6
convalescent	T50.Z11	T50.Z12	T50.Z13	T50.Z14	T50.Z15	T50.Z16
hemolytic complement	T45.8X1	T45.8X2	T45.8X3	T45.8X4	T45.8X5	T45.8X6
immune (human)	T50.Z11	T50.Z12	T50.Z13	T50.Z14	T50.Z15	T50.Z16
protective NEC	T50.Z11	T50.Z12	T50.Z13	T50.Z14	T50.Z15	T50.Z16
Setastine	T45.0X1	T45.0X2	T45.0X3	T45.0X4	T45.0X5	T45.0X6
Setoperone	T43.591	T43.592	T43.593	T43.594	T43.595	T43.596
Sewer gas	T59.91	T59.92	T59.93	T59.94	—	—
Shampoo	T55.0X1	T55.0X2	T55.0X3	T55.0X4	—	—
Shellfish, noxious, nonbacterial	T61.781	T61.782	T61.783	T61.784	—	—
Sildenafil	T46.7X1	T46.7X2	T46.7X3	T46.7X4	T46.7X5	T46.7X6
Silibinin	T50.991	T50.992	T50.993	T50.994	T50.995	T50.996
Silicone NEC	T65.891	T65.892	T65.893	T65.894	—	—
medicinal	T49.3X1	T49.3X2	T49.3X3	T49.3X4	T49.3X5	T49.3X6
Silvadene	T49.0X1	T49.0X2	T49.0X3	T49.0X4	T49.0X5	T49.0X6
Silver	T49.0X1	T49.0X2	T49.0X3	T49.0X4	T49.0X5	T49.0X6
anti-infectives	T49.0X1	T49.0X2	T49.0X3	T49.0X4	T49.0X5	T49.0X6
arsphenamine	T37.8X1	T37.8X2	T37.8X3	T37.8X4	T37.8X5	T37.8X6

Substance	Poisoning, Accidental (Unintentional)	Poisoning, Intentional Self-Harm	Poisoning, Assault	Poisoning, Undetermined	Adverse Effect	Underdosing
Silver (Continued)						
colloidal	T49.0X1	T49.0X2	T49.0X3	T49.0X4	T49.0X5	T49.0X6
nitrate	T49.0X1	T49.0X2	T49.0X3	T49.0X4	T49.0X5	T49.0X6
ophthalmic preparation	T49.5X1	T49.5X2	T49.5X3	T49.5X4	T49.5X5	T49.5X6
toughened (keratolytic)	T49.4X1	T49.4X2	T49.4X3	T49.4X4	T49.4X5	T49.4X6
nonmedicinal (dust)	T56.891	T56.892	T56.893	T56.894	—	—
protein	T49.5X1	T49.5X2	T49.5X3	T49.5X4	T49.5X5	T49.5X6
salvarsan	T37.8X1	T37.8X2	T37.8X3	T37.8X4	T37.8X5	T37.8X6
sulfadiazine	T49.4X1	T49.4X2	T49.4X3	T49.4X4	T49.4X5	T49.4X6
Silymarin	T50.991	T50.992	T50.993	T50.994	T50.995	T50.996
Simaldrate	T47.1X1	T47.1X2	T47.1X3	T47.1X4	T47.1X5	T47.1X6
Simazine	T60.3X1	T60.3X2	T60.3X3	T60.3X4	—	—
Simethicone	T47.1X1	T47.1X2	T47.1X3	T47.1X4	T47.1X5	T47.1X6
Simfibrate	T46.6X1	T46.6X2	T46.6X3	T46.6X4	T46.6X5	T46.6X6
Simvastatin	T46.6X1	T46.6X2	T46.6X3	T46.6X4	T46.6X5	T46.6X6
Sincalide	T50.8X1	T50.8X2	T50.8X3	T50.8X4	T50.8X5	T50.8X6
Sinequan	T43.011	T43.012	T43.013	T43.014	T43.015	T43.016
Singoserp	T46.5X1	T46.5X2	T46.5X3	T46.5X4	T46.5X5	T46.5X6
Sintrom	T45.511	T45.512	T45.513	T45.514	T45.515	T45.516
Sisomicin	T36.5X1	T36.5X2	T36.5X3	T36.5X4	T36.5X5	T36.5X6
Sitosterols	T46.6X1	T46.6X2	T46.6X3	T46.6X4	T46.6X5	T46.6X6
Skeletal muscle relaxants	T48.1X1	T48.1X2	T48.1X3	T48.1X4	T48.1X5	T48.1X6
Skin						
agents (external)	T49.91	T49.92	T49.93	T49.94	T49.95	T49.96
specified NEC	T49.8X1	T49.8X2	T49.8X3	T49.8X4	T49.8X5	T49.8X6
test antigen	T50.8X1	T50.8X2	T50.8X3	T50.8X4	T50.8X5	T50.8X6
Sleep-eze	T45.0X1	T45.0X2	T45.0X3	T45.0X4	T45.0X5	T45.0X6
Sleeping draught, pill	T42.71	T42.72	T42.73	T42.74	T42.75	T42.76
Smallpox vaccine	T50.B11	T50.B12	T50.B13	T50.B14	T50.B15	T50.B16
Smelter fumes NEC	T56.91	T56.92	T56.93	T56.94	—	—
Smog	T59.1X1	T59.1X2	T59.1X3	T59.1X4	—	—
Smoke NEC	T59.811	T59.812	T59.813	T59.814	—	—
Smooth muscle relaxant	T44.3X1	T44.3X2	T44.3X3	T44.3X4	T44.3X5	T44.3X6
Snail killer NEC	T60.8X1	T60.8X2	T60.8X3	T60.8X4	—	—
Snake venom or bite	T63.001	T63.002	T63.003	T63.004	—	—
hemocoagulase	T45.7X1	T45.7X2	T45.7X3	T45.7X4	T45.7X5	T45.7X6
Snuff	T65.211	T65.212	T65.213	T65.214	—	—
Soap (powder) (product)	T55.0X1	T55.0X2	T55.0X3	T55.0X4	—	—
enema	T47.4X1	T47.4X2	T47.4X3	T47.4X4	T47.4X5	T47.4X6
medicinal, soft	T49.2X1	T49.2X2	T49.2X3	T49.2X4	T49.2X5	T49.2X6
superfatted	T49.2X1	T49.2X2	T49.2X3	T49.2X4	T49.2X5	T49.2X6
Sobrerol	T48.4X1	T48.4X2	T48.4X3	T48.4X4	T48.4X5	T48.4X6

◀ New   ◀ Revised   ~~deleted~~ Deleted

	External Cause (T-Code)					
Substance	Poisoning, Accidental (Unintentional)	Poisoning, Intentional Self-Harm	Poisoning, Assault	Poisoning, Undetermined	Adverse Effect	Underdosing
Soda (caustic)	T54.3X1	T54.3X2	T54.3X3	T54.3X4	—	—
bicarb	T47.1X1	T47.1X2	T47.1X3	T47.1X4	T47.1X5	T47.1X6
chlorinated — see Sodium, hypochlorite						
Sodium						
acetosulfone	T37.1X1	T37.1X2	T37.1X3	T37.1X4	T37.1X5	T37.1X6
acetrizoate	T50.8X1	T50.8X2	T50.8X3	T50.8X4	T50.8X5	T50.8X6
acid phosphate	T50.3X1	T50.3X2	T50.3X3	T50.3X4	T50.3X5	T50.3X6
alginate	T47.8X1	T47.8X2	T47.8X3	T47.8X4	T47.8X5	T47.8X6
amidotrizoate	T50.8X1	T50.8X2	T50.8X3	T50.8X4	T50.8X5	T50.8X6
aminopterin	T45.1X1	T45.1X2	T45.1X3	T45.1X4	T45.1X5	T45.1X6
amylosulfate	T47.8X1	T47.8X2	T47.8X3	T47.8X4	T47.8X5	T47.8X6
amytal	T42.3X1	T42.3X2	T42.3X3	T42.3X4	T42.3X5	T42.3X6
antimony gluconate	T37.3X1	T37.3X2	T37.3X3	T37.3X4	T37.3X5	T37.3X6
arsenate	T57.0X1	T57.0X2	T57.0X3	T57.0X4	—	—
aurothiomalate	T39.4X1	T39.4X2	T39.4X3	T39.4X4	T39.4X5	T39.4X6
aurothiosulfate	T39.4X1	T39.4X2	T39.4X3	T39.4X4	T39.4X5	T39.4X6
barbiturate	T42.3X1	T42.3X2	T42.3X3	T42.3X4	T42.3X5	T42.3X6
basic phosphate	T47.4X1	T47.4X2	T47.4X3	T47.4X4	T47.4X5	T47.4X6
bicarbonate	T47.1X1	T47.1X2	T47.1X3	T47.1X4	T47.1X5	T47.1X6
bichromate	T57.8X1	T57.8X2	T57.8X3	T57.8X4	—	—
biphosphate	T50.3X1	T50.3X2	T50.3X3	T50.3X4	T50.3X5	T50.3X6
bisulfate	T65.891	T65.892	T65.893	T65.894	—	—
borate						
cleanser	T57.8X1	T57.8X2	T57.8X3	T57.8X4	—	—
eye	T49.5X1	T49.5X2	T49.5X3	T49.5X4	T49.5X5	T49.5X6
therapeutic	T49.8X1	T49.8X2	T49.8X3	T49.8X4	T49.8X5	T49.8X6
bromide	T42.6X1	T42.6X2	T42.6X3	T42.6X4	T42.6X5	T42.6X6
cacodylate (nonmedicinal) NEC	T50.8X1	T50.8X2	T50.8X3	T50.8X4	T50.8X5	T50.8X6
anti-infective	T37.8X1	T37.8X2	T37.8X3	T37.8X4	T37.8X5	T37.8X6
herbicide	T60.3X1	T60.3X2	T60.3X3	T60.3X4	—	—
calcium edetate	T45.8X1	T45.8X2	T45.8X3	T45.8X4	T45.8X5	T45.8X6
carbonate NEC	T54.3X1	T54.3X2	T54.3X3	T54.3X4	—	—
chlorate NEC	T65.891	T65.892	T65.893	T65.894	—	—
herbicide	T54.91	T54.92	T54.93	T54.94	—	—
chloride	T50.3X1	T50.3X2	T50.3X3	T50.3X4	T50.3X5	T50.3X6
with glucose	T50.3X1	T50.3X2	T50.3X3	T50.3X4	T50.3X5	T50.3X6
chromate	T65.891	T65.892	T65.893	T65.894	—	—
citrate	T50.991	T50.992	T50.993	T50.994	T50.995	T50.996
cromoglicate	T48.6X1	T48.6X2	T48.6X3	T48.6X4	T48.6X5	T48.6X6
cyanide	T65.0X1	T65.0X2	T65.0X3	T65.0X4	—	—
cyclamate	T50.3X1	T50.3X2	T50.3X3	T50.3X4	T50.3X5	T50.3X6

	External Cause (T-Code)					
Substance	Poisoning, Accidental (Unintentional)	Poisoning, Intentional Self-Harm	Poisoning, Assault	Poisoning, Undetermined	Adverse Effect	Underdosing
Sodium (Continued)						
dehydrocholate	T45.8X1	T45.8X2	T45.8X3	T45.8X4	T45.8X5	T45.8X6
diatrizoate	T50.8X1	T50.8X2	T50.8X3	T50.8X4	T50.8X5	T50.8X6
dibunate	T48.4X1	T48.4X2	T48.4X3	T48.4X4	T48.4X5	T48.4X6
dioctyl sulfosuccinate	T47.4X1	T47.4X2	T47.4X3	T47.4X4	T47.4X5	T47.4X6
dipantoyl ferrate	T45.8X1	T45.8X2	T45.8X3	T45.8X4	T45.8X5	T45.8X6
edetate	T45.8X1	T45.8X2	T45.8X3	T45.8X4	T45.8X5	T45.8X6
ethacrynate	T50.1X1	T50.1X2	T50.1X3	T50.1X4	T50.1X5	T50.1X6
feredetate	T45.8X1	T45.8X2	T45.8X3	T45.8X4	T45.8X5	T45.8X6
Fluoride — see Fluoride						
fluoroacetate (dust) (pesticide)	T60.4X1	T60.4X2	T60.4X3	T60.4X4	—	—
free salt	T50.3X1	T50.3X2	T50.3X3	T50.3X4	T50.3X5	T50.3X6
fusidate	T36.8X1	T36.8X2	T36.8X3	T36.8X4	T36.8X5	T36.8X6
glucaldrate	T47.1X1	T47.1X2	T47.1X3	T47.1X4	T47.1X5	T47.1X6
glucosulfone	T37.1X1	T37.1X2	T37.1X3	T37.1X4	T37.1X5	T37.1X6
glutamate	T45.8X1	T45.8X2	T45.8X3	T45.8X4	T45.8X5	T45.8X6
hydrogen carbonate	T50.3X1	T50.3X2	T50.3X3	T50.3X4	T50.3X5	T50.3X6
hydroxide	T54.3X1	T54.3X2	T54.3X3	T54.3X4	—	—
hypochlorite (bleach) NEC	T54.3X1	T54.3X2	T54.3X3	T54.3X4	—	—
disinfectant	T54.3X1	T54.3X2	T54.3X3	T54.3X4	—	—
medicinal (anti-infective) (external)	T49.0X1	T49.0X2	T49.0X3	T49.0X4	T49.0X5	T49.0X6
vapor	T54.3X1	T54.3X2	T54.3X3	T54.3X4	—	—
hyposulfite	T49.0X1	T49.0X2	T49.0X3	T49.0X4	T49.0X5	T49.0X6
indigotin disulfonate	T50.8X1	T50.8X2	T50.8X3	T50.8X4	T50.8X5	T50.8X6
iodide	T50.991	T50.992	T50.993	T50.994	T50.995	T50.996
I-131	T50.8X1	T50.8X2	T50.8X3	T50.8X4	T50.8X5	T50.8X6
therapeutic	T38.2X1	T38.2X2	T38.2X3	T38.2X4	T38.2X5	T38.2X6
iodohippurate (131I)	T50.8X1	T50.8X2	T50.8X3	T50.8X4	T50.8X5	T50.8X6
iopodate	T50.8X1	T50.8X2	T50.8X3	T50.8X4	T50.8X5	T50.8X6
iothalamate	T50.8X1	T50.8X2	T50.8X3	T50.8X4	T50.8X5	T50.8X6
iron edetate	T45.4X1	T45.4X2	T45.4X3	T45.4X4	T45.4X5	T45.4X6
lactate (compound solution)	T45.8X1	T45.8X2	T45.8X3	T45.8X4	T45.8X5	T45.8X6
lauryl (sulfate)	T49.2X1	T49.2X2	T49.2X3	T49.2X4	T49.2X5	T49.2X6
(L)-triiodothyronine	T38.1X1	T38.1X2	T38.1X3	T38.1X4	T38.1X5	T38.1X6
magnesium citrate	T50.991	T50.992	T50.993	T50.994	T50.995	T50.996
mersalate	T50.2X1	T50.2X2	T50.2X3	T50.2X4	T50.2X5	T50.2X6
metasilicate	T65.891	T65.892	T65.893	T65.894	—	—
metrizoate	T50.8X1	T50.8X2	T50.8X3	T50.8X4	T50.8X5	T50.8X6
monofluoroacetate (pesticide)	T60.1X1	T60.1X2	T60.1X3	T60.1X4	—	—
morrhuate	T46.8X1	T46.8X2	T46.8X3	T46.8X4	T46.8X5	T46.8X6
nafcillin	T36.0X1	T36.0X2	T36.0X3	T36.0X4	T36.0X5	T36.0X6

◀ New　◀| Revised　deleted Deleted

Substance	External Cause (T-Code)					
	Poisoning, Accidental (Unintentional)	Poisoning, Intentional Self-Harm	Poisoning, Assault	Poisoning, Undetermined	Adverse Effect	Underdosing
Sodium (Continued)						
nitrate (oxidizing agent)	T65.891	T65.892	T65.893	T65.894	—	—
nitrite	T50.6X1	T50.6X2	T50.6X3	T50.6X4	T50.6X5	T50.6X6
nitroferricyanide	T46.5X1	T46.5X2	T46.5X3	T46.5X4	T46.5X5	T46.5X6
nitroprusside	T46.5X1	T46.5X2	T46.5X3	T46.5X4	T46.5X5	T46.5X6
oxalate	T65.891	T65.892	T65.893	T65.894	—	—
oxide/peroxide	T65.891	T65.892	T65.893	T65.894	—	—
oxybate	T41.291	T41.292	T41.293	T41.294	T41.295	T41.296
para-aminohippurate	T50.8X1	T50.8X2	T50.8X3	T50.8X4	T50.8X5	T50.8X6
perborate (nonmedicinal) NEC	T65.891	T65.892	T65.893	T65.894	—	—
medicinal	T49.0X1	T49.0X2	T49.0X3	T49.0X4	T49.0X5	T49.0X6
soap	T55.0X1	T55.0X2	T55.0X3	T55.0X4	—	—
percarbonate — see Sodium, perborate						
pertechnetate Tc99m	T50.8X1	T50.8X2		T50.8X4	T50.8X5	T50.8X6
phosphate						
cellulose	T45.8X1	T45.8X2	T45.8X3	T45.8X4	T45.8X5	T45.8X6
dibasic	T47.2X1	T47.2X2	T47.2X3	T47.2X4	T47.2X5	T47.2X6
monobasic	T47.2X1	T47.2X2	T47.2X3	T47.2X4	T47.2X5	T47.2X6
phytate	T50.6X1	T50.6X2	T50.6X3	T50.6X4	T50.6X5	T50.6X6
picosulfate	T47.2X1	T47.2X2	T47.2X3	T47.2X4	T47.2X5	T47.2X6
polyhydroxyaluminium monocarbonate	T47.1X1	T47.1X2	T47.1X3	T47.1X4	T47.1X5	T47.1X6
polystyrene sulfonate	T50.3X1	T50.3X2	T50.3X3	T50.3X4	T50.3X5	T50.3X6
propionate	T49.0X1	T49.0X2	T49.0X3	T49.0X4	T49.0X5	T49.0X6
propyl hydroxybenzoate	T50.991	T50.992	T50.993	T50.994	T50.995	T50.996
psylliate	T46.8X1	T46.8X2	T46.8X3	T46.8X4	T46.8X5	T46.8X6
removing resins	T50.3X1	T50.3X2	T50.3X3	T50.3X4	T50.3X5	T50.3X6
salicylate	T39.091	T39.092	T39.093	T39.094	T39.095	T39.096
salt NEC	T50.3X1	T50.3X2	T50.3X3	T50.3X4	T50.3X5	T50.3X6
selenate	T60.2X1	T60.2X2	T60.2X3	T60.2X4	—	—
stibogluconate	T37.3X1	T37.3X2	T37.3X3	T37.3X4	T37.3X5	T37.3X6
sulfate	T47.4X1	T47.4X2	T47.4X3	T47.4X4	T47.4X5	T47.4X6
sulfoxone	T37.1X1	T37.1X2	T37.1X3	T37.1X4	T37.1X5	T37.1X6
tetradecyl sulfate	T46.8X1	T46.8X2	T46.8X3	T46.8X4	T46.8X5	T46.8X6
thiopental	T41.1X1	T41.1X2	T41.1X3	T41.1X4	T41.1X5	T41.1X6
thiosalicylate	T39.091	T39.092	T39.093	T39.094	T39.095	T39.096
thiosulfate	T50.6X1	T50.6X2	T50.6X3	T50.6X4	T50.6X5	T50.6X6
tolbutamide	T38.3X1	T38.3X2	T38.3X3	T38.3X4	T38.3X5	T38.3X6
l-triiodothyronine	T38.1X1	T38.1X2	T38.1X3	T38.1X4	T38.1X5	T38.1X6
tyropanoate	T50.8X1	T50.8X2	T50.8X3	T50.8X4	T50.8X5	T50.8X6
valproate	T42.6X1	T42.6X2	T42.6X3	T42.6X4	T42.6X5	T42.6X6
versenate	T50.6X1	T50.6X2	T50.6X3	T50.6X4	T50.6X5	T50.6X6

Substance	External Cause (T-Code)					
	Poisoning, Accidental (Unintentional)	Poisoning, Intentional Self-Harm	Poisoning, Assault	Poisoning, Undetermined	Adverse Effect	Underdosing
Sodium-free salt	T50.901	T50.902	T50.903	T50.904	T50.905	T50.906
Sodium-removing resin	T50.3X1	T50.3X2	T50.3X3	T50.3X4	T50.3X5	T50.3X6
Soft soap	T55.0X1	T55.0X2	T55.0X3	T55.0X4	—	—
Solanine	T62.2X1	T62.2X2	T62.2X3	T62.2X4		
berries	T62.1X1	T62.1X2	T62.1X3	T62.1X4		
Solanum dulcamara	T62.2X1	T62.2X2	T62.2X3	T62.2X4		
berries	T62.1X1	T62.1X2	T62.1X3	T62.1X4		
Solapsone	T37.1X1	T37.1X2	T37.1X3	T37.1X4	T37.1X5	T37.1X6
Solar lotion	T49.3X1	T49.3X2	T49.3X3	T49.3X4	T49.3X5	T49.3X6
Solasulfone	T37.1X1	T37.1X2	T37.1X3	T37.1X4	T37.1X5	T37.1X6
Soldering fluid	T65.891	T65.892	T65.893	T65.894	—	—
Solid substance	T65.91	T65.92	T65.93	T65.94		
specified NEC	T65.891	T65.892	T65.893	T65.894		
Solvent, industrial NEC	T52.91	T52.92	T52.93	T52.94	—	—
naphtha	T52.0X1	T52.0X2	T52.0X3	T52.0X4	—	—
petroleum	T52.0X1	T52.0X2	T52.0X3	T52.0X4	—	—
specified NEC	T52.8X1	T52.8X2	T52.8X3	T52.8X4	—	—
Soma	T42.8X1	T42.8X2	T42.8X3	T42.8X4	T42.8X5	T42.8X6
Somatorelin	T38.891	T38.892	T38.893	T38.894	T38.895	T38.896
Somatostatin	T38.991	T38.992	T38.993	T38.994	T38.995	T38.996
Somatotropin	T38.811	T38.812	T38.813	T38.814	T38.815	T38.816
Somatrem	T38.811	T38.812	T38.813	T38.814	T38.815	T38.816
Somatropin	T38.811	T38.812	T38.813	T38.814	T38.815	T38.816
Sominex	T45.0X1	T45.0X2	T45.0X3	T45.0X4	T45.0X5	T45.0X6
Somnos	T42.6X1	T42.6X2	T42.6X3	T42.6X4	T42.6X5	T42.6X6
Somonal	T42.3X1	T42.3X2	T42.3X3	T42.3X4	T42.3X5	T42.3X6
Soneryl	T42.3X1	T42.3X2	T42.3X3	T42.3X4	T42.3X5	T42.3X6
Soothing syrup	T50.901	T50.902	T50.903	T50.904	T50.905	T50.906
Sopor	T42.6X1	T42.6X2	T42.6X3	T42.6X4	T42.6X5	T42.6X6
Soporific	T42.71	T42.72	T42.73	T42.74	T42.75	T42.76
Soporific drug	T42.71	T42.72	T42.73	T42.74	T42.75	T42.76
specified type NEC	T42.6X1	T42.6X2	T42.6X3	T42.6X4	T42.6X5	T42.6X6
Sorbide nitrate	T46.3X1	T46.3X2	T46.3X3	T46.3X4	T46.3X5	T46.3X6
Sorbitol	T47.4X1	T47.4X2	T47.4X3	T47.4X4	T47.4X5	T47.4X6
Sotalol	T44.7X1	T44.7X2	T44.7X3	T44.7X4	T44.7X5	T44.7X6
Sotradecol	T46.8X1	T46.8X2	T46.8X3	T46.8X4	T46.8X5	T46.8X6
Soysterol	T46.6X1	T46.6X2	T46.6X3	T46.6X4	T46.6X5	T46.6X6
Spacoline	T44.3X1	T44.3X2	T44.3X3	T44.3X4	T44.3X5	T44.3X6
Spanish fly	T49.8X1	T49.8X2	T49.8X3	T49.8X4	T49.8X5	T49.8X6
Sparine	T43.3X1	T43.3X2	T43.3X3	T43.3X4	T43.3X5	T43.3X6
Sparteine	T48.0X1	T48.0X2	T48.0X3	T48.0X4	T48.0X5	T48.0X6

◀ New   ◀ Revised   deleted Deleted

Substance	Poisoning, Accidental (Unintentional)	Poisoning, Intentional Self-Harm	Poisoning, Assault	Poisoning, Undetermined	Adverse Effect	Underdosing
Spasmolytic						
anticholinergics	T44.3X1	T44.3X2	T44.3X3	T44.3X4	T44.3X5	T44.3X6
autonomic	T44.3X1	T44.3X2	T44.3X3	T44.3X4	T44.3X5	T44.3X6
bronchial NEC	T48.6X1	T48.6X2	T48.6X3	T48.6X4	T48.6X5	T48.6X6
quaternary ammonium	T44.3X1	T44.3X2	T44.3X3	T44.3X4	T44.3X5	T44.3X6
skeletal muscle NEC	T48.1X1	T48.1X2	T48.1X3	T48.1X4	T48.1X5	T48.1X6
Spectinomycin	T36.5X1	T36.5X2	T36.5X3	T36.5X4	T36.5X5	T36.5X6
Speed	T43.621	T43.622	T43.623	T43.624	T43.625	T43.626
Spermicide	T49.8X1	T49.8X2	T49.8X3	T49.8X4	T49.8X5	T49.8X6
Spider (bite) (venom)	T63.391	T63.392	T63.393	T63.394	—	—
antivenin	T50.Z11	T50.Z12	T50.Z13	T50.Z14	T50.Z15	T50.Z16
Spigelia (root)	T37.4X1	T37.4X2	T37.4X3	T37.4X4	T37.4X5	T37.4X6
Spindle inactivator	T50.4X1	T50.4X2	T50.4X3	T50.4X4	T50.4X5	T50.4X6
Spiperone	T43.4X1	T43.4X2	T43.4X3	T43.4X4	T43.4X5	T43.4X6
Spiramycin	T36.3X1	T36.3X2	T36.3X3	T36.3X4	T36.3X5	T36.3X6
Spirapril	T46.4X1	T46.4X2	T46.4X3	T46.4X4	T46.4X5	T46.4X6
Spirilene	T43.591	T43.592	T43.593	T43.594	T43.595	T43.596
Spirit(s) (neutral) NEC	T51.0X1	T51.0X2	T51.0X3	T51.0X4	—	—
beverage	T51.0X1	T51.0X2	T51.0X3	T51.0X4	—	—
industrial	T51.0X1	T51.0X2	T51.0X3	T51.0X4	—	—
mineral	T52.0X1	T52.0X2	T52.0X3	T52.0X4	—	—
of salt — see Hydrochloric acid						
surgical	T51.0X1	T51.0X2	T51.0X3	T51.0X4	—	—
Spironolactone	T50.0X1	T50.0X2	T50.0X3	T50.0X4	T50.0X5	T50.0X6
Spiroperidol	T43.4X1	T43.4X2	T43.4X3	T43.4X4	T43.4X5	T43.4X6
Sponge, absorbable (gelatin)	T45.7X1	T45.7X2	T45.7X3	T45.7X4	T45.7X5	T45.7X6
Sporostacin	T49.0X1	T49.0X2	T49.0X3	T49.0X4	T49.0X5	T49.0X6
Spray (aerosol)	T65.91	T65.92	T65.93	T65.94	—	—
cosmetic	T65.891	T65.892	T65.893	T65.894	—	—
medicinal NEC	T50.901	T50.902	T50.903	T50.904	T50.905	T50.906
pesticides — see Pesticides						
specified content — see specific substance						
Spurge flax	T62.2X1	T62.2X2	T62.2X3	T62.2X4	—	—
Spurges	T62.2X1	T62.2X2	T62.2X3	T62.2X4	—	—
Sputum viscosity-lowering drug	T48.4X1	T48.4X2	T48.4X3	T48.4X4	T48.4X5	T48.4X6
Squill	T46.0X1	T46.0X2	T46.0X3	T46.0X4	T46.0X5	T46.0X6
rat poison	T60.4X1	T60.4X2	T60.4X3	T60.4X4	—	—
Squirting cucumber (cathartic)	T47.2X1	T47.2X2	T47.2X3	T47.2X4	T47.2X5	T47.2X6
Stains	T65.6X1	T65.6X2	T65.6X3	T65.6X4	—	—
Stannous fluoride	T49.7X1	T49.7X2	T49.7X3	T49.7X4	T49.7X5	T49.7X6
Stanolone	T38.7X1	T38.7X2	T38.7X3	T38.7X4	T38.7X5	T38.7X6

Substance	Poisoning, Accidental (Unintentional)	Poisoning, Intentional Self-Harm	Poisoning, Assault	Poisoning, Undetermined	Adverse Effect	Underdosing
Stanozolol	T38.7X1	T38.7X2	T38.7X3	T38.7X4	T38.7X5	T38.7X6
Staphisagria or stavesacre (pediculicide)	T49.0X1	T49.0X2	T49.0X3	T49.0X4	T49.0X5	T49.0X6
Starch	T50.901	T50.902	T50.903	T50.904	T50.905	T50.906
Stelazine	T43.3X1	T43.3X2	T43.3X3	T43.3X4	T43.3X5	T43.3X6
Stemetil	T43.3X1	T43.3X2	T43.3X3	T43.3X4	T43.3X5	T43.3X6
Stepronin	T48.4X1	T48.4X2	T48.4X3	T48.4X4	T48.4X5	T48.4X6
Sterculia	T47.4X1	T47.4X2	T47.4X3	T47.4X4	T47.4X5	T47.4X6
Sternutator gas	T59.891	T59.892	T59.893	T59.894	—	—
Steroid	T38.0X1	T38.0X2	T38.0X3	T38.0X4	T38.0X5	T38.0X6
anabolic	T38.7X1	T38.7X2	T38.7X3	T38.7X4	T38.7X5	T38.7X6
androgenic	T38.7X1	T38.7X2	T38.7X3	T38.7X4	T38.7X5	T38.7X6
antineoplastic, hormone	T38.7X1	T38.7X2	T38.7X3	T38.7X4	T38.7X5	T38.7X6
estrogen	T38.5X1	T38.5X2	T38.5X3	T38.5X4	T38.5X5	T38.5X6
ENT agent	T49.6X1	T49.6X2	T49.6X3	T49.6X4	T49.6X5	T49.6X6
ophthalmic preparation	T49.5X1	T49.5X2	T49.5X3	T49.5X4	T49.5X5	T49.5X6
topical NEC	T49.0X1	T49.0X2	T49.0X3	T49.0X4	T49.0X5	T49.0X6
Stibine	T56.891	T56.892	T56.893	T56.894	—	—
Stibogluconate	T37.3X1	T37.3X2	T37.3X3	T37.3X4	T37.3X5	T37.3X6
Stibophen	T37.4X1	T37.4X2	T37.4X3	T37.4X4	T37.4X5	T37.4X6
Stilbamidine (isetionate)	T37.3X1	T37.3X2	T37.3X3	T37.3X4	T37.3X5	T37.3X6
Stilbestrol	T38.5X1	T38.5X2	T38.5X3	T38.5X4	T38.5X5	T38.5X6
Stilboestrol	T38.5X1	T38.5X2	T38.5X3	T38.5X4	T38.5X5	T38.5X6
Stimulant						
central nervous system — see also Psychostimulant	T43.601	T43.602	T43.603	T43.604	T43.605	T43.606
analeptics	T50.7X1	T50.7X2	T50.7X3	T50.7X4	T50.7X5	T50.7X6
opiate antagonist	T50.7X1	T50.7X2	T50.7X3	T50.7X4	T50.7X5	T50.7X6
psychotherapeutic NEC — see also Psychotherapeutic drug	T43.601	T43.602	T43.603	T43.604	T43.605	T43.606
specified NEC	T43.691	T43.692	T43.693	T43.694	T43.695	T43.696
respiratory	T48.901	T48.902	T48.903	T48.904	T48.905	T48.906
Stone-dissolving drug	T50.901	T50.902	T50.903	T50.904	T50.905	T50.906
Storage battery (cells) (acid)	T54.2X1	T54.2X2	T54.2X3	T54.2X4	—	—
Stovaine	T41.3X1	T41.3X2	T41.3X3	T41.3X4	T41.3X5	T41.3X6
infiltration (subcutaneous)	T41.3X1	T41.3X2	T41.3X3	T41.3X4	T41.3X5	T41.3X6
nerve block (peripheral) (plexus)	T41.3X1	T41.3X2	T41.3X3	T41.3X4	T41.3X5	T41.3X6
spinal	T41.3X1	T41.3X2	T41.3X3	T41.3X4	T41.3X5	T41.3X6
topical (surface)	T41.3X1	T41.3X2	T41.3X3	T41.3X4	T41.3X5	T41.3X6
Stovarsal	T37.8X1	T37.8X2	T37.8X3	T37.8X4	T37.8X5	T37.8X6
Stove gas — see Gas, stove	T57.91	T57.92	T57.93	T57.94	—	—

◀ New ◀ Revised ~~deleted~~ Deleted

TABLE OF DRUGS AND CHEMICALS

Substance	Poisoning, Accidental (Unintentional)	Poisoning, Intentional Self-Harm	Poisoning, Assault	Poisoning, Undetermined	Adverse Effect	Underdosing
Stoxil	T49.5X1	T49.5X2	T49.5X3	T49.5X4	T49.5X5	T49.5X6
Stramonium	T48.6X1	T48.6X2	T48.6X3	T48.6X4	T48.6X5	T48.6X6
natural state	T62.2X1	T62.2X2	T62.2X3	T62.2X4	—	—
Streptodornase	T45.3X1	T45.3X2	T45.3X3	T45.3X4	T45.3X5	T45.3X6
Streptoduocin	T36.5X1	T36.5X2	T36.5X3	T36.5X4	T36.5X5	T36.5X6
Streptokinase	T45.611	T45.612	T45.613	T45.614	T45.615	T45.616
Streptomycin (derivative)	T36.5X1	T36.5X2	T36.5X3	T36.5X4	T36.5X5	T36.5X6
Streptonivicin	T36.5X1	T36.5X2	T36.5X3	T36.5X4	T36.5X5	T36.5X6
Streptovarycin	T36.5X1	T36.5X2	T36.5X3	T36.5X4	T36.5X5	T36.5X6
Streptozocin	T45.1X1	T45.1X2	T45.1X3	T45.1X4	T45.1X5	T45.1X6
Streptozotocin	T45.1X1	T45.1X2	T45.1X3	T45.1X4	T45.1X5	T45.1X6
Stripper (paint) (solvent)	T52.8X1	T52.8X2	T52.8X3	T52.8X4	—	—
Strobane	T60.1X1	T60.1X2	T60.1X3	T60.1X4	—	—
Strofantina	T46.0X1	T46.0X2	T46.0X3	T46.0X4	T46.0X5	T46.0X6
Strophanthin (g) (k)	T46.0X1	T46.0X2	T46.0X3	T46.0X4	T46.0X5	T46.0X6
Strophanthus	T46.0X1	T46.0X2	T46.0X3	T46.0X4	T46.0X5	T46.0X6
Strophantin	T46.0X1	T46.0X2	T46.0X3	T46.0X4	T46.0X5	T46.0X6
Strophantin-g	T46.0X1	T46.0X2	T46.0X3	T46.0X4	T46.0X5	T46.0X6
Strychnine (nonmedicinal) (pesticide) (salts)	T65.1X1	T65.1X2	T65.1X3	T65.1X4	—	—
medicinal	T48.291	T48.292	T48.293	T48.294	T48.295	T48.296
Strychnos (ignatii) — see Strychnine						
Styramate	T42.8X1	T42.8X2	T42.8X3	T42.8X4	T42.8X5	T42.8X6
Styrene	T65.891	T65.892	T65.893	T65.894	—	—
Succinimide, antiepileptic or anticonvulsant	T42.2X1	T42.2X2	T42.2X3	T42.2X4	T42.2X5	T42.2X6
mercuric — see Mercury						
Succinylcholine	T48.1X1	T48.1X2	T48.1X3	T48.1X4	T48.1X5	T48.1X6
Succinylsulfathiazole	T37.0X1	T37.0X2	T37.0X3	T37.0X4	T37.0X5	T37.0X6
Sucralfate	T47.1X1	T47.1X2	T47.1X3	T47.1X4	T47.1X5	T47.1X6
Sucrose	T50.3X1	T50.3X2	T50.3X3	T50.3X4	T50.3X5	T50.3X6
Sufentanil	T40.4X1	T40.4X2	T40.4X3	T40.4X4	T40.4X5	T40.4X6
Sulbactam	T36.0X1	T36.0X2	T36.0X3	T36.0X4	T36.0X5	T36.0X6
Sulbenicillin	T36.0X1	T36.0X2	T36.0X3	T36.0X4	T36.0X5	T36.0X6
Sulbentine	T49.0X1	T49.0X2	T49.0X3	T49.0X4	T49.0X5	T49.0X6
Sulfacetamide	T49.0X1	T49.0X2	T49.0X3	T49.0X4	T49.0X5	T49.0X6
ophthalmic preparation	T49.5X1	T49.5X2	T49.5X3	T49.5X4	T49.5X5	T49.5X6
Sulfachlorpyridazine	T37.0X1	T37.0X2	T37.0X3	T37.0X4	T37.0X5	T37.0X6
Sulfacitine	T37.0X1	T37.0X2	T37.0X3	T37.0X4	T37.0X5	T37.0X6
Sulfadiasulfone sodium	T37.0X1	T37.0X2	T37.0X3	T37.0X4	T37.0X5	T37.0X6
Sulfadiazine	T37.0X1	T37.0X2	T37.0X3	T37.0X4	T37.0X5	T37.0X6
silver (topical)	T49.0X1	T49.0X2	T49.0X3	T49.0X4	T49.0X5	T49.0X6

Substance	Poisoning, Accidental (Unintentional)	Poisoning, Intentional Self-Harm	Poisoning, Assault	Poisoning, Undetermined	Adverse Effect	Underdosing
Sulfadimethoxine	T37.0X1	T37.0X2	T37.0X3	T37.0X4	T37.0X5	T37.0X6
Sulfadimidine	T37.0X1	T37.0X2	T37.0X3	T37.0X4	T37.0X5	T37.0X6
Sulfadoxine	T37.0X1	T37.0X2	T37.0X3	T37.0X4	T37.0X5	T37.0X6
with pyrimethamine	T37.2X1	T37.2X2	T37.2X3	T37.2X4	T37.2X5	T37.2X6
Sulfaethidole	T37.0X1	T37.0X2	T37.0X3	T37.0X4	T37.0X5	T37.0X6
Sulfafurazole	T37.0X1	T37.0X2	T37.0X3	T37.0X4	T37.0X5	T37.0X6
Sulfaguanidine	T37.0X1	T37.0X2	T37.0X3	T37.0X4	T37.0X5	T37.0X6
Sulfalene	T37.0X1	T37.0X2	T37.0X3	T37.0X4	T37.0X5	T37.0X6
Sulfaloxate	T37.0X1	T37.0X2	T37.0X3	T37.0X4	T37.0X5	T37.0X6
Sulfaloxic acid	T37.0X1	T37.0X2	T37.0X3	T37.0X4	T37.0X5	T37.0X6
Sulfamazone	T39.2X1	T39.2X2	T39.2X3	T39.2X4	T39.2X5	T39.2X6
Sulfamerazine	T37.0X1	T37.0X2	T37.0X3	T37.0X4	T37.0X5	T37.0X6
Sulfameter	T37.0X1	T37.0X2	T37.0X3	T37.0X4	T37.0X5	T37.0X6
Sulfamethazine	T37.0X1	T37.0X2	T37.0X3	T37.0X4	T37.0X5	T37.0X6
Sulfamethizole	T37.0X1	T37.0X2	T37.0X3	T37.0X4	T37.0X5	T37.0X6
Sulfamethoxazole	T37.0X1	T37.0X2	T37.0X3	T37.0X4	T37.0X5	T37.0X6
with trimethoprim	T36.8X1	T36.8X2	T36.8X3	T36.8X4	T36.8X5	T36.8X6
Sulfamethoxydiazine	T37.0X1	T37.0X2	T37.0X3	T37.0X4	T37.0X5	T37.0X6
Sulfamethoxypyridazine	T37.0X1	T37.0X2	T37.0X3	T37.0X4	T37.0X5	T37.0X6
Sulfamethylthiazole	T37.0X1	T37.0X2	T37.0X3	T37.0X4	T37.0X5	T37.0X6
Sulfametoxydiazine	T37.0X1	T37.0X2	T37.0X3	T37.0X4	T37.0X5	T37.0X6
Sulfamidopyrine	T39.2X1	T39.2X2	T39.2X3	T39.2X4	T39.2X5	T39.2X6
Sulfamonomethoxine	T37.0X1	T37.0X2	T37.0X3	T37.0X4	T37.0X5	T37.0X6
Sulfamoxole	T37.0X1	T37.0X2	T37.0X3	T37.0X4	T37.0X5	T37.0X6
Sulfamylon	T49.0X1	T49.0X2	T49.0X3	T49.0X4	T49.0X5	T49.0X6
Sulfan blue (diagnostic dye)	T50.8X1	T50.8X2	T50.8X3	T50.8X4	T50.8X5	T50.8X6
Sulfanilamide	T37.0X1	T37.0X2	T37.0X3	T37.0X4	T37.0X5	T37.0X6
Sulfanilylguanidine	T37.0X1	T37.0X2	T37.0X3	T37.0X4	T37.0X5	T37.0X6
Sulfaperin	T37.0X1	T37.0X2	T37.0X3	T37.0X4	T37.0X5	T37.0X6
Sulfaphenazole	T37.0X1	T37.0X2	T37.0X3	T37.0X4	T37.0X5	T37.0X6
Sulfaphenylthiazole	T37.0X1	T37.0X2	T37.0X3	T37.0X4	T37.0X5	T37.0X6
Sulfaproxyline	T37.0X1	T37.0X2	T37.0X3	T37.0X4	T37.0X5	T37.0X6
Sulfapyridine	T37.0X1	T37.0X2	T37.0X3	T37.0X4	T37.0X5	T37.0X6
Sulfapyrimidine	T37.0X1	T37.0X2	T37.0X3	T37.0X4	T37.0X5	T37.0X6
Sulfarsphenamine	T37.8X1	T37.8X2	T37.8X3	T37.8X4	T37.8X5	T37.8X6
Sulfasalazine	T37.0X1	T37.0X2	T37.0X3	T37.0X4	T37.0X5	T37.0X6
Sulfasuxidine	T37.0X1	T37.0X2	T37.0X3	T37.0X4	T37.0X5	T37.0X6
Sulfasymazine	T37.0X1	T37.0X2	T37.0X3	T37.0X4	T37.0X5	T37.0X6
Sulfated amylopectin	T47.8X1	T47.8X2	T47.8X3	T47.8X4	T47.8X5	T47.8X6
Sulfathiazole	T37.0X1	T37.0X2	T37.0X3	T37.0X4	T37.0X5	T37.0X6
Sulfatostearate	T49.2X1	T49.2X2	T49.2X3	T49.2X4	T49.2X5	T49.2X6
Sulfinpyrazone	T50.4X1	T50.4X2	T50.4X3	T50.4X4	T50.4X5	T50.4X6

◀ New   ◀ Revised   ~~deleted~~ Deleted

	External Cause (T-Code)					
Substance	Poisoning, Accidental (Unintentional)	Poisoning, Intentional Self-Harm	Poisoning, Assault	Poisoning, Undetermined	Adverse Effect	Underdosing
Sulfiram	T49.0X1	T49.0X2	T49.0X3	T49.0X4	T49.0X5	T49.0X6
Sulfisomidine	T37.0X1	T37.0X2	T37.0X3	T37.0X4	T37.0X5	T37.0X6
Sulfisoxazole	T37.0X1	T37.0X2	T37.0X3	T37.0X4	T37.0X5	T37.0X6
ophthalmic preparation	T49.5X1	T49.5X2	T49.5X3	T49.5X4	T49.5X5	T49.5X6
Sulfobromophthalein (sodium)	T50.8X1	T50.8X2	T50.8X3	T50.8X4	T50.8X5	T50.8X6
Sulfobromphthalein	T50.8X1	T50.8X2	T50.8X3	T50.8X4	T50.8X5	T50.8X6
Sulfogaiacol	T48.4X1	T48.4X2	T48.4X3	T48.4X4	T48.4X5	T48.4X6
Sulfomyxin	T36.8X1	T36.8X2	T36.8X3	T36.8X4	T36.8X5	T36.8X6
Sulfonal	T42.6X1	T42.6X2	T42.6X3	T42.6X4	T42.6X5	T42.6X6
Sulfonamide NEC	T37.0X1	T37.0X2	T37.0X3	T37.0X4	T37.0X5	T37.0X6
eye	T49.5X1	T49.5X2	T49.5X3	T49.5X4	T49.5X5	T49.5X6
Sulfonazide	T37.1X1	T37.1X2	T37.1X3	T37.1X4	T37.1X5	T37.1X6
Sulfones	T37.1X1	T37.1X2	T37.1X3	T37.1X4	T37.1X5	T37.1X6
Sulfonethylmethane	T42.6X1	T42.6X2	T42.6X3	T42.6X4	T42.6X5	T42.6X6
Sulfonmethane	T42.6X1	T42.6X2	T42.6X3	T42.6X4	T42.6X5	T42.6X6
Sulfonphthal, sulfonphthol	T50.8X1	T50.8X2	T50.8X3	T50.8X4	T50.8X5	T50.8X6
Sulfonylurea derivatives, oral	T38.3X1	T38.3X2	T38.3X3	T38.3X4	T38.3X5	T38.3X6
Sulforidazine	T43.3X1	T43.3X2	T43.3X3	T43.3X4	T43.3X5	T43.3X6
Sulfoxone	T37.1X1	T37.1X2	T37.1X3	T37.1X4	T37.1X5	T37.1X6
Sulfur, sulfurated, sulfuric, sulfurous, sulfuryl (compounds NEC) (medicinal)	T49.4X1	T49.4X2	T49.4X3	T49.4X4	T49.4X5	T49.4X6
acid	T54.2X1	T54.2X2	T54.2X3	T54.2X4	—	—
dioxide (gas)	T59.1X1	T59.1X2	T59.1X3	T59.1X4	—	—
ether — see Ether(s)						
hydrogen	T59.6X1	T59.6X2	T59.6X3	T59.6X4		
medicinal (keratolytic) (ointment) NEC	T49.4X1	T49.4X2	T49.4X3	T49.4X4	T49.4X5	T49.4X6
ointment	T49.0X1	T49.0X2	T49.0X3	T49.0X4	T49.0X5	T49.0X6
pesticide (vapor)	T60.91	T60.92	T60.93	T60.94	—	—
vapor NEC	T59.891	T59.892	T59.893	T59.894	—	—
Sulfuric acid	T54.2X1	T54.2X2	T54.2X3	T54.2X4	—	—
Sulglicotide	T47.1X1	T47.1X2	T47.1X3	T47.1X4	T47.1X5	T47.1X6
Sulindac	T39.391	T39.392	T39.393	T39.394	T39.395	T39.396
Sulisatin	T47.2X1	T47.2X2	T47.2X3	T47.2X4	T47.2X5	T47.2X6
Sulisobenzone	T49.3X1	T49.3X2	T49.3X3	T49.3X4	T49.3X5	T49.3X6
Sulkowitch's reagent	T50.8X1	T50.8X2	T50.8X3	T50.8X4	T50.8X5	T50.8X6
Sulmetozine	T44.3X1	T44.3X2	T44.3X3	T44.3X4	T44.3X5	T44.3X6
Suloctidil	T46.7X1	T46.7X2	T46.7X3	T46.7X4	T46.7X5	T46.7X6
Sulph — see also Sulf-						
Sulphadiazine	T37.0X1	T37.0X2	T37.0X3	T37.0X4	T37.0X5	T37.0X6

	External Cause (T-Code)					
Substance	Poisoning, Accidental (Unintentional)	Poisoning, Intentional Self-Harm	Poisoning, Assault	Poisoning, Undetermined	Adverse Effect	Underdosing
Sulphadimethoxine	T37.0X1	T37.0X2	T37.0X3	T37.0X4	T37.0X5	T37.0X6
Sulphadimidine	T37.0X1	T37.0X2	T37.0X3	T37.0X4	T37.0X5	T37.0X6
Sulphadione	T37.1X1	T37.1X2	T37.1X3	T37.1X4	T37.1X5	T37.1X6
Sulphafurazole	T37.0X1	T37.0X2	T37.0X3	T37.0X4	T37.0X5	T37.0X6
Sulphamethizole	T37.0X1	T37.0X2	T37.0X3	T37.0X4	T37.0X5	T37.0X6
Sulphamethoxazole	T37.0X1	T37.0X2	T37.0X3	T37.0X4	T37.0X5	T37.0X6
Sulphan blue	T50.8X1	T50.8X2	T50.8X3	T50.8X4	T50.8X5	T50.8X6
Sulphaphenazole	T37.0X1	T37.0X2	T37.0X3	T37.0X4	T37.0X5	T37.0X6
Sulphapyridine	T37.0X1	T37.0X2	T37.0X3	T37.0X4	T37.0X5	T37.0X6
Sulphasalazine	T37.0X1	T37.0X2	T37.0X3	T37.0X4	T37.0X5	T37.0X6
Sulphinpyrazone	T50.4X1	T50.4X2	T50.4X3	T50.4X4	T50.4X5	T50.4X6
Sulpiride	T43.591	T43.592	T43.593	T43.594	T43.595	T43.596
Sulprostone	T48.0X1	T48.0X2	T48.0X3	T48.0X4	T48.0X5	T48.0X6
Sulpyrine	T39.2X1	T39.2X2	T39.2X3	T39.2X4	T39.2X5	T39.2X6
Sultamicillin	T36.0X1	T36.0X2	T36.0X3	T36.0X4	T36.0X5	T36.0X6
Sulthiame	T42.6X1	T42.6X2	T42.6X3	T42.6X4	T42.6X5	T42.6X6
Sultiame	T42.6X1	T42.6X2	T42.6X3	T42.6X4	T42.6X5	T42.6X6
Sultopride	T43.591	T43.592	T43.593	T43.594	T43.595	T43.596
Sumatriptan	T39.8X1	T39.8X2	T39.8X3	T39.8X4	T39.8X5	T39.8X6
Sunflower seed oil	T46.6X1	T46.6X2	T46.6X3	T46.6X4	T46.6X5	T46.6X6
Superinone	T48.4X1	T48.4X2	T48.4X3	T48.4X4	T48.4X5	T48.4X6
Suprofen	T39.311	T39.312	T39.313	T39.314	T39.315	T39.316
Suramin (sodium)	T37.4X1	T37.4X2	T37.4X3	T37.4X4	T37.4X5	T37.4X6
Surfacaine	T41.3X1	T41.3X2	T41.3X3	T41.3X4	T41.3X5	T41.3X6
Surital	T41.1X1	T41.1X2	T41.1X3	T41.1X4	T41.1X5	T41.1X6
Sutilains	T45.3X1	T45.3X2	T45.3X3	T45.3X4	T45.3X5	T45.3X6
Suxamethonium (chloride)	T48.1X1	T48.1X2	T48.1X3	T48.1X4	T48.1X5	T48.1X6
Suxethonium (chloride)	T48.1X1	T48.1X2	T48.1X3	T48.1X4	T48.1X5	T48.1X6
Suxibuzone	T39.2X1	T39.2X2	T39.2X3	T39.2X4	T39.2X5	T39.2X6
Sweet oil (birch)	T49.3X1	T49.3X2	T49.3X3	T49.3X4	T49.3X5	T49.3X6
Sweet niter spirit	T46.3X1	T46.3X2	T46.3X3	T46.3X4	T46.3X5	T46.3X6
Sweetener	T50.901	T50.902	T50.903	T50.904	T50.905	T50.906
Sym-dichloroethyl ether	T53.6X1	T53.6X2	T53.6X3	T53.6X4	—	—
Sympatholytic NEC	T44.8X1	T44.8X2	T44.8X3	T44.8X4	T44.8X5	T44.8X6
haloalkylamine	T44.8X1	T44.8X2	T44.8X3	T44.8X4	T44.8X5	T44.8X6
Sympathomimetic NEC	T44.901	T44.902	T44.903	T44.904	T44.905	T44.906
anti-common-cold	T48.5X1	T48.5X2	T48.5X3	T48.5X4	T48.5X5	T48.5X6
bronchodilator	T48.6X1	T48.6X2	T48.6X3	T48.6X4	T48.6X5	T48.6X6
specified NEC	T44.991	T44.992	T44.993	T44.994	T44.995	T44.996
Synagis	T50.B91	T50.B92	T50.B93	T50.B94	T50.B95	T50.B96
Synalar	T49.0X1	T49.0X2	T49.0X3	T49.0X4	T49.0X5	T49.0X6
Synthroid	T38.1X1	T38.1X2	T38.1X3	T38.1X4	T38.1X5	T38.1X6

◀ New   ◀❚ Revised   ~~deleted~~ Deleted

Substance	Poisoning, Accidental (Unintentional)	Poisoning, Intentional Self-Harm	Poisoning, Assault	Poisoning, Undetermined	Adverse Effect	Underdosing
Syntocinon	T48.0X1	T48.0X2	T48.0X3	T48.0X4	T48.0X5	T48.0X6
Syrosingopine	T46.5X1	T46.5X2	T46.5X3	T46.5X4	T46.5X5	T46.5X6
Systemic drug	T45.91	T45.92	T45.93	T45.94	T45.95	T45.96
specified NEC	T45.8X1	T45.8X2	T45.8X3	T45.8X4	T45.8X5	T45.8X6
2,4,5-T	T60.3X1	T60.3X2	T60.3X3	T60.3X4	—	—
T						
Tablets — see also specified substance	T50.901	T50.902	T50.903	T50.904	T50.905	T50.906
Tace	T38.5X1	T38.5X2	T38.5X3	T38.5X4	T38.5X5	T38.5X6
Tacrine	T44.0X1	T44.0X2	T44.0X3	T44.0X4	T44.0X5	T44.0X6
Tadalafil	T46.7X1	T46.7X2	T46.7X3	T46.7X4	T46.7X5	T46.7X6
Talampicillin	T36.0X1	T36.0X2	T36.0X3	T36.0X4	T36.0X5	T36.0X6
Talbutal	T42.3X1	T42.3X2	T42.3X3	T42.3X4	T42.3X5	T42.3X6
Talc powder	T49.3X1	T49.3X2	T49.3X3	T49.3X4	T49.3X5	T49.3X6
Talcum	T49.3X1	T49.3X2	T49.3X3	T49.3X4	T49.3X5	T49.3X6
Taleranol	T38.6X1	T38.6X2	T38.6X3	T38.6X4	T38.6X5	T38.6X6
Tamoxifen	T38.6X1	T38.6X2	T38.6X3	T38.6X4	T38.6X5	T38.6X6
Tamsulosin	T44.6X1	T44.6X2	T44.6X3	T44.6X4	T44.6X5	T44.6X6
Tandearil, tanderil	T39.2X1	T39.2X2	T39.2X3	T39.2X4	T39.2X5	T39.2X6
Tannic acid	T49.2X1	T49.2X2	T49.2X3	T49.2X4	T49.2X5	T49.2X6
medicinal (astringent)	T49.2X1	T49.2X2	T49.2X3	T49.2X4	T49.2X5	T49.2X6
Tannin — see Tannic acid						
Tansy	T62.2X1	T62.2X2	T62.2X3	T62.2X4	—	—
TAO	T36.3X1	T36.3X2	T36.3X3	T36.3X4	T36.3X5	T36.3X6
Tapazole	T38.2X1	T38.2X2	T38.2X3	T38.2X4	T38.2X5	T38.2X6
Tar NEC	T52.0X1	T52.0X2	T52.0X3	T52.0X4		
camphor	T60.1X1	T60.1X2	T60.1X3	T60.1X4	—	—
distillate	T49.1X1	T49.1X2	T49.1X3	T49.1X4	T49.1X5	T49.1X6
fumes	T59.891	T59.892	T59.893	T59.894	—	—
medicinal	T49.1X1	T49.1X2	T49.1X3	T49.1X4	T49.1X5	T49.1X6
ointment	T49.1X1	T49.1X2	T49.1X3	T49.1X4	T49.1X5	T49.1X6
Taractan	T43.591	T43.592	T43.593	T43.594	T43.595	T43.596
Tarantula (venomous)	T63.321	T63.322	T63.323	T63.324	—	—
Tartar emetic	T37.8X1	T37.8X2	T37.8X3	T37.8X4	T37.8X5	T37.8X6
Tartaric acid	T65.891	T65.892	T65.893	T65.894		
Tartrated antimony (anti-infective)	T37.8X1	T37.8X2	T37.8X3	T37.8X4	T37.8X5	T37.8X6
Tartrate, laxative	T47.4X1	T47.4X2	T47.4X3	T47.4X4	T47.4X5	T47.4X6
Tauromustine	T45.1X1	T45.1X2	T45.1X3	T45.1X4	T45.1X5	T45.1X6
TCA — see Trichloroacetic acid						
TCDD	T53.7X1	T53.7X2	T53.7X3	T53.7X4	—	—
TDI (vapor)	T65.0X1	T65.0X2	T65.0X3	T65.0X4	—	—

Substance	Poisoning, Accidental (Unintentional)	Poisoning, Intentional Self-Harm	Poisoning, Assault	Poisoning, Undetermined	Adverse Effect	Underdosing
Tear						
gas	T59.3X1	T59.3X2	T59.3X3	T59.3X4	—	—
solution	T49.5X1	T49.5X2	T49.5X3	T49.5X4	T49.5X5	T49.5X6
Teclothiazide	T50.2X1	T50.2X2	T50.2X3	T50.2X4	T50.2X5	T50.2X6
Teclozan	T37.3X1	T37.3X2	T37.3X3	T37.3X4	T37.3X5	T37.3X6
Tegafur	T45.1X1	T45.1X2	T45.1X3	T45.1X4	T45.1X5	T45.1X6
Tegretol	T42.1X1	T42.1X2	T42.1X3	T42.1X4	T42.1X5	T42.1X6
Teicoplanin	T36.8X1	T36.8X2	T36.8X3	T36.8X4	T36.8X5	T36.8X6
Telepaque	T50.8X1	T50.8X2	T50.8X3	T50.8X4	T50.8X5	T50.8X6
Tellurium	T56.891	T56.892	T56.893	T56.894	—	—
fumes	T56.891	T56.892	T56.893	T56.894	—	—
TEM	T45.1X1	T45.1X2	T45.1X3	T45.1X4	T45.1X5	T45.1X6
Temazepam	T42.4X1	T42.4X2	T42.4X3	T42.4X4	T42.4X5	T42.4X6
Temocillin	T36.0X1	T36.0X2	T36.0X3	T36.0X4	T36.0X5	T36.0X6
Tenamfetamine	T43.621	T43.622	T43.623	T43.624	T43.625	T43.626
Teniposide	T45.1X1	T45.1X2	T45.1X3	T45.1X4	T45.1X5	T45.1X6
Tenitramine	T46.3X1	T46.3X2	T46.3X3	T46.3X4	T46.3X5	T46.3X6
Tenoglicin	T48.4X1	T48.4X2	T48.4X3	T48.4X4	T48.4X5	T48.4X6
Tenonitrozole	T37.3X1	T37.3X2	T37.3X3	T37.3X4	T37.3X5	T37.3X6
Tenoxicam	T39.391	T39.392	T39.393	T39.394	T39.395	T39.396
TEPA	T45.1X1	T45.1X2	T45.1X3	T45.1X4	T45.1X5	T45.1X6
TEPP	T60.0X1	T60.0X2	T60.0X3	T60.0X4	—	—
Teprotide	T46.5X1	T46.5X2	T46.5X3	T46.5X4	T46.5X5	T46.5X6
Terazosin	T44.6X1	T44.6X2	T44.6X3	T44.6X4	T44.6X5	T44.6X6
Terbufos	T60.0X1	T60.0X2	T60.0X3	T60.0X4	—	—
Terbutaline	T48.6X1	T48.6X2	T48.6X3	T48.6X4	T48.6X5	T48.6X6
Terconazole	T49.0X1	T49.0X2	T49.0X3	T49.0X4	T49.0X5	T49.0X6
Terfenadine	T45.0X1	T45.0X2	T45.0X3	T45.0X4	T45.0X5	T45.0X6
Teriparatide (acetate)	T50.991	T50.992	T50.993	T50.994	T50.995	T50.996
Terizidone	T37.1X1	T37.1X2	T37.1X3	T37.1X4	T37.1X5	T37.1X6
Terlipressin	T38.891	T38.892	T38.893	T38.894	T38.895	T38.896
Terodiline	T46.3X1	T46.3X2	T46.3X3	T46.3X4	T46.3X5	T46.3X6
Teroxalene	T37.4X1	T37.4X2	T37.4X3	T37.4X4	T37.4X5	T37.4X6
Terpin(cis) hydrate	T48.4X1	T48.4X2	T48.4X3	T48.4X4	T48.4X5	T48.4X6
Terramycin	T36.4X1	T36.4X2	T36.4X3	T36.4X4	T36.4X5	T36.4X6
Tertatolol	T44.7X1	T44.7X2	T44.7X3	T44.7X4	T44.7X5	T44.7X6
Tessalon	T48.3X1	T48.3X2	T48.3X3	T48.3X4	T48.3X5	T48.3X6
Testolactone	T38.7X1	T38.7X2	T38.7X3	T38.7X4	T38.7X5	T38.7X6
Testosterone	T38.7X1	T38.7X2	T38.7X3	T38.7X4	T38.7X5	T38.7X6
Tetanus toxoid or vaccine	T50.A91	T50.A92	T50.A93	T50.A94	T50.A95	T50.A96
antitoxin	T50.Z11	T50.Z12	T50.Z13	T50.Z14	T50.Z15	T50.Z16
immune globulin (human)	T50.Z11	T50.Z12	T50.Z13	T50.Z14	T50.Z15	T50.Z16

◀ New　◀|| Revised　~~deleted~~ Deleted

Substance	Poisoning, Accidental (Unintentional)	Poisoning, Intentional Self-Harm	Poisoning, Assault	Poisoning, Undetermined	Adverse Effect	Underdosing
Tetanus toxoid or vaccine (Continued)						
toxoid	T50.A91	T50.A92	T50.A93	T50.A94	T50.A95	T50.A96
with diphtheria toxoid	T50.A21	T50.A22	T50.A23	T50.A24	T50.A25	T50.A26
with pertussis	T50.A11	T50.A12	T50.A13	T50.A14	T50.A15	T50.A16
Tetrabenazine	T43.591	T43.592	T43.593	T43.594	T43.595	T43.596
Tetracaine	T41.3X1	T41.3X2	T41.3X3	T41.3X4	T41.3X5	T41.3X6
nerve block (peripheral) (plexus)	T41.3X1	T41.3X2	T41.3X3	T41.3X4	T41.3X5	T41.3X6
regional	T41.3X1	T41.3X2	T41.3X3	T41.3X4	T41.3X5	T41.3X6
spinal	T41.3X1	T41.3X2	T41.3X3	T41.3X4	T41.3X5	T41.3X6
Tetrachlorethylene — see Tetrachloroethylene						
Tetrachlormethiazide	T50.2X1	T50.2X2	T50.2X3	T50.2X4	T50.2X5	T50.2X6
2,3,7,8-Tetrachlorodibenzo-p-dioxin	T53.7X1	T53.7X2	T53.7X3	T53.7X4	—	—
Tetrachloroethane	T53.6X1	T53.6X2	T53.6X3	T53.6X4	—	—
vapor	T53.6X1	T53.6X2	T53.6X3	T53.6X4	—	—
paint or varnish	T53.6X1	T53.6X2	T53.6X3	T53.6X4	—	—
Tetrachloroethylene (liquid)	T53.3X1	T53.3X2	T53.3X3	T53.3X4	—	—
medicinal	T37.4X1	T37.4X2	T37.4X3	T37.4X4	T37.4X5	T37.4X6
vapor	T53.3X1	T53.3X2	T53.3X3	T53.3X4	—	—
Tetrachloromethane — see Carbon tetrachloride						
Tetracosactide	T38.811	T38.812	T38.813	T38.814	T38.815	T38.816
Tetracosactrin	T38.811	T38.812	T38.813	T38.814	T38.815	T38.816
Tetracycline	T36.4X1	T36.4X2	T36.4X3	T36.4X4	T36.4X5	T36.4X6
ophthalmic preparation	T49.5X1	T49.5X2	T49.5X3	T49.5X4	T49.5X5	T49.5X6
topical NEC	T49.0X1	T49.0X2	T49.0X3	T49.0X4	T49.0X5	T49.0X6
Tetradifon	T60.8X1	T60.8X2	T60.8X3	T60.8X4	—	—
Tetradotoxin	T61.771	T61.772	T61.773	T61.774	—	—
Tetraethyl						
lead	T56.0X1	T56.0X2	T56.0X3	T56.0X4	—	—
pyrophosphate	T60.0X1	T60.0X2	T60.0X3	T60.0X4	—	—
Tetraethylammonium chloride	T44.2X1	T44.2X2	T44.2X3	T44.2X4	T44.2X5	T44.2X6
Tetraethylthiuram disulfide	T50.6X1	T50.6X2	T50.6X3	T50.6X4	T50.6X5	T50.6X6
Tetrahydroaminoacridine	T44.0X1	T44.0X2	T44.0X3	T44.0X4	T44.0X5	T44.0X6
Tetrahydrocannabinol	T40.7X1	T40.7X2	T40.7X3	T40.7X4	T40.7X5	T40.7X6
Tetrahydrofuran	T52.8X1	T52.8X2	T52.8X3	T52.8X4	—	—
Tetrahydronaphthalene	T52.8X1	T52.8X2	T52.8X3	T52.8X4	—	—
Tetrahydrozoline	T49.5X1	T49.5X2	T49.5X3	T49.5X4	T49.5X5	T49.5X6
Tetralin	T52.8X1	T52.8X2	T52.8X3	T52.8X4	—	—
Tetramethrin	T60.2X1	T60.2X2	T60.2X3	T60.2X4	—	—

Substance	Poisoning, Accidental (Unintentional)	Poisoning, Intentional Self-Harm	Poisoning, Assault	Poisoning, Undetermined	Adverse Effect	Underdosing
Tetramethylthiuram (disulfide) NEC	T60.3X1	T60.3X2	T60.3X3	T60.3X4	—	—
medicinal	T49.0X1	T49.0X2	T49.0X3	T49.0X4	T49.0X5	T49.0X6
Tetramisole	T37.4X1	T37.4X2	T37.4X3	T37.4X4	T37.4X5	T37.4X6
Tetranicotinoyl fructose	T46.7X1	T46.7X2	T46.7X3	T46.7X4	T46.7X5	T46.7X6
Tetronal	T42.6X1	T42.6X2	T42.6X3	T42.6X4	T42.6X5	T42.6X6
Tetrazepam	T42.4X1	T42.4X2	T42.4X3	T42.4X4	T42.4X5	T42.4X6
Tetryl	T65.3X1	T65.3X2	T65.3X3	T65.3X4	—	—
Tetrylammonium chloride	T44.2X1	T44.2X2	T44.2X3	T44.2X4	T44.2X5	T44.2X6
Tetryzoline	T49.5X1	T49.5X2	T49.5X3	T49.5X4	T49.5X5	T49.5X6
Thalidomide	T45.1X1	T45.1X2	T45.1X3	T45.1X4	T45.1X5	T45.1X6
Thallium (compounds) (dust) NEC	T56.811	T56.812	T56.813	T56.814	—	—
pesticide	T60.4X1	T60.4X2	T60.4X3	T60.4X4	—	—
THC	T40.7X1	T40.7X2	T40.7X3	T40.7X4	T40.7X5	T40.7X6
Thebacon	T48.3X1	T48.3X2	T48.3X3	T48.3X4	T48.3X5	T48.3X6
Thebaine	T40.2X1	T40.2X2	T40.2X3	T40.2X4	T40.2X5	T40.2X6
Thenoic acid	T49.6X1	T49.6X2	T49.6X3	T49.6X4	T49.6X5	T49.6X6
Thenyldiamine	T45.0X1	T45.0X2	T45.0X3	T45.0X4	T45.0X5	T45.0X6
Theobromine (calcium salicylate)	T48.6X1	T48.6X2	T48.6X3	T48.6X4	T48.6X5	T48.6X6
sodium salicylate	T48.6X1	T48.6X2	T48.6X3	T48.6X4	T48.6X5	T48.6X6
Theophyllamine	T48.6X1	T48.6X2	T48.6X3	T48.6X4	T48.6X5	T48.6X6
Theophylline	T48.6X1	T48.6X2	T48.6X3	T48.6X4	T48.6X5	T48.6X6
aminobenzoic acid	T48.6X1	T48.6X2	T48.6X3	T48.6X4	T48.6X5	T48.6X6
ethylenediamine	T48.6X1	T48.6X2	T48.6X3	T48.6X4	T48.6X5	T48.6X6
piperazine p-amino-benzoate	T48.6X1	T48.6X2	T48.6X3	T48.6X4	T48.6X5	T48.6X6
Thiabendazole	T37.4X1	T37.4X2	T37.4X3	T37.4X4	T37.4X5	T37.4X6
Thialbarbital	T41.1X1	T41.1X2	T41.1X3	T41.1X4	T41.1X5	T41.1X6
Thiamazole	T38.2X1	T38.2X2	T38.2X3	T38.2X4	T38.2X5	T38.2X6
Thiambutosine	T37.1X1	T37.1X2	T37.1X3	T37.1X4	T37.1X5	T37.1X6
Thiamine	T45.2X1	T45.2X2	T45.2X3	T45.2X4	T45.2X5	T45.2X6
Thiamphenicol	T36.2X1	T36.2X2	T36.2X3	T36.2X4	T36.2X5	T36.2X6
Thiamylal	T41.1X1	T41.1X2	T41.1X3	T41.1X4	T41.1X5	T41.1X6
sodium	T41.1X1	T41.1X2	T41.1X3	T41.1X4	T41.1X5	T41.1X6
Thiazesim	T43.291	T43.292	T43.293	T43.294	T43.295	T43.296
Thiazides (diuretics)	T50.2X1	T50.2X2	T50.2X3	T50.2X4	T50.2X5	T50.2X6
Thiazinamium metilsulfate	T43.3X1	T43.3X2	T43.3X3	T43.3X4	T43.3X5	T43.3X6
Thiethylperazine	T43.3X1	T43.3X2	T43.3X3	T43.3X4	T43.3X5	T43.3X6
Thimerosal	T49.0X1	T49.0X2	T49.0X3	T49.0X4	T49.0X5	T49.0X6
ophthalmic preparation	T49.5X1	T49.5X2	T49.5X3	T49.5X4	T49.5X5	T49.5X6
Thioacetazone	T37.1X1	T37.1X2	T37.1X3	T37.1X4	T37.1X5	T37.1X6
with isoniazid	T37.1X1	T37.1X2	T37.1X3	T37.1X4	T37.1X5	T37.1X6
Thiobarbital sodium	T41.1X1	T41.1X2	T41.1X3	T41.1X4	T41.1X5	T41.1X6

◀ New ◀◀ Revised deleted Deleted

TABLE OF DRUGS AND CHEMICALS

TABLE OF DRUGS AND CHEMICALS

Substance	External Cause (T-Code)					
	Poisoning, Accidental (Unintentional)	Poisoning, Intentional Self-Harm	Poisoning, Assault	Poisoning, Undetermined	Adverse Effect	Underdosing
Thiobarbiturate anesthetic	T41.1X1	T41.1X2	T41.1X3	T41.1X4	T41.1X5	T41.1X6
Thiobismol	T37.8X1	T37.8X2	T37.8X3	T37.8X4	T37.8X5	T37.8X6
Thiobutabarbital sodium	T41.1X1	T41.1X2	T41.1X3	T41.1X4	T41.1X5	T41.1X6
Thiocarbamate (insecticide)	T60.0X1	T60.0X2	T60.0X3	T60.0X4	—	—
Thiocarbamide	T38.2X1	T38.2X2	T38.2X3	T38.2X4	T38.2X5	T38.2X6
Thiocarbarsone	T37.8X1	T37.8X2	T37.8X3	T37.8X4	T37.8X5	T37.8X6
Thiocarlide	T37.1X1	T37.1X2	T37.1X3	T37.1X4	T37.1X5	T37.1X6
Thioctamide	T50.991	T50.992	T50.993	T50.994	T50.995	T50.996
Thioctic acid	T50.991	T50.992	T50.993	T50.994	T50.995	T50.996
Thiofos	T60.0X1	T60.0X2	T60.0X3	T60.0X4	—	—
Thioglycolate	T49.4X1	T49.4X2	T49.4X3	T49.4X4	T49.4X5	T49.4X6
Thioglycolic acid	T65.891	T65.892	T65.893	T65.894	—	—
Thioguanine	T45.1X1	T45.1X2	T45.1X3	T45.1X4	T45.1X5	T45.1X6
Thiomercaptomerin	T50.2X1	T50.2X2	T50.2X3	T50.2X4	T50.2X5	T50.2X6
Thiomerin	T50.2X1	T50.2X2	T50.2X3	T50.2X4	T50.2X5	T50.2X6
Thiomersal	T49.0X1	T49.0X2	T49.0X3	T49.0X4	T49.0X5	T49.0X6
Thionazin	T60.0X1	T60.0X2	T60.0X3	T60.0X4	—	—
Thiopental (sodium)	T41.1X1	T41.1X2	T41.1X3	T41.1X4	T41.1X5	T41.1X6
Thiopentone (sodium)	T41.1X1	T41.1X2	T41.1X3	T41.1X4	T41.1X5	T41.1X6
Thiopropazate	T43.3X1	T43.3X2	T43.3X3	T43.3X4	T43.3X5	T43.3X6
Thioproperazine	T43.3X1	T43.3X2	T43.3X3	T43.3X4	T43.3X5	T43.3X6
Thioridazine	T43.3X1	T43.3X2	T43.3X3	T43.3X4	T43.3X5	T43.3X6
Thiosinamine	T49.3X1	T49.3X2	T49.3X3	T49.3X4	T49.3X5	T49.3X6
Thiotepa	T45.1X1	T45.1X2	T45.1X3	T45.1X4	T45.1X5	T45.1X6
Thiothixene	T43.4X1	T43.4X2	T43.4X3	T43.4X4	T43.4X5	T43.4X6
Thiouracil (benzyl) (methyl) (propyl)	T38.2X1	T38.2X2	T38.2X3	T38.2X4	T38.2X5	T38.2X6
Thiourea	T38.2X1	T38.2X2	T38.2X3	T38.2X4	T38.2X5	T38.2X6
Thiphenamil	T44.3X1	T44.3X2	T44.3X3	T44.3X4	T44.3X5	T44.3X6
Thiram	T60.3X1	T60.3X2	T60.3X3	T60.3X4	—	—
medicinal	T49.2X1	T49.2X2	T49.2X3	T49.2X4	T49.2X5	T49.2X6
Thonzylamine (systemic)	T45.0X1	T45.0X2	T45.0X3	T45.0X4	T45.0X5	T45.0X6
mucosal decongestant	T48.5X1	T48.5X2	T48.5X3	T48.5X4	T48.5X5	T48.5X6
Thorazine	T43.3X1	T43.3X2	T43.3X3	T43.3X4	T43.3X5	T43.3X6
Thorium dioxide suspension	T50.8X1	T50.8X2	T50.8X3	T50.8X4	T50.8X5	T50.8X6
Thornapple	T62.2X1	T62.2X2	T62.2X3	T62.2X4	—	—
Throat drug NEC	T49.6X1	T49.6X2	T49.6X3	T49.6X4	T49.6X5	T49.6X6
Thrombin	T45.7X1	T45.7X2	T45.7X3	T45.7X4	T45.7X5	T45.7X6
Thrombolysin	T45.611	T45.612	T45.613	T45.614	T45.615	T45.616
Thromboplastin	T45.7X1	T45.7X2	T45.7X3	T45.7X4	T45.7X5	T45.7X6
Thurfyl nicotinate	T46.7X1	T46.7X2	T46.7X3	T46.7X4	T46.7X5	T46.7X6
Thymol	T49.0X1	T49.0X2	T49.0X3	T49.0X4	T49.0X5	T49.0X6

Substance	External Cause (T-Code)					
	Poisoning, Accidental (Unintentional)	Poisoning, Intentional Self-Harm	Poisoning, Assault	Poisoning, Undetermined	Adverse Effect	Underdosing
Thymopentin	T37.5X1	T37.5X2	T37.5X3	T37.5X4	T37.5X5	T37.5X6
Thymoxamine	T46.7X1	T46.7X2	T46.7X3	T46.7X4	T46.7X5	T46.7X6
Thymus extract	T38.891	T38.892	T38.893	T38.894	T38.895	T38.896
Thyreotrophic hormone	T38.811	T38.812	T38.813	T38.814	T38.815	T38.816
Thyroglobulin	T38.1X1	T38.1X2	T38.1X3	T38.1X4	T38.1X5	T38.1X6
Thyroid (hormone)	T38.1X1	T38.1X2	T38.1X3	T38.1X4	T38.1X5	T38.1X6
Thyrolar	T38.1X1	T38.1X2	T38.1X3	T38.1X4	T38.1X5	T38.1X6
Thyrotrophin	T38.811	T38.812	T38.813	T38.814	T38.815	T38.816
Thyrotropic hormone	T38.811	T38.812	T38.813	T38.814	T38.815	T38.816
Thyroxine	T38.1X1	T38.1X2	T38.1X3	T38.1X4	T38.1X5	T38.1X6
Tiabendazole	T37.4X1	T37.4X2	T37.4X3	T37.4X4	T37.4X5	T37.4X6
Tiamizide	T50.2X1	T50.2X2	T50.2X3	T50.2X4	T50.2X5	T50.2X6
Tianeptine	T43.291	T43.292	T43.293	T43.294	T43.295	T43.296
Tiapamil	T46.1X1	T46.1X2	T46.1X3	T46.1X4	T46.1X5	T46.1X6
Tiapride	T43.591	T43.592	T43.593	T43.594	T43.595	T43.596
Tiaprofenic acid	T39.311	T39.312	T39.313	T39.314	T39.315	T39.316
Tiaramide	T39.8X1	T39.8X2	T39.8X3	T39.8X4	T39.8X5	T39.8X6
Ticarcillin	T36.0X1	T36.0X2	T36.0X3	T36.0X4	T36.0X5	T36.0X6
Ticlatone	T49.0X1	T49.0X2	T49.0X3	T49.0X4	T49.0X5	T49.0X6
Ticlopidine	T45.521	T45.522	T45.523	T45.524	T45.525	T45.526
Ticrynafen	T50.1X1	T50.1X2	T50.1X3	T50.1X4	T50.1X5	T50.1X6
Tidiacic	T50.991	T50.992	T50.993	T50.994	T50.995	T50.996
Tiemonium	T44.3X1	T44.3X2	T44.3X3	T44.3X4	T44.3X5	T44.3X6
iodide	T44.3X1	T44.3X2	T44.3X3	T44.3X4	T44.3X5	T44.3X6
Tienilic acid	T50.1X1	T50.1X2	T50.1X3	T50.1X4	T50.1X5	T50.1X6
Tifenamil	T44.3X1	T44.3X2	T44.3X3	T44.3X4	T44.3X5	T44.3X6
Tigan	T45.0X1	T45.0X2	T45.0X3	T45.0X4	T45.0X5	T45.0X6
Tigloidine	T44.3X1	T44.3X2	T44.3X3	T44.3X4	T44.3X5	T44.3X6
Tilactase	T47.5X1	T47.5X2	T47.5X3	T47.5X4	T47.5X5	T47.5X6
Tiletamine	T41.291	T41.292	T41.293	T41.294	T41.295	T41.296
Tilidine	T40.4X1	T40.4X2	T40.4X3	T40.4X4	—	—
Timepidium bromide	T44.3X1	T44.3X2	T44.3X3	T44.3X4	T44.3X5	T44.3X6
Timiperone	T43.4X1	T43.4X2	T43.4X3	T43.4X4	T43.4X5	T43.4X6
Timolol	T44.7X1	T44.7X2	T44.7X3	T44.7X4	T44.7X5	T44.7X6
Tin (chloride) (dust) (oxide) NEC	T56.6X1	T56.6X2	T56.6X3	T56.6X4	—	—
anti-infectives	T37.8X1	T37.8X2	T37.8X3	T37.8X4	T37.8X5	T37.8X6
Tincture, iodine — see Iodine						
Tindal	T43.3X1	T43.3X2	T43.3X3	T43.3X4	T43.3X5	T43.3X6
Tinidazole	T37.3X1	T37.3X2	T37.3X3	T37.3X4	T37.3X5	T37.3X6
Tinoridine	T39.8X1	T39.8X2	T39.8X3	T39.8X4	T39.8X5	T39.8X6
Tiocarlide	T37.1X1	T37.1X2	T37.1X3	T37.1X4	T37.1X5	T37.1X6
Tioclomarol	T45.511	T45.512	T45.513	T45.514	T45.515	T45.516

◀ New ◀ Revised ~~deleted~~ Deleted

Substance	Poisoning, Accidental (Unintentional)	Poisoning, Intentional Self-Harm	Poisoning, Assault	Poisoning, Undetermined	Adverse Effect	Underdosing
	External Cause (T-Code)					
Tioconazole	T49.0X1	T49.0X2	T49.0X3	T49.0X4	T49.0X5	T49.0X6
Tioguanine	T45.1X1	T45.1X2	T45.1X3	T45.1X4	T45.1X5	T45.1X6
Tiopronin	T50.991	T50.992	T50.993	T50.994	T50.995	T50.996
Tiotixene	T43.4X1	T43.4X2	T43.4X3	T43.4X4	T43.4X5	T43.4X6
Tioxolone	T49.4X1	T49.4X2	T49.4X3	T49.4X4	T49.4X5	T49.4X6
Tipepidine	T48.3X1	T48.3X2	T48.3X3	T48.3X4	T48.3X5	T48.3X6
Tiquizium bromide	T44.3X1	T44.3X2	T44.3X3	T44.3X4	T44.3X5	T44.3X6
Tiratricol	T38.1X1	T38.1X2	T38.1X3	T38.1X4	T38.1X5	T38.1X6
Tisopurine	T50.4X1	T50.4X2	T50.4X3	T50.4X4	T50.4X5	T50.4X6
Titanium (compounds) (vapor)	T56.891	T56.892	T56.893	T56.894	—	—
dioxide	T49.3X1	T49.3X2	T49.3X3	T49.3X4	T49.3X5	T49.3X6
ointment	T49.3X1	T49.3X2	T49.3X3	T49.3X4	T49.3X5	T49.3X6
oxide	T49.3X1	T49.3X2	T49.3X3	T49.3X4	T49.3X5	T49.3X6
tetrachloride	T56.891	T56.892	T56.893	T56.894	—	—
Titanocene	T56.891	T56.892	T56.893	T56.894	—	—
Titroid	T38.1X1	T38.1X2	T38.1X3	T38.1X4	T38.1X5	T38.1X6
Tizanidine	T42.8X1	T42.8X2	T42.8X3	T42.8X4	T42.8X5	T42.8X6
TMTD	T60.3X1	T60.3X2	T60.3X3	T60.3X4		
TNT (fumes)	T65.3X1	T65.3X2	T65.3X3	T65.3X4		
Toadstool	T62.0X1	T62.0X2	T62.0X3	T62.0X4	—	—
Tobacco NEC	T65.291	T65.292	T65.293	T65.294		
cigarettes	T65.221	T65.222	T65.223	T65.224		
Indian	T62.2X1	T62.2X2	T62.2X3	T62.2X4	—	—
smoke, second-hand	T65.221	T65.222	T65.223	T65.224	—	—
Tobramycin	T36.5X1	T36.5X2	T36.5X3	T36.5X4	T36.5X5	T36.5X6
Tocainide	T46.2X1	T46.2X2	T46.2X3	T46.2X4	T46.2X5	T46.2X6
Tocoferol	T45.2X1	T45.2X2	T45.2X3	T45.2X4	T45.2X5	T45.2X6
Tocopherol	T45.2X1	T45.2X2	T45.2X3	T45.2X4	T45.2X5	T45.2X6
acetate	T45.2X1	T45.2X2	T45.2X3	T45.2X4	T45.2X5	T45.2X6
Tocosamine	T48.0X1	T48.0X2	T48.0X3	T48.0X4	T48.0X5	T48.0X6
Todralazine	T46.5X1	T46.5X2	T46.5X3	T46.5X4	T46.5X5	T46.5X6
Tofisopam	T42.4X1	T42.4X2	T42.4X3	T42.4X4	T42.4X5	T42.4X6
Tofranil	T43.011	T43.012	T43.013	T43.014	T43.015	T43.016
Toilet deodorizer	T65.891	T65.892	T65.893	T65.894	—	—
Tolamolol	T44.7X1	T44.7X2	T44.7X3	T44.7X4	T44.7X5	T44.7X6
Tolazamide	T38.3X1	T38.3X2	T38.3X3	T38.3X4	T38.3X5	T38.3X6
Tolazoline	T46.7X1	T46.7X2	T46.7X3	T46.7X4	T46.7X5	T46.7X6
Tolbutamide (sodium)	T38.3X1	T38.3X2	T38.3X3	T38.3X4	T38.3X5	T38.3X6
Tolciclate	T49.0X1	T49.0X2	T49.0X3	T49.0X4	T49.0X5	T49.0X6
Tolmetin	T39.391	T39.392	T39.393	T39.394	T39.395	T39.396
Tolnaftate	T49.0X1	T49.0X2	T49.0X3	T49.0X4	T49.0X5	T49.0X6
Tolonidine	T46.5X1	T46.5X2	T46.5X3	T46.5X4	T46.5X5	T46.5X6

Substance	Poisoning, Accidental (Unintentional)	Poisoning, Intentional Self-Harm	Poisoning, Assault	Poisoning, Undetermined	Adverse Effect	Underdosing
	External Cause (T-Code)					
Toloxatone	T42.6X1	T42.6X2	T42.6X3	T42.6X4	T42.6X5	T42.6X6
Tolperisone	T44.3X1	T44.3X2	T44.3X3	T44.3X4	T44.3X5	T44.3X6
Tolserol	T42.8X1	T42.8X2	T42.8X3	T42.8X4	T42.8X5	T42.8X6
Toluene (liquid)	T52.2X1	T52.2X2	T52.2X3	T52.2X4	—	—
diisocyanate	T65.0X1	T65.0X2	T65.0X3	T65.0X4	—	—
Toluidine	T65.891	T65.892	T65.893	T65.894		
vapor	T59.891	T59.892	T59.893	T59.894		
Toluol (liquid)	T52.2X1	T52.2X2	T52.2X3	T52.2X4	—	—
vapor	T52.2X1	T52.2X2	T52.2X3	T52.2X4		
Toluylenediamine	T65.3X1	T65.3X2	T65.3X3	T65.3X4		
Tolylene-2,4-diisocyanate	T65.0X1	T65.0X2	T65.0X3	T65.0X4	—	—
Tonic NEC	T50.901	T50.902	T50.903	T50.904	T50.905	T50.906
Topical action drug NEC	T49.91	T49.92	T49.93	T49.94	T49.95	T49.96
ear, nose or throat	T49.6X1	T49.6X2	T49.6X3	T49.6X4	T49.6X5	T49.6X6
eye	T49.5X1	T49.5X2	T49.5X3	T49.5X4	T49.5X5	T49.5X6
skin	T49.91	T49.92	T49.93	T49.94	T49.95	T49.96
specified NEC	T49.8X1	T49.8X2	T49.8X3	T49.8X4	T49.8X5	T49.8X6
Toquizine	T44.3X1	T44.3X2	T44.3X3	T44.3X4	T44.3X5	T44.3X6
Toremifene	T38.6X1	T38.6X2	T38.6X3	T38.6X4	T38.6X5	T38.6X6
Tosylchloramide sodium	T49.8X1	T49.8X2	T49.8X3	T49.8X4	T49.8X5	T49.8X6
Toxaphene (dust) (spray)	T60.1X1	T60.1X2	T60.1X3	T60.1X4	—	—
Toxin, diphtheria (Schick Test)	T50.8X1	T50.8X2	T50.8X3	T50.8X4	T50.8X5	T50.8X6
Toxoid						
combined	T50.A21	T50.A22	T50.A23	T50.A24	T50.A25	T50.A26
diphtheria	T50.A91	T50.A92	T50.A93	T50.A94	T50.A95	T50.A96
tetanus	T50.A91	T50.A92	T50.A93	T50.A94	T50.A95	T50.A96
Trace element NEC	T45.8X1	T45.8X2	T45.8X3	T45.8X4	T45.8X5	T45.8X6
Tractor fuel NEC	T52.0X1	T52.0X2	T52.0X3	T52.0X4	—	—
Tragacanth	T50.991	T50.992	T50.993	T50.994	T50.995	T50.996
Tramadol	T40.4X1	T40.4X2	T40.4X3	T40.4X4	T40.4X5	T40.4X6
Tramazoline	T48.5X1	T48.5X2	T48.5X3	T48.5X4	T48.5X5	T48.5X6
Tranexamic acid	T45.621	T45.622	T45.623	T45.624	T45.625	T45.626
Tranilast	T45.0X1	T45.0X2	T45.0X3	T45.0X4	T45.0X5	T45.0X6
Tranquilizer NEC	T43.501	T43.502	T43.503	T43.504	T43.505	T43.506
with hypnotic or sedative	T42.6X1	T42.6X2	T42.6X3	T42.6X4	T42.6X5	T42.6X6
benzodiazepine NEC	T42.4X1	T42.4X2	T42.4X3	T42.4X4	T42.4X5	T42.4X6
butyrophenone NEC	T43.4X1	T43.4X2	T43.4X3	T43.4X4	T43.4X5	T43.4X6
carbamate	T43.591	T43.592	T43.593	T43.594	T43.595	T43.596
dimethylamine	T43.3X1	T43.3X2	T43.3X3	T43.3X4	T43.3X5	T43.3X6
ethylamine	T43.3X1	T43.3X2	T43.3X3	T43.3X4	T43.3X5	T43.3X6
hydroxyzine	T43.591	T43.592	T43.593	T43.594	T43.595	T43.596
major NEC	T43.501	T43.502	T43.503	T43.504	T43.505	T43.506

◀ New　◀▪ Revised　~~deleted~~ Deleted

Substance	External Cause (T-Code)					
	Poisoning, Accidental (Unintentional)	Poisoning, Intentional Self-Harm	Poisoning, Assault	Poisoning, Undetermined	Adverse Effect	Underdosing
Tranquilizer NEC *(Continued)*						
penothiazine NEC	T43.3X1	T43.3X2	T43.3X3	T43.3X4	T43.3X5	T43.3X6
phenothiazine-based	T43.3X1	T43.3X2	T43.3X3	T43.3X4	T43.3X5	T43.3X6
piperazine NEC	T43.3X1	T43.3X2	T43.3X3	T43.3X4	T43.3X5	T43.3X6
piperidine	T43.3X1	T43.3X2	T43.3X3	T43.3X4	T43.3X5	T43.3X6
propylamine	T43.3X1	T43.3X2	T43.3X3	T43.3X4	T43.3X5	T43.3X6
specified NEC	T43.591	T43.592	T43.593	T43.594	T43.595	T43.596
thioxanthene NEC	T43.591	T43.592	T43.593	T43.594	T43.595	T43.596
Tranxene	T42.4X1	T42.4X2	T42.4X3	T42.4X4	T42.4X5	T42.4X6
Tranylcypromine	T43.1X1	T43.1X2	T43.1X3	T43.1X4	T43.1X5	T43.1X6
Trapidil	T46.3X1	T46.3X2	T46.3X3	T46.3X4	T46.3X5	T46.3X6
Trasentine	T44.3X1	T44.3X2	T44.3X3	T44.3X4	T44.3X5	T44.3X6
Travert	T50.3X1	T50.3X2	T50.3X3	T50.3X4	T50.3X5	T50.3X6
Trazodone	T43.211	T43.212	T43.213	T43.214	T43.215	T43.216
Trecator	T37.1X1	T37.1X2	T37.1X3	T37.1X4	T37.1X5	T37.1X6
Treosulfan	T45.1X1	T45.1X2	T45.1X3	T45.1X4	T45.1X5	T45.1X6
Tretamine	T45.1X1	T45.1X2	T45.1X3	T45.1X4	T45.1X5	T45.1X6
Tretinoin	T49.0X1	T49.0X2	T49.0X3	T49.0X4	T49.0X5	T49.0X6
Tretoquinol	T48.6X1	T48.6X2	T48.6X3	T48.6X4	T48.6X5	T48.6X6
Triacetin	T49.0X1	T49.0X2	T49.0X3	T49.0X4	T49.0X5	T49.0X6
Triacetoxyanthracene	T49.4X1	T49.4X2	T49.4X3	T49.4X4	T49.4X5	T49.4X6
Triacetyloleandomycin	T36.3X1	T36.3X2	T36.3X3	T36.3X4	T36.3X5	T36.3X6
Triamcinolone	T38.0X1	T38.0X2	T38.0X3	T38.0X4	T38.0X5	T38.0X6
ENT agent	T49.6X1	T49.6X2	T49.6X3	T49.6X4	T49.6X5	T49.6X6
hexacetonide	T49.0X1	T49.0X2	T49.0X3	T49.0X4	T49.0X5	T49.0X6
ophthalmic preparation	T49.5X1	T49.5X2	T49.5X3	T49.5X4	T49.5X5	T49.5X6
topical NEC	T49.0X1	T49.0X2	T49.0X3	T49.0X4	T49.0X5	T49.0X6
Triampyzine	T44.3X1	T44.3X2	T44.3X3	T44.3X4	T44.3X5	T44.3X6
Triamterene	T50.2X1	T50.2X2	T50.2X3	T50.2X4	T50.2X5	T50.2X6
Triazine (herbicide)	T60.3X1	T60.3X2	T60.3X3	T60.3X4	—	—
Triaziquone	T45.1X1	T45.1X2	T45.1X3	T45.1X4	T45.1X5	T45.1X6
Triazolam	T42.4X1	T42.4X2	T42.4X3	T42.4X4	T42.4X5	T42.4X6
Triazole (herbicide)	T60.3X1	T60.3X2	T60.3X3	T60.3X4	—	—
Tribenoside	T46.991	T46.992	T46.993	T46.994	T46.995	T46.996
Tribromacetaldehyde	T42.6X1	T42.6X2	T42.6X3	T42.6X4	T42.6X5	T42.6X6
Tribromoethanol, rectal	T41.291	T41.292	T41.293	T41.294	T41.295	T41.296
Tribromomethane	T42.6X1	T42.6X2	T42.6X3	T42.6X4	T42.6X5	T42.6X6
Trichlorethane	T53.2X1	T53.2X2	T53.2X3	T53.2X4	—	—
Trichlorethylene	T53.2X1	T53.2X2	T53.2X3	T53.2X4	—	—
Trichlorfon	T60.0X1	T60.0X2	T60.0X3	T60.0X4	—	—
Trichlormethiazide	T50.2X1	T50.2X2	T50.2X3	T50.2X4	T50.2X5	T50.2X6
Trichlormethine	T45.1X1	T45.1X2	T45.1X3	T45.1X4	T45.1X5	T45.1X6

Substance	External Cause (T-Code)					
	Poisoning, Accidental (Unintentional)	Poisoning, Intentional Self-Harm	Poisoning, Assault	Poisoning, Undetermined	Adverse Effect	Underdosing
Trichloroacetic acid, Trichloracetic acid	T54.2X1	T54.2X2	T54.2X3	T54.2X4	—	—
medicinal	T49.4X1	T49.4X2	T49.4X3	T49.4X4	T49.4X5	T49.4X6
Trichloroethane	T53.2X1	T53.2X2	T53.2X3	T53.2X4	—	—
Trichloroethanol	T42.6X1	T42.6X2	T42.6X3	T42.6X4	T42.6X5	T42.6X6
Trichloroethylene (liquid) (vapor)	T53.2X1	T53.2X2	T53.2X3	T53.2X4	—	—
anesthetic (gas)	T41.0X1	T41.0X2	T41.0X3	T41.0X4	T41.0X5	T41.0X6
vapor NEC	T53.2X1	T53.2X2	T53.2X3	T53.2X4	—	—
Trichloroethyl phosphate	T42.6X1	T42.6X2	T42.6X3	T42.6X4	T42.6X5	T42.6X6
Trichlorofluoromethane NEC	T53.5X1	T53.5X2	T53.5X3	T53.5X4	—	—
Trichloronate	T60.0X1	T60.0X2	T60.0X3	T60.0X4	—	—
2,4,5-Trichlorophen-oxyacetic acid	T60.3X1	T60.3X2	T60.3X3	T60.3X4	—	—
Trichloropropane	T53.6X1	T53.6X2	T53.6X3	T53.6X4	—	—
Trichlorotriethylamine	T45.1X1	T45.1X2	T45.1X3	T45.1X4	T45.1X5	T45.1X6
Trichomonacides NEC	T37.3X1	T37.3X2	T37.3X3	T37.3X4	T37.3X5	T37.3X6
Trichomycin	T36.7X1	T36.7X2	T36.7X3	T36.7X4	T36.7X5	T36.7X6
Triclobisonium chloride	T49.0X1	T49.0X2	T49.0X3	T49.0X4	T49.0X5	T49.0X6
Triclocarban	T49.0X1	T49.0X2	T49.0X3	T49.0X4	T49.0X5	T49.0X6
Triclofos	T42.6X1	T42.6X2	T42.6X3	T42.6X4	T42.6X5	T42.6X6
Triclosan	T49.0X1	T49.0X2	T49.0X3	T49.0X4	T49.0X5	T49.0X6
Tricresyl phosphate	T65.891	T65.892	T65.893	T65.894	—	—
solvent	T52.91	T52.92	T52.93	T52.94	—	—
Tricyclamol chloride	T44.3X1	T44.3X2	T44.3X3	T44.3X4	T44.3X5	T44.3X6
Tridesilon	T49.0X1	T49.0X2	T49.0X3	T49.0X4	T49.0X5	T49.0X6
Tridihexethyl iodide	T44.3X1	T44.3X2	T44.3X3	T44.3X4	T44.3X5	T44.3X6
Tridione	T42.2X1	T42.2X2	T42.2X3	T42.2X4	T42.2X5	T42.2X6
Trientine	T45.8X1	T45.8X2	T45.8X3	T45.8X4	T45.8X5	T45.8X6
Triethanolamine NEC	T54.3X1	T54.3X2	T54.3X3	T54.3X4	—	—
detergent	T54.3X1	T54.3X2	T54.3X3	T54.3X4	—	—
trinitrate (biphosphate)	T46.3X1	T46.3X2	T46.3X3	T46.3X4	T46.3X5	T46.3X6
Triethanomelamine	T45.1X1	T45.1X2	T45.1X3	T45.1X4	T45.1X5	T45.1X6
Triethylenemelamine	T45.1X1	T45.1X2	T45.1X3	T45.1X4	T45.1X5	T45.1X6
Triethylenephosphoramide	T45.1X1	T45.1X2	T45.1X3	T45.1X4	T45.1X5	T45.1X6
Triethylenethiophosphoramide	T45.1X1	T45.1X2	T45.1X3	T45.1X4	T45.1X5	T45.1X6
Trifluoperazine	T43.3X1	T43.3X2	T43.3X3	T43.3X4	T43.3X5	T43.3X6
Trifluoroethyl vinyl ether	T41.0X1	T41.0X2	T41.0X3	T41.0X4	T41.0X5	T41.0X6
Trifluperidol	T43.4X1	T43.4X2	T43.4X3	T43.4X4	T43.4X5	T43.4X6
Triflupromazine	T43.3X1	T43.3X2	T43.3X3	T43.3X4	T43.3X5	T43.3X6
Trifluridine	T37.5X1	T37.5X2	T37.5X3	T37.5X4	T37.5X5	T37.5X6
Triflusal	T45.521	T45.522	T45.523	T45.524	T45.525	T45.526
Trihexyphenidyl	T44.3X1	T44.3X2	T44.3X3	T44.3X4	T44.3X5	T44.3X6
Triiodothyronine	T38.1X1	T38.1X2	T38.1X3	T38.1X4	T38.1X5	T38.1X6

◀ New ◀ Revised ~~deleted~~ Deleted

Substance	Poisoning, Accidental (Unintentional)	Poisoning, Intentional Self-Harm	Poisoning, Assault	Poisoning, Undetermined	Adverse Effect	Underdosing
Trilene	T41.0X1	T41.0X2	T41.0X3	T41.0X4	T41.0X5	T41.0X6
Trilostane	T38.991	T38.992	T38.993	T38.994	T38.995	T38.996
Trimebutine	T44.3X1	T44.3X2	T44.3X3	T44.3X4	T44.3X5	T44.3X6
Trimecaine	T41.3X1	T41.3X2	T41.3X3	T41.3X4	T41.3X5	T41.3X6
Trimeprazine (tartrate)	T44.3X1	T44.3X2	T44.3X3	T44.3X4	T44.3X5	T44.3X6
Trimetaphan camsilate	T44.2X1	T44.2X2	T44.2X3	T44.2X4	T44.2X5	T44.2X6
Trimetazidine	T46.7X1	T46.7X2	T46.7X3	T46.7X4	T46.7X5	T46.7X6
Trimethadione	T42.2X1	T42.2X2	T42.2X3	T42.2X4	T42.2X5	T42.2X6
Trimethaphan	T44.2X1	T44.2X2	T44.2X3	T44.2X4	T44.2X5	T44.2X6
Trimethidinium	T44.2X1	T44.2X2	T44.2X3	T44.2X4	T44.2X5	T44.2X6
Trimethobenzamide	T45.0X1	T45.0X2	T45.0X3	T45.0X4	T45.0X5	T45.0X6
Trimethoprim	T37.8X1	T37.8X2	T37.8X3	T37.8X4	T37.8X5	T37.8X6
with sulfamethoxazole	T36.8X1	T36.8X2	T36.8X3	T36.8X4	T36.8X5	T36.8X6
Trimethylcarbinol	T51.3X1	T51.3X2	T51.3X3	T51.3X4	—	—
Trimethylpsoralen	T49.3X1	T49.3X2	T49.3X3	T49.3X4	T49.3X5	T49.3X6
Trimeton	T45.0X1	T45.0X2	T45.0X3	T45.0X4	T45.0X5	T45.0X6
Trimetrexate	T45.1X1	T45.1X2	T45.1X3	T45.1X4	T45.1X5	T45.1X6
Trimipramine	T43.011	T43.012	T43.013	T43.014	T43.015	T43.016
Trimustine	T45.1X1	T45.1X2	T45.1X3	T45.1X4	T45.1X5	T45.1X6
Trinitrine	T46.3X1	T46.3X2	T46.3X3	T46.3X4	T46.3X5	T46.3X6
Trinitrobenzol	T65.3X1	T65.3X2	T65.3X3	T65.3X4	—	—
Trinitrophenol	T65.3X1	T65.3X2	T65.3X3	T65.3X4	—	—
Trinitrotoluene (fumes)	T65.3X1	T65.3X2	T65.3X3	T65.3X4	—	—
Trional	T42.6X1	T42.6X2	T42.6X3	T42.6X4	T42.6X5	T42.6X6
Triorthocresyl phosphate	T65.891	T65.892	T65.893	T65.894		
Trioxide of arsenic	T57.0X1	T57.0X2	T57.0X3	T57.0X4	—	—
Trioxysalen	T49.4X1	T49.4X2	T49.4X3	T49.4X4	T49.4X5	T49.4X6
Tripamide	T50.2X1	T50.2X2	T50.2X3	T50.2X4	T50.2X5	T50.2X6
Triparanol	T46.6X1	T46.6X2	T46.6X3	T46.6X4	T46.6X5	T46.6X6
Tripelennamine	T45.0X1	T45.0X2	T45.0X3	T45.0X4	T45.0X5	T45.0X6
Triperiden	T44.3X1	T44.3X2	T44.3X3	T44.3X4	T44.3X5	T44.3X6
Triperidol	T43.4X1	T43.4X2	T43.4X3	T43.4X4	T43.4X5	T43.4X6
Triphenylphosphate	T65.891	T65.892	T65.893	T65.894	—	—
Triple						
bromides	T42.6X1	T42.6X2	T42.6X3	T42.6X4	T42.6X5	T42.6X6
carbonate	T47.1X1	T47.1X2	T47.1X3	T47.1X4	T47.1X5	T47.1X6
vaccine						
DPT	T50.A11	T50.A12	T50.A13	T50.A14	T50.A15	T50.A16
including pertussis	T50.A11	T50.A12	T50.A13	T50.A14	T50.A15	T50.A16
MMR	T50.B91	T50.B92	—	—	—	—
Triprolidine	T45.0X1	T45.0X2	T45.0X3	T45.0X4	T45.0X5	T45.0X6
Trisodium hydrogen edetate	T50.6X1	T50.6X2	T50.6X3	T50.6X4	T50.6X5	T50.6X6

Substance	Poisoning, Accidental (Unintentional)	Poisoning, Intentional Self-Harm	Poisoning, Assault	Poisoning, Undetermined	Adverse Effect	Underdosing
Trisoralen	T49.3X1	T49.3X2	T49.3X3	T49.3X4	T49.3X5	T49.3X6
Trisulfapyrimidines	T37.0X1	T37.0X2	T37.0X3	T37.0X4	T37.0X5	T37.0X6
Trithiozine	T44.3X1	T44.3X2	T44.3X3	T44.3X4	T44.3X5	T44.3X6
Tritiozine	T44.3X1	T44.3X2	T44.3X3	T44.3X4	T44.3X5	T44.3X6
Tritoqualine	T45.0X1	T45.0X2	T45.0X3	T45.0X4	T45.0X5	T45.0X6
Trofosfamide	T45.1X1	T45.1X2	T45.1X3	T45.1X4	T45.1X5	T45.1X6
Troleandomycin	T36.3X1	T36.3X2	T36.3X3	T36.3X4	T36.3X5	T36.3X6
Trolnitrate (phosphate)	T46.3X1	T46.3X2	T46.3X3	T46.3X4	T46.3X5	T46.3X6
Tromantadine	T37.5X1	T37.5X2	T37.5X3	T37.5X4	T37.5X5	T37.5X6
Trometamol	T50.2X1	T50.2X2	T50.2X3	T50.2X4	T50.2X5	T50.2X6
Tromethamine	T50.2X1	T50.2X2	T50.2X3	T50.2X4	T50.2X5	T50.2X6
Tronothane	T41.3X1	T41.3X2	T41.3X3	T41.3X4	T41.3X5	T41.3X6
Tropacine	T44.3X1	T44.3X2	T44.3X3	T44.3X4	T44.3X5	T44.3X6
Tropatepine	T44.3X1	T44.3X2	T44.3X3	T44.3X4	T44.3X5	T44.3X6
Tropicamide	T44.3X1	T44.3X2	T44.3X3	T44.3X4	T44.3X5	T44.3X6
Trospium chloride	T44.3X1	T44.3X2	T44.3X3	T44.3X4	T44.3X5	T44.3X6
Troxerutin	T46.991	T46.992	T46.993	T46.994	T46.995	T46.996
Troxidone	T42.2X1	T42.2X2	T42.2X3	T42.2X4	T42.2X5	T42.2X6
Tryparsamide	T37.3X1	T37.3X2	T37.3X3	T37.3X4	T37.3X5	T37.3X6
Trypsin	T45.3X1	T45.3X2	T45.3X3	T45.3X4	T45.3X5	T45.3X6
Tryptizol	T43.011	T43.012	T43.013	T43.014	T43.015	T43.016
TSH	T38.811	T38.812	T38.813	T38.814	T38.815	T38.816
Tuaminoheptane	T48.5X1	T48.5X2	T48.5X3	T48.5X4	T48.5X5	T48.5X6
Tuberculin, purified protein derivative (PPD)	T50.8X1	T50.8X2	T50.8X3	T50.8X4	T50.8X5	T50.8X6
Tubocurare	T48.1X1	T48.1X2	T48.1X3	T48.1X4	T48.1X5	T48.1X6
Tubocurarine (chloride)	T48.1X1	T48.1X2	T48.1X3	T48.1X4	T48.1X5	T48.1X6
Tulobuterol	T48.6X1	T48.6X2	T48.6X3	T48.6X4	T48.6X5	T48.6X6
Turpentine (spirits of)	T52.8X1	T52.8X2	T52.8X3	T52.8X4	—	—
vapor	T52.8X1	T52.8X2	T52.8X3	T52.8X4	—	—
Tybamate	T43.591	T43.592	T43.593	T43.594	T43.595	T43.596
Tyloxapol	T48.4X1	T48.4X2	T48.4X3	T48.4X4	T48.4X5	T48.4X6
Tymazoline	T48.5X1	T48.5X2	T48.5X3	T48.5X4	T48.5X5	T48.5X6
Typhoid-paratyphoid vaccine	T50.A91	T50.A92	T50.A93	T50.A94	T50.A95	T50.A96
Typhus vaccine	T50.A91	T50.A92	T50.A93	T50.A94	T50.A95	T50.A96
Tyropanoate	T50.8X1	T50.8X2	T50.8X3	T50.8X4	T50.8X5	T50.8X6
Tyrothricin	T49.6X1	T49.6X2	T49.6X3	T49.6X4	T49.6X5	T49.6X6
ENT agent	T49.6X1	T49.6X2	T49.6X3	T49.6X4	T49.6X5	T49.6X6
ophthalmic preparation	T49.5X1	T49.5X2	T49.5X3	T49.5X4	T49.5X5	T49.5X6
U						
Ufenamate	T39.391	T39.392	T39.393	T39.394	T39.395	T39.396
Ultraviolet light protectant	T49.3X1	T49.3X2	T49.3X3	T49.3X4	T49.3X5	T49.3X6

◀ New   ◀◀ Revised   ~~deleted~~ Deleted

TABLE OF DRUGS AND CHEMICALS

Substance	External Cause (T-Code)					
	Poisoning, Accidental (Unintentional)	Poisoning, Intentional Self-Harm	Poisoning, Assault	Poisoning, Undetermined	Adverse Effect	Underdosing
Undecenoic acid	T49.0X1	T49.0X2	T49.0X3	T49.0X4	T49.0X5	T49.0X6
Undecoylium	T49.0X1	T49.0X2	T49.0X3	T49.0X4	T49.0X5	T49.0X6
Undecylenic acid (derivatives)	T49.0X1	T49.0X2	T49.0X3	T49.0X4	T49.0X5	T49.0X6
Unna's boot	T49.3X1	T49.3X2	T49.3X3	T49.3X4	T49.3X5	T49.3X6
Unsaturated fatty acid	T46.6X1	T46.6X2	T46.6X3	T46.6X4	T46.6X5	T46.6X6
Uracil mustard	T45.1X1	T45.1X2	T45.1X3	T45.1X4	T45.1X5	T45.1X6
Uramustine	T45.1X1	T45.1X2	T45.1X3	T45.1X4	T45.1X5	T45.1X6
Urapidil	T46.5X1	T46.5X2	T46.5X3	T46.5X4	T46.5X5	T46.5X6
Urari	T48.1X1	T48.1X2	T48.1X3	T48.1X4	T48.1X5	T48.1X6
Urate oxidase	T50.4X1	T50.4X2	T50.4X3	T50.4X4	T50.4X5	T50.4X6
Urea	T47.3X1	T47.3X2	T47.3X3	T47.3X4	T47.3X5	T47.3X6
peroxide	T49.0X1	T49.0X2	T49.0X3	T49.0X4	T49.0X5	T49.0X6
stibamine	T37.4X1	T37.4X2	T37.4X3	T37.4X4	T37.4X5	T37.4X6
topical	T49.8X1	T49.8X2	T49.8X3	T49.8X4	T49.8X5	T49.8X6
Urethane	T45.1X1	T45.1X2	T45.1X3	T45.1X4	T45.1X5	T45.1X6
Urginea (maritima) (scilla) —see Squill						
Uric acid metabolism drug NEC	T50.4X1	T50.4X2	T50.4X3	T50.4X4	T50.4X5	T50.4X6
Uricosuric agent	T50.4X1	T50.4X2	T50.4X3	T50.4X4	T50.4X5	T50.4X6
Urinary anti-infective	T37.8X1	T37.8X2	T37.8X3	T37.8X4	T37.8X5	T37.8X6
Urofollitropin	T38.811	T38.812	T38.813	T38.814	T38.815	T38.816
Urokinase	T45.611	T45.612	T45.613	T45.614	T45.615	T45.616
Urokon	T50.8X1	T50.8X2	T50.8X3	T50.8X4	T50.8X5	T50.8X6
Ursodeoxycholic acid	T50.991	T50.992	T50.993	T50.994	T50.995	T50.996
Ursodiol	T50.991	T50.992	T50.993	T50.994	T50.995	T50.996
Urtica	T62.2X1	T62.2X2	T62.2X3	T62.2X4	—	—
Utility gas — see Gas, utility						
V						
Vaccine NEC	T50.Z91	T50.Z92	T50.Z93	T50.Z94	T50.Z95	T50.Z96
antineoplastic	T50.Z91	T50.Z92	T50.Z93	T50.Z94	T50.Z95	T50.Z96
bacterial NEC	T50.A91	T50.A92	T50.A93	T50.A94	T50.A95	T50.A96
with						
other bacterial component	T50.A91	T50.A92	T50.A93	T50.A94	T50.A95	T50.A96
pertussis component	T50.A91	T50.A92	T50.A93	T50.A94	T50.A95	T50.A96
viral-rickettsial component	T50.A91	T50.A92	T50.A93	T50.A94	T50.A95	T50.A96
mixed NEC	T50.A91	T50.A92	T50.A93	T50.A94	T50.A95	T50.A96
BCG	T50.A91	T50.A92	T50.A93	T50.A94	T50.A95	T50.A96
cholera	T50.A91	T50.A92	T50.A93	T50.A94	T50.A95	T50.A96
diphtheria	T50.A91	T50.A92	T50.A93	T50.A94	T50.A95	T50.A96
with tetanus	T50.A21	T50.A22	T50.A23	T50.A24	T50.A25	T50.A26
and pertussis	T50.A11	T50.A12	T50.A13	T50.A14	T50.A15	T50.A16

Substance	External Cause (T-Code)					
	Poisoning, Accidental (Unintentional)	Poisoning, Intentional Self-Harm	Poisoning, Assault	Poisoning, Undetermined	Adverse Effect	Underdosing
Vaccine NEC *(Continued)*						
influenza	T50.B91	T50.B92	T50.B93	T50.B94	T50.B95	T50.B96
measles	T50.B91	T50.B92	T50.B93	T50.B94	T50.B95	T50.B96
with mumps and rubella	T50.B91	T50.B92	T50.B93	T50.B94	T50.B95	T50.B96
meningococcal	T50.A91	T50.A92	T50.A93	T50.A94	T50.A95	T50.A96
mumps	T50.B91	T50.B92	T50.B93	T50.B94	T50.B95	T50.B96
paratyphoid	T50.A91	T50.A92	T50.A93	T50.A94	T50.A95	T50.A96
pertussis	T50.A11	T50.A12	T50.A13	T50.A14	T50.A15	T50.A16
with diphtheria	T50.A11	T50.A12	T50.A13	T50.A14	T50.A15	T50.A16
and tetanus	T50.A11	T50.A12	T50.A13	T50.A14	T50.A15	T50.A16
plague	T50.A91	T50.A92	T50.A93	T50.A94	T50.A95	T50.A96
poliomyelitis	T50.B91	T50.B92	T50.B93	T50.B94	T50.B95	T50.B96
poliovirus	T50.B91	T50.B92	T50.B93	T50.B94	T50.B95	T50.B96
rabies	T50.B91	T50.B92	T50.B93	T50.B94	T50.B95	T50.B96
respiratory syncytial virus	T50.B91	T50.B92	T50.B93	T50.B94	T50.B95	T50.B96
rickettsial NEC	T50.A91	T50.A92	T50.A93	T50.A94	T50.A95	T50.A96
with						
bacterial component	T50.A21	T50.A22	T50.A23	T50.A24	T50.A25	T50.A26
Rocky Mountain spotted fever	T50.A91	T50.A92	T50.A93	T50.A94	T50.A95	T50.A96
rubella	T50.B91	T50.B92	T50.B93	T50.B94	T50.B95	T50.B96
sabin oral	T50.B91	T50.B92	T50.B93	T50.B94	T50.B95	T50.B96
smallpox	T50.B11	T50.B12	T50.B13	T50.B14	T50.B15	T50.B16
TAB	T50.A91	T50.A92	T50.A93	T50.A94	T50.A95	T50.A96
tetanus	T50.A91	T50.A92	T50.A93	T50.A94	T50.A95	T50.A96
typhoid	T50.A91	T50.A92	T50.A93	T50.A94	T50.A95	T50.A96
typhus	T50.A91	T50.A92	T50.A93	T50.A94	T50.A95	T50.A96
viral NEC	T50.B91	T50.B92	T50.B93	T50.B94	T50.B95	T50.B96
yellow fever	T50.B91	T50.B92	T50.B93	T50.B94	T50.B95	T50.B96
Vaccinia immune globulin	T50.Z11	T50.Z12	T50.Z13	T50.Z14	T50.Z15	T50.Z16
Vaginal contraceptives	T49.8X1	T49.8X2	T49.8X3	T49.8X4	T49.8X5	T49.8X6
Valerian						
root	T42.6X1	T42.6X2	T42.6X3	T42.6X4	T42.6X5	T42.6X6
tincture	T42.6X1	T42.6X2	T42.6X3	T42.6X4	T42.6X5	T42.6X6
Valethamate bromide	T44.3X1	T44.3X2	T44.3X3	T44.3X4	T44.3X5	T44.3X6
Valisone	T49.0X1	T49.0X2	T49.0X3	T49.0X4	T49.0X5	T49.0X6
Valium	T42.4X1	T42.4X2	T42.4X3	T42.4X4	T42.4X5	T42.4X6
Valmid	T42.6X1	T42.6X2	T42.6X3	T42.6X4	T42.6X5	T42.6X6
Valnoctamide	T42.6X1	T42.6X2	T42.6X3	T42.6X4	T42.6X5	T42.6X6
Valproate (sodium)	T42.6X1	T42.6X2	T42.6X3	T42.6X4	T42.6X5	T42.6X6
Valproic acid	T42.6X1	T42.6X2	T42.6X3	T42.6X4	T42.6X5	T42.6X6
Valpromide	T42.6X1	T42.6X2	T42.6X3	T42.6X4	T42.6X5	T42.6X6
Vanadium	T56.891	T56.892	T56.893	T56.894	—	—

◄ New ◄╍ Revised ~~deleted~~ Deleted

Substance	External Cause (T-Code)					
	Poisoning, Accidental (Unintentional)	Poisoning, Intentional Self-Harm	Poisoning, Assault	Poisoning, Undetermined	Adverse Effect	Underdosing
Vancomycin	T36.8X1	T36.8X2	T36.8X3	T36.8X4	T36.8X5	T36.8X6
Vapor—*see also Gas*	T59.91	T59.92	T59.93	T59.94	—	—
kiln (carbon monoxide)	T58.8X1	T58.8X2	T58.8X3	T58.8X4		
lead—*see lead*						
specified source NEC	T59.891	T59.892	T59.893	T59.894	—	—
Vardenafil	T46.7X1	T46.7X2	T46.7X3	T46.7X4	T46.7X5	T46.7X6
Varicose reduction drug	T46.8X1	T46.8X2	T46.8X3	T46.8X4	T46.8X5	T46.8X6
Varnish	T65.4X1	T65.4X2	T65.4X3	T65.4X4		
cleaner	T52.91	T52.92	T52.93	T52.94	—	—
Vaseline	T49.3X1	T49.3X2	T49.3X3	T49.3X4	T49.3X5	T49.3X6
Vasodilan	T46.7X1	T46.7X2	T46.7X3	T46.7X4	T46.7X5	T46.7X6
Vasodilator						
coronary NEC	T46.3X1	T46.3X2	T46.3X3	T46.3X4	T46.3X5	T46.3X6
peripheral NEC	T46.7X1	T46.7X2	T46.7X3	T46.7X4	T46.7X5	T46.7X6
Vasopressin	T38.891	T38.892	T38.893	T38.894	T38.895	T38.896
Vasopressor drugs	T38.891	T38.892	T38.893	T38.894	T38.895	T38.896
Vecuronium bromide	T48.1X1	T48.1X2	T48.1X3	T48.1X4	T48.1X5	T48.1X6
Vegetable extract, astringent	T49.2X1	T49.2X2	T49.2X3	T49.2X4	T49.2X5	T49.2X6
Venlafaxine	T43.211	T43.212	T43.213	T43.214	T43.215	T43.216
Venom, venomous (bite) (sting)	T63.91	T63.92	T63.93	T63.94	—	—
amphibian NEC	T63.831	T63.832	T63.833	T63.834	—	—
animal NEC	T63.891	T63.892	T63.893	T63.894	—	—
ant	T63.421	T63.422	T63.423	T63.424	—	—
arthropod NEC	T63.481	T63.482	T63.483	T63.484	—	—
bee	T63.441	T63.442	T63.443	T63.444	—	—
centipede	T63.411	T63.412	T63.413	T63.414	—	—
fish	T63.591	T63.592	T63.593	T63.594	—	—
frog	T63.811	T63.812	T63.813	T63.814	—	—
hornet	T63.451	T63.452	T63.453	T63.454	—	—
insect NEC	T63.481	T63.482	T63.483	T63.484	—	—
lizard	T63.121	T63.122	T63.123	T63.124	—	—
marine						
animals	T63.691	T63.692	T63.693	T63.694	—	—
bluebottle	T63.611	T63.612	T63.613	T63.614	—	—
jellyfish NEC	T63.621	T63.622	T63.623	T63.624	—	—
Portugese Man-o-war	T63.611	T63.612	T63.613	T63.614	—	—
sea anemone	T63.631	T63.632	T63.633	T63.634	—	—
specified NEC	T63.691	T63.692	T63.693	T63.694	—	—
fish	T63.591	T63.592	T63.593	T63.594	—	—
plants	T63.711	T63.712	T63.713	T63.714	—	—
sting ray	T63.511	T63.512	T63.513	T63.514	—	—

Substance	External Cause (T-Code)					
	Poisoning, Accidental (Unintentional)	Poisoning, Intentional Self-Harm	Poisoning, Assault	Poisoning, Undetermined	Adverse Effect	Underdosing
Venom, venomous *(Continued)*						
millipede (tropical)	T63.411	T63.412	T63.413	T63.414	—	—
plant NEC	T63.791	T63.792	T63.793	T63.794	—	—
marine	T63.711	T63.712	T63.713	T63.714	—	—
reptile	T63.191	T63.192	T63.193	T63.194	—	—
gila monster	T63.111	T63.112	T63.113	T63.114	—	—
lizard NEC	T63.121	T63.122	T63.123	T63.124	—	—
scorpion	T63.2X1	T63.2X2	T63.2X3	T63.2X4	—	—
snake	T63.001	T63.002	T63.003	T63.004	—	—
African NEC	T63.081	T63.082	T63.083	T63.084	—	—
American (North) (South) NEC	T63.061	T63.062	T63.063	T63.064	—	—
Asian	T63.081	T63.082	T63.083	T63.084	—	—
Australian	T63.071	T63.072	T63.073	T63.074	—	—
cobra	T63.041	T63.042	T63.043	T63.044	—	—
coral snake	T63.021	T63.022	T63.023	T63.024	—	—
rattlesnake	T63.011	T63.012	T63.013	T63.014	—	—
specified NEC	T63.091	T63.092	T63.093	T63.094	—	—
taipan	T63.031	T63.032	T63.033	T63.034	—	—
specified NEC	T63.891	T63.892	T63.893	T63.894	—	—
spider	T63.301	T63.302	T63.303	T63.304	—	—
black widow	T63.311	T63.312	T63.313	T63.314	—	—
brown recluse	T63.331	T63.332	T63.333	T63.334	—	—
specified NEC	T63.391	T63.392	T63.393	T63.394	—	—
tarantula	T63.321	T63.322	T63.323	T63.324	—	—
sting ray	T63.511	T63.512	T63.513	T63.514	—	—
toad	T63.821	T63.822	T63.823	T63.824	—	—
wasp	T63.461	T63.462	T63.463	T63.464	—	—
Venous sclerosing drug NEC	T46.8X1	T46.8X2	T46.8X3	T46.8X4	T46.8X5	T46.8X6
Ventolin—*see Albuterol*						
Verapamil	T46.1X1	T46.1X2	T46.1X3	T46.1X4	T46.1X5	T46.1X6
Veramon	T42.3X1	T42.3X2	T42.3X3	T42.3X4	T42.3X5	T42.3X6
Veratrine	T46.5X1	T46.5X2	T46.5X3	T46.5X4	T46.5X5	T46.5X6
Veratrum						
album	T62.2X1	T62.2X2	T62.2X3	T62.2X4	—	—
alkaloids	T46.5X1	T46.5X2	T46.5X3	T46.5X4	T46.5X5	T46.5X6
viride	T62.2X1	T62.2X2	T62.2X3	T62.2X4	—	—
Verdigris	T60.3X1	T60.3X2	T60.3X3	T60.3X4	—	—
Veronal	T42.3X1	T42.3X2	T42.3X3	T42.3X4	T42.3X5	T42.3X6
Veroxil	T37.4X1	T37.4X2	T37.4X3	T37.4X4	T37.4X5	T37.4X6
Versenate	T50.6X1	T50.6X2	T50.6X3	T50.6X4	T50.6X5	T50.6X6

TABLE OF DRUGS AND CHEMICALS

TABLE OF DRUGS AND CHEMICALS

Substance	External Cause (T-Code)					
	Poisoning, Accidental (Unintentional)	Poisoning, Intentional Self-Harm	Poisoning, Assault	Poisoning, Undetermined	Adverse Effect	Underdosing
Versidyne	T39.8X1	T39.8X2	T39.8X3	T39.8X4	T39.8X5	T39.8X6
Vetrabutine	T48.0X1	T48.0X2	T48.0X3	T48.0X4	T48.0X5	T48.0X6
Vidarabine	T37.5X1	T37.5X2	T37.5X3	T37.5X4	T37.5X5	T37.5X6
Vienna						
green	T57.0X1	T57.0X2	T57.0X3	T57.0X4	—	—
insecticide	T60.2X1	T60.2X2	T60.2X3	T60.2X4		
red	T57.0X1	T57.0X2	T57.0X3	T57.0X4	—	—
pharmaceutical dye	T50.991	T50.992	T50.993	T50.994	T50.995	T50.996
Vigabatrin	T42.6X1	T42.6X2	T42.6X3	T42.6X4	T42.6X5	T42.6X6
Viloxazine	T43.291	T43.292	T43.293	T43.294	T43.295	T43.296
Viminol	T39.8X1	T39.8X2	T39.8X3	T39.8X4	T39.8X5	T39.8X6
Vinbarbital, vinbarbitone	T42.3X1	T42.3X2	T42.3X3	T42.3X4	T42.3X5	T42.3X6
Vinblastine	T45.1X1	T45.1X2	T45.1X3	T45.1X4	T45.1X5	T45.1X6
Vinburnine	T46.7X1	T46.7X2	T46.7X3	T46.7X4	T46.7X5	T46.7X6
Vincamine	T45.1X1	T45.1X2	T45.1X3	T45.1X4	T45.1X5	T45.1X6
Vincristine	T45.1X1	T45.1X2	T45.1X3	T45.1X4	T45.1X5	T45.1X6
Vindesine	T45.1X1	T45.1X2	T45.1X3	T45.1X4	T45.1X5	T45.1X6
Vinesthene, vinethene	T41.0X1	T41.0X2	T41.0X3	T41.0X4	T41.0X5	T41.0X6
Vinorelbine tartrate	T45.1X1	T45.1X2	T45.1X3	T45.1X4	T45.1X5	T45.1X6
Vinpocetine	T46.7X1	T46.7X2	T46.7X3	T46.7X4	T46.7X5	T46.7X6
Vinyl						
acetate	T65.891	T65.892	T65.893	T65.894	—	—
bital	T42.3X1	T42.3X2	T42.3X3	T42.3X4	T42.3X5	T42.3X6
bromide	T65.891	T65.892	T65.893	T65.894	—	—
chloride	T59.891	T59.892	T59.893	T59.894		
ether	T41.0X1	T41.0X2	T41.0X3	T41.0X4	T41.0X5	T41.0X6
Vinylbital	T42.3X1	T42.3X2	T42.3X3	T42.3X4	T42.3X5	T42.3X6
Vinylidene chloride	T65.891	T65.892	T65.893	T65.894	—	—
Vioform	T37.8X1	T37.8X2	T37.8X3	T37.8X4	T37.8X5	T37.8X6
topical	T49.0X1	T49.0X2	T49.0X3	T49.0X4	T49.0X5	T49.0X6
Viomycin	T36.8X1	T36.8X2	T36.8X3	T36.8X4	T36.8X5	T36.8X6
Viosterol	T45.2X1	T45.2X2	T45.2X3	T45.2X4	T45.2X5	T45.2X6
Viper (venom)	T63.091	T63.092	T63.093	T63.094	—	—
Viprynium	T37.4X1	T37.4X2	T37.4X3	T37.4X4	T37.4X5	T37.4X6
Viquidil	T46.7X1	T46.7X2	T46.7X3	T46.7X4	T46.7X5	T46.7X6
Viral vaccine NEC	T50.B91	T50.B92	T50.B93	T50.B94	T50.B95	T50.B96
Virginiamycin	T36.8X1	T36.8X2	T36.8X3	T36.8X4	T36.8X5	T36.8X6
Virugon	T37.5X1	T37.5X2	T37.5X3	T37.5X4	T37.5X5	T37.5X6
Viscous agent	T50.901	T50.902	T50.903	T50.904	T50.905	T50.906
Visine	T49.5X1	T49.5X2	T49.5X3	T49.5X4	T49.5X5	T49.5X6
Visnadine	T46.3X1	T46.3X2	T46.3X3	T46.3X4	T46.3X5	T46.3X6

Substance	External Cause (T-Code)					
	Poisoning, Accidental (Unintentional)	Poisoning, Intentional Self-Harm	Poisoning, Assault	Poisoning, Undetermined	Adverse Effect	Underdosing
Vitamin NEC	T45.2X1	T45.2X2	T45.2X3	T45.2X4	T45.2X5	T45.2X6
A	T45.2X1	T45.2X2	T45.2X3	T45.2X4	T45.2X5	T45.2X6
B NEC	T45.2X1	T45.2X2	T45.2X3	T45.2X4	T45.2X5	T45.2X6
nicotinic acid	T46.7X1	T46.7X2	T46.7X3	T46.7X4	T46.7X5	T46.7X6
B1	T45.2X1	T45.2X2	T45.2X3	T45.2X4	T45.2X5	T45.2X6
B2	T45.2X1	T45.2X2	T45.2X3	T45.2X4	T45.2X5	T45.2X6
B6	T45.2X1	T45.2X2	T45.2X3	T45.2X4	T45.2X5	T45.2X6
B12	T45.2X1	T45.2X2	T45.2X3	T45.2X4	T45.2X5	T45.2X6
B15	T45.2X1	T45.2X2	T45.2X3	T45.2X4	T45.2X5	T45.2X6
C	T45.2X1	T45.2X2	T45.2X3	T45.2X4	T45.2X5	T45.2X6
D	T45.2X1	T45.2X2	T45.2X3	T45.2X4	T45.2X5	T45.2X6
D2	T45.2X1	T45.2X2	T45.2X3	T45.2X4	T45.2X5	T45.2X6
D3	T45.2X1	T45.2X2	T45.2X3	T45.2X4	T45.2X5	T45.2X6
E	T45.2X1	T45.2X2	T45.2X3	T45.2X4	T45.2X5	T45.2X6
E acetate	T45.2X1	T45.2X2	T45.2X3	T45.2X4	T45.2X5	T45.2X6
hematopoietic	T45.8X1	T45.8X2	T45.8X3	T45.8X4	T45.8X5	T45.8X6
K NEC	T45.7X1	T45.7X2	T45.7X3	T45.7X4	T45.7X5	T45.7X6
K1	T45.7X1	T45.7X2	T45.7X3	T45.7X4	T45.7X5	T45.7X6
K2	T45.7X1	T45.7X2	T45.7X3	T45.7X4	T45.7X5	T45.7X6
PP	T45.2X1	T45.2X2	T45.2X3	T45.2X4	T45.2X5	T45.2X6
ulceroprotectant	T47.1X1	T47.1X2	T47.1X3	T47.1X4	T47.1X5	T47.1X6
Vleminckx's solution	T49.4X1	T49.4X2	T49.4X3	T49.4X4	T49.4X5	T49.4X6
Voltaren — see Diclofenac sodium						
W						
Warfarin	T45.511	T45.512	T45.513	T45.514	T45.515	T45.516
rodenticide	T60.4X1	T60.4X2	T60.4X3	T60.4X4	—	—
sodium	T45.511	T45.512	T45.513	T45.514	T45.515	T45.516
Wasp (sting)	T63.461	T63.462	T63.463	T63.464	—	—
Water						
balance drug	T50.3X1	T50.3X2	T50.3X3	T50.3X4	T50.3X5	T50.3X6
distilled	T50.3X1	T50.3X2	T50.3X3	T50.3X4	T50.3X5	T50.3X6
gas — see Gas, water						
incomplete combustion of — see Carbon, monoxide, fuel, utility						
hemlock	T62.2X1	T62.2X2	T62.2X3	T62.2X4	—	—
moccasin (venom)	T63.061	T63.062	T63.063	T63.064	—	—
purified	T50.3X1	T50.3X2	T50.3X3	T50.3X4	T50.3X5	T50.3X6
Wax (paraffin) (petroleum)	T52.0X1	T52.0X2	T52.0X3	T52.0X4	—	—
automobile	T65.891	T65.892	T65.893	T65.894	—	—
floor	T52.0X1	T52.0X2	T52.0X3	T52.0X4	—	—

◀ New   ◀ Revised   ~~deleted~~ Deleted

Substance	External Cause (T-Code)					
	Poisoning, Accidental (Unintentional)	Poisoning, Intentional Self-Harm	Poisoning, Assault	Poisoning, Undetermined	Adverse Effect	Underdosing
Weed killers NEC	T60.3X1	T60.3X2	T60.3X3	T60.3X4	—	—
Welldorm	T42.6X1	T42.6X2	T42.6X3	T42.6X4	T42.6X5	T42.6X6
White						
arsenic	T57.0X1	T57.0X2	T57.0X3	T57.0X4	—	—
hellebore	T62.2X1	T62.2X2	T62.2X3	T62.2X4	—	—
lotion (keratolytic)	T49.4X1	T49.4X2	T49.4X3	T49.4X4	T49.4X5	T49.4X6
spirit	T52.0X1	T52.0X2	T52.0X3	T52.0X4	—	—
Whitewash	T65.891	T65.892	T65.893	T65.894	—	—
Whole blood (human)	T45.8X1	T45.8X2	T45.8X3	T45.8X4	T45.8X5	T45.8X6
Wild						
black cherry	T62.2X1	T62.2X2	T62.2X3	T62.2X4	—	—
poisonous plants NEC	T62.2X1	T62.2X2	T62.2X3	T62.2X4	—	—
Window cleaning fluid	T65.891	T65.892	T65.893	T65.894	—	—
Wintergreen (oil)	T49.3X1	T49.3X2	T49.3X3	T49.3X4	T49.3X5	T49.3X6
Wisterine	T62.2X1	T62.2X2	T62.2X3	T62.2X4	—	—
Witch hazel	T49.2X1	T49.2X2	T49.2X3	T49.2X4	T49.2X5	T49.2X6
Wood alcohol or spirit	T51.1X1	T51.1X2	T51.1X3	T51.1X4	—	—
Wool fat (hydrous)	T49.3X1	T49.3X2	T49.3X3	T49.3X4	T49.3X5	T49.3X6
Woorali	T48.1X1	T48.1X2	T48.1X3	T48.1X4	T48.1X5	T48.1X6
Wormseed, American	T37.4X1	T37.4X2	T37.4X3	T37.4X4	T37.4X5	T37.4X6
X						
Xamoterol	T44.5X1	T44.5X2	T44.5X3	T44.5X4	T44.5X5	T44.5X6
Xanthine diuretics	T50.2X1	T50.2X2	T50.2X3	T50.2X4	T50.2X5	T50.2X6
Xanthinol nicotinate	T46.7X1	T46.7X2	T46.7X3	T46.7X4	T46.7X5	T46.7X6
Xanthotoxin	T49.3X1	T49.3X2	T49.3X3	T49.3X4	T49.3X5	T49.3X6
Xantinol nicotinate	T46.7X1	T46.7X2	T46.7X3	T46.7X4	T46.7X5	T46.7X6
Xantocillin	T36.0X1	T36.0X2	T36.0X3	T36.0X4	T36.0X5	T36.0X6
Xenon (127Xe) (133Xe)	T50.8X1	T50.8X2	T50.8X3	T50.8X4	T50.8X5	T50.8X6
Xenysalate	T49.4X1	T49.4X2	T49.4X3	T49.4X4	T49.4X5	T49.4X6
Xibornol	T37.8X1	T37.8X2	T37.8X3	T37.8X4	T37.8X5	T37.8X6
Xigris	T45.511	T45.512	T45.513	T45.514	T45.515	T45.516
Xipamide	T50.2X1	T50.2X2	T50.2X3	T50.2X4	T50.2X5	T50.2X6
Xylene (vapor)	T52.2X1	T52.2X2	T52.2X3	T52.2X4	—	—
Xylocaine (infiltration) (topical)	T41.3X1	T41.3X2	T41.3X3	T41.3X4	T41.3X5	T41.3X6
nerve block (peripheral) (plexus)	T41.3X1	T41.3X2	T41.3X3	T41.3X4	T41.3X5	T41.3X6
spinal	T41.3X1	T41.3X2	T41.3X3	T41.3X4	T41.3X5	T41.3X6
Xylol (vapor)	T52.2X1	T52.2X2	T52.2X3	T52.2X4	—	—
Xylometazoline	T48.5X1	T48.5X2	T48.5X3	T48.5X4	T48.5X5	T48.5X6

Substance	External Cause (T-Code)					
	Poisoning, Accidental (Unintentional)	Poisoning, Intentional Self-Harm	Poisoning, Assault	Poisoning, Undetermined	Adverse Effect	Underdosing
Y						
Yeast	T45.2X1	T45.2X2	T45.2X3	T45.2X4	T45.2X5	T45.2X6
dried	T45.2X1	T45.2X2	T45.2X3	T45.2X4	T45.2X5	T45.2X6
Yellow						
fever vaccine	T50.B91	T50.B92	T50.B93	T50.B94	T50.B95	T50.B96
jasmine	T62.2X1	T62.2X2	T62.2X3	T62.2X4	—	—
phenolphthalein	T47.2X1	T47.2X2	T47.2X3	T47.2X4	T47.2X5	T47.2X6
Yew	T62.2X1	T62.2X2	T62.2X3	T62.2X4	—	—
Yohimbic acid	T40.991	T40.992	T40.993	T40.994	T40.995	T40.996
Z						
Zactane	T39.8X1	T39.8X2	T39.8X3	T39.8X4	T39.8X5	T39.8X6
Zalcitabine	T37.5X1	T37.5X2	T37.5X3	T37.5X4	T37.5X5	T37.5X6
Zaroxolyn	T50.2X1	T50.2X2	T50.2X3	T50.2X4	T50.2X5	T50.2X6
Zephiran (topical)	T49.0X1	T49.0X2	T49.0X3	T49.0X4	T49.0X5	T49.0X6
ophthalmic preparation	T49.5X1	T49.5X2	T49.5X3	T49.5X4	T49.5X5	T49.5X6
Zeranol	T38.7X1	T38.7X2	T38.7X3	T38.7X4	T38.7X5	T38.7X6
Zerone	T51.1X1	T51.1X2	T51.1X3	T51.1X4	—	—
Zidovudine	T37.5X1	T37.5X2	T37.5X3	T37.5X4	T37.5X5	T37.5X6
Zimeldine	T43.221	T43.222	T43.223	T43.224	T43.225	T43.226
Zinc (compounds) (fumes) (vapor) NEC	T56.5X1	T56.5X2	T56.5X3	T56.5X4	—	—
anti-infectives	T49.0X1	T49.0X2	T49.0X3	T49.0X4	T49.0X5	T49.0X6
antivaricose	T46.8X1	T46.8X2	T46.8X3	T46.8X4	T46.8X5	T46.8X6
bacitracin	T49.0X1	T49.0X2	T49.0X3	T49.0X4	T49.0X5	T49.0X6
chloride (mouthwash)	T49.6X1	T49.6X2	T49.6X3	T49.6X4	T49.6X5	T49.6X6
chromate	T56.5X1	T56.5X2	T56.5X3	T56.5X4	—	—
gelatin	T49.3X1	T49.3X2	T49.3X3	T49.3X4	T49.3X5	T49.3X6
oxide	T49.3X1	T49.3X2	T49.3X3	T49.3X4	T49.3X5	T49.3X6
plaster	T49.3X1	T49.3X2	T49.3X3	T49.3X4	T49.3X5	T49.3X6
peroxide	T49.0X1	T49.0X2	T49.0X3	T49.0X4	T49.0X5	T49.0X6
pesticides	T56.5X1	T56.5X2	T56.5X3	T56.5X4	—	—
phosphide	T60.4X1	T60.4X2	T60.4X3	T60.4X4	—	—
pyrithionate	T49.4X1	T49.4X2	T49.4X3	T49.4X4	T49.4X5	T49.4X6
stearate	T49.3X1	T49.3X2	T49.3X3	T49.3X4	T49.3X5	T49.3X6
sulfate	T49.5X1	T49.5X2	T49.5X3	T49.5X4	T49.5X5	T49.5X6
ENT agent	T49.6X1	T49.6X2	T49.6X3	T49.6X4	T49.6X5	T49.6X6
ophthalmic solution	T49.5X1	T49.5X2	T49.5X3	T49.5X4	T49.5X5	T49.5X6
topical NEC	T49.0X1	T49.0X2	T49.0X3	T49.0X4	T49.0X5	T49.0X6
undecylenate	T49.0X1	T49.0X2	T49.0X3	T49.0X4	T49.0X5	T49.0X6

◀ New   ◀ Revised   ~~deleted~~ Deleted

Substance	External Cause (T-Code)					
	Poisoning, Accidental (Unintentional)	Poisoning, Intentional Self-Harm	Poisoning, Assault	Poisoning, Undetermined	Adverse Effect	Underdosing
Zineb	T60.0X1	T60.0X2	T60.0X3	T60.0X4	—	—
Zinostatin	T45.1X1	T45.1X2	T45.1X3	T45.1X4	T45.1X5	T45.1X6
Zipeprol	T48.3X1	T48.3X2	T48.3X3	T48.3X4	T48.3X5	T48.3X6
Zofenopril	T46.4X1	T46.4X2	T46.4X3	T46.4X4	T46.4X5	T46.4X6
Zolpidem	T42.6X1	T42.6X2	T42.6X3	T42.6X4	T42.6X5	T42.6X6
Zomepirac	T39.391	T39.392	T39.393	T39.394	T39.395	T39.396
Zopiclone	T42.6X1	T42.6X2	T42.6X3	T42.6X4	T42.6X5	T42.6X6

Substance	External Cause (T-Code)					
	Poisoning, Accidental (Unintentional)	Poisoning, Intentional Self-Harm	Poisoning, Assault	Poisoning, Undetermined	Adverse Effect	Underdosing
Zorubicin	T45.1X1	T45.1X2	T45.1X3	T45.1X4	T45.1X5	T45.1X6
Zotepine	T43.591	T43.592	T43.593	T43.594	T43.595	T43.596
Zovant	T45.511	T45.512	T45.513	T45.514	T45.515	T45.516
Zoxazolamine	T42.8X1	T42.8X2	T42.8X3	T42.8X4	T42.8X5	T42.8X6
Zuclopenthixol	T43.4X1	T43.4X2	T43.4X3	T43.4X4	T43.4X5	T43.4X6
Zygadenus (venenosus)	T62.2X1	T62.2X2	T62.2X3	T62.2X4	—	—
Zyprexa	T43.591	T43.592	T43.593	T43.594	T43.595	T43.596

◄ New   ◀▌ Revised   ~~deleted~~ Deleted

External Cause
of Injuries Index

A

Abandonment (causing exposure to weather conditions) (with intent to injure or kill) NEC X58

Abuse (adult) (child) (mental) (physical) (sexual) X58

Accident (to) X58
 aircraft (in transit) (powered) —*see also* Accident, transport, aircraft
  due to, caused by cataclysm —*see* Forces of nature, by type
 animal-drawn vehicle —*see* Accident, transport, animal-drawn vehicle occupant
 animal-rider —*see* Accident, transport, animal-rider
 automobile —*see* Accident, transport, car occupant
 bare foot water skiier V94.4
 boat, boating —*see also* Accident, watercraft
  striking swimmer
   powered V94.11
   unpowered V94.12
 bus —*see* Accident, transport, bus occupant
 cable car, not on rails V98.0
  on rails —*see* Accident, transport, streetcar occupant
 car —*see* Accident, transport, car occupant
 caused by, due to
  animal NEC W64
  chain hoist W24.0
  cold (excessive) —*see* Exposure, cold
  corrosive liquid, substance —*see* Table of Drugs and Chemicals
  cutting or piercing instrument —*see* Contact, with, by type of instrument
  drive belt W24.0
  electric
   current —*see* Exposure, electric current
   motor —*see also* Contact, with, by type of machine W31.3
    current (of) W86.8
  environmental factor NEC X58
  explosive material —*see* Explosion
  fire, flames —*see* Exposure, fire
  firearm missile —*see* Discharge, firearm by type
  heat (excessive) —*see* Heat
  hot —*see* Contact, with, hot
  ignition —*see* Ignition
  lifting device W24.0
  lightning —*see* subcategory T75.0
   causing fire —*see* Exposure, fire
  machine, machinery —*see* Contact, with, by type of machine
  natural factor NEC X58
  pulley (block) W24.0
  radiation —*see* Radiation
  steam X13.1
   inhalation X13.0
   pipe X16
  thunderbolt —*see* subcategory T75.0
   causing fire —*see* Exposure, fire
  transmission device W24.1
 coach —*see* Accident, transport, bus occupant
 coal car —*see* Accident, transport, industrial vehicle occupant
 diving —*see also* Fall, into, water
  with
   drowning or submersion —*see* Drowning
 forklift —*see* Accident, transport, industrial vehicle occupant
 heavy transport vehicle NOS —*see* Accident, transport, truck occupant
 ice yacht V98.2

Accident (*Continued*)
 in
  medical, surgical procedure
   as, or due to misadventure —*see* Misadventure
   causing an abnormal reaction or later complication without mention of misadventure —*see also* Complication of or following, by type of procedure Y84.9
 land yacht V98.1
 late effect of —*see* W00-X58 with 7th character S
 logging car —*see* Accident, transport, industrial vehicle occupant
 machine, machinery —*see also* Contact, with, by type of machine
  on board watercraft V93.69
   explosion —*see* Explosion, in, watercraft
   fire —*see* Burn, on board watercraft
   powered craft V93.63
    ferry boat V93.61
    fishing boat V93.62
    jetskis V93.63
    liner V93.61
    merchant ship V93.60
    passenger ship V93.61
    sailboat V93.64
 mine tram —*see* Accident, transport, industrial vehicle occupant
 mobility scooter (motorized) —*see* Accident, transport, pedestrian, conveyance, specified type NEC
 motor scooter —*see* Accident, transport, motorcyclist
 motor vehicle NOS (traffic) —*see also* Accident, transport V89.2
  nontraffic V89.0
  three-wheeled NOS —*see* Accident, transport, three-wheeled motor vehicle occupant
 motorcycle NOS —*see* Accident, transport, motorcyclist
 nonmotor vehicle NOS (nontraffic) —*see also* Accident, transport V89.1
  traffic NOS V89.3
 nontraffic (victim's mode of transport NOS) V88.9
  collision (between) V88.7
   bus and truck V88.5
   car and:
    bus V88.3
    pickup V88.2
    three-wheeled motor vehicle V88.0
    train V88.6
    truck V88.4
    two-wheeled motor vehicle V88.0
    van V88.2
   specified vehicle NEC and:
    three-wheeled motor vehicle V88.1
    two-wheeled motor vehicle V88.1
  known mode of transport —*see* Accident, transport, by type of vehicle
  noncollision V88.8
 on board watercraft V93.89
  powered craft V93.83
   ferry boat V93.81
   fishing boat V93.82
   jetskis V93.83
   liner V93.81
   merchant ship V93.80
   passenger ship V93.81
  unpowered craft V93.88
   canoe V93.85
   inflatable V93.86
    in tow
     recreational V94.31
     specified NEC V94.32
   kayak V93.85

Accident (*Continued*)
 on board watercraft (*Continued*)
  unpowered craft (*Continued*)
   sailboat V93.84
   surf-board V93.88
   water skis V93.87
   windsurfer V93.88
 parachutist V97.29
  entangled in object V97.21
  injured on landing V97.22
 pedal cycle —*see* Accident, transport, pedal cyclist
 pedestrian (on foot)
  with
   another pedestrian W51
    with fall W03
     due to ice or snow W00.0
     on pedestrian conveyance NEC V00.09
   roller skater (in-line) V00.01
   skate boarder V00.02
   transport vehicle —*see* Accident, transport
  on pedestrian conveyance —*see* Accident, transport, pedestrian, conveyance
 pick-up truck or van —*see* Accident, transport, pickup truck occupant
 quarry truck —*see* Accident, transport, industrial vehicle occupant
 railway vehicle (any) (in motion) —*see* Accident, transport, railway vehicle occupant
  due to cataclysm —*see* Forces of nature, by type
 scooter (non-motorized) —*see* Accident, transport, pedestrian, conveyance, scooter
 sequelae of —*see* W00-X58 with 7th character S
 skateboard —*see* Accident, transport, pedestrian, conveyance, skateboard
 ski (ing) —*see* Accident, transport, pedestrian, conveyance
  lift V98.3
 specified cause NEC X58
 streetcar —*see* Accident, transport, streetcar occupant
 traffic (victim's mode of transport NOS) V87.9
  collision (between) V87.7
   bus and truck V87.5
   car and:
    bus V87.3
    pickup V87.2
    three-wheeled motor vehicle V87.0
    train V87.6
    truck V87.4
    two-wheeled motor vehicle V87.0
    van V87.2
   specified vehicle NEC and:
    three-wheeled motor vehicle V87.1
    two-wheeled motor vehicle V87.1
  known mode of transport —*see* Accident, transport, by type of vehicle
  noncollision V87.8
 transport (involving injury to) V99
  18 wheeler —*see* Accident, transport, truck occupant
  agricultural vehicle occupant (nontraffic) V84.9
   driver V84.5
   hanger-on V84.7
   passenger V84.6
   traffic V84.3
    driver V84.0
    hanger-on V84.2
    passenger V84.1
   while boarding or alighting V84.4

Accident *(Continued)*
transport *(Continued)*
aircraft NEC V97.89
military NEC V97.818
with civilian aircraft V97.810
civilian injured by V97.811
occupant injured (in)
nonpowered craft accident
V96.9
balloon V96.00
collision V96.03
crash V96.01
explosion V96.05
fire V96.04
forced landing V96.02
specified type NEC V96.09
glider V96.20
collision V96.23
crash V96.21
explosion V96.25
fire V96.24
forced landing V96.22
specified type NEC V96.29
hang glider V96.10
collision V96.13
crash V96.11
explosion V96.15
fire V96.14
forced landing V96.12
specified type NEC V96.19
specified craft NEC V96.8
powered craft accident V95.9
fixed wing NEC
commercial V95.30
collision V95.33
crash V95.31
explosion V95.35
fire V95.34
forced landing V95.32
specified type NEC
V95.39
private V95.20
collision V95.23
crash V95.21
explosion V95.25
fire V95.24
forced landing V95.22
specified type NEC
V95.29
glider V95.10
collision V95.13
crash V95.11
explosion V95.15
fire V95.14
forced landing V95.12
specified type NEC V95.19
helicopter V95.00
collision V95.03
crash V95.01
explosion V95.05
fire V95.04
forced landing V95.02
specified type NEC V95.09
spacecraft V95.40
collision V95.43
crash V95.41
explosion V95.45
fire V95.44
forced landing V95.42
specified type NEC V95.49
specified craft NEC V95.8
ultralight V95.10
collision V95.13
crash V95.11
explosion V95.15
fire V95.14
forced landing V95.12
specified type NEC V95.19
specified accident NEC V97.0
while boarding or alighting
V97.1

Accident *(Continued)*
transport *(Continued)*
aircraft NEC *(Continued)*
person (injured by)
falling from, in or on aircraft V97.0
machinery on aircraft V97.89
on ground with aircraft involvement
V97.39
rotating propeller V97.32
struck by object falling from aircraft
V97.31
sucked into aircraft jet V97.33
while boarding or alighting aircraft
V97.1
airport (battery-powered) passenger
vehicle —*see* Accident, transport,
industrial vehicle occupant
⟹all-terrain vehicle occupant (nontraffic)
V86.95
⟹driver V86.55
dune buggy —*see* Accident, transport,
dune buggy occupant
⟹hanger-on V86.75
⟹passenger V86.65
snowmobile —*see* Accident, transport,
snowmobile occupant
▶specified type NEC V86.99
⟹traffic V86.35
⟹driver V86.05
⟹hanger-on V86.25
⟹passenger V86.15
⟹while boarding or alighting V86.45
ambulance occupant (traffic) V86.31
driver V86.01
hanger-on V86.21
nontraffic V86.91
driver V86.51
hanger-on V86.71
passenger V86.61
passenger V86.11
while boarding or alighting V86.41
animal-drawn vehicle occupant (in)
V80.929
collision (with)
animal V80.12
being ridden V80.711
animal-drawn vehicle V80.721
bus V80.42
car V80.42
fixed or stationary object V80.82
military vehicle V80.920
nonmotor vehicle V80.791
pedal cycle V80.22
pedestrian V80.12
pickup V80.42
railway train or vehicle V80.62
specified motor vehicle NEC V80.52
streetcar V80.731
truck V80.42
two-or three-wheeled motor vehicle
V80.32
van V80.42
noncollision V80.02
specified circumstance NEC V80. 928
animal-rider V80.919
collision (with)
animal V80.11
being ridden V80.710
animal-drawn vehicle V80.720
bus V80.41
car V80.41
fixed or stationary object V80.81
military vehicle V80.910
nonmotor vehicle V80.790
pedal cycle V80.21
pedestrian V80.11
pickup V80.41
railway train or vehicle V80.61
specified motor vehicle NEC V80.51
streetcar V80.730
truck V80.41

Accident *(Continued)*
transport *(Continued)*
animal-rider *(Continued)*
collision *(Continued)*
two- or three-wheeled motor vehicle
V80.31
van V80.41
noncollision V80.018
specified as horse rider V80.010
specified circumstance NEC V80.918
armored car —*see* Accident, transport,
truck occupant
battery-powered truck (baggage) (mail) —
see Accident, transport, industrial
vehicle occupant
bus occupant V79.9
collision (with)
animal (traffic) V70.9
being ridden (traffic) V76.9
nontraffic V76.3
while boarding or alighting V76.4
nontraffic V70.3
while boarding or alighting V70.4
animal-drawn vehicle (traffic) V76.9
nontraffic V76.3
while boarding or alighting V76.4
bus (traffic) V74.9
nontraffic V74.3
while boarding or alighting V74.4
car (traffic) V73.9
nontraffic V73.3
while boarding or alighting V73.4
motor vehicle NOS (traffic) V79.60
nontraffic V79.20
specified type NEC (traffic) V79.69
nontraffic V79.29
pedal cycle (traffic) V71.9
nontraffic V71.3
while boarding or alighting V71.4
pickup truck (traffic) V73.9
nontraffic V73.3
while boarding or alighting V73.4
railway vehicle (traffic) V75.9
nontraffic V75.3
while boarding or alighting V75.4
specified vehicle NEC (traffic) V76.9
nontraffic V76.3
while boarding or alighting V76.4
stationary object (traffic) V77.9
nontraffic V77.3
while boarding or alighting V77.4
streetcar (traffic) V76.9
nontraffic V76.3
while boarding or alighting V76.4
three wheeled motor vehicle (traffic)
V72.9
nontraffic V72.3
while boarding or alighting V72.4
truck (traffic) V74.9
nontraffic V74.3
while boarding or alighting V74.4
two wheeled motor vehicle (traffic)
V72.9
nontraffic V72.3
while boarding or alighting V72.4
van (traffic) V73.9
nontraffic V73.3
while boarding or alighting V73.4
driver
collision (with)
animal (traffic) V70.5
being ridden (traffic) V76.5
nontraffic V76.0
nontraffic V70.0
animal-drawn vehicle (traffic)
V76.5
nontraffic V76.0
bus (traffic) V74.5
nontraffic V74.0
car (traffic) V73.5
nontraffic V73.0

Accident *(Continued)*
  transport *(Continued)*
    bus occupant *(Continued)*
      driver *(Continued)*
        collision *(Continued)*
          motor vehicle NOS (traffic) V79.40
            nontraffic V79.00
            specified type NEC (traffic)
              V79.49
              nontraffic V79.09
          pedal cycle (traffic) V71.5
            nontraffic V71.0
          pickup truck (traffic) V73.5
            nontraffic V73.0
          railway vehicle (traffic) V75.5
            nontraffic V75.0
          specified vehicle NEC (traffic)
            V76.5
            nontraffic V76.0
          stationary object (traffic) V77.5
            nontraffic V77.0
          streetcar (traffic) V76.5
            nontraffic V76.0
          three wheeled motor vehicle
            (traffic) V72.5
            nontraffic V72.0
          truck (traffic) V74.5
            nontraffic V74.0
          two wheeled motor vehicle (traffic)
            V72.5
            nontraffic V72.0
          van (traffic) V73.5
            nontraffic V73.0
        noncollision accident (traffic) V78.5
          nontraffic V78.0
      hanger-on
        collision (with)
          animal (traffic) V70.7
            being ridden (traffic) V76.7
              nontraffic V76.2
            nontraffic V70.2
          animal-drawn vehicle (traffic) V76.7
            nontraffic V76.2
          bus (traffic) V74.7
            nontraffic V74.2
          car (traffic) V73.7
            nontraffic V73.2
          pedal cycle (traffic) V71.7
            nontraffic V71.2
          pickup truck (traffic) V73.7
            nontraffic V73.2
          railway vehicle (traffic) V75.7
            nontraffic V75.2
          specified vehicle NEC (traffic) V76.7
            nontraffic V76.2
          stationary object (traffic) V77.7
            nontraffic V77.2
          streetcar (traffic) V76.7
            nontraffic V76.2
          three wheeled motor vehicle
            (traffic) V72.7
            nontraffic V72.2
          truck (traffic) V74.7
            nontraffic V74.2
          two wheeled motor vehicle (traffic)
            V72.7
            nontraffic V72.2
          van (traffic) V73.7
            nontraffic V73.2
        noncollision accident (traffic) V78.7
          nontraffic V78.2
      noncollision accident (traffic) V78.9
        nontraffic V78.3
        while boarding or alighting V78.4
      nontraffic V79.3
      passenger
        collision (with)
          animal (traffic) V70.6
            being ridden (traffic) V76.6
              nontraffic V76.1
            nontraffic V70.1

Accident *(Continued)*
  transport *(Continued)*
    bus occupant *(Continued)*
      passenger *(Continued)*
        collision *(Continued)*
          animal-drawn vehicle (traffic) V76.6
            nontraffic V76.1
          bus (traffic) V74.6
            nontraffic V74.1
          car (traffic) V73.6
            nontraffic V73.1
          motor vehicle NOS (traffic) V79.50
            nontraffic V79.10
            specified type NEC (traffic)
              V79.59
              nontraffic V79.19
          pedal cycle (traffic) V71.6
            nontraffic V71.1
          pickup truck (traffic) V73.6
            nontraffic V73.1
          railway vehicle (traffic) V75.6
            nontraffic V75.1
          specified vehicle NEC (traffic) V76.6
            nontraffic V76.1
          stationary object (traffic) V77.6
            nontraffic V77.1
          streetcar (traffic) V76.6
            nontraffic V76.1
          three wheeled motor vehicle
            (traffic) V72.6
            nontraffic V72.1
          truck (traffic) V74.6
            nontraffic V74.1
          two wheeled motor vehicle (traffic)
            V72.6
            nontraffic V72.1
          van (traffic) V73.6
            nontraffic V73.1
        noncollision accident (traffic) V78.6
          nontraffic V78.1
      specified type NEC V79.88
      military vehicle V79.81
    cable car, not on rails V98.0
      on rails —*see* Accident, transport,
        streetcar occupant
    car occupant V49.9
      ambulance occupant —*see* Accident,
        transport, ambulance occupant
      collision (with)
        animal (traffic) V40.9
          being ridden (traffic) V46.9
            nontraffic V46.3
            while boarding or alighting
              V46.4
          nontraffic V40.3
          while boarding or alighting V40.4
        animal-drawn vehicle (traffic) V46.9
          nontraffic V46.3
          while boarding or alighting V46.4
        bus (traffic) V44.9
          nontraffic V44.3
          while boarding or alighting V44.4
        car (traffic) V43.92
          nontraffic V43.32
          while boarding or alighting V43.42
        motor vehicle NOS (traffic) V49.60
          nontraffic V49.20
          specified type NEC (traffic) V49.69
            nontraffic V49.29
        pedal cycle (traffic) V41.9
          nontraffic V41.3
          while boarding or alighting V41.4
        pickup truck (traffic) V43.93
          nontraffic V43.33
          while boarding or alighting V43.43
        railway vehicle (traffic) V45.9
          nontraffic V45.3
          while boarding or alighting V45.4
        specified vehicle NEC (traffic) V46.9
          nontraffic V46.3
          while boarding or alighting V46.4

Accident *(Continued)*
  transport *(Continued)*
    car occupant *(Continued)*
      collision *(Continued)*
        sport utility vehicle (traffic) V43.91
          nontraffic V43.31
          while boarding or alighting V43.41
        ➠stationary object (traffic) V47.9
          ➠nontraffic V47.3
          while boarding or alighting V47.4
        streetcar (traffic) V46.9
          nontraffic V46.3
          while boarding or alighting V46.4
        three wheeled motor vehicle (traffic)
          V42.9
          nontraffic V42.3
          while boarding or alighting V42.4
        truck (traffic) V44.9
          nontraffic V44.3
          while boarding or alighting V44.4
        two wheeled motor vehicle (traffic)
          V42.9
          nontraffic V42.3
          while boarding or alighting V42.4
        van (traffic) V43.94
          nontraffic V43.34
          while boarding or alighting V43.44
    driver
      collision (with)
        animal (traffic) V40.5
          being ridden (traffic) V46.5
            nontraffic V46.0
          nontraffic V40.0
        animal-drawn vehicle (traffic) V46.5
          nontraffic V46.0
        bus (traffic) V44.5
          nontraffic V44.0
        car (traffic) V43.52
          nontraffic V43.02
        motor vehicle NOS (traffic) V49.40
          nontraffic V49.00
          specified type NEC (traffic)
            V49.49
            nontraffic V49.09
        pedal cycle (traffic) V41.5
          nontraffic V41.0
        pickup truck (traffic) V43.53
          nontraffic V43.03
        railway vehicle (traffic) V45.5
          nontraffic V45.0
        specified vehicle NEC (traffic) V46.5
          nontraffic V46.0
        sport utility vehicle (traffic) V43.51
          nontraffic V43.01
        ➠stationary object (traffic) V47.5
          ➠nontraffic V47.0
        streetcar (traffic) V46.5
          nontraffic V46.0
        three wheeled motor vehicle
          (traffic) V42.5
          nontraffic V42.0
        truck (traffic) V44.5
          nontraffic V44.0
        two wheeled motor vehicle (traffic)
          V42.5
          nontraffic V42.0
        van (traffic) V43.54
          nontraffic V43.04
       noncollision accident (traffic) V48.5
         nontraffic V48.0
    hanger-on
      collision (with)
        animal (traffic) V40.7
          being ridden (traffic) V46.7
            nontraffic V46.2
          nontraffic V40.2
        animal-drawn vehicle (traffic)
          V46.7
          nontraffic V46.2
        bus (traffic) V44.7
          nontraffic V44.2

▶ New   ➠ Revised   ~~deleted~~ Deleted   ● Use Additional Character(s)

Accident *(Continued)*
  transport *(Continued)*
    car occupant *(Continued)*
      hanger-on *(Continued)*
        collision *(Continued)*
          car (traffic) V43.72
            nontraffic V43.22
          pedal cycle (traffic) V41.7
            nontraffic V41.2
          pickup truck (traffic) V43.73
            nontraffic V43.23
          railway vehicle (traffic) V45.7
            nontraffic V45.2
          specified vehicle NEC (traffic) V46.7
            nontraffic V46.2
          sport utility vehicle (traffic) V43.71
            nontraffic V43.21
          stationary object (traffic) V47.7
            nontraffic V47.2
          streetcar (traffic) V46.7
            nontraffic V46.2
          three wheeled motor vehicle
              (traffic) V42.7
            nontraffic V42.2
          truck (traffic) V44.7
            nontraffic V44.2
          two wheeled motor vehicle (traffic)
              V42.7
            nontraffic V42.2
          van (traffic) V43.74
            nontraffic V43.24
        noncollision accident (traffic) V48.7
          nontraffic V48.2
      noncollision accident (traffic) V48.9
        nontraffic V48.3
        while boarding or alighting V48.4
      nontraffic V49.3
      passenger
        collision (with)
          animal (traffic) V40.6
            being ridden (traffic) V46.6
              nontraffic V46.1
            nontraffic V40.1
          animal-drawn vehicle (traffic) V46.6
            nontraffic V46.1
          bus (traffic) V44.6
            nontraffic V44.1
          car (traffic) V43.62
            nontraffic V43.12
          motor vehicle NOS (traffic) V49.50
            nontraffic V49.10
            specified type NEC (traffic) V49.59
              nontraffic V49.19
          pedal cycle (traffic) V41.6
            nontraffic V41.1
          pickup truck (traffic) V43.63
            nontraffic V43.13
          railway vehicle (traffic) V45.6
            nontraffic V45.1
          specified vehicle NEC (traffic) V46.6
            nontraffic V46.1
          sport utility vehicle (traffic) V43.61
            nontraffic V43.11
          ➡stationary object (traffic) V47.6
            ➡nontraffic V47.1
          streetcar (traffic) V46.6
            nontraffic V46.1
          three wheeled motor vehicle
              (traffic) V42.6
            nontraffic V42.1
          truck (traffic) V44.6
            nontraffic V44.1
          two wheeled motor vehicle (traffic)
              V42.6
            nontraffic V42.1
          van (traffic) V43.64
            nontraffic V43.14
        noncollision accident (traffic) V48.6
          nontraffic V48.1
      specified type NEC V49.88
        military vehicle V49.81

Accident *(Continued)*
  transport *(Continued)*
    coal car —*see* Accident, transport,
        industrial vehicle occupant
    construction vehicle occupant (nontraffic)
        V85.9
      driver V85.5
      hanger-on V85.7
      passenger V85.6
      traffic V85.3
        driver V85.0
        hanger-on V85.2
        passenger V85.1
      while boarding or alighting V85.4
    ➤dirt bike rider (nontraffic) V86.96
      ➤driver V86.56
      ➤hanger-on V86.76
      ➤passenger V86.66
      ➤traffic V86.36
        ➤driver V86.06
        ➤hanger-on V86.26
        ➤passenger V86.16
      ➤while boarding or alighting V86.46
    due to cataclysm —*see* Forces of nature,
        by type
    dune buggy occupant (nontraffic) V86.93
      driver V86.53
      hanger-on V86.73
      passenger V86.63
      traffic V86.33
        driver V86.03
        hanger-on V86.23
        passenger V86.13
      while boarding or alighting V86.43
    forklift —*see* Accident, transport,
        industrial vehicle occupant
    go cart —*see* Accident, transport, all-terrain
        vehicle occupant
    golf cart —*see* Accident, transport,
        all-terrain vehicle occupant
    heavy transport vehicle occupant —
        see Accident, transport, truck occupant
    ice yacht V98.2
    industrial vehicle occupant (nontraffic)
        V83.9
      driver V83.5
      hanger-on V83.7
      passenger V83.6
      traffic V83.3
        driver V83.0
        hanger-on V83.2
        passenger V83.1
      while boarding or alighting V83.4
    interurban electric car —*see* Accident,
        transport, streetcar
    land yacht V98.1
    logging car —*see* Accident, transport,
        industrial vehicle occupant
    military vehicle occupant (traffic) V86.34
      driver V86.04
      hanger-on V86.24
      nontraffic V86.94
        driver V86.54
        hanger-on V86.74
        passenger V86.64
      passenger V86.14
      while boarding or alighting V86.44
    mine tram —*see* Accident, transport,
        industrial vehicle occupant
    motor vehicle NEC occupant (traffic) V89.2
    motorcoach —*see* Accident, transport,
        bus occupant
    ➤motor/cross bike rider —*see also* Accident,
        transport, dirt bike rider V86.96
    motorcyclist V29.9
      collision (with)
        animal (traffic) V20.9
          being ridden (traffic) V26.9
            nontraffic V26.2
            while boarding or alighting V26.3
          nontraffic V20.2
          while boarding or alighting V20.3

Accident *(Continued)*
  transport *(Continued)*
    motorcyclist *(Continued)*
      collision *(Continued)*
        animal-drawn vehicle (traffic) V26.9
          nontraffic V26.2
          while boarding or alighting V26.3
        bus (traffic) V24.9
          nontraffic V24.2
          while boarding or alighting V24.3
        car (traffic) V23.9
          nontraffic V23.2
          while boarding or alighting V23.3
        motor vehicle NOS (traffic) V29.60
          nontraffic V29.20
          specified type NEC (traffic) V29.69
            nontraffic V29.29
        pedal cycle (traffic) V21.9
          nontraffic V21.2
          while boarding or alighting V21.3
        pickup truck (traffic) V23.9
          nontraffic V23.2
          while boarding or alighting V23.3
        railway vehicle (traffic) V25.9
          nontraffic V25.2
          while boarding or alighting V25.3
        specified vehicle NEC (traffic) V26.9
          nontraffic V26.2
          while boarding or alighting V26.3
        stationary object (traffic) V27.9
          nontraffic V27.2
          while boarding or alighting V27.3
        streetcar (traffic) V26.9
          nontraffic V26.2
          while boarding or alighting V26.3
        three wheeled motor vehicle (traffic)
            V22.9
          nontraffic V22.2
          while boarding or alighting V22.3
        truck (traffic) V24.9
          nontraffic V24.2
          while boarding or alighting V24.3
        two wheeled motor vehicle (traffic)
            V22.9
          nontraffic V22.2
          while boarding or alighting V22.3
        van (traffic) V23.9
          nontraffic V23.2
          while boarding or alighting V23.3
      driver
        collision (with)
          animal (traffic) V20.4
            being ridden (traffic) V26.4
              nontraffic V26.0
            nontraffic V20.0
          animal-drawn vehicle (traffic) V26.4
            nontraffic V26.0
          bus (traffic) V24.4
            nontraffic V24.0
          car (traffic) V23.4
            nontraffic V23.0
          motor vehicle NOS (traffic) V29.40
            nontraffic V29.00
            specified type NEC (traffic)
                V29.49
              nontraffic V29.09
          pedal cycle (traffic) V21.4
            nontraffic V21.0
          pickup truck (traffic) V23.4
            nontraffic V23.0
          railway vehicle (traffic) V25.4
            nontraffic V25.0
          specified vehicle NEC (traffic) V26.4
            nontraffic V26.0
          stationary object (traffic) V27.4
            nontraffic V27.0
          streetcar (traffic) V26.4
            nontraffic V26.0
          three wheeled motor vehicle
              (traffic) V22.4
            nontraffic V22.0

A

Accident *(Continued)*
  transport *(Continued)*
    motorcyclist *(Continued)*
     driver *(Continued)*
      collision *(Continued)*
       truck (traffic) V24.4
        nontraffic V24.0
       two wheeled motor vehicle (traffic) V22.4
        nontraffic V22.0
       van (traffic) V23.4
        nontraffic V23.0
      noncollision accident (traffic) V28.4
       nontraffic V28.0
     noncollision accident (traffic) V28.9
      nontraffic V28.2
      while boarding or alighting V28.3
     nontraffic V29.3
     passenger
      collision (with)
       animal (traffic) V20.5
        being ridden (traffic) V26.5
         nontraffic V26.1
        nontraffic V20.1
       animal-drawn vehicle (traffic) V26.5
        nontraffic V26.1
       bus (traffic) V24.5
        nontraffic V24.1
       car (traffic) V23.5
        nontraffic V23.1
       motor vehicle NOS (traffic) V29.50
        nontraffic V29.10
        specified type NEC (traffic) V29.59
         nontraffic V29.19
       pedal cycle (traffic) V21.5
        nontraffic V21.1
       pickup truck (traffic) V23.5
        nontraffic V23.1
       railway vehicle (traffic) V25.5
        nontraffic V25.1
       specified vehicle NEC (traffic) V26.5
        nontraffic V26.1
       stationary object (traffic) V27.5
        nontraffic V27.1
       streetcar (traffic) V26.5
        nontraffic V26.1
       three wheeled motor vehicle (traffic) V22.5
        nontraffic V22.1
       truck (traffic) V24.5
        nontraffic V24.1
       two wheeled motor vehicle (traffic) V22.5
        nontraffic V22.1
       van (traffic) V23.5
        nontraffic V23.1
      noncollision accident (traffic) V28.5
       nontraffic V28.1
    specified type NEC V29.88
    military vehicle V29.81
   occupant (of)
    aircraft (powered) V95.9
     fixed wing
      commercial —*see* Accident, transport, aircraft, occupant, powered, fixed wing, commercial
      private —*see* Accident, transport, aircraft, occupant, powered, fixed wing, private
     nonpowered V96.9
     specified NEC V95.8
    airport battery-powered vehicle —*see* Accident, transport, industrial vehicle occupant
    all-terrain vehicle (ATV) —*see* Accident, transport, all-terrain vehicle occupant
    animal-drawn vehicle —*see* Accident, transport, animal-drawn vehicle occupant

Accident *(Continued)*
  transport *(Continued)*
   occupant *(Continued)*
    automobile —*see* Accident, transport, car occupant
    balloon V96.00
    battery-powered vehicle —*see* Accident, transport, industrial vehicle occupant
    bicycle —*see* Accident, transport, pedal cyclist
     motorized —*see* Accident, transport, motorcycle rider
    boat NEC —*see* Accident, watercraft
    bulldozer —*see* Accident, transport, construction vehicle occupant
    bus —*see* Accident, transport, bus occupant
    cable car (on rails) —*see also* Accident, transport, streetcar occupant
     not on rails V98.0
    car —*see also* Accident, transport, car occupant
     cable (on rails) —*see also* Accident, transport, streetcar occupant
     not on rails V98.0
    coach —*see* Accident, transport, bus occupant
    coal-car —*see* Accident, transport, industrial vehicle occupant
    digger —*see* Accident, transport, construction vehicle occupant
    dump truck —*see* Accident, transport, construction vehicle occupant
    earth-leveler —*see* Accident, transport, construction vehicle occupant
    farm machinery (self-propelled) —*see* Accident, transport, agricultural vehicle occupant
    forklift —*see* Accident, transport, industrial vehicle occupant
    glider (unpowered) V96.20
     hang V96.10
     powered (microlight) (ultralight) —*see* Accident, transport, aircraft, occupant, powered, glider
    glider (unpowered) NEC V96.20
    hang-glider V96.10
    harvester —*see* Accident, transport, agricultural vehicle occupant
    heavy (transport) vehicle —*see* Accident, transport, truck occupant
    helicopter —*see* Accident, transport, aircraft, occupant, helicopter
    ice-yacht V98.2
    kite (carrying person) V96.8
    land-yacht V98.1
    logging car —*see* Accident, transport, industrial vehicle occupant
    mechanical shovel —*see* Accident, transport, construction vehicle occupant
    microlight —*see* Accident, transport, aircraft, occupant, powered, glider
    minibus —*see* Accident, transport, pickup truck occupant
    minivan —*see* Accident, transport, pickup truck occupant
    moped —*see* Accident, transport, motorcycle
    motor scooter —*see* Accident, transport, motorcycle
    motorcycle (with sidecar) —*see* Accident, transport, motorcycle
    ▶off-road motor-vehicle —*see also* Accident, transport, all-terrain vehicle occupant V86.99
    pedal cycle —*see also* Accident, transport, pedal cyclist
    pick-up (truck) —*see* Accident, transport, pickup truck occupant

Accident *(Continued)*
  transport *(Continued)*
   occupant *(Continued)*
    railway (train) (vehicle) (subterranean) (elevated) —*see* Accident, transport, railway vehicle occupant
    rickshaw —*see* Accident, transport, pedal cycle
     pedal driven —*see* Accident, transport, pedal cyclist
    road-roller —*see* Accident, transport, construction vehicle occupant
    ship NOS V94.9
    ski-lift (chair) (gondola) V98.3
    snowmobile —*see* Accident, transport, snowmobile occupant
    spacecraft, spaceship —*see* Accident, transport, aircraft, occupant, spacecraft
    sport utility vehicle —*see* Accident, transport, pickup truck occupant
    streetcar (interurban) (operating on public street or highway) —*see* Accident, transport, streetcar occupant
    SUV —*see* Accident, transport, pickup truck occupant
    téléférique V98.0
    three-wheeled vehicle (motorized) —*see also* Accident, transport, three-wheeled motor vehicle occupant
     nonmotorized —*see* Accident, transport, pedal cycle
    tractor (farm) (and trailer) —*see* Accident, transport, agricultural vehicle occupant
    train —*see* Accident, transport, railway vehicle occupant
    tram —*see* Accident, transport, streetcar occupant
     in mine or quarry —*see* Accident, transport, industrial vehicle occupant
    tricycle —*see* Accident, transport, pedal cycle
     motorized —*see* Accident, transport, three-wheeled motor vehicle
    trolley —*see* Accident, transport, streetcar occupant
     in mine or quarry —*see* Accident, transport, industrial vehicle occupant
    tub, in mine or quarry —*see* Accident, transport, industrial vehicle occupant
    ultralight —*see* Accident, transport, aircraft, occupant, powered, glider
    van —*see* Accident, transport, van occupant
    vehicle NEC V89.9
     heavy transport —*see* Accident, transport, truck occupant
     motor (traffic) NEC V89.2
      nontraffic NEC V89.0
    watercraft NOS V94.9
     causing drowning —*see* Drowning, resulting from accident to boat
   ▶off-road motor-vehicle —*see also* Accident, transport, all-terrain vehicle occupant V86.99
   parachutist V97.29
    after accident to aircraft —*see* Accident, transport, aircraft
    entangled in object V97.21
    injured on landing V97.22
   pedal cyclist V19.9
    collision (with)
     animal (traffic) V10.9
      being ridden (traffic) V16.9
       nontraffic V16.2
       while boarding or alighting V16.3

▶ New   ⇒ Revised   ~~deleted~~ Deleted   ● Use Additional Character(s)

Accident *(Continued)*
 transport *(Continued)*
  pedal cyclist *(Continued)*
   collision *(Continued)*
    animal (traffic) V10.9 *(Continued)*
     nontraffic V10.2
     while boarding or alighting V10.3
    animal-drawn vehicle (traffic) V16.9
     nontraffic V16.2
     while boarding or alighting V16.3
    bus (traffic) V14.9
     nontraffic V14.2
     while boarding or alighting V14.3
    car (traffic) V13.9
     nontraffic V13.2
     while boarding or alighting V13.3
    motor vehicle NOS (traffic) V19.60
     nontraffic V19.20
     specified type NEC (traffic) V19.69
      nontraffic V19.29
    pedal cycle (traffic) V11.9
     nontraffic V11.2
     while boarding or alighting V11.3
    pickup truck (traffic) V13.9
     nontraffic V13.2
     while boarding or alighting V13.3
    railway vehicle (traffic) V15.9
     nontraffic V15.2
     while boarding or alighting V15.3
    specified vehicle NEC (traffic) V16.9
     nontraffic V16.2
     while boarding or alighting V16.3
    stationary object (traffic) V17.9
     nontraffic V17.2
     while boarding or alighting V17.3
    streetcar (traffic) V16.9
     nontraffic V16.2
     while boarding or alighting V16.3
    three wheeled motor vehicle (traffic)
      V12.9
     nontraffic V12.2
     while boarding or alighting V12.3
    truck (traffic) V14.9
     nontraffic V14.2
     while boarding or alighting V14.3
    two wheeled motor vehicle (traffic)
      V12.9
     nontraffic V12.2
     while boarding or alighting V12.3
    van (traffic) V13.9
     nontraffic V13.2
     while boarding or alighting V13.3
   driver
    collision (with)
     animal (traffic) V10.4
      being ridden (traffic) V16.4
       nontraffic V16.1
      nontraffic V10.0
     animal-drawn vehicle (traffic) V16.4
      nontraffic V16.0
     bus (traffic) V14.4
      nontraffic V14.0
     car (traffic) V13.4
      nontraffic V13.0
     motor vehicle NOS (traffic) V19.40
      nontraffic V19.00
      specified type NEC (traffic) V19.49
       nontraffic V19.09
     pedal cycle (traffic) V11.4
      nontraffic V11.0
     pickup truck (traffic) V13.4
      nontraffic V13.0
     railway vehicle (traffic) V15.4
      nontraffic V15.0
     specified vehicle NEC (traffic) V16.4
      nontraffic V16.0
     stationary object (traffic) V17.4
      nontraffic V17.0
     streetcar (traffic) V16.4
      nontraffic V16.0
     three wheeled motor vehicle
       (traffic) V12.4
      nontraffic V12.0

Accident *(Continued)*
 transport *(Continued)*
  pedal cyclist *(Continued)*
   driver *(Continued)*
    collision *(Continued)*
     truck (traffic) V14.4
      nontraffic V14.0
     two wheeled motor vehicle (traffic)
       V12.4
      nontraffic V12.0
     van (traffic) V13.4
      nontraffic V13.0
    noncollision accident (traffic) V18.4
     nontraffic V18.0
   noncollision accident (traffic) V18.9
    nontraffic V18.2
    while boarding or alighting V18.3
   nontraffic V19.3
   passenger
    collision (with)
     animal (traffic) V10.5
      being ridden (traffic) V16.5
       nontraffic V16.1
      nontraffic V10.1
     animal-drawn vehicle (traffic) V16.5
      nontraffic V16.1
     bus (traffic) V14.5
      nontraffic V14.1
     car (traffic) V13.5
      nontraffic V13.1
     motor vehicle NOS (traffic) V19.50
      nontraffic V19.10
      specified type NEC (traffic)
       V19.59
       nontraffic V19.19
     pedal cycle (traffic) V11.5
      nontraffic V11.1
     pickup truck (traffic) V13.5
      nontraffic V13.1
     railway vehicle (traffic) V15.5
      nontraffic V15.1
     specified vehicle NEC (traffic) V16.5
      nontraffic V16.1
     stationary object (traffic) V17.5
      nontraffic V17.1
     streetcar (traffic) V16.5
      nontraffic V16.1
     three wheeled motor vehicle
       (traffic) V12.5
      nontraffic V12.1
     truck (traffic) V14.5
      nontraffic V14.1
     two wheeled motor vehicle (traffic)
       V12.5
      nontraffic V12.1
     van (traffic) V13.5
      nontraffic V13.1
    noncollision accident (traffic) V18.5
     nontraffic V18.1
   specified type NEC V19.88
    military vehicle V19.81
  pedestrian
   conveyance (occupant) V09.9
    babystroller V00.828
     collision (with) V09.9
      animal being ridden or animal
        drawn vehicle V06.99
       nontraffic V06.09
       traffic V06.19
      bus or heavy transport V04.99
       nontraffic V04.09
       traffic V04.19
      car V03.99
       nontraffic V03.09
       traffic V03.19
      pedal cycle V01.99
       nontraffic V01.09
       traffic V01.19
      pick-up truck or van V03.99
       nontraffic V03.09
       traffic V03.19

Accident *(Continued)*
 transport *(Continued)*
  pedestrian *(Continued)*
   conveyance *(Continued)*
    babystroller *(Continued)*
     collision *(Continued)*
      railway (train) (vehicle) V05.99
       nontraffic V05.09
       traffic V05.19
      stationary object V00.822
      streetcar V06.99
       nontraffic V06.09
       traffic V06.19
      two- or three-wheeled motor
        vehicle V02.99
       nontraffic V02.09
       traffic V02.19
      vehicle V09.9
       animal-drawn V06.99
        nontraffic V06.09
        traffic V06.19
       motor
        nontraffic V09.00
        traffic V09.20
     fall V00.821
     nontraffic V09.1
      involving motor vehicle NEC
        V09.00
     traffic V09.3
      involving motor vehicle NEC
        V09.20
    flat-bottomed NEC V00.388
     collision (with) V09.9
      animal being ridden or animal
        drawn vehicle V06.99
       nontraffic V06.09
       traffic V06.19
      bus or heavy transport V04.99
       nontraffic V04.09
       traffic V04.19
      car V03.99
       nontraffic V03.09
       traffic V03.19
      pedal cycle V01.99
       nontraffic V01.09
       traffic V01.19
      pick-up truck or van V03.99
       nontraffic V03.09
       traffic V03.19
      railway (train) (vehicle) V05.99
       nontraffic V05.09
       traffic V05.19
      stationary object V00.382
      streetcar V06.99
       nontraffic V06.09
       traffic V06.19
      two-or three-wheeled motor
        vehicle V02.99
       nontraffic V02.09
       traffic V02.19
      vehicle V09.9
       animal-drawn V06.99
        nontraffic V06.09
        traffic V06.19
       motor
        nontraffic V09.00
        traffic V09.20
     fall V00.381
     nontraffic V09.1
      involving motor vehicle NEC
        V09.00
     snow
      board —*see* Accident, transport,
        pedestrian, conveyance,
        snow board
      ski —*see* Accident, transport,
        pedestrian, conveyance, skis
        (snow)
     traffic V09.3
      involving motor vehicle NEC
        V09.20

Accident *(Continued)*
  transport *(Continued)*
    pedestrian *(Continued)*
      conveyance *(Continued)*
        gliding type NEC V00.288
          collision (with) V09.9
            animal being ridden or animal
              drawn vehicle V06.99
              nontraffic V06.09
              traffic V06.19
            bus or heavy transport
              V04.99
              nontraffic V04.09
              traffic V04.19
            car V03.99
              nontraffic V03.09
              traffic V03.19
            pedal cycle V01.99
              nontraffic V01.09
              traffic V01.19
            pick-up truck or van V03.99
              nontraffic V03.09
              traffic V03.19
            railway (train) (vehicle) V05.99
              nontraffic V05.09
              traffic V05.19
            stationary object V00.282
            streetcar V06.99
              nontraffic V06.09
              traffic V06.19
            two- or three-wheeled motor
              vehicle V02.99
              nontraffic V02.09
              traffic V02.19
            vehicle V09.9
              animal-drawn V06.99
                nontraffic V06.09
                traffic V06.19
              motor
                nontraffic V09.00
                traffic V09.20
        fall V00.281
        heelies —*see* Accident, transport,
          pedestrian, conveyance,
          heelies
        ice skate —*see* Accident, transport,
          pedestrian, conveyance, ice
          skate
        nontraffic V09.1
          involving motor vehicle NEC
            V09.00
        sled —*see* Accident, transport,
          pedestrian, conveyance, sled
        traffic V09.3
          involving motor vehicle NEC
            V09.20
        wheelies —*see* Accident,
          transport, pedestrian,
          conveyance, heelies
      heelies V00.158
        colliding with stationary object
          V00.152
        fall V00.151
      ice skates V00.218
        collision (with) V09.9
          animal being ridden or animal
            drawn vehicle V06.99
            nontraffic V06.09
            traffic V06.19
          bus or heavy transport V04.99
            nontraffic V04.09
            traffic V04.19
          car V03.99
            nontraffic V03.09
            traffic V03.19
          pedal cycle V01.99
            nontraffic V01.09
            traffic V01.19
          pick-up truck or van V03.99
            nontraffic V03.09
            traffic V03.19

Accident *(Continued)*
  transport *(Continued)*
    pedestrian *(Continued)*
      conveyance *(Continued)*
        ice skates *(Continued)*
          collision *(Continued)*
            railway (train) (vehicle)
              V05.99
              nontraffic V05.09
              traffic V05.19
            stationary object V00.212
            streetcar V06.99
              nontraffic V06.09
              traffic V06.19
            two- or three-wheeled motor
              vehicle V02.99
              nontraffic V02.09
              traffic V02.19
            vehicle V09.9
              animal-drawn V06.99
                nontraffic V06.09
                traffic V06.19
              motor
                nontraffic V09.00
                traffic V09.20
        fall V00.211
        nontraffic V09.1
          involving motor vehicle NEC
            V09.00
        traffic V09.3
          involving motor vehicle NEC
            V09.20
        motorized mobility scooter
          V00.838
          collision with stationary object
            V00.832
          fall from V00.831
        nontraffic V09.1
          involving motor vehicle
            V09.00
          military V09.01
          specified type NEC V09.09
        roller skates (non in-line) V00.128
          collision (with) V09.9
            animal being ridden or animal
              drawn vehicle V06.91
              nontraffic V06.01
              traffic V06.11
            bus or heavy transport
              V04.91
              nontraffic V04.01
              traffic V04.11
            car V03.91
              nontraffic V03.01
              traffic V03.11
            pedal cycle V01.91
              nontraffic V01.01
              traffic V01.11
            pick-up truck or van V03.91
              nontraffic V03.01
              traffic V03.11
            railway (train) (vehicle)
              V05.91
              nontraffic V05.01
              traffic V05.11
            stationary object V00.122
            streetcar V06.91
              nontraffic V06.01
              traffic V06.11
            two- or three-wheeled motor
              vehicle V02.91
              nontraffic V02.01
              traffic V02.11
            vehicle V09.9
              animal-drawn V06.91
                nontraffic V06.01
                traffic V06.11
              motor
                nontraffic V09.00
                traffic V09.20
        fall V00.121

Accident *(Continued)*
  transport *(Continued)*
    pedestrian *(Continued)*
      conveyance *(Continued)*
        roller skates *(Continued)*
          in-line V00.118
            collision —*see also* Accident,
              transport, pedestrian,
              conveyance occupant, roller
              skates, collision
              with stationary object
                V00.112
            fall V00.111
            nontraffic V09.1
              involving motor vehicle NEC
                V09.00
            traffic V09.3
              involving motor vehicle NEC
                V09.20
        rolling shoes V00.158
          colliding with stationary object
            V00.152
          fall V00.151
        rolling type NEC V00.188
          collision (with) V09.9
            animal being ridden or animal
              drawn vehicle V06.99
              nontraffic V06.09
              traffic V06.19
            bus or heavy transport V04.99
              nontraffic V04.09
              traffic V04.19
            car V03.99
              nontraffic V03.09
              traffic V03.19
            pedal cycle V01.99
              nontraffic V01.09
              traffic V01.19
            pick-up truck or van V03.99
              nontraffic V03.09
              traffic V03.19
            railway (train) (vehicle)
              V05.99
              nontraffic V05.09
              traffic V05.19
            stationary object V00.182
            streetcar V06.99
              nontraffic V06.09
              traffic V06.19
            two- or three-wheeled motor
              vehicle V02.99
              nontraffic V02.09
              traffic V02.19
            vehicle V09.9
              animal-drawn V06.99
                nontraffic V06.09
                traffic V06.19
              motor
                nontraffic V09.00
                traffic V09.20
        fall V00.181
        in-line roller skate —*see* Accident,
          transport, pedestrian,
          conveyance, roller skate,
          in-line
        nontraffic V09.1
          involving motor vehicle NEC
            V09.00
        roller skate —*see* Accident,
          transport, pedestrian,
          conveyance, roller skate
        scooter (non-motorized) —
          see Accident, transport,
          pedestrian, conveyance,
          scooter
        skateboard —*see* Accident,
          transport, pedestrian,
          conveyance, skateboard
        traffic V09.3
          involving motor vehicle NEC
            V09.20

    ▶ New   ➡ Revised   ~~deleted~~ Deleted   ● Use Additional Character(s)

Accident *(Continued)*
  transport *(Continued)*
    pedestrian *(Continued)*
      conveyance *(Continued)*
        scooter (non-motorized) V00.148
          collision (with) V09.9
            animal being ridden or animal
                drawn vehicle V06.99
              nontraffic V06.09
              traffic V06.19
            bus or heavy transport
                V04.99
              nontraffic V04.09
              traffic V04.19
            car V03.99
              nontraffic V03.09
              traffic V03.19
            pedal cycle V01.99
              nontraffic V01.09
              traffic V01.19
            pick-up truck or van V03.99
              nontraffic V03.09
              traffic V03.19
            railway (train) (vehicle)
                V05.99
              nontraffic V05.09
              traffic V05.19
            stationary object V00.142
            streetcar V06.99
              nontraffic V06.09
              traffic V06.19
            two- or three-wheeled motor
                vehicle V02.99
              nontraffic V02.09
              traffic V02.19
            vehicle V09.9
              animal-drawn V06.99
                nontraffic V06.09
                traffic V06.19
              motor
                nontraffic V09.00
                traffic V09.20
          fall V00.141
          nontraffic V09.1
            involving motor vehicle NEC
                V09.00
          traffic V09.3
            involving motor vehicle NEC
                V09.20
        skate board V00.138
          collision (with) V09.9
            animal being ridden or
                animal drawn vehicle
                V06.92
              nontraffic V06.02
              traffic V06.12
            bus or heavy transport
                V04.92
              nontraffic V04.02
              traffic V04.12
            car V03.92
              nontraffic V03.02
              traffic V03.12
            pedal cycle V01.92
              nontraffic V01.02
              traffic V01.12
            pick-up truck or van V03.92
              nontraffic V03.02
              traffic V03.12
            railway (train) (vehicle)
                V05.92
              nontraffic V05.02
              traffic V05.12
            stationary object V00.132
            streetcar V06.92
              nontraffic V06.02
              traffic V06.12
            two- or three-wheeled motor
                vehicle V02.92
              nontraffic V02.02
              traffic V02.12

Accident *(Continued)*
  transport *(Continued)*
    pedestrian *(Continued)*
      conveyance *(Continued)*
        skate board *(Continued)*
          collision *(Continued)*
            vehicle V09.9
              animal-drawn V06.92
                nontraffic V06.02
                traffic V06.12
              motor
                nontraffic V09.00
                traffic V09.20
          fall V00.131
          nontraffic V09.1
            involving motor vehicle NEC
                V09.00
          traffic V09.3
            involving motor vehicle NEC
                V09.20
        skis (snow) V00.328
          collision (with) V09.9
            animal being ridden or animal
                drawn vehicle V06.99
              nontraffic V06.09
              traffic V06.19
            bus or heavy transport V04.99
              nontraffic V04.09
              traffic V04.19
            car V03.99
              nontraffic V03.09
              traffic V03.19
            pedal cycle V01.99
              nontraffic V01.09
              traffic V01.19
            pick-up truck or van V03.99
              nontraffic V03.09
              traffic V03.19
            railway (train) (vehicle) V05.99
              nontraffic V05.09
              traffic V05.19
            stationary object V00.322
            streetcar V06.99
              nontraffic V06.09
              traffic V06.19
            two- or three-wheeled motor
                vehicle V02.99
              nontraffic V02.09
              traffic V02.19
            vehicle V09.9
              animal-drawn V06.99
                nontraffic V06.09
                traffic V06.19
              motor
                nontraffic V09.00
                traffic V09.20
          fall V00.321
          nontraffic V09.1
            involving motor vehicle NEC
                V09.00
          traffic V09.3
            involving motor vehicle NEC
                V09.20
        sled V00.228
          collision (with) V09.9
            animal being ridden or animal
                drawn vehicle V06.99
              nontraffic V06.09
              traffic V06.19
            bus or heavy transport V04.99
              nontraffic V04.09
              traffic V04.19
            car V03.99
              nontraffic V03.09
              traffic V03.19
            pedal cycle V01.99
              nontraffic V01.09
              traffic V01.19
            pick-up truck or van V03.99
              nontraffic V03.09
              traffic V03.19

Accident *(Continued)*
  transport *(Continued)*
    pedestrian *(Continued)*
      conveyance *(Continued)*
        sled *(Continued)*
          collision *(Continued)*
            railway (train) (vehicle)
                V05.99
              nontraffic V05.09
              traffic V05.19
            stationary object V00.222
            streetcar V06.99
              nontraffic V06.09
              traffic V06.19
            two- or three-wheeled motor
                vehicle V02.99
              nontraffic V02.09
              traffic V02.19
            vehicle V09.9
              animal-drawn V06.99
                nontraffic V06.09
                traffic V06.19
              motor
                nontraffic V09.00
                traffic V09.20
          fall V00.221
          nontraffic V09.1
            involving motor vehicle NEC
                V09.00
          traffic V09.3
            involving motor vehicle NEC
                V09.20
        snow board V00.318
          collision (with) V09.9
            animal being ridden or animal
                drawn vehicle V06.99
              nontraffic V06.09
              traffic V06.19
            bus or heavy transport V04.99
              nontraffic V04.09
              traffic V04.19
            car V03.99
              nontraffic V03.09
              traffic V03.19
            pedal cycle V01.99
              nontraffic V01.09
              traffic V01.19
            pick-up truck or van V03.99
              nontraffic V03.09
              traffic V03.19
            railway (train) (vehicle) V05.99
              nontraffic V05.09
              traffic V05.19
            stationary object V00.312
            streetcar V06.99
              nontraffic V06.09
              traffic V06.19
            two- or three-wheeled motor
                vehicle V02.99
              nontraffic V02.09
              traffic V02.19
            vehicle V09.9
              animal-drawn V06.99
                nontraffic V06.09
                traffic V06.19
              motor
                nontraffic V09.00
                traffic V09.20
          fall V00.311
          nontraffic V09.1
            involving motor vehicle NEC
                V09.00
          traffic V09.3
            involving motor vehicle NEC
                V09.20
        specified type NEC V00.898
          collision (with) V09.9
            animal being ridden or animal
                drawn vehicle V06.99
              nontraffic V06.09
              traffic V06.19

Accident (Continued)
 transport (Continued)
  pedestrian (Continued)
   conveyance (Continued)
    specified type NEC (Continued)
     collision (Continued)
      bus or heavy transport
       V04.99
       nontraffic V04.09
       traffic V04.19
      car V03.99
       nontraffic V03.09
       traffic V03.19
      pedal cycle V01.99
       nontraffic V01.09
       traffic V01.19
      pick-up truck or van V03.99
       nontraffic V03.09
       traffic V03.19
      railway (train) (vehicle)
       V05.99
       nontraffic V05.09
       traffic V05.19
      stationary object V00.892
      streetcar V06.99
       nontraffic V06.09
       traffic V06.19
      two- or three-wheeled motor
       vehicle V02.99
       nontraffic V02.09
       traffic V02.19
      vehicle V09.9
       animal-drawn V06.99
        nontraffic V06.09
        traffic V06.19
       motor
        nontraffic V09.00
        traffic V09.20
     fall V00.891
     nontraffic V09.1
      involving motor vehicle NEC
       V09.00
     traffic V09.3
      involving motor vehicle NEC
       V09.20
    traffic V09.3
     involving motor vehicle V09.20
      military V09.21
      specified type NEC V09.29
   wheelchair (powered) V00.818
    collision (with) V09.9
     animal being ridden or
      animal drawn vehicle
       V06.99
       nontraffic V06.09
       traffic V06.19
     bus or heavy transport
      V04.99
      nontraffic V04.09
      traffic V04.19
     car V03.99
      nontraffic V03.09
      traffic V03.19
     pedal cycle V01.99
      nontraffic V01.09
      traffic V01.19
     pick-up truck or van V03.99
      nontraffic V03.09
      traffic V03.19
     railway (train) (vehicle)
      V05.99
      nontraffic V05.09
      traffic V05.19
     stationary object V00.812
     streetcar V06.99
      nontraffic V06.09
      traffic V06.19
     two- or three-wheeled motor
      vehicle V02.99
      nontraffic V02.09
      traffic V02.19

Accident (Continued)
 transport (Continued)
  pedestrian (Continued)
   conveyance (Continued)
    wheelchair (Continued)
     collision (Continued)
      vehicle V09.9
       animal-drawn V06.99
        nontraffic V06.09
        traffic V06.19
       motor
        nontraffic V09.00
        traffic V09.20
     fall V00.811
     nontraffic V09.1
      involving motor vehicle NEC
       V09.00
     traffic V09.3
      involving motor vehicle NEC
       V09.20
    wheeled shoe V00.158
     colliding with stationary object
      V00.152
     fall V00.151
  on foot —see also Accident, pedestrian
   collision (with)
    animal being ridden or animal
     drawn vehicle V06.90
     nontraffic V06.00
     traffic V06.10
    bus or heavy transport V04.90
     nontraffic V04.00
     traffic V04.10
    car V03.90
     nontraffic V03.00
     traffic V03.10
    pedal cycle V01.90
     nontraffic V01.00
     traffic V01.10
    pick-up truck or van V03.90
     nontraffic V03.00
     traffic V03.10
    railway (train) (vehicle) V05.90
     nontraffic V05.00
     traffic V05.10
    streetcar V06.90
     nontraffic V06.00
     traffic V06.10
    two- or three-wheeled motor
     vehicle V02.90
     nontraffic V02.00
     traffic V02.10
    vehicle V09.9
     animal-drawn V06.90
      nontraffic V06.00
      traffic V06.10
     motor
      nontraffic V09.00
      traffic V09.20
    nontraffic V09.1
     involving motor vehicle V09.00
      military V09.01
      specified type NEC V09.09
    traffic V09.3
     involving motor vehicle V09.20
      military V09.21
      specified type NEC V09.29
  person NEC (unknown way or
   transportation) V99
   collision (between)
    bus (with)
     heavy transport vehicle (traffic)
      V87.5
     nontraffic V88.5
    car (with)
     nontraffic V88.5
     bus (traffic) V87.3
      nontraffic V88.3
     heavy transport vehicle (traffic)
      V87.4
      nontraffic V88.4

Accident (Continued)
 transport (Continued)
  person NEC (Continued)
   collision (Continued)
    car (Continued)
     pick-up truck or van (traffic) V87.2
      nontraffic V88.2
     train or railway vehicle (traffic)
      V87.6
      nontraffic V88.6
     two- or three-wheeled motor
      vehicle (traffic) V87.0
      nontraffic V88.0
     motor vehicle (traffic) NEC V87.7
      nontraffic V88.7
     two- or three-wheeled vehicle (with)
      (traffic)
      motor vehicle NEC V87.1
      nontraffic V88.1
    nonmotor vehicle (collision)
     (noncollision) (traffic) V87.9
     nontraffic V88.9
   pickup truck occupant V59.9
    collision (with)
     animal (traffic) V50.9
      being ridden (traffic) V56.9
       nontraffic V56.3
       while boarding or alighting V56.4
      nontraffic V50.3
      while boarding or alighting V50.4
     animal-drawn vehicle (traffic) V56.9
      nontraffic V56.3
      while boarding or alighting V56.4
     bus (traffic) V54.9
      nontraffic V54.3
      while boarding or alighting V54.4
     car (traffic) V53.9
      nontraffic V53.3
      while boarding or alighting V53.4
     motor vehicle NOS (traffic) V59.60
      nontraffic V59.20
      specified type NEC (traffic) V59.69
       nontraffic V59.29
     pedal cycle (traffic) V51.9
      nontraffic V51.3
      while boarding or alighting V51.4
     pickup truck (traffic) V53.9
      nontraffic V53.3
      while boarding or alighting V53.4
     railway vehicle (traffic) V55.9
      nontraffic V55.3
      while boarding or alighting V55.4
     specified vehicle NEC (traffic) V56.9
      nontraffic V56.3
      while boarding or alighting V56.4
     stationary object (traffic) V57.9
      nontraffic V57.3
      while boarding or alighting V57.4
     streetcar (traffic) V56.9
      nontraffic V56.3
      while boarding or alighting V56.4
     three wheeled motor vehicle (traffic)
      V52.9
      nontraffic V52.3
      while boarding or alighting V52.4
     truck (traffic) V54.9
      nontraffic V54.3
      while boarding or alighting V54.4
     two wheeled motor vehicle (traffic)
      V52.9
      nontraffic V52.3
      while boarding or alighting V52.4
     van (traffic) V53.9
      nontraffic V53.3
      while boarding or alighting V53.4
    driver
     collision (with)
      animal (traffic) V50.5
       being ridden (traffic) V56.5
        nontraffic V56.0
       nontraffic V50.0

▶ New   ➡ Revised   ~~deleted~~ Deleted   ● Use Additional Character(s)

Accident (Continued)
  transport (Continued)
    pickup truck occupant (Continued)
      driver (Continued)
        collision (Continued)
          animal-drawn vehicle (traffic)
            V56.5
            nontraffic V56.0
          bus (traffic) V54.5
            nontraffic V54.0
          car (traffic) V53.5
            nontraffic V53.0
          motor vehicle NOS (traffic) V59.40
            nontraffic V59.00
            specified type NEC (traffic)
              V59.49
              nontraffic V59.09
          pedal cycle (traffic) V51.5
            nontraffic V51.0
          pickup truck (traffic) V53.5
            nontraffic V53.0
          railway vehicle (traffic) V55.5
            nontraffic V55.0
          specified vehicle NEC (traffic) V56.5
            nontraffic V56.0
          stationary object (traffic) V57.5
            nontraffic V57.0
          streetcar (traffic) V56.5
            nontraffic V56.0
          three wheeled motor vehicle
            (traffic) V52.5
            nontraffic V52.0
          truck (traffic) V54.5
            nontraffic V54.0
          two wheeled motor vehicle (traffic)
            V52.5
            nontraffic V52.0
          van (traffic) V53.5
            nontraffic V53.0
        noncollision accident (traffic) V58.5
         nontraffic V58.0
      hanger-on
        collision (with)
          animal (traffic) V50.7
            being ridden (traffic) V56.7
              nontraffic V56.2
            nontraffic V50.2
          animal-drawn vehicle (traffic) V56.7
            nontraffic V56.2
          bus (traffic) V54.7
            nontraffic V54.2
          car (traffic) V53.7
            nontraffic V53.2
          pedal cycle (traffic) V51.7
            nontraffic V51.2
          pickup truck (traffic) V53.7
            nontraffic V53.2
          railway vehicle (traffic) V55.7
            nontraffic V55.2
          specified vehicle NEC (traffic) V56.7
            nontraffic V56.2
          stationary object (traffic) V57.7
            nontraffic V57.2
          streetcar (traffic) V56.7
            nontraffic V56.2
          three wheeled motor vehicle
            (traffic) V52.7
            nontraffic V52.2
          truck (traffic) V54.7
            nontraffic V54.2
          two wheeled motor vehicle (traffic)
            V52.7
            nontraffic V52.2
          van (traffic) V53.7
            nontraffic V53.2
        noncollision accident (traffic) V58.7
         nontraffic V58.2
      noncollision accident (traffic) V58.9
        nontraffic V58.3
        while boarding or alighting V58.4
      nontraffic V59.3

Accident (Continued)
  transport (Continued)
    pickup truck occupant (Continued)
      passenger
        collision (with)
          animal (traffic) V50.6
            being ridden (traffic) V56.6
              nontraffic V56.1
            nontraffic V50.1
          animal-drawn vehicle (traffic)
            V56.6
            nontraffic V56.1
          bus (traffic) V54.6
            nontraffic V54.1
          car (traffic) V53.6
            nontraffic V53.1
          motor vehicle NOS (traffic) V59.50
            nontraffic V59.10
            specified type NEC (traffic)
              V59.59
              nontraffic V59.19
          pedal cycle (traffic) V51.6
            nontraffic V51.1
          pickup truck (traffic) V53.6
            nontraffic V53.1
          railway vehicle (traffic) V55.6
            nontraffic V55.1
          specified vehicle NEC (traffic) V56.6
            nontraffic V56.1
          stationary object (traffic) V57.6
            nontraffic V57.1
          streetcar (traffic) V56.6
            nontraffic V56.1
          three wheeled motor vehicle
            (traffic) V52.6
            nontraffic V52.1
          truck (traffic) V54.6
            nontraffic V54.1
          two wheeled motor vehicle (traffic)
            V52.6
            nontraffic V52.1
          van (traffic) V53.6
            nontraffic V53.1
        noncollision accident (traffic) V58.6
         nontraffic V58.1
      specified type NEC V59.88
        military vehicle V59.81
    quarry truck —see Accident, transport,
      industrial vehicle occupant
    race car —see Accident, transport, motor
      vehicle NEC occupant
    railway vehicle occupant V81.9
      collision (with) V81.3
        motor vehicle (non-military) (traffic)
          V81.1
          military V81.83
          nontraffic V81.0
        rolling stock V81.2
        specified object NEC V81.3
      during derailment V81.7
        with antecedent collision —see
          Accident, transport, railway
          vehicle occupant, collision
      explosion V81.81
      fall (in railway vehicle) V81.5
        during derailment V81.7
          with antecedent collision —see
            Accident, transport, railway
            vehicle occupant, collision
        from railway vehicle V81.6
          during derailment V81.7
            with antecedent collision —see
              Accident, transport,
              railway vehicle occupant,
              collision
        while boarding or alighting V81.4
      fire V81.81
      object falling onto train V81.82
      specified type NEC V81.89
      while boarding or alighting V81.4
    ski lift V98.3

Accident (Continued)
  transport (Continued)
    snowmobile occupant (nontraffic)
      V86.92
      driver V86.52
      hanger-on V86.72
      passenger V86.62
      traffic V86.32
        driver V86.02
        hanger-on V86.22
        passenger V86.12
      while boarding or alighting V86.42
    specified NEC V98.8
    sport utility vehicle occupant —see also
      Accident, transport, pickup truck
      occupant
    streetcar occupant V82.9
      collision (with) V82.3
        motor vehicle (traffic) V82.1
          nontraffic V82.0
        rolling stock V82.2
      during derailment V82.7
        with antecedent collision —see
          Accident, transport, streetcar
          occupant, collision
      fall (in streetcar) V82.5
        during derailment V82.7
          with antecedent collision —see
            Accident, transport, streetcar
            occupant, collision
        from streetcar V82.6
          during derailment V82.7
            with antecedent collision —see
              Accident, transport, streetcar
              occupant, collision
          while boarding or alighting
            V82.4
        while boarding or alighting V82.4
      specified type NEC V82.8
      while boarding or alighting V82.4
    three-wheeled motor vehicle occupant
      V39.9
      collision (with)
        animal (traffic) V30.9
          being ridden (traffic) V36.9
            nontraffic V36.3
            while boarding or alighting
              V36.4
          nontraffic V30.3
            while boarding or alighting
             V30.4
        animal-drawn vehicle (traffic)
          V36.9
          nontraffic V36.3
            while boarding or alighting
             V36.4
        bus (traffic) V34.9
          nontraffic V34.3
            while boarding or alighting
             V34.4
        car (traffic) V33.9
          nontraffic V33.3
            while boarding or alighting
             V33.4
        motor vehicle NOS (traffic) V39.60
          nontraffic V39.20
          specified type NEC (traffic)
            V39.69
            nontraffic V39.29
        pedal cycle (traffic) V31.9
          nontraffic V31.3
            while boarding or alighting
             V31.4
        pickup truck (traffic) V33.9
          nontraffic V33.3
            while boarding or alighting
             V33.4
        railway vehicle (traffic) V35.9
          nontraffic V35.3
            while boarding or alighting
             V35.4

A

Accident *(Continued)*
 transport *(Continued)*
  three-wheeled motor vehicle occupant
    (Continued)
   collision *(Continued)*
    specified vehicle NEC (traffic) V36.9
     nontraffic V36.3
      while boarding or alighting V36.4
    stationary object (traffic) V37.9
     nontraffic V37.3
      while boarding or alighting V37.4
    streetcar (traffic) V36.9
     nontraffic V36.3
      while boarding or alighting V36.4
    three wheeled motor vehicle (traffic)
      V32.9
     nontraffic V32.3
      while boarding or alighting V32.4
    truck (traffic) V34.9
     nontraffic V34.3
      while boarding or alighting V34.4
    two wheeled motor vehicle (traffic)
      V32.9
     nontraffic V32.3
      while boarding or alighting V32.4
    van (traffic) V33.9
     nontraffic V33.3
      while boarding or alighting V33.4
   driver
    collision (with)
     animal (traffic) V30.5
      being ridden (traffic) V36.5
       nontraffic V36.0
      nontraffic V30.0
     animal-drawn vehicle (traffic) V36.5
      nontraffic V36.0
     bus (traffic) V34.5
      nontraffic V34.0
     car (traffic) V33.5
      nontraffic V33.0
     motor vehicle NOS (traffic) V39.40
      nontraffic V39.00
       specified type NEC (traffic)
         V39.49
        nontraffic V39.09
     pedal cycle (traffic) V31.5
      nontraffic V31.0
     pickup truck (traffic) V33.5
      nontraffic V33.0
     railway vehicle (traffic) V35.5
      nontraffic V35.0
     specified vehicle NEC (traffic) V36.5
      nontraffic V36.0
     stationary object (traffic) V37.5
      nontraffic V37.0
     streetcar (traffic) V36.5
      nontraffic V36.0
     three wheeled motor vehicle
       (traffic) V32.5
      nontraffic V32.0
     truck (traffic) V34.5
      nontraffic V34.0
     two wheeled motor vehicle (traffic)
       V32.5
      nontraffic V32.0
     van (traffic) V33.5
      nontraffic V33.0
    noncollision accident (traffic) V38.5
     nontraffic V38.0
   hanger-on
    collision (with)
     animal (traffic) V30.7
      being ridden (traffic) V36.7
       nontraffic V36.2
      nontraffic V30.2
     animal-drawn vehicle (traffic) V36.7
      nontraffic V36.2
     bus (traffic) V34.7
      nontraffic V34.2
     car (traffic) V33.7
      nontraffic V33.2

Accident *(Continued)*
 transport *(Continued)*
  three-wheeled motor vehicle occupant
    (Continued)
   hanger-on *(Continued)*
    collision *(Continued)*
     pedal cycle (traffic) V31.7
      nontraffic V31.2
     pickup truck (traffic) V33.7
      nontraffic V33.2
     railway vehicle (traffic) V35.7
      nontraffic V35.2
     specified vehicle NEC (traffic) V36.7
      nontraffic V36.2
     stationary object (traffic) V37.7
      nontraffic V37.2
     streetcar (traffic) V36.7
      nontraffic V36.2
     three wheeled motor vehicle
       (traffic) V32.7
      nontraffic V32.2
     truck (traffic) V34.7
      nontraffic V34.2
     two wheeled motor vehicle (traffic)
       V32.7
      nontraffic V32.2
     van (traffic) V33.7
      nontraffic V33.2
    noncollision accident (traffic) V38.7
     nontraffic V38.2
   noncollision accident (traffic) V38.9
    nontraffic V38.3
    while boarding or alighting V38.4
   nontraffic V39.3
   passenger
    collision (with)
     animal (traffic) V30.6
      being ridden (traffic) V36.6
       nontraffic V36.1
      nontraffic V30.1
     animal-drawn vehicle (traffic) V36.6
      nontraffic V36.1
     bus (traffic) V34.6
      nontraffic V34.1
     car (traffic) V33.6
      nontraffic V33.1
     motor vehicle NOS (traffic) V39.50
      nontraffic V39.10
       specified type NEC (traffic)
         V39.59
        nontraffic V39.19
     pedal cycle (traffic) V31.6
      nontraffic V31.1
     pickup truck (traffic) V33.6
      nontraffic V33.1
     railway vehicle (traffic) V35.6
      nontraffic V35.1
     specified vehicle NEC (traffic)
       V36.6
      nontraffic V36.1
     stationary object (traffic) V37.6
      nontraffic V37.1
     streetcar (traffic) V36.6
      nontraffic V36.1
     three wheeled motor vehicle
       (traffic) V32.6
      nontraffic V32.1
     truck (traffic) V34.6
      nontraffic V34.1
     two wheeled motor vehicle (traffic)
       V32.6
      nontraffic V32.1
     van (traffic) V33.6
      nontraffic V33.1
    noncollision accident (traffic) V38.6
     nontraffic V38.1
   specified type NEC V39.89
   military vehicle V39.81
  tractor (farm) (and trailer) —*see* Accident,
    transport, agricultural vehicle
    occupant

Accident *(Continued)*
 transport *(Continued)*
  tram —*see* Accident, transport, streetcar
   in mine or quarry —*see* Accident,
     transport, industrial vehicle
     occupant
  trolley —*see* Accident, transport, streetcar
   in mine or quarry —*see* Accident,
     transport, industrial vehicle
     occupant
  truck (heavy) occupant V69.9
   collision (with)
    animal (traffic) V60.9
     being ridden (traffic) V66.9
      nontraffic V66.3
       while boarding or alighting V66.4
     nontraffic V60.3
      while boarding or alighting V60.4
    animal-drawn vehicle (traffic) V66.9
     nontraffic V66.3
      while boarding or alighting V66.4
    bus (traffic) V64.9
     nontraffic V64.3
      while boarding or alighting V64.4
    car (traffic) V63.9
     nontraffic V63.3
      while boarding or alighting V63.4
    motor vehicle NOS (traffic) V69.60
     nontraffic V69.20
      specified type NEC (traffic) V69.69
       nontraffic V69.29
    pedal cycle (traffic) V61.9
     nontraffic V61.3
      while boarding or alighting V61.4
    pickup truck (traffic) V63.9
     nontraffic V63.3
      while boarding or alighting V63.4
    railway vehicle (traffic) V65.9
     nontraffic V65.3
      while boarding or alighting V65.4
    specified vehicle NEC (traffic) V66.9
     nontraffic V66.3
      while boarding or alighting V66.4
    stationary object (traffic) V67.9
     nontraffic V67.3
      while boarding or alighting V67.4
    streetcar (traffic) V66.9
     nontraffic V66.3
      while boarding or alighting V66.4
    three wheeled motor vehicle (traffic)
      V62.9
     nontraffic V62.3
      while boarding or alighting V62.4
    truck (traffic) V64.9
     nontraffic V64.3
      while boarding or alighting V64.4
    two wheeled motor vehicle (traffic)
      V62.9
     nontraffic V62.3
      while boarding or alighting V62.4
    van (traffic) V63.9
     nontraffic V63.3
      while boarding or alighting V63.4
   driver
    collision (with)
     animal (traffic) V60.5
      being ridden (traffic) V66.5
       nontraffic V66.0
      nontraffic V60.0
     animal-drawn vehicle (traffic)
       V66.5
      nontraffic V66.0
     bus (traffic) V64.5
      nontraffic V64.0
     car (traffic) V63.5
      nontraffic V63.0
     motor vehicle NOS (traffic) V69.40
      nontraffic V69.00
       specified type NEC (traffic)
         V69.49
        nontraffic V69.09

▶ New   ⇒ Revised   ~~deleted~~ Deleted   ● Use Additional Character(s)

Accident *(Continued)*
  transport *(Continued)*
    truck occupant *(Continued)*
      driver *(Continued)*
        collision *(Continued)*
          pedal cycle (traffic) V61.5
            nontraffic V61.0
          pickup truck (traffic) V63.5
            nontraffic V63.0
          railway vehicle (traffic) V65.5
            nontraffic V65.0
          specified vehicle NEC (traffic) V66.5
            nontraffic V66.0
          stationary object (traffic) V67.5
            nontraffic V67.0
          streetcar (traffic) V66.5
            nontraffic V66.0
          three wheeled motor vehicle
            (traffic) V62.5
            nontraffic V62.0
          truck (traffic) V64.5
            nontraffic V64.0
          two wheeled motor vehicle (traffic)
            V62.5
            nontraffic V62.0
          van (traffic) V63.5
            nontraffic V63.0
        noncollision accident (traffic) V68.5
          nontraffic V68.0
      dump —*see* Accident, transport,
        construction vehicle occupant
      hanger-on
        collision (with)
          animal (traffic) V60.7
            being ridden (traffic) V66.7
              nontraffic V66.2
            nontraffic V60.2
          animal-drawn vehicle (traffic) V66.7
            nontraffic V66.2
          bus (traffic) V64.7
            nontraffic V64.2
          car (traffic) V63.7
            nontraffic V63.2
          pedal cycle (traffic) V61.7
            nontraffic V61.2
          pickup truck (traffic) V63.7
            nontraffic V63.2
          railway vehicle (traffic) V65.7
            nontraffic V65.2
          specified vehicle NEC (traffic) V66.7
            nontraffic V66.2
          stationary object (traffic) V67.7
            nontraffic V67.2
          streetcar (traffic) V66.7
            nontraffic V66.2
          three wheeled motor vehicle
            (traffic) V62.7
            nontraffic V62.2
          truck (traffic) V64.7
            nontraffic V64.2
          two wheeled motor vehicle (traffic)
            V62.7
            nontraffic V62.2
          van (traffic) V63.7
            nontraffic V63.2
        noncollision accident (traffic) V68.7
          nontraffic V68.2
      noncollision accident (traffic) V68.9
        nontraffic V68.3
        while boarding or alighting V68.4
      nontraffic V69.3
      passenger
        collision (with)
          animal (traffic) V60.6
            being ridden (traffic) V66.6
              nontraffic V66.1
            nontraffic V60.1
          animal-drawn vehicle (traffic) V66.6
            nontraffic V66.1
          bus (traffic) V64.6
            nontraffic V64.1

Accident *(Continued)*
  transport *(Continued)*
    truck occupant *(Continued)*
      passenger *(Continued)*
        collision *(Continued)*
          car (traffic) V63.6
            nontraffic V63.1
          motor vehicle NOS (traffic) V69.50
            nontraffic V69.10
            specified type NEC (traffic)
              V69.59
              nontraffic V69.19
          pedal cycle (traffic) V61.6
            nontraffic V61.1
          pickup truck (traffic) V63.6
            nontraffic V63.1
          railway vehicle (traffic) V65.6
            nontraffic V65.1
          specified vehicle NEC (traffic)
            V66.6
            nontraffic V66.1
          stationary object (traffic) V67.6
            nontraffic V67.1
          streetcar (traffic) V66.6
            nontraffic V66.1
          three wheeled motor vehicle
            (traffic) V62.6
            nontraffic V62.1
          truck (traffic) V64.6
            nontraffic V64.1
          two wheeled motor vehicle (traffic)
            V62.6
            nontraffic V62.1
          van (traffic) V63.6
            nontraffic V63.1
        noncollision accident (traffic) V68.6
          nontraffic V68.1
      pickup —*see* Accident, transport, pickup
        truck occupant
      specified type NEC V69.88
        military vehicle V69.81
    van occupant V59.9
      collision (with)
        animal (traffic) V50.9
          being ridden (traffic) V56.9
            nontraffic V56.3
            while boarding or alighting
              V56.4
          nontraffic V50.3
          while boarding or alighting V50.4
        animal-drawn vehicle (traffic) V56.9
          nontraffic V56.3
          while boarding or alighting V56.4
        bus (traffic) V54.9
          nontraffic V54.3
          while boarding or alighting V54.4
        car (traffic) V53.9
          nontraffic V53.3
          while boarding or alighting V53.4
        motor vehicle NOS (traffic) V59.60
          nontraffic V59.20
          specified type NEC (traffic) V59.69
            nontraffic V59.29
        pedal cycle (traffic) V51.9
          nontraffic V51.3
          while boarding or alighting V51.4
        pickup truck (traffic) V53.9
          nontraffic V53.3
          while boarding or alighting V53.4
        railway vehicle (traffic) V55.9
          nontraffic V55.3
          while boarding or alighting V55.4
        specified vehicle NEC (traffic) V56.9
          nontraffic V56.3
          while boarding or alighting V56.4
        stationary object (traffic) V57.9
          nontraffic V57.3
          while boarding or alighting V57.4
        streetcar (traffic) V56.9
          nontraffic V56.3
          while boarding or alighting V56.4

Accident *(Continued)*
  transport *(Continued)*
    van occupant *(Continued)*
      collision *(Continued)*
        three wheeled motor vehicle (traffic)
          V52.9
          nontraffic V52.3
          while boarding or alighting V52.4
        truck (traffic) V54.9
          nontraffic V54.3
          while boarding or alighting V54.4
        two wheeled motor vehicle (traffic)
          V52.9
          nontraffic V52.3
          while boarding or alighting V52.4
        van (traffic) V53.9
          nontraffic V53.3
          while boarding or alighting V53.4
      driver
        collision (with)
          animal (traffic) V50.5
            being ridden (traffic) V56.5
              nontraffic V56.0
            nontraffic V50.0
          animal-drawn vehicle (traffic) V56.5
            nontraffic V56.0
          bus (traffic) V54.5
            nontraffic V54.0
          car (traffic) V53.5
            nontraffic V53.0
          motor vehicle NOS (traffic) V59.40
            nontraffic V59.00
            specified type NEC (traffic)
              V59.49
              nontraffic V59.09
          pedal cycle (traffic) V51.5
            nontraffic V51.0
          pickup truck (traffic) V53.5
            nontraffic V53.0
          railway vehicle (traffic) V55.5
            nontraffic V55.0
          specified vehicle NEC (traffic) V56.5
            nontraffic V56.0
          stationary object (traffic) V57.5
            nontraffic V57.0
          streetcar (traffic) V56.5
            nontraffic V56.0
          three wheeled motor vehicle
            (traffic) V52.5
            nontraffic V52.0
          truck (traffic) V54.5
            nontraffic V54.0
          two wheeled motor vehicle (traffic)
            V52.5
            nontraffic V52.0
          van (traffic) V53.5
            nontraffic V53.0
        noncollision accident (traffic) V58.5
          nontraffic V58.0
      hanger-on
        collision (with)
          animal (traffic) V50.7
            being ridden (traffic) V56.7
              nontraffic V56.2
            nontraffic V50.2
          animal-drawn vehicle (traffic) V56.7
            nontraffic V56.2
          bus (traffic) V54.7
            nontraffic V54.2
          car (traffic) V53.7
            nontraffic V53.2
          pedal cycle (traffic) V51.7
            nontraffic V51.2
          pickup truck (traffic) V53.7
            nontraffic V53.2
          railway vehicle (traffic) V55.7
            nontraffic V55.2
          specified vehicle NEC (traffic) V56.7
            nontraffic V56.2
          stationary object (traffic) V57.7
            nontraffic V57.2

Accident (Continued)
  transport (Continued)
    van occupant (Continued)
      hanger-on (Continued)
        collision (Continued)
          streetcar (traffic) V56.7
            nontraffic V56.2
          three wheeled motor vehicle
              (traffic) V52.7
            nontraffic V52.2
          truck (traffic) V54.7
            nontraffic V54.2
          two wheeled motor vehicle (traffic)
              V52.7
            nontraffic V52.2
          van (traffic) V53.7
            nontraffic V53.2
        noncollision accident (traffic) V58.7
          nontraffic V58.2
      noncollision accident (traffic) V58.9
        nontraffic V58.3
        while boarding or alighting V58.4
      nontraffic V59.3
      passenger
        collision (with)
          animal (traffic) V50.6
            being ridden (traffic) V56.6
              nontraffic V56.1
            nontraffic V50.1
          animal-drawn vehicle (traffic) V56.6
            nontraffic V56.1
          bus (traffic) V54.6
            nontraffic V54.1
          car (traffic) V53.6
            nontraffic V53.1
          motor vehicle NOS (traffic) V59.50
            nontraffic V59.10
            specified type NEC (traffic) V59.59
              nontraffic V59.19
          pedal cycle (traffic) V51.6
            nontraffic V51.1
          pickup truck (traffic) V53.6
            nontraffic V53.1
          railway vehicle (traffic) V55.6
            nontraffic V55.1
          specified vehicle NEC (traffic) V56.6
            nontraffic V56.1
          stationary object (traffic) V57.6
            nontraffic V57.1
          streetcar (traffic) V56.6
            nontraffic V56.1
          three wheeled motor vehicle
              (traffic) V52.6
            nontraffic V52.1
          truck (traffic) V54.6
            nontraffic V54.1
          two wheeled motor vehicle (traffic)
              V52.6
            nontraffic V52.1
          van (traffic) V53.6
            nontraffic V53.1
        noncollision accident (traffic) V58.6
          nontraffic V58.1
      specified type NEC V59.88
        military vehicle V59.81
    watercraft occupant —see Accident,
        watercraft
    vehicle NEC V89.9
    animal-drawn NEC —see Accident,
        transport, animal-drawn vehicle
        occupant
    special
      agricultural —see Accident, transport,
          agricultural vehicle occupant
      construction —see Accident, transport,
          construction vehicle occupant
      industrial —see Accident, transport,
          industrial vehicle occupant
      three-wheeled NEC (motorized) —see
          Accident, transport, three-wheeled
          motor vehicle occupant

Accident (Continued)
  watercraft V94.9
    causing
      drowning —see Drowning, due to,
          accident to, watercraft
      injury NEC V91.89
        crushed between craft and object
            V91.19
          powered craft V91.13
            ferry boat V91.11
            fishing boat V91.12
            jetskis V91.13
            liner V91.11
            merchant ship V91.10
            passenger ship V91.11
          unpowered craft V91.18
            canoe V91.15
            inflatable V91.16
            kayak V91.15
            sailboat V91.14
            surf-board V91.18
            windsurfer V91.18
        fall on board V91.29
          powered craft V91.23
            ferry boat V91.21
            fishing boat V91.22
            jetskis V91.23
            liner V91.21
            merchant ship V91.20
            passenger ship V91.21
          unpowered craft
            canoe V91.25
            inflatable V91.26
            kayak V91.25
            sailboat V91.24
        fire on board causing burn V91.09
          powered craft V91.03
            ferry boat V91.01
            fishing boat V91.02
            jetskis V91.03
            liner V91.01
            merchant ship V91.00
            passenger ship V91.01
          unpowered craft V91.08
            canoe V91.05
            inflatable V91.06
            kayak V91.05
            sailboat V91.04
            surf-board V91.08
            water skis V91.07
            windsurfer V91.08
        hit by falling object V91.39
          powered craft V91.33
            ferry boat V91.31
            fishing boat V91.32
            jetskis V91.33
            liner V91.31
            merchant ship V91.30
            passenger ship V91.31
          unpowered craft V91.38
            canoe V91.35
            inflatable V91.36
            kayak V91.35
            sailboat V91.34
            surf-board V91.38
            water skis V91.37
            windsurfer V91.38
        specified type NEC V91.89
          powered craft V91.83
            ferry boat V91.81
            fishing boat V91.82
            jetskis V91.83
            liner V91.81
            merchant ship V91.80
            passenger ship V91.81
          unpowered craft V91.88
            canoe V91.85
            inflatable V91.86
            kayak V91.85
            sailboat V91.84
            surf-board V91.88

Accident (Continued)
  watercraft (Continued)
    causing (Continued)
      injury NEC (Continued)
        specified type NEC (Continued)
          unpowered craft (Continued)
            water skis V91.87
            windsurfer V91.88
      due to, caused by cataclysm —see Forces of
          nature, by type
      military NEC V94.818
        with civilian watercraft V94.810
          civilian in water injured by V94.811
      nonpowered, struck by
        nonpowered vessel V94.22
        powered vessel V94.21
      specified type NEC V94.89
      striking swimmer
        powered V94.11
        unpowered V94.12
Acid throwing (assault) Y08.89
Activity (involving) (of victim at time of event)
    Y93.9
  aerobic and step exercise (class) Y93.A3
  alpine skiing Y93.23
  animal care NEC Y93.K9
  arts and handcrafts NEC Y93.D9
  athletics NEC Y93.79
  athletics played as a team or group NEC
      Y93.69
  athletics played individually NEC Y93.59
  baking Y93.G3
  ballet Y93.41
  barbells Y93.B3
  BASE (Building, Antenna, Span, Earth)
      jumping Y93.33
  baseball Y93.64
  basketball Y93.67
  bathing (personal) Y93.E1
  beach volleyball Y93.68
  bike riding Y93.55
  blackout game Y93.85
  boogie boarding Y93.18
  bowling Y93.54
  boxing Y93.71
  brass instrument playing Y93.J4
  building construction Y93.H3
  bungee jumping Y93.34
  calisthenics Y93.A2
  canoeing (in calm and turbulent water) Y93.16
  capture the flag Y93.6A
  cardiorespiratory exercise NEC Y93.A9
  caregiving (providing) NEC Y93.F9
    bathing Y93.F1
    lifting Y93.F2
  cellular
    communication device Y93.C2
    telephone Y93.C2
  challenge course Y93.A5
  cheerleading Y93.45
  choking game Y93.85
  circuit training Y93.A4
  cleaning
    floor Y93.E5
  climbing NEC Y93.39
    mountain Y93.31
    rock Y93.31
    wall Y93.31
  clothing care and maintenance NEC Y93.E9
  combatives Y93.75
  computer
    keyboarding Y93.C1
    technology NEC Y93.C9
  confidence course Y93.A5
  construction (building) Y93.H3
  cooking and baking Y93.G3
  cool down exercises Y93.A2
  cricket Y93.69
  crocheting Y93.D1
  cross country skiing Y93.24
  dancing (all types) Y93.41

▶ New   ⇒ Revised   ~~deleted~~ Deleted   ● Use Additional Character(s)

A

▶ New   ➡ Revised   ~~deleted~~ Deleted   ● Use Additional Character(s)

Aerosinusitis —*see* Air, pressure
After-effect, late —*see* Sequelae
Air
  blast in war operations —*see* War operations,
    air blast
  pressure
    change, rapid
      during
        ascent W94.29
          while (in) (surfacing from)
            aircraft W94.23
            deep water diving W94.21
            underground W94.22
        descent W94.39
          in
            aircraft W94.31
            water W94.32
    high, prolonged W94.0
    low, prolonged W94.12
      due to residence or long visit at high
        altitude W94.11
Alpine sickness W94.11
Altitude sickness W94.11
Anaphylactic shock, anaphylaxis —*see* Table of
  Drugs and Chemicals
Andes disease W94.11
Arachnidism, arachnoidism X58
Arson (with intent to injure or kill) X97
Asphyxia, asphyxiation
  by
    food (bone) (seed) —*see* categories T17
      and T18
    gas —*see also* Table of Drugs and
      Chemicals
      legal
        execution —*see* Legal, intervention,
          gas
        intervention —*see* Legal, intervention,
          gas
  from
    fire —*see also* Exposure, fire
      in war operations —*see* War operations,
        fire
    ignition —*see* Ignition
    vomitus T17.81
  in war operations —*see* War operations,
    restriction of airway
Aspiration
  food (any type) (into respiratory tract) (with
    asphyxia, obstruction respiratory tract,
    suffocation) —*see* categories T17 and T18
  foreign body —*see* Foreign body, aspiration
  vomitus (with asphyxia, obstruction
    respiratory tract, suffocation) T17.81
Assassination (attempt) —*see* Assault
Assault (homicidal) (by) (in) Y09
  arson X97
  bite (of human being) Y04.1
  bodily force Y04.8
    bite Y04.1
    bumping into Y04.2
    sexual —*see* subcategories T74.0, T76.0
    unarmed fight Y04.0

Assault *(Continued)*
  bomb X96.9
    antipersonnel X96.0
    fertilizer X96.3
    gasoline X96.1
    letter X96.2
    petrol X96.1
    pipe X96.3
    specified NEC X96.8
  brawl (hand) (fists) (foot) (unarmed) Y04.0
  burning, burns (by fire) NEC X97
    acid Y08.89
    caustic, corrosive substance Y08.89
    chemical from swallowing caustic,
      corrosive substance —*see* Table of
        Drugs and Chemicals
    cigarette(s) X97
    hot object X98.9
      fluid NEC X98.2
      household appliance X98.3
      specified NEC X98.8
      steam X98.0
      tap water X98.1
      vapors X98.0
    scalding —*see* Assault, burning
    steam X98.0
    vitriol Y08.89
  caustic, corrosive substance (gas) Y08.89
  crashing of
    aircraft Y08.81
    motor vehicle Y03.8
      pushed in front of Y02.0
      run over Y03.0
      specified NEC Y03.8
  cutting or piercing instrument X99.9
    dagger X99.2
    glass X99.0
    knife X99.1
    specified NEC X99.8
    sword X99.2
  dagger X99.2
  drowning (in) X92.9
    bathtub X92.0
    natural water X92.3
    specified NEC X92.8
    swimming pool X92.1
      following fall X92.2
  dynamite X96.8
  explosive(s) (material) X96.9
  fight (hand) (fists) (foot) (unarmed) Y04.0
    with weapon —*see* Assault, by type of
      weapon
  fire X97
  firearm X95.9
    airgun X95.01
    handgun X93
    hunting rifle X94.1
    larger X94.9
      specified NEC X94.8
    machine gun X94.2
    shotgun X94.0
    specified NEC X95.8

Assault *(Continued)*
  from high place Y01
  gunshot (wound) NEC —*see* Assault, firearm,
    by type
  incendiary device X97
  injury Y09
    to child due to criminal abortion attempt
      NEC Y08.89
  knife X99.1
  late effect of —*see* X92-Y08 with 7th character
    S
  placing before moving object NEC Y02.8
    motor vehicle Y02.0
  poisoning —*see* categories T36-T65 with 7th
    character S
  puncture, any part of body —*see* Assault,
    cutting or piercing instrument
  pushing
    before moving object NEC Y02.8
      motor vehicle Y02.0
      subway train Y02.1
      train Y02.1
  rape T74.2-●
  scalding —*see* Assault, burning
  sequelae of —*see* X92-Y08 with 7th character S
  sexual (by bodily force) T74.2-●
  shooting —*see* Assault, firearm
  specified means NEC Y08.89
  stab, any part of body —*see* Assault, cutting
    or piercing instrument
  steam X98.0
  striking against
    other person Y04.2
    sports equipment Y08.09
      baseball bat Y08.02
      hockey stick Y08.01
  struck by
    sports equipment Y08.09
      baseball bat Y08.02
      hockey stick Y08.01
  submersion —*see* Assault, drowning
  violence Y09
  weapon Y09
    blunt Y00
    cutting or piercing —*see* Assault, cutting or
      piercing instrument
    firearm —*see* Assault, firearm
  wound Y09
    cutting —*see* Assault, cutting or piercing
      instrument
    gunshot —*see* Assault, firearm
    knife X99.1
    piercing —*see* Assault, cutting or piercing
      instrument
    puncture —*see* Assault, cutting or piercing
      instrument
    stab —*see* Assault, cutting or piercing
      instrument
Attack by mammals NEC W55.89
Avalanche —*see* Landslide
Aviator's disease —*see* Air, pressure

B

Barotitis, barodontalgia, barosinusitis, barotrauma (otitic) (sinus) —*see* Air, pressure
Battered (baby) (child) (person) (syndrome) X58
Bayonet wound W26.1
  in
    legal intervention —*see* Legal, intervention, sharp object, bayonet
    war operations —*see* War operations, combat
  stated as undetermined whether accidental or intentional Y28.8
  suicide (attempt) X78.2
Bean in nose —*see* categories T17 and T18
Bed set on fire NEC —*see* Exposure, fire, uncontrolled, building, bed
Beheading (by guillotine)
  homicide X99.9
  legal execution —*see* Legal, intervention
Bending, injury in (prolonged) (static) X50.1
Bends —*see* Air, pressure, change
Bite, bitten by
  alligator W58.01
  arthropod (nonvenomous) NEC W57
  bull W55.21
  cat W55.01
  cow W55.21
  crocodile W58.11
  dog W54.0
  goat W55.31
  hoof stock NEC W55.31
  horse W55.11
  human being (accidentally) W50.3
    with intent to injure or kill Y04.1
    as, or caused by, a crowd or human stampede (with fall) W52
    assault Y04.1
    homicide (attempt) Y04.1
    in
      fight Y04.1
  insect (nonvenomous) W57
  lizard (nonvenomous) W59.01
  mammal NEC W55.81
    marine W56.31
  marine animal (nonvenomous) W56.81
  millipede W57
  moray eel W56.51
  mouse W53.01
  person(s) (accidentally) W50.3
    with intent to injure or kill Y04.1
    as, or caused by, a crowd or human stampede (with fall) W52
    assault Y04.1
    homicide (attempt) Y04.1
    in
      fight Y04.1
  pig W55.41
  raccoon W55.51
  rat W53.11
  reptile W59.81
    lizard W59.01
    snake W59.11
    turtle W59.21
      terrestrial W59.81
  rodent W53.81
    mouse W53.01
    rat W53.11
    specified NEC W53.81
    squirrel W53.21
  shark W56.41
  sheep W55.31
  snake (nonvenomous) W59.11
  spider (nonvenomous) W57
  squirrel W53.21
Blast (air) in war operations —*see* War operations, blast
Blizzard X37.2

Blood alcohol level Y90.9
  20-39mg/100ml Y90.1
  40-59mg/100ml Y90.2
  60-79mg/100ml Y90.3
  80-99mg/100ml Y90.4
  100-119mg/100ml Y90.5
  120-199mg/100ml Y90.6
  200-239mg/100ml Y90.7
  less than 20mg/100ml Y90.0
  presence in blood, level not specified Y90.9
Blow X58
  by law-enforcing agent, police (on duty) —*see* Legal, intervention, manhandling
    blunt object —*see* Legal, intervention, blunt object
Blowing up —*see* Explosion
Brawl (hand) (fists) (foot) Y04.0
Breakage (accidental) (part of)
  ladder (causing fall) W11
  scaffolding (causing fall) W12
Broken
  glass, contact with —*see* Contact, with, glass
  power line (causing electric shock) W85
Bumping against, into (accidentally)
  object NEC W22.8
    with fall —*see* Fall, due to, bumping against, object
    caused by crowd or human stampede (with fall) W52
    sports equipment W21.9
  person(s) W51
    with fall W03
      due to ice or snow W00.0
    assault Y04.2
    caused by, a crowd or human stampede (with fall) W52
    homicide (attempt) Y04.2
  sports equipment W21.9
Burn, burned, burning (accidental) (by) (from) (on)
  acid NEC —*see* Table of Drugs and Chemicals
  bed linen —*see* Exposure, fire, uncontrolled, in building, bed
  blowtorch X08.8
    with ignition of clothing NEC X06.2
      nightwear X05
  bonfire, campfire (controlled) —*see also* Exposure, fire, controlled, not in building
    uncontrolled —*see* Exposure, fire, uncontrolled, not in building
  candle X08.8
    with ignition of clothing NEC X06.2
      nightwear X05
  caustic liquid, substance (external) (internal) NEC —*see* Table of Drugs and Chemicals
  chemical (external) (internal) —*see also* Table of Drugs and Chemicals
    in war operations —*see* War operations, fire
  cigar(s) or cigarette(s) X08.8
    with ignition of clothing NEC X06.2
      nightwear X05
  clothes, clothing NEC (from controlled fire) X06.2
    with conflagration —*see* Exposure, fire, uncontrolled, building
    not in building or structure —*see* Exposure, fire, uncontrolled, not in building
  cooker (hot) X15.8
    stated as undetermined whether accidental or intentional Y27.3
    suicide (attempt) X77.3
  electric blanket X16
  engine (hot) X17
  fire, flames —*see* Exposure, fire
  flare, Very pistol —*see* Discharge, firearm NEC

Burn, burned, burning (*Continued*)
  heat
    from appliance (electrical) (household) X15.8
      cooker X15.8
      hotplate X15.2
      kettle X15.8
      light bulb X15.8
      saucepan X15.3
      skillet X15.3
      stated as undetermined whether accidental or intentional Y27.3
      stove X15.0
      suicide (attempt) X77.3
      toaster X15.1
    in local application or packing during medical or surgical procedure Y63.5
  heating
    appliance, radiator or pipe X16
  homicide (attempt) —*see* Assault, burning
  hot
    air X14.1
    cooker X15.8
    drink X10.0
    engine X17
    fat X10.2
    fluid NEC X12
    food X10.1
    gases X14.1
    heating appliance X16
    household appliance NEC X15.8
    kettle X15.8
    liquid NEC X12
    machinery X17
    metal (molten) (liquid) NEC X18
    object (not producing fire or flames) NEC X19
    oil (cooking) X10.2
    pipe(s) X16
    radiator X16
    saucepan (glass) (metal) X15.3
    stove (kitchen) X15.0
    substance NEC X19
      caustic or corrosive NEC —*see* Table of Drugs and Chemicals
    toaster X15.1
    tool X17
    vapor X13.1
    water (tap) —*see* Contact, with, hot, tap water
  hotplate X15.2
    suicide (attempt) X77.3
  ignition —*see* Ignition
  in war operations —*see* War operations, fire
  inflicted by other person X97
    by hot objects, hot vapor, and steam —*see* Assault, burning, hot object
  internal, from swallowed caustic, corrosive liquid, substance —*see* Table of Drugs and Chemicals
  iron (hot) X15.8
    stated as undetermined whether accidental or intentional Y27.3
    suicide (attempt) X77.3
  kettle (hot) X15.8
    stated as undetermined whether accidental or intentional Y27.3
    suicide (attempt) X77.3
  lamp (flame) X08.8
    with ignition of clothing NEC X06.2
      nightwear X05
  lighter (cigar) (cigarette) X08.8
    with ignition of clothing NEC X06.2
      nightwear X05
  lightning —*see* subcategory T75.0
    causing fire —*see* Exposure, fire
  liquid (boiling) (hot) NEC X12
    stated as undetermined whether accidental or intentional Y27.2
    suicide (attempt) X77.2

Burn, burned, burning (Continued)
  local application of externally applied
    substance in medical or surgical care
    Y63.5
  machinery (hot) X17
  matches X08.8
    with ignition of clothing NEC X06.2
      nightwear X05
  mattress —see Exposure, fire, uncontrolled,
    building, bed
  medicament, externally applied Y63.5
  metal (hot) (liquid) (molten) NEC X18
  nightwear (nightclothes, nightdress, gown,
    pajamas, robe) X05
  object (hot) NEC X19
  on board watercraft
    due to
      accident to watercraft V91.09
        powered craft V91.03
          ferry boat V91.01
          fishing boat V91.02
          jetskis V91.03
          liner V91.01
          merchant ship V91.00
          passenger ship V91.01
        unpowered craft V91.08
          canoe V91.05
          inflatable V91.06
          kayak V91.05
          sailboat V91.04
          surf-board V91.08
          water skis V91.07
          windsurfer V91.08
      fire on board V93.09
        ferry boat V93.01
        fishing boat V93.02
        jetskis V93.03
        liner V93.01
        merchant ship V93.00
        passenger ship V93.01
        powered craft NEC V93.03
        sailboat V93.04

Burn, burned, burning (Continued)
  on board watercraft (Continued)
    due to (Continued)
      specified heat source NEC on board
        V93.19
      ferry boat V93.11
      fishing boat V93.12
      jetskis V93.13
      liner V93.11
      merchant ship V93.10
      passenger ship V93.11
      powered craft NEC V93.13
      sailboat V93.14
  pipe (hot) X16
    smoking X08.8
      with ignition of clothing NEC X06.2
        nightwear X05
  powder —see Powder burn
  radiator (hot) X16
  saucepan (hot) (glass) (metal) X15.3
    stated as undetermined whether
      accidental or intentional
      Y27.3
    suicide (attempt) X77.3
  self-inflicted X76
    stated as undetermined whether
      accidental or intentional
      Y26
  stated as undetermined whether
    accidental or intentional Y27.0
  steam X13.1
    pipe X16
      stated as undetermined whether
        accidental or intentional
        Y27.8
    stated as undetermined whether
      accidental or intentional Y27.0
    suicide (attempt) X77.0
  stove (hot) (kitchen) X15.0
    stated as undetermined whether
      accidental or intentional Y27.3
    suicide (attempt) X77.3

Burn, burned, burning (Continued)
  substance (hot) NEC X19
    boiling X12
      stated as undetermined whether
        accidental or intentional Y27.2
      suicide (attempt) X77.2
    molten (metal) X18
  suicide (attempt) NEC X76
    hot
      household appliance X77.3
      object X77.9
  stated as undetermined whether accidental or
    intentional Y27.0
  therapeutic misadventure
    heat in local application or packing during
      medical or surgical procedure Y63.5
    overdose of radiation Y63.2
  toaster (hot) X15.1
    stated as undetermined whether accidental
      or intentional Y27.3
    suicide (attempt) X77.3
  tool (hot) X17
  torch, welding X08.8
    with ignition of clothing NEC X06.2
      nightwear X05
  trash fire (controlled) —see Exposure, fire,
    controlled, not in building
    uncontrolled —see Exposure, fire,
      uncontrolled, not in building
  vapor (hot) X13.1
    stated as undetermined whether accidental
      or intentional Y27.0
    suicide (attempt) X77.0
  Very pistol —see Discharge, firearm NEC
Butted by animal W55.82
  bull W55.22
  cow W55.22
  goat W55.32
  horse W55.12
  pig W55.42
  sheep W55.32

B

▶ New   ➠ Revised   ~~deleted~~ Deleted   ● Use Additional Character(s)

C

Caisson disease —*see* Air, pressure, change
Campfire (exposure to) (controlled) —*see also* Exposure, fire, controlled, not in building
  uncontrolled —*see* Exposure, fire, uncontrolled, not in building
Capital punishment (any means) —*see* Legal, intervention
Car sickness T75.3
Casualty (not due to war) NEC X58
  war —*see* War operations
Cat
  bite W55.01
  scratch W55.03
Cataclysm, cataclysmic (any injury) NEC —*see* Forces of nature
Catching fire —*see* Exposure, fire
Caught
  between
    folding object W23.0
    objects (moving) (stationary and moving) W23.0
    and machinery —*see* Contact, with, by type of machine
      stationary W23.1
    sliding door and door frame W23.0
  by, in
    machinery (moving parts of) —*see* Contact, with, by type of machine
    washing-machine wringer W23.0
  under packing crate (due to losing grip) W23.1
Cave-in caused by cataclysmic earth surface movement or eruption —*see* Landslide
Change(s) in air pressure —*see* Air, pressure, change
Choked, choking (on) (any object except food or vomitus)
  food (bone) (seed) —*see* categories T17 and T18
  vomitus T17.81-●
Civil insurrection —*see* War operations
Cloudburst (any injury) X37.8
Cold, exposure to (accidental) (excessive) (extreme) (natural) (place) NEC —*see* Exposure, cold
Collapse
  building W20.1
    burning (uncontrolled fire) X00.2
  dam or man-made structure (causing earth movement) X36.0
  machinery —*see* Contact, with, by type of machine
  structure W20.1
    burning (uncontrolled fire) X00.2
Collision (accidental) NEC —*see also* Accident, transport V89.9
  pedestrian W51
    with fall W03
      due to ice or snow W00.0
      involving pedestrian conveyance —*see* Accident, transport, pedestrian, conveyance
    and
      crowd or human stampede (with fall) W52
      object W22.8
        with fall —*see* Fall, due to, bumping against, object
  person(s) —*see* Collision, pedestrian
  transport vehicle NEC V89.9
    and
      avalanche, fallen or not moving —*see* Accident, transport
        falling or moving —*see* Landslide
      landslide, fallen or not moving —*see* Accident, transport
        falling or moving —*see* Landslide

Collision NEC (Continued)
  transport vehicle NEC (Continued)
    due to cataclysm —*see* Forces of nature, by type
    intentional, purposeful suicide (attempt) —*see* Suicide, collision
Combustion, spontaneous —*see* Ignition
Complication (delayed) of or following (medical or surgical procedure) Y84.9
  with misadventure —*see* Misadventure
  amputation of limb(s) Y83.5
  anastomosis (arteriovenous) (blood vessel) (gastrojejunal) (tendon) (natural or artificial material) Y83.2
  aspiration (of fluid) Y84.4
    tissue Y84.8
  biopsy Y84.8
  blood
    sampling Y84.7
    transfusion
      procedure Y84.8
  bypass Y83.2
  catheterization (urinary) Y84.6
    cardiac Y84.0
  colostomy Y83.3
  cystostomy Y83.3
  dialysis (kidney) Y84.1
  drug —*see* Table of Drugs and Chemicals
  due to misadventure —*see* Misadventure
  duodenostomy Y83.3
  electroshock therapy Y84.3
  external stoma, creation of Y83.3
  formation of external stoma Y83.3
  gastrostomy Y83.3
  graft Y83.2
  hypothermia (medically-induced) Y84.8
  implant, implantation (of)
    artificial
      internal device (cardiac pacemaker) (electrodes in brain) (heart valve prosthesis) (orthopedic) Y83.1
      material or tissue (for anastomosis or bypass) Y83.2
        with creation of external stoma Y83.3
    natural tissues (for anastomosis or bypass) Y83.2
      with creation of external stoma Y83.3
  infusion
    procedure Y84.8
  injection —*see* Table of Drugs and Chemicals
    procedure Y84.8
  insertion of gastric or duodenal sound Y84.5
  insulin-shock therapy Y84.3
  paracentesis (abdominal) (thoracic) (aspirative) Y84.4
  procedures other than surgical operation —*see* Complication of or following, by type of procedure
  radiological procedure or therapy Y84.2
  removal of organ (partial) (total) NEC Y83.6
  sampling
    blood Y84.7
    fluid NEC Y84.4
    tissue Y84.8
  shock therapy Y84.3
  surgical operation NEC —*see also* Complication of or following, by type of operation Y83.9
    reconstructive NEC Y83.4
    with
      anastomosis, bypass or graft Y83.2
      formation of external stoma Y83.3
    specified NEC Y83.8
  transfusion —*see also* Table of Drugs and Chemicals
    procedure Y84.8
  transplant, transplantation (heart) (kidney) (liver) (whole organ, any) Y83.0
    partial organ Y83.4
  ureterostomy Y83.3

Complication of or following (Continued)
  vaccination —*see also* Table of Drugs and Chemicals
    procedure Y84.8
Compression
  divers' squeeze —*see* Air, pressure, change
  trachea by
    food (lodged in esophagus) —*see* categories T17 and T18
    vomitus (lodged in esophagus) T17.81-●
Conflagration —*see* Exposure, fire, uncontrolled
Constriction (external)
  hair W49.01
  jewelry W49.04
  ring W49.04
  rubber band W49.03
  specified item NEC W49.09
  string W49.02
  thread W49.02
Contact (accidental)
  with
    abrasive wheel (metalworking) W31.1
    alligator W58.09
      bite W58.01
      crushing W58.03
      strike W58.02
    amphibian W62.9
      frog W62.0
      toad W62.1
    animal (nonvenomous) NEC W64
      marine W56.89
        bite W56.81
        dolphin —*see* Contact, with, dolphin
        fish NEC —*see* Contact, with, fish
        mammal —*see* Contact, with, mammal, marine
        orca —*see* Contact, with, orca
        sea lion —*see* Contact, with, sea lion
        shark —*see* Contact, with, shark
        strike W56.82
    animate mechanical force NEC W64
    arrow W21.89
      not thrown, projected or falling W45.8
    arthropods (nonvenomous) W57
    axe W27.0
    band-saw (industrial) W31.2
    bayonet —*see* Bayonet wound
    bee(s) X58
    bench-saw (industrial) W31.2
    bird W61.99
      bite W61.91
      chicken —*see* Contact, with, chicken
      duck —*see* Contact, with, duck
      goose —*see* Contact, with, goose
      macaw —*see* Contact, with, macaw
      parrot —*see* Contact, with, parrot
      psittacine —*see* Contact, with, psittacine
      strike W61.92
      turkey —*see* Contact, with, turkey
    blender W29.0
    boiling water X12
      stated as undetermined whether accidental or intentional Y27.2
      suicide (attempt) X77.2
    bore, earth-drilling or mining (land) (seabed) W31.0
    buffalo —*see* Contact, with, hoof stock NEC
    bull W55.29
      bite W55.21
      gored W55.22
      strike W55.22
    bumper cars W31.81
    camel —*see* Contact, with, hoof stock NEC
    can
      lid W26.8
      opener W27.4
        powered W29.0
    cat W55.09
      bite W55.01
      scratch W55.03
    caterpillar (venomous) X58

Contact *(Continued)*
  with *(Continued)*
    centipede (venomous) X58
    chain
      hoist W24.0
        agricultural operations W30.89
      saw W29.3
    chicken W61.39
      peck W61.33
      strike W61.32
    chisel W27.0
    circular saw W31.2
    cobra X58
    combine (harvester) W30.0
    conveyer belt W24.1
    cooker (hot) X15.8
      stated as undetermined whether
          accidental or intentional Y27.3
      suicide (attempt) X77.3
    coral X58
    cotton gin W31.82
    cow W55.29
      bite W55.21
      strike W55.22
    crane W24.0
      agricultural operations W30.89
    crocodile W58.19
      bite W58.11
      crushing W58.13
      strike W58.12
    dagger W26.1
      stated as undetermined whether
          accidental or intentional Y28.2
      suicide (attempt) X78.2
    dairy equipment W31.82
    dart W21.89
      not thrown, projected or falling W45.8
    deer —*see* Contact, with, hoof stock
        NEC
    derrick W24.0
      agricultural operations W30.89
        hay W30.2
    dog W54.8
      bite W54.0
      strike W54.1
    dolphin W56.09
      bite W56.01
      strike W56.02
    donkey —*see* Contact, with, hoof stock
        NEC
    drill (powered) W29.8
      earth (land) (seabed) W31.0
      nonpowered W27.8
    drive belt W24.0
      agricultural operations W30.89
    dry ice —*see* Exposure, cold, man-made
    dryer (clothes) (powered) (spin) W29.2
    duck W61.69
      bite W61.61
      strike W61.62
    earth(-)
      drilling machine (industrial) W31.0
      scraping machine in stationary use
          W31.83
    edge of stiff paper W26.2
    electric
      beater W29.0
      blanket X16
      fan W29.2
        commercial W31.82
      knife W29.1
      mixer W29.0
    elevator (building) W24.0
      agricultural operations W30.89
        grain W30.3
    engine(s), hot NEC X17
    excavating machine W31.0
    farm machine W30.9
    feces —*see* Contact, with, by type of
        animal
    fer de lance X58

Contact *(Continued)*
  with *(Continued)*
    fish W56.59
      bite W56.51
      shark —*see* Contact, with, shark
      strike W56.52
    flying horses W31.81
    forging (metalworking) machine
        W31.1
    fork W27.4
    forklift (truck) W24.0
      agricultural operations W30.89
    frog W62.0
    garden
      cultivator (powered) W29.3
        riding W30.89
      fork W27.1
    gas turbine W31.3
    Gila monster X58
    giraffe —*see* Contact, with, hoof stock
        NEC
    glass (sharp) (broken) W25
      with subsequent fall W18.02
      assault X99.0
      due to fall —*see* Fall, by type
      stated as undetermined whether
          accidental or intentional Y28. 0
      suicide (attempt) X78.0
    goat W55.39
      bite W55.31
      strike W55.32
    goose W61.59
      bite W61.51
      strike W61.52
    hand
      saw W27.0
      tool (not powered) NEC W27.8
        powered W29.8
    harvester W30.0
    hay-derrick W30.2
    heat NEC X19
      from appliance (electrical)
          (household) —*see* Contact, with,
          hot, household appliance
      heating appliance X16
    heating
      appliance (hot) X16
      pad (electric) X16
    hedge-trimmer (powered) W29.3
    hoe W27.1
    hoist (chain) (shaft) NEC W24.0
      agricultural W30.89
    hoof stock NEC W55.39
      bite W55.31
      strike W55.32
    hornet(s) X58
    horse W55.19
      bite W55.11
      strike W55.12
    hot
      air X14.1
        inhalation X14.0
      cooker X15.8
      drinks X10.0
      engine X17
      fats X10.2
      fluids NEC X12
        assault X98.2
        suicide (attempt) X77.2
        undetermined whether accidental or
            intentional Y27.2
      food X10.1
      gases X14.1
        inhalation X14.0
      heating appliance X16
      household appliance X15.8
        assault X98.3
        cooker X15.8
        hotplate X15.2
        kettle X15.8
        light bulb X15.8

Contact *(Continued)*
  with *(Continued)*
    hot *(Continued)*
      household appliance *(Continued)*
        object NEC X19
          assault X98.8
          stated as undetermined whether
              accidental or intentional Y27.9
          suicide (attempt) X77.8
        saucepan X15.3
        skillet X15.3
        stated as undetermined whether
            accidental or intentional Y27.3
        stove X15.0
        suicide (attempt) X77.3
        toaster X15.1
      kettle X15.8
      light bulb X15.8
      liquid NEC —*see also* Burn X12
        drinks X10.0
        stated as undetermined whether
            accidental or intentional Y27.2
        suicide (attempt) X77.2
        tap water X11.8
          stated as undetermined whether
              accidental or intentional Y27.1
          suicide (attempt) X77.1
      machinery X17
      metal (molten) (liquid) NEC X18
      object (not producing fire or flames)
          NEC X19
      oil (cooking) X10.2
      pipe X16
      plate X15.2
      radiator X16
      saucepan (glass) (metal) X15.3
      skillet X15.3
      stove (kitchen) X15.0
      substance NEC X19
      tap-water X11.8
        assault X98.1
        heated on stove X12
          stated as undetermined whether
              accidental or intentional Y27.2
          suicide (attempt) X77.2
        in bathtub X11.0
        running X11.1
        stated as undetermined whether
            accidental or intentional Y27.1
        suicide (attempt) X77.1
      toaster X15.1
      tool X17
      vapors X13.1
        inhalation X13.0
      water (tap) X11.8
        boiling X12
          stated as undetermined whether
              accidental or intentional Y27.2
          suicide (attempt) X77.2
        heated on stove X12
          stated as undetermined whether
              accidental or intentional Y27.2
          suicide (attempt) X77.2
        in bathtub X11.0
        running X11.1
        stated as undetermined whether
            accidental or intentional Y27.1
        suicide (attempt) X77.1
    hotplate X15.2
    ice-pick W27.4
    insect (nonvenomous) NEC W57
    kettle (hot) X15.8
    knife W26.0
      assault X99.1
      electric W29.1
      stated as undetermined whether
          accidental or intentional Y28.1
      suicide (attempt) X78.1
    lathe (metalworking) W31.1
      turnings W45.8
      woodworking W31.2

▶ New   ➡ Revised   ~~deleted~~ Deleted   ● Use Additional Character(s)

Contact *(Continued)*
  with *(Continued)*
    lawnmower (powered) (ridden) W28
      causing electrocution W86.8
        suicide (attempt) X83.1
      unpowered W27.1
    lift, lifting (devices) W24.0
      agricultural operations W30.89
      shaft W24.0
    liquefied gas —*see* Exposure, cold, man-made
    liquid air, hydrogen, nitrogen —*see* Exposure, cold, man-made
    lizard (nonvenomous) W59.09
      bite W59.01
      strike W59.02
    llama —*see* Contact, with, hoof stock NEC
    macaw W61.19
      bite W61.11
      strike W61.12
    machine, machinery W31.9
      abrasive wheel W31.1
      agricultural including animal-powered W30.9
        combine harvester W30.0
        grain storage elevator W30.3
        hay derrick W30.2
        power take-off device W30.1
        reaper W30.0
        specified NEC W30.89
        thresher W30.0
        transport vehicle, stationary W30.81
      band saw W31.2
      bench saw W31.2
      circular saw W31.2
      commercial NEC W31.82
      drilling, metal (industrial) W31.1
      earth-drilling W31.0
      earthmoving or scraping W31.89
      excavating W31.89
      forging machine W31.1
      gas turbine W31.3
      hot X17
      internal combustion engine W31.3
      land drill W31.0
      lathe W31.1
      lifting (devices) W24.0
      metal drill W31.1
      metalworking (industrial) W31.1
      milling, metal W31.1
      mining W31.0
      molding W31.2
      overhead plane W31.2
      power press, metal W31.1
      prime mover W31.3
      printing W31.89
      radial saw W31.2
      recreational W31.81
      roller-coaster W31.81
      rolling mill, metal W31.1
      sander W31.2
      seabed drill W31.0
      shaft
        hoist W31.0
        lift W31.0
      specified NEC W31.89
      spinning W31.89
      steam engine W31.3
      transmission W24.1
      undercutter W31.0
      water driven turbine W31.3
      weaving W31.89
      woodworking or forming (industrial) W31.2
    mammal (feces) (urine) W55.89
      bull —*see* Contact, with, bull
      cat —*see* Contact, with, cat
      cow —*see* Contact, with, cow
      goat —*see* Contact, with, goat
      hoof stock —*see* Contact, with, hoof stock

Contact *(Continued)*
  with *(Continued)*
    mammal *(Continued)*
      horse —*see* Contact, with, horse
      marine W56.39
        dolphin —*see* Contact, with, dolphin
        orca —*see* Contact, with, orca
        sea lion —*see* Contact, with, sea lion
        specified NEC W56.39
          bite W56.31
          strike W56.32
      pig —*see* Contact, with, pig
      raccoon —*see* Contact, with, raccoon
      rodent —*see* Contact, with, rodent
      sheep —*see* Contact, with, sheep
      specified NEC W55.89
        bite W55.81
        strike W55.82
    marine
      animal W56.89
        bite W56.81
        dolphin —*see* Contact, with, dolphin
        fish NEC —*see* Contact, with, fish
        mammal —*see* Contact, with, mammal, marine
        orca —*see* Contact, with, orca
        sea lion —*see* Contact, with, sea lion
        shark —*see* Contact, with, shark
        strike W56.82
    meat
      grinder (domestic) W29.0
        industrial W31.82
        nonpowered W27.4
      slicer (domestic) W29.0
        industrial W31.82
    merry go round W31.81
    metal, (hot) (liquid) (molten) NEC X18
    millipede W57
    nail W45.0
      gun W29.4
    needle (sewing) W27.3
      hypodermic W46.0
        contaminated W46.1
    object (blunt) NEC
      hot NEC X19
      legal intervention —*see* Legal, intervention, blunt object
      sharp NEC W45.8
        inflicted by other person NEC W45.8 stated as
          intentional homicide (attempt) — *see* Assault, cutting or piercing instrument
        legal intervention —*see* Legal, intervention, sharp object
        self-inflicted X78.9
    orca W56.29
      bite W56.21
      strike W56.22
    overhead plane W31.2
    paper (as sharp object) W26.2
    paper-cutter W27.5
    parrot W61.09
      bite W61.01
      strike W61.02
    pig W55.49
      bite W55.41
      strike W55.42
    pipe, hot X16
    pitchfork W27.1
    plane (metal) (wood) W27.0
      overhead W31.2
    plant thorns, spines, sharp leaves or other mechanisms W60
    powered
      garden cultivator W29.3
      household appliance, implement, or machine W29.8
      saw (industrial) W31.2
        hand W29.8
    printing machine W31.89

Contact *(Continued)*
  with *(Continued)*
    psittacine bird W61.29
      bite W61.21
      macaw —*see* Contact, with, macaw
      parrot —*see* Contact, with, parrot
      strike W61.22
    pulley (block) (transmission) W24.0
      agricultural operations W30.89
    raccoon W55.59
      bite W55.51
      strike W55.52
    radial-saw (industrial) W31.2
    radiator (hot) X16
    rake W27.1
    rattlesnake X58
    reaper W30.0
    reptile W59.89
      lizard —*see* Contact, with, lizard
      snake —*see* Contact, with, snake
      specified NEC W59.89
        bite W59.81
        crushing W59.83
        strike W59.82
      turtle —*see* Contact, with, turtle
    rivet gun (powered) W29.4
    road scraper —*see* Accident, transport, construction vehicle
    rodent (feces) (urine) W53.89
      bite W53.81
      mouse W53.09
        bite W53.01
      rat W53.19
        bite W53.11
      specified NEC W53.89
        bite W53.81
      squirrel W53.29
        bite W53.21
    roller coaster W31.81
    rope NEC W24.0
      agricultural operations W30.89
    saliva —*see* Contact, with, by type of animal
    sander W29.8
      industrial W31.2
    saucepan (hot) (glass) (metal) X15.3
    saw W27.0
      band (industrial) W31.2
      bench (industrial) W31.2
      chain W29.3
      hand W27.0
    sawing machine, metal W31.1
    scissors W27.2
    scorpion X58
    screwdriver W27.0
      powered W29.8
    sea
      anemone, cucumber or urchin (spine) X58
      lion W56.19
        bite W56.11
        strike W56.12
    serpent —*see* Contact, with, snake, by type
    sewing-machine (electric) (powered) W29.2
      not powered W27.8
    shaft (hoist) (lift) (transmission) NEC W24.0
      agricultural W30.89
    shark W56.49
      bite W56.41
      strike W56.42
    sharp object(s) W26.9
      specified NEC W26.8
    shears (hand) W27.2
      powered (industrial) W31.1
        domestic W29.2
    sheep W55.39
      bite W55.31
      strike W55.32
    shovel W27.8
      steam —*see* Accident, transport, construction vehicle

Contact *(Continued)*
  with *(Continued)*
    snake (nonvenomous) W59.19
      bite W59.11
      crushing W59.13
      strike W59.12
    spade W27.1
    spider (venomous) X58
    spin-drier W29.2
    spinning machine W31.89
    splinter W45.8
    sports equipment W21.9
    staple gun (powered) W29.8
    steam X13.1
      engine W31.3
      inhalation X13.0
      pipe X16
      shovel W31.89
    stove (hot) (kitchen) X15.0
    substance, hot NEC X19
      molten (metal) X18
    sword W26.1
      assault X99.2
      stated as undetermined whether
        accidental or intentional
        Y28.2
      suicide (attempt) X78.2
    tarantula X58
    thresher W30.0
    tin can lid W26.8
    toad W62.1
    toaster (hot) X15.1
    tool W27.8
      hand (not powered) W27.8
        auger W27.0
        axe W27.0
        can opener W27.4
        chisel W27.0
        fork W27.4
        garden W27.1
        handsaw W27.0
        hoe W27.1
        ice-pick W27.4
        kitchen utensil W27.4
        manual
          lawn mower W27.1
          sewing machine W27.8
        meat grinder W27.4
        needle (sewing) W27.3
          hypodermic W46.0
            contaminated W46.1
        paper cutter W27.5
        pitchfork W27.1
        rake W27.1
        scissors W27.2
        screwdriver W27.0
        specified NEC W27.8
        workbench W27.0
      hot X17
      powered W29.8
        blender W29.0
          commercial W31.82
        can opener W29.0
          commercial W31.82
        chainsaw W29.3
        clothes dryer W29.2
          commercial W31.82
        dishwasher W29.2
          commercial W31.82
        edger W29.3
        electric fan W29.2
          commercial W31.82
        electric knife W29.1
        food processor W29.0
          commercial W31.82
        garbage disposal W29.0
          commercial W31.82

Contact *(Continued)*
  with *(Continued)*
    tool *(Continued)*
      powered *(Continued)*
        garden tool W29.3
        hedge trimmer W29.3
        ice maker W29.0
          commercial W31.82
        kitchen appliance W29.0
          commercial W31.82
        lawn mower W28
        meat grinder W29.0
          commercial W31.82
        mixer W29.0
          commercial W31.82
        rototiller W29.3
        sewing machine W29.2
          commercial W31.82
        washing machine W29.2
          commercial W31.82
    transmission device (belt, cable, chain,
      gear, pinion, shaft) W24.1
      agricultural operations W30.89
    turbine (gas) (water-driven) W31.3
    turkey W61.49
      peck W61.43
      strike W61.42
    turtle (nonvenomous) W59.29
      bite W59.21
      strike W59.22
      terrestrial W59.89
        bite W59.81
        crushing W59.83
        strike W59.82
    under-cutter W31.0
    urine —*see* Contact, with, by type of animal
    vehicle
      agricultural use (transport) —*see*
        Accident, transport, agricultural
        vehicle
        not on public highway W30.81
      industrial use (transport) —*see*
        Accident, transport, industrial
        vehicle
        not on public highway W31.83
      off-road use (transport) —*see* Accident,
        transport, all-terrain or off-road
        vehicle
        not on public highway W31.83
      special construction use (transport) —*see*
        Accident, transport, construction
        vehicle
        not on public highway W31.83
    venomous
      animal X58
      arthropods X58
      lizard X58
      marine animal NEC X58
      marine plant NEC X58
      millipedes (tropical) X58
      plant(s) X58
      snake X58
      spider X58
      viper X58
    washing-machine (powered) W29.2
    wasp X58
    weaving-machine W31.89
    winch W24.0
      agricultural operations W30.89
    wire NEC W24.0
      agricultural operations W30.89
    wood slivers W45.8
    yellow jacket X58
    zebra —*see* Contact, with, hoof stock NEC
  pressure X50.9
  stress X50.9
Coup de soleil X32

Crash
  aircraft (in transit) (powered) V95.9
    balloon V96.01
    fixed wing NEC (private) V95.21
      commercial V95.31
    glider V96.21
      hang V96.11
      powered V95.11
    helicopter V95.01
    in war operations —*see* War operations,
      destruction of aircraft
    microlight V95.11
    nonpowered V96.9
      specified NEC V96.8
    powered NEC V95.8
    stated as
      homicide (attempt) Y08.81
      suicide (attempt) X83.0
    ultralight V95.11
  spacecraft V95.41
  transport vehicle NEC —*see also* Accident,
    transport V89.9
    homicide (attempt) Y03.8
    motor NEC (traffic) V89.2
      homicide (attempt) Y03.8
      suicide (attempt) —*see* Suicide, collision
Cruelty (mental) (physical) (sexual) X58
Crushed (accidentally) X58
  between objects (moving) (stationary and
    moving) W23.0
    stationary W23.1
  by
    alligator W58.03
    avalanche NEC —*see* Landslide
    cave-in W20.0
      caused by cataclysmic earth surface
        movement —*see* Landslide
    crocodile W58.13
    crowd or human stampede W52
    falling
      aircraft V97.39
        in war operations —*see* War
          operations, destruction of aircraft
      earth, material W20.0
        caused by cataclysmic earth surface
          movement —*see* Landslide
      object NEC W20.8
    landslide NEC —*see* Landslide
    lizard (nonvenomous) W59.09
    machinery —*see* Contact, with, by type of
      machine
    reptile NEC W59.89
    snake (nonvenomous) W59.13
  in
    machinery —*see* Contact, with, by type of
      machine
Cut, cutting (any part of body) (accidental) —
    see also Contact, with, by object or machine
  during medical or surgical treatment as
    misadventure —*see* Index to Diseases
    and Injuries, Complications
  homicide (attempt) —*see* Assault, cutting or
    piercing instrument
  inflicted by other person —*see* Assault,
    cutting or piercing instrument
  legal
    execution —*see* Legal, intervention
    intervention —*see* Legal, intervention,
      sharp object
  machine NEC —*see also* Contact, with, by
    type of machine W31.9
  self-inflicted —*see* Suicide, cutting or piercing
    instrument
  suicide (attempt) —*see* Suicide, cutting or
    piercing instrument
Cyclone (any injury) X37.1

▶ New   ⟹ Revised   ~~deleted~~ Deleted   ● Use Additional Character(s)

D

Decapitation (accidental circumstances)
  NEC X58
  homicide X99.9
  legal execution —*see* Legal, intervention
Dehydration from lack of water X58
Deprivation X58
Derailment (accidental)
  railway (rolling stock) (train) (vehicle)
    (without antecedent collision) V81.7
    with antecedent collision —*see* Accident,
      transport, railway vehicle occupant
  streetcar (without antecedent collision)
    V82.7
    with antecedent collision —*see* Accident,
      transport, streetcar occupant
Descent
  parachute (voluntary) (without accident to
    aircraft) V97.29
    due to accident to aircraft —*see* Accident,
      transport, aircraft
Desertion X58
Destitution X58
Disability, late effect or sequela of injury —*see*
  Sequelae
Discharge (accidental)
  airgun W34.010
    assault X95.01
    homicide (attempt) X95.01
    stated as undetermined whether accidental
      or intentional Y24.0
    suicide (attempt) X74.01
  BB gun —*see* Discharge, airgun
  firearm (accidental) W34.00
    assault X95.9
    handgun (pistol) (revolver) W32.0
      assault X93
      homicide (attempt) X93
      legal intervention —*see* Legal,
        intervention, firearm, handgun
      stated as undetermined whether
        accidental or intentional Y22
      suicide (attempt) X72
    homicide (attempt) X95.9
    hunting rifle W33.02
      assault X94.1
      homicide (attempt) X94.1
      legal intervention
        injuring
          bystander Y35.032
          law enforcement personnel
            Y35.031
          suspect Y35.033
      stated as undetermined whether
        accidental or intentional Y23.1
      suicide (attempt) X73.1
    larger W33.00
      assault X94.9
      homicide (attempt) X94.9
      hunting rifle —*see* Discharge, firearm,
        hunting rifle
      legal intervention —*see* Legal,
        intervention, firearm by type of
        firearm
      machine gun —*see* Discharge, firearm,
        machine gun
      shotgun —*see* Discharge, firearm,
        shotgun
      specified NEC W33.09
        assault X94.8
        homicide (attempt) X94.8
        legal intervention
          injuring
            bystander Y35.092
            law enforcement personnel
              Y35.091
            suspect Y35.093
        stated as undetermined whether
          accidental or intentional Y23.8
        suicide (attempt) X73.8

Discharge (Continued)
  firearm (Continued)
    larger (Continued)
      stated as undetermined whether
        accidental or intentional Y23.9
      suicide (attempt) X73.9
    legal intervention
      injuring
        bystander Y35.002
        law enforcement personnel Y35.001
        suspect Y35.03
      using rubber bullet
        injuring
          bystander Y35.042
          law enforcement personnel
            Y35.041
          suspect Y35.043
    machine gun W33.03
      assault X94.2
      homicide (attempt) X94.2
      legal intervention —*see* Legal,
        intervention, firearm, machine gun
      stated as undetermined whether
        accidental or intentional Y23.3
      suicide (attempt) X73.2
    pellet gun —*see* Discharge, airgun
    shotgun W33.01
      assault X94.0
      homicide (attempt) X94.0
      legal intervention —*see* Legal,
        intervention, firearm, specified NEC
      stated as undetermined whether
        accidental or intentional Y23.0
      suicide (attempt) X73.0
    specified NEC W34.09
      assault X95.8
      homicide (attempt) X95.8
      legal intervention —*see* Legal,
        intervention, firearm, specified NEC
      stated as undetermined whether
        accidental or intentional Y24.8
      suicide (attempt) X74.8
    stated as undetermined whether accidental
      or intentional Y24.9
    suicide (attempt) X74.9
    Very pistol W34.09
      assault X95.8
      homicide (attempt) X95.8
      stated as undetermined whether
        accidental or intentional Y24.8
      suicide (attempt) X74.8
  firework(s) W39
    stated as undetermined whether accidental
      or intentional Y25
  gas-operated gun NEC W34.018
    airgun —*see* Discharge, airgun
    assault X95.09
    homicide (attempt) X95.09
    paintball gun —*see* Discharge, paintball
      gun
    stated as undetermined whether accidental
      or intentional Y24.8
    suicide (attempt) X74.09
  gun NEC —*see also* Discharge, firearm NEC
    air —*see* Discharge, airgun
    BB —*see* Discharge, airgun
    for single hand use —*see* Discharge,
      firearm, handgun
    hand —*see* Discharge, firearm, handgun
    machine —*see* Discharge, firearm, machine
      gun
    other specified —*see* Discharge, firearm
      NEC
    paintball —*see* Discharge, paintball gun
    pellet —*see* Discharge, airgun
  handgun —*see* Discharge, firearm, handgun
  machine gun —*see* Discharge, firearm,
    machine gun
  paintball gun W34.011
    assault X95.02
    homicide (attempt) X95.02

Discharge (Continued)
  paintball gun (Continued)
    stated as undetermined whether accidental
      or intentional Y24.8
    suicide (attempt) X74.02
  pistol —*see* Discharge, firearm, handgun
    flare —*see* Discharge, firearm, Very pistol
    pellet —*see* Discharge, airgun
    Very —*see* Discharge, firearm, Very pistol
  revolver —*see* Discharge, firearm, handgun
  rifle (hunting) —*see* Discharge, firearm,
    hunting rifle
  shotgun —*see* Discharge, firearm, shotgun
  spring-operated gun NEC W34.018
    assault X95.09
    homicide (attempt) X95.09
    stated as undetermined whether accidental
      or intentional Y24.8
    suicide (attempt) X74.09
Disease
  Andes W94.11
  aviator's —*see* Air, pressure
  range W94.11
Diver's disease, palsy, paralysis, squeeze —*see*
  Air, pressure
Diving (into water) —*see* Accident, diving
Dog bite W54.0
Dragged by transport vehicle NEC —*see also*
  Accident, transport V09.9
Drinking poison (accidental) —*see* Table of
  Drugs and Chemicals
Dropped (accidentally) **while being carried or**
  supported by other person W04
Drowning (accidental) W74
  assault X92.9
  due to
    accident (to)
      machinery —*see* Contact, with, by type
        of machine
      watercraft V90.89
        burning V90.29
          powered V90.23
            fishing boat V90.22
            jetskis V90.23
            merchant ship V90.20
            passenger ship V90.21
          unpowered V90.28
            canoe V90.25
            inflatable V90.26
            kayak V90.25
            sailboat V90.24
            water skis V90.27
        crushed V90.39
          powered V90.33
            fishing boat V90.32
            jetskis V90.33
            merchant ship V90.30
            passenger ship V90.31
          unpowered V90.38
            canoe V90.35
            inflatable V90.36
            kayak V90.35
            sailboat V90.34
            water skis V90.37
        overturning V90.09
          powered V90.03
            fishing boat V90.02
            jetskis V90.03
            merchant ship V90.00
            passenger ship V90.01
          unpowered V90.08
            canoe V90.05
            inflatable V90.06
            kayak V90.05
            sailboat V90.04
        sinking V90.19
          powered V90.13
            fishing boat V90.12
            jetskis V90.13
            merchant ship V90.10
            passenger ship V90.11

Drowning *(Continued)*
  due to *(Continued)*
    accident *(Continued)*
      watercraft *(Continued)*
        sinking *(Continued)*
          unpowered V90.18
            canoe V90.15
            inflatable V90.16
            kayak V90.15
            sailboat V90.14
          specified type NEC V90.89
          powered V90.83
            fishing boat V90.82
            jetskis V90.83
            merchant ship V90.80
            passenger ship V90.81
          unpowered V90.88
            canoe V90.85
            inflatable V90.86
            kayak V90.85
            sailboat V90.84
            water skis V90.87
    avalanche —*see* Landslide
    cataclysmic
      earth surface movement NEC —*see*
        Forces of nature, earth movement
      storm —*see* Forces of nature, cataclysmic
        storm
    cloudburst X37.8
    cyclone X37.1
    fall overboard (from) V92.09
      powered craft V92.03
        ferry boat V92.01
        fishing boat V92.02
        jetskis V92.03
        liner V92.01
        merchant ship V92.00
        passenger ship V92.01
      resulting from
        accident to watercraft —*see* Drowning,
          due to, accident to, watercraft
        being washed overboard (from)
          V92.29
          powered craft V92.23
            ferry boat V92.21
             fishing boat V92.22
             jetskis V92.23
             liner V92.21
             merchant ship V92.20
             passenger ship V92.21
          unpowered craft V92.28
            canoe V92.25
            inflatable V92.26
            kayak V92.25
            sailboat V92.24
            surf-board V92.28
            water skis V92.27
            windsurfer V92.28
        motion of watercraft V92.19
          powered craft V92.13
            ferry boat V92.11
            fishing boat V92.12
            jetskis V92.13
            liner V92.11
            merchant ship V92.10
            passenger ship V92.11
          unpowered craft
            canoe V92.15
            inflatable V92.16
            kayak V92.15
            sailboat V92.14
      unpowered craft V92.08
        canoe V92.05
        inflatable V92.06
        kayak V92.05

Drowning *(Continued)*
  due to *(Continued)*
    fall overboard *(Continued)*
      unpowered craft *(Continued)*
        sailboat V92.04
        surf-board V92.08
        water skis V92.07
        windsurfer V92.08
    hurricane X37.0
    jumping into water from watercraft
      (involved in accident) —*see also*
      Drowning, due to, accident to,
      watercraft
      without accident to or on watercraft
        W16.711
    tidal wave NEC —*see* Forces of nature,
      tidal wave
    torrential rain X37.8
  following
    fall
      into
        bathtub W16.211
        bucket W16.221
        fountain —*see* Drowning, following,
          fall, into, water, specified NEC
        quarry —*see* Drowning, following,
          fall, into, water, specified NEC
        reservoir —*see* Drowning, following,
          fall, into, water, specified NEC
        swimming-pool W16.011
          stated as undetermined whether
            accidental or intentional
            Y21.3
          striking
            bottom W16.021
            wall W16.031
          suicide (attempt) X71.2
        water NOS W16.41
          natural (lake) (open sea) (river)
            (stream) (pond) W16.111
            striking
              bottom W16.121
              side W16.131
          specified NEC W16.311
            striking
             bottom W16.321
             wall W16.331
      overboard NEC —*see* Drowning, due to,
        fall overboard
    jump or dive
      from boat W16.711
        striking bottom W16.721
      into
        fountain —*see* Drowning, following,
          jump or dive, into, water,
          specified NEC
        quarry —*see* Drowning, following,
          jump or dive, into, water,
          specified NEC
        reservoir —*see* Drowning, following,
          jump or dive, into, water,
          specified NEC
        swimming-pool W16.511
          striking
            bottom W16.521
            wall W16.531
          suicide (attempt) X71.2
        water NOS W16.91
          natural (lake) (open sea) (river)
            (stream) (pond) W16.611
          specified NEC W16.811
            striking
             bottom W16.821
             wall W16.831
          striking bottom W16.621

Drowning *(Continued)*
  homicide (attempt) X92.9
  in
    bathtub (accidental) W65
      assault X92.0
      following fall W16.211
        stated as undetermined whether
          accidental or intentional
          Y21.1
      stated as undetermined whether
        accidental or intentional Y21.0
      suicide (attempt) X71.0
    lake —*see* Drowning, in, natural water
    natural water (lake) (open sea) (river)
      (stream) (pond) W69
      assault X92.3
      following
        dive or jump W16.611
          striking bottom W16.621
        fall W16.111
          striking
            bottom W16.121
            side W16.131
      stated as undetermined whether
        accidental or intentional Y21.4
      suicide (attempt) X71.3
    quarry —*see* Drowning, in, specified place
      NEC
    quenching tank —*see* Drowning, in,
      specified place NEC
    reservoir —*see* Drowning, in, specified
      place NEC
    river —*see* Drowning, in, natural water
    sea —*see* Drowning, in, natural water
    specified place NEC W73
      assault X92.8
      following
        dive or jump W16.811
          striking
            bottom W16.821
            wall W16.831
        fall W16.311
          striking
            bottom W16.321
            wall W16.331
      stated as undetermined whether
        accidental or intentional Y21.8
      suicide (attempt) X71.8
    stream —*see* Drowning, in, natural water
    swimming-pool W67
      assault X92.1
        following fall X92.2
      following
        dive or jump W16.511
          striking
            bottom W16.521
            wall W16.531
        fall W16.011
          striking
            bottom W16.021
            wall W16.031
      stated as undetermined whether
        accidental or intentional Y21.2
        following fall Y21.3
      suicide (attempt) X71.1
        following fall X71.2
    war operations —*see* War operations,
      restriction of airway
  resulting from accident to watercraft —*see*
    Drowning, due to, accident, watercraft
  self-inflicted X71.9
  stated as undetermined whether accidental or
    intentional Y21.9
  suicide (attempt) X71.9

▶ New   ➡ Revised   ~~deleted~~ Deleted   ● Use Additional Character(s)

E

Earth (surface) movement NEC —*see* Forces of nature, earth movement
Earth falling (on) W20.0
  caused by cataclysmic earth surface movement or eruption —*see* Landslide
Earthquake (any injury) X34
Effect(s) (adverse) of
  air pressure (any) —*see* Air, pressure
  cold, excessive (exposure to) —*see* Exposure, cold
  heat (excessive) —*see* Heat
  hot place (weather) —*see* Heat
  insolation X30
  late —*see* Sequelae
  motion —*see* Motion
  nuclear explosion or weapon in war operations —*see* War operations, nuclear weapon
  radiation —*see* Radiation
  travel —*see* Travel
Electric shock (accidental) (by) (in) —*see* Exposure, electric current
Electrocution (accidental) —*see* Exposure, electric current
Endotracheal tube wrongly placed during anesthetic procedure Y65.3
Entanglement
  in
    bed linen, causing suffocation —*see* category T71
    wheel of pedal cycle V19.88
Entry of foreign body or material —*see* Foreign body
Environmental pollution related condition — *see* Z57
Execution, legal (any method) —*see* Legal, intervention
Exhaustion
  cold —*see* Exposure, cold
  due to excessive exertion —*see also* Overexertion X50.9
  heat —*see* Heat
Explosion (accidental) (of) (with secondary fire) W40.9
  acetylene W40.1
  aerosol can W36.1
  air tank (compressed) (in machinery) W36.2
  aircraft (in transit) (powered) NEC V95.9
    balloon V96.05
    fixed wing NEC (private) V95.25
      commercial V95.35
    glider V96.25
      hang V96.15
      powered V95.15
    helicopter V95.05
    in war operations —*see* War operations, destruction of aircraft
    microlight V95.15
    nonpowered V96.9
      specified NEC V96.8
    powered NEC V95.8
    stated as
      homicide (attempt) Y03.8
      suicide (attempt) X83.0
    ultralight V95.15
  anesthetic gas in operating room W40.1
  antipersonnel bomb W40.8
    assault X96.0
    homicide (attempt) X96.0
    suicide (attempt) X75
  assault X96.9
  bicycle tire W37.0
  blasting (cap) (materials) W40.0
  boiler (machinery), not on transport vehicle W35
    on watercraft —*see* Explosion, in, watercraft
  butane W40.1
  caused by other person X96.9
  coal gas W40.1

Explosion *(Continued)*
  detonator W40.0
  dump (munitions) W40.8
  dynamite W40.0
    in
      assault X96.8
      homicide (attempt) X96.8
      legal intervention
        injuring
          bystander Y35.112
          law enforcement personnel Y35.111
          suspect Y35.113
      suicide (attempt) X75
  explosive (material) W40.9
    gas W40.1
    in blasting operation W40.0
    specified NEC W40.8
      in
        assault X96.8
        homicide (attempt) X96.8
        legal intervention
          injuring
            bystander Y35.192
            law enforcement personnel Y35.191
            suspect Y35.193
        suicide (attempt) X75
  factory (munitions) W40.8
  fertilizer bomb W40.8
    assault X96.3
    homicide (attempt) X96.3
    suicide (attempt) X75
  fire-damp W40.1
  firearm (parts) NEC W34.19
    airgun W34.110
    BB gun W34.110
    gas, air or spring-operated gun NEC W34.118
    handgun W32.1
    hunting rifle W33.12
    larger firearm W33.10
      specified NEC W33.19
    machine gun W33.13
    paintball gun W34.111
    pellet gun W34.110
    shotgun W33.11
    Very pistol [flare] W34.19
  fireworks W39
  gas (coal) (explosive) W40.1
    cylinder W36.9
      aerosol can W36.1
      air tank W36.2
      pressurized W36.3
      specified NEC W36.8
  gasoline (fumes) (tank) not in moving motor vehicle W40.1
    bomb W40.8
      assault X96.1
      homicide (attempt) X96.1
      suicide (attempt) X75
    in motor vehicle —*see* Accident, transport, by type of vehicle
  grain store W40.8
  grenade W40.8
    in
      assault X96.8
      homicide (attempt) X96.8
      legal intervention
        injuring
          bystander Y35.192
          law enforcement personnel Y35.191
          suspect Y35.193
      suicide (attempt) X75
  handgun (parts) —*see* Explosion, firearm, handgun (parts)
  homicide (attempt) X96.9
    antipersonnel bomb —*see* Explosion, antipersonnel bomb
    fertilizer bomb —*see* Explosion, fertilizer bomb

Explosion *(Continued)*
  homicide *(Continued)*
    gasoline bomb —*see* Explosion, gasoline bomb
    letter bomb —*see* Explosion, letter bomb
    pipe bomb —*see* Explosion, pipe bomb
    specified NEC X96.8
  hose, pressurized W37.8
  hot water heater, tank (in machinery) W35
    on watercraft —*see* Explosion, in, watercraft
  in, on
    dump W40.8
    factory W40.8
    mine (of explosive gases) NEC W40.1
    watercraft V93.59
      powered craft V93.53
        ferry boat V93.51
        fishing boat V93.52
        jetskis V93.53
        liner V93.51
        merchant ship V93.50
        passenger ship V93.51
        sailboat V93.54
  letter bomb W40.8
    assault X96.2
    homicide (attempt) X96.2
    suicide (attempt) X75
  machinery —*see also* Contact, with, by type of machine
    on board watercraft —*see* Explosion, in, watercraft
    pressure vessel —*see* Explosion, by type of vessel
  methane W40.1
  mine W40.1
  missile NEC W40.8
  mortar bomb W40.8
    in
      assault X96.8
      homicide (attempt) X96.8
      legal intervention
        injuring
          bystander Y35.192
          law enforcement personnel Y35.191
          suspect Y35.193
      suicide (attempt) X75
  munitions (dump) (factory) W40.8
  pipe, pressurized W37.8
    bomb W40.8
      assault X96.4
      homicide (attempt) X96.4
      suicide (attempt) X75
  pressure, pressurized
    cooker W38
    gas tank (in machinery) W36.3
    hose W37.8
    pipe W37.8
    specified device NEC W38
    tire W37.8
      bicycle W37.0
    vessel (in machinery) W38
  propane W40.1
  self-inflicted X75
  shell (artillery) NEC W40.8
    during war operations —*see* War operations, explosion
    in
      legal intervention
        injuring
          bystander Y35.122
          law enforcement personnel Y35.121
          suspect Y35.123
    war —*see* War operations, explosion
  spacecraft V95.45
  stated as undetermined whether accidental or intentional Y25
  steam or water lines (in machinery) W37.8
  stove W40.9
  suicide (attempt) X75

Explosion (Continued)
- tire, pressurized W37.8
  - bicycle W37.0
- undetermined whether accidental or intentional Y25
- vehicle tire NEC W37.8
  - bicycle W37.0
- war operations —see War operations, explosion

Exposure (to) X58
- air pressure change —see Air, pressure
- cold (accidental) (excessive) (extreme) (natural) (place) X31
  - assault Y08.89
  - due to
    - man-made conditions W93.8
      - dry ice (contact) W93.01
        - inhalation W93.02
      - liquid air (contact) (hydrogen) (nitrogen) W93.11
        - inhalation W93.12
      - refrigeration unit (deep freeze) W93.2
    - suicide (attempt) X83.2
    - weather (conditions) X31
  - homicide (attempt) Y08.89
  - self-inflicted X83.2
- due to abandonment or neglect X58
- electric current W86.8
  - appliance (faulty) W86.8
    - domestic W86.0
  - caused by other person Y08.89
  - conductor (faulty) W86.1
  - control apparatus (faulty) W86.1
  - electric power generating plant, distribution station W86.1
  - electroshock gun —see Exposure, electric current, taser
  - high-voltage cable W85
  - homicide (attempt) Y08.89
  - legal execution —see Legal, intervention, specified means NEC
  - lightning —see subcategory T75.0
  - live rail W86.8
  - misadventure in medical or surgical procedure in electroshock therapy Y63.4
  - motor (electric) (faulty) W86.8
    - domestic W86.0
  - self-inflicted X83.1
  - specified NEC W86.8
    - domestic W86.0
  - stun gun —see Exposure, electric current, taser
  - suicide (attempt) X83.1
  - taser W86.8
    - assault Y08.89
    - legal intervention —see category Y35
    - self-harm (intentional) X83.8
    - undetermined intent Y33
  - third rail W86.8
  - transformer (faulty) W86.1
  - transmission lines W85
- environmental tobacco smoke X58
- excessive
  - cold —see Exposure, cold
  - heat (natural) NEC X30
    - man-made W92
- factor(s) NOS X58
  - environmental NEC X58
  - man-made NEC W99
  - natural NEC —see Forces of nature
  - specified NEC X58
- fire, flames (accidental) X08.8
  - assault X97
  - campfire —see Exposure, fire, controlled, not in building
  - controlled (in)
    - with ignition (of) clothing —see also Ignition, clothes X06.2
      - nightwear X05

Exposure (Continued)
- fire, flames (Continued)
  - controlled (Continued)
    - bonfire —see Exposure, fire, controlled, not in building
    - brazier (in building or structure) —see also Exposure, fire, controlled, building
      - not in building or structure —see Exposure, fire, controlled, not in building
    - building or structure X02.0
      - with
        - fall from building X02.3
        - from building X02.5
        - injury due to building collapse X02.2
        - smoke inhalation X02.1
      - hit by object from building X02.4
      - specified mode of injury NEC X02.8
    - fireplace, furnace or stove —see Exposure, fire, controlled, building
    - not in building or structure X03.0
      - with
        - fall X03.3
        - smoke inhalation X03.1
      - hit by object X03.4
      - specified mode of injury NEC X03.8
    - trash —see Exposure, fire, controlled, not in building
  - fireplace —see Exposure, fire, controlled, building
  - fittings or furniture (in building or structure) (uncontrolled) —see Exposure, fire, uncontrolled, building
  - forest (uncontrolled) —see Exposure, fire, uncontrolled, not in building
  - grass (uncontrolled) —see Exposure, fire, uncontrolled, not in building
  - hay (uncontrolled) —see Exposure, fire, uncontrolled, not in building
  - homicide (attempt) X97
  - ignition of highly flammable material X04
  - in, of, on, starting in
    - machinery —see Contact, with, by type of machine
    - motor vehicle (in motion) —see also Accident, transport, occupant by type of vehicle V87.8
      - with collision —see Collision
    - railway rolling stock, train, vehicle V81.81
      - with collision —see Accident, transport, railway vehicle occupant
    - street car (in motion) V82.8
      - with collision —see Accident, transport, streetcar occupant
    - transport vehicle NEC —see also Accident, transport
      - with collision —see Collision
    - war operations —see also War operations, fire
      - from nuclear explosion —see War operations, nuclear weapons
    - watercraft (in transit) (not in transit) V91.09
      - localized —see Burn, on board watercraft, due to, fire on board
      - powered craft V91.03
        - ferry boat V91.01
        - fishing boat V91.02
        - jet skis V91.03
        - liner V91.01
        - merchant ship V91.00
        - passenger ship V91.01
      - unpowered craft V91.08
        - canoe V91.05
        - inflatable V91.06
        - kayak V91.05
        - sailboat V91.04

Exposure (Continued)
- fire, flames (Continued)
  - in, of, on, starting in (Continued)
    - watercraft (Continued)
      - unpowered craft (Continued)
        - surf-board V91.08
        - waterskis V91.07
        - windsurfer V91.08
    - lumber (uncontrolled) —see Exposure, fire, uncontrolled, not in building
    - mine (uncontrolled) —see Exposure, fire, uncontrolled, not in building
    - prairie (uncontrolled) —see Exposure, fire, uncontrolled, not in building
  - resulting from
    - explosion —see Explosion
    - lightning X08.8
  - self-inflicted X76
  - specified NEC X08.8
  - started by other person X97
  - stated as undetermined whether accidental or intentional Y26
  - stove —see Exposure, fire, controlled, building
  - suicide (attempt) X76
  - tunnel (uncontrolled) —see Exposure, fire, uncontrolled, not in building
  - uncontrolled
    - in building or structure X00.0
      - with
        - fall from building X00.3
        - injury due to building collapse X00.2
        - jump from building X00.5
        - smoke inhalation X00.1
      - bed X08.00
        - due to
          - cigarette X08.01
          - specified material NEC X08.09
        - furniture NEC X08.20
          - due to
            - cigarette X08.21
            - specified material NEC X08.29
        - hit by object from building X00.4
        - sofa X08.10
          - due to
            - cigarette X08.11
            - specified material NEC X08.19
        - specified mode of injury NEC X00.8
    - not in building or structure (any) X01.0
      - with
        - fall X01.3
        - smoke inhalation X01.1
      - hit by object X01.4
      - specified mode of injury NEC X01.8
  - undetermined whether accidental or intentional Y26
- forces of nature NEC —see Forces of nature
- G-forces (abnormal) W49.9
- gravitational forces (abnormal) W49.9
- heat (natural) NEC —see Heat
- high-pressure jet (hydraulic) (pneumatic) W49.9
- hydraulic jet W49.9
- inanimate mechanical force W49.9
- jet, high-pressure (hydraulic) (pneumatic) W49.9
- lightning —see subcategory T75.0
  - causing fire —see Exposure, fire
- mechanical forces NEC W49.9
  - animate NEC W64
  - inanimate NEC W49.9
- noise W42.9
  - supersonic W42.0
- noxious substance —see Table of Drugs and Chemicals
- pneumatic jet W49.9

▶ New   ⇒ Revised   ~~deleted~~ Deleted   ● Use Additional Character(s)

Exposure *(Continued)*
    prolonged in deep-freeze unit or refrigerator
        W93.2
    radiation —*see* Radiation
    smoke —*see also* Exposure, fire
        tobacco, second hand Z77.22
    specified factors NEC X58
    sunlight X32
        man-made (sun lamp) W89.8
            tanning bed W89.1
    supersonic waves W42.0
    transmission line(s), electric W85
    vibration W49.9

Exposure *(Continued)*
    waves
        infrasound W49.9
        sound W42.9
        supersonic W42.0
    weather NEC —*see* Forces of nature
External cause status Y99.9
    child assisting in compensated work for
        family Y99.8
    civilian activity done for financial or other
        compensation Y99.0
    civilian activity done for income or pay
        Y99.0

External cause status *(Continued)*
    family member assisting in compensated
        work for other family member Y99.8
    hobby not done for income Y99.8
    leisure activity Y99.8
    military activity Y99.1
    off-duty activity of military personnel Y99.8
    recreation or sport not for income or while a
        student Y99.8
    specified NEC Y99.8
    student activity Y99.8
    volunteer activity Y99.2

F

Factors, supplemental
  alcohol
    blood level
      less than 20mg/100ml Y90.0
      presence in blood, level not specified
        Y90.9
      20-39mg/100ml Y90.1
      40-59mg/100ml Y90.2
      60-79mg/100ml Y90.3
      80-99mg/100ml Y90.4
      100-119mg/100ml Y90.5
      120-199mg/100ml Y90.6
      200-239mg/100ml Y90.7
      240mg/100ml or more Y90.8
      presence in blood, but level not specified
        Y90.9
  environmental-pollution-related condition —
    see Z57
  nosocomial condition Y95
  work-related condition Y99.0
Failure
  in suture or ligature during surgical
    procedure Y65.2
  mechanical, of instrument or apparatus
    (any) (during any medical or surgical
    procedure) Y65.8
  sterile precautions (during medical and
    surgical care) —see Misadventure,
    failure, sterile precautions, by type of
    procedure
  to
    introduce tube or instrument Y65.4
      endotracheal tube during anesthesia Y65.3
    make curve (transport vehicle) NEC —see
      Accident, transport
    remove tube or instrument Y65.4
Fall, falling (accidental) W19
  building W20.1
    burning (uncontrolled fire) X00.3
  down
    embankment W17.81
    escalator W10.0
    hill W17.81
    ladder W11
    ramp W10.2
    stairs, steps W10.9
  due to
    bumping against
      object W18.00
        sharp glass W18.02
        specified NEC W18.09
        sports equipment W18.01
      person W03
        due to ice or snow W00.0
        on pedestrian conveyance —see
          Accident, transport, pedestrian,
          conveyance
    collision with another person W03
      due to ice or snow W00.0
      involving pedestrian conveyance —see
        Accident, transport, pedestrian,
        conveyance
    grocery cart tipping over W17.82
    ice or snow W00.9
      from one level to another W00.2
        on stairs or steps W00.1
      involving pedestrian conveyance —see
        Accident, transport, pedestrian,
        conveyance
      on same level W00.0
    slipping (on moving sidewalk) W01.0
      with subsequent striking against object
        W01.10
        furniture W01.190
        sharp object W01.119
          glass W01.110
          power tool or machine W01.111
          specified NEC W01.118
        specified NEC W01.198

Fall, falling (Continued)
  due to (Continued)
    striking against
      object W18.00
        sharp glass W18.02
        specified NEC W18.09
        sports equipment W18.01
      person W03
        due to ice or snow W00.0
        on pedestrian conveyance —see
          Accident, transport, pedestrian,
          conveyance
  earth (with asphyxia or suffocation (by
    pressure)) —see Earth, falling
  from, off, out of
    aircraft NEC (with accident to aircraft
      NEC) V97.0
      while boarding or alighting V97.1
    balcony W13.0
    bed W06
    boat, ship, watercraft NEC (with
      drowning or submersion) —
      see Drowning, due to, fall
      overboard
      with hitting bottom or object V94.0
    bridge W13.1
    building W13.9
      burning (uncontrolled fire) X00.3
    cavity W17.2
    chair W07
    cherry picker W17.89
    cliff W15
    dock W17.4
    embankment W17.81
    escalator W10.0
    flagpole W13.8
    furniture NEC W08
    grocery cart W17.82
    haystack W17.89
    high place NEC W17.89
      stated as undetermined whether
        accidental or intentional Y30
    hole W17.2
    incline W10.2
    ladder W11
    lifting device W17.89
    machine, machinery —see also Contact,
      with, by type of machine
      not in operation W17.89
    manhole W17.1
    mobile elevated work platform [MEWP]
      W17.89
    motorized mobility scooter W05.2
    one level to another NEC W17.89
      intentional, purposeful, suicide
        (attempt) X80
      stated as undetermined whether
        accidental or intentional Y30
    pit W17.2
    playground equipment W09.8
      jungle gym W09.2
      slide W09.0
      swing W09.1
    quarry W17.89
    railing W13.9
    ramp W10.2
    roof W13.2
    scaffolding W12
    scooter (nonmotorized) W05.1
      motorized mobility W05.2
    sky lift W17.89
    stairs, steps W10.9
      curb W10.1
      due to ice or snow W00.1
      escalator W10.0
      incline W10.2
      ramp W10.2
      sidewalk curb W10.1
      specified NEC W10.8
    stepladder W11
    storm drain W17.1

Fall, falling (Continued)
  from, off, out of (Continued)
    streetcar NEC V82.6
      with antecedent collision —see
        Accident, transport, streetcar
        occupant
      while boarding or alighting V82.4
    structure NEC W13.8
      burning (uncontrolled fire) X00.3
    table W08
    toilet W18.11
      with subsequent striking against object
        W18.12
    train NEC V81.6
      during derailment (without antecedent
        collision) V81.7
      with antecedent collision —see
        Accident, transport, railway
        vehicle occupant
      while boarding or alighting V81.4
    transport vehicle after collision —see
      Accident, transport, by type of
      vehicle, collision
    tree W14
    vehicle (in motion) NEC —see also
      Accident, transport V89.9
      motor NEC —see also Accident,
        transport, occupant, by type of
        vehicle V87.8
      stationary W17.89
        while boarding or alighting —see
          Accident, transport, by type of
          vehicle, while boarding or
          alighting
    viaduct W13.8
    wall W13.8
    watercraft —see also Drowning, due to, fall
      overboard
      with hitting bottom or object V94.0
    well W17.0
    wheelchair, non-moving W05.0
      powered —see Accident, transport,
        pedestrian, conveyance occupant,
        specified type NEC
    window W13.4
  in, on
    aircraft NEC V97.0
      with accident to aircraft V97.0
      while boarding or alighting
        V97.1
    bathtub (empty) W18.2
      filled W16.212
        causing drowning W16.211
    escalator W10.0
    incline W10.2
    ladder W11
    machine, machinery —see Contact, with,
      by type of machine
    object, edged, pointed or sharp (with
      cut) —see Fall, by type
    playground equipment W09.8
      jungle gym W09.2
      slide W09.0
      swing W09.1
    ramp W10.2
    scaffolding W12
    shower W18.2
      causing drowning W16.211
    staircase, stairs, steps W10.9
      curb W10.1
      due to ice or snow W00.1
      escalator W10.0
      incline W10.2
      specified NEC W10.8
    streetcar (without antecedent collision)
      V82.5
      with antecedent collision —see
        Accident, transport, streetcar
        occupant
      while boarding or alighting
        V82.4

Fall, falling *(Continued)*
  in, on *(Continued)*
    train (without antecedent collision) V81.5
      with antecedent collision —*see* Accident,
        transport, railway vehicle occupant
      during derailment (without antecedent
        collision) V81.7
        with antecedent collision —*see*
          Accident, transport, railway
          vehicle occupant
      while boarding or alighting V81.4
    transport vehicle after collision —*see*
      Accident, transport, by type of
      vehicle, collision
    watercraft V93.39
      due to
        accident to craft V91.29
          powered craft V91.23
            ferry boat V91.21
            fishing boat V91.22
            jetskis V91.23
            liner V91.21
            merchant ship V91.20
            passenger ship V91.21
          unpowered craft
            canoe V91.25
            inflatable V91.26
            kayak V91.25
            sailboat V91.24
        powered craft V93.33
          ferry boat V93.31
          fishing boat V93.32
          jetskis V93.33
          liner V93.31
          merchant ship V93.30
          passenger ship V93.31
        unpowered craft V93.38
          canoe V93.35
          inflatable V93.36
          kayak V93.35
          sailboat V93.34
          surf-board V93.38
          windsurfer V93.38
  into
    cavity W17.2
    dock W17.4
    fire —*see* Exposure, fire, by type
    haystack W17.89
    hole W17.2
    manhole W17.1
    moving part of machinery —*see* Contact,
      with, by type of machine
    ocean —*see* Fall, into, water
    opening in surface NEC W17.89
    pit W17.2
    pond —*see* Fall, into, water
    quarry W17.89
    river —*see* Fall, into, water
    shaft W17.89
    storm drain W17.1
    stream —*see* Fall, into, water
    swimming pool —*see also* Fall, into, water,
      in, swimming pool
      empty W17.3
    tank W17.89
    water W16.42
      causing drowning W16.41
      from watercraft —*see* Drowning, due to,
        fall overboard
      hitting diving board W21.4
      in
        bathtub W16.212
          causing drowning W16.211
        bucket W16.222
          causing drowning W16.221
        natural body of water W16.112
          causing drowning W16.111
          striking
            bottom W16.122
              causing drowning
                W16.121

Fall, falling *(Continued)*
  into *(Continued)*
    water *(Continued)*
      in *(Continued)*
        natural body of water *(Continued)*
          striking *(Continued)*
            side W16.132
              causing drowning W16.131
        specified water NEC W16.312
          causing drowning W16.311
          striking
            bottom W16.322
              causing drowning W16.321
            wall W16.332
              causing drowning W16.331
        swimming pool W16.012
          causing drowning W16.011
          striking
            bottom W16.022
              causing drowning W16.021
            wall W16.032
              causing drowning W16.031
        utility bucket W16.222
          causing drowning W16.221
    well W17.0
  involving
    bed W06
    chair W07
    furniture NEC W08
    glass —*see* Fall, by type
    playground equipment W09.8
      jungle gym W09.2
      slide W09.0
      swing W09.1
    roller blades —*see* Accident, transport,
      pedestrian, conveyance
    skateboard(s) —*see* Accident, transport,
      pedestrian, conveyance
    skates (ice) (in line) (roller) —*see*
      Accident, transport, pedestrian,
      conveyance
    skis —*see* Accident, transport, pedestrian,
      conveyance
    table W08
    wheelchair, non-moving W05.0
      powered —*see* Accident, transport,
        pedestrian, conveyance, specified
        type NEC
  object —*see* Struck by, object, falling
  off
    toilet W18.11
      with subsequent striking against object
        W18.12
  on same level W18.30
    due to
      specified NEC W18.39
      stepping on an object W18.31
  out of
    bed W06
    building NEC W13.8
    chair W07
    furniture NEC W08
    wheelchair, non-moving W05.0
      powered —*see* Accident, transport,
        pedestrian, conveyance, specified
        type NEC
    window W13.4
  over
    animal W01.0
    cliff W15
    embankment W17.81
    small object W01.0
  rock W20.8
  same level W18.30
    from
      being crushed, pushed, or stepped on
        by a crowd or human stampede
        W52
      collision, pushing, shoving, by or with
        other person W03
      slipping, stumbling, tripping W01.0

Fall, falling *(Continued)*
  same level *(Continued)*
    involving ice or snow W00.0
      involving skates (ice) (roller),
        skateboard, skis —*see* Accident,
        transport, pedestrian, conveyance
    snowslide (avalanche) —*see* Landslide
    stone W20.8
    structure W20.1
      burning (uncontrolled fire) X00.3
    through
      bridge W13.1
      floor W13.3
      roof W13.2
      wall W13.8
      window W13.4
    timber W20.8
    tree (caused by lightning) W20.8
    while being carried or supported by other
      person(s) W04
Fallen on by
  animal (not being ridden) NEC W55.89
Felo-de-se —*see* Suicide
Fight (hand) (fists) (foot) —*see* Assault, fight
Fire (accidental) —*see* Exposure, fire
Firearm discharge —*see* Discharge, firearm
**Fireball effects from nuclear explosion in war
  operations** —*see* War operations, nuclear
  weapons
Fireworks (explosion) W39
Flash burns from explosion —*see* Explosion
Flood (any injury) (caused by) X38
  collapse of man-made structure causing earth
    movement X36.0
  tidal wave —*see* Forces of nature, tidal wave
Food (any type) in
  air passages (with asphyxia, obstruction, or
    suffocation) —*see* categories T17 and T18
  alimentary tract causing asphyxia (due to
    compression of trachea) —*see* categories
    T17 and T18
Forces of nature X39.8
  avalanche X36.1
    causing transport accident —*see* Accident,
      transport, by type of vehicle
  blizzard X37.2
  cataclysmic storm X37.9
    with flood X38
    blizzard X37.2
    cloudburst X37.8
    cyclone X37.1
    dust storm X37.3
    hurricane X37.0
    specified storm NEC X37.8
    storm surge X37.0
    tornado X37.1
    twister X37.1
    typhoon X37.0
  cloudburst X37.8
  cold (natural) X31
  cyclone X37.1
  dam collapse causing earth movement X36.0
  dust storm X37.3
  earth movement X36.1
    caused by dam or structure collapse X36.0
    earthquake X34
  earthquake X34
  flood (caused by) X38
    dam collapse X36.0
    tidal wave —*see* Forces of nature, tidal
      wave
  heat (natural) X30
  hurricane X37.0
  landslide X36.1
    causing transport accident —*see* Accident,
      transport, by type of vehicle
  lightning —*see* subcategory T75.0
    causing fire —*see* Exposure, fire
  mudslide X36.1
    causing transport accident —*see* Accident,
      transport, by type of vehicle

Forces of nature *(Continued)*
 radiation (natural) X39.Ø8
  radon X39.Ø1
 radon X39.Ø1
 specified force NEC X39.8
 storm surge X37.Ø
 structure collapse causing
   earth movement
   X36.Ø
 sunlight X32
 tidal wave X37.41
  due to
   earthquake X37.41
   landslide X37.43
   storm X37.42
   volcanic eruption X37.41
 tornado X37.1

Forces of nature *(Continued)*
 tsunami X37.41
 twister X37.1
 typhoon X37.Ø
 volcanic eruption X35
Foreign body
 aspiration —*see* Index to Diseases and
   Injuries, Foreign body, respitory
   tract
 embedded in skin W45
 entering through skin W45.8
  can lid W26.2
  nail W45.Ø
  paper W26.2
  specified NEC 45.8
  splinter W45.8

Forest fire (exposure to) —*see* Exposure, fire,
   uncontrolled, not in building
Found injured X58
 from exposure (to) —*see* Exposure
 on
   highway, road(way), street V89.9
   railway right of way V81.9
Fracture (circumstances unknown or
   unspecified) X58
 due to specified cause NEC X58
Freezing —*see* Exposure, cold
Frostbite X31
 due to man-made conditions —*see* Exposure,
   cold, man-made
Frozen —*see* Exposure, cold

G

Gored by bull W55.22
Gunshot wound W34.ØØ

H

Hailstones, injured by X39.8
Hanged herself or himself —*see* Hanging,
 self-inflicted
Hanging (accidental) —*see also* category T71
 legal execution —*see* Legal, intervention,
   specified means NEC
Heat (effects of) (excessive) X3Ø
 due to
   man-made conditions W92
    on board watercraft V93.29
     fishing boat V93.22
     merchant ship V93.2Ø
     passenger ship V93.21
     sailboat V93.24
     specified powered craft NEC V93.23
   weather (conditions) X3Ø

Heat *(Continued)*
 from
   electric heating apparatus causing
    burning X16
   nuclear explosion in war operations —
    see War operations, nuclear
    weapons
 inappropriate in local application or
   packing in medical or surgical
   procedure Y63.5
Hemorrhage
 delayed following medical or surgical
   treatment without mention of
   misadventure —*see* Index to Diseases
   and Injuries, Complication(s)
 during medical or surgical treatment as
   misadventure —*see* Index to Diseases
   and Injuries, Complication(s)

High
 altitude (effects) —*see* Air, pressure, low
 level of radioactivity, effects —*see* Radiation
 pressure (effects) —*see* Air, pressure, high
 temperature, effects —*see* Heat
Hit, hitting (accidental) by —*see* Struck by
Hitting against —*see* Striking against
Homicide (attempt) (justifiable) —*see* Assault
Hot
 place, effects —*see also* Heat
 weather, effects X3Ø
House fire (uncontrolled) —*see* Exposure, fire,
   uncontrolled, building
Humidity, causing problem X39.8
Hunger X58
Hurricane (any injury) X37.Ø
Hypobarism, hypobaropathy —*see* Air,
   pressure, low

▶ New   ⇒ Revised   ~~deleted~~ Deleted   ● Use Additional Character(s)

F, G, & H

I

Ictus
caloris —see also Heat
solaris X30
Ignition (accidental) —see also Exposure, fire
X08.8
anesthetic gas in operating room W40.1
apparel X06.2
from highly flammable material X04
nightwear X05
bed linen (sheets) (spreads) (pillows)
(mattress) —see Exposure, fire,
uncontrolled, building, bed
benzine X04
clothes, clothing NEC (from controlled fire)
X06.2
from
highly flammable material X04
ether X04
in operating room W40.1
explosive material —see Explosion
gasoline X04
jewelry (plastic) (any) X06.0
kerosene X04
material
explosive —see Explosion
highly flammable with secondary
explosion X04
nightwear X05
paraffin X04
petrol X04
Immersion (accidental) —see also Drowning
hand or foot due to cold (excessive) X31
Implantation of quills of porcupine
W55.89
Inanition (from) (hunger) X58
thirst X58.8
Inappropriate operation performed
correct operation on wrong side or body
part (wrong side) (wrong site)
Y65.53
operation intended for another patient done
on wrong patient Y65.52
wrong operation performed on correct
patient Y65.51
Inattention after, at birth (homicidal intent)
(infanticidal intent) X58
Incident, adverse
device
anesthesiology Y70.8
accessory Y70.2
diagnostic Y70.0
miscellaneous Y70.8
monitoring Y70.0
prosthetic Y70.2
rehabilitative Y70.1
surgical Y70.3
therapeutic Y70.1
cardiovascular Y71.8
accessory Y71.2
diagnostic Y71.0
miscellaneous Y71.8
monitoring Y71.0
prosthetic Y71.2
rehabilitative Y71.1
surgical Y71.3
therapeutic Y71.1
gastroenterology Y73.8
accessory Y73.2
diagnostic Y73.0
miscellaneous Y73.8
monitoring Y73.0
prosthetic Y73.2
rehabilitative Y73.1
surgical Y73.3
therapeutic Y73.1
general
hospital Y74.8
accessory Y74.2
diagnostic Y74.0

Incident, adverse (Continued)
device (Continued)
general (Continued)
hospital (Continued)
miscellaneous Y74.8
monitoring Y74.0
prosthetic Y74.2
rehabilitative Y74.1
surgical Y74.3
therapeutic Y74.1
surgical Y81.8
accessory Y81.2
diagnostic Y81.0
miscellaneous Y81.8
monitoring Y81.0
prosthetic Y81.2
rehabilitative Y81.1
surgical Y81.3
therapeutic Y81.1
gynecological Y76.8
accessory Y76.2
diagnostic Y76.0
miscellaneous Y76.8
monitoring Y76.0
prosthetic Y76.2
rehabilitative Y76.1
surgical Y76.3
therapeutic Y76.1
medical Y82.9
specified type NEC Y82.8
neurological Y75.8
accessory Y75.2
diagnostic Y75.0
miscellaneous Y75.8
monitoring Y75.0
prosthetic Y75.2
rehabilitative Y75.1
surgical Y75.3
therapeutic Y75.1
obstetrical Y76.8
accessory Y76.2
diagnostic Y76.0
miscellaneous Y76.8
monitoring Y76.0
prosthetic Y76.2
rehabilitative Y76.1
surgical Y76.3
therapeutic Y76.1
ophthalmic Y77.8
accessory Y77.2
diagnostic Y77.0
miscellaneous Y77.8
monitoring Y77.0
prosthetic Y77.2
rehabilitative Y77.1
surgical Y77.3
therapeutic Y77.1
orthopedic Y79.8
accessory Y79.2
diagnostic Y79.0
miscellaneous Y79.8
monitoring Y79.0
prosthetic Y79.2
rehabilitative Y79.1
surgical Y79.3
therapeutic Y79.1
otorhinolaryngological Y72.8
accessory Y72.2
diagnostic Y72.0
miscellaneous Y72.8
monitoring Y72.0
prosthetic Y72.2
rehabilitative Y72.1
surgical Y72.3
therapeutic Y72.1
personal use Y74.8
accessory Y74.2
diagnostic Y74.0
miscellaneous Y74.8
monitoring Y74.0
prosthetic Y74.2

Incident, adverse (Continued)
device (Continued)
personal use (Continued)
rehabilitative Y74.1
surgical Y74.3
therapeutic Y74.1
physical medicine Y80.8
accessory Y80.2
diagnostic Y80.0
miscellaneous Y80.8
monitoring Y80.0
prosthetic Y80.2
rehabilitative Y80.1
surgical Y80.3
therapeutic Y80.1
plastic surgical Y81.8
accessory Y81.2
diagnostic Y81.0
miscellaneous Y81.8
monitoring Y81.0
prosthetic Y81.2
rehabilitative Y81.1
surgical Y81.3
therapeutic Y81.1
radiological Y78.8
accessory Y78.2
diagnostic Y78.0
miscellaneous Y78.8
monitoring Y78.0
prosthetic Y78.2
rehabilitative Y78.1
surgical Y78.3
therapeutic Y78.1
urology Y73.8
accessory Y73.2
diagnostic Y73.0
miscellaneous Y73.8
monitoring Y73.0
prosthetic Y73.2
rehabilitative Y73.1
surgical Y73.3
therapeutic Y73.1
Incineration (accidental) —see Exposure, fire
Infanticide —see Assault
Infrasound waves (causing injury) W49.9
Ingestion
foreign body (causing injury) (with
obstruction) —see Foreign body,
alimentary canal
poisonous
plant(s) X58
substance NEC —see Table of Drugs and
Chemicals
Inhalation
excessively cold substance, man-made —see
Exposure, cold, man-made
food (any type) (into respiratory tract) (with
asphyxia, obstruction respiratory tract,
suffocation) —see categories T17 and T18
foreign body —see Foreign body, aspiration
gastric contents (with asphyxia, obstruction
respiratory passage, suffocation) T17.81-●
hot air or gases X14.0
liquid air, hydrogen, nitrogen W93.12
suicide (attempt) X83.2
steam X13.0
assault X98.0
stated as undetermined whether accidental
or intentional Y27.0
suicide (attempt) X77.0
toxic gas —see Table of Drugs and
Chemicals
vomitus (with asphyxia, obstruction
respiratory passage, suffocation) T17.81-●
Injury, injured (accidental(ly)) **NOS** X58
by, caused by, from
assault —see Assault
law-enforcing agent, police, in course
of legal intervention —see Legal
intervention
suicide (attempt) X83.8

▶ New ⟹ Revised ~~deleted~~ Deleted ● Use Additional Character(s)

587

I, J, & K

Injury, injured NOS *(Continued)*
  due to, in
    civil insurrection —*see* War
        operations
    fight —*see also* Assault, fight
        Y04.0
    war operations —*see* War
        operations
  homicide —*see also* Assault Y09
  inflicted (by)
    in course of arrest (attempted), suppression
        of disturbance, maintenance of order,
        by law-enforcing agents —*see* Legal
        intervention

Injury, injured NOS *(Continued)*
  inflicted *(Continued)*
    other person
      stated as
        accidental X58
        intentional, homicide (attempt) —*see*
            Assault
        undetermined whether accidental or
            intentional Y33
    purposely (inflicted) by other person(s) —*see*
        Assault
    self-inflicted X83.8
      stated as accidental X58
    specified cause NEC X58

Injury, injured NOS *(Continued)*
  undetermined whether accidental or
      intentional Y33
Insolation, effects X30
Insufficient nourishment X58
Interruption of respiration (by)
  food (lodged in esophagus) —*see* categories
      T17 and T18
  vomitus (lodged in esophagus) T17.81-●
Intervention, legal —*see* Legal intervention
Intoxication
  drug —*see* Table of Drugs and Chemicals
  poison —*see* Table of Drugs and
      Chemicals

J

Jammed (accidentally)
  between objects (moving) (stationary and
      moving) W23.0
    stationary W23.1
Jumped, jumping
  before moving object NEC X81.8
    motor vehicle X81.0
    subway train X81.1
    train X81.1
    undetermined whether accidental or
        intentional Y31
  from
    boat (into water) voluntarily,
        without accident (to or on boat)
        W16.712
      with
        accident to or on boat —*see* Accident,
            watercraft
        drowning or submersion W16.711
          suicide (attempt) X71.3

Jumped, jumping *(Continued)*
  from *(Continued)*
    boat voluntarily, without accident
        (Continued)
      striking bottom W16.722
        causing drowning W16.721
    building —*see also* Jumped, from,
        high place W13.9
      burning (uncontrolled fire)
          X00.5
    high place NEC W17.89
      suicide (attempt) X80
      undetermined whether accidental or
          intentional Y30
    structure —*see also* Jumped, from, high
        place W13.9
      burning (uncontrolled fire)
          X00.5
  into water W16.92
    causing drowning W16.91
    from, off watercraft —*see* Jumped, from,
        boat

Jumped, jumping *(Continued)*
  into water *(Continued)*
    in
      natural body W16.612
        causing drowning W16.611
        striking bottom W16.622
          causing drowning W16.621
      specified place NEC W16.812
        causing drowning W16.811
        striking
          bottom W16.822
            causing drowning W16.821
          wall W16.832
            causing drowning W16.831
      swimming pool W16.512
        causing drowning W16.511
        striking
          bottom W16.522
            causing drowning W16.521
          wall W16.532
            causing drowning W16.531
    suicide (attempt) X71.3

K

Kicked by
  animal NEC W55.82
  person(s) (accidentally) W50.1
    with intent to injure or kill Y04.0
    as, or caused by, a crowd or human
        stampede (with fall) W52
    assault Y04.0
    homicide (attempt) Y04.0
    in
      fight Y04.0
      legal intervention
        injuring
          bystander Y35.812
          law enforcement personnel
              Y35.811
          suspect Y35.813

Kicking
  against
    object W22.8
      sports equipment W21.9
      stationary W22.09
        sports equipment W21.89
    person —*see* Striking against, person
    sports equipment W21.9
  carpet stretcher with knee X50.3
Killed, killing (accidentally) NOS —*see also*
    Injury X58
  in
    action —*see* War operations
    brawl, fight (hand) (fists) (foot) Y04.0
      by weapon —*see also* Assault
        cutting, piercing —*see* Assault, cutting
            or piercing instrument
        firearm —*see* Discharge, firearm, by
            type, homicide

Killed, killing NOS *(Continued)*
  self
    stated as
      accident NOS X58
      suicide —*see* Suicide
      undetermined whether accidental or
          intentional Y33
Kneeling (prolonged) (static) X50.1
Knocked down (accidentally) (by) NOS X58
  animal (not being ridden) NEC —*see also*
      Struck by, by type of animal
  crowd or human stampede W52
  person W51
    in brawl, fight Y04.0
  transport vehicle NEC —*see also* Accident,
      transport V09.9

▶ New   ➡ Revised   ~~deleted~~ Deleted   ● Use Additional Character(s)

L

Laceration NEC —see Injury
Lack of
care (helpless person) (infant) (newborn) X58
food except as result of abandonment or
   neglect X58
   due to abandonment or neglect X58
water except as result of transport accident X58
   due to transport accident —see Accident,
     transport, by type
helpless person, infant, newborn X58
Landslide (falling on transport vehicle) X36.1
caused by collapse of man-made structure
   X36.0
Late effect —see Sequelae
Legal
execution (any method) —see Legal,
   intervention
intervention (by)
baton —see Legal, intervention, blunt
   object, baton
bayonet —see Legal, intervention, sharp
   object, bayonet
blow —see Legal, intervention,
   manhandling
blunt object
  baton
   injuring
    bystander Y35.312
    law enforcement personnel Y35.311
    suspect Y35.313
  injuring
   bystander Y35.302
   law enforcement personnel Y35.301
   suspect Y35.303
  specified NEC
   injuring
    bystander Y35.392
    law enforcement personnel Y35.391
    suspect Y35.393
  stave
   injuring
    bystander Y35.392
    law enforcement personnel Y35.391
    suspect Y35.393
bomb —see Legal, intervention, explosive
cutting or piercing instrument —see Legal,
   intervention, sharp object
dynamite —see Legal, intervention,
   explosive, dynamite
explosive(s)
  dynamite
   injuring
    bystander Y35.112
    law enforcement personnel Y35.111
    suspect Y35.113
  grenade
   injuring
    bystander Y35.192
    law enforcement personnel Y35.191
    suspect Y35.193
  injuring
   bystander Y35.102
   law enforcement personnel Y35.101
   suspect Y35.103

Legal (Continued)
intervention (Continued)
explosive (Continued)
  mortar bomb
   injuring
    bystander Y35.192
    law enforcement personnel
     Y35.191
    suspect Y35.193
  shell
   injuring
    bystander Y35.122
    law enforcement personnel Y35.121
    suspect Y35.123
  specified NEC
   injuring
    bystander Y35.192
    law enforcement personnel Y35.191
    suspect Y35.193
firearm(s) (discharge)
  handgun
   injuring
    bystander Y35.022
    law enforcement personnel Y35.021
    suspect Y35.023
  injuring
   bystander Y35.002
   law enforcement personnel Y35.001
   suspect Y35.003
  machine gun
   injuring
    bystander Y35.012
    law enforcement personnel Y35.011
    suspect Y35.013
  rifle pellet
   injuring
    bystander Y35.032
    law enforcement personnel Y35.031
    suspect Y35.033
  rubber bullet
   injuring
    bystander Y35.042
    law enforcement personnel Y35.041
    suspect Y35.043
  shotgun —see Legal, intervention,
   firearm, specified NEC
  specified NEC
   injuring
    bystander Y35.092
    law enforcement personnel Y35.091
    suspect Y35.093
gas (asphyxiation) (poisoning)
  injuring
   bystander Y35.202
   law enforcement personnel Y35.201
   suspect Y35.203
  specified NEC
   injuring
    bystander Y35.292
    law enforcement personnel Y35.291
    suspect Y35.293
  tear gas
   injuring
    bystander Y35.212
    law enforcement personnel Y35.211
    suspect Y35.213

Legal (Continued)
intervention (Continued)
grenade —see Legal, intervention,
   explosive, grenade
injuring
  bystander Y35.92
  law enforcement personnel Y35.91
  suspect Y35.93
late effect (of) —see with 7th character S
  Y35
manhandling
  injuring
   bystander Y35.812
   law enforcement personnel Y35.811
   suspect Y35.813
sequelae (of) —see with 7th character S
  Y35
sharp objects
  bayonet
   injuring
    bystander Y35.412
    law enforcement personnel
     Y35.411
    suspect Y35.413
  injuring
   bystander Y35.402
   law enforcement personnel Y35.401
   suspect Y35.403
  specified NEC
   injuring
    bystander Y35.492
    law enforcement personnel Y35.491
    suspect Y35.493
specified means NEC
  injuring
   bystander Y35.892
   law enforcement personnel Y35.891
   suspect Y35.893
stabbing —see Legal, intervention, sharp
  object
stave —see Legal, intervention, blunt
  object, stave
tear gas —see Legal, intervention, gas, tear
  gas
truncheon —see Legal, intervention, blunt
  object, stave
Lifting —see also Overexertion
heavy objects X50.0
weights X50.0
Lightning (shock) (stroke) (struck by) —see
  subcategory T75.0
causing fire —see Exposure, fire
Loss of control (transport vehicle) NEC —see
  Accident, transport
Lost at sea NOS —see Drowning, due to, fall
  overboard
Low
pressure (effects) —see Air, pressure, low
temperature (effects) —see Exposure, cold
Lying before train, vehicle or other moving
  object X81.8
subway train X81.1
train X81.1
undetermined whether accidental or
  intentional Y31
Lynching —see Assault

M

Malfunction (mechanism or component) (of)
  firearm
    airgun W34.10
    BB gun W34.110
    gas, air or spring-operated gun NEC
      W34.118
    handgun W32.1
    hunting rifle W33.12
    larger firearm W33.10
      specified NEC W33.19
    machine gun W33.13
    paintball gun W34.111
    pellet gun W34.110
    shotgun W33.11
    specified NEC W34.19
    Very pistol [flare] W34.19
  handgun —see Malfunction, firearm,
    handgun
Maltreatment —see Perpetrator
Mangled (accidentally) **NOS** X58
Manhandling (in brawl, fight) Y04.0
  legal intervention —see Legal, intervention,
    manhandling
Manslaughter (nonaccidental) —see Assault
Mauled by animal NEC W55.89
Medical procedure, complication of
    (delayed or as an abnormal reaction
    without mention of misadventure) —see
    Complication of or following, by specified
    type of procedure
  due to or as a result of misadventure —see
    Misadventure
Melting (due to fire) —see also Exposure, fire
  apparel NEC X06.3
  clothes, clothing NEC X06.3
    nightwear X05
  fittings or furniture (burning building)
    (uncontrolled fire) X00.8
  nightwear X05
  plastic jewelry X06.1
Mental cruelty X58
Military operations (injuries to military and
    civilians occuring during peacetime on
    military property and during routine
    military exercises and operations) (by)
    (from) (involving) Y37.90-●
  air blast Y37.20-●
  aircraft
    destruction —see Military operations,
      destruction of aircraft
    airway restriction —see Military operations,
      restriction of airways
  asphyxiation —see Military operations,
    restriction of airways
  biological weapons Y37.6X-●
  blast Y37.20-●
  blast fragments Y37.20-●
  blast wave Y37.20-●
  blast wind Y37.20-●
  bomb Y37.20-●
    dirty Y37.50-●
    gasoline Y37.31-●
    incendiary Y37.31-●
    petrol Y37.31-●
  bullet Y37.43-●
    incendiary Y37.32-●
    rubber Y37.41-●
  chemical weapons Y37.7X-●
  combat
    hand to hand (unarmed) combat
      Y37.44-●
    using blunt or piercing object Y37.45-●
  conflagration —see Military operations, fire
  conventional warfare NEC Y37.49-●
  depth-charge Y37.01-●
  destruction of aircraft Y37.10-●
    due to
      air to air missile Y37.11-●
      collision with other aircraft Y37.12-●

Military operations (Continued)
  destruction of aircraft (Continued)
    due to (Continued)
      detonation (accidental) of onboard
        munitions and explosives Y37.14-●
      enemy fire or explosives Y37.11-●
      explosive placed on aircraft Y37.11-●
      onboard fire Y37.13-●
      rocket propelled grenade [RPG] Y37.11-●
      small arms fire Y37.11-●
      surface to air missile Y37.11-●
    specified NEC Y37.19-●
  detonation (accidental) of
    onboard marine weapons Y37.05-●
    own munitions or munitions launch device
      Y37.24-●
  dirty bomb Y37.50-●
  explosion (of) Y37.20-●
    aerial bomb Y37.21-●
    bomb NOS —see also Military operations,
      bomb(s) Y37.20-●
    fragments Y37.20-●
    grenade Y37.29-●
    guided missile Y37.22-●
    improvised explosive device [IED]
      (person-borne) (roadside) (vehicle-
      borne) Y37.23-●
    land mine Y37.29-●
    marine mine (at sea) (in harbor) Y37.02-●
    marine weapon Y37.00-●
      specified NEC Y37.09-●
    own munitions or munitions launch device
      (accidental) Y37.24-●
    sea-based artillery shell Y37.03-●
    specified NEC Y37.29-●
    torpedo Y37.04-●
  fire Y37.30-●
    specified NEC Y37.39-●
  firearms
    discharge Y37.43-●
    pellets Y37.42-●
  flamethrower Y37.33-●
  fragments (from) (of)
    improvised explosive device [IED]
      (person-borne) (roadside) (vehicle-
      borne) Y37.26-●
    munitions Y37.25-●
    specified NEC Y37.29-●
    weapons Y37.27-●
  friendly fire Y37.92-●
  hand to hand (unarmed) combat Y37.44-●
  hot substances —see Military operations, fire
  incendiary bullet Y37.32-●
  nuclear weapon (effects of) Y37.50-●
    acute radiation exposure Y37.54-●
    blast pressure Y37.51-●
    direct blast Y37.51-●
    direct heat Y37.53-●
    fallout exposure Y37.54-●
    fireball Y37.53-●
    indirect blast (struck or crushed by blast
      debris) (being thrown by blast)
      Y37.52-●
    ionizing radiation (immediate exposure)
      Y37.54-●
    nuclear radiation Y37.54-●
    radiation
      ionizing (immediate exposure) Y37.54-●
      nuclear Y37.54-●
      thermal Y37.53-●
    secondary effects Y37.54-●
    specified NEC Y37.59-●
    thermal radiation Y37.53-●
  restriction of air (airway)
    intentional Y37.46-●
    unintentional Y37.47-●
  rubber bullets Y37.41-●
  shrapnel NOS Y37.29-●
  suffocation —see Military operations,
    restriction of airways
  unconventional warfare NEC Y37.7X-●

Military operations (Continued)
  underwater blast NOS Y37.00-●
  warfare
    conventional NEC Y37.49-●
    unconventional NEC Y37.7X-●
  weapon of mass destruction [WMD]
    Y37.91-●
  weapons
    biological weapons Y37.6X-●
    chemical Y37.7X-●
    nuclear (effects of) Y37.50-●
      acute radiation exposure Y37.54-●
      blast pressure Y37.51-●
      direct blast Y37.51-●
      direct heat Y37.53-●
      fallout exposure Y37.54-●
      fireball Y37.53-●
      radiation
        ionizing (immediate exposure)
          Y37.54-●
        nuclear Y37.54-●
        thermal Y37.53-●
      secondary effects Y37.54-●
      specified NEC Y37.59-●
    of mass destruction [WMD] Y37.91-●
**Misadventure(s) to patient(s) during surgical
    or medical care** Y69
  contaminated medical or biological substance
    (blood, drug, fluid) Y64.9
    administered (by) NEC Y64.9
      immunization Y64.1
      infusion Y64.0
      injection Y64.1
      specified means NEC Y64.8
      transfusion Y64.0
      vaccination Y64.1
  excessive amount of blood or other fluid
    during transfusion or infusion Y63.0
  failure
    in dosage Y63.9
      electroshock therapy Y63.4
      inappropriate temperature (too hot or
        too cold) in local application and
        packing Y63.5
      infusion
        excessive amount of fluid Y63.0
        incorrect dilution of fluid Y63.1
      insulin-shock therapy Y63.4
      nonadministration of necessary drug or
        biological substance Y63.6
      overdose —see Table of Drugs and
        Chemicals
        radiation, in therapy Y63.2
      radiation
        overdose Y63.2
      specified procedure NEC Y63.8
      transfusion
        excessive amount of blood Y63.0
    mechanical, of instrument or apparatus
      (any) (during any procedure) Y65.8
    sterile precautions (during procedure)
      Y62.9
      aspiration of fluid or tissue (by puncture
        or catheterization, except heart)
        Y62.6
      biopsy (except needle aspiration)
        Y62.8
        needle (aspirating) Y62.6
      blood sampling Y62.6
      catheterization Y62.6
        heart Y62.5
      dialysis (kidney) Y62.2
      endoscopic examination Y62.4
      enema Y62.8
      immunization Y62.3
      infusion Y62.1
      injection Y62.3
      needle biopsy Y62.6
      paracentesis (abdominal) (thoracic)
        Y62.6
      perfusion Y62.2

Misadventure(s) to patient(s) during surgical or medical care *(Continued)*
failure *(Continued)*
  sterile precautions *(Continued)*
    puncture (lumbar) Y62.6
    removal of catheter or packing Y62.8
    specified procedure NEC Y62.8
    surgical operation Y62.0
    transfusion Y62.1
    vaccination Y62.3
  suture or ligature during surgical procedure Y65.2
  to introduce or to remove tube or instrument —*see* Failure, to
hemorrhage —*see* Index to Diseases and Injuries, Complication(s)
inadvertent exposure of patient to radiation Y63.3
inappropriate
  operation performed —*see* Inappropriate operation performed
  temperature (too hot or too cold) in local application or packing Y63.5

Misadventure(s) to patient(s) during surgical or medical care *(Continued)*
infusion —*see also* Misadventure, by type, infusion Y69
  excessive amount of fluid Y63.0
  incorrect dilution of fluid Y63.1
  wrong fluid Y65.1
mismatched blood in transfusion Y65.0
nonadministration of necessary drug or biological substance Y63.6
overdose —*see* Table of Drugs and Chemicals
  radiation (in therapy) Y63.2
perforation —*see* Index to Diseases and Injuries, Complication(s)
performance of inappropriate operation —*see* Inappropriate operation performed
puncture —*see* Index to Diseases and Injuries, Complication(s)
specified type NEC Y65.8
  failure
    suture or ligature during surgical operation Y65.2
    to introduce or to remove tube or instrument —*see* Failure, to
  infusion of wrong fluid Y65.1

Misadventure(s) to patient(s) during surgical or medical care *(Continued)*
specified type NEC *(Continued)*
  performance of inappropriate operation —*see* Inappropriate operation performed
  transfusion of mismatched blood Y65.0
  wrong
    fluid in infusion Y65.1
    placement of endotracheal tube during anesthetic procedure Y65.3
transfusion —*see* Misadventure, by type, transfusion
  excessive amount of blood Y63.0
  mismatched blood Y65.0
wrong
  drug given in error —*see* Table of Drugs and Chemicals
  fluid in infusion Y65.1
  placement of endotracheal tube during anesthetic procedure Y65.3
Mismatched blood in transfusion Y65.0
Motion sickness T75.3
Mountain sickness W94.11
Mudslide (of cataclysmic nature) —*see* Landslide
Murder (attempt) —*see* Assault

N

Nail
contact with W45.0
  gun W29.4
embedded in skin W45.0
Neglect (criminal) (homicidal intent) X58

Noise (causing injury) (pollution) W42.9
  supersonic W42.0
Nonadministration (of)
drug or biological substance (necessary) Y63.6
surgical and medical care Y66
Nosocomial condition Y95

O

Object
falling
  from, in, on, hitting
    machinery —*see* Contact, with, by type of machine
set in motion by
  accidental explosion or rupture of pressure vessel W38
  firearm —*see* Discharge, firearm, by type
  machine (ry) —*see* Contact, with, by type of machine
Overdose (drug) —*see* Table of Drugs and Chemicals
radiation Y63.2

Overexertion X50.9
from
  prolonged static or awkward postures X50.1
  repetitive movements X50.3
  specified strenuous movements or postures NEC X50.9
  strenuous movement or load X50.0
Overexposure (accidental) (to)
cold —*see also* Exposure, cold X31
  due to man-made conditions —*see* Exposure, cold, man-made
heat —*see also* Heat X30
radiation —*see* Radiation
radioactivity W88.0
sun (sunburn) X32

Overexposure *(Continued)*
weather NEC —*see* Forces of nature
wind NEC —*see* Forces of nature
Overheated —*see* Heat
Overturning (accidental)
machinery —*see* Contact, with, by type of machine
transport vehicle NEC —*see also* Accident, transport V89.9
watercraft (causing drowning, submersion) —*see also* Drowning, due to, accident to, watercraft, overturning
  causing injury except drowning or submersion —*see* Accident, watercraft, causing, injury NEC

M, N, & O

P

Parachute descent (voluntary) (without accident to aircraft) V97.29
  due to accident to aircraft —*see* Accident, transport, aircraft
Pecked by bird W61.99
Perforation during medical or surgical treatment as misadventure —*see* Index to Diseases and Injuries, Complication(s)
Perpetrator, perpetration, of assault, maltreatment and neglect (by) Y07.9
  boyfriend Y07.03
  brother Y07.410
    stepbrother Y07.435
  coach Y07.53
  cousin
    female Y07.491
    male Y07.490
  daycare provider Y07.519
    at-home
      adult care Y07.512
      childcare Y07.510
    care center
      adult care Y07.513
      childcare Y07.511
  family member NEC Y07.499
  father Y07.11
    adoptive Y07.13
    foster Y07.420
    stepfather Y07.430
  foster father Y07.420
  foster mother Y07.421
  girl friend Y07.04
  healthcare provider Y07.529
    mental health Y07.521
    specified NEC Y07.528
  husband Y07.01
  instructor Y07.53
  mother Y07.12
    adoptive Y07.14
    foster Y07.421
    stepmother Y07.433
  nonfamily member Y07.50
    specified NEC Y07.59
  nurse Y07.528
  occupational therapist Y07.528
  partner of parent
    female Y07.434
    male Y07.432
  physical therapist Y07.528
  sister Y07.411
  speech therapist Y07.528
  stepbrother Y07.435
  stepfather Y07.430
  stepmother Y07.433
  stepsister Y07.436
  teacher Y07.53
  wife Y07.02
Piercing —*see* Contact, with, by type of object or machine
Pinched
  between objects (moving) (stationary and moving) W23.0
    stationary W23.1
Pinned under machine (ry) —*see* Contact, with, by type of machine
Place of occurrence Y92.9
  abandoned house Y92.89
  airplane Y92.813
  airport Y92.520
  ambulatory health services establishment NEC Y92.538
  ambulatory surgery center Y92.530
  amusement park Y92.831
  apartment (co-op) —*see* Place of occurrence, residence, apartment
  assembly hall Y92.29
  bank Y92.510
  barn Y92.71
  baseball field Y92.320

Place of occurrence (*Continued*)
  basketball court Y92.310
  beach Y92.832
  boarding house —*see* Place of occurrence, residence, boarding house
  boat Y92.814
  bowling alley Y92.39
  bridge Y92.89
  building under construction Y92.61
  bus Y92.811
    station Y92.521
  cafe Y92.511
  campsite Y92.833
  campus —*see* Place of occurrence, school
  canal Y92.89
  car Y92.810
  casino Y92.59
  children's home —*see* Place of occurrence, residence, institutional, orphanage
  church Y92.22
  cinema Y92.26
  clubhouse Y92.29
  coal pit Y92.64
  college (community) Y92.214
  condominium —*see* Place of occurrence, residence, apartment
  construction area —*see* Place of occurrence, industrial and construction area
  convalescent home —*see* Place of occurrence, residence, institutional, nursing home
  court-house Y92.240
  cricket ground Y92.328
  cultural building Y92.258
    art gallery Y92.250
    museum Y92.251
    music hall Y92.252
    opera house Y92.253
    specified NEC Y92.258
    theater Y92.254
  dancehall Y92.252
  day nursery Y92.210
  dentist office Y92.531
  derelict house Y92.89
  desert Y92.820
  dock NOS Y92.89
  dockyard Y92.62
  doctor's office Y92.531
  dormitory —*see* Place of occurrence, residence, institutional, school dormitory
  dry dock Y92.62
  factory (building) (premises) Y92.63
  farm (land under cultivation) (outbuildings) Y92.79
    barn Y92.71
    chicken coop Y92.72
    field Y92.73
    hen house Y92.72
    house —*see* Place of occurrence, residence, house
    orchard Y92.74
    specified NEC Y92.79
  football field Y92.321
  forest Y92.821
  freeway Y92.411
  gallery Y92.250
  garage (commercial) Y92.59
    boarding house Y92.044
    military base Y92.135
    mobile home Y92.025
    nursing home Y92.124
    orphanage Y92.114
    private house Y92.015
    reform school Y92.155
  gas station Y92.524
  gasworks Y92.69
  golf course Y92.39
  gravel pit Y92.64
  grocery Y92.512
  gymnasium Y92.39
  handball court Y92.318
  harbor Y92.89

Place of occurrence (*Continued*)
  harness racing course Y92.39
  healthcare provider office Y92.531
  highway (interstate) Y92.411
  hill Y92.828
  hockey rink Y92.330
  home —*see* Place of occurrence, residence
  hospice —*see* Place of occurrence, residence, institutional, nursing home
  hospital Y92.239
    cafeteria Y92.233
    corridor Y92.232
    operating room Y92.234
    patient
      bathroom Y92.231
      room Y92.230
    specified NEC Y92.238
  hotel Y92.59
  house —*see also* Place of occurrence, residence
    abandoned Y92.89
    under construction Y92.61
  industrial and construction area (yard) Y92.69
    building under construction Y92.61
    dock Y92.62
    dry dock Y92.62
    factory Y92.63
    gasworks Y92.69
    mine Y92.64
    oil rig Y92.65
    pit Y92.64
    power station Y92.69
    shipyard Y92.62
    specified NEC Y92.69
    tunnel under construction Y92.69
    workshop Y92.69
  kindergarten Y92.211
  lacrosse field Y92.328
  lake Y92.828
  library Y92.241
  mall Y92.59
  market Y92.512
  marsh Y92.828
  military
    base —*see* Place of occurrence, residence, institutional, military base
    training ground Y92.84
  mine Y92.64
  mosque Y92.22
  motel Y92.59
  motorway (interstate) Y92.411
  mountain Y92.828
  movie-house Y92.26
  museum Y92.251
  music-hall Y92.252
  not applicable Y92.9
  nuclear power station Y92.69
  nursing home —*see* Place of occurrence, residence, institutional, nursing home
  office building Y92.59
  offshore installation Y92.65
  oil rig Y92.65
  old people's home —*see* Place of occurrence, residence, institutional, specified NEC
  opera-house Y92.253
  orphanage —*see* Place of occurrence, residence, institutional, orphanage
  outpatient surgery center Y92.530
  park (public) Y92.830
    amusement Y92.831
  parking garage Y92.89
    lot Y92.481
  pavement Y92.480
  physician office Y92.531
  polo field Y92.328
  pond Y92.828
  post office Y92.242
  power station Y92.69
  prairie Y92.828
  prison —*see* Place of occurrence, residence, institutional, prison

▶ New   ➡ Revised   ~~deleted~~ Deleted   ● Use Additional Character(s)

Place of occurrence *(Continued)*
- public
  - administration building Y92.248
    - city hall Y92.243
    - courthouse Y92.240
    - library Y92.241
    - post office Y92.242
    - specified NEC Y92.248
  - building NEC Y92.29
  - hall Y92.29
  - place NOS Y92.89
- race course Y92.39
- radio station Y92.59
- railway line (bridge) Y92.85
- ranch (outbuildings) —*see* Place of occurrence, farm
- recreation area Y92.838
  - amusement park Y92.831
  - beach Y92.832
  - campsite Y92.833
  - park (public) Y92.830
  - seashore Y92.832
  - specified NEC Y92.838
- reform school —*see* Place of occurrence, residence, institutional, reform school
- religious institution Y92.22
- residence (non-institutional) (private) Y92.009
  - apartment Y92.039
    - bathroom Y92.031
    - bedroom Y92.032
    - kitchen Y92.030
    - specified NEC Y92.038
  - bathroom Y92.002
  - bedroom Y92.003
  - boarding house Y92.049
    - bathroom Y92.041
    - bedroom Y92.042
    - driveway Y92.043
    - garage Y92.044
    - garden Y92.046
    - kitchen Y92.040
    - specified NEC Y92.048
    - swimming pool Y92.045
    - yard Y92.046
  - dining room Y92.001
  - garden Y92.007
  - home Y92.009
  - house, single family Y92.019
    - bathroom Y92.012
    - bedroom Y92.013
    - dining room Y92.011
    - driveway Y92.014
    - garage Y92.015
    - garden Y92.017
    - kitchen Y92.010
    - specified NEC Y92.018
    - swimming pool Y92.016
    - yard Y92.017
  - institutional Y92.10
    - children's home —*see* Place of occurrence, residence, institutional, orphanage
    - hospice —*see* Place of occurrence, residence, institutional, nursing home
    - military base Y92.139
      - barracks Y92.133
      - garage Y92.135
      - garden Y92.137
      - kitchen Y92.130
      - mess hall Y92.131
      - specified NEC Y92.138
      - swimming pool Y92.136
      - yard Y92.137
    - nursing home Y92.129
      - bathroom Y92.121
      - bedroom Y92.122
      - driveway Y92.123
      - garage Y92.124
      - garden Y92.126
      - kitchen Y92.120

Place of occurrence *(Continued)*
- residence *(Continued)*
  - institutional *(Continued)*
    - nursing home *(Continued)*
      - specified NEC Y92.128
      - swimming pool Y92.125
      - yard Y92.126
    - orphanage Y92.119
      - bathroom Y92.111
      - bedroom Y92.112
      - driveway Y92.113
      - garage Y92.114
      - garden Y92.116
      - kitchen Y92.110
      - specified NEC Y92.118
      - swimming pool Y92.115
      - yard Y92.116
    - prison Y92.149
      - bathroom Y92.142
      - cell Y92.143
      - courtyard Y92.147
      - dining room Y92.141
      - kitchen Y92.140
      - specified NEC Y92.148
      - swimming pool Y92.146
    - reform school Y92.159
      - bathroom Y92.152
      - bedroom Y92.153
      - dining room Y92.151
      - driveway Y92.154
      - garage Y92.155
      - garden Y92.157
      - kitchen Y92.150
      - specified NEC Y92.158
      - swimming pool Y92.156
      - yard Y92.157
    - school dormitory Y92.169
      - bathroom Y92.162
      - bedroom Y92.163
      - dining room Y92.161
      - kitchen Y92.160
      - specified NEC Y92.168
    - specified NEC Y92.199
      - bathroom Y92.192
      - bedroom Y92.193
      - dining room Y92.191
      - driveway Y92.194
      - garage Y92.195
      - garden Y92.197
      - kitchen Y92.190
      - specified NEC Y92.198
      - swimming pool Y92.196
      - yard Y92.197
  - kitchen Y92.000
  - mobile home Y92.029
    - bathroom Y92.022
    - bedroom Y92.023
    - dining room Y92.021
    - driveway Y92.024
    - garage Y92.025
    - garden Y92.027
    - kitchen Y92.020
    - specified NEC Y92.028
    - swimming pool Y92.026
    - yard Y92.027
  - specified place in residence NEC Y92.008
  - specified residence type NEC Y92.099
    - bathroom Y92.091
    - bedroom Y92.092
    - driveway Y92.093
    - garage Y92.094
    - garden Y92.096
    - kitchen Y92.090
    - specified NEC Y92.098
    - swimming pool Y92.095
    - yard Y92.096
  - restaurant Y92.511
  - riding school Y92.39
  - river Y92.828
  - road Y92.488
  - rodeo ring Y92.39

Place of occurrence *(Continued)*
- rugby field Y92.328
- same day surgery center Y92.530
- sand pit Y92.64
- school (private) (public) (state) Y92.219
  - college Y92.214
  - daycare center Y92.210
  - elementary school Y92.211
  - high school Y92.213
  - kindergarten Y92.211
  - middle school Y92.212
  - specified NEC Y92.218
  - trace school Y92.215
  - university Y92.214
  - vocational school Y92.215
- sea (shore) Y92.832
- senior citizen center Y92.29
- service area
  - airport Y92.520
  - bus station Y92.521
  - gas station Y92.524
  - highway rest stop Y92.523
  - railway station Y92.522
- shipyard Y92.62
- shop(commercial) Y92.513
- sidewalk Y92.480
- silo Y92.79
- skating rink (roller) Y92.331
  - ice Y92.330
- slaughter house Y92.86
- soccer field Y92.322
- specified place NEC Y92.89
- sports area Y92.39
  - athletic
    - court Y92.318
      - basketball Y92.310
      - specified NEC Y92.318
      - squash Y92.311
      - tennis Y92.312
    - field Y92.328
      - baseball Y92.320
      - cricket ground Y92.328
      - football Y92.321
      - hockey Y92.328
      - soccer Y92.322
      - specified NEC Y92.328
  - golf course Y92.39
  - gymnasium Y92.39
  - riding school Y92.39
  - skating rink (roller) Y92.331
    - ice Y92.330
  - stadium Y92.39
  - swimming pool Y92.34
- squash court Y92.311
- stadium Y92.39
- steeplechasing course Y92.39
- store Y92.512
- stream Y92.828
- street and highway Y92.410
  - bike path Y92.482
  - freeway Y92.411
  - highway ramp Y92.415
  - interstate highway Y92.411
  - local residential or business street Y92.414
  - motorway Y92.411
  - parking lot Y92.481
  - parkway Y92.412
  - sidewalk Y92.480
  - specified NEC Y92.488
  - state road Y92.413
- subway car Y92.816
- supermarket Y92.512
- swamp Y92.828
- swimming pool (public) Y92.34
  - private (at) Y92.095
    - boarding house Y92.045
    - military base Y92.136
    - mobile home Y92.026
    - nursing home Y92.125
    - orphanage Y92.115

Place of occurrence (Continued)
  swimming pool (Continued)
    private (Continued)
      prison Y92.146
      reform school Y92.156
      single family residence
        Y92.016
  synagogue Y92.22
  television station Y92.59
  tennis court Y92.312
  theater Y92.254
  trade area Y92.59
    bank Y92.510
    cafe Y92.511
    casino Y92.59
    garage Y92.59
    hotel Y92.59
    market Y92.512
    office building Y92.59
    radio station Y92.59
    restaurant Y92.511
    shop Y92.513
    shopping mall Y92.59
    store Y92.512
    supermarket Y92.512
    television station Y92.59
    warehouse Y92.59
  trailer park, residential —see Place of
    occurrence, residence, mobile
    home
  trailer site NOS Y92.89
  train Y92.815
    station Y92.522
  truck Y92.812
  tunnel under construction Y92. 69
  university Y92.214
  urgent (health) care center Y92.532
  vehicle (transport) Y92.818
    airplane Y92.813
    boat Y92.814
    bus Y92.811
    car Y92.810
    specified NEC Y92.818
    subway car Y92.816
    train Y92.815
    truck Y92.812
  warehouse Y92.59
  water reservoir Y92.89
  wilderness area Y92.828
    desert Y92.820
    forest Y92.821
    marsh Y92.828
    mountain Y92.828
    prairie Y92.828
    specified NEC Y92.828
    swamp Y92.828
  workshop Y92.69
  yard, private Y92.096
    boarding house Y92.046
    mobile home Y92.027
    single family house Y92.017

Place of occurrence (Continued)
  youth center Y92.29
  zoo (zoological garden) Y92.834
Plumbism —see Table of Drugs and Chemicals,
  lead
Poisoning (accidental) (by) —see also Table of
  Drugs and Chemicals
  by plant, thorns, spines, sharp leaves or other
    mechanisms NEC X58
  carbon monoxide
    generated by
      motor vehicle —see Accident, transport
      watercraft (in transit) (not in transit)
        V93.89
        ferry boat V93.81
        fishing boat V93.82
        jet skis V93.83
        liner V93.81
        merchant ship V93.80
        passenger ship V93.81
        powered craft NEC V93.83
  caused by injection of poisons into skin by
    plant thorns, spines, sharp leaves X58
    marine or sea plants (venomous) X58
  exhaust gas
    generated by
      motor vehicle —see Accident, transport
      watercraft (in transit) (not in transit)
        V93.89
        ferry boat V93.81
        fishing boat V93.82
        jet skis V93.83
        liner V93.81
        merchant ship V93.80
        passenger ship V93.81
        powered craft NEC V93.83
  fumes or smoke due to
    explosion —see also Explosion W40.9
    fire —see Exposure, fire
    ignition —see Ignition
  gas
    in legal intervention —see Legal,
      intervention, gas
    legal execution —see Legal, intervention,
      gas
  in war operations —see War operations
  legal
    execution —see Legal, intervention, gas
    intervention
      by gas —see Legal, intervention, gas
      other specified means —see Legal,
        intervention, specified means
        NEC
Powder burn (by) (from)
  airgun W34.110
  BB gun W34.110
  firearm NEC W34.19
  gas, air or spring-operated gun NEC
    W34.118
  handgun W32.1
  hunting rifle W33.12

Powder burn (Continued)
  larger firearm W33.10
    specified NEC W33.19
  machine gun W33.13
  paintball gun W34.111
  pellet gun W34.110
  shotgun W33.11
  Very pistol [flare] W34.19
Premature cessation (of) surgical and medical
  care Y66
Privation (food) (water) X58
Procedure (operation)
  correct, on wrong side or body part (wrong
    side) (wrong site) Y65.53
  intended for another patient done on wrong
    patient Y65.52
  performed on patient not scheduled for
    surgery Y65.52
  performed on wrong patient Y65.52
  wrong, performed on correct patient Y65.51
Prolonged
  sitting in transport vehicle —see Travel, by
    type of vehicle
  stay in
    high altitude as cause of anoxia,
      barodontalgia, barotitis or hypoxia
      W94.11
    weightless environment X52
Pulling, excessive —see also Overexertion
  X50.9
Puncture, puncturing —see also Contact, with,
  by type of object or machine
  by
    plant thorns, spines, sharp leaves or other
      mechanisms NEC W60
  during medical or surgical treatment as
    misadventure —see Index to Diseases
    and Injuries, Complication(s)
Pushed, pushing (accidental) (injury in)
  by other person(s) (accidental) W51
    with fall W03
      due to ice or snow W00.0
    as, or caused by, a crowd or human
      stampede (with fall) W52
    before moving object NEC Y02.8
      motor vehicle Y02.0
      subway train Y02.1
      train Y02.1
    from
      high place NEC
        in accidental circumstances W17.89
        stated as
          intentional, homicide (attempt) Y01
          undetermined whether accidental
            or intentional Y30
        transport vehicle NEC —see also
          Accident, transport V89.9
        stated as
          intentional, homicide (attempt)
            Y08.89
      overexertion X50.9

▶ New   ⇒ Revised   ~~deleted~~ Deleted   ● Use Additional Character(s)

R

Radiation (exposure to)
arc lamps W89.0
atomic power plant (malfunction) NEC
    W88.1
complication of or abnormal reaction to
    medical radiotherapy Y84.2
electromagnetic, ionizing W88.0
gamma rays W88.1
in
    war operations (from or following
        nuclear explosion) —*see also* War
        operations
inadvertent exposure of patient (receiving
    test or therapy) Y63.3
infrared (heaters and lamps) W90.1
    excessive heat from W92
ionized, ionizing (particles, artificially
        accelerated)
    radioisotopes W88.1
    specified NEC W88.8
    x-rays W88.0
isotopes, radioactive —*see* Radiation,
    radioactive isotopes
laser(s) W90.2
    in war operations —*see* War operations
    misadventure in medical care Y63.2
light sources (man-made visible and
        ultraviolet) W89.9
    natural X32
    specified NEC W89.8
    tanning bed W89.1
    welding light W89.0
man-made visible light W89.9
    specified NEC W89.8
    tanning bed W89.1
    welding light W89.0
microwave W90.8
misadventure in medical or surgical
    procedure Y63.2

Radiation (*Continued*)
natural NEC X39.08
    radon X39.01
overdose (in medical or surgical procedure)
        Y63.2
radar W90.0
radioactive isotopes (any) W88.1
    atomic power plant malfunction W88.1
    misadventure in medical or surgical
        treatment Y63.2
radiofrequency W90.0
radium NEC W88.1
sun X32
ultraviolet (light) (man-made) W89.9
    natural X32
    specified NEC W89.8
    tanning bed W89.1
    welding light W89.0
welding arc, torch, or light W89.0
    excessive heat from W92
x-rays (hard) (soft) W88.0
Range disease W94.11
Rape (attempted) T74.2-●
Rat bite W53.11
Reaching (prolonged) (static) X50.1
Reaction, abnormal to medical procedure —*see
    also* Complication of or following, by type
    of procedure Y84.9
with misadventure —*see* Misadventure
biologicals —*see* Table of Drugs and
    Chemicals
drugs —*see* Table of Drugs and Chemicals
vaccine —*see* Table of Drugs and
    Chemicals
Recoil
airgun W34.110
BB gun W34.110
firearm NEC W34.19
gas, air or spring-operated gun NEC W34.118

Recoil (*Continued*)
handgun W32.1
hunting rifle W33.12
larger firearm W33.10
    specified NEC W33.19
machine gun W33.13
paintball gun W34.111
pellet W34.110
shotgun W33.11
Very pistol [flare] W34.19
Reduction in
atmospheric pressure —*see* Air, pressure,
    change
Rock falling on or hitting (accidentally)
    (person) W20.8
in cave-in W20.0
Run over (accidentally) (by)
animal (not being ridden) NEC W55.89
machinery —*see* Contact, with, by specified
    type of machine
transport vehicle NEC —*see also* Accident,
    transport V09.9
    intentional homicide (attempt) Y03.0
    motor NEC V09.20
        intentional homicide (attempt) Y03.0
Running
before moving object X81.8
    motor vehicle X81.0
Running off, away
animal (being ridden) —*see also* Accident,
    transport V80.918
    not being ridden W55.89
animal-drawn vehicle NEC —*see also*
    Accident, transport V80.928
highway, road(way), street
    transport vehicle NEC —*see also* Accident,
        transport V89.9
Rupture pressurized devices —*see* Explosion,
    by type of device

S

Saturnism —see Table of Drugs and Chemicals, lead
Scald, scalding (accidental) (by) (from) (in) X19
  air (hot) X14.1
  gases (hot) X14.1
  homicide (attempt) —see Assault, burning, hot object
  inflicted by other person
    stated as intentional, homicide (attempt) —see Assault, burning, hot object
  liquid (boiling) (hot) NEC X12
    stated as undetermined whether accidental or intentional Y27.2
    suicide (attempt) X77.2
  local application of externally applied substance in medical or surgical care Y63.5
  metal (molten) (liquid) (hot) NEC X18
  self-inflicted X77.9
  stated as undetermined whether accidental or intentional Y27.8
  steam X13.1
    assault X98.0
    stated as undetermined whether accidental or intentional Y27.0
    suicide (attempt) X77.0
  suicide (attempt) X77.9
  vapor (hot) X13.1
    assault X98.0
    stated as undetermined whether accidental or intentional Y27.0
    suicide (attempt) X77.0
Scratched by
  cat W55.03
  person(s) (accidentally) W50.4
    with intent to injure or kill Y04.0
    as, or caused by, a crowd or human stampede (with fall) W52
    assault Y04.0
    homicide (attempt) Y04.0
    in
      fight Y04.0
      legal intervention
        injuring
          bystander Y35.892
          law enforcement personnel Y35.891
          suspect Y35.893
Seasickness T75.3
Self-harm NEC —see also External cause by type, undetermined whether accidental or intentional
  intentional —see Suicide
  poisoning NEC —see Table of drugs and biologicals, accident
Self-inflicted (injury) NEC —see also External cause by type, undetermined whether accidental or intentional
  intentional —see Suicide
  poisoning NEC —see Table of drugs and biologicals, accident
Sequelae (of)
  accident NEC —see W00-X58 with 7th character S
  assault (homicidal) (any means) —see X92-Y08 with 7th character S
  homicide, attempt (any means) —see X92-Y08 with 7th character S
  injury undetermined whether accidentally or purposely inflicted —see Y21-Y33 with 7th character S
  intentional self-harm (classifiable to X71-X83) —see X71-X83 with 7th character S
  legal intervention (see with 7th character S Y35)
  motor vehicle accident —see V00-V99 with 7th character S
  suicide, attempt (any means) —see X71-X83 with 7th character S

Sequelae (Continued)
  transport accident —see V00-V99 with 7th character S
  war operations —see War operations
Shock
  electric —see Exposure, electric current
  from electric appliance (any) (faulty) W86.8
    domestic W86.0
    suicide (attempt) X83.1
Shooting, shot (accidental (ly)) —see also Discharge, firearm, by type
  herself or himself —see Discharge, firearm by type, self-inflicted
  homicide (attempt) —see Discharge, firearm by type, homicide
  in war operations —see War operations
  inflicted by other person —see Discharge, firearm by type, homicide
    accidental —see Discharge, firearm, by type of firearm
  legal
    execution —see Legal, intervention, firearm
    intervention —see Legal, intervention, firearm
  self-inflicted —see Discharge, firearm by type, suicide
    accidental —see Discharge, firearm, by type of firearm
  suicide (attempt) —see Discharge, firearm by type, suicide
Shoving (accidentally) by other person —see Pushed, by other person
Sickness
  alpine W94.11
  motion —see Motion
  mountain W94.11
Sinking (accidental)
  watercraft (causing drowning, submersion) —see also Drowning, due to, accident to, watercraft, sinking
    causing injury except drowning or submersion —see Accident, watercraft, causing, injury NEC
Siriasis X32
Sitting (prolonged) (static) X50.1
Slashed wrists —see Cut, self-inflicted
Slipping (accidental) (on same level) (with fall) W01.0
  without fall W18.40
    due to
      specified NEC W18.49
      stepping from one level to another W18.43
      stepping into hole or opening W18.42
      stepping on object W18.41
  on
    ice W00.0
      with skates —see Accident, transport, pedestrian, conveyance
    mud W01.0
    oil W01.0
    snow W00.0
      with skis —see Accident, transport, pedestrian, conveyance
    surface (slippery) (wet) NEC W01.0
Sliver, wood, contact with W45.8
Smoldering (due to fire) —see Exposure, fire
Sodomy (attempted) by force T74.2-●
Sound waves (causing injury) W42.9
  supersonic W42.0
Splinter, contact with W45.8
Stab, stabbing —see Cut
Standing (prolonged) (static) X50.1
Starvation X58
Status of external cause Y99.9
  child assisting in compensated work for family Y99.8
  civilian activity done for financial or other compensation Y99.0
  civilian activity done for income or pay Y99.0

Status of external cause (Continued)
  family member assisting in compensated work for other family member Y99.8
  hobby not done for income Y99.8
  leisure activity Y99.8
  military activity Y99.1
  off-duty activity of military personnel Y99.8
  recreation or sport not for income or while a student Y99.8
  specified NEC Y99.8
  student activity Y99.8
  volunteer activity Y99.2
Stepped on
  by
    animal (not being ridden) NEC W55.89
    crowd or human stampede W52
    person W50.0
Stepping on
  object W22.8
    with fall W18.31
    sports equipment W21.9
    stationary W22.09
      sports equipment W21.89
  person W51
    by crowd or human stampede W52
  sports equipment W21.9
Sting
  arthropod, nonvenomous W57
  insect, nonvenomous W57
Storm (cataclysmic) —see Forces of nature, cataclysmic storm
Straining, excessive —see also Overexertion X50.9
Strangling —see Strangulation
Strangulation (accidental) —see category T71
Strenuous movements —see also Overexertion X50.9
Striking against
  airbag (automobile) W22.10
    driver side W22.11
    front passenger side W22.12
    specified NEC W22.19
  bottom when
    diving or jumping into water (in) W16.822
      causing drowning W16.821
      from boat W16.722
        causing drowning W16.721
      natural body W16.622
        causing drowning W16.821
      swimming pool W16.522
        causing drowning W16.521
    falling into water (in) W16.322
      causing drowning W16.321
      fountain —see Striking against, bottom when, falling into water, specified NEC
      natural body W16.122
        causing drowning W16.121
      reservoir —see Striking against, bottom when, falling into water, specified NEC
      specified NEC W16.322
        causing drowning W16.321
      swimming pool W16.022
        causing drowning W16.021
  diving board (swimming-pool) W21.4
  object W22.8
    with
      drowning or submersion —see Drowning
      fall —see Fall, due to, bumping against, object
    caused by crowd or human stampede (with fall) W52
    furniture W22.03
    lamppost W22.02
    sports equipment W21.9
    stationary W22.09
      sports equipment W21.89
    wall W22.01

▶ New   ⇒ Revised   ~~deleted~~ Deleted   ● Use Additional Character(s)

Striking against *(Continued)*
  person(s) W51
    with fall W03
      due to ice or snow W00.0
    as, or caused by, a crowd or human
      stampede (with fall) W52
    assault Y04.2
    homicide (attempt) Y04.2
  sports equipment W21.9
  wall (when) W22.01
    diving or jumping into water (in) W16.832
      causing drowning W16.831
      swimming pool W16.532
        causing drowning W16.531
    falling into water (in) W16.332
      causing drowning W16.331
      fountain —*see* Striking against, wall
        when, falling into water, specified
        NEC
      natural body W16.132
        causing drowning W16.131
      reservoir —*see* Striking against, wall
        when, falling into water, specified
        NEC
      specified NEC W16.332
        causing drowning W16.331
      swimming pool W16.032
        causing drowning W16.031
    swimming pool (when) W22.042
      causing drowning W22.041
      diving or jumping into water W16.532
        causing drowning W16.531
      falling into water W16.032
        causing drowning W16.031
Struck (accidentally) by
  airbag (automobile) W22.10
    driver side W22.11
    front passenger side W22.12
    specified NEC W22.19
  alligator W58.02
  animal (not being ridden) NEC W55.89
  avalanche —*see* Landslide
  ball (hit) (thrown) W21.00
    assault Y08.09
    baseball W21.03
    basketball W21.05
    football W21.01
    golf ball W21.04
    football W21.01
    soccer W21.02
    softball W21.07
    specified NEC W21.09
    volleyball W21.06
  bat or racquet
    baseball bat W21.11
      assault Y08.02
    golf club W21.13
      assault Y08.09
    specified NEC W21.19
      assault Y08.09
    tennis racquet W21.12
      assault Y08.09
  bullet —*see also* Discharge, firearm by type
    in war operations —*see* War operations
  crocodile W58.12
  dog W54.1
  flare, Very pistol —*see* Discharge, firearm
    NEC
  hailstones X39.8
  hockey (ice)
    field
      puck W21.221
      stick W21.211
    puck W21.220
    stick W21.210
      assault Y08.01
  landslide —*see* Landslide
  law-enforcement agent (on duty) —*see* Legal,
    intervention, manhandling
    with blunt object —*see* Legal, intervention,
      blunt object

Struck by *(Continued)*
  lightning —*see* subcategory T75.0
    causing fire —*see* Exposure, fire
  machine —*see* Contact, with, by type of
    machine
  mammal NEC W55.89
    marine W56.32
  marine animal W56.82
  missile
    firearm —*see* Discharge, firearm by type
    in war operations —*see* War operations,
      missile
  object W22.8
    blunt W22.8
      assault Y00
      suicide (attempt) X79
      undetermined whether accidental or
        intentional Y29
    falling W20.8
      from, in, on
        building W20.1
          burning (uncontrolled fire) X00.4
        cataclysmic
          earth surface movement NEC —*see*
            Landslide
          storm —*see* Forces of nature,
            cataclysmic storm
        cave-in W20.0
        earthquake X34
        machine (in operation) —*see* Contact,
          with, by type of machine
        structure W20.1
          burning X00.4
        transport vehicle (in motion) —*see*
          Accident, transport, by type of
          vehicle
        watercraft V93.49
          due to
            accident to craft V91.39
              powered craft V91.33
                ferry boat V91.31
                fishing boat V91.32
                jetskis V91.33
                liner V91.31
                merchant ship V91.30
                passenger ship V91.31
             unpowered craft V91.38
                canoe V91.35
                inflatable V91.36
                kayak V91.35
                sailboat V91.34
                surf-board V91.38
                windsurfer V91.38
            powered craft V93.43
              ferry boat V93.41
              fishing boat V93.42
              jetskis V93.43
              liner V93.41
              merchant ship V93.40
              passenger ship V93.41
            unpowered craft V93.48
              sailboat V93.44
              surf-board V93.48
              windsurfer V93.48
    moving NEC W20.8
    projected W20.8
      assault Y00
      in sports W21.9
        assault Y08.09
        ball W21.00
          baseball W21.03
          basketball W21.05
          football W21.01
          golf ball W21.04
          soccer W21.02
          softball W21.07
          specified NEC W21.09
          volleyball W21.06
        bat or racquet
          baseball bat W21.11
            assault Y08.02

Struck by *(Continued)*
  object *(Continued)*
    projected *(Continued)*
      in sports *(Continued)*
        bat or racquet *(Continued)*
          golf club W21.13
            assault Y08.09-•
          specified NEC W21.19
            assault Y08.09
          tennis racquet W21.12
            assault Y08.09
        hockey (ice)
          field
            puck W21.221
            stick W21.211
          puck W21.220
          stick W21.210
            assault Y08.01
        specified NEC W21.89
    set in motion by explosion —*see* Explosion
    thrown W20.8
      assault Y00
      in sports W21.9
        assault Y08.09
        ball W21.00
          baseball W21.03
          basketball W21.05
          football W21.01
          golf ball W21.04
          soccer W21.02
          soft ball W21.07
          specified NEC W21.09
          volleyball W21.06
        bat or racquet
          baseball bat W21.11
            assault Y08.02
          golf club W21.13
            assault Y08.09
          specified NEC W21.19
            assault Y08.09
          tennis racquet W21.12
            assault Y08.09
        hockey (ice)
          field
            puck W21.221
            stick W21.211
          puck W21.220
          stick W21.210
            assault Y08.01
        specified NEC W21.89
  other person(s) W50.0
    with
      blunt object W22.8
        intentional, homicide (attempt) Y00
        sports equipment W21.9
        undetermined whether accidental or
          intentional Y29
      fall W03
        due to ice or snow W00.0
    as, or caused by, a crowd or human
      stampede (with fall) W52
    assault Y04.2
    homicide (attempt) Y04.2
    in legal intervention
      injuring
        bystander Y35.812
        law enforcement personnel Y35.811
        suspect Y35.813
    sports equipment W21.9
  police (on duty) —*see* Legal, intervention,
    manhandling
    with blunt object —*see* Legal, intervention,
      blunt object
  sports equipment W21.9
    assault Y08.09
    ball W21.00
      baseball W21.03
      basketball W21.05
      football W21.01
      golf ball W21.04
      soccer W21.02

▶ New   ⇒ Revised   ~~deleted~~ Deleted   • Use Additional Character(s)

Struck by (Continued)
  sports equipment (Continued)
    ball (Continued)
      soft ball W21.07
      specified NEC W21.09
      volleyball W21.06
    bat or racquet
      baseball bat W21.11
        assault Y08.02
      golf club W21.13
        assault Y08.09
      specified NEC W21.19
      tennis racquet W21.12
        assault Y08.09
    cleats (shoe) W21.31
    foot wear NEC W21.39
    football helmet W21.81
    hockey (ice)
      field
        puck W21.221
        stick W21.211
      puck W21.220
      stick W21.210
        assault Y08.01
    skate blades W21.32
    specified NEC W21.89
      assault Y08.09
  thunderbolt —see subcategory
    T75.0
  causing fire —see Exposure, fire
  transport vehicle NEC —see also Accident,
    transport V09.9
    intentional, homicide (attempt) Y03.0
    motor NEC —see also Accident, transport
      V09.20
      homicide Y03.0
  vehicle (transport) NEC —see Accident,
    transport, by type of vehicle
    stationary (falling from jack,
      hydraulic lift, ramp)
      W20.8
Stumbling
  without fall W18.40
    due to
      specified NEC W18.49
      stepping from one level to another
        W18.43
      stepping into hole or opening W18.42
      stepping on object W18.41
  over
    animal NEC W01.0
      with fall W18.09
    carpet, rug or (small) object W22.8
      with fall W18.09
    person W51
      with fall W03
        due to ice or snow W00.0

Submersion (accidental) —see Drowning
Suffocation (accidental) (by external means)
    (by pressure) (mechanical) —see also
    category T71
  due to, by
    avalanche —see Landslide
    explosion —see Explosion
    fire —see Exposure, fire
    food, any type (aspiration) (ingestion)
      (inhalation) —see categories T17 and
      T18
    ignition —see Ignition
    landslide —see Landslide
    machine (ry) —see Contact, with, by type
      of machine
    vomitus (aspiration) (inhalation)
      T17.81-●
  in
    burning building X00.8
Suicide, suicidal (attempted) (by) X83.8
  blunt object X79
  burning, burns X76
    hot object X77.9
      fluid NEC X77.2
      household appliance X77.3
      specified NEC X77.8
      steam X77.0
      tap water X77.1
      vapors X77.0
  caustic substance —see Table of Drugs and
    Chemicals
  cold, extreme X83.2
  collision of motor vehicle with
    motor vehicle X82.0
    specified NEC X82.8
    train X82.1
    tree X82.2
  crashing of aircraft X83.0
  cut (any part of body) X78.9
  cutting or piercing instrument X78.9
    dagger X78.2
    glass X78.0
    knife X78.1
    specified NEC X78.8
    sword X78.2
  drowning (in) X71.9
    bathtub X71.0
    natural water X71.3
    specified NEC X71.8
    swimming pool X71.1
      following fall X71.2
  electrocution X83.1
  explosive(s) (material) X75
  fire, flames X76
  firearm X74.9
    airgun X74.01
    handgun X72

Suicide, suicidal (Continued)
  firearm (Continued)
    hunting rifle X73.1
    larger X73.9
      specified NEC X73.8
    machine gun X73.2
    shotgun X73.0
    specified NEC X74.8
  hanging X83.8
  hot object —see Suicide, burning, hot object
  jumping
    before moving object X81.8
      motor vehicle X81.0
      subway train X81.1
      train X81.1
    from high place X80
  late effect of attempt —see X71-X83 with 7th
    character S
  lying before moving object, train, vehicle X81.8
  poisoning —see Table of Drugs and
    Chemicals
  puncture (any part of body) —see Suicide,
    cutting or piercing instrument
  scald —see Suicide, burning, hot object
  sequelae of attempt —see X71-X83 with 7th
    character S
  sharp object (any) —see Suicide, cutting or
    piercing instrument
  shooting —see Suicide, firearm
  specified means NEC X83.8
  stab (any part of body) —see Suicide, cutting
    or piercing instrument
  steam, hot vapors X77.0
  strangulation X83.8
  submersion —see Suicide, drowning
  suffocation X83.8
  wound NEC X83.8
Sunstroke X32
Supersonic waves (causing injury) W42.0
Surgical procedure, complication of (delayed
    or as an abnormal reaction without
    mention of misadventure) —see also
    Complication of or following, by type of
    procedure
  due to or as a result of misadventure —see
    Misadventure
Swallowed, swallowing
  foreign body —see Foreign body, alimentary
    canal
  poison —see Table of Drugs and Chemicals
  substance
    caustic or corrosive —see Table of Drugs
      and Chemicals
      poisonous —see Table of Drugs and
        Chemicals

T

Tackle in sport W03
Terrorism (involving) Y38.80
  biological weapons Y38.6X-●
  chemical weapons Y38.7X-●
  conflagration Y38.3X-●
  drowning and submersion Y38.89-●
  explosion Y38.2X-●
    destruction of aircraft Y38.1X-●
    marine weapons Y38.0X-●
  fire Y38.3X-●
  firearms Y38.4X-●
  hot substances Y38.3X-●
  lasers Y38.89-●
  nuclear weapons Y38.5X-●
  piercing or stabbing instruments
    Y38.89-●
  secondary effects Y38.9X-●
  specified method NEC Y38.89-●
  suicide bomber Y38.81-●
Thirst X58
Threat to breathing
  aspiration —*see* Aspiration
  due to cave-in, falling earth or substance
    NEC —*see* category T71
Thrown (accidentally)
  against part (any) of or object in transport
    vehicle (in motion) NEC —*see also*
    Accident, transport

Thrown *(Continued)*
  from
    high place, homicide (attempt) Y01
    machinery —*see* Contact, with, by type of
      machine
    transport vehicle NEC —*see also* Accident,
      transport V89.9
  off —*see* Thrown, from
Thunderbolt —*see* subcategory T75.0
  causing fire —*see* Exposure, fire
Tidal wave (any injury) NEC —*see* Forces of
  nature, tidal wave
Took
  overdose (drug) —*see* Table of Drugs and
    Chemicals
  poison —*see* Table of Drugs and
    Chemicals
Tornado (any injury) X37.1
Torrential rain (any injury) X37.8
Torture X58
Trampled by animal NEC W55.89
Trapped (accidentally)
  between objects (moving) (stationary and
    moving) —*see* Caught
  by part (any) of
    motorcycle V29.88
    pedal cycle V19.88
    transport vehicle NEC —*see also* Accident,
      transport V89.9
Travel (effects) (sickness) T75.3

Tree falling on or hitting (accidentally)
  (person) W20.8
Tripping
  without fall W18.40
    due to
      specified NEC W18.49
      stepping from one level to another
        W18.43
      stepping into hole or opening
        W18.42
      stepping on object W18.41
  over
    animal W01.0
      with fall W01.0
    carpet, rug or (small) object W22.8
      with fall W18.09
    person W51
      with fall W03
        due to ice or snow W00.0
Twisted by person(s) (accidentally) W50.2
  with intent to injure or kill Y04.0
  as, or caused by, a crowd or human stampede
    (with fall) W52
  assault Y04.0
  homicide (attempt) Y04.0
  in
    fight Y04.0
    legal intervention —*see* Legal, intervention,
      manhandling
Twisting (prolonged) (static) X50.1

U

Underdosing of necessary drugs, medicaments
  or biological substances Y63.6
Undetermined intent (contact)
  (exposure)
    automobile collision Y32
  blunt object Y29
  drowning (submersion) (in) Y21.9
    bathtub Y21.0
      after fall Y21.1
    natural water (lake) (ocean) (pond) (river)
      (stream) Y21.4
    specified place NEC Y21.8
    swimming pool Y21.2
      after fall Y21.3
  explosive material Y25
  fall, jump or push from high place Y30
  falling, lying or running before moving object
    Y31
  fire Y26

Undetermined intent *(Continued)*
  firearm discharge Y24.9
    airgun (BB) (pellet) Y24.0
    handgun (pistol) (revolver)
      Y22
    hunting rifle Y23.1
    larger Y23.9
      hunting rifle Y23.1
      machine gun Y23.3
      military Y23.2
      shotgun Y23.0
      specified type NEC Y23.8
    machine gun Y23.3
    military Y23.2
    shotgun Y23.0
    specified type NEC Y24.8
    Very pistol Y24.8
  hot object Y27.9
    fluid NEC Y27.2
    household appliance Y27.3
    specified object NEC Y27.8

Undetermined intent *(Continued)*
  hot object *(Continued)*
    steam Y27.0
    tap water Y27.1
    vapor Y27.0
  jump, fall or push from high place Y30
  lying, falling or running before moving object
    Y31
  motor vehicle crash Y32
  push, fall or jump from high place Y30
  running, falling or lying before moving object
    Y31
  sharp object Y28.9
    dagger Y28.2
    glass Y28.0
    knife Y28.1
    specified object NEC Y28.8
    sword Y28.2
  smoke Y26
  specified event NEC Y33
Use of hand as hammer X50.3

V

Vibration (causing injury) W49.9
Victim (of)
  avalanche —*see* Landslide
  earth movements NEC —*see* Forces of nature,
    earth movement
  earthquake X34

Victim *(Continued)*
  flood —*see* Flood
  landslide —*see* Landslide
  lightning —*see* subcategory T75.0
    causing fire —*see* Exposure, fire
  storm (cataclysmic) NEC —*see* Forces of
    nature, cataclysmic storm
  volcanic eruption X35

Volcanic eruption (any injury) X35
Vomitus, gastric contents in air passages (with
  asphyxia, obstruction or
  suffocation) T17.81-●

▶ New   ⮕ Revised   ~~deleted~~ Deleted   ● Use Additional Character(s)

W

Walked into stationary object (any) W22.09
  furniture W22.03
  lamppost W22.02
  wall W22.01
War operations (injuries to military personnel
    and civilians during war, civil insurrection
    and peacekeeping missions) (by) (from)
    (involving) Y36.90-•
  after cessation of hostilities Y36.89-•
    explosion (of)
      bomb placed during war operations
        Y36.82-•
      mine placed during war operations
        Y36.81-•
    specified NEC Y36.88-•
  air blast Y36.20-•
  aircraft
    destruction —see War operations,
      destruction of aircraft
  airway restriction —see War operations,
    restriction of airways
  asphyxiation —see War operations, restriction
    of airways
  biological weapons Y36.6X-•
  blast Y36.20-•
  blast fragments Y36.20-•
  blast wave Y36.20-•
  blast wind Y36.20-•
  bomb Y36.20-•
    dirty Y36.50-•
    gasoline Y36.31-•
    incendiary Y36.31-•
    petrol Y36.31-•
  bullet Y36.43-•
    incendiary Y36.32-•
    rubber Y36.41-•
  chemical weapons Y36.7X-•
  combat
    hand to hand (unarmed) combat Y36.44-•
    using blunt or piercing object Y36.45-•
  conflagration —see War operations, fire
  conventional warfare NEC Y36.49-•
  depth-charge Y36.01-•
  destruction of aircraft Y36.10-•
    due to
      air to air missile Y36.11-•
      collision with other aircraft Y36.12-•
      detonation (accidental) of onboard
        munitions and explosives Y36.14-•
      enemy fire or explosives Y36.11-•
      explosive placed on aircraft Y36.11-•
      onboard fire Y36.13-•
      rocket propelled grenade [RPG] Y36.11-•
      small arms fire Y36.11-•
      surface to air missile Y36.11-•
    specified NEC Y36.19-•
  detonation (accidental) of
    onboard marine weapons Y36.05-•
    own munitions or munitions launch device
      Y36.24-•

War operations (Continued)
  dirty bomb Y36.50-•
  explosion (of) Y36.20-•
    aerial bomb Y36.21-•
    after cessation of hostilities
      bomb placed during war operations
        Y36.82-•
      mine placed during war operations
        Y36.81-•
    bomb NOS —see also War operations,
      bomb(s) Y36.20-•
    fragments Y36.20-•
    grenade Y36.29-•
    guided missile Y36.22-•
    improvised explosive device [IED]
      (person-borne) (roadside)
      (vehicle-borne) Y36.23-•
    land mine Y36.29-•
    marine mine (at sea) (in harbor)
      Y36.02-•
    marine weapon Y36.00-•
      specified NEC Y36.09-•
    own munitions or munitions launch
      device (accidental) Y36.24-•
    sea-based artillery shell Y36.03-•
    specified NEC Y36.29-•
    torpedo Y36.04-•
  fire Y36.30-•
    specified NEC Y36.39-•
  firearms
    discharge Y36.43-•
    pellets Y36.42-•
  flamethrower Y36.33-•
  fragments (from) (of)
    improvised explosive device [IED]
      (person-borne) (roadside)
      (vehicle-borne) Y36.26-•
    munitions Y36.25-•
    specified NEC Y36.29-•
    weapons Y36.27-•
  friendly fire Y36.92
  hand to hand (unarmed) combat
    Y36.44-•
  hot substances —see War operations,
    fire
  incendiary bullet Y36.32-•
  nuclear weapon (effects of) Y36.50-•
    acute radiation exposure Y36.54-•
    blast pressure Y36.51-•
    direct blast Y36.51-•
    direct heat Y36.53-•
    fallout exposure Y36.54-•
    fireball Y36.53-•
    indirect blast (struck or crushed by blast
      debris) (being thrown by blast)
      Y36.52-•
    ionizing radiation (immediate exposure)
      Y36.54-•
    nuclear radiation Y36.54-•
    radiation
      ionizing (immediate exposure)
        Y36.54-•

War operations (Continued)
  nuclear weapon (Continued)
    radiation (Continued)
      nuclear Y36.54-•
      thermal Y36.53-•
    secondary effects Y36.54-•
    specified NEC Y36.59-•
    thermal radiation Y36.53-•
  restriction of air (airway)
    intentional Y36.46-•
    unintentional Y36.47-•
  rubber bullets Y36.41-•
  shrapnel NOS Y36.29-•
  suffocation —see War operations, restriction
    of airways
  unconventional warfare NEC Y36.7X-•
  underwater blast NOS Y36.00-•
  warfare
    conventional NEC Y36.49-•
    unconventional NEC Y36.7X-•
  weapon of mass destruction [WMD] Y36.91
  weapons
    biological weapons Y36.6X-•
    chemical Y36.7X-•
    nuclear (effects of) Y36.50-•
      acute radiation exposure Y36.54-•
      blast pressure Y36.51-•
      direct blast Y36.51-•
      direct heat Y36.53-•
      fallout exposure Y36.54-•
      fireball Y36.53-•
      radiation
        ionizing (immediate exposure)
          Y36.54-•
        nuclear Y36.54-•
        thermal Y36.53-•
      secondary effects Y36.54-•
      specified NEC Y36.59-•
    of mass destruction [WMD] Y36.91-•
Washed
  away by flood —see Flood
  off road by storm (transport vehicle) —see
    Forces of nature, cataclysmic storm
Weather exposure NEC —see Forces of nature
Weightlessness (causing injury) (effects of) (in
    spacecraft, real or simulated) X52
Work related condition Y99.0
Wound (accidental) NEC —see also Injury X58
  battle —see also War operations Y36.90
  gunshot —see Discharge, firearm by type
Wreck transport vehicle NEC —see also
  Accident, transport V89.9
Wrong
  device implanted into correct surgical site
    Y65.51
  fluid in infusion Y65.1
  patient, procedure performed on Y65.52
  procedure (operation) on correct patient
    Y65.51

▶ New   ⇒ Revised   ~~deleted~~ Deleted   • Use Additional Character(s)

PART III

ICD-10-CM Tabular List of Diseases and Injuries

CHAPTER 1

CERTAIN INFECTIOUS AND PARASITIC DISEASES (A00-B99)

OGCR Chapter-Specific Coding Guidelines

1. **Chapter 1: Certain Infectious and Parasitic Diseases (A00-B99)**

   a. **Human Immunodeficiency Virus (HIV) Infections**

      1) **Code only confirmed cases**

      Code only confirmed cases of HIV infection/illness. This is an exception to the hospital inpatient guideline Section II, H.

      In this context, "confirmation" does not require documentation of positive serology or culture for HIV; the provider's diagnostic statement that the patient is HIV positive, or has an HIV-related illness is sufficient.

      2) **Selection and sequencing of HIV codes**

         (a) **Patient admitted for HIV-related condition**

         If a patient is admitted for an HIV-related condition, the principal diagnosis should be B20, Human immunodeficiency virus [HIV] disease followed by additional diagnosis codes for all reported HIV-related conditions.

         (b) **Patient with HIV disease admitted for unrelated condition**

         If a patient with HIV disease is admitted for an unrelated condition (such as a traumatic injury), the code for the unrelated condition (e.g., the nature of injury code) should be the principal diagnosis. Other diagnoses would be B20 followed by additional diagnosis codes for all reported HIV-related conditions.

         (c) **Whether the patient is newly diagnosed**

         Whether the patient is newly diagnosed or has had previous admissions/encounters for HIV conditions is irrelevant to the sequencing decision.

         (d) **Asymptomatic human immunodeficiency virus**

         Z21, Asymptomatic human immunodeficiency virus [HIV] infection status, is to be applied when the patient without any documentation of symptoms is listed as being "HIV positive," "known HIV," "HIV test positive," or similar terminology. Do not use this code if the term "AIDS" is used or if the patient is treated for any HIV-related illness or is described as having any condition(s) resulting from his/her HIV positive status; use B20 in these cases.

         (e) **Patients with inconclusive HIV serology**

         Patients with inconclusive HIV serology, but no definitive diagnosis or manifestations of the illness, may be assigned code R75, Inconclusive laboratory evidence of human immunodeficiency virus [HIV].

         (f) **Previously diagnosed HIV-related illness**

         Patients with any known prior diagnosis of an HIV-related illness should be coded to B20. Once a patient has developed an HIV-related illness, the patient should always be assigned code B20 on every subsequent admission/encounter. Patients previously diagnosed with any HIV illness (B20) should never be assigned to R75 or Z21, Asymptomatic human immunodeficiency virus [HIV] infection status.

         (g) **HIV Infection in Pregnancy, Childbirth and the Puerperium**

         During pregnancy, childbirth or the puerperium, a patient admitted (or presenting for a health care encounter) because of an HIV-related illness should receive a principal diagnosis code of O98.7-, Human immunodeficiency [HIV] disease complicating pregnancy, childbirth and the puerperium, followed by B20 and the code(s) for the HIV-related illness(es). Codes from Chapter 15 always take sequencing priority.

         Patients with asymptomatic HIV infection status admitted (or presenting for a health care encounter) during pregnancy, childbirth, or the puerperium should receive codes of O98.7- and Z21.

         (h) **Encounters for testing for HIV**

         If a patient is being seen to determine his/her HIV status, use code Z11.4, Encounter for screening for human immunodeficiency virus [HIV]. Use additional codes for any associated high risk behavior.

         If a patient with signs or symptoms is being seen for HIV testing, code the signs and symptoms. An additional counseling code Z71.7, Human immunodeficiency virus [HIV] counseling, may be used if counseling is provided during the encounter for the test.

         When a patient returns to be informed of his/her HIV test results and the test result is negative, use code Z71.7, Human immunodeficiency virus [HIV] counseling.

         If the results are positive, see previous guidelines and assign codes as appropriate.

   b. **Infectious agents as the cause of diseases classified to other chapters**

   Certain infections are classified in chapters other than Chapter 1 and no organism is identified as part of the infection code. In these instances, it is necessary to use an additional code from Chapter 1 to identify the organism. A code from category B95, Streptococcus, Staphylococcus, and Enterococcus as the cause of diseases classified to other chapters, B96, Other bacterial agents as the cause of diseases classified to other chapters, or B97, Viral agents as the cause of diseases classified to other chapters, is to be used as an additional code to identify the organism. An instructional note will be found at the infection code advising that an additional organism code is required.

   c. **Infections resistant to antibiotics**

   Many bacterial infections are resistant to current antibiotics. It is necessary to identify all infections documented as antibiotic resistant. Assign a code from category Z16, Resistance to antimicrobial drugs, following the infection code only if the infection code does not identify drug resistance.

   d. **Sepsis, Severe Sepsis, and Septic Shock**

      1) **Coding of Sepsis and Severe Sepsis**

         (a) **Sepsis**

         For a diagnosis of sepsis, assign the appropriate code for the underlying systemic infection. If the type of infection or causal organism is not further specified, assign code A41.9, Sepsis, unspecified organism.

         A code from subcategory R65.2, Severe sepsis, should not be assigned unless severe sepsis or an associated acute organ dysfunction is documented.

            (i) Negative or inconclusive blood cultures and sepsis

            Negative or inconclusive blood cultures do not preclude a diagnosis of sepsis in patients with clinical evidence of the condition, however, the provider should be queried.

            (ii) Urosepsis

            The term urosepsis is a nonspecific term. It is not to be considered synonymous with sepsis. It has no default code in the Alphabetic Index. Should a provider use this term, he/she must be queried for clarification.

            (iii) Sepsis with organ dysfunction

            If a patient has sepsis and associated acute organ dysfunction or multiple organ dysfunction (MOD), follow the instructions for coding severe sepsis.

            (iv) Acute organ dysfunction that is not clearly associated with the sepsis

            If a patient has sepsis and an acute organ dysfunction, but the medical record documentation indicates that the acute organ dysfunction is related to a medical condition other than the sepsis, do not assign a code from subcategory R65.2, Severe sepsis. An acute organ dysfunction must be associated with the sepsis in order to assign the severe sepsis code. If the documentation is not clear as to whether an acute organ dysfunction is related to the sepsis or another medical condition, query the provider.

         (b) **Severe sepsis**

         The coding of severe sepsis requires a minimum of 2 codes: first a code for the underlying systemic infection, followed by a code from subcategory R65.2, Severe sepsis. If the causal organism is not documented, assign code A41.9, Sepsis, unspecified organism, for the infection. Additional code(s) for the associated acute organ dysfunction are also required.

         Due to the complex nature of severe sepsis, some cases may require querying the provider prior to assignment of the codes.

2) Septic shock

    (a) Septic shock generally refers to circulatory failure associated with severe sepsis, and therefore, it represents a type of acute organ dysfunction.

For all cases of septic shock, the code for the systemic infection should be sequenced first, followed by code R65.21, Severe sepsis with septic shock or code T81.12, Postprocedural septic shock. Any additional codes for the other acute organ dysfunctions should also be assigned. As noted in the sequencing instructions in the Tabular List, the code for septic shock cannot be assigned as a principal diagnosis.

3) Sequencing of severe sepsis

If severe sepsis is present on admission, and meets the definition of principal diagnosis, the underlying systemic infection should be assigned as principal diagnosis followed by the appropriate code from subcategory R65.2 as required by the sequencing rules in the Tabular List. A code from subcategory R65.2 can never be assigned as a principal diagnosis.

    When severe sepsis develops during an encounter (it was not present on admission) the underlying systemic infection and the appropriate code from subcategory R65.2 should be assigned as secondary diagnoses.

    Severe sepsis may be present on admission but the diagnosis may not be confirmed until sometime after admission. If the documentation is not clear whether severe sepsis was present on admission, the provider should be queried.

4) Sepsis and severe sepsis with a localized infection

If the reason for admission is both sepsis or severe sepsis and a localized infection, such as pneumonia or cellulitis, a code(s) for the underlying systemic infection should be assigned first and the code for the localized infection should be assigned as a secondary diagnosis. If the patient has severe sepsis, a code from subcategory R65.2 should also be assigned as a secondary diagnosis. If the patient is admitted with a localized infection, such as pneumonia, and sepsis/severe sepsis doesn't develop until after admission, the localized infection should be assigned first, followed by the appropriate sepsis/severe sepsis codes.

5) Sepsis due to a postprocedural infection

    (a) Documentation of causal relationship

As with all postprocedural complications, code assignment is based on the provider's documentation of the relationship between the infection and the procedure.

    (b) Sepsis due to a postprocedural infection

For such cases, the postprocedural infection code, such as, T80.2, Infections following infusion, transfusion, and therapeutic injection, T81.4, Infection following a procedure, T88.0, Infection following immunization, or O86.0, Infection of obstetric surgical wound, should be coded first, followed by the code for the specific infection. If the patient has severe sepsis the appropriate code from subcategory R65.2 should also be assigned with the additional code(s) for any acute organ dysfunction.

    (c) Postprocedural infection and postprocedural septic shock

In cases where a postprocedural infection has occurred and has resulted in severe sepsis the code for the precipitating complication such as code T81.4, Infection following a procedure, or O86.0, Infection of obstetrical surgical wound should be coded first followed by code R65.20, Severe sepsis without septic shock. A Code for the systemic infection should also be assigned.

    If a postprocedural infection has resulted in postprocedural septic shock, the code for the precipitating complication such as code T81.4, Infection following a procedure, or O86.0, Infection of obstetrical surgical wound should be coded first followed by code T81.12-, Postprocedural septic shock. A code for the systemic infection should also be assigned.

6) Sepsis and severe sepsis associated with a noninfectious process (condition)

In some cases a noninfectious process (condition), such as trauma, may lead to an infection which can result in sepsis or severe sepsis. If sepsis or severe sepsis is documented as associated with a noninfectious condition, such as a burn or serious injury, and this condition meets the definition for principal diagnosis, the code for the noninfectious condition should be sequenced first, followed by the code for the resulting infection. If severe sepsis is present, a code from subcategory R65.2 should also be assigned with any associated organ dysfunction(s) codes. It is not necessary to assign a code from subcategory R65.1, Systemic inflammatory response syndrome (SIRS) of non-infectious origin, for these cases.

    If the infection meets the definition of principal diagnosis it should be sequenced before the non-infectious condition. When both the associated non-infectious condition and the infection meet the definition of principal diagnosis either may be assigned as principal diagnosis.

    Only one code from category R65, Symptoms and signs specifically associated with systemic inflammation and infection, should be assigned. Therefore, when a non-infectious condition leads to an infection resulting in severe sepsis, assign the appropriate code from subcategory R65.2, Severe sepsis. Do not additionally assign a code from subcategory R65.1, Systemic inflammatory response syndrome (SIRS) of non-infectious origin.

    See Section I.C.18. SIRS due to non-infectious process

7) Sepsis and septic shock complicating abortion, pregnancy, childbirth, and the puerperium

See Section I.C.15. Sepsis and septic shock complicating abortion, pregnancy, childbirth and the puerperium

8) Newborn sepsis

See Section I.C.16. f. Bacterial sepsis of Newborn

e. Methicillin Resistant Staphylococcus aureus (MRSA) Conditions

    1) Selection and sequencing of MRSA codes

        (a) Combination codes for MRSA infection

When a patient is diagnosed with an infection that is due to methicillin resistant *Staphylococcus aureus* (MRSA), and that infection has a combination code that includes the causal organism (e.g., sepsis, pneumonia) assign the appropriate combination code for the condition (e.g., code A41.02, Sepsis due to Methicillin resistant Staphylococcus aureus or code J15.212, Pneumonia due to Methicillin resistant Staphylococcus aureus). Do not assign code B95.62, Methicillin resistant Staphylococcus aureus infection as the cause of diseases classified elsewhere, as an additional code because the combination code includes the type of infection and the MRSA organism. Do not assign a code from subcategory Z16.11, Resistance to penicillins, as an additional diagnosis.

    See Section C.1. for instructions on coding and sequencing of sepsis and severe sepsis.

        (b) Other codes for MRSA infection

When there is documentation of a current infection (e.g., wound infection, stitch abscess, urinary tract infection) due to MRSA, and that infection does not have a combination code that includes the causal organism, assign the appropriate code to identify the condition along with code B95.62, Methicillin resistant Staphylococcus aureus infection as the cause of diseases classified elsewhere for the MRSA infection. Do not assign a code from subcategory Z16.11, Resistance to penicillins.

        (c) Methicillin susceptible Staphylococcus aureus (MSSA) and MRSA colonization

The condition or state of being colonized or carrying MSSA or MRSA is called colonization or carriage, while an individual person is described as being colonized or being a carrier. Colonization means that MSSA or MSRA is present on or in the body without necessarily causing illness. A positive MRSA colonization test might be documented by the provider as "MRSA screen positive" or "MRSA nasal swab positive".

    Assign code Z22.322, Carrier or suspected carrier of Methicillin resistant Staphylococcus aureus, for patients documented as having MRSA colonization. Assign code Z22.321, Carrier or suspected carrier of Methicillin susceptible Staphylococcus aureus, for patient documented as having MSSA colonization. Colonization is not necessarily indicative of a disease process or as the cause of a specific condition the patient may have unless documented as such by the provider.

        (d) MRSA colonization and infection

If a patient is documented as having both MRSA colonization and infection during a hospital admission, code Z22.322, Carrier or suspected carrier of Methicillin resistant Staphylococcus aureus, and a code for the MRSA infection may both be assigned.

f. Zika virus infections

    1) Code only confirmed cases

Code only a confirmed diagnosis of Zika virus (A92.5, Zika virus disease) as documented by the provider. This is an exception to the hospital inpatient guideline Section II, H.

    In this context, "confirmation" does not require documentation of the type of test performed; the physician's diagnostic statement that the condition is confirmed is sufficient. This code should be assigned regardless of the stated mode of transmission.

    If the provider documents "suspected", "possible" or "probable" Zika, do not assign code A92.5. Assign a code(s) explaining the reason for encounter (such as fever, rash, or joint pain) or Z20.828, Contact with and (suspected) exposure to other viral communicable diseases.

CHAPTER 1

CERTAIN INFECTIOUS AND PARASITIC DISEASES (A00-B99)

Includes   diseases generally recognized as communicable or transmissible

Use additional code to identify resistance to antimicrobial drugs (Z16.-)

Excludes1   certain localized infections - see body system-related chapters

Excludes2   carrier or suspected carrier of infectious disease (Z22.-)

infectious and parasitic diseases complicating pregnancy, childbirth and the puerperium (O98.-)

infectious and parasitic diseases specific to the perinatal period (P35-P39)

influenza and other acute respiratory infections (J00-J22)

This chapter contains the following blocks:

A00-A09	Intestinal infectious diseases
A15-A19	Tuberculosis
A20-A28	Certain zoonotic bacterial diseases
A30-A49	Other bacterial diseases
A50-A64	Infections with a predominantly sexual mode of transmission
A65-A69	Other spirochetal diseases
A70-A74	Other diseases caused by chlamydiae
A75-A79	Rickettsioses
A80-A89	Viral and prion infections of the central nervous system
A90-A99	Arthropod-borne viral fevers and viral hemorrhagic fevers
B00-B09	Viral infections characterized by skin and mucous membrane lesions
B10	Other human herpesviruses
B15-B19	Viral hepatitis
B20	Human immunodeficiency virus [HIV] disease
B25-B34	Other viral diseases
B35-B49	Mycoses
B50-B64	Protozoal diseases
B65-B83	Helminthiases
B85-B89	Pediculosis, acariasis and other infestations
B90-B94	Sequelae of infectious and parasitic diseases
B95-B97	Bacterial and viral infectious agents
B99	Other infectious diseases

INTESTINAL INFECTIOUS DISEASES (A00-A09)

● **A00**   **Cholera**
A serious, often deadly, infectious disease of the small intestine

    A00.0   **Cholera due to Vibrio cholerae 01, biovar cholerae**
      Classical cholera

    A00.1   **Cholera due to Vibrio cholerae 01, biovar eltor**
      Cholera eltor

    A00.9   **Cholera, unspecified**

● **A01**   **Typhoid and paratyphoid fevers**
Caused by Salmonella typhi and Salmonella paratyphi A, B, and C bacteria

   ● **A01.0**   **Typhoid fever**
      Infection due to Salmonella typhi

      A01.00   **Typhoid fever, unspecified**

      A01.01   **Typhoid meningitis**

      A01.02   **Typhoid fever with heart involvement**
        Typhoid endocarditis
        Typhoid myocarditis

      A01.03   **Typhoid pneumonia**

      A01.04   **Typhoid arthritis**

      A01.05   **Typhoid osteomyelitis**

      A01.09   **Typhoid fever with other complications**

      A01.1   **Paratyphoid fever A**

      A01.2   **Paratyphoid fever B**

      A01.3   **Paratyphoid fever C**

      A01.4   **Paratyphoid fever, unspecified**
        Infection due to Salmonella paratyphi NOS

● **A02**   **Other salmonella infections**
    Includes   infection or foodborne intoxication due to any Salmonella species other than S. typhi and S. paratyphi

    A02.0   **Salmonella enteritis**
      Salmonellosis

    A02.1   **Salmonella sepsis**

   ● **A02.2**   **Localized salmonella infections**

      A02.20   **Localized salmonella infection, unspecified**
        Specified in the documentation as localized, but unspecified as to type

      A02.21   **Salmonella meningitis**
        Specified as localized in the meninges

      A02.22   **Salmonella pneumonia**
        Specified as localized in the lungs

      A02.23   **Salmonella arthritis**
        Specified as localized in the joints

      A02.24   **Salmonella osteomyelitis**
        Specified as localized in bone

      A02.25   **Salmonella pyelonephritis**
        Salmonella tubulo-interstitial nephropathy

      A02.29   **Salmonella with other localized infection**
        Specified as localized (because it is still under localized heading) but does not assign into any of the above codes

    A02.8   **Other specified salmonella infections**
      Any specified salmonella infection which does NOT assign into any of the above codes (not specified as localized)

    A02.9   **Salmonella infection, unspecified**
      Unspecified in the documentation as to specific type of salmonella

● **A03**   **Shigellosis**
    An infectious disease caused by bacteria (Shigella)

    A03.0   **Shigellosis due to Shigella dysenteriae**
      Group A shigellosis [Shiga-Kruse dysentery]

    A03.1   **Shigellosis due to Shigella flexneri**
      Group B shigellosis

    A03.2   **Shigellosis due to Shigella boydii**
      Group C shigellosis

    A03.3   **Shigellosis due to Shigella sonnei**
      Group D shigellosis

    A03.8   **Other shigellosis**

    A03.9   **Shigellosis, unspecified**
      Bacillary dysentery NOS

Item 1-1   **Salmonella** is a bacterium that lives in the intestines of fowl and mammals and can spread to humans through improper food preparation and cooking. Salmonellosis is an infection with the bacterium. Symptoms include diarrhea, fever, and abdominal cramps 12 to 72 hours after infection. The illness usually lasts 4 to 7 days, and most persons recover without treatment. The diarrhea may be so severe that the patient needs to be hospitalized. Patients with immunocompromised systems in chronic, ill health are more likely to have the infection invade their bloodstream with life-threatening results. For example, patients with sickle cell disease are more prone to salmonella osteomyelitis than others.

▶ New   ⇒ Revised   ~~deleted~~ Deleted   OGCR Official Guidelines   X Assign placeholder X   ● Use Additional Character(s)

Excludes 1   Excludes 2   Includes   Use additional   Code first   Code also   Key words

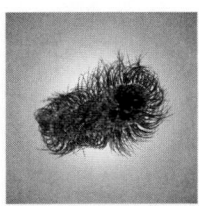

Figure 1-1 Electron micrograph of escherichia coli (E. coli) expressing P fimbriae. (Getty Image)

Item 1–2 *Escherichia coli [E. coli]* is a gram-negative bacterium found in the intestinal tracts of humans and animals and is usually nonpathogenic. Pathogenic strains can cause diarrhea or pyogenic (pus-producing) infections. Can be a threat to food safety.

● **A04   Other bacterial intestinal infections**
> **Excludes1**   bacterial foodborne intoxications, NEC (A05.-)
> tuberculous enteritis (A18.32)

A04.0   Enteropathogenic Escherichia coli infection
Pertaining to or producing intestinal disease

A04.1   Enterotoxigenic Escherichia coli infection
Producing or containing intestinal toxin

A04.2   Enteroinvasive Escherichia coli infection
Capable of penetrating and spreading through intestinal mucosal epithelium

A04.3   Enterohemorrhagic Escherichia coli infection
Causing bloody diarrhea, resulting from microorganisms

A04.4   Other intestinal Escherichia coli infections
Escherichia coli enteritis NOS

A04.5   Campylobacter enteritis
Spiral shaped bacterium

A04.6   Enteritis due to Yersinia enterocolitica
> **Excludes1**   extraintestinal yersiniosis (A28.2)
Transmitted by infected food /water and person-to-person contact, affecting intestinal tract

● **A04.7   Enterocolitis due to Clostridium difficile**
Foodborne intoxication by Clostridium difficile
Pseudomembraneous colitis
Marked by fibrinous deposit (false membrane) with enmeshed necrotic cells

▶ **A04.71   Enterocolitis due to Clostridium difficile, recurrent**

▶ **A04.72   Enterocolitis due to Clostridium difficile, not specified as recurrent**

A04.8   Other specified bacterial intestinal infections

A04.9   Bacterial intestinal infection, unspecified
Bacterial enteritis NOS

● **A05   Other bacterial foodborne intoxications, not elsewhere classified**
> ⇒ **Excludes1**   Clostridium difficile foodborne intoxication and infection (A04.7-)
> Escherichia coli infection (A04.0-A04.4)
> listeriosis (A32.-)
> salmonella foodborne intoxication and infection (A02.-)
> toxic effect of noxious foodstuffs (T61-T62)

A05.0   Foodborne staphylococcal intoxication

A05.1   Botulism food poisoning
Botulism NOS
Classical foodborne intoxication due to Clostridium botulinum
> **Excludes1**   infant botulism (A48.51)
> wound botulism (A48.52)

A05.2   Foodborne Clostridium perfringens [Clostridium welchii] intoxication
Type A causes gas gangrene and necrotizing colitis; major cause of food poisoning in humans
Enteritis necroticans
Pig-bel

A05.3   Foodborne Vibrio parahaemolyticus intoxication
Organism that survives only in high salt environment (halophilic), major cause of gastroenteritis due to consumption of raw or improperly cooked fish/seafood

A05.4   Foodborne Bacillus cereus intoxication
Spore-forming species commonly found in soil, causes food poisoning from formation of intestinal toxins in contaminated foods

A05.5   Foodborne Vibrio vulnificus intoxication
Species that survives in high salt environment (halophilic) with infection by eating raw seafood causes septicemia and cellulitis

A05.8   Other specified bacterial foodborne intoxications

A05.9   Bacterial foodborne intoxication, unspecified

● **A06   Amebiasis**
An intestinal illness caused by the microscopic parasite Entamoeba histolytica
> **Includes**   infection due to Entamoeba histolytica
> **Excludes1**   other protozoal intestinal diseases (A07.-)
> **Excludes2**   acanthamebiasis (B60.1-)
> Naegleriasis (B60.2)

A06.0   Acute amebic dysentery
Acute amebiasis
Intestinal amebiasis NOS

A06.1   Chronic intestinal amebiasis

A06.2   Amebic nondysenteric colitis
Pertaining to single cell microorganism

A06.3   Ameboma of intestine
Tumorlike mass produced by localized inflammation often in intestine
Ameboma NOS

A06.4   Amebic liver abscess
Hepatic amebiasis

A06.5   Amebic lung abscess
Amebic abscess of lung (and liver)

A06.6   Amebic brain abscess
Amebic abscess of brain (and liver) (and lung)

A06.7   Cutaneous amebiasis

● **A06.8   Amebic infection of other sites**
A06.81   Amebic cystitis
A06.82   Other amebic genitourinary infections
Amebic balanitis
Amebic vesiculitis
Amebic vulvovaginitis

A06.89   Other amebic infections
Amebic appendicitis
Amebic splenic abscess

A06.9   Amebiasis, unspecified

● **A07   Other protozoal intestinal diseases**
A07.0   Balantidiasis
Balantidial dysentery
Infection by protozoa that may cause diarrhea and dysentery, with ulceration of colonic mucous membranes

A07.1   Giardiasis [lambliasis]
Common infection in small intestine spread by contaminated food, water, or direct person-to-person contact

A07.2   Cryptosporidiosis
Human infection with protozoa usually seen as self-limited diarrhea in those who work with cattle

CHAPTER 1 (A00-B99)

A07.3   Isosporiasis
Human intestinal disease caused by protozoa
Infection due to Isospora belli and Isospora hominis
Intestinal coccidiosis
Isosporosis

A07.4   Cyclosporiasis
Infection by protozoa with most common species infecting humans being C cayetanensis

A07.8   Other specified protozoal intestinal diseases
Intestinal microsporidiosis
Intestinal trichomoniasis
Sarcocystosis
Sarcosporidiosis

A07.9   Protozoal intestinal disease, unspecified
Flagellate diarrhea
Protozoal colitis
Protozoal diarrhea
Protozoal dysentery

● **A08   Viral and other specified intestinal infections**
     Excludes1   influenza with involvement of gastrointestinal
                  tract (J09.X3, J10.2, J11.2)

   A08.0   Rotaviral enteritis

● **A08.1   Acute gastroenteropathy due to Norwalk agent and other small round viruses**
     A08.11   Acute gastroenteropathy due to Norwalk agent
           Acute gastroenteropathy due to Norovirus
           Acute gastroenteropathy due to Norwalk-like agent
     A08.19   Acute gastroenteropathy due to other small round viruses
           Acute gastroenteropathy due to small round virus [SRV] NOS

   A08.2   Adenoviral enteritis

● **A08.3   Other viral enteritis**
     A08.31   Calicivirus enteritis
     A08.32   Astrovirus enteritis
     A08.39   Other viral enteritis
           Coxsackie virus enteritis
           Echovirus enteritis
           Enterovirus enteritis NEC
           Torovirus enteritis

   A08.4   Viral intestinal infection, unspecified
     Viral enteritis NOS
     Viral gastroenteritis NOS
     Viral gastroenteropathy NOS

   A08.8   Other specified intestinal infections

A09   Infectious gastroenteritis and colitis, unspecified
   Infectious colitis NOS
   Infectious enteritis NOS
   Infectious gastroenteritis NOS
     Excludes1   colitis NOS (K52.9)
               diarrhea NOS (R19.7)
               enteritis NOS (K52.9)
               gastroenteritis NOS (K52.9)
               noninfective gastroenteritis and colitis, unspecified (K52.9)

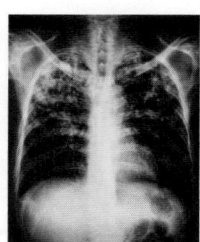

Figure 1-2   Far advanced bilateral pulmonary tuberculosis before and after 8 months of treatment with streptomycin, PAS, and isoniazid. (Getty Image)

Item 1-3   Tuberculosis is a common and deadly infectious disease caused by the *Mycobacterium tuberculosis* organism. The first tuberculosis infection is called the **primary infection** and most commonly attacks the lungs but can affect the central nervous system, lymphatic system, circulatory system, genitourinary system, bones, joints, and even the skin. A **Ghon** lesion is the **initial lesion.** A **secondary lesion** occurs when the tubercle bacilli are carried to other areas.

Item 1-4   Although it primarily affects the lungs, the bacteria *Mycobacterium tuberculosis* can travel from the pulmonary circulation to virtually any organ in the body, much as a cancer metastasizes to a secondary site. If the immune system becomes compromised by age or disease, what would otherwise be a self-limiting primary tuberculosis in the lungs will develop in other organs. These are known as extrapulmonary sites.

TUBERCULOSIS (A15-A19)

Includes   infections due to Mycobacterium tuberculosis and Mycobacterium bovis
Excludes1   congenital tuberculosis (P37.0)
     nonspecific reaction to test for tuberculosis without active tuberculosis (R76.1-)
     pneumoconiosis associated with tuberculosis, any type in A15 (J65)
     positive PPD (R76.11)
     positive tuberculin skin test without active tuberculosis (R76.11)
     sequelae of tuberculosis (B90.-)
     silicotuberculosis (J65)

● **A15   Respiratory tuberculosis**
   A15.0   Tuberculosis of lung
     Tuberculous bronchiectasis
     Chronic dilatation of bronchi
     Tuberculous fibrosis of lung
     Tuberculous pneumonia
     Tuberculous pneumothorax

   A15.4   Tuberculosis of intrathoracic lymph nodes
     Tuberculosis of hilar lymph nodes
     Tuberculosis of mediastinal lymph nodes
     Tuberculosis of tracheobronchial lymph nodes
     Excludes1   tuberculosis specified as primary (A15.7)

   A15.5   Tuberculosis of larynx, trachea and bronchus
     Tuberculosis of bronchus
     Tuberculosis of glottis
     Tuberculosis of larynx
     Tuberculosis of trachea

   A15.6   Tuberculous pleurisy
     Tuberculosis of pleura
     Tuberculous empyema
     Excludes1   primary respiratory tuberculosis (A15.7)

   A15.7   Primary respiratory tuberculosis

   A15.8   Other respiratory tuberculosis
     Mediastinal tuberculosis
     Nasopharyngeal tuberculosis
     Tuberculosis of nose
     Tuberculosis of sinus [any nasal]

   A15.9   Respiratory tuberculosis unspecified

▶ New   ⇒ Revised   ~~deleted~~ Deleted   **OGCR** Official Guidelines   X Assign placeholder X   ● Use Additional Character(s)

Excludes 1   Excludes 2   Includes   Use additional   Code first   Code also   Key words

● **A17 Tuberculosis of nervous system**

  A17.0 Tuberculous meningitis
    Tuberculosis of meninges (cerebral) (spinal)
    Tuberculous leptomeningitis
    Excludes1 tuberculous meningoencephalitis (A17.82)

  A17.1 Meningeal tuberculoma
    Tuberculoma of meninges (cerebral) (spinal)
    Excludes2 tuberculoma of brain and spinal cord (A17.81)

  ● **A17.8 Other tuberculosis of nervous system**

    A17.81 Tuberculoma of brain and spinal cord
      Tuberculous abscess of brain and spinal cord

    A17.82 Tuberculous meningoencephalitis
      Inflammation of brain and meninges; AKA cerebromeningitis and encephalomeningitis
      Tuberculous myelitis

    A17.83 Tuberculous neuritis
      Tuberculous mononeuropathy

    A17.89 Other tuberculosis of nervous system
      Tuberculous polyneuropathy

  A17.9 Tuberculosis of nervous system, unspecified

● **A18 Tuberculosis of other organs**

  ● **A18.0 Tuberculosis of bones and joints**

    A18.01 Tuberculosis of spine
      Pott's disease or curvature of spine
      Tuberculous arthritis
      Tuberculous osteomyelitis of spine
      Tuberculous spondylitis

    A18.02 Tuberculous arthritis of other joints
      Tuberculosis of hip (joint)
      Tuberculosis of knee (joint)

    A18.03 Tuberculosis of other bones
      Tuberculous mastoiditis
      Tuberculous osteomyelitis

    A18.09 Other musculoskeletal tuberculosis
      Tuberculous myositis
      Tuberculous synovitis
      Tuberculous tenosynovitis

  ● **A18.1 Tuberculosis of genitourinary system**

    A18.10 Tuberculosis of genitourinary system, unspecified

    A18.11 Tuberculosis of kidney and ureter

    A18.12 Tuberculosis of bladder

    A18.13 Tuberculosis of other urinary organs
      Tuberculous urethritis

    A18.14 Tuberculosis of prostate

    A18.15 Tuberculosis of other male genital organs

    A18.16 Tuberculosis of cervix

    A18.17 Tuberculous female pelvic inflammatory disease
      Tuberculous endometritis
      Tuberculous oophoritis and salpingitis
      Oophoritis = inflammation of ovary
      Salpingitis = inflammation of fallopian tube

    A18.18 Tuberculosis of other female genital organs
      Tuberculous ulceration of vulva

  A18.2 Tuberculous peripheral lymphadenopathy
    Tuberculous adenitis
    Excludes2 tuberculosis of bronchial and mediastinal lymph nodes (A15.4)
      tuberculosis of mesenteric and retroperitoneal lymph nodes (A18.39)
      tuberculous tracheobronchial adenopathy (A15.4)

● **A18.3 Tuberculosis of intestines, peritoneum and mesenteric glands**

  A18.31 Tuberculous peritonitis
    Tuberculous ascites

  A18.32 Tuberculous enteritis
    Tuberculosis of anus and rectum
    Tuberculosis of intestine (large) (small)

  A18.39 Retroperitoneal tuberculosis
    Tuberculosis of mesenteric glands
    Tuberculosis of retroperitoneal (lymph glands)

A18.4 Tuberculosis of skin and subcutaneous tissue
  Erythema induratum, tuberculous
  Lupus excedens
  Lupus vulgaris NOS
  Lupus vulgaris of eyelid
    Cutaneous tuberculosis characterized by reddish brown plaque on skin surrounded by papules and nodules
  Scrofuloderma
    Type of cutaneous tuberculosis, with direct extension of tuberculosis into skin from underlying structures; AKA tuberculosis colliquativa
  Tuberculosis of external ear
  Excludes2 lupus erythematosus (L93.-)
    lupus NOS (M32.9)
    systemic (M32.-)

● **A18.5 Tuberculosis of eye**
  Excludes2 lupus vulgaris of eyelid (A18.4)

  A18.50 Tuberculosis of eye, unspecified

  A18.51 Tuberculous episcleritis
    Inflammation of episclera and adjacent tissues

  A18.52 Tuberculous keratitis
    Tuberculous interstitial keratitis
    Tuberculous keratoconjunctivitis (interstitial) (phlyctenular)
    Inflammation of cornea and conjunctiva

  A18.53 Tuberculous chorioretinitis
    Inflammation of choroid and retina; retinochoroiditis

  A18.54 Tuberculous iridocyclitis
    Inflammation of iris and ciliary body

  A18.59 Other tuberculosis of eye
    Tuberculous conjunctivitis

A18.6 Tuberculosis of (inner) (middle) ear
  Tuberculous otitis media
  Excludes2 tuberculosis of external ear (A18.4)
    tuberculous mastoiditis (A18.03)

A18.7 Tuberculosis of adrenal glands
  Tuberculous Addison's disease

● **A18.8 Tuberculosis of other specified organs**

  A18.81 Tuberculosis of thyroid gland

  A18.82 Tuberculosis of other endocrine glands
    Tuberculosis of pituitary gland
    Tuberculosis of thymus gland

  A18.83 Tuberculosis of digestive tract organs, not elsewhere classified
    Excludes1 tuberculosis of intestine (A18.32)

  A18.84 Tuberculosis of heart
    Tuberculous cardiomyopathy
    Tuberculous endocarditis
    Tuberculous myocarditis
    Tuberculous pericarditis

  A18.85 Tuberculosis of spleen

  A18.89 Tuberculosis of other sites
    Tuberculosis of muscle
    Tuberculous cerebral arteritis

CHAPTER 1 (A00-B99)

▶ New ➡ Revised ~~deleted~~ Deleted **OGCR** Official Guidelines **X** Assign placeholder X ● Use Additional Character(s)

Excludes 1 Excludes 2 Includes Use additional Code first Code also Key words

Item 1–5 Miliary tuberculosis can be a life-threatening condition. If a tuberculous lesion enters a blood vessel, immense dissemination of tuberculous organisms can occur if the immune system is weak. High-risk populations—children under 4 years of age, the elderly, or the immunocompromised—are particularly prone to this type of infection. The lesions will have a millet seedlike appearance on chest x-ray. Bronchial washings and biopsy may aid in diagnosis.

● **A19 Miliary tuberculosis**

    Includes   disseminated tuberculosis
                      generalized tuberculosis
                      tuberculous polyserositis

    A19.0 Acute miliary tuberculosis of a single specified site
    A19.1 Acute miliary tuberculosis of multiple sites
    A19.2 Acute miliary tuberculosis, unspecified
    A19.8 Other miliary tuberculosis
    A19.9 Miliary tuberculosis, unspecified

CERTAIN ZOONOTIC BACTERIAL DISEASES (A20-A28)

● **A20 Plague**
    Infectious disease caused by a Yersinia pestis bacterium, transmitted by a rodent flea bite or handling of infected animal

    Includes   infection due to Yersinia pestis

    A20.0 Bubonic plague
    A20.1 Cellulocutaneous plague
           Skin and subcutaneous tissue plague
    A20.2 Pneumonic plague
    A20.3 Plague meningitis
    A20.7 Septicemic plague
    A20.8 Other forms of plague
           Abortive plague
           Asymptomatic plague
           Pestis minor
               Systemic bacterial disease
    A20.9 Plague, unspecified

● **A21 Tularemia**
    Caused by Francisella tularensis bacterium found in rodents, rabbits, and hares and transmitted to humans by contact with infected animal tissues or by ticks, biting flies, or mosquitoes

    Includes   deer-fly fever
                infection due to Francisella tularensis
                rabbit fever

    A21.0 Ulceroglandular tularemia
           Most common form of tularemia in humans is painful, swollen, erythematous papule at point of inoculation that ruptures to form shallow ulcer
    A21.1 Oculoglandular tularemia
           Primary site of entry is conjunctival sac, results in granulomatous corneal lesions
           Ophthalmic tularemia
    A21.2 Pulmonary tularemia
    A21.3 Gastrointestinal tularemia
           Abdominal tularemia
    A21.7 Generalized tularemia
    A21.8 Other forms of tularemia
    A21.9 Tularemia, unspecified

Item 1-6 Brucellosis: An infectious disease caused by the bacterium Brucella. Humans are infected by contact with contaminated animals or animal products. In humans brucellosis symptoms that are similar to the flu include fever, sweats, headaches, back pains, and physical weakness. Severe infections of the central nervous system or lining of the heart may occur. Brucellosis can also cause chronic symptoms that include recurrent fevers, joint pain, and fatigue.

● **A22 Anthrax**
    An acute infectious disease caused by the spore-forming Bacillus anthracis; occurs in humans exposed to infected animals or tissue from infected animals

    Includes   infection due to Bacillus anthracis

    A22.0 Cutaneous anthrax
           Malignant carbuncle
           Malignant pustule
    A22.1 Pulmonary anthrax
           Inhalation anthrax
           Ragpicker's disease
           Woolsorter's disease
    A22.2 Gastrointestinal anthrax
    A22.7 Anthrax sepsis
           Infectious bacterial disease
    A22.8 Other forms of anthrax
           Anthrax meningitis
    A22.9 Anthrax, unspecified

● **A23 Brucellosis**

    Includes   Malta fever
                Mediterranean fever
                undulant fever

    A23.0 Brucellosis due to Brucella melitensis
           Resulting in flu-like symptoms that may lead to chronic symptoms that include recurrent fevers, joint pain, and fatigue
    A23.1 Brucellosis due to Brucella abortus
           Most common cause of brucellosis in humans; AKA Bang bacillus
    A23.2 Brucellosis due to Brucella suis
           Species found primarily in pigs, rabbits, and reindeer
    A23.3 Brucellosis due to Brucella canis
            Species that causes respiratory tract infection in humans
    A23.8 Other brucellosis
    A23.9 Brucellosis, unspecified

● **A24 Glanders and melioidosis**
    Infection, usually of rodents, which spreads to other animals and humans, caused by Burkholderia pseudomallei through break in skin contaminated with infested soil or water

    A24.0 Glanders
           Infection due to Pseudomonas mallei
           Malleus
    A24.1 Acute and fulminating melioidosis
           Melioidosis pneumonia
           Melioidosis sepsis
    A24.2 Subacute and chronic melioidosis
    A24.3 Other melioidosis
    A24.9 Melioidosis, unspecified
           Infection due to Pseudomonas pseudomallei NOS
           Whitmore's disease

▶ New   ⇒ Revised   ~~deleted~~ Deleted   **OGCR** Official Guidelines   X Assign placeholder X   ● Use Additional Character(s)

Excludes 1   Excludes 2   Includes   Use additional   Code first   Code also   Key words

● **A25 Rat-bite fevers**
RBF, infectious disease caused by Streptobacillus moniliformis or Spirillum minus.

A25.0 Spirillosis
Any disease condition caused by spirilla
Sodoku

A25.1 Streptobacillosis
Acute, febrile human illness caused by bacteria transmitted by rats in most cases, passed from rodent to human via rodent's urine or mucous secretions; AKA rat fever
Epidemic arthritic erythema
Haverhill fever
Streptobacillary rat-bite fever

A25.9 Rat-bite fever, unspecified

● **A26 Erysipeloid**
Infection with Erysipelothrix rhusiopathiae, occurring often as occupational disease resulting from handling infected fish, shellfish, meat, or poultry

A26.0 Cutaneous erysipeloid
Erythema migrans

A26.7 Erysipelothrix sepsis

A26.8 Other forms of erysipeloid

A26.9 Erysipeloid, unspecified

● **A27 Leptospirosis**
Occurs most commonly in the tropics

A27.0 Leptospirosis icterohemorrhagica
Leptospiral or spirochetal jaundice (hemorrhagic)
Weil's disease

● **A27.8 Other forms of leptospirosis**
A27.81 Aseptic meningitis in leptospirosis
A27.89 Other forms of leptospirosis

A27.9 Leptospirosis, unspecified

● **A28 Other zoonotic bacterial diseases, not elsewhere classified**

A28.0 Pasteurellosis
Infection of humans or other animals by species of Pasteurella

A28.1 Cat-scratch disease
Cat-scratch fever

A28.2 Extraintestinal yersiniosis
Infection from Yersinia enterocolitica; AKA enteric yersiniosis, intestinal yersiniosis, Yersinia enteritis
Excludes1 enteritis due to Yersinia enterocolitica (A04.6)
plague (A20.-)

A28.8 Other specified zoonotic bacterial diseases, not elsewhere classified

A28.9 Zoonotic bacterial disease, unspecified

OTHER BACTERIAL DISEASES (A30-A49)

● **A30 Leprosy [Hansen's disease]**
Chronic infectious disease attacking the skin, peripheral nerves, and mucous membranes
Includes infection due to Mycobacterium leprae
Excludes1 sequelae of leprosy (B92)

A30.0 Indeterminate leprosy
I leprosy

A30.1 Tuberculoid leprosy
TT leprosy

A30.2 Borderline tuberculoid leprosy
BT leprosy

A30.3 Borderline leprosy
BB leprosy

A30.4 Borderline lepromatous leprosy
BL leprosy

A30.5 Lepromatous leprosy
LL leprosy

A30.8 Other forms of leprosy

A30.9 Leprosy, unspecified

● **A31 Infection due to other mycobacteria**
Excludes2 leprosy (A30.-)
tuberculosis (A15-A19)

A31.0 Pulmonary mycobacterial infection
Infection due to Mycobacterium avium
Infection due to Mycobacterium intracellulare [Battey bacillus]
Infection due to Mycobacterium kansasii

A31.1 Cutaneous mycobacterial infection
Buruli ulcer
Infection due to Mycobacterium marinum
Infection due to Mycobacterium ulcerans

A31.2 Disseminated mycobacterium avium-intracellulare complex (DMAC)
MAC sepsis

A31.8 Other mycobacterial infections

A31.9 Mycobacterial infection, unspecified
Atypical mycobacterial infection NOS
Mycobacteriosis NOS

● **A32 Listeriosis**
Infection caused by Listeria monocytogenes
Includes listerial foodborne infection
Excludes1 neonatal (disseminated) listeriosis (P37.2)

A32.0 Cutaneous listeriosis

● **A32.1 Listerial meningitis and meningoencephalitis**
A32.11 Listerial meningitis
A32.12 Listerial meningoencephalitis

A32.7 Listerial sepsis

● **A32.8 Other forms of listeriosis**
A32.81 Oculoglandular listeriosis
Primary infection site is conjunctival sac, which if untreated may result in perforation of cornea and optic atrophy
A32.82 Listerial endocarditis
Exudative and proliferative inflammatory condition of endocardium caused by listeria bacteria
A32.89 Other forms of listeriosis
Listerial cerebral arteritis

A32.9 Listeriosis, unspecified

A33 Tetanus neonatorum
Neonate = newborn

A34 Obstetrical tetanus

A35 Other tetanus
Tetanus NOS
Excludes1 tetanus neonatorum (A33)
obstetrical tetanus (A34)

● **A36 Diphtheria**
A36.0 Pharyngeal diphtheria
Diphtheritic membranous angina
Tonsillar diphtheria

A36.1 Nasopharyngeal diphtheria

A36.2 Laryngeal diphtheria
Diphtheritic laryngotracheitis

A36.3 Cutaneous diphtheria
Excludes2 erythrasma (L08.1)

Item 1-7 Diptheria: A highly contagious bacterial disease that results in the formation of an adherent membrane in the throat that may lead to suffocation. In its most poisonous form, it attacks the heart and lungs. It is spread by direct physical contact or breathing the aerosolized secretions of infected individuals. The exact location is specified in the codes.

CHAPTER 1 (A00-B99)

▶ New   ⟹ Revised   ~~deleted~~ Deleted   **OGCR** Official Guidelines   X Assign placeholder X   ● Use Additional Character(s)
Excludes 1   Excludes 2   Includes   Use additional   Code first   Code also   Key words

CHAPTER 1 (A00-B99)

● **A36.8** **Other diphtheria**
    A36.81 Diphtheritic **cardiomyopathy**
        Diphtheritic myocarditis
    A36.82 Diphtheritic **radiculomyelitis**
    A36.83 Diphtheritic **polyneuritis**
    A36.84 Diphtheritic **tubulo-interstitial nephropathy**
    A36.85 Diphtheritic **cystitis**
    A36.86 Diphtheritic **conjunctivitis**
    A36.89 **Other** diphtheritic complications
        Diphtheritic peritonitis
  A36.9 Diphtheria, **unspecified**

● **A37** **Whooping cough**
   Pertussis is a highly contagious disease caused by the bacterium
   Bordetella pertussis and results in a whooping sounding cough.
  ● **A37.0** **Whooping cough due to** **Bordetella pertussis**
    A37.00 Whooping cough due to Bordetella pertussis **without pneumonia**
    A37.01 Whooping cough due to Bordetella pertussis **with pneumonia**
  ● **A37.1** Whooping cough due to **Bordetella parapertussis**
    A37.10 Whooping cough due to Bordetella parapertussis **without pneumonia**
    A37.11 Whooping cough due to Bordetella parapertussis **with pneumonia**
  ● **A37.8** Whooping cough due to **other** Bordetella species
    A37.80 Whooping cough due to other Bordetella species **without pneumonia**
    A37.81 Whooping cough due to other Bordetella species **with pneumonia**
  ● **A37.9** Whooping cough, **unspecified** species
    A37.90 Whooping cough, unspecified species **without pneumonia**
    A37.91 Whooping cough, unspecified species **with pneumonia**

● **A38** **Scarlet fever**
   Most commonly caused by the bacteria Streptococcus pneumoniae and
   Neisseria meningitides
     Includes   scarlatina
     Excludes2 streptococcal sore throat (J02.0)
  A38.0 Scarlet fever with **otitis media**
  A38.1 Scarlet fever with **myocarditis**
  A38.8 Scarlet fever with **other complications**
  A38.9 Scarlet fever, **uncomplicated**
    Scarlet fever, NOS

● **A39** **Meningococcal infection**
   Most commonly caused by the bacteria Streptococcus pneumoniae and
   Neisseria meningitides
  A39.0 **Meningococcal** **meningitis**
  A39.1 **Waterhouse-Friderichsen** syndrome
    Fulminating complication of meningococcemia
    Meningococcal hemorrhagic adrenalitis
    Meningococcic adrenal syndrome
  A39.2 **Acute** meningococcemia
  A39.3 **Chronic** meningococcemia
  A39.4 Meningococcemia, **unspecified**
  ● **A39.5** **Meningococcal heart disease**
    A39.50 Meningococcal **carditis, unspecified**
    A39.51 Meningococcal **endocarditis**
    A39.52 Meningococcal **myocarditis**
    A39.53 Meningococcal **pericarditis**

● **A39.8** **Other meningococcal infections**
    A39.81 Meningococcal **encephalitis**
    A39.82 Meningococcal **retrobulbar neuritis**
       Optic neuritis in portion of optic nerve posterior to
       eyeball; AKA postocular optic neuritis
    A39.83 Meningococcal **arthritis**
    A39.84 **Postmeningococcal arthritis**
    A39.89 **Other meningococcal infections**
       Meningococcal conjunctivitis
  A39.9 Meningococcal infection, **unspecified**
    Meningococcal disease NOS

● **A40** **Streptococcal sepsis**
   Code first
    postprocedural streptococcal sepsis (T81.4-)
    streptococcal sepsis during labor (O75.3)
    streptococcal sepsis following abortion or ectopic or molar
      pregnancy (O03-O07, O08.0)
    streptococcal sepsis following immunization (T88.0)
    streptococcal sepsis following infusion, transfusion or
      therapeutic injection (T80.2-)
    Excludes1 neonatal (P36.0-P36.1)
              puerperal sepsis (O85)
              sepsis due to Streptococcus, group D (A41.81)
  A40.0 Sepsis due to streptococcus, group **A**
  A40.1 Sepsis due to streptococcus, group **B**
  A40.3 Sepsis due to Streptococcus **pneumoniae**
    Pneumococcal sepsis
  A40.8 **Other** streptococcal sepsis
  A40.9 Streptococcal sepsis, **unspecified**

● **A41** **Other sepsis**
   Code first
    postprocedural sepsis (T81.4-)
    sepsis during labor (O75.3)
    sepsis following abortion, ectopic or molar pregnancy
      (O03-O07, O08.0)
    sepsis following immunization (T88.0)
    sepsis following infusion, transfusion or therapeutic injection
      (T80.2-)
    Excludes1 bacteremia NOS (R78.81)
              neonatal (P36.-)
              puerperal sepsis (O85)
              streptococcal sepsis (A40.-)
    Excludes2 sepsis (due to) (in) actinomycotic (A42.7)
              sepsis (due to) (in) anthrax (A22.7)
              sepsis (due to) (in) candidal (B37.7)
              sepsis (due to) (in) Erysipelothrix (A26.7)
              sepsis (due to) (in) extraintestinal yersiniosis
                (A28.2)
              sepsis (due to) (in) gonococcal (A54.86)
              sepsis (due to) (in) herpesviral (B00.7)
              sepsis (due to) (in) listerial (A32.7)
              sepsis (due to) (in) melioidosis (A24.1)
              sepsis (due to) (in) meningococcal (A39.2-A39.4)
              sepsis (due to) (in) plague (A20.7)
              sepsis (due to) (in) tularemia (A21.7)
              toxic shock syndrome (A48.3)
  ● **A41.0** **Sepsis due to Staphylococcus aureus**
    A41.01 Sepsis due to Methicillin **susceptible** Staphylococcus aureus
       MSSA sepsis
       Staphylococcus aureus sepsis NOS
    A41.02 Sepsis due to Methicillin **resistant** Staphylococcus aureus
  A41.1 Sepsis due to **other** specified staphylococcus
    Coagulase negative staphylococcus sepsis
  A41.2 Sepsis due to **unspecified** staphylococcus
  A41.3 Sepsis due to **Hemophilus influenzae**
  A41.4 Sepsis due to **anaerobes**
    Excludes1 gas gangrene (A48.0)

▶ New   ⇒ Revised   ~~deleted~~ Deleted   **OGCR** Official Guidelines   X Assign placeholder X   ● Use Additional Character(s)

Excludes 1   Excludes 2   Includes   Use additional   Code first   Code also   Key words

● **A41.5 Sepsis due to other Gram-negative organisms**
    A41.50 Gram-negative sepsis, unspecified
        Gram-negative sepsis NOS
    A41.51 Sepsis due to Escherichia coli [E. coli]
    A41.52 Sepsis due to Pseudomonas
        Pseudomonas aeroginosa
    A41.53 Sepsis due to Serratia
    A41.59 Other Gram-negative sepsis
● **A41.8 Other specified sepsis**
    A41.81 Sepsis due to Enterococcus
    A41.89 Other specified sepsis
  A41.9 Sepsis, unspecified organism
    Septicemia NOS

● **A42 Actinomycosis**
    | Excludes1 | actinomycetoma (B47.1)
  A42.0 Pulmonary actinomycosis
  A42.1 Abdominal actinomycosis
  A42.2 Cervicofacial actinomycosis
  A42.7 Actinomycotic sepsis
● **A42.8 Other forms of actinomycosis**
    A42.81 Actinomycotic meningitis
    A42.82 Actinomycotic encephalitis
    A42.89 Other forms of actinomycosis
  A42.9 Actinomycosis, unspecified

● **A43 Nocardiosis**
  A43.0 Pulmonary nocardiosis
  A43.1 Cutaneous nocardiosis
  A43.8 Other forms of nocardiosis
  A43.9 Nocardiosis, unspecified

● **A44 Bartonellosis**
  A44.0 Systemic bartonellosis
    Oroya fever
  A44.1 Cutaneous and mucocutaneous bartonellosis
    Verruga peruana
  A44.8 Other forms of bartonellosis
  A44.9 Bartonellosis, unspecified

  A46 Erysipelas
    | Excludes1 | postpartum or puerperal erysipelas (O86.89)

● **A48 Other bacterial diseases, not elsewhere classified**
    | Excludes1 | actinomycetoma (B47.1)
  A48.0 Gas gangrene
    Clostridial cellulitis
    Clostridial myonecrosis
  A48.1 Legionnaires' disease
  A48.2 Nonpneumonic Legionnaires' disease [Pontiac fever]
  A48.3 Toxic shock syndrome
    Use additional code to identify the organism (B95, B96)
    | Excludes1 | endotoxic shock NOS (R57.8)
        sepsis NOS (A41.9)
  A48.4 Brazilian purpuric fever
    Systemic Hemophilus aegyptius infection

● **A48.5 Other specified botulism**
    Non-foodborne intoxication due to toxins of
        Clostridium botulinum [C. botulinum]
    | Excludes1 | food poisoning due to toxins of
        Clostridium botulinum (A05.1)
  A48.51 Infant botulism
  A48.52 Wound botulism
    Non-foodborne botulism NOS
    Use additional code for associated wound
  A48.8 Other specified bacterial diseases

● **A49 Bacterial infection of unspecified site**
    | Excludes1 | bacterial agents as the cause of diseases classified
        elsewhere (B95-B96)
        chlamydial infection NOS (A74.9)
        meningococcal infection NOS (A39.9)
        rickettsial infection NOS (A79.9)
        spirochetal infection NOS (A69.9)
● **A49.0 Staphylococcal infection, unspecified site**
    A49.01 Methicillin susceptible Staphylococcus aureus infection, unspecified site
        Methicillin susceptible Staphylococcus aureus (MSSA) infection
        Staphylococcus aureus infection NOS
    A49.02 Methicillin resistant Staphylococcus aureus infection, unspecified site
        Methicillin resistant Staphylococcus aureus (MRSA) infection
  A49.1 Streptococcal infection, unspecified site
  A49.2 Hemophilus influenzae infection, unspecified site
    Any of seven bacterium of genus Haemophilus
  A49.3 Mycoplasma infection, unspecified site
    Bacterium of class Mollicutes, unusual group of bacteria distinguished by absence of cell wall
  A49.8 Other bacterial infections of unspecified site
  A49.9 Bacterial infection, unspecified
    | Excludes1 | bacteremia NOS (R78.81)

INFECTIONS WITH A PREDOMINANTLY SEXUAL MODE OF TRANSMISSION (A50-A64)

    | Excludes1 | human immunodeficiency virus [HIV] disease (B20)
        nonspecific and nongonococcal urethritis (N34.1)
        Reiter's disease (M02.3-)

● **A50 Congenital syphilis**
  ● **A50.0 Early congenital syphilis, symptomatic**
    Any congenital syphilitic condition specified as early or manifest less than two years after birth
    A50.01 Early congenital syphilitic oculopathy
    A50.02 Early congenital syphilitic osteochondropathy
    A50.03 Early congenital syphilitic pharyngitis
        Early congenital syphilitic laryngitis
    A50.04 Early congenital syphilitic pneumonia
    A50.05 Early congenital syphilitic rhinitis
    A50.06 Early cutaneous congenital syphilis
    A50.07 Early mucocutaneous congenital syphilis
    A50.08 Early visceral congenital syphilis
    A50.09 Other early congenital syphilis, symptomatic
  A50.1 Early congenital syphilis, latent
    Congenital syphilis without clinical manifestations, with positive serological reaction and negative spinal fluid test, less than two years after birth
  A50.2 Early congenital syphilis, unspecified
    Congenital syphilis NOS less than two years after birth

Item 1-8 Gas gangrene is a necrotizing subcutaneous infection that will cause tissue death. Patients with poor circulation (e.g., diabetes, peripheral nephropathy) will have low oxygen content in their tissues (hypoxia), which allows the Clostridium bacteria to flourish. Gas gangrene often occurs at the site of a surgical wound or trauma. Onset is sudden and dramatic. Treatment can include debridement, amputation, and/or hyperbaric oxygen treatments.

CHAPTER 1 (A00-B99)

▶ New ⟹ Revised ~~deleted~~ Deleted **OGCR** Official Guidelines X Assign placeholder X ● Use Additional Character(s)

| Excludes 1 | | Excludes 2 | Includes Use additional Code first Code also Key words

Figure 1-3 Chancre of primary syphilis. (From James WD, Berger TG, Elston DM: Andrews' Diseases of the Skin: Clinical Dermatology, Philadelphia, Saunders Elsevier, 2006)

Item 1–9 Syphilis, also known as lues, is the most serious of the venereal diseases caused by *Treponema pallidum*. The **primary** stage is characterized by an ulceration known as **chancre,** which usually appears on the genitals but can also develop on the anus, lips, tonsils, breasts, or fingers. Syphilis is easy to cure in its early stages. A single intramuscular injection of penicillin will usually cure a person who has had syphilis for less than a year.

The **secondary** stage is characterized by a rash that can affect any area of the body. **Latent** syphilis is divided into **early,** which is diagnosed within two years of infection, and **late,** which is diagnosed two years or more after infection. Additional doses of penicillin or another antibiotic are needed to treat someone who has had syphilis for longer than a year. For those allergic to penicillin, there are other antibiotic treatments. **Congenital** syphilis is also labeled **early** or **late** based on the time of diagnosis.

● **A50.3   Late congenital syphilitic oculopathy**
    Excludes1   Hutchinson's triad (A50.53)

    A50.30   Late congenital syphilitic oculopathy, unspecified

    A50.31   Late congenital syphilitic interstitial keratitis

    A50.32   Late congenital syphilitic chorioretinitis

    A50.39   Other late congenital syphilitic oculopathy

● **A50.4   Late congenital neurosyphilis [juvenile neurosyphilis]**
    Use additional code to identify any associated mental disorder
    Excludes1   Hutchinson's triad (A50.53)

    A50.40   Late congenital neurosyphilis, unspecified
        Juvenile neurosyphilis NOS

    A50.41   Late congenital syphilitic meningitis

    A50.42   Late congenital syphilitic encephalitis

    A50.43   Late congenital syphilitic polyneuropathy

    A50.44   Late congenital syphilitic optic nerve atrophy

    A50.45   Juvenile general paresis
        Dementia paralytica juvenilis
        Juvenile tabetoparetic neurosyphilis

    A50.49   Other late congenital neurosyphilis
        Juvenile tabes dorsalis

● **A50.5   Other late congenital syphilis, symptomatic**
    Any congenital syphilitic condition specified as late or manifest two years or more after birth

    A50.51   Clutton's joints

    A50.52   Hutchinson's teeth

    A50.53   Hutchinson's triad

    A50.54   Late congenital cardiovascular syphilis

    A50.55   Late congenital syphilitic arthropathy

    A50.56   Late congenital syphilitic osteochondropathy

    A50.57   Syphilitic saddle nose

    A50.59   Other late congenital syphilis, symptomatic

   A50.6   Late congenital syphilis, latent
    Congenital syphilis without clinical manifestations, with positive serological reaction and negative spinal fluid test, two years or more after birth.

   A50.7   Late congenital syphilis, unspecified
    Congenital syphilis NOS two years or more after birth.

   A50.9   Congenital syphilis, unspecified

● **A51   Early syphilis**

   A51.0   Primary genital syphilis
    Syphilitic chancre NOS

   A51.1   Primary anal syphilis

   A51.2   Primary syphilis of other sites

● **A51.3   Secondary syphilis of skin and mucous membranes**

    A51.31   Condyloma latum

    A51.32   Syphilitic alopecia

    A51.39   Other secondary syphilis of skin
        Syphilitic leukoderma
        Syphilitic mucous patch
        Excludes1   late syphilitic leukoderma (A52.79)

● **A51.4   Other secondary syphilis**

    A51.41   Secondary syphilitic meningitis

    A51.42   Secondary syphilitic female pelvic disease

    A51.43   Secondary syphilitic oculopathy
        Secondary syphilitic chorioretinitis
        Secondary syphilitic iridocyclitis, iritis
        Secondary syphilitic uveitis

    A51.44   Secondary syphilitic nephritis

    A51.45   Secondary syphilitic hepatitis

    A51.46   Secondary syphilitic osteopathy

    A51.49   Other secondary syphilitic conditions
        Secondary syphilitic lymphadenopathy
        Secondary syphilitic myositis

   A51.5   Early syphilis, latent
    Syphilis (acquired) without clinical manifestations, with positive serological reaction and negative spinal fluid test, less than two years after infection.

   A51.9   Early syphilis, unspecified

● **A52   Late syphilis**

● **A52.0   Cardiovascular and cerebrovascular syphilis**

    A52.00   Cardiovascular syphilis, unspecified

    A52.01   Syphilitic aneurysm of aorta

    A52.02   Syphilitic aortitis

    A52.03   Syphilitic endocarditis
        Syphilitic aortic valve incompetence or stenosis
        Syphilitic mitral valve stenosis
        Syphilitic pulmonary valve regurgitation

    A52.04   Syphilitic cerebral arteritis

    A52.05   Other cerebrovascular syphilis
        Syphilitic cerebral aneurysm (ruptured) (non-ruptured)
        Syphilitic cerebral thrombosis

    A52.06   Other syphilitic heart involvement
        Syphilitic coronary artery disease
        Syphilitic myocarditis
        Syphilitic pericarditis

    A52.09   Other cardiovascular syphilis

● **A52.1   Symptomatic neurosyphilis**

    A52.10   Symptomatic neurosyphilis, unspecified

    A52.11   Tabes dorsalis
        Cognitive decline with progressive degeneration of posterior columns, roots, and ganglia of spinal cord, occur 15-20 years after initial infection of syphilis; AKA Duchenne disease
        Locomotor ataxia (progressive)
        Tabetic neurosyphilis

    A52.12   Other cerebrospinal syphilis

    A52.13   Late syphilitic meningitis

    A52.14   Late syphilitic encephalitis

A52.15   Late syphilitic neuropathy
　　Late syphilitic acoustic neuritis
　　Late syphilitic optic (nerve) atrophy
　　Late syphilitic polyneuropathy
　　Late syphilitic retrobulbar neuritis

A52.16   Charcôt's arthropathy (tabetic)
　　Progressive musculoskeletal condition characterized by joint dislocation, fractures, and deformities, results in progressive destruction of bone and soft tissue of weight-bearing joints

A52.17   General paresis
　　Chronic meningoencephalitis results in loss of cortical function, or progressive dementia and generalized paralysis, occurring 10-20 years after initial infection of syphilis; AKA Bayle disease, dementia paralytica, paralytic dementiaparetic neurosyphilis, syphilitic meningoencephalitis
　　Dementia paralytica

A52.19   Other symptomatic neurosyphilis
　　Syphilitic parkinsonism

A52.2   Asymptomatic neurosyphilis

A52.3   Neurosyphilis, unspecified
　　Gumma (syphilitic)
　　Destructive lesions of syphilis
　　Syphilis (late)
　　Syphiloma

● **A52.7   Other symptomatic late syphilis**

A52.71   Late syphilitic oculopathy
　　Late syphilitic chorioretinitis
　　Late syphilitic episcleritis

A52.72   Syphilis of lung and bronchus

A52.73   Symptomatic late syphilis of other respiratory organs

A52.74   Syphilis of liver and other viscera
　　Late syphilitic peritonitis

A52.75   Syphilis of kidney and ureter
　　Syphilitic glomerular disease

A52.76   Other genitourinary symptomatic late syphilis
　　Late syphilitic female pelvic inflammatory disease

A52.77   Syphilis of bone and joint

A52.78   Syphilis of other musculoskeletal tissue
　　Late syphilitic bursitis
　　Syphilis [stage unspecified] of bursa
　　Syphilis [stage unspecified] of muscle
　　Syphilis [stage unspecified] of synovium
　　Syphilis [stage unspecified] of tendon

A52.79   Other symptomatic late syphilis
　　Late syphilitic leukoderma
　　Syphilis of adrenal gland
　　Syphilis of pituitary gland
　　Syphilis of thyroid gland
　　Syphilitic splenomegaly
　　Excludes1　syphilitic leukoderma (secondary) (A51.39)

A52.8   Late syphilis, latent
　　Syphilis (acquired) without clinical manifestations, with positive serological reaction and negative spinal fluid test, two years or more after infection

A52.9   Late syphilis, unspecified

● **A53   Other and unspecified syphilis**

A53.0   Latent syphilis, unspecified as early or late
　　Latent syphilis NOS
　　Positive serological reaction for syphilis

A53.9   Syphilis, unspecified
　　Infection due to Treponema pallidum NOS
　　Syphilis (acquired) NOS
　　Excludes1　syphilis NOS under two years of age (A50.2)

Item 1-10 An STD (sexually transmitted disease) caused by **Neisseria gonorrhoeae** that flourishes in the warm, moist areas of the reproductive tract. Untreated gonorrhea spreads to other parts of the body, causing inflammation of the testes or prostate or pelvic inflammatory disease (PID).

● **A54   Gonococcal infection**

● **A54.0   Gonococcal infection of lower genitourinary tract without periurethral or accessory gland abscess**
　　Excludes1　gonococcal infection with genitourinary gland abscess (A54.1)
　　　　gonococcal infection with periurethral abscess (A54.1)

A54.00   Gonococcal infection of lower genitourinary tract, unspecified

A54.01   Gonococcal cystitis and urethritis, unspecified

A54.02   Gonococcal vulvovaginitis, unspecified

A54.03   Gonococcal cervicitis, unspecified

A54.09   Other gonococcal infection of lower genitourinary tract

A54.1   Gonococcal infection of lower genitourinary tract with periurethral and accessory gland abscess
　　Gonococcal Bartholin's gland abscess

● **A54.2   Gonococcal pelviperitonitis and other gonococcal genitourinary infection**

A54.21   Gonococcal infection of kidney and ureter

A54.22   Gonococcal prostatitis

A54.23   Gonococcal infection of other male genital organs
　　Gonococcal epididymitis
　　Gonococcal orchitis

A54.24   Gonococcal female pelvic inflammatory disease
　　Gonococcal pelviperitonitis
　　Excludes1　gonococcal peritonitis (A54.85)

A54.29   Other gonococcal genitourinary infections

● **A54.3   Gonococcal infection of eye**

A54.30   Gonococcal infection of eye, unspecified

A54.31   Gonococcal conjunctivitis
　　Form of bacterial conjunctivitis contracted by newborns during delivery; AKA neonatal conjunctivitis
　　Ophthalmia neonatorum due to gonococcus

A54.32   Gonococcal iridocyclitis
　　Inflammation of iris and of ciliary body due to gonococcal infection

A54.33   Gonococcal keratitis
　　Inflammation of cornea due to gonococcal infection; AKA keratoconjunctivitis, keratopathy

A54.39   Other gonococcal eye infection
　　Gonococcal endophthalmia

● **A54.4   Gonococcal infection of musculoskeletal system**

A54.40   Gonococcal infection of musculoskeletal system, unspecified

A54.41   Gonococcal spondylopathy
　　Disorder of vertebrae due to gonococcal infection; AKA rachiopathy

A54.42   Gonococcal arthritis
　　Excludes2　gonococcal infection of spine (A54.41)

A54.43   Gonococcal osteomyelitis
　　Excludes2　gonococcal infection of spine (A54.41)

A54.49   Gonococcal infection of other musculoskeletal tissue
　　Gonococcal bursitis
　　Gonococcal myositis
　　Gonococcal synovitis
　　Gonococcal tenosynovitis

▶ New　➡ Revised　~~deleted~~ Deleted　**OGCR** Official Guidelines　X Assign placeholder X　● Use Additional Character(s)

| Excludes 1 | Excludes 2 | Includes | Use additional | Code first | Code also | Key words |

A54.5   Gonococcal pharyngitis

A54.6   Gonococcal infection of anus and rectum

● A54.8   Other gonococcal infections

     A54.81   Gonococcal meningitis

     A54.82   Gonococcal brain abscess

     A54.83   Gonococcal heart infection
            Gonococcal endocarditis
            Gonococcal myocarditis
            Gonococcal pericarditis

     A54.84   Gonococcal pneumonia

     A54.85   Gonococcal peritonitis
         Excludes1   gonococcal pelviperitonitis (A54.24)

     A54.86   Gonococcal sepsis

     A54.89   Other gonococcal infections
            Gonococcal keratoderma
            Gonococcal lymphadenitis

A54.9   Gonococcal infection, unspecified

A55   Chlamydial lymphogranuloma (venereum)
     Climatic or tropical bubo
     Durand-Nicolas-Favre disease
     Esthiomene
     Lymphogranuloma inguinale

● A56   Other sexually transmitted chlamydial diseases
     Includes   sexually transmitted diseases due to Chlamydia trachomatis
     Excludes1   neonatal chlamydial conjunctivitis (P39.1)
            neonatal chlamydial pneumonia (P23.1)
     Excludes2   chlamydial lymphogranuloma (A55)
            conditions classified to A74.-

● A56.0   Chlamydial infection of lower genitourinary tract

     A56.00   Chlamydial infection of lower genitourinary tract, unspecified

     A56.01   Chlamydial cystitis and urethritis

     A56.02   Chlamydial vulvovaginitis

     A56.09   Other chlamydial infection of lower genitourinary tract
            Chlamydial cervicitis

● A56.1   Chlamydial infection of pelviperitoneum and other genitourinary organs

     A56.11   Chlamydial female pelvic inflammatory disease

     A56.19   Other chlamydial genitourinary infection
            Chlamydial epididymitis
            Chlamydial orchitis

A56.2   Chlamydial infection of genitourinary tract, unspecified

A56.3   Chlamydial infection of anus and rectum

A56.4   Chlamydial infection of pharynx

A56.8   Sexually transmitted chlamydial infection of other sites

A57   Chancroid
     Ulcus molle
     Sexually transmitted infection caused by bacteria, Haemophilus ducreyi

A58   Granuloma inguinale
     Chronic, progressive, ulcerative granulomatous disease
     Donovanosis

● A59   Trichomoniasis
     Excludes2   intestinal trichomoniasis (A07.8)
     A common STD caused by a parasite, Trichomonas vaginalis

● A59.0   Urogenital trichomoniasis

     A59.00   Urogenital trichomoniasis, unspecified
            Fluor (vaginalis) due to Trichomonas
            Leukorrhea (vaginalis) due to Trichomonas

     A59.01   Trichomonal vulvovaginitis

     A59.02   Trichomonal prostatitis

     A59.03   Trichomonal cystitis and urethritis

     A59.09   Other urogenital trichomoniasis
         Common sexually transmitted disease (STD) caused by single-celled protozoan parasite; AKA trich
            Trichomonas cervicitis

A59.8   Trichomoniasis of other sites

A59.9   Trichomoniasis, unspecified

● A60   Anogenital herpesviral [herpes simplex] infections

● A60.0   Herpesviral infection of genitalia and urogenital tract

     A60.00   Herpesviral infection of urogenital system, unspecified

     A60.01   Herpesviral infection of penis

     A60.02   Herpesviral infection of other male genital organs

     A60.03   Herpesviral cervicitis

     A60.04   Herpesviral vulvovaginitis
            Herpesviral [herpes simplex] ulceration
            Herpesviral [herpes simplex] vaginitis
            Herpesviral [herpes simplex] vulvitis

     A60.09   Herpesviral infection of other urogenital tract

A60.1   Herpesviral infection of perianal skin and rectum

A60.9   Anogenital herpesviral infection, unspecified

● A63   Other predominantly sexually transmitted diseases, not elsewhere classified
     Excludes2   molluscum contagiosum (B08.1)
            papilloma of cervix (D26.0)

     A63.0   Anogenital (venereal) warts
         Anogenital warts due to (human) papillomavirus [HPV]
         Condyloma acuminatum

     A63.8   Other specified predominantly sexually transmitted diseases

A64   Unspecified sexually transmitted disease

OTHER SPIROCHETAL DISEASES (A65-A69)

     Excludes2   leptospirosis (A27.-)
            syphilis (A50-A53)

A65   Nonvenereal syphilis
     Bejel
     Endemic syphilis
     Njovera

● A66   Yaws
     Endemic, infectious, tropical disease caused by spirochete, spread by direct contact; AKA frambesia, framboesia, frambesia tropica
     Includes   bouba
            frambesia (tropica)
            pian

     A66.0   Initial lesions of yaws
         Chancre of yaws
         Frambesia, initial or primary
         Initial frambesial ulcer
         Mother yaw

     A66.1   Multiple papillomata and wet crab yaws
         Frambesioma
         Pianoma
         Plantar or palmar papilloma of yaws

A66.2   **Other early skin lesions** of yaws
     Cutaneous yaws, less than five years after infection
     Early yaws (cutaneous)(macular)(maculopapular)
         (micropapular)(papular)
     Frambeside of early yaws

A66.3   **Hyperkeratosis** of yaws
     Hypertrophy of stratum corneum of skin in which there are
         small, hard, verrucous scales
     Ghoul hand
     Hyperkeratosis, palmar or plantar (early) (late) due to
         yaws
     Worm-eaten soles

A66.4   **Gummata and ulcers** of yaws
     Small, rubbery granuloma with necrotic center and inflamed
         characteristic of advanced stage of syphilis; AKA
         syphiloma
     Gummatous frambeside
     Nodular late yaws (ulcerated)

A66.5   Gangosa
     Manifestation of yaws that develops in the soft palate and
         spreads eroding bone, cartilage, and soft tissue
     Rhinopharyngitis mutilans

A66.6   **Bone and joint lesions** of yaws
     Yaws ganglion
     Yaws goundou
     Yaws gumma, bone
     Yaws gummatous osteitis or periostitis
     Yaws hydrarthrosis
     Yaws osteitis
     Yaws periostitis (hypertrophic)

A66.7   **Other** manifestations of yaws
     Juxta-articular nodules of yaws
     Mucosal yaws

A66.8   **Latent** yaws
     Yaws without clinical manifestations, with positive
         serology

A66.9   Yaws, **unspecified**

● A67   Pinta [carate]
     Group of nonvenereal diseases caused by Treponema species

A67.0   **Primary** lesions of pinta
     Chancre (primary) of pinta
     Papule (primary) of pinta

A67.1   **Intermediate** lesions of pinta
     Erythematous plaques of pinta
     Hyperchromic lesions of pinta
     Hyperkeratosis of pinta
     Pintids

A67.2   **Late** lesions of pinta
     Achromic skin lesions of pinta
     Cicatricial skin lesions of pinta
     Dyschromic skin lesions of pinta

A67.3   **Mixed** lesions of pinta
     Achromic with hyperchromic skin lesions of pinta
         [carate]

A67.9   Pinta, **unspecified**

● A68   **Relapsing fevers**
     Includes   recurrent fever
     Excludes2   Lyme disease (A69.2-)

A68.0   **Louse-borne** relapsing fever
     Relapsing fever due to Borrelia recurrentis

A68.1   **Tick-borne** relapsing fever
     Relapsing fever due to any Borrelia species other than
         Borrelia recurrentis

A68.9   Relapsing fever, **unspecified**

Item 1-11 Cancrum oris, also known as **noma** or **gangrenous
stomatitis,** begins as an ulcer of the gingiva and results in a progressive
gangrenous process.

● A69   Other spirochetal infections

A69.0   **Necrotizing ulcerative stomatitis**
     Cancrum oris
     Fusospirochetal gangrene
     Noma
     Stomatitis gangrenosa

A69.1   **Other Vincent's infections**
     Fusospirochetal pharyngitis
     Necrotizing ulcerative (acute) gingivitis
     Necrotizing ulcerative (acute) gingivostomatitis
     Spirochetal stomatitis
     Trench mouth
     Vincent's angina
     Vincent's gingivitis

● A69.2   Lyme disease
     Erythema chronicum migrans due to Borrelia
         burgdorferi

     A69.20   **Lyme disease, unspecified**

     A69.21   **Meningitis** due to Lyme disease

     A69.22   **Other neurologic disorders** in Lyme disease
         Cranial neuritis
         Meningoencephalitis
         Polyneuropathy

     A69.23   **Arthritis** due to Lyme disease

     A69.29   **Other conditions** associated with Lyme disease
         Myopericarditis due to Lyme disease

A69.8   **Other specified** spirochetal infections

A69.9   Spirochetal infection, **unspecified**

OTHER DISEASES CAUSED BY CHLAMYDIAE (A70-A74)

Excludes1   sexually transmitted chlamydial diseases
         (A55-A56)

A70   Chlamydia psittaci infections
     Ornithosis
     Parrot fever
     Psittacosis

● A71   Trachoma
     Excludes1   sequelae of trachoma (B94.0)

A71.0   **Initial stage** of trachoma
     Trachoma dubium

A71.1   **Active stage** of trachoma
     Granular conjunctivitis (trachomatous)
     Trachomatous follicular conjunctivitis
     Trachomatous pannus

A71.9   Trachoma, **unspecified**

● A74   Other diseases caused by chlamydiae
     Excludes1   neonatal chlamydial conjunctivitis (P39.1)
         neonatal chlamydial pneumonia (P23.1)
         Reiter's disease (M02.3-)
         sexually transmitted chlamydial diseases
         (A55-A56)
     Excludes2   chlamydial pneumonia (J16.0)

A74.0   **Chlamydial conjunctivitis**
     Paratrachoma

● A74.8   Other chlamydial diseases

     A74.81   Chlamydial **peritonitis**

     A74.89   **Other** chlamydial diseases

A74.9   Chlamydial infection, **unspecified**
     Chlamydiosis NOS

▶ New   ⇒ Revised   ~~deleted~~ Deleted   **OGCR** Official Guidelines   X Assign placeholder X   ● Use Additional Character(s)

| Excludes 1 | Excludes 2 | Includes | Use additional | Code first | Code also | Key words |

Item 1–12 Rickettsioses are diseases spread from ticks, lice, fleas, or mites to humans.

Typhus is spread to humans chiefly by the fleas of rats.

Endemic identifies a disease as being present in low numbers of humans at all times, whereas **epidemic** identifies a disease as being present in high numbers of humans at a specific time. Morbidity (death) is higher in epidemic diseases.

Brill's disease, also known as **Brill-Zinsser disease,** is spread from human to human by body lice and also from the lice of flying squirrels. **Scrub typhus** is spread in the same ways as Brill's disease.

Malaria is spread to humans by mosquitoes.

RICKETTSIOSES (A75-A79)

● **A75 Typhus fever**
Excludes1 rickettsiosis due to Ehrlichia sennetsu (A79.81)

A75.0 Epidemic louse-borne typhus fever due to Rickettsia prowazekii
Organisms transmitted between humans via louse
Classical typhus (fever)
Epidemic (louse-borne) typhus

A75.1 Recrudescent typhus [Brill's disease]
Brill-Zinsser disease

A75.2 Typhus fever due to Rickettsia typhi
Murine (flea-borne) typhus

A75.3 Typhus fever due to Rickettsia tsutsugamushi
Scrub (mite-borne) typhus
Tsutsugamushi fever

A75.9 Typhus fever, unspecified
Typhus (fever) NOS

● **A77 Spotted fever [tick-borne rickettsioses]**

A77.0 Spotted fever due to Rickettsia rickettsii
Rocky Mountain spotted fever
Sao Paulo fever

A77.1 Spotted fever due to Rickettsia conorii
African tick typhus
Boutonneuse fever
India tick typhus
Kenya tick typhus
Marseilles fever
Mediterranean tick fever

A77.2 Spotted fever due to Rickettsia siberica
North Asian tick fever
Siberian tick typhus

A77.3 Spotted fever due to Rickettsia australis
Queensland tick typhus

● **A77.4 Ehrlichiosis**
Type of tick-borne fever caused by bacteria infection
Excludes1 Rickettsiosis due to Ehrlichia sennetsu (A79.81)

A77.40 Ehrlichiosis, unspecified
A77.41 Ehrlichiosis chafeensis [E. chafeensis]
A77.49 Other ehrlichiosis

A77.8 Other spotted fevers

A77.9 Spotted fever, unspecified
Tick-borne typhus NOS

A78 Q fever
Infection due to Coxiella burnetii
Nine Mile fever
Quadrilateral fever

● **A79 Other rickettsioses**

A79.0 Trench fever
Quintan fever
Wolhynian fever

A79.1 Rickettsialpox due to Rickettsia akari
Kew Garden fever
Vesicular rickettsiosis

● **A79.8 Other specified rickettsioses**
A79.81 Rickettsiosis due to Ehrlichia sennetsu
A79.89 Other specified rickettsioses

A79.9 Rickettsiosis, unspecified
Rickettsial infection NOS

Item 1–13 Acute Poliomyelitis: Also called infantile paralysis and is caused by the poliovirus, which enters the body orally and infects the intestinal wall and then enters the blood stream and central nervous system, causing muscle weakness and paralysis. This disease has been nearly eradicated with the polio vaccine.

VIRAL AND PRION INFECTIONS OF THE CENTRAL NERVOUS SYSTEM (A80-A89)

Excludes1 postpolio syndrome (G14)
sequelae of poliomyelitis (B91)
sequelae of viral encephalitis (B94.1)

● **A80 Acute poliomyelitis**
A80.0 Acute paralytic poliomyelitis, vaccine-associated
A80.1 Acute paralytic poliomyelitis, wild virus, imported
A80.2 Acute paralytic poliomyelitis, wild virus, indigenous
● **A80.3 Acute paralytic poliomyelitis, other and unspecified**
A80.30 Acute paralytic poliomyelitis, unspecified
A80.39 Other acute paralytic poliomyelitis
A80.4 Acute nonparalytic poliomyelitis
A80.9 Acute poliomyelitis, unspecified

● **A81 Atypical virus infections of central nervous system**
Includes diseases of the central nervous system caused by prions
Use additional code to identify:
dementia with behavioral disturbance (F02.81)
dementia without behavioral disturbance (F02.80)

● **A81.0 Creutzfeldt-Jakob disease**
A81.00 Creutzfeldt-Jakob disease, unspecified
Jakob-Creutzfeldt disease, unspecified
A81.01 Variant Creutzfeldt-Jakob disease
vCJD
A81.09 Other Creutzfeldt-Jakob disease
CJD
Familial Creutzfeldt-Jakob disease
Iatrogenic Creutzfeldt-Jakob disease
Sporadic Creutzfeldt-Jakob disease
Subacute spongiform encephalopathy (with dementia)

A81.1 Subacute sclerosing panencephalitis
Type of viral encephalitis that causes parenchymatous lesions in gray and white matter of brain
Dawson's inclusion body encephalitis
Van Bogaert's sclerosing leukoencephalopathy

A81.2 Progressive multifocal leukoencephalopathy
Group of diseases affecting white matter of brain
Multifocal leukoencephalopathy NOS

● **A81.8 Other atypical virus infections of central nervous system**
A81.81 Kuru
A81.82 Gerstmann-Sträussler-Scheinker syndrome
GSS syndrome
A81.83 Fatal familial insomnia
FFI
A81.89 Other atypical virus infections of central nervous system
A81.9 Atypical virus infection of central nervous system, unspecified
Prion diseases of the central nervous system NOS

● **A82 Rabies**
Viral disease affecting the central nervous system and transmitted from infected mammals to man.
A82.0 Sylvatic rabies
A82.1 Urban rabies
A82.9 Rabies, unspecified

▶ New ⇒ Revised ~~deleted~~ Deleted **OGCR** Official Guidelines **X** Assign placeholder X ● Use Additional Character(s)
Excludes 1 | Excludes 2 | Includes | Use additional | Code first | Code also | Key words

Item 1-14   **Encephalitis** is an inflammation of the brain most often caused by a virus but may also be caused by a bacteria and most commonly transmitted by a mosquito. **Myelitis** is an inflammation of the spinal cord that may disrupt CNS function. Untreated myelitis may rapidly lead to permanent damage to the spinal cord. **Encephalomyelitis** is a general term for an inflammation of the brain and spinal cord.

● **A83**   **Mosquito-borne viral encephalitis**
    Inflammation of the brain caused most commonly by Herpes Simplex virus.

    | **Includes** | mosquito-borne viral meningoencephalitis |
    | **Excludes2** | Venezuelan equine encephalitis (A92.2) |
    West Nile fever (A92.3-)
    West Nile virus (A92.3-)

    A83.0   **Japanese** encephalitis

    A83.1   **Western equine** encephalitis

    A83.2   **Eastern equine** encephalitis

    A83.3   **St. Louis** encephalitis

    A83.4   **Australian** encephalitis
         Kunjin virus disease

    A83.5   **California** encephalitis
         California meningoencephalitis
         La Crosse encephalitis

    A83.6   **Rocio virus disease**
         Mosquito-borne virus

    A83.8   **Other** mosquito-borne viral encephalitis

    A83.9   Mosquito-borne viral encephalitis, **unspecified**

● **A84**   **Tick-borne viral encephalitis**

    | **Includes** | tick-borne viral meningoencephalitis |

    A84.0   **Far Eastern** tick-borne encephalitis [Russian spring-summer encephalitis]

    A84.1   **Central European** tick-borne encephalitis

    A84.8   **Other** tick-borne viral encephalitis
         Louping ill
         Powassan virus disease

    A84.9   Tick-borne viral encephalitis, **unspecified**

● **A85**   **Other viral encephalitis, not elsewhere classified**

    | **Includes** | specified viral encephalomyelitis NEC |
    specified viral meningoencephalitis NEC

    | **Excludes1** | benign myalgic encephalomyelitis (G93.3) |
    encephalitis due to cytomegalovirus (B25.8)
    encephalitis due to herpesvirus NEC (B10.0-)
    encephalitis due to herpesvirus [herpes simplex] (B00.4)
    encephalitis due to measles virus (B05.0)
    encephalitis due to mumps virus (B26.2)
    encephalitis due to poliomyelitis virus (A80.-)
    encephalitis due to zoster (B02.0)
    lymphocytic choriomeningitis (A87.2)

    A85.0   **Enteroviral** encephalitis
         Enteroviral encephalomyelitis

    A85.1   **Adenoviral** encephalitis
         Adenoviral meningoencephalitis

    A85.2   **Arthropod-borne viral** encephalitis, **unspecified**

        | **Excludes1** | West nile virus with encephalitis (A92.31) |

    A85.8   **Other** specified viral encephalitis
         Encephalitis lethargica
         Von Economo-Cruchet disease

    A86   **Unspecified** viral encephalitis
         Viral encephalomyelitis NOS
         Viral meningoencephalitis NOS

● **A87**   **Viral meningitis**

    | **Excludes1** | meningitis due to herpesvirus [herpes simplex] (B00.3) |
    meningitis due to measles virus (B05.1)
    meningitis due to mumps virus (B26.1)
    meningitis due to poliomyelitis virus (A80.-)
    meningitis due to zoster (B02.1)

    A87.0   **Enteroviral** meningitis
         Group of common viruses responsible for the majority of viral meningitis
         Coxsackievirus meningitis
         Echovirus meningitis

    A87.1   **Adenoviral** meningitis

    A87.2   **Lymphocytic** choriomeningitis
         Lymphocytic meningoencephalitis

    A87.8   **Other** viral meningitis

    A87.9   Viral meningitis, **unspecified**

● **A88**   **Other viral infections of central nervous system, not elsewhere classified**

    | **Excludes1** | viral encephalitis NOS (A86) |
    viral meningitis NOS (A87.9)

    A88.0   **Enteroviral exanthematous fever [Boston exanthem]**
         Infectious skin eruption

    A88.1   **Epidemic vertigo**

    A88.8   **Other specified viral infections of central nervous system**

    A89   **Unspecified** viral infection of central nervous system

ARTHROPOD-BORNE VIRAL FEVERS AND VIRAL HEMORRHAGIC FEVERS (A90-A99)

    A90   **Dengue fever [classical dengue]**
         Acute, self-limited disease, characterized by fever, prostration, severe muscle pains, headache, rash, lymphadenopathy, and leukopenia, caused by dengue virus; AKA breakbone, dandy

        | **Excludes1** | dengue hemorrhagic fever (A91) |

    A91   **Dengue hemorrhagic fever**
         Serious follow-up to regular dengue, with symptoms of hemorrhage

● **A92**   **Other mosquito-borne viral fevers**
    | **Excludes1** | Ross River disease (B33.1) |

    A92.0   **Chikungunya virus disease**
         Transmitted by mosquitoes
         Chikungunya (hemorrhagic) fever

    A92.1   **O'nyong-nyong fever**
         Acute, nonfatal febrile disease transmitted by mosquitoes, which clinically resembles dengue and chikungunya

    A92.2   **Venezuelan equine fever**
         Venezuelan equine encephalitis
         Venezuelan equine encephalomyelitis virus disease

    ● **A92.3**   **West Nile virus infection**
         West Nile fever

        A92.30   **West Nile virus infection, unspecified**
             West Nile fever NOS
             West Nile fever without complications
             West Nile virus NOS

        A92.31   **West Nile virus infection with encephalitis**
             West Nile encephalitis
             West Nile encephalomyelitis

        A92.32   **West Nile virus infection with other neurologic manifestation**
             Use additional code to specify the neurologic manifestation

        A92.39   **West Nile virus infection with other complications**
             Use additional code to specify the other conditions

CHAPTER 1 (A00-B99)

OGCR Section I. C.1.f.

Certain Infectious and Parasitic Diseases (A00-B99)

Zika virus infections

Code only confirmed cases

Code only a confirmed diagnosis of Zika virus (A92.5, Zika virus disease) as documented by the provider. This is an exception to the hospital inpatient guideline Section II, H.

In this context, "confirmation" does not require documentation of the type of test performed; the physician's diagnostic statement that the condition is confirmed is sufficient. This code should be assigned regardless of the stated mode of transmission.

If the provider documents "suspected", "possible" or "probable" Zika, do not assign code A92.5. Assign a code(s) explaining the reason for encounter (such as fever, rash, or joint pain) or Z20.828, Contact with and (suspected) exposure to other viral communicable diseases.

  A92.4   **Rift Valley fever**

  A92.5   **Zika virus disease**
       Zika virus fever
       Zika virus infection
       Zika NOS

  A92.8   **Other specified mosquito-borne viral fevers**

  A92.9   **Mosquito-borne viral fever, unspecified**

● **A93**   **Other arthropod-borne viral fevers, not elsewhere classified**

  A93.0   **Oropouche virus disease**
       Tropical viral infection
       Oropouche fever

  A93.1   **Sandfly fever**
       Pappataci fever
       Phlebotomus fever

  A93.2   **Colorado tick fever**

  A93.8   **Other specified arthropod-borne viral fevers**
       Piry virus disease
       Vesicular stomatitis virus disease [Indiana fever]

  A94   **Unspecified arthropod-borne viral fever**
       Arboviral fever NOS
       Arbovirus infection NOS

● **A95**   **Yellow fever**
       Acute infectious disease transmitted by mosquitoes

  A95.0   **Sylvatic yellow fever**
       Jungle yellow fever

  A95.1   **Urban yellow fever**

  A95.9   **Yellow fever, unspecified**

● **A96**   **Arenaviral hemorrhagic fever**
       Virus that causes various hemorrhagic fevers

  A96.0   **Junin hemorrhagic fever**
       Argentinian hemorrhagic fever

  A96.1   **Machupo hemorrhagic fever**
       Transmitted by contact with infected rodents
       Bolivian hemorrhagic fever

  A96.2   **Lassa fever**
       Acute type of hemorrhagic fever caused by contact with
       disease carrying mouse or person

  A96.8   **Other arenaviral hemorrhagic fevers**

  A96.9   **Arenaviral hemorrhagic fever, unspecified**

● **A98**   **Other viral hemorrhagic fevers, not elsewhere classified**
     Excludes1   chikungunya hemorrhagic fever (A92.0)
                dengue hemorrhagic fever (A91)

  A98.0   **Crimean-Congo hemorrhagic fever**
       Virus transmitted by ticks and contact with blood, secretions,
       or fluids from infected humans or animals
       Central Asian hemorrhagic fever

  A98.1   **Omsk hemorrhagic fever**
       Transmitted to humans by bites of infected ticks or contact
       with infected muskrats

  A98.2   **Kyasanur Forest disease**
       Transmitted via infected monkeys, voles, ticks

  A98.3   **Marburg virus disease**
       Rare, acute, often fatal type of hemorrhagic fever

  A98.4   **Ebola virus disease**

  A98.5   **Hemorrhagic fever with renal syndrome**
       Epidemic hemorrhagic fever
       Korean hemorrhagic fever
       Russian hemorrhagic fever
       Hantaan virus disease
       Hantavirus disease with renal manifestations
       Nephropathia epidemica
       Songo fever
     Excludes1   hantavirus (cardio)-pulmonary syndrome
                (B33.4)

  A98.8   **Other specified viral hemorrhagic fevers**

  A99   **Unspecified viral hemorrhagic fever**

VIRAL INFECTIONS CHARACTERIZED BY SKIN AND MUCOUS MEMBRANE LESIONS (B00-B09)

● **B00**   **Herpesviral [herpes simplex] infections**
     Excludes1   congenital herpesviral infections (P35.2)
     Excludes2   anogenital herpesviral infection (A60.-)
                gammaherpesviral mononucleosis (B27.0-)
                herpangina (B08.5)

  B00.0   **Eczema herpeticum**
       Cutaneous eruption caused by herpes simplex virus (HSV)
       type 1, HSV-2, coxsackievirus A16, or vaccinia virus
       Kaposi's varicelliform eruption

  B00.1   **Herpesviral vesicular dermatitis**
       Vesicle formation; characteristics include formation of blisters
       and scabs on feet and legs
       Herpes simplex facialis
       Herpes simplex labialis
       Herpes simplex otitis externa
       Vesicular dermatitis of ear
       Vesicular dermatitis of lip

  B00.2   **Herpesviral gingivostomatitis and pharyngotonsillitis**
       Inflammation involving both gingivae and oral mucosa
       Herpesviral pharyngitis
       Inflammation of pharynx and tonsils; AKA
       tonsillopharyngitis

  B00.3   **Herpesviral meningitis**

  B00.4   **Herpesviral encephalitis**
       Herpesviral meningoencephalitis
       Simian B disease
     Excludes1   herpesviral encephalitis due to herpesvirus 6
                and 7 (B10.01, B10.09)
                non-simplex herpesviral encephalitis
                (B10.0-)

● **B00.5**   **Herpesviral ocular disease**

  B00.50   **Herpesviral ocular disease, unspecified**

  B00.51   **Herpesviral iridocyclitis**
       Herpesviral iritis
       Herpesviral uveitis, anterior

  B00.52   **Herpesviral keratitis**
       Herpesviral keratoconjunctivitis

  B00.53   **Herpesviral conjunctivitis**

  B00.59   **Other herpesviral disease of eye**
       Herpesviral dermatitis of eyelid

Figure 1-4 Primary herpes simplex in and around the mouth. The infection is usually acquired from siblings or parents and is readily transmitted to other direct contacts. (Getty Image)

Item 1-15 **Herpes** is a viral disease for which there is no cure. There are two types of the herpes simplex virus: **Type I** causes **cold sores** or **fever blisters,** and **Type II** causes **genital herpes.** The virus can be spread from a sore on the lips to the genitals or from the genitals to the lips.

▶ New   ⇒ Revised   ~~deleted~~ Deleted   **OGCR** Official Guidelines   X Assign placeholder X   ● Use Additional Character(s)

Excludes 1   Excludes 2   Includes   Use additional   Code first   Code also   Key words

B00.7 Disseminated herpesviral disease
Herpesviral sepsis

● **B00.8 Other forms of herpesviral infections**

     B00.81 Herpesviral hepatitis

     B00.82 Herpes simplex myelitis

     B00.89 Other herpesviral infection
         Herpesviral whitlow

B00.9 Herpesviral infection, unspecified
Herpes simplex infection NOS

● **B01 Varicella [chickenpox]**
Very contagious disease caused by the varicella zoster virus that results in an itchy outbreak of skin blisters (varicella). The same virus causes shingles (zoster).

B01.0 Varicella meningitis

● **B01.1 Varicella encephalitis, myelitis and encephalomyelitis**
Postchickenpox encephalitis, myelitis and encephalomyelitis

     B01.11 Varicella encephalitis and encephalomyelitis
         Postchickenpox encephalitis and encephalomyelitis

     B01.12 Varicella myelitis
         Postchickenpox myelitis

B01.2 Varicella pneumonia

● **B01.8 Varicella with other complications**

     B01.81 Varicella keratitis

     B01.89 Other varicella complications

B01.9 Varicella without complication
Varicella NOS

● **B02 Zoster [herpes zoster]**

     Includes   shingles
                 zona

B02.0 Zoster encephalitis
Zoster meningoencephalitis

B02.1 Zoster meningitis

● **B02.2 Zoster with other nervous system involvement**

     B02.21 Postherpetic geniculate ganglionitis

     B02.22 Postherpetic trigeminal neuralgia

     B02.23 Postherpetic polyneuropathy

     B02.24 Postherpetic myelitis
         Herpes zoster myelitis

     B02.29 Other postherpetic nervous system involvement
         Postherpetic radiculopathy

● **B02.3 Zoster ocular disease**

     B02.30 Zoster ocular disease, unspecified

     B02.31 Zoster conjunctivitis

     B02.32 Zoster iridocyclitis

     B02.33 Zoster keratitis
         Herpes zoster keratoconjunctivitis

     B02.34 Zoster scleritis

     B02.39 Other herpes zoster eye disease
         Zoster blepharitis

B02.7 Disseminated zoster

B02.8 Zoster with other complications
Herpes zoster otitis externa

B02.9 Zoster without complications
Zoster NOS

Figure 1-5 Photograph of eyelids with marginal blepharitis. (From Hoyt CS, Taylor D: Pediatric Ophthalmology and Strabismus, London, Elsevier Saunders, 2005)

Item 1–17 Blepharitis is a common condition in which the eyelid is swollen and yellow scaling and conjunctivitis develop. Usually the hair on the scalp and brow is involved.

B03 Smallpox
Note: In 1980 the 33rd World Health Assembly declared that smallpox had been eradicated. The classification is maintained for surveillance purposes.

B04 Monkeypox
Disease occurring in captive monkeys and other mammals that may be transmitted to humans, clinically similar to smallpox

● **B05 Measles**

     Includes   morbilli

     Excludes1   subacute sclerosing panencephalitis (A81.1)

     B05.0 Measles complicated by encephalitis
         Postmeasles encephalitis

     B05.1 Measles complicated by meningitis
         Postmeasles meningitis

     B05.2 Measles complicated by pneumonia
         Postmeasles pneumonia

     B05.3 Measles complicated by otitis media
         Postmeasles otitis media

     B05.4 Measles with intestinal complications

●   **B05.8 Measles with other complications**

         B05.81 Measles keratitis and keratoconjunctivitis

         B05.89 Other measles complications

     B05.9 Measles without complication
         Measles NOS

● **B06 Rubella [German measles]**

     Excludes1   congenital rubella (P35.0)

●   **B06.0 Rubella with neurological complications**

         B06.00 Rubella with neurological complication, unspecified

         B06.01 Rubella encephalitis
             Rubella meningoencephalitis

         B06.02 Rubella meningitis

         B06.09 Other neurological complications of rubella

●   **B06.8 Rubella with other complications**

         B06.81 Rubella pneumonia

         B06.82 Rubella arthritis

         B06.89 Other rubella complications

     B06.9 Rubella without complication
         Rubella NOS

● **B07 Viral warts**

     Includes   verruca simplex
                 verruca vulgaris
                 viral warts due to human papillomavirus

     Excludes2   anogenital (venereal) warts (A63.0)
                  papilloma of bladder (D41.4)
                  papilloma of cervix (D26.0)
                  papilloma larynx (D14.1)

     B07.0 Plantar wart
         Verruca plantaris

     B07.8 Other viral warts
         Common wart
         Flat wart
         Verruca plana

     B07.9 Viral wart, unspecified

Item 1-16 Zoster: Also known as *shingles* and is caused by the same virus as chickenpox. After exposure, the virus lies dormant in nerve tissue and is activated by factors including aging, stress, suppression of the immune system, and certain medication. It begins as a unilateral rash that leads to blisters and sores on the skin. It may involve the nerve pathways of the eye, forehead, nose, and eyelids and may be very painful with long-term systemic effects.

▶ New   ⇒ Revised   ~~deleted~~ Deleted   **OGCR** Official Guidelines   X Assign placeholder X   ● Use Additional Character(s)

Excludes 1   Excludes 2   Includes   Use additional   Code first   Code also   Key words

CHAPTER 1 (A00-B99)

CHAPTER 1 (A00-B99)

● **B08**   **Other viral infections characterized by skin and mucous membrane lesions, not elsewhere classified**

     Excludes1   vesicular stomatitis virus disease (A93.8)

  ● **B08.0**   **Other orthopoxvirus infections**

      Excludes2   monkeypox (B04)

    ● **B08.01**   **Cowpox and vaccinia not from vaccine**

        B08.010   **Cowpox**

        B08.011   **Vaccinia not from vaccine**

           Excludes1   vaccinia (from vaccination) (generalized) (T88.1)

       B08.02   **Orf virus disease**
           Contagious pustular dermatitis
           Ecthyma contagiosum

       B08.03   **Pseudocowpox [milker's node]**

       B08.04   **Paravaccinia, unspecified**

       B08.09   **Other orthopoxvirus infections**
           Orthopoxvirus infection NOS

  ● **B08.1**   **Molluscum contagiosum**
       Various skin diseases characterized by soft, rounded, cutaneous lesions

  ● **B08.2**   **Exanthema subitum [sixth disease] Roseola infantum**
       Acute, short-lived high fever in infants and young children followed by a rash mainly on the trunk, caused by human herpesvirus 6

       B08.20   **Exanthema subitum [sixth disease], unspecified Roseola infantum, unspecified**

       B08.21   **Exanthema subitum [sixth disease] due to human herpesvirus 6 Roseola infantum due to human herpesvirus 6**
           Virus results in sudden rash; infection results in lifelong persistence

       B08.22   **Exanthema subitum [sixth disease] due to human herpesvirus 7 Roseola infantum due to human herpesvirus 7**

  ● **B08.3**   **Erythema infectiosum [fifth disease]**
       Moderately contagious, epidemic disease in children caused by B19 virus; onset of rash that begins as redness of cheeks, later there is rash on trunk and limbs; when this fades, there may be central clearing that leaves lacelike pattern

  ● **B08.4**   **Enteroviral vesicular stomatitis with exanthem**
       Hand, foot and mouth disease
       Check your documentation—this code is HAND, foot, and mouth disease. Code B08.8 is foot and mouth disease.

  ● **B08.5**   **Enteroviral vesicular pharyngitis**
       Herpangina

  ● **B08.6**   **Parapoxvirus infections**

       B08.60   **Parapoxvirus infection, unspecified**

       B08.61   **Bovine stomatitis**

       B08.62   **Sealpox**

       B08.69   **Other parapoxvirus infections**

  ● **B08.7**   **Yatapoxvirus infections**

       B08.70   **Yatapoxvirus infection, unspecified**

       B08.71   **Tanapox virus disease**

       B08.72   **Yaba pox virus disease**
           Yaba monkey tumor disease

       B08.79   **Other yatapoxvirus infections**

  ● **B08.8**   **Other specified viral infections characterized by skin and mucous membrane lesions**
       Enteroviral lymphonodular pharyngitis
       Foot-and-mouth disease
       Check your documentation. Code B08.4 is for HAND, foot, and mouth disease.
       Poxvirus NEC

B09   **Unspecified viral infection characterized by skin and mucous membrane lesions**
       Viral enanthema NOS
       Viral exanthema NOS

OTHER HUMAN HERPESVIRUSES (B10)

● **B10**   **Other human herpesviruses**

     Excludes2   cytomegalovirus (B25.9)
           Epstein-Barr virus (B27.0-)
           herpes NOS (B00.9)
           herpes simplex (B00.-)
           herpes zoster (B02.-)
           human herpesvirus NOS (B00.-)
           human herpesvirus 1 and 2 (B00.-)
           human herpesvirus 3 (B01.-, B02.-)
           human herpesvirus 4 (B27.0-)
           human herpesvirus 5 (B25.-)
           varicella (B01.-)
           zoster (B02.-)

  ● **B10.0**   **Other human herpesvirus encephalitis**

      Excludes2   herpes encephalitis NOS (B00.4)
           herpes simplex encephalitis (B00.4)
           human herpesvirus encephalitis (B00.4)
           simian B herpes virus encephalitis (B00.4)

       B10.01   **Human herpesvirus 6 encephalitis**
           Sudden rash or roseola

       B10.09   **Other human herpesvirus encephalitis**
           Human herpesvirus 7 encephalitis
           Virus closely related to human herpesvirus 6, but not known to cause any disease

  ● **B10.8**   **Other human herpesvirus infection**

       B10.81   **Human herpesvirus 6 infection**
           Causative agent of exanthema subitum that results in sudden rash

       B10.82   **Human herpesvirus 7 infection**
           Closely related to human herpesvirus 6, but not known cause any disease

       B10.89   **Other human herpesvirus infection**
           Human herpesvirus 8 infection
           May be the cause of Kaposi sarcoma, a malignant tumor
           Kaposi's sarcoma-associated herpesvirus infection

VIRAL HEPATITIS (B15-B19)

     Excludes1   sequelae of viral hepatitis (B94.2)
     Excludes2   cytomegaloviral hepatitis (B25.1)
           herpesviral [herpes simplex] hepatitis (B00.81)

● **B15**   **Acute hepatitis A**

     B15.0   **Hepatitis A with hepatic coma**

     B15.9   **Hepatitis A without hepatic coma**
       Hepatitis A (acute) (viral) NOS

Figure 1-6   Hepatitis B viral infection. **A.** Liver parenchyma showing hepatocytes with diffuse granular cytoplasm, so-called ground glass hepatocytes (H&E). **B.** Immunoperoxidase stains from the same case, showing cytoplasmic inclusions of viral particles. (From Kumar: Robbins and Cotran: Pathologic Basis of Disease, ed 8, Saunders, An Imprint of Elsevier, 2009)

Item 1–18   **Hepatitis A (HAV)** was formerly called epidemic, infectious, short-incubation, or acute catarrhal jaundice hepatitis. The primary transmission mode is the oral–fecal route. **Hepatitis B (HBV)** was formerly called long-incubation period, serum, or homologous serum hepatitis. Transmission modes are through blood from infected persons and from body fluids of infected mother to neonate. **Hepatitis C (HCV),** caused by the hepatitis C virus, is primarily transfusion associated. **Hepatitis D (HDV),** also called delta hepatitis, is caused by the hepatitis D virus in patients formerly or currently infected with hepatitis B. **Hepatitis E (HEV)** is also called enterically transmitted non-A, non-B hepatitis. The primary transmission mode is the oral–fecal route, usually through contaminated water.

▶ New   ⇒ Revised   ~~deleted~~ Deleted   **OGCR** Official Guidelines   X Assign placeholder X   ● Use Additional Character(s)

Excludes 1   Excludes 2   Includes   Use additional   Code first   Code also   Key words

● **B16**   **Acute hepatitis B**
    B16.0   **Acute hepatitis B with delta-agent with hepatic coma**
    B16.1   **Acute hepatitis B with delta-agent without hepatic coma**
    B16.2   **Acute hepatitis B without delta-agent with hepatic coma**
    B16.9   **Acute hepatitis B without delta-agent and without hepatic coma**
            Hepatitis B (acute) (viral) NOS

● **B17**   **Other acute viral hepatitis**
    B17.0   **Acute delta-(super) infection of hepatitis B carrier**
  ● **B17.1**   **Acute hepatitis C**
        B17.10   **Acute hepatitis C without hepatic coma**
               Acute hepatitis C NOS
        B17.11   **Acute hepatitis C with hepatic coma**
    B17.2   **Acute hepatitis E**
    B17.8   **Other specified acute viral hepatitis**
            Hepatitis non-A non-B (acute) (viral) NEC
    B17.9   **Acute viral hepatitis, unspecified**
            Acute hepatitis NOS
            Acute infectious hepatitis NOS

● **B18**   **Chronic viral hepatitis**
    Includes   Carrier of viral hepatitis
    B18.0   **Chronic viral hepatitis B with delta-agent**
    B18.1   **Chronic viral hepatitis B without delta-agent**
            Carrier of viral hepatitis B
            Chronic (viral) hepatitis B
    B18.2   **Chronic viral hepatitis C**
            Carrier of viral hepatitis C
    B18.8   **Other chronic viral hepatitis**
            Carrier of other viral hepatitis
    B18.9   **Chronic viral hepatitis, unspecified**
            Carrier of unspecified viral hepatitis

● **B19**   **Unspecified viral hepatitis**
    B19.0   **Unspecified viral hepatitis with hepatic coma**
  ● **B19.1**   **Unspecified viral hepatitis B**
        B19.10   **Unspecified viral hepatitis B without hepatic coma**
               Unspecified viral hepatitis B NOS
        B19.11   **Unspecified viral hepatitis B with hepatic coma**
  ● **B19.2**   **Unspecified viral hepatitis C**
        B19.20   **Unspecified viral hepatitis C without hepatic coma**
               Viral hepatitis C NOS
        B19.21   **Unspecified viral hepatitis C with hepatic coma**
    B19.9   **Unspecified viral hepatitis without hepatic coma**
            Viral hepatitis NOS

OGCR   Section I. C.1.a.

Certain Infectious and Parasitic Diseases (A00-B99)

a. Human Immunodeficiency Virus (HIV) Infections

  1) Code only confirmed cases

    Code only confirmed cases of HIV infection illness. This is an exception to the hospital inpatient guideline Section II, H.

    In this context, "confirmation" does not require documentation of positive serology or culture for HIV; the provider's diagnostic statement that the patient is HIV positive, or has an HIV-related illness is sufficient.

HUMAN IMMUNODEFICIENCY VIRUS [HIV] DISEASE (B20)

B20   **Human immunodeficiency virus [HIV] disease**
    Includes   acquired immune deficiency syndrome [AIDS]
               AIDS-related complex [ARC]
               HIV infection, symptomatic
    Code first Human immunodeficiency virus [HIV] disease complicating pregnancy, childbirth and the puerperium, if applicable (O98.7-)
    Use additional code(s) to identify all manifestations of HIV infection
    Excludes1   asymptomatic human immunodeficiency virus [HIV] infection status (Z21)
               exposure to HIV virus (Z20.6)
               inconclusive serologic evidence of HIV (R75)

OTHER VIRAL DISEASES (B25-B34)

● **B25**   **Cytomegaloviral disease**
    AKA: HCMV or Human Herpesvirus 5 (HHV-5)
    Excludes1   congenital cytomegalovirus infection (P35.1)
               cytomegaloviral mononucleosis (B27.1-)
    B25.0   **Cytomegaloviral pneumonitis**
    B25.1   **Cytomegaloviral hepatitis**
    B25.2   **Cytomegaloviral pancreatitis**
    B25.8   **Other cytomegaloviral diseases**
            Cytomegaloviral encephalitis
    B25.9   **Cytomegaloviral disease, unspecified**

● **B26**   **Mumps**
    Includes   epidemic parotitis
               infectious parotitis
    Acute, contagious, viral disease
    B26.0   **Mumps orchitis**
    B26.1   **Mumps meningitis**
    B26.2   **Mumps encephalitis**
    B26.3   **Mumps pancreatitis**
  ● **B26.8**   **Mumps with other complications**
        B26.81   **Mumps hepatitis**
        B26.82   **Mumps myocarditis**
        B26.83   **Mumps nephritis**
        B26.84   **Mumps polyneuropathy**
        B26.85   **Mumps arthritis**
        B26.89   **Other mumps complications**
    B26.9   **Mumps without complication**
            Mumps NOS
            Mumps parotitis NOS

Figure 1-7 Kaposi's sarcoma. There are large confluent hyperpigmented patch-stage lesions with lymphedema. (From Kanski, JJ: Clinical Diagnosis in Ophthalmology, London, Elsevier Mosby, 2006)

Item 1-19   **AIDS** (acquired immune deficiency syndrome) is caused by **HIV** (human immunodeficiency virus). HIV affects certain white blood cells (T-4 lymphocytes) and destroys the ability of the cells to fight infections, making patients susceptible to a host of infectious diseases (e.g., ***Pneumocystis carinii pneumonia (PCP), Kaposi's sarcoma,*** and **lymphoma**). ***AIDS-related complex (ARC)*** is an early stage of AIDS in which tests for HIV are positive but the symptoms are mild.

▶ New   ⇒ Revised   ~~deleted~~ Deleted   **OGCR** Official Guidelines   X Assign placeholder X   ● Use Additional Character(s)

| Excludes 1 | Excludes 2 | Includes | Use additional | Code first | Code also | Key words |

● **B27 Infectious mononucleosis**
> **Includes** glandular fever
> monocytic angina
> Pfeiffer's disease

● **B27.0 Gammaherpesviral mononucleosis**
AKA: Pfeiffer's disease, infective mononucleosis
Mononucleosis due to Epstein-Barr virus

- **B27.00 Gammaherpesviral mononucleosis without complication**
Infective mononucleosis
- **B27.01 Gammaherpesviral mononucleosis with polyneuropathy**
- **B27.02 Gammaherpesviral mononucleosis with meningitis**
- **B27.09 Gammaherpesviral mononucleosis with other complications**
Hepatomegaly in gammaherpesviral mononucleosis

● **B27.1 Cytomegaloviral mononucleosis**
Infectious disease resembling infectious mononucleosis

- **B27.10 Cytomegaloviral mononucleosis without complications**
- **B27.11 Cytomegaloviral mononucleosis with polyneuropathy**
- **B27.12 Cytomegaloviral mononucleosis with meningitis**
- **B27.19 Cytomegaloviral mononucleosis with other complication**
Hepatomegaly in cytomegaloviral mononucleosis

● **B27.8 Other infectious mononucleosis**

- **B27.80 Other infectious mononucleosis without complication**
- **B27.81 Other infectious mononucleosis with polyneuropathy**
- **B27.82 Other infectious mononucleosis with meningitis**
- **B27.89 Other infectious mononucleosis with other complication**
Hepatomegaly in other infectious mononucleosis

● **B27.9 Infectious mononucleosis, unspecified**

- **B27.90 Infectious mononucleosis, unspecified without complication**
- **B27.91 Infectious mononucleosis, unspecified with polyneuropathy**
- **B27.92 Infectious mononucleosis, unspecified with meningitis**
- **B27.99 Infectious mononucleosis, unspecified with other complication**
Hepatomegaly in unspecified infectious mononucleosis

● **B30 Viral conjunctivitis**
> **Excludes1** herpesviral [herpes simplex] ocular disease (B00.5)
> ocular zoster (B02.3)

B30.0 Keratoconjunctivitis due to adenovirus
Epidemic keratoconjunctivitis
Shipyard eye

B30.1 Conjunctivitis due to adenovirus
Acute adenoviral follicular conjunctivitis
Swimming-pool conjunctivitis

B30.2 Viral pharyngoconjunctivitis

B30.3 Acute epidemic hemorrhagic conjunctivitis (enteroviral)
Conjunctivitis due to coxsackievirus 24
Conjunctivitis due to enterovirus 70
Hemorrhagic conjunctivitis (acute)(epidemic)

B30.8 Other viral conjunctivitis
Newcastle conjunctivitis

B30.9 Viral conjunctivitis, unspecified

● **B33 Other viral diseases, not elsewhere classified**

B33.0 Epidemic myalgia
Acute infectious disease, caused by group A coxsackie viruses or other enteroviruses with symptoms that include sudden pain in chest or upper abdomen with fever
Bornholm disease

B33.1 Ross River disease
Epidemic polyarthritis and exanthema
Ross River fever

● **B33.2 Viral carditis**
Coxsackie (virus) carditis

- **B33.20 Viral carditis, unspecified**
- **B33.21 Viral endocarditis**
- **B33.22 Viral myocarditis**
- **B33.23 Viral pericarditis**
- **B33.24 Viral cardiomyopathy**

B33.3 Retrovirus infections, not elsewhere classified
Retrovirus infection NOS

B33.4 Hantavirus (cardio)-pulmonary syndrome [HPS] [HCPS]
Hantavirus disease with pulmonary manifestations
Sin nombre virus disease
> **Use additional** code to identify any associated acute kidney failure (N17.9)
> **Excludes1** hantavirus disease with renal manifestations (A98.5)
> hemorrhagic fever with renal manifestations (A98.5)

B33.8 Other specified viral diseases
> **Excludes1** anogenital human papillomavirus infection (A63.0)
> viral warts due to human papillomavirus infection (B07)

● **B34 Viral infection of unspecified site**
> **Excludes1** anogenital human papillomavirus infection (A63.0)
> cytomegaloviral disease NOS (B25.9)
> herpesvirus [herpes simplex] infection NOS (B00.9)
> retrovirus infection NOS (B33.3)
> viral agents as the cause of diseases classified elsewhere (B97.-)
> viral warts due to human papillomavirus infection (B07)

B34.0 Adenovirus infection, unspecified

B34.1 Enterovirus infection, unspecified
Intestinal tract infection
Coxsackievirus infection NOS
Echovirus infection NOS

B34.2 Coronavirus infection, unspecified
> **Excludes1** pneumonia due to SARS-associated coronavirus (J12.81)

B34.3 Parvovirus infection, unspecified

B34.4 Papovavirus infection, unspecified

B34.8 Other viral infections of unspecified site

B34.9 Viral infection, unspecified
Viremia NOS

▶ New   ⇒ Revised   ~~deleted~~ Deleted   **OGCR** Official Guidelines   X Assign placeholder X   ● Use Additional Character(s)
Excludes 1   Excludes 2   Includes   Use additional   Code first   Code also   Key words

MYCOSES (B35-B49)

Excludes2　hypersensitivity pneumonitis due to organic dust (J67.-)

mycosis fungoides (C84.0-)

● **B35** **Dermatophytosis**

AKA tinea or ringworm

Includes　favus

infections due to species of Epidermophyton, Micro-sporum and Trichophyton

tinea, any type except those in B36.-

B35.0 **Tinea barbae and tinea capitis**

Beard ringworm

Kerion

Scalp ringworm

Sycosis, mycotic

B35.1 **Tinea unguium**

White patches or pits on surface or edges of nails, followed by infection under nail plate

Dermatophytic onychia

Dermatophytosis of nail

Onychomycosis

Ringworm of nails

B35.2 **Tinea manuum**

Tinea of hands

Dermatophytosis of hand

Hand ringworm

B35.3 **Tinea pedis**

Tinea affecting feet

Athlete's foot

Dermatophytosis of foot

Foot ringworm

B35.4 **Tinea corporis**

Infecting skin areas other than hands

Ringworm of the body

B35.5 **Tinea imbricata**

Chronic tropical tinea corporis; AKA Oriental ringworm, tinea inguinalis, tinea cruris

Tokelau

B35.6 **Tinea cruris**

In groin or perineal area, spreading to adjacent regions; AKA jock itch, eczema marginatum, ringworm of groin, or t inguinalis

Dhobi itch

Groin ringworm

Jock itch

B35.8 **Other dermatophytoses**

Disseminated dermatophytosis

Granulomatous dermatophytosis

B35.9 **Dermatophytosis, unspecified**

Ringworm NOS

● **B36** **Other superficial mycoses**

B36.0 **Pityriasis versicolor**

Common, chronic, symptomless disorder that includes macular patches of various sizes and shapes; AKA liver spots

Tinea flava

Tinea versicolor

B36.1 **Tinea nigra**

Minor fungal infection, with dark lesions, usually on skin of hands

Keratomycosis nigricans palmaris

Microsporosis nigra

Pityriasis nigra

B36.2 **White piedra**

White to light brown nodules on hair of beard, axilla, or groin; AKA trichosporosis

Tinea blanca

B36.3 **Black piedra**

Characterized by small black or brown nodules on shafts of scalp hair

B36.8 **Other specified superficial mycoses**

B36.9 **Superficial mycosis, unspecified**

Figure 1-8 Oral candidiasis (thrush). (From James WD, Berger T, Elston D: Andrews' Diseases of the Skin: Clinical Dermatology, 11e, Saunders, 2011)

Item 1–20 Candidiasis, also called oidiomycosis or moniliasis, is a fungal infection. It most often appears on moist cutaneous areas of the body but can also be responsible for a variety of systemic infections such as endocarditis, meningitis, arthritis, and myositis. Antifungal medications cure most yeast infections.

● **B37** **Candidiasis**

Includes　candidosis

moniliasis

Excludes1　neonatal candidiasis (P37.5)

B37.0 **Candidal stomatitis**

Oral thrush

B37.1 **Pulmonary candidiasis**

Candidal bronchitis

Candidal pneumonia

B37.2 **Candidiasis of skin and nail**

Candidal onychia

Candidal paronychia

Excludes2　diaper dermatitis (L22)

B37.3 **Candidiasis of vulva and vagina**

Candidal vulvovaginitis

Monilial vulvovaginitis

Vaginal thrush

● **B37.4** **Candidiasis of other urogenital sites**

B37.41 **Candidal cystitis and urethritis**

B37.42 **Candidal balanitis**

Male condition only

B37.49 **Other urogenital candidiasis**

Candidal pyelonephritis

B37.5 **Candidal meningitis**

B37.6 **Candidal endocarditis**

B37.7 **Candidal sepsis**

Disseminated candidiasis systemic candidiasis

● **B37.8** **Candidiasis of other sites**

B37.81 **Candidal esophagitis**

B37.82 **Candidal enteritis**

Candidal proctitis

B37.83 **Candidal cheilitis**

Inflammation affecting lip

B37.84 **Candidal otitis externa**

Inflammation of external auditory canal

B37.89 **Other sites of candidiasis**

Infection manifested by invasive candidiasis

Candidal osteomyelitis

B37.9 **Candidiasis, unspecified**

Thrush NOS

● **B38** **Coccidioidomycosis**

Fungal disease; AKA coccidioidosis, coccidioidal granuloma, Posadas, or Posadas-Wernicke disease

B38.0 **Acute pulmonary coccidioidomycosis**

B38.1 **Chronic pulmonary coccidioidomycosis**

B38.2 **Pulmonary coccidioidomycosis, unspecified**

B38.3 **Cutaneous coccidioidomycosis**

B38.4 **Coccidioidomycosis meningitis**

B38.7 **Disseminated coccidioidomycosis**

Generalized coccidioidomycosis

● **B38.8** **Other forms of coccidioidomycosis**

B38.81 **Prostatic coccidioidomycosis**

B38.89 **Other forms of coccidioidomycosis**

B38.9 **Coccidioidomycosis, unspecified**

▶ New　➡ Revised　~~deleted~~ Deleted　**OGCR** Official Guidelines　X Assign placeholder X　● Use Additional Character(s)

Excludes 1　Excludes 2　Includes　Use additional　Code first　Code also　Key words

Item 1–21 Bird and bat droppings that fall into the soil give rise to a fungus that can spread airborne spores. When inhaled into the lungs, these spores divide and multiply into lesions. Histoplasmosis capsulatum takes three forms: primary (lodged in the lungs only), chronic (resembles TB), and disseminated (infection has moved to other organs). This is an opportunistic infection in immunosuppressed patients.

● **B39   Histoplasmosis**

Infection resulting from inhalation or ingestion of spores; AKA Darling disease

Code first *associated AIDS (B20)*

Use additional *code for any associated manifestations, such as:*
    endocarditis (I39)
    meningitis (G02)
    pericarditis (I32)
    retinitits (H32)

    B39.0   Acute pulmonary histoplasmosis capsulati
    B39.1   Chronic pulmonary histoplasmosis capsulati
    B39.2   Pulmonary histoplasmosis capsulati, unspecified
    B39.3   Disseminated histoplasmosis capsulati
          Generalized histoplasmosis capsulati
    B39.4   Histoplasmosis capsulati, unspecified
          American histoplasmosis
    B39.5   Histoplasmosis duboisii
          African histoplasmosis
    B39.9   Histoplasmosis, unspecified

● **B40   Blastomycosis**

Rare and potentially fatal infection caused by inhaling fungus found in moist soil in temperate climates.

   Excludes1   Brazilian blastomycosis (B41.-)
                keloidal blastomycosis (B48.0)

    B40.0   Acute pulmonary blastomycosis
    B40.1   Chronic pulmonary blastomycosis
    B40.2   Pulmonary blastomycosis, unspecified
    B40.3   Cutaneous blastomycosis
    B40.7   Disseminated blastomycosis
          Generalized blastomycosis
  ● B40.8   Other forms of blastomycosis
        B40.81   Blastomycotic meningoencephalitis
              Meningomyelitis due to blastomycosis
        B40.89   Other forms of blastomycosis
    B40.9   Blastomycosis, unspecified

● **B41   Paracoccidioidomycosis**

Fungal infection usually chronic that begins in lungs, spreads to mucocutaneous areas which may extend to skin, tonsils, gastrointestinal lymphatics, liver, and spleen; AKA Almeida or Lutz-Splendore-Almeida disease, Brazilian or South American blastomycosis, or paracoccidioidal granuloma

   Includes   Brazilian blastomycosis
             Lutz' disease

    B41.0   Pulmonary paracoccidioidomycosis
    B41.7   Disseminated paracoccidioidomycosis
          Generalized paracoccidioidomycosis
    B41.8   Other forms of paracoccidioidomycosis
    B41.9   Paracoccidioidomycosis, unspecified

● **B42   Sporotrichosis**

Chronic fungal infection with nodular lesions

    B42.0   Pulmonary sporotrichosis
    B42.1   Lymphocutaneous sporotrichosis
    B42.7   Disseminated sporotrichosis
          Generalized sporotrichosis
  ● B42.8   Other forms of sporotrichosis
        B42.81   Cerebral sporotrichosis
              Meningitis due to sporotrichosis
        B42.82   Sporotrichosis arthritis
        B42.89   Other forms of sporotrichosis
    B42.9   Sporotrichosis, unspecified

● **B43   Chromomycosis and pheomycotic abscess**

Chronic fungal infection of skin, initiated at site of puncture affecting lower limb or foot (mossy foot)

    B43.0   Cutaneous chromomycosis
          Dermatitis verrucosa
    B43.1   Pheomycotic brain abscess
          Cerebral chromomycosis
    B43.2   Subcutaneous pheomycotic abscess and cyst
    B43.8   Other forms of chromomycosis
    B43.9   Chromomycosis, unspecified

● **B44   Aspergillosis**

Infection marked by inflammatory lesions in skin, ear, orbit, nasal sinuses, lungs, and occasionally bones and meninges

   Includes   aspergilloma

    B44.0   Invasive pulmonary aspergillosis
    B44.1   Other pulmonary aspergillosis
    B44.2   Tonsillar aspergillosis
    B44.7   Disseminated aspergillosis
          Generalized aspergillosis
  ● B44.8   Other forms of aspergillosis
        B44.81   Allergic bronchopulmonary aspergillosis
        B44.89   Other forms of aspergillosis
    B44.9   Aspergillosis, unspecified

● **B45   Cryptococcosis**

Infection in the immunocompromised and fatal if left untreated; AKA torulosis, Buschke, or Busse-Buschke disease

    B45.0   Pulmonary cryptococcosis
    B45.1   Cerebral cryptococcosis
          Cryptococcal meningitis
          Cryptococcosis meningocerebralis
    B45.2   Cutaneous cryptococcosis
    B45.3   Osseous cryptococcosis
    B45.7   Disseminated cryptococcosis
          Generalized cryptococcosis
    B45.8   Other forms of cryptococcosis
    B45.9   Cryptococcosis, unspecified

● **B46   Zygomycosis**

Fungal infections including subcutaneous lesions and infection of sinuses, brain, or lungs

    B46.0   Pulmonary mucormycosis
          Fungal infection affecting lung
    B46.1   Rhinocerebral mucormycosis
    B46.2   Gastrointestinal mucormycosis
    B46.3   Cutaneous mucormycosis
          Subcutaneous mucormycosis
    B46.4   Disseminated mucormycosis
          Generalized mucormycosis
    B46.5   Mucormycosis, unspecified
    B46.8   Other zygomycoses
          Entomophthoromycosis
    B46.9   Zygomycosis, unspecified
          Phycomycosis NOS

● **B47   Mycetoma**

Slow progressive, destructive fungal infection of cutaneous and subcutaneous tissues, fascia, and bone, primarily seen in foot (Madura foot) or leg

    B47.0   Eumycetoma
          Madura foot, mycotic Maduromycosis
    B47.1   Actinomycetoma
    B47.9   Mycetoma, unspecified
          Madura foot NOS

CHAPTER 1 (A00-B99)

▶ New   ⟹ Revised   ~~deleted~~ Deleted   **OGCR** Official Guidelines   X Assign placeholder X   ● Use Additional Character(s)

Excludes 1   Excludes 2   Includes   Use additional   Code first   Code also   Key words

- **B48   Other mycoses, not elsewhere classified**

  B48.0   Lobomycosis
  Infection with symptoms of red, smooth, hard cutaneous nodules resembling keloids
  Keloidal blastomycosis
  Lobo's disease

  B48.1   Rhinosporidiosis
  Chronic, localized granulomatous fungal infection, affecting mucocutaneous tissues, usually of nose characterized by polyps, papillomas, and wartlike lesions

  B48.2   Allescheriasis
  Fungal infection
  Infection due to Pseudallescheria boydii
  | **Excludes1** | eumycetoma (B47.0) |

  B48.3   Geotrichosis
  Fungal infection usually of bronchi, lungs, mouth, or intestinal tract
  Geotrichum stomatitis

  B48.4   Penicillosis
  Fungal infection

  B48.8   Other specified mycoses
  Adiaspiromycosis
  Infection of tissue and organs by Alternaria
  Infection of tissue and organs by Drechslera
  Infection of tissue and organs by Fusarium
  Infection of tissue and organs by saprophytic fungi NEC

- **B49   Unspecified mycosis**
  Fungemia NOS

PROTOZOAL DISEASES (B50-B64)

| **Excludes1** | amebiasis (A06.-) |
| | other protozoal intestinal diseases (A07.-) |

- **B50   Plasmodium falciparum malaria**
  Severe form of malaria that can be fatal
  | **Includes** | mixed infections of Plasmodium falciparum with any other Plasmodium species |

  B50.0   Plasmodium falciparum malaria with cerebral complications
  Cerebral malaria NOS

  B50.8   Other severe and complicated Plasmodium falciparum malaria
  Severe or complicated Plasmodium falciparum malaria NOS

  B50.9   Plasmodium falciparum malaria, unspecified

- **B51   Plasmodium vivax malaria**
  | **Includes** | mixed infections of Plasmodium vivax with other Plasmodium species, except Plasmodium falciparum |
  | **Excludes1** | plasmodium vivav with Plasmodium falciparum (B50.-) |

  B51.0   Plasmodium vivax malaria with rupture of spleen

  B51.8   Plasmodium vivax malaria with other complications

  B51.9   Plasmodium vivax malaria without complication
  Plasmodium vivax malaria NOS

- **B52   Plasmodium malariae malaria**
  Causes fever that recurs at approximately three-day intervals (quartan fever), longer than two-day (tertian) intervals of other malarial parasites
Includes	mixed infections of Plasmodium malariae with other Plasmodium species, except Plasmodium falciparum and Plasmodium vivax
Excludes1	plasmodium falciparum (B50.-)
	plasmodium vivax (B51.-)

  B52.0   Plasmodium malariae malaria with nephropathy

  B52.8   Plasmodium malariae malaria with other complications

  B52.9   Plasmodium malariae malaria without complication
  Plasmodium malariae malaria NOS

- **B53   Other specified malaria**

  B53.0   Plasmodium ovale malaria
  Least diagnosed type of malaria spread by female mosquitoes of rare species
Excludes1	plasmodium ovale with Plasmodium falciparum (B50.-)
	plasmodium ovale with Plasmodium malariae (B52.-)
	plasmodium ovale with Plasmodium vivax (B51.-)

  B53.1   Malaria due to simian plasmodia
  Malaria-like disease (parasite infection)
Excludes1	malaria due to simian plasmodia with Plasmodium falciparum (B50.-)
	malaria due to simian plasmodia with Plasmodium malariae (B52.-)
	malaria due to simian plasmodia with Plasmodium ovale (B53.0)
	malaria due to simian plasmodia with Plasmodium vivax (B51.-)

  B53.8   Other malaria, not elsewhere classified

- **B54   Unspecified malaria**

- **B55   Leishmaniasis**
  Protozoal infection

  B55.0   Visceral leishmaniasis
  Kala-azar
  Post-kala-azar dermal leishmaniasis

  B55.1   Cutaneous leishmaniasis

  B55.2   Mucocutaneous leishmaniasis

  B55.9   Leishmaniasis, unspecified

- **B56   African trypanosomiasis**
  Human African trypanosomiasis (HAT) is transmitted by fly bites

  B56.0   Gambiense trypanosomiasis
  Infection due to Trypanosoma brucei gambiense
  West African sleeping sickness

  B56.1   Rhodesiense trypanosomiasis
  East African sleeping sickness
  Infection due to Trypanosoma brucei rhodesiense

  B56.9   African trypanosomiasis, unspecified
  Sleeping sickness NOS

- **B57   Chagas' disease**
  Tropical parasitic disease
  | **Includes** | American trypanosomiasis |
  | | infection due to Trypanosoma cruzi |

  B57.0   Acute Chagas' disease with heart involvement
  Acute Chagas' disease with myocarditis

  B57.1   Acute Chagas' disease without heart involvement
  Acute Chagas' disease NOS

  B57.2   Chagas' disease (chronic) with heart involvement
  American trypanosomiasis NOS
  Chagas' disease (chronic) NOS
  Chagas' disease (chronic) with myocarditis
  Trypanosomiasis NOS

- **B57.3   Chagas' disease (chronic) with digestive system involvement**

  B57.30   Chagas' disease with digestive system involvement, unspecified

  B57.31   Megaesophagus in Chagas' disease

  B57.32   Megacolon in Chagas' disease

  B57.39   Other digestive system involvement in Chagas' disease

- **B57.4   Chagas' disease (chronic) with nervous system involvement**

  B57.40   Chagas' disease with nervous system involvement, unspecified

  B57.41   Meningitis in Chagas' disease

  B57.42   Meningoencephalitis in Chagas' disease

  B57.49   Other nervous system involvement in Chagas' disease

  B57.5   Chagas' disease (chronic) with other organ involvement

CHAPTER 1 (A00-B99)

▶ New   ⇒ Revised   ~~deleted~~ Deleted   **OGCR** Official Guidelines   X Assign placeholder X   ● Use Additional Character(s)

| Excludes 1 | Excludes 2 | Includes | Use additional | Code first | Code also | Key words |

CHAPTER 1 (A00-B99)

Item 1–22 Toxoplasmosis is caused by the protozoa **Toxoplasma gondii,** of which the house cat can be a host. Human infection occurs when contact is made with materials containing the pathogen, such as feces, contaminated soil, or ingestion of infected lamb, goat, or pork. Of the infected, very few have symptoms because a healthy person's immune system keeps the parasite from causing illness. When the immune system is compromised, symptoms may occur. Clinical symptoms include flu-like symptoms, but the disease progresses to include the eyes and the brain in babies.

● **B58**   **Toxoplasmosis**
    Infection by protozoon transmitted in cysts in feces of cats
    Includes   infection due to Toxoplasma gondii
    Excludes1   congenital toxoplasmosis (P37.1)

   ● **B58.0**   **Toxoplasma oculopathy**
     B58.00   **Toxoplasma oculopathy, unspecified**
     B58.01   **Toxoplasma chorioretinitis**
     B58.09   **Other toxoplasma oculopathy**
       Toxoplasma uveitis

   B58.1   **Toxoplasma hepatitis**
   B58.2   **Toxoplasma meningoencephalitis**
   B58.3   **Pulmonary toxoplasmosis**

   ● **B58.8**   **Toxoplasmosis with other organ involvement**
     B58.81   **Toxoplasma myocarditis**
     B58.82   **Toxoplasma myositis**
     B58.83   **Toxoplasma tubulo-interstitial nephropathy**
       Toxoplasma pyelonephritis
     B58.89   **Toxoplasmosis with other organ involvement**

   B58.9   **Toxoplasmosis, unspecified**

  B59   **Pneumocystosis**
    Caused by fungus
    Pneumonia due to Pneumocystis carinii
    Pneumonia due to Pneumocystis jiroveci

● **B60**   **Other protozoal diseases, not elsewhere classified**
    Excludes1   cryptosporidiosis (A07.2)
            intestinal microsporidiosis (A07.8)
            isosporiasis (A07.3)

   B60.0   **Babesiosis**
     Tickborne disease caused by microscopic organisms
     Piroplasmosis

   ● **B60.1**   **Acanthamebiasis**
     B60.10   **Acanthamebiasis, unspecified**
     B60.11   **Meningoencephalitis due to Acanthamoeba (culbertsoni)**
     B60.12   **Conjunctivitis due to Acanthamoeba**
     B60.13   **Keratoconjunctivitis due to Acanthamoeba**
     B60.19   **Other acanthamebic disease**

   B60.2   **Naegleriasis**
     Infection with microscopic organisms
     Primary amebic meningoencephalitis

   B60.8   **Other specified protozoal diseases**
     Microsporidiosis

  B64   **Unspecified protozoal disease**

HELMINTHIASES (B65-B83)

Diseases or infestations caused by parasitic worms

● **B65**   **Schistosomiasis [bilharziasis]**
    Infection with flukes (flat parasitic worms)
    Includes   snail fever

   B65.0   **Schistosomiasis due to Schistosoma haematobium [urinary schistosomiasis]**
   B65.1   **Schistosomiasis due to Schistosoma mansoni [intestinal schistosomiasis]**
   B65.2   **Schistosomiasis due to Schistosoma japonicum**
     Asiatic schistosomiasis

   B65.3   **Cercarial dermatitis**
     Swimmer's itch
   B65.8   **Other schistosomiasis**
     Infection due to Schistosoma intercalatum
     Infection due to Schistosoma mattheei
     Infection due to Schistosoma mekongi
   B65.9   **Schistosomiasis, unspecified**

● **B66**   **Other fluke infections**
    Trematode (parasitic worms)

   B66.0   **Opisthorchiasis**
     Infection due to cat liver fluke
     Infection due to Opisthorchis (felineus)(viverrini)
   B66.1   **Clonorchiasis**
     Chinese liver fluke disease
     Infection due to Clonorchis sinensis
     Oriental liver fluke disease
   B66.2   **Dicroceliasis**
     Liver fluke
     Infection due to Dicrocoelium dendriticum
     Lancet fluke infection
   B66.3   **Fascioliasis**
     Infection due to Fasciola gigantica
     Infection due to Fasciola hepatica
     Infection due to Fasciola indica
     Sheep liver fluke disease
   B66.4   **Paragonimiasis**
     Infection due to Paragonimus species
     Lung fluke disease
     Pulmonary distomiasis
   B66.5   **Fasciolopsiasis**
     Largest intestinal fluke in humans
     Infection due to Fasciolopsis buski
     Intestinal distomiasis
   B66.8   **Other specified fluke infections**
     Echinostomiasis
     Heterophyiasis
     Metagonimiasis
     Nanophyetiasis
     Watsoniasis
   B66.9   **Fluke infection, unspecified**

● **B67**   **Echinococcosis**
    Larval forms of tapeworms usually of liver or lungs
    Includes   hydatidosis

   B67.0   **Echinococcus granulosus infection of liver**
   B67.1   **Echinococcus granulosus infection of lung**
   B67.2   **Echinococcus granulosus infection of bone**
   ● **B67.3**   **Echinococcus granulosus infection, other and multiple sites**
     B67.31   **Echinococcus granulosus infection, thyroid gland**
     B67.32   **Echinococcus granulosus infection, multiple sites**
     B67.39   **Echinococcus granulosus infection, other sites**
   B67.4   **Echinococcus granulosus infection, unspecified**
     Dog tapeworm (infection)
   B67.5   **Echinococcus multilocularis infection of liver**
   ● **B67.6**   **Echinococcus multilocularis infection, other and multiple sites**
     B67.61   **Echinococcus multilocularis infection, multiple sites**
     B67.69   **Echinococcus multilocularis infection, other sites**

Item 1-23 Echinococcosis: Also known as hydatid disease; is caused by Echinococcus granulosus, E. multilocularis, and E. vogeli tapeworms; and is contracted from infected food. Found in southern South America, the Mediterranean, the Middle East, central Asia, and Africa and uncommon in the United States but has been reported in California, New Mexico, Arizona and Utah. The disease is treated with medication over a long course as it is resistive.

▶ New   ⇒ Revised   ~~deleted~~ Deleted   **OGCR** Official Guidelines   X Assign placeholder X   ● Use Additional Character(s)

Excludes 1   Excludes 2   Includes   Use additional   Code first   Code also   Key words

B67.7   Echinococcus multilocularis infection, unspecified

B67.8   Echinococcosis, unspecified, of liver

● **B67.9**   Echinococcosis, other and unspecified

      B67.90   Echinococcosis, unspecified
                   Echinococcosis NOS

      B67.99   Other echinococcosis

● **B68**   **Taeniasis**

Intestinal tapeworm (cestode) infection from raw or undercooked meat of infected animal

    Excludes1   cysticercosis (B69.-)

B68.0   Taenia solium taeniasis
          Pork tapeworm (infection)

B68.1   Taenia saginata taeniasis
          Beef tapeworm (infection)
          Infection due to adult tapeworm Taenia saginata

B68.9   Taeniasis, unspecified

● **B69**   **Cysticercosis**

Systemic illness caused by the larvae of pork tapeworm

    Includes   cysticerciasis infection due to larval form of Taenia solium

B69.0   Cysticercosis of central nervous system

B69.1   Cysticercosis of eye

● **B69.8**   Cysticercosis of other sites

      B69.81   Myositis in cysticercosis

      B69.89   Cysticercosis of other sites

B69.9   Cysticercosis, unspecified

● **B70**   **Diphyllobothriasis and sparganosis**

Infection with tapeworms seen most often from inadequately cooked fish

B70.0   Diphyllobothriasis
          Diphyllobothrium (adult) (latum) (pacificum) infection
          Fish tapeworm (infection)
      Excludes2   larval diphyllobothriasis (B70.1)

B70.1   Sparganosis
          Infection with migrating tapeworm larvae, which invade subcutaneous tissues, causing inflammation and fibrosis that resembles cellulitis
          Infection due to Sparganum (mansoni) (proliferum)
          Infection due to Spirometra larva
          Larval diphyllobothriasis
          Spirometrosis

● **B71**   **Other cestode infections**

B71.0   Hymenolepiasis
          Intestinal infestation with tapeworms
          Dwarf tapeworm infection
          Rat tapeworm (infection)

B71.1   Dipylidiasis
          Infection with tapeworm common to dogs and cats and seen in children having close contact with infected pets

B71.8   Other specified cestode infections
          Infection by the larval stage of a tapeworm, usually through fruit or vegetables
          Coenurosis

B71.9   Cestode infection, unspecified
          Tapeworm (infection) NOS

B72   **Dracunculiasis**

Infection with roundworms

    Includes   guinea worm infection
          infection due to Dracunculus medinensis

● **B73**   **Onchocerciasis**

Infection with parasitic worm

    Includes   onchocerca volvulus infection
          onchocercosis
          river blindness

● **B73.0**   Onchocerciasis with eye disease

      B73.00   Onchocerciasis with eye involvement, unspecified

      B73.01   Onchocerciasis with endophthalmitis

      B73.02   Onchocerciasis with glaucoma

      B73.09   Onchocerciasis with other eye involvement
              Infestation of eyelid due to onchocerciasis

B73.1   Onchocerciasis without eye disease

● **B74**   **Filariasis**

Infestation with slender threadlike worms

    Excludes2   onchocerciasis (B73)
          tropical (pulmonary) eosinophilia NOS (J82)

B74.0   Filariasis due to Wuchereria bancrofti
          Bancroftian elephantiasis
          Bancroftian filariasis

B74.1   Filariasis due to Brugia malayi

B74.2   Filariasis due to Brugia timori

B74.3   Loiasis
          Infection with round worms growing in subcutaneous connective tissue
          Calabar swelling
          Eyeworm disease of Africa
          Loa loa infection

B74.4   Mansonelliasis
          Infection with filarial parasite
          Infection due to Mansonella ozzardi
          Infection due to Mansonella perstans
          Infection due to Mansonella streptocerca

B74.8   Other filariases
          Dirofilariasis

B74.9   Filariasis, unspecified

B75   **Trichinellosis**

Infestation with parasitic roundworms ingested in undercooked contaminated meat

    Includes   infection due to Trichinella species trichiniasis

● **B76**   **Hookworm diseases**

Occurs in hot, humid parts of world where larvae are soil borne, enter digestive tract through skin of feet/legs or in contaminated food/water; AKA ground itch

    Includes   uncinariasis

B76.0   Ancylostomiasis
          Infection due to Ancylostoma species

B76.1   Necatoriasis
          Infection due to Necator americanus

B76.8   Other hookworm diseases

B76.9   Hookworm disease, unspecified
          Cutaneous larva migrans NOS

● **B77**   **Ascariasis**

Infection by roundworm in small intestine

    Includes   ascaridiasis
          roundworm infection

B77.0   Ascariasis with intestinal complications

● **B77.8**   Ascariasis with other complications

      B77.81   Ascariasis pneumonia

      B77.89   Ascariasis with other complications

B77.9   Ascariasis, unspecified

CHAPTER 1 (A00-B99)

▶ New   ⇨ Revised   ~~deleted~~ Deleted   **OGCR** Official Guidelines   X Assign placeholder X   ● Use Additional Character(s)

Excludes 1   Excludes 2   Includes   Use additional   Code first   Code also   Key words

CHAPTER 1 (A00–B99)

● **B78 Strongyloidiasis**
      Infection with adult female roundworms
       Excludes1   trichostrongyliasis (B81.2)

    B78.0 Intestinal strongyloidiasis
    B78.1 Cutaneous strongyloidiasis
    B78.7 Disseminated strongyloidiasis
    B78.9 Strongyloidiasis, unspecified

  B79 Trichuriasis
      Intestinal infection with roundworms
       Includes   trichocephaliasis
                 whipworm (disease)(infection)

  B80 Enterobiasis
      Intestinal infection with pinworms
       Includes   oxyuriasis
                 pinworm infection
                 threadworm infection

● **B81 Other intestinal helminthiases, not elsewhere classified**
      Diseases or infestations caused by parasitic worms
       Excludes1 ➡ angiostrongyliasis due to:
                 ▶ Angiostrongylus cantonensis (B83.2)
                 ▶ Parastrongylus cantonensis (B83.2)

    B81.0 Anisakiasis
        Roundworm infection via contaminated undercooked infected
          fish or marine mammals
        Infection due to Anisakis larva

    B81.1 Intestinal capillariasis
        Infestation with of parasites (nematodes)
        Capillariasis NOS
        Infection due to Capillaria philippinensis
         Excludes2   hepatic capillariasis (B83.8)

    B81.2 Trichostrongyliasis

    B81.3 Intestinal angiostrongyliasis
        ➡ Angiostrongyliasis due to:
           ▶ Angiostrongylus costaricensis (B83.2)
           ▶ Parastrongylus costaricensis (B83.2)

    B81.4 Mixed intestinal helminthiases
        Infection due to intestinal helminths classified to more
          than one of the categories B65.0-B81.3 and B81.8
        Mixed helminthiasis NOS

    B81.8 Other specified intestinal helminthiases
        Infection due to Oesophagostomum species
          [esophagostomiasis]
        Infection due to Ternidens diminutus [ternidensiasis]

● **B82 Unspecified intestinal parasitism**
    B82.0 Intestinal helminthiasis, unspecified
        Infected with worms
    B82.9 Intestinal parasitism, unspecified

● **B83 Other helminthiases**
      Caused by parasitic worms
       Excludes1   capillariasis NOS (B81.1)
       Excludes2   intestinal capillariasis (B81.1)

    B83.0 Visceral larva migrans
        Prolonged migration of nematode larvae
        Toxocariasis

    B83.1 Gnathostomiasis
        Infection with nematode occurring from ingested undercooked
          fish contaminated with larvae; larvae migrate to
          subcutaneous tissue or deeper tissues, results are
          abscesses
        Wandering swelling

    B83.2 Angiostrongyliasis due to Parastrongylus cantonensis
        Nematode infection caused by eating contaminated raw
          snails, slugs, or paratenic hosts such as prawns or
          crabs; larval worms migrate to central nervous system
          resulting in eosinophilic meningitis
        Eosinophilic meningoencephalitis due to
          Parastrongylus cantonensis
         Excludes2   intestinal angiostrongyliasis (B81.3)

    B83.3 Syngamiasis
        Infestation with gapeworm from turkey, pheasant, guinea fowl,
          goose, and wild birds
        Syngamosis

    B83.4 Internal hirudiniasis
        Infestation by leeches
         Excludes2   external hirudiniasis (B88.3)

    B83.8 Other specified helminthiases
        Parasitic worm infestation
        Acanthocephaliasis
        Gongylonemiasis
        Hepatic capillariasis
        Metastrongyliasis
        Thelaziasis

    B83.9 Helminthiasis, unspecified
        Worms NOS
         Excludes1   intestinal helminthiasis NOS (B82.0)

PEDICULOSIS, ACARIASIS AND OTHER INFESTATIONS (B85-B89)

● **B85 Pediculosis and phthiriasis**
      Infestation of lice

    B85.0 Pediculosis due to Pediculus humanus capitis
        Head-louse infestation

    B85.1 Pediculosis due to Pediculus humanus corporis
        Body-louse infestation

    B85.2 Pediculosis, unspecified

    B85.3 Phthiriasis
        Crab or pubic lice
        Infestation by crab-louse
        Infestation by Phthirus pubis

    B85.4 Mixed pediculosis and phthiriasis
        Infestation classifiable to more than one of the
          categories B85.0-B85.3

  B86 Scabies
      Contagious dermatitis caused by mites
      Sarcoptic itch

● **B87 Myiasis**
      Infestation by fly maggots
       Includes   infestation by larva of flies

    B87.0 Cutaneous myiasis
        Creeping myiasis

    B87.1 Wound myiasis
        Traumatic myiasis

    B87.2 Ocular myiasis

    B87.3 Nasopharyngeal myiasis
        Laryngeal myiasis

    B87.4 Aural myiasis

●   **B87.8 Myiasis of other sites**
      B87.81 Genitourinary myiasis
      B87.82 Intestinal myiasis
      B87.89 Myiasis of other sites

    B87.9 Myiasis, unspecified

▶ New   ➡ Revised   ~~deleted~~ Deleted   **OGCR** Official Guidelines   X Assign placeholder X   ● Use Additional Character(s)

Excludes 1   Excludes 2   Includes   Use additional   Code first   Code also   Key words

● **B88   Other infestations**

   B88.0   Other acariasis
         Acarine dermatitis
         Dermatitis due to Demodex species
         Dermatitis due to Dermanyssus gallinae
         Dermatitis due to Liponyssoides sanguineus
         Trombiculosis
         Excludes2   scabies (B86)

   B88.1   Tungiasis [sandflea infestation]
         Inflammatory skin disease caused by infestation of fleas

   B88.2   Other arthropod infestations
         Scarabiasis

   B88.3   External hirudiniasis
         Leech infestation NOS
         Excludes2   internal hirudiniasis (B83.4)

   B88.8   Other specified infestations
         Infection of topical fresh water fish parasite
         Ichthyoparasitism due to Vandellia cirrhosa
         Linguatulosis
         Porocephaliasis

   B88.9   Infestation, unspecified
         Infestation (skin) NOS
         Infestation by mites NOS
         Skin parasites NOS

● **B89   Unspecified parasitic disease**

SEQUELAE OF INFECTIOUS AND PARASITIC DISEASES (B90-B94)

Note: Categories B90-B94 are to be used to indicate conditions
   in categories A00-B89 as the cause of sequelae, which are
   themselves classified elsewhere. The 'sequelae' include
   conditions specified as such; they also include residuals
   of diseases classifiable to the above categories if there
   is evidence that the disease itself is no longer present.
   Codes from these categories are not to be used for chronic
   infections. Code chronic current infections to active infectious
   disease as appropriate.

*Code first condition resulting from (sequela) the infectious or parasitic
   disease*

● **B90   Sequelae of tuberculosis**
         Condition resulting from tuberculosis

   B90.0   Sequelae of central nervous system tuberculosis

   B90.1   Sequelae of genitourinary tuberculosis

   B90.2   Sequelae of tuberculosis of bones and joints

   B90.8   Sequelae of tuberculosis of other organs
         Excludes2   sequelae of respiratory tuberculosis
                  (B90.9)

   B90.9   Sequelae of respiratory and unspecified tuberculosis
         Sequelae of tuberculosis NOS

   B91   Sequelae of poliomyelitis
         Excludes1   postpolio syndrome (G14)

   B92   Sequelae of leprosy

● **B94   Sequelae of other and unspecified infectious and parasitic
      diseases**

   B94.0   Sequelae of trachoma

   B94.1   Sequelae of viral encephalitis

   B94.2   Sequelae of viral hepatitis

   **B94.8   Sequelae of other specified infectious and parasitic
         diseases**

   B94.9   Sequelae of unspecified infectious and parasitic disease

OGCR   Section I.C.1.b.

Certain infectious and parasitic diseases
Infectious agents as the cause of diseases classified to other chapters
Certain infections are classified in chapters other than Chapter 1 and no
organism is identified as part of the infection code. In these instances,
it is necessary to use an additional code from Chapter 1 to identify the
organism. A code from category B95, Streptococcus, Staphylococcus,
and Enterococcus as the cause of diseases classified to other chapters,
B96, Other bacterial agents as the cause of diseases classified to other
chapters, or B97, Viral agents as the cause of diseases classified to other
chapters, is to be used as an additional code to identify the organism.
An instructional note will be found at the infection code advising that an
additional organism code is required.

BACTERIAL AND VIRAL INFECTIOUS AGENTS (B95-B97)

Note: These categories are provided for use as supplementary or
   additional codes to identify the infectious agent(s) in diseases
   classified elsewhere.
   *Code the disease first, then the bacterium. Do not report codes from
   B95-B97 for sepsis.*

● **B95   Streptococcus, Staphylococcus, and Enterococcus as the cause of
      diseases classified elsewhere**

   **B95.0   Streptococcus, group A, as the cause of diseases
         classified elsewhere**

   **B95.1   Streptococcus, group B, as the cause of diseases
         classified elsewhere**

   **B95.2   Enterococcus as the cause of diseases classified
         elsewhere**

   **B95.3   Streptococcus pneumoniae as the cause of diseases
         classified elsewhere**

   **B95.4   Other streptococcus as the cause of diseases classified
         elsewhere**

   **B95.5   Unspecified streptococcus as the cause of diseases
         classified elsewhere**

● **B95.6   Staphylococcus aureus as the cause of diseases classified
         elsewhere**

      **B95.61   Methicillin susceptible Staphylococcus aureus
            infection as the cause of diseases classified
            elsewhere**
            Methicillin susceptible Staphylococcus aureus
               (MSSA) infection as the cause of diseases
               classified elsewhere
            Staphylococcus aureus infection NOS as the
               cause of diseases classified elsewhere

      **B95.62   Methicillin resistant Staphylococcus aureus
            infection as the cause of diseases classified
            elsewhere**
            Methicillin resistant staphylococcus aureus
               (MRSA) infection as the cause of diseases
               classified elsewhere

   **B95.7   Other staphylococcus as the cause of diseases classified
         elsewhere**

   **B95.8   Unspecified staphylococcus as the cause of diseases
         classified elsewhere**

▶ New   ⇒ Revised   ~~deleted~~ Deleted   **OGCR** Official Guidelines   X Assign placeholder X   ● Use Additional Character(s)

Excludes 1   Excludes 2   Includes   Use additional   Code first   Code also   Key words

● **B96**   **Other bacterial agents as the cause of diseases classified elsewhere**

    B96.0   **Mycoplasma** pneumoniae [M. pneumoniae] as the cause of diseases classified elsewhere

       Pleuro-pneumonia-like-organism [PPLO]

    B96.1   **Klebsiella** pneumoniae [K. pneumoniae] as the cause of diseases classified elsewhere

   ● **B96.2**   **Escherichia coli** [E. coli] as the cause of diseases classified elsewhere

       B96.20   **Unspecified** Escherichia coli [E. coli] as the cause of diseases classified elsewhere

          Escherichia coli [E. coli] NOS

       B96.21   **Shiga toxin-producing** Escherichia coli [E. coli] (STEC) O157 as the cause of diseases classified elsewhere

          E. coli O157:H- (nonmotile) with confirmation of Shiga toxin

          E. coli O157 with confirmation of Shiga toxin when H antigen is unknown, or is not H7

          O157:H7 Escherichia coli [E.coli] with or without confirmation of Shiga toxin-production

          Shiga toxin-producing Escherichia coli [E.coli] O157:H7 with or without confirmation of Shiga toxin-production

          STEC O157:H7 with or without confirmation of Shiga toxin-production

       B96.22   **Other specified Shiga toxin-producing** Escherichia coli [E. coli] (STEC) as the cause of diseases classified elsewhere

          Non-O157 Shiga toxin-producing Escherichia coli [E.coli]

          Non-O157 Shiga toxin-producing Escherichia coli [E.coli] with known O group

       B96.23   **Unspecified Shiga toxin-producing** Escherichia coli [E. coli] (STEC) as the cause of diseases classified elsewhere

          Shiga toxin-producing Escherichia coli [E. coli] with unspecified O group

          STEC NOS

       B96.29   **Other** Escherichia coli [E. coli] as the cause of diseases classified elsewhere

          Non-Shiga toxin-producing E. coli

    B96.3   **Hemophilus influenzae** [H. influenzae] as the cause of diseases classified elsewhere

    B96.4   **Proteus** (mirabilis) (morganii) as the cause of diseases classified elsewhere

    B96.5   **Pseudomonas** (aeruginosa) (mallei) (pseudomallei) as the cause of diseases classified elsewhere

    B96.6   **Bacteroides fragilis** [B. fragilis] as the cause of diseases classified elsewhere

    B96.7   **Clostridium perfringens** [C. perfringens] as the cause of diseases classified elsewhere

   ● **B96.8**   **Other specified bacterial agents as the cause of diseases classified elsewhere**

       B96.81   **Helicobacter pylori** [H. pylori] as the cause of diseases classified elsewhere

       B96.82   **Vibrio vulnificus** as the cause of diseases classified elsewhere

       B96.89   **Other** specified bacterial agents as the cause of diseases classified elsewhere

● **B97**   **Viral agents as the cause of diseases classified elsewhere**

    B97.0   **Adenovirus** as the cause of diseases classified elsewhere

   ● **B97.1**   **Enterovirus** as the cause of diseases classified elsewhere

       B97.10   **Unspecified** enterovirus as the cause of diseases classified elsewhere

       B97.11   **Coxsackievirus** as the cause of diseases classified elsewhere

       B97.12   **Echovirus** as the cause of diseases classified elsewhere

       B97.19   **Other** enterovirus as the cause of diseases classified elsewhere

Item 1–24   **Retrovirus** develops by copying its RNA, genetic materials, into the DNA, which then produces new virus particles. It is from the Retroviridae virus family. **Human T-cell lymphotropic virus, Type I (HTLV-I)** is also called human T-cell leukemia virus, Type I, and is a retrovirus thought to cause T-cell leukemia/lymphoma. **Human T-cell lymphotropic virus, Type II (HTLV-II),** is also called human T-cell leukemia virus, Type II, and is a retrovirus associated with hematologic disorders.

    HIV-2 is one of the serotypes of HIV and is usually confined to West Africa, whereas HIV-**1** is found worldwide.

   ● **B97.2**   **Coronavirus** as the cause of diseases classified elsewhere

       B97.21   **SARS**-associated coronavirus as the cause of diseases classified elsewhere

          Excludes1   pneumonia due to SARS-associated coronavirus (J12.81)

       B97.29   **Other** coronavirus as the cause of diseases classified elsewhere

   ● **B97.3**   **Retrovirus** as the cause of diseases classified elsewhere

       Excludes1   human immunodeficiency virus [HIV] disease (B20)

       B97.30   **Unspecified** retrovirus as the cause of diseases classified elsewhere

       B97.31   **Lentivirus** as the cause of diseases classified elsewhere

       B97.32   **Oncovirus** as the cause of diseases classified elsewhere

       B97.33   **Human T-cell lymphotrophic virus, type I [HTLV-I]** as the cause of diseases classified elsewhere

       B97.34   **Human T-cell lymphotrophic virus, type II [HTLV-II]** as the cause of diseases classified elsewhere

       B97.35   **Human immunodeficiency virus, type 2 [HIV 2]** as the cause of diseases classified elsewhere

       B97.39   **Other** retrovirus as the cause of diseases classified elsewhere

    B97.4   **Respiratory syncytial** virus as the cause of diseases classified elsewhere

    B97.5   **Reovirus** as the cause of diseases classified elsewhere

    B97.6   **Parvovirus** as the cause of diseases classified elsewhere

    B97.7   **Papillomavirus** as the cause of diseases classified elsewhere

   ● **B97.8**   **Other** viral agents as the cause of diseases classified elsewhere

       B97.81   **Human metapneumovirus** as the cause of diseases classified elsewhere

       B97.89   **Other** viral agents as the cause of diseases classified elsewhere

OTHER INFECTIOUS DISEASES (B99)

● **B99**   **Other and unspecified infectious diseases**

    B99.8   **Other** infectious disease

    B99.9   **Unspecified** infectious disease

▶ New   ⇒ Revised   ~~deleted~~ Deleted   **OGCR** Official Guidelines   X Assign placeholder X   ● Use Additional Character(s)

Excludes 1   Excludes 2   Includes   Use additional   Code first   Code also   Key words

CHAPTER 2

NEOPLASMS (C00-D49)

OGCR Chapter-Specific Coding Guidelines

2. Chapter 2: Neoplasms (C00-D49)
General guidelines
Chapter 2 of the ICD-10-CM contains the codes for most benign and all malignant neoplasms. Certain benign neoplasms, such as prostatic adenomas, may be found in the specific body system chapters. To properly code a neoplasm it is necessary to determine from the record if the neoplasm is benign, in-situ, malignant, or of uncertain histologic behavior. If malignant, any secondary (metastatic) sites should also be determined.

Primary malignant neoplasms overlapping site boundaries
A primary malignant neoplasm that overlaps two or more contiguous (next to each other) sites should be classified to the subcategory/code .8 ('overlapping lesion'), unless the combination is specifically indexed elsewhere. For multiple neoplasms of the same site that are not contiguous such as tumors in different quadrants of the same breast, codes for each site should be assigned.

Malignant neoplasm of ectopic tissue
Malignant neoplasms of ectopic tissue are to be coded to the site of origin mentioned, e.g., ectopic pancreatic malignant neoplasms involving the stomach are coded to **malignant neoplasm of** pancreas, unspecified (C25.9).

The neoplasm table in the Alphabetic Index should be referenced first. However, if the histological term is documented, that term should be referenced first, rather than going immediately to the Neoplasm Table, in order to determine which column in the Neoplasm Table is appropriate. For example, if the documentation indicates "adenoma," refer to the term in the Alphabetic Index to review the entries under this term and the instructional note to "see also neoplasm, by site, benign." The table provides the proper code based on the type of neoplasm and the site. It is important to select the proper column in the table that corresponds to the type of neoplasm. The Tabular List should then be referenced to verify that the correct code has been selected from the table and that a more specific site code does not exist.

See Section I.C.21. Factors influencing health status and contact with health services, Status, for information regarding Z15.0, codes for genetic susceptibility to cancer.

a. Treatment directed at the malignancy
If the treatment is directed at the malignancy, designate the malignancy as the principal diagnosis.

The only exception to this guideline is if a patient admission/encounter is solely for the administration of chemotherapy, immunotherapy or **external beam** radiation therapy, assign the appropriate Z51.— code as the first-listed or principal diagnosis, and the diagnosis or problem for which the service is being performed as a secondary diagnosis.

b. Treatment of secondary site
When a patient is admitted because of a primary neoplasm with metastasis and treatment is directed toward the secondary site only, the secondary neoplasm is designated as the principal diagnosis even though the primary malignancy is still present.

c. Coding and sequencing of complications
Coding and sequencing of complications associated with the malignancies or with the therapy thereof are subject to the following guidelines:

1) Anemia associated with malignancy
When admission/encounter is for management of an anemia associated with the malignancy, and the treatment is only for anemia, the appropriate code for the malignancy is sequenced as the principal or first-listed diagnosis followed by the appropriate code for the anemia (such as code D63.0, Anemia in neoplastic disease).

2) Anemia associated with chemotherapy, immunotherapy and radiation therapy
When the admission/encounter is for management of an anemia associated with an adverse effect of the administration of chemotherapy or immunotherapy and the only treatment is for the anemia, the anemia code is sequenced first followed by the appropriate codes for the neoplasm and the adverse effect

(T45.1X5, Adverse effect of antineoplastic and immunosuppressive drugs).

When the admission/encounter is for management of an anemia associated with an adverse effect of radiotherapy, the anemia code should be sequenced first, followed by the appropriate neoplasm code and code Y84.2, Radiological procedure and radiotherapy as the cause of abnormal reaction of the patient, or of later complication, without mention of misadventure at the time of the procedure.

3) Management of dehydration due to the malignancy
When the admission/encounter is for management of dehydration due to the malignancy and only the dehydration is being treated (intravenous rehydration), the dehydration is sequenced first, followed by the code(s) for the malignancy.

4) Treatment of a complication resulting from a surgical procedure
When the admission/encounter is for treatment of a complication resulting from a surgical procedure, designate the complication as the principal or first-listed diagnosis if treatment is directed at resolving the complication.

d. Primary malignancy previously excised
When a primary malignancy has been previously excised or eradicated from its site and there is no further treatment directed to that site and there is no evidence of any existing primary malignancy, a code from category Z85, Personal history of malignant neoplasm, should be used to indicate the former site of the malignancy. Any mention of extension, invasion, or metastasis to another site is coded as a secondary malignant neoplasm to that site. The secondary site may be the principal or first-listed with the Z85 code used as a secondary code.

e. Admissions/Encounters involving chemotherapy, immunotherapy and radiation therapy

1) Episode of care involves surgical removal of neoplasm
When an episode of care involves the surgical removal of a neoplasm, primary or secondary site, followed by adjunct chemotherapy or radiation treatment during the same episode of care, the code for the neoplasm should be assigned as principal or first-listed diagnosis.

2) Patient admission/encounter solely for administration of chemotherapy, immunotherapy and radiation therapy
If a patient admission/encounter is solely for the administration of chemotherapy, immunotherapy or **external beam** radiation therapy assign code Z51.0, Encounter for antineoplastic radiation therapy, or Z51.11, Encounter for antineoplastic chemotherapy, or Z51.12, Encounter for antineoplastic immunotherapy as the first-listed or principal diagnosis. If a patient receives more than one of these therapies during the same admission more than one of these codes may be assigned, in any sequence.

The malignancy for which the therapy is being administered should be assigned as a secondary diagnosis.

If a patient admission/encounter is for the insertion or implantation of radioactive elements (e.g., brachytherapy) the appropriate code for the malignancy is sequenced as the principal or first-listed diagnosis. Code Z51.0 should not be assigned.

3) Patient admitted for radiation therapy, chemotherapy or immunotherapy and develops complications
When a patient is admitted for the purpose of **external beam** radiotherapy, immunotherapy or chemotherapy and develops complications such as uncontrolled nausea and vomiting or dehydration, the principal or first-listed diagnosis is Z51.0, Encounter for antineoplastic radiation therapy, or Z51.11, Encounter for antineoplastic chemotherapy, or Z51.12, Encounter for antineoplastic immunotherapy followed by any codes for the complications.

When a patient is admitted for the purpose of insertion or implantation of radioactive elements (e.g., brachytherapy) and develops complications such as uncontrolled nausea and vomiting or dehydration, the principal or first-listed diagnosis is the appropriate code for the malignancy followed by any codes for the complications.

f. Admission/encounter to determine extent of malignancy
When the reason for admission/encounter is to determine the extent of the malignancy, or for a procedure such as paracentesis or thoracentesis, the primary malignancy or appropriate metastatic site is designated as the principal or first-listed

diagnosis, even though chemotherapy or radiotherapy is administered.

g. Symptoms, signs, and abnormal findings listed in Chapter 18 associated with neoplasms

Symptoms, signs, and ill-defined conditions listed in Chapter 18 characteristic of, or associated with, an existing primary or secondary site malignancy cannot be used to replace the malignancy as principal or first-listed diagnosis, regardless of the number of admissions or encounters for treatment and care of the neoplasm.

See section I.C.21. Factors influencing health status and contact with health services, Encounter for prophylactic organ removal.

h. Admission/encounter for pain control/management

See Section I.C.6. for information on coding admission/encounter for pain control/management.

i. Malignancy in two or more noncontiguous sites

A patient may have more than one malignant tumor in the same organ. These tumors may represent different primaries or metastatic disease, depending on the site. Should the documentation be unclear, the provider should be queried as to the status of each tumor so that the correct codes can be assigned.

j. Disseminated malignant neoplasm, unspecified

Code C80.0, Disseminated malignant neoplasm, unspecified, is for use only in those cases where the patient has advanced metastatic disease and no known primary or secondary sites are specified. It should not be used in place of assigning codes for the primary site and all known secondary sites.

k. Malignant neoplasm without specification of site

Code C80.1, Malignant (primary) neoplasm, unspecified, equates to Cancer, unspecified. This code should only be used when no determination can be made as to the primary site of a malignancy. This code should rarely be used in the inpatient setting.

l. Sequencing of neoplasm codes

1) Encounter for treatment of primary malignancy

If the reason for the encounter is for treatment of a primary malignancy, assign the malignancy as the principal/first-listed diagnosis. The primary site is to be sequenced first, followed by any metastatic sites.

2) Encounter for treatment of secondary malignancy

When an encounter is for a primary malignancy with metastasis and treatment is directed toward the metastatic (secondary) site(s) only, the metastatic site(s) is designated as the principal/first-listed diagnosis. The primary malignancy is coded as an additional code.

3) Malignant neoplasm in a pregnant patient

When a pregnant woman has a malignant neoplasm, a code from subcategory O9A.1-, Malignant neoplasm complicating pregnancy, childbirth, and the puerperium, should be sequenced first, followed by the appropriate code from Chapter 2 to indicate the type of neoplasm.

4) Encounter for complication associated with a neoplasm

When an encounter is for management of a complication associated with a neoplasm, such as dehydration, and the treatment is only for the complication, the complication is coded first, followed by the appropriate code(s) for the neoplasm.

The exception to this guideline is anemia. When the admission/encounter is for management of an anemia associated with the malignancy, and the treatment is only for anemia, the appropriate code for the malignancy is sequenced as the principal or first-listed diagnosis followed by code D63.0, Anemia in neoplastic disease.

5) Complication from surgical procedure for treatment of a neoplasm

When an encounter is for treatment of a complication resulting from a surgical procedure performed for the treatment of the neoplasm, designate the complication as the principal/first-listed diagnosis. See guideline regarding the coding of a current malignancy versus personal history to determine if the code for the neoplasm should also be assigned.

6) Pathologic fracture due to a neoplasm

When an encounter is for a pathological fracture due to a neoplasm, and the focus of treatment is the fracture, a code from subcategory M84.5, Pathological fracture in neoplastic disease, should be sequenced first, followed by the code for the neoplasm.

If the focus of treatment is the neoplasm with an associated pathological fracture, the neoplasm code should be sequenced first, followed by a code from M84.5 for the pathological fracture.

m. Current malignancy versus personal history of malignancy

When a primary malignancy has been excised but further treatment, such as an additional surgery for the malignancy, radiation therapy or chemotherapy is directed to that site, the primary malignancy code should be used until treatment is completed.

When a primary malignancy has been previously excised or eradicated from its site, there is no further treatment (of the malignancy) directed to that site, and there is no evidence of any existing primary malignancy, a code from category Z85, Personal history of malignant neoplasm, should be used to indicate the former site of the malignancy.

See Section I.C.21. Factors influencing health status and contact with health services, History (of)

n. Leukemia, Multiple Myeloma, and Malignant Plasma Cell Neoplasms in remission versus personal history

The categories for leukemia, and category C90, Multiple myeloma and malignant plasma cell neoplasms, have codes indicating whether or not the leukemia has achieved remission. There are also codes Z85.6, Personal history of leukemia, and Z85.79, Personal history of other malignant neoplasms of lymphoid, hematopoietic and related tissues. If the documentation is unclear, as to whether the leukemia has achieved remission, the provider should be queried.

See Section I.C.21. Factors influencing health status and contact with health services, History (of)

o. Aftercare following surgery for neoplasm
See Section I.C.21. Factors influencing health status and contact with health services, Aftercare

p. Follow-up care for completed treatment of a malignancy
See Section I.C.21. Factors influencing health status and contact with health services, Follow-up

q. Prophylactic organ removal for prevention of malignancy
See Section I.C. 21, Factors influencing health status and contact with health services, Prophylactic organ removal

r. Malignant neoplasm associated with transplanted organ

A malignant neoplasm of a transplanted organ should be coded as a transplant complication. Assign first the appropriate code from category T86.-, Complications of transplanted organs and tissue, followed by code C80.2, Malignant neoplasm associated with transplanted organ. Use an additional code for the specific malignancy.

Item 2-1 Neoplasm: Neo = new, plasm = growth, development, formation. This new growth (mass, tumor) can be malignant or benign, which is confirmed by the pathology report. Do not assign a code to a neoplasm until you review the pathology report. Certain CPT codes will specify benign or malignant lesion, so be certain the diagnosis code supports the procedure code.

CHAPTER 2

NEOPLASMS (C00-D49)

This chapter contains the following blocks:

C00-C14	Malignant neoplasms of lip, oral cavity and pharynx
C15-C26	Malignant neoplasms of digestive organs
C30-C39	Malignant neoplasms of respiratory and intrathoracic organs
C40-C41	Malignant neoplasms of bone and articular cartilage
C43-C44	Melanoma and other malignant neoplasms of skin
C45-C49	Malignant neoplasms of mesothelial and soft tissue
C50	Malignant neoplasms of breast
C51-C58	Malignant neoplasms of female genital organs
C60-C63	Malignant neoplasms of male genital organs
C64-C68	Malignant neoplasms of urinary tract
C69-C72	Malignant neoplasms of eye, brain and other parts of central nervous system
C73-C75	Malignant neoplasms of thyroid and other endocrine glands
C7A	Malignant neuroendocrine tumors
C7B	Secondary neuroendocrine tumors
C76-C80	Malignant neoplasms of ill-defined, other secondary and unspecified sites
C81-C96	Malignant neoplasms of lymphoid, hematopoietic and related tissue
D00-D09	In situ neoplasms
D10-D36	Benign neoplasms, except benign neuroendocrine tumors
D3A	Benign neuroendocrine tumors
D37-D48	Neoplasms of uncertain behavior, polycythemia vera and myelodysplastic syndromes
D49	Neoplasms of unspecified behavior

Notes: Functional activity

All neoplasms are classified in this chapter, whether they are functionally active or not. An additional code from Chapter 4 may be used, to identify functional activity associated with any neoplasm.

Morphology [Histology]

Chapter 2 classifies neoplasms primarily by site (topography), with broad groupings for behavior, malignant, in situ, benign, etc. The Table of Neoplasms should be used to identify the correct topography code. In a few cases, such as for malignant melanoma and certain neuroendocrine tumors, the morphology (histologic type) is included in the category and codes.

Primary malignant neoplasms overlapping site boundaries

A primary malignant neoplasm that overlaps two or more contiguous (next to each other) sites should be classified to the subcategory/code .8 ('overlapping lesion'), unless the combination is specifically indexed elsewhere. For multiple neoplasms of the same site that are not contiguous, such as tumors in different quadrants of the same breast, codes for each site should be assigned.

Malignant neoplasm of ectopic tissue

Malignant neoplasms of ectopic tissue are to be coded to the site mentioned, e.g., ectopic pancreatic malignant neoplasms are coded to pancreas, unspecified (C25.9).

MALIGNANT NEOPLASMS (C00-C96)

MALIGNANT NEOPLASMS, STATED OR PRESUMED TO BE PRIMARY (OF SPECIFIED SITES), AND CERTAIN SPECIFIED HISTOLOGIES, EXCEPT NEUROENDOCRINE, AND OF LYMPHOID, HEMATOPOIETIC AND RELATED TISSUE (C00-C75)

MALIGNANT NEOPLASMS OF LIP, ORAL CAVITY AND PHARYNX (C00-C14)

● **C00   Malignant neoplasm of lip**

Use additional code to identify:
alcohol abuse and dependence (F10.-)
history of tobacco dependence (Z87.891)
tobacco dependence (F17.-)
tobacco use (Z72.0)

Excludes1   malignant melanoma of lip (C43.0)
Merkel cell carcinoma of lip (C4A.0)
other and unspecified malignant neoplasm of skin of lip (C44.0-)

C00.0   Malignant neoplasm of external upper lip
Malignant neoplasm of lipstick area of upper lip
Malignant neoplasm of upper lip NOS
Malignant neoplasm of vermilion border of upper lip

C00.1   Malignant neoplasm of external lower lip
Malignant neoplasm of lower lip NOS
Malignant neoplasm of lipstick area of lower lip
Malignant neoplasm of vermilion border of lower lip

C00.2   Malignant neoplasm of external lip, unspecified
Malignant neoplasm of vermilion border of lip NOS

C00.3   Malignant neoplasm of upper lip, inner aspect
Malignant neoplasm of buccal aspect of upper lip
Malignant neoplasm of frenulum of upper lip
Malignant neoplasm of mucosa of upper lip
Malignant neoplasm of oral aspect of upper lip

C00.4   Malignant neoplasm of lower lip, inner aspect
Malignant neoplasm of buccal aspect of lower lip
Malignant neoplasm of frenulum of lower lip
Malignant neoplasm of mucosa of lower lip
Malignant neoplasm of oral aspect of lower lip

C00.5   Malignant neoplasm of lip, unspecified, inner aspect
Malignant neoplasm of buccal aspect of lip, unspecified
Malignant neoplasm of frenulum of lip, unspecified
Malignant neoplasm of mucosa of lip, unspecified
Malignant neoplasm of oral aspect of lip, unspecified

C00.6   Malignant neoplasm of commissure of lip, unspecified
Commissure: Site of union of corresponding parts

C00.8   Malignant neoplasm of overlapping sites of lip

C00.9   Malignant neoplasm of lip, unspecified

▶ New   ⇒ Revised   deleted Deleted   OGCR Official Guidelines   X Assign placeholder X   ● Use Additional Character(s)
Excludes 1   Excludes 2   Includes   Use additional   Code first   Code also   Key words
633

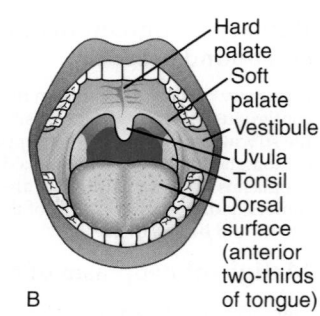

Transitional or vermilion surfaces

Lips are connected to
A the gums by frenulum

B

Hard palate
Soft palate
Vestibule
Uvula
Tonsil
Dorsal surface (anterior two-thirds of tongue)

Ventral surface

Lingual frenum

C

Figure 2-1 Anatomical structures of the mouth and lips. **A.** Transitional or vermilion borders. Lips are connected to the gums by frenulum. **B.** Dorsal surface. **C.** Ventral surface.

C01   **Malignant neoplasm of base of tongue**
     Malignant neoplasm of dorsal surface of base of tongue
     Malignant neoplasm of fixed part of tongue NOS
     Malignant neoplasm of posterior third of tongue
     Use additional code to identify:
        alcohol abuse and dependence (F10.-)
        history of tobacco dependence (Z87.891)
        tobacco dependence (F17.-)
        tobacco use (Z72.0)

● **C02**   **Malignant neoplasm of other and unspecified parts of tongue**
     Use additional code to identify:
        alcohol abuse and dependence (F10.-)
        history of tobacco dependence (Z87.891)
        tobacco dependence (F17.-)
        tobacco use (Z72.0)

    C02.0   **Malignant neoplasm of dorsal surface of tongue**
        Malignant neoplasm of anterior two-thirds of tongue, dorsal surface
        Excludes2   malignant neoplasm of dorsal surface of base of tongue (C01)

    C02.1   **Malignant neoplasm of border of tongue**
        Malignant neoplasm of tip of tongue

    C02.2   **Malignant neoplasm of ventral surface of tongue**
        Malignant neoplasm of anterior two-thirds of tongue, ventral surface
        Malignant neoplasm of frenulum linguae

    C02.3   **Malignant neoplasm of anterior two-thirds of tongue, part unspecified**
        Malignant neoplasm of middle third of tongue NOS
        Malignant neoplasm of mobile part of tongue NOS

    C02.4   **Malignant neoplasm of lingual tonsil**
        Lingual tonsil: Aggregation of lymph follicles at root of tongue
        Excludes2   malignant neoplasm of tonsil NOS (C09.9)

    C02.8   **Malignant neoplasm of overlapping sites of tongue**
        Malignant neoplasm of two or more contiguous sites of tongue

    C02.9   **Malignant neoplasm of tongue, unspecified**

● **C03**   **Malignant neoplasm of gum**
    Includes   malignant neoplasm of alveolar (ridge) mucosa
                   malignant neoplasm of gingiva
    Use additional code to identify:
        alcohol abuse and dependence (F10.-)
        history of tobacco dependence (Z87.891)
        tobacco dependence (F17.-)
        tobacco use (Z72.0)
    Excludes2   malignant odontogenic neoplasms (C41.0-C41.1)

    C03.0   **Malignant neoplasm of upper gum**
    C03.1   **Malignant neoplasm of lower gum**
    C03.9   **Malignant neoplasm of gum, unspecified**

● **C04**   **Malignant neoplasm of floor of mouth**
    Use additional code to identify:
        alcohol abuse and dependence (F10.-)
        history of tobacco dependence (Z87.891)
        tobacco dependence (F17.-)
        tobacco use (Z72.0)

    C04.0   **Malignant neoplasm of anterior floor of mouth**
        Malignant neoplasm of anterior to the premolar-canine junction

    C04.1   **Malignant neoplasm of lateral floor of mouth**
    C04.8   **Malignant neoplasm of overlapping sites of floor of mouth**
    C04.9   **Malignant neoplasm of floor of mouth, unspecified**

● **C05**   **Malignant neoplasm of palate**
    Use additional code to identify:
        alcohol abuse and dependence (F10.-)
        history of tobacco dependence (Z87.891)
        tobacco dependence (F17.-)
        tobacco use (Z72.0)
    Excludes1   Kaposi's sarcoma of palate (C46.2)

    C05.0   **Malignant neoplasm of hard palate**
    C05.1   **Malignant neoplasm of soft palate**
        Excludes2   malignant neoplasm of nasopharyngeal surface of soft palate (C11.3)

    C05.2   **Malignant neoplasm of uvula**
    C05.8   **Malignant neoplasm of overlapping sites of palate**
    C05.9   **Malignant neoplasm of palate, unspecified**
        Malignant neoplasm of roof of mouth

● **C06**   **Malignant neoplasm of other and unspecified parts of mouth**
    Use additional code to identify:
        alcohol abuse and dependence (F10.-)
        history of tobacco dependence (Z87.891)
        tobacco dependence (F17.-)
        tobacco use (Z72.0)

    C06.0   **Malignant neoplasm of cheek mucosa**
        Malignant neoplasm of buccal mucosa NOS
        Malignant neoplasm of internal cheek

    C06.1   **Malignant neoplasm of vestibule of mouth**
        Malignant neoplasm of buccal sulcus (upper) (lower)
        Malignant neoplasm of labial sulcus (upper) (lower)

    C06.2   **Malignant neoplasm of retromolar area**

● **C06.8**   **Malignant neoplasm of overlapping sites of other and unspecified parts of mouth**

        C06.80   **Malignant neoplasm of overlapping sites of unspecified parts of mouth**

        C06.89   **Malignant neoplasm of overlapping sites of other parts of mouth**
            'book leaf' neoplasm [ventral surface of tongue and floor of mouth]

    C06.9   **Malignant neoplasm of mouth, unspecified**
        Malignant neoplasm of minor salivary gland, unspecified site
        Malignant neoplasm of oral cavity NOS

▶ New   ⇨ Revised   ~~deleted~~ Deleted   **OGCR** Official Guidelines   X Assign placeholder X   ● Use Additional Character(s)

Excludes 1   Excludes 2   Includes   Use additional   Code first   Code also   Key words

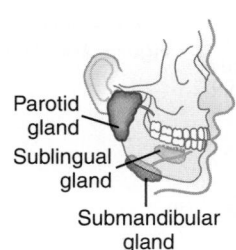

Parotid gland

Sublingual gland

Submandibular gland

Figure 2-2   Major salivary glands.

C07   **Malignant neoplasm of parotid gland**
     Use additional code to identify:
         alcohol abuse and dependence (F10.-)
         exposure to environmental tobacco smoke (Z77.22)
         exposure to tobacco smoke in the perinatal period (P96.81)
         history of tobacco dependence (Z87.891)
         occupational exposure to environmental tobacco smoke
             (Z57.31)
         tobacco dependence (F17.-)
         tobacco use (Z72.0)

● **C08**   **Malignant neoplasm of other and unspecified major salivary glands**
     Includes   malignant neoplasm of salivary ducts
     Use additional code to identify:
         alcohol abuse and dependence (F10.-)
         exposure to environmental tobacco smoke (Z77.22)
         exposure to tobacco smoke in the perinatal period (P96.81)
         history of tobacco dependence (Z87.891)
         occupational exposure to environmental tobacco smoke
             (Z57.31)
         tobacco dependence (F17.-)
         tobacco use (Z72.0)
     Excludes1   malignant neoplasms of specified minor salivary
            glands which are classified according to their
            anatomical location
     Excludes2   malignant neoplasms of minor salivary glands
            NOS (C06.9)
            malignant neoplasm of parotid gland (C07)

C08.0   **Malignant neoplasm of submandibular gland**
     Malignant neoplasm of submaxillary gland

C08.1   **Malignant neoplasm of sublingual gland**

C08.9   **Malignant neoplasm of major salivary gland, unspecified**
     Malignant neoplasm of salivary gland (major) NOS

★**(See Plate 61 on page 73.)**

● **C09**   **Malignant neoplasm of tonsil**
     Use additional code to identify:
         alcohol abuse and dependence (F10.-)
         exposure to environmental tobacco smoke (Z77.22)
         exposure to tobacco smoke in the perinatal period (P96.81)
         history of tobacco dependence (Z87.891)
         occupational exposure to environmental tobacco smoke
             (Z57.31)
         tobacco dependence (F17.-)
         tobacco use (Z72.0)
     Excludes2   malignant neoplasm of lingual tonsil (C02.4)
            malignant neoplasm of pharyngeal tonsil (C11.1)

C09.0   **Malignant neoplasm of tonsillar fossa**
     Surface of palatine (two masses of lymphatic tissue on sides of
         throat) tonsils

C09.1   **Malignant neoplasm of tonsillar pillar (anterior) (posterior)**
     Extension from palatine (two masses of lymphatic tissue on
         sides of throat) tonsils

C09.8   **Malignant neoplasm of overlapping sites of tonsil**

C09.9   **Malignant neoplasm of tonsil, unspecified**
     Malignant neoplasm of tonsil NOS
     Malignant neoplasm of faucial tonsils
     Malignant neoplasm of palatine tonsils

● **C10**   **Malignant neoplasm of oropharynx**
     Area of throat at back of mouth
     Use additional code to identify:
         alcohol abuse and dependence (F10.-)
         exposure to environmental tobacco smoke (Z77.22)
         exposure to tobacco smoke in the perinatal period (P96.81)
         history of tobacco dependence (Z87.891)
         occupational exposure to environmental tobacco smoke
             (Z57.31)
         tobacco dependence (F17.-)
         tobacco use (Z72.0)
     Excludes2   malignant neoplasm of tonsil (C09.-)

C10.0   **Malignant neoplasm of vallecula**
     Vallecula, depression or furrow

C10.1   **Malignant neoplasm of anterior surface of epiglottis**
     Malignant neoplasm of epiglottis, free border [margin]
     Malignant neoplasm of glossoepiglottic fold(s)
     Excludes2   malignant neoplasm of epiglottis
            (suprahyoid portion) NOS (C32.1)

C10.2   **Malignant neoplasm of lateral wall of oropharynx**

C10.3   **Malignant neoplasm of posterior wall of oropharynx**

C10.4   **Malignant neoplasm of branchial cleft**
     Congenital slitlike openings formed between branchial arches
         pharyngeal groove
     Malignant neoplasm of branchial cyst [site of neoplasm]

C10.8   **Malignant neoplasm of overlapping sites of oropharynx**
     Malignant neoplasm of junctional region of oropharynx

C10.9   **Malignant neoplasm of oropharynx, unspecified**

● **C11**   **Malignant neoplasm of nasopharynx**
     Use additional code to identify:
         exposure to environmental tobacco smoke (Z77.22)
         exposure to tobacco smoke in the perinatal period (P96.81)
         history of tobacco dependence (Z87.891)
         occupational exposure to environmental tobacco smoke
             (Z57.31)
         tobacco dependence (F17.-)
         tobacco use (Z72.0)

C11.0   **Malignant neoplasm of superior wall of nasopharynx**
     Part of pharynx that lies above soft palate
     Malignant neoplasm of roof of nasopharynx

C11.1   **Malignant neoplasm of posterior wall of nasopharynx**
     Malignant neoplasm of adenoid
     Malignant neoplasm of pharyngeal tonsil

C11.2   **Malignant neoplasm of lateral wall of nasopharynx**
     Malignant neoplasm of fossa of Rosenmüller
     Malignant neoplasm of opening of auditory tube
     Malignant neoplasm of pharyngeal recess

C11.3   **Malignant neoplasm of anterior wall of nasopharynx**
     Malignant neoplasm of floor of nasopharynx
     Malignant neoplasm of nasopharyngeal (anterior)
         (posterior) surface of soft palate
     Malignant neoplasm of posterior margin of nasal
         choana
     Malignant neoplasm of posterior margin of nasal
         septum

C11.8   **Malignant neoplasm of overlapping sites of nasopharynx**

C11.9   **Malignant neoplasm of nasopharynx, unspecified**
     Malignant neoplasm of nasopharyngeal wall NOS

C12   **Malignant neoplasm of pyriform sinus**
     Malignant neoplasm of pyriform fossa
     Use additional code to identify:
         exposure to environmental tobacco smoke (Z77.22)
         exposure to tobacco smoke in the perinatal period (P96.81)
         history of tobacco dependence (Z87.891)
         occupational exposure to environmental tobacco smoke
             (Z57.31)
         tobacco dependence (F17.-)
         tobacco use (Z72.0)

CHAPTER 2 (C00-D49)

● **C13 Malignant neoplasm of hypopharynx**

Use additional code to identify:

exposure to environmental tobacco smoke (Z77.22)
exposure to tobacco smoke in the perinatal period (P96.81)
history of tobacco dependence (Z87.891)
occupational exposure to environmental tobacco smoke (Z57.31)
tobacco dependence (F17.-)
tobacco use (Z72.0)

Excludes2   malignant neoplasm of pyriform sinus (C12)

C13.0 Malignant neoplasm of postcricoid region
Behind the cricoid cartilage of neck

C13.1 Malignant neoplasm of aryepiglottic fold, hypopharyngeal aspect
Arytenoepiglottic fold, triangular opening between side of epiglottis and apex of arytenoid cartilage
Malignant neoplasm of aryepiglottic fold, marginal zone
Malignant neoplasm of aryepiglottic fold NOS
Malignant neoplasm of interarytenoid fold, marginal zone
Malignant neoplasm of interarytenoid fold NOS

Excludes2   malignant neoplasm of aryepiglottic fold or interarytenoid fold, laryngeal aspect (C32.1)

C13.2 Malignant neoplasm of posterior wall of hypopharynx

C13.8 Malignant neoplasm of overlapping sites of hypopharynx

C13.9 Malignant neoplasm of hypopharynx, unspecified
Malignant neoplasm of hypopharyngeal wall NOS

● **C14 Malignant neoplasm of other and ill-defined sites in the lip, oral cavity and pharynx**

Use additional code to identify:

alcohol abuse and dependence (F10.-)
exposure to environmental tobacco smoke (Z77.22)
exposure to tobacco smoke in the perinatal period (P96.81)
history of tobacco dependence (Z87.891)
occupational exposure to environmental tobacco smoke (Z57.31)
tobacco dependence (F17.-)
tobacco use (Z72.0)

Excludes1   malignant neoplasm of oral cavity NOS (C06.9)

C14.0 Malignant neoplasm of pharynx, unspecified

C14.2 Malignant neoplasm of Waldeyer's ring

C14.8 Malignant neoplasm of overlapping sites of lip, oral cavity and pharynx
Primary malignant neoplasm of two or more contiguous sites of lip, oral cavity and pharynx

Excludes1   'book leaf' neoplasm [ventral surface of tongue and floor of mouth] (C06.89)

CERVICAL ESOPHAGUS
Left subclavian artery
First rib
Arch of aorta
Diaphragm
THORACIC ESOPHAGUS
Stomach
ABDOMINAL ESOPHAGUS

Figure 2-3 The esophagus is the muscular tube that connects the pharynx and the stomach. The 10 inch (25 cm) long esophagus is divided into three parts: **cervical, thoracic,** and **abdominal.**

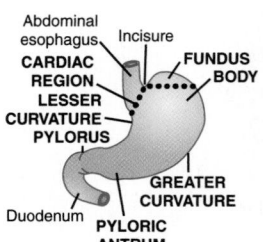

Abdominal esophagus   Incisure
CARDIAC REGION   **FUNDUS**   **BODY**
LESSER CURVATURE
PYLORUS
GREATER CURVATURE
Duodenum   **PYLORIC ANTRUM**

Figure 2-4 Parts of the stomach.

Item 2-2 The esophagus opens into the stomach through the **cardiac orifice,** also called the **cardioesophageal junction.** The **cardia** is adjacent to the cardiac orifice. The stomach widens into the **greater** and **lesser curvatures.** The **pyloric antrum** precedes the **pylorus,** which opens to the duodenum.

MALIGNANT NEOPLASM OF DIGESTIVE ORGANS (C15-C26)

Excludes1   Kaposi's sarcoma of gastrointestinal sites (C46.4)

Excludes2   gastrointestinal stromal tumors (C49.A-)

● **C15 Malignant neoplasms of esophagus**

Use additional code to identify:
alcohol abuse and dependence (F10.-)

C15.3 Malignant neoplasm of upper third of esophagus

C15.4 Malignant neoplasm of middle third of esophagus

C15.5 Malignant neoplasm of lower third of esophagus

Excludes1   malignant neoplasm of cardio-esophageal junction (C16.0)

C15.8 Malignant neoplasm of overlapping sites of esophagus

C15.9 Malignant neoplasm of esophagus, unspecified

● **C16 Malignant neoplasm of stomach**

Use additional code to identify:
alcohol abuse and dependence (F10.-)

Excludes2   malignant carcinoid tumor of the stomach (C7A.092)

C16.0 Malignant neoplasm of cardia
Malignant neoplasm of cardiac orifice
Malignant neoplasm of cardio-esophageal junction
Malignant neoplasm of esophagus and stomach
Malignant neoplasm of gastro-esophageal junction

C16.1 Malignant neoplasm of fundus of stomach

C16.2 Malignant neoplasm of body of stomach

C16.3 Malignant neoplasm of pyloric antrum
Malignant neoplasm of gastric antrum

C16.4 Malignant neoplasm of pylorus
Malignant neoplasm of prepylorus
Malignant neoplasm of pyloric canal

C16.5 Malignant neoplasm of lesser curvature of stomach, unspecified
Malignant neoplasm of lesser curvature of stomach, not classifiable to C16.1-C16.4

C16.6 Malignant neoplasm of greater curvature of stomach, unspecified
Malignant neoplasm of greater curvature of stomach, not classifiable to C16.0-C16.4

C16.8 Malignant neoplasm of overlapping sites of stomach

C16.9 Malignant neoplasm of stomach, unspecified
Gastric cancer NOS

▶ New   ⇒ Revised   ~~deleted~~ Deleted   OGCR Official Guidelines   X Assign placeholder X   ● Use Additional Character(s)

Excludes 1   Excludes 2   Includes   Use additional   Code first   Code also   Key words

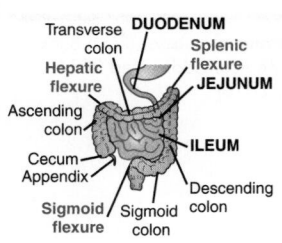

Figure 2-5   Small intestine and colon.

● **C17   Malignant neoplasm of small intestine**
>   **Excludes1**   malignant carcinoid tumor of the small intestine
>   (C7A.Ø1)

C17.Ø   Malignant neoplasm of duodenum
First or proximal portion of small intestine, extending from pylorus to jejunum

C17.1   Malignant neoplasm of jejunum
Second section of small intestine, extending from duodenum to ileum

C17.2   Malignant neoplasm of ileum
Distal and longest portion of small intestine, extending from jejunum to cecum
>   **Excludes1**   malignant neoplasm of ileocecal valve
>   (C18.Ø)

C17.3   Meckel's diverticulum, malignant
Appendage of ileum
>   **Excludes1**   Meckel's diverticulum, congenital (Q43.Ø)

C17.8   Malignant neoplasm of overlapping sites of small intestine

C17.9   Malignant neoplasm of small intestine, unspecified

● **C18   Malignant neoplasm of colon**
>   **Excludes1**   malignant carcinoid tumors of the colon (C7A.Ø2)

C18.Ø   Malignant neoplasm of cecum
First section of large intestine
Malignant neoplasm of ileocecal valve

C18.1   Malignant neoplasm of appendix
Blind ended tube connected to the cecum; AKA vermiform appendix

C18.2   Malignant neoplasm of ascending colon
Ascending colon is between cecum and right colic flexure

C18.3   Malignant neoplasm of hepatic flexure
A flexure is a bending in a structure or organ. Note the three flexures illustrated in Figure 2–5.

C18.4   Malignant neoplasm of transverse colon
Portion of colon that runs transversely across upper part of abdomen, between right and left colic flexures

C18.5   Malignant neoplasm of splenic flexure
Bend at junction of transverse and descending colon

C18.6   Malignant neoplasm of descending colon
Portion between left colic flexure and sigmoid colon at pelvic brim; AKA iliac colon

C18.7   Malignant neoplasm of sigmoid colon
S-shaped part of colon extending from pelvic brim to third segment of sacrum
Malignant neoplasm of sigmoid (flexure)
>   **Excludes1**   malignant neoplasm of rectosigmoid junction (C19)

C18.8   Malignant neoplasm of overlapping sites of colon

C18.9   Malignant neoplasm of colon, unspecified
Malignant neoplasm of large intestine NOS

● **C19   Malignant neoplasm of rectosigmoid junction**
Malignant neoplasm of colon with rectum
Malignant neoplasm of rectosigmoid (colon)
>   **Excludes1**   malignant carcinoid tumors of the colon
>   (C7A.Ø2-)

● **C20   Malignant neoplasm of rectum**
Malignant neoplasm of rectal ampulla
>   **Excludes1**   malignant carcinoid tumor of the rectum
>   (C7A.Ø26)

● **C21   Malignant neoplasm of anus and anal canal**
>   **Excludes2**   malignant carcinoid tumors of the colon
>   (C7A.Ø2-)
>   malignant melanoma of anal margin (C43.51)
>   malignant melanoma of anal skin (C43.51)
>   malignant melanoma of perianal skin (C43.51)
>   other and unspecified malignant neoplasm of anal margin (C44.5ØØ, C44.51Ø, C44.52Ø, C44.59Ø)
>   other and unspecified malignant neoplasm of anal skin (C44.5ØØ, C44.51Ø, C44.52Ø, C44.59Ø)
>   other and unspecified malignant neoplasm of perianal skin (C44.5ØØ, C44.51Ø, C44.52Ø, C44.59Ø)

C21.Ø   Malignant neoplasm of anus, unspecified

C21.1   Malignant neoplasm of anal canal
Terminal part of large intestine
Malignant neoplasm of anal sphincter

C21.2   Malignant neoplasm of cloacogenic zone

C21.8   Malignant neoplasm of overlapping sites of rectum, anus and anal canal
Malignant neoplasm of anorectal junction
Malignant neoplasm of anorectum
Primary malignant neoplasm of two or more contiguous sites of rectum, anus and anal canal

● **C22   Malignant neoplasm of liver and intrahepatic bile ducts**
Intrahepatic: Within liver
Use additional code to identify:
alcohol abuse and dependence (F1Ø.-)
hepatitis B (B16.-, B18.Ø-B18.1) hepatitis C (B17.1-, B18.2)
>   **Excludes1**   malignant neoplasm of biliary tract NOS (C24.9)
>   secondary malignant neoplasm of liver and intrahepatic bile duct (C78.7)

C22.Ø   Liver cell carcinoma
Hepatocellular carcinoma
Hepatoma

C22.1   Intrahepatic bile duct carcinoma
Cholangiocarcinoma
Adenocarcinoma (cancer that originates in glandular tissue) arising from epithelium of intrahepatic bile ducts
>   **Excludes1**   malignant neoplasm of hepatic duct
>   (C24.Ø)

C22.2   Hepatoblastoma
Malignant intrahepatic tumor

C22.3   Angiosarcoma of liver
Kupffer cell sarcoma

C22.4   Other sarcomas of liver

C22.7   Other specified carcinomas of liver

C22.8   Malignant neoplasm of liver, primary, unspecified as to type

C22.9   Malignant neoplasm of liver, not specified as primary or secondary

▶ New   ⇒ Revised   ~~deleted~~ Deleted   **OGCR** Official Guidelines   X Assign placeholder X   ● Use Additional Character(s)
| Excludes 1 | Excludes 2 | Includes | Use additional | Code first | Code also | Key words |

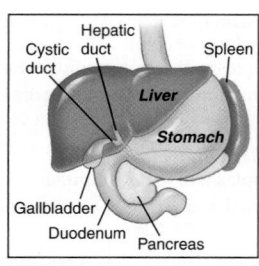

Figure 2-6 Diagram of liver, gallbladder, hepatic duct, pancreas, and spleen. (From Thibodeau and Patton: Anatomy and Physiology, ed 7, Mosby, 2010)

C23   Malignant neoplasm of gallbladder

● **C24   Malignant neoplasm of other and unspecified parts of biliary tract**
    Excludes1   malignant neoplasm of intrahepatic bile duct (C22.1)

C24.0   Malignant neoplasm of extrahepatic bile duct
    Extrahepatic = outside the liver
    Malignant neoplasm of biliary duct or passage NOS
    Malignant neoplasm of common bile duct
    Malignant neoplasm of cystic duct
    Malignant neoplasm of hepatic duct

C24.1   Malignant neoplasm of ampulla of Vater
    Union of pancreatic duct and common bile duct

C24.8   Malignant neoplasm of overlapping sites of biliary tract
    Malignant neoplasm involving both intrahepatic and extrahepatic bile ducts
    Primary malignant neoplasm of two or more contiguous sites of biliary tract

C24.9   Malignant neoplasm of biliary tract, unspecified

● **C25   Malignant neoplasm of pancreas**
    Check documentation for specific site.
    Code also exocrine pancreatic insufficiency (K86.81)
    Use additional code to identify:
        alcohol abuse and dependence (F10.-)

C25.0   Malignant neoplasm of head of pancreas
C25.1   Malignant neoplasm of body of pancreas
C25.2   Malignant neoplasm of tail of pancreas
C25.3   Malignant neoplasm of pancreatic duct
C25.4   Malignant neoplasm of endocrine pancreas
    Malignant neoplasm of islets of Langerhans
    That part of the pancreas that acts as endocrine gland and consists of islets of Langerhans
    Use additional code to identify any functional activity.

C25.7   Malignant neoplasm of other parts of pancreas
    Malignant neoplasm of neck of pancreas
C25.8   Malignant neoplasm of overlapping sites of pancreas
C25.9   Malignant neoplasm of pancreas, unspecified

Item 2–3   Islets of Langerhans (endocrine producing cells comprising 1% to 2% of the pancreatic mass) make and secrete hormones that regulate the body's production of insulin, glucagon, and stomach acid. Breakdown of the insulin-producing cells can cause diabetes mellitus. Islet cell tumors can be benign or malignant and include glucagonomas, insulinomas, gastrinomas, and neuroendocrine tumor. The neoplasm table must be consulted for the correct neoplasm code.

Figure 2-7 Paranasal sinuses. (From Buck CJ: Step-by-Step Medical Coding, ed 2016, St. Louis, Elsevier, 2016)

● **C26   Malignant neoplasm of other and ill-defined digestive organs**
    Excludes1   malignant neoplasm of peritoneum and retroperitoneum (C48.-)

C26.0   Malignant neoplasm of intestinal tract, part unspecified
    Malignant neoplasm of intestine NOS

C26.1   Malignant neoplasm of spleen
    Excludes1   Hodgkin lymphoma (C81.-)
        non-Hodgkin lymphoma (C82-C85)

C26.9   Malignant neoplasm of ill-defined sites within the digestive system
    Malignant neoplasm of alimentary canal or tract NOS
    Malignant neoplasm of gastrointestinal tract NOS
    Excludes1   malignant neoplasm of abdominal NOS (C76.2)
        malignant neoplasm of intra-abdominal NOS (C76.2)

MALIGNANT NEOPLASMS OF RESPIRATORY AND INTRATHORACIC ORGANS (C30-C39)

    Includes   malignant neoplasm of middle ear
    Excludes1   mesothelioma (C45.-)

● **C30   Malignant neoplasm of nasal cavity and middle ear**
C30.0   Malignant neoplasm of nasal cavity
    Malignant neoplasm of cartilage of nose
    Malignant neoplasm of nasal concha
    Malignant neoplasm of internal nose
    Malignant neoplasm of septum of nose
    Malignant neoplasm of vestibule of nose
    Anterior part of nasal cavity
    Excludes1   malignant neoplasm of nasal bone (C41.0)
        malignant neoplasm of nose NOS (C76.0)
        malignant neoplasm of olfactory bulb (C72.2-)
        malignant neoplasm of posterior margin of nasal septum and choana (C11.3)
        malignant melanoma of skin of nose (C43.31)
        malignant neoplasm of turbinates (C41.0)
        other and unspecified malignant neoplasm of skin of nose C44.301, C44.311, C44.321, C44.391)

C30.1   Malignant neoplasm of middle ear
    Malignant neoplasm of antrum tympanicum
    Boney cavity or chamber
    Malignant neoplasm of auditory tube
    Malignant neoplasm of eustachian tube
    Malignant neoplasm of inner ear
    Malignant neoplasm of mastoid air cells
    Malignant neoplasm of tympanic cavity
    Excludes1   malignant neoplasm of auricular canal (external) (C43.2-, C44.2-)
        malignant neoplasm of bone of ear (meatus) (C41.0)
        malignant neoplasm of cartilage of ear (C49.0)
        malignant melanoma of skin of (external) ear (C43.2-)
        other and unspecified malignant neoplasm of skin of (external) ear (C44.2-)

▶ New   ⇒ Revised   ~~deleted~~ Deleted   **OGCR** Official Guidelines   **X** Assign placeholder X   ● Use Additional Character(s)

Excludes 1   Excludes 2   Includes   Use additional   Code first   Code also   Key words

● **C31** **Malignant neoplasm of accessory sinuses**
 Paired sinuses in bones of face
 C31.0 **Malignant neoplasm of maxillary sinus**
  Malignant neoplasm of antrum (Highmore) (maxillary)
 C31.1 **Malignant neoplasm of ethmoidal sinus**
 C31.2 **Malignant neoplasm of frontal sinus**
 C31.3 **Malignant neoplasm of sphenoid sinus**
 C31.8 **Malignant neoplasm of overlapping sites of accessory sinuses**
 C31.9 **Malignant neoplasm of accessory sinus, unspecified**

● **C32** **Malignant neoplasm of larynx**
 Use additional code to identify:
  alcohol abuse and dependence (F10.-)
  exposure to environmental tobacco smoke (Z77.22)
  exposure to tobacco smoke in the perinatal period (P96.81)
  history of tobacco dependence (Z87.891)
  occupational exposure to environmental tobacco smoke (Z57.31)
  tobacco dependence (F17.-)
  tobacco use (Z72.0)
 C32.0 **Malignant neoplasm of glottis**
  Vocal apparatus of larynx, consisting of true vocal cords (plicae vocales) and opening between them (rima glottidis)
  Malignant neoplasm of intrinsic larynx
  Malignant neoplasm of laryngeal commissure (anterior) (posterior)
  Malignant neoplasm of vocal cord (true) NOS
   True vocal cords ("lower vocal folds") produce vocalization when air from the lungs passes between them. Check your documentation. Code C32.1 is for malignant neoplasm of the false vocal cords.
 C32.1 **Malignant neoplasm of supraglottis**
  Area of pharynx above glottis
  Malignant neoplasm of aryepiglottic fold or interarytenoid fold, laryngeal aspect
  Malignant neoplasm of epiglottis (suprahyoid portion) NOS
  Malignant neoplasm of extrinsic larynx
  Malignant neoplasm of false vocal cord
   False vocal cords ("upper vocal folds") are not involved in vocalization. Check your documentation. Code C32.0 is for true vocal cords.
  Malignant neoplasm of posterior (laryngeal) surface of epiglottis
  Malignant neoplasm of ventricular bands
  Excludes2 malignant neoplasm of anterior surface of epiglottis (C10.1)
   malignant neoplasm of aryepiglottic fold or interarytenoid fold, hypopharyngeal aspect (C13.1)
   malignant neoplasm of aryepiglottic fold or interarytenoid fold, marginal zone (C13.1)
   malignant neoplasm of aryepiglottic fold or interarytenoid fold NOS (C13.1)
 C32.2 **Malignant neoplasm of subglottis**
  Lowest part of larynx from just below vocal cords down to top of trachea
 C32.3 **Malignant neoplasm of laryngeal cartilage**
  Cartilages of larynx, including cricoid, thyroid, and epiglottic, and two each of arytenoid, corniculate, and cuneiform
 C32.8 **Malignant neoplasm of overlapping sites of larynx**
 C32.9 **Malignant neoplasm of larynx, unspecified**

● **C33** **Malignant neoplasm of trachea**
 Use additional code to identify:
  exposure to environmental tobacco smoke (Z77.22)
  exposure to tobacco smoke in the perinatal period (P96.81)
  history of tobacco dependence (Z87.891)
  occupational exposure to environmental tobacco smoke (Z57.31)
  tobacco dependence (F17.-)
  tobacco use (Z72.0)

● **C34** **Malignant neoplasm of bronchus and lung**
 Use additional code to identify:
  exposure to environmental tobacco smoke (Z77.22)
  exposure to tobacco smoke in the perinatal period (P96.81)
  history of tobacco dependence (Z87.891)
  occupational exposure to environmental tobacco smoke (Z57.31)
  tobacco dependence (F17.-)
  tobacco use (Z72.0)
 Excludes1 Kaposi's sarcoma of lung (C46.5-)
   malignant carcinoid tumor of the bronchus and lung (C7A.090)
 ● **C34.0** **Malignant neoplasm of main bronchus**
  Malignant neoplasm of carina
  Ridgelike structure
  Malignant neoplasm of hilus (of lung)
  Anatomic depression or pit
  C34.00 **Malignant neoplasm of unspecified main bronchus**
  C34.01 **Malignant neoplasm of right main bronchus**
  C34.02 **Malignant neoplasm of left main bronchus**
 ● **C34.1** **Malignant neoplasm of upper lobe, bronchus or lung**
  C34.10 **Malignant neoplasm of unspecified bronchus or lung**
  C34.11 **Malignant neoplasm of upper lobe, right bronchus or lung**
  C34.12 **Malignant neoplasm of upper lobe, left bronchus or lung**
  C34.2 **Malignant neoplasm of middle lobe, bronchus or lung**
 ● **C34.3** **Malignant neoplasm of lower lobe, bronchus or lung**
  C34.30 **Malignant neoplasm of lower lobe, unspecified bronchus or lung**
  C34.31 **Malignant neoplasm of lower lobe, right bronchus or lung**
  C34.32 **Malignant neoplasm of lower lobe, left bronchus or lung**
 ● **C34.8** **Malignant neoplasm of overlapping sites of bronchus and lung**
  C34.80 **Malignant neoplasm of overlapping sites of unspecified bronchus and lung**
  C34.81 **Malignant neoplasm of overlapping sites of right bronchus and lung**
  C34.82 **Malignant neoplasm of overlapping sites of left bronchus and lung**
 ● **C34.9** **Malignant neoplasm of unspecified part of bronchus or lung**
  C34.90 **Malignant neoplasm of unspecified part of unspecified bronchus or lung**
   Lung cancer NOS
  C34.91 **Malignant neoplasm of unspecified part of right bronchus or lung**
  C34.92 **Malignant neoplasm of unspecified part of left bronchus or lung**

CHAPTER 2 (C00-D49)

▶ New ⟹ Revised ~~deleted~~ Deleted **OGCR** Official Guidelines X Assign placeholder X ● Use Additional Character(s)
Excludes 1 Excludes 2 Includes Use additional Code first Code also Key words

C37   Malignant neoplasm of thymus

> **Excludes1**   malignant carcinoid tumor of the thymus (C7A.091)

● **C38   Malignant neoplasm of heart, mediastinum and pleura**

> **Excludes1**   mesothelioma (C45.-)

C38.0   Malignant neoplasm of heart
Malignant neoplasm of pericardium

> **Excludes1**   malignant neoplasm of great vessels (C49.3)

C38.1   Malignant neoplasm of anterior mediastinum

C38.2   Malignant neoplasm of posterior mediastinum

C38.3   Malignant neoplasm of mediastinum, part unspecified

C38.4   Malignant neoplasm of pleura

C38.8   Malignant neoplasm of overlapping sites of heart, mediastinum and pleura

> *Pleura are comprised of serous membrane that lines the thoracic cavity (parietal) and covers the lungs (visceral).*

● **C39   Malignant neoplasm of other and ill-defined sites in the respiratory system and intrathoracic organs**

> *Intrathoracic: within thorax/chest*

Use additional code to identify:
exposure to environmental tobacco smoke (Z77.22)
exposure to tobacco smoke in the perinatal period (P96.81)
history of tobacco dependence (Z87.891)
occupational exposure to environmental tobacco smoke (Z57.31)
tobacco dependence (F17.-)
tobacco use (Z72.0)

> **Excludes1**   intrathoracic malignant neoplasm NOS (C76.1)
> thoracic malignant neoplasm NOS (C76.1)

C39.0   Malignant neoplasm of upper respiratory tract, part unspecified

C39.9   Malignant neoplasm of lower respiratory tract, part unspecified
Malignant neoplasm of respiratory tract NOS

MALIGNANT NEOPLASMS OF BONE AND ARTICULAR CARTILAGE (C40-C41)

> **Includes**   malignant neoplasm of cartilage (articular) (joint)
> malignant neoplasm of periosteum

> **Excludes1**   malignant neoplasm of bone marrow NOS (C96.9)
> malignant neoplasm of synovia (C49.-)

● **C40   Malignant neoplasm of bone and articular cartilage of limbs**
Use additional code to identify major osseous defect, if applicable (M89.7-)

● **C40.0   Malignant neoplasm of scapula and long bones of upper limb**

C40.00   Malignant neoplasm of scapula and long bones of unspecified upper limb

C40.01   Malignant neoplasm of scapula and long bones of right upper limb

C40.02   Malignant neoplasm of scapula and long bones of left upper limb

● **C40.1   Malignant neoplasm of short bones of upper limb**

C40.10   Malignant neoplasm of short bones of unspecified upper limb

C40.11   Malignant neoplasm of short bones of right upper limb

C40.12   Malignant neoplasm of short bones of left upper limb

● **C40.2   Malignant neoplasm of long bones of lower limb**

C40.20   Malignant neoplasm of long bones of unspecified lower limb

C40.21   Malignant neoplasm of long bones of right lower limb

C40.22   Malignant neoplasm of long bones of left lower limb

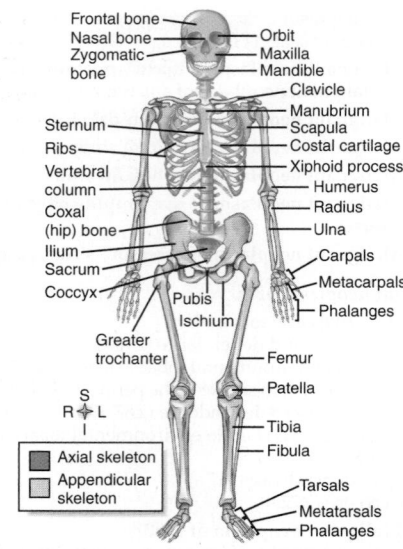

Figure 2-8   Diagram of skeleton of trunk and limbs with bones labeled. (From Thibodeau and Patton: Anatomy and Physiology, ed 7, Mosby, 2010)

● **C40.3   Malignant neoplasm of short bones of lower limb**

C40.30   Malignant neoplasm of short bones of unspecified lower limb

C40.31   Malignant neoplasm of short bones of right lower limb

C40.32   Malignant neoplasm of short bones of left lower limb

● **C40.8   Malignant neoplasm of overlapping sites of bone and articular cartilage of limb**

C40.80   Malignant neoplasm of overlapping sites of bone and articular cartilage of unspecified limb

C40.81   Malignant neoplasm of overlapping sites of bone and articular cartilage of right limb

C40.82   Malignant neoplasm of overlapping sites of bone and articular cartilage of left limb

● **C40.9   Malignant neoplasm of unspecified bones and articular cartilage of limb**

C40.90   Malignant neoplasm of unspecified bones and articular cartilage of unspecified limb

C40.91   Malignant neoplasm of unspecified bones and articular cartilage of right limb

C40.92   Malignant neoplasm of unspecified bones and articular cartilage of left limb

● **C41   Malignant neoplasm of bone and articular cartilage of other and unspecified sites**

> **Excludes1**   malignant neoplasm of bones of limbs (C40.-)
> malignant neoplasm of cartilage of ear (C49.0)
> malignant neoplasm of cartilage of eyelid (C49.0)
> malignant neoplasm of cartilage of larynx (C32.3)
> malignant neoplasm of cartilage of limbs (C40.-)
> malignant neoplasm of cartilage of nose (C30.0)

C41.0   Malignant neoplasm of bones of skull and face
Malignant neoplasm of maxilla (superior)
Malignant neoplasm of orbital bone

> **Excludes2**   carcinoma, any type except intraosseous or odontogenic of:
> maxillary sinus (C31.0)
> upper jaw (C03.0)
> malignant neoplasm of jaw bone (lower) (C41.1)

▶ New   ⇒ Revised   ~~deleted~~ Deleted   **OGCR** Official Guidelines   X Assign placeholder X   ● Use Additional Character(s)

Excludes 1   Excludes 2   Includes   Use additional   Code first   Code also   Key words

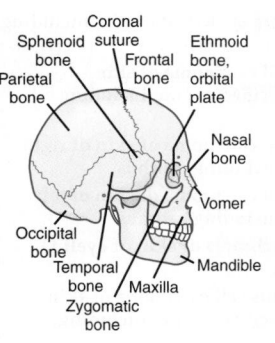

Figure 2-9   Bones of the skull.

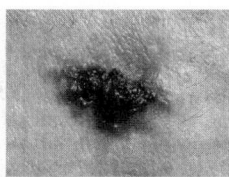

Figure 2-10   Malignant melanoma of skin. (Getty Image)

Item 2–4   Malignant melanoma is a serious form of skin cancer that affects the melanocytes (pigment-forming cells) and is caused by ultraviolet (UV) rays from the sun that damage skin. It is most commonly seen in the 40- to 60-year-olds with fair skin, blue or green eyes, and red or blond hair who sunburn easily.

    Melanoma can spread very rapidly and is the most deadly form of skin cancer. It is less common than other types of skin cancer. The rate of melanoma is increasing and currently is the leading cause of death from skin disease.

C41.1   Malignant neoplasm of mandible
     Malignant neoplasm of inferior maxilla
     Malignant neoplasm of lower jaw bone
     Excludes2   carcinoma, any type except intraosseous or odontogenic of:
       jaw NOS (C03.9)
       lower (C03.1)
       malignant neoplasm of upper jaw bone (C41.0)

C41.2   Malignant neoplasm of vertebral column
     Excludes1   malignant neoplasm of sacrum and coccyx (C41.4)

C41.3   Malignant neoplasm of ribs, sternum and clavicle

C41.4   Malignant neoplasm of pelvic bones, sacrum and coccyx

C41.9   Malignant neoplasm of bone and articular cartilage, unspecified

MELANOMA AND OTHER MALIGNANT NEOPLASMS OF SKIN (C43-C44)

● **C43**   Malignant melanoma of skin
     Excludes1   melanoma in situ (D03.-)
     Excludes2   malignant melanoma of skin of genital organs (C51-C52, C60.-, C63.-)
       Merkel cell carcinoma (C4A.-)
       sites other than skin-code to malignant neoplasm of the site

C43.0   Malignant melanoma of lip
     Excludes1   malignant neoplasm of vermilion border of lip (C00.0-C00.2)

● **C43.1**   Malignant melanoma of eyelid, including canthus
     Canthus: Either corner of eye where upper and lower eyelids meet
     C43.10   Malignant melanoma of unspecified eyelid, including canthus
     C43.11   Malignant melanoma of right eyelid, including canthus
     C43.12   Malignant melanoma of left eyelid, including canthus

● **C43.2**   Malignant melanoma of ear and external auricular canal
     C43.20   Malignant melanoma of unspecified ear and external auricular canal
     C43.21   Malignant melanoma of right ear and external auricular canal
     C43.22   Malignant melanoma of left ear and external auricular canal

● **C43.3**   Malignant melanoma of other and unspecified parts of face
     C43.30   Malignant melanoma of unspecified part of face
     C43.31   Malignant melanoma of nose
     C43.39   Malignant melanoma of other parts of face

C43.4   Malignant melanoma of scalp and neck

● **C43.5**   Malignant melanoma of trunk
     Excludes2   malignant neoplasm of anus NOS (C21.0)
       malignant neoplasm of scrotum (C63.2)
     C43.51   Malignant melanoma of anal skin
       Malignant melanoma of anal margin
       Malignant melanoma of perianal skin
     C43.52   Malignant melanoma of skin of breast
     C43.59   Malignant melanoma of other part of trunk

● **C43.6**   Malignant melanoma of upper limb, including shoulder
     C43.60   Malignant melanoma of upper limb, including shoulder, unspecified side
     C43.61   Malignant melanoma of right upper limb, including shoulder
     C43.62   Malignant melanoma of left upper limb, including shoulder

● **C43.7**   Malignant melanoma of lower limb, including hip
     C43.70   Malignant melanoma of unspecified lower limb, including hip
     C43.71   Malignant melanoma of right lower limb, including hip
     C43.72   Malignant melanoma of left lower limb, including hip

C43.8   Malignant melanoma of overlapping sites of skin

C43.9   Malignant melanoma of skin, unspecified
     Malignant melanoma of unspecified site of skin
     Melanoma (malignant) NOS

● **C4A**   Merkel cell carcinoma
C4A.0   Merkel cell carcinoma of lip
     Excludes1   malignant neoplasm of vermilion border of lip (C00.0-C00.2)

● **C4A.1**   Merkel cell carcinoma of eyelid, including canthus
     C4A.10   Merkel cell carcinoma of unspecified eyelid, including canthus
     C4A.11   Merkel cell carcinoma of right eyelid, including canthus
     C4A.12   Merkel cell carcinoma of left eyelid, including canthus

● **C4A.2**   Merkel cell carcinoma of ear and external auricular canal
     C4A.20   Merkel cell carcinoma of unspecified ear and external auricular canal
     C4A.21   Merkel cell carcinoma of right ear and external auricular canal
     C4A.22   Merkel cell carcinoma of left ear and external auricular canal

CHAPTER 2 (C00-D49)

● C4A.3 Merkel cell carcinoma of other and unspecified parts of face

    C4A.30 Merkel cell carcinoma of unspecified part of face

    C4A.31 Merkel cell carcinoma of nose

    C4A.39 Merkel cell carcinoma of other parts of face

  C4A.4 Merkel cell carcinoma of scalp and neck

● C4A.5 Merkel cell carcinoma of trunk

    Excludes2 malignant neoplasm of anus NOS (C21.0)
              malignant neoplasm of scrotum (C63.2)

    C4A.51 Merkel cell carcinoma of anal skin
          Merkel cell carcinoma of anal margin
          Merkel cell carcinoma of perianal skin

    C4A.52 Merkel cell carcinoma of skin of breast

    C4A.59 Merkel cell carcinoma of other part of trunk

● C4A.6 Merkel cell carcinoma of upper limb, including shoulder

    C4A.60 Merkel cell carcinoma of unspecified upper limb, including shoulder

    C4A.61 Merkel cell carcinoma of right upper limb, including shoulder

    C4A.62 Merkel cell carcinoma of left upper limb, including shoulder

● C4A.7 Merkel cell carcinoma of lower limb, including hip

    C4A.70 Merkel cell carcinoma of unspecified lower limb, including hip

    C4A.71 Merkel cell carcinoma of right lower limb, including hip

    C4A.72 Merkel cell carcinoma of left lower limb, including hip

  C4A.8 Merkel cell carcinoma of overlapping sites

  C4A.9 Merkel cell carcinoma, unspecified
       Merkel cell carcinoma of unspecified site
       Merkel cell carcinoma NOS

● C44 Other and unspecified malignant neoplasm of skin

    Includes malignant neoplasm of sebaceous glands
             malignant neoplasm of sweat glands

    Excludes1 Kaposi's sarcoma of skin (C46.0)
          malignant melanoma of skin (C43.-)
          malignant neoplasm of skin of genital organs
            (C51-C52, C60.-, C63.2)
          Merkel cell carcinoma (C4A.-)

● C44.0 Other and unspecified malignant neoplasm of skin of lip

    Excludes1 malignant neoplasm of lip (C00.-)

    C44.00 Unspecified malignant neoplasm of skin of lip

    C44.01 Basal cell carcinoma of skin of lip

    C44.02 Squamous cell carcinoma of skin of lip

    C44.09 Other specified malignant neoplasm of skin of lip

● C44.1 Other and unspecified malignant neoplasm of skin of eyelid, including canthus

    Excludes1 connective tissue of eyelid (C49.0)

  ● C44.10 Unspecified malignant neoplasm of skin of eyelid, including canthus

    C44.101 Unspecified malignant neoplasm of skin of unspecified eyelid, including canthus

    C44.102 Unspecified malignant neoplasm of skin of right eyelid, including canthus

    C44.109 Unspecified malignant neoplasm of skin of left eyelid, including canthus

● C44.11 Basal cell carcinoma of skin of eyelid, including canthus

    C44.111 Basal cell carcinoma of skin of unspecified eyelid, including canthus

    C44.112 Basal cell carcinoma of skin of right eyelid, including canthus

    C44.119 Basal cell carcinoma of skin of left eyelid, including canthus

● C44.12 Squamous cell carcinoma of skin of eyelid, including canthus

    C44.121 Squamous cell carcinoma of skin of unspecified eyelid, including canthus

    C44.122 Squamous cell carcinoma of skin of right eyelid, including canthus

    C44.129 Squamous cell carcinoma of skin of left eyelid, including canthus

● C44.19 Other specified malignant neoplasm of skin of eyelid, including canthus

    C44.191 Other specified malignant neoplasm of skin of unspecified eyelid, including canthus

    C44.192 Other specified malignant neoplasm of skin of right eyelid, including canthus

    C44.199 Other specified malignant neoplasm of skin of left eyelid, including canthus

● C44.2 Other and unspecified malignant neoplasm of skin of ear and external auricular canal

    Excludes1 connective tissue of ear (C49.0)

● C44.20 Unspecified malignant neoplasm of skin of ear and external auricular canal

    C44.201 Unspecified malignant neoplasm of skin of unspecified ear and external auricular canal

    C44.202 Unspecified malignant neoplasm of skin of right ear and external auricular canal

    C44.209 Unspecified malignant neoplasm of skin of left ear and external auricular canal

● C44.21 Basal cell carcinoma of skin of ear and external auricular canal

    C44.211 Basal cell carcinoma of skin of unspecified ear and external auricular canal

    C44.212 Basal cell carcinoma of skin of right ear and external auricular canal

    C44.219 Basal cell carcinoma of skin of left ear and external auricular canal

● C44.22 Squamous cell carcinoma of skin of ear and external auricular canal

    C44.221 Squamous cell carcinoma of skin of unspecified ear and external auricular canal

    C44.222 Squamous cell carcinoma of skin of right ear and external auricular canal

    C44.229 Squamous cell carcinoma of skin of left ear and external auricular canal

● C44.29 Other specified malignant neoplasm of skin of ear and external auricular canal

    C44.291 Other specified malignant neoplasm of skin of unspecified ear and external auricular canal

    C44.292 Other specified malignant neoplasm of skin of right ear and external auricular canal

    C44.299 Other specified malignant neoplasm of skin of left ear and external auricular canal

▶ New   ⫸ Revised   ~~deleted~~ Deleted   **OGCR** Official Guidelines   X Assign placeholder X   ● Use Additional Character(s)

Excludes 1   Excludes 2   Includes   Use additional   Code first   Code also   Key words

● **C44.3**   **Other and unspecified malignant neoplasm of skin of other and unspecified parts of face**
- ● **C44.30**   Unspecified malignant neoplasm of skin of other and unspecified parts of face
  - **C44.300**   Unspecified malignant neoplasm of skin of unspecified part of face
  - **C44.301**   Unspecified malignant neoplasm of skin of nose
  - **C44.309**   Unspecified malignant neoplasm of skin of other parts of face
- ● **C44.31**   Basal cell carcinoma of skin of other and unspecified parts of face
  - **C44.310**   Basal cell carcinoma of skin of unspecified parts of face
  - **C44.311**   Basal cell carcinoma of skin of nose
  - **C44.319**   Basal cell carcinoma of skin of other parts of face
- ● **C44.32**   Squamous cell carcinoma of skin of other and unspecified parts of face
  - **C44.320**   Squamous cell carcinoma of skin of unspecified parts of face
  - **C44.321**   Squamous cell carcinoma of skin of nose
  - **C44.329**   Squamous cell carcinoma of skin of other parts of face
- ● **C44.39**   Other specified malignant neoplasm of skin of other and unspecified parts of face
  - **C44.390**   Other specified malignant neoplasm of skin of unspecified parts of face
  - **C44.391**   Other specified malignant neoplasm of skin of nose
  - **C44.399**   Other specified malignant neoplasm of skin of other parts of face

● **C44.4**   **Other and unspecified malignant neoplasm of skin of scalp and neck**
- **C44.40**   Unspecified malignant neoplasm of skin of scalp and neck
- **C44.41**   Basal cell carcinoma of skin of scalp and neck
- **C44.42**   Squamous cell carcinoma of skin of scalp and neck
- **C44.49**   Other specified malignant neoplasm of skin of scalp and neck

● **C44.5**   **Other and unspecified malignant neoplasm of skin of trunk**

     | Excludes1 | anus NOS (C21.0)
                   scrotum (C63.2)

- ● **C44.50**   Unspecified malignant neoplasm of skin of trunk
  - **C44.500**   Unspecified malignant neoplasm of anal skin
    - Unspecified malignant neoplasm of anal margin
    - Unspecified malignant neoplasm of perianal skin
  - **C44.501**   Unspecified malignant neoplasm of skin of breast
  - **C44.509**   Unspecified malignant neoplasm of skin of other part of trunk
- ● **C44.51**   Basal cell carcinoma of skin of trunk
  - **C44.510**   Basal cell carcinoma of anal skin
    - Basal cell carcinoma of anal margin
    - Basal cell carcinoma of perianal skin
  - **C44.511**   Basal cell carcinoma of skin of breast
  - **C44.519**   Basal cell carcinoma of skin of other part of trunk

- ● **C44.52**   Squamous cell carcinoma of skin of trunk
  - **C44.520**   Squamous cell carcinoma of anal skin
    - Squamous cell carcinoma of anal margin
    - Squamous cell carcinoma of perianal skin
  - **C44.521**   Squamous cell carcinoma of skin of breast
  - **C44.529**   Squamous cell carcinoma of skin of other part of trunk
- ● **C44.59**   Other specified malignant neoplasm of skin of trunk
  - **C44.590**   Other specified malignant neoplasm of anal skin
    - Other specified malignant neoplasm of anal margin
    - Other specified malignant neoplasm of perianal skin
  - **C44.591**   Other specified malignant neoplasm of skin of breast
  - **C44.599**   Other specified malignant neoplasm of skin of other part of trunk

● **C44.6**   **Other and unspecified malignant neoplasm of skin of upper limb, including shoulder**
- ● **C44.60**   Unspecified malignant neoplasm of skin of upper limb, including shoulder
  - **C44.601**   Unspecified malignant neoplasm of skin of unspecified upper limb, including shoulder
  - **C44.602**   Unspecified malignant neoplasm of skin of right upper limb, including shoulder
  - **C44.609**   Unspecified malignant neoplasm of skin of left upper limb, including shoulder
- ● **C44.61**   Basal cell carcinoma of skin of upper limb, including shoulder
  - **C44.611**   Basal cell carcinoma of skin of unspecified upper limb, including shoulder
  - **C44.612**   Basal cell carcinoma of skin of right upper limb, including shoulder
  - **C44.619**   Basal cell carcinoma of skin of left upper limb, including shoulder
- ● **C44.62**   Squamous cell carcinoma of skin of upper limb, including shoulder
  - **C44.621**   Squamous cell carcinoma of skin of unspecified upper limb, including shoulder
  - **C44.622**   Squamous cell carcinoma of skin of right upper limb, including shoulder
  - **C44.629**   Squamous cell carcinoma of skin of left upper limb, including shoulder
- ● **C44.69**   Other specified malignant neoplasm of skin of upper limb, including shoulder
  - **C44.691**   Other specified malignant neoplasm of skin of unspecified upper limb, including shoulder
  - **C44.692**   Other specified malignant neoplasm of skin of right upper limb, including shoulder
  - **C44.699**   Other specified malignant neoplasm of skin of left upper limb, including shoulder

● **C44.7**   **Other and unspecified malignant neoplasm of skin of lower limb, including hip**
  ● **C44.70**   Unspecified malignant neoplasm of skin of lower limb, including hip
     C44.701   Unspecified malignant neoplasm of skin of unspecified lower limb, including hip
     C44.702   Unspecified malignant neoplasm of skin of right lower limb, including hip
     C44.709   Unspecified malignant neoplasm of skin of left lower limb, including hip
  ● **C44.71**   Basal cell carcinoma of skin of lower limb, including hip
     C44.711   Basal cell carcinoma of skin of unspecified lower limb, including hip
     C44.712   Basal cell carcinoma of skin of right lower limb, including hip
     C44.719   Basal cell carcinoma of skin of left lower limb, including hip
  ● **C44.72**   Squamous cell carcinoma of skin of lower limb, including hip
     C44.721   Squamous cell carcinoma of skin of unspecified lower limb, including hip
     C44.722   Squamous cell carcinoma of skin of right lower limb, including hip
     C44.729   Squamous cell carcinoma of skin of left lower limb, including hip
  ● **C44.79**   Other specified malignant neoplasm of skin of lower limb, including hip
     C44.791   Other specified malignant neoplasm of skin of unspecified lower limb, including hip
     C44.792   Other specified malignant neoplasm of skin of right lower limb, including hip
     C44.799   Other specified malignant neoplasm of skin of left lower limb, including hip
● **C44.8**   **Other and unspecified malignant neoplasm of overlapping sites of skin**
   C44.80   Unspecified malignant neoplasm of overlapping sites of skin
   C44.81   Basal cell carcinoma of overlapping sites of skin
   C44.82   Squamous cell carcinoma of overlapping sites of skin
   C44.89   Other specified malignant neoplasm of overlapping sites of skin
● **C44.9**   **Other and unspecified malignant neoplasm of skin, unspecified**
   C44.90   Unspecified malignant neoplasm of skin, unspecified
     Malignant neoplasm of unspecified site of skin
   C44.91   Basal cell carcinoma of skin, unspecified
   C44.92   Squamous cell carcinoma of skin, unspecified
   C44.99   Other specified malignant neoplasm of skin, unspecified

MALIGNANT NEOPLASMS OF MESOTHELIAL AND SOFT TISSUE (C45-C49)

● **C45**   **Mesothelioma**
   Malignant cells develop in protective lining that covers internal organs (mesothelium) caused by exposure to asbestos
   C45.0   **Mesothelioma of pleura**
     Excludes1   other malignant neoplasm of pleura (C38.4)
   C45.1   **Mesothelioma of peritoneum**
     Mesothelioma of cul-de-sac
     Mesothelioma of mesentery
     Mesothelioma of mesocolon
     Mesothelioma of omentum
     Mesothelioma of peritoneum (parietal) (pelvic)
     Excludes1   other malignant neoplasm of soft tissue of peritoneum (C48.-)
   C45.2   **Mesothelioma of pericardium**
     Excludes1   other malignant neoplasm of pericardium (C38.0)
   C45.7   **Mesothelioma of other sites**
   C45.9   **Mesothelioma, unspecified**

● **C46**   **Kaposi's sarcoma**
   Code first any human immunodeficiency virus [HIV] disease (B20)
   C46.0   **Kaposi's sarcoma of skin**
   C46.1   **Kaposi's sarcoma of soft tissue**
     Kaposi's sarcoma of blood vessel
     Kaposi's sarcoma of connective tissue
     Kaposi's sarcoma of fascia
     Kaposi's sarcoma of ligament
     Kaposi's sarcoma of lymphatic(s) NEC
     Kaposi's sarcoma of muscle
     Excludes2   Kaposi's sarcoma of lymph glands and nodes (C46.3)
   C46.2   **Kaposi's sarcoma of palate**
   C46.3   **Kaposi's sarcoma of lymph nodes**
   C46.4   **Kaposi's sarcoma of gastrointestinal sites**
  ● **C46.5**   **Kaposi's sarcoma of lung**
     C46.50   Kaposi's sarcoma of unspecified lung
     C46.51   Kaposi's sarcoma of right lung
     C46.52   Kaposi's sarcoma of left lung
   C46.7   **Kaposi's sarcoma of other sites**
   C46.9   **Kaposi's sarcoma, unspecified**
     Kaposi's sarcoma of unspecified site

Figure 2-11   Kaposi's sarcoma. There are large confluent hyperpigmented patch-stage lesions with lymphedema. (From Goldman L, Ausiello D, Arend W, Armitage J, Clemmons D, Drazen J, Griggs R, et al: Cecil Medicine: Expert Consult, 23e, Saunders, 2007)

Item 2–5   Kaposi's sarcoma is a cancer that causes patches of abnormal tissue to grow under the skin; in the lining of the mouth, nose, and throat; or in other organs, often beginning and spreading to other organs. Patients who have had organ transplants or patients with AIDS are at high risk for this malignancy.

● **C47**   **Malignant neoplasm of peripheral nerves and autonomic nervous system**

> **Includes**   malignant neoplasm of sympathetic and parasympathetic nerves and ganglia

> **Excludes1**   Kaposi's sarcoma of soft tissue (C46.1)

C47.0   **Malignant neoplasm of peripheral nerves of head, face and neck**

> **Excludes1**   malignant neoplasm of peripheral nerves of orbit (C69.6-)

● **C47.1**   **Malignant neoplasm of peripheral nerves of upper limb, including shoulder**

     C47.10   **Malignant neoplasm of peripheral nerves of unspecified upper limb, including shoulder**

     C47.11   **Malignant neoplasm of peripheral nerves of right upper limb, including shoulder**

     C47.12   **Malignant neoplasm of peripheral nerves of left upper limb, including shoulder**

● **C47.2**   **Malignant neoplasm of peripheral nerves of lower limb, including hip**

     C47.20   **Malignant neoplasm of peripheral nerves of unspecified lower limb, including hip**

     C47.21   **Malignant neoplasm of peripheral nerves of right lower limb, including hip**

     C47.22   **Malignant neoplasm of peripheral nerves of left lower limb, including hip**

C47.3   **Malignant neoplasm of peripheral nerves of thorax**

C47.4   **Malignant neoplasm of peripheral nerves of abdomen**

C47.5   **Malignant neoplasm of peripheral nerves of pelvis**

C47.6   **Malignant neoplasm of peripheral nerves of trunk, unspecified**

> Malignant neoplasm of peripheral nerves of unspecified part of trunk

C47.8   **Malignant neoplasm of overlapping sites of peripheral nerves and autonomic nervous system**

C47.9   **Malignant neoplasm of peripheral nerves and autonomic nervous system, unspecified**

> Malignant neoplasm of unspecified site of peripheral nerves and autonomic nervous system

● **C48**   **Malignant neoplasm of retroperitoneum and peritoneum**

> **Excludes1**   Kaposi's sarcoma of connective tissue (C46.1)
> mesothelioma (C45.-)

C48.0   **Malignant neoplasm of retroperitoneum**

> *Behind/outside of peritoneum*

C48.1   **Malignant neoplasm of specified parts of peritoneum**

> *Serous membrane lining abdominopelvic walls and covering viscera*
> Malignant neoplasm of cul-de-sac
> Malignant neoplasm of mesentery
> Malignant neoplasm of mesocolon
> Malignant neoplasm of omentum
> Malignant neoplasm of parietal peritoneum
> Malignant neoplasm of pelvic peritoneum

C48.2   **Malignant neoplasm of peritoneum, unspecified**

C48.8   **Malignant neoplasm of overlapping sites of retroperitoneum and peritoneum**

● **C49**   **Malignant neoplasm of other connective and soft tissue**

> **Includes**   malignant neoplasm of blood vessel
> malignant neoplasm of bursa
> malignant neoplasm of cartilage
> malignant neoplasm of fascia
> malignant neoplasm of fat
> malignant neoplasm of ligament, except uterine
> malignant neoplasm of lymphatic vessel
> malignant neoplasm of muscle
> malignant neoplasm of synovia
> malignant neoplasm of tendon (sheath)

> **Excludes1**   malignant neoplasm of cartilage (of):
> articular (C40-C41)
> larynx (C32.3)
> nose (C30.0)
> malignant neoplasm of connective tissue of breast (C50.-)

> **Excludes2**   Kaposi's sarcoma of soft tissue (C46.1)
> malignant neoplasm of heart (C38.0)
> malignant neoplasm of peripheral nerves and autonomic nervous system (C47.-)
> malignant neoplasm of peritoneum (C48.2)
> malignant neoplasm of retroperitoneum (C48.0)
> malignant neoplasm of uterine ligament (C57.3)
> mesothelioma (C45.-)

C49.0   **Malignant neoplasm of connective and soft tissue of head, face and neck**

> Malignant neoplasm of connective tissue of ear
> Malignant neoplasm of connective tissue of eyelid

> **Excludes1**   connective tissue of orbit (C69.6-)

● **C49.1**   **Malignant neoplasm of connective and soft tissue of upper limb, including shoulder**

     C49.10   **Malignant neoplasm of connective and soft tissue of unspecified upper limb, including shoulder**

     C49.11   **Malignant neoplasm of connective and soft tissue of right upper limb, including shoulder**

     C49.12   **Malignant neoplasm of connective and soft tissue of left upper limb, including shoulder**

● **C49.2**   **Malignant neoplasm of connective and soft tissue of lower limb, including hip**

     C49.20   **Malignant neoplasm of connective and soft tissue of unspecified lower limb, including hip**

     C49.21   **Malignant neoplasm of connective and soft tissue of right lower limb, including hip**

     C49.22   **Malignant neoplasm of connective and soft tissue of left lower limb, including hip**

C49.3   **Malignant neoplasm of connective and soft tissue of thorax**

> Malignant neoplasm of axilla
> Malignant neoplasm of diaphragm
> Malignant neoplasm of great vessels

> **Excludes1**   malignant neoplasm of breast (C50.-)
> malignant neoplasm of heart (C38.0)
> malignant neoplasm of mediastinum (C38.1-C38.3)
> malignant neoplasm of thymus (C37)

C49.4   **Malignant neoplasm of connective and soft tissue of abdomen**

> Malignant neoplasm of abdominal wall
> Malignant neoplasm of hypochondrium

C49.5   **Malignant neoplasm of connective and soft tissue of pelvis**

> Malignant neoplasm of buttock
> Malignant neoplasm of groin
> Malignant neoplasm of perineum

▶ New   ⇒ Revised   ~~deleted~~ Deleted   **OGCR** Official Guidelines   X Assign placeholder X   ● Use Additional Character(s)

Excludes 1   Excludes 2   Includes   Use additional   Code first   Code also   Key words

C49.6   **Malignant neoplasm of connective and soft tissue of trunk, unspecified**
       Malignant neoplasm of back NOS

C49.8   **Malignant neoplasm of overlapping sites of connective and soft tissue**
       Primary malignant neoplasm of two or more contiguous sites of connective and soft tissue

C49.9   **Malignant neoplasm of connective and soft tissue, unspecified**

● C49.A   **Gastrointestinal stromal tumor**

      C49.A0   Gastrointestinal stromal tumor, **unspecified** site

      C49.A1   Gastrointestinal stromal tumor of **esophagus**

      C49.A2   Gastrointestinal stromal tumor of **stomach**

      C49.A3   Gastrointestinal stromal tumor of **small intestine**

      C49.A4   Gastrointestinal stromal tumor of **large intestine**

      C49.A5   Gastrointestinal stromal tumor of **rectum**

      C49.A9   Gastrointestinal stromal tumor of **other sites**

MALIGNANT NEOPLASMS OF BREAST (C50)

● C50   **Malignant neoplasm of breast**

     Includes   connective tissue of breast
                Paget's disease of breast
                Paget's disease of nipple
                Intraductal carcinoma of breast characterized by eczema-like inflammatory skin changes

     Use additional code to identify estrogen receptor status (Z17.0, Z17.1)

     Excludes1   skin of breast (C44.501, C44.511, C44.521, C44.591)

   ● C50.0   **Malignant neoplasm of nipple and areola**

     ● C50.01   Malignant neoplasm of nipple and areola, **female**

         C50.011   Malignant neoplasm of nipple and areola, **right** female breast

         C50.012   Malignant neoplasm of nipple and areola, **left** female breast

         C50.019   Malignant neoplasm of nipple and areola, **unspecified** female breast

     ● C50.02   Malignant neoplasm of nipple and areola, **male**

         C50.021   Malignant neoplasm of nipple and areola, **right** male breast

         C50.022   Malignant neoplasm of nipple and areola, **left** male breast

         C50.029   Malignant neoplasm of nipple and areola, **unspecified** male breast

   ● C50.1   **Malignant neoplasm of central portion of breast**

     ● C50.11   Malignant neoplasm of central portion of breast, **female**

         C50.111   Malignant neoplasm of central portion of **right** female breast

         C50.112   Malignant neoplasm of central portion of **left** female breast

         C50.119   Malignant neoplasm of central portion of **unspecified** female breast

     ● C50.12   Malignant neoplasm of central portion of breast, **male**

         C50.121   Malignant neoplasm of central portion of **right** male breast

         C50.122   Malignant neoplasm of central portion of **left** male breast

         C50.129   Malignant neoplasm of central portion of **unspecified** male breast

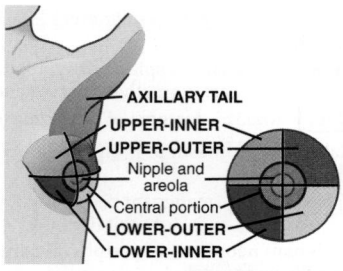

Figure 2-12   Female breast quadrants and axillary tail.

   ● C50.2   **Malignant neoplasm of upper-inner quadrant of breast**

     ● C50.21   Malignant neoplasm of upper-inner quadrant of breast, **female**

         C50.211   Malignant neoplasm of upper-inner quadrant of **right** female breast

         C50.212   Malignant neoplasm of upper-inner quadrant of **left** female breast

         C50.219   Malignant neoplasm of upper-inner quadrant of **unspecified** female breast

     ● C50.22   Malignant neoplasm of upper-inner quadrant of breast, **male**

         C50.221   Malignant neoplasm of upper-inner quadrant of **right** male breast

         C50.222   Malignant neoplasm of upper-inner quadrant of **left** male breast

         C50.229   Malignant neoplasm of upper-inner quadrant of **unspecified** male breast

   ● C50.3   **Malignant neoplasm of lower-inner quadrant of breast**

     ● C50.31   Malignant neoplasm of lower-inner quadrant of breast, **female**

         C50.311   Malignant neoplasm of lower-inner quadrant of **right** female breast

         C50.312   Malignant neoplasm of lower-inner quadrant of **left** female breast

         C50.319   Malignant neoplasm of lower-inner quadrant of **unspecified** female breast

     ● C50.32   Malignant neoplasm of lower-inner quadrant of breast, **male**

         C50.321   Malignant neoplasm of lower-inner quadrant of **right** male breast

         C50.322   Malignant neoplasm of lower-inner quadrant of **left** male breast

         C50.329   Malignant neoplasm of lower-inner quadrant of **unspecified** male breast

   ● C50.4   **Malignant neoplasm of upper-outer quadrant of breast**

     ● C50.41   Malignant neoplasm of upper-outer quadrant of breast, **female**

         C50.411   Malignant neoplasm of upper-outer quadrant of **right** female breast

         C50.412   Malignant neoplasm of upper-outer quadrant of **left** female breast

         C50.419   Malignant neoplasm of upper-outer quadrant of **unspecified** female breast

     ● C50.42   Malignant neoplasm of upper-outer quadrant of breast, **male**

         C50.421   Malignant neoplasm of upper-outer quadrant of **right** male breast

         C50.422   Malignant neoplasm of upper-outer quadrant of **left** male breast

         C50.429   Malignant neoplasm of upper-outer quadrant of **unspecified** male breast

● **C50.5   Malignant neoplasm of lower-outer quadrant of breast**
  ● **C50.51   Malignant neoplasm of lower-outer quadrant of breast, female**
       C50.511   Malignant neoplasm of lower-outer quadrant of right female breast
       C50.512   Malignant neoplasm of lower-outer quadrant of left female breast
       C50.519   Malignant neoplasm of lower-outer quadrant of unspecified female breast
  ● **C50.52   Malignant neoplasm of lower-outer quadrant of breast, male**
       C50.521   Malignant neoplasm of lower-outer quadrant of right male breast
       C50.522   Malignant neoplasm of lower-outer quadrant of left male breast
       C50.529   Malignant neoplasm of lower-outer quadrant of unspecified male breast
● **C50.6   Malignant neoplasm of axillary tail of breast**
  ● **C50.61   Malignant neoplasm of axillary tail of breast, female**
       C50.611   Malignant neoplasm of axillary tail of right female breast
       C50.612   Malignant neoplasm of axillary tail of left female breast
       C50.619   Malignant neoplasm of axillary tail of unspecified female breast
  ● **C50.62   Malignant neoplasm of axillary tail of breast, male**
       C50.621   Malignant neoplasm of axillary tail of right male breast
       C50.622   Malignant neoplasm of axillary tail of left male breast
       C50.629   Malignant neoplasm of axillary tail of unspecified male breast
● **C50.8   Malignant neoplasm of overlapping sites of breast**
  ● **C50.81   Malignant neoplasm of overlapping sites of breast, female**
       C50.811   Malignant neoplasm of overlapping sites of right female breast
       C50.812   Malignant neoplasm of overlapping sites of left female breast
       C50.819   Malignant neoplasm of overlapping sites of unspecified female breast
  ● **C50.82   Malignant neoplasm of overlapping sites of breast, male**
       C50.821   Malignant neoplasm of overlapping sites of right male breast
       C50.822   Malignant neoplasm of overlapping sites of left male breast
       C50.829   Malignant neoplasm of overlapping sites of unspecified male breast
● **C50.9   Malignant neoplasm of breast of unspecified site**
  ● **C50.91   Malignant neoplasm of breast of unspecified site, female**
       C50.911   Malignant neoplasm of unspecified site of right female breast
       C50.912   Malignant neoplasm of unspecified site of left female breast
       C50.919   Malignant neoplasm of unspecified site of unspecified female breast
  ● **C50.92   Malignant neoplasm of breast of unspecified site, male**
       C50.921   Malignant neoplasm of unspecified site of right male breast
       C50.922   Malignant neoplasm of unspecified site of left male breast
       C50.929   Malignant neoplasm of unspecified site of unspecified male breast

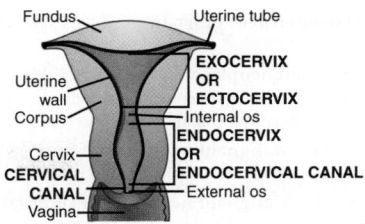

Figure 2-13   Cervix uteri.

MALIGNANT NEOPLASMS OF FEMALE GENITAL ORGANS (C51-C58)

  Includes   malignant neoplasm of skin of female genital organs

● **C51   Malignant neoplasm of vulva**
      Excludes1   carcinoma in situ of vulva (D07.1)
   C51.0   Malignant neoplasm of labium majus
            Outer folds of skin external female genitalia
            Malignant neoplasm of Bartholin's [greater vestibular] gland
   C51.1   Malignant neoplasm of labium minus
            Two inner folds surrounding vulva in female genitalia
   C51.2   Malignant neoplasm of clitoris
   C51.8   Malignant neoplasm of overlapping sites of vulva
   C51.9   Malignant neoplasm of vulva, unspecified
            Malignant neoplasm of external female genitalia NOS
            Malignant neoplasm of pudendum

  C52   Malignant neoplasm of vagina
      Excludes1   carcinoma in situ of vagina (D07.2)

● **C53   Malignant neoplasm of cervix uteri**
      Excludes1   carcinoma in situ of cervix uteri (D06.-)
   C53.0   Malignant neoplasm of endocervix
            Inside the cervix
   C53.1   Malignant neoplasm of exocervix
            Outside the cervix
   C53.8   Malignant neoplasm of overlapping sites of cervix uteri
   C53.9   Malignant neoplasm of cervix uteri, unspecified

● **C54   Malignant neoplasm of corpus uteri**
   C54.0   Malignant neoplasm of isthmus uteri
            Constricted part of uterus between cervix and body
            Malignant neoplasm of lower uterine segment
   C54.1   Malignant neoplasm of endometrium
            Lining of uterus
   C54.2   Malignant neoplasm of myometrium
            Middle layer of uterine wall consisting of smooth muscle supporting stromal and vascular tissue
   C54.3   Malignant neoplasm of fundus uteri
            Top rounded portion of uterus
   C54.8   Malignant neoplasm of overlapping sites of corpus uteri
            Main body of uterus
   C54.9   Malignant neoplasm of corpus uteri, unspecified

  C55   Malignant neoplasm of uterus, part unspecified

● **C56   Malignant neoplasm of ovary**
      Use additional code to identify any functional activity
   C56.1   Malignant neoplasm of right ovary
   C56.2   Malignant neoplasm of left ovary
   C56.9   Malignant neoplasm of unspecified ovary

▶ New   ⇒ Revised   ~~deleted~~ Deleted   **OGCR** Official Guidelines   X Assign placeholder X   ● Use Additional Character(s)

| Excludes 1 | Excludes 2 | Includes | Use additional | Code first | Code also | Key words |

CHAPTER 2 (C00-D49)

● **C57**   **Malignant neoplasm of other and unspecified female genital organs**

   ● **C57.0**   **Malignant neoplasm of fallopian tube**
         Malignant neoplasm of oviduct
         Malignant neoplasm of uterine tube

      C57.00   Malignant neoplasm of unspecified fallopian tube

      C57.01   Malignant neoplasm of right fallopian tube

      C57.02   Malignant neoplasm of left fallopian tube

   ● **C57.1**   **Malignant neoplasm of broad ligament**

      C57.10   Malignant neoplasm of unspecified broad ligament

      C57.11   Malignant neoplasm of right broad ligament

      C57.12   Malignant neoplasm of left broad ligament

   ● **C57.2**   **Malignant neoplasm of round ligament**

      C57.20   Malignant neoplasm of unspecified round ligament

      C57.21   Malignant neoplasm of right round ligament

      C57.22   Malignant neoplasm of left round ligament

   C57.3   **Malignant neoplasm of parametrium**
        Malignant neoplasm of uterine ligament NOS

   C57.4   **Malignant neoplasm of uterine adnexa, unspecified**

   C57.7   **Malignant neoplasm of other specified female genital organs**
        Malignant neoplasm of wolffian body or duct

   C57.8   **Malignant neoplasm of overlapping sites of female genital organs**
        Primary malignant neoplasm of two or more contiguous sites of the female genital organs whose point of origin cannot be determined
        Primary tubo-ovarian malignant neoplasm whose point of origin cannot be determined
        Primary utero-ovarian malignant neoplasm whose point of origin cannot be determined

   C57.9   **Malignant neoplasm of female genital organ, unspecified**
        Malignant neoplasm of female genitourinary tract NOS

C58   **Malignant neoplasm of placenta**
   | **Includes** | choriocarcinoma NOS |
                 chorionepithelioma NOS
   | **Excludes1** | chorioadenoma (destruens) (D39.2) |
                 hydatidiform mole NOS (O01.9)
                 invasive hydatidiform mole (D39.2)
                 male choriocarcinoma NOS (C62.9-)
                 malignant hydatidiform mole (D39.2)

MALIGNANT NEOPLASMS OF MALE GENITAL ORGANS (C60-C63)

   | **Includes** | malignant neoplasm of skin of male genital organs |

● **C60**   **Malignant neoplasm of penis**

   C60.0   **Malignant neoplasm of prepuce**
        Malignant neoplasm of foreskin

   C60.1   **Malignant neoplasm of glans penis**

   C60.2   **Malignant neoplasm of body of penis**
        Malignant neoplasm of corpus cavernosum

   C60.8   **Malignant neoplasm of overlapping sites of penis**

   C60.9   **Malignant neoplasm of penis, unspecified**
        Malignant neoplasm of skin of penis NOS

C61   **Malignant neoplasm of prostate**
   Use additional code to identify:
     hormone sensitivity status (Z19.1-Z19.2)
     rising PSA following treatment for malignant neoplasm of prostate (R97.21)
   | **Excludes1** | malignant neoplasm of seminal vesicle (C63.7) |

Figure 2-14   Penis and other male genital organs.

● **C62**   **Malignant neoplasm of testis**
   Use additional code to identify any functional activity.

   ● **C62.0**   **Malignant neoplasm of undescended testis**
        Malignant neoplasm of ectopic testis
        Malignant neoplasm of retained testis

      C62.00   Malignant neoplasm of unspecified undescended testis

      C62.01   Malignant neoplasm of undescended right testis

      C62.02   Malignant neoplasm of undescended left testis

   ● **C62.1**   **Malignant neoplasm of descended testis**
        Malignant neoplasm of scrotal testis

      C62.10   Malignant neoplasm of unspecified descended testis, unspecified side

      C62.11   Malignant neoplasm of descended right testis

      C62.12   Malignant neoplasm of descended left testis

   ● **C62.9**   **Malignant neoplasm of testis, unspecified whether descended or undescended**

      C62.90   Malignant neoplasm of unspecified testis, unspecified whether descended or undescended
           Malignant neoplasm of testis NOS

      C62.91   Malignant neoplasm of right testis, unspecified whether descended or undescended

      C62.92   Malignant neoplasm of left testis, unspecified whether descended or undescended

● **C63**   **Malignant neoplasm of other and unspecified male genital organs**

   ● **C63.0**   **Malignant neoplasm of epididymis**

      C63.00   Malignant neoplasm of unspecified epididymis

      C63.01   Malignant neoplasm of right epididymis

      C63.02   Malignant neoplasm of left epididymis

   ● **C63.1**   **Malignant neoplasm of spermatic cord**

      C63.10   Malignant neoplasm of unspecified spermatic cord

      C63.11   Malignant neoplasm of right spermatic cord

      C63.12   Malignant neoplasm of left spermatic cord

   C63.2   **Malignant neoplasm of scrotum**
        Malignant neoplasm of skin of scrotum

   C63.7   **Malignant neoplasm of other specified male genital organs**
        Malignant neoplasm of seminal vesicle
        Malignant neoplasm of tunica vaginalis

   C63.8   **Malignant neoplasm of overlapping sites of male genital organs**
        Primary malignant neoplasm of two or more contiguous sites of male genital organs whose point of origin cannot be determined

   C63.9   **Malignant neoplasm of male genital organ, unspecified**
        Malignant neoplasm of male genitourinary tract NOS

▶ New   ➡ Revised   ~~deleted~~ Deleted   **OGCR** Official Guidelines   X Assign placeholder X   ● Use Additional Character(s)

| Excludes 1 | Excludes 2 | Includes | Use additional | Code first | Code also | Key words |

MALIGNANT NEOPLASMS OF URINARY TRACT (C64-C68)

● **C64** Malignant neoplasm of kidney, except renal pelvis

     Excludes1   malignant carcinoid tumor of the kidney (C7A.093)

             malignant neoplasm of renal calyces (C65.-)

             malignant neoplasm of renal pelvis (C65.-)

   C64.1   Malignant neoplasm of right kidney, except renal pelvis

   C64.2   Malignant neoplasm of left kidney, except renal pelvis

   C64.9   Malignant neoplasm of unspecified kidney, except renal pelvis

● **C65** Malignant neoplasm of renal pelvis

     Includes   malignant neoplasm of pelviureteric junction

             malignant neoplasm of renal calyces

   C65.1   Malignant neoplasm of right renal pelvis

   C65.2   Malignant neoplasm of left renal pelvis

   C65.9   Malignant neoplasm of unspecified renal pelvis

● **C66** Malignant neoplasm of ureter

     Excludes1   malignant neoplasm of ureteric orifice of bladder (C67.6)

   C66.1   Malignant neoplasm of right ureter

   C66.2   Malignant neoplasm of left ureter

   C66.9   Malignant neoplasm of unspecified ureter

● **C67** Malignant neoplasm of bladder

   C67.0   Malignant neoplasm of trigone of bladder
        Triangular area formed by three openings in the floor of urinary bladder

   C67.1   Malignant neoplasm of dome of bladder
        Vaulted roof

   C67.2   Malignant neoplasm of lateral wall of bladder
        Side walls

   C67.3   Malignant neoplasm of anterior wall of bladder
        Front wall

   C67.4   Malignant neoplasm of posterior wall of bladder
        Back wall

   C67.5   Malignant neoplasm of bladder neck
        Joining of bladder and urethra
        Malignant neoplasm of internal urethral orifice

   C67.6   Malignant neoplasm of ureteric orifice
        Opening from bladder to ureters

   C67.7   Malignant neoplasm of urachus
        Embryonic canal that connects the urinary bladder with the structure that forms the umbilical cord (allantois)

   C67.8   Malignant neoplasm of overlapping sites of bladder

   C67.9   Malignant neoplasm of bladder, unspecified

● **C68** Malignant neoplasm of other and unspecified urinary organs

     Excludes1   malignant neoplasm of female genitourinary tract NOS (C57.9)

             malignant neoplasm of male genitourinary tract NOS (C63.9)

   C68.0   Malignant neoplasm of urethra

       Excludes1   malignant neoplasm of urethral orifice of bladder (C67.5)

   C68.1   Malignant neoplasm of paraurethral glands
        Group of glands of female urethra drained by paraurethral ducts; AKA Skene glands, female prostate

   C68.8   Malignant neoplasm of overlapping sites of urinary organs
        Primary malignant neoplasm of two or more contiguous sites of urinary organs whose point of origin cannot be determined

   C68.9   Malignant neoplasm of urinary organ, unspecified
        Malignant neoplasm of urinary system NOS

MALIGNANT NEOPLASMS OF EYE, BRAIN AND OTHER PARTS OF CENTRAL NERVOUS SYSTEM (C69-C72)

● **C69** Malignant neoplasm of eye and adnexa

     Excludes1   malignant neoplasm of connective tissue of eyelid (C49.0)

             malignant neoplasm of eyelid (skin) (C43.1-, C44.1-)

             malignant neoplasm of optic nerve (C72.3-)

● C69.0   Malignant neoplasm of conjunctiva

   C69.00   Malignant neoplasm of unspecified conjunctiva

   C69.01   Malignant neoplasm of right conjunctiva

   C69.02   Malignant neoplasm of left conjunctiva

● C69.1   Malignant neoplasm of cornea

   C69.10   Malignant neoplasm of unspecified cornea

   C69.11   Malignant neoplasm of right cornea

   C69.12   Malignant neoplasm of left cornea

● C69.2   Malignant neoplasm of retina

     Excludes1   dark area on retina (D49.81)

             neoplasm of unspecified behavior of retina and choroid (D49.81)

             retinal freckle (D49.81)

   C69.20   Malignant neoplasm of unspecified retina

   C69.21   Malignant neoplasm of right retina

   C69.22   Malignant neoplasm of left retina

● C69.3   Malignant neoplasm of choroid

   C69.30   Malignant neoplasm of unspecified choroid

   C69.31   Malignant neoplasm of right choroid

   C69.32   Malignant neoplasm of left choroid

● C69.4   Malignant neoplasm of ciliary body

   C69.40   Malignant neoplasm of unspecified ciliary body

   C69.41   Malignant neoplasm of right ciliary body

   C69.42   Malignant neoplasm of left ciliary body

● C69.5   Malignant neoplasm of lacrimal gland and duct
        Malignant neoplasm of lacrimal sac
        Malignant neoplasm of nasolacrimal duct

   C69.50   Malignant neoplasm of unspecified lacrimal gland and duct

   C69.51   Malignant neoplasm of right lacrimal gland and duct

   C69.52   Malignant neoplasm of left lacrimal gland and duct

● C69.6   Malignant neoplasm of orbit
        Malignant neoplasm of connective tissue of orbit
        Malignant neoplasm of extraocular muscle
        Malignant neoplasm of peripheral nerves of orbit
        Malignant neoplasm of retrobulbar tissue
        Malignant neoplasm of retro-ocular tissue

     Excludes1   malignant neoplasm of orbital bone (C41.0)

   C69.60   Malignant neoplasm of unspecified orbit

   C69.61   Malignant neoplasm of right orbit

   C69.62   Malignant neoplasm of left orbit

● C69.8   Malignant neoplasm of overlapping sites of eye and adnexa

   C69.80   Malignant neoplasm of overlapping sites of unspecified eye and adnexa

   C69.81   Malignant neoplasm of overlapping sites of right eye and adnexa

   C69.82   Malignant neoplasm of overlapping sites of left eye and adnexa

● C69.9   Malignant neoplasm of unspecified site of eye
        Malignant neoplasm of eyeball

   C69.90   Malignant neoplasm of unspecified site of unspecified eye

   C69.91   Malignant neoplasm of unspecified site of right eye

   C69.92   Malignant neoplasm of unspecified site of left eye

CHAPTER 2 (C00-D49)

▶ New   ⟹ Revised   ~~deleted~~ Deleted   **OGCR** Official Guidelines   **X** Assign placeholder X   ● Use Additional Character(s)

 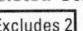

Excludes 1   Excludes 2   Includes   Use additional   Code first   Code also   Key words

Figure 2-15 The brain.

● **C70** Malignant neoplasm of meninges
- **C70.0** Malignant neoplasm of cerebral meninges
- **C70.1** Malignant neoplasm of spinal meninges
- **C70.9** Malignant neoplasm of meninges, unspecified

● **C71** Malignant neoplasm of brain
> **Excludes1** malignant neoplasm of cranial nerves (C72.2-C72.5)
> retrobulbar malignant neoplasm (C69.6-)

- **C71.0** Malignant neoplasm of cerebrum, except lobes and ventricles
  Malignant neoplasm of supratentorial NOS
- **C71.1** Malignant neoplasm of frontal lobe
- **C71.2** Malignant neoplasm of temporal lobe
- **C71.3** Malignant neoplasm of parietal lobe
- **C71.4** Malignant neoplasm of occipital lobe
- **C71.5** Malignant neoplasm of cerebral ventricle
  > **Excludes1** malignant neoplasm of fourth cerebral ventricle (C71.7)
- **C71.6** Malignant neoplasm of cerebellum
- **C71.7** Malignant neoplasm of brain stem
  Malignant neoplasm of fourth cerebral ventricle
  Infratentorial malignant neoplasm NOS
- **C71.8** Malignant neoplasm of overlapping sites of brain
- **C71.9** Malignant neoplasm of brain, unspecified

● **C72** Malignant neoplasm of spinal cord, cranial nerves and other parts of central nervous system
> **Excludes1** malignant neoplasm of meninges (C70.-)
> malignant neoplasm of peripheral nerves and autonomic nervous system (C47.-)

- **C72.0** Malignant neoplasm of spinal cord
- **C72.1** Malignant neoplasm of cauda equina
  Lower end of spinal column
- ● **C72.2** Malignant neoplasm of olfactory nerve
  Malignant neoplasm of olfactory bulb
  - **C72.20** Malignant neoplasm of unspecified olfactory nerve
  - **C72.21** Malignant neoplasm of right olfactory nerve
  - **C72.22** Malignant neoplasm of left olfactory nerve
- ● **C72.3** Malignant neoplasm of optic nerve
  - **C72.30** Malignant neoplasm of unspecified optic nerve
  - **C72.31** Malignant neoplasm of right optic nerve
  - **C72.32** Malignant neoplasm of left optic nerve
- ● **C72.4** Malignant neoplasm of acoustic nerve
  - **C72.40** Malignant neoplasm of unspecified acoustic nerve
  - **C72.41** Malignant neoplasm of right acoustic nerve
  - **C72.42** Malignant neoplasm of left acoustic nerve

● **C72.5** Malignant neoplasm of other and unspecified cranial nerves
- **C72.50** Malignant neoplasm of unspecified cranial nerve
  Malignant neoplasm of cranial nerve NOS
- **C72.59** Malignant neoplasm of other cranial nerves
- **C72.9** Malignant neoplasm of central nervous system, unspecified
  Malignant neoplasm of unspecified site of central nervous system
  Malignant neoplasm of nervous system NOS

MALIGNANT NEOPLASMS OF THYROID AND OTHER ENDOCRINE GLANDS (C73-C75)

C73 Malignant neoplasm of thyroid gland
Use additional code to identify any functional activity

● **C74** Malignant neoplasm of adrenal gland
- ● **C74.0** Malignant neoplasm of cortex of adrenal gland
  - **C74.00** Malignant neoplasm of cortex of unspecified adrenal gland
  - **C74.01** Malignant neoplasm of cortex of right adrenal gland
  - **C74.02** Malignant neoplasm of cortex of left adrenal gland
- ● **C74.1** Malignant neoplasm of medulla of adrenal gland
  Pair of glands situated on top of or above each kidney ("suprarenal")
  - **C74.10** Malignant neoplasm of medulla of unspecified adrenal gland
  - **C74.11** Malignant neoplasm of medulla of right adrenal gland
  - **C74.12** Malignant neoplasm of medulla of left adrenal gland
- ● **C74.9** Malignant neoplasm of unspecified part of adrenal gland
  - **C74.90** Malignant neoplasm of unspecified part of unspecified adrenal gland
  - **C74.91** Malignant neoplasm of unspecified part of right adrenal gland
  - **C74.92** Malignant neoplasm of unspecified part of left adrenal gland

● **C75** Malignant neoplasm of other endocrine glands and related structures
> **Excludes1** malignant carcinoid tumors (C7A.0-)
> malignant neoplasm of adrenal gland (C74.-)
> malignant neoplasm of endocrine pancreas (C25.4)
> malignant neoplasm of islets of Langerhans (C25.4)
> malignant neoplasm of ovary (C56.-)
> malignant neoplasm of testis (C62.-)
> malignant neoplasm of thymus (C37)
> malignant neoplasm of thyroid gland (C73)
> malignant neuroendocrine tumors (C7A.-)

- **C75.0** Malignant neoplasm of parathyroid gland
- **C75.1** Malignant neoplasm of pituitary gland
- **C75.2** Malignant neoplasm of craniopharyngeal duct
- **C75.3** Malignant neoplasm of pineal gland
- **C75.4** Malignant neoplasm of carotid body
- **C75.5** Malignant neoplasm of aortic body and other paraganglia
- **C75.8** Malignant neoplasm with pluriglandular involvement, unspecified
- **C75.9** Malignant neoplasm of endocrine gland, unspecified

▶ New   ⇒ Revised   ~~deleted~~ Deleted   **OGCR** Official Guidelines   **X** Assign placeholder X   ● Use Additional Character(s)

Excludes 1   Excludes 2   Includes   Use additional   Code first   Code also   Key words

CHAPTER 2 (C00-D49)

MALIGNANT NEUROENDOCRINE TUMORS (C7A)

● **C7A**   Malignant neuroendocrine tumors

Code also any associated multiple endocrine neoplasia [MEN] syndromes (E31.2-)

Use additional code to identify any associated endocrine syndrome, such as:
carcinoid syndrome (E34.0)

> **Excludes2**   malignant pancreatic islet cell tumors (C25.4)
> Merkel cell carcinoma (C4A.-)

● **C7A.0**   Malignant carcinoid tumors

C7A.00   Malignant carcinoid tumor of unspecified site

● **C7A.01**   Malignant carcinoid tumors of the small intestine

C7A.010   Malignant carcinoid tumor of the duodenum

C7A.011   Malignant carcinoid tumor of the jejunum

C7A.012   Malignant carcinoid tumor of the ileum

C7A.019   Malignant carcinoid tumor of the small intestine, unspecified portion

● **C7A.02**   Malignant carcinoid tumors of the appendix, large intestine, and rectum

C7A.020   Malignant carcinoid tumor of the appendix

C7A.021   Malignant carcinoid tumor of the cecum

C7A.022   Malignant carcinoid tumor of the ascending colon

C7A.023   Malignant carcinoid tumor of the transverse colon

C7A.024   Malignant carcinoid tumor of the descending colon

C7A.025   Malignant carcinoid tumor of the sigmoid colon

C7A.026   Malignant carcinoid tumor of the rectum

C7A.029   Malignant carcinoid tumor of the large intestine, unspecified portion
Malignant carcinoid tumor of the colon NOS

● **C7A.09**   Malignant carcinoid tumors of other sites

C7A.090   Malignant carcinoid tumor of the bronchus and lung

C7A.091   Malignant carcinoid tumor of the thymus

C7A.092   Malignant carcinoid tumor of the stomach

C7A.093   Malignant carcinoid tumor of the kidney

C7A.094   Malignant carcinoid tumor of the foregut, unspecified

C7A.095   Malignant carcinoid tumor of the midgut, unspecified

C7A.096   Malignant carcinoid tumor of the hindgut, unspecified

C7A.098   Malignant carcinoid tumors of other sites

C7A.1   Malignant poorly differentiated neuroendocrine tumors
Malignant poorly differentiated neuroendocrine tumor NOS
Malignant poorly differentiated neuroendocrine carcinoma, any site
High grade neuroendocrine carcinoma, any site

C7A.8   Other malignant neuroendocrine tumors
Secondary neuroendocrine tumors (C7B)

SECONDARY NEUROENDOCRINE TUMORS (C7B)

● **C7B**   Secondary neuroendocrine tumors

Use additional code to identify any functional activity

● **C7B.0**   Secondary carcinoid tumors

C7B.00   Secondary carcinoid tumors, unspecified site

C7B.01   Secondary carcinoid tumors of distant lymph nodes

C7B.02   Secondary carcinoid tumors of liver

C7B.03   Secondary carcinoid tumors of bone

C7B.04   Secondary carcinoid tumors of peritoneum
Mesentary metastasis of carcinoid tumor

C7B.09   Secondary carcinoid tumors of other sites

C7B.1   Secondary Merkel cell carcinoma
Merkel cell carcinoma nodal presentation
Merkel cell carcinoma visceral metastatic presentation

C7B.8   Other secondary neuroendocrine tumors

MALIGNANT NEOPLASMS OF ILL-DEFINED, OTHER SECONDARY AND UNSPECIFIED SITES (C76-C80)

● **C76**   Malignant neoplasm of other and ill-defined sites

> **Excludes1**   malignant neoplasm of female genitourinary tract NOS (C57.9)
> malignant neoplasm of male genitourinary tract NOS (C63.9)
> malignant neoplasm of lymphoid, hematopoietic and related tissue (C81-C96)
> malignant neoplasm of skin (C44.-)
> malignant neoplasm of unspecified site NOS (C80.1)

C76.0   Malignant neoplasm of head, face and neck
Malignant neoplasm of cheek NOS
Malignant neoplasm of nose NOS

C76.1   Malignant neoplasm of thorax
Intrathoracic malignant neoplasm NOS
Malignant neoplasm of axilla NOS
Thoracic malignant neoplasm NOS

C76.2   Malignant neoplasm of abdomen

C76.3   Malignant neoplasm of pelvis
Malignant neoplasm of groin NOS
Malignant neoplasm of sites overlapping systems within the pelvis
Rectovaginal (septum) malignant neoplasm
Between rectum and vagina
Rectovesical (septum) malignant neoplasm
Between rectum and urinary bladder; AKA vesicorectal

● **C76.4**   Malignant neoplasm of upper limb

C76.40   Malignant neoplasm of unspecified upper limb

C76.41   Malignant neoplasm of right upper limb

C76.42   Malignant neoplasm of left upper limb

● **C76.5**   Malignant neoplasm of lower limb

C76.50   Malignant neoplasm of unspecified lower limb

C76.51   Malignant neoplasm of right lower limb

C76.52   Malignant neoplasm of left lower limb

C76.8   Malignant neoplasm of other specified ill-defined sites
Malignant neoplasm of overlapping ill-defined sites

CHAPTER 2 (C00-D49)

● **C77** Secondary and unspecified malignant neoplasm of lymph nodes

> **Excludes1** malignant neoplasm of lymph nodes, specified as primary (C81-C86, C88, C96.-)
> mesentary metastasis of carcinoid tumor (C7B.04)
> secondary carcinoid tumors of distant lymph nodes (C7B.01)

C77.0 Secondary and unspecified malignant neoplasm of lymph nodes of head, face and neck

> Secondary and unspecified malignant neoplasm of supraclavicular lymph nodes

C77.1 Secondary and unspecified malignant neoplasm of intrathoracic lymph nodes

C77.2 Secondary and unspecified malignant neoplasm of intra-abdominal lymph nodes

C77.3 Secondary and unspecified malignant neoplasm of axilla and upper limb lymph nodes

> Secondary and unspecified malignant neoplasm of pectoral lymph nodes

C77.4 Secondary and unspecified malignant neoplasm of inguinal and lower limb lymph nodes

C77.5 Secondary and unspecified malignant neoplasm of intrapelvic lymph nodes

C77.8 Secondary and unspecified malignant neoplasm of lymph nodes of multiple regions

C77.9 Secondary and unspecified malignant neoplasm of lymph node, unspecified

● **C78** Secondary malignant neoplasm of respiratory and digestive organs

> **Excludes1** secondary carcinoid tumors of liver (C7B.02)
> secondary carcinoid tumors of peritoneum (C7B.04)

> **Excludes2** lymph node metastases (C77.0)

● **C78.0** Secondary malignant neoplasm of lung

C78.00 Secondary malignant neoplasm of unspecified lung

C78.01 Secondary malignant neoplasm of right lung

C78.02 Secondary malignant neoplasm of left lung

C78.1 Secondary malignant neoplasm of mediastinum

> *Thoracic cavity between pleural cavities*

C78.2 Secondary malignant neoplasm of pleura

> *Serous membrane covering lungs and lining thoracic cavity*

● **C78.3** Secondary malignant neoplasm of other and unspecified respiratory organs

C78.30 Secondary malignant neoplasm of unspecified respiratory organ

C78.39 Secondary malignant neoplasm of other respiratory organs

C78.4 Secondary malignant neoplasm of small intestine

C78.5 Secondary malignant neoplasm of large intestine and rectum

C78.6 Secondary malignant neoplasm of retroperitoneum and peritoneum

C78.7 Secondary malignant neoplasm of liver and intrahepatic bile duct

● **C78.8** Secondary malignant neoplasm of other and unspecified digestive organs

C78.80 Secondary malignant neoplasm of unspecified digestive organ

C78.89 Secondary malignant neoplasm of other digestive organs

> Code also exocrine pancreatic insufficiency (K86.81)

Item 2-6 The adrenal glands are a pair of glands situated on top of or above each kidney ("suprarenal") and chiefly responsible for regulating the stress response through the synthesis of corticosteroids and catecholamines, including cortisol and adrenaline.

● **C79** Secondary malignant neoplasm of other and unspecified sites

> **Excludes1** secondary carcinoid tumors (C7B.-)
> secondary neuroendocrine tumors (C7B.-)

> **Excludes2** ~~lymph node metastases (C77.0)~~

● **C79.0** Secondary malignant neoplasm of kidney and renal pelvis

C79.00 Secondary malignant neoplasm of unspecified kidney and renal pelvis

C79.01 Secondary malignant neoplasm of right kidney and renal pelvis

C79.02 Secondary malignant neoplasm of left kidney and renal pelvis

● **C79.1** Secondary malignant neoplasm of bladder and other and unspecified urinary organs

C79.10 Secondary malignant neoplasm of unspecified urinary organs

C79.11 Secondary malignant neoplasm of bladder

> ▶ **Excludes2** lymph node metastases (C77.0)

C79.19 Secondary malignant neoplasm of other urinary organs

C79.2 Secondary malignant neoplasm of skin

> **Excludes1** secondary Merkel cell carcinoma (C7B.1)

● **C79.3** Secondary malignant neoplasm of brain and cerebral meninges

C79.31 Secondary malignant neoplasm of brain

C79.32 Secondary malignant neoplasm of cerebral meninges

● **C79.4** Secondary malignant neoplasm of other and unspecified parts of nervous system

C79.40 Secondary malignant neoplasm of unspecified part of nervous system

C79.49 Secondary malignant neoplasm of other parts of nervous system

● **C79.5** Secondary malignant neoplasm of bone and bone marrow

> **Excludes1** secondary carcinoid tumors of bone (C7B.03)

C79.51 Secondary malignant neoplasm of bone

C79.52 Secondary malignant neoplasm of bone marrow

● **C79.6** Secondary malignant neoplasm of ovary

C79.60 Secondary malignant neoplasm of unspecified ovary

C79.61 Secondary malignant neoplasm of right ovary

C79.62 Secondary malignant neoplasm of left ovary

● **C79.7** Secondary malignant neoplasm of adrenal gland

C79.70 Secondary malignant neoplasm of unspecified adrenal gland

C79.71 Secondary malignant neoplasm of right adrenal gland

C79.72 Secondary malignant neoplasm of left adrenal gland

● **C79.8** Secondary malignant neoplasm of other specified sites

C79.81 Secondary malignant neoplasm of breast

C79.82 Secondary malignant neoplasm of genital organs

C79.89 Secondary malignant neoplasm of other specified sites

C79.9 Secondary malignant neoplasm of unspecified site

> Metastatic cancer NOS
> Metastatic disease NOS

> **Excludes1** carcinomatosis NOS (C80.0)
> generalized cancer NOS (C80.0)
> malignant (primary) neoplasm of unspecified site (C80.1)

▶ New   ➡ Revised   ~~deleted~~ Deleted   **OGCR** Official Guidelines   X Assign placeholder X   ● Use Additional Character(s)

Excludes 1   Excludes 2   Includes   Use additional   Code first   Code also   Key words

OGCR Section I.C.2.j and k

Disseminated malignant neoplasm, unspecified

j. Code C80.0, Disseminated malignant neoplasm, unspecified, is for use only in those cases where the patient has advanced metastatic disease and no known primary or secondary sites are specified. It should not be used in place of assigning codes for the primary site and all known secondary sites.

Malignant neoplasm without specification of site

k. Code C80.1, Malignant (primary) neoplasm, unspecified, equates to Cancer, unspecified. This code should only be used when no determination can be made as to the primary site of a malignancy. This code should rarely be used in the inpatient setting.

● **C80** Malignant neoplasm without specification of site

 Excludes1 malignant carcinoid tumor of unspecified site (C7A.00)

   malignant neoplasm of specified multiple sites-code to each site

 C80.0 Disseminated malignant neoplasm, unspecified

  Carcinomatosis NOS

  Generalized cancer, unspecified site (primary) (secondary)

  Generalized malignancy, unspecified site (primary) (secondary)

 C80.1 Malignant (primary) neoplasm, unspecified

  Cancer NOS

  Cancer unspecified site (primary)

  Carcinoma unspecified site (primary)

  Malignancy unspecified site (primary)

  Excludes1 secondary malignant neoplasm of unspecified site (C79.9)

 C80.2 Malignant neoplasm associated with transplanted organ

  Code first complication of transplanted organ (T86.-)

  Use additional code to identify the specific malignancy

★ **(See Plate 315 on page 49.)**

MALIGNANT NEOPLASMS OF LYMPHOID, HEMATOPOIETIC AND RELATED TISSUE (C81-C96)

 Excludes2 Kaposi's sarcoma of lymph nodes (C46.3)

  secondary and unspecified neoplasm of lymph nodes (C77.-)

  secondary neoplasm of bone marrow (C79.52)

  secondary neoplasm of spleen (C78.89)

● **C81** Hodgkin lymphoma

 Form of malignant lymphoma with four types, nodular sclerosis, mixed cellularity, lymphocyte depleted, and lymphocyte predominant

 Excludes1 personal history of Hodgkin lymphoma (Z85.71)

 ● **C81.0** Nodular lymphocyte predominant Hodgkin lymphoma

  Least aggressive, least common, typically no symptoms

  Lymphocytic-histiocytic predominance Hodgkin's disease

  C81.00 Nodular lymphocyte predominant Hodgkin lymphoma, unspecified site

  C81.01 Nodular lymphocyte predominant Hodgkin lymphoma, lymph nodes of head, face, and neck

  C81.02 Nodular lymphocyte predominant Hodgkin lymphoma, intrathoracic lymph nodes

  C81.03 Nodular lymphocyte predominant Hodgkin lymphoma, intra-abdominal lymph nodes

C81.04 Nodular lymphocyte predominant Hodgkin lymphoma, lymph nodes of axilla and upper limb

C81.05 Nodular lymphocyte predominant Hodgkin lymphoma, lymph nodes of inguinal region and lower limb

C81.06 Nodular lymphocyte predominant Hodgkin lymphoma, intrapelvic lymph nodes

C81.07 Nodular lymphocyte predominant Hodgkin lymphoma, spleen

C81.08 Nodular lymphocyte predominant Hodgkin lymphoma, lymph nodes of multiple sites

C81.09 Nodular lymphocyte predominant Hodgkin lymphoma, extranodal and solid organ sites

● **C81.1** Nodular sclerosis Hodgkin lymphoma

 Nodular sclerosis classical Hodgkin lymphoma

 Moderately aggressive; most common in young adults

 C81.10 Nodular sclerosis Hodgkin lymphoma, unspecified site

 C81.11 Nodular sclerosis Hodgkin lymphoma, lymph nodes of head, face, and neck

 C81.12 Nodular sclerosis Hodgkin lymphoma, intrathoracic lymph nodes

 C81.13 Nodular sclerosis Hodgkin lymphoma, intra-abdominal lymph nodes

 C81.14 Nodular sclerosis Hodgkin lymphoma, lymph nodes of axilla and upper limb

 C81.15 Nodular sclerosis Hodgkin lymphoma, lymph nodes of inguinal region and lower limb

 C81.16 Nodular sclerosis Hodgkin lymphoma, intrapelvic lymph nodes

 C81.17 Nodular sclerosis Hodgkin lymphoma, spleen

 C81.18 Nodular sclerosis Hodgkin lymphoma, lymph nodes of multiple sites

 C81.19 Nodular sclerosis Hodgkin lymphoma, extranodal and solid organ sites

● **C81.2** Mixed cellularity Hodgkin lymphoma

 Mixed cellularity classical Hodgkin lymphoma

 A type of Hodgkin's that is moderately aggressive with mixed cell types

 C81.20 Mixed cellularity Hodgkin lymphoma, unspecified site

 C81.21 Mixed cellularity Hodgkin lymphoma, lymph nodes of head, face, and neck

 C81.22 Mixed cellularity Hodgkin lymphoma, intrathoracic lymph nodes

 C81.23 Mixed cellularity Hodgkin lymphoma, intra-abdominal lymph nodes

 C81.24 Mixed cellularity Hodgkin lymphoma, lymph nodes of axilla and upper limb

 C81.25 Mixed cellularity Hodgkin lymphoma, lymph nodes of inguinal region and lower limb

 C81.26 Mixed cellularity Hodgkin lymphoma, intrapelvic lymph nodes

 C81.27 Mixed cellularity Hodgkin lymphoma, spleen

 C81.28 Mixed cellularity Hodgkin lymphoma, lymph nodes of multiple sites

 C81.29 Mixed cellularity Hodgkin lymphoma, extranodal and solid organ sites

▶ New ⟹ Revised ~~deleted~~ Deleted **OGCR** Official Guidelines X Assign placeholder X ● Use Additional Character(s)

Excludes 1 Excludes 2 Includes Use additional Code first Code also Key words

653

CHAPTER 2 (C00-D49)

● **C81.3 Lymphocyte depleted Hodgkin lymphoma**
Lymphocyte depleted classical Hodgkin lymphoma
Most aggressive type with poor prognosis

C81.30   Lymphocyte depleted Hodgkin lymphoma, unspecified site

C81.31   Lymphocyte depleted Hodgkin lymphoma, lymph nodes of head, face, and neck

C81.32   Lymphocyte depleted Hodgkin lymphoma, intrathoracic lymph nodes

C81.33   Lymphocyte depleted Hodgkin lymphoma, intra-abdominal lymph nodes

C81.34   Lymphocyte depleted Hodgkin lymphoma, lymph nodes of axilla and upper limb

C81.35   Lymphocyte depleted Hodgkin lymphoma, lymph nodes of inguinal region and lower limb

C81.36   Lymphocyte depleted Hodgkin lymphoma, intrapelvic lymph nodes

C81.37   Lymphocyte depleted Hodgkin lymphoma, spleen

C81.38   Lymphocyte depleted Hodgkin lymphoma, lymph nodes of multiple sites

C81.39   Lymphocyte depleted Hodgkin lymphoma, extranodal and solid organ sites

● **C81.4 Lymphocyte-rich Hodgkin lymphoma**
Lymphocyte-rich classical Hodgkin lymphoma

Excludes1   nodular lymphocyte predominant Hodgkin lymphoma (C81.0-)

C81.40   Lymphocyte-rich Hodgkin lymphoma, unspecified site

C81.41   Lymphocyte-rich Hodgkin lymphoma, lymph nodes of head, face, and neck

C81.42   Lymphocyte-rich Hodgkin lymphoma, intrathoracic lymph nodes

C81.43   Lymphocyte-rich Hodgkin lymphoma, intra-abdominal lymph nodes

C81.44   Lymphocyte-rich Hodgkin lymphoma, lymph nodes of axilla and upper limb

C81.45   Lymphocyte-rich Hodgkin lymphoma, lymph nodes of inguinal region and lower limb

C81.46   Lymphocyte-rich Hodgkin lymphoma, intrapelvic lymph nodes

C81.47   Lymphocyte-rich Hodgkin lymphoma, spleen

C81.48   Lymphocyte-rich Hodgkin lymphoma, lymph nodes of multiple sites

C81.49   Lymphocyte-rich Hodgkin lymphoma, extranodal and solid organ sites

● **C81.7 Other Hodgkin lymphoma**
Classical Hodgkin lymphoma NOS
Other classical Hodgkin lymphoma

C81.70   Other Hodgkin lymphoma, unspecified site

C81.71   Other Hodgkin lymphoma, lymph nodes of head, face, and neck

C81.72   Other Hodgkin lymphoma, intrathoracic lymph nodes

C81.73   Other Hodgkin lymphoma, intra-abdominal lymph nodes

C81.74   Other Hodgkin lymphoma, lymph nodes of axilla and upper limb

C81.75   Other Hodgkin lymphoma, lymph nodes of inguinal region and lower limb

C81.76   Other Hodgkin lymphoma, intrapelvic lymph nodes

C81.77   Other Hodgkin lymphoma, spleen

C81.78   Other Hodgkin lymphoma, lymph nodes of multiple sites

C81.79   Other Hodgkin lymphoma, extranodal and solid organ sites

● **C81.9 Hodgkin lymphoma, unspecified**

C81.90   Hodgkin lymphoma, unspecified, unspecified site

C81.91   Hodgkin lymphoma, unspecified, lymph nodes of head, face, and neck

C81.92   Hodgkin lymphoma, unspecified, intrathoracic lymph nodes

C81.93   Hodgkin lymphoma, unspecified, intra-abdominal lymph nodes

C81.94   Hodgkin lymphoma, unspecified, lymph nodes of axilla and upper limb

C81.95   Hodgkin lymphoma, unspecified, lymph nodes of inguinal region and lower limb

C81.96   Hodgkin lymphoma, unspecified, intrapelvic lymph nodes

C81.97   Hodgkin lymphoma, unspecified, spleen

C81.98   Hodgkin lymphoma, unspecified, lymph nodes of multiple sites

C81.99   Hodgkin lymphoma, unspecified, extranodal and solid organ sites

● **C82 Follicular lymphoma**
Group of malignant lymphomas

Includes   follicular lymphoma with or without diffuse areas

Excludes1   mature T/NK-cell lymphomas (C84.-)
personal history of non-Hodgkin lymphoma (Z85.72)

● **C82.0 Follicular lymphoma grade I**

C82.00   Follicular lymphoma grade I, unspecified site

C82.01   Follicular lymphoma grade I, lymph nodes of head, face, and neck

C82.02   Follicular lymphoma grade I, intrathoracic lymph nodes

C82.03   Follicular lymphoma grade I, intra-abdominal lymph nodes

C82.04   Follicular lymphoma grade I, lymph nodes of axilla and upper limb

C82.05   Follicular lymphoma grade I, lymph nodes of inguinal region and lower limb

C82.06   Follicular lymphoma grade I, intrapelvic lymph nodes

C82.07   Follicular lymphoma grade I, spleen

C82.08   Follicular lymphoma grade I, lymph nodes of multiple sites

C82.09   Follicular lymphoma grade I, extranodal and solid organ sites

● **C82.1 Follicular lymphoma grade II**

C82.10   Follicular lymphoma grade II, unspecified site

C82.11   Follicular lymphoma grade II, lymph nodes of head, face, and neck

C82.12   Follicular lymphoma grade II, intrathoracic lymph nodes

C82.13   Follicular lymphoma grade II, intra-abdominal lymph nodes

C82.14   Follicular lymphoma grade II, lymph nodes of axilla and upper limb

C82.15   Follicular lymphoma grade II, lymph nodes of inguinal region and lower limb

C82.16   Follicular lymphoma grade II, intrapelvic lymph nodes

C82.17   Follicular lymphoma grade II, spleen

C82.18   Follicular lymphoma grade II, lymph nodes of multiple sites

C82.19   Follicular lymphoma grade II, extranodal and solid organ sites

▶ New   ⟹ Revised   ~~deleted~~ Deleted   **OGCR** Official Guidelines   X Assign placeholder X   ● Use Additional Character(s)

Excludes 1   Excludes 2   Includes   Use additional   Code first   Code also   Key words

● C82.2   Follicular lymphoma grade III, unspecified

     C82.20   Follicular lymphoma grade III, unspecified, unspecified site

     C82.21   Follicular lymphoma grade III, unspecified, lymph nodes of head, face, and neck

     C82.22   Follicular lymphoma grade III, unspecified, intrathoracic lymph nodes

     C82.23   Follicular lymphoma grade III, unspecified, intra-abdominal lymph nodes

     C82.24   Follicular lymphoma grade III, unspecified, lymph nodes of axilla and upper limb

     C82.25   Follicular lymphoma grade III, unspecified, lymph nodes of inguinal region and lower limb

     C82.26   Follicular lymphoma grade III, unspecified, intrapelvic lymph nodes

     C82.27   Follicular lymphoma grade III, unspecified, spleen

     C82.28   Follicular lymphoma grade III, unspecified, lymph nodes of multiple sites

     C82.29   Follicular lymphoma grade III, unspecified, extranodal and solid organ sites

● C82.3   Follicular lymphoma grade IIIa

     C82.30   Follicular lymphoma grade IIIa, unspecified site

     C82.31   Follicular lymphoma grade IIIa, lymph nodes of head, face, and neck

     C82.32   Follicular lymphoma grade IIIa, intrathoracic lymph nodes

     C82.33   Follicular lymphoma grade IIIa, intra-abdominal lymph nodes

     C82.34   Follicular lymphoma grade IIIa, lymph nodes of axilla and upper limb

     C82.35   Follicular lymphoma grade IIIa, lymph nodes of inguinal region and lower limb

     C82.36   Follicular lymphoma grade IIIa, intrapelvic lymph nodes

     C82.37   Follicular lymphoma grade IIIa, spleen

     C82.38   Follicular lymphoma grade IIIa, lymph nodes of multiple sites

     C82.39   Follicular lymphoma grade IIIa, extranodal and solid organ sites

● C82.4   Follicular lymphoma grade IIIb

     C82.40   Follicular lymphoma grade IIIb, unspecified site

     C82.41   Follicular lymphoma grade IIIb, lymph nodes of head, face, and neck

     C82.42   Follicular lymphoma grade IIIb, intrathoracic lymph nodes

     C82.43   Follicular lymphoma grade IIIb, intra-abdominal lymph nodes

     C82.44   Follicular lymphoma grade IIIb, lymph nodes of axilla and upper limb

     C82.45   Follicular lymphoma grade IIIb, lymph nodes of inguinal region and lower limb

     C82.46   Follicular lymphoma grade IIIb, intrapelvic lymph nodes

     C82.47   Follicular lymphoma grade IIIb, spleen

     C82.48   Follicular lymphoma grade IIIb, lymph nodes of multiple sites

     C82.49   Follicular lymphoma grade IIIb, extranodal and solid organ sites

● C82.5   Diffuse follicle center lymphoma

     C82.50   Diffuse follicle center lymphoma, unspecified site

     C82.51   Diffuse follicle center lymphoma, lymph nodes of head, face, and neck

     C82.52   Diffuse follicle center lymphoma, intrathoracic lymph nodes

     C82.53   Diffuse follicle center lymphoma, intra-abdominal lymph nodes

     C82.54   Diffuse follicle center lymphoma, lymph nodes of axilla and upper limb

     C82.55   Diffuse follicle center lymphoma, lymph nodes of inguinal region and lower limb

     C82.56   Diffuse follicle center lymphoma, intrapelvic lymph nodes

     C82.57   Diffuse follicle center lymphoma, spleen

     C82.58   Diffuse follicle center lymphoma, lymph nodes of multiple sites

     C82.59   Diffuse follicle center lymphoma, extranodal and solid organ sites

● C82.6   Cutaneous follicle center lymphoma

     C82.60   Cutaneous follicle center lymphoma, unspecified site

     C82.61   Cutaneous follicle center lymphoma, lymph nodes of head, face, and neck

     C82.62   Cutaneous follicle center lymphoma, intrathoracic lymph nodes

     C82.63   Cutaneous follicle center lymphoma, intra-abdominal lymph nodes

     C82.64   Cutaneous follicle center lymphoma, lymph nodes of axilla and upper limb

     C82.65   Cutaneous follicle center lymphoma, lymph nodes of inguinal region and lower limb

     C82.66   Cutaneous follicle center lymphoma, intrapelvic lymph nodes

     C82.67   Cutaneous follicle center lymphoma, spleen

     C82.68   Cutaneous follicle center lymphoma, lymph nodes of multiple sites

     C82.69   Cutaneous follicle center lymphoma, extranodal and solid organ sites

● C82.8   Other types of follicular lymphoma

     C82.80   Other types of follicular lymphoma, unspecified site

     C82.81   Other types of follicular lymphoma, lymph nodes of head, face, and neck

     C82.82   Other types of follicular lymphoma, intrathoracic lymph nodes

     C82.83   Other types of follicular lymphoma, intra-abdominal lymph nodes

     C82.84   Other types of follicular lymphoma, lymph nodes of axilla and upper limb

     C82.85   Other types of follicular lymphoma, lymph nodes of inguinal region and lower limb

     C82.86   Other types of follicular lymphoma, intrapelvic lymph nodes

     C82.87   Other types of follicular lymphoma, spleen

     C82.88   Other types of follicular lymphoma, lymph nodes of multiple sites

     C82.89   Other types of follicular lymphoma, extranodal and solid organ sites

CHAPTER 2 (C00-D49)

CHAPTER 2 (C00-D49)

● C82.9 Follicular lymphoma, unspecified

C82.90 Follicular lymphoma, unspecified, unspecified site

C82.91 Follicular lymphoma, unspecified, lymph nodes of head, face, and neck

C82.92 Follicular lymphoma, unspecified, intrathoracic lymph nodes

C82.93 Follicular lymphoma, unspecified, intra-abdominal lymph nodes

C82.94 Follicular lymphoma, unspecified, lymph nodes of axilla and upper limb

C82.95 Follicular lymphoma, unspecified, lymph nodes of inguinal region and lower limb

C82.96 Follicular lymphoma, unspecified, intrapelvic lymph nodes

C82.97 Follicular lymphoma, unspecified, spleen

C82.98 Follicular lymphoma, unspecified, lymph nodes of multiple sites

C82.99 Follicular lymphoma, unspecified, extranodal and solid organ sites

● C83 Non-follicular lymphoma

Excludes1 personal history of non-Hodgkin lymphoma (Z85.72)

● C83.0 Small cell B-cell lymphoma

Lymphoplasmacytic lymphoma
Nodal marginal zone lymphoma
Non-leukemic variant of B-CLL
Splenic marginal zone lymphoma

Excludes1 chronic lymphocytic leukemia (C91.1)
mature T/NK-cell lymphomas (C84.-)
Waldenström macroglobulinemia (C88.0)

C83.00 Small cell B-cell lymphoma, unspecified site

C83.01 Small cell B-cell lymphoma, lymph nodes of head, face, and neck

C83.02 Small cell B-cell lymphoma, intrathoracic lymph nodes

C83.03 Small cell B-cell lymphoma, intra-abdominal lymph nodes

C83.04 Small cell B-cell lymphoma, lymph nodes of axilla and upper limb

C83.05 Small cell B-cell lymphoma, lymph nodes of inguinal region and lower limb

C83.06 Small cell B-cell lymphoma, intrapelvic lymph nodes

C83.07 Small cell B-cell lymphoma, spleen

C83.08 Small cell B-cell lymphoma, lymph nodes of multiple sites

C83.09 Small cell B-cell lymphoma, extranodal and solid organ sites

● C83.1 Mantle cell lymphoma

Centrocytic lymphoma
Malignant lymphomatous polyposis

C83.10 Mantle cell lymphoma, unspecified site

C83.11 Mantle cell lymphoma, lymph nodes of head, face, and neck

C83.12 Mantle cell lymphoma, intrathoracic lymph nodes

C83.13 Mantle cell lymphoma, intra-abdominal lymph nodes

C83.14 Mantle cell lymphoma, lymph nodes of axilla and upper limb

C83.15 Mantle cell lymphoma, lymph nodes of inguinal region and lower limb

C83.16 Mantle cell lymphoma, intrapelvic lymph nodes

C83.17 Mantle cell lymphoma, spleen

C83.18 Mantle cell lymphoma, lymph nodes of multiple sites

C83.19 Mantle cell lymphoma, extranodal and solid organ sites

● C83.3 Diffuse large B-cell lymphoma

Anaplastic diffuse large B-cell lymphoma
CD30-positive diffuse large B-cell lymphoma
Centroblastic diffuse large B-cell lymphoma
Diffuse large B-cell lymphoma, subtype not specified
Immunoblastic diffuse large B-cell lymphoma
Plasmablastic diffuse large B-cell lymphoma
Diffuse large B-cell lymphoma, subtype not specified
T-cell rich diffuse large B-cell lymphoma

Excludes1 mediastinal (thymic) large B-cell lymphoma (C85.2-)
mature T/NK-cell lymphomas (C84.-)

C83.30 Diffuse large B-cell lymphoma, unspecified site

C83.31 Diffuse large B-cell lymphoma, lymph nodes of head, face, and neck

C83.32 Diffuse large B-cell lymphoma, intrathoracic lymph nodes

C83.33 Diffuse large B-cell lymphoma, intra-abdominal lymph nodes

C83.34 Diffuse large B-cell lymphoma, lymph nodes of axilla and upper limb

C83.35 Diffuse large B-cell lymphoma, lymph nodes of inguinal region and lower limb

C83.36 Diffuse large B-cell lymphoma, intrapelvic lymph nodes

C83.37 Diffuse large B-cell lymphoma, spleen

C83.38 Diffuse large B-cell lymphoma, lymph nodes of multiple sites

C83.39 Diffuse large B-cell lymphoma, extranodal and solid organ sites

● C83.5 Lymphoblastic (diffuse) lymphoma

Highly malignant type of non-Hodgkin lymphoma with diffuse infiltration
B-precursor lymphoma
Lymphoblastic B-cell lymphoma
Lymphoblastic lymphoma NOS
Lymphoblastic T-cell lymphoma
T-precursor lymphoma

C83.50 Lymphoblastic (diffuse) lymphoma, unspecified site

C83.51 Lymphoblastic (diffuse) lymphoma, lymph nodes of head, face, and neck

C83.52 Lymphoblastic (diffuse) lymphoma, intrathoracic lymph nodes

C83.53 Lymphoblastic (diffuse) lymphoma, intra-abdominal lymph nodes

C83.54 Lymphoblastic (diffuse) lymphoma, lymph nodes of axilla and upper limb

C83.55 Lymphoblastic (diffuse) lymphoma, lymph nodes of inguinal region and lower limb

C83.56 Lymphoblastic (diffuse) lymphoma, intrapelvic lymph nodes

C83.57 Lymphoblastic (diffuse) lymphoma, spleen

C83.58 Lymphoblastic (diffuse) lymphoma, lymph nodes of multiple sites

C83.59 Lymphoblastic (diffuse) lymphoma, extranodal and solid organ sites

▶ New   ⇒ Revised   ~~deleted~~ Deleted   **OGCR** Official Guidelines   X Assign placeholder X   ● Use Additional Character(s)

| Excludes 1 | Excludes 2 | Includes | Use additional | Code first | Code also | Key words |

● **C83.7　Burkitt lymphoma**
Form of small cell lymphoma
Atypical Burkitt lymphoma
Burkitt-like lymphoma

　　Excludes1　mature B-cell leukemia Burkitt type (C91.A-)

C83.70　Burkitt lymphoma, unspecified site

C83.71　Burkitt lymphoma, lymph nodes of head, face, and neck

C83.72　Burkitt lymphoma, intrathoracic lymph nodes

C83.73　Burkitt lymphoma, intra-abdominal lymph nodes

C83.74　Burkitt lymphoma, lymph nodes of axilla and upper limb

C83.75　Burkitt lymphoma, lymph nodes of inguinal region and lower limb

C83.76　Burkitt lymphoma, intrapelvic lymph nodes

C83.77　Burkitt lymphoma, spleen

C83.78　Burkitt lymphoma, lymph nodes of multiple sites

C83.79　Burkitt lymphoma, extranodal and solid organ sites

● **C83.8　Other non-follicular lymphoma**
Intravascular large B-cell lymphoma
Lymphoid granulomatosis
Primary effusion B-cell lymphoma

　　Excludes1　mediastinal (thymic) large B-cell lymphoma (C85.2-)
　　　　　　　T-cell rich B-cell lymphoma (C83.3-)

C83.80　Other non-follicular lymphoma, unspecified site

C83.81　Other non-follicular lymphoma, lymph nodes of head, face, and neck

C83.82　Other non-follicular lymphoma, intrathoracic lymph nodes

C83.83　Other non-follicular lymphoma, intra-abdominal lymph nodes

C83.84　Other non-follicular lymphoma, lymph nodes of axilla and upper limb

C83.85　Other non-follicular lymphoma, lymph nodes of inguinal region and lower limb

C83.86　Other non-follicular lymphoma, intrapelvic lymph nodes

C83.87　Other non-follicular lymphoma, spleen

C83.88　Other non-follicular lymphoma, lymph nodes of multiple sites

C83.89　Other non-follicular lymphoma, extranodal and solid organ sites

● **C83.9　Non-follicular (diffuse) lymphoma, unspecified**

C83.90　Non-follicular (diffuse) lymphoma, unspecified, unspecified site

C83.91　Non-follicular (diffuse) lymphoma, unspecified, lymph nodes of head, face, and neck

C83.92　Non-follicular (diffuse) lymphoma, unspecified, intrathoracic lymph nodes

C83.93　Non-follicular (diffuse) lymphoma, unspecified, intra-abdominal lymph nodes

C83.94　Non-follicular (diffuse) lymphoma, unspecified, lymph nodes of axilla and upper limb

C83.95　Non-follicular (diffuse) lymphoma, unspecified, lymph nodes of inguinal region and lower limb

C83.96　Non-follicular (diffuse) lymphoma, unspecified, intrapelvic lymph nodes

C83.97　Non-follicular (diffuse) lymphoma, unspecified, spleen

C83.98　Non-follicular (diffuse) lymphoma, unspecified, lymph nodes of multiple sites

C83.99　Non-follicular (diffuse) lymphoma, unspecified, extranodal and solid organ sites

● **C84　Mature T/NK-cell lymphomas**

　　Excludes1　personal history of non-Hodgkin lymphoma (Z85.72)

● **C84.0　Mycosis fungoides**
Chronic or rapidly progressive form of cutaneous T-cell lymphoma; AKA granuloma fungoides

　　Excludes1　peripheral T-cell lymphoma, not classified (C84.4-)

C84.00　Mycosis fungoides, unspecified site

C84.01　Mycosis fungoides, lymph nodes of head, face, and neck

C84.02　Mycosis fungoides, intrathoracic lymph nodes

C84.03　Mycosis fungoides, intra-abdominal lymph nodes

C84.04　Mycosis fungoides, lymph nodes of axilla and upper limb

C84.05　Mycosis fungoides, lymph nodes of inguinal region and lower limb

C84.06　Mycosis fungoides, intrapelvic lymph nodes

C84.07　Mycosis fungoides, spleen

C84.08　Mycosis fungoides, lymph nodes of multiple sites

C84.09　Mycosis fungoides, extranodal and solid organ sites

● **C84.1　Sézary disease**
Type of cutaneous lymphoma affecting T-cells

C84.10　Sézary disease, unspecified site

C84.11　Sézary disease, lymph nodes of head, face, and neck

C84.12　Sézary disease, intrathoracic lymph nodes

C84.13　Sézary disease, intra-abdominal lymph nodes

C84.14　Sézary disease, lymph nodes of axilla and upper limb

C84.15　Sézary disease, lymph nodes of inguinal region and lower limb

C84.16　Sézary disease, intrapelvic lymph nodes

C84.17　Sézary disease, spleen

C84.18　Sézary disease, lymph nodes of multiple sites

C84.19　Sézary disease, extranodal and solid organ sites

● **C84.4　Peripheral T-cell lymphoma, not classified**
Diverse group of blood carcinomas originating from T-cells, requiring aggressive chemotherapy
Lennert's lymphoma
Lymphoepithelioid lymphoma
Mature T-cell lymphoma, not elsewhere classified

C84.40　Peripheral T-cell lymphoma, not classified, unspecified site

C84.41　Peripheral T-cell lymphoma, not classified, lymph nodes of head, face, and neck

C84.42　Peripheral T-cell lymphoma, not classified, intrathoracic lymph nodes

C84.43　Peripheral T-cell lymphoma, not classified, intra-abdominal lymph nodes

C84.44　Peripheral T-cell lymphoma, not classified, lymph nodes of axilla and upper limb

C84.45　Peripheral T-cell lymphoma, not classified, lymph nodes of inguinal region and lower limb

C84.46　Peripheral T-cell lymphoma, not classified, intrapelvic lymph nodes

C84.47　Peripheral T-cell lymphoma, not classified, spleen

C84.48　Peripheral T-cell lymphoma, not classified, lymph nodes of multiple sites

C84.49　Peripheral T-cell lymphoma, not classified, extranodal and solid organ sites

CHAPTER 2 (C00-D49)

▶ New　⮕ Revised　~~deleted~~ Deleted　**OGCR** Official Guidelines　X Assign placeholder X　● Use Additional Character(s)

| Excludes 1 | Excludes 2 | Includes | Use additional | Code first | Code also | Key words |

CHAPTER 2 (C00-D49)

● **C84.6** **Anaplastic large cell lymphoma, ALK-positive**
Anaplastic large cell lymphoma, CD30-positive

C84.60 Anaplastic large cell lymphoma, ALK-positive, unspecified site

C84.61 Anaplastic large cell lymphoma, ALK-positive, lymph nodes of head, face, and neck

C84.62 Anaplastic large cell lymphoma, ALK-positive, intrathoracic lymph nodes

C84.63 Anaplastic large cell lymphoma, ALK-positive, intra-abdominal lymph nodes

C84.64 Anaplastic large cell lymphoma, ALK-positive, lymph nodes of axilla and upper limb

C84.65 Anaplastic large cell lymphoma, ALK-positive, lymph nodes of inguinal region and lower limb

C84.66 Anaplastic large cell lymphoma, ALK-positive, intrapelvic lymph nodes

C84.67 Anaplastic large cell lymphoma, ALK-positive, spleen

C84.68 Anaplastic large cell lymphoma, ALK-positive, lymph nodes of multiple sites

C84.69 Anaplastic large cell lymphoma, ALK-positive, extranodal and solid organ sites

● **C84.7** **Anaplastic large cell lymphoma, ALK-negative**
| Excludes1 | primary cutaneous CD30-positive T-cell proliferations (C86.6-)

C84.70 Anaplastic large cell lymphoma, ALK-negative, unspecified site

C84.71 Anaplastic large cell lymphoma, ALK-negative, lymph nodes of head, face, and neck

C84.72 Anaplastic large cell lymphoma, ALK-negative, intrathoracic lymph nodes

C84.73 Anaplastic large cell lymphoma, ALK-negative, intra-abdominal lymph nodes

C84.74 Anaplastic large cell lymphoma, ALK-negative, lymph nodes of axilla and upper limb

C84.75 Anaplastic large cell lymphoma, ALK-negative, lymph nodes of inguinal region and lower limb

C84.76 Anaplastic large cell lymphoma, ALK-negative, intrapelvic lymph nodes

C84.77 Anaplastic large cell lymphoma, ALK-negative, spleen

C84.78 Anaplastic large cell lymphoma, ALK-negative, lymph nodes of multiple sites

C84.79 Anaplastic large cell lymphoma, ALK-negative, extranodal and solid organ sites

● **C84.A** **Cutaneous T-cell lymphoma, unspecified**

C84.A0 Cutaneous T-cell lymphoma, unspecified, unspecified site

C84.A1 Cutaneous T-cell lymphoma, unspecified lymph nodes of head, face, and neck

C84.A2 Cutaneous T-cell lymphoma, unspecified, intrathoracic lymph nodes

C84.A3 Cutaneous T-cell lymphoma, unspecified, intra-abdominal lymph nodes

C84.A4 Cutaneous T-cell lymphoma, unspecified, lymph nodes of axilla and upper limb

C84.A5 Cutaneous T-cell lymphoma, unspecified, lymph nodes of inguinal region and lower limb

C84.A6 Cutaneous T-cell lymphoma, unspecified, intrapelvic lymph nodes

C84.A7 Cutaneous T-cell lymphoma, unspecified, spleen

C84.A8 Cutaneous T-cell lymphoma, unspecified, lymph nodes of multiple sites

C84.A9 Cutaneous T-cell lymphoma, unspecified, extranodal and solid organ sites

● **C84.Z** **Other mature T/NK-cell lymphomas**
Note: If T-cell lineage or involvement is mentioned in conjunction with a specific lymphoma, code to the more specific description.
| Excludes1 | angioimmunoblastic T-cell lymphoma (C86.5)
blastic NK-cell lymphoma (C86.4)
enteropathy-type T-cell lymphoma (C86.2)
extranodal NK-cell lymphoma, nasal type (C86.0)
hepatosplenic T-cell lymphoma (C86.1)
primary cutaneous CD30-positive T-cell proliferations (C86.6)
subcutaneous panniculitis-like T-cell lymphoma (C86.3)
T-cell leukemia (C91.1-)

C84.Z0 Other mature T/NK-cell lymphomas, unspecified site

C84.Z1 Other mature T/NK-cell lymphomas, lymph nodes of head, face, and neck

C84.Z2 Other mature T/NK-cell lymphomas, intrathoracic lymph nodes

C84.Z3 Other mature T/NK-cell lymphomas, intra-abdominal lymph nodes

C84.Z4 Other mature T/NK-cell lymphomas, lymph nodes of axilla and upper limb

C84.Z5 Other mature T/NK-cell lymphomas, lymph nodes of inguinal region and lower limb

C84.Z6 Other mature T/NK-cell lymphomas, intrapelvic lymph nodes

C84.Z7 Other mature T/NK-cell lymphomas, spleen

C84.Z8 Other mature T/NK-cell lymphomas, lymph nodes of multiple sites

C84.Z9 Other mature T/NK-cell lymphomas, extranodal and solid organ sites

● **C84.9** **Mature T/NK-cell lymphomas, unspecified**
NK/T cell lymphoma NOS
| Excludes1 | mature T-cell lymphoma, not elsewhere classified (C84.4-)

C84.90 Mature T/NK-cell lymphomas, unspecified, unspecified site

C84.91 Mature T/NK-cell lymphomas, unspecified, lymph nodes of head, face, and neck

C84.92 Mature T/NK-cell lymphomas, unspecified, intrathoracic lymph nodes

C84.93 Mature T/NK-cell lymphomas, unspecified, intra-abdominal lymph nodes

C84.94 Mature T/NK-cell lymphomas, unspecified, lymph nodes of axilla and upper limb

C84.95 Mature T/NK-cell lymphomas, unspecified, lymph nodes of inguinal region and lower limb

C84.96 Mature T/NK-cell lymphomas, unspecified, intrapelvic lymph nodes

C84.97 Mature T/NK-cell lymphomas, unspecified, spleen

C84.98 Mature T/NK-cell lymphomas, unspecified, lymph nodes of multiple sites

C84.99 Mature T/NK-cell lymphomas, unspecified, extranodal and solid organ sites

▶ New   ⇒ Revised   ~~deleted~~ Deleted   **OGCR** Official Guidelines   X Assign placeholder X   ● Use Additional Character(s)
| Excludes 1 | | Excludes 2 | Includes   Use additional   Code first   Code also   Key words

● **C85   Other specified and unspecified types of non-Hodgkin lymphoma**

> | Excludes1 | other specified types of T/NK-cell lymphoma (C86.-) |
> | | personal history of non-Hodgkin lymphoma (Z85.72) |

● **C85.1   Unspecified B-cell lymphoma**

> **Note:** If B-cell lineage or involvement is mentioned in conjunction with a specific lymphoma, code to the more specific description.

C85.10   Unspecified B-cell lymphoma, unspecified site

C85.11   Unspecified B-cell lymphoma, lymph nodes of head, face, and neck

C85.12   Unspecified B-cell lymphoma, intrathoracic lymph nodes

C85.13   Unspecified B-cell lymphoma, intra-abdominal lymph nodes

C85.14   Unspecified B-cell lymphoma, lymph nodes of axilla and upper limb

C85.15   Unspecified B-cell lymphoma, lymph nodes of inguinal region and lower limb

C85.16   Unspecified B-cell lymphoma, intrapelvic lymph nodes

C85.17   Unspecified B-cell lymphoma, spleen

C85.18   Unspecified B-cell lymphoma, lymph nodes of multiple sites

C85.19   Unspecified B-cell lymphoma, extranodal and solid organ sites

● **C85.2   Mediastinal (thymic) large B-cell lymphoma**

C85.20   Mediastinal (thymic) large B-cell lymphoma, unspecified site

C85.21   Mediastinal (thymic) large B-cell lymphoma, lymph nodes of head, face, and neck

C85.22   Mediastinal (thymic) large B-cell lymphoma, intrathoracic lymph nodes

C85.23   Mediastinal (thymic) large B-cell lymphoma, intra-abdominal lymph nodes

C85.24   Mediastinal (thymic) large B-cell lymphoma, lymph nodes of axilla and upper limb

C85.25   Mediastinal (thymic) large B-cell lymphoma, lymph nodes of inguinal region and lower limb

C85.26   Mediastinal (thymic) large B-cell lymphoma, intrapelvic lymph nodes

C85.27   Mediastinal (thymic) large B-cell lymphoma, spleen

C85.28   Mediastinal (thymic) large B-cell lymphoma, lymph nodes of multiple sites

C85.29   Mediastinal (thymic) large B-cell lymphoma, extranodal and solid organ sites

● **C85.8   Other specified types of non-Hodgkin lymphoma**

C85.80   Other specified types of non-Hodgkin lymphoma, unspecified site

C85.81   Other specified types of non-Hodgkin lymphoma, lymph nodes of head, face, and neck

C85.82   Other specified types of non-Hodgkin lymphoma, intrathoracic lymph nodes

C85.83   Other specified types of non-Hodgkin lymphoma, intra-abdominal lymph nodes

C85.84   Other specified types of non-Hodgkin lymphoma, lymph nodes of axilla and upper limb

C85.85   Other specified types of non-Hodgkin lymphoma, lymph nodes of inguinal region and lower limb

Item 2–7   Lymphosarcoma, also known as malignant lymphoma, is a cancer of the lymph system exhibiting abnormal cells encompassing an entire lymph node creating a diffuse pattern without any definite organization. Diffuse pattern lymphoma has a more unfavorable survival outlook than those with a follicular or nodular pattern. Reticulosarcoma is the most common aggressive form of non-Hodgkin's lymphoma.

C85.86   Other specified types of non-Hodgkin lymphoma, intrapelvic lymph nodes

C85.87   Other specified types of non-Hodgkin lymphoma, spleen

C85.88   Other specified types of non-Hodgkin lymphoma, lymph nodes of multiple sites

C85.89   Other specified types of non-Hodgkin lymphoma, extranodal and solid organ sites

● **C85.9   Non-Hodgkin lymphoma, unspecified**
Lymphoma NOS
Malignant lymphoma NOS
Non-Hodgkin lymphoma NOS

C85.90   Non-Hodgkin lymphoma, unspecified, unspecified site

C85.91   Non-Hodgkin lymphoma, unspecified, lymph nodes of head, face, and neck

C85.92   Non-Hodgkin lymphoma, unspecified, intrathoracic lymph nodes

C85.93   Non-Hodgkin lymphoma, unspecified, intra-abdominal lymph nodes

C85.94   Non-Hodgkin lymphoma, unspecified, lymph nodes of axilla and upper limb

C85.95   Non-Hodgkin lymphoma, unspecified, lymph nodes of inguinal region and lower limb

C85.96   Non-Hodgkin lymphoma, unspecified, intrapelvic lymph nodes

C85.97   Non-Hodgkin lymphoma, unspecified, spleen

C85.98   Non-Hodgkin lymphoma, unspecified, lymph nodes of multiple sites

C85.99   Non-Hodgkin lymphoma, unspecified, extranodal and solid organ sites

● **C86   Other specified types of T/NK-cell lymphoma**

> | Excludes1 | anaplastic large cell lymphoma, ALK negative (C84.7-) |
> | | anaplastic large cell lymphoma, ALK positive (C84.6-) |
> | | mature T/NK-cell lymphomas (C84.-) |
> | | other specified types of non-Hodgkin lymphoma (C85.8-) |

C86.0   Extranodal NK/T-cell lymphoma, nasal type

C86.1   **Hepatosplenic T-cell lymphoma**
Alpha-beta and gamma delta types

C86.2   **Enteropathy-type (intestinal) T-cell lymphoma**
Enteropathy associated T-cell lymphoma

C86.3   **Subcutaneous panniculitis-like T-cell lymphoma**

C86.4   **Blastic NK-cell lymphoma**
▶Blastic plasmacytoid dendritic cell neoplasm (BPDCN)

C86.5   **Angioimmunoblastic T-cell lymphoma**
Angioimmunoblastic lymphadenopathy with dysproteinemia (AILD)

C86.6   **Primary cutaneous CD30-positive T-cell proliferations**
Lymphomatoid papulosis
Primary cutaneous anaplastic large cell lymphoma
Primary cutaneous CD30-positive large T-cell lymphoma

CHAPTER 2 (C00-D49)

● C88 **Malignant immunoproliferative diseases and certain other B-cell lymphomas**
Diseases involving immune system

> **Excludes1** B-cell lymphoma, unspecified (C85.1-)
> personal history of other malignant neoplasms of lymphoid, hematopoietic and related tissues (Z85.79)

C88.0 **Waldenström's macroglobulinemia**
Lymphoplasmacytic lymphoma with IgM-production
Macroglobulinemia (idiopathic) (primary)

> **Excludes1** small cell B-cell lymphoma (C83.0)

C88.2 **Heavy chain disease**
Franklin disease
Gamma heavy chain disease
Mu heavy chain disease

C88.3 **Immunoproliferative small intestinal disease**
Alpha heavy chain disease
Mediterranean lymphoma

C88.4 **Extranodal marginal zone B-cell lymphoma of mucosa-associated lymphoid tissue [MALT-lymphoma]**
Lymphoma of skin-associated lymphoid tissue [SALT-lymphoma]
Lymphoma of bronchial-associated lymphoid tissue [BALT-lymphoma]

> **Excludes1** high malignant (diffuse large B-cell) lymphoma (C83.3-)

C88.8 **Other malignant immunoproliferative diseases**

C88.9 **Malignant immunoproliferative disease, unspecified**
Immunoproliferative disease NOS

● C90 **Multiple myeloma and malignant plasma cell neoplasms**

> **Excludes1** personal history of other malignant neoplasms of lymphoid, hematopoietic and related tissues (Z85.79)

● C90.0 **Multiple myeloma**
Kahler's disease
Medullary plasmacytoma
Myelomatosis
Plasma cell myeloma

> **Excludes1** solitary myeloma (C90.3-)
> solitary plasmacytoma (C90.3-)

C90.00 **Multiple myeloma not having achieved remission**
Multiple myeloma with failed remission
Multiple myeloma NOS

C90.01 **Multiple myeloma in remission**

C90.02 **Multiple myeloma in relapse**

● C90.1 **Plasma cell leukemia**
Rare type of acute leukemia
Plasmacytic leukemia

C90.10 **Plasma cell leukemia not having achieved remission**
Plasma cell leukemia with failed remission
Plasma cell leukemia NOS

C90.11 **Plasma cell leukemia in remission**

C90.12 **Plasma cell leukemia in relapse**

● C90.2 **Extramedullary plasmacytoma**
Malignant monoclonal plasma cell tumor growing in soft tissue; AKA plasma cell dyscrasias

C90.20 **Extramedullary plasmacytoma not having achieved remission**
Extramedullary plasmacytoma with failed remission
Extramedullary plasmacytoma NOS

C90.21 **Extramedullary plasmacytoma in remission**

C90.22 **Extramedullary plasmacytoma in relapse**

● C90.3 **Solitary plasmacytoma**
Localized malignant plasma cell tumor NOS
Plasmacytoma NOS
Solitary myeloma

C90.30 **Solitary plasmacytoma not having achieved remission**
Solitary plasmacytoma with failed remission
Solitary plasmacytoma NOS

C90.31 **Solitary plasmacytoma in remission**

C90.32 **Solitary plasmacytoma in relapse**

● C91 **Lymphoid leukemia**
Type of leukemia affecting circulating cells of lymphoid origin

> **Excludes1** personal history of leukemia (Z85.6)

● C91.0 **Acute lymphoblastic leukemia [ALL]**
> **Note:** Code C91.0 should only be used for T-cell and B-cell precursor leukemia

C91.00 **Acute lymphoblastic leukemia not having achieved remission**
Acute lymphoblastic leukemia with failed remission
Acute lymphoblastic leukemia NOS

C91.01 **Acute lymphoblastic leukemia, in remission**

C91.02 **Acute lymphoblastic leukemia, in relapse**

● C91.1 **Chronic lymphocytic leukemia of B-cell type**
Lymphoplasmacytic leukemia
Richter syndrome

> **Excludes1** lymphoplasmacytic lymphoma (C83.0-)

C91.10 **Chronic lymphocytic leukemia of B-cell type not having achieved remission**
Chronic lymphocytic leukemia of B-cell type with failed remission
Chronic lymphocytic leukemia of B-cell type NOS

C91.11 **Chronic lymphocytic leukemia of B-cell type in remission**

C91.12 **Chronic lymphocytic leukemia of B-cell type in relapse**

● C91.3 **Prolymphocytic leukemia of B-cell type**
Chronic leukemia with symptoms of large number of circulating lymphocytes

C91.30 **Prolymphocytic leukemia of B-cell type not having achieved remission**
Prolymphocytic leukemia of B-cell type with failed remission
Prolymphocytic leukemia of B-cell type NOS

C91.31 **Prolymphocytic leukemia of B-cell type, in remission**

C91.32 **Prolymphocytic leukemia of B-cell type, in relapse**

● C91.4 **Hairy cell leukemia**
Chronic leukemia with splenomegaly and excessive number of abnormal large mononuclear cells covered by hairlike villi
Leukemic reticuloendotheliosis

C91.40 **Hairy cell leukemia not having achieved remission**
Hairy cell leukemia with failed remission
Hairy cell leukemia NOS

C91.41 **Hairy cell leukemia, in remission**

C91.42 **Hairy cell leukemia, in relapse**

Item 2-8 Multiple myeloma is a cancer of a plasma cell (a type of white blood cell) and is an incurable but treatable disease. Immunoproliferative neoplasm is a term for diseases (mostly cancers) in which the immune system cells proliferate.

Item 2-9 Leukemia is a cancer (acute or chronic) of the blood-forming tissues of the bone marrow. Blood cells all start out as stem cells. They mature and become red cells, white cells, or platelets. There are three main types of leukocytes (white cells that fight infection): monocytes, lymphocytes, and granulocytes. **Acute monocytic leukemia** (AML) affects monocytes. **Acute lymphoid leukemia** (ALL) affects lymphocytes, and **acute myeloid leukemia** (AML) affects cells that typically develop into white blood cells (not lymphocytes), though it may develop in other blood cells.

▶ New   ⇒ Revised   ~~deleted~~ Deleted   **OGCR** Official Guidelines   X Assign placeholder X   ● Use Additional Character(s)

| Excludes 1 | Excludes 2 | Includes | Use additional | Code first | Code also | Key words |

- **C91.5 Adult T-cell lymphoma/leukemia (HTLV-1-associated)**
  Acute variant of adult T-cell lymphoma/leukemia (HTLV-1-associated)
  Chronic variant of adult T-cell lymphoma/leukemia (HTLV-1-associated)
  Lymphomatoid variant of adult T-cell lymphoma/leukemia (HTLV-1-associated)
  Smouldering variant of adult T-cell lymphoma/leukemia (HTLV-1-associated)

  C91.50 Adult T-cell lymphoma/leukemia (HTLV-1-associated) not having achieved remission
    Adult T-cell lymphoma/leukemia (HTLV-1-associated) with failed remission
    Adult T-cell lymphoma/leukemia (HTLV-1-associated) NOS

  C91.51 Adult T-cell lymphoma/leukemia (HTLV-1-associated), in remission

  C91.52 Adult T-cell lymphoma/leukemia (HTLV-1-associated), in relapse

- **C91.6 Prolymphocytic leukemia of T-cell type**

  C91.60 Prolymphocytic leukemia of T-cell type not having achieved remission
    Prolymphocytic leukemia of T-cell type with failed remission
    Prolymphocytic leukemia of T-cell type NOS

  C91.61 Prolymphocytic leukemia of T-cell type, in remission

  C91.62 Prolymphocytic leukemia of T-cell type, in relapse

- **C91.A Mature B-cell leukemia Burkitt-type**

Excludes1	Burkitt lymphoma (C83.7-)

  C91.A0 Mature B-cell leukemia Burkitt-type not having achieved remission
    Mature B-cell leukemia Burkitt-type with failed remission
    Mature B-cell leukemia Burkitt-type NOS

  C91.A1 Mature B-cell leukemia Burkitt-type, in remission

  C91.A2 Mature B-cell leukemia Burkitt-type, in relapse

- **C91.Z Other lymphoid leukemia**
  T-cell large granular lymphocytic leukemia (associated with rheumatoid arthritis)

  C91.Z0 Other lymphoid leukemia not having achieved remission
    Other lymphoid leukemia with failed remission
    Other lymphoid leukemia NOS

  C91.Z1 Other lymphoid leukemia, in remission

  C91.Z2 Other lymphoid leukemia, in relapse

- **C91.9 Lymphoid leukemia, unspecified**

  C91.90 Lymphoid leukemia, unspecified not having achieved remission
    Lymphoid leukemia with failed remission
    Lymphoid leukemia NOS

  C91.91 Lymphoid leukemia, unspecified, in remission

  C91.92 Lymphoid leukemia, unspecified, in relapse

- **C92 Myeloid leukemia**

Includes	granulocytic leukemia
	myelogenous leukemia

Excludes1	personal history of leukemia (Z85.6)

- **C92.0 Acute myeloblastic leukemia**
  Acute myeloblastic leukemia, minimal differentiation
  Acute myeloblastic leukemia (with maturation)
  Acute myeloblastic leukemia 1/ETO
  Acute myeloblastic leukemia M0
  Acute myeloblastic leukemia M1
  Acute myeloblastic leukemia M2
  Acute myeloblastic leukemia with t(8;21)
  Acute myeloblastic leukemia (without a FAB classification) NOS
  Refractory anemia with excess blasts in transformation [RAEB T]

Excludes1	acute exacerbation of chronic myeloid leukemia (C92.10)
	refractory anemia with excess of blasts not in transformation (D46.2-)

  C92.00 Acute myeloblastic leukemia, not having achieved remission
    Acute myeloblastic leukemia with failed remission
    Acute myeloblastic leukemia NOS

  C92.01 Acute myeloblastic leukemia, in remission

  C92.02 Acute myeloblastic leukemia, in relapse

- **C92.1 Chronic myeloid leukemia, BCR/ABL-positive**
  Chronic myelogenous leukemia, Philadelphia chromosome (Ph1) positive
  Chronic myelogenous leukemia, t(9;22) (q34;q11)
  Chronic myelogenous leukemia with crisis of blast cells

Excludes1	atypical chronic myeloid leukemia BCR/ABL-negative (C92.2-)
	chronic myelomonocytic leukemia (C93.1-)
	chronic myeloproliferative disease (D47.1)

  C92.10 Chronic myeloid leukemia, BCR/ABL-positive, not having achieved remission
    Chronic myeloid leukemia, BCR/ABL-positive with failed remission
    Chronic myeloid leukemia, BCR/ABL-positive NOS

  C92.11 Chronic myeloid leukemia, BCR/ABL-positive, in remission

  C92.12 Chronic myeloid leukemia, BCR/ABL-positive, in relapse

- **C92.2 Atypical chronic myeloid leukemia, BCR/ABL-negative**

  C92.20 Atypical chronic myeloid leukemia, BCR/ABL-negative, not having achieved remission
    Atypical chronic myeloid leukemia, BCR/ABL-negative with failed remission
    Atypical chronic myeloid leukemia, BCR/ABL-negative NOS

  C92.21 Atypical chronic myeloid leukemia, BCR/ABL-negative, in remission

  C92.22 Atypical chronic myeloid leukemia, BCR/ABL-negative, in relapse

CHAPTER 2 (C00-D49)

CHAPTER 2 (C00-D49)

● **C92.3** **Myeloid sarcoma**
A malignant tumor of immature myeloid cells
Chloroma
Granulocytic sarcoma

  C92.30 **Myeloid sarcoma, not having achieved remission**
Myeloid sarcoma with failed remission
Myeloid sarcoma NOS

  C92.31 **Myeloid sarcoma, in remission**

  C92.32 **Myeloid sarcoma, in relapse**

● **C92.4** **Acute promyelocytic leukemia**
AML M3
AML Me with t(15;17) and variants

  C92.40 **Acute promyelocytic leukemia, not having achieved remission**
Acute promyelocytic leukemia with failed remission
Acute promyelocytic leukemia NOS

  C92.41 **Acute promyelocytic leukemia, in remission**

  C92.42 **Acute promyelocytic leukemia, in relapse**

● **C92.5** **Acute myelomonocytic leukemia**
AML M4
AML M4 Eo with inv(16) or t(16;16)

  C92.50 **Acute myelomonocytic leukemia, not having achieved remission**
Acute myelomonocytic leukemia with failed remission
Acute myelomonocytic leukemia NOS

  C92.51 **Acute myelomonocytic leukemia, in remission**

  C92.52 **Acute myelomonocytic leukemia, in relapse**

● **C92.6** **Acute myeloid leukemia with 11q23-abnormality**
Acute myeloid leukemia with variation of MLL-gene

  C92.60 **Acute myeloid leukemia with 11q23-abnormality not having achieved remission**
Acute myeloid leukemia with 11q23-abnormality with failed remission
Acute myeloid leukemia with 11q23-abnormality NOS

  C92.61 **Acute myeloid leukemia with 11q23-abnormality in remission**

  C92.62 **Acute myeloid leukemia with 11q23-abnormality in relapse**

● **C92.A** **Acute myeloid leukemia with multilineage dysplasia**
Acute myeloid leukemia with dysplasia of remaining hematopoesis and/or myelodysplastic disease in its history

  C92.A0 **Acute myeloid leukemia with multilineage dysplasia, not having achieved remission**
Acute myeloid leukemia with multilineage dysplasia with failed remission
Acute myeloid leukemia with multilineage dysplasia NOS

  C92.A1 **Acute myeloid leukemia with multilineage dysplasia, in remission**

  C92.A2 **Acute myeloid leukemia with multilineage dysplasia, in relapse**

● **C92.Z** **Other myeloid leukemia**

  C92.Z0 **Other myeloid leukemia not having achieved remission**
Myeloid leukemia NEC with failed remission
Myeloid leukemia NEC

  C92.Z1 **Other myeloid leukemia, in remission**

  C92.Z2 **Other myeloid leukemia, in relapse**

● **C92.9** **Myeloid leukemia, unspecified**

  C92.90 **Myeloid leukemia, unspecified, not having achieved remission**
Myeloid leukemia, unspecified with failed remission
Myeloid leukemia, unspecified NOS

  C92.91 **Myeloid leukemia, unspecified in remission**

  C92.92 **Myeloid leukemia, unspecified in relapse**

● **C93** **Monocytic leukemia**
  Includes   monocytoid leukemia
  Excludes1   personal history of leukemia (Z85.6)

● **C93.0** **Acute monoblastic/monocytic leukemia**
AML M5
AML M5a
AML M5b

  C93.00 **Acute monoblastic/monocytic leukemia, not having achieved remission**
Acute monoblastic/monocytic leukemia with failed remission
Acute monoblastic/monocytic leukemia NOS

  C93.01 **Acute monoblastic/monocytic leukemia, in remission**

  C93.02 **Acute monoblastic/monocytic leukemia, in relapse**

● **C93.1** **Chronic myelomonocytic leukemia**
Chronic monocytic leukemia
CMML-1
CMML-2
CMML with eosinophilia

  C93.10 **Chronic myelomonocytic leukemia not having achieved remission**
Chronic myelomonocytic leukemia with failed remission
Chronic myelomonocytic leukemia NOS

  C93.11 **Chronic myelomonocytic leukemia, in remission**

  C93.12 **Chronic myelomonocytic leukemia, in relapse**

● **C93.3** **Juvenile myelomonocytic leukemia**

  C93.30 **Juvenile myelomonocytic leukemia, not having achieved remission**
Juvenile myelomonocytic leukemia with failed remission
Juvenile myelomonocytic leukemia NOS

  C93.31 **Juvenile myelomonocytic leukemia, in remission**

  C93.32 **Juvenile myelomonocytic leukemia, in relapse**

● **C93.Z** **Other monocytic leukemia**

  C93.Z0 **Other monocytic leukemia, not having achieved remission**
Other monocytic leukemia NOS

  C93.Z1 **Other monocytic leukemia, in remission**

  C93.Z2 **Other monocytic leukemia, in relapse**

● **C93.9** **Monocytic leukemia, unspecified**

  C93.90 **Monocytic leukemia, unspecified, not having achieved remission**
Monocytic leukemia, unspecified with failed remission
Monocytic leukemia, unspecified NOS

  C93.91 **Monocytic leukemia, unspecified in remission**

  C93.92 **Monocytic leukemia, unspecified in relapse**

● **C94** **Other leukemias of specified cell type**
  Excludes1   leukemic reticuloendotheliosis (C91.4-)
  myelodysplastic syndromes (D46.-)
  personal history of leukemia (Z85.6)
  plasma cell leukemia (C90.1-)

● **C94.0** **Acute erythroid leukemia**
Acute myeloid leukemia M6(a)(b)
Erythroleukemia

  C94.00 **Acute erythroid leukemia, not having achieved remission**
Acute erythroid leukemia with failed remission
Acute erythroid leukemia NOS

  C94.01 **Acute erythroid leukemia, in remission**

  C94.02 **Acute erythroid leukemia, in relapse**

▶ New   ⇒ Revised   ~~deleted~~ Deleted   **OGCR** Official Guidelines   X Assign placeholder X   ● Use Additional Character(s)

Excludes 1   **Excludes 2**   Includes   Use additional   Code first   Code also   Key words

● C94.2 **Acute megakaryoblastic leukemia**
    Acute myeloid leukemia M7
    Acute megakaryocytic leukemia

    C94.20 **Acute megakaryoblastic leukemia not having achieved remission**
        Acute megakaryoblastic leukemia with failed remission
        Acute megakaryoblastic leukemia NOS

    C94.21 **Acute megakaryoblastic leukemia, in remission**

    C94.22 **Acute megakaryoblastic leukemia, in relapse**

● C94.3 **Mast cell leukemia**

    C94.30 **Mast cell leukemia not having achieved remission**
        Mast cell leukemia with failed remission
        Mast cell leukemia NOS

    C94.31 **Mast cell leukemia, in remission**

    C94.32 **Mast cell leukemia, in relapse**

● C94.4 **Acute panmyelosis with myelofibrosis**
    Acute myelofibrosis

    Excludes1 myelofibrosis NOS (D75.81)
        secondary myelofibrosis NOS (D75.81)

    C94.40 **Acute panmyelosis with myelofibrosis not having achieved remission**
        Acute myelofibrosis NOS
        Acute panmyelosis with myelofibrosis with failed remission
        Acute panmyelosis NOS

    C94.41 **Acute panmyelosis with myelofibrosis, in remission**

    C94.42 **Acute panmyelosis with myelofibrosis, in relapse**

  C94.6 **Myelodysplastic disease, not classified**
    Myeloproliferative disease, not classified

● C94.8 **Other specified leukemias**
    Aggressive NK-cell leukemia
    Acute basophilic leukemia

    C94.80 **Other specified leukemias not having achieved remission**
        Other specified leukemia with failed remission
        Other specified leukemias NOS

    C94.81 **Other specified leukemias, in remission**

    C94.82 **Other specified leukemias, in relapse**

● C95 **Leukemia of unspecified cell type**

    Excludes1 personal history of leukemia (Z85.6)

● C95.0 **Acute leukemia of unspecified cell type**
    Acute bilineal leukemia
    Acute mixed lineage leukemia
    Biphenotypic acute leukemia
    Stem cell leukemia of unclear lineage

    Excludes1 acute exacerbation of unspecified chronic leukemia (C95.10)

    C95.00 **Acute leukemia of unspecified cell type not having achieved remission**
        Acute leukemia of unspecified cell type with failed remission
        Acute leukemia NOS

    C95.01 **Acute leukemia of unspecified cell type, in remission**

    C95.02 **Acute leukemia of unspecified cell type, in relapse**

● C95.1 **Chronic leukemia of unspecified cell type**

    C95.10 **Chronic leukemia of unspecified cell type not having achieved remission**
        Chronic leukemia of unspecified cell type with failed remission
        Chronic leukemia NOS

    C95.11 **Chronic leukemia of unspecified cell type, in remission**

    C95.12 **Chronic leukemia of unspecified cell type, in relapse**

● C95.9 **Leukemia, unspecified**

    C95.90 **Leukemia, unspecified not having achieved remission**
        Leukemia, unspecified with failed remission
        Leukemia NOS

    C95.91 **Leukemia, unspecified, in remission**

    C95.92 **Leukemia, unspecified, in relapse**

● C96 **Other and unspecified malignant neoplasms of lymphoid, hematopoietic and related tissue**

    Excludes1 personal history of other malignant neoplasms of lymphoid, hematopoietic and related tissues (Z85.79)

  C96.0 **Multifocal and multisystemic (disseminated) Langerhans-cell histiocytosis**
    Histiocytosis X, multisystemic
    Letterer-Siwe disease

    Excludes1 adult pulmonary Langerhans cell histiocytosis (J84.82)
        multifocal and unisystemic Langerhans-cell histiocytosis (C96.5)
        unifocal Langerhans-cell histiocytosis (C96.6)

➡● C96.2 **Malignant mast cell neoplasm**
    ~~Aggressive systemic mastocytosis~~
    ~~Mast cell sarcoma~~

    Excludes1 ➡indolent mastocytosis (D47.02)
        mast cell leukemia (C94.30)
        mastocytosis (congenital) (cutaneous) (Q82.2)

    ▶ C96.20 **Malignant mast cell neoplasm, unspecified**

    ▶ C96.21 **Aggressive systemic mastocytosis**

    ▶ C96.22 **Mast cell sarcoma**

    ▶ C96.29 **Other malignant mast cell neoplasm**

  C96.4 **Sarcoma of dendritic cells (accessory cells)**
    Follicular dendritic cell sarcoma
    Interdigitating dendritic cell sarcoma
    Langerhans cell sarcoma

  C96.5 **Multifocal and unisystemic Langerhans-cell histiocytosis**
    Hand-Schüller-Christian disease
    Histiocytosis X, multifocal

    Excludes1 multifocal and multisystemic (disseminated) Langerhans-cell histiocytosis (C96.0)
        unifocal Langerhans-cell histiocytosis (C96.6)

  C96.6 **Unifocal Langerhans-cell histiocytosis**
    Eosinophilic granuloma
    Histiocytosis X, unifocal
    Histiocytosis X NOS
    Langerhans-cell histiocytosis NOS

    Excludes1 multifocal and multisysemic (disseminated) Langerhans-cell histiocytosis (C96.0)
        multifocal and unisystemic Langerhans-cell histiocytosis (C96.5)

  C96.A **Histiocytic sarcoma**
    Malignant histiocytosis

  C96.Z **Other specified malignant neoplasms of lymphoid, hematopoietic and related tissue**

  C96.9 **Malignant neoplasm of lymphoid, hematopoietic and related tissue, unspecified**

CHAPTER 2 (C00-D49)

IN SITU NEOPLASMS (D00-D09)

In situ is carcinoma involving cells in localized tissues that has not spread to nearby tissues

> **Includes**　Bowen's disease
> erythroplasia
> grade III intraepithelial neoplasia
> Queyrat's erythroplasia

● **D00** **Carcinoma in situ of oral cavity, esophagus and stomach**
　　Excludes1　melanoma in situ (D03.-)

● **D00.0** **Carcinoma in situ of lip, oral cavity and pharynx**
　　Use additional code to identify:
　　exposure to environmental tobacco smoke (Z77.22)
　　exposure to tobacco smoke in the perinatal period (P96.81)
　　history of tobacco dependence (Z87.891)
　　occupational exposure to environmental tobacco smoke (Z57.31)
　　tobacco dependence (F17.-)
　　tobacco use (Z72.0)
　　Excludes1　carcinoma in situ of aryepiglottic fold or interarytenoid fold, laryngeal aspect (D02.0)
　　carcinoma in situ of epiglottis NOS (D02.0)
　　carcinoma in situ of epiglottis suprahyoid portion (D02.0)
　　carcinoma in situ of skin of lip (D03.0, D04.0)

　　D00.00 **Carcinoma in situ of oral cavity, unspecified site**
　　D00.01 **Carcinoma in situ of labial mucosa and vermilion border**
　　D00.02 **Carcinoma in situ of buccal mucosa**
　　D00.03 **Carcinoma in situ of gingiva and edentulous alveolar ridge**
　　D00.04 **Carcinoma in situ of soft palate**
　　D00.05 **Carcinoma in situ of hard palate**
　　D00.06 **Carcinoma in situ of floor of mouth**
　　D00.07 **Carcinoma in situ of tongue**
　　D00.08 **Carcinoma in situ of pharynx**
　　　　Carcinoma in situ of aryepiglottic fold NOS
　　　　Carcinoma in situ of hypopharyngeal aspect of aryepiglottic fold
　　　　Carcinoma in situ of marginal zone of aryepiglottic fold

　D00.1 **Carcinoma in situ of esophagus**
　D00.2 **Carcinoma in situ of stomach**

● **D01** **Carcinoma in situ of other and unspecified digestive organs**
　　Excludes1　melanoma in situ (D03.-)

　D01.0 **Carcinoma in situ of colon**
　　Excludes1　carcinoma in situ of rectosigmoid junction (D01.1)

　D01.1 **Carcinoma in situ of rectosigmoid junction**
　D01.2 **Carcinoma in situ of rectum**
　D01.3 **Carcinoma in situ of anus and anal canal**
　　　Anal intraepithelial neoplasia III [AIN III]
　　　Severe dysplasia of anus
　　　Excludes1　anal intraepithelial neoplasia I and II [AIN I and AIN II] (K62.82)
　　　carcinoma in situ of anal margin (D04.5)
　　　carcinoma in situ of anal skin (D04.5)
　　　carcinoma in situ of perianal skin (D04.5)

● **D01.4** **Carcinoma in situ of other and unspecified parts of intestine**
　　Excludes1　carcinoma in situ of ampulla of Vater (D01.5)

　　D01.40 **Carcinoma in situ of unspecified part of intestine**
　　D01.49 **Carcinoma in situ of other parts of intestine**

　D01.5 **Carcinoma in situ of liver, gallbladder and bile ducts**
　　　Carcinoma in situ of ampulla of Vater

　D01.7 **Carcinoma in situ of other specified digestive organs**
　　　Carcinoma in situ of pancreas

　D01.9 **Carcinoma in situ of digestive organ, unspecified**

● **D02** **Carcinoma in situ of middle ear and respiratory system**
　　Use additional code to identify:
　　exposure to environmental tobacco smoke (Z77.22)
　　exposure to tobacco smoke in the perinatal period (P96.81)
　　history of tobacco dependence (Z87.891)
　　occupational exposure to environmental tobacco smoke (Z57.31)
　　tobacco dependence (F17.-)
　　tobacco use (Z72.0)
　　Excludes1　melanoma in situ (D03.-)

　D02.0 **Carcinoma in situ of larynx**
　　　Carcinoma in situ of aryepiglottic fold or interarytenoid fold, laryngeal aspect
　　　Carcinoma in situ of epiglottis (suprahyoid portion)
　　　Excludes1　carcinoma in situ of aryepiglottic fold or interarytenoid fold NOS (D00.08)
　　　carcinoma in situ of hypopharyngeal aspect (D00.08)
　　　carcinoma in situ of marginal zone (D00.08)

　D02.1 **Carcinoma in situ of trachea**
● **D02.2** **Carcinoma in situ of bronchus and lung**
　　D02.20 **Carcinoma in situ of unspecified bronchus and lung**
　　D02.21 **Carcinoma in situ of right bronchus and lung**
　　D02.22 **Carcinoma in situ of left bronchus and lung**
　D02.3 **Carcinoma in situ of other parts of respiratory system**
　　　Carcinoma in situ of accessory sinuses
　　　Carcinoma in situ of middle ear
　　　Carcinoma in situ of nasal cavities
　　　Excludes1　carcinoma in situ of ear (external) (skin) (D04.2-)
　　　carcinoma in situ of nose NOS (D09.8)
　　　carcinoma in situ of skin of nose (D04.3)

　D02.4 **Carcinoma in situ of respiratory system, unspecified**

● **D03** **Melanoma in situ**
　D03.0 **Melanoma in situ of lip**
● **D03.1** **Melanoma in situ of eyelid, including canthus**
　　D03.10 **Melanoma in situ of unspecified eyelid, including canthus**
　　D03.11 **Melanoma in situ of right eyelid, including canthus**
　　D03.12 **Melanoma in situ of left eyelid, including canthus**
● **D03.2** **Melanoma in situ of ear and external auricular canal**
　　D03.20 **Melanoma in situ of unspecified ear and external auricular canal**
　　D03.21 **Melanoma in situ of right ear and external auricular canal**
　　D03.22 **Melanoma in situ of left ear and external auricular canal**

▶ New　⇒ Revised　~~deleted~~ Deleted　**OGCR** Official Guidelines　X Assign placeholder X　● Use Additional Character(s)

Excludes 1　Excludes 2　Includes　Use additional　Code first　Code also　Key words

● **D03.3**   Melanoma in situ of other and unspecified parts of face
     D03.30   Melanoma in situ of unspecified part of face
     D03.39   Melanoma in situ of other parts of face
   D03.4   Melanoma in situ of scalp and neck
● **D03.5**   Melanoma in situ of trunk
     D03.51   Melanoma in situ of anal skin
           Melanoma in situ of anal margin
           Melanoma in situ of perianal skin
     D03.52   Melanoma in situ of breast (skin) (soft tissue)
     D03.59   Melanoma in situ of other part of trunk
● **D03.6**   Melanoma in situ of upper limb, including shoulder
     D03.60   Melanoma in situ of unspecified upper limb, including shoulder
     D03.61   Melanoma in situ of right upper limb, including shoulder
     D03.62   Melanoma in situ of left upper limb, including shoulder
● **D03.7**   Melanoma in situ of lower limb, including hip
     D03.70   Melanoma in situ of unspecified lower limb, including hip
     D03.71   Melanoma in situ of right lower limb, including hip
     D03.72   Melanoma in situ of left lower limb, including hip
   D03.8   Melanoma in situ of other sites
           Melanoma in situ of scrotum
         Excludes1   carcinoma in situ of scrotum (D07.61)
   D03.9   Melanoma in situ, unspecified

● **D04**   Carcinoma in situ of skin
     Excludes1   erythroplasia of Queyrat (penis) NOS (D07.4)
                melanoma in situ (D03.-)
   D04.0   Carcinoma in situ of skin of lip
     Excludes1   carcinoma in situ of vermilion border of lip (D00.01)
● **D04.1**   Carcinoma in situ of skin of eyelid, including canthus
     D04.10   Carcinoma in situ of skin of unspecified eyelid, including canthus
     D04.11   Carcinoma in situ of skin of right eyelid, including canthus
     D04.12   Carcinoma in situ of skin of left eyelid, including canthus
● **D04.2**   Carcinoma in situ of skin of ear and external auricular canal
     D04.20   Carcinoma in situ of skin of unspecified ear and external auricular canal
     D04.21   Carcinoma in situ of skin of right ear and external auricular canal
     D04.22   Carcinoma in situ of skin of left ear and external auricular canal
● **D04.3**   Carcinoma in situ of skin of other and unspecified parts of face
     D04.30   Carcinoma in situ of skin of unspecified part of face
     D04.39   Carcinoma in situ of skin of other parts of face
   D04.4   Carcinoma in situ of skin of scalp and neck
   D04.5   Carcinoma in situ of skin of trunk
           Carcinoma in situ of anal margin
           Carcinoma in situ of anal skin
           Carcinoma in situ of perianal skin
           Carcinoma in situ of skin of breast
         Excludes1   carcinoma in situ of anus NOS (D01.3)
                carcinoma in situ of scrotum (D07.61)
                carcinoma in situ of skin of genital organs (D07.-)

● **D04.6**   Carcinoma in situ of skin of upper limb, including shoulder
     D04.60   Carcinoma in situ of skin of unspecified upper limb, including shoulder
     D04.61   Carcinoma in situ of skin of right upper limb, including shoulder
     D04.62   Carcinoma in situ of skin of left upper limb, including shoulder
● **D04.7**   Carcinoma in situ of skin of lower limb, including hip
     D04.70   Carcinoma in situ of skin of unspecified lower limb, including hip
     D04.71   Carcinoma in situ of skin of right lower limb, including hip
     D04.72   Carcinoma in situ of skin of left lower limb, including hip
   D04.8   Carcinoma in situ of skin of other sites
   D04.9   Carcinoma in situ of skin, unspecified

● **D05**   Carcinoma in situ of breast
     Excludes1   carcinoma in situ of skin of breast (D04.5)
                melanoma in situ of breast (skin) (D03.5)
                Paget's disease of breast or nipple (C50.-)
● **D05.0**   Lobular carcinoma in situ of breast
     D05.00   Lobular carcinoma in situ of unspecified breast
     D05.01   Lobular carcinoma in situ of right breast
     D05.02   Lobular carcinoma in situ of left breast
● **D05.1**   Intraductal carcinoma in situ of breast
     D05.10   Intraductal carcinoma in situ of unspecified breast
     D05.11   Intraductal carcinoma in situ of right breast
     D05.12   Intraductal carcinoma in situ of left breast
● **D05.8**   Other specified type of carcinoma in situ of breast
     D05.80   Other specified type of carcinoma in situ of unspecified breast
     D05.81   Other specified type of carcinoma in situ of right breast
     D05.82   Other specified type of carcinoma in situ of left breast
● **D05.9**   Unspecified type of carcinoma in situ of breast
     D05.90   Unspecified type of carcinoma in situ of unspecified breast
     D05.91   Unspecified type of carcinoma in situ of right breast
     D05.92   Unspecified type of carcinoma in situ of left breast

● **D06**   Carcinoma in situ of cervix uteri
     Includes   cervical adenocarcinoma in situ
                cervical intraepithelial glandular neoplasia
                cervical intraepithelial neoplasia III [CIN III]
                severe dysplasia of cervix uteri
     Excludes1   cervical intraepithelial neoplasia II [CIN II] (N87.1)
                cytologic evidence of malignancy of cervix without histologic confirmation (R87.614)
                high grade squamous intraepithelial lesion (HGSIL) of cervix (R87.613)
                melanoma in situ of cervix (D03.5)
                moderate cervical dysplasia (N87.1)
   D06.0   Carcinoma in situ of endocervix
   D06.1   Carcinoma in situ of exocervix
   D06.7   Carcinoma in situ of other parts of cervix
   D06.9   Carcinoma in situ of cervix, unspecified

CHAPTER 2 (C00-D49)

● **D07** Carcinoma in situ of other and unspecified genital organs
> **Excludes1** melanoma in situ of trunk (D03.5)

D07.0 Carcinoma in situ of endometrium

D07.1 Carcinoma in situ of vulva
Severe dysplasia of vulva
Vulvar intraepithelial neoplasia III [VIN III]
> **Excludes1** moderate dysplasia of vulva (N90.1)
> vulvar intraepithelial neoplasia II [VIN II] (N90.1)

D07.2 Carcinoma in situ of vagina
Severe dysplasia of vagina
Vaginal intraepithelial neoplasia III [VIN III]
> **Excludes1** moderate dysplasia of vagina (N89.1)
> vaginal intraepithelial neoplasia II [VIN II] (N89.1)

● **D07.3** Carcinoma in situ of other and unspecified female genital organs

    D07.30 Carcinoma in situ of unspecified female genital organs

    D07.39 Carcinoma in situ of other female genital organs

D07.4 Carcinoma in situ of penis
Erythroplasia of Queyrat NOS

D07.5 Carcinoma in situ of prostate
Prostatic intraepithelial neoplasia III (PIN III)
Severe dysplasia of prostate
> **Excludes1** dysplasia (mild) (moderate) of prostate (N42.3-)
> prostatic intraepithelial neoplasia II [PIN II] (N42.3-)

● **D07.6** Carcinoma in situ of other and unspecified male genital organs

    D07.60 Carcinoma in situ of unspecified male genital organs

    D07.61 Carcinoma in situ of scrotum

    D07.69 Carcinoma in situ of other male genital organs

● **D09** Carcinoma in situ of other and unspecified sites
> **Excludes1** melanoma in situ (D03.-)

D09.0 Carcinoma in situ of bladder

● **D09.1** Carcinoma in situ of other and unspecified urinary organs

    D09.10 Carcinoma in situ of unspecified urinary organ

    D09.19 Carcinoma in situ of other urinary organs

● **D09.2** Carcinoma in situ of eye
> **Excludes1** carcinoma in situ of skin of eyelid (D04.1-)

    D09.20 Carcinoma in situ of unspecified eye

    D09.21 Carcinoma in situ of right eye

    D09.22 Carcinoma in situ of left eye

D09.3 Carcinoma in situ of thyroid and other endocrine glands
> **Excludes1** carcinoma in situ of endocrine pancreas (D01.7)
> carcinoma in situ of ovary (D07.39)
> carcinoma in situ of testis (D07.69)

D09.8 Carcinoma in situ of other specified sites

D09.9 Carcinoma in situ, unspecified

BENIGN NEOPLASMS, EXCEPT BENIGN NEUROENDOCRINE TUMORS (D10-D36)

● **D10** Benign neoplasm of mouth and pharynx

D10.0 Benign neoplasm of lip
Benign neoplasm of lip (frenulum) (inner aspect) (mucosa) (vermilion border)
> **Excludes1** benign neoplasm of skin of lip (D22.0, D23.0)

D10.1 Benign neoplasm of tongue
Benign neoplasm of lingual tonsil

D10.2 Benign neoplasm of floor of mouth

● **D10.3** Benign neoplasm of other and unspecified parts of mouth

    D10.30 Benign neoplasm of unspecified part of mouth

    D10.39 Benign neoplasm of other parts of mouth
    Benign neoplasm of minor salivary gland NOS
> **Excludes1** benign odontogenic neoplasms (D16.4-D16.5)
> benign neoplasm of mucosa of lip (D10.0)
> benign neoplasm of nasopharyngeal surface of soft palate (D10.6)

D10.4 Benign neoplasm of tonsil
Benign neoplasm of tonsil (faucial) (palatine)
> **Excludes1** benign neoplasm of lingual tonsil (D10.1)
> benign neoplasm of pharyngeal tonsil (D10.6)
> benign neoplasm of tonsillar fossa (D10.5)
> benign neoplasm of tonsillar pillars (D10.5)

D10.5 Benign neoplasm of other parts of oropharynx
Division of pharynx lying between soft palate and upper edge of epiglottis
Benign neoplasm of epiglottis, anterior aspect
Benign neoplasm of tonsillar fossa
Benign neoplasm of tonsillar pillars
Benign neoplasm of vallecula
> **Excludes1** benign neoplasm of epiglottis NOS (D14.1)
> benign neoplasm of epiglottis, suprahyoid portion (D14.1)

D10.6 Benign neoplasm of nasopharynx
Segment of pharynx that lies above soft palate
Benign neoplasm of pharyngeal tonsil
Benign neoplasm of posterior margin of septum and choanae

D10.7 Benign neoplasm of hypopharynx
Segment of pharynx that lies below upper edge of epiglottis and opens into larynx and esophagus

D10.9 Benign neoplasm of pharynx, unspecified

Figure 2-16 The esophagus is the muscular tube that connects the pharynx and the stomach. The 10 inch (25 cm) long esophagus is divided into three parts: **cervical, thoracic,** and **abdominal.**

▶ New   ⇒ Revised   ~~deleted~~ Deleted   **OGCR** Official Guidelines   X Assign placeholder X   ● Use Additional Character(s)

Excludes 1   Excludes 2   Includes   Use additional   Code first   Code also   Key words

● **D11**   **Benign neoplasm of major salivary glands**

> **Excludes1**   benign neoplasms of specified minor salivary glands which are classified according to their anatomical location
> benign neoplasms of minor salivary glands NOS (D10.39)

D11.0   **Benign neoplasm of parotid gland**

D11.7   **Benign neoplasm of other major salivary glands**
Benign neoplasm of sublingual salivary gland
Benign neoplasm of submandibular salivary gland

D11.9   **Benign neoplasm of major salivary gland, unspecified**

● **D12**   **Benign neoplasm of colon, rectum, anus and anal canal**

> **Excludes1**   benign carcinoid tumors of the large intestine, and rectum (D3A.02-)

D12.0   **Benign neoplasm of cecum**
Benign neoplasm of ileocecal valve

D12.1   **Benign neoplasm of appendix**

> **Excludes1**   benign carcinoid tumor of the appendix (D3A.020)

D12.2   **Benign neoplasm of ascending colon**

D12.3   **Benign neoplasm of transverse colon**
Benign neoplasm of hepatic flexure
Benign neoplasm of splenic flexure
Flexure is a bending in a structure or organ. Note the three flexures illustrated in Figure 2–17. Hepatic = liver, sigmoid = colon, splenic = spleen.

D12.4   **Benign neoplasm of descending colon**

D12.5   **Benign neoplasm of sigmoid colon**

D12.6   **Benign neoplasm of colon, unspecified**
Adenomatosis of colon
Benign neoplasm of large intestine NOS
Polyposis (hereditary) of colon

> **Excludes1**   inflammatory polyp of colon (K51.4-)
> polyp of colon NOS (K63.5)

D12.7   **Benign neoplasm of rectosigmoid junction**
Angle where sigmoid colon becomes rectum

D12.8   **Benign neoplasm of rectum**

> **Excludes1**   benign carcinoid tumor of the rectum (D3A.026)

D12.9   **Benign neoplasm of anus and anal canal**
Benign neoplasm of anus NOS

> **Excludes1**   benign neoplasm of anal margin (D22.5, D23.5)
> benign neoplasm of anal skin (D22.5, D23.5)
> benign neoplasm of perianal skin (D22.5, D23.5)

● **D13**   **Benign neoplasm of other and ill-defined parts of digestive system**

> **Excludes1**   benign stromal tumors of digestive system (D21.4)

D13.0   **Benign neoplasm of esophagus**

D13.1   **Benign neoplasm of stomach**

> **Excludes1**   benign carcinoid tumor of the stomach (D3A.092)

D13.2   **Benign neoplasm of duodenum**

> **Excludes1**   benign carcinoid tumor of the duodenum (D3A.010)

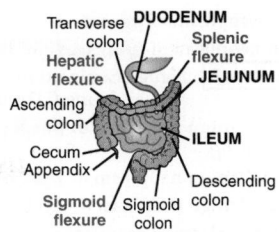

Figure 2-17   Small intestine and colon.

● **D13.3**   **Benign neoplasm of other and unspecified parts of small intestine**

> **Excludes1**   benign carcinoid tumors of the small intestine (D3A.01-)
> benign neoplasm of ileocecal valve (D12.0)

D13.30   **Benign neoplasm of unspecified part of small intestine**

D13.39   **Benign neoplasm of other parts of small intestine**

D13.4   **Benign neoplasm of liver**
Benign neoplasm of intrahepatic bile ducts

D13.5   **Benign neoplasm of extrahepatic bile ducts**
Extensions of common hepatic bile duct (tube that collects bile from liver)

D13.6   **Benign neoplasm of pancreas**

> **Excludes1**   benign neoplasm of endocrine pancreas (D13.7)

D13.7   **Benign neoplasm of endocrine pancreas**
Pancreatic islets: Cells scattered throughout pancreas
Islet cell tumor
Benign neoplasm of islets of Langerhans
Use additional code to identify any functional activity.

D13.9   **Benign neoplasm of ill-defined sites within the digestive system**
Benign neoplasm of digestive system NOS
Benign neoplasm of intestine NOS
Benign neoplasm of spleen

● **D14**   **Benign neoplasm of middle ear and respiratory system**

D14.0   **Benign neoplasm of middle ear, nasal cavity and accessory sinuses**
Benign neoplasm of cartilage of nose

> **Excludes1**   benign neoplasm of auricular canal (external) (D22.2-, D23.2-)
> benign neoplasm of bone of ear (D16.4)
> benign neoplasm of bone of nose (D16.4)
> benign neoplasm of cartilage of ear (D21.0)
> benign neoplasm of ear (external) (skin) (D22.2-, D23.2-)
> benign neoplasm of nose NOS (D36.7)
> benign neoplasm of skin of nose (D22.39, D23.39)
> benign neoplasm of olfactory bulb (D33.3)
> benign neoplasm of posterior margin of septum and choanae (D10.6)
> polyp of accessory sinus (J33.8)
> polyp of ear (middle) (H74.4)
> polyp of nasal (cavity) (J33.-)

D14.1   **Benign neoplasm of larynx**
Adenomatous polyp of larynx
Benign neoplasm of epiglottis (suprahyoid portion)
Horseshoe shaped bone in anterior midline of neck between chin and thyroid cartilage

> **Excludes1**   benign neoplasm of epiglottis, anterior aspect (D10.5)
> polyp (nonadenomatous) of vocal cord or larynx (J38.1)

CHAPTER 2 (C00-D49)

D14.2   Benign neoplasm of trachea

● D14.3   Benign neoplasm of bronchus and lung

     Excludes1   benign carcinoid tumor of the bronchus and lung (D3A.090)

     D14.30   Benign neoplasm of unspecified bronchus and lung

     D14.31   Benign neoplasm of right bronchus and lung

     D14.32   Benign neoplasm of left bronchus and lung

D14.4   Benign neoplasm of respiratory system, unspecified

● D15   Benign neoplasm of other and unspecified intrathoracic organs

     Excludes1   benign neoplasm of mesothelial tissue (D19.-)

D15.0   Benign neoplasm of thymus

     Excludes1   benign carcinoid tumor of the thymus (D3A.091)

D15.1   Benign neoplasm of heart

     Excludes1   benign neoplasm of great vessels (D21.3)

D15.2   Benign neoplasm of mediastinum

D15.7   Benign neoplasm of other specified intrathoracic organs

D15.9   Benign neoplasm of intrathoracic organ, unspecified

● D16   Benign neoplasm of bone and articular cartilage

     Excludes1   benign neoplasm of connective tissue of ear (D21.0)

                  benign neoplasm of connective tissue of eyelid (D21.0)

                  benign neoplasm of connective tissue of larynx (D14.1)

                  benign neoplasm of connective tissue of nose (D14.0)

                  benign neoplasm of synovia (D21.-)

● D16.0   Benign neoplasm of scapula and long bones of upper limb

     D16.00   Benign neoplasm of scapula and long bones of unspecified upper limb

     D16.01   Benign neoplasm of scapula and long bones of right upper limb

     D16.02   Benign neoplasm of scapula and long bones of left upper limb

● D16.1   Benign neoplasm of short bones of upper limb

     D16.10   Benign neoplasm of short bones of unspecified upper limb

     D16.11   Benign neoplasm of short bones of right upper limb

     D16.12   Benign neoplasm of short bones of left upper limb

● D16.2   Benign neoplasm of long bones of lower limb

     D16.20   Benign neoplasm of long bones of unspecified lower limb

     D16.21   Benign neoplasm of long bones of right lower limb

     D16.22   Benign neoplasm of long bones of left lower limb

● D16.3   Benign neoplasm of short bones of lower limb

     D16.30   Benign neoplasm of short bones of unspecified lower limb

     D16.31   Benign neoplasm of short bones of right lower limb

     D16.32   Benign neoplasm of short bones of left lower limb

D16.4   Benign neoplasm of bones of skull and face

     Benign neoplasm of maxilla (superior)

     Benign neoplasm of orbital bone

     Cavity or socket of skull in which eye and its appendages are located

     Keratocyst of maxilla

     Keratocystic odontogenic tumor of maxilla

     Excludes2   benign neoplasm of lower jaw bone (D16.5)

D16.5   Benign neoplasm of lower jaw bone

     Keratocyst of mandible

     Keratocystic odontogenic tumor of mandible

D16.6   Benign neoplasm of vertebral column

     Excludes1   benign neoplasm of sacrum and coccyx (D16.8)

D16.7   Benign neoplasm of ribs, sternum and clavicle

D16.8   Benign neoplasm of pelvic bones, sacrum and coccyx

D16.9   Benign neoplasm of bone and articular cartilage, unspecified

● D17   Benign lipomatous neoplasm

     Slow-growing benign tumors (rubbery masses) of mature fat cells enclosed in a thin fibrous capsule

D17.0   Benign lipomatous neoplasm of skin and subcutaneous tissue of head, face and neck

D17.1   Benign lipomatous neoplasm of skin and subcutaneous tissue of trunk

● D17.2   Benign lipomatous neoplasm of skin and subcutaneous tissue of limb

     D17.20   Benign lipomatous neoplasm of skin and subcutaneous tissue of unspecified limb

     D17.21   Benign lipomatous neoplasm of skin and subcutaneous tissue of right arm

     D17.22   Benign lipomatous neoplasm of skin and subcutaneous tissue of left arm

     D17.23   Benign lipomatous neoplasm of skin and subcutaneous tissue of right leg

     D17.24   Benign lipomatous neoplasm of skin and subcutaneous tissue of left leg

● D17.3   Benign lipomatous neoplasm of skin and subcutaneous tissue of other and unspecified sites

     D17.30   Benign lipomatous neoplasm of skin and subcutaneous tissue of unspecified sites

     D17.39   Benign lipomatous neoplasm of skin and subcutaneous tissue of other sites

D17.4   Benign lipomatous neoplasm of intrathoracic organs

D17.5   Benign lipomatous neoplasm of intra-abdominal organs

     Excludes1   benign lipomatous neoplasm of peritoneum and retroperitoneum (D17.79)

D17.6   Benign lipomatous neoplasm of spermatic cord

● D17.7   Benign lipomatous neoplasm of other sites

     D17.71   Benign lipomatous neoplasm of kidney

     D17.72   Benign lipomatous neoplasm of other genitourinary organ

     D17.79   Benign lipomatous neoplasm of other sites

                  Benign lipomatous neoplasm of peritoneum

                  Benign lipomatous neoplasm of retroperitoneum

D17.9   Benign lipomatous neoplasm, unspecified

     Lipoma NOS

Figure 2-18 Hemangioma of skin and subcutaneous tissue. (Getty Image)

Item 2–10 Hemangiomas are abnormally dense collections of dilated capillaries that occur on the skin or in internal organs. Hemangiomas are both deep and superficial and undergo a rapid growth phase when the size increases rapidly, followed by a rest phase, in which the tumor changes very little, followed by an involutional phase in which the tumor begins to and can disappear altogether. **Lymphangiomas** or cystic hygroma are benign collections of overgrown lymph vessels and, although rare, may occur anywhere but most commonly on the head and neck of children and infants. Visceral organs, lungs, and gastrointestinal tract may also be involved.

● **D18   Hemangioma and lymphangioma, any site**
> **Excludes1**   benign neoplasm of glomus jugulare (D35.6)
> blue or pigmented nevus (D22.-)
> nevus NOS (D22.-)
> vascular nevus (Q82.5)

● **D18.0   Hemangioma**
> *Common type of vascular malformation*
> Angioma NOS
> Cavernous nevus

> **D18.00   Hemangioma unspecified site**

> **D18.01   Hemangioma of skin and subcutaneous tissue**

> **D18.02   Hemangioma of intracranial structures**

> **D18.03   Hemangioma of intra-abdominal structures**

> **D18.09   Hemangioma of other sites**

> **D18.1   Lymphangioma, any site**

● **D19   Benign neoplasm of mesothelial tissue**
> *Mesothelial tissue is the membrane lining several body cavities*

> **D19.0   Benign neoplasm of mesothelial tissue of pleura**

> **D19.1   Benign neoplasm of mesothelial tissue of peritoneum**

> **D19.7   Benign neoplasm of mesothelial tissue of other sites**

> **D19.9   Benign neoplasm of mesothelial tissue, unspecified**
> Benign mesothelioma NOS

● **D20   Benign neoplasm of soft tissue of retroperitoneum and peritoneum**
> **Excludes1**   benign lipomatous neoplasm of peritoneum and retroperitoneum (D17.79)
> benign neoplasm of mesothelial tissue (D19.-)

> **D20.0   Benign neoplasm of soft tissue of retroperitoneum**

> **D20.1   Benign neoplasm of soft tissue of peritoneum**

● **D21   Other benign neoplasms of connective and other soft tissue**
> **Includes**   benign neoplasm of blood vessel
> benign neoplasm of bursa
> benign neoplasm of cartilage
> benign neoplasm of fascia
> benign neoplasm of fat
> benign neoplasm of ligament, except uterine
> benign neoplasm of lymphatic channel
> benign neoplasm of muscle
> benign neoplasm of synovia
> benign neoplasm of tendon (sheath)
> benign stromal tumors

> **Excludes1**   benign neoplasm of articular cartilage (D16.-)
> benign neoplasm of cartilage of larynx (D14.1)
> benign neoplasm of cartilage of nose (D14.0)
> benign neoplasm of connective tissue of breast (D24.-)
> benign neoplasm of peripheral nerves and autonomic nervous system (D36.1-)
> benign neoplasm of peritoneum (D20.1)
> benign neoplasm of retroperitoneum (D20.0)
> benign neoplasm of uterine ligament, any (D28.2)
> benign neoplasm of vascular tissue (D18.-)
> hemangioma (D18.0-)
> lipomatous neoplasm (D17.-)
> lymphangioma (D18.1)
> uterine leiomyoma (D25.-)

> **D21.0   Benign neoplasm of connective and other soft tissue of head, face and neck**
> Benign neoplasm of connective tissue of ear
> Benign neoplasm of connective tissue of eyelid
>> **Excludes1**   benign neoplasm of connective tissue of orbit (D31.6-)

● **D21.1   Benign neoplasm of connective and other soft tissue of upper limb, including shoulder**

> **D21.10   Benign neoplasm of connective and other soft tissue of unspecified upper limb, including shoulder**

> **D21.11   Benign neoplasm of connective and other soft tissue of right upper limb, including shoulder**

> **D21.12   Benign neoplasm of connective and other soft tissue of left upper limb, including shoulder**

● **D21.2   Benign neoplasm of connective and other soft tissue of lower limb, including hip**

> **D21.20   Benign neoplasm of connective and other soft tissue of unspecified lower limb, including hip**

> **D21.21   Benign neoplasm of connective and other soft tissue of right lower limb, including hip**

> **D21.22   Benign neoplasm of connective and other soft tissue of left lower limb, including hip**

> **D21.3   Benign neoplasm of connective and other soft tissue of thorax**
> Benign neoplasm of axilla
> Benign neoplasm of diaphragm
> Benign neoplasm of great vessels
>> **Excludes1**   benign neoplasm of heart (D15.1)
>> benign neoplasm of mediastinum (D15.2)
>> benign neoplasm of thymus (D15.0)

> **D21.4   Benign neoplasm of connective and other soft tissue of abdomen**
> Benign stromal tumors of abdomen

> **D21.5   Benign neoplasm of connective and other soft tissue of pelvis**
>> **Excludes1**   benign neoplasm of any uterine ligament (D28.2)
>> uterine leiomyoma (D25.-)

> **D21.6   Benign neoplasm of connective and other soft tissue of trunk, unspecified**
> Benign neoplasm of back NOS

> **D21.9   Benign neoplasm of connective and other soft tissue, unspecified**

▶ New   ⇒ Revised   ~~deleted~~ Deleted   **OGCR** Official Guidelines   X Assign placeholder X   ● Use Additional Character(s)

| Excludes 1 | Excludes 2 | Includes | Use additional | Code first | Code also | Key words |

● **D22 Melanocytic nevi**

> **Includes**   atypical nevus
> blue hairy pigmented nevus
> nevus NOS

D22.0 Melanocytic nevi of lip
Skin lesions composed of nests of nevus cells with macules/ papules

● **D22.1 Melanocytic nevi of eyelid, including canthus**

D22.10 Melanocytic nevi of unspecified eyelid, including canthus

D22.11 Melanocytic nevi of right eyelid, including canthus

D22.12 Melanocytic nevi of left eyelid, including canthus

● **D22.2 Melanocytic nevi of ear and external auricular canal**

D22.20 Melanocytic nevi of unspecified ear and external auricular canal

D22.21 Melanocytic nevi of right ear and external auricular canal

D22.22 Melanocytic nevi of left ear and external auricular canal

● **D22.3 Melanocytic nevi of other and unspecified parts of face**

D22.30 Melanocytic nevi of unspecified part of face

D22.39 Melanocytic nevi of other parts of face

D22.4 Melanocytic nevi of scalp and neck

D22.5 Melanocytic nevi of trunk
Melanocytic nevi of anal margin
Melanocytic nevi of anal skin
Melanocytic nevi of perianal skin
Melanocytic nevi of skin of breast

● **D22.6 Melanocytic nevi of upper limb, including shoulder**

D22.60 Melanocytic nevi of unspecified upper limb, including shoulder

D22.61 Melanocytic nevi of right upper limb, including shoulder

D22.62 Melanocytic nevi of left upper limb, including shoulder

● **D22.7 Melanocytic nevi of lower limb, including hip**

D22.70 Melanocytic nevi of unspecified lower limb, including hip

D22.71 Melanocytic nevi of right lower limb, including hip

D22.72 Melanocytic nevi of left lower limb, including hip

D22.9 Melanocytic nevi, unspecified

● **D23 Other benign neoplasms of skin**

> **Includes**   benign neoplasm of hair follicles
> benign neoplasm of sebaceous glands
> benign neoplasm of sweat glands

> **Excludes1**   benign lipomatous neoplasms of skin (D17.0-D17.3)
> melanocytic nevi (D22.-)

D23.0 Other benign neoplasm of skin of lip

> **Excludes1**   benign neoplasm of vermilion border of lip (D10.0)

● **D23.1 Other benign neoplasm of skin of eyelid, including canthus**

D23.10 Other benign neoplasm of skin unspecified of eyelid, including canthus

D23.11 Other benign neoplasm of skin of right eyelid, including canthus

D23.12 Other benign neoplasm of skin of left eyelid, including canthus

● **D23.2 Other benign neoplasm of skin of ear and external auricular canal**

D23.20 Other benign neoplasm of skin of unspecified ear and external auricular canal

D23.21 Other benign neoplasm of skin of right ear and external auricular canal

D23.22 Other benign neoplasm of skin of left ear and external auricular canal

● **D23.3 Other benign neoplasm of skin of other and unspecified parts of face**

D23.30 Other benign neoplasm of skin of unspecified part of face

D23.39 Other benign neoplasm of skin of other parts of face

D23.4 Other benign neoplasm of skin of scalp and neck

D23.5 Other benign neoplasm of skin of trunk
Other benign neoplasm of anal margin
Other benign neoplasm of anal skin
Other benign neoplasm of perianal skin
Other benign neoplasm of skin of breast

> **Excludes1**   benign neoplasm of anus NOS (D12.9)

● **D23.6 Other benign neoplasm of skin of upper limb, including shoulder**

D23.60 Other benign neoplasm of skin of unspecified upper limb, including shoulder

D23.61 Other benign neoplasm of skin of right upper limb, including shoulder

D23.62 Other benign neoplasm of skin of left upper limb, including shoulder

● **D23.7 Other benign neoplasm of skin of lower limb, including hip**

D23.70 Other benign neoplasm of skin of unspecified lower limb, including hip

D23.71 Other benign neoplasm of skin of right lower limb, including hip

D23.72 Other benign neoplasm of skin of left lower limb, including hip

D23.9 Other benign neoplasm of skin, unspecified

● **D24 Benign neoplasm of breast**

> **Includes**   benign neoplasm of connective tissue of breast
> benign neoplasm of soft parts of breast
> fibroadenoma of breast

> **Excludes2**   adenofibrosis of breast (N60.2)
> benign cyst of breast (N60.-)
> benign mammary dysplasia (N60.-)
> benign neoplasm of skin of breast (D22.5, D23.5)
> fibrocystic disease of breast (N60.-)

D24.1 Benign neoplasm of right breast

D24.2 Benign neoplasm of left breast

D24.9 Benign neoplasm of unspecified breast

● **D25 Leiomyoma of uterus**
Benign tumors or nodules of the uterine wall

> **Includes**   uterine fibroid
> uterine fibromyoma
> uterine myoma

D25.0 Submucous leiomyoma of uterus

D25.1 Intramural leiomyoma of uterus
Interstitial leiomyoma of uterus

D25.2 Subserosal leiomyoma of uterus
Subperitoneal leiomyoma of uterus

D25.9 Leiomyoma of uterus, unspecified

▶ New   ⇨ Revised   ~~deleted~~ Deleted   **OGCR** Official Guidelines   X Assign placeholder X   ● Use Additional Character(s)
Excludes 1   Excludes 2   Includes   Use additional   Code first   Code also   Key words

● **D26**   Other benign neoplasms of uterus

     D26.0   Other benign neoplasm of cervix uteri

     D26.1   Other benign neoplasm of corpus uteri

     D26.7   Other benign neoplasm of other parts of uterus

     D26.9   Other benign neoplasm of uterus, unspecified

● **D27**   Benign neoplasm of ovary

     Use additional code to identify any functional activity.

     Excludes2   corpus albicans cyst (N83.2-)
                     corpus luteum cyst (N83.1-)
                     endometrial cyst (N80.1)
                     follicular (atretic) cyst (N83.0-)
                     graafian follicle cyst (N83.0-)
                     ovarian cyst NEC (N83.2-)
                     ovarian retention cyst (N83.2-)

     D27.0   Benign neoplasm of right ovary

     D27.1   Benign neoplasm of left ovary

     D27.9   Benign neoplasm of unspecified ovary
              Ovarian teratoma

● **D28**   Benign neoplasm of other and unspecified female genital organs

     Includes   adenomatous polyp
                  benign neoplasm of skin of female genital organs
                  benign teratoma

     Excludes1   epoophoron cyst (Q50.5)
                    fimbrial cyst (Q50.4)
                    Gartner's duct cyst (Q52.4)
                    parovarian cyst (Q50.5)

     D28.0   Benign neoplasm of vulva

     D28.1   Benign neoplasm of vagina

     D28.2   Benign neoplasm of uterine tubes and ligaments
              Benign neoplasm of fallopian tube
              Benign neoplasm of uterine ligament (broad) (round)

     D28.7   Benign neoplasm of other specified female genital organs

     D28.9   Benign neoplasm of female genital organ, unspecified

● **D29**   Benign neoplasm of male genital organs

     Includes   benign neoplasm of skin of male genital organs

     D29.0   Benign neoplasm of penis

     D29.1   Benign neoplasm of prostate

         Excludes1   enlarged prostate (N40.-)

●   D29.2   Benign neoplasm of testis

         Use additional code to identify any functional activity.

         D29.20   Benign neoplasm of unspecified testis

         D29.21   Benign neoplasm of right testis

         D29.22   Benign neoplasm of left testis

●   D29.3   Benign neoplasm of epididymis

         D29.30   Benign neoplasm of unspecified epididymis

         D29.31   Benign neoplasm of right epididymis

         D29.32   Benign neoplasm of left epididymis

     D29.4   Benign neoplasm of scrotum
              Benign neoplasm of skin of scrotum

     D29.8   Benign neoplasm of other specified male genital organs
              Benign neoplasm of seminal vesicle
              Benign neoplasm of spermatic cord
              Benign neoplasm of tunica vaginalis

     D29.9   Benign neoplasm of male genital organ, unspecified

● **D30**   Benign neoplasm of urinary organs

●   D30.0   Benign neoplasm of kidney

         Excludes1   benign carcinoid tumor of the kidney (D3A.093)
                     benign neoplasm of renal calyces (D30.1-)
                     benign neoplasm of renal pelvis (D30.1-)

         D30.00   Benign neoplasm of unspecified kidney

         D30.01   Benign neoplasm of right kidney

         D30.02   Benign neoplasm of left kidney

●   D30.1   Benign neoplasm of renal pelvis

         D30.10   Benign neoplasm of unspecified renal pelvis

         D30.11   Benign neoplasm of right renal pelvis

         D30.12   Benign neoplasm of left renal pelvis

●   D30.2   Benign neoplasm of ureter

         Excludes1   benign neoplasm of ureteric orifice of bladder (D30.3)

         D30.20   Benign neoplasm of unspecified ureter

         D30.21   Benign neoplasm of right ureter

         D30.22   Benign neoplasm of left ureter

     D30.3   Benign neoplasm of bladder
              Benign neoplasm of ureteric orifice of bladder
              Benign neoplasm of urethral orifice of bladder

     D30.4   Benign neoplasm of urethra

         Excludes1   benign neoplasm of urethral orifice of bladder (D30.3)

     D30.8   Benign neoplasm of other specified urinary organs
              Benign neoplasm of paraurethral glands

     D30.9   Benign neoplasm of urinary organ, unspecified
              Benign neoplasm of urinary system NOS

● **D31**   Benign neoplasm of eye and adnexa

     Excludes1   benign neoplasm of connective tissue of eyelid (D21.0)
                  benign neoplasm of optic nerve (D33.3)
                  benign neoplasm of skin of eyelid (D22.1-, D23.1-)

●   D31.0   Benign neoplasm of conjunctiva

         D31.00   Benign neoplasm of unspecified conjunctiva

         D31.01   Benign neoplasm of right conjunctiva

         D31.02   Benign neoplasm of left conjunctiva

●   D31.1   Benign neoplasm of cornea

         D31.10   Benign neoplasm of unspecified cornea

         D31.11   Benign neoplasm of right cornea

         D31.12   Benign neoplasm of left cornea

●   D31.2   Benign neoplasm of retina

         Excludes1   dark area on retina (D49.81)
                  hemangioma of retina (D49.81)
                  neoplasm of unspecified behavior of retina and choroid (D49.81)
                  retinal freckle (D49.81)

         D31.20   Benign neoplasm of unspecified retina

         D31.21   Benign neoplasm of right retina

         D31.22   Benign neoplasm of left retina

●   D31.3   Benign neoplasm of choroid

         D31.30   Benign neoplasm of unspecified choroid

         D31.31   Benign neoplasm of right choroid

         D31.32   Benign neoplasm of left choroid

●   D31.4   Benign neoplasm of ciliary body

         D31.40   Benign neoplasm of unspecified ciliary body

         D31.41   Benign neoplasm of right ciliary body

         D31.42   Benign neoplasm of left ciliary body

●   D31.5   Benign neoplasm of lacrimal gland and duct
              Benign neoplasm of lacrimal sac
              Benign neoplasm of nasolacrimal duct

         D31.50   Benign neoplasm of unspecified lacrimal gland and duct

         D31.51   Benign neoplasm of right lacrimal gland and duct

         D31.52   Benign neoplasm of left lacrimal gland and duct

---

Item 2-11   Teratoma: terat = monster, oma = mass, tumor. Alternate terms: dermoid cyst of the ovary, ovarian teratoma. Teratomas are neoplasms and arise from germ cells (ovaries in female and testes in male) and can be benign or malignant. Teratomas have been known to contain hair, nails, and teeth, giving them a bizarre ("monster") appearance.

● **D31.6** **Benign neoplasm of unspecified site of orbit**
Benign neoplasm of connective tissue of orbit
Benign neoplasm of extraocular muscle
Benign neoplasm of peripheral nerves of orbit
Benign neoplasm of retrobulbar tissue
Benign neoplasm of retro-ocular tissue
> **Excludes1**   benign neoplasm of orbital bone (D16.4)

     D31.60 **Benign neoplasm of unspecified site of unspecified orbit**

     D31.61 **Benign neoplasm of unspecified site of right orbit**

     D31.62 **Benign neoplasm of unspecified site of left orbit**

● **D31.9** **Benign neoplasm of unspecified part of eye**
Benign neoplasm of eyeball

     D31.90 **Benign neoplasm of unspecified part of unspecified eye**

     D31.91 **Benign neoplasm of unspecified part of right eye**

     D31.92 **Benign neoplasm of unspecified part of left eye**

● **D32** **Benign neoplasm of meninges**

     D32.0 **Benign neoplasm of cerebral meninges**

     D32.1 **Benign neoplasm of spinal meninges**

     D32.9 **Benign neoplasm of meninges, unspecified**
Meningioma NOS

● **D33** **Benign neoplasm of brain and other parts of central nervous system**
> **Excludes1**   angioma (D18.0-)
> benign neoplasm of meninges (D32.-)
> benign neoplasm of peripheral nerves and autonomic nervous system (D36.1-)
> hemangioma (D18.0-)
> neurofibromatosis (Q85.0-)
> retro-ocular benign neoplasm (D31.6-)

     D33.0 **Benign neoplasm of brain, supratentorial**
Benign neoplasm of cerebral ventricle
Benign neoplasm of cerebrum
Benign neoplasm of frontal lobe
Benign neoplasm of occipital lobe
Benign neoplasm of parietal lobe
Benign neoplasm of temporal lobe
> **Excludes1**   benign neoplasm of fourth ventricle (D33.1)

     D33.1 **Benign neoplasm of brain, infratentorial**
Benign neoplasm of brain stem
Benign neoplasm of cerebellum
Benign neoplasm of fourth ventricle

     D33.2 **Benign neoplasm of brain, unspecified**

     D33.3 **Benign neoplasm of cranial nerves**
Benign neoplasm of olfactory bulb

     D33.4 **Benign neoplasm of spinal cord**

     D33.7 **Benign neoplasm of other specified parts of central nervous system**

     D33.9 **Benign neoplasm of central nervous system, unspecified**
Benign neoplasm of nervous system (central) NOS

● **D34** **Benign neoplasm of thyroid gland**
Use additional code to identify any functional activity.

● **D35** **Benign neoplasm of other and unspecified endocrine glands**
Use additional code to identify any functional activity.
> **Excludes1**   benign neoplasm of endocrine pancreas (D13.7)
> benign neoplasm of ovary (D27.-)
> benign neoplasm of testis (D29.2.-)
> benign neoplasm of thymus (D15.0)

     ● **D35.0** **Benign neoplasm of adrenal gland**

         D35.00 **Benign neoplasm of unspecified adrenal gland**

         D35.01 **Benign neoplasm of right adrenal gland**

         D35.02 **Benign neoplasm of left adrenal gland**

     D35.1 **Benign neoplasm of parathyroid gland**

     D35.2 **Benign neoplasm of pituitary gland**

     D35.3 **Benign neoplasm of craniopharyngeal duct**

     D35.4 **Benign neoplasm of pineal gland**

     D35.5 **Benign neoplasm of carotid body**

     D35.6 **Benign neoplasm of aortic body and other paraganglia**
Benign tumor of glomus jugulare

     D35.7 **Benign neoplasm of other specified endocrine glands**

     D35.9 **Benign neoplasm of endocrine gland, unspecified**
Benign neoplasm of unspecified endocrine gland

● **D36** **Benign neoplasm of other and unspecified sites**

     D36.0 **Benign neoplasm of lymph nodes**
> **Excludes1**   lymphangioma (D18.1)

     ● **D36.1** **Benign neoplasm of peripheral nerves and autonomic nervous system**
> **Excludes1**   benign neoplasm of peripheral nerves of orbit (D31.6-)
> neurofibromatosis (Q85.0-)

         D36.10 **Benign neoplasm of peripheral nerves and autonomic nervous system, unspecified**

         D36.11 **Benign neoplasm of peripheral nerves and autonomic nervous system of face, head, and neck**

         D36.12 **Benign neoplasm of peripheral nerves and autonomic nervous system, upper limb, including shoulder**

         D36.13 **Benign neoplasm of peripheral nerves and autonomic nervous system of lower limb, including hip**

         D36.14 **Benign neoplasm of peripheral nerves and autonomic nervous system of thorax**

         D36.15 **Benign neoplasm of peripheral nerves and autonomic nervous system of abdomen**

         D36.16 **Benign neoplasm of peripheral nerves and autonomic nervous system of pelvis**

         D36.17 **Benign neoplasm of peripheral nerves and autonomic nervous system of trunk, unspecified**

     D36.7 **Benign neoplasm of other specified sites**
Benign neoplasm of nose NOS

     D36.9 **Benign neoplasm, unspecified site**

▶ New   ⟹ Revised   ~~deleted~~ Deleted   **OGCR** Official Guidelines   X Assign placeholder X   ● Use Additional Character(s)

Excludes 1   Excludes 2   Includes   Use additional   Code first   Code also   Key words

BENIGN NEUROENDOCRINE TUMORS (D3A)

● **D3A Benign neuroendocrine tumors**
  Code also any associated multiple endocrine neoplasia [MEN] syndromes (E31.2-)
  Use additional code to identify any associated endocrine syndrome, such as:
  carcinoid syndrome (E34.0)
  Excludes2 benign pancreatic islet cell tumors (D13.7)

● **D3A.0 Benign carcinoid tumors**

     D3A.00 Benign carcinoid tumor of unspecified site
  Carcinoid tumor NOS

●   **D3A.01 Benign carcinoid tumors of the small intestine**

         D3A.010 Benign carcinoid tumor of the duodenum

         D3A.011 Benign carcinoid tumor of the jejunum

         D3A.012 Benign carcinoid tumor of the ileum

         D3A.019 Benign carcinoid tumor of the small intestine, unspecified portion

●   **D3A.02 Benign carcinoid tumors of the appendix, large intestine, and rectum**

         D3A.020 Benign carcinoid tumor of the appendix

         D3A.021 Benign carcinoid tumor of the cecum

         D3A.022 Benign carcinoid tumor of the ascending colon

         D3A.023 Benign carcinoid tumor of the transverse colon

         D3A.024 Benign carcinoid tumor of the descending colon

         D3A.025 Benign carcinoid tumor of the sigmoid colon

         D3A.026 Benign carcinoid tumor of the rectum

         D3A.029 Benign carcinoid tumor of the large intestine, unspecified portion
  Benign carcinoid tumor of the colon NOS

●   **D3A.09 Benign carcinoid tumors of other sites**

         D3A.090 Benign carcinoid tumor of the bronchus and lung

         D3A.091 Benign carcinoid tumor of the thymus

         D3A.092 Benign carcinoid tumor of the stomach

         D3A.093 Benign carcinoid tumor of the kidney

         D3A.094 Benign carcinoid tumor of the foregut, unspecified

         D3A.095 Benign carcinoid tumor of the midgut, unspecified

         D3A.096 Benign carcinoid tumor of the hindgut, unspecified

         D3A.098 Benign carcinoid tumors of other sites

D3A.8 Other benign neuroendocrine tumors
  Neuroendocrine tumor NOS

Figure 2-19 Major salivary glands.

Parotid gland
Sublingual gland
Submandibular gland

NEOPLASMS OF UNCERTAIN BEHAVIOR, POLYCYTHEMIA VERA AND MYELODYSPLASTIC SYNDROMES (D37-D48)

Note: Categories D37-D44, and D48 classify by site neoplasms of uncertain behavior, i.e., histologic confirmation whether the neoplasm is malignant or benign cannot be made.
  Excludes1 neoplasms of unspecified behavior (D49.-)

● **D37 Neoplasm of uncertain behavior of oral cavity and digestive organs**
  Excludes1 stromal tumors of uncertain behavior of digestive system (D48.1)

●   **D37.0 Neoplasm of uncertain behavior of lip, oral cavity and pharynx**
  Excludes1 neoplasm of uncertain behavior of aryepiglottic fold or interarytenoid fold, laryngeal aspect (D38.0)
  neoplasm of uncertain behavior of epiglottis NOS (D38.0)
  neoplasm of uncertain behavior of skin of lip (D48.5)
  neoplasm of uncertain behavior of suprahyoid portion of epiglottis (D38.0)

     D37.01 Neoplasm of uncertain behavior of lip
  Neoplasm of uncertain behavior of vermilion border of lip

     D37.02 Neoplasm of uncertain behavior of tongue

●   **D37.03 Neoplasm of uncertain behavior of the major salivary glands**

         D37.030 Neoplasm of uncertain behavior of the parotid salivary glands

         D37.031 Neoplasm of uncertain behavior of the sublingual salivary glands

         D37.032 Neoplasm of uncertain behavior of the submandibular salivary glands

         D37.039 Neoplasm of uncertain behavior of the major salivary glands, unspecified

     D37.04 Neoplasm of uncertain behavior of the minor salivary glands
  Neoplasm of uncertain behavior of submucosal salivary glands of lip
  Neoplasm of uncertain behavior of submucosal salivary glands of cheek
  Neoplasm of uncertain behavior of submucosal salivary glands of hard palate
  Neoplasm of uncertain behavior of submucosal salivary glands of soft palate

     D37.05 Neoplasm of uncertain behavior of pharynx
  Neoplasm of uncertain behavior of aryepiglottic fold of pharynx NOS
  Neoplasm of uncertain behavior of hypopharyngeal aspect of aryepiglottic fold of pharynx
  Neoplasm of uncertain behavior of marginal zone of aryepiglottic fold of pharynx

     D37.09 Neoplasm of uncertain behavior of other specified sites of the oral cavity

CHAPTER 2 (C00-D49)

▶ New   ⇒ Revised   ~~deleted~~ Deleted   **OGCR** Official Guidelines   X Assign placeholder X   ● Use Additional Character(s)

Excludes 1   Excludes 2   Includes   Use additional   Code first   Code also   Key words

D37.1   **Neoplasm of uncertain behavior of stomach**

D37.2   **Neoplasm of uncertain behavior of small intestine**

D37.3   **Neoplasm of uncertain behavior of appendix**

D37.4   **Neoplasm of uncertain behavior of colon**

D37.5   **Neoplasm of uncertain behavior of rectum**
Neoplasm of uncertain behavior of rectosigmoid junction
Rectosigmoid junction: Angle where sigmoid colon becomes rectum

D37.6   **Neoplasm of uncertain behavior of liver, gallbladder and bile ducts**
Neoplasm of uncertain behavior of ampulla of Vater
Ampulla of Vater: Enlarged segment of ducts from liver and pancreas at entry point to small intestine

D37.8   **Neoplasm of uncertain behavior of other specified digestive organs**
Neoplasm of uncertain behavior of anal canal
Neoplasm of uncertain behavior of anal sphincter
Neoplasm of uncertain behavior of anus NOS
Neoplasm of uncertain behavior of esophagus
Neoplasm of uncertain behavior of intestine NOS
Neoplasm of uncertain behavior of pancreas
Excludes1 neoplasm of uncertain behavior of anal margin (D48.5)
neoplasm of uncertain behavior of anal skin (D48.5)
neoplasm of uncertain behavior of perianal skin (D48.5)

D37.9   **Neoplasm of uncertain behavior of digestive organ, unspecified**

● D38   **Neoplasm of uncertain behavior of middle ear and respiratory and intrathoracic organs**
Excludes1 neoplasm of uncertain behavior of heart (D48.7)

D38.0   **Neoplasm of uncertain behavior of larynx**
Neoplasm of uncertain behavior of aryepiglottic fold or interarytenoid fold, laryngeal aspect
Neoplasm of uncertain behavior of epiglottis (suprahyoid portion)
Excludes1 neoplasm of uncertain behavior of aryepiglottic fold or interarytenoid fold NOS (D37.05)
neoplasm of uncertain behavior of hypopharyngeal aspect of aryepiglottic fold (D37.05)
neoplasm of uncertain behavior of marginal zone of aryepiglottic fold (D37.05)

D38.1   **Neoplasm of uncertain behavior of trachea, bronchus and lung**

D38.2   **Neoplasm of uncertain behavior of pleura**

D38.3   **Neoplasm of uncertain behavior of mediastinum**

D38.4   **Neoplasm of uncertain behavior of thymus**

D38.5   **Neoplasm of uncertain behavior of other respiratory organs**
Neoplasm of uncertain behavior of accessory sinuses
Neoplasm of uncertain behavior of cartilage of nose
Neoplasm of uncertain behavior of middle ear
Neoplasm of uncertain behavior of nasal cavities
Excludes1 neoplasm of uncertain behavior of ear (external) (skin) (D48.5)
neoplasm of uncertain behavior of nose NOS (D48.7)
neoplasm of uncertain behavior of skin of nose (D48.5)

D38.6   **Neoplasm of uncertain behavior of respiratory organ, unspecified**

● D39   **Neoplasm of uncertain behavior of female genital organs**

D39.0   **Neoplasm of uncertain behavior of uterus**

● D39.1   **Neoplasm of uncertain behavior of ovary**
Use additional code to identify any functional activity.

    D39.10   **Neoplasm of uncertain behavior of unspecified ovary**

    D39.11   **Neoplasm of uncertain behavior of right ovary**

    D39.12   **Neoplasm of uncertain behavior of left ovary**

D39.2   **Neoplasm of uncertain behavior of placenta**
Chorioadenoma destruens
Invasive hydatidiform mole
Malignant hydatidiform mole
Excludes1 hydatidiform mole NOS (O01.9)

D39.8   **Neoplasm of uncertain behavior of other specified female genital organs**
Neoplasm of uncertain behavior of skin of female genital organs

D39.9   **Neoplasm of uncertain behavior of female genital organ, unspecified**

● D40   **Neoplasm of uncertain behavior of male genital organs**

D40.0   **Neoplasm of uncertain behavior of prostate**

● D40.1   **Neoplasm of uncertain behavior of testis**

    D40.10   **Neoplasm of uncertain behavior of unspecified testis**

    D40.11   **Neoplasm of uncertain behavior of right testis**

    D40.12   **Neoplasm of uncertain behavior of left testis**

D40.8   **Neoplasm of uncertain behavior of other specified male genital organs**
Neoplasm of uncertain behavior of skin of male genital organs

D40.9   **Neoplasm of uncertain behavior of male genital organ, unspecified**

● D41   **Neoplasm of uncertain behavior of urinary organs**

● D41.0   **Neoplasm of uncertain behavior of kidney**
Excludes1 neoplasm of uncertain behavior of renal pelvis (D41.1-)

    D41.00   **Neoplasm of uncertain behavior of unspecified kidney**

    D41.01   **Neoplasm of uncertain behavior of right kidney**

    D41.02   **Neoplasm of uncertain behavior of left kidney**

● D41.1   **Neoplasm of uncertain behavior of renal pelvis**

    D41.10   **Neoplasm of uncertain behavior of unspecified renal pelvis**

    D41.11   **Neoplasm of uncertain behavior of right renal pelvis**

    D41.12   **Neoplasm of uncertain behavior of left renal pelvis**

● D41.2   **Neoplasm of uncertain behavior of ureter**

    D41.20   **Neoplasm of uncertain behavior of unspecified ureter**

    D41.21   **Neoplasm of uncertain behavior of right ureter**

    D41.22   **Neoplasm of uncertain behavior of left ureter**

D41.3   **Neoplasm of uncertain behavior of urethra**

D41.4   **Neoplasm of uncertain behavior of bladder**

D41.8   **Neoplasm of uncertain behavior of other specified urinary organs**

D41.9   **Neoplasm of uncertain behavior of unspecified urinary organ**

► New   ⇒ Revised   ~~deleted~~ Deleted   **OGCR** Official Guidelines   X Assign placeholder X   ● Use Additional Character(s)
Excludes 1   Excludes 2   Includes   Use additional   Code first   Code also   Key words

● **D42 Neoplasm of uncertain behavior of meninges**
  D42.0 Neoplasm of uncertain behavior of cerebral meninges
  D42.1 Neoplasm of uncertain behavior of spinal meninges
  D42.9 Neoplasm of uncertain behavior of meninges, unspecified

● **D43 Neoplasm of uncertain behavior of brain and central nervous system**
  Excludes1 neoplasm of uncertain behavior of peripheral nerves and autonomic nervous system (D48.2)

  D43.0 Neoplasm of uncertain behavior of brain, supratentorial
    Superior to tentorium of cerebellum
    Neoplasm of uncertain behavior of cerebral ventricle
    Neoplasm of uncertain behavior of cerebrum
    Neoplasm of uncertain behavior of frontal lobe
    Neoplasm of uncertain behavior of occipital lobe
    Neoplasm of uncertain behavior of parietal lobe
    Neoplasm of uncertain behavior of temporal lobe
    Excludes1 neoplasm of uncertain behavior of fourth ventricle (D43.1)

  D43.1 Neoplasm of uncertain behavior of brain, infratentorial
    Beneath the tentorium of cerebellum
    Neoplasm of uncertain behavior of brain stem
    Neoplasm of uncertain behavior of cerebellum
    Neoplasm of uncertain behavior of fourth ventricle

  D43.2 Neoplasm of uncertain behavior of brain, unspecified
  D43.3 Neoplasm of uncertain behavior of cranial nerves
  D43.4 Neoplasm of uncertain behavior of spinal cord
  D43.8 Neoplasm of uncertain behavior of other specified parts of central nervous system
  D43.9 Neoplasm of uncertain behavior of central nervous system, unspecified
    Neoplasm of uncertain behavior of nervous system (central) NOS

● **D44 Neoplasm of uncertain behavior of endocrine glands**
  Excludes1 multiple endocrine adenomatosis (E31.2-)
    multiple endocrine neoplasia (E31.2-)
    neoplasm of uncertain behavior of endocrine pancreas (D37.8)
    neoplasm of uncertain behavior of ovary (D39.1-)
    neoplasm of uncertain behavior of testis (D40.1-)
    neoplasm of uncertain behavior of thymus (D38.4)

  D44.0 Neoplasm of uncertain behavior of thyroid gland
  ● **D44.1 Neoplasm of uncertain behavior of adrenal gland**
    Use additional code to identify any functional activity.
    D44.10 Neoplasm of uncertain behavior of unspecified adrenal gland
    D44.11 Neoplasm of uncertain behavior of right adrenal gland
    D44.12 Neoplasm of uncertain behavior of left adrenal gland
  D44.2 Neoplasm of uncertain behavior of parathyroid gland
  D44.3 Neoplasm of uncertain behavior of pituitary gland
    Use additional code to identify any functional activity.
  D44.4 Neoplasm of uncertain behavior of craniopharyngeal duct
  D44.5 Neoplasm of uncertain behavior of pineal gland
  D44.6 Neoplasm of uncertain behavior of carotid body
  D44.7 Neoplasm of uncertain behavior of aortic body and other paraganglia
  D44.9 Neoplasm of uncertain behavior of unspecified endocrine gland

● **D45 Polycythemia vera**
  Excludes1 familial polycythemia (D75.0)
    secondary polycythemia (D75.1)
  Primary polycythemia. Secondary polycythemia is D75.1. Check your documentation. Polycythemia is caused by too many red blood cells, which increase the thickness of blood (viscosity). This can cause engorgement of the spleen (splenomegaly) with extra RBCs and potential clot formation.

● **D46 Myelodysplastic syndromes**
  Use additional code for adverse effect, if applicable, to identify drug (T36-T50 with fifth or sixth character 5)
  Excludes2 drug-induced aplastic anemia (D61.1)

  D46.0 Refractory anemia without ring sideroblasts, so stated
    Refractory anemia without sideroblasts, without excess of blasts
  D46.1 Refractory anemia with ring sideroblasts RARS
  ● **D46.2 Refractory anemia with excess of blasts [RAEB]**
    Form of myelodysplasia with increased immature white blood cells (blasts) in bone marrow
    D46.20 Refractory anemia with excess of blasts, unspecified RAEB NOS
    D46.21 Refractory anemia with excess of blasts 1 RAEB 1
      Bone marrow disease which results in insufficient RBCs (anemia) in which level of blasts is less than 10%
    D46.22 Refractory anemia with excess of blasts 2 RAEB 2
      Bone marrow disease manifested by insufficient numbers of RBCs (anemia) with level of blasts 10-20%
  D46.A Refractory cytopenia with multilineage dysplasia
  D46.B Refractory cytopenia with multilineage dysplasia and ring sideroblasts
    RCMD RS
  D46.C Myelodysplastic syndrome with isolated del(5q) chromosomal abnormality
    Myelodysplastic syndrome with 5q deletion
    5q minus syndrome NOS
  D46.4 Refractory anemia, unspecified
  D46.Z Other myelodysplastic syndromes
    Excludes1 chronic myelomonocytic leukemia (C93.1-)
  D46.9 Myelodysplastic syndrome, unspecified
    Myelodysplasia NOS

● **D47 Other neoplasms of uncertain behavior of lymphoid, hematopoietic and related tissue**
  ⇒● **D47.0 Mast cell neoplasms of uncertain behavior**
    ~~Indolent systemic mastocytosis~~
    ~~Mast cell tumor NOS~~
    ~~Mastocytoma NOS~~
    Excludes1 ~~malignant mast cell tumor (C96.2)~~
      ~~mastocytosis (congenital) (cutaneous) (Q82.2)~~
      ▶congenital cutaneous mastocytosis (Q82.2-)
      ▶histiocytic neoplasms of uncertain behavior (D47.Z9)
      ▶malignant mast cell neoplasm (C96.2-)

    ▶ **D47.01 Cutaneous mastocytosis**
      ▶Diffuse cutaneous mastocytosis
      ▶Maculopapular cutaneous mastocytosis
      ▶Solitary mastocytoma
      ▶Telangiectasia macularis eruptiva perstans
      ▶Urticaria pigmentosa
      ▶ **Excludes1** congenital (diffuse) (maculopapular) cutaneous mastocytosis (Q82.2)
        ▶congenital urticaria pigmentosa (Q82.2)
        ▶extracutaneous mastocytoma (D47.09)

CHAPTER 2 (C00-D49)

▶ **D47.02 Systemic mastocytosis**
▶ Indolent systemic mastocytosis
▶ Isolated bone marrow mastocytosis
▶ Smoldering systemic mastocytosis
▶ Systemic mastocytosis, with an associated hematological non-mast cell lineage disease (SM-AHNMD)
▶ Code also if applicable, any associated hematological non-mast cell lineage disease, such as:
▶ acute myeloid leukemia (C92.6-, C92.A-)
▶ chronic myelomonocytic leukemia (C93.1-)
▶ essential thrombocytosis (D47.3)
▶ hypereosinophilic syndrome (D72.1)
▶ myelodysplastic syndrome (D46.9)
▶ myeloproliferative syndrome (D47.1)
▶ non-Hodgkin lymphoma (C82-C85)
▶ plasma cell myeloma (C90.0-)
▶ polycythemia vera (D45)
▶ **Excludes1** aggressive systemic mastocytosis (C96.21)
▶ mast cell leukemia (C94.3-)

▶ **D47.09 Other mast cell neoplasms of uncertain behavior**
▶ Extracutaneous mastocytoma
▶ Mast cell tumor NOS
▶ Mastocytoma NOS
▶ Mastocytosis NOS

D47.1 Chronic myeloproliferative disease
Chronic neutrophilic leukemia
Myeloproliferative disease, unspecified
Excludes1 atypical chronic myeloid leukemia BCR/ABL-negative (C92.2-)
chronic myeloid leukemia BCR/ABL-positive (C92.1-)
myelofibrosis NOS (D75.81)
myelophthisic anemia (D61.82)
myelophthisis (D61.82)
secondary myelofibrosis NOS (D75.81)

D47.2 Monoclonal gammopathy
Monoclonal gammopathy of undetermined significance [MGUS]

D47.3 Essential (hemorrhagic) thrombocythemia
Essential thrombocytosis
Idiopathic hemorrhagic thrombocythemia

D47.4 Osteomyelofibrosis
Chronic idiopathic myelofibrosis
Myelofibrosis (idiopathic) (with myeloid metaplasia)
Myelosclerosis (megakaryocytic) with myeloid metaplasia
Secondary myelofibrosis in myeloproliferative disease
Excludes1 acute myelofibrosis (C94.4-)

● **D47.Z Other specified neoplasms of uncertain behavior of lymphoid, hematopoietic and related tissue**
D47.Z1 Post-transplant lymphoproliferative disorder (PTLD)
Code first complications of transplanted organs and tissue (T86.-)

D47.Z2 Castleman disease
Code also if applicable human herpesvirus 8 infection (B10.89)
Excludes2 Kaposi's sarcoma (C46-)

D47.Z9 Other specified neoplasms of uncertain behavior of lymphoid, hematopoietic and related tissue
Histiocytic tumors of uncertain behavior

D47.9 Neoplasm of uncertain behavior of lymphoid, hematopoietic and related tissue, unspecified
Lymphoproliferative disease NOS

● **D48 Neoplasm of uncertain behavior of other and unspecified sites**
Excludes1 neurofibromatosis (nonmalignant) (Q85.0-)

D48.0 Neoplasm of uncertain behavior of bone and articular cartilage
Excludes1 neoplasm of uncertain behavior of cartilage of ear (D48.1)
neoplasm of uncertain behavior of cartilage of larynx (D38.0)
neoplasm of uncertain behavior of cartilage of nose (D38.5)
neoplasm of uncertain behavior of connective tissue of eyelid (D48.1)
neoplasm of uncertain behavior of synovia (D48.1)

D48.1 Neoplasm of uncertain behavior of connective and other soft tissue
Neoplasm of uncertain behavior of connective tissue of ear
Neoplasm of uncertain behavior of connective tissue of eyelid
Stromal tumors of uncertain behavior of digestive system
Excludes1 neoplasm of uncertain behavior of articular cartilage (D48.0)
neoplasm of uncertain behavior of cartilage of larynx (D38.0)
neoplasm of uncertain behavior of cartilage of nose (D38.5)
neoplasm of uncertain behavior of connective tissue of breast (D48.6-)

D48.2 Neoplasm of uncertain behavior of peripheral nerves and autonomic nervous system
Excludes1 neoplasm of uncertain behavior of peripheral nerves of orbit (D48.7)

D48.3 Neoplasm of uncertain behavior of retroperitoneum

D48.4 Neoplasm of uncertain behavior of peritoneum

D48.5 Neoplasm of uncertain behavior of skin
Neoplasm of uncertain behavior of anal margin
Neoplasm of uncertain behavior of anal skin
Neoplasm of uncertain behavior of perianal skin
Neoplasm of uncertain behavior of skin of breast
Excludes1 neoplasm of uncertain behavior of anus NOS (D37.8)
neoplasm of uncertain behavior of skin of genital organs (D39.8, D40.8)
neoplasm of uncertain behavior of vermilion border of lip (D37.0)

● **D48.6 Neoplasm of uncertain behavior of breast**
Neoplasm of uncertain behavior of connective tissue of breast
Cystosarcoma phyllodes
Excludes1 neoplasm of uncertain behavior of skin of breast (D48.5)

D48.60 Neoplasm of uncertain behavior of unspecified breast

D48.61 Neoplasm of uncertain behavior of right breast

D48.62 Neoplasm of uncertain behavior of left breast

D48.7 Neoplasm of uncertain behavior of other specified sites
Neoplasm of uncertain behavior of eye
Neoplasm of uncertain behavior of heart
Neoplasm of uncertain behavior of peripheral nerves of orbit
Excludes1 neoplasm of uncertain behavior of connective tissue (D48.1)
neoplasm of uncertain behavior of skin of eyelid (D48.5)

D48.9 Neoplasm of uncertain behavior, unspecified

▶ New ⇒ Revised ~~deleted~~ Deleted **OGCR** Official Guidelines X Assign placeholder X ● Use Additional Character(s)

Excludes 1 | Excludes 2 | Includes | Use additional | Code first | Code also | Key words

● **D49 Neoplasms of unspecified behavior**

> **Note:** Category D49 classifies by site neoplasms of unspecified morphology and behavior. The term 'mass,' unless otherwise stated, is not to be regarded as a neoplastic growth.

> **Includes** 'growth' NOS
> neoplasm NOS
> new growth NOS
> tumor NOS

> **Excludes1** neoplasms of uncertain behavior (D37-D44, D48)

D49.0 Neoplasm of unspecified behavior of digestive system

> **Excludes1** neoplasm of unspecified behavior of margin of anus (D49.2)
> neoplasm of unspecified behavior of perianal skin (D49.2)
> neoplasm of unspecified behavior of skin of anus (D49.2)

D49.1 Neoplasm of unspecified behavior of respiratory system

D49.2 Neoplasm of unspecified behavior of bone, soft tissue, and skin

> **Excludes1** neoplasm of unspecified behavior of anal canal (D49.0)
> neoplasm of unspecified behavior of anus NOS (D49.0)
> neoplasm of unspecified behavior of bone marrow (D49.89)
> neoplasm of unspecified behavior of cartilage of larynx (D49.1)
> neoplasm of unspecified behavior of cartilage of nose (D49.1)
> neoplasm of unspecified behavior of connective tissue of breast (D49.3)
> neoplasm of unspecified behavior of skin of genital organs (D49.59)
> neoplasm of unspecified behavior of vermilion border of lip (D49.0)

D49.3 Neoplasm of unspecified behavior of breast

> **Excludes1** neoplasm of unspecified behavior of skin of breast (D49.2)

D49.4 Neoplasm of unspecified behavior of bladder

● **D49.5 Neoplasm of unspecified behavior of other genitourinary organs**

> ● **D49.51 Neoplasm of unspecified behavior of kidney**
>
> > **D49.511 Neoplasm of unspecified behavior of right kidney**
> >
> > **D49.512 Neoplasm of unspecified behavior of left kidney**
> >
> > **D49.519 Neoplasm of unspecified behavior of unspecified kidney**
>
> **D49.59 Neoplasm of unspecified behavior of other genitourinary organ**

D49.6 Neoplasm of unspecified behavior of brain

> **Excludes1** neoplasm of unspecified behavior of cerebral meninges (D49.7)
> neoplasm of unspecified behavior of cranial nerves (D49.7)

D49.7 Neoplasm of unspecified behavior of endocrine glands and other parts of nervous system

> **Excludes1** neoplasm of unspecified behavior of peripheral, sympathetic, and parasympathetic nerves and ganglia (D49.2)

● **D49.8 Neoplasm of unspecified behavior of other specified sites**

> **Excludes1** neoplasm of unspecified behavior of eyelid (skin) (D49.2)
> neoplasm of unspecified behavior of eyelid cartilage (D49.2)
> neoplasm of unspecified behavior of great vessels (D49.2)
> neoplasm of unspecified behavior of optic nerve (D49.7)

> **D49.81 Neoplasm of unspecified behavior of retina and choroid**
> Dark area on retina
> Retinal freckle

> **D49.89 Neoplasm of unspecified behavior of other specified sites**

D49.9 Neoplasm of unspecified behavior of unspecified site

OGCR Chapter-Specific Coding Guidelines

3. **Chapter 3: Disease of the blood and blood-forming organs and certain disorders involving the immune mechanism (D50-D89)**
Reserved for future guideline expansion

CHAPTER 3

DISEASES OF THE BLOOD AND BLOOD-FORMING ORGANS AND CERTAIN DISORDERS INVOLVING THE IMMUNE MECHANISM (D50-D89)

| Excludes2 | autoimmune disease (systemic) NOS (M35.9) |

certain conditions originating in the perinatal period (P00-P96)
complications of pregnancy, childbirth and the puerperium (O00-O9A)
congenital malformations, deformations and chromosomal abnormalities (Q00-Q99)
endocrine, nutritional and metabolic diseases (E00-E88)
human immunodeficiency virus [HIV] disease (B20)
injury, poisoning and certain other consequences of external causes (S00-T88)
neoplasms (C00-D49)
symptoms, signs and abnormal clinical and laboratory findings, not elsewhere classified (R00-R94)

This chapter contains the following blocks:

D50-D53	Nutritional anemias
D55-D59	Hemolytic anemias
D60-D64	Aplastic and other anemias and other bone marrow failure syndromes
D65-D69	Coagulation defects, purpura and other hemorrhagic conditions
D70-D77	Other disorders of blood and blood-forming organs
D78	Intraoperative and postprocedural complications of the spleen
D80-D89	Certain disorders involving the immune mechanism

NUTRITIONAL ANEMIAS (D50-D53)

● **D50** **Iron** deficiency anemia
A disease characterized by a decrease in the number of red cells (hemoglobin) in the blood.

Includes asiderotic anemia
hypochromic anemia

D50.0 Iron deficiency anemia **secondary to blood loss (chronic)**
Posthemorrhagic anemia (chronic)

Excludes1 acute posthemorrhagic anemia (D62)
congenital anemia from fetal blood loss (P61.3)

D50.1 **Sideropenic dysphagia**
Web-like growth of membranes in throat that makes swallowing difficult
Kelly-Paterson syndrome
Plummer-Vinson syndrome

D50.8 **Other iron deficiency anemias**
Iron deficiency anemia due to inadequate dietary iron intake

D50.9 Iron deficiency anemia, **unspecified**

● **D51** **Vitamin B12 deficiency anemia**

Excludes1 vitamin B12 deficiency (E53.8)

D51.0 Vitamin B12 deficiency anemia due to **intrinsic factor deficiency**
Addison anemia
Biermer anemia
Pernicious (congenital) anemia
Congenital intrinsic factor deficiency

D51.1 Vitamin B12 deficiency anemia due to **selective vitamin B12 malabsorption with proteinuria**
Imerslund (Gräsbeck) syndrome
Megaloblastic hereditary anemia

D51.2 **Transcobalamin II deficiency**

D51.3 **Other dietary vitamin B12 deficiency anemia**
Vegan anemia

D51.8 **Other vitamin B12 deficiency anemias**

D51.9 **Vitamin B12 deficiency anemia, unspecified**

● **D52** **Folate deficiency anemia**

Excludes1 folate deficiency without anemia (E53.8)

D52.0 **Dietary folate deficiency anemia**
Nutritional megaloblastic anemia

D52.1 **Drug-induced** folate deficiency anemia
Use additional code for adverse effect, if applicable, to identify drug (T36-T50 with fifth or sixth character 5)

D52.8 **Other folate deficiency anemias**

D52.9 **Folate deficiency anemia, unspecified**
Folic acid deficiency anemia NOS

● **D53** **Other nutritional anemias**

Includes megaloblastic anemia unresponsive to vitamin B12 or folate therapy

D53.0 **Protein deficiency anemia**
Amino-acid deficiency anemia
Orotaciduric anemia

Excludes1 Lesch-Nyhan syndrome (E79.1)

D53.1 **Other megaloblastic anemias, not elsewhere classified**
Megaloblastic anemia NOS

Excludes1 Di Guglielmo's disease (C94.0)

D53.2 **Scorbutic anemia**
Anemia resulting from deficiency of ascorbic acid (vitamin C)

Excludes1 scurvy (E54)

D53.8 **Other specified nutritional anemias**
Anemia associated with deficiency of copper
Anemia associated with deficiency of molybdenum
Anemia associated with deficiency of zinc

Excludes1 nutritional deficiencies without anemia, such as:
copper deficiency NOS (E61.0)
molybdenum deficiency NOS (E61.5)
zinc deficiency NOS (E60)

D53.9 **Nutritional anemia, unspecified**
Simple chronic anemia

Excludes1 anemia NOS (D64.9)

▶ New　⇛ Revised　~~deleted~~ Deleted　**OGCR** Official Guidelines　X Assign placeholder X　● Use Additional Character(s)

| Excludes 1 | Excludes 2 | Includes | Use additional | Code first | Code also | Key words |

HEMOLYTIC ANEMIAS (D55-D59)

● **D55** **Anemia due to enzyme disorders**

     | **Excludes1** | drug-induced enzyme deficiency anemia (D59.2) |

  D55.0 **Anemia due to glucose-6-phosphate dehydrogenase [G6PD] deficiency**
      Favism
      G6PD deficiency anemia

  D55.1 **Anemia due to other disorders of glutathione metabolism**
      Anemia (due to) enzyme deficiencies, except G6PD, related to the hexose monophosphate [HMP] shunt pathway
      Anemia (due to) hemolytic nonspherocytic (hereditary), type I

  D55.2 **Anemia due to disorders of glycolytic enzymes**
      Hemolytic nonspherocytic (hereditary) anemia, type II
      Hexokinase deficiency anemia
      Pyruvate kinase [PK] deficiency anemia
      Triose-phosphate isomerase deficiency anemia

      | **Excludes1** | disorders of glycolysis not associated with anemia (E74.8) |

  D55.3 **Anemia due to disorders of nucleotide metabolism**

  D55.8 **Other anemias due to enzyme disorders**

  D55.9 **Anemia due to enzyme disorder, unspecified**

● **D56** **Thalassemia**
    Hereditary disorders characterized by low production of hemoglobin or excessive destruction of red blood cells

     | **Excludes1** | sickle-cell thalassemia (D57.4-) |

  D56.0 **Alpha thalassemia**
      Alpha thalassemia major
      Hemoglobin H Constant Spring
      Hemoglobin H disease
      Hydrops fetalis due to alpha thalassemia
      Severe alpha thalassemia
      Triple gene defect alpha thalassemia

      Use additional code, if applicable, for hydrops fetalis due to alpha thalassemia (P56.99)

      | **Excludes1** | alpha thalassemia trait or minor (D56.3) |
      | | asymptomatic alpha thalassemia (D56.3) |
      | | hydrops fetalis due to isoimmunization (P56.0) |
      | | hydrops fetalis not due to immune hemolysis (P83.2) |

  D56.1 **Beta thalassemia**
      Beta thalassemia major
      Cooley's anemia
      Homozygous beta thalassemia
      Severe beta thalassemia
      Thalassemia intermedia
      Thalassemia major

      | **Excludes1** | beta thalassemia minor (D56.3) |
      | | beta thalassemia trait (D56.3) |
      | | delta-beta thalassemia (D56.2) |
      | | hemoglobin E-beta thalassemia (D56.5) |
      | | sickle-cell beta thalassemia (D57.4-) |

  D56.2 **Delta-beta thalassemia**
      Homozygous delta-beta thalassemia

      | **Excludes1** | delta-beta thalassemia minor (D56.3) |
      | | delta-beta thalassemia trait (D56.3) |

  D56.3 **Thalassemia minor**
    Genetic disorders that have in common defective production of hemoglobin
      Alpha thalassemia minor
      Alpha thalassemia silent carrier
      Alpha thalassemia trait
      Beta thalassemia minor
      Beta thalassemia trait
      Delta-beta thalassemia minor
      Delta-beta thalassemia trait
      Thalassemia trait NOS

      | **Excludes1** | alpha thalassemia (D56.0) |
      | | beta thalassemia (D56.1) |
      | | delta-beta thalassemia (D56.2) |
      | | hemoglobin E-beta thalassemia (D56.5) |
      | | sickle-cell trait (D57.3) |

  D56.4 **Hereditary persistence of fetal hemoglobin [HPFH]**
    Persistent production of hemoglobin

  D56.5 **Hemoglobin E-beta thalassemia**

      | **Excludes1** | beta thalassemia (D56.1) |
      | | beta thalassemia minor (D56.3) |
      | | beta thalassemia trait (D56.3) |
      | | delta-beta thalassemia (D56.2) |
      | | delta-beta thalassemia trait (D56.3) |
      | | hemoglobin E disease (D58.2) |
      | | other hemoglobinopathies (D58.2) |
      | | sickle-cell beta thalassemia (D57.4-) |

  D56.8 **Other thalassemias**
      Dominant thalassemia
      Hemoglobin C thalassemia
      Mixed thalassemia
      Thalassemia with other hemoglobinopathy

      | **Excludes1** | hemoglobin C disease (D58.2) |
      | | hemoglobin E disease (D58.2) |
      | | other hemoglobinopathies (D58.2) |
      | | sickle cell anemia (D57.-) |
      | | sickle-cell thalassemia (D57.4) |

  D56.9 **Thalassemia, unspecified**
      Mediterranean anemia (with other hemoglobinopathy)

● **D57** **Sickle-cell disorders**
    Inherited disease in which red blood cells, normally disc-shaped, become crescent shaped

    Use additional code for any associated fever (R50.81)

     | **Excludes1** | other hemoglobinopathies (D58.-) |

  ● **D57.0** **Hb-SS disease with crisis**
      Sickle-cell disease NOS with crisis
      Hb-SS disease with vasoocclusive pain

    D57.00 **Hb-SS disease with crisis, unspecified**

    D57.01 **Hb-SS disease with acute chest syndrome**

    D57.02 **Hb-SS disease with splenic sequestration**

  D57.1 **Sickle-cell disease without crisis Hb-SS disease without crisis**
      Sickle-cell anemia NOS
      Sickle-cell disease NOS
      Sickle-cell disorder NOS

  ● **D57.2** **Sickle-cell/Hb-C disease**
      Hb-SC disease
      Hb-S/Hb-C disease

    D57.20 **Sickle-cell/Hb-C disease without crisis**

    ● **D57.21** **Sickle-cell/Hb-C disease with crisis**

        D57.211 **Sickle-cell/Hb-C disease with acute chest syndrome**

        D57.212 **Sickle-cell/Hb-C disease with splenic sequestration**

        D57.219 **Sickle-cell/Hb-C disease with crisis, unspecified**
          Sickle-cell/Hb-C disease with crisis NOS

CHAPTER 3 (D50-D89)

D57.3 Sickle-cell trait
Hb-S trait
Heterozygous hemoglobin S

● **D57.4 Sickle-cell thalassemia**
Sickle-cell beta thalassemia
Thalassemia Hb-S disease

D57.40 Sickle-cell thalassemia without crisis
Microdrepanocytosis
Sickle-cell thalassemia NOS

● **D57.41 Sickle-cell thalassemia with crisis**
Sickle-cell "crisis" is precipitated when abnormally crescent-shaped red blood cells form clots and interrupt blood flow to major organs, causing severe pain and organ damage.
Sickle-cell thalassemia with vasoocclusive pain

D57.411 Sickle-cell thalassemia with acute chest syndrome

D57.412 Sickle-cell thalassemia with splenic sequestration

D57.419 Sickle-cell thalassemia with crisis, unspecified
Sickle-cell thalassemia with crisis NOS

● **D57.8 Other sickle-cell disorders**
Hb-SD disease
Hb-SE disease

D57.80 Other sickle-cell disorders without crisis

● **D57.81 Other sickle-cell disorders with crisis**

D57.811 Other sickle-cell disorders with acute chest syndrome

D57.812 Other sickle-cell disorders with splenic sequestration

D57.819 Other sickle-cell disorders with crisis, unspecified
Other sickle-cell disorders with crisis NOS

● **D58 Other hereditary hemolytic anemias**
Genetic condition in which bone marrow is unable to compensate for premature destruction of red blood cells
Excludes1 hemolytic anemia of the newborn (P55.-)

D58.0 Hereditary spherocytosis
Presence of spherocytes (spherically shaped red blood cells)
Acholuric (familial) jaundice
Congenital (spherocytic) hemolytic icterus
Minkowski-Chauffard syndrome

D58.1 Hereditary elliptocytosis
Presence of large numbers of elliptocytes in blood
Elliptocytosis (congenital)
Ovalocytosis (congenital) (hereditary)

D58.2 Other hemoglobinopathies
Abnormal hemoglobin NOS
Congenital Heinz body anemia
Hb-C disease
Hb-D disease
Hb-E disease
Hemoglobinopathy NOS
Unstable hemoglobin hemolytic disease
Excludes1 familial polycythemia (D75.0)
Hb-M disease (D74.0)
hemoglobin E-beta thalassemia (D56.5)
hereditary persistence of fetal hemoglobin [HPFH] (D56.4)
high-altitude polycythemia (D75.1)
methemoglobinemia (D74.-)
other hemoglobinopathies with thalassemia (D56.8)

D58.8 Other specified hereditary hemolytic anemias
Stomatocytosis

D58.9 Hereditary hemolytic anemia, unspecified

● **D59 Acquired hemolytic anemia**

D59.0 Drug-induced autoimmune hemolytic anemia
Use additional code for adverse effect, if applicable, to identify drug (T36-T50 with fifth or sixth character 5)

D59.1 Other autoimmune hemolytic anemias
Autoimmune hemolytic disease (cold type) (warm type)
Chronic cold hemagglutinin disease
Cold agglutinin disease
Cold agglutinin hemoglobinuria
Cold type (secondary) (symptomatic) hemolytic anemia
Warm type (secondary) (symptomatic) hemolytic anemia
Excludes1 Evans syndrome (D69.41)
hemolytic disease of newborn (P55.-)
paroxysmal cold hemoglobinuria (D59.6)

D59.2 Drug-induced nonautoimmune hemolytic anemia
Drug-induced enzyme deficiency anemia
Use additional code for adverse effect, if applicable, to identify drug (T36-T50 with fifth or sixth character 5)

D59.3 Hemolytic-uremic syndrome
Use additional code to identify associated:
E. coli infection (B96.2-)
Pneumococcal pneumonia (J13)
Shigella dysenteriae (A03.9)

D59.4 Other nonautoimmune hemolytic anemias
Mechanical hemolytic anemia
Microangiopathic hemolytic anemia
Toxic hemolytic anemia

D59.5 Paroxysmal nocturnal hemoglobinuria [Marchiafava-Micheli]
Excludes1 hemoglobinuria NOS (R82.3)

D59.6 Hemoglobinuria due to hemolysis from other external causes
Hemoglobinuria from exertion
March hemoglobinuria
Paroxysmal cold hemoglobinuria
Use additional code (Chapter 20) to identify external cause
Excludes1 hemoglobinuria NOS (R82.3)

D59.8 Other acquired hemolytic anemias

D59.9 Acquired hemolytic anemia, unspecified
Idiopathic hemolytic anemia, chronic

APLASTIC AND OTHER ANEMIAS AND OTHER BONE MARROW FAILURE SYNDROMES (D60-D64)

● **D60 Acquired pure red cell aplasia [erythroblastopenia]**
Deficiency of erythroblasts
Includes red cell aplasia (acquired) (adult) (with thymoma)
Excludes1 congenital red cell aplasia (D61.01)

D60.0 Chronic acquired pure red cell aplasia
Lack of development of blood cell

D60.1 Transient acquired pure red cell aplasia

D60.8 Other acquired pure red cell aplasias

D60.9 Acquired pure red cell aplasia, unspecified

● **D61 Other aplastic anemias and other bone marrow failure syndromes**
Excludes1 neutropenia (D70.-)

● **D61.0 Constitutional aplastic anemia**
Condition where bone marrow is unable to produce blood cells

D61.01 Constitutional (pure) red blood cell aplasia
Blackfan-Diamond syndrome
Congenital (pure) red cell aplasia
Familial hypoplastic anemia
Primary (pure) red cell aplasia
Red cell (pure) aplasia of infants
Excludes1 acquired red cell aplasia (D60.9)

D61.09 Other constitutional aplastic anemia
Fanconi's anemia
Pancytopenia with malformations

D61.1 Drug-induced aplastic anemia
Use additional code for adverse effect, if applicable, to identify drug (T36-T50 with fifth or sixth character 5)

D61.2 Aplastic anemia due to other external agents
Code first, if applicable, toxic effects of substances chiefly nonmedicinal as to source (T51-T65)

D61.3 Idiopathic aplastic anemia

● **D61.8 Other specified aplastic anemias and other bone marrow failure syndromes**

● **D61.81 Pancytopenia**
Marked deficiency of all the blood elements: Red blood cells (erythrocytes), white blood cells (leukocytes), and platelets (thrombocytes). Check laboratory results.

Excludes1 pancytopenia (due to) (with) aplastic anemia (D61.9)
pancytopenia (due to) (with) bone marrow infiltration (D61.82)
pancytopenia (due to) (with) congenital (pure) red cell aplasia (D61.01)
pancytopenia (due to) (with) hairy cell leukemia (C91.4-)
pancytopenia (due to) (with) human immunodeficiency virus disease (B20.-)
pancytopenia (due to) (with) leukoerythroblastic anemia (D61.82)
pancytopenia (due to) (with) myeloproliferative disease (D47.1)

Excludes2 pancytopenia (due to) (with) myelodysplastic syndromes (D46.-)

D61.810 Antineoplastic chemotherapy induced pancytopenia
Excludes2 aplastic anemia due to antineoplastic chemotherapy (D61.1)

D61.811 Other drug-induced pancytopenia
Excludes2 aplastic anemia due to drugs (D61.1)

D61.818 Other pancytopenia

D61.82 Myelophthisis
Leukoerythroblastic anemia
Myelophthisic anemia
Panmyelophthisis
Code also the underlying disorder, such as:
malignant neoplasm of breast (C50.-)
tuberculosis (A15.-)
Excludes1 idiopathic myelofibrosis (D47.1)
myelofibrosis NOS (D75.81)
myelofibrosis with myeloid metaplasia (D47.4)
primary myelofibrosis (D47.1)
secondary myelofibrosis (D75.81)

D61.89 Other specified aplastic anemias and other bone marrow failure syndromes

D61.9 Aplastic anemia, unspecified
Hypoplastic anemia NOS
Medullary hypoplasia

D62 Acute posthemorrhagic anemia
Excludes1 anemia due to chronic blood loss (D50.0)
blood loss anemia NOS (D50.0)
congenital anemia from fetal blood loss (P61.3)

● **D63 Anemia in chronic diseases classified elsewhere**

D63.0 Anemia in neoplastic disease
Code first neoplasm (C00-D49)
Excludes1 ~~anemia due to antineoplastic chemotherapy (D64.81)~~
aplastic anemia due to antineoplastic chemotherapy (D61.1)
▶ **Excludes2** anemia due to antineoplastic chemotherapy (D64.81)

OGCR Section I.C.2.e.2.

2) Anemia associated with chemotherapy, immunotherapy and radiation therapy
When the admission/encounter is for management of an anemia associated with an adverse effect of the administration of chemotherapy or immunotherapy and the only treatment is for the anemia, the anemia code is sequenced first followed by the appropriate codes for the neoplasm and the adverse effect (T45.1X5, Adverse effect of antineoplastic and immunosuppressive drugs).

D63.1 Anemia in chronic kidney disease
Erythropoietin resistant anemia (EPO resistant anemia)
Code first underlying chronic kidney disease (CKD) (N18.-)

D63.8 Anemia in other chronic diseases classified elsewhere
Code first underlying disease, such as:
diphyllobothriasis (B70.0)
hookworm disease (B76.0-B76.9)
hypothyroidism (E00.0-E03.9)
malaria (B50.0-B54)
symptomatic late syphilis (A52.79)
tuberculosis (A18.89)

● **D64 Other anemias**
Excludes1 refractory anemia (D46.-)
refractory anemia with excess blasts in transformation [RAEB T] (C92.0-)

D64.0 Hereditary sideroblastic anemia
Abnormal production RBCs (erythrocytes)
Sex-linked hypochromic sideroblastic anemia

D64.1 Secondary sideroblastic anemia due to disease
Code first underlying disease

D64.2 Secondary sideroblastic anemia due to drugs and toxins
Code first poisoning due to drug or toxin, if applicable (T36-T65 with fifth or sixth character 1-4 or 6)
Use additional code for adverse effect, if applicable, to identify drug (T36-T50 with fifth or sixth character 5)

D64.3 Other sideroblastic anemias
Sideroblastic anemia NOS
Pyridoxine-responsive sideroblastic anemia NEC

D64.4 Congenital dyserythropoietic anemia
Any of several rare hereditary anemias, mostly types of macrocytic anemia
Dyshematopoietic anemia (congenital)
Excludes1 Blackfan-Diamond syndrome (D61.01)
Di Guglielmo's disease (C94.0)

● **D64.8 Other specified anemias**
D64.81 Anemia due to antineoplastic chemotherapy
Antineoplastic chemotherapy induced anemia
Excludes1 aplastic anemia due to antineoplastic chemotherapy (D61.1)
Excludes2 anemia in neoplastic disease (D63.0)

D64.89 Other specified anemias
Infantile pseudoleukemia

D64.9 Anemia, unspecified

CHAPTER 3 (D50-D89)

CHAPTER 3 (D50-D89)

COAGULATION DEFECTS, PURPURA AND OTHER HEMORRHAGIC CONDITIONS (D65-D69)

D65   Disseminated intravascular coagulation [defibrination syndrome]
Blood clots form and consume all coagulation proteins and platelets and disrupt normal coagulation, resulting in abnormal bleeding
Afibrinogenemia, acquired
Consumption coagulopathy
Diffuse or disseminated intravascular coagulation [DIC]
Fibrinolytic hemorrhage, acquired
Fibrinolytic purpura
Purpura fulminans

> **Excludes1**   disseminated intravascular coagulation (complicating):
> abortion or ectopic or molar pregnancy (O00-O07, O08.1)
> in newborn (P60)
> pregnancy, childbirth and the puerperium (O45.0, O46.0, O67.0, O72.3)

D66   Hereditary factor VIII deficiency
Inherited coagulation disorder carried by females but most often affecting males
Classical hemophilia
Deficiency factor VIII (with functional defect)
Hemophilia NOS
Hemophilia A

> **Excludes1**   factor VIII deficiency with vascular defect (D68.0)

D67   Hereditary factor IX deficiency
Christmas disease
Factor IX deficiency (with functional defect)
Hemophilia B
Plasma thromboplastin component [PTC] deficiency

● D68   Other coagulation defects

> **Excludes1**   abnormal coagulation profile (R79.1)
> coagulation defects complicating abortion or ectopic or molar pregnancy (O00-O07, O08.1)
> coagulation defects complicating pregnancy, childbirth and the puerperium (O45.0, O46.0, O67.0, O72.3)

D68.0   Von Willebrand's disease
Congenital bleeding disorder
Angiohemophilia
Factor VIII deficiency with vascular defect
Vascular hemophilia

> **Excludes1**   capillary fragility (hereditary) (D69.8)
> factor VIII deficiency NOS (D66)
> factor VIII deficiency with functional defect (D66)

D68.1   Hereditary factor XI deficiency
Deficiency of blood coagulation resulting in systemic blood-clotting defect
Hemophilia C
Plasma thromboplastin antecedent [PTA] deficiency
Rosenthal's disease

D68.2   Hereditary deficiency of other clotting factors
Blood clotting disorders caused by hereditary deficiencies of one or more clotting factors
AC globulin deficiency
Congenital afibrinogenemia
Deficiency of factor I [fibrinogen]
Deficiency of factor II [prothrombin]
Deficiency of factor V [labile]
Deficiency of factor VII [stable]
Deficiency of factor X [Stuart-Prower]
Deficiency of factor XII [Hageman]
Deficiency of factor XIII [fibrin stabilizing]
Dysfibrinogenemia (congenital)
Hypoproconvertinemia
Owren's disease
Proaccelerin deficiency

● D68.3   Hemorrhagic disorder due to circulating anticoagulants
Blood clotting disorders caused by anticoagulants (warfarin and heparin)

● D68.31   Hemorrhagic disorder due to intrinsic circulating anticoagulants, antibodies, or inhibitors

D68.311   Acquired hemophilia
Autoimmune hemophilia
Autoimmune inhibitors to clotting factors
Secondary hemophilia

D68.312   Antiphospholipid antibody with hemorrhagic disorder
Lupus anticoagulant (LAC) with hemorrhagic disorder
Systemic lupus erythematosus [SLE] inhibitor with hemorrhagic disorder

> **Excludes1**   antiphospholipid antibody, finding without diagnosis (R76.0)
> antiphospholipid antibody syndrome (D68.61)
> antiphospholipid antibody with hypercoagulable state (D68.61)
> lupus anticoagulant (LAC) finding without diagnosis (R76.0)
> lupus anticoagulant (LAC) with hypercoagulable state (D68.62)
> systemic lupus erythematosus [SLE] inhibitor finding without diagnosis (R76.0)
> systemic lupus erythematosus [SLE] inhibitor with hypercoagulable state (D68.62)

D68.318   Other hemorrhagic disorder due to intrinsic circulating anticoagulants, antibodies, or inhibitors
Antithromboplastinemia
Antithromboplastinogenemia
Hemorrhagic disorder due to intrinsic increase in antithrombin
Hemorrhagic disorder due to intrinsic increase in anti-VIIIa
Hemorrhagic disorder due to intrinsic increase in anti-IXa
Hemorrhagic disorder due to intrinsic increase in anti-XIa

D68.32   Hemorrhagic disorder due to extrinsic circulating anticoagulants
Drug-induced hemorrhagic disorder
Hemorrhagic disorder due to increase in anti-IIa
Hemorrhagic disorder due to increase in anti-Xa
Hyperheparinemia

> Use additional code for adverse effect, if applicable, to identify drug (T45.515, T45.525)

D68.4　Acquired coagulation factor deficiency
　　　Deficiency of coagulation factor due to liver disease
　　　Deficiency of coagulation factor due to vitamin K
　　　　deficiency
　　　| Excludes1 |　vitamin K deficiency of newborn (P53)

● **D68.5　Primary thrombophilia**
　　　AKA idiopathic thrombocytopenia, may be acquired or
　　　congenital and is a common cause of coagulation
　　　disorders.
　　　Primary hypercoagulable states
　　　| Excludes1 |　antiphospholipid syndrome (D68.61)
　　　　　　　　lupus anticoagulant (D68.62)
　　　　　　　　secondary activated protein C resistance
　　　　　　　　　(D68.69)
　　　　　　　　secondary antiphospholipid antibody
　　　　　　　　　syndrome (D68.69)
　　　　　　　　secondary lupus anticoagulant with
　　　　　　　　　hypercoagulable state (D68.69)
　　　　　　　　secondary systemic lupus erythematosus
　　　　　　　　　[SLE] inhibitor with hypercoagulable
　　　　　　　　　state (D68.69)
　　　　　　　　systemic lupus erythematosus [SLE]
　　　　　　　　　inhibitor finding without diagnosis
　　　　　　　　　(R76.0)
　　　　　　　　systemic lupus erythematosus [SLE]
　　　　　　　　　inhibitor with hemorrhagic disorder
　　　　　　　　　(D68.312)
　　　　　　　　thrombotic thrombocytopenic purpura
　　　　　　　　　(M31.1)

　　D68.51　Activated protein C resistance
　　　　　Factor V Leiden mutation

　　D68.52　Prothrombin gene mutation

　　D68.59　Other primary thrombophilia
　　　　　Antithrombin III deficiency
　　　　　Hypercoagulable state NOS
　　　　　Primary hypercoagulable state NEC
　　　　　Primary thrombophilia NEC
　　　　　Protein C deficiency
　　　　　Protein S deficiency
　　　　　Thrombophilia NOS

● **D68.6　Other thrombophilia**
　　　Other hypercoagulable states
　　　| Excludes1 |　diffuse or disseminated intravascular
　　　　　　　　coagulation [DIC] (D65)
　　　　　　　　heparin induced thrombocytopenia (HIT)
　　　　　　　　　(D75.82)
　　　　　　　　hyperhomocysteinemia (E72.11)

　　D68.61　Antiphospholipid syndrome
　　　　　Anticardiolipin syndrome
　　　　　Antiphospholipid antibody syndrome
　　　　　| Excludes1 |　anti-phospholipid antibody,
　　　　　　　　　finding without diagnosis
　　　　　　　　　(R76.0)
　　　　　　　　　anti-phospholipid antibody
　　　　　　　　　with hemorrhagic disorder
　　　　　　　　　(D68.312)
　　　　　　　　　lupus anticoagulant syndrome
　　　　　　　　　(D68.62)

　　D68.62　Lupus anticoagulant syndrome
　　　　　Lupus anticoagulant
　　　　　Presence of systemic lupus erythematosus
　　　　　　[SLE] inhibitor
　　　　　| Excludes1 |　anticardiolipin syndrome
　　　　　　　　　(D68.61)
　　　　　　　　　antiphospholipid syndrome
　　　　　　　　　(D68.61)
　　　　　　　　　lupus anticoagulant (LAC)
　　　　　　　　　finding without diagnosis
　　　　　　　　　(R76.0)
　　　　　　　　　lupus anticoagulant (LAC)
　　　　　　　　　with hemorrhagic disorder
　　　　　　　　　(D68.312)

　　D68.69　Other thrombophilia
　　　　　Hypercoagulable states NEC
　　　　　Secondary hypercoagulable state NOS

D68.8　Other specified coagulation defects
　　　| Excludes1 |　hemorrhagic disease of newborn (P53)

D68.9　Coagulation defect, unspecified

● **D69　Purpura and other hemorrhagic conditions**
　　Group of conditions characterized by small hemorrhages in skin,
　　　mucous membranes, or serosal surfaces
　　　| Excludes1 |　benign hypergammaglobulinemic purpura
　　　　　　　　(D89.0)
　　　　　　　　cryoglobulinemic purpura (D89.1)
　　　　　　　　essential (hemorrhagic) thrombocythemia (D47.3)
　　　　　　　　hemorrhagic thrombocythemia (D47.3)
　　　　　　　　purpura fulminans (D65)
　　　　　　　　thrombotic thrombocytopenic purpura (M31.1)
　　　　　　　　Waldenström hypergammaglobulinemic purpura
　　　　　　　　　(D89.0)

D69.0　Allergic purpura
　　　Allergic vasculitis
　　　Nonthrombocytopenic hemorrhagic purpura
　　　Nonthrombocytopenic idiopathic purpura
　　　Purpura anaphylactoid
　　　Purpura Henoch(-Schönlein)
　　　Purpura rheumatica
　　　Vascular purpura
　　　| Excludes1 |　thrombocytopenic hemorrhagic purpura
　　　　　　　　(D69.3)

D69.1　Qualitative platelet defects
　　　Bernard-Soulier [giant platelet] syndrome
　　　Glanzmann's disease
　　　Grey platelet syndrome
　　　Thromboasthenia (hemorrhagic) (hereditary)
　　　Thrombocytopathy
　　　| Excludes1 |　von Willebrand's disease (D68.0)

D69.2　Other nonthrombocytopenic purpura
　　　Purpura NOS
　　　Purpura simplex
　　　Senile purpura

D69.3　Immune thrombocytopenic purpura
　　　Hemorrhagic (thrombocytopenic) purpura
　　　Idiopathic thrombocytopenic purpura
　　　Tidal platelet dysgenesis

● **D69.4　Other primary thrombocytopenia**
　　　| Excludes1 |　transient neonatal thrombocytopenia
　　　　　　　　(P61.0)
　　　　　　　　Wiskott-Aldrich syndrome (D82.0)

　　D69.41　Evans syndrome
　　　　　Acquired hemolytic anemia and thrombocytopenia

　　D69.42　Congenital and hereditary thrombocytopenia
　　　　purpura
　　　　　Congenital thrombocytopenia
　　　　　Hereditary thrombocytopenia
　　　　　Code first congential or hereditary disorder,
　　　　　　such as:
　　　　　　thrombocytopenia with absent radius (TAR
　　　　　　　syndrome) (Q87.2)

　　D69.49　Other primary thrombocytopenia
　　　　　Megakaryocytic hypoplasia
　　　　　Primary thrombocytopenia NOS

● **D69.5　Secondary thrombocytopenia**
　　　Acquired reduction of number of platelets required for blood
　　　　clotting
　　　| Excludes1 |　heparin induced thrombocytopenia (HIT)
　　　　　　　　(D75.82)
　　　　　　　　transient thrombocytopenia of newborn
　　　　　　　　　(P61.0)

　　D69.51　Posttransfusion purpura
　　　　　Posttransfusion purpura from whole blood
　　　　　　(fresh) or blood products PTP

　　D69.59　Other secondary thrombocytopenia

D69.6　Thrombocytopenia, unspecified

D69.8　Other specified hemorrhagic conditions
　　　Capillary fragility (hereditary)
　　　Vascular pseudohemophilia

D69.9　Hemorrhagic condition, unspecified

OTHER DISORDERS OF BLOOD AND BLOOD-FORMING ORGANS (D70-D77)

● **D70 Neutropenia**
Decrease in number of neutrophils (type of white blood cell)

Includes   agranulocytosis
decreased absolute neurophile count (ANC)

Use additional code for any associated:
fever (R50.81)
mucositis (J34.81, K12.3-, K92.81, N76.81)

Excludes1   neutropenic splenomegaly (D73.81)
transient neonatal neutropenia (P61.5)

D70.0 Congenital agranulocytosis
Reduced numbers of neutrophils (type of white blood cell)
Congenital neutropenia
Infantile genetic agranulocytosis
Kostmann's disease

D70.1 Agranulocytosis secondary to cancer chemotherapy
Decreased numbers of granulocytes (type of white blood cell)
Code also *underlying neoplasm*
Use additional code for adverse effect, if applicable, to identify drug (T45.1X5)

D70.2 Other drug-induced agranulocytosis
Use additional code for adverse effect, if applicable, to identify drug (T36-T50 with fifth or sixth character 5)

D70.3 Neutropenia due to infection

D70.4 Cyclic neutropenia
Chronic neutropenia (low number of type of white blood cell)
Cyclic hematopoiesis
Periodic neutropenia

D70.8 Other neutropenia

D70.9 Neutropenia, unspecified

D71 Functional disorders of polymorphonuclear neutrophils
Polymorphonuclear: varying shapes of nucleus; AKA PMNs
Cell membrane receptor complex [CR3] defect
Chronic (childhood) granulomatous disease
Congenital dysphagocytosis
Progressive septic granulomatosis

● **D72 Other disorders of white blood cells**

Excludes1   basophilia (D72.824)
immunity disorders (D80-D89)
neutropenia (D70)
preleukemia (syndrome) (D46.9)

D72.0 Genetic anomalies of leukocytes
Alder (granulation) (granulocyte) anomaly
Alder syndrome
Hereditary leukocytic hypersegmentation
Hereditary leukocytic hyposegmentation
Hereditary leukomelanopathy
May-Hegglin (granulation) (granulocyte) anomaly
May-Hegglin syndrome
Pelger-Huët (granulation) (granulocyte) anomaly
Pelger-Huët syndrome

Excludes1   Chédiak (-Steinbrinck)-Higashi syndrome (E70.330)

D72.1 Eosinophilia
Formation and accumulation of high number of white cells in blood/tissue
Allergic eosinophilia
Hereditary eosinophilia

Excludes1   Löffler's syndrome (J82)
pulmonary eosinophilia (J82)

● **D72.8 Other specified disorders of white blood cells**
Excludes1   leukemia (C91-C95)

● **D72.81 Decreased white blood cell count**
Excludes1   neutropenia (D70.-)

D72.810 Lymphocytopenia
Decreased lymphocytes
Reduction in number of lympho cytes in blood

D72.818 Other decreased white blood cell count
Basophilic leukopenia
Eosinophilic leukopenia
Monocytopenia
Other decreased leukocytes
Plasmacytopenia

D72.819 Decreased white blood cell count, unspecified
Decreased leukocytes, unspecified
Leukocytopenia, unspecified
Leukopenia
Excludes1   malignant leukopenia (D70.9)

● **D72.82 Elevated white blood cell count**
Excludes1   eosinophilia (D72.1)

D72.820 Lymphocytosis (symptomatic)
Elevated lymphocytes
Excess of normal lymphocytes

D72.821 Monocytosis (symptomatic)
Excludes1   infectious mononucleosis (B27.-)

D72.822 Plasmacytosis
Presence of excess plasma cells

D72.823 Leukemoid reaction
Basophilic leukemoid reaction
Leukemoid reaction NOS
Lymphocytic leukemoid reaction
Monocytic leukemoid reaction
Myelocytic leukemoid reaction
Neutrophilic leukemoid reaction

D72.824 Basophilia
Increase of basophils in blood

D72.825 Bandemia
Bandemia without diagnosis of specific infection
Excess number of band cells (immature white blood cells) released by bone marrow
Excludes1   confirmed infection -code to infection leukemia (C91.-, C92.-, C93.-, C94.-, C95.-)

D72.828 Other elevated white blood cell count

D72.829 Elevated white blood cell count, unspecified
Elevated leukocytes, unspecified
Leukocytosis, unspecified

D72.89 Other specified disorders of white blood cells
Abnormality of white blood cells NEC

D72.9 Disorder of white blood cells, unspecified
Abnormal leukocyte differential NOS

● **D73   Diseases of spleen**

D73.0   Hyposplenism
Diminished functioning of spleen
Atrophy of spleen

Excludes1	asplenia (congenital) (Q89.Ø1)
	postsurgical absence of spleen (Z9Ø.81)

D73.1   Hypersplenism
Accelerated function of spleen

Excludes1	neutropenic splenomegaly (D73.81)
	primary splenic neutropenia (D73.81)
	splenitis, splenomegaly in late syphilis (A52.79)
	splenitis, splenomegaly in tuberculosis (A18.85)
	splenomegaly NOS (R16.1)
	splenomegaly congenital (Q89.Ø)

D73.2   Chronic congestive splenomegaly
Enlargement of spleen

D73.3   Abscess of spleen

D73.4   Cyst of spleen

D73.5   Infarction of spleen
Splenic rupture, nontraumatic
Torsion of spleen

Excludes1	rupture of spleen due to Plasmodium vivax malaria (B51.Ø)
	traumatic rupture of spleen (S36.Ø3-)

● **D73.8   Other diseases of spleen**

D73.81   Neutropenic splenomegaly
Werner-Schultz disease
Enlarged spleen responding to inadequate number of neutrophils

D73.89   Other diseases of spleen
Fibrosis of spleen NOS
Perisplenitis
Splenitis NOS

D73.9   Disease of spleen, unspecified

● **D74   Methemoglobinemia**
Excessive methemoglobin (form of hemoglobin)

D74.0   Congenital methemoglobinemia
Congenital NADH-methemoglobin reductase deficiency
Hemoglobin-M [Hb-M] disease
Methemoglobinemia, hereditary

D74.8   Other methemoglobinemias
Acquired methemoglobinemia (with sulfhemoglobinemia)
Toxic methemoglobinemia

D74.9   Methemoglobinemia, unspecified

● **D75   Other and unspecified diseases of blood and blood-forming organs**

Excludes2	acute lymphadenitis (LØ4.-)
	chronic lymphadenitis (I88.1)
	enlarged lymph nodes (R59.-)
	hypergammaglobulinemia NOS (D89.2)
	lymphadenitis NOS (I88.9)
	mesenteric lymphadenitis (acute) (chronic) (I88.Ø)

D75.0   Familial erythrocytosis
Genetic mutation of gene that results in increased circulating RBCs
Benign polycythemia
Familial polycythemia

Excludes1	hereditary ovalocytosis (D58.1)

D75.1   Secondary polycythemia
Increase in total red cell mass
Acquired polycythemia
Emotional polycythemia
Erythrocytosis NOS
Hypoxemic polycythemia
Nephrogenous polycythemia
Polycythemia due to erythropoietin
Polycythemia due to fall in plasma volume
Polycythemia due to high altitude
Polycythemia due to stress
Polycythemia NOS
Relative polycythemia

Excludes1	polycythemia neonatorum (P61.1)
	polycythemia vera (D45)

● **D75.8   Other specified diseases of blood and blood-forming organs**

D75.81   Myelofibrosis
Replacing bone marrow by fibrous tissue
Myelofibrosis NOS
Secondary myelofibrosis NOS

Code first the underlying disorder, such as:
malignant neoplasm of breast (C5Ø.-)

Use additional code, if applicable, for associated therapy-related myelodysplastic syndrome (D46.-)

Use additional code for adverse effect, if applicable, to identify drug (T45.1X5)

Excludes1	acute myelofibrosis (C94.4-)
	idiopathic myelofibrosis (D47.1)
	leukoerythroblastic anemia (D61.82)
	myelofibrosis with myeloid metaplasia (D47.4)
	myelophthisic anemia (D61.82)
	myelophthisis (D61.82)
	primary myelofibrosis (D47.1)

D75.82   Heparin induced thrombocytopenia (HIT)

D75.89   Other specified diseases of blood and blood-forming organs

D75.9   Disease of blood and blood-forming organs, unspecified

● **D76   Other specified diseases with participation of lymphoreticular and reticulohistiocytic tissue**

Excludes1	(Abt-) Letterer-Siwe disease (C96.Ø)
	eosinophilic granuloma (C96.6)
	Hand-Schüller-Christian disease (C96.5)
	histiocytic medullary reticulosis (C96.9)
	histiocytic sarcoma (C96.A)
	histiocytosis X, multifocal (C96.5)
	histiocytosis X, unifocal (C96.6)
	Langerhans-cell histiocytosis, multifocal (C96.5)
	Langerhans-cell histiocytosis NOS (C96.6)
	Langerhans-cell histiocytosis, unifocal (C96.6)
	leukemic reticuloendotheliosis (C91.4-)
	lipomelanotic reticulosis (I89.8)
	malignant histiocytosis (C96.A)
	malignant reticulosis (C86.Ø)
	nonlipid reticuloendotheliosis (C96.Ø)

D76.1   Hemophagocytic lymphohistiocytosis
Familial hemophagocytic reticulosis
Histiocytoses of mononuclear phagocytes

D76.2   Hemophagocytic syndrome, infection-associated
Use additional code to identify infectious agent or disease.

D76.3   Other histiocytosis syndromes
Reticulohistiocytoma (giant-cell)
Sinus histiocytosis with massive lymphadenopathy
Xanthogranuloma

CHAPTER 3 (D5Ø-D89)

D77   **Other disorders of blood and blood-forming organs in diseases classified elsewhere**

     Code first underlying disease, such as:
       amyloidosis (E85.-)
       congenital early syphilis (A50.0)
       echinococcosis (B67.0-B67.9)
       malaria (B50.0-B54)
       schistosomiasis [bilharziasis] (B65.0-B65.9)
       vitamin C deficiency (E54)

     Excludes1   rupture of spleen due to Plasmodium vivax malaria (B51.0)
               splenitis, splenomegaly in late syphilis (A52.79)
               splenitis, splenomegaly in tuberculosis (A18.85)

INTRAOPERATIVE AND POSTPROCEDURAL COMPLICATIONS OF THE SPLEEN (D78)

● D78   **Intraoperative and postprocedural complications of the spleen**

    ● D78.0   **Intraoperative hemorrhage and hematoma of the spleen complicating a procedure**

       Excludes1   intraoperative hemorrhage and hematoma of the spleen due to accidental puncture or laceration during a procedure (D78.1-)

       D78.01   Intraoperative hemorrhage and hematoma of the spleen complicating a procedure on the spleen

       D78.02   Intraoperative hemorrhage and hematoma of the spleen complicating other procedure

    ● D78.1   **Accidental puncture and laceration of the spleen during a procedure**

       D78.11   Accidental puncture and laceration of the spleen during a procedure on the spleen

       D78.12   Accidental puncture and laceration of the spleen during other procedure

    ● D78.2   **Postprocedural hemorrhage of the spleen following a procedure**

       D78.21   Postprocedural hemorrhage of the spleen following a procedure on the spleen

       D78.22   Postprocedural hemorrhage of the spleen following other procedure

    ● D78.3   **Postprocedural hematoma and seroma of the spleen following a procedure**

       D78.31   Postprocedural hematoma of the spleen following a procedure on the spleen

       D78.32   Postprocedural hematoma of the spleen following other procedure

       D78.33   Postprocedural seroma of the spleen following a procedure on the spleen

       D78.34   Postprocedural seroma of the spleen following other procedure

    ● D78.8   **Other intraoperative and postprocedural complications of the spleen**

       Use additional code, if applicable, to further specify disorder

       D78.81   Other intraoperative complications of the spleen

       D78.89   Other postprocedural complications of the spleen

CERTAIN DISORDERS INVOLVING THE IMMUNE MECHANISM (D80-D89)

    Includes   defects in the complement system
             immunodeficiency disorders, except human immunodeficiency virus [HIV] disease
             sarcoidosis

    Excludes1   autoimmune disease (systemic) NOS (M35.9)
             functional disorders of polymorphonuclear neutrophils (D71)
             human immunodeficiency virus [HIV] disease (B20)

● D80   **Immunodeficiency with predominantly antibody defects**

    D80.0   **Hereditary hypogammaglobulinemia**
       Autosomal recessive agammaglobulinemia (Swiss type)
       X-linked agammaglobulinemia [Bruton] (with growth hormone deficiency)

    D80.1   **Nonfamilial hypogammaglobulinemia**
       Abnormally low levels of all classes of immunoglobulins
       Agammaglobulinemia with immunoglobulin-bearing B-lymphocytes
       Common variable agammaglobulinemia [CVAgamma]
       Hypogammaglobulinemia NOS

    D80.2   **Selective deficiency of immunoglobulin A [IgA]**

    D80.3   **Selective deficiency of immunoglobulin G [IgG] subclasses**

    D80.4   **Selective deficiency of immunoglobulin M [IgM]**

    D80.5   **Immunodeficiency with increased immunoglobulin M [IgM]**

    D80.6   **Antibody deficiency with near-normal immunoglobulins or with hyperimmunoglobulinemia**
       Abnormally high levels of immunoglobulins in serum

    D80.7   **Transient hypogammaglobulinemia of infancy**

    D80.8   **Other immunodeficiencies with predominantly antibody defects**
       Kappa light chain deficiency

    D80.9   **Immunodeficiency with predominantly antibody defects, unspecified**

● D81   **Combined immunodeficiencies**

    Excludes1   autosomal recessive agammaglobulinemia (Swiss type) (D80.0)

    D81.0   **Severe combined immunodeficiency [SCID] with reticular dysgenesis**

    D81.1   **Severe combined immunodeficiency [SCID] with low T- and B-cell numbers**

    D81.2   **Severe combined immunodeficiency [SCID] with low or normal B-cell numbers**

    D81.3   **Adenosine deaminase [ADA] deficiency**

    D81.4   **Nezelof's syndrome**

    D81.5   **Purine nucleoside phosphorylase [PNP] deficiency**

    D81.6   **Major histocompatibility complex class I deficiency**
       Bare lymphocyte syndrome

    D81.7   **Major histocompatibility complex class II deficiency**

▶ New   ⇒ Revised   ~~deleted~~ Deleted   **OGCR** Official Guidelines   X Assign placeholder X   ● Use Additional Character(s)

Excludes 1   Excludes 2   Includes   Use additional   Code first   Code also   Key words

- **D81.8**   **Other combined immunodeficiencies**
  - **D81.81**   **Biotin-dependent carboxylase deficiency**
    Multiple carboxylase deficiency
    > **Excludes1**   biotin-dependent carboxylase deficiency due to dietary deficiency of biotin (E53.8)
    - **D81.810**   **Biotinidase deficiency**
    - **D81.818**   **Other biotin-dependent carboxylase deficiency**
      Holocarboxylase synthetase deficiency
      Other multiple carboxylase deficiency
    - **D81.819**   **Biotin-dependent carboxylase deficiency, unspecified**
      Multiple carboxylase deficiency, unspecified
  - **D81.89**   **Other combined immunodeficiencies**
  - **D81.9**   **Combined immunodeficiency, unspecified**
    Severe combined immunodeficiency disorder [SCID] NOS

- **D82**   **Immunodeficiency associated with other major defects**
  > **Excludes1**   ataxia telangiectasia [Louis-Bar] (G11.3)
  - **D82.0**   **Wiskott-Aldrich syndrome**
    X-linked immunodeficiency
    Immunodeficiency with thrombocytopenia and eczema
  - **D82.1**   **Di George's syndrome**
    Congenital disorder with defective development of third and fourth pharyngeal pouches
    Pharyngeal pouch syndrome
    Thymic alymphoplasia
    Thymic aplasia or hypoplasia with immunodeficiency
  - **D82.2**   **Immunodeficiency with short-limbed stature**
  - **D82.3**   **Immunodeficiency following hereditary defective response to Epstein-Barr virus**
    X-linked lymphoproliferative disease
  - **D82.4**   **Hyperimmunoglobulin E [IgE] syndrome**
    Suspected genetic defect that produces high levels of antibody immunoglobulin (IgE) that causes skin and lung infections and eczema
  - **D82.8**   **Immunodeficiency associated with other specified major defects**
  - **D82.9**   **Immunodeficiency associated with major defect, unspecified**

- **D83**   **Common variable immunodeficiency**
  - **D83.0**   **Common variable immunodeficiency with predominant abnormalities of B-cell numbers and function**
  - **D83.1**   **Common variable immunodeficiency with predominant immunoregulatory T-cell disorders**
  - **D83.2**   **Common variable immunodeficiency with autoantibodies to B- or T-cells**
  - **D83.8**   **Other common variable immunodeficiencies**
  - **D83.9**   **Common variable immunodeficiency, unspecified**

- **D84**   **Other immunodeficiencies**
  - **D84.0**   **Lymphocyte function antigen-1 [LFA-1] defect**
  - **D84.1**   **Defects in the complement system**
    C1 esterase inhibitor [C1-INH] deficiency
  - **D84.8**   **Other specified immunodeficiencies**
  - **D84.9**   **Immunodeficiency, unspecified**

Item 3-1 Sarcoidosis: A symptom of an inflammation producing tiny lumps of cells (granulomas) in various organs, most commonly the lungs and lymph nodes, that affect organ function. Cause is unknown occurring primarily in 20- to 40-year-olds, African-American, especially women, and those of Asian, German, Irish, Scandinavian, and Puerto Rican heritage.

- **D86**   **Sarcoidosis**
  - **D86.0**   **Sarcoidosis of lung**
  - **D86.1**   **Sarcoidosis of lymph nodes**
  - **D86.2**   **Sarcoidosis of lung with sarcoidosis of lymph nodes**
  - **D86.3**   **Sarcoidosis of skin**
  - **D86.8**   **Sarcoidosis of other sites**
    - **D86.81**   **Sarcoid meningitis**
    - **D86.82**   **Multiple cranial nerve palsies in sarcoidosis**
    - **D86.83**   **Sarcoid iridocyclitis**
      Rare large tumor with irregular surface of iris
    - **D86.84**   **Sarcoid pyelonephritis**
      Systemic disease of unknown etiology characterized by chronic granulomatous inflammation with tissue destruction of pelvis kidney
      Tubulo-interstitial nephropathy in sarcoidosis
    - **D86.85**   **Sarcoid myocarditis**
    - **D86.86**   **Sarcoid arthropathy**
      Polyarthritis in sarcoidosis
    - **D86.87**   **Sarcoid myositis**
      Granumloma of muscle
    - **D86.89**   **Sarcoidosis of other sites**
      Hepatic granuloma
      Uveoparotid fever [Heerfordt]
  - **D86.9**   **Sarcoidosis, unspecified**

- **D89**   **Other disorders involving the immune mechanism, not elsewhere classified**
  > **Excludes1**   hyperglobulinemia NOS (R77.1)
  > monoclonal gammopathy (of undetermined significance) (D47.2)
  > **Excludes2**   transplant failure and rejection (T86.-)
  - **D89.0**   **Polyclonal hypergammaglobulinemia**
    Benign hypergammaglobulinemic purpura
    Polyclonal gammopathy NOS
  - **D89.1**   **Cryoglobulinemia**
    Cryoglobulin (proteins) in blood that precipitate temperatures below 98.6° F; usually symptomatic of underlying disease
    Cryoglobulinemic purpura
    Cryoglobulinemic vasculitis
    Essential cryoglobulinemia
    Idiopathic cryoglobulinemia
    Mixed cryoglobulinemia
    Primary cryoglobulinemia
    Secondary cryoglobulinemia
  - **D89.2**   **Hypergammaglobulinemia, unspecified**
  - **D89.3**   **Immune reconstitution syndrome**
    Immune reconstitution inflammatory syndrome [IRIS]
    Use additional code for adverse effect, if applicable, to identify drug (T36-T50 with fifth or sixth character 5)

CHAPTER 3 (D50-D89)

● **D89.4   Mast cell activation syndrome and related disorders**

> ⇛ **Excludes1**   aggressive systemic mastocytosis (C96.21)
> ⇛ congenital cutaneous mastocytosis (Q82.2)
> ~~indolent systemic mastocytosis (D47.0)~~
> ~~malignant mastocytoma (C96.2)~~
> ▶(non-congenital) cutaneous mastocytosis (D47.01)
> ▶(indolent) systemic mastocytosis (D47.02)
> ▶malignant mast cell neoplasm (C96.2-)
> ▶malignant mastocytoma (C96.29)
> mast cell leukemia (C94.3-)
> ~~mastocytoma (D47.0)~~
> ~~systemic mastocytosis associated with a clonal hematologic non-mast cell lineage disease (SM-AHNMD) (D47.0)~~
> ▶mast cell sarcoma (C96.22)
> ▶mastocytoma NOS (D47.09)
> ▶other mast cell neoplasms of uncertain behavior (D47.09)
> ▶systemic mastocytosis associated with a clonal hematologic non-mast cell lineage disease (SM-AHNMD) (D47.02)

D89.40   **Mast cell activation, unspecified**
Mast cell activation disorder, unspecified
Mast cell activation syndrome, NOS

D89.41   **Monoclonal mast cell activation syndrome**

D89.42   **Idiopathic mast cell activation syndrome**

D89.43   **Secondary mast cell activation**
Secondary mast cell activation syndrome
Code also underlying etiology, if known

D89.49   **Other mast cell activation disorder**
Other mast cell activation syndrome

● **D89.8   Other specified disorders involving the immune mechanism, not elsewhere classified**

● **D89.81   Graft-versus-host disease**

Code first underlying cause, such as:
complications of transplanted organs and tissue (T86.-)
complications of blood transfusion (T80.89)
Use additional code to identify associated manifestations, such as:
desquamative dermatitis (L30.8)
diarrhea (R19.7)
elevated bilirubin (R17)
hair loss (L65.9)

D89.810   **Acute graft-versus-host disease**

D89.811   **Chronic graft-versus-host disease**

D89.812   **Acute on chronic graft-versus-host disease**

D89.813   **Graft-versus-host disease, unspecified**

D89.82   **Autoimmune lymphoproliferative syndrome [ALPS]**

D89.89   **Other specified disorders involving the immune mechanism, not elsewhere classified**

> **Excludes1**   human immunodeficiency virus disease (B20)

D89.9   **Disorder involving the immune mechanism, unspecified**
Immune disease NOS

CHAPTER 3 (D50-D89)

▶ New   ⇛ Revised   ~~deleted~~ Deleted   **OGCR** Official Guidelines   X Assign placeholder X   ● Use Additional Character(s)
Excludes 1   Excludes 2   Includes   Use additional   Code first   Code also   Key words

CHAPTER 4

ENDOCRINE, NUTRITIONAL AND METABOLIC DISEASES (E00-E89)

OGCR Chapter-Specific Coding Guidelines

4. **Chapter 4: Endocrine, Nutritional, and Metabolic Diseases (E00-E89)**

   a. **Diabetes mellitus**

   The diabetes mellitus codes are combination codes that include the type of diabetes mellitus, the body system affected, and the complications affecting that body system. As many codes within a particular category as are necessary to describe all of the complications of the disease may be used. They should be sequenced based on the reason for a particular encounter. Assign as many codes from categories E08 – E13 as needed to identify all of the associated conditions that the patient has.

   1) **Type of diabetes**

   The age of a patient is not the sole determining factor, though most type 1 diabetics develop the condition before reaching puberty. For this reason type 1 diabetes mellitus is also referred to as juvenile diabetes.

   2) **Type of diabetes mellitus not documented**

   If the type of diabetes mellitus is not documented in the medical record the default is E11.-, Type 2 diabetes mellitus.

   3) **Diabetes mellitus and the use of insulin oral hypoglycemics**

   If the documentation in a medical record does not indicate the type of diabetes but does indicate that the patient uses insulin, code E11, Type 2 diabetes mellitus, should be assigned. **An additional code should be assigned from category Z79 to identify the long-term (current) use of insulin or oral hypoglycemic drugs. If the patient is treated with both oral medications and insulin, only the code for long-term (current) use of insulin should be assigned. Code Z79.4 should not be assigned if insulin is given temporarily to bring a type 2 patient's blood sugar under control during an encounter.**

   4) **Diabetes mellitus in pregnancy and gestational diabetes**
   See Section I.C.15. Diabetes mellitus in pregnancy.
   See Section I.C.15. Gestational (pregnancy induced) diabetes

   5) **Complications due to insulin pump malfunction**

      (a) **Underdose of insulin due to insulin pump failure**
   An underdose of insulin due to an insulin pump failure should be assigned to a code from subcategory T85.6, Mechanical complication of other specified internal and external prosthetic devices, implants and grafts, that specifies the type of pump malfunction, as the principal or first-listed code, followed by code T38.3X6-, Underdosing of insulin and oral hypoglycemic [antidiabetic] drugs. Additional codes for the type of diabetes mellitus and any associated complications due to the underdosing should also be assigned.

      (b) **Overdose of insulin due to insulin pump failure**
   The principal or first-listed code for an encounter due to an insulin pump malfunction resulting in an overdose of insulin, should also be T85.6-, Mechanical complication of other specified internal and external prosthetic devices, implants and grafts, followed by code T38.3X1-, Poisoning by insulin and oral hypoglycemic [antidiabetic] drugs, accidental (unintentional).

   6) **Secondary diabetes mellitus**
   Codes under categories E08, Diabetes mellitus due to underlying condition, E09, Drug or chemical induced diabetes mellitus and E13, Other specified diabetes mellitus, identify complications/manifestations associated with secondary diabetes mellitus. Secondary diabetes is always caused by another condition or event (e.g., cystic fibrosis, malignant neoplasm of pancreas, pancreatectomy, adverse effect of drug, or poisoning).

      (a) **Secondary diabetes mellitus and the use of insulin or hypoglycemic drugs**
   For patients with secondary diabetes mellitus who routinely use insulin or oral hypoglycemic drugs, an additional code from category Z79 should be assigned to identify the long-term (current) use of insulin or oral hypoglycemic drugs. If the patient is treated with both oral medications and insulin, only the code for long-term (current) use of insulin should be assigned. Code Z79.4 should not be assigned if insulin is given temporarily to bring a secondary diabetic patient's blood sugar under control during an encounter.

      (b) **Assigning and sequencing secondary diabetes codes and its causes**
   The sequencing of the secondary diabetes codes in relationship to codes for the cause of the diabetes is based on the Tabular List instructions for categories E08, E09 and E13.

         (i) **Secondary diabetes mellitus due to pancreatectomy** For postpancreatectomy diabetes mellitus (lack of insulin due to the surgical removal of all or part of the pancreas), assign code E89.1, Postprocedural hypoinsulinemia. Assign a code from category E13 and a code from subcategory Z90.41-, Acquired absence of pancreas, as additional codes.

         (ii) **Secondary diabetes due to drugs** Secondary diabetes may be caused by an adverse effect of correctly administered medications, poisoning or sequela of poisoning.
   See section I.C.19.e for coding of adverse effects and poisoning, and section I.C.20 for external cause code reporting.

Figure 4-1 The endocrine system. (From Buck CJ: Step-by-Step Medical Coding, ed 2016, St. Louis, Elsevier, 2016)

CHAPTER 4

ENDOCRINE, NUTRITIONAL AND METABOLIC DISEASES (E00-E89)

All neoplasms, whether functionally active or not, are classified in Chapter 2. Appropriate codes in this chapter (i.e., E05.8, E07.0, E16-E31, E34.-) may be used as additional codes to indicate either functional activity by neoplasms and ectopic endocrine tissue or hyperfunction and hypofunction of endocrine glands associated with neoplasms and other conditions classified elsewhere.

| **Excludes1** | transitory endocrine and metabolic disorders specific to newborn (P70-P74) |

This chapter contains the following blocks:

E00-E07	Disorders of thyroid gland
E08-E13	Diabetes mellitus
E15-E16	Other disorders of glucose regulation and pancreatic internal secretion
E20-E35	Disorders of other endocrine glands
E36	Intraoperative complications of endocrine system
E40-E46	Malnutrition
E50-E64	Other nutritional deficiencies
E65-E68	Overweight, obesity and other hyperalimentation
E70-E88	Metabolic disorders
E89	Postprocedural endocrine and metabolic complications and disorders, not elsewhere classified

DISORDERS OF THYROID GLAND (E00-E07)

● **E00**   **Congenital iodine-deficiency syndrome**

Use additional code (F70-F79) to identify associated intellectual disabilities.

| **Excludes1** | subclinical iodine-deficiency hypothyroidism (E02) |

E00.0   **Congenital iodine-deficiency syndrome, neurological type**
Endemic cretinism, neurological type

E00.1   **Congenital iodine-deficiency syndrome, myxedematous type**
Dry, waxy type of swelling (nonpitting edema) with abnormal deposits of mucin in skin (mucinosis) and other tissues
Endemic hypothyroid cretinism
Endemic cretinism, myxedematous type

E00.2   **Congenital iodine-deficiency syndrome, mixed type**
Endemic cretinism, mixed type

E00.9   **Congenital iodine-deficiency syndrome, unspecified**
Congenital iodine-deficiency hypothyroidism NOS
Endemic cretinism NOS

Figure 4-2 **Goiter** is an enlargement of the thyroid gland.

Item 4-1 **Simple** goiter indicates no nodules are present. The most common type of goiter is a **diffuse colloidal,** also called a **nontoxic** or **endemic** goiter.

● **E01**   **Iodine-deficiency related thyroid disorders and allied conditions**

| **Excludes1** | congenital iodine-deficiency syndrome (E00.-) subclinical iodine-deficiency hypothyroidism (E02) |

E01.0   **Iodine-deficiency related diffuse (endemic) goiter**
Thyroid gland is enlarged

E01.1   **Iodine-deficiency related multinodular (endemic) goiter**
Iodine-deficiency related nodular goiter

E01.2   **Iodine-deficiency related (endemic) goiter, unspecified**
Endemic goiter NOS

E01.8   **Other iodine-deficiency related thyroid disorders and allied conditions**
Acquired iodine-deficiency hypothyroidism NOS

   E02   **Subclinical iodine-deficiency hypothyroidism**

● **E03**   **Other hypothyroidism**

| **Excludes1** | iodine-deficiency related hypothyroidism (E00-E02) postprocedural hypothyroidism (E89.0) |

E03.0   **Congenital hypothyroidism with diffuse goiter**
Congenital parenchymatous goiter (nontoxic)
Congenital goiter (nontoxic) NOS

| **Excludes1** | transitory congenital goiter with normal function (P72.0) |

E03.1   **Congenital hypothyroidism without goiter**
Aplasia of thyroid (with myxedema)
Congenital atrophy of thyroid
Congenital hypothyroidism NOS

E03.2   **Hypothyroidism due to medicaments and other exogenous substances**

Code first poisoning due to drug or toxin, if applicable (T36-T65 with fifth or sixth character 1-4 or 6)

Use additional code for adverse effect, if applicable, to identify drug (T36-T50 with fifth or sixth character 5)

E03.3   **Postinfectious hypothyroidism**

E03.4   **Atrophy of thyroid (acquired)**

| **Excludes1** | congenital atrophy of thyroid (E03.1) |

E03.5   **Myxedema coma**
Often fatal complication of long-term hypothyroidism

E03.8   **Other specified hypothyroidism**

E03.9   **Hypothyroidism, unspecified**
Myxedema NOS

Item 4-2 **Hypothyroidism** is a condition in which there are insufficient levels of thyroxine. **Cretinism** is congenital hypothyroidism, which can result in mental and physical retardation.

● **E04　Other nontoxic goiter**
　　[Excludes1]　congenital goiter (NOS) (diffuse)
　　　　　　　　　　(parenchymatous) (E03.0)
　　　　　　　　iodine-deficiency related goiter (E00-E02)

E04.0　Nontoxic diffuse goiter
　　　Thyroid gland is enlarged
　　　Diffuse (colloid) nontoxic goiter
　　　Simple nontoxic goiter

E04.1　Nontoxic single thyroid nodule
　　　Colloid nodule (cystic) (thyroid)
　　　Nontoxic uninodular goiter
　　　Thyroid (cystic) nodule NOS

E04.2　Nontoxic multinodular goiter
　　　Enlarged thyroid gland with multiple nodules
　　　Cystic goiter NOS
　　　Multinodular (cystic) goiter NOS

E04.8　Other specified nontoxic goiter

E04.9　Nontoxic goiter, unspecified
　　　Goiter NOS
　　　Nodular goiter (nontoxic) NOS

● **E05　Thyrotoxicosis [hyperthyroidism]**
　　Enlarged thyroid gland with multiple nodules
　　[Excludes1]　chronic thyroiditis with transient thyrotoxicosis
　　　　　　　　　(E06.2)
　　　　　　　　neonatal thyrotoxicosis (P72.1)

● **E05.0　Thyrotoxicosis with diffuse goiter**
　　　Exophthalmic or toxic goiter NOS
　　　Graves' disease
　　　Toxic diffuse goiter

　　E05.00　Thyrotoxicosis with diffuse goiter without thyrotoxic crisis or storm

　　E05.01　Thyrotoxicosis with diffuse goiter with thyrotoxic crisis or storm

● **E05.1　Thyrotoxicosis with toxic single thyroid nodule**
　　　Thyrotoxicosis with toxic uninodular goiter

　　E05.10　Thyrotoxicosis with toxic single thyroid nodule without thyrotoxic crisis or storm

　　E05.11　Thyrotoxicosis with toxic single thyroid nodule with thyrotoxic crisis or storm

● **E05.2　Thyrotoxicosis with toxic multinodular goiter**
　　　Toxic nodular goiter NOS

　　E05.20　Thyrotoxicosis with toxic multinodular goiter without thyrotoxic crisis or storm

　　E05.21　Thyrotoxicosis with toxic multinodular goiter with thyrotoxic crisis or storm

● **E05.3　Thyrotoxicosis from ectopic thyroid tissue**

　　E05.30　Thyrotoxicosis from ectopic thyroid tissue without thyrotoxic crisis or storm

　　E05.31　Thyrotoxicosis from ectopic thyroid tissue with thyrotoxic crisis or storm

● **E05.4　Thyrotoxicosis factitia**

　　E05.40　Thyrotoxicosis factitia without thyrotoxic crisis or storm

　　E05.41　Thyrotoxicosis factitia with thyrotoxic crisis or storm

● **E05.8　Other thyrotoxicosis**
　　　Overproduction of thyroid-stimulating hormone

　　E05.80　Other thyrotoxicosis without thyrotoxic crisis or storm

　　E05.81　Other thyrotoxicosis with thyrotoxic crisis or storm

● **E05.9　Thyrotoxicosis, unspecified**
　　　Hyperthyroidism NOS

　　E05.90　Thyrotoxicosis, unspecified without thyrotoxic crisis or storm

　　E05.91　Thyrotoxicosis, unspecified with thyrotoxic crisis or storm

● **E06　Thyroiditis**
　　An inflammation of the thyroid gland which results in an inability to convert iodine into thyroid hormone
　　[Excludes1]　postpartum thyroiditis (O90.5)

E06.0　Acute thyroiditis
　　　Abscess of thyroid
　　　Pyogenic thyroiditis
　　　Suppurative thyroiditis
　　　Use additional code (B95-B97) to identify infectious agent.

E06.1　Subacute thyroiditis
　　　Inflammation of thyroid gland following viral upper respiratory infection
　　　de Quervain thyroiditis
　　　Giant-cell thyroiditis
　　　Granulomatous thyroiditis
　　　Nonsuppurative thyroiditis
　　　Viral thyroiditis
　　　[Excludes1]　autoimmune thyroiditis (E06.3)

E06.2　Chronic thyroiditis with transient thyrotoxicosis
　　　Chronic inflammation of thyroid gland with intermittent overproduction of thyroid hormone
　　　[Excludes1]　autoimmune thyroiditis (E06.3)

E06.3　Autoimmune thyroiditis
　　　Hashimoto's thyroiditis
　　　Hashitoxicosis (transient)
　　　Lymphadenoid goiter
　　　Lymphocytic thyroiditis
　　　Struma lymphomatosa

E06.4　Drug-induced thyroiditis
　　　Use additional code for adverse effect, if applicable, to identify drug (T36-T50 with fifth or sixth character 5)

E06.5　Other chronic thyroiditis
　　　Chronic fibrous thyroiditis
　　　Chronic thyroiditis NOS
　　　Ligneous thyroiditis
　　　Riedel thyroiditis

E06.9　Thyroiditis, unspecified

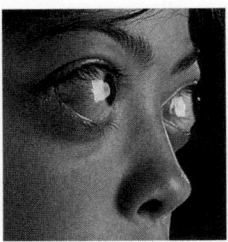

Figure 4-3　Graves' disease. In Graves' disease, exophthalmos often looks more pronounced than it actually is because of the extreme lid retraction that may occur. This patient, for instance, had minimal proptosis of the left eye but marked lid retraction. (From Lissauer T, Clayden G, and Craft A: Illustrated Textbook of Paediatrics, Edinburgh, Mosby, 2015)

Item 4–3　Thyrotoxicosis is a condition caused by excessive amounts of the thyroid hormone thyroxine production or hyperthyroidism. **Graves' disease is associated with hyperthyroidism** (known as **Basedow's disease** in Europe).

▶ New　➡ Revised　~~deleted~~ Deleted　**OGCR** Official Guidelines　X Assign placeholder X　● Use Additional Character(s)

Excludes 1　Excludes 2　Includes　Use additional　Code first　Code also　Key words

CHAPTER 4 (E00-E90)

● **E07   Other disorders of thyroid**

     E07.0   Hypersecretion of calcitonin
         C-cell hyperplasia of thyroid
         Hypersecretion of thyrocalcitonin

     E07.1   Dyshormogenetic goiter
         Group of several types of goiter resulting from enzyme defects
         in hormone synthesis
         Familial dyshormogenetic goiter
         Pendred's syndrome

         | Excludes1 | transitory congenital goiter with normal
                            function (P72.0)

   ● **E07.8   Other specified disorders of thyroid**

     E07.81   Sick-euthyroid syndrome
         Euthyroid sick-syndrome

     E07.89   Other specified disorders of thyroid
         Abnormality of thyroid-binding globulin
         Hemorrhage of thyroid
         Infarction of thyroid

     E07.9   Disorder of thyroid, unspecified
     OGCR   Section I.C.4.a.

> Diabetes mellitus
>
> The diabetes mellitus codes are combination codes that include the type of diabetes mellitus, body system affected, and the complications affecting that body system. As many codes within a particular category as are necessary to describe all of the complications of the disease may be used. They should be sequenced based on the reason for a particular visit. Assign as many codes from categories E08–E13 as needed to identify all of the associated conditions that the patient has.

DIABETES MELLITUS (E08-E13)
A metabolic disease that results in persistent hyperglycemia.

● **E08   Diabetes mellitus due to underlying condition**

     Code first the underlying condition, such as:
         congenital rubella (P35.0)
         Cushing's syndrome (E24.-)
         cystic fibrosis (E84.-)
         malignant neoplasm (C00-C96)
         malnutrition (E40-E46)
         pancreatitis and other diseases of the pancreas (K85-K86.-)

     Use additional code to identify control using:
         insulin (Z79.4)
         oral antidiabetic drugs (Z79.84)
         oral hypoglycemic drugs (Z79.84)

     | Excludes1 | drug or chemical induced diabetes mellitus
                        (E09.-)
                        gestational diabetes (O24.4-)
                        neonatal diabetes mellitus (P70.2)
                        postpancreatectomy diabetes mellitus (E13.-)
                        postprocedural diabetes mellitus (E13.-)
                        secondary diabetes mellitus NEC (E13.-)
                        type 1 diabetes mellitus (E10.-)
                        type 2 diabetes mellitus (E11.-)

   ● **E08.0   Diabetes mellitus due to underlying condition with hyperosmolarity**

     E08.00   Diabetes mellitus due to underlying condition with hyperosmolarity without nonketotic hyperglycemic-hyperosmolar coma (NKHHC)

     E08.01   Diabetes mellitus due to underlying condition with hyperosmolarity with coma

   ● **E08.1   Diabetes mellitus due to underlying condition with ketoacidosis**

     E08.10   Diabetes mellitus due to underlying condition with ketoacidosis without coma

     E08.11   Diabetes mellitus due to underlying condition with ketoacidosis with coma

   ● **E08.2   Diabetes mellitus due to underlying condition with kidney complications**

     E08.21   Diabetes mellitus due to underlying condition with diabetic nephropathy
         Diabetes mellitus due to underlying condition with intercapillary glomerulosclerosis
         Diabetes mellitus due to underlying condition with intracapillary glomerulonephrosis
         Diabetes mellitus due to underlying condition with Kimmelstiel-Wilson disease

     E08.22   Diabetes mellitus due to underlying condition with diabetic chronic kidney disease
         Use additional code to identify stage of chronic kidney disease (N18.1-N18.6)

     E08.29   Diabetes mellitus due to underlying condition with other diabetic kidney complication
         Renal tubular degeneration in diabetes mellitus due to underlying condition

   ● **E08.3   Diabetes mellitus due to underlying condition with ophthalmic complications**
     Changes in blood vessels of retina in which blood vessels swell and leak fluid into retinal surface.

   ● **E08.31   Diabetes mellitus due to underlying condition with unspecified diabetic retinopathy**

     E08.311   Diabetes mellitus due to underlying condition with unspecified diabetic retinopathy with macular edema

     E08.319   Diabetes mellitus due to underlying condition with unspecified diabetic retinopathy without macular edema

   ● **E08.32   Diabetes mellitus due to underlying condition with mild nonproliferative diabetic retinopathy**
         Diabetes mellitus due to underlying condition with nonproliferative diabetic retinopathy NOS

     One of the following 7th characters is to be assigned to codes in subcategory E08.32 to designate laterality of the disease:

1	right eye
2	left eye
3	bilateral
9	unspecified eye

   ● **E08.321   Diabetes mellitus due to underlying condition with mild nonproliferative diabetic retinopathy with macular edema**

   ● **E08.329   Diabetes mellitus due to underlying condition with mild nonproliferative diabetic retinopathy without macular edema**

   ● **E08.33   Diabetes mellitus due to underlying condition with moderate nonproliferative diabetic retinopathy**

     One of the following 7th characters is to be assigned to codes in subcategory E08.33 to designate laterality of the disease:

1	right eye
2	left eye
3	bilateral
9	unspecified eye

   ● **E08.331   Diabetes mellitus due to underlying condition with moderate nonproliferative diabetic retinopathy with macular edema**

   ● **E08.339   Diabetes mellitus due to underlying condition with moderate nonproliferative diabetic retinopathy without macular edema**

▶ New   ➡ Revised   ~~deleted~~ Deleted   **OGCR** Official Guidelines   X Assign placeholder X   ● Use Additional Character(s)

| Excludes 1 | | Excludes 2 | Includes   Use additional   Code first   Code also   Key words

● **E08.34** **Diabetes mellitus due to underlying condition with severe nonproliferative diabetic retinopathy**

One of the following 7th characters is to be assigned to codes in subcategory E08.34 to designate laterality of the disease:

> 1   right eye
> 2   left eye
> 3   bilateral
> 9   unspecified eye

  ● **E08.341** **Diabetes mellitus due to underlying condition with severe nonproliferative diabetic retinopathy with macular edema**

  ● **E08.349** **Diabetes mellitus due to underlying condition with severe nonproliferative diabetic retinopathy without macular edema**

● **E08.35** **Diabetes mellitus due to underlying condition with proliferative diabetic retinopathy**

One of the following 7th characters is to be assigned to codes in subcategory E08.35 to designate laterality of the disease:

> 1   right eye
> 2   left eye
> 3   bilateral
> 9   unspecified eye

  ● **E08.351** **Diabetes mellitus due to underlying condition with proliferative diabetic retinopathy with macular edema**

  ● **E08.352** **Diabetes mellitus due to underlying condition with proliferative diabetic retinopathy with traction retinal detachment involving the macula**

  ● **E08.353** **Diabetes mellitus due to underlying condition with proliferative diabetic retinopathy with traction retinal detachment not involving the macula**

  ● **E08.354** **Diabetes mellitus due to underlying condition with proliferative diabetic retinopathy with combined traction retinal detachment and rhegmatogenous retinal detachment**

  ● **E08.355** **Diabetes mellitus due to underlying condition with stable proliferative diabetic retinopathy**

  ● **E08.359** **Diabetes mellitus due to underlying condition with proliferative diabetic retinopathy without macular edema**

 E08.36 **Diabetes mellitus due to underlying condition with diabetic cataract**

X ● **E08.37** **Diabetes mellitus due to underlying condition with diabetic macular edema, resolved following treatment**

One of the following 7th characters is to be assigned to code E08.37 to designate laterality of the disease:

> 1   right eye
> 2   left eye
> 3   bilateral
> 9   unspecified eye

 E08.39 **Diabetes mellitus due to underlying condition with other diabetic ophthalmic complication**

Use additional code to identify manifestation, such as:
diabetic glaucoma (H40-H42)

● **E08.4** **Diabetes mellitus due to underlying condition with neurological complications**

 E08.40 **Diabetes mellitus due to underlying condition with diabetic neuropathy, unspecified**

 E08.41 **Diabetes mellitus due to underlying condition with diabetic mononeuropathy**

 E08.42 **Diabetes mellitus due to underlying condition with diabetic polyneuropathy**

Diabetes mellitus due to underlying condition with diabetic neuralgia

 E08.43 **Diabetes mellitus due to underlying condition with diabetic autonomic (poly)neuropathy**

Diabetes mellitus due to underlying condition with diabetic gastroparesis

 E08.44 **Diabetes mellitus due to underlying condition with diabetic amyotrophy**

 E08.49 **Diabetes mellitus due to underlying condition with other diabetic neurological complication**

● **E08.5** **Diabetes mellitus due to underlying condition with circulatory complications**

 E08.51 **Diabetes mellitus due to underlying condition with diabetic peripheral angiopathy without gangrene**

 E08.52 **Diabetes mellitus due to underlying condition with diabetic peripheral angiopathy with gangrene**

Diabetes mellitus due to underlying condition with diabetic gangrene

 E08.59 **Diabetes mellitus due to underlying condition with other circulatory complications**

● **E08.6** **Diabetes mellitus due to underlying condition with other specified complications**

 ● **E08.61** **Diabetes mellitus due to underlying condition with diabetic arthropathy**

  E08.610 **Diabetes mellitus due to underlying condition with diabetic neuropathic arthropathy**

Diabetes mellitus due to underlying condition with Charcôt's joints

  E08.618 **Diabetes mellitus due to underlying condition with other diabetic arthropathy**

 ● **E08.62** **Diabetes mellitus due to underlying condition with skin complications**

  E08.620 **Diabetes mellitus due to underlying condition with diabetic dermatitis**

Diabetes mellitus due to underlying condition with diabetic necrobiosis lipoidica

  E08.621 **Diabetes mellitus due to underlying condition with foot ulcer**

Use additional code to identify site of ulcer (L97.4-, L97.5-)

  E08.622 **Diabetes mellitus due to underlying condition with other skin ulcer**

Use additional code to identify site of ulcer (L97.1-L97.9, L98.41-L98.49)

  E08.628 **Diabetes mellitus due to underlying condition with other skin complications**

 ● **E08.63** **Diabetes mellitus due to underlying condition with oral complications**

  E08.630 **Diabetes mellitus due to underlying condition with periodontal disease**

  E08.638 **Diabetes mellitus due to underlying condition with other oral complications**

CHAPTER 4 (E00-E90)

● E08.64 Diabetes mellitus due to underlying condition with hypoglycemia

E08.641 Diabetes mellitus due to underlying condition with hypoglycemia with coma

E08.649 Diabetes mellitus due to underlying condition with hypoglycemia without coma

E08.65 Diabetes mellitus due to underlying condition with hyperglycemia

E08.69 Diabetes mellitus due to underlying condition with other specified complication

Use additional code to identify complication

E08.8 Diabetes mellitus due to underlying condition with unspecified complications

E08.9 Diabetes mellitus due to underlying condition without complications

● E09 Drug or chemical induced diabetes mellitus

Code first poisoning due to drug or toxin, if applicable (T36-T65 with fifth or sixth character 1-4 or 6)

Use additional code for adverse effect, if applicable, to identify drug (T36-T50 with fifth or sixth character 5)

Use additional code to identify control using:
insulin (Z79.4)
oral antidiabetic drugs (Z79.84)
oral hypoglycemic drugs (Z79.84)

Excludes1 diabetes mellitus due to underlying condition (E08.-)
gestational diabetes (O24.4-)
neonatal diabetes mellitus (P70.2)
postpancreatectomy diabetes mellitus (E13.-)
postprocedural diabetes mellitus (E13.-)
secondary diabetes mellitus NEC (E13.-)
type 1 diabetes mellitus (E10.-)
type 2 diabetes mellitus (E11.-)

● E09.0 Drug or chemical induced diabetes mellitus with hyperosmolarity

E09.00 Drug or chemical induced diabetes mellitus with hyperosmolarity without nonketotic hyperglycemic-hyperosmolar coma (NKHHC)

E09.01 Drug or chemical induced diabetes mellitus with hyperosmolarity with coma

● E09.1 Drug or chemical induced diabetes mellitus with ketoacidosis

E09.10 Drug or chemical induced diabetes mellitus with ketoacidosis without coma

E09.11 Drug or chemical induced diabetes mellitus with ketoacidosis with coma

● E09.2 Drug or chemical induced diabetes mellitus with kidney complications

E09.21 Drug or chemical induced diabetes mellitus with diabetic nephropathy
Drug or chemical induced diabetes mellitus with intercapillary glomerulosclerosis
Drug or chemical induced diabetes mellitus with intracapillary glomerulonephrosis
Drug or chemical induced diabetes mellitus with Kimmelstiel-Wilson disease

E09.22 Drug or chemical induced diabetes mellitus with diabetic chronic kidney disease
Use additional code to identify stage of chronic kidney disease (N18.1-N18.6)

E09.29 Drug or chemical induced diabetes mellitus with other diabetic kidney complication
Drug or chemical induced diabetes mellitus with renal tubular degeneration

● E09.3 Drug or chemical induced diabetes mellitus with ophthalmic complications

● E09.31 Drug or chemical induced diabetes mellitus with unspecified diabetic retinopathy

E09.311 Drug or chemical induced diabetes mellitus with unspecified diabetic retinopathy with macular edema

E09.319 Drug or chemical induced diabetes mellitus with unspecified diabetic retinopathy without macular edema

● E09.32 Drug or chemical induced diabetes mellitus with mild nonproliferative diabetic retinopathy
Drug or chemical induced diabetes mellitus with nonproliferative diabetic retinopathy NOS

One of the following 7th characters is to be assigned to codes in subcategory E09.32 to designate laterality of the disease:

1	right eye
2	left eye
3	bilateral
9	unspecified eye

● E09.321 Drug or chemical induced diabetes mellitus with mild nonproliferative diabetic retinopathy with macular edema

● E09.329 Drug or chemical induced diabetes mellitus with mild nonproliferative diabetic retinopathy without macular edema

● E09.33 Drug or chemical induced diabetes mellitus with moderate nonproliferative diabetic retinopathy

One of the following 7th characters is to be assigned to codes in subcategory E09.33 to designate laterality of the disease:

1	right eye
2	left eye
3	bilateral
9	unspecified eye

● E09.331 Drug or chemical induced diabetes mellitus with moderate nonproliferative diabetic retinopathy with macular edema

● E09.339 Drug or chemical induced diabetes mellitus with moderate nonproliferative diabetic retinopathy without macular edema

● E09.34 Drug or chemical induced diabetes mellitus with severe nonproliferative diabetic retinopathy

One of the following 7th characters is to be assigned to codes in subcategory E09.34 to designate laterality of the disease:

1	right eye
2	left eye
3	bilateral
9	unspecified eye

● E09.341 Drug or chemical induced diabetes mellitus with severe nonproliferative diabetic retinopathy with macular edema

● E09.349 Drug or chemical induced diabetes mellitus with severe nonproliferative diabetic retinopathy without macular edema

▶ New   ⇒ Revised   ~~deleted~~ Deleted   **OGCR** Official Guidelines   X Assign placeholder X   ● Use Additional Character(s)

Excludes 1   Excludes 2   Includes   Use additional   Code first   Code also   Key words

● **E09.35** Drug or chemical induced diabetes mellitus with proliferative diabetic retinopathy

One of the following 7th characters is to be assigned to codes in subcategory E09.35 to designate laterality of the disease:

1	right eye
2	left eye
3	bilateral
9	unspecified eye

  ● **E09.351** Drug or chemical induced diabetes mellitus with proliferative diabetic retinopathy with macular edema

  ● **E09.352** Drug or chemical induced diabetes mellitus with proliferative diabetic retinopathy with traction retinal detachment involving the macula

  ● **E09.353** Drug or chemical induced diabetes mellitus with proliferative diabetic retinopathy with traction retinal detachment not involving the macula

  ● **E09.354** Drug or chemical induced diabetes mellitus with proliferative diabetic retinopathy with combined traction retinal detachment and rhegmatogenous retinal detachment

  ● **E09.355** Drug or chemical induced diabetes mellitus with stable proliferative diabetic retinopathy

  ● **E09.359** Drug or chemical induced diabetes mellitus with proliferative diabetic retinopathy without macular edema

E09.36 Drug or chemical induced diabetes mellitus with diabetic cataract

X ● **E09.37** Drug or chemical induced diabetes mellitus with diabetic macular edema, resolved following treatment

One of the following 7th characters is to be assigned to code E09.37 to designate laterality of the disease:

1	right eye
2	left eye
3	bilateral
9	unspecified eye

E09.39 Drug or chemical induced diabetes mellitus with other diabetic ophthalmic complication

Use additional code to identify manifestation, such as:
diabetic glaucoma (H40-H42)

● **E09.4** Drug or chemical induced diabetes mellitus with neurological complications

E09.40 Drug or chemical induced diabetes mellitus with neurological complications with diabetic neuropathy, unspecified

E09.41 Drug or chemical induced diabetes mellitus with neurological complications with diabetic mononeuropathy

E09.42 Drug or chemical induced diabetes mellitus with neurological complications with diabetic polyneuropathy

Drug or chemical induced diabetes mellitus with diabetic neuralgia

E09.43 Drug or chemical induced diabetes mellitus with neurological complications with diabetic autonomic (poly)neuropathy

Drug or chemical induced diabetes mellitus with diabetic gastroparesis

E09.44 Drug or chemical induced diabetes mellitus with neurological complications with diabetic amyotrophy

E09.49 Drug or chemical induced diabetes mellitus with neurological complications with other diabetic neurological complication

● **E09.5** Drug or chemical induced diabetes mellitus with circulatory complications

E09.51 Drug or chemical induced diabetes mellitus with diabetic peripheral angiopathy without gangrene

E09.52 Drug or chemical induced diabetes mellitus with diabetic peripheral angiopathy with gangrene

Drug or chemical induced diabetes mellitus with diabetic gangrene

E09.59 Drug or chemical induced diabetes mellitus with other circulatory complications

● **E09.6** Drug or chemical induced diabetes mellitus with other specified complications

  ● **E09.61** Drug or chemical induced diabetes mellitus with diabetic arthropathy

    E09.610 Drug or chemical induced diabetes mellitus with diabetic neuropathic arthropathy

Drug or chemical induced diabetes mellitus with Charcôt's joints
Progressive degeneration of weight-bearing joint

    E09.618 Drug or chemical induced diabetes mellitus with other diabetic arthropathy

  ● **E09.62** Drug or chemical induced diabetes mellitus with skin complications

    E09.620 Drug or chemical induced diabetes mellitus with diabetic dermatitis

Drug or chemical induced diabetes mellitus with diabetic necrobiosis lipoidica
Necrotizing skin condition

    E09.621 Drug or chemical induced diabetes mellitus with foot ulcer

Use additional code to identify site of ulcer (L97.4-, L97.5-)

    E09.622 Drug or chemical induced diabetes mellitus with other skin ulcer

Use additional code to identify site of ulcer (L97.1-L97.9, L98.41-L98.49)

    E09.628 Drug or chemical induced diabetes mellitus with other skin complications

  ● **E09.63** Drug or chemical induced diabetes mellitus with oral complications

    E09.630 Drug or chemical induced diabetes mellitus with periodontal disease

    E09.638 Drug or chemical induced diabetes mellitus with other oral complications

  ● **E09.64** Drug or chemical induced diabetes mellitus with hypoglycemia

    E09.641 Drug or chemical induced diabetes mellitus with hypoglycemia with coma

    E09.649 Drug or chemical induced diabetes mellitus with hypoglycemia without coma

E09.65 Drug or chemical induced diabetes mellitus with hyperglycemia

E09.69 Drug or chemical induced diabetes mellitus with other specified complication

Use additional code to identify complication

E09.8 Drug or chemical induced diabetes mellitus with unspecified complications

E09.9 Drug or chemical induced diabetes mellitus without complications

---

▶ New   ➭ Revised   ~~deleted~~ Deleted   **OGCR** Official Guidelines   X Assign placeholder X   ● Use Additional Character(s)

Excludes 1   Excludes 2   Includes   Use additional   Code first   Code also   Key words

● E10　Type 1 diabetes mellitus

Includes　brittle diabetes (mellitus)
　　　　　　diabetes (mellitus) due to autoimmune process
　　　　　　diabetes (mellitus) due to immune mediated
　　　　　　　　pancreatic islet beta-cell destruction
　　　　　　idiopathic diabetes (mellitus)
　　　　　　juvenile onset diabetes (mellitus)
　　　　　　ketosis-prone diabetes (mellitus)

Excludes1　diabetes mellitus due to underlying condition
　　　　　　　　(E08.-)
　　　　　　drug or chemical induced diabetes mellitus (E09.-)
　　　　　　gestational diabetes (O24.4-)
　　　　　　hyperglycemia NOS (R73.9)
　　　　　　neonatal diabetes mellitus (P70.2)
　　　　　　postpancreatectomy diabetes mellitus (E13.-)
　　　　　　postprocedural diabetes mellitus (E13.-)
　　　　　　secondary diabetes mellitus NEC (E13.-)
　　　　　　type 2 diabetes mellitus (E11.-)

● E10.1　Type 1 diabetes mellitus with ketoacidosis
*Acidosis accompanied by accumulation of ketone bodies
(ketosis) in body tissues and fluids*

　**E10.10　Type 1 diabetes mellitus with ketoacidosis
without coma**

　**E10.11　Type 1 diabetes mellitus with ketoacidosis with
coma**

● E10.2　Type 1 diabetes mellitus with kidney complications
　**E10.21　Type 1 diabetes mellitus with diabetic
nephropathy**
　　　Type 1 diabetes mellitus with intercapillary
　　　　glomerulosclerosis
　　　Type 1 diabetes mellitus with intracapillary
　　　　glomerulonephrosis
　　　Type 1 diabetes mellitus with Kimmelstiel-
　　　　Wilson disease

　**E10.22　Type 1 diabetes mellitus with diabetic chronic
kidney disease**
　　　Use additional code to identify stage of chronic
　　　　kidney disease (N18.1-N18.6)

　**E10.29　Type 1 diabetes mellitus with other diabetic
kidney complication**
　　　Type 1 diabetes mellitus with renal tubular
　　　　degeneration

● E10.3　Type 1 diabetes mellitus with ophthalmic complications
　**● E10.31　Type 1 diabetes mellitus with unspecified
diabetic retinopathy**
　　**E10.311　Type 1 diabetes mellitus
　　　　with unspecified diabetic retinopathy
　　　　with macular edema**
　　**E10.319　Type 1 diabetes mellitus
　　　　with unspecified diabetic retinopathy
　　　　without macular edema**

　**● E10.32　Type 1 diabetes mellitus with mild
nonproliferative diabetic retinopathy**
　　　Type 1 diabetes mellitus with nonproliferative
　　　　diabetic retinopathy NOS

　　One of the following 7th characters is to be
　　assigned to codes in subcategory E10.32 to
　　designate laterality of the disease:

1	right eye
2	left eye
3	bilateral
9	unspecified eye

　　**● E10.321　Type 1 diabetes mellitus with mild
　　　　nonproliferative diabetic retinopathy
　　　　with macular edema**
　　**● E10.329　Type 1 diabetes mellitus with mild
　　　　nonproliferative diabetic retinopathy
　　　　without macular edema**

**● E10.33　Type 1 diabetes mellitus with moderate
nonproliferative diabetic retinopathy**

　　One of the following 7th characters is to be
　　assigned to codes in subcategory E10.33 to
　　designate laterality of the disease:

1	right eye
2	left eye
3	bilateral
9	unspecified eye

　**● E10.331　Type 1 diabetes mellitus with
　　　moderate nonproliferative diabetic
　　　retinopathy with macular edema**
　**● E10.339　Type 1 diabetes mellitus with
　　　moderate nonproliferative diabetic
　　　retinopathy without macular edema**

**● E10.34　Type 1 diabetes mellitus with severe
nonproliferative diabetic retinopathy**

　　One of the following 7th characters is to be
　　assigned to codes in subcategory E10.34 to
　　designate laterality of the disease:

1	right eye
2	left eye
3	bilateral
9	unspecified eye

　**● E10.341　Type 1 diabetes mellitus with severe
　　　nonproliferative diabetic retinopathy
　　　with macular edema**
　**● E10.349　Type 1 diabetes mellitus with severe
　　　nonproliferative diabetic retinopathy
　　　without macular edema**

**● E10.35　Type 1 diabetes mellitus with proliferative
diabetic retinopathy**

　　One of the following 7th characters is to be
　　assigned to codes in subcategory E10.35 to
　　designate laterality of the disease:

1	right eye
2	left eye
3	bilateral
9	unspecified eye

　**● E10.351　Type 1 diabetes mellitus with
　　　proliferative diabetic retinopathy
　　　with macular edema**
　**● E10.352　Type 1 diabetes mellitus with
　　　proliferative diabetic retinopathy
　　　with traction retinal detachment
　　　involving the macula**
　**● E10.353　Type 1 diabetes mellitus with
　　　proliferative diabetic retinopathy
　　　with traction retinal detachment not
　　　involving the macula**
　**● E10.354　Type 1 diabetes mellitus with
　　　proliferative diabetic retinopathy
　　　with combined traction retinal
　　　detachment and rhegmatogenous
　　　retinal detachment**
　**● E10.355　Type 1 diabetes mellitus with stable
　　　proliferative diabetic retinopathy**
　**● E10.359　Type 1 diabetes mellitus with
　　　proliferative diabetic retinopathy
　　　without macular edema**

E10.36   Type 1 diabetes mellitus with diabetic cataract

X● E10.37   Type 1 diabetes mellitus with diabetic macular edema, resolved following treatment

     One of the following 7th characters is to be assigned to code E10.37 to designate laterality of the disease:

1	right eye
2	left eye
3	bilateral
9	unspecified eye

E10.39   Type 1 diabetes mellitus with other diabetic ophthalmic complication

     Use additional code to identify manifestation, such as:
     diabetic glaucoma (H40-H42)

● E10.4   Type 1 diabetes mellitus with neurological complications

E10.40   Type 1 diabetes mellitus with diabetic neuropathy, unspecified

E10.41   Type 1 diabetes mellitus with diabetic mononeuropathy

E10.42   Type 1 diabetes mellitus with diabetic polyneuropathy
     Type 1 diabetes mellitus with diabetic neuralgia

E10.43   Type 1 diabetes mellitus with diabetic autonomic (poly)neuropathy
     Type 1 diabetes mellitus with diabetic gastroparesis

E10.44   Type 1 diabetes mellitus with diabetic amyotrophy

E10.49   Type 1 diabetes mellitus with other diabetic neurological complication

● E10.5   Type 1 diabetes mellitus with circulatory complications

E10.51   Type 1 diabetes mellitus with diabetic peripheral angiopathy without gangrene

E10.52   Type 1 diabetes mellitus with diabetic peripheral angiopathy with gangrene
     Type 1 diabetes mellitus with diabetic gangrene

E10.59   Type 1 diabetes mellitus with other circulatory complications

● E10.6   Type 1 diabetes mellitus with other specified complications

 ● E10.61   Type 1 diabetes mellitus with diabetic arthropathy

E10.610   Type 1 diabetes mellitus with diabetic neuropathic arthropathy
     Type 1 diabetes mellitus with Charcôt's joints

E10.618   Type 1 diabetes mellitus with other diabetic arthropathy

 ● E10.62   Type 1 diabetes mellitus with skin complications

E10.620   Type 1 diabetes mellitus with diabetic dermatitis
     Type 1 diabetes mellitus with diabetic necrobiosis lipoidica

E10.621   Type 1 diabetes mellitus with foot ulcer
     Use additional code to identify site of ulcer (L97.4-, L97.5-)

E10.622   Type 1 diabetes mellitus with other skin ulcer
     Use additional code to identify site of ulcer (L97.1-L97.9, L98.41-L98.49)

E10.628   Type 1 diabetes mellitus with other skin complications

● E10.63   Type 1 diabetes mellitus with oral complications

E10.630   Type 1 diabetes mellitus with periodontal disease

E10.638   Type 1 diabetes mellitus with other oral complications

● E10.64   Type 1 diabetes mellitus with hypoglycemia

E10.641   Type 1 diabetes mellitus with hypoglycemia with coma

E10.649   Type 1 diabetes mellitus with hypoglycemia without coma

E10.65   Type 1 diabetes mellitus with hyperglycemia

E10.69   Type 1 diabetes mellitus with other specified complication
     Use additional code to identify complication

E10.8   Type 1 diabetes mellitus with unspecified complications

E10.9   Type 1 diabetes mellitus without complications

● E11   Type 2 diabetes mellitus

     Includes   diabetes (mellitus) due to insulin secretory defect
     diabetes NOS
     insulin resistant diabetes (mellitus)

     Use additional code to identify control using:
     insulin (Z79.4)
     oral antidiabetic drugs (Z79.84)
     oral hypoglycemic drugs (Z79.84)

     Excludes1   diabetes mellitus due to underlying condition (E08.-)
     drug or chemical induced diabetes mellitus (E09.-)
     gestational diabetes (O24.4-)
     neonatal diabetes mellitus (P70.2)
     postpancreatectomy diabetes mellitus (E13.-)
     postprocedural diabetes mellitus (E13.-)
     secondary diabetes mellitus NEC (E13.-)
     type 1 diabetes mellitus (E10.-)

● E11.0   Type 2 diabetes mellitus with hyperosmolarity

E11.00   Type 2 diabetes mellitus with hyperosmolarity without nonketotic hyperglycemic-hyperosmolar coma (NKHHC)

E11.01   Type 2 diabetes mellitus with hyperosmolarity with coma

▶● E11.1   Type 2 diabetes mellitus with ketoacidosis

▶ E11.10   Type 2 diabetes mellitus with ketoacidosis without coma

▶ E11.11   Type 2 diabetes mellitus with ketoacidosis with coma

● E11.2   Type 2 diabetes mellitus with kidney complications

E11.21   Type 2 diabetes mellitus with diabetic nephropathy
     Type 2 diabetes mellitus with intercapillary glomerulosclerosis
     Type 2 diabetes mellitus with intracapillary glomerulonephrosis
     Type 2 diabetes mellitus with Kimmelstiel-Wilson disease

E11.22   Type 2 diabetes mellitus with diabetic chronic kidney disease
     Use additional code to identify stage of chronic kidney disease (N18.1-N18.6)

E11.29   Type 2 diabetes mellitus with other diabetic kidney complication
     Type 2 diabetes mellitus with renal tubular degeneration

● E11.3   Type 2 diabetes mellitus with ophthalmic complications

 ● E11.31   Type 2 diabetes mellitus with unspecified diabetic retinopathy

E11.311   Type 2 diabetes mellitus with unspecified diabetic retinopathy with macular edema

E11.319   Type 2 diabetes mellitus with unspecified diabetic retinopathy without macular edema

CHAPTER 4 (E00-E90)

● **E11.32** **Type 2 diabetes mellitus with mild nonproliferative diabetic retinopathy**
Type 2 diabetes mellitus with nonproliferative diabetic retinopathy NOS

One of the following 7th characters is to be assigned to codes in subcategory E11.32 to designate laterality of the disease:

1	right eye
2	left eye
3	bilateral
9	unspecified eye

● **E11.321** **Type 2 diabetes mellitus with mild nonproliferative diabetic retinopathy with macular edema**
● **E11.329** **Type 2 diabetes mellitus with mild nonproliferative diabetic retinopathy without macular edema**

● **E11.33** **Type 2 diabetes mellitus with moderate nonproliferative diabetic retinopathy**

One of the following 7th characters is to be assigned to codes in subcategory E11.33 to designate laterality of the disease:

1	right eye
2	left eye
3	bilateral
9	unspecified eye

● **E11.331** **Type 2 diabetes mellitus with moderate nonproliferative diabetic retinopathy with macular edema**
● **E11.339** **Type 2 diabetes mellitus with moderate nonproliferative diabetic retinopathy without macular edema**

● **E11.34** **Type 2 diabetes mellitus with severe nonproliferative diabetic retinopathy**

One of the following 7th characters is to be assigned to codes in subcategory E11.34 to designate laterality of the disease:

1	right eye
2	left eye
3	bilateral
9	unspecified eye

● **E11.341** **Type 2 diabetes mellitus with severe nonproliferative diabetic retinopathy with macular edema**
● **E11.349** **Type 2 diabetes mellitus with severe nonproliferative diabetic retinopathy without macular edema**

● **E11.35** **Type 2 diabetes mellitus with proliferative diabetic retinopathy**

One of the following 7th characters is to be assigned to codes in subcategory E11.35 to designate laterality of the disease:

1	right eye
2	left eye
3	bilateral
9	unspecified eye

● **E11.351** **Type 2 diabetes mellitus with proliferative diabetic retinopathy with macular edema**
● **E11.352** **Type 2 diabetes mellitus with proliferative diabetic retinopathy with traction retinal detachment involving the macula**

● **E11.353** **Type 2 diabetes mellitus with proliferative diabetic retinopathy with traction retinal detachment not involving the macula**
● **E11.354** **Type 2 diabetes mellitus with proliferative diabetic retinopathy with combined traction retinal detachment and rhegmatogenous retinal detachment**
● **E11.355** **Type 2 diabetes mellitus with stable proliferative diabetic retinopathy**
● **E11.359** **Type 2 diabetes mellitus with proliferative diabetic retinopathy without macular edema**

E11.36 **Type 2 diabetes mellitus with diabetic cataract**
X ● **E11.37** **Type 2 diabetes mellitus with diabetic macular edema, resolved following treatment**

One of the following 7th characters is to be assigned to code E11.37 to designate laterality of the disease:

1	right eye
2	left eye
3	bilateral
9	unspecified eye

E11.39 **Type 2 diabetes mellitus with other diabetic ophthalmic complication**
Use additional code to identify manifestation, such as:
diabetic glaucoma (H40-H42)

● **E11.4** **Type 2 diabetes mellitus with neurological complications**
E11.40 **Type 2 diabetes mellitus with diabetic neuropathy, unspecified**
E11.41 **Type 2 diabetes mellitus with diabetic mononeuropathy**
E11.42 **Type 2 diabetes mellitus with diabetic polyneuropathy**
Type 2 diabetes mellitus with diabetic neuralgia
E11.43 **Type 2 diabetes mellitus with diabetic autonomic (poly)neuropathy**
Type 2 diabetes mellitus with diabetic gastroparesis
E11.44 **Type 2 diabetes mellitus with diabetic amyotrophy**
E11.49 **Type 2 diabetes mellitus with other diabetic neurological complication**

● **E11.5** **Type 2 diabetes mellitus with circulatory complications**
E11.51 **Type 2 diabetes mellitus with diabetic peripheral angiopathy without gangrene**
E11.52 **Type 2 diabetes mellitus with diabetic peripheral angiopathy with gangrene**
Type 2 diabetes mellitus with diabetic gangrene
E11.59 **Type 2 diabetes mellitus with other circulatory complications**

● **E11.6** **Type 2 diabetes mellitus with other specified complications**
● **E11.61** **Type 2 diabetes mellitus with diabetic arthropathy**
E11.610 **Type 2 diabetes mellitus with diabetic neuropathic arthropathy**
Type 2 diabetes mellitus with Charcôt's joints
E11.618 **Type 2 diabetes mellitus with other diabetic arthropathy**

▶ New   ⮕ Revised   ~~deleted~~ Deleted   **OGCR** Official Guidelines   X Assign placeholder X   ● Use Additional Character(s)

Excludes 1   Excludes 2   Includes   Use additional   Code first   Code also   Key words

● **E11.62**   **Type 2 diabetes mellitus with skin complications**

     E11.620   **Type 2 diabetes mellitus with diabetic dermatitis**

          Type 2 diabetes mellitus with diabetic necrobiosis lipoidica

     E11.621   **Type 2 diabetes mellitus with foot ulcer**

          Use additional code to identify site of ulcer (L97.4-, L97.5-)

     E11.622   **Type 2 diabetes mellitus with other skin ulcer**

          Use additional code to identify site of ulcer (L97.1-L97.9, L98.41-L98.49)

     E11.628   **Type 2 diabetes mellitus with other skin complications**

● **E11.63**   **Type 2 diabetes mellitus with oral complications**

     E11.630   **Type 2 diabetes mellitus with periodontal disease**

     E11.638   **Type 2 diabetes mellitus with other oral complications**

● **E11.64**   **Type 2 diabetes mellitus with hypoglycemia**

     E11.641   **Type 2 diabetes mellitus with hypoglycemia with coma**

     E11.649   **Type 2 diabetes mellitus with hypoglycemia without coma**

   E11.65   **Type 2 diabetes mellitus with hyperglycemia**

   E11.69   **Type 2 diabetes mellitus with other specified complication**

       Use additional code to identify complication

       Use this code with E11.65 to report DKA in a Type 2 patient

   E11.8   **Type 2 diabetes mellitus with unspecified complications**

   E11.9   **Type 2 diabetes mellitus without complications**

● **E13**   **Other specified diabetes mellitus**

     Includes   diabetes mellitus due to genetic defects of beta-cell function

          diabetes mellitus due to genetic defects in insulin action

          postpancreatectomy diabetes mellitus

          postprocedural diabetes mellitus

          secondary diabetes mellitus NEC

     Use additional code to identify control using:

       insulin (Z79.4)

       oral antidiabetic drugs (Z79.84)

       oral hypoglycemic drugs (Z79.84)

     Excludes1   diabetes (mellitus) due to autoimmune process (E10.-)

          diabetes (mellitus) due to immune mediated pancreatic islet beta-cell destruction (E10.-)

          diabetes mellitus due to underlying condition (E08.-)

          drug or chemical induced diabetes mellitus (E09.-)

          gestational diabetes (O24.4-)

          neonatal diabetes mellitus (P70.2)

          type 1 diabetes mellitus (E10.-)

          type 2 diabetes mellitus (E11.-)

● **E13.0**   **Other specified diabetes mellitus with hyperosmolarity**

     E13.00   **Other specified diabetes mellitus with hyperosmolarity without nonketotic hyperglycemic-hyperosmolar coma (NKHHC)**

       ▶ **Excludes2**   type 2 diabetes mellitus (E11.-)

     E13.01   **Other specified diabetes mellitus with hyperosmolarity with coma**

● **E13.1**   **Other specified diabetes mellitus with ketoacidosis**

     E13.10   **Other specified diabetes mellitus with ketoacidosis without coma**

     E13.11   **Other specified diabetes mellitus with ketoacidosis with coma**

● **E13.2**   **Other specified diabetes mellitus with kidney complications**

     E13.21   **Other specified diabetes mellitus with diabetic nephropathy**

          Other specified diabetes mellitus with intercapillary glomerulosclerosis

          Other specified diabetes mellitus with intracapillary glomerulonephrosis

          Other specified diabetes mellitus with Kimmelstiel-Wilson disease

     E13.22   **Other specified diabetes mellitus with diabetic chronic kidney disease**

          Use additional code to identify stage of chronic kidney disease (N18.1-N18.6)

     E13.29   **Other specified diabetes mellitus with other diabetic kidney complication**

          Other specified diabetes mellitus with renal tubular degeneration

● **E13.3**   **Other specified diabetes mellitus with ophthalmic complications**

     ● **E13.31**   **Other specified diabetes mellitus with unspecified diabetic retinopathy**

         E13.311   **Other specified diabetes mellitus with unspecified diabetic retinopathy with macular edema**

         E13.319   **Other specified diabetes mellitus with unspecified diabetic retinopathy without macular edema**

     ● **E13.32**   **Other specified diabetes mellitus with mild nonproliferative diabetic retinopathy**

         Other specified diabetes mellitus with nonproliferative diabetic retinopathy NOS

         One of the following 7th characters is to be assigned to codes in subcategory E13.32 to designate laterality of the disease:

1	right eye
2	left eye
3	bilateral
9	unspecified eye

     ● **E13.321**   **Other specified diabetes mellitus with mild nonproliferative diabetic retinopathy with macular edema**

     ● **E13.329**   **Other specified diabetes mellitus with mild nonproliferative diabetic retinopathy without macular edema**

     ● **E13.33**   **Other specified diabetes mellitus with moderate nonproliferative diabetic retinopathy**

         One of the following 7th characters is to be assigned to codes in subcategory E13.33 to designate laterality of the disease:

1	right eye
2	left eye
3	bilateral
9	unspecified eye

     ● **E13.331**   **Other specified diabetes mellitus with moderate nonproliferative diabetic retinopathy with macular edema**

     ● **E13.339**   **Other specified diabetes mellitus with moderate nonproliferative diabetic retinopathy without macular edema**

CHAPTER 4 (E00-E90)

● **E13.34** **Other specified diabetes mellitus with severe nonproliferative diabetic retinopathy**

One of the following 7th characters is to be assigned to codes in subcategory E13.34 to designate laterality of the disease:

1	right eye
2	left eye
3	bilateral
9	unspecified eye

● **E13.341** **Other specified diabetes mellitus with severe nonproliferative diabetic retinopathy with macular edema**

● **E13.349** **Other specified diabetes mellitus with severe nonproliferative diabetic retinopathy without macular edema**

● **E13.35** **Other specified diabetes mellitus with proliferative diabetic retinopathy**

One of the following 7th characters is to be assigned to codes in subcategory E13.35 to designate laterality of the disease:

1	right eye
2	left eye
3	bilateral
9	unspecified eye

● **E13.351** **Other specified diabetes mellitus with proliferative diabetic retinopathy with macular edema**

● **E13.352** **Other specified diabetes mellitus with proliferative diabetic retinopathy with traction retinal detachment involving the macula**

● **E13.353** **Other specified diabetes mellitus with proliferative diabetic retinopathy with traction retinal detachment not involving the macula**

● **E13.354** **Other specified diabetes mellitus with proliferative diabetic retinopathy with combined traction retinal detachment and rhegmatogenous retinal detachment**

● **E13.355** **Other specified diabetes mellitus with stable proliferative diabetic retinopathy**

● **E13.359** **Other specified diabetes mellitus with proliferative diabetic retinopathy without macular edema**

E13.36 **Other specified diabetes mellitus with diabetic cataract**

X ● **E13.37** **Other specified diabetes mellitus with diabetic macular edema, resolved following treatment**

One of the following 7th characters is to be assigned to code E13.37 to designate laterality of the disease:

1	right eye
2	left eye
3	bilateral
9	unspecified eye

E13.39 **Other specified diabetes mellitus with other diabetic ophthalmic complication**

Use additional code to identify manifestation, such as:
diabetic glaucoma (H40-H42)

● **E13.4** **Other specified diabetes mellitus with neurological complications**

E13.40 **Other specified diabetes mellitus with diabetic neuropathy, unspecified**

E13.41 **Other specified diabetes mellitus with diabetic mononeuropathy**

E13.42 **Other specified diabetes mellitus with diabetic polyneuropathy**

Other specified diabetes mellitus with diabetic neuralgia

E13.43 **Other specified diabetes mellitus with diabetic autonomic (poly)neuropathy**

Other specified diabetes mellitus with diabetic gastroparesis

E13.44 **Other specified diabetes mellitus with diabetic amyotrophy**

E13.49 **Other specified diabetes mellitus with other diabetic neurological complication**

● **E13.5** **Other specified diabetes mellitus with circulatory complications**

E13.51 **Other specified diabetes mellitus with diabetic peripheral angiopathy without gangrene**

E13.52 **Other specified diabetes mellitus with diabetic peripheral angiopathy with gangrene**

Other specified diabetes mellitus with diabetic gangrene

E13.59 **Other specified diabetes mellitus with other circulatory complications**

● **E13.6** **Other specified diabetes mellitus with other specified complications**

● **E13.61** **Other specified diabetes mellitus with diabetic arthropathy**

E13.610 **Other specified diabetes mellitus with diabetic neuropathic arthropathy**

Other specified diabetes mellitus with Charcôt's joints

E13.618 **Other specified diabetes mellitus with other diabetic arthropathy**

● **E13.62** **Other specified diabetes mellitus with skin complications**

E13.620 **Other specified diabetes mellitus with diabetic dermatitis**

Other specified diabetes mellitus with diabetic necrobiosis lipoidica

E13.621 **Other specified diabetes mellitus with foot ulcer**

Use additional code to identify site of ulcer (L97.4-, L97.5-)

E13.622 **Other specified diabetes mellitus with other skin ulcer**

Use additional code to identify site of ulcer (L97.1-L97.9, L98.41-L98.49)

E13.628 **Other specified diabetes mellitus with other skin complications**

● **E13.63** **Other specified diabetes mellitus with oral complications**

E13.630 **Other specified diabetes mellitus with periodontal disease**

E13.638 **Other specified diabetes mellitus with other oral complications**

● **E13.64**   **Other specified diabetes mellitus with hypoglycemia**
     E13.641   **Other specified diabetes mellitus with hypoglycemia with coma**
     E13.649   **Other specified diabetes mellitus with hypoglycemia without coma**
   E13.65   **Other specified diabetes mellitus with hyperglycemia**
   E13.69   **Other specified diabetes mellitus with other specified complication**
     Use additional code to identify complication
 E13.8   **Other specified diabetes mellitus with unspecified complications**
 E13.9   **Other specified diabetes mellitus without complications**

OTHER DISORDERS OF GLUCOSE REGULATION AND PANCREATIC INTERNAL SECRETION (E15-E16)

E15   **Nondiabetic hypoglycemic coma**
   Includes   drug-induced insulin coma in nondiabetic
     hyperinsulinism with hypoglycemic coma
     hypoglycemic coma NOS

● **E16**   **Other disorders of pancreatic internal secretion**
   E16.0   **Drug-induced hypoglycemia without coma**
     Excludes1   diabetes with hypoglycemia without coma (E09.649)
     Use additional code for adverse effect, if applicable, to identify drug (T36-T50 with fifth or sixth character 5)
   E16.1   **Other hypoglycemia**
     Functional hyperinsulinism
     Functional nonhyperinsulinemic hypoglycemia
     Hyperinsulinism NOS
     Hyperplasia of pancreatic islet beta cells NOS
     Excludes1   diabetes with hypoglycemia (E08.649, E10.649, E11.649, E13.649)
       hypoglycemia in infant of diabetic mother (P70.1)
       neonatal hypoglycemia (P70.4)
   E16.2   **Hypoglycemia, unspecified**
     Excludes1   diabetes with hypoglycemia (E08.649, E10.649, E11.649, E13.649)
   E16.3   **Increased secretion of glucagon**
     Hyperplasia of pancreatic endocrine cells with glucagon excess
   E16.4   **Increased secretion of gastrin**
     Hypergastrinemia
     Hyperplasia of pancreatic endocrine cells with gastrin excess
     Zollinger-Ellison syndrome
   E16.8   **Other specified disorders of pancreatic internal secretion**
     Increased secretion from endocrine pancreas of growth hormone-releasing hormone
     Increased secretion from endocrine pancreas of pancreatic polypeptide
     Increased secretion from endocrine pancreas of somatostatin
     Increased secretion from endocrine pancreas of vasoactive-intestinal polypeptide
   E16.9   **Disorder of pancreatic internal secretion, unspecified**
     Islet-cell hyperplasia NOS
     Pancreatic endocrine cell hyperplasia NOS

DISORDERS OF OTHER ENDOCRINE GLANDS (E20-E35)

   Excludes1   galactorrhea (N64.3)
     gynecomastia (N62)

● **E20**   **Hypoparathyroidism**
     Greatly reduced function of parathyroid glands; AKA parathyroid insufficiency
   Excludes1   Di George's syndrome (D82.1)
     postprocedural hypoparathyroidism (E89.2)
     tetany NOS (R29.0)
     transitory neonatal hypoparathyroidism (P71.4)
   E20.0   **Idiopathic hypoparathyroidism**
     Rare condition, unknown cause; short dwarf-like with round face
   E20.1   **Pseudohypoparathyroidism**
     Hereditary condition resembling hypoparathyroidism, but caused by inability to respond to parathyroid hormone
   E20.8   **Other hypoparathyroidism**
   E20.9   **Hypoparathyroidism, unspecified**
     Parathyroid tetany

● **E21**   **Hyperparathyroidism and other disorders of parathyroid gland**
   Excludes1   adult osteomalacia (M83.-)
     ectopic hyperparathyroidism (E34.2)
     familial hypocalciuric hypercalcemia (E83.52)
     hungry bone syndrome (E83.81)
     infantile and juvenile osteomalacia (E55.0)
   E21.0   **Primary hyperparathyroidism**
     Hyperplasia of parathyroid
     Osteitis fibrosa cystica generalisata [von Recklinghausen's disease of bone]
   E21.1   **Secondary hyperparathyroidism, not elsewhere classified**
     Excludes1   secondary hyperparathyroidism of renal origin (N25.81)
   E21.2   **Other hyperparathyroidism**
     Tertiary hyperparathyroidism
     Excludes1   familial hypocalciuric hypercalcemia (E83.52)
   E21.3   **Hyperparathyroidism, unspecified**
   E21.4   **Other specified disorders of parathyroid gland**
   E21.5   **Disorder of parathyroid gland, unspecified**

Item 4–4 Hyperparathyroidism is an overactive parathyroid gland that secretes excessive parathormone, causing increased levels of circulating calcium. This results in a loss of calcium in the bone (osteoporosis).

Hypoparathyroidism is an underactive parathyroid gland that results in decreased levels of circulating calcium. The primary manifestation is **tetany,** a continuous muscle spasm.

Figure 4-4 Tetany caused by hypoparathyroidism.

CHAPTER 4 (E00-E90)

Item 4–5 **Hyperadrenalism** is overactivity of the adrenal cortex, which secretes corticosteroid hormones. Excessive glucocorticoid hormone results in hyperglycemia **(Cushing's syndrome)**, and excessive aldosterone results in **Conn's syndrome. Adrenogenital syndrome** is the result of excessive secretion of androgens, male hormones, which stimulates premature sexual development. **Hypoadrenalism, Addison's disease,** is a condition in which the adrenal glands atrophy.

Figure 4-5 Centripetal and generalized obesity and dorsal kyphosis in a woman with Cushing's disease. (From Salvo SG: Mosby's Pathology for Massage Therapists, St. Louis, MO: Mosby/Elsevier, 2009)

● **E22**   **Hyperfunction of pituitary gland**
      Excludes1 Cushing's syndrome (E24.-)
                Nelson's syndrome (E24.1)
                overproduction of ACTH not associated with
                    Cushing's disease (E27.0)
                overproduction of pituitary ACTH (E24.0)
                overproduction of thyroid-stimulating hormone
                    (E05.8-)

    E22.0   **Acromegaly and pituitary gigantism**
          Chronic disease caused by hypersecretion of growth hormone
          Overproduction of growth hormone
          Excludes1 constitutional gigantism (E34.4)
                      constitutional tall stature (E34.4)
                      increased secretion from endocrine
                          pancreas of growth hormone-
                          releasing hormone (E16.8)

    E22.1   **Hyperprolactinemia**
          Increased levels of prolactin
          Use additional code for adverse effect, if applicable,
             to identify drug (T36-T50 with fifth or sixth
             character 5)

    E22.2   **Syndrome of inappropriate secretion of antidiuretic hormone**

    E22.8   **Other hyperfunction of pituitary gland**
          Central precocious puberty

    E22.9   **Hyperfunction of pituitary gland, unspecified**

● **E23**   **Hypofunction and other disorders of the pituitary gland**
      Includes the listed conditions whether the disorder is in
              the pituitary or the hypothalamus
      Excludes1 postprocedural hypopituitarism (E89.3)

    E23.0   **Hypopituitarism**
          Fertile eunuch syndrome
          Hypogonadotropic hypogonadism
          Idiopathic growth hormone deficiency
          Isolated deficiency of gonadotropin
          Isolated deficiency of growth hormone
          Isolated deficiency of pituitary hormone
          Kallmann's syndrome
          Lorain-Levi short stature
          Necrosis of pituitary gland (postpartum)
          Panhypopituitarism
          Pituitary cachexia
          Pituitary insufficiency NOS
          Pituitary short stature
          Sheehan's syndrome
          Simmonds' disease

    E23.1   **Drug-induced hypopituitarism**
          Use additional code for adverse effect, if applicable,
             to identify drug (T36-T50 with fifth or sixth
             character 5)

    E23.2   **Diabetes insipidus**
          Excludes1 nephrogenic diabetes insipidus (N25.1)

    E23.3   **Hypothalamic dysfunction, not elsewhere classified**
          Excludes1 Prader-Willi syndrome (Q87.1)
                   Russell-Silver syndrome (Q87.1)

    E23.6   **Other disorders of pituitary gland**
          Abscess of pituitary
          Adiposogenital dystrophy

    E23.7   **Disorder of pituitary gland, unspecified**

● **E24**   **Cushing's syndrome**
      Excludes1 congenital adrenal hyperplasia (E25.0)

    E24.0   **Pituitary-dependent Cushing's disease**
          Overproduction of pituitary ACTH
          Pituitary-dependent hypercorticalism

    E24.1   **Nelson's syndrome**

    E24.2   **Drug-induced Cushing's syndrome**
          Use additional code for adverse effect, if applicable,
             to identify drug (T36-T50 with fifth or sixth
             character 5)

    E24.3   **Ectopic ACTH syndrome**

    E24.4   **Alcohol-induced pseudo-Cushing's syndrome**

    E24.8   **Other Cushing's syndrome**

    E24.9   **Cushing's syndrome, unspecified**

● **E25**   **Adrenogenital disorders**
      Disorder of production of steroid hormone in adrenal gland
      Includes adrenogenital syndromes, virilizing or
                feminizing, whether acquired or due to
                adrenal hyperplasia consequent on inborn
                enzyme defects in hormone synthesis
              female adrenal pseudohermaphroditism
              female heterosexual precocious pseudopuberty
              male isosexual precocious pseudopuberty
              male macrogenitosomia praecox
              male sexual precocity with adrenal hyperplasia
              male virilization (female)
      Excludes1 indeterminate sex and pseudohermaphroditism
                (Q56)
              chromosomal abnormalities (Q90-Q99)

    E25.0   **Congenital adrenogenital disorders associated with enzyme deficiency**
          Congenital adrenal hyperplasia
          21-Hydroxylase deficiency
          Salt-losing congenital adrenal hyperplasia

    E25.8   **Other adrenogenital disorders**
          Idiopathic adrenogenital disorder
          Use additional code for adverse effect, if applicable,
             to identify drug (T36-T50 with fifth or sixth
             character 5)

    E25.9   **Adrenogenital disorder, unspecified**
          Adrenogenital syndrome NOS

● **E26**   **Hyperaldosteronism**
      Abnormality of electrolyte metabolism caused by excessive secretion of aldosterone

  ● **E26.0**   **Primary hyperaldosteronism**
      E26.01   **Conn's syndrome**
             Code also adrenal adenoma (D35.0-)

      E26.02   **Glucocorticoid-remediable aldosteronism**
             Familial aldosteronism type I

      E26.09   **Other primary hyperaldosteronism**
             Primary aldosteronism due to adrenal
               hyperplasia (bilateral)

▶ New   ⇒ Revised   deleted Deleted   **OGCR** Official Guidelines   X Assign placeholder X   ● Use Additional Character(s)

Excludes 1   Excludes 2   Includes   Use additional   Code first   Code also   Key words

E26.1   Secondary hyperaldosteronism
- E26.8   Other hyperaldosteronism
     E26.81   Bartter's syndrome
     E26.89   Other hyperaldosteronism
E26.9   Hyperaldosteronism, unspecified
     Aldosteronism NOS
     Hyperaldosteronism NOS

- **E27**   Other disorders of adrenal gland
   E27.0   Other adrenocortical overactivity
     Overproduction of ACTH, not associated with
       Cushing's disease
     Premature adrenarche
     | Excludes1 | Cushing's syndrome (E24.-)
   E27.1   Primary adrenocortical insufficiency
     Addison's disease
     Autoimmune adrenalitis
     | Excludes1 | Addison only phenotype
          adrenoleukodystrophy (E71.528)
          amyloidosis (E85.-)
          tuberculous Addison's disease (A18.7)
          Waterhouse-Friderichsen syndrome
            (A39.1)
   E27.2   Addisonian crisis
     Acute onset of adrenocortical insufficiency
     Adrenal crisis
     Adrenocortical crisis
   E27.3   Drug-induced adrenocortical insufficiency
     Use additional code for adverse effect, if applicable,
       to identify drug (T36-T50 with fifth or sixth
       character 5)
- E27.4   Other and unspecified adrenocortical insufficiency
     | Excludes1 | adrenoleukodystrophy [Addison-
          Schilder] (E71.528)
          Waterhouse-Friderichsen syndrome
            (A39.1)
     E27.40   Unspecified adrenocortical insufficiency
       Adrenocortical insufficiency NOS
       Hypoaldosteronism
     E27.49   Other adrenocortical insufficiency
       Adrenal hemorrhage
       Adrenal infarction
   E27.5   Adrenomedullary hyperfunction
     Adrenomedullary hyperplasia
     Catecholamine hypersecretion
   E27.8   Other specified disorders of adrenal gland
     Abnormality of cortisol-binding globulin
   E27.9   Disorder of adrenal gland, unspecified

- **E28**   Ovarian dysfunction
   | Excludes1 | isolated gonadotropin deficiency (E23.0)
          postprocedural ovarian failure (E89.4-)
   E28.0   Estrogen excess
     Use additional code for adverse effect, if applicable,
       to identify drug (T36-T50 with fifth or sixth
       character 5)
   E28.1   Androgen excess
     Hypersecretion of ovarian androgens
     Use additional code for adverse effect, if applicable,
       to identify drug (T36-T50 with fifth or sixth
       character 5)
   E28.2   Polycystic ovarian syndrome
     Sclerocystic ovary syndrome
     Stein-Leventhal syndrome

- E28.3   Primary ovarian failure
     | Excludes1 | pure gonadal dysgenesis (Q99.1)
          Turner's syndrome (Q96.-)
     ● E28.31   Premature menopause
       E28.310   Symptomatic premature menopause
         Symptoms such as flushing,
           sleeplessness, headache, lack of
           concentration, associated with
           premature menopause
       E28.319   Asymptomatic premature menopause
         Premature menopause NOS
     E28.39   Other primary ovarian failure
       Decreased estrogen
       Resistant ovary syndrome
   E28.8   Other ovarian dysfunction
     Ovarian hyperfunction NOS
     | Excludes1 | postprocedural ovarian failure (E89.4-)
   E28.9   Ovarian dysfunction, unspecified

- **E29**   Testicular dysfunction
   | Excludes1 | androgen insensitivity syndrome (E34.5-)
          azoospermia or oligospermia NOS (N46.0-N46.1)
          isolated gonadotropin deficiency (E23.0)
          Klinefelter's syndrome (Q98.0-Q98.1, Q98.4)
   E29.0   Testicular hyperfunction
     Hypersecretion of testicular hormones
   E29.1   Testicular hypofunction
     Defective biosynthesis of testicular androgen NOS
     5-delta-Reductase deficiency (with male
       pseudohermaphroditism)
     Testicular hypogonadism NOS
     Use additional code for adverse effect, if applicable,
       to identify drug (T36-T50 with fifth or sixth
       character 5)
     | Excludes1 | postprocedural testicular hypofunction
          (E89.5)
   E29.8   Other testicular dysfunction
   E29.9   Testicular dysfunction, unspecified

- **E30**   Disorders of puberty, not elsewhere classified
   E30.0   Delayed puberty
     Constitutional delay of puberty
     Delayed sexual development
   E30.1   Precocious puberty
     Sexual maturation at earlier age than normal, or before age
       8 in girls and 9 in boys, usually hormonal; AKA sexual
       precocity or pubertas praecox
     Precocious menstruation
     | Excludes1 | Albright (-McCune) (-Sternberg)
          syndrome (Q78.1)
          central precocious puberty (E22.8)
          congenital adrenal hyperplasia (E25.0)
          female heterosexual precocious
            pseudopuberty (E25.-)
          male isosexual precocious pseudopuberty
            (E25.-)
   E30.8   Other disorders of puberty
     Premature thelarche
   E30.9   Disorder of puberty, unspecified

CHAPTER 4 (E00-E90)

● **E31**   **Polyglandular dysfunction**
> **Excludes1**   ataxia telangiectasia [Louis-Bar] (G11.3)
> dystrophia myotonica [Steinert] (G71.11)
> pseudohypoparathyroidism (E20.1)

E31.0   **Autoimmune polyglandular failure**
Schmidt's syndrome

E31.1   **Polyglandular hyperfunction**
> **Excludes1**   multiple endocrine adenomatosis (E31.2-)
> multiple endocrine neoplasia (E31.2-)

● **E31.2**   **Multiple endocrine neoplasia [MEN] syndromes**
Adenomatous hyperplasia and malignant tumors in endocrine glands
Multiple endocrine adenomatosis
Code also any associated malignancies and other conditions associated with the syndromes

E31.20   **Multiple endocrine neoplasia [MEN] syndrome, unspecified**
Multiple endocrine adenomatosis NOS
Multiple endocrine neoplasia [MEN] syndrome NOS

E31.21   **Multiple endocrine neoplasia [MEN] type I**
Wermer's syndrome

E31.22   **Multiple endocrine neoplasia [MEN] type IIA**
Sipple's syndrome

E31.23   **Multiple endocrine neoplasia [MEN] type IIB**

E31.8   **Other polyglandular dysfunction**

E31.9   **Polyglandular dysfunction, unspecified**

● **E32**   **Diseases of thymus**
> **Excludes1**   aplasia or hypoplasia of thymus with immunodeficiency (D82.1)
> myasthenia gravis (G70.0)

E32.0   **Persistent hyperplasia of thymus**
Hypertrophy of thymus

E32.1   **Abscess of thymus**

E32.8   **Other diseases of thymus**
> **Excludes1**   aplasia or hypoplasia with immunodeficiency (D82.1)
> thymoma (D15.0)

E32.9   **Disease of thymus, unspecified**

● **E34**   **Other endocrine disorders**
> **Excludes1**   pseudohypoparathyroidism (E20.1)

E34.0   **Carcinoid syndrome**
Note: May be used as an additional code to identify functional activity associated with a carcinoid tumor.

E34.1   **Other hypersecretion of intestinal hormones**

E34.2   **Ectopic hormone secretion, not elsewhere classified**
> **Excludes1**   ectopic ACTH syndrome (E24.3)

E34.3   **Short stature due to endocrine disorder**
Constitutional short stature
Laron-type short stature
> **Excludes1**   achondroplastic short stature (Q77.4)
> hypochondroplastic short stature (Q77.4)
> nutritional short stature (E45)
> pituitary short stature (E23.0)
> progeria (E34.8)
> renal short stature (N25.0)
> Russell-Silver syndrome (Q87.1)
> short-limbed stature with immunodeficiency (D82.2)
> short stature in specific dysmorphic syndromes - code to syndrome - see Alphabetical Index
> short stature NOS (R62.52)

E34.4   **Constitutional tall stature**
Constitutional gigantism

● **E34.5**   **Androgen insensitivity syndrome**

E34.50   **Androgen insensitivity syndrome, unspecified**
Androgen insensitivity NOS

E34.51   **Complete androgen insensitivity syndrome**
Complete androgen insensitivity
de Quervain syndrome
Goldberg-Maxwell syndrome

E34.52   **Partial androgen insensitivity syndrome**
Partial androgen insensitivity
Reifenstein syndrome

E34.8   **Other specified endocrine disorders**
Pineal gland dysfunction
Progeria
> **Excludes2**   pseudohypoparathyroidism (E20.1)

E34.9   **Endocrine disorder, unspecified**
Endocrine disturbance NOS
Hormone disturbance NOS

E35   **Disorders of endocrine glands in diseases classified elsewhere**
Code first underlying disease, such as:
late congenital syphilis of thymus gland [Dubois disease] (A50.5)
Use additional code, if applicable, to identify:
sequelae of tuberculosis of other organs (B90.8)
> **Excludes1**   Echinococcus granulosus infection of thyroid gland (B67.3)
> meningococcal hemorrhagic adrenalitis (A39.1)
> syphilis of endocrine gland (A52.79)
> tuberculosis of adrenal gland, except calcification (A18.7)
> tuberculosis of endocrine gland NEC (A18.82)
> tuberculosis of thyroid gland (A18.81)
> Waterhouse-Friderichsen syndrome (A39.1)

INTRAOPERATIVE COMPLICATIONS OF ENDOCRINE SYSTEM (E36)

● **E36**   **Intraoperative complications of endocrine system**
> **Excludes2**   postprocedural endocrine and metabolic complications and disorders, not elsewhere classified (E89.-)

● **E36.0**   **Intraoperative hemorrhage and hematoma of an endocrine system organ or structure complicating a procedure**
> **Excludes1**   intraoperative hemorrhage and hematoma of an endocrine system organ or structure due to accidental puncture or laceration during a procedure (E36.1-)

E36.01   **Intraoperative hemorrhage and hematoma of an endocrine system organ or structure complicating an endocrine system procedure**

E36.02   **Intraoperative hemorrhage and hematoma of an endocrine system organ or structure complicating other procedure**

● **E36.1**   **Accidental puncture and laceration of an endocrine system organ or structure during a procedure**

E36.11   **Accidental puncture and laceration of an endocrine system organ or structure during an endocrine system procedure**

E36.12   **Accidental puncture and laceration of an endocrine system organ or structure during other procedure**

E36.8   **Other intraoperative complications of endocrine system**
Use additional code, if applicable, to further specify disorder

MALNUTRITION (E40-E46)

Excludes1	intestinal malabsorption (K90.-)
	sequelae of protein-calorie malnutrition (E64.0)
Excludes2	nutritional anemias (D50-D53)
	starvation (T73.0)

E40 Kwashiorkor
Malnutrition produced by severe protein deficiency
Severe malnutrition with nutritional edema with dyspigmentation of skin and hair

| **Excludes1** | marasmic kwashiorkor (E42) |

E41 Nutritional marasmus
Severe malnutrition with marasmus

| **Excludes1** | marasmic kwashiorkor (E42) |

E42 Marasmic kwashiorkor
Severe protein malnutrition
Intermediate form severe protein-calorie malnutrition
Severe protein-calorie malnutrition with signs of both kwashiorkor and marasmus

E43 Unspecified severe protein-calorie malnutrition
Starvation edema

● **E44 Protein-calorie malnutrition of moderate and mild degree**
    E44.0 Moderate protein-calorie malnutrition
    E44.1 Mild protein-calorie malnutrition

E45 Retarded development following protein-calorie malnutrition
Nutritional short stature
Nutritional stunting
Physical retardation due to malnutrition

E46 Unspecified protein-calorie malnutrition
Malnutrition NOS
Protein-calorie imbalance NOS

| **Excludes1** | nutritional deficiency NOS (E63.9) |

OTHER NUTRITIONAL DEFICIENCIES (E50-E64)

| **Excludes2** | nutritional anemias (D50-D53) |

● **E50 Vitamin A deficiency**

| **Excludes1** | sequelae of vitamin A deficiency (E64.1) |

    E50.0 Vitamin A deficiency with conjunctival xerosis
    E50.1 Vitamin A deficiency with Bitot's spot and conjunctival xerosis
        Bitot's spot in the young child
    E50.2 Vitamin A deficiency with corneal xerosis
    E50.3 Vitamin A deficiency with corneal ulceration and xerosis
    E50.4 Vitamin A deficiency with keratomalacia
        Eye disorder that results in dry cornea caused by vitamin A deficiency
    E50.5 Vitamin A deficiency with night blindness
    E50.6 Vitamin A deficiency with xerophthalmic scars of cornea
        Abnormal dryness and thickening of conjunctiva and cornea due to vitamin A deficiency
    E50.7 Other ocular manifestations of vitamin A deficiency
        Xerophthalmia NOS

    E50.8 Other manifestations of vitamin A deficiency
        Follicular keratosis
        Xeroderma
    E50.9 Vitamin A deficiency, unspecified
        Hypovitaminosis A NOS

● **E51 Thiamine deficiency**

| **Excludes1** | sequelae of thiamine deficiency (E64.8) |

●   **E51.1 Beriberi**
        E51.11 Dry beriberi
          Thiamine deficiency with nervous system manifestation most often caused by excessive alcohol consumption
          Beriberi NOS
          Beriberi with polyneuropathy
        E51.12 Wet beriberi
          Thiamine deficiency with cardiovascular manifestation most often caused by excessive alcohol consumption
          Beriberi with cardiovascular manifestations
          Cardiovascular beriberi
          Shoshin disease
    E51.2 Wernicke's encephalopathy
        Acute disease of brain due to thiamine deficiency most often associated with excessive alcohol consumption
    E51.8 Other manifestations of thiamine deficiency
    E51.9 Thiamine deficiency, unspecified

E52 Niacin deficiency [pellagra]
Niacin (-tryptophan) deficiency
Nicotinamide deficiency
Pellagra (alcoholic)

| **Excludes1** | sequelae of niacin deficiency (E64.8) |

● **E53 Deficiency of other B group vitamins**

| **Excludes1** | sequelae of vitamin B deficiency (E64.8) |

    E53.0 Riboflavin deficiency
        Ariboflavinosis
        Vitamin B2 deficiency
    E53.1 Pyridoxine deficiency
        Vitamin B6 deficiency

| **Excludes1** | pyridoxine-responsive sideroblastic anemia (D64.3) |

    E53.8 Deficiency of other specified B group vitamins
        Biotin deficiency
        Cyanocobalamin deficiency
        Folate deficiency
        Folic acid deficiency
        Pantothenic acid deficiency
        Vitamin B12 deficiency

| **Excludes1** | folate deficiency anemia (D52.-) |
| | vitamin B12 deficiency anemia (D51.-) |

    E53.9 Vitamin B deficiency, unspecified

E54 Ascorbic acid deficiency
Deficiency of vitamin C
Scurvy

| **Excludes1** | scorbutic anemia (D53.2) |
| | sequelae of vitamin C deficiency (E64.2) |

Item 4-6 Bitot's spots are the result of a buildup of keratin debris found on the superficial surface the conjunctiva; oval, triangular, or irregular in shape; and a sign of vitamin A deficiency and associated with night blindness. The disease may progress to **keratomalacia,** which can result in eventual prolapse of the iris and loss of the lens.

Figure 4-6 Bitot's spot on the conjunctiva.

Figure 4-7 The sharply demarcated, characteristic scaling dermatitis of pellagra. (From James WD, Berger TG, Elston DM: Andrews' Diseases of the Skin: Clinical Dermatology, Philadelphia, Saunders Elsevier, 2006)

Item 4-7 Pellagra is associated with a deficiency of niacin and its precursor, **tryptophan.** Characteristics of the condition include diarrhea, dermatitis on exposed skin surfaces, dementia, and death. It is prevalent in developing countries where nutrition is inadequate. **Beriberi** is associated with thiamine deficiency.

▶ New ⇒ Revised ~~deleted~~ Deleted **OGCR** Official Guidelines **X** Assign placeholder X ● Use Additional Character(s)

| Excludes 1 | Excludes 2 | Includes | Use additional | Code first | Code also | Key words |

CHAPTER 4 (E00-E90)

CHAPTER 4 (E00-E90)

● **E55   Vitamin D deficiency**
- **Excludes1**   adult osteomalacia (M83.-)
  osteoporosis (M80.-)
  sequelae of rickets (E64.3)

    E55.0   Rickets, active
       Infantile osteomalacia
       Juvenile osteomalacia
       Softening of bone
- **Excludes1**   celiac rickets (K90.0)
  Crohn's rickets (K50.-)
  hereditary vitamin D-dependent rickets (E83.32)
  inactive rickets (E64.3)
  renal rickets (N25.0)
  sequelae of rickets (E64.3)
  vitamin D-resistant rickets (E83.31)

    E55.9   Vitamin D deficiency, unspecified
       Avitaminosis D

● **E56   Other vitamin deficiencies**
- **Excludes1**   sequelae of other vitamin deficiencies (E64.8)

    E56.0   Deficiency of vitamin E
    E56.1   Deficiency of vitamin K
- **Excludes1**   deficiency of coagulation factor due to vitamin K deficiency (D68.4)
  vitamin K deficiency of newborn (P53)

    E56.8   Deficiency of other vitamins
    E56.9   Vitamin deficiency, unspecified

   E58   Dietary calcium deficiency
- **Excludes1**   disorders of calcium metabolism (E83.5-)
  sequelae of calcium deficiency (E64.8)

   E59   Dietary selenium deficiency
      Keshan disease
- **Excludes1**   sequelae of selenium deficiency (E64.8)

   E60   Dietary zinc deficiency

● **E61   Deficiency of other nutrient elements**
     Use additional code for adverse effect, if applicable, to identify drug (T36-T50 with fifth or sixth character 5)
- **Excludes1**   disorders of mineral metabolism (E83.-)
  iodine deficiency related thyroid disorders (E00-E02)
  sequelae of malnutrition and other nutritional deficiencies (E64.-)

    E61.0   Copper deficiency
    E61.1   Iron deficiency
- **Excludes1**   iron deficiency anemia (D50.-)

    E61.2   Magnesium deficiency
    E61.3   Manganese deficiency
    E61.4   Chromium deficiency
    E61.5   Molybdenum deficiency
    E61.6   Vanadium deficiency
    E61.7   Deficiency of multiple nutrient elements
    E61.8   Deficiency of other specified nutrient elements
    E61.9   Deficiency of nutrient element, unspecified

● **E63   Other nutritional deficiencies**
- **Excludes1**   dehydration (E86.0)
  failure to thrive, adult (R62.7)
  failure to thrive, child (R62.51)
  feeding problems in newborn (P92.-)
  sequelae of malnutrition and other nutritional deficiencies (E64.-)

    E63.0   Essential fatty acid [EFA] deficiency
    E63.1   Imbalance of constituents of food intake
    E63.8   Other specified nutritional deficiencies
    E63.9   Nutritional deficiency, unspecified

● **E64   Sequelae of malnutrition and other nutritional deficiencies**
    Pathological condition resulting from disease, injury, or other trauma
    Note: This category is to be used to indicate conditions in categories E43, E44, E46, E50-E63 as the cause of sequelae, which are themselves classified elsewhere. The 'sequelae' include conditions specified as such; they also include the late effects of diseases classifiable to the above categories if the disease itself is no longer present
    Code first condition resulting from (sequela) of malnutrition and other nutritional deficiencies

    E64.0   Sequelae of protein-calorie malnutrition
- **Excludes2**   retarded development following protein-calorie malnutrition (E45)

    E64.1   Sequelae of vitamin A deficiency
    E64.2   Sequelae of vitamin C deficiency
    E64.3   Sequelae of rickets
    E64.8   Sequelae of other nutritional deficiencies
    E64.9   Sequelae of unspecified nutritional deficiency

OVERWEIGHT, OBESITY AND OTHER HYPERALIMENTATION (E65-E68)

   E65   Localized adiposity
      Fat pad

● **E66   Overweight and obesity**
    Code first obesity complicating pregnancy, childbirth and the puerperium, if applicable (O99.21-)
    Use additional code to identify body mass index (BMI), if known (Z68.-)
- **Excludes1**   adiposogenital dystrophy (E23.6)
  lipomatosis NOS (E88.2)
  lipomatosis dolorosa [Dercum] (E88.2)
  Prader-Willi syndrome (Q87.1)

●   **E66.0   Obesity due to excess calories**
      E66.01   Morbid (severe) obesity due to excess calories
- **Excludes1**   morbid (severe) obesity with alveolar hypoventilation (E66.2)

      E66.09   Other obesity due to excess calories
    E66.1   Drug-induced obesity
      Use additional code for adverse effect, if applicable, to identify drug (T36-T50 with fifth or sixth character 5)

    E66.2   Morbid (severe) obesity with alveolar hypoventilation
      Uncommon condition of unknown cause leading to inadequate ventilation in lungs, even though lungs and airways are normal
      Obesity hypoventilation syndrome (OHS)
      Pickwickian syndrome

    E66.3   Overweight
    E66.8   Other obesity
    E66.9   Obesity, unspecified
      Obesity NOS

● **E67   Other hyperalimentation**
    Ingestion of more than optimal amount of nutrients
- **Excludes1**   hyperalimentation NOS (R63.2)
  sequelae of hyperalimentation (E68)

    E67.0   Hypervitaminosis A
    E67.1   Hypercarotinemia
    E67.2   Megavitamin-B6 syndrome
    E67.3   Hypervitaminosis D
    E67.8   Other specified hyperalimentation

   E68   Sequelae of hyperalimentation
    Code first condition resulting from (sequela) of hyperalimentation

METABOLIC DISORDERS (E70-E88)

> **Excludes1**
> androgen insensitivity syndrome (E34.5-)
> congenital adrenal hyperplasia (E25.0)
> Ehlers-Danlos syndrome (Q79.6)
> hemolytic anemias attributable to enzyme
>   disorders (D55.-)
> Marfan's syndrome (Q87.4)
> 5-alpha-reductase deficiency (E29.1)

● **E70   Disorders of aromatic amino-acid metabolism**

E70.0   Classical phenylketonuria
Inherited disorder that increases to harmful levels amino acid phenylalanine

E70.1   Other hyperphenylalaninemias

● **E70.2   Disorders of tyrosine metabolism**

> **Excludes1**   transitory tyrosinemia of newborn (P74.5)

E70.20   Disorder of tyrosine metabolism, unspecified
Tyrosine: Nonessential amino acid occurring in most proteins

E70.21   Tyrosinemia
Congenital amino acid metabolism
Hypertyrosinemia

E70.29   Other disorders of tyrosine metabolism
Alkaptonuria
Ochronosis

● **E70.3   Albinism**
Congenital condition of reduced or absent pigment in eyes, skin, and hair

E70.30   Albinism, unspecified

● **E70.31   Ocular albinism**

E70.310   X-linked ocular albinism

E70.311   Autosomal recessive ocular albinism

E70.318   Other ocular albinism

E70.319   Ocular albinism, unspecified

● **E70.32   Oculocutaneous albinism**
Partial or total lack of melanin pigment in eyes

> **Excludes1**   Chediak-Higashi syndrome
>   (E70.330)
> Hermansky-Pudlak syndrome
>   (E70.331)

E70.320   Tyrosinase negative oculocutaneous albinism
Albinism I
Oculocutaneous albinism ty-neg

E70.321   Tyrosinase positive oculocutaneous albinism
Albinism II
Oculocutaneous albinism ty-pos

E70.328   Other oculocutaneous albinism
Cross syndrome

E70.329   Oculocutaneous albinism, unspecified

● **E70.33   Albinism with hematologic abnormality**

E70.330   Chediak-Higashi syndrome

E70.331   Hermansky-Pudlak syndrome

E70.338   Other albinism with hematologic abnormality

E70.339   Albinism with hematologic abnormality, unspecified

E70.39   Other specified albinism
Piebaldism

● **E70.4   Disorders of histidine metabolism**

E70.40   Disorders of histidine metabolism, unspecified

E70.41   Histidinemia

E70.49   Other disorders of histidine metabolism

E70.5   Disorders of tryptophan metabolism

E70.8   Other disorders of aromatic amino-acid metabolism

E70.9   Disorder of aromatic amino-acid metabolism, unspecified

● **E71   Disorders of branched-chain amino-acid metabolism and fatty-acid metabolism**

E71.0   Maple-syrup-urine disease
Due to defect in amino acid catabolism, causing severe ketoacidosis with smell of maple syrup in urine and on body

● **E71.1   Other disorders of branched-chain amino-acid metabolism**

● **E71.11   Branched-chain organic acidurias**

E71.110   Isovaleric acidemia

E71.111   3-methylglutaconic aciduria

E71.118   Other branched-chain organic acidurias

● **E71.12   Disorders of propionate metabolism**

E71.120   Methylmalonic acidemia

E71.121   Propionic acidemia

E71.128   Other disorders of propionate metabolism

E71.19   Other disorders of branched-chain amino-acid metabolism
Hyperleucine-isoleucinemia
Hypervalinemia

E71.2   Disorder of branched-chain amino-acid metabolism, unspecified

● **E71.3   Disorders of fatty-acid metabolism**

> **Excludes1**   peroxisomal disorders (E71.5)
> Refsum's disease (G60.1)
> Schilder's disease (G37.0)

> **Excludes2**   carnitine deficiency due to inborn error of metabolism (E71.42)

E71.30   Disorder of fatty-acid metabolism, unspecified

● **E71.31   Disorders of fatty-acid oxidation**

E71.310   Long chain/very long chain acyl CoA dehydrogenase deficiency
LCAD
VLCAD

E71.311   Medium chain acyl CoA dehydrogenase deficiency
MCAD

E71.312   Short chain acyl CoA dehydrogenase deficiency
SCAD

E71.313   Glutaric aciduria type II
Glutaric aciduria type II A
Glutaric aciduria type II B
Glutaric aciduria type II C

> **Excludes1**   glutaric aciduria (type 1) NOS (E72.3)

E71.314   Muscle carnitine palmitoyltransferase deficiency

E71.318   Other disorders of fatty-acid oxidation

E71.32   Disorders of ketone metabolism

E71.39   Other disorders of fatty-acid metabolism

● **E71.4   Disorders of carnitine metabolism**

> **Excludes1**   muscle carnitine palmitoyltransferase deficiency (E71.314)

E71.40   Disorder of carnitine metabolism, unspecified

E71.41   Primary carnitine deficiency

E71.42   Carnitine deficiency due to inborn errors of metabolism
Code also associated inborn error or metabolism

E71.43   Iatrogenic carnitine deficiency
Iatrogenic: Outcomes from activity of physicians
Carnitine deficiency due to hemodialysis
Carnitine deficiency due to Valproic acid therapy

● **E71.44   Other secondary carnitine deficiency**

E71.440   Ruvalcaba-Myhre-Smith syndrome

E71.448   Other secondary carnitine deficiency

▶ New   ⇒ Revised   ~~deleted~~ Deleted   **OGCR** Official Guidelines   X Assign placeholder X   ● Use Additional Character(s)

| Excludes 1 | Excludes 2 | Includes | Use additional | Code first | Code also | Key words |

CHAPTER 4 (E00-E90)

● **E71.5 Peroxisomal disorders**
Class of conditions which lead to disorders of lipid metabolism
> **Excludes1** Schilder's disease (G37.0)

E71.50 Peroxisomal disorder, unspecified

● **E71.51 Disorders of peroxisome biogenesis**
Group 1 peroxisomal disorders
> **Excludes1** Refsum's disease (G60.1)

E71.510 Zellweger syndrome

E71.511 Neonatal adrenoleukodystrophy
> **Excludes1** X-linked adrenoleuko-dystrophy (E71.42-)

E71.518 Other disorders of peroxisome biogenesis

● **E71.52 X-linked adrenoleukodystrophy**

E71.520 Childhood cerebral X-linked adrenoleukodystrophy

E71.521 Adolescent X-linked adrenoleukodystrophy

E71.522 Adrenomyeloneuropathy

E71.528 Other X-linked adrenoleukodystrophy
Addison only phenotype adrenoleukodystrophy
Addison-Schilder adrenoleukodystrophy

E71.529 X-linked adrenoleukodystrophy, unspecified type

E71.53 Other group 2 peroxisomal disorders

● **E71.54 Other peroxisomal disorders**

E71.540 Rhizomelic chondrodysplasia punctata
Rare, severe, inherited disorder with limb shortening, bone and cartilage abnormalities, abnormal facial appearance, severe mental retardation, psychomotor retardation, and cataracts
> **Excludes1** chondrodysplasia punctata NOS (Q77.3)

E71.541 Zellweger-like syndrome

E71.542 Other group 3 peroxisomal disorders

E71.548 Other peroxisomal disorders

● **E72 Other disorders of amino-acid metabolism**
> **Excludes1** disorders of:
> aromatic amino-acid metabolism (E70.-)
> branched-chain amino-acid metabolism (E71.0-E71.2)
> fatty-acid metabolism (E71.3)
> purine and pyrimidine metabolism (E79.-)
> gout (M1A.-, M10.-)

● **E72.0 Disorders of amino-acid transport**
> **Excludes1** disorders of tryptophan metabolism (E70.5)

E72.00 Disorders of amino-acid transport, unspecified

E72.01 Cystinuria
Hereditary aminoaciduria due to impairment of renal transport with predominant symptom of urinary cystine calculi

E72.02 Hartnup's disease
Inborn error of metabolism

E72.03 Lowe's syndrome
X-linked disorder with rickets, hydrophthalmia, congenital glaucoma, cataracts, mental retardation, and renal tubule dysfunction
Use additional code for associated glaucoma (H42)

E72.04 Cystinosis
Genetic disease with excessive depostits of amino acid cystine in cells
Fanconi (-de Toni) (-Debré) syndrome with cystinosis
> **Excludes1** Fanconi (-de Toni) (-Debré) syndrome without cystinosis (E72.09)

E72.09 Other disorders of amino-acid transport
Fanconi (-de Toni) (-Debré) syndrome, unspecified

● **E72.1 Disorders of sulfur-bearing amino-acid metabolism**
> **Excludes1** cystinosis (E72.04)
> cystinuria (E72.01)
> transcobalamin II deficiency (D51.2)

E72.10 Disorders of sulfur-bearing amino-acid metabolism, unspecified

E72.11 Homocystinuria
Cystathionine synthase deficiency

E72.12 Methylenetetrahydrofolate reductase deficiency

E72.19 Other disorders of sulfur-bearing amino-acid metabolism
Cystathioninuria
Methioninemia
Sulfite oxidase deficiency

● **E72.2 Disorders of urea cycle metabolism**
> **Excludes1** disorders of ornithine metabolism (E72.4)

E72.20 Disorder of urea cycle metabolism, unspecified
Hyperammonemia
Elevated levels of ammonia
> **Excludes1** hyperammonemia-hyperornithinemia-homocitrullinemia syndrome E72.4
> transient hyperammonemia of newborn (P74.6)

E72.21 Argininemia
Disorder in which deficiency of enzyme arginase causes build up of arginine and ammonia in blood

E72.22 Arginosuccinic aciduria
Gene disorder of urea cycle resulting accumulation of ammonia

E72.23 Citrullinemia
Urea cycle disorder that causes ammonia and other toxic substances to accumulate in blood

E72.29 Other disorders of urea cycle metabolism

E72.3 Disorders of lysine and hydroxylysine metabolism
Glutaric aciduria NOS
Glutaric aciduria (type I)
Hydroxylysinemia
Hyperlysinemia
> **Excludes1** glutaric aciduria type II (E71.313)
> Refsum's disease (G60.1)
> Zellweger syndrome (E71.510)

E72.4 Disorders of ornithine metabolism
Hyperammonemia-Hyperornithinemia-Homocitrullinemia syndrome
Ornithinemia (types I, II)
Ornithine transcarbamylase deficiency
> **Excludes1** hereditary choroidal dystrophy (H31.2-)

● **E72.5 Disorders of glycine metabolism**

E72.50 Disorder of glycine metabolism, unspecified

E72.51 Non-ketotic hyperglycinemia

E72.52 Trimethylaminuria

E72.53 Hyperoxaluria
Oxalosis
Oxaluria

E72.59 Other disorders of glycine metabolism
D-glycericacidemia
Hyperhydroxyprolinemia
Hyperprolinemia (types I, II)
Sarcosinemia

▶ New   ⇒ Revised   ~~deleted~~ Deleted   **OGCR** Official Guidelines   X Assign placeholder X   ● Use Additional Character(s)

| Excludes 1 | Excludes 2 | Includes | Use additional | Code first | Code also | Key words |

E72.8   **Other** specified disorders of amino-acid metabolism
    Disorders of beta-amino-acid metabolism
    Disorders of gamma-glutamyl cycle

E72.9   Disorder of amino-acid metabolism, **unspecified**

● E73   Lactose intolerance
    Intolerance for lactose, due to inherited deficiency of lactase activity in intestinal mucosa

E73.0   **Congenital** lactase deficiency

E73.1   **Secondary** lactase deficiency

E73.8   **Other** lactose intolerance

E73.9   Lactose intolerance, **unspecified**

● E74   Other disorders of carbohydrate metabolism
    Excludes1   diabetes mellitus (E08-E13)
     hypoglycemia NOS (E16.2)
     increased secretion of glucagon (E16.3)
     mucopolysaccharidosis (E76.0-E76.3)

● E74.0   Glycogen storage disease

   E74.00   Glycogen storage disease, **unspecified**

   E74.01   **von Gierke's disease**
     Type I glycogen storage disease

   E74.02   **Pompe disease**
     Cardiac glycogenosis
     Type II glycogen storage disease

   E74.03   **Cori disease**
     Forbes' disease
     Type III glycogen storage disease

   E74.04   **McArdle disease**
     Type V glycogen storage disease

   E74.09   **Other** glycogen storage disease
     Andersen disease
     Hers disease
     Tauri disease
     Glycogen storage disease, types 0, IV, VI-XI
     Liver phosphorylase deficiency
     Muscle phosphofructokinase deficiency

● E74.1   Disorders of fructose metabolism
    Excludes1   muscle phosphofructokinase deficiency (E74.09)

   E74.10   Disorder of fructose metabolism, **unspecified**

   E74.11   **Essential** fructosuria
     Fructokinase deficiency

   E74.12   **Hereditary** fructose intolerance
     Fructosemia

   E74.19   **Other** disorders of fructose metabolism
     Fructose-1, 6-diphosphatase deficiency

● E74.2   Disorders of galactose metabolism

   E74.20   Disorders of galactose metabolism, **unspecified**

   E74.21   **Galactosemia**
     Genetic disorders resulting from defective simple sugar (galactose) metabolism

   E74.29   **Other** disorders of galactose metabolism
     Galactokinase deficiency

● E74.3   Other disorders of intestinal carbohydrate absorption
    Excludes2   lactose intolerance (E73.-)

   E74.31   **Sucrase-isomaltase deficiency**
     Deficiency in metabolism in intestinal mucosa results in malabsorption of sucrose and starch

   E74.39   **Other** disorders of intestinal carbohydrate absorption
     Disorder of intestinal carbohydrate absorption NOS
     Glucose-galactose malabsorption
     Sucrase deficiency

E74.4   Disorders of pyruvate metabolism and gluconeogenesis
    Deficiency of phosphoenolpyruvate carboxykinase
    Deficiency of pyruvate carboxylase
    Deficiency of pyruvate dehydrogenase
    Excludes1   disorders of pyruvate metabolism and gluconeogenesis with anemia (D55.-)
     Leigh's syndrome (G31.82)

E74.8   **Other** specified disorders of carbohydrate metabolism
    Essential pentosuria
    Renal glycosuria

E74.9   Disorder of carbohydrate metabolism, **unspecified**

● E75   Disorders of sphingolipid metabolism and other lipid storage disorders
    Excludes1   mucolipidosis, types I-III (E77.0-E77.1)
     Refsum's disease (G60.1)

● E75.0   GM2 gangliosidosis
    Rare metabolic disorder that causes destruction of nerve cells of brain and spinal cord

   E75.00   GM2 gangliosidosis, **unspecified**

   E75.01   **Sandhoff** disease

   E75.02   **Tay-Sachs** disease

   E75.09   **Other** GM2 gangliosidosis
     Adult GM2 gangliosidosis
     Juvenile GM2 gangliosidosis

● E75.1   Other and unspecified gangliosidosis

   E75.10   **Unspecified** gangliosidosis
     Gangliosidosis NOS

   E75.11   **Mucolipidosis IV**
     Disorder with symptoms of psychomotor retardation and severe visual impairment

   E75.19   **Other** gangliosidosis
     GM1 gangliosidosis
     GM3 gangliosidosis

● E75.2   Other sphingolipidosis
    Lysosomal (a particle in a cytoplasm cell that contains digestive enzymes) storage diseases with symptoms of abnormal storage of amino acids
    Excludes1   adrenoleukodystrophy [Addison-Schilder] (E71.528)

   E75.21   **Fabry (-Anderson) disease**

   E75.22   **Gaucher disease**

   E75.23   **Krabbe disease**

●   E75.24   **Niemann-Pick disease**

    E75.240   Niemann-Pick disease type A

    E75.241   Niemann-Pick disease type B

    E75.242   Niemann-Pick disease type C

    E75.243   Niemann-Pick disease type D

    E75.248   Other Niemann-Pick disease

    E75.249   Niemann-Pick disease, **unspecified**

   E75.25   Metachromatic leukodystrophy

   E75.29   Other sphingolipidosis
     Farber's syndrome
     Sulfatase deficiency
     Sulfatide lipidosis

E75.3   Sphingolipidosis, **unspecified**

E75.4   Neuronal ceroid lipofuscinosis
    Batten disease
    Bielschowsky-Jansky disease
    Kufs disease
    Spielmeyer-Vogt disease

E75.5   Other lipid storage disorders
    Cerebrotendinous cholesterosis [van Bogaert-Scherer-Epstein]
    Wolman's disease

E75.6   Lipid storage disorder, **unspecified**

Item 4–8 Leukodystrophy is characterized by degeneration and/or failure of the myelin formation of the central nervous system and sometimes of the peripheral nervous system. The disease is inherited and progressive.

CHAPTER 4 (E00-E90)

▶ New   ⇒ Revised   ~~deleted~~ Deleted   **OGCR** Official Guidelines   X Assign placeholder X   ● Use Additional Character(s)
Excludes 1   Excludes 2   Includes   Use additional   Code first   Code also   Key words
709

● E76　Disorders of glycosaminoglycan metabolism
　● E76.0　Mucopolysaccharidosis, type I
　　　*Inborn metabolic disorder of enzymes that break down
　　　carbohydrates*
　　　E76.01　Hurler's syndrome
　　　E76.02　Hurler-Scheie syndrome
　　　E76.03　Scheie's syndrome
　　E76.1　Mucopolysaccharidosis, type II
　　　*Inborn metabolic disorder of enzymes that break down
　　　carbohydrates occurs in 2-4 year old males*
　　　Hunter's syndrome
　● E76.2　Other mucopolysaccharidoses
　　● E76.21　Morquio mucopolysaccharidoses
　　　　E76.210　Morquio A mucopolysaccharidoses
　　　　　　　Classic Morquio syndrome
　　　　　　　Morquio syndrome A
　　　　　　　Mucopolysaccharidosis, type IVA
　　　　E76.211　Morquio B mucopolysaccharidoses
　　　　　　　Morquio-like
　　　　　　　　mucopolysaccharidoses
　　　　　　　Morquio-like syndrome
　　　　　　　Morquio syndrome B
　　　　　　　Mucopolysaccharidosis, type IVB
　　　　E76.219　Morquio mucopolysaccharidoses,
　　　　　　　unspecified
　　　　　　　Morquio syndrome
　　　　　　　Mucopolysaccharidosis, type IV
　　　E76.22　Sanfilippo mucopolysaccharidoses
　　　　　　Mucopolysaccharidosis, type III (A) (B) (C) (D)
　　　　　　Sanfilippo A syndrome
　　　　　　Sanfilippo B syndrome
　　　　　　Sanfilippo C syndrome
　　　　　　Sanfilippo D syndrome
　　　E76.29　Other mucopolysaccharidoses
　　　　　　beta-Glucuronidase deficiency
　　　　　　Maroteaux-Lamy (mild) (severe) syndrome
　　　　　　Mucopolysaccharidosis, types VI, VII
　　E76.3　Mucopolysaccharidosis, unspecified
　　E76.8　Other disorders of glycosaminoglycan metabolism
　　E76.9　Glucosaminoglycan metabolism disorder, unspecified

● E77　Disorders of glycoprotein metabolism
　　E77.0　Defects in post-translational modification of lysosomal
　　　　　enzymes
　　　　　Mucolipidosis II [I-cell disease]
　　　　　Mucolipidosis III [pseudo-Hurler polydystrophy]
　　E77.1　Defects in glycoprotein degradation
　　　　　Aspartylglucosaminuria
　　　　　Fucosidosis
　　　　　Mannosidosis
　　　　　Sialidosis [mucolipidosis I]
　　E77.8　Other disorders of glycoprotein metabolism
　　E77.9　Disorder of glycoprotein metabolism, unspecified

● E78　Disorders of lipoprotein metabolism and other lipidemias
　　　Excludes1　sphingolipidosis (E75.0-E75.3)
　● E78.0　Pure hypercholesterolemia
　　　E78.00　Pure hypercholesterolemia, unspecified
　　　　　　Fredrickson's hyperlipoproteinemia, type IIa
　　　　　　Hyperbetalipoproteinemia
　　　　　　Low-density-lipoprotein-type [LDL]
　　　　　　　hyperlipoproteinemia
　　　　▶(Pure) hypercholesterolemia NOS
　　　E78.01　Familial hypercholesterolemia

　　E78.1　Pure hyperglyceridemia
　　　　　Elevated fasting triglycerides
　　　　　Endogenous hyperglyceridemia
　　　　　Fredrickson's hyperlipoproteinemia, type IV
　　　　　Hyperlipidemia, group B
　　　　　Hyperprebetalipoproteinemia
　　　　　Very-low-density-lipoprotein-type [VLDL]
　　　　　　hyperlipoproteinemia
　　E78.2　Mixed hyperlipidemia
　　　　　Broad- or floating-betalipoproteinemia
　　　　　Combined hyperlipidemia NOS
　　　　　Elevated cholesterol with elevated triglycerides NEC
　　　　　Fredrickson's hyperlipoproteinemia, type IIb or III
　　　　　Hyperbetalipoproteinemia with prebetalipoproteinemia
　　　　　Hypercholesteremia with endogenous
　　　　　　hyperglyceridemia
　　　　　Hyperlipidemia, group C
　　　　　Tubo-eruptive xanthoma
　　　　　Xanthoma tuberosum
　　　　　Excludes1　cerebrotendinous cholesterosis [van
　　　　　　　Bogaert-Scherer-Epstein] (E75.5)
　　　　　　　familial combined hyperlipidemia (E78.4)
　　E78.3　Hyperchylomicronemia
　　　　　Chylomicron retention disease
　　　　　Fredrickson's hyperlipoproteinemia, type I or V
　　　　　Hyperlipidemia, group D
　　　　　Mixed hyperglyceridemia
　　E78.4　Other hyperlipidemia
　　　　　Familial combined hyperlipidemia
　　E78.5　Hyperlipidemia, unspecified
　　E78.6　Lipoprotein deficiency
　　　　　Abetalipoproteinemia
　　　　　Depressed HDL cholesterol
　　　　　High-density lipoprotein deficiency
　　　　　Hypoalphalipoproteinemia
　　　　　Hypobetalipoproteinemia (familial)
　　　　　Lecithin cholesterol acyltransferase deficiency
　　　　　Tangier disease
　● E78.7　Disorders of bile acid and cholesterol metabolism
　　　　Excludes1　Niemann-Pick disease type C (E75.242)
　　　E78.70　Disorder of bile acid and cholesterol
　　　　　　metabolism, unspecified
　　　E78.71　Barth syndrome
　　　E78.72　Smith-Lemli-Opitz syndrome
　　　E78.79　Other disorders of bile acid and cholesterol
　　　　　　metabolism
　● E78.8　Other disorders of lipoprotein metabolism
　　　E78.81　Lipoid dermatoarthritis
　　　E78.89　Other lipoprotein metabolism disorders
　　E78.9　Disorder of lipoprotein metabolism, unspecified

● E79　Disorders of purine and pyrimidine metabolism
　　　Purines, along with pyrimidines, signal RNA and DNA production
　　　Excludes1　Ataxia-telangiectasia (Q87.1)
　　　　　Bloom's syndrome (Q82.8)
　　　　　Cockayne's syndrome (Q87.1)
　　　　　calculus of kidney (N20.0)
　　　　　combined immunodeficiency disorders (D81.-)
　　　　　Fanconi's anemia (D61.09)
　　　　　gout (M1A.-, M10.-)
　　　　　orotaciduric anemia (D53.0)
　　　　　progeria (E34.8)
　　　　　Werner's syndrome (E34.8)
　　　　　xeroderma pigmentosum (Q82.1)
　　E79.0　Hyperuricemia without signs of inflammatory arthritis
　　　　　and tophaceous disease
　　　　　Asymptomatic hyperuricemia
　　E79.1　Lesch-Nyhan syndrome
　　　　　HGPRT deficiency
　　E79.2　Myoadenylate deaminase deficiency
　　E79.8　Other disorders of purine and pyrimidine metabolism
　　　　　Hereditary xanthinuria
　　E79.9　Disorder of purine and pyrimidine
　　　　　metabolism, unspecified

▶ New　⟹ Revised　~~deleted~~ Deleted　**OGCR** Official Guidelines　X Assign placeholder X　● Use Additional Character(s)
Excludes 1　Excludes 2　Includes　Use additional　Code first　Code also　Key words

● **E80**   **Disorders of porphyrin and bilirubin metabolism**
Group of chemical compounds in RBC's that combine with iron to form heme

     Includes   defects of catalase and peroxidase

   E80.0   **Hereditary erythropoietic porphyria**
       Congenital erythropoietic porphyria
       Erythropoietic protoporphyria

   E80.1   **Porphyria cutanea tarda**

●   **E80.2**   **Other and unspecified porphyria**

     E80.20   **Unspecified porphyria**
         Porphyria NOS

     E80.21   **Acute intermittent (hepatic) porphyria**

     E80.29   **Other porphyria**
         Hereditary coproporphyria

   E80.3   **Defects of catalase and peroxidase**
       Acatalasia [Takahara]

   E80.4   **Gilbert syndrome**

   E80.5   **Crigler-Najjar syndrome**

   E80.6   **Other disorders of bilirubin metabolism**
       Dubin-Johnson syndrome
       Rotor's syndrome

   E80.7   **Disorder of bilirubin metabolism, unspecified**

● **E83**   **Disorders of mineral metabolism**

     Excludes1   dietary mineral deficiency (E58-E61)
            parathyroid disorders (E20-E21)
            vitamin D deficiency (E55.-)

●   **E83.0**   **Disorders of copper metabolism**

     E83.00   **Disorder of copper metabolism, unspecified**

     E83.01   **Wilson's disease**

         Code also associated Kayser Fleischer ring (H18.04-)

     E83.09   **Other disorders of copper metabolism**
         Menkes' (kinky hair) (steely hair) disease

●   **E83.1**   **Disorders of iron metabolism**

     Excludes1   iron deficiency anemia (D50.-)
            sideroblastic anemia (D64.0-D64.3)

     E83.10   **Disorder of iron metabolism, unspecified**

●   **E83.11**   **Hemochromatosis**

       ▶ **Excludes1**   GALD (P78.84)
             ▶Gestational alloimmune liver disease (P78.84)
             ▶Neonatal hemochromatosis (P78.84)

       E83.110   **Hereditary hemochromatosis**
           Bronzed diabetes
           Pigmentary cirrhosis (of liver)
           Primary (hereditary) hemochromatosis

       E83.111   **Hemochromatosis due to repeated red blood cell transfusions**
           Iron overload due to repeated red blood cell transfusions
           Transfusion (red blood cell) associated hemochromatosis

       E83.118   **Other hemochromatosis**

       E83.119   **Hemochromatosis, unspecified**

     E83.19   **Other disorders of iron metabolism**

         Use additional code, if applicable, for idiopathic pulmonary hemosiderosis (J84.03)

   E83.2   **Disorders of zinc metabolism**
       Acrodermatitis enteropathica

●   **E83.3**   **Disorders of phosphorus metabolism and phosphatases**

     Excludes1   adult osteomalacia (M83.-)
            osteoporosis (M80.-)

     E83.30   **Disorder of phosphorus metabolism, unspecified**

     E83.31   **Familial hypophosphatemia**
         Vitamin D-resistant osteomalacia
         Vitamin D-resistant rickets

         Excludes1   vitamin D-deficiency rickets (E55.0)

     E83.32   **Hereditary vitamin D-dependent rickets (type 1) (type 2)**
         25-hydroxyvitamin D 1-alpha-hydroxylase deficiency
         Pseudovitamin D deficiency
         Vitamin D receptor defect

     E83.39   **Other disorders of phosphorus metabolism**
         Acid phosphatase deficiency
         Hypophosphatasia

●   **E83.4**   **Disorders of magnesium metabolism**

     E83.40   **Disorders of magnesium metabolism, unspecified**

     E83.41   **Hypermagnesemia**

     E83.42   **Hypomagnesemia**

     E83.49   **Other disorders of magnesium metabolism**

●   **E83.5**   **Disorders of calcium metabolism**

     Excludes1   chondrocalcinosis (M11.1-M11.2)
            hungry bone syndrome (E83.81)
            hyperparathyroidism (E21.0-E21.3)

     E83.50   **Unspecified disorder of calcium metabolism**

     E83.51   **Hypocalcemia**

     E83.52   **Hypercalcemia**
         Familial hypocalciuric hypercalcemia

     E83.59   **Other disorders of calcium metabolism**
         Idiopathic hypercalciuria

●   **E83.8**   **Other disorders of mineral metabolism**

     E83.81   **Hungry bone syndrome**

     E83.89   **Other disorders of mineral metabolism**

   E83.9   **Disorder of mineral metabolism, unspecified**

● **E84**   **Cystic fibrosis**

     Includes   mucoviscidosis

     Code also exocrine pancreatic insufficiency (K86.81)

   E84.0   **Cystic fibrosis with pulmonary manifestations**

       Use additional code to identify any infectious organism present, such as:
       Pseudomonas (B96.5)

●   **E84.1**   **Cystic fibrosis with intestinal manifestations**

     E84.11   **Meconium ileus in cystic fibrosis**

         Excludes1   meconium ileus not due to cystic fibrosis (P76.0)

     E84.19   **Cystic fibrosis with other intestinal manifestations**
         Distal intestinal obstruction syndrome

   E84.8   **Cystic fibrosis with other manifestations**

   E84.9   **Cystic fibrosis, unspecified**

▶ New   ⇒ Revised   ~~deleted~~ Deleted   **OGCR** Official Guidelines   X Assign placeholder X   ● Use Additional Character(s)

Excludes 1   Excludes 2   Includes   Use additional   Code first   Code also   Key words

● **E85   Amyloidosis**
*A disorder resulting from the abnormal deposition of a particular
protein (amyloid) into tissues of the body*
~~Excludes1~~   ~~Alzheimer's disease (G30.0-)~~
▶ Excludes2   Alzheimer's disease (G30.0-)
E85.0   Non-neuropathic heredofamilial amyloidosis
Hereditary amyloid nephropathy
▶Code also associated disorders, such as:
▶autoinflammatory syndromes (M04.-)
▶ Excludes2   Transthyretin-related (ATTR) familial
amyloid cardiomyopathy (E85.4)
E85.1   Neuropathic heredofamilial amyloidosis
Amyloid polyneuropathy (Portuguese)
▶Transthyretin-related (ATTR) familial amyloid
polyneuropathy
E85.2   Heredofamilial amyloidosis, unspecified
E85.3   Secondary systemic amyloidosis
Hemodialysis-associated amyloidosis
E85.4   Organ-limited amyloidosis
Localized amyloidosis
▶Transthyretin-related (ATTR) familial amyloid
cardiomyopathy
● **E85.8   Other amyloidosis**
▶ **E85.81   Light chain (AL) amyloidosis**
▶ **E85.82   Wild-type transthyretin-related (ATTR)
amyloidosis**
▶Senile systemic amyloidosis (SSA)
▶ **E85.89   Other amyloidosis**
E85.9   Amyloidosis, unspecified

● **E86   Volume depletion**
Excludes1   dehydration of newborn (P74.1)
hypovolemic shock NOS (R57.1)
postprocedural hypovolemic shock (T81.19)
traumatic hypovolemic shock (T79.4)
Use additional code(s) for any associated disorders of
electrolyte and acid-base balance (E87.-)
E86.0   Dehydration
Excessive loss of body water
E86.1   Hypovolemia
Diminished volume of circulating blood
Depletion of volume of plasma
E86.9   Volume depletion, unspecified

● **E87   Other disorders of fluid, electrolyte and acid-base balance**
Excludes1   diabetes insipidus (E23.2)
electrolyte imbalance associated with
hyperemesis gravidarum (O21.1)
electrolyte imbalance following ectopic or molar
pregnancy (O08.5)
familial periodic paralysis (G72.3)
E87.0   Hyperosmolality and hypernatremia
Sodium [Na] excess
Sodium [Na] overload
E87.1   Hypo-osmolality and hyponatremia
Sodium [Na] deficiency
Excludes1   syndrome of inappropriate secretion of
antidiuretic hormone (E22.2)
E87.2   Acidosis
Acidosis NOS
Lactic acidosis
Metabolic acidosis
Respiratory acidosis
Excludes1   diabetic acidosis - see categories E08-E10,
E13 with ketoacidosis

Item 4–9   Circulating fluid volume is regulated by the amount of water and
sodium ingested, excreted by the kidneys into the urine, and lost through the
gastrointestinal tract, lungs, and skin. To maintain blood volume within a normal
range, the kidneys regulate the amount of water and sodium lost into the urine.
Too much (**fluid overload**) or too little fluid volume (**volume depletion**)
will affect blood pressure. Severe cases of vomiting, diarrhea, bleeding, and
burns (fluid loss through exposed burn surface area) can contribute to fluid
loss. Internal body environment must maintain a precise balance (homeostasis)
between too much fluid and too little fluid. This complex balancing mechanism
is critical to good health.

E87.3   Alkalosis
Alkalosis NOS
Metabolic alkalosis
Respiratory alkalosis
E87.4   Mixed disorder of acid-base balance
E87.5   Hyperkalemia
Potassium [K] excess
Potassium [K] overload
E87.6   Hypokalemia
Potassium [K] deficiency
● **E87.7   Fluid overload**
Excludes1   edema NOS (R60.9)
fluid retention (R60.9)
E87.70   Fluid overload, unspecified
E87.71   Transfusion associated circulatory overload
Fluid overload due to transfusion (blood)
(blood components) TACO
E87.79   Other fluid overload
**E87.8   Other disorders of electrolyte and fluid balance, not
elsewhere classified**
Electrolyte imbalance NOS
Hyperchloremia
Hypochloremia

● **E88   Other and unspecified metabolic disorders**
Use additional codes for associated conditions
Excludes1   histiocytosis X (chronic) (C96.6)
● **E88.0   Disorders of plasma-protein metabolism, not elsewhere
classified**
Excludes1   disorder of lipoprotein metabolism (E78.-)
monoclonal gammopathy (of
undetermined significance) (D47.2)
polyclonal hypergammaglobulinemia
(D89.0)
Waldenström macroglobulinemia (C88.0)
E88.01   Alpha-1-antitrypsin deficiency AAT deficiency
**E88.09   Other disorders of plasma-protein metabolism,
not elsewhere classified**
Bisalbuminemia
E88.1   Lipodystrophy, not elsewhere classified
*Defective fat metabolism resulting in absence of subcutaneous
fat*
Lipodystrophy NOS
Excludes1   Whipple's disease (K90.81)
E88.2   Lipomatosis, not elsewhere classified
Abnormal tumorlike accumulations of fat in tissue
Lipomatosis NOS
Lipomatosis (Check) dolorosa [Dercum]
E88.3   Tumor lysis syndrome
Tumor lysis syndrome (spontaneous)
Tumor lysis syndrome following antineoplastic drug
chemotherapy
Use additional code for adverse effect, if applicable, to
identify drug (T45.1X5)

▶ New   ⇒ Revised   ~~deleted~~ Deleted   **OGCR** Official Guidelines   X Assign placeholder X   ● Use Additional Character(s)

Excludes 1   Excludes 2   Includes   Use additional   Code first   Code also   Key words

● **E88.4** **Mitochondrial metabolism disorders**
Congenital disorder of metabolism

> **Excludes1** disorders of pyruvate metabolism (E74.4)
> Kearns-Sayre syndrome (H49.81)
> Leber's disease (H47.22)
> Leigh's encephalopathy (G31.82)
> Mitochondrial myopathy, NEC (G71.3)
> Reye's syndrome (G93.7)

E88.40 **Mitochondrial metabolism disorder, unspecified**

E88.41 **MELAS syndrome**
Mitochondrial myopathy, encephalopathy, lactic acidosis and stroke-like episodes

E88.42 **MERRF syndrome**
Myoclonic epilepsy associated with ragged-red fibers

> Code also progressive myoclonic epilepsy (G40.3-)

E88.49 **Other mitochondrial metabolism disorders**

● **E88.8** **Other specified metabolic disorders**

E88.81 **Metabolic syndrome**
Dysmetabolic syndrome X

> Use additional codes for associated manifestations, such as:
> obesity (E66.-)

E88.89 **Other specified metabolic disorders**
Launois-Bensaude adenolipomatosis

> **Excludes1** adult pulmonary Langerhans cell histiocytosis (J84.82)

E88.9 **Metabolic disorder, unspecified**

POSTPROCEDURAL ENDOCRINE AND METABOLIC COMPLICATIONS AND DISORDERS, NOT ELSEWHERE CLASSIFIED (E89)

● **E89** **Postprocedural endocrine and metabolic complications and disorders, not elsewhere classified**

> **Excludes2** intraoperative complications of endocrine system organ or structure (E36.0-, E36.1-, E36.8)

E89.0 **Postprocedural hypothyroidism**
Postirradiation hypothyroidism
Postsurgical hypothyroidism

E89.1 **Postprocedural hypoinsulinemia**
Postpancreatectomy hyperglycemia
Postsurgical hypoinsulinemia

> Use additional code, if applicable, to identify:
> acquired absence of pancreas (Z90.41-)
> diabetes mellitus (postpancreatectomy) (postprocedural) (E13.-)
> insulin use (Z79.4)

> **Excludes1** transient postprocedural hyperglycemia (R73.9)
> transient postprocedural hypoglycemia (E16.2)

E89.2 **Postprocedural hypoparathyroidism**
Parathyroprival tetany

E89.3 **Postprocedural hypopituitarism**
Postirradiation hypopituitarism

● **E89.4** **Postprocedural ovarian failure**

E89.40 **Asymptomatic postprocedural ovarian failure**
Postprocedural ovarian failure NOS

E89.41 **Symptomatic postprocedural ovarian failure**
Symptoms such as flushing, sleeplessness, headache, lack of concentration, associated with postprocedural menopause

E89.5 **Postprocedural testicular hypofunction**

E89.6 **Postprocedural adrenocortical (-medullary) hypofunction**

● **E89.8** **Other postprocedural endocrine and metabolic complications and disorders**

● E89.81 **Postprocedural hemorrhage of an endocrine system organ or structure following a procedure**

E89.810 Postprocedural hemorrhage of an endocrine system organ or structure following an endocrine system procedure

E89.811 Postprocedural hemorrhage of an endocrine system organ or structure following other procedure

● E89.82 **Postprocedural hematoma and seroma of an endocrine system organ or structure**

E89.820 Postprocedural hematoma of an endocrine system organ or structure following an endocrine system procedure

E89.821 Postprocedural hematoma of an endocrine system organ or structure following other procedure

E89.822 Postprocedural seroma of an endocrine system organ or structure following an endocrine system procedure

E89.823 Postprocedural seroma of an endocrine system organ or structure following other procedure

E89.89 **Other postprocedural endocrine and metabolic complications and disorders**

> Use additional code, if applicable, to further specify disorder

CHAPTER 4 (E00-E90)

▶ New　⇒ Revised　~~deleted~~ Deleted　**OGCR** Official Guidelines　**X** Assign placeholder X　● Use Additional Character(s)

Excludes 1　Excludes 2　Includes　Use additional　Code first　Code also　Key words

713

CHAPTER 5

MENTAL, BEHAVIORAL AND NEURODEVELOPMENTAL DISORDERS (F01-F99)

OGCR Chapter-Specific Coding Guidelines

5. **Chapter 5: Mental, Behavioral and Neurodevelopmental disorders (F01 – F99)**

a. **Pain disorders related to psychological factors**
Assign code F45.41, for pain that is exclusively related to psychological disorders. As indicated by the Excludes 1 note under category G89, a code from category G89 should not be assigned with code F45.41

Code F45.42, Pain disorders with related psychological factors, should be used with a code from category G89, Pain, not elsewhere classified, if there is documentation of a psychological component for a patient with acute or chronic pain.

See Section I.C.6. Pain

c. **Mental and behavioral disorders due to psychoactive substance use**

1) **In Remission**
Selection of codes for "in remission" for categories F10-F19, Mental and behavioral disorders due to psychoactive substance use (categories F10-F19 with -.11, -.21) requires the provider's clinical judgment. The appropriate codes for "in remission" are assigned only on the basis of provider documentation (as defined in the Official Guidelines for Coding and Reporting), **unless otherwise instructed by the classification.**

Mild substance use disorders in early or sustained remission are classified to the appropriate codes for substance abuse in remission, and moderate or severe substance use disorders in early or sustained remission are classified to the appropriate codes for substance dependence in remission.

2) **Psychoactive Substance Use, Abuse and Dependence**
When the provider documentation refers to use, abuse and dependence of the same substance (e.g. alcohol, opioid, cannabis, etc.), only one code should be assigned to identify the pattern of use based on the following hierarchy:
- If both use and abuse are documented, assign only the code for abuse
- If both abuse and dependence are documented, assign only the code for dependence
- If use, abuse and dependence are all documented, assign only the code for dependence
- If both use and dependence are documented, assign only the code for dependence.

3) **Psychoactive Substance Use** *Disorders*
As with all other diagnoses, the codes for psychoactive substance use **disorders** (F10.9-, F11.9-, F12.9-, F13.9-, F14.9-, F15.9-, F16.9-) should only be assigned based on provider documentation and when they meet the definition of a reportable diagnosis (see Section III, Reporting Additional Diagnoses). The codes are to be used only when the psychoactive substance use is associated with a **physical,** mental or behavioral disorder, and such a relationship is documented by the provider.

CHAPTER 5

MENTAL, BEHAVIORAL AND NEURODEVELOPMENTAL DISORDERS (F01-F99)

Includes disorders of psychological development

Excludes2 symptoms, signs and abnormal clinical laboratory findings, not elsewhere classified (R00-R99)

This chapter contains the following blocks:

F01-F09	Mental disorders due to known physiological conditions
F10-F19	Mental and behavioral disorders due to psychoactive substance use
F20-F29	Schizophrenia, schizotypal, delusional, and other non-mood psychotic disorders
F30-F39	Mood [affective] disorders
F40-F48	Anxiety, dissociative, stress-related, somatoform and other nonpsychotic mental disorders
F50-F59	Behavioral syndromes associated with physiological disturbances and physical factors
F60-F69	Disorders of adult personality and behavior
F70-F79	Intellectual disabilities
F80-F89	Pervasive and specific developmental disorders
F90-F98	Behavioral and emotional disorders with onset usually occurring in childhood and adolescence
F99	Unspecified mental disorder

MENTAL DISORDERS DUE TO KNOWN PHYSIOLOGICAL CONDITIONS (F01-F09)

This block comprises a range of mental disorders grouped together on the basis of their having in common a demonstrable etiology in cerebral disease, brain injury, or other insult leading to cerebral dysfunction. The dysfunction may be primary, as in diseases, injuries, and insults that affect the brain directly and selectively; or secondary, as in systemic diseases and disorders that attack the brain only as one of the multiple organs or systems of the body that are involved.

● **F01   Vascular dementia**
Vascular dementia as a result of infarction of the brain due to vascular disease, including hypertensive cerebrovascular disease.

Includes arteriosclerotic dementia

Code first the underlying physiological condition or sequelae of cerebrovascular disease.

● **F01.5   Vascular dementia**

F01.50   Vascular dementia without behavioral disturbance
Major neurocognitive disorder without behavioral disturbance

F01.51   Vascular dementia with behavioral disturbance
Major neurocognitive disorder due to vascular disease, with behavioral disturbance
Major neurocognitive disorder with aggressive behavior
Major neurocognitive disorder with combative behavior
Major neurocognitive disorder with violent behavior
Vascular dementia with aggressive behavior
Vascular dementia with combative behavior
Vascular dementia with violent behavior
Use additional code, if applicable, to identify wandering in vascular dementia (Z91.83)

▶ New   ⇒ Revised   ~~deleted~~ Deleted   **OGCR** Official Guidelines   X Assign placeholder X   ● Use Additional Character(s)
| Excludes 1 | | Excludes 2 | | Includes | | Use additional | | Code first | | Code also | | Key words |

● **F02   Dementia in other diseases classified elsewhere**

    Code first the underlying physiological condition, such as:
       Alzheimer's (G30.-)
       cerebral lipidosis (E75.4)
       Creutzfeldt-Jakob disease (A81.0-)
       dementia with Lewy bodies (G31.83)
       dementia with Parkinsonism (G31.83)
       epilepsy and recurrent seizures (G40.-)
       frontotemporal dementia (G31.09)
       hepatolenticular degeneration (E83.0)
       human immunodeficiency virus [HIV] disease (B20)
       Huntington's disease (G10)
       hypercalcemia (E83.52)
       hypothyroidism, acquired (E00-E03.-)
       intoxications (T36-T65)
       Jakob-Creutzfeldt disease (A81.0-)
       multiple sclerosis (G35)
       neurosyphilis (A52.17)
       niacin deficiency [pellagra] (E52)
       Parkinson's disease (G20)
       Pick's disease (G31.01)
       polyarteritis nodosa (M30.0)
       prion disease (A81.9)
       systemic lupus erythematosus (M32.-)
       traumatic brain injury (S06.-)
       trypanosomiasis (B56.-, B57.-)
       vitamin B deficiency (E53.8)

    Includes   Major neurocognitive disorder in other diseases classified elsewhere

    Excludes2   dementia in alcohol and psychoactive substance disorders (F10-F19, with .17, .27, .97)
                vascular dementia (F01.5-)

● **F02.8   Dementia in other diseases classified elsewhere**

    F02.80   **Dementia in other diseases classified elsewhere without behavioral disturbance**
          Dementia in other diseases classified elsewhere NOS
          Major neurocognitive disorder in other diseases classified elsewhere

    F02.81   **Dementia in other diseases classified elsewhere with behavioral disturbance**
          Dementia in other diseases classified elsewhere with aggressive behavior
          Dementia in other diseases classified elsewhere with combative behavior
          Dementia in other diseases classified elsewhere with violent behavior
          Major neurocognitive disorder in other diseases classified elsewhere with aggressive behavior
          Major neurocognitive disorder in other diseases classified elsewhere with combative behavior
          Major neurocognitive disorder in other diseases classified elsewhere with violent behavior
          Use additional code, if applicable, to identify wandering in dementia in conditions classified elsewhere (Z91.83)

Item 5-1 Psychosis was a term formerly applied to any mental disorder but is now restricted to disturbances of a great magnitude in which there is a personality disintegration and loss of contact with reality.

● **F03   Unspecified dementia**
       Presenile dementia NOS
       Presenile psychosis NOS
       Primary degenerative dementia NOS
       Senile dementia NOS
       Senile dementia depressed or paranoid type
       Senile psychosis NOS

    Excludes1   senility NOS (R41.81)
    Excludes2   mild memory disturbance due to known physiological condition (F06.8)
             senile dementia with delirium or acute confusional state (F05)

  ● **F03.9   Unspecified dementia**

    F03.90   **Unspecified dementia without behavioral disturbance**
          Dementia NOS

    F03.91   **Unspecified dementia with behavioral disturbance**
          Unspecified dementia with aggressive behavior
          Unspecified dementia with combative behavior
          Unspecified dementia with violent behavior
          Use additional code, if applicable, to identify wandering in unspecified dementia (Z91.83)

F04   Amnestic disorder due to known physiological condition
       Korsakov's psychosis or syndrome, nonalcoholic

    Code first the underlying physiological condition
    Excludes1   amnesia NOS (R41.3)
             anterograde amnesia (R41.1)
             dissociative amnesia (F44.0)
             retrograde amnesia (R41.2)
    Excludes2   alcohol-induced or unspecified Korsakov's syndrome (F10.26, F10.96)
             Korsakov's syndrome induced by other psychoactive substances (F13.26, F13.96, F19.16, F19.26, F19.96)

F05   Delirium due to known physiological condition
       Acute or subacute brain syndrome
       Acute or subacute confusional state (nonalcoholic)
       Acute or subacute infective psychosis
       Acute or subacute organic reaction
       Acute or subacute psycho-organic syndrome
       Delirium of mixed etiology
       Delirium superimposed on dementia
       Sundowning

    Code first the underlying physiological condition
    Excludes1   delirium NOS (R41.0)
    Excludes2   delirium tremens alcohol-induced or unspecified (F10.231, F10.921)

CHAPTER 5 (F01-F99)

CHAPTER 5 (F01-F99)

● **F06**   **Other mental disorders** due to known physiological condition

     Includes   mental disorders due to endocrine disorder
                  mental disorders due to exogenous hormone
                  mental disorders due to exogenous toxic
                      substance
                  mental disorders due to primary cerebral disease
                  mental disorders due to somatic illness
                  mental disorders due to systemic disease
                      affecting the brain

     Code first the underlying physiological condition
     Excludes1   unspecified dementia (F03)
     Excludes2   delirium due to known physiological condition
                      (F05)
                      dementia as classified in F01-F02
                      other mental disorders associated with alcohol
                         and other psychoactive substances (F10-F19)

     F06.0   **Psychotic disorder with hallucinations** due to known
             physiological condition
             Organic hallucinatory state (nonalcoholic)
             Excludes2   hallucinations and perceptual disturbance
                         induced by alcohol and other
                         psychoactive substances (F10-F19
                         with .151, .251, .951)
                         schizophrenia (F20.-)

     F06.1   **Catatonic** disorder due to known physiological
             condition
             Catatonia associated with another mental disorder
             Catatonia NOS
             Excludes1   catatonic stupor (R40.1)
                       stupor NOS (R40.1)
             Excludes2   catatonic schizophrenia (F20.2)
                       dissociative stupor (F44.2)

     F06.2   **Psychotic disorder with delusions** due to known
             physiological condition
             Paranoid and paranoid-hallucinatory organic states
             Schizophrenia-like psychosis in epilepsy
             Excludes2   alcohol and drug-induced psychotic
                         disorder (F10-F19 with .150, .250,
                         .950)
                       brief psychotic disorder (F23)
                       delusional disorder (F22)
                       schizophrenia (F20.-)

● **F06.3**   **Mood disorder** due to known physiological condition
             Excludes2   mood disorders due to alcohol and other
                         psychoactive
                         substances (F10-F19 with .14, .24, .94)
                       mood disorders, not due to known
                         physiological condition or
                         unspecified (F30-F39)

     F06.30   **Mood disorder** due to known physiological
              condition, **unspecified**

     F06.31   **Mood disorder** due to known physiological
              condition **with depressive features**
             ▶Depressive disorder due to known
                  physiological condition, with depressive
                  features

     F06.32   **Mood disorder** due to known physiological
              condition **with major depressive-like episode**
             ▶Depressive disorder due to known
                  physiological condition, with major
                  depressive-like episode

     F06.33   **Mood disorder** due to known physiological
              condition **with manic features**
             ▶Bipolar and related disorder due to a known
                  physiological condition, with manic
                  features
             ▶Bipolar and related disorder due to known
                  physiological condition, with manic- or
                  hypomanic-like episodes

     F06.34   **Mood disorder** due to known physiological
              condition **with mixed features**
             ▶Bipolar and related disorder due to known
                  physiological condition, with mixed
                  features
             ▶Depressive disorder due to known
                  physiological condition, with mixed
                  features

     F06.4   **Anxiety disorder** due to known physiological condition
             Excludes2   anxiety disorders due to alcohol and
                       other psychoactive substances
                       (F10-F19 with .180, .280, .980)
                       anxiety disorders, not due to known
                       physiological condition or
                       unspecified (F40.-, F41.-)

     F06.8   **Other** specified mental disorders due to known
             physiological condition
             Epileptic psychosis NOS
             ▶Obsessive-compulsive and related disorder due to a
                  known physiological condition
             Organic dissociative disorder
             Organic emotionally labile [asthenic] disorder

● **F07**   **Personality and behavioral disorders** due to known
physiological condition

     Code first the underlying physiological condition

     F07.0   **Personality** change due to known physiological
             condition
             Frontal lobe syndrome
             Limbic epilepsy personality syndrome
             Lobotomy syndrome
             Organic personality disorder
             Organic pseudopsychopathic personality
             Organic pseudoretarded personality
             Postleucotomy syndrome
             Code first underlying physiological condition
             Excludes1   mild cognitive impairment (G31.84)
                       postconcussional syndrome (F07.81)
                       postencephalitic syndrome (F07.89)
                       signs and symptoms involving emotional
                         state (R45.-)
             Excludes2   specific personality disorder (F60.-)

● **F07.8**   **Other personality and behavioral disorders** due to
known physiological condition

     F07.81   **Postconcussional** syndrome
             Postcontusional syndrome (encephalopathy)
             Post-traumatic brain syndrome, nonpsychotic
             Use additional code to identify associated
                  post-traumatic headache, if applicable
                  (G44.3-)
             Excludes1   current concussion (brain) (S06.0-)
                       postencephalitic syndrome
                         (F07.89)

     F07.89   **Other** personality and behavioral disorders due
             to known physiological condition
             Postencephalitic syndrome
             Damage to temporal brain lobes with memory
                loss and abnormal behavior
             Right hemispheric organic affective disorder

     F07.9   **Unspecified** personality and behavioral disorder due to
             known physiological condition
             Organic psychosyndrome
             Due to exposure to organic solvents

F09   **Unspecified mental disorder** due to known physiological
condition
     Mental disorder NOS due to known physiological condition
     Organic brain syndrome NOS
     Organic mental disorder NOS
     Organic psychosis NOS
     Symptomatic psychosis NOS
     Code first the underlying physiological condition
     Excludes1   psychosis NOS (F29)

▶ New   ⇨ Revised   ~~deleted~~ Deleted   **OGCR** Official Guidelines   X Assign placeholder X   ● Use Additional Character(s)

Excludes 1   Excludes 2   Includes   Use additional   Code first   Code also   Key words

MENTAL AND BEHAVIORAL DISORDERS DUE TO PSYCHOACTIVE SUBSTANCE USE (F10-F19)

● **F10   Alcohol related disorders**

Use additional code for blood alcohol level, if applicable (Y90.-)

● **F10.1   Alcohol abuse**

Excludes1   alcohol dependence (F10.2-)
alcohol use, unspecified (F10.9-)

F10.10   Alcohol abuse, uncomplicated
Alcohol use disorder, mild

▶ **F10.11   Alcohol abuse, in remission**
▶Alcohol use disorder, mild, in early remission
▶Alcohol use disorder, mild, in sustained remission

● **F10.12   Alcohol abuse with intoxication**

F10.120   Alcohol abuse with intoxication, uncomplicated

F10.121   Alcohol abuse with intoxication, delirium

F10.129   Alcohol abuse with intoxication, unspecified

F10.14   Alcohol abuse with alcohol-induced mood disorder
Alcohol use disorder, mild, with alcohol-induced bipolar or related disorder
Alcohol use disorder, mild, with alcohol-induced depressive disorder

● **F10.15   Alcohol abuse with alcohol-induced psychotic disorder**

F10.150   Alcohol abuse with alcohol-induced psychotic disorder with delusions

F10.151   Alcohol abuse with alcohol-induced psychotic disorder with hallucinations

F10.159   Alcohol abuse with alcohol-induced psychotic disorder, unspecified

● **F10.18   Alcohol abuse with other alcohol-induced disorders**

F10.180   Alcohol abuse with alcohol-induced anxiety disorder

F10.181   Alcohol abuse with alcohol-induced sexual dysfunction

F10.182   Alcohol abuse with alcohol-induced sleep disorder

F10.188   Alcohol abuse with other alcohol-induced disorder

F10.19   Alcohol abuse with unspecified alcohol-induced disorder

● **F10.2   Alcohol dependence**

Excludes1   alcohol abuse (F10.1-)
alcohol use, unspecified (F10.9-)

Excludes2   toxic effect of alcohol (T51.0-)

F10.20   Alcohol dependence, uncomplicated
Alcohol use disorder, moderate
Alcohol use disorder, severe

F10.21   Alcohol dependence, in remission
▶Alcohol use disorder, moderate, in early remission
▶Alcohol use disorder, moderate, in sustained remission
▶Alcohol use disorder, severe, in early remission
▶Alcohol use disorder, severe, in sustained remission

● **F10.22   Alcohol dependence with intoxication**
Acute drunkenness (in alcoholism)

Excludes2   alcohol dependence with withdrawal (F10.23-)

F10.220   Alcohol dependence with intoxication, uncomplicated

F10.221   Alcohol dependence with intoxication delirium

F10.229   Alcohol dependence with intoxication, unspecified

● **F10.23   Alcohol dependence with withdrawal**

Excludes2   alcohol dependence with intoxication (F10.22-)

F10.230   Alcohol dependence with withdrawal, uncomplicated

F10.231   Alcohol dependence with withdrawal delirium

F10.232   Alcohol dependence with withdrawal with perceptual disturbance

F10.239   Alcohol dependence with withdrawal, unspecified

F10.24   Alcohol dependence with alcohol-induced mood disorder
Alcohol use disorder, moderate, with alcohol-induced bipolar or related disorder
Alcohol use disorder, moderate, with alcohol-induced depressive disorder
Alcohol use disorder, severe, with alcohol-induced bipolar or related disorder
Alcohol use disorder, severe, with alcohol-induced depressive disorder

● **F10.25   Alcohol dependence with alcohol-induced psychotic disorder**

F10.250   Alcohol dependence with alcohol-induced psychotic disorder with delusions

F10.251   Alcohol dependence with alcohol-induced psychotic disorder with hallucinations

F10.259   Alcohol dependence with alcohol-induced psychotic disorder, unspecified

F10.26   Alcohol dependence with alcohol-induced persisting amnestic disorder
Alcohol use disorder, moderate, with alcohol-induced major neurocognitive disorder, amnestic-confabulatory type
Alcohol use disorder, severe, with alcohol-induced major neurocognitive disorder, amnestic-confabulatory type

F10.27   Alcohol dependence with alcohol-induced persisting dementia
Alcohol use disorder, moderate, with alcohol-induced major neurocognitive disorder, nonamnestic-confabulatory type
Alcohol use disorder, severe, with alcohol-induced major neurocognitive disorder, nonamnestic-confabulatory type

● **F10.28** **Alcohol dependence with other alcohol-induced disorders**

    F10.280 **Alcohol dependence with alcohol-induced anxiety disorder**

    F10.281 **Alcohol dependence with alcohol-induced sexual dysfunction**

    F10.282 **Alcohol dependence with alcohol-induced sleep disorder**

    F10.288 **Alcohol dependence with other alcohol-induced disorder**
        Alcohol use disorder, moderate, with alcohol-induced mild neurocognitive disorder
        Alcohol use disorder, severe, with alcohol-induced mild neurocognitive disorder

    F10.29 **Alcohol dependence with unspecified alcohol-induced disorder**

● **F10.9** **Alcohol use, unspecified**

    Excludes1   alcohol abuse (F10.1-)
                alcohol dependence (F10.2-)

● **F10.92** **Alcohol use, unspecified with intoxication**

    F10.920 **Alcohol use, unspecified with intoxication, uncomplicated**

    F10.921 **Alcohol use, unspecified with intoxication delirium**

    F10.929 **Alcohol use, unspecified with intoxication, unspecified**

    F10.94 **Alcohol use, unspecified with alcohol-induced mood disorder**
        Alcohol-induced bipolar or related disorder, without use disorder
        Alcohol-induced depressive disorder, without use disorder

● **F10.95** **Alcohol use, unspecified with alcohol-induced psychotic disorder**

    F10.950 **Alcohol use, unspecified with alcohol-induced psychotic disorder with delusions**

    F10.951 **Alcohol use, unspecified with alcohol-induced psychotic disorder with hallucinations**

    F10.959 **Alcohol use, unspecified with alcohol-induced psychotic disorder, unspecified**
        Alcohol-induced psychotic disorder without use disorder

    F10.96 **Alcohol use, unspecified with alcohol-induced persisting amnestic disorder**
        Alcohol-induced major neurocognitive disorder, amnestic-confabulatory type, without use disorder

    F10.97 **Alcohol use, unspecified with alcohol-induced persisting dementia**
        Alcohol-induced major neurocognitive disorder, nonamnestic-confabulatory type, without use disorder

● **F10.98** **Alcohol use, unspecified with other alcohol-induced disorders**

    F10.980 **Alcohol use, unspecified with alcohol-induced anxiety disorder**
        Alcohol-induced anxiety disorder, without use disorder

    F10.981 **Alcohol use, unspecified with alcohol-induced sexual dysfunction**
        Alcohol-induced sexual dysfunction, without use disorder

    F10.982 **Alcohol use, unspecified with alcohol-induced sleep disorder**
        Alcohol-induced sleep disorder, without use disorder

    F10.988 **Alcohol use, unspecified with other alcohol-induced disorder**
        Alcohol-induced mild neurocognitive disorder, without use disorder

    F10.99 **Alcohol use, unspecified with unspecified alcohol-induced disorder**

● **F11** **Opioid related disorders**

● **F11.1** **Opioid abuse**

    Excludes1   opioid dependence (F11.2-)
                opioid use, unspecified (F11.9-)

    F11.10 **Opioid abuse, uncomplicated**
        Opioid use disorder, mild

▶ **F11.11** **Opioid abuse, in remission**
    ▶Opioid use disorder, mild, in early remission
    ▶Opioid use disorder, mild, in sustained remission

● **F11.12** **Opioid abuse with intoxication**

    F11.120 **Opioid abuse with intoxication, uncomplicated**

    F11.121 **Opioid abuse with intoxication delirium**

    F11.122 **Opioid abuse with intoxication with perceptual disturbance**

    F11.129 **Opioid abuse with intoxication, unspecified**

    F11.14 **Opioid abuse with opioid-induced mood disorder**
        Opioid use disorder, mild, with opioid-induced depressive disorder

● **F11.15** **Opioid abuse with opioid-induced psychotic disorder**

    F11.150 **Opioid abuse with opioid-induced psychotic disorder with delusions**

    F11.151 **Opioid abuse with opioid-induced psychotic disorder with hallucinations**

    F11.159 **Opioid abuse with opioid-induced psychotic disorder, unspecified**

● **F11.18** **Opioid abuse with other opioid-induced disorder**

    F11.181 **Opioid abuse with opioid-induced sexual dysfunction**

    F11.182 **Opioid abuse with opioid-induced sleep disorder**

    F11.188 **Opioid abuse with other opioid-induced disorder**

    F11.19 **Opioid abuse with unspecified opioid-induced disorder**

● **F11.2** **Opioid dependence**

    Excludes1   opioid abuse (F11.1-)
                opioid use, unspecified (F11.9-)

    Excludes2   opioid poisoning (T40.0--T40.2-)

    F11.20 **Opioid dependence, uncomplicated**
        Opioid use disorder, moderate
        Opioid use disorder, severe

    F11.21 **Opioid dependence, in remission**
    ▶Opioid use disorder, moderate, in early remission
    ▶Opioid use disorder, moderate, in sustained remission
    ▶Opioid use disorder, severe, in early remission
    ▶Opioid use disorder, severe, in sustained remission

▶ New   ⇒ Revised   ~~deleted~~ Deleted   **OGCR** Official Guidelines   X Assign placeholder X   ● Use Additional Character(s)

Excludes 1   Excludes 2   Includes   Use additional   Code first   Code also   Key words

● F11.22   Opioid dependence with intoxication
    Excludes1   opioid dependence with
                    withdrawal (F11.23)
    F11.220   Opioid dependence with intoxication,
                uncomplicated
    F11.221   Opioid dependence with intoxication
                delirium
    F11.222   Opioid dependence with intoxication
                with perceptual disturbance
    F11.229   Opioid dependence with
                intoxication, unspecified
F11.23   Opioid dependence with withdrawal
    Excludes1   opioid dependence with
                    intoxication (F11.22-)
F11.24   Opioid dependence with opioid-induced mood
            disorder
                Opioid use disorder, moderate, with
                    opioid-induced depressive disorder
● F11.25   Opioid dependence with opioid-induced
            psychotic disorder
    F11.250   Opioid dependence with opioid-
                induced psychotic disorder with
                delusions
    F11.251   Opioid dependence with opioid-
                induced psychotic disorder with
                hallucinations
    F11.259   Opioid dependence with opioid-
                induced psychotic disorder,
                unspecified
● F11.28   Opioid dependence with other opioid-induced
            disorder
    F11.281   Opioid dependence with opioid-
                induced sexual dysfunction
    F11.282   Opioid dependence with opioid-
                induced sleep disorder
    F11.288   Opioid dependence with other
                opioid-induced disorder
F11.29   Opioid dependence with unspecified opioid-
            induced disorder
● F11.9   Opioid use, unspecified
    Excludes1   opioid abuse (F11.1-)
                    opioid dependence (F11.2-)
F11.90   Opioid use, unspecified, uncomplicated
● F11.92   Opioid use, unspecified with intoxication
    Excludes1   opioid use, unspecified with
                    withdrawal (F11.93)
    F11.920   Opioid use, unspecified with
                intoxication, uncomplicated
    F11.921   Opioid use, unspecified with
                intoxication delirium
                    Opioid-induced delirium
    F11.922   Opioid use, unspecified with
                intoxication with perceptual
                disturbance
    F11.929   Opioid use, unspecified with
                intoxication, unspecified
F11.93   Opioid use, unspecified with withdrawal
    Excludes1   opioid use, unspecified with
                    intoxication (F11.92-)
F11.94   Opioid use, unspecified with opioid-induced
            mood disorder
                Opioid-induced depressive disorder, without
                    use disorder

● F11.95   Opioid use, unspecified with opioid-induced
            psychotic disorder
    F11.950   Opioid use, unspecified with opioid-
                induced psychotic disorder with
                delusions
    F11.951   Opioid use, unspecified with opioid-
                induced psychotic disorder with
                hallucinations
    F11.959   Opioid use, unspecified with
                opioid-induced psychotic disorder,
                unspecified
● F11.98   Opioid use, unspecified with other specified
            opioid-induced disorder
    F11.981   Opioid use, unspecified with opioid-
                induced sexual dysfunction
                    Opioid-induced sexual dysfunction,
                        without use disorder
    F11.982   Opioid use, unspecified with opioid-
                induced sleep disorder
                    Opioid-induced sleep disorder,
                        without use disorder
    F11.988   Opioid use, unspecified with other
                opioid-induced disorder
                    Opioid-induced anxiety disorder,
                        without use disorder
F11.99   Opioid use, unspecified with unspecified
            opioid-induced disorder
● F12   Cannabis related disorders
    Includes   marijuana
● F12.1   Cannabis abuse
    Excludes1   cannabis dependence (F12.2-)
                    cannabis use, unspecified (F12.9-)
    F12.10   Cannabis abuse, uncomplicated
                    Cannabis use disorder, mild
    ▶ F12.11   Cannabis abuse, in remission
                ▶Cannabis use disorder, mild, in early remission
                ▶Cannabis use disorder, mild, in sustained
                    remission
● F12.12   Cannabis abuse with intoxication
    F12.120   Cannabis abuse with intoxication,
                uncomplicated
    F12.121   Cannabis abuse with intoxication
                delirium
    F12.122   Cannabis abuse with intoxication
                with perceptual disturbance
    F12.129   Cannabis abuse with
                intoxication, unspecified
● F12.15   Cannabis abuse with psychotic disorder
    F12.150   Cannabis abuse with psychotic
                disorder with delusions
    F12.151   Cannabis abuse with psychotic
                disorder with hallucinations
    F12.159   Cannabis abuse with psychotic
                disorder, unspecified
● F12.18   Cannabis abuse with other cannabis-induced
            disorder
    F12.180   Cannabis abuse with cannabis-
                induced anxiety disorder
    F12.188   Cannabis abuse with other cannabis-
                induced disorder
                    Cannabis use disorder, mild,
                        with cannabis-induced sleep
                        disorder
F12.19   Cannabis abuse with unspecified cannabis-
            induced disorder

CHAPTER 5 (F01-F99)

● **F12.2 Cannabis dependence**

> **Excludes1**   cannabis abuse (F12.1-)
>   cannabis use, unspecified (F12.9-)
>
> **Excludes2**   cannabis poisoning (T40.7-)

    F12.20   **Cannabis dependence, uncomplicated**
              Cannabis use disorder, moderate
              Cannabis use disorder, severe

    F12.21   **Cannabis dependence, in remission**
        ▶Cannabis use disorder, moderate, in early remission
        ▶Cannabis use disorder, moderate, in sustained remission
        ▶Cannabis use disorder, severe, in early remission
        ▶Cannabis use disorder, severe, in sustained remission

   ● F12.22   **Cannabis dependence with intoxication**

      F12.220   **Cannabis dependence with intoxication, uncomplicated**

      F12.221   **Cannabis dependence with intoxication delirium**

      F12.222   **Cannabis dependence with intoxication with perceptual disturbance**

      F12.229   **Cannabis dependence with intoxication, unspecified**

   ● F12.25   **Cannabis dependence with psychotic disorder**

      F12.250   **Cannabis dependence with psychotic disorder with delusions**

      F12.251   **Cannabis dependence with psychotic disorder with hallucinations**

      F12.259   **Cannabis dependence with psychotic disorder, unspecified**

   ● F12.28   **Cannabis dependence with other cannabis-induced disorder**

      F12.280   **Cannabis dependence with cannabis-induced anxiety disorder**

      F12.288   **Cannabis dependence with other cannabis-induced disorder**
                Cannabis use disorder, moderate, with cannabis-induced sleep disorder
                Cannabis use disorder, severe, with cannabis-induced sleep disorder
                Cannabis withdrawal

    F12.29   **Cannabis dependence with unspecified cannabis-induced disorder**

● **F12.9 Cannabis use, unspecified**

> **Excludes1**   cannabis abuse (F12.1-)
>   cannabis dependence (F12.2-)

    F12.90   **Cannabis use, unspecified, uncomplicated**

   ● F12.92   **Cannabis use, unspecified with intoxication**

      F12.920   **Cannabis use, unspecified with intoxication, uncomplicated**

      F12.921   **Cannabis use, unspecified with intoxication delirium**

      F12.922   **Cannabis use, unspecified with intoxication with perceptual disturbance**

      F12.929   **Cannabis use, unspecified with intoxication, unspecified**

   ● F12.95   **Cannabis use, unspecified with psychotic disorder**

      F12.950   **Cannabis use, unspecified with psychotic disorder with delusions**

      F12.951   **Cannabis use, unspecified with psychotic disorder with hallucinations**

      F12.959   **Cannabis use, unspecified with psychotic disorder, unspecified**
                Cannabis-induced psychotic disorder, without use disorder

   ● F12.98   **Cannabis use, unspecified with other cannabis-induced disorder**

      F12.980   **Cannabis use, unspecified with anxiety disorder**
                Cannabis-induced anxiety disorder, without use disorder

      F12.988   **Cannabis use, unspecified with other cannabis-induced disorder**
                Cannabis-induced sleep disorder, without use disorder

    F12.99   **Cannabis use, unspecified with unspecified cannabis-induced disorder**

● **F13 Sedative, hypnotic, or anxiolytic related disorders**

   ● **F13.1 Sedative, hypnotic or anxiolytic-related abuse**

> **Excludes1**   sedative, hypnotic or anxiolytic-related dependence (F13.2-)
>   sedative, hypnotic, or anxiolytic use, unspecified (F13.9-)

    F13.10   **Sedative, hypnotic or anxiolytic abuse, uncomplicated**
              Sedative, hypnotic, or anxiolytic use disorder, mild

  ▶ F13.11   **Sedative, hypnotic or anxiolytic abuse, in remission**
        ▶Sedative, hypnotic or anxiolytic use disorder, mild, in early remission
        ▶Sedative, hypnotic or anxiolytic use disorder, mild, in sustained remission

   ● F13.12   **Sedative, hypnotic or anxiolytic abuse with intoxication**

      F13.120   **Sedative, hypnotic or anxiolytic abuse with intoxication, uncomplicated**

      F13.121   **Sedative, hypnotic or anxiolytic abuse with intoxication delirium**

      F13.129   **Sedative, hypnotic or anxiolytic abuse with intoxication, unspecified**

    F13.14   **Sedative, hypnotic or anxiolytic abuse with sedative, hypnotic or anxiolytic-induced mood disorder**
        ⇒Sedative, hypnotic, or anxiolytic use disorder, mild, with sedative, hypnotic, or anxiolytic-induced bipolar or related disorder
        ⇒Sedative, hypnotic, or anxiolytic use disorder, mild, with sedative, hypnotic, or anxiolytic-induced depressive disorder

   ● F13.15   **Sedative, hypnotic or anxiolytic abuse with sedative, hypnotic or anxiolytic-induced psychotic disorder**

      F13.150   **Sedative, hypnotic or anxiolytic abuse with sedative, hypnotic or anxiolytic-induced psychotic disorder with delusions**

      F13.151   **Sedative, hypnotic or anxiolytic abuse with sedative, hypnotic or anxiolytic-induced psychotic disorder with hallucinations**

      F13.159   **Sedative, hypnotic or anxiolytic abuse with sedative, hypnotic or anxiolytic-induced psychotic disorder, unspecified**

   ● F13.18   **Sedative, hypnotic or anxiolytic abuse with other sedative, hypnotic or anxiolytic-induced disorders**

      F13.180   **Sedative, hypnotic or anxiolytic abuse with sedative, hypnotic or anxiolytic-induced anxiety disorder**

      F13.181   **Sedative, hypnotic or anxiolytic abuse with sedative, hypnotic or anxiolytic-induced sexual dysfunction**

F13.182   Sedative, hypnotic or anxiolytic abuse with sedative, hypnotic or anxiolytic-induced sleep disorder

F13.188   Sedative, hypnotic or anxiolytic abuse with other sedative, hypnotic or anxiolytic-induced disorder

F13.19   Sedative, hypnotic or anxiolytic abuse with unspecified sedative, hypnotic or anxiolytic-induced disorder

● **F13.2   Sedative, hypnotic or anxiolytic-related dependence**

Excludes1   sedative, hypnotic or anxiolytic-related abuse (F13.1-)
sedative, hypnotic, or anxiolytic use, unspecified (F13.9-)

Excludes2   sedative, hypnotic, or anxiolytic poisoning (T42.-)

F13.20   Sedative, hypnotic or anxiolytic dependence, uncomplicated

F13.21   Sedative, hypnotic or anxiolytic dependence, in remission
▶Sedative, hypnotic or anxiolytic use disorder, moderate, in early remission
▶Sedative, hypnotic or anxiolytic use disorder, moderate, in sustained remission
▶Sedative, hypnotic or anxiolytic use disorder, severe, in early remission
▶Sedative, hypnotic or anxiolytic use disorder, severe, in sustained remission

● F13.22   Sedative, hypnotic or anxiolytic dependence with intoxication

Excludes1   sedative, hypnotic or anxiolytic dependence with withdrawal (F13.23-)

F13.220   Sedative, hypnotic or anxiolytic dependence with intoxication, uncomplicated

F13.221   Sedative, hypnotic or anxiolytic dependence with intoxication delirium

F13.229   Sedative, hypnotic or anxiolytic dependence with intoxication, unspecified

● F13.23   Sedative, hypnotic or anxiolytic dependence with withdrawal
Sedative, hypnotic, or anxiolytic use disorder, moderate
Sedative, hypnotic, or anxiolytic use disorder, severe

Excludes1   sedative, hypnotic or anxiolytic dependence with intoxication (F13.22-)

F13.230   Sedative, hypnotic or anxiolytic dependence with withdrawal, uncomplicated

F13.231   Sedative, hypnotic or anxiolytic dependence with withdrawal delirium

F13.232   Sedative, hypnotic or anxiolytic dependence with withdrawal with perceptual disturbance
Sedative, hypnotic, or anxiolytic withdrawal with perceptual disturbances

F13.239   Sedative, hypnotic or anxiolytic dependence with withdrawal, unspecified
Sedative, hypnotic, or anxiolytic withdrawal without perceptual disturbances

F13.24   Sedative, hypnotic or anxiolytic dependence with sedative, hypnotic or anxiolytic-induced mood disorder
➠Sedative, hypnotic, or anxiolytic use disorder, moderate, with sedative, hypnotic, or anxiolytic-induced bipolar or related disorder
➠Sedative, hypnotic, or anxiolytic use disorder, moderate, with sedative, hypnotic, or anxiolytic-induced depressive disorder
Sedative, hypnotic, or anxiolytic use disorder, severe, with sedative, hypnotic, or anxiolytic-induced bipolar or related disorder
➠Sedative, hypnotic, or anxiolytic use disorder, severe, with sedative, hypnotic, or anxiolytic-induced depressive disorder

● F13.25   Sedative, hypnotic or anxiolytic dependence with sedative, hypnotic or anxiolytic-induced psychotic disorder

F13.250   Sedative, hypnotic or anxiolytic dependence with sedative, hypnotic or anxiolytic-induced psychotic disorder with delusions

F13.251   Sedative, hypnotic or anxiolytic dependence with sedative, hypnotic or anxiolytic-induced psychotic disorder with hallucinations

F13.259   Sedative, hypnotic or anxiolytic dependence with sedative, hypnotic or anxiolytic-induced psychotic disorder, unspecified

F13.26   Sedative, hypnotic or anxiolytic dependence with sedative, hypnotic or anxiolytic-induced persisting amnestic disorder

F13.27   Sedative, hypnotic or anxiolytic dependence with sedative, hypnotic or anxiolytic-induced persisting dementia
➠Sedative, hypnotic, or anxiolytic use disorder, moderate, with sedative, hypnotic, or anxiolytic-induced major neurocognitive disorder
Sedative, hypnotic, or anxiolytic use disorder, severe, with sedative, hypnotic, or anxiolytic-induced major neurocognitive disorder

● F13.28   Sedative, hypnotic or anxiolytic dependence with other sedative, hypnotic or anxiolytic-induced disorders

F13.280   Sedative, hypnotic or anxiolytic dependence with sedative, hypnotic or anxiolytic-induced anxiety disorder

F13.281   Sedative, hypnotic or anxiolytic dependence with sedative, hypnotic or anxiolytic-induced sexual dysfunction

F13.282   Sedative, hypnotic or anxiolytic dependence with sedative, hypnotic or anxiolytic-induced sleep disorder

F13.288   Sedative, hypnotic or anxiolytic dependence with other sedative, hypnotic or anxiolytic-induced disorder
➠Sedative, hypnotic, or anxiolytic use disorder, moderate, with sedative, hypnotic, or anxiolytic-induced mild neurocognitive disorder
➠Sedative, hypnotic, or anxiolytic use disorder, severe, with sedative, hypnotic, or anxiolytic-induced mild neurocognitive disorder

F13.29   Sedative, hypnotic or anxiolytic dependence with unspecified sedative, hypnotic or anxiolytic-induced disorder

● F13.9　Sedative, hypnotic or anxiolytic-related use, unspecified

　　Excludes1　sedative, hypnotic or anxiolytic-related abuse (F13.1-)
　　　　　　　sedative, hypnotic or anxiolytic-related dependence (F13.2-)

　F13.90　Sedative, hypnotic, or anxiolytic use, unspecified, uncomplicated

● F13.92　Sedative, hypnotic or anxiolytic use, unspecified with intoxication

　　Excludes1　sedative, hypnotic or anxiolytic use, unspecified with withdrawal (F13.93-)

　F13.920　Sedative, hypnotic or anxiolytic use, unspecified with intoxication, uncomplicated

　F13.921　Sedative, hypnotic or anxiolytic use, unspecified with intoxication delirium
　　　　　Sedative, hypnotic, or anxiolytic-induced delirium

　F13.929　Sedative, hypnotic or anxiolytic use, unspecified with intoxication, unspecified

● F13.93　Sedative, hypnotic or anxiolytic use, unspecified with withdrawal

　　Excludes1　sedative, hypnotic or anxiolytic use, unspecified with intoxication (F13.92-)

　F13.930　Sedative, hypnotic or anxiolytic use, unspecified with withdrawal, uncomplicated

　F13.931　Sedative, hypnotic or anxiolytic use, unspecified with withdrawal delirium

　F13.932　Sedative, hypnotic or anxiolytic use, unspecified with withdrawal with perceptual disturbances

　F13.939　Sedative, hypnotic or anxiolytic use, unspecified with withdrawal, unspecified

　F13.94　Sedative, hypnotic or anxiolytic use, unspecified with sedative, hypnotic or anxiolytic-induced mood disorder
　　　　Sedative, hypnotic, or anxiolytic-induced bipolar or related disorder, without use disorder
　　　　Sedative, hypnotic, or anxiolytic-induced depressive disorder, without use disorder

● F13.95　Sedative, hypnotic or anxiolytic use, unspecified with sedative, hypnotic or anxiolytic-induced psychotic disorder

　F13.950　Sedative, hypnotic or anxiolytic use, unspecified with sedative, hypnotic or anxiolytic-induced psychotic disorder with delusions

　F13.951　Sedative, hypnotic or anxiolytic use, unspecified with sedative, hypnotic or anxiolytic-induced psychotic disorder with hallucinations

　F13.959　Sedative, hypnotic or anxiolytic use, unspecified with sedative, hypnotic or anxiolytic-induced psychotic disorder, unspecified
　　　　➠Sedative, hypnotic, or anxiolytic-induced psychotic disorder, without use disorder

　F13.96　Sedative, hypnotic or anxiolytic use, unspecified with sedative, hypnotic or anxiolytic-induced persisting amnestic disorder

　F13.97　Sedative, hypnotic or anxiolytic use, unspecified with sedative, hypnotic or anxiolytic-induced persisting dementia
　　　　➠Sedative, hypnotic, or anxiolytic-induced major neurocognitive disorder, without use disorder

● F13.98　Sedative, hypnotic or anxiolytic use, unspecified with other sedative, hypnotic or anxiolytic-induced disorders

　F13.980　Sedative, hypnotic or anxiolytic use, unspecified with sedative, hypnotic or anxiolytic-induced anxiety disorder
　　　　➠Sedative, hypnotic, or anxiolytic-induced anxiety disorder, without use disorder

　F13.981　Sedative, hypnotic or anxiolytic use, unspecified with sedative, hypnotic or anxiolytic-induced sexual dysfunction
　　　　➠Sedative, hypnotic, or anxiolytic-induced sexual dysfunction disorder, without use disorder

　F13.982　Sedative, hypnotic or anxiolytic use, unspecified with sedative, hypnotic or anxiolytic-induced sleep disorder
　　　　➠Sedative, hypnotic, or anxiolytic-induced sleep disorder, without use disorder

　F13.988　Sedative, hypnotic or anxiolytic use, unspecified with other sedative, hypnotic or anxiolytic-induced disorder
　　　　➠Sedative, hypnotic, or anxiolytic-induced mild neurocognitive disorder

　F13.99　Sedative, hypnotic or anxiolytic use, unspecified with unspecified sedative, hypnotic or anxiolytic-induced disorder

● F14　Cocaine related disorders

　　Excludes2　other stimulant-related disorders (F15.-)

● F14.1　Cocaine abuse

　　Excludes1　cocaine dependence (F14.2-)
　　　　　　　cocaine use, unspecified (F14.9-)

　F14.10　Cocaine abuse, uncomplicated
　　　　Cocaine use disorder, mild

▶ F14.11　Cocaine abuse, in remission
　　　　▶Cocaine use disorder, mild, in early remission
　　　　▶Cocaine use disorder, mild, in sustained remission

● F14.12　Cocaine abuse with intoxication

　F14.120　Cocaine abuse with intoxication, uncomplicated

　F14.121　Cocaine abuse with intoxication with delirium

　F14.122　Cocaine abuse with intoxication with perceptual disturbance

　F14.129　Cocaine abuse with intoxication, unspecified

　F14.14　Cocaine abuse with cocaine-induced mood disorder
　　　　Cocaine use disorder, mild, with cocaine-induced bipolar or related disorder
　　　　Cocaine use disorder, mild, with cocaine-induced depressive disorder

● F14.15　Cocaine abuse with cocaine-induced psychotic disorder

　F14.150　Cocaine abuse with cocaine-induced psychotic disorder with delusions

　F14.151　Cocaine abuse with cocaine-induced psychotic disorder with hallucinations

　F14.159　Cocaine abuse with cocaine-induced psychotic disorder, unspecified

▶ New　　➠ Revised　　d̶e̶l̶e̶t̶e̶d̶ Deleted　　OGCR Official Guidelines　　X Assign placeholder X　　● Use Additional Character(s)

Excludes 1　　Excludes 2　　Includes　　Use additional　　Code first　　Code also　　Key words

● **F14.18**   Cocaine abuse with other cocaine-induced disorder

    F14.180   Cocaine abuse with cocaine-induced anxiety disorder

    F14.181   Cocaine abuse with cocaine-induced sexual dysfunction

    F14.182   Cocaine abuse with cocaine-induced sleep disorder

    F14.188   Cocaine abuse with other cocaine-induced disorder

       Cocaine use disorder, mild, with cocaine-induced obsessive-compulsive or related disorder

   F14.19   Cocaine abuse with unspecified cocaine-induced disorder

● **F14.2**   Cocaine dependence

   Excludes1   cocaine abuse (F14.1-)

              cocaine use, unspecified (F14.9-)

   Excludes2   cocaine poisoning (T40.5-)

   F14.20   Cocaine dependence, uncomplicated

       Cocaine use disorder, moderate

       Cocaine use disorder, severe

   F14.21   Cocaine dependence, in remission

     ▶Cocaine use disorder, moderate, in early remission

     ▶Cocaine use disorder, moderate, in sustained remission

     ▶Cocaine use disorder, severe, in early remission

     ▶Cocaine use disorder, severe, in sustained remission

● **F14.22**   Cocaine dependence with intoxication

    Excludes1   cocaine dependence with withdrawal (F14.23)

    F14.220   Cocaine dependence with intoxication, uncomplicated

    F14.221   Cocaine dependence with intoxication delirium

    F14.222   Cocaine dependence with intoxication with perceptual disturbance

    F14.229   Cocaine dependence with intoxication, unspecified

   F14.23   Cocaine dependence with withdrawal

    Excludes1   cocaine dependence with intoxication (F14.22-)

   F14.24   Cocaine dependence with cocaine-induced mood disorder

       Cocaine use disorder, moderate, with cocaine-induced bipolar or related disorder

       Cocaine use disorder, moderate, with cocaine-induced depressive disorder

       Cocaine use disorder, severe, with cocaine-induced bipolar or related disorder

       Cocaine use disorder, severe, with cocaine-induced depressive disorder

● **F14.25**   Cocaine dependence with cocaine-induced psychotic disorder

    F14.250   Cocaine dependence with cocaine-induced psychotic disorder with delusions

    F14.251   Cocaine dependence with cocaine-induced psychotic disorder with hallucinations

    F14.259   Cocaine dependence with cocaine-induced psychotic disorder, unspecified

● **F14.28**   Cocaine dependence with other cocaine-induced disorder

    F14.280   Cocaine dependence with cocaine-induced anxiety disorder

    F14.281   Cocaine dependence with cocaine-induced sexual dysfunction

    F14.282   Cocaine dependence with cocaine-induced sleep disorder

    F14.288   Cocaine dependence with other cocaine-induced disorder

       Cocaine use disorder, moderate, with cocaine-induced obsessive-compulsive or related disorder

       Cocaine use disorder, severe, with cocaine-induced obsessive-compulsive or related disorder

   F14.29   Cocaine dependence with unspecified cocaine-induced disorder

● **F14.9**   Cocaine use, unspecified

   Excludes1   cocaine abuse (F14.1-)

              cocaine dependence (F14.2-)

   F14.90   Cocaine use, unspecified, uncomplicated

● **F14.92**   Cocaine use, unspecified with intoxication

    F14.920   Cocaine use, unspecified with intoxication, uncomplicated

    F14.921   Cocaine use, unspecified with intoxication delirium

    F14.922   Cocaine use, unspecified with intoxication with perceptual disturbance

    F14.929   Cocaine use, unspecified with intoxication, unspecified

   F14.94   Cocaine use, unspecified with cocaine-induced mood disorder

       Cocaine-induced bipolar or related disorder, without use disorder

       Cocaine-induced depressive disorder, without use disorder

● **F14.95**   Cocaine use, unspecified with cocaine-induced psychotic disorder

    F14.950   Cocaine use, unspecified with cocaine-induced psychotic disorder with delusions

    F14.951   Cocaine use, unspecified with cocaine-induced psychotic disorder with hallucinations

    F14.959   Cocaine use, unspecified with cocaine-induced psychotic disorder, unspecified

       Cocaine-induced psychotic disorder, without use disorder

● **F14.98**   Cocaine use, unspecified with other specified cocaine-induced disorder

    F14.980   Cocaine use, unspecified with cocaine-induced anxiety disorder

       Cocaine-induced anxiety disorder, without use disorder

    F14.981   Cocaine use, unspecified with cocaine-induced sexual dysfunction

       Cocaine-induced sexual dysfunction, without use disorder

    F14.982   Cocaine use, unspecified with cocaine-induced sleep disorder

       Cocaine-induced sleep disorder, without use disorder

    F14.988   Cocaine use, unspecified with other cocaine-induced disorder

       Cocaine-induced obsessive-compulsive or related disorder

   F14.99   Cocaine use, unspecified with unspecified cocaine-induced disorder

▶ New   ⇒ Revised   ~~deleted~~ Deleted   **OGCR** Official Guidelines   X Assign placeholder X   ● Use Additional Character(s)

   | Excludes 1 | | Excludes 2 | | Includes | | Use additional | | Code first | | Code also | | Key words |

CHAPTER 5 (F01-F99)

● F15   **Other stimulant related disorders**

Includes   amphetamine-related disorders
caffeine

Excludes2   cocaine-related disorders (F14.-)

● F15.1   **Other stimulant abuse**

Excludes1   other stimulant dependence (F15.2-)
other stimulant use, unspecified (F15.9-)

F15.10   **Other stimulant abuse, uncomplicated**
Amphetamine type substance use disorder, mild
Other or unspecified stimulant use disorder, mild

▶F15.11   **Other stimulant abuse, in remission**
▶Amphetamine type substance use disorder, mild, in early remission
▶Amphetamine type substance use disorder, mild, in sustained remission
▶Other or unspecified stimulant use disorder, mild, in early remission
▶Other or unspecified stimulant use disorder, mild, in sustained remission

● F15.12   **Other stimulant abuse with intoxication**

F15.120   **Other stimulant abuse with intoxication, uncomplicated**

F15.121   **Other stimulant abuse with intoxication delirium**

F15.122   **Other stimulant abuse with intoxication with perceptual disturbance**
Amphetamine or other stimulant use disorder, mild, with amphetamine or other stimulant intoxication, with perceptual disturbances

F15.129   **Other stimulant abuse with intoxication, unspecified**
Amphetamine or other stimulant use disorder, mild, with amphetamine or other stimulant intoxication, without perceptual disturbances

F15.14   **Other stimulant abuse with stimulant-induced mood disorder**
Amphetamine or other stimulant use disorder, mild, with amphetamine or other stimulant-induced bipolar or related disorder
Amphetamine or other stimulant use disorder, mild, with amphetamine or other stimulant-induced depressive disorder

● F15.15   **Other stimulant abuse with stimulant-induced psychotic disorder**

F15.150   **Other stimulant abuse with stimulant-induced psychotic disorder with delusions**

F15.151   **Other stimulant abuse with stimulant-induced psychotic disorder with hallucinations**

F15.159   **Other stimulant abuse with stimulant-induced psychotic disorder, unspecified**

● F15.18   **Other stimulant abuse with other stimulant-induced disorder**

F15.180   **Other stimulant abuse with stimulant-induced anxiety disorder**

F15.181   **Other stimulant abuse with stimulant-induced sexual dysfunction**

F15.182   **Other stimulant abuse with stimulant-induced sleep disorder**

F15.188   **Other stimulant abuse with other stimulant-induced disorder**
Amphetamine or other stimulant use disorder, mild, with amphetamine or other stimulant-induced obsessive-compulsive or related disorder

F15.19   **Other stimulant abuse with unspecified stimulant-induced disorder**

● F15.2   **Other stimulant dependence**

Excludes1   other stimulant abuse (F15.1-)
other stimulant use, unspecified (F15.9-)

F15.20   **Other stimulant dependence, uncomplicated**
Amphetamine type substance use disorder, moderate
Amphetamine type substance use disorder, severe
Other or unspecified stimulant use disorder, moderate
Other or unspecified stimulant use disorder, severe

F15.21   **Other stimulant dependence, in remission**
▶Amphetamine type substance use disorder, moderate, in early remission
▶Amphetamine type substance use disorder, moderate, in sustained remission
▶Amphetamine type substance use disorder, severe, in early remission
▶Amphetamine type substance use disorder, severe, in sustained remission
▶Other or unspecified stimulant use disorder, moderate, in early remission
▶Other or unspecified stimulant use disorder, moderate, in sustained remission
▶Other or unspecified stimulant use disorder, severe, in early remission
▶Other or unspecified stimulant use disorder, severe, in sustained remission

● F15.22   **Other stimulant dependence with intoxication**

Excludes1   other stimulant dependence with withdrawal (F15.23)

F15.220   **Other stimulant dependence with intoxication, uncomplicated**

F15.221   **Other stimulant dependence with intoxication delirium**

F15.222   **Other stimulant dependence with intoxication with perceptual disturbance**
Amphetamine or other stimulant use disorder, moderate, with amphetamine or other stimulant intoxication, with perceptual disturbances
Amphetamine or other stimulant use disorder, severe, with amphetamine or other stimulant intoxication, with perceptual disturbances

F15.229   **Other stimulant dependence with intoxication, unspecified**
Amphetamine or other stimulant use disorder, moderate, with amphetamine or other stimulant intoxication, without perceptual disturbances
Amphetamine or other stimulant use disorder, severe, with amphetamine or other stimulant intoxication, without perceptual disturbances

▶ New   ⇒ Revised   ~~deleted~~ Deleted   **OGCR** Official Guidelines   X Assign placeholder X   ● Use Additional Character(s)

Excludes 1   Excludes 2   Includes   Use additional   Code first   Code also   Key words

F15.23   Other stimulant dependence with withdrawal
Amphetamine or other stimulant withdrawal
> **Excludes1**   other stimulant dependence with
> intoxication (F15.22-)

F15.24   Other stimulant dependence with stimulant-induced mood disorder
Amphetamine or other stimulant use disorder, moderate, with amphetamine or other stimulant-induced bipolar or related disorder
Amphetamine or other stimulant use disorder, moderate, with amphetamine or other stimulant-induced depressive disorder
Amphetamine or other stimulant use disorder, severe, with amphetamine or other stimulant-induced bipolar or related disorder
Amphetamine or other stimulant use disorder, severe, with amphetamine or other stimulant-induced depressive disorder

● **F15.25**   Other stimulant dependence with stimulant-induced psychotic disorder

     F15.250   Other stimulant dependence with stimulant-induced psychotic disorder with delusions

     F15.251   Other stimulant dependence with stimulant-induced psychotic disorder with hallucinations

     F15.259   Other stimulant dependence with stimulant-induced psychotic disorder, unspecified

● **F15.28**   Other stimulant dependence with other stimulant-induced disorder

     F15.280   Other stimulant dependence with stimulant-induced anxiety disorder

     F15.281   Other stimulant dependence with stimulant-induced sexual dysfunction

     F15.282   Other stimulant dependence with stimulant-induced sleep disorder

     F15.288   Other stimulant dependence with other stimulant-induced disorder
➡ Amphetamine or other stimulant use disorder, moderate, with amphetamine or other stimulant-induced obsessive-compulsive or related disorder
➡ Amphetamine or other stimulant use disorder, severe, with amphetamine or other stimulant-induced obsessive-compulsive or related disorder

F15.29   Other stimulant dependence with unspecified stimulant-induced disorder

● **F15.9**   Other stimulant use, unspecified
> **Excludes1**   other stimulant abuse (F15.1-)
> other stimulant dependence (F15.2-)

F15.90   Other stimulant use, unspecified, uncomplicated

● **F15.92**   Other stimulant use, unspecified with intoxication
> **Excludes1**   other stimulant use, unspecified
> with withdrawal (F15.93)

     F15.920   Other stimulant use, unspecified with intoxication, uncomplicated

     F15.921   Other stimulant use, unspecified with intoxication delirium
Amphetamine or other stimulant-induced delirium

     F15.922   Other stimulant use, unspecified with intoxication with perceptual disturbance

     F15.929   Other stimulant use, unspecified with intoxication, unspecified
Caffeine intoxication

F15.93   Other stimulant use, unspecified with withdrawal
Caffeine withdrawal
> **Excludes1**   other stimulant use, unspecified
> with intoxication (F15.92-)

F15.94   Other stimulant use, unspecified with stimulant-induced mood disorder
Amphetamine or other stimulant-induced bipolar or related disorder, without use disorder
Amphetamine or other stimulant-induced depressive disorder, without use disorder

● **F15.95**   Other stimulant use, unspecified with stimulant-induced psychotic disorder

     F15.950   Other stimulant use, unspecified with stimulant-induced psychotic disorder with delusions

     F15.951   Other stimulant use, unspecified with stimulant-induced psychotic disorder with hallucinations

     F15.959   Other stimulant use, unspecified with stimulant-induced psychotic disorder, unspecified
➡ Amphetamine or other stimulant-induced psychotic disorder, without use disorder

● **F15.98**   Other stimulant use, unspecified with other stimulant-induced disorder

     F15.980   Other stimulant use, unspecified with stimulant-induced anxiety disorder
Amphetamine or other stimulant-induced anxiety disorder, without use disorder
Caffeine-induced anxiety disorder, without use disorder

     F15.981   Other stimulant use, unspecified with stimulant-induced sexual dysfunction
Amphetamine or other stimulant-induced sexual dysfunction, without use disorder

     F15.982   Other stimulant use, unspecified with stimulant-induced sleep disorder
Amphetamine or other stimulant-induced sleep disorder, without use disorder
Caffeine-induced sleep disorder, without use disorder

     F15.988   Other stimulant use, unspecified with other stimulant-induced disorder
Amphetamine or other stimulant-induced obsessive-compulsive or related disorder, without use disorder

F15.99   Other stimulant use, unspecified with unspecified stimulant-induced disorder

● **F16**   **Hallucinogen related disorders**
> **Includes**   ecstasy
> PCP
> phencyclidine

● **F16.1**   **Hallucinogen abuse**
> **Excludes1**   hallucinogen dependence (F16.2-)
> hallucinogen use, unspecified (F16.9-)

     F16.10   Hallucinogen abuse, uncomplicated
Other hallucinogen use disorder, mild
Phencyclidine use disorder, mild

▶ **F16.11**   Hallucinogen abuse, in remission
▶ Other hallucinogen use disorder, mild, in early remission
▶ Other hallucinogen use disorder, mild, in sustained remission
▶ Phencyclidine use disorder, mild, in early remission
▶ Phencyclidine use disorder, mild, in sustained remission

▶ New   ➡ Revised   ~~deleted~~ Deleted   **OGCR** Official Guidelines   X Assign placeholder X   ● Use Additional Character(s)

| Excludes 1 | Excludes 2 | Includes | Use additional | Code first | Code also | Key words |

● F16.12   Hallucinogen abuse with intoxication
   F16.120   Hallucinogen abuse with intoxication, uncomplicated
   F16.121   Hallucinogen abuse with intoxication with delirium
   F16.122   Hallucinogen abuse with intoxication with perceptual disturbance
   F16.129   Hallucinogen abuse with intoxication, unspecified
F16.14   Hallucinogen abuse with hallucinogen-induced mood disorder
   Other hallucinogen use disorder, mild, with other hallucinogen-induced bipolar or related disorder
   Other hallucinogen use disorder, mild, with other hallucinogen-induced depressive disorder
   Phencyclidine use disorder, mild, with phencyclidine-induced bipolar or related disorder
   Phencyclidine use disorder, mild, with phencyclidine-induced depressive disorder
● F16.15   Hallucinogen abuse with hallucinogen-induced psychotic disorder
   F16.150   Hallucinogen abuse with hallucinogen-induced psychotic disorder with delusions
   F16.151   Hallucinogen abuse with hallucinogen-induced psychotic disorder with hallucinations
   F16.159   Hallucinogen abuse with hallucinogen-induced psychotic disorder, unspecified
● F16.18   Hallucinogen abuse with other hallucinogen-induced disorder
   F16.180   Hallucinogen abuse with hallucinogen-induced anxiety disorder
   F16.183   Hallucinogen abuse with hallucinogen persisting perception disorder (flashbacks)
   F16.188   Hallucinogen abuse with other hallucinogen-induced disorder
F16.19   Hallucinogen abuse with unspecified hallucinogen-induced disorder
● F16.2   Hallucinogen dependence
   Excludes1   hallucinogen abuse (F16.1-)
                 hallucinogen use, unspecified (F16.9-)
F16.20   Hallucinogen dependence, uncomplicated
   Other hallucinogen use disorder, moderate
   Other hallucinogen use disorder, severe
   Phencyclidine use disorder, moderate
   Phencyclidine use disorder, severe
F16.21   Hallucinogen dependence, in remission
   ▶Other hallucinogen use disorder, moderate, in early remission
   ▶Other hallucinogen use disorder, moderate, in sustained remission
   ▶Other hallucinogen use disorder, severe, in early remission
   ▶Other hallucinogen use disorder, severe, in sustained remission
   ▶Phencyclidine use disorder, moderate, in early remission
   ▶Phencyclidine use disorder, moderate, in sustained remission
   ▶Phencyclidine use disorder, severe, in early remission
   ▶Phencyclidine use disorder, severe, in sustained remission

● F16.22   Hallucinogen dependence with intoxication
   F16.220   Hallucinogen dependence with intoxication, uncomplicated
   F16.221   Hallucinogen dependence with intoxication with delirium
   F16.229   Hallucinogen dependence with intoxication, unspecified
F16.24   Hallucinogen dependence with hallucinogen-induced mood disorder
   Other hallucinogen use disorder, moderate, with other hallucinogen-induced bipolar or related disorder
   Other hallucinogen use disorder, moderate, with other hallucinogen-induced depressive disorder
   Other hallucinogen use disorder, severe, with other hallucinogen-induced bipolar or related disorder
   Other hallucinogen use disorder, severe, with other hallucinogen-induced depressive disorder
   Phencyclidine use disorder, moderate, with phencyclidine-induced bipolar or related disorder
   Phencyclidine use disorder, moderate, with phencyclidine-induced depressive disorder
   Phencyclidine use disorder, severe, with phencyclidine-induced bipolar or related disorder
   Phencyclidine use disorder, severe, with phencyclidine-induced depressive disorder
● F16.25   Hallucinogen dependence with hallucinogen-induced psychotic disorder
   F16.250   Hallucinogen dependence with hallucinogen-induced psychotic disorder with delusions
   F16.251   Hallucinogen dependence with hallucinogen-induced psychotic disorder with hallucinations
   F16.259   Hallucinogen dependence with hallucinogen-induced psychotic disorder, unspecified
● F16.28   Hallucinogen dependence with other hallucinogen-induced disorder
   F16.280   Hallucinogen dependence with hallucinogen-induced anxiety disorder
   F16.283   Hallucinogen dependence with hallucinogen persisting perception disorder (flashbacks)
   F16.288   Hallucinogen dependence with other hallucinogen-induced disorder
F16.29   Hallucinogen dependence with unspecified hallucinogen-induced disorder
● F16.9   Hallucinogen use, unspecified
   Excludes1   hallucinogen abuse (F16.1-)
                 hallucinogen dependence (F16.2-)
F16.90   Hallucinogen use, unspecified, uncomplicated
● F16.92   Hallucinogen use, unspecified with intoxication
   F16.920   Hallucinogen use, unspecified with intoxication, uncomplicated
   F16.921   Hallucinogen use, unspecified with intoxication with delirium
             Other hallucinogen intoxication delirium
   F16.929   Hallucinogen use, unspecified with intoxication, unspecified

CHAPTER 5 (F01-F99)

▶ New   ⇒ Revised   deleted Deleted   OGCR Official Guidelines   X Assign placeholder X   ● Use Additional Character(s)
Excludes 1   Excludes 2   Includes   Use additional   Code first   Code also   Key words

F16.94　Hallucinogen use, unspecified with hallucinogen-induced mood disorder
　　　　Other hallucinogen-induced bipolar or related disorder, without use disorder
　　　　Other hallucinogen-induced depressive disorder, without use disorder
　　　　Phencyclidine-induced bipolar or related disorder, without use disorder
　　　　Phencyclidine-induced depressive disorder, without use disorder

● F16.95　Hallucinogen use, unspecified with hallucinogen-induced psychotic disorder
　　F16.950　Hallucinogen use, unspecified with hallucinogen-induced psychotic disorder with delusions
　　F16.951　Hallucinogen use, unspecified with hallucinogen-induced psychotic disorder with hallucinations
　　F16.959　Hallucinogen use, unspecified with hallucinogen-induced psychotic disorder, unspecified
　　　　Other hallucinogen-induced psychotic disorder, without use disorder
　　　　Phencyclidine-induced psychotic disorder, without use disorder

● F16.98　Hallucinogen use, unspecified with other specified hallucinogen-induced disorder
　　F16.980　Hallucinogen use, unspecified with hallucinogen-induced anxiety disorder
　　　　Other hallucinogen-induced anxiety disorder, without use disorder
　　　　Phencyclidine-induced anxiety disorder, without use disorder
　　F16.983　Hallucinogen use, unspecified with hallucinogen persisting perception disorder (flashbacks)
　　F16.988　Hallucinogen use, unspecified with other hallucinogen-induced disorder

F16.99　Hallucinogen use, unspecified with unspecified hallucinogen-induced disorder

● F17　Nicotine dependence
　　Excludes1　history of tobacco dependence (Z87.891)
　　　　tobacco use NOS (Z72.0)
　　Excludes2　tobacco use (smoking) during pregnancy, childbirth and the puerperium (O99.33-)
　　　　toxic effect of nicotine (T65.2-)

● F17.2　Nicotine dependence
　● F17.20　Nicotine dependence, unspecified
　　F17.200　Nicotine dependence, unspecified, uncomplicated
　　　　Tobacco use disorder, mild
　　　　Tobacco use disorder, moderate
　　　　Tobacco use disorder, severe
　　F17.201　Nicotine dependence, unspecified, in remission
　　　▶Tobacco use disorder, mild, in early remission
　　　▶Tobacco use disorder, mild, in sustained remission
　　　▶Tobacco use disorder, moderate, in early remission
　　　▶Tobacco use disorder, moderate, in sustained remission
　　　▶Tobacco use disorder, severe, in early remission
　　　▶Tobacco use disorder, severe, in sustained remission

F17.203　Nicotine dependence unspecified, with withdrawal
　　　Tobacco withdrawal
F17.208　Nicotine dependence, unspecified, with other nicotine-induced disorders
F17.209　Nicotine dependence, unspecified, with unspecified nicotine-induced disorders

● F17.21　Nicotine dependence, cigarettes
　　F17.210　Nicotine dependence, cigarettes, uncomplicated
　　F17.211　Nicotine dependence, cigarettes, in remission
　　　▶Tobacco use disorder, cigarettes, mild, in early remission
　　　▶Tobacco use disorder, cigarettes, mild, in sustained remission
　　　▶Tobacco use disorder, cigarettes, moderate, in early remission
　　　▶Tobacco use disorder, cigarettes, moderate, in sustained remission
　　　▶Tobacco use disorder, cigarettes, severe, in early remission
　　　▶Tobacco use disorder, cigarettes, severe, in sustained remission
　　F17.213　Nicotine dependence, cigarettes, with withdrawal
　　F17.218　Nicotine dependence, cigarettes, with other nicotine-induced disorders
　　F17.219　Nicotine dependence, cigarettes, with unspecified nicotine-induced disorders

● F17.22　Nicotine dependence, chewing tobacco
　　F17.220　Nicotine dependence, chewing tobacco, uncomplicated
　　F17.221　Nicotine dependence, chewing tobacco, in remission
　　　▶Tobacco use disorder, chewing tobacco, mild, in early remission
　　　▶Tobacco use disorder, chewing tobacco, mild, in sustained remission
　　　▶Tobacco use disorder, chewing tobacco, moderate, in early remission
　　　▶Tobacco use disorder, chewing tobacco, moderate, in sustained remission
　　　▶Tobacco use disorder, chewing tobacco, severe, in early remission
　　　▶Tobacco use disorder, chewing tobacco, severe, in sustained remission
　　F17.223　Nicotine dependence, chewing tobacco, with withdrawal
　　F17.228　Nicotine dependence, chewing tobacco, with other nicotine-induced disorders
　　F17.229　Nicotine dependence, chewing tobacco, with unspecified nicotine-induced disorders

CHAPTER 5 (F01-F99)

▶ New　⇒ Revised　~~deleted~~ Deleted　OGCR Official Guidelines　X Assign placeholder X　● Use Additional Character(s)

Excludes 1　Excludes 2　Includes　Use additional·　Code first　Code also　Key words

● F17.29   Nicotine dependence, other tobacco product

F17.290   Nicotine dependence, other tobacco product, uncomplicated

F17.291   Nicotine dependence, other tobacco product, in remission
▶ Tobacco use disorder, other tobacco product, mild, in early remission
▶ Tobacco use disorder, other tobacco product, mild, in sustained remission
▶ Tobacco use disorder, other tobacco product, moderate, in early remission
▶ Tobacco use disorder, other tobacco product, moderate, in sustained remission
▶ Tobacco use disorder, other tobacco product, severe, in early remission
▶ Tobacco use disorder, other tobacco product, severe, in sustained remission

F17.293   Nicotine dependence, other tobacco product, with withdrawal

F17.298   Nicotine dependence, other tobacco product, with other nicotine-induced disorders

F17.299   Nicotine dependence, other tobacco product, with unspecified nicotine-induced disorders

● F18   Inhalant related disorders
Includes   volatile solvents

● F18.1   Inhalant abuse
Excludes1   inhalant dependence (F18.2-)
inhalant use, unspecified (F18.9-)

F18.10   Inhalant abuse, uncomplicated
Inhalant use disorder, mild

▶ F18.11   Inhalant abuse, in remission
▶ Inhalant use disorder, mild, in early remission
▶ Inhalant use disorder, mild, in sustained remission

● F18.12   Inhalant abuse with intoxication

F18.120   Inhalant abuse with intoxication, uncomplicated

F18.121   Inhalant abuse with intoxication delirium

F18.129   Inhalant abuse with intoxication, unspecified

F18.14   Inhalant abuse with inhalant-induced mood disorder
Inhalant use disorder, mild, with inhalant-induced depressive disorder

● F18.15   Inhalant abuse with inhalant-induced psychotic disorder

F18.150   Inhalant abuse with inhalant-induced psychotic disorder with delusions

F18.151   Inhalant abuse with inhalant-induced psychotic disorder with hallucinations

F18.159   Inhalant abuse with inhalant-induced psychotic disorder, unspecified

F18.17   Inhalant abuse with inhalant-induced dementia
Inhalant use disorder, mild, with inhalant-induced major neurocognitive disorder

● F18.18   Inhalant abuse with other inhalant-induced disorders

F18.180   Inhalant abuse with inhalant-induced anxiety disorder

F18.188   Inhalant abuse with other inhalant-induced disorder
Inhalant use disorder, mild, with inhalant-induced mild neurocognitive disorder

F18.19   Inhalant abuse with unspecified inhalant-induced disorder

● F18.2   Inhalant dependence
Excludes1   inhalant abuse (F18.1-)
inhalant use, unspecified (F18.9-)

F18.20   Inhalant dependence, uncomplicated
Inhalant use disorder, moderate
Inhalant use disorder, severe

F18.21   Inhalant dependence, in remission
▶ Inhalant use disorder, moderate, in early remission
▶ Inhalant use disorder, moderate, in sustained remission
▶ Inhalant use disorder, severe, in early remission
▶ Inhalant use disorder, severe, in sustained remission

● F18.22   Inhalant dependence with intoxication

F18.220   Inhalant dependence with intoxication, uncomplicated

F18.221   Inhalant dependence with intoxication delirium

F18.229   Inhalant dependence with intoxication, unspecified

F18.24   Inhalant dependence with inhalant-induced mood disorder
Inhalant use disorder, moderate, with inhalant-induced depressive disorder
Inhalant use disorder, severe, with inhalant-induced depressive disorder

● F18.25   Inhalant dependence with inhalant-induced psychotic disorder

F18.250   Inhalant dependence with inhalant-induced psychotic disorder with delusions

F18.251   Inhalant dependence with inhalant-induced psychotic disorder with hallucinations

F18.259   Inhalant dependence with inhalant-induced psychotic disorder, unspecified

F18.27   Inhalant dependence with inhalant-induced dementia
Inhalant use disorder, moderate, with inhalant-induced major neurocognitive disorder
Inhalant use disorder, severe, with inhalant-induced major neurocognitive disorder

● F18.28   Inhalant dependence with other inhalant-induced disorders

F18.280   Inhalant dependence with inhalant-induced anxiety disorder

F18.288   Inhalant dependence with other inhalant-induced disorder
Inhalant use disorder, moderate, with inhalant-induced mild neurocognitive disorder
Inhalant use disorder, severe, with inhalant-induced mild neurocognitive disorder

F18.29   Inhalant dependence with unspecified inhalant-induced disorder

▶ New   ⇒ Revised   ~~deleted~~ Deleted   OGCR Official Guidelines   X Assign placeholder X   ● Use Additional Character(s)

Excludes 1   Excludes 2   Includes   Use additional   Code first   Code also   Key words

● **F18.9**   **Inhalant use, unspecified**
> **Excludes1**   inhalant abuse (F18.1-)
> inhalant dependence (F18.2-)

F18.90   Inhalant use, unspecified, uncomplicated

● **F18.92**   Inhalant use, unspecified with intoxication

F18.920   Inhalant use, unspecified with intoxication, uncomplicated

F18.921   Inhalant use, unspecified with intoxication with delirium

F18.929   Inhalant use, unspecified with intoxication, unspecified

F18.94   Inhalant use, unspecified with inhalant-induced mood disorder
> Inhalant-induced depressive disorder

● **F18.95**   Inhalant use, unspecified with inhalant-induced psychotic disorder

F18.950   Inhalant use, unspecified with inhalant-induced psychotic disorder with delusions

F18.951   Inhalant use, unspecified with inhalant-induced psychotic disorder with hallucinations

F18.959   Inhalant use, unspecified with inhalant-induced psychotic disorder, unspecified

F18.97   Inhalant use, unspecified with inhalant-induced persisting dementia
> Inhalant-induced major neurocognitive disorder

● **F18.98**   Inhalant use, unspecified with other inhalant-induced disorders

F18.980   Inhalant use, unspecified with inhalant-induced anxiety disorder

F18.988   Inhalant use, unspecified with other inhalant-induced disorder
> Inhalant-induced mild neurocognitive disorder

F18.99   Inhalant use, unspecified with unspecified inhalant-induced disorder

● **F19**   **Other psychoactive substance related disorders**
> **Includes**   polysubstance drug use (indiscriminate drug use)

● **F19.1**   **Other psychoactive substance abuse**
> **Excludes1**   other psychoactive substance dependence (F19.2-)
> other psychoactive substance use, unspecified (F19.9-)

F19.10   Other psychoactive substance abuse, uncomplicated
> Other (or unknown) substance use disorder, mild

▶ **F19.11**   Other psychoactive substance abuse, in remission
> ▶Other (or unknown) substance use disorder, mild, in early remission
> ▶Other (or unknown) substance use disorder, mild, in sustained remission

● **F19.12**   Other psychoactive substance abuse with intoxication

F19.120   Other psychoactive substance abuse with intoxication, uncomplicated

F19.121   Other psychoactive substance abuse with intoxication delirium

F19.122   Other psychoactive substance abuse with intoxication with perceptual disturbances

F19.129   Other psychoactive substance abuse with intoxication, unspecified

F19.14   Other psychoactive substance abuse with psychoactive substance-induced mood disorder
> Other (or unknown) substance use disorder, mild, with other (or unknown) substance-induced bipolar or related disorder
> Other (or unknown) substance use disorder, mild, with other (or unknown) substance-induced depressive disorder

● **F19.15**   Other psychoactive substance abuse with psychoactive substance-induced psychotic disorder

F19.150   Other psychoactive substance abuse with psychoactive substance-induced psychotic disorder with delusions

F19.151   Other psychoactive substance abuse with psychoactive substance-induced psychotic disorder with hallucinations

F19.159   Other psychoactive substance abuse with psychoactive substance-induced psychotic disorder, unspecified

F19.16   Other psychoactive substance abuse with psychoactive substance-induced persisting amnestic disorder

F19.17   Other psychoactive substance abuse with psychoactive substance-induced persisting dementia
> Other (or unknown) substance use disorder, mild, with other (or unknown) substance-induced major neurocognitive disorder

● **F19.18**   Other psychoactive substance abuse with other psychoactive substance-induced disorders

F19.180   Other psychoactive substance abuse with psychoactive substance-induced anxiety disorder

F19.181   Other psychoactive substance abuse with psychoactive substance-induced sexual dysfunction

F19.182   Other psychoactive substance abuse with psychoactive substance-induced sleep disorder

F19.188   Other psychoactive substance abuse with other psychoactive substance-induced disorder
> Other (or unknown) substance use disorder, mild, with other (or unknown) substance-induced mild neurocognitive disorder
> Other (or unknown) substance use disorder, mild, with other (or unknown) substance-induced obsessive-compulsive or related disorder

F19.19   Other psychoactive substance abuse with unspecified psychoactive substance-induced disorder

● **F19.2**   **Other psychoactive substance dependence**
> **Excludes1**   other psychoactive substance abuse (F19.1-)
> other psychoactive substance use, unspecified (F19.9-)

F19.20   Other psychoactive substance dependence, uncomplicated
> Other (or unknown) substance use disorder, moderate
> Other (or unknown) substance use disorder, severe

F19.21   Other psychoactive substance dependence, in remission
> ▶Other (or unknown) substance use disorder, moderate, in early remission
> ▶Other (or unknown) substance use disorder, moderate, in sustained remission
> ▶Other (or unknown) substance use disorder, severe, in early remission
> ▶Other (or unknown) substance use, severe, in sustained remission

---

▶ New   ⇒ Revised   ~~deleted~~ Deleted   **OGCR** Official Guidelines   X Assign placeholder X   ● Use Additional Character(s)

Excludes 1   Excludes 2   Includes   Use additional   Code first   Code also   Key words

● F19.22   **Other psychoactive substance dependence with intoxication**
> **Excludes1**   other psychoactive substance dependence with withdrawal (F19.23-)

    F19.220   **Other psychoactive substance dependence with intoxication, uncomplicated**

    F19.221   **Other psychoactive substance dependence with intoxication delirium**

    F19.222   **Other psychoactive substance dependence with intoxication with perceptual disturbance**

    F19.229   **Other psychoactive substance dependence with intoxication, unspecified**

● F19.23   **Other psychoactive substance dependence with withdrawal**
> **Excludes1**   other psychoactive substance dependence with intoxication (F19.22-)

    F19.230   **Other psychoactive substance dependence with withdrawal, uncomplicated**

    F19.231   **Other psychoactive substance dependence with withdrawal delirium**

    F19.232   **Other psychoactive substance dependence with withdrawal with perceptual disturbance**

    F19.239   **Other psychoactive substance dependence with withdrawal, unspecified**

   F19.24   **Other psychoactive substance dependence with psychoactive substance-induced mood disorder**
Other (or unknown) substance use disorder, moderate, with other (or unknown) substance-induced bipolar or related disorder
Other (or unknown) substance use disorder, moderate, with other (or unknown) substance-induced depressive disorder
Other (or unknown) substance use disorder, severe, with other (or unknown) substance-induced bipolar or related disorder
Other (or unknown) substance use disorder, severe, with other (or unknown) substance-induced depressive disorder

● F19.25   **Other psychoactive substance dependence with psychoactive substance-induced psychotic disorder**

    F19.250   **Other psychoactive substance dependence with psychoactive substance-induced psychotic disorder with delusions**

    F19.251   **Other psychoactive substance dependence with psychoactive substance-induced psychotic disorder with hallucinations**

    F19.259   **Other psychoactive substance dependence with psychoactive substance-induced psychotic disorder, unspecified**

   F19.26   **Other psychoactive substance dependence with psychoactive substance-induced persisting amnestic disorder**

   F19.27   **Other psychoactive substance dependence with psychoactive substance-induced persisting dementia**
Other (or unknown) substance use disorder, moderate, with other (or unknown) substance-induced major neurocognitive disorder
Other (or unknown) substance use disorder, severe, with other (or unknown) substance-induced major neurocognitive disorder

● F19.28   **Other psychoactive substance dependence with other psychoactive substance-induced disorders**

    F19.280   **Other psychoactive substance dependence with psychoactive substance-induced anxiety disorder**

    F19.281   **Other psychoactive substance dependence with psychoactive substance-induced sexual dysfunction**

    F19.282   **Other psychoactive substance dependence with psychoactive substance-induced sleep disorder**

    F19.288   **Other psychoactive substance dependence with other psychoactive substance-induced disorder**
Other (or unknown) substance use disorder, moderate, with other (or unknown) substance-induced mild neurocognitive disorder
Other (or unknown) substance use disorder, severe, with other (or unknown) substance-induced mild neurocognitive disorder
Other (or unknown) substance use disorder, moderate, with other (or unknown) substance-induced obsessive-compulsive or related disorder
Other (or unknown) substance use disorder, severe, with other (or unknown) substance-induced obsessive-compulsive or related disorder

   F19.29   **Other psychoactive substance dependence with unspecified psychoactive substance-induced disorder**

● F19.9   **Other psychoactive substance use, unspecified**
> **Excludes1**   other psychoactive substance abuse (F19.1-)
>   other psychoactive substance dependence (F19.2-)

    F19.90   **Other psychoactive substance use, unspecified, uncomplicated**

● F19.92   **Other psychoactive substance use, unspecified with intoxication**
> **Excludes1**   other psychoactive substance use, unspecified with withdrawal (F19.93)

    F19.920   **Other psychoactive substance use, unspecified with intoxication, uncomplicated**

    F19.921   **Other psychoactive substance use, unspecified with intoxication with delirium**
Other (or unknown) substance-induced delirium

    F19.922   **Other psychoactive substance use, unspecified with intoxication with perceptual disturbance**

    F19.929   **Other psychoactive substance use, unspecified with intoxication, unspecified**

● **F19.93** **Other psychoactive substance use, unspecified with withdrawal**

> | **Excludes1** | other psychoactive substance use, unspecified with intoxication (F19.92-) |

     F19.930 **Other psychoactive substance use, unspecified with withdrawal, uncomplicated**

     F19.931 **Other psychoactive substance use, unspecified with withdrawal delirium**

     F19.932 **Other psychoactive substance use, unspecified with withdrawal with perceptual disturbance**

     F19.939 **Other psychoactive substance use, unspecified with withdrawal, unspecified**

F19.94 **Other psychoactive substance use, unspecified with psychoactive substance-induced mood disorder**

> Other (or unknown) substance-induced bipolar or related disorder, without use disorder
> Other (or unknown) substance-induced depressive disorder, without use disorder

● **F19.95** **Other psychoactive substance use, unspecified with psychoactive substance-induced psychotic disorder**

     F19.950 **Other psychoactive substance use, unspecified with psychoactive substance-induced psychotic disorder with delusions**

     F19.951 **Other psychoactive substance use, unspecified with psychoactive substance-induced psychotic disorder with hallucinations**

     F19.959 **Other psychoactive substance use, unspecified with psychoactive substance-induced psychotic disorder, unspecified**

> Other or unknown substance-induced psychotic disorder, without use disorder

F19.96 **Other psychoactive substance use, unspecified with psychoactive substance-induced persisting amnestic disorder**

F19.97 **Other psychoactive substance use, unspecified with psychoactive substance-induced persisting dementia**

> Other (or unknown) substance-induced major neurocognitive disorder, without use disorder

● **F19.98** **Other psychoactive substance use, unspecified with other psychoactive substance-induced disorders**

     F19.980 **Other psychoactive substance use, unspecified with psychoactive substance-induced anxiety disorder**

> Other (or unknown) substance-induced anxiety disorder, without use disorder

     F19.981 **Other psychoactive substance use, unspecified with psychoactive substance-induced sexual dysfunction**

> Other (or unknown) substance-induced sexual dysfunction, without use disorder

     F19.982 **Other psychoactive substance use, unspecified with psychoactive substance-induced sleep disorder**

> Other (or unknown) substance-induced sleep disorder, without use disorder

     F19.988 **Other psychoactive substance use, unspecified with other psychoactive substance-induced disorder**

> Other (or unknown) substance-induced mild neurocognitive disorder, without use disorder
> Other (or unknown) substance-induced obsessive-compulsive or related disorder, without use disorder

     F19.99 **Other psychoactive substance use, unspecified with unspecified psychoactive substance-induced disorder**

SCHIZOPHRENIA, SCHIZOTYPAL, DELUSIONAL, AND OTHER NON-MOOD PSYCHOTIC DISORDERS (F20-F29)

● **F20** **Schizophrenia**

> *Personality disorders characterized by multiple mental and behavioral irregularities (may exhibit disorganized thinking, delusions, and auditory hallucinations)*

> | **Excludes1** | brief psychotic disorder (F23) |
> | | cyclic schizophrenia (F25.0) |
> | | mood [affective] disorders with psychotic symptoms (F30.2, F31.2, F31.5, F31.64, F32.3, F33.3) |
> | | schizoaffective disorder (F25.-) |
> | | schizophrenic reaction NOS (F23) |

> | **Excludes2** | schizophrenic reaction in: |
> | | alcoholism (F10.15-, F10.25-, F10.95-) |
> | | brain disease (F06.2) |
> | | epilepsy (F06.2) |
> | | psychoactive drug use (F11-F19 with .15, .25, .95) |
> | | schizotypal disorder (F21) |

F20.0 **Paranoid schizophrenia**

> Paraphrenic schizophrenia

> | **Excludes1** | involutional paranoid state (F22) |
> | | paranoia (F22) |

F20.1 **Disorganized schizophrenia**

> Hebephrenic schizophrenia
> Hebephrenia

F20.2 **Catatonic schizophrenia**

> Schizophrenic catalepsy
> Schizophrenic catatonia
> Schizophrenic flexibilitas cerea

> | **Excludes1** | catatonic stupor (R40.1) |

F20.3 **Undifferentiated schizophrenia**

> Atypical schizophrenia

> | **Excludes1** | acute schizophrenia-like psychotic disorder (F23) |

> | **Excludes2** | post-schizophrenic depression (F32.89) |

F20.5 **Residual schizophrenia**

> Restzustand (schizophrenic)
> Schizophrenic residual state

● **F20.8** **Other schizophrenia**

     F20.81 **Schizophreniform disorder**

> Schizophreniform psychosis NOS

     F20.89 **Other schizophrenia**

> Cenesthopathic schizophrenia
> Simple schizophrenia

F20.9 **Schizophrenia, unspecified**

F21   Schizotypal disorder
Personality disorder characterized by need for social isolation, odd behavior and thinking, and often unconventional beliefs
Borderline schizophrenia
Latent schizophrenia
Latent schizophrenic reaction
Prepsychotic schizophrenia
Prodromal schizophrenia
Pseudoneurotic schizophrenia
Pseudopsychopathic schizophrenia
Schizotypal personality disorder
| Excludes2 | Asperger's syndrome (F84.5) |
schizoid personality disorder (F60.1)

F22   Delusional disorders
Delusional dysmorphophobia
Involutional paranoid state
Paranoia
Paranoia querulans
Paranoid psychosis
Paranoid state
Paraphrenia (late)
Sensitiver Beziehungswahn
| Excludes1 | mood [affective] disorders with psychotic symptoms (F30.2, F31.2, F31.5, F31.64, F32.3, F33.3) |
paranoid schizophrenia (F20.0)
| Excludes2 | paranoid personality disorder (F60.0) |
paranoid psychosis, psychogenic (F23)
paranoid reaction (F23)

F23   Brief psychotic disorder
Paranoid reaction
Psychogenic paranoid psychosis
| Excludes2 | mood [affective] disorders with psychotic symptoms (F30.2, F31.2, F31.5, F31.64, F32.3, F33.3) |

F24   Shared psychotic disorder
Folie à deux
Induced paranoid disorder
Induced psychotic disorder

● **F25   Schizoaffective disorders**
Mental disorder exhibiting major depressive episode, manic episode, or mixed episode occurs with symptoms of schizophrenia, and mood disorder
| Excludes1 | mood [affective] disorders with psychotic symptoms (F30.2, F31.2, F31.5, F31.64, F32.3, F33.3) |
schizophrenia (F20.-)

F25.0   Schizoaffective disorder, bipolar type
Cyclic schizophrenia
Schizoaffective disorder, manic type
Schizoaffective disorder, mixed type
Schizoaffective psychosis, bipolar type
~~Schizophreniform psychosis, manic type~~

F25.1   Schizoaffective disorder, depressive type
Schizoaffective psychosis, depressive type
~~Schizophreniform psychosis, depressive type~~

F25.8   Other schizoaffective disorders

F25.9   Schizoaffective disorder, unspecified
Schizoaffective psychosis NOS

F28   Other psychotic disorder not due to a substance or known physiological condition
Chronic hallucinatory psychosis
▶Other specified schizophrenia spectrum and other psychotic disorder

F29   Unspecified psychosis not due to a substance or known physiological condition
Psychosis NOS
▶Unspecified schizophrenia spectrum and other psychotic disorder
| Excludes1 | mental disorder NOS (F99) |
unspecified mental disorder due to known physiological condition (F09)

MOOD [AFFECTIVE] DISORDERS (F30-F39)

● **F30   Manic episode**
Elevated, expansive, or irritable mood
| Includes | bipolar disorder, single manic episode |
mixed affective episode
| Excludes1 | bipolar disorder (F31.-) |
major depressive disorder, single episode (F32.-)
major depressive disorder, recurrent (F33.-)

● **F30.1   Manic episode without psychotic symptoms**

F30.10   Manic episode without psychotic symptoms, unspecified

F30.11   Manic episode without psychotic symptoms, mild

F30.12   Manic episode without psychotic symptoms, moderate

F30.13   Manic episode, severe, without psychotic symptoms

F30.2   Manic episode, severe with psychotic symptoms
Manic stupor
Mania with mood-congruent psychotic symptoms
Mania with mood-incongruent psychotic symptoms

F30.3   Manic episode in partial remission

F30.4   Manic episode in full remission

F30.8   Other manic episodes
Abnormality of mood resembling mania but less intense
Hypomania

F30.9   Manic episode, unspecified
Mania NOS

● **F31   Bipolar disorder**
Mood disorders with history of manic, mixed, or hypomanic episodes
| Includes | ▶bipolar I disorder |
▶bipolar type I disorder
manic-depressive illness
manic-depressive psychosis
manic-depressive reaction
| Excludes1 | bipolar disorder, single manic episode (F30.-) |
major depressive disorder, single episode (F32.-)
major depressive disorder, recurrent (F33.-)
| Excludes2 | cyclothymia (F34.0) |

F31.0   Bipolar disorder, current episode hypomanic

● **F31.1   Bipolar disorder, current episode manic without psychotic features**

F31.10   Bipolar disorder, current episode manic without psychotic features, unspecified

F31.11   Bipolar disorder, current episode manic without psychotic features, mild

F31.12   Bipolar disorder, current episode manic without psychotic features, moderate

F31.13   Bipolar disorder, current episode manic without psychotic features, severe

F31.2   Bipolar disorder, current episode manic severe with psychotic features
Bipolar disorder, current episode manic with mood-congruent psychotic symptoms
Bipolar disorder, current episode manic with mood-incongruent psychotic symptoms
▶Bipolar I disorder, current or most recent episode manic with psychotic features

▶ New   ⇒ Revised   ~~deleted~~ Deleted   **OGCR** Official Guidelines   X Assign placeholder X   ● Use Additional Character(s)
| Excludes 1 | | Excludes 2 | Includes   Use additional   Code first   Code also   Key words

● F31.3   Bipolar disorder, current episode depressed, mild or moderate severity

    F31.30   Bipolar disorder, current episode depressed, mild or moderate severity, unspecified

    F31.31   Bipolar disorder, current episode depressed, mild

    F31.32   Bipolar disorder, current episode depressed, moderate

F31.4   Bipolar disorder, current episode depressed, severe, without psychotic features

F31.5   Bipolar disorder, current episode depressed, severe, with psychotic features
    Bipolar disorder, current episode depressed with mood-incongruent psychotic symptoms
    Bipolar disorder, current episode depressed with mood-congruent psychotic symptoms
    ▶Bipolar I disorder, current or most recent episode depressed, with psychotic features

● F31.6   Bipolar disorder, current episode mixed

    F31.60   Bipolar disorder, current episode mixed, unspecified

    F31.61   Bipolar disorder, current episode mixed, mild

    F31.62   Bipolar disorder, current episode mixed, moderate

    F31.63   Bipolar disorder, current episode mixed, severe, without psychotic features

    F31.64   Bipolar disorder, current episode mixed, severe, with psychotic features
        Bipolar disorder, current episode mixed with mood-congruent psychotic symptoms
        Bipolar disorder, current episode mixed with mood-incongruent psychotic symptoms

● F31.7   Bipolar disorder, currently in remission

    F31.70   Bipolar disorder, currently in remission, most recent episode unspecified

    F31.71   Bipolar disorder, in partial remission, most recent episode hypomanic

    F31.72   Bipolar disorder, in full remission, most recent episode hypomanic

    F31.73   Bipolar disorder, in partial remission, most recent episode manic

    F31.74   Bipolar disorder, in full remission, most recent episode manic

    F31.75   Bipolar disorder, in partial remission, most recent episode depressed

    F31.76   Bipolar disorder, in full remission, most recent episode depressed

    F31.77   Bipolar disorder, in partial remission, most recent episode mixed

    F31.78   Bipolar disorder, in full remission, most recent episode mixed

● F31.8   Other bipolar disorders

    F31.81   Bipolar II disorder
        ▶Bipolar disorder, type 2

    F31.89   Other bipolar disorder
        Recurrent manic episodes NOS

F31.9   Bipolar disorder, unspecified
    ▶Manic depression

● F32   Major depressive disorder, single episode

    Includes   single episode of agitated depression
             single episode of depressive reaction
             single episode of major depression
             single episode of psychogenic depression
             single episode of reactive depression
             single episode of vital depression

    Excludes1   bipolar disorder (F31.-)
             manic episode (F30.-)
             recurrent depressive disorder (F33.-)

    Excludes2   adjustment disorder (F43.2)

F32.0   Major depressive disorder, single episode, mild

F32.1   Major depressive disorder, single episode, moderate

F32.2   Major depressive disorder, single episode, severe without psychotic features

F32.3   Major depressive disorder, single episode, severe with psychotic features
    Single episode of major depression with mood-congruent psychotic symptoms
    Single episode of major depression with mood-incongruent psychotic symptoms
    Single episode of major depression with psychotic symptoms
    Single episode of psychogenic depressive psychosis
    Single episode of psychotic depression
    Single episode of reactive depressive psychosis

F32.4   Major depressive disorder, single episode, in partial remission

F32.5   Major depressive disorder, single episode, in full remission

● F32.8   Other depressive episodes

    F32.81   Premenstrual dysphoric disorder
        Excludes1   premenstrual tension syndrome (N94.3)

    F32.89   Other specified depressive episodes
        Atypical depression
        Post-schizophrenic depression
        Single episode of 'masked' depression NOS

F32.9   Major depressive disorder, single episode, unspecified
    Depression NOS
    Depressive disorder NOS
    Major depression NOS

● F33   Major depressive disorder, recurrent

    Includes   recurrent episodes of depressive reaction
             recurrent episodes of endogenous depression
             recurrent episodes of major depression
             recurrent episodes of psychogenic depression
             recurrent episodes of reactive depression
             recurrent episodes of seasonal depressive disorder
             recurrent episodes of vital depression

    Excludes1   bipolar disorder (F31.-)
             manic episode (F30.-)

F33.0   Major depressive disorder, recurrent, mild

F33.1   Major depressive disorder, recurrent, moderate

F33.2   Major depressive disorder, recurrent severe without psychotic features

F33.3   Major depressive disorder, recurrent, severe with psychotic symptoms
    Endogenous depression with psychotic symptoms
    ▶Major depressive disorder, recurrent, with psychotic features
    Recurrent severe episodes of major depression with mood-congruent psychotic symptoms
    Recurrent severe episodes of major depression with mood-incongruent psychotic symptoms
    Recurrent severe episodes of major depression with psychotic symptoms
    Recurrent severe episodes of psychogenic depressive psychosis
    Recurrent severe episodes of psychotic depression
    Recurrent severe episodes of reactive depressive psychosis

● F33.4   Major depressive disorder, recurrent, in remission

    F33.40   Major depressive disorder, recurrent, in remission, unspecified

    F33.41   Major depressive disorder, recurrent, in partial remission

    F33.42   Major depressive disorder, recurrent, in full remission

F33.8   Other recurrent depressive disorders
    Recurrent brief depressive episodes

F33.9   Major depressive disorder, recurrent, unspecified
    Monopolar depression NOS

CHAPTER 5 (F01–F99)

▶ New   ⇒ Revised   ~~deleted~~ Deleted   **OGCR** Official Guidelines   X Assign placeholder X   ● Use Additional Character(s)

| Excludes 1 | Excludes 2 | Includes | Use additional | Code first | Code also | Key words |

Figure 5-1 PET scan of depressed individual's brain before and after recovery. (From Fortinash KM: Psychiatric Mental Health Nursing, ed 4, St. Louis, Mosby, 2008)

● **F34   Persistent mood [affective] disorders**

    F34.0   Cyclothymic disorder
        Affective personality disorder
        Cycloid personality
        Cyclothymia
        Cyclothymic personality

    F34.1   Dysthymic disorder
        Depressive neurosis
        Depressive personality disorder
        Dysthymia
        Neurotic depression
        Persistent anxiety depression
        Persistent depressive disorder
        | Excludes2 | anxiety depression (mild or not persistent) (F41.8) |

● **F34.8   Other persistent mood [affective] disorders**
        F34.81   Disruptive mood dysregulation disorder
        F34.89   Other specified persistent mood disorders

    F34.9   Persistent mood [affective] disorder, unspecified

F39   Unspecified mood [affective] disorder
    Affective psychosis NOS

ANXIETY, DISSOCIATIVE, STRESS-RELATED, SOMATOFORM AND OTHER NONPSYCHOTIC MENTAL DISORDERS (F40-F48)

● **F40   Phobic anxiety disorders**
    Irrational fear with avoidance of the feared subject, activity, or situation even though the individual knows that the reaction is excessive

● **F40.0   Agoraphobia**
        Intense, irrational fear of open spaces
        F40.00   Agoraphobia, unspecified
        F40.01   Agoraphobia with panic disorder
            Panic disorder with agoraphobia
            | Excludes1 | panic disorder without agoraphobia (F41.0) |
        F40.02   Agoraphobia without panic disorder

● **F40.1   Social phobias**
        Anthropophobia
        ▶Social anxiety disorder
        Social anxiety disorder of childhood
        Social neurosis
        F40.10   Social phobia, unspecified
        F40.11   Social phobia, generalized

● **F40.2   Specific (isolated) phobias**
        | Excludes2 | dysmorphophobia (nondelusional) (F45.22) |
                nosophobia (F45.22)

● **F40.21   Animal type phobia**
        F40.210   Arachnophobia
                Fear of spiders
        F40.218   Other animal type phobia

● **F40.22   Natural environment type phobia**
        F40.220   Fear of thunderstorms
        F40.228   Other natural environment type phobia

● **F40.23   Blood, injection, injury type phobia**
        F40.230   Fear of blood
        F40.231   Fear of injections and transfusions
        F40.232   Fear of other medical care
        F40.233   Fear of injury

● **F40.24   Situational type phobia**
        F40.240   Claustrophobia
                Fear of closed spaces
        F40.241   Acrophobia
                Fear of heights
        F40.242   Fear of bridges
        F40.243   Fear of flying
        F40.248   Other situational type phobia

● **F40.29   Other specified phobia**
        F40.290   Androphobia
                Fear of men
        F40.291   Gynephobia
                Fear of women
        F40.298   Other specified phobia

    F40.8   Other phobic anxiety disorders
        Phobic anxiety disorder of childhood

    F40.9   Phobic anxiety disorder, unspecified
        Phobia NOS
        Phobic state NOS

● **F41   Other anxiety disorders**
    | Excludes2 | anxiety in: |
            acute stress reaction (F43.0)
            transient adjustment reaction (F43.2)
            neurasthenia (F48.8)
            psychophysiologic disorders (F45.-)
            separation anxiety (F93.0)

⇒ **F41.0   Panic disorder [episodic paroxysmal anxiety]**
        Panic attack
        Panic state
        | Excludes1 | panic disorder with agoraphobia (F40.01) |

    F41.1   Generalized anxiety disorder
        Anxiety neurosis
        Anxiety reaction
        Anxiety state
        Overanxious disorder
        | Excludes2 | neurasthenia (F48.8) |

    F41.3   Other mixed anxiety disorders

    F41.8   Other specified anxiety disorders
        Anxiety depression (mild or not persistent)
        Anxiety hysteria
        Mixed anxiety and depressive disorder

    F41.9   Anxiety disorder, unspecified
        Anxiety NOS

● **F42   Obsessive-compulsive disorder**
  Anxiety disorder with recurrent obsessions or compulsions
  Excludes2   obsessive-compulsive personality (disorder)
                       (F60.5)
                   obsessive-compulsive symptoms occurring in
                       depression (F32-F33)
                   obsessive-compulsive symptoms occurring in
                       schizophrenia (F20.-)
  F42.2   Mixed obsessional thoughts and acts
  F42.3   Hoarding disorder
  F42.4   Excoriation (skin-picking) disorder
           Excludes1   factitial dermatitis (L98.1)
                           other specified behavioral and emotional
                               disorders with onset usually
                               occurring in early childhood and
                               adolescence (F98.8)
  F42.8   Other obsessive-compulsive disorder
           Anancastic neurosis
           Obsessive-compulsive neurosis
  F42.9   Obsessive-compulsive disorder, unspecified

● **F43   Reaction to severe stress and adjustment disorders**
  F43.0   Acute stress reaction
           Acute crisis reaction
           Acute reaction to stress
           Combat and operational stress reaction
           Combat fatigue
           Crisis state
           Psychic shock
  ● **F43.1   Post-traumatic stress disorder (PTSD)**
           Traumatic neurosis
           F43.10   Post-traumatic stress disorder, unspecified
           F43.11   Post-traumatic stress disorder, acute
           F43.12   Post-traumatic stress disorder, chronic
  ● **F43.2   Adjustment disorders**
           Culture shock
           Grief reaction
           Hospitalism in children
           Excludes2   separation anxiety disorder of childhood
                               (F93.0)
           F43.20   Adjustment disorder, unspecified
           F43.21   Adjustment disorder with depressed mood
           F43.22   Adjustment disorder with anxiety
           **F43.23   Adjustment disorder with mixed anxiety and
                       depressed mood**
           **F43.24   Adjustment disorder with disturbance of
                       conduct**
           **F43.25   Adjustment disorder with mixed disturbance of
                       emotions and conduct**
           F43.29   Adjustment disorder with other symptoms
  F43.8   Other reactions to severe stress
           Other specified trauma and stressor-related disorder
  F43.9   Reaction to severe stress, unspecified
           Trauma and stressor-related disorder, NOS

● **F44   Dissociative and conversion disorders**
       Includes   conversion hysteria
                       conversion reaction
                       hysteria
                       hysterical psychosis
       Excludes2   malingering [conscious simulation] (Z76.5)
  F44.0   Dissociative amnesia
           Sudden loss of memory for personal information
           Excludes1   amnesia NOS (R41.3)
                           anterograde amnesia (R41.1)
                           dissociative amnesia with dissociative
                               fugue (F44.1)
                           retrograde amnesia (R41.2)
           Excludes2   alcohol-or other psychoactive substance-
                               induced amnestic disorder (F10, F13,
                               F19 with .26, .96)
                           amnestic disorder due to known
                               physiological condition (F04)
                           postictal amnesia in epilepsy (G40.-)
  F44.1   Dissociative fugue
           *Characterized by episode of sudden, unexpected travel with
           amnesia for past and partial to total confusion about
           identity or assumption of new identity*
           Dissociative amnesia with dissociative fugue
           Excludes2   postictal fugue in epilepsy (G40.-)
  F44.2   Dissociative stupor
           *Profound diminution or absence of voluntary movement and
           responsiveness to external stimuli*
           Excludes1   catatonic stupor (R40.1)
                           stupor NOS (R40.1)
           Excludes2   catatonic disorder due to known
                               physiological condition (F06.1)
                           depressive stupor (F32, F33)
                           manic stupor (F30, F31)
  F44.4   Conversion disorder with motor symptom or deficit
           ▶Conversion disorder with abnormal movement
           ▶Conversion disorder with speech symptoms
           ▶Conversion disorder with swallowing symptoms
           ▶Conversion disorder with weakness/paralysis
           Dissociative motor disorders
           Psychogenic aphonia
           Psychogenic dysphonia
  F44.5   Conversion disorder with seizures or convulsions
           ▶Conversion disorder with attacks or seizures
           Dissociative convulsions
  F44.6   Conversion disorder with sensory symptom or deficit
           ▶Conversion disorder with anesthesia or sensory loss
           ▶Conversion disorder with special sensory symptoms
           Dissociative anesthesia and sensory loss
           Psychogenic deafness
  F44.7   Conversion disorder with mixed symptom presentation
  ● **F44.8   Other dissociative and conversion disorders**
           F44.81   Dissociative identity disorder
                       Multiple personality disorder
           F44.89   Other dissociative and conversion disorders
                       Ganser's syndrome
                       Psychogenic confusion
                       Psychogenic twilight state
                       Trance and possession disorders
  F44.9   Dissociative and conversion disorder, unspecified
           Dissociative disorder NOS

▶ New   ⟹ Revised   ~~deleted~~ Deleted   **OGCR** Official Guidelines   X Assign placeholder X   ● Use Additional Character(s)
| Excludes 1 | Excludes 2 | Includes   Use additional   Code first   Code also   Key words

OGCR Section I.C.5.a.

> Pain disorders related to psychological factors
>
> Assign code F45.41, for pain that is exclusively related to psychological disorders. As indicated by the Excludes 1 note under category G89, a code from category G89 should not be assigned with code F45.41 Code F45.42, Pain disorders with related psychological factors, should be used with a code from category G89, Pain, not elsewhere classified, if there is documentation of a psychological component for a patient with acute or chronic pain.
>
> *See Section I.C.6. Pain*

● **F45   Somatoform disorders**

Mental disorders characterized by symptoms suggesting general medical condition

    Excludes2   dissociative and conversion disorders (F44.-)
                factitious disorders (F68.1-)
                hair-plucking (F63.3)
                lalling (F80.0)
                lisping (F80.0)
                malingering [conscious simulation] (Z76.5)
                nail-biting (F98.8)
                psychological or behavioral factors associated with disorders or diseases classified elsewhere (F54)
                sexual dysfunction, not due to a substance or known physiological condition (F52.-)
                thumb-sucking (F98.8)
                tic disorders (in childhood and adolescence) (F95.-)
                Tourette's syndrome (F95.2)
                trichotillomania (F63.3)

   F45.0   Somatization disorder
        Briquet's disorder
        Multiple psychosomatic disorder

   F45.1   Undifferentiated somatoform disorder
        Somatic symptom disorder
        Undifferentiated psychosomatic disorder

● **F45.2   Hypochondriacal disorders**

Persistent, unrealistic preoccupation with possibility of having serious disease

    Excludes2   delusional dysmorphophobia (F22)
                fixed delusions about bodily functions or shape (F22)

   F45.20   Hypochondriacal disorder, unspecified

   F45.21   Hypochondriasis
        Hypochondriacal neurosis
        Illness anxiety disorder

   F45.22   Body dysmorphic disorder
        Dysmorphophobia (nondelusional)
        Nosophobia

   F45.29   Other hypochondriacal disorders

● **F45.4   Pain disorders related to psychological factors**
    Excludes1   pain NOS (R52)

   F45.41   Pain disorder exclusively related to psychological factors
        Somatoform pain disorder (persistent)

   F45.42   Pain disorder with related psychological factors
        Code also associated acute or chronic pain (G89.-)

   F45.8   Other somatoform disorders
        Psychogenic dysmenorrhea
        Psychogenic dysphagia, including 'globus hystericus'
        Psychogenic pruritus
        Psychogenic torticollis
        Somatoform autonomic dysfunction
        Teeth grinding
    Excludes1   sleep related teeth grinding (G47.63)

   F45.9   Somatoform disorder, unspecified
        Psychosomatic disorder NOS

● **F48   Other nonpsychotic mental disorders**

   F48.1   Depersonalization-derealization syndrome

   F48.2   Pseudobulbar affect
        Involuntary emotional expression disorder
        Code first underlying cause, if known, such as:
          amyotrophic lateral sclerosis (G12.21)
          multiple sclerosis (G35)
          sequelae of cerebrovascular disease (I69.-)
          sequelae of traumatic intracranial injury (S06.-)

   F48.8   Other specified nonpsychotic mental disorders
        Dhat syndrome
        Neurasthenia
        Occupational neurosis, including writer's cramp
        Psychasthenia
        Psychasthenic neurosis
        Psychogenic syncope

   F48.9   Nonpsychotic mental disorder, unspecified
        Neurosis NOS

BEHAVIORAL SYNDROMES ASSOCIATED WITH PHYSIOLOGICAL DISTURBANCES AND PHYSICAL FACTORS (F50-F59)

● **F50   Eating disorders**
    Excludes1   anorexia NOS (R63.0)
                feeding difficulties (R63.3)
                ▶feeding problems of newborn (P92.-)
                polyphagia (R63.2)
    Excludes2   feeding disorder in infancy or childhood (F98.2-)

● **F50.0   Anorexia nervosa**
    Excludes1   loss of appetite (R63.0)
                psychogenic loss of appetite (F50.89)

   F50.00   Anorexia nervosa, unspecified

   F50.01   Anorexia nervosa, restricting type

   F50.02   Anorexia nervosa, binge eating/purging type
    Excludes1   bulimia nervosa (F50.2)

   F50.2   Bulimia nervosa
        Bulimia NOS
        Hyperorexia nervosa
    Excludes1   anorexia nervosa, binge eating/purging type (F50.02)

● **F50.8   Other eating disorders**
    Excludes2   pica of infancy and childhood (F98.3)

   F50.81   Binge eating disorder

▶ **F50.82   Avoidant/restrictive food intake disorder**

   F50.89   Other specified eating disorder
        Pica in adults
        Psychogenic loss of appetite

   F50.9   Eating disorder, unspecified
        Atypical anorexia nervosa
        Atypical bulimia nervosa
        ▶Feeding or eating disorder, unspecified
        ▶Other specified feeding disorder

● **F51   Sleep disorders not due to a substance or known physiological condition**
> **Excludes2**   organic sleep disorders (G47.-)

● **F51.0   Insomnia not due to a substance or known physiological condition**
> **Excludes2**   alcohol related insomnia (F10.182, F10.282, F10.982)
> drug-related insomnia (F11.182, F11.282, F11.982, F13.182, F13.282, F13.982, F14.182, F14.282, F14.982, F15.182, F15.282, F15.982, F19.182, F19.282, F19.982)
> insomnia NOS (G47.0-)
> insomnia due to known physiological condition (G47.0-)
> organic insomnia (G47.0-)
> sleep deprivation (Z72.820)

F51.01   Primary insomnia
Idiopathic insomnia

F51.02   Adjustment insomnia

F51.03   Paradoxical insomnia

F51.04   Psychophysiologic insomnia

F51.05   Insomnia due to other mental disorder
Code also associated mental disorder

F51.09   Other insomnia not due to a substance or known physiological condition

● **F51.1   Hypersomnia not due to a substance or known physiological condition**
Hypersomnia: Excessive sleeping/sleepiness
> **Excludes2**   alcohol related hypersomnia (F10.182, F10.282, F10.982)
> drug-related hypersomnia (F11.182, F11.282, F11.982, F13.182, F13.282, F13.982, F14.182, F14.282, F14.982, F15.182, F15.282, F15.982, F19.182, F19.282, F19.982)
> hypersomnia NOS (G47.10)
> hypersomnia due to known physiological condition (G47.10)
> idiopathic hypersomnia (G47.11, G47.12)
> narcolepsy (G47.4-)

F51.11   Primary hypersomnia

F51.12   Insufficient sleep syndrome
> **Excludes1**   sleep deprivation (Z72.820)

F51.13   Hypersomnia due to other mental disorder
Code also associated mental disorder

F51.19   Other hypersomnia not due to a substance or known physiological condition

F51.3   Sleepwalking [somnambulism]
▶Non-rapid eye movement sleep arousal disorders, sleepwalking type

F51.4   Sleep terrors [night terrors]
▶Non-rapid eye movement sleep arousal disorders, sleep terror type

F51.5   Nightmare disorder
Dream anxiety disorder

F51.8   Other sleep disorders not due to a substance or known physiological condition

F51.9   Sleep disorder not due to a substance or known physiological condition, unspecified
Emotional sleep disorder NOS

● **F52   Sexual dysfunction not due to a substance or known physiological condition**
> **Excludes2**   Dhat syndrome (F48.8)

F52.0   Hypoactive sexual desire disorder
Total loss of feeling of sexual pleasure
Lack or loss of sexual desire
▶Male hypoactive sexual desire disorder
Sexual anhedonia
> **Excludes1**   decreased libido (R68.82)

F52.1   Sexual aversion disorder
Sexual aversion and lack of sexual enjoyment

● **F52.2   Sexual arousal disorders**
Failure of genital response

F52.21   Male erectile disorder
▶Erectile disorder
Psychogenic impotence
> **Excludes1**   impotence of organic origin (N52.-)
> impotence NOS (N52.-)

F52.22   Female sexual arousal disorder
▶Female sexual interest/arousal disorder

● **F52.3   Orgasmic disorder**
Inhibited orgasm
Psychogenic anorgasmy

F52.31   Female orgasmic disorder

F52.32   Male orgasmic disorder
Delayed ejaculation

F52.4   Premature ejaculation

F52.5   Vaginismus not due to a substance or known physiological condition
Psychogenic vaginismus
> **Excludes2**   vaginismus (due to a known physiological condition) (N94.2)

F52.6   Dyspareunia not due to a substance or known physiological condition
Dyspareunia: Difficult or painful sexual intercourse
Genito-pelvic pain penetration disorder
Psychogenic dyspareunia
> **Excludes2**   dyspareunia (due to a known physiological condition) (N94.1-)

F52.8   Other sexual dysfunction not due to a substance or known physiological condition
Excessive sexual drive
Nymphomania
Satyriasis

F52.9   Unspecified sexual dysfunction not due to a substance or known physiological condition
Sexual dysfunction NOS

F53   Puerperal psychosis
Postpartum depression
Acute mental illness with sudden onset following childbirth with symptoms of affective psychosis, disorientation, and confusion are prevalent
> **Excludes1**   mood disorders with psychotic features (F30.2, F31.2, F31.5, F31.64, F32.3, F33.3)
> postpartum dysphoria (O90.6)
> psychosis in schizophrenia, schizotypal, delusional, and other psychotic disorders (F20-F29)

F54   Psychological and behavioral factors associated with disorders or diseases classified elsewhere
Psychological factors affecting physical conditions
Code first the associated physical disorder, such as:
asthma (J45.-)
dermatitis (L23-L25)
gastric ulcer (K25.-)
mucous colitis (K58.-)
ulcerative colitis (K51.-)
urticaria (L50.-)
> **Excludes2**   tension-type headache (G44.2)

CHAPTER 5 (F01-F99)

CHAPTER 5 (F01-F99)

● **F55 Abuse of non-psychoactive substances**
  Excludes2 abuse of psychoactive substances (F10-F19)
  F55.0 Abuse of antacids
  F55.1 Abuse of herbal or folk remedies
  F55.2 Abuse of laxatives
  F55.3 Abuse of steroids or hormones
  F55.4 Abuse of vitamins
  F55.8 Abuse of other non-psychoactive substances

F59 Unspecified behavioral syndromes associated with physiological disturbances and physical factors
  Psychogenic physiological dysfunction NOS

DISORDERS OF ADULT PERSONALITY AND BEHAVIOR (F60-F69)

● **F60 Specific personality disorders**
  Long-term patterns of thoughts and behaviors causing serious problems with relationships and work.
  F60.0 Paranoid personality disorder
    Hostile, devious, and combative response to disappointments
    Expansive paranoid personality (disorder)
    Fanatic personality (disorder)
    Querulant personality (disorder)
    Paranoid personality (disorder)
    Sensitive paranoid personality (disorder)
    Excludes2 paranoia (F22)
      paranoia querulans (F22)
      paranoid psychosis (F22)
      paranoid schizophrenia (F20.0)
      paranoid state (F22)

  F60.1 Schizoid personality disorder
    Detachment from social relationships with minimal emotional experiences and expressions
    Excludes2 Asperger's syndrome (F84.5)
      delusional disorder (F22)
      schizoid disorder of childhood (F84.5)
      schizophrenia (F20.-)
      schizotypal disorder (F21)

  F60.2 Antisocial personality disorder
    Continuous and chronic antisocial behavior
    Amoral personality (disorder)
    Asocial personality (disorder)
    Dissocial personality disorder
    Psychopathic personality (disorder)
    Sociopathic personality (disorder)
    Excludes1 conduct disorders (F91.-)
    Excludes2 borderline personality disorder (F60.3)

  F60.3 Borderline personality disorder
    Instability of mood, self-image or sense of self, and interpersonal relationships
    Aggressive personality (disorder)
    Emotionally unstable personality disorder
    Explosive personality (disorder)
    Excludes2 antisocial personality disorder (F60.2)

  F60.4 Histrionic personality disorder
    Personality disorder with excessive emotional and attention-seeking behavior
    Hysterical personality (disorder)
    Psychoinfantile personality (disorder)

  F60.5 Obsessive-compulsive personality disorder
    Anankastic personality (disorder)
    Compulsive personality (disorder)
    Obsessional personality (disorder)
    Excludes2 obsessive-compulsive disorder (F42-)

  F60.6 Avoidant personality disorder
    Anxious personality disorder

  F60.7 Dependent personality disorder
    Asthenic personality (disorder)
    Inadequate personality (disorder)
    Passive personality (disorder)

● **F60.8 Other specific personality disorders**
  F60.81 Narcissistic personality disorder
    Vanity, conceit, egotism or indifference to plight of others

  F60.89 Other specific personality disorders
    Eccentric personality disorder
    'Haltlose' type personality disorder
    Immature personality disorder
    Passive-aggressive personality disorder
    Psychoneurotic personality disorder
    Self-defeating personality disorder

  F60.9 Personality disorder, unspecified
    Character disorder NOS
    Character neurosis NOS
    Pathological personality NOS

● **F63 Impulse disorders**
  Excludes2 habitual excessive use of alcohol or psychoactive substances (F10-F19)
    impulse disorders involving sexual behavior (F65.-)
  F63.0 Pathological gambling
    Compulsive gambling
    ▶Gambling disorder
    Excludes1 gambling and betting NOS (Z72.6)
    Excludes2 excessive gambling by manic patients (F30, F31)
      gambling in antisocial personality disorder (F60.2)

  F63.1 Pyromania
    Pathological fire-setting
    Excludes2 fire-setting (by) (in):
      adult with antisocial personality disorder (F60.2)
      alcohol or psychoactive substance intoxication (F10-F19)
      conduct disorders (F91.-)
      mental disorders due to known physiological condition (F01-F09)
      schizophrenia (F20.-)

  F63.2 Kleptomania
    Pathological stealing
    Excludes1 shoplifting as the reason for observation for suspected mental disorder (Z03.8)
    Excludes2 depressive disorder with stealing (F31-F33)
      stealing due to underlying mental condition-code to mental condition
      stealing in mental disorders due to known physiological condition (F01-F09)

  F63.3 Trichotillomania
    Hair plucking
    Excludes2 other stereotyped movement disorder (F98.4)

● **F63.8 Other impulse disorders**
  F63.81 Intermittent explosive disorder
  F63.89 Other impulse disorders

  F63.9 Impulse disorder, unspecified
    Impulse control disorder NOS

▶ New   ⇒ Revised   ~~deleted~~ Deleted   **OGCR** Official Guidelines   X Assign placeholder X   ● Use Additional Character(s)

Excludes 1   Excludes 2   Includes   Use additional   Code first   Code also   Key words

● **F64 Gender identity disorders**

  F64.0 Transsexualism
    Gender identity disorder in adolescence and
      adulthood
    Gender dysphoria in adolescents and adults

  F64.1 Dual role transvestism
    Use additional code to identify sex reassignment status
      (Z87.890)
    | Excludes1 | gender identity disorder in childhood (F64.2) |
    | Excludes2 | fetishistic transvestism (F65.1) |

  F64.2 Gender identity disorder of childhood
    Gender dysphoria in children
    | Excludes1 | gender identity disorder in adolescence and adulthood (F64.0) |
    | Excludes2 | sexual maturation disorder (F66) |

  F64.8 Other gender identity disorders
    ▶Other specified gender dysphoria

  F64.9 Gender identity disorder, unspecified
    ▶Gender dysphoria, unspecified
    Gender-role disorder NOS

● **F65 Paraphilias**

  F65.0 Fetishism
    Intense sexual urges and arousing fantasies using inanimate objects
    ▶Fetishistic disorder

  F65.1 Transvestic fetishism
    Intense sexual urges, arousal, or orgasm associated with fantasized/actual cross-dressing
    Fetishistic transvestism
    ▶Transvestic disorder

  F65.2 Exhibitionism
    ▶Exhibitionistic disorder

  F65.3 Voyeurism
    Sexual urges or arousal involving real or fantasized observation of unsuspecting people who are naked, disrobing, or engaging in sexual activity
    ▶Voyeuristic disorder

  F65.4 Pedophilia
    ▶Pedophilic disorder

● **F65.5 Sadomasochism**

    F65.50 Sadomasochism, unspecified

    F65.51 Sexual masochism
      ▶Sexual masochism disorder

    F65.52 Sexual sadism
      ▶Sexual sadism disorder

● **F65.8 Other paraphilias**

    F65.81 Frotteurism
      Sexual arousal or orgasm is achieved by rubbing up against another person (or fantasies of), in crowded place with unsuspecting victim
      ▶Frotteuristic disorder

    F65.89 Other paraphilias
      Necrophilia
      ▶Other specified paraphilic disorder

  F65.9 Paraphilia, unspecified
    ▶Paraphilic disorder, unspecified
    Sexual deviation NOS

  F66 Other sexual disorders
    Sexual maturation disorder
    Sexual relationship disorder

● **F68 Other disorders of adult personality and behavior**

  ● **F68.1 Factitious disorder**
    Compensation neurosis
    Elaboration of physical symptoms for psychological
      reasons
    Hospital hopper syndrome
    Münchhausen's syndrome
    Peregrinating patient
    | Excludes2 | factitial dermatitis (L98.1) |
    | | person feigning illness (with obvious motivation) (Z76.5) |

    F68.10 Factitious disorder, unspecified

    F68.11 Factitious disorder with predominantly psychological signs and symptoms

    F68.12 Factitious disorder with predominantly physical signs and symptoms

    F68.13 Factitious disorder with combined psychological and physical signs and symptoms

  F68.8 Other specified disorders of adult personality and behavior

  F69 Unspecified disorder of adult personality and behavior

INTELLECTUAL DISABILITIES (F70-F79)

Code first any associated physical or developmental disorders
| Excludes1 | borderline intellectual functioning, IQ above 70 to 84 (R41.83) |

  F70 Mild intellectual disabilities
    IQ level 50-55 to approximately 70
    Mild mental subnormality

  F71 Moderate intellectual disabilities
    IQ level 35-40 to 50-55
    Moderate mental subnormality

  F72 Severe intellectual disabilities
    IQ 20-25 to 35-40
    Severe mental subnormality

  F73 Profound intellectual disabilities
    IQ level below 20-25
    Profound mental subnormality

  F78 Other intellectual disabilities

  F79 Unspecified intellectual disabilities
    Mental deficiency NOS
    Mental subnormality NOS

PERVASIVE AND SPECIFIC DEVELOPMENTAL DISORDERS (F80-F89)

● **F80 Specific developmental disorders of speech and language**

  F80.0 Phonological disorder
    Communication disorder of unknown cause, characterized by failure to use age-appropriate sounds
    Dyslalia
    Functional speech articulation disorder
    Lalling
    Lisping
    Phonological developmental disorder
    Speech articulation developmental disorder
    Speech-sound disorder
    | Excludes1 | speech articulation impairment due to aphasia NOS (R47.01) |
    | | speech articulation impairment due to apraxia (R48.2) |
    | Excludes2 | speech articulation impairment due to hearing loss (F80.4) |
    | | speech articulation impairment due to intellectual disabilities (F70-F79) |
    | | speech articulation impairment with expressive language developmental disorder (F80.1) |
    | | speech articulation impairment with mixed receptive expressive language developmental disorder (F80.2) |

▶ New   ⇒ Revised   ~~deleted~~ Deleted   **OGCR** Official Guidelines   X Assign placeholder X   ● Use Additional Character(s)

| Excludes 1 | Excludes 2 | Includes | Use additional | Code first | Code also | Key words |

F80.1   **Expressive language disorder**
Developmental dysphasia or aphasia, expressive type

> Excludes1   mixed receptive-expressive language disorder (F80.2)
> dysphasia and aphasia NOS (R47.-)

> Excludes2   acquired aphasia with epilepsy [Landau-Kleffner] (G40.80-)
> intellectual disabilities (F70-F79)
> pervasive developmental disorders (F84.-)
> selective mutism (F94.0)

F80.2   **Mixed receptive-expressive language disorder**
Developmental dysphasia or aphasia, receptive type
Developmental Wernicke's aphasia

> Excludes1   central auditory processing disorder (H93.25)
> dysphasia or aphasia NOS (R47.-)
> expressive language disorder (F80.1)
> expressive type dysphasia or aphasia (F80.1)
> word deafness (H93.25)

> Excludes2   acquired aphasia with epilepsy [Landau-Kleffner] (G40.80-)
> intellectual disabilities (F70-F79)
> pervasive developmental disorders (F84.-)
> selective mutism (F94.0)

F80.4   **Speech and language development delay due to hearing loss**
Code also type of hearing loss (H90.-, H91.-)

● **F80.8**   **Other developmental disorders of speech or language**

    F80.81   **Childhood onset fluency disorder**
       Cluttering NOS
       Stuttering NOS

> Excludes1   adult onset fluency disorder (F98.5)
> fluency disorder in conditions classified elsewhere (R47.82)
> fluency disorder (stuttering) following cerebrovascular disease (I69. with final characters -23)

    F80.82   **Social pragmatic communication disorder**

> Excludes1   Asperger's syndrome (F84.5)
> autistic disorder (F84.0)

    F80.89   **Other developmental disorders of speech and language**

F80.9   **Developmental disorder of speech and language, unspecified**
Communication disorder NOS
Language disorder NOS

● **F81**   **Specific developmental disorders of scholastic skills**

    F81.0   **Specific reading disorder**
       'Backward reading'
       Developmental dyslexia
       ▶Specific learning disorder, with impairment in reading
       Specific reading retardation

> Excludes1   alexia NOS (R48.0)
> dyslexia NOS (R48.0)

    F81.2   **Mathematics disorder**
       Developmental acalculia
       Developmental arithmetical disorder
       Developmental Gerstmann's syndrome
       ▶Specific learning disorder, with impairment in mathematics

> Excludes1   acalculia NOS (R48.8)

> Excludes2   arithmetical difficulties associated with a reading disorder (F81.0)
> arithmetical difficulties associated with a spelling disorder (F81.81)
> arithmetical difficulties due to inadequate teaching (Z55.8)

● **F81.8**   **Other developmental disorders of scholastic skills**

    F81.81   **Disorder of written expression**
       ▶Specific learning disorder, with impairment in written expression
       Specific spelling disorder

    F81.89   **Other developmental disorders of scholastic skills**

F81.9   **Developmental disorder of scholastic skills, unspecified**
Knowledge acquisition disability NOS
Learning disability NOS
Learning disorder NOS

F82   **Specific developmental disorder of motor function**
Clumsy child syndrome
Developmental coordination disorder
Developmental dyspraxia

> Excludes1   abnormalities of gait and mobility (R26.-)
> lack of coordination (R27.-)

> Excludes2   lack of coordination secondary to intellectual disabilities (F70-F79)

● **F84**   **Pervasive developmental disorders**
Use additional code to identify any associated medical condition and intellectual disabilities.

    F84.0   **Autistic disorder**
       Autism spectrum disorder
       Infantile autism
       Infantile psychosis
       Kanner's syndrome

> Excludes1   Asperger's syndrome (F84.5)

    F84.2   **Rett's syndrome**
       Neurodevelopmental disorder

> Excludes1   Asperger's syndrome (F84.5)
> Autistic disorder (F84.0)
> other childhood disintegrative disorder (F84.3)

    F84.3   **Other childhood disintegrative disorder**
       Dementia infantilis
       At least two years of normal development followed by significant loss of language abilities, social skills, bowel/bladder control, motor skills
       Disintegrative psychosis
       Heller's syndrome
       At least two years of normal development followed by significant loss of language abilities, social skills, bowel/bladder control, motor skills
       Symbiotic psychosis
       Abnormal relationship to mothering figure, characterized by intense separation anxiety, severe regression, giving up of useful speech, and autism
       Use additional code to identify any associated neurological condition.

> Excludes1   Asperger's syndrome (F84.5)
> Autistic disorder (F84.0)
> Rett's syndrome (F84.2)

    F84.5   **Asperger's syndrome**
       Developmental disorder
       Asperger's disorder
       Autistic psychopathy
       Schizoid disorder of childhood

    F84.8   **Other pervasive developmental disorders**
       Overactive disorder associated with intellectual disabilities and stereotyped movements

    F84.9   **Pervasive developmental disorder, unspecified**
       Atypical autism

F88   **Other disorders of psychological development**
Developmental agnosia
Global developmental delay
Other specified neurodevelopmental disorder

F89   **Unspecified disorder of psychological development**
Developmental disorder NOS
Neurodevelopmental disorder NOS

▶ New   ⇒ Revised   ~~deleted~~ Deleted   **OGCR** Official Guidelines   X Assign placeholder X   ● Use Additional Character(s)

Excludes 1   Excludes 2   Includes   Use additional   Code first   Code also   Key words

BEHAVIORAL AND EMOTIONAL DISORDERS WITH ONSET USUALLY OCCURRING IN CHILDHOOD AND ADOLESCENCE (F90-F98)

Note: Codes within categories F90-F98 may be used regardless of the age of a patient. These disorders generally have onset within the childhood or adolescent years, but may continue throughout life or not be diagnosed until adulthood.

● **F90　Attention-deficit hyperactivity disorders**
　　Attention deficit disorder with hyperactivity=ADHD
　　Includes　　attention deficit disorder with hyperactivity
　　　　　　　　　　attention deficit syndrome with hyperactivity
　　Excludes2　　anxiety disorders (F40.-, F41.-)
　　　　　　　　　　mood [affective] disorders (F30-F39)
　　　　　　　　　　pervasive developmental disorders (F84.-)
　　　　　　　　　　schizophrenia (F20.-)

　F90.0　Attention-deficit hyperactivity disorder, predominantly inattentive type
　　　　▶Attention-deficit/hyperactivity disorder, predominantly inattentive presentation

　F90.1　Attention-deficit hyperactivity disorder, predominantly hyperactive type
　　　　▶Attention-deficit/hyperactivity disorder, predominantly hyperactive impulsive presentation

　F90.2　Attention-deficit hyperactivity disorder, combined type
　　　　▶Attention-deficit/hyperactivity disorder, combined presentation

　F90.8　Attention-deficit hyperactivity disorder, other type

　F90.9　Attention-deficit hyperactivity disorder, unspecified type
　　　　Attention-deficit hyperactivity disorder of childhood or adolescence NOS
　　　　Attention-deficit hyperactivity disorder NOS

● **F91　Conduct disorders**
　　Childhood/adolescence disruptive behavior disorder
　　Excludes1　　antisocial behavior (Z72.81-)
　　　　　　　　　　antisocial personality disorder (F60.2)
　　Excludes2　　conduct problems associated with attention-deficit hyperactivity disorder (F90.-)
　　　　　　　　　　mood [affective] disorders (F30-F39)
　　　　　　　　　　pervasive developmental disorders (F84.-)
　　　　　　　　　　schizophrenia (F20.-)

　F91.0　Conduct disorder confined to family context

　F91.1　Conduct disorder, childhood-onset type
　　　　Unsocialized conduct disorder
　　　　Conduct disorder, solitary aggressive type
　　　　Unsocialized aggressive disorder

　F91.2　Conduct disorder, adolescent-onset type
　　　　Socialized conduct disorder
　　　　Conduct disorder, group type

　F91.3　Oppositional defiant disorder

　F91.8　Other conduct disorders
　　　　Other specified conduct disorder
　　　　Other specified disruptive disorder

　F91.9　Conduct disorder, unspecified
　　　　Behavioral disorder NOS
　　　　Conduct disorder NOS
　　　　Disruptive behavior disorder NOS
　　　　Disruptive disorder NOS

● **F93　Emotional disorders with onset specific to childhood**

　F93.0　Separation anxiety disorder of childhood
　　　　Excludes2　　mood [affective] disorders (F30-F39)
　　　　　　　　　　　　nonpsychotic mental disorders (F40-F48)
　　　　　　　　　　　　phobic anxiety disorder of childhood (F40.8)
　　　　　　　　　　　　social phobia (F40.1)

　F93.8　Other childhood emotional disorders
　　　　Identity disorder
　　　　Excludes2　　gender identity disorder of childhood (F64.2)

　F93.9　Childhood emotional disorder, unspecified

● **F94　Disorders of social functioning with onset specific to childhood and adolescence**

　F94.0　Selective mutism
　　　　Elective mutism
　　　　Excludes2　　pervasive developmental disorders (F84.-)
　　　　　　　　　　　　schizophrenia (F20.-)
　　　　　　　　　　　　specific developmental disorders of speech and language (F80.-)
　　　　　　　　　　　　transient mutism as part of separation anxiety in young children (F93.0)

　F94.1　Reactive attachment disorder of childhood
　　　　Use additional code to identify any associated failure to thrive or growth retardation
　　　　Excludes1　　disinhibited attachment disorder of childhood (F94.2)
　　　　　　　　　　　　normal variation in pattern of selective attachment
　　　　Excludes2　　Asperger's syndrome (F84.5)
　　　　　　　　　　　　maltreatment syndromes (T74.-)
　　　　　　　　　　　　sexual or physical abuse in childhood, resulting in psychosocial problems (Z62.81-)

　F94.2　Disinhibited attachment disorder of childhood
　　　　Affectionless psychopathy
　　　　Institutional syndrome
　　　　Excludes1　　reactive attachment disorder of childhood (F94.1)
　　　　Excludes2　　Asperger's syndrome (F84.5)
　　　　　　　　　　　　attention-deficit hyperactivity disorders (F90.-)
　　　　　　　　　　　　hospitalism in children (F43.2-)

　F94.8　Other childhood disorders of social functioning

　F94.9　Childhood disorder of social functioning, unspecified

● **F95　Tic disorder**
　　Involuntary twitch

　F95.0　Transient tic disorder
　　　　Provisional tic disorder

　F95.1　Chronic motor or vocal tic disorder

　F95.2　Tourette's disorder
　　　　Combined vocal and multiple motor tic disorder [de la Tourette]
　　　　Tourette's syndrome

　F95.8　Other tic disorders

　F95.9　Tic disorder, unspecified
　　　　Tic NOS

● **F98　Other behavioral and emotional disorders with onset usually occurring in childhood and adolescence**
　　Excludes2　　breath-holding spells (R06.89)
　　　　　　　　　　gender identity disorder of childhood (F64.2)
　　　　　　　　　　Kleine-Levin syndrome (G47.13)
　　　　　　　　　　obsessive-compulsive disorder (F42-)
　　　　　　　　　　sleep disorders not due to a substance or known physiological condition (F51.-)

　F98.0　Enuresis not due to a substance or known physiological condition
　　　　Enuresis: Urinary incontinence
　　　　Enuresis (primary) (secondary) of nonorganic origin
　　　　Functional enuresis
　　　　Psychogenic enuresis
　　　　Urinary incontinence of nonorganic origin
　　　　Excludes1　　enuresis NOS (R32)

　F98.1　Encopresis not due to a substance or known physiological condition
　　　　Encopresis: Fecal incontinence
　　　　Functional encopresis
　　　　Incontinence of feces of nonorganic origin
　　　　Psychogenic encopresis
　　　　Use additional code to identify the cause of any coexisting constipation.
　　　　Excludes1　　encopresis NOS (R15.-)

▶ New　　⇒ Revised　　~~deleted~~ Deleted　　**OGCR** Official Guidelines　　X Assign placeholder X　　● Use Additional Character(s)

| Excludes 1 | Excludes 2 | Includes | Use additional | Code first | Code also | Key words |

Item 5–2 Enuresis: Bed wetting by children at night. Causes can be either psychological or medical (diabetes, urinary tract infections, or abnormalities). **Encopresis:** Overflow incontinence of bowels sometimes resulting from chronic constipation or fecal impaction. Check the documentation for additional diagnoses.

●F98.2 **Other feeding disorders of infancy and childhood**
     Excludes1 feeding difficulties (R63.3)
     Excludes2 anorexia nervosa and other eating disorders (F50.-)
              feeding problems of newborn (P92.-)
              pica of infancy or childhood (F98.3)

   F98.21 **Rumination disorder of infancy**

   F98.29 **Other feeding disorders of infancy and early childhood**

F98.3 **Pica of infancy and childhood**
     Craving and eating substances such as paint, clay, or dirt to replace a nutritional deficit in the body.

F98.4 **Stereotyped movement disorders**
     Stereotype/habit disorder
     Excludes1 abnormal involuntary movements (R25.-)
     Excludes2 compulsions in obsessive-compulsive disorder (F42-)
              hair plucking (F63.3)
              movement disorders of organic origin (G20-G25)
              nail-biting (F98.8)
              nose-picking (F98.8)
              stereotypies that are part of a broader psychiatric condition (F01-F95)
              thumb-sucking (F98.8)
              tic disorders (F95.-)
              trichotillomania (F63.3)

F98.5 **Adult onset fluency disorder**
     Excludes1 childhood onset fluency disorder (F80.81)
              dysphasia (R47.02)
              fluency disorder in conditions classified elsewhere (R47.82)
              fluency disorder (stuttering) following cerebrovascular disease (I69. with final characters -23)
              tic disorders (F95.-)

F98.8 **Other specified behavioral and emotional disorders with onset usually occurring in childhood and adolescence**
     Excessive masturbation
     Nail-biting
     Nose-picking
     Thumb-sucking

F98.9 **Unspecified behavioral and emotional disorders with onset usually occurring in childhood and adolescence**

UNSPECIFIED MENTAL DISORDER (F99)

F99 **Mental disorder, not otherwise specified**
     Mental illness NOS
     Excludes1 unspecified mental disorder due to known physiological condition (F09)

▶ New   ⟹ Revised   ~~deleted~~ Deleted   **OGCR** Official Guidelines   X Assign placeholder X   ● Use Additional Character(s)

| Excludes 1 | Excludes 2 | Includes | Use additional | Code first | Code also | Key words |

CHAPTER 6

DISEASES OF THE NERVOUS SYSTEM (G00-G99)

OGCR Chapter-Specific Coding Guidelines

6. **Chapter 6: Diseases of the Nervous System (G00-G99)**

   a. **Dominant/nondominant side**

   Codes from category G81, Hemiplegia and hemiparesis, and subcategories, G83.1, Monoplegia of lower limb, G83.2, Monoplegia of upper limb, and G83.3, Monoplegia, unspecified, identify whether the dominant or nondominant side is affected. Should the affected side be documented, but not specified as dominant or nondominant, and the classification system does not indicate a default, code selection is as follows:

   - For ambidextrous patients, the default should be dominant.
   - If the left side is affected, the default is non-dominant.
   - If the right side is affected, the default is dominant.

   b. **Pain - Category G89**

   1) **General coding information**

   Codes in category G89, Pain, not elsewhere classified, may be used in conjunction with codes from other categories and chapters to provide more detail about acute or chronic pain and neoplasm-related pain, unless otherwise indicated below.

   If the pain is not specified as acute or chronic, post-thoracotomy, postprocedural, or neoplasm-related, do not assign codes from category G89.

   A code from category G89 should not be assigned if the underlying (definitive) diagnosis is known, unless the reason for the encounter is pain control/management and not management of the underlying condition.

   When an admission or encounter is for a procedure aimed at treating the underlying condition (e.g., spinal fusion, kyphoplasty), a code for the underlying condition (e.g., vertebral fracture, spinal stenosis) should be assigned as the principal diagnosis. No code from category G89 should be assigned.

   (a) **Category G89 Codes as Principal or First-Listed Diagnosis**

   Category G89 codes are acceptable as principal diagnosis or the first-listed code:

   - When pain control or pain management is the reason for the admission/encounter (e.g., a patient with displaced intervertebral disc, nerve impingement and severe back pain presents for injection of steroid into the spinal canal). The underlying cause of the pain should be reported as an additional diagnosis, if known.
   - When a patient is admitted for the insertion of a neurostimulator for pain control, assign the appropriate pain code as the principal or first-listed diagnosis. When an admission or encounter is for a procedure aimed at treating the underlying condition and a neurostimulator is inserted for pain control during the same admission/encounter, a code for the underlying condition should be assigned as the principal diagnosis and the appropriate pain code should be assigned as a secondary diagnosis.

   (b) **Use of Category G89 Codes in Conjunction with Site Specific Pain Codes**

   (i) **Assigning Category G89 and Site-Specific Pain Codes**

   Codes from category G89 may be used in conjunction with codes that identify the site of pain (including codes from chapter 18) if the category G89 code provides additional information. For example, if the code describes the site of the pain, but does not fully describe whether the pain is acute or chronic, then both codes should be assigned.

   (ii) **Sequencing of Category G89 Codes with Site-Specific Pain Codes**

The sequencing of category G89 codes with site-specific pain codes (including chapter 18 codes), is dependent on the circumstances of the encounter/admission as follows:

- If the encounter is for pain control or pain management, assign the code from category G89 followed by the code identifying the specific site of pain (e.g., encounter for pain management for acute neck pain from trauma is assigned code G89.11, Acute pain due to trauma, followed by code M54.2, Cervicalgia, to identify the site of pain).
- If the encounter is for any other reason except pain control or pain management, and a related definitive diagnosis has not been established (confirmed) by the provider, assign the code for the specific site of pain first, followed by the appropriate code from category G89.

   2) **Pain due to devices, implants and grafts**
   See Section I.C.19. Pain due to medical devices

   3) **Postoperative Pain**
   The provider's documentation should be used to guide the coding of postoperative pain, as well as *Section III. Reporting Additional Diagnoses* and *Section IV. Diagnostic Coding and Reporting in the Outpatient Setting.*

   The default for post-thoracotomy and other postoperative pain not specified as acute or chronic is the code for the acute form.

   Routine or expected postoperative pain immediately after surgery should not be coded.

   (a) **Postoperative pain not associated with specific postoperative complication**
   Postoperative pain not associated with a specific postoperative complication is assigned to the appropriate postoperative pain code in category G89.

   (b) **Postoperative pain associated with specific postoperative complication**
   Postoperative pain associated with a specific postoperative complication (such as painful wire sutures) is assigned to the appropriate code(s) found in Chapter 19, Injury, poisoning, and certain other consequences of external causes. If appropriate, use additional code(s) from category G89 to identify acute or chronic pain (G89.18 or G89.28).

   4) **Chronic pain**
   Chronic pain is classified to subcategory G89.2. There is no time frame defining when pain becomes chronic pain. The provider's documentation should be used to guide use of these codes.

   5) **Neoplasm Related Pain**
   Code G89.3 is assigned to pain documented as being related, associated or due to cancer, primary or secondary malignancy, or tumor. This code is assigned regardless of whether the pain is acute or chronic.

   This code may be assigned as the principal or first-listed code when the stated reason for the admission/encounter is documented as pain control/pain management. The underlying neoplasm should be reported as an additional diagnosis.

   When the reason for the admission/encounter is management of the neoplasm and the pain associated with the neoplasm is also documented, code G89.3 may be assigned as an additional diagnosis. It is not necessary to assign an additional code for the site of the pain.

   See Section I.C.2 for instructions on the sequencing of neoplasms for all other stated reasons for the admission/encounter (except for pain control/pain management).

   6) **Chronic pain syndrome**
   Central pain syndrome (G89.0) and chronic pain syndrome (G89.4) are different than the term "chronic pain," and therefore codes should only be used when the provider has specifically documented this condition.

   See Section I.C.5. Pain disorders related to psychological factors

743

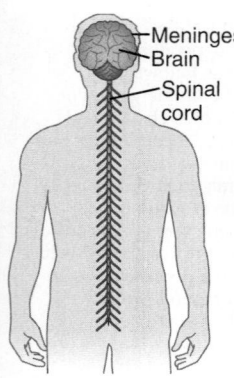

Meninges
Brain
Spinal cord

Figure 6-1 The brain and spinal cord make up the central nervous system.

Item 6-1 The two major classifications of the nervous system are the peripheral nervous system and the central nervous system (CNS). The central nervous system is comprised of the brain and the spinal cord. The peripheral nervous system is comprised of the parasympathetic and sympathetic systems. **Encephalitis** is the swelling of the brain. **Meningitis** is swelling of the covering of the brain, the meninges. Types and causes of brain infections are:

Type	Cause
purulent	bacterial
aseptic/abacterial	viral
chronic meningitis	mycobacterial and fungal

CHAPTER 6

DISEASES OF THE NERVOUS SYSTEM
(G00-G99)

Excludes2   certain conditions originating in the perinatal period (P04-P96)
certain infectious and parasitic diseases (A00-B99)
complications of pregnancy, childbirth and the puerperium (O00-O9A)
congenital malformations, deformations, and chromosomal abnormalities (Q00-Q99)
endocrine, nutritional and metabolic diseases (E00-E88)
injury, poisoning and certain other consequences of external causes (S00-T88)
neoplasms (C00-D49)
symptoms, signs and abnormal clinical and laboratory findings, not elsewhere classified (R00-R94)

This chapter contains the following blocks:

G00-G09	Inflammatory diseases of the central nervous system
G10-G14	Systemic atrophies primarily affecting the central nervous system
G20-G26	Extrapyramidal and movement disorders
G30-G32	Other degenerative diseases of the nervous system
G35-G37	Demyelinating diseases of the central nervous system
G40-G47	Episodic and paroxysmal disorders
G50-G59	Nerve, nerve root and plexus disorders
G60-G65	Polyneuropathies and other disorders of the peripheral nervous system
G70-G73	Diseases of myoneural junction and muscle
G80-G83	Cerebral palsy and other paralytic syndromes
G89-G99	Other disorders of the nervous system

INFLAMMATORY DISEASES OF THE CENTRAL NERVOUS SYSTEM (G00-G09)

● **G00   Bacterial meningitis, not elsewhere classified**
An infection of the cerebrospinal fluid surrounding the spinal cord and brain.

Includes   bacterial arachnoiditis
bacterial leptomeningitis
bacterial meningitis
bacterial pachymeningitis

➡ Excludes1   bacterial meningoencephalitis (G04.2)
➡ bacterial meningomyelitis (G04.2)
~~meningomyelitis (G04.2)~~

G00.0   Hemophilus meningitis
Meningitis due to Hemophilus influenzae

G00.1   Pneumococcal meningitis
Meningitis due to Streptococcal pneumoniae

G00.2   Streptococcal meningitis
Use additional code to further identify organism (B95.0-B95.5)

G00.3   Staphylococcal meningitis
Use additional code to further identify organism (B95.61-B95.8)

G00.8   Other bacterial meningitis
Meningitis due to Escherichia coli
Meningitis due to Friedländer bacillus
Meningitis due to Klebsiella
Use additional code to further identify organism (B96.-)

G00.9   Bacterial meningitis, unspecified
Meningitis due to gram-negative bacteria, unspecified
Purulent meningitis NOS
Pyogenic meningitis NOS
Suppurative meningitis NOS

G01   Meningitis in bacterial diseases classified elsewhere
Code first underlying disease
Excludes1   meningitis (in):
gonococcal (A54.81)
leptospirosis (A27.81)
listeriosis (A32.11)
Lyme disease (A69.21)
meningococcal (A39.0)
neurosyphilis (A52.13)
tuberculosis (A17.0)
meningoencephalitis and meningomyelitis in bacterial diseases classified elsewhere (G05)

G02   Meningitis in other infectious and parasitic diseases classified elsewhere
Code first underlying disease, such as:
African trypanosomiasis (B56.-)
poliovirus infection (A80.-)
Excludes1   candidal meningitis (B37.5)
coccidioidomycosis meningitis (B38.4)
cryptococcal meningitis (B45.1)
herpesviral [herpes simplex] meningitis (B00.3)
infectious mononucleosis complicated by meningitis (B27.- with fourth character 2)
measles complicated by meningitis (B05.1)
meningoencephalitis and meningomyelitis in other infectious and parasitic diseases classified elsewhere (G05)
mumps meningitis (B26.1)
rubella meningitis (B06.02)
varicella [chickenpox] meningitis (B01.0)
zoster meningitis (B02.1)

▶ New   ⇒ Revised   ~~deleted~~ Deleted   **OGCR** Official Guidelines   X Assign placeholder X   ● Use Additional Character(s)

Excludes 1   Excludes 2   Includes   Use additional   Code first   Code also   Key words

● **G03   Meningitis due to other and unspecified causes**
> **Includes**   arachnoiditis NOS
> leptomeningitis NOS
> meningitis NOS
> pachymeningitis NOS
>
> **Excludes1**   meningoencephalitis (G04.-)
> meningomyelitis (G04.-)

G03.0   Nonpyogenic meningitis
> Aseptic meningitis
> Nonbacterial meningitis

G03.1   Chronic meningitis

G03.2   Benign recurrent meningitis [Mollaret]

G03.8   Meningitis due to other specified causes

G03.9   Meningitis, unspecified
> Arachnoiditis (spinal) NOS

● **G04   Encephalitis, myelitis and encephalomyelitis**
> **Includes**   acute ascending myelitis
> meningoencephalitis
> meningomyelitis
>
> **Excludes1**   encephalopathy NOS (G93.40)
> other noninfectious acute disseminated
> encephalomyelitis (noninfectious ADEM)
> (G04.81)
>
> **Excludes2**   acute transverse myelitis (G37.3-)
> alcoholic encephalopathy (G31.2)
> benign myalgic encephalomyelitis (G93.3)
> multiple sclerosis (G35)
> subacute necrotizing myelitis (G37.4)
> toxic encephalitis (G92)
> toxic encephalopathy (G92)

● **G04.0   Acute disseminated encephalitis and encephalomyelitis (ADEM)**
> **Excludes1**   acute necrotizing hemorrhagic
> encephalopathy (G04.3-)

G04.00   Acute disseminated encephalitis and encephalomyelitis, unspecified

G04.01   Postinfectious acute disseminated encephalitis and encephalomyelitis (postinfectious ADEM)
> **Excludes1**   post chickenpox encephalitis
> (B01.1)
> post measles encephalitis (B05.0)
> post measles myelitis (B05.1)

G04.02   Postimmunization acute disseminated encephalitis, myelitis and encephalomyelitis
> Encephalitis, post immunization
> Encephalomyelitis, post immunization
> Use additional code to identify the vaccine
> (T50.A-, T50.B-, T50.Z-)

G04.1   Tropical spastic paraplegia

G04.2   Bacterial meningoencephalitis and meningomyelitis, not elsewhere classified

● **G04.3   Acute necrotizing hemorrhagic encephalopathy**
> *Sudden and severe CNS disease with pathology of hemorrhages and necrosis of white matter*
> **Excludes1**   acute disseminated encephalitis and
> encephalomyelitis (G04.0-)

G04.30   Acute necrotizing hemorrhagic encephalopathy, unspecified

G04.31   Postinfectious acute necrotizing hemorrhagic encephalopathy

G04.32   Postimmunization acute necrotizing hemorrhagic encephalopathy
> Use additional code to identify vaccine
> (T50.A-, T50.B-, T50.Z-)

G04.39   Other acute necrotizing hemorrhagic encephalopathy
> Code also underlying etiology, if applicable

● **G04.8   Other encephalitis, myelitis and encephalomyelitis**
> Code also any associated seizure (G40.-, R56.9)

G04.81   Other encephalitis and encephalomyelitis
> Noninfectious acute disseminated
> encephalomyelitis (noninfectious ADEM)

G04.89   Other myelitis

● **G04.9   Encephalitis, myelitis and encephalomyelitis, unspecified**

G04.90   Encephalitis and encephalomyelitis, unspecified
> Ventriculitis (cerebral) NOS

G04.91   Myelitis, unspecified

● **G05   Encephalitis, myelitis and encephalomyelitis in diseases classified elsewhere**
> *Code first underlying disease, such as:*
> human immunodeficiency virus [HIV] disease (B20)
> poliovirus (A80.-)
> suppurative otitis media (H66.01-H66.4)
> trichinellosis (B75)
>
> **Excludes1**   adenoviral encephalitis, myelitis and
> encephalomyelitis (A85.1)
> congenital toxoplasmosis encephalitis, myelitis
> and encephalomyelitis (P37.1)
> cytomegaloviral encephalitis, myelitis and
> encephalomyelitis (B25.8)
> encephalitis, myelitis and encephalomyelitis (in)
> measles (B05.0)
> encephalitis, myelitis and encephalomyelitis (in)
> systemic lupus erythematosus (M32.19)
> enteroviral encephalitis, myelitis and
> encephalomyelitis (A85.0)
> eosinophilic meningoencephalitis (B83.2)
> herpesviral [herpes simplex] encephalitis,
> myelitis and encephalomyelitis (B00.4)
> listerial encephalitis, myelitis and
> encephalomyelitis (A32.12)
> meningococcal encephalitis, myelitis and
> encephalomyelitis (A39.81)
> mumps encephalitis, myelitis and
> encephalomyelitis (B26.2)
> postchickenpox encephalitis, myelitis and
> encephalomyelitis (B01.1-)
> rubella encephalitis, myelitis and
> encephalomyelitis (B06.01)
> toxoplasmosis encephalitis, myelitis and
> encephalomyelitis (B58.2)
> zoster encephalitis, myelitis and
> encephalomyelitis (B02.0)

G05.3   Encephalitis and encephalomyelitis in diseases classified elsewhere
> Meningoencephalitis in diseases classified elsewhere

G05.4   Myelitis in diseases classified elsewhere
> Meningomyelitis in diseases classified elsewhere

● **G06   Intracranial and intraspinal abscess and granuloma**
> *An accumulation of pus in either the brain or spinal cord*
> Use additional code (B95-B97) to identify infectious agent.

G06.0   Intracranial abscess and granuloma
> Brain [any part] abscess (embolic)
> Cerebellar abscess (embolic)
> Cerebral abscess (embolic)
> Intracranial epidural abscess or granuloma
> Intracranial extradural abscess or granuloma
> Intracranial subdural abscess or granuloma
> Otogenic abscess (embolic)
> **Excludes1**   tuberculous intracranial abscess and
> granuloma (A17.81)

G06.1   Intraspinal abscess and granuloma
> Abscess (embolic) of spinal cord [any part]
> Intraspinal epidural abscess or granuloma
> Intraspinal extradural abscess or granuloma
> Intraspinal subdural abscess or granuloma
> **Excludes1**   tuberculous intraspinal abscess and
> granuloma (A17.81)

G06.2   Extradural and subdural abscess, unspecified

CHAPTER 6 (G00-G99)

▶ New   ⮕ Revised   ~~deleted~~ Deleted   **OGCR** Official Guidelines   X Assign placeholder X   ● Use Additional Character(s)

| Excludes 1 | Excludes 2 | Includes | Use additional | Code first | Code also | Key words |

G07   Intracranial and intraspinal abscess and granuloma in diseases classified elsewhere

> *Code first* underlying disease, such as:
> schistosomiasis granuloma of brain (B65.-)
>
> **Excludes1**   abscess of brain:
>   amebic (A06.6)
>   chromomycotic (B43.1)
>   gonococcal (A54.82)
>   tuberculous (A17.81)
>   tuberculoma of meninges (A17.1)

G08   Intracranial and intraspinal phlebitis and thrombophlebitis

> Septic embolism of intracranial or intraspinal venous sinuses and veins
> Septic endophlebitis of intracranial or intraspinal venous sinuses and veins
> Septic phlebitis of intracranial or intraspinal venous sinuses and veins
> Septic thrombophlebitis of intracranial or intraspinal venous sinuses and veins
> Septic thrombosis of intracranial or intraspinal venous sinuses and veins
>
> **Excludes1**   intracranial phlebitis and thrombophlebitis complicating:
>   abortion, ectopic or molar pregnancy (O00-O07, O08.7)
>   pregnancy, childbirth and the puerperium (O22.5, O87.3)
>   nonpyogenic intracranial phlebitis and thrombophlebitis (I67.6)
>
> **Excludes2**   intracranial phlebitis and thrombophlebitis complicating nonpyogenic intraspinal phlebitis and thrombophlebitis (G95.1)

G09   Sequelae of inflammatory diseases of central nervous system

> **Note:**   Category G09 is to be used to indicate conditions whose primary classification is to G00-G08 as the cause of sequelae, themselves classifiable elsewhere. The 'sequelae' include conditions specified as residuals.
>
> *Code first* condition resulting from (sequela) of inflammatory diseases of central nervous system

---

SYSTEMIC ATROPHIES PRIMARILY AFFECTING THE CENTRAL NERVOUS SYSTEM (G10-G14)

G10   Huntington's disease

> *Genetic disease with degeneration of cells of the nervous system, including brain*
> Huntington's chorea
> Huntington's dementia
>
> ▶ Code also dementia in other diseases classified elsewhere without behavioral disturbance (F02.80)

● **G11   Hereditary ataxia**

> *Genetic neurological disorder affecting coordination*
>
> **Excludes2**   cerebral palsy (G80.-)
>   hereditary and idiopathic neuropathy (G60.-)
>   metabolic disorders (E70-E88)

> **G11.0   Congenital nonprogressive ataxia**

> **G11.1   Early-onset cerebellar ataxia**
>   Early-onset cerebellar ataxia with essential tremor
>   Early-onset cerebellar ataxia with myoclonus [Hunt's ataxia]
>   Early-onset cerebellar ataxia with retained tendon reflexes
>   Friedreich's ataxia (autosomal recessive)
>   X-linked recessive spinocerebellar ataxia

> **G11.2   Late-onset cerebellar ataxia**

> **G11.3   Cerebellar ataxia with defective DNA repair**
>   Ataxia telangiectasia [Louis-Bar]
>   **Excludes2**   Cockayne's syndrome (Q87.1)
>   other disorders of purine and pyrimidine metabolism (E79.-)
>   xeroderma pigmentosum (Q82.1)

> **G11.4   Hereditary spastic paraplegia**

> **G11.8   Other hereditary ataxias**

> **G11.9   Hereditary ataxia, unspecified**
>   Hereditary cerebellar ataxia NOS
>   Hereditary cerebellar degeneration
>   Hereditary cerebellar disease
>   Hereditary cerebellar syndrome

● **G12   Spinal muscular atrophy and related syndromes**

> **G12.0   Infantile spinal muscular atrophy, type I [Werdnig-Hoffman]**

> **G12.1   Other inherited spinal muscular atrophy**
>   Adult form spinal muscular atrophy
>   Childhood form, type II spinal muscular atrophy
>   Distal spinal muscular atrophy
>   Juvenile form, type III spinal muscular atrophy [Kugelberg-Welander]
>   Progressive bulbar palsy of childhood [Fazio-Londe]
>   Scapuloperoneal form spinal muscular atrophy

● **G12.2   Motor neuron disease**
> *Progressive disease of motor neurons that carry impulses to muscles to move*

>   **G12.20   Motor neuron disease, unspecified**

>   **G12.21   Amyotrophic lateral sclerosis**
>   *Lou Gehrig's disease (ALS)*
>   ~~Progressive spinal muscle atrophy~~

>   **G12.22   Progressive bulbar palsy**
> ▶   **G12.23   Primary lateral sclerosis**
> ▶   **G12.24   Familial motor neuron disease**
> ▶   **G12.25   Progressive spinal muscle atrophy**
>   **G12.29   Other motor neuron disease**
>   ~~Familial motor neuron disease~~
>   ~~Primary lateral sclerosis~~

> **G12.8   Other spinal muscular atrophies and related syndromes**

> **G12.9   Spinal muscular atrophy, unspecified**

● **G13   Systemic atrophies primarily affecting central nervous system in diseases classified elsewhere**

> **G13.0   Paraneoplastic neuromyopathy and neuropathy**
>   Carcinomatous neuromyopathy
>   Sensorial paraneoplastic neuropathy [Denny Brown]
>   *Code first* underlying neoplasm (C00-D49)

> **G13.1   Other systemic atrophy primarily affecting central nervous system in neoplastic disease**
>   Paraneoplastic limbic encephalopathy
>   *Code first* underlying neoplasm (C00-D49)

> **G13.2   Systemic atrophy primarily affecting the central nervous system in myxedema**
>   *Code first* underlying disease, such as:
>   hypothyroidism (E03.-)
>   myxedematous congenital iodine deficiency (E00.1)

> **G13.8   Systemic atrophy primarily affecting central nervous system in other diseases classified elsewhere**
>   *Code first* underlying disease

G14   Postpolio syndrome

> **Includes**   Postpolio myelitic syndrome
> **Excludes1**   sequelae of poliomyelitis (B91)

Item 6–2 Huntington's chorea is an inherited degenerative disorder of the central nervous system and is characterized by ceaseless, jerky movements and progressive cognitive and behavioral deterioration.

▶ New   ⇒ Revised   ~~deleted~~ Deleted   **OGCR** Official Guidelines   X Assign placeholder X   ● Use Additional Character(s)

Excludes 1   Excludes 2   Includes   Use additional   Code first   Code also   Key words

EXTRAPYRAMIDAL AND MOVEMENT DISORDERS (G20-G26)

G20   Parkinson's disease
Progressive disease of the nervous system that affects muscle coordination
Hemiparkinsonism
Idiopathic Parkinsonism or Parkinson's disease
Paralysis agitans
Parkinsonism or Parkinson's disease NOS
Primary Parkinsonism or Parkinson's disease
> **Excludes1**   dementia with Parkinsonism (G31.83)

● G21   Secondary parkinsonism
Symptoms of Parkinson's caused by medicines, illness, or other nervous system disorder
> **Excludes1**   dementia with Parkinsonism (G31.83)
> Huntington's disease (G10)
> Shy-Drager syndrome (G90.3)
> syphilitic Parkinsonism (A52.19)

G21.0   Malignant neuroleptic syndrome
Use additional code for adverse effect, if applicable, to identify drug (T43.3X5, T43.4X5, T43.505, T43.595)
> **Excludes1**   neuroleptic induced parkinsonism (G21.11)

● G21.1   Other drug-induced secondary parkinsonism

    G21.11   Neuroleptic induced parkinsonism
Use additional code for adverse effect, if applicable, to identify drug (T43.3X5, T43.4X5, T43.505, T43.595)
> **Excludes1**   malignant neuroleptic syndrome (G21.0)

    G21.19   Other drug induced secondary parkinsonism
▶Other medication-induced parkinsonism
Use additional code for adverse effect, if applicable, to identify drug (T36-T50 with fifth or sixth character 5)

G21.2   Secondary parkinsonism due to other external agents
Code first (T51-T65) to identify external agent

G21.3   Postencephalitic parkinsonism
G21.4   Vascular parkinsonism
G21.8   Other secondary parkinsonism
G21.9   Secondary parkinsonism, unspecified

● G23   Other degenerative diseases of basal ganglia
> **Excludes2**   multi-system degeneration of the autonomic nervous system (G90.3)

G23.0   Hallervorden-Spatz disease
Pigmentary pallidal degeneration
G23.1   Progressive supranuclear ophthalmoplegia [Steele-Richardson-Olszewski]
Progressive supranuclear palsy
G23.2   Striatonigral degeneration
G23.8   Other specified degenerative diseases of basal ganglia
Calcification of basal ganglia
G23.9   Degenerative disease of basal ganglia, unspecified

● G24   Dystonia
Involuntary movements
> **Includes**   dyskinesia
> **Excludes2**   athetoid cerebral palsy (G80.3)

● G24.0   Drug induced dystonia
Use additional code for adverse effect, if applicable, to identify drug (T36-T50 with fifth or sixth character 5)

    G24.01   Drug induced subacute dyskinesia
Drug induced blepharospasm
Drug induced orofacial dyskinesia
Neuroleptic induced tardive dyskinesia
Tardive dyskinesia

    G24.02   Drug induced acute dystonia
Acute dystonic reaction to drugs
Neuroleptic induced acute dystonia

    G24.09   Other drug induced dystonia

G24.1   Genetic torsion dystonia
Dystonia deformans progressiva
Dystonia musculorum deformans
Familial torsion dystonia
Idiopathic familial dystonia
Idiopathic (torsion) dystonia NOS
(Schwalbe-) Ziehen-Oppenheim disease

G24.2   Idiopathic nonfamilial dystonia

G24.3   Spasmodic torticollis
Head tilts toward one side and chin is elevated and turned toward opposite side (wry neck)
> **Excludes1**   congenital torticollis (Q68.0)
> hysterical torticollis (F44.4)
> ocular torticollis (R29.891)
> psychogenic torticollis (F45.8)
> torticollis NOS (M43.6)
> traumatic recurrent torticollis (S13.4)

G24.4   Idiopathic orofacial dystonia
Orofacial dyskinesia
> **Excludes1**   drug induced orofacial dyskinesia (G24.01)

G24.5   Blepharospasm
Tonic spasm of orbicularis oculi muscle, producing closure of eyelids
> **Excludes1**   drug induced blepharospasm (G24.01)

G24.8   Other dystonia
Acquired torsion dystonia NOS

G24.9   Dystonia, unspecified
Dyskinesia NOS

● G25   Other extrapyramidal and movement disorders
Extrapyramidal: Other than pyramidal tracts
> **Excludes2**   sleep related movement disorders (G47.6-)

G25.0   Essential tremor
Familial tremor
> **Excludes1**   tremor NOS (R25.1)

G25.1   Drug-induced tremor
Use additional code for adverse effect, if applicable, to identify drug (T36-T50 with fifth or sixth character 5)

G25.2   Other specified forms of tremor
Intention tremor

G25.3   Myoclonus
Shocklike contractions muscle(s)
Drug-induced myoclonus
Palatal myoclonus
Use additional code for adverse effect, if applicable, to identify drug (T36-T50 with fifth or sixth character 5)
> **Excludes1**   facial myokymia (G51.4)
> myoclonic epilepsy (G40.-)

G25.4   Drug-induced chorea
Use additional code for adverse effect, if applicable, to identify drug (T36-T50 with fifth or sixth character 5)

G25.5   Other chorea
Continual, involuntary, jerky, movements
Chorea NOS
> **Excludes1**   chorea NOS with heart involvement (I02.0)
> Huntington's chorea (G10)
> rheumatic chorea (I02.-)
> Sydenham's chorea (I02.-)

● G25.6   Drug induced tics and other tics of organic origin

    G25.61   Drug induced tics
Use additional code for adverse effect, if applicable, to identify drug (T36-T50 with fifth or sixth character 5)

    G25.69   Other tics of organic origin
> **Excludes1**   habit spasm (F95.9)
> tic NOS (F95.9)
> Tourette's syndrome (F95.2)

CHAPTER 6 (G00-G99)

▶ New   ⟹ Revised   ~~deleted~~ Deleted   **OGCR** Official Guidelines   X Assign placeholder X   ● Use Additional Character(s)

| Excludes 1 | Excludes 2 | Includes | Use additional | Code first | Code also | Key words |

● **G25.7 Other and unspecified drug induced movement disorders**

> Use additional code for adverse effect, if applicable, to identify drug (T36-T50 with fifth or sixth character 5)

    G25.70 Drug induced movement disorder, unspecified

    G25.71 Drug induced akathisia
        Drug induced acathisia
        Neuroleptic induced acute akathisia
        ▶Tardive akathisia

    G25.79 Other drug induced movement disorders

● **G25.8 Other specified extrapyramidal and movement disorders**

    G25.81 Restless legs syndrome

    G25.82 Stiff-man syndrome

    G25.83 Benign shuddering attacks

    G25.89 Other specified extrapyramidal and movement disorders

G25.9 Extrapyramidal and movement disorder, unspecified

G26 Extrapyramidal and movement disorders in diseases classified elsewhere

> *Code first* underlying disease

OTHER DEGENERATIVE DISEASES OF THE NERVOUS SYSTEM (G30-G32)

● **G30 Alzheimer's disease**

> *Progressive central neurodegenerative disorder*

> **Includes** Alzheimer's dementia senile and presenile forms

> Use additional code to identify:
>   delirium, if applicable (F05)
>   dementia with behavioral disturbance (F02.81)
>   dementia without behavioral disturbance (F02.80)

> **Excludes1** senile degeneration of brain NEC (G31.1)
>   senile dementia NOS (F03)
>   senility NOS (R41.81)

G30.0 Alzheimer's disease with early onset

G30.1 Alzheimer's disease with late onset

G30.8 Other Alzheimer's disease

G30.9 Alzheimer's disease, unspecified

● **G31 Other degenerative diseases of nervous system, not elsewhere classified**

> Use additional code to identify:
>   dementia with behavioral disturbance (F02.81)
>   dementia without behavioral disturbance (F02.80)

> **Excludes2** Reye's syndrome (G93.7)

● **G31.Ø Frontotemporal dementia**

    G31.Ø1 Pick's disease
        Primary progressive aphasia
        Progressive isolated aphasia

    G31.Ø9 Other frontotemporal dementia
        Frontal dementia

G31.1 Senile degeneration of brain, not elsewhere classified

> **Excludes1** Alzheimer's disease (G3Ø.-)
>   senility NOS (R41.81)

G31.2 Degeneration of nervous system due to alcohol
    Alcoholic cerebellar ataxia
    Alcoholic cerebellar degeneration
    Alcoholic cerebral degeneration
    Alcoholic encephalopathy
    Dysfunction of the autonomic nervous system due to alcohol

> Code also associated alcoholism (F1Ø.-)

● **G31.8 Other specified degenerative diseases of nervous system**

    G31.81 Alpers' disease
>   *Rare neuronal degeneration of cerebral cortex disease of young children*
        Grey-matter degeneration

    G31.82 Leigh's disease
>   *Rare neurometabolic disorder that affects central nervous system*
        Subacute necrotizing encephalopathy

    G31.83 Dementia with Lewy bodies
>   *Closely allied to Parkinson's Disease*
        Dementia with Parkinsonism
        Lewy body dementia
        Lewy body disease

    G31.84 Mild cognitive impairment, so stated
        ▶Mild neurocognitive disorder

> **Excludes1** age related cognitive decline (R41.81)
>   altered mental status (R41.82)
>   cerebral degeneration (G31.9)
>   change in mental status (R41.82)
>   cognitive deficits following (sequelae of) cerebral hemorrhage or infarction (I69.Ø1-, I69.11-, I69.21-, I69.31-, I69.81-, I69.91-)
>   cognitive impairment due to intracranial or head injury (SØ6.-)
>   dementia (FØ1.-, FØ2.-, FØ3)
>   mild memory disturbance (FØ6.8)
>   neurologic neglect syndrome (R41.4)
>   personality change, nonpsychotic (F68.8)

    G31.85 Corticobasal degeneration

    G31.89 Other specified degenerative diseases of nervous system

G31.9 Degenerative disease of nervous system, unspecified

● **G32 Other degenerative disorders of nervous system in diseases classified elsewhere**

    G32.Ø Subacute combined degeneration of spinal cord in diseases classified elsewhere
        Dana-Putnam syndrome
        Sclerosis of spinal cord (combined) (dorsolateral) (posterolateral)

>   *Code first* underlying disease, such as:
>   anemia (D51.9)
>   dietary (D51.3)
>   pernicious (D51.Ø)
>   vitamin B12 deficiency (E53.8)

> **Excludes1** syphilitic combined degeneration of spinal cord (A52.11)

● **G32.8   Other specified degenerative disorders of nervous system in diseases classified elsewhere**
Code first underlying disease, such as:
amyloidosis cerebral degeneration (E85.-)
cerebral degeneration (due to) hypothyroidism (E00.0-E03.9)
cerebral degeneration (due to) neoplasm (C00-D49)
cerebral degeneration (due to) vitamin B deficiency, except thiamine (E52-E53.-)
| Excludes1 | superior hemorrhagic polioencephalitis [Wernicke's encephalopathy] (E51.2) |

G32.81   Cerebellar ataxia in diseases classified elsewhere
Code first underlying disease, such as:
celiac disease (with gluten ataxia) (K90.0)
cerebellar ataxia (in) neoplastic disease (paraneoplastic cerebellar degeneration) (C00-D49)
non-celiac gluten ataxia (M35.9)
| Excludes1 | systemic atrophy primarily affecting the central nervous system in alcoholic cerebellar ataxia (G31.2) |
| | systemic atrophy primarily affecting the central nervous system in myxedema (G13.2) |

G32.89   Other specified degenerative disorders of nervous system in diseases classified elsewhere
Degenerative encephalopathy in diseases classified elsewhere

DEMYELINATING DISEASES OF THE CENTRAL NERVOUS SYSTEM (G35-G37)

G35   Multiple sclerosis
Destruction of central nervous system; four types: relapsing remitting, secondary progressive, primary progressive, and progressive relapsing
Disseminated multiple sclerosis
Generalized multiple sclerosis
Multiple sclerosis NOS
Multiple sclerosis of brain stem
Multiple sclerosis of cord

● **G36   Other acute disseminated demyelination**
| Excludes1 | postinfectious encephalitis and encephalomyelitis NOS (G04.01) |

G36.0   Neuromyelitis optica [Devic]
Inflammatory disorder in which immune system attacks optic nerves and spinal cord producing inflammation of optic nerve (optic neuritis) and spinal cord (myelitis)
Demyelination in optic neuritis
| Excludes1 | optic neuritis NOS (H46) |

G36.1   Acute and subacute hemorrhagic leukoencephalitis [Hurst]

G36.8   Other specified acute disseminated demyelination

G36.9   Acute disseminated demyelination, unspecified

● **G37   Other demyelinating diseases of central nervous system**
Destruction of central nervous system

G37.0   Diffuse sclerosis of central nervous system
Periaxial encephalitis
Schilder's disease
| Excludes1 | X linked adrenoleukodystrophy (E71.52-) |

G37.1   Central demyelination of corpus callosum

G37.2   Central pontine myelinolysis

G37.3   Acute transverse myelitis in demyelinating disease of central nervous system
Acute transverse myelitis NOS
Acute transverse myelopathy
| Excludes1 | multiple sclerosis (G35) |
| | neuromyelitis optica [Devic] (G36.0) |

G37.4   Subacute necrotizing myelitis of central nervous system

G37.5   Concentric sclerosis [Baló] of central nervous system

G37.8   Other specified demyelinating diseases of central nervous system

G37.9   Demyelinating disease of central nervous system, unspecified

EPISODIC AND PAROXYSMAL DISORDERS (G40-G47)

● **G40   Epilepsy and recurrent seizures**
Note: The following terms are to be considered equivalent to intractable: pharmacoresistant (pharmacologically resistant), treatment resistant, refractory (medically) and poorly controlled
Excludes1	conversion disorder with seizures (F44.5)
	convulsions NOS (R56.9)
	post traumatic seizures (R56.1)
	seizure (convulsive) NOS (R56.9)
	seizure of newborn (P90)
Excludes2	hippocampal sclerosis (G93.81)
	mesial temporal sclerosis (G93.81)
	temporal sclerosis (G93.81)
	Todd's paralysis (G83.84)

● **G40.0   Localization-related (focal) (partial) idiopathic epilepsy and epileptic syndromes with seizures of localized onset**
Benign childhood epilepsy with centrotemporal EEG spikes
Childhood epilepsy with occipital EEG paroxysms
| Excludes1 | adult onset localization-related epilepsy (G40.1-, G40.2-) |

● **G40.00   Localization-related (focal) (partial) idiopathic epilepsy and epileptic syndromes with seizures of localized onset, not intractable**
Localization-related (focal) (partial) idiopathic epilepsy and epileptic syndromes with seizures of localized onset without intractability

G40.001   Localization-related (focal) (partial) idiopathic epilepsy and epileptic syndromes with seizures of localized onset, not intractable, with status epilepticus

G40.009   Localization-related (focal) (partial) idiopathic epilepsy and epileptic syndromes with seizures of localized onset, not intractable, without status epilepticus
Localization-related (focal) (partial) idiopathic epilepsy and epileptic syndromes with seizures of localized onset NOS

● **G40.01   Localization-related (focal) (partial) idiopathic epilepsy and epileptic syndromes with seizures of localized onset, intractable**

G40.011   Localization-related (focal) (partial) idiopathic epilepsy and epileptic syndromes with seizures of localized onset, intractable, with status epilepticus

G40.019   Localization-related (focal) (partial) idiopathic epilepsy and epileptic syndromes with seizures of localized onset, intractable, without status epilepticus

Item 6-3   Multiple sclerosis (MS) is a nervous system disease affecting the brain and spinal cord by damaging the myelin sheath surrounding and protecting nerve cells. The damage slows down/blocks messages between the brain and body. Symptoms are: visual disturbances, muscle weakness, coordination and balance issues, numbness, prickling, thinking and memory problems. The cause is unknown, though it is thought that it may be an autoimmune disease. It affects women more than men, between 20 and 40 years of age. MS can be mild, but it may cause the loss of ability to write, walk, and speak. There is no cure, but medication may slow or control symptoms.

CHAPTER 6 (G00-G99)

▶ New   ⇒ Revised   ~~deleted~~ Deleted   **OGCR** Official Guidelines   X Assign placeholder X   ● Use Additional Character(s)

| Excludes 1 | Excludes 2 | Includes | Use additional | Code first | Code also | Key words |

CHAPTER 6 (G00-G99)

● **G40.1   Localization-related (focal) (partial) symptomatic epilepsy and epileptic syndromes with simple** partial seizures

Attacks without alteration of consciousness
Epilepsia partialis continua [Kozhevnikof]
Simple partial seizures developing into secondarily generalized seizures

    ● **G40.10   Localization-related (focal) (partial) symptomatic epilepsy and epileptic syndromes with simple partial seizures,** not intractable

        Localization-related (focal) (partial) symptomatic epilepsy and epileptic syndromes with simple partial seizures without intractability

        G40.101   Localization-related (focal) (partial) symptomatic epilepsy and epileptic syndromes with simple partial seizures, not intractable, with status epilepticus

        G40.109   Localization-related (focal) (partial) symptomatic epilepsy and epileptic syndromes with simple partial seizures, not intractable, without status epilepticus

            Localization-related (focal) (partial) symptomatic epilepsy and epileptic syndromes with simple partial seizures NOS

    ● **G40.11   Localization-related (focal) (partial) symptomatic epilepsy and epileptic syndromes with simple partial seizures,** intractable

        G40.111   Localization-related (focal) (partial) symptomatic epilepsy and epileptic syndromes with simple partial seizures, intractable, with status epilepticus

        G40.119   Localization-related (focal) (partial) symptomatic epilepsy and epileptic syndromes with simple partial seizures, intractable, without status epilepticus

● **G40.2   Localization-related (focal) (partial) symptomatic epilepsy and epileptic syndromes with complex** partial seizures

Attacks with alteration of consciousness, often with automatisms
Complex partial seizures developing into secondarily generalized seizures

    ● **G40.20   Localization-related (focal) (partial) symptomatic epilepsy and epileptic syndromes with complex partial seizures,** not intractable

        Localization-related (focal) (partial) symptomatic epilepsy and epileptic syndromes with complex partial seizures without intractability

        G40.201   Localization-related (focal) (partial) symptomatic epilepsy and epileptic syndromes with complex partial seizures, not intractable, with status epilepticus

        G40.209   Localization-related (focal) (partial) symptomatic epilepsy and epileptic syndromes with complex partial seizures, not intractable, without status epilepticus

            Localization-related (focal) (partial) symptomatic epilepsy and epileptic syndromes with complex partial seizures NOS

    ● **G40.21   Localization-related (focal) (partial) symptomatic epilepsy and epileptic syndromes with complex partial seizures,** intractable

        G40.211   Localization-related (focal) (partial) symptomatic epilepsy and epileptic syndromes with complex partial seizures, intractable, with status epilepticus

        G40.219   Localization-related (focal) (partial) symptomatic epilepsy and epileptic syndromes with complex partial seizures, intractable, without status epilepticus

● **G40.3   ** Generalized **idiopathic epilepsy and epileptic syndromes**

Code also MERRF syndrome, if applicable (E88.42)

    ● **G40.30   Generalized idiopathic epilepsy and epileptic syndromes,** not intractable

        Generalized idiopathic epilepsy and epileptic syndromes without intractability

        G40.301   Generalized idiopathic epilepsy and epileptic syndromes, not intractable, with status epilepticus

        G40.309   Generalized idiopathic epilepsy and epileptic syndromes, not intractable, without status epilepticus

            Generalized idiopathic epilepsy and epileptic syndromes NOS

    ● **G40.31   Generalized idiopathic epilepsy and epileptic syndromes,** intractable

        G40.311   Generalized idiopathic epilepsy and epileptic syndromes, intractable, with status epilepticus

        G40.319   Generalized idiopathic epilepsy and epileptic syndromes, intractable, without status epilepticus

● **G40.A   ** Absence **epileptic syndrome**

Childhood absence epilepsy [pyknolepsy]
Juvenile absence epilepsy
Absence epileptic syndrome, NOS

    ● **G40.A0   Absence epileptic syndrome,** not intractable

        G40.A01   Absence epileptic syndrome, not intractable, with status epilepticus

        G40.A09   Absence epileptic syndrome, not intractable, without status epilepticus

    ● **G40.A1   Absence epileptic syndrome,** intractable

        G40.A11   Absence epileptic syndrome, intractable, with status epilepticus

        G40.A19   Absence epileptic syndrome, intractable, without status epilepticus

● **G40.B   ** Juvenile myoclonic **epilepsy [impulsive petit mal]**

    ● **G40.B0   Juvenile myoclonic epilepsy,** not intractable

        G40.B01   Juvenile myoclonic epilepsy, not intractable, with status epilepticus

        G40.B09   Juvenile myoclonic epilepsy, not intractable, without status epilepticus

    ● **G40.B1   Juvenile myoclonic epilepsy,** intractable

        G40.B11   Juvenile myoclonic epilepsy, intractable, with status epilepticus

        G40.B19   Juvenile myoclonic epilepsy, intractable, without status epilepticus

▶ New   ⇛ Revised   ~~deleted~~ Deleted   **OGCR** Official Guidelines   X Assign placeholder X   ● Use Additional Character(s)

Excludes 1   Excludes 2   Includes   Use additional   Code first   Code also   Key words

● **G40.4 Other generalized epilepsy and epileptic syndromes**
     Epilepsy with grand mal seizures on awakening
     Epilepsy with myoclonic absences
     Epilepsy with myoclonic-astatic seizures
     Grand mal seizure NOS
     Nonspecific atonic epileptic seizures
     Nonspecific clonic epileptic seizures
     Nonspecific myoclonic epileptic seizures
     Nonspecific tonic epileptic seizures
     Nonspecific tonic-clonic epileptic seizures
     Symptomatic early myoclonic encephalopathy

     ● **G40.40 Other generalized epilepsy and epileptic syndromes, not intractable**
         Other generalized epilepsy and epileptic syndromes without intractability
         Other generalized epilepsy and epileptic syndromes NOS

         G40.401 Other generalized epilepsy and epileptic syndromes, not intractable, with status epilepticus

         G40.409 Other generalized epilepsy and epileptic syndromes, not intractable, without status epilepticus

     ● **G40.41 Other generalized epilepsy and epileptic syndromes, intractable**

         G40.411 Other generalized epilepsy and epileptic syndromes, intractable, with status epilepticus

         G40.419 Other generalized epilepsy and epileptic syndromes, intractable, without status epilepticus

● **G40.5 Epileptic seizures related to external causes**
     Epileptic seizures related to alcohol
     Epileptic seizures related to drugs
     Epileptic seizures related to hormonal changes
     Epileptic seizures related to sleep deprivation
     Epileptic seizures related to stress
     Code also, if applicable, associated epilepsy and recurrent seizures (G40.-)
     Use additional code for adverse effect, if applicable, to identify drug (T36-T50 with fifth or sixth character 5)

     ● **G40.50 Epileptic seizures related to external causes, not intractable**

         G40.501 Epileptic seizures related to external causes, not intractable, with status epilepticus

         G40.509 Epileptic seizures related to external causes, not intractable, without status epilepticus
            Epileptic seizures related to external causes, NOS

● **G40.8 Other epilepsy and recurrent seizures**
     Epilepsies and epileptic syndromes undetermined as to whether they are focal or generalized
     Landau-Kleffner syndrome

     ● **G40.80 Other epilepsy**

         G40.801 Other epilepsy, not intractable, with status epilepticus
            Other epilepsy without intractability with status epilepticus

         G40.802 Other epilepsy, not intractable, without status epilepticus
            Other epilepsy NOS
            Other epilepsy without intractability without status epilepticus

         G40.803 Other epilepsy, intractable, with status epilepticus

         G40.804 Other epilepsy, intractable, without status epilepticus

● **G40.81 Lennox-Gastaut syndrome**

         G40.811 Lennox-Gastaut syndrome, not intractable, with status epilepticus

         G40.812 Lennox-Gastaut syndrome, not intractable, without status epilepticus

         G40.813 Lennox-Gastaut syndrome, intractable, with status epilepticus

         G40.814 Lennox-Gastaut syndrome, intractable, without status epilepticus

● **G40.82 Epileptic spasms**
     Infantile spasms
     Salaam attacks
     West's syndrome

         G40.821 Epileptic spasms, not intractable, with status epilepticus

         G40.822 Epileptic spasms, not intractable, without status epilepticus

         G40.823 Epileptic spasms, intractable, with status epilepticus

         G40.824 Epileptic spasms, intractable, without status epilepticus

     G40.89 Other seizures
         Excludes1   post traumatic seizures (R56.1)
                    recurrent seizures NOS (G40.909)
                    seizure NOS (R56.9)

● **G40.9 Epilepsy, unspecified**

     ● **G40.90 Epilepsy, unspecified, not intractable**
         Epilepsy, unspecified, without intractability

         G40.901 Epilepsy, unspecified, not intractable, with status epilepticus

         G40.909 Epilepsy, unspecified, not intractable, without status epilepticus
            Epilepsy NOS
            Epileptic convulsions NOS
            Epileptic fits NOS
            Epileptic seizures NOS
            Recurrent seizures NOS
            Seizure disorder NOS

     ● **G40.91 Epilepsy, unspecified, intractable**
         Intractable seizure disorder NOS

         G40.911 Epilepsy, unspecified, intractable, with status epilepticus

         G40.919 Epilepsy, unspecified, intractable, without status epilepticus

● **G43 Migraine**
     Note: The following terms are to be considered equivalent to intractable: pharmacoresistant (pharmacologically resistant), treatment resistant, refractory (medically) and poorly controlled
     Use additional code for adverse effect, if applicable, to identify drug (T36-T50 with fifth or sixth character 5)
     Excludes1   headache NOS (R51)
                  lower half migraine (G44.00)
     Excludes2   headache syndromes (G44.-)

● **G43.0 Migraine without aura**
     Neurological disorder, generally recurring headaches without early symptom (aura)
     Common migraine
     Excludes1   chronic migraine without aura (G43.7-)

     ● **G43.00 Migraine without aura, not intractable**
         Neurological disorder, generally recurring headaches without early symptom (aura); resistant to cure, relief, or control
         Migraine without aura without mention of refractory migraine

         G43.001 Migraine without aura, not intractable, with status migrainosus

         G43.009 Migraine without aura, not intractable, without status migrainosus
            Migraine without aura NOS

Item 6–4 Migraine headache is described as an intense pulsing or throbbing pain in one area of the head. It can be accompanied by extreme sensitivity to light (photophobic) and sound and is three times more common in women than in men. Symptoms include nausea and vomiting. Research indicates migraine headaches are caused by inherited abnormalities in genes that control the activities of certain cell populations in the brain.

● **G43.Ø1   Migraine without aura, intractable**
> *Intractable migraine: Not easily cured or managed; relentless pain from a migraine*
> Migraine without aura with refractory migraine

    G43.Ø11   Migraine without aura, intractable, with status migrainosus

    G43.Ø19   Migraine without aura, intractable, without status migrainosus

● **G43.1   Migraine with aura**
> Basilar migraine
> Classical migraine
> Migraine equivalents
> Migraine preceded or accompanied by transient focal neurological phenomena
> Migraine triggered seizures
> Migraine with acute-onset aura
> Migraine with aura without headache (migraine equivalents)
> Migraine with prolonged aura
> Migraine with typical aura
> Retinal migraine
>
> Code also any associated seizure (G40.-, R56.9)
>
> **Excludes1**   persistent migraine aura (G43.5-, G43.6-)

● **G43.1Ø   Migraine with aura, not intractable**
> Migraine with aura without mention of refractory migraine

    G43.1Ø1   Migraine with aura, not intractable, with status migrainosus

    G43.1Ø9   Migraine with aura, not intractable, without status migrainosus
> Migraine with aura NOS

● **G43.11   Migraine with aura, intractable**
> Migraine with aura with refractory migraine

    G43.111   Migraine with aura, intractable, with status migrainosus

    G43.119   Migraine with aura, intractable, without status migrainosus

● **G43.4   Hemiplegic migraine**
> *Inherited migraine disorder causing temporary paralysis of one side of body followed by severe headache and nausea*
> Familial migraine
> Sporadic migraine

● **G43.4Ø   Hemiplegic migraine, not intractable**
> Hemiplegic migraine without refractory migraine

    G43.4Ø1   Hemiplegic migraine, not intractable, with status migrainosus

    G43.4Ø9   Hemiplegic migraine, not intractable, without status migrainosus
> Hemiplegic migraine NOS

● **G43.41   Hemiplegic migraine, intractable**
> Hemiplegic migraine with refractory migraine

    G43.411   Hemiplegic migraine, intractable, with status migrainosus

    G43.419   Hemiplegic migraine, intractable, without status migrainosus

● **G43.5   Persistent migraine aura without cerebral infarction**

● **G43.5Ø   Persistent migraine aura without cerebral infarction, not intractable**
> Persistent migraine aura without cerebral infarction, without refractory migraine

    G43.5Ø1   Persistent migraine aura without cerebral infarction, not intractable, with status migrainosus

    G43.5Ø9   Persistent migraine aura without cerebral infarction, not intractable, without status migrainosus
> Persistent migraine aura NOS

● **G43.51   Persistent migraine aura without cerebral infarction, intractable**
> Persistent migraine aura without cerebral infarction, with refractory migraine

    G43.511   Persistent migraine aura without cerebral infarction, intractable, with status migrainosus

    G43.519   Persistent migraine aura without cerebral infarction, intractable, without status migrainosus

● **G43.6   Persistent migraine aura with cerebral infarction**
> *Visual, motor, or psychic disturbances, paresthesias, and related neurologic abnormalities accompanying migraine*
> Code also the type of cerebral infarction (I63.-)

● **G43.6Ø   Persistent migraine aura with cerebral infarction, not intractable**
> Persistent migraine aura with cerebral infarction, without refractory migraine

    G43.6Ø1   Persistent migraine aura with cerebral infarction, not intractable, with status migrainosus

    G43.6Ø9   Persistent migraine aura with cerebral infarction, not intractable, without status migrainosus

● **G43.61   Persistent migraine aura with cerebral infarction, intractable**
> Persistent migraine aura with cerebral infarction, with refractory migraine

    G43.611   Persistent migraine aura with cerebral infarction, intractable, with status migrainosus

    G43.619   Persistent migraine aura with cerebral infarction, intractable, without status migrainosus

● **G43.7   Chronic migraine without aura**
> Transformed migraine
>
> **Excludes1**   migraine without aura (G43.Ø-)

● **G43.7Ø   Chronic migraine without aura, not intractable**
> Chronic migraine without aura, without refractory migraine

    G43.7Ø1   Chronic migraine without aura, not intractable, with status migrainosus

    G43.7Ø9   Chronic migraine without aura, not intractable, without status migrainosus
> Chronic migraine without aura NOS

● **G43.71   Chronic migraine without aura, intractable**
> Chronic migraine without aura, with refractory migraine

    G43.711   Chronic migraine without aura, intractable, with status migrainosus

    G43.719   Chronic migraine without aura, intractable, without status migrainosus

▶ New   ⥤ Revised   ~~deleted~~ Deleted   **OGCR** Official Guidelines   X Assign placeholder X   ● Use Additional Character(s)

Excludes 1   Excludes 2   Includes   Use additional   Code first   Code also   Key words

● **G43.A   Cyclical vomiting**
    G43.A0   Cyclical vomiting, not intractable
        Cyclical vomiting, without refractory migraine
    G43.A1   Cyclical vomiting, intractable
        Cyclical vomiting, with refractory migraine
● **G43.B   Ophthalmoplegic migraine**
    G43.B0   Ophthalmoplegic migraine, not intractable
        Ophthalmoplegic migraine, without refractory migraine
    G43.B1   Ophthalmoplegic migraine, intractable
        Ophthalmoplegic migraine, with refractory migraine
● **G43.C   Periodic headache syndromes in child or adult**
    G43.C0   Periodic headache syndromes in child or adult, not intractable
        Periodic headache syndromes in child or adult, without refractory migraine
    G43.C1   Periodic headache syndromes in child or adult, intractable
        Periodic headache syndromes in child or adult, with refractory migraine
● **G43.D   Abdominal migraine**
    G43.D0   Abdominal migraine, not intractable
        Abdominal migraine, without refractory migraine
    G43.D1   Abdominal migraine, intractable
        Abdominal migraine, with refractory migraine
● **G43.8   Other migraine**
    ● **G43.80   Other migraine, not intractable**
        Other migraine, without refractory migraine
        G43.801   Other migraine, not intractable, with status migrainosus
        G43.809   Other migraine, not intractable, without status migrainosus
    ● **G43.81   Other migraine, intractable**
        Other migraine, with refractory migraine
        G43.811   Other migraine, intractable, with status migrainosus
        G43.819   Other migraine, intractable, without status migrainosus
    ● **G43.82   Menstrual migraine, not intractable**
        Menstrual headache, not intractable
        Menstrual migraine, without refractory migraine
        Menstrually related migraine, not intractable
        Pre-menstrual headache, not intractable
        Pre-menstrual migraine, not intractable
        Pure menstrual migraine, not intractable
        Code also associated premenstrual tension syndrome (N94.3)
        G43.821   Menstrual migraine, not intractable, with status migrainosus
        G43.829   Menstrual migraine, not intractable, without status migrainosus
            Menstrual migraine NOS
    ● **G43.83   Menstrual migraine, intractable**
        Menstrual headache, intractable
        Menstrual migraine, with refractory migraine
        Menstrually related migraine, intractable
        Pre-menstrual headache, intractable
        Pre-menstrual migraine, intractable
        Pure menstrual migraine, intractable
        Code also associated premenstrual tension syndrome (N94.3)
        G43.831   Menstrual migraine, intractable, with status migrainosus
        G43.839   Menstrual migraine, intractable, without status migrainosus

● **G43.9   Migraine, unspecified**
    ● **G43.90   Migraine, unspecified, not intractable**
        Migraine, unspecified, without refractory migraine
        G43.901   Migraine, unspecified, not intractable, with status migrainosus
            Status migrainosus NOS
        G43.909   Migraine, unspecified, not intractable, without status migrainosus
            Migraine NOS
    ● **G43.91   Migraine, unspecified, intractable**
        Migraine, unspecified, with refractory migraine
        G43.911   Migraine, unspecified, intractable, with status migrainosus
        G43.919   Migraine, unspecified, intractable, without status migrainosus

● **G44   Other headache syndromes**
    Excludes1   headache NOS (R51)
    Excludes2   atypical facial pain (G50.1)
        headache due to lumbar puncture (G97.1)
        migraines (G43.-)
        trigeminal neuralgia (G50.0)
● **G44.0   Cluster headaches and other trigeminal autonomic cephalgias (TAC)**
    ● **G44.00   Cluster headache syndrome, unspecified**
        Ciliary neuralgia
        Cluster headache NOS
        Histamine cephalgia
        Lower half migraine
        Migrainous neuralgia
        G44.001   Cluster headache syndrome, unspecified, intractable
        G44.009   Cluster headache syndrome, unspecified, not intractable
            Cluster headache syndrome NOS
    ● **G44.01   Episodic cluster headache**
        G44.011   Episodic cluster headache, intractable
        G44.019   Episodic cluster headache, not intractable
            Episodic cluster headache NOS
    ● **G44.02   Chronic cluster headache**
        G44.021   Chronic cluster headache, intractable
        G44.029   Chronic cluster headache, not intractable
            Chronic cluster headache NOS
    ● **G44.03   Episodic paroxysmal hemicrania**
        Paroxysmal hemicrania NOS
        G44.031   Episodic paroxysmal hemicrania, intractable
        G44.039   Episodic paroxysmal hemicrania, not intractable
            Episodic paroxysmal hemicrania NOS
    ● **G44.04   Chronic paroxysmal hemicrania**
        Unilateral headache
        G44.041   Chronic paroxysmal hemicrania, intractable
        G44.049   Chronic paroxysmal hemicrania, not intractable
            Chronic paroxysmal hemicrania NOS

CHAPTER 6 (G00-G99)

● **G44.05** **Short lasting unilateral** neuralgiform headache with conjunctival injection and tearing (SUNCT)

     G44.051 Short lasting unilateral neuralgiform headache with conjunctival injection and tearing (SUNCT), **intractable**

     G44.059 Short lasting unilateral neuralgiform headache with conjunctival injection and tearing (SUNCT), **not intractable**

         Short lasting unilateral neuralgiform headache with conjunctival injection and tearing (SUNCT) NOS

● **G44.09** **Other** trigeminal autonomic cephalgias (TAC)

     Cluster headaches

     G44.091 Other trigeminal autonomic cephalgias (TAC), **intractable**

     G44.099 Other trigeminal autonomic cephalgias (TAC), **not intractable**

G44.1 **Vascular** headache, not elsewhere classified

     Excludes2   cluster headache (G44.0)
complicated headache syndromes (G44.5-)
drug-induced headache (G44.4-)
migraine (G43.-)
other specified headache syndromes (G44.8-)
post-traumatic headache (G44.3-)
tension-type headache (G44.2-)

● **G44.2** **Tension-type** headache

 ● **G44.20** Tension-type headache, **unspecified**

     G44.201 Tension-type headache, unspecified, **intractable**

     G44.209 Tension-type headache, unspecified, **not intractable**

         Tension headache NOS

 ● **G44.21** **Episodic** tension-type headache

     G44.211 Episodic tension-type headache, **intractable**

     G44.219 Episodic tension-type headache, **not intractable**

         Episodic tension-type headache NOS

 ● **G44.22** **Chronic** tension-type headache

     G44.221 Chronic tension-type headache, **intractable**

     G44.229 Chronic tension-type headache, **not intractable**

         Chronic tension-type headache NOS

● **G44.3** **Post-traumatic** headache

 ● **G44.30** Post-traumatic headache, **unspecified**

     G44.301 Post-traumatic headache, unspecified, **intractable**

     G44.309 Post-traumatic headache, unspecified, **not intractable**

         Post-traumatic headache NOS

 ● **G44.31** **Acute** post-traumatic headache

     G44.311 Acute post-traumatic headache, **intractable**

     G44.319 Acute post-traumatic headache, **not intractable**

         Acute post-traumatic headache NOS

 ● **G44.32** **Chronic** post-traumatic headache

     G44.321 Chronic post-traumatic headache, **intractable**

     G44.329 Chronic post-traumatic headache, **not intractable**

         Chronic post-traumatic headache NOS

● **G44.4** **Drug-induced** headache, not elsewhere classified

     Medication overuse headache

     Use additional code for adverse effect, if applicable, to identify drug (T36-T50 with fifth or sixth character 5)

     G44.40 Drug-induced headache, not elsewhere classified, **not intractable**

     G44.41 Drug-induced headache, not elsewhere classified, **intractable**

● **G44.5** **Complicated** headache syndromes

     G44.51 Hemicrania continua

         Persistent unilateral headache

     G44.52 New daily persistent headache (NDPH)

     G44.53 Primary thunderclap headache

     G44.59 Other complicated headache syndrome

● **G44.8** **Other** specified headache syndromes

     G44.81 **Hypnic** headache

         Benign primary headaches

     G44.82 Headache associated with **sexual activity**

         Orgasmic headache
         Preorgasmic headache

     G44.83 Primary **cough** headache

     G44.84 Primary **exertional** headache

     G44.85 Primary **stabbing** headache

     G44.89 **Other** headache syndrome

● **G45** **Transient cerebral ischemic attacks and related syndromes**

     Excludes1   neonatal cerebral ischemia (P91.0)
transient retinal artery occlusion (H34.0-)

     G45.0 Vertebro-basilar artery syndrome

     G45.1 Carotid artery syndrome (hemispheric)

     G45.2 Multiple and bilateral precerebral artery syndromes

     G45.3 Amaurosis fugax

         Transient visual loss in one eye

     G45.4 Transient global amnesia

         Episode of short-term memory loss, nonrecurrent, lasting few hours

         Excludes1   amnesia NOS (R41.3)

     G45.8 Other transient cerebral ischemic attacks and related syndromes

     G45.9 Transient cerebral ischemic attack, **unspecified**

         Spasm of cerebral artery
         TIA
         Transient cerebral ischemia NOS

● **G46** **Vascular syndromes of brain in cerebrovascular diseases**

     Code first underlying cerebrovascular disease (I60-I69)

     G46.0 **Middle** cerebral artery syndrome

     G46.1 **Anterior** cerebral artery syndrome

     G46.2 **Posterior** cerebral artery syndrome

     G46.3 **Brain stem stroke** syndrome

         Benedikt syndrome
         Claude syndrome
         Foville syndrome
         Millard-Gubler syndrome
         Wallenberg syndrome
         Weber syndrome

     G46.4 **Cerebellar stroke** syndrome

     G46.5 **Pure motor lacunar** syndrome

         Occlusion of single deep penetrating artery

     G46.6 **Pure sensory lacunar** syndrome

     G46.7 **Other lacunar** syndromes

     G46.8 **Other** vascular syndromes of brain in cerebrovascular diseases

▶ New   ⇒ Revised   ~~deleted~~ Deleted   **OGCR** Official Guidelines   X Assign placeholder X   ● Use Additional Character(s)

Excludes 1   Excludes 2   Includes   Use additional   Code first   Code also   Key words

● **G47   Sleep disorders**
    Excludes2   nightmares (F51.5)
                nonorganic sleep disorders (F51.-)
                sleep terrors (F51.4)
                sleepwalking (F51.3)

● **G47.0   Insomnia**
    Excludes2   alcohol related insomnia (F10.182,
                   F10.282, F10.982)
              drug-related insomnia (F11.182, F11.282,
                   F11.982, F13.182, F13.282, F13.982,
                   F14.182, F14.282, F14.982, F15.182,
                   F15.282, F15.982, F19.182, F19.282,
                   F19.982)
              idiopathic insomnia (F51.01)
              insomnia due to a mental disorder (F51.05)
              insomnia not due to a substance or known
                   physiological condition (F51.0-)
              nonorganic insomnia (F51.0-)
              primary insomnia (F51.01)
              sleep apnea (G47.3-)

    G47.00   Insomnia, unspecified
             Insomnia NOS

    G47.01   Insomnia due to medical condition
             Code also associated medical condition

    G47.09   Other insomnia

● **G47.1   Hypersomnia**
    Excludes2   alcohol-related hypersomnia (F10.182,
                   F10.282, F10.982)
              drug-related hypersomnia (F11.182,
                   F11.282, F11.982, F13.182, F13.282,
                   F13.982, F14.182, F14.282, F14.982,
                   F15.182, F15.282, F15.982, F19.182,
                   F19.282, F19.982)
              hypersomnia due to a mental disorder
                   (F51.13)
              hypersomnia not due to a substance
                   or known physiological condition
                   (F51.1-)
              primary hypersomnia (F51.11)
              sleep apnea (G47.3-)

    G47.10   Hypersomnia, unspecified
             Hypersomnia NOS

    G47.11   Idiopathic hypersomnia with long sleep time
             Idiopathic hypersomnia NOS

    G47.12   Idiopathic hypersomnia without long sleep time

    G47.13   Recurrent hypersomnia
             Kleine-Levin syndrome
             Menstrual related hypersomnia

    G47.14   Hypersomnia due to medical condition
             Code also associated medical condition

    G47.19   Other hypersomnia

● **G47.2   Circadian rhythm sleep disorders**
          Disorders of the sleep wake schedule
          Inversion of nyctohemeral rhythm
          Inversion of sleep rhythm

    G47.20   Circadian rhythm sleep disorder, unspecified type
             Sleep wake schedule disorder NOS

    G47.21   Circadian rhythm sleep disorder, delayed sleep phase type
             Delayed sleep phase syndrome

    G47.22   Circadian rhythm sleep disorder, advanced sleep phase type

    G47.23   Circadian rhythm sleep disorder, irregular sleep wake type
             Irregular sleep-wake pattern

    G47.24   Circadian rhythm sleep disorder, free running type
             ▶Circadian rhythm sleep disorder, non-24-hour
               sleep-wake type

    G47.25   Circadian rhythm sleep disorder, jet lag type

    G47.26   Circadian rhythm sleep disorder, shift work type

    G47.27   Circadian rhythm sleep disorder in conditions classified elsewhere
             Code first underlying condition

    G47.29   Other circadian rhythm sleep disorder

● **G47.3   Sleep apnea**
          Characterized by episodes in which breathing stops during sleep
          Code also any associated underlying condition
    Excludes1   apnea NOS (R06.81)
              Cheyne-Stokes breathing (R06.3)
              pickwickian syndrome (E66.2)
              sleep apnea of newborn (P28.3)

    G47.30   Sleep apnea, unspecified
             Sleep apnea NOS

    G47.31   Primary central sleep apnea
             ▶Idiopathic central sleep apnea

    G47.32   High altitude periodic breathing

    G47.33   Obstructive sleep apnea (adult) (pediatric)
             ▶Obstructive sleep apnea hypopnea
        Excludes1   obstructive sleep apnea of
                   newborn (P28.3)

    G47.34   Idiopathic sleep related nonobstructive alveolar hypoventilation
             Sleep related hypoxia

    G47.35   Congenital central alveolar hypoventilation syndrome

    G47.36   Sleep related hypoventilation in conditions classified elsewhere
             Sleep related hypoxemia in conditions
                classified elsewhere
             Code first underlying condition

    G47.37   Central sleep apnea in conditions classified elsewhere
             Code first underlying condition

    G47.39   Other sleep apnea

● **G47.4   Narcolepsy and cataplexy**
          *Cataplexy is a disorder evidenced by seizures including minor slacking of the facial muscles to complete collapse and often affects people who have **narcolepsy**, a disorder in which there is great difficulty remaining awake during the daytime.*

    ● **G47.41   Narcolepsy**

        G47.411   Narcolepsy with cataplexy

        G47.419   Narcolepsy without cataplexy
                 Narcolepsy NOS

    ● **G47.42   Narcolepsy in conditions classified elsewhere**
             Code first underlying condition

        G47.421   Narcolepsy in conditions classified elsewhere with cataplexy

        G47.429   Narcolepsy in conditions classified elsewhere without cataplexy

● **G47.5   Parasomnia**
    Excludes1   alcohol induced parasomnia (F10.182,
                   F10.282, F10.982)
              drug induced parasomnia (F11.182,
                   F11.282, F11.982, F13.182, F13.282,
                   F13.982, F14.182, F14.282, F14.982,
                   F15.182, F15.282, F15.982, F19.182,
                   F19.282, F19.982)
              parasomnia not due to a substance or
                   known physiological condition (F51.8)

    G47.50   Parasomnia, unspecified
             Parasomnia NOS

    G47.51   Confusional arousals

    G47.52   REM sleep behavior disorder

    G47.53   Recurrent isolated sleep paralysis

    G47.54   Parasomnia in conditions classified elsewhere
             Code first underlying condition

    G47.59   Other parasomnia

CHAPTER 6 (G00-G99)

▶ New   ⇒ Revised   ~~deleted~~ Deleted   **OGCR** Official Guidelines   X Assign placeholder X   ● Use Additional Character(s)

  Includes   Use additional   Code first   Code also   Key words

CHAPTER 6 (G00-G99)

● G47.6   Sleep related movement disorders
    Excludes2   restless legs syndrome (G25.81)
   G47.61   Periodic limb movement disorder
      ~~Periodic limb movement disorder~~
   G47.62   Sleep related leg cramps
   G47.63   Sleep related bruxism
      Excludes1   psychogenic bruxism (F45.8)
   G47.69   Other sleep related movement disorders
  G47.8   Other sleep disorders
    ▶Other specified sleep-wake disorder
  G47.9   Sleep disorder, unspecified
    Sleep disorder NOS
    ▶Unspecified sleep-wake disorder

★ (See Plate 118 on page 54.)

NERVE, NERVE ROOT AND PLEXUS DISORDERS (G50-G59)

Excludes1   current traumatic nerve, nerve root and plexus
       disorders - see Injury, nerve by body region
     neuralgia NOS (M79.2)
     neuritis NOS (M79.2)
     peripheral neuritis in pregnancy (O26.82-)
     radiculitis NOS (M54.1-)

● G50   Disorders of trigeminal nerve
    Includes   disorders of 5th cranial nerve
   G50.0   Trigeminal neuralgia
     Syndrome of paroxysmal facial pain
     Tic douloureux
   G50.1   Atypical facial pain
   G50.8   Other disorders of trigeminal nerve
   G50.9   Disorder of trigeminal nerve, unspecified

● G51   Facial nerve disorders
    Includes   disorders of 7th cranial nerve
   G51.0   Bell's palsy
     Facial palsy
   G51.1   Geniculate ganglionitis
     Rare disorder with symptoms of severe pain deep in ear,
     spreading to ear canal, outer ear, mastoid or eye regions
     Excludes1   postherpetic geniculate ganglionitis
         (B02.21)
   G51.2   Melkersson's syndrome
     Melkersson-Rosenthal syndrome
   G51.3   Clonic hemifacial spasm
   G51.4   Facial myokymia
     Involuntary facial muscle movement
   G51.8   Other disorders of facial nerve
   G51.9   Disorder of facial nerve, unspecified

● G52   Disorders of other cranial nerves
    Excludes2   disorders of acoustic [8th] nerve (H93.3)
      disorders of optic [2nd] nerve (H46, H47.0)
      paralytic strabismus due to nerve palsy
       (H49.0-H49.2)
   G52.0   Disorders of olfactory nerve
     Disorders of 1st cranial nerve
   G52.1   Disorders of glossopharyngeal nerve
     Disorder of 9th cranial nerve
     Glossopharyngeal neuralgia
   G52.2   Disorders of vagus nerve
     Disorders of pneumogastric [10th] nerve
   G52.3   Disorders of hypoglossal nerve
     Disorders of 12th cranial nerve
   G52.7   Disorders of multiple cranial nerves
     Polyneuritis cranialis
   G52.8   Disorders of other specified cranial nerves
   G52.9   Cranial nerve disorder, unspecified

  G53   Cranial nerve disorders in diseases classified elsewhere
    Code first underlying disease, such as:
    neoplasm (C00-D49)
    Excludes1   multiple cranial nerve palsy in sarcoidosis
       (D86.82)
      multiple cranial nerve palsy in syphilis (A52.15)
      postherpetic geniculate ganglionitis (B02.21)
      postherpetic trigeminal neuralgia (B02.22)

● G54   Nerve root and plexus disorders
    Raiculopathy (nerve root disorder) caused by pressure on nerve root,
    most common cause is herniation of intervertebral disk. Plexus
    disorders (plexopathies) are due to compression or injury.
    Excludes1   current traumatic nerve root and plexus disorders
       - see nerve injury by body region
      intervertebral disc disorders (M50-M51)
      neuralgia or neuritis NOS (M79.2)
      neuritis or radiculitis brachial NOS (M54.13)
      neuritis or radiculitis lumbar NOS (M54.16)
      neuritis or radiculitis lumbosacral NOS (M54.17)
      neuritis or radiculitis thoracic NOS (M54.14)
      radiculitis NOS (M54.10)
      radiculopathy NOS (M54.10)
      spondylosis (M47.-)
   G54.0   Brachial plexus disorders
     Thoracic outlet syndrome
   G54.1   Lumbosacral plexus disorders
   G54.2   Cervical root disorders, not elsewhere classified
   G54.3   Thoracic root disorders, not elsewhere classified
   G54.4   Lumbosacral root disorders, not elsewhere classified
   G54.5   Neuralgic amyotrophy
     Parsonage-Aldren-Turner syndrome
     Shoulder-girdle neuritis
     Excludes1   neuralgic amyotrophy in diabetes
         mellitus (E08-E13 with .44)
   G54.6   Phantom limb syndrome with pain
     Sensations (cramping, itching) in a limb that no longer
     exists
   G54.7   Phantom limb syndrome without pain
     Phantom limb syndrome NOS
   G54.8   Other nerve root and plexus disorders
   G54.9   Nerve root and plexus disorder, unspecified

  G55   Nerve root and plexus compressions in diseases classified elsewhere
    Code first underlying disease, such as:
    neoplasm (C00-D49)
    Excludes1   nerve root compression (due to) (in) ankylosing
       spondylitis (M45.-)
      nerve root compression (due to) (in)dorsopathies
       (M53.-, M54.-)
      nerve root compression (due to) (in)intervertebral
       disc disorders (M50.1.-, M51.1.-)
      nerve root compression (due to) (in)
       spondylopathies (M46.-, M48.-)

Item 6–5   Trigeminal neuralgia, tic douloureux, is a pain syndrome diagnosed from the patient's history alone. The condition is characterized by pain and a brief facial spasm or tic. Pain is unilateral and follows the sensory distribution of cranial nerve V, typically radiating to the maxillary (V2) or mandibular (V3) area.

Item 6–6   The most common facial nerve disorder is **Bell's Palsy,** which occurs suddenly and results in facial drooping unilaterally. This disorder is the result of a reaction to a virus that causes the facial nerve in the ear to swell resulting in pressure in the bony canal.

▶ New   ⇒ Revised   ~~deleted~~ Deleted   OGCR Official Guidelines   X Assign placeholder X   ● Use Additional Character(s)

| Excludes 1 | Excludes 2 | Includes | Use additional | Code first | Code also | Key words |

★ **(See Plates 472 and 473 on pages 56 and 57.)**

● **G56   Mononeuropathies of upper limb**
> **Excludes1**   current traumatic nerve disorder - see nerve injury by body region

● **G56.0   Carpal tunnel syndrome**
> G56.00   Carpal tunnel syndrome, unspecified upper limb
> G56.01   Carpal tunnel syndrome, right upper limb
> G56.02   Carpal tunnel syndrome, left upper limb
> G56.03   Carpal tunnel syndrome, bilateral upper limbs

● **G56.1   Other lesions of median nerve**
> G56.10   Other lesions of median nerve, unspecified side
> G56.11   Other lesions of median nerve, right upper limb
> G56.12   Other lesions of median nerve, left upper limb
> G56.13   Other lesions of median nerve, bilateral upper limbs

● **G56.2   Lesion of ulnar nerve**
> Tardy ulnar nerve palsy
> G56.20   Lesion of ulnar nerve, unspecified upper limb
> G56.21   Lesion of ulnar nerve, right upper limb
> G56.22   Lesion of ulnar nerve, left upper limb
> G56.23   Lesion of ulnar nerve, bilateral upper limbs

● **G56.3   Lesion of radial nerve**
> G56.30   Lesion of radial nerve, unspecified upper limb
> G56.31   Lesion of radial nerve, right upper limb
> G56.32   Lesion of radial nerve, left upper limb
> G56.33   Lesion of radial nerve, bilateral upper limbs

● **G56.4   Causalgia of upper limb**
> *Intense burning pain and sensitivity to slight touch*
> Complex regional pain syndrome II of upper limb
> **Excludes1**   complex regional pain syndrome I of lower limb (G90.52-)
> complex regional pain syndrome I of upper limb (G90.51-)
> complex regional pain syndrome II of lower limb (G57.7-)
> reflex sympathetic dystrophy of lower limb (G90.52-)
> reflex sympathetic dystrophy (G90.51-)
> G56.40   Causalgia of unspecified upper limb
> G56.41   Causalgia of right upper limb
> G56.42   Causalgia of left upper limb
> G56.43   Causalgia of bilateral upper limbs

● **G56.8   Other specified mononeuropathies of upper limb**
> *Disease of a single nerve*
> Interdigital neuroma of upper limb
> G56.80   Other specified mononeuropathies of unspecified upper limb
> G56.81   Other specified mononeuropathies of right upper limb
> G56.82   Other specified mononeuropathies of left upper limb
> G56.83   Other specified mononeuropathies of bilateral upper limbs

● **G56.9   Unspecified mononeuropathy of upper limb**
> *Disease of a single nerve*
> G56.90   Unspecified mononeuropathy of unspecified upper limb
> G56.91   Unspecified mononeuropathy of right upper limb
> G56.92   Unspecified mononeuropathy of left upper limb
> G56.93   Unspecified mononeuropathy of bilateral upper limbs

● **G57   Mononeuropathies of lower limb**
> **Excludes1**   current traumatic nerve disorder - see nerve injury by body region

★ **(See Plates 544 and 545 on pages 58 and 59.)**

● **G57.0   Lesion of sciatic nerve**
> **Excludes1**   sciatica NOS (M54.3-)
> **Excludes2**   sciatica attributed to intervertebral disc disorder (M51.1.-)
> G57.00   Lesion of sciatic nerve, unspecified lower limb
> G57.01   Lesion of sciatic nerve, right lower limb
> G57.02   Lesion of sciatic nerve, left lower limb
> G57.03   Lesion of sciatic nerve, bilateral lower limbs

● **G57.1   Meralgia paresthetica**
> *Numbness or pain in outer thigh caused by injury to nerve*
> Lateral cutaneous nerve of thigh syndrome
> G57.10   Meralgia paresthetica, unspecified lower limb
> G57.11   Meralgia paresthetica, right lower limb
> G57.12   Meralgia paresthetica, left lower limb
> G57.13   Meralgia paresthetica, bilateral lower limbs

● **G57.2   Lesion of femoral nerve**
> G57.20   Lesion of femoral nerve, unspecified lower limb
> G57.21   Lesion of femoral nerve, right lower limb
> G57.22   Lesion of femoral nerve, left lower limb
> G57.23   Lesion of femoral nerve, bilateral lower limbs

● **G57.3   Lesion of lateral popliteal nerve**
> Peroneal nerve palsy
> G57.30   Lesion of lateral popliteal nerve, unspecified lower limb
> G57.31   Lesion of lateral popliteal nerve, right lower limb
> G57.32   Lesion of lateral popliteal nerve, left lower limb
> G57.33   Lesion of lateral popliteal nerve, bilateral lower limbs

● **G57.4   Lesion of medial popliteal nerve**
> G57.40   Lesion of medial popliteal nerve, unspecified lower limb
> G57.41   Lesion of medial popliteal nerve, right lower limb
> G57.42   Lesion of medial popliteal nerve, left lower limb
> G57.43   Lesion of medial popliteal nerve, bilateral lower limbs

● **G57.5   Tarsal tunnel syndrome**
> G57.50   Tarsal tunnel syndrome, unspecified lower limb
> G57.51   Tarsal tunnel syndrome, right lower limb
> G57.52   Tarsal tunnel syndrome, left lower limb
> G57.53   Tarsal tunnel syndrome, bilateral lower limbs

● **G57.6   Lesion of plantar nerve**
> Morton's metatarsalgia
> G57.60   Lesion of plantar nerve, unspecified lower limb
> G57.61   Lesion of plantar nerve, right lower limb
> G57.62   Lesion of plantar nerve, left lower limb
> G57.63   Lesion of plantar nerve, bilateral lower limbs

● **G57.7   Causalgia of lower limb**
> Complex regional pain syndrome II of lower limb
> **Excludes1**   complex regional pain syndrome I of lower limb (G90.52-)
> complex regional pain syndrome I of upper limb (G90.51-)
> complex regional pain syndrome II of upper limb (G56.4-)
> reflex sympathetic dystrophy of lower limb (G90.52-)
> reflex sympathetic dystrophy of upper limb (G90.51-)
> G57.70   Causalgia of unspecified lower limb
> G57.71   Causalgia of right lower limb
> G57.72   Causalgia of left lower limb
> G57.73   Causalgia of bilateral lower limbs

CHAPTER 6 (G00-G99)

- **G57.8** Other specified mononeuropathies of lower limb
  - Interdigital neuroma of lower limb
  - **G57.80** Other specified mononeuropathies of unspecified lower limb
  - **G57.81** Other specified mononeuropathies of right lower limb
  - **G57.82** Other specified mononeuropathies of left lower limb
  - **G57.83** Other specified mononeuropathies of bilateral lower limbs
- **G57.9** Unspecified mononeuropathy of lower limb
  - **G57.90** Unspecified mononeuropathy of unspecified lower limb
  - **G57.91** Unspecified mononeuropathy of right lower limb
  - **G57.92** Unspecified mononeuropathy of left lower limb
  - **G57.93** Unspecified mononeuropathy of bilateral lower limbs
- **G58** Other mononeuropathies
  - **G58.0** Intercostal neuropathy
  - **G58.7** Mononeuritis multiplex
  - **G58.8** Other specified mononeuropathies
  - **G58.9** Mononeuropathy, unspecified
- **G59** Mononeuropathy in diseases classified elsewhere
  - *Code first underlying disease*
  - **Excludes1** diabetic mononeuropathy (E08-E13 with .41)
    syphilitic nerve paralysis (A52.19)
    syphilitic neuritis (A52.15)
    tuberculous mononeuropathy (A17.83)

POLYNEUROPATHIES AND OTHER DISORDERS OF THE PERIPHERAL NERVOUS SYSTEM (G60-G65)

Excludes1 neuralgia NOS (M79.2)
neuritis NOS (M79.2)
peripheral neuritis in pregnancy (O26.82-)
radiculitis NOS (M54.10)

- **G60** Hereditary and idiopathic neuropathy
  - **G60.0** Hereditary motor and sensory neuropathy
    Charcot-Marie-Tooth disease
    Déjerine-Sottas disease
    Hereditary motor and sensory neuropathy, types I-IV
    Hypertrophic neuropathy of infancy
    Peroneal muscular atrophy (axonal type) (hypertrophic type)
    Roussy-Lévy syndrome
  - **G60.1** Refsum's disease
    Genetic disorder affecting fatty acid metabolism
    Infantile Refsum disease
  - **G60.2** Neuropathy in association with hereditary ataxia
  - **G60.3** Idiopathic progressive neuropathy
  - **G60.8** Other hereditary and idiopathic neuropathies
    Dominantly inherited sensory neuropathy
    Morvan's disease
    Nelaton's syndrome
    Recessively inherited sensory neuropathy
  - **G60.9** Hereditary and idiopathic neuropathy, unspecified

Figure 6-2 Actions of parasympathetic and sympathetic nerves. (From Chabner: The Language of Medicine, ed 9, St. Louis, Saunders, 2011)

Item 6–7 The **peripheral nervous system** consists of 31 pairs of spinal nerves, 12 pairs of cranial nerves, and the autonomic nerves, which are divided into the parasympathetic and sympathetic nerves. The cranial nerves are: olfactory (I), optic (II), oculomotor (III), trochlear (IV), trigeminal (V), abducens (VI), facial (VII), vestibulocochlear (VIII), glossopharyngeal (IX), vagus (X), accessory (XI), and hypoglossal (XII).

- **G61** Inflammatory polyneuropathy
  - **G61.0** Guillain-Barré syndrome
    Autoimmune disease affecting peripheral nervous system
    Acute (post-)infective polyneuritis
    Miller Fisher Syndrome
  - **G61.1** Serum neuropathy
    Use additional code for adverse effect, if applicable, to identify serum (T50.-)
  - **G61.8** Other inflammatory polyneuropathies
    - **G61.81** Chronic inflammatory demyelinating polyneuritis
    - **G61.82** Multifocal motor neuropathy
      MMN
    - **G61.89** Other inflammatory polyneuropathies
  - **G61.9** Inflammatory polyneuropathy, unspecified

▶ New ⇒ Revised ~~deleted~~ Deleted **OGCR** Official Guidelines X Assign placeholder X ● Use Additional Character(s)

Excludes 1 Excludes 2 Includes Use additional Code first Code also Key words

● **G62   Other and unspecified polyneuropathies**
   G62.0   Drug-induced polyneuropathy
     Use additional code for adverse effect, if applicable, to identify drug (T36-T50 with fifth or sixth character 5)
   G62.1   Alcoholic polyneuropathy
     Malfunction of many peripheral nerves throughout the body
   G62.2   Polyneuropathy due to other toxic agents
     Code first (T51-T65) to identify toxic agent
 ● **G62.8   Other specified polyneuropathies**
     G62.81   Critical illness polyneuropathy
       Acute motor neuropathy
     G62.82   Radiation-induced polyneuropathy
       Use additional external cause code (W88-W90, X39.0-) to identify cause
     G62.89   Other specified polyneuropathies
   G62.9   Polyneuropathy, unspecified
     Neuropathy NOS

   G63   Polyneuropathy in diseases classified elsewhere
     Code first underlying disease, such as:
       amyloidosis (E85.-)
       endocrine disease, except diabetes (E00-E07, E15-E16, E20-E34)
       metabolic diseases (E70-E88)
       neoplasm (C00-D49)
       nutritional deficiency (E40-E64)
     Excludes1   polyneuropathy (in):
       diabetes mellitus (E08-E13 with .42)
       diphtheria (A36.83)
       infectious mononucleosis (B27.0-B27.9 with 1)
       Lyme disease (A69.22)
       mumps (B26.84)
       postherpetic (B02.23)
       rheumatoid arthritis (M05.33)
       scleroderma (M34.83)
       systemic lupus erythematosus (M32.19)

   G64   Other disorders of peripheral nervous system
     Disorder of peripheral nervous system NOS

● **G65   Sequelae of inflammatory and toxic polyneuropathies**
     Code first condition resulting from (sequela) of inflammatory and toxic polyneuropathies
   G65.0   Sequelae of Guillain-Barré syndrome
   G65.1   Sequelae of other inflammatory polyneuropathy
   G65.2   Sequelae of toxic polyneuropathy

DISEASES OF MYONEURAL JUNCTION AND MUSCLE (G70-G73)

● **G70   Myasthenia gravis and other myoneural disorders**
     Excludes1   botulism (A05.1, A48.51-A48.52)
       transient neonatal myasthenia gravis (P94.0)
 ● **G70.0   Myasthenia gravis**
     Acquired and results in fatigable muscle weakness exacerbated by activity and improved with rest
     G70.00   Myasthenia gravis without (acute) exacerbation
       Myasthenia gravis NOS
     G70.01   Myasthenia gravis with (acute) exacerbation
       Myasthenia gravis in crisis
   G70.1   Toxic myoneural disorders
     Dysfunction at junction of muscle and motor nerve (myoneural junction)
     Code first (T51-T65) to identify toxic agent
   G70.2   Congenital and developmental myasthenia

● **G70.8   Other specified myoneural disorders**
     G70.80   Lambert-Eaton syndrome, unspecified
       Lambert-Eaton syndrome NOS
     G70.81   Lambert-Eaton syndrome in disease classified elsewhere
       Code first underlying disease
       Excludes1   Lambert-Eaton syndrome in neoplastic disease (G73.1)
     G70.89   Other specified myoneural disorders
   G70.9   Myoneural disorder, unspecified

● **G71   Primary disorders of muscles**
     Excludes2   arthrogryposis multiplex congenita (Q74.3)
       metabolic disorders (E70-E88)
       myositis (M60.-)
   G71.0   Muscular dystrophy
     Autosomal recessive, childhood type, muscular dystrophy resembling Duchenne or Becker muscular dystrophy
     Benign [Becker] muscular dystrophy
     Benign scapuloperoneal muscular dystrophy with early contractures [Emery-Dreifuss]
     Congenital muscular dystrophy NOS
     Congenital muscular dystrophy with specific morphological abnormalities of the muscle fiber
     Distal muscular dystrophy
     Facioscapulohumeral muscular dystrophy
     Limb-girdle muscular dystrophy
     Ocular muscular dystrophy
     Oculopharyngeal muscular dystrophy
     Scapuloperoneal muscular dystrophy
     Severe [Duchenne] muscular dystrophy
 ● **G71.1   Myotonic disorders**
     Inherited disorder that affects muscles tone
     G71.11   Myotonic muscular dystrophy
       Dystrophia myotonica [Steinert]
       Myotonia atrophica
       Myotonic dystrophy
       Proximal myotonic myopathy (PROMM)
       Steinert disease
     G71.12   Myotonia congenita
       Acetazolamide responsive myotonia congenita
       Dominant myotonia congenita [Thomsen disease]
       Myotonia levior
       Recessive myotonia congenita [Becker disease]
     G71.13   Myotonic chondrodystrophy
       Chondrodystrophic myotonia
       Congenital myotonic chondrodystrophy
       Schwartz-Jampel disease
     G71.14   Drug induced myotonia
       Use additional code for adverse effect, if applicable, to identify drug (T36-T50 with fifth or sixth character 5)
     G71.19   Other specified myotonic disorders
       Myotonia fluctuans
       Myotonia permanens
       Neuromyotonia [Isaacs]
       Paramyotonia congenita (of von Eulenburg)
       Pseudomyotonia
       Symptomatic myotonia

CHAPTER 6 (G00-G99)

Item 6-8 Muscular dystrophies (MD) are a group of rare inherited muscle diseases. Voluntary muscles become progressively weaker. In the late stages of MD, fat and connective tissue replace muscle fibers. In some types of muscular dystrophy, heart muscles, other involuntary muscles, and other organs are affected. **Myopathies** is a general term for neuromuscular diseases in which the muscle fibers dysfunction for any one of many reasons, resulting in muscular weakness.

▶ New   ⇨ Revised   ~~deleted~~ Deleted   **OGCR** Official Guidelines   **X** Assign placeholder X   ● Use Additional Character(s)
Excludes 1   Excludes 2   Includes   Use additional   Code first   Code also   Key words

G71.2 **Congenital** myopathies
  Central core disease
  Fiber-type disproportion
  Minicore disease
  Multicore disease
  Myotubular (centronuclear) myopathy
  Nemaline myopathy
  > **Excludes1** arthrogryposis multiplex congenita
  >   (Q74.3)

G71.3 **Mitochondrial myopathy,** not elsewhere classified
  Myopathies associated with increased number of enlarged,
  often abnormal, mitochondria in muscle fibers
  > **Excludes1** Kearns-Sayre syndrome (H49.81)
  >   Leber's disease (H47.21)
  >   Leigh's encephalopathy (G31.82)
  >   mitochondrial metabolism disorders
  >   (E88.4.-)
  >   Reye's syndrome (G93.7)

G71.8 **Other** primary disorders of muscles

G71.9 **Primary** disorder of muscle, **unspecified**
  Hereditary myopathy NOS

● **G72** **Other and unspecified myopathies**
  > **Excludes1** arthrogryposis multiplex congenita (Q74.3)
  >   dermatopolymyositis (M33.-)
  >   ischemic infarction of muscle (M62.2-)
  >   myositis (M60.-)
  >   polymyositis (M33.2.-)

G72.0 **Drug-induced** myopathy
  Use additional code for adverse effect, if applicable,
  to identify drug (T36-T50 with fifth or sixth
  character 5)

G72.1 **Alcoholic myopathy**
  Use additional code to identify alcoholism (F10.-)

G72.2 **Myopathy due to** other toxic agents
  Code first (T51-T65) to identify toxic agent

G72.3 **Periodic paralysis**
  Familial periodic paralysis
  Hyperkalemic periodic paralysis (familial)
  Hypokalemic periodic paralysis (familial)
  Myotonic periodic paralysis (familial)
  Normokalemic paralysis (familial)
  Potassium sensitive periodic paralysis
  > **Excludes1** paramyotonia congenita (of von
  >   Eulenburg) (G71.19)

● **G72.4** **Inflammatory and immune myopathies,** not elsewhere classified
  G72.41 **Inclusion body myositis [IBM]**
  G72.49 **Other inflammatory and immune myopathies,**
            not elsewhere classified
            Inflammatory myopathy NOS

● **G72.8** **Other specified myopathies**
  G72.81 **Critical illness** myopathy
            Acute necrotizing myopathy
            Acute quadriplegic myopathy
            Intensive care (ICU) myopathy
            Myopathy of critical illness
  G72.89 **Other specified myopathies**

G72.9 **Myopathy, unspecified**

● **G73** **Disorders of myoneural junction and muscle in diseases
      classified elsewhere**
  G73.1 **Lambert-Eaton syndrome in neoplastic disease**
    Rare autoimmune disorder affecting calcium channels of
    nerve-muscle (neuromuscular) junction
    Code first underlying neoplasm (C00-D49)
    > **Excludes1** Lambert-Eaton syndrome not associated
    >   with neoplasm (G70.80-G70.81)
  G73.3 **Myasthenic syndromes in other diseases classified
        elsewhere**
    Code first underlying disease, such as:
      neoplasm (C00-D49)
      thyrotoxicosis (E05.-)
  G73.7 **Myopathy in diseases classified elsewhere**
    Code first underlying disease, such as:
      hyperparathyroidism (E21.0, E21.3)
      hypoparathyroidism (E20.-)
      glycogen storage disease (E74.0)
      lipid storage disorders (E75.-)
    > **Excludes1** myopathy in:
    >   rheumatoid arthritis (M05.32)
    >   sarcoidosis (D86.87)
    >   scleroderma (M34.82)
    >   sicca syndrome [Sjögren] (M35.03)
    >   systemic lupus erythematosus (M32.19)

CEREBRAL PALSY AND OTHER PARALYTIC SYNDROMES (G80-G83)

● **G80** **Cerebral palsy**
  > **Excludes1** hereditary spastic paraplegia (G11.4)
  G80.0 **Spastic quadriplegic** cerebral palsy
            Congenital spastic paralysis (cerebral)
  G80.1 **Spastic diplegic** cerebral palsy
            Spastic cerebral palsy NOS
  G80.2 **Spastic hemiplegic** cerebral palsy
  G80.3 **Athetoid** cerebral palsy
            Result of damage to cerebellum or basal ganglia responsible
            for processing neuromuscular signals
            Double athetosis (syndrome)
            Dyskinetic cerebral palsy
            Dystonic cerebral palsy
            Vogt disease
  G80.4 **Ataxic cerebral palsy**
            Poor muscle tone and coordination
  G80.8 **Other** cerebral palsy
            Mixed cerebral palsy syndromes
  G80.9 **Cerebral palsy, unspecified**
            Cerebral palsy NOS

● **G81** **Hemiplegia and hemiparesis**
  Note: This category is to be used only when hemiplegia
           (complete)(incomplete) is reported without further
           specification, or is stated to be old or longstanding but of
           unspecified cause. The category is also for use in multiple
           coding to identify these types of hemiplegia resulting
           from any cause.
  > **Excludes1** congenital cerebral palsy (G80.-)
  >   hemiplegia and hemiparesis due to sequela of
  >   cerebrovascular disease (I69.05-, I69.15-,
  >   I69.25-, I69.35-, I69.85-, I69.95-)

● **G81.0** **Flaccid hemiplegia**
    Paralysis of half of body with loss of tone of muscles of
    paralyzed part and absence of tendon reflexes
    G81.00 Flaccid hemiplegia affecting **unspecified** side
    G81.01 Flaccid hemiplegia affecting **right dominant**
              side
    G81.02 Flaccid hemiplegia affecting **left dominant** side
    G81.03 Flaccid hemiplegia affecting **right nondominant**
              side
    G81.04 Flaccid hemiplegia affecting **left nondominant**
              side

Item 6–9 **Hemiplegia** is complete paralysis of one side of the body—arm, leg, and trunk. **Hemiparesis** is a generalized weakness or incomplete paralysis of one side of the body. If most activities (eating, writing) are performed with the right hand, the right is the dominant side, and the left is the nondominant side. **Quadriplegia,** also called tetraplegia, is the complete paralysis of all four limbs. **Quadriparesis** is the incomplete paralysis of all four limbs. Nerve damage in C1–C4 is associated with lower limb paralysis, and C5–C7 damage is associated with upper limb paralysis. **Diplegia** is the paralysis of the upper limbs. **Monoplegia** is the complete paralysis of one limb.

OGCR Section I.C.6.a.

Dominant/nondominant side

Codes from category G81, Hemiplegia and hemiparesis, and subcategories, G83.1, Monoplegia of lower limb, G83.2, Monoplegia of upper limb, and G83.3, Monoplegia, unspecified, identify whether the dominant and nondominant side is affected. Should the affected side be documented, but not specified as dominant or nondominant, and the classification system does not indicate a default, code selection is as follows:
- For ambidextrous patients, the default should be dominant.
- If the left side is affected, the default is non-dominant.
- If the right side is affected, the default is dominant.

● **G81.1** **Spastic hemiplegia**
Paralysis of half of body with spasticity of muscles of paralyzed part and increased tendon reflexes

G81.10　Spastic hemiplegia affecting **unspecified** side
G81.11　Spastic hemiplegia affecting **right dominant** side
G81.12　Spastic hemiplegia affecting **left dominant** side
G81.13　Spastic hemiplegia affecting **right nondominant** side
G81.14　Spastic hemiplegia affecting **left nondominant** side

● **G81.9** **Hemiplegia, unspecified**
G81.90　Hemiplegia, unspecified affecting **unspecified** side
G81.91　Hemiplegia, unspecified affecting **right dominant** side
G81.92　Hemiplegia, unspecified affecting **left dominant** side
G81.93　Hemiplegia, unspecified affecting **right nondominant** side
G81.94　Hemiplegia, unspecified affecting **left nondominant** side

● **G82** **Paraplegia (paraparesis) and quadriplegia (quadriparesis)**
Note: This category is to be used only when the listed conditions are reported without further specification, or are stated to be old or longstanding but of unspecified cause. The category is also for use in multiple coding to identify these conditions resulting from any cause.
Excludes1　congenital cerebral palsy (G80.-)
　　　　　　functional quadriplegia (R53.2)
　　　　　　hysterical paralysis (F44.4)

● **G82.2** **Paraplegia**
Paralysis of both lower limbs NOS
Paraparesis (lower) NOS
Paraplegia (lower) NOS
G82.20　Paraplegia, **unspecified**
G82.21　Paraplegia, **complete**
G82.22　Paraplegia, **incomplete**

● **G82.5** **Quadriplegia**
Paralysis of all limbs; AKA tetraplegia
G82.50　Quadriplegia, **unspecified**
G82.51　Quadriplegia, **C1-C4 complete**
G82.52　Quadriplegia, **C1-C4 incomplete**
G82.53　Quadriplegia, **C5-C7 complete**
G82.54　Quadriplegia, **C5-C7 incomplete**

● **G83** **Other paralytic syndromes**
Note: This category is to be used only when the listed conditions are reported without further specification, or are stated to be old or longstanding but of unspecified cause. The category is also for use in multiple coding to identify these conditions resulting from any cause.
Includes　paralysis (complete) (incomplete), except as in G80-G82

G83.0 **Diplegia of upper limbs**
Paralysis affecting limbs on both sides; AKA bilateral paralysis
Diplegia (upper)
Paralysis of both upper limbs

● **G83.1** **Monoplegia of lower limb**
Paralysis of limb on one side
Paralysis of lower limb
Excludes1　monoplegia of lower limbs due to sequela of cerebrovascular disease (I69.04-, I69.14-, I69.24-, I69.34-, I69.84-, I69.94-)
G83.10　Monoplegia of lower limb affecting **unspecified** side
G83.11　Monoplegia of lower limb affecting **right dominant** side
G83.12　Monoplegia of lower limb affecting **left dominant** side
G83.13　Monoplegia of lower limb affecting **right nondominant** side
G83.14　Monoplegia of lower limb affecting **left nondominant** side

● **G83.2** **Monoplegia of upper limb**
Paralysis of upper limb
Excludes1　monoplegia of upper limbs due to sequela of cerebrovascular disease (I69.03-, I69.13-, I69.23-, I69.33-, I69.83-, I69.93-)
G83.20　Monoplegia of upper limb affecting **unspecified** side
G83.21　Monoplegia of upper limb affecting **right dominant** side
G83.22　Monoplegia of upper limb affecting **left dominant** side
G83.23　Monoplegia of upper limb affecting **right nondominant** side
G83.24　Monoplegia of upper limb affecting **left nondominant** side

● **G83.3** **Monoplegia, unspecified**
G83.30　Monoplegia, unspecified affecting **unspecified** side
G83.31　Monoplegia, unspecified affecting **right dominant** side
G83.32　Monoplegia, unspecified affecting **left dominant** side
G83.33　Monoplegia, unspecified affecting **right nondominant** side
G83.34　Monoplegia, unspecified affecting **left nondominant** side

G83.4 **Cauda equina syndrome**
Aching pain due to compression of spinal nerve roots
Neurogenic bladder due to cauda equina syndrome
Excludes1　cord bladder NOS (G95.89)
　　　　　　neurogenic bladder NOS (N31.9)

G83.5 **Locked-in state**

CHAPTER 6 (G00-G99)

▶ New　⇒ Revised　~~deleted~~ Deleted　OGCR Official Guidelines　X Assign placeholder X　● Use Additional Character(s)
Excludes 1　Excludes 2　Includes　Use additional　Code first　Code also　Key words
761

● G83.8   Other specified paralytic syndromes
    | Excludes1 | paralytic syndromes due to current spinal cord injury-code to spinal cord injury (S14, S24, S34) |

    G83.81   Brown-Séquard syndrome
    G83.82   Anterior cord syndrome
    G83.83   Posterior cord syndrome
    G83.84   Todd's paralysis (postepileptic)
    G83.89   Other specified paralytic syndromes
  G83.9   Paralytic syndrome, unspecified

OTHER DISORDERS OF THE NERVOUS SYSTEM (G89-G99)

● G89   Pain, not elsewhere classified
    Code also related psychological factors associated with pain (F45.42)
    | Excludes1 | generalized pain NOS (R52) |
    | | pain disorders exclusively related to psychological factors (F45.41) |
    | | pain NOS (R52) |
    | Excludes2 | atypical face pain (G50.1) |
    | | headache syndromes (G44.-) |
    | | localized pain, unspecified type - code to pain by site, such as: |
    | | abdomen pain (R10.-) |
    | | back pain (M54.9) |
    | | breast pain (N64.4) |
    | | chest pain (R07.1-R07.9) |
    | | ear pain (H92.0-) |
    | | eye pain (H57.1) |
    | | headache (R51) |
    | | joint pain (M25.5-) |
    | | limb pain (M79.6-) |
    | | lumbar region pain (M54.5) |
    | | painful urination (R30.9) |
    | | pelvic and perineal pain (R10.2) |
    | | shoulder pain (M25.51-) |
    | | spine pain (M54.-) |
    | | throat pain (R07.0) |
    | | tongue pain (K14.6) |
    | | tooth pain (K08.8) |
    | | renal colic (N23) |
    | | migraines (G43.-) |
    | | myalgia (M79.1) |
    | | pain from prosthetic devices, implants, and grafts (T82.84, T83.84, T84.84, T85.84-) |
    | | phantom limb syndrome with pain (G54.6) |
    | | vulvar vestibulitis (N94.810) |
    | | vulvodynia (N94.81-) |

    G89.0   Central pain syndrome
        Neurological condition causing intractable pain resulting from damage to CNS
        Déjérine-Roussy syndrome
        Myelopathic pain syndrome
        Thalamic pain syndrome (hyperesthetic)
● G89.1   Acute pain, not elsewhere classified
    G89.11   Acute pain due to trauma
    G89.12   Acute post-thoracotomy pain
        Post-thoracotomy pain NOS
    G89.18   Other acute postprocedural pain
        Postoperative pain NOS
        Postprocedural pain NOS

● G89.2   Chronic pain, not elsewhere classified
    | Excludes1 | causalgia, lower limb (G57.7-) |
    | | causalgia, upper limb (G56.4-) |
    | | central pain syndrome (G89.0) |
    | | chronic pain syndrome (G89.4) |
    | | complex regional pain syndrome II, lower limb (G57.7-) |
    | | complex regional pain syndrome II, upper limb (G56.4-) |
    | | neoplasm related chronic pain (G89.3) |
    | | reflex sympathetic dystrophy (G90.5-) |

    G89.21   Chronic pain due to trauma
    G89.22   Chronic post-thoracotomy pain
    G89.28   Other chronic postprocedural pain
        Other chronic postoperative pain
    G89.29   Other chronic pain
    G89.3   Neoplasm related pain (acute) (chronic)
        Cancer associated pain
        Pain due to malignancy (primary) (secondary)
        Tumor associated pain
    G89.4   Chronic pain syndrome
        Chronic pain associated with significant psychosocial dysfunction

● G90   Disorders of autonomic nervous system
    | Excludes1 | dysfunction of the autonomic nervous system due to alcohol (G31.2) |

● G90.0   Idiopathic peripheral autonomic neuropathy
    G90.01   Carotid sinus syncope
        Carotid sinus syndrome
    G90.09   Other idiopathic peripheral autonomic neuropathy
        Idiopathic peripheral autonomic neuropathy NOS
    G90.1   Familial dysautonomia [Riley-Day]
        Inherited disorder that affects nerve function
    G90.2   Horner's syndrome
        Due to damage of the sympathetic nervous system
        Bernard(-Horner) syndrome
        Cervical sympathetic dystrophy or paralysis
    G90.3   Multi-system degeneration of the autonomic nervous system
        Neurogenic orthostatic hypotension [Shy-Drager]
        | Excludes1 | orthostatic hypotension NOS (I95.1) |
    G90.4   Autonomic dysreflexia
        Syndrome resulting from lesions of spinal cord
        Use additional code to identify the cause, such as:
          fecal impaction (K56.41)
          pressure ulcer (pressure area) (L89.-)
          urinary tract infection (N39.0)
● G90.5   Complex regional pain syndrome I (CRPS I)
        Reflex sympathetic dystrophy
        | Excludes1 | causalgia of lower limb (G57.7-) |
        | | causalgia of upper limb (G56.4-) |
        | | complex regional pain syndrome II of lower limb (G57.7-) |
        | | complex regional pain syndrome II of upper limb (G56.4-) |

    G90.50   Complex regional pain syndrome I, unspecified
● G90.51   Complex regional pain syndrome I of upper limb
        G90.511   Complex regional pain syndrome I of right upper limb
        G90.512   Complex regional pain syndrome I of left upper limb
        G90.513   Complex regional pain syndrome I of upper limb, bilateral
        G90.519   Complex regional pain syndrome I of unspecified upper limb

CHAPTER 6 (G00-G99)

▶ New   ⇒ Revised   ~~deleted~~ Deleted   **OGCR** Official Guidelines   X Assign placeholder X   ● Use Additional Character(s)

| Excludes 1 | Excludes 2 | Includes | Use additional | Code first | Code also | Key words |

● G90.52 **Complex regional pain syndrome I of lower limb**

    G90.521 **Complex regional pain syndrome I of right lower limb**

    G90.522 **Complex regional pain syndrome I of left lower limb**

    G90.523 **Complex regional pain syndrome I of lower limb, bilateral**

    G90.529 **Complex regional pain syndrome I of unspecified lower limb**

  G90.59 **Complex regional pain syndrome I of other specified site**

G90.8 **Other disorders of autonomic nervous system**

G90.9 **Disorder of the autonomic nervous system, unspecified**

● **G91 Hydrocephalus**

Dilatation of cerebral ventricles, accompanied by accumulation of cerebrospinal fluid

  Includes acquired hydrocephalus

  Excludes1 Arnold-Chiari syndrome with hydrocephalus (Q07.-)
      congenital hydrocephalus (Q03.-)
      spina bifida with hydrocephalus (Q05.-)

G91.0 **Communicating hydrocephalus**
    Secondary normal pressure hydrocephalus

G91.1 **Obstructive hydrocephalus**

G91.2 **(Idiopathic) normal pressure hydrocephalus**
    Normal pressure hydrocephalus NOS

G91.3 **Post-traumatic hydrocephalus, unspecified**

G91.4 **Hydrocephalus in diseases classified elsewhere**
    Code first underlying condition, such as:
      congenital syphilis (A50.4-)
      neoplasm (C00-D49)

    Excludes1 hydrocephalus due to congenital toxoplasmosis (P37.1)

G91.8 **Other hydrocephalus**

G91.9 **Hydrocephalus, unspecified**

G92 **Toxic encephalopathy**
Disorder or disease of brain caused by chemicals
  Toxic encephalitis
  Toxic metabolic encephalopathy

▶ *Code first if applicable, drug induced (T36-T50) (T51-T65) to identify toxic agent*

● G93 **Other disorders of brain**

G93.0 **Cerebral cysts**
  Arachnoid cyst
  Porencephalic cyst, acquired

  Excludes1 acquired periventricular cysts of newborn (P91.1)
      congenital cerebral cysts (Q04.6)

G93.1 **Anoxic brain damage, not elsewhere classified**
Permanent brain damage by lack of oxygen perfusion through brain tissues.

  Excludes1 cerebral anoxia due to anesthesia during labor and delivery (O74.3)
      cerebral anoxia due to anesthesia during the puerperium (O89.2)
      neonatal anoxia (P84)

G93.2 **Benign intracranial hypertension**
  Excludes1 hypertensive encephalopathy (I67.4)

G93.3 **Postviral fatigue syndrome**
  Benign myalgic encephalomyelitis
  Excludes1 chronic fatigue syndrome NOS (R53.82)

● G93.4 **Other and unspecified encephalopathy**
  Excludes1 alcoholic encephalopathy (G31.2)
      encephalopathy in diseases classified elsewhere (G94)
      hypertensive encephalopathy (I67.4)
      toxic (metabolic) encephalopathy (G92)

  G93.40 **Encephalopathy, unspecified**

  G93.41 **Metabolic encephalopathy**
    Septic encephalopathy

  G93.49 **Other encephalopathy**
    Encephalopathy NEC

G93.5 **Compression of brain**
  Arnold-Chiari type 1 compression of brain
  Compression of brain (stem)
  Herniation of brain (stem)

  Excludes1 diffuse traumatic compression of brain (S06.2-)
      focal traumatic compression of brain (S06.3-)

G93.6 **Cerebral edema**
  Excludes1 cerebral edema due to birth injury (P11.0)
      traumatic cerebral edema (S06.1-)

G93.7 **Reye's syndrome**
Life-threatening neurological condition, usually follows viral illness

▶ *Code first (poisoning due to salicylates, if applicable (T39.0-, with sixth character 1-4)*
  ~~(T39.0-), if salicylates-induced~~

▶ *Use additional code for adverse effect due to salicylates, if applicable (T39.0-, with sixth character 5)*

● G93.8 **Other specified disorders of brain**

  G93.81 **Temporal sclerosis**
    Hippocampal sclerosis
    Mesial temporal sclerosis

  G93.82 **Brain death**

  G93.89 **Other specified disorders of brain**
    Postradiation encephalopathy

G93.9 **Disorder of brain, unspecified**

G94 **Other disorders of brain in diseases classified elsewhere**
Code first underlying disease

  Excludes1 encephalopathy in congenital syphilis (A50.49)
      encephalopathy in influenza (J09.X9, J10.81, J11.81)
      encephalopathy in syphilis (A52.19)
      hydrocephalus in diseases classified elsewhere (G91.4)

● G95 **Other and unspecified diseases of spinal cord**
  Excludes2 myelitis (G04.-)

G95.0 **Syringomyelia and syringobulbia**

● G95.1 **Vascular myelopathies**
  Excludes2 intraspinal phlebitis and thrombophlebitis, except non-pyogenic (G08)

  G95.11 **Acute infarction of spinal cord (embolic) (nonembolic)**
    Anoxia of spinal cord
    Arterial thrombosis of spinal cord

  G95.19 **Other vascular myelopathies**
    Edema of spinal cord
    Hematomyelia
    Nonpyogenic intraspinal phlebitis and thrombophlebitis
    Subacute necrotic myelopathy

● G95.2 **Other and unspecified cord compression**

  G95.20 **Unspecified cord compression**

  G95.29 **Other cord compression**

CHAPTER 6 (G00-G99)

● **G95.8** **Other specified diseases of spinal cord**
> **Excludes1**   neurogenic bladder NOS (N31.9)
> neurogenic bladder due to cauda equina syndrome (G83.4)
> neuromuscular dysfunction of bladder without spinal cord lesion (N31.-)

    G95.81 **Conus medullaris syndrome**
> *Damage to gray matter and/or nerve roots in lower end of spinal cord*

    G95.89 **Other specified diseases of spinal cord**
Cord bladder NOS
Drug-induced myelopathy
Radiation-induced myelopathy
> **Excludes1**   myelopathy NOS (G95.9)

G95.9 **Disease of spinal cord, unspecified**
Myelopathy NOS

● **G96** **Other disorders of central nervous system**

G96.0 **Cerebrospinal fluid leak**
> **Excludes1**   cerebrospinal fluid leak from spinal puncture (G97.0)

● **G96.1** **Disorders of meninges, not elsewhere classified**

    G96.11 **Dural tear**
> **Excludes1**   accidental puncture or laceration of dura during a procedure (G97.41)

    G96.12 **Meningeal adhesions (cerebral) (spinal)**

    G96.19 **Other disorders of meninges, not elsewhere classified**

G96.8 **Other specified disorders of central nervous system**

G96.9 **Disorder of central nervous system, unspecified**

● **G97** **Intraoperative and postprocedural complications and disorders of nervous system, not elsewhere classified**
> **Excludes2**   intraoperative and postprocedural cerebrovascular infarction (I97.81-, I97.82-)

G97.0 **Cerebrospinal fluid leak from spinal puncture**

G97.1 **Other reaction to spinal and lumbar puncture**
Headache due to lumbar puncture

G97.2 **Intracranial hypotension following ventricular shunting**

● **G97.3** **Intraoperative hemorrhage and hematoma of a nervous system organ or structure complicating a procedure**
> **Excludes1**   intraoperative hemorrhage and hematoma of a nervous system organ or structure due to accidental puncture and laceration during a procedure (G97.4-)

    G97.31 **Intraoperative hemorrhage and hematoma of a nervous system organ or structure complicating a nervous system procedure**

    G97.32 **Intraoperative hemorrhage and hematoma of a nervous system organ or structure complicating other procedure**

● **G97.4** **Accidental puncture and laceration of a nervous system organ or structure during a procedure**

    G97.41 **Accidental puncture or laceration of dura during a procedure**
Incidental (inadvertent) durotomy

    G97.48 **Accidental puncture and laceration of other nervous system organ or structure during a nervous system procedure**

    G97.49 **Accidental puncture and laceration of other nervous system organ or structure during other procedure**

● **G97.5** **Postprocedural hemorrhage of a nervous system organ or structure following a procedure**

    G97.51 **Postprocedural hemorrhage of a nervous system organ or structure following a nervous system procedure**

    G97.52 **Postprocedural hemorrhage of a nervous system organ or structure following other procedure**

● **G97.6** **Postprocedural hematoma and seroma of a nervous system organ or structure following a procedure**

    G97.61 **Postprocedural hematoma of a nervous system organ or structure following a nervous system procedure**

    G97.62 **Postprocedural hematoma of a nervous system organ or structure following other procedure**

    G97.63 **Postprocedural seroma of a nervous system organ or structure following a nervous system procedure**

    G97.64 **Postprocedural seroma of a nervous system organ or structure following other procedure**

● **G97.8** **Other intraoperative and postprocedural complications and disorders of nervous system**
> Use additional code to further specify disorder

    G97.81 **Other intraoperative complications of nervous system**

    G97.82 **Other postprocedural complications and disorders of nervous system**

● **G98** **Other disorders of nervous system not elsewhere classified**
> **Includes**   nervous system disorder NOS

G98.0 **Neurogenic arthritis, not elsewhere classified**
Nonsyphilitic neurogenic arthropathy NEC
Nonsyphilitic neurogenic spondylopathy NEC
> **Excludes1**   spondylopathy (in):
> syringomyelia and syringobulbia (G95.0)
> tabes dorsalis (A52.11)

G98.8 **Other disorders of nervous system**
Nervous system disorder NOS

● **G99** **Other disorders of nervous system in diseases classified elsewhere**

G99.0 **Autonomic neuropathy in diseases classified elsewhere**
> *Code first underlying disease, such as:*
> amyloidosis (E85.-)
> gout (M1A.-, M10.-)
> hyperthyroidism (E05.-)
> **Excludes1**   diabetic autonomic neuropathy (E08-E13 with .43)

G99.2 **Myelopathy in diseases classified elsewhere**
> *Code first underlying disease, such as:*
> neoplasm (C00-D49)
> **Excludes1**   myelopathy in:
> intervertebral disease (M50.0-, M51.0-)
> spondylosis (M47.0-, M47.1-)

G99.8 **Other specified disorders of nervous system in diseases classified elsewhere**
> *Code first underlying disorder, such as:*
> amyloidosis (E85.-)
> avitaminosis (E56.9)
> **Excludes1**   nervous system involvement in:
> cysticercosis (B69.0)
> rubella (B06.0-)
> syphilis (A52.1-)

▶ New   ⇛ Revised   ~~deleted~~ Deleted   **OGCR** Official Guidelines   X Assign placeholder X   ● Use Additional Character(s)

Excludes 1   Excludes 2   Includes   Use additional   Code first   Code also   Key words

CHAPTER 7

DISEASES OF THE EYE AND ADNEXA
(H00-H59)

7. Chapter 7: Diseases of the Eye and Adnexa (H00-H59)

a. Glaucoma

1) **Assigning Glaucoma Codes**

Assign as many codes from category H40, Glaucoma, as needed to identify the type of glaucoma, the affected eye, and the glaucoma stage.

2) **Bilateral glaucoma with same type and stage**

When a patient has bilateral glaucoma and both eyes are documented as being the same type and stage, and there is a code for bilateral glaucoma, report only the code for the type of glaucoma, bilateral, with the seventh character for the stage.

When a patient has bilateral glaucoma and both eyes are documented as being the same type and stage, and the classification does not provide a code for bilateral glaucoma (i.e. subcategories H40.10, H40.11 and H40.20) report only one code for the type of glaucoma with the appropriate seventh character for the stage.

3) **Bilateral glaucoma stage with different types or stages**

When a patient has bilateral glaucoma and each eye is documented as having a different type or stage, and the classification distinguishes laterality, assign the appropriate code for each eye rather than the code for bilateral glaucoma.

When a patient has bilateral glaucoma and each eye is documented as having a different type, and the classification does not distinguish laterality (i.e. subcategories H40.10, H40.11 and H40.20), assign one code for each type of glaucoma with the appropriate seventh character for the stage.

When a patient has bilateral glaucoma and each eye is documented as having the same type, but different stage, and the classification does not distinguish laterality (i.e. subcategories H40.10, H40.11 and H40.20), assign a code for the type of glaucoma for each eye with the seventh character for the specific glaucoma stage documented for each eye.

4) **Patient admitted with glaucoma and stage evolves during the admission**

If a patient is admitted with glaucoma and the stage progresses during the admission, assign the code for highest stage documented.

5) **Indeterminate stage glaucoma**

Assignment of the seventh character "4" for "indeterminate stage" should be based on the clinical documentation. The seventh character "4" is used for glaucomas whose stage cannot be clinically determined. This seventh character should not be confused with the seventh character "0", unspecified, which should be assigned when there is no documentation regarding the stage of the glaucoma.

b. Blindness

If "blindness" or "low vision" of both eyes is documented but the visual impairment category is not documented, assign code H54.3, Unqualified visual loss, both eyes. If "blindness" or "low vision" in one eye is documented but the visual impairment category is not documented, assign a code from H54.6-, Unqualified visual loss, one eye. If "blindness" or "visual loss" is documented without any information about whether one or both eyes are affected, assign code H54.7, Unspecified visual loss.

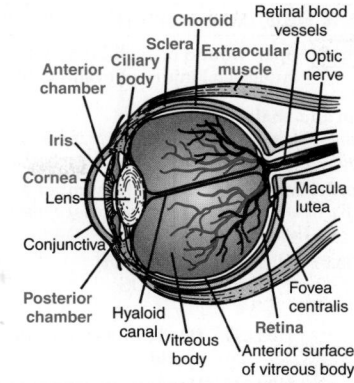

Figure 7-1 Eye and ocular adnexa. (From Buck CJ: Step-by-Step Medical Coding, ed 2016, St. Louis, Elsevier, 2016)

★**(See Plate 87 on page 63.)**

CHAPTER 7

DISEASES OF THE EYE AND ADNEXA
(H00-H59)

Note: Use an external cause code following the code for the eye condition, if applicable, to identify the cause of the eye condition

Excludes2
certain conditions originating in the perinatal period (P04-P96)
certain infectious and parasitic diseases (A00-B99)
complications of pregnancy, childbirth and the puerperium (O00-O9A)
congenital malformations, deformations, and chromosomal abnormalities (Q00-Q99)
diabetes mellitus related eye conditions (E09.3-, E10.3-, E11.3-, E13.3-)
endocrine, nutritional and metabolic diseases (E00-E88)
injury (trauma) of eye and orbit (S05.-)
injury, poisoning and certain other consequences of external causes (S00-T88)
neoplasms (C00-D49)
symptoms, signs and abnormal clinical and laboratory findings, not elsewhere classified (R00-R94)
syphilis related eye disorders (A50.01, A50.3-, A51.43, A52.71)

This chapter contains the following blocks:

H00-H05	Disorders of eyelid, lacrimal system and orbit
H10-H11	Disorders of conjunctiva
H15-H22	Disorders of sclera, cornea, iris and ciliary body
H25-H28	Disorders of lens
H30-H36	Disorders of choroid and retina
H40-H42	Glaucoma
H43-H44	Disorders of vitreous body and globe
H46-H47	Disorders of optic nerve and visual pathways
H49-H52	Disorders of ocular muscles, binocular movement, accommodation and refraction
H53-H54	Visual disturbances and blindness
H55-H57	Other disorders of eye and adnexa
H59	Intraoperative and postprocedural complications and disorders of eye and adnexa, not elsewhere classified

DISORDERS OF EYELID, LACRIMAL SYSTEM AND ORBIT (H00-H05)

Excludes2   open wound of eyelid (S01.1-)
                  superficial injury of eyelid (S00.1-, S00.2-)

● **H00**   **Hordeolum and chalazion**
Hordeolum: inflammatory staphylococcal infection of sebaceous glands of eyelids; AKA stye. Chalazion: eyelid mass

● **H00.0**   **Hordeolum (externum) (internum) of eyelid**
Bacterial infection (staphylococcus) of the sebaceous gland of the eyelid (stye)

● **H00.01**   **Hordeolum externum**
Hordeolum NOS
Stye

     H00.011   Hordeolum externum right upper eyelid

     H00.012   Hordeolum externum right lower eyelid

     H00.013   Hordeolum externum right eye, unspecified eyelid

     H00.014   Hordeolum externum left upper eyelid

     H00.015   Hordeolum externum left lower eyelid

     H00.016   Hordeolum externum left eye, unspecified eyelid

     H00.019   Hordeolum externum unspecified eye, unspecified eyelid

● **H00.02**   **Hordeolum internum**
Infection of meibomian gland

     H00.021   Hordeolum internum right upper eyelid

     H00.022   Hordeolum internum right lower eyelid

     H00.023   Hordeolum internum right eye, unspecified eyelid

     H00.024   Hordeolum internum left upper eyelid

     H00.025   Hordeolum internum left lower eyelid

     H00.026   Hordeolum internum left eye, unspecified eyelid

     H00.029   Hordeolum internum unspecified eye, unspecified eyelid

● **H00.03**   **Abscess of eyelid**
Furuncle of eyelid

     H00.031   Abscess of right upper eyelid

     H00.032   Abscess of right lower eyelid

     H00.033   Abscess of eyelid right eye, unspecified eyelid

     H00.034   Abscess of left upper eyelid

     H00.035   Abscess of left lower eyelid

     H00.036   Abscess of eyelid left eye, unspecified eyelid

     H00.039   Abscess of eyelid unspecified eye, unspecified eyelid

● **H00.1**   **Chalazion**
Often caused by accumulation of meibomian gland secretions resulting from a blockage of duct.
Meibomian (gland) cyst

Excludes2   infected meibomian gland (H00.02-)

     H00.11   Chalazion right upper eyelid

     H00.12   Chalazion right lower eyelid

     H00.13   Chalazion right eye, unspecified eyelid

     H00.14   Chalazion left upper eyelid

     H00.15   Chalazion left lower eyelid

     H00.16   Chalazion left eye, unspecified eyelid

     H00.19   Chalazion unspecified eye, unspecified eyelid

● **H01**   **Other inflammation of eyelid**

● **H01.0**   **Blepharitis**
Inflammation of eyelids

Excludes1   blepharoconjunctivitis (H10.5-)

● **H01.00**   **Unspecified blepharitis**

     H01.001   Unspecified blepharitis right upper eyelid

     H01.002   Unspecified blepharitis right lower eyelid

     H01.003   Unspecified blepharitis right eye, unspecified eyelid

     H01.004   Unspecified blepharitis left upper eyelid

     H01.005   Unspecified blepharitis left lower eyelid

     H01.006   Unspecified blepharitis left eye, unspecified eyelid

     H01.009   Unspecified blepharitis unspecified eye, unspecified eyelid

● **H01.01**   **Ulcerative blepharitis**

     H01.011   Ulcerative blepharitis right upper eyelid

     H01.012   Ulcerative blepharitis right lower eyelid

     H01.013   Ulcerative blepharitis right eye, unspecified eyelid

     H01.014   Ulcerative blepharitis left upper eyelid

     H01.015   Ulcerative blepharitis left lower eyelid

     H01.016   Ulcerative blepharitis left eye, unspecified eyelid

     H01.019   Ulcerative blepharitis unspecified eye, unspecified eyelid

● **H01.02**   **Squamous blepharitis**

     H01.021   Squamous blepharitis right upper eyelid

     H01.022   Squamous blepharitis right lower eyelid

     H01.023   Squamous blepharitis right eye, unspecified eyelid

     H01.024   Squamous blepharitis left upper eyelid

     H01.025   Squamous blepharitis left lower eyelid

     H01.026   Squamous blepharitis left eye, unspecified eyelid

     H01.029   Squamous blepharitis unspecified eye, unspecified eyelid

● **H01.1**   **Noninfectious dermatoses of eyelid**

● **H01.11**   **Allergic dermatitis of eyelid**
Contact dermatitis of eyelid

     H01.111   Allergic dermatitis of right upper eyelid

     H01.112   Allergic dermatitis of right lower eyelid

     H01.113   Allergic dermatitis of right eye, unspecified eyelid

     H01.114   Allergic dermatitis of left upper eyelid

     H01.115   Allergic dermatitis of left lower eyelid

     H01.116   Allergic dermatitis of left eye, unspecified eyelid

     H01.119   Allergic dermatitis of unspecified eye, unspecified eyelid

▶ New   ⇒ Revised   ~~deleted~~ Deleted   **OGCR** Official Guidelines   X Assign placeholder X   ● Use Additional Character(s)

Excludes 1   Excludes 2   Includes   Use additional   Code first   Code also   Key words

● **H01.12   Discoid lupus erythematosus of eyelid**
   H01.121   Discoid lupus erythematosus of right upper eyelid
   H01.122   Discoid lupus erythematosus of right lower eyelid
   H01.123   Discoid lupus erythematosus of right eye, unspecified eyelid
   H01.124   Discoid lupus erythematosus of left upper eyelid
   H01.125   Discoid lupus erythematosus of left lower eyelid
   H01.126   Discoid lupus erythematosus of left eye, unspecified eyelid
   H01.129   Discoid lupus erythematosus of unspecified eye, unspecified eyelid

● **H01.13   Eczematous dermatitis of eyelid**
   H01.131   Eczematous dermatitis of right upper eyelid
   H01.132   Eczematous dermatitis of right lower eyelid
   H01.133   Eczematous dermatitis of right eye, unspecified eyelid
   H01.134   Eczematous dermatitis of left upper eyelid
   H01.135   Eczematous dermatitis of left lower eyelid
   H01.136   Eczematous dermatitis of left eye, unspecified eyelid
   H01.139   Eczematous dermatitis of unspecified eye, unspecified eyelid

● **H01.14   Xeroderma of eyelid**
   Abnormally dry
   H01.141   Xeroderma of right upper eyelid
   H01.142   Xeroderma of right lower eyelid
   H01.143   Xeroderma of right eye, unspecified eyelid
   H01.144   Xeroderma of left upper eyelid
   H01.145   Xeroderma of left lower eyelid
   H01.146   Xeroderma of left eye, unspecified eyelid
   H01.149   Xeroderma of unspecified eye, unspecified eyelid

H01.8   **Other specified inflammations of eyelid**
H01.9   **Unspecified inflammation of eyelid**
   Inflammation of eyelid NOS

● **H02   Other disorders of eyelid**
   Turning inward (inversion) of eyelid margin and ingrowing eyelashes
   Excludes1   congenital malformations of eyelid (Q10.0-Q10.3)

● **H02.0   Entropion and trichiasis of eyelid**
  ● **H02.00   Unspecified entropion of eyelid**
    H02.001   Unspecified entropion of right upper eyelid
    H02.002   Unspecified entropion of right lower eyelid
    H02.003   Unspecified entropion of right eye, unspecified eyelid
    H02.004   Unspecified entropion of left upper eyelid

    H02.005   Unspecified entropion of left lower eyelid
    H02.006   Unspecified entropion of left eye, unspecified eyelid
    H02.009   Unspecified entropion of unspecified eye, unspecified eyelid

● **H02.01   Cicatricial entropion of eyelid**
   Scar
   H02.011   Cicatricial entropion of right upper eyelid
   H02.012   Cicatricial entropion of right lower eyelid
   H02.013   Cicatricial entropion of right eye, unspecified eyelid
   H02.014   Cicatricial entropion of left upper eyelid
   H02.015   Cicatricial entropion of left lower eyelid
   H02.016   Cicatricial entropion of left eye, unspecified eyelid
   H02.019   Cicatricial entropion of unspecified eye, unspecified eyelid

● **H02.02   Mechanical entropion of eyelid**
   Turning inward (inversion) of eyelid margin due to lack of support
   H02.021   Mechanical entropion of right upper eyelid
   H02.022   Mechanical entropion of right lower eyelid
   H02.023   Mechanical entropion of right eye, unspecified eyelid
   H02.024   Mechanical entropion of left upper eyelid
   H02.025   Mechanical entropion of left lower eyelid
   H02.026   Mechanical entropion of left eye, unspecified eyelid
   H02.029   Mechanical entropion of unspecified eye, unspecified eyelid

● **H02.03   Senile entropion of eyelid**
   Turning inward (inversion) of eyelid margin due to aging
   H02.031   Senile entropion of right upper eyelid
   H02.032   Senile entropion of right lower eyelid
   H02.033   Senile entropion of right eye, unspecified eyelid
   H02.034   Senile entropion of left upper eyelid
   H02.035   Senile entropion of left lower eyelid
   H02.036   Senile entropion of left eye, unspecified eyelid
   H02.039   Senile entropion of unspecified eye, unspecified eyelid

● **H02.04   Spastic entropion of eyelid**
   Turning inward (inversion) of eyelid margin caused by spasm of muscle
   H02.041   Spastic entropion of right upper eyelid
   H02.042   Spastic entropion of right lower eyelid
   H02.043   Spastic entropion of right eye, unspecified eyelid
   H02.044   Spastic entropion of left upper eyelid
   H02.045   Spastic entropion of left lower eyelid
   H02.046   Spastic entropion of left eye, unspecified eyelid
   H02.049   Spastic entropion of unspecified eye, unspecified eyelid

CHAPTER 7 (H00-H59)

Figure 7-2   Right lower eyelid entropion. Note the inward rotation of the tarsal plate about the horizontal axis and the resultant contact between the mucocutaneous junction and ocular surface. (From Glynn M, Drake WM, Hutchison R: Hutchison's Clinical Methods: An Integrated Approach to Clinical Practice, Edinburgh, Saunders/Elsevier, 2012)

▶ New   ➡ Revised   ~~deleted~~ Deleted   **OGCR** Official Guidelines   X Assign placeholder X   ● Use Additional Character(s)

Excludes 1   Excludes 2   Includes   Use additional   Code first   Code also   Key words

CHAPTER 7 (H00-H59)

▶● **H02.05**   **Trichiasis without entropion**
       Ingrowing hairs of eyelashes

➡ **H02.051**   Trichiasis without entropion right upper eyelid

➡ **H02.052**   Trichiasis without entropion right lower eyelid

➡ **H02.053**   Trichiasis without entropion right eye, unspecified eyelid

➡ **H02.054**   Trichiasis without entropion left upper eyelid

➡ **H02.055**   Trichiasis without entropion left lower eyelid

➡ **H02.056**   Trichiasis without entropion left eye, unspecified eyelid

➡ **H02.059**   Trichiasis without entropion unspecified eye, unspecified eyelid

● **H02.1**   **Ectropion of eyelid**
       Eversion (pulling away) of eyelid

● **H02.10**   **Unspecified** ectropion of eyelid

     H02.101   Unspecified ectropion of right upper eyelid

     H02.102   Unspecified ectropion of right lower eyelid

     H02.103   Unspecified ectropion of right eye, unspecified eyelid

     H02.104   Unspecified ectropion of left upper eyelid

     H02.105   Unspecified ectropion of left lower eyelid

     H02.106   Unspecified ectropion of left eye, unspecified eyelid

     H02.109   Unspecified ectropion of unspecified eye, unspecified eyelid

● **H02.11**   **Cicatricial** ectropion of eyelid
       Pulling of eyelid down and away from eye due to scar or tightening

     H02.111   Cicatricial ectropion of right upper eyelid

     H02.112   Cicatricial ectropion of right lower eyelid

     H02.113   Cicatricial ectropion of right eye, unspecified eyelid

     H02.114   Cicatricial ectropion of left upper eyelid

     H02.115   Cicatricial ectropion of left lower eyelid

     H02.116   Cicatricial ectropion of left eye, unspecified eyelid

     H02.119   Cicatricial ectropion of unspecified eye, unspecified eyelid

● **H02.12**   **Mechanical** ectropion of eyelid
       Eversion (pulling away) of eyelid due to lack of support

     H02.121   Mechanical ectropion of right upper eyelid

     H02.122   Mechanical ectropion of right lower eyelid

     H02.123   Mechanical ectropion of right eye, unspecified eyelid

     H02.124   Mechanical ectropion of left upper eyelid

     H02.125   Mechanical ectropion of left lower eyelid

     H02.126   Mechanical ectropion of left eye, unspecified eyelid

     H02.129   Mechanical ectropion of unspecified eye, unspecified eyelid

● **H02.13**   **Senile** ectropion of eyelid
       Eversion (pulling away) of eyelid due to age

     H02.131   Senile ectropion of right upper eyelid

     H02.132   Senile ectropion of right lower eyelid

     H02.133   Senile ectropion of right eye, unspecified eyelid

     H02.134   Senile ectropion of left upper eyelid

     H02.135   Senile ectropion of left lower eyelid

     H02.136   Senile ectropion of left eye, unspecified eyelid

     H02.139   Senile ectropion of unspecified eye, unspecified eyelid

● **H02.14**   **Spastic** ectropion of eyelid
       Eversion (pulling away) of eyelid due to tonic muscle spasm

     H02.141   Spastic ectropion of right upper eyelid

     H02.142   Spastic ectropion of right lower eyelid

     H02.143   Spastic ectropion of right eye, unspecified eyelid

     H02.144   Spastic ectropion of left upper eyelid

     H02.145   Spastic ectropion of left lower eyelid

     H02.146   Spastic ectropion of left eye, unspecified eyelid

     H02.149   Spastic ectropion of unspecified eye, unspecified eyelid

● **H02.2**   **Lagophthalmos**
       Condition in which eye cannot completely close

● **H02.20**   **Unspecified** lagophthalmos

     H02.201   Unspecified lagophthalmos right upper eyelid

     H02.202   Unspecified lagophthalmos right lower eyelid

     H02.203   Unspecified lagophthalmos right eye, unspecified eyelid

     H02.204   Unspecified lagophthalmos left upper eyelid

     H02.205   Unspecified lagophthalmos left lower eyelid

     H02.206   Unspecified lagophthalmos left eye, unspecified eyelid

     H02.209   Unspecified lagophthalmos unspecified eye, unspecified eyelid

● **H02.21**   **Cicatricial** lagophthalmos
       Upper or lower eyelid does not close due to scar or tightening

     H02.211   Cicatricial lagophthalmos right upper eyelid

     H02.212   Cicatricial lagophthalmos right lower eyelid

     H02.213   Cicatricial lagophthalmos right eye, unspecified eyelid

     H02.214   Cicatricial lagophthalmos left upper eyelid

     H02.215   Cicatricial lagophthalmos left lower eyelid

     H02.216   Cicatricial lagophthalmos left eye, unspecified eyelid

     H02.219   Cicatricial lagophthalmos unspecified eye, unspecified eyelid

▶ New   ➡ Revised   ~~deleted~~ Deleted   OGCR Official Guidelines   X Assign placeholder X   ● Use Additional Character(s)

Excludes 1   Excludes 2   Includes   Use additional   Code first   Code also   Key words

● **H02.22**   Mechanical lagophthalmos
     Inability to close lids due to structural disorder
     H02.221   Mechanical lagophthalmos right upper eyelid
     H02.222   Mechanical lagophthalmos right lower eyelid
     H02.223   Mechanical lagophthalmos right eye, unspecified eyelid
     H02.224   Mechanical lagophthalmos left upper eyelid
     H02.225   Mechanical lagophthalmos left lower eyelid
     H02.226   Mechanical lagophthalmos left eye, unspecified eyelid
     H02.229   Mechanical lagophthalmos unspecified eye, unspecified eyelid

● **H02.23**   Paralytic lagophthalmos
     Eyelids do not close due to paralysis
     H02.231   Paralytic lagophthalmos right upper eyelid
     H02.232   Paralytic lagophthalmos right lower eyelid
     H02.233   Paralytic lagophthalmos right eye, unspecified eyelid
     H02.234   Paralytic lagophthalmos left upper eyelid
     H02.235   Paralytic lagophthalmos left lower eyelid
     H02.236   Paralytic lagophthalmos left eye, unspecified eyelid
     H02.239   Paralytic lagophthalmos unspecified eye, unspecified eyelid

★ **(See Plate 81, middle, on page 65.)**

● **H02.3**   Blepharochalasis
     Relaxation of skin of eyelid, due to atrophy of intercellular tissue
     Pseudoptosis
     H02.30   Blepharochalasis unspecified eye, unspecified eyelid
     H02.31   Blepharochalasis right upper eyelid
     H02.32   Blepharochalasis right lower eyelid
     H02.33   Blepharochalasis right eye, unspecified eyelid
     H02.34   Blepharochalasis left upper eyelid
     H02.35   Blepharochalasis left lower eyelid
     H02.36   Blepharochalasis left eye, unspecified eyelid

● **H02.4**   Ptosis of eyelid
     Falling forward, drooping, sagging of eyelid
  ● **H02.40**   Unspecified ptosis of eyelid
     H02.401   Unspecified ptosis of right eyelid
     H02.402   Unspecified ptosis of left eyelid
     H02.403   Unspecified ptosis of bilateral eyelids
     H02.409   Unspecified ptosis of unspecified eyelid
  ● **H02.41**   Mechanical ptosis of eyelid
     H02.411   Mechanical ptosis of right eyelid
     H02.412   Mechanical ptosis of left eyelid
     H02.413   Mechanical ptosis of bilateral eyelids
     H02.419   Mechanical ptosis of unspecified eyelid

Item 7–1   Ptosis of eyelid is drooping of the upper eyelid over the pupil when the eyes are fully opened resulting from nerve or muscle damage, which may require surgical correction.

  ● **H02.42**   Myogenic ptosis of eyelid
     H02.421   Myogenic ptosis of right eyelid
     H02.422   Myogenic ptosis of left eyelid
     H02.423   Myogenic ptosis of bilateral eyelids
     H02.429   Myogenic ptosis of unspecified eyelid
  ● **H02.43**   Paralytic ptosis of eyelid
     Neurogenic ptosis of eyelid
     H02.431   Paralytic ptosis of right eyelid
     H02.432   Paralytic ptosis of left eyelid
     H02.433   Paralytic ptosis of bilateral eyelids
     H02.439   Paralytic ptosis unspecified eyelid

● **H02.5**   Other disorders affecting eyelid function
     | Excludes2 | blepharospasm (G24.5)
           organic tic (G25.69)
           psychogenic tic (F95.-)
  ● **H02.51**   Abnormal innervation syndrome
     H02.511   Abnormal innervation syndrome right upper eyelid
     H02.512   Abnormal innervation syndrome right lower eyelid
     H02.513   Abnormal innervation syndrome right eye, unspecified eyelid
     H02.514   Abnormal innervation syndrome left upper eyelid
     H02.515   Abnormal innervation syndrome left lower eyelid
     H02.516   Abnormal innervation syndrome left eye, unspecified eyelid
     H02.519   Abnormal innervation syndrome unspecified eye, unspecified eyelid
  ● **H02.52**   Blepharophimosis
     Drooping of eyelid with reduced lid size
     Ankyloblepharon
     H02.521   Blepharophimosis right upper eyelid
     H02.522   Blepharophimosis right lower eyelid
     H02.523   Blepharophimosis right eye, unspecified eyelid
     H02.524   Blepharophimosis left upper eyelid
     H02.525   Blepharophimosis left lower eyelid
     H02.526   Blepharophimosis left eye, unspecified eyelid
     H02.529   Blepharophimosis unspecified eye, unspecified lid
  ● **H02.53**   Eyelid retraction
     Eyelid lag
     H02.531   Eyelid retraction right upper eyelid
     H02.532   Eyelid retraction right lower eyelid
     H02.533   Eyelid retraction right eye, unspecified eyelid
     H02.534   Eyelid retraction left upper eyelid
     H02.535   Eyelid retraction left lower eyelid
     H02.536   Eyelid retraction left eye, unspecified eyelid
     H02.539   Eyelid retraction unspecified eye, unspecified lid
     H02.59   Other disorders affecting eyelid function
         Deficient blink reflex
         Sensory disorders

Figure 7-3   Ptosis of eyelid. (From Kanski JJ: Clinical Diagnosis in Ophthalmology, London, Elsevier Mosby, 2006)

CHAPTER 7 (H00-H59)

▶ New   ⇒ Revised   ~~deleted~~ Deleted   **OGCR** Official Guidelines   X Assign placeholder X   ● Use Additional Character(s)

| Excludes 1 | | Excludes 2 | Includes   Use additional   Code first   Code also   Key words

CHAPTER 7 (H00-H59)

● H02.6 **Xanthelasma** of eyelid
      Yellow-to-orange patches or pimples clustered together on eyelid
    H02.60 Xanthelasma of **unspecified eye, unspecified eyelid**
    H02.61 Xanthelasma of **right upper** eyelid
    H02.62 Xanthelasma of **right lower** eyelid
    H02.63 Xanthelasma of **right eye, unspecified** eyelid
    H02.64 Xanthelasma of **left upper** eyelid
    H02.65 Xanthelasma of **left lower** eyelid
    H02.66 Xanthelasma of **left eye, unspecified** eyelid

● H02.7 Other and unspecified degenerative disorders of eyelid and periocular area
    H02.70 **Unspecified** degenerative disorders of eyelid and periocular area
   ● H02.71 **Chloasma** of eyelid and periocular area
       Dyspigmentation of eyelid
       Hyperpigmentation of eyelid
    H02.711 Chloasma of **right upper** eyelid and periocular area
    H02.712 Chloasma of **right lower** eyelid and periocular area
    H02.713 Chloasma of **right eye, unspecified** eyelid and periocular area
    H02.714 Chloasma of **left upper** eyelid and periocular area
    H02.715 Chloasma of **left lower** eyelid and periocular area
    H02.716 Chloasma of **left eye, unspecified** eyelid and periocular area
    H02.719 Chloasma of **unspecified** eye, **unspecified** eyelid and periocular area
   ● H02.72 **Madarosis** of eyelid and periocular area
       Loss of eyelashes and/or eyebrows
       Hypotrichosis of eyelid
    H02.721 Madarosis of **right upper** eyelid and periocular area
    H02.722 Madarosis of **right lower** eyelid and periocular area
    H02.723 Madarosis of **right eye, unspecified** eyelid and periocular area
    H02.724 Madarosis of **left upper** eyelid and periocular area
    H02.725 Madarosis of **left lower** eyelid and periocular area
    H02.726 Madarosis of **left eye, unspecified** eyelid and periocular area
    H02.729 Madarosis of **unspecified** eye, **unspecified** eyelid and periocular area
   ● H02.73 **Vitiligo** of eyelid and periocular area
       Skin pigmentation disease characterized by white patches
       Hypopigmentation of eyelid
    H02.731 Vitiligo of **right upper** eyelid and periocular area
    H02.732 Vitiligo of **right lower** eyelid and periocular area
    H02.733 Vitiligo of **right eye, unspecified** eyelid and periocular area
    H02.734 Vitiligo of **left upper** eyelid and periocular area
    H02.735 Vitiligo of **left lower** eyelid and periocular area
    H02.736 Vitiligo of **left eye, unspecified** eyelid and periocular area
    H02.739 Vitiligo of **unspecified** eye, **unspecified** eyelid and periocular area
    H02.79 **Other** degenerative disorders of eyelid and periocular area

● H02.8 Other specified disorders of eyelid
   ● H02.81 **Retained foreign body in eyelid**
       Use additional code to identify the type of retained foreign body (Z18.-)
       Excludes1 laceration of eyelid with foreign body (S01.12-)
             retained intraocular foreign body (H44.6-, H44.7-)
             superficial foreign body of eyelid and periocular area (S00.25-)
    H02.811 Retained foreign body in **right upper** eyelid
    H02.812 Retained foreign body in **right lower** eyelid
    H02.813 Retained foreign body in **right eye, unspecified** eyelid
    H02.814 Retained foreign body in **left upper** eyelid
    H02.815 Retained foreign body in **left lower** eyelid
    H02.816 Retained foreign body in **left eye, unspecified** eyelid
    H02.819 Retained foreign body in **unspecified** eye, **unspecified** eyelid
   ● H02.82 **Cysts** of eyelid
       Sebaceous cyst of eyelid
    H02.821 Cysts of **right upper** eyelid
    H02.822 Cysts of **right lower** eyelid
    H02.823 Cysts of **right eye, unspecified** eyelid
    H02.824 Cysts of **left upper** eyelid
    H02.825 Cysts of **left lower** eyelid
    H02.826 Cysts of **left eye, unspecified** eyelid
    H02.829 Cysts of **unspecified eye, unspecified** eyelid
   ● H02.83 **Dermatochalasis** of eyelid
       Skin is inelastic and hangs loosely in folds
    H02.831 Dermatochalasis of **right upper** eyelid
    H02.832 Dermatochalasis of **right lower** eyelid
    H02.833 Dermatochalasis of **right eye, unspecified** eyelid
    H02.834 Dermatochalasis of **left upper** eyelid
    H02.835 Dermatochalasis of **left lower** eyelid
    H02.836 Dermatochalasis of **left eye, unspecified** eyelid
    H02.839 Dermatochalasis of **unspecified eye, unspecified** eyelid
   ● H02.84 **Edema** of eyelid
       Hyperemia of eyelid
    H02.841 Edema of **right upper** eyelid
    H02.842 Edema of **right lower** eyelid
    H02.843 Edema of **right eye, unspecified** eyelid
    H02.844 Edema of **left upper** eyelid
    H02.845 Edema of **left lower** eyelid
    H02.846 Edema of **left eye, unspecified** eyelid
    H02.849 Edema of **unspecified eye, unspecified** eyelid
   ● H02.85 **Elephantiasis** of eyelid
       Massive secondary lymphedema with hypertrophy of skin and subcutaneous tissues (pachyderma)
    H02.851 Elephantiasis of **right upper** eyelid
    H02.852 Elephantiasis of **right lower** eyelid
    H02.853 Elephantiasis of **right eye, unspecified** eyelid
    H02.854 Elephantiasis of **left upper** eyelid
    H02.855 Elephantiasis of **left lower** eyelid

▶ New   ⇛ Revised   ~~deleted~~ Deleted   **OGCR** Official Guidelines   X Assign placeholder X   ● Use Additional Character(s)

Excludes 1   Excludes 2   Includes   Use additional   Code first   Code also   Key words

H02.856   Elephantiasis of left eye, unspecified eyelid

H02.859   Elephantiasis of unspecified eye, unspecified eyelid

● H02.86   Hypertrichosis of eyelid
Excessive growth of hair

H02.861   Hypertrichosis of right upper eyelid

H02.862   Hypertrichosis of right lower eyelid

H02.863   Hypertrichosis of right eye, unspecified eyelid

H02.864   Hypertrichosis of left upper eyelid

H02.865   Hypertrichosis of left lower eyelid

H02.866   Hypertrichosis of left eye, unspecified eyelid

H02.869   Hypertrichosis of unspecified eye, unspecified eyelid

● H02.87   Vascular anomalies of eyelid

H02.871   Vascular anomalies of right upper eyelid

H02.872   Vascular anomalies of right lower eyelid

H02.873   Vascular anomalies of right eye, unspecified eyelid

H02.874   Vascular anomalies of left upper eyelid

H02.875   Vascular anomalies of left lower eyelid

H02.876   Vascular anomalies of left eye, unspecified eyelid

H02.879   Vascular anomalies of unspecified eye, unspecified eyelid

H02.89   Other specified disorders of eyelid
Hemorrhage of eyelid

H02.9   Unspecified disorder of eyelid
Disorder of eyelid NOS

● H04   Disorders of lacrimal system
Excludes1   congenital malformations of lacrimal system (Q10.4-Q10.6)

● H04.0   Dacryoadenitis
Inflammation of lacrimal gland

● H04.00   Unspecified dacryoadenitis

H04.001   Unspecified dacryoadenitis, right lacrimal gland

H04.002   Unspecified dacryoadenitis, left lacrimal gland

H04.003   Unspecified dacryoadenitis, bilateral lacrimal glands

H04.009   Unspecified dacryoadenitis, unspecified lacrimal gland

● H04.01   Acute dacryoadenitis

H04.011   Acute dacryoadenitis, right lacrimal gland

H04.012   Acute dacryoadenitis, left lacrimal gland

H04.013   Acute dacryoadenitis, bilateral lacrimal glands

H04.019   Acute dacryoadenitis, unspecified lacrimal gland

★ **(See Plate 82 on page 67.)**

● H04.02   Chronic dacryoadenitis

H04.021   Chronic dacryoadenitis, right lacrimal gland

H04.022   Chronic dacryoadenitis, left lacrimal gland

H04.023   Chronic dacryoadenitis, bilateral lacrimal gland

H04.029   Chronic dacryoadenitis, unspecified lacrimal gland

● H04.03   Chronic enlargement of lacrimal gland

H04.031   Chronic enlargement of right lacrimal gland

H04.032   Chronic enlargement of left lacrimal gland

H04.033   Chronic enlargement of bilateral lacrimal glands

H04.039   Chronic enlargement of unspecified lacrimal gland

● H04.1   Other disorders of lacrimal gland

● H04.11   Dacryops
Watery eye or distention of lacrimal duct due to fluid

H04.111   Dacryops of right lacrimal gland

H04.112   Dacryops of left lacrimal gland

H04.113   Dacryops of bilateral lacrimal glands

H04.119   Dacryops of unspecified lacrimal gland

● H04.12   Dry eye syndrome
Tear film insufficiency, NOS

H04.121   Dry eye syndrome of right lacrimal gland

H04.122   Dry eye syndrome of left lacrimal gland

H04.123   Dry eye syndrome of bilateral lacrimal glands

H04.129   Dry eye syndrome of unspecified lacrimal gland

● H04.13   Lacrimal cyst
Lacrimal cystic degeneration

H04.131   Lacrimal cyst right lacrimal gland

H04.132   Lacrimal cyst left lacrimal gland

H04.133   Lacrimal cyst bilateral lacrimal glands

H04.139   Lacrimal cyst unspecified lacrimal gland

● H04.14   Primary lacrimal gland atrophy

H04.141   Primary lacrimal gland atrophy, right lacrimal gland

H04.142   Primary lacrimal gland atrophy, left lacrimal gland

H04.143   Primary lacrimal gland atrophy, bilateral lacrimal glands

H04.149   Primary lacrimal gland atrophy, unspecified lacrimal gland

● H04.15   Secondary lacrimal gland atrophy

H04.151   Secondary lacrimal gland atrophy, right lacrimal gland

H04.152   Secondary lacrimal gland atrophy, left lacrimal gland

H04.153   Secondary lacrimal gland atrophy, bilateral lacrimal glands

H04.159   Secondary lacrimal gland atrophy, unspecified lacrimal gland

CHAPTER 7 (H00-H59)

Figure 7-4   Lacrimal apparatus. (From Buck CJ: Step-by-Step Medical Coding, 2016, St. Louis, Elsevier, 2016)

▶ New   ⇒ Revised   ~~deleted~~ Deleted   **OGCR** Official Guidelines   X Assign placeholder X   ● Use Additional Character(s)

| Excludes 1 | Excludes 2 | Includes | Use additional | Code first | Code also | Key words |

● **H04.16**   Lacrimal gland dislocation

    H04.161   Lacrimal gland dislocation, right lacrimal gland

    H04.162   Lacrimal gland dislocation, left lacrimal gland

    H04.163   Lacrimal gland dislocation, bilateral lacrimal glands

    H04.169   Lacrimal gland dislocation, unspecified lacrimal gland

  H04.19   Other specified disorders of lacrimal gland

● **H04.2**   Epiphora

    Overflow of tears due to stricture of lacrimal passages; AKA lacrimation

  ● **H04.20**   Unspecified epiphora

    H04.201   Unspecified epiphora, right lacrimal gland

    H04.202   Unspecified epiphora, left lacrimal gland

    H04.203   Unspecified epiphora, bilateral lacrimal glands

    H04.209   Unspecified epiphora, unspecified lacrimal gland

  ● **H04.21**   Epiphora due to excess lacrimation

    H04.211   Epiphora due to excess lacrimation, right lacrimal gland

    H04.212   Epiphora due to excess lacrimation, left lacrimal gland

    H04.213   Epiphora due to excess lacrimation, bilateral lacrimal glands

    H04.219   Epiphora due to excess lacrimation, unspecified lacrimal gland

  ● **H04.22**   Epiphora due to insufficient drainage

    H04.221   Epiphora due to insufficient drainage, right lacrimal gland

    H04.222   Epiphora due to insufficient drainage, left lacrimal gland

    H04.223   Epiphora due to insufficient drainage, bilateral lacrimal glands

    H04.229   Epiphora due to insufficient drainage, unspecified lacrimal gland

● **H04.3**   Acute and unspecified inflammation of lacrimal passages

    Excludes1   neonatal dacryocystitis (P39.1)

  ● **H04.30**   Unspecified dacryocystitis

    H04.301   Unspecified dacryocystitis of right lacrimal passage

    H04.302   Unspecified dacryocystitis of left lacrimal passage

    H04.303   Unspecified dacryocystitis of bilateral lacrimal passages

    H04.309   Unspecified dacryocystitis of unspecified lacrimal passage

  ● **H04.31**   Phlegmonous dacryocystitis

    Cellulitis of lacrimal sac

    H04.311   Phlegmonous dacryocystitis of right lacrimal passage

    H04.312   Phlegmonous dacryocystitis of left lacrimal passage

    H04.313   Phlegmonous dacryocystitis of bilateral lacrimal passages

    H04.319   Phlegmonous dacryocystitis of unspecified lacrimal passage

● **H04.32**   Acute dacryocystitis

    Acute dacryopericystitis

    H04.321   Acute dacryocystitis of right lacrimal passage

    H04.322   Acute dacryocystitis of left lacrimal passage

    H04.323   Acute dacryocystitis of bilateral lacrimal passages

    H04.329   Acute dacryocystitis of unspecified lacrimal passage

● **H04.33**   Acute lacrimal canaliculitis

    H04.331   Acute lacrimal canaliculitis of right lacrimal passage

    H04.332   Acute lacrimal canaliculitis of left lacrimal passage

    H04.333   Acute lacrimal canaliculitis of bilateral lacrimal passages

    H04.339   Acute lacrimal canaliculitis of unspecified lacrimal passage

● **H04.4**   Chronic inflammation of lacrimal passages

  ● **H04.41**   Chronic dacryocystitis

    Inflammation of lacrimal sac

    H04.411   Chronic dacryocystitis of right lacrimal passage

    H04.412   Chronic dacryocystitis of left lacrimal passage

    H04.413   Chronic dacryocystitis of bilateral lacrimal passages

    H04.419   Chronic dacryocystitis of unspecified lacrimal passage

  ● **H04.42**   Chronic lacrimal canaliculitis

    Inflammation of lacrimal ducts

    H04.421   Chronic lacrimal canaliculitis of right lacrimal passage

    H04.422   Chronic lacrimal canaliculitis of left lacrimal passage

    H04.423   Chronic lacrimal canaliculitis of bilateral lacrimal passages

    H04.429   Chronic lacrimal canaliculitis of unspecified lacrimal passage

  ● **H04.43**   Chronic lacrimal mucocele

    Accumulation of mucous secretion

    H04.431   Chronic lacrimal mucocele of right lacrimal passage

    H04.432   Chronic lacrimal mucocele of left lacrimal passage

    H04.433   Chronic lacrimal mucocele of bilateral lacrimal passages

    H04.439   Chronic lacrimal mucocele of unspecified lacrimal passage

● **H04.5**   Stenosis and insufficiency of lacrimal passages

  ● **H04.51**   Dacryolith

    Concretion in lacrimal sac/duct; AKA lacrimal calculus

    H04.511   Dacryolith of right lacrimal passage

    H04.512   Dacryolith of left lacrimal passage

    H04.513   Dacryolith of bilateral lacrimal passages

    H04.519   Dacryolith of unspecified lacrimal passage

  ● **H04.52**   Eversion of lacrimal punctum

    Turning out of lacrimal drainage opening

    H04.521   Eversion of right lacrimal punctum

    H04.522   Eversion of left lacrimal punctum

    H04.523   Eversion of bilateral lacrimal punctum

    H04.529   Eversion of unspecified lacrimal punctum

● **H04.53** Neonatal obstruction of nasolacrimal duct

    | Excludes1 | congenital stenosis and stricture of lacrimal duct (Q10.5)

    H04.531 Neonatal obstruction of right nasolacrimal duct

    H04.532 Neonatal obstruction of left nasolacrimal duct

    H04.533 Neonatal obstruction of bilateral nasolacrimal duct

    H04.539 Neonatal obstruction of unspecified nasolacrimal duct

● **H04.54** Stenosis of lacrimal canaliculi

    H04.541 Stenosis of right lacrimal canaliculi

    H04.542 Stenosis of left lacrimal canaliculi

    H04.543 Stenosis of bilateral lacrimal canaliculi

    H04.549 Stenosis of unspecified lacrimal canaliculi

● **H04.55** Acquired stenosis of nasolacrimal duct

    H04.551 Acquired stenosis of right nasolacrimal duct

    H04.552 Acquired stenosis of left nasolacrimal duct

    H04.553 Acquired stenosis of bilateral nasolacrimal duct

    H04.559 Acquired stenosis of unspecified nasolacrimal duct

● **H04.56** Stenosis of lacrimal punctum

    H04.561 Stenosis of right lacrimal punctum

    H04.562 Stenosis of left lacrimal punctum

    H04.563 Stenosis of bilateral lacrimal punctum

    H04.569 Stenosis of unspecified lacrimal punctum

● **H04.57** Stenosis of lacrimal sac

    H04.571 Stenosis of right lacrimal sac

    H04.572 Stenosis of left lacrimal sac

    H04.573 Stenosis of bilateral lacrimal sac

    H04.579 Stenosis of unspecified lacrimal sac

● **H04.6** Other changes of lacrimal passages

   ● **H04.61** Lacrimal fistula

    H04.611 Lacrimal fistula right lacrimal passage

    H04.612 Lacrimal fistula left lacrimal passage

    H04.613 Lacrimal fistula bilateral lacrimal passages

    H04.619 Lacrimal fistula unspecified lacrimal passage

   H04.69 Other changes of lacrimal passages

● **H04.8** Other disorders of lacrimal system

   ● **H04.81** Granuloma of lacrimal passages

    Inflammatory response due to infectious or noninfectious agents

    H04.811 Granuloma of right lacrimal passage

    H04.812 Granuloma of left lacrimal passage

    H04.813 Granuloma of bilateral lacrimal passages

    H04.819 Granuloma of unspecified lacrimal passage

   H04.89 Other disorders of lacrimal system

   H04.9 Disorder of lacrimal system, unspecified

● **H05** Disorders of orbit

    | Excludes1 | congenital malformation of orbit (Q10.7)

  ● **H05.0** Acute inflammation of orbit

    H05.00 Unspecified acute inflammation of orbit

   ● **H05.01** Cellulitis of orbit

    Infection of soft tissue of orbit
    Abscess of orbit

    H05.011 Cellulitis of right orbit

    H05.012 Cellulitis of left orbit

    H05.013 Cellulitis of bilateral orbits

    H05.019 Cellulitis of unspecified orbit

   ● **H05.02** Osteomyelitis of orbit

    Infection of boney orbit of eye

    H05.021 Osteomyelitis of right orbit

    H05.022 Osteomyelitis of left orbit

    H05.023 Osteomyelitis of bilateral orbits

    H05.029 Osteomyelitis of unspecified orbit

   ● **H05.03** Periostitis of orbit

    Inflammation of periosteum (membrane covering bone surface)

    H05.031 Periostitis of right orbit

    H05.032 Periostitis of left orbit

    H05.033 Periostitis of bilateral orbits

    H05.039 Periostitis of unspecified orbit

   ● **H05.04** Tenonitis of orbit

    Inflammation of tenon capsule (space enclosing fascia of Tenon between eyeball and fat of orbit)

    H05.041 Tenonitis of right orbit

    H05.042 Tenonitis of left orbit

    H05.043 Tenonitis of bilateral orbits

    H05.049 Tenonitis of unspecified orbit

  ● **H05.1** Chronic inflammatory disorders of orbit

    H05.10 Unspecified chronic inflammatory disorders of orbit

   ● **H05.11** Granuloma of orbit

    Pseudotumor (inflammatory) of orbit

    H05.111 Granuloma of right orbit

    H05.112 Granuloma of left orbit

    H05.113 Granuloma of bilateral orbits

    H05.119 Granuloma of unspecified orbit

   ● **H05.12** Orbital myositis

    Inflammation of extraocular muscles of orbit

    H05.121 Orbital myositis, right orbit

    H05.122 Orbital myositis, left orbit

    H05.123 Orbital myositis, bilateral

    H05.129 Orbital myositis, unspecified orbit

  ● **H05.2** Exophthalmic conditions

    Bulging eyes

    H05.20 Unspecified exophthalmos

   ● **H05.21** Displacement (lateral) of globe

    H05.211 Displacement (lateral) of globe, right eye

    H05.212 Displacement (lateral) of globe, left eye

    H05.213 Displacement (lateral) of globe, bilateral

    H05.219 Displacement (lateral) of globe, unspecified eye

   ● **H05.22** Edema of orbit

    Orbital congestion

    H05.221 Edema of right orbit

    H05.222 Edema of left orbit

    H05.223 Edema of bilateral orbit

    H05.229 Edema of unspecified orbit

CHAPTER 7 (H00-H59)

Figure 7-5 Exophthalmos. (From Black JM, Hokanson JH: Medical-Surgical Nursing: Clinical Management for Positive Outcomes, St. Louis, Saunders Elsevier, 2009)

● H05.23   Hemorrhage of orbit
     H05.231   Hemorrhage of right orbit
     H05.232   Hemorrhage of left orbit
     H05.233   Hemorrhage of bilateral orbit
     H05.239   Hemorrhage of unspecified orbit
● H05.24   Constant exophthalmos
     Constant bulging eyes, often symptom of Graves disease
     H05.241   Constant exophthalmos, right eye
     H05.242   Constant exophthalmos, left eye
     H05.243   Constant exophthalmos, bilateral
     H05.249   Constant exophthalmos, unspecified eye
● H05.25   Intermittent exophthalmos
     Intermittent bulging eye occurring with bending forward or sharp turning of head
     H05.251   Intermittent exophthalmos, right eye
     H05.252   Intermittent exophthalmos, left eye
     H05.253   Intermittent exophthalmos, bilateral
     H05.259   Intermittent exophthalmos, unspecified eye
● H05.26   Pulsating exophthalmos
     Bulging eyes with pulsation and bruit, often due to aneurysm pushing eye forward
     H05.261   Pulsating exophthalmos, right eye
     H05.262   Pulsating exophthalmos, left eye
     H05.263   Pulsating exophthalmos, bilateral
     H05.269   Pulsating exophthalmos, unspecified eye
● H05.3   Deformity of orbit
     Excludes1   congenital deformity of orbit (Q10.7)
              hypertelorism (Q75.2)
     H05.30   Unspecified deformity of orbit
●   H05.31   Atrophy of orbit
     H05.311   Atrophy of right orbit
     H05.312   Atrophy of left orbit
     H05.313   Atrophy of bilateral orbit
     H05.319   Atrophy of unspecified orbit
● H05.32   Deformity of orbit due to bone disease
     Code also associated bone disease
     H05.321   Deformity of right orbit due to bone disease
     H05.322   Deformity of left orbit due to bone disease
     H05.323   Deformity of bilateral orbits due to bone disease
     H05.329   Deformity of unspecified orbit due to bone disease

● H05.33   Deformity of orbit due to trauma or surgery
     H05.331   Deformity of right orbit due to trauma or surgery
     H05.332   Deformity of left orbit due to trauma or surgery
     H05.333   Deformity of bilateral orbits due to trauma or surgery
     H05.339   Deformity of unspecified orbit due to trauma or surgery
● H05.34   Enlargement of orbit
     H05.341   Enlargement of right orbit
     H05.342   Enlargement of left orbit
     H05.343   Enlargement of bilateral orbits
     H05.349   Enlargement of unspecified orbit
● H05.35   Exostosis of orbit
     H05.351   Exostosis of right orbit
     H05.352   Exostosis of left orbit
     H05.353   Exostosis of bilateral orbits
     H05.359   Exostosis of unspecified orbit
● H05.4   Enophthalmos
     Recessed eyeball into orbit
●   H05.40   Unspecified enophthalmos
     H05.401   Unspecified enophthalmos, right eye
     H05.402   Unspecified enophthalmos, left eye
     H05.403   Unspecified enophthalmos, bilateral
     H05.409   Unspecified enophthalmos, unspecified eye
● H05.41   Enophthalmos due to atrophy of orbital tissue
     H05.411   Enophthalmos due to atrophy of orbital tissue, right eye
     H05.412   Enophthalmos due to atrophy of orbital tissue, left eye
     H05.413   Enophthalmos due to atrophy of orbital tissue, bilateral
     H05.419   Enophthalmos due to atrophy of orbital tissue, unspecified eye
● H05.42   Enophthalmos due to trauma or surgery
     H05.421   Enophthalmos due to trauma or surgery, right eye
     H05.422   Enophthalmos due to trauma or surgery, left eye
     H05.423   Enophthalmos due to trauma or surgery, bilateral
     H05.429   Enophthalmos due to trauma or surgery, unspecified eye
● H05.5   Retained (old) foreign body following penetrating wound of orbit
     Retrobulbar foreign body
     Use additional code to identify the type of retained foreign body (Z18.-)
     Excludes1   current penetrating wound of orbit (S05.4-)
     Excludes2   retained foreign body of eyelid (H02.81-)
              retained intraocular foreign body (H44.6-, H44.7-)
     H05.50   Retained (old) foreign body following penetrating wound of unspecified orbit
     H05.51   Retained (old) foreign body following penetrating wound of right orbit
     H05.52   Retained (old) foreign body following penetrating wound of left orbit
     H05.53   Retained (old) foreign body following penetrating wound of bilateral orbits

▶ New   ⇒ Revised   ~~deleted~~ Deleted   **OGCR** Official Guidelines   X Assign placeholder X   ● Use Additional Character(s)

Excludes 1   Excludes 2   Includes   Use additional   Code first   Code also   Key words

● **H05.8**   Other disorders of orbit
- ● **H05.81**   Cyst of orbit
  Encephalocele of orbit
  - H05.811   Cyst of right orbit
  - H05.812   Cyst of left orbit
  - H05.813   Cyst of bilateral orbits
  - H05.819   Cyst of unspecified orbit
- ● **H05.82**   Myopathy of extraocular muscles
  Weakness of muscles of eye
  - H05.821   Myopathy of extraocular muscles, right orbit
  - H05.822   Myopathy of extraocular muscles, left orbit
  - H05.823   Myopathy of extraocular muscles, bilateral
  - H05.829   Myopathy of extraocular muscles, unspecified orbit
- **H05.89**   Other disorders of orbit
- **H05.9**   Unspecified disorder of orbit

DISORDERS OF CONJUNCTIVA (H10-H11)

★**(See Plate 81, upper, on page 66.)**

● **H10**   Conjunctivitis
Inflammation of membrane of the inside of the eyelid or on surface of eye (conjunctiva)
> Excludes1   keratoconjunctivitis (H16.2-)
- ● **H10.0**   Mucopurulent conjunctivitis
  - ● **H10.01**   Acute follicular conjunctivitis
    - H10.011   Acute follicular conjunctivitis, right eye
    - H10.012   Acute follicular conjunctivitis, left eye
    - H10.013   Acute follicular conjunctivitis, bilateral
    - H10.019   Acute follicular conjunctivitis, unspecified eye
  - ● **H10.02**   Other mucopurulent conjunctivitis
    - H10.021   Other mucopurulent conjunctivitis, right eye
    - H10.022   Other mucopurulent conjunctivitis, left eye
    - H10.023   Other mucopurulent conjunctivitis, bilateral
    - H10.029   Other mucopurulent conjunctivitis, unspecified eye
- ● **H10.1**   Acute atopic conjunctivitis
  Acute papillary conjunctivitis
  - H10.10   Acute atopic conjunctivitis, unspecified eye
  - H10.11   Acute atopic conjunctivitis, right eye
  - H10.12   Acute atopic conjunctivitis, left eye
  - H10.13   Acute atopic conjunctivitis, bilateral
- ● **H10.2**   Other acute conjunctivitis
  - ● **H10.21**   Acute toxic conjunctivitis
    Acute chemical conjunctivitis
    > *Code first (T51-T65) to identify chemical and intent*
    > Excludes1   burn and corrosion of eye and adnexa (T26.-)
    - H10.211   Acute toxic conjunctivitis, right eye
    - H10.212   Acute toxic conjunctivitis, left eye
    - H10.213   Acute toxic conjunctivitis, bilateral
    - H10.219   Acute toxic conjunctivitis, unspecified eye

- ● **H10.22**   Pseudomembranous conjunctivitis
  - H10.221   Pseudomembranous conjunctivitis, right eye
  - H10.222   Pseudomembranous conjunctivitis, left eye
  - H10.223   Pseudomembranous conjunctivitis, bilateral
  - H10.229   Pseudomembranous conjunctivitis, unspecified eye
- ● **H10.23**   Serous conjunctivitis, except viral
  > Excludes1   viral conjunctivitis (B30.-)
  - H10.231   Serous conjunctivitis, except viral, right eye
  - H10.232   Serous conjunctivitis, except viral, left eye
  - H10.233   Serous conjunctivitis, except viral, bilateral
  - H10.239   Serous conjunctivitis, except viral, unspecified eye
- ● **H10.3**   Unspecified acute conjunctivitis
  > Excludes1   ophthalmia neonatorum NOS (P39.1)
  - H10.30   Unspecified acute conjunctivitis, unspecified eye
  - H10.31   Unspecified acute conjunctivitis, right eye
  - H10.32   Unspecified acute conjunctivitis, left eye
  - H10.33   Unspecified acute conjunctivitis, bilateral
- ● **H10.4**   Chronic conjunctivitis
  - ● **H10.40**   Unspecified chronic conjunctivitis
    - H10.401   Unspecified chronic conjunctivitis, right eye
    - H10.402   Unspecified chronic conjunctivitis, left eye
    - H10.403   Unspecified chronic conjunctivitis, bilateral
    - H10.409   Unspecified chronic conjunctivitis, unspecified eye
  - ● **H10.41**   Chronic giant papillary conjunctivitis
    Inflammation of membrane of the inside of the eyelid or on surface of eye often associated with contact lens wear
    - H10.411   Chronic giant papillary conjunctivitis, right eye
    - H10.412   Chronic giant papillary conjunctivitis, left eye
    - H10.413   Chronic giant papillary conjunctivitis, bilateral
    - H10.419   Chronic giant papillary conjunctivitis, unspecified eye
  - ● **H10.42**   Simple chronic conjunctivitis
    - H10.421   Simple chronic conjunctivitis, right eye
    - H10.422   Simple chronic conjunctivitis, left eye
    - H10.423   Simple chronic conjunctivitis, bilateral
    - H10.429   Simple chronic conjunctivitis, unspecified eye
  - ● **H10.43**   Chronic follicular conjunctivitis
    Inflammation of membrane of the inside of the eyelid or on surface of eye due to topical medications or infection
    - H10.431   Chronic follicular conjunctivitis, right eye
    - H10.432   Chronic follicular conjunctivitis, left eye
    - H10.433   Chronic follicular conjunctivitis, bilateral
    - H10.439   Chronic follicular conjunctivitis, unspecified eye

CHAPTER 7 (H00-H59)

H10.44   **Vernal** conjunctivitis
Affecting children, especially boys in which there are flattened papules with thick, gelatinous exudate on conjunctivae on inside of upper lid

Excludes1   vernal keratoconjunctivitis with limbar and corneal involvement (H16.26-)

H10.45   **Other chronic** allergic conjunctivitis

● H10.5   **Blepharoconjunctivitis**
Inflammation of eyelids and conjunctiva

● H10.50   **Unspecified** blepharoconjunctivitis

H10.501   Unspecified blepharoconjunctivitis, **right eye**

H10.502   Unspecified blepharoconjunctivitis, **left eye**

H10.503   Unspecified blepharoconjunctivitis, **bilateral**

H10.509   Unspecified blepharoconjunctivitis, **unspecified** eye

● H10.51   **Ligneous** conjunctivitis

H10.511   Ligneous conjunctivitis, **right eye**

H10.512   Ligneous conjunctivitis, **left eye**

H10.513   Ligneous conjunctivitis, **bilateral**

H10.519   Ligneous conjunctivitis, **unspecified** eye

● H10.52   **Angular** blepharoconjunctivitis

H10.521   Angular blepharoconjunctivitis, **right** eye

H10.522   Angular blepharoconjunctivitis, **left** eye

H10.523   Angular blepharoconjunctivitis, **bilateral**

H10.529   Angular blepharoconjunctivitis, **unspecified** eye

● H10.53   **Contact** blepharoconjunctivitis

H10.531   Contact blepharoconjunctivitis, **right** eye

H10.532   Contact blepharoconjunctivitis, **left** eye

H10.533   Contact blepharoconjunctivitis, **bilateral**

H10.539   Contact blepharoconjunctivitis, **unspecified** eye

● H10.8   **Other** conjunctivitis

● H10.81   **Pingueculitis**
Inflammation of a yellow, raised thickening on the white of the eye associated with chronic dry eyes

Excludes1   pinguecula (H11.15-)

H10.811   Pingueculitis, **right eye**

H10.812   Pingueculitis, **left eye**

H10.813   Pingueculitis, **bilateral**

H10.819   Pingueculitis, **unspecified** eye

H10.89   **Other** conjunctivitis

H10.9   **Unspecified** conjunctivitis

● H11   **Other disorders of conjunctiva**

Excludes1   keratoconjunctivitis (H16.2-)

● H11.0   **Pterygium of eye**

Excludes1   pseudopterygium (H11.81-)

● H11.00   **Unspecified** pterygium of eye

H11.001   Unspecified pterygium of **right** eye

H11.002   Unspecified pterygium of **left** eye

H11.003   Unspecified pterygium of eye, **bilateral**

H11.009   Unspecified pterygium of **unspecified** eye

Figure 7-6 Double pterygium. Note both nasal and temporal pterygia in a 57-year-old farmer. (From Brightbill FS, McDonnell PJ: Corneal Surgery: Theory, Technique and Tissue, S.l., Mosby Elsevier, 2009)

Item 7–2 **Pterygium** is Greek for batlike. The condition is characterized by a membrane that extends from the limbus to the center of the cornea and resembles a wing.

● H11.01   **Amyloid** pterygium

H11.011   Amyloid pterygium of **right** eye

H11.012   Amyloid pterygium of **left** eye

H11.013   Amyloid pterygium of eye, **bilateral**

H11.019   Amyloid pterygium of **unspecified** eye

● H11.02   **Central** pterygium of eye

H11.021   Central pterygium of **right** eye

H11.022   Central pterygium of **left** eye

H11.023   Central pterygium of eye, **bilateral**

H11.029   Central pterygium of **unspecified** eye

● H11.03   **Double** pterygium of eye

H11.031   Double pterygium of **right** eye

H11.032   Double pterygium of **left** eye

H11.033   Double pterygium of eye, **bilateral**

H11.039   Double pterygium of **unspecified eye**

● H11.04   **Peripheral** pterygium of eye, **stationary**

H11.041   Peripheral pterygium, stationary, **right** eye

H11.042   Peripheral pterygium, stationary, **left** eye

H11.043   Peripheral pterygium, stationary, **bilateral**

H11.049   Peripheral pterygium, stationary, **unspecified** eye

● H11.05   **Peripheral** pterygium of eye, **progressive**

H11.051   Peripheral pterygium, progressive, **right** eye

H11.052   Peripheral pterygium, progressive, **left** eye

H11.053   Peripheral pterygium, progressive, **bilateral**

H11.059   Peripheral pterygium, progressive, **unspecified** eye

● H11.06   **Recurrent** pterygium of eye

H11.061   Recurrent pterygium of **right** eye

H11.062   Recurrent pterygium of **left** eye

H11.063   Recurrent pterygium of eye, **bilateral**

H11.069   Recurrent pterygium of **unspecified** eye

● H11.1   **Conjunctival degenerations and deposits**

Excludes2   pseudopterygium (H11.81)

H11.10   **Unspecified** conjunctival degenerations

● H11.11   **Conjunctival deposits**

H11.111   Conjunctival deposits, **right eye**

H11.112   Conjunctival deposits, **left eye**

H11.113   Conjunctival deposits, **bilateral**

H11.119   Conjunctival deposits, **unspecified** eye

● H11.12   **Conjunctival concretions**
White to yellow nodules within or beneath conjunctiva

H11.121   Conjunctival concretions, **right eye**

H11.122   Conjunctival concretions, **left eye**

H11.123   Conjunctival concretions, **bilateral**

H11.129   Conjunctival concretions, **unspecified** eye

▶ New   ⟹ Revised   ~~deleted~~ Deleted   **OGCR** Official Guidelines   X Assign placeholder X   ● Use Additional Character(s)

Excludes 1   Excludes 2   Includes   Use additional   Code first   Code also   Key words

● **H11.13** Conjunctival **pigmentations**
Conjunctival argyrosis [argyria]
   H11.131 Conjunctival pigmentations, **right eye**
   H11.132 Conjunctival pigmentations, **left eye**
   H11.133 Conjunctival pigmentations, **bilateral**
   H11.139 Conjunctival pigmentations, **unspecified** eye

● **H11.14** Conjunctival xerosis, **unspecified**
   Excludes1   xerosis of conjunctiva due to vitamin A deficiency (E50.0, E50.1)
   H11.141 Conjunctival xerosis, unspecified, **right eye**
   H11.142 Conjunctival xerosis, unspecified, **left** eye
   H11.143 Conjunctival xerosis, unspecified, **bilateral**
   H11.149 Conjunctival xerosis, unspecified, **unspecified** eye

● **H11.15** Pinguecula
Yellowish spot near sclerocorneal junction, usually on nasal side; associated with aging
   Excludes1   pingueculitis (H10.81-)
   H11.151 Pinguecula, **right eye**
   H11.152 Pinguecula, **left eye**
   H11.153 Pinguecula, **bilateral**
   H11.159 Pinguecula, **unspecified** eye

● **H11.2** Conjunctival scars
 ● **H11.21** Conjunctival **adhesions and strands** (localized)
   H11.211 Conjunctival adhesions and strands (localized), **right eye**
   H11.212 Conjunctival adhesions and strands (localized), **left eye**
   H11.213 Conjunctival adhesions and strands (localized), **bilateral**
   H11.219 Conjunctival adhesions and strands (localized), **unspecified** eye

 ● **H11.22** Conjunctival **granuloma**
   H11.221 Conjunctival granuloma, **right eye**
   H11.222 Conjunctival granuloma, **left eye**
   H11.223 Conjunctival granuloma, **bilateral**
   H11.229 Conjunctival granuloma, **unspecified**

 ● **H11.23** Symblepharon
Adhesion between tarsal conjunctiva and bulbar conjunctiva
   H11.231 Symblepharon, **right eye**
   H11.232 Symblepharon, **left eye**
   H11.233 Symblepharon, **bilateral**
   H11.239 Symblepharon, **unspecified** eye

 ● **H11.24** Scarring of conjunctiva
   H11.241 Scarring of conjunctiva, **right eye**
   H11.242 Scarring of conjunctiva, **left eye**
   H11.243 Scarring of conjunctiva, **bilateral**
   H11.249 Scarring of conjunctiva, **unspecified** eye

● **H11.3** Conjunctival **hemorrhage**
Subconjunctival hemorrhage
   H11.30 Conjunctival hemorrhage, **unspecified** eye
   H11.31 Conjunctival hemorrhage, **right eye**
   H11.32 Conjunctival hemorrhage, **left eye**
   H11.33 Conjunctival hemorrhage, **bilateral**

● **H11.4** Other conjunctival vascular disorders and cysts
 ● **H11.41** Vascular **abnormalities** of conjunctiva
Conjunctival aneurysm
   H11.411 Vascular abnormalities of conjunctiva, **right eye**
   H11.412 Vascular abnormalities of conjunctiva, **left eye**
   H11.413 Vascular abnormalities of conjunctiva, **bilateral**
   H11.419 Vascular abnormalities of conjunctiva, **unspecified** eye

 ● **H11.42** Conjunctival **edema**
   H11.421 Conjunctival edema, **right eye**
   H11.422 Conjunctival edema, **left eye**
   H11.423 Conjunctival edema, **bilateral**
   H11.429 Conjunctival edema, **unspecified** eye

 ● **H11.43** Conjunctival **hyperemia**
   H11.431 Conjunctival hyperemia, **right eye**
   H11.432 Conjunctival hyperemia, **left eye**
   H11.433 Conjunctival hyperemia, **bilateral**
   H11.439 Conjunctival hyperemia, **unspecified** eye

 ● **H11.44** Conjunctival **cysts**
   H11.441 Conjunctival cysts, **right eye**
   H11.442 Conjunctival cysts, **left eye**
   H11.443 Conjunctival cysts, **bilateral**
   H11.449 Conjunctival cysts, **unspecified** eye

● **H11.8** Other specified disorders of conjunctiva
 ● **H11.81** Pseudopterygium of conjunctiva
Conjunctival scar attached to cornea
   H11.811 Pseudopterygium of conjunctiva, **right eye**
   H11.812 Pseudopterygium of conjunctiva, **left** eye
   H11.813 Pseudopterygium of conjunctiva, **bilateral**
   H11.819 Pseudopterygium of conjunctiva, **unspecified** eye

 ● **H11.82** Conjunctivochalasis
Conjunctiva bulges over eyelid margin or covers lower punctum
   H11.821 Conjunctivochalasis, **right eye**
   H11.822 Conjunctivochalasis, **left eye**
   H11.823 Conjunctivochalasis, **bilateral**
   H11.829 Conjunctivochalasis, **unspecified** eye

   H11.89 Other specified disorders of conjunctiva
  H11.9 Unspecified disorder of conjunctiva

DISORDERS OF SCLERA, CORNEA, IRIS AND CILIARY BODY (H15-H22)

● **H15** Disorders of sclera
 ● **H15.0** Scleritis
Inflammation of the white (sclera and episclera) of the eye.
 ● **H15.00** Unspecified scleritis
   H15.001 Unspecified scleritis, **right eye**
   H15.002 Unspecified scleritis, **left eye**
   H15.003 Unspecified scleritis, **bilateral**
   H15.009 Unspecified scleritis, **unspecified** eye

 ● **H15.01** Anterior scleritis
   H15.011 Anterior scleritis, **right eye**
   H15.012 Anterior scleritis, **left eye**
   H15.013 Anterior scleritis, **bilateral**
   H15.019 Anterior scleritis, **unspecified** eye

CHAPTER 7 (H00-H59)

● H15.02 **Brawny** scleritis
  Swelling around the cornea that is gelantinous in appearance
  H15.021 Brawny scleritis, **right** eye
  H15.022 Brawny scleritis, **left** eye
  H15.023 Brawny scleritis, **bilateral**
  H15.029 Brawny scleritis, **unspecified** eye
● H15.03 **Posterior** scleritis
  Sclerotenonitis
  H15.031 Posterior scleritis, **right** eye
  H15.032 Posterior scleritis, **left** eye
  H15.033 Posterior scleritis, **bilateral**
  H15.039 Posterior scleritis, **unspecified** eye
● H15.04 Scleritis with **corneal involvement**
  H15.041 Scleritis with corneal involvement, **right** eye
  H15.042 Scleritis with corneal involvement, **left** eye
  H15.043 Scleritis with corneal involvement, **bilateral**
  H15.049 Scleritis with corneal involvement, **unspecified** eye
● H15.05 Scleromalacia **perforans**
  Necrotic without inflammation; usually associated with rheumatoid arthritis
  H15.051 Scleromalacia perforans, **right** eye
  H15.052 Scleromalacia perforans, **left** eye
  H15.053 Scleromalacia perforans, **bilateral**
  H15.059 Scleromalacia perforans, **unspecified** eye
● H15.09 **Other scleritis**
  Scleral abscess
  H15.091 Other scleritis, **right** eye
  H15.092 Other scleritis, **left** eye
  H15.093 Other scleritis, **bilateral**
  H15.099 Other scleritis, **unspecified** eye
● H15.1 **Episcleritis**
  Inflammation of the white (sclera and episclera) of the eye.
● H15.10 **Unspecified** episcleritis
  H15.101 Unspecified episcleritis, **right** eye
  H15.102 Unspecified episcleritis, **left** eye
  H15.103 Unspecified episcleritis, **bilateral**
  H15.109 Unspecified episcleritis, unspecified eye
● H15.11 Episcleritis **periodica fugax**
  Transient, recurrent inflammation of portion of episclera (connective tissue on the surface of the sclera)
  H15.111 Episcleritis periodica fugax, **right** eye
  H15.112 Episcleritis periodica fugax, **left** eye
  H15.113 Episcleritis periodica fugax, **bilateral**
  H15.119 Episcleritis periodica fugax, **unspecified** eye
● H15.12 **Nodular** episcleritis
  Characterized by tender, localized, moveable nodule within inflamed area
  H15.121 Nodular episcleritis, **right** eye
  H15.122 Nodular episcleritis, **left** eye
  H15.123 Nodular episcleritis, **bilateral**
  H15.129 Nodular episcleritis, **unspecified** eye

● H15.8 **Other** disorders of sclera
  | Excludes2 | blue sclera (Q13.5)
  | | degenerative myopia (H44.2-)
● H15.81 **Equatorial** staphyloma
  H15.811 Equatorial staphyloma, **right** eye
  H15.812 Equatorial staphyloma, **left** eye
  H15.813 Equatorial staphyloma, **bilateral**
  H15.819 Equatorial staphyloma, **unspecified** eye
● H15.82 **Localized anterior** staphyloma
  H15.821 Localized anterior staphyloma, **right** eye
  H15.822 Localized anterior staphyloma, **left** eye
  H15.823 Localized anterior staphyloma, **bilateral**
  H15.829 Localized anterior staphyloma, **unspecified** eye
● H15.83 Staphyloma **posticum**
  H15.831 Staphyloma posticum, **right** eye
  H15.832 Staphyloma posticum, **left** eye
  H15.833 Staphyloma posticum, **bilateral**
  H15.839 Staphyloma posticum, **unspecified** eye
● H15.84 Scleral **ectasia**
  H15.841 Scleral ectasia, **right** eye
  H15.842 Scleral ectasia, **left** eye
  H15.843 Scleral ectasia, **bilateral**
  H15.849 Scleral ectasia, **unspecified** eye
● H15.85 Ring staphyloma
  H15.851 Ring staphyloma, **right** eye
  H15.852 Ring staphyloma, **left** eye
  H15.853 Ring staphyloma, **bilateral**
  H15.859 Ring staphyloma, **unspecified** eye
  H15.89 **Other** disorders of sclera
  H15.9 **Unspecified** disorder of sclera
● H16 **Keratitis**
● H16.0 **Corneal ulcer**
● H16.00 **Unspecified** corneal ulcer
  H16.001 Unspecified corneal ulcer, **right** eye
  H16.002 Unspecified corneal ulcer, **left** eye
  H16.003 Unspecified corneal ulcer, **bilateral**
  H16.009 Unspecified corneal ulcer, **unspecified** eye
● H16.01 **Central** corneal ulcer
  H16.011 Central corneal ulcer, **right** eye
  H16.012 Central corneal ulcer, **left** eye
  H16.013 Central corneal ulcer, **bilateral**
  H16.019 Central corneal ulcer, **unspecified** eye
● H16.02 **Ring** corneal ulcer
  H16.021 Ring corneal ulcer, **right** eye
  H16.022 Ring corneal ulcer, **left** eye
  H16.023 Ring corneal ulcer, **bilateral**
  H16.029 Ring corneal ulcer, **unspecified** eye
● H16.03 Corneal ulcer with **hypopyon**
  H16.031 Corneal ulcer with hypopyon, **right** eye
  H16.032 Corneal ulcer with hypopyon, **left** eye
  H16.033 Corneal ulcer with hypopyon, **bilateral**
  H16.039 Corneal ulcer with hypopyon, **unspecified** eye

▶ New   ⇛ Revised   ~~deleted~~ Deleted   **OGCR** Official Guidelines   X Assign placeholder X   ● Use Additional Character(s)
| Excludes 1 | | Excludes 2 | Includes   Use additional   Code first   Code also   Key words

Figure 7-7 Corneal ulcers: marginal, ring, central corneal, rosacea, and Mooren's.

Item 7–3 An infected ulcer is usually called a **serpiginous** or **hypopyon** ulcer which is a pus sac in the anterior chamber of the eye. **Marginal** ulcers are usually asymptomatic, not primary, and are often superficial and simple. More severe marginal ulcers spread to form a ring ulcer. **Ring** ulcers can extend around the entire corneal periphery. **Central corneal** ulcers develop when there is an abrasion to the epithelium and an infection develops in the eroded area. The **pyocyaneal** ulcer is the most serious corneal infection, which, if left untreated, can lead to loss of the eye.

● H16.04　Marginal corneal ulcer
　　　H16.041　Marginal corneal ulcer, right eye
　　　H16.042　Marginal corneal ulcer, left eye
　　　H16.043　Marginal corneal ulcer, bilateral
　　　H16.049　Marginal corneal ulcer, unspecified eye
● H16.05　Mooren's corneal ulcer
　　　H16.051　Mooren's corneal ulcer, right eye
　　　H16.052　Mooren's corneal ulcer, left eye
　　　H16.053　Mooren's corneal ulcer, bilateral
　　　H16.059　Mooren's corneal ulcer, unspecified eye
● H16.06　Mycotic corneal ulcer
　　　H16.061　Mycotic corneal ulcer, right eye
　　　H16.062　Mycotic corneal ulcer, left eye
　　　H16.063　Mycotic corneal ulcer, bilateral
　　　H16.069　Mycotic corneal ulcer, unspecified eye
● H16.07　Perforated corneal ulcer
　　　H16.071　Perforated corneal ulcer, right eye
　　　H16.072　Perforated corneal ulcer, left eye
　　　H16.073　Perforated corneal ulcer, bilateral
　　　H16.079　Perforated corneal ulcer, unspecified eye
● H16.1　Other and unspecified superficial keratitis without conjunctivitis
　● H16.10　Unspecified superficial keratitis
　　　H16.101　Unspecified superficial keratitis, right eye
　　　H16.102　Unspecified superficial keratitis, left eye
　　　H16.103　Unspecified superficial keratitis, bilateral
　　　H16.109　Unspecified superficial keratitis, unspecified eye
　● H16.11　Macular keratitis
　　　　Areolar keratitis
　　　　Nummular keratitis
　　　　Stellate keratitis
　　　　Striate keratitis
　　　H16.111　Macular keratitis, right eye
　　　H16.112　Macular keratitis, left eye
　　　H16.113　Macular keratitis, bilateral
　　　H16.119　Macular keratitis, unspecified eye
　● H16.12　Filamentary keratitis
　　　H16.121　Filamentary keratitis, right eye
　　　H16.122　Filamentary keratitis, left eye
　　　H16.123　Filamentary keratitis, bilateral
　　　H16.129　Filamentary keratitis, unspecified eye

● H16.13　Photokeratitis
　　　　Snow blindness
　　　　Welders' keratitis
　　　H16.131　Photokeratitis, right eye
　　　H16.132　Photokeratitis, left eye
　　　H16.133　Photokeratitis, bilateral
　　　H16.139　Photokeratitis, unspecified eye
● H16.14　Punctate keratitis
　　　H16.141　Punctate keratitis, right eye
　　　H16.142　Punctate keratitis, left eye
　　　H16.143　Punctate keratitis, bilateral
　　　H16.149　Punctate keratitis, unspecified eye
● H16.2　Keratoconjunctivitis
　● H16.20　Unspecified keratoconjunctivitis
　　　　Superficial keratitis with conjunctivitis NOS
　　　H16.201　Unspecified keratoconjunctivitis, right eye
　　　H16.202　Unspecified keratoconjunctivitis, left eye
　　　H16.203　Unspecified keratoconjunctivitis, bilateral
　　　H16.209　Unspecified keratoconjunctivitis, unspecified eye
　● H16.21　Exposure keratoconjunctivitis
　　　H16.211　Exposure keratoconjunctivitis, right eye
　　　H16.212　Exposure keratoconjunctivitis, left eye
　　　H16.213　Exposure keratoconjunctivitis, bilateral
　　　H16.219　Exposure keratoconjunctivitis, unspecified eye
　● H16.22　Keratoconjunctivitis sicca, not specified as Sjögren's
　　　　Excludes1　Sjogren's syndrome (M35.01)
　　　H16.221　Keratoconjunctivitis sicca, not specified as Sjögren's, right eye
　　　H16.222　Keratoconjunctivitis sicca, not specified as Sjögren's, left eye
　　　H16.223　Keratoconjunctivitis sicca, not specified as Sjögren's, bilateral
　　　H16.229　Keratoconjunctivitis sicca, not specified as Sjögren's, unspecified eye
　● H16.23　Neurotrophic keratoconjunctivitis
　　　H16.231　Neurotrophic keratoconjunctivitis, right eye
　　　H16.232　Neurotrophic keratoconjunctivitis, left eye
　　　H16.233　Neurotrophic keratoconjunctivitis, bilateral
　　　H16.239　Neurotrophic keratoconjunctivitis, unspecified eye
　● H16.24　Ophthalmia nodosa
　　　H16.241　Ophthalmia nodosa, right eye
　　　H16.242　Ophthalmia nodosa, left eye
　　　H16.243　Ophthalmia nodosa, bilateral
　　　H16.249　Ophthalmia nodosa, unspecified eye
　● H16.25　Phlyctenular keratoconjunctivitis
　　　H16.251　Phlyctenular keratoconjunctivitis, right eye
　　　H16.252　Phlyctenular keratoconjunctivitis, left eye
　　　H16.253　Phlyctenular keratoconjunctivitis, bilateral
　　　H16.259　Phlyctenular keratoconjunctivitis, unspecified eye

▶ New　　⇒ Revised　　deleted Deleted　　OGCR Official Guidelines　　X Assign placeholder X　　● Use Additional Character(s)

Excludes 1　　Excludes 2　　Includes　　Use additional　　Code first　　Code also　　Key words

CHAPTER 7 (H00–H59)

● H16.26   Vernal keratoconjunctivitis, with limbar and corneal involvement

    Excludes1   vernal conjunctivitis without limbar and corneal involvement (H10.44)

    H16.261   Vernal keratoconjunctivitis, with limbar and corneal involvement, right eye

    H16.262   Vernal keratoconjunctivitis, with limbar and corneal involvement, left eye

    H16.263   Vernal keratoconjunctivitis, with limbar and corneal involvement, bilateral

    H16.269   Vernal keratoconjunctivitis, with limbar and corneal involvement, unspecified eye

● H16.29   Other keratoconjunctivitis

    H16.291   Other keratoconjunctivitis, right eye

    H16.292   Other keratoconjunctivitis, left eye

    H16.293   Other keratoconjunctivitis, bilateral

    H16.299   Other keratoconjunctivitis, unspecified eye

● H16.3   Interstitial and deep keratitis

● H16.30   Unspecified interstitial keratitis

    H16.301   Unspecified interstitial keratitis, right eye

    H16.302   Unspecified interstitial keratitis, left eye

    H16.303   Unspecified interstitial keratitis, bilateral

    H16.309   Unspecified interstitial keratitis, unspecified eye

● H16.31   Corneal abscess

    H16.311   Corneal abscess, right eye

    H16.312   Corneal abscess, left eye

    H16.313   Corneal abscess, bilateral

    H16.319   Corneal abscess, unspecified eye

● H16.32   Diffuse interstitial keratitis
      Cogan's syndrome

    H16.321   Diffuse interstitial keratitis, right eye

    H16.322   Diffuse interstitial keratitis, left eye

    H16.323   Diffuse interstitial keratitis, bilateral

    H16.329   Diffuse interstitial keratitis, unspecified eye

● H16.33   Sclerosing keratitis

    H16.331   Sclerosing keratitis, right eye

    H16.332   Sclerosing keratitis, left eye

    H16.333   Sclerosing keratitis, bilateral

    H16.339   Sclerosing keratitis, unspecified eye

● H16.39   Other interstitial and deep keratitis

    H16.391   Other interstitial and deep keratitis, right eye

    H16.392   Other interstitial and deep keratitis, left eye

    H16.393   Other interstitial and deep keratitis, bilateral

    H16.399   Other interstitial and deep keratitis, unspecified eye

● H16.4   Corneal neovascularization

● H16.40   Unspecified corneal neovascularization

    H16.401   Unspecified corneal neovascularization, right eye

    H16.402   Unspecified corneal neovascularization, left eye

    H16.403   Unspecified corneal neovascularization, bilateral

    H16.409   Unspecified corneal neovascularization, unspecified eye

● H16.41   Ghost vessels (corneal)

    H16.411   Ghost vessels (corneal), right eye

    H16.412   Ghost vessels (corneal), left eye

    H16.413   Ghost vessels (corneal), bilateral

    H16.419   Ghost vessels (corneal), unspecified eye

● H16.42   Pannus (corneal)

    H16.421   Pannus (corneal), right eye

    H16.422   Pannus (corneal), left eye

    H16.423   Pannus (corneal), bilateral

    H16.429   Pannus (corneal), unspecified eye

● H16.43   Localized vascularization of cornea

    H16.431   Localized vascularization of cornea, right eye

    H16.432   Localized vascularization of cornea, left eye

    H16.433   Localized vascularization of cornea, bilateral

    H16.439   Localized vascularization of cornea, unspecified eye

● H16.44   Deep vascularization of cornea

    H16.441   Deep vascularization of cornea, right eye

    H16.442   Deep vascularization of cornea, left eye

    H16.443   Deep vascularization of cornea, bilateral

    H16.449   Deep vascularization of cornea, unspecified eye

H16.8   Other keratitis

H16.9   Unspecified keratitis

● H17   Corneal scars and opacities

● H17.0   Adherent leukoma

    H17.00   Adherent leukoma, unspecified eye

    H17.01   Adherent leukoma, right eye

    H17.02   Adherent leukoma, left eye

    H17.03   Adherent leukoma, bilateral

● H17.1   Central corneal opacity

    H17.10   Central corneal opacity, unspecified eye

    H17.11   Central corneal opacity, right eye

    H17.12   Central corneal opacity, left eye

    H17.13   Central corneal opacity, bilateral

● H17.8   Other corneal scars and opacities

● H17.81   Minor opacity of cornea
      Corneal nebula

    H17.811   Minor opacity of cornea, right eye

    H17.812   Minor opacity of cornea, left eye

    H17.813   Minor opacity of cornea, bilateral

    H17.819   Minor opacity of cornea, unspecified eye

● H17.82   Peripheral opacity of cornea

    H17.821   Peripheral opacity of cornea, right eye

    H17.822   Peripheral opacity of cornea, left eye

    H17.823   Peripheral opacity of cornea, bilateral

    H17.829   Peripheral opacity of cornea, unspecified eye

H17.89   Other corneal scars and opacities

H17.9   Unspecified corneal scar and opacity

● H18   Other disorders of cornea

● H18.0   Corneal pigmentations and deposits

● H18.00   Unspecified corneal deposit

    H18.001   Unspecified corneal deposit, right eye

    H18.002   Unspecified corneal deposit, left eye

    H18.003   Unspecified corneal deposit, bilateral

    H18.009   Unspecified corneal deposit, unspecified eye

▶ New   ⇒ Revised   ~~deleted~~ Deleted   **OGCR** Official Guidelines   X Assign placeholder X   ● Use Additional Character(s)

Excludes 1   Excludes 2   Includes   Use additional   Code first   Code also   Key words

● H18.01　Anterior corneal pigmentations
　　　　　Staehli's line
　　　H18.011　Anterior corneal pigmentations, right eye
　　　H18.012　Anterior corneal pigmentations, left eye
　　　H18.013　Anterior corneal pigmentations, bilateral
　　　H18.019　Anterior corneal pigmentations, unspecified eye

● H18.02　Argentous corneal deposits
　　　H18.021　Argentous corneal deposits, right eye
　　　H18.022　Argentous corneal deposits, left eye
　　　H18.023　Argentous corneal deposits, bilateral
　　　H18.029　Argentous corneal deposits, unspecified eye

● H18.03　Corneal deposits in metabolic disorders
　　　　　Code also associated metabolic disorder
　　　H18.031　Corneal deposits in metabolic disorders, right eye
　　　H18.032　Corneal deposits in metabolic disorders, left eye
　　　H18.033　Corneal deposits in metabolic disorders, bilateral
　　　H18.039　Corneal deposits in metabolic disorders, unspecified eye

● H18.04　Kayser-Fleischer ring
　　　　　Code also associated Wilson's disease (E83.01)
　　　H18.041　Kayser-Fleischer ring, right eye
　　　H18.042　Kayser-Fleischer ring, left eye
　　　H18.043　Kayser-Fleischer ring, bilateral
　　　H18.049　Kayser-Fleischer ring, unspecified eye

● H18.05　Posterior corneal pigmentations
　　　　　Krukenberg's spindle
　　　H18.051　Posterior corneal pigmentations, right eye
　　　H18.052　Posterior corneal pigmentations, left eye
　　　H18.053　Posterior corneal pigmentations, bilateral
　　　H18.059　Posterior corneal pigmentations, unspecified eye

● H18.06　Stromal corneal pigmentations
　　　　　Hematocornea
　　　H18.061　Stromal corneal pigmentations, right eye
　　　H18.062　Stromal corneal pigmentations, left eye
　　　H18.063　Stromal corneal pigmentations, bilateral
　　　H18.069　Stromal corneal pigmentations, unspecified eye

● H18.1　Bullous keratopathy
　　　H18.10　Bullous keratopathy, unspecified eye
　　　H18.11　Bullous keratopathy, right eye
　　　H18.12　Bullous keratopathy, left eye
　　　H18.13　Bullous keratopathy, bilateral

● H18.2　Other and unspecified corneal edema
　　　H18.20　Unspecified corneal edema
● 　　H18.21　Corneal edema secondary to contact lens
　　　　　　Excludes2　other corneal disorders due to contact lens (H18.82-)
　　　H18.211　Corneal edema secondary to contact lens, right eye
　　　H18.212　Corneal edema secondary to contact lens, left eye
　　　H18.213　Corneal edema secondary to contact lens, bilateral
　　　H18.219　Corneal edema secondary to contact lens, unspecified eye

● H18.22　Idiopathic corneal edema
　　　H18.221　Idiopathic corneal edema, right eye
　　　H18.222　Idiopathic corneal edema, left eye
　　　H18.223　Idiopathic corneal edema, bilateral
　　　H18.229　Idiopathic corneal edema, unspecified eye

● H18.23　Secondary corneal edema
　　　H18.231　Secondary corneal edema, right eye
　　　H18.232　Secondary corneal edema, left eye
　　　H18.233　Secondary corneal edema, bilateral
　　　H18.239　Secondary corneal edema, unspecified eye

● H18.3　Changes of corneal membranes
　　　H18.30　Unspecified corneal membrane change
● 　　H18.31　Folds and rupture in Bowman's membrane
　　　H18.311　Folds and rupture in Bowman's membrane, right eye
　　　H18.312　Folds and rupture in Bowman's membrane, left eye
　　　H18.313　Folds and rupture in Bowman's membrane, bilateral
　　　H18.319　Folds and rupture in Bowman's membrane, unspecified eye
● 　　H18.32　Folds in Descemet's membrane
　　　H18.321　Folds in Descemet's membrane, right eye
　　　H18.322　Folds in Descemet's membrane, left eye
　　　H18.323　Folds in Descemet's membrane, bilateral
　　　H18.329　Folds in Descemet's membrane, unspecified eye
● 　　H18.33　Rupture in Descemet's membrane
　　　H18.331　Rupture in Descemet's membrane, right eye
　　　H18.332　Rupture in Descemet's membrane, left eye
　　　H18.333　Rupture in Descemet's membrane, bilateral
　　　H18.339　Rupture in Descemet's membrane, unspecified eye

● H18.4　Corneal degeneration
　　　Excludes1　Mooren's ulcer (H16.0-)
　　　　　　　　recurrent erosion of cornea (H18.83-)
　　　H18.40　Unspecified corneal degeneration
● 　　H18.41　Arcus senilis
　　　　　Senile corneal changes
　　　H18.411　Arcus senilis, right eye
　　　H18.412　Arcus senilis, left eye
　　　H18.413　Arcus senilis, bilateral
　　　H18.419　Arcus senilis, unspecified eye
● 　　H18.42　Band keratopathy
　　　H18.421　Band keratopathy, right eye
　　　H18.422　Band keratopathy, left eye
　　　H18.423　Band keratopathy, bilateral
　　　H18.429　Band keratopathy, unspecified eye
　　　H18.43　Other calcerous corneal degeneration
● 　　H18.44　Keratomalacia
　　　　　Excludes1　keratomalacia due to vitamin A deficiency (E50.4)
　　　H18.441　Keratomalacia, right eye
　　　H18.442　Keratomalacia, left eye
　　　H18.443　Keratomalacia, bilateral
　　　H18.449　Keratomalacia, unspecified eye

CHAPTER 7 (H00-H59)

- H18.45 Nodular corneal degeneration
  - H18.451 Nodular corneal degeneration, right eye
  - H18.452 Nodular corneal degeneration, left eye
  - H18.453 Nodular corneal degeneration, bilateral
  - H18.459 Nodular corneal degeneration, unspecified eye
- H18.46 Peripheral corneal degeneration
  - H18.461 Peripheral corneal degeneration, right eye
  - H18.462 Peripheral corneal degeneration, left eye
  - H18.463 Peripheral corneal degeneration, bilateral
  - H18.469 Peripheral corneal degeneration, unspecified eye
  - H18.49 Other corneal degeneration
- H18.5 Hereditary corneal dystrophies
  - H18.50 Unspecified hereditary corneal dystrophies
  - H18.51 Endothelial corneal dystrophy
    Fuchs' dystrophy
  - H18.52 Epithelial (juvenile) corneal dystrophy
  - H18.53 Granular corneal dystrophy
  - H18.54 Lattice corneal dystrophy
  - H18.55 Macular corneal dystrophy
  - H18.59 Other hereditary corneal dystrophies
- H18.6 Keratoconus
  - H18.60 Keratoconus, unspecified
    - H18.601 Keratoconus, unspecified, right eye
    - H18.602 Keratoconus, unspecified, left eye
    - H18.603 Keratoconus, unspecified, bilateral
    - H18.609 Keratoconus, unspecified, unspecified eye
  - H18.61 Keratoconus, stable
    - H18.611 Keratoconus, stable, right eye
    - H18.612 Keratoconus, stable, left eye
    - H18.613 Keratoconus, stable, bilateral
    - H18.619 Keratoconus, stable, unspecified eye
  - H18.62 Keratoconus, unstable
    Acute hydrops
    - H18.621 Keratoconus, unstable, right eye
    - H18.622 Keratoconus, unstable, left eye
    - H18.623 Keratoconus, unstable, bilateral
    - H18.629 Keratoconus, unstable, unspecified eye

Figure 7-8 Lateral view of the displacement of the cone apex in keratoconus. (From Yanoff: Ophthalmology, ed 3, Mosby, Inc., 2008)

- H18.7 Other and unspecified corneal deformities
  - Excludes1 congenital malformations of cornea (Q13.3-Q13.4)
  - H18.70 Unspecified corneal deformity
  - H18.71 Corneal ectasia
    - H18.711 Corneal ectasia, right eye
    - H18.712 Corneal ectasia, left eye
    - H18.713 Corneal ectasia, bilateral
    - H18.719 Corneal ectasia, unspecified eye
  - H18.72 Corneal staphyloma
    - H18.721 Corneal staphyloma, right eye
    - H18.722 Corneal staphyloma, left eye
    - H18.723 Corneal staphyloma, bilateral
    - H18.729 Corneal staphyloma, unspecified eye
  - H18.73 Descemetocele
    - H18.731 Descemetocele, right eye
    - H18.732 Descemetocele, left eye
    - H18.733 Descemetocele, bilateral
    - H18.739 Descemetocele, unspecified eye
  - H18.79 Other corneal deformities
    - H18.791 Other corneal deformities, right eye
    - H18.792 Other corneal deformities, left eye
    - H18.793 Other corneal deformities, bilateral
    - H18.799 Other corneal deformities, unspecified eye
- H18.8 Other specified disorders of cornea
  - H18.81 Anesthesia and hypoesthesia of cornea
    - H18.811 Anesthesia and hypoesthesia of cornea, right eye
    - H18.812 Anesthesia and hypoesthesia of cornea, left eye
    - H18.813 Anesthesia and hypoesthesia of cornea, bilateral
    - H18.819 Anesthesia and hypoesthesia of cornea, unspecified eye
  - H18.82 Corneal disorder due to contact lens
    - Excludes2 corneal edema due to contact lens (H18.21-)
    - H18.821 Corneal disorder due to contact lens, right eye
    - H18.822 Corneal disorder due to contact lens, left eye
    - H18.823 Corneal disorder due to contact lens, bilateral
    - H18.829 Corneal disorder due to contact lens, unspecified eye
  - H18.83 Recurrent erosion of cornea
    - H18.831 Recurrent erosion of cornea, right eye
    - H18.832 Recurrent erosion of cornea, left eye
    - H18.833 Recurrent erosion of cornea, bilateral
    - H18.839 Recurrent erosion of cornea, unspecified eye
  - H18.89 Other specified disorders of cornea
    - H18.891 Other specified disorders of cornea, right eye
    - H18.892 Other specified disorders of cornea, left eye
    - H18.893 Other specified disorders of cornea, bilateral
    - H18.899 Other specified disorders of cornea, unspecified eye
- H18.9 Unspecified disorder of cornea

Item 7–4 Keratoconus results in corneal degeneration that begins in childhood, gradually changes the cornea from a round to cone shape, decreasing visual acuity. Treatment includes contact lenses. In severe cases the need for corneal transplant may be the treatment of choice; however, newer technologies may use high frequency radio energy to shrink the edges of the cornea, pulling the central area back to a more normal shape. It can help delay or avoid the need for a corneal transplantation.

▶ New   ⟹ Revised   ~~deleted~~ Deleted   **OGCR** Official Guidelines   X Assign placeholder X   ● Use Additional Character(s)

Excludes 1   Excludes 2   Includes   Use additional   Code first   Code also   Key words

CHAPTER 7 (H00-H59)

● **H20**   **Iridocyclitis**
  ● **H20.0**   Acute and subacute iridocyclitis
    Acute anterior uveitis
    Acute cyclitis
    Acute iritis
    Subacute anterior uveitis
    Subacute cyclitis
    Subacute iritis
    Excludes1   iridocyclitis, iritis, uveitis (due to) (in) diabetes mellitus (E08-E13 with .39)
        iridocyclitis, iritis, uveitis (due to) (in) diphtheria (A36.89)
        iridocyclitis, iritis, uveitis (due to) (in) gonococcal (A54.32)
        iridocyclitis, iritis, uveitis (due to) (in) herpes (simplex) (B00.51)
        iridocyclitis, iritis, uveitis (due to) (in) herpes zoster (B02.32)
        iridocyclitis, iritis, uveitis (due to) (in) late congenital syphilis (A50.39)
        iridocyclitis, iritis, uveitis (due to) (in) late syphilis (A52.71)
        iridocyclitis, iritis, uveitis (due to) (in) sarcoidosis (D86.83)
        iridocyclitis, iritis, uveitis (due to) (in) syphilis (A51.43)
        iridocyclitis, iritis, uveitis (due to) (in) toxoplasmosis (B58.09)
        iridocyclitis, iritis, uveitis (due to) (in) tuberculosis (A18.54)

    H20.00   Unspecified acute and subacute iridocyclitis
  ● **H20.01**   Primary iridocyclitis
    H20.011   Primary iridocyclitis, right eye
    H20.012   Primary iridocyclitis, left eye
    H20.013   Primary iridocyclitis, bilateral
    H20.019   Primary iridocyclitis, unspecified eye
  ● **H20.02**   Recurrent acute iridocyclitis
    H20.021   Recurrent acute iridocyclitis, right eye
    H20.022   Recurrent acute iridocyclitis, left eye
    H20.023   Recurrent acute iridocyclitis, bilateral
    H20.029   Recurrent acute iridocyclitis, unspecified eye
  ● **H20.03**   Secondary infectious iridocyclitis
    H20.031   Secondary infectious iridocyclitis, right eye
    H20.032   Secondary infectious iridocyclitis, left eye
    H20.033   Secondary infectious iridocyclitis, bilateral
    H20.039   Secondary infectious iridocyclitis, unspecified eye
  ● **H20.04**   Secondary noninfectious iridocyclitis
    H20.041   Secondary noninfectious iridocyclitis, right eye
    H20.042   Secondary noninfectious iridocyclitis, left eye
    H20.043   Secondary noninfectious iridocyclitis, bilateral
    H20.049   Secondary noninfectious iridocyclitis, unspecified eye
  ● **H20.05**   Hypopyon
    H20.051   Hypopyon, right eye
    H20.052   Hypopyon, left eye
    H20.053   Hypopyon, bilateral
    H20.059   Hypopyon, unspecified eye

● **H20.1**   Chronic iridocyclitis
    Use additional code for any associated cataract (H26.21-)
    Excludes2   posterior cyclitis (H30.2-)
    H20.10   Chronic iridocyclitis, unspecified eye
    H20.11   Chronic iridocyclitis, right eye
    H20.12   Chronic iridocyclitis, left eye
    H20.13   Chronic iridocyclitis, bilateral
● **H20.2**   Lens-induced iridocyclitis
    H20.20   Lens-induced iridocyclitis, unspecified eye
    H20.21   Lens-induced iridocyclitis, right eye
    H20.22   Lens-induced iridocyclitis, left eye
    H20.23   Lens-induced iridocyclitis, bilateral
● **H20.8**   Other iridocyclitis
    Excludes2   glaucomatocyclitis crises (H40.4-)
        posterior cyclitis (H30.2-)
        sympathetic uveitis (H44.13-)
  ● **H20.81**   Fuchs' heterochromic cyclitis
    H20.811   Fuchs' heterochromic cyclitis, right eye
    H20.812   Fuchs' heterochromic cyclitis, left eye
    H20.813   Fuchs' heterochromic cyclitis, bilateral
    H20.819   Fuchs' heterochromic cyclitis, unspecified eye
  ● **H20.82**   Vogt-Koyanagi syndrome
    H20.821   Vogt-Koyanagi syndrome, right eye
    H20.822   Vogt-Koyanagi syndrome, left eye
    H20.823   Vogt-Koyanagi syndrome, bilateral
    H20.829   Vogt-Koyanagi syndrome, unspecified eye
  H20.9   Unspecified iridocyclitis
    Uveitis NOS

● **H21**   **Other disorders of iris and ciliary body**
    Excludes2   sympathetic uveitis (H44.1-)
  ● **H21.0**   Hyphema
    Excludes1   traumatic hyphema (S05.1-)
    H21.00   Hyphema, unspecified eye
    H21.01   Hyphema, right eye
    H21.02   Hyphema, left eye
    H21.03   Hyphema, bilateral
  ● **H21.1**   Other vascular disorders of iris and ciliary body
    Neovascularization of iris or ciliary body
    Rubeosis iridis
    Rubeosis of iris
  ● **H21.1X**   Other vascular disorders of iris and ciliary body
    H21.1X1   Other vascular disorders of iris and ciliary body, right eye
    H21.1X2   Other vascular disorders of iris and ciliary body, left eye
    H21.1X3   Other vascular disorders of iris and ciliary body, bilateral
    H21.1X9   Other vascular disorders of iris and ciliary body, unspecified eye
  ● **H21.2**   Degeneration of iris and ciliary body
  ● **H21.21**   Degeneration of chamber angle
    H21.211   Degeneration of chamber angle, right eye
    H21.212   Degeneration of chamber angle, left eye
    H21.213   Degeneration of chamber angle, bilateral
    H21.219   Degeneration of chamber angle, unspecified eye

CHAPTER 7 (H00-H59)

● H21.22 Degeneration of ciliary body
  H21.221 Degeneration of ciliary body, right eye
  H21.222 Degeneration of ciliary body, left eye
  H21.223 Degeneration of ciliary body, bilateral
  H21.229 Degeneration of ciliary body, unspecified eye
● H21.23 Degeneration of iris (pigmentary)
         Translucency of iris
  H21.231 Degeneration of iris (pigmentary), right eye
  H21.232 Degeneration of iris (pigmentary), left eye
  H21.233 Degeneration of iris (pigmentary), bilateral
  H21.239 Degeneration of iris (pigmentary), unspecified eye
● H21.24 Degeneration of pupillary margin
  H21.241 Degeneration of pupillary margin, right eye
  H21.242 Degeneration of pupillary margin, left eye
  H21.243 Degeneration of pupillary margin, bilateral
  H21.249 Degeneration of pupillary margin, unspecified eye
● H21.25 Iridoschisis
  H21.251 Iridoschisis, right eye
  H21.252 Iridoschisis, left eye
  H21.253 Iridoschisis, bilateral
  H21.259 Iridoschisis, unspecified eye
● H21.26 Iris atrophy (essential) (progressive)
  H21.261 Iris atrophy (essential) (progressive), right eye
  H21.262 Iris atrophy (essential) (progressive), left eye
  H21.263 Iris atrophy (essential) (progressive), bilateral
  H21.269 Iris atrophy (essential) (progressive), unspecified eye
● H21.27 Miotic pupillary cyst
  H21.271 Miotic pupillary cyst, right eye
  H21.272 Miotic pupillary cyst, left eye
  H21.273 Miotic pupillary cyst, bilateral
  H21.279 Miotic pupillary cyst, unspecified eye
  H21.29 Other iris atrophy
● H21.3 Cyst of iris, ciliary body and anterior chamber
         Excludes2 miotic pupillary cyst (H21.27-)
● H21.30 Idiopathic cysts of iris, ciliary body or anterior chamber
         Cyst of iris, ciliary body or anterior chamber NOS
  H21.301 Idiopathic cysts of iris, ciliary body or anterior chamber, right eye
  H21.302 Idiopathic cysts of iris, ciliary body or anterior chamber, left eye
  H21.303 Idiopathic cysts of iris, ciliary body or anterior chamber, bilateral
  H21.309 Idiopathic cysts of iris, ciliary body or anterior chamber, unspecified eye
● H21.31 Exudative cysts of iris or anterior chamber
  H21.311 Exudative cysts of iris or anterior chamber, right eye
  H21.312 Exudative cysts of iris or anterior chamber, left eye
  H21.313 Exudative cysts of iris or anterior chamber, bilateral
  H21.319 Exudative cysts of iris or anterior chamber, unspecified eye

● H21.32 Implantation cysts of iris, ciliary body or anterior chamber
  H21.321 Implantation cysts of iris, ciliary body or anterior chamber, right eye
  H21.322 Implantation cysts of iris, ciliary body or anterior chamber, left eye
  H21.323 Implantation cysts of iris, ciliary body or anterior chamber, bilateral
  H21.329 Implantation cysts of iris, ciliary body or anterior chamber, unspecified eye
● H21.33 Parasitic cyst of iris, ciliary body or anterior chamber
  H21.331 Parasitic cyst of iris, ciliary body or anterior chamber, right eye
  H21.332 Parasitic cyst of iris, ciliary body or anterior chamber, left eye
  H21.333 Parasitic cyst of iris, ciliary body or anterior chamber, bilateral
  H21.339 Parasitic cyst of iris, ciliary body or anterior chamber, unspecified eye
● H21.34 Primary cyst of pars plana
  H21.341 Primary cyst of pars plana, right eye
  H21.342 Primary cyst of pars plana, left eye
  H21.343 Primary cyst of pars plana, bilateral
  H21.349 Primary cyst of pars plana, unspecified eye
● H21.35 Exudative cyst of pars plana
  H21.351 Exudative cyst of pars plana, right eye
  H21.352 Exudative cyst of pars plana, left eye
  H21.353 Exudative cyst of pars plana, bilateral
  H21.359 Exudative cyst of pars plana, unspecified eye
● H21.4 Pupillary membranes
         Iris bombé
         Pupillary occlusion
         Pupillary seclusion
         Excludes1 congenital pupillary membranes (Q13.8)
  H21.40 Pupillary membranes, unspecified eye
  H21.41 Pupillary membranes, right eye
  H21.42 Pupillary membranes, left eye
  H21.43 Pupillary membranes, bilateral
● H21.5 Other and unspecified adhesions and disruptions of iris and ciliary body
         Excludes1 corectopia (Q13.2)
● H21.50 Unspecified adhesions of iris
         Synechia (iris) NOS
  H21.501 Unspecified adhesions of iris, right eye
  H21.502 Unspecified adhesions of iris, left eye
  H21.503 Unspecified adhesions of iris, bilateral
  H21.509 Unspecified adhesions of iris and ciliary body, unspecified eye
● H21.51 Anterior synechiae (iris)
  H21.511 Anterior synechiae (iris), right eye
  H21.512 Anterior synechiae (iris), left eye
  H21.513 Anterior synechiae (iris), bilateral
  H21.519 Anterior synechiae (iris), unspecified eye
● H21.52 Goniosynechiae
  H21.521 Goniosynechiae, right eye
  H21.522 Goniosynechiae, left eye
  H21.523 Goniosynechiae, bilateral
  H21.529 Goniosynechiae, unspecified eye

▶ New   ⇨ Revised   ~~deleted~~ Deleted   OGCR Official Guidelines   X Assign placeholder X   ● Use Additional Character(s)

Excludes 1   Excludes 2   Includes   Use additional   Code first   Code also   Key words

● **H21.53**   **Iridodialysis**
     H21.531   Iridodialysis, right eye
     H21.532   Iridodialysis, left eye
     H21.533   Iridodialysis, bilateral
     H21.539   Iridodialysis, unspecified eye

● **H21.54**   **Posterior synechiae (iris)**
     H21.541   Posterior synechiae (iris), right eye
     H21.542   Posterior synechiae (iris), left eye
     H21.543   Posterior synechiae (iris), bilateral
     H21.549   Posterior synechiae (iris), unspecified eye

● **H21.55**   **Recession of chamber angle**
     H21.551   Recession of chamber angle, right eye
     H21.552   Recession of chamber angle, left eye
     H21.553   Recession of chamber angle, bilateral
     H21.559   Recession of chamber angle, unspecified eye

● **H21.56**   **Pupillary abnormalities**
     Deformed pupil
     Ectopic pupil
     Rupture of sphincter, pupil
     Excludes1   congenital deformity of pupil (Q13.2-)
     H21.561   Pupillary abnormality, right eye
     H21.562   Pupillary abnormality, left eye
     H21.563   Pupillary abnormality, bilateral
     H21.569   Pupillary abnormality, unspecified eye

● **H21.8**   **Other specified disorders of iris and ciliary body**
     H21.81   Floppy iris syndrome
         Intraoperative floppy iris syndrome (IFIS)
         Use additional code for adverse effect, if applicable, to identify drug (T36-T50 with fifth or sixth character 5)
     H21.82   Plateau iris syndrome (post-iridectomy) (postprocedural)
     H21.89   Other specified disorders of iris and ciliary body
   H21.9   Unspecified disorder of iris and ciliary body

H22   **Disorders of iris and ciliary body in diseases classified elsewhere**
     Code first underlying disease, such as:
     gout (M1A.-, M10.-)
     leprosy (A30.-)
     parasitic disease (B89)

DISORDERS OF LENS (H25-H28)

● **H25**   **Age-related cataract**
     Senile cataract
     Excludes2   capsular glaucoma with pseudoexfoliation of lens (H40.1-)

● **H25.0**   **Age-related incipient cataract**
   ● **H25.01**   Cortical age-related cataract
     H25.011   Cortical age-related cataract, right eye
     H25.012   Cortical age-related cataract, left eye
     H25.013   Cortical age-related cataract, bilateral
     H25.019   Cortical age-related cataract, unspecified eye
   ● **H25.03**   Anterior subcapsular polar age-related cataract
     H25.031   Anterior subcapsular polar age-related cataract, right eye
     H25.032   Anterior subcapsular polar age-related cataract, left eye
     H25.033   Anterior subcapsular polar age-related cataract, bilateral
     H25.039   Anterior subcapsular polar age-related cataract, unspecified eye

Figure 7-9   Age-related cataract. Nuclear sclerosis and cortical lens opacities are present. (From Ignatavicius DD, Workman ML: Medical-Surgical Nursing: Patient-Centered Collaborative Care, St. Louis, MO, Saunders/Elsevier, 2010)

Item 7–5 Senile cataracts are linked to the aging process. The most common area for the formation of a cataract is the cortical area of the lens. **Polar cataracts** can be either anterior or posterior. **Anterior polar cataracts** are more common and are small, white, capsular cataracts located on the anterior portion of the lens. **Total cataracts**, also called **complete** or **mature**, cause an opacity of all fibers of the lens. **Hypermature** describes a mature cataract with a swollen, milky cortex that covers the entire lens. **Immature**, also called **incipient**, cataracts have a clear cortex and are only slightly opaque. Treatment for all cataracts is the removal of the lens.

   ● **H25.04**   Posterior subcapsular polar age-related cataract
     H25.041   Posterior subcapsular polar age-related cataract, right eye
     H25.042   Posterior subcapsular polar age-related cataract, left eye
     H25.043   Posterior subcapsular polar age-related cataract, bilateral
     H25.049   Posterior subcapsular polar age-related cataract, unspecified eye
   ● **H25.09**   Other age-related incipient cataract
     Coronary age-related cataract
     Punctate age-related cataract
     Water clefts
     H25.091   Other age-related incipient cataract, right eye
     H25.092   Other age-related incipient cataract, left eye
     H25.093   Other age-related incipient cataract, bilateral
     H25.099   Other age-related incipient cataract, unspecified eye

● **H25.1**   **Age-related nuclear cataract**
     Cataracta brunescens
     Nuclear sclerosis cataract
     H25.10   Age-related nuclear cataract, unspecified eye
     H25.11   Age-related nuclear cataract, right eye
     H25.12   Age-related nuclear cataract, left eye
     H25.13   Age-related nuclear cataract, bilateral

● **H25.2**   **Age-related cataract, morgagnian type**
     Age-related hypermature cataract
     H25.20   Age-related cataract, morgagnian type, unspecified eye
     H25.21   Age-related cataract, morgagnian type, right eye
     H25.22   Age-related cataract, morgagnian type, left eye
     H25.23   Age-related cataract, morgagnian type, bilateral

● **H25.8**   **Other age-related cataract**
   ● **H25.81**   Combined forms of age-related cataract
     H25.811   Combined forms of age-related cataract, right eye
     H25.812   Combined forms of age-related cataract, left eye
     H25.813   Combined forms of age-related cataract, bilateral
     H25.819   Combined forms of age-related cataract, unspecified eye
     H25.89   Other age-related cataract
   H25.9   Unspecified age-related cataract

CHAPTER 7 (H00-H59)

▶ New   ⇒ Revised   ~~deleted~~ Deleted   **OGCR** Official Guidelines   X Assign placeholder X   ● Use Additional Character(s)

Excludes 1   Excludes 2   Includes   Use additional   Code first   Code also   Key words

● **H26**   **Other cataract**
    Excludes1   congenital cataract (Q12.0)
   ● **H26.0**   **Infantile and juvenile cataract**
     ● **H26.00**   Unspecified infantile and juvenile cataract
       H26.001   Unspecified infantile and juvenile cataract, right eye
       H26.002   Unspecified infantile and juvenile cataract, left eye
       H26.003   Unspecified infantile and juvenile cataract, bilateral
       H26.009   Unspecified infantile and juvenile cataract, unspecified eye
     ● **H26.01**   Infantile and juvenile cortical, lamellar, or zonular cataract
       H26.011   Infantile and juvenile cortical, lamellar, or zonular cataract, right eye
       H26.012   Infantile and juvenile cortical, lamellar, or zonular cataract, left eye
       H26.013   Infantile and juvenile cortical, lamellar, or zonular cataract, bilateral
       H26.019   Infantile and juvenile cortical, lamellar, or zonular cataract, unspecified eye
     ● **H26.03**   Infantile and juvenile nuclear cataract
       H26.031   Infantile and juvenile nuclear cataract, right eye
       H26.032   Infantile and juvenile nuclear cataract, left eye
       H26.033   Infantile and juvenile nuclear cataract, bilateral
       H26.039   Infantile and juvenile nuclear cataract, unspecified eye
     ● **H26.04**   Anterior subcapsular polar infantile and juvenile cataract
       H26.041   Anterior subcapsular polar infantile and juvenile cataract, right eye
       H26.042   Anterior subcapsular polar infantile and juvenile cataract, left eye
       H26.043   Anterior subcapsular polar infantile and juvenile cataract, bilateral
       H26.049   Anterior subcapsular polar infantile and juvenile cataract, unspecified eye
     ● **H26.05**   Posterior subcapsular polar infantile and juvenile cataract
       H26.051   Posterior subcapsular polar infantile and juvenile cataract, right eye
       H26.052   Posterior subcapsular polar infantile and juvenile cataract, left eye
       H26.053   Posterior subcapsular polar infantile and juvenile cataract, bilateral
       H26.059   Posterior subcapsular polar infantile and juvenile cataract, unspecified eye
     ● **H26.06**   Combined forms of infantile and juvenile cataract
       H26.061   Combined forms of infantile and juvenile cataract, right eye
       H26.062   Combined forms of infantile and juvenile cataract, left eye
       H26.063   Combined forms of infantile and juvenile cataract bilateral
       H26.069   Combined forms of infantile and juvenile cataract, unspecified eye
     H26.09   Other infantile and juvenile cataract

   ● **H26.1**   **Traumatic cataract**
     Use additional code (Chapter 20) to identify external cause
     ● **H26.10**   Unspecified traumatic cataract
       H26.101   Unspecified traumatic cataract, right eye
       H26.102   Unspecified traumatic cataract, left eye
       H26.103   Unspecified traumatic cataract, bilateral
       H26.109   Unspecified traumatic cataract, unspecified eye
     ● **H26.11**   Localized traumatic opacities
       H26.111   Localized traumatic opacities, right eye
       H26.112   Localized traumatic opacities, left eye
       H26.113   Localized traumatic opacities, bilateral
       H26.119   Localized traumatic opacities, unspecified eye
     ● **H26.12**   Partially resolved traumatic cataract
       H26.121   Partially resolved traumatic cataract, right eye
       H26.122   Partially resolved traumatic cataract, left eye
       H26.123   Partially resolved traumatic cataract, bilateral
       H26.129   Partially resolved traumatic cataract, unspecified eye
     ● **H26.13**   Total traumatic cataract
       H26.131   Total traumatic cataract, right eye
       H26.132   Total traumatic cataract, left eye
       H26.133   Total traumatic cataract, bilateral
       H26.139   Total traumatic cataract, unspecified eye

   ● **H26.2**   **Complicated cataract**
     H26.20   Unspecified complicated cataract
       Cataracta complicata NOS
     ● **H26.21**   Cataract with neovascularization
       Code also associated condition, such as: chronic iridocyclitis (H20.1-)
       H26.211   Cataract with neovascularization, right eye
       H26.212   Cataract with neovascularization, left eye
       H26.213   Cataract with neovascularization, bilateral
       H26.219   Cataract with neovascularization, unspecified eye
     ● **H26.22**   Cataract secondary to ocular disorders (degenerative) (inflammatory)
       Code also associated ocular disorder
       H26.221   Cataract secondary to ocular disorders (degenerative) (inflammatory), right eye
       H26.222   Cataract secondary to ocular disorders (degenerative) (inflammatory), left eye
       H26.223   Cataract secondary to ocular disorders (degenerative) (inflammatory), bilateral
       H26.229   Cataract secondary to ocular disorders (degenerative) (inflammatory), unspecified eye

▶ New   ⇒ Revised   ~~deleted~~ Deleted   **OGCR** Official Guidelines   X Assign placeholder X   ● Use Additional Character(s)

Excludes 1   Excludes 2   Includes   Use additional   Code first   Code also   Key words

● H26.23 **Glaucomatous flecks** (subcapsular)
Code first underlying glaucoma (H40-H42)
   H26.231   Glaucomatous flecks (subcapsular), **right** eye
   H26.232   Glaucomatous flecks (subcapsular), **left** eye
   H26.233   Glaucomatous flecks (subcapsular), **bilateral**
   H26.239   Glaucomatous flecks (subcapsular), **unspecified** eye

● H26.3   **Drug-induced** cataract
   Toxic cataract
   Use additional code for adverse effect, if applicable, to identify drug (T36-T50 with fifth or sixth character 5)
   H26.30   Drug-induced cataract, **unspecified** eye
   H26.31   Drug-induced cataract, **right** eye
   H26.32   Drug-induced cataract, **left** eye
   H26.33   Drug-induced cataract, **bilateral**

● H26.4   **Secondary** cataract
   H26.40   **Unspecified** secondary cataract
 ● H26.41   **Soemmering's ring**
    H26.411   Soemmering's ring, **right** eye
    H26.412   Soemmering's ring, **left** eye
    H26.413   Soemmering's ring, **bilateral**
    H26.419   Soemmering's ring, **unspecified** eye
 ● H26.49   **Other** secondary cataract
    H26.491   Other secondary cataract, **right** eye
    H26.492   Other secondary cataract, **left** eye
    H26.493   Other secondary cataract, **bilateral**
    H26.499   Other secondary cataract, **unspecified** eye

H26.8   **Other** specified cataract
H26.9   **Unspecified** cataract

● H27   Other disorders of lens
  Excludes1   congenital lens malformations (Q12.-)
     mechanical complications of intraocular lens implant (T85.2)
     pseudophakia (Z96.1)

● H27.0   Aphakia
   Acquired absence of lens
   Acquired aphakia
   Aphakia due to trauma
   Excludes1   cataract extraction status (Z98.4-)
     congenital absence of lens (Q12.3)
     congenital aphakia (Q12.3)
   H27.00   Aphakia, **unspecified** eye
   H27.01   Aphakia, **right** eye
   H27.02   Aphakia, **left** eye
   H27.03   Aphakia, **bilateral**

● H27.1   Dislocation of lens
   H27.10   **Unspecified** dislocation of lens
 ● H27.11   **Subluxation** of lens
    H27.111   Subluxation of lens, **right** eye
    H27.112   Subluxation of lens, **left** eye
    H27.113   Subluxation of lens, **bilateral**
    H27.119   Subluxation of lens, **unspecified** eye
 ● H27.12   **Anterior** dislocation of lens
    H27.121   Anterior dislocation of lens, **right** eye
    H27.122   Anterior dislocation of lens, **left** eye
    H27.123   Anterior dislocation of lens, **bilateral**
    H27.129   Anterior dislocation of lens, **unspecified** eye

● H27.13   **Posterior** dislocation of lens
   H27.131   Posterior dislocation of lens, **right** eye
   H27.132   Posterior dislocation of lens, **left** eye
   H27.133   Posterior dislocation of lens, **bilateral**
   H27.139   Posterior dislocation of lens, **unspecified** eye

H27.8   **Other** specified disorders of lens
H27.9   **Unspecified** disorder of lens

H28   Cataract in diseases classified elsewhere
  Code first underlying disease, such as:
   hypoparathyroidism (E20.-)
   myotonia (G71.1-)
   myxedema (E03.-)
   protein-calorie malnutrition (E40-E46)
  Excludes1   cataract in diabetes mellitus (E08.36, E09.36, E10.36, E11.36, E13.36)

DISORDERS OF CHOROID AND RETINA (H30-H36)

★ **(See Plate 90 on page 64.)**

● H30   Chorioretinal inflammation
 ● H30.0   **Focal** chorioretinal inflammation
   Focal chorioretinitis
   Focal choroiditis
   Focal retinitis
   Focal retinochoroiditis
 ● H30.00   **Unspecified** focal chorioretinal inflammation
   Focal chorioretinitis NOS
   Focal choroiditis NOS
   Focal retinitis NOS
   Focal retinochoroiditis NOS
    H30.001   Unspecified focal chorioretinal inflammation, **right** eye
    H30.002   Unspecified focal chorioretinal inflammation, **left** eye
    H30.003   Unspecified focal chorioretinal inflammation, **bilateral**
    H30.009   Unspecified focal chorioretinal inflammation, **unspecified** eye
 ● H30.01   Focal chorioretinal inflammation, **juxtapapillary**
    H30.011   Focal chorioretinal inflammation, juxtapapillary, **right** eye
    H30.012   Focal chorioretinal inflammation, juxtapapillary, **left** eye
    H30.013   Focal chorioretinal inflammation, juxtapapillary, **bilateral**
    H30.019   Focal chorioretinal inflammation, juxtapapillary, **unspecified** eye
 ● H30.02   Focal chorioretinal inflammation of **posterior pole**
    H30.021   Focal chorioretinal inflammation of posterior pole, **right** eye
    H30.022   Focal chorioretinal inflammation of posterior pole, **left** eye
    H30.023   Focal chorioretinal inflammation of posterior pole, **bilateral**
    H30.029   Focal chorioretinal inflammation of posterior pole, **unspecified** eye
 ● H30.03   Focal chorioretinal inflammation, **peripheral**
    H30.031   Focal chorioretinal inflammation, peripheral, **right** eye
    H30.032   Focal chorioretinal inflammation, peripheral, **left** eye
    H30.033   Focal chorioretinal inflammation, peripheral, **bilateral**
    H30.039   Focal chorioretinal inflammation, peripheral, **unspecified** eye

---

▶ New   ⇒ Revised   ~~deleted~~ Deleted   **OGCR** Official Guidelines   X Assign placeholder X   ● Use Additional Character(s)

| Excludes 1 | Excludes 2 | Includes | Use additional | Code first | Code also | Key words |

● **H30.04** Focal chorioretinal inflammation, macular or paramacular

    H30.041 Focal chorioretinal inflammation, macular or paramacular, right eye

    H30.042 Focal chorioretinal inflammation, macular or paramacular, left eye

    H30.043 Focal chorioretinal inflammation, macular or paramacular, bilateral

    H30.049 Focal chorioretinal inflammation, macular or paramacular, unspecified eye

● **H30.1** Disseminated chorioretinal inflammation

    Disseminated chorioretinitis
    Disseminated choroiditis
    Disseminated retinitis
    Disseminated retinochoroiditis

    Excludes2   exudative retinopathy (H35.02-)

  ● **H30.10** Unspecified disseminated chorioretinal inflammation

    Disseminated chorioretinitis NOS
    Disseminated choroiditis NOS
    Disseminated retinitis NOS
    Disseminated retinochoroiditis NOS

    H30.101 Unspecified disseminated chorioretinal inflammation, right eye

    H30.102 Unspecified disseminated chorioretinal inflammation, left eye

    H30.103 Unspecified disseminated chorioretinal inflammation, bilateral

    H30.109 Unspecified disseminated chorioretinal inflammation, unspecified eye

  ● **H30.11** Disseminated chorioretinal inflammation of posterior pole

    H30.111 Disseminated chorioretinal inflammation of posterior pole, right eye

    H30.112 Disseminated chorioretinal inflammation of posterior pole, left eye

    H30.113 Disseminated chorioretinal inflammation of posterior pole, bilateral

    H30.119 Disseminated chorioretinal inflammation of posterior pole, unspecified eye

  ● **H30.12** Disseminated chorioretinal inflammation, peripheral

    H30.121 Disseminated chorioretinal inflammation, peripheral right eye

    H30.122 Disseminated chorioretinal inflammation, peripheral, left eye

    H30.123 Disseminated chorioretinal inflammation, peripheral, bilateral

    H30.129 Disseminated chorioretinal inflammation, peripheral, unspecified eye

  ● **H30.13** Disseminated chorioretinal inflammation, generalized

    H30.131 Disseminated chorioretinal inflammation, generalized, right eye

    H30.132 Disseminated chorioretinal inflammation, generalized, left eye

    H30.133 Disseminated chorioretinal inflammation, generalized, bilateral

    H30.139 Disseminated chorioretinal inflammation, generalized, unspecified eye

● **H30.14** Acute posterior multifocal placoid pigment epitheliopathy

    H30.141 Acute posterior multifocal placoid pigment epitheliopathy, right eye

    H30.142 Acute posterior multifocal placoid pigment epitheliopathy, left eye

    H30.143 Acute posterior multifocal placoid pigment epitheliopathy, bilateral

    H30.149 Acute posterior multifocal placoid pigment epitheliopathy, unspecified eye

● **H30.2** Posterior cyclitis

    Pars planitis

    H30.20 Posterior cyclitis, unspecified eye

    H30.21 Posterior cyclitis, right eye

    H30.22 Posterior cyclitis, left eye

    H30.23 Posterior cyclitis, bilateral

● **H30.8** Other chorioretinal inflammations

  ● **H30.81** Harada's disease

    H30.811 Harada's disease, right eye

    H30.812 Harada's disease, left eye

    H30.813 Harada's disease, bilateral

    H30.819 Harada's disease, unspecified eye

  ● **H30.89** Other chorioretinal inflammations

    H30.891 Other chorioretinal inflammations, right eye

    H30.892 Other chorioretinal inflammations, left eye

    H30.893 Other chorioretinal inflammations, bilateral

    H30.899 Other chorioretinal inflammations, unspecified eye

● **H30.9** Unspecified chorioretinal inflammation

    Chorioretinitis NOS
    Choroiditis NOS
    Neuroretinitis NOS
    Retinitis NOS
    Retinochoroiditis NOS

    H30.90 Unspecified chorioretinal inflammation, unspecified eye

    H30.91 Unspecified chorioretinal inflammation, right eye

    H30.92 Unspecified chorioretinal inflammation, left eye

    H30.93 Unspecified chorioretinal inflammation, bilateral

● **H31** Other disorders of choroid

  ● **H31.0** Chorioretinal scars

    Excludes2   postsurgical chorioretinal scars (H59.81-)

  ● **H31.00** Unspecified chorioretinal scars

    H31.001 Unspecified chorioretinal scars, right eye

    H31.002 Unspecified chorioretinal scars, left eye

    H31.003 Unspecified chorioretinal scars, bilateral

    H31.009 Unspecified chorioretinal scars, unspecified eye

▶ New   ⇒ Revised   ~~deleted~~ Deleted   **OGCR** Official Guidelines   X Assign placeholder X   ● Use Additional Character(s)

Excludes 1   Excludes 2   Includes   Use additional   Code first   Code also   Key words

● **H31.01 Macula scars of posterior pole (postinflammatory) (post-traumatic)**

     Excludes1   postprocedural chorioretinal scar (H59.81-)

     H31.011   Macula scars of posterior pole (postinflammatory) (post-traumatic), **right** eye

     H31.012   Macula scars of posterior pole (postinflammatory) (post-traumatic), **left** eye

     H31.013   Macula scars of posterior pole (postinflammatory) (post-traumatic), **bilateral**

     H31.019   Macula scars of posterior pole (postinflammatory) (post-traumatic), **unspecified** eye

● **H31.02 Solar retinopathy**

     H31.021   Solar retinopathy, **right** eye

     H31.022   Solar retinopathy, **left** eye

     H31.023   Solar retinopathy, **bilateral**

     H31.029   Solar retinopathy, **unspecified** eye

● **H31.09 Other chorioretinal scars**

     H31.091   Other chorioretinal scars, **right** eye

     H31.092   Other chorioretinal scars, **left** eye

     H31.093   Other chorioretinal scars, **bilateral**

     H31.099   Other chorioretinal scars, **unspecified** eye

● **H31.1 Choroidal degeneration**

     Excludes2   angioid streaks of macula (H35.33)

● **H31.10 Unspecified choroidal degeneration**
     Choroidal sclerosis NOS

     H31.101   Choroidal degeneration, unspecified, **right** eye

     H31.102   Choroidal degeneration, unspecified, **left** eye

     H31.103   Choroidal degeneration, unspecified, **bilateral**

     H31.109   Choroidal degeneration, unspecified, **unspecified** eye

● **H31.11 Age-related choroidal atrophy**

     H31.111   Age-related choroidal atrophy, **right** eye

     H31.112   Age-related choroidal atrophy, **left** eye

     H31.113   Age-related choroidal atrophy, **bilateral**

     H31.119   Age-related choroidal atrophy, **unspecified** eye

● **H31.12 Diffuse secondary atrophy of choroid**

     H31.121   Diffuse secondary atrophy of choroid, **right** eye

     H31.122   Diffuse secondary atrophy of choroid, **left** eye

     H31.123   Diffuse secondary atrophy of choroid, **bilateral**

     H31.129   Diffuse secondary atrophy of choroid, **unspecified** eye

● **H31.2 Hereditary choroidal dystrophy**

     Excludes2   hyperornithinemia (E72.4)
                   ornithinemia (E72.4)

     H31.20   Hereditary choroidal dystrophy, **unspecified**

     H31.21   Choroideremia

     H31.22   Choroidal dystrophy (central areolar) (generalized) (peripapillary)

     H31.23   Gyrate atrophy, choroid

     H31.29   Other hereditary choroidal dystrophy

● **H31.3 Choroidal hemorrhage and rupture**

● **H31.30 Unspecified choroidal hemorrhage**

     H31.301   Unspecified choroidal hemorrhage, **right** eye

     H31.302   Unspecified choroidal hemorrhage, **left** eye

     H31.303   Unspecified choroidal hemorrhage, **bilateral**

     H31.309   Unspecified choroidal hemorrhage, **unspecified** eye

● **H31.31 Expulsive choroidal hemorrhage**

     H31.311   Expulsive choroidal hemorrhage, **right** eye

     H31.312   Expulsive choroidal hemorrhage, **left** eye

     H31.313   Expulsive choroidal hemorrhage, **bilateral**

     H31.319   Expulsive choroidal hemorrhage, **unspecified** eye

● **H31.32 Choroidal rupture**

     H31.321   Choroidal rupture, **right** eye

     H31.322   Choroidal rupture, **left** eye

     H31.323   Choroidal rupture, **bilateral**

     H31.329   Choroidal rupture, **unspecified** eye

● **H31.4 Choroidal detachment**

● **H31.40 Unspecified choroidal detachment**

     H31.401   Unspecified choroidal detachment, **right** eye

     H31.402   Unspecified choroidal detachment, **left** eye

     H31.403   Unspecified choroidal detachment, **bilateral**

     H31.409   Unspecified choroidal detachment, **unspecified** eye

● **H31.41 Hemorrhagic choroidal detachment**

     H31.411   Hemorrhagic choroidal detachment, **right** eye

     H31.412   Hemorrhagic choroidal detachment, **left** eye

     H31.413   Hemorrhagic choroidal detachment, **bilateral**

     H31.419   Hemorrhagic choroidal detachment, **unspecified** eye

● **H31.42 Serous choroidal detachment**

     H31.421   Serous choroidal detachment, **right** eye

     H31.422   Serous choroidal detachment, **left eye**

     H31.423   Serous choroidal detachment, **bilateral**

     H31.429   Serous choroidal detachment, **unspecified** eye

     H31.8   **Other** specified disorders of choroid

     H31.9   **Unspecified** disorder of choroid

H32 Chorioretinal disorders in diseases classified elsewhere

Code first underlying disease, such as:
     congenital toxoplasmosis (P37.1)
     histoplasmosis (B39.-)
     leprosy (A30.-)

     Excludes1   chorioretinitis (in):
                   toxoplasmosis (acquired) (B58.01)
                   tuberculosis (A18.53)

CHAPTER 7 (H00-H59)

▶ New   ⇒ Revised   ~~deleted~~ Deleted   **OGCR** Official Guidelines   X Assign placeholder X   ● Use Additional Character(s)

Excludes 1   Excludes 2   Includes   Use additional   Code first   Code also   Key words

NON-RHEGMATOGENOUS
RETINAL DETACHMENT

- Vitreous
- Retina
- Protein-rich fluid in sub-retinal space
- Retinal pigment epithelium

VITREOUS DETACHMENT

- Vitreous
- Posterior hyaloid
- Internal limiting membrane

RHEGMATOGENOUS
RETINAL
DETACHMENT

Blood

- Vitreous
- Posterior hyaloid
- Retina
- Retinal tear
- Liquified vitreous
- Retinal pigment epithelium

Figure 7-10   Retinal detachment. (From Kumar: Robbins and Cotran: Pathologic Basis of Disease, ed 7, Saunders, 2005)

Item 7–6   Retinal detachments and defects are conditions of the eye in which the retina separates from the underlying tissue. Initial detachment may be localized, requiring rapid treatment (medical emergency) to avoid the entire retina from detaching which leads to vision loss and blindness.

● H33   **Retinal detachments and breaks**

    Excludes1   detachment of retinal pigment epithelium (H35.72-, H35.73-)

   ● H33.0   **Retinal detachment with retinal break**
      Rhegmatogenous retinal detachment

      Excludes1   serous retinal detachment (without retinal break) (H33.2-)

    ● H33.00   **Unspecified retinal detachment with retinal break**

      H33.001   Unspecified retinal detachment with retinal break, **right** eye

      H33.002   Unspecified retinal detachment with retinal break, **left** eye

      H33.003   Unspecified retinal detachment with retinal break, **bilateral**

      H33.009   Unspecified retinal detachment with retinal break, **unspecified** eye

    ● H33.01   **Retinal detachment with single break**

      H33.011   Retinal detachment with single break, **right** eye

      H33.012   Retinal detachment with single break, **left** eye

      H33.013   Retinal detachment with single break, **bilateral**

      H33.019   Retinal detachment with single break, **unspecified** eye

   ● H33.02   **Retinal detachment with multiple breaks**

      H33.021   Retinal detachment with multiple breaks, **right** eye

      H33.022   Retinal detachment with multiple breaks, **left** eye

      H33.023   Retinal detachment with multiple breaks, **bilateral**

      H33.029   Retinal detachment with multiple breaks, **unspecified** eye

   ● H33.03   **Retinal detachment with giant retinal tear**

      H33.031   Retinal detachment with giant retinal tear, **right** eye

      H33.032   Retinal detachment with giant retinal tear, **left** eye

      H33.033   Retinal detachment with giant retinal tear, **bilateral**

      H33.039   Retinal detachment with giant retinal tear, **unspecified** eye

   ● H33.04   **Retinal detachment with retinal dialysis**

      H33.041   Retinal detachment with retinal dialysis, **right** eye

      H33.042   Retinal detachment with retinal dialysis, **left** eye

      H33.043   Retinal detachment with retinal dialysis, **bilateral**

      H33.049   Retinal detachment with retinal dialysis, **unspecified** eye

   ● H33.05   **Total retinal detachment**

      H33.051   Total retinal detachment, **right** eye

      H33.052   Total retinal detachment, **left** eye

      H33.053   Total retinal detachment, **bilateral**

      H33.059   Total retinal detachment, **unspecified** eye

● H33.1   **Retinoschisis and retinal cysts**

    Excludes1   congenital retinoschisis (Q14.1)
         microcystoid degeneration of retina (H35.42-)

   ● H33.10   **Unspecified retinoschisis**

      H33.101   Unspecified retinoschisis, **right** eye

      H33.102   Unspecified retinoschisis, **left** eye

      H33.103   Unspecified retinoschisis, **bilateral**

      H33.109   Unspecified retinoschisis, **unspecified** eye

   ● H33.11   **Cyst of ora serrata**

      H33.111   Cyst of ora serrata, **right** eye

      H33.112   Cyst of ora serrata, **left** eye

      H33.113   Cyst of ora serrata, **bilateral**

      H33.119   Cyst of ora serrata, **unspecified** eye

   ● H33.12   **Parasitic cyst of retina**

      H33.121   Parasitic cyst of retina, **right** eye

      H33.122   Parasitic cyst of retina, **left** eye

      H33.123   Parasitic cyst of retina, **bilateral**

      H33.129   Parasitic cyst of retina, **unspecified** eye

   ● H33.19   **Other retinoschisis and retinal cysts**
       Pseudocyst of retina

      H33.191   Other retinoschisis and retinal cysts, **right** eye

      H33.192   Other retinoschisis and retinal cysts, **left** eye

      H33.193   Other retinoschisis and retinal cysts, **bilateral**

      H33.199   Other retinoschisis and retinal cysts, **unspecified** eye

▶ New   ⮕ Revised   ~~deleted~~ Deleted   **OGCR** Official Guidelines   X Assign placeholder X   ● Use Additional Character(s)

Excludes 1   Excludes 2   Includes   Use additional   Code first   Code also   Key words

● H33.2 Serous retinal detachment
    Retinal detachment NOS
    Retinal detachment without retinal break
    Excludes1   central serous chorioretinopathy
                     (H35.71-)
    H33.20 Serous retinal detachment, unspecified eye
    H33.21 Serous retinal detachment, right eye
    H33.22 Serous retinal detachment, left eye
    H33.23 Serous retinal detachment, bilateral

● H33.3 Retinal breaks without detachment
    Excludes1   chorioretinal scars after surgery for
                     detachment (H59.81-)
                     peripheral retinal degeneration without
                     break (H35.4-)
  ● H33.30 Unspecified retinal break
    H33.301 Unspecified retinal break, right eye
    H33.302 Unspecified retinal break, left eye
    H33.303 Unspecified retinal break, bilateral
    H33.309 Unspecified retinal break, unspecified
               eye
  ● H33.31 Horseshoe tear of retina without detachment
    Operculum of retina without detachment
    H33.311 Horseshoe tear of retina without
               detachment, right eye
    H33.312 Horseshoe tear of retina without
               detachment, left eye
    H33.313 Horseshoe tear of retina without
               detachment, bilateral
    H33.319 Horseshoe tear of retina without
               detachment, unspecified eye
  ● H33.32 Round hole of retina without detachment
    H33.321 Round hole, right eye
    H33.322 Round hole, left eye
    H33.323 Round hole, bilateral
    H33.329 Round hole, unspecified eye
  ● H33.33 Multiple defects of retina without detachment
    H33.331 Multiple defects of retina without
               detachment, right eye
    H33.332 Multiple defects of retina without
               detachment, left eye
    H33.333 Multiple defects of retina without
               detachment, bilateral
    H33.339 Multiple defects of retina without
               detachment, unspecified eye

● H33.4 Traction detachment of retina
    Proliferative vitreo-retinopathy with retinal
        detachment
    H33.40 Traction detachment of retina, unspecified eye
    H33.41 Traction detachment of retina, right eye
    H33.42 Traction detachment of retina, left eye
    H33.43 Traction detachment of retina, bilateral
  H33.8 Other retinal detachments

● H34 Retinal vascular occlusions
    Blockage in vessel of the retina
    Excludes1   amaurosis fugax (G45.3)
● H34.0 Transient retinal artery occlusion
    H34.00 Transient retinal artery occlusion, unspecified
            eye
    H34.01 Transient retinal artery occlusion, right eye
    H34.02 Transient retinal artery occlusion, left eye
    H34.03 Transient retinal artery occlusion, bilateral
● H34.1 Central retinal artery occlusion
    H34.10 Central retinal artery occlusion, unspecified eye
    H34.11 Central retinal artery occlusion, right eye
    H34.12 Central retinal artery occlusion, left eye
    H34.13 Central retinal artery occlusion, bilateral

● H34.2 Other retinal artery occlusions
  ● H34.21 Partial retinal artery occlusion
    Hollenhorst's plaque
    Retinal microembolism
    H34.211 Partial retinal artery occlusion, right
               eye
    H34.212 Partial retinal artery occlusion, left
               eye
    H34.213 Partial retinal artery occlusion,
               bilateral
    H34.219 Partial retinal artery occlusion,
               unspecified eye
  ● H34.23 Retinal artery branch occlusion
    H34.231 Retinal artery branch occlusion, right
               eye
    H34.232 Retinal artery branch occlusion, left
               eye
    H34.233 Retinal artery branch occlusion,
               bilateral
    H34.239 Retinal artery branch occlusion,
               unspecified eye

● H34.8 Other retinal vascular occlusions
  ● H34.81 Central retinal vein occlusion
    One of the following 7th characters is to
      be assigned to codes in subcategory
      H34.81 to designate the severity of the
      occlusion:

    Ø   with macular edema
    1   with retinal neovascularization
    2   stable
        Old central retinal vein occlusion

   ● H34.811 Central retinal vein occlusion, right
               eye
   ● H34.812 Central retinal vein occlusion, left eye
   ● H34.813 Central retinal vein occlusion,
               bilateral
   ● H34.819 Central retinal vein occlusion,
               unspecified eye
  ● H34.82 Venous engorgement
    Incipient retinal vein occlusion
    Partial retinal vein occlusion
    H34.821 Venous engorgement, right eye
    H34.822 Venous engorgement, left eye
    H34.823 Venous engorgement, bilateral
    H34.829 Venous engorgement, unspecified eye
  ● H34.83 Tributary (branch) retinal vein occlusion
    One of the following 7th characters is to
      be assigned to codes in subcategory
      H34.83 to designate the severity of the
      occlusion:

    Ø   with macular edema
    1   with retinal neovascularization
    2   stable
        Old tributary (branch) retinal vein
        occlusion

   ● H34.831 Tributary (branch) retinal vein
               occlusion, right eye
   ● H34.832 Tributary (branch) retinal vein
               occlusion, left eye
   ● H34.833 Tributary (branch) retinal vein
               occlusion, bilateral
   ● H34.839 Tributary (branch) retinal vein
               occlusion, unspecified eye
  H34.9 Unspecified retinal vascular occlusion

▶ New   ⇒ Revised   ~~deleted~~ Deleted   **OGCR** Official Guidelines   X Assign placeholder X   ● Use Additional Character(s)

Excludes 1   Excludes 2   Includes   Use additional   Code first   Code also   Key words

● **H35   Other retinal disorders**

> Excludes2   diabetic retinal disorders (E08.311-E08.359,
> E09.311-E09.359, E10.311-E10.359,
> E11.311-E11.359, E13.311-E13.359)

● **H35.0   Background retinopathy and retinal vascular changes**
> Code also any associated hypertension (I10.-)

OGCR   Section I. C.9.a.5.

> Hypertensive Retinopathy
> Subcategory H35.0, Background retinopathy and
> retinal vascular changes, should be used with a
> code from category I10–I15, Hypertensive disease to
> include the systemic hypertension. The sequencing is
> based on the reason for the encounter.

 H35.00   Unspecified background retinopathy

● H35.01   Changes in retinal vascular appearance
    Retinal vascular sheathing

   H35.011   Changes in retinal vascular appearance, right eye

   H35.012   Changes in retinal vascular appearance, left eye

   H35.013   Changes in retinal vascular appearance, bilateral

   H35.019   Changes in retinal vascular appearance, unspecified eye

● H35.02   Exudative retinopathy
    Coats retinopathy

   H35.021   Exudative retinopathy, right eye

   H35.022   Exudative retinopathy, left eye

   H35.023   Exudative retinopathy, bilateral

   H35.029   Exudative retinopathy, unspecified eye

● H35.03   Hypertensive retinopathy

   H35.031   Hypertensive retinopathy, right eye

   H35.032   Hypertensive retinopathy, left eye

   H35.033   Hypertensive retinopathy, bilateral

   H35.039   Hypertensive retinopathy, unspecified eye

● H35.04   Retinal micro-aneurysms, unspecified

   H35.041   Retinal micro-aneurysms, unspecified, right eye

   H35.042   Retinal micro-aneurysms, unspecified, left eye

   H35.043   Retinal micro-aneurysms, unspecified, bilateral

   H35.049   Retinal micro-aneurysms, unspecified, unspecified eye

● H35.05   Retinal neovascularization, unspecified

   H35.051   Retinal neovascularization, unspecified, right eye

   H35.052   Retinal neovascularization, unspecified, left eye

   H35.053   Retinal neovascularization, unspecified, bilateral

   H35.059   Retinal neovascularization, unspecified, unspecified eye

● H35.06   Retinal vasculitis
    Eales disease
    Retinal perivasculitis

   H35.061   Retinal vasculitis, right eye

   H35.062   Retinal vasculitis, left eye

   H35.063   Retinal vasculitis, bilateral

   H35.069   Retinal vasculitis, unspecified eye

 H35.07   Retinal telangiectasis

   H35.071   Retinal telangiectasis, right eye

   H35.072   Retinal telangiectasis, left eye

   H35.073   Retinal telangiectasis, bilateral

   H35.079   Retinal telangiectasis, unspecified eye

 H35.09   Other intraretinal microvascular abnormalities
    Retinal varices

● **H35.1   Retinopathy of prematurity**

● H35.10   Retinopathy of prematurity, unspecified
    Retinopathy of prematurity NOS

   H35.101   Retinopathy of prematurity, unspecified, right eye

   H35.102   Retinopathy of prematurity, unspecified, left eye

   H35.103   Retinopathy of prematurity, unspecified, bilateral

   H35.109   Retinopathy of prematurity, unspecified, unspecified eye

● H35.11   Retinopathy of prematurity, stage 0

   H35.111   Retinopathy of prematurity, stage 0, right eye

   H35.112   Retinopathy of prematurity, stage 0, left eye

   H35.113   Retinopathy of prematurity, stage 0, bilateral

   H35.119   Retinopathy of prematurity, stage 0, unspecified eye

● H35.12   Retinopathy of prematurity, stage 1

   H35.121   Retinopathy of prematurity, stage 1, right eye

   H35.122   Retinopathy of prematurity, stage 1, left eye

   H35.123   Retinopathy of prematurity, stage 1, bilateral

   H35.129   Retinopathy of prematurity, stage 1, unspecified eye

● H35.13   Retinopathy of prematurity, stage 2

   H35.131   Retinopathy of prematurity, stage 2, right eye

   H35.132   Retinopathy of prematurity, stage 2, left eye

   H35.133   Retinopathy of prematurity, stage 2, bilateral

   H35.139   Retinopathy of prematurity, stage 2, unspecified eye

● H35.14   Retinopathy of prematurity, stage 3

   H35.141   Retinopathy of prematurity, stage 3, right eye

   H35.142   Retinopathy of prematurity, stage 3, left eye

   H35.143   Retinopathy of prematurity, stage 3, bilateral

   H35.149   Retinopathy of prematurity, stage 3, unspecified eye

● H35.15   Retinopathy of prematurity, stage 4

   H35.151   Retinopathy of prematurity, stage 4, right eye

   H35.152   Retinopathy of prematurity, stage 4, left eye

   H35.153   Retinopathy of prematurity, stage 4, bilateral

   H35.159   Retinopathy of prematurity, stage 4, unspecified eye

▶ New ➡ Revised ~~deleted~~ Deleted **OGCR** Official Guidelines X Assign placeholder X ● Use Additional Character(s)

Excludes 1 Excludes 2 Includes Use additional Code first Code also Key words

● H35.16 Retinopathy of prematurity, stage 5
    H35.161 Retinopathy of prematurity, stage 5, right eye
    H35.162 Retinopathy of prematurity, stage 5, left eye
    H35.163 Retinopathy of prematurity, stage 5, bilateral
    H35.169 Retinopathy of prematurity, stage 5, unspecified eye
● H35.17 Retrolental fibroplasia
    H35.171 Retrolental fibroplasia, right eye
    H35.172 Retrolental fibroplasia, left eye
    H35.173 Retrolental fibroplasia, bilateral
    H35.179 Retrolental fibroplasia, unspecified eye
● H35.2 Other non-diabetic proliferative retinopathy
    Proliferative vitreo-retinopathy

> **Excludes1** proliferative vitreo-retinopathy with retinal detachment (H33.4-)

    H35.20 Other non-diabetic proliferative retinopathy, unspecified eye
    H35.21 Other non-diabetic proliferative retinopathy, right eye
    H35.22 Other non-diabetic proliferative retinopathy, left eye
    H35.23 Other non-diabetic proliferative retinopathy, bilateral
● H35.3 Degeneration of macula and posterior pole
    H35.30 Unspecified macular degeneration
        Age-related macular degeneration
● H35.31 Nonexudative age-related macular degeneration
    Atrophic age-related macular degeneration
    Dry age-related macular degeneration
    One of the following 7th characters is to be assigned to codes in subcategory H35.31 to designate the stage of the disease:

Ø	stage unspecified
1	early dry stage
2	intermediate dry stage
3	advanced atrophic without subfoveal involvement
	advanced dry stage
4	advanced atrophic with subfoveal involvement

    ● H35.311 Nonexudative age-related macular degeneration, right eye
    ● H35.312 Nonexudative age-related macular degeneration, left eye
    ● H35.313 Nonexudative age-related macular degeneration, bilateral
    ● H35.319 Nonexudative age-related macular degeneration, unspecified eye

● H35.32 Exudative age-related macular degeneration
    Wet age-related macular degeneration
    One of the following 7th characters is to be assigned to codes in subcategory H35.32 to designate the stage of the disease:

Ø	stage unspecified
1	with active choroidal neovascularization
2	with inactive choroidal neovascularization
	with involuted or regressed neovascularization
3	with inactive scar

    ● H35.321 Exudative age-related macular degeneration, right eye
    ● H35.322 Exudative age-related macular degeneration, left eye
    ● H35.323 Exudative age-related macular degeneration, bilateral
    ● H35.329 Exudative age-related macular degeneration, unspecified eye
  H35.33 Angioid streaks of macula
● H35.34 Macular cyst, hole, or pseudohole
    H35.341 Macular cyst, hole, or pseudohole, right eye
    H35.342 Macular cyst, hole, or pseudohole, left eye
    H35.343 Macular cyst, hole, or pseudohole, bilateral
    H35.349 Macular cyst, hole, or pseudohole, unspecified eye
● H35.35 Cystoid macular degeneration

> **Excludes1** cystoid macular edema following cataract surgery (H59.03-)

    H35.351 Cystoid macular degeneration, right eye
    H35.352 Cystoid macular degeneration, left eye
    H35.353 Cystoid macular degeneration, bilateral
    H35.359 Cystoid macular degeneration, unspecified eye
● H35.36 Drusen (degenerative) of macula
    H35.361 Drusen (degenerative) of macula, right eye
    H35.362 Drusen (degenerative) of macula, left eye
    H35.363 Drusen (degenerative) of macula, bilateral
    H35.369 Drusen (degenerative) of macula, unspecified eye
● H35.37 Puckering of macula
    H35.371 Puckering of macula, right eye
    H35.372 Puckering of macula, left eye
    H35.373 Puckering of macula, bilateral
    H35.379 Puckering of macula, unspecified eye

CHAPTER 7 (HØØ-H59)

Item 7–7 Macular degeneration is typically age-related, chronic, and is evidenced by deterioration of the macula (the part of the retina that provides for central field vision), resulting in blurred vision or a blind spot in the center of visual field while not affecting peripheral vision.

▶ New ⇒ Revised ~~deleted~~ Deleted **OGCR** Official Guidelines X Assign placeholder X ● Use Additional Character(s)

| Excludes 1 | Excludes 2 | Includes | Use additional | Code first | Code also | Key words |

● **H35.38 Toxic maculopathy**

> *Code first poisoning due to drug or toxin, if applicable (T36-T65 with fifth or sixth character 1-4 or 6)*

Use additional code for adverse effect, if applicable, to identify drug (T36-T50 with fifth or sixth character 5)

H35.381 Toxic maculopathy, right eye

H35.382 Toxic maculopathy, left eye

H35.383 Toxic maculopathy, bilateral

H35.389 Toxic maculopathy, unspecified eye

● **H35.4 Peripheral retinal degeneration**

Excludes1   hereditary retinal degeneration (dystrophy) (H35.5-)

peripheral retinal degeneration with retinal break (H33.3-)

H35.40 Unspecified peripheral retinal degeneration

● **H35.41 Lattice degeneration of retina**

Palisade degeneration of retina

H35.411 Lattice degeneration of retina, right eye

H35.412 Lattice degeneration of retina, left eye

H35.413 Lattice degeneration of retina, bilateral

H35.419 Lattice degeneration of retina, unspecified eye

● **H35.42 Microcystoid degeneration of retina**

H35.421 Microcystoid degeneration of retina, right eye

H35.422 Microcystoid degeneration of retina, left eye

H35.423 Microcystoid degeneration of retina, bilateral

H35.429 Microcystoid degeneration of retina, unspecified eye

● **H35.43 Paving stone degeneration of retina**

H35.431 Paving stone degeneration of retina, right eye

H35.432 Paving stone degeneration of retina, left eye

H35.433 Paving stone degeneration of retina, bilateral

H35.439 Paving stone degeneration of retina, unspecified eye

● **H35.44 Age-related reticular degeneration of retina**

H35.441 Age-related reticular degeneration of retina, right eye

H35.442 Age-related reticular degeneration of retina, left eye

H35.443 Age-related reticular degeneration of retina, bilateral

H35.449 Age-related reticular degeneration of retina, unspecified eye

● **H35.45 Secondary pigmentary degeneration**

H35.451 Secondary pigmentary degeneration, right eye

H35.452 Secondary pigmentary degeneration, left eye

H35.453 Secondary pigmentary degeneration, bilateral

H35.459 Secondary pigmentary degeneration, unspecified eye

● **H35.46 Secondary vitreoretinal degeneration**

H35.461 Secondary vitreoretinal degeneration, right eye

H35.462 Secondary vitreoretinal degeneration, left eye

H35.463 Secondary vitreoretinal degeneration, bilateral

H35.469 Secondary vitreoretinal degeneration, unspecified eye

● **H35.5 Hereditary retinal dystrophy**

Excludes1   dystrophies primarily involving Bruch's membrane (H31.1-)

H35.50 Unspecified hereditary retinal dystrophy

H35.51 Vitreoretinal dystrophy

H35.52 Pigmentary retinal dystrophy

Albipunctate retinal dystrophy

Retinitis pigmentosa

Tapetoretinal dystrophy

H35.53 Other dystrophies primarily involving the sensory retina

Stargardt's disease

H35.54 Dystrophies primarily involving the retinal pigment epithelium

Vitelliform retinal dystrophy

● **H35.6 Retinal hemorrhage**

H35.60 Retinal hemorrhage, unspecified eye

H35.61 Retinal hemorrhage, right eye

H35.62 Retinal hemorrhage, left eye

H35.63 Retinal hemorrhage, bilateral

● **H35.7 Separation of retinal layers**

Excludes1   retinal detachment (serous) (H33.2-)

rhegmatogenous retinal detachment (H33.0-)

H35.70 Unspecified separation of retinal layers

● **H35.71 Central serous chorioretinopathy**

H35.711 Central serous chorioretinopathy, right eye

H35.712 Central serous chorioretinopathy, left eye

H35.713 Central serous chorioretinopathy, bilateral

H35.719 Central serous chorioretinopathy, unspecified eye

● **H35.72 Serous detachment of retinal pigment epithelium**

H35.721 Serous detachment of retinal pigment epithelium, right eye

H35.722 Serous detachment of retinal pigment epithelium, left eye

H35.723 Serous detachment of retinal pigment epithelium, bilateral

H35.729 Serous detachment of retinal pigment epithelium, unspecified eye

● **H35.73 Hemorrhagic detachment of retinal pigment epithelium**

H35.731 Hemorrhagic detachment of retinal pigment epithelium, right eye

H35.732 Hemorrhagic detachment of retinal pigment epithelium, left eye

H35.733 Hemorrhagic detachment of retinal pigment epithelium, bilateral

H35.739 Hemorrhagic detachment of retinal pigment epithelium, unspecified eye

▶ New   ⇒ Revised   ~~deleted~~ Deleted   **OGCR** Official Guidelines   X Assign placeholder X   ● Use Additional Character(s)

Excludes 1   Excludes 2   Includes   Use additional   Code first   Code also   Key words

● H35.8　Other specified retinal disorders
　　　　| Excludes2 | retinal hemorrhage (H35.6-)
　　H35.81　Retinal edema
　　　　　　Retinal cotton wool spots
　　H35.82　Retinal ischemia
　　H35.89　Other specified retinal disorders
　H35.9　Unspecified retinal disorder

H36　Retinal disorders in diseases classified elsewhere
　　　Code first underlying disease, such as:
　　　　lipid storage disorders (E75.-)
　　　　sickle-cell disorders (D57.-)
　　　| Excludes1 | arteriosclerotic retinopathy (H35.0-)
　　　　　　diabetic retinopathy (E08.3-, E09.3-, E10.3-,
　　　　　　　E11.3-, E13.3-)

GLAUCOMA (H40-H42)

● H40　Glaucoma
　　　Intraocular pressure (IOP) that is too high results from too much
　　　aqueous humor and because of excess production or inadequate
　　　drainage, optic nerve damage and vision loss may occur.
　　　| Excludes1 | absolute glaucoma (H44.51-)
　　　　　　congenital glaucoma (Q15.0)
　　　　　　traumatic glaucoma due to birth injury (P15.3)
　● H40.0　Glaucoma suspect
　　● H40.00　Preglaucoma, unspecified
　　　　H40.001　Preglaucoma, unspecified, right eye
　　　　H40.002　Preglaucoma, unspecified, left eye
　　　　H40.003　Preglaucoma, unspecified, bilateral
　　　　H40.009　Preglaucoma, unspecified, unspecified eye
　　● H40.01　Open angle with borderline findings, low risk
　　　　　　Open angle, low risk
　　　　H40.011　Open angle with borderline findings, low risk, right eye
　　　　H40.012　Open angle with borderline findings, low risk, left eye
　　　　H40.013　Open angle with borderline findings, low risk, bilateral
　　　　H40.019　Open angle with borderline findings, low risk, unspecified eye
　　● H40.02　Open angle with borderline findings, high risk
　　　　　　Open angle, high risk
　　　　H40.021　Open angle with borderline findings, high risk, right eye
　　　　H40.022　Open angle with borderline findings, high risk, left eye
　　　　H40.023　Open angle with borderline findings, high risk, bilateral
　　　　H40.029　Open angle with borderline findings, high risk, unspecified eye
　　● H40.03　Anatomical narrow angle
　　　　　　Primary angle closure suspect
　　　　H40.031　Anatomical narrow angle, right eye
　　　　H40.032　Anatomical narrow angle, left eye
　　　　H40.033　Anatomical narrow angle, bilateral
　　　　H40.039　Anatomical narrow angle, unspecified eye
　　● H40.04　Steroid responder
　　　　H40.041　Steroid responder, right eye
　　　　H40.042　Steroid responder, left eye
　　　　H40.043　Steroid responder, bilateral
　　　　H40.049　Steroid responder, unspecified eye

● H40.05　Ocular hypertension
　　H40.051　Ocular hypertension, right eye
　　H40.052　Ocular hypertension, left eye
　　H40.053　Ocular hypertension, bilateral
　　H40.059　Ocular hypertension, unspecified eye
● H40.06　Primary angle closure without glaucoma damage
　　H40.061　Primary angle closure without glaucoma damage, right eye
　　H40.062　Primary angle closure without glaucoma damage, left eye
　　H40.063　Primary angle closure without glaucoma damage, bilateral
　　H40.069　Primary angle closure without glaucoma damage, unspecified eye
● H40.1　Open-angle glaucoma
　X ● H40.10　Unspecified open-angle glaucoma
　　　　One of the following 7th characters is to be assigned to code H40.10 to designate the stage of glaucoma

0	stage unspecified
1	mild stage
2	moderate stage
3	severe stage
4	indeterminate stage

　● H40.11　Primary open-angle glaucoma
　　　　Chronic simple glaucoma
　　　　One of the following 7th characters is to be assigned to each code in subcategory H40.11 to designate the stage of glaucoma

0	stage unspecified
1	mild stage
2	moderate stage
3	severe stage
4	indeterminate stage

　　● H40.111　Primary open-angle glaucoma, right eye
　　● H40.112　Primary open-angle glaucoma, left eye
　　● H40.113　Primary open-angle glaucoma, bilateral
　　● H40.119　Primary open-angle glaucoma, unspecified eye
　● H40.12　Low-tension glaucoma
　　　　One of the following 7th characters is to be assigned to each code in subcategory H40.12 to designate the stage of glaucoma

0	stage unspecified
1	mild stage
2	moderate stage
3	severe stage
4	indeterminate stage

　　● H40.121　Low-tension glaucoma, right eye
　　● H40.122　Low-tension glaucoma, left eye
　　● H40.123　Low-tension glaucoma, bilateral
　　● H40.129　Low-tension glaucoma, unspecified eye

CHAPTER 7 (H00-H59)

● **H40.13**   **Pigmentary** glaucoma

One of the following 7th characters is to be assigned to each code in subcategory H40.13 to designate the stage of glaucoma

Ø	stage unspecified
1	mild stage
2	moderate stage
3	severe stage
4	indeterminate stage

  ● **H40.131**   Pigmentary glaucoma, **right** eye
  ● **H40.132**   Pigmentary glaucoma, **left** eye
  ● **H40.133**   Pigmentary glaucoma, **bilateral**
  ● **H40.139**   Pigmentary glaucoma, **unspecified** eye

● **H40.14**   **Capsular** glaucoma **with pseudoexfoliation** of lens

One of the following 7th characters is to be assigned to each code in subcategory H40.14 to designate the stage of glaucoma

Ø	stage unspecified
1	mild stage
2	moderate stage
3	severe stage
4	indeterminate stage

  ● **H40.141**   Capsular glaucoma with pseudoexfoliation of lens, **right** eye
  ● **H40.142**   Capsular glaucoma with pseudoexfoliation of lens, **left** eye
  ● **H40.143**   Capsular glaucoma with pseudoexfoliation of lens, **bilateral**
  ● **H40.149**   Capsular glaucoma with pseudoexfoliation of lens, **unspecified** eye

● **H40.15**   **Residual stage** of open-angle glaucoma
  H40.151   Residual stage of open-angle glaucoma, **right** eye
  H40.152   Residual stage of open-angle glaucoma, **left** eye
  H40.153   Residual stage of open-angle glaucoma, **bilateral**
  H40.159   Residual stage of open-angle glaucoma, **unspecified** eye

● **H40.2**   **Primary** angle-closure glaucoma
  Excludes1   aqueous misdirection (H40.83-)
              malignant glaucoma (H40.83-)

X ● **H40.20**   **Unspecified** primary angle-closure glaucoma

One of the following 7th characters is to be assigned to code H40.20 to designate the stage of glaucoma

Ø	stage unspecified
1	mild stage
2	moderate stage
3	severe stage
4	indeterminate stage

● **H40.21**   **Acute** angle-closure glaucoma
Acute angle-closure glaucoma attack
Acute angle-closure glaucoma crisis
  H40.211   Acute angle-closure glaucoma, **right** eye
  H40.212   Acute angle-closure glaucoma, **left** eye
  H40.213   Acute angle-closure glaucoma, **bilateral**
  H40.219   Acute angle-closure glaucoma, **unspecified** eye

● **H40.22**   **Chronic** angle-closure glaucoma
Chronic primary angle closure glaucoma

One of the following 7th characters is to be assigned to each code in subcategory H40.22 to designate the stage of glaucoma

Ø	stage unspecified
1	mild stage
2	moderate stage
3	severe stage
4	indeterminate stage

  ● **H40.221**   Chronic angle-closure glaucoma, **right** eye
  ● **H40.222**   Chronic angle-closure glaucoma, **left** eye
  ● **H40.223**   Chronic angle-closure glaucoma, **bilateral**
  ● **H40.229**   Chronic angle-closure glaucoma, **unspecified** eye

● **H40.23**   **Intermittent** angle-closure glaucoma
  H40.231   Intermittent angle-closure glaucoma, **right** eye
  H40.232   Intermittent angle-closure glaucoma, **left** eye
  H40.233   Intermittent angle-closure glaucoma, **bilateral**
  H40.239   Intermittent angle-closure glaucoma, **unspecified** eye

● **H40.24**   **Residual stage** of angle-closure glaucoma
  H40.241   Residual stage of angle-closure glaucoma, **right** eye
  H40.242   Residual stage of angle-closure glaucoma, **left** eye
  H40.243   Residual stage of angle-closure glaucoma, **bilateral**
  H40.249   Residual stage of angle-closure glaucoma, **unspecified** eye

● **H40.3**   Glaucoma **secondary** to eye **trauma**
Code also underlying condition

One of the following 7th characters is to be assigned to each code in subcategory H40.3 to designate the stage of glaucoma

Ø	stage unspecified
1	mild stage
2	moderate stage
3	severe stage
4	indeterminate stage

X ● **H40.30**   Glaucoma secondary to eye trauma, **unspecified** eye
X ● **H40.31**   Glaucoma secondary to eye trauma, **right** eye
X ● **H40.32**   Glaucoma secondary to eye trauma, **left** eye
X ● **H40.33**   Glaucoma secondary to eye trauma, **bilateral**

► New   ⇒ Revised   ~~deleted~~ Deleted   **OGCR** Official Guidelines   X Assign placeholder X   ● Use Additional Character(s)

Excludes 1   Excludes 2   Includes   Use additional   Code first   Code also   Key words

CHAPTER 7 (H00-H59)

● **H40.4**   Glaucoma secondary to eye inflammation

     Code also underlying condition

     One of the following 7th characters is to be assigned to each code in subcategory H40.4 to designate the stage of glaucoma

0	stage unspecified
1	mild stage
2	moderate stage
3	severe stage
4	indeterminate stage

   X● **H40.40**   Glaucoma secondary to eye inflammation, unspecified eye

   X● **H40.41**   Glaucoma secondary to eye inflammation, right eye

   X● **H40.42**   Glaucoma secondary to eye inflammation, left eye

   X● **H40.43**   Glaucoma secondary to eye inflammation, bilateral

● **H40.5**   Glaucoma secondary to other eye disorders

     Code also underlying eye disorder

     One of the following 7th characters is to be assigned to each code in subcategory H40.5 to designate the stage of glaucoma

0	stage unspecified
1	mild stage
2	moderate stage
3	severe stage
4	indeterminate stage

   X● **H40.50**   Glaucoma secondary to other eye disorders, unspecified eye

   X● **H40.51**   Glaucoma secondary to other eye disorders, right eye

   X● **H40.52**   Glaucoma secondary to other eye disorders, left eye

   X● **H40.53**   Glaucoma secondary to other eye disorders, bilateral

● **H40.6**   Glaucoma secondary to drugs

     Use additional code for adverse effect, if applicable, to identify drug (T36-T50 with fifth or sixth character 5)

     One of the following 7th characters is to be assigned to each code in subcategory H40.6 to designate the stage of glaucoma

0	stage unspecified
1	mild stage
2	moderate stage
3	severe stage
4	indeterminate stage

   X● **H40.60**   Glaucoma secondary to drugs, unspecified eye

   X● **H40.61**   Glaucoma secondary to drugs, right eye

   X● **H40.62**   Glaucoma secondary to drugs, left eye

   X● **H40.63**   Glaucoma secondary to drugs, bilateral

● **H40.8**   Other glaucoma

   ● **H40.81**   Glaucoma with increased episcleral venous pressure

       H40.811   Glaucoma with increased episcleral venous pressure, right eye

       H40.812   Glaucoma with increased episcleral venous pressure, left eye

       H40.813   Glaucoma with increased episcleral venous pressure, bilateral

       H40.819   Glaucoma with increased episcleral venous pressure, unspecified eye

● **H40.82**   Hypersecretion glaucoma

       H40.821   Hypersecretion glaucoma, right eye

       H40.822   Hypersecretion glaucoma, left eye

       H40.823   Hypersecretion glaucoma, bilateral

       H40.829   Hypersecretion glaucoma, unspecified eye

● **H40.83**   Aqueous misdirection

     Malignant glaucoma

       H40.831   Aqueous misdirection, right eye

       H40.832   Aqueous misdirection, left eye

       H40.833   Aqueous misdirection, bilateral

       H40.839   Aqueous misdirection, unspecified eye

   H40.89   Other specified glaucoma

  H40.9   Unspecified glaucoma

  H42   Glaucoma in diseases classified elsewhere

     Code first underlying condition, such as:

       amyloidosis (E85.-)

       aniridia (Q13.1)

     ▶ glaucoma (in) diabetes mellitus (E08.39, E09.39, E10.39, E11.39, E13.39)

       Lowe's syndrome (E72.03)

       Reiger's anomaly (Q13.81)

       specified metabolic disorder (E70-E88)

     | **Excludes1** | glaucoma (in) onchocerciasis (B73.02)

                   glaucoma (in) syphilis (A52.71)

                   glaucoma (in) tuberculous (A18.59)

     | ~~Excludes2~~ | ~~glaucoma (in) diabetes mellitus (E08.39, E09.39, E10.39, E11.39, E13.39)~~

DISORDERS OF VITREOUS BODY AND GLOBE (H43-H44)

● **H43**   Disorders of vitreous body

   ● **H43.0**   Vitreous prolapse

     | **Excludes1** | vitreous syndrome following cataract surgery (H59.0-)

                   traumatic vitreous prolapse (S05.2-)

       H43.00   Vitreous prolapse, unspecified eye

       H43.01   Vitreous prolapse, right eye

       H43.02   Vitreous prolapse, left eye

       H43.03   Vitreous prolapse, bilateral

   ● **H43.1**   Vitreous hemorrhage

       H43.10   Vitreous hemorrhage, unspecified eye

       H43.11   Vitreous hemorrhage, right eye

       H43.12   Vitreous hemorrhage, left eye

       H43.13   Vitreous hemorrhage, bilateral

   ● **H43.2**   Crystalline deposits in vitreous body

       H43.20   Crystalline deposits in vitreous body, unspecified eye

       H43.21   Crystalline deposits in vitreous body, right eye

       H43.22   Crystalline deposits in vitreous body, left eye

       H43.23   Crystalline deposits in vitreous body, bilateral

   ● **H43.3**   Other vitreous opacities

     ● **H43.31**   Vitreous membranes and strands

       H43.311   Vitreous membranes and strands, right eye

       H43.312   Vitreous membranes and strands, left eye

       H43.313   Vitreous membranes and strands, bilateral

       H43.319   Vitreous membranes and strands, unspecified eye

---

CHAPTER 7 (H00-H59)

● H43.39   Other vitreous opacities
     Vitreous floaters
     Small clumps of cells that float in the vitreous of the eye, appearing as black specks or dots in the field of vision and common in the aging eye.

     H43.391   Other vitreous opacities, right eye
     H43.392   Other vitreous opacities, left eye
     H43.393   Other vitreous opacities, bilateral
     H43.399   Other vitreous opacities, unspecified eye

● H43.8   Other disorders of vitreous body
     Excludes1   proliferative vitreo-retinopathy with retinal detachment (H33.4)
     Excludes2   vitreous abscess (H44.02-)

   ● H43.81   Vitreous degeneration
     Vitreous detachment
     H43.811   Vitreous degeneration, right eye
     H43.812   Vitreous degeneration, left eye
     H43.813   Vitreous degeneration, bilateral
     H43.819   Vitreous degeneration, unspecified eye

   ● H43.82   Vitreomacular adhesion
     Vitreomacular traction
     H43.821   Vitreomacular adhesion, right eye
     H43.822   Vitreomacular adhesion, left eye
     H43.823   Vitreomacular adhesion, bilateral
     H43.829   Vitreomacular adhesion, unspecified eye

   H43.89   Other disorders of vitreous body
   H43.9   Unspecified disorder of vitreous body

● H44   Disorders of globe
     Includes   disorders affecting multiple structures of eye

   ● H44.0   Purulent endophthalmitis
     Use additional code to identify organism
     Excludes1   bleb associated endophthalmitis (H59.4-)

   ● H44.00   Unspecified purulent endophthalmitis
     H44.001   Unspecified purulent endophthalmitis, right eye
     H44.002   Unspecified purulent endophthalmitis, left eye
     H44.003   Unspecified purulent endophthalmitis, bilateral
     H44.009   Unspecified purulent endophthalmitis, unspecified eye

   ● H44.01   Panophthalmitis (acute)
     H44.011   Panophthalmitis (acute), right eye
     H44.012   Panophthalmitis (acute), left eye
     H44.013   Panophthalmitis (acute), bilateral
     H44.019   Panophthalmitis (acute), unspecified eye

   ● H44.02   Vitreous abscess (chronic)
     H44.021   Vitreous abscess (chronic), right eye
     H44.022   Vitreous abscess (chronic), left eye
     H44.023   Vitreous abscess (chronic), bilateral
     H44.029   Vitreous abscess (chronic), unspecified eye

● H44.1   Other endophthalmitis
     Excludes1   bleb associated endophthalmitis (H59.4-)
     Excludes2   ophthalmia nodosa (H16.2-)

   ● H44.11   Panuveitis
     H44.111   Panuveitis, right eye
     H44.112   Panuveitis, left eye
     H44.113   Panuveitis, bilateral
     H44.119   Panuveitis, unspecified eye

   ● H44.12   Parasitic endophthalmitis, unspecified
     H44.121   Parasitic endophthalmitis, unspecified, right eye
     H44.122   Parasitic endophthalmitis, unspecified, left eye
     H44.123   Parasitic endophthalmitis, unspecified, bilateral
     H44.129   Parasitic endophthalmitis, unspecified, unspecified eye

   ● H44.13   Sympathetic uveitis
     H44.131   Sympathetic uveitis, right eye
     H44.132   Sympathetic uveitis, left eye
     H44.133   Sympathetic uveitis, bilateral
     H44.139   Sympathetic uveitis, unspecified eye

   H44.19   Other endophthalmitis

● H44.2   Degenerative myopia
     Malignant myopia
     H44.20   Degenerative myopia, unspecified eye
     H44.21   Degenerative myopia, right eye
     H44.22   Degenerative myopia, left eye
     H44.23   Degenerative myopia, bilateral

   ▶● H44.2A   Degenerative myopia with choroidal neovascularization
     ▶ Use Additional code for any associated choroid disorders (H31.-)
     ▶ H44.2A1   Degenerative myopia with choroidal neovascularization, right eye
     ▶ H44.2A2   Degenerative myopia with choroidal neovascularization, left eye
     ▶ H44.2A3   Degenerative myopia with choroidal neovascularization, bilateral eye
     ▶ H44.2A9   Degenerative myopia with choroidal neovascularization, unspecified eye

   ▶● H44.2B   Degenerative myopia with macular hole
     ▶ H44.2B1   Degenerative myopia with macular hole, right eye
     ▶ H44.2B2   Degenerative myopia with macular hole, left eye
     ▶ H44.2B3   Degenerative myopia with macular hole, bilateral eye
     ▶ H44.2B9   Degenerative myopia with macular hole, unspecified eye

   ▶● H44.2C   Degenerative myopia with retinal detachment
     ▶ Use Additional code to identify the retinal detachment (H33.-)
     ▶ H44.2C1   Degenerative myopia with retinal detachment, right eye
     H44.2C2   Degenerative myopia with retinal detachment, left eye
     ▶ H44.2C3   Degenerative myopia with retinal detachment, bilateral eye
     ▶ H44.2C9   Degenerative myopia with retinal detachment, unspecified eye

▶ New   ⇒ Revised   ~~deleted~~ Deleted   **OGCR** Official Guidelines   X Assign placeholder X   ● Use Additional Character(s)

Excludes 1   Excludes 2   Includes   Use additional   Code first   Code also   Key words

▶●H44.2D Degenerative myopia with foveoschisis
    ▶ H44.2D1 Degenerative myopia with foveoschisis, right eye
    ▶ H44.2D2 Degenerative myopia with foveoschisis, left eye
    ▶ H44.2D3 Degenerative myopia with foveoschisis, bilateral eye
    ▶ H44.2D9 Degenerative myopia with foveoschisis, unspecified eye
▶●H44.2E Degenerative myopia with other maculopathy
    ▶ H44.2E1 Degenerative myopia with other maculopathy, right eye
    ▶ H44.2E2 Degenerative myopia with other maculopathy, left eye
    ▶ H44.2E3 Degenerative myopia with other maculopathy, bilateral eye
    ▶ H44.2E9 Degenerative myopia with other maculopathy, unspecified eye
●H44.3 Other and unspecified degenerative disorders of globe
    H44.30 Unspecified degenerative disorder of globe
    ●H44.31 Chalcosis
        H44.311 Chalcosis, right eye
        H44.312 Chalcosis, left eye
        H44.313 Chalcosis, bilateral
        H44.319 Chalcosis, unspecified eye
    ●H44.32 Siderosis of eye
        H44.321 Siderosis of eye, right eye
        H44.322 Siderosis of eye, left eye
        H44.323 Siderosis of eye, bilateral
        H44.329 Siderosis of eye, unspecified eye
    ●H44.39 Other degenerative disorders of globe
        H44.391 Other degenerative disorders of globe, right eye
        H44.392 Other degenerative disorders of globe, left eye
        H44.393 Other degenerative disorders of globe, bilateral
        H44.399 Other degenerative disorders of globe, unspecified eye
●H44.4 Hypotony of eye
    H44.40 Unspecified hypotony of eye
    ●H44.41 Flat anterior chamber hypotony of eye
        H44.411 Flat anterior chamber hypotony of right eye
        H44.412 Flat anterior chamber hypotony of left eye
        H44.413 Flat anterior chamber hypotony of eye, bilateral
        H44.419 Flat anterior chamber hypotony of unspecified eye
    ●H44.42 Hypotony of eye due to ocular fistula
        H44.421 Hypotony of right eye due to ocular fistula
        H44.422 Hypotony of left eye due to ocular fistula
        H44.423 Hypotony of eye due to ocular fistula, bilateral
        H44.429 Hypotony of unspecified eye due to ocular fistula
    ●H44.43 Hypotony of eye due to other ocular disorders
        H44.431 Hypotony of eye due to other ocular disorders, right eye
        H44.432 Hypotony of eye due to other ocular disorders, left eye
        H44.433 Hypotony of eye due to other ocular disorders, bilateral
        H44.439 Hypotony of eye due to other ocular disorders, unspecified eye

●H44.44 Primary hypotony of eye
    H44.441 Primary hypotony of right eye
    H44.442 Primary hypotony of left eye
    H44.443 Primary hypotony of eye, bilateral
    H44.449 Primary hypotony of unspecified eye
●H44.5 Degenerated conditions of globe
    H44.50 Unspecified degenerated conditions of globe
    ●H44.51 Absolute glaucoma
        H44.511 Absolute glaucoma, right eye
        H44.512 Absolute glaucoma, left eye
        H44.513 Absolute glaucoma, bilateral
        H44.519 Absolute glaucoma, unspecified eye
    ●H44.52 Atrophy of globe
        Phthisis bulbi
        H44.521 Atrophy of globe, right eye
        H44.522 Atrophy of globe, left eye
        H44.523 Atrophy of globe, bilateral
        H44.529 Atrophy of globe, unspecified eye
    ●H44.53 Leucocoria
        H44.531 Leucocoria, right eye
        H44.532 Leucocoria, left eye
        H44.533 Leucocoria, bilateral
        H44.539 Leucocoria, unspecified eye
●H44.6 Retained (old) intraocular foreign body, magnetic

    Use additional code to identify magnetic foreign body (Z18.11)

> **Excludes1** current intraocular foreign body (S05.-)
>
> **Excludes2** retained foreign body in eyelid (H02.81-)
> retained (old) foreign body following penetrating wound of orbit (H05.5-)
> retained (old) intraocular foreign body, nonmagnetic (H44.7-)

    ●H44.60 Unspecified retained (old) intraocular foreign body, magnetic
        H44.601 Unspecified retained (old) intraocular foreign body, magnetic, right eye
        H44.602 Unspecified retained (old) intraocular foreign body, magnetic, left eye
        H44.603 Unspecified retained (old) intraocular foreign body, magnetic, bilateral
        H44.609 Unspecified retained (old) intraocular foreign body, magnetic, unspecified eye
    ●H44.61 Retained (old) magnetic foreign body in anterior chamber
        H44.611 Retained (old) magnetic foreign body in anterior chamber, right eye
        H44.612 Retained (old) magnetic foreign body in anterior chamber, left eye
        H44.613 Retained (old) magnetic foreign body in anterior chamber, bilateral
        H44.619 Retained (old) magnetic foreign body in anterior chamber, unspecified eye
    ●H44.62 Retained (old) magnetic foreign body in iris or ciliary body
        H44.621 Retained (old) magnetic foreign body in iris or ciliary body, right eye
        H44.622 Retained (old) magnetic foreign body in iris or ciliary body, left eye
        H44.623 Retained (old) magnetic foreign body in iris or ciliary body, bilateral
        H44.629 Retained (old) magnetic foreign body in iris or ciliary body, unspecified eye

● H44.63   Retained (old) magnetic foreign body in lens

     H44.631   Retained (old) magnetic foreign body in lens, right eye

     H44.632   Retained (old) magnetic foreign body in lens, left eye

     H44.633   Retained (old) magnetic foreign body in lens, bilateral

     H44.639   Retained (old) magnetic foreign body in lens, unspecified eye

● H44.64   Retained (old) magnetic foreign body in posterior wall of globe

     H44.641   Retained (old) magnetic foreign body in posterior wall of globe, right eye

     H44.642   Retained (old) magnetic foreign body in posterior wall of globe, left eye

     H44.643   Retained (old) magnetic foreign body in posterior wall of globe, bilateral

     H44.649   Retained (old) magnetic foreign body in posterior wall of globe, unspecified eye

● H44.65   Retained (old) magnetic foreign body in vitreous body

     H44.651   Retained (old) magnetic foreign body in vitreous body, right eye

     H44.652   Retained (old) magnetic foreign body in vitreous body, left eye

     H44.653   Retained (old) magnetic foreign body in vitreous body, bilateral

     H44.659   Retained (old) magnetic foreign body in vitreous body, unspecified eye

● H44.69   Retained (old) intraocular foreign body, magnetic, in other or multiple sites

     H44.691   Retained (old) intraocular foreign body, magnetic, in other or multiple sites, right eye

     H44.692   Retained (old) intraocular foreign body, magnetic, in other or multiple sites, left eye

     H44.693   Retained (old) intraocular foreign body, magnetic, in other or multiple sites, bilateral

     H44.699   Retained (old) intraocular foreign body, magnetic, in other or multiple sites, unspecified eye

● H44.7   Retained (old) intraocular foreign body, nonmagnetic

Use additional code to identify nonmagnetic foreign body (Z18.01-Z18.10, Z18.12, Z18.2-Z18.9)

> **Excludes1**   current intraocular foreign body (S05.-)
>
> **Excludes2**   retained foreign body in eyelid (H02.81-)
> retained (old) foreign body following penetrating wound of orbit (H05.5-)
> retained (old) intraocular foreign body, magnetic (H44.6-)

● H44.70   Unspecified retained (old) intraocular foreign body, nonmagnetic

     H44.701   Unspecified retained (old) intraocular foreign body, nonmagnetic, right eye

     H44.702   Unspecified retained (old) intraocular foreign body, nonmagnetic, left eye

     H44.703   Unspecified retained (old) intraocular foreign body, nonmagnetic, bilateral

     H44.709   Unspecified retained (old) intraocular foreign body, nonmagnetic, unspecified eye

           Retained (old) intraocular foreign body NOS

● H44.71   Retained (nonmagnetic) (old) foreign body in anterior chamber

     H44.711   Retained (nonmagnetic) (old) foreign body in anterior chamber, right eye

     H44.712   Retained (nonmagnetic) (old) foreign body in anterior chamber, left eye

     H44.713   Retained (nonmagnetic) (old) foreign body in anterior chamber, bilateral

     H44.719   Retained (nonmagnetic) (old) foreign body in anterior chamber, unspecified eye

● H44.72   Retained (nonmagnetic) (old) foreign body in iris or ciliary body

     H44.721   Retained (nonmagnetic) (old) foreign body in iris or ciliary body, right eye

     H44.722   Retained (nonmagnetic) (old) foreign body in iris or ciliary body, left eye

     H44.723   Retained (nonmagnetic) (old) foreign body in iris or ciliary body, bilateral

     H44.729   Retained (nonmagnetic) (old) foreign body in iris or ciliary body, unspecified eye

● H44.73   Retained (nonmagnetic) (old) foreign body in lens

     H44.731   Retained (nonmagnetic) (old) foreign body in lens, right eye

     H44.732   Retained (nonmagnetic) (old) foreign body in lens, left eye

     H44.733   Retained (nonmagnetic) (old) foreign body in lens, bilateral

     H44.739   Retained (nonmagnetic) (old) foreign body in lens, unspecified eye

● H44.74   Retained (nonmagnetic) (old) foreign body in posterior wall of globe

     H44.741   Retained (nonmagnetic) (old) foreign body in posterior wall of globe, right eye

     H44.742   Retained (nonmagnetic) (old) foreign body in posterior wall of globe, left eye

     H44.743   Retained (nonmagnetic) (old) foreign body in posterior wall of globe, bilateral

     H44.749   Retained (nonmagnetic) (old) foreign body in posterior wall of globe, unspecified eye

● H44.75   Retained (nonmagnetic) (old) foreign body in vitreous body

     H44.751   Retained (nonmagnetic) (old) foreign body in vitreous body, right eye

     H44.752   Retained (nonmagnetic) (old) foreign body in vitreous body, left eye

     H44.753   Retained (nonmagnetic) (old) foreign body in vitreous body, bilateral

     H44.759   Retained (nonmagnetic) (old) foreign body in vitreous body, unspecified eye

● H44.79   Retained (old) intraocular foreign body, nonmagnetic, in other or multiple sites

     H44.791   Retained (old) intraocular foreign body, nonmagnetic, in other or multiple sites, right eye

     H44.792   Retained (old) intraocular foreign body, nonmagnetic, in other or multiple sites, left eye

     H44.793   Retained (old) intraocular foreign body, nonmagnetic, in other or multiple sites, bilateral

     H44.799   Retained (old) intraocular foreign body, nonmagnetic, in other or multiple sites, unspecified eye

▶ New   ⇒ Revised   ~~deleted~~ Deleted   **OGCR** Official Guidelines   X Assign placeholder X   ● Use Additional Character(s)

Excludes 1   Excludes 2   Includes   Use additional   Code first   Code also   Key words

● **H44.8**   Other disorders of globe
    ● **H44.81**   Hemophthalmos
       H44.811   Hemophthalmos, right eye
       H44.812   Hemophthalmos, left eye
       H44.813   Hemophthalmos, bilateral
       H44.819   Hemophthalmos, unspecified eye
    ● **H44.82**   Luxation of globe
       H44.821   Luxation of globe, right eye
       H44.822   Luxation of globe, left eye
       H44.823   Luxation of globe, bilateral
       H44.829   Luxation of globe, unspecified eye
    H44.89   Other disorders of globe
  H44.9   Unspecified disorder of globe

★ **(See Plate 86 on page 55.)**

DISORDERS OF OPTIC NERVE AND VISUAL PATHWAYS (H46-H47)

● **H46**   Optic neuritis
    Excludes2   ischemic optic neuropathy (H47.01-)
              neuromyelitis optica [Devic] (G36.0)
    ● **H46.0**   Optic papillitis
       H46.00   Optic papillitis, unspecified eye
       H46.01   Optic papillitis, right eye
       H46.02   Optic papillitis, left eye
       H46.03   Optic papillitis, bilateral
    ● **H46.1**   Retrobulbar neuritis
       Retrobulbar neuritis NOS
       Excludes1   syphilitic retrobulbar neuritis (A52.15)
       H46.10   Retrobulbar neuritis, unspecified eye
       H46.11   Retrobulbar neuritis, right eye
       H46.12   Retrobulbar neuritis, left eye
       H46.13   Retrobulbar neuritis, bilateral
    H46.2   Nutritional optic neuropathy
    H46.3   Toxic optic neuropathy
       Code first (T51-T65) to identify cause
    H46.8   Other optic neuritis
    H46.9   Unspecified optic neuritis

● **H47**   Other disorders of optic [2nd] nerve and visual pathways
    ● **H47.0**   Disorders of optic nerve, not elsewhere classified
       ● **H47.01**   Ischemic optic neuropathy
          H47.011   Ischemic optic neuropathy, right eye
          H47.012   Ischemic optic neuropathy, left eye
          H47.013   Ischemic optic neuropathy, bilateral
          H47.019   Ischemic optic neuropathy, unspecified eye
       ● **H47.02**   Hemorrhage in optic nerve sheath
          H47.021   Hemorrhage in optic nerve sheath, right eye
          H47.022   Hemorrhage in optic nerve sheath, left eye
          H47.023   Hemorrhage in optic nerve sheath, bilateral
          H47.029   Hemorrhage in optic nerve sheath, unspecified eye
       ● **H47.03**   Optic nerve hypoplasia
          H47.031   Optic nerve hypoplasia, right eye
          H47.032   Optic nerve hypoplasia, left eye
          H47.033   Optic nerve hypoplasia, bilateral
          H47.039   Optic nerve hypoplasia, unspecified eye

Figure 7-11   Stages of papilledema according to the Frisén grading scale. **A,** Very eary papilledema (Frisén stage 1). **B,** Early papilledema (Frisén stage 2). **C,** Moderate papilledema (Frisén stage 3). **D,** Marked papilledema (Frisén stage 4). **E,** Severe papilledema. (From Youmans JR, Winn HR: Youmans Neurological Surgery, Philadelphia, PA, Elsevier/Saunders, 2011)

Item 7–8   Papilledema is swelling of the optic disc caused by increased intracranial pressure. It is most often bilateral and occurs quickly (hours) or over weeks of time. It is a common symptom of a brain tumor. The term should not be used to describe optic disc swelling with underlying infectious, infiltrative, or inflammatory etiologies.

       ● **H47.09**   Other disorders of optic nerve, not elsewhere classified
          Compression of optic nerve
          H47.091   Other disorders of optic nerve, not elsewhere classified, right eye
          H47.092   Other disorders of optic nerve, not elsewhere classified, left eye
          H47.093   Other disorders of optic nerve, not elsewhere classified, bilateral
          H47.099   Other disorders of optic nerve, not elsewhere classified, unspecified eye
    ● **H47.1**   Papilledema
       H47.10   Unspecified papilledema
       H47.11   Papilledema associated with increased intracranial pressure
       H47.12   Papilledema associated with decreased ocular pressure
       H47.13   Papilledema associated with retinal disorder
       ● **H47.14**   Foster-Kennedy syndrome
          H47.141   Foster-Kennedy syndrome, right eye
          H47.142   Foster-Kennedy syndrome, left eye
          H47.143   Foster-Kennedy syndrome, bilateral
          H47.149   Foster-Kennedy syndrome, unspecified eye
    ● **H47.2**   Optic atrophy
       H47.20   Unspecified optic atrophy
       ● **H47.21**   Primary optic atrophy
          H47.211   Primary optic atrophy, right eye
          H47.212   Primary optic atrophy, left eye
          H47.213   Primary optic atrophy, bilateral
          H47.219   Primary optic atrophy, unspecified eye
       H47.22   Hereditary optic atrophy
          Leber's optic atrophy
       ● **H47.23**   Glaucomatous optic atrophy
          H47.231   Glaucomatous optic atrophy, right eye
          H47.232   Glaucomatous optic atrophy, left eye
          H47.233   Glaucomatous optic atrophy, bilateral
          H47.239   Glaucomatous optic atrophy, unspecified eye

- H47.29 **Other** optic atrophy
  - Temporal pallor of optic disc
  - H47.291 Other optic atrophy, **right** eye
  - H47.292 Other optic atrophy, **left** eye
  - H47.293 Other optic atrophy, **bilateral**
  - H47.299 Other optic atrophy, **unspecified** eye
- H47.3 Other disorders of optic disc
  - H47.31 **Coloboma** of optic disc
    - H47.311 Coloboma of optic disc, **right** eye
    - H47.312 Coloboma of optic disc, **left** eye
    - H47.313 Coloboma of optic disc, **bilateral**
    - H47.319 Coloboma of optic disc, **unspecified** eye
  - H47.32 **Drusen** of optic disc
    - H47.321 Drusen of optic disc, **right** eye
    - H47.322 Drusen of optic disc, **left** eye
    - H47.323 Drusen of optic disc, **bilateral**
    - H47.329 Drusen of optic disc, **unspecified** eye
  - H47.33 **Pseudopapilledema** of optic disc
    - H47.331 Pseudopapilledema of optic disc, **right** eye
    - H47.332 Pseudopapilledema of optic disc, **left** eye
    - H47.333 Pseudopapilledema of optic disc, **bilateral**
    - H47.339 Pseudopapilledema of optic disc, **unspecified** eye
  - H47.39 **Other** disorders of optic disc
    - H47.391 Other disorders of optic disc, **right** eye
    - H47.392 Other disorders of optic disc, **left** eye
    - H47.393 Other disorders of optic disc, **bilateral**
    - H47.399 Other disorders of optic disc, **unspecified** eye
- H47.4 Disorders of optic chiasm
  - **Code also** underlying condition
  - H47.41 Disorders of optic chiasm in (due to) **inflammatory disorders**
  - H47.42 Disorders of optic chiasm in (due to) **neoplasm**
  - H47.43 Disorders of optic chiasm in (due to) **vascular disorders**
  - H47.49 Disorders of optic chiasm in (due to) **other** disorders
- H47.5 Disorders of other visual pathways
  - Disorders of optic tracts, geniculate nuclei and optic radiations
  - **Code also** underlying condition
  - H47.51 Disorders of visual pathways in (due to) **inflammatory disorders**
    - H47.511 Disorders of visual pathways in (due to) inflammatory disorders, **right** side
    - H47.512 Disorders of visual pathways in (due to) inflammatory disorders, **left** side
    - H47.519 Disorders of visual pathways in (due to) inflammatory disorders, **unspecified** side
  - H47.52 Disorders of visual pathways in (due to) **neoplasm**
    - H47.521 Disorders of visual pathways in (due to) neoplasm, **right** side
    - H47.522 Disorders of visual pathways in (due to) neoplasm, **left** side
    - H47.529 Disorders of visual pathways in (due to) neoplasm, **unspecified** side

- H47.53 Disorders of visual pathways in (due to) **vascular disorders**
  - H47.531 Disorders of visual pathways in (due to) vascular disorders, **right** side
  - H47.532 Disorders of visual pathways in (due to) vascular disorders, **left** side
  - H47.539 Disorders of visual pathways in (due to) vascular disorders, **unspecified** side
- H47.6 Disorders of visual cortex
  - **Code also** underlying condition
  - **Excludes1** injury to visual cortex S04.04
  - H47.61 **Cortical blindness**
    - H47.611 Cortical blindness, **right** side of brain
    - H47.612 Cortical blindness, **left** side of brain
    - H47.619 Cortical blindness, **unspecified** side of brain
  - H47.62 Disorders of visual cortex in (due to) **inflammatory disorders**
    - H47.621 Disorders of visual cortex in (due to) inflammatory disorders, **right** side of brain
    - H47.622 Disorders of visual cortex in (due to) inflammatory disorders, **left** side of brain
    - H47.629 Disorders of visual cortex in (due to) inflammatory disorders, **unspecified** side of brain
  - H47.63 Disorders of visual cortex in (due to) **neoplasm**
    - H47.631 Disorders of visual cortex in (due to) neoplasm, **right** side of brain
    - H47.632 Disorders of visual cortex in (due to) neoplasm, **left** side of brain
    - H47.639 Disorders of visual cortex in (due to) neoplasm, **unspecified** side of brain
  - H47.64 Disorders of visual cortex in (due to) **vascular disorders**
    - H47.641 Disorders of visual cortex in (due to) vascular disorders, **right** side of brain
    - H47.642 Disorders of visual cortex in (due to) vascular disorders, **left** side of brain
    - H47.649 Disorders of visual cortex in (due to) vascular disorders, **unspecified** side of brain
- H47.9 **Unspecified** disorder of visual pathways

DISORDERS OF OCULAR MUSCLES, BINOCULAR MOVEMENT, ACCOMMODATION AND REFRACTION (H49-H52)

Excludes2 nystagmus and other irregular eye movements (H55)

- H49 Paralytic strabismus
  - **Excludes2** internal ophthalmoplegia (H52.51-)
    - internuclear ophthalmoplegia (H51.2-)
    - progressive supranuclear ophthalmoplegia (G23.1)
  - H49.0 **Third [oculomotor] nerve palsy**
    - H49.00 Third [oculomotor] nerve palsy, **unspecified** eye
    - H49.01 Third [oculomotor] nerve palsy, **right** eye
    - H49.02 Third [oculomotor] nerve palsy, **left** eye
    - H49.03 Third [oculomotor] nerve palsy, **bilateral**
  - H49.1 **Fourth [trochlear] nerve palsy**
    - H49.10 Fourth [trochlear] nerve palsy, **unspecified** eye
    - H49.11 Fourth [trochlear] nerve palsy, **right** eye
    - H49.12 Fourth [trochlear] nerve palsy, **left** eye
    - H49.13 Fourth [trochlear] nerve palsy, **bilateral**

▶ New   ⟹ Revised   ~~deleted~~ Deleted   **OGCR** Official Guidelines   X Assign placeholder X   ● Use Additional Character(s)

Excludes 1   Excludes 2   Includes   Use additional   Code first   Code also   Key words

Item 7–9 Strabismus or esotropia (crossed eyes) is a condition of the extraocular eye muscles, resulting in an inability of the eyes to focus and also affects depth perception.

Figure 7-12 A. Image of strabismus. **B.** Exotropia. (**A** from Yanoff: *Ophthalmology*, ed 3, Mosby, Inc., 2008. **B** from Zitelli BJ, Davis HW, *Pediatric Physical Diagnosis: Atlas of Pediatric Physical Diagnosis*, Philadelphia, Elsevier Saunders, 2012)

● H49.2   Sixth [abducent] nerve palsy
    H49.20   Sixth [abducent] nerve palsy, unspecified eye
    H49.21   Sixth [abducent] nerve palsy, right eye
    H49.22   Sixth [abducent] nerve palsy, left eye
    H49.23   Sixth [abducent] nerve palsy, bilateral
● H49.3   Total (external) ophthalmoplegia
    H49.30   Total (external) ophthalmoplegia, unspecified eye
    H49.31   Total (external) ophthalmoplegia, right eye
    H49.32   Total (external) ophthalmoplegia, left eye
    H49.33   Total (external) ophthalmoplegia, bilateral
● H49.4   Progressive external ophthalmoplegia
    Excludes1   Kearns-Sayre syndrome (H49.81-)
    H49.40   Progressive external ophthalmoplegia, unspecified eye
    H49.41   Progressive external ophthalmoplegia, right eye
    H49.42   Progressive external ophthalmoplegia, left eye
    H49.43   Progressive external ophthalmoplegia, bilateral
● H49.8   Other paralytic strabismus
   ● H49.81   Kearns-Sayre syndrome
       Progressive external ophthalmoplegia with pigmentary retinopathy
       Use additional code for other manifestation, such as:
         heart block (I45.9)
      H49.811   Kearns-Sayre syndrome, right eye
      H49.812   Kearns-Sayre syndrome, left eye
      H49.813   Kearns-Sayre syndrome, bilateral
      H49.819   Kearns-Sayre syndrome, unspecified eye
   ● H49.88   Other paralytic strabismus
       External ophthalmoplegia NOS
      H49.881   Other paralytic strabismus, right eye
      H49.882   Other paralytic strabismus, left eye
      H49.883   Other paralytic strabismus, bilateral
      H49.889   Other paralytic strabismus, unspecified eye
    H49.9   Unspecified paralytic strabismus

● H50   Other strabismus
   ● H50.0   Esotropia
       Convergent concomitant strabismus
      Excludes1   intermittent esotropia (H50.31-, H50.32)
     H50.00   Unspecified esotropia
   ● H50.01   Monocular esotropia
      H50.011   Monocular esotropia, right eye
      H50.012   Monocular esotropia, left eye

   ● H50.02   Monocular esotropia with A pattern
      H50.021   Monocular esotropia with A pattern, right eye
      H50.022   Monocular esotropia with A pattern, left eye
   ● H50.03   Monocular esotropia with V pattern
      H50.031   Monocular esotropia with V pattern, right eye
      H50.032   Monocular esotropia with V pattern, left eye
   ● H50.04   Monocular esotropia with other noncomitancies
      H50.041   Monocular esotropia with other noncomitancies, right eye
      H50.042   Monocular esotropia with other noncomitancies, left eye
     H50.05   Alternating esotropia
     H50.06   Alternating esotropia with A pattern
     H50.07   Alternating esotropia with V pattern
     H50.08   Alternating esotropia with other noncomitancies
● H50.1   Exotropia
     Misalignment in which one eye deviates outward (away from nose) while the other fixates normally
     Divergent concomitant strabismus
     Excludes1   intermittent exotropia (H50.33-, H50.34)
    H50.10   Unspecified exotropia
   ● H50.11   Monocular exotropia
      H50.111   Monocular exotropia, right eye
      H50.112   Monocular exotropia, left eye
   ● H50.12   Monocular exotropia with A pattern
      H50.121   Monocular exotropia with A pattern, right eye
      H50.122   Monocular exotropia with A pattern, left eye
   ● H50.13   Monocular exotropia with V pattern
      H50.131   Monocular exotropia with V pattern, right eye
      H50.132   Monocular exotropia with V pattern, left eye
   ● H50.14   Monocular exotropia with other noncomitancies
      H50.141   Monocular exotropia with other noncomitancies, right eye
      H50.142   Monocular exotropia with other noncomitancies, left eye
     H50.15   Alternating exotropia
     H50.16   Alternating exotropia with A pattern
     H50.17   Alternating exotropia with V pattern
     H50.18   Alternating exotropia with other noncomitancies
● H50.2   Vertical strabismus
     Hypertropia
    H50.21   Vertical strabismus, right eye
    H50.22   Vertical strabismus, left eye
● H50.3   Intermittent heterotropia
     Displacement of an organ or part of an organ from its normal position
    H50.30   Unspecified intermittent heterotropia
   ● H50.31   Intermittent monocular esotropia
      H50.311   Intermittent monocular esotropia, right eye
      H50.312   Intermittent monocular esotropia, left eye
     H50.32   Intermittent alternating esotropia
   ● H50.33   Intermittent monocular exotropia
      H50.331   Intermittent monocular exotropia, right eye
      H50.332   Intermittent monocular exotropia, left eye
     H50.34   Intermittent alternating exotropia

▶ New   ⇒ Revised   ~~deleted~~ Deleted   **OGCR** Official Guidelines   X Assign placeholder X   ● Use Additional Character(s)

| Excludes 1 | Excludes 2 | Includes | Use additional | Code first | Code also | Key words |

CHAPTER 7 (H00–H59)

● H50.4   **Other and unspecified heterotropia**
     H50.40   Unspecified heterotropia
   ● H50.41   Cyclotropia
        H50.411   Cyclotropia, right eye
        H50.412   Cyclotropia, left eye
     H50.42   Monofixation syndrome
     H50.43   Accommodative component in esotropia
● H50.5   **Heterophoria**
     One or both eyes wander away from the position where both
     eyes are looking together in the same direction
     H50.50   Unspecified heterophoria
     H50.51   Esophoria
        Eye deviates inward (toward the nose)
     H50.52   Exophoria
        Eye deviates outward (toward the ear)
     H50.53   Vertical heterophoria
     H50.54   Cyclophoria
     H50.55   Alternating heterophoria
● H50.6   **Mechanical strabismus**
     H50.60   Mechanical strabismus, unspecified
   ● H50.61   Brown's sheath syndrome
        H50.611   Brown's sheath syndrome, right eye
        H50.612   Brown's sheath syndrome, left eye
     H50.69   Other mechanical strabismus
        Strabismus due to adhesions
        Traumatic limitation of duction of eye muscle
● H50.8   **Other specified strabismus**
   ● H50.81   Duane's syndrome
        H50.811   Duane's syndrome, right eye
        H50.812   Duane's syndrome, left eye
     H50.89   Other specified strabismus
     H50.9   Unspecified strabismus

● H51   **Other disorders of binocular movement**
     H51.0   Palsy (spasm) of conjugate gaze
   ● H51.1   Convergence insufficiency and excess
     H51.11   Convergence insufficiency
     H51.12   Convergence excess
   ● H51.2   Internuclear ophthalmoplegia
     H51.20   Internuclear ophthalmoplegia, unspecified eye
     H51.21   Internuclear ophthalmoplegia, right eye
     H51.22   Internuclear ophthalmoplegia, left eye
     H51.23   Internuclear ophthalmoplegia, bilateral
     H51.8   Other specified disorders of binocular movement
     H51.9   Unspecified disorder of binocular movement

● H52   **Disorders of refraction and accommodation**
   ● H52.0   Hypermetropia
     H52.00   Hypermetropia, unspecified eye
     H52.01   Hypermetropia, right eye
     H52.02   Hypermetropia, left eye
     H52.03   Hypermetropia, bilateral
   ● H52.1   Myopia
       Excludes1   degenerative myopia (H44.2-)
     H52.10   Myopia, unspecified eye
     H52.11   Myopia, right eye
     H52.12   Myopia, left eye
     H52.13   Myopia, bilateral

● H52.2   **Astigmatism**
   ● H52.20   Unspecified astigmatism
     H52.201   Unspecified astigmatism, right eye
     H52.202   Unspecified astigmatism, left eye
     H52.203   Unspecified astigmatism, bilateral
     H52.209   Unspecified astigmatism, unspecified eye
   ● H52.21   Irregular astigmatism
     H52.211   Irregular astigmatism, right eye
     H52.212   Irregular astigmatism, left eye
     H52.213   Irregular astigmatism, bilateral
     H52.219   Irregular astigmatism, unspecified eye
   ● H52.22   Regular astigmatism
     H52.221   Regular astigmatism, right eye
     H52.222   Regular astigmatism, left eye
     H52.223   Regular astigmatism, bilateral
     H52.229   Regular astigmatism, unspecified eye
● H52.3   **Anisometropia and aniseikonia**
     H52.31   Anisometropia
     H52.32   Aniseikonia
     H52.4   Presbyopia
● H52.5   **Disorders of accommodation**
   ● H52.51   Internal ophthalmoplegia (complete) (total)
     H52.511   Internal ophthalmoplegia (complete) (total), right eye
     H52.512   Internal ophthalmoplegia (complete) (total), left eye
     H52.513   Internal ophthalmoplegia (complete) (total), bilateral
     H52.519   Internal ophthalmoplegia (complete) (total), unspecified eye
   ● H52.52   Paresis of accommodation
     H52.521   Paresis of accommodation, right eye
     H52.522   Paresis of accommodation, left eye
     H52.523   Paresis of accommodation, bilateral
     H52.529   Paresis of accommodation, unspecified eye
   ● H52.53   Spasm of accommodation
     H52.531   Spasm of accommodation, right eye
     H52.532   Spasm of accommodation, left eye
     H52.533   Spasm of accommodation, bilateral
     H52.539   Spasm of accommodation, unspecified eye
     H52.6   Other disorders of refraction
     H52.7   Unspecified disorder of refraction

VISUAL DISTURBANCES AND BLINDNESS (H53-H54)

◐ H53   **Visual disturbances**
   ● H53.0   Amblyopia ex anopsia
     Excludes1   amblyopia due to vitamin A deficiency (E50.5)
   ● H53.00   Unspecified amblyopia
     H53.001   Unspecified amblyopia, right eye
     H53.002   Unspecified amblyopia, left eye
     H53.003   Unspecified amblyopia, bilateral
     H53.009   Unspecified amblyopia, unspecified eye
   ● H53.01   Deprivation amblyopia
     H53.011   Deprivation amblyopia, right eye
     H53.012   Deprivation amblyopia, left eye
     H53.013   Deprivation amblyopia, bilateral
     H53.019   Deprivation amblyopia, unspecified eye

Item 7-10 Disorders of refraction: **Hypermetropia,** or farsightedness, means focus at a distance is adequate but not on close objects. **Myopia** is near-sightedness or short-sightedness and means the focus on nearby objects is clear but distant objects appear blurred. **Astigmatism** is warping of the curvature of the cornea so light rays entering do not meet a single focal point, resulting in a distorted image. **Anisometropia** is unequal refractive power in which one eye may be myopic (near-sighted) and the other hyperopic (far-sighted). **Presbyopia** is the loss of focus on near objects, which occurs with age because the lens loses elasticity.

▶ New   ➡ Revised   ~~deleted~~ Deleted   OGCR Official Guidelines   X Assign placeholder X   ● Use Additional Character(s)

Excludes 1   Excludes 2   Includes   Use additional   Code first   Code also   Key words

● **H53.02** Refractive amblyopia
    H53.021   Refractive amblyopia, **right** eye
    H53.022   Refractive amblyopia, **left** eye
    H53.023   Refractive amblyopia, **bilateral**
    H53.029   Refractive amblyopia, **unspecified** eye
● **H53.03** Strabismic amblyopia
    Excludes1   strabismus (H50.-)
    H53.031   Strabismic amblyopia, **right** eye
    H53.032   Strabismic amblyopia, **left** eye
    H53.033   Strabismic amblyopia, **bilateral**
    H53.039   Strabismic amblyopia, **unspecified** eye
● **H53.04** Amblyopia suspect
    H53.041   Amblyopia suspect, **right** eye
    H53.042   Amblyopia suspect, **left** eye
    H53.043   Amblyopia suspect, **bilateral**
    H53.049   Amblyopia suspect, **unspecified** eye
● **H53.1** Subjective visual disturbances
    Excludes1   subjective visual disturbances due to vitamin A deficiency (E50.5)
                   visual hallucinations (R44.1)
    H53.10   **Unspecified** subjective visual disturbances
    H53.11   **Day blindness**
         Hemeralopia
    H53.12   **Transient** visual loss
         Scintillating scotoma
        Excludes1   amaurosis fugax (G45.3-)
                    transient retinal artery occlusion (H34.0-)
        H53.121   Transient visual loss, **right** eye
        H53.122   Transient visual loss, **left** eye
        H53.123   Transient visual loss, **bilateral**
        H53.129   Transient visual loss, **unspecified** eye
● **H53.13** Sudden visual loss
    H53.131   Sudden visual loss, **right** eye
    H53.132   Sudden visual loss, **left** eye
    H53.133   Sudden visual loss, **bilateral**
    H53.139   Sudden visual loss, **unspecified** eye
● **H53.14** Visual discomfort
         Asthenopia
         Photophobia
    H53.141   Visual discomfort, **right** eye
    H53.142   Visual discomfort, **left** eye
    H53.143   Visual discomfort, **bilateral**
    H53.149   Visual discomfort, **unspecified**
    H53.15   Visual distortions of shape and size
         Metamorphopsia
    H53.16   **Psychophysical** visual disturbances
    H53.19   **Other** subjective visual disturbances
         Visual halos
   H53.2 Diplopia
         Double vision
● **H53.3** Other and unspecified disorders of binocular vision
    H53.30   **Unspecified** disorder of binocular vision
    H53.31   Abnormal retinal correspondence
    H53.32   Fusion with defective stereopsis
    H53.33   Simultaneous visual perception without fusion
    H53.34   Suppression of binocular vision

● **H53.4** Visual field defects
    H53.40   **Unspecified** visual field defects
● **H53.41** Scotoma involving central area
         Central scotoma
    H53.411   Scotoma involving central area, **right** eye
    H53.412   Scotoma involving central area, **left** eye
    H53.413   Scotoma involving central area, **bilateral**
    H53.419   Scotoma involving central area, **unspecified** eye
● **H53.42** Scotoma of blind spot area
         Enlarged blind spot
    H53.421   Scotoma of blind spot area, **right** eye
    H53.422   Scotoma of blind spot area, **left** eye
    H53.423   Scotoma of blind spot area, **bilateral**
    H53.429   Scotoma of blind spot area, **unspecified** eye
● **H53.43** Sector or arcuate defects
         Arcuate scotoma
         Bjerrum scotoma
    H53.431   Sector or arcuate defects, **right** eye
    H53.432   Sector or arcuate defects, **left** eye
    H53.433   Sector or arcuate defects, **bilateral**
    H53.439   Sector or arcuate defects, **unspecified** eye
● **H53.45** Other localized visual field defect
         Peripheral visual field defect
         Ring scotoma NOS
         Scotoma NOS
    H53.451   Other localized visual field defect, **right** eye
    H53.452   Other localized visual field defect, **left** eye
    H53.453   Other localized visual field defect, **bilateral**
    H53.459   Other localized visual field defect, **unspecified** eye
● **H53.46** Homonymous bilateral field defects
         Homonymous hemianopia
         Homonymous hemianopsia
         Quadrant anopia
         Quadrant anopsia
    H53.461   Homonymous bilateral field defects, **right side**
    H53.462   Homonymous bilateral field defects, **left side**
    H53.469   Homonymous bilateral field defects, **unspecified side**
         Homonymous bilateral field defects NOS
    H53.47   **Heteronymous** bilateral field defects
         Heteronymous hemianop(s)ia
● **H53.48** Generalized contraction of visual field
    H53.481   Generalized contraction of visual field, **right** eye
    H53.482   Generalized contraction of visual field, **left** eye
    H53.483   Generalized contraction of visual field, **bilateral**
    H53.489   Generalized contraction of visual field, **unspecified** eye

CHAPTER 7 (H00-H59)

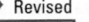

H53.5 **Color vision deficiencies**
Color blindness
Excludes2 day blindness (H53.11)

H53.50 **Unspecified color vision deficiencies**
Color blindness NOS

H53.51 **Achromatopsia**

H53.52 **Acquired color vision deficiency**

H53.53 **Deuteranomaly**
Deuteranopia

H53.54 **Protanomaly**
Protanopia

H53.55 **Tritanomaly**
Tritanopia

H53.59 **Other color vision deficiencies**

H53.6 **Night blindness**
Excludes1 night blindness due to vitamin A deficiency (E50.5)

H53.60 **Unspecified night blindness**

H53.61 **Abnormal dark adaptation curve**

H53.62 **Acquired night blindness**

H53.63 **Congenital night blindness**

H53.69 **Other night blindness**

H53.7 **Vision sensitivity deficiencies**

H53.71 **Glare sensitivity**

H53.72 **Impaired contrast sensitivity**

H53.8 **Other visual disturbances**

H53.9 **Unspecified visual disturbance**

H54 **Blindness and low vision**
Note: For definition of visual impairment categories see table below.
Code first any associated underlying cause of the blindness
Excludes1 amaurosis fugax (G45.3)

H54.0 **Blindness, both eyes**
Visual impairment categories 3, 4, 5 in both eyes.

▶● H54.0X **Blindness, both eyes, different category levels**

▶ H54.0X3 **Blindness right eye, category 3**

▶ H54.0X33 **Blindness right eye category 3, blindness left eye category 3**

▶ H54.0X34 **Blindness right eye category 3, blindness left eye category 4**

▶ H54.0X35 **Blindness right eye category 3, blindness left eye category 5**

▶ H54.0X4 **Blindness right eye, category 4**

▶ H54.0X43 **Blindness right eye category 4, blindness left eye category 3**

▶ H54.0X44 **Blindness right eye category 4, blindness left eye category 4**

▶ H54.0X45 **Blindness right eye category 4, blindness left eye category 5**

▶● H54.0X5 **Blindness right eye, category 5**

▶ H54.0X53 **Blindness right eye category 5, blindness left eye category 3**

▶ H54.0X54 **Blindness right eye category 5, blindness left eye category 4**

▶ H54.0X55 **Blindness right eye category 5, blindness left eye category 5**

H54.1 **Blindness, one eye, low vision other eye**
Visual impairment categories 3, 4, 5 in one eye, with categories 1 or 2 in the other eye.

H54.10 **Blindness, one eye, low vision other eye, unspecified eyes**

● H54.11 **Blindness, right eye, low vision left eye**

▶● H54.113 **Blindness right eye category 3, low vision left eye**

▶ H54.1131 **Blindness right eye category 3, low vision left eye category 1**

▶ H54.1132 **Blindness right eye category 3, low vision left eye category 2**

▶● H54.114 **Blindness right eye category 4, low vision left eye**

▶ H54.1141 **Blindness right eye category 4, low vision left eye category 1**

▶ H54.1142 **Blindness right eye category 4, low vision left eye category 2**

▶● H54.115 **Blindness right eye category 5, low vision left eye**

▶ H54.1151 **Blindness right eye category 5, low vision left eye category 1**

▶ H54.1152 **Blindness right eye category 5, low vision left eye category 2**

● H54.12 **Blindness, left eye, low vision right eye**

▶● H54.121 **Low vision right eye category 1, blindness left eye**

▶ H54.1213 **Low vision right eye category 1, blindness left eye category 3**

▶ H54.1214 **Low vision right eye category 1, blindness left eye category 4**

▶ H54.1215 **Low vision right eye category 1, blindness left eye category 5**

▶● H54.122 **Low vision right eye category 2, blindness left eye**

▶ H54.1223 **Low vision right eye category 2, blindness left eye category 3**

▶ H54.1224 **Low vision right eye category 2, blindness left eye category 4**

▶ H54.1225 **Low vision right eye category 2, blindness left eye category 5**

● H54.2 **Low vision, both eyes**
Visual impairment categories 1 or 2 in both eyes.

▶● H54.2X **Low vision, both eyes, different category levels**

▶● H54.2X1 **Low vision, right eye, category 1**

▶ H54.2X11 **Low vision right eye category 1, low vision left eye category 1**

▶ H54.2X12 **Low vision right eye category 1, low vision left eye category 2**

▶● **H54.2X2**　Low vision, right eye, category 2
　　　▶ **H54.2X21**　Low vision right eye category 2, low vision left eye category 1
　　　▶ **H54.2X22**　Low vision right eye category 2, low vision left eye category 2
H54.3　Unqualified visual loss, both eyes
　　　Visual impairment category 9 in both eyes.
● **H54.4**　Blindness, one eye
　　　Visual impairment categories 3, 4, 5 in one eye [normal vision in other eye]
　　H54.40　Blindness, one eye, unspecified eye
　● **H54.41**　Blindness, right eye, normal vision left eye
　　▶● **H54.413**　Blindness, right eye, category 3
　　　　▶ **H54.413A**　Blindness right eye category 3, normal vision left eye
　　▶● **H54.414**　Blindness, right eye, category 4
　　　　▶ **H54.414A**　Blindness right eye category 4, normal vision left eye
　　▶● **H54.415**　Blindness, right eye, category 5
　　　　▶ **H54.415A**　Blindness right eye category 5, normal vision left eye
　● **H54.42**　Blindness, left eye, normal vision right eye
　　▶● **H54.42A**　Blindness, left eye, category 3-5
　　　　▶ **H54.42A3**　Blindness left eye category 3, normal vision right eye
　　　　▶ **H54.42A4**　Blindness left eye category 4, normal vision right eye
　　　　▶ **H54.42A5**　Blindness left eye category 5, normal vision right eye
● **H54.5**　Low vision, one eye
　　　Visual impairment categories 1 or 2 in one eye [normal vision in other eye].
　　H54.50　Low vision, one eye, unspecified eye
　● **H54.51**　Low vision, right eye, normal vision left eye
　　▶● **H54.511**　Low vision, right eye, category 1-2
　　　　▶ **H54.511A**　Low vision right eye category 1, normal vision left eye
　　　　▶ **H54.512A**　Low vision right eye category 2, normal vision left eye
　　H54.52　Low vision, left eye, normal vision right eye
　　▶● **H54.52A**　Low vision, left eye, category 1-2
　　　　▶ **H54.52A1**　Low vision left eye category 1, normal vision right eye
　　　　▶ **H54.52A2**　Low vision left eye category 2, normal vision right eye
● **H54.6**　Unqualified visual loss, one eye
　　　Visual impairment category 9 in one eye [normal vision in other eye].
　　H54.60　Unqualified visual loss, one eye, unspecified
　　H54.61　Unqualified visual loss, right eye, normal vision left eye
　　H54.62　Unqualified visual loss, left eye, normal vision right eye

OGCR　Section I.C.7.b.

Blindness
If "blindness" or "low vision" of both eyes is documented but the visual impairment category is not documented, assign code H54.3, Unqualified visual loss, both eyes. If "blindness" or "low vision" in one eye is documented but the visual impairment category is not documented, assign a code from H54.6-, Unqualified visual loss, one eye. If "blindness" or "visual loss" is documented without any information about whether one or both eyes are affected, assign code H54.7, Unspecified visual loss.

H54.7　Unspecified visual loss
　　　Visual impairment category 9 NOS
H54.8　Legal blindness, as defined in USA
　　　Blindness NOS according to USA definition
　　　Excludes1　legal blindness with specification of impairment level (H54.0-H54.7)
　　Note:　The table below gives a classification of severity of visual impairment recommended by a WHO Study Group on the Prevention of Blindness, Geneva, 6-10 November 1972.

The term 'low vision' in category H54 comprises categories 1 and 2 of the table, the term 'blindness' categories 3, 4 and 5, and the term 'unqualified visual loss' category 9.

If the extent of the visual field is taken into account, patients with a field no greater than 10 but greater than 5 around central fixation should be placed in category 3 and patients with a field no greater than 5 around central fixation should be placed in category 4, even if the central acuity is not impaired.

(Document 508 compliance requires all cells in the following table to be filled.)

Category of visual impairment	Visual acuity with best possible correction	
	Maximum less than:	**Minimum equal to or better than:**
—	6/18	6/60
3/10 (0.3)	1/10 (0.1)	—
20/70	20/200	
—	6/60	3/60
1/10 (0.1)	1/20 (0.05)	—
20/200	20/400	
—	3/60	1/60 (finger counting at one meter)
1/20 (0.05)	1/50 (0.02)	—
20/400	5/300 (20/1200)	
—	1/60 (finger counting at one meter)	Light perception
1/50 (0.02)	—	—
5/300	—	
—	No light perception	—
—	Undetermined or unspecified	—

OTHER DISORDERS OF EYE AND ADNEXA (H55-H57)

● **H55**　Nystagmus and other irregular eye movements
　● **H55.0**　Nystagmus
　　　Rapid, involuntary movements of the eyes in the horizontal or vertical direction
　　H55.00　Unspecified nystagmus
　　H55.01　Congenital nystagmus
　　H55.02　Latent nystagmus
　　H55.03　Visual deprivation nystagmus
　　H55.04　Dissociated nystagmus
　　H55.09　Other forms of nystagmus
　● **H55.8**　Other irregular eye movements
　　H55.81　Saccadic eye movements
　　H55.89　Other irregular eye movements

▶ New　⇒ Revised　~~deleted~~ Deleted　**OGCR** Official Guidelines　X Assign placeholder X　● Use Additional Character(s)

Excludes 1　Excludes 2　Includes　Use additional　Code first　Code also　Key words

CHAPTER 7 (H00-H59)

● H57   Other disorders of eye and adnexa
  ● H57.0   Anomalies of pupillary function
     H57.00   Unspecified anomaly of pupillary function
     H57.01   Argyll Robertson pupil, atypical
         Excludes1   syphilitic Argyll Robertson pupil (A52.19)
     H57.02   Anisocoria
     H57.03   Miosis
     H57.04   Mydriasis
   ● H57.05   Tonic pupil
       H57.051   Tonic pupil, right eye
       H57.052   Tonic pupil, left eye
       H57.053   Tonic pupil, bilateral
       H57.059   Tonic pupil, unspecified eye
     H57.09   Other anomalies of pupillary function
  ● H57.1   Ocular pain
     H57.10   Ocular pain, unspecified eye
     H57.11   Ocular pain, right eye
     H57.12   Ocular pain, left eye
     H57.13   Ocular pain, bilateral
   H57.8   Other specified disorders of eye and adnexa
   H57.9   Unspecified disorder of eye and adnexa

INTRAOPERATIVE AND POSTPROCEDURAL COMPLICATIONS AND DISORDERS OF EYE AND ADNEXA, NOT ELSEWHERE CLASSIFIED (H59)

● H59   Intraoperative and postprocedural complications and disorders of eye and adnexa, not elsewhere classified
     Excludes1   mechanical complication of intraocular lens (T85.2)
         mechanical complication of other ocular prosthetic devices, implants and grafts (T85.3)
         pseudophakia (Z96.1)
         secondary cataracts (H26.4-)
  ● H59.0   Disorders of the eye following cataract surgery
   ● H59.01   Keratopathy (bullous aphakic) following cataract surgery
       Vitreal corneal syndrome
       Vitreous (touch) syndrome
       H59.011   Keratopathy (bullous aphakic) following cataract surgery, right eye
       H59.012   Keratopathy (bullous aphakic) following cataract surgery, left eye
       H59.013   Keratopathy (bullous aphakic) following cataract surgery, bilateral
       H59.019   Keratopathy (bullous aphakic) following cataract surgery, unspecified eye
   ● H59.02   Cataract (lens) fragments in eye following cataract surgery
       H59.021   Cataract (lens) fragments in eye following cataract surgery, right eye
       H59.022   Cataract (lens) fragments in eye following cataract surgery, left eye
       H59.023   Cataract (lens) fragments in eye following cataract surgery, bilateral
       H59.029   Cataract (lens) fragments in eye following cataract surgery, unspecified eye
   ● H59.03   Cystoid macular edema following cataract surgery
       H59.031   Cystoid macular edema following cataract surgery, right eye
       H59.032   Cystoid macular edema following cataract surgery, left eye
       H59.033   Cystoid macular edema following cataract surgery, bilateral
       H59.039   Cystoid macular edema following cataract surgery, unspecified eye

● H59.09   Other disorders of the eye following cataract surgery
       H59.091   Other disorders of the right eye following cataract surgery
       H59.092   Other disorders of the left eye following cataract surgery
       H59.093   Other disorders of the eye following cataract surgery, bilateral
       H59.099   Other disorders of unspecified eye following cataract surgery
● H59.1   Intraoperative hemorrhage and hematoma of eye and adnexa complicating a procedure
     Excludes1   intraoperative hemorrhage and hematoma of eye and adnexa due to accidental puncture or laceration during a procedure (H59.2-)
  ● H59.11   Intraoperative hemorrhage and hematoma of eye and adnexa complicating an ophthalmic procedure
       H59.111   Intraoperative hemorrhage and hematoma of right eye and adnexa complicating an ophthalmic procedure
       H59.112   Intraoperative hemorrhage and hematoma of left eye and adnexa complicating an ophthalmic procedure
       H59.113   Intraoperative hemorrhage and hematoma of eye and adnexa complicating an ophthalmic procedure, bilateral
       H59.119   Intraoperative hemorrhage and hematoma of unspecified eye and adnexa complicating an ophthalmic procedure
  ● H59.12   Intraoperative hemorrhage and hematoma of eye and adnexa complicating other procedure
       H59.121   Intraoperative hemorrhage and hematoma of right eye and adnexa complicating other procedure
       H59.122   Intraoperative hemorrhage and hematoma of left eye and adnexa complicating other procedure
       H59.123   Intraoperative hemorrhage and hematoma of eye and adnexa complicating other procedure, bilateral
       H59.129   Intraoperative hemorrhage and hematoma of unspecified eye and adnexa complicating other procedure
● H59.2   Accidental puncture and laceration of eye and adnexa during a procedure
  ● H59.21   Accidental puncture and laceration of eye and adnexa during an ophthalmic procedure
       H59.211   Accidental puncture and laceration of right eye and adnexa during an ophthalmic procedure
       H59.212   Accidental puncture and laceration of left eye and adnexa during an ophthalmic procedure
       H59.213   Accidental puncture and laceration of eye and adnexa during an ophthalmic procedure, bilateral
       H59.219   Accidental puncture and laceration of unspecified eye and adnexa during an ophthalmic procedure

---

▶ New   ⇒ Revised   ~~deleted~~ Deleted   **OGCR** Official Guidelines   X Assign placeholder X   ● Use Additional Character(s)

Excludes 1   Excludes 2   Includes   Use additional   Code first   Code also   Key words

● H59.22   Accidental puncture and laceration of eye and adnexa during other procedure

   H59.221   Accidental puncture and laceration of right eye and adnexa during other procedure

   H59.222   Accidental puncture and laceration of left eye and adnexa during other procedure

   H59.223   Accidental puncture and laceration of eye and adnexa during other procedure, bilateral

   H59.229   Accidental puncture and laceration of unspecified eye and adnexa during other procedure

● H59.3   Postprocedural hemorrhage, hematoma, and seroma of eye and adnexa following other procedure

   ● H59.31   Postprocedural hemorrhage of eye and adnexa following an ophthalmic procedure

      H59.311   Postprocedural hemorrhage of right eye and adnexa following an ophthalmic procedure

      H59.312   Postprocedural hemorrhage of left eye and adnexa following an ophthalmic procedure

      H59.313   Postprocedural hemorrhage of eye and adnexa following an ophthalmic procedure, bilateral

      H59.319   Postprocedural hemorrhage of unspecified eye and adnexa following an ophthalmic procedure

   ● H59.32   Postprocedural hemorrhage of eye and adnexa following other procedure

      H59.321   Postprocedural hemorrhage of right eye and adnexa following other procedure

      H59.322   Postprocedural hemorrhage of left eye and adnexa following other procedure

      H59.323   Postprocedural hemorrhage of eye and adnexa following other procedure, bilateral

      H59.329   Postprocedural hemorrhage of unspecified eye and adnexa following other procedure

   ● H59.33   Postprocedural hematoma of eye and adnexa following an ophthalmic procedure

      H59.331   Postprocedural hematoma of right eye and adnexa following an ophthalmic procedure

      H59.332   Postprocedural hematoma of left eye and adnexa following an ophthalmic procedure

      H59.333   Postprocedural hematoma of eye and adnexa following an ophthalmic procedure, bilateral

      H59.339   Postprocedural hematoma of unspecified eye and adnexa following an ophthalmic procedure

   ● H59.34   Postprocedural hematoma of eye and adnexa following other procedure

      H59.341   Postprocedural hematoma of right eye and adnexa following other procedure

      H59.342   Postprocedural hematoma of left eye and adnexa following other procedure

      H59.343   Postprocedural hematoma of eye and adnexa following other procedure, bilateral

      H59.349   Postprocedural hematoma of unspecified eye and adnexa following other procedure

● H59.35   Postprocedural seroma of eye and adnexa following an ophthalmic procedure

   H59.351   Postprocedural seroma of right eye and adnexa following an ophthalmic procedure

   H59.352   Postprocedural seroma of left eye and adnexa following an ophthalmic procedure

   H59.353   Postprocedural seroma of eye and adnexa following an ophthalmic procedure, bilateral

   H59.359   Postprocedural seroma of unspecified eye and adnexa following an ophthalmic procedure

● H59.36   Postprocedural seroma of eye and adnexa following other procedure

   H59.361   Postprocedural seroma of right eye and adnexa following other procedure

   H59.362   Postprocedural seroma of left eye and adnexa following other procedure

   H59.363   Postprocedural seroma of eye and adnexa following other procedure, bilateral

   H59.369   Postprocedural seroma of unspecified eye and adnexa following other procedure

● H59.4   Inflammation (infection) of postprocedural bleb
          Postprocedural blebitis

   > Excludes1   filtering (vitreous) bleb after glaucoma surgery status (Z98.83)

   H59.40   Inflammation (infection) of postprocedural bleb, unspecified

   H59.41   Inflammation (infection) of postprocedural bleb, stage 1

   H59.42   Inflammation (infection) of postprocedural bleb, stage 2

   H59.43   Inflammation (infection) of postprocedural bleb, stage 3
            Bleb endophthalmitis

● H59.8   Other intraoperative and postprocedural complications and disorders of eye and adnexa, not elsewhere classified

   ● H59.81   Chorioretinal scars after surgery for detachment

      H59.811   Chorioretinal scars after surgery for detachment, right eye

      H59.812   Chorioretinal scars after surgery for detachment, left eye

      H59.813   Chorioretinal scars after surgery for detachment, bilateral

      H59.819   Chorioretinal scars after surgery for detachment, unspecified eye

   H59.88   Other intraoperative complications of eye and adnexa, not elsewhere classified

   H59.89   Other postprocedural complications and disorders of eye and adnexa, not elsewhere classified

▶ New   ⟹ Revised   ~~deleted~~ Deleted   OGCR Official Guidelines   X Assign placeholder X   ● Use Additional Character(s)

Excludes 1   Excludes 2   Includes   Use additional   Code first   Code also   Key words

CHAPTER 8

DISEASES OF THE EAR AND MASTOID PROCESS (H60-H95)

OGCR Chapter-Specific Coding Guidelines

> 8. **Chapter 8: Diseases of the Ear and Mastoid Process (H60-H95)**
> Reserved for future guideline expansion

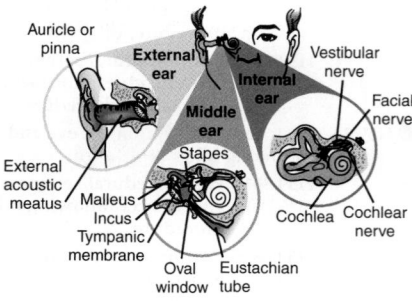

Figure 8-1 Auditory system. (From Buck CJ: Step-by-Step Medical Coding, ed 2016, St. Louis, Elsevier, 2016)

★**(See Plate 92 on page 68.)**

CHAPTER 8

DISEASES OF THE EAR AND MASTOID PROCESS (H60-H95)

Note: Use an external cause code following the code for the ear condition, if applicable, to identify the cause of the ear condition

Excludes2 certain conditions originating in the perinatal period (P04-P96)
certain infectious and parasitic diseases (A00-B99)
complications of pregnancy, childbirth and the puerperium (O00-O9A)
congenital malformations, deformations and chromosomal abnormalities (Q00-Q99)
endocrine, nutritional and metabolic diseases (E00-E88)
injury, poisoning and certain other consequences of external causes (S00-T88)
neoplasms (C00-D49)
symptoms, signs and abnormal clinical and laboratory findings, not elsewhere classified (R00-R94)

This chapter contains the following blocks:

H60-H62	Diseases of external ear
H65-H75	Diseases of middle ear and mastoid
H80-H83	Diseases of inner ear
H90-H94	Other disorders of ear
H95	Intraoperative and postprocedural complications and disorders of ear and mastoid process, not elsewhere classified

DISEASES OF EXTERNAL EAR (H60-H62)

● **H60** Otitis externa
  ● **H60.0** Abscess of external ear
        Boil of external ear
        Carbuncle of auricle or external auditory canal
        Furuncle of external ear
      H60.00 Abscess of external ear, unspecified ear
      H60.01 Abscess of right external ear
      H60.02 Abscess of left external ear
      H60.03 Abscess of external ear, bilateral

● **H60.1** Cellulitis of external ear
        Cellulitis of auricle
        Cellulitis of external auditory canal
      H60.10 Cellulitis of external ear, unspecified ear
      H60.11 Cellulitis of right external ear
      H60.12 Cellulitis of left external ear
      H60.13 Cellulitis of external ear, bilateral
  ● **H60.2** Malignant otitis externa
      H60.20 Malignant otitis externa, unspecified ear
      H60.21 Malignant otitis externa, right ear
      H60.22 Malignant otitis externa, left ear
      H60.23 Malignant otitis externa, bilateral
  ● **H60.3** Other infective otitis externa
    ● **H60.31** Diffuse otitis externa
        H60.311 Diffuse otitis externa, right ear
        H60.312 Diffuse otitis externa, left ear
        H60.313 Diffuse otitis externa, bilateral
        H60.319 Diffuse otitis externa, unspecified ear
    ● **H60.32** Hemorrhagic otitis externa
        H60.321 Hemorrhagic otitis externa, right ear
        H60.322 Hemorrhagic otitis externa, left ear
        H60.323 Hemorrhagic otitis externa, bilateral
        H60.329 Hemorrhagic otitis externa, unspecified ear
    ● **H60.33** Swimmer's ear
        H60.331 Swimmer's ear, right ear
        H60.332 Swimmer's ear, left ear
        H60.333 Swimmer's ear, bilateral
        H60.339 Swimmer's ear, unspecified ear
    ● **H60.39** Other infective otitis externa
        H60.391 Other infective otitis externa, right ear
        H60.392 Other infective otitis externa, left ear
        H60.393 Other infective otitis externa, bilateral
        H60.399 Other infective otitis externa, unspecified ear
  ● **H60.4** Cholesteatoma of external ear
        Keratosis obturans of external ear (canal)
        Excludes2 cholesteatoma of middle ear (H71.-)
                recurrent cholesteatoma of postmastoidectomy cavity (H95.0-)
      H60.40 Cholesteatoma of external ear, unspecified ear
      H60.41 Cholesteatoma of right external ear
      H60.42 Cholesteatoma of left external ear
      H60.43 Cholesteatoma of external ear, bilateral
  ● **H60.5** Acute noninfective otitis externa
    ● **H60.50** Unspecified acute noninfective otitis externa
        Acute otitis externa NOS
        H60.501 Unspecified acute noninfective otitis externa, right ear
        H60.502 Unspecified acute noninfective otitis externa, left ear
        H60.503 Unspecified acute noninfective otitis externa, bilateral
        H60.509 Unspecified acute noninfective otitis externa, unspecified ear
    ● **H60.51** Acute actinic otitis externa
        H60.511 Acute actinic otitis externa, right ear
        H60.512 Acute actinic otitis externa, left ear
        H60.513 Acute actinic otitis externa, bilateral
        H60.519 Acute actinic otitis externa, unspecified ear

● **H60.52**   Acute chemical otitis externa

    H60.521   Acute chemical otitis externa, right ear

    H60.522   Acute chemical otitis externa, left ear

    H60.523   Acute chemical otitis externa, bilateral

    H60.529   Acute chemical otitis externa, unspecified ear

● **H60.53**   Acute contact otitis externa

    H60.531   Acute contact otitis externa, right ear

    H60.532   Acute contact otitis externa, left ear

    H60.533   Acute contact otitis externa, bilateral

    H60.539   Acute contact otitis externa, unspecified ear

● **H60.54**   Acute eczematoid otitis externa

    H60.541   Acute eczematoid otitis externa, right ear

    H60.542   Acute eczematoid otitis externa, left ear

    H60.543   Acute eczematoid otitis externa, bilateral

    H60.549   Acute eczematoid otitis externa, unspecified ear

● **H60.55**   Acute reactive otitis externa

    H60.551   Acute reactive otitis externa, right ear

    H60.552   Acute reactive otitis externa, left ear

    H60.553   Acute reactive otitis externa, bilateral

    H60.559   Acute reactive otitis externa, unspecified ear

● **H60.59**   Other noninfective acute otitis externa

    H60.591   Other noninfective acute otitis externa, right ear

    H60.592   Other noninfective acute otitis externa, left ear

    H60.593   Other noninfective acute otitis externa, bilateral

    H60.599   Other noninfective acute otitis externa, unspecified ear

● **H60.6**   Unspecified chronic otitis externa

    H60.60   Unspecified chronic otitis externa, unspecified ear

    H60.61   Unspecified chronic otitis externa, right ear

    H60.62   Unspecified chronic otitis externa, left ear

    H60.63   Unspecified chronic otitis externa, bilateral

● **H60.8**   Other otitis externa

   ● H60.8X   Other otitis externa

    H60.8X1   Other otitis externa, right ear

    H60.8X2   Other otitis externa, left ear

    H60.8X3   Other otitis externa, bilateral

    H60.8X9   Other otitis externa, unspecified ear

● **H60.9**   Unspecified otitis externa

    H60.90   Unspecified otitis externa, unspecified ear

    H60.91   Unspecified otitis externa, right ear

    H60.92   Unspecified otitis externa, left ear

    H60.93   Unspecified otitis externa, bilateral

● **H61**   Other disorders of external ear

   ● H61.0   Chondritis and perichondritis of external ear

     Chondrodermatitis nodularis chronica helicis

     Perichondritis of auricle

     Perichondritis of pinna

    ● H61.00   Unspecified perichondritis of external ear

     H61.001   Unspecified perichondritis of right external ear

     H61.002   Unspecified perichondritis of left external ear

     H61.003   Unspecified perichondritis of external ear, bilateral

     H61.009   Unspecified perichondritis of external ear, unspecified ear

● **H61.01**   Acute perichondritis of external ear

    H61.011   Acute perichondritis of right external ear

    H61.012   Acute perichondritis of left external ear

    H61.013   Acute perichondritis of external ear, bilateral

    H61.019   Acute perichondritis of external ear, unspecified ear

● **H61.02**   Chronic perichondritis of external ear

    H61.021   Chronic perichondritis of right external ear

    H61.022   Chronic perichondritis of left external ear

    H61.023   Chronic perichondritis of external ear, bilateral

    H61.029   Chronic perichondritis of external ear, unspecified ear

● **H61.03**   Chondritis of external ear

     Chondritis of auricle

     Chondritis of pinna

    H61.031   Chondritis of right external ear

    H61.032   Chondritis of left external ear

    H61.033   Chondritis of external ear, bilateral

    H61.039   Chondritis of external ear, unspecified ear

● **H61.1**   Noninfective disorders of pinna

    Excludes2   cauliflower ear (M95.1-)

          gouty tophi of ear (M1A.-)

   ● H61.10   Unspecified noninfective disorders of pinna

     Disorder of pinna NOS

    H61.101   Unspecified noninfective disorders of pinna, right ear

    H61.102   Unspecified noninfective disorders of pinna, left ear

    H61.103   Unspecified noninfective disorders of pinna, bilateral

    H61.109   Unspecified noninfective disorders of pinna, unspecified ear

● **H61.11**   Acquired deformity of pinna

     Acquired deformity of auricle

    Excludes2   cauliflower ear (M95.1-)

    H61.111   Acquired deformity of pinna, right ear

    H61.112   Acquired deformity of pinna, left ear

    H61.113   Acquired deformity of pinna, bilateral

    H61.119   Acquired deformity of pinna, unspecified ear

● **H61.12**   Hematoma of pinna

     Hematoma of auricle

    H61.121   Hematoma of pinna, right ear

    H61.122   Hematoma of pinna, left ear

    H61.123   Hematoma of pinna, bilateral

    H61.129   Hematoma of pinna, unspecified ear

● **H61.19**   Other noninfective disorders of pinna

    H61.191   Noninfective disorders of pinna, right ear

    H61.192   Noninfective disorders of pinna, left ear

    H61.193   Noninfective disorders of pinna, bilateral

    H61.199   Noninfective disorders of pinna, unspecified ear

CHAPTER 8 (H60-H95)

▶ New   ⇒ Revised   ~~deleted~~ Deleted   **OGCR** Official Guidelines   X Assign placeholder X   ● Use Additional Character(s)

Excludes 1   Excludes 2   Includes   Use additional   Code first   Code also   Key words

CHAPTER 8 (H60–H95)

- **H61.2 Impacted cerumen**
  Wax in ear
  - H61.20   Impacted cerumen, unspecified ear
  - H61.21   Impacted cerumen, right ear
  - H61.22   Impacted cerumen, left ear
  - H61.23   Impacted cerumen, bilateral
- **H61.3 Acquired stenosis of external ear canal**
  Collapse of external ear canal
  > **Excludes1**   postprocedural stenosis of external ear canal (H95.81-)
  - **H61.30   Acquired stenosis of external ear canal, unspecified**
    - H61.301   Acquired stenosis of right external ear canal, unspecified
    - H61.302   Acquired stenosis of left external ear canal, unspecified
    - H61.303   Acquired stenosis of external ear canal, unspecified, bilateral
    - H61.309   Acquired stenosis of external ear canal, unspecified, unspecified ear
  - **H61.31   Acquired stenosis of external ear canal secondary to trauma**
    - H61.311   Acquired stenosis of right external ear canal secondary to trauma
    - H61.312   Acquired stenosis of left external ear canal secondary to trauma
    - H61.313   Acquired stenosis of external ear canal secondary to trauma, bilateral
    - H61.319   Acquired stenosis of external ear canal secondary to trauma, unspecified ear
  - **H61.32   Acquired stenosis of external ear canal secondary to inflammation and infection**
    - H61.321   Acquired stenosis of right external ear canal secondary to inflammation and infection
    - H61.322   Acquired stenosis of left external ear canal secondary to inflammation and infection
    - H61.323   Acquired stenosis of external ear canal secondary to inflammation and infection, bilateral
    - H61.329   Acquired stenosis of external ear canal secondary to inflammation and infection, unspecified ear
  - **H61.39   Other acquired stenosis of external ear canal**
    - H61.391   Other acquired stenosis of right external ear canal
    - H61.392   Other acquired stenosis of left external ear canal
    - H61.393   Other acquired stenosis of external ear canal, bilateral
    - H61.399   Other acquired stenosis of external ear canal, unspecified ear
- **H61.8 Other specified disorders of external ear**
  - **H61.81   Exostosis of external canal**
    - H61.811   Exostosis of right external canal
    - H61.812   Exostosis of left external canal
    - H61.813   Exostosis of external canal, bilateral
    - H61.819   Exostosis of external canal, unspecified ear
  - **H61.89   Other specified disorders of external ear**
    - H61.891   Other specified disorders of right external ear
    - H61.892   Other specified disorders of left external ear
    - H61.893   Other specified disorders of external ear, bilateral
    - H61.899   Other specified disorders of external ear, unspecified ear

- **H61.9 Disorder of external ear, unspecified**
  - H61.90   Disorder of external ear, unspecified, unspecified ear
  - H61.91   Disorder of right external ear, unspecified
  - H61.92   Disorder of left external ear, unspecified
  - H61.93   Disorder of external ear, unspecified, bilateral
- **H62   Disorders of external ear in diseases classified elsewhere**
  - **H62.4   Otitis externa in other diseases classified elsewhere**
    Code first underlying disease, such as:
      erysipelas (A46)
      impetigo (L01.0)
    > **Excludes1**   otitis externa (in):
    >   candidiasis (B37.84)
    >   herpes viral [herpes simplex] (B00.1)
    >   herpes zoster (B02.8)
    - H62.40   Otitis externa in other diseases classified elsewhere, unspecified ear
    - H62.41   Otitis externa in other diseases classified elsewhere, right ear
    - H62.42   Otitis externa in other diseases classified elsewhere, left ear
    - H62.43   Otitis externa in other diseases classified elsewhere, bilateral
  - **H62.8   Other disorders of external ear in diseases classified elsewhere**
    Code first underlying disease, such as:
      gout (M1A.-, M10.-)
    - **H62.8X   Other disorders of external ear in diseases classified elsewhere**
      - H62.8X1   Other disorders of right external ear in diseases classified elsewhere
      - H62.8X2   Other disorders of left external ear in diseases classified elsewhere
      - H62.8X3   Other disorders of external ear in diseases classified elsewhere, bilateral
      - H62.8X9   Other disorders of external ear in diseases classified elsewhere, unspecified ear

---

DISEASES OF MIDDLE EAR AND MASTOID (H65–H75)

★ **(See Plate 94 on page 69.)**

- **H65   Nonsuppurative otitis media**
  Bacterial or viral infection or inflammation of the middle ear; may result in fluid accumulation with pain and temporary hearing loss.
  > **Includes**   nonsuppurative otitis media with myringitis

  Use additional code for any associated perforated tympanic membrane (H72.-)
  Use additional code to identify:
    exposure to environmental tobacco smoke (Z77.22)
    exposure to tobacco smoke in the perinatal period (P96.81)
    history of tobacco dependence (Z87.891)
    occupational exposure to environmental tobacco smoke (Z57.31)
    tobacco dependence (F17.-)
    tobacco use (Z72.0)
  - **H65.0   Acute serous otitis media**
    Acute and subacute secretory otitis
    - H65.00   Acute serous otitis media, unspecified ear
    - H65.01   Acute serous otitis media, right ear
    - H65.02   Acute serous otitis media, left ear
    - H65.03   Acute serous otitis media, bilateral
    - H65.04   Acute serous otitis media, recurrent, right ear
    - H65.05   Acute serous otitis media, recurrent, left ear
    - H65.06   Acute serous otitis media, recurrent, bilateral
    - H65.07   Acute serous otitis media, recurrent, unspecified ear

▶ New   ⇒ Revised   ~~deleted~~ Deleted   **OGCR** Official Guidelines   X Assign placeholder X   ● Use Additional Character(s)

Excludes 1   Excludes 2   Includes   Use additional   Code first   Code also   Key words

● **H65.1**   **Other acute** nonsuppurative otitis media

> **Excludes1**   otitic barotrauma (T70.0)
>   otitis media (acute) NOS (H66.9)

● **H65.11**   **Acute and subacute allergic** otitis media (mucoid) (sanguinous) (serous)

     H65.111   Acute and subacute allergic otitis media (mucoid) (sanguinous) (serous), **right ear**

     H65.112   Acute and subacute allergic otitis media (mucoid) (sanguinous) (serous), **left ear**

     H65.113   Acute and subacute allergic otitis media (mucoid) (sanguinous) (serous), **bilateral**

     H65.114   Acute and subacute allergic otitis media (mucoid) (sanguinous) (serous), **recurrent, right ear**

     H65.115   Acute and subacute allergic otitis media (mucoid) (sanguinous) (serous), **recurrent, left ear**

     H65.116   Acute and subacute allergic otitis media (mucoid) (sanguinous) (serous), **recurrent, bilateral**

     H65.117   Acute and subacute allergic otitis media (mucoid) (sanguinous) (serous), **recurrent, unspecified** ear

     H65.119   Acute and subacute allergic otitis media (mucoid) (sanguinous) (serous), **unspecified** ear

● **H65.19**   **Other acute** nonsuppurative otitis media

> Acute and subacute mucoid otitis media
> Acute and subacute nonsuppurative otitis media NOS
> Acute and subacute sanguinous otitis media
> Acute and subacute seromucinous otitis media

     H65.191   Other acute nonsuppurative otitis media, **right ear**

     H65.192   Other acute nonsuppurative otitis media, **left ear**

     H65.193   Other acute nonsuppurative otitis media, **bilateral**

     H65.194   Other acute nonsuppurative otitis media, **recurrent, right ear**

     H65.195   Other acute nonsuppurative otitis media, **recurrent, left ear**

     H65.196   Other acute nonsuppurative otitis media, **recurrent, bilateral**

     H65.197   Other acute nonsuppurative otitis media **recurrent, unspecified** ear

     H65.199   Other acute nonsuppurative otitis media, **unspecified** ear

● **H65.2**   **Chronic serous** otitis media

> Chronic tubotympanal catarrh

     H65.20   Chronic serous otitis media, **unspecified** ear

     H65.21   Chronic serous otitis media, **right ear**

     H65.22   Chronic serous otitis media, **left ear**

     H65.23   Chronic serous otitis media, **bilateral**

● **H65.3**   **Chronic mucoid** otitis media

> Chronic mucinous otitis media
> Chronic secretory otitis media
> Chronic transudative otitis media
> Glue ear

> **Excludes1**   adhesive middle ear disease (H74.1)

     H65.30   Chronic mucoid otitis media, **unspecified** ear

     H65.31   Chronic mucoid otitis media, **right ear**

     H65.32   Chronic mucoid otitis media, **left ear**

     H65.33   Chronic mucoid otitis media, **bilateral**

● **H65.4**   **Other chronic nonsuppurative** otitis media

   ● **H65.41**   Chronic **allergic** otitis media

     H65.411   Chronic allergic otitis media, **right ear**

     H65.412   Chronic allergic otitis media, **left ear**

     H65.413   Chronic allergic otitis media, **bilateral**

     H65.419   Chronic allergic otitis media, **unspecified** ear

   ● **H65.49**   **Other chronic** nonsuppurative otitis media

> Chronic exudative otitis media
> Chronic nonsuppurative otitis media NOS
> Chronic otitis media with effusion (nonpurulent)
> Chronic seromucinous otitis media

     H65.491   Other chronic nonsuppurative otitis media, **right ear**

     H65.492   Other chronic nonsuppurative otitis media, **left ear**

     H65.493   Other chronic nonsuppurative otitis media, **bilateral**

     H65.499   Other chronic nonsuppurative otitis media, **unspecified** ear

● **H65.9**   **Unspecified** nonsuppurative otitis media

> Allergic otitis media NOS
> Catarrhal otitis media NOS
> Exudative otitis media NOS
> Mucoid otitis media NOS
> Otitis media with effusion (nonpurulent) NOS
> Secretory otitis media NOS
> Seromucinous otitis media NOS
> Serous otitis media NOS
> Transudative otitis media NOS

     H65.90   Unspecified nonsuppurative otitis media, **unspecified** ear

     H65.91   Unspecified nonsuppurative otitis media, **right** ear

     H65.92   Unspecified nonsuppurative otitis media, **left** ear

     H65.93   Unspecified nonsuppurative otitis media, **bilateral**

● **H66**   Suppurative and unspecified otitis media

> *Suppurative: Discharging pus*

> **Includes**   suppurative and unspecified otitis media with myringitis

> Use additional code to identify:
>   exposure to environmental tobacco smoke (Z77.22)
>   exposure to tobacco smoke in the perinatal period (P96.81)
>   history of tobacco dependence (Z87.891)
>   occupational exposure to environmental tobacco smoke (Z57.31)
>   tobacco dependence (F17.-)
>   tobacco use (Z72.0)

   ● **H66.0**   **Acute suppurative** otitis media

     ● **H66.00**   Acute suppurative otitis media **without spontaneous rupture of ear drum**

       H66.001   Acute suppurative otitis media without spontaneous rupture of ear drum, **right ear**

       H66.002   Acute suppurative otitis media without spontaneous rupture of ear drum, **left ear**

       H66.003   Acute suppurative otitis media without spontaneous rupture of ear drum, **bilateral**

       H66.004   Acute suppurative otitis media without spontaneous rupture of ear drum, **recurrent, right ear**

       H66.005   Acute suppurative otitis media without spontaneous rupture of ear drum, **recurrent, left ear**

       H66.006   Acute suppurative otitis media without spontaneous rupture of ear drum, **recurrent, bilateral**

H66.007 Acute suppurative otitis media without spontaneous rupture of ear drum, recurrent, unspecified ear

H66.009 Acute suppurative otitis media without spontaneous rupture of ear drum, unspecified ear

● **H66.01** Acute suppurative otitis media with spontaneous rupture of ear drum

H66.011 Acute suppurative otitis media with spontaneous rupture of ear drum, right ear

H66.012 Acute suppurative otitis media with spontaneous rupture of ear drum, left ear

H66.013 Acute suppurative otitis media with spontaneous rupture of ear drum, bilateral

H66.014 Acute suppurative otitis media with spontaneous rupture of ear drum, recurrent, right ear

H66.015 Acute suppurative otitis media with spontaneous rupture of ear drum, recurrent, left ear

H66.016 Acute suppurative otitis media with spontaneous rupture of ear drum, recurrent, bilateral

H66.017 Acute suppurative otitis media with spontaneous rupture of ear drum, recurrent, unspecified ear

H66.019 Acute suppurative otitis media with spontaneous rupture of ear drum, unspecified ear

● **H66.1** Chronic tubotympanic suppurative otitis media
Benign chronic suppurative otitis media
Chronic tubotympanic disease
Use additional code for any associated perforated tympanic membrane (H72.-)

H66.10 Chronic tubotympanic suppurative otitis media, unspecified

H66.11 Chronic tubotympanic suppurative otitis media, right ear

H66.12 Chronic tubotympanic suppurative otitis media, left ear

H66.13 Chronic tubotympanic suppurative otitis media, bilateral

● **H66.2** Chronic atticoantral suppurative otitis media
Chronic atticoantral disease
Use additional code for any associated perforated tympanic membrane (H72.-)

H66.20 Chronic atticoantral suppurative otitis media, unspecified ear

H66.21 Chronic atticoantral suppurative otitis media, right ear

H66.22 Chronic atticoantral suppurative otitis media, left ear

H66.23 Chronic atticoantral suppurative otitis media, bilateral

● **H66.3** Other chronic suppurative otitis media
Chronic suppurative otitis media NOS
Use additional code for any associated perforated tympanic membrane (H72.-)
Excludes1   tuberculous otitis media (A18.6)

● **H66.3X** Other chronic suppurative otitis media

H66.3X1 Other chronic suppurative otitis media, right ear

H66.3X2 Other chronic suppurative otitis media, left ear

H66.3X3 Other chronic suppurative otitis media, bilateral

H66.3X9 Other chronic suppurative otitis media, unspecified ear

● **H66.4** Suppurative otitis media, unspecified
Purulent otitis media NOS
Use additional code for any associated perforated tympanic membrane (H72.-)

H66.40 Suppurative otitis media, unspecified, unspecified ear

H66.41 Suppurative otitis media, unspecified, right ear

H66.42 Suppurative otitis media, unspecified, left ear

H66.43 Suppurative otitis media, unspecified, bilateral

● **H66.9** Otitis media, unspecified
Otitis media NOS
Acute otitis media NOS
Chronic otitis media NOS
Use additional code for any associated perforated tympanic membrane (H72.-)

H66.90 Otitis media, unspecified, unspecified ear

H66.91 Otitis media, unspecified, right ear

H66.92 Otitis media, unspecified, left ear

H66.93 Otitis media, unspecified, bilateral

● **H67** Otitis media in diseases classified elsewhere
Code first underlying disease, such as:
viral disease NEC (B00-B34)
Use additional code for any associated perforated tympanic membrane (H72.-)
Excludes1   otitis media in:
influenza (J09.X9, J10.83, J11.83)
measles (B05.3)
scarlet fever (A38.0)
tuberculosis (A18.6)

H67.1 Otitis media in diseases classified elsewhere, right ear

H67.2 Otitis media in diseases classified elsewhere, left ear

H67.3 Otitis media in diseases classified elsewhere, bilateral

H67.9 Otitis media in diseases classified elsewhere, unspecified ear

● **H68** Eustachian salpingitis and obstruction

● **H68.0** Eustachian salpingitis

● **H68.00** Unspecified Eustachian salpingitis

H68.001 Unspecified Eustachian salpingitis, right ear

H68.002 Unspecified Eustachian salpingitis, left ear

H68.003 Unspecified Eustachian salpingitis, bilateral

H68.009 Unspecified Eustachian salpingitis, unspecified ear

● **H68.01** Acute Eustachian salpingitis

H68.011 Acute Eustachian salpingitis, right ear

H68.012 Acute Eustachian salpingitis, left ear

H68.013 Acute Eustachian salpingitis, bilateral

H68.019 Acute Eustachian salpingitis, unspecified ear

● **H68.02** Chronic Eustachian salpingitis

H68.021 Chronic Eustachian salpingitis, right ear

H68.022 Chronic Eustachian salpingitis, left ear

H68.023 Chronic Eustachian salpingitis, bilateral

H68.029 Chronic Eustachian salpingitis, unspecified ear

▶ New   ⇒ Revised   ~~deleted~~ Deleted   **OGCR** Official Guidelines   X Assign placeholder X   ● Use Additional Character(s)
Excludes 1   Excludes 2   Includes   Use additional   Code first   Code also   Key words

● **H68.1 Obstruction of Eustachian tube**
    Stenosis of Eustachian tube
    Stricture of Eustachian tube

  ● **H68.10 Unspecified obstruction of Eustachian tube**
      H68.101   Unspecified obstruction of Eustachian tube, **right** ear
      H68.102   Unspecified obstruction of Eustachian tube, **left** ear
      H68.103   Unspecified obstruction of Eustachian tube, **bilateral**
      H68.109   Unspecified obstruction of Eustachian tube, **unspecified** ear

  ● **H68.11 Osseous obstruction of Eustachian tube**
      H68.111   Osseous obstruction of Eustachian tube, **right** ear
      H68.112   Osseous obstruction of Eustachian tube, **left** ear
      H68.113   Osseous obstruction of Eustachian tube, **bilateral**
      H68.119   Osseous obstruction of Eustachian tube, **unspecified** ear

  ● **H68.12 Intrinsic cartilagenous obstruction of Eustachian tube**
      H68.121   Intrinsic cartilagenous obstruction of Eustachian tube, **right** ear
      H68.122   Intrinsic cartilagenous obstruction of Eustachian tube, **left** ear
      H68.123   Intrinsic cartilagenous obstruction of Eustachian tube, **bilateral**
      H68.129   Intrinsic cartilagenous obstruction of Eustachian tube, **unspecified** ear

  ● **H68.13 Extrinsic cartilagenous obstruction of Eustachian tube**
    Compression of Eustachian tube
      H68.131   Extrinsic cartilagenous obstruction of Eustachian tube, **right** ear
      H68.132   Extrinsic cartilagenous obstruction of Eustachian tube, **left** ear
      H68.133   Extrinsic cartilagenous obstruction of Eustachian tube, **bilateral**
      H68.139   Extrinsic cartilagenous obstruction of Eustachian tube, **unspecified** ear

● **H69 Other and unspecified disorders of Eustachian tube**

  ● **H69.0 Patulous Eustachian tube**
      H69.00   Patulous Eustachian tube, **unspecified** ear
      H69.01   Patulous Eustachian tube, **right** ear
      H69.02   Patulous Eustachian tube, **left** ear
      H69.03   Patulous Eustachian tube, **bilateral**

  ● **H69.8 Other specified disorders of Eustachian tube**
      H69.80   Other specified disorders of Eustachian tube, **unspecified** ear
      H69.81   Other specified disorders of Eustachian tube, **right** ear
      H69.82   Other specified disorders of Eustachian tube, **left** ear
      H69.83   Other specified disorders of Eustachian tube, **bilateral**

  ● **H69.9 Unspecified Eustachian tube disorder**
      H69.90   Unspecified Eustachian tube disorder, **unspecified** ear
      H69.91   Unspecified Eustachian tube disorder, **right** ear
      H69.92   Unspecified Eustachian tube disorder, **left** ear
      H69.93   Unspecified Eustachian tube disorder, **bilateral**

● **H70 Mastoiditis and related conditions**
  ● **H70.0 Acute mastoiditis**
    Abscess of mastoid
    Empyema of mastoid

    ● **H70.00 Acute mastoiditis without complications**
      H70.001   Acute mastoiditis without complications, **right** ear
      H70.002   Acute mastoiditis without complications, **left** ear
      H70.003   Acute mastoiditis without complications, **bilateral**
      H70.009   Acute mastoiditis without complications, **unspecified** ear

    ● **H70.01 Subperiosteal abscess of mastoid**
      H70.011   Subperiosteal abscess of mastoid, **right** ear
      H70.012   Subperiosteal abscess of mastoid, **left** ear
      H70.013   Subperiosteal abscess of mastoid, **bilateral**
      H70.019   Subperiosteal abscess of mastoid, **unspecified** ear

    ● **H70.09 Acute mastoiditis with other complications**
      H70.091   Acute mastoiditis with other complications, **right** ear
      H70.092   Acute mastoiditis with other complications, **left** ear
      H70.093   Acute mastoiditis with other complications, **bilateral**
      H70.099   Acute mastoiditis with other complications, **unspecified** ear

  ● **H70.1 Chronic mastoiditis**
    Caries of mastoid
    Fistula of mastoid
    Excludes1   tuberculous mastoiditis (A18.03)
    H70.10   Chronic mastoiditis, **unspecified** ear
    H70.11   Chronic mastoiditis, **right** ear
    H70.12   Chronic mastoiditis, **left** ear
    H70.13   Chronic mastoiditis, **bilateral**

  ● **H70.2 Petrositis**
    Inflammation of petrous bone

    ● **H70.20 Unspecified petrositis**
      H70.201   Unspecified petrositis, **right** ear
      H70.202   Unspecified petrositis, **left** ear
      H70.203   Unspecified petrositis, **bilateral**
      H70.209   Unspecified petrositis, **unspecified** ear

    ● **H70.21 Acute petrositis**
      H70.211   Acute petrositis, **right** ear
      H70.212   Acute petrositis, **left** ear
      H70.213   Acute petrositis, **bilateral**
      H70.219   Acute petrositis, **unspecified** ear

    ● **H70.22 Chronic petrositis**
      H70.221   Chronic petrositis, **right** ear
      H70.222   Chronic petrositis, **left** ear
      H70.223   Chronic petrositis, **bilateral**
      H70.229   Chronic petrositis, **unspecified** ear

Item 8–1 Mastoiditis is an infection of the portion of the temporal bone of the skull that is behind the ear (mastoid process) caused by an untreated otitis media, leading to an infection of the surrounding structures which may include the brain.

▶ New   ⇒ Revised   ~~deleted~~ Deleted   **OGCR** Official Guidelines   X Assign placeholder X   ● Use Additional Character(s)

Excludes 1   Excludes 2   Includes   Use additional   Code first   Code also   Key words

CHAPTER 8 (H60-H95)

● **H70.8**   **Other mastoiditis and related conditions**
> **Excludes1**   preauricular sinus and cyst (Q18.1)
> sinus, fistula, and cyst of branchial cleft
> (Q18.0)

  ● **H70.81**   Postauricular fistula
     H70.811   Postauricular fistula, right ear
     H70.812   Postauricular fistula, left ear
     H70.813   Postauricular fistula, bilateral
     H70.819   Postauricular fistula, unspecified ear

  ● **H70.89**   Other mastoiditis and related conditions
     H70.891   Other mastoiditis and related conditions, right ear
     H70.892   Other mastoiditis and related conditions, left ear
     H70.893   Other mastoiditis and related conditions, bilateral
     H70.899   Other mastoiditis and related conditions, unspecified ear

● **H70.9**   Unspecified mastoiditis
     H70.90   Unspecified mastoiditis, unspecified ear
     H70.91   Unspecified mastoiditis, right ear
     H70.92   Unspecified mastoiditis, left ear
     H70.93   Unspecified mastoiditis, bilateral

● **H71**   **Cholesteatoma of middle ear**
> **Excludes2**   cholesteatoma of external ear (H60.4-)
> recurrent cholesteatoma of postmastoidectomy
> cavity (H95.0-)

● **H71.0**   Cholesteatoma of attic
     H71.00   Cholesteatoma of attic, unspecified ear
     H71.01   Cholesteatoma of attic, right ear
     H71.02   Cholesteatoma of attic, left ear
     H71.03   Cholesteatoma of attic, bilateral

● **H71.1**   Cholesteatoma of tympanum
     H71.10   Cholesteatoma of tympanum, unspecified ear
     H71.11   Cholesteatoma of tympanum, right ear
     H71.12   Cholesteatoma of tympanum, left ear
     H71.13   Cholesteatoma of tympanum, bilateral

● **H71.2**   Cholesteatoma of mastoid
     H71.20   Cholesteatoma of mastoid, unspecified ear
     H71.21   Cholesteatoma of mastoid, right ear
     H71.22   Cholesteatoma of mastoid, left ear
     H71.23   Cholesteatoma of mastoid, bilateral

● **H71.3**   Diffuse cholesteatosis
     H71.30   Diffuse cholesteatosis, unspecified ear
     H71.31   Diffuse cholesteatosis, right ear
     H71.32   Diffuse cholesteatosis, left ear
     H71.33   Diffuse cholesteatosis, bilateral

● **H71.9**   Unspecified cholesteatoma
     H71.90   Unspecified cholesteatoma, unspecified ear
     H71.91   Unspecified cholesteatoma, right ear
     H71.92   Unspecified cholesteatoma, left ear
     H71.93   Unspecified cholesteatoma, bilateral

★ **(See Plate 93 on page 69.)**

● **H72**   **Perforation of tympanic membrane**
Hole or rupture in ear drum
> **Includes**   persistent post-traumatic perforation of ear drum
> postinflammatory perforation of ear drum

Code first any associated otitis media (H65.-, H66.1-, H66.2-, H66.3-, H66.4-, H66.9-, H67.-)
> **Excludes1**   acute suppurative otitis media with rupture of
> the tympanic membrane (H66.01-)
> traumatic rupture of ear drum (S09.2-)

● **H72.0**   Central perforation of tympanic membrane
     H72.00   Central perforation of tympanic membrane, unspecified ear
     H72.01   Central perforation of tympanic membrane, right ear
     H72.02   Central perforation of tympanic membrane, left ear
     H72.03   Central perforation of tympanic membrane, bilateral

● **H72.1**   Attic perforation of tympanic membrane
Perforation of pars flaccida
     H72.10   Attic perforation of tympanic membrane, unspecified ear
     H72.11   Attic perforation of tympanic membrane, right ear
     H72.12   Attic perforation of tympanic membrane, left ear
     H72.13   Attic perforation of tympanic membrane, bilateral

● **H72.2**   Other marginal perforations of tympanic membrane
  ● **H72.2X**   Other marginal perforations of tympanic membrane
     H72.2X1   Other marginal perforations of tympanic membrane, right ear
     H72.2X2   Other marginal perforations of tympanic membrane, left ear
     H72.2X3   Other marginal perforations of tympanic membrane, bilateral
     H72.2X9   Other marginal perforations of tympanic membrane, unspecified ear

● **H72.8**   Other perforations of tympanic membrane
  ● **H72.81**   Multiple perforations of tympanic membrane
     H72.811   Multiple perforations of tympanic membrane, right ear
     H72.812   Multiple perforations of tympanic membrane, left ear
     H72.813   Multiple perforations of tympanic membrane, bilateral
     H72.819   Multiple perforations of tympanic membrane, unspecified ear

  ● **H72.82**   Total perforations of tympanic membrane
     H72.821   Total perforations of tympanic membrane, right ear
     H72.822   Total perforations of tympanic membrane, left ear
     H72.823   Total perforations of tympanic membrane, bilateral
     H72.829   Total perforations of tympanic membrane, unspecified ear

● **H72.9**   Unspecified perforation of tympanic membrane
     H72.90   Unspecified perforation of tympanic membrane, unspecified ear
     H72.91   Unspecified perforation of tympanic membrane, right ear
     H72.92   Unspecified perforation of tympanic membrane, left ear
     H72.93   Unspecified perforation of tympanic membrane, bilateral

CHAPTER 8 (H60-H95)

▶ New   ➡ Revised   ~~deleted~~ Deleted   **OGCR** Official Guidelines   X Assign placeholder X   ● Use Additional Character(s)

Excludes 1   Excludes 2   Includes   Use additional   Code first   Code also   Key words

● **H73**   Other disorders of tympanic membrane
  ● **H73.0**   Acute myringitis
     Excludes1   acute myringitis with otitis media (H65, H66)
    ● **H73.00**   Unspecified acute myringitis
       Acute tympanitis NOS
       H73.001   Acute myringitis, right ear
       H73.002   Acute myringitis, left ear
       H73.003   Acute myringitis, bilateral
       H73.009   Acute myringitis, unspecified ear
    ● **H73.01**   Bullous myringitis
       H73.011   Bullous myringitis, right ear
       H73.012   Bullous myringitis, left ear
       H73.013   Bullous myringitis, bilateral
       H73.019   Bullous myringitis, unspecified ear
    ● **H73.09**   Other acute myringitis
       H73.091   Other acute myringitis, right ear
       H73.092   Other acute myringitis, left ear
       H73.093   Other acute myringitis, bilateral
       H73.099   Other acute myringitis, unspecified ear
  ● **H73.1**   Chronic myringitis
     Chronic tympanitis
     Excludes1   chronic myringitis with otitis media (H65, H66)
     H73.10   Chronic myringitis, unspecified ear
     H73.11   Chronic myringitis, right ear
     H73.12   Chronic myringitis, left ear
     H73.13   Chronic myringitis, bilateral
  ● **H73.2**   Unspecified myringitis
     H73.20   Unspecified myringitis, unspecified ear
     H73.21   Unspecified myringitis, right ear
     H73.22   Unspecified myringitis, left ear
     H73.23   Unspecified myringitis, bilateral
  ● **H73.8**   Other specified disorders of tympanic membrane
    ● **H73.81**   Atrophic flaccid tympanic membrane
       H73.811   Atrophic flaccid tympanic membrane, right ear
       H73.812   Atrophic flaccid tympanic membrane, left ear
       H73.813   Atrophic flaccid tympanic membrane, bilateral
       H73.819   Atrophic flaccid tympanic membrane, unspecified ear
    ● **H73.82**   Atrophic nonflaccid tympanic membrane
       H73.821   Atrophic nonflaccid tympanic membrane, right ear
       H73.822   Atrophic nonflaccid tympanic membrane, left ear
       H73.823   Atrophic nonflaccid tympanic membrane, bilateral
       H73.829   Atrophic nonflaccid tympanic membrane, unspecified ear
    ● **H73.89**   Other specified disorders of tympanic membrane
       H73.891   Other specified disorders of tympanic membrane, right ear
       H73.892   Other specified disorders of tympanic membrane, left ear
       H73.893   Other specified disorders of tympanic membrane, bilateral
       H73.899   Other specified disorders of tympanic membrane, unspecified ear

● **H73.9**   Unspecified disorder of tympanic membrane
     H73.90   Unspecified disorder of tympanic membrane, unspecified ear
     H73.91   Unspecified disorder of tympanic membrane, right ear
     H73.92   Unspecified disorder of tympanic membrane, left ear
     H73.93   Unspecified disorder of tympanic membrane, bilateral

● **H74**   Other disorders of middle ear mastoid
     Excludes2   mastoiditis (H70.-)
  ● **H74.0**   Tympanosclerosis
     H74.01   Tympanosclerosis, right ear
     H74.02   Tympanosclerosis, left ear
     H74.03   Tympanosclerosis, bilateral
     H74.09   Tympanosclerosis, unspecified ear
  ● **H74.1**   Adhesive middle ear disease
     Adhesive otitis
     Excludes1   glue ear (H65.3-)
     H74.11   Adhesive right middle ear disease
     H74.12   Adhesive left middle ear disease
     H74.13   Adhesive middle ear disease, bilateral
     H74.19   Adhesive middle ear disease, unspecified ear
  ● **H74.2**   Discontinuity and dislocation of ear ossicles
     H74.20   Discontinuity and dislocation of ear ossicles, unspecified ear
     H74.21   Discontinuity and dislocation of right ear ossicles
     H74.22   Discontinuity and dislocation of left ear ossicles
     H74.23   Discontinuity and dislocation of ear ossicles, bilateral
  ● **H74.3**   Other acquired abnormalities of ear ossicles
    ● **H74.31**   Ankylosis of ear ossicles
       H74.311   Ankylosis of ear ossicles, right ear
       H74.312   Ankylosis of ear ossicles, left ear
       H74.313   Ankylosis of ear ossicles, bilateral
       H74.319   Ankylosis of ear ossicles, unspecified ear
    ● **H74.32**   Partial loss of ear ossicles
       H74.321   Partial loss of ear ossicles, right ear
       H74.322   Partial loss of ear ossicles, left ear
       H74.323   Partial loss of ear ossicles, bilateral
       H74.329   Partial loss of ear ossicles, unspecified ear
    ● **H74.39**   Other acquired abnormalities of ear ossicles
       H74.391   Other acquired abnormalities of right ear ossicles
       H74.392   Other acquired abnormalities of left ear ossicles
       H74.393   Other acquired abnormalities of ear ossicles, bilateral
       H74.399   Other acquired abnormalities of ear ossicles, unspecified ear
  ● **H74.4**   Polyp of middle ear
     H74.40   Polyp of middle ear, unspecified ear
     H74.41   Polyp of right middle ear
     H74.42   Polyp of left middle ear
     H74.43   Polyp of middle ear, bilateral

CHAPTER 8 (H60–H95)

● H74.8　Other specified disorders of middle ear and mastoid

　● H74.8X　Other specified disorders of middle ear and mastoid

　　　H74.8X1　Other specified disorders of right middle ear and mastoid

　　　H74.8X2　Other specified disorders of left middle ear and mastoid

　　　H74.8X3　Other specified disorders of middle ear and mastoid, bilateral

　　　H74.8X9　Other specified disorders of middle ear and mastoid, unspecified ear

● H74.9　Unspecified disorder of middle ear and mastoid

　　H74.90　Unspecified disorder of middle ear and mastoid, unspecified ear

　　H74.91　Unspecified disorder of right middle ear and mastoid

　　H74.92　Unspecified disorder of left middle ear and mastoid

　　H74.93　Unspecified disorder of middle ear and mastoid, bilateral

● H75　Other disorders of middle ear and mastoid in diseases classified elsewhere

　　　Code first underlying disease

　● H75.0　Mastoiditis in infectious and parasitic diseases classified elsewhere

　　　　Excludes1　mastoiditis (in):
　　　　　　　syphilis (A52.77)
　　　　　　　tuberculosis (A18.03)

　　　H75.00　Mastoiditis in infectious and parasitic diseases classified elsewhere, unspecified ear

　　　H75.01　Mastoiditis in infectious and parasitic diseases classified elsewhere, right ear

　　　H75.02　Mastoiditis in infectious and parasitic diseases classified elsewhere, left ear

　　　H75.03　Mastoiditis in infectious and parasitic diseases classified elsewhere, bilateral

　● H75.8　Other specified disorders of middle ear and mastoid in diseases classified elsewhere

　　　H75.80　Other specified disorders of middle ear and mastoid in diseases classified elsewhere, unspecified ear

　　　H75.81　Other specified disorders of right middle ear and mastoid in diseases classified elsewhere

　　　H75.82　Other specified disorders of left middle ear and mastoid in diseases classified elsewhere

　　　H75.83　Other specified disorders of middle ear and mastoid in diseases classified elsewhere, bilateral

DISEASES OF INNER EAR (H80-H83)

★ **(See Plate 95 on page 69.)**

● H80　Otosclerosis

　　　Inherited middle ear spongelike bone growth causing hearing loss

　　　Includes　Otospongiosis

　● H80.0　Otosclerosis involving oval window, nonobliterative

　　　H80.00　Otosclerosis involving oval window, nonobliterative, unspecified ear

　　　H80.01　Otosclerosis involving oval window, nonobliterative, right ear

　　　H80.02　Otosclerosis involving oval window, nonobliterative, left ear

　　　H80.03　Otosclerosis involving oval window, nonobliterative, bilateral

● H80.1　Otosclerosis involving oval window, obliterative

　　H80.10　Otosclerosis involving oval window, obliterative, unspecified ear

　　H80.11　Otosclerosis involving oval window, obliterative, right ear

　　H80.12　Otosclerosis involving oval window, obliterative, left ear

　　H80.13　Otosclerosis involving oval window, obliterative, bilateral

● H80.2　Cochlear otosclerosis

　　　Otosclerosis involving otic capsule
　　　Otosclerosis involving round window

　　H80.20　Cochlear otosclerosis, unspecified ear

　　H80.21　Cochlear otosclerosis, right ear

　　H80.22　Cochlear otosclerosis, left ear

　　H80.23　Cochlear otosclerosis, bilateral

● H80.8　Other otosclerosis

　　H80.80　Other otosclerosis, unspecified ear

　　H80.81　Other otosclerosis, right ear

　　H80.82　Other otosclerosis, left ear

　　H80.83　Other otosclerosis, bilateral

● H80.9　Unspecified otosclerosis

　　H80.90　Unspecified otosclerosis, unspecified ear

　　H80.91　Unspecified otosclerosis, right ear

　　H80.92　Unspecified otosclerosis, left ear

　　H80.93　Unspecified otosclerosis, bilateral

● H81　Disorders of vestibular function

　　　Excludes1　epidemic vertigo (A88.1)
　　　　　　　vertigo NOS (R42)

　● H81.0　Ménière's disease

　　　　Vestibular disorder that produces recurring symptoms including severe and intermittent hearing loss including the feeling of ear pressure or pain
　　　Labyrinthine hydrops
　　　Ménière's syndrome or vertigo

　　　H81.01　Ménière's disease, right ear

　　　H81.02　Ménière's disease, left ear

　　　H81.03　Ménière's disease, bilateral

　　　H81.09　Ménière's disease, unspecified ear

　● H81.1　Benign paroxysmal vertigo

　　　H81.10　Benign paroxysmal vertigo, unspecified ear

　　　H81.11　Benign paroxysmal vertigo, right ear

　　　H81.12　Benign paroxysmal vertigo, left ear

　　　H81.13　Benign paroxysmal vertigo, bilateral

　● H81.2　Vestibular neuronitis

　　　H81.20　Vestibular neuronitis, unspecified ear

　　　H81.21　Vestibular neuronitis, right ear

　　　H81.22　Vestibular neuronitis, left ear

　　　H81.23　Vestibular neuronitis, bilateral

　● H81.3　Other peripheral vertigo

　　● H81.31　Aural vertigo

　　　　H81.311　Aural vertigo, right ear

　　　　H81.312　Aural vertigo, left ear

　　　　H81.313　Aural vertigo, bilateral

　　　　H81.319　Aural vertigo, unspecified ear

　　● H81.39　Other peripheral vertigo

　　　　Lermoyez' syndrome
　　　　Otogenic vertigo
　　　　Peripheral vertigo NOS

　　　　H81.391　Other peripheral vertigo, right ear

　　　　H81.392　Other peripheral vertigo, left ear

　　　　H81.393　Other peripheral vertigo, bilateral

　　　　H81.399　Other peripheral vertigo, unspecified ear

▶ New　⇒ Revised　~~deleted~~ Deleted　**OGCR** Official Guidelines　X Assign placeholder X　● Use Additional Character(s)

Excludes 1　Excludes 2　Includes　Use additional　Code first　Code also　Key words

● H81.4   **Vertigo of central origin**
     Central positional nystagmus
   H81.41   Vertigo of central origin, right ear
   H81.42   Vertigo of central origin, left ear
   H81.43   Vertigo of central origin, bilateral
   H81.49   Vertigo of central origin, unspecified ear

● H81.8   **Other disorders of vestibular function**
   ● H81.8X   Other disorders of vestibular function
     H81.8X1   Other disorders of vestibular function, right ear
     H81.8X2   Other disorders of vestibular function, left ear
     H81.8X3   Other disorders of vestibular function, bilateral
     H81.8X9   Other disorders of vestibular function, unspecified ear

● H81.9   **Unspecified disorder of vestibular function**
     Vertiginous syndrome NOS
   H81.90   Unspecified disorder of vestibular function, unspecified ear
   H81.91   Unspecified disorder of vestibular function, right ear
   H81.92   Unspecified disorder of vestibular function, left ear
   H81.93   Unspecified disorder of vestibular function, bilateral

● H82   **Vertiginous syndromes in diseases classified elsewhere**
     Code first underlying disease
     Excludes1   epidemic vertigo (A88.1)
   H82.1   Vertiginous syndromes in diseases classified elsewhere, right ear
   H82.2   Vertiginous syndromes in diseases classified elsewhere, left ear
   H82.3   Vertiginous syndromes in diseases classified elsewhere, bilateral
   H82.9   Vertiginous syndromes in diseases classified elsewhere, unspecified ear

● H83   **Other diseases of inner ear**
   ● H83.0   Labyrinthitis
     Balance disorder that follows URI or head injury
     H83.01   Labyrinthitis, right ear
     H83.02   Labyrinthitis, left ear
     H83.03   Labyrinthitis, bilateral
     H83.09   Labyrinthitis, unspecified ear
   ● H83.1   Labyrinthine fistula
     H83.11   Labyrinthine fistula, right ear
     H83.12   Labyrinthine fistula, left ear
     H83.13   Labyrinthine fistula, bilateral
     H83.19   Labyrinthine fistula, unspecified ear
   ● H83.2   Labyrinthine dysfunction
     Labyrinthine hypersensitivity
     Labyrinthine hypofunction
     Labyrinthine loss of function
     ● H83.2X   Labyrinthine dysfunction
       H83.2X1   Labyrinthine dysfunction, right ear
       H83.2X2   Labyrinthine dysfunction, left ear
       H83.2X3   Labyrinthine dysfunction, bilateral
       H83.2X9   Labyrinthine dysfunction, unspecified ear
   ● H83.3   Noise effects on inner ear
     Acoustic trauma of inner ear
     Noise-induced hearing loss of inner ear
     ● H83.3X   Noise effects on inner ear
       H83.3X1   Noise effects on right inner ear
       H83.3X2   Noise effects on left inner ear
       H83.3X3   Noise effects on inner ear, bilateral
       H83.3X9   Noise effects on inner ear, unspecified ear

● H83.8   **Other specified diseases of inner ear**
   ● H83.8X   Other specified diseases of inner ear
     H83.8X1   Other specified diseases of right inner ear
     H83.8X2   Other specified diseases of left inner ear
     H83.8X3   Other specified diseases of inner ear, bilateral
     H83.8X9   Other specified diseases of inner ear, unspecified ear

● H83.9   **Unspecified disease of inner ear**
   H83.90   Unspecified disease of inner ear, unspecified ear
   H83.91   Unspecified disease of right inner ear
   H83.92   Unspecified disease of left inner ear
   H83.93   Unspecified disease of inner ear, bilateral

OTHER DISORDERS OF EAR (H90-H94)

● H90   **Conductive and sensorineural hearing loss**
     Excludes1   deaf nonspeaking NEC (H91.3)
              deafness NOS (H91.9-)
              hearing loss NOS (H91.9-)
              noise-induced hearing loss (H83.3-)
              ototoxic hearing loss (H91.0-)
              sudden (idiopathic) hearing loss (H91.2-)
   H90.0   Conductive hearing loss, bilateral
   ● H90.1   Conductive hearing loss, unilateral with unrestricted hearing on the contralateral side
     H90.11   Conductive hearing loss, unilateral, right ear, with unrestricted hearing on the contralateral side
     H90.12   Conductive hearing loss, unilateral, left ear, with unrestricted hearing on the contralateral side
   H90.2   Conductive hearing loss, unspecified
     Conductive deafness NOS
   H90.3   Sensorineural hearing loss, bilateral
   ● H90.4   Sensorineural hearing loss, unilateral with unrestricted hearing on the contralateral side
     H90.41   Sensorineural hearing loss, unilateral, right ear, with unrestricted hearing on the contralateral side
     H90.42   Sensorineural hearing loss, unilateral, left ear, with unrestricted hearing on the contralateral side
   H90.5   Unspecified sensorineural hearing loss
     Central hearing loss NOS
     Congenital deafness NOS
     Neural hearing loss NOS
     Perceptive hearing loss NOS
     Sensorineural deafness NOS
     Sensory hearing loss NOS
     Excludes1   abnormal auditory perception (H93.2-)
              psychogenic deafness (F44.6)
   H90.6   Mixed conductive and sensorineural hearing loss, bilateral
   ● H90.7   Mixed conductive and sensorineural hearing loss, unilateral with unrestricted hearing on the contralateral side
     H90.71   Mixed conductive and sensorineural hearing loss, unilateral, right ear, with unrestricted hearing on the contralateral side
     H90.72   Mixed conductive and sensorineural hearing loss, unilateral, left ear, with unrestricted hearing on the contralateral side
   H90.8   Mixed conductive and sensorineural hearing loss, unspecified

CHAPTER 8 (H60-H95)

● H90.A Conductive and sensorineural hearing loss with restricted hearing on the contralateral side
  ● H90.A1 Conductive hearing loss, unilateral, with restricted hearing on the contralateral side
    H90.A11 Conductive hearing loss, unilateral, right ear with restricted hearing on the contralateral side
    H90.A12 Conductive hearing loss, unilateral, left ear with restricted hearing on the contralateral side
  ● H90.A2 Sensorineural hearing loss, unilateral, with restricted hearing on the contralateral side
    H90.A21 Sensorineural hearing loss, unilateral, right ear, with restricted hearing on the contralateral side
    H90.A22 Sensorineural hearing loss, unilateral, left ear, with restricted hearing on the contralateral side
  ● H90.A3 Mixed conductive and sensorineural hearing loss, unilateral with restricted hearing on the contralateral side
    H90.A31 Mixed conductive and sensorineural hearing loss, unilateral, right ear with restricted hearing on the contralateral side
    H90.A32 Mixed conductive and sensorineural hearing loss, unilateral, left ear with restricted hearing on the contralateral side

● H91 Other and unspecified hearing loss
  Excludes1 abnormal auditory perception (H93.2-)
    hearing loss as classified in H90.-
    impacted cerumen (H61.2-)
    noise-induced hearing loss (H83.3-)
    psychogenic deafness (F44.6)
    transient ischemic deafness (H93.01-)
  ● H91.0 Ototoxic hearing loss
    Code first poisoning due to drug or toxin, if applicable (T36-T65 with fifth or sixth character 1-4 or 6)
    Use additional code for adverse effect, if applicable, to identify drug (T36-T50 with fifth or sixth character 5)
    H91.01 Ototoxic hearing loss, right ear
    H91.02 Ototoxic hearing loss, left ear
    H91.03 Ototoxic hearing loss, bilateral
    H91.09 Ototoxic hearing loss, unspecified ear
  ● H91.1 Presbycusis
    Presbyacusia
    H91.10 Presbycusis, unspecified ear
    H91.11 Presbycusis, right ear
    H91.12 Presbycusis, left ear
    H91.13 Presbycusis, bilateral
  ● H91.2 Sudden idiopathic hearing loss
    Sudden hearing loss NOS
    H91.20 Sudden idiopathic hearing loss, unspecified ear
    H91.21 Sudden idiopathic hearing loss, right ear
    H91.22 Sudden idiopathic hearing loss, left ear
    H91.23 Sudden idiopathic hearing loss, bilateral
  H91.3 Deaf nonspeaking, not elsewhere classified
  ● H91.8 Other specified hearing loss
    ● H91.8X Other specified hearing loss
      H91.8X1 Other specified hearing loss, right ear
      H91.8X2 Other specified hearing loss, left ear
      H91.8X3 Other specified hearing loss, bilateral
      H91.8X9 Other specified hearing loss, unspecified ear

● H91.9 Unspecified hearing loss
  Deafness NOS
  High frequency deafness
  Low frequency deafness
  H91.90 Unspecified hearing loss, unspecified ear
  H91.91 Unspecified hearing loss, right ear
  H91.92 Unspecified hearing loss, left ear
  H91.93 Unspecified hearing loss, bilateral

● H92 Otalgia and effusion of ear
  ● H92.0 Otalgia
    H92.01 Otalgia, right ear
    H92.02 Otalgia, left ear
    H92.03 Otalgia, bilateral
    H92.09 Otalgia, unspecified ear
  ● H92.1 Otorrhea
    Excludes1 leakage of cerebrospinal fluid through ear (G96.0)
    H92.10 Otorrhea, unspecified ear
    H92.11 Otorrhea, right ear
    H92.12 Otorrhea, left ear
    H92.13 Otorrhea, bilateral
  ● H92.2 Otorrhagia
    Excludes1 traumatic otorrhagia - code to injury
    H92.20 Otorrhagia, unspecified ear
    H92.21 Otorrhagia, right ear
    H92.22 Otorrhagia, left ear
    H92.23 Otorrhagia, bilateral

● H93 Other disorders of ear, not elsewhere classified
  ● H93.0 Degenerative and vascular disorders of ear
    Excludes1 presbycusis (H91.1)
    ● H93.01 Transient ischemic deafness
      H93.011 Transient ischemic deafness, right ear
      H93.012 Transient ischemic deafness, left ear
      H93.013 Transient ischemic deafness, bilateral
      H93.019 Transient ischemic deafness, unspecified ear
    ● H93.09 Unspecified degenerative and vascular disorders of ear
      H93.091 Unspecified degenerative and vascular disorders of right ear
      H93.092 Unspecified degenerative and vascular disorders of left ear
      H93.093 Unspecified degenerative and vascular disorders of ear, bilateral
      H93.099 Unspecified degenerative and vascular disorders of unspecified ear
  ● H93.1 Tinnitus
    Perception of sound (ringing, buzzing, humming, whistling tunes, or singing)
    H93.11 Tinnitus, right ear
    H93.12 Tinnitus, left ear
    H93.13 Tinnitus, bilateral
    H93.19 Tinnitus, unspecified ear
  ● H93.A Pulsatile tinnitus
    H93.A1 Pulsatile tinnitus, right ear
    H93.A2 Pulsatile tinnitus, left ear
    H93.A3 Pulsatile tinnitus, bilateral
    H93.A9 Pulsatile tinnitus, unspecified ear

▶ New   ⇒ Revised   ~~deleted~~ Deleted   OGCR Official Guidelines   X Assign placeholder X   ● Use Additional Character(s)

Excludes 1   Excludes 2   Includes   Use additional   Code first   Code also   Key words

● **H93.2   Other abnormal auditory perceptions**
     Excludes2   auditory hallucinations (R44.0)
     ● **H93.21   Auditory recruitment**
         H93.211   Auditory recruitment, **right** ear
         H93.212   Auditory recruitment, **left** ear
         H93.213   Auditory recruitment, **bilateral**
         H93.219   Auditory recruitment, **unspecified** ear
     ● **H93.22   Diplacusis**
         H93.221   Diplacusis, **right** ear
         H93.222   Diplacusis, **left** ear
         H93.223   Diplacusis, **bilateral**
         H93.229   Diplacusis, **unspecified** ear
     ● **H93.23   Hyperacusis**
         H93.231   Hyperacusis, **right** ear
         H93.232   Hyperacusis, **left** ear
         H93.233   Hyperacusis, **bilateral**
         H93.239   Hyperacusis, **unspecified** ear
     ● **H93.24   Temporary auditory threshold shift**
         H93.241   Temporary auditory threshold shift, **right** ear
         H93.242   Temporary auditory threshold shift, **left** ear
         H93.243   Temporary auditory threshold shift, **bilateral**
         H93.249   Temporary auditory threshold shift, **unspecified** ear
     H93.25   Central auditory processing disorder
         Congenital auditory imperception
         Word deafness
         Excludes1   mixed receptive-expressive language disorder (F80.2)
     ● **H93.29   Other abnormal auditory perceptions**
         H93.291   Other abnormal auditory perceptions, **right** ear
         H93.292   Other abnormal auditory perceptions, **left** ear
         H93.293   Other abnormal auditory perceptions, **bilateral**
         H93.299   Other abnormal auditory perceptions, **unspecified** ear

● **H93.3   Disorders of acoustic nerve**
     Disorder of 8th cranial nerve
     Excludes1   acoustic neuroma (D33.3)
                 syphilitic acoustic neuritis (A52.15)
     ● **H93.3X   Disorders of acoustic nerve**
         H93.3X1   Disorders of **right** acoustic nerve
         H93.3X2   Disorders of **left** acoustic nerve
         H93.3X3   Disorders of **bilateral** acoustic nerves
         H93.3X9   Disorders of **unspecified** acoustic nerve

● **H93.8   Other specified disorders of ear**
     ● **H93.8X   Other specified disorders of ear**
         H93.8X1   Other specified disorders of **right** ear
         H93.8X2   Other specified disorders of **left** ear
         H93.8X3   Other specified disorders of ear, **bilateral**
         H93.8X9   Other specified disorders of ear, **unspecified** ear

● **H93.9   Unspecified disorder of ear**
     H93.90   Unspecified disorder of ear, **unspecified** ear
     H93.91   Unspecified disorder of **right** ear
     H93.92   Unspecified disorder of **left** ear
     H93.93   Unspecified disorder of ear, **bilateral**

● **H94   Other disorders of ear in diseases classified elsewhere**
     ● **H94.0   Acoustic neuritis in infectious and parasitic diseases classified elsewhere**
         Code first underlying disease, such as:
         parasitic disease (B65-B89)
         Excludes1   acoustic neuritis (in):
                 herpes zoster (B02.29)
                 syphilis (A52.15)
         H94.00   Acoustic neuritis in infectious and parasitic diseases classified elsewhere, **unspecified** ear
         H94.01   Acoustic neuritis in infectious and parasitic diseases classified elsewhere, **right** ear
         H94.02   Acoustic neuritis in infectious and parasitic diseases classified elsewhere, **left** ear
         H94.03   Acoustic neuritis in infectious and parasitic diseases classified elsewhere, **bilateral**
     ● **H94.8   Other specified disorders of ear in diseases classified elsewhere**
         Code first underlying disease, such as:
         congenital syphilis (A50.0)
         Excludes1   aural myiasis (B87.4)
                 syphilitic labyrinthitis (A52.79)
         H94.80   Other specified disorders of ear in diseases classified elsewhere, **unspecified** ear
         H94.81   Other specified disorders of **right** ear in diseases classified elsewhere
         H94.82   Other specified disorders of **left** ear in diseases classified elsewhere
         H94.83   Other specified disorders of ear in diseases classified elsewhere, **bilateral**

● **H95   Intraoperative and postprocedural complications and disorders of ear and mastoid process, not elsewhere classified**
     ● **H95.0   Recurrent cholesteatoma of postmastoidectomy cavity**
         H95.00   Recurrent cholesteatoma of postmastoidectomy cavity, **unspecified** ear
         H95.01   Recurrent cholesteatoma of postmastoidectomy cavity, **right** ear
         H95.02   Recurrent cholesteatoma of postmastoidectomy cavity, **left** ear
         H95.03   Recurrent cholesteatoma of postmastoidectomy cavity, **bilateral** ears
     ● **H95.1   Other disorders of ear and mastoid process following mastoidectomy**
         ● **H95.11   Chronic inflammation of postmastoidectomy cavity**
                 H95.111   Chronic inflammation of postmastoidectomy cavity, **right** ear
                 H95.112   Chronic inflammation of postmastoidectomy cavity, **left** ear
                 H95.113   Chronic inflammation of postmastoidectomy cavity, **bilateral** ears
                 H95.119   Chronic inflammation of postmastoidectomy cavity, **unspecified** ear
         ● **H95.12   Granulation of postmastoidectomy cavity**
                 H95.121   Granulation of postmastoidectomy cavity, **right** ear
                 H95.122   Granulation of postmastoidectomy cavity, **left** ear
                 H95.123   Granulation of postmastoidectomy cavity, **bilateral** ears
                 H95.129   Granulation of postmastoidectomy cavity, **unspecified** ear

● H95.13   Mucosal cyst of postmastoidectomy cavity

     H95.131   Mucosal cyst of postmastoidectomy cavity, right ear

     H95.132   Mucosal cyst of postmastoidectomy cavity, left ear

     H95.133   Mucosal cyst of postmastoidectomy cavity, bilateral ears

     H95.139   Mucosal cyst of postmastoidectomy cavity, unspecified ear

● H95.19   Other disorders following mastoidectomy

     H95.191   Other disorders following mastoidectomy, right ear

     H95.192   Other disorders following mastoidectomy, left ear

     H95.193   Other disorders following mastoidectomy, bilateral ears

     H95.199   Other disorders following mastoidectomy, unspecified ear

● H95.2   Intraoperative hemorrhage and hematoma of ear and mastoid process complicating a procedure

     Excludes1   intraoperative hemorrhage and hematoma of ear and mastoid process due to accidental puncture or laceration during a procedure (H95.3-)

     H95.21   Intraoperative hemorrhage and hematoma of ear and mastoid process complicating a procedure on the ear and mastoid process

     H95.22   Intraoperative hemorrhage and hematoma of ear and mastoid process complicating other procedure

● H95.3   Accidental puncture and laceration of ear and mastoid process during a procedure

     H95.31   Accidental puncture and laceration of the ear and mastoid process during a procedure on the ear and mastoid process

     H95.32   Accidental puncture and laceration of the ear and mastoid process during other procedure

● H95.4   Postprocedural hemorrhage of ear and mastoid process following a procedure

     H95.41   Postprocedural hemorrhage of ear and mastoid process following a procedure on the ear and mastoid process

     H95.42   Postprocedural hemorrhage of ear and mastoid process following other procedure

● H95.5   Postprocedural hematoma and seroma of ear and mastoid process following a procedure

     H95.51   Postprocedural hematoma of ear and mastoid process following a procedure on the ear and mastoid process

     H95.52   Postprocedural hematoma of ear and mastoid process following other procedure

     H95.53   Postprocedural seroma of ear and mastoid process following a procedure on the ear and mastoid process

     H95.54   Postprocedural seroma of ear and mastoid process following other procedure

● H95.8   Other intraoperative and postprocedural complications and disorders of the ear and mastoid process, not elsewhere classified

     Excludes2   postprocedural complications and disorders following mastoidectomy (H95.0-, H95.1-)

● H95.81   Postprocedural stenosis of external ear canal

     H95.811   Postprocedural stenosis of right external ear canal

     H95.812   Postprocedural stenosis of left external ear canal

     H95.813   Postprocedural stenosis of external ear canal, bilateral

     H95.819   Postprocedural stenosis of unspecified external ear canal

     H95.88   Other intraoperative complications and disorders of the ear and mastoid process, not elsewhere classified

       Use additional code, if applicable, to further specify disorder

     H95.89   Other postprocedural complications and disorders of the ear and mastoid process, not elsewhere classified

       Use additional code, if applicable, to further specify disorder

▶ New   ⟹ Revised   ~~deleted~~ Deleted   **OGCR** Official Guidelines   X Assign placeholder X   ● Use Additional Character(s)

Excludes 1   Excludes 2   Includes   Use additional   Code first   Code also   Key words

CHAPTER 9

DISEASES OF THE CIRCULATORY SYSTEM
(I00-I99)

OGCR Chapter-Specific Coding Guidelines

9. **Chapter 9: Diseases of the Circulatory System (I00-I99)**

a. **Hypertension**

The classification presumes a causal relationship between hypertension and heart involvement and between hypertension and kidney involvement, as the two conditions are linked by the term "with" in the Alphabetic Index. These conditions should be coded as related even in the absence of provider documentation explicitly linking them, unless the documentation clearly states the conditions are unrelated.

For hypertension and conditions not specifically linked by relational terms such as "with," "associated with" or "due to" in the classification, provider documentation must link the conditions in order to code them as related.

1) **Hypertension with Heart Disease**

Hypertension with heart conditions classified to I50.- or I51.4-I51.9, are assigned to, a code from category I11, Hypertensive heart disease. Use additional code(s) from category I50, Heart failure, to identify the type(s) of heart failure in those patients with heart failure.

The same heart conditions (I50.-, I51.4-I51.9) with hypertension, are coded separately if the provider has specifically documented a different cause. Sequence according to the circumstances of the admission/encounter.

2) **Hypertensive Chronic Kidney Disease**

Assign codes from category I12, Hypertensive chronic kidney disease, when both hypertension and a condition classifiable to category N18, Chronic kidney disease (CKD), are present. CKD should not be coded as hypertensive if the physician has specifically documented a different cause.

The appropriate code from category N18 should be used as a secondary code with a code from category I12 to identify the stage of chronic kidney disease.

See Section I.C.14. Chronic kidney disease.

If a patient has hypertensive chronic kidney disease and acute renal failure, an additional code for the acute renal failure is required.

3) **Hypertensive Heart and Chronic Kidney Disease**

Assign codes from combination category I13, Hypertensive heart and chronic kidney disease, when there is hypertension with both heart and kidney involvement. If heart failure is present, assign an additional code from category I50 to identify the type of heart failure.

The appropriate code from category N18, Chronic kidney disease, should be used as a secondary code with a code from category I13 to identify the stage of chronic kidney disease.

See Section I.C.14. Chronic kidney disease.

The codes in category I13, Hypertensive heart and chronic kidney disease, are combination codes that include hypertension, heart disease and chronic kidney disease. The Includes note at I13 specifies that the conditions included at I11 and I12 are included together in I13. If a patient has hypertension, heart disease and chronic kidney disease then a code from I13 should be used, not individual codes for hypertension, heart disease and chronic kidney disease, or codes from I11 or I12.

For patients with both acute renal failure and chronic kidney disease an additional code for acute renal failure is required.

4) **Hypertensive Cerebrovascular Disease**

For hypertensive cerebrovascular disease, first assign the appropriate code from categories I60-I69, followed by the appropriate hypertension code.

5) **Hypertensive Retinopathy**

Subcategory H35.0, Background retinopathy and retinal vascular changes, should be used with a code from category I10 – I15, Hypertensive disease to include the systemic hypertension. The sequencing is based on the reason for the encounter.

6) **Hypertension, Secondary**

Secondary hypertension is due to an underlying condition. Two codes are required: one to identify the underlying etiology and one from category I15 to identify the hypertension. Sequencing of codes is determined by the reason for admission/encounter.

7) **Hypertension, Transient**

Assign code R03.0, Elevated blood pressure reading without diagnosis of hypertension, unless patient has an established diagnosis of hypertension. Assign code O13.-, Gestational [pregnancy-induced] hypertension without significant proteinuria, or O14.-, Pre-eclampsia, for transient hypertension of pregnancy.

8) **Hypertension, Controlled**

This diagnostic statement usually refers to an existing state of hypertension under control by therapy. Assign the appropriate code from categories I10-I15, Hypertensive diseases.

9) **Hypertension, Uncontrolled**

Uncontrolled hypertension may refer to untreated hypertension or hypertension not responding to current therapeutic regimen. In either case, assign the appropriate code from categories I10-I15, Hypertensive diseases.

10) **Hypertensive Crisis**

Assign a code from category I16, Hypertensive crisis, for documented hypertensive urgency, hypertensive emergency or unspecified hypertensive crisis. Code also any identified hypertensive disease (I10-I15). The sequencing is based on the reason for the encounter.

11) **Pulmonary Hypertension**

Pulmonary hypertension is classified to category I27, Other pulmonary heart diseases. For secondary pulmonary hypertension (I27.1, I27.2-), code also any associated conditions or adverse effects of drugs or toxins. The sequencing is based on the reason for the encounter.

b. **Atherosclerotic Coronary Artery Disease and Angina**

ICD-10-CM has combination codes for atherosclerotic heart disease with angina pectoris. The subcategories for these codes are I25.11, Atherosclerotic heart disease of native coronary artery with angina pectoris and I25.7, Atherosclerosis of coronary artery bypass graft(s) and coronary artery of transplanted heart with angina pectoris.

When using one of these combination codes it is not necessary to use an additional code for angina pectoris. A causal relationship can be assumed in a patient with both atherosclerosis and angina pectoris, unless the documentation indicates the angina is due to something other than the atherosclerosis.

If a patient with coronary artery disease is admitted due to an acute myocardial infarction (AMI), the AMI should be sequenced before the coronary artery disease.

See Section I.C.9. Acute myocardial infarction (AMI)

c. **Intraoperative and Postprocedural Cerebrovascular Accident**

Medical record documentation should clearly specify the cause-and-effect relationship between the medical intervention and the cerebrovascular accident in order to assign a code for intraoperative or postprocedural cerebrovascular accident.

Proper code assignment depends on whether it was an infarction or hemorrhage and whether it occurred intraoperatively or postoperatively. If it was a cerebral hemorrhage, code assignment depends on the type of procedure performed.

d. **Sequelae of Cerebrovascular Disease**

1) **Category I69, Sequelae of Cerebrovascular disease**

Category I69 is used to indicate conditions classifiable to categories I60-I67 as the causes of sequela (neurologic deficits), themselves classified elsewhere. These "late effects" include neurologic deficits that persist after initial onset of conditions classifiable to categories I60-I67. The neurologic deficits caused by cerebrovascular disease may be present from the onset or may arise at any time after the onset of the condition classifiable to categories I60-I67.

Codes from category I69, Sequelae of cerebrovascular disease, that specify hemiplegia, hemiparesis and monoplegia identify whether the dominant or nondominant side is affected. Should the affected side be documented, but not specified as dominant or nondominant, and the classification system does not indicate a default, code selection is as follows:

- For ambidextrous patients, the default should be dominant.
- If the left side is affected, the default is non-dominant.
- If the right side is affected, the default is dominant.

2) **Codes from category I69 with codes from I60-I67**

Codes from category I69 may be assigned on a health care record with codes from I60-I67, if the patient has a current cerebrovascular disease and deficits from an old cerebrovascular disease.

3) **Codes from category I69 and Personal history of transient ischemic attack (TIA) and cerebral infarction (Z86.73)**
Codes from category I69 should not be assigned if the patient does not have neurologic deficits.
See Section I.C.21. 4. History (of) for use of personal history codes

e. **Acute myocardial infarction (AMI)**

1) **Type 1 ST elevation myocardial infarction (STEMI) and non ST elevation myocardial infarction (NSTEMI)**
The ICD-10-CM codes for acute **type 1** myocardial infarction (AMI) identify the site, such as anterolateral wall or true posterior wall. Subcategories I21.0-I21.2 and code I21.3 are used for **type 1** ST elevation myocardial infarction (STEMI). Code I21.4, Non-ST elevation (NSTEMI) myocardial infarction, is used for **type 1** non ST elevation myocardial infarction (NSTEMI) and nontransmural MIs.
If **a type 1** NSTEMI evolves to STEMI, assign the STEMI code. If **a type 1** STEMI converts to NSTEMI due to thrombolytic therapy, it is still coded as STEMI.
For encounters occurring while the myocardial infarction is equal to, or less than, four weeks old, including transfers to another acute setting or a postacute setting, and the myocardial infarction meets the definition for "other diagnoses" (see Section III, Reporting Additional Diagnoses), codes from category I21 may continue to be reported. For encounters after the 4 week time frame and the patient is still receiving care related to the myocardial infarction, the appropriate aftercare code should be assigned, rather than a code from category I21. For old or healed myocardial infarctions not requiring further care, code I25.2, Old myocardial infarction, may be assigned.

2) **Acute myocardial infarction, unspecified**
Code **I21.9, Acute myocardial infarction, unspecified,** is the default for unspecified acute myocardial infarction **or unspecified type**. If only **type 1** STEMI or transmural MI without the site is documented, assign code I21.3, **ST elevation (STEMI) myocardial infarction of unspecified site.**

3) **AMI documented as nontransmural or subendocardial but site provided**
If an AMI is documented as nontransmural or subendocardial, but the site is provided, it is still coded as a subendocardial AMI.
See Section I.C.21.3 for information on coding status post administration of tPA in a different facility within the last 24 hours.

4) **Subsequent acute myocardial infarction**
A code from category I22, Subsequent ST elevation (STEMI) and non ST elevation (NSTEMI) myocardial infarction, is to be used when a patient who has suffered **a type 1 or unspecified** AMI has a new AMI within the 4 week time frame of the initial AMI. A code from category I22 must be used in conjunction with a code from category I21. The sequencing of the I22 and I21 codes depends on the circumstances of the encounter.
Do not assign code I22 for subsequent myocardial infarctions other than type 1 or unspecified. For subsequent type 2 AMI assign only code I21.A1. For subsequent type 4 or type 5 AMI, assign only code I21.A9.

5) Other Types of Myocardial Infarction
The ICD-10-CM provides codes for different types of myocardial infarction. Type 1 myocardial infarctions are assigned to codes I21.0-I21.4.
Type 2 myocardial infarction, and myocardial infarction due to demand ischemia or secondary to ischemic balance, is assigned to code I21.A1, Myocardial infarction type 2 with a code for the underlying cause. Do not assign code I24.8, Other forms of acute ischemic heart disease for the demand ischemia. Sequencing of type 2 AMI or the underlying cause is dependent on the circumstances of admission. When a type 2 AMI code is described as NSTEMI or STEMI, only assign code I21.A1. Codes I21.01-I21.4 should only be assigned for type 1 AMIs.
Acute myocardial infarctions type 3, 4a, 4b, 4c and 5 are assigned to code I21.A9, Other myocardial infarction type.
The "Code also" and "Code first" notes should be followed related to complications, and for coding of postprocedural myocardial infarctions during or following cardiac surgery.

Figure 9-1   Cardiovascular valves.

Item 9–1 Rheumatic fever is the inflammation of the valve(s) of the heart, usually the mitral or aortic, which leads to valve damage. Rheumatic heart inflammations are usually **pericarditis** (sac surrounding heart), **endocarditis** (heart cavity), or **myocarditis** (heart muscle).

CHAPTER 9

DISEASES OF THE CIRCULATORY SYSTEM
(I00–I99)

| Excludes2 | certain conditions originating in the perinatal period (P04-P96)
certain infectious and parasitic diseases (A00-B99)
complications of pregnancy, childbirth and the puerperium (O00-O9A)
congenital malformations, deformations, and chromosomal abnormalities (Q00-Q99)
endocrine, nutritional and metabolic diseases (E00-E88)
injury, poisoning and certain other consequences of external causes (S00-T88)
neoplasms (C00-D49)
symptoms, signs and abnormal clinical and laboratory findings, not elsewhere classified (R00-R94)
systemic connective tissue disorders (M30-M36)
transient cerebral ischemic attacks and related syndromes (G45.-)

This chapter contains the following blocks:

I00-I02	Acute rheumatic fever
I05-I09	Chronic rheumatic heart diseases
I10-I16	Hypertensive diseases
I20-I25	Ischemic heart diseases
I26-I28	Pulmonary heart disease and diseases of pulmonary circulation
I30-I52	Other forms of heart disease
I60-I69	Cerebrovascular diseases
I70-I79	Diseases of arteries, arterioles and capillaries
I80-I89	Diseases of veins, lymphatic vessels and lymph nodes, not elsewhere classified
I95-I99	Other and unspecified disorders of the circulatory system

ACUTE RHEUMATIC FEVER (I00-I02)

I00   Rheumatic fever without heart involvement
     Includes   arthritis, rheumatic, acute or subacute
     Excludes1   rheumatic fever with heart involvement (I01.0-I01.9)

● **I01   Rheumatic fever with heart involvement**
     Excludes1   chronic diseases of rheumatic origin (I05-I09) unless rheumatic fever is also present or there is evidence of reactivation or activity of the rheumatic process.

     I01.0   Acute rheumatic pericarditis
         Any condition in I00 with pericarditis
         Rheumatic pericarditis (acute)
         Excludes1   acute pericarditis not specified as rheumatic (I30.-)

     I01.1   Acute rheumatic endocarditis
         Any condition in I00 with endocarditis or valvulitis
         Acute rheumatic valvulitis

     I01.2   Acute rheumatic myocarditis
         Any condition in I00 with myocarditis

▶ New   ⟹ Revised   ~~deleted~~ Deleted   **OGCR** Official Guidelines   X Assign placeholder X   ● Use Additional Character(s)

Excludes 1   Excludes 2   Includes   Use additional   Code first   Code also   Key words

Item 9–2 Rheumatic chorea, also called Sydenham's, juvenile, minor, simple, or St. Vitus' dance, is a major symptom of rheumatic fever and is characterized by ceaseless, involuntary, jerky, purposeless movements.

I01.8   **Other acute rheumatic heart disease**
     Any condition in I00 with other or multiple types of heart involvement
     Acute rheumatic pancarditis

I01.9   **Acute rheumatic heart disease, unspecified**
     Any condition in I00 with unspecified type of heart involvement
     Rheumatic carditis, acute
     Rheumatic heart disease, active or acute

● **I02**   **Rheumatic chorea**

     Includes   Sydenham's chorea
     Excludes1   chorea NOS (G25.5)
                Huntington's chorea (G10)

I02.0   **Rheumatic chorea with heart involvement**
     Chorea NOS with heart involvement
     Rheumatic chorea with heart involvement of any type classifiable under I01.-

I02.9   **Rheumatic chorea without heart involvement**
     Rheumatic chorea NOS

CHRONIC RHEUMATIC HEART DISEASES (I05-I09)

● **I05**   **Rheumatic mitral valve diseases**

     Includes   conditions classifiable to both I05.0 and I05.2-I05.9, whether specified as rheumatic or not

     Excludes1   mitral valve disease specified as nonrheumatic (I34.-)
                mitral valve disease with aortic and/or tricuspid valve involvement (I08.-)

I05.0   **Rheumatic mitral stenosis**
     Mitral (valve) obstruction (rheumatic)

I05.1   **Rheumatic mitral insufficiency**
     Rheumatic mitral incompetence
     Rheumatic mitral regurgitation
     Excludes1   mitral insufficiency not specified as rheumatic (I34.0)

I05.2   **Rheumatic mitral stenosis with insufficiency**
     Rheumatic mitral stenosis with incompetence or regurgitation

I05.8   **Other rheumatic mitral valve diseases**
     Rheumatic mitral (valve) failure

I05.9   **Rheumatic mitral valve disease, unspecified**
     Rheumatic mitral (valve) disorder (chronic) NOS

● **I06**   **Rheumatic aortic valve diseases**

     Excludes1   aortic valve disease not specified as rheumatic (I35.-)
                aortic valve disease with mitral and/or tricuspid valve involvement (I08.-)

I06.0   **Rheumatic aortic stenosis**
     Rheumatic aortic (valve) obstruction

I06.1   **Rheumatic aortic insufficiency**
     Rheumatic aortic incompetence
     Rheumatic aortic regurgitation

★ **(See Plate 244 on page 78.)**

I06.2   **Rheumatic aortic stenosis with insufficiency**
     Rheumatic aortic stenosis with incompetence or regurgitation

I06.8   **Other rheumatic aortic valve diseases**

I06.9   **Rheumatic aortic valve disease, unspecified**
     Rheumatic aortic (valve) disease NOS

● **I07**   **Rheumatic tricuspid valve diseases**

     Includes   rheumatic tricuspid valve diseases specified as rheumatic or unspecified

     Excludes1   tricuspid valve disease specified as nonrheumatic (I36.-)
                tricuspid valve disease with aortic and/or mitral valve involvement (I08.-)

I07.0   **Rheumatic tricuspid stenosis**
     Tricuspid (valve) stenosis (rheumatic)

I07.1   **Rheumatic tricuspid insufficiency**
     Tricuspid (valve) insufficiency (rheumatic)

I07.2   **Rheumatic tricuspid stenosis and insufficiency**

I07.8   **Other rheumatic tricuspid valve diseases**

I07.9   **Rheumatic tricuspid valve disease, unspecified**
     Rheumatic tricuspid valve disorder NOS

● **I08**   **Multiple valve diseases**

     Includes   multiple valve diseases specified as rheumatic or unspecified

     Excludes1   endocarditis, valve unspecified (I38)
                multiple valve disease specified a nonrheumatic (I34.-, I35.-, I36.-, I37.-, I38.-, Q22.-, Q23.-, Q24.8-)
                rheumatic valve disease NOS (I09.1)

I08.0   **Rheumatic disorders of both mitral and aortic valves**
     Involvement of both mitral and aortic valves specified as rheumatic or unspecified

I08.1   **Rheumatic disorders of both mitral and tricuspid valves**

I08.2   **Rheumatic disorders of both aortic and tricuspid valves**

I08.3   **Combined rheumatic disorders of mitral, aortic and tricuspid valves**

I08.8   **Other rheumatic multiple valve diseases**

I08.9   **Rheumatic multiple valve disease, unspecified**

● **I09**   **Other rheumatic heart diseases**

I09.0   **Rheumatic myocarditis**
     Excludes1   myocarditis not specified as rheumatic (I51.4)

I09.1   **Rheumatic diseases of endocardium, valve unspecified**
     Rheumatic endocarditis (chronic)
     Rheumatic valvulitis (chronic)
     Excludes1   endocarditis, valve unspecified (I38)

I09.2   **Chronic rheumatic pericarditis**
     Adherent pericardium, rheumatic
     Chronic rheumatic mediastinopericarditis
     Chronic rheumatic myopericarditis
     Excludes1   chronic pericarditis not specified as rheumatic (I31.-)

● I09.8   **Other specified rheumatic heart diseases**

I09.81   **Rheumatic heart failure**
     Use additional code to identify type of heart failure (I50.-)

I09.89   **Other specified rheumatic heart diseases**
     Rheumatic disease of pulmonary valve

I09.9   **Rheumatic heart disease, unspecified**
     Rheumatic carditis
     Excludes1   rheumatoid carditis (M05.31)

Item 9–3 Mitral stenosis is the narrowing of the mitral valve separating the left atrium from the left ventricle. **Mitral insufficiency** is the improper closure of the mitral valve which may lead to enlargement (hypertrophy) of the left atrium.

Item 9–4 Aortic stenosis is the narrowing of the aortic valve located between the left ventricle and the aorta. **Aortic insufficiency** is the improper closure of the aortic valve which may lead to enlargement (hypertrophy) of the left ventricle.

CHAPTER 9 (I00-I99)

▶ New   ⇒ Revised   ~~deleted~~ Deleted   **OGCR** Official Guidelines   X Assign placeholder X   ● Use Additional Character(s)

Excludes 1   Excludes 2   Includes   Use additional   Code first   Code also   Key words

Item 9–5 Hypertension is caused by high arterial blood pressure in the arteries. **Essential, primary,** or **idiopathic** hypertension occurs without identifiable organic cause. **Secondary** hypertension is that which has an organic cause. **Malignant** hypertension is severely elevated blood pressure. **Benign** hypertension is mildly elevated blood pressure.

HYPERTENSIVE DISEASES (I10-I16)

Use additional code to identify:
  exposure to environmental tobacco smoke (Z77.22)
  history of tobacco dependence (Z87.891)
  occupational exposure to environmental tobacco
    smoke (Z57.31)
  tobacco dependence (F17.-)
  tobacco use (Z72.Ø)

| Excludes1 | neonatal hypertension (P29.2) |
| | primary pulmonary hypertension (I27.Ø) |

Excludes2	hypertensive disease complicating pregnancy,
	childbirth and the puerperium (O1Ø-O11,
	O13-O16)

I10   Essential (primary) hypertension

Includes	high blood pressure
	hypertension (arterial) (benign) (essential)
	(malignant) (primary) (systemic)

Excludes1	hypertensive disease complicating pregnancy,
	childbirth and the puerperium (O1Ø-O11,
	O13-O16)

Excludes2	essential (primary) hypertension involving
	vessels of brain (I6Ø-I69)
	essential (primary) hypertension involving
	vessels of eye (H35.Ø-)

● **I11   Hypertensive heart disease**

➡ | Includes | any condition in I5Ø.-, I51.4-I51.9 due to |
| | hypertension |

   I11.Ø   Hypertensive heart disease with heart failure
          Hypertensive heart failure
          Use additional code to identify type of heart failure (I5Ø.-)

   I11.9   Hypertensive heart disease without heart failure
          Hypertensive heart disease NOS

   OGCR   Section I.C.9.a.2.

> Hypertensive Chronic Kidney Disease
> Assign codes from category I12, Hypertensive chronic kidney disease, when both hypertension and a condition classifiable to category N18, Chronic kidney disease (CKD), are present. **CKD should not be coded as hypertensive if the physician has specifically documented a different cause.**
>
> The appropriate code from category N18 should be used as a secondary code with a code from category I12 to identify the stage of chronic kidney disease.
> *See Section I.C.14. Chronic kidney disease.*
>
> If a patient has hypertensive chronic kidney disease and acute renal failure, an additional code for the acute renal failure is required.

● **I12   Hypertensive chronic kidney disease**

Includes	any condition in N18 and N26 - due to hypertension
	arteriosclerosis of kidney
	arteriosclerotic nephritis (chronic) (interstitial)
	hypertensive nephropathy
	nephrosclerosis

Excludes1	hypertension due to kidney disease (I15.Ø, I15.1)
	renovascular hypertension (I15.Ø)
	secondary hypertension (I15.-)

| Excludes2 | acute kidney failure (N17.-) |

   I12.Ø   Hypertensive chronic kidney disease with stage 5 chronic kidney disease or end stage renal disease
          Use additional code to identify the stage of chronic kidney disease (N18.5, N18.6)

   I12.9   Hypertensive chronic kidney disease with stage 1 through stage 4 chronic kidney disease, or unspecified chronic kidney disease
          Hypertensive chronic kidney disease NOS
          Hypertensive renal disease NOS
          Use additional code to identify the stage of chronic kidney disease (N18.1-N18.4, N18.9)

   OGCR   Section I.c.9.a.3.

> Hypertensive Heart and Chronic Kidney Disease
> Assign codes from combination category I13, Hypertensive heart and chronic kidney disease, when **there is hypertension with both heart and kidney involvement.** If heart failure is present, assign an additional code from category I5Ø to identify the type of heart failure.
>
> The appropriate code from category N18, Chronic kidney disease, should be used as a secondary code with a code from category I13 to identify the stage of chronic kidney disease.
> *See Section I.C.14. Chronic kidney disease.*
>
> The codes in category I13, Hypertensive heart and chronic kidney disease, are combination codes that include hypertension, heart disease and chronic kidney disease. The Includes note at I13 specifies that the conditions included at I11 and I12 are included together in I13. If a patient has hypertension, heart disease and chronic kidney disease then a code from I13 should be used, not individual codes for hypertension, heart disease and chronic kidney disease, or codes from I11 or I12.
>
> For patients with both acute renal failure and chronic kidney disease an additional code for acute renal failure is required.

● **I13   Hypertensive heart and chronic kidney disease**

Includes	any condition in I11.- with any condition in I12.-
	cardiorenal disease
	cardiovascular renal disease

   I13.Ø   Hypertensive heart and chronic kidney disease with heart failure and stage 1 through stage 4 chronic kidney disease, or unspecified chronic kidney disease
          Use additional code to identify type of heart failure (I5Ø.-)
          Use additional code to identify stage of chronic kidney disease (N18.1-N18.4, N18.9)

● **I13.1   Hypertensive heart and chronic kidney disease without heart failure**

   I13.10   Hypertensive heart and chronic kidney disease without heart failure, with stage 1 through stage 4 chronic kidney disease, or unspecified chronic kidney disease
          Hypertensive heart disease and hypertensive chronic kidney disease NOS
          Use additional code to identify the stage of chronic kidney disease (N18.1-N18.4, N18.9)

   I13.11   Hypertensive heart and chronic kidney disease without heart failure, with stage 5 chronic kidney disease, or end stage renal disease
          Use additional code to identify the stage of chronic kidney disease (N18.5, N18.6)

   I13.2   Hypertensive heart and chronic kidney disease with heart failure and with stage 5 chronic kidney disease, or end stage renal disease
          Use additional code to identify type of heart failure (I5Ø.-)
          Use additional code to identify the stage of chronic kidney disease (N18.5, N18.6)

▶ New   ➡ Revised   ~~deleted~~ Deleted   **OGCR** Official Guidelines   X Assign placeholder X   ● Use Additional Character(s)

Excludes 1   Excludes 2   Includes   Use additional   Code first   Code also   Key words

OGCR Section I.9.a.6.

Hypertension, Secondary
Secondary hypertension is due to an underlying condition. Two codes are required: one to identify the underlying etiology and one from category I15 to identify the hypertension. Sequencing of codes is determined by the reason for admission/encounter.

● **I15   Secondary hypertension**
    Code also underlying condition
    Excludes1   postprocedural hypertension (I97.3)
    Excludes2   secondary hypertension involving vessels of brain (I60-I69)
                  secondary hypertension involving vessels of eye (H35.0-)

    I15.0   Renovascular hypertension
    I15.1   Hypertension secondary to other renal disorders
    I15.2   Hypertension secondary to endocrine disorders
    I15.8   Other secondary hypertension
    I15.9   Secondary hypertension, unspecified

● **I16   Hypertensive crisis**
    Code also any identified hypertensive disease (I10-I15)
    I16.0   Hypertensive urgency
    I16.1   Hypertensive emergency
    I16.9   Hypertensive crisis, unspecified

ISCHEMIC HEART DISEASES (I20-I25)

Use additional code to identify presence of hypertension (I10-I16)

● **I20   Angina pectoris**
    Chest pain/discomfort due to lack of oxygen to the heart muscle. Principal symptom of myocardial infarction.
    Use additional code to identify:
        exposure to environmental tobacco smoke (Z77.22)
        history of tobacco dependence (Z87.891)
        occupational exposure to environmental tobacco smoke (Z57.31)
        tobacco dependence (F17.-)
        tobacco use (Z72.0)
    Excludes1   angina pectoris with atherosclerotic heart disease of native coronary arteries (I25.1-)
                atherosclerosis of coronary artery bypass graft(s) and coronary artery of transplanted heart with angina pectoris (I25.7-)
                postinfarction angina (I23.7)

    I20.0   Unstable angina
        Accelerated angina
        Crescendo angina
        De novo effort angina
        Intermediate coronary syndrome
        Preinfarction syndrome
        Worsening effort angina

    I20.1   Angina pectoris with documented spasm
        Angiospastic angina
        Prinzmetal angina
        Spasm-induced angina
        Variant angina

    I20.8   Other forms of angina pectoris
        Angina equivalent
        Angina of effort
        Coronary slow flow syndrome
        Stable angina
        Stenocardia
        Use additional code(s) for symptoms associated with angina equivalent

    I20.9   Angina pectoris, unspecified
        Angina NOS
        Anginal syndrome
        Cardiac angina
        Ischemic chest pain

➡ **I21   Acute myocardial infarction**
    Includes   cardiac infarction
              coronary (artery) embolism
              coronary (artery) occlusion
              coronary (artery) rupture
              coronary (artery) thrombosis
              infarction of heart, myocardium, or ventricle
              myocardial infarction specified as acute or with a stated duration of 4 weeks (28 days) or less from onset
    Use additional code, if applicable, to identify:
        exposure to environmental tobacco smoke (Z77.22)
        history of tobacco dependence (Z87.891)
        occupational exposure to environmental tobacco smoke (Z57.31)
        status post administration of tPA (rtPA) in a different facility within the last 24 hours prior to admission to current facility (Z92.82)
        tobacco dependence (F17.-)
        tobacco use (Z72.0)
    Excludes2   old myocardial infarction (I25.2)
                postmyocardial infarction syndrome (I24.1)
        ➡ subsequent type 1 myocardial infarction (I22.-)

● **I21.0   ST elevation (STEMI) myocardial infarction of anterior wall**
    ▶ Type 1 ST elevation myocardial infarction of anterior wall
    I21.01   ST elevation (STEMI) myocardial infarction involving left main coronary artery
    I21.02   ST elevation (STEMI) myocardial infarction involving left anterior descending coronary artery
            ST elevation (STEMI) myocardial infarction involving diagonal coronary artery
    I21.09   ST elevation (STEMI) myocardial infarction involving other coronary artery of anterior wall
            Acute transmural myocardial infarction of anterior wall
            Anteroapical transmural (Q wave) infarction (acute)
            Anterolateral transmural (Q wave) infarction (acute)
            Anteroseptal transmural (Q wave) infarction (acute)
            Transmural (Q wave) infarction (acute) (of) anterior (wall) NOS

● **I21.1   ST elevation (STEMI) myocardial infarction of inferior wall**
    ▶ Type 1 ST elevation myocardial infarction of inferior wall
    I21.11   ST elevation (STEMI) myocardial infarction involving right coronary artery
            Inferoposterior transmural (Q wave) infarction (acute)
    I21.19   ST elevation (STEMI) myocardial infarction involving other coronary artery of inferior wall
            Acute transmural myocardial infarction of inferior wall
            Inferolateral transmural (Q wave) infarction (acute)
            Transmural (Q wave) infarction (acute) (of) diaphragmatic wall
            Transmural (Q wave) infarction (acute) (of) inferior (wall) NOS
        Excludes2   ST elevation (STEMI) myocardial infarction involving left circumflex coronary artery (I21.21)

CHAPTER 9 (I00-I99)

CHAPTER 9 (I00-I99)

● **I21.2 ST elevation (STEMI) myocardial infarction of other sites**
> ▶ Type 1 ST elevation myocardial infarction of other sites

  I21.21 ST elevation (STEMI) myocardial infarction involving left circumflex coronary artery
      ST elevation (STEMI) myocardial infarction involving oblique marginal coronary artery

  I21.29 ST elevation (STEMI) myocardial infarction involving other sites
      Acute transmural myocardial infarction of other sites
      Apical-lateral transmural (Q wave) infarction (acute)
      Basal-lateral transmural (Q wave) infarction (acute)
      High lateral transmural (Q wave) infarction (acute)
      Lateral (wall) NOS transmural (Q wave) infarction (acute)
      Posterior (true) transmural (Q wave) infarction (acute)
      Posterobasal transmural (Q wave) infarction (acute)
      Posterolateral transmural (Q wave) infarction (acute)
      Posteroseptal transmural (Q wave) infarction (acute)
      Septal transmural (Q wave) infarction (acute) NOS

OGCR Section I.c.9.e.2.

> Acute myocardial infarction, unspecified
>
> Code **I21.9, Acute myocardial infarction, unspecified,** is the default for unspecified acute myocardial infarction **or unspecified type.** If only **type 1** STEMI or transmural MI without the site is documented, assign I21.3, **ST elevation (STEMI) myocardial infarction of unspecified site.**

I21.3 ST elevation (STEMI) myocardial infarction of unspecified site
    Acute transmural myocardial infarction of unspecified site
    ~~Myocardial infarction (acute) NOS~~
    Transmural (Q wave) myocardial infarction NOS
    ▶ Type 1 ST elevation myocardial infarction of unspecified site

I21.4 Non-ST elevation (NSTEMI) myocardial infarction
    Acute subendocardial myocardial infarction
    Non-Q wave myocardial infarction NOS
    Nontransmural myocardial infarction NOS
    ▶ Type 1 non-ST elevation myocardial infarction

▶ **I21.9 Acute myocardial infarction, unspecified**
    ▶ Myocardial infarction (acute) NOS

▶● **I21.A Other type of myocardial infarction**

  ▶ **I21.A1 Myocardial infarction type 2**
    ▶ Myocardial infarction due to demand ischemia
    ▶ Myocardial infarction secondary to ischemic imbalance

    ▶ **Code also** the underlying cause, if known and applicable, such as:
    ▶ anemia (D50.0-D64.9)
    ▶ chronic obstructive pulmonary disease (J44.-)
    ▶ heart failure (I50.-)
    ▶ paroxysmal tachycardia (I47.0-I47.9)
    ▶ renal failure (N17.0-N19)
    ▶ shock (R57.0-R57.9)

▶ **I21.A9 Other myocardial infarction type**
    ▶ Myocardial infarction associated with revascularization procedure
    ▶ Myocardial infarction type 3
    ▶ Myocardial infarction type 4a
    ▶ Myocardial infarction type 4b
    ▶ Myocardial infarction type 4c
    ▶ Myocardial infarction type 5

    ▶ *Code first, if applicable, postprocedural infarction following cardiac surgery (I97.190), or postprocedural myocardial infarction during cardiac surgery (I97.790)*

    ▶ **Code also** complication, if known and applicable, such as:
    ▶ (acute) stent occlusion (T82.897-)
    ▶ (acute) stent stenosis (T82.857-)
    ▶ (acute) stent thrombosis (T82.867-)
    ▶ cardiac arrest due to underlying cardiac condition (I46.2)
    ▶ complication of percutaneous coronary intervention (PCI) (I97.89)
    ▶ occlusion of coronary artery bypass graft (T82.218-)

● **I22 Subsequent ST elevation (STEMI) and non-ST elevation (NSTEMI) myocardial infarction**

  Includes   acute myocardial infarction occurring within four weeks (28 days) of a previous acute myocardial infarction, regardless of site
          cardiac infarction
          coronary (artery) embolism
          coronary (artery) occlusion
          coronary (artery) rupture
          coronary (artery) thrombosis
          infarction of heart, myocardium, or ventricle
          recurrent myocardial infarction
          reinfarction of myocardium
          rupture of heart, myocardium, or ventricle
          ▶ subsequent type 1 myocardial infarction

▶ **Excludes1**   subsequent myocardial infarction, type 2 (I21.A1)
         subsequent myocardial infarction of other type (type 3) (type 4) (type 5) (I21.A9)

Use additional code, if applicable, to identify:
  exposure to environmental tobacco smoke (Z77.22)
  history of tobacco dependence (Z87.891)
  occupational exposure to environmental tobacco smoke (Z57.31)
  status post administration of tPA (rtPA) in a different facility within the last 24 hours prior to admission to current facility (Z92.82)
  tobacco dependence (F17.-)
  tobacco use (Z72.0)

I22.0 Subsequent ST elevation (STEMI) myocardial infarction of anterior wall
    Subsequent acute transmural myocardial infarction of anterior wall
    Subsequent transmural (Q wave) infarction (acute)(of) anterior (wall) NOS
    Subsequent anteroapical transmural (Q wave) infarction (acute)
    Subsequent anterolateral transmural (Q wave) infarction (acute)
    Subsequent anteroseptal transmural (Q wave) infarction (acute)

I22.1 Subsequent ST elevation (STEMI) myocardial infarction of inferior wall
    Subsequent acute transmural myocardial infarction of inferior wall
    Subsequent transmural (Q wave) infarction (acute)(of) diaphragmatic wall
    Subsequent transmural (Q wave) infarction (acute)(of) inferior (wall) NOS
    Subsequent inferolateral transmural (Q wave) infarction (acute)
    Subsequent inferoposterior transmural (Q wave) infarction (acute)

I22.2   **Subsequent non-ST elevation (NSTEMI) myocardial infarction**
Subsequent acute subendocardial myocardial infarction
Subsequent non-Q wave myocardial infarction NOS
Subsequent nontransmural myocardial infarction NOS

I22.8   **Subsequent ST elevation (STEMI) myocardial infarction of other sites**
Subsequent acute transmural myocardial infarction of other sites
Subsequent apical-lateral transmural (Q wave) myocardial infarction (acute)
Subsequent basal-lateral transmural (Q wave) myocardial infarction (acute)
Subsequent high lateral transmural (Q wave) myocardial infarction (acute)
Subsequent transmural (Q wave) myocardial infarction (acute)(of) lateral (wall) NOS
Subsequent posterior (true) transmural (Q wave) myocardial infarction (acute)
Subsequent posterobasal transmural (Q wave) myocardial infarction (acute)
Subsequent posterolateral transmural (Q wave) myocardial infarction (acute)
Subsequent posteroseptal transmural (Q wave) myocardial infarction (acute)
Subsequent septal NOS transmural (Q wave) myocardial infarction (acute)

I22.9   **Subsequent ST elevation (STEMI) myocardial infarction of unspecified site**
Subsequent acute myocardial infarction of unspecified site
Subsequent myocardial infarction (acute) NOS

● I23   **Certain current complications following ST elevation (STEMI) and non-ST elevation (NSTEMI) myocardial infarction (within the 28 day period)**

I23.0   **Hemopericardium as current complication following acute myocardial infarction**
| Excludes1 | hemopericardium not specified as current complication following acute myocardial infarction (I31.2) |

I23.1   **Atrial septal defect as current complication following acute myocardial infarction**
| Excludes1 | acquired atrial septal defect not specified as current complication following acute myocardial infarction (I51.0) |

I23.2   **Ventricular septal defect as current complication following acute myocardial infarction**
| Excludes1 | acquired ventricular septal defect not specified as current complication following acute myocardial infarction (I51.0) |

I23.3   **Rupture of cardiac wall without hemopericardium as current complication following acute myocardial infarction**

I23.4   **Rupture of chordae tendineae as current complication following acute myocardial infarction**
| Excludes1 | rupture of chordae tendineae not specified as current complication following acute myocardial infarction (I51.1) |

I23.5   **Rupture of papillary muscle as current complication following acute myocardial infarction**
| Excludes1 | rupture of papillary muscle not specified as current complication following acute myocardial infarction (I51.2) |

I23.6   **Thrombosis of atrium, auricular appendage, and ventricle as current complications following acute myocardial infarction**
| Excludes1 | thrombosis of atrium, auricular appendage, and ventricle not specified as current complication following acute myocardial infarction (I51.3) |

I23.7   **Postinfarction angina**

I23.8   **Other current complications following acute myocardial infarction**

● I24   **Other acute ischemic heart diseases**
| Excludes1 | angina pectoris (I20.-) |
| | transient myocardial ischemia in newborn (P29.4) |

I24.0   **Acute coronary thrombosis not resulting in myocardial infarction**
Acute coronary (artery) (vein) embolism not resulting in myocardial infarction
Acute coronary (artery) (vein) occlusion not resulting in myocardial infarction
Acute coronary (artery) (vein) thromboembolism not resulting in myocardial infarction
| Excludes1 | atherosclerotic heart disease (I25.1-) |

I24.1   **Dressler's syndrome**
Postmyocardial infarction syndrome
| Excludes1 | postinfarction angina (I23.7) |

I24.8   **Other forms of acute ischemic heart disease**
▶ | Excludes1 | myocardial infarction due to demand ischemia (I21.A1) |

I24.9   **Acute ischemic heart disease, unspecified**
| Excludes1 | ischemic heart disease (chronic) NOS (I25.9) |

● I25   **Chronic ischemic heart disease**
Use additional code to identify:
chronic total occlusion of coronary artery (I25.82)
exposure to environmental tobacco smoke (Z77.22)
history of tobacco dependence (Z87.891)
occupational exposure to environmental tobacco smoke (Z57.31)
tobacco dependence (F17.-)
tobacco use (Z72.0)

★ **(See Plates 218 and 219 on pages 74 and 75.)**

● I25.1   **Atherosclerotic heart disease of native coronary artery**
Disease in which fatty deposits form on the walls of arteries
Atherosclerotic cardiovascular disease
Coronary (artery) atheroma
Coronary (artery) atherosclerosis
Coronary (artery) disease
Coronary (artery) sclerosis
Use additional code, if applicable, to identify:
coronary atherosclerosis due to calcified coronary lesion (I25.84)
coronary atherosclerosis due to lipid rich plaque (I25.83)
| Excludes2 | atheroembolism (I75.-) |
| | atherosclerosis of coronary artery bypass graft(s) and transplanted heart (I25.7-) |

I25.10   **Atherosclerotic heart disease of native coronary artery without angina pectoris**
Atherosclerotic heart disease NOS

Item 9–6 Classification is based on the location of the atherosclerosis. **"Of native coronary artery"** indicates the atherosclerosis is within an original heart artery. **"Of autologous vein bypass graft"** indicates that the atherosclerosis is within a vein graft that was taken from within the patient. **"Of nonautologous biological bypass graft"** indicates the atherosclerosis is within a vessel grafted from other than the patient. **"Of artery bypass graft"** indicates the atherosclerosis is within an artery that was grafted from within the patient.

Figure 9-2 Atherosclerotic plaque.

Atherosclerotic plaque (atheromas)

OGCR See Section I.9.b.

Atherosclerotic Coronary Artery Disease and Angina

ICD-10-CM has combination codes for atherosclerotic heart disease with angina pectoris. The subcategories for these codes are I25.11, Atherosclerotic heart disease of native coronary artery with angina pectoris and I25.7, Atherosclerosis of coronary artery bypass graft(s) and coronary artery of transplanted heart with angina pectoris.

When using one of these combination codes it is not necessary to use an additional code for angina pectoris. A causal relationship can be assumed in a patient with both atherosclerosis and angina pectoris, unless the documentation indicates the angina is due to something other than the atherosclerosis.

If a patient with coronary artery disease is admitted due to an acute myocardial infarction (AMI), the AMI should be sequenced before the coronary artery disease.

See Section I.C.9. Acute myocardial infarction (AMI)

● **I25.11**   **Atherosclerotic heart disease of native coronary artery with angina pectoris**

     I25.110   **Atherosclerotic heart disease of native coronary artery with unstable angina pectoris**

         Excludes1   unstable angina without atherosclerotic heart disease (I20.0)

     I25.111   **Atherosclerotic heart disease of native coronary artery with angina pectoris with documented spasm**

         Excludes1   angina pectoris with documented spasm without atherosclerotic heart disease (I20.1)

     I25.118   **Atherosclerotic heart disease of native coronary artery with other forms of angina pectoris**

         Excludes1   other forms of angina pectoris without atherosclerotic heart disease (I20.8)

     I25.119   **Atherosclerotic heart disease of native coronary artery with unspecified angina pectoris**

         Atherosclerotic heart disease with angina NOS

         Atherosclerotic heart disease with ischemic chest pain

         Excludes1   unspecified angina pectoris without atherosclerotic heart disease (I20.9)

I25.2   **Old myocardial infarction**

     Healed myocardial infarction

     Past myocardial infarction diagnosed by ECG or other investigation, but currently presenting no symptoms

I25.3   **Aneurysm of heart**

     Mural aneurysm

     Ventricular aneurysm

● **I25.4**   **Coronary artery aneurysm and dissection**

     I25.41   **Coronary artery aneurysm**

         Coronary arteriovenous fistula, acquired

         Excludes1   congenital coronary (artery) aneurysm (Q24.5)

     I25.42   **Coronary artery dissection**

I25.5   **Ischemic cardiomyopathy**

     Excludes2   coronary atherosclerosis (I25.1-, I25.7-)

I25.6   **Silent myocardial ischemia**

● **I25.7**   **Atherosclerosis of coronary artery bypass graft(s) and coronary artery of transplanted heart with angina pectoris**

     Use additional code, if applicable, to identify:

         coronary atherosclerosis due to calcified coronary lesion (I25.84)

         coronary atherosclerosis due to lipid rich plaque (I25.83)

     Excludes1   atherosclerosis of bypass graft(s) of transplanted heart without angina pectoris (I25.812)

         atherosclerosis of coronary artery bypass graft(s) without angina pectoris (I25.810)

         atherosclerosis of native coronary artery of transplanted heart without angina pectoris (I25.811)

         ~~embolism or thrombus of coronary artery bypass graft(s) (T82.8-)~~

● **I25.70**   **Atherosclerosis of coronary artery bypass graft(s), unspecified, with angina pectoris**

     I25.700   **Atherosclerosis of coronary artery bypass graft(s), unspecified, with unstable angina pectoris**

         Excludes1   unstable angina pectoris without atherosclerosis of coronary artery bypass graft (I20.0)

     I25.701   **Atherosclerosis of coronary artery bypass graft(s), unspecified, with angina pectoris with documented spasm**

         Excludes1   angina pectoris with documented spasm without atherosclerosis of coronary artery bypass graft (I20.1)

     I25.708   **Atherosclerosis of coronary artery bypass graft(s), unspecified, with other forms of angina pectoris**

         Excludes1   other forms of angina pectoris without atherosclerosis of coronary artery bypass graft (I20.8)

     I25.709   **Atherosclerosis of coronary artery bypass graft(s), unspecified, with unspecified angina pectoris**

         Excludes1   unspecified angina pectoris without atherosclerosis of coronary artery bypass graft (I20.9)

▶ New   ➡ Revised   ~~deleted~~ Deleted   **OGCR** Official Guidelines   X Assign placeholder X   ● Use Additional Character(s)

Excludes 1   Excludes 2   Includes   Use additional   Code first   Code also   Key words

● **I25.71**   **Atherosclerosis of autologous vein coronary artery bypass graft(s) with angina pectoris**

     I25.710   **Atherosclerosis of autologous vein coronary artery bypass graft(s) with unstable angina pectoris**

         Excludes1   unstable angina without atherosclerosis of autologous vein coronary artery bypass graft(s) (I20.0)

         ▶ Excludes2   embolism or thrombus of coronary artery bypass graft(s) (T82.8-)

     I25.711   **Atherosclerosis of autologous vein coronary artery bypass graft(s) with angina pectoris with documented spasm**

         Excludes1   angina pectoris with documented spasm without atherosclerosis of autologous vein coronary artery bypass graft(s) (I20.1)

     I25.718   **Atherosclerosis of autologous vein coronary artery bypass graft(s) with other forms of angina pectoris**

         Excludes1   other forms of angina pectoris without atherosclerosis of autologous vein coronary artery bypass graft(s) (I20.8)

     I25.719   **Atherosclerosis of autologous vein coronary artery bypass graft(s) with unspecified angina pectoris**

         Excludes1   unspecified angina pectoris without atherosclerosis of autologous vein coronary artery bypass graft(s) (I20.9)

● **I25.72**   **Atherosclerosis of autologous artery coronary artery bypass graft(s) with angina pectoris**

     Atherosclerosis of internal mammary artery graft with angina pectoris

     I25.720   **Atherosclerosis of autologous artery coronary artery bypass graft(s) with unstable angina pectoris**

         Excludes1   unstable angina without atherosclerosis of autologous artery coronary artery bypass graft(s) (I20.0)

     I25.721   **Atherosclerosis of autologous artery coronary artery bypass graft(s) with angina pectoris with documented spasm**

         Excludes1   angina pectoris with documented spasm without atherosclerosis of autologous artery coronary artery bypass graft(s) (I20.1)

     I25.728   **Atherosclerosis of autologous artery coronary artery bypass graft(s) with other forms of angina pectoris**

         Excludes1   other forms of angina pectoris without atherosclerosis of autologous artery coronary artery bypass graft(s) (I20.8)

     I25.729   **Atherosclerosis of autologous artery coronary artery bypass graft(s) with unspecified angina pectoris**

         Excludes1   unspecified angina pectoris without atherosclerosis of autologous artery coronary artery bypass graft(s) (I20.9)

● **I25.73**   **Atherosclerosis of nonautologous biological coronary artery bypass graft(s) with angina pectoris**

     I25.730   **Atherosclerosis of nonautologous biological coronary artery bypass graft(s) with unstable angina pectoris**

         Excludes1   unstable angina without atherosclerosis of nonautologous biological coronary artery bypass graft(s) (I20.0)

     I25.731   **Atherosclerosis of nonautologous biological coronary artery bypass graft(s) with angina pectoris with documented spasm**

         Excludes1   angina pectoris with documented spasm without atherosclerosis of nonautologous biological coronary artery bypass graft(s) (I20.1)

     I25.738   **Atherosclerosis of nonautologous biological coronary artery bypass graft(s) with other forms of angina pectoris**

         Excludes1   other forms of angina pectoris without atherosclerosis of nonautologous biological coronary artery bypass graft(s) (I20.8)

     I25.739   **Atherosclerosis of nonautologous biological coronary artery bypass graft(s) with unspecified angina pectoris**

         Excludes1   unspecified angina pectoris without atherosclerosis of nonautologous biological coronary artery bypass graft(s) (I20.9)

CHAPTER 9 (I00-I99)

● **I25.75** **Atherosclerosis of native coronary artery of transplanted heart with angina pectoris**

> **Excludes1**   atherosclerosis of native coronary artery of transplanted heart without angina pectoris (I25.811)

    I25.750 **Atherosclerosis of native coronary artery of transplanted heart with unstable angina**

    I25.751 **Atherosclerosis of native coronary artery of transplanted heart with angina pectoris with documented spasm**

    I25.758 **Atherosclerosis of native coronary artery of transplanted heart with other forms of angina pectoris**

    I25.759 **Atherosclerosis of native coronary artery of transplanted heart with unspecified angina pectoris**

● **I25.76** **Atherosclerosis of bypass graft of coronary artery of transplanted heart with angina pectoris**

> **Excludes1**   atherosclerosis of bypass graft of coronary artery of transplanted heart without angina pectoris (I25.812)

    I25.760 **Atherosclerosis of bypass graft of coronary artery of transplanted heart with unstable angina**

    I25.761 **Atherosclerosis of bypass graft of coronary artery of transplanted heart with angina pectoris with documented spasm**

    I25.768 **Atherosclerosis of bypass graft of coronary artery of transplanted heart with other forms of angina pectoris**

    I25.769 **Atherosclerosis of bypass graft of coronary artery of transplanted heart with unspecified angina pectoris**

● **I25.79** **Atherosclerosis of other coronary artery bypass graft(s) with angina pectoris**

    I25.790 **Atherosclerosis of other coronary artery bypass graft(s) with unstable angina pectoris**

> **Excludes1**   unstable angina without atherosclerosis of other coronary artery bypass graft(s) (I20.0)

    I25.791 **Atherosclerosis of other coronary artery bypass graft(s) with angina pectoris with documented spasm**

> **Excludes1**   angina pectoris with documented spasm without atherosclerosis of other coronary artery bypass graft(s) (I20.1)

    I25.798 **Atherosclerosis of other coronary artery bypass graft(s) with other forms of angina pectoris**

> **Excludes1**   other forms of angina pectoris without atherosclerosis of other coronary artery bypass graft(s) (I20.8)

    I25.799 **Atherosclerosis of other coronary artery bypass graft(s) with unspecified angina pectoris**

> **Excludes1**   unspecified angina pectoris without atherosclerosis of other coronary artery bypass graft(s) (I20.9)

● **I25.8** **Other forms of chronic ischemic heart disease**

● **I25.81** **Atherosclerosis of other coronary vessels without angina pectoris**

> Use additional code, if applicable, to identify:
> coronary atherosclerosis due to calcified coronary lesion (I25.84)
> coronary atherosclerosis due to lipid rich plaque (I25.83)

> **Excludes1**   atherosclerotic heart disease of native coronary artery without angina pectoris (I25.10)

    I25.810 **Atherosclerosis of coronary artery bypass graft(s) without angina pectoris**

> Atherosclerosis of coronary artery bypass graft NOS

> **Excludes1**   atherosclerosis of coronary bypass graft(s) with angina pectoris (I25.70- -I25.73-, I25.79-)

    I25.811 **Atherosclerosis of native coronary artery of transplanted heart without angina pectoris**

> Atherosclerosis of native coronary artery of transplanted heart NOS

> **Excludes1**   atherosclerosis of native coronary artery of transplanted heart with angina pectoris (I25.75-)

    I25.812 **Atherosclerosis of bypass graft of coronary artery of transplanted heart without angina pectoris**

> Atherosclerosis of bypass graft of transplanted heart NOS

> **Excludes1**   atherosclerosis of bypass graft of transplanted heart with angina pectoris (I25.76)

▶ New   ⇒ Revised   ~~deleted~~ Deleted   **OGCR** Official Guidelines   X Assign placeholder X   ● Use Additional Character(s)

Excludes 1   Excludes 2   Includes   Use additional   Code first   Code also   Key words

I25.82   Chronic total occlusion of coronary artery
        Complete occlusion of coronary artery
        Total occlusion of coronary artery
        *Code first coronary atherosclerosis (I25.1-, I25.7-,
            I25.81-)*
        | Excludes1 | ⇒acute coronary occlusion with
                        myocardial infarction
                        (I21.0-I21.9, I22.-)
                      ⇒acute coronary occlusion without
                        myocardial infarction (I24.0)

**I25.83   Coronary atherosclerosis due to lipid rich
            plaque**
        *Code first coronary atherosclerosis (I25.1-, I25.7-,
            I25.81-)*

**I25.84   Coronary atherosclerosis due to calcified
            coronary lesion**
        Coronary atherosclerosis due to severely
            calcified coronary lesion
        *Code first coronary atherosclerosis (I25.1-, I25.7-,
            I25.81-)*

I25.89   Other forms of chronic ischemic heart disease

I25.9   Chronic ischemic heart disease, unspecified
        Ischemic heart disease (chronic) NOS

PULMONARY HEART DISEASE AND DISEASES OF PULMONARY CIRCULATION (I26-I28)

● **I26   Pulmonary embolism**
    | Includes | pulmonary (acute)(artery)(vein) infarction
                    pulmonary (acute)(artery)(vein)
                        thromboembolism
                    pulmonary (acute)(artery)(vein) thrombosis
    | Excludes2 | chronic pulmonary embolism (I27.82)
                    personal history of pulmonary embolism
                        (Z86.711)
                    pulmonary embolism due to trauma (T79.0,
                        T79.1)
                    pulmonary embolism due to complications of
                        surgical and medical care (T80.0, T81.7-,
                        T82.8-)
                    pulmonary embolism complicating abortion,
                        ectopic or molar pregnancy (O00-O07, O08.2)
                    pulmonary embolism complicating pregnancy,
                        childbirth and the puerperium (O88.-)
                    septic (non-pulmonary) arterial embolism (I76)

● **I26.0 Pulmonary embolism with acute cor pulmonale**
    **I26.01   Septic pulmonary embolism with acute cor
               pulmonale**
            Code first underlying infection

    **I26.02   Saddle embolus of pulmonary artery with acute
               cor pulmonale**

    **I26.09   Other pulmonary embolism with acute cor
               pulmonale**
            Acute cor pulmonale NOS

● **I26.9 Pulmonary embolism without acute cor pulmonale**
    **I26.90   Septic pulmonary embolism without acute cor
               pulmonale**
            Code first underlying infection

    **I26.92   Saddle embolus of pulmonary artery without
               acute cor pulmonale**

    **I26.99   Other pulmonary embolism without acute cor
               pulmonale**
            Acute pulmonary embolism NOS
            Pulmonary embolism NOS

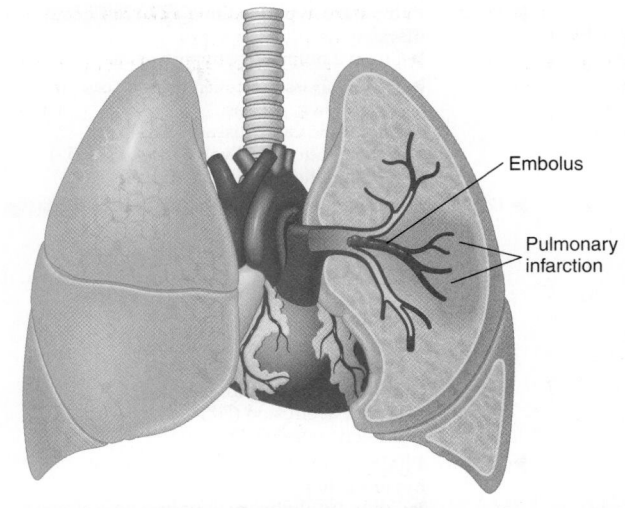

Figure 9-3   Pulmonary Embolism. (From Chabner: The Language of
Medicine, ed 8, St. Louis, Saunders, 2007)

Item 9–7   Pulmonary heart disease or **cor pulmonale** is right ventricle
hypertrophy or RVH as a result of a respiratory disorder increasing back flow
pressure to the right ventricle. Left untreated, cor pulmonale leads to right-heart
failure and death.

● **I27   Other pulmonary heart diseases**
    I27.0   Primary pulmonary hypertension
        ▶Heritable pulmonary arterial hypertension
        ▶Idiopathic pulmonary arterial hypertension
        ▶Primary group 1 pulmonary hypertension
        ▶Primary pulmonary arterial hypertension
        | Excludes1 | ~~pulmonary hypertension NOS (I27.2)~~
                        ~~secondary pulmonary hypertension (I27.2)~~
                        ▶persistent pulmonary hypertension of
                            newborn (P29.30)
                        ▶pulmonary hypertension NOS (I27.20)
                        ▶secondary pulmonary arterial
                            hypertension (I27.21)
                        ▶secondary pulmonary hypertension
                            (I27.29)

    I27.1   Kyphoscoliotic heart disease
● **I27.2   Other secondary pulmonary hypertension**
        ~~Pulmonary hypertension NOS~~
        Code also associated underlying condition
        ▶ | Excludes1 | Eisenmenger's syndrome (I27.83)

    ▶ **I27.20   Pulmonary hypertension, unspecified**
            ▶Pulmonary hypertension NOS

    ▶ **I27.21   Secondary pulmonary arterial hypertension**
            ▶(Associated) (drug-induced) (toxin-induced)
                pulmonary arterial hypertension NOS
            ▶(Associated) (drug-induced) (toxin-induced)
                (secondary) group 1 pulmonary
                hypertension
            ▶*Code also associated conditions if applicable, or
                adverse effects of drugs or toxins, such as:*
            ▶adverse effect of appetite depressants
                (T50.5X5)
            ▶congenital heart disease (Q20-Q28)
            ▶human immunodeficiency virus [HIV]
                disease (B20)
            ▶polymyositis (M33.2-)
            ▶portal hypertension (K76.6)
            ▶rheumatoid arthritis (M05.-)
            ▶schistosomiasis (B65.-)
            ▶Sjögren syndrome (M35.0-)
            ▶systemic sclerosis (M34.-)

▶ **I27.22** Pulmonary hypertension due to left heart disease
- ▶Group 2 pulmonary hypertension
- ▶ Code also associated left heart disease, if known, such as:
  - ▶multiple valve disease (I08.-)
  - ▶rheumatic mitral valve diseases (I05.-)
  - ▶rheumatic aortic valve diseases (I06.-)

▶ **I27.23** Pulmonary hypertension due to lung diseases and hypoxia
- ▶Group 3 pulmonary hypertension
- ▶ Code also associated lung disease, if known, such as:
  - ▶bronchiectasis (J47.-)
  - ▶cystic fibrosis with pulmonary manifestations (E84.0)
  - ▶interstitial lung disease (J84.-)
  - ▶pleural effusion (J90)
  - ▶sleep apnea (G47.3-)

▶ **I27.24** Chronic thromboembolic pulmonary hypertension
- ▶Group 4 pulmonary hypertension
- ▶ Code also associated pulmonary embolism, if applicable (I26.-, I27.82)

▶ **I27.29** Other secondary pulmonary hypertension
- ▶Group 5 pulmonary hypertension
- ▶Pulmonary hypertension with unclear multifactorial mechanisms
- ▶Pulmonary hypertension due to hematologic disorders
- ▶Pulmonary hypertension due to metabolic disorders
- ▶Pulmonary hypertension due to other systemic disorders
- ▶ Code also other associated disorders, if known, such as:
  - ▶chronic myeloid leukemia (C92.10- C92.22)
  - ▶essential thrombocythemia (D47.3)
  - ▶Gaucher disease (E75.22)
  - ▶hypertensive chronic kidney disease with end stage renal disease (I12.0, I12.11, I13.2)
  - ▶hyperthyroidism (E05.-)
  - ▶hypothyroidism (E00-E03)
  - ▶polycythemia vera (D45)
  - ▶sarcoidosis (D86.-)

● **I27.8** Other specified pulmonary heart diseases

I27.81 Cor pulmonale (chronic)
- Cor pulmonale NOS
  - **Excludes1** acute cor pulmonale (I26.0-)

I27.82 Chronic pulmonary embolism
- Use additional code, if applicable, for associated long-term (current) use of anticoagulants (Z79.01)
  - **Excludes1** personal history of pulmonary embolism (Z86.711)

▶ **I27.83** Eisenmenger's syndrome
- ▶Eisenmenger's complex
- ▶(Irreversible) Eisenmenger's disease
- ▶Pulmonary hypertension with right to left shunt related to congenital heart disease
- ▶ Code also underlying heart defect, if known, such as:
  - ▶atrial septal defect (Q21.1)
  - ▶Eisenmenger's defect (Q21.8)
  - ▶patent ductus arteriosus (Q25.0)
  - ▶ventricular septal defect (Q21.0)

I27.89 Other specified pulmonary heart diseases
- ~~Eisenmenger's complex~~
- ~~Eisenmenger's syndrome~~
  - **Excludes1** ~~Eisenmenger's defect (Q21.8)~~

I27.9 Pulmonary heart disease, unspecified
- Chronic cardiopulmonary disease

● **I28** Other diseases of pulmonary vessels

I28.0 Arteriovenous fistula of pulmonary vessels
- **Excludes1** congenital arteriovenous fistula (Q25.72)

I28.1 Aneurysm of pulmonary artery
- **Excludes1** congenital aneurysm (Q25.79)
  - congenital arteriovenous aneurysm (Q25.72)

I28.8 Other diseases of pulmonary vessels
- Pulmonary arteritis
- Pulmonary endarteritis
- Rupture of pulmonary vessels
- Stenosis of pulmonary vessels
- Stricture of pulmonary vessels

I28.9 Disease of pulmonary vessels, unspecified

OTHER FORMS OF HEART DISEASE (I30-I52)

● **I30** Acute pericarditis
Inflammation of pericardium (sac surrounding the heart) caused by an infection
- **Includes** acute mediastinopericarditis
  - acute myopericarditis
  - acute pericardial effusion
  - acute pleuropericarditis
  - acute pneumopericarditis
- **Excludes1** Dressler's syndrome (I24.1)
  - rheumatic pericarditis (acute) (I01.0)
  - ▶viral pericarditis due to Coxsakie virus (B33.23)

I30.0 Acute nonspecific idiopathic pericarditis

I30.1 Infective pericarditis
- Pneumococcal pericarditis
- Pneumopyopericardium
- Purulent pericarditis
- Pyopericarditis
- Pyopericardium
- Pyopneumopericardium
- Staphylococcal pericarditis
- Streptococcal pericarditis
- Suppurative pericarditis
- Viral pericarditis
  - Use additional code (B95-B97) to identify infectious agent

I30.8 Other forms of acute pericarditis

I30.9 Acute pericarditis, unspecified

● **I31** Other diseases of pericardium
- **Excludes1** diseases of pericardium specified as rheumatic (I09.2)
  - postcardiotomy syndrome (I97.0)
  - traumatic injury to pericardium (S26.-)

I31.0 Chronic adhesive pericarditis
- Accretio cordis
- Adherent pericardium
- Adhesive mediastinopericarditis

I31.1 Chronic constrictive pericarditis
- Concretio cordis
- Pericardial calcification

I31.2 Hemopericardium, not elsewhere classified
- **Excludes1** hemopericardium as current complication following acute myocardial infarction (I23.0)

I31.3 Pericardial effusion (noninflammatory)
- Chylopericardium
  - **Excludes1** acute pericardial effusion (I30.9)

I31.4 Cardiac tamponade
- *Code first underlying cause*

I31.8 Other specified diseases of pericardium
- Epicardial plaques
- Focal pericardial adhesions

I31.9 Disease of pericardium, unspecified
- Pericarditis (chronic) NOS

▶ New   ⇨ Revised   ~~deleted~~ Deleted   **OGCR** Official Guidelines   X Assign placeholder X   ● Use Additional Character(s)

Excludes 1   Excludes 2   Includes   Use additional   Code first   Code also   Key words

I32   Pericarditis in diseases classified elsewhere
Code first underlying disease
Excludes1   pericarditis (in):
coxsackie (virus) (B33.23)
gonococcal (A54.83)
meningococcal (A39.53)
rheumatoid (arthritis) (M05.31)
syphilitic (A52.06)
systemic lupus erythematosus (M32.12)
tuberculosis (A18.84)

● **I33   Acute and subacute endocarditis**
Inflammation/infection of lining of heart, affecting heart valves
including replacement valves and is usually caused by a
bacterial infection
Excludes1   acute rheumatic endocarditis (I01.1)
endocarditis NOS (I38)

I33.0   **Acute and subacute infective endocarditis**
Bacterial endocarditis (acute) (subacute)
Infective endocarditis (acute) (subacute) NOS
Endocarditis lenta (acute) (subacute)
Malignant endocarditis (acute) (subacute)
Purulent endocarditis (acute) (subacute)
Septic endocarditis (acute) (subacute)
Ulcerative endocarditis (acute) (subacute)
Vegetative endocarditis (acute) (subacute)
Use additional code (B95-B97) to identify infectious
agent

I33.9   **Acute and subacute endocarditis, unspecified**
Acute endocarditis NOS
Acute myoendocarditis NOS
Acute periendocarditis NOS
Subacute endocarditis NOS
Subacute myoendocarditis NOS
Subacute periendocarditis NOS

● **I34   Nonrheumatic mitral valve disorders**
Excludes1   mitral valve disease (I05.9)
mitral valve failure (I05.8)
mitral valve stenosis (I05.0)
mitral valve disorder of unspecified cause with
diseases of aortic and/or tricuspid valve(s)
(I08.-)
mitral valve disorder of unspecified cause with
mitral stenosis or obstruction (I05.0)
➡ mitral valve disorder specified as congenital
(Q23.2, Q23.9)
mitral valve disorder specified as rheumatic
(I05.-)

I34.0   **Nonrheumatic mitral (valve) insufficiency**
Nonrheumatic mitral (valve) incompetence NOS
Nonrheumatic mitral (valve) regurgitation NOS

I34.1   **Nonrheumatic mitral (valve) prolapse**
Floppy nonrheumatic mitral valve syndrome
Excludes1   Marfan's syndrome (Q87.4-)

I34.2   **Nonrheumatic mitral (valve) stenosis**

I34.8   **Other nonrheumatic mitral valve disorders**

I34.9   **Nonrheumatic mitral valve disorder, unspecified**

● **I35   Nonrheumatic aortic valve disorders**
Excludes1   aortic valve disorder of unspecified cause but
with diseases of mitral and/or tricuspid
valve(s) (I08.-)
aortic valve disorder specified as congenital
(Q23.0, Q23.1)
aortic valve disorder specified as rheumatic (I06.-)
hypertrophic subaortic stenosis (I42.1)

I35.0   **Nonrheumatic aortic (valve) stenosis**

I35.1   **Nonrheumatic aortic (valve) insufficiency**
Nonrheumatic aortic (valve) incompetence NOS
Nonrheumatic aortic (valve) regurgitation NOS

I35.2   **Nonrheumatic aortic (valve) stenosis with insufficiency**

I35.8   **Other nonrheumatic aortic valve disorders**

I35.9   **Nonrheumatic aortic valve disorder, unspecified**

● **I36   Nonrheumatic tricuspid valve disorders**
Excludes1   tricuspid valve disorders of unspecified cause
(I07.-)
tricuspid valve disorders specified as congenital
(Q22.4, Q22.8, Q22.9)
tricuspid valve disorders specified as rheumatic
(I07.-)
tricuspid valve disorders with aortic and/or
mitral valve involvement (I08.-)

I36.0   **Nonrheumatic tricuspid (valve) stenosis**

I36.1   **Nonrheumatic tricuspid (valve) insufficiency**
Nonrheumatic tricuspid (valve) incompetence
Nonrheumatic tricuspid (valve) regurgitation

I36.2   **Nonrheumatic tricuspid (valve) stenosis with insufficiency**

I36.8   **Other nonrheumatic tricuspid valve disorders**

I36.9   **Nonrheumatic tricuspid valve disorder, unspecified**

● **I37   Nonrheumatic pulmonary valve disorders**
Excludes1   pulmonary valve disorder specified as congenital
(Q22.1, Q22.2, Q22.3)
pulmonary valve disorder specified as rheumatic
(I09.89)

I37.0   **Nonrheumatic pulmonary valve stenosis**

I37.1   **Nonrheumatic pulmonary valve insufficiency**
Nonrheumatic pulmonary valve incompetence
Nonrheumatic pulmonary valve regurgitation

I37.2   **Nonrheumatic pulmonary valve stenosis with insufficiency**

I37.8   **Other nonrheumatic pulmonary valve disorders**

I37.9   **Nonrheumatic pulmonary valve disorder, unspecified**

I38   **Endocarditis, valve unspecified**
Includes   endocarditis (chronic) NOS
valvular incompetence NOS
valvular insufficiency NOS
valvular regurgitation NOS
valvular stenosis NOS
valvulitis (chronic) NOS
Excludes1   congenital insufficiency of cardiac valve NOS
(Q24.8)
congenital stenosis of cardiac valve NOS (Q24.8)
endocardial fibroelastosis (I42.4)
endocarditis specified as rheumatic (I09.1)

I39   **Endocarditis and heart valve disorders in diseases classified**
elsewhere
Code first underlying disease, such as:
Q fever (A78)
Excludes1   endocardial involvement in:
candidiasis (B37.6)
gonococcal infection (A54.83)
Libman-Sacks disease (M32.11)
listerosis (A32.82)
meningococcal infection (A39.51)
rheumatoid arthritis (M05.31)
syphilis (A52.03)
tuberculosis (A18.84)
typhoid fever (A01.02)

● **I40   Acute myocarditis**
Inflammation of heart muscle due to infection (viral/bacterial)
Includes   subacute myocarditis
Excludes1   acute rheumatic myocarditis (I01.2)

I40.0   **Infective myocarditis**
Septic myocarditis
Use additional code (B95-B97) to identify infectious
agent

I40.1   **Isolated myocarditis**
Fiedler's myocarditis
Giant cell myocarditis
Idiopathic myocarditis

I40.8   **Other acute myocarditis**

I40.9   **Acute myocarditis, unspecified**

CHAPTER 9 (I00-I99)

I41   **Myocarditis in diseases classified elsewhere**
Code first underlying disease, such as:
     typhus (A75.0-A75.9)

Excludes1	myocarditis (in):

           Chagas' disease (chronic) (B57.2)
           acute (B57.0)
           coxsackie (virus) infection (B33.22)
           diphtheritic (A36.81)
           gonococcal (A54.83)
           influenzal (J09.X9, J10.82, J11.82)
           meningococcal (A39.52)
           mumps (B26.82)
           rheumatoid arthritis (M05.31)
           sarcoid (D86.85)
           syphilis (A52.06)
           toxoplasmosis (B58.81)
           tuberculous (A18.84)

● **I42**   **Cardiomyopathy**
Disease of the heart muscle resulting in an abnormally enlarged, weakened, thickened, and/or stiffened muscles

Includes	myocardiopathy

Code first pre-existing cardiomyopathy complicating pregnancy and puerperium (O99.4)

Excludes2	ischemic cardiomyopathy (I25.5)

           peripartum cardiomyopathy (O90.3)
           ventricular hypertrophy (I51.7)

   I42.0   **Dilated cardiomyopathy**
           Congestive cardiomyopathy

   I42.1   **Obstructive hypertrophic cardiomyopathy**
           Hypertrophic subaortic stenosis (idiopathic)

   I42.2   **Other hypertrophic cardiomyopathy**
           Nonobstructive hypertrophic cardiomyopathy

   I42.3   **Endomyocardial (eosinophilic) disease**
           Endomyocardial (tropical) fibrosis
           Löffler's endocarditis

   I42.4   **Endocardial fibroelastosis**
           Congenital cardiomyopathy
           Elastomyofibrosis

   I42.5   **Other restrictive cardiomyopathy**
           Constrictive cardiomyopathy NOS

   I42.6   **Alcoholic cardiomyopathy**
           Code also presence of alcoholism (F10.-)

   I42.7   **Cardiomyopathy due to drug and external agent**
           Code first poisoning due to drug or toxin, if applicable (T36-T65 with fifth or sixth character 1-4 or 6)
           Use additional code for adverse effect, if applicable, to identify drug (T36-T50 with fifth or sixth character 5)

   I42.8   **Other cardiomyopathies**

   I42.9   **Cardiomyopathy, unspecified**
           Cardiomyopathy (primary) (secondary) NOS

I43   **Cardiomyopathy in diseases classified elsewhere**
Code first underlying disease, such as:
     amyloidosis (E85.-)
     glycogen storage disease (E74.0)
     gout (M10.0-)
     thyrotoxicosis (E05.0-E05.9-)

Excludes1	cardiomyopathy (in):

           coxsackie (virus) (B33.24)
           diphtheria (A36.81)
           sarcoidosis (D86.85)
           tuberculosis (A18.84)

● **I44**   **Atrioventricular and left bundle-branch block**
Conduction problem resulting in arrhythmias/dysrhythmias due to a lack of electrical impulses being transmitted normally through the heart

   I44.0   **Atrioventricular block, first degree**

   I44.1   **Atrioventricular block, second degree**
           Atrioventricular block, type I and II
           Möbitz block, type I and II
           Second degree block, type I and II
           Wenckebach's block

   I44.2   **Atrioventricular block, complete**
           Complete heart block NOS
           Third degree block

●   **I44.3**   **Other and unspecified atrioventricular block**
           Atrioventricular block NOS

     I44.30   **Unspecified atrioventricular block**

     I44.39   **Other atrioventricular block**

   I44.4   **Left anterior fascicular block**

   I44.5   **Left posterior fascicular block**

●   **I44.6**   **Other and unspecified fascicular block**

     I44.60   **Unspecified fascicular block**
           Left bundle-branch hemiblock NOS

     I44.69   **Other fascicular block**

   I44.7   **Left bundle-branch block, unspecified**

● **I45**   **Other conduction disorders**

   I45.0   **Right fascicular block**

●   **I45.1**   **Other and unspecified right bundle-branch block**

     I45.10   **Unspecified right bundle-branch block**
           Right bundle-branch block NOS

     I45.19   **Other right bundle-branch block**

   I45.2   **Bifascicular block**

   I45.3   **Trifascicular block**

   I45.4   **Nonspecific intraventricular block**
           Bundle-branch block NOS

   I45.5   **Other specified heart block**
           Sinoatrial block
           Sinoauricular block

Excludes1	heart block NOS (I45.9)

   I45.6   **Pre-excitation syndrome**
           Accelerated atrioventricular conduction
           Accessory atrioventricular conduction
           Anomalous atrioventricular excitation
           Lown-Ganong-Levine syndrome
           Pre-excitation atrioventricular conduction
           Wolff-Parkinson-White syndrome

●   **I45.8**   **Other specified conduction disorders**

     I45.81   **Long QT syndrome**

     I45.89   **Other specified conduction disorders**
           Atrioventricular [AV] dissociation
           Interference dissociation
           Isorhythmic dissociation
           Nonparoxysmal AV nodal tachycardia

   I45.9   **Conduction disorder, unspecified**
           Heart block NOS
           Stokes-Adams syndrome

● **I46**　**Cardiac arrest**
　　Excludes1　cardiogenic shock (R57.0)
　I46.2　**Cardiac arrest due to underlying cardiac condition**
　　　　Code first underlying cardiac condition
　I46.8　**Cardiac arrest due to other underlying condition**
　　　　Code first underlying condition
　I46.9　**Cardiac arrest, cause unspecified**

● **I47**　**Paroxysmal tachycardia**
　　Code first tachycardia complicating:
　　　abortion or ectopic or molar pregnancy (O00-O07, O08.8)
　　　obstetric surgery and procedures (O75.4)
　　Excludes1　tachycardia NOS (R00.0)
　　　　　　sinoauricular tachycardia NOS (R00.0)
　　　　　　sinus [sinusal] tachycardia NOS (R00.0)
　I47.0　**Re-entry ventricular arrhythmia**
　I47.1　**Supraventricular tachycardia**
　　　Atrial (paroxysmal) tachycardia
　　　Atrioventricular [AV] (paroxysmal) tachycardia
　　　Atrioventricular re-entrant (nodal) tachycardia
　　　　[AVNRT] [AVRT]
　　　Junctional (paroxysmal) tachycardia
　　　Nodal (paroxysmal) tachycardia
　I47.2　**Ventricular tachycardia**
　I47.9　**Paroxysmal tachycardia, unspecified**
　　　Bouveret (-Hoffman) syndrome

● **I48**　**Atrial fibrillation and flutter**
　　Most common abnormal heart rhythm (arrhythmia) presenting
　　　as irregular, rapid beating (tachycardia) of the heart's upper
　　　chamber.
　I48.0　**Paroxysmal atrial fibrillation**
　I48.1　**Persistent atrial fibrillation**
　　　Rapid contractions of the upper heart chamber
　I48.2　**Chronic atrial fibrillation**
　　　Permanent atrial fibrillation
　I48.3　**Typical atrial flutter**
　　　Type I atrial flutter
　I48.4　**Atypical atrial flutter**
　　　Type II atrial flutter
　● **I48.9**　**Unspecified atrial fibrillation and atrial flutter**
　　　I48.91　**Unspecified atrial fibrillation**
　　　I48.92　**Unspecified atrial flutter**

● **I49**　**Other cardiac arrhythmias**
　　Code first cardiac arrhythmia complicating:
　　　abortion or ectopic or molar pregnancy (O00-O07, O08.8)
　　　obstetric surgery and procedures (O75.4)
　　Excludes1　~~bradycardia NOS (R00.1)~~
　　　　　　neonatal dysrhythmia (P29.1-)
　　　　　　sinoatrial bradycardia (R00.1)
　　　　　　sinus bradycardia (R00.1)
　　　　　　vagal bradycardia (R00.1)
　　▶ **Excludes2**　bradycardia NOS (R00.1)
　● **I49.0**　**Ventricular fibrillation and flutter**
　　　I49.01　**Ventricular fibrillation**
　　　I49.02　**Ventricular flutter**
　I49.1　**Atrial premature depolarization**
　　　Atrial premature beats
　I49.2　**Junctional premature depolarization**

I49.3　**Ventricular premature depolarization**
● **I49.4**　**Other and unspecified premature depolarization**
　I49.40　**Unspecified premature depolarization**
　　　Premature beats NOS
　I49.49　**Other premature depolarization**
　　　Ectopic beats
　　　Extrasystoles
　　　Extrasystolic arrhythmias
　　　Premature contractions
I49.5　**Sick sinus syndrome**
　　Tachycardia-bradycardia syndrome
I49.8　**Other specified cardiac arrhythmias**
　　▶Brugada syndrome
　　Coronary sinus rhythm disorder
　　Ectopic rhythm disorder
　　Nodal rhythm disorder
I49.9　**Cardiac arrhythmia, unspecified**
　　Arrhythmia (cardiac) NOS

● **I50**　**Heart failure**
　　Code first heart failure complicating abortion or ectopic or molar
　　　pregnancy (O00-O07, O08.8)
　　　heart failure due to hypertension (I11.0)
　　　heart failure due to hypertension with chronic kidney disease
　　　　(I13.-)
　　　heart failure following surgery (I97.13-)
　　　obstetric surgery and procedures (O75.4)
　　　rheumatic heart failure (I09.81)
　　Excludes1　neonatal cardiac failure (P29.0)
　　Excludes2　cardiac arrest (I46.-)
　⇒ **I50.1**　**Left ventricular failure, unspecified**
　　　Cardiac asthma
　　　Edema of lung with heart disease NOS
　　　Edema of lung with heart failure
　　　Left heart failure
　　　Pulmonary edema with heart disease NOS
　　　Pulmonary edema with heart failure
　　Excludes1　edema of lung without heart disease or
　　　　　　heart failure (J81.-)
　　　　　　pulmonary edema without heart disease
　　　　　　or failure (J81.-)
　● **I50.2**　**Systolic (congestive) heart failure**
　　　▶Heart failure with reduced ejection fraction [HFrEF]
　　　▶Systolic left ventricular heart failure
　　　▶ Code also end stage heart failure, if applicable (I50.84)
　　　Excludes1　combined systolic (congestive) and
　　　　　　diastolic (congestive) heart failure
　　　　　　(I50.4-)
　　I50.20　**Unspecified systolic (congestive) heart failure**
　　I50.21　**Acute systolic (congestive) heart failure**
　　　　Presenting a short and relatively severe episode
　　I50.22　**Chronic systolic (congestive) heart failure**
　　　　Long-lasting, presenting over time
　　I50.23　**Acute on chronic systolic (congestive) heart**
　　　　failure
　　　　　Combination code. What was a chronic condition
　　　　　　now has an acute exacerbation (to make more
　　　　　　severe).

Item 9-8 Congestive heart failure (CHF) is a condition in which the left ventricle of the heart cannot pump enough blood to the body. The blood flow from the heart slows or returns to the heart from the venous system (back flow) resulting in congestion (fluid accumulation) particularly in the abdomen. Most commonly, fluid collects in the lungs and results in shortness of breath, especially when in a reclining position.

▶ New　⇒ Revised　~~deleted~~ Deleted　**OGCR** Official Guidelines　X Assign placeholder X　● Use Additional Character(s)
　　　　Excludes 1　Excludes 2　Includes　Use additional　Code first　Code also　Key words

CHAPTER 9 (I00-I99)

CHAPTER 9 (I00-I99)

● **I50.3** **Diastolic (congestive) heart failure**
▶Diastolic left ventricular heart failure
▶Heart failure with normal ejection fraction
▶Heart failure with preserved ejection fraction [HFpEF]
▶ Code also end stage heart failure, if applicable (I50.84)
Excludes1 combined systolic (congestive) and diastolic (congestive) heart failure (I50.4-)

I50.30 **Unspecified** diastolic (congestive) heart failure
I50.31 **Acute** diastolic (congestive) heart failure
I50.32 **Chronic** diastolic (congestive) heart failure
I50.33 **Acute on chronic** diastolic (congestive) heart failure

● **I50.4** **Combined systolic (congestive) and diastolic (congestive) heart failure**
▶Combined systolic and diastolic left ventricular heart failure
▶Heart failure with reduced ejection fraction and diastolic dysfunction
▶ Code also end stage heart failure, if applicable (I50.84)

I50.40 **Unspecified** combined systolic (congestive) and diastolic (congestive) heart failure
I50.41 **Acute** combined systolic (congestive) and diastolic (congestive) heart failure
I50.42 **Chronic** combined systolic (congestive) and diastolic (congestive) heart failure
I50.43 **Acute on chronic** combined systolic (congestive) and diastolic (congestive) heart failure

▶● **I50.8** **Other heart failure**
▶● **I50.81** **Right heart failure**
▶Right ventricular failure

I50.810 **Right heart failure, unspecified**
▶Right heart failure without mention of left heart failure
▶Right ventricular failure NOS

I50.811 **Acute** right heart failure
▶Acute isolated right heart failure
▶Acute (isolated) right ventricular failure

I50.812 **Chronic** right heart failure
▶Chronic isolated right heart failure
▶Chronic (isolated) right ventricular failure

I50.813 **Acute on chronic** right heart failure
▶Acute on chronic isolated right heart failure
▶Acute on chronic (isolated) right ventricular failure
▶Acute decompensation of chronic (isolated) right ventricular failure
▶Acute exacerbation of chronic (isolated) right ventricular failure

I50.814 **Right heart failure due to left heart failure**
▶Right ventricular failure secondary to left ventricular failure
▶ Code also the type of left ventricular failure, if known (I50.2-I50.43)
▶ **Excludes1** Right heart failure with but not due to left heart failure (I50.82)

▶ **I50.82** **Biventricular heart failure**
▶ Code also the type of left ventricular failure as systolic, diastolic, or combined, if known (I50.2-I50.43)
▶ **I50.83** **High output heart failure**
▶ **I50.84** **End stage heart failure**
▶Stage D heart failure
▶ Code also the type of heart failure as systolic, diastolic, or combined, if known (I50.2-I50.43)
▶ **I50.89** **Other heart failure**
I50.9 **Heart failure, unspecified**
~~Biventricular (heart) failure NOS~~
Cardiac, heart or myocardial failure NOS
Congestive heart disease
Congestive heart failure NOS
~~Right ventricular failure (secondary to left heart failure)~~
Excludes2 fluid overload (E87.70)

● **I51** **Complications and ill-defined descriptions of heart disease**
Excludes1 any condition in I51.4-I51.9 due to hypertension (I11.-)
any condition in I51.4-I51.9 due to hypertension and chronic kidney disease (I13.-)
heart disease specified as rheumatic (I00-I09)

I51.0 **Cardiac septal defect, acquired**
Acquired septal atrial defect (old)
Acquired septal auricular defect (old)
Acquired septal ventricular defect (old)
Excludes1 cardiac septal defect as current complication following acute myocardial infarction (I23.1, I23.2)

I51.1 **Rupture of chordae tendineae, not elsewhere classified**
Excludes1 rupture of chordae tendineae as current complication following acute myocardial infarction (I23.4)

I51.2 **Rupture of papillary muscle, not elsewhere classified**
Excludes1 rupture of papillary muscle as current complication following acute myocardial infarction (I23.5)

I51.3 **Intracardiac thrombosis, not elsewhere classified**
Apical thrombosis (old)
Atrial thrombosis (old)
Auricular thrombosis (old)
Mural thrombosis (old)
Ventricular thrombosis (old)
Excludes1 intracardiac thrombosis as current complication following acute myocardial infarction (I23.6)

I51.4 **Myocarditis, unspecified**
Chronic (interstitial) myocarditis
Myocardial fibrosis
Myocarditis NOS
Excludes1 acute or subacute myocarditis (I40.-)

I51.5 **Myocardial degeneration**
Fatty degeneration of heart or myocardium
Myocardial disease
Senile degeneration of heart or myocardium

I51.7 **Cardiomegaly**
Cardiac dilatation
Cardiac hypertrophy
Ventricular dilatation

▶ New   ⟹ Revised   ~~deleted~~ Deleted   **OGCR** Official Guidelines   X Assign placeholder X   ● Use Additional Character(s)
Excludes 1   Excludes 2   Includes   Use additional   Code first   Code also   Key words

● **I51.8** **Other ill-defined heart diseases**
    I51.81 **Takotsubo syndrome**
        Reversible left ventricular dysfunction following sudden emotional stress
        Stress induced cardiomyopathy
        Takotsubo cardiomyopathy
        Transient left ventricular apical ballooning syndrome
    I51.89 **Other ill-defined heart diseases**
        Carditis (acute)(chronic)
        Pancarditis (acute)(chronic)

  I51.9 **Heart disease, unspecified**

I52 **Other heart disorders in diseases classified elsewhere**
    Code first underlying disease, such as:
      congenital syphilis (A50.5)
      mucopolysaccharidosis (E76.3)
      schistosomiasis (B65.0-B65.9)
    Excludes1 heart disease (in):
      gonococcal infection (A54.83)
      meningococcal infection (A39.50)
      rheumatoid arthritis (M05.31)
      syphilis (A52.06)

CEREBROVASCULAR DISEASES (I60-I69)

Use additional code to identify presence of:
  alcohol abuse and dependence (F10.-)
  exposure to environmental tobacco smoke (Z77.22)
  history of tobacco dependence (Z87.891)
  hypertension (I10-I15)
  occupational exposure to environmental tobacco smoke (Z57.31)
  tobacco dependence (F17.-)
  tobacco use (Z72.0)
Excludes1 ~~transient cerebral ischemic attacks and related syndromes (G45.-)~~
      traumatic intracranial hemorrhage (S06.-)

● **I60** **Nontraumatic subarachnoid hemorrhage**
    ~~Includes ruptured cerebral aneurysm~~
    Excludes1 syphilitic ruptured cerebral aneurysm (A52.05)
    Excludes2 sequelae of subarachnoid hemorrhage (I69.0-)

● **I60.0** **Nontraumatic subarachnoid hemorrhage from carotid siphon and bifurcation**
    I60.00 **Nontraumatic subarachnoid hemorrhage from unspecified carotid siphon and bifurcation**
    I60.01 **Nontraumatic subarachnoid hemorrhage from right carotid siphon and bifurcation**
    I60.02 **Nontraumatic subarachnoid hemorrhage from left carotid siphon and bifurcation**

● **I60.1** **Nontraumatic subarachnoid hemorrhage from middle cerebral artery**
    I60.10 **Nontraumatic subarachnoid hemorrhage from unspecified middle cerebral artery**
    I60.11 **Nontraumatic subarachnoid hemorrhage from right middle cerebral artery**
    I60.12 **Nontraumatic subarachnoid hemorrhage from left middle cerebral artery**

  I60.2 **Nontraumatic subarachnoid hemorrhage from anterior communicating artery**

● **I60.3** **Nontraumatic subarachnoid hemorrhage from posterior communicating artery**
    I60.30 **Nontraumatic subarachnoid hemorrhage from unspecified posterior communicating artery**
    I60.31 **Nontraumatic subarachnoid hemorrhage from right posterior communicating artery**
    I60.32 **Nontraumatic subarachnoid hemorrhage from left posterior communicating artery**

  I60.4 **Nontraumatic subarachnoid hemorrhage from basilar artery**

● **I60.5** **Nontraumatic subarachnoid hemorrhage from vertebral artery**
    I60.50 **Nontraumatic subarachnoid hemorrhage from unspecified vertebral artery**
    I60.51 **Nontraumatic subarachnoid hemorrhage from right vertebral artery**
    I60.52 **Nontraumatic subarachnoid hemorrhage from left vertebral artery**

  I60.6 **Nontraumatic subarachnoid hemorrhage from other intracranial arteries**

  I60.7 **Nontraumatic subarachnoid hemorrhage from unspecified intracranial artery**
    Ruptured (congenital) berry aneurysm
    Ruptured (congenital) cerebral aneurysm
    Subarachnoid hemorrhage (nontraumatic) from cerebral artery NOS
    Subarachnoid hemorrhage (nontraumatic) from communicating artery NOS
    Excludes1 berry aneurysm, nonruptured (I67.1)

  I60.8 **Other nontraumatic subarachnoid hemorrhage**
    Meningeal hemorrhage
    Rupture of cerebral arteriovenous malformation

  I60.9 **Nontraumatic subarachnoid hemorrhage, unspecified**

● **I61** **Nontraumatic intracerebral hemorrhage**
    Excludes2 sequelae of intracerebral hemorrhage (I69.1-)

  I61.0 **Nontraumatic intracerebral hemorrhage in hemisphere, subcortical**
    Deep intracerebral hemorrhage (nontraumatic)

  I61.1 **Nontraumatic intracerebral hemorrhage in hemisphere, cortical**
    Cerebral lobe hemorrhage (nontraumatic)
    Superficial intracerebral hemorrhage (nontraumatic)

  I61.2 **Nontraumatic intracerebral hemorrhage in hemisphere, unspecified**

  I61.3 **Nontraumatic intracerebral hemorrhage in brain stem**

  I61.4 **Nontraumatic intracerebral hemorrhage in cerebellum**

  I61.5 **Nontraumatic intracerebral hemorrhage, intraventricular**

  I61.6 **Nontraumatic intracerebral hemorrhage, multiple localized**

  I61.8 **Other nontraumatic intracerebral hemorrhage**

  I61.9 **Nontraumatic intracerebral hemorrhage, unspecified**

● **I62** **Other and unspecified nontraumatic intracranial hemorrhage**
    Excludes2 sequelae of intracranial hemorrhage (I69.2)

● **I62.0** **Nontraumatic subdural hemorrhage**
    I62.00 **Nontraumatic subdural hemorrhage, unspecified**
    I62.01 **Nontraumatic acute subdural hemorrhage**
    I62.02 **Nontraumatic subacute subdural hemorrhage**
    I62.03 **Nontraumatic chronic subdural hemorrhage**

  I62.1 **Nontraumatic extradural hemorrhage**
    Nontraumatic epidural hemorrhage

  I62.9 **Nontraumatic intracranial hemorrhage, unspecified**

Cerebral embolus

Cerebral hemorrhage

Cerebral thrombosis

Figure 9-4   Events causing a stroke. (From Shiland: Mastering Healthcare Terminology, ed 1, St. Louis, Mosby, 2003)

★ **(See Plate 141 on page 76.)**

● I63   Cerebral infarction

     Includes   occlusion and stenosis of cerebral and precerebral arteries, resulting in cerebral infarction

     Use additional code, if applicable, to identify status post administration of tPA (rtPA) in a different facility within the last 24 hours prior to admission to current facility (Z92.82)

     Use additional code, if known, to indicate National Institutes of Health Stroke Scale (NIHSS) score (R29.7-)

     Excludes2   sequelae of cerebral infarction (I69.3-)

● I63.0   Cerebral infarction due to thrombosis of precerebral arteries

     I63.00   Cerebral infarction due to thrombosis of unspecified precerebral artery

     ● I63.01   Cerebral infarction due to thrombosis of vertebral artery

         I63.011   Cerebral infarction due to thrombosis of right vertebral artery

         I63.012   Cerebral infarction due to thrombosis of left vertebral artery

         I63.013   Cerebral infarction due to thrombosis of bilateral vertebral arteries

         I63.019   Cerebral infarction due to thrombosis of unspecified vertebral artery

     I63.02   Cerebral infarction due to thrombosis of basilar artery

     ● I63.03   Cerebral infarction due to thrombosis of carotid artery

         I63.031   Cerebral infarction due to thrombosis of right carotid artery

         I63.032   Cerebral infarction due to thrombosis of left carotid artery

         I63.033   Cerebral infarction due to thrombosis of bilateral carotid arteries

         I63.039   Cerebral infarction due to thrombosis of unspecified carotid artery

     I63.09   Cerebral infarction due to thrombosis of other precerebral artery

● I63.1   Cerebral infarction due to embolism of precerebral arteries

     I63.10   Cerebral infarction due to embolism of unspecified precerebral artery

     ● I63.11   Cerebral infarction due to embolism of vertebral artery

         I63.111   Cerebral infarction due to embolism of right vertebral artery

         I63.112   Cerebral infarction due to embolism of left vertebral artery

         I63.113   Cerebral infarction due to embolism of bilateral vertebral arteries

         I63.119   Cerebral infarction due to embolism of unspecified vertebral artery

     I63.12   Cerebral infarction due to embolism of basilar artery

     ● I63.13   Cerebral infarction due to embolism of carotid artery

         I63.131   Cerebral infarction due to embolism of right carotid artery

         I63.132   Cerebral infarction due to embolism of left carotid artery

         I63.133   Cerebral infarction due to embolism of bilateral carotid arteries

         I63.139   Cerebral infarction due to embolism of unspecified carotid artery

     I63.19   Cerebral infarction due to embolism of other precerebral artery

● I63.2   Cerebral infarction due to unspecified occlusion or stenosis of precerebral arteries

     I63.20   Cerebral infarction due to unspecified occlusion or stenosis of unspecified precerebral arteries

     ● I63.21   Cerebral infarction due to unspecified occlusion or stenosis of vertebral arteries

         ⇒ I63.211   Cerebral infarction due to unspecified occlusion or stenosis of right vertebral artery

         ⇒ I63.212   Cerebral infarction due to unspecified occlusion or stenosis of left vertebral artery

         I63.213   Cerebral infarction due to unspecified occlusion or stenosis of bilateral vertebral arteries

         I63.219   Cerebral infarction due to unspecified occlusion or stenosis of unspecified vertebral arteries

     ⇒ I63.22   Cerebral infarction due to unspecified occlusion or stenosis of basilar artery

     ● I63.23   Cerebral infarction due to unspecified occlusion or stenosis of carotid arteries

         I63.231   Cerebral infarction due to unspecified occlusion or stenosis of right carotid arteries

         I63.232   Cerebral infarction due to unspecified occlusion or stenosis of left carotid arteries

         I63.233   Cerebral infarction due to unspecified occlusion or stenosis of bilateral carotid arteries

         I63.239   Cerebral infarction due to unspecified occlusion or stenosis of unspecified carotid arteries

     I63.29   Cerebral infarction due to unspecified occlusion or stenosis of other precerebral arteries

CHAPTER 9 (I00-I99)

▶ New   ⇒ Revised   ~~deleted~~ Deleted   **OGCR** Official Guidelines   X Assign placeholder X   ● Use Additional Character(s)

Excludes 1   Excludes 2   Includes   Use additional   Code first   Code also   Key words

● **I63.3** Cerebral infarction due to thrombosis of cerebral arteries

   I63.30   Cerebral infarction due to thrombosis of unspecified cerebral artery

● I63.31   Cerebral infarction due to thrombosis of middle cerebral artery

      I63.311   Cerebral infarction due to thrombosis of right middle cerebral artery

      I63.312   Cerebral infarction due to thrombosis of left middle cerebral artery

      I63.313   Cerebral infarction due to thrombosis of bilateral middle cerebral arteries

      I63.319   Cerebral infarction due to thrombosis of unspecified middle cerebral artery

● I63.32   Cerebral infarction due to thrombosis of anterior cerebral artery

      I63.321   Cerebral infarction due to thrombosis of right anterior cerebral artery

      I63.322   Cerebral infarction due to thrombosis of left anterior cerebral artery

    ➠ I63.323   Cerebral infarction due to thrombosis of bilateral anterior cerebral arteries

      I63.329   Cerebral infarction due to thrombosis of unspecified anterior cerebral artery

● I63.33   Cerebral infarction due to thrombosis of posterior cerebral artery

      I63.331   Cerebral infarction due to thrombosis of right posterior cerebral artery

      I63.332   Cerebral infarction due to thrombosis of left posterior cerebral artery

    ➠ I63.333   Cerebral infarction to thrombosis of bilateral posterior cerebral arteries

      I63.339   Cerebral infarction due to thrombosis of unspecified posterior cerebral artery

● I63.34   Cerebral infarction due to thrombosis of cerebellar artery

      I63.341   Cerebral infarction due to thrombosis of right cerebellar artery

      I63.342   Cerebral infarction due to thrombosis of left cerebellar artery

      I63.343   Cerebral infarction to thrombosis of bilateral cerebellar arteries

      I63.349   Cerebral infarction due to thrombosis of unspecified cerebellar artery

   I63.39   Cerebral infarction due to thrombosis of other cerebral artery

● **I63.4** Cerebral infarction due to embolism of cerebral arteries

   I63.40   Cerebral infarction due to embolism of unspecified cerebral artery

● I63.41   Cerebral infarction due to embolism of middle cerebral artery

      I63.411   Cerebral infarction due to embolism of right middle cerebral artery

      I63.412   Cerebral infarction due to embolism of left middle cerebral artery

      I63.413   Cerebral infarction due to embolism of bilateral middle cerebral arteries

      I63.419   Cerebral infarction due to embolism of unspecified middle cerebral artery

● I63.42   Cerebral infarction due to embolism of anterior cerebral artery

      I63.421   Cerebral infarction due to embolism of right anterior cerebral artery

      I63.422   Cerebral infarction due to embolism of left anterior cerebral artery

      I63.423   Cerebral infarction due to embolism of bilateral anterior cerebral arteries

      I63.429   Cerebral infarction due to embolism of unspecified anterior cerebral artery

● I63.43   Cerebral infarction due to embolism of posterior cerebral artery

      I63.431   Cerebral infarction due to embolism of right posterior cerebral artery

      I63.432   Cerebral infarction due to embolism of left posterior cerebral artery

      I63.433   Cerebral infarction due to embolism of bilateral posterior cerebral arteries

      I63.439   Cerebral infarction due to embolism of unspecified posterior cerebral artery

● I63.44   Cerebral infarction due to embolism of cerebellar artery

      I63.441   Cerebral infarction due to embolism of right cerebellar artery

      I63.442   Cerebral infarction due to embolism of left cerebellar artery

      I63.443   Cerebral infarction due to embolism of bilateral cerebellar arteries

      I63.449   Cerebral infarction due to embolism of unspecified cerebellar artery

   I63.49   Cerebral infarction due to embolism of other cerebral artery

● **I63.5** Cerebral infarction due to unspecified occlusion or stenosis of cerebral arteries

   I63.50   Cerebral infarction due to unspecified occlusion or stenosis of unspecified cerebral artery

● I63.51   Cerebral infarction due to unspecified occlusion or stenosis of middle cerebral artery

      I63.511   Cerebral infarction due to unspecified occlusion or stenosis of right middle cerebral artery

      I63.512   Cerebral infarction due to unspecified occlusion or stenosis of left middle cerebral artery

    ➠ I63.513   Cerebral infarction due to unspecified occlusion or stenosis of bilateral middle cerebral arteries

      I63.519   Cerebral infarction due to unspecified occlusion or stenosis of unspecified middle cerebral artery

● I63.52   Cerebral infarction due to unspecified occlusion or stenosis of anterior cerebral artery

      I63.521   Cerebral infarction due to unspecified occlusion or stenosis of right anterior cerebral artery

      I63.522   Cerebral infarction due to unspecified occlusion or stenosis of left anterior cerebral artery

    ➠ I63.523   Cerebral infarction due to unspecified occlusion or stenosis of bilateral anterior cerebral arteries

      I63.529   Cerebral infarction due to unspecified occlusion or stenosis of unspecified anterior cerebral artery

▶ New   ➠ Revised   ~~deleted~~ Deleted   **OGCR** Official Guidelines   X Assign placeholder X   ● Use Additional Character(s)

Excludes 1   Excludes 2   Includes   Use additional   Code first   Code also   Key words

● I63.53   Cerebral infarction due to unspecified occlusion or stenosis of posterior cerebral artery

    I63.531   Cerebral infarction due to unspecified occlusion or stenosis of right posterior cerebral artery

    I63.532   Cerebral infarction due to unspecified occlusion or stenosis of left posterior cerebral artery

    ⮕ I63.533   Cerebral infarction due to unspecified occlusion or stenosis of bilateral posterior cerebral arteries

    I63.539   Cerebral infarction due to unspecified occlusion or stenosis of unspecified posterior cerebral artery

● I63.54   Cerebral infarction due to unspecified occlusion or stenosis of cerebellar artery

    I63.541   Cerebral infarction due to unspecified occlusion or stenosis of right cerebellar artery

    I63.542   Cerebral infarction due to unspecified occlusion or stenosis of left cerebellar artery

    I63.543   Cerebral infarction due to unspecified occlusion or stenosis of bilateral cerebellar arteries

    I63.549   Cerebral infarction due to unspecified occlusion or stenosis of unspecified cerebellar artery

I63.59   Cerebral infarction due to unspecified occlusion or stenosis of other cerebral artery

I63.6   Cerebral infarction due to cerebral venous thrombosis, nonpyogenic

I63.8   Other cerebral infarction

I63.9   Cerebral infarction, unspecified
    Stroke NOS
    ▶ **Excludes2**   transient cerebral ischemic attacks and related syndromes (G45.-)

● I65   Occlusion and stenosis of precerebral arteries, not resulting in cerebral infarction

    Includes   embolism of precerebral artery
       narrowing of precerebral artery
       obstruction (complete) (partial) of precerebral artery
       thrombosis of precerebral artery

    Excludes1   insufficiency, NOS, of precerebral artery (G45.-)
       insufficiency of precerebral arteries causing cerebral infarction (I63.0-I63.2)

● I65.0   Occlusion and stenosis of vertebral artery

    I65.01   Occlusion and stenosis of right vertebral artery

    I65.02   Occlusion and stenosis of left vertebral artery

    I65.03   Occlusion and stenosis of bilateral vertebral arteries

    I65.09   Occlusion and stenosis of unspecified vertebral artery

I65.1   Occlusion and stenosis of basilar artery

● I65.2   Occlusion and stenosis of carotid artery

    I65.21   Occlusion and stenosis of right carotid artery

    I65.22   Occlusion and stenosis of left carotid artery

    I65.23   Occlusion and stenosis of bilateral carotid arteries

    I65.29   Occlusion and stenosis of unspecified carotid artery

I65.8   Occlusion and stenosis of other precerebral arteries

I65.9   Occlusion and stenosis of unspecified precerebral artery
    Occlusion and stenosis of precerebral artery NOS

● I66   Occlusion and stenosis of cerebral arteries, not resulting in cerebral infarction

    Includes   embolism of cerebral artery
       narrowing of cerebral artery
       obstruction (complete) (partial) of cerebral artery
       thrombosis of cerebral artery

    Excludes1   occlusion and stenosis of cerebral artery causing cerebral infarction (I63.3-I63.5)

● I66.0   Occlusion and stenosis of middle cerebral artery

    I66.01   Occlusion and stenosis of right middle cerebral artery

    I66.02   Occlusion and stenosis of left middle cerebral artery

    I66.03   Occlusion and stenosis of bilateral middle cerebral arteries

    I66.09   Occlusion and stenosis of unspecified middle cerebral artery

● I66.1   Occlusion and stenosis of anterior cerebral artery

    I66.11   Occlusion and stenosis of right anterior cerebral artery

    I66.12   Occlusion and stenosis of left anterior cerebral artery

    I66.13   Occlusion and stenosis of bilateral anterior cerebral arteries

    I66.19   Occlusion and stenosis of unspecified anterior cerebral artery

● I66.2   Occlusion and stenosis of posterior cerebral artery

    I66.21   Occlusion and stenosis of right posterior cerebral artery

    I66.22   Occlusion and stenosis of left posterior cerebral artery

    I66.23   Occlusion and stenosis of bilateral posterior cerebral arteries

    I66.29   Occlusion and stenosis of unspecified posterior cerebral artery

I66.3   Occlusion and stenosis of cerebellar arteries

I66.8   Occlusion and stenosis of other cerebral arteries
    Occlusion and stenosis of perforating arteries

I66.9   Occlusion and stenosis of unspecified cerebral artery

● I67   Other cerebrovascular diseases
    Excludes2   sequelae of the listed conditions (I69.8)

I67.0   Dissection of cerebral arteries, nonruptured
    Excludes1   ruptured cerebral arteries (I60.7)

I67.1   Cerebral aneurysm, nonruptured
    Cerebral aneurysm NOS
    Cerebral arteriovenous fistula, acquired
    Internal carotid artery aneurysm, intracranial portion
    Internal carotid artery aneurysm, NOS
    Excludes1   congenital cerebral aneurysm, nonruptured (Q28.-)
       ruptured cerebral aneurysm (I60.7)

I67.2   Cerebral atherosclerosis
    Atheroma of cerebral and precerebral arteries

I67.3   Progressive vascular leukoencephalopathy
    Binswanger's disease

I67.4   Hypertensive encephalopathy
    ▶ **Excludes2**   insufficiency, NOS, of precerebral arteries (G45.2)

I67.5   Moyamoya disease

I67.6   Nonpyogenic thrombosis of intracranial venous system
    Nonpyogenic thrombosis of cerebral vein
    Nonpyogenic thrombosis of intracranial venous sinus
    Excludes1   nonpyogenic thrombosis of intracranial venous system causing infarction (I63.6)

I67.7   Cerebral arteritis, not elsewhere classified
    Granulomatous angiitis of the nervous system
    Excludes1   allergic granulomatous angiitis (M30.1)

▶ New   ⮕ Revised   ~~deleted~~ Deleted   **OGCR** Official Guidelines   X Assign placeholder X   ● Use Additional Character(s)

Excludes 1   Excludes 2   Includes   Use additional   Code first   Code also   Key words

OGCR Section I.c.9.d.

Sequelae of Cerebrovascular Disease

1) Category I69, Sequelae of Cerebrovascular disease

Category 169 is used to indicate conditions classifiable to categories I60-I67 as the causes of sequela (neurologic deficits), themselves classified elsewhere. These "late effects" include neurologic deficits that persist after initial onset of conditions classifiable to categories I60-I67. The neurologic deficits caused by cerebrovascular disease may be present from the onset of may arise at any time after the onset of the condition classifiable to categories I60-I67.

Codes from category I69, Sequelae of cerebrovascular disease, that specify hemiplegia, hemiparesis and monoplegia identify whether the dominant or nondominant side is affected. Should the affected side be documented, but not specified as dominant or nondominant, and the classification system does not indicate a default, code selection is as follows:

For ambidextrous patients, the default should be dominant.

If the left side is affected, the default is non-dominant.

If the right side is affected, the default is dominant.

2) Codes from category I69 with codes from I60-I67

Codes from category I69 may be assigned on a health care record with codes from I60-I67, if the patient has a current cerebrovascular disease and deficits from an old cerebrovascular disease.

- ● **I67.8**   **Other specified cerebrovascular diseases**
  - **I67.81**   **Acute cerebrovascular insufficiency**
    - Acute cerebrovascular insufficiency unspecified as to location or reversibility
  - **I67.82**   **Cerebral ischemia**
    - Chronic cerebral ischemia
  - **I67.83**   **Posterior reversible encephalopathy syndrome**
    - PRES
  - ● **I67.84**   **Cerebral vasospasm and vasoconstriction**
    - **I67.841**   **Reversible cerebrovascular vasoconstriction syndrome**
      - Call-Fleming syndrome
      - *Code first underlying condition, if applicable, such as eclampsia (O15.00-O15.9)*
    - **I67.848**   **Other cerebrovascular vasospasm and vasoconstriction**
  - **I67.89**   **Other cerebrovascular disease**
- **I67.9**   **Cerebrovascular disease, unspecified**

- ● **I68**   **Cerebrovascular disorders in diseases classified elsewhere**
  - **I68.0**   **Cerebral amyloid angiopathy**
    - *Code first underlying amyloidosis (E85.-)*
  - **I68.2**   **Cerebral arteritis in other diseases classified elsewhere**
    - *Code first underlying disease*
    - **Excludes1**   cerebral arteritis (in):
      - listerosis (A32.89)
      - systemic lupus erythematosus (M32.19)
      - syphilis (A52.04)
      - tuberculosis (A18.89)
  - **I68.8**   **Other cerebrovascular disorders in diseases classified elsewhere**
    - *Code first underlying disease*
    - **Excludes1**   syphilitic cerebral aneurysm (A52.05)

- ● **I69**   **Sequelae of cerebrovascular disease**
  - **Note:** Category I69 is to be used to indicate conditions in I60-I67 as the cause of sequelae. The 'sequelae' include conditions specified as such or as residuals which may occur at any time after the onset of the causal condition.
  - **Excludes1**   personal history of cerebral infarction without residual deficit (Z86.73)
    - personal history of prolonged reversible ischemic neurologic deficit (PRIND) (Z86.73)
    - personal history of reversible ischemic neurologcial deficit (RIND) (Z86.73)
    - sequelae of traumatic intracranial injury (S06.-)
    - ~~transient ischemic attack (TIA) (G45.9)~~
  - ● **I69.0**   **Sequelae of nontraumatic subarachnoid hemorrhage**
    - **I69.00**   **Unspecified sequelae of nontraumatic subarachnoid hemorrhage**
    - ● **I69.01**   **Cognitive deficits following nontraumatic subarachnoid hemorrhage**
      - **I69.010**   **Attention and concentration** deficit following nontraumatic subarachnoid hemorrhage
      - **I69.011**   **Memory** deficit following nontraumatic subarachnoid hemorrhage
      - **I69.012**   **Visuospatial** deficit and spatial neglect following nontraumatic subarachnoid hemorrhage
      - **I69.013**   **Psychomotor** deficit following nontraumatic subarachnoid hemorrhage
      - **I69.014**   **Frontal lobe and executive function** deficit following nontraumatic subarachnoid hemorrhage
      - **I69.015**   **Cognitive social or emotional** deficit following nontraumatic subarachnoid hemorrhage
      - **I69.018**   **Other symptoms and signs** involving cognitive functions following nontraumatic subarachnoid hemorrhage
      - **I69.019**   **Unspecified** symptoms and signs involving cognitive functions following nontraumatic subarachnoid hemorrhage
    - ● **I69.02**   **Speech and language deficits** following nontraumatic subarachnoid hemorrhage
      - **I69.020**   **Aphasia** following nontraumatic subarachnoid hemorrhage
      - **I69.021**   **Dysphasia** following nontraumatic subarachnoid hemorrhage
      - **I69.022**   **Dysarthria** following nontraumatic subarachnoid hemorrhage
      - **I69.023**   **Fluency disorder** following nontraumatic subarachnoid hemorrhage
        - Stuttering following nontraumatic subarachnoid hemorrhage
      - **I69.028**   **Other** speech and language deficits following nontraumatic subarachnoid hemorrhage

CHAPTER 9 (I00-I99)

● **I69.03** Monoplegia of upper limb following nontraumatic subarachnoid hemorrhage

   I69.031 Monoplegia of upper limb following nontraumatic subarachnoid hemorrhage affecting right dominant side

   I69.032 Monoplegia of upper limb following nontraumatic subarachnoid hemorrhage affecting left dominant side

   I69.033 Monoplegia of upper limb following nontraumatic subarachnoid hemorrhage affecting right non-dominant side

   I69.034 Monoplegia of upper limb following nontraumatic subarachnoid hemorrhage affecting left non-dominant side

   I69.039 Monoplegia of upper limb following nontraumatic subarachnoid hemorrhage affecting unspecified side

● **I69.04** Monoplegia of lower limb following nontraumatic subarachnoid hemorrhage

   I69.041 Monoplegia of lower limb following nontraumatic subarachnoid hemorrhage affecting right dominant side

   I69.042 Monoplegia of lower limb following nontraumatic subarachnoid hemorrhage affecting left dominant side

   I69.043 Monoplegia of lower limb following nontraumatic subarachnoid hemorrhage affecting right non-dominant side

   I69.044 Monoplegia of lower limb following nontraumatic subarachnoid hemorrhage affecting left non-dominant side

   I69.049 Monoplegia of lower limb following nontraumatic subarachnoid hemorrhage affecting unspecified side

● **I69.05** Hemiplegia and hemiparesis following nontraumatic subarachnoid hemorrhage

   I69.051 Hemiplegia and hemiparesis following nontraumatic subarachnoid hemorrhage affecting right dominant side

   I69.052 Hemiplegia and hemiparesis following nontraumatic subarachnoid hemorrhage affecting left dominant side

   I69.053 Hemiplegia and hemiparesis following nontraumatic subarachnoid hemorrhage affecting right non-dominant side

   I69.054 Hemiplegia and hemiparesis following nontraumatic subarachnoid hemorrhage affecting left non-dominant side

   I69.059 Hemiplegia and hemiparesis following nontraumatic subarachnoid hemorrhage affecting unspecified side

● **I69.06** Other paralytic syndrome following nontraumatic subarachnoid hemorrhage

   Use additional code to identify type of paralytic syndrome, such as:
   locked-in state (G83.5)
   quadriplegia (G82.5-)

   Excludes1 hemiplegia/hemiparesis following nontraumatic subarachnoid hemorrhage (I69.05-)
     monoplegia of lower limb following nontraumatic subarachnoid hemorrhage (I69.04-)
     monoplegia of upper limb following nontraumatic subarachnoid hemorrhage (I69.03-)

   I69.061 Other paralytic syndrome following nontraumatic subarachnoid hemorrhage affecting right dominant side

   I69.062 Other paralytic syndrome following nontraumatic subarachnoid hemorrhage affecting left dominant side

   I69.063 Other paralytic syndrome following nontraumatic subarachnoid hemorrhage affecting right non-dominant side

   I69.064 Other paralytic syndrome following nontraumatic subarachnoid hemorrhage affecting left non-dominant side

   I69.065 Other paralytic syndrome following nontraumatic subarachnoid hemorrhage, bilateral

   I69.069 Other paralytic syndrome following nontraumatic subarachnoid hemorrhage affecting unspecified side

● **I69.09** Other sequelae of nontraumatic subarachnoid hemorrhage

   I69.090 Apraxia following nontraumatic subarachnoid hemorrhage

   I69.091 Dysphagia following nontraumatic subarachnoid hemorrhage

     Use additional code to identify the type of dysphagia, if known (R13.1-)

   I69.092 Facial weakness following nontraumatic subarachnoid hemorrhage

     Facial droop following nontraumatic subarachnoid hemorrhage

   I69.093 Ataxia following nontraumatic subarachnoid hemorrhage

   I69.098 Other sequelae following nontraumatic subarachnoid hemorrhage

     Alterations of sensation following nontraumatic subarachnoid hemorrhage
     Disturbance of vision following nontraumatic subarachnoid hemorrhage
     Use additional code to identify the sequelae

▶ New   ➡ Revised   ~~deleted~~ Deleted   **OGCR** Official Guidelines   X Assign placeholder X   ● Use Additional Character(s)

Excludes 1   Excludes 2   Includes   Use additional   Code first   Code also   Key words

● **I69.1**　**Sequelae** of nontraumatic **intracerebral** hemorrhage

　　I69.10　**Unspecified** sequelae of nontraumatic intracerebral hemorrhage

　● **I69.11**　**Cognitive deficits** following nontraumatic intracerebral hemorrhage

　　　I69.110　**Attention and concentration** deficit following nontraumatic intracerebral hemorrhage

　　　I69.111　**Memory** deficit following nontraumatic intracerebral hemorrhage

　　　I69.112　**Visuospatial** deficit and spatial neglect following nontraumatic intracerebral hemorrhage

　　　I69.113　**Psychomotor** deficit following nontraumatic intracerebral hemorrhage

　　　I69.114　**Frontal lobe and executive function** deficit following nontraumatic intracerebral hemorrhage

　　　I69.115　**Cognitive social or emotional** deficit following nontraumatic intracerebral hemorrhage

　　　I69.118　**Other symptoms and signs** involving cognitive functions following nontraumatic intracerebral hemorrhage

　　　I69.119　**Unspecified** symptoms and signs involving cognitive functions following nontraumatic intracerebral hemorrhage

　● **I69.12**　**Speech and language deficits** following nontraumatic intracerebral hemorrhage

　　　I69.120　**Aphasia** following nontraumatic intracerebral hemorrhage

　　　I69.121　**Dysphasia** following nontraumatic intracerebral hemorrhage

　　　I69.122　**Dysarthria** following nontraumatic intracerebral hemorrhage

　　　I69.123　**Fluency disorder** following nontraumatic intracerebral hemorrhage
　　　　　　　Stuttering following nontraumatic intracerebral hemorrhage

　　　I69.128　**Other** speech and language deficits following nontraumatic intracerebral hemorrhage

　● **I69.13**　**Monoplegia of upper limb** following nontraumatic intracerebral hemorrhage

　　　I69.131　Monoplegia of upper limb following nontraumatic intracerebral hemorrhage affecting **right dominant side**

　　　I69.132　Monoplegia of upper limb following nontraumatic intracerebral hemorrhage affecting **left dominant side**

　　　I69.133　Monoplegia of upper limb following nontraumatic intracerebral hemorrhage affecting **right non-dominant side**

　　　I69.134　Monoplegia of upper limb following nontraumatic intracerebral hemorrhage affecting left **non-dominant side**

　　　I69.139　Monoplegia of upper limb following nontraumatic intracerebral hemorrhage affecting **unspecified** side

● **I69.14**　**Monoplegia of lower limb** following nontraumatic intracerebral hemorrhage

　　I69.141　Monoplegia of lower limb following nontraumatic intracerebral hemorrhage affecting **right dominant side**

　　I69.142　Monoplegia of lower limb following nontraumatic intracerebral hemorrhage affecting **left dominant side**

　　I69.143　Monoplegia of lower limb following nontraumatic intracerebral hemorrhage affecting **right non-dominant side**

　　I69.144　Monoplegia of lower limb following nontraumatic intracerebral hemorrhage affecting **left non-dominant side**

　　I69.149　Monoplegia of lower limb following nontraumatic intracerebral hemorrhage affecting **unspecified** side

● **I69.15**　**Hemiplegia and hemiparesis** following nontraumatic intracerebral hemorrhage

　　I69.151　Hemiplegia and hemiparesis following nontraumatic intracerebral hemorrhage affecting **right dominant side**

　　I69.152　Hemiplegia and hemiparesis following nontraumatic intracerebral hemorrhage affecting **left dominant side**

　　I69.153　Hemiplegia and hemiparesis following nontraumatic intracerebral hemorrhage affecting **right non-dominant side**

　　I69.154　Hemiplegia and hemiparesis following nontraumatic intracerebral hemorrhage affecting **left non-dominant side**

　　I69.159　Hemiplegia and hemiparesis following nontraumatic intracerebral hemorrhage affecting **unspecified** side

● **I69.16**　**Other paralytic syndrome** following nontraumatic intracerebral hemorrhage

　　Use additional code to identify type of paralytic syndrome, such as:
　　locked-in state (G83.5)
　　quadriplegia (G82.5-)

　　| **Excludes1** | hemiplegia/hemiparesis following nontraumatic intracerebral hemorrhage (I69.15-)
　　　　　　　monoplegia of lower limb following nontraumatic intracerebral hemorrhage (I69.14-)
　　　　　　　monoplegia of upper limb following nontraumatic intracerebral hemorrhage (I69.13-)

　　I69.161　Other paralytic syndrome following nontraumatic intracerebral hemorrhage affecting **right dominant side**

　　I69.162　Other paralytic syndrome following nontraumatic intracerebral hemorrhage affecting **left dominant side**

　　I69.163　Other paralytic syndrome following nontraumatic intracerebral hemorrhage affecting **right non-dominant side**

　　I69.164　Other paralytic syndrome following nontraumatic intracerebral hemorrhage affecting **left non-dominant side**

　　I69.165　Other paralytic syndrome following nontraumatic intracerebral hemorrhage, **bilateral**

　　I69.169　Other paralytic syndrome following nontraumatic intracerebral hemorrhage affecting **unspecified** side

---

▶ New　⇒ Revised　~~deleted~~ Deleted　**OGCR** Official Guidelines　X Assign placeholder X　● Use Additional Character(s)

Excludes 1　Excludes 2　Includes　Use additional　Code first　Code also　Key words

● **I69.19**   **Other** sequelae of nontraumatic intracerebral hemorrhage

    I69.190   **Apraxia** following nontraumatic intracerebral hemorrhage

    I69.191   **Dysphagia** following nontraumatic intracerebral hemorrhage

       Use additional code to identify the type of dysphagia, if known (R13.1-)

    I69.192   **Facial weakness** following nontraumatic intracerebral hemorrhage

       Facial droop following nontraumatic intracerebral hemorrhage

    I69.193   **Ataxia** following nontraumatic intracerebral hemorrhage

    I69.198   **Other** sequelae of nontraumatic intracerebral hemorrhage

       Alteration of sensations following nontraumatic intracerebral hemorrhage

       Disturbance of vision following nontraumatic intracerebral hemorrhage

       Use additional code to identify the sequelae

● **I69.2**   Sequelae of other nontraumatic **intracranial** hemorrhage

    I69.20   **Unspecified** sequelae of other nontraumatic intracranial hemorrhage

●   I69.21   **Cognitive deficits** following other nontraumatic intracranial hemorrhage

    I69.210   **Attention and concentration** deficit following other nontraumatic intracranial hemorrhage

    I69.211   **Memory** deficit following other nontraumatic intracranial hemorrhage

    I69.212   **Visuospatial** deficit and spatial neglect following other nontraumatic intracranial hemorrhage

    I69.213   **Psychomotor** deficit following other nontraumatic intracranial hemorrhage

    I69.214   **Frontal lobe and executive function** deficit following other nontraumatic intracranial hemorrhage

    I69.215   **Cognitive social or emotional** deficit following other nontraumatic intracranial hemorrhage

    I69.218   **Other** symptoms and signs involving cognitive functions following other nontraumatic intracranial hemorrhage

    I69.219   **Unspecified** symptoms and signs involving cognitive functions following other nontraumatic intracranial hemorrhage

●   I69.22   **Speech and language deficits** following other nontraumatic intracranial hemorrhage

    I69.220   **Aphasia** following other nontraumatic intracranial hemorrhage

    I69.221   **Dysphasia** following other nontraumatic intracranial hemorrhage

    I69.222   **Dysarthria** following other nontraumatic intracranial hemorrhage

    I69.223   **Fluency disorder** following other nontraumatic intracranial hemorrhage

       Stuttering following other nontraumatic intracranial hemorrhage

    I69.228   **Other** speech and language deficits following other nontraumatic intracranial hemorrhage

● **I69.23**   **Monoplegia of upper limb** following other nontraumatic intracranial hemorrhage

    I69.231   Monoplegia of upper limb following other nontraumatic intracranial hemorrhage affecting **right dominant side**

    I69.232   Monoplegia of upper limb following other nontraumatic intracranial hemorrhage affecting **left dominant side**

    I69.233   Monoplegia of upper limb following other nontraumatic intracranial hemorrhage affecting **right non-dominant side**

    I69.234   Monoplegia of upper limb following other nontraumatic intracranial hemorrhage affecting **left non-dominant side**

    I69.239   Monoplegia of upper limb following other nontraumatic intracranial hemorrhage affecting **unspecified** side

● **I69.24**   **Monoplegia of lower limb** following other nontraumatic intracranial hemorrhage

    I69.241   Monoplegia of lower limb following other nontraumatic intracranial hemorrhage affecting **right dominant side**

    I69.242   Monoplegia of lower limb following other nontraumatic intracranial hemorrhage affecting **left dominant side**

    I69.243   Monoplegia of lower limb following other nontraumatic intracranial hemorrhage affecting **right non-dominant side**

    I69.244   Monoplegia of lower limb following other nontraumatic intracranial hemorrhage affecting **left non-dominant side**

    I69.249   Monoplegia of lower limb following other nontraumatic intracranial hemorrhage affecting **unspecified** side

● **I69.25**   **Hemiplegia and hemiparesis** following other nontraumatic intracranial hemorrhage

    I69.251   Hemiplegia and hemiparesis following other nontraumatic intracranial hemorrhage affecting **right dominant side**

    I69.252   Hemiplegia and hemiparesis following other nontraumatic intracranial hemorrhage affecting **left dominant side**

    I69.253   Hemiplegia and hemiparesis following other nontraumatic intracranial hemorrhage affecting **right non-dominant side**

    I69.254   Hemiplegia and hemiparesis following other nontraumatic intracranial hemorrhage affecting **left non-dominant side**

    I69.259   Hemiplegia and hemiparesis following other nontraumatic intracranial hemorrhage affecting **unspecified** side

▶ New   ⇒ Revised   ~~deleted~~ Deleted   **OGCR** Official Guidelines   X Assign placeholder X   ● Use Additional Character(s)

Excludes 1   Excludes 2   Includes   Use additional   Code first   Code also   Key words

● **I69.26**   **Other** paralytic syndrome following other nontraumatic intracranial hemorrhage

> Use additional code to identify type of paralytic syndrome, such as:
> locked-in state (G83.5)
> quadriplegia (G82.5-)

> Excludes1   hemiplegia/hemiparesis following other nontraumatic intracranial hemorrhage (I69.25-)
> monoplegia of lower limb following other nontraumatic intracranial hemorrhage (I69.24-)
> monoplegia of upper limb following other nontraumatic intracranial hemorrhage (I69.23-)

     I69.261   Other paralytic syndrome following other nontraumatic intracranial hemorrhage affecting **right dominant side**

     I69.262   Other paralytic syndrome following other nontraumatic intracranial hemorrhage affecting **left dominant side**

     I69.263   Other paralytic syndrome following other nontraumatic intracranial hemorrhage affecting **right non-dominant side**

     I69.264   Other paralytic syndrome following other nontraumatic intracranial hemorrhage affecting **left non-dominant side**

     I69.265   Other paralytic syndrome following other nontraumatic intracranial hemorrhage, **bilateral**

     I69.269   Other paralytic syndrome following other nontraumatic intracranial hemorrhage affecting **unspecified** side

● **I69.29**   **Other** sequelae of other nontraumatic intracranial hemorrhage

     I69.290   **Apraxia** following other nontraumatic intracranial hemorrhage

     I69.291   **Dysphagia** following other nontraumatic intracranial hemorrhage

> Use additional code to identify the type of dysphagia, if known (R13.1-)

     I69.292   **Facial weakness** following other nontraumatic intracranial hemorrhage
> Facial droop following other nontraumatic intracranial hemorrhage

     I69.293   **Ataxia** following other nontraumatic intracranial hemorrhage

     I69.298   **Other** sequelae of other nontraumatic intracranial hemorrhage
> Alteration of sensation following other nontraumatic intracranial hemorrhage
> Disturbance of vision following other nontraumatic intracranial hemorrhage
> Use additional code to identify the sequelae

● **I69.3**   Sequelae of **cerebral infarction**
> Sequelae of stroke NOS

     I69.30   **Unspecified** sequelae of cerebral infarction

● **I69.31**   **Cognitive deficits** following cerebral infarction

     I69.310   **Attention and concentration** deficit following cerebral infarction

     I69.311   **Memory** deficit following cerebral infarction

     I69.312   **Visuospatial** deficit and spatial neglect following cerebral infarction

     I69.313   **Psychomotor** deficit following cerebral infarction

     I69.314   **Frontal lobe and executive function** deficit following cerebral infarction

     I69.315   **Cognitive social or emotional** deficit following cerebral infarction

     I69.318   **Other** symptoms and signs involving cognitive functions following cerebral infarction

     I69.319   **Unspecified** symptoms and signs involving cognitive functions following cerebral infarction

● **I69.32**   **Speech and language** deficits following cerebral infarction

     I69.320   **Aphasia** following cerebral infarction

     I69.321   **Dysphasia** following cerebral infarction

     I69.322   **Dysarthria** following cerebral infarction

> ▶ Excludes2   transient ischemic attack (TIA) (G45.9)

     I69.323   **Fluency disorder** following cerebral infarction
> Stuttering following cerebral infarction

     I69.328   **Other** speech and language deficits following cerebral infarction

● **I69.33**   **Monoplegia of upper limb** following cerebral infarction

     I69.331   Monoplegia of upper limb following cerebral infarction affecting **right dominant side**

     I69.332   Monoplegia of upper limb following cerebral infarction affecting **left dominant side**

     I69.333   Monoplegia of upper limb following cerebral infarction affecting **right non-dominant side**

     I69.334   Monoplegia of upper limb following cerebral infarction affecting **left non-dominant side**

     I69.339   Monoplegia of upper limb following cerebral infarction affecting **unspecified** side

● I69.34 **Monoplegia of lower limb** following cerebral infarction

I69.341 Monoplegia of lower limb following cerebral infarction affecting **right dominant side**

I69.342 Monoplegia of lower limb following cerebral infarction affecting **left dominant side**

I69.343 Monoplegia of lower limb following cerebral infarction affecting **right non-dominant side**

I69.344 Monoplegia of lower limb following cerebral infarction affecting **left non-dominant side**

I69.349 Monoplegia of lower limb following cerebral infarction affecting **unspecified** side

● I69.35 **Hemiplegia and hemiparesis** following cerebral infarction

I69.351 Hemiplegia and hemiparesis following cerebral infarction affecting **right dominant side**

   ▶ **Excludes2**   transient ischemic attack (TIA) (G45.9)

I69.352 Hemiplegia and hemiparesis following cerebral infarction affecting **left dominant side**

I69.353 Hemiplegia and hemiparesis following cerebral infarction affecting **right non-dominant side**

I69.354 Hemiplegia and hemiparesis following cerebral infarction affecting **left non-dominant side**

I69.359 Hemiplegia and hemiparesis following cerebral infarction affecting **unspecified** side

● I69.36 **Other** paralytic syndrome following cerebral infarction

Use additional code to identify type of paralytic syndrome, such as:
locked-in state (G83.5)
quadriplegia (G82.5-)

Excludes1   hemiplegia/hemiparesis following cerebral infarction (I69.35-)
monoplegia of lower limb following cerebral infarction (I69.34-)
monoplegia of upper limb following cerebral infarction (I69.33-)

I69.361 Other paralytic syndrome following cerebral infarction affecting **right dominant side**

I69.362 Other paralytic syndrome following cerebral infarction affecting **left dominant side**

I69.363 Other paralytic syndrome following cerebral infarction affecting **right non-dominant side**

I69.364 Other paralytic syndrome following cerebral infarction affecting **left non-dominant side**

I69.365 Other paralytic syndrome following cerebral infarction, **bilateral**

I69.369 Other paralytic syndrome following cerebral infarction affecting **unspecified** side

● I69.39 **Other** sequelae of cerebral infarction

I69.390 **Apraxia** following cerebral infarction

I69.391 **Dysphagia** following cerebral infarction

Use additional code to identify the type of dysphagia, if known (R13.1-)

I69.392 **Facial weakness** following cerebral infarction
Facial droop following cerebral infarction

I69.393 **Ataxia** following cerebral infarction

I69.398 **Other** sequelae of cerebral infarction
Alteration of sensation following cerebral infarction
Disturbance of vision following cerebral infarction
Use additional code to identify the sequelae

● I69.8 **Sequelae of** other cerebrovascular diseases

Excludes1   sequelae of traumatic intracranial injury (S06.-)

I69.80 **Unspecified** sequelae of other cerebrovascular disease

● I69.81 **Cognitive deficits** following other cerebrovascular disease

I69.810 **Attention and concentration** deficit following other cerebrovascular disease

I69.811 **Memory** deficit following other cerebrovascular disease

I69.812 **Visuospatial** deficit and spatial neglect following other cerebrovascular disease

I69.813 **Psychomotor** deficit following other cerebrovascular disease

I69.814 **Frontal lobe and executive function** deficit following other cerebrovascular disease

I69.815 **Cognitive social or emotional** deficit following other cerebrovascular disease

I69.818 **Other symptoms and signs** involving cognitive functions following other cerebrovascular disease

I69.819 **Unspecified** symptoms and signs involving cognitive functions following other cerebrovascular disease

▶ New   ⇒ Revised   ~~deleted~~ Deleted   **OGCR** Official Guidelines   X Assign placeholder X   ● Use Additional Character(s)
Excludes 1   Excludes 2   Includes   Use additional   Code first   Code also   Key words

● I69.82 **Speech and language** deficits following other cerebrovascular disease

    I69.820   **Aphasia** following other cerebrovascular disease

    I69.821   **Dysphasia** following other cerebrovascular disease

    I69.822   **Dysarthria** following other cerebrovascular disease

    I69.823   **Fluency** disorder following other cerebrovascular disease

         Stuttering following other cerebrovascular disease

    I69.828   **Other** speech and language deficits following other cerebrovascular disease

● I69.83 **Monoplegia of upper limb** following other cerebrovascular disease

    I69.831   Monoplegia of upper limb following other cerebrovascular disease affecting **right dominant side**

    I69.832   Monoplegia of upper limb following other cerebrovascular disease affecting **left dominant side**

    I69.833   Monoplegia of upper limb following other cerebrovascular disease affecting **right non-dominant side**

    I69.834   Monoplegia of upper limb following other cerebrovascular disease affecting **left non-dominant side**

    I69.839   Monoplegia of upper limb following other cerebrovascular disease affecting **unspecified** side

● I69.84 **Monoplegia of lower limb** following other cerebrovascular disease

    I69.841   Monoplegia of lower limb following other cerebrovascular disease affecting **right dominant side**

    I69.842   Monoplegia of lower limb following other cerebrovascular disease affecting **left dominant side**

    I69.843   Monoplegia of lower limb following other cerebrovascular disease affecting **right non-dominant side**

    I69.844   Monoplegia of lower limb following other cerebrovascular disease affecting **left non-dominant side**

    I69.849   Monoplegia of lower limb following other cerebrovascular disease affecting **unspecified** side

● I69.85 **Hemiplegia and hemiparesis** following other cerebrovascular disease

    I69.851   Hemiplegia and hemiparesis following other cerebrovascular disease affecting **right dominant side**

    I69.852   Hemiplegia and hemiparesis following other cerebrovascular disease affecting **left dominant side**

    I69.853   Hemiplegia and hemiparesis following other cerebrovascular disease affecting **right non-dominant side**

    I69.854   Hemiplegia and hemiparesis following other cerebrovascular disease affecting **left non-dominant side**

    I69.859   Hemiplegia and hemiparesis following other cerebrovascular disease affecting **unspecified** side

● I69.86 **Other paralytic syndrome** following other cerebrovascular disease

    Use additional code to identify type of paralytic syndrome, such as:
    locked-in state (G83.5)
    quadriplegia (G82.5-)

    Excludes1   hemiplegia/hemiparesis following other cerebrovascular disease (I69.85-)
         monoplegia of lower limb following other cerebrovascular disease (I69.84-)
         monoplegia of upper limb following other cerebrovascular disease (I69.83-)

    I69.861   Other paralytic syndrome following other cerebrovascular disease affecting **right dominant side**

    I69.862   Other paralytic syndrome following other cerebrovascular disease affecting **left dominant side**

    I69.863   Other paralytic syndrome following other cerebrovascular disease affecting **right non-dominant side**

    I69.864   Other paralytic syndrome following other cerebrovascular disease affecting **left non-dominant side**

    I69.865   Other paralytic syndrome following other cerebrovascular disease, **bilateral**

    I69.869   Other paralytic syndrome following other cerebrovascular disease affecting **unspecified** side

● I69.89 **Other** sequelae of other cerebrovascular disease

    I69.890   **Apraxia** following other cerebrovascular disease

    I69.891   **Dysphagia** following other cerebrovascular disease

         Use additional code to identify the type of dysphagia, if known (R13.1-)

    I69.892   **Facial weakness** following other cerebrovascular disease

         Facial droop following other cerebrovascular disease

    I69.893   **Ataxia** following other cerebrovascular disease

    I69.898   **Other** sequelae of other cerebrovascular disease

         Alteration of sensation following other cerebrovascular disease
         Disturbance of vision following other cerebrovascular disease

         Use additional code to identify the sequelae

CHAPTER 9 (I00-I99)

● I69.9 Sequelae of unspecified cerebrovascular diseases

  Excludes1 sequelae of stroke (I69.3)
        sequelae of traumatic intracranial injury
         (S06.-)

 I69.90 Unspecified sequelae of unspecified
     cerebrovascular disease

● I69.91 Cognitive deficits following unspecified
    cerebrovascular disease

  I69.910 Attention and concentration deficit
     following unspecified cerebrovascular
     disease

  I69.911 Memory deficit following unspecified
     cerebrovascular disease

  I69.912 Visuospatial deficit and spatial
     neglect following unspecified
     cerebrovascular disease

  I69.913 Psychomotor deficit following
     unspecified cerebrovascular
     disease

  I69.914 Frontal lobe and executive function
     deficit following unspecified
     cerebrovascular disease

  I69.915 Cognitive social or emotional deficit
     following unspecified cerebrovascular
     disease

  I69.918 Other symptoms and signs involving
     cognitive functions following
     unspecified cerebrovascular
     disease

  I69.919 Unspecified symptoms and signs
     involving cognitive functions
     following unspecified cerebrovascular
     disease

● I69.92 Speech and language deficits following
    unspecified cerebrovascular disease

  I69.920 Aphasia following unspecified
     cerebrovascular disease

  I69.921 Dysphasia following unspecified
     cerebrovascular disease

  I69.922 Dysarthria following unspecified
     cerebrovascular disease

  I69.923 Fluency disorder following
     unspecified cerebrovascular disease
      Stuttering following unspecified
       cerebrovascular disease

  I69.928 Other speech and language deficits
     following unspecified cerebrovascular
     disease

● I69.93 Monoplegia of upper limb following
    unspecified cerebrovascular disease

  I69.931 Monoplegia of upper limb following
     unspecified cerebrovascular disease
     affecting right dominant side

  I69.932 Monoplegia of upper limb following
     unspecified cerebrovascular disease
     affecting left dominant side

  I69.933 Monoplegia of upper limb following
     unspecified cerebrovascular disease
     affecting right non-dominant side

  I69.934 Monoplegia of upper limb following
     unspecified cerebrovascular disease
     affecting left non-dominant side

  I69.939 Monoplegia of upper limb following
     unspecified cerebrovascular disease
     affecting unspecified side

● I69.94 Monoplegia of lower limb following
    unspecified cerebrovascular disease

  I69.941 Monoplegia of lower limb following
     unspecified cerebrovascular disease
     affecting right dominant side

  I69.942 Monoplegia of lower limb following
     unspecified cerebrovascular disease
     affecting left dominant side

  I69.943 Monoplegia of lower limb following
     unspecified cerebrovascular disease
     affecting right non-dominant side

  I69.944 Monoplegia of lower limb following
     unspecified cerebrovascular disease
     affecting left non-dominant side

  I69.949 Monoplegia of lower limb following
     unspecified cerebrovascular disease
     affecting unspecified side

● I69.95 Hemiplegia and hemiparesis following
    unspecified cerebrovascular disease

  I69.951 Hemiplegia and hemiparesis
     following unspecified cerebrovascular
     disease affecting right dominant side

  I69.952 Hemiplegia and hemiparesis
     following unspecified cerebrovascular
     disease affecting left dominant side

  I69.953 Hemiplegia and hemiparesis
     following unspecified cerebrovascular
     disease affecting right non-dominant
     side

  I69.954 Hemiplegia and hemiparesis
     following unspecified cerebrovascular
     disease affecting left non-dominant
     side

  I69.959 Hemiplegia and hemiparesis
     following unspecified cerebrovascular
     disease affecting unspecified side

● I69.96 Other paralytic syndrome following
    unspecified cerebrovascular disease

  Use additional code to identify type of
    paralytic syndrome, such as:
    locked-in state (G83.5)
    quadriplegia (G82.5-)

  Excludes1 hemiplegia/hemiparesis
       following unspecified
       cerebrovascular disease
       (I69.95-)
      monoplegia of lower limb
       following unspecified
       cerebrovascular disease
       (I69.94-)
      monoplegia of upper limb
       following unspecified
       cerebrovascular disease
       (I69.93-)

  I69.961 Other paralytic syndrome following
     unspecified cerebrovascular disease
     affecting right dominant side

  I69.962 Other paralytic syndrome following
     unspecified cerebrovascular disease
     affecting left dominant side

  I69.963 Other paralytic syndrome following
     unspecified cerebrovascular disease
     affecting right non-dominant side

  I69.964 Other paralytic syndrome following
     unspecified cerebrovascular disease
     affecting left non-dominant side

  I69.965 Other paralytic syndrome following
     unspecified cerebrovascular disease,
     bilateral

  I69.969 Other paralytic syndrome following
     unspecified cerebrovascular disease
     affecting unspecified side

▶ New ⇒ Revised ~~deleted~~ Deleted **OGCR** Official Guidelines X Assign placeholder X ● Use Additional Character(s)

Excludes 1 Excludes 2 Includes Use additional Code first Code also Key words

● **I69.99**   **Other sequelae of unspecified cerebrovascular disease**

    I69.990   **Apraxia following unspecified cerebrovascular disease**

    I69.991   **Dysphagia following unspecified cerebrovascular disease**

       Use additional code to identify the type of dysphagia, if known (R13.1-)

    I69.992   **Facial weakness following unspecified cerebrovascular disease**

       Facial droop following unspecified cerebrovascular disease

    I69.993   **Ataxia following unspecified cerebrovascular disease**

    I69.998   **Other sequelae following unspecified cerebrovascular disease**

       Alteration in sensation following unspecified cerebrovascular disease

       Disturbance of vision following unspecified cerebrovascular disease

       Use additional code to identify the sequelae

DISEASES OF ARTERIES, ARTERIOLES AND CAPILLARIES (I70-I79)

● **I70**   **Atherosclerosis**

   Includes   arteriolosclerosis
             arterial degeneration
             arteriosclerosis
             arteriosclerotic vascular disease
             arteriovascular degeneration
             atheroma
             endarteritis deformans or obliterans
             senile arteritis
             senile endarteritis
             vascular degeneration

   Use additional code to identify:
     exposure to environmental tobacco smoke (Z77.22)
     history of tobacco dependence (Z87.891)
     occupational exposure to environmental tobacco smoke (Z57.31)
     tobacco dependence (F17.-)
     tobacco use (Z72.0)

   Excludes2   arteriosclerotic cardiovascular disease (I25.1-)
                 arteriosclerotic heart disease (I25.1-)
                 atheroembolism (I75.-)
                 cerebral atherosclerosis (I67.2)
                 coronary atherosclerosis (I25.1-)
                 mesenteric atherosclerosis (K55.1)
                 precerebral atherosclerosis (I67.2)
                 primary pulmonary atherosclerosis (I27.0)

  I70.0   **Atherosclerosis of aorta**

  I70.1   **Atherosclerosis of renal artery**
     Goldblatt's kidney
     Excludes2   atherosclerosis of renal arterioles (I12.-)

★**(See Plates 500, 501, and 502 on pages 60 – 62.)**

  ● **I70.2**   **Atherosclerosis of native arteries of the extremities**
     Mönckeberg's (medial) sclerosis
     Use additional code, if applicable, to identify chronic total occlusion of artery of extremity (I70.92)
     Excludes2   atherosclerosis of bypass graft of extremities (I70.30-I70.79)

   ● **I70.20**   **Unspecified atherosclerosis of native arteries of extremities**

     I70.201   **Unspecified atherosclerosis of native arteries of extremities, right leg**

     I70.202   **Unspecified atherosclerosis of native arteries of extremities, left leg**

     I70.203   Unspecified atherosclerosis of native arteries of extremities, **bilateral legs**

     I70.208   Unspecified atherosclerosis of native arteries of extremities, **other extremity**

     I70.209   Unspecified atherosclerosis of native arteries of extremities, **unspecified extremity**

   ● **I70.21**   **Atherosclerosis of native arteries of extremities with intermittent claudication**

     I70.211   **Atherosclerosis of native arteries of extremities with intermittent claudication, right leg**

     I70.212   **Atherosclerosis of native arteries of extremities with intermittent claudication, left leg**

     I70.213   **Atherosclerosis of native arteries of extremities with intermittent claudication, bilateral legs**

     I70.218   **Atherosclerosis of native arteries of extremities with intermittent claudication, other extremity**

     I70.219   **Atherosclerosis of native arteries of extremities with intermittent claudication, unspecified extremity**

   ● **I70.22**   **Atherosclerosis of native arteries of extremities with rest pain**
     Includes   any condition classifiable to I70.21-

     I70.221   **Atherosclerosis of native arteries of extremities with rest pain, right leg**

     I70.222   **Atherosclerosis of native arteries of extremities with rest pain, left leg**

     I70.223   **Atherosclerosis of native arteries of extremities with rest pain, bilateral legs**

     I70.228   **Atherosclerosis of native arteries of extremities with rest pain, other extremity**

     I70.229   **Atherosclerosis of native arteries of extremities with rest pain, unspecified extremity**

   ● **I70.23**   **Atherosclerosis of native arteries of right leg with ulceration**
     Includes   any condition classifiable to I70.211 and I70.221
     Use additional code to identify severity of ulcer (L97.-)

     I70.231   **Atherosclerosis of native arteries of right leg with ulceration of thigh**

     I70.232   **Atherosclerosis of native arteries of right leg with ulceration of calf**

     I70.233   **Atherosclerosis of native arteries of right leg with ulceration of ankle**

     I70.234   **Atherosclerosis of native arteries of right leg with ulceration of heel and midfoot**
       Atherosclerosis of native arteries of right leg with ulceration of plantar surface of midfoot

     I70.235   **Atherosclerosis of native arteries of right leg with ulceration of other part of foot**
       Atherosclerosis of native arteries of right leg extremities with ulceration of toe

     I70.238   **Atherosclerosis of native arteries of right leg with ulceration of other part of lower right leg**

     I70.239   **Atherosclerosis of native arteries of right leg with ulceration of unspecified site**

● **I70.24   Atherosclerosis of native arteries of left leg with ulceration**

     Includes   any condition classifiable to I70.212 and I70.222

     Use additional code to identify severity of ulcer (L97.-)

     I70.241   Atherosclerosis of native arteries of left leg with ulceration of thigh

     I70.242   Atherosclerosis of native arteries of left leg with ulceration of calf

     I70.243   Atherosclerosis of native arteries of left leg with ulceration of ankle

     I70.244   Atherosclerosis of native arteries of left leg with ulceration of heel and midfoot

           Atherosclerosis of native arteries of left leg with ulceration of plantar surface of midfoot

     I70.245   Atherosclerosis of native arteries of left leg with ulceration of other part of foot

           Atherosclerosis of native arteries of left leg extremities with ulceration of toe

     I70.248   Atherosclerosis of native arteries of left leg with ulceration of other part of lower left leg

     I70.249   Atherosclerosis of native arteries of left leg with ulceration of unspecified site

● **I70.25   Atherosclerosis of native arteries of other extremities with ulceration**

     Includes   any condition classifiable to I70.218 and I70.228

     Use additional code to identify the severity of the ulcer (L98.49-)

● **I70.26   Atherosclerosis of native arteries of extremities with gangrene**

     Includes   any condition classifiable to I70.21-, I70.22-, I70.23-, I70.24-, and I70.25-

     Use additional code to identify the severity of any ulcer (L97.-, L98.49-), if applicable

     I70.261   Atherosclerosis of native arteries of extremities with gangrene, right leg

     I70.262   Atherosclerosis of native arteries of extremities with gangrene, left leg

     I70.263   Atherosclerosis of native arteries of extremities with gangrene, bilateral legs

     I70.268   Atherosclerosis of native arteries of extremities with gangrene, other extremity

     I70.269   Atherosclerosis of native arteries of extremities with gangrene, unspecified extremity

● **I70.29   Other atherosclerosis of native arteries of extremities**

     I70.291   Other atherosclerosis of native arteries of extremities, right leg

     I70.292   Other atherosclerosis of native arteries of extremities, left leg

     I70.293   Other atherosclerosis of native arteries of extremities, bilateral legs

     I70.298   Other atherosclerosis of native arteries of extremities, other extremity

     I70.299   Other atherosclerosis of native arteries of extremities, unspecified extremity

● **I70.3   Atherosclerosis of unspecified type of bypass graft(s) of the extremities**

     Use additional code, if applicable, to identify chronic total occlusion of artery of extremity (I70.92)

     Excludes1   embolism or thrombus of bypass graft(s) of extremities (T82.8-)

● **I70.30   Unspecified atherosclerosis of unspecified type of bypass graft(s) of the extremities**

     70.301   Unspecified atherosclerosis of unspecified type of bypass graft(s) of the extremities, right leg

     I70.302   Unspecified atherosclerosis of unspecified type of bypass graft(s) of the extremities, left leg

     I70.303   Unspecified atherosclerosis of unspecified type of bypass graft(s) of the extremities, bilateral legs

     I70.308   Unspecified atherosclerosis of unspecified type of bypass graft(s) of the extremities, other extremity

     I70.309   Unspecified atherosclerosis of unspecified type of bypass graft(s) of the extremities, unspecified extremity

● **I70.31   Atherosclerosis of unspecified type of bypass graft(s) of the extremities with intermittent claudication**

     I70.311   Atherosclerosis of unspecified type of bypass graft(s) of the extremities with intermittent claudication, right leg

     I70.312   Atherosclerosis of unspecified type of bypass graft(s) of the extremities with intermittent claudication, left leg

     I70.313   Atherosclerosis of unspecified type of bypass graft(s) of the extremities with intermittent claudication, bilateral legs

     I70.318   Atherosclerosis of unspecified type of bypass graft(s) of the extremities with intermittent claudication, other extremity

     I70.319   Atherosclerosis of unspecified type of bypass graft(s) of the extremities with intermittent claudication, unspecified extremity

● **I70.32   Atherosclerosis of unspecified type of bypass graft(s) of the extremities with rest pain**

     Includes   any condition classifiable to I70.31-

     I70.321   Atherosclerosis of unspecified type of bypass graft(s) of the extremities with rest pain, right leg

     I70.322   Atherosclerosis of unspecified type of bypass graft(s) of the extremities with rest pain, left leg

     I70.323   Atherosclerosis of unspecified type of bypass graft(s) of the extremities with rest pain, bilateral legs

     I70.328   Atherosclerosis of unspecified type of bypass graft(s) of the extremities with rest pain, other extremity

     I70.329   Atherosclerosis of unspecified type of bypass graft(s) of the extremities with rest pain, unspecified extremity

▶ New   ⇒ Revised   ~~deleted~~ Deleted   **OGCR** Official Guidelines   X Assign placeholder X   ● Use Additional Character(s)

Excludes 1   Excludes 2   Includes   Use additional   Code first   Code also   Key words

● **I70.33**   **Atherosclerosis of unspecified type of bypass graft(s) of the right leg with ulceration**

> Includes   any condition classifiable to I70.311 and I70.321

> Use additional code to identify severity of ulcer (L97.-)

    I70.331   Atherosclerosis of unspecified type of bypass graft(s) of the right leg with ulceration of thigh

    I70.332   Atherosclerosis of unspecified type of bypass graft(s) of the right leg with ulceration of calf

    I70.333   Atherosclerosis of unspecified type of bypass graft(s) of the right leg with ulceration of ankle

    I70.334   Atherosclerosis of unspecified type of bypass graft(s) of the right leg with ulceration of heel and midfoot

> Atherosclerosis of unspecified type of bypass graft(s) of right leg with ulceration of plantar surface of midfoot

    I70.335   Atherosclerosis of unspecified type of bypass graft(s) of the right leg with ulceration of other part of foot

> Atherosclerosis of unspecified type of bypass graft(s) of the right leg with ulceration of toe

    I70.338   Atherosclerosis of unspecified type of bypass graft(s) of the right leg with ulceration of other part of lower leg

    I70.339   Atherosclerosis of unspecified type of bypass graft(s) of the right leg with ulceration of unspecified site

● **I70.34**   **Atherosclerosis of unspecified type of bypass graft(s) of the left leg with ulceration**

> Includes   any condition classifiable to I70.312 and I70.322

> Use additional code to identify severity of ulcer (L97.-)

    I70.341   Atherosclerosis of unspecified type of bypass graft(s) of the left leg with ulceration of thigh

    I70.342   Atherosclerosis of unspecified type of bypass graft(s) of the left leg with ulceration of calf

    I70.343   Atherosclerosis of unspecified type of bypass graft(s) of the left leg with ulceration of ankle

    I70.344   Atherosclerosis of unspecified type of bypass graft(s) of the left leg with ulceration of heel and midfoot

> Atherosclerosis of unspecified type of bypass graft(s) of left leg with ulceration of plantar surface of midfoot

    I70.345   Atherosclerosis of unspecified type of bypass graft(s) of the left leg with ulceration of other part of foot

> Atherosclerosis of unspecified type of bypass graft(s) of the left leg with ulceration of toe

    I70.348   Atherosclerosis of unspecified type of bypass graft(s) of the left leg with ulceration of other part of lower leg

    I70.349   Atherosclerosis of unspecified type of bypass graft(s) of the left leg with ulceration of unspecified site

I70.35   **Atherosclerosis of unspecified type of bypass graft(s) of other extremity with ulceration**

> Includes   any condition classifiable to I70.318 and I70.328

> Use additional code to identify severity of ulcer (L98.49-)

● **I70.36**   **Atherosclerosis of unspecified type of bypass graft(s) of the extremities with gangrene**

> Includes   any condition classifiable to I70.31-, I70.32-, I70.33-, I70.34-, I70.35

> Use additional code to identify the severity of any ulcer (L97.-, L98.49-), if applicable

    I70.361   Atherosclerosis of unspecified type of bypass graft(s) of the extremities with gangrene, right leg

    I70.362   Atherosclerosis of unspecified type of bypass graft(s) of the extremities with gangrene, left leg

    I70.363   Atherosclerosis of unspecified type of bypass graft(s) of the extremities with gangrene, bilateral legs

    I70.368   Atherosclerosis of unspecified type of bypass graft(s) of the extremities with gangrene, other extremity

    I70.369   Atherosclerosis of unspecified type of bypass graft(s) of the extremities with gangrene, unspecified extremity

● **I70.39**   **Other atherosclerosis of unspecified type of bypass graft(s) of the extremities**

    I70.391   Other atherosclerosis of unspecified type of bypass graft(s) of the extremities, right leg

    I70.392   Other atherosclerosis of unspecified type of bypass graft(s) of the extremities, left leg

    I70.393   Other atherosclerosis of unspecified type of bypass graft(s) of the extremities, bilateral legs

    I70.398   Other atherosclerosis of unspecified type of bypass graft(s) of the extremities, other extremity

    I70.399   Other atherosclerosis of unspecified type of bypass graft(s) of the extremities, unspecified extremity

● **I70.4**   **Atherosclerosis of autologous vein bypass graft(s) of the extremities**

> Use additional code, if applicable, to identify chronic total occlusion of artery of extremity (I70.92)

● **I70.40**   **Unspecified atherosclerosis of autologous vein bypass graft(s) of the extremities**

    I70.401   Unspecified atherosclerosis of autologous vein bypass graft(s) of the extremities, right leg

    I70.402   Unspecified atherosclerosis of autologous vein bypass graft(s) of the extremities, left leg

    I70.403   Unspecified atherosclerosis of autologous vein bypass graft(s) of the extremities, bilateral legs

    I70.408   Unspecified atherosclerosis of autologous vein bypass graft(s) of the extremities, other extremity

    I70.409   Unspecified atherosclerosis of autologous vein bypass graft(s) of the extremities, unspecified extremity

● **I70.41** **Atherosclerosis of autologous vein bypass graft(s) of the extremities with intermittent claudication**

     I70.411   Atherosclerosis of autologous vein bypass graft(s) of the extremities with intermittent claudication, right leg

     I70.412   Atherosclerosis of autologous vein bypass graft(s) of the extremities with intermittent claudication, left leg

     I70.413   Atherosclerosis of autologous vein bypass graft(s) of the extremities with intermittent claudication, bilateral legs

     I70.418   Atherosclerosis of autologous vein bypass graft(s) of the extremities with intermittent claudication, other extremity

     I70.419   Atherosclerosis of autologous vein bypass graft(s) of the extremities with intermittent claudication, unspecified extremity

● **I70.42** **Atherosclerosis of autologous vein bypass graft(s) of the extremities with rest pain**

     Includes   any condition classifiable to I70.41-

     I70.421   Atherosclerosis of autologous vein bypass graft(s) of the extremities with rest pain, right leg

     I70.422   Atherosclerosis of autologous vein bypass graft(s) of the extremities with rest pain, left leg

     I70.423   Atherosclerosis of autologous vein bypass graft(s) of the extremities with rest pain, bilateral legs

     I70.428   Atherosclerosis of autologous vein bypass graft(s) of the extremities with rest pain, other extremity

     I70.429   Atherosclerosis of autologous vein bypass graft(s) of the extremities with rest pain, unspecified extremity

● **I70.43** **Atherosclerosis of autologous vein bypass graft(s) of the right leg with ulceration**

     Includes   any condition classifiable to I70.411 and I70.421

     Use additional code to identify severity of ulcer (L97.-)

     I70.431   Atherosclerosis of autologous vein bypass graft(s) of the right leg with ulceration of thigh

     I70.432   Atherosclerosis of autologous vein bypass graft(s) of the right leg with ulceration of calf

     I70.433   Atherosclerosis of autologous vein bypass graft(s) of the right leg with ulceration of ankle

     I70.434   Atherosclerosis of autologous vein bypass graft(s) of the right leg with ulceration of heel and midfoot

       Atherosclerosis of autologous vein bypass graft(s) of right leg with ulceration of plantar surface of midfoot

     I70.435   Atherosclerosis of autologous vein bypass graft(s) of the right leg with ulceration of other part of foot

       Atherosclerosis of autologous vein bypass graft(s) of right leg with ulceration of toe

     I70.438   Atherosclerosis of autologous vein bypass graft(s) of the right leg with ulceration of other part of lower leg

     I70.439   Atherosclerosis of autologous vein bypass graft(s) of the right leg with ulceration of unspecified site

● **I70.44** **Atherosclerosis of autologous vein bypass graft(s) of the left leg with ulceration**

     Includes   any condition classifiable to I70.412 and I70.422

     Use additional code to identify severity of ulcer (L97.-)

     I70.441   Atherosclerosis of autologous vein bypass graft(s) of the left leg with ulceration of thigh

     I70.442   Atherosclerosis of autologous vein bypass graft(s) of the left leg with ulceration of calf

     I70.443   Atherosclerosis of autologous vein bypass graft(s) of the left leg with ulceration of ankle

     I70.444   Atherosclerosis of autologous vein bypass graft(s) of the left leg with ulceration of heel and midfoot

       Atherosclerosis of autologous vein bypass graft(s) of left leg with ulceration of plantar surface of midfoot

     I70.445   Atherosclerosis of autologous vein bypass graft(s) of the left leg with ulceration of other part of foot

       Atherosclerosis of autologous vein bypass graft(s) of left leg with ulceration of toe

     I70.448   Atherosclerosis of autologous vein bypass graft(s) of the left leg with ulceration of other part of lower leg

     I70.449   Atherosclerosis of autologous vein bypass graft(s) of the left leg with ulceration of unspecified site

     I70.45   **Atherosclerosis of autologous vein bypass graft(s) of other extremity with ulceration**

     Includes   any condition classifiable to I70.418, I70.428, and I70.438

     Use additional code to identify severity of ulcer (L98.49-)

● **I70.46** **Atherosclerosis of autologous vein bypass graft(s) of the extremities with gangrene**

     Includes   any condition classifiable to I70.41-, I70.42-, and I70.43-, I70.44-, I70.45

     Use additional code to identify the severity of any ulcer (L97.-, L98.49-), if applicable

     I70.461   Atherosclerosis of autologous vein bypass graft(s) of the extremities with gangrene, right leg

     I70.462   Atherosclerosis of autologous vein bypass graft(s) of the extremities with gangrene, left leg

     I70.463   Atherosclerosis of autologous vein bypass graft(s) of the extremities with gangrene, bilateral legs

     I70.468   Atherosclerosis of autologous vein bypass graft(s) of the extremities with gangrene, other extremity

     I70.469   Atherosclerosis of autologous vein bypass graft(s) of the extremities with gangrene, unspecified extremity

● **I70.49** **Other atherosclerosis of autologous vein bypass graft(s) of the extremities**

     I70.491   Other atherosclerosis of autologous vein bypass graft(s) of the extremities, right leg

     I70.492   Other atherosclerosis of autologous vein bypass graft(s) of the extremities, left leg

     I70.493   Other atherosclerosis of autologous vein bypass graft(s) of the extremities, bilateral legs

▶ New   ⇒ Revised   ~~deleted~~ Deleted   **OGCR** Official Guidelines   X Assign placeholder X   ● Use Additional Character(s)

Excludes 1   Excludes 2   Includes   Use additional   Code first   Code also   Key words

I70.498 Other atherosclerosis of autologous vein bypass graft(s) of the extremities, other extremity

I70.499 Other atherosclerosis of autologous vein bypass graft(s) of the extremities, unspecified extremity

● **I70.5** Atherosclerosis of nonautologous biological bypass graft(s) of the extremities

Use additional code, if applicable, to identify chronic total occlusion of artery of extremity (I70.92)

● **I70.50** Unspecified atherosclerosis of nonautologous biological bypass graft(s) of the extremities

I70.501 Unspecified atherosclerosis of nonautologous biological bypass graft(s) of the extremities, right leg

I70.502 Unspecified atherosclerosis of nonautologous biological bypass graft(s) of the extremities, left leg

I70.503 Unspecified atherosclerosis of nonautologous biological bypass graft(s) of the extremities, bilateral legs

I70.508 Unspecified atherosclerosis of nonautologous biological bypass graft(s) of the extremities, other extremity

I70.509 Unspecified atherosclerosis of nonautologous biological bypass graft(s) of the extremities, unspecified extremity

● **I70.51** Atherosclerosis of nonautologous biological bypass graft(s) of the extremities intermittent claudication

I70.511 Atherosclerosis of nonautologous biological bypass graft(s) of the extremities with intermittent claudication, right leg

I70.512 Atherosclerosis of nonautologous biological bypass graft(s) of the extremities with intermittent claudication, left leg

I70.513 Atherosclerosis of nonautologous biological bypass graft(s) of the extremities with intermittent claudication, bilateral legs

I70.518 Atherosclerosis of nonautologous biological bypass graft(s) of the extremities with intermittent claudication, other extremity

I70.519 Atherosclerosis of nonautologous biological bypass graft(s) of the extremities with intermittent claudication, unspecified extremity

● **I70.52** Atherosclerosis of nonautologous biological bypass graft(s) of the extremities with rest pain

Includes   any condition classifiable to I70.51-

I70.521 Atherosclerosis of nonautologous biological bypass graft(s) of the extremities with rest pain, right leg

I70.522 Atherosclerosis of nonautologous biological bypass graft(s) of the extremities with rest pain, left leg

I70.523 Atherosclerosis of nonautologous biological bypass graft(s) of the extremities with rest pain, bilateral legs

I70.528 Atherosclerosis of nonautologous biological bypass graft(s) of the extremities with rest pain, other extremity

I70.529 Atherosclerosis of nonautologous biological bypass graft(s) of the extremities with rest pain, unspecified extremity

● **I70.53** Atherosclerosis of nonautologous biological bypass graft(s) of the right leg with ulceration

Includes   any condition classifiable to I70.511 and I70.521

Use additional code to identify severity of ulcer (L97.-)

I70.531 Atherosclerosis of nonautologous biological bypass graft(s) of the right leg with ulceration of thigh

I70.532 Atherosclerosis of nonautologous biological bypass graft(s) of the right leg with ulceration of calf

I70.533 Atherosclerosis of nonautologous biological bypass graft(s) of the right leg with ulceration of ankle

I70.534 Atherosclerosis of nonautologous biological bypass graft(s) of the right leg with ulceration of heel and midfoot

Atherosclerosis of nonautologous biological bypass graft(s) of right leg with ulceration of plantar surface of midfoot

I70.535 Atherosclerosis of nonautologous biological bypass graft(s) of the right leg with ulceration of other part of foot

Atherosclerosis of nonautologous biological bypass graft(s) of the right leg with ulceration of toe

I70.538 Atherosclerosis of nonautologous biological bypass graft(s) of the right leg with ulceration of other part of lower leg

I70.539 Atherosclerosis of nonautologous biological bypass graft(s) of the right leg with ulceration of unspecified site

● **I70.54** Atherosclerosis of nonautologous biological bypass graft(s) of the left leg with ulceration

Includes   any condition classifiable to I70.512 and I70.522

Use additional code to identify severity of ulcer (L97.-)

I70.541 Atherosclerosis of nonautologous biological bypass graft(s) of the left leg with ulceration of thigh

I70.542 Atherosclerosis of nonautologous biological bypass graft(s) of the left leg with ulceration of calf

I70.543 Atherosclerosis of nonautologous biological bypass graft(s) of the left leg with ulceration of ankle

I70.544 Atherosclerosis of nonautologous biological bypass graft(s) of the left leg with ulceration of heel and midfoot

Atherosclerosis of nonautologous biological bypass graft(s) of left leg with ulceration of plantar surface of midfoot

I70.545 Atherosclerosis of nonautologous biological bypass graft(s) of the left leg with ulceration of other part of foot

Atherosclerosis of nonautologous biological bypass graft(s) of the left leg with ulceration of toe

I70.548 Atherosclerosis of nonautologous biological bypass graft(s) of the left leg with ulceration of other part of lower leg

I70.549 Atherosclerosis of nonautologous biological bypass graft(s) of the left leg with ulceration of unspecified site

CHAPTER 9 (I00-I99)

I70.55   Atherosclerosis of nonautologous biological bypass graft(s) of other extremity with ulceration

Includes   any condition classifiable to I70.518, I70.528, and I70.538

Use additional code to identify severity of ulcer (L98.49)

● I70.56   Atherosclerosis of nonautologous biological bypass graft(s) of the extremities with gangrene

Includes   any condition classifiable to I70.51-, I70.52-, and I70.53-, I70.54-, I70.55

Use additional code to identify the severity of any ulcer (L97.-, L98.49-), if applicable

I70.561   Atherosclerosis of nonautologous biological bypass graft(s) of the extremities with gangrene, right leg

I70.562   Atherosclerosis of nonautologous biological bypass graft(s) of the extremities with gangrene, left leg

I70.563   Atherosclerosis of nonautologous biological bypass graft(s) of the extremities with gangrene, bilateral legs

I70.568   Atherosclerosis of nonautologous biological bypass graft(s) of the extremities with gangrene, other extremity

I70.569   Atherosclerosis of nonautologous biological bypass graft(s) of the extremities with gangrene, unspecified extremity

● I70.59   Other atherosclerosis of nonautologous biological bypass graft(s) of the extremities

I70.591   Other atherosclerosis of nonautologous biological bypass graft(s) of the extremities, right leg

I70.592   Other atherosclerosis of nonautologous biological bypass graft(s) of the extremities, left leg

I70.593   Other atherosclerosis of nonautologous biological bypass graft(s) of the extremities, bilateral legs

I70.598   Other atherosclerosis of nonautologous biological bypass graft(s) of the extremities, other extremity

I70.599   Other atherosclerosis of nonautologous biological bypass graft(s) of the extremities, unspecified extremity

● I70.6   Atherosclerosis of nonbiological bypass graft(s) of the extremities

Use additional code, if applicable, to identify chronic total occlusion of artery of extremity (I70.92)

● I70.60   Unspecified atherosclerosis of nonbiological bypass graft(s) of the extremities

I70.601   Unspecified atherosclerosis of nonbiological bypass graft(s) of the extremities, right leg

I70.602   Unspecified atherosclerosis of nonbiological bypass graft(s) of the extremities, left leg

I70.603   Unspecified atherosclerosis of nonbiological bypass graft(s) of the extremities, bilateral legs

I70.608   Unspecified atherosclerosis of nonbiological bypass graft(s) of the extremities, other extremity

I70.609   Unspecified atherosclerosis of nonbiological bypass graft(s) of the extremities, unspecified extremity

● I70.61   Atherosclerosis of nonbiological bypass graft(s) of the extremities with intermittent claudication

I70.611   Atherosclerosis of nonbiological bypass graft(s) of the extremities with intermittent claudication, right leg

I70.612   Atherosclerosis of nonbiological bypass graft(s) of the extremities with intermittent claudication, left leg

I70.613   Atherosclerosis of nonbiological bypass graft(s) of the extremities with intermittent claudication, bilateral legs

I70.618   Atherosclerosis of nonbiological bypass graft(s) of the extremities with intermittent claudication, other extremity

I70.619   Atherosclerosis of nonbiological bypass graft(s) of the extremities with intermittent claudication, unspecified extremity

● I70.62   Atherosclerosis of nonbiological bypass graft(s) of the extremities with rest pain

Includes   any condition classifiable to I70.61-

I70.621   Atherosclerosis of nonbiological bypass graft(s) of the extremities with rest pain, right leg

I70.622   Atherosclerosis of nonbiological bypass graft(s) of the extremities with rest pain, left leg

I70.623   Atherosclerosis of nonbiological bypass graft(s) of the extremities with rest pain, bilateral legs

I70.628   Atherosclerosis of nonbiological bypass graft(s) of the extremities with rest pain, other extremity

I70.629   Atherosclerosis of nonbiological bypass graft(s) of the extremities with rest pain, unspecified extremity

● I70.63   Atherosclerosis of nonbiological bypass graft(s) of the right leg with ulceration

Includes   any condition classifiable to I70.611 and I70.621

Use additional code to identify severity of ulcer (L97.-)

I70.631   Atherosclerosis of nonbiological bypass graft(s) of the right leg with ulceration of thigh

I70.632   Atherosclerosis of nonbiological bypass graft(s) of the right leg with ulceration of calf

I70.633   Atherosclerosis of nonbiological bypass graft(s) of the right leg with ulceration of ankle

I70.634   Atherosclerosis of nonbiological bypass graft(s) of the right leg with ulceration of heel and midfoot
   Atherosclerosis of nonbiological bypass graft(s) of right leg with ulceration of plantar surface of midfoot

I70.635   Atherosclerosis of nonbiological bypass graft(s) of the right leg with ulceration of other part of foot
   Atherosclerosis of nonbiological bypass graft(s) of the right leg with ulceration of toe

I70.638   Atherosclerosis of nonbiological bypass graft(s) of the right leg with ulceration of other part of lower leg

I70.639   Atherosclerosis of nonbiological bypass graft(s) of the right leg with ulceration of unspecified site

▶ New   ⇒ Revised   deleted Deleted   OGCR Official Guidelines   X Assign placeholder X   ● Use Additional Character(s)
Excludes 1   Excludes 2   Includes   Use additional   Code first   Code also   Key words

● **I70.64**   **Atherosclerosis of nonbiological bypass graft(s) of the left leg with ulceration**

       Includes   any condition classifiable to I70.612 and I70.622

       Use additional code to identify severity of ulcer (L97.-)

     I70.641   Atherosclerosis of nonbiological bypass graft(s) of the left leg with ulceration of thigh

     I70.642   Atherosclerosis of nonbiological bypass graft(s) of the left leg with ulceration of calf

     I70.643   Atherosclerosis of nonbiological bypass graft(s) of the left leg with ulceration of ankle

     I70.644   Atherosclerosis of nonbiological bypass graft(s) of the left leg with ulceration of heel and midfoot

           Atherosclerosis of nonbiological bypass graft(s) of left leg with ulceration of plantar surface of midfoot

     I70.645   Atherosclerosis of nonbiological bypass graft(s) of the left leg with ulceration of other part of foot

           Atherosclerosis of nonbiological bypass graft(s) of the left leg with ulceration of toe

     I70.648   Atherosclerosis of nonbiological bypass graft(s) of the left leg with ulceration of other part of lower leg

     I70.649   Atherosclerosis of nonbiological bypass graft(s) of the left leg with ulceration of unspecified site

I70.65   **Atherosclerosis of nonbiological bypass graft(s) of other extremity with ulceration**

       Includes   any condition classifiable to I70.618 and I70.628

       Use additional code to identify severity of ulcer (L98.49-)

● **I70.66**   **Atherosclerosis of nonbiological bypass graft(s) of the extremities with gangrene**

       Includes   any condition classifiable to I70.61-, I70.62-, I70.63-, I70.64-, I70.65

       Use additional code to identify the severity of any ulcer (L97.-, L98.49-), if applicable

     I70.661   Atherosclerosis of nonbiological bypass graft(s) of the extremities with gangrene, right leg

     I70.662   Atherosclerosis of nonbiological bypass graft(s) of the extremities with gangrene, left leg

     I70.663   Atherosclerosis of nonbiological bypass graft(s) of the extremities with gangrene, bilateral legs

     I70.668   Atherosclerosis of nonbiological bypass graft(s) of the extremities with gangrene, other extremity

     I70.669   Atherosclerosis of nonbiological bypass graft(s) of the extremities with gangrene, unspecified extremity

● **I70.69**   **Other atherosclerosis of nonbiological bypass graft(s) of the extremities**

     I70.691   Other atherosclerosis of nonbiological bypass graft(s) of the extremities, right leg

     I70.692   Other atherosclerosis of nonbiological bypass graft(s) of the extremities, left leg

     I70.693   Other atherosclerosis of nonbiological bypass graft(s) of the extremities, bilateral legs

     I70.698   Other atherosclerosis of nonbiological bypass graft(s) of the extremities, other extremity

     I70.699   Other atherosclerosis of nonbiological bypass graft(s) of the extremities, unspecified extremity

● **I70.7**   **Atherosclerosis of other type of bypass graft(s) of the extremities**

       Use additional code, if applicable, to identify chronic total occlusion of artery of extremity (I70.92)

● **I70.70**   **Unspecified atherosclerosis of other type of bypass graft(s) of the extremities**

     I70.701   Unspecified atherosclerosis of other type of bypass graft(s) of the extremities, right leg

     I70.702   Unspecified atherosclerosis of other type of bypass graft(s) of the extremities, left leg

     I70.703   Unspecified atherosclerosis of other type of bypass graft(s) of the extremities, bilateral legs

     I70.708   Unspecified atherosclerosis of other type of bypass graft(s) of the extremities, other extremity

     I70.709   Unspecified atherosclerosis of other type of bypass graft(s) of the extremities, unspecified extremity

● **I70.71**   **Atherosclerosis of other type of bypass graft(s) of the extremities with intermittent claudication**

     I70.711   Atherosclerosis of other type of bypass graft(s) of the extremities with intermittent claudication, right leg

     I70.712   Atherosclerosis of other type of bypass graft(s) of the extremities with intermittent claudication, left leg

     I70.713   Atherosclerosis of other type of bypass graft(s) of the extremities with intermittent claudication, bilateral legs

     I70.718   Atherosclerosis of other type of bypass graft(s) of the extremities with intermittent claudication, other extremity

     I70.719   Atherosclerosis of other type of bypass graft(s) of the extremities with intermittent claudication, unspecified extremity

● **I70.72**   **Atherosclerosis of other type of bypass graft(s) of the extremities with rest pain**

       Includes   any condition classifiable to I70.71-

     I70.721   Atherosclerosis of other type of bypass graft(s) of the extremities with rest pain, right leg

     I70.722   Atherosclerosis of other type of bypass graft(s) of the extremities with rest pain, left leg

     I70.723   Atherosclerosis of other type of bypass graft(s) of the extremities with rest pain, bilateral legs

     I70.728   Atherosclerosis of other type of bypass graft(s) of the extremities with rest pain, other extremity

     I70.729   Atherosclerosis of other type of bypass graft(s) of the extremities with rest pain, unspecified extremity

---

▶ New   ⇒ Revised   ~~deleted~~ Deleted   **OGCR** Official Guidelines   X Assign placeholder X   ● Use Additional Character(s)

| Excludes 1 | Excludes 2 | Includes | Use additional | Code first | Code also | Key words |

● **I70.73**   **Atherosclerosis of other type of bypass graft(s) of the right leg with ulceration**

> **Includes**   any condition classifiable to I70.711 and I70.721

Use additional code to identify severity of ulcer (L97.-)

I70.731   Atherosclerosis of other type of bypass graft(s) of the right leg with ulceration of **thigh**

I70.732   Atherosclerosis of other type of bypass graft(s) of the right leg with ulceration of **calf**

I70.733   Atherosclerosis of other type of bypass graft(s) of the right leg with ulceration of **ankle**

I70.734   Atherosclerosis of other type of bypass graft(s) of the right leg with ulceration of **heel and midfoot**
> Atherosclerosis of other type of bypass graft(s) of right leg with ulceration of plantar surface of midfoot

I70.735   Atherosclerosis of other type of bypass graft(s) of the right leg with ulceration of **other part of foot**
> Atherosclerosis of other type of bypass graft(s) of right leg with ulceration of toe

I70.738   Atherosclerosis of other type of bypass graft(s) of the right leg with ulceration of **other part of lower leg**

I70.739   Atherosclerosis of other type of bypass graft(s) of the right leg with ulceration of **unspecified** site

● **I70.74**   **Atherosclerosis of other type of bypass graft(s) of the left leg with ulceration**

> **Includes**   any condition classifiable to I70.712 and I70.722

Use additional code to identify severity of ulcer (L97.-)

I70.741   Atherosclerosis of other type of bypass graft(s) of the left leg with ulceration of **thigh**

I70.742   Atherosclerosis of other type of bypass graft(s) of the left leg with ulceration of **calf**

I70.743   Atherosclerosis of other type of bypass graft(s) of the left leg with ulceration of ankle

I70.744   Atherosclerosis of other type of bypass graft(s) of the left leg with ulceration of **heel and midfoot**
> Atherosclerosis of other type of bypass graft(s) of left leg with ulceration of plantar surface of midfoot

I70.745   Atherosclerosis of other type of bypass graft(s) of the left leg with ulceration of **other part of foot**
> Atherosclerosis of other type of bypass graft(s) of left leg with ulceration of toe

I70.748   Atherosclerosis of other type of bypass graft(s) of the left leg with ulceration of **other part of lower leg**

I70.749   Atherosclerosis of other type of bypass graft(s) of the left leg with ulceration of **unspecified** site

I70.75   Atherosclerosis of other type of bypass graft(s) of **other extremity with ulceration**

> **Includes**   any condition classifiable to I70.718 and I70.728

Use additional code to identify severity of ulcer (L98.49)

● **I70.76**   **Atherosclerosis of other type of bypass graft(s) of the extremities with gangrene**

> **Includes**   any condition classifiable to I70.71-, I70.72-, I70.73-, I70.74-, I70.75

Use additional code to identify the severity of any ulcer (L97.-, L98.49-), if applicable

I70.761   Atherosclerosis of other type of bypass graft(s) of the extremities with gangrene, **right leg**

I70.762   Atherosclerosis of other type of bypass graft(s) of the extremities with gangrene, **left leg**

I70.763   Atherosclerosis of other type of bypass graft(s) of the extremities with gangrene, **bilateral legs**

I70.768   Atherosclerosis of other type of bypass graft(s) of the extremities with gangrene, **other extremity**

I70.769   Atherosclerosis of other type of bypass graft(s) of the extremities with gangrene, **unspecified extremity**

● **I70.79**   **Other** atherosclerosis of other type of bypass graft(s) of the extremities

I70.791   Other atherosclerosis of other type of bypass graft(s) of the extremities, **right leg**

I70.792   Other atherosclerosis of other type of bypass graft(s) of the extremities, **left leg**

I70.793   Other atherosclerosis of other type of bypass graft(s) of the extremities, **bilateral legs**

I70.798   Other atherosclerosis of other type of bypass graft(s) of the extremities, **other extremity**

I70.799   Other atherosclerosis of other type of bypass graft(s) of the extremities, **unspecified extremity**

I70.8   Atherosclerosis of **other arteries**

● **I70.9**   **Other and unspecified atherosclerosis**

I70.90   **Unspecified** atherosclerosis

I70.91   **Generalized** atherosclerosis

I70.92   **Chronic total occlusion** of artery of the extremities
> Complete occlusion of artery of the extremities
> Total occlusion of artery of the extremities
>
> *Code first atherosclerosis of arteries of the extremities (I70.2-, I70.3-, I70.4-, I70.5-, I70.6-, I70.7-)*

▶ New   ⇒ Revised   ~~deleted~~ Deleted   **OGCR** Official Guidelines   **X** Assign placeholder X   ● Use Additional Character(s)

Excludes 1   Excludes 2   Includes   Use additional   Code first   Code also   Key words

● **I71**   **Aortic aneurysm and dissection**

> **Excludes1**   aortic ectasia (I77.81-)
> syphilitic aortic aneurysm (A52.01)
> traumatic aortic aneurysm (S25.09, S35.09)

  ● **I71.0**   **Dissection of aorta**

      I71.00   **Dissection of unspecified site of aorta**

      I71.01   **Dissection of thoracic aorta**

      I71.02   **Dissection of abdominal aorta**

      I71.03   **Dissection of thoracoabdominal aorta**

  I71.1   **Thoracic aortic aneurysm, ruptured**

  I71.2   **Thoracic aortic aneurysm, without rupture**

  I71.3   **Abdominal aortic aneurysm, ruptured**

  I71.4   **Abdominal aortic aneurysm, without rupture**

  I71.5   **Thoracoabdominal aortic aneurysm, ruptured**

  I71.6   **Thoracoabdominal aortic aneurysm, without rupture**

  I71.8   **Aortic aneurysm of unspecified site, ruptured**
      Rupture of aorta NOS

  I71.9   **Aortic aneurysm of unspecified site, without rupture**
      Aneurysm of aorta
      Dilatation of aorta
      Hyaline necrosis of aorta

● **I72**   **Other aneurysm**

> **Includes**   aneurysm (cirsoid) (false) (ruptured)
> **Excludes2**   acquired aneurysm (I77.0)
> aneurysm (of) aorta (I71.-)
> aneurysm (of) arteriovenous NOS (Q27.3-)
> carotid artery dissection (I77.71)
> cerebral (nonruptured) aneurysm (I67.1)
> coronary aneurysm (I25.4)
> coronary artery dissection (I25.42)
> dissection of artery NEC (I77.79)
> dissection of precerebral artery, congenital (nonruptured) (Q28.1)
> heart aneurysm (I25.3)
> iliac artery dissection (I77.72)
> ▶precerebral artery, congential (nonruptured) (Q28.1)
> pulmonary artery aneurysm (I28.1)
> renal artery dissection (I77.73)
> retinal aneurysm (H35.0)
> ruptured cerebral aneurysm (I60.7)
> varicose aneurysm (I77.0)
> vertebral artery dissection (I77.74)

  I72.0   **Aneurysm of carotid artery**
      Aneurysm of common carotid artery
      Aneurysm of external carotid artery
      Aneurysm of internal carotid artery, extracranial portion

> **Excludes1**   aneurysm of internal carotid artery, intracranial portion (I67.1)
> aneurysm of internal carotid artery NOS (I67.1)

  I72.1   **Aneurysm of artery of upper extremity**

  I72.2   **Aneurysm of renal artery**

  I72.3   **Aneurysm of iliac artery**

  I72.4   **Aneurysm of artery of lower extremity**

  I72.5   **Aneurysm of other precerebral arteries**
      Aneurysm of basilar artery (trunk)

> **Excludes2**   aneurysm of carotid artery (I72.0)
> aneurysm of vertebral artery (I72.6)
> dissection of carotid artery (I77.71)
> dissection of other precerebral arteries (I77.75)
> dissection of vertebral artery (I77.74)

  I72.6   **Aneurysm of vertebral artery**

> **Excludes2**   dissection of vertebral artery (I77.74)

  I72.8   **Aneurysm of other specified arteries**

  I72.9   **Aneurysm of unspecified site**

● **I73**   **Other peripheral vascular diseases**

> **Excludes2**   chilblains (T69.1)
> frostbite (T33-T34)
> immersion hand or foot (T69.0-)
> spasm of cerebral artery (G45.9)

  ● **I73.0**   **Raynaud's syndrome**
      Diminishing oxygen supply to fingers, toes, nose, and ears when exposed to temperature changes or stress
      Raynaud's disease
      Raynaud's phenomenon (secondary)

      I73.00   **Raynaud's syndrome without gangrene**

      I73.01   **Raynaud's syndrome with gangrene**

  I73.1   **Thromboangiitis obliterans [Buerger's disease]**
      Inflammatory occlusive disease resulting in poor circulation to the legs, feet, and sometimes the hands due to progressive inflammatory narrowing and eventually obliteration of the small arteries

  ● **I73.8**   **Other specified peripheral vascular diseases**

> **Excludes1**   diabetic (peripheral) angiopathy (E08-E13 with .51-.52)

      I73.81   **Erythromelalgia**

      I73.89   **Other specified peripheral vascular diseases**
        Acrocyanosis
        Erythrocyanosis
        Simple acroparesthesia [Schultze's type]
        Vasomotor acroparesthesia [Nothnagel's type]

  I73.9   **Peripheral vascular disease, unspecified**
      Intermittent claudication
      Peripheral angiopathy NOS
      Spasm of artery

> **Excludes1**   atherosclerosis of the extremities (I70.2--I70.7-)

Figure 9-5 Raynaud's syndrome. (From Hallett: Comprehensive Vascular and Endovascular Surgery, ed 2, Philadelphia, Mosby Ltd., 2010)

CHAPTER 9 (I00-I99)

▶ New   ⇒ Revised   ~~deleted~~ Deleted   **OGCR** Official Guidelines   X Assign placeholder X   ● Use Additional Character(s)

Excludes 1   Excludes 2   Includes   Use additional   Code first   Code also   Key words

Item 9-9 An **embolus** is a mass of undissolved matter present in the blood that is transported by the blood current. A **thrombus** is a blood clot that occludes or shuts off a vessel. When a thrombus is dislodged, it becomes an embolus.

Embolus

Figure 9-6 An arterial embolus.

● I74   Arterial embolism and thrombosis

Includes	embolic infarction

embolic infarction
embolic occlusion
thrombotic infarction
thrombotic occlusion

Code first embolism and thrombosis complicating abortion or ectopic or molar pregnancy (O00-O07, O08.2)
embolism and thrombosis complicating pregnancy, childbirth and the puerperium (O88.-)

Excludes2 atheroembolism (I75.-)
basilar embolism and thrombosis (I63.0-I63.2, I65.1)
carotid embolism and thrombosis (I63.0-I63.2, I65.2)
cerebral embolism and thrombosis (I63.3-I63.5, I66.-)
coronary embolism and thrombosis (I21-I25)
mesenteric embolism and thrombosis (K55.0-)
ophthalmic embolism and thrombosis (H34.-)
precerebral embolism and thrombosis NOS (I63.0-I63.2, I65.9)
pulmonary embolism and thrombosis (I26.-)
renal embolism and thrombosis (N28.0)
retinal embolism and thrombosis (H34.-)
septic embolism and thrombosis (I76)
vertebral embolism and thrombosis (I63.0-I63.2, I65.0)

● I74.0   Embolism and thrombosis of abdominal aorta
    I74.01   Saddle embolus of abdominal aorta
    I74.09   Other arterial embolism and thrombosis of abdominal aorta
        Aortic bifurcation syndrome
        Aortoiliac obstruction
        Leriche's syndrome

● I74.1   Embolism and thrombosis of other and unspecified parts of aorta
    I74.10   Embolism and thrombosis of unspecified parts of aorta
    I74.11   Embolism and thrombosis of thoracic aorta
    I74.19   Embolism and thrombosis of other parts of aorta

    I74.2   Embolism and thrombosis of arteries of the upper extremities
    I74.3   Embolism and thrombosis of arteries of the lower extremities
    I74.4   Embolism and thrombosis of arteries of extremities, unspecified
        Peripheral arterial embolism NOS
    I74.5   Embolism and thrombosis of iliac artery
    I74.8   Embolism and thrombosis of other arteries
    I74.9   Embolism and thrombosis of unspecified artery

● I75   Atheroembolism

Includes	atherothrombotic microembolism

atherothrombotic microembolism
cholesterol embolism

● I75.0   Atheroembolism of extremities
    ● I75.01   Atheroembolism of upper extremity
        I75.011   Atheroembolism of right upper extremity
        I75.012   Atheroembolism of left upper extremity
        I75.013   Atheroembolism of bilateral upper extremities
        I75.019   Atheroembolism of unspecified upper extremity
    ● I75.02   Atheroembolism of lower extremity
        I75.021   Atheroembolism of right lower extremity
        I75.022   Atheroembolism of left lower extremity
        I75.023   Atheroembolism of bilateral lower extremities
        I75.029   Atheroembolism of unspecified lower extremity

● I75.8   Atheroembolism of other sites
    I75.81   Atheroembolism of kidney
        Use additional code for any associated acute kidney failure and chronic kidney disease (N17.-, N18.-)
    I75.89   Atheroembolism of other site

I76   Septic arterial embolism
    Code first underlying infection, such as:
        infective endocarditis (I33.0)
        lung abscess (J85.-)
    Use additional code to identify the site of the embolism (I74.-)
    Excludes2 septic pulmonary embolism (I26.01, I26.90)

● I77   Other disorders of arteries and arterioles
    Excludes2 collagen (vascular) diseases (M30-M36)
        hypersensitivity angiitis (M31.0)
        pulmonary artery (I28.-)

    I77.0   Arteriovenous fistula, acquired
        Aneurysmal varix
        Arteriovenous aneurysm, acquired
        Excludes1 arteriovenous aneurysm NOS (Q27.3-)
            presence of arteriovenous shunt (fistula) for dialysis (Z99.2)
            traumatic - see injury of blood vessel by body region
        Excludes2 cerebral (I67.1)
            coronary (I25.4)

    I77.1   Stricture of artery
        Narrowing of artery
    I77.2   Rupture of artery
        Erosion of artery
        Fistula of artery
        Ulcer of artery
        Excludes1 traumatic rupture of artery - see injury of blood vessel by body region
    I77.3   Arterial fibromuscular dysplasia
        Fibromuscular hyperplasia (of) carotid artery
        Fibromuscular hyperplasia (of) renal artery
    I77.4   Celiac artery compression syndrome
    I77.5   Necrosis of artery

▶ New   ⇒ Revised   ~~deleted~~ Deleted   **OGCR** Official Guidelines   X Assign placeholder X   ● Use Additional Character(s)

Excludes 1   Excludes 2   Includes   Use additional   Code first   Code also   Key words

I77.6   **Arteritis, unspecified**
Aortitis NOS
Endarteritis NOS
> Excludes1   arteritis or endarteritis:
> aortic arch (M31.4)
> cerebral NEC (I67.7)
> coronary (I25.89)
> deformans (I70.-)
> giant cell (M31.5., M31.6)
> obliterans (I70.-)
> senile (I70.-)

● **I77.7**   **Other arterial dissection**
> Excludes2   dissection of aorta (I71.0-)
> dissection of coronary artery (I25.42)

I77.70   Dissection of unspecified artery

I77.71   Dissection of carotid artery

I77.72   Dissection of iliac artery

I77.73   Dissection of renal artery

I77.74   Dissection of vertebral artery
> Excludes2   aneurysm of vertebral artery
> (I72.6)

I77.75   Dissection of other precerebral arteries
Dissection of basilar artery (trunk)
> Excludes2   aneurysm of carotid artery
> (I72.0)
> aneurysm of other precerebral
> arteries (I72.5)
> aneurysm of vertebral artery
> (I72.6)
> dissection of carotid artery
> (I77.71)
> dissection of vertebral artery
> (I77.74)

I77.76   Dissection of artery of upper extremity

I77.77   Dissection of artery of lower extremity

I77.79   Dissection of other specified artery

● **I77.8**   **Other specified disorders of arteries and arterioles**

I77.81   Aortic ectasia
Ectasis aorta
> Excludes1   aortic aneurysm and dissection
> (I71.0-)

I77.810   Thoracic aortic ectasia

I77.811   Abdominal aortic ectasia

I77.812   Thoracoabdominal aortic ectasia

I77.819   Aortic ectasia, unspecified site

I77.89   Other specified disorders of arteries and arterioles

I77.9   **Disorder of arteries and arterioles, unspecified**

● **I78**   **Diseases of capillaries**

I78.0   **Hereditary hemorrhagic telangiectasia**
Rendu-Osler-Weber disease

I78.1   **Nevus, non-neoplastic**
Araneus nevus   Spider nevus
Senile nevus   Stellar nevus
> Excludes1   nevus NOS (D22.-)
> vascular NOS (Q82.5)
> Excludes2   blue nevus (D22.-)
> flammeus nevus (Q82.5)
> hairy nevus (D22.-)
> melanocytic nevus (D22.-)
> pigmented nevus (D22.-)
> portwine nevus (Q82.5)
> sanguineous nevus (Q82.5)
> strawberry nevus (Q82.5)
> verrucous nevus (Q82.5)

I78.8   **Other diseases of capillaries**

I78.9   **Disease of capillaries, unspecified**

● **I79**   **Disorders of arteries, arterioles and capillaries in diseases classified elsewhere**

I79.0   **Aneurysm of aorta in diseases classified elsewhere**
Code first underlying disease
> Excludes1   syphilitic aneurysm (A52.01)

I79.1   **Aortitis in diseases classified elsewhere**
Code first underlying disease
> Excludes1   syphilitic aortitis (A52.02)

I79.8   **Other disorders of arteries, arterioles and capillaries in diseases classified elsewhere**
Code first underlying disease, such as:
amyloidosis (E85.-)
> Excludes1   diabetic (peripheral) angiopathy
> (E08-E13 with .51-.52)
> syphilitic endarteritis (A52.09)
> tuberculous endarteritis (A18.89)

DISEASES OF VEINS, LYMPHATIC VESSELS AND LYMPH NODES, NOT ELSEWHERE CLASSIFIED (I80-I89)

● **I80**   **Phlebitis and thrombophlebitis**
Inflammation of a vein with infiltration of walls (phlebitis).
> Includes   endophlebitis
> inflammation, vein
> periphlebitis
> suppurative phlebitis

Code first phlebitis and thrombophlebitis complicating
abortion, ectopic or molar pregnancy (O00-O07, O08.7)
phlebitis and thrombophlebitis complicating pregnancy,
childbirth and the puerperium (O22.-, O87.-)
> Excludes1   venous embolism and thrombosis of lower
> extremities (I82.4-, I82.5-, I82.81-)

● **I80.0**   **Phlebitis and thrombophlebitis of superficial vessels of lower extremities**
Phlebitis and thrombophlebitis of femoropopliteal vein

I80.00   Phlebitis and thrombophlebitis of superficial vessels of unspecified lower extremity

I80.01   Phlebitis and thrombophlebitis of superficial vessels of right lower extremity

I80.02   Phlebitis and thrombophlebitis of superficial vessels of left lower extremity

I80.03   Phlebitis and thrombophlebitis of superficial vessels of lower extremities, bilateral

● **I80.1**   **Phlebitis and thrombophlebitis of femoral vein**

I80.10   Phlebitis and thrombophlebitis of unspecified femoral vein

I80.11   Phlebitis and thrombophlebitis of right femoral vein

I80.12   Phlebitis and thrombophlebitis of left femoral vein

I80.13   Phlebitis and thrombophlebitis of femoral vein, bilateral

● **I80.2**   **Phlebitis and thrombophlebitis of other and unspecified deep vessels of lower extremities**

● **I80.20**   Phlebitis and thrombophlebitis of unspecified deep vessels of lower extremities

I80.201   Phlebitis and thrombophlebitis of unspecified deep vessels of right lower extremity

I80.202   Phlebitis and thrombophlebitis of unspecified deep vessels of left lower extremity

I80.203   Phlebitis and thrombophlebitis of unspecified deep vessels of lower extremities, bilateral

I80.209   Phlebitis and thrombophlebitis of unspecified deep vessels of unspecified lower extremity

---

● **I80.21**   Phlebitis and thrombophlebitis of iliac vein

     I80.211   Phlebitis and thrombophlebitis of right iliac vein

     I80.212   Phlebitis and thrombophlebitis of left iliac vein

     I80.213   Phlebitis and thrombophlebitis of iliac vein, bilateral

     I80.219   Phlebitis and thrombophlebitis of unspecified iliac vein

● **I80.22**   Phlebitis and thrombophlebitis of popliteal vein

     I80.221   Phlebitis and thrombophlebitis of right popliteal vein

     I80.222   Phlebitis and thrombophlebitis of left popliteal vein

     I80.223   Phlebitis and thrombophlebitis of popliteal vein, bilateral

     I80.229   Phlebitis and thrombophlebitis of unspecified popliteal vein

● **I80.23**   Phlebitis and thrombophlebitis of tibial vein

     I80.231   Phlebitis and thrombophlebitis of right tibial vein

     I80.232   Phlebitis and thrombophlebitis of left tibial vein

     I80.233   Phlebitis and thrombophlebitis of tibial vein, bilateral

     I80.239   Phlebitis and thrombophlebitis of unspecified tibial vein

● **I80.29**   Phlebitis and thrombophlebitis of other deep vessels of lower extremities

     I80.291   Phlebitis and thrombophlebitis of other deep vessels of right lower extremity

     I80.292   Phlebitis and thrombophlebitis of other deep vessels of left lower extremity

     I80.293   Phlebitis and thrombophlebitis of other deep vessels of lower extremity, bilateral

     I80.299   Phlebitis and thrombophlebitis of other deep vessels of unspecified lower extremity

I80.3   Phlebitis and thrombophlebitis of lower extremities, unspecified

I80.8   Phlebitis and thrombophlebitis of other sites

I80.9   Phlebitis and thrombophlebitis of unspecified site

I81   **Portal vein thrombosis**
Portal (vein) obstruction

> **Excludes2**   hepatic vein thrombosis (I82.0)
> phlebitis of portal vein (K75.1)

● **I82**   **Other venous embolism and thrombosis**

Code first venous embolism and thrombosis complicating:
abortion, ectopic or molar pregnancy (O00-O07, O08.7)
pregnancy, childbirth and the puerperium (O22.-, O87.-)

> **Excludes2**   venous embolism and thrombosis (of):
> cerebral (I63.6, I67.6)
> coronary (I21-I25)
> intracranial and intraspinal, septic or NOS (G08)
> intracranial, nonpyogenic (I67.6)
> intraspinal, nonpyogenic (G95.1)
> mesenteric (K55.0-)
> portal (I81)
> pulmonary (I26.-)

I82.0   **Budd-Chiari syndrome**
Hepatic vein thrombosis

I82.1   **Thrombophlebitis migrans**
"White leg" is the other term to describe a migrating thrombus.

● **I82.2**   Embolism and thrombosis of vena cava and other thoracic veins

   ● **I82.21**   Embolism and thrombosis of superior vena cava

     I82.210   Acute embolism and thrombosis of superior vena cava
Embolism and thrombosis of superior vena cava NOS

     I82.211   Chronic embolism and thrombosis of superior vena cava

   ● **I82.22**   Embolism and thrombosis of inferior vena cava

     I82.220   Acute embolism and thrombosis of inferior vena cava
Embolism and thrombosis of inferior vena cava NOS

     I82.221   Chronic embolism and thrombosis of inferior vena cava

   ● **I82.29**   Embolism and thrombosis of other thoracic veins
Embolism and thrombosis of brachiocephalic (innominate) vein

     I82.290   Acute embolism and thrombosis of other thoracic veins

     I82.291   Chronic embolism and thrombosis of other thoracic veins

I82.3   Embolism and thrombosis of renal vein

● **I82.4**   Acute embolism and thrombosis of deep veins of lower extremity

     I82.40   Acute embolism and thrombosis of unspecified deep veins of lower extremity
Deep vein thrombosis NOS
DVT NOS

> **Excludes1**   acute embolism and thrombosis of unspecified deep veins of distal lower extremity (I82.4Z-)
> acute embolism and thrombosis of unspecified deep veins of proximal lower extremity (I82.4Y-)

     I82.401   Acute embolism and thrombosis of unspecified deep veins of right lower extremity

     I82.402   Acute embolism and thrombosis of unspecified deep veins of left lower extremity

     I82.403   Acute embolism and thrombosis of unspecified deep veins of lower extremity, bilateral

     I82.409   Acute embolism and thrombosis of unspecified deep veins of unspecified lower extremity

   ● **I82.41**   Acute embolism and thrombosis of femoral vein

     I82.411   Acute embolism and thrombosis of right femoral vein

     I82.412   Acute embolism and thrombosis of left femoral vein

     I82.413   Acute embolism and thrombosis of femoral vein, bilateral

     I82.419   Acute embolism and thrombosis of unspecified femoral vein

   ● **I82.42**   Acute embolism and thrombosis of iliac vein

     I82.421   Acute embolism and thrombosis of right iliac vein

     I82.422   Acute embolism and thrombosis of left iliac vein

     I82.423   Acute embolism and thrombosis of iliac vein, bilateral

     I82.429   Acute embolism and thrombosis of unspecified iliac vein

▶ New   ➡ Revised   ~~deleted~~ Deleted   **OGCR** Official Guidelines   X Assign placeholder X   ● Use Additional Character(s)

Excludes 1   Excludes 2   Includes   Use additional   Code first   Code also   Key words

● I82.43 Acute embolism and thrombosis of popliteal vein

  I82.431 Acute embolism and thrombosis of right popliteal vein

  I82.432 Acute embolism and thrombosis of left popliteal vein

  I82.433 Acute embolism and thrombosis of popliteal vein, bilateral

  I82.439 Acute embolism and thrombosis of unspecified popliteal vein

● I82.44 Acute embolism and thrombosis of tibial vein

  I82.441 Acute embolism and thrombosis of right tibial vein

  I82.442 Acute embolism and thrombosis of left tibial vein

  I82.443 Acute embolism and thrombosis of tibial vein, bilateral

  I82.449 Acute embolism and thrombosis of unspecified tibial vein

● I82.49 Acute embolism and thrombosis of other specified deep vein of lower extremity

  I82.491 Acute embolism and thrombosis of other specified deep vein of right lower extremity

  I82.492 Acute embolism and thrombosis of other specified deep vein of left lower extremity

  I82.493 Acute embolism and thrombosis of other specified deep vein of lower extremity, bilateral

  I82.499 Acute embolism and thrombosis of other specified deep vein of unspecified lower extremity

● I82.4Y Acute embolism and thrombosis of unspecified deep veins of proximal lower extremity
  Acute embolism and thrombosis of deep vein of thigh NOS
  Acute embolism and thrombosis of deep vein of upper leg NOS

  I82.4Y1 Acute embolism and thrombosis of unspecified deep veins of right proximal lower extremity

  I82.4Y2 Acute embolism and thrombosis of unspecified deep veins of left proximal lower extremity

  I82.4Y3 Acute embolism and thrombosis of unspecified deep veins of proximal lower extremity, bilateral

  I82.4Y9 Acute embolism and thrombosis of unspecified deep veins of unspecified proximal lower extremity

● I82.4Z Acute embolism and thrombosis of unspecified deep veins of distal lower extremity
  Acute embolism and thrombosis of deep vein of calf NOS
  Acute embolism and thrombosis of deep vein of lower leg NOS

  I82.4Z1 Acute embolism and thrombosis of unspecified deep veins of right distal lower extremity

  I82.4Z2 Acute embolism and thrombosis of unspecified deep veins of left distal lower extremity

  I82.4Z3 Acute embolism and thrombosis of unspecified deep veins of distal lower extremity, bilateral

  I82.4Z9 Acute embolism and thrombosis of unspecified deep veins of unspecified distal lower extremity

● I82.5 Chronic embolism and thrombosis of deep veins of lower extremity
  Use additional code, if applicable, for associated long-term (current) use of anticoagulants (Z79.01)
  Excludes1 personal history of venous embolism and thrombosis (Z86.718)

● I82.50 Chronic embolism and thrombosis of unspecified deep veins of lower extremity
  Excludes1 chronic embolism and thrombosis of unspecified deep veins of distal lower extremity (I82.5Z-)
           chronic embolism and thrombosis of unspecified deep veins of proximal lower extremity (I82.5Y-)

  I82.501 Chronic embolism and thrombosis of unspecified deep veins of right lower extremity

  I82.502 Chronic embolism and thrombosis of unspecified deep veins of left lower extremity

  I82.503 Chronic embolism and thrombosis of unspecified deep veins of lower extremity, bilateral

  I82.509 Chronic embolism and thrombosis of unspecified deep veins of unspecified lower extremity

● I82.51 Chronic embolism and thrombosis of femoral vein

  I82.511 Chronic embolism and thrombosis of right femoral vein

  I82.512 Chronic embolism and thrombosis of left femoral vein

  I82.513 Chronic embolism and thrombosis of femoral vein, bilateral

  I82.519 Chronic embolism and thrombosis of unspecified femoral vein

● I82.52 Chronic embolism and thrombosis of iliac vein

  I82.521 Chronic embolism and thrombosis of right iliac vein

  I82.522 Chronic embolism and thrombosis of left iliac vein

  I82.523 Chronic embolism and thrombosis of iliac vein, bilateral

  I82.529 Chronic embolism and thrombosis of unspecified iliac vein

● I82.53 Chronic embolism and thrombosis of popliteal vein

  I82.531 Chronic embolism and thrombosis of right popliteal vein

  I82.532 Chronic embolism and thrombosis of left popliteal vein

  I82.533 Chronic embolism and thrombosis of popliteal vein, bilateral

  I82.539 Chronic embolism and thrombosis of unspecified popliteal vein

● I82.54 Chronic embolism and thrombosis of tibial vein

  I82.541 Chronic embolism and thrombosis of right tibial vein

  I82.542 Chronic embolism and thrombosis of left tibial vein

  I82.543 Chronic embolism and thrombosis of tibial vein, bilateral

  I82.549 Chronic embolism and thrombosis of unspecified tibial vein

CHAPTER 9 (I00-I99)

▶ New   ⇒ Revised   ~~deleted~~ Deleted   OGCR Official Guidelines   X Assign placeholder X   ● Use Additional Character(s)

Excludes 1   Excludes 2   Includes   Use additional   Code first   Code also   Key words

CHAPTER 9 (I00-I99)

● **I82.59**   Chronic embolism and thrombosis of other specified deep vein of lower extremity

     I82.591   Chronic embolism and thrombosis of other specified deep vein of right lower extremity

     I82.592   Chronic embolism and thrombosis of other specified deep vein of left lower extremity

     I82.593   Chronic embolism and thrombosis of other specified deep vein of lower extremity, bilateral

     I82.599   Chronic embolism and thrombosis of other specified deep vein of unspecified lower extremity

● **I82.5Y**   Chronic embolism and thrombosis of unspecified deep veins of proximal lower extremity

     Chronic embolism and thrombosis of deep veins of thigh NOS

     Chronic embolism and thrombosis of deep veins of upper leg NOS

     I82.5Y1   Chronic embolism and thrombosis of unspecified deep veins of right proximal lower extremity

     I82.5Y2   Chronic embolism and thrombosis of unspecified deep veins of left proximal lower extremity

     I82.5Y3   Chronic embolism and thrombosis of unspecified deep veins of proximal lower extremity, bilateral

     I82.5Y9   Chronic embolism and thrombosis of unspecified deep veins of unspecified proximal lower extremity

● **I82.5Z**   Chronic embolism and thrombosis of unspecified deep veins of distal lower extremity

     Chronic embolism and thrombosis of deep veins of calf NOS

     Chronic embolism and thrombosis of deep veins of lower leg NOS

     I82.5Z1   Chronic embolism and thrombosis of unspecified deep veins of right distal lower extremity

     I82.5Z2   Chronic embolism and thrombosis of unspecified deep veins of left distal lower extremity

     I82.5Z3   Chronic embolism and thrombosis of unspecified deep veins of distal lower extremity, bilateral

     I82.5Z9   Chronic embolism and thrombosis of unspecified deep veins of unspecified distal lower extremity

Item 9–10 Varicose/Varicosities (varix = singular, varices = plural): Enlarged, engorged, tortuous, twisted vascular vessels (veins, arteries, lymphatics). As such, the condition can present in various parts of the body, although the most familiar locations are the lower extremities. A common complication of varices is thrombophlebitis. Varicosities of the anus and rectum are called hemorrhoids.

Figure 9-7   Varicose veins of the legs. (Getty Image)

● **I82.6**   Acute embolism and thrombosis of veins of upper extremity

● **I82.60**   Acute embolism and thrombosis of unspecified veins of upper extremity

     I82.601   Acute embolism and thrombosis of unspecified veins of right upper extremity

     I82.602   Acute embolism and thrombosis of unspecified veins of left upper extremity

     I82.603   Acute embolism and thrombosis of unspecified veins of upper extremity, bilateral

     I82.609   Acute embolism and thrombosis of unspecified veins of unspecified upper extremity

● **I82.61**   Acute embolism and thrombosis of superficial veins of upper extremity

     Acute embolism and thrombosis of antecubital vein

     Acute embolism and thrombosis of basilic vein

     Acute embolism and thrombosis of cephalic vein

     I82.611   Acute embolism and thrombosis of superficial veins of right upper extremity

     I82.612   Acute embolism and thrombosis of superficial veins of left upper extremity

     I82.613   Acute embolism and thrombosis of superficial veins of upper extremity, bilateral

     I82.619   Acute embolism and thrombosis of superficial veins of unspecified upper extremity

● **I82.62**   Acute embolism and thrombosis of deep veins of upper extremity

     Acute embolism and thrombosis of brachial vein

     Acute embolism and thrombosis of radial vein

     Acute embolism and thrombosis of ulnar vein

     I82.621   Acute embolism and thrombosis of deep veins of right upper extremity

     I82.622   Acute embolism and thrombosis of deep veins of left upper extremity

     I82.623   Acute embolism and thrombosis of deep veins of upper extremity, bilateral

     I82.629   Acute embolism and thrombosis of deep veins of unspecified upper extremity

● **I82.7**   Chronic embolism and thrombosis of veins of upper extremity

     Use additional code, if applicable, for associated long-term (current) use of anticoagulants (Z79.01)

     Excludes1   personal history of venous embolism and thrombosis (Z86.718)

● **I82.70**   Chronic embolism and thrombosis of unspecified veins of upper extremity

     I82.701   Chronic embolism and thrombosis of unspecified veins of right upper extremity

     I82.702   Chronic embolism and thrombosis of unspecified veins of left upper extremity

     I82.703   Chronic embolism and thrombosis of unspecified veins of upper extremity, bilateral

     I82.709   Chronic embolism and thrombosis of unspecified veins of unspecified upper extremity

▶ New   ⇒ Revised   ~~deleted~~ Deleted   **OGCR** Official Guidelines   X Assign placeholder X   ● Use Additional Character(s)

Excludes 1   Excludes 2   Includes   Use additional   Code first   Code also   Key words

● **I82.71** **Chronic embolism and thrombosis of superficial veins of upper extremity**
Chronic embolism and thrombosis of antecubital vein
Chronic embolism and thrombosis of basilic vein
Chronic embolism and thrombosis of cephalic vein

- **I82.711** Chronic embolism and thrombosis of superficial veins of right upper extremity
- **I82.712** Chronic embolism and thrombosis of superficial veins of left upper extremity
- **I82.713** Chronic embolism and thrombosis of superficial veins of upper extremity, bilateral
- **I82.719** Chronic embolism and thrombosis of superficial veins of unspecified upper extremity

● **I82.72** **Chronic embolism and thrombosis of deep veins of upper extremity**
Chronic embolism and thrombosis of brachial vein
Chronic embolism and thrombosis of radial vein
Chronic embolism and thrombosis of ulnar vein

- **I82.721** Chronic embolism and thrombosis of deep veins of right upper extremity
- **I82.722** Chronic embolism and thrombosis of deep veins of left upper extremity
- **I82.723** Chronic embolism and thrombosis of deep veins of upper extremity, bilateral
- **I82.729** Chronic embolism and thrombosis of deep veins of unspecified upper extremity

● **I82.A** **Embolism and thrombosis of axillary vein**
● **I82.A1** Acute embolism and thrombosis of axillary vein
- **I82.A11** Acute embolism and thrombosis of right axillary vein
- **I82.A12** Acute embolism and thrombosis of left axillary vein
- **I82.A13** Acute embolism and thrombosis of axillary vein, bilateral
- **I82.A19** Acute embolism and thrombosis of unspecified axillary vein

● **I82.A2** Chronic embolism and thrombosis of axillary vein
- **I82.A21** Chronic embolism and thrombosis of right axillary vein
- **I82.A22** Chronic embolism and thrombosis of left axillary vein
- **I82.A23** Chronic embolism and thrombosis of axillary vein, bilateral
- **I82.A29** Chronic embolism and thrombosis of unspecified axillary vein

● **I82.B** **Embolism and thrombosis of subclavian vein**
● **I82.B1** Acute embolism and thrombosis of subclavian vein
- **I82.B11** Acute embolism and thrombosis of right subclavian vein
- **I82.B12** Acute embolism and thrombosis of left subclavian vein
- **I82.B13** Acute embolism and thrombosis of subclavian vein, bilateral
- **I82.B19** Acute embolism and thrombosis of unspecified subclavian vein

● **I82.B2** Chronic embolism and thrombosis of subclavian vein
- **I82.B21** Chronic embolism and thrombosis of right subclavian vein
- **I82.B22** Chronic embolism and thrombosis of left subclavian vein
- **I82.B23** Chronic embolism and thrombosis of subclavian vein, bilateral
- **I82.B29** Chronic embolism and thrombosis of unspecified subclavian vein

● **I82.C** **Embolism and thrombosis of internal jugular vein**
● **I82.C1** Acute embolism and thrombosis of internal jugular vein
- **I82.C11** Acute embolism and thrombosis of right internal jugular vein
- **I82.C12** Acute embolism and thrombosis of left internal jugular vein
- **I82.C13** Acute embolism and thrombosis of internal jugular vein, bilateral
- **I82.C19** Acute embolism and thrombosis of unspecified internal jugular vein

● **I82.C2** Chronic embolism and thrombosis of internal jugular vein
- **I82.C21** Chronic embolism and thrombosis of right internal jugular vein
- **I82.C22** Chronic embolism and thrombosis of left internal jugular vein
- **I82.C23** Chronic embolism and thrombosis of internal jugular vein, bilateral
- **I82.C29** Chronic embolism and thrombosis of unspecified internal jugular vein

● **I82.8** **Embolism and thrombosis of other specified veins**
Use additional code, if applicable, for associated long-term (current) use of anticoagulants (Z79.01)

● **I82.81** **Embolism and thrombosis of superficial veins of lower extremities**
Embolism and thrombosis of saphenous vein (greater) (lesser)
- ⇒ **I82.811** Embolism and thrombosis of superficial veins of right lower extremity
- ⇒ **I82.812** Embolism and thrombosis of superficial veins of left lower extremity
- **I82.813** Embolism and thrombosis of superficial veins of lower extremities, bilateral
- ⇒ **I82.819** Embolism and thrombosis of superficial veins of unspecified lower extremity

● **I82.89** **Embolism and thrombosis of other specified veins**
- **I82.890** Acute embolism and thrombosis of other specified veins
- **I82.891** Chronic embolism and thrombosis of other specified veins

● **I82.9** **Embolism and thrombosis of unspecified vein**
- **I82.90** Acute embolism and thrombosis of unspecified vein
Embolism of vein NOS
Thrombosis (vein) NOS
- **I82.91** Chronic embolism and thrombosis of unspecified vein

CHAPTER 9 (I00-I99)

● **I83**   **Varicose veins of lower extremities**

> **Excludes1**   varicose veins complicating pregnancy (O22.0-)
> varicose veins complicating the puerperium
> (O87.4)

● **I83.0**   **Varicose veins of lower extremities with ulcer**

> Use additional code to identify severity of ulcer (L97.-)

  ● **I83.00**   **Varicose veins of unspecified lower extremity with ulcer**

     I83.001   Varicose veins of unspecified lower extremity with ulcer of **thigh**

     I83.002   Varicose veins of unspecified lower extremity with ulcer of **calf**

     I83.003   Varicose veins of unspecified lower extremity with ulcer of **ankle**

     I83.004   Varicose veins of unspecified lower extremity with ulcer of **heel and midfoot**

> Varicose veins of unspecified lower extremity with ulcer of plantar surface of midfoot

     I83.005   Varicose veins of unspecified lower extremity with ulcer **other part of foot**

> Varicose veins of unspecified lower extremity with ulcer of toe

     I83.008   Varicose veins of unspecified lower extremity with ulcer **other part of lower leg**

     I83.009   Varicose veins of unspecified lower extremity with ulcer of **unspecified** site

  ● **I83.01**   **Varicose veins of right lower extremity with ulcer**

     I83.011   Varicose veins of right lower extremity with ulcer of **thigh**

     I83.012   Varicose veins of right lower extremity with ulcer of **calf**

     I83.013   Varicose veins of right lower extremity with ulcer of **ankle**

     I83.014   Varicose veins of right lower extremity with ulcer of **heel and midfoot**

> Varicose veins of right lower extremity with ulcer of plantar surface of midfoot

     I83.015   Varicose veins of right lower extremity with ulcer **other part of foot**

> Varicose veins of right lower extremity with ulcer of toe

     I83.018   Varicose veins of right lower extremity with ulcer **other part of lower leg**

     I83.019   Varicose veins of right lower extremity with ulcer of **unspecified** site

  ● **I83.02**   **Varicose veins of left lower extremity with ulcer**

     I83.021   Varicose veins of left lower extremity with ulcer of **thigh**

     I83.022   Varicose veins of left lower extremity with ulcer of **calf**

     I83.023   Varicose veins of left lower extremity with ulcer of **ankle**

     I83.024   Varicose veins of left lower extremity with ulcer of **heel and midfoot**

> Varicose veins of left lower extremity with ulcer of plantar surface of midfoot

     I83.025   Varicose veins of left lower extremity with ulcer **other part of foot**

> Varicose veins of left lower extremity with ulcer of toe

     I83.028   Varicose veins of left lower extremity with ulcer **other part of lower leg**

     I83.029   Varicose veins of left lower extremity with ulcer of **unspecified** site

● **I83.1**   **Varicose veins of lower extremities with inflammation**

     I83.10   Varicose veins of **unspecified** lower extremity with inflammation

     I83.11   Varicose veins of **right** lower extremity with inflammation

     I83.12   Varicose veins of **left** lower extremity with inflammation

● **I83.2**   **Varicose veins of lower extremities with both ulcer and inflammation**

> Use additional code to identify severity of ulcer (L97.-)

  ● **I83.20**   **Varicose veins of unspecified lower extremity with both ulcer and inflammation**

     I83.201   Varicose veins of unspecified lower extremity with both ulcer of **thigh** and inflammation

     I83.202   Varicose veins of unspecified lower extremity with both ulcer of **calf** and inflammation

     I83.203   Varicose veins of unspecified lower extremity with both ulcer of **ankle** and inflammation

     I83.204   Varicose veins of unspecified lower extremity with both ulcer of **heel and midfoot** and inflammation

> Varicose veins of unspecified lower extremity with both ulcer of plantar surface of midfoot and inflammation

     I83.205   Varicose veins of unspecified lower extremity with both ulcer **other part of foot** and inflammation

> Varicose veins of unspecified lower extremity with both ulcer of toe and inflammation

     I83.208   Varicose veins of unspecified lower extremity with both ulcer of **other part of lower extremity** and inflammation

     I83.209   Varicose veins of unspecified lower extremity with both ulcer of **unspecified site** and inflammation

  ● **I83.21**   **Varicose veins of right lower extremity with both ulcer and inflammation**

     I83.211   Varicose veins of right lower extremity with both ulcer of **thigh** and inflammation

     I83.212   Varicose veins of right lower extremity with both ulcer of **calf** and inflammation

     I83.213   Varicose veins of right lower extremity with both ulcer of **ankle** and inflammation

     I83.214   Varicose veins of right lower extremity with both ulcer of **heel and midfoot** and inflammation

> Varicose veins of right lower extremity with both ulcer of plantar surface of midfoot and inflammation

▶ New   ⇒ Revised   ~~deleted~~ Deleted   **OGCR** Official Guidelines   X Assign placeholder X   ● Use Additional Character(s)

Excludes 1   Excludes 2   Includes   Use additional   Code first   Code also   Key words

I83.215   Varicose veins of right lower extremity with both ulcer other part of foot and inflammation
    Varicose veins of right lower extremity with both ulcer of toe and inflammation

I83.218   Varicose veins of right lower extremity with both ulcer of other part of lower extremity and inflammation

I83.219   Varicose veins of right lower extremity with both ulcer of unspecified site and inflammation

● I83.22   Varicose veins of left lower extremity with both ulcer and inflammation

I83.221   Varicose veins of left lower extremity with both ulcer of thigh and inflammation

I83.222   Varicose veins of left lower extremity with both ulcer of calf and inflammation

I83.223   Varicose veins of left lower extremity with both ulcer of ankle and inflammation

I83.224   Varicose veins of left lower extremity with both ulcer of heel and midfoot and inflammation
    Varicose veins of left lower extremity with both ulcer of plantar surface of midfoot and inflammation

I83.225   Varicose veins of left lower extremity with both ulcer other part of foot and inflammation
    Varicose veins of left lower extremity with both ulcer of toe and inflammation

I83.228   Varicose veins of left lower extremity with both ulcer of other part of lower extremity and inflammation

I83.229   Varicose veins of left lower extremity with both ulcer of unspecified site and inflammation

● I83.8   Varicose veins of lower extremities with other complications

● I83.81   Varicose veins of lower extremities with pain

⇒ I83.811   Varicose veins of right lower extremity with pain

⇒ I83.812   Varicose veins of left lower extremity with pain

I83.813   Varicose veins of bilateral lower extremities with pain

⇒ I83.819   Varicose veins of unspecified lower extremity with pain

● I83.89   Varicose veins of lower extremities with other complications
    Varicose veins of lower extremities with edema
    Varicose veins of lower extremities with swelling

⇒ I83.891   Varicose veins of right lower extremity with other complications

⇒ I83.892   Varicose veins of left lower extremity with other complications

I83.893   Varicose veins of bilateral lower extremities with other complications

⇒ I83.899   Varicose veins of unspecified lower extremity with other complications

● I83.9   Asymptomatic varicose veins of lower extremities
    Phlebectasia of lower extremities
    Varicose veins of lower extremities
    Varix of lower extremities

I83.90   Asymptomatic varicose veins of unspecified lower extremity
    Varicose veins NOS

I83.91   Asymptomatic varicose veins of right lower extremity

I83.92   Asymptomatic varicose veins of left lower extremity

I83.93   Asymptomatic varicose veins of bilateral lower extremities

● I85   **Esophageal varices**
    Use additional code to identify:
    alcohol abuse and dependence (F10.-)

● I85.0   Esophageal varices
    Idiopathic esophageal varices
    Primary esophageal varices

I85.00   Esophageal varices without bleeding
    Esophageal varices NOS

I85.01   Esophageal varices with bleeding

● I85.1   Secondary esophageal varices
    Esophageal varices secondary to alcoholic liver disease
    Esophageal varices secondary to cirrhosis of liver
    Esophageal varices secondary to schistosomiasis
    Esophageal varices secondary to toxic liver disease
    Code first underlying disease

I85.10   Secondary esophageal varices without bleeding

I85.11   Secondary esophageal varices with bleeding

● I86   **Varicose veins of other sites**
    Excludes1   varicose veins of unspecified site (I83.9-)
    Excludes2   retinal varices (H35.0-)

I86.0   Sublingual varices

I86.1   Scrotal varices
    Varicocele

I86.2   Pelvic varices

I86.3   Vulval varices
    Excludes1   vulval varices complicating childbirth and the puerperium (O87.8)
    vulval varices complicating pregnancy (O22.1-)

I86.4   Gastric varices

I86.8   Varicose veins of other specified sites
    Varicose ulcer of nasal septum

● I87   **Other disorders of veins**

● I87.0   Postthrombotic syndrome
    Chronic venous hypertension due to deep vein thrombosis
    Postphlebitic syndrome
    Excludes1   chronic venous hypertension without deep vein thrombosis (I87.3-)

● I87.00   Postthrombotic syndrome without complications
    Asymptomatic Postthrombotic syndrome

I87.001   Postthrombotic syndrome without complications of right lower extremity

I87.002   Postthrombotic syndrome without complications of left lower extremity

I87.003   Postthrombotic syndrome without complications of bilateral lower extremity

I87.009   Postthrombotic syndrome without complications of unspecified extremity
    Postthrombotic syndrome NOS

● **I87.01**   **Postthrombotic syndrome with ulcer**
Use additional code to specify site and severity of ulcer (L97.-)

    I87.011   **Postthrombotic syndrome with ulcer of right lower extremity**

    I87.012   **Postthrombotic syndrome with ulcer of left lower extremity**

    I87.013   **Postthrombotic syndrome with ulcer of bilateral lower extremity**

    I87.019   **Postthrombotic syndrome with ulcer of unspecified lower extremity**

● **I87.02**   **Postthrombotic syndrome with inflammation**

    I87.021   **Postthrombotic syndrome with inflammation of right lower extremity**

    I87.022   **Postthrombotic syndrome with inflammation of left lower extremity**

    I87.023   **Postthrombotic syndrome with inflammation of bilateral lower extremity**

    I87.029   **Postthrombotic syndrome with inflammation of unspecified lower extremity**

● **I87.03**   **Postthrombotic syndrome with ulcer and inflammation**
Use additional code to specify site and severity of ulcer (L97.-)

    I87.031   **Postthrombotic syndrome with ulcer and inflammation of right lower extremity**

    I87.032   **Postthrombotic syndrome with ulcer and inflammation of left lower extremity**

    I87.033   **Postthrombotic syndrome with ulcer and inflammation of bilateral lower extremity**

    I87.039   **Postthrombotic syndrome with ulcer and inflammation of unspecified lower extremity**

● **I87.09**   **Postthrombotic syndrome with other complications**

    I87.091   **Postthrombotic syndrome with other complications of right lower extremity**

    I87.092   **Postthrombotic syndrome with other complications of left lower extremity**

    I87.093   **Postthrombotic syndrome with other complications of bilateral lower extremity**

    I87.099   **Postthrombotic syndrome with other complications of unspecified lower extremity**

I87.1   **Compression of vein**
Stricture of vein
Vena cava syndrome (inferior) (superior)
| Excludes2 | compression of pulmonary vein (I28.8)

I87.2   **Venous insufficiency (chronic) (peripheral)**
Stasis dermatitis
| Excludes1 | stasis dermatitis with varicose veins of lower extremities (I83.1-, I83.2-)

● **I87.3**   **Chronic venous hypertension (idiopathic)**
Stasis edema
| Excludes1 | chronic venous hypertension due to deep vein thrombosis (I87.0-)
varicose veins of lower extremities (I83.-)

● **I87.30**   **Chronic venous hypertension (idiopathic) without complications**
Asymptomatic chronic venous hypertension (idiopathic)

    I87.301   **Chronic venous hypertension (idiopathic) without complications of right lower extremity**

    I87.302   **Chronic venous hypertension (idiopathic) without complications of left lower extremity**

    I87.303   **Chronic venous hypertension (idiopathic) without complications of bilateral lower extremity**

    I87.309   **Chronic venous hypertension (idiopathic) without complications of unspecified lower extremity**
Chronic venous hypertension NOS

● **I87.31**   **Chronic venous hypertension (idiopathic) with ulcer**
Use additional code to specify site and severity of ulcer (L97.-)

    I87.311   **Chronic venous hypertension (idiopathic) with ulcer of right lower extremity**

    I87.312   **Chronic venous hypertension (idiopathic) with ulcer of left lower extremity**

    I87.313   **Chronic venous hypertension (idiopathic) with ulcer of bilateral lower extremity**

    I87.319   **Chronic venous hypertension (idiopathic) with ulcer of unspecified lower extremity**

● **I87.32**   **Chronic venous hypertension (idiopathic) with inflammation**

    I87.321   **Chronic venous hypertension (idiopathic) with inflammation of right lower extremity**

    I87.322   **Chronic venous hypertension (idiopathic) with inflammation of left lower extremity**

    I87.323   **Chronic venous hypertension (idiopathic) with inflammation of bilateral lower extremity**

    I87.329   **Chronic venous hypertension (idiopathic) with inflammation of unspecified lower extremity**

● **I87.33**   **Chronic venous hypertension (idiopathic) with ulcer and inflammation**
Use additional code to specify site and severity of ulcer (L97.-)

    I87.331   **Chronic venous hypertension (idiopathic) with ulcer and inflammation of right lower extremity**

    I87.332   **Chronic venous hypertension (idiopathic) with ulcer and inflammation of left lower extremity**

    I87.333   **Chronic venous hypertension (idiopathic) with ulcer and inflammation of bilateral lower extremity**

    I87.339   **Chronic venous hypertension (idiopathic) with ulcer and inflammation of unspecified lower extremity**

▶ New   ⇒ Revised   ~~deleted~~ Deleted   **OGCR** Official Guidelines   X Assign placeholder X   ● Use Additional Character(s)

| Excludes 1 | | Excludes 2 | | Includes | | Use additional | | Code first | | Code also | | Key words |

● **I87.39** **Chronic venous hypertension (idiopathic) with other complications**

    I87.391 **Chronic venous hypertension (idiopathic) with other complications of right lower extremity**

    I87.392 **Chronic venous hypertension (idiopathic) with other complications of left lower extremity**

    I87.393 **Chronic venous hypertension (idiopathic) with other complications of bilateral lower extremity**

    I87.399 **Chronic venous hypertension (idiopathic) with other complications of unspecified lower extremity**

I87.8 **Other specified disorders of veins**
Phlebosclerosis
Venofibrosis

I87.9 **Disorder of vein, unspecified**

● **I88** **Nonspecific lymphadenitis**
> **Excludes1**   acute lymphadenitis, except mesenteric (L04.-)
> enlarged lymph nodes NOS (R59.-)
> human immunodeficiency virus [HIV] disease resulting in generalized lymphadenopathy (B20)

I88.0 **Nonspecific mesenteric lymphadenitis**
Mesenteric lymphadenitis (acute)(chronic)

I88.1 **Chronic lymphadenitis, except mesenteric**
Adenitis
Lymphadenitis

I88.8 **Other nonspecific lymphadenitis**

I88.9 **Nonspecific lymphadenitis, unspecified**
Lymphadenitis NOS

● **I89** **Other noninfective disorders of lymphatic vessels and lymph nodes**
> **Excludes1**   chylocele, tunica vaginalis (nonfilarial) NOS (N50.89)
> enlarged lymph nodes NOS (R59.-)
> filarial chylocele (B74.-)
> hereditary lymphedema (Q82.0)

I89.0 **Lymphedema, not elsewhere classified**
Elephantiasis (nonfilarial) NOS
Lymphangiectasis
Obliteration, lymphatic vessel
Praecox lymphedema
Secondary lymphedema
> **Excludes1**   postmastectomy lymphedema (I97.2)

I89.1 **Lymphangitis**
Chronic lymphangitis
Lymphangitis NOS
Subacute lymphangitis
> **Excludes1**   acute lymphangitis (L03.-)

I89.8 **Other specified noninfective disorders of lymphatic vessels and lymph nodes**
Chylocele (nonfilarial)
Chylous ascites
Chylous cyst
Lipomelanotic reticulosis
Lymph node or vessel fistula
Lymph node or vessel infarction
Lymph node or vessel rupture

I89.9 **Noninfective disorder of lymphatic vessels and lymph nodes, unspecified**
Disease of lymphatic vessels NOS

OTHER AND UNSPECIFIED DISORDERS OF THE CIRCULATORY SYSTEM (I95-I99)

● **I95** **Hypotension**
Subnormal arterial blood pressure
> **Excludes1**   cardiovascular collapse (R57.9)
> maternal hypotension syndrome (O26.5-)
> nonspecific low blood pressure reading NOS (R03.1)

I95.0 **Idiopathic hypotension**

I95.1 **Orthostatic hypotension**
Hypotension, postural
Moving from a sitting or reclining position to a standing position precipitates a sudden drop in blood pressure (hypotension).
> **Excludes1**   neurogenic orthostatic hypotension [Shy-Drager] (G90.3)
> orthostatic hypotension due to drugs (I95.2)

I95.2 **Hypotension due to drugs**
Orthostatic hypotension due to drugs
Use additional code for adverse effect, if applicable, to identify drug (T36-T50 with fifth or sixth character 5)

I95.3 **Hypotension of hemodialysis**
Intra-dialytic hypotension

● **I95.8** **Other hypotension**
I95.81 **Postprocedural hypotension**
I95.89 **Other hypotension**
Chronic hypotension

I95.9 **Hypotension, unspecified**

● **I96** **Gangrene, not elsewhere classified**
Gangrenous cellulitis
> **Excludes1**   gangrene in atherosclerosis of native arteries of the extremities (I70.26)
> gangrene of certain specified sites - *see* Alphabetical Index
> ~~gangrene in diabetes mellitus (E08-E13 with .52)~~
> gangrene in hernia (K40.1, K40.4, K41.1, K41.4, K42.1, K43.1-, K44.1, K45.1, K46.1)
> gangrene in other peripheral vascular diseases (I73.-)
> gas gangrene (A48.0)
> pyoderma gangrenosum (L88)

> ▶ **Excludes2**   gangrene in diabetes mellitus (E08-E13 with .52)

● **I97** **Intraoperative and postprocedural complications and disorders of circulatory system, not elsewhere classified**
> **Excludes2**   postprocedural shock (T81.1-)

I97.0 **Postcardiotomy syndrome**

● **I97.1** **Other postprocedural cardiac functional disturbances**
> **Excludes2**   acute pulmonary insufficiency following thoracic surgery (J95.1)
> intraoperative cardiac functional disturbances (I97.7-)

  ● **I97.11** **Postprocedural cardiac insufficiency**
    I97.110 **Postprocedural cardiac insufficiency following cardiac surgery**
    I97.111 **Postprocedural cardiac insufficiency following other surgery**

  ● **I97.12** **Postprocedural cardiac arrest**
    I97.120 **Postprocedural cardiac arrest following cardiac surgery**
    I97.121 **Postprocedural cardiac arrest following other surgery**

CHAPTER 9 (I00-I99)

● **I97.13**   **Postprocedural heart failure**
Use additional code to identify the heart failure (I50.-)

     I97.130   **Postprocedural heart failure following cardiac surgery**

     I97.131   **Postprocedural heart failure following other surgery**

● **I97.19**   **Other postprocedural cardiac functional disturbances**
Use additional code, if applicable, to further specify disorder

     I97.190   **Other postprocedural cardiac functional disturbances following cardiac surgery**
▶ Use Additional code, if applicable, for type 4 or type 5 myocardial infarction, to further specify disorder

     I97.191   **Other postprocedural cardiac functional disturbances following other surgery**

I97.2   **Postmastectomy lymphedema syndrome**
Elephantiasis due to mastectomy
Obliteration of lymphatic vessels

I97.3   **Postprocedural hypertension**

● **I97.4**   **Intraoperative hemorrhage and hematoma of a circulatory system organ or structure complicating a procedure**

   Excludes1   intraoperative hemorrhage and hematoma of a circulatory system organ or structure due to accidental puncture and laceration during a procedure (I97.5-)

   Excludes2   intraoperative cerebrovascular hemorrhage complicating a procedure (G97.3-)

● **I97.41**   **Intraoperative hemorrhage and hematoma of a circulatory system organ or structure complicating a circulatory system procedure**

     I97.410   **Intraoperative hemorrhage and hematoma of a circulatory system organ or structure complicating a cardiac catheterization**

     I97.411   **Intraoperative hemorrhage and hematoma of a circulatory system organ or structure complicating a cardiac bypass**

     I97.418   **Intraoperative hemorrhage and hematoma of a circulatory system organ or structure complicating other circulatory system procedure**

I97.42   **Intraoperative hemorrhage and hematoma of a circulatory system organ or structure complicating other procedure**

● **I97.5**   **Accidental puncture and laceration of a circulatory system organ or structure during a procedure**

   Excludes2   accidental puncture and laceration of brain during a procedure (G97.4-)

I97.51   **Accidental puncture and laceration of a circulatory system organ or structure during a circulatory system procedure**

I97.52   **Accidental puncture and laceration of a circulatory system organ or structure during other procedure**

● **I97.6**   **Postprocedural hemorrhage, hematoma and seroma of a circulatory system organ or structure following a procedure**

   Excludes2   postprocedural cerebrovascular hemorrhage complicating a procedure (G97.5-)

● **I97.61**   **Postprocedural hemorrhage of a circulatory system organ or structure following a circulatory system procedure**

     I97.610   **Postprocedural hemorrhage of a circulatory system organ or structure following a cardiac catheterization**

     I97.611   **Postprocedural hemorrhage of a circulatory system organ or structure following cardiac bypass**

     I97.618   **Postprocedural hemorrhage of a circulatory system organ or structure following other circulatory system procedure**

● **I97.62**   **Postprocedural hemorrhage, hematoma and seroma of a circulatory system organ or structure following other procedure**

     I97.620   **Postprocedural hemorrhage of a circulatory system organ or structure following other procedure**

     I97.621   **Postprocedural hematoma of a circulatory system organ or structure following other procedure**

     I97.622   **Postprocedural seroma of a circulatory system organ or structure following other procedure**

● **I97.63**   **Postprocedural hematoma of a circulatory system organ or structure following a circulatory system procedure**

     I97.630   **Postprocedural hematoma of a circulatory system organ or structure following a cardiac catheterization**

     I97.631   **Postprocedural hematoma of a circulatory system organ or structure following cardiac bypass**

     I97.638   **Postprocedural hematoma of a circulatory system organ or structure following other circulatory system procedure**

● **I97.64**   **Postprocedural seroma of a circulatory system organ or structure following a circulatory system procedure**

     I97.640   **Postprocedural seroma of a circulatory system organ or structure following a cardiac catheterization**

     I97.641   **Postprocedural seroma of a circulatory system organ or structure following cardiac bypass**

     I97.648   **Postprocedural seroma of a circulatory system organ or structure following other circulatory system procedure**

● **I97.7**   **Intraoperative cardiac functional disturbances**

> Excludes2   acute pulmonary insufficiency following thoracic surgery (J95.1)
> postprocedural cardiac functional disturbances (I97.1-)

  ● **I97.71**   **Intraoperative cardiac arrest**

    I97.710   **Intraoperative cardiac arrest during cardiac surgery**

    I97.711   **Intraoperative cardiac arrest during other surgery**

  ● **I97.79**   **Other intraoperative cardiac functional disturbances**

> Use additional code, if applicable, to further specify disorder

    I97.790   **Other intraoperative cardiac functional disturbances during cardiac surgery**

    I97.791   **Other intraoperative cardiac functional disturbances during other surgery**

● **I97.8**   **Other intraoperative and postprocedural complications and disorders of the circulatory system, not elsewhere classified**

> Use additional code, if applicable, to further specify disorder

  ● **I97.81**   **Intraoperative cerebrovascular infarction**

    I97.810   **Intraoperative cerebrovascular infarction during cardiac surgery**

    I97.811   **Intraoperative cerebrovascular infarction during other surgery**

  ● **I97.82**   **Postprocedural cerebrovascular infarction**

    I97.820   **Postprocedural cerebrovascular infarction following cardiac surgery**

    I97.821   **Postprocedural cerebrovascular infarction following other surgery**

    I97.88   **Other intraoperative complications of the circulatory system, not elsewhere classified**

    I97.89   **Other postprocedural complications and disorders of the circulatory system, not elsewhere classified**

● **I99**   **Other and unspecified disorders of circulatory system**

  I99.8   **Other disorder of circulatory system**

  I99.9   **Unspecified disorder of circulatory system**

CHAPTER 10

DISEASES OF THE RESPIRATORY SYSTEM (J00-J99)

OGCR Chapter-Specific Coding Guidelines

10. **Chapter 10: Diseases of the Respiratory System (J00-J99)**

a. **Chronic Obstructive Pulmonary Disease [COPD] and Asthma**

1) **Acute exacerbation of chronic obstructive bronchitis and asthma**

The codes in categories J44 and J45 distinguish between uncomplicated cases and those in acute exacerbation. An acute exacerbation is a worsening or a decompensation of a chronic condition. An acute exacerbation is not equivalent to an infection superimposed on a chronic condition, though an exacerbation may be triggered by an infection.

b. **Acute Respiratory Failure**

1) **Acute respiratory failure as principal diagnosis**

A code from subcategory J96.0, Acute respiratory failure, or subcategory J96.2, Acute and chronic respiratory failure, may be assigned as a principal diagnosis when it is the condition established after study to be chiefly responsible for occasioning the admission to the hospital, and the selection is supported by the Alphabetic Index and Tabular List. However, chapter-specific coding guidelines (such as obstetrics, poisoning, HIV, newborn) that provide sequencing direction take precedence.

2) **Acute respiratory failure as secondary diagnosis**

Respiratory failure may be listed as a secondary diagnosis if it occurs after admission, or if it is present on admission, but does not meet the definition of principal diagnosis.

3) **Sequencing of acute respiratory failure and another acute condition**

When a patient is admitted with respiratory failure and another acute condition, (e.g., myocardial infarction, cerebrovascular accident, aspiration pneumonia), the principal diagnosis will not be the same in every situation. This applies whether the other acute condition is a respiratory or nonrespiratory condition. Selection of the principal diagnosis will be dependent on the circumstances of admission. If both the respiratory failure and the other acute condition are equally responsible for occasioning the admission to the hospital, and there are no chapter-specific sequencing rules, the guideline regarding two or more diagnoses that equally meet the definition for principal diagnosis (*Section II, C.*) may be applied in these situations.

If the documentation is not clear as to whether acute respiratory failure and another condition are equally responsible for occasioning the admission, query the provider for clarification.

c. **Influenza due to certain identified influenza viruses**

Code only confirmed cases of influenza due to certain identified influenza viruses (category J09), and due to other identified influenza virus (category J10). This is an exception to the hospital inpatient guideline Section II, H. (Uncertain Diagnosis).

In this context, "confirmation" does not require documentation of positive laboratory testing specific for avian or other novel influenza A or other identified influenza virus. However, coding should be based on the provider's diagnostic statement that the patient has avian influenza, or other novel influenza A, for category J09, or has another particular identified strain of influenza, such as H1N1 or H3N2, but not identified as novel or variant, for category J10.

If the provider records "suspected" or "possible" or "probable" avian influenza, or novel influenza, or other identified influenza, then the appropriate influenza code from category J11, Influenza due to unidentified influenza virus, should be assigned. A code from category J09, Influenza due to certain identified influenza viruses, should not be assigned nor should a code from category J10, Influenza due to other identified influenza virus.

d. **Ventilator associated Pneumonia**

1) **Documentation of Ventilator associated Pneumonia**

As with all procedural or postprocedural complications, code assignment is based on the provider's documentation of the relationship between the condition and the procedure.

Code J95.851, Ventilator associated pneumonia, should be assigned only when the provider has documented ventilator associated pneumonia (VAP). An additional code to identify the organism (e.g., Pseudomonas aeruginosa, code B96.5) should also be assigned. Do not assign an additional code from categories J12-J18 to identify the type of pneumonia.

Code J95.851 should not be assigned for cases where the patient has pneumonia and is on a mechanical ventilator and the provider has not specifically stated that the pneumonia is ventilator-associated pneumonia. If the documentation is unclear as to whether the patient has a pneumonia that is a complication attributable to the mechanical ventilator, query the provider.

2) **Ventilator associated Pneumonia Develops after Admission**

A patient may be admitted with one type of pneumonia (e.g., code J13, Pneumonia due to Streptococcus pneumonia) and subsequently develop VAP. In this instance, the principal diagnosis would be the appropriate code from categories J12-J18 for the pneumonia diagnosed at the time of admission. Code J95.851, Ventilator associated pneumonia, would be assigned as an additional diagnosis when the provider has also documented the presence of ventilator associated pneumonia.

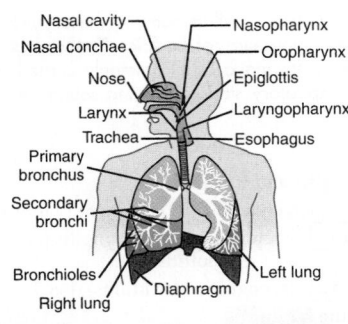

Figure 10-1 Respiratory system. (From Buck CJ: Step-by-Step Medical Coding, ed 2016, St. Louis, Elsevier, 2016)

Figure 10-2 Paranasal sinuses. (From Buck CJ: Step-by-Step Medical Coding, ed 2016, St. Louis, Elsevier, 2016)

Item 10-1 Pharyngitis is painful inflammation of the pharynx (sore throat). Ninety percent of the infections are caused by a virus with the remaining being bacterial and rarely a fungus (candidiasis). Other irritants such as pollutants, chemicals, or smoke may cause similar symptoms.

CHAPTER 10

DISEASES OF THE RESPIRATORY SYSTEM (J00-J99)

Note: When a respiratory condition is described as occurring in more than one site and is not specifically indexed, it should be classified to the lower anatomic site (e.g., tracheobronchitis to bronchitis in J40).

Use additional code, where applicable, to identify:
exposure to environmental tobacco smoke (Z77.22)
exposure to tobacco smoke in the perinatal period (P96.81)
history of tobacco dependence (Z87.891)
occupational exposure to environmental tobacco smoke (Z57.31)
tobacco dependence (F17.-)
tobacco use (Z72.0)

Excludes2　certain conditions originating in the perinatal period (P04-P96)
certain infectious and parasitic diseases (A00-B99)
complications of pregnancy, childbirth and the puerperium (O00-O99A)
congenital malformations, deformations and chromosomal abnormalities (Q00-Q99)
endocrine, nutritional and metabolic diseases (E00-E88)
injury, poisoning and certain other consequences of external causes (S00-T88)
neoplasms (C00-D49)
smoke inhalation (T59.81-)
symptoms, signs and abnormal clinical and laboratory findings, not elsewhere classified (R00-R94)

This chapter contains the following blocks:

J00-J06	Acute upper respiratory infections
J09-J18	Influenza and pneumonia
J20-J22	Other acute lower respiratory infections
J30-J39	Other diseases of upper respiratory tract
J40-J47	Chronic lower respiratory diseases
J60-J70	Lung diseases due to external agents
J80-J84	Other respiratory diseases principally affecting the interstitium
J85-J86	Suppurative and necrotic conditions of the lower respiratory tract
J90-J94	Other diseases of the pleura
J95	Intraoperative and postprocedural complications and disorders of respiratory system, not elsewhere classified
J96-J99	Other diseases of the respiratory system

ACUTE UPPER RESPIRATORY INFECTIONS (J00-J06)

Excludes1　chronic obstructive pulmonary disease with acute lower respiratory infection (J44.0)
influenza virus with other respiratory manifestations (J09.X2, J10.1, J11.1)

J00　Acute nasopharyngitis [common cold]
Acute rhinitis
Coryza (acute)
Infective nasopharyngitis NOS
Infective rhinitis
Nasal catarrh, acute
Nasopharyngitis NOS

Excludes1　acute pharyngitis (J02.-)
acute sore throat NOS (J02.9)
pharyngitis NOS (J02.9)
rhinitis NOS (J31.0)
sore throat NOS (J02.9)

Excludes2　allergic rhinitis (J30.1-J30.9)
chronic pharyngitis (J31.2)
chronic rhinitis (J31.0)
chronic sore throat (J31.2)
nasopharyngitis, chronic (J31.1)
vasomotor rhinitis (J30.0)

★ **(See Plate 49 on page 72.)**

● J01　Acute sinusitis
Includes　acute abscess of sinus
acute empyema of sinus
acute infection of sinus
acute inflammation of sinus
acute suppuration of sinus

Use additional code (B95-B97) to identify infectious agent.

Excludes1　sinusitis NOS (J32.9)
Excludes2　chronic sinusitis (J32.0-J32.8)

● J01.0　Acute maxillary sinusitis
Acute antritis
　　J01.00　Acute maxillary sinusitis, unspecified
　　J01.01　Acute recurrent maxillary sinusitis

● J01.1　Acute frontal sinusitis
　　J01.10　Acute frontal sinusitis, unspecified
　　J01.11　Acute recurrent frontal sinusitis

● J01.2　Acute ethmoidal sinusitis
　　J01.20　Acute ethmoidal sinusitis, unspecified
　　J01.21　Acute recurrent ethmoidal sinusitis

● J01.3　Acute sphenoidal sinusitis
　　J01.30　Acute sphenoidal sinusitis, unspecified
　　J01.31　Acute recurrent sphenoidal sinusitis

● J01.4　Acute pansinusitis
　　J01.40　Acute pansinusitis, unspecified
　　J01.41　Acute recurrent pansinusitis

● **J01.8** Other acute sinusitis

    J01.80 Other acute sinusitis
        Acute sinusitis involving more than one sinus but not pansinusitis

    J01.81 Other acute recurrent sinusitis
        Acute recurrent sinusitis involving more than one sinus but not pansinusitis

● **J01.9** Acute sinusitis, unspecified

    J01.90 Acute sinusitis, unspecified

    J01.91 Acute recurrent sinusitis, unspecified

● **J02** Acute pharyngitis

    Includes acute sore throat

    Excludes1 acute laryngopharyngitis (J06.0)
        peritonsillar abscess (J36)
        pharyngeal abscess (J39.1)
        retropharyngeal abscess (J39.0)

    Excludes2 chronic pharyngitis (J31.2)

    J02.0 Streptococcal pharyngitis
        Septic pharyngitis
        Streptococcal sore throat

        Excludes2 scarlet fever (A38.-)

    J02.8 Acute pharyngitis due to other specified organisms
        Use additional code (B95-B97) to identify infectious agent

        Excludes1 pharyngitis due to coxsackie virus (B08.5)
            pharyngitis due to gonococcus (A54.5)
            acute pharyngitis due to herpes [simplex] virus (B00.2)
            acute pharyngitis due to infectious mononucleosis (B27.-)
            enteroviral vesicular pharyngitis (B08.5)

    J02.9 Acute pharyngitis, unspecified
        Gangrenous pharyngitis (acute)
        Infective pharyngitis (acute) NOS
        Pharyngitis (acute) NOS
        Sore throat (acute) NOS
        Suppurative pharyngitis (acute)
        Ulcerative pharyngitis (acute)

● **J03** Acute tonsillitis

    Inflammation of pharyngeal tonsils caused by virus or bacteria

    Excludes1 acute sore throat (J02.-)
        hypertrophy of tonsils (J35.1)
        peritonsillar abscess (J36)
        sore throat NOS (J02.9)
        streptococcal sore throat (J02.0)

    Excludes2 chronic tonsillitis (J35.0)

  ● **J03.0** Streptococcal tonsillitis

    J03.00 Acute streptococcal tonsillitis, unspecified

    J03.01 Acute recurrent streptococcal tonsillitis

  ● **J03.8** Acute tonsillitis due to other specified organisms
    Use additional code (B95-B97) to identify infectious agent.

    Excludes1 diphtheritic tonsillitis (A36.0)
        herpesviral pharyngotonsillitis (B00.2)
        streptococcal tonsillitis (J03.0)
        tuberculous tonsillitis (A15.8)
        Vincent's tonsillitis (A69.1)

    J03.80 Acute tonsillitis due to other specified organisms

    J03.81 Acute recurrent tonsillitis due to other specified organisms

  ● **J03.9** Acute tonsillitis, unspecified
    Follicular tonsillitis (acute)
    Gangrenous tonsillitis (acute)
    Infective tonsillitis (acute)
    Tonsillitis (acute) NOS
    Ulcerative tonsillitis (acute)

    J03.90 Acute tonsillitis, unspecified

    J03.91 Acute recurrent tonsillitis, unspecified

Item 10–2 **Laryngitis** is an inflammation of the larynx (voice box) resulting in hoarse voice or the complete loss of the voice. **Tracheitis** is an inflammation of the trachea (often following a URI) commonly caused by *staphylococcus aureus* resulting in inspiratory stridor (crowing sound on inspiration) and a croup like cough.

● **J04** Acute laryngitis and tracheitis
    Use additional code (B95-B97) to identify infectious agent.

    Excludes1 acute obstructive laryngitis [croup] and epiglottitis (J05.-)

    Excludes2 laryngismus (stridulus) (J38.5)

    J04.0 Acute laryngitis
        Edematous laryngitis (acute)
        Laryngitis (acute) NOS
        Subglottic laryngitis (acute)
        Suppurative laryngitis (acute)
        Ulcerative laryngitis (acute)

        Excludes1 acute obstructive laryngitis (J05.0)
        Excludes2 chronic laryngitis (J37.0)

  ● **J04.1** Acute tracheitis
        Acute viral tracheitis
        Catarrhal tracheitis (acute)
        Tracheitis (acute) NOS

        Excludes2 chronic tracheitis (J42)

    J04.10 Acute tracheitis without obstruction

    J04.11 Acute tracheitis with obstruction

    J04.2 Acute laryngotracheitis
        Laryngotracheitis NOS
        Tracheitis (acute) with laryngitis (acute)

        Excludes1 acute obstructive laryngotracheitis (J05.0)
        Excludes2 chronic laryngotracheitis (J37.1)

  ● **J04.3** Supraglottitis, unspecified

    J04.30 Supraglottitis, unspecified, without obstruction

    J04.31 Supraglottitis, unspecified, with obstruction

● **J05** Acute obstructive laryngitis [croup] and epiglottitis
    Use additional code (B95-B97) to identify infectious agent.

    J05.0 Acute obstructive laryngitis [croup]
        Obstructive laryngitis (acute) NOS
        Obstructive laryngotracheitis NOS

  ● **J05.1** Acute epiglottitis

    Excludes2 epiglottitis, chronic (J37.0)

    J05.10 Acute epiglottitis without obstruction
        Epiglottitis NOS

    J05.11 Acute epiglottitis with obstruction

● **J06** Acute upper respiratory infections of multiple and unspecified sites

    Excludes1 acute respiratory infection NOS (J22)
        streptococcal pharyngitis (J02.0)

    J06.0 Acute laryngopharyngitis

    J06.9 Acute upper respiratory infection, unspecified
        Upper respiratory disease, acute
        Upper respiratory infection NOS

▶ New　⇒ Revised　~~deleted~~ Deleted　**OGCR** Official Guidelines　X Assign placeholder X　● Use Additional Character(s)

Excludes 1　Excludes 2　Includes　Use additional　Code first　Code also　Key words

INFLUENZA AND PNEUMONIA (JØ9-J18)

> **Excludes2**　allergic or eosinophilic pneumonia (J82)
> aspiration pneumonia NOS (J69.Ø)
> meconium pneumonia (P24.Ø1)
> neonatal aspiration pneumonia (P24.-)
> pneumonia due to solids and liquids (J69.-)
> congenital pneumonia (P23.9)
> lipid pneumonia (J69.1)
> rheumatic pneumonia (IØØ)
> ventilator associated pneumonia (J95.851)

● **JØ9**　**Influenza due to certain identified influenza viruses**

> **Excludes1** ▶ influenza A/H1N1 (J10.-)
> influenza due to other influenza viruses (J10.-)
> influenza due to unidentified influenza virus (J11.-)
> seasonal influenza due to other identified influenza virus (J10.-)
> seasonal influenza due to unidentified influenza virus (J11.-)

● **JØ9.X**　**Influenza due to identified novel influenza A virus**
> Avian influenza
> Bird influenza
> Influenza A/H5N1
> Influenza of other animal origin, not bird or swine
> Swine influenza virus (viruses that normally cause infections in pigs)

　　JØ9.X1　**Influenza due to identified novel influenza A virus with pneumonia**
> Code also , if applicable, associated:
> lung abscess (J85.1)
> other specified type of pneumonia

　　JØ9.X2　**Influenza due to identified novel influenza A virus with other respiratory manifestations**
> Influenza due to identified novel influenza A virus NOS
> Influenza due to identified novel influenza A virus with laryngitis
> Influenza due to identified novel influenza A virus with pharyngitis
> Influenza due to identified novel influenza A virus with upper respiratory symptoms
> Use additional code, if applicable, for associated:
> pleural effusion (J91.8)
> sinusitis (JØ1.-)

　　JØ9.X3　**Influenza due to identified novel influenza A virus with gastrointestinal manifestations**
> Influenza due to identified novel influenza A virus gastroenteritis
> > **Excludes1**　'intestinal flu' [viral gastroenteritis] (AØ8.-)

　　JØ9.X9　**Influenza due to identified novel influenza A virus with other manifestations**
> Influenza due to identified novel influenza A virus with encephalopathy
> Influenza due to identified novel influenza A virus with myocarditis
> Influenza due to identified novel influenza A virus with otitis media
> Use additional code to identify manifestation

● **J10**　**Influenza due to other identified influenza virus**

> **Excludes1**　influenza due to avian influenza virus (JØ9.X-)
> influenza due to swine flu (JØ9.X-)
> influenza due to unidentified influenza virus (J11.-)

● **J10.Ø**　**Influenza due to other identified influenza virus with pneumonia**
> Code also associated lung abscess, if applicable (J85.1)

　　J10.ØØ　**Influenza due to other identified influenza virus with unspecified type of pneumonia**

　　J10.Ø1　**Influenza due to other identified influenza virus with the same other identified influenza virus pneumonia**

　　J10.Ø8　**Influenza due to other identified influenza virus with other specified pneumonia**
> Code also other specified type of pneumonia

　　J10.1　**Influenza due to other identified influenza virus with other respiratory manifestations**
> Influenza due to other identified influenza virus NOS
> Influenza due to other identified influenza virus with laryngitis
> Influenza due to other identified influenza virus with pharyngitis
> Influenza due to other identified influenza virus with upper respiratory symptoms
> Use additional code for associated pleural effusion, if applicable (J91.8)
> Use additional code for associated sinusitis, if applicable (JØ1.-)

　　J10.2　**Influenza due to other identified influenza virus with gastrointestinal manifestations**
> Influenza due to other identified influenza virus gastroenteritis
> > **Excludes1**　'intestinal flu' [viral gastroenteritis] (AØ8.-)

● **J10.8**　**Influenza due to other identified influenza virus with other manifestations**

　　J10.81　**Influenza due to other identified influenza virus with encephalopathy**

　　J10.82　**Influenza due to other identified influenza virus with myocarditis**

　　J10.83　**Influenza due to other identified influenza virus with otitis media**
> Use additional code for any associated perforated tympanic membrane (H72.-)

　　J10.89　**Influenza due to other identified influenza virus with other manifestations**
> Use additional codes to identify the manifestations

● **J11**　**Influenza due to unidentified influenza virus**

● **J11.Ø**　**Influenza due to unidentified influenza virus with pneumonia**
> Code also associated lung abscess, if applicable (J85.1)

　　J11.ØØ　**Influenza due to unidentified influenza virus with unspecified type of pneumonia**
> Influenza with pneumonia NOS

　　J11.Ø8　**Influenza due to unidentified influenza virus with specified pneumonia**
> Code also other specified type of pneumonia

CHAPTER 1Ø (JØØ-J99)

▶ New　⟹ Revised　~~deleted~~ Deleted　**OGCR** Official Guidelines　X Assign placeholder X　● Use Additional Character(s)

Excludes 1　Excludes 2　Includes　Use additional　Code first　Code also　Key words

J11.1 Influenza due to unidentified influenza virus with other respiratory manifestations
    Influenza NOS
    Influenzal laryngitis NOS
    Influenzal pharyngitis NOS
    Influenza with upper respiratory symptoms NOS
    Use additional code for associated pleural effusion, if applicable (J91.8)
    Use additional code for associated sinusitis, if applicable (J01.-)

J11.2 Influenza due to unidentified influenza virus with gastrointestinal manifestations
    Influenza gastroenteritis NOS
    Excludes1 'intestinal flu' [viral gastroenteritis] (A08.-)

● **J11.8 Influenza due to unidentified influenza virus with other manifestations**

    J11.81 Influenza due to unidentified influenza virus with encephalopathy
        Influenzal encephalopathy NOS

    J11.82 Influenza due to unidentified influenza virus with myocarditis
        Influenzal myocarditis NOS

    J11.83 Influenza due to unidentified influenza virus with otitis media
        Influenzal otitis media NOS
        Use additional code for any associated perforated tympanic membrane (H72.-)

    J11.89 Influenza due to unidentified influenza virus with other manifestations
        Use additional codes to identify the manifestations

● **J12 Viral pneumonia, not elsewhere classified**
    Includes bronchopneumonia due to viruses other than influenza viruses
    Code first associated influenza, if applicable (J09.X1, J10.0-, J11.0-)
    Code also associated abscess, if applicable (J85.1)
    Excludes1 aspiration pneumonia due to anesthesia during labor and delivery (O74.0)
        aspiration pneumonia due to anesthesia during pregnancy (O29)
        aspiration pneumonia due to anesthesia during puerperium (O89.0)
        aspiration pneumonia due to solids and liquids (J69.-)
        aspiration pneumonia NOS (J69.0)
        congenital pneumonia (P23.0)
        congenital rubella pneumonitis (P35.0)
        interstitial pneumonia NOS (J84.9)
        lipid pneumonia (J69.1)
        neonatal aspiration pneumonia (P24.-)

    J12.0 Adenoviral pneumonia
    J12.1 Respiratory syncytial virus pneumonia
    J12.2 Parainfluenza virus pneumonia
    J12.3 Human metapneumovirus pneumonia
●   **J12.8 Other viral pneumonia**

    J12.81 Pneumonia due to SARS-associated coronavirus
        Severe acute respiratory syndrome NOS

    J12.89 Other viral pneumonia

    J12.9 Viral pneumonia, unspecified

Item 10-3 Pneumonia is an infection of the lungs, caused by a variety of microorganisms, including viruses, most commonly the Streptococcus pneumoniae (pneumococcus) bacteria, fungi, and parasites. Pneumonia occurs when the immune system is weakened, often by a URI or influenza.

J13 Pneumonia due to Streptococcus pneumoniae
    Bronchopneumonia due to S. pneumoniae
    Code first associated influenza, if applicable (J09.X1, J10.0-, J11.0-)
    Code also associated abscess, if applicable (J85.1)
    Excludes1 congenital pneumonia due to S. pneumoniae (P23.6)
        lobar pneumonia, unspecified organism (J18.1)
        pneumonia due to other streptococci (J15.3-J15.4)

J14 Pneumonia due to Hemophilus influenzae
    Bronchopneumonia due to H. influenzae
    Code first associated influenza, if applicable (J09.X1, J10.0-, J11.0-)
    Code also associated abscess, if applicable (J85.1)
    Excludes1 congenital pneumonia due to H. influenzae (P23.6)

● **J15 Bacterial pneumonia, not elsewhere classified**
    Includes bronchopneumonia due to bacteria other than S. pneumoniae and H. influenzae
    Code first associated influenza, if applicable (J09.X1, J10.0-, J11.0-)
    Code also associated abscess, if applicable (J85.1)
    Excludes1 chlamydial pneumonia (J16.0)
        congenital pneumonia (P23.-)
        Legionnaires' disease (A48.1)
        spirochetal pneumonia (A69.8)

    J15.0 Pneumonia due to Klebsiella pneumoniae
    J15.1 Pneumonia due to Pseudomonas
●   **J15.2 Pneumonia due to staphylococcus**

    J15.20 Pneumonia due to staphylococcus, unspecified
●   **J15.21 Pneumonia due to staphylococcus aureus**

        J15.211 Pneumonia due to Methicillin susceptible Staphylococcus aureus
            MSSA pneumonia
            Pneumonia due to Staphylococcus aureus NOS

        J15.212 Pneumonia due to Methicillin resistant Staphylococcus aureus

    J15.29 Pneumonia due to other staphylococcus

    J15.3 Pneumonia due to streptococcus, group B
    J15.4 Pneumonia due to other streptococci
    Excludes1 pneumonia due to streptococcus, group B (J15.3)
        pneumonia due to Streptococcus pneumoniae (J13)

    J15.5 Pneumonia due to Escherichia coli
⇒   **J15.6 Pneumonia due to other Gram-negative bacteria**
    ▶Pneumonia due to other aerobic Gram-negative bacteria
    Pneumonia due to Serratia marcescens

    J15.7 Pneumonia due to Mycoplasma pneumoniae
    J15.8 Pneumonia due to other specified bacteria
    J15.9 Unspecified bacterial pneumonia
        Pneumonia due to gram-positive bacteria

▶ New   ⇒ Revised   ~~deleted~~ Deleted   **OGCR** Official Guidelines   X Assign placeholder X   ● Use Additional Character(s)

Excludes 1   Excludes 2   Includes   Use additional   Code first   Code also   Key words

● **J16**   **Pneumonia due to other infectious organisms, not elsewhere classified**

> *Code first* associated influenza, if applicable (J09.X1, J10.0-, J11.0-)
>
> Code also associated abscess, if applicable (J85.1)
>
> **Excludes1**   congenital pneumonia (P23.-)
> ornithosis (A70)
> pneumocystosis (B59)
> pneumonia NOS (J18.9)

J16.0   **Chlamydial pneumonia**

J16.8   **Pneumonia due to other specified infectious organisms**

J17   **Pneumonia in diseases classified elsewhere**

> *Code first* underlying disease, such as:
> Q fever (A78)
> rheumatic fever (I00)
> schistosomiasis (B65.0-B65.9)
>
> **Excludes1**   candidial pneumonia (B37.1)
> chlamydial pneumonia (J16.0)
> gonorrheal pneumonia (A54.84)
> histoplasmosis pneumonia (B39.0-B39.2)
> measles pneumonia (B05.2)
> nocardiosis pneumonia (A43.0)
> pneumocystosis (B59)
> pneumonia due to Pneumocystis carinii (B59)
> pneumonia due to Pneumocystis jiroveci (B59)
> pneumonia in actinomycosis (A42.0)
> pneumonia in anthrax (A22.1)
> pneumonia in ascariasis (B77.81)
> pneumonia in aspergillosis (B44.0-B44.1)
> pneumonia in coccidioidomycosis (B38.0-B38.2)
> pneumonia in cytomegalovirus disease (B25.0)
> pneumonia in toxoplasmosis (B58.3)
> rubella pneumonia (B06.81)
> salmonella pneumonia (A02.22)
> spirochetal infection NEC with pneumonia (A69.8)
> tularemia pneumonia (A21.2)
> typhoid fever with pneumonia (A01.03)
> varicella pneumonia (B01.2)
> whooping cough with pneumonia (A37 with fifth-character 1)

● **J18**   **Pneumonia, unspecified organism**

> *Code first* associated influenza, if applicable (J09.X1, J10.0-, J11.0-)
>
> **Excludes1**   abscess of lung with pneumonia (J85.1)
> aspiration pneumonia due to anesthesia during labor and delivery (O74.0)
> aspiration pneumonia due to anesthesia during pregnancy (O29)
> aspiration pneumonia due to anesthesia during puerperium (O89.0)
> aspiration pneumonia due to solids and liquids (J69.-)
> aspiration pneumonia NOS (J69.0)
> congenital pneumonia (P23.0)
> drug-induced interstitial lung disorder (J70.2-J70.4)
> interstitial pneumonia NOS (J84.9)
> lipid pneumonia (J69.1)
> neonatal aspiration pneumonia (P24.-)
> pneumonitis due to external agents (J67-J70)
> pneumonitis due to fumes and vapors (J68.0)
> usual interstitial pneumonia (J84.17)

J18.0   **Bronchopneumonia, unspecified organism**

> **Excludes1**   hypostatic bronchopneumonia (J18.2)
> lipid pneumonia (J69.1)
>
> **Excludes2**   acute bronchiolitis (J21.-)
> chronic bronchiolitis (J44.9)

J18.1   **Lobar pneumonia, unspecified organism**

J18.2   **Hypostatic pneumonia, unspecified organism**
> Hypostatic bronchopneumonia
> Passive pneumonia

J18.8   **Other pneumonia, unspecified organism**

J18.9   **Pneumonia, unspecified organism**

OTHER ACUTE LOWER RESPIRATORY INFECTIONS (J20-J22)

> **Excludes2**   chronic obstructive pulmonary disease with acute lower respiratory infection (J44.0)

● **J20**   **Acute bronchitis**

> *Inflammation/irritation of the bronchial tubes lasting 2-3 weeks, most commonly caused by a virus*
>
> **Includes**   acute and subacute bronchitis (with) bronchospasm
> acute and subacute bronchitis (with) tracheitis
> acute and subacute bronchitis (with) tracheobronchitis, acute
> acute and subacute fibrinous bronchitis
> acute and subacute membranous bronchitis
> acute and subacute purulent bronchitis
> acute and subacute septic bronchitis
>
> **Excludes1**   bronchitis NOS (J40)
> tracheobronchitis NOS (J40)
>
> **Excludes2**   acute bronchitis with bronchiectasis (J47.0)
> acute bronchitis with chronic obstructive asthma (J44.0)
> acute bronchitis with chronic obstructive pulmonary disease (J44.0)
> allergic bronchitis NOS (J45.909-)
> bronchitis due to chemicals, fumes and vapors (J68.0)
> chronic bronchitis NOS (J42)
> chronic mucopurulent bronchitis (J41.1)
> chronic obstructive bronchitis (J44.-)
> chronic obstructive tracheobronchitis (J44.-)
> chronic simple bronchitis (J41.0)
> chronic tracheobronchitis (J42)

J20.0   **Acute bronchitis due to Mycoplasma pneumoniae**

J20.1   **Acute bronchitis due to Hemophilus influenzae**

J20.2   **Acute bronchitis due to streptococcus**

J20.3   **Acute bronchitis due to coxsackievirus**

J20.4   **Acute bronchitis due to parainfluenza virus**

J20.5   **Acute bronchitis due to respiratory syncytial virus**

J20.6   **Acute bronchitis due to rhinovirus**

J20.7   **Acute bronchitis due to echovirus**

J20.8   **Acute bronchitis due to other specified organisms**

J20.9   **Acute bronchitis, unspecified**

● **J21**   **Acute bronchiolitis**

> *Bronchiolitis obliterans with organizing pneumonia (BOOP) inflammation of bronchioles and surrounding tissue in lung*
>
> **Includes**   acute bronchiolitis with bronchospasm
> **Excludes2**   respiratory bronchiolitis interstitial lung disease (J84.115)

J21.0   **Acute bronchiolitis due to respiratory syncytial virus**

J21.1   **Acute bronchiolitis due to human metapneumovirus**

J21.8   **Acute bronchiolitis due to other specified organisms**

J21.9   **Acute bronchiolitis, unspecified**
> Bronchiolitis (acute)
>
> **Excludes1**   chronic bronchiolitis (J44.-)

J22   **Unspecified acute lower respiratory infection**
> Acute (lower) respiratory (tract) infection NOS
>
> **Excludes1**   upper respiratory infection (acute) (J06.9)

CHAPTER 10 (J00-J99)

OTHER DISEASES OF UPPER RESPIRATORY TRACT (J30–J39)

● **J30**   **Vasomotor and allergic rhinitis**
> **Includes**   spasmodic rhinorrhea
> **Excludes1**   allergic rhinitis with asthma (bronchial) (J45.909)
> rhinitis NOS (J31.0)

J30.0   **Vasomotor rhinitis**

J30.1   **Allergic rhinitis due to pollen**
> Allergy NOS due to pollen
> Hay fever
> Pollinosis

J30.2   **Other seasonal allergic rhinitis**

J30.5   **Allergic rhinitis due to food**

● **J30.8**   **Other allergic rhinitis**

    J30.81   **Allergic rhinitis due to animal (cat) (dog) hair and dander**

    J30.89   **Other allergic rhinitis**
> Perennial allergic rhinitis

J30.9   **Allergic rhinitis, unspecified**

● **J31**   **Chronic rhinitis, nasopharyngitis and pharyngitis**
> Use additional code to identify:
> exposure to environmental tobacco smoke (Z77.22)
> exposure to tobacco smoke in the perinatal period (P96.81)
> history of tobacco dependence (Z87.891)
> occupational exposure to environmental tobacco smoke (Z57.31)
> tobacco dependence (F17.-)
> tobacco use (Z72.0)

J31.0   **Chronic rhinitis**
> Atrophic rhinitis (chronic)
> Granulomatous rhinitis (chronic)
> Hypertrophic rhinitis (chronic)
> Obstructive rhinitis (chronic)
> Ozena
> Purulent rhinitis (chronic)
> Rhinitis (chronic) NOS
> Ulcerative rhinitis (chronic)
> **Excludes1**   allergic rhinitis (J30.1-J30.9)
> vasomotor rhinitis (J30.0)

J31.1   **Chronic nasopharyngitis**
> **Excludes2**   acute nasopharyngitis (J00)

J31.2   **Chronic pharyngitis**
> Chronic sore throat
> Atrophic pharyngitis (chronic)
> Granular pharyngitis (chronic)
> Hypertrophic pharyngitis (chronic)
> **Excludes2**   acute pharyngitis (J02.9)

● **J32**   **Chronic sinusitis**
> **Includes**   sinus abscess
> sinus empyema
> sinus infection
> sinus suppuration
> Use additional code to identify:
> exposure to environmental tobacco smoke (Z77.22)
> exposure to tobacco smoke in the perinatal period (P96.81)
> history of tobacco dependence (Z87.891)
> infectious agent (B95-B97)
> occupational exposure to environmental tobacco smoke (Z57.31)
> tobacco dependence (F17.-)
> tobacco use (Z72.0)
> **Excludes2**   acute sinusitis (J01.-)

J32.0   **Chronic maxillary sinusitis**
> Antritis (chronic)
> Maxillary sinusitis NOS

J32.1   **Chronic frontal sinusitis**
> Frontal sinusitis NOS

> **Item 10–4**   **Nasal polyps** are an abnormal growth of tissue (tumor) projecting from a mucous membrane and attached to the surface by a narrow elongated stalk (pedunculated). Nasal polyps usually originate in the ethmoid sinus but also may occur in the maxillary sinus. Symptoms are nasal block, sinusitis, anosmia, and secondary infections.

J32.2   **Chronic ethmoidal sinusitis**
> Ethmoidal sinusitis NOS
> **Excludes1**   Woakes' ethmoiditis (J33.1)

J32.3   **Chronic sphenoidal sinusitis**
> Sphenoidal sinusitis NOS

J32.4   **Chronic pansinusitis**
> Pansinusitis NOS

J32.8   **Other chronic sinusitis**
> Sinusitis (chronic) involving more than one sinus but not pansinusitis

J32.9   **Chronic sinusitis, unspecified**
> Sinusitis (chronic) NOS

● **J33**   **Nasal polyp**
> Use additional code to identify:
> exposure to environmental tobacco smoke (Z77.22)
> exposure to tobacco smoke in the perinatal period (P96.81)
> history of tobacco dependence (Z87.891)
> occupational exposure to environmental tobacco smoke (Z57.31)
> tobacco dependence (F17.-)
> tobacco use (Z72.0)
> **Excludes1**   adenomatous polyps (D14.0)

J33.0   **Polyp of nasal cavity**
> Choanal polyp
> Nasopharyngeal polyp

J33.1   **Polypoid sinus degeneration**
> Woakes' syndrome or ethmoiditis

J33.8   **Other polyp of sinus**
> Accessory polyp of sinus
> Ethmoidal polyp of sinus
> Maxillary polyp of sinus
> Sphenoidal polyp of sinus

J33.9   **Nasal polyp, unspecified**

● **J34**   **Other and unspecified disorders of nose and nasal sinuses**
> **Excludes2**   varicose ulcer of nasal septum (I86.8)

J34.0   **Abscess, furuncle and carbuncle of nose**
> Cellulitis of nose
> Necrosis of nose
> Ulceration of nose

J34.1   **Cyst and mucocele of nose and nasal sinus**

J34.2   **Deviated nasal septum**
> Deflection or deviation of septum (nasal) (acquired)
> **Excludes1**   congenital deviated nasal septum (Q67.4)

J34.3   **Hypertrophy of nasal turbinates**

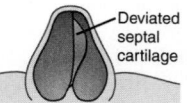
Deviated septal cartilage

Figure 10-3   Deviated nasal septum.

> **Item 10–5**   A **deviated nasal septum** is the displacement of the septal cartilage that separates the nares. This displacement causes obstructed air flow through the nasal passages. A child can be born with this displacement (congenital), or the condition may be acquired through trauma, such as a sports injury. Symptoms include nasal block, sinusitis, and related secondary infections. Septoplasty is surgical repair of this condition.

▶ New   ⇒ Revised   ~~deleted~~ Deleted   **OGCR** Official Guidelines   X Assign placeholder X   ● Use Additional Character(s)

Excludes 1   Excludes 2   Includes   Use additional   Code first   Code also   Key words

● **J34.8   Other specified disorders of nose and nasal sinuses**

  J34.81   Nasal mucositis (ulcerative)

  Code also type of associated therapy, such as:
  antineoplastic and immunosuppressive
      drugs (T45.1X-)
  radiological procedure and radiotherapy
      (Y84.2)

  | Excludes2 | gastrointestinal mucositis
  (ulcerative) (K92.81)
  mucositis (ulcerative) of vagina
      and vulva (N76.81)
  oral mucositis (ulcerative)
      (K12.3-)

  **J34.89   Other specified disorders of nose and nasal
  sinuses**

  Perforation of nasal septum NOS
  Rhinolith

  J34.9   Unspecified disorder of nose and nasal sinuses

● **J35   Chronic diseases of tonsils and adenoids**

  Use additional code to identify:
  exposure to environmental tobacco smoke (Z77.22)
  exposure to tobacco smoke in the perinatal period (P96.81)
  history of tobacco dependence (Z87.891)
  occupational exposure to environmental tobacco smoke
      (Z57.31)
  tobacco dependence (F17.-)
  tobacco use (Z72.0)

● **J35.0   Chronic tonsillitis and adenoiditis**

  | Excludes2 | acute tonsillitis (J03.-)

  J35.01   Chronic tonsillitis

  J35.02   Chronic adenoiditis

  J35.03   Chronic tonsillitis and adenoiditis

  J35.1   Hypertrophy of tonsils
  Enlargement of tonsils

  | Excludes1 | hypertrophy of tonsils with tonsillitis
      (J35.0-)

  J35.2   Hypertrophy of adenoids
  Enlargement of adenoids

  | Excludes1 | hypertrophy of adenoids with adenoiditis
      (J35.0-)

  J35.3   Hypertrophy of tonsils with hypertrophy of adenoids

  | Excludes1 | hypertrophy of tonsils and adenoids with
      tonsillitis and adenoiditis (J35.03)

  J35.8   Other chronic diseases of tonsils and adenoids
  Adenoid vegetations
  Amygdalolith
  Calculus, tonsil
  Cicatrix of tonsil (and adenoid)
  Tonsillar tag
  Ulcer of tonsil

  J35.9   Chronic disease of tonsils and adenoids, unspecified
  Disease (chronic) of tonsils and adenoids NOS

J36   Peritonsillar abscess

  | Includes | abscess of tonsil
  peritonsillar cellulitis
  quinsy

  Use additional code (B95-B97) to identify infectious agent.

  | Excludes1 | acute tonsillitis (J03.-)
  chronic tonsillitis (J35.0)
  retropharyngeal abscess (J39.0)
  tonsillitis NOS (J03.9-)

● **J37   Chronic laryngitis and laryngotracheitis**

  Use additional code to identify:
  exposure to environmental tobacco smoke (Z77.22)
  exposure to tobacco smoke in the perinatal period (P96.81)
  history of tobacco dependence (Z87.891)
  infectious agent (B95-B97)
  occupational exposure to environmental tobacco smoke
      (Z57.31)
  tobacco dependence (F17.-)
  tobacco use (Z72.0)

  J37.0   Chronic laryngitis
  Catarrhal laryngitis
  Hypertrophic laryngitis
  Sicca laryngitis

  | Excludes2 | acute laryngitis (J04.0)
  obstructive (acute) laryngitis (J05.0)

  J37.1   Chronic laryngotracheitis
  Laryngitis, chronic, with tracheitis (chronic)
  Tracheitis, chronic, with laryngitis

  | Excludes1 | chronic tracheitis (J42)
  | Excludes2 | acute laryngotracheitis (J04.2)
  acute tracheitis (J04.1)

● **J38   Diseases of vocal cords and larynx, not elsewhere classified**

  Use additional code to identify:
  exposure to environmental tobacco smoke (Z77.22)
  exposure to tobacco smoke in the perinatal period (P96.81)
  history of tobacco dependence (Z87.891)
  occupational exposure to environmental tobacco smoke
      (Z57.31)
  tobacco dependence (F17.-)
  tobacco use (Z72.0)

  | Excludes1 | congenital laryngeal stridor (P28.89)
  obstructive laryngitis (acute) (J05.0)
  postprocedural subglottic stenosis (J95.5)
  stridor (R06.1)
  ulcerative laryngitis (J04.0)

● **J38.0   Paralysis of vocal cords and larynx**
  Laryngoplegia
  Paralysis of glottis

  J38.00   Paralysis of vocal cords and larynx, unspecified

  J38.01   Paralysis of vocal cords and larynx, unilateral

  J38.02   Paralysis of vocal cords and larynx, bilateral

  J38.1   Polyp of vocal cord and larynx

  | Excludes1 | adenomatous polyps (D14.1)

  J38.2   Nodules of vocal cords
  Chorditis (fibrinous)(nodosa)(tuberosa)
  Singer's nodes
  Teacher's nodes

Figure 10-4 Coronal section of the larynx.

Item 10–6 The **larynx** extends from the tongue to the trachea and is
divided into an upper and lower portion separated by folds. The framework
of the larynx is cartilage composed of the single cricoid, thyroid, and epiglottic
cartilages, and the paired arytenoid, cuneiform, and corniculate cartilages.

▶ New   ⇛ Revised   ~~deleted~~ Deleted   **OGCR** Official Guidelines   X Assign placeholder X   ● Use Additional Character(s)

| Excludes 1 | | Excludes 2 | | Includes | | Use additional | | Code first | | Code also | | Key words |

J38.3 **Other** diseases of vocal cords
    Abscess of vocal cords
    Cellulitis of vocal cords
    Granuloma of vocal cords
    Leukokeratosis of vocal cords
    Leukoplakia of vocal cords

J38.4 **Edema** of larynx
    Edema (of) glottis
    Subglottic edema
    Supraglottic edema
    Excludes1 acute obstructive laryngitis [croup] (J05.0)
           edematous laryngitis (J04.0)

J38.5 **Laryngeal spasm**
    Laryngismus (stridulus)

J38.6 **Stenosis** of larynx

J38.7 **Other** diseases of larynx
    Abscess of larynx
    Cellulitis of larynx
    Disease of larynx NOS
    Necrosis of larynx
    Pachyderma of larynx
    Perichondritis of larynx
    Ulcer of larynx

● **J39** Other diseases of upper respiratory tract
    Excludes1 acute respiratory infection NOS (J22)
           acute upper respiratory infection (J06.9)
           upper respiratory inflammation due to chemicals, gases, fumes or vapors (J68.2)

J39.0 **Retropharyngeal and parapharyngeal abscess**
    Peripharyngeal abscess
    Excludes1 peritonsillar abscess (J36)

J39.1 **Other abscess** of pharynx
    Cellulitis of pharynx
    Nasopharyngeal abscess

J39.2 **Other diseases** of pharynx
    Cyst of pharynx
    Edema of pharynx
    Excludes2 chronic pharyngitis (J31.2)
           ulcerative pharyngitis (J02.9)

J39.3 **Upper respiratory tract hypersensitivity reaction, site unspecified**
    Excludes1 hypersensitivity reaction of upper respiratory tract, such as:
           extrinsic allergic alveolitis (J67.9)
           pneumoconiosis (J60-J67.9)

J39.8 **Other specified diseases** of upper respiratory tract

J39.9 **Disease of upper respiratory tract, unspecified**

Item 10–8 **Chronic bronchitis** is usually defined as being present in any patient who has persistent cough with sputum production for at least three months in at least two consecutive years. **Simple chronic bronchitis** is marked by a productive cough but no pathological airflow obstruction. **Chronic obstructive pulmonary disease (COPD)** is a group of conditions—bronchitis, emphysema, asthma, bronchiectasis, allergic alveolitis—marked by dyspnea. **Catarrhal** bronchitis is an acute form of bronchitis marked by profuse mucus and pus production (**mucopurulent** discharge). **Croupous** bronchitis, also known as pseudomembranous, fibrinous, plastic, exudative, or membranous, is marked by a violent cough and dyspnea.

CHRONIC LOWER RESPIRATORY DISEASES (J40-J47)

    Excludes1 bronchitis due to chemicals, gases, fumes and vapors (J68.0)
    Excludes2 cystic fibrosis (E84.-)

J40 **Bronchitis, not specified as acute or chronic**
    Bronchitis NOS
    Catarrhal bronchitis
    Bronchitis with tracheitis NOS
    Tracheobronchitis NOS
    Use additional code to identify:
        exposure to environmental tobacco smoke (Z77.22)
        exposure to tobacco smoke in the perinatal period (P96.81)
        history of tobacco dependence (Z87.891)
        occupational exposure to environmental tobacco smoke (Z57.31)
        tobacco dependence (F17.-)
        tobacco use (Z72.0)
    Excludes1 acute bronchitis (J20.-)
           allergic bronchitis NOS (J45.909-)
           asthmatic bronchitis NOS (J45.9-)
           bronchitis due to chemicals, fumes and vapors (J68.0)

● **J41** Simple and mucopurulent chronic bronchitis
    Use additional code to identify:
        exposure to environmental tobacco smoke (Z77.22)
        exposure to tobacco smoke in the perinatal period (P96.81)
        history of tobacco dependence (Z87.891)
        occupational exposure to environmental tobacco smoke (Z57.31)
        tobacco dependence (F17.-)
        tobacco use (Z72.0)
    Excludes1 chronic bronchitis NOS (J42)
           chronic obstructive bronchitis (J44.-)

J41.0 **Simple chronic bronchitis**

J41.1 **Mucopurulent chronic bronchitis**

J41.8 **Mixed simple and mucopurulent chronic bronchitis**

J42 **Unspecified chronic bronchitis**
    Chronic bronchitis NOS
    Chronic tracheitis
    Chronic tracheobronchitis
    Use additional code to identify:
        exposure to environmental tobacco smoke (Z77.22)
        exposure to tobacco smoke in the perinatal period (P96.81)
        history of tobacco dependence (Z87.891)
        occupational exposure to environmental tobacco smoke (Z57.31)
        tobacco dependence (F17.-)
        tobacco use (Z72.0)
    Excludes1 chronic asthmatic bronchitis (J44.-)
           chronic bronchitis with airways obstruction (J44.-)
           chronic emphysematous bronchitis (J44.-)
           chronic obstructive pulmonary disease NOS (J44.9)
           simple and mucopurulent chronic bronchitis (J41.-)

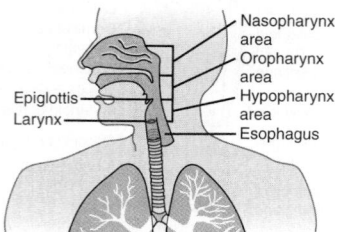

Figure 10-5 The pharynx.

Item 10–7 The **pharynx** is the passage for both food and air between the mouth and the esophagus and is divided into three areas: nasopharynx, oropharynx, and hypopharynx. The hypopharynx branches into the esophagus and the voice box.

▶ New   ⇒ Revised   ~~deleted~~ Deleted   **OGCR** Official Guidelines   X Assign placeholder X   ● Use Additional Character(s)

Excludes 1   Excludes 2   Includes   Use additional   Code first   Code also   Key words

● **J43   Emphysema**

> Use additional code to identify:
>> exposure to environmental tobacco smoke (Z77.22)
>> history of tobacco dependence (Z87.891)
>> occupational exposure to environmental tobacco smoke
>>   (Z57.31)
>> tobacco dependence (F17.-)
>> tobacco use (Z72.Ø)

> **Excludes1**   compensatory emphysema (J98.3)
>> emphysema due to inhalation of chemicals, gases,
>>   fumes or vapors (J68.4)
>> emphysema with chronic (obstructive) bronchitis
>>   (J44.-)
>> emphysematous (obstructive) bronchitis (J44.-)
>> interstitial emphysema (J98.2)
>> mediastinal emphysema (J98.2)
>> neonatal interstitial emphysema (P25.Ø)
>> surgical (subcutaneous) emphysema (T81.82)
>> traumatic subcutaneous emphysema (T79.7)

**J43.Ø   Unilateral pulmonary emphysema [MacLeod's
          syndrome]**
> Swyer-James syndrome
> Unilateral emphysema
> Unilateral hyperlucent lung
> Unilateral pulmonary artery functional hypoplasia
> Unilateral transparency of lung

J43.1   Panlobular emphysema
> Panacinar emphysema

J43.2   Centrilobular emphysema

J43.8   Other emphysema

J43.9   Emphysema, unspecified
> Bullous emphysema (lung)(pulmonary)
> Emphysema (lung)(pulmonary) NOS
> Emphysematous bleb
> Vesicular emphysema (lung)(pulmonary)

● **J44   Other chronic obstructive pulmonary disease**

> **Includes**   asthma with chronic obstructive pulmonary
>>   disease
>> chronic asthmatic (obstructive) bronchitis
>> chronic bronchitis with airways obstruction
>> chronic bronchitis with emphysema
>> chronic emphysematous bronchitis
>> chronic obstructive asthma
>> chronic obstructive bronchitis
>> chronic obstructive tracheobronchitis

> Code also type of asthma, if applicable (J45.-)
> Use additional code to identify:
>> exposure to environmental tobacco smoke (Z77.22)
>> history of tobacco dependence (Z87.891)
>> occupational exposure to environmental tobacco smoke
>>   (Z57.31)
>> tobacco dependence (F17.-)
>> tobacco use (Z72.Ø)

> **Excludes1**   bronchiectasis (J47.-)
>> chronic bronchitis NOS (J42)
>> chronic simple and mucopurulent bronchitis (J41.-)
>> chronic tracheitis (J42)
>> chronic tracheobronchitis (J42)
>> emphysema without chronic bronchitis (J43.-)

> ~~Excludes2~~   ~~lung diseases due to external agents (J6Ø-J7Ø)~~

**J44.Ø   Chronic obstructive pulmonary disease with acute lower
          respiratory infection**
> ~~Use additional code to identify the infection~~
> ▶ Code also to identify the infection

**J44.1   Chronic obstructive pulmonary disease with (acute)
          exacerbation**
> Decompensated COPD
> Decompensated COPD with (acute) exacerbation

> **Excludes2**   chronic obstructive pulmonary disease
>>   [COPD] with acute bronchitis (J44.Ø)
>> ▶lung diseases due to external agents
>>   (J6Ø-J7Ø)

J44.9   Chronic obstructive pulmonary disease, unspecified
> Chronic obstructive airway disease NOS
> Chronic obstructive lung disease NOS

> ▶ **Excludes2**   lung diseases due to external agents
>>   (J6Ø-J7Ø)

● **J45   Asthma**
> Allergic (predominantly) asthma
> Allergic bronchitis NOS
> Allergic rhinitis with asthma
> Atopic asthma
> Extrinsic allergic asthma
> Hay fever with asthma
> Idiosyncratic asthma
> Intrinsic nonallergic asthma
> Nonallergic asthma

> Use additional code to identify:
>> exposure to environmental tobacco smoke (Z77.22)
>> exposure to tobacco smoke in the perinatal period (P96.81)
>> history of tobacco dependence (Z87.891)
>> occupational exposure to environmental tobacco smoke (Z57.31)
>> tobacco dependence (F17.-)
>> tobacco use (Z72.Ø)

> **Excludes1**   detergent asthma (J69.8)
>> eosinophilic asthma (J82)
>> ~~lung diseases due to external agents (J6Ø-J7Ø)~~
>> miner's asthma (J6Ø)
>> wheezing NOS (RØ6.2)
>> wood asthma (J67.8)

> **Excludes2**   asthma with chronic obstructive pulmonary
>>   disease (J44.9)
>> chronic asthmatic (obstructive) bronchitis (J44.9)
>> chronic obstructive asthma (J44.9)

● **J45.2   Mild intermittent asthma**

> **J45.2Ø   Mild intermittent asthma, uncomplicated**
>> Mild intermittent asthma NOS

> **J45.21   Mild intermittent asthma with (acute)
>   exacerbation**

> **J45.22   Mild intermittent asthma with status
>   asthmaticus**

Item 10–9   Asthma is a bronchial condition marked by airway obstruction,
hyper-responsiveness, and inflammation. **Extrinsic** asthma, also known as allergic
asthma, is characterized by the same symptoms that occur with exposure to allergens
and is divided into the following types: **atopic, occupational, and allergic
bronchopulmonary aspergillosis. Intrinsic** asthma occurs in patients
who have no history of allergy or sensitivities to allergens and is divided into the
following types: **nonreaginic and pharmacologic. Status asthmaticus** is
the most severe form of asthma attack and can last for days or weeks.

CHAPTER 1Ø (JØØ-J99)

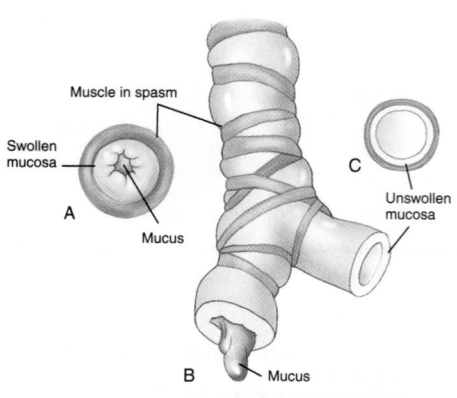

Figure 10-7 Factors causing expiratory obstruction in asthma. **A.** Cross section of a bronchiole occluded by muscle spasm, swollen mucosa, and mucus. **B.** Longitudinal section of an obstructed bronchiole. **C.** Cross-section of a clear bronchiole. (From Shiland: Mastering Healthcare Terminology, ed 1, St. Louis, Mosby, 2003)

● **J45.3**   **Mild persistent asthma**
     J45.30   **Mild persistent asthma, uncomplicated**
         Mild persistent asthma NOS
     J45.31   **Mild persistent asthma with (acute) exacerbation**
     J45.32   **Mild persistent asthma with status asthmaticus**

● **J45.4**   **Moderate persistent asthma**
     J45.40   **Moderate persistent asthma, uncomplicated**
         Moderate persistent asthma NOS
     J45.41   **Moderate persistent asthma with (acute) exacerbation**
     J45.42   **Moderate persistent asthma with status asthmaticus**

● **J45.5**   **Severe persistent asthma**
     J45.50   **Severe persistent asthma, uncomplicated**
         Severe persistent asthma NOS
     J45.51   **Severe persistent asthma with (acute) exacerbation**
     J45.52   **Severe persistent asthma with status asthmaticus**

● **J45.9**   **Other and unspecified asthma**
   ● **J45.90**   **Unspecified asthma**
         Asthmatic bronchitis NOS
         Childhood asthma NOS
         Late onset asthma
         J45.901   **Unspecified asthma with (acute) exacerbation**
         J45.902   **Unspecified asthma with status asthmaticus**
         J45.909   **Unspecified asthma, uncomplicated**
           Asthma NOS
           ▶ **Excludes2**   lung diseases due to external agents (J60-J70)

   ● **J45.99**   **Other asthma**
         J45.990   **Exercise induced bronchospasm**
         J45.991   **Cough variant asthma**
         J45.998   **Other asthma**

● **J47**   **Bronchiectasis**
     Includes   bronchiolectasis
     Use additional code to identify:
       exposure to environmental tobacco smoke (Z77.22)
       exposure to tobacco smoke in the perinatal period (P96.81)
       history of tobacco dependence (Z87.891)
       occupational exposure to environmental tobacco smoke (Z57.31)
       tobacco dependence (F17.-)
       tobacco use (Z72.0)
     Excludes1   congenital bronchiectasis (Q33.4)
                  tuberculous bronchiectasis (current disease) (A15.0)
     J47.0   **Bronchiectasis with acute lower respiratory infection**
         Bronchiectasis with acute bronchitis
         Use additional code to identify the infection
     J47.1   **Bronchiectasis with (acute) exacerbation**
     J47.9   **Bronchiectasis, uncomplicated**
         Bronchiectasis NOS

LUNG DISEASES DUE TO EXTERNAL AGENTS (J60-J70)

     Excludes2   asthma (J45.-)
                  malignant neoplasm of bronchus and lung (C34.-)

J60   **Coalworker's pneumoconiosis**
     Anthracosilicosis
     Anthracosis
     Black lung disease
     Coalworker's lung
     Excludes1   coalworker pneumoconiosis with tuberculosis, any type in A15 (J65)

J61   **Pneumoconiosis due to asbestos and other mineral fibers**
     Asbestosis
     Excludes1   pleural plaque with asbestosis (J92.0)
                  pneumoconiosis with tuberculosis, any type in A15 (J65)

● **J62**   **Pneumoconiosis due to dust containing silica**
     Includes   silicotic fibrosis (massive) of lung
     Excludes1   pneumoconiosis with tuberculosis, any type in A15 (J65)
     J62.0   **Pneumoconiosis due to talc dust**
     J62.8   **Pneumoconiosis due to other dust containing silica**
         Silicosis NOS

● **J63**   **Pneumoconiosis due to other inorganic dusts**
     Excludes1   pneumoconiosis with tuberculosis, any type in A15 (J65)
     J63.0   **Aluminosis (of lung)**
     J63.1   **Bauxite fibrosis (of lung)**
     J63.2   **Berylliosis**
     J63.3   **Graphite fibrosis (of lung)**
     J63.4   **Siderosis**
     J63.5   **Stannosis**
     J63.6   **Pneumoconiosis due to other specified inorganic dusts**

Figure 10-8 Progressive massive fibrosis superimposed on coal workers' pneumoconiosis. The large, blackened scars are located principally in the upper lobe. (From Frazier MS, Drzymkowski JW: Essentials of Human Diseases and Conditions, St. Louis, MO, Saunders, 2004)

Item 10–10 Pneumoconiosis refers to a lung condition resulting from exposure to inorganic or organic airborne particles, such as coal dust or moldy hay, as well as chemical fumes and vapors, such as insecticides. In this condition, the lungs retain the airborne particles.

▶ New   ⇒ Revised   ~~deleted~~ Deleted   **OGCR** Official Guidelines   X Assign placeholder X   ● Use Additional Character(s)

Excludes 1   Excludes 2   Includes   Use additional   Code first   Code also   Key words

J64   **Unspecified pneumoconiosis**
> **Excludes1**   pneumonoconiosis with tuberculosis, any type in A15 (J65)

J65   **Pneumoconiosis associated with tuberculosis**
> Any condition in J60-J64 with tuberculosis, any type in A15
> Silicotuberculosis

● **J66**   **Airway disease due to specific organic dust**
> **Excludes2**   allergic alveolitis (J67.-)
> asbestosis (J61)
> bagassosis (J67.1)
> farmer's lung (J67.0)
> hypersensitivity pneumonitis due to organic dust (J67.-)
> reactive airways dysfunction syndrome (J68.3)

J66.0   **Byssinosis**
> Airway disease due to cotton dust

J66.1   **Flax-dressers' disease**

J66.2   **Cannabinosis**

J66.8   **Airway disease due to other specific organic dusts**

● **J67**   **Hypersensitivity pneumonitis due to organic dust**
> **Includes**   allergic alveolitis and pneumonitis due to inhaled organic dust and particles of fungal, actinomycetic or other origin
> **Excludes1**   pneumonitis due to inhalation of chemicals, gases, fumes or vapors (J68.0)

J67.0   **Farmer's lung**
> Harvester's lung
> Haymaker's lung
> Moldy hay disease

J67.1   **Bagassosis**
> Bagasse disease
> Bagasse pneumonitis

J67.2   **Bird fancier's lung**
> Budgerigar fancier's disease or lung
> Pigeon fancier's disease or lung

J67.3   **Suberosis**
> Corkhandler's disease or lung
> Corkworker's disease or lung

J67.4   **Maltworker's lung**
> Alveolitis due to Aspergillus clavatus

J67.5   **Mushroom-worker's lung**

J67.6   **Maple-bark-stripper's lung**
> Alveolitis due to Cryptostroma corticale
> Cryptostromosis

J67.7   **Air conditioner and humidifier lung**
> Allergic alveolitis due to fungal, thermophilic actinomycetes and other organisms growing in ventilation [air conditioning] systems

J67.8   **Hypersensitivity pneumonitis due to other organic dusts**
> Cheese-washer's lung
> Coffee-worker's lung
> Fish-meal worker's lung
> Furrier's lung
> Sequoiosis

J67.9   **Hypersensitivity pneumonitis due to unspecified organic dust**
> Allergic alveolitis (extrinsic) NOS
> Hypersensitivity pneumonitis NOS

● **J68**   **Respiratory conditions due to inhalation of chemicals, gases, fumes and vapors**
> *Code first (T51-T65) to identify cause*
> Use additional code to identify associated respiratory conditions, such as:
> acute respiratory failure (J96.0-)

J68.0   **Bronchitis and pneumonitis due to chemicals, gases, fumes and vapors**
> Chemical bronchitis (acute)

J68.1   **Pulmonary edema due to chemicals, gases, fumes and vapors**
> Chemical pulmonary edema (acute) (chronic)
> **Excludes1**   pulmonary edema (acute) (chronic) NOS (J81.-)

J68.2   **Upper respiratory inflammation due to chemicals, gases, fumes and vapors, not elsewhere classified**

J68.3   **Other acute and subacute respiratory conditions due to chemicals, gases, fumes and vapors**
> Reactive airways dysfunction syndrome

J68.4   **Chronic respiratory conditions due to chemicals, gases, fumes and vapors**
> Emphysema (diffuse) (chronic) due to inhalation of chemicals, gases, fumes and vapors
> Obliterative bronchiolitis (chronic) (subacute) due to inhalation of chemicals, gases, fumes and vapors
> Pulmonary fibrosis (chronic) due to inhalation of chemicals, gases, fumes and vapors
> **Excludes1**   chronic pulmonary edema due to chemicals, gases, fumes and vapors (J68.1)

J68.8   **Other respiratory conditions due to chemicals, gases, fumes and vapors**

J68.9   **Unspecified respiratory condition due to chemicals, gases, fumes and vapors**

● **J69**   **Pneumonitis due to solids and liquids**
> **Excludes1**   neonatal aspiration syndromes (P24.-)
> postprocedural pneumonitis (J95.4)

J69.0   **Pneumonitis due to inhalation of food and vomit**
> Aspiration pneumonia NOS
> Aspiration pneumonia (due to) food (regurgitated)
> Aspiration pneumonia (due to) gastric secretions
> Aspiration pneumonia (due to) milk
> Aspiration pneumonia (due to) vomit
> Code also any associated foreign body in respiratory tract (T17.-)
> **Excludes1**   chemical pneumonitis due to anesthesia (J95.4)
> obstetric aspiration pneumonitis (O74.0)

J69.1   **Pneumonitis due to inhalation of oils and essences**
> Exogenous lipoid pneumonia
> Lipid pneumonia NOS
> *Code first (T51-T65) to identify substance*
> **Excludes1**   endogenous lipoid pneumonia (J84.89)

J69.8   **Pneumonitis due to inhalation of other solids and liquids**
> Pneumonitis due to aspiration of blood
> Pneumonitis due to aspiration of detergent
> *Code first (T51-T65) to identify substance*

CHAPTER 10 (J00-J99)

● **J70**   **Respiratory conditions due to other external agents**

    J70.0   **Acute pulmonary manifestations due to radiation**
          Radiation pneumonitis
          Use additional code (W88-W90, X39.0-) to identify the
            external cause

    J70.1   **Chronic and other pulmonary manifestations due to radiation**
          Fibrosis of lung following radiation
          Use additional code (W88-W90, X39.0-) to identify the
            external cause

    J70.2   **Acute drug-induced interstitial lung disorders**
          Use additional code for adverse effect, if applicable,
            to identify drug (T36-T50 with fifth or sixth
            character 5)
          Excludes1   interstitial pneumonia NOS (J84.9)
                        lymphoid interstitial pneumonia (J84.2)

    J70.3   **Chronic drug-induced interstitial lung disorders**
          Use additional code for adverse effect, if applicable,
            to identify drug (T36-T50 with fifth or sixth
            character 5)
          Excludes1   interstitial pneumonia NOS (J84.9)
                        lymphoid interstitial pneumonia (J84.2)

    J70.4   **Drug-induced interstitial lung disorders, unspecified**
          Use additional code for adverse effect, if applicable,
            to identify drug (T36-T50 with fifth or sixth
            character 5)
          Excludes1   interstitial pneumonia NOS (J84.9)
                        lymphoid interstitial pneumonia (J84.2)

    J70.5   **Respiratory conditions due to smoke inhalation**
          Smoke inhalation NOS
          Excludes1   smoke inhalation due to chemicals, gases,
                        fumes and vapors (J68.9)

    J70.8   **Respiratory conditions due to other specified external agents**
          Code first (T51-T65) to identify the external agent

    J70.9   **Respiratory conditions due to unspecified external agent**
          Code first (T51-T65) to identify the external agent

---

OTHER RESPIRATORY DISEASES PRINCIPALLY AFFECTING THE INTERSTITIUM (J80-J84)

J80   **Acute respiratory distress syndrome**
      Acute respiratory distress syndrome in adult or child
      Adult hyaline membrane disease
      Excludes1   respiratory distress syndrome in newborn
                 (perinatal) (P22.0)

● **J81**   **Pulmonary edema**
      Use additional code to identify:
        exposure to environmental tobacco smoke (Z77.22)
        history of tobacco dependence (Z87.891)
        occupational exposure to environmental tobacco smoke
           (Z57.31)
        tobacco dependence (F17.-)
        tobacco use (Z72.0)
      Excludes1   chemical (acute) pulmonary edema (J68.1)
                 hypostatic pneumonia (J18.2)
                 passive pneumonia (J18.2)
                 pulmonary edema due to external agents (J60-J70)
                 pulmonary edema with heart disease NOS (I50.1)
                 pulmonary edema with heart failure (I50.1)

    J81.0   **Acute pulmonary edema**
          Acute edema of lung

    J81.1   **Chronic pulmonary edema**
          Pulmonary congestion (chronic) (passive)
          Pulmonary edema NOS

Figure 10-9   Bullous emphysema with large subpleural bullae *(upper left)*. (From Kumar: Robbins and Cotran: Pathologic Basis of Disease, ed 8, Saunders, An Imprint of Elsevier, 2009)

J82   **Pulmonary eosinophilia, not elsewhere classified**
      Allergic pneumonia
      Eosinophilic asthma
      Eosinophilic pneumonia
      Löffler's pneumonia
      Tropical (pulmonary) eosinophilia NOS
      Excludes1   pulmonary eosinophilia due to aspergillosis
                 (B44.-)
                 pulmonary eosinophilia due to drugs (J70.2-J70.4)
                 pulmonary eosinophilia due to specified parasitic
                    infection (B50-B83)
                 pulmonary eosinophilia due to systemic
                    connective tissue disorders (M30-M36)
                 pulmonary infiltrate NOS (R91.8)

● **J84**   **Other interstitial pulmonary diseases**
      Excludes1   drug-induced interstitial lung disorders
                 (J70.2-J70.4)
                 interstitial emphysema (J98.2)
                 ~~lung diseases due to external agents (J60-J70)~~
    ▶ **Excludes2**   lung diseases due to external agents (J60-J70)

●   **J84.0**   **Alveolar and parieto-alveolar conditions**
        J84.01   **Alveolar proteinosis**
        J84.02   **Pulmonary alveolar microlithiasis**
        J84.03   **Idiopathic pulmonary hemosiderosis**
             Essential brown induration of lung
             Code first underlying disease, such as:
               disorders of iron metabolism (E83.1-)
             Excludes1   acute idiopathic pulmonary
                      hemorrhage in infants
                      [AIPHI] (R04.81)
        J84.09   **Other alveolar and parieto-alveolar conditions**
●   **J84.1**   **Other interstitial pulmonary diseases with fibrosis**
        Excludes1   pulmonary fibrosis (chronic) due to
                   inhalation of chemicals, gases, fumes
                   or vapors (J68.4)
                 pulmonary fibrosis (chronic) following
                   radiation (J70.1)

        J84.10   **Pulmonary fibrosis, unspecified**
             Capillary fibrosis of lung
             Cirrhosis of lung (chronic) NOS
             Fibrosis of lung (atrophic) (chronic) (confluent)
               (massive) (perialveolar) (peribronchial)
               NOS
             Induration of lung (chronic) NOS
             Postinflammatory pulmonary fibrosis

▶ New   ➡ Revised   ~~deleted~~ Deleted   **OGCR** Official Guidelines   X Assign placeholder X   ● Use Additional Character(s)

Excludes 1   Excludes 2   Includes   Use additional   Code first   Code also   Key words

● **J84.11 Idiopathic interstitial pneumonia**

> Excludes1 lymphoid interstitial pneumonia (J84.2)
> pneumocystis pneumonia (B59)

J84.111 **Idiopathic interstitial pneumonia, not otherwise specified**

J84.112 **Idiopathic pulmonary fibrosis**
Cryptogenic fibrosing alveolitis
Idiopathic fibrosing alveolitis

J84.113 **Idiopathic non-specific interstitial pneumonitis**

> Excludes1 non-specific interstitial pneumonia NOS, or due to known underlying cause (J84.89)

J84.114 **Acute interstitial pneumonitis**
Hamman-Rich syndrome

> Excludes1 pneumocystis pneumonia (B59)

J84.115 **Respiratory bronchiolitis interstitial lung disease**

J84.116 **Cryptogenic organizing pneumonia**

> Excludes1 organizing pneumonia NOS, or due to known underlying cause (J84.89)

J84.117 **Desquamative interstitial pneumonia**

J84.17 **Other interstitial pulmonary diseases with fibrosis in diseases classified elsewhere**
Interstitial pneumonia (nonspecific) (usual) due to collagen vascular disease
Interstitial pneumonia (nonspecific) (usual) in diseases classified elsewhere
Organizing pneumonia due to collagen vascular disease
Organizing pneumonia in diseases classified elsewhere

> *Code first* underlying disease, such as:
> progressive systemic sclerosis (M34.0)
> rheumatoid arthritis (M05.00-M06.9)
> systemic lupus erythematosis (M32.0-M32.9)

J84.2 **Lymphoid interstitial pneumonia**
Lymphoid interstitial pneumonitis

● J84.8 **Other specified interstitial pulmonary diseases**

> Excludes1 exogenous lipoid pneumonia (J69.1)
> unspecified lipoid pneumonia (J69.1)

J84.81 **Lymphangioleiomyomatosis**
Lymphangiomyomatosis

J84.82 **Adult pulmonary Langerhans cell histiocytosis**
Adult PLCH

J84.83 **Surfactant mutations of the lung**

● J84.84 **Other interstitial lung diseases of childhood**

J84.841 **Neuroendocrine cell hyperplasia of infancy**

J84.842 **Pulmonary interstitial glycogenosis**

J84.843 **Alveolar capillary dysplasia with vein misalignment**

J84.848 **Other interstitial lung diseases of childhood**

J84.89 **Other specified interstitial pulmonary diseases**
Endogenous lipoid pneumonia
Interstitial pneumonitis
Non-specific interstitial pneumonitis NOS
Organizing pneumonia NOS

> *Code first, if applicable:*
> poisoning due to drug or toxin (T51-T65 with fifth or sixth character to indicate intent), for toxic pneumonopathy underlying cause of pneumonopathy, if known

> Use additional code, for adverse effect, to identify drug (T36-T50 with fifth or sixth character 5), if drug-induced

> Excludes1 cryptogenic organizing pneumonia (J84.116)
> idiopathic non-specific interstitial pneumonia (J84.113)
> lipoid pneumonia, exogenous or unspecified (J69.1)
> lymphoid interstitial pneumonia (J84.2)

J84.9 **Interstitial pulmonary disease, unspecified**
Interstitial pneumonia NOS

SUPPURATIVE AND NECROTIC CONDITIONS OF THE LOWER RESPIRATORY TRACT (J85-J86)

● **J85 Abscess of lung and mediastinum**

> Use additional code (B95-B97) to identify infectious agent.

J85.0 **Gangrene and necrosis of lung**

J85.1 **Abscess of lung with pneumonia**

> Code also the type of pneumonia

J85.2 **Abscess of lung without pneumonia**
Abscess of lung NOS

J85.3 **Abscess of mediastinum**

Item 10–11 Empyema is a condition in which pus accumulates in a body cavity. Empyema **with fistula** occurs when the pus passes from one cavity to another organ or structure.

● **J86 Pyothorax**

> Use additional code (B95-B97) to identify infectious agent.

> Excludes1 abscess of lung (J85.-)
> pyothorax due to tuberculosis (A15.6)

J86.0 **Pyothorax with fistula**
Bronchocutaneous fistula
Bronchopleural fistula
Hepatopleural fistula
Mediastinal fistula
Pleural fistula
Thoracic fistula
Any condition classifiable to J86.9 with fistula

J86.9 **Pyothorax without fistula**
Abscess of pleura
Abscess of thorax
Empyema (chest) (lung) (pleura)
Fibrinopurulent pleurisy
Purulent pleurisy
Pyopneumothorax
Septic pleurisy
Seropurulent pleurisy
Suppurative pleurisy

CHAPTER 10 (J00-J99)

OTHER DISEASES OF THE PLEURA (J90-J94)

J90 Pleural effusion, not elsewhere classified
Encysted pleurisy
Pleural effusion NOS
Pleurisy with effusion (exudative) (serous)
Excludes1 chylous (pleural) effusion (J94.0)
malignant pleural effusion (J91.0))
pleurisy NOS (R09.1)
tuberculous pleural effusion (A15.6)

●**J91** Pleural effusion in conditions classified elsewhere
Excludes2 pleural effusion in heart failure (I50.-)
pleural effusion in systemic lupus erythematosus (M32.13)

J91.0 Malignant pleural effusion
Code first underlying neoplasm

J91.8 Pleural effusion in other conditions classified elsewhere
Code first underlying disease, such as:
filariasis (B74.0-B74.9)
influenza (J09.X2, J10.1, J11.1)

●**J92** Pleural plaque
Includes pleural thickening
J92.0 Pleural plaque with presence of asbestos
J92.9 Pleural plaque without asbestos
Pleural plaque NOS

●**J93** Pneumothorax and air leak
Collapsed lung
Excludes1 congenital or perinatal pneumothorax (P25.1)
postprocedural air leak (J95.812)
postprocedural pneumothorax (J95.811)
traumatic pneumothorax (S27.0)
tuberculous (current disease) pneumothorax (A15.-)
pyopneumothorax (J86.-)

J93.0 Spontaneous tension pneumothorax
Tension pneumothorax (most serious type) occurs when air (positive pressure) collects in the pleural space

●**J93.1** Other spontaneous pneumothorax
J93.11 Primary spontaneous pneumothorax
J93.12 Secondary spontaneous pneumothorax
Code first underlying condition, such as:
catamenial pneumothorax due to endometriosis (N80.8)
cystic fibrosis (E84.-)
eosinophilic pneumonia (J82)
lymphangioleiomyomatosis (J84.81)
malignant neoplasm of bronchus and lung (C34.-)
Marfan's syndrome (Q87.4)
pneumonia due to Pneumocystis carinii (B59)
secondary malignant neoplasm of lung (C78.0-)
spontaneous rupture of the esophagus (K22.3)

●**J93.8** Other pneumothorax and air leak
J93.81 Chronic pneumothorax
J93.82 Other air leak
Persistent air leak
J93.83 Other pneumothorax
Acute pneumothorax
Spontaneous pneumothorax NOS
J93.9 Pneumothorax, unspecified
Pneumothorax NOS

●**J94** Other pleural conditions
Excludes1 pleurisy NOS (R09.1)
traumatic hemopneumothorax (S27.2)
traumatic hemothorax (S27.1)
tuberculous pleural conditions (current disease) (A15.-)

J94.0 Chylous effusion
Chyliform effusion
J94.1 Fibrothorax
J94.2 Hemothorax
Hemopneumothorax
J94.8 Other specified pleural conditions
Hydropneumothorax
Hydrothorax
J94.9 Pleural condition, unspecified

INTRAOPERATIVE AND POSTPROCEDURAL COMPLICATIONS AND DISORDERS OF RESPIRATORY SYSTEM, NOT ELSEWHERE CLASSIFIED (J95)

●**J95** Intraoperative and postprocedural complications and disorders of respiratory system, not elsewhere classified
Excludes2 aspiration pneumonia (J69.-)
emphysema (subcutaneous) resulting from a procedure (T81.82)
hypostatic pneumonia (J18.2)
pulmonary manifestations due to radiation (J70.0- J70.1)

●**J95.0** Tracheostomy complications
J95.00 Unspecified tracheostomy complication
J95.01 Hemorrhage from tracheostomy stoma
J95.02 Infection of tracheostomy stoma
Use additional code to identify type of infection, such as:
➡cellulitis of neck (L03.221)
sepsis (A40, A41.-)
J95.03 Malfunction of tracheostomy stoma
Mechanical complication of tracheostomy stoma
Obstruction of tracheostomy airway
Tracheal stenosis due to tracheostomy
J95.04 Tracheo-esophageal fistula following tracheostomy
J95.09 Other tracheostomy complication
J95.1 Acute pulmonary insufficiency following thoracic surgery
Excludes2 functional disturbances following cardiac surgery (I97.0, I97.1-)
J95.2 Acute pulmonary insufficiency following nonthoracic surgery
Excludes2 functional disturbances following cardiac surgery (I97.0, I97.1-)
J95.3 Chronic pulmonary insufficiency following surgery
Excludes2 functional disturbances following cardiac surgery (I97.0, I97.1-)
J95.4 Chemical pneumonitis due to anesthesia
Mendelson's syndrome
Postprocedural aspiration pneumonia
Use additional code for adverse effect, if applicable, to identify drug (T41.- with fifth or sixth character 5)
Excludes1 aspiration pneumonitis due to anesthesia complicating labor and delivery (O74.0)
aspiration pneumonitis due to anesthesia complicating pregnancy (O29)
aspiration pneumonitis due to anesthesia complicating the puerperium (O89.01)

J95.5   Postprocedural subglottic stenosis

● **J95.6**   Intraoperative hemorrhage and hematoma of a respiratory system organ or structure complicating a procedure

> **Excludes1**   intraoperative hemorrhage and hematoma of a respiratory system organ or structure due to accidental puncture and laceration during procedure (J95.7-)

    J95.61   Intraoperative hemorrhage and hematoma of a respiratory system organ or structure complicating a respiratory system procedure

    J95.62   Intraoperative hemorrhage and hematoma of a respiratory system organ or structure complicating other procedure

● **J95.7**   Accidental puncture and laceration of a respiratory system organ or structure during a procedure

> **Excludes2**   postprocedural pneumothorax (J95.811)

    J95.71   Accidental puncture and laceration of a respiratory system organ or structure during a respiratory system procedure

    J95.72   Accidental puncture and laceration of a respiratory system organ or structure during other procedure

● **J95.8**   Other intraoperative and postprocedural complications and disorders of respiratory system, not elsewhere classified

   ● **J95.81**   Postprocedural pneumothorax and air leak

      J95.811   Postprocedural pneumothorax

      J95.812   Postprocedural air leak

   ● **J95.82**   Postprocedural respiratory failure

> **Excludes1**   Respiratory failure in other conditions (J96.-)

      J95.821   Acute postprocedural respiratory failure
> Postprocedural respiratory failure NOS

      J95.822   Acute and chronic postprocedural respiratory failure

   ● **J95.83**   Postprocedural hemorrhage of a respiratory system organ or structure following a procedure

      J95.830   Postprocedural hemorrhage of a respiratory system organ or structure following a respiratory system procedure

      J95.831   Postprocedural hemorrhage of a respiratory system organ or structure following other procedure

    J95.84   Transfusion-related acute lung injury (TRALI)

   ● **J95.85**   Complication of respirator [ventilator]

      J95.850   Mechanical complication of respirator

> **Excludes1**   encounter for respirator [ventilator] dependence during power failure (Z99.12)

      J95.851   Ventilator associated pneumonia
> Ventilator associated pneumonitis
> Use additional code to identify the organism, if known (B95.-, B96.-, B97.-)

> **Excludes1**   ventilator lung in newborn (P27.8)

      J95.859   Other complication of respirator [ventilator]

● **J95.86**   Postprocedural hematoma and seroma of a respiratory system organ or structure following a procedure

    J95.860   Postprocedural hematoma of a respiratory system organ or structure following a respiratory system procedure

    J95.861   Postprocedural hematoma of a respiratory system organ or structure following other procedure

    J95.862   Postprocedural seroma of a respiratory system organ or structure following a respiratory system procedure

    J95.863   Postprocedural seroma of a respiratory system organ or structure following other procedure

    J95.88   Other intraoperative complications of respiratory system, not elsewhere classified

    J95.89   Other postprocedural complications and disorders of respiratory system, not elsewhere classified

> Use additional code to identify disorder, such as:
> aspiration pneumonia (J69.-)
> bacterial or viral pneumonia (J12-J18)

> **Excludes2**   acute pulmonary insufficiency following thoracic surgery (J95.1)
> postprocedural subglottic stenosis (J95.5)

OTHER DISEASES OF THE RESPIRATORY SYSTEM (J96-J99)

● **J96**   Respiratory failure, not elsewhere classified

> **Excludes1**   acute respiratory distress syndrome (J80)
> cardiorespiratory failure (R09.2)
> newborn respiratory distress syndrome (P22.0)
> postprocedural respiratory failure (J95.82-)
> respiratory arrest (R09.2)
> respiratory arrest of newborn (P28.81)
> respiratory failure of newborn (P28.5)

   ● **J96.0**   Acute respiratory failure

      J96.00   Acute respiratory failure, unspecified whether with hypoxia or hypercapnia

      J96.01   Acute respiratory failure with hypoxia

      J96.02   Acute respiratory failure with hypercapnia

   ● **J96.1**   Chronic respiratory failure

      J96.10   Chronic respiratory failure, unspecified whether with hypoxia or hypercapnia

      J96.11   Chronic respiratory failure with hypoxia

      J96.12   Chronic respiratory failure with hypercapnia

   ● **J96.2**   Acute and chronic respiratory failure
> Acute on chronic respiratory failure

      J96.20   Acute and chronic respiratory failure, unspecified whether with hypoxia or hypercapnia

      J96.21   Acute and chronic respiratory failure with hypoxia

      J96.22   Acute and chronic respiratory failure with hypercapnia

   ● **J96.9**   Respiratory failure, unspecified

      J96.90   Respiratory failure, unspecified, unspecified whether with hypoxia or hypercapnia

      J96.91   Respiratory failure, unspecified with hypoxia

      J96.92   Respiratory failure, unspecified with hypercapnia

CHAPTER 10 (J00-J99)

● J98   Other respiratory disorders

Use additional code to identify:

exposure to environmental tobacco smoke (Z77.22)

exposure to tobacco smoke in the perinatal period (P96.81)

history of tobacco dependence (Z87.891)

occupational exposure to environmental tobacco smoke (Z57.31)

tobacco dependence (F17.-)

tobacco use (Z72.Ø)

Excludes1   newborn apnea (P28.4)

newborn sleep apnea (P28.3)

Excludes2   apnea NOS (RØ6.81)

sleep apnea (G47.3-)

● J98.Ø   Diseases of bronchus, not elsewhere classified

     J98.Ø1   **Acute bronchospasm**

         Excludes1   acute bronchiolitis with bronchospasm (J21.-)

acute bronchitis with bronchospasm (J2Ø.-)

asthma (J45.-)

exercise induced bronchospasm (J45.99Ø)

     J98.Ø9   **Other diseases of bronchus, not elsewhere classified**

Broncholithiasis

Calcification of bronchus

Stenosis of bronchus

Tracheobronchial collapse

Tracheobronchial dyskinesia

Ulcer of bronchus

● J98.1   Pulmonary collapse

Excludes1   therapeutic collapse of lung status (Z98.3)

     J98.11   **Atelectasis**

         Excludes1   newborn atelectasis

tuberculous atelectasis (current disease) (A15)

     J98.19   **Other pulmonary collapse**

   J98.2   **Interstitial emphysema**

Mediastinal emphysema

Excludes1   emphysema NOS (J43.9)

emphysema in newborn (P25.Ø)

surgical emphysema (subcutaneous) (T81.82)

traumatic subcutaneous emphysema (T79.7)

   J98.3   **Compensatory emphysema**

   J98.4   **Other disorders of lung**

Calcification of lung

Cystic lung disease (acquired)

Lung disease NOS

Pulmolithiasis

Excludes1   acute interstitial pneumonitis (J84.114)

pulmonary insufficiency following surgery (J95.1-J95.2)

● J98.5   Diseases of mediastinum, not elsewhere classified

Excludes2   abscess of mediastinum (J85.3)

     J98.51   **Mediastinitis**

Code first underlying condition, if applicable, such as postoperative mediastinitis (T81.-)

     J98.59   **Other diseases of mediastinum, not elsewhere classified**

Fibrosis of mediastinum

Hernia of mediastinum

Retraction of mediastinum

   J98.6   **Disorders of diaphragm**

Diaphragmatitis

Paralysis of diaphragm

Relaxation of diaphragm

Excludes1   congenital malformation of diaphragm NEC (Q79.1)

congenital diaphragmatic hernia (Q79.Ø)

Excludes2   diaphragmatic hernia (K44.-)

   J98.8   **Other specified respiratory disorders**

   J98.9   **Respiratory disorder, unspecified**

Respiratory disease (chronic) NOS

J99   Respiratory disorders in diseases classified elsewhere

Code first underlying disease, such as:

amyloidosis (E85.-)

ankylosing spondylitis (M45)

congenital syphilis (A5Ø.5)

cryoglobulinemia (D89.1)

early congenital syphilis (A5Ø.Ø)

schistosomiasis (B65.Ø-B65.9)

Excludes1   respiratory disorders in:

amebiasis (AØ6.5)

blastomycosis (B4Ø.Ø-B4Ø.2)

candidiasis (B37.1)

coccidioidomycosis (B38.Ø-B38.2)

cystic fibrosis with pulmonary manifestations (E84.Ø)

dermatomyositis (M33.Ø1, M33.11)

histoplasmosis (B39.Ø-B39.2)

late syphilis (A52.72, A52.73)

polymyositis (M33.21)

sicca syndrome (M35.Ø2)

systemic lupus erythematosus (M32.13)

systemic sclerosis (M34.81)

Wegener's granulomatosis (M31.3Ø-M31.31)

CHAPTER 11

DISEASES OF THE DIGESTIVE SYSTEM
(K00-K95)

OGCR Chapter-Specific Coding Guidelines

> 11. Chapter 11: Diseases of the Digestive System (K00-K95)
> Reserved for future guideline expansion

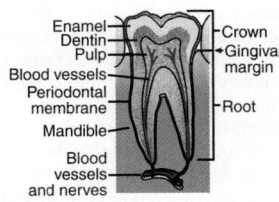

Figure 11-1 Anatomy of a tooth.

Item 11-1 Anodontia is the congenital absence of teeth. **Hypodontia** is partial anodontia. **Oligodontia** is the congenital absence of some teeth, whereas **supernumerary** is having more teeth than the normal number. **Mesiodens** are small extra teeth that often appear in pairs, although single small teeth are not uncommon.

CHAPTER 11

DISEASES OF THE DIGESTIVE SYSTEM
(K00-K95)

Excludes2 certain conditions originating in the perinatal period (P04-P96)
certain infectious and parasitic diseases (A00-B99)
complications of pregnancy, childbirth and the puerperium (O00-O9A)
congenital malformations, deformations and chromosomal abnormalities (Q00-Q99)
endocrine, nutritional and metabolic diseases (E00-E88)
injury, poisoning and certain other consequences of external causes (S00-T88)
neoplasms (C00-D49)
symptoms, signs and abnormal clinical and laboratory findings, not elsewhere classified (R00-R94)

This chapter contains the following blocks:

K00-K14	Diseases of oral cavity and salivary glands
K20-K31	Diseases of esophagus, stomach and duodenum
K35-K38	Diseases of appendix
K40-K46	Hernia
K50-K52	Noninfective enteritis and colitis
K55-K64	Other diseases of intestines
K65-K68	Diseases of peritoneum and retroperitoneum
K70-K77	Diseases of liver
K80-K87	Disorders of gallbladder, biliary tract and pancreas
K90-K95	Other diseases of the digestive system

DISEASES OF ORAL CAVITY AND SALIVARY GLANDS (K00-K14)

● **K00 Disorders of tooth development and eruption**
> **Excludes2** embedded and impacted teeth (K01.-)

K00.0 Anodontia
Hypodontia
Oligodontia
> **Excludes1** acquired absence of teeth (K08.1-)

K00.1 Supernumerary teeth
Distomolar
Fourth molar
Mesiodens
Paramolar
Supplementary teeth
> **Excludes2** supernumerary roots (K00.2)

K00.2 Abnormalities of size and form of teeth
Concrescence of teeth
Fusion of teeth
Gemination of teeth
Dens evaginatus
Dens in dente
Dens invaginatus
Enamel pearls
Macrodontia
Microdontia
Peg-shaped [conical] teeth
Supernumerary roots
Taurodontism
Tuberculum paramolare
> **Excludes1** abnormalities of teeth due to congenital syphilis (A50.5)
> tuberculum Carabelli, which is regarded as a normal variation and should not be coded

K00.3 Mottled teeth
Dental fluorosis
Mottling of enamel
Nonfluoride enamel opacities
> **Excludes2** deposits [accretions] on teeth (K03.6)

K00.4 Disturbances in tooth formation
Aplasia and hypoplasia of cementum
Dilaceration of tooth
Enamel hypoplasia (neonatal) (postnatal) (prenatal)
Regional odontodysplasia
Turner's tooth
> **Excludes1** Hutchinson's teeth and mulberry molars in congenital syphilis (A50.5)
> **Excludes2** mottled teeth (K00.3)

K00.5 Hereditary disturbances in tooth structure, not elsewhere classified
Amelogenesis imperfecta
Dentinogenesis imperfecta
Odontogenesis imperfecta
Dentinal dysplasia
Shell teeth

K00.6 Disturbances in tooth eruption
Dentia praecox
Natal tooth
Neonatal tooth
Premature eruption of tooth
Premature shedding of primary [deciduous] tooth
Prenatal teeth
Retained [persistent] primary tooth
> **Excludes2** embedded and impacted teeth (K01.-)

K00.7 Teething syndrome

K00.8 Other disorders of tooth development
Color changes during tooth formation
Intrinsic staining of teeth NOS
> **Excludes2** posteruptive color changes (K03.7)

K00.9 Disorder of tooth development, unspecified
Disorder of odontogenesis NOS

● **K01 Embedded and impacted teeth**
> **Excludes1** abnormal position of fully erupted teeth (M26.3-)

K01.0 Embedded teeth

K01.1 Impacted teeth

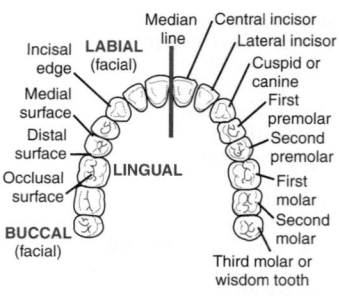

Figure 11-2 The permanent teeth within the dental arch.

Item 11–2 Each dental arch (jaw) normally contains 16 teeth. Tooth decay or **dental caries** is a disease of the enamel, dentin, and cementum of the tooth and can result in a cavity.

● **K02   Dental caries**
Includes	caries of dentine
	dental cavities
	early childhood caries
	pre-eruptive caries
	recurrent caries (dentino enamel junction)
	(enamel) (to the pulp)
	tooth decay

  K02.3   Arrested dental caries
    Arrested coronal and root caries
● **K02.5   Dental caries on pit and fissure surface**
    Dental caries on chewing surface of tooth
    K02.51   Dental caries on pit and fissure surface limited to enamel
      White spot lesions [initial caries] on pit and fissure surface of tooth
    K02.52   Dental caries on pit and fissure surface penetrating into dentin
      Primary dental caries, cervical origin
    K02.53   Dental caries on pit and fissure surface penetrating into pulp
● **K02.6   Dental caries on smooth surface**
    K02.61   Dental caries on smooth surface limited to enamel
      White spot lesions [initial caries] on smooth surface of tooth
    K02.62   Dental caries on smooth surface penetrating into dentin
    K02.63   Dental caries on smooth surface penetrating into pulp
  K02.7   Dental root caries
  K02.9   Dental caries, unspecified

● **K03   Other diseases of hard tissues of teeth**
Excludes2	bruxism (F45.8)
	dental caries (K02.-)
	teeth-grinding NOS (F45.8)

  K03.0   Excessive attrition of teeth
    Approximal wear of teeth
    Occlusal wear of teeth
  K03.1   Abrasion of teeth
    Dentifrice abrasion of teeth
    Habitual abrasion of teeth
    Occupational abrasion of teeth
    Ritual abrasion of teeth
    Traditional abrasion of teeth
    Wedge defect NOS
  K03.2   Erosion of teeth
    Erosion of teeth due to diet
    Erosion of teeth due to drugs and medicaments
    Erosion of teeth due to persistent vomiting
    Erosion of teeth NOS
    Idiopathic erosion of teeth
    Occupational erosion of teeth

  K03.3   Pathological resorption of teeth
    Internal granuloma of pulp
    Resorption of teeth (external)
  K03.4   Hypercementosis
    Cementation hyperplasia
  K03.5   Ankylosis of teeth
  K03.6   Deposits [accretions] on teeth
    Betel deposits [accretions] on teeth
    Black deposits [accretions] on teeth
    Extrinsic staining of teeth NOS
    Green deposits [accretions] on teeth
    Materia alba deposits [accretions] on teeth
    Orange deposits [accretions] on teeth
    Staining of teeth NOS
    Subgingival dental calculus
    Supragingival dental calculus
    Tobacco deposits [accretions] on teeth
  K03.7   Posteruptive color changes of dental hard tissues
Excludes2	deposits [accretions] on teeth (K03.6)
● **K03.8   Other specified diseases of hard tissues of teeth**
    K03.81   Cracked tooth
Excludes1	asymptomatic craze lines in enamel - omit code
	broken or fractured tooth due to trauma (S02.5)
    K03.89   Other specified diseases of hard tissues of teeth
  K03.9   Disease of hard tissues of teeth, unspecified

  K04   Diseases of pulp and periapical tissues
● **K04.0   Pulpitis**
    Acute pulpitis
    Chronic (hyperplastic) (ulcerative) pulpitis
    K04.01   Reversible pulpitis
    K04.02   Irreversible pulpitis
  K04.1   Necrosis of pulp
    Pulpal gangrene
  K04.2   Pulp degeneration
    Denticles
    Pulpal calcifications
    Pulpal stones
  K04.3   Abnormal hard tissue formation in pulp
    Secondary or irregular dentine
  K04.4   Acute apical periodontitis of pulpal origin
    Acute apical periodontitis NOS
Excludes1	acute periodontitis (K05.2-)
  K04.5   Chronic apical periodontitis
    Apical or periapical granuloma
    Apical periodontitis NOS
Excludes1	chronic periodontitis (K05.3-)
  K04.6   Periapical abscess with sinus
    Dental abscess with sinus
    Dentoalveolar abscess with sinus
  K04.7   Periapical abscess without sinus
    Dental abscess without sinus
    Dentoalveolar abscess without sinus
    ~~Periapical abscess without sinus~~
  K04.8   Radicular cyst
    Apical (periodontal) cyst
    Periapical cyst
    Residual radicular cyst
Excludes2	lateral periodontal cyst (K09.0)
● **K04.9   Other and unspecified diseases of pulp and periapical tissues**
    K04.90   Unspecified diseases of pulp and periapical tissues
    K04.99   Other diseases of pulp and periapical tissues

CHAPTER 11 (K00-K95)

Item 11–3 Acute gingivitis, also known as orilitis or ulitis, is the short-term, severe inflammation of the gums (gingiva) caused by bacteria. **Chronic gingivitis** is persistent inflammation of the gums. When the gingivitis moves into the periodontium it is called periodontitis, also known as paradentitis.

● **K05   Gingivitis and periodontal diseases**
    Use additional code to identify:
      alcohol abuse and dependence (F10.-)
      exposure to environmental tobacco smoke (Z77.22)
      exposure to tobacco smoke in the perinatal period (P96.81)
      history of tobacco dependence (Z87.891)
      occupational exposure to environmental tobacco smoke (Z57.31)
      tobacco dependence (F17.-)
      tobacco use (Z72.0)

● **K05.0   Acute gingivitis**
    Excludes1   acute necrotizing ulcerative gingivitis (A69.1)
             herpesviral [herpes simplex] gingivostomatitis (B00.2)

    K05.00   Acute gingivitis, plaque induced
      Acute gingivitis NOS
      Plaque induced gingival disease

    K05.01   Acute gingivitis, non-plaque induced

● **K05.1   Chronic gingivitis**
    Desquamative gingivitis (chronic)
    Gingivitis (chronic) NOS
    Hyperplastic gingivitis (chronic)
    Pregnancy associated gingivitis
    Simple marginal gingivitis (chronic)
    Ulcerative gingivitis (chronic)

    Code first, if applicable, diseases of the digestive system complicating pregnancy (O99.61-)

    K05.10   Chronic gingivitis, plaque induced
      Chronic gingivitis NOS
      Gingivitis NOS

    K05.11   Chronic gingivitis, non-plaque induced

● **K05.2   Aggressive periodontitis**
    Acute pericoronitis
    Excludes1   acute apical periodontitis (K04.4)
             periapical abscess (K04.7)
             periapical abscess with sinus (K04.6)

    K05.20   Aggressive periodontitis, unspecified

●   **K05.21   Aggressive periodontitis, localized**
      Periodontal abscess

      K05.211   Aggressive periodontitis, localized, slight

      K05.212   Aggressive periodontitis, localized, moderate

      K05.213   Aggressive periodontitis, localized, severe

      K05.219   Aggressive periodontitis, localized, unspecified severity

●   **K05.22   Aggressive periodontitis, generalized**

      K05.221   Aggressive periodontitis, generalized, slight

      K05.222   Aggressive periodontitis, generalized, moderate

      K05.223   Aggressive periodontitis, generalized, severe

      K05.229   Aggressive periodontitis, generalized, unspecified severity

● **K05.3   Chronic periodontitis**
    Chronic pericoronitis
    Complex periodontitis
    Periodontitis NOS
    Simplex periodontitis
    Excludes1   chronic apical periodontitis (K04.5)

    K05.30   Chronic periodontitis, unspecified

●   **K05.31   Chronic periodontitis, localized**

      K05.311   Chronic periodontitis, localized, slight

      K05.312   Chronic periodontitis, localized, moderate

      K05.313   Chronic periodontitis, localized, severe

      K05.319   Chronic periodontitis, localized, unspecified severity

●   **K05.32   Chronic periodontitis, generalized**

      K05.321   Chronic periodontitis, generalized, slight

      K05.322   Chronic periodontitis, generalized, moderate

      K05.323   Chronic periodontitis, generalized, severe

      K05.329   Chronic periodontitis, generalized, unspecified severity

   K05.4   Periodontosis
    Juvenile periodontosis

   K05.5   Other periodontal diseases
    Combined periodontic-endodontic lesion
    Narrow gingival width (of periodontal soft tissue)
    Excludes2   leukoplakia of gingiva (K13.21)

   K05.6   Periodontal disease, unspecified

● **K06   Other disorders of gingiva and edentulous alveolar ridge**
    Excludes2   acute gingivitis (K05.0)
             atrophy of edentulous alveolar ridge (K08.2)
             chronic gingivitis (K05.1)
             gingivitis NOS (K05.1)

● **K06.0   Gingival recession**
    ⟹ Gingival recession (postinfective) (postprocedural)

▶●   **K06.01   Gingival recession, localized**

     ▶ **K06.010   Localized gingival recession, unspecified**
          Localized gingival recession, NOS

     ▶ **K06.011   Localized gingival recession, minimal**

     ▶ **K06.012   Localized gingival recession, moderate**

     ▶ **K06.013   Localized gingival recession, severe**

▶●   **K06.02   Gingival recession, generalized**

     ▶ **K06.020   Generalized gingival recession, unspecified**
          Generalized gingival recession, NOS

     ▶ **K06.021   Generalized gingival recession, minimal**

     ▶ **K06.022   Generalized gingival recession, moderate**

     ▶ **K06.023   Generalized gingival recession, severe**

   K06.1   Gingival enlargement
    Gingival fibromatosis

   K06.2   Gingival and edentulous alveolar ridge lesions associated with trauma
    Irritative hyperplasia of edentulous ridge [denture hyperplasia]
    Use additional code (Chapter 20) to identify external cause or denture status (Z97.2)

K06.3   Horizontal alveolar bone loss

K06.8   Other specified disorders of gingiva and edentulous alveolar ridge
   Fibrous epulis
   Flabby alveolar ridge
   Giant cell epulis
   Peripheral giant cell granuloma of gingiva
   Pyogenic granuloma of gingiva
   Vertical ridge deficiency
   Excludes2   gingival cyst (K09.0)

K06.9   Disorder of gingiva and edentulous alveolar ridge, unspecified

● K08   Other disorders of teeth and supporting structures
   Excludes2   dentofacial anomalies [including malocclusion] (M26.-)
            disorders of jaw (M27.-)

K08.0   Exfoliation of teeth due to systemic causes
   Code also underlying systemic condition

● K08.1   Complete loss of teeth
   Acquired loss of teeth, complete
   Excludes1   congenital absence of teeth (K00.0)
            exfoliation of teeth due to systemic causes (K08.0)
            partial loss of teeth (K08.4-)

● K08.10   Complete loss of teeth, unspecified cause
   K08.101   Complete loss of teeth, unspecified cause, class I
   K08.102   Complete loss of teeth, unspecified cause, class II
   K08.103   Complete loss of teeth, unspecified cause, class III
   K08.104   Complete loss of teeth, unspecified cause, class IV
   K08.109   Complete loss of teeth, unspecified cause, unspecified class
           Edentulism NOS

● K08.11   Complete loss of teeth due to trauma
   K08.111   Complete loss of teeth due to trauma, class I
   K08.112   Complete loss of teeth due to trauma, class II
   K08.113   Complete loss of teeth due to trauma, class III
   K08.114   Complete loss of teeth due to trauma, class IV
   K08.119   Complete loss of teeth due to trauma, unspecified class

● K08.12   Complete loss of teeth due to periodontal diseases
   K08.121   Complete loss of teeth due to periodontal diseases, class I
   K08.122   Complete loss of teeth due to periodontal diseases, class II
   K08.123   Complete loss of teeth due to periodontal diseases, class III
   K08.124   Complete loss of teeth due to periodontal diseases, class IV
   K08.129   Complete loss of teeth due to periodontal diseases, unspecified class

● K08.13   Complete loss of teeth due to caries
   K08.131   Complete loss of teeth due to caries, class I
   K08.132   Complete loss of teeth due to caries, class II
   K08.133   Complete loss of teeth due to caries, class III
   K08.134   Complete loss of teeth due to caries, class IV
   K08.139   Complete loss of teeth due to caries, unspecified class

● K08.19   Complete loss of teeth due to other specified cause
   K08.191   Complete loss of teeth due to other specified cause, class I
   K08.192   Complete loss of teeth due to other specified cause, class II
   K08.193   Complete loss of teeth due to other specified cause, class III
   K08.194   Complete loss of teeth due to other specified cause, class IV
   K08.199   Complete loss of teeth due to other specified cause, unspecified class

● K08.2   Atrophy of edentulous alveolar ridge
   K08.20   Unspecified atrophy of edentulous alveolar ridge
           Atrophy of the mandible NOS
           Atrophy of the maxilla NOS
   K08.21   Minimal atrophy of the mandible
           Minimal atrophy of the edentulous mandible
   K08.22   Moderate atrophy of the mandible
           Moderate atrophy of the edentulous mandible
   K08.23   Severe atrophy of the mandible
           Severe atrophy of the edentulous mandible
   K08.24   Minimal atrophy of maxilla
           Minimal atrophy of the edentulous maxilla
   K08.25   Moderate atrophy of the maxilla
           Moderate atrophy of the edentulous maxilla
   K08.26   Severe atrophy of the maxilla
           Severe atrophy of the edentulous maxilla

K08.3   Retained dental root

● K08.4   Partial loss of teeth
   Acquired loss of teeth, partial
   Excludes1   complete loss of teeth (K08.1-)
            congenital absence of teeth (K00.0)
   Excludes2   exfoliation of teeth due to systemic causes (K08.0)

● K08.40   Partial loss of teeth, unspecified cause
   K08.401   Partial loss of teeth, unspecified cause, class I
   K08.402   Partial loss of teeth, unspecified cause, class II
   K08.403   Partial loss of teeth, unspecified cause, class III
   K08.404   Partial loss of teeth, unspecified cause, class IV
   K08.409   Partial loss of teeth, unspecified cause, unspecified class
           Tooth extraction status NOS

● K08.41   Partial loss of teeth due to trauma
   K08.411   Partial loss of teeth due to trauma, class I
   K08.412   Partial loss of teeth due to trauma, class II
   K08.413   Partial loss of teeth due to trauma, class III
   K08.414   Partial loss of teeth due to trauma, class IV
   K08.419   Partial loss of teeth due to trauma, unspecified class

● K08.42   Partial loss of teeth due to periodontal diseases
   K08.421   Partial loss of teeth due to periodontal diseases, class I
   K08.422   Partial loss of teeth due to periodontal diseases, class II
   K08.423   Partial loss of teeth due to periodontal diseases, class III
   K08.424   Partial loss of teeth due to periodontal diseases, class IV
   K08.429   Partial loss of teeth due to periodontal diseases, unspecified class

▶ New   ⇒ Revised   ~~deleted~~ Deleted   OGCR Official Guidelines   X Assign placeholder X   ● Use Additional Character(s)

Excludes 1   Excludes 2   Includes   Use additional   Code first   Code also   Key words

● K08.43   Partial loss of teeth due to caries
    K08.431   Partial loss of teeth due to caries,
           class I
    K08.432   Partial loss of teeth due to caries,
           class II
    K08.433   Partial loss of teeth due to caries,
           class III
    K08.434   Partial loss of teeth due to caries,
           class IV
    K08.439   Partial loss of teeth due to caries,
           unspecified class

● K08.49   Partial loss of teeth due to other specified cause
    K08.491   Partial loss of teeth due to other
           specified cause, class I
    K08.492   Partial loss of teeth due to other
           specified cause, class II
    K08.493   Partial loss of teeth due to other
           specified cause, class III
    K08.494   Partial loss of teeth due to other
           specified cause, class IV
    K08.499   Partial loss of teeth due to other
           specified cause, unspecified class

● K08.5   Unsatisfactory restoration of tooth
    Defective bridge, crown, filling
    Defective dental restoration

    Excludes1   dental restoration status (Z98.811)
    Excludes2   endosseous dental implant failure
                (M27.6-)
                unsatisfactory endodontic treatment
                (M27.5-)

    K08.50   Unsatisfactory restoration of tooth, unspecified
           Defective dental restoration NOS

    K08.51   Open restoration margins of tooth
           Dental restoration failure of marginal integrity
           Open margin on tooth restoration
           Poor gingival margin to tooth restoration

    K08.52   Unrepairable overhanging of dental restorative materials
           Overhanging of tooth restoration

● K08.53   Fractured dental restorative material

    Excludes1   cracked tooth (K03.81)
                traumatic fracture of tooth
                (S02.5)

    K08.530   Fractured dental restorative material without loss of material
    K08.531   Fractured dental restorative material with loss of material
    K08.539   Fractured dental restorative material, unspecified

    K08.54   Contour of existing restoration of tooth biologically incompatible with oral health
           Dental restoration failure of periodontal
              anatomical integrity
           Unacceptable contours of existing restoration
              of tooth
           Unacceptable morphology of existing
              restoration of tooth

    K08.55   Allergy to existing dental restorative material
           Use additional code to identify the specific
              type of allergy

    K08.56   Poor aesthetic of existing restoration of tooth
           Dental restoration aesthetically inadequate or
              displeasing

    K08.59   Other unsatisfactory restoration of tooth
           Other defective dental restoration

● K08.8   Other specified disorders of teeth and supporting structures
    K08.81   Primary occlusal trauma
    K08.82   Secondary occlusal trauma
    K08.89   Other specified disorders of teeth and supporting structures
           Enlargement of alveolar ridge NOS
           Insufficient anatomic crown height
           Insufficient clinical crown length
           Irregular alveolar process
           Toothache NOS

    K08.9   Disorder of teeth and supporting structures, unspecified

● K09   Cysts of oral region, not elsewhere classified

    Includes   lesions showing histological features both of
                aneurysmal cyst and of another fibro-
                osseous lesion

    Excludes2   cysts of jaw (M27.0-, M27.4-)
                radicular cyst (K04.8)

    K09.0   Developmental odontogenic cysts
           Dentigerous cyst
           Eruption cyst
           Follicular cyst
           Gingival cyst
           Lateral periodontal cyst
           Primordial cyst

    Excludes2   keratocysts (D16.4, D16.5)
                odontogenic keratocystic tumors
                (D16.4, D16.5)

    K09.1   Developmental (nonodontogenic) cysts of oral region
           Cyst (of) incisive canal
           Cyst (of) palatine of papilla
           Globulomaxillary cyst
           Median palatal cyst
           Nasoalveolar cyst
           Nasolabial cyst
           Nasopalatine duct cyst

    K09.8   Other cysts of oral region, not elsewhere classified
           Dermoid cyst
           Epidermoid cyst
           Lymphoepithelial cyst
           Epstein's pearl

    K09.9   Cyst of oral region, unspecified

★ **(See Plate 61 on page 73.)**

● K11   Diseases of salivary glands
    Use additional code to identify:
        alcohol abuse and dependence (F10.-)
        exposure to environmental tobacco smoke (Z77.22)
        exposure to tobacco smoke in the perinatal period (P96.81)
        history of tobacco dependence (Z87.891)
        occupational exposure to environmental tobacco smoke
           (Z57.31)
        tobacco dependence (F17.-)
        tobacco use (Z72.0)

    K11.0   Atrophy of salivary gland
    K11.1   Hypertrophy of salivary gland

Item 11–4 Atrophy is wasting away of a tissue or organ, whereas **hypertrophy** is overdevelopment or enlargement of a tissue or organ. **Sialoadenitis** is salivary gland inflammation. **Parotitis** is the inflammation of the parotid gland. In the epidemic form, parotitis is also known as mumps. **Sialolithiasis** is the formation of calculus within a salivary gland. **Mucocele** is a polyp composed of mucus.

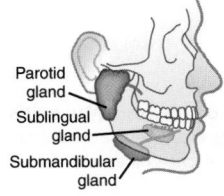

Figure 11-3 Major salivary glands.

Parotid gland
Sublingual gland
Submandibular gland

● **K11.2 Sialoadenitis**
  Parotitis
  | Excludes1 | epidemic parotitis (B26.-)
              | mumps (B26.-)
              | uveoparotid fever [Heerfordt] (D86.89)

  K11.20 Sialoadenitis, unspecified
  K11.21 Acute sialoadenitis
           | Excludes1 | acute recurrent sialoadenitis
                       | (K11.22)

  K11.22 Acute recurrent sialoadenitis
  K11.23 Chronic sialoadenitis

K11.3 Abscess of salivary gland
K11.4 Fistula of salivary gland
        | Excludes1 | congenital fistula of salivary gland (Q38.4)

K11.5 Sialolithiasis
  Calculus of salivary gland or duct
  Stone of salivary gland or duct

K11.6 Mucocele of salivary gland
  Mucous extravasation cyst of salivary gland
  Mucous retention cyst of salivary gland
  Ranula

K11.7 Disturbances of salivary secretion
  Hypoptyalism
  Ptyalism
  Xerostomia
  | Excludes2 | dry mouth NOS (R68.2)

K11.8 Other diseases of salivary glands
  Benign lymphoepithelial lesion of salivary gland
  Mikulicz' disease
  Necrotizing sialometaplasia
  Sialectasia
  Stenosis of salivary duct
  Stricture of salivary duct
  | Excludes1 | sicca syndrome [Sjögren] (M35.0-)

K11.9 Disease of salivary gland, unspecified
  Sialoadenopathy NOS

● **K12 Stomatitis and related lesions**
  Use additional code to identify:
  alcohol abuse and dependence (F10.-)
  exposure to environmental tobacco smoke (Z77.22)
  exposure to tobacco smoke in the perinatal period (P96.81)
  history of tobacco dependence (Z87.891)
  occupational exposure to environmental tobacco smoke (Z57.31)
  tobacco dependence (F17.-)
  tobacco use (Z72.0)
  | Excludes1 | cancrum oris (A69.0)
              | cheilitis (K13.0)
              | gangrenous stomatitis (A69.0)
              | herpesviral [herpes simplex] gingivostomatitis
              | (B00.2)
              | noma (A69.0)

  K12.0 Recurrent oral aphthae
    Aphthous stomatitis (major) (minor)
    Bednar's aphthae
    Periadenitis mucosa necrotica recurrens
    Recurrent aphthous ulcer
    Stomatitis herpetiformis

  K12.1 Other forms of stomatitis
    Stomatitis NOS
    Denture stomatitis
    Ulcerative stomatitis
    Vesicular stomatitis
    | Excludes1 | acute necrotizing ulcerative stomatitis
                | (A69.1)
                | Vincent's stomatitis (A69.1)

K12.2 Cellulitis and abscess of mouth
  Cellulitis of mouth (floor)
  Submandibular abscess
  | Excludes2 | abscess of salivary gland (K11.3)
              | abscess of tongue (K14.0)
              | periapical abscess (K04.6-K04.7)
              | periodontal abscess (K05.21)
              | peritonsillar abscess (J36)

● **K12.3 Oral mucositis (ulcerative)**
  Mucositis (oral) (oropharyneal)
  | Excludes2 | gastrointestinal mucositis (ulcerative)
              | (K92.81)
              | mucositis (ulcerative) of vagina and vulva
              | (N76.81)
              | nasal mucositis (ulcerative) (J34.81)

  K12.30 Oral mucositis (ulcerative), unspecified
  **K12.31 Oral mucositis (ulcerative) due to antineoplastic
            therapy**
            Use additional code for adverse effect, if
              applicable, to identify antineoplastic and
              immunosuppressive drugs (T45.1X5)
            Use additional code for other antineoplastic
              therapy, such as:
              radiological procedure and radiotherapy
                (Y84.2)

  K12.32 Oral mucositis (ulcerative) due to other drugs
            Use additional code for adverse effect, if
              applicable, to identify drug (T36-T50 with
              fifth or sixth character 5)

  K12.33 Oral mucositis (ulcerative) due to radiation
            Use additional external cause code (W88-W90,
              X39.0-) to identify cause

  K12.39 Other oral mucositis (ulcerative)
            Viral oral mucositis (ulcerative)

● **K13 Other diseases of lip and oral mucosa**
  | Includes | epithelial disturbances of tongue
  Use additional code to identify:
  alcohol abuse and dependence (F10.-)
  exposure to environmental tobacco smoke (Z77.22)
  exposure to tobacco smoke in the perinatal period (P96.81)
  history of tobacco dependence (Z87.891)
  occupational exposure to environmental tobacco smoke
    (Z57.31)
  tobacco dependence (F17.-)
  tobacco use (Z72.0)
  | Excludes2 | certain disorders of gingiva and edentulous
              | alveolar ridge (K05-K06)
              | cysts of oral region (K09.-)
              | diseases of tongue (K14.-)
              | stomatitis and related lesions (K12.-)

  K13.0 Diseases of lips
    Abscess of lips   Exfoliative cheilitis
    Angular cheilitis   Fistula of lips
    Cellulitis of lips   Glandular cheilitis
    Cheilitis NOS   Hypertrophy of lips
    Cheilodynia   Perlèche NEC
    Cheilosis
    | Excludes1 | ariboflavinosis (E53.0)
                | cheilitis due to radiation-related disorders
                | (L55-L59)
                | congenital fistula of lips (Q38.0)
                | congenital hypertrophy of lips (Q18.6)
                | Perlèche due to candidiasis (B37.83)
                | Perlèche due to riboflavin deficiency
                | (E53.0)

  K13.1 Cheek and lip biting

Item 11-5 Stomatitis is the inflammation of the oral mucosa. **Mucositis** is the inflammation of the mucous membranes lining the digestive tract from the mouth to the anus. It is a common side effect of chemotherapy and of radiotherapy that involves any part of the digestive tract.

▶ New   ⇒ Revised   ~~deleted~~ Deleted   **OGCR** Official Guidelines   X Assign placeholder X   ● Use Additional Character(s)

| Excludes 1 | | Excludes 2 | Includes   Use additional   Code first   Code also   Key words

Figure 11-4 Oral leukoplakia and associated. (From Swartz MH: Textbook of Physical Diagnosis: History and Examination, Philadelphia, PA, Saunders/Elsevier, 2010)

● **K13.2 Leukoplakia and other disturbances of oral epithelium, including tongue**

> **Excludes1** carcinoma in situ of oral epithelium (D00.0-)
> hairy leukoplakia (K13.3)

K13.21 Leukoplakia of oral mucosa, including tongue
Considered precancerous and evidenced by thickened white patches of epithelium on mucous membranes
Leukokeratosis of oral mucosa
Leukoplakia of gingiva, lips, tongue

> **Excludes1** hairy leukoplakia (K13.3)
> leukokeratosis nicotina palati (K13.24)

K13.22 Minimal keratinized residual ridge mucosa
Minimal keratinization of alveolar ridge mucosa

K13.23 Excessive keratinized residual ridge mucosa
Excessive keratinization of alveolar ridge mucosa

K13.24 Leukokeratosis nicotina palati
Smoker's palate

K13.29 Other disturbances of oral epithelium, including tongue
Erythroplakia of mouth or tongue
Focal epithelial hyperplasia of mouth or tongue
Leukoedema of mouth or tongue
Other oral epithelium disturbances

K13.3 Hairy leukoplakia

K13.4 Granuloma and granuloma-like lesions of oral mucosa
Eosinophilic granuloma
Granuloma pyogenicum
Verrucous xanthoma

K13.5 Oral submucous fibrosis
Submucous fibrosis of tongue

K13.6 Irritative hyperplasia of oral mucosa

> **Excludes2** irritative hyperplasia of edentulous ridge [denture hyperplasia] (K06.2)

● **K13.7 Other and unspecified lesions of oral mucosa**

K13.70 Unspecified lesions of oral mucosa

K13.79 Other lesions of oral mucosa
Focal oral mucinosis

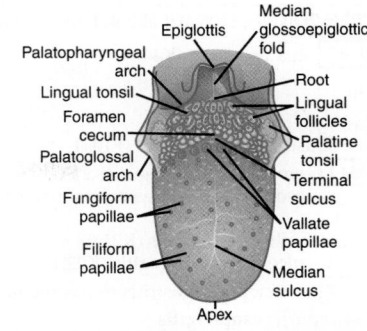

Median
Epiglottis   glossoepiglottic
fold
Palatopharyngeal
arch   Root
Lingual tonsil   Lingual
Foramen   follicles
cecum   Palatine
Palatoglossal   tonsil
arch   Terminal
Fungiform   sulcus
papillae   Vallate
papillae
Filiform
papillae   Median
sulcus
Apex

Figure 11-5 Structure of the tongue.

★**(See Plate 58 on page 71.)**

● **K14 Diseases of tongue**
Use additional code to identify:
alcohol abuse and dependence (F10.-)
exposure to environmental tobacco smoke (Z77.22)
history of tobacco dependence (Z87.891)
occupational exposure to environmental tobacco smoke (Z57.31)
tobacco dependence (F17.-)
tobacco use (Z72.0)

> **Excludes2** erythroplakia (K13.29)
> focal epithelial hyperplasia (K13.29)
> leukedema of tongue (K13.29)
> leukoplakia of tongue (K13.21)
> hairy leukoplakia (K13.3)
> macroglossia (congenital) (Q38.2)
> submucous fibrosis of tongue (K13.5)

K14.0 Glossitis
Abscess of tongue
Ulceration (traumatic) of tongue

> **Excludes1** atrophic glossitis (K14.4)

K14.1 Geographic tongue
Benign migratory glossitis
Glossitis areata exfoliativa

K14.2 Median rhomboid glossitis

K14.3 Hypertrophy of tongue papillae
Black hairy tongue
Coated tongue
Hypertrophy of foliate papillae
Lingua villosa nigra

K14.4 Atrophy of tongue papillae
Atrophic glossitis

K14.5 Plicated tongue
Fissured tongue   Scrotal tongue
Furrowed tongue

> **Excludes1** fissured tongue, congenital (Q38.3)

K14.6 Glossodynia
Glossopyrosis   Painful tongue

K14.8 Other diseases of tongue
Atrophy of tongue   Glossocele
Crenated tongue   Glossoptosis
Enlargement of tongue   Hypertrophy of tongue

K14.9 Disease of tongue, unspecified
Glossopathy NOS

CHAPTER 11 (K00-K95)

DISEASES OF ESOPHAGUS, STOMACH AND DUODENUM (K20-K31)

> **Excludes2**   hiatus hernia (K44.-)

● **K20**   **Esophagitis**
> Use additional code to identify:
>   alcohol abuse and dependence (F10.-)
> **Excludes1**   erosion of esophagus (K22.1-)
>   esophagitis with gastro-esophageal reflux disease
>   (K21.0)
>   reflux esophagitis (K21.0)
>   ulcerative esophagitis (K22.1-)
> **Excludes2**   eosinophilic gastritis or gastroenteritis (K52.81)

   K20.0   **Eosinophilic esophagitis**

   K20.8   **Other esophagitis**
>   Abscess of esophagus

   K20.9   **Esophagitis, unspecified**
>   Esophagitis NOS

● **K21**   **Gastro-esophageal reflux disease**
> **Excludes1**   newborn esophageal reflux (P78.83)

   K21.0   **Gastro-esophageal reflux disease with esophagitis**
>   Reflux esophagitis

   K21.9   **Gastro-esophageal reflux disease without esophagitis**
>   Esophageal reflux NOS

● **K22**   **Other diseases of esophagus**
> **Excludes2**   esophageal varices (I85.-)

   K22.0   **Achalasia of cardia**
>   Achalasia NOS
>   Cardiospasm
> **Excludes1**   congenital cardiospasm (Q39.5)

   ● **K22.1**   **Ulcer of esophagus**
>   Barrett's ulcer
>   Erosion of esophagus
>   Fungal ulcer of esophagus
>   Peptic ulcer of esophagus
>   Ulcer of esophagus due to ingestion of chemicals
>   Ulcer of esophagus due to ingestion of drugs and
>   medicaments
>   Ulcerative esophagitis
> *Code first poisoning due to drug or toxin, if applicable*
> *   (T36-T65 with fifth or sixth character 1-4 or 6)*
> Use additional code for adverse effect, if applicable,
>   to identify drug (T36-T50 with fifth or sixth
>   character 5)
> **Excludes1**   Barrett's esophagus (K22.87-)

     K22.10   **Ulcer of esophagus without bleeding**
>   Ulcer of esophagus NOS

     K22.11   **Ulcer of esophagus with bleeding**
>   **Excludes2**   bleeding esophageal varices
>   (I85.01, I85.11)

   K22.2   **Esophageal obstruction**
>   Compression of esophagus
>   Constriction of esophagus
>   Stenosis of esophagus
>   Stricture of esophagus
> **Excludes1**   congenital stenosis or stricture of
>   esophagus (Q39.3)

   K22.3   **Perforation of esophagus**
>   Rupture of esophagus
> **Excludes1**   traumatic perforation of (thoracic)
>   esophagus (S27.8-)

CERVICAL ESOPHAGUS
First rib
Left subclavian artery
Arch of aorta
Diaphragm
THORACIC ESOPHAGUS
ABDOMINAL ESOPHAGUS
Stomach

Figure 11-6 The esophagus is the muscular tube that connects the pharynx and the stomach. The 10 inch (25 cm) long esophagus is divided into three parts: **cervical, thoracic,** and **abdominal.**

Item 11-7 Achalasia is a condition in which the smooth muscle fibers of the esophagus do not relax. Most frequently, this condition occurs at the esophagogastric sphincter. **Cardiospasm,** also known as **megaesophagus,** is achalasia of the thoracic esophagus.

   K22.4   **Dyskinesia of esophagus**
>   *Difficulty in moving*
>   Corkscrew esophagus
>   Diffuse esophageal spasm
>   Spasm of esophagus
> **Excludes1**   cardiospasm (K22.0)

   K22.5   **Diverticulum of esophagus, acquired**
>   Esophageal pouch, acquired
> **Excludes1**   diverticulum of esophagus (congenital)
>   (Q39.6)

   K22.6   **Gastro-esophageal laceration-hemorrhage syndrome**
>   Mallory-Weiss syndrome

   ● **K22.7**   **Barrett's esophagus**
>   Barrett's disease
>   Barrett's syndrome
> **Excludes1**   Barrett's ulcer (K22.1)
>   malignant neoplasm of esophagus
>   (C15.-)

     K22.70   **Barrett's esophagus without dysplasia**
>   Barrett's esophagus NOS

     ● **K22.71**   **Barrett's esophagus with dysplasia**

       K22.710   **Barrett's esophagus with low grade dysplasia**

       K22.711   **Barrett's esophagus with high grade dysplasia**

       K22.719   **Barrett's esophagus with dysplasia, unspecified**

   K22.8   **Other specified diseases of esophagus**
>   Hemorrhage of esophagus NOS
> **Excludes2**   esophageal varices (I85.-)
>   Paterson-Kelly syndrome (D50.1)

   K22.9   **Disease of esophagus, unspecified**

● **K23**   **Disorders of esophagus in diseases classified elsewhere**
> *Code first underlying disease, such as:*
>   congenital syphilis (A50.5)
> **Excludes1**   late syphilis (A52.79)
>   megaesophagus due to Chagas' disease (B57.31)
>   tuberculosis (A18.83)

Item 11-6 Esophageal reflux is the return flow of the contents of the stomach to the esophagus and is referred to as GERD and/or "heartburn." **Gastroesophageal reflux** is the return flow of the contents of the stomach and duodenum to the esophagus. **Esophageal leukoplakia** are white areas on the mucous membrane of the esophagus for which no specific cause can be identified.

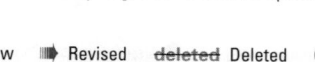

▶ New   ⇒ Revised   ~~deleted~~ Deleted   **OGCR** Official Guidelines   X Assign placeholder X   ● Use Additional Character(s)

Excludes 1   Excludes 2   Includes   Use additional   Code first   Code also   Key words

Figure 11-7 A. Ulcer. **B.** Perforated ulcer. **C.** Laparoscopic view of a perforated duodenal ulcer *(arrow)* with fibrinous exudate on the adjacent peritoneum. (**C** from Feldman: Sleisenger & Fordtran's Gastrointestinal and Liver Disease, ed 8, Saunders, An Imprint of Elsevier, 2006)

Item 11–8   Gastric ulcers are lesions of the stomach that result in the death of the tissue and a defect of the surface. **Perforated ulcers** are those in which the lesion penetrates the gastric wall, leaving a hole. **Peptic ulcers** are lesions of the stomach or the duodenum. **Peptic** refers to the gastric juice, pepsin.

● **K25   Gastric ulcer**

> **Includes**   erosion (acute) of stomach
> pylorus ulcer (peptic)
> stomach ulcer (peptic)
>
> Use additional code to identify:
> alcohol abuse and dependence (F10.-)
>
> **Excludes1**   acute gastritis (K29.0-)
> peptic ulcer NOS (K27.-)

K25.0   Acute gastric ulcer with hemorrhage
K25.1   Acute gastric ulcer with perforation
K25.2   Acute gastric ulcer with both hemorrhage and perforation
K25.3   Acute gastric ulcer without hemorrhage or perforation
K25.4   Chronic or unspecified gastric ulcer with hemorrhage
K25.5   Chronic or unspecified gastric ulcer with perforation
K25.6   Chronic or unspecified gastric ulcer with both hemorrhage and perforation
K25.7   Chronic gastric ulcer without hemorrhage or perforation
K25.9   Gastric ulcer, unspecified as acute or chronic, without hemorrhage or perforation

● **K26   Duodenal ulcer**

> **Includes**   erosion (acute) of duodenum
> duodenum ulcer (peptic)
> postpyloric ulcer (peptic)
>
> Use additional code to identify:
> alcohol abuse and dependence (F10.-)
>
> **Excludes1**   peptic ulcer NOS (K27.-)

K26.0   Acute duodenal ulcer with hemorrhage
K26.1   Acute duodenal ulcer with perforation
K26.2   Acute duodenal ulcer with both hemorrhage and perforation
K26.3   Acute duodenal ulcer without hemorrhage or perforation
K26.4   Chronic or unspecified duodenal ulcer with hemorrhage
K26.5   Chronic or unspecified duodenal ulcer with perforation
K26.6   Chronic or unspecified duodenal ulcer with both hemorrhage and perforation
K26.7   Chronic duodenal ulcer without hemorrhage or perforation
K26.9   Duodenal ulcer, unspecified as acute or chronic, without hemorrhage or perforation

● **K27   Peptic ulcer, site unspecified**

> **Includes**   gastroduodenal ulcer NOS
> peptic ulcer NOS
>
> Use additional code to identify:
> alcohol abuse and dependence (F10.-)
>
> **Excludes1**   peptic ulcer of newborn (P78.82)

K27.0   Acute peptic ulcer, site unspecified, with hemorrhage
K27.1   Acute peptic ulcer, site unspecified, with perforation
K27.2   Acute peptic ulcer, site unspecified, with both hemorrhage and perforation
K27.3   Acute peptic ulcer, site unspecified, without hemorrhage or perforation
K27.4   Chronic or unspecified peptic ulcer, site unspecified, with hemorrhage
K27.5   Chronic or unspecified peptic ulcer, site unspecified, with perforation
K27.6   Chronic or unspecified peptic ulcer, site unspecified, with both hemorrhage and perforation
K27.7   Chronic peptic ulcer, site unspecified, without hemorrhage or perforation
K27.9   Peptic ulcer, site unspecified, unspecified as acute or chronic, without hemorrhage or perforation

● **K28   Gastrojejunal ulcer**

> **Includes**   anastomotic ulcer (peptic) or erosion
> gastrocolic ulcer (peptic) or erosion
> gastrointestinal ulcer (peptic) or erosion
> gastrojejunal ulcer (peptic) or erosion
> jejunal ulcer (peptic) or erosion
> marginal ulcer (peptic) or erosion
> stomal ulcer (peptic) or erosion
>
> Use additional code to identify:
> alcohol abuse and dependence (F10.-)
>
> **Excludes1**   primary ulcer of small intestine (K63.3)

K28.0   Acute gastrojejunal ulcer with hemorrhage
K28.1   Acute gastrojejunal ulcer with perforation
K28.2   Acute gastrojejunal ulcer with both hemorrhage and perforation
K28.3   Acute gastrojejunal ulcer without hemorrhage or perforation
K28.4   Chronic or unspecified gastrojejunal ulcer with hemorrhage
K28.5   Chronic or unspecified gastrojejunal ulcer with perforation
K28.6   Chronic or unspecified gastrojejunal ulcer with both hemorrhage and perforation
K28.7   Chronic gastrojejunal ulcer without hemorrhage or perforation
K28.9   Gastrojejunal ulcer, unspecified as acute or chronic, without hemorrhage or perforation

● **K29   Gastritis and duodenitis**

> **Excludes1**   eosinophilic gastritis or gastroenteritis (K52.81)
> Zollinger-Ellison syndrome (E16.4)

● **K29.0   Acute gastritis**

> Use additional code to identify:
> alcohol abuse and dependence (F10.-)
>
> **Excludes1**   erosion (acute) of stomach (K25.-)

K29.00   Acute gastritis without bleeding
K29.01   Acute gastritis with bleeding

● **K29.2   Alcoholic gastritis**

> Use additional code to identify:
> alcohol abuse and dependence (F10.-)

K29.20   Alcoholic gastritis without bleeding
K29.21   Alcoholic gastritis with bleeding

CHAPTER 11 (K00-K95)

● K29.3   Chronic superficial gastritis
     K29.30   Chronic superficial gastritis without bleeding
     K29.31   Chronic superficial gastritis with bleeding

● K29.4   Chronic atrophic gastritis
     Gastric atrophy
     K29.40   Chronic atrophic gastritis without bleeding
     K29.41   Chronic atrophic gastritis with bleeding

● K29.5   Unspecified chronic gastritis
     Chronic antral gastritis
     Chronic fundal gastritis
     K29.50   Unspecified chronic gastritis without bleeding
     K29.51   Unspecified chronic gastritis with bleeding

● K29.6   Other gastritis
     Giant hypertrophic gastritis
     Granulomatous gastritis
     Ménétrier's disease
     K29.60   Other gastritis without bleeding
     K29.61   Other gastritis with bleeding

● K29.7   Gastritis, unspecified
     K29.70   Gastritis, unspecified, without bleeding
     K29.71   Gastritis, unspecified, with bleeding

● K29.8   Duodenitis
     K29.80   Duodenitis without bleeding
     K29.81   Duodenitis with bleeding

● K29.9   Gastroduodenitis, unspecified
     K29.90   Gastroduodenitis, unspecified, without bleeding
     K29.91   Gastroduodenitis, unspecified, with bleeding

K30   Functional dyspepsia
     Indigestion
     Excludes1   dyspepsia NOS (R10.13)
                 heartburn (R12)
                 nervous dyspepsia (F45.8)
                 neurotic dyspepsia (F45.8)
                 psychogenic dyspepsia (F45.8)

● K31   Other diseases of stomach and duodenum
     Includes   functional disorders of stomach
     Excludes2   diabetic gastroparesis (E08.43, E09.43, E10.43, E11.43, E13.43)
                 diverticulum of duodenum (K57.00-K57.13)

     K31.0   Acute dilatation of stomach
          Acute distention of stomach

     K31.1   Adult hypertrophic pyloric stenosis
          Pyloric stenosis NOS
          Excludes1   congenital or infantile pyloric stenosis (Q40.0)

     K31.2   Hourglass stricture and stenosis of stomach
          Excludes1   congenital hourglass stomach (Q40.2)
                 hourglass contraction of stomach (K31.89)

     K31.3   Pylorospasm, not elsewhere classified
          Excludes1   congenital or infantile pylorospasm (Q40.0)
                 neurotic pylorospasm (F45.8)
                 psychogenic pylorospasm (F45.8)

     K31.4   Gastric diverticulum
          Excludes1   congenital diverticulum of stomach (Q40.2)

     K31.5   Obstruction of duodenum
          Constriction of duodenum
          Duodenal ileus (chronic)
          Stenosis of duodenum
             Narrowing
          Stricture of duodenum
             Narrowing
          Volvulus of duodenum
             Twisting/knotting
          Excludes1   congenital stenosis of duodenum (Q41.0)

     K31.6   Fistula of stomach and duodenum
          Gastrocolic fistula
          Gastrojejunocolic fistula

     K31.7   Polyp of stomach and duodenum
          Excludes1   adenomatous polyp of stomach (D13.1)

● K31.8   Other specified diseases of stomach and duodenum
     ● K31.81   Angiodysplasia of stomach and duodenum
          K31.811   Angiodysplasia of stomach and duodenum with bleeding
          K31.819   Angiodysplasia of stomach and duodenum without bleeding
                 Angiodysplasia of stomach and duodenum NOS

     K31.82   Dieulafoy lesion (hemorrhagic) of stomach and duodenum
          Excludes2   Dieulafoy lesion of intestine (K63.81)

     K31.83   Achlorhydria
     K31.84   Gastroparesis
          Gastroparalysis
          Code first underlying disease, if known, such as:
          anorexia nervosa (F50.0-)
          diabetes mellitus (E08.43, E09.43, E10.43, E11.43, E13.43)
          scleroderma (M34.-)

     K31.89   Other diseases of stomach and duodenum
     K31.9   Disease of stomach and duodenum, unspecified

DISEASES OF APPENDIX (K35-K38)

● K35   Acute appendicitis
     K35.2   Acute appendicitis with generalized peritonitis
          Appendicitis (acute) with generalized (diffuse) peritonitis following rupture or perforation of appendix
          Perforated appendix NOS
          Ruptured appendix NOS

     K35.3   Acute appendicitis with localized peritonitis
          Acute appendicitis with or without perforation or rupture with peritonitis NOS
          Acute appendicitis with or without perforation or rupture with localized peritonitis
          Acute appendicitis with peritoneal abscess

● K35.8   Other and unspecified acute appendicitis
     K35.80   Unspecified acute appendicitis
          Acute appendicitis NOS
          Acute appendicitis without (localized) (generalized) peritonitis
     K35.89   Other acute appendicitis

Item 11–10 Achlorhydria, also known as gastric anacidity, is the absence of gastric acid.

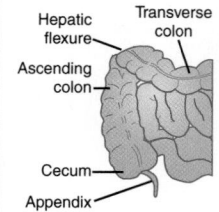

Figure 11-8 Acute appendicitis is the inflammation of the appendix, usually associated with obstruction. Most often this is a disease of adolescents and young adults.

Item 11–9 Gastritis is a severe inflammation of the stomach. **Atrophic gastritis** is a chronic inflammation of the stomach that results in destruction of the cells of the mucosa of the stomach. Duodenitis is an inflammation of the duodenum, the first section of the small intestine.

▶ New   ➡ Revised   ~~deleted~~ Deleted   **OGCR** Official Guidelines   X Assign placeholder X   ● Use Additional Character(s)

Excludes 1   Excludes 2   Includes   Use additional   Code first   Code also   Key words

K36 Other appendicitis
     Chronic appendicitis
     Recurrent appendicitis

K37 Unspecified appendicitis
     Excludes1 -unspecified appendicitis with peritonitis
         (K35.2-K35.3)

● **K38 Other diseases of appendix**
     K38.0 Hyperplasia of appendix
     K38.1 Appendicular concretions
         Fecalith of appendix
         Stercolith of appendix
     K38.2 Diverticulum of appendix
     K38.3 Fistula of appendix
     K38.8 Other specified diseases of appendix
         Intussusception of appendix
     K38.9 Disease of appendix, unspecified

HERNIA (K40-K46)

     Note: Hernia with both gangrene and obstruction is classified
         to hernia with gangrene.
     Includes   acquired hernia
               congenital [except diaphragmatic or hiatus]
                 hernia
               recurrent hernia

● **K40 Inguinal hernia**
     Includes   bubonocele
               direct inguinal hernia
               double inguinal hernia
               indirect inguinal hernia
               inguinal hernia NOS
               oblique inguinal hernia
               scrotal hernia

   ● **K40.0 Bilateral inguinal hernia, with obstruction, without gangrene**
         Inguinal hernia (bilateral) causing obstruction without
             gangrene
         Incarcerated inguinal hernia (bilateral) without
             gangrene
         Irreducible inguinal hernia (bilateral) without gangrene
         Strangulated inguinal hernia (bilateral) without
             gangrene
     K40.00 Bilateral inguinal hernia, with obstruction, without gangrene, not specified as recurrent
         Bilateral inguinal hernia, with obstruction,
             without gangrene NOS
     K40.01 Bilateral inguinal hernia, with obstruction, without gangrene, recurrent
   ● **K40.1 Bilateral inguinal hernia, with gangrene**
     K40.10 Bilateral inguinal hernia, with gangrene, not specified as recurrent
         Bilateral inguinal hernia, with gangrene NOS
     K40.11 Bilateral inguinal hernia, with gangrene, recurrent
   ● **K40.2 Bilateral inguinal hernia, without obstruction or gangrene**
     K40.20 Bilateral inguinal hernia, without obstruction or gangrene, not specified as recurrent
         Bilateral inguinal hernia NOS
     K40.21 Bilateral inguinal hernia, without obstruction or gangrene, recurrent

Item 11–11 **Hernias** of the groin are the most common type, accounting for 80 percent of all hernias. There are two major types of inguinal hernias: indirect (oblique) affecting men only and direct. **Indirect inguinal hernias** result when the intestines emerge through the abdominal wall in an indirect fashion through the inguinal canal. **Direct inguinal hernias** penetrate through the abdominal wall in a direct fashion. **Femoral hernias** occur at the femoral ring where the femoral vessels enter the thigh and is most common in women. An abdominal wall hernia is also called a ventral or epigastric hernia and occurs in both sexes. Classification is based on location of the hernia and whether there is obstruction or gangrene.

     Ventral, epigastric, or incisional hernia occurs on the abdominal surface caused by musculature weakness or a tear at a previous surgical site and is evidenced by a bulge that changes in size, becoming larger with exertion. An **incarcerated** hernia is one in which the intestines become trapped in the hernia. A **strangulated** hernia is one in which the blood supply to the intestines is lost. **Hiatal hernia** occurs when a loop of the stomach protrudes upward through the small opening in the diaphragm through which the esophagus passes, leaving the abdominal cavity and entering the chest. It occurs in both sexes.

Figure 11-9 Inguinal hernias are those that are located in the inguinal or iliac areas of the abdomen.

   ● **K40.3 Unilateral inguinal hernia, with obstruction, without gangrene**
         Inguinal hernia (unilateral) causing obstruction without
             gangrene
         Incarcerated inguinal hernia (unilateral) without
             gangrene
         Irreducible inguinal hernia (unilateral) without gangrene
         Strangulated inguinal hernia (unilateral) without
             gangrene
     K40.30 Unilateral inguinal hernia, with obstruction, without gangrene, not specified as recurrent
         Inguinal hernia, with obstruction NOS
         Unilateral inguinal hernia, with obstruction,
             without gangrene NOS
     K40.31 Unilateral inguinal hernia, with obstruction, without gangrene, recurrent
   ● **K40.4 Unilateral inguinal hernia, with gangrene**
     K40.40 Unilateral inguinal hernia, with gangrene, not specified as recurrent
         Inguinal hernia with gangrene NOS
         Unilateral inguinal hernia with gangrene NOS
     K40.41 Unilateral inguinal hernia, with gangrene, recurrent
   ● **K40.9 Unilateral inguinal hernia, without obstruction or gangrene**
     K40.90 Unilateral inguinal hernia, without obstruction or gangrene, not specified as recurrent
         Inguinal hernia NOS
         Unilateral inguinal hernia NOS
     K40.91 Unilateral inguinal hernia, without obstruction or gangrene, recurrent

---

▶ New   ⇢ Revised   ~~deleted~~ Deleted   **OGCR** Official Guidelines   X Assign placeholder X   ● Use Additional Character(s)

Excludes 1   Excludes 2   Includes   Use additional   Code first   Code also   Key words

● **K41**   **Femoral hernia**

  ● **K41.0**   **Bilateral femoral hernia, with obstruction, without gangrene**

    Femoral hernia (bilateral) causing obstruction, without gangrene

    Incarcerated femoral hernia (bilateral), without gangrene

    Irreducible femoral hernia (bilateral), without gangrene

    Strangulated femoral hernia (bilateral), without gangrene

    K41.00   **Bilateral femoral hernia, with obstruction, without gangrene, not specified as recurrent**

      Bilateral femoral hernia, with obstruction, without gangrene NOS

    K41.01   **Bilateral femoral hernia, with obstruction, without gangrene, recurrent**

  ● **K41.1**   **Bilateral femoral hernia, with gangrene**

    K41.10   **Bilateral femoral hernia, with gangrene, not specified as recurrent**

      Bilateral femoral hernia, with gangrene NOS

    K41.11   **Bilateral femoral hernia, with gangrene, recurrent**

  ● **K41.2**   **Bilateral femoral hernia, without obstruction or gangrene**

    K41.20   **Bilateral femoral hernia, without obstruction or gangrene, not specified as recurrent**

      Bilateral femoral hernia NOS

    K41.21   **Bilateral femoral hernia, without obstruction or gangrene, recurrent**

  ● **K41.3**   **Unilateral femoral hernia, with obstruction, without gangrene**

    Femoral hernia (unilateral) causing obstruction, without gangrene

    Incarcerated femoral hernia (unilateral), without gangrene

    Irreducible femoral hernia (unilateral), without gangrene

    Strangulated femoral hernia (unilateral), without gangrene

    K41.30   **Unilateral femoral hernia, with obstruction, without gangrene, not specified as recurrent**

      Femoral hernia, with obstruction NOS

      Unilateral femoral hernia, with obstruction NOS

    K41.31   **Unilateral femoral hernia, with obstruction, without gangrene, recurrent**

  ● **K41.4**   **Unilateral femoral hernia, with gangrene**

    K41.40   **Unilateral femoral hernia, with gangrene, not specified as recurrent**

      Femoral hernia, with gangrene NOS

      Unilateral femoral hernia, with gangrene NOS

    K41.41   **Unilateral femoral hernia, with gangrene, recurrent**

  ● **K41.9**   **Unilateral femoral hernia, without obstruction or gangrene**

    K41.90   **Unilateral femoral hernia, without obstruction or gangrene, not specified as recurrent**

      Femoral hernia NOS

      Unilateral femoral hernia NOS

    K41.91   **Unilateral femoral hernia, without obstruction or gangrene, recurrent**

● **K42**   **Umbilical hernia**

    Includes   paraumbilical hernia

    Excludes1   omphalocele (Q79.2)

  K42.0   **Umbilical hernia with obstruction, without gangrene**

    Umbilical hernia causing obstruction, without gangrene

    Incarcerated umbilical hernia, without gangrene

    Irreducible umbilical hernia, without gangrene

    Strangulated umbilical hernia, without gangrene

  K42.1   **Umbilical hernia with gangrene**

    Gangrenous umbilical hernia

  K42.9   **Umbilical hernia without obstruction or gangrene**

    Umbilical hernia NOS

● **K43**   **Ventral hernia**

  K43.0   **Incisional hernia with obstruction, without gangrene**

    Incisional hernia causing obstruction, without gangrene

    Incarcerated incisional hernia, without gangrene

    Irreducible incisional hernia, without gangrene

    Strangulated incisional hernia, without gangrene

  K43.1   **Incisional hernia with gangrene**

    Gangrenous incisional hernia

  K43.2   **Incisional hernia without obstruction or gangrene**

    Incisional hernia NOS

  K43.3   **Parastomal hernia with obstruction, without gangrene**

    Incarcerated parastomal hernia, without gangrene

    Irreducible parastomal hernia, without gangrene

    Parastomal hernia causing obstruction, without gangrene

    Strangulated parastomal hernia, without gangrene

  K43.4   **Parastomal hernia with gangrene**

    Gangrenous parastomal hernia

  K43.5   **Parastomal hernia without obstruction or gangrene**

    Parastomal hernia NOS

  K43.6   **Other and unspecified ventral hernia with obstruction, without gangrene**

    Epigastric hernia causing obstruction, without gangrene

    Hypogastric hernia causing obstruction, without gangrene

    Incarcerated epigastric hernia without gangrene

    Incarcerated hypogastric hernia without gangrene

    Incarcerated midline hernia without gangrene

    Incarcerated spigelian hernia without gangrene

    Incarcerated subxiphoid hernia without gangrene

    Irreducible epigastric hernia without gangrene

    Irreducible hypogastric hernia without gangrene

    Irreducible midline hernia without gangrene

    Irreducible spigelian hernia without gangrene

    Irreducible subxiphoid hernia without gangrene

    Midline hernia causing obstruction, without gangrene

    Spigelian hernia causing obstruction, without gangrene

    Strangulated epigastric hernia without gangrene

    Strangulated hypogastric hernia without gangrene

    Strangulated midline hernia without gangrene

    Strangulated spigelian hernia without gangrene

    Strangulated subxiphoid hernia without gangrene

    Subxiphoid hernia causing obstruction, without gangrene

  K43.7   **Other and unspecified ventral hernia with gangrene**

    Any condition listed under K43.6 specified as gangrenous

  K43.9   **Ventral hernia without obstruction or gangrene**

    Epigastric hernia

    Ventral hernia NOS

● **K44**   **Diaphragmatic hernia**

    Includes   hiatus hernia (esophageal) (sliding)

      paraesophageal hernia

    Excludes1   congenital diaphragmatic hernia (Q79.0)

      congenital hiatus hernia (Q40.1)

  K44.0   **Diaphragmatic hernia with obstruction, without gangrene**

    Diaphragmatic hernia causing obstruction

    Incarcerated diaphragmatic hernia

    Irreducible diaphragmatic hernia

    Strangulated diaphragmatic hernia

  K44.1   **Diaphragmatic hernia with gangrene**

    Gangrenous diaphragmatic hernia

  K44.9   **Diaphragmatic hernia without obstruction or gangrene**

    Diaphragmatic hernia NOS

● **K45   Other abdominal hernia**
         Includes   abdominal hernia, specified site NEC
                           lumbar hernia
                           obturator hernia
                           pudendal hernia
                           retroperitoneal hernia
                           sciatic hernia
    K45.0   Other specified abdominal hernia with obstruction, without gangrene
                 Other specified abdominal hernia causing obstruction
                 Other specified incarcerated abdominal hernia
                 Other specified irreducible abdominal hernia
                 Other specified strangulated abdominal hernia
    K45.1   Other specified abdominal hernia with gangrene
                 Any condition listed under K45 specified as gangrenous
    K45.8   Other specified abdominal hernia without obstruction or gangrene

● **K46   Unspecified abdominal hernia**
         Includes   enterocele
                           epiplocele
                           hernia NOS
                           interstitial hernia
                           intestinal hernia
                           intra-abdominal hernia
         Excludes1   vaginal enterocele (N81.5)
    K46.0   Unspecified abdominal hernia with obstruction, without gangrene
                 Unspecified abdominal hernia causing obstruction
                 Unspecified incarcerated abdominal hernia
                 Unspecified irreducible abdominal hernia
                 Unspecified strangulated abdominal hernia
    K46.1   Unspecified abdominal hernia with gangrene
                 Any condition listed under K46 specified as gangrenous
    K46.9   Unspecified abdominal hernia without obstruction or gangrene
                 Abdominal hernia NOS

★ **(See Plate 284 on page 77.)**

NONINFECTIVE ENTERITIS AND COLITIS (K50-K52)

         Includes   noninfective inflammatory bowel disease
         Excludes1   irritable bowel syndrome (K58.-)
                           megacolon (K59.3-)

● **K50   Crohn's disease [regional enteritis]**
         Includes   granulomatous enteritis
         Use additional code to identify manifestations, such as:
         pyoderma gangrenosum (L88)
         Excludes1   ulcerative colitis (K51.-)
    ● **K50.0   Crohn's disease of small intestine**
                 Crohn's disease [regional enteritis] of duodenum
                 Crohn's disease [regional enteritis] of ileum
                 Crohn's disease [regional enteritis] of jejunum
                 Regional ileitis
                 Terminal ileitis
                 Excludes1   Crohn's disease of both small and large
                                 intestine (K50.8-)
         K50.00   Crohn's disease of small intestine without complications
       ● **K50.01   Crohn's disease of small intestine with complications**
                 K50.011   Crohn's disease of small intestine with rectal bleeding
                 K50.012   Crohn's disease of small intestine with intestinal obstruction
                 K50.013   Crohn's disease of small intestine with fistula
                 K50.014   Crohn's disease of small intestine with abscess
                 K50.018   Crohn's disease of small intestine with other complication
                 K50.019   Crohn's disease of small intestine with unspecified complications

Item 11–12 Crohn's disease, also known as **regional enteritis,** is a chronic inflammatory disease of the intestines. Classification is based on location in the small (duodenum, ileum, jejunum) or large (cecum, colon, rectum, anal canal) intestine.

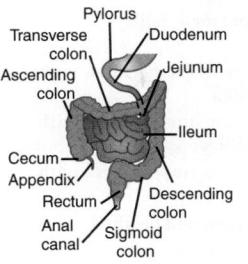

Figure 11-10 Small and large intestines.

● **K50.1   Crohn's disease of large intestine**
                 Crohn's disease [regional enteritis] of colon
                 Crohn's disease [regional enteritis] of large bowel
                 Crohn's disease [regional enteritis] of rectum
                 Granulomatous colitis
                 Regional colitis
         Excludes1   Crohn's disease of both small and large
                         intestine (K50.8)
         K50.10   Crohn's disease of large intestine without complications
       ● **K50.11   Crohn's disease of large intestine with complications**
                 K50.111   Crohn's disease of large intestine with rectal bleeding
                 K50.112   Crohn's disease of large intestine with intestinal obstruction
                 K50.113   Crohn's disease of large intestine with fistula
                 K50.114   Crohn's disease of large intestine with abscess
                 K50.118   Crohn's disease of large intestine with other complication
                 K50.119   Crohn's disease of large intestine with unspecified complications
    ● **K50.8   Crohn's disease of both small and large intestine**
         K50.80   Crohn's disease of both small and large intestine without complications
       ● **K50.81   Crohn's disease of both small and large intestine with complications**
                 K50.811   Crohn's disease of both small and large intestine with rectal bleeding
                 K50.812   Crohn's disease of both small and large intestine with intestinal obstruction
                 K50.813   Crohn's disease of both small and large intestine with fistula
                 K50.814   Crohn's disease of both small and large intestine with abscess
                 K50.818   Crohn's disease of both small and large intestine with other complication
                 K50.819   Crohn's disease of both small and large intestine with unspecified complications

● **K50.9 Crohn's disease, unspecified**

    K50.90 Crohn's disease, unspecified, without complications
        Crohn's disease NOS
        Regional enteritis NOS

    ● **K50.91 Crohn's disease, unspecified, with complications**

        K50.911 Crohn's disease, unspecified, with rectal bleeding

        K50.912 Crohn's disease, unspecified, with intestinal obstruction

        K50.913 Crohn's disease, unspecified, with fistula

        K50.914 Crohn's disease, unspecified, with abscess

        K50.918 Crohn's disease, unspecified, with other complication

        K50.919 Crohn's disease, unspecified, with unspecified complications

● **K51 Ulcerative colitis**

    Use additional code to identify manifestations, such as: pyoderma gangrenosum (L88)

    Excludes1 Crohn's disease [regional enteritis] (K50.-)

    ● **K51.0 Ulcerative (chronic) pancolitis**
        Backwash ileitis

        K51.00 Ulcerative (chronic) pancolitis without complications
            Ulcerative (chronic) pancolitis NOS

        ● **K51.01 Ulcerative (chronic) pancolitis with complications**

            K51.011 Ulcerative (chronic) pancolitis with rectal bleeding

            K51.012 Ulcerative (chronic) pancolitis with intestinal obstruction

            K51.013 Ulcerative (chronic) pancolitis with fistula

            K51.014 Ulcerative (chronic) pancolitis with abscess

            K51.018 Ulcerative (chronic) pancolitis with other complication

            K51.019 Ulcerative (chronic) pancolitis with unspecified complications

    ● **K51.2 Ulcerative (chronic) proctitis**

        K51.20 Ulcerative (chronic) proctitis without complications
            Ulcerative (chronic) proctitis NOS

        ● **K51.21 Ulcerative (chronic) proctitis with complications**

            K51.211 Ulcerative (chronic) proctitis with rectal bleeding

            K51.212 Ulcerative (chronic) proctitis with intestinal obstruction

            K51.213 Ulcerative (chronic) proctitis with fistula

            K51.214 Ulcerative (chronic) proctitis with abscess

            K51.218 Ulcerative (chronic) proctitis with other complication

            K51.219 Ulcerative (chronic) proctitis with unspecified complications

● **K51.3 Ulcerative (chronic) rectosigmoiditis**

    K51.30 Ulcerative (chronic) rectosigmoiditis without complications
        Ulcerative (chronic) rectosigmoiditis NOS

    ● **K51.31 Ulcerative (chronic) rectosigmoiditis with complications**

        K51.311 Ulcerative (chronic) rectosigmoiditis with rectal bleeding

        K51.312 Ulcerative (chronic) rectosigmoiditis with intestinal obstruction

        K51.313 Ulcerative (chronic) rectosigmoiditis with fistula

        K51.314 Ulcerative (chronic) rectosigmoiditis with abscess

        K51.318 Ulcerative (chronic) rectosigmoiditis with other complication

        K51.319 Ulcerative (chronic) rectosigmoiditis with unspecified complications

● **K51.4 Inflammatory polyps of colon**

    Excludes1 adenomatous polyp of colon (D12.6)
               polyposis of colon (D12.6)
               polyps of colon NOS (K63.5)

    K51.40 Inflammatory polyps of colon without complications
        Inflammatory polyps of colon NOS

    ● **K51.41 Inflammatory polyps of colon with complications**

        K51.411 Inflammatory polyps of colon with rectal bleeding

        K51.412 Inflammatory polyps of colon with intestinal obstruction

        K51.413 Inflammatory polyps of colon with fistula

        K51.414 Inflammatory polyps of colon with abscess

        K51.418 Inflammatory polyps of colon with other complication

        K51.419 Inflammatory polyps of colon with unspecified complications

● **K51.5 Left sided colitis**
    Left hemicolitis

    K51.50 Left sided colitis without complications
        Left sided colitis NOS

    ● **K51.51 Left sided colitis with complications**

        K51.511 Left sided colitis with rectal bleeding

        K51.512 Left sided colitis with intestinal obstruction

        K51.513 Left sided colitis with fistula

        K51.514 Left sided colitis with abscess

        K51.518 Left sided colitis with other complication

        K51.519 Left sided colitis with unspecified complications

● **K51.8 Other ulcerative colitis**

    K51.80 Other ulcerative colitis without complications

    ● **K51.81 Other ulcerative colitis with complications**

        K51.811 Other ulcerative colitis with rectal bleeding

        K51.812 Other ulcerative colitis with intestinal obstruction

        K51.813 Other ulcerative colitis with fistula

        K51.814 Other ulcerative colitis with abscess

        K51.818 Other ulcerative colitis with other complication

        K51.819 Other ulcerative colitis with unspecified complications

Item 11-13 Ulcerative colitis attacks the colonic mucosa and forms abscesses. The disease involves the intestines. Classification is based on the location:
- Enterocolitis: large and small intestine
- Ileocolitis: ileum and colon
- Proctitis: rectum
- Proctosigmoiditis: sigmoid colon and rectum

▶ New   ⇒ Revised   ~~deleted~~ Deleted   **OGCR** Official Guidelines   X Assign placeholder X   ● Use Additional Character(s)

Excludes 1   Excludes 2   Includes   Use additional   Code first   Code also   Key words

● **K51.9**   Ulcerative colitis, unspecified

     K51.90   Ulcerative colitis, unspecified, without complications

    ● **K51.91**   Ulcerative colitis, unspecified, with complications

       K51.911   Ulcerative colitis, unspecified with rectal bleeding

       K51.912   Ulcerative colitis, unspecified with intestinal obstruction

       K51.913   Ulcerative colitis, unspecified with fistula

       K51.914   Ulcerative colitis, unspecified with abscess

       K51.918   Ulcerative colitis, unspecified with other complication

       K51.919   Ulcerative colitis, unspecified with unspecified complications

● **K52**   Other and unspecified noninfective gastroenteritis and colitis

     K52.0   Gastroenteritis and colitis due to radiation

     K52.1   Toxic gastroenteritis and colitis

       Drug-induced gastroenteritis and colitis

       Code first (T51-T65) to identify toxic agent

       Use additional code for adverse effect, if applicable, to identify drug (T36-T50 with fifth or sixth character 5)

    ● **K52.2**   Allergic and dietetic gastroenteritis and colitis

       Food hypersensitivity gastroenteritis or colitis

       Use additional code to identify type of food allergy (Z91.01-, Z91.02-)

       | Excludes2 | allergic eosinophilic colitis (K52.82)
                           allergic eosinophilic esophagitis (K20.0)
                           allergic eosinophilic gastritis (K52.81)
                           allergic eosinophilic gastroenteritis (K52.81)
                           food protein-induced proctocolitis (K52.82)

       K52.21   Food protein-induced enterocolitis syndrome

          Use additional code for hypovolemic shock, if present (R57.1)

       K52.22   Food protein-induced enteropathy

       K52.29   Other allergic and dietetic gastroenteritis and colitis

          Food hypersensitivity gastroenteritis or colitis

          Immediate gastrointestinal hypersensitivity

     K52.3   Indeterminate colitis

       Colonic inflammatory bowel disease unclassified (IBDU)

       | Excludes1 | unspecified colitis (K52.9)

    ● **K52.8**   Other specified noninfective gastroenteritis and colitis

       K52.81   Eosinophilic gastritis or gastroenteritis

          Eosinophilic enteritis

          | Excludes2 | eosinophilic esophagitis (K20.0)

       K52.82   Eosinophilic colitis

          Allergic proctocolitis

          Food-induced eosinophilic proctocolitis

          Food protein-induced proctocolitis

          Milk protein-induced proctocolitis

     K52.83   Microscopic colitis

       K52.831   Collagenous colitis

       K52.832   Lymphocytic colitis

       K52.838   Other microscopic colitis

       K52.839   Microscopic colitis, unspecified

     K52.89   Other specified noninfective gastroenteritis and colitis

     K52.9   Noninfective gastroenteritis and colitis, unspecified

       Colitis NOS   Ileitis NOS

       Enteritis NOS   Jejunitis NOS

       Gastroenteritis NOS   Sigmoiditis NOS

       | Excludes1 | diarrhea NOS (R19.7)
                          functional diarrhea (K59.1)
                          infectious gastroenteritis and colitis NOS (A09)
                          neonatal diarrhea (noninfective) (P78.3)
                          psychogenic diarrhea (F45.8)

OTHER DISEASES OF INTESTINES (K55-K64)

● **K55**   Vascular disorders of intestine

     | Excludes1 | necrotizing enterocolitis of newborn (P77.-)

    ● **K55.0**   Acute vascular disorders of intestine

       Infarction of appendices epiploicae

       Mesenteric (artery) (vein) embolism

       Mesenteric (artery) (vein) infarction

       Mesenteric (artery) (vein) thrombosis

    ● **K55.01**   Acute (reversible) ischemia of small intestine

       K55.011   Focal (segmental) acute (reversible) ischemia of small intestine

       K55.012   Diffuse acute (reversible) ischemia of small intestine

       K55.019   Acute (reversible) ischemia of small intestine, extent unspecified

    ● **K55.02**   Acute infarction of small intestine

       Gangrene of small intestine

       Necrosis of small intestine

       K55.021   Focal (segmental) acute infarction of small intestine

       K55.022   Diffuse acute infarction of small intestine

       K55.029   Acute infarction of small intestine, extent unspecified

    ● **K55.03**   Acute (reversible) ischemia of large intestine

       Acute fulminant ischemic colitis

       Subacute ischemic colitis

       K55.031   Focal (segmental) acute (reversible) ischemia of large intestine

       K55.032   Diffuse acute (reversible) ischemia of large intestine

       K55.039   Acute (reversible) ischemia of large intestine, extent unspecified

    ● **K55.04**   Acute infarction of large intestine

       Gangrene of large intestine

       Necrosis of large intestine

       K55.041   Focal (segmental) acute infarction of large intestine

       K55.042   Diffuse acute infarction of large intestine

       K55.049   Acute infarction of large intestine, extent unspecified

CHAPTER 11 (K00-K95)

● **K55.05 Acute (reversible) ischemia of intestine, part unspecified**

    K55.051 Focal (segmental) acute (reversible) ischemia of intestine, part unspecified

    K55.052 Diffuse acute (reversible) ischemia of intestine, part unspecified

    K55.059 Acute (reversible) ischemia of intestine, part and extent unspecified

● **K55.06 Acute infarction of intestine, part unspecified**
    Acute intestinal infarction
    Gangrene of intestine
    Necrosis of intestine

    K55.061 Focal (segmental) acute infarction of intestine, part unspecified

    K55.062 Diffuse acute infarction of intestine, part unspecified

    K55.069 Acute infarction of intestine, part and extent unspecified

K55.1 Chronic vascular disorders of intestine
    Chronic ischemic colitis
    Chronic ischemic enteritis
    Chronic ischemic enterocolitis
    Ischemic stricture of intestine
    Mesenteric atherosclerosis
    Mesenteric vascular insufficiency

● **K55.2 Angiodysplasia of colon**

    K55.20 Angiodysplasia of colon without hemorrhage

    K55.21 Angiodysplasia of colon with hemorrhage

● **K55.3 Necrotizing enterocolitis**

    Excludes1   necrotizing enterocolitis of newborn (P77.-)

    Excludes2   necrotizing enterocolitis due to Clostridium difficile (A04.7-)

    K55.30 Necrotizing enterocolitis, unspecified
      Necrotizing enterocolitis, NOS

    K55.31 Stage 1 necrotizing enterocolitis
      Necrotizing enterocolitis without pneumatosis, without perforation

    K55.32 Stage 2 necrotizing enterocolitis
      Necrotizing enterocolitis with pneumatosis, without perforation

    K55.33 Stage 3 necrotizing enterocolitis
      Necrotizing enterocolitis with perforation
      Necrotizing enterocolitis with pneumatosis and perforation

K55.8 Other vascular disorders of intestine

K55.9 Vascular disorder of intestine, unspecified
    Ischemic colitis
    Ischemic enteritis
    Ischemic enterocolitis

● **K56 Paralytic ileus and intestinal obstruction without hernia**

    Excludes1   congenital stricture or stenosis of intestine (Q41-Q42)
      cystic fibrosis with meconium ileus (E84.11)
      ischemic stricture of intestine (K55.1)
      meconium ileus NOS (P76.0)
      neonatal intestinal obstructions classifiable to P76.-
      obstruction of duodenum (K31.5)
      postprocedural intestinal obstruction (K91.3-)
      stenosis of anus or rectum (K62.4)
      ~~intestinal obstruction with hernia (K40-K46)~~

K56.0 Paralytic ileus
    Paralysis of bowel
    Paralysis of colon
    Paralysis of intestine

    Excludes1   gallstone ileus (K56.3)
      ileus NOS (K56.7)
      obstructive ileus NOS (K56.69-)

Figure 11-11   Types of intussusception.

Item 11–14 Intussusception is the prolapse (telescoping) of a part of the intestine into another adjacent part of the intestine. Intussusception may be enteric (ileoileal, jejunoileal, jejunojejunal), colic (colocolic), or intracolic (ileocecal, ileocolic).

Item 11–15 Volvulus is the twisting of a segment of the intestine, resulting in obstruction. Paralytic ileus is paralysis of the intestine. It need not be a complete paralysis, but it must prohibit the passage of food through the intestine and lead to intestinal blockage. It is a common aftermath of some types of surgery.

K56.1 Intussusception
    Intussusception or invagination of bowel
    Intussusception or invagination of colon
    Intussusception or invagination of intestine
    Intussusception or invagination of rectum

    Excludes2   intussusception of appendix (K38.8)

K56.2 Volvulus
    Strangulation of colon or intestine
    Torsion of colon or intestine
    Twist of colon or intestine

    Excludes2   volvulus of duodenum (K31.5)

K56.3 Gallstone ileus
    Obstruction of intestine by gallstone

● **K56.4 Other impaction of intestine**

    K56.41 Fecal impaction

      Excludes1   constipation (K59.0-)
        incomplete defecation (R15.0)

    K56.49 Other impaction of intestine

● **K56.5 Intestinal adhesions [bands] with obstruction (postinfection)**
    Abdominal hernia due to adhesions with obstruction
    Peritoneal adhesions [bands] with intestinal obstruction (postinfection)

    ▶ **K56.50 Intestinal adhesions [bands], unspecified as to partial versus complete obstruction**
      ▶ Intestinal adhesions with obstruction NOS

    ▶ **K56.51 Intestinal adhesions [bands], with partial obstruction**
      ▶ Intestinal adhesions with incomplete obstruction

    ▶ **K56.52 Intestinal adhesions [bands] with complete obstruction**

▶ New   ➡ Revised   ~~deleted~~ Deleted   **OGCR** Official Guidelines   X Assign placeholder X   ● Use Additional Character(s)

Excludes 1   Excludes 2   Includes   Use additional   Code first   Code also   Key words

● **K56.6   Other and unspecified intestinal obstruction**
    ● **K56.60   Unspecified intestinal obstruction**
       ~~Intestinal obstruction NOS~~
       | Excludes1 | intestinal obstruction due to specified condition-code to condition

       ▶ **K56.600   Partial intestinal obstruction, unspecified as to cause**
          ▶Incomplete intestinal obstruction, NOS

       ▶ **K56.601   Complete intestinal obstruction, unspecified as to cause**

       ▶ **K56.609   Unspecified intestinal obstruction, unspecified as to partial versus complete obstruction**
          ▶Intestinal obstruction NOS

    ● **K56.69   Other intestinal obstruction**
       Enterostenosis NOS
       Obstructive ileus NOS
       Occlusion of colon or intestine NOS
       Stenosis of colon or intestine NOS
       Stricture of colon or intestine NOS
       | Excludes1 | intestinal obstruction due to specified condition-code to condition

       ▶ **K56.690   Other partial intestinal obstruction**
          ▶Other incomplete intestinal obstruction

       ▶ **K56.691   Other complete intestinal obstruction**

       ▶ **K56.699   Other intestinal obstruction unspecified as to partial versus complete obstruction**
          ▶Other intestinal obstruction, NEC

   K56.7   Ileus, unspecified
       ⇒| Excludes1 | obstructive ileus (K56.69-)
       ▶| Excludes2 | intestinal obstruction with hernia (K40-K46)

● **K57   Diverticular disease of intestine**
       | Excludes1 | congenital diverticulum of intestine (Q43.8)
                  Meckel's diverticulum (Q43.0)
       | Excludes2 | diverticulum of appendix (K38.2)

   ● **K57.0   Diverticulitis of small intestine with perforation and abscess**
       Diverticulitis of small intestine with peritonitis
       | Excludes1 | diverticulitis of both small and large intestine with perforation and abscess (K57.4-)

      K57.00   Diverticulitis of small intestine with perforation and abscess without bleeding

      K57.01   Diverticulitis of small intestine with perforation and abscess with bleeding

   ● **K57.1   Diverticular disease of small intestine without perforation or abscess**
       | Excludes1 | diverticular disease of both small and large intestine without perforation or abscess (K57.5-)

      K57.10   Diverticulosis of small intestine without perforation or abscess without bleeding
       Diverticular disease of small intestine NOS

      K57.11   Diverticulosis of small intestine without perforation or abscess with bleeding

      K57.12   Diverticulitis of small intestine without perforation or abscess without bleeding

      K57.13   Diverticulitis of small intestine without perforation or abscess with bleeding

Figure 11-12   Diverticulosis. (From Shiland: Mastering Healthcare Terminology, ed 4, St. Louis, Mosby, 2012)

Item 11–16   Diverticula of the intestines are acquired herniations of the mucosa. Diverticulum (singular): Pocket or pouch that bulges outward through a weak spot (herniation) in the colon. Diverticula (plural). **Diverticulosis** is the condition of having diverticula. **Diverticulitis** is inflammation of these pouches or herniations. Classification is based on location (small intestine or colon) and whether it occurs with or without hemorrhage.

   ● **K57.2   Diverticulitis of large intestine with perforation and abscess**
       Diverticulitis of colon with peritonitis
       | Excludes1 | diverticulitis of both small and large intestine with perforation and abscess (K57.4-)

      K57.20   Diverticulitis of large intestine with perforation and abscess without bleeding

      K57.21   Diverticulitis of large intestine with perforation and abscess with bleeding

   ● **K57.3   Diverticular disease of large intestine without perforation or abscess**
       | Excludes1 | diverticular disease of both small and large intestine without perforation or abscess (K57.5-)

      K57.30   Diverticulosis of large intestine without perforation or abscess without bleeding
       Diverticular disease of colon NOS

      K57.31   Diverticulosis of large intestine without perforation or abscess with bleeding

      K57.32   Diverticulitis of large intestine without perforation or abscess without bleeding

      K57.33   Diverticulitis of large intestine without perforation or abscess with bleeding

   ● **K57.4   Diverticulitis of both small and large intestine with perforation and abscess**
       Diverticulitis of both small and large intestine with peritonitis

      K57.40   Diverticulitis of both small and large intestine with perforation and abscess without bleeding

      K57.41   Diverticulitis of both small and large intestine with perforation and abscess with bleeding

   ● **K57.5   Diverticular disease of both small and large intestine without perforation or abscess**

      K57.50   Diverticulosis of both small and large intestine without perforation or abscess without bleeding
       Diverticular disease of both small and large intestine NOS

      K57.51   Diverticulosis of both small and large intestine without perforation or abscess with bleeding

      K57.52   Diverticulitis of both small and large intestine without perforation or abscess without bleeding

      K57.53   Diverticulitis of both small and large intestine without perforation or abscess with bleeding

▶ New   ⇒ Revised   ~~deleted~~ Deleted   **OGCR** Official Guidelines   **X** Assign placeholder X   ● Use Additional Character(s)

| Excludes 1 | | Excludes 2 | | Includes | | Use additional | | Code first | | Code also | | Key words |

905

CHAPTER 11 (K00-K95)

● **K57.8 Diverticulitis of intestine, part unspecified, with perforation and abscess**
Diverticulitis of intestine NOS with peritonitis

     K57.80 Diverticulitis of intestine, part unspecified, with perforation and abscess without bleeding

     K57.81 Diverticulitis of intestine, part unspecified, with perforation and abscess with bleeding

● **K57.9 Diverticular disease of intestine, part unspecified, without perforation or abscess**

     K57.90 Diverticulosis of intestine, part unspecified, without perforation or abscess without bleeding
Diverticular disease of intestine NOS

     K57.91 Diverticulosis of intestine, part unspecified, without perforation or abscess with bleeding

     K57.92 Diverticulitis of intestine, part unspecified, without perforation or abscess without bleeding

     K57.93 Diverticulitis of intestine, part unspecified, without perforation or abscess with bleeding

● **K58 Irritable bowel syndrome**
     Includes   irritable colon
                 spastic colon

     K58.0 Irritable bowel syndrome with diarrhea

     K58.1 Irritable bowel syndrome with constipation

     K58.2 Mixed irritable bowel syndrome

     K58.8 Other irritable bowel syndrome

     K58.9 Irritable bowel syndrome without diarrhea
Irritable bowel syndrome NOS

● **K59 Other functional intestinal disorders**
     Excludes1   change in bowel habit NOS (R19.4)
                 intestinal malabsorption (K90.-)
                 psychogenic intestinal disorders (F45.8)
     Excludes2   functional disorders of stomach (K31.-)

● **K59.0 Constipation**
     Use additional code for adverse effect, if applicable, to identify drug (T36-T50 with fifth or sixth character 5)
     Excludes1   fecal impaction (K56.41)
                 incomplete defecation (R15.0)

     K59.00 Constipation, unspecified

     K59.01 Slow transit constipation

     K59.02 Outlet dysfunction constipation

     K59.03 Drug induced constipation
        Use additional code for adverse effect, if applicable, to identify drug (T36-T50 with fifth or sixth character 5)

     K59.04 Chronic idiopathic constipation
Functional constipation

     K59.09 Other constipation
Chronic constipation

   K59.1 Functional diarrhea
     Excludes1   diarrhea NOS (R19.7)
                 irritable bowel syndrome with diarrhea (K58.0)

   K59.2 Neurogenic bowel, not elsewhere classified

● **K59.3 Megacolon, not elsewhere classified**
Dilatation of colon
Code first, if applicable (T51-T65) to identify toxic agent
     Excludes1   congenital megacolon (aganglionic) (Q43.1)
                 megacolon (due to) (in) Chagas' disease (B57.32)
       ⇒ megacolon (due to) (in) Clostridium difficile (A04.7-)
                 megacolon (due to) (in) Hirschsprung's disease (Q43.1)

     K59.31 Toxic megacolon

     K59.39 Other megacolon
Megacolon NOS

   K59.4 Anal spasm
Proctalgia fugax

   K59.8 Other specified functional intestinal disorders
Atony of colon Pseudo-obstruction (acute) (chronic) of intestine

   K59.9 Functional intestinal disorder, unspecified

● **K60 Fissure and fistula of anal and rectal regions**
     Excludes1   fissure and fistula of anal and rectal regions with abscess or cellulitis (K61.-)
     Excludes2   anal sphincter tear (healed) (nontraumatic) (old) (K62.81)

   K60.0 Acute anal fissure

   K60.1 Chronic anal fissure

   K60.2 Anal fissure, unspecified

   K60.3 Anal fistula

   K60.4 Rectal fistula
Fistula of rectum to skin
     Excludes1   rectovaginal fistula (N82.3)
                 vesicorectal fistula (N32.1)

   K60.5 Anorectal fistula

● **K61 Abscess of anal and rectal regions**
     Includes   abscess of anal and rectal regions
                 cellulitis of anal and rectal regions

   K61.0 Anal abscess
Perianal abscess
     Excludes1   intrasphincteric abscess (K61.4)

   K61.1 Rectal abscess
Perirectal abscess
     Excludes1   ischiorectal abscess (K61.3)

   K61.2 Anorectal abscess

   K61.3 Ischiorectal abscess
Abscess of ischiorectal fossa

   K61.4 Intrasphincteric abscess

● **K62 Other diseases of anus and rectum**
     Includes   anal canal
     Excludes2   colostomy and enterostomy malfunction (K94.0-, K91.4-)
                 fecal incontinence (R15.-)
                 hemorrhoids (K64.-)

   K62.0 Anal polyp

   K62.1 Rectal polyp
     Excludes1   adenomatous polyp (D12.8)

   K62.2 Anal prolapse
Prolapse of anal canal

   K62.3 Rectal prolapse
Prolapse of rectal mucosa

   K62.4 Stenosis of anus and rectum
Stricture of anus (sphincter)

   K62.5 Hemorrhage of anus and rectum
     Excludes1   gastrointestinal bleeding NOS (K92.2)
                 melena (K92.1)
                 neonatal rectal hemorrhage (P54.2)

Item 11-17 A **fissure** is a groove in the surface, whereas a **fistula** is an abnormal passage. An **abscess** is an accumulation of pus in a tissue cavity resulting from a bacterial or parasitic infection.

▶ New   ⇒ Revised   ~~deleted~~ Deleted   **OGCR** Official Guidelines   X Assign placeholder X   ● Use Additional Character(s)
Excludes 1   Excludes 2   Includes   Use additional   Code first   Code also   Key words

K62.6 Ulcer of anus and rectum
Solitary ulcer of anus and rectum
Stercoral ulcer of anus and rectum
Excludes1 fissure and fistula of anus and rectum (K60.-)
ulcerative colitis (K51.-)

K62.7 Radiation proctitis
Use additional code to identify the type of radiation (W90.-)

● **K62.8 Other specified diseases of anus and rectum**
Excludes2 ulcerative proctitis (K51.2)

K62.81 Anal sphincter tear (healed) (nontraumatic) (old)
Tear of anus, nontraumatic
Use additional code for any associated fecal incontinence (R15.-)
Excludes2 anal fissure (K60.-)
anal sphincter tear (healed) (old) complicating delivery (O34.7-)
traumatic tear of anal sphincter (S31.831)

K62.82 Dysplasia of anus
Anal intraepithelial neoplasia I and II (AIN I and II) (histologically confirmed)
Dysplasia of anus NOS
Mild and moderate dysplasia of anus (histologically confirmed)
Excludes1 abnormal results from anal cytologic examination without histologic confirmation (R85.61-)
anal intraepithelial neoplasia III (D01.3)
carcinoma in situ of anus (D01.3)
HGSIL of anus (R85.613)
severe dysplasia of anus (D01.3)

K62.89 Other specified diseases of anus and rectum
Proctitis NOS
Use additional code for any associated fecal incontinence (R15.-)

K62.9 Disease of anus and rectum, unspecified

● **K63 Other diseases of intestine**

K63.0 Abscess of intestine
Excludes1 abscess of intestine with Crohn's disease (K50.014, K50.114, K50.814, K50.914)
abscess of intestine with diverticular disease (K57.0, K57.2, K57.4, K57.8)
abscess of intestine with ulcerative colitis (K51.014, K51.214, K51.314, K51.414, K51.514, K51.814, K51.914)
Excludes2 abscess of anal and rectal regions (K61.-)
abscess of appendix (K35.3)

K63.1 Perforation of intestine (nontraumatic)
Perforation (nontraumatic) of rectum
Excludes1 perforation (nontraumatic) of duodenum (K26.-)
perforation (nontraumatic) of intestine with diverticular disease (K57.0, K57.2, K57.4, K57.8)
Excludes2 perforation (nontraumatic) of appendix (K35.2, K35.3)

K63.2 Fistula of intestine
Excludes1 fistula of duodenum (K31.6)
fistula of intestine with Crohn's disease (K50.013, K50.113, K50.813, K50.913)
fistula of intestine with ulcerative colitis (K51.013, K51.213, K51.313, K51.413, K51.513, K51.813, K51.913)
Excludes2 fistula of anal and rectal regions (K60.-)
fistula of appendix (K38.3)
intestinal-genital fistula, female (N82.2-N82.4)
vesicointestinal fistula (N32.1)

K63.3 Ulcer of intestine
Primary ulcer of small intestine
Excludes1 duodenal ulcer (K26.-)
gastrointestinal ulcer (K28.-)
gastrojejunal ulcer (K28.-)
jejunal ulcer (K28.-)
peptic ulcer, site unspecified (K27.-)
ulcer of intestine with perforation (K63.1)
ulcer of anus or rectum (K62.6)
ulcerative colitis (K51.-)

K63.4 Enteroptosis

K63.5 Polyp of colon
Excludes1 adenomatous polyp of colon (D12.6)
inflammatory polyp of colon (K51.4-)
polyposis of colon (D12.6)

● **K63.8 Other specified diseases of intestine**

K63.81 Dieulafoy lesion of intestine
Excludes2 Dieulafoy lesion of stomach and duodenum (K31.82)

K63.89 Other specified diseases of intestine

K63.9 Disease of intestine, unspecified

● **K64 Hemorrhoids and perianal venous thrombosis**
Includes piles
Excludes1 hemorrhoids complicating childbirth and the puerperium (O87.2)
hemorrhoids complicating pregnancy (O22.4)

K64.0 First degree hemorrhoids
Grade/stage I hemorrhoids
Hemorrhoids (bleeding) without prolapse outside of anal canal

K64.1 Second degree hemorrhoids
Grade/stage II hemorrhoids
Hemorrhoids (bleeding) that prolapse with straining, but retract spontaneously

K64.2 Third degree hemorrhoids
Grade/stage III hemorrhoids
Hemorrhoids (bleeding) that prolapse with straining and require manual replacement back inside anal canal

K64.3 Fourth degree hemorrhoids
Grade/stage IV hemorrhoids
Hemorrhoids (bleeding) with prolapsed tissue that cannot be manually replaced

K64.4 Residual hemorrhoidal skin tags
External hemorrhoids, NOS
Skin tags of anus

K64.5 Perianal venous thrombosis
External hemorrhoids with thrombosis
Perianal hematoma
Thrombosed hemorrhoids NOS

K64.8 Other hemorrhoids
Internal hemorrhoids, without mention of degree
Prolapsed hemorrhoids, degree not specified

K64.9 Unspecified hemorrhoids
Hemorrhoids (bleeding) NOS
Hemorrhoids (bleeding) without mention of degree

CHAPTER 11 (K00-K95)

▶ New ⇒ Revised ~~deleted~~ Deleted **OGCR** Official Guidelines X Assign placeholder X ● Use Additional Character(s)
Excludes 1 | Excludes 2 | Includes | Use additional | Code first | Code also | Key words
907

Item 11–18 Peritonitis is an inflammation of the lining (peritoneum) of the abdominal cavity and surface of the intestines.

Item 11–19 Retroperitoneal infections occur between the posterior parietal peritoneum and posterior abdominal wall where the kidneys, adrenal glands, ureters, duodenum, ascending colon, descending colon, pancreas, and the large vessels and nerves are located.

DISEASES OF PERITONEUM AND RETROPERITONEUM (K65-K68)

● **K65 Peritonitis**
Use additional code (B95-B97), to identify infectious agent
Excludes1   acute appendicitis with generalized peritonitis (K35.2)
aseptic peritonitis (T81.6)
benign paroxysmal peritonitis (E85.0)
chemical peritonitis (T81.6)
diverticulitis of both small and large intestine with peritonitis (K57.4-)
diverticulitis of colon with peritonitis (K57.2-)
diverticulitis of intestine, NOS, with peritonitis (K57.8-)
diverticulitis of small intestine with peritonitis (K57.0-)
gonococcal peritonitis (A54.85)
neonatal peritonitis (P78.0-P78.1)
pelvic peritonitis, female (N73.3-N73.5)
periodic familial peritonitis (E85.0)
peritonitis due to talc or other foreign substance (T81.6)
peritonitis in chlamydia (A74.81)
peritonitis in diphtheria (A36.89)
peritonitis in syphilis (late) (A52.74)
peritonitis in tuberculosis (A18.31)
peritonitis with or following abortion or ectopic or molar pregnancy (O00-O07, O08.0)
peritonitis with or following appendicitis (K35.-)
peritonitis with or following diverticular disease of intestine (K57.-)
puerperal peritonitis (O85)
retroperitoneal infections (K68.-)

K65.0 Generalized (acute) peritonitis
Pelvic peritonitis (acute), male
Subphrenic peritonitis (acute)
Suppurative peritonitis (acute)

K65.1 Peritoneal abscess
Abdominopelvic abscess
Abscess (of) omentum
Abscess (of) peritoneum
Mesenteric abscess
Retrocecal abscess
Subdiaphragmatic abscess
Subhepatic abscess
Subphrenic abscess

K65.2 Spontaneous bacterial peritonitis
Excludes1   bacterial peritonitis NOS (K65.9)

K65.3 Choleperitonitis
Peritonitis due to bile

K65.4 Sclerosing mesenteritis
Fat necrosis of peritoneum
(Idiopathic) sclerosing mesenteric fibrosis
Mesenteric lipodystrophy
Mesenteric panniculitis
Retractile mesenteritis

K65.8 Other peritonitis
Chronic proliferative peritonitis
Peritonitis due to urine

K65.9 Peritonitis, unspecified
Bacterial peritonitis NOS

● **K66 Other disorders of peritoneum**
Excludes2   ascites (R18.-)
peritoneal effusion (chronic) (R18.8)

K66.0 Peritoneal adhesions (postprocedural) (postinfection)
Adhesions (of) abdominal (wall)
Adhesions (of) diaphragm
Adhesions (of) intestine
Adhesions (of) male pelvis
Adhesions (of) omentum
Adhesions (of) stomach
Adhesive bands
Mesenteric adhesions
Excludes1   female pelvic adhesions [bands] (N73.6)
➡ peritoneal adhesions with intestinal obstruction (K56.5-)

K66.1 Hemoperitoneum
Excludes1   traumatic hemoperitoneum (S36.8-)

K66.8 Other specified disorders of peritoneum

K66.9 Disorder of peritoneum, unspecified

K67 Disorders of peritoneum in infectious diseases classified elsewhere
Code first underlying disease, such as:
congenital syphilis (A50.0)
helminthiasis (B65.0-B83.9)
Excludes1   peritonitis in chlamydia (A74.81)
peritonitis in diphtheria (A36.89)
peritonitis in gonococcal (A54.85)
peritonitis in syphilis (late) (A52.74)
peritonitis in tuberculosis (A18.31)

● **K68 Disorders of retroperitoneum**
● **K68.1 Retroperitoneal abscess**
K68.11 Postprocedural retroperitoneal abscess
K68.12 Psoas muscle abscess
K68.19 Other retroperitoneal abscess
K68.9 Other disorders of retroperitoneum

DISEASES OF LIVER (K70-K77)

Excludes1   jaundice NOS (R17)
Excludes2   hemochromatosis (E83.11-)
Reye's syndrome (G93.7)
viral hepatitis (B15-B19)
Wilson's disease (E83.0)

● **K70 Alcoholic liver disease**
Use additional code to identify:
alcohol abuse and dependence (F10.-)
K70.0 Alcoholic fatty liver
● **K70.1 Alcoholic hepatitis**
K70.10 Alcoholic hepatitis without ascites
K70.11 Alcoholic hepatitis with ascites
K70.2 Alcoholic fibrosis and sclerosis of liver
● **K70.3 Alcoholic cirrhosis of liver**
Alcoholic cirrhosis NOS
K70.30 Alcoholic cirrhosis of liver without ascites
K70.31 Alcoholic cirrhosis of liver with ascites
● **K70.4 Alcoholic hepatic failure**
Acute alcoholic hepatic failure
Alcoholic hepatic failure NOS
Chronic alcoholic hepatic failure
Subacute alcoholic hepatic failure
K70.40 Alcoholic hepatic failure without coma
K70.41 Alcoholic hepatic failure with coma
K70.9 Alcoholic liver disease, unspecified

Item 11–20 Cirrhosis is the progressive fibrosis of the liver resulting in loss of liver function. The main causes of cirrhosis of the liver are alcohol abuse, chronic hepatitis (inflammation of the liver), biliary disease, and excessive amounts of iron. **Alcoholic cirrhosis of the liver** is also called portal, Laënnec's, or fatty nutritional cirrhosis.

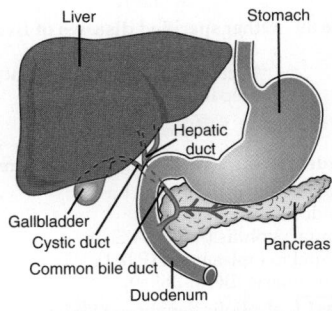

Figure 11-13 Liver and bile ducts.

● **K71 Toxic liver disease**

> **Includes** drug-induced idiosyncratic (unpredictable) liver disease
> drug-induced toxic (predictable) liver disease

> *Code first poisoning due to drug or toxin, if applicable (T36-T65 with fifth or sixth character 1-4 or 6)*

> Use additional code for adverse effect, if applicable, to identify drug (T36-T50 with fifth or sixth character 5)

> **Excludes2** alcoholic liver disease (K70.-)
> Budd-Chiari syndrome (I82.0)

K71.0 Toxic liver disease with cholestasis
> Cholestasis with hepatocyte injury
> 'Pure' cholestasis

● **K71.1 Toxic liver disease with hepatic necrosis**
> Hepatic failure (acute) (chronic) due to drugs

> **K71.10 Toxic liver disease with hepatic necrosis, without coma**

> **K71.11 Toxic liver disease with hepatic necrosis, with coma**

K71.2 Toxic liver disease with acute hepatitis

K71.3 Toxic liver disease with chronic persistent hepatitis

K71.4 Toxic liver disease with chronic lobular hepatitis

● **K71.5 Toxic liver disease with chronic active hepatitis**
> Toxic liver disease with lupoid hepatitis

> **K71.50 Toxic liver disease with chronic active hepatitis without ascites**

> **K71.51 Toxic liver disease with chronic active hepatitis with ascites**

K71.6 Toxic liver disease with hepatitis, not elsewhere classified

K71.7 Toxic liver disease with fibrosis and cirrhosis of liver

K71.8 Toxic liver disease with other disorders of liver
> Toxic liver disease with focal nodular hyperplasia
> Toxic liver disease with hepatic granulomas
> Toxic liver disease with peliosis hepatis
> Toxic liver disease with veno-occlusive disease of liver

K71.9 Toxic liver disease, unspecified

● **K72 Hepatic failure, not elsewhere classified**

> **Includes** fulminant hepatitis NEC, with hepatic failure
> hepatic encephalopathy NOS
> liver (cell) necrosis with hepatic failure
> malignant hepatitis NEC, with hepatic failure
> yellow liver atrophy or dystrophy

> **Excludes1** alcoholic hepatic failure (K70.4)
> hepatic failure with toxic liver disease (K71.1-)
> icterus of newborn (P55-P59)
> postprocedural hepatic failure (K91.82)

> **Excludes2** hepatic failure complicating abortion or ectopic or molar pregnancy (O00-O07, O08.8)
> hepatic failure complicating pregnancy, childbirth and the puerperium (O26.6-)
> viral hepatitis with hepatic coma (B15-B19)

● **K72.0 Acute and subacute hepatic failure**
> Acute non-viral hepatitis NOS

> **K72.00 Acute and subacute hepatic failure without coma**

> **K72.01 Acute and subacute hepatic failure with coma**

● **K72.1 Chronic hepatic failure**
> **K72.10 Chronic hepatic failure without coma**
> **K72.11 Chronic hepatic failure with coma**

● **K72.9 Hepatic failure, unspecified**
> **K72.90 Hepatic failure, unspecified without coma**
> **K72.91 Hepatic failure, unspecified with coma**
> Hepatic coma NOS

● **K73 Chronic hepatitis, not elsewhere classified**
> **Excludes1** alcoholic hepatitis (chronic) (K70.1-)
> drug-induced hepatitis (chronic) (K71.-)
> granulomatous hepatitis (chronic) NEC (K75.3)
> reactive, nonspecific hepatitis (chronic) (K75.2)
> viral hepatitis (chronic) (B15-B19)

> **K73.0 Chronic persistent hepatitis, not elsewhere classified**
> **K73.1 Chronic lobular hepatitis, not elsewhere classified**
> **K73.2 Chronic active hepatitis, not elsewhere classified**
> **K73.8 Other chronic hepatitis, not elsewhere classified**
> **K73.9 Chronic hepatitis, unspecified**

● **K74 Fibrosis and cirrhosis of liver**
> *Code also, if applicable, viral hepatitis (acute) (chronic) (B15-B19)*

> **Excludes1** alcoholic cirrhosis (of liver) (K70.3)
> alcoholic fibrosis of liver (K70.2)
> cardiac sclerosis of liver (K76.1)
> cirrhosis (of liver) with toxic liver disease (K71.7)
> congenital cirrhosis (of liver) (P78.81)
> pigmentary cirrhosis (of liver) (E83.110)

> **K74.0 Hepatic fibrosis**
> **K74.1 Hepatic sclerosis**
> **K74.2 Hepatic fibrosis with hepatic sclerosis**
> **K74.3 Primary biliary cirrhosis**
> Chronic nonsuppurative destructive cholangitis
> **K74.4 Secondary biliary cirrhosis**
> **K74.5 Biliary cirrhosis, unspecified**

● **K74.6 Other and unspecified cirrhosis of liver**
> **K74.60 Unspecified cirrhosis of liver**
> Cirrhosis (of liver) NOS

> **K74.69 Other cirrhosis of liver**
> Cryptogenic cirrhosis (of liver)
> Macronodular cirrhosis (of liver)
> Micronodular cirrhosis (of liver)
> Mixed type cirrhosis (of liver)
> Portal cirrhosis (of liver)
> Postnecrotic cirrhosis (of liver)

▶ New   ➡ Revised   ~~deleted~~ Deleted   **OGCR** Official Guidelines   X Assign placeholder X   ● Use Additional Character(s)

Excludes 1   Excludes 2   Includes   Use additional   Code first   Code also   Key words

● **K75** **Other inflammatory liver diseases**
> **Excludes2**   toxic liver disease (K71.-)

  K75.0 **Abscess of liver**
    Cholangitic hepatic abscess
    Hematogenic hepatic abscess
    Hepatic abscess NOS
    Lymphogenic hepatic abscess
    Pylephlebitic hepatic abscess
> **Excludes1**   amebic liver abscess (A06.4)
> cholangitis without liver abscess (K83.0)
> pylephlebitis without liver abscess (K75.1)

> **Excludes2**   acute or subacute hepatitis NOS (B17.9)
> acute or subacute non-viral hepatitis (K72.0)
> chronic hepatitis NEC (K73.8)

  K75.1 **Phlebitis of portal vein**
    Pylephlebitis
> **Excludes1**   pylephlebitic liver abscess (K75.0)

  K75.2 **Nonspecific reactive hepatitis**
> **Excludes1**   acute or subacute hepatitis (K72.0-)
> chronic hepatitis NEC (K73.-)
> viral hepatitis (B15-B19)

  K75.3 **Granulomatous hepatitis, not elsewhere classified**
> **Excludes1**   acute or subacute hepatitis (K72.0-)
> chronic hepatitis NEC (K73.-)
> viral hepatitis (B15-B19)

  K75.4 **Autoimmune hepatitis**
    Lupoid hepatitis NEC

● **K75.8** **Other specified inflammatory liver diseases**
    K75.81 **Nonalcoholic steatohepatitis (NASH)**
    K75.89 **Other specified inflammatory liver diseases**

  K75.9 **Inflammatory liver disease, unspecified**
    Hepatitis NOS
> **Excludes1**   acute or subacute hepatitis (K72.0-)
> chronic hepatitis NEC (K73.-)
> viral hepatitis (B15-B19)

● **K76** **Other diseases of liver**
> **Excludes2**   alcoholic liver disease (K70.-)
> amyloid degeneration of liver (E85.-)
> cystic disease of liver (congenital) (Q44.6)
> hepatic vein thrombosis (I82.0)
> hepatomegaly NOS (R16.0)
> pigmentary cirrhosis (of liver) (E83.110)
> portal vein thrombosis (I81)
> toxic liver disease (K71.-)

  K76.0 **Fatty (change of) liver, not elsewhere classified**
    Nonalcoholic fatty liver disease (NAFLD)
> **Excludes1**   nonalcoholic steatohepatitis (NASH) (K75.81)

  K76.1 **Chronic passive congestion of liver**
    Cardiac cirrhosis
    Cardiac sclerosis

  K76.2 **Central hemorrhagic necrosis of liver**
> **Excludes1**   liver necrosis with hepatic failure (K72.-)

  K76.3 **Infarction of liver**

  K76.4 **Peliosis hepatis**
    Hepatic angiomatosis

  K76.5 **Hepatic veno-occlusive disease**
> **Excludes1**   Budd-Chiari syndrome (I82.0)

  K76.6 **Portal hypertension**
> Use additional code for any associated complications, such as:
> portal hypertensive gastropathy (K31.89)

  K76.7 **Hepatorenal syndrome**
> **Excludes1**   hepatorenal syndrome following labor and delivery (O90.4)
> postprocedural hepatorenal syndrome (K91.83)

● **K76.8** **Other specified diseases of liver**
  K76.81 **Hepatopulmonary syndrome**
> *Code first underlying liver disease, such as:*
> alcoholic cirrhosis of liver (K70.3-)
> cirrhosis of liver without mention of alcohol (K74.6-)

  K76.89 **Other specified diseases of liver**
    Cyst (simple) of liver
    Focal nodular hyperplasia of liver
    Hepatoptosis

  K76.9 **Liver disease, unspecified**

K77 **Liver disorders in diseases classified elsewhere**
> *Code first underlying disease, such as:*
> amyloidosis (E85.-)
> congenital syphilis (A50.0, A50.5)
> congenital toxoplasmosis (P37.1)
> schistosomiasis (B65.0-B65.9)

> **Excludes1**   alcoholic hepatitis (K70.1-)
> alcoholic liver disease (K70.-)
> cytomegaloviral hepatitis (B25.1)
> herpesviral [herpes simplex] hepatitis (B00.81)
> infectious mononucleosis with liver disease (B27.0-B27.9 with .9)
> mumps hepatitis (B26.81)
> sarcoidosis with liver disease (D86.89)
> secondary syphilis with liver disease (A51.45)
> syphilis (late) with liver disease (A52.74)
> toxoplasmosis (acquired) hepatitis (B58.1)
> tuberculosis with liver disease (A18.83)

DISORDERS OF GALLBLADDER, BILIARY TRACT AND PANCREAS (K80–K87)

● **K80** **Cholelithiasis**
> *Presence or formation of gallstones*
> **Excludes1**   retained cholelithiasis following cholecystectomy (K91.86)

● **K80.0** **Calculus of gallbladder with acute cholecystitis**
  Any condition listed in K80.2 with acute cholecystitis
> *Check documentation for acute/chronic gallbladder/common bile duct either with or without obstruction.*

  K80.00 **Calculus of gallbladder with acute cholecystitis without obstruction**

  K80.01 **Calculus of gallbladder with acute cholecystitis with obstruction**

● **K80.1** **Calculus of gallbladder with other cholecystitis**
  K80.10 **Calculus of gallbladder with chronic cholecystitis without obstruction**
    Cholelithiasis with cholecystitis NOS

  K80.11 **Calculus of gallbladder with chronic cholecystitis with obstruction**

  K80.12 **Calculus of gallbladder with acute and chronic cholecystitis without obstruction**

  K80.13 **Calculus of gallbladder with acute and chronic cholecystitis with obstruction**

  K80.18 **Calculus of gallbladder with other cholecystitis without obstruction**

  K80.19 **Calculus of gallbladder with other cholecystitis with obstruction**

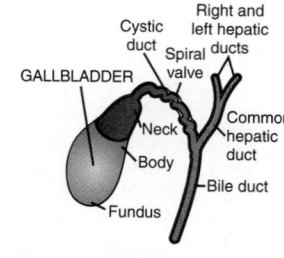
Figure 11-14   Gallbladder and bile ducts.

▶ New   ⇛ Revised   ~~deleted~~ Deleted   **OGCR** Official Guidelines   X Assign placeholder X   ● Use Additional Character(s)
Excludes 1   Excludes 2   Includes   Use additional   Code first   Code also   Key words

CHAPTER 11 (K00-K95)

● **K80.2   Calculus of gallbladder without cholecystitis**
    Cholecystolithiasis without cholecystitis
    Cholelithiasis (without cholecystitis)
    Colic (recurrent) of gallbladder (without cholecystitis)
    Gallstone (impacted) of cystic duct (without cholecystitis)
    Gallstone (impacted) of gallbladder (without cholecystitis)

    K80.20   Calculus of gallbladder without cholecystitis without obstruction

    K80.21   Calculus of gallbladder without cholecystitis with obstruction

● **K80.3   Calculus of bile duct with cholangitis**
    Any condition listed in K80.5 with cholangitis

    K80.30   Calculus of bile duct with cholangitis, unspecified, without obstruction

    K80.31   Calculus of bile duct with cholangitis, unspecified, with obstruction

    K80.32   Calculus of bile duct with acute cholangitis without obstruction

    K80.33   Calculus of bile duct with acute cholangitis with obstruction

    K80.34   Calculus of bile duct with chronic cholangitis without obstruction

    K80.35   Calculus of bile duct with chronic cholangitis with obstruction

    K80.36   Calculus of bile duct with acute and chronic cholangitis without obstruction

    K80.37   Calculus of bile duct with acute and chronic cholangitis with obstruction

● **K80.4   Calculus of bile duct with cholecystitis**
    Any condition listed in K80.5 with cholecystitis (with cholangitis)

    K80.40   Calculus of bile duct with cholecystitis, unspecified, without obstruction

    K80.41   Calculus of bile duct with cholecystitis, unspecified, with obstruction

    K80.42   Calculus of bile duct with acute cholecystitis without obstruction

    K80.43   Calculus of bile duct with acute cholecystitis with obstruction

    K80.44   Calculus of bile duct with chronic cholecystitis without obstruction

    K80.45   Calculus of bile duct with chronic cholecystitis with obstruction

    K80.46   Calculus of bile duct with acute and chronic cholecystitis without obstruction

    K80.47   Calculus of bile duct with acute and chronic cholecystitis with obstruction

● **K80.5   Calculus of bile duct without cholangitis or cholecystitis**
    Choledocholithiasis (without cholangitis or cholecystitis)
    Gallstone (impacted) of bile duct NOS (without cholangitis or cholecystitis)
    Gallstone (impacted) of common duct (without cholangitis or cholecystitis)
    Gallstone (impacted) of hepatic duct (without cholangitis or cholecystitis)
    Hepatic cholelithiasis (without cholangitis or cholecystitis)
    Hepatic colic (recurrent) (without cholangitis or cholecystitis)

    K80.50   Calculus of bile duct without cholangitis or cholecystitis without obstruction

    K80.51   Calculus of bile duct without cholangitis or cholecystitis with obstruction

● **K80.6   Calculus of gallbladder and bile duct with cholecystitis**

    K80.60   Calculus of gallbladder and bile duct with cholecystitis, unspecified, without obstruction

    K80.61   Calculus of gallbladder and bile duct with cholecystitis, unspecified, with obstruction

    K80.62   Calculus of gallbladder and bile duct with acute cholecystitis without obstruction

    K80.63   Calculus of gallbladder and bile duct with acute cholecystitis with obstruction

    K80.64   Calculus of gallbladder and bile duct with chronic cholecystitis without obstruction

    K80.65   Calculus of gallbladder and bile duct with chronic cholecystitis with obstruction

    K80.66   Calculus of gallbladder and bile duct with acute and chronic cholecystitis without obstruction

    K80.67   Calculus of gallbladder and bile duct with acute and chronic cholecystitis with obstruction

● **K80.7   Calculus of gallbladder and bile duct without cholecystitis**

    K80.70   Calculus of gallbladder and bile duct without cholecystitis without obstruction

    K80.71   Calculus of gallbladder and bile duct without cholecystitis with obstruction

● **K80.8   Other cholelithiasis**

    K80.80   Other cholelithiasis without obstruction

    K80.81   Other cholelithiasis with obstruction

● **K81   Cholecystitis**
    Chronic or acute inflammation of the gallbladder

    Excludes1   cholecystitis with cholelithiasis (K80.-)

    K81.0   Acute cholecystitis
        Abscess of gallbladder
        Angiocholecystitis
        Emphysematous (acute) cholecystitis
        Empyema of gallbladder
        Gangrene of gallbladder
        Gangrenous cholecystitis
        Suppurative cholecystitis

    K81.1   Chronic cholecystitis

    K81.2   Acute cholecystitis with chronic cholecystitis

    K81.9   Cholecystitis, unspecified

● **K82   Other diseases of gallbladder**

    Excludes1   nonvisualization of gallbladder (R93.2)
                  postcholecystectomy syndrome (K91.5)

    K82.0   Obstruction of gallbladder
        Occlusion of cystic duct or gallbladder without cholelithiasis
        Stenosis of cystic duct or gallbladder without cholelithiasis
        Stricture of cystic duct or gallbladder without cholelithiasis

        Excludes1   obstruction of gallbladder with cholelithiasis (K80.-)

    K82.1   Hydrops of gallbladder
        Mucocele of gallbladder

    K82.2   Perforation of gallbladder
        Rupture of cystic duct or gallbladder

    K82.3   Fistula of gallbladder
        Cholecystocolic fistula
        Cholecystoduodenal fistula

    K82.4   Cholesterolosis of gallbladder
        Strawberry gallbladder

        Excludes1   cholesterolosis of gallbladder with cholecystitis (K81.-)
                  cholesterolosis of gallbladder with cholelithiasis (K80.-)

    K82.8   Other specified diseases of gallbladder
        Adhesions of cystic duct or gallbladder
        Atrophy of cystic duct or gallbladder
        Cyst of cystic duct or gallbladder
        Dyskinesia of cystic duct or gallbladder
        Hypertrophy of cystic duct or gallbladder
        Nonfunctioning of cystic duct or gallbladder
        Ulcer of cystic duct or gallbladder

    K82.9   Disease of gallbladder, unspecified

▶ New   ⇒ Revised   ~~deleted~~ Deleted   **OGCR** Official Guidelines   X Assign placeholder X   ● Use Additional Character(s)

Excludes 1   Excludes 2   Includes   Use additional   Code first   Code also   Key words

● **K83** **Other diseases of biliary tract**

> **Excludes1** postcholecystectomy syndrome (K91.5)
> **Excludes2** conditions involving the gallbladder (K81-K82)
> conditions involving the cystic duct (K81-K82)

K83.0 **Cholangitis**
Ascending cholangitis
Cholangitis NOS
Primary cholangitis
Recurrent cholangitis
Sclerosing cholangitis
Secondary cholangitis
Stenosing cholangitis
Suppurative cholangitis

> **Excludes1** cholangitic liver abscess (K75.0)
> cholangitis with choledocholithiasis (K80.3-, K80.4-)
> chronic nonsuppurative destructive cholangitis (K74.3)

K83.1 **Obstruction of bile duct**
Occlusion of bile duct without cholelithiasis
Stenosis of bile duct without cholelithiasis
Stricture of bile duct without cholelithiasis

> **Excludes1** congenital obstruction of bile duct (Q44.3)
> obstruction of bile duct with cholelithiasis (K80.-)

K83.2 **Perforation of bile duct**
Rupture of bile duct

K83.3 **Fistula of bile duct**
Choledochoduodenal fistula

K83.4 **Spasm of sphincter of Oddi**

K83.5 **Biliary cyst**

K83.8 **Other specified diseases of biliary tract**
Adhesions of biliary tract
Atrophy of biliary tract
Hypertrophy of biliary tract
Ulcer of biliary tract

K83.9 **Disease of biliary tract, unspecified**

● **K85** **Acute pancreatitis**
Inflammatory process in which pancreatic enzymes autodigest the gland

> **Includes** acute (recurrent) pancreatitis
> subacute pancreatitis

● **K85.0** **Idiopathic acute pancreatitis**

K85.00 **Idiopathic acute pancreatitis without necrosis or infection**

K85.01 **Idiopathic acute pancreatitis with uninfected necrosis**

K85.02 **Idiopathic acute pancreatitis with infected necrosis**

● **K85.1** **Biliary acute pancreatitis**
Gallstone pancreatitis

K85.10 **Biliary acute pancreatitis without necrosis or infection**

K85.11 **Biliary acute pancreatitis with uninfected necrosis**

K85.12 **Biliary acute pancreatitis with infected necrosis**

● **K85.2** **Alcohol induced acute pancreatitis**

> **Excludes2** alcohol induced chronic pancreatitis (K86.0)

K85.20 **Alcohol induced acute pancreatitis without necrosis or infection**

K85.21 **Alcohol induced acute pancreatitis with uninfected necrosis**

K85.22 **Alcohol induced acute pancreatitis with infected necrosis**

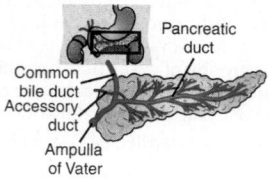
Pancreatic duct
Common bile duct
Accessory duct
Ampulla of Vater

● **K85.3** **Drug induced acute pancreatitis**

> Use additional code for adverse effect, if applicable, to identify drug (T36-T50 with fifth or sixth character 5)
> Use additional code to identify drug abuse and dependence (F11.-F17.-)

K85.30 **Drug induced acute pancreatitis without necrosis or infection**

K85.31 **Drug induced acute pancreatitis with uninfected necrosis**

K85.32 **Drug induced acute pancreatitis with infected necrosis**

● **K85.8** **Other acute pancreatitis**

K85.80 **Other acute pancreatitis without necrosis or infection**

K85.81 **Other acute pancreatitis with uninfected necrosis**

K85.82 **Other acute pancreatitis with infected necrosis**

● **K85.9** **Acute pancreatitis, unspecified**
Pancreatitis NOS

K85.90 **Acute pancreatitis without necrosis or infection, unspecified**

K85.91 **Acute pancreatitis with uninfected necrosis, unspecified**

K85.92 **Acute pancreatitis with infected necrosis, unspecified**

● **K86** **Other diseases of pancreas**

> **Excludes2** fibrocystic disease of pancreas (E84.-)
> islet cell tumor (of pancreas) (D13.7)
> pancreatic steatorrhea (K90.3)

K86.0 **Alcohol-induced chronic pancreatitis**

> Use additional code to identify:
> alcohol abuse and dependence (F10.-)
> Code also exocrine pancreatic insufficiency (K86.81)
> **Excludes2** alcohol induced acute pancreatitis (K85.2-)

K86.1 **Other chronic pancreatitis**
Chronic pancreatitis NOS
Infectious chronic pancreatitis
Recurrent chronic pancreatitis
Relapsing chronic pancreatitis

> Code also exocrine pancreatic insufficiency (K86.81)

K86.2 **Cyst of pancreas**

K86.3 **Pseudocyst of pancreas**

● **K86.8** **Other specified diseases of pancreas**

K86.81 **Exocrine pancreatic insufficiency**

K86.89 **Other specified diseases of pancreas**
Aseptic pancreatic necrosis, unrelated to acute pancreatitis
Atrophy of pancreas
Calculus of pancreas
Cirrhosis of pancreas
Fibrosis of pancreas
Pancreatic fat necrosis, unrelated to acute pancreatitis
Pancreatic infantilism
Pancreatic necrosis NOS, unrelated to acute pancreatitis

K86.9 **Disease of pancreas, unspecified**

K87 **Disorders of gallbladder, biliary tract and pancreas in diseases classified elsewhere**

> *Code first underlying disease*
> **Excludes1** cytomegaloviral pancreatitis (B25.2)
> mumps pancreatitis (B26.3)
> syphilitic gallbladder (A52.74)
> syphilitic pancreas (A52.74)
> tuberculosis of gallbladder (A18.83)
> tuberculosis of pancreas (A18.83)

Figure 11-15 Pancreatic ductal system.

▶ New   ⇒ Revised   ~~deleted~~ Deleted   **OGCR** Official Guidelines   X Assign placeholder X   ● Use Additional Character(s)

Excludes 1   Excludes 2   Includes   Use additional   Code first   Code also   Key words

OTHER DISEASES OF THE DIGESTIVE SYSTEM (K90-K95)

● **K90   Intestinal malabsorption**
  Excludes1 intestinal malabsorption following
                 gastrointestinal surgery (K91.2)

  K90.0   Celiac disease
          Celiac disease with steatorrhea
      ⇒ Celiac gluten-sensitive enteropathy
          Nontropical sprue
          Use additional code for associated disorders including:
              dermatitis herpetiformis (L13.0)
              gluten ataxia (G32.81)
          Code also exocrine pancreatic insufficiency (K86.81)

  K90.1   Tropical sprue
          Sprue NOS
          Tropical steatorrhea

  K90.2   Blind loop syndrome, not elsewhere classified
          Blind loop syndrome NOS
          Excludes1 congenital blind loop syndrome (Q43.8)
                         postsurgical blind loop syndrome (K91.2)

  K90.3   Pancreatic steatorrhea
● **K90.4   Other malabsorption due to intolerance**
      ⇒ **Excludes2** celiac gluten-sensitive enteropathy
                        (K90.0)
                        lactose intolerance (E73.-)

      K90.41   Non-celiac gluten sensitivity
              Gluten sensitivity NOS
              Non-celiac gluten sensitive enteropathy

      **K90.49   Malabsorption due to intolerance, not
                  elsewhere classified**
              Malabsorption due to intolerance to
                  carbohydrate
              Malabsorption due to intolerance to fat
              Malabsorption due to intolerance to protein
              Malabsorption due to intolerance to starch

● **K90.8   Other intestinal malabsorption**
      K90.81   Whipple's disease
      K90.89   Other intestinal malabsorption
  K90.9   Intestinal malabsorption, unspecified

● **K91   Intraoperative and postprocedural complications and disorders
           of digestive system, not elsewhere classified**
  Excludes2 complications of artificial opening of digestive
                 system (K94.-)
                 complications of bariatric procedures (K95.-)
                 gastrojejunal ulcer (K28.-)
                 postprocedural (radiation) retroperitoneal abscess
                     (K68.11)
                 radiation colitis (K52.0)
                 radiation gastroenteritis (K52.0)
                 radiation proctitis (K62.7)

  K91.0   Vomiting following gastrointestinal surgery
  K91.1   Postgastric surgery syndromes
          Dumping syndrome
          Postgastrectomy syndrome
          Postvagotomy syndrome

  K91.2   Postsurgical malabsorption, not elsewhere classified
          Postsurgical blind loop syndrome
          Excludes1 malabsorption osteomalacia in adults
                         (M83.2)
                         malabsorption osteoporosis, postsurgical
                         (M80.8-, M81.8)

● **K91.3   Postprocedural intestinal obstruction**
  ▶ **K91.30   Postprocedural intestinal obstruction,
                unspecified as to partial versus complete**
      ▶ Postprocedural intestinal obstruction NOS

  ▶ **K91.31   Postprocedural partial intestinal obstruction**
      ▶ Postprocedural incomplete intestinal
          obstruction

  ▶ **K91.32   Postprocedural complete intestinal obstruction**

  K91.5   Postcholecystectomy syndrome
● **K91.6   Intraoperative hemorrhage and hematoma of a digestive
           system organ or structure complicating a procedure**
      Excludes1 intraoperative hemorrhage and
                     hematoma of a digestive system
                     organ or structure due to accidental
                     puncture and laceration during a
                     procedure (K91.7-)

      **K91.61   Intraoperative hemorrhage and hematoma of a
                  digestive system organ or structure complicating
                  a digestive system procedure**
      **K91.62   Intraoperative hemorrhage and hematoma
                  of a digestive system organ or structure
                  complicating other procedure**

● **K91.7   Accidental puncture and laceration of a digestive system
           organ or structure during a procedure**
      **K91.71   Accidental puncture and laceration of a
                  digestive system organ or structure during a
                  digestive system procedure**
      **K91.72   Accidental puncture and laceration of a
                  digestive system organ or structure during
                  other procedure**

● **K91.8   Other intraoperative and postprocedural complications
           and disorders of digestive system**
      **K91.81   Other intraoperative complications of digestive
                  system**
      K91.82   Postprocedural hepatic failure
      K91.83   Postprocedural hepatorenal syndrome
  ● **K91.84   Postprocedural hemorrhage of a digestive
                system organ or structure following a
                procedure**
          **K91.840   Postprocedural hemorrhage of a
                      digestive system organ or structure
                      following a digestive system
                      procedure**
          **K91.841   Postprocedural hemorrhage of a
                      digestive system organ or structure
                      following other procedure**
  ● **K91.85   Complications of intestinal pouch**
          K91.850   Pouchitis
                      Inflammation of internal ileoanal
                      pouch
          **K91.858   Other complications of intestinal
                      pouch**
      **K91.86   Retained cholelithiasis following
                  cholecystectomy**
  ● **K91.87   Postprocedural hematoma and seroma of a
                digestive system organ or structure following a
                procedure**
          **K91.870   Postprocedural hematoma of a
                      digestive system organ or structure
                      following a digestive system
                      procedure**
          **K91.871   Postprocedural hematoma of a
                      digestive system organ or structure
                      following other procedure**
          **K91.872   Postprocedural seroma of a digestive
                      system organ or structure following a
                      digestive system procedure**
          **K91.873   Postprocedural seroma of a digestive
                      system organ or structure following
                      other procedure**
      **K91.89   Other postprocedural complications and
                  disorders of digestive system**
              Use additional code, if applicable, to further
                  specify disorder
              Excludes2 postprocedural retroperitoneal
                             abscess (K68.11)

▶ New   ⇒ Revised   ~~deleted~~ Deleted   **OGCR** Official Guidelines   X Assign placeholder X   ● Use Additional Character(s)

Excludes 1   Excludes 2   Includes   Use additional   Code first   Code also   Key words

● **K92   Other diseases of digestive system**
> **Excludes1**   neonatal gastrointestinal hemorrhage (P54.0-P54.3)

K92.0   Hematemesis

K92.1   Melena
> **Excludes1**   occult blood in feces (R19.5)

K92.2   Gastrointestinal hemorrhage, unspecified
Gastric hemorrhage NOS
Intestinal hemorrhage NOS
> **Excludes1**   acute hemorrhagic gastritis (K29.01)
> hemorrhage of anus and rectum (K62.5)
> angiodysplasia of stomach with hemorrhage (K31.811)
> diverticular disease with hemorrhage (K57.-)
> gastritis and duodenitis with hemorrhage (K29.-)
> peptic ulcer with hemorrhage (K25-K28)

● **K92.8   Other specified diseases of the digestive system**

K92.81   Gastrointestinal mucositis (ulcerative)
Code also type of associated therapy, such as:
antineoplastic and immunosuppressive drugs (T45.1X-)
radiological procedure and radiotherapy (Y84.2)
> **Excludes2**   mucositis (ulcerative) of vagina and vulva (N76.81)
> nasal mucositis (ulcerative) (J34.81)
> oral mucositis (ulcerative) (K12.3-)

K92.89   Other specified diseases of the digestive system

K92.9   Disease of digestive system, unspecified

● **K94   Complications of artificial openings of the digestive system**

● **K94.0   Colostomy complications**
K94.00   Colostomy complication, unspecified
K94.01   Colostomy hemorrhage
K94.02   Colostomy infection
Use additional code to specify type of infection, such as:
cellulitis of abdominal wall (L03.311)
sepsis (A40.-, A41.-)
K94.03   Colostomy malfunction
Mechanical complication of colostomy
K94.09   Other complications of colostomy

● **K94.1   Enterostomy complications**
K94.10   Enterostomy complication, unspecified
K94.11   Enterostomy hemorrhage
K94.12   Enterostomy infection
Use additional code to specify type of infection, such as:
cellulitis of abdominal wall (L03.311)
sepsis (A40.-, A41.-)
K94.13   Enterostomy malfunction
Mechanical complication of enterostomy
K94.19   Other complications of enterostomy

● **K94.2   Gastrostomy complications**
K94.20   Gastrostomy complication, unspecified
K94.21   Gastrostomy hemorrhage
K94.22   Gastrostomy infection
Use additional code to specify type of infection, such as:
cellulitis of abdominal wall (L03.311)
sepsis (A40.-, A41.-)
K94.23   Gastrostomy malfunction
Mechanical complication of gastrostomy
K94.29   Other complications of gastrostomy

● **K94.3   Esophagostomy complications**
K94.30   Esophagostomy complications, unspecified
K94.31   Esophagostomy hemorrhage
K94.32   Esophagostomy infection
Use additional code to identify the infection
K94.33   Esophagostomy malfunction
Mechanical complication of esophagostomy
K94.39   Other complications of esophagostomy

● **K95   Complications of bariatric procedures**

● **K95.0   Complications of gastric band procedure**
K95.01   Infection due to gastric band procedure
Use additional code to specify type of infection or organism, such as:
bacterial and viral infectious agents (B95.-, B96.-)
cellulitis of abdominal wall (L03.311)
sepsis (A40.-, A41.-)
K95.09   Other complications of gastric band procedure
Use additional code, if applicable, to further specify complication

● **K95.8   Complications of other bariatric procedure**
> **Excludes1**   complications of gastric band surgery (K95.0-)

K95.81   Infection due to other bariatric procedure
Use additional code to specify type of infection or organism, such as:
bacterial and viral infectious agents (B95.-, B96.-)
cellulitis of abdominal wall (L03.311)
sepsis (A40.-, A41.-)
K95.89   Other complications of other bariatric procedure
Use additional code, if applicable, to further specify complication

CHAPTER 12

DISEASES OF THE SKIN AND SUBCUTANEOUS TISSUE (L00-L99)

OGCR Chapter-Specific Coding Guidelines

12. **Chapter 12: Diseases of the Skin and Subcutaneous Tissue (L00-L99)**

   a. **Pressure ulcer stage codes**

   1) **Pressure ulcer stages**
   Codes from category L89, Pressure ulcer, identify the site of the pressure ulcer as well as the stage of the ulcer.
   The ICD-10-CM classifies pressure ulcer stages based on severity, which is designated by stages 1-4, unspecified stage and unstageable.
   Assign as many codes from category L89 as needed to identify all the pressure ulcers the patient has, if applicable.

   2) **Unstageable pressure ulcers**
   Assignment of the code for unstageable pressure ulcer (L89.--0) should be based on the clinical documentation. These codes are used for pressure ulcers whose stage cannot be clinically determined (e.g., the ulcer is covered by eschar or has been treated with a skin or muscle graft) and pressure ulcers that are documented as deep tissue injury but not documented as due to trauma. This code should not be confused with the codes for unspecified stage (L89.--9). When there is no documentation regarding the stage of the pressure ulcer, assign the appropriate code for unspecified stage (L89.--9).

   3) **Documented pressure ulcer stage**
   Assignment of the pressure ulcer stage code should be guided by clinical documentation of the stage or documentation of the terms found in the Alphabetic Index. For clinical terms describing the stage that are not found in the Alphabetic Index, and there is no documentation of the stage, the provider should be queried.

   4) **Patients admitted with pressure ulcers documented as healed**
   No code is assigned if the documentation states that the pressure ulcer is completely healed.

   5) **Patients admitted with pressure ulcers documented as healing**
   Pressure ulcers described as healing should be assigned the appropriate pressure ulcer stage code based on the documentation in the medical record. If the documentation does not provide information about the stage of the healing pressure ulcer, assign the appropriate code for unspecified stage.
   If the documentation is unclear as to whether the patient has a current (new) pressure ulcer or if the patient is being treated for a healing pressure ulcer, query the provider.
   For ulcers that were present on admission but healed at the time of discharge, assign the code for the site and stage of the pressure ulcer at the time of admission.

   6) **Patient admitted with pressure ulcer evolving into another stage during the admission**
   If a patient is admitted to an inpatient hospital with a pressure ulcer at one stage and it progresses to a higher stage, two separate codes should be assigned: one code for the site and stage of the ulcer on admission and a second code for the same ulcer site and the highest stage reported during the stay.

   b. *Non-Pressure Chronic Ulcers*

   1) *Patients admitted with non-pressure ulcers documented as healed*
   No code is assigned if the documentation states that the non-pressure ulcer is completely healed.

   2) *Patients admitted with non-pressure ulcers documented as healing*
   Non-pressure ulcers described as healing should be assigned the appropriate non-pressure ulcer code based on the documentation in the medical record. If the documentation does not provide information about the severity of the healing non-pressure ulcer, assign the appropriate code for unspecified severity.
   If the documentation is unclear as to whether the patient has a current (new) non-pressure ulcer or if the patient is being treated for a healing non-pressure ulcer, query the provider.
   For ulcers that were present on admission but healed at the time of discharge, assign the code for the site and severity of the non-pressure ulcer at the time of admission.

   3) *Patient admitted with non-pressure ulcer that progresses to another severity level during the admission*
   If a patient is admitted to an inpatient hospital with a non-pressure ulcer at one severity level and it progresses to a higher severity level, two separate codes should be assigned: one code for the site and severity level of the ulcer on admission and a second code for the same ulcer site and the highest severity level reported during the stay.

Figure 12-1 Furuncle, also known as a boil, is a staphylococcal infection. The organism enters the body through a hair follicle and so furuncles usually appear in hairy areas of the body. A cluster of furuncles is known as a carbuncle and involves infection into the deep subcutaneous fascia. These usually appear on the back and neck. (**B** from Habif TP, Binnick AN, Meyerson LB: Clinical Dermatology: A Color Guide to Diagnosis and Therapy, S.l., Mosby Elsevier, 2010)

CHAPTER 12

DISEASES OF THE SKIN AND SUBCUTANEOUS TISSUE (L00-L99)

Excludes2 certain conditions originating in the perinatal period (P04-P96)
certain infectious and parasitic diseases (A00-B99)
complications of pregnancy, childbirth and the puerperium (O00-O9A)
congenital malformations, deformations, and chromosomal abnormalities (Q00-Q99)
endocrine, nutritional and metabolic diseases (E00-E88)
lipomelanotic reticulosis (I89.8)
neoplasms (C00-D49)
symptoms, signs and abnormal clinical and laboratory findings, not elsewhere classified (R00-R94)
systemic connective tissue disorders (M30-M36)
viral warts (B07.-)

This chapter contains the following blocks:

L00-L08	Infections of the skin and subcutaneous tissue
L10-L14	Bullous disorders
L20-L30	Dermatitis and eczema
L40-L45	Papulosquamous disorders
L49-L54	Urticaria and erythema
L55-L59	Radiation-related disorders of the skin and subcutaneous tissue
L60-L75	Disorders of skin appendages
L76	Intraoperative and postprocedural complications of skin and subcutaneous tissue
L80-L99	Other disorders of the skin and subcutaneous tissue

▶ New   ⟹ Revised   ~~deleted~~ Deleted   **OGCR** Official Guidelines   X Assign placeholder X   ● Use Additional Character(s)

Excludes 1   Excludes 2   Includes   Use additional   Code first   Code also   Key words

Figure 12-2 Impetigo. A thick, honey-yellow adherent crust covers the entire eroded surface. (From James WD, Elston DM, Berger TG, Andrews GC: Andrews' Diseases of the Skin: Clinical Dermatology, London, Saunders/Elsevier, 2011)

INFECTIONS OF THE SKIN AND SUBCUTANEOUS TISSUE (L00-L08)

Use additional code (B95-B97) to identify infectious agent.

Excludes2　hordeolum (H00.0)
infective dermatitis (L30.3)
local infections of skin classified in Chapter 1
lupus panniculitis (L93.2)
panniculitis NOS (M79.3)
panniculitis of neck and back (M54.0-)
Perlèche NOS (K13.0)
Perlèche due to candidiasis (B37.0)
Perlèche due to riboflavin deficiency (E53.0)
pyogenic granuloma (L98.0)
relapsing panniculitis [Weber-Christian] (M35.6)
viral warts (B07.-)
zoster (B02.-)

L00　**Staphylococcal scalded skin syndrome**
Ritter's disease
Use additional code to identify percentage of skin exfoliation (L49.-)

Excludes1　bullous impetigo (L01.03)
pemphigus neonatorum (L01.03)
toxic epidermal necrolysis [Lyell] (L51.2)

● L01　**Impetigo**
Contagious skin infection caused by a streptococcus or staphylococcus aureus, common skin infections among children

Excludes1　impetigo herpetiformis (L40.1)

● L01.0　**Impetigo**
Impetigo contagiosa
Impetigo vulgaris

L01.00　**Impetigo, unspecified**
Impetigo NOS

L01.01　**Non-bullous impetigo**

L01.02　**Bockhart's impetigo**
Impetigo follicularis
Perifolliculitis NOS
Superficial pustular perifolliculitis

L01.03　**Bullous impetigo**
Impetigo neonatorum
Pemphigus neonatorum
Neonate = newborn

L01.09　**Other impetigo**
Ulcerative impetigo

L01.1　**Impetiginization of other dermatoses**

● L02　**Cutaneous abscess, furuncle and carbuncle**
Use additional code to identify organism (B95-B96)

Excludes2　abscess of anus and rectal regions (K61.-)
abscess of female genital organs (external) (N76.4)
abscess of male genital organs (external) (N48.2, N49.-)

● L02.0　**Cutaneous abscess, furuncle and carbuncle of face**

Excludes2　abscess of ear, external (H60.0)
abscess of eyelid (H00.0)
abscess of head [any part, except face] (L02.8)
abscess of lacrimal gland (H04.0)
abscess of lacrimal passages (H04.3)
abscess of mouth (K12.2)
abscess of nose (J34.0)
abscess of orbit (H05.0)
submandibular abscess (K12.2)

L02.01　**Cutaneous abscess of face**

L02.02　**Furuncle of face**
Boil of face
Folliculitis of face

L02.03　**Carbuncle of face**

● L02.1　Cutaneous abscess, furuncle and carbuncle of **neck**

L02.11　**Cutaneous abscess of neck**

L02.12　**Furuncle of neck**
Boil of neck
Folliculitis of neck

L02.13　**Carbuncle of neck**

● L02.2　Cutaneous abscess, furuncle and carbuncle of **trunk**

Excludes1　non-newborn omphalitis (L08.82)
omphalitis of newborn (P38.-)

Excludes2　abscess of breast (N61.1)
abscess of buttocks (L02.3)
abscess of female external genital organs (N76.4)
abscess of male external genital organs (N48.2, N49.-)
abscess of hip (L02.4)

● L02.21　**Cutaneous abscess of trunk**

L02.211　Cutaneous abscess of **abdominal wall**

L02.212　Cutaneous abscess of **back** [any part, except buttock]

L02.213　Cutaneous abscess of **chest wall**

L02.214　Cutaneous abscess of **groin**

L02.215　Cutaneous abscess of **perineum**

L02.216　Cutaneous abscess of **umbilicus**

L02.219　Cutaneous abscess of **trunk, unspecified**

● L02.22　**Furuncle of trunk**
Boil of trunk
Folliculitis of trunk

L02.221　Furuncle of **abdominal wall**

L02.222　Furuncle of **back** [any part, except buttock]

L02.223　Furuncle of **chest wall**

L02.224　Furuncle of **groin**

L02.225　Furuncle of **perineum**

L02.226　Furuncle of **umbilicus**

L02.229　Furuncle of trunk, **unspecified**

● L02.23　**Carbuncle of trunk**

L02.231　Carbuncle of **abdominal wall**

L02.232　Carbuncle of **back** [any part, except buttock]

L02.233　Carbuncle of **chest wall**

L02.234　Carbuncle of **groin**

L02.235　Carbuncle of **perineum**

L02.236　Carbuncle of **umbilicus**

L02.239　Carbuncle of trunk, **unspecified**

● L02.3　Cutaneous abscess, furuncle and carbuncle of **buttock**

Excludes1　pilonidal cyst with abscess (L05.01)

L02.31　**Cutaneous abscess of buttock**
Cutaneous abscess of gluteal region

L02.32　**Furuncle of buttock**
Boil of buttock
Folliculitis of buttock
Furuncle of gluteal region

L02.33　**Carbuncle of buttock**
Carbuncle of gluteal region

▶ New　⇒ Revised　~~deleted~~ Deleted　**OGCR** Official Guidelines　X Assign placeholder X　● Use Additional Character(s)

Excludes 1　Excludes 2　Includes　Use additional　Code first　Code also　Key words

● **L02.4**   **Cutaneous abscess, furuncle and carbuncle of limb**
> **Excludes2**   Cutaneous abscess, furuncle and carbuncle of groin (L02.214, L02.224, L02.234)
> Cutaneous abscess, furuncle and carbuncle of hand (L02.5-)
> Cutaneous abscess, furuncle and carbuncle of foot (L02.6-)

● **L02.41**   **Cutaneous abscess of limb**
    L02.411   Cutaneous abscess of right axilla
    L02.412   Cutaneous abscess of left axilla
    L02.413   Cutaneous abscess of right upper limb
    L02.414   Cutaneous abscess of left upper limb
    L02.415   Cutaneous abscess of right lower limb
    L02.416   Cutaneous abscess of left lower limb
    L02.419   Cutaneous abscess of limb, unspecified

● **L02.42**   **Furuncle of limb**
> Boil of limb
> Folliculitis of limb

    L02.421   Furuncle of right axilla
    L02.422   Furuncle of left axilla
    L02.423   Furuncle of right upper limb
    L02.424   Furuncle of left upper limb
    L02.425   Furuncle of right lower limb
    L02.426   Furuncle of left lower limb
    L02.429   Furuncle of limb, unspecified

● **L02.43**   **Carbuncle of limb**
    L02.431   Carbuncle of right axilla
    L02.432   Carbuncle of left axilla
    L02.433   Carbuncle of right upper limb
    L02.434   Carbuncle of left upper limb
    L02.435   Carbuncle of right lower limb
    L02.436   Carbuncle of left lower limb
    L02.439   Carbuncle of limb, unspecified

● **L02.5**   **Cutaneous abscess, furuncle and carbuncle of hand**

● **L02.51**   **Cutaneous abscess of hand**
    L02.511   Cutaneous abscess of right hand
    L02.512   Cutaneous abscess of left hand
    L02.519   Cutaneous abscess of unspecified hand

● **L02.52**   **Furuncle hand**
> Boil of hand
> Folliculitis of hand

    L02.521   Furuncle right hand
    L02.522   Furuncle left hand
    L02.529   Furuncle unspecified hand

● **L02.53**   **Carbuncle of hand**
    L02.531   Carbuncle of right hand
    L02.532   Carbuncle of left hand
    L02.539   Carbuncle of unspecified hand

● **L02.6**   **Cutaneous abscess, furuncle and carbuncle of foot**

● **L02.61**   **Cutaneous abscess of foot**
    L02.611   Cutaneous abscess of right foot
    L02.612   Cutaneous abscess of left foot
    L02.619   Cutaneous abscess of unspecified foot

● **L02.62**   **Furuncle of foot**
> Boil of foot
> Folliculitis of foot

    L02.621   Furuncle of right foot
    L02.622   Furuncle of left foot
    L02.629   Furuncle of unspecified foot

● **L02.63**   **Carbuncle of foot**
    L02.631   Carbuncle of right foot
    L02.632   Carbuncle of left foot
    L02.639   Carbuncle of unspecified foot

● **L02.8**   **Cutaneous abscess, furuncle and carbuncle of other sites**

● **L02.81**   **Cutaneous abscess of other sites**
    L02.811   Cutaneous abscess of head [any part, except face]
    L02.818   Cutaneous abscess of other sites

● **L02.82**   **Furuncle of other sites**
> Boil of other sites
> Folliculitis of other sites

    L02.821   Furuncle of head [any part, except face]
    L02.828   Furuncle of other sites

● **L02.83**   **Carbuncle of other sites**
    L02.831   Carbuncle of head [any part, except face]
    L02.838   Carbuncle of other sites

● **L02.9**   **Cutaneous abscess, furuncle and carbuncle, unspecified**
    L02.91   Cutaneous abscess, unspecified
    L02.92   Furuncle, unspecified
> Boil NOS
> Furunculosis NOS

    L02.93   Carbuncle, unspecified

● **L03**   **Cellulitis and acute lymphangitis**
> **Excludes2**   cellulitis of anal and rectal region (K61.-)
> cellulitis of external auditory canal (H60.1)
> cellulitis of eyelid (H00.0)
> cellulitis of female external genital organs (N76.4)
> cellulitis of lacrimal apparatus (H04.3)
> cellulitis of male external genital organs (N48.2, N49.-)
> cellulitis of mouth (K12.2)
> cellulitis of nose (J34.0)
> eosinophilic cellulitis [Wells] (L98.3)
> febrile neutrophilic dermatosis [Sweet] (L98.2)
> lymphangitis (chronic) (subacute) (I89.1)

● **L03.0**   **Cellulitis and acute lymphangitis of finger and toe**
> Infection of nail
> Onychia
> Paronychia
> Perionychia

● **L03.01**   **Cellulitis of finger**
> Felon
> Whitlow
> **Excludes1**   herpetic whitlow (B00.89)

    L03.011   Cellulitis of right finger
    L03.012   Cellulitis of left finger
    L03.019   Cellulitis of unspecified finger

● **L03.02**   **Acute lymphangitis of finger**
> Hangnail with lymphangitis of finger

    L03.021   Acute lymphangitis of right finger
    L03.022   Acute lymphangitis of left finger
    L03.029   Acute lymphangitis of unspecified finger

● **L03.03**   **Cellulitis of toe**
    L03.031   Cellulitis of right toe
    L03.032   Cellulitis of left toe
    L03.039   Cellulitis of unspecified toe

● **L03.04**   **Acute lymphangitis of toe**
> Hangnail with lymphangitis of toe

    L03.041   Acute lymphangitis of right toe
    L03.042   Acute lymphangitis of left toe
    L03.049   Acute lymphangitis of unspecified toe

Item 12-1   **Onychia** is an inflammation of the tissue surrounding the nail with pus accumulation and loss of the nail, resulting from microscopic pathogens entering through small wounds. **Paronychia** is a nail disease also known as felon or whitlow and is a bacterial or fungal infection.

CHAPTER 12 (L00-L99)

▶ New   ⟹ Revised   ~~deleted~~ Deleted   **OGCR** Official Guidelines   **X** Assign placeholder X   ● Use Additional Character(s)

Excludes 1   Excludes 2   Includes   Use additional   Code first   Code also   Key words

Item 12-2 Cellulitis is an acute spreading bacterial infection below the surface of the skin characterized by redness (erythema), warmth, swelling, pain, fever, chills, and enlarged lymph nodes ("swollen glands").

● **L03.1** Cellulitis and acute lymphangitis of other parts of limb
  ● **L03.11** Cellulitis of other parts of limb
    Excludes2 cellulitis of fingers (L03.01-)
                cellulitis of toes (L03.03-)
                groin (L03.314)
    L03.111 Cellulitis of right axilla
    L03.112 Cellulitis of left axilla
    L03.113 Cellulitis of right upper limb
    L03.114 Cellulitis of left upper limb
    L03.115 Cellulitis of right lower limb
    L03.116 Cellulitis of left lower limb
    L03.119 Cellulitis of unspecified part of limb
  ● **L03.12** Acute lymphangitis of other parts of limb
    Excludes2 acute lymphangitis of fingers
                (L03.2-)
                acute lymphangitis of toes
                (L03.04-)
                acute lymphangitis of groin
                (L03.324)
    L03.121 Acute lymphangitis of right axilla
    L03.122 Acute lymphangitis of left axilla
    L03.123 Acute lymphangitis of right upper limb
    L03.124 Acute lymphangitis of left upper limb
    L03.125 Acute lymphangitis of right lower limb
    L03.126 Acute lymphangitis of left lower limb
    L03.129 Acute lymphangitis of unspecified part of limb
● **L03.2** Cellulitis and acute lymphangitis of face and neck
  ● **L03.21** Cellulitis and acute lymphangitis of face
    L03.211 Cellulitis of face
             Excludes2 abscess of orbit
                        (H05.01-)
                        cellulitis of ear
                        (H60.1-)
                        cellulitis of eyelid
                        (H00.0-)
                        cellulitis of head
                        (L03.81)
                        cellulitis of lacrimal
                        apparatus (H04.3)
                        cellulitis of lip (K13.0)
                        cellulitis of mouth
                        (K12.2)
                        cellulitis of nose
                        (internal) (J34.0)
                        cellulitis of orbit
                        (H05.01-)
                        cellulitis of scalp
                        (L03.81)
    L03.212 Acute lymphangitis of face
    L03.213 Periorbital cellulitis
             Preseptal cellulitis
  ● **L03.22** Cellulitis and acute lymphangitis of neck
    L03.221 Cellulitis of neck
    L03.222 Acute lymphangitis of neck

● **L03.3** Cellulitis and acute lymphangitis of trunk
  ● **L03.31** Cellulitis of trunk
    Excludes2 cellulitis of anal and rectal
                regions (K61.-)
                cellulitis of breast NOS
                (N61.0)
                cellulitis of female external
                genital organs (N76.4)
                cellulitis of male external genital
                organs (N48.2, N49.-)
                omphalitis of newborn (P38.-)
                puerperal cellulitis of breast
                (O91.2)
    L03.311 Cellulitis of abdominal wall
             Excludes2 cellulitis of umbilicus
                        (L03.316)
                        cellulitis of groin
                        (L03.314)
    L03.312 Cellulitis of back [any part except buttock]
    L03.313 Cellulitis of chest wall
    L03.314 Cellulitis of groin
    L03.315 Cellulitis of perineum
    L03.316 Cellulitis of umbilicus
    L03.317 Cellulitis of buttock
    L03.319 Cellulitis of trunk, unspecified
  ● **L03.32** Acute lymphangitis of trunk
    L03.321 Acute lymphangitis of abdominal wall
    L03.322 Acute lymphangitis of back [any part except buttock]
    L03.323 Acute lymphangitis of chest wall
    L03.324 Acute lymphangitis of groin
    L03.325 Acute lymphangitis of perineum
    L03.326 Acute lymphangitis of umbilicus
    L03.327 Acute lymphangitis of buttock
    L03.329 Acute lymphangitis of trunk, unspecified
● **L03.8** Cellulitis and acute lymphangitis of other sites
  ● **L03.81** Cellulitis of other sites
    L03.811 Cellulitis of head [any part, except face]
             Cellulitis of scalp
             Excludes2 cellulitis of face
                        (L03.211)
    L03.818 Cellulitis of other sites
  ● **L03.89** Acute lymphangitis of other sites
    L03.891 Acute lymphangitis of head [any part, except face]
    L03.898 Acute lymphangitis of other sites
● **L03.9** Cellulitis and acute lymphangitis, unspecified
  L03.90 Cellulitis, unspecified
  L03.91 Acute lymphangitis, unspecified
          Excludes1 lymphangitis NOS (I89.1)

▶ New   ⟹ Revised   ~~deleted~~ Deleted   **OGCR** Official Guidelines   X Assign placeholder X   ● Use Additional Character(s)

Excludes 1   Excludes 2   Includes   Use additional   Code first   Code also   Key words

Item 12–3 **Abscess** is a localized collection of pus in tissues or organs and is a sign of infection resulting in swelling and inflammation.

Item 12–4 **Pilonidal cyst,** also called a coccygeal cyst, is the result of a disorder called pilonidal disease. The cyst usually contains hair and pus.

● **L04** **Acute lymphadenitis**
Short-term inflammation of lymph nodes which can be regionalized to involve a given area of the lymph system or systemic involving much of the body
> **Includes** abscess (acute) of lymph nodes, except mesenteric
> acute lymphadenitis, except mesenteric
> **Excludes1** chronic or subacute lymphadenitis, except mesenteric (I88.1)
> enlarged lymph nodes (R59.-)
> human immunodeficiency virus [HIV] disease resulting in generalized lymphadenopathy (B20)
> lymphadenitis NOS (I88.9)
> nonspecific mesenteric lymphadenitis (I88.0)

L04.0 **Acute lymphadenitis of face, head and neck**
L04.1 **Acute lymphadenitis of trunk**
L04.2 **Acute lymphadenitis of upper limb**
Acute lymphadenitis of axilla
Acute lymphadenitis of shoulder
L04.3 **Acute lymphadenitis of lower limb**
Acute lymphadenitis of hip
> **Excludes2** acute lymphadenitis of groin (L04.1)
L04.8 **Acute lymphadenitis of other sites**
L04.9 **Acute lymphadenitis, unspecified**

● **L05** **Pilonidal cyst and sinus**
● **L05.0** **Pilonidal cyst and sinus with abscess**
L05.01 **Pilonidal cyst with abscess**
Pilonidal abscess
Pilonidal dimple with abscess
Postanal dimple with abscess
> **Excludes2** congenital sacral dimple (Q82.6)
> parasacral dimple (Q82.6)
L05.02 **Pilonidal sinus with abscess**
Coccygeal fistula with abscess
Coccygeal sinus with abscess
Pilonidal fistula with abscess
● **L05.9** **Pilonidal cyst and sinus without abscess**
L05.91 **Pilonidal cyst without abscess**
Pilonidal dimple
Postanal dimple
Pilonidal cyst NOS
> **Excludes2** congenital sacral dimple (Q82.6)
> parasacral dimple (Q82.6)
L05.92 **Pilonidal sinus without abscess**
Coccygeal fistula
Coccygeal sinus without abscess
Pilonidal fistula

● **L08** **Other local infections of skin and subcutaneous tissue**
L08.0 **Pyoderma**
Dermatitis gangrenosa
Purulent dermatitis
Septic dermatitis
Suppurative dermatitis
> **Excludes1** pyoderma gangrenosum (L88)
> pyoderma vegetans (L08.81)
L08.1 **Erythrasma**

● **L08.8** **Other specified local infections of the skin and subcutaneous tissue**
L08.81 **Pyoderma vegetans**
> **Excludes1** pyoderma gangrenosum (L88)
> pyoderma NOS (L08.0)
L08.82 **Omphalitis not of newborn**
> **Excludes1** omphalitis of newborn (P38.-)
L08.89 **Other specified local infections of the skin and subcutaneous tissue**
L08.9 **Local infection of the skin and subcutaneous tissue, unspecified**

BULLOUS DISORDERS (L10-L14)
> **Excludes1** benign familial pemphigus [Hailey-Hailey] (Q82.8)
> staphylococcal scalded skin syndrome (L00)
> toxic epidermal necrolysis [Lyell] (L51.2)

● **L10** **Pemphigus**
> **Excludes1** pemphigus neonatorum (L01.03)
L10.0 **Pemphigus vulgaris**
L10.1 **Pemphigus vegetans**
L10.2 **Pemphigus foliaceus**
L10.3 **Brazilian pemphigus [fogo selvagem]**
L10.4 **Pemphigus erythematosus**
Senear-Usher syndrome
L10.5 **Drug-induced pemphigus**
> Use additional code for adverse effect, if applicable, to identify drug (T36-T50 with fifth or sixth character 5)
● **L10.8** **Other pemphigus**
L10.81 **Paraneoplastic pemphigus**
L10.89 **Other pemphigus**
L10.9 **Pemphigus, unspecified**

● **L11** **Other acantholytic disorders**
L11.0 **Acquired keratosis follicularis**
> **Excludes1** keratosis follicularis (congenital) [Darier-White] (Q82.8)
L11.1 **Transient acantholytic dermatosis [Grover]**
L11.8 **Other specified acantholytic disorders**
L11.9 **Acantholytic disorder, unspecified**

● **L12** **Pemphigoid**
> **Excludes1** herpes gestationis (O26.4-)
> impetigo herpetiformis (L40.1)
L12.0 **Bullous pemphigoid**
L12.1 **Cicatricial pemphigoid**
Benign mucous membrane pemphigoid
L12.2 **Chronic bullous disease of childhood**
Juvenile dermatitis herpetiformis
● **L12.3** **Acquired epidermolysis bullosa**
> **Excludes1** epidermolysis bullosa (congenital) (Q81.-)
L12.30 **Acquired epidermolysis bullosa, unspecified**
L12.31 **Epidermolysis bullosa due to drug**
> Use additional code for adverse effect, if applicable, to identify drug (T36-T50 with fifth or sixth character 5)
L12.35 **Other acquired epidermolysis bullosa**
L12.8 **Other pemphigoid**
L12.9 **Pemphigoid, unspecified**

CHAPTER 12 (L00-L99)

▶ New   ➡ Revised   ~~deleted~~ Deleted   **OGCR** Official Guidelines   X Assign placeholder X   ● Use Additional Character(s)
Excludes 1   Excludes 2   Includes   Use additional   Code first   Code also   Key words
919

Item 12–5 Dermatitis herpetiformis, also known as Duhring's disease, is a systemic disease characterized by small blisters (3 to 5 mm) and occasionally large bullae (> 5 mm).

Figure 12-3 Dermatitis herpetiformis. (From Terhorst D: BASICS Dermatologie, München, Elsevier, Urban & Fischer, 2011)

● **L13 Other bullous disorders**

L13.0 Dermatitis herpetiformis
Duhring's disease
Hydroa herpetiformis
Excludes1 | juvenile dermatitis herpetiformis (L12.2)
senile dermatitis herpetiformis (L12.0)

L13.1 Subcorneal pustular dermatitis
Sneddon-Wilkinson disease

L13.8 Other specified bullous disorders

L13.9 Bullous disorder, unspecified

L14 Bullous disorders in diseases classified elsewhere
Code first underlying disease

DERMATITIS AND ECZEMA (L20-L30)

Note: In this block the terms dermatitis and eczema are used synonymously and interchangeably.

Excludes2 | chronic (childhood) granulomatous disease (D71)
dermatitis gangrenosa (L08.0)
dermatitis herpetiformis (L13.0)
dry skin dermatitis (L85.3)
factitial dermatitis (L98.1)
perioral dermatitis (L71.0)
radiation-related disorders of the skin and
subcutaneous tissue (L55-L59)
stasis dermatitis (I87.2)

● **L20 Atopic dermatitis**

L20.0 Besnier's prurigo

● **L20.8 Other atopic dermatitis**
Excludes2 | circumscribed neurodermatitis (L28.0)

L20.81 Atopic neurodermatitis
Diffuse neurodermatitis

L20.82 Flexural eczema

L20.83 Infantile (acute) (chronic) eczema

L20.84 Intrinsic (allergic) eczema

L20.89 Other atopic dermatitis

L20.9 Atopic dermatitis, unspecified

● **L21 Seborrheic dermatitis**
Excludes2 | infective dermatitis (L30.3)
seborrheic keratosis (L82.-)

L21.0 Seborrhea capitis
Cradle cap

L21.1 Seborrheic infantile dermatitis

L21.8 Other seborrheic dermatitis

L21.9 Seborrheic dermatitis, unspecified
Seborrhea NOS

Item 12–7 Atopic dermatitis, also known as atopic eczema, infantile eczema, disseminated neuro dermatitis, flexural eczema, and *prurigo diathesique* (Besnier), is characterized by intense itching and is often hereditary.

Figure 12-5 Atopic dermatitis. (From Chabner D-E: The Language of Medicine, St. Louis, MO, Saunders/Elsevier, 2007)

L22 Diaper dermatitis
Diaper erythema
Diaper rash
Psoriasiform diaper rash

● **L23 Allergic contact dermatitis**
Excludes1 | allergy NOS (T78.40)
contact dermatitis NOS (L25.9)
dermatitis NOS (L30.9)
Excludes2 | dermatitis due to substances taken internally
(L27.-)
dermatitis of eyelid (H01.1-)
diaper dermatitis (L22)
eczema of external ear (H60.5-)
irritant contact dermatitis (L24.-)
perioral dermatitis (L71.0)
radiation-related disorders of the skin and
subcutaneous tissue (L55-L59)

L23.0 Allergic contact dermatitis due to metals
Allergic contact dermatitis due to chromium
Allergic contact dermatitis due to nickel

L23.1 Allergic contact dermatitis due to adhesives

L23.2 Allergic contact dermatitis due to cosmetics

L23.3 Allergic contact dermatitis due to drugs in contact with skin
Use additional code for adverse effect, if applicable, to identify drug (T36-T50 with fifth or sixth character 5)
Excludes2 | dermatitis due to ingested drugs and medicaments (L27.0-L27.1)

L23.4 Allergic contact dermatitis due to dyes

L23.5 Allergic contact dermatitis due to other chemical products
Allergic contact dermatitis due to cement
Allergic contact dermatitis due to insecticide
Allergic contact dermatitis due to plastic
Allergic contact dermatitis due to rubber

L23.6 Allergic contact dermatitis due to food in contact with the skin
Excludes2 | dermatitis due to ingested food (L27.2)

L23.7 Allergic contact dermatitis due to plants, except food
Excludes2 | allergy NOS due to pollen (J30.1)

● **L23.8 Allergic contact dermatitis due to other agents**

L23.81 Allergic contact dermatitis due to animal (cat) (dog) dander
Allergic contact dermatitis due to animal (cat) (dog) hair

L23.89 Allergic contact dermatitis due to other agents

L23.9 Allergic contact dermatitis, unspecified cause
Allergic contact eczema NOS

Item 12–6 Seborrheic dermatitis is characterized by greasy, scaly, red patches and is associated with oily skin and scalp.

Figure 12-4 Seborrheic dermatitis. (Getty Image)

▶ New ➡ Revised ~~deleted~~ Deleted **OGCR** Official Guidelines **X** Assign placeholder X ● Use Additional Character(s)
Excludes 1 | Excludes 2 | Includes | Use additional | Code first | Code also | Key words

● **L24   Irritant contact dermatitis**

> **Excludes1**   allergy NOS (T78.4Ø)
> contact dermatitis NOS (L25.9)
> dermatitis NOS (L3Ø.9)

> **Excludes2**   allergic contact dermatitis (L23.-)
> dermatitis due to substances taken internally
> (L27.-)
> dermatitis of eyelid (HØ1.1-)
> diaper dermatitis (L22)
> eczema of external ear (H6Ø.5-)
> perioral dermatitis (L71.Ø)
> radiation-related disorders of the skin and
> subcutaneous tissue (L55-L59)

L24.Ø   Irritant contact dermatitis due to detergents

L24.1   Irritant contact dermatitis due to oils and greases

L24.2   Irritant contact dermatitis due to solvents
> Irritant contact dermatitis due to chlorocompound
> Irritant contact dermatitis due to cyclohexane
> Irritant contact dermatitis due to ester
> Irritant contact dermatitis due to glycol
> Irritant contact dermatitis due to hydrocarbon
> Irritant contact dermatitis due to ketone

L24.3   Irritant contact dermatitis due to cosmetics

L24.4   Irritant contact dermatitis due to drugs in contact with skin
> Use additional code for adverse effect, if applicable,
> to identify drug (T36-T5Ø with fifth or sixth
> character 5)

L24.5   Irritant contact dermatitis due to other chemical products
> Irritant contact dermatitis due to cement
> Irritant contact dermatitis due to insecticide
> Irritant contact dermatitis due to plastic
> Irritant contact dermatitis due to rubber

L24.6   Irritant contact dermatitis due to food in contact with skin
> **Excludes2**   dermatitis due to ingested food (L27.2)

L24.7   Irritant contact dermatitis due to plants, except food
> **Excludes2**   allergy NOS to pollen (J3Ø.1)

● **L24.8   Irritant contact dermatitis due to other agents**

> **L24.81   Irritant contact dermatitis due to metals**
> Irritant contact dermatitis due to chromium
> Irritant contact dermatitis due to nickel

> **L24.89   Irritant contact dermatitis due to other agents**
> Irritant contact dermatitis due to dyes

L24.9   Irritant contact dermatitis, unspecified cause
> Irritant contact eczema NOS

● **L25   Unspecified contact dermatitis**

> **Excludes1**   allergic contact dermatitis (L23.-)
> allergy NOS (T78.4Ø)
> dermatitis NOS (L3Ø.9)
> irritant contact dermatitis (L24.-)

> **Excludes2**   dermatitis due to ingested substances (L27.-)
> dermatitis of eyelid (HØ1.1-)
> eczema of external ear (H6Ø.5-)
> perioral dermatitis (L71.Ø)
> radiation-related disorders of the skin and
> subcutaneous tissue (L55-L59)

L25.Ø   Unspecified contact dermatitis due to cosmetics

L25.1   Unspecified contact dermatitis due to drugs in contact with skin
> Use additional code for adverse effect, if applicable,
> to identify drug (T36-T5Ø with fifth or sixth
> character 5)
> **Excludes2**   dermatitis due to ingested drugs and
> medicaments (L27.Ø-L27.1)

L25.2   Unspecified contact dermatitis due to dyes

L25.3   Unspecified contact dermatitis due to other chemical products
> Unspecified contact dermatitis due to cement
> Unspecified contact dermatitis due to insecticide

L25.4   Unspecified contact dermatitis due to food in contact with skin
> **Excludes2**   dermatitis due to ingested food (L27.2)

L25.5   Unspecified contact dermatitis due to plants, except food
> **Excludes1**   nettle rash (L5Ø.9)
> **Excludes2**   allergy NOS due to pollen (J3Ø.1)

L25.8   Unspecified contact dermatitis due to other agents

L25.9   Unspecified contact dermatitis, unspecified cause
> Contact dermatitis (occupational) NOS
> Contact eczema (occupational) NOS

L26   Exfoliative dermatitis
> Hebra's pityriasis
> **Excludes1**   Ritter's disease (LØØ)

● **L27   Dermatitis due to substances taken internally**
> **Excludes1**   allergy NOS (T78.4Ø)
> **Excludes2**   adverse food reaction, except dermatitis
> (T78.Ø-T78.1)
> contact dermatitis (L23-L25)
> drug photoallergic response (L56.1)
> drug phototoxic response (L56.Ø)
> urticaria (L5Ø.-)

L27.Ø   Generalized skin eruption due to drugs and medicaments taken internally
> Use additional code for adverse effect, if applicable,
> to identify drug (T36-T5Ø with fifth or sixth
> character 5)

L27.1   Localized skin eruption due to drugs and medicaments taken internally
> Use additional code for adverse effect, if applicable,
> to identify drug (T36-T5Ø with fifth or sixth
> character 5)

L27.2   Dermatitis due to ingested food
> **Excludes2**   dermatitis due to food in contact with
> skin (L23.6, L24.6, L25.4)

L27.8   Dermatitis due to other substances taken internally

L27.9   Dermatitis due to unspecified substance taken internally

● **L28   Lichen simplex chronicus and prurigo**

L28.Ø   Lichen simplex chronicus
> Circumscribed neurodermatitis
> Lichen NOS

L28.1   Prurigo nodularis

L28.2   Other prurigo
> Prurigo NOS   Prurigo mitis
> Prurigo Hebra   Urticaria papulosa

● **L29   Pruritus**
> **Excludes1**   neurotic excoriation (L98.1)
> psychogenic pruritus (F45.8)

L29.Ø   Pruritus ani

L29.1   Pruritus scroti

L29.2   Pruritus vulvae

L29.3   Anogenital pruritus, unspecified

L29.8   Other pruritus

L29.9   Pruritus, unspecified
> Itch NOS

CHAPTER 12 (LØØ-L99)

●L30 Other and unspecified dermatitis
> Excludes2   contact dermatitis (L23-L25)
> dry skin dermatitis (L85.3)
> small plaque parapsoriasis (L41.3)
> stasis dermatitis (I87.2)

L30.0 Nummular dermatitis

L30.1 Dyshidrosis [pompholyx]

L30.2 Cutaneous autosensitization
Candidid [levurid]   Eczematid
Dermatophytid

L30.3 Infective dermatitis
Infectious eczematoid dermatitis

L30.4 Erythema intertrigo

L30.5 Pityriasis alba

L30.8 Other specified dermatitis

L30.9 Dermatitis, unspecified
Eczema NOS

PAPULOSQUAMOUS DISORDERS (L40-L45)

●L40 Psoriasis

L40.0 Psoriasis vulgaris
Nummular psoriasis   Plaque psoriasis

L40.1 Generalized pustular psoriasis
Impetigo herpetiformis
Von Zumbusch's disease

L40.2 Acrodermatitis continua

L40.3 Pustulosis palmaris et plantaris

L40.4 Guttate psoriasis

●L40.5 Arthropathic psoriasis
L40.50   Arthropathic psoriasis, unspecified
L40.51   Distal interphalangeal psoriatic arthropathy
L40.52   Psoriatic arthritis mutilans
L40.53   Psoriatic spondylitis
L40.54   Psoriatic juvenile arthropathy
L40.59   Other psoriatic arthropathy

L40.8 Other psoriasis
Flexural psoriasis

L40.9 Psoriasis, unspecified

●L41 Parapsoriasis
> Excludes1   poikiloderma vasculare atrophicans (L94.5)

L41.0 Pityriasis lichenoides et varioliformis acuta
Mucha-Habermann disease

L41.1 Pityriasis lichenoides chronica

L41.3 Small plaque parapsoriasis

L41.4 Large plaque parapsoriasis

L41.5 Retiform parapsoriasis

L41.8 Other parapsoriasis

L41.9 Parapsoriasis, unspecified

L42 Pityriasis rosea

●L43 Lichen planus
> Excludes1   lichen planopilaris (L66.1)

L43.0 Hypertrophic lichen planus

L43.1 Bullous lichen planus

L43.2 Lichenoid drug reaction
Use additional code for adverse effect, if applicable, to identify drug (T36-T50 with fifth or sixth character 5)

L43.3 Subacute (active) lichen planus
Lichen planus tropicus

L43.8 Other lichen planus

L43.9 Lichen planus, unspecified

●L44 Other papulosquamous disorders

L44.0 Pityriasis rubra pilaris

L44.1 Lichen nitidus

L44.2 Lichen striatus

L44.3 Lichen ruber moniliformis

L44.4 Infantile papular acrodermatitis [Gianotti-Crosti]

L44.8 Other specified papulosquamous disorders

L44.9 Papulosquamous disorder, unspecified

L45 Papulosquamous disorders in diseases classified elsewhere
Code first underlying disease

URTICARIA AND ERYTHEMA (L49-L54)

> Excludes1   Lyme disease (A69.2-)
> rosacea (L71.-)

●L49 Exfoliation due to erythematous conditions according to extent of body surface involved
Code first erythematous condition causing exfoliation, such as:
Ritter's disease (L00)
(Staphylococcal) scalded skin syndrome (L00)
Stevens-Johnson syndrome (L51.1)
Stevens-Johnson syndrome-toxic epidermal necrolysis overlap syndrome (L51.3)
Toxic epidermal necrolysis (L51.2)

L49.0 Exfoliation due to erythematous condition involving less than 10 percent of body surface
Exfoliation due to erythematous condition NOS

L49.1 Exfoliation due to erythematous condition involving 10-19 percent of body surface

L49.2 Exfoliation due to erythematous condition involving 20-29 percent of body surface

L49.3 Exfoliation due to erythematous condition involving 30-39 percent of body surface

L49.4 Exfoliation due to erythematous condition involving 40-49 percent of body surface

L49.5 Exfoliation due to erythematous condition involving 50-59 percent of body surface

L49.6 Exfoliation due to erythematous condition involving 60-69 percent of body surface

L49.7 Exfoliation due to erythematous condition involving 70-79 percent of body surface

L49.8 Exfoliation due to erythematous condition involving 80-89 percent of body surface

L49.9 Exfoliation due to erythematous condition involving 90 or more percent of body surface

Item 12-8 Psoriasis is a chronic, recurrent inflammatory skin disease characterized by small patches covered with thick silvery scales. **Parapsoriasis** is a treatment-resistant erythroderma. **Pityriasis rosea** is characterized by a herald patch that is a single large lesion and that usually appears on the trunk and is followed by scattered, smaller lesions.

Figure 12-6 Erythematous plaques with silvery scales in a patient with psoriasis. (Getty Image)

▶ New   ⇒ Revised   ~~deleted~~ Deleted   **OGCR** Official Guidelines   X Assign placeholder X   ● Use Additional Character(s)

Excludes 1   Excludes 2   Includes   Use additional   Code first   Code also   Key words

Figure 12-7 Urticaria (hives). *(Courtesy of David Effron, MD.) (Getty Image)*

Item 12–9 Urticaria is a vascular reaction in which wheals surrounded by a red halo appear and cause severe itching. The causes of urticaria or hives are extensive and varied (e.g., food, heat, cold, drugs, stress, infections).

● **L50 Urticaria**
> Excludes1 allergic contact dermatitis (L23.-)
> angioneurotic edema (T78.3)
> giant urticaria (T78.3)
> hereditary angio-edema (D84.1)
> Quincke's edema (T78.3)
> serum urticaria (T80.6-)
> solar urticaria (L56.3)
> urticaria neonatorum (P83.8)
> urticaria papulosa (L28.2)
> urticaria pigmentosa (Q82.2)

  L50.0 Allergic urticaria
  L50.1 Idiopathic urticaria
  L50.2 Urticaria due to cold and heat
> Excludes2 familial cold urticaria (M04.2)

  L50.3 Dermatographic urticaria
  L50.4 Vibratory urticaria
  L50.5 Cholinergic urticaria
  L50.6 Contact urticaria
  L50.8 Other urticaria
> Chronic urticaria
> Recurrent periodic urticaria

  L50.9 Urticaria, unspecified

● **L51 Erythema multiforme**
> Use additional code for adverse effect, if applicable, to identify drug (T36-T50 with fifth or sixth character 5)
> Use additional code to identify associated manifestations, such as:
> arthropathy associated with dermatological disorders (M14.8-)
> conjunctival edema (H11.42)
> conjunctivitis (H10.22-)
> corneal scars and opacities (H17.-)
> corneal ulcer (H16.0-)
> edema of eyelid (H02.84)
> inflammation of eyelid (H01.8)
> keratoconjunctivitis sicca (H16.22-)
> mechanical lagophthalmos (H02.22-)
> stomatitis (K12.-)
> symblepharon (H11.23-)
> Use additional code to identify percentage of skin exfoliation (L49.-)
> Excludes1 staphylococcal scalded skin syndrome (L00)
> Ritter's disease (L00)

  L51.0 Nonbullous erythema multiforme
  L51.1 Stevens-Johnson syndrome
  L51.2 Toxic epidermal necrolysis [Lyell]
  L51.3 Stevens-Johnson syndrome-toxic epidermal necrolysis overlap syndrome
> SJS-TEN overlap syndrome

  L51.8 Other erythema multiforme
  L51.9 Erythema multiforme, unspecified
> Erythema iris
> Erythema multiforme major NOS
> Erythema multiforme minor NOS
> Herpes iris

L52 Erythema nodosum
> Excludes1 tuberculous erythema nodosum (A18.4)

L53 Other erythematous conditions
> Excludes1 erythema ab igne (L59.0)
> erythema due to external agents in contact with skin (L23-L25)
> erythema intertrigo (L30.4)

  L53.0 Toxic erythema
> *Code first poisoning due to drug or toxin, if applicable (T36-T65 with fifth or sixth character 1-4 or 6)*
> Use additional code for adverse effect, if applicable, to identify drug (T36-T50 with fifth or sixth character 5)
> Excludes1 neonatal erythema toxicum (P83.1)

  L53.1 Erythema annulare centrifugum
  L53.2 Erythema marginatum
  L53.3 Other chronic figurate erythema
  L53.8 Other specified erythematous conditions
  L53.9 Erythematous condition, unspecified
> Erythema NOS
> Erythroderma NOS

L54 Erythema in diseases classified elsewhere
> *Code first underlying disease*

RADIATION-RELATED DISORDERS OF THE SKIN AND SUBCUTANEOUS TISSUE (L55-L59)

● **L55 Sunburn**
  L55.0 Sunburn of first degree
  L55.1 Sunburn of second degree
  L55.2 Sunburn of third degree
  L55.9 Sunburn, unspecified

● **L56 Other acute skin changes due to ultraviolet radiation**
> Use additional code to identify the source of the ultraviolet radiation (W89, X32)

  L56.0 Drug phototoxic response
> Use additional code for adverse effect, if applicable, to identify drug (T36-T50 with fifth or sixth character 5)

  L56.1 Drug photoallergic response
> Use additional code for adverse effect, if applicable, to identify drug (T36-T50 with fifth or sixth character 5)

  L56.2 Photocontact dermatitis [berloque dermatitis]
  L56.3 Solar urticaria
  L56.4 Polymorphous light eruption
  L56.5 Disseminated superficial actinic porokeratosis (DSAP)
  L56.8 Other specified acute skin changes due to ultraviolet radiation
  L56.9 Acute skin change due to ultraviolet radiation, unspecified

● **L57 Skin changes due to chronic exposure to nonionizing radiation**
> ⇒ Use additional code to identify the source of the ultraviolet radiation (W89)

  L57.0 Actinic keratosis
> Keratosis NOS   Solar keratosis
> Senile keratosis

  L57.1 Actinic reticuloid
  L57.2 Cutis rhomboidalis nuchae
  L57.3 Poikiloderma of Civatte
  L57.4 Cutis laxa senilis
> Elastosis senilis

  L57.5 Actinic granuloma
  L57.8 Other skin changes due to chronic exposure to nonionizing radiation
> Farmer's skin   Solar dermatitis
> Sailor's skin

  L57.9 Skin changes due to chronic exposure to nonionizing radiation, unspecified

● **L58   Radiodermatitis**

Use additional code to identify the source of the radiation (W88, W90)

L58.0   Acute radiodermatitis

L58.1   Chronic radiodermatitis

L58.9   Radiodermatitis, unspecified

● **L59   Other disorders of skin and subcutaneous tissue related to radiation**

L59.0   Erythema ab igne [dermatitis ab igne]

L59.8   Other specified disorders of the skin and subcutaneous tissue related to radiation

L59.9   Disorder of the skin and subcutaneous tissue related to radiation, unspecified

DISORDERS OF SKIN APPENDAGES (L60-L75)

Excludes1   congenital malformations of integument (Q84.-)

● **L60   Nail disorders**

Excludes2   clubbing of nails (R68.3)
onychia and paronychia (L03.0-)

L60.0   Ingrowing nail

L60.1   Onycholysis

L60.2   Onychogryphosis

L60.3   Nail dystrophy

L60.4   Beau's lines

L60.5   Yellow nail syndrome

L60.8   Other nail disorders

L60.9   Nail disorder, unspecified

L62   Nail disorders in diseases classified elsewhere

Code first underlying disease, such as:
pachydermoperiostosis (M89.4-)

● **L63   Alopecia areata**

L63.0   Alopecia (capitis) totalis

L63.1   Alopecia universalis

L63.2   Ophiasis

L63.8   Other alopecia areata

L63.9   Alopecia areata, unspecified

● **L64   Androgenic alopecia**

Includes   male-pattern baldness

L64.0   Drug-induced androgenic alopecia

Use additional code for adverse effect, if applicable, to identify drug (T36-T50 with fifth or sixth character 5)

L64.8   Other androgenic alopecia

L64.9   Androgenic alopecia, unspecified

● **L65   Other nonscarring hair loss**

Use additional code for adverse effect, if applicable, to identify drug (T36-T50 with fifth or sixth character 5)

Excludes1   trichotillomania (F63.3)

L65.0   Telogen effluvium

L65.1   Anagen effluvium

L65.2   Alopecia mucinosa

L65.8   Other specified nonscarring hair loss

L65.9   Nonscarring hair loss, unspecified
Alopecia NOS

● **L66   Cicatricial alopecia [scarring hair loss]**

L66.0   Pseudopelade

L66.1   Lichen planopilaris
Follicular lichen planus

L66.2   Folliculitis decalvans

L66.3   Perifolliculitis capitis abscedens

L66.4   Folliculitis ulerythematosa reticulata

L66.8   Other cicatricial alopecia

L66.9   Cicatricial alopecia, unspecified

● **L67   Hair color and hair shaft abnormalities**

Excludes1   monilethrix (Q84.1)
pili annulati (Q84.1)
telogen effluvium (L65.0)

L67.0   Trichorrhexis nodosa

L67.1   Variations in hair color
Canities
Greyness, hair (premature)
Heterochromia of hair
Poliosis circumscripta, acquired
Poliosis NOS

L67.8   Other hair color and hair shaft abnormalities
Fragilitas crinium

L67.9   Hair color and hair shaft abnormality, unspecified

● **L68   Hypertrichosis**

Includes   excess hair

Excludes1   congenital hypertrichosis (Q84.2)
persistent lanugo (Q84.2)

L68.0   Hirsutism
Excessive growth of hair

L68.1   Acquired hypertrichosis lanuginosa

L68.2   Localized hypertrichosis

L68.3   Polytrichia

L68.8   Other hypertrichosis

L68.9   Hypertrichosis, unspecified

Item 12–10   Alopecia is lack of hair and takes many forms. The most common is male pattern alopecia, also known as **androgenetic alopecia. Telogen effluvium** is early and excessive loss of hair resulting from a trauma to the hair follicle (fever, drugs, surgery, etc.).

Figure 12-8   Male pattern alopecia.

▶ New   ⇒ Revised   ~~deleted~~ Deleted   **OGCR** Official Guidelines   X Assign placeholder X   ● Use Additional Character(s)

Excludes 1   Excludes 2   Includes   Use additional   Code first   Code also   Key words

● **L70   Acne**

> **Excludes2**   acne keloid (L73.0)

L70.0   Acne vulgaris

L70.1   Acne conglobata

L70.2   Acne varioliformis
Acne necrotica miliaris

L70.3   Acne tropica

L70.4   Infantile acne

L70.5   Acné excoriée
Acné excoriée des jeunes filles
Picker's acne

L70.8   Other acne

L70.9   Acne, unspecified

● **L71   Rosacea**

> Use additional code for adverse effect, if applicable, to identify drug (T36-T50 with fifth or sixth character 5)

L71.0   Perioral dermatitis

L71.1   Rhinophyma

L71.8   Other rosacea

L71.9   Rosacea, unspecified

● **L72   Follicular cysts of skin and subcutaneous tissue**

L72.0   Epidermal cyst

● **L72.1   Pilar and trichodermal cyst**

L72.11   Pilar cyst

L72.12   Trichodermal cyst
Trichilemmal (proliferating) cyst

L72.3   Sebaceous cyst

> **Excludes2**   pilar cyst (L72.11)
> trichilemmal (proliferating) cyst (L72.12)

L72.2   Steatocystoma multiplex

L72.8   Other follicular cysts of the skin and subcutaneous tissue

L72.9   Follicular cyst of the skin and subcutaneous tissue, unspecified

● **L73   Other follicular disorders**

L73.0   Acne keloid

L73.1   Pseudofolliculitis barbae

L73.2   Hidradenitis suppurativa

L73.8   Other specified follicular disorders
Sycosis barbae

L73.9   Follicular disorder, unspecified

● **L74   Eccrine sweat disorders**

> **Excludes2**   generalized hyperhidrosis (R61)

L74.0   Miliaria rubra

L74.1   Miliaria crystallina

L74.2   Miliaria profunda
Miliaria tropicalis

L74.3   Miliaria, unspecified

L74.4   Anhidrosis
Hypohidrosis

● **L74.5   Focal hyperhidrosis**

● **L74.51   Primary focal hyperhidrosis**

L74.510   Primary focal hyperhidrosis, axilla

L74.511   Primary focal hyperhidrosis, face

L74.512   Primary focal hyperhidrosis, palms

L74.513   Primary focal hyperhidrosis, soles

L74.519   Primary focal hyperhidrosis, unspecified

L74.52   Secondary focal hyperhidrosis
Frey's syndrome

L74.8   Other eccrine sweat disorders

L74.9   Eccrine sweat disorder, unspecified
Sweat gland disorder NOS

● **L75   Apocrine sweat disorders**

> **Excludes1**   dyshidrosis (L30.1)
> hidradenitis suppurativa (L73.2)

L75.0   Bromhidrosis

L75.1   Chromhidrosis

L75.2   Apocrine miliaria
Fox-Fordyce disease

L75.8   Other apocrine sweat disorders

L75.9   Apocrine sweat disorder, unspecified
Intraoperative and postprocedural complications of skin and subcutaneous tissue (L76)

INTRAOPERATIVE AND POSTPROCEDURAL COMPLICATIONS OF SKIN AND SUBCUTANEOUS TISSUE (L76)

● **L76   Intraoperative and postprocedural complications of skin and subcutaneous tissue**

● **L76.0   Intraoperative hemorrhage and hematoma of skin and subcutaneous tissue complicating a procedure**

> **Excludes1**   intraoperative hemorrhage and hematoma of skin and subcutaneous tissue due to accidental puncture and laceration during a procedure (L76.1-)

L76.01   Intraoperative hemorrhage and hematoma of skin and subcutaneous tissue complicating a dermatologic procedure

L76.02   Intraoperative hemorrhage and hematoma of skin and subcutaneous tissue complicating other procedure

● **L76.1   Accidental puncture and laceration of skin and subcutaneous tissue during a procedure**

L76.11   Accidental puncture and laceration of skin and subcutaneous tissue during a dermatologic procedure

L76.12   Accidental puncture and laceration of skin and subcutaneous tissue during other procedure

● **L76.2   Postprocedural hemorrhage of skin and subcutaneous tissue following a procedure**

L76.21   Postprocedural hemorrhage of skin and subcutaneous tissue following a dermatologic procedure

L76.22   Postprocedural hemorrhage of skin and subcutaneous tissue following other procedure

● **L76.3   Postprocedural hematoma and seroma of skin and subcutaneous tissue following a procedure**

L76.31   Postprocedural hematoma of skin and subcutaneous tissue following a dermatologic procedure

L76.32   Postprocedural hematoma of skin and subcutaneous tissue following other procedure

L76.33   Postprocedural seroma of skin and subcutaneous tissue following a dermatologic procedure

L76.34   Postprocedural seroma of skin and subcutaneous tissue following other procedure

● **L76.8   Other intraoperative and postprocedural complications of skin and subcutaneous tissue**

> Use additional code, if applicable, to further specify disorder

L76.81   Other intraoperative complications of skin and subcutaneous tissue

L76.82   Other postprocedural complications of skin and subcutaneous tissue

OTHER DISORDERS OF THE SKIN AND SUBCUTANEOUS TISSUE (L80-L99)

L80   Vitiligo
> **Excludes2**   vitiligo of eyelids (H02.73-)
>   vitiligo of vulva (N90.89)

● **L81   Other disorders of pigmentation**
> **Excludes1**   birthmark NOS (Q82.5)
>   Peutz-Jeghers syndrome (Q85.8)
> **Excludes2**   nevus - see Alphabetical Index

   L81.0   Postinflammatory hyperpigmentation

   L81.1   Chloasma

   L81.2   Freckles

   L81.3   Café au lait spots

   L81.4   Other melanin hyperpigmentation
        Lentigo

   L81.5   Leukoderma, not elsewhere classified

   L81.6   Other disorders of diminished melanin formation

   L81.7   Pigmented purpuric dermatosis
        Angioma serpiginosum

   L81.8   Other specified disorders of pigmentation
        Iron pigmentation
        Tattoo pigmentation

   L81.9   Disorder of pigmentation, unspecified

● **L82   Seborrheic keratosis**
> **Includes**   basal cell papilloma
>   dermatosis papulosa nigra
>   Leser-Trélat disease
> **Excludes2**   seborrheic dermatitis (L21.-)

   L82.0   Inflamed seborrheic keratosis

   L82.1   Other seborrheic keratosis
        Seborrheic keratosis NOS

● **L83   Acanthosis nigricans**
      Confluent and reticulated papillomatosis

L84   Corns and callosities
      Callus
      Clavus

● **L85   Other epidermal thickening**
> **Excludes2**   hypertrophic disorders of the skin (L91.-)

   L85.0   Acquired ichthyosis
> **Excludes1**   congenital ichthyosis (Q80.-)

   L85.1   Acquired keratosis [keratoderma] palmaris et plantaris
> **Excludes1**   inherited keratosis palmaris et plantaris (Q82.8)

   L85.2   Keratosis punctata (palmaris et plantaris)

   L85.3   Xerosis cutis
        Dry skin dermatitis

   L85.8   Other specified epidermal thickening
        Cutaneous horn

   L85.9   Epidermal thickening, unspecified

L86   Keratoderma in diseases classified elsewhere
Firm horny papules that have a cobblestone appearance.
Code first underlying disease, such as:
      Reiter's disease (M02.3-)
> **Excludes1**   gonococcal keratoderma (A54.89)
>   gonococcal keratosis (A54.89)
>   keratoderma due to vitamin A deficiency (E50.8)
>   keratosis due to vitamin A deficiency (E50.8)
>   xeroderma due to vitamin A deficiency (E50.8)

● **L87   Transepidermal elimination disorders**
> **Excludes1**   granuloma annulare (perforating) (L92.0)

   L87.0   Keratosis follicularis et parafollicularis in cutem penetrans
        Kyrle disease
        Hyperkeratosis follicularis penetrans

   L87.1   Reactive perforating collagenosis

   L87.2   Elastosis perforans serpiginosa

   L87.8   Other transepidermal elimination disorders

   L87.9   Transepidermal elimination disorder, unspecified

L88   Pyoderma gangrenosum
      Phagedenic pyoderma
> **Excludes1**   dermatitis gangrenosa (L08.0)

OGCR   Section I.B.14.

> General Coding Guidelines
>
> Documentation for BMI, *Depth of* Non-pressure ulcers, Pressure Ulcer Stages, **Coma Scale, and** *NIH Stroke Scale*
>
> For the Body Mass Index (BMI), depth of non-pressure chronic ulcers, pressure ulcer stage, **coma scale, and NIH stroke scale (NIHSS) codes,** code assignment may be based on medical record documentation from clinicians who are not the patient's provider (i.e., physician or other qualified healthcare practitioner legally accountable for establishing the patient's diagnosis), since this information is typically documented by other clinicians involved in the care of the patient (e.g., a dietitian often documents the BMI, a nurse often documents the pressure ulcer stages, **and an emergency medical technician often documents the coma scale**). However, the associated diagnosis (such as overweight, obesity, **acute stroke,** or pressure ulcer) must be documented by the patient's provider. If there is conflicting medical record documentation, either from the same clinician or different clinicians, the patient's attending provider should be queried for clarification.
>
> The BMI, **coma scale, and NHSS** codes should only be reported as secondary diagnoses.

● **L89   Pressure ulcer**
> **Includes**   bed sore   pressure area
>   decubitus ulcer   pressure sore
>   plaster ulcer

Code first any associated gangrene (I96)

> **Excludes2**   decubitus (trophic) ulcer of cervix (uteri) (N86)
>   diabetic ulcers (E08.621, E08.622, E09.621,
>   E09.622, E10.621, E10.622, E11.621, E11.622,
>   E13.621, E13.622)
>   non-pressure chronic ulcer of skin (L97.-)
>   skin infections (L00-L08)
>   varicose ulcer (I83.0, I83.2)

● **L89.0   Pressure ulcer of elbow**

   ● **L89.00   Pressure ulcer of unspecified elbow**

      L89.000   Pressure ulcer of unspecified elbow, unstageable

      L89.001   Pressure ulcer of unspecified elbow, stage 1
          Healing pressure ulcer of unspecified elbow, stage 1
          Pressure pre-ulcer skin changes limited to persistent focal edema, unspecified elbow

      L89.002   Pressure ulcer of unspecified elbow, stage 2
          Healing pressure ulcer of unspecified elbow, stage 2
          Pressure ulcer with abrasion, blister, partial thickness skin loss involving epidermis and/or dermis, unspecified elbow

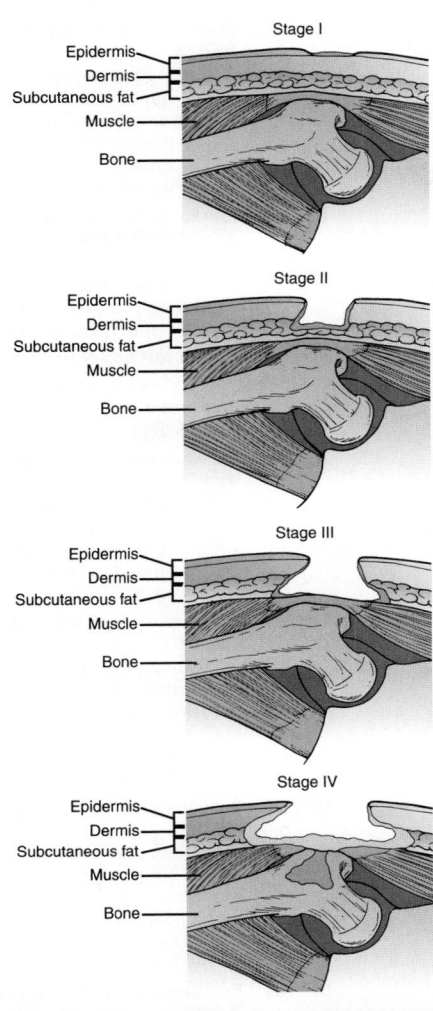

Stage I

Epidermis
Dermis
Subcutaneous fat
Muscle
Bone

Stage II

Epidermis
Dermis
Subcutaneous fat
Muscle
Bone

Stage III

Epidermis
Dermis
Subcutaneous fat
Muscle
Bone

Stage IV

Epidermis
Dermis
Subcutaneous fat
Muscle
Bone

Figure 12-9 Stage I, II, III, and IV of pressure ulcers.

L89.003 **Pressure ulcer of unspecified elbow, stage 3**
    Healing pressure ulcer of unspecified elbow, stage 3
    Pressure ulcer with full thickness skin loss involving damage or necrosis of subcutaneous tissue, unspecified elbow

L89.004 **Pressure ulcer of unspecified elbow, stage 4**
    Healing pressure ulcer of unspecified elbow, stage 4
    Pressure ulcer with necrosis of soft tissues through to underlying muscle, tendon, or bone, unspecified elbow

L89.009 **Pressure ulcer of unspecified elbow, unspecified stage**
    Healing pressure ulcer of elbow NOS
    Healing pressure ulcer of unspecified elbow, unspecified stage

● **L89.01** **Pressure ulcer of right elbow**
   L89.010 **Pressure ulcer of right elbow, unstageable**
   L89.011 **Pressure ulcer of right elbow, stage 1**
      Healing pressure ulcer of right elbow, stage 1
      Pressure pre-ulcer skin changes limited to persistent focal edema, right elbow
   L89.012 **Pressure ulcer of right elbow, stage 2**
      Healing pressure ulcer of right elbow, stage 2
      Pressure ulcer with abrasion, blister, partial thickness skin loss involving epidermis and/or dermis, right elbow
   L89.013 **Pressure ulcer of right elbow, stage 3**
      Healing pressure ulcer of right elbow, stage 3
      Pressure ulcer with full thickness skin loss involving damage or necrosis of subcutaneous tissue, right elbow
   L89.014 **Pressure ulcer of right elbow, stage 4**
      Healing pressure ulcer of right elbow, stage 4
      Pressure ulcer with necrosis of soft tissues through to underlying muscle, tendon, or bone, right elbow
   L89.019 **Pressure ulcer of right elbow, unspecified stage**
      Healing pressure right of elbow NOS
      ➠Healing pressure ulcer of right elbow, unspecified stage

● **L89.02** **Pressure ulcer of left elbow**
   L89.020 **Pressure ulcer of left elbow, unstageable**
   L89.021 **Pressure ulcer of left elbow, stage 1**
      Healing pressure ulcer of left elbow, stage 1
      Pressure pre-ulcer skin changes limited to persistent focal edema, left elbow
   L89.022 **Pressure ulcer of left elbow, stage 2**
      Healing pressure ulcer of left elbow, stage 2
      Pressure ulcer with abrasion, blister, partial thickness skin loss involving epidermis and/or dermis, left elbow
   L89.023 **Pressure ulcer of left elbow, stage 3**
      Healing pressure ulcer of left elbow, stage 3
      Pressure ulcer with full thickness skin loss involving damage or necrosis of subcutaneous tissue, left elbow
   L89.024 **Pressure ulcer of left elbow, stage 4**
      Healing pressure ulcer of left elbow, stage 4
      Pressure ulcer with necrosis of soft tissues through to underlying muscle, tendon, or bone, left elbow
   L89.029 **Pressure ulcer of left elbow, unspecified stage**
      Healing pressure ulcer of left of elbow NOS
      ➠Healing pressure ulcer of left elbow, unspecified stage

CHAPTER 12 (L00-L99)

CHAPTER 12 (L00-L99)

● **L89.1**   Pressure ulcer of back
    ● **L89.10**   Pressure ulcer of unspecified part of back
        L89.100   Pressure ulcer of unspecified part of back, **unstageable**
        L89.101   Pressure ulcer of unspecified part of back, **stage 1**
               Healing pressure ulcer of unspecified part of back, stage 1
               Pressure pre-ulcer skin changes limited to persistent focal edema, unspecified part of back
        L89.102   Pressure ulcer of unspecified part of back, **stage 2**
               Healing pressure ulcer of unspecified part of back, stage 2
               Pressure ulcer with abrasion, blister, partial thickness skin loss involving epidermis and/or dermis, unspecified part of back
        L89.103   Pressure ulcer of unspecified part of back, **stage 3**
               Healing pressure ulcer of unspecified part of back, stage 3
               Pressure ulcer with full thickness skin loss involving damage or necrosis of subcutaneous tissue, unspecified part of back
        L89.104   Pressure ulcer of unspecified part of back, **stage 4**
               Healing pressure ulcer of unspecified part of back, stage 4
               Pressure ulcer with necrosis of soft tissues through to underlying muscle, tendon, or bone, unspecified part of back
        L89.109   Pressure ulcer of unspecified part of back, **unspecified stage**
               Healing pressure ulcer of unspecified part of back NOS
               Healing pressure ulcer of unspecified part of back, unspecified stage
    ● **L89.11**   Pressure ulcer of right upper back
            Pressure ulcer of right shoulder blade
        L89.110   Pressure ulcer of right upper back, **unstageable**
        L89.111   Pressure ulcer of right upper back, **stage 1**
               Healing pressure ulcer of right upper back, stage 1
               Pressure pre-ulcer skin changes limited to persistent focal edema, right upper back
        L89.112   Pressure ulcer of right upper back, **stage 2**
               Healing pressure ulcer of right upper back, stage 2
               Pressure ulcer with abrasion, blister, partial thickness skin loss involving epidermis and/or dermis, right upper back
        L89.113   Pressure ulcer of right upper back, **stage 3**
               Healing pressure ulcer of right upper back, stage 3
               Pressure ulcer with full thickness skin loss involving damage or necrosis of subcutaneous tissue, right upper back

        L89.114   Pressure ulcer of right upper back, **stage 4**
               Healing pressure ulcer of right upper back, stage 4
               Pressure ulcer with necrosis of soft tissues through to underlying muscle, tendon, or bone, right upper back
        L89.119   Pressure ulcer of right upper back, **unspecified stage**
               Healing pressure ulcer of right upper back NOS
               Healing pressure ulcer of right upper back, unspecified stage
    ● **L89.12**   Pressure ulcer of left upper back
            Pressure ulcer of left shoulder blade
        L89.120   Pressure ulcer of left upper back, **unstageable**
        L89.121   Pressure ulcer of left upper back, **stage 1**
               Healing pressure ulcer of left upper back, stage 1
               Pressure pre-ulcer skin changes limited to persistent focal edema, left upper back
        L89.122   Pressure ulcer of left upper back, **stage 2**
               Healing pressure ulcer of left upper back, stage 2
               Pressure ulcer with abrasion, blister, partial thickness skin loss involving epidermis and/or dermis, left upper back
        L89.123   Pressure ulcer of left upper back, **stage 3**
               Healing pressure ulcer of left upper back, stage 3
               Pressure ulcer with full thickness skin loss involving damage or necrosis of subcutaneous tissue, left upper back
        L89.124   Pressure ulcer of left upper back, **stage 4**
               Healing pressure ulcer of left upper back, stage 4
               Pressure ulcer with necrosis of soft tissues through to underlying muscle, tendon, or bone, left upper back
        L89.129   Pressure ulcer of left upper back, **unspecified stage**
               Healing pressure ulcer of left upper back NOS
               Healing pressure ulcer of left upper back, unspecified stage
    ● **L89.13**   Pressure ulcer of right lower back
        L89.130   Pressure ulcer of right lower back, **unstageable**
        L89.131   Pressure ulcer of right lower back, **stage 1**
               Healing pressure ulcer of right lower back, stage 1
               Pressure pre-ulcer skin changes limited to persistent focal edema, right lower back
        L89.132   Pressure ulcer of right lower back, **stage 2**
               Healing pressure ulcer of right lower back, stage 2
               Pressure ulcer with abrasion, blister, partial thickness skin loss involving epidermis and/or dermis, right lower back

▶ New   ⟹ Revised   ~~deleted~~ Deleted   **OGCR** Official Guidelines   X Assign placeholder X   ● Use Additional Character(s)

Excludes 1   Excludes 2   Includes   Use additional   Code first   Code also   Key words

L89.133   **Pressure ulcer of right lower back, stage 3**
       Healing pressure ulcer of right lower back, stage 3
       Pressure ulcer with full thickness skin loss involving damage or necrosis of subcutaneous tissue, right lower back

L89.134   **Pressure ulcer of right lower back, stage 4**
       Healing pressure ulcer of right lower back, stage 4
       Pressure ulcer with necrosis of soft tissues through to underlying muscle, tendon, or bone, right lower back

L89.139   **Pressure ulcer of right lower back, unspecified stage**
       Healing pressure ulcer of right lower back NOS
       Healing pressure ulcer of right lower back, unspecified stage

● **L89.14   Pressure ulcer of left lower back**

L89.140   **Pressure ulcer of left lower back, unstageable**

L89.141   **Pressure ulcer of left lower back, stage 1**
       Healing pressure ulcer of left lower back, stage 1
       Pressure pre-ulcer skin changes limited to persistent focal edema, left lower back

L89.142   **Pressure ulcer of left lower back, stage 2**
       Healing pressure ulcer of left lower back, stage 2
       Pressure ulcer with abrasion, blister, partial thickness skin loss involving epidermis and/or dermis, left lower back

L89.143   **Pressure ulcer of left lower back, stage 3**
       Healing pressure ulcer of left lower back, stage 3
       Pressure ulcer with full thickness skin loss involving damage or necrosis of subcutaneous tissue, left lower back

L89.144   **Pressure ulcer of left lower back, stage 4**
       Healing pressure ulcer of left lower back, stage 4
       Pressure ulcer with necrosis of soft tissues through to underlying muscle, tendon, or bone, left lower back

L89.149   **Pressure ulcer of left lower back, unspecified stage**
       Healing pressure ulcer of left lower back NOS
       Healing pressure ulcer of left lower back, unspecified stage

● **L89.15   Pressure ulcer of sacral region**
     Pressure ulcer of coccyx
     Pressure ulcer of tailbone

L89.150   **Pressure ulcer of sacral region, unstageable**

L89.151   **Pressure ulcer of sacral region, stage 1**
       Healing pressure ulcer of sacral region, stage 1
       Pressure pre-ulcer skin changes limited to persistent focal edema, sacral region

L89.152   **Pressure ulcer of sacral region, stage 2**
       Healing pressure ulcer of sacral region, stage 2
       Pressure ulcer with abrasion, blister, partial thickness skin loss involving epidermis and/or dermis, sacral region

L89.153   **Pressure ulcer of sacral region, stage 3**
       Healing pressure ulcer of sacral region, stage 3
       Pressure ulcer with full thickness skin loss involving damage or necrosis of subcutaneous tissue, sacral region

L89.154   **Pressure ulcer of sacral region, stage 4**
       Healing pressure ulcer of sacral region, stage 4
       Pressure ulcer with necrosis of soft tissues through to underlying muscle, tendon, or bone, sacral region

L89.159   **Pressure ulcer of sacral region, unspecified stage**
       Healing pressure ulcer of sacral region NOS
       Healing pressure ulcer of sacral region, unspecified stage

● **L89.2   Pressure ulcer of hip**

● **L89.20   Pressure ulcer of unspecified hip**

L89.200   **Pressure ulcer of unspecified hip, unstageable**

L89.201   **Pressure ulcer of unspecified hip, stage 1**
       Healing pressure ulcer of unspecified hip back, stage 1
       Pressure pre-ulcer skin changes limited to persistent focal edema, unspecified hip

L89.202   **Pressure ulcer of unspecified hip, stage 2**
       Healing pressure ulcer of unspecified hip, stage 2
       Pressure ulcer with abrasion, blister, partial thickness skin loss involving epidermis and/or dermis, unspecified hip

L89.203   **Pressure ulcer of unspecified hip, stage 3**
       Healing pressure ulcer of unspecified hip, stage 3
       Pressure ulcer with full thickness skin loss involving damage or necrosis of subcutaneous tissue, unspecified hip

L89.204   **Pressure ulcer of unspecified hip, stage 4**
       Healing pressure ulcer of unspecified hip, stage 4
       Pressure ulcer with necrosis of soft tissues through to underlying muscle, tendon, or bone, unspecified hip

L89.209   **Pressure ulcer of unspecified hip, unspecified stage**
       Healing pressure ulcer of unspecified hip NOS
       Healing pressure ulcer of unspecified hip, unspecified stage

CHAPTER 12 (L00-L99)

▶ New   ➡ Revised   ~~deleted~~ Deleted   **OGCR** Official Guidelines   **X** Assign placeholder X   ● Use Additional Character(s)

Excludes 1   Excludes 2   Includes   Use additional   Code first   Code also   Key words

929

● **L89.21** **Pressure ulcer of right hip**
   L89.210 **Pressure ulcer of right hip, unstageable**
   L89.211 **Pressure ulcer of right hip, stage 1**
      Healing pressure ulcer of right hip back, stage 1
      Pressure pre-ulcer skin changes limited to persistent focal edema, right hip
   L89.212 **Pressure ulcer of right hip, stage 2**
      Healing pressure ulcer of right hip, stage 2
      Pressure ulcer with abrasion, blister, partial thickness skin loss involving epidermis and/or dermis, right hip
   L89.213 **Pressure ulcer of right hip, stage 3**
      Healing pressure ulcer of right hip, stage 3
      Pressure ulcer with full thickness skin loss involving damage or necrosis of subcutaneous tissue, right hip
   L89.214 **Pressure ulcer of right hip, stage 4**
      Healing pressure ulcer of right hip, stage 4
      Pressure ulcer with necrosis of soft tissues through to underlying muscle, tendon, or bone, right hip
   L89.219 **Pressure ulcer of right hip, unspecified stage**
      Healing pressure ulcer of right hip NOS
      Healing pressure ulcer of right hip, unspecified stage

● **L89.22** **Pressure ulcer of left hip**
   L89.220 **Pressure ulcer of left hip, unstageable**
   L89.221 **Pressure ulcer of left hip, stage 1**
      Healing pressure ulcer of left hip back, stage 1
      Pressure pre-ulcer skin changes limited to persistent focal edema, left hip
   L89.222 **Pressure ulcer of left hip, stage 2**
      Healing pressure ulcer of left hip, stage 2
      Pressure ulcer with abrasion, blister, partial thickness skin loss involving epidermis and/or dermis, left hip
   L89.223 **Pressure ulcer of left hip, stage 3**
      Healing pressure ulcer of left hip, stage 3
      Pressure ulcer with full thickness skin loss involving damage or necrosis of subcutaneous tissue, left hip
   L89.224 **Pressure ulcer of left hip, stage 4**
      Healing pressure ulcer of left hip, stage 4
      Pressure ulcer with necrosis of soft tissues through to underlying muscle, tendon, or bone, left hip
   L89.229 **Pressure ulcer of left hip, unspecified stage**
      Healing pressure ulcer of left hip NOS
      Healing pressure ulcer of left hip, unspecified stage

● **L89.3** **Pressure ulcer of buttock**
  ● **L89.30** **Pressure ulcer of unspecified buttock**
   L89.300 **Pressure ulcer of unspecified buttock, unstageable**
   L89.301 **Pressure ulcer of unspecified buttock, stage 1**
      Healing pressure ulcer of unspecified buttock, stage 1
      Pressure pre-ulcer skin changes limited to persistent focal edema, unspecified buttock
   L89.302 **Pressure ulcer of unspecified buttock, stage 2**
      Healing pressure ulcer of unspecified buttock, stage 2
      Pressure ulcer with abrasion, blister, partial thickness skin loss involving epidermis and/or dermis, unspecified buttock
   L89.303 **Pressure ulcer of unspecified buttock, stage 3**
      Healing pressure ulcer of unspecified buttock, stage 3
      Pressure ulcer with full thickness skin loss involving damage or necrosis of subcutaneous tissue, unspecified buttock
   L89.304 **Pressure ulcer of unspecified buttock, stage 4**
      Healing pressure ulcer of unspecified buttock, stage 4
      Pressure ulcer with necrosis of soft tissues through to underlying muscle, tendon, or bone, unspecified buttock
   L89.309 **Pressure ulcer of unspecified buttock, unspecified stage**
      Healing pressure ulcer of unspecified buttock NOS
      Healing pressure ulcer of unspecified buttock, unspecified stage

  ● **L89.31** **Pressure ulcer of right buttock**
   L89.310 **Pressure ulcer of right buttock, unstageable**
   L89.311 **Pressure ulcer of right buttock, stage 1**
      Healing pressure ulcer of right buttock, stage 1
      Pressure pre-ulcer skin changes limited to persistent focal edema, right buttock
   L89.312 **Pressure ulcer of right buttock, stage 2**
      Healing pressure ulcer of right buttock, stage 2
      Pressure ulcer with abrasion, blister, partial thickness skin loss involving epidermis and/or dermis, right buttock
   L89.313 **Pressure ulcer of right buttock, stage 3**
      Healing pressure ulcer of right buttock, stage 3
      Pressure ulcer with full thickness skin loss involving damage or necrosis of subcutaneous tissue, right buttock

▶ New　⇒ Revised　~~deleted~~ Deleted　**OGCR** Official Guidelines　X Assign placeholder X　● Use Additional Character(s)

Excludes 1　Excludes 2　Includes　Use additional　Code first　Code also　Key words

L89.314   **Pressure ulcer of right buttock, stage 4**
Healing pressure ulcer of right buttock, stage 4
Pressure ulcer with necrosis of soft tissues through to underlying muscle, tendon, or bone, right buttock

L89.319   **Pressure ulcer of right buttock, unspecified stage**
Healing pressure ulcer of right buttock NOS
Healing pressure ulcer of right buttock, unspecified stage

● **L89.32   Pressure ulcer of left buttock**

L89.320   **Pressure ulcer of left buttock, unstageable**

L89.321   **Pressure ulcer of left buttock, stage 1**
Healing pressure ulcer of left buttock, stage 1
Pressure pre-ulcer skin changes limited to persistent focal edema, left buttock

L89.322   **Pressure ulcer of left buttock, stage 2**
Healing pressure ulcer of left buttock, stage 2
Pressure ulcer with abrasion, blister, partial thickness skin loss involving epidermis and/or dermis, left buttock

L89.323   **Pressure ulcer of left buttock, stage 3**
Healing pressure ulcer of left buttock, stage 3
Pressure ulcer with full thickness skin loss involving damage or necrosis of subcutaneous tissue, left buttock

L89.324   **Pressure ulcer of left buttock, stage 4**
Healing pressure ulcer of left buttock, stage 4
Pressure ulcer with necrosis of soft tissues through to underlying muscle, tendon, or bone, left buttock

L89.329   **Pressure ulcer of left buttock, unspecified stage**
Healing pressure ulcer of left buttock NOS
Healing pressure ulcer of left buttock, unspecified stage

● **L89.4   Pressure ulcer of contiguous site of back, buttock and hip**

L89.40   **Pressure ulcer of contiguous site of back, buttock and hip, unspecified stage**
Healing pressure ulcer of contiguous site of back, buttock and hip NOS
Healing pressure ulcer of contiguous site of back, buttock and hip, unspecified stage

L89.41   **Pressure ulcer of contiguous site of back, buttock and hip, stage 1**
Healing pressure ulcer of contiguous site of back, buttock and hip, stage 1
Pressure pre-ulcer skin changes limited to persistent focal edema, contiguous site of back, buttock and hip

L89.42   **Pressure ulcer of contiguous site of back, buttock and hip, stage 2**
Healing pressure ulcer of contiguous site of back, buttock and hip, stage 2
Pressure ulcer with abrasion, blister, partial thickness skin loss involving epidermis and/or dermis, contiguous site of back, buttock and hip

L89.43   **Pressure ulcer of contiguous site of back, buttock and hip, stage 3**
Healing pressure ulcer of contiguous site of back, buttock and hip, stage 3
Pressure ulcer with full thickness skin loss involving damage or necrosis of subcutaneous tissue, contiguous site of back, buttock and hip

L89.44   **Pressure ulcer of contiguous site of back, buttock and hip, stage 4**
Healing pressure ulcer of contiguous site of back, buttock and hip, stage 4
Pressure ulcer with necrosis of soft tissues through to underlying muscle, tendon, or bone, contiguous site of back, buttock and hip

L89.45   **Pressure ulcer of contiguous site of back, buttock and hip, unstageable**

● **L89.5   Pressure ulcer of ankle**

● **L89.50   Pressure ulcer of unspecified ankle**

L89.500   **Pressure ulcer of unspecified ankle, unstageable**

L89.501   **Pressure ulcer of unspecified ankle, stage 1**
Healing pressure ulcer of unspecified ankle, stage 1
Pressure pre-ulcer skin changes limited to persistent focal edema, unspecified ankle

L89.502   **Pressure ulcer of unspecified ankle, stage 2**
Healing pressure ulcer of unspecified ankle, stage 2
Pressure ulcer with abrasion, blister, partial thickness skin loss involving epidermis and/or dermis, unspecified ankle

L89.503   **Pressure ulcer of unspecified ankle, stage 3**
Healing pressure ulcer of unspecified ankle, stage 3
Pressure ulcer with full thickness skin loss involving damage or necrosis of subcutaneous tissue, unspecified ankle

L89.504   **Pressure ulcer of unspecified ankle, stage 4**
Healing pressure ulcer of unspecified ankle, stage 4
Pressure ulcer with necrosis of soft tissues through to underlying muscle, tendon, or bone, unspecified ankle

L89.509   **Pressure ulcer of unspecified ankle, unspecified stage**
Healing pressure ulcer of unspecified ankle NOS
Healing pressure ulcer of unspecified ankle, unspecified stage

CHAPTER 12 (L00-L99)

CHAPTER 12 (L00-L99)

● **L89.51　Pressure ulcer of right ankle**

　L89.510　Pressure ulcer of right ankle, unstageable

　L89.511　Pressure ulcer of right ankle, stage 1
　　　　Healing pressure ulcer of right ankle, stage 1
　　　　Pressure pre-ulcer skin changes limited to persistent focal edema, right ankle

　L89.512　Pressure ulcer of right ankle, stage 2
　　　　Healing pressure ulcer of right ankle, stage 2
　　　　Pressure ulcer with abrasion, blister, partial thickness skin loss involving epidermis and/or dermis, right ankle

　L89.513　Pressure ulcer of right ankle, stage 3
　　　　Healing pressure ulcer of right ankle, stage 3
　　　　Pressure ulcer with full thickness skin loss involving damage or necrosis of subcutaneous tissue, right ankle

　L89.514　Pressure ulcer of right ankle, stage 4
　　　　Healing pressure ulcer of right ankle, stage 4
　　　　Pressure ulcer with necrosis of soft tissues through to underlying muscle, tendon, or bone, right ankle

　L89.519　Pressure ulcer of right ankle, unspecified stage
　　　　Healing pressure ulcer of right ankle NOS
　　　　Healing pressure ulcer of right ankle, unspecified stage

● **L89.52　Pressure ulcer of left ankle**

　L89.520　Pressure ulcer of left ankle, unstageable

　L89.521　Pressure ulcer of left ankle, stage 1
　　　　Healing pressure ulcer of left ankle, stage 1
　　　　Pressure pre-ulcer skin changes limited to persistent focal edema, left ankle

　L89.522　Pressure ulcer of left ankle, stage 2
　　　　Healing pressure ulcer of left ankle, stage 2
　　　　Pressure ulcer with abrasion, blister, partial thickness skin loss involving epidermis and/or dermis, left ankle

　L89.523　Pressure ulcer of left ankle, stage 3
　　　　Healing pressure ulcer of left ankle, stage 3
　　　　Pressure ulcer with full thickness skin loss involving damage or necrosis of subcutaneous tissue, left ankle

　L89.524　Pressure ulcer of left ankle, stage 4
　　　　Healing pressure ulcer of left ankle, stage 4
　　　　Pressure ulcer with necrosis of soft tissues through to underlying muscle, tendon, or bone, left ankle

　L89.529　Pressure ulcer of left ankle, unspecified stage
　　　　Healing pressure ulcer of left ankle NOS
　　　　Healing pressure ulcer of left ankle, unspecified stage

● **L89.6　Pressure ulcer of heel**

● **L89.60　Pressure ulcer of unspecified heel**

　L89.600　Pressure ulcer of unspecified heel, unstageable

　L89.601　Pressure ulcer of unspecified heel, stage 1
　　　　Healing pressure ulcer of unspecified heel, stage 1
　　　　Pressure pre-ulcer skin changes limited to persistent focal edema, unspecified heel

　L89.602　Pressure ulcer of unspecified heel, stage 2
　　　　Healing pressure ulcer of unspecified heel, stage 2
　　　　Pressure ulcer with abrasion, blister, partial thickness skin loss involving epidermis and/or dermis, unspecified heel

　L89.603　Pressure ulcer of unspecified heel, stage 3
　　　　Healing pressure ulcer of unspecified heel, stage 3
　　　　Pressure ulcer with full thickness skin loss involving damage or necrosis of subcutaneous tissue, unspecified heel

　L89.604　Pressure ulcer of unspecified heel, stage 4
　　　　Healing pressure ulcer of unspecified heel, stage 4
　　　　Pressure ulcer with necrosis of soft tissues through to underlying muscle, tendon, or bone, unspecified heel

　L89.609　Pressure ulcer of unspecified heel, unspecified stage
　　　　Healing pressure ulcer of unspecified heel NOS
　　　　Healing pressure ulcer of unspecified heel, unspecified stage

● **L89.61　Pressure ulcer of right heel**

　L89.610　Pressure ulcer of right heel, unstageable

　L89.611　Pressure ulcer of right heel, stage 1
　　　　Healing pressure ulcer of right heel, stage 1
　　　　Pressure pre-ulcer skin changes limited to persistent focal edema, right heel

　L89.612　Pressure ulcer of right heel, stage 2
　　　　Healing pressure ulcer of right heel, stage 2
　　　　Pressure ulcer with abrasion, blister, partial thickness skin loss involving epidermis and/or dermis, right heel

　L89.613　Pressure ulcer of right heel, stage 3
　　　　Healing pressure ulcer of right heel, stage 3
　　　　Pressure ulcer with full thickness skin loss involving damage or necrosis of subcutaneous tissue, right heel

　L89.614　Pressure ulcer of right heel, stage 4
　　　　Healing pressure ulcer of right heel, stage 4
　　　　Pressure ulcer with necrosis of soft tissues through to underlying muscle, tendon, or bone, right heel

　L89.619　Pressure ulcer of right heel, unspecified stage
　　　　Healing pressure ulcer of right heel NOS
　　　⇒　Healing pressure ulcer of right heel, unspecified stage

▶ New　⇒ Revised　~~deleted~~ Deleted　**OGCR** Official Guidelines　X Assign placeholder X　● Use Additional Character(s)

Excludes 1　Excludes 2　Includes　Use additional　Code first　Code also　Key words

● **L89.62   Pressure ulcer of left heel**

     L89.620   Pressure ulcer of left heel, unstageable

     L89.621   Pressure ulcer of left heel, stage 1
         Healing pressure ulcer of left heel, stage 1
         Pressure pre-ulcer skin changes limited to persistent focal edema, left heel

     L89.622   Pressure ulcer of left heel, stage 2
         Healing pressure ulcer of left heel, stage 2
         Pressure ulcer with abrasion, blister, partial thickness skin loss involving epidermis and/or dermis, left heel

     L89.623   Pressure ulcer of left heel, stage 3
         Healing pressure ulcer of left heel, stage 3
         Pressure ulcer with full thickness skin loss involving damage or necrosis of subcutaneous tissue, left heel

     L89.624   Pressure ulcer of left heel, stage 4
         Healing pressure ulcer of left heel, stage 4
         Pressure ulcer with necrosis of soft tissues through to underlying muscle, tendon, or bone, left heel

     L89.629   Pressure ulcer of left heel, unspecified stage
         Healing pressure ulcer of left heel NOS
         Healing pressure ulcer of left heel, unspecified stage

● **L89.8   Pressure ulcer of other site**

● **L89.81   Pressure ulcer of head**
     Pressure ulcer of face

     L89.810   Pressure ulcer of head, unstageable

     L89.811   Pressure ulcer of head, stage 1
         Healing pressure ulcer of head, stage 1
         Pressure pre-ulcer skin changes limited to persistent focal edema, head

     L89.812   Pressure ulcer of head, stage 2
         Healing pressure ulcer of head, stage 2
         Pressure ulcer with abrasion, blister, partial thickness skin loss involving epidermis and/or dermis, head

     L89.813   Pressure ulcer of head, stage 3
         Healing pressure ulcer of head, stage 3
         Pressure ulcer with full thickness skin loss involving damage or necrosis of subcutaneous tissue, head

     L89.814   Pressure ulcer of head, stage 4
         Healing pressure ulcer of head, stage 4
         Pressure ulcer with necrosis of soft tissues through to underlying muscle, tendon, or bone, head

     L89.819   Pressure ulcer of head, unspecified stage
         Healing pressure ulcer of head NOS
         Healing pressure ulcer of head, unspecified stage

● **L89.89   Pressure ulcer of other site**

     L89.890   Pressure ulcer of other site, unstageable

     L89.891   Pressure ulcer of other site, stage 1
         Healing pressure ulcer of other site, stage 1
         Pressure pre-ulcer skin changes limited to persistent focal edema, other site

     L89.892   Pressure ulcer of other site, stage 2
         Healing pressure ulcer of other site, stage 2
         Pressure ulcer with abrasion, blister, partial thickness skin loss involving epidermis and/or dermis, other site

     L89.893   Pressure ulcer of other site, stage 3
         Healing pressure ulcer of other site, stage 3
         Pressure ulcer with full thickness skin loss involving damage or necrosis of subcutaneous tissue, other site

     L89.894   Pressure ulcer of other site, stage 4
         Healing pressure ulcer of other site, stage 4
         Pressure ulcer with necrosis of soft tissues through to underlying muscle, tendon, or bone, other site

     L89.899   Pressure ulcer of other site, unspecified stage
         Healing pressure ulcer of other site NOS
         Healing pressure ulcer of other site, unspecified stage

● **L89.9   Pressure ulcer of unspecified site**

     L89.90   Pressure ulcer of unspecified site, unspecified stage
         Healing pressure ulcer of unspecified site NOS
         Healing pressure ulcer of unspecified site, unspecified stage

     L89.91   Pressure ulcer of unspecified site, stage 1
         Healing pressure ulcer of unspecified site, stage 1
         Pressure pre-ulcer skin changes limited to persistent focal edema, unspecified site

     L89.92   Pressure ulcer of unspecified site, stage 2
         Healing pressure ulcer of unspecified site, stage 2
         Pressure ulcer with abrasion, blister, partial thickness skin loss involving epidermis and/or dermis, unspecified site

     L89.93   Pressure ulcer of unspecified site, stage 3
         Healing pressure ulcer of unspecified site, stage 3
         Pressure ulcer with full thickness skin loss involving damage or necrosis of subcutaneous tissue, unspecified site

     L89.94   Pressure ulcer of unspecified site, stage 4
         Healing pressure ulcer of unspecified site, stage 4
         Pressure ulcer with necrosis of soft tissues through to underlying muscle, tendon, or bone, unspecified site

     L89.95   Pressure ulcer of unspecified site, unstageable

CHAPTER 12 (L00-L99)

CHAPTER 12 (L00-L99)

● **L90 Atrophic disorders of skin**

L90.0 Lichen sclerosus et atrophicus

> **Excludes2**   lichen sclerosus of external female genital
> organs (N90.4)
> lichen sclerosus of external male genital
> organs (N48.0)

L90.1 Anetoderma of Schweninger-Buzzi

L90.2 Anetoderma of Jadassohn-Pellizzari

L90.3 Atrophoderma of Pasini and Pierini

L90.4 Acrodermatitis chronica atrophicans

L90.5 Scar conditions and fibrosis of skin
Adherent scar (skin)
Cicatrix
Disfigurement of skin due to scar
Fibrosis of skin NOS
Scar NOS

> **Excludes2**   hypertrophic scar (L91.0)
> keloid scar (L91.0)

L90.6 Striae atrophicae

L90.8 Other atrophic disorders of skin

L90.9 Atrophic disorder of skin, unspecified

● **L91 Hypertrophic disorders of skin**

L91.0 Keloid scar
Hypertrophic scar
Keloid

> **Excludes2**   acne keloid (L73.0)
> scar NOS (L90.5)

L91.8 Other hypertrophic disorders of the skin

L91.9 Hypertrophic disorder of the skin, unspecified

● **L92 Granulomatous disorders of skin and subcutaneous tissue**

> **Excludes2**   actinic granuloma (L57.5)

L92.0 Granuloma annulare
Perforating granuloma annulare

L92.1 Necrobiosis lipoidica, not elsewhere classified

> **Excludes1**   necrobiosis lipoidica associated with
> diabetes mellitus (E08-E13 with .620)

L92.2 Granuloma faciale [eosinophilic granuloma of skin]

L92.3 Foreign body granuloma of the skin and subcutaneous tissue

> Use additional code to identify the type of retained
> foreign body (Z18.-)

L92.8 Other granulomatous disorders of the skin and subcutaneous tissue

L92.9 Granulomatous disorder of the skin and subcutaneous tissue, unspecified

> ▶ **Excludes2**   umbilical granuloma (P83.81)

● **L93 Lupus erythematosus**

> Use additional code for adverse effect, if applicable, to identify
> drug (T36-T50 with fifth or sixth character 5)

> **Excludes1**   lupus exedens (A18.4)
> lupus vulgaris (A18.4)
> scleroderma (M34.-)
> systemic lupus erythematosus (M32.-)

L93.0 Discoid lupus erythematosus
Lupus erythematosus NOS

L93.1 Subacute cutaneous lupus erythematosus

L93.2 Other local lupus erythematosus
Lupus erythematosus profundus
Lupus panniculitis

● **L94 Other localized connective tissue disorders**

> **Excludes1**   systemic connective tissue disorders (M30-M36)

L94.0 Localized scleroderma [morphea]
Circumscribed scleroderma

L94.1 Linear scleroderma
En coup de sabre lesion

L94.2 Calcinosis cutis

L94.3 Sclerodactyly

L94.4 Gottron's papules

L94.5 Poikiloderma vasculare atrophicans

L94.6 Ainhum

L94.8 Other specified localized connective tissue disorders

L94.9 Localized connective tissue disorder, unspecified

● **L95 Vasculitis limited to skin, not elsewhere classified**

> **Excludes1**   angioma serpiginosum (L81.7)
> Henoch(-Schönlein) purpura (D69.0)
> hypersensitivity angiitis (M31.0)
> lupus panniculitis (L93.2)
> panniculitis NOS (M79.3)
> panniculitis of neck and back (M54.0-)
> polyarteritis nodosa (M30.0)
> relapsing panniculitis (M35.6)
> rheumatoid vasculitis (M05.2)
> serum sickness (T80.6-)
> urticaria (L50.-)
> Wegener's granulomatosis (M31.3-)

L95.0 Livedoid vasculitis
Atrophie blanche (en plaque)

L95.1 Erythema elevatum diutinum

L95.8 Other vasculitis limited to the skin

L95.9 Vasculitis limited to the skin, unspecified

● **L97 Non-pressure chronic ulcer of lower limb, not elsewhere classified**

> **Includes**   chronic ulcer of skin of lower limb NOS
> non-healing ulcer of skin
> non-infected sinus of skin
> trophic ulcer NOS
> tropical ulcer NOS
> ulcer of skin of lower limb NOS

> *Code first any associated underlying condition, such as:*
> any associated gangrene (I96)
> atherosclerosis of the lower extremities (I70.23-, I70.24-,
> I70.33-, I70.34-, I70.43-, I70.44-, I70.53-, I70.54-, I70.63-,
> I70.64-, I70.73-, I70.74-)
> chronic venous hypertension (I87.31-, I87.33-)
> diabetic ulcers (E08.621, E08.622, E09.621, E09.622, E10.621,
> E10.622, E11.621, E11.622, E13.621, E13.622)
> postphlebitic syndrome (I87.01-, I87.03-)
> postthrombotic syndrome (I87.01-, I87.03-)
> varicose ulcer (I83.0-, I83.2-)

> **Excludes2**   pressure ulcer (pressure area) (L89.-)
> skin infections (L00-L08)
> specific infections classified to A00-B99

● **L97.1 Non-pressure chronic ulcer of thigh**

> ● **L97.10 Non-pressure chronic ulcer of unspecified thigh**

L97.101 Non-pressure chronic ulcer of unspecified thigh limited to breakdown of skin

L97.102 Non-pressure chronic ulcer of unspecified thigh with fat layer exposed

L97.103 Non-pressure chronic ulcer of unspecified thigh with necrosis of muscle

L97.104 Non-pressure chronic ulcer of unspecified thigh with necrosis of bone

▶ **L97.105 Non-pressure chronic ulcer of unspecified thigh with muscle involvement without evidence of necrosis**

Item 12-11 Scleroderma means hard skin. It is a group of diseases that causes abnormal growth of connective tissues that support the skin and organs. There are two types: localized scleroderma affecting the skin and systemic scleroderma affecting blood vessels and internal organs and the skin.

▶ New   ⇒ Revised   ~~deleted~~ Deleted   **OGCR** Official Guidelines   X Assign placeholder X   ● Use Additional Character(s)

Excludes 1   Excludes 2   Includes   Use additional   Code first   Code also   Key words

▶ **L97.106**   Non-pressure chronic ulcer of unspecified thigh with bone involvement without evidence of necrosis

▶ **L97.108**   Non-pressure chronic ulcer of unspecified thigh with other specified severity

L97.109   Non-pressure chronic ulcer of unspecified thigh with unspecified severity

● **L97.11**   Non-pressure chronic ulcer of right thigh

L97.111   Non-pressure chronic ulcer of right thigh limited to breakdown of skin

L97.112   Non-pressure chronic ulcer of right thigh with fat layer exposed

L97.113   Non-pressure chronic ulcer of right thigh with necrosis of muscle

L97.114   Non-pressure chronic ulcer of right thigh with necrosis of bone

▶ **L97.115**   Non-pressure chronic ulcer of right thigh with muscle involvement without evidence of necrosis

▶ **L97.116**   Non-pressure chronic ulcer of right thigh with bone involvement without evidence of necrosis

▶ **L97.118**   Non-pressure chronic ulcer of right thigh with other specified severity

L97.119   Non-pressure chronic ulcer of right thigh with unspecified severity

● **L97.12**   Non-pressure chronic ulcer of left thigh

L97.121   Non-pressure chronic ulcer of left thigh limited to breakdown of skin

L97.122   Non-pressure chronic ulcer of left thigh with fat layer exposed

L97.123   Non-pressure chronic ulcer of left thigh with necrosis of muscle

L97.124   Non-pressure chronic ulcer of left thigh with necrosis of bone

▶ **L97.125**   Non-pressure chronic ulcer of left thigh with muscle involvement without evidence of necrosis

▶ **L97.126**   Non-pressure chronic ulcer of left thigh with bone involvement without evidence of necrosis

▶ **L97.128**   Non-pressure chronic ulcer of left thigh with other specified severity

L97.129   Non-pressure chronic ulcer of left thigh with unspecified severity

● **L97.2**   Non-pressure chronic ulcer of calf

● **L97.20**   Non-pressure chronic ulcer of unspecified calf

L97.201   Non-pressure chronic ulcer of unspecified calf limited to breakdown of skin

L97.202   Non-pressure chronic ulcer of unspecified calf with fat layer exposed

L97.203   Non-pressure chronic ulcer of unspecified calf with necrosis of muscle

L97.204   Non-pressure chronic ulcer of unspecified calf with necrosis of bone

▶ **L97.205**   Non-pressure chronic ulcer of unspecified calf with muscle involvement without evidence of necrosis

▶ **L97.206**   Non-pressure chronic ulcer of unspecified calf with bone involvement without evidence of necrosis

▶ **L97.208**   Non-pressure chronic ulcer of unspecified calf with other specified severity

L97.209   Non-pressure chronic ulcer of unspecified calf with unspecified severity

● **L97.21**   Non-pressure chronic ulcer of right calf

L97.211   Non-pressure chronic ulcer of right calf limited to breakdown of skin

L97.212   Non-pressure chronic ulcer of right calf with fat layer exposed

L97.213   Non-pressure chronic ulcer of right calf with necrosis of muscle

L97.214   Non-pressure chronic ulcer of right calf with necrosis of bone

▶ **L97.215**   Non-pressure chronic ulcer of right calf with muscle involvement without evidence of necrosis

▶ **L97.216**   Non-pressure chronic ulcer of right calf with bone involvement without evidence of necrosis

▶ **L97.218**   Non-pressure chronic ulcer of right calf with other specified severity

L97.219   Non-pressure chronic ulcer of right calf with unspecified severity

● **L97.22**   Non-pressure chronic ulcer of left calf

L97.221   Non-pressure chronic ulcer of left calf limited to breakdown of skin

L97.222   Non-pressure chronic ulcer of left calf with fat layer exposed

L97.223   Non-pressure chronic ulcer of left calf with necrosis of muscle

L97.224   Non-pressure chronic ulcer of left calf with necrosis of bone

▶ **L97.225**   Non-pressure chronic ulcer of left calf with muscle involvement without evidence of necrosis

▶ **L97.226**   Non-pressure chronic ulcer of left calf with bone involvement without evidence of necrosis

▶ **L97.228**   Non-pressure chronic ulcer of left calf with other specified severity

L97.229   Non-pressure chronic ulcer of left calf with unspecified severity

● **L97.3**   Non-pressure chronic ulcer of ankle

● **L97.30**   Non-pressure chronic ulcer of unspecified ankle

L97.301   Non-pressure chronic ulcer of unspecified ankle limited to breakdown of skin

L97.302   Non-pressure chronic ulcer of unspecified ankle with fat layer exposed

L97.303   Non-pressure chronic ulcer of unspecified ankle with necrosis of muscle

L97.304   Non-pressure chronic ulcer of unspecified ankle with necrosis of bone

▶ **L97.305**   Non-pressure chronic ulcer of unspecified ankle with muscle involvement without evidence of necrosis

▶ **L97.306**   Non-pressure chronic ulcer of unspecified ankle with bone involvement without evidence of necrosis

▶ **L97.308**   Non-pressure chronic ulcer of unspecified ankle with other specified severity

L97.309   Non-pressure chronic ulcer of unspecified ankle with unspecified severity

---

▶ New   ⇒ Revised   ~~deleted~~ Deleted   **OGCR** Official Guidelines   X Assign placeholder X   ● Use Additional Character(s)

Excludes 1   Excludes 2   Includes   Use additional   Code first   Code also   Key words

CHAPTER 12 (L00-L99)

● **L97.31** Non-pressure chronic ulcer of right ankle

　　L97.311　Non-pressure chronic ulcer of right ankle limited to breakdown of skin

　　L97.312　Non-pressure chronic ulcer of right ankle with fat layer exposed

　　L97.313　Non-pressure chronic ulcer of right ankle with necrosis of muscle

　　L97.314　Non-pressure chronic ulcer of right ankle with necrosis of bone

▶ L97.315　Non-pressure chronic ulcer of right ankle with muscle involvement without evidence of necrosis

▶ L97.316　Non-pressure chronic ulcer of right ankle with bone involvement without evidence of necrosis

▶ L97.318　Non-pressure chronic ulcer of right ankle with other specified severity

　　L97.319　Non-pressure chronic ulcer of right ankle with unspecified severity

● **L97.32** Non-pressure chronic ulcer of left ankle

　　L97.321　Non-pressure chronic ulcer of left ankle limited to breakdown of skin

　　L97.322　Non-pressure chronic ulcer of left ankle with fat layer exposed

　　L97.323　Non-pressure chronic ulcer of left ankle with necrosis of muscle

　　L97.324　Non-pressure chronic ulcer of left ankle with necrosis of bone

▶ L97.325　Non-pressure chronic ulcer of left ankle with muscle involvement without evidence of necrosis

▶ L97.326　Non-pressure chronic ulcer of left ankle with bone involvement without evidence of necrosis

▶ L97.328　Non-pressure chronic ulcer of left ankle with other specified severity

　　L97.329　Non-pressure chronic ulcer of left ankle with unspecified severity

● **L97.4** Non-pressure chronic ulcer of heel and midfoot

Non-pressure chronic ulcer of plantar surface of midfoot

● **L97.40** Non-pressure chronic ulcer of unspecified heel and midfoot

　　L97.401　Non-pressure chronic ulcer of unspecified heel and midfoot limited to breakdown of skin

　　L97.402　Non-pressure chronic ulcer of unspecified heel and midfoot with fat layer exposed

　　L97.403　Non-pressure chronic ulcer of unspecified heel and midfoot with necrosis of muscle

　　L97.404　Non-pressure chronic ulcer of unspecified heel and midfoot with necrosis of bone

▶ L97.405　Non-pressure chronic ulcer of unspecified heel and midfoot with muscle involvement without evidence of necrosis

▶ L97.406　Non-pressure chronic ulcer of unspecified heel and midfoot with bone involvement without evidence of necrosis

▶ L97.408　Non-pressure chronic ulcer of unspecified heel and midfoot with other specified severity

　　L97.409　Non-pressure chronic ulcer of unspecified heel and midfoot with unspecified severity

● **L97.41** Non-pressure chronic ulcer of right heel and midfoot

　　L97.411　Non-pressure chronic ulcer of right heel and midfoot limited to breakdown of skin

　　L97.412　Non-pressure chronic ulcer of right heel and midfoot with fat layer exposed

　　L97.413　Non-pressure chronic ulcer of right heel and midfoot with necrosis of muscle

　　L97.414　Non-pressure chronic ulcer of right heel and midfoot with necrosis of bone

▶ L97.415　Non-pressure chronic ulcer of right heel and midfoot with muscle involvement without evidence of necrosis

▶ L97.416　Non-pressure chronic ulcer of right heel and midfoot with bone involvement without evidence of necrosis

▶ L97.418　Non-pressure chronic ulcer of right heel and midfoot with other specified severity

　　L97.419　Non-pressure chronic ulcer of right heel and midfoot with unspecified severity

● **L97.42** Non-pressure chronic ulcer of left heel and midfoot

　　L97.421　Non-pressure chronic ulcer of left heel and midfoot limited to breakdown of skin

　　L97.422　Non-pressure chronic ulcer of left heel and midfoot with fat layer exposed

　　L97.423　Non-pressure chronic ulcer of left heel and midfoot with necrosis of muscle

　　L97.424　Non-pressure chronic ulcer of left heel and midfoot with necrosis of bone

▶ L97.425　Non-pressure chronic ulcer of left heel and midfoot with muscle involvement without evidence of necrosis

▶ L97.426　Non-pressure chronic ulcer of left heel and midfoot with bone involvement without evidence of necrosis

▶ L97.428　Non-pressure chronic ulcer of left heel and midfoot with other specified severity

　　L97.429　Non-pressure chronic ulcer of left heel and midfoot with unspecified severity

● **L97.5** Non-pressure chronic ulcer of other part of foot

Non-pressure chronic ulcer of toe

● **L97.50** Non-pressure chronic ulcer of other part of unspecified foot

　　L97.501　Non-pressure chronic ulcer of other part of unspecified foot limited to breakdown of skin

　　L97.502　Non-pressure chronic ulcer of other part of unspecified foot with fat layer exposed

---

▶ New　⇒ Revised　~~deleted~~ Deleted　**OGCR** Official Guidelines　X Assign placeholder X　● Use Additional Character(s)

Excludes 1　Excludes 2　Includes　Use additional　Code first　Code also　Key words

L97.503   Non-pressure chronic ulcer of other part of unspecified foot with necrosis of muscle

L97.504   Non-pressure chronic ulcer of other part of unspecified foot with necrosis of bone

▶ L97.505   Non-pressure chronic ulcer of other part of unspecified foot with muscle involvement without evidence of necrosis

▶ L97.506   Non-pressure chronic ulcer of other part of unspecified foot with bone involvement without evidence of necrosis

▶ L97.508   Non-pressure chronic ulcer of other part of unspecified foot with other specified severity

L97.509   Non-pressure chronic ulcer of other part of unspecified foot with unspecified severity

● L97.51   Non-pressure chronic ulcer of other part of right foot

L97.511   Non-pressure chronic ulcer of other part of right foot limited to breakdown of skin

L97.512   Non-pressure chronic ulcer of other part of right foot with fat layer exposed

L97.513   Non-pressure chronic ulcer of other part of right foot with necrosis of muscle

L97.514   Non-pressure chronic ulcer of other part of right foot with necrosis of bone

▶ L97.515   Non-pressure chronic ulcer of other part of right foot with muscle involvement without evidence of necrosis

▶ L97.516   Non-pressure chronic ulcer of other part of right foot with bone involvement without evidence of necrosis

▶ L97.518   Non-pressure chronic ulcer of other part of right foot with other specified severity

L97.519   Non-pressure chronic ulcer of other part of right foot with unspecified severity

● L97.52   Non-pressure chronic ulcer of other part of left foot

L97.521   Non-pressure chronic ulcer of other part of left foot limited to breakdown of skin

L97.522   Non-pressure chronic ulcer of other part of left foot with fat layer exposed

L97.523   Non-pressure chronic ulcer of other part of left foot with necrosis of muscle

L97.524   Non-pressure chronic ulcer of other part of left foot with necrosis of bone

▶ L97.525   Non-pressure chronic ulcer of other part of left foot with muscle involvement without evidence of necrosis

▶ L97.526   Non-pressure chronic ulcer of other part of left foot with bone involvement without evidence of necrosis

▶ L97.528   Non-pressure chronic ulcer of other part of left foot with other specified severity

L97.529   Non-pressure chronic ulcer of other part of left foot with unspecified severity

● L97.8   Non-pressure chronic ulcer of other part of lower leg

  ● L97.80   Non-pressure chronic ulcer of other part of unspecified lower leg

L97.801   Non-pressure chronic ulcer of other part of unspecified lower leg limited to breakdown of skin

L97.802   Non-pressure chronic ulcer of other part of unspecified lower leg with fat layer exposed

L97.803   Non-pressure chronic ulcer of other part of unspecified lower leg with necrosis of muscle

L97.804   Non-pressure chronic ulcer of other part of unspecified lower leg with necrosis of bone

▶ L97.805   Non-pressure chronic ulcer of other part of unspecified lower leg with muscle involvement without evidence of necrosis

▶ L97.806   Non-pressure chronic ulcer of other part of unspecified lower leg with bone involvement without evidence of necrosis

▶ L97.808   Non-pressure chronic ulcer of other part of unspecified lower leg with other specified severity

L97.809   Non-pressure chronic ulcer of other part of unspecified lower leg with unspecified severity

  ● L97.81   Non-pressure chronic ulcer of other part of right lower leg

L97.811   Non-pressure chronic ulcer of other part of right lower leg limited to breakdown of skin

L97.812   Non-pressure chronic ulcer of other part of right lower leg with fat layer exposed

L97.813   Non-pressure chronic ulcer of other part of right lower leg with necrosis of muscle

L97.814   Non-pressure chronic ulcer of other part of right lower leg with necrosis of bone

▶ L97.815   Non-pressure chronic ulcer of other part of right lower leg with muscle involvement without evidence of necrosis

▶ L97.816   Non-pressure chronic ulcer of other part of right lower leg with bone involvement without evidence of necrosis

▶ L97.818   Non-pressure chronic ulcer of other part of right lower leg with other specified severity

L97.819   Non-pressure chronic ulcer of other part of right lower leg with unspecified severity

▶ New   ⇒ Revised   ~~deleted~~ Deleted   **OGCR** Official Guidelines   **X** Assign placeholder X   ● Use Additional Character(s)

| Excludes 1 | Excludes 2 | Includes | Use additional | Code first | Code also | Key words |

CHAPTER 12 (L00-L99)

● **L97.82** Non-pressure chronic ulcer of other part of left lower leg

     L97.821 Non-pressure chronic ulcer of other part of left lower leg limited to breakdown of skin

     L97.822 Non-pressure chronic ulcer of other part of left lower leg with fat layer exposed

     L97.823 Non-pressure chronic ulcer of other part of left lower leg with necrosis of muscle

     L97.824 Non-pressure chronic ulcer of other part of left lower leg with necrosis of bone

     ▶ L97.825 Non-pressure chronic ulcer of other part of left lower leg with muscle involvement without evidence of necrosis

     ▶ L97.826 Non-pressure chronic ulcer of other part of left lower leg with bone involvement without evidence of necrosis

     ▶ L97.828 Non-pressure chronic ulcer of other part of left lower leg with other specified severity

     L97.829 Non-pressure chronic ulcer of other part of left lower leg with unspecified severity

● **L97.9** Non-pressure chronic ulcer of unspecified part of lower leg

     ● **L97.90** Non-pressure chronic ulcer of unspecified part of unspecified lower leg

         L97.901 Non-pressure chronic ulcer of unspecified part of unspecified lower leg limited to breakdown of skin

         L97.902 Non-pressure chronic ulcer of unspecified part of unspecified lower leg with fat layer exposed

         L97.903 Non-pressure chronic ulcer of unspecified part of unspecified lower leg with necrosis of muscle

         L97.904 Non-pressure chronic ulcer of unspecified part of unspecified lower leg with necrosis of bone

         ▶ L97.905 Non-pressure chronic ulcer of unspecified part of unspecified lower leg with muscle involvement without evidence of necrosis

         ▶ L97.906 Non-pressure chronic ulcer of unspecified part of unspecified lower leg with bone involvement without evidence of necrosis

         ▶ L97.908 Non-pressure chronic ulcer of unspecified part of unspecified lower leg with other specified severity

         L97.909 Non-pressure chronic ulcer of unspecified part of unspecified lower leg with unspecified severity

     ● **L97.91** Non-pressure chronic ulcer of unspecified part of right lower leg

         L97.911 Non-pressure chronic ulcer of unspecified part of right lower leg limited to breakdown of skin

         L97.912 Non-pressure chronic ulcer of unspecified part of right lower leg with fat layer exposed

     L97.913 Non-pressure chronic ulcer of unspecified part of right lower leg with necrosis of muscle

     L97.914 Non-pressure chronic ulcer of unspecified part of right lower leg with necrosis of bone

     ▶ L97.915 Non-pressure chronic ulcer of unspecified part of right lower leg with muscle involvement without evidence of necrosis

     ▶ L97.916 Non-pressure chronic ulcer of unspecified part of right lower leg with bone involvement without evidence of necrosis

     ▶ L97.918 Non-pressure chronic ulcer of unspecified part of right lower leg with other specified severity

     L97.919 Non-pressure chronic ulcer of unspecified part of right lower leg with unspecified severity

● **L97.92** Non-pressure chronic ulcer of unspecified part of left lower leg

     L97.921 Non-pressure chronic ulcer of unspecified part of left lower leg limited to breakdown of skin

     L97.922 Non-pressure chronic ulcer of unspecified part of left lower leg with fat layer exposed

     L97.923 Non-pressure chronic ulcer of unspecified part of left lower leg with necrosis of muscle

     L97.924 Non-pressure chronic ulcer of unspecified part of left lower leg with necrosis of bone

     ▶ L97.925 Non-pressure chronic ulcer of unspecified part of left lower leg with muscle involvement without evidence of necrosis

     ▶ L97.926 Non-pressure chronic ulcer of unspecified part of left lower leg with bone involvement without evidence of necrosis

     ▶ L97.928 Non-pressure chronic ulcer of unspecified part of left lower leg with other specified severity

     L97.929 Non-pressure chronic ulcer of unspecified part of left lower leg with unspecified severity

● **L98** Other disorders of skin and subcutaneous tissue, not elsewhere classified

     L98.0 Pyogenic granuloma

         Excludes2   pyogenic granuloma of gingiva (K06.8)
                     pyogenic granuloma of maxillary alveolar ridge (K04.5)
                     pyogenic granuloma of oral mucosa (K13.4)

     L98.1 Factitial dermatitis
         Neurotic excoriation
         Excludes1   Excoriation (skin-picking) disorder (F42.4)

     L98.2 Febrile neutrophilic dermatosis [Sweet]

     L98.3 Eosinophilic cellulitis [Wells]

▶ New   ⇨ Revised   ~~deleted~~ Deleted   **OGCR** Official Guidelines   X Assign placeholder X   ● Use Additional Character(s)

Excludes 1   Excludes 2   Includes   Use additional   Code first   Code also   Key words

● **L98.4**   **Non-pressure chronic ulcer of skin, not elsewhere classified**
     Chronic ulcer of skin NOS
     Tropical ulcer NOS
     Ulcer of skin NOS
     Excludes2   pressure ulcer (pressure area) (L89.-)
                 gangrene (I96)
                 skin infections (L00-L08)
                 specific infections classified to A00-B99
                 ulcer of lower limb NEC (L97.-)
                 varicose ulcer (I83.0-I82.2)

● **L98.41**   **Non-pressure chronic ulcer of buttock**

     L98.411   Non-pressure chronic ulcer of buttock limited to breakdown of skin

     L98.412   Non-pressure chronic ulcer of buttock with fat layer exposed

     L98.413   Non-pressure chronic ulcer of buttock with necrosis of muscle

     L98.414   Non-pressure chronic ulcer of buttock with necrosis of bone

▶ **L98.415**   Non-pressure chronic ulcer of buttock with muscle involvement without evidence of necrosis

▶ **L98.416**   Non-pressure chronic ulcer of buttock with bone involvement without evidence of necrosis

▶ **L98.418**   Non-pressure chronic ulcer of buttock with other specified severity

     L98.419   Non-pressure chronic ulcer of buttock with unspecified severity

● **L98.42**   **Non-pressure chronic ulcer of back**

     L98.421   Non-pressure chronic ulcer of back limited to breakdown of skin

     L98.422   Non-pressure chronic ulcer of back with fat layer exposed

     L98.423   Non-pressure chronic ulcer of back with necrosis of muscle

     L98.424   Non-pressure chronic ulcer of back with necrosis of bone

▶ **L98.425**   Non-pressure chronic ulcer of back with muscle involvement without evidence of necrosis

▶ **L98.426**   Non-pressure chronic ulcer of back with bone involvement without evidence of necrosis

▶ **L98.428**   Non-pressure chronic ulcer of back with other specified severity

     L98.429   Non-pressure chronic ulcer of back with unspecified severity

● **L98.49**   **Non-pressure chronic ulcer of skin of other sites**
     Non-pressure chronic ulcer of skin NOS

     L98.491   Non-pressure chronic ulcer of skin of other sites limited to breakdown of skin

     L98.492   Non-pressure chronic ulcer of skin of other sites with fat layer exposed

     L98.493   Non-pressure chronic ulcer of skin of other sites with necrosis of muscle

     L98.494   Non-pressure chronic ulcer of skin of other sites with necrosis of bone

▶ **L98.495**   Non-pressure chronic ulcer of other sites with muscle involvement without evidence of necrosis

▶ **L98.496**   Non-pressure chronic ulcer of other sites with bone involvement without evidence of necrosis

▶ **L98.498**   Non-pressure chronic ulcer of other sites with other specified severity

     L98.499   Non-pressure chronic ulcer of skin of other sites with unspecified severity

L98.5   **Mucinosis of the skin**
     Focal mucinosis
     Lichen myxedematosus
     Reticular erythematous mucinosis
     Excludes1   focal oral mucinosis (K13.79)
                 myxedema (E03.9)

L98.6   **Other infiltrative disorders of the skin and subcutaneous tissue**
     Excludes1   hyalinosis cutis et mucosae (E78.89)

L98.7   **Excessive and redundant skin and subcutaneous tissue**
     Loose or sagging skin following bariatric surgery weight loss
     Loose or sagging skin following dietary weight loss
     Loose or sagging skin, NOS
     Excludes2   acquired excess or redundant skin of eyelid (H02.3-)
                 congenital excess or redundant skin of eyelid (Q10.3)
                 skin changes due to chronic exposure to nonionizing radiation (L57.-)

L98.8   **Other specified disorders of the skin and subcutaneous tissue**

L98.9   **Disorder of the skin and subcutaneous tissue, unspecified**

L99   **Other disorders of skin and subcutaneous tissue in diseases classified elsewhere**
     Code first underlying disease, such as:
     amyloidosis (E85.-)
     Excludes1   skin disorders in diabetes (E08-E13 with .62)
                 skin disorders in gonorrhea (A54.89)
                 skin disorders in syphilis (A51.31, A52.79)

CHAPTER 12 (L00-L99)

▶ New   ⇒ Revised   ~~deleted~~ Deleted   **OGCR** Official Guidelines   X Assign placeholder X   ● Use Additional Character(s)

Excludes 1   Excludes 2   Includes   Use additional   Code first   Code also   Key words

CHAPTER 13

DISEASES OF THE MUSCULOSKELETAL SYSTEM AND CONNECTIVE TISSUE (M00-M99)

OGCR Chapter-Specific Coding Guidelines

13. **Chapter 13: Diseases of the Musculoskeletal System and Connective Tissue (M00-M99)**

a. **Site and laterality**

Most of the codes within Chapter 13 have site and laterality designations. The site represents the bone, joint or the muscle involved. For some conditions where more than one bone, joint or muscle is usually involved, such as osteoarthritis, there is a "multiple sites" code available. For categories where no multiple site code is provided and more than one bone, joint or muscle is involved, multiple codes should be used to indicate the different sites involved.

1) **Bone versus joint**

For certain conditions, the bone may be affected at the upper or lower end, (e.g., avascular necrosis of bone, M87, Osteoporosis, M80, M81). Though the portion of the bone affected may be at the joint, the site designation will be the bone, not the joint.

b. **Acute traumatic versus chronic or recurrent musculoskeletal conditions**

Many musculoskeletal conditions are a result of previous injury or trauma to a site, or are recurrent conditions. Bone, joint or muscle conditions that are the result of a healed injury are usually found in chapter 13. Recurrent bone, joint or muscle conditions are also usually found in chapter 13. Any current, acute injury should be coded to the appropriate injury code from chapter 19. Chronic or recurrent conditions should generally be coded with a code from chapter 13. If it is difficult to determine from the documentation in the record which code is best to describe a condition, query the provider.

c. **Coding of Pathologic Fractures**

7th character A is for use as long as the patient is receiving active treatment for the fracture. While the patient may be seen by a new or different provider over the course of treatment for a pathological fracture, assignment of the 7th character is based on whether the patient is undergoing active treatment and not whether the provider is seeing the patient for the first time.

7th character, D is to be used for encounters after the patient has completed active treatment **for the fracture and is receiving routine care for the fracture during the healing or recovery phase.** The other 7th characters, listed under each subcategory in the Tabular List, are to be used for subsequent encounters for treatment of problems associated with the healing, such as malunions, nonunions, and sequelae.

Care for complications of surgical treatment for fracture repairs during the healing or recovery phase should be coded with the appropriate complication codes.

See Section I.C.19. Coding of traumatic fractures.

d. **Osteoporosis**

Osteoporosis is a systemic condition, meaning that all bones of the musculoskeletal system are affected. Therefore, site is not a component of the codes under category M81, Osteoporosis without current pathological fracture. The site codes under category M80, Osteoporosis with current pathological fracture, identify the site of the fracture, not the osteoporosis.

1) **Osteoporosis without pathological fracture**

Category M81, Osteoporosis without current pathological fracture, is for use for patients with osteoporosis who do not currently have a pathologic fracture due to the osteoporosis, even if they have had a fracture in the past. For patients with a history of osteoporosis fractures, status code Z87.310, Personal history of (healed) osteoporosis fracture, should follow the code from M81.

2) **Osteoporosis with current pathological fracture**

Category M80, Osteoporosis with current pathological fracture, is for patients who have a current pathologic fracture at the time of an encounter. The codes under M80 identify the site of the fracture. A code from category M80, not a traumatic fracture code, should be used for any patient with known osteoporosis who suffers a fracture, even if the patient had a minor fall or trauma, if that fall or trauma would not usually break a normal, healthy bone.

CHAPTER 13

DISEASES OF THE MUSCULOSKELETAL SYSTEM AND CONNECTIVE TISSUE (M00-M99)

Note: Use an external cause code following the code for the musculoskeletal condition, if applicable, to identify the cause of the musculoskeletal condition

Excludes2 arthropathic psoriasis (L40.5-)

certain conditions originating in the perinatal period (P04-P96)

certain infectious and parasitic diseases (A00-B99)

compartment syndrome (traumatic) (T79.A-)

complications of pregnancy, childbirth and the puerperium (O00-O9A)

congenital malformations, deformations, and chromosomal abnormalities (Q00-Q99)

endocrine, nutritional and metabolic diseases (E00-E88)

injury, poisoning and certain other consequences of external causes (S00-T88)

neoplasms (C00-D49)

symptoms, signs and abnormal clinical and laboratory findings, not elsewhere classified (R00-R94)

This chapter contains the following blocks:

M00-M02	Infectious arthropathies
~~M04~~	~~Autoinflammatory syndromes~~
M05-M14	Inflammatory polyarthropathies
M15-M19	Osteoarthritis
M20-M25	Other joint disorders
M26-M27	Dentofacial anomalies [including malocclusion] and other disorders of jaw
M30-M36	Systemic connective tissue disorders
M40-M43	Deforming dorsopathies
M45-M49	Spondylopathies
M50-M54	Other dorsopathies
M60-M63	Disorders of muscles
M65-M67	Disorders of synovium and tendon
M70-M79	Other soft tissue disorders
M80-M85	Disorders of bone density and structure
M86-M90	Other osteopathies
M91-M94	Chondropathies
M95	Other disorders of the musculoskeletal system and connective tissue
M96	Intraoperative and postprocedural complications and disorders of musculoskeletal system, not elsewhere classified
~~M97~~	~~Periprosthetic fracture around internal prosthetic joint~~
M99	Biomechanical lesions, not elsewhere classified

ARTHROPATHIES (M00-M25)

Includes Disorders affecting predominantly peripheral (limb) joints

INFECTIOUS ARTHROPATHIES (M00-M02)

Note: This block comprises arthropathies due to microbiological agents.

Distinction is made between the following types of etiological relationship:

a) direct infection of joint, where organisms invade synovial tissue and microbial antigen is present in the joint;

b) indirect infection, which may be of two types: a reactive arthropathy, where microbial infection of the body is established but neither organisms nor antigens can be identified in the joint, and a postinfective arthropathy, where microbial antigen is present but recovery of an organism is inconstant and evidence of local multiplication is lacking.

▶ New   ➡ Revised   ~~deleted~~ Deleted   **OGCR** Official Guidelines   X Assign placeholder X   ● Use Additional Character(s)

Excludes 1 · Excludes 2 · Includes · Use additional · Code first · Code also · Key words

● **M00   Pyogenic arthritis**
   ● **M00.0   Staphylococcal arthritis and polyarthritis**
     Use additional code (B95.61-B95.8) to identify bacterial agent
     Excludes2   infection and inflammatory reaction due to internal joint prosthesis (T84.5-)
     M00.00   Staphylococcal arthritis, unspecified joint
     ● M00.01   Staphylococcal arthritis, shoulder
       M00.011   Staphylococcal arthritis, right shoulder
       M00.012   Staphylococcal arthritis, left shoulder
       M00.019   Staphylococcal arthritis, unspecified shoulder
     ● M00.02   Staphylococcal arthritis, elbow
       M00.021   Staphylococcal arthritis, right elbow
       M00.022   Staphylococcal arthritis, left elbow
       M00.029   Staphylococcal arthritis, unspecified elbow
     ● M00.03   Staphylococcal arthritis, wrist
       Staphylococcal arthritis of carpal bones
       M00.031   Staphylococcal arthritis, right wrist
       M00.032   Staphylococcal arthritis, left wrist
       M00.039   Staphylococcal arthritis, unspecified wrist
     ● M00.04   Staphylococcal arthritis, hand
       Staphylococcal arthritis of metacarpus and phalanges
       M00.041   Staphylococcal arthritis, right hand
       M00.042   Staphylococcal arthritis, left hand
       M00.049   Staphylococcal arthritis, unspecified hand
     ● M00.05   Staphylococcal arthritis, hip
       M00.051   Staphylococcal arthritis, right hip
       M00.052   Staphylococcal arthritis, left hip
       M00.059   Staphylococcal arthritis, unspecified hip
     ● M00.06   Staphylococcal arthritis, knee
       M00.061   Staphylococcal arthritis, right knee
       M00.062   Staphylococcal arthritis, left knee
       M00.069   Staphylococcal arthritis, unspecified knee
     ● M00.07   Staphylococcal arthritis, ankle and foot
       Staphylococcal arthritis, tarsus, metatarsus and phalanges
       M00.071   Staphylococcal arthritis, right ankle and foot
       M00.072   Staphylococcal arthritis, left ankle and foot
       M00.079   Staphylococcal arthritis, unspecified ankle and foot
     M00.08   Staphylococcal arthritis, vertebrae
     M00.09   Staphylococcal polyarthritis
   ● **M00.1   Pneumococcal arthritis and polyarthritis**
     M00.10   Pneumococcal arthritis, unspecified joint
     ● M00.11   Pneumococcal arthritis, shoulder
       M00.111   Pneumococcal arthritis, right shoulder
       M00.112   Pneumococcal arthritis, left shoulder
       M00.119   Pneumococcal arthritis, unspecified shoulder
     ● M00.12   Pneumococcal arthritis, elbow
       M00.121   Pneumococcal arthritis, right elbow
       M00.122   Pneumococcal arthritis, left elbow
       M00.129   Pneumococcal arthritis, unspecified elbow

     ● M00.13   Pneumococcal arthritis, wrist
       Pneumococcal arthritis of carpal bones
       M00.131   Pneumococcal arthritis, right wrist
       M00.132   Pneumococcal arthritis, left wrist
       M00.139   Pneumococcal arthritis, unspecified wrist
     ● M00.14   Pneumococcal arthritis, hand
       Pneumococcal arthritis of metacarpus and phalanges
       M00.141   Pneumococcal arthritis, right hand
       M00.142   Pneumococcal arthritis, left hand
       M00.149   Pneumococcal arthritis, unspecified hand
     ● M00.15   Pneumococcal arthritis, hip
       M00.151   Pneumococcal arthritis, right hip
       M00.152   Pneumococcal arthritis, left hip
       M00.159   Pneumococcal arthritis, unspecified hip
     ● M00.16   Pneumococcal arthritis, knee
       M00.161   Pneumococcal arthritis, right knee
       M00.162   Pneumococcal arthritis, left knee
       M00.169   Pneumococcal arthritis, unspecified knee
     ● M00.17   Pneumococcal arthritis, ankle and foot
       Pneumococcal arthritis, tarsus, metatarsus and phalanges
       M00.171   Pneumococcal arthritis, right ankle and foot
       M00.172   Pneumococcal arthritis, left ankle and foot
       M00.179   Pneumococcal arthritis, unspecified ankle and foot
     M00.18   Pneumococcal arthritis, vertebrae
     M00.19   Pneumococcal polyarthritis
   ● **M00.2   Other streptococcal arthritis and polyarthritis**
     Use additional code (B95.0-B95.2, B95.4-B95.5) to identify bacterial agent
     M00.20   Other streptococcal arthritis, unspecified joint
     ● M00.21   Other streptococcal arthritis, shoulder
       M00.211   Other streptococcal arthritis, right shoulder
       M00.212   Other streptococcal arthritis, left shoulder
       M00.219   Other streptococcal arthritis, unspecified shoulder
     ● M00.22   Other streptococcal arthritis, elbow
       M00.221   Other streptococcal arthritis, right elbow
       M00.222   Other streptococcal arthritis, left elbow
       M00.229   Other streptococcal arthritis, unspecified elbow
     ● M00.23   Other streptococcal arthritis, wrist
       Other streptococcal arthritis of carpal bones
       M00.231   Other streptococcal arthritis, right wrist
       M00.232   Other streptococcal arthritis, left wrist
       M00.239   Other streptococcal arthritis, unspecified wrist
     ● M00.24   Other streptococcal arthritis, hand
       Other streptococcal arthritis metacarpus and phalanges
       M00.241   Other streptococcal arthritis, right hand
       M00.242   Other streptococcal arthritis, left hand
       M00.249   Other streptococcal arthritis, unspecified hand

● **M00.25 Other streptococcal arthritis, hip**
     M00.251   Other streptococcal arthritis, right hip
     M00.252   Other streptococcal arthritis, left hip
     M00.259   Other streptococcal arthritis, unspecified hip

● **M00.26 Other streptococcal arthritis, knee**
     M00.261   Other streptococcal arthritis, right knee
     M00.262   Other streptococcal arthritis, left knee
     M00.269   Other streptococcal arthritis, unspecified knee

● **M00.27 Other streptococcal arthritis, ankle and foot**
     Other streptococcal arthritis, tarsus, metatarsus and phalanges
     M00.271   Other streptococcal arthritis, right ankle and foot
     M00.272   Other streptococcal arthritis, left ankle and foot
     M00.279   Other streptococcal arthritis, unspecified ankle and foot

     M00.28   Other streptococcal arthritis, vertebrae
     M00.29   Other streptococcal polyarthritis

● **M00.8 Arthritis and polyarthritis due to other bacteria**
     Use additional code (B96) to identify bacteria
     M00.80   Arthritis due to other bacteria, unspecified joint

●   M00.81   Arthritis due to other bacteria, shoulder
     M00.811   Arthritis due to other bacteria, right shoulder
     M00.812   Arthritis due to other bacteria, left shoulder
     M00.819   Arthritis due to other bacteria, unspecified shoulder

●   M00.82   Arthritis due to other bacteria, elbow
     M00.821   Arthritis due to other bacteria, right elbow
     M00.822   Arthritis due to other bacteria, left elbow
     M00.829   Arthritis due to other bacteria, unspecified elbow

●   M00.83   Arthritis due to other bacteria, wrist
     Arthritis due to other bacteria, carpal bones
     M00.831   Arthritis due to other bacteria, right wrist
     M00.832   Arthritis due to other bacteria, left wrist
     M00.839   Arthritis due to other bacteria, unspecified wrist

●   M00.84   Arthritis due to other bacteria, hand
     Arthritis due to other bacteria, metacarpus and phalanges
     M00.841   Arthritis due to other bacteria, right hand
     M00.842   Arthritis due to other bacteria, left hand
     M00.849   Arthritis due to other bacteria, unspecified hand

●   M00.85   Arthritis due to other bacteria, hip
     M00.851   Arthritis due to other bacteria, right hip
     M00.852   Arthritis due to other bacteria, left hip
     M00.859   Arthritis due to other bacteria, unspecified hip

●   M00.86   Arthritis due to other bacteria, knee
     M00.861   Arthritis due to other bacteria, right knee
     M00.862   Arthritis due to other bacteria, left knee
     M00.869   Arthritis due to other bacteria, unspecified knee

●   M00.87   Arthritis due to other bacteria, ankle and foot
     Arthritis due to other bacteria, tarsus, metatarsus, and phalanges
     M00.871   Arthritis due to other bacteria, right ankle and foot
     M00.872   Arthritis due to other bacteria, left ankle and foot
     M00.879   Arthritis due to other bacteria, unspecified ankle and foot

     M00.88   Arthritis due to other bacteria, vertebrae
     M00.89   Polyarthritis due to other bacteria

     M00.9   Pyogenic arthritis, unspecified
     Infective arthritis NOS

● **M01 Direct infections of joint in infectious and parasitic diseases classified elsewhere**
     Code first underlying disease, such as:
     leprosy [Hansen's disease] (A30.-)
     mycoses (B35-B49)
     O'nyong-nyong fever (A92.1)
     paratyphoid fever (A01.1-A01.4)
     Excludes1   arthropathy in Lyme disease (A69.23)
         gonococcal arthritis (A54.42)
         meningococcal arthritis (A39.83)
         mumps arthritis (B26.85)
         postinfective arthropathy (M02.-)
         postmeningococcal arthritis (A39.84)
         reactive arthritis (M02.3)
         rubella arthritis (B06.82)
         sarcoidosis arthritis (D86.86)
         typhoid fever arthritis (A01.04)
         tuberculosis arthritis (A18.01-A18.02)

● **M01.X Direct infection of joint in infectious and parasitic diseases classified elsewhere**
     M01.X0   Direct infection of unspecified joint in infectious and parasitic diseases classified elsewhere

●   M01.X1   Direct infection of shoulder joint in infectious and parasitic diseases classified elsewhere
     M01.X11   Direct infection of right shoulder in infectious and parasitic diseases classified elsewhere
     M01.X12   Direct infection of left shoulder in infectious and parasitic diseases classified elsewhere
     M01.X19   Direct infection of unspecified shoulder in infectious and parasitic diseases classified elsewhere

●   M01.X2   Direct infection of elbow in infectious and parasitic diseases classified elsewhere
     M01.X21   Direct infection of right elbow in infectious and parasitic diseases classified elsewhere
     M01.X22   Direct infection of left elbow in infectious and parasitic diseases classified elsewhere
     M01.X29   Direct infection of unspecified elbow in infectious and parasitic diseases classified elsewhere

▶ New   ⇒ Revised   ~~deleted~~ Deleted   **OGCR** Official Guidelines   X Assign placeholder X   ● Use Additional Character(s)

Excludes 1   Excludes 2   Includes   Use additional   Code first   Code also   Key words

● **M01.X3**   Direct infection of wrist in infectious and parasitic diseases classified elsewhere
     Direct infection of carpal bones in infectious and parasitic diseases classified elsewhere

     M01.X31   Direct infection of right wrist in infectious and parasitic diseases classified elsewhere

     M01.X32   Direct infection of left wrist in infectious and parasitic diseases classified elsewhere

     M01.X39   Direct infection of unspecified wrist in infectious and parasitic diseases classified elsewhere

● **M01.X4**   Direct infection of hand in infectious and parasitic diseases classified elsewhere
     Direct infection of metacarpus and phalanges in infectious and parasitic diseases classified elsewhere

     M01.X41   Direct infection of right hand in infectious and parasitic diseases classified elsewhere

     M01.X42   Direct infection of left hand in infectious and parasitic diseases classified elsewhere

     M01.X49   Direct infection of unspecified hand in infectious and parasitic diseases classified elsewhere

● **M01.X5**   Direct infection of hip in infectious and parasitic diseases classified elsewhere

     M01.X51   Direct infection of right hip in infectious and parasitic diseases classified elsewhere

     M01.X52   Direct infection of left hip in infectious and parasitic diseases classified elsewhere

     M01.X59   Direct infection of unspecified hip in infectious and parasitic diseases classified elsewhere

● **M01.X6**   Direct infection of knee in infectious and parasitic diseases classified elsewhere

     M01.X61   Direct infection of right knee in infectious and parasitic diseases classified elsewhere

     M01.X62   Direct infection of left knee in infectious and parasitic diseases classified elsewhere

     M01.X69   Direct infection of unspecified knee in infectious and parasitic diseases classified elsewhere

● **M01.X7**   Direct infection of ankle and foot in infectious and parasitic diseases classified elsewhere
     Direct infection of tarsus, metatarsus and phalanges in infectious and parasitic diseases classified elsewhere

     M01.X71   Direct infection of right ankle and foot in infectious and parasitic diseases classified elsewhere

     M01.X72   Direct infection of left ankle and foot in infectious and parasitic diseases classified elsewhere

     M01.X79   Direct infection of unspecified ankle and foot in infectious and parasitic diseases classified elsewhere

   M01.X8   Direct infection of vertebrae in infectious and parasitic diseases classified elsewhere

   M01.X9   Direct infection of multiple joints in infectious and parasitic diseases classified elsewhere

● **M02**   Postinfective and reactive arthropathies

     Code first underlying disease, such as:
       congenital syphilis [Clutton's joints] (A50.5)
       enteritis due to Yersinia enterocolitica (A04.6)
       infective endocarditis (I33.0)
       viral hepatitis (B15-B19)

     | Excludes 1 | Behçet's disease (M35.2)
       direct infections of joint in infectious and parasitic diseases classified elsewhere (M01.-)
       postmeningococcal arthritis (A39.84)
       mumps arthritis (B26.85)
       rubella arthritis (B06.82)
       syphilis arthritis (late) (A52.77)
       rheumatic fever (I00)
       tabetic arthropathy [Charcôt's] (A52.16)

● **M02.0**   Arthropathy following intestinal bypass

     M02.00   Arthropathy following intestinal bypass, unspecified site

     ● **M02.01**   Arthropathy following intestinal bypass, shoulder

       M02.011   Arthropathy following intestinal bypass, right shoulder

       M02.012   Arthropathy following intestinal bypass, left shoulder

       M02.019   Arthropathy following intestinal bypass, unspecified shoulder

     ● **M02.02**   Arthropathy following intestinal bypass, elbow

       M02.021   Arthropathy following intestinal bypass, right elbow

       M02.022   Arthropathy following intestinal bypass, left elbow

       M02.029   Arthropathy following intestinal bypass, unspecified elbow

     ● **M02.03**   Arthropathy following intestinal bypass, wrist
       Arthropathy following intestinal bypass, carpal bones

       M02.031   Arthropathy following intestinal bypass, right wrist

       M02.032   Arthropathy following intestinal bypass, left wrist

       M02.039   Arthropathy following intestinal bypass, unspecified wrist

     ● **M02.04**   Arthropathy following intestinal bypass, hand
       Arthropathy following intestinal bypass, metacarpals and phalanges

       M02.041   Arthropathy following intestinal bypass, right hand

       M02.042   Arthropathy following intestinal bypass, left hand

       M02.049   Arthropathy following intestinal bypass, unspecified hand

     ● **M02.05**   Arthropathy following intestinal bypass, hip

       M02.051   Arthropathy following intestinal bypass, right hip

       M02.052   Arthropathy following intestinal bypass, left hip

       M02.059   Arthropathy following intestinal bypass, unspecified hip

     ● **M02.06**   Arthropathy following intestinal bypass, knee

       M02.061   Arthropathy following intestinal bypass, right knee

       M02.062   Arthropathy following intestinal bypass, left knee

       M02.069   Arthropathy following intestinal bypass, unspecified knee

CHAPTER 13 (M00-M99)

● M02.07 Arthropathy following intestinal bypass, ankle and foot
    Arthropathy following intestinal bypass, tarsus, metatarsus and phalanges
    M02.071 Arthropathy following intestinal bypass, right ankle and foot
    M02.072 Arthropathy following intestinal bypass, left ankle and foot
    M02.079 Arthropathy following intestinal bypass, unspecified ankle and foot

M02.08 Arthropathy following intestinal bypass, vertebrae

M02.09 Arthropathy following intestinal bypass, multiple sites

● M02.1 Postdysenteric arthropathy
M02.10 Postdysenteric arthropathy, unspecified site
● M02.11 Postdysenteric arthropathy, shoulder
    M02.111 Postdysenteric arthropathy, right shoulder
    M02.112 Postdysenteric arthropathy, left shoulder
    M02.119 Postdysenteric arthropathy, unspecified shoulder
● M02.12 Postdysenteric arthropathy, elbow
    M02.121 Postdysenteric arthropathy, right elbow
    M02.122 Postdysenteric arthropathy, left elbow
    M02.129 Postdysenteric arthropathy, unspecified elbow
● M02.13 Postdysenteric arthropathy, wrist
    Postdysenteric arthropathy, carpal bones
    M02.131 Postdysenteric arthropathy, right wrist
    M02.132 Postdysenteric arthropathy, left wrist
    M02.139 Postdysenteric arthropathy, unspecified wrist
● M02.14 Postdysenteric arthropathy, hand
    Postdysenteric arthropathy, metacarpus and phalanges
    M02.141 Postdysenteric arthropathy, right hand
    M02.142 Postdysenteric arthropathy, left hand
    M02.149 Postdysenteric arthropathy, unspecified hand
● M02.15 Postdysenteric arthropathy, hip
    M02.151 Postdysenteric arthropathy, right hip
    M02.152 Postdysenteric arthropathy, left hip
    M02.159 Postdysenteric arthropathy, unspecified hip
● M02.16 Postdysenteric arthropathy, knee
    M02.161 Postdysenteric arthropathy, right knee
    M02.162 Postdysenteric arthropathy, left knee
    M02.169 Postdysenteric arthropathy, unspecified knee
● M02.17 Postdysenteric arthropathy, ankle and foot
    Postdysenteric arthropathy, tarsus, metatarsus and phalanges
    M02.171 Postdysenteric arthropathy, right ankle and foot
    M02.172 Postdysenteric arthropathy, left ankle and foot
    M02.179 Postdysenteric arthropathy, unspecified ankle and foot

M02.18 Postdysenteric arthropathy, vertebrae

M02.19 Postdysenteric arthropathy, multiple sites

● M02.2 Postimmunization arthropathy
M02.20 Postimmunization arthropathy, unspecified site
● M02.21 Postimmunization arthropathy, shoulder
    M02.211 Postimmunization arthropathy, right shoulder
    M02.212 Postimmunization arthropathy, left shoulder
    M02.219 Postimmunization arthropathy, unspecified shoulder
● M02.22 Postimmunization arthropathy, elbow
    M02.221 Postimmunization arthropathy, right elbow
    M02.222 Postimmunization arthropathy, left elbow
    M02.229 Postimmunization arthropathy, unspecified elbow
● M02.23 Postimmunization arthropathy, wrist
    Postimmunization arthropathy, carpal bones
    M02.231 Postimmunization arthropathy, right wrist
    M02.232 Postimmunization arthropathy, left wrist
    M02.239 Postimmunization arthropathy, unspecified wrist
● M02.24 Postimmunization arthropathy, hand
    Postimmunization arthropathy, metacarpus and phalanges
    M02.241 Postimmunization arthropathy, right hand
    M02.242 Postimmunization arthropathy, left hand
    M02.249 Postimmunization arthropathy, unspecified hand
● M02.25 Postimmunization arthropathy, hip
    M02.251 Postimmunization arthropathy, right hip
    M02.252 Postimmunization arthropathy, left hip
    M02.259 Postimmunization arthropathy, unspecified hip
● M02.26 Postimmunization arthropathy, knee
    M02.261 Postimmunization arthropathy, right knee
    M02.262 Postimmunization arthropathy, left knee
    M02.269 Postimmunization arthropathy, unspecified knee
● M02.27 Postimmunization arthropathy, ankle and foot
    Postimmunization arthropathy, tarsus, metatarsus and phalanges
    M02.271 Postimmunization arthropathy, right ankle and foot
    M02.272 Postimmunization arthropathy, left ankle and foot
    M02.279 Postimmunization arthropathy, unspecified ankle and foot

M02.28 Postimmunization arthropathy, vertebrae

M02.29 Postimmunization arthropathy, multiple sites

● M02.3 Reiter's disease
    Reactive arthritis
M02.30 Reiter's disease, unspecified site
● M02.31 Reiter's disease, shoulder
    M02.311 Reiter's disease, right shoulder
    M02.312 Reiter's disease, left shoulder
    M02.319 Reiter's disease, unspecified shoulder

● M02.32   Reiter's disease, elbow
     M02.321   Reiter's disease, right elbow
     M02.322   Reiter's disease, left elbow
     M02.329   Reiter's disease, unspecified elbow

● M02.33   Reiter's disease, wrist
     Reiter's disease, carpal bones
     M02.331   Reiter's disease, right wrist
     M02.332   Reiter's disease, left wrist
     M02.339   Reiter's disease, unspecified wrist

● M02.34   Reiter's disease, hand
     Reiter's disease, metacarpus and phalanges
     M02.341   Reiter's disease, right hand
     M02.342   Reiter's disease, left hand
     M02.349   Reiter's disease, unspecified hand

● M02.35   Reiter's disease, hip
     M02.351   Reiter's disease, right hip
     M02.352   Reiter's disease, left hip
     M02.359   Reiter's disease, unspecified hip

● M02.36   Reiter's disease, knee
     M02.361   Reiter's disease, right knee
     M02.362   Reiter's disease, left knee
     M02.369   Reiter's disease, unspecified knee

● M02.37   Reiter's disease, ankle and foot
     Reiter's disease, tarsus, metatarsus and
     phalanges
     M02.371   Reiter's disease, right ankle and foot
     M02.372   Reiter's disease, left ankle and foot
     M02.379   Reiter's disease, unspecified ankle
     and foot

     M02.38   Reiter's disease, vertebrae
     M02.39   Reiter's disease, multiple sites

● M02.8   Other reactive arthropathies
     M02.80   Other reactive arthropathies, unspecified site

● M02.81   Other reactive arthropathies, shoulder
     M02.811   Other reactive arthropathies, right
     shoulder
     M02.812   Other reactive arthropathies, left
     shoulder
     M02.819   Other reactive arthropathies,
     unspecified shoulder

● M02.82   Other reactive arthropathies, elbow
     M02.821   Other reactive arthropathies, right
     elbow
     M02.822   Other reactive arthropathies, left
     elbow
     M02.829   Other reactive arthropathies,
     unspecified elbow

● M02.83   Other reactive arthropathies, wrist
     Other reactive arthropathies, carpal bones
     M02.831   Other reactive arthropathies, right
     wrist
     M02.832   Other reactive arthropathies, left
     wrist
     M02.839   Other reactive arthropathies,
     unspecified wrist

● M02.84   Other reactive arthropathies, hand
     Other reactive arthropathies, metacarpus and
     phalanges
     M02.841   Other reactive arthropathies, right
     hand
     M02.842   Other reactive arthropathies, left
     hand
     M02.849   Other reactive arthropathies,
     unspecified hand

● M02.85   Other reactive arthropathies, hip
     M02.851   Other reactive arthropathies, right hip
     M02.852   Other reactive arthropathies, left hip
     M02.859   Other reactive arthropathies,
     unspecified hip

● M02.86   Other reactive arthropathies, knee
     M02.861   Other reactive arthropathies, right
     knee
     M02.862   Other reactive arthropathies, left knee
     M02.869   Other reactive arthropathies,
     unspecified knee

● M02.87   Other reactive arthropathies, ankle and foot
     Other reactive arthropathies, tarsus,
     metatarsus and phalanges
     M02.871   Other reactive arthropathies, right
     ankle and foot
     M02.872   Other reactive arthropathies, left
     ankle and foot
     M02.879   Other reactive arthropathies,
     unspecified ankle and foot

     M02.88   Other reactive arthropathies, vertebrae
     M02.89   Other reactive arthropathies, multiple sites

M02.9   Reactive arthropathy, unspecified

AUTOINFLAMMATORY SYNDROMES (M04)

● M04   Autoinflammatory syndromes
     Excludes2   Crohn's disease (K50.-)

     M04.1   Periodic fever syndromes
         Familial Mediterranean fever
         Hyperimmunoglobin D syndrome
         Mevalonate kinase deficiency
         Tumor necrosis factor receptor associated periodic
         syndrome [TRAPS]

     M04.2   Cryopyrin-associated periodic syndromes
         Chronic infantile neurological, cutaneous and articular
         syndrome [CINCA]
         Familial cold autoinflammatory syndrome
         Familial cold urticaria
         Muckle-Wells syndrome
         Neonatal onset multisystemic inflammatory disorder
         [NOMID]

     M04.8   Other autoinflammatory syndromes
         Blau syndrome
         Deficiency of interleukin 1 receptor antagonist [DIRA]
         Majeed syndrome
         Periodic fever, aphthous stomatitis, pharyngitis, and
         adenopathy syndrome [PFAPA]
         Pyogenic arthritis, pyoderma gangrenosum, and acne
         syndrome [PAPA]

     M04.9   Autoinflammatory syndrome, unspecified

INFLAMMATORY POLYARTHROPATHIES (M05-M14)

● M05   Rheumatoid arthritis with rheumatoid factor
     Excludes1   rheumatic fever (I00)
         juvenile rheumatoid arthritis (M08.-)
         rheumatoid arthritis of spine (M45.-)

● M05.0   Felty's syndrome
     Rheumatoid arthritis with splenoadenomegaly and
     leukopenia
     M05.00   Felty's syndrome, unspecified site

● M05.01   Felty's syndrome, shoulder
     M05.011   Felty's syndrome, right shoulder
     M05.012   Felty's syndrome, left shoulder
     M05.019   Felty's syndrome, unspecified
     shoulder

● M05.02   Felty's syndrome, elbow
     M05.021   Felty's syndrome, right elbow
     M05.022   Felty's syndrome, left elbow
     M05.029   Felty's syndrome, unspecified elbow

CHAPTER 13 (M00-M99)

CHAPTER 13 (M00-M99)

Item 13-1   Rheumatoid arthritis (RA) is a chronic systemic inflammatory autoimmune disease of undetermined etiology involving primarily the synovial membranes and articular structures of multiple joints. It can also affect other organs, including the eyes, blood vessels, heart, and lungs. The disease is often progressive. In late stages, deformity, ankylosis, and other **inflammatory polyarthropathies** develop.

- **M05.03   Felty's syndrome, wrist**
  Felty's syndrome, carpal bones
    - M05.031   Felty's syndrome, right wrist
    - M05.032   Felty's syndrome, left wrist
    - M05.039   Felty's syndrome, unspecified wrist
- **M05.04   Felty's syndrome, hand**
  Felty's syndrome, metacarpus and phalanges
    - M05.041   Felty's syndrome, right hand
    - M05.042   Felty's syndrome, left hand
    - M05.049   Felty's syndrome, unspecified hand
- **M05.05   Felty's syndrome, hip**
    - M05.051   Felty's syndrome, right hip
    - M05.052   Felty's syndrome, left hip
    - M05.059   Felty's syndrome, unspecified hip
- **M05.06   Felty's syndrome, knee**
    - M05.061   Felty's syndrome, right knee
    - M05.062   Felty's syndrome, left knee
    - M05.069   Felty's syndrome, unspecified knee
- **M05.07   Felty's syndrome, ankle and foot**
  Felty's syndrome, tarsus, metatarsus and phalanges
    - M05.071   Felty's syndrome, right ankle and foot
    - M05.072   Felty's syndrome, left ankle and foot
    - M05.079   Felty's syndrome, unspecified ankle and foot
  - M05.09   Felty's syndrome, multiple sites
- **M05.1   Rheumatoid lung disease with rheumatoid arthritis**
    - M05.10   Rheumatoid lung disease with rheumatoid arthritis of unspecified site
  - **M05.11   Rheumatoid lung disease with rheumatoid arthritis of shoulder**
    - M05.111   Rheumatoid lung disease with rheumatoid arthritis of right shoulder
    - M05.112   Rheumatoid lung disease with rheumatoid arthritis of left shoulder
    - M05.119   Rheumatoid lung disease with rheumatoid arthritis of unspecified shoulder
  - **M05.12   Rheumatoid lung disease with rheumatoid arthritis of elbow**
    - M05.121   Rheumatoid lung disease with rheumatoid arthritis of right elbow
    - M05.122   Rheumatoid lung disease with rheumatoid arthritis of left elbow
    - M05.129   Rheumatoid lung disease with rheumatoid arthritis of unspecified elbow
  - **M05.13   Rheumatoid lung disease with rheumatoid arthritis of wrist**
    Rheumatoid lung disease with rheumatoid arthritis, carpal bones
    - M05.131   Rheumatoid lung disease with rheumatoid arthritis of right wrist
    - M05.132   Rheumatoid lung disease with rheumatoid arthritis of left wrist
    - M05.139   Rheumatoid lung disease with rheumatoid arthritis of unspecified wrist

- **M05.14   Rheumatoid lung disease with rheumatoid arthritis of hand**
  Rheumatoid lung disease with rheumatoid arthritis, metacarpus and phalanges
    - M05.141   Rheumatoid lung disease with rheumatoid arthritis of right hand
    - M05.142   Rheumatoid lung disease with rheumatoid arthritis of left hand
    - M05.149   Rheumatoid lung disease with rheumatoid arthritis of unspecified hand
- **M05.15   Rheumatoid lung disease with rheumatoid arthritis of hip**
    - M05.151   Rheumatoid lung disease with rheumatoid arthritis of right hip
    - M05.152   Rheumatoid lung disease with rheumatoid arthritis of left hip
    - M05.159   Rheumatoid lung disease with rheumatoid arthritis of unspecified hip
- **M05.16   Rheumatoid lung disease with rheumatoid arthritis of knee**
    - M05.161   Rheumatoid lung disease with rheumatoid arthritis of right knee
    - M05.162   Rheumatoid lung disease with rheumatoid arthritis of left knee
    - M05.169   Rheumatoid lung disease with rheumatoid arthritis of unspecified knee
- **M05.17   Rheumatoid lung disease with rheumatoid arthritis of ankle and foot**
  Rheumatoid lung disease with rheumatoid arthritis, tarsus, metatarsus and phalanges
    - M05.171   Rheumatoid lung disease with rheumatoid arthritis of right ankle and foot
    - M05.172   Rheumatoid lung disease with rheumatoid arthritis of left ankle and foot
    - M05.179   Rheumatoid lung disease with rheumatoid arthritis of unspecified ankle and foot
  - M05.19   Rheumatoid lung disease with rheumatoid arthritis of multiple sites
- **M05.2   Rheumatoid vasculitis with rheumatoid arthritis**
    - M05.20   Rheumatoid vasculitis with rheumatoid arthritis of unspecified site
  - **M05.21   Rheumatoid vasculitis with rheumatoid arthritis of shoulder**
    - M05.211   Rheumatoid vasculitis with rheumatoid arthritis of right shoulder
    - M05.212   Rheumatoid vasculitis with rheumatoid arthritis of left shoulder
    - M05.219   Rheumatoid vasculitis with rheumatoid arthritis of unspecified shoulder
  - **M05.22   Rheumatoid vasculitis with rheumatoid arthritis of elbow**
    - M05.221   Rheumatoid vasculitis with rheumatoid arthritis of right elbow
    - M05.222   Rheumatoid vasculitis with rheumatoid arthritis of left elbow
    - M05.229   Rheumatoid vasculitis with rheumatoid arthritis of unspecified elbow

▶ New   ⇒ Revised   ~~deleted~~ Deleted   OGCR Official Guidelines   X Assign placeholder X   ● Use Additional Character(s)

Excludes 1   Excludes 2   Includes   Use additional   Code first   Code also   Key words

● M05.23   Rheumatoid vasculitis with rheumatoid arthritis of wrist
> Rheumatoid vasculitis with rheumatoid arthritis, carpal bones

    M05.231   Rheumatoid vasculitis with rheumatoid arthritis of right wrist

    M05.232   Rheumatoid vasculitis with rheumatoid arthritis of left wrist

    M05.239   Rheumatoid vasculitis with rheumatoid arthritis of unspecified wrist

● M05.24   Rheumatoid vasculitis with rheumatoid arthritis of hand
> Rheumatoid vasculitis with rheumatoid arthritis, metacarpus and phalanges

    M05.241   Rheumatoid vasculitis with rheumatoid arthritis of right hand

    M05.242   Rheumatoid vasculitis with rheumatoid arthritis of left hand

    M05.249   Rheumatoid vasculitis with rheumatoid arthritis of unspecified hand

● M05.25   Rheumatoid vasculitis with rheumatoid arthritis of hip

    M05.251   Rheumatoid vasculitis with rheumatoid arthritis of right hip

    M05.252   Rheumatoid vasculitis with rheumatoid arthritis of left hip

    M05.259   Rheumatoid vasculitis with rheumatoid arthritis of unspecified hip

● M05.26   Rheumatoid vasculitis with rheumatoid arthritis of knee

    M05.261   Rheumatoid vasculitis with rheumatoid arthritis of right knee

    M05.262   Rheumatoid vasculitis with rheumatoid arthritis of left knee

    M05.269   Rheumatoid vasculitis with rheumatoid arthritis of unspecified knee

● M05.27   Rheumatoid vasculitis with rheumatoid arthritis of ankle and foot
> Rheumatoid vasculitis with rheumatoid arthritis, tarsus, metatarsus and phalanges

    M05.271   Rheumatoid vasculitis with rheumatoid arthritis of right ankle and foot

    M05.272   Rheumatoid vasculitis with rheumatoid arthritis of left ankle and foot

    M05.279   Rheumatoid vasculitis with rheumatoid arthritis of unspecified ankle and foot

   M05.29   Rheumatoid vasculitis with rheumatoid arthritis of multiple sites

● M05.3   Rheumatoid heart disease with rheumatoid arthritis
> Rheumatoid carditis
> Rheumatoid endocarditis
> Rheumatoid myocarditis
> Rheumatoid pericarditis

   M05.30   Rheumatoid heart disease with rheumatoid arthritis of unspecified site

● M05.31   Rheumatoid heart disease with rheumatoid arthritis of shoulder

    M05.311   Rheumatoid heart disease with rheumatoid arthritis of right shoulder

    M05.312   Rheumatoid heart disease with rheumatoid arthritis of left shoulder

    M05.319   Rheumatoid heart disease with rheumatoid arthritis of unspecified shoulder

● M05.32   Rheumatoid heart disease with rheumatoid arthritis of elbow

    M05.321   Rheumatoid heart disease with rheumatoid arthritis of right elbow

    M05.322   Rheumatoid heart disease with rheumatoid arthritis of left elbow

    M05.329   Rheumatoid heart disease with rheumatoid arthritis of unspecified elbow

● M05.33   Rheumatoid heart disease with rheumatoid arthritis of wrist
> Rheumatoid heart disease with rheumatoid arthritis, carpal bones

    M05.331   Rheumatoid heart disease with rheumatoid arthritis of right wrist

    M05.332   Rheumatoid heart disease with rheumatoid arthritis of left wrist

    M05.339   Rheumatoid heart disease with rheumatoid arthritis of unspecified wrist

● M05.34   Rheumatoid heart disease with rheumatoid arthritis of hand
> Rheumatoid heart disease with rheumatoid arthritis, metacarpus and phalanges

    M05.341   Rheumatoid heart disease with rheumatoid arthritis of right hand

    M05.342   Rheumatoid heart disease with rheumatoid arthritis of left hand

    M05.349   Rheumatoid heart disease with rheumatoid arthritis of unspecified hand

● M05.35   Rheumatoid heart disease with rheumatoid arthritis of hip

    M05.351   Rheumatoid heart disease with rheumatoid arthritis of right hip

    M05.352   Rheumatoid heart disease with rheumatoid arthritis of left hip

    M05.359   Rheumatoid heart disease with rheumatoid arthritis of unspecified hip

● M05.36   Rheumatoid heart disease with rheumatoid arthritis of knee

    M05.361   Rheumatoid heart disease with rheumatoid arthritis of right knee

    M05.362   Rheumatoid heart disease with rheumatoid arthritis of left knee

    M05.369   Rheumatoid heart disease with rheumatoid arthritis of unspecified knee

● M05.37   Rheumatoid heart disease with rheumatoid arthritis of ankle and foot
> Rheumatoid heart disease with rheumatoid arthritis, tarsus, metatarsus and phalanges

    M05.371   Rheumatoid heart disease with rheumatoid arthritis of right ankle and foot

    M05.372   Rheumatoid heart disease with rheumatoid arthritis of left ankle and foot

    M05.379   Rheumatoid heart disease with rheumatoid arthritis of unspecified ankle and foot

   M05.39   Rheumatoid heart disease with rheumatoid arthritis of multiple sites

▶ New   ⇒ Revised   ~~deleted~~ Deleted   **OGCR** Official Guidelines   X Assign placeholder X   ● Use Additional Character(s)

| Excludes 1 | Excludes 2 | Includes | Use additional | Code first | Code also | Key words |

● **M05.4** Rheumatoid myopathy with rheumatoid arthritis

    M05.40 Rheumatoid myopathy with rheumatoid arthritis of unspecified site

● **M05.41** Rheumatoid myopathy with rheumatoid arthritis of shoulder

    M05.411 Rheumatoid myopathy with rheumatoid arthritis of right shoulder

    M05.412 Rheumatoid myopathy with rheumatoid arthritis of left shoulder

    M05.419 Rheumatoid myopathy with rheumatoid arthritis of unspecified shoulder

● **M05.42** Rheumatoid myopathy with rheumatoid arthritis of elbow

    M05.421 Rheumatoid myopathy with rheumatoid arthritis of right elbow

    M05.422 Rheumatoid myopathy with rheumatoid arthritis of left elbow

    M05.429 Rheumatoid myopathy with rheumatoid arthritis of unspecified elbow

● **M05.43** Rheumatoid myopathy with rheumatoid arthritis of wrist

    Rheumatoid myopathy with rheumatoid arthritis, carpal bones

    M05.431 Rheumatoid myopathy with rheumatoid arthritis of right wrist

    M05.432 Rheumatoid myopathy with rheumatoid arthritis of left wrist

    M05.439 Rheumatoid myopathy with rheumatoid arthritis of unspecified wrist

● **M05.44** Rheumatoid myopathy with rheumatoid arthritis of hand

    Rheumatoid myopathy with rheumatoid arthritis, metacarpus and phalanges

    M05.441 Rheumatoid myopathy with rheumatoid arthritis of right hand

    M05.442 Rheumatoid myopathy with rheumatoid arthritis of left hand

    M05.449 Rheumatoid myopathy with rheumatoid arthritis of unspecified hand

● **M05.45** Rheumatoid myopathy with rheumatoid arthritis of hip

    M05.451 Rheumatoid myopathy with rheumatoid arthritis of right hip

    M05.452 Rheumatoid myopathy with rheumatoid arthritis of left hip

    M05.459 Rheumatoid myopathy with rheumatoid arthritis of unspecified hip

● **M05.46** Rheumatoid myopathy with rheumatoid arthritis of knee

    M05.461 Rheumatoid myopathy with rheumatoid arthritis of right knee

    M05.462 Rheumatoid myopathy with rheumatoid arthritis of left knee

    M05.469 Rheumatoid myopathy with rheumatoid arthritis of unspecified knee

● **M05.47** Rheumatoid myopathy with rheumatoid arthritis of ankle and foot

    Rheumatoid myopathy with rheumatoid arthritis, tarsus, metatarsus and phalanges

    M05.471 Rheumatoid myopathy with rheumatoid arthritis of right ankle and foot

    M05.472 Rheumatoid myopathy with rheumatoid arthritis of left ankle and foot

    M05.479 Rheumatoid myopathy with rheumatoid arthritis of unspecified ankle and foot

    M05.49 Rheumatoid myopathy with rheumatoid arthritis of multiple sites

● **M05.5** Rheumatoid polyneuropathy with rheumatoid arthritis

    M05.50 Rheumatoid polyneuropathy with rheumatoid arthritis of unspecified site

● **M05.51** Rheumatoid polyneuropathy with rheumatoid arthritis of shoulder

    M05.511 Rheumatoid polyneuropathy with rheumatoid arthritis of right shoulder

    M05.512 Rheumatoid polyneuropathy with rheumatoid arthritis of left shoulder

    M05.519 Rheumatoid polyneuropathy with rheumatoid arthritis of unspecified shoulder

● **M05.52** Rheumatoid polyneuropathy with rheumatoid arthritis of elbow

    M05.521 Rheumatoid polyneuropathy with rheumatoid arthritis of right elbow

    M05.522 Rheumatoid polyneuropathy with rheumatoid arthritis of left elbow

    M05.529 Rheumatoid polyneuropathy with rheumatoid arthritis of unspecified elbow

● **M05.53** Rheumatoid polyneuropathy with rheumatoid arthritis of wrist

    Rheumatoid polyneuropathy with rheumatoid arthritis, carpal bones

    M05.531 Rheumatoid polyneuropathy with rheumatoid arthritis of right wrist

    M05.532 Rheumatoid polyneuropathy with rheumatoid arthritis of left wrist

    M05.539 Rheumatoid polyneuropathy with rheumatoid arthritis of unspecified wrist

● **M05.54** Rheumatoid polyneuropathy with rheumatoid arthritis of hand

    Rheumatoid polyneuropathy with rheumatoid arthritis, metacarpus and phalanges

    M05.541 Rheumatoid polyneuropathy with rheumatoid arthritis of right hand

    M05.542 Rheumatoid polyneuropathy with rheumatoid arthritis of left hand

    M05.549 Rheumatoid polyneuropathy with rheumatoid arthritis of unspecified hand

● **M05.55** Rheumatoid polyneuropathy with rheumatoid arthritis of hip

    M05.551 Rheumatoid polyneuropathy with rheumatoid arthritis of right hip

    M05.552 Rheumatoid polyneuropathy with rheumatoid arthritis of left hip

    M05.559 Rheumatoid polyneuropathy with rheumatoid arthritis of unspecified hip

▶ New   ⇨ Revised   ~~deleted~~ Deleted   **OGCR** Official Guidelines   X Assign placeholder X   ● Use Additional Character(s)

Excludes 1   Excludes 2   Includes   Use additional   Code first   Code also   Key words

● M05.56   Rheumatoid polyneuropathy with rheumatoid arthritis of knee

     M05.561   Rheumatoid polyneuropathy with rheumatoid arthritis of right knee

     M05.562   Rheumatoid polyneuropathy with rheumatoid arthritis of left knee

     M05.569   Rheumatoid polyneuropathy with rheumatoid arthritis of unspecified knee

● M05.57   Rheumatoid polyneuropathy with rheumatoid arthritis of ankle and foot

     Rheumatoid polyneuropathy with rheumatoid arthritis, tarsus, metatarsus and phalanges

     M05.571   Rheumatoid polyneuropathy with rheumatoid arthritis of right ankle and foot

     M05.572   Rheumatoid polyneuropathy with rheumatoid arthritis of left ankle and foot

     M05.579   Rheumatoid polyneuropathy with rheumatoid arthritis of unspecified ankle and foot

   M05.59   Rheumatoid polyneuropathy with rheumatoid arthritis of multiple sites

● M05.6   Rheumatoid arthritis with involvement of other organs and systems

     M05.60   Rheumatoid arthritis of unspecified site with involvement of other organs and systems

● M05.61   Rheumatoid arthritis of shoulder with involvement of other organs and systems

     M05.611   Rheumatoid arthritis of right shoulder with involvement of other organs and systems

     M05.612   Rheumatoid arthritis of left shoulder with involvement of other organs and systems

     M05.619   Rheumatoid arthritis of unspecified shoulder with involvement of other organs and systems

● M05.62   Rheumatoid arthritis of elbow with involvement of other organs and systems

     M05.621   Rheumatoid arthritis of right elbow with involvement of other organs and systems

     M05.622   Rheumatoid arthritis of left elbow with involvement of other organs and systems

     M05.629   Rheumatoid arthritis of unspecified elbow with involvement of other organs and systems

● M05.63   Rheumatoid arthritis of wrist with involvement of other organs and systems

     Rheumatoid arthritis of carpal bones with involvement of other organs and systems

     M05.631   Rheumatoid arthritis of right wrist with involvement of other organs and systems

     M05.632   Rheumatoid arthritis of left wrist with involvement of other organs and systems

     M05.639   Rheumatoid arthritis of unspecified wrist with involvement of other organs and systems

● M05.64   Rheumatoid arthritis of hand with involvement of other organs and systems

     Rheumatoid arthritis of metacarpus and phalanges with involvement of other organs and systems

     M05.641   Rheumatoid arthritis of right hand with involvement of other organs and systems

     M05.642   Rheumatoid arthritis of left hand with involvement of other organs and systems

     M05.649   Rheumatoid arthritis of unspecified hand with involvement of other organs and systems

● M05.65   Rheumatoid arthritis of hip with involvement of other organs and systems

     M05.651   Rheumatoid arthritis of right hip with involvement of other organs and systems

     M05.652   Rheumatoid arthritis of left hip with involvement of other organs and systems

     M05.659   Rheumatoid arthritis of unspecified hip with involvement of other organs and systems

● M05.66   Rheumatoid arthritis of knee with involvement of other organs and systems

     M05.661   Rheumatoid arthritis of right knee with involvement of other organs and systems

     M05.662   Rheumatoid arthritis of left knee with involvement of other organs and systems

     M05.669   Rheumatoid arthritis of unspecified knee with involvement of other organs and systems

● M05.67   Rheumatoid arthritis of ankle and foot with involvement of other organs and systems

     Rheumatoid arthritis of tarsus, metatarsus and phalanges with involvement of other organs and systems

     M05.671   Rheumatoid arthritis of right ankle and foot with involvement of other organs and systems

     M05.672   Rheumatoid arthritis of left ankle and foot with involvement of other organs and systems

     M05.679   Rheumatoid arthritis of unspecified ankle and foot with involvement of other organs and systems

   M05.69   Rheumatoid arthritis of multiple sites with involvement of other organs and systems

● M05.7   Rheumatoid arthritis with rheumatoid factor without organ or systems involvement

     M05.70   Rheumatoid arthritis with rheumatoid factor of unspecified site without organ or systems involvement

● M05.71   Rheumatoid arthritis with rheumatoid factor of shoulder without organ or systems involvement

     M05.711   Rheumatoid arthritis with rheumatoid factor of right shoulder without organ or systems involvement

     M05.712   Rheumatoid arthritis with rheumatoid factor of left shoulder without organ or systems involvement

     M05.719   Rheumatoid arthritis with rheumatoid factor of unspecified shoulder without organ or systems involvement

CHAPTER 13 (M00-M99)

CHAPTER 13 (M00-M99)

● M05.72　Rheumatoid arthritis with rheumatoid factor of elbow without organ or systems involvement
　　　M05.721　Rheumatoid arthritis with rheumatoid factor of right elbow without organ or systems involvement
　　　M05.722　Rheumatoid arthritis with rheumatoid factor of left elbow without organ or systems involvement
　　　M05.729　Rheumatoid arthritis with rheumatoid factor of unspecified elbow without organ or systems involvement
● M05.73　Rheumatoid arthritis with rheumatoid factor of wrist without organ or systems involvement
　　　M05.731　Rheumatoid arthritis with rheumatoid factor of right wrist without organ or systems involvement
　　　M05.732　Rheumatoid arthritis with rheumatoid factor of left wrist without organ or systems involvement
　　　M05.739　Rheumatoid arthritis with rheumatoid factor of unspecified wrist without organ or systems involvement
● M05.74　Rheumatoid arthritis with rheumatoid factor of hand without organ or systems involvement
　　　M05.741　Rheumatoid arthritis with rheumatoid factor of right hand without organ or systems involvement
　　　M05.742　Rheumatoid arthritis with rheumatoid factor of left hand without organ or systems involvement
　　　M05.749　Rheumatoid arthritis with rheumatoid factor of unspecified hand without organ or systems involvement
● M05.75　Rheumatoid arthritis with rheumatoid factor of hip without organ or systems involvement
　　　M05.751　Rheumatoid arthritis with rheumatoid factor of right hip without organ or systems involvement
　　　M05.752　Rheumatoid arthritis with rheumatoid factor of left hip without organ or systems involvement
　　　M05.759　Rheumatoid arthritis with rheumatoid factor of unspecified hip without organ or systems involvement
● M05.76　Rheumatoid arthritis with rheumatoid factor of knee without organ or systems involvement
　　　M05.761　Rheumatoid arthritis with rheumatoid factor of right knee without organ or systems involvement
　　　M05.762　Rheumatoid arthritis with rheumatoid factor of left knee without organ or systems involvement
　　　M05.769　Rheumatoid arthritis with rheumatoid factor of unspecified knee without organ or systems involvement

● M05.77　Rheumatoid arthritis with rheumatoid factor of ankle and foot without organ or systems involvement
　　　M05.771　Rheumatoid arthritis with rheumatoid factor of right ankle and foot without organ or systems involvement
　　　M05.772　Rheumatoid arthritis with rheumatoid factor of left ankle and foot without organ or systems involvement
　　　M05.779　Rheumatoid arthritis with rheumatoid factor of unspecified ankle and foot without organ or systems involvement
　　　M05.79　Rheumatoid arthritis with rheumatoid factor of multiple sites without organ or systems involvement
● M05.8　Other rheumatoid arthritis with rheumatoid factor
　　　M05.80　Other rheumatoid arthritis with rheumatoid factor of unspecified site
● M05.81　Other rheumatoid arthritis with rheumatoid factor of shoulder
　　　M05.811　Other rheumatoid arthritis with rheumatoid factor of right shoulder
　　　M05.812　Other rheumatoid arthritis with rheumatoid factor of left shoulder
　　　M05.819　Other rheumatoid arthritis with rheumatoid factor of unspecified shoulder
● M05.82　Other rheumatoid arthritis with rheumatoid factor of elbow
　　　M05.821　Other rheumatoid arthritis with rheumatoid factor of right elbow
　　　M05.822　Other rheumatoid arthritis with rheumatoid factor of left elbow
　　　M05.829　Other rheumatoid arthritis with rheumatoid factor of unspecified elbow
● M05.83　Other rheumatoid arthritis with rheumatoid factor of wrist
　　　M05.831　Other rheumatoid arthritis with rheumatoid factor of right wrist
　　　M05.832　Other rheumatoid arthritis with rheumatoid factor of left wrist
　　　M05.839　Other rheumatoid arthritis with rheumatoid factor of unspecified wrist
● M05.84　Other rheumatoid arthritis with rheumatoid factor of hand
　　　M05.841　Other rheumatoid arthritis with rheumatoid factor of right hand
　　　M05.842　Other rheumatoid arthritis with rheumatoid factor of left hand
　　　M05.849　Other rheumatoid arthritis with rheumatoid factor of unspecified hand
● M05.85　Other rheumatoid arthritis with rheumatoid factor of hip
　　　M05.851　Other rheumatoid arthritis with rheumatoid factor of right hip
　　　M05.852　Other rheumatoid arthritis with rheumatoid factor of left hip
　　　M05.859　Other rheumatoid arthritis with rheumatoid factor of unspecified hip

▶ New　⮕ Revised　deleted Deleted　OGCR Official Guidelines　X Assign placeholder X　● Use Additional Character(s)
Excludes 1　Excludes 2　Includes　Use additional　Code first　Code also　Key words

● M05.86 Other rheumatoid arthritis with rheumatoid factor of knee

    M05.861 Other rheumatoid arthritis with rheumatoid factor of right knee

    M05.862 Other rheumatoid arthritis with rheumatoid factor of left knee

    M05.869 Other rheumatoid arthritis with rheumatoid factor of unspecified knee

● M05.87 Other rheumatoid arthritis with rheumatoid factor of ankle and foot

    M05.871 Other rheumatoid arthritis with rheumatoid factor of right ankle and foot

    M05.872 Other rheumatoid arthritis with rheumatoid factor of left ankle and foot

    M05.879 Other rheumatoid arthritis with rheumatoid factor of unspecified ankle and foot

  M05.89 Other rheumatoid arthritis with rheumatoid factor of multiple sites

  M05.9 Rheumatoid arthritis with rheumatoid factor, unspecified

● M06 Other rheumatoid arthritis

  ● M06.0 Rheumatoid arthritis without rheumatoid factor

    M06.00 Rheumatoid arthritis without rheumatoid factor, unspecified site

    ● M06.01 Rheumatoid arthritis without rheumatoid factor, shoulder

      M06.011 Rheumatoid arthritis without rheumatoid factor, right shoulder

      M06.012 Rheumatoid arthritis without rheumatoid factor, left shoulder

      M06.019 Rheumatoid arthritis without rheumatoid factor, unspecified shoulder

    ● M06.02 Rheumatoid arthritis without rheumatoid factor, elbow

      M06.021 Rheumatoid arthritis without rheumatoid factor, right elbow

      M06.022 Rheumatoid arthritis without rheumatoid factor, left elbow

      M06.029 Rheumatoid arthritis without rheumatoid factor, unspecified elbow

    ● M06.03 Rheumatoid arthritis without rheumatoid factor, wrist

      M06.031 Rheumatoid arthritis without rheumatoid factor, right wrist

      M06.032 Rheumatoid arthritis without rheumatoid factor, left wrist

      M06.039 Rheumatoid arthritis without rheumatoid factor, unspecified wrist

    ● M06.04 Rheumatoid arthritis without rheumatoid factor, hand

      M06.041 Rheumatoid arthritis without rheumatoid factor, right hand

      M06.042 Rheumatoid arthritis without rheumatoid factor, left hand

      M06.049 Rheumatoid arthritis without rheumatoid factor, unspecified hand

    ● M06.05 Rheumatoid arthritis without rheumatoid factor, hip

      M06.051 Rheumatoid arthritis without rheumatoid factor, right hip

      M06.052 Rheumatoid arthritis without rheumatoid factor, left hip

      M06.059 Rheumatoid arthritis without rheumatoid factor, unspecified hip

● M06.06 Rheumatoid arthritis without rheumatoid factor, knee

    M06.061 Rheumatoid arthritis without rheumatoid factor, right knee

    M06.062 Rheumatoid arthritis without rheumatoid factor, left knee

    M06.069 Rheumatoid arthritis without rheumatoid factor, unspecified knee

● M06.07 Rheumatoid arthritis without rheumatoid factor, ankle and foot

    M06.071 Rheumatoid arthritis without rheumatoid factor, right ankle and foot

    M06.072 Rheumatoid arthritis without rheumatoid factor, left ankle and foot

    M06.079 Rheumatoid arthritis without rheumatoid factor, unspecified ankle and foot

  M06.08 Rheumatoid arthritis without rheumatoid factor, vertebrae

  M06.09 Rheumatoid arthritis without rheumatoid factor, multiple sites

  M06.1 Adult-onset Still's disease

    Excludes1   Still's disease NOS (M08.2-)

● M06.2 Rheumatoid bursitis

  M06.20 Rheumatoid bursitis, unspecified site

  ● M06.21 Rheumatoid bursitis, shoulder

    M06.211 Rheumatoid bursitis, right shoulder

    M06.212 Rheumatoid bursitis, left shoulder

    M06.219 Rheumatoid bursitis, unspecified shoulder

  ● M06.22 Rheumatoid bursitis, elbow

    M06.221 Rheumatoid bursitis, right elbow

    M06.222 Rheumatoid bursitis, left elbow

    M06.229 Rheumatoid bursitis, unspecified elbow

  ● M06.23 Rheumatoid bursitis, wrist

    M06.231 Rheumatoid bursitis, right wrist

    M06.232 Rheumatoid bursitis, left wrist

    M06.239 Rheumatoid bursitis, unspecified wrist

  ● M06.24 Rheumatoid bursitis, hand

    M06.241 Rheumatoid bursitis, right hand

    M06.242 Rheumatoid bursitis, left hand

    M06.249 Rheumatoid bursitis, unspecified hand

  ● M06.25 Rheumatoid bursitis, hip

    M06.251 Rheumatoid bursitis, right hip

    M06.252 Rheumatoid bursitis, left hip

    M06.259 Rheumatoid bursitis, unspecified hip

  ● M06.26 Rheumatoid bursitis, knee

    M06.261 Rheumatoid bursitis, right knee

    M06.262 Rheumatoid bursitis, left knee

    M06.269 Rheumatoid bursitis, unspecified knee

  ● M06.27 Rheumatoid bursitis, ankle and foot

    M06.271 Rheumatoid bursitis, right ankle and foot

    M06.272 Rheumatoid bursitis, left ankle and foot

    M06.279 Rheumatoid bursitis, unspecified ankle and foot

  M06.28 Rheumatoid bursitis, vertebrae

  M06.29 Rheumatoid bursitis, multiple sites

▶ New   ⇨ Revised   ~~deleted~~ Deleted   **OGCR** Official Guidelines   X Assign placeholder X   ● Use Additional Character(s)

Excludes 1   Excludes 2   Includes   Use additional   Code first   Code also   Key words

● M06.3　Rheumatoid nodule
　　M06.30　Rheumatoid nodule, unspecified site
　● M06.31　Rheumatoid nodule, shoulder
　　　M06.311　Rheumatoid nodule, right shoulder
　　　M06.312　Rheumatoid nodule, left shoulder
　　　M06.319　Rheumatoid nodule, unspecified shoulder
　● M06.32　Rheumatoid nodule, elbow
　　　M06.321　Rheumatoid nodule, right elbow
　　　M06.322　Rheumatoid nodule, left elbow
　　　M06.329　Rheumatoid nodule, unspecified elbow
　● M06.33　Rheumatoid nodule, wrist
　　　M06.331　Rheumatoid nodule, right wrist
　　　M06.332　Rheumatoid nodule, left wrist
　　　M06.339　Rheumatoid nodule, unspecified wrist
　● M06.34　Rheumatoid nodule, hand
　　　M06.341　Rheumatoid nodule, right hand
　　　M06.342　Rheumatoid nodule, left hand
　　　M06.349　Rheumatoid nodule, unspecified hand
　● M06.35　Rheumatoid nodule, hip
　　　M06.351　Rheumatoid nodule, right hip
　　　M06.352　Rheumatoid nodule, left hip
　　　M06.359　Rheumatoid nodule, unspecified hip
　● M06.36　Rheumatoid nodule, knee
　　　M06.361　Rheumatoid nodule, right knee
　　　M06.362　Rheumatoid nodule, left knee
　　　M06.369　Rheumatoid nodule, unspecified knee
　● M06.37　Rheumatoid nodule, ankle and foot
　　　M06.371　Rheumatoid nodule, right ankle and foot
　　　M06.372　Rheumatoid nodule, left ankle and foot
　　　M06.379　Rheumatoid nodule, unspecified ankle and foot
　　M06.38　Rheumatoid nodule, vertebrae
　　M06.39　Rheumatoid nodule, multiple sites
　M06.4　Inflammatory polyarthropathy
　　　Excludes1　polyarthritis NOS (M13.0)
● M06.8　Other specified rheumatoid arthritis
　　M06.80　Other specified rheumatoid arthritis, unspecified site
　● M06.81　Other specified rheumatoid arthritis, shoulder
　　　M06.811　Other specified rheumatoid arthritis, right shoulder
　　　M06.812　Other specified rheumatoid arthritis, left shoulder
　　　M06.819　Other specified rheumatoid arthritis, unspecified shoulder
　● M06.82　Other specified rheumatoid arthritis, elbow
　　　M06.821　Other specified rheumatoid arthritis, right elbow
　　　M06.822　Other specified rheumatoid arthritis, left elbow
　　　M06.829　Other specified rheumatoid arthritis, unspecified elbow
　● M06.83　Other specified rheumatoid arthritis, wrist
　　　M06.831　Other specified rheumatoid arthritis, right wrist
　　　M06.832　Other specified rheumatoid arthritis, left wrist
　　　M06.839　Other specified rheumatoid arthritis, unspecified wrist

● M06.84　Other specified rheumatoid arthritis, hand
　　　M06.841　Other specified rheumatoid arthritis, right hand
　　　M06.842　Other specified rheumatoid arthritis, left hand
　　　M06.849　Other specified rheumatoid arthritis, unspecified hand
　● M06.85　Other specified rheumatoid arthritis, hip
　　　M06.851　Other specified rheumatoid arthritis, right hip
　　　M06.852　Other specified rheumatoid arthritis, left hip
　　　M06.859　Other specified rheumatoid arthritis, unspecified hip
　● M06.86　Other specified rheumatoid arthritis, knee
　　　M06.861　Other specified rheumatoid arthritis, right knee
　　　M06.862　Other specified rheumatoid arthritis, left knee
　　　M06.869　Other specified rheumatoid arthritis, unspecified knee
　● M06.87　Other specified rheumatoid arthritis, ankle and foot
　　　M06.871　Other specified rheumatoid arthritis, right ankle and foot
　　　M06.872　Other specified rheumatoid arthritis, left ankle and foot
　　　M06.879　Other specified rheumatoid arthritis, unspecified ankle and foot
　　M06.88　Other specified rheumatoid arthritis, vertebrae
　　M06.89　Other specified rheumatoid arthritis, multiple sites
　M06.9　Rheumatoid arthritis, unspecified

● M07　Enteropathic arthropathies
　　Code also associated enteropathy, such as:
　　　regional enteritis [Crohn's disease] (K50.-)
　　　ulcerative colitis (K51.-)
　　　Excludes1　psoriatic arthropathies (L40.5-)
　● M07.6　Enteropathic arthropathies
　　M07.60　Enteropathic arthropathies, unspecified site
　● M07.61　Enteropathic arthropathies, shoulder
　　　M07.611　Enteropathic arthropathies, right shoulder
　　　M07.612　Enteropathic arthropathies, left shoulder
　　　M07.619　Enteropathic arthropathies, unspecified shoulder
　● M07.62　Enteropathic arthropathies, elbow
　　　M07.621　Enteropathic arthropathies, right elbow
　　　M07.622　Enteropathic arthropathies, left elbow
　　　M07.629　Enteropathic arthropathies, unspecified elbow
　● M07.63　Enteropathic arthropathies, wrist
　　　M07.631　Enteropathic arthropathies, right wrist
　　　M07.632　Enteropathic arthropathies, left wrist
　　　M07.639　Enteropathic arthropathies, unspecified wrist
　● M07.64　Enteropathic arthropathies, hand
　　　M07.641　Enteropathic arthropathies, right hand
　　　M07.642　Enteropathic arthropathies, left hand
　　　M07.649　Enteropathic arthropathies, unspecified hand

● M07.65 Enteropathic arthropathies, hip
    M07.651 Enteropathic arthropathies, right hip
    M07.652 Enteropathic arthropathies, left hip
    M07.659 Enteropathic arthropathies, unspecified hip
● M07.66 Enteropathic arthropathies, knee
    M07.661 Enteropathic arthropathies, right knee
    M07.662 Enteropathic arthropathies, left knee
    M07.669 Enteropathic arthropathies, unspecified knee
● M07.67 Enteropathic arthropathies, ankle and foot
    M07.671 Enteropathic arthropathies, right ankle and foot
    M07.672 Enteropathic arthropathies, left ankle and foot
    M07.679 Enteropathic arthropathies, unspecified ankle and foot
  M07.68 Enteropathic arthropathies, vertebrae
  M07.69 Enteropathic arthropathies, multiple sites

● M08 Juvenile arthritis
    Code also any associated underlying condition, such as:
      regional enteritis [Crohn's disease] (K50.-)
      ulcerative colitis (K51.-)
    Excludes1 arthropathy in Whipple's disease (M14.8)
               Felty's syndrome (M05.0)
               juvenile dermatomyositis (M33.0-)
               psoriatic juvenile arthropathy (L40.54)
● M08.0 Unspecified juvenile rheumatoid arthritis
    Juvenile rheumatoid arthritis with or without rheumatoid factor
    M08.00 Unspecified juvenile rheumatoid arthritis of unspecified site
● M08.01 Unspecified juvenile rheumatoid arthritis, shoulder
    M08.011 Unspecified juvenile rheumatoid arthritis, right shoulder
    M08.012 Unspecified juvenile rheumatoid arthritis, left shoulder
    M08.019 Unspecified juvenile rheumatoid arthritis, unspecified shoulder
● M08.02 Unspecified juvenile rheumatoid arthritis of elbow
    M08.021 Unspecified juvenile rheumatoid arthritis, right elbow
    M08.022 Unspecified juvenile rheumatoid arthritis, left elbow
    M08.029 Unspecified juvenile rheumatoid arthritis, unspecified elbow
● M08.03 Unspecified juvenile rheumatoid arthritis, wrist
    M08.031 Unspecified juvenile rheumatoid arthritis, right wrist
    M08.032 Unspecified juvenile rheumatoid arthritis, left wrist
    M08.039 Unspecified juvenile rheumatoid arthritis, unspecified wrist
● M08.04 Unspecified juvenile rheumatoid arthritis, hand
    M08.041 Unspecified juvenile rheumatoid arthritis, right hand
    M08.042 Unspecified juvenile rheumatoid arthritis, left hand
    M08.049 Unspecified juvenile rheumatoid arthritis, unspecified hand

● M08.05 Unspecified juvenile rheumatoid arthritis, hip
    M08.051 Unspecified juvenile rheumatoid arthritis, right hip
    M08.052 Unspecified juvenile rheumatoid arthritis, left hip
    M08.059 Unspecified juvenile rheumatoid arthritis, unspecified hip
● M08.06 Unspecified juvenile rheumatoid arthritis, knee
    M08.061 Unspecified juvenile rheumatoid arthritis, right knee
    M08.062 Unspecified juvenile rheumatoid arthritis, left knee
    M08.069 Unspecified juvenile rheumatoid arthritis, unspecified knee
● M08.07 Unspecified juvenile rheumatoid arthritis, ankle and foot
    M08.071 Unspecified juvenile rheumatoid arthritis, right ankle and foot
    M08.072 Unspecified juvenile rheumatoid arthritis, left ankle and foot
    M08.079 Unspecified juvenile rheumatoid arthritis, unspecified ankle and foot
  M08.08 Unspecified juvenile rheumatoid arthritis, vertebrae
  M08.09 Unspecified juvenile rheumatoid arthritis, multiple sites
  M08.1 Juvenile ankylosing spondylitis
    Excludes1 ankylosing spondylitis in adults (M45.0-)
● M08.2 Juvenile rheumatoid arthritis with systemic onset
    Still's disease NOS
    Excludes1 adult-onset Still's disease (M06.1-)
    M08.20 Juvenile rheumatoid arthritis with systemic onset, unspecified site
● M08.21 Juvenile rheumatoid arthritis with systemic onset, shoulder
    M08.211 Juvenile rheumatoid arthritis with systemic onset, right shoulder
    M08.212 Juvenile rheumatoid arthritis with systemic onset, left shoulder
    M08.219 Juvenile rheumatoid arthritis with systemic onset, unspecified shoulder
● M08.22 Juvenile rheumatoid arthritis with systemic onset, elbow
    M08.221 Juvenile rheumatoid arthritis with systemic onset, right elbow
    M08.222 Juvenile rheumatoid arthritis with systemic onset, left elbow
    M08.229 Juvenile rheumatoid arthritis with systemic onset, unspecified elbow
● M08.23 Juvenile rheumatoid arthritis with systemic onset, wrist
    M08.231 Juvenile rheumatoid arthritis with systemic onset, right wrist
    M08.232 Juvenile rheumatoid arthritis with systemic onset, left wrist
    M08.239 Juvenile rheumatoid arthritis with systemic onset, unspecified wrist
● M08.24 Juvenile rheumatoid arthritis with systemic onset, hand
    M08.241 Juvenile rheumatoid arthritis with systemic onset, right hand
    M08.242 Juvenile rheumatoid arthritis with systemic onset, left hand
    M08.249 Juvenile rheumatoid arthritis with systemic onset, unspecified hand

CHAPTER 13 (M00-M99)

CHAPTER 13 (M00-M99)

● M08.25   Juvenile rheumatoid arthritis with systemic onset, hip
- M08.251   Juvenile rheumatoid arthritis with systemic onset, right hip
- M08.252   Juvenile rheumatoid arthritis with systemic onset, left hip
- M08.259   Juvenile rheumatoid arthritis with systemic onset, unspecified hip

● M08.26   Juvenile rheumatoid arthritis with systemic onset, knee
- M08.261   Juvenile rheumatoid arthritis with systemic onset, right knee
- M08.262   Juvenile rheumatoid arthritis with systemic onset, left knee
- M08.269   Juvenile rheumatoid arthritis with systemic onset, unspecified knee

● M08.27   Juvenile rheumatoid arthritis with systemic onset, ankle and foot
- M08.271   Juvenile rheumatoid arthritis with systemic onset, right ankle and foot
- M08.272   Juvenile rheumatoid arthritis with systemic onset, left ankle and foot
- M08.279   Juvenile rheumatoid arthritis with systemic onset, unspecified ankle and foot

M08.28   Juvenile rheumatoid arthritis with systemic onset, vertebrae

M08.29   Juvenile rheumatoid arthritis with systemic onset, multiple sites

M08.3   Juvenile rheumatoid polyarthritis (seronegative)

● M08.4   Pauciarticular juvenile rheumatoid arthritis

M08.40   Pauciarticular juvenile rheumatoid arthritis, unspecified site

● M08.41   Pauciarticular juvenile rheumatoid arthritis, shoulder
- M08.411   Pauciarticular juvenile rheumatoid arthritis, right shoulder
- M08.412   Pauciarticular juvenile rheumatoid arthritis, left shoulder
- M08.419   Pauciarticular juvenile rheumatoid arthritis, unspecified shoulder

● M08.42   Pauciarticular juvenile rheumatoid arthritis, elbow
- M08.421   Pauciarticular juvenile rheumatoid arthritis, right elbow
- M08.422   Pauciarticular juvenile rheumatoid arthritis, left elbow
- M08.429   Pauciarticular juvenile rheumatoid arthritis, unspecified elbow

● M08.43   Pauciarticular juvenile rheumatoid arthritis, wrist
- M08.431   Pauciarticular juvenile rheumatoid arthritis, right wrist
- M08.432   Pauciarticular juvenile rheumatoid arthritis, left wrist
- M08.439   Pauciarticular juvenile rheumatoid arthritis, unspecified wrist

● M08.44   Pauciarticular juvenile rheumatoid arthritis, hand
- M08.441   Pauciarticular juvenile rheumatoid arthritis, right hand
- M08.442   Pauciarticular juvenile rheumatoid arthritis, left hand
- M08.449   Pauciarticular juvenile rheumatoid arthritis, unspecified hand

● M08.45   Pauciarticular juvenile rheumatoid arthritis, hip
- M08.451   Pauciarticular juvenile rheumatoid arthritis, right hip
- M08.452   Pauciarticular juvenile rheumatoid arthritis, left hip
- M08.459   Pauciarticular juvenile rheumatoid arthritis, unspecified hip

● M08.46   Pauciarticular juvenile rheumatoid arthritis, knee
- M08.461   Pauciarticular juvenile rheumatoid arthritis, right knee
- M08.462   Pauciarticular juvenile rheumatoid arthritis, left knee
- M08.469   Pauciarticular juvenile rheumatoid arthritis, unspecified knee

● M08.47   Pauciarticular juvenile rheumatoid arthritis, ankle and foot
- M08.471   Pauciarticular juvenile rheumatoid arthritis, right ankle and foot
- M08.472   Pauciarticular juvenile rheumatoid arthritis, left ankle and foot
- M08.479   Pauciarticular juvenile rheumatoid arthritis, unspecified ankle and foot

M08.48   Pauciarticular juvenile rheumatoid arthritis, vertebrae

● M08.8   Other juvenile arthritis

M08.80   Other juvenile arthritis, unspecified site

● M08.81   Other juvenile arthritis, shoulder
- M08.811   Other juvenile arthritis, right shoulder
- M08.812   Other juvenile arthritis, left shoulder
- M08.819   Other juvenile arthritis, unspecified shoulder

● M08.82   Other juvenile arthritis, elbow
- M08.821   Other juvenile arthritis, right elbow
- M08.822   Other juvenile arthritis, left elbow
- M08.829   Other juvenile arthritis, unspecified elbow

● M08.83   Other juvenile arthritis, wrist
- M08.831   Other juvenile arthritis, right wrist
- M08.832   Other juvenile arthritis, left wrist
- M08.839   Other juvenile arthritis, unspecified wrist

● M08.84   Other juvenile arthritis, hand
- M08.841   Other juvenile arthritis, right hand
- M08.842   Other juvenile arthritis, left hand
- M08.849   Other juvenile arthritis, unspecified hand

● M08.85   Other juvenile arthritis, hip
- M08.851   Other juvenile arthritis, right hip
- M08.852   Other juvenile arthritis, left hip
- M08.859   Other juvenile arthritis, unspecified hip

● M08.86   Other juvenile arthritis, knee
- M08.861   Other juvenile arthritis, right knee
- M08.862   Other juvenile arthritis, left knee
- M08.869   Other juvenile arthritis, unspecified knee

▶ New   ⇒ Revised   ~~deleted~~ Deleted   **OGCR** Official Guidelines   X Assign placeholder X   ● Use Additional Character(s)

Excludes 1   Excludes 2   Includes   Use additional   Code first   Code also   Key words

● M08.87 Other juvenile arthritis, ankle and foot
    M08.871 Other juvenile arthritis, right ankle and foot
    M08.872 Other juvenile arthritis, left ankle and foot
    M08.879 Other juvenile arthritis, unspecified ankle and foot
    M08.88 Other juvenile arthritis, other specified site
       Other juvenile arthritis, vertebrae
    M08.89 Other juvenile arthritis, multiple sites
● M08.9 Juvenile arthritis, unspecified
    Excludes1   juvenile rheumatoid arthritis, unspecified (M08.0-)
    M08.90 Juvenile arthritis, unspecified, unspecified site
● M08.91 Juvenile arthritis, unspecified, shoulder
    M08.911 Juvenile arthritis, unspecified, right shoulder
    M08.912 Juvenile arthritis, unspecified, left shoulder
    M08.919 Juvenile arthritis, unspecified, unspecified shoulder
● M08.92 Juvenile arthritis, unspecified, elbow
    M08.921 Juvenile arthritis, unspecified, right elbow
    M08.922 Juvenile arthritis, unspecified, left elbow
    M08.929 Juvenile arthritis, unspecified, unspecified elbow
● M08.93 Juvenile arthritis, unspecified, wrist
    M08.931 Juvenile arthritis, unspecified, right wrist
    M08.932 Juvenile arthritis, unspecified, left wrist
    M08.939 Juvenile arthritis, unspecified, unspecified wrist
● M08.94 Juvenile arthritis, unspecified, hand
    M08.941 Juvenile arthritis, unspecified, right hand
    M08.942 Juvenile arthritis, unspecified, left hand
    M08.949 Juvenile arthritis, unspecified, unspecified hand
● M08.95 Juvenile arthritis, unspecified, hip
    M08.951 Juvenile arthritis, unspecified, right hip
    M08.952 Juvenile arthritis, unspecified, left hip
    M08.959 Juvenile arthritis, unspecified, unspecified hip
● M08.96 Juvenile arthritis, unspecified, knee
    M08.961 Juvenile arthritis, unspecified, right knee
    M08.962 Juvenile arthritis, unspecified, left knee
    M08.969 Juvenile arthritis, unspecified, unspecified knee
● M08.97 Juvenile arthritis, unspecified, ankle and foot
    M08.971 Juvenile arthritis, unspecified, right ankle and foot
    M08.972 Juvenile arthritis, unspecified, left ankle and foot
    M08.979 Juvenile arthritis, unspecified, unspecified ankle and foot
    M08.98 Juvenile arthritis, unspecified, vertebrae
    M08.99 Juvenile arthritis, unspecified, multiple sites

● M1A Chronic gout
    Use additional code to identify:
    Autonomic neuropathy in diseases classified elsewhere (G99.0)
    Calculus of urinary tract in diseases classified elsewhere (N22)
    Cardiomyopathy in diseases classified elsewhere (I43)
    Disorders of external ear in diseases classified elsewhere (H61.1-, H62.8-)
    Disorders of iris and ciliary body in diseases classified elsewhere (H22)
    Glomerular disorders in diseases classified elsewhere (N08)
    Excludes1   gout NOS (M10.-)
    Excludes2   acute gout (M10.-)
    The appropriate 7th character is to be added to each code from category M1A

> Ø   without tophus (tophi)
> 1   with tophus (tophi)

● M1A.0 Idiopathic chronic gout
    Chronic gouty bursitis
    Primary chronic gout
  X ● M1A.00 Idiopathic chronic gout, unspecified site
    ● M1A.01 Idiopathic chronic gout, shoulder
      ● M1A.011 Idiopathic chronic gout, right shoulder
      ● M1A.012 Idiopathic chronic gout, left shoulder
      ● M1A.019 Idiopathic chronic gout, unspecified shoulder
    ● M1A.02 Idiopathic chronic gout, elbow
      ● M1A.021 Idiopathic chronic gout, right elbow
      ● M1A.022 Idiopathic chronic gout, left elbow
      ● M1A.029 Idiopathic chronic gout, unspecified elbow
    ● M1A.03 Idiopathic chronic gout, wrist
      ● M1A.031 Idiopathic chronic gout, right wrist
      ● M1A.032 Idiopathic chronic gout, left wrist
      ● M1A.039 Idiopathic chronic gout, unspecified wrist
    ● M1A.04 Idiopathic chronic gout, hand
      ● M1A.041 Idiopathic chronic gout, right hand
      ● M1A.042 Idiopathic chronic gout, left hand
      ● M1A.049 Idiopathic chronic gout, unspecified hand
    ● M1A.05 Idiopathic chronic gout, hip
      ● M1A.051 Idiopathic chronic gout, right hip
      ● M1A.052 Idiopathic chronic gout, left hip
      ● M1A.059 Idiopathic chronic gout, unspecified hip
    ● M1A.06 Idiopathic chronic gout, knee
      ● M1A.061 Idiopathic chronic gout, right knee
      ● M1A.062 Idiopathic chronic gout, left knee
      ● M1A.069 Idiopathic chronic gout, unspecified knee
    ● M1A.07 Idiopathic chronic gout, ankle and foot
      ● M1A.071 Idiopathic chronic gout, right ankle and foot
      ● M1A.072 Idiopathic chronic gout, left ankle and foot
      ● M1A.079 Idiopathic chronic gout, unspecified ankle and foot
  X ● M1A.08 Idiopathic chronic gout, vertebrae
  X ● M1A.09 Idiopathic chronic gout, multiple sites

CHAPTER 13 (M00-M99)

● M1A.1 Lead-induced chronic gout
    Code first toxic effects of lead and its compounds (T56.0-)
X ● M1A.10 Lead-induced chronic gout, unspecified site
● M1A.11 Lead-induced chronic gout, shoulder
    ● M1A.111 Lead-induced chronic gout, right shoulder
    ● M1A.112 Lead-induced chronic gout, left shoulder
    ● M1A.119 Lead-induced chronic gout, unspecified shoulder
● M1A.12 Lead-induced chronic gout, elbow
    ● M1A.121 Lead-induced chronic gout, right elbow
    ● M1A.122 Lead-induced chronic gout, left elbow
    ● M1A.129 Lead-induced chronic gout, unspecified elbow
● M1A.13 Lead-induced chronic gout, wrist
    ● M1A.131 Lead-induced chronic gout, right wrist
    ● M1A.132 Lead-induced chronic gout, left wrist
    ● M1A.139 Lead-induced chronic gout, unspecified wrist
● M1A.14 Lead-induced chronic gout, hand
    ● M1A.141 Lead-induced chronic gout, right hand
    ● M1A.142 Lead-induced chronic gout, left hand
    ● M1A.149 Lead-induced chronic gout, unspecified hand
● M1A.15 Lead-induced chronic gout, hip
    ● M1A.151 Lead-induced chronic gout, right hip
    ● M1A.152 Lead-induced chronic gout, left hip
    ● M1A.159 Lead-induced chronic gout, unspecified hip
● M1A.16 Lead-induced chronic gout, knee
    ● M1A.161 Lead-induced chronic gout, right knee
    ● M1A.162 Lead-induced chronic gout, left knee
    ● M1A.169 Lead-induced chronic gout, unspecified knee
● M1A.17 Lead-induced chronic gout, ankle and foot
    ● M1A.171 Lead-induced chronic gout, right ankle and foot
    ● M1A.172 Lead-induced chronic gout, left ankle and foot
    ● M1A.179 Lead-induced chronic gout, unspecified ankle and foot
X ● M1A.18 Lead-induced chronic gout, vertebrae
X ● M1A.19 Lead-induced chronic gout, multiple sites
● M1A.2 Drug-induced chronic gout
    Use additional code for adverse effect, if applicable, to identify drug (T36-T50 with fifth or sixth character 5)
X ● M1A.20 Drug-induced chronic gout, unspecified site
● M1A.21 Drug-induced chronic gout, shoulder
    ● M1A.211 Drug-induced chronic gout, right shoulder
    ● M1A.212 Drug-induced chronic gout, left shoulder
    ● M1A.219 Drug-induced chronic gout, unspecified shoulder
● M1A.22 Drug-induced chronic gout, elbow
    ● M1A.221 Drug-induced chronic gout, right elbow
    ● M1A.222 Drug-induced chronic gout, left elbow
    ● M1A.229 Drug-induced chronic gout, unspecified elbow

● M1A.23 Drug-induced chronic gout, wrist
    ● M1A.231 Drug-induced chronic gout, right wrist
    ● M1A.232 Drug-induced chronic gout, left wrist
    ● M1A.239 Drug-induced chronic gout, unspecified wrist
● M1A.24 Drug-induced chronic gout, hand
    ● M1A.241 Drug-induced chronic gout, right hand
    ● M1A.242 Drug-induced chronic gout, left hand
    ● M1A.249 Drug-induced chronic gout, unspecified hand
● M1A.25 Drug-induced chronic gout, hip
    ● M1A.251 Drug-induced chronic gout, right hip
    ● M1A.252 Drug-induced chronic gout, left hip
    ● M1A.259 Drug-induced chronic gout, unspecified hip
● M1A.26 Drug-induced chronic gout, knee
    ● M1A.261 Drug-induced chronic gout, right knee
    ● M1A.262 Drug-induced chronic gout, left knee
    ● M1A.269 Drug-induced chronic gout, unspecified knee
● M1A.27 Drug-induced chronic gout, ankle and foot
    ● M1A.271 Drug-induced chronic gout, right ankle and foot
    ● M1A.272 Drug-induced chronic gout, left ankle and foot
    ● M1A.279 Drug-induced chronic gout, unspecified ankle and foot
X ● M1A.28 Drug-induced chronic gout, vertebrae
X ● M1A.29 Drug-induced chronic gout, multiple sites
● M1A.3 Chronic gout due to renal impairment
    Code first associated renal disease
X ● M1A.30 Chronic gout due to renal impairment, unspecified site
● M1A.31 Chronic gout due to renal impairment, shoulder
    ● M1A.311 Chronic gout due to renal impairment, right shoulder
    ● M1A.312 Chronic gout due to renal impairment, left shoulder
    ● M1A.319 Chronic gout due to renal impairment, unspecified shoulder
● M1A.32 Chronic gout due to renal impairment, elbow
    ● M1A.321 Chronic gout due to renal impairment, right elbow
    ● M1A.322 Chronic gout due to renal impairment, left elbow
    ● M1A.329 Chronic gout due to renal impairment, unspecified elbow
● M1A.33 Chronic gout due to renal impairment, wrist
    ● M1A.331 Chronic gout due to renal impairment, right wrist
    ● M1A.332 Chronic gout due to renal impairment, left wrist
    ● M1A.339 Chronic gout due to renal impairment, unspecified wrist
● M1A.34 Chronic gout due to renal impairment, hand
    ● M1A.341 Chronic gout due to renal impairment, right hand
    ● M1A.342 Chronic gout due to renal impairment, left hand
    ● M1A.349 Chronic gout due to renal impairment, unspecified hand

▶ New   ➡ Revised   ~~deleted~~ Deleted   **OGCR** Official Guidelines   X Assign placeholder X   ● Use Additional Character(s)

Excludes 1   Excludes 2   Includes   Use additional   Code first   Code also   Key words

● M1A.35 Chronic gout due to renal impairment, hip
  ● M1A.351 Chronic gout due to renal impairment, right hip
  ● M1A.352 Chronic gout due to renal impairment, left hip
  ● M1A.359 Chronic gout due to renal impairment, unspecified hip
● M1A.36 Chronic gout due to renal impairment, knee
  ● M1A.361 Chronic gout due to renal impairment, right knee
  ● M1A.362 Chronic gout due to renal impairment, left knee
  ● M1A.369 Chronic gout due to renal impairment, unspecified knee
● M1A.37 Chronic gout due to renal impairment, ankle and foot
  ● M1A.371 Chronic gout due to renal impairment, right ankle and foot
  ● M1A.372 Chronic gout due to renal impairment, left ankle and foot
  ● M1A.379 Chronic gout due to renal impairment, unspecified ankle and foot
X ● M1A.38 Chronic gout due to renal impairment, vertebrae
X ● M1A.39 Chronic gout due to renal impairment, multiple sites
● M1A.4 Other secondary chronic gout
  Code first associated condition
X ● M1A.40 Other secondary chronic gout, unspecified site
● M1A.41 Other secondary chronic gout, shoulder
  ● M1A.411 Other secondary chronic gout, right shoulder
  ● M1A.412 Other secondary chronic gout, left shoulder
  ● M1A.419 Other secondary chronic gout, unspecified shoulder
● M1A.42 Other secondary chronic gout, elbow
  ● M1A.421 Other secondary chronic gout, right elbow
  ● M1A.422 Other secondary chronic gout, left elbow
  ● M1A.429 Other secondary chronic gout, unspecified elbow
● M1A.43 Other secondary chronic gout, wrist
  ● M1A.431 Other secondary chronic gout, right wrist
  ● M1A.432 Other secondary chronic gout, left wrist
  ● M1A.439 Other secondary chronic gout, unspecified wrist
● M1A.44 Other secondary chronic gout, hand
  ● M1A.441 Other secondary chronic gout, right hand
  ● M1A.442 Other secondary chronic gout, left hand
  ● M1A.449 Other secondary chronic gout, unspecified hand
● M1A.45 Other secondary chronic gout, hip
  ● M1A.451 Other secondary chronic gout, right hip
  ● M1A.452 Other secondary chronic gout, left hip
  ● M1A.459 Other secondary chronic gout, unspecified hip

● M1A.46 Other secondary chronic gout, knee
  ● M1A.461 Other secondary chronic gout, right knee
  ● M1A.462 Other secondary chronic gout, left knee
  ● M1A.469 Other secondary chronic gout, unspecified knee
● M1A.47 Other secondary chronic gout, ankle and foot
  ● M1A.471 Other secondary chronic gout, right ankle and foot
  ● M1A.472 Other secondary chronic gout, left ankle and foot
  ● M1A.479 Other secondary chronic gout, unspecified ankle and foot
X ● M1A.48 Other secondary chronic gout, vertebrae
X ● M1A.49 Other secondary chronic gout, multiple sites
X ● M1A.9 Chronic gout, unspecified

● M10 Gout
  Accumulation of uric acid that results in swollen, red, hot, painful, stiff joints
  Acute gout
  Gout attack
  Gout flare
  Podagra
  Use additional code to identify:
    Autonomic neuropathy in diseases classified elsewhere (G99.0)
    Calculus of urinary tract in diseases classified elsewhere (N22)
    Cardiomyopathy in diseases classified elsewhere (I43)
    Disorders of external ear in diseases classified elsewhere (H61.1-, H62.8-)
    Disorders of iris and ciliary body in diseases classified elsewhere (H22)
    Glomerular disorders in diseases classified elsewhere (N08)
  Excludes2   chronic gout (M1A.-)
  ● M10.0 Idiopathic gout
    Gouty bursitis
    Primary gout
    M10.00 Idiopathic gout, unspecified site
    ● M10.01 Idiopathic gout, shoulder
      M10.011 Idiopathic gout, right shoulder
      M10.012 Idiopathic gout, left shoulder
      M10.019 Idiopathic gout, unspecified shoulder
    ● M10.02 Idiopathic gout, elbow
      M10.021 Idiopathic gout, right elbow
      M10.022 Idiopathic gout, left elbow
      M10.029 Idiopathic gout, unspecified elbow
    ● M10.03 Idiopathic gout, wrist
      M10.031 Idiopathic gout, right wrist
      M10.032 Idiopathic gout, left wrist
      M10.039 Idiopathic gout, unspecified wrist
    ● M10.04 Idiopathic gout, hand
      M10.041 Idiopathic gout, right hand
      M10.042 Idiopathic gout, left hand
      M10.049 Idiopathic gout, unspecified hand
    ● M10.05 Idiopathic gout, hip
      M10.051 Idiopathic gout, right hip
      M10.052 Idiopathic gout, left hip
      M10.059 Idiopathic gout, unspecified hip
    ● M10.06 Idiopathic gout, knee
      M10.061 Idiopathic gout, right knee
      M10.062 Idiopathic gout, left knee
      M10.069 Idiopathic gout, unspecified knee

CHAPTER 13 (M00-M99)

● M10.07 Idiopathic gout, ankle and foot
    M10.071 Idiopathic gout, right ankle and foot
    M10.072 Idiopathic gout, left ankle and foot
    M10.079 Idiopathic gout, unspecified ankle and foot
  M10.08 Idiopathic gout, vertebrae
  M10.09 Idiopathic gout, multiple sites

● M10.1 Lead-induced gout
    Code first toxic effects of lead and its compounds (T56.0-)
  M10.10 Lead-induced gout, unspecified site
 ● M10.11 Lead-induced gout, shoulder
    M10.111 Lead-induced gout, right shoulder
    M10.112 Lead-induced gout, left shoulder
    M10.119 Lead-induced gout, unspecified shoulder
 ● M10.12 Lead-induced gout, elbow
    M10.121 Lead-induced gout, right elbow
    M10.122 Lead-induced gout, left elbow
    M10.129 Lead-induced gout, unspecified elbow
 ● M10.13 Lead-induced gout, wrist
    M10.131 Lead-induced gout, right wrist
    M10.132 Lead-induced gout, left wrist
    M10.139 Lead-induced gout, unspecified wrist
 ● M10.14 Lead-induced gout, hand
    M10.141 Lead-induced gout, right hand
    M10.142 Lead-induced gout, left hand
    M10.149 Lead-induced gout, unspecified hand
 ● M10.15 Lead-induced gout, hip
    M10.151 Lead-induced gout, right hip
    M10.152 Lead-induced gout, left hip
    M10.159 Lead-induced gout, unspecified hip
 ● M10.16 Lead-induced gout, knee
    M10.161 Lead-induced gout, right knee
    M10.162 Lead-induced gout, left knee
    M10.169 Lead-induced gout, unspecified knee
 ● M10.17 Lead-induced gout, ankle and foot
    M10.171 Lead-induced gout, right ankle and foot
    M10.172 Lead-induced gout, left ankle and foot
    M10.179 Lead-induced gout, unspecified ankle and foot
  M10.18 Lead-induced gout, vertebrae
  M10.19 Lead-induced gout, multiple sites

● M10.2 Drug-induced gout
    Use additional code for adverse effect, if applicable, to identify drug (T36-T50 with fifth or sixth character 5)
  M10.20 Drug-induced gout, unspecified site
 ● M10.21 Drug-induced gout, shoulder
    M10.211 Drug-induced gout, right shoulder
    M10.212 Drug-induced gout, left shoulder
    M10.219 Drug-induced gout, unspecified shoulder
 ● M10.22 Drug-induced gout, elbow
    M10.221 Drug-induced gout, right elbow
    M10.222 Drug-induced gout, left elbow
    M10.229 Drug-induced gout, unspecified elbow
 ● M10.23 Drug-induced gout, wrist
    M10.231 Drug-induced gout, right wrist
    M10.232 Drug-induced gout, left wrist
    M10.239 Drug-induced gout, unspecified wrist

● M10.24 Drug-induced gout, hand
    M10.241 Drug-induced gout, right hand
    M10.242 Drug-induced gout, left hand
    M10.249 Drug-induced gout, unspecified hand
● M10.25 Drug-induced gout, hip
    M10.251 Drug-induced gout, right hip
    M10.252 Drug-induced gout, left hip
    M10.259 Drug-induced gout, unspecified hip
● M10.26 Drug-induced gout, knee
    M10.261 Drug-induced gout, right knee
    M10.262 Drug-induced gout, left knee
    M10.269 Drug-induced gout, unspecified knee
● M10.27 Drug-induced gout, ankle and foot
    M10.271 Drug-induced gout, right ankle and foot
    M10.272 Drug-induced gout, left ankle and foot
    M10.279 Drug-induced gout, unspecified ankle and foot
  M10.28 Drug-induced gout, vertebrae
  M10.29 Drug-induced gout, multiple sites

● M10.3 Gout due to renal impairment
    Code also associated renal disease
  M10.30 Gout due to renal impairment, unspecified site
 ● M10.31 Gout due to renal impairment, shoulder
    M10.311 Gout due to renal impairment, right shoulder
    M10.312 Gout due to renal impairment, left shoulder
    M10.319 Gout due to renal impairment, unspecified shoulder
 ● M10.32 Gout due to renal impairment, elbow
    M10.321 Gout due to renal impairment, right elbow
    M10.322 Gout due to renal impairment, left elbow
    M10.329 Gout due to renal impairment, unspecified elbow
 ● M10.33 Gout due to renal impairment, wrist
    M10.331 Gout due to renal impairment, right wrist
    M10.332 Gout due to renal impairment, left wrist
    M10.339 Gout due to renal impairment, unspecified wrist
 ● M10.34 Gout due to renal impairment, hand
    M10.341 Gout due to renal impairment, right hand
    M10.342 Gout due to renal impairment, left hand
    M10.349 Gout due to renal impairment, unspecified hand
 ● M10.35 Gout due to renal impairment, hip
    M10.351 Gout due to renal impairment, right hip
    M10.352 Gout due to renal impairment, left hip
    M10.359 Gout due to renal impairment, unspecified hip
 ● M10.36 Gout due to renal impairment, knee
    M10.361 Gout due to renal impairment, right knee
    M10.362 Gout due to renal impairment, left knee
    M10.369 Gout due to renal impairment, unspecified knee

▶ New   ⇒ Revised   ~~deleted~~ Deleted   **OGCR** Official Guidelines   X Assign placeholder X   ● Use Additional Character(s)

Excludes 1   Excludes 2   Includes   Use additional   Code first   Code also   Key words

● M10.37   Gout due to renal impairment, ankle and foot
     M10.371   Gout due to renal impairment, right ankle and foot
     M10.372   Gout due to renal impairment, left ankle and foot
     M10.379   Gout due to renal impairment, unspecified ankle and foot
   M10.38   Gout due to renal impairment, vertebrae
   M10.39   Gout due to renal impairment, multiple sites
● M10.4   Other secondary gout
     Code first associated condition
   M10.40   Other secondary gout, unspecified site
● M10.41   Other secondary gout, shoulder
     M10.411   Other secondary gout, right shoulder
     M10.412   Other secondary gout, left shoulder
     M10.419   Other secondary gout, unspecified shoulder
● M10.42   Other secondary gout, elbow
     M10.421   Other secondary gout, right elbow
     M10.422   Other secondary gout, left elbow
     M10.429   Other secondary gout, unspecified elbow
● M10.43   Other secondary gout, wrist
     M10.431   Other secondary gout, right wrist
     M10.432   Other secondary gout, left wrist
     M10.439   Other secondary gout, unspecified wrist
● M10.44   Other secondary gout, hand
     M10.441   Other secondary gout, right hand
     M10.442   Other secondary gout, left hand
     M10.449   Other secondary gout, unspecified hand
● M10.45   Other secondary gout, hip
     M10.451   Other secondary gout, right hip
     M10.452   Other secondary gout, left hip
     M10.459   Other secondary gout, unspecified hip
● M10.46   Other secondary gout, knee
     M10.461   Other secondary gout, right knee
     M10.462   Other secondary gout, left knee
     M10.469   Other secondary gout, unspecified knee
● M10.47   Other secondary gout, ankle and foot
     M10.471   Other secondary gout, right ankle and foot
     M10.472   Other secondary gout, left ankle and foot
     M10.479   Other secondary gout, unspecified ankle and foot
   M10.48   Other secondary gout, vertebrae
   M10.49   Other secondary gout, multiple sites
M10.9   Gout, unspecified
     Gout NOS

● M11   Other crystal arthropathies
● M11.0   Hydroxyapatite deposition disease
   M11.00   Hydroxyapatite deposition disease, unspecified site
● M11.01   Hydroxyapatite deposition disease, shoulder
     M11.011   Hydroxyapatite deposition disease, right shoulder
     M11.012   Hydroxyapatite deposition disease, left shoulder
     M11.019   Hydroxyapatite deposition disease, unspecified shoulder

● M11.02   Hydroxyapatite deposition disease, elbow
     M11.021   Hydroxyapatite deposition disease, right elbow
     M11.022   Hydroxyapatite deposition disease, left elbow
     M11.029   Hydroxyapatite deposition disease, unspecified elbow
● M11.03   Hydroxyapatite deposition disease, wrist
     M11.031   Hydroxyapatite deposition disease, right wrist
     M11.032   Hydroxyapatite deposition disease, left wrist
     M11.039   Hydroxyapatite deposition disease, unspecified wrist
● M11.04   Hydroxyapatite deposition disease, hand
     M11.041   Hydroxyapatite deposition disease, right hand
     M11.042   Hydroxyapatite deposition disease, left hand
     M11.049   Hydroxyapatite deposition disease, unspecified hand
● M11.05   Hydroxyapatite deposition disease, hip
     M11.051   Hydroxyapatite deposition disease, right hip
     M11.052   Hydroxyapatite deposition disease, left hip
     M11.059   Hydroxyapatite deposition disease, unspecified hip
● M11.06   Hydroxyapatite deposition disease, knee
     M11.061   Hydroxyapatite deposition disease, right knee
     M11.062   Hydroxyapatite deposition disease, left knee
     M11.069   Hydroxyapatite deposition disease, unspecified knee
● M11.07   Hydroxyapatite deposition disease, ankle and foot
     M11.071   Hydroxyapatite deposition disease, right ankle and foot
     M11.072   Hydroxyapatite deposition disease, left ankle and foot
     M11.079   Hydroxyapatite deposition disease, unspecified ankle and foot
   M11.08   Hydroxyapatite deposition disease, vertebrae
   M11.09   Hydroxyapatite deposition disease, multiple sites
● M11.1   Familial chondrocalcinosis
   M11.10   Familial chondrocalcinosis, unspecified site
● M11.11   Familial chondrocalcinosis, shoulder
     M11.111   Familial chondrocalcinosis, right shoulder
     M11.112   Familial chondrocalcinosis, left shoulder
     M11.119   Familial chondrocalcinosis, unspecified shoulder
● M11.12   Familial chondrocalcinosis, elbow
     M11.121   Familial chondrocalcinosis, right elbow
     M11.122   Familial chondrocalcinosis, left elbow
     M11.129   Familial chondrocalcinosis, unspecified elbow
● M11.13   Familial chondrocalcinosis, wrist
     M11.131   Familial chondrocalcinosis, right wrist
     M11.132   Familial chondrocalcinosis, left wrist
     M11.139   Familial chondrocalcinosis, unspecified wrist

CHAPTER 13 (M00-M99)

● M11.14 Familial chondrocalcinosis, hand

    M11.141 Familial chondrocalcinosis, right hand

    M11.142 Familial chondrocalcinosis, left hand

    M11.149 Familial chondrocalcinosis, unspecified hand

● M11.15 Familial chondrocalcinosis, hip

    M11.151 Familial chondrocalcinosis, right hip

    M11.152 Familial chondrocalcinosis, left hip

    M11.159 Familial chondrocalcinosis, unspecified hip

● M11.16 Familial chondrocalcinosis, knee

    M11.161 Familial chondrocalcinosis, right knee

    M11.162 Familial chondrocalcinosis, left knee

    M11.169 Familial chondrocalcinosis, unspecified knee

● M11.17 Familial chondrocalcinosis, ankle and foot

    M11.171 Familial chondrocalcinosis, right ankle and foot

    M11.172 Familial chondrocalcinosis, left ankle and foot

    M11.179 Familial chondrocalcinosis, unspecified ankle and foot

    M11.18 Familial chondrocalcinosis, vertebrae

    M11.19 Familial chondrocalcinosis, multiple sites

● M11.2 Other chondrocalcinosis
    Chondrocalcinosis NOS

    M11.20 Other chondrocalcinosis, unspecified site

● M11.21 Other chondrocalcinosis, shoulder

    M11.211 Other chondrocalcinosis, right shoulder

    M11.212 Other chondrocalcinosis, left shoulder

    M11.219 Other chondrocalcinosis, unspecified shoulder

● M11.22 Other chondrocalcinosis, elbow

    M11.221 Other chondrocalcinosis, right elbow

    M11.222 Other chondrocalcinosis, left elbow

    M11.229 Other chondrocalcinosis, unspecified elbow

● M11.23 Other chondrocalcinosis, wrist

    M11.231 Other chondrocalcinosis, right wrist

    M11.232 Other chondrocalcinosis, left wrist

    M11.239 Other chondrocalcinosis, unspecified wrist

● M11.24 Other chondrocalcinosis, hand

    M11.241 Other chondrocalcinosis, right hand

    M11.242 Other chondrocalcinosis, left hand

    M11.249 Other chondrocalcinosis, unspecified hand

● M11.25 Other chondrocalcinosis, hip

    M11.251 Other chondrocalcinosis, right hip

    M11.252 Other chondrocalcinosis, left hip

    M11.259 Other chondrocalcinosis, unspecified hip

● M11.26 Other chondrocalcinosis, knee

    M11.261 Other chondrocalcinosis, right knee

    M11.262 Other chondrocalcinosis, left knee

    M11.269 Other chondrocalcinosis, unspecified knee

● M11.27 Other chondrocalcinosis, ankle and foot

    M11.271 Other chondrocalcinosis, right ankle and foot

    M11.272 Other chondrocalcinosis, left ankle and foot

    M11.279 Other chondrocalcinosis, unspecified ankle and foot

    M11.28 Other chondrocalcinosis, vertebrae

    M11.29 Other chondrocalcinosis, multiple sites

● M11.8 Other specified crystal arthropathies

    M11.80 Other specified crystal arthropathies, unspecified site

● M11.81 Other specified crystal arthropathies, shoulder

    M11.811 Other specified crystal arthropathies, right shoulder

    M11.812 Other specified crystal arthropathies, left shoulder

    M11.819 Other specified crystal arthropathies, unspecified shoulder

● M11.82 Other specified crystal arthropathies, elbow

    M11.821 Other specified crystal arthropathies, right elbow

    M11.822 Other specified crystal arthropathies, left elbow

    M11.829 Other specified crystal arthropathies, unspecified elbow

● M11.83 Other specified crystal arthropathies, wrist

    M11.831 Other specified crystal arthropathies, right wrist

    M11.832 Other specified crystal arthropathies, left wrist

    M11.839 Other specified crystal arthropathies, unspecified wrist

● M11.84 Other specified crystal arthropathies, hand

    M11.841 Other specified crystal arthropathies, right hand

    M11.842 Other specified crystal arthropathies, left hand

    M11.849 Other specified crystal arthropathies, unspecified hand

● M11.85 Other specified crystal arthropathies, hip

    M11.851 Other specified crystal arthropathies, right hip

    M11.852 Other specified crystal arthropathies, left hip

    M11.859 Other specified crystal arthropathies, unspecified hip

● M11.86 Other specified crystal arthropathies, knee

    M11.861 Other specified crystal arthropathies, right knee

    M11.862 Other specified crystal arthropathies, left knee

    M11.869 Other specified crystal arthropathies, unspecified knee

● M11.87 Other specified crystal arthropathies, ankle and foot

    M11.871 Other specified crystal arthropathies, right ankle and foot

    M11.872 Other specified crystal arthropathies, left ankle and foot

    M11.879 Other specified crystal arthropathies, unspecified ankle and foot

    M11.88 Other specified crystal arthropathies, vertebrae

    M11.89 Other specified crystal arthropathies, multiple sites

    M11.9 Crystal arthropathy, unspecified

▶ New   ⇒ Revised   ~~deleted~~ Deleted   OGCR Official Guidelines   X Assign placeholder X   ● Use Additional Character(s)

Excludes 1   Excludes 2   Includes   Use additional   Code first   Code also   Key words

● **M12**   Other and unspecified arthropathy

    Excludes1   arthrosis (M15-M19)
                cricoarytenoid arthropathy (J38.7)

    ● **M12.0**   Chronic postrheumatic arthropathy [Jaccoud]

       M12.00   Chronic postrheumatic arthropathy [Jaccoud], unspecified site

       ● **M12.01**   Chronic postrheumatic arthropathy [Jaccoud], shoulder

           M12.011   Chronic postrheumatic arthropathy [Jaccoud], right shoulder

           M12.012   Chronic postrheumatic arthropathy [Jaccoud], left shoulder

           M12.019   Chronic postrheumatic arthropathy [Jaccoud], unspecified shoulder

       ● **M12.02**   Chronic postrheumatic arthropathy [Jaccoud], elbow

           M12.021   Chronic postrheumatic arthropathy [Jaccoud], right elbow

           M12.022   Chronic postrheumatic arthropathy [Jaccoud], left elbow

           M12.029   Chronic postrheumatic arthropathy [Jaccoud], unspecified elbow

       ● **M12.03**   Chronic postrheumatic arthropathy [Jaccoud], wrist

           M12.031   Chronic postrheumatic arthropathy [Jaccoud], right wrist

           M12.032   Chronic postrheumatic arthropathy [Jaccoud], left wrist

           M12.039   Chronic postrheumatic arthropathy [Jaccoud], unspecified wrist

       ● **M12.04**   Chronic postrheumatic arthropathy [Jaccoud], hand

           M12.041   Chronic postrheumatic arthropathy [Jaccoud], right hand

           M12.042   Chronic postrheumatic arthropathy [Jaccoud], left hand

           M12.049   Chronic postrheumatic arthropathy [Jaccoud], unspecified hand

       ● **M12.05**   Chronic postrheumatic arthropathy [Jaccoud], hip

           M12.051   Chronic postrheumatic arthropathy [Jaccoud], right hip

           M12.052   Chronic postrheumatic arthropathy [Jaccoud], left hip

           M12.059   Chronic postrheumatic arthropathy [Jaccoud], unspecified hip

       ● **M12.06**   Chronic postrheumatic arthropathy [Jaccoud], knee

           M12.061   Chronic postrheumatic arthropathy [Jaccoud], right knee

           M12.062   Chronic postrheumatic arthropathy [Jaccoud], left knee

           M12.069   Chronic postrheumatic arthropathy [Jaccoud], unspecified knee

       ● **M12.07**   Chronic postrheumatic arthropathy [Jaccoud], ankle and foot

           M12.071   Chronic postrheumatic arthropathy [Jaccoud], right ankle and foot

           M12.072   Chronic postrheumatic arthropathy [Jaccoud], left ankle and foot

           M12.079   Chronic postrheumatic arthropathy [Jaccoud], unspecified ankle and foot

       M12.08   Chronic postrheumatic arthropathy [Jaccoud], other specified site

           Chronic postrheumatic arthropathy [Jaccoud], vertebrae

       M12.09   Chronic postrheumatic arthropathy [Jaccoud], multiple sites

● **M12.1**   Kaschin-Beck disease

     Osteochondroarthrosis deformans endemica

       M12.10   Kaschin-Beck disease, unspecified site

       ● **M12.11**   Kaschin-Beck disease, shoulder

           M12.111   Kaschin-Beck disease, right shoulder

           M12.112   Kaschin-Beck disease, left shoulder

           M12.119   Kaschin-Beck disease, unspecified shoulder

       ● **M12.12**   Kaschin-Beck disease, elbow

           M12.121   Kaschin-Beck disease, right elbow

           M12.122   Kaschin-Beck disease, left elbow

           M12.129   Kaschin-Beck disease, unspecified elbow

       ● **M12.13**   Kaschin-Beck disease, wrist

           M12.131   Kaschin-Beck disease, right wrist

           M12.132   Kaschin-Beck disease, left wrist

           M12.139   Kaschin-Beck disease, unspecified wrist

       ● **M12.14**   Kaschin-Beck disease, hand

           M12.141   Kaschin-Beck disease, right hand

           M12.142   Kaschin-Beck disease, left hand

           M12.149   Kaschin-Beck disease, unspecified hand

       ● **M12.15**   Kaschin-Beck disease, hip

           M12.151   Kaschin-Beck disease, right hip

           M12.152   Kaschin-Beck disease, left hip

           M12.159   Kaschin-Beck disease, unspecified hip

       ● **M12.16**   Kaschin-Beck disease, knee

           M12.161   Kaschin-Beck disease, right knee

           M12.162   Kaschin-Beck disease, left knee

           M12.169   Kaschin-Beck disease, unspecified knee

       ● **M12.17**   Kaschin-Beck disease, ankle and foot

           M12.171   Kaschin-Beck disease, right ankle and foot

           M12.172   Kaschin-Beck disease, left ankle and foot

           M12.179   Kaschin-Beck disease, unspecified ankle and foot

       M12.18   Kaschin-Beck disease, vertebrae

       M12.19   Kaschin-Beck disease, multiple sites

● **M12.2**   Villonodular synovitis (pigmented)

       M12.20   Villonodular synovitis (pigmented), unspecified site

       ● **M12.21**   Villonodular synovitis (pigmented), shoulder

           M12.211   Villonodular synovitis (pigmented), right shoulder

           M12.212   Villonodular synovitis (pigmented), left shoulder

           M12.219   Villonodular synovitis (pigmented), unspecified shoulder

       ● **M12.22**   Villonodular synovitis (pigmented), elbow

           M12.221   Villonodular synovitis (pigmented), right elbow

           M12.222   Villonodular synovitis (pigmented), left elbow

           M12.229   Villonodular synovitis (pigmented), unspecified elbow

       ● **M12.23**   Villonodular synovitis (pigmented), wrist

           M12.231   Villonodular synovitis (pigmented), right wrist

           M12.232   Villonodular synovitis (pigmented), left wrist

           M12.239   Villonodular synovitis (pigmented), unspecified wrist

▶ New   ⇒ Revised   ~~deleted~~ Deleted   **OGCR** Official Guidelines   **X** Assign placeholder X   ● Use Additional Character(s)

Excludes 1   Excludes 2   Includes   Use additional   Code first   Code also   Key words

● M12.24　Villonodular synovitis (pigmented), hand
　　　M12.241　Villonodular synovitis (pigmented), right hand
　　　M12.242　Villonodular synovitis (pigmented), left hand
　　　M12.249　Villonodular synovitis (pigmented), unspecified hand
● M12.25　Villonodular synovitis (pigmented), hip
　　　M12.251　Villonodular synovitis (pigmented), right hip
　　　M12.252　Villonodular synovitis (pigmented), left hip
　　　M12.259　Villonodular synovitis (pigmented), unspecified hip
● M12.26　Villonodular synovitis (pigmented), knee
　　　M12.261　Villonodular synovitis (pigmented), right knee
　　　M12.262　Villonodular synovitis (pigmented), left knee
　　　M12.269　Villonodular synovitis (pigmented), unspecified knee
● M12.27　Villonodular synovitis (pigmented), ankle and foot
　　　M12.271　Villonodular synovitis (pigmented), right ankle and foot
　　　M12.272　Villonodular synovitis (pigmented), left ankle and foot
　　　M12.279　Villonodular synovitis (pigmented), unspecified ankle and foot
　　M12.28　Villonodular synovitis (pigmented), other specified site
　　　　　Villonodular synovitis (pigmented), vertebrae
　　M12.29　Villonodular synovitis (pigmented), multiple sites
● M12.3　Palindromic rheumatism
　　M12.30　Palindromic rheumatism, unspecified site
● M12.31　Palindromic rheumatism, shoulder
　　　M12.311　Palindromic rheumatism, right shoulder
　　　M12.312　Palindromic rheumatism, left shoulder
　　　M12.319　Palindromic rheumatism, unspecified shoulder
● M12.32　Palindromic rheumatism, elbow
　　　M12.321　Palindromic rheumatism, right elbow
　　　M12.322　Palindromic rheumatism, left elbow
　　　M12.329　Palindromic rheumatism, unspecified elbow
● M12.33　Palindromic rheumatism, wrist
　　　M12.331　Palindromic rheumatism, right wrist
　　　M12.332　Palindromic rheumatism, left wrist
　　　M12.339　Palindromic rheumatism, unspecified wrist
● M12.34　Palindromic rheumatism, hand
　　　M12.341　Palindromic rheumatism, right hand
　　　M12.342　Palindromic rheumatism, left hand
　　　M12.349　Palindromic rheumatism, unspecified hand
● M12.35　Palindromic rheumatism, hip
　　　M12.351　Palindromic rheumatism, right hip
　　　M12.352　Palindromic rheumatism, left hip
　　　M12.359　Palindromic rheumatism, unspecified hip

● M12.36　Palindromic rheumatism, knee
　　　M12.361　Palindromic rheumatism, right knee
　　　M12.362　Palindromic rheumatism, left knee
　　　M12.369　Palindromic rheumatism, unspecified knee
● M12.37　Palindromic rheumatism, ankle and foot
　　　M12.371　Palindromic rheumatism, right ankle and foot
　　　M12.372　Palindromic rheumatism, left ankle and foot
　　　M12.379　Palindromic rheumatism, unspecified ankle and foot
　　M12.38　Palindromic rheumatism, other specified site
　　　　　Palindromic rheumatism, vertebrae
　　M12.39　Palindromic rheumatism, multiple sites
● M12.4　Intermittent hydrarthrosis
　　M12.40　Intermittent hydrarthrosis, unspecified site
● M12.41　Intermittent hydrarthrosis, shoulder
　　　M12.411　Intermittent hydrarthrosis, right shoulder
　　　M12.412　Intermittent hydrarthrosis, left shoulder
　　　M12.419　Intermittent hydrarthrosis, unspecified shoulder
● M12.42　Intermittent hydrarthrosis, elbow
　　　M12.421　Intermittent hydrarthrosis, right elbow
　　　M12.422　Intermittent hydrarthrosis, left elbow
　　　M12.429　Intermittent hydrarthrosis, unspecified elbow
● M12.43　Intermittent hydrarthrosis, wrist
　　　M12.431　Intermittent hydrarthrosis, right wrist
　　　M12.432　Intermittent hydrarthrosis, left wrist
　　　M12.439　Intermittent hydrarthrosis, unspecified wrist
● M12.44　Intermittent hydrarthrosis, hand
　　　M12.441　Intermittent hydrarthrosis, right hand
　　　M12.442　Intermittent hydrarthrosis, left hand
　　　M12.449　Intermittent hydrarthrosis, unspecified hand
● M12.45　Intermittent hydrarthrosis, hip
　　　M12.451　Intermittent hydrarthrosis, right hip
　　　M12.452　Intermittent hydrarthrosis, left hip
　　　M12.459　Intermittent hydrarthrosis, unspecified hip
● M12.46　Intermittent hydrarthrosis, knee
　　　M12.461　Intermittent hydrarthrosis, right knee
　　　M12.462　Intermittent hydrarthrosis, left knee
　　　M12.469　Intermittent hydrarthrosis, unspecified knee
● M12.47　Intermittent hydrarthrosis, ankle and foot
　　　M12.471　Intermittent hydrarthrosis, right ankle and foot
　　　M12.472　Intermittent hydrarthrosis, left ankle and foot
　　　M12.479　Intermittent hydrarthrosis, unspecified ankle and foot
　　M12.48　Intermittent hydrarthrosis, other site
　　M12.49　Intermittent hydrarthrosis, multiple sites

▶ New　⇒ Revised　~~deleted~~ Deleted　OGCR Official Guidelines　X Assign placeholder X　● Use Additional Character(s)

Excludes 1　Excludes 2　Includes　Use additional　Code first　Code also　Key words

● **M12.5**   Traumatic arthropathy
     Excludes1   current injury-see Alphabetic Index
         post-traumatic osteoarthritis of first
           carpometacarpal joint (M18.2-M18.3)
         post-traumatic osteoarthritis of hip
           (M16.4-M16.5)
         post-traumatic osteoarthritis of knee
           (M17.2-M17.3)
         post-traumatic osteoarthritis NOS
           (M19.1-)
         post-traumatic osteoarthritis of other
           single joints (M19.1-)

     M12.50   Traumatic arthropathy, unspecified site
●   M12.51   Traumatic arthropathy, shoulder
        M12.511   Traumatic arthropathy, right shoulder
        M12.512   Traumatic arthropathy, left shoulder
        M12.519   Traumatic arthropathy, unspecified
               shoulder
●   M12.52   Traumatic arthropathy, elbow
        M12.521   Traumatic arthropathy, right elbow
        M12.522   Traumatic arthropathy, left elbow
        M12.529   Traumatic arthropathy, unspecified
               elbow
●   M12.53   Traumatic arthropathy, wrist
        M12.531   Traumatic arthropathy, right wrist
        M12.532   Traumatic arthropathy, left wrist
        M12.539   Traumatic arthropathy, unspecified
               wrist
●   M12.54   Traumatic arthropathy, hand
        M12.541   Traumatic arthropathy, right hand
        M12.542   Traumatic arthropathy, left hand
        M12.549   Traumatic arthropathy, unspecified
               hand
●   M12.55   Traumatic arthropathy, hip
        M12.551   Traumatic arthropathy, right hip
        M12.552   Traumatic arthropathy, left hip
        M12.559   Traumatic arthropathy, unspecified
               hip
●   M12.56   Traumatic arthropathy, knee
        M12.561   Traumatic arthropathy, right knee
        M12.562   Traumatic arthropathy, left knee
        M12.569   Traumatic arthropathy, unspecified
               knee
●   M12.57   Traumatic arthropathy, ankle and foot
        M12.571   Traumatic arthropathy, right ankle
               and foot
        M12.572   Traumatic arthropathy, left ankle and
               foot
        M12.579   Traumatic arthropathy, unspecified
               ankle and foot
     M12.58   Traumatic arthropathy, other specified site
          Traumatic arthropathy, vertebrae
     M12.59   Traumatic arthropathy, multiple sites
● **M12.8**   Other specific arthropathies, not elsewhere classified
         Transient arthropathy
     M12.80   Other specific arthropathies, not elsewhere
            classified, unspecified site
●   M12.81   Other specific arthropathies, not elsewhere
            classified, shoulder
        M12.811   Other specific arthropathies, not
               elsewhere classified, right shoulder
        M12.812   Other specific arthropathies, not
               elsewhere classified, left shoulder
        M12.819   Other specific arthropathies, not
               elsewhere classified, unspecified
               shoulder

●   M12.82   Other specific arthropathies, not elsewhere
            classified, elbow
        M12.821   Other specific arthropathies, not
               elsewhere classified, right elbow
        M12.822   Other specific arthropathies, not
               elsewhere classified, left elbow
        M12.829   Other specific arthropathies, not
               elsewhere classified, unspecified
               elbow
●   M12.83   Other specific arthropathies, not elsewhere
            classified, wrist
        M12.831   Other specific arthropathies, not
               elsewhere classified, right wrist
        M12.832   Other specific arthropathies, not
               elsewhere classified, left wrist
        M12.839   Other specific arthropathies, not
               elsewhere classified, unspecified wrist
●   M12.84   Other specific arthropathies, not elsewhere
            classified, hand
        M12.841   Other specific arthropathies, not
               elsewhere classified, right hand
        M12.842   Other specific arthropathies, not
               elsewhere classified, left hand
        M12.849   Other specific arthropathies, not
               elsewhere classified, unspecified hand
●   M12.85   Other specific arthropathies, not elsewhere
            classified, hip
        M12.851   Other specific arthropathies, not
               elsewhere classified, right hip
        M12.852   Other specific arthropathies, not
               elsewhere classified, left hip
        M12.859   Other specific arthropathies, not
               elsewhere classified, unspecified hip
●   M12.86   Other specific arthropathies, not elsewhere
            classified, knee
        M12.861   Other specific arthropathies, not
               elsewhere classified, right knee
        M12.862   Other specific arthropathies, not
               elsewhere classified, left knee
        M12.869   Other specific arthropathies, not
               elsewhere classified, unspecified knee
●   M12.87   Other specific arthropathies, not elsewhere
            classified, ankle and foot
        M12.871   Other specific arthropathies, not
               elsewhere classified, right ankle and
               foot
        M12.872   Other specific arthropathies, not
               elsewhere classified, left ankle and
               foot
        M12.879   Other specific arthropathies, not
               elsewhere classified, unspecified
               ankle and foot
     M12.88   Other specific arthropathies, not elsewhere
            classified, other specified site
          Other specific arthropathies, not elsewhere
            classified, vertebrae
     M12.89   Other specific arthropathies, not elsewhere
            classified, multiple sites
    M12.9   Arthropathy, unspecified

CHAPTER 13 (M00-M99)

CHAPTER 13 (M00-M99)

- ● **M13** **Other** arthritis
  - **Excludes1**   arthrosis (M15-M19)
    - osteoarthritis (M15-M19)
  - **M13.0** **Polyarthritis, unspecified**
  - ● **M13.1** **Monoarthritis, not elsewhere classified**
    - **M13.10** Monoarthritis, not elsewhere classified, **unspecified** site
    - ● **M13.11** Monoarthritis, not elsewhere classified, **shoulder**
      - **M13.111** Monoarthritis, not elsewhere classified, **right** shoulder
      - **M13.112** Monoarthritis, not elsewhere classified, **left** shoulder
      - **M13.119** Monoarthritis, not elsewhere classified, **unspecified** shoulder
    - ● **M13.12** Monoarthritis, not elsewhere classified, **elbow**
      - **M13.121** Monoarthritis, not elsewhere classified, **right** elbow
      - **M13.122** Monoarthritis, not elsewhere classified, **left** elbow
      - **M13.129** Monoarthritis, not elsewhere classified, **unspecified** elbow
    - ● **M13.13** Monoarthritis, not elsewhere classified, **wrist**
      - **M13.131** Monoarthritis, not elsewhere classified, **right** wrist
      - **M13.132** Monoarthritis, not elsewhere classified, **left** wrist
      - **M13.139** Monoarthritis, not elsewhere classified, **unspecified** wrist
    - ● **M13.14** Monoarthritis, not elsewhere classified, **hand**
      - **M13.141** Monoarthritis, not elsewhere classified, **right** hand
      - **M13.142** Monoarthritis, not elsewhere classified, **left** hand
      - **M13.149** Monoarthritis, not elsewhere classified, **unspecified** hand
    - ● **M13.15** Monoarthritis, not elsewhere classified, **hip**
      - **M13.151** Monoarthritis, not elsewhere classified, **right** hip
      - **M13.152** Monoarthritis, not elsewhere classified, **left** hip
      - **M13.159** Monoarthritis, not elsewhere classified, **unspecified** hip
    - ● **M13.16** Monoarthritis, not elsewhere classified, **knee**
      - **M13.161** Monoarthritis, not elsewhere classified, **right** knee
      - **M13.162** Monoarthritis, not elsewhere classified, **left** knee
      - **M13.169** Monoarthritis, not elsewhere classified, **unspecified** knee
    - ● **M13.17** Monoarthritis, not elsewhere classified, **ankle and foot**
      - **M13.171** Monoarthritis, not elsewhere classified, **right** ankle and foot
      - **M13.172** Monoarthritis, not elsewhere classified, **left** ankle and foot
      - **M13.179** Monoarthritis, not elsewhere classified, **unspecified** ankle and foot
  - ● **M13.8** **Other specified** arthritis
    - Allergic arthritis
    - **Excludes1**   osteoarthritis (M15-M19)
    - **M13.80** Other specified arthritis, **unspecified** site
    - ● **M13.81** Other specified arthritis, **shoulder**
      - **M13.811** Other specified arthritis, **right** shoulder
      - **M13.812** Other specified arthritis, **left** shoulder
      - **M13.819** Other specified arthritis, **unspecified** shoulder
    - ● **M13.82** Other specified arthritis, **elbow**
      - **M13.821** Other specified arthritis, **right** elbow
      - **M13.822** Other specified arthritis, **left** elbow
      - **M13.829** Other specified arthritis, **unspecified** elbow
    - ● **M13.83** Other specified arthritis, **wrist**
      - **M13.831** Other specified arthritis, **right** wrist
      - **M13.832** Other specified arthritis, **left** wrist
      - **M13.839** Other specified arthritis, **unspecified** wrist
    - ● **M13.84** Other specified arthritis, **hand**
      - **M13.841** Other specified arthritis, **right** hand
      - **M13.842** Other specified arthritis, **left** hand
      - **M13.849** Other specified arthritis, **unspecified** hand
    - ● **M13.85** Other specified arthritis, **hip**
      - **M13.851** Other specified arthritis, **right** hip
      - **M13.852** Other specified arthritis, **left** hip
      - **M13.859** Other specified arthritis, **unspecified** hip
    - ● **M13.86** Other specified arthritis, **knee**
      - **M13.861** Other specified arthritis, **right** knee
      - **M13.862** Other specified arthritis, **left** knee
      - **M13.869** Other specified arthritis, **unspecified** knee
    - ● **M13.87** Other specified arthritis, **ankle and foot**
      - **M13.871** Other specified arthritis, **right** ankle and foot
      - **M13.872** Other specified arthritis, **left** ankle and foot
      - **M13.879** Other specified arthritis, **unspecified** ankle and foot
    - **M13.88** Other specified arthritis, **other site**
    - **M13.89** Other specified arthritis, **multiple sites**
- ● **M14** **Arthropathies in other diseases classified elsewhere**
  - **Excludes1**   arthropathy in:
    - diabetes mellitus (E08-E13 with .61-)
    - hematological disorders (M36.2-M36.3)
    - hypersensitivity reactions (M36.4)
    - neoplastic disease (M36.1)
    - neurosyphillis (A52.16)
    - sarcoidosis (D86.86)
    - enteropathic arthropathies (M07.0-)
    - juvenile psoriatic arthropathy (L40.54)
    - lipoid dermatoarthritis (E78.81)
  - ● **M14.6** **Charcôt's joint**
    - Neuropathic arthropathy
    - **Excludes1**   Charcôt's joint in diabetes mellitus (E08-E13 with .610)
      - Charcôt's joint in tabes dorsalis (A52.16)
    - **M14.60** Charcôt's joint, **unspecified** site
    - ● **M14.61** Charcôt's joint, **shoulder**
      - **M14.611** Charcôt's joint, **right** shoulder
      - **M14.612** Charcôt's joint, **left** shoulder
      - **M14.619** Charcôt's joint, **unspecified** shoulder
    - ● **M14.62** Charcôt's joint, **elbow**
      - **M14.621** Charcôt's joint, **right** elbow
      - **M14.622** Charcôt's joint, **left** elbow
      - **M14.629** Charcôt's joint, **unspecified** elbow
    - ● **M14.63** Charcôt's joint, **wrist**
      - **M14.631** Charcôt's joint, **right** wrist
      - **M14.632** Charcôt's joint, **left** wrist
      - **M14.639** Charcôt's joint, **unspecified** wrist

▶ New   ⇒ Revised   deleted Deleted   **OGCR** Official Guidelines   X Assign placeholder X   ● Use Additional Character(s)

Excludes 1   Excludes 2   Includes   Use additional   Code first   Code also   Key words

● **M14.64 Charcôt's joint, hand**
     M14.641 Charcôt's joint, right hand
     M14.642 Charcôt's joint, left hand
     M14.649 Charcôt's joint, unspecified hand

● **M14.65 Charcôt's joint, hip**
     M14.651 Charcôt's joint, right hip
     M14.652 Charcôt's joint, left hip
     M14.659 Charcôt's joint, unspecified hip

● **M14.66 Charcôt's joint, knee**
     M14.661 Charcôt's joint, right knee
     M14.662 Charcôt's joint, left knee
     M14.669 Charcôt's joint, unspecified knee

● **M14.67 Charcôt's joint, ankle and foot**
     M14.671 Charcôt's joint, right ankle and foot
     M14.672 Charcôt's joint, left ankle and foot
     M14.679 Charcôt's joint, unspecified ankle and foot

   M14.68 Charcôt's joint, vertebrae
   M14.69 Charcôt's joint, multiple sites

● **M14.8 Arthropathies in other specified diseases classified elsewhere**

     Code first underlying disease, such as:
       amyloidosis (E85.-)
       erythema multiforme (L51.-)
       erythema nodosum (L52)
       hemochromatosis (E83.11-)
       hyperparathyroidism (E21.-)
       hypothyroidism (E00-E03)
       sickle-cell disorders (D57.-)
       thyrotoxicosis [hyperthyroidism] (E05.-)
       Whipple's disease (K90.81)

   M14.80 Arthropathies in other specified diseases classified elsewhere, unspecified site

● **M14.81 Arthropathies in other specified diseases classified elsewhere, shoulder**
     M14.811 Arthropathies in other specified diseases classified elsewhere, right shoulder
     M14.812 Arthropathies in other specified diseases classified elsewhere, left shoulder
     M14.819 Arthropathies in other specified diseases classified elsewhere, unspecified shoulder

● **M14.82 Arthropathies in other specified diseases classified elsewhere, elbow**
     M14.821 Arthropathies in other specified diseases classified elsewhere, right elbow
     M14.822 Arthropathies in other specified diseases classified elsewhere, left elbow
     M14.829 Arthropathies in other specified diseases classified elsewhere, unspecified elbow

● **M14.83 Arthropathies in other specified diseases classified elsewhere, wrist**
     M14.831 Arthropathies in other specified diseases classified elsewhere, right wrist
     M14.832 Arthropathies in other specified diseases classified elsewhere, left wrist
     M14.839 Arthropathies in other specified diseases classified elsewhere, unspecified wrist

● **M14.84 Arthropathies in other specified diseases classified elsewhere, hand**
     M14.841 Arthropathies in other specified diseases classified elsewhere, right hand
     M14.842 Arthropathies in other specified diseases classified elsewhere, left hand
     M14.849 Arthropathies in other specified diseases classified elsewhere, unspecified hand

● **M14.85 Arthropathies in other specified diseases classified elsewhere, hip**
     M14.851 Arthropathies in other specified diseases classified elsewhere, right hip
     M14.852 Arthropathies in other specified diseases classified elsewhere, left hip
     M14.859 Arthropathies in other specified diseases classified elsewhere, unspecified hip

● **M14.86 Arthropathies in other specified diseases classified elsewhere, knee**
     M14.861 Arthropathies in other specified diseases classified elsewhere, right knee
     M14.862 Arthropathies in other specified diseases classified elsewhere, left knee
     M14.869 Arthropathies in other specified diseases classified elsewhere, unspecified knee

● **M14.87 Arthropathies in other specified diseases classified elsewhere, ankle and foot**
     M14.871 Arthropathies in other specified diseases classified elsewhere, right ankle and foot
     M14.872 Arthropathies in other specified diseases classified elsewhere, left ankle and foot
     M14.879 Arthropathies in other specified diseases classified elsewhere, unspecified ankle and foot

   M14.88 Arthropathies in other specified diseases classified elsewhere, vertebrae
   M14.89 Arthropathies in other specified diseases classified elsewhere, multiple sites

---

OSTEOARTHRITIS (M15-M19)

Osteoarthritis is the most common degenerative joint disease and form of arthritis that breaks down the cartilage causing pain, swelling, and reduced motion in the joints.

   Excludes2   osteoarthritis of spine (M47.-)

● **M15 Polyosteoarthritis**
   Includes   arthritis of multiple sites
   Excludes1   bilateral involvement of single joint (M16-M19)

   M15.0 Primary generalized (osteo)arthritis
   M15.1 Heberden's nodes (with arthropathy)
     Interphalangeal distal osteoarthritis
   M15.2 Bouchard's nodes (with arthropathy)
     Juxtaphalangeal distal osteoarthritis
   M15.3 Secondary multiple arthritis
     Post-traumatic polyosteoarthritis
   M15.4 Erosive (osteo)arthritis
   M15.8 Other polyosteoarthritis
   M15.9 Polyosteoarthritis, unspecified
     Generalized osteoarthritis NOS

CHAPTER 13 (M00-M99)

● M16 Osteoarthritis of hip
   M16.0 Bilateral primary osteoarthritis of hip
   ● M16.1 Unilateral primary osteoarthritis of hip
      Primary osteoarthritis of hip NOS
      M16.10 Unilateral primary osteoarthritis, unspecified hip
      M16.11 Unilateral primary osteoarthritis, right hip
      M16.12 Unilateral primary osteoarthritis, left hip
   M16.2 Bilateral osteoarthritis resulting from hip dysplasia
   ● M16.3 Unilateral osteoarthritis resulting from hip dysplasia
      Dysplastic osteoarthritis of hip NOS
      M16.30 Unilateral osteoarthritis resulting from hip dysplasia, unspecified hip
      M16.31 Unilateral osteoarthritis resulting from hip dysplasia, right hip
      M16.32 Unilateral osteoarthritis resulting from hip dysplasia, left hip
   M16.4 Bilateral post-traumatic osteoarthritis of hip
   ● M16.5 Unilateral post-traumatic osteoarthritis of hip
      Post-traumatic osteoarthritis of hip NOS
      M16.50 Unilateral post-traumatic osteoarthritis, unspecified hip
      M16.51 Unilateral post-traumatic osteoarthritis, right hip
      M16.52 Unilateral post-traumatic osteoarthritis, left hip
   M16.6 Other bilateral secondary osteoarthritis of hip
   M16.7 Other unilateral secondary osteoarthritis of hip
      Secondary osteoarthritis of hip NOS
   M16.9 Osteoarthritis of hip, unspecified

● M17 Osteoarthritis of knee
   M17.0 Bilateral primary osteoarthritis of knee
   ● M17.1 Unilateral primary osteoarthritis of knee
      Primary osteoarthritis of knee NOS
      M17.10 Unilateral primary osteoarthritis, unspecified knee
      M17.11 Unilateral primary osteoarthritis, right knee
      M17.12 Unilateral primary osteoarthritis, left knee
   M17.2 Bilateral post-traumatic osteoarthritis of knee
   ● M17.3 Unilateral post-traumatic osteoarthritis of knee
      Post-traumatic osteoarthritis of knee NOS
      M17.30 Unilateral post-traumatic osteoarthritis, unspecified knee
      M17.31 Unilateral post-traumatic osteoarthritis, right knee
      M17.32 Unilateral post-traumatic osteoarthritis, left knee
   M17.4 Other bilateral secondary osteoarthritis of knee
   M17.5 Other unilateral secondary osteoarthritis of knee
      Secondary osteoarthritis of knee NOS
   M17.9 Osteoarthritis of knee, unspecified

● M18 Osteoarthritis of first carpometacarpal joint
   M18.0 Bilateral primary osteoarthritis of first carpometacarpal joints
   ● M18.1 Unilateral primary osteoarthritis of first carpometacarpal joint
      Primary osteoarthritis of first carpometacarpal joint NOS
      M18.10 Unilateral primary osteoarthritis of first carpometacarpal joint, unspecified hand
      M18.11 Unilateral primary osteoarthritis of first carpometacarpal joint, right hand
      M18.12 Unilateral primary osteoarthritis of first carpometacarpal joint, left hand
   M18.2 Bilateral post-traumatic osteoarthritis of first carpometacarpal joints

● M18.3 Unilateral post-traumatic osteoarthritis of first carpometacarpal joint
      Post-traumatic osteoarthritis of first carpometacarpal joint NOS
      M18.30 Unilateral post-traumatic osteoarthritis of first carpometacarpal joint, unspecified hand
      M18.31 Unilateral post-traumatic osteoarthritis of first carpometacarpal joint, right hand
      M18.32 Unilateral post-traumatic osteoarthritis of first carpometacarpal joint, left hand
   M18.4 Other bilateral secondary osteoarthritis of first carpometacarpal joints
   ● M18.5 Other unilateral secondary osteoarthritis of first carpometacarpal joint
      Secondary osteoarthritis of first carpometacarpal joint NOS
      M18.50 Other unilateral secondary osteoarthritis of first carpometacarpal joint, unspecified hand
      M18.51 Other unilateral secondary osteoarthritis of first carpometacarpal joint, right hand
      M18.52 Other unilateral secondary osteoarthritis of first carpometacarpal joint, left hand
   M18.9 Osteoarthritis of first carpometacarpal joint, unspecified

● M19 Other and unspecified osteoarthritis
   | Excludes1 | polyarthritis (M15.-) |
   | Excludes2 | arthrosis of spine (M47.-) |
      hallux rigidus (M20.2)
      osteoarthritis of spine (M47.-)
   ● M19.0 Primary osteoarthritis of other joints
      ● M19.01 Primary osteoarthritis, shoulder
         M19.011 Primary osteoarthritis, right shoulder
         M19.012 Primary osteoarthritis, left shoulder
         M19.019 Primary osteoarthritis, unspecified shoulder
      ● M19.02 Primary osteoarthritis, elbow
         M19.021 Primary osteoarthritis, right elbow
         M19.022 Primary osteoarthritis, left elbow
         M19.029 Primary osteoarthritis, unspecified elbow
      ● M19.03 Primary osteoarthritis, wrist
         M19.031 Primary osteoarthritis, right wrist
         M19.032 Primary osteoarthritis, left wrist
         M19.039 Primary osteoarthritis, unspecified wrist
      ● M19.04 Primary osteoarthritis, hand
         | Excludes2 | primary osteoarthritis of first carpometacarpal joint (M18.0-, M18.1-) |
         M19.041 Primary osteoarthritis, right hand
         M19.042 Primary osteoarthritis, left hand
         M19.049 Primary osteoarthritis, unspecified hand
      ● M19.07 Primary osteoarthritis ankle and foot
         M19.071 Primary osteoarthritis, right ankle and foot
         M19.072 Primary osteoarthritis, left ankle and foot
         M19.079 Primary osteoarthritis, unspecified ankle and foot
   ● M19.1 Post-traumatic osteoarthritis of other joints
      ● M19.11 Post-traumatic osteoarthritis, shoulder
         M19.111 Post-traumatic osteoarthritis, right shoulder
         M19.112 Post-traumatic osteoarthritis, left shoulder
         M19.119 Post-traumatic osteoarthritis, unspecified shoulder

▶ New   ⇒ Revised   ~~deleted~~ Deleted   **OGCR** Official Guidelines   X Assign placeholder X   ● Use Additional Character(s)

| Excludes 1 | Excludes 2 | Includes | Use additional | Code first | Code also | Key words |

● M19.12　Post-traumatic osteoarthritis, elbow

　　M19.121　Post-traumatic osteoarthritis, right elbow

　　M19.122　Post-traumatic osteoarthritis, left elbow

　　M19.129　Post-traumatic osteoarthritis, unspecified elbow

● M19.13　Post-traumatic osteoarthritis, wrist

　　M19.131　Post-traumatic osteoarthritis, right wrist

　　M19.132　Post-traumatic osteoarthritis, left wrist

　　M19.139　Post-traumatic osteoarthritis, unspecified wrist

● M19.14　Post-traumatic osteoarthritis, hand

　　Excludes2　post-traumatic osteoarthritis of first carpometacarpal joint (M18.2-, M18.3-)

　　M19.141　Post-traumatic osteoarthritis, right hand

　　M19.142　Post-traumatic osteoarthritis, left hand

　　M19.149　Post-traumatic osteoarthritis, unspecified hand

● M19.17　Post-traumatic osteoarthritis, ankle and foot

　　M19.171　Post-traumatic osteoarthritis, right ankle and foot

　　M19.172　Post-traumatic osteoarthritis, left ankle and foot

　　M19.179　Post-traumatic osteoarthritis, unspecified ankle and foot

● M19.2　Secondary osteoarthritis of other joints

　● M19.21　Secondary osteoarthritis, shoulder

　　　M19.211　Secondary osteoarthritis, right shoulder

　　　M19.212　Secondary osteoarthritis, left shoulder

　　　M19.219　Secondary osteoarthritis, unspecified shoulder

　● M19.22　Secondary osteoarthritis, elbow

　　　M19.221　Secondary osteoarthritis, right elbow

　　　M19.222　Secondary osteoarthritis, left elbow

　　　M19.229　Secondary osteoarthritis, unspecified elbow

　● M19.23　Secondary osteoarthritis, wrist

　　　M19.231　Secondary osteoarthritis, right wrist

　　　M19.232　Secondary osteoarthritis, left wrist

　　　M19.239　Secondary osteoarthritis, unspecified wrist

　● M19.24　Secondary osteoarthritis, hand

　　　M19.241　Secondary osteoarthritis, right hand

　　　M19.242　Secondary osteoarthritis, left hand

　　　M19.249　Secondary osteoarthritis, unspecified hand

　● M19.27　Secondary osteoarthritis, ankle and foot

　　　M19.271　Secondary osteoarthritis, right ankle and foot

　　　M19.272　Secondary osteoarthritis, left ankle and foot

　　　M19.279　Secondary osteoarthritis, unspecified ankle and foot

● M19.9　Osteoarthritis, unspecified site

　　M19.90　Unspecified osteoarthritis, unspecified site
　　　　Arthrosis NOS
　　　　Arthritis NOS
　　　　Osteoarthritis NOS

　　M19.91　Primary osteoarthritis, unspecified site
　　　　Primary osteoarthritis NOS

　　M19.92　Post-traumatic osteoarthritis, unspecified site
　　　　Post-traumatic osteoarthritis NOS

　　M19.93　Secondary osteoarthritis, unspecified site
　　　　Secondary osteoarthritis NOS

OTHER JOINT DISORDERS (M20-M25)

Excludes2　joints of the spine (M40-M54)

● M20　Acquired deformities of fingers and toes

　　Excludes1　acquired absence of fingers and toes (Z89.-)
　　　　congenital absence of fingers and toes (Q71.3-, Q72.3-)
　　　　congenital deformities and malformations of fingers and toes (Q66.-, Q68-Q70, Q74.-)

● M20.0　Deformity of finger(s)

　　Excludes1　clubbing of fingers (R68.3)
　　　　palmar fascial fibromatosis [Dupuytren] (M72.0)
　　　　trigger finger (M65.3)

　● M20.00　Unspecified deformity of finger(s)

　　　M20.001　Unspecified deformity of right finger(s)

　　　M20.002　Unspecified deformity of left finger(s)

　　　M20.009　Unspecified deformity of unspecified finger(s)

　● M20.01　Mallet finger

　　　M20.011　Mallet finger of right finger(s)

　　　M20.012　Mallet finger of left finger(s)

　　　M20.019　Mallet finger of unspecified finger(s)

　● M20.02　Boutonnière deformity

　　　M20.021　Boutonnière deformity of right finger(s)

　　　M20.022　Boutonnière deformity of left finger(s)

　　　M20.029　Boutonnière deformity of unspecified finger(s)

　● M20.03　Swan-neck deformity

　　　M20.031　Swan-neck deformity of right finger(s)

　　　M20.032　Swan-neck deformity of left finger(s)

　　　M20.039　Swan-neck deformity of unspecified finger(s)

　● M20.09　Other deformity of finger(s)

　　　M20.091　Other deformity of right finger(s)

　　　M20.092　Other deformity of left finger(s)

　　　M20.099　Other deformity of finger(s), unspecified finger(s)

● M20.1　Hallux valgus (acquired)

　　Excludes2　bunion (M21.6-)

　　M20.10　Hallux valgus (acquired), unspecified foot

　　M20.11　Hallux valgus (acquired), right foot

　　M20.12　Hallux valgus (acquired), left foot

● M20.2　Hallux rigidus

　　M20.20　Hallux rigidus, unspecified foot

　　M20.21　Hallux rigidus, right foot

　　M20.22　Hallux rigidus, left foot

Figure 13-1   Hallux valgus.

Item 13–2   **Hallux valgus** is a sometimes painful structural deformity caused by an inflammation of the bursal sac at the base of the metatarsophalangeal joint (big toe). **Hallus varus** is a deviation of the great toe to the inner side of the foot or away from the next toe.

● M20.3   Hallux varus (acquired)
- M20.30   Hallux varus (acquired), unspecified foot
- M20.31   Hallux varus (acquired), right foot
- M20.32   Hallux varus (acquired), left foot

● M20.4   Other hammer toe(s) (acquired)
- M20.40   Other hammer toe(s) (acquired), unspecified foot
- M20.41   Other hammer toe(s) (acquired), right foot
- M20.42   Other hammer toe(s) (acquired), left foot

● M20.5   Other deformities of toe(s) (acquired)
- ● M20.5X   Other deformities of toe(s) (acquired)
  - M20.5X1   Other deformities of toe(s) (acquired), right foot
  - M20.5X2   Other deformities of toe(s) (acquired), left foot
  - M20.5X9   Other deformities of toe(s) (acquired), unspecified foot

● M20.6   Acquired deformities of toe(s), unspecified
- M20.60   Acquired deformities of toe(s), unspecified, unspecified foot
- M20.61   Acquired deformities of toe(s), unspecified, right foot
- M20.62   Acquired deformities of toe(s), unspecified, left foot

● M21   Other acquired deformities of limbs

> **Excludes1**   acquired absence of limb (Z89.-)
> congenital absence of limbs (Q71-Q73)
> congenital deformities and malformations of limbs (Q65-Q66, Q68-Q74)

> **Excludes2**   acquired deformities of fingers or toes (M20.-)
> coxa plana (M91.2)

● M21.0   Valgus deformity, not elsewhere classified

> **Excludes1**   metatarsus valgus (Q66.6)
> talipes calcaneovalgus (Q66.4)

- M21.00   Valgus deformity, not elsewhere classified, unspecified site
- ● M21.02   Valgus deformity, not elsewhere classified, elbow
  - Cubitus valgus
  - M21.021   Valgus deformity, not elsewhere classified, right elbow
  - M21.022   Valgus deformity, not elsewhere classified, left elbow
  - M21.029   Valgus deformity, not elsewhere classified, unspecified elbow

Item 13–3   **Cubitus valgus** is a deformity of the elbow resulting in an increased carrying angle in which the arm extends at the side and the palm faces forward, which results in the forearm and hand extended at a greater than 15 degrees.

Item 13–4   **Cubitus varus** is a deformity of the elbow resulting in the arm extended at the side and the palm facing forward so that the forearm and hand are held at less than 5 degrees, decreasing the carrying angle.

● M21.05   Valgus deformity, not elsewhere classified, hip
- M21.051   Valgus deformity, not elsewhere classified, right hip
- M21.052   Valgus deformity, not elsewhere classified, left hip
- M21.059   Valgus deformity, not elsewhere classified, unspecified hip

● M21.06   Valgus deformity, not elsewhere classified, knee
- Genu valgum
- Knock knee
  - M21.061   Valgus deformity, not elsewhere classified, right knee
  - M21.062   Valgus deformity, not elsewhere classified, left knee
  - M21.069   Valgus deformity, not elsewhere classified, unspecified knee

● M21.07   Valgus deformity, not elsewhere classified, ankle
- M21.071   Valgus deformity, not elsewhere classified, right ankle
- M21.072   Valgus deformity, not elsewhere classified, left ankle
- M21.079   Valgus deformity, not elsewhere classified, unspecified ankle

● M21.1   Varus deformity, not elsewhere classified

> **Excludes1**   metatarsus varus (Q66.22)
> tibia vara (M92.5)

- M21.10   Varus deformity, not elsewhere classified, unspecified site
- ● M21.12   Varus deformity, not elsewhere classified, elbow
  - Cubitus varus, elbow
  - M21.121   Varus deformity, not elsewhere classified, right elbow
  - M21.122   Varus deformity, not elsewhere classified, left elbow
  - M21.129   Varus deformity, not elsewhere classified, unspecified elbow
- ● M21.15   Varus deformity, not elsewhere classified, hip
  - M21.151   Varus deformity, not elsewhere classified, right hip
  - M21.152   Varus deformity, not elsewhere classified, left hip
  - M21.159   Varus deformity, not elsewhere classified, unspecified
- ● M21.16   Varus deformity, not elsewhere classified, knee
  - Bow leg
  - Genu varum
  - M21.161   Varus deformity, not elsewhere classified, right knee
  - M21.162   Varus deformity, not elsewhere classified, left knee
  - M21.169   Varus deformity, not elsewhere classified, unspecified knee
- ● M21.17   Varus deformity, not elsewhere classified, ankle
  - M21.171   Varus deformity, not elsewhere classified, right ankle
  - M21.172   Varus deformity, not elsewhere classified, left ankle
  - M21.179   Varus deformity, not elsewhere classified, unspecified ankle

▶ New   ⮞ Revised   ~~deleted~~ Deleted   **OGCR** Official Guidelines   **X** Assign placeholder X   ● Use Additional Character(s)

Excludes 1   Excludes 2   Includes   Use additional   Code first   Code also   Key words

● **M21.2** **Flexion** deformity
   M21.20 Flexion deformity, **unspecified** site
   ● **M21.21** Flexion deformity, **shoulder**
     M21.211 Flexion deformity, **right** shoulder
     M21.212 Flexion deformity, **left** shoulder
     M21.219 Flexion deformity, **unspecified** shoulder
   ● **M21.22** Flexion deformity, **elbow**
     M21.221 Flexion deformity, **right** elbow
     M21.222 Flexion deformity, **left** elbow
     M21.229 Flexion deformity, **unspecified** elbow
   ● **M21.23** Flexion deformity, **wrist**
     M21.231 Flexion deformity, **right** wrist
     M21.232 Flexion deformity, **left** wrist
     M21.239 Flexion deformity, **unspecified** wrist
   ● **M21.24** Flexion deformity, **finger joints**
     M21.241 Flexion deformity, **right** finger joints
     M21.242 Flexion deformity, **left** finger joints
     M21.249 Flexion deformity, **unspecified** finger joints
   ● **M21.25** Flexion deformity, **hip**
     M21.251 Flexion deformity, **right** hip
     M21.252 Flexion deformity, **left** hip
     M21.259 Flexion deformity, **unspecified** hip
   ● **M21.26** Flexion deformity, **knee**
     M21.261 Flexion deformity, **right** knee
     M21.262 Flexion deformity, **left** knee
     M21.269 Flexion deformity, **unspecified** knee
   ● **M21.27** Flexion deformity, **ankle and toes**
     M21.271 Flexion deformity, **right** ankle and toes
     M21.272 Flexion deformity, **left** ankle and toes
     M21.279 Flexion deformity, **unspecified** ankle and toes
● **M21.3** Wrist or foot **drop** (acquired)
   ● **M21.33** **Wrist** drop (acquired)
     M21.331 Wrist drop, **right** wrist
     M21.332 Wrist drop, **left** wrist
     M21.339 Wrist drop, **unspecified** wrist
   ● **M21.37** **Foot** drop (acquired)
     M21.371 Foot drop, **right** foot
     M21.372 Foot drop, **left** foot
     M21.379 Foot drop, **unspecified** foot
● **M21.4** **Flat foot** [pes planus] (acquired)
   Excludes1   congenital pes planus (Q66.5-)
   M21.40 Flat foot [pes planus] (acquired), **unspecified** foot
   M21.41 Flat foot [pes planus] (acquired), **right** foot
   M21.42 Flat foot [pes planus] (acquired), **left** foot
● **M21.5** **Acquired** clawhand, clubhand, clawfoot and clubfoot
   Excludes1   clubfoot, not specified as acquired (Q66.89)
   ● **M21.51** Acquired **clawhand**
     M21.511 Acquired clawhand, **right** hand
     M21.512 Acquired clawhand, **left** hand
     M21.519 Acquired clawhand, **unspecified** hand
   ● **M21.52** Acquired **clubhand**
     M21.521 Acquired clubhand, **right** hand
     M21.522 Acquired clubhand, **left** hand
     M21.529 Acquired clubhand, **unspecified** hand
   ● **M21.53** Acquired **clawfoot**
     M21.531 Acquired clawfoot, **right** foot
     M21.532 Acquired clawfoot, **left** foot
     M21.539 Acquired clawfoot, **unspecified** foot

   ● **M21.54** Acquired **clubfoot**
     M21.541 Acquired clubfoot, **right** foot
     M21.542 Acquired clubfoot, **left** foot
     M21.549 Acquired clubfoot, **unspecified** foot
● **M21.6** **Other acquired** deformities of foot
   Excludes2   deformities of toe (acquired) (M20.1-M20.6-)
   ● **M21.61** **Bunion**
     M21.611 Bunion of **right** foot
     M21.612 Bunion of **left** foot
     M21.619 Bunion of **unspecified** foot
   ● **M21.62** **Bunionette**
     M21.621 Bunionette of **right** foot
     M21.622 Bunionette of **left** foot
     M21.629 Bunionette of **unspecified** foot
   ● **M21.6X** **Other** acquired deformities of foot
     M21.6X1 Other acquired deformities of **right** foot
     M21.6X2 Other acquired deformities of **left** foot
     M21.6X9 Other acquired deformities of **unspecified** foot
● **M21.7** **Unequal limb length** (acquired)
   Note: The site used should correspond to the shorter limb.
   M21.70 Unequal limb length (acquired), **unspecified** site
   ● **M21.72** Unequal limb length (acquired), **humerus**
     M21.721 Unequal limb length (acquired), **right** humerus
     M21.722 Unequal limb length (acquired), **left** humerus
     M21.729 Unequal limb length (acquired), **unspecified** humerus
   ● **M21.73** Unequal limb length (acquired), **ulna and radius**
     M21.731 Unequal limb length (acquired), **right** ulna
     M21.732 Unequal limb length (acquired), **left** ulna
     M21.733 Unequal limb length (acquired), **right** radius
     M21.734 Unequal limb length (acquired), **left** radius
     M21.739 Unequal limb length (acquired), **unspecified** ulna and radius
   ● **M21.75** Unequal limb length (acquired), **femur**
     M21.751 Unequal limb length (acquired), **right** femur
     M21.752 Unequal limb length (acquired), **left** femur
     M21.759 Unequal limb length (acquired), **unspecified** femur
   ● **M21.76** Unequal limb length (acquired), **tibia and fibula**
     M21.761 Unequal limb length (acquired), **right** tibia
     M21.762 Unequal limb length (acquired), **left** tibia
     M21.763 Unequal limb length (acquired), **right** fibula
     M21.764 Unequal limb length (acquired), **left** fibula
     M21.769 Unequal limb length (acquired), **unspecified** tibia and fibula

CHAPTER 13 (M00-M99)

▶ New   ⇒ Revised   ~~deleted~~ Deleted   **OGCR** Official Guidelines   **X** Assign placeholder X   ● Use Additional Character(s)

Excludes 1   Excludes 2   Includes   Use additional   Code first   Code also   Key words

● M21.8 Other specified acquired deformities of limbs
    Excludes2 coxa plana (M91.2)
    M21.80 Other specified acquired deformities of unspecified limb
  ● M21.82 Other specified acquired deformities of upper arm
    M21.821 Other specified acquired deformities of right upper arm
    M21.822 Other specified acquired deformities of left upper arm
    M21.829 Other specified acquired deformities of unspecified upper arm
  ● M21.83 Other specified acquired deformities of forearm
    M21.831 Other specified acquired deformities of right forearm
    M21.832 Other specified acquired deformities of left forearm
    M21.839 Other specified acquired deformities of unspecified forearm
  ● M21.85 Other specified acquired deformities of thigh
    M21.851 Other specified acquired deformities of right thigh
    M21.852 Other specified acquired deformities of left thigh
    M21.859 Other specified acquired deformities of unspecified thigh
  ● M21.86 Other specified acquired deformities of lower leg
    M21.861 Other specified acquired deformities of right lower leg
    M21.862 Other specified acquired deformities of left lower leg
    M21.869 Other specified acquired deformities of unspecified lower leg
● M21.9 Unspecified acquired deformity of limb and hand
    M21.90 Unspecified acquired deformity of unspecified limb
  ● M21.92 Unspecified acquired deformity of upper arm
    M21.921 Unspecified acquired deformity of right upper arm
    M21.922 Unspecified acquired deformity of left upper arm
    M21.929 Unspecified acquired deformity of unspecified upper arm
  ● M21.93 Unspecified acquired deformity of forearm
    M21.931 Unspecified acquired deformity of right forearm
    M21.932 Unspecified acquired deformity of left forearm
    M21.939 Unspecified acquired deformity of unspecified forearm
  ● M21.94 Unspecified acquired deformity of hand
    M21.941 Unspecified acquired deformity of hand, right hand
    M21.942 Unspecified acquired deformity of hand, left hand
    M21.949 Unspecified acquired deformity of hand, unspecified hand

● M21.95 Unspecified acquired deformity of thigh
    M21.951 Unspecified acquired deformity of right thigh
    M21.952 Unspecified acquired deformity of left thigh
    M21.959 Unspecified acquired deformity of unspecified thigh
● M21.96 Unspecified acquired deformity of lower leg
    M21.961 Unspecified acquired deformity of right lower leg
    M21.962 Unspecified acquired deformity of left lower leg
    M21.969 Unspecified acquired deformity of unspecified lower leg

● M22 Disorder of patella
    Excludes1 traumatic dislocation of patella (S83.0-)
  ● M22.0 Recurrent dislocation of patella
    M22.00 Recurrent dislocation of patella, unspecified knee
    M22.01 Recurrent dislocation of patella, right knee
    M22.02 Recurrent dislocation of patella, left knee
  ● M22.1 Recurrent subluxation of patella
    Incomplete dislocation of patella
    M22.10 Recurrent subluxation of patella, unspecified knee
    M22.11 Recurrent subluxation of patella, right knee
    M22.12 Recurrent subluxation of patella, left knee
  ● M22.2 Patellofemoral disorders
    ● M22.2X Patellofemoral disorders
      M22.2X1 Patellofemoral disorders, right knee
      M22.2X2 Patellofemoral disorders, left knee
      M22.2X9 Patellofemoral disorders, unspecified knee
  ● M22.3 Other derangements of patella
    ● M22.3X Other derangements of patella
      M22.3X1 Other derangements of patella, right knee
      M22.3X2 Other derangements of patella, left knee
      M22.3X9 Other derangements of patella, unspecified knee
  ● M22.4 Chondromalacia patellae
    M22.40 Chondromalacia patellae, unspecified knee
    M22.41 Chondromalacia patellae, right knee
    M22.42 Chondromalacia patellae, left knee
  ● M22.8 Other disorders of patella
    ● M22.8X Other disorders of patella
      M22.8X1 Other disorders of patella, right knee
      M22.8X2 Other disorders of patella, left knee
      M22.8X9 Other disorders of patella, unspecified knee
  ● M22.9 Unspecified disorder of patella
    M22.90 Unspecified disorder of patella, unspecified knee
    M22.91 Unspecified disorder of patella, right knee
    M22.92 Unspecified disorder of patella, left knee

▶ New ⇒ Revised deleted Deleted OGCR Official Guidelines X Assign placeholder X ● Use Additional Character(s)

Excludes 1 Excludes 2 Includes Use additional Code first Code also Key words

● M23 **Internal derangement of knee**

Excludes1 | ankylosis (M24.66)
current injury - see injury of knee and lower leg (S80-S89)
deformity of knee (M21.-)
osteochondritis dissecans (M93.2)
recurrent dislocation or subluxation of joints (M24.4)
recurrent dislocation or subluxation of patella (M22.0-M22.1)

● M23.0 **Cystic meniscus**

● M23.00 **Cystic meniscus, unspecified meniscus**
Cystic meniscus, unspecified lateral meniscus
Cystic meniscus, unspecified medial meniscus

M23.000 Cystic meniscus, unspecified lateral meniscus, right knee

M23.001 Cystic meniscus, unspecified lateral meniscus, left knee

M23.002 Cystic meniscus, unspecified lateral meniscus, unspecified knee

M23.003 Cystic meniscus, unspecified medial meniscus, right knee

M23.004 Cystic meniscus, unspecified medial meniscus, left knee

M23.005 Cystic meniscus, unspecified medial meniscus, unspecified knee

M23.006 Cystic meniscus, unspecified meniscus, right knee

M23.007 Cystic meniscus, unspecified meniscus, left knee

M23.009 Cystic meniscus, unspecified meniscus, unspecified knee

● M23.01 **Cystic meniscus, anterior horn of medial meniscus**

M23.011 Cystic meniscus, anterior horn of medial meniscus, right knee

M23.012 Cystic meniscus, anterior horn of medial meniscus, left knee

M23.019 Cystic meniscus, anterior horn of medial meniscus, unspecified knee

● M23.02 **Cystic meniscus, posterior horn of medial meniscus**

M23.021 Cystic meniscus, posterior horn of medial meniscus, right knee

M23.022 Cystic meniscus, posterior horn of medial meniscus, left knee

M23.029 Cystic meniscus, posterior horn of medial meniscus, unspecified knee

● M23.03 **Cystic meniscus, other medial meniscus**

M23.031 Cystic meniscus, other medial meniscus, right knee

M23.032 Cystic meniscus, other medial meniscus, left knee

M23.039 Cystic meniscus, other medial meniscus, unspecified knee

● M23.04 **Cystic meniscus, anterior horn of lateral meniscus**

M23.041 Cystic meniscus, anterior horn of lateral meniscus, right knee

M23.042 Cystic meniscus, anterior horn of lateral meniscus, left knee

M23.049 Cystic meniscus, anterior horn of lateral meniscus, unspecified knee

● M23.05 **Cystic meniscus, posterior horn of lateral meniscus**

M23.051 Cystic meniscus, posterior horn of lateral meniscus, right knee

M23.052 Cystic meniscus, posterior horn of lateral meniscus, left knee

M23.059 Cystic meniscus, posterior horn of lateral meniscus, unspecified knee

● M23.06 **Cystic meniscus, other lateral meniscus**

M23.061 Cystic meniscus, other lateral meniscus, right knee

M23.062 Cystic meniscus, other lateral meniscus, left knee

M23.069 Cystic meniscus, other lateral meniscus, unspecified knee

★ **(See Plate 509 on page 79.)**

● M23.2 **Derangement of meniscus due to old tear or injury**
Old bucket-handle tear

● M23.20 **Derangement of unspecified meniscus due to old tear or injury**
Derangement of unspecified lateral meniscus due to old tear or injury
Derangement of unspecified medial meniscus due to old tear or injury

M23.200 Derangement of unspecified lateral meniscus due to old tear or injury, right knee

M23.201 Derangement of unspecified lateral meniscus due to old tear or injury, left knee

M23.202 Derangement of unspecified lateral meniscus due to old tear or injury, unspecified knee

M23.203 Derangement of unspecified medial meniscus due to old tear or injury, right knee

M23.204 Derangement of unspecified medial meniscus due to old tear or injury, left knee

M23.205 Derangement of unspecified medial meniscus due to old tear or injury, unspecified knee

M23.206 Derangement of unspecified meniscus due to old tear or injury, right knee

M23.207 Derangement of unspecified meniscus due to old tear or injury, left knee

M23.209 Derangement of unspecified meniscus due to old tear or injury, unspecified knee

● M23.21 **Derangement of anterior horn of medial meniscus due to old tear or injury**

M23.211 Derangement of anterior horn of medial meniscus due to old tear or injury, right knee

M23.212 Derangement of anterior horn of medial meniscus due to old tear or injury, left knee

M23.219 Derangement of anterior horn of medial meniscus due to old tear or injury, unspecified knee

● M23.22 Derangement of posterior horn of medial meniscus due to old tear or injury

    M23.221 Derangement of posterior horn of medial meniscus due to old tear or injury, right knee

    M23.222 Derangement of posterior horn of medial meniscus due to old tear or injury, left knee

    M23.229 Derangement of posterior horn of medial meniscus due to old tear or injury, unspecified knee

● M23.23 Derangement of other medial meniscus due to old tear or injury

    M23.231 Derangement of other medial meniscus due to old tear or injury, right knee

    M23.232 Derangement of other medial meniscus due to old tear or injury, left knee

    M23.239 Derangement of other medial meniscus due to old tear or injury, unspecified knee

● M23.24 Derangement of anterior horn of lateral meniscus due to old tear or injury

    M23.241 Derangement of anterior horn of lateral meniscus due to old tear or injury, right knee

    M23.242 Derangement of anterior horn of lateral meniscus due to old tear or injury, left knee

    M23.249 Derangement of anterior horn of lateral meniscus due to old tear or injury, unspecified knee

● M23.25 Derangement of posterior horn of lateral meniscus due to old tear or injury

    M23.251 Derangement of posterior horn of lateral meniscus due to old tear or injury, right knee

    M23.252 Derangement of posterior horn of lateral meniscus due to old tear or injury, left knee

    M23.259 Derangement of posterior horn of lateral meniscus due to old tear or injury, unspecified knee

● M23.26 Derangement of other lateral meniscus due to old tear or injury

    M23.261 Derangement of other lateral meniscus due to old tear or injury, right knee

    M23.262 Derangement of other lateral meniscus due to old tear or injury, left knee

    M23.269 Derangement of other lateral meniscus due to old tear or injury, unspecified knee

● M23.3 Other meniscus derangements
    Degenerate meniscus
    Detached meniscus
    Retained meniscus

● M23.30 Other meniscus derangements, unspecified meniscus
    Other meniscus derangements, unspecified lateral meniscus
    Other meniscus derangements, unspecified medial meniscus

    M23.300 Other meniscus derangements, unspecified lateral meniscus, right knee

    M23.301 Other meniscus derangements, unspecified lateral meniscus, left knee

    M23.302 Other meniscus derangements, unspecified lateral meniscus, unspecified knee

    M23.303 Other meniscus derangements, unspecified medial meniscus, right knee

    M23.304 Other meniscus derangements, unspecified medial meniscus, left knee

    M23.305 Other meniscus derangements, unspecified medial meniscus, unspecified knee

    M23.306 Other meniscus derangements, unspecified meniscus, right knee

    M23.307 Other meniscus derangements, unspecified meniscus, left knee

    M23.309 Other meniscus derangements, unspecified meniscus, unspecified knee

● M23.31 Other meniscus derangements, anterior horn of medial meniscus

    M23.311 Other meniscus derangements, anterior horn of medial meniscus, right knee

    M23.312 Other meniscus derangements, anterior horn of medial meniscus, left knee

    M23.319 Other meniscus derangements, anterior horn of medial meniscus, unspecified knee

● M23.32 Other meniscus derangements, posterior horn of medial meniscus

    M23.321 Other meniscus derangements, posterior horn of medial meniscus, right knee

    M23.322 Other meniscus derangements, posterior horn of medial meniscus, left knee

    M23.329 Other meniscus derangements, posterior horn of medial meniscus, unspecified knee

● M23.33 Other meniscus derangements, other medial meniscus

    M23.331 Other meniscus derangements, other medial meniscus, right knee

    M23.332 Other meniscus derangements, other medial meniscus, left knee

    M23.339 Other meniscus derangements, other medial meniscus, unspecified knee

● M23.34 Other meniscus derangements, anterior horn of lateral meniscus

    M23.341 Other meniscus derangements, anterior horn of lateral meniscus, right knee

    M23.342 Other meniscus derangements, anterior horn of lateral meniscus, left knee

    M23.349 Other meniscus derangements, anterior horn of lateral meniscus, unspecified knee

● M23.35 Other meniscus derangements, posterior horn of lateral meniscus

    M23.351 Other meniscus derangements, posterior horn of lateral meniscus, right knee

    M23.352 Other meniscus derangements, posterior horn of lateral meniscus, left knee

    M23.359 Other meniscus derangements, posterior horn of lateral meniscus, unspecified knee

▶ New   ⇒ Revised   ~~deleted~~ Deleted   OGCR Official Guidelines   X Assign placeholder X   ● Use Additional Character(s)

Excludes 1   Excludes 2   Includes   Use additional   Code first   Code also   Key words

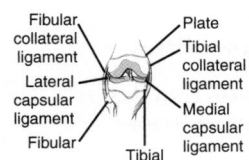

Figure 13-2 Collateral and cruciate ligament of knee. (From DeLee: DeLee and Drez's Orthopaedic Sports Medicine, ed 3, Saunders, 2009)

● M23.36 Other meniscus derangements, other lateral meniscus

    M23.361 Other meniscus derangements, other lateral meniscus, right knee

    M23.362 Other meniscus derangements, other lateral meniscus, left knee

    M23.369 Other meniscus derangements, other lateral meniscus, unspecified knee

● M23.4 Loose body in knee

    M23.40 Loose body in knee, unspecified knee

    M23.41 Loose body in knee, right knee

    M23.42 Loose body in knee, left knee

● M23.5 Chronic instability of knee

    M23.50 Chronic instability of knee, unspecified knee

    M23.51 Chronic instability of knee, right knee

    M23.52 Chronic instability of knee, left knee

● M23.6 Other spontaneous disruption of ligament(s) of knee

    ● M23.60 Other spontaneous disruption of unspecified ligament of knee

        M23.601 Other spontaneous disruption of unspecified ligament of right knee

        M23.602 Other spontaneous disruption of unspecified ligament of left knee

        M23.609 Other spontaneous disruption of unspecified ligament of unspecified knee

    ● M23.61 Other spontaneous disruption of anterior cruciate ligament of knee

        M23.611 Other spontaneous disruption of anterior cruciate ligament of right knee

        M23.612 Other spontaneous disruption of anterior cruciate ligament of left knee

        M23.619 Other spontaneous disruption of anterior cruciate ligament of unspecified knee

    ● M23.62 Other spontaneous disruption of posterior cruciate ligament of knee

        M23.621 Other spontaneous disruption of posterior cruciate ligament of right knee

        M23.622 Other spontaneous disruption of posterior cruciate ligament of left knee

        M23.629 Other spontaneous disruption of posterior cruciate ligament of unspecified knee

    ● M23.63 Other spontaneous disruption of medial collateral ligament of knee

        M23.631 Other spontaneous disruption of medial collateral ligament of right knee

        M23.632 Other spontaneous disruption of medial collateral ligament of left knee

        M23.639 Other spontaneous disruption of medial collateral ligament of unspecified knee

    ● M23.64 Other spontaneous disruption of lateral collateral ligament of knee

        M23.641 Other spontaneous disruption of lateral collateral ligament of right knee

        M23.642 Other spontaneous disruption of lateral collateral ligament of left knee

        M23.649 Other spontaneous disruption of lateral collateral ligament of unspecified knee

    ● M23.67 Other spontaneous disruption of capsular ligament of knee

        M23.671 Other spontaneous disruption of capsular ligament of right knee

        M23.672 Other spontaneous disruption of capsular ligament of left knee

        M23.679 Other spontaneous disruption of capsular ligament of unspecified knee

● M23.8 Other internal derangements of knee

    Laxity of ligament of knee

    Snapping knee

    ● M23.8X Other internal derangements of knee

        M23.8X1 Other internal derangements of right knee

        M23.8X2 Other internal derangements of left knee

        M23.8X9 Other internal derangements of unspecified knee

● M23.9 Unspecified internal derangement of knee

    M23.90 Unspecified internal derangement of unspecified knee

    M23.91 Unspecified internal derangement of right knee

    M23.92 Unspecified internal derangement of left knee

● M24 Other specific joint derangements

    Excludes1 current injury - see injury of joint by body region

    Excludes2 ganglion (M67.4)

                snapping knee (M23.8-)

                temporomandibular joint disorders (M26.6-)

● M24.0 Loose body in joint

    Excludes2 loose body in knee (M23.4)

    M24.00 Loose body in unspecified joint

    ● M24.01 Loose body in shoulder

        M24.011 Loose body in right shoulder

        M24.012 Loose body in left shoulder

        M24.019 Loose body in unspecified shoulder

    ● M24.02 Loose body in elbow

        M24.021 Loose body in right elbow

        M24.022 Loose body in left elbow

        M24.029 Loose body in unspecified elbow

    ● M24.03 Loose body in wrist

        M24.031 Loose body in right wrist

        M24.032 Loose body in left wrist

        M24.039 Loose body in unspecified wrist

    ● M24.04 Loose body in finger joints

        M24.041 Loose body in right finger joint(s)

        M24.042 Loose body in left finger joint(s)

        M24.049 Loose body in unspecified finger joint(s)

    ● M24.05 Loose body in hip

        M24.051 Loose body in right hip

        M24.052 Loose body in left hip

        M24.059 Loose body in unspecified hip

▶ New   ⇒ Revised   ~~deleted~~ Deleted   **OGCR** Official Guidelines   X Assign placeholder X   ● Use Additional Character(s)

| Excludes 1 | Excludes 2 | Includes | Use additional | Code first | Code also | Key words |

● M24.07 Loose body in ankle and toe joints
    M24.071 Loose body in right ankle
    M24.072 Loose body in left ankle
    M24.073 Loose body in unspecified ankle
    M24.074 Loose body in right toe joint(s)
    M24.075 Loose body in left toe joint(s)
    M24.076 Loose body in unspecified toe joints
  M24.08 Loose body, other site
● M24.1 Other articular cartilage disorders
    Excludes2   chondrocalcinosis (M11.1, M11.2-)
               internal derangement of knee (M23.-)
               metastatic calcification (E83.5)
               ochronosis (E70.2)
  M24.10 Other articular cartilage disorders, unspecified site
● M24.11 Other articular cartilage disorders, shoulder
    M24.111 Other articular cartilage disorders, right shoulder
    M24.112 Other articular cartilage disorders, left shoulder
    M24.119 Other articular cartilage disorders, unspecified shoulder
● M24.12 Other articular cartilage disorders, elbow
    M24.121 Other articular cartilage disorders, right elbow
    M24.122 Other articular cartilage disorders, left elbow
    M24.129 Other articular cartilage disorders, unspecified elbow
● M24.13 Other articular cartilage disorders, wrist
    M24.131 Other articular cartilage disorders, right wrist
    M24.132 Other articular cartilage disorders, left wrist
    M24.139 Other articular cartilage disorders, unspecified wrist
● M24.14 Other articular cartilage disorders, hand
    M24.141 Other articular cartilage disorders, right hand
    M24.142 Other articular cartilage disorders, left hand
    M24.149 Other articular cartilage disorders, unspecified hand
● M24.15 Other articular cartilage disorders, hip
    M24.151 Other articular cartilage disorders, right hip
    M24.152 Other articular cartilage disorders, left hip
    M24.159 Other articular cartilage disorders, unspecified hip
● M24.17 Other articular cartilage disorders, ankle and foot
    M24.171 Other articular cartilage disorders, right ankle
    M24.172 Other articular cartilage disorders, left ankle
    M24.173 Other articular cartilage disorders, unspecified ankle
    M24.174 Other articular cartilage disorders, right foot
    M24.175 Other articular cartilage disorders, left foot
    M24.176 Other articular cartilage disorders, unspecified foot

● M24.2 Disorder of ligament
  Instability secondary to old ligament injury
  Ligamentous laxity NOS
    Excludes1 familial ligamentous laxity (M35.7)
    Excludes2 internal derangement of knee (M23.5-M23.89)
  M24.20 Disorder of ligament, unspecified site
● M24.21 Disorder of ligament, shoulder
    M24.211 Disorder of ligament, right shoulder
    M24.212 Disorder of ligament, left shoulder
    M24.219 Disorder of ligament, unspecified shoulder
● M24.22 Disorder of ligament, elbow
    M24.221 Disorder of ligament, right elbow
    M24.222 Disorder of ligament, left elbow
    M24.229 Disorder of ligament, unspecified elbow
● M24.23 Disorder of ligament, wrist
    M24.231 Disorder of ligament, right wrist
    M24.232 Disorder of ligament, left wrist
    M24.239 Disorder of ligament, unspecified wrist
● M24.24 Disorder of ligament, hand
    M24.241 Disorder of ligament, right hand
    M24.242 Disorder of ligament, left hand
    M24.249 Disorder of ligament, unspecified hand
● M24.25 Disorder of ligament, hip
    M24.251 Disorder of ligament, right hip
    M24.252 Disorder of ligament, left hip
    M24.259 Disorder of ligament, unspecified hip
● M24.27 Disorder of ligament, ankle and foot
    M24.271 Disorder of ligament, right ankle
    M24.272 Disorder of ligament, left ankle
    M24.273 Disorder of ligament, unspecified ankle
    M24.274 Disorder of ligament, right foot
    M24.275 Disorder of ligament, left foot
    M24.276 Disorder of ligament, unspecified foot
  M24.28 Disorder of ligament, vertebrae
● M24.3 Pathological dislocation of joint, not elsewhere classified
    Excludes1 congenital dislocation or displacement of joint - see congenital malformations and deformations of the musculoskeletal system (Q65-Q79)
               current injury - see injury of joints and ligaments by body region
               recurrent dislocation of joint (M24.4-)
  M24.30 Pathological dislocation of unspecified joint, not elsewhere classified
● M24.31 Pathological dislocation of shoulder, not elsewhere classified
    M24.311 Pathological dislocation of right shoulder, not elsewhere classified
    M24.312 Pathological dislocation of left shoulder, not elsewhere classified
    M24.319 Pathological dislocation of unspecified shoulder, not elsewhere classified
● M24.32 Pathological dislocation of elbow, not elsewhere classified
    M24.321 Pathological dislocation of right elbow, not elsewhere classified
    M24.322 Pathological dislocation of left elbow, not elsewhere classified
    M24.329 Pathological dislocation of unspecified elbow, not elsewhere classified

▶ New ⇒ Revised ~~deleted~~ Deleted **OGCR** Official Guidelines X Assign placeholder X ● Use Additional Character(s)
Excludes 1 Excludes 2 Includes Use additional Code first Code also Key words

● **M24.33** Pathological dislocation of wrist, not elsewhere classified

    M24.331 Pathological dislocation of right wrist, not elsewhere classified

    M24.332 Pathological dislocation of left wrist, not elsewhere classified

    M24.339 Pathological dislocation of unspecified wrist, not elsewhere classified

● **M24.34** Pathological dislocation of hand, not elsewhere classified

    M24.341 Pathological dislocation of right hand, not elsewhere classified

    M24.342 Pathological dislocation of left hand, not elsewhere classified

    M24.349 Pathological dislocation of unspecified hand, not elsewhere classified

● **M24.35** Pathological dislocation of hip, not elsewhere classified

    M24.351 Pathological dislocation of right hip, not elsewhere classified

    M24.352 Pathological dislocation of left hip, not elsewhere classified

    M24.359 Pathological dislocation of unspecified hip, not elsewhere classified

● **M24.36** Pathological dislocation of knee, not elsewhere classified

    M24.361 Pathological dislocation of right knee, not elsewhere classified

    M24.362 Pathological dislocation of left knee, not elsewhere classified

    M24.369 Pathological dislocation of unspecified knee, not elsewhere classified

● **M24.37** Pathological dislocation of ankle and foot, not elsewhere classified

    M24.371 Pathological dislocation of right ankle, not elsewhere classified

    M24.372 Pathological dislocation of left ankle, not elsewhere classified

    M24.373 Pathological dislocation of unspecified ankle, not elsewhere classified

    M24.374 Pathological dislocation of right foot, not elsewhere classified

    M24.375 Pathological dislocation of left foot, not elsewhere classified

    M24.376 Pathological dislocation of unspecified foot, not elsewhere classified

● **M24.4** Recurrent dislocation of joint

    Recurrent subluxation of joint

    Excludes2 recurrent dislocation of patella (M22.0-M22.1)

                recurrent vertebral dislocation (M43.3-, M43.4, M43.5-)

    M24.40 Recurrent dislocation, unspecified joint

● **M24.41** Recurrent dislocation, shoulder

    M24.411 Recurrent dislocation, right shoulder

    M24.412 Recurrent dislocation, left shoulder

    M24.419 Recurrent dislocation, unspecified shoulder

● **M24.42** Recurrent dislocation, elbow

    M24.421 Recurrent dislocation, right elbow

    M24.422 Recurrent dislocation, left elbow

    M24.429 Recurrent dislocation, unspecified elbow

● **M24.43** Recurrent dislocation, wrist

    M24.431 Recurrent dislocation, right wrist

    M24.432 Recurrent dislocation, left wrist

    M24.439 Recurrent dislocation, unspecified wrist

● **M24.44** Recurrent dislocation, hand and finger(s)

    M24.441 Recurrent dislocation, right hand

    M24.442 Recurrent dislocation, left hand

    M24.443 Recurrent dislocation, unspecified hand

    M24.444 Recurrent dislocation, right finger

    M24.445 Recurrent dislocation, left finger

    M24.446 Recurrent dislocation, unspecified finger

● **M24.45** Recurrent dislocation, hip

    M24.451 Recurrent dislocation, right hip

    M24.452 Recurrent dislocation, left hip

    M24.459 Recurrent dislocation, unspecified hip

● **M24.46** Recurrent dislocation, knee

    M24.461 Recurrent dislocation, right knee

    M24.462 Recurrent dislocation, left knee

    M24.469 Recurrent dislocation, unspecified knee

● **M24.47** Recurrent dislocation, ankle, foot and toes

    M24.471 Recurrent dislocation, right ankle

    M24.472 Recurrent dislocation, left ankle

    M24.473 Recurrent dislocation, unspecified ankle

    M24.474 Recurrent dislocation, right foot

    M24.475 Recurrent dislocation, left foot

    M24.476 Recurrent dislocation, unspecified foot

    M24.477 Recurrent dislocation, right toe(s)

    M24.478 Recurrent dislocation, left toe(s)

    M24.479 Recurrent dislocation, unspecified toe(s)

● **M24.5** Contracture of joint

    Excludes1 contracture of muscle without contracture of joint (M62.4-)

                contracture of tendon (sheath) without contracture of joint (M62.4-)

                Dupuytren's contracture (M72.0)

    Excludes2 acquired deformities of limbs (M20-M21)

    M24.50 Contracture, unspecified joint

● **M24.51** Contracture, shoulder

    M24.511 Contracture, right shoulder

    M24.512 Contracture, left shoulder

    M24.519 Contracture, unspecified shoulder

● **M24.52** Contracture, elbow

    M24.521 Contracture, right elbow

    M24.522 Contracture, left elbow

    M24.529 Contracture, unspecified elbow

● **M24.53** Contracture, wrist

    M24.531 Contracture, right wrist

    M24.532 Contracture, left wrist

    M24.539 Contracture, unspecified wrist

● **M24.54** Contracture, hand

    M24.541 Contracture, right hand

    M24.542 Contracture, left hand

    M24.549 Contracture, unspecified hand

● **M24.55** Contracture, hip

    M24.551 Contracture, right hip

    M24.552 Contracture, left hip

    M24.559 Contracture, unspecified hip

CHAPTER 13 (M00-M99)

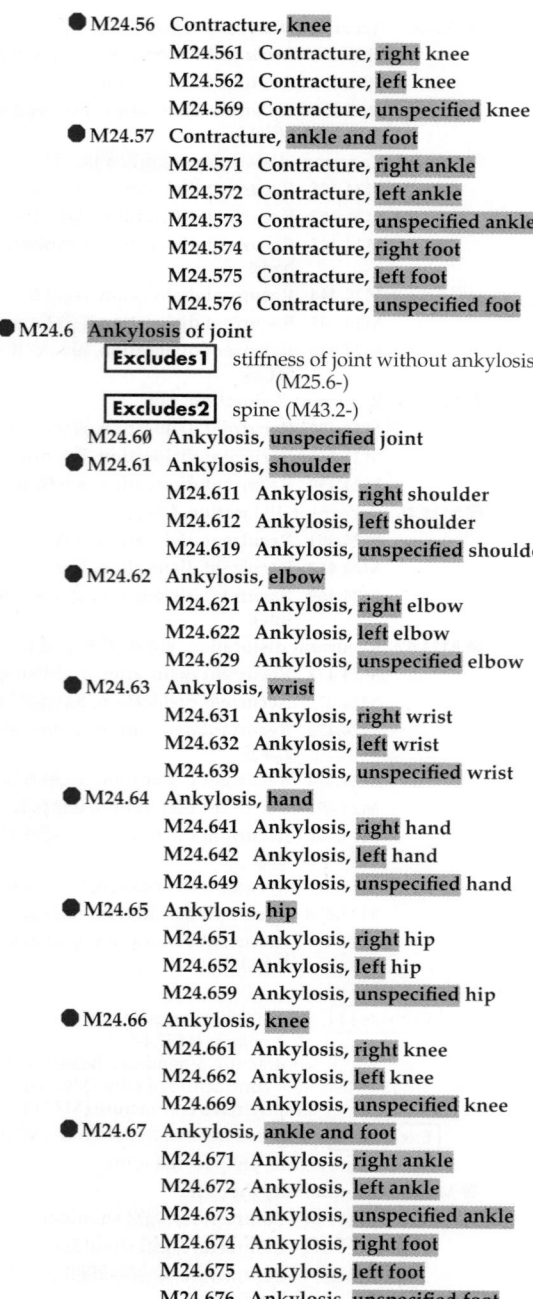

● M24.56   Contracture, knee
     M24.561   Contracture, right knee
     M24.562   Contracture, left knee
     M24.569   Contracture, unspecified knee
● M24.57   Contracture, ankle and foot
     M24.571   Contracture, right ankle
     M24.572   Contracture, left ankle
     M24.573   Contracture, unspecified ankle
     M24.574   Contracture, right foot
     M24.575   Contracture, left foot
     M24.576   Contracture, unspecified foot
● M24.6   Ankylosis of joint

> **Excludes1**   stiffness of joint without ankylosis (M25.6-)

> **Excludes2**   spine (M43.2-)

     M24.60   Ankylosis, unspecified joint
● M24.61   Ankylosis, shoulder
     M24.611   Ankylosis, right shoulder
     M24.612   Ankylosis, left shoulder
     M24.619   Ankylosis, unspecified shoulder
● M24.62   Ankylosis, elbow
     M24.621   Ankylosis, right elbow
     M24.622   Ankylosis, left elbow
     M24.629   Ankylosis, unspecified elbow
● M24.63   Ankylosis, wrist
     M24.631   Ankylosis, right wrist
     M24.632   Ankylosis, left wrist
     M24.639   Ankylosis, unspecified wrist
● M24.64   Ankylosis, hand
     M24.641   Ankylosis, right hand
     M24.642   Ankylosis, left hand
     M24.649   Ankylosis, unspecified hand
● M24.65   Ankylosis, hip
     M24.651   Ankylosis, right hip
     M24.652   Ankylosis, left hip
     M24.659   Ankylosis, unspecified hip
● M24.66   Ankylosis, knee
     M24.661   Ankylosis, right knee
     M24.662   Ankylosis, left knee
     M24.669   Ankylosis, unspecified knee
● M24.67   Ankylosis, ankle and foot
     M24.671   Ankylosis, right ankle
     M24.672   Ankylosis, left ankle
     M24.673   Ankylosis, unspecified ankle
     M24.674   Ankylosis, right foot
     M24.675   Ankylosis, left foot
     M24.676   Ankylosis, unspecified foot

Item 13–5   Ankylosis or arthrokleisis is a consolidation of a joint due to disease, injury, or surgical procedure. Spondylosis is the degeneration of the vertebral processes and formation of osteophytes and commonly occurs with age. **Spondylitis** or ankylosing spondylitis is a type of arthritis that affects the spine or backbone causing back pain and stiffness.

M24.7   Protrusio acetabuli
● M24.8   Other specific joint derangements, not elsewhere classified

> **Excludes2**   iliotibial band syndrome (M76.3)

     M24.80   Other specific joint derangements of unspecified joint, not elsewhere classified
● M24.81   Other specific joint derangements of shoulder, not elsewhere classified
     M24.811   Other specific joint derangements of right shoulder, not elsewhere classified
     M24.812   Other specific joint derangements of left shoulder, not elsewhere classified
     M24.819   Other specific joint derangements of unspecified shoulder, not elsewhere classified
● M24.82   Other specific joint derangements of elbow, not elsewhere classified
     M24.821   Other specific joint derangements of right elbow, not elsewhere classified
     M24.822   Other specific joint derangements of left elbow, not elsewhere classified
     M24.829   Other specific joint derangements of unspecified elbow, not elsewhere classified
● M24.83   Other specific joint derangements of wrist, not elsewhere classified
     M24.831   Other specific joint derangements of right wrist, not elsewhere classified
     M24.832   Other specific joint derangements of left wrist, not elsewhere classified
     M24.839   Other specific joint derangements of unspecified wrist, not elsewhere classified
● M24.84   Other specific joint derangements of hand, not elsewhere classified
     M24.841   Other specific joint derangements of right hand, not elsewhere classified
     M24.842   Other specific joint derangements of left hand, not elsewhere classified
     M24.849   Other specific joint derangements of unspecified hand, not elsewhere classified
● M24.85   Other specific joint derangements of hip, not elsewhere classified
     Irritable hip
     M24.851   Other specific joint derangements of right hip, not elsewhere classified
     M24.852   Other specific joint derangements of left hip, not elsewhere classified
     M24.859   Other specific joint derangements of unspecified hip, not elsewhere classified
● M24.87   Other specific joint derangements of ankle and foot, not elsewhere classified
     M24.871   Other specific joint derangements of right ankle, not elsewhere classified
     M24.872   Other specific joint derangements of left ankle, not elsewhere classified
     M24.873   Other specific joint derangements of unspecified ankle, not elsewhere classified
     M24.874   Other specific joint derangements of right foot, not elsewhere classified
     M24.875   Other specific joint derangements left foot, not elsewhere classified
     M24.876   Other specific joint derangements of unspecified foot, not elsewhere classified

M24.9   Joint derangement, unspecified

▶ New   ⇒ Revised   ~~deleted~~ Deleted   **OGCR** Official Guidelines   X Assign placeholder X   ● Use Additional Character(s)

Excludes 1   Excludes 2   Includes   Use additional   Code first   Code also   Key words

● M25 **Other joint disorder, not elsewhere classified**
      Excludes2   abnormality of gait and mobility (R26.-)
                 acquired deformities of limb (M20-M21)
                 calcification of bursa (M71.4-)
                 calcification of shoulder (joint) (M75.3)
                 calcification of tendon (M65.2-)
                 difficulty in walking (R26.2)
                 temporomandibular joint disorder (M26.6-)

● M25.0 **Hemarthrosis**
      Excludes1   current injury - see injury of joint by body
                        region
                 hemophilic arthropathy (M36.2)
      M25.00 Hemarthrosis, unspecified joint
   ● M25.01 Hemarthrosis, shoulder
         M25.011 Hemarthrosis, right shoulder
         M25.012 Hemarthrosis, left shoulder
         M25.019 Hemarthrosis, unspecified shoulder
   ● M25.02 Hemarthrosis, elbow
         M25.021 Hemarthrosis, right elbow
         M25.022 Hemarthrosis, left elbow
         M25.029 Hemarthrosis, unspecified elbow
   ● M25.03 Hemarthrosis, wrist
         M25.031 Hemarthrosis, right wrist
         M25.032 Hemarthrosis, left wrist
         M25.039 Hemarthrosis, unspecified wrist
   ● M25.04 Hemarthrosis, hand
         M25.041 Hemarthrosis, right hand
         M25.042 Hemarthrosis, left hand
         M25.049 Hemarthrosis, unspecified hand
   ● M25.05 Hemarthrosis, hip
         M25.051 Hemarthrosis, right hip
         M25.052 Hemarthrosis, left hip
         M25.059 Hemarthrosis, unspecified hip
   ● M25.06 Hemarthrosis, knee
         M25.061 Hemarthrosis, right knee
         M25.062 Hemarthrosis, left knee
         M25.069 Hemarthrosis, unspecified knee
   ● M25.07 Hemarthrosis, ankle and foot
         M25.071 Hemarthrosis, right ankle
         M25.072 Hemarthrosis, left ankle
         M25.073 Hemarthrosis, unspecified ankle
         M25.074 Hemarthrosis, right foot
         M25.075 Hemarthrosis, left foot
         M25.076 Hemarthrosis, unspecified foot
      M25.08 Hemarthrosis, other specified site
              Hemarthrosis, vertebrae
● M25.1 **Fistula of joint**
      M25.10 Fistula, unspecified joint
   ● M25.11 Fistula, shoulder
         M25.111 Fistula, right shoulder
         M25.112 Fistula, left shoulder
         M25.119 Fistula, unspecified shoulder
   ● M25.12 Fistula, elbow
         M25.121 Fistula, right elbow
         M25.122 Fistula, left elbow
         M25.129 Fistula, unspecified elbow
   ● M25.13 Fistula, wrist
         M25.131 Fistula, right wrist
         M25.132 Fistula, left wrist
         M25.139 Fistula, unspecified wrist
   ● M25.14 Fistula, hand
         M25.141 Fistula, right hand
         M25.142 Fistula, left hand
         M25.149 Fistula, unspecified hand

   ● M25.15 Fistula, hip
         M25.151 Fistula, right hip
         M25.152 Fistula, left hip
         M25.159 Fistula, unspecified hip
   ● M25.16 Fistula, knee
         M25.161 Fistula, right knee
         M25.162 Fistula, left knee
         M25.169 Fistula, unspecified knee
   ● M25.17 Fistula, ankle and foot
         M25.171 Fistula, right ankle
         M25.172 Fistula, left ankle
         M25.173 Fistula, unspecified ankle
         M25.174 Fistula, right foot
         M25.175 Fistula, left foot
         M25.176 Fistula, unspecified foot
      M25.18 Fistula, other specified site
            Fistula, vertebrae
● M25.2 **Flail joint**
      M25.20 Flail joint, unspecified joint
   ● M25.21 Flail joint, shoulder
         M25.211 Flail joint, right shoulder
         M25.212 Flail joint, left shoulder
         M25.219 Flail joint, unspecified shoulder
   ● M25.22 Flail joint, elbow
         M25.221 Flail joint, right elbow
         M25.222 Flail joint, left elbow
         M25.229 Flail joint, unspecified elbow
   ● M25.23 Flail joint, wrist
         M25.231 Flail joint, right wrist
         M25.232 Flail joint, left wrist
         M25.239 Flail joint, unspecified wrist
   ● M25.24 Flail joint, hand
         M25.241 Flail joint, right hand
         M25.242 Flail joint, left hand
         M25.249 Flail joint, unspecified hand
   ● M25.25 Flail joint, hip
         M25.251 Flail joint, right hip
         M25.252 Flail joint, left hip
         M25.259 Flail joint, unspecified hip
   ● M25.26 Flail joint, knee
         M25.261 Flail joint, right knee
         M25.262 Flail joint, left knee
         M25.269 Flail joint, unspecified knee
   ● M25.27 Flail joint, ankle and foot
         M25.271 Flail joint, right ankle and foot
         M25.272 Flail joint, left ankle and foot
         M25.279 Flail joint, unspecified ankle and foot
      M25.28 Flail joint, other site
● M25.3 **Other instability of joint**
      Excludes1   instability of joint secondary to old
                      ligament injury (M24.2-)
                 instability of joint secondary to removal
                      of joint prosthesis (M96.8-)
      Excludes2   spinal instabilities (M53.2-)
      M25.30 Other instability, unspecified joint
   ● M25.31 Other instability, shoulder
         M25.311 Other instability, right shoulder
         M25.312 Other instability, left shoulder
         M25.319 Other instability, unspecified
                 shoulder
   ● M25.32 Other instability, elbow
         M25.321 Other instability, right elbow
         M25.322 Other instability, left elbow
         M25.329 Other instability, unspecified elbow

▶ New   ⇒ Revised   ~~deleted~~ Deleted   **OGCR** Official Guidelines   X Assign placeholder X   ● Use Additional Character(s)

| Excludes 1 | Excludes 2 | Includes | Use additional | Code first | Code also | Key words |

● M25.33　Other instability, wrist
　　　M25.331　Other instability, right wrist
　　　M25.332　Other instability, left wrist
　　　M25.339　Other instability, unspecified wrist
● M25.34　Other instability, hand
　　　M25.341　Other instability, right hand
　　　M25.342　Other instability, left hand
　　　M25.349　Other instability, unspecified hand
● M25.35　Other instability, hip
　　　M25.351　Other instability, right hip
　　　M25.352　Other instability, left hip
　　　M25.359　Other instability, unspecified hip
● M25.36　Other instability, knee
　　　M25.361　Other instability, right knee
　　　M25.362　Other instability, left knee
　　　M25.369　Other instability, unspecified knee
● M25.37　Other instability, ankle and foot
　　　M25.371　Other instability, right ankle
　　　M25.372　Other instability, left ankle
　　　M25.373　Other instability, unspecified ankle
　　　M25.374　Other instability, right foot
　　　M25.375　Other instability, left foot
　　　M25.376　Other instability, unspecified foot
● M25.4　Effusion of joint
　　　Excludes1　hydrarthrosis in yaws (A66.6)
　　　　　　　　intermittent hydrarthrosis (M12.4-)
　　　　　　　　other infective (teno)synovitis (M65.1-)
　　M25.40　Effusion, unspecified joint
● M25.41　Effusion, shoulder
　　　M25.411　Effusion, right shoulder
　　　M25.412　Effusion, left shoulder
　　　M25.419　Effusion, unspecified shoulder
● M25.42　Effusion, elbow
　　　M25.421　Effusion, right elbow
　　　M25.422　Effusion, left elbow
　　　M25.429　Effusion, unspecified elbow
● M25.43　Effusion, wrist
　　　M25.431　Effusion, right wrist
　　　M25.432　Effusion, left wrist
　　　M25.439　Effusion, unspecified wrist
● M25.44　Effusion, hand
　　　M25.441　Effusion, right hand
　　　M25.442　Effusion, left hand
　　　M25.449　Effusion, unspecified hand
● M25.45　Effusion, hip
　　　M25.451　Effusion, right hip
　　　M25.452　Effusion, left hip
　　　M25.459　Effusion, unspecified hip
● M25.46　Effusion, knee
　　　M25.461　Effusion, right knee
　　　M25.462　Effusion, left knee
　　　M25.469　Effusion, unspecified knee
● M25.47　Effusion, ankle and foot
　　　M25.471　Effusion, right ankle
　　　M25.472　Effusion, left ankle
　　　M25.473　Effusion, unspecified ankle
　　　M25.474　Effusion, right foot
　　　M25.475　Effusion, left foot
　　　M25.476　Effusion, unspecified foot
　　M25.48　Effusion, other site

● M25.5　Pain in joint
　　　Excludes2　pain in hand (M79.64-)
　　　　　　　　pain in fingers (M79.64-)
　　　　　　　　pain in foot (M79.67-)
　　　　　　　　pain in limb (M79.6-)
　　　　　　　　pain in toes (M79.67-)
　　M25.50　Pain in unspecified joint
● M25.51　Pain in shoulder
　　　M25.511　Pain in right shoulder
　　　M25.512　Pain in left shoulder
　　　M25.519　Pain in unspecified shoulder
● M25.52　Pain in elbow
　　　M25.521　Pain in right elbow
　　　M25.522　Pain in left elbow
　　　M25.529　Pain in unspecified elbow
● M25.53　Pain in wrist
　　　M25.531　Pain in right wrist
　　　M25.532　Pain in left wrist
　　　M25.539　Pain in unspecified wrist
● M25.54　Pain in joints of hand
　　　M25.541　Pain in joints of right hand
　　　M25.542　Pain in joints of left hand
　　　M25.549　Pain in joints of unspecified hand
　　　　　　　　Pain in joints of hand NOS
● M25.55　Pain in hip
　　　M25.551　Pain in right hip
　　　M25.552　Pain in left hip
　　　M25.559　Pain in unspecified hip
● M25.56　Pain in knee
　　　M25.561　Pain in right knee
　　　M25.562　Pain in left knee
　　　M25.569　Pain in unspecified knee
● M25.57　Pain in ankle and joints of foot
　　　M25.571　Pain in right ankle and joints of right foot
　　　M25.572　Pain in left ankle and joints of left foot
　　　M25.579　Pain in unspecified ankle and joints of unspecified foot
● M25.6　Stiffness of joint, not elsewhere classified
　　　Excludes1　ankylosis of joint (M24.6-)
　　　　　　　　contracture of joint (M24.5-)
　　M25.60　Stiffness of unspecified joint, not elsewhere classified
● M25.61　Stiffness of shoulder, not elsewhere classified
　　　M25.611　Stiffness of right shoulder, not elsewhere classified
　　　M25.612　Stiffness of left shoulder, not elsewhere classified
　　　M25.619　Stiffness of unspecified shoulder, not elsewhere classified
● M25.62　Stiffness of elbow, not elsewhere classified
　　　M25.621　Stiffness of right elbow, not elsewhere classified
　　　M25.622　Stiffness of left elbow, not elsewhere classified
　　　M25.629　Stiffness of unspecified elbow, not elsewhere classified
● M25.63　Stiffness of wrist, not elsewhere classified
　　　M25.631　Stiffness of right wrist, not elsewhere classified
　　　M25.632　Stiffness of left wrist, not elsewhere classified
　　　M25.639　Stiffness of unspecified wrist, not elsewhere classified

▶ New　⟹ Revised　deleted Deleted　OGCR Official Guidelines　X Assign placeholder X　● Use Additional Character(s)
Excludes 1　Excludes 2　Includes　Use additional　Code first　Code also　Key words

● M25.64 Stiffness of hand, not elsewhere classified
    M25.641 Stiffness of right hand, not elsewhere classified
    M25.642 Stiffness of left hand, not elsewhere classified
    M25.649 Stiffness of unspecified hand, not elsewhere classified
● M25.65 Stiffness of hip, not elsewhere classified
    M25.651 Stiffness of right hip, not elsewhere classified
    M25.652 Stiffness of left hip, not elsewhere classified
    M25.659 Stiffness of unspecified hip, not elsewhere classified
● M25.66 Stiffness of knee, not elsewhere classified
    M25.661 Stiffness of right knee, not elsewhere classified
    M25.662 Stiffness of left knee, not elsewhere classified
    M25.669 Stiffness of unspecified knee, not elsewhere classified
● M25.67 Stiffness of ankle and foot, not elsewhere classified
    M25.671 Stiffness of right ankle, not elsewhere classified
    M25.672 Stiffness of left ankle, not elsewhere classified
    M25.673 Stiffness of unspecified ankle, not elsewhere classified
    M25.674 Stiffness of right foot, not elsewhere classified
    M25.675 Stiffness of left foot, not elsewhere classified
    M25.676 Stiffness of unspecified foot, not elsewhere classified
● M25.7 Osteophyte
    M25.70 Osteophyte, unspecified joint
● M25.71 Osteophyte, shoulder
    M25.711 Osteophyte, right shoulder
    M25.712 Osteophyte, left shoulder
    M25.719 Osteophyte, unspecified shoulder
● M25.72 Osteophyte, elbow
    M25.721 Osteophyte, right elbow
    M25.722 Osteophyte, left elbow
    M25.729 Osteophyte, unspecified elbow
● M25.73 Osteophyte, wrist
    M25.731 Osteophyte, right wrist
    M25.732 Osteophyte, left wrist
    M25.739 Osteophyte, unspecified wrist
● M25.74 Osteophyte, hand
    M25.741 Osteophyte, right hand
    M25.742 Osteophyte, left hand
    M25.749 Osteophyte, unspecified hand
● M25.75 Osteophyte, hip
    M25.751 Osteophyte, right hip
    M25.752 Osteophyte, left hip
    M25.759 Osteophyte, unspecified hip
● M25.76 Osteophyte, knee
    M25.761 Osteophyte, right knee
    M25.762 Osteophyte, left knee
    M25.769 Osteophyte, unspecified knee

● M25.77 Osteophyte, ankle and foot
    M25.771 Osteophyte, right ankle
    M25.772 Osteophyte, left ankle
    M25.773 Osteophyte, unspecified ankle
    M25.774 Osteophyte, right foot
    M25.775 Osteophyte, left foot
    M25.776 Osteophyte, unspecified foot
    M25.78 Osteophyte, vertebrae
● M25.8 Other specified joint disorders
    M25.80 Other specified joint disorders, unspecified joint
● M25.81 Other specified joint disorders, shoulder
    M25.811 Other specified joint disorders, right shoulder
    M25.812 Other specified joint disorders, left shoulder
    M25.819 Other specified joint disorders, unspecified shoulder
● M25.82 Other specified joint disorders, elbow
    M25.821 Other specified joint disorders, right elbow
    M25.822 Other specified joint disorders, left elbow
    M25.829 Other specified joint disorders, unspecified elbow
● M25.83 Other specified joint disorders, wrist
    M25.831 Other specified joint disorders, right wrist
    M25.832 Other specified joint disorders, left wrist
    M25.839 Other specified joint disorders, unspecified wrist
● M25.84 Other specified joint disorders, hand
    M25.841 Other specified joint disorders, right hand
    M25.842 Other specified joint disorders, left hand
    M25.849 Other specified joint disorders, unspecified hand
● M25.85 Other specified joint disorders, hip
    M25.851 Other specified joint disorders, right hip
    M25.852 Other specified joint disorders, left hip
    M25.859 Other specified joint disorders, unspecified hip
● M25.86 Other specified joint disorders, knee
    M25.861 Other specified joint disorders, right knee
    M25.862 Other specified joint disorders, left knee
    M25.869 Other specified joint disorders, unspecified knee
● M25.87 Other specified joint disorders, ankle and foot
    M25.871 Other specified joint disorders, right ankle and foot
    M25.872 Other specified joint disorders, left ankle and foot
    M25.879 Other specified joint disorders, unspecified ankle and foot
    M25.9 Joint disorder, unspecified

CHAPTER 13 (M00-M99)

Figure 13-3   Dentofacial malocclusion.

Item 13–6 Hyperplasia is a condition of overdevelopment, whereas **hypoplasia** is a condition of underdevelopment. **Macrogenia** is overdevelopment of the chin, whereas **microgenia** is underdevelopment of the chin.

DENTOFACIAL ANOMALIES [INCLUDING MALOCCLUSION] AND OTHER DISORDERS OF JAW (M26-M27)

> **Excludes1**   hemifacial atrophy or hypertrophy (Q67.4)
> unilateral condylar hyperplasia or hypoplasia (M27.8)

● **M26**   Dentofacial anomalies [including malocclusion]

   ● **M26.0**   Major anomalies of jaw size

> **Excludes1**   acromegaly (E22.0)
> Robin's syndrome (Q87.0)

     M26.00   Unspecified anomaly of jaw size

     M26.01   Maxillary hyperplasia

     M26.02   Maxillary hypoplasia

     M26.03   Mandibular hyperplasia

     M26.04   Mandibular hypoplasia

     M26.05   Macrogenia

     M26.06   Microgenia

     M26.07   Excessive tuberosity of jaw
              Entire maxillary tuberosity

     M26.09   Other specified anomalies of jaw size

   ● **M26.1**   Anomalies of jaw-cranial base relationship

     M26.10   Unspecified anomaly of jaw-cranial base relationship

     M26.11   Maxillary asymmetry

     M26.12   Other jaw asymmetry

     M26.19   Other specified anomalies of jaw-cranial base relationship

   ● **M26.2**   Anomalies of dental arch relationship

     M26.20   Unspecified anomaly of dental arch relationship

     ● **M26.21**   Malocclusion, Angle's class

       M26.211   Malocclusion, Angle's class I
                Neutro-occlusion

       M26.212   Malocclusion, Angle's class II
                Disto-occlusion Division I
                Disto-occlusion Division II

       M26.213   Malocclusion, Angle's class III
                Mesio-occlusion

       M26.219   Malocclusion, Angle's class, unspecified

     ● **M26.22**   Open occlusal relationship

       M26.220   Open anterior occlusal relationship
                Anterior openbite

       M26.221   Open posterior occlusal relationship
                Posterior openbite

     M26.23   Excessive horizontal overlap
              Excessive horizontal overjet

     M26.24   Reverse articulation
              Crossbite (anterior) (posterior)

     M26.25   Anomalies of interarch distance

     M26.29   Other anomalies of dental arch relationship
              Midline deviation of dental arch
              Overbite (excessive) deep
              Overbite (excessive) horizontal
              Overbite (excessive) vertical
              Posterior lingual occlusion of mandibular teeth

   ● **M26.3**   Anomalies of tooth position of fully erupted tooth or teeth

> **Excludes2**   embedded and impacted teeth (K01.-)

     M26.30   Unspecified anomaly of tooth position of fully erupted tooth or teeth
              Abnormal spacing of fully erupted tooth or teeth NOS
              Displacement of fully erupted tooth or teeth NOS
              Transposition of fully erupted tooth or teeth NOS

     M26.31   Crowding of fully erupted teeth

     M26.32   Excessive spacing of fully erupted teeth
              Diastema of fully erupted tooth or teeth NOS

     M26.33   Horizontal displacement of fully erupted tooth or teeth
              Tipped tooth or teeth
              Tipping of fully erupted tooth

     M26.34   Vertical displacement of fully erupted tooth or teeth
              Extruded tooth
              Infraeruption of tooth or teeth
              Supraeruption of tooth or teeth

     M26.35   Rotation of fully erupted tooth or teeth

     M26.36   Insufficient interocclusal distance of fully erupted teeth (ridge)
              Lack of adequate intermaxillary vertical dimension of fully erupted teeth

     M26.37   Excessive interocclusal distance of fully erupted teeth
              Excessive intermaxillary vertical dimension of fully erupted teeth
              Loss of occlusal vertical dimension of fully erupted teeth

     M26.39   Other anomalies of tooth position of fully erupted tooth or teeth

   M26.4   Malocclusion, unspecified

   ● **M26.5**   Dentofacial functional abnormalities

> **Excludes1**   bruxism (F45.8)
> teeth-grinding NOS (F45.8)

     M26.50   Dentofacial functional abnormalities, unspecified

     M26.51   Abnormal jaw closure

     M26.52   Limited mandibular range of motion

     M26.53   Deviation in opening and closing of the mandible

     M26.54   Insufficient anterior guidance
              Insufficient anterior occlusal guidance

     M26.55   Centric occlusion maximum intercuspation discrepancy

> **Excludes1**   centric occlusion NOS (M26.59)

     M26.56   Non-working side interference
              Balancing side interference

     M26.57   Lack of posterior occlusal support

     M26.59   Other dentofacial functional abnormalities
              Centric occlusion (of teeth) NOS
              Malocclusion due to abnormal swallowing
              Malocclusion due to mouth breathing
              Malocclusion due to tongue, lip or finger habits

▶ New   ➡ Revised   ~~deleted~~ Deleted   **OGCR** Official Guidelines   X Assign placeholder X   ● Use Additional Character(s)

Excludes 1   Excludes 2   Includes   Use additional   Code first   Code also   Key words

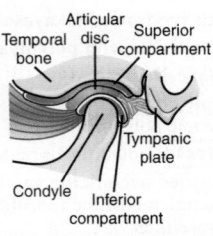

Figure 13-4   Temporomandibular joint.

Item 13–7 Dysfunction of the temporomandibular joint is termed **temporomandibular joint (TMJ) syndrome** and is characterized by pain and tenderness/spasm of the muscles of mastication, joint noise, and in the later stages, limited mandibular movement.

● **M26.6 Temporomandibular joint disorders**
     Excludes2   current temporomandibular joint
                   dislocation (S03.0)
                   current temporomandibular joint sprain
                   (S03.4)

   ● **M26.60 Temporomandibular joint disorder, unspecified**
         M26.601 Right temporomandibular joint disorder, unspecified
         M26.602 Left temporomandibular joint disorder, unspecified
         M26.603 Bilateral temporomandibular joint disorder, unspecified
         M26.609 Unspecified temporomandibular joint disorder, unspecified side
                 Temporomandibular joint disorder NOS

   ● **M26.61 Adhesions and ankylosis of temporomandibular joint**
         M26.611 Adhesions and ankylosis of right temporomandibular joint
         M26.612 Adhesions and ankylosis of left temporomandibular joint
         M26.613 Adhesions and ankylosis of bilateral temporomandibular joint
         M26.619 Adhesions and ankylosis of temporomandibular joint, unspecified side

   ● **M26.62 Arthralgia of temporomandibular joint**
         M26.621 Arthralgia of right temporomandibular joint
         M26.622 Arthralgia of left temporomandibular joint
         M26.623 Arthralgia of bilateral temporomandibular joint
         M26.629 Arthralgia of temporomandibular joint, unspecified side

   ● **M26.63 Articular disc disorder of temporomandibular joint**
         M26.631 Articular disc disorder of right temporomandibular joint
         M26.632 Articular disc disorder of left temporomandibular joint
         M26.633 Articular disc disorder of bilateral temporomandibular joint
         M26.639 Articular disc disorder of temporomandibular joint, unspecified side
     M26.69 Other specified disorders of temporomandibular joint

● **M26.7 Dental alveolar anomalies**
     M26.70 Unspecified alveolar anomaly
     M26.71 Alveolar maxillary hyperplasia
     M26.72 Alveolar mandibular hyperplasia
     M26.73 Alveolar maxillary hypoplasia
     M26.74 Alveolar mandibular hypoplasia
     M26.79 Other specified alveolar anomalies
● **M26.8 Other dentofacial anomalies**
     M26.81 Anterior soft tissue impingement
           Anterior soft tissue impingement on teeth
     M26.82 Posterior soft tissue impingement
           Posterior soft tissue impingement on teeth
     M26.89 Other dentofacial anomalies
     M26.9 Dentofacial anomaly, unspecified
● **M27 Other diseases of jaws**
     M27.0 Developmental disorders of jaws
           Latent bone cyst of jaw
           Stafne's cyst
           Torus mandibularis
           Torus palatinus
     M27.1 Giant cell granuloma, central
           Giant cell granuloma NOS
         Excludes1   peripheral giant cell granuloma (K06.8)
     M27.2 Inflammatory conditions of jaws
           Osteitis of jaw(s)
           Osteomyelitis (neonatal) jaw(s)
           Osteoradionecrosis jaw(s)
           Periostitis jaw(s)
           Sequestrum of jaw bone
         Use additional code (W88-W90, X39.0) to identify
           radiation, if radiation-induced
         Excludes2   osteonecrosis of jaw due to drug
                   (M87.180)
     M27.3 Alveolitis of jaws
           Alveolar osteitis
           Dry socket
● **M27.4 Other and unspecified cysts of jaw**
         Excludes1   cysts of oral region (K09.-)
                   latent bone cyst of jaw (M27.0)
                   Stafne's cyst (M27.0)
     M27.40 Unspecified cyst of jaw
           Cyst of jaw NOS
     M27.49 Other cysts of jaw
           Aneurysmal cyst of jaw
           Hemorrhagic cyst of jaw
           Traumatic cyst of jaw
● **M27.5 Periradicular pathology associated with previous endodontic treatment**
     M27.51 Perforation of root canal space due to endodontic treatment
     M27.52 Endodontic overfill
     M27.53 Endodontic underfill
     M27.59 Other periradicular pathology associated with previous endodontic treatment
● **M27.6 Endosseous dental implant failure**
     M27.61 Osseointegration failure of dental implant
           Hemorrhagic complications of dental implant placement
           Iatrogenic osseointegration failure of dental implant
           Osseointegration failure of dental implant due to complications of systemic disease
           Osseointegration failure of dental implant due to poor bone quality
           Pre-integration failure of dental implant NOS
           Pre-osseointegration failure of dental implant

CHAPTER 13 (M00-M99)

M27.62 **Post-osseointegration biological** failure of dental implant
     Failure of dental implant due to lack of attached gingiva
     Failure of dental implant due to occlusal trauma (caused by poor prosthetic design)
     Failure of dental implant due to parafunctional habits
     Failure of dental implant due to periodontal infection (peri–implantitis)
     Failure of dental implant due to poor oral hygiene
     Iatrogenic post-osseointegration failure of dental implant
     Post-osseointegration failure of dental implant due to complications of systemic disease

M27.63 **Post-osseointegration mechanical** failure of dental implant
     Failure of dental prosthesis causing loss of dental implant
     Fracture of dental implant
     Excludes2   cracked tooth (K03.81)
                 fractured dental restorative material with loss of material (K08.531)
                 fractured dental restorative material without loss of material (K08.530)
                 fractured tooth (S02.5)

M27.69 **Other endosseous dental implant failure**
     Dental implant failure NOS

M27.8 **Other** specified diseases of jaws
     Cherubism
     Exostosis
     Fibrous dysplasia
     Unilateral condylar hyperplasia
     Unilateral condylar hypoplasia
     Excludes1   jaw pain (R68.84)

M27.9 Disease of jaws, **unspecified**

SYSTEMIC CONNECTIVE TISSUE DISORDERS (M30-M36)

Includes   autoimmune disease NOS
           collagen (vascular) disease NOS
           systemic autoimmune disease
           systemic collagen (vascular) disease

Excludes1   autoimmune disease, single organ or single cell-type - code to relevant condition category

● M30   Polyarteritis nodosa and related conditions
     Excludes1   microscopic polyarteritis (M31.7)

M30.0   Polyarteritis nodosa

M30.1   Polyarteritis with **lung involvement** [Churg-Strauss]
     Allergic granulomatous angiitis

M30.2   **Juvenile** polyarteritis

M30.3   Mucocutaneous lymph node syndrome [Kawasaki]

M30.8   **Other** conditions related to polyarteritis nodosa
     Polyangiitis overlap syndrome

● M31   Other necrotizing vasculopathies

M31.0   Hypersensitivity angiitis
     Goodpasture's syndrome

M31.1   Thrombotic microangiopathy
     Thrombotic thrombocytopenic purpura

M31.2   Lethal midline granuloma

● M31.3   Wegener's granulomatosis
     Necrotizing respiratory granulomatosis

M31.30   Wegener's granulomatosis **without renal involvement**
     Wegener's granulomatosis NOS

M31.31   Wegener's granulomatosis **with renal involvement**

M31.4   Aortic arch syndrome [Takayasu]

M31.5   Giant cell arteritis with polymyalgia rheumatica

M31.6   Other giant cell arteritis

M31.7   Microscopic polyangiitis
     Microscopic polyarteritis
     Excludes1   polyarteritis nodosa (M30.0)

M31.8   Other specified necrotizing vasculopathies
     Hypocomplementemic vasculitis
     Septic vasculitis

M31.9   Necrotizing vasculopathy, **unspecified**

● M32   Systemic lupus erythematosus (SLE)
     Autoimmune inflammatory connective tissue disease of unknown cause that occurs most often in women
     Excludes1   lupus erythematosus (discoid) (NOS) (L93.0)

M32.0   **Drug-induced** systemic lupus erythematosus
     Use additional code for adverse effect, if applicable, to identify drug (T36-T50 with fifth or sixth character 5)

● M32.1   Systemic lupus erythematosus **with organ or system involvement**

M32.10   Systemic lupus erythematosus, organ or system involvement **unspecified**

M32.11   **Endocarditis** in systemic lupus erythematosus
     Libman-Sacks disease

M32.12   **Pericarditis** in systemic lupus erythematosus
     Lupus pericarditis

M32.13   **Lung** involvement in systemic lupus erythematosus
     Pleural effusion due to systemic lupus erythematosus

M32.14   **Glomerular disease** in systemic lupus erythematosus
     Lupus renal disease NOS

M32.15   **Tubulo-interstitial nephropathy** in systemic lupus erythematosus

M32.19   **Other** organ or system involvement in systemic lupus erythematosus

M32.8   **Other forms** of systemic lupus erythematosus

M32.9   Systemic lupus erythematosus, **unspecified**
     SLE NOS
     Systemic lupus erythematosus NOS
     Systemic lupus erythematosus without organ involvement

● M33   Dermatopolymyositis

⇒● M33.0   **Juvenile** dermatomyositis

⇒ M33.00   Juvenile dermatomyositis, organ involvement **unspecified**

⇒ M33.01   Juvenile dermatomyositis with **respiratory** involvement

⇒ M33.02   Juvenile dermatomyositis with **myopathy**

▶ M33.03   Juvenile dermatomyositis **without myopathy**

⇒ M33.09   Juvenile dermatomyositis **with other organ** involvement

⇒● M33.1   **Other dermatomyositis**
     ▶Adult dermatomyositis

⇒ M33.10   Other dermatomyositis, organ involvement **unspecified**

⇒ M33.11   Other dermatomyositis with **respiratory** involvement

⇒ M33.12   Other dermatomyositis with **myopathy**

▶ M33.13   Other dermatomyositis **without myopathy**
     ▶Dermatomyositis NOS

⇒ M33.19   Other dermatomyositis with **other organ** involvement

---

▶ New   ⇒ Revised   ~~deleted~~ Deleted   **OGCR** Official Guidelines   X Assign placeholder X   ● Use Additional Character(s)

| Excludes 1 | Excludes 2 | Includes | Use additional | Code first | Code also | Key words |

Item 13–8 Polymyalgia rheumatica is a syndrome characterized by aching and morning stiffness and is related to aging and hereditary predisposition.

- ● **M33.2 Polymyositis**
  - M33.20 Polymyositis, organ involvement unspecified
  - M33.21 Polymyositis with respiratory involvement
  - M33.22 Polymyositis with myopathy
  - M33.29 Polymyositis with other organ involvement
- ● **M33.9 Dermatopolymyositis, unspecified**
  - M33.90 Dermatopolymyositis, unspecified, organ involvement unspecified
  - M33.91 Dermatopolymyositis, unspecified with respiratory involvement
  - M33.92 Dermatopolymyositis, unspecified with myopathy
  - ▶ M33.93 Dermatopolymyositis, unspecified without myopathy
  - M33.99 Dermatopolymyositis, unspecified with other organ involvement
- ● **M34 Systemic sclerosis [scleroderma]**
  - **Excludes1**   circumscribed scleroderma (L94.0)
    neonatal scleroderma (P83.8)
  - M34.0 Progressive systemic sclerosis
  - M34.1 CR(E)ST syndrome
    - Combination of calcinosis, Raynaud's phenomenon, esophageal dysfunction, sclerodactyly, telangiectasia
  - M34.2 Systemic sclerosis induced by drug and chemical
    - *Code first* poisoning due to drug or toxin, if applicable (T36-T65 with fifth or sixth character 1-4 or 6)
    - Use additional code for adverse effect, if applicable, to identify drug (T36-T50 with fifth or sixth character 5)
  - ● M34.8 Other forms of systemic sclerosis
    - M34.81 Systemic sclerosis with lung involvement
    - M34.82 Systemic sclerosis with myopathy
    - M34.83 Systemic sclerosis with polyneuropathy
    - M34.89 Other systemic sclerosis
  - M34.9 Systemic sclerosis, unspecified
- ● **M35 Other systemic involvement of connective tissue**
  - **Excludes1**   reactive perforating collagenosis (L87.1)
  - ● M35.0 Sicca syndrome [Sjögren]
    - M35.00 Sicca syndrome, unspecified
    - M35.01 Sicca syndrome with keratoconjunctivitis
    - M35.02 Sicca syndrome with lung involvement
    - M35.03 Sicca syndrome with myopathy
    - M35.04 Sicca syndrome with tubulo-interstitial nephropathy
      - Renal tubular acidosis in sicca syndrome
    - M35.09 Sicca syndrome with other organ involvement
  - M35.1 Other overlap syndromes
    - Mixed connective tissue disease
    - **Excludes1**   polyangiitis overlap syndrome (M30.8)
  - M35.2 Behçet's disease
  - M35.3 Polymyalgia rheumatica
    - **Excludes1**   polymyalgia rheumatica with giant cell arteritis (M31.5)

- M35.4 Diffuse (eosinophilic) fasciitis
- M35.5 Multifocal fibrosclerosis
- M35.6 Relapsing panniculitis [Weber-Christian]
  - **Excludes1**   lupus panniculitis (L93.2)
    panniculitis NOS (M79.3-)
- M35.7 Hypermobility syndrome
  - Familial ligamentous laxity
  - **Excludes1**   Ehlers-Danlos syndrome (Q79.6)
    ligamentous laxity, NOS (M24.2-)
- M35.8 Other specified systemic involvement of connective tissue
- M35.9 Systemic involvement of connective tissue, unspecified
  - Autoimmune disease (systemic) NOS
  - Collagen (vascular) disease NOS
- ● **M36 Systemic disorders of connective tissue in diseases classified elsewhere**
  - **Excludes2**   arthropathies in diseases classified elsewhere (M14.-)
  - M36.0 Dermato(poly)myositis in neoplastic disease
    - *Code first* underlying neoplasm (C00-D49)
  - M36.1 Arthropathy in neoplastic disease
    - *Code first* underlying neoplasm, such as:
      - leukemia (C91-C95)
      - malignant histiocytosis (C96.A)
      - multiple myeloma (C90.0)
  - M36.2 Hemophilic arthropathy
    - Hemarthrosis in hemophilic arthropathy
    - *Code first* underlying disease, such as:
      - factor VIII deficiency (D66)
      - with vascular defect (D68.0)
      - factor IX deficiency (D67)
      - hemophilia (classical) (D66)
      - hemophilia B (D67)
      - hemophilia C (D68.1)
  - M36.3 Arthropathy in other blood disorders
  - M36.4 Arthropathy in hypersensitivity reactions classified elsewhere
    - *Code first* underlying disease, such as:
      - Henoch (-Schönlein) purpura (D69.0)
      - serum sickness (T80.6-)
  - M36.8 Systemic disorders of connective tissue in other diseases classified elsewhere
    - *Code first* underlying disease, such as:
      - alkaptonuria (E70.2)
      - hypogammaglobulinemia (D80.-)
      - ochronosis (E70.2)

DORSOPATHIES (M40-M54)

DEFORMING DORSOPATHIES (M40-M43)

- ● **M40 Kyphosis and lordosis**
  - **Excludes1**   congenital kyphosis and lordosis (Q76.4)
    kyphoscoliosis (M41.-)
    postprocedural kyphosis and lordosis (M96.-)
  - ● M40.0 Postural kyphosis
    - **Excludes1**   osteochondrosis of spine (M42.-)
    - M40.00 Postural kyphosis, site unspecified
    - M40.03 Postural kyphosis, cervicothoracic region
    - M40.04 Postural kyphosis, thoracic region
    - M40.05 Postural kyphosis, thoracolumbar region

CHAPTER 13 (M00-M99)

▶ New   ⇒ Revised   ~~deleted~~ Deleted   **OGCR** Official Guidelines   X Assign placeholder X   ● Use Additional Character(s)

Excludes 1   Excludes 2   Includes   Use additional   Code first   Code also   Key words

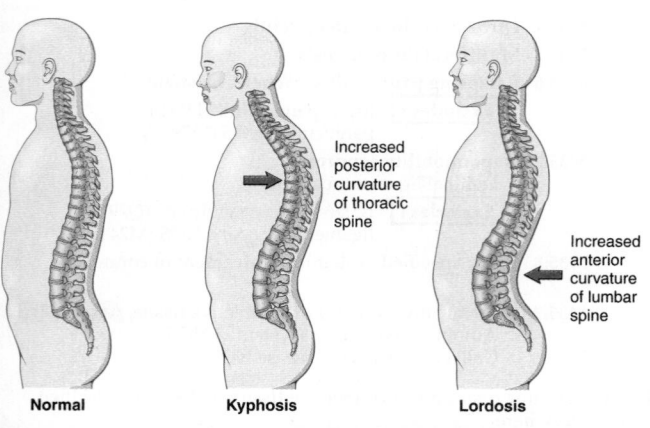

Normal   **Kyphosis**   **Lordosis**

Increased posterior curvature of thoracic spine

Increased anterior curvature of lumbar spine

Figure 13-5   Kyphosis, Lordosis, Scoliosis. (From Chabner: The Language of Medicine, ed 8, St. Louis, Saunders, 2007)

Item 13–9 Kyphosis is an abnormal curvature of the spine. **Senile kyphosis** is a result of disc degeneration causing ossification (turning to bone). **Adolescent** or **juvenile** kyphosis is also known as **Scheuermann's disease,** a condition in which the discs of the lower thoracic spine herniate, causing the disc space to narrow and the spine to tilt forward. This condition is attributed to poor posture. **Lordosis or swayback** is an abnormal curvature of the spine resulting in an inward curve of the lumbar spine just above the buttocks. **Scoliosis** causes a sideways curve to the spine. The curves are S- or C-shaped, and it is most commonly acquired in late childhood and early teen years, when growth is fast.

- M40.1   Other secondary kyphosis
  - M40.10   Other secondary kyphosis, site unspecified
  - M40.12   Other secondary kyphosis, cervical region
  - M40.13   Other secondary kyphosis, cervicothoracic region
  - M40.14   Other secondary kyphosis, thoracic region
  - M40.15   Other secondary kyphosis, thoracolumbar region
- M40.2   Other and unspecified kyphosis
  - M40.20   Unspecified kyphosis
    - M40.202   Unspecified kyphosis, cervical region
    - M40.203   Unspecified kyphosis, cervicothoracic region
    - M40.204   Unspecified kyphosis, thoracic region
    - M40.205   Unspecified kyphosis, thoracolumbar region
    - M40.209   Unspecified kyphosis, site unspecified
  - M40.29   Other kyphosis
    - M40.292   Other kyphosis, cervical region
    - M40.293   Other kyphosis, cervicothoracic region
    - M40.294   Other kyphosis, thoracic region
    - M40.295   Other kyphosis, thoracolumbar region
    - M40.299   Other kyphosis, site unspecified
- M40.3   Flatback syndrome
  - M40.30   Flatback syndrome, site unspecified
  - M40.35   Flatback syndrome, thoracolumbar region
  - M40.36   Flatback syndrome, lumbar region
  - M40.37   Flatback syndrome, lumbosacral region

- M40.4   Postural lordosis
  Abnormal increase in the normal curvature of the lumbar spine (sway back)
  Acquired lordosis
  - M40.40   Postural lordosis, site unspecified
  - M40.45   Postural lordosis, thoracolumbar region
  - M40.46   Postural lordosis, lumbar region
  - M40.47   Postural lordosis, lumbosacral region
- M40.5   Lordosis, unspecified
  - M40.50   Lordosis, unspecified, site unspecified
  - M40.55   Lordosis, unspecified, thoracolumbar region
  - M40.56   Lordosis, unspecified, lumbar region
  - M40.57   Lordosis, unspecified, lumbosacral region
- M41   Scoliosis
  - **Includes**   kyphoscoliosis
  - **Excludes1**   congenital scoliosis NOS (Q67.5)
    congenital scoliosis due to bony malformation (Q76.3)
    postural congenital scoliosis (Q67.5)
    kyphoscoliotic heart disease (I27.1)
    postprocedural scoliosis (M96.-)
  - M41.0   Infantile idiopathic scoliosis
    - M41.00   Infantile idiopathic scoliosis, site unspecified
    - M41.02   Infantile idiopathic scoliosis, cervical region
    - M41.03   Infantile idiopathic scoliosis, cervicothoracic region
    - M41.04   Infantile idiopathic scoliosis, thoracic region
    - M41.05   Infantile idiopathic scoliosis, thoracolumbar region
    - M41.06   Infantile idiopathic scoliosis, lumbar region
    - M41.07   Infantile idiopathic scoliosis, lumbosacral region
    - M41.08   Infantile idiopathic scoliosis, sacral and sacrococcygeal region
  - M41.1   Juvenile and adolescent idiopathic scoliosis
    - M41.11   Juvenile idiopathic scoliosis
      - M41.112   Juvenile idiopathic scoliosis, cervical region
      - M41.113   Juvenile idiopathic scoliosis, cervicothoracic region
      - M41.114   Juvenile idiopathic scoliosis, thoracic region
      - M41.115   Juvenile idiopathic scoliosis, thoracolumbar region
      - M41.116   Juvenile idiopathic scoliosis, lumbar region
      - M41.117   Juvenile idiopathic scoliosis, lumbosacral region
      - M41.119   Juvenile idiopathic scoliosis, site unspecified
    - M41.12   Adolescent scoliosis
      - M41.122   Adolescent idiopathic scoliosis, cervical region
      - M41.123   Adolescent idiopathic scoliosis, cervicothoracic region
      - M41.124   Adolescent idiopathic scoliosis, thoracic region
      - M41.125   Adolescent idiopathic scoliosis, thoracolumbar region
      - M41.126   Adolescent idiopathic scoliosis, lumbar region
      - M41.127   Adolescent idiopathic scoliosis, lumbosacral region
      - M41.129   Adolescent idiopathic scoliosis, site unspecified

▶ New   ⇒ Revised   ~~deleted~~ Deleted   **OGCR** Official Guidelines   X Assign placeholder X   ● Use Additional Character(s)

Excludes 1   Excludes 2   Includes   Use additional   Code first   Code also   Key words

● **M41.2** Other idiopathic scoliosis

     M41.20   Other idiopathic scoliosis, site unspecified

     M41.22   Other idiopathic scoliosis, cervical region

     M41.23   Other idiopathic scoliosis, cervicothoracic region

     M41.24   Other idiopathic scoliosis, thoracic region

     M41.25   Other idiopathic scoliosis, thoracolumbar region

     M41.26   Other idiopathic scoliosis, lumbar region

     M41.27   Other idiopathic scoliosis, lumbosacral region

● **M41.3** Thoracogenic scoliosis

     M41.30   Thoracogenic scoliosis, site unspecified

     M41.34   Thoracogenic scoliosis, thoracic region

     M41.35   Thoracogenic scoliosis, thoracolumbar region

● **M41.4** Neuromuscular scoliosis

     Scoliosis secondary to cerebral palsy, Friedreich's ataxia, poliomyelitis and other neuromuscular disorders

     Code also underlying condition

     M41.40   Neuromuscular scoliosis, site unspecified

     M41.41   Neuromuscular scoliosis, occipito-atlanto-axial region

     M41.42   Neuromuscular scoliosis, cervical region

     M41.43   Neuromuscular scoliosis, cervicothoracic region

     M41.44   Neuromuscular scoliosis, thoracic region

     M41.45   Neuromuscular scoliosis, thoracolumbar region

     M41.46   Neuromuscular scoliosis, lumbar region

     M41.47   Neuromuscular scoliosis, lumbosacral region

● **M41.5** Other secondary scoliosis

     M41.50   Other secondary scoliosis, site unspecified

     M41.52   Other secondary scoliosis, cervical region

     M41.53   Other secondary scoliosis, cervicothoracic region

     M41.54   Other secondary scoliosis, thoracic region

     M41.55   Other secondary scoliosis, thoracolumbar region

     M41.56   Other secondary scoliosis, lumbar region

     M41.57   Other secondary scoliosis, lumbosacral region

● **M41.8** Other forms of scoliosis

     M41.80   Other forms of scoliosis, site unspecified

     M41.82   Other forms of scoliosis, cervical region

     M41.83   Other forms of scoliosis, cervicothoracic region

     M41.84   Other forms of scoliosis, thoracic region

     M41.85   Other forms of scoliosis, thoracolumbar region

     M41.86   Other forms of scoliosis, lumbar region

     M41.87   Other forms of scoliosis, lumbosacral region

     M41.9   Scoliosis, unspecified

● **M42** Spinal osteochondrosis

● **M42.0** Juvenile osteochondrosis of spine

     Calvé's disease

     Scheuermann's disease

     Excludes1   postural kyphosis (M40.0)

     M42.00   Juvenile osteochondrosis of spine, site unspecified

     M42.01   Juvenile osteochondrosis of spine, occipito-atlanto-axial region

     M42.02   Juvenile osteochondrosis of spine, cervical region

     M42.03   Juvenile osteochondrosis of spine, cervicothoracic region

     M42.04   Juvenile osteochondrosis of spine, thoracic region

     M42.05   Juvenile osteochondrosis of spine, thoracolumbar region

     M42.06   Juvenile osteochondrosis of spine, lumbar region

     M42.07   Juvenile osteochondrosis of spine, lumbosacral region

     M42.08   Juvenile osteochondrosis of spine, sacral and sacrococcygeal region

     M42.09   Juvenile osteochondrosis of spine, multiple sites in spine

● **M42.1** Adult osteochondrosis of spine

     M42.10   Adult osteochondrosis of spine, site unspecified

     M42.11   Adult osteochondrosis of spine, occipitoatlanto-axial region

     M42.12   Adult osteochondrosis of spine, cervical region

     M42.13   Adult osteochondrosis of spine, cervicothoracic region

     M42.14   Adult osteochondrosis of spine, thoracic region

     M42.15   Adult osteochondrosis of spine, thoracolumbar region

     M42.16   Adult osteochondrosis of spine, lumbar region

     M42.17   Adult osteochondrosis of spine, lumbosacral region

     M42.18   Adult osteochondrosis of spine, sacral and sacrococcygeal region

     M42.19   Adult osteochondrosis of spine, multiple sites in spine

     M42.9   Spinal osteochondrosis, unspecified

● **M43** Other deforming dorsopathies

     Excludes1   congenital spondylolysis and spondylolisthesis (Q76.2)

         hemivertebra (Q76.3-Q76.4)

         Klippel-Feil syndrome (Q76.1)

         lumbarization and sacralization (Q76.4)

         platyspondylisis (Q76.4)

         spina bifida occulta (Q76.0)

         spinal curvature in osteoporosis (M80.-)

         spinal curvature in Paget's disease of bone [osteitis deformans] (M88.-)

● **M43.0** Spondylolysis

     Excludes1   congenital spondylolysis (Q76.2)

         spondylolisthesis (M43.1)

     M43.00   Spondylolysis, site unspecified

     M43.01   Spondylolysis, occipito-atlanto-axial region

     M43.02   Spondylolysis, cervical region

     M43.03   Spondylolysis, cervicothoracic region

     M43.04   Spondylolysis, thoracic region

     M43.05   Spondylolysis, thoracolumbar region

     M43.06   Spondylolysis, lumbar region

     M43.07   Spondylolysis, lumbosacral region

     M43.08   Spondylolysis, sacral and sacrococcygeal region

     M43.09   Spondylolysis, multiple sites in spine

▶ New   ⇒ Revised   ~~deleted~~ Deleted   **OGCR** Official Guidelines   **X** Assign placeholder X   ● Use Additional Character(s)

Excludes 1   Excludes 2   Includes   Use additional   Code first   Code also   Key words

985

Item 13–10 **Spondylolisthesis** is a condition caused by the slipping forward of one disc over another.

- **M43.1** Spondylolisthesis
    - **Excludes1**   acute traumatic of lumbosacral region (S33.1)
    - acute traumatic of sites other than lumbosacral - code to Fracture, vertebra, by region
    - congenital spondylolisthesis (Q76.2)
    - M43.10   Spondylolisthesis, site unspecified
    - M43.11   Spondylolisthesis, occipito-atlanto-axial region
    - M43.12   Spondylolisthesis, cervical region
    - M43.13   Spondylolisthesis, cervicothoracic region
    - M43.14   Spondylolisthesis, thoracic region
    - M43.15   Spondylolisthesis, thoracolumbar region
    - M43.16   Spondylolisthesis, lumbar region
    - M43.17   Spondylolisthesis, lumbosacral region
    - M43.18   Spondylolisthesis, sacral and sacrococcygeal region
    - M43.19   Spondylolisthesis, multiple sites in spine
- **M43.2** Fusion of spine
    - Ankylosis of spinal joint
    - **Excludes1**   ankylosing spondylitis (M45.0-)
    - congenital fusion of spine (Q76.4)
    - **Excludes2**   arthrodesis status (Z98.1)
    - pseudoarthrosis after fusion or arthrodesis (M96.0)
    - M43.20   Fusion of spine, site unspecified
    - M43.21   Fusion of spine, occipito-atlanto-axial region
    - M43.22   Fusion of spine, cervical region
    - M43.23   Fusion of spine, cervicothoracic region
    - M43.24   Fusion of spine, thoracic region
    - M43.25   Fusion of spine, thoracolumbar region
    - M43.26   Fusion of spine, lumbar region
    - M43.27   Fusion of spine, lumbosacral region
    - M43.28   Fusion of spine, sacral and sacrococcygeal region
- M43.3   Recurrent atlantoaxial dislocation with myelopathy
- M43.4   Other recurrent atlantoaxial dislocation
- **M43.5** Other recurrent vertebral dislocation
    - **Excludes1**   biomechanical lesions NEC (M99.-)
    - **M43.5X** Other recurrent vertebral dislocation
        - M43.5X2   Other recurrent vertebral dislocation, cervical region
        - M43.5X3   Other recurrent vertebral dislocation, cervicothoracic region
        - M43.5X4   Other recurrent vertebral dislocation, thoracic region
        - M43.5X5   Other recurrent vertebral dislocation, thoracolumbar region
        - M43.5X6   Other recurrent vertebral dislocation, lumbar region
        - M43.5X7   Other recurrent vertebral dislocation, lumbosacral region
        - M43.5X8   Other recurrent vertebral dislocation, sacral and sacrococcygeal region
        - M43.5X9   Other recurrent vertebral dislocation, site unspecified
- M43.6   Torticollis
    - **Excludes1**   congenital (sternomastoid) torticollis (Q68.0)
    - current injury - see Injury, of spine, by body region ocular torticollis (R29.891)
    - psychogenic torticollis (F45.8)
    - spasmodic torticollis (G24.3)
    - torticollis due to birth injury (P15.2)

- **M43.8** Other specified deforming dorsopathies
    - **Excludes2**   kyphosis and lordosis (M40.-)
    - scoliosis (M41.-)
    - **M43.8X** Other specified deforming dorsopathies
        - M43.8X1   Other specified deforming dorsopathies, occipito-atlanto-axial region
        - M43.8X2   Other specified deforming dorsopathies, cervical region
        - M43.8X3   Other specified deforming dorsopathies, cervicothoracic region
        - M43.8X4   Other specified deforming dorsopathies, thoracic region
        - M43.8X5   Other specified deforming dorsopathies, thoracolumbar region
        - M43.8X6   Other specified deforming dorsopathies, lumbar region
        - M43.8X7   Other specified deforming dorsopathies, lumbosacral region
        - M43.8X8   Other specified deforming dorsopathies, sacral and sacrococcygeal region
        - M43.8X9   Other specified deforming dorsopathies, site unspecified
- M43.9   Deforming dorsopathy, unspecified
    - Curvature of spine NOS

SPONDYLOPATHIES (M45-M49)

- **M45** Ankylosing spondylitis
    - Rheumatoid arthritis of spine
    - **Excludes1**   arthropathy in Reiter's disease (M02.3-)
    - juvenile (ankylosing) spondylitis (M08.1)
    - **Excludes2**   Behçet's disease (M35.2)
    - M45.0   Ankylosing spondylitis of multiple sites in spine
    - M45.1   Ankylosing spondylitis of occipito-atlanto-axial region
    - M45.2   Ankylosing spondylitis of cervical region
    - M45.3   Ankylosing spondylitis of cervicothoracic region
    - M45.4   Ankylosing spondylitis of thoracic region
    - M45.5   Ankylosing spondylitis of thoracolumbar region
    - M45.6   Ankylosing spondylitis lumbar region
    - M45.7   Ankylosing spondylitis of lumbosacral region
    - M45.8   Ankylosing spondylitis sacral and sacrococcygeal region
    - M45.9   Ankylosing spondylitis of unspecified sites in spine
- **M46** Other inflammatory spondylopathies
    - **M46.0** Spinal enthesopathy
        - Disorder of ligamentous or muscular attachments of spine
        - M46.00   Spinal enthesopathy, site unspecified
        - M46.01   Spinal enthesopathy, occipito-atlanto-axial region
        - M46.02   Spinal enthesopathy, cervical region
        - M46.03   Spinal enthesopathy, cervicothoracic region
        - M46.04   Spinal enthesopathy, thoracic region
        - M46.05   Spinal enthesopathy, thoracolumbar region
        - M46.06   Spinal enthesopathy, lumbar region
        - M46.07   Spinal enthesopathy, lumbosacral region
        - M46.08   Spinal enthesopathy, sacral and sacrococcygeal region
        - M46.09   Spinal enthesopathy, multiple sites in spine
    - M46.1   Sacroiliitis, not elsewhere classified

▶ New   ⇒ Revised   ~~deleted~~ Deleted   **OGCR** Official Guidelines   X Assign placeholder X   ● Use Additional Character(s)

Excludes 1   Excludes 2   Includes   Use additional   Code first   Code also   Key words

● **M46.2 Osteomyelitis of vertebra**
    M46.2Ø Osteomyelitis of vertebra, site unspecified
    M46.21 Osteomyelitis of vertebra, occipito-atlanto-axial region
    M46.22 Osteomyelitis of vertebra, cervical region
    M46.23 Osteomyelitis of vertebra, cervicothoracic region
    M46.24 Osteomyelitis of vertebra, thoracic region
    M46.25 Osteomyelitis of vertebra, thoracolumbar region
    M46.26 Osteomyelitis of vertebra, lumbar region
    M46.27 Osteomyelitis of vertebra, lumbosacral region
    M46.28 Osteomyelitis of vertebra, sacral and sacrococcygeal region

● **M46.3 Infection of intervertebral disc (pyogenic)**
    Use additional code (B95-B97) to identify infectious agent
    M46.3Ø Infection of intervertebral disc (pyogenic), site unspecified
    M46.31 Infection of intervertebral disc (pyogenic), occipito-atlanto-axial region
    M46.32 Infection of intervertebral disc (pyogenic), cervical region
    M46.33 Infection of intervertebral disc (pyogenic), cervicothoracic region
    M46.34 Infection of intervertebral disc (pyogenic), thoracic region
    M46.35 Infection of intervertebral disc (pyogenic), thoracolumbar region
    M46.36 Infection of intervertebral disc (pyogenic), lumbar region
    M46.37 Infection of intervertebral disc (pyogenic), lumbosacral region
    M46.38 Infection of intervertebral disc (pyogenic), sacral and sacrococcygeal region
    M46.39 Infection of intervertebral disc (pyogenic), multiple sites in spine

● **M46.4 Discitis, unspecified**
    M46.4Ø Discitis, unspecified, site unspecified
    M46.41 Discitis, unspecified, occipito-atlanto-axial region
    M46.42 Discitis, unspecified, cervical region
    M46.43 Discitis, unspecified, cervicothoracic region
    M46.44 Discitis, unspecified, thoracic region
    M46.45 Discitis, unspecified, thoracolumbar region
    M46.46 Discitis, unspecified, lumbar region
    M46.47 Discitis, unspecified, lumbosacral region
    M46.48 Discitis, unspecified, sacral and sacrococcygeal region
    M46.49 Discitis, unspecified, multiple sites in spine

● **M46.5 Other infective spondylopathies**
    M46.5Ø Other infective spondylopathies, site unspecified
    M46.51 Other infective spondylopathies, occipitoatlanto-axial region
    M46.52 Other infective spondylopathies, cervical region
    M46.53 Other infective spondylopathies, cervicothoracic region
    M46.54 Other infective spondylopathies, thoracic region
    M46.55 Other infective spondylopathies, thoracolumbar region
    M46.56 Other infective spondylopathies, lumbar region
    M46.57 Other infective spondylopathies, lumbosacral region
    M46.58 Other infective spondylopathies, sacral and sacrococcygeal region
    M46.59 Other infective spondylopathies, multiple sites in spine

● **M46.8 Other specified inflammatory spondylopathies**
    M46.8Ø Other specified inflammatory spondylopathies, site unspecified
    M46.81 Other specified inflammatory spondylopathies, occipito-atlanto-axial region
    M46.82 Other specified inflammatory spondylopathies, cervical region
    M46.83 Other specified inflammatory spondylopathies, cervicothoracic region
    M46.84 Other specified inflammatory spondylopathies, thoracic region
    M46.85 Other specified inflammatory spondylopathies, thoracolumbar region
    M46.86 Other specified inflammatory spondylopathies, lumbar region
    M46.87 Other specified inflammatory spondylopathies, lumbosacral region
    M46.88 Other specified inflammatory spondylopathies, sacral and sacrococcygeal region
    M46.89 Other specified inflammatory spondylopathies, multiple sites in spine

● **M46.9 Unspecified inflammatory spondylopathy**
    M46.9Ø Unspecified inflammatory spondylopathy, site unspecified
    M46.91 Unspecified inflammatory spondylopathy, occipito-atlanto-axial region
    M46.92 Unspecified inflammatory spondylopathy, cervical region
    M46.93 Unspecified inflammatory spondylopathy, cervicothoracic region
    M46.94 Unspecified inflammatory spondylopathy, thoracic region
    M46.95 Unspecified inflammatory spondylopathy, thoracolumbar region
    M46.96 Unspecified inflammatory spondylopathy, lumbar region
    M46.97 Unspecified inflammatory spondylopathy, lumbosacral region
    M46.98 Unspecified inflammatory spondylopathy, sacral and sacrococcygeal region
    M46.99 Unspecified inflammatory spondylopathy, multiple sites in spine

● **M47 Spondylosis**
    Includes arthrosis or osteoarthritis of spine
                 degeneration of facet joints
  ● **M47.Ø Anterior spinal and vertebral artery compression syndromes**
    ● **M47.Ø1 Anterior spinal artery compression syndromes**
        M47.Ø11 Anterior spinal artery compression syndromes, occipito-atlanto-axial region
        M47.Ø12 Anterior spinal artery compression syndromes, cervical region
        M47.Ø13 Anterior spinal artery compression syndromes, cervicothoracic region
        M47.Ø14 Anterior spinal artery compression syndromes, thoracic region
        M47.Ø15 Anterior spinal artery compression syndromes, thoracolumbar region
        M47.Ø16 Anterior spinal artery compression syndromes, lumbar region
        M47.Ø19 Anterior spinal artery compression syndromes, site unspecified

● M47.02   Vertebral artery compression syndromes

     M47.021   Vertebral artery compression syndromes, occipito-atlanto-axial region

     M47.022   Vertebral artery compression syndromes, cervical region

     M47.029   Vertebral artery compression syndromes, site unspecified

● M47.1   Other spondylosis with myelopathy

     Spondylogenic compression of spinal cord

     Excludes1   vertebral subluxation (M43.3-M43.59)

     M47.10   Other spondylosis with myelopathy, site unspecified

     M47.11   Other spondylosis with myelopathy, occipito-atlanto-axial region

     M47.12   Other spondylosis with myelopathy, cervical region

     M47.13   Other spondylosis with myelopathy, cervicothoracic region

     M47.14   Other spondylosis with myelopathy, thoracic region

     M47.15   Other spondylosis with myelopathy, thoracolumbar region

     M47.16   Other spondylosis with myelopathy, lumbar region

● M47.2   Other spondylosis with radiculopathy

     M47.20   Other spondylosis with radiculopathy, site unspecified

     M47.21   Other spondylosis with radiculopathy, occipito-atlanto-axial region

     M47.22   Other spondylosis with radiculopathy, cervical region

     M47.23   Other spondylosis with radiculopathy, cervicothoracic region

     M47.24   Other spondylosis with radiculopathy, thoracic region

     M47.25   Other spondylosis with radiculopathy, thoracolumbar region

     M47.26   Other spondylosis with radiculopathy, lumbar region

     M47.27   Other spondylosis with radiculopathy, lumbosacral region

     M47.28   Other spondylosis with radiculopathy, sacral and sacrococcygeal region

● M47.8   Other spondylosis

  ● M47.81   Spondylosis without myelopathy or radiculopathy

     M47.811   Spondylosis without myelopathy or radiculopathy, occipito-atlanto-axial region

     M47.812   Spondylosis without myelopathy or radiculopathy, cervical region

     M47.813   Spondylosis without myelopathy or radiculopathy, cervicothoracic region

     M47.814   Spondylosis without myelopathy or radiculopathy, thoracic region

     M47.815   Spondylosis without myelopathy or radiculopathy, thoracolumbar region

     M47.816   Spondylosis without myelopathy or radiculopathy, lumbar region

     M47.817   Spondylosis without myelopathy or radiculopathy, lumbosacral region

     M47.818   Spondylosis without myelopathy or radiculopathy, sacral and sacrococcygeal region

     M47.819   Spondylosis without myelopathy or radiculopathy, site unspecified

● M47.89   Other spondylosis

     M47.891   Other spondylosis, occipito-atlanto-axial region

     M47.892   Other spondylosis, cervical region

     M47.893   Other spondylosis, cervicothoracic region

     M47.894   Other spondylosis, thoracic region

     M47.895   Other spondylosis, thoracolumbar region

     M47.896   Other spondylosis, lumbar region

     M47.897   Other spondylosis, lumbosacral region

     M47.898   Other spondylosis, sacral and sacrococcygeal region

     M47.899   Other spondylosis, site unspecified

M47.9   Spondylosis, unspecified

● M48   Other spondylopathies

  ● M48.0   Spinal stenosis

     Caudal stenosis

     M48.00   Spinal stenosis, site unspecified

     M48.01   Spinal stenosis, occipito-atlanto-axial region

     M48.02   Spinal stenosis, cervical region

     M48.03   Spinal stenosis, cervicothoracic region

     M48.04   Spinal stenosis, thoracic region

     M48.05   Spinal stenosis, thoracolumbar region

  ● M48.06   Spinal stenosis, lumbar region

    ▶ M48.061   Spinal stenosis, lumbar region without neurogenic claudication
      ▶ Spinal stenosis, lumbar region NOS

    ▶ M48.062   Spinal stenosis, lumbar region with neurogenic claudication

     M48.07   Spinal stenosis, lumbosacral region

     M48.08   Spinal stenosis, sacral and sacrococcygeal region

  ● M48.1   Ankylosing hyperostosis [Forestier]

     Diffuse idiopathic skeletal hyperostosis [DISH]

     M48.10   Ankylosing hyperostosis [Forestier], site unspecified

     M48.11   Ankylosing hyperostosis [Forestier], occipito-atlanto-axial region

     M48.12   Ankylosing hyperostosis [Forestier], cervical region

     M48.13   Ankylosing hyperostosis [Forestier], cervicothoracic region

     M48.14   Ankylosing hyperostosis [Forestier], thoracic region

     M48.15   Ankylosing hyperostosis [Forestier], thoracolumbar region

     M48.16   Ankylosing hyperostosis [Forestier], lumbar region

     M48.17   Ankylosing hyperostosis [Forestier], lumbosacral region

     M48.18   Ankylosing hyperostosis [Forestier], sacral and sacrococcygeal region

     M48.19   Ankylosing hyperostosis [Forestier], multiple sites in spine

● **M48.2** **Kissing spine**

    M48.20 Kissing spine, site unspecified

    M48.21 Kissing spine, occipito-atlanto-axial region

    M48.22 Kissing spine, cervical region

    M48.23 Kissing spine, cervicothoracic region

    M48.24 Kissing spine, thoracic region

    M48.25 Kissing spine, thoracolumbar region

    M48.26 Kissing spine, lumbar region

    M48.27 Kissing spine, lumbosacral region

● **M48.3** **Traumatic spondylopathy**

    M48.30 Traumatic spondylopathy, site unspecified

    M48.31 Traumatic spondylopathy, occipito-atlanto-axial region

    M48.32 Traumatic spondylopathy, cervical region

    M48.33 Traumatic spondylopathy, cervicothoracic region

    M48.34 Traumatic spondylopathy, thoracic region

    M48.35 Traumatic spondylopathy, thoracolumbar region

    M48.36 Traumatic spondylopathy, lumbar region

    M48.37 Traumatic spondylopathy, lumbosacral region

    M48.38 Traumatic spondylopathy, sacral and sacrococcygeal region

● **M48.4** **Fatigue fracture of vertebra**

    Stress fracture of vertebra

    Excludes 1 pathological fracture NOS (M84.4-)

                  pathological fracture of vertebra due to neoplasm (M84.58)

                  pathological fracture of vertebra due to other diagnosis (M84.68)

                  pathological fracture of vertebra due to osteoporosis (M80.-)

                  traumatic fracture of vertebrae (S12.0-S12.3-, S22.0-, S32.0-)

    The appropriate 7th character is to be added to each code from subcategory M48.4:

    A initial encounter for fracture
    D subsequent encounter for fracture with routine healing
    G subsequent encounter for fracture with delayed healing
    S sequela of fracture

X ● M48.40 Fatigue fracture of vertebra, site unspecified

X ● M48.41 Fatigue fracture of vertebra, occipitoatlanto-axial region

X ● M48.42 Fatigue fracture of vertebra, cervical region

X ● M48.43 Fatigue fracture of vertebra, cervicothoracic region

X ● M48.44 Fatigue fracture of vertebra, thoracic region

X ● M48.45 Fatigue fracture of vertebra, thoracolumbar region

X ● M48.46 Fatigue fracture of vertebra, lumbar region

X ● M48.47 Fatigue fracture of vertebra, lumbosacral region

X ● M48.48 Fatigue fracture of vertebra, sacral and sacrococcygeal region

● **M48.5** **Collapsed vertebra, not elsewhere classified**

    Collapsed vertebra NOS

    Compression fracture of vertebra NOS

    Wedging of vertebra NOS

    Excludes 1 current injury - see Injury of spine, by body region

                  fatigue fracture of vertebra (M48.4)

                  pathological fracture of vertebra due to neoplasm (M84.58)

                  pathological fracture of vertebra due to other diagnosis (M84.68)

                  pathological fracture of vertebra due to osteoporosis (M80.-)

                  pathological fracture NOS (M84.4-)

                  stress fracture of vertebra (M48.4-)

                  traumatic fracture of vertebra (S12.-, S22.-, S32.-)

    The appropriate 7th character is to be added to each code from subcategory M48.5:

    A initial encounter for fracture
    D subsequent encounter for fracture with routine healing
    G subsequent encounter for fracture with delayed healing
    S sequela of fracture

X ● M48.50 Collapsed vertebra, not elsewhere classified, site unspecified

X ● M48.51 Collapsed vertebra, not elsewhere classified, occipito-atlanto-axial region

X ● M48.52 Collapsed vertebra, not elsewhere classified, cervical region

X ● M48.53 Collapsed vertebra, not elsewhere classified, cervicothoracic region

X ● M48.54 Collapsed vertebra, not elsewhere classified, thoracic region

X ● M48.55 Collapsed vertebra, not elsewhere classified, thoracolumbar region

X ● M48.56 Collapsed vertebra, not elsewhere classified, lumbar region

X ● M48.57 Collapsed vertebra, not elsewhere classified, lumbosacral region

X ● M48.58 Collapsed vertebra, not elsewhere classified, sacral and sacrococcygeal region

● **M48.8** **Other specified spondylopathies**

    Ossification of posterior longitudinal ligament

  ● M48.8X Other specified spondylopathies

      M48.8X1 Other specified spondylopathies, occipito-atlanto-axial region

      M48.8X2 Other specified spondylopathies, cervical region

      M48.8X3 Other specified spondylopathies, cervicothoracic region

      M48.8X4 Other specified spondylopathies, thoracic region

      M48.8X5 Other specified spondylopathies, thoracolumbar region

      M48.8X6 Other specified spondylopathies, lumbar region

      M48.8X7 Other specified spondylopathies, lumbosacral region

      M48.8X8 Other specified spondylopathies, sacral and sacrococcygeal region

      M48.8X9 Other specified spondylopathies, site unspecified

  M48.9 **Spondylopathy, unspecified**

▶ New   ⇒ Revised   ~~deleted~~ Deleted   **OGCR** Official Guidelines   X Assign placeholder X   ● Use Additional Character(s)

Excludes 1   Excludes 2   Includes   Use additional   Code first   Code also   Key words

● M49　Spondylopathies in diseases classified elsewhere
>　Includes　curvature of spine in diseases classified elsewhere
>　　deformity of spine in diseases classified
>　　　elsewhere
>　　kyphosis in diseases classified elsewhere
>　　scoliosis in diseases classified elsewhere
>　　spondylopathy in diseases classified elsewhere

>　*Code first* underlying disease, such as:
>　　brucellosis (A23.-)
>　　Charcot-Marie-Tooth disease (G60.0)
>　　enterobacterial infections (A01-A04)
>　　osteitis fibrosa cystica (E21.0)

>　Excludes1　curvature of spine in tuberculosis [Pott's]
>　　　(A18.01)
>　　enteropathic arthropathies (M07.-)
>　　gonococcal spondylitis (A54.41)
>　　neuropathic [tabes dorsalis] spondylitis (A52.11)
>　　neuropathic spondylopathy in syringomyelia
>　　　(G95.0)
>　　neuropathic spondylopathy in tabes dorsalis
>　　　(A52.11)
>　　nonsyphilitic neuropathic spondylopathy NEC
>　　　(G98.0)
>　　spondylitis in syphilis (acquired) (A52.77)
>　　tuberculous spondylitis (A18.01)
>　　typhoid fever spondylitis (A01.05)

●　M49.8　Spondylopathy in diseases classified elsewhere

　　M49.80　Spondylopathy in diseases classified elsewhere, site unspecified

　　M49.81　Spondylopathy in diseases classified elsewhere, occipito-atlanto-axial region

　　M49.82　Spondylopathy in diseases classified elsewhere, cervical region

　　M49.83　Spondylopathy in diseases classified elsewhere, cervicothoracic region

　　M49.84　Spondylopathy in diseases classified elsewhere, thoracic region

　　M49.85　Spondylopathy in diseases classified elsewhere, thoracolumbar region

　　M49.86　Spondylopathy in diseases classified elsewhere, lumbar region

　　M49.87　Spondylopathy in diseases classified elsewhere, lumbosacral region

　　M49.88　Spondylopathy in diseases classified elsewhere, sacral and sacrococcygeal region

　　M49.89　Spondylopathy in diseases classified elsewhere, multiple sites in spine

OTHER DORSOPATHIES (M50-M54)

>　Excludes1　current injury - see injury of spine by body region
>　　discitis NOS (M46.4-)

● M50　Cervical disc disorders
>　**Note:** Code to the most superior level of disorder.
>　Includes　cervicothoracic disc disorders with cervicalgia
>　　cervicothoracic disc disorders

●　M50.0　Cervical disc disorder with myelopathy

　　M50.00　Cervical disc disorder with myelopathy, unspecified cervical region

　　M50.01　Cervical disc disorder with myelopathy, high cervical region
　　　　C2-C3 disc disorder with myelopathy
　　　　C3-C4 disc disorder with myelopathy

●　M50.02　Cervical disc disorder with myelopathy, mid-cervical region

　　M50.020　Cervical disc disorder with myelopathy, mid-cervical region, unspecified level

　　M50.021　Cervical disc disorder at C4-C5 level with myelopathy
　　　　C4-C5 disc disorder with myelopathy

　　M50.022　Cervical disc disorder at C5-C6 level with myelopathy
　　　　C5-C6 disc disorder with myelopathy

　　M50.023　Cervical disc disorder at C6-C7 level with myelopathy
　　　　C6-C7 disc disorder with myelopathy

　　M50.03　Cervical disc disorder with myelopathy, cervicothoracic region
　　　　C7-T1 disc disorder with myelopathy

●　M50.1　Cervical disc disorder with radiculopathy
>　　Excludes2　brachial radiculitis NOS (M54.13)

　　M50.10　Cervical disc disorder with radiculopathy, unspecified cervical region

　　M50.11　Cervical disc disorder with radiculopathy, high cervical region
　　　　C2-C3 disc disorder with radiculopathy
　　　　C3 radiculopathy due to disc disorder
　　　　C3-C4 disc disorder with radiculopathy
　　　　C4 radiculopathy due to disc disorder

●　M50.12　Cervical disc disorder with radiculopathy, mid-cervical region

　　M50.120　Mid-cervical disc disorder, unspecified

　　M50.121　Cervical disc disorder at C4-C5 level with radiculopathy
　　　　C4-C5 disc disorder with radiculopathy
　　　　C5 radiculopathy due to disc disorder

　　M50.122　Cervical disc disorder at C5-C6 level with radiculopathy
　　　　C5-C6 disc disorder with radiculopathy
　　　　C6 radiculopathy due to disc disorder

　　M50.123　Cervical disc disorder at C6-C7 level with radiculopathy
　　　　C6-C7 disc disorder with radiculopathy
　　　　C7 radiculopathy due to disc disorder

　　M50.13　Cervical disc disorder with radiculopathy, cervicothoracic region
　　　　C7-T1 disc disorder with radiculopathy
　　　　C8 radiculopathy due to disc disorder

●　M50.2　Other cervical disc displacement

　　M50.20　Other cervical disc displacement, unspecified cervical region

　　M50.21　Other cervical disc displacement, high cervical region
　　　　Other C2-C3 cervical disc displacement
　　　　Other C3-C4 cervical disc displacement

▶ New　⇒ Revised　~~deleted~~ Deleted　**OGCR** Official Guidelines　X Assign placeholder X　● Use Additional Character(s)

Excludes 1　Excludes 2　Includes　Use additional　Code first　Code also　Key words

● M50.22   Other cervical disc displacement, mid-cervical region

    M50.220   Other cervical disc displacement, mid-cervical region, unspecified level

    M50.221   Other cervical disc displacement at C4-C5 level
       Other C4-C5 cervical disc displacement

    M50.222   Other cervical disc displacement at C5-C6 level
       Other C5-C6 cervical disc displacement

    M50.223   Other cervical disc displacement at C6-C7 level
       Other C6-C7 cervical disc displacement

  M50.23   Other cervical disc displacement, cervicothoracic region
     Other C7-T1 cervical disc displacement

● M50.3   Other cervical disc degeneration

  M50.30   Other cervical disc degeneration, unspecified cervical region

  M50.31   Other cervical disc degeneration, high cervical region
     Other C2-C3 cervical disc degeneration
     Other C3-C4 cervical disc degeneration

● M50.32   Other cervical disc degeneration, mid-cervical region

    M50.320   Other cervical disc degeneration, mid-cervical region, unspecified level

    M50.321   Other cervical disc degeneration at C4-C5 level
       Other C4-C5 cervical disc degeneration

    M50.322   Other cervical disc degeneration at C5-C6 level
       Other C5-C6 cervical disc degeneration

    M50.323   Other cervical disc degeneration at C6-C7 level
       Other C6-C7 cervical disc degeneration

  M50.33   Other cervical disc degeneration, cervicothoracic region
     Other C7-T1 cervical disc degeneration

● M50.8   Other cervical disc disorders

  M50.80   Other cervical disc disorders, unspecified cervical region

  M50.81   Other cervical disc disorders, high cervical region
     Other C2-C3 cervical disc disorders
     Other C3-C4 cervical disc disorders

● M50.82   Other cervical disc disorders, mid-cervical region

    M50.820   Other cervical disc disorders, mid-cervical region, unspecified level

    M50.821   Other cervical disc disorders at C4-C5 level
       Other C4-C5 cervical disc disorders

    M50.822   Other cervical disc disorders at C5-C6 level
       Other C5-C6 cervical disc disorders

    M50.823   Other cervical disc disorders at C6-C7 level
       Other C6-C7 cervical disc disorders

  M50.83   Other cervical disc disorders, cervicothoracic region
     Other C7-T1 cervical disc disorders

● M50.9   Cervical disc disorder, unspecified

  M50.90   Cervical disc disorder, unspecified, unspecified cervical region

  M50.91   Cervical disc disorder, unspecified, high cervical region
     C2-C3 cervical disc disorder, unspecified
     C3-C4 cervical disc disorder, unspecified

● M50.92   Cervical disc disorder, unspecified, mid-cervical region

    M50.920   Unspecified cervical disc disorder, mid-cervical region, unspecified level

    M50.921   Unspecified cervical disc disorder at C4-C5 level
       Unspecified C4-C5 cervical disc disorder

    M50.922   Unspecified cervical disc disorder at C5-C6 level
       Unspecified C5-C6 cervical disc disorder

    M50.923   Unspecified cervical disc disorder at C6-C7 level
       Unspecified C6-C7 cervical disc disorder

  M50.93   Cervical disc disorder, unspecified, cervicothoracic region
     C7-T1 cervical disc disorder, unspecified

● M51   Thoracic, thoracolumbar, and lumbosacral intervertebral disc disorders

   Excludes2   cervical and cervicothoracic disc disorders (M50.-)
         sacral and sacrococcygeal disorders (M53.3)

● M51.0   Thoracic, thoracolumbar and lumbosacral intervertebral disc disorders with myelopathy

  M51.04   Intervertebral disc disorders with myelopathy, thoracic region

  M51.05   Intervertebral disc disorders with myelopathy, thoracolumbar region

  M51.06   Intervertebral disc disorders with myelopathy, lumbar region

● M51.1   Thoracic, thoracolumbar and lumbosacral intervertebral disc disorders with radiculopathy
    Sciatica due to intervertebral disc disorder

   Excludes1   lumbar radiculitis NOS (M54.16)
         sciatica NOS (M54.3)

  M51.14   Intervertebral disc disorders with radiculopathy, thoracic region

  M51.15   Intervertebral disc disorders with radiculopathy, thoracolumbar region

  M51.16   Intervertebral disc disorders with radiculopathy, lumbar region

  M51.17   Intervertebral disc disorders with radiculopathy, lumbosacral region

CHAPTER 13 (M00-M99)

● **M51.2** Other thoracic, thoracolumbar and lumbosacral intervertebral disc displacement
     Lumbago due to displacement of intervertebral disc

     M51.24   Other intervertebral disc displacement, thoracic region

     M51.25   Other intervertebral disc displacement, thoracolumbar region

     M51.26   Other intervertebral disc displacement, lumbar region

     M51.27   Other intervertebral disc displacement, lumbosacral region

● **M51.3** Other thoracic, thoracolumbar and lumbosacral intervertebral disc degeneration

     M51.34   Other intervertebral disc degeneration, thoracic region

     M51.35   Other intervertebral disc degeneration, thoracolumbar region

     M51.36   Other intervertebral disc degeneration, lumbar region

     M51.37   Other intervertebral disc degeneration, lumbosacral region

● **M51.4** Schmorl's nodes

     M51.44   Schmorl's nodes, thoracic region

     M51.45   Schmorl's nodes, thoracolumbar region

     M51.46   Schmorl's nodes, lumbar region

     M51.47   Schmorl's nodes, lumbosacral region

● **M51.8** Other thoracic, thoracolumbar and lumbosacral intervertebral disc disorders

     M51.84   Other intervertebral disc disorders, thoracic region

     M51.85   Other intervertebral disc disorders, thoracolumbar region

     M51.86   Other intervertebral disc disorders, lumbar region

     M51.87   Other intervertebral disc disorders, lumbosacral region

     M51.9 Unspecified thoracic, thoracolumbar and lumbosacral intervertebral disc disorder

● **M53** Other and unspecified dorsopathies, not elsewhere classified

     M53.0 Cervicocranial syndrome
         Posterior cervical sympathetic syndrome

     M53.1 Cervicobrachial syndrome

         Excludes2   cervical disc disorder (M50.-)
                   thoracic outlet syndrome (G54.0)

● **M53.2** Spinal instabilities

     ● **M53.2X** Spinal instabilities

         M53.2X1   Spinal instabilities, occipito-atlanto-axial region

         M53.2X2   Spinal instabilities, cervical region

         M53.2X3   Spinal instabilities, cervicothoracic region

         M53.2X4   Spinal instabilities, thoracic region

         M53.2X5   Spinal instabilities, thoracolumbar region

         M53.2X6   Spinal instabilities, lumbar region

         M53.2X7   Spinal instabilities, lumbosacral region

         M53.2X8   Spinal instabilities, sacral and sacrococcygeal region

         M53.2X9   Spinal instabilities, site unspecified

     M53.3 Sacrococcygeal disorders, not elsewhere classified
         Coccygodynia

● **M53.8** Other specified dorsopathies

     M53.80   Other specified dorsopathies, site unspecified

     M53.81   Other specified dorsopathies, occipito-atlanto-axial region

     M53.82   Other specified dorsopathies, cervical region

     M53.83   Other specified dorsopathies, cervicothoracic region

     M53.84   Other specified dorsopathies, thoracic region

     M53.85   Other specified dorsopathies, thoracolumbar region

     M53.86   Other specified dorsopathies, lumbar region

     M53.87   Other specified dorsopathies, lumbosacral region

     M53.88   Other specified dorsopathies, sacral and sacrococcygeal region

     M53.9 Dorsopathy, unspecified

● **M54** Dorsalgia

     Excludes1   psychogenic dorsalgia (F45.41)

● **M54.0** Panniculitis affecting regions of neck and back

     Excludes1   lupus panniculitis (L93.2)
                 panniculitis NOS (M79.3)
                 relapsing [Weber-Christian] panniculitis (M35.6)

     M54.00   Panniculitis affecting regions of neck and back, site unspecified

     M54.01   Panniculitis affecting regions of neck and back, occipito-atlanto-axial region

     M54.02   Panniculitis affecting regions of neck and back, cervical region

     M54.03   Panniculitis affecting regions of neck and back, cervicothoracic region

     M54.04   Panniculitis affecting regions of neck and back, thoracic region

     M54.05   Panniculitis affecting regions of neck and back, thoracolumbar region

     M54.06   Panniculitis affecting regions of neck and back, lumbar region

     M54.07   Panniculitis affecting regions of neck and back, lumbosacral region

     M54.08   Panniculitis affecting regions of neck and back, sacral and sacrococcygeal region

     M54.09   Panniculitis affecting regions, neck and back, multiple sites in spine

● **M54.1** Radiculopathy
     Brachial neuritis or radiculitis NOS
     Lumbar neuritis or radiculitis NOS
     Lumbosacral neuritis or radiculitis NOS
     Thoracic neuritis or radiculitis NOS
     Radiculitis NOS

     Excludes1   neuralgia and neuritis NOS (M79.2)
                 radiculopathy with cervical disc disorder (M50.1)
                 radiculopathy with lumbar and other intervertebral disc disorder (M51.1-)
                 radiculopathy with spondylosis (M47.2-)

     M54.10   Radiculopathy, site unspecified

     M54.11   Radiculopathy, occipito-atlanto-axial region

     M54.12   Radiculopathy, cervical region

     M54.13   Radiculopathy, cervicothoracic region

     M54.14   Radiculopathy, thoracic region

     M54.15   Radiculopathy, thoracolumbar region

     M54.16   Radiculopathy, lumbar region

     M54.17   Radiculopathy, lumbosacral region

     M54.18   Radiculopathy, sacral and sacrococcygeal region

M54.2 **Cervicalgia**
- **Excludes1** cervicalgia due to intervertebral cervical disc disorder (M50.-)

● M54.3 **Sciatica**
- **Excludes1** lesion of sciatic nerve (G57.0)
  sciatica due to intervertebral disc disorder (M51.1-)
  sciatica with lumbago (M54.4-)

  M54.30 Sciatica, unspecified side
  M54.31 Sciatica, right side
  M54.32 Sciatica, left side

● M54.4 **Lumbago with sciatica**
- **Excludes1** lumbago with sciatica due to intervertebral disc disorder (M51.1-)

  M54.40 Lumbago with sciatica, unspecified side
  M54.41 Lumbago with sciatica, right side
  M54.42 Lumbago with sciatica, left side

M54.5 **Low back pain**
  Loin pain
  Lumbago NOS
- **Excludes1** low back strain (S39.012)
  lumbago due to intervertebral disc displacement (M51.2-)
  lumbago with sciatica (M54.4-)

M54.6 **Pain in thoracic spine**
- **Excludes1** pain in thoracic spine due to intervertebral disc disorder (M51.)

● M54.8 **Other dorsalgia**
- **Excludes1** dorsalgia in thoracic region (M54.6)
  low back pain (M54.5)

  M54.81 Occipital neuralgia
  M54.89 Other dorsalgia
M54.9 **Dorsalgia, unspecified**
  Backache NOS
  Back pain NOS

SOFT TISSUE DISORDERS (M60-M79)

DISORDERS OF MUSCLES (M60-M63)

- **Excludes1** dermatopolymyositis (M33.-)
  muscular dystrophies and myopathies (G71-G72)
  myopathy in amyloidosis (E85.-)
  myopathy in polyarteritis nodosa (M30.0)
  myopathy in rheumatoid arthritis (M05.32)
  myopathy in scleroderma (M34.-)
  myopathy in Sjögren's syndrome (M35.03)
  myopathy in systemic lupus erythematosus (M32.-)

● **M60 Myositis**
- **Excludes2** inclusion body myositis [IBM] (G72.41)
● M60.0 **Infective myositis**
  Tropical pyomyositis
  Use additional code (B95-B97) to identify infectious agent

  ● M60.00 Infective myositis, unspecified site
    M60.000 Infective myositis, unspecified right arm
      Infective myositis, right upper limb NOS
    M60.001 Infective myositis, unspecified left arm
      Infective myositis, left upper limb NOS
    M60.002 Infective myositis, unspecified arm
      Infective myositis, upper limb NOS

    M60.003 Infective myositis, unspecified right leg
      Infective myositis, right lower limb NOS
    M60.004 Infective myositis, unspecified left leg
      Infective myositis, left lower limb NOS
    M60.005 Infective myositis, unspecified leg
      Infective myositis, lower limb NOS
    M60.009 Infective myositis, unspecified site
  ● M60.01 Infective myositis, shoulder
    M60.011 Infective myositis, right shoulder
    M60.012 Infective myositis, left shoulder
    M60.019 Infective myositis, unspecified shoulder
  ● M60.02 Infective myositis, upper arm
    M60.021 Infective myositis, right upper arm
    M60.022 Infective myositis, left upper arm
    M60.029 Infective myositis, unspecified upper arm
  ● M60.03 Infective myositis, forearm
    M60.031 Infective myositis, right forearm
    M60.032 Infective myositis, left forearm
    M60.039 Infective myositis, unspecified forearm
  ● M60.04 Infective myositis, hand and fingers
    M60.041 Infective myositis, right hand
    M60.042 Infective myositis, left hand
    M60.043 Infective myositis, unspecified hand
    M60.044 Infective myositis, right finger(s)
    M60.045 Infective myositis, left finger(s)
    M60.046 Infective myositis, unspecified finger(s)
  ● M60.05 Infective myositis, thigh
    M60.051 Infective myositis, right thigh
    M60.052 Infective myositis, left thigh
    M60.059 Infective myositis, unspecified thigh
  ● M60.06 Infective myositis, lower leg
    M60.061 Infective myositis, right lower leg
    M60.062 Infective myositis, left lower leg
    M60.069 Infective myositis, unspecified lower leg
  ● M60.07 Infective myositis, ankle, foot and toes
    M60.070 Infective myositis, right ankle
    M60.071 Infective myositis, left ankle
    M60.072 Infective myositis, unspecified ankle
    M60.073 Infective myositis, right foot
    M60.074 Infective myositis, left foot
    M60.075 Infective myositis, unspecified foot
    M60.076 Infective myositis, right toe(s)
    M60.077 Infective myositis, left toe(s)
    M60.078 Infective myositis, unspecified toe(s)
  M60.08 Infective myositis, other site
  M60.09 Infective myositis, multiple sites
● M60.1 **Interstitial myositis**
  M60.10 Interstitial myositis of unspecified site
  ● M60.11 Interstitial myositis, shoulder
    M60.111 Interstitial myositis, right shoulder
    M60.112 Interstitial myositis, left shoulder
    M60.119 Interstitial myositis, unspecified shoulder

● M60.12   Interstitial myositis, upper arm
     M60.121   Interstitial myositis, right upper arm
     M60.122   Interstitial myositis, left upper arm
     M60.129   Interstitial myositis, unspecified upper arm
● M60.13   Interstitial myositis, forearm
     M60.131   Interstitial myositis, right forearm
     M60.132   Interstitial myositis, left forearm
     M60.139   Interstitial myositis, unspecified forearm
● M60.14   Interstitial myositis, hand
     M60.141   Interstitial myositis, right hand
     M60.142   Interstitial myositis, left hand
     M60.149   Interstitial myositis, unspecified hand
● M60.15   Interstitial myositis, thigh
     M60.151   Interstitial myositis, right thigh
     M60.152   Interstitial myositis, left thigh
     M60.159   Interstitial myositis, unspecified thigh
● M60.16   Interstitial myositis, lower leg
     M60.161   Interstitial myositis, right lower leg
     M60.162   Interstitial myositis, left lower leg
     M60.169   Interstitial myositis, unspecified lower leg
● M60.17   Interstitial myositis, ankle and foot
     M60.171   Interstitial myositis, right ankle and foot
     M60.172   Interstitial myositis, left ankle and foot
     M60.179   Interstitial myositis, unspecified ankle and foot
     M60.18   Interstitial myositis, other site
     M60.19   Interstitial myositis, multiple sites
● M60.2   Foreign body granuloma of soft tissue, not elsewhere classified

Use additional code to identify the type of retained foreign body (Z18.-)

Excludes1   foreign body granuloma of skin and subcutaneous tissue (L92.3)

     M60.20   Foreign body granuloma of soft tissue, not elsewhere classified, unspecified site
● M60.21   Foreign body granuloma of soft tissue, not elsewhere classified, shoulder
     M60.211   Foreign body granuloma of soft tissue, not elsewhere classified, right shoulder
     M60.212   Foreign body granuloma of soft tissue, not elsewhere classified, left shoulder
     M60.219   Foreign body granuloma of soft tissue, not elsewhere classified, unspecified shoulder
● M60.22   Foreign body granuloma of soft tissue, not elsewhere classified, upper arm
     M60.221   Foreign body granuloma of soft tissue, not elsewhere classified, right upper arm
     M60.222   Foreign body granuloma of soft tissue, not elsewhere classified, left upper arm
     M60.229   Foreign body granuloma of soft tissue, not elsewhere classified, unspecified upper arm

● M60.23   Foreign body granuloma of soft tissue, not elsewhere classified, forearm
     M60.231   Foreign body granuloma of soft tissue, not elsewhere classified, right forearm
     M60.232   Foreign body granuloma of soft tissue, not elsewhere classified, left forearm
     M60.239   Foreign body granuloma of soft tissue, not elsewhere classified, unspecified forearm
● M60.24   Foreign body granuloma of soft tissue, not elsewhere classified, hand
     M60.241   Foreign body granuloma of soft tissue, not elsewhere classified, right hand
     M60.242   Foreign body granuloma of soft tissue, not elsewhere classified, left hand
     M60.249   Foreign body granuloma of soft tissue, not elsewhere classified, unspecified hand
● M60.25   Foreign body granuloma of soft tissue, not elsewhere classified, thigh
     M60.251   Foreign body granuloma of soft tissue, not elsewhere classified, right thigh
     M60.252   Foreign body granuloma of soft tissue, not elsewhere classified, left thigh
     M60.259   Foreign body granuloma of soft tissue, not elsewhere classified, unspecified thigh
● M60.26   Foreign body granuloma of soft tissue, not elsewhere classified, lower leg
     M60.261   Foreign body granuloma of soft tissue, not elsewhere classified, right lower leg
     M60.262   Foreign body granuloma of soft tissue, not elsewhere classified, left lower leg
     M60.269   Foreign body granuloma of soft tissue, not elsewhere classified, unspecified lower leg
● M60.27   Foreign body granuloma of soft tissue, not elsewhere classified, ankle and foot
     M60.271   Foreign body granuloma of soft tissue, not elsewhere classified, right ankle and foot
     M60.272   Foreign body granuloma of soft tissue, not elsewhere classified, left ankle and foot
     M60.279   Foreign body granuloma of soft tissue, not elsewhere classified, unspecified ankle and foot
     M60.28   Foreign body granuloma of soft tissue, not elsewhere classified, other site
● M60.8   Other myositis
     M60.80   Other myositis, unspecified site
● M60.81   Other myositis shoulder
     M60.811   Other myositis, right shoulder
     M60.812   Other myositis, left shoulder
     M60.819   Other myositis, unspecified shoulder
● M60.82   Other myositis, upper arm
     M60.821   Other myositis, right upper arm
     M60.822   Other myositis, left upper arm
     M60.829   Other myositis, unspecified upper arm

▶ New   ⇒ Revised   ~~deleted~~ Deleted   **OGCR** Official Guidelines   X Assign placeholder X   ● Use Additional Character(s)

Excludes 1   Excludes 2   Includes   Use additional   Code first   Code also   Key words

● M60.83   Other myositis, forearm
     M60.831   Other myositis, right forearm
     M60.832   Other myositis, left forearm
     M60.839   Other myositis, unspecified forearm

● M60.84   Other myositis, hand
     M60.841   Other myositis, right hand
     M60.842   Other myositis, left hand
     M60.849   Other myositis, unspecified hand

● M60.85   Other myositis, thigh
     M60.851   Other myositis, right thigh
     M60.852   Other myositis, left thigh
     M60.859   Other myositis, unspecified thigh

● M60.86   Other myositis, lower leg
     M60.861   Other myositis, right lower leg
     M60.862   Other myositis, left lower leg
     M60.869   Other myositis, unspecified lower leg

● M60.87   Other myositis, ankle and foot
     M60.871   Other myositis, right ankle and foot
     M60.872   Other myositis, left ankle and foot
     M60.879   Other myositis, unspecified ankle and foot

     M60.88   Other myositis, other site
     M60.89   Other myositis, multiple sites
M60.9   Myositis, unspecified

● M61   Calcification and ossification of muscle
  ● M61.0   Myositis ossificans traumatica
     M61.00   Myositis ossificans traumatica, unspecified site

  ● M61.01   Myositis ossificans traumatica, shoulder
     M61.011   Myositis ossificans traumatica, right shoulder
     M61.012   Myositis ossificans traumatica, left shoulder
     M61.019   Myositis ossificans traumatica, unspecified shoulder

  ● M61.02   Myositis ossificans traumatica, upper arm
     M61.021   Myositis ossificans traumatica, right upper arm
     M61.022   Myositis ossificans traumatica, left upper arm
     M61.029   Myositis ossificans traumatica, unspecified upper arm

  ● M61.03   Myositis ossificans traumatica, forearm
     M61.031   Myositis ossificans traumatica, right forearm
     M61.032   Myositis ossificans traumatica, left forearm
     M61.039   Myositis ossificans traumatica, unspecified forearm

  ● M61.04   Myositis ossificans traumatica, hand
     M61.041   Myositis ossificans traumatica, right hand
     M61.042   Myositis ossificans traumatica, left hand
     M61.049   Myositis ossificans traumatica, unspecified hand

  ● M61.05   Myositis ossificans traumatica, thigh
     M61.051   Myositis ossificans traumatica, right thigh
     M61.052   Myositis ossificans traumatica, left thigh
     M61.059   Myositis ossificans traumatica, unspecified thigh

● M61.06   Myositis ossificans traumatica, lower leg
     M61.061   Myositis ossificans traumatica, right lower leg
     M61.062   Myositis ossificans traumatica, left lower leg
     M61.069   Myositis ossificans traumatica, unspecified lower leg

● M61.07   Myositis ossificans traumatica, ankle and foot
     M61.071   Myositis ossificans traumatica, right ankle and foot
     M61.072   Myositis ossificans traumatica, left ankle and foot
     M61.079   Myositis ossificans traumatica, unspecified ankle and foot

     M61.08   Myositis ossificans traumatica, other site
     M61.09   Myositis ossificans traumatica, multiple sites

● M61.1   Myositis ossificans progressiva
     Fibrodysplasia ossificans progressiva
     M61.10   Myositis ossificans progressiva, unspecified site

● M61.11   Myositis ossificans progressiva, shoulder
     M61.111   Myositis ossificans progressiva, right shoulder
     M61.112   Myositis ossificans progressiva, left shoulder
     M61.119   Myositis ossificans progressiva, unspecified shoulder

● M61.12   Myositis ossificans progressiva, upper arm
     M61.121   Myositis ossificans progressiva, right upper arm
     M61.122   Myositis ossificans progressiva, left upper arm
     M61.129   Myositis ossificans progressiva, unspecified arm

● M61.13   Myositis ossificans progressiva, forearm
     M61.131   Myositis ossificans progressiva, right forearm
     M61.132   Myositis ossificans progressiva, left forearm
     M61.139   Myositis ossificans progressiva, unspecified forearm

● M61.14   Myositis ossificans progressiva, hand and finger(s)
     M61.141   Myositis ossificans progressiva, right hand
     M61.142   Myositis ossificans progressiva, left hand
     M61.143   Myositis ossificans progressiva, unspecified hand
     M61.144   Myositis ossificans progressiva, right finger(s)
     M61.145   Myositis ossificans progressiva, left finger(s)
     M61.146   Myositis ossificans progressiva, unspecified finger(s)

● M61.15   Myositis ossificans progressiva, thigh
     M61.151   Myositis ossificans progressiva, right thigh
     M61.152   Myositis ossificans progressiva, left thigh
     M61.159   Myositis ossificans progressiva, unspecified thigh

● M61.16   Myositis ossificans progressiva, lower leg
     M61.161   Myositis ossificans progressiva, right lower leg
     M61.162   Myositis ossificans progressiva, left lower leg
     M61.169   Myositis ossificans progressiva, unspecified lower leg

CHAPTER 13 (M00-M99)

▶ New   ⟹ Revised   ~~deleted~~ Deleted   **OGCR** Official Guidelines   X Assign placeholder X   ● Use Additional Character(s)

Excludes 1   Excludes 2   Includes   Use additional   Code first   Code also   Key words

● M61.17   Myositis ossificans progressiva, ankle, foot and toe(s)

     M61.171   Myositis ossificans progressiva, right ankle

     M61.172   Myositis ossificans progressiva, left ankle

     M61.173   Myositis ossificans progressiva, unspecified ankle

     M61.174   Myositis ossificans progressiva, right foot

     M61.175   Myositis ossificans progressiva, left foot

     M61.176   Myositis ossificans progressiva, unspecified foot

     M61.177   Myositis ossificans progressiva, right toe(s)

     M61.178   Myositis ossificans progressiva, left toe(s)

     M61.179   Myositis ossificans progressiva, unspecified toe(s)

   M61.18   Myositis ossificans progressiva, other site

   M61.19   Myositis ossificans progressiva, multiple sites

● M61.2   Paralytic calcification and ossification of muscle

    Myositis ossificans associated with quadriplegia or paraplegia

   M61.20   Paralytic calcification and ossification of muscle, unspecified site

● M61.21   Paralytic calcification and ossification of muscle, shoulder

     M61.211   Paralytic calcification and ossification of muscle, right shoulder

     M61.212   Paralytic calcification and ossification of muscle, left shoulder

     M61.219   Paralytic calcification and ossification of muscle, unspecified shoulder

● M61.22   Paralytic calcification and ossification of muscle, upper arm

     M61.221   Paralytic calcification and ossification of muscle, right upper arm

     M61.222   Paralytic calcification and ossification of muscle, left upper arm

     M61.229   Paralytic calcification and ossification of muscle, unspecified upper arm

● M61.23   Paralytic calcification and ossification of muscle, forearm

     M61.231   Paralytic calcification and ossification of muscle, right forearm

     M61.232   Paralytic calcification and ossification of muscle, left forearm

     M61.239   Paralytic calcification and ossification of muscle, unspecified forearm

● M61.24   Paralytic calcification and ossification of muscle, hand

     M61.241   Paralytic calcification and ossification of muscle, right hand

     M61.242   Paralytic calcification and ossification of muscle, left hand

     M61.249   Paralytic calcification and ossification of muscle, unspecified hand

● M61.25   Paralytic calcification and ossification of muscle, thigh

     M61.251   Paralytic calcification and ossification of muscle, right thigh

     M61.252   Paralytic calcification and ossification of muscle, left thigh

     M61.259   Paralytic calcification and ossification of muscle, unspecified thigh

● M61.26   Paralytic calcification and ossification of muscle, lower leg

     M61.261   Paralytic calcification and ossification of muscle, right lower leg

     M61.262   Paralytic calcification and ossification of muscle, left lower leg

     M61.269   Paralytic calcification and ossification of muscle, unspecified lower leg

● M61.27   Paralytic calcification and ossification of muscle, ankle and foot

     M61.271   Paralytic calcification and ossification of muscle, right ankle and foot

     M61.272   Paralytic calcification and ossification of muscle, left ankle and foot

     M61.279   Paralytic calcification and ossification of muscle, unspecified ankle and foot

   M61.28   Paralytic calcification and ossification of muscle, other site

   M61.29   Paralytic calcification and ossification of muscle, multiple sites

● M61.3   Calcification and ossification of muscles associated with burns

    Myositis ossificans associated with burns

   M61.30   Calcification and ossification of muscles associated with burns, unspecified site

● M61.31   Calcification and ossification of muscles associated with burns, shoulder

     M61.311   Calcification and ossification of muscles associated with burns, right shoulder

     M61.312   Calcification and ossification of muscles associated with burns, left shoulder

     M61.319   Calcification and ossification of muscles associated with burns, unspecified shoulder

● M61.32   Calcification and ossification of muscles associated with burns, upper arm

     M61.321   Calcification and ossification of muscles associated with burns, right upper arm

     M61.322   Calcification and ossification of muscles associated with burns, left upper arm

     M61.329   Calcification and ossification of muscles associated with burns, unspecified upper arm

● M61.33   Calcification and ossification of muscles associated with burns, forearm

     M61.331   Calcification and ossification of muscles associated with burns, right forearm

     M61.332   Calcification and ossification of muscles associated with burns, left forearm

     M61.339   Calcification and ossification of muscles associated with burns, unspecified forearm

● M61.34   Calcification and ossification of muscles associated with burns, hand

     M61.341   Calcification and ossification of muscles associated with burns, right hand

     M61.342   Calcification and ossification of muscles associated with burns, left hand

     M61.349   Calcification and ossification of muscles associated with burns, unspecified hand

▶ New   ⇢ Revised   ~~deleted~~ Deleted   **OGCR** Official Guidelines   X Assign placeholder X   ● Use Additional Character(s)

Excludes 1   Excludes 2   Includes   Use additional   Code first   Code also   Key words

● M61.35 Calcification and ossification of muscles associated with burns, thigh

    M61.351 Calcification and ossification of muscles associated with burns, right thigh

    M61.352 Calcification and ossification of muscles associated with burns, left thigh

    M61.359 Calcification and ossification of muscles associated with burns, unspecified thigh

● M61.36 Calcification and ossification of muscles associated with burns, lower leg

    M61.361 Calcification and ossification of muscles associated with burns, right lower leg

    M61.362 Calcification and ossification of muscles associated with burns, left lower leg

    M61.369 Calcification and ossification of muscles associated with burns, unspecified lower leg

● M61.37 Calcification and ossification of muscles associated with burns, ankle and foot

    M61.371 Calcification and ossification of muscles associated with burns, right ankle and foot

    M61.372 Calcification and ossification of muscles associated with burns, left ankle and foot

    M61.379 Calcification and ossification of muscles associated with burns, unspecified ankle and foot

  M61.38 Calcification and ossification of muscles associated with burns, other site

  M61.39 Calcification and ossification of muscles associated with burns, multiple sites

● M61.4 Other calcification of muscle

    Excludes1 calcific tendinitis NOS (M65.2-)
                calcific tendinitis of shoulder (M75.3)

  M61.40 Other calcification of muscle, unspecified site

● M61.41 Other calcification of muscle, shoulder

    M61.411 Other calcification of muscle, right shoulder

    M61.412 Other calcification of muscle, left shoulder

    M61.419 Other calcification of muscle, unspecified shoulder

● M61.42 Other calcification of muscle, upper arm

    M61.421 Other calcification of muscle, right upper arm

    M61.422 Other calcification of muscle, left upper arm

    M61.429 Other calcification of muscle, unspecified upper arm

● M61.43 Other calcification of muscle, forearm

    M61.431 Other calcification of muscle, right forearm

    M61.432 Other calcification of muscle, left forearm

    M61.439 Other calcification of muscle, unspecified forearm

● M61.44 Other calcification of muscle, hand

    M61.441 Other calcification of muscle, right hand

    M61.442 Other calcification of muscle, left hand

    M61.449 Other calcification of muscle, unspecified hand

● M61.45 Other calcification of muscle, thigh

    M61.451 Other calcification of muscle, right thigh

    M61.452 Other calcification of muscle, left thigh

    M61.459 Other calcification of muscle, unspecified thigh

● M61.46 Other calcification of muscle, lower leg

    M61.461 Other calcification of muscle, right lower leg

    M61.462 Other calcification of muscle, left lower leg

    M61.469 Other calcification of muscle, unspecified lower leg

● M61.47 Other calcification of muscle, ankle and foot

    M61.471 Other calcification of muscle, right ankle and foot

    M61.472 Other calcification of muscle, left ankle and foot

    M61.479 Other calcification of muscle, unspecified ankle and foot

  M61.48 Other calcification of muscle, other site

  M61.49 Other calcification of muscle, multiple sites

● M61.5 Other ossification of muscle

  M61.50 Other ossification of muscle, unspecified site

● M61.51 Other ossification of muscle, shoulder

    M61.511 Other ossification of muscle, right shoulder

    M61.512 Other ossification of muscle, left shoulder

    M61.519 Other ossification of muscle, unspecified shoulder

● M61.52 Other ossification of muscle, upper arm

    M61.521 Other ossification of muscle, right upper arm

    M61.522 Other ossification of muscle, left upper arm

    M61.529 Other ossification of muscle, unspecified upper arm

● M61.53 Other ossification of muscle, forearm

    M61.531 Other ossification of muscle, right forearm

    M61.532 Other ossification of muscle, left forearm

    M61.539 Other ossification of muscle, unspecified forearm

● M61.54 Other ossification of muscle, hand

    M61.541 Other ossification of muscle, right hand

    M61.542 Other ossification of muscle, left hand

    M61.549 Other ossification of muscle, unspecified hand

● M61.55 Other ossification of muscle, thigh

    M61.551 Other ossification of muscle, right thigh

    M61.552 Other ossification of muscle, left thigh

    M61.559 Other ossification of muscle, unspecified thigh

● M61.56 Other ossification of muscle, lower leg

    M61.561 Other ossification of muscle, right lower leg

    M61.562 Other ossification of muscle, left lower leg

    M61.569 Other ossification of muscle, unspecified lower leg

CHAPTER 13 (M00-M99)

▶ New   ⟹ Revised   ~~deleted~~ Deleted   **OGCR** Official Guidelines   X Assign placeholder X   ● Use Additional Character(s)

Excludes 1   Excludes 2   Includes   Use additional   Code first   Code also   Key words

● **M61.57 Other ossification of muscle, ankle and foot**

     M61.571 Other ossification of muscle, right ankle and foot

     M61.572 Other ossification of muscle, left ankle and foot

     M61.579 Other ossification of muscle, unspecified ankle and foot

   M61.58 Other ossification of muscle, other site

   M61.59 Other ossification of muscle, multiple sites

  M61.9 Calcification and ossification of muscle, unspecified

● **M62 Other disorders of muscle**

   Excludes1   alcoholic myopathy (G72.1)
               cramp and spasm (R25.2)
               drug-induced myopathy (G72.0)
               myalgia (M79.1)
               stiff-man syndrome (G25.82)

   Excludes2   nontraumatic hematoma of muscle (M79.81)

● **M62.0 Separation of muscle (nontraumatic)**

   Diastasis of muscle

   Excludes1   diastasis recti complicating pregnancy, labor and delivery (O71.8)
               traumatic separation of muscle - see strain of muscle by body region

   M62.00 Separation of muscle (nontraumatic), unspecified site

●   M62.01 Separation of muscle (nontraumatic), shoulder

     M62.011 Separation of muscle (nontraumatic), right shoulder

     M62.012 Separation of muscle (nontraumatic), left shoulder

     M62.019 Separation of muscle (nontraumatic), unspecified shoulder

●   M62.02 Separation of muscle (nontraumatic), upper arm

     M62.021 Separation of muscle (nontraumatic), right upper arm

     M62.022 Separation of muscle (nontraumatic), left upper arm

     M62.029 Separation of muscle (nontraumatic), unspecified upper arm

●   M62.03 Separation of muscle (nontraumatic), forearm

     M62.031 Separation of muscle (nontraumatic), right forearm

     M62.032 Separation of muscle (nontraumatic), left forearm

     M62.039 Separation of muscle (nontraumatic), unspecified forearm

●   M62.04 Separation of muscle (nontraumatic), hand

     M62.041 Separation of muscle (nontraumatic), right hand

     M62.042 Separation of muscle (nontraumatic), left hand

     M62.049 Separation of muscle (nontraumatic), unspecified hand

●   M62.05 Separation of muscle (nontraumatic), thigh

     M62.051 Separation of muscle (nontraumatic), right thigh

     M62.052 Separation of muscle (nontraumatic), left thigh

     M62.059 Separation of muscle (nontraumatic), unspecified thigh

●   M62.06 Separation of muscle (nontraumatic), lower leg

     M62.061 Separation of muscle (nontraumatic), right lower leg

     M62.062 Separation of muscle (nontraumatic), left lower leg

     M62.069 Separation of muscle (nontraumatic), unspecified lower leg

●   M62.07 Separation of muscle (nontraumatic), ankle and foot

     M62.071 Separation of muscle (nontraumatic), right ankle and foot

     M62.072 Separation of muscle (nontraumatic), left ankle and foot

     M62.079 Separation of muscle (nontraumatic), unspecified ankle and foot

   M62.08 Separation of muscle (nontraumatic), other site

● **M62.1 Other rupture of muscle (nontraumatic)**

   Excludes1   traumatic rupture of muscle - see strain of muscle by body region

   Excludes2   rupture of tendon (M66.-)

   M62.10 Other rupture of muscle (nontraumatic), unspecified site

●   M62.11 Other rupture of muscle (nontraumatic), shoulder

     M62.111 Other rupture of muscle (nontraumatic), right shoulder

     M62.112 Other rupture of muscle (nontraumatic), left shoulder

     M62.119 Other rupture of muscle (nontraumatic), unspecified shoulder

●   M62.12 Other rupture of muscle (nontraumatic), upper arm

     M62.121 Other rupture of muscle (nontraumatic), right upper arm

     M62.122 Other rupture of muscle (nontraumatic), left upper arm

     M62.129 Other rupture of muscle (nontraumatic), unspecified upper arm

●   M62.13 Other rupture of muscle (nontraumatic), forearm

     M62.131 Other rupture of muscle (nontraumatic), right forearm

     M62.132 Other rupture of muscle (nontraumatic), left forearm

     M62.139 Other rupture of muscle (nontraumatic), unspecified forearm

●   M62.14 Other rupture of muscle (nontraumatic), hand

     M62.141 Other rupture of muscle (nontraumatic), right hand

     M62.142 Other rupture of muscle (nontraumatic), left hand

     M62.149 Other rupture of muscle (nontraumatic), unspecified hand

●   M62.15 Other rupture of muscle (nontraumatic), thigh

     M62.151 Other rupture of muscle (nontraumatic), right thigh

     M62.152 Other rupture of muscle (nontraumatic), left thigh

     M62.159 Other rupture of muscle (nontraumatic), unspecified thigh

●   M62.16 Other rupture of muscle (nontraumatic), lower leg

     M62.161 Other rupture of muscle (nontraumatic), right lower leg

     M62.162 Other rupture of muscle (nontraumatic), left lower leg

     M62.169 Other rupture of muscle (nontraumatic), unspecified lower leg

●   M62.17 Other rupture of muscle (nontraumatic), ankle and foot

     M62.171 Other rupture of muscle (nontraumatic), right ankle and foot

     M62.172 Other rupture of muscle (nontraumatic), left ankle and foot

     M62.179 Other rupture of muscle (nontraumatic), unspecified ankle and foot

   M62.18 Other rupture of muscle (nontraumatic), other site

▶ New   ⇒ Revised   ~~deleted~~ Deleted   **OGCR** Official Guidelines   X Assign placeholder X   ● Use Additional Character(s)

Excludes 1   Excludes 2   Includes   Use additional   Code first   Code also   Key words

● M62.2   Nontraumatic ischemic infarction of muscle

> **Excludes1**   compartment syndrome (traumatic) (T79.A-)
> nontraumatic compartment syndrome (M79.A-)
> traumatic ischemia of muscle (T79.6)
> rhabdomyolysis (M62.82)
> Volkmann's ischemic contracture (T79.6)

   M62.20   Nontraumatic ischemic infarction of muscle, unspecified site

● M62.21   Nontraumatic ischemic infarction of muscle, shoulder

     M62.211   Nontraumatic ischemic infarction of muscle, right shoulder

     M62.212   Nontraumatic ischemic infarction of muscle, left shoulder

     M62.219   Nontraumatic ischemic infarction of muscle, unspecified shoulder

● M62.22   Nontraumatic ischemic infarction of muscle, upper arm

     M62.221   Nontraumatic ischemic infarction of muscle, right upper arm

     M62.222   Nontraumatic ischemic infarction of muscle, left upper arm

     M62.229   Nontraumatic ischemic infarction of muscle, unspecified upper arm

● M62.23   Nontraumatic ischemic infarction of muscle, forearm

     M62.231   Nontraumatic ischemic infarction of muscle, right forearm

     M62.232   Nontraumatic ischemic infarction of muscle, left forearm

     M62.239   Nontraumatic ischemic infarction of muscle, unspecified forearm

● M62.24   Nontraumatic ischemic infarction of muscle, hand

     M62.241   Nontraumatic ischemic infarction of muscle, right hand

     M62.242   Nontraumatic ischemic infarction of muscle, left hand

     M62.249   Nontraumatic ischemic infarction of muscle, unspecified hand

● M62.25   Nontraumatic ischemic infarction of muscle, thigh

     M62.251   Nontraumatic ischemic infarction of muscle, right thigh

     M62.252   Nontraumatic ischemic infarction of muscle, left thigh

     M62.259   Nontraumatic ischemic infarction of muscle, unspecified thigh

● M62.26   Nontraumatic ischemic infarction of muscle, lower leg

     M62.261   Nontraumatic ischemic infarction of muscle, right lower leg

     M62.262   Nontraumatic ischemic infarction of muscle, left lower leg

     M62.269   Nontraumatic ischemic infarction of muscle, unspecified lower leg

● M62.27   Nontraumatic ischemic infarction of muscle, ankle and foot

     M62.271   Nontraumatic ischemic infarction of muscle, right ankle and foot

     M62.272   Nontraumatic ischemic infarction of muscle, left ankle and foot

     M62.279   Nontraumatic ischemic infarction of muscle, unspecified ankle and foot

   M62.28   Nontraumatic ischemic infarction of muscle, other site

M62.3   Immobility syndrome (paraplegic)

M62.4   Contracture of muscle

> Contracture of tendon (sheath)

> **Excludes1**   contracture of joint (M24.5-)

   M62.40   Contracture of muscle, unspecified site

● M62.41   Contracture of muscle, shoulder

     M62.411   Contracture of muscle, right shoulder

     M62.412   Contracture of muscle, left shoulder

     M62.419   Contracture of muscle, unspecified shoulder

● M62.42   Contracture of muscle, upper arm

     M62.421   Contracture of muscle, right upper arm

     M62.422   Contracture of muscle, left upper arm

     M62.429   Contracture of muscle, unspecified upper arm

● M62.43   Contracture of muscle, forearm

     M62.431   Contracture of muscle, right forearm

     M62.432   Contracture of muscle, left forearm

     M62.439   Contracture of muscle, unspecified forearm

● M62.44   Contracture of muscle, hand

     M62.441   Contracture of muscle, right hand

     M62.442   Contracture of muscle, left hand

     M62.449   Contracture of muscle, unspecified hand

● M62.45   Contracture of muscle, thigh

     M62.451   Contracture of muscle, right thigh

     M62.452   Contracture of muscle, left thigh

     M62.459   Contracture of muscle, unspecified thigh

● M62.46   Contracture of muscle, lower leg

     M62.461   Contracture of muscle, right lower leg

     M62.462   Contracture of muscle, left lower leg

     M62.469   Contracture of muscle, unspecified lower leg

● M62.47   Contracture of muscle, ankle and foot

     M62.471   Contracture of muscle, right ankle and foot

     M62.472   Contracture of muscle, left ankle and foot

     M62.479   Contracture of muscle, unspecified ankle and foot

   M62.48   Contracture of muscle, other site

   M62.49   Contracture of muscle, multiple sites

● M62.5   Muscle wasting and atrophy, not elsewhere classified

> Disuse atrophy NEC

> **Excludes1**   neuralgic amyotrophy (G54.5)
> ⇒ progressive muscular atrophy (G12.21)
> sarcopenia (M62.84)

> **Excludes2**   pelvic muscle wasting (N81.84)

   M62.50   Muscle wasting and atrophy, not elsewhere classified, unspecified site

● M62.51   Muscle wasting and atrophy, not elsewhere classified, shoulder

     M62.511   Muscle wasting and atrophy, not elsewhere classified, right shoulder

     M62.512   Muscle wasting and atrophy, not elsewhere classified, left shoulder

     M62.519   Muscle wasting and atrophy, not elsewhere classified, unspecified shoulder

● M62.52 Muscle wasting and atrophy, not elsewhere classified, upper arm
  M62.521 Muscle wasting and atrophy, not elsewhere classified, right upper arm
  M62.522 Muscle wasting and atrophy, not elsewhere classified, left upper arm
  M62.529 Muscle wasting and atrophy, not elsewhere classified, unspecified upper arm

● M62.53 Muscle wasting and atrophy, not elsewhere classified, forearm
  M62.531 Muscle wasting and atrophy, not elsewhere classified, right forearm
  M62.532 Muscle wasting and atrophy, not elsewhere classified, left forearm
  M62.539 Muscle wasting and atrophy, not elsewhere classified, unspecified forearm

● M62.54 Muscle wasting and atrophy, not elsewhere classified, hand
  M62.541 Muscle wasting and atrophy, not elsewhere classified, right hand
  M62.542 Muscle wasting and atrophy, not elsewhere classified, left hand
  M62.549 Muscle wasting and atrophy, not elsewhere classified, unspecified hand

● M62.55 Muscle wasting and atrophy, not elsewhere classified, thigh
  M62.551 Muscle wasting and atrophy, not elsewhere classified, right thigh
  M62.552 Muscle wasting and atrophy, not elsewhere classified, left thigh
  M62.559 Muscle wasting and atrophy, not elsewhere classified, unspecified thigh

● M62.56 Muscle wasting and atrophy, not elsewhere classified, lower leg
  M62.561 Muscle wasting and atrophy, not elsewhere classified, right lower leg
  M62.562 Muscle wasting and atrophy, not elsewhere classified, left lower leg
  M62.569 Muscle wasting and atrophy, not elsewhere classified, unspecified lower leg

● M62.57 Muscle wasting and atrophy, not elsewhere classified, ankle and foot
  M62.571 Muscle wasting and atrophy, not elsewhere classified, right ankle and foot
  M62.572 Muscle wasting and atrophy, not elsewhere classified, left ankle and foot
  M62.579 Muscle wasting and atrophy, not elsewhere classified, unspecified ankle and foot

M62.58 Muscle wasting and atrophy, not elsewhere classified, other site
M62.59 Muscle wasting and atrophy, not elsewhere classified, multiple sites

● M62.8 Other specified disorders of muscle
  Excludes2 nontraumatic hematoma of muscle (M79.81)
  M62.81 Muscle weakness (generalized)
    Excludes1 muscle weakness in sarcopenia (M62.84)
  M62.82 Rhabdomyolysis
    Excludes1 traumatic rhabdomyolysis (T79.6)

● M62.83 Muscle spasm
  M62.830 Muscle spasm of back
  M62.831 Muscle spasm of calf
          Charley-horse
  M62.838 Other muscle spasm
M62.84 Sarcopenia
        Age-related sarcopenia
        Code first underlying disease, if applicable, such as:
          disorders of myoneural junction and muscle disease in diseases classified elsewhere (G73.-)
          other and unspecified myopathies (G72.-)
          primary disorders of muscles (G71.-)
M62.89 Other specified disorders of muscle
        Muscle (sheath) hernia
M62.9 Disorder of muscle, unspecified

● M63 Disorders of muscle in diseases classified elsewhere
  Code first underlying disease, such as:
    leprosy (A30.-)
    neoplasm (C49.-, C79.89, D21.-, D48.1)
    schistosomiasis (B65.-)
    trichinellosis (B75)
  Excludes1 myopathy in cysticercosis (B69.81)
             myopathy in endocrine diseases (G73.7)
             myopathy in metabolic diseases (G73.7)
             myopathy in sarcoidosis (D86.87)
             myopathy in secondary syphilis (A51.49)
             myopathy in syphilis (late) (A52.78)
             myopathy in toxoplasmosis (B58.82)
             myopathy in tuberculosis (A18.09)

● M63.8 Disorders of muscle in diseases classified elsewhere
  M63.80 Disorders of muscle in diseases classified elsewhere, unspecified site
  ● M63.81 Disorders of muscle in diseases classified elsewhere, shoulder
    M63.811 Disorders of muscle in diseases classified elsewhere, right shoulder
    M63.812 Disorders of muscle in diseases classified elsewhere, left shoulder
    M63.819 Disorders of muscle in diseases classified elsewhere, unspecified shoulder
  ● M63.82 Disorders of muscle in diseases classified elsewhere, upper arm
    M63.821 Disorders of muscle in diseases classified elsewhere, right upper arm
    M63.822 Disorders of muscle in diseases classified elsewhere, left upper arm
    M63.829 Disorders of muscle in diseases classified elsewhere, unspecified upper arm
  ● M63.83 Disorders of muscle in diseases classified elsewhere, forearm
    M63.831 Disorders of muscle in diseases classified elsewhere, right forearm
    M63.832 Disorders of muscle in diseases classified elsewhere, left forearm
    M63.839 Disorders of muscle in diseases classified elsewhere, unspecified forearm
  ● M63.84 Disorders of muscle in diseases classified elsewhere, hand
    M63.841 Disorders of muscle in diseases classified elsewhere, right hand
    M63.842 Disorders of muscle in diseases classified elsewhere, left hand
    M63.849 Disorders of muscle in diseases classified elsewhere, unspecified hand

● **M63.85**   Disorders of muscle in diseases classified elsewhere, thigh

    M63.851   Disorders of muscle in diseases classified elsewhere, right thigh

    M63.852   Disorders of muscle in diseases classified elsewhere, left thigh

    M63.859   Disorders of muscle in diseases classified elsewhere, unspecified thigh

● **M63.86**   Disorders of muscle in diseases classified elsewhere, lower leg

    M63.861   Disorders of muscle in diseases classified elsewhere, right lower leg

    M63.862   Disorders of muscle in diseases classified elsewhere, left lower leg

    M63.869   Disorders of muscle in diseases classified elsewhere, unspecified lower leg

● **M63.87**   Disorders of muscle in diseases classified elsewhere, ankle and foot

    M63.871   Disorders of muscle in diseases classified elsewhere, right ankle and foot

    M63.872   Disorders of muscle in diseases classified elsewhere, left ankle and foot

    M63.879   Disorders of muscle in diseases classified elsewhere, unspecified ankle and foot

   M63.88   Disorders of muscle in diseases classified elsewhere, other site

   M63.89   Disorders of muscle in diseases classified elsewhere, multiple sites

DISORDERS OF SYNOVIUM AND TENDON (M65-M67)

● **M65**   **Synovitis and tenosynovitis**

   Excludes1   chronic crepitant synovitis of hand and wrist (M70.0-)

          current injury - see injury of ligament or tendon by body region

          soft tissue disorders related to use, overuse and pressure (M70.-)

● **M65.0**   **Abscess of tendon sheath**

     Use additional code (B95-B96) to identify bacterial agent

   M65.00   Abscess of tendon sheath, unspecified site

● **M65.01**   Abscess of tendon sheath, shoulder

    M65.011   Abscess of tendon sheath, right shoulder

    M65.012   Abscess of tendon sheath, left shoulder

    M65.019   Abscess of tendon sheath, unspecified shoulder

● **M65.02**   Abscess of tendon sheath, upper arm

    M65.021   Abscess of tendon sheath, right upper arm

    M65.022   Abscess of tendon sheath, left upper arm

    M65.029   Abscess of tendon sheath, unspecified upper arm

● **M65.03**   Abscess of tendon sheath, forearm

    M65.031   Abscess of tendon sheath, right forearm

    M65.032   Abscess of tendon sheath, left forearm

    M65.039   Abscess of tendon sheath, unspecified forearm

Item 13-11 Synovitis is an inflammation of a synovial membrane resulting in pain on motion and is characterized by fluctuating swelling due to effusion in a synovial sac. **Tenosynovitis** is an inflammation of a tendon sheath and occurs most commonly in the wrists, hands, and feet. Bursitis is inflammation of a bursa (fluid filled sac) caused by repetitive use, trauma, infection, or systemic inflammatory disease. Bursae act as protectors and facilitate movement between bones and overlapping muscles (deep bursae) or between bones and tendons/skin (superficial bursae).

● **M65.04**   Abscess of tendon sheath, hand

    M65.041   Abscess of tendon sheath, right hand

    M65.042   Abscess of tendon sheath, left hand

    M65.049   Abscess of tendon sheath, unspecified hand

● **M65.05**   Abscess of tendon sheath, thigh

    M65.051   Abscess of tendon sheath, right thigh

    M65.052   Abscess of tendon sheath, left thigh

    M65.059   Abscess of tendon sheath, unspecified thigh

● **M65.06**   Abscess of tendon sheath, lower leg

    M65.061   Abscess of tendon sheath, right lower leg

    M65.062   Abscess of tendon sheath, left lower leg

    M65.069   Abscess of tendon sheath, unspecified lower leg

● **M65.07**   Abscess of tendon sheath, ankle and foot

    M65.071   Abscess of tendon sheath, right ankle and foot

    M65.072   Abscess of tendon sheath, left ankle and foot

    M65.079   Abscess of tendon sheath, unspecified ankle and foot

   M65.08   Abscess of tendon sheath, other site

● **M65.1**   Other infective (teno)synovitis

   M65.10   Other infective (teno)synovitis, unspecified site

● **M65.11**   Other infective (teno)synovitis, shoulder

    M65.111   Other infective (teno)synovitis, right shoulder

    M65.112   Other infective (teno)synovitis, left shoulder

    M65.119   Other infective (teno)synovitis, unspecified shoulder

● **M65.12**   Other infective (teno)synovitis, elbow

    M65.121   Other infective (teno)synovitis, right elbow

    M65.122   Other infective (teno)synovitis, left elbow

    M65.129   Other infective (teno)synovitis, unspecified elbow

● **M65.13**   Other infective (teno)synovitis, wrist

    M65.131   Other infective (teno)synovitis, right wrist

    M65.132   Other infective (teno)synovitis, left wrist

    M65.139   Other infective (teno)synovitis, unspecified wrist

● **M65.14**   Other infective (teno)synovitis, hand

    M65.141   Other infective (teno)synovitis, right hand

    M65.142   Other infective (teno)synovitis, left hand

    M65.149   Other infective (teno)synovitis, unspecified hand

● M65.15   Other infective (teno)synovitis, hip
  - M65.151   Other infective (teno)synovitis, right hip
  - M65.152   Other infective (teno)synovitis, left hip
  - M65.159   Other infective (teno)synovitis, unspecified hip

● M65.16   Other infective (teno)synovitis, knee
  - M65.161   Other infective (teno)synovitis, right knee
  - M65.162   Other infective (teno)synovitis, left knee
  - M65.169   Other infective (teno)synovitis, unspecified knee

● M65.17   Other infective (teno)synovitis, ankle and foot
  - M65.171   Other infective (teno)synovitis, right ankle and foot
  - M65.172   Other infective (teno)synovitis, left ankle and foot
  - M65.179   Other infective (teno)synovitis, unspecified ankle and foot

M65.18   Other infective (teno)synovitis, other site

M65.19   Other infective (teno)synovitis, multiple sites

● M65.2   Calcific tendinitis

> **Excludes1**   tendinitis as classified in M75-M77
> calcified tendinitis of shoulder (M75.3)

M65.20   Calcific tendinitis, unspecified site

● M65.22   Calcific tendinitis, upper arm
  - M65.221   Calcific tendinitis, right upper arm
  - M65.222   Calcific tendinitis, left upper arm
  - M65.229   Calcific tendinitis, unspecified upper arm

● M65.23   Calcific tendinitis, forearm
  - M65.231   Calcific tendinitis, right forearm
  - M65.232   Calcific tendinitis, left forearm
  - M65.239   Calcific tendinitis, unspecified forearm

● M65.24   Calcific tendinitis, hand
  - M65.241   Calcific tendinitis, right hand
  - M65.242   Calcific tendinitis, left hand
  - M65.249   Calcific tendinitis, unspecified hand

● M65.25   Calcific tendinitis, thigh
  - M65.251   Calcific tendinitis, right thigh
  - M65.252   Calcific tendinitis, left thigh
  - M65.259   Calcific tendinitis, unspecified thigh

● M65.26   Calcific tendinitis, lower leg
  - M65.261   Calcific tendinitis, right lower leg
  - M65.262   Calcific tendinitis, left lower leg
  - M65.269   Calcific tendinitis, unspecified lower leg

● M65.27   Calcific tendinitis, ankle and foot
  - M65.271   Calcific tendinitis, right ankle and foot
  - M65.272   Calcific tendinitis, left ankle and foot
  - M65.279   Calcific tendinitis, unspecified ankle and foot

M65.28   Calcific tendinitis, other site

M65.29   Calcific tendinitis, multiple sites

● M65.3   Trigger finger
  Nodular tendinous disease

M65.30   Trigger finger, unspecified finger

● M65.31   Trigger thumb
  - M65.311   Trigger thumb, right thumb
  - M65.312   Trigger thumb, left thumb
  - M65.319   Trigger thumb, unspecified thumb

● M65.32   Trigger finger, index finger
  - M65.321   Trigger finger, right index finger
  - M65.322   Trigger finger, left index finger
  - M65.329   Trigger finger, unspecified index finger

● M65.33   Trigger finger, middle finger
  - M65.331   Trigger finger, right middle finger
  - M65.332   Trigger finger, left middle finger
  - M65.339   Trigger finger, unspecified middle finger

● M65.34   Trigger finger, ring finger
  - M65.341   Trigger finger, right ring finger
  - M65.342   Trigger finger, left ring finger
  - M65.349   Trigger finger, unspecified ring finger

● M65.35   Trigger finger, little finger
  - M65.351   Trigger finger, right little finger
  - M65.352   Trigger finger, left little finger
  - M65.359   Trigger finger, unspecified little finger

M65.4   Radial styloid tenosynovitis [de Quervain]

● M65.8   Other synovitis and tenosynovitis

M65.80   Other synovitis and tenosynovitis, unspecified site

● M65.81   Other synovitis and tenosynovitis, shoulder
  - M65.811   Other synovitis and tenosynovitis, right shoulder
  - M65.812   Other synovitis and tenosynovitis, left shoulder
  - M65.819   Other synovitis and tenosynovitis, unspecified shoulder

● M65.82   Other synovitis and tenosynovitis, upper arm
  - M65.821   Other synovitis and tenosynovitis, right upper arm
  - M65.822   Other synovitis and tenosynovitis, left upper arm
  - M65.829   Other synovitis and tenosynovitis, unspecified upper arm

● M65.83   Other synovitis and tenosynovitis, forearm
  - M65.831   Other synovitis and tenosynovitis, right forearm
  - M65.832   Other synovitis and tenosynovitis, left forearm
  - M65.839   Other synovitis and tenosynovitis, unspecified forearm

● M65.84   Other synovitis and tenosynovitis, hand
  - M65.841   Other synovitis and tenosynovitis, right hand
  - M65.842   Other synovitis and tenosynovitis, left hand
  - M65.849   Other synovitis and tenosynovitis, unspecified hand

● M65.85   Other synovitis and tenosynovitis, thigh
  - M65.851   Other synovitis and tenosynovitis, right thigh
  - M65.852   Other synovitis and tenosynovitis, left thigh
  - M65.859   Other synovitis and tenosynovitis, unspecified thigh

▶ New   ➡ Revised   ~~deleted~~ Deleted   **OGCR** Official Guidelines   X Assign placeholder X   ● Use Additional Character(s)

Excludes 1   Excludes 2   Includes   Use additional   Code first   Code also   Key words

● M65.86   Other synovitis and tenosynovitis, lower leg
     M65.861   Other synovitis and tenosynovitis, right lower leg
     M65.862   Other synovitis and tenosynovitis, left lower leg
     M65.869   Other synovitis and tenosynovitis, unspecified lower leg
● M65.87   Other synovitis and tenosynovitis, ankle and foot
     M65.871   Other synovitis and tenosynovitis, right ankle and foot
     M65.872   Other synovitis and tenosynovitis, left ankle and foot
     M65.879   Other synovitis and tenosynovitis, unspecified ankle and foot
   M65.88   Other synovitis and tenosynovitis, other site
   M65.89   Other synovitis and tenosynovitis, multiple sites
  M65.9   Synovitis and tenosynovitis, unspecified

● M66   Spontaneous rupture of synovium and tendon

Includes	rupture that occurs when a normal force is applied to tissues that are inferred to have less than normal strength
Excludes2	rotator cuff syndrome (M75.1-)
	rupture where an abnormal force is applied to normal tissue - see injury of tendon by body region

  M66.0   Rupture of popliteal cyst
● M66.1   Rupture of synovium
     Rupture of synovial cyst

Excludes2	rupture of popliteal cyst (M66.0)

   M66.10   Rupture of synovium, unspecified joint
● M66.11   Rupture of synovium, shoulder
     M66.111   Rupture of synovium, right shoulder
     M66.112   Rupture of synovium, left shoulder
     M66.119   Rupture of synovium, unspecified shoulder
● M66.12   Rupture of synovium, elbow
     M66.121   Rupture of synovium, right elbow
     M66.122   Rupture of synovium, left elbow
     M66.129   Rupture of synovium, unspecified elbow
● M66.13   Rupture of synovium, wrist
     M66.131   Rupture of synovium, right wrist
     M66.132   Rupture of synovium, left wrist
     M66.139   Rupture of synovium, unspecified wrist
● M66.14   Rupture of synovium, hand and fingers
     M66.141   Rupture of synovium, right hand
     M66.142   Rupture of synovium, left hand
     M66.143   Rupture of synovium, unspecified hand
     M66.144   Rupture of synovium, right finger(s)
     M66.145   Rupture of synovium, left finger(s)
     M66.146   Rupture of synovium, unspecified finger(s)
● M66.15   Rupture of synovium, hip
     M66.151   Rupture of synovium, right hip
     M66.152   Rupture of synovium, left hip
     M66.159   Rupture of synovium, unspecified hip

● M66.17   Rupture of synovium, ankle, foot and toes
     M66.171   Rupture of synovium, right ankle
     M66.172   Rupture of synovium, left ankle
     M66.173   Rupture of synovium, unspecified ankle
     M66.174   Rupture of synovium, right foot
     M66.175   Rupture of synovium, left foot
     M66.176   Rupture of synovium, unspecified foot
     M66.177   Rupture of synovium, right toe(s)
     M66.178   Rupture of synovium, left toe(s)
     M66.179   Rupture of synovium, unspecified toe(s)
   M66.18   Rupture of synovium, other site
● M66.2   Spontaneous rupture of extensor tendons
   M66.20   Spontaneous rupture of extensor tendons, unspecified site
● M66.21   Spontaneous rupture of extensor tendons, shoulder
     M66.211   Spontaneous rupture of extensor tendons, right shoulder
     M66.212   Spontaneous rupture of extensor tendons, left shoulder
     M66.219   Spontaneous rupture of extensor tendons, unspecified shoulder
● M66.22   Spontaneous rupture of extensor tendons, upper arm
     M66.221   Spontaneous rupture of extensor tendons, right upper arm
     M66.222   Spontaneous rupture of extensor tendons, left upper arm
     M66.229   Spontaneous rupture of extensor tendons, unspecified upper arm
● M66.23   Spontaneous rupture of extensor tendons, forearm
     M66.231   Spontaneous rupture of extensor tendons, right forearm
     M66.232   Spontaneous rupture of extensor tendons, left forearm
     M66.239   Spontaneous rupture of extensor tendons, unspecified forearm
● M66.24   Spontaneous rupture of extensor tendons, hand
     M66.241   Spontaneous rupture of extensor tendons, right hand
     M66.242   Spontaneous rupture of extensor tendons, left hand
     M66.249   Spontaneous rupture of extensor tendons, unspecified hand
● M66.25   Spontaneous rupture of extensor tendons, thigh
     M66.251   Spontaneous rupture of extensor tendons, right thigh
     M66.252   Spontaneous rupture of extensor tendons, left thigh
     M66.259   Spontaneous rupture of extensor tendons, unspecified thigh
● M66.26   Spontaneous rupture of extensor tendons, lower leg
     M66.261   Spontaneous rupture of extensor tendons, right lower leg
     M66.262   Spontaneous rupture of extensor tendons, left lower leg
     M66.269   Spontaneous rupture of extensor tendons, unspecified lower leg

● M66.27   Spontaneous rupture of extensor tendons, ankle and foot

     M66.271   Spontaneous rupture of extensor tendons, right ankle and foot

     M66.272   Spontaneous rupture of extensor tendons, left ankle and foot

     M66.279   Spontaneous rupture of extensor tendons, unspecified ankle and foot

   M66.28   Spontaneous rupture of extensor tendons, other site

   M66.29   Spontaneous rupture of extensor tendons, multiple sites

● M66.3   Spontaneous rupture of flexor tendons

   M66.30   Spontaneous rupture of flexor tendons, unspecified site

● M66.31   Spontaneous rupture of flexor tendons, shoulder

     M66.311   Spontaneous rupture of flexor tendons, right shoulder

     M66.312   Spontaneous rupture of flexor tendons, left shoulder

     M66.319   Spontaneous rupture of flexor tendons, unspecified shoulder

● M66.32   Spontaneous rupture of flexor tendons, upper arm

     M66.321   Spontaneous rupture of flexor tendons, right upper arm

     M66.322   Spontaneous rupture of flexor tendons, left upper arm

     M66.329   Spontaneous rupture of flexor tendons, unspecified upper arm

● M66.33   Spontaneous rupture of flexor tendons, forearm

     M66.331   Spontaneous rupture of flexor tendons, right forearm

     M66.332   Spontaneous rupture of flexor tendons, left forearm

     M66.339   Spontaneous rupture of flexor tendons, unspecified forearm

● M66.34   Spontaneous rupture of flexor tendons, hand

     M66.341   Spontaneous rupture of flexor tendons, right hand

     M66.342   Spontaneous rupture of flexor tendons, left hand

     M66.349   Spontaneous rupture of flexor tendons, unspecified hand

● M66.35   Spontaneous rupture of flexor tendons, thigh

     M66.351   Spontaneous rupture of flexor tendons, right thigh

     M66.352   Spontaneous rupture of flexor tendons, left thigh

     M66.359   Spontaneous rupture of flexor tendons, unspecified thigh

● M66.36   Spontaneous rupture of flexor tendons, lower leg

     M66.361   Spontaneous rupture of flexor tendons, right lower leg

     M66.362   Spontaneous rupture of flexor tendons, left lower leg

     M66.369   Spontaneous rupture of flexor tendons, unspecified lower leg

● M66.37   Spontaneous rupture of flexor tendons, ankle and foot

     M66.371   Spontaneous rupture of flexor tendons, right ankle and foot

     M66.372   Spontaneous rupture of flexor tendons, left ankle and foot

     M66.379   Spontaneous rupture of flexor tendons, unspecified ankle and foot

   M66.38   Spontaneous rupture of flexor tendons, other site

   M66.39   Spontaneous rupture of flexor tendons, multiple sites

● M66.8   Spontaneous rupture of other tendons

   M66.80   Spontaneous rupture of other tendons, unspecified site

● M66.81   Spontaneous rupture of other tendons, shoulder

     M66.811   Spontaneous rupture of other tendons, right shoulder

     M66.812   Spontaneous rupture of other tendons, left shoulder

     M66.819   Spontaneous rupture of other tendons, unspecified shoulder

● M66.82   Spontaneous rupture of other tendons, upper arm

     M66.821   Spontaneous rupture of other tendons, right upper arm

     M66.822   Spontaneous rupture of other tendons, left upper arm

     M66.829   Spontaneous rupture of other tendons, unspecified upper arm

● M66.83   Spontaneous rupture of other tendons, forearm

     M66.831   Spontaneous rupture of other tendons, right forearm

     M66.832   Spontaneous rupture of other tendons, left forearm

     M66.839   Spontaneous rupture of other tendons, unspecified forearm

● M66.84   Spontaneous rupture of other tendons, hand

     M66.841   Spontaneous rupture of other tendons, right hand

     M66.842   Spontaneous rupture of other tendons, left hand

     M66.849   Spontaneous rupture of other tendons, unspecified hand

● M66.85   Spontaneous rupture of other tendons, thigh

     M66.851   Spontaneous rupture of other tendons, right thigh

     M66.852   Spontaneous rupture of other tendons, left thigh

     M66.859   Spontaneous rupture of other tendons, unspecified thigh

● M66.86   Spontaneous rupture of other tendons, lower leg

     M66.861   Spontaneous rupture of other tendons, right lower leg

     M66.862   Spontaneous rupture of other tendons, left lower leg

     M66.869   Spontaneous rupture of other tendons, unspecified lower leg

● M66.87   Spontaneous rupture of other tendons, ankle and foot

     M66.871   Spontaneous rupture of other tendons, right ankle and foot

     M66.872   Spontaneous rupture of other tendons, left ankle and foot

     M66.879   Spontaneous rupture of other tendons, unspecified ankle and foot

   M66.88   Spontaneous rupture of other tendons, other

   M66.89   Spontaneous rupture of other tendons, multiple sites

M66.9   Spontaneous rupture of unspecified tendon

     Rupture at musculotendinous junction, nontraumatic

▶ New   ⟹ Revised   ~~deleted~~ Deleted   **OGCR** Official Guidelines   X Assign placeholder X   ● Use Additional Character(s)

Excludes 1   Excludes 2   Includes   Use additional   Code first   Code also   Key words

● **M67   Other disorders of synovium and tendon**

> **Excludes1**   palmar fascial fibromatosis [Dupuytren] (M72.0)
> tendinitis NOS (M77.9-)
> xanthomatosis localized to tendons (E78.2)

● **M67.0   Short Achilles tendon (acquired)**

     M67.00   Short Achilles tendon (acquired), unspecified ankle

     M67.01   Short Achilles tendon (acquired), right ankle

     M67.02   Short Achilles tendon (acquired), left ankle

● **M67.2   Synovial hypertrophy, not elsewhere classified**

> **Excludes1**   villonodular synovitis (pigmented) (M12.2-)

     M67.20   Synovial hypertrophy, not elsewhere classified, unspecified site

     ● **M67.21   Synovial hypertrophy, not elsewhere classified, shoulder**

         M67.211   Synovial hypertrophy, not elsewhere classified, right shoulder

         M67.212   Synovial hypertrophy, not elsewhere classified, left shoulder

         M67.219   Synovial hypertrophy, not elsewhere classified, unspecified shoulder

     ● **M67.22   Synovial hypertrophy, not elsewhere classified, upper arm**

         M67.221   Synovial hypertrophy, not elsewhere classified, right upper arm

         M67.222   Synovial hypertrophy, not elsewhere classified, left upper arm

         M67.229   Synovial hypertrophy, not elsewhere classified, unspecified upper arm

     ● **M67.23   Synovial hypertrophy, not elsewhere classified, forearm**

         M67.231   Synovial hypertrophy, not elsewhere classified, right forearm

         M67.232   Synovial hypertrophy, not elsewhere classified, left forearm

         M67.239   Synovial hypertrophy, not elsewhere classified, unspecified forearm

     ● **M67.24   Synovial hypertrophy, not elsewhere classified, hand**

         M67.241   Synovial hypertrophy, not elsewhere classified, right hand

         M67.242   Synovial hypertrophy, not elsewhere classified, left hand

         M67.249   Synovial hypertrophy, not elsewhere classified, unspecified hand

     ● **M67.25   Synovial hypertrophy, not elsewhere classified, thigh**

         M67.251   Synovial hypertrophy, not elsewhere classified, right thigh

         M67.252   Synovial hypertrophy, not elsewhere classified, left thigh

         M67.259   Synovial hypertrophy, not elsewhere classified, unspecified thigh

     ● **M67.26   Synovial hypertrophy, not elsewhere classified, lower leg**

         M67.261   Synovial hypertrophy, not elsewhere classified, right lower leg

         M67.262   Synovial hypertrophy, not elsewhere classified, left lower leg

         M67.269   Synovial hypertrophy, not elsewhere classified, unspecified lower leg

     ● **M67.27   Synovial hypertrophy, not elsewhere classified, ankle and foot**

         M67.271   Synovial hypertrophy, not elsewhere classified, right ankle and foot

         M67.272   Synovial hypertrophy, not elsewhere classified, left ankle and foot

         M67.279   Synovial hypertrophy, not elsewhere classified, unspecified ankle and foot

     M67.28   Synovial hypertrophy, not elsewhere classified, other site

     M67.29   Synovial hypertrophy, not elsewhere classified, multiple sites

● **M67.3   Transient synovitis**

     Toxic synovitis

> **Excludes1**   palindromic rheumatism (M12.3-)

     M67.30   Transient synovitis, unspecified site

     ● **M67.31   Transient synovitis, shoulder**

         M67.311   Transient synovitis, right shoulder

         M67.312   Transient synovitis, left shoulder

         M67.319   Transient synovitis, unspecified shoulder

     ● **M67.32   Transient synovitis, elbow**

         M67.321   Transient synovitis, right elbow

         M67.322   Transient synovitis, left elbow

         M67.329   Transient synovitis, unspecified elbow

     ● **M67.33   Transient synovitis, wrist**

         M67.331   Transient synovitis, right wrist

         M67.332   Transient synovitis, left wrist

         M67.339   Transient synovitis, unspecified wrist

     ● **M67.34   Transient synovitis, hand**

         M67.341   Transient synovitis, right hand

         M67.342   Transient synovitis, left hand

         M67.349   Transient synovitis, unspecified hand

     ● **M67.35   Transient synovitis, hip**

         M67.351   Transient synovitis, right hip

         M67.352   Transient synovitis, left hip

         M67.359   Transient synovitis, unspecified hip

     ● **M67.36   Transient synovitis, knee**

         M67.361   Transient synovitis, right knee

         M67.362   Transient synovitis, left knee

         M67.369   Transient synovitis, unspecified knee

     ● **M67.37   Transient synovitis, ankle and foot**

         M67.371   Transient synovitis, right ankle and foot

         M67.372   Transient synovitis, left ankle and foot

         M67.379   Transient synovitis, unspecified ankle and foot

     M67.38   Transient synovitis, other site

     M67.39   Transient synovitis, multiple sites

● **M67.4   Ganglion**

     Ganglion of joint or tendon (sheath)

> **Excludes1**   ganglion in yaws (A66.6)
> **Excludes2**   cyst of bursa (M71.2-M71.3)
> cyst of synovium (M71.2-M71.3)

     M67.40   Ganglion, unspecified site

     ● **M67.41   Ganglion, shoulder**

         M67.411   Ganglion, right shoulder

         M67.412   Ganglion, left shoulder

         M67.419   Ganglion, unspecified shoulder

     ● **M67.42   Ganglion, elbow**

         M67.421   Ganglion, right elbow

         M67.422   Ganglion, left elbow

         M67.429   Ganglion, unspecified elbow

     ● **M67.43   Ganglion, wrist**

         M67.431   Ganglion, right wrist

         M67.432   Ganglion, left wrist

         M67.439   Ganglion, unspecified wrist

     ● **M67.44   Ganglion, hand**

         M67.441   Ganglion, right hand

         M67.442   Ganglion, left hand

         M67.449   Ganglion, unspecified hand

CHAPTER 13 (M00-M99)

● M67.45 Ganglion, hip
    M67.451 Ganglion, right hip
    M67.452 Ganglion, left hip
    M67.459 Ganglion, unspecified hip
● M67.46 Ganglion, knee
    M67.461 Ganglion, right knee
    M67.462 Ganglion, left knee
    M67.469 Ganglion, unspecified knee
● M67.47 Ganglion, ankle and foot
    M67.471 Ganglion, right ankle and foot
    M67.472 Ganglion, left ankle and foot
    M67.479 Ganglion, unspecified ankle and foot
  M67.48 Ganglion, other site
  M67.49 Ganglion, multiple sites
● M67.5 Plica syndrome
    Plica knee
  M67.50 Plica syndrome, unspecified knee
  M67.51 Plica syndrome, right knee
  M67.52 Plica syndrome, left knee
● M67.8 Other specified disorders of synovium and tendon
  M67.80 Other specified disorders of synovium and tendon, unspecified site
● M67.81 Other specified disorders of synovium and tendon, shoulder
    M67.811 Other specified disorders of synovium, right shoulder
    M67.812 Other specified disorders of synovium, left shoulder
    M67.813 Other specified disorders of tendon, right shoulder
    M67.814 Other specified disorders of tendon, left shoulder
    M67.819 Other specified disorders of synovium and tendon, unspecified shoulder
● M67.82 Other specified disorders of synovium and tendon, elbow
    M67.821 Other specified disorders of synovium, right elbow
    M67.822 Other specified disorders of synovium, left elbow
    M67.823 Other specified disorders of tendon, right elbow
    M67.824 Other specified disorders of tendon, left elbow
    M67.829 Other specified disorders of synovium and tendon, unspecified elbow
● M67.83 Other specified disorders of synovium and tendon, wrist
    M67.831 Other specified disorders of synovium, right wrist
    M67.832 Other specified disorders of synovium, left wrist
    M67.833 Other specified disorders of tendon, right wrist
    M67.834 Other specified disorders of tendon, left wrist
    M67.839 Other specified disorders of synovium and tendon, unspecified forearm
● M67.84 Other specified disorders of synovium and tendon, hand
    M67.841 Other specified disorders of synovium, right hand
    M67.842 Other specified disorders of synovium, left hand
    M67.843 Other specified disorders of tendon, right hand
    M67.844 Other specified disorders of tendon, left hand
    M67.849 Other specified disorders of synovium and tendon, unspecified hand
● M67.85 Other specified disorders of synovium and tendon, hip
    M67.851 Other specified disorders of synovium, right hip
    M67.852 Other specified disorders of synovium, left hip
    M67.853 Other specified disorders of tendon, right hip
    M67.854 Other specified disorders of tendon, left hip
    M67.859 Other specified disorders of synovium and tendon, unspecified hip
● M67.86 Other specified disorders of synovium and tendon, knee
    M67.861 Other specified disorders of synovium, right knee
    M67.862 Other specified disorders of synovium, left knee
    M67.863 Other specified disorders of tendon, right knee
    M67.864 Other specified disorders of tendon, left knee
    M67.869 Other specified disorders of synovium and tendon, unspecified knee
● M67.87 Other specified disorders of synovium and tendon, ankle and foot
    M67.871 Other specified disorders of synovium, right ankle and foot
    M67.872 Other specified disorders of synovium, left ankle and foot
    M67.873 Other specified disorders of tendon, right ankle and foot
    M67.874 Other specified disorders of tendon, left ankle and foot
    M67.879 Other specified disorders of synovium and tendon, unspecified ankle and foot
  M67.88 Other specified disorders of synovium and tendon, other site
  M67.89 Other specified disorders of synovium and tendon, multiple sites
● M67.9 Unspecified disorder of synovium and tendon
  M67.90 Unspecified disorder of synovium and tendon, unspecified site
● M67.91 Unspecified disorder of synovium and tendon, shoulder
    M67.911 Unspecified disorder of synovium and tendon, right shoulder
    M67.912 Unspecified disorder of synovium and tendon, left shoulder
    M67.919 Unspecified disorder of synovium and tendon, unspecified shoulder
● M67.92 Unspecified disorder of synovium and tendon, upper arm
    M67.921 Unspecified disorder of synovium and tendon, right upper arm
    M67.922 Unspecified disorder of synovium and tendon, left upper arm
    M67.929 Unspecified disorder of synovium and tendon, unspecified upper arm

● M67.93   Unspecified disorder of synovium and tendon, forearm

    M67.931   Unspecified disorder of synovium and tendon, right forearm

    M67.932   Unspecified disorder of synovium and tendon, left forearm

    M67.939   Unspecified disorder of synovium and tendon, unspecified forearm

● M67.94   Unspecified disorder of synovium and tendon, hand

    M67.941   Unspecified disorder of synovium and tendon, right hand

    M67.942   Unspecified disorder of synovium and tendon, left hand

    M67.949   Unspecified disorder of synovium and tendon, unspecified hand

● M67.95   Unspecified disorder of synovium and tendon, thigh

    M67.951   Unspecified disorder of synovium and tendon, right thigh

    M67.952   Unspecified disorder of synovium and tendon, left thigh

    M67.959   Unspecified disorder of synovium and tendon, unspecified thigh

● M67.96   Unspecified disorder of synovium and tendon, lower leg

    M67.961   Unspecified disorder of synovium and tendon, right lower leg

    M67.962   Unspecified disorder of synovium and tendon, left lower leg

    M67.969   Unspecified disorder of synovium and tendon, unspecified lower leg

● M67.97   Unspecified disorder of synovium and tendon, ankle and foot

    M67.971   Unspecified disorder of synovium and tendon, right ankle and foot

    M67.972   Unspecified disorder of synovium and tendon, left ankle and foot

    M67.979   Unspecified disorder of synovium and tendon, unspecified ankle and foot

    M67.98   Unspecified disorder of synovium and tendon, other site

    M67.99   Unspecified disorder of synovium and tendon, multiple sites

OTHER SOFT TISSUE DISORDERS (M70-M79)

● M70   Soft tissue disorders related to use, overuse and pressure

   Includes   soft tissue disorders of occupational origin

   Use additional external cause code to identify activity causing disorder (Y93.-)

   Excludes1   bursitis NOS (M71.9-)

   Excludes2   bursitis of shoulder (M75.5)
             enthesopathies (M76-M77)
             pressure ulcer (pressure area) (L89.-)

● M70.0   Crepitant synovitis (acute) (chronic) of hand and wrist

   ● M70.03   Crepitant synovitis (acute) (chronic), wrist

     M70.031   Crepitant synovitis (acute) (chronic), right wrist

     M70.032   Crepitant synovitis (acute) (chronic), left wrist

     M70.039   Crepitant synovitis (acute) (chronic), unspecified wrist

   ● M70.04   Crepitant synovitis (acute) (chronic), hand

     M70.041   Crepitant synovitis (acute) (chronic), right hand

     M70.042   Crepitant synovitis (acute) (chronic), left hand

     M70.049   Crepitant synovitis (acute) (chronic), unspecified hand

● M70.1   Bursitis of hand

    M70.10   Bursitis, unspecified hand

    M70.11   Bursitis, right hand

    M70.12   Bursitis, left hand

● M70.2   Olecranon bursitis

    M70.20   Olecranon bursitis, unspecified elbow

    M70.21   Olecranon bursitis, right elbow

    M70.22   Olecranon bursitis, left elbow

● M70.3   Other bursitis of elbow

    M70.30   Other bursitis of elbow, unspecified elbow

    M70.31   Other bursitis of elbow, right elbow

    M70.32   Other bursitis of elbow, left elbow

● M70.4   Prepatellar bursitis

    M70.40   Prepatellar bursitis, unspecified knee

    M70.41   Prepatellar bursitis, right knee

    M70.42   Prepatellar bursitis, left knee

● M70.5   Other bursitis of knee

    M70.50   Other bursitis of knee, unspecified knee

    M70.51   Other bursitis of knee, right knee

    M70.52   Other bursitis of knee, left knee

● M70.6   Trochanteric bursitis
       Trochanteric tendinitis

    M70.60   Trochanteric bursitis, unspecified hip

    M70.61   Trochanteric bursitis, right hip

    M70.62   Trochanteric bursitis, left hip

● M70.7   Other bursitis of hip
       Ischial bursitis

    M70.70   Other bursitis of hip, unspecified hip

    M70.71   Other bursitis of hip, right hip

    M70.72   Other bursitis of hip, left hip

● M70.8   Other soft tissue disorders related to use, overuse and pressure

    M70.80   Other soft tissue disorders related to use, overuse and pressure of unspecified site

   ● M70.81   Other soft tissue disorders related to use, overuse and pressure of shoulder

     M70.811   Other soft tissue disorders related to use, overuse and pressure, right shoulder

     M70.812   Other soft tissue disorders related to use, overuse and pressure, left shoulder

     M70.819   Other soft tissue disorders related to use, overuse and pressure, unspecified shoulder

   ● M70.82   Other soft tissue disorders related to use, overuse and pressure of upper arm

     M70.821   Other soft tissue disorders related to use, overuse and pressure, right upper arm

     M70.822   Other soft tissue disorders related to use, overuse and pressure, left upper arm

     M70.829   Other soft tissue disorders related to use, overuse and pressure, unspecified upper arms

   ● M70.83   Other soft tissue disorders related to use, overuse and pressure of forearm

     M70.831   Other soft tissue disorders related to use, overuse and pressure, right forearm

     M70.832   Other soft tissue disorders related to use, overuse and pressure, left forearm

     M70.839   Other soft tissue disorders related to use, overuse and pressure, unspecified forearm

● M70.84   Other soft tissue disorders related to use, overuse and pressure of hand

     M70.841   Other soft tissue disorders related to use, overuse and pressure, right hand

     M70.842   Other soft tissue disorders related to use, overuse and pressure, left hand

     M70.849   Other soft tissue disorders related to use, overuse and pressure, unspecified hand

● M70.85   Other soft tissue disorders related to use, overuse and pressure of thigh

     M70.851   Other soft tissue disorders related to use, overuse and pressure, right thigh

     M70.852   Other soft tissue disorders related to use, overuse and pressure, left thigh

     M70.859   Other soft tissue disorders related to use, overuse and pressure, unspecified thigh

● M70.86   Other soft tissue disorders related to use, overuse and pressure lower leg

     M70.861   Other soft tissue disorders related to use, overuse and pressure, right lower leg

     M70.862   Other soft tissue disorders related to use, overuse and pressure, left lower leg

     M70.869   Other soft tissue disorders related to use, overuse and pressure, unspecified leg

● M70.87   Other soft tissue disorders related to use, overuse and pressure of ankle and foot

     M70.871   Other soft tissue disorders related to use, overuse and pressure, right ankle and foot

     M70.872   Other soft tissue disorders related to use, overuse and pressure, left ankle and foot

     M70.879   Other soft tissue disorders related to use, overuse and pressure, unspecified ankle and foot

   M70.88   Other soft tissue disorders related to use, overuse and pressure other site

   M70.89   Other soft tissue disorders related to use, overuse and pressure multiple sites

● M70.9   Unspecified soft tissue disorder related to use, overuse and pressure

   M70.90   Unspecified soft tissue disorder related to use, overuse and pressure of unspecified site

● M70.91   Unspecified soft tissue disorder related to use, overuse and pressure of shoulder

     M70.911   Unspecified soft tissue disorder related to use, overuse and pressure, right shoulder

     M70.912   Unspecified soft tissue disorder related to use, overuse and pressure, left shoulder

     M70.919   Unspecified soft tissue disorder related to use, overuse and pressure, unspecified shoulder

● M70.92   Unspecified soft tissue disorder related to use, overuse and pressure of upper arm

     M70.921   Unspecified soft tissue disorder related to use, overuse and pressure, right upper arm

     M70.922   Unspecified soft tissue disorder related to use, overuse and pressure, left upper arm

     M70.929   Unspecified soft tissue disorder related to use, overuse and pressure, unspecified upper arm

● M70.93   Unspecified soft tissue disorder related to use, overuse and pressure of forearm

     M70.931   Unspecified soft tissue disorder related to use, overuse and pressure, right forearm

     M70.932   Unspecified soft tissue disorder related to use, overuse and pressure, left forearm

     M70.939   Unspecified soft tissue disorder related to use, overuse and pressure, unspecified forearm

● M70.94   Unspecified soft tissue disorder related to use, overuse and pressure of hand

     M70.941   Unspecified soft tissue disorder related to use, overuse and pressure, right hand

     M70.942   Unspecified soft tissue disorder related to use, overuse and pressure, left hand

     M70.949   Unspecified soft tissue disorder related to use, overuse and pressure, unspecified hand

● M70.95   Unspecified soft tissue disorder related to use, overuse and pressure of thigh

     M70.951   Unspecified soft tissue disorder related to use, overuse and pressure, right thigh

     M70.952   Unspecified soft tissue disorder related to use, overuse and pressure, left thigh

     M70.959   Unspecified soft tissue disorder related to use, overuse and pressure, unspecified thigh

● M70.96   Unspecified soft tissue disorder related to use, overuse and pressure lower leg

     M70.961   Unspecified soft tissue disorder related to use, overuse and pressure, right lower leg

     M70.962   Unspecified soft tissue disorder related to use, overuse and pressure, left lower leg

     M70.969   Unspecified soft tissue disorder related to use, overuse and pressure, unspecified lower leg

● M70.97   Unspecified soft tissue disorder related to use, overuse and pressure of ankle and foot

     M70.971   Unspecified soft tissue disorder related to use, overuse and pressure, right ankle and foot

     M70.972   Unspecified soft tissue disorder related to use, overuse and pressure, left ankle and foot

     M70.979   Unspecified soft tissue disorder related to use, overuse and pressure, unspecified ankle and foot

   M70.98   Unspecified soft tissue disorder related to use, overuse and pressure other

   M70.99   Unspecified soft tissue disorder related to use, overuse and pressure multiple sites

● M71   Other bursopathies

   Excludes1   bunion (M20.1)
           bursitis related to use, overuse or pressure (M70.-)
           enthesopathies (M76-M77)

● M71.0   Abscess of bursa

     Use additional code (B95.-, B96.-) to identify causative organism

     M71.00   Abscess of bursa, unspecified site

●   M71.01   Abscess of bursa, shoulder

     M71.011   Abscess of bursa, right shoulder

     M71.012   Abscess of bursa, left shoulder

     M71.019   Abscess of bursa, unspecified shoulder

▶ New   ⇒ Revised   ~~deleted~~ Deleted   **OGCR** Official Guidelines   X Assign placeholder X   ● Use Additional Character(s)

Excludes 1   Excludes 2   Includes   Use additional   Code first   Code also   Key words

● M71.02 Abscess of bursa, elbow
    M71.021 Abscess of bursa, right elbow
    M71.022 Abscess of bursa, left elbow
    M71.029 Abscess of bursa, unspecified elbow
● M71.03 Abscess of bursa, wrist
    M71.031 Abscess of bursa, right wrist
    M71.032 Abscess of bursa, left wrist
    M71.039 Abscess of bursa, unspecified wrist
● M71.04 Abscess of bursa, hand
    M71.041 Abscess of bursa, right hand
    M71.042 Abscess of bursa, left hand
    M71.049 Abscess of bursa, unspecified hand
● M71.05 Abscess of bursa, hip
    M71.051 Abscess of bursa, right hip
    M71.052 Abscess of bursa, left hip
    M71.059 Abscess of bursa, unspecified hip
● M71.06 Abscess of bursa, knee
    M71.061 Abscess of bursa, right knee
    M71.062 Abscess of bursa, left knee
    M71.069 Abscess of bursa, unspecified knee
● M71.07 Abscess of bursa, ankle and foot
    M71.071 Abscess of bursa, right ankle and foot
    M71.072 Abscess of bursa, left ankle and foot
    M71.079 Abscess of bursa, unspecified ankle and foot
  M71.08 Abscess of bursa, other site
  M71.09 Abscess of bursa, multiple sites

● M71.1 Other infective bursitis
    Use additional code (B95.-, B96.-) to identify causative organism
  M71.10 Other infective bursitis, unspecified site
● M71.11 Other infective bursitis, shoulder
    M71.111 Other infective bursitis, right shoulder
    M71.112 Other infective bursitis, left shoulder
    M71.119 Other infective bursitis, unspecified shoulder
● M71.12 Other infective bursitis, elbow
    M71.121 Other infective bursitis, right elbow
    M71.122 Other infective bursitis, left elbow
    M71.129 Other infective bursitis, unspecified elbow
● M71.13 Other infective bursitis, wrist
    M71.131 Other infective bursitis, right wrist
    M71.132 Other infective bursitis, left wrist
    M71.139 Other infective bursitis, unspecified wrist
● M71.14 Other infective bursitis, hand
    M71.141 Other infective bursitis, right hand
    M71.142 Other infective bursitis, left hand
    M71.149 Other infective bursitis, unspecified hand
● M71.15 Other infective bursitis, hip
    M71.151 Other infective bursitis, right hip
    M71.152 Other infective bursitis, left hip
    M71.159 Other infective bursitis, unspecified hip
● M71.16 Other infective bursitis, knee
    M71.161 Other infective bursitis, right knee
    M71.162 Other infective bursitis, left knee
    M71.169 Other infective bursitis, unspecified knee

● M71.17 Other infective bursitis, ankle and foot
    M71.171 Other infective bursitis, right ankle and foot
    M71.172 Other infective bursitis, left ankle and foot
    M71.179 Other infective bursitis, unspecified ankle and foot
  M71.18 Other infective bursitis, other site
  M71.19 Other infective bursitis, multiple sites
● M71.2 Synovial cyst of popliteal space [Baker]
    Popliteal space = popliteal cavity, popliteal fossa. Depression in the posterior aspect of the knee (behind the knee).
    Excludes1 synovial cyst of popliteal space with rupture (M66.0)
  M71.20 Synovial cyst of popliteal space [Baker], unspecified knee
  M71.21 Synovial cyst of popliteal space [Baker], right knee
  M71.22 Synovial cyst of popliteal space [Baker], left knee
● M71.3 Other bursal cyst
    Synovial cyst NOS
    Excludes1 synovial cyst with rupture (M66.1-)
  M71.30 Other bursal cyst, unspecified site
● M71.31 Other bursal cyst, shoulder
    M71.311 Other bursal cyst, right shoulder
    M71.312 Other bursal cyst, left shoulder
    M71.319 Other bursal cyst, unspecified shoulder
● M71.32 Other bursal cyst, elbow
    M71.321 Other bursal cyst, right elbow
    M71.322 Other bursal cyst, left elbow
    M71.329 Other bursal cyst, unspecified elbow
● M71.33 Other bursal cyst, wrist
    M71.331 Other bursal cyst, right wrist
    M71.332 Other bursal cyst, left wrist
    M71.339 Other bursal cyst, unspecified wrist
● M71.34 Other bursal cyst, hand
    M71.341 Other bursal cyst, right hand
    M71.342 Other bursal cyst, left hand
    M71.349 Other bursal cyst, unspecified hand
● M71.35 Other bursal cyst, hip
    M71.351 Other bursal cyst, right hip
    M71.352 Other bursal cyst, left hip
    M71.359 Other bursal cyst, unspecified hip
● M71.37 Other bursal cyst, ankle and foot
    M71.371 Other bursal cyst, right ankle and foot
    M71.372 Other bursal cyst, left ankle and foot
    M71.379 Other bursal cyst, unspecified ankle and foot
  M71.38 Other bursal cyst, other site
  M71.39 Other bursal cyst, multiple sites
● M71.4 Calcium deposit in bursa
    Excludes2 calcium deposit in bursa of shoulder (M75.3)
  M71.40 Calcium deposit in bursa, unspecified site
● M71.42 Calcium deposit in bursa, elbow
    M71.421 Calcium deposit in bursa, right elbow
    M71.422 Calcium deposit in bursa, left elbow
    M71.429 Calcium deposit in bursa, unspecified elbow
● M71.43 Calcium deposit in bursa, wrist
    M71.431 Calcium deposit in bursa, right wrist
    M71.432 Calcium deposit in bursa, left wrist
    M71.439 Calcium deposit in bursa, unspecified wrist

▶ New   ⇒ Revised   ~~deleted~~ Deleted   **OGCR** Official Guidelines   X Assign placeholder X   ● Use Additional Character(s)

| Excludes 1 | Excludes 2 | Includes | Use additional | Code first | Code also | Key words |

- M71.44 Calcium deposit in bursa, hand
  - M71.441 Calcium deposit in bursa, right hand
  - M71.442 Calcium deposit in bursa, left hand
  - M71.449 Calcium deposit in bursa, unspecified hand
- M71.45 Calcium deposit in bursa, hip
  - M71.451 Calcium deposit in bursa, right hip
  - M71.452 Calcium deposit in bursa, left hip
  - M71.459 Calcium deposit in bursa, unspecified hip
- M71.46 Calcium deposit in bursa, knee
  - M71.461 Calcium deposit in bursa, right knee
  - M71.462 Calcium deposit in bursa, left knee
  - M71.469 Calcium deposit in bursa, unspecified knee
- M71.47 Calcium deposit in bursa, ankle and foot
  - M71.471 Calcium deposit in bursa, right ankle and foot
  - M71.472 Calcium deposit in bursa, left ankle and foot
  - M71.479 Calcium deposit in bursa, unspecified ankle and foot
  - M71.48 Calcium deposit in bursa, other site
  - M71.49 Calcium deposit in bursa, multiple sites
- M71.5 Other bursitis, not elsewhere classified

  Excludes1 bursitis NOS (M71.9-)
  Excludes2 bursitis of shoulder (M75.5)
  bursitis of tibial collateral [Pellegrini-Stieda] (M76.4-)

  - M71.50 Other bursitis, not elsewhere classified, unspecified site
- M71.52 Other bursitis, not elsewhere classified, elbow
  - M71.521 Other bursitis, not elsewhere classified, right elbow
  - M71.522 Other bursitis, not elsewhere classified, left elbow
  - M71.529 Other bursitis, not elsewhere classified, unspecified elbow
- M71.53 Other bursitis, not elsewhere classified, wrist
  - M71.531 Other bursitis, not elsewhere classified, right wrist
  - M71.532 Other bursitis, not elsewhere classified, left wrist
  - M71.539 Other bursitis, not elsewhere classified, unspecified wrist
- M71.54 Other bursitis, not elsewhere classified, hand
  - M71.541 Other bursitis, not elsewhere classified, right hand
  - M71.542 Other bursitis, not elsewhere classified, left hand
  - M71.549 Other bursitis, not elsewhere classified, unspecified hand
- M71.55 Other bursitis, not elsewhere classified, hip
  - M71.551 Other bursitis, not elsewhere classified, right hip
  - M71.552 Other bursitis, not elsewhere classified, left hip
  - M71.559 Other bursitis, not elsewhere classified, unspecified hip
- M71.56 Other bursitis, not elsewhere classified, knee
  - M71.561 Other bursitis, not elsewhere classified, right knee
  - M71.562 Other bursitis, not elsewhere classified, left knee
  - M71.569 Other bursitis, not elsewhere classified, unspecified knee
- M71.57 Other bursitis, not elsewhere classified, ankle and foot
  - M71.571 Other bursitis, not elsewhere classified, right ankle and foot
  - M71.572 Other bursitis, not elsewhere classified, left ankle and foot
  - M71.579 Other bursitis, not elsewhere classified, unspecified ankle and foot
  - M71.58 Other bursitis, not elsewhere classified, other site
- M71.8 Other specified bursopathies
  - M71.80 Other specified bursopathies, unspecified site
- M71.81 Other specified bursopathies, shoulder
  - M71.811 Other specified bursopathies, right shoulder
  - M71.812 Other specified bursopathies, left shoulder
  - M71.819 Other specified bursopathies, unspecified shoulder
- M71.82 Other specified bursopathies, elbow
  - M71.821 Other specified bursopathies, right elbow
  - M71.822 Other specified bursopathies, left elbow
  - M71.829 Other specified bursopathies, unspecified elbow
- M71.83 Other specified bursopathies, wrist
  - M71.831 Other specified bursopathies, right wrist
  - M71.832 Other specified bursopathies, left wrist
  - M71.839 Other specified bursopathies, unspecified wrist
- M71.84 Other specified bursopathies, hand
  - M71.841 Other specified bursopathies, right hand
  - M71.842 Other specified bursopathies, left hand
  - M71.849 Other specified bursopathies, unspecified hand
- M71.85 Other specified bursopathies, hip
  - M71.851 Other specified bursopathies, right hip
  - M71.852 Other specified bursopathies, left hip
  - M71.859 Other specified bursopathies, unspecified hip
- M71.86 Other specified bursopathies, knee
  - M71.861 Other specified bursopathies, right knee
  - M71.862 Other specified bursopathies, left knee
  - M71.869 Other specified bursopathies, unspecified knee
- M71.87 Other specified bursopathies, ankle and foot
  - M71.871 Other specified bursopathies, right ankle and foot
  - M71.872 Other specified bursopathies, left ankle and foot
  - M71.879 Other specified bursopathies, unspecified ankle and foot
  - M71.88 Other specified bursopathies, other site
  - M71.89 Other specified bursopathies, multiple sites
- M71.9 Bursopathy, unspecified
  Bursitis NOS

▶ New   ⇒ Revised   ~~deleted~~ Deleted   OGCR Official Guidelines   X Assign placeholder X   ● Use Additional Character(s)

Excludes 1   Excludes 2   Includes   Use additional   Code first   Code also   Key words

● **M72 Fibroblastic disorders**

> **Excludes2**   retroperitoneal fibromatosis (D48.3)

M72.0 Palmar fascial fibromatosis [Dupuytren]

M72.1 Knuckle pads

M72.2 Plantar fascial fibromatosis
> Plantar fasciitis

M72.4 Pseudosarcomatous fibromatosis
> Nodular fasciitis

M72.6 Necrotizing fasciitis
> Use additional code (B95.-, B96.-) to identify causative organism

M72.8 Other fibroblastic disorders
> Abscess of fascia
> Fasciitis NEC
> Other infective fasciitis
> Use additional code to (B95.-, B96.-) identify causative organism

> > **Excludes1**   diffuse (eosinophilic) fasciitis (M35.4)
> > necrotizing fasciitis (M72.6)
> > nodular fasciitis (M72.4)
> > perirenal fasciitis NOS (N13.5)
> > perirenal fasciitis with infection (N13.6)
> > plantar fasciitis (M72.2)

M72.9 Fibroblastic disorder, unspecified
> Fasciitis NOS
> Fibromatosis NOS

● **M75 Shoulder lesions**

> **Excludes2**   shoulder-hand syndrome (M89.0-)

● **M75.0 Adhesive capsulitis of shoulder**
> Frozen shoulder
> Periarthritis of shoulder

M75.00 Adhesive capsulitis of unspecified shoulder

M75.01 Adhesive capsulitis of right shoulder

M75.02 Adhesive capsulitis of left shoulder

● **M75.1 Rotator cuff tear or rupture, not specified as traumatic**
> Rotator cuff syndrome
> Supraspinatus syndrome
> Supraspinatus tear or rupture, not specified as traumatic

> > **Excludes1**   tear of rotator cuff, traumatic (S46.01-)
> > *Gradual onset due to repetitive stress to rotator cuff*

● **M75.10 Unspecified rotator cuff tear or rupture, not specified as traumatic**

M75.100 Unspecified rotator cuff tear or rupture of unspecified shoulder, not specified as traumatic

M75.101 Unspecified rotator cuff tear or rupture of right shoulder, not specified as traumatic

M75.102 Unspecified rotator cuff tear or rupture of left shoulder, not specified as traumatic

● **M75.11 Incomplete rotator cuff tear or rupture not specified as traumatic**

M75.110 Incomplete rotator cuff tear or rupture of unspecified shoulder, not specified as traumatic

M75.111 Incomplete rotator cuff tear or rupture of right shoulder, not specified as traumatic

M75.112 Incomplete rotator cuff tear or rupture of left shoulder, not specified as traumatic

● **M75.12 Complete rotator cuff tear or rupture not specified as traumatic**

M75.120 Complete rotator cuff tear or rupture of unspecified shoulder, not specified as traumatic

M75.121 Complete rotator cuff tear or rupture of right shoulder, not specified as traumatic

M75.122 Complete rotator cuff tear or rupture of left shoulder, not specified as traumatic

● **M75.2 Bicipital tendinitis**

M75.20 Bicipital tendinitis, unspecified shoulder

M75.21 Bicipital tendinitis, right shoulder

M75.22 Bicipital tendinitis, left shoulder

● **M75.3 Calcific tendinitis of shoulder**
> Calcified bursa of shoulder

M75.30 Calcific tendinitis of unspecified shoulder

M75.31 Calcific tendinitis of right shoulder

M75.32 Calcific tendinitis of left shoulder

● **M75.4 Impingement syndrome of shoulder**

M75.40 Impingement syndrome of unspecified shoulder

M75.41 Impingement syndrome of right shoulder

M75.42 Impingement syndrome of left shoulder

● **M75.5 Bursitis of shoulder**

M75.50 Bursitis of unspecified shoulder

M75.51 Bursitis of right shoulder

M75.52 Bursitis of left shoulder

● **M75.8 Other shoulder lesions**

M75.80 Other shoulder lesions, unspecified shoulder

M75.81 Other shoulder lesions, right shoulder

M75.82 Other shoulder lesions, left shoulder

● **M75.9 Shoulder lesion, unspecified**

M75.90 Shoulder lesion, unspecified, unspecified shoulder

M75.91 Shoulder lesion, unspecified, right shoulder

M75.92 Shoulder lesion, unspecified, left shoulder

● **M76 Enthesopathies, lower limb, excluding foot**

> **Excludes2**   bursitis due to use, overuse and pressure (M70.-)
> enthesopathies of ankle and foot (M77.5-)

● **M76.0 Gluteal tendinitis**

M76.00 Gluteal tendinitis, unspecified hip

M76.01 Gluteal tendinitis, right hip

M76.02 Gluteal tendinitis, left hip

● **M76.1 Psoas tendinitis**

M76.10 Psoas tendinitis, unspecified hip

M76.11 Psoas tendinitis, right hip

M76.12 Psoas tendinitis, left hip

● **M76.2 Iliac crest spur**

M76.20 Iliac crest spur, unspecified hip

M76.21 Iliac crest spur, right hip

M76.22 Iliac crest spur, left hip

● **M76.3 Iliotibial band syndrome**

M76.30 Iliotibial band syndrome, unspecified leg

M76.31 Iliotibial band syndrome, right leg

M76.32 Iliotibial band syndrome, left leg

● **M76.4 Tibial collateral bursitis [Pellegrini-Stieda]**

M76.40 Tibial collateral bursitis [Pellegrini-Stieda], unspecified leg

M76.41 Tibial collateral bursitis [Pellegrini-Stieda], right leg

M76.42 Tibial collateral bursitis [Pellegrini-Stieda], left leg

- M76.5   **Patellar** tendinitis
  - M76.50   Patellar tendinitis, **unspecified** knee
  - M76.51   Patellar tendinitis, **right** knee
  - M76.52   Patellar tendinitis, **left** knee
- M76.6   **Achilles** tendinitis
  - Achilles bursitis
  - M76.60   Achilles tendinitis, **unspecified** leg
  - M76.61   Achilles tendinitis, **right** leg
  - M76.62   Achilles tendinitis, **left** leg
- M76.7   **Peroneal** tendinitis
  - M76.70   Peroneal tendinitis, **unspecified** leg
  - M76.71   Peroneal tendinitis, **right** leg
  - M76.72   Peroneal tendinitis, **left** leg
- M76.8   Other specified enthesopathies of lower limb, excluding foot
  - M76.81   **Anterior** tibial syndrome
    - M76.811   Anterior tibial syndrome, **right** leg
    - M76.812   Anterior tibial syndrome, **left** leg
    - M76.819   Anterior tibial syndrome, **unspecified** leg
  - M76.82   **Posterior** tibial tendinitis
    - M76.821   Posterior tibial tendinitis, **right** leg
    - M76.822   Posterior tibial tendinitis, **left** leg
    - M76.829   Posterior tibial tendinitis, **unspecified** leg
  - M76.89   **Other** specified enthesopathies of lower limb, excluding foot
    - M76.891   Other specified enthesopathies of **right** lower limb, excluding foot
    - M76.892   Other specified enthesopathies of **left** lower limb, excluding foot
    - M76.899   Other specified enthesopathies of **unspecified** lower limb, excluding foot
- M76.9   **Unspecified** enthesopathy, lower limb, excluding foot

- M77   Other enthesopathies
  - **Excludes1**   bursitis NOS (M71.9-)
  - **Excludes2**   bursitis due to use, overuse and pressure (M70.-)
    - osteophyte (M25.7)
    - spinal enthesopathy (M46.0-)
  - M77.0   **Medial** epicondylitis
    - M77.00   Medial epicondylitis, **unspecified** elbow
    - M77.01   Medial epicondylitis, **right** elbow
    - M77.02   Medial epicondylitis, **left** elbow
  - M77.1   **Lateral** epicondylitis
    - Tennis elbow
    - M77.10   Lateral epicondylitis, **unspecified** elbow
    - M77.11   Lateral epicondylitis, **right** elbow
    - M77.12   Lateral epicondylitis, **left** elbow
  - M77.2   **Periarthritis of wrist**
    - M77.20   Periarthritis, **unspecified** wrist
    - M77.21   Periarthritis, **right** wrist
    - M77.22   Periarthritis, **left** wrist
  - M77.3   **Calcaneal spur**
    - M77.30   Calcaneal spur, **unspecified** foot
    - M77.31   Calcaneal spur, **right** foot
    - M77.32   Calcaneal spur, **left** foot
  - M77.4   **Metatarsalgia**
    - **Excludes1**   Morton's metatarsalgia (G57.6)
    - M77.40   Metatarsalgia, **unspecified** foot
    - M77.41   Metatarsalgia, **right** foot
    - M77.42   Metatarsalgia, **left** foot

- M77.5   **Other** enthesopathy of **foot**
  - M77.50   Other enthesopathy of **unspecified** foot
  - M77.51   Other enthesopathy of **right** foot
  - M77.52   Other enthesopathy of **left** foot
- M77.8   **Other** enthesopathies, not elsewhere classified
- M77.9   Enthesopathy, **unspecified**
  - Bone spur NOS
  - Capsulitis NOS
  - Periarthritis NOS
  - Tendinitis NOS

- M79   Other and unspecified soft tissue disorders, not elsewhere classified
  - **Excludes1**   psychogenic rheumatism (F45.8)
    - soft tissue pain, psychogenic (F45.41)
  - M79.0   Rheumatism, **unspecified**
    - **Excludes1**   fibromyalgia (M79.7)
      - palindromic rheumatism (M12.3-)
  - M79.1   Myalgia
    - Myofascial pain syndrome
    - **Excludes1**   fibromyalgia (M79.7)
      - myositis (M60.-)
  - M79.2   Neuralgia and neuritis, **unspecified**
    - **Excludes1**   brachial radiculitis NOS (M54.1)
      - lumbosacral radiculitis NOS (M54.1)
      - mononeuropathies (G56-G58)
      - radiculitis NOS (M54.1)
      - sciatica (M54.3-M54.4)
  - M79.3   Panniculitis, **unspecified**
    - **Excludes1**   lupus panniculitis (L93.2)
      - neck and back panniculitis (M54.0-)
      - relapsing [Weber-Christian] panniculitis (M35.6)
  - M79.4   Hypertrophy of (infrapatellar) fat pad
  - M79.5   Residual foreign body in soft tissue
    - **Excludes1**   foreign body granuloma of skin and subcutaneous tissue (L92.3)
      - foreign body granuloma of soft tissue (M60.2-)
- M79.6   Pain in limb, hand, foot, fingers and toes
  - **Excludes2**   pain in joint (M25.5-)
  - M79.60   Pain in limb, **unspecified**
    - M79.601   Pain in **right arm**
      - Pain in right upper limb NOS
    - M79.602   Pain in **left arm**
      - Pain in left upper limb NOS
    - M79.603   Pain in arm, **unspecified**
      - Pain in upper limb NOS
    - M79.604   Pain in **right leg**
      - Pain in right lower limb NOS
    - M79.605   Pain in **left leg**
      - Pain in left lower limb NOS
    - M79.606   Pain in leg, **unspecified**
      - Pain in lower limb NOS
    - M79.609   Pain in **unspecified limb**
      - Pain in limb NOS
  - M79.62   Pain in **upper arm**
    - Pain in axillary region
    - M79.621   Pain in **right** upper arm
    - M79.622   Pain in **left** upper arm
    - M79.629   Pain in **unspecified** upper arm
  - M79.63   Pain in **forearm**
    - M79.631   Pain in **right** forearm
    - M79.632   Pain in **left** forearm
    - M79.639   Pain in **unspecified** forearm

● **M79.64 Pain in hand and fingers**
  M79.641 Pain in right hand
  M79.642 Pain in left hand
  M79.643 Pain in unspecified hand
  M79.644 Pain in right finger(s)
  M79.645 Pain in left finger(s)
  M79.646 Pain in unspecified finger(s)
● **M79.65 Pain in thigh**
  M79.651 Pain in right thigh
  M79.652 Pain in left thigh
  M79.659 Pain in unspecified thigh
● **M79.66 Pain in lower leg**
  M79.661 Pain in right lower leg
  M79.662 Pain in left lower leg
  M79.669 Pain in unspecified lower leg
● **M79.67 Pain in foot and toes**
  M79.671 Pain in right foot
  M79.672 Pain in left foot
  M79.673 Pain in unspecified foot
  M79.674 Pain in right toe(s)
  M79.675 Pain in left toe(s)
  M79.676 Pain in unspecified toe(s)

M79.7 Fibromyalgia
Fibromyositis
Fibrositis
Myofibrositis

● **M79.A Nontraumatic compartment syndrome**
Code first, if applicable, associated postprocedural complication
Excludes1   compartment syndrome NOS (T79.A-)
   fibromyalgia (M79.7) nontraumatic ischemic infarction of muscle (M62.2-)
   traumatic compartment syndrome (T79.A-)

● **M79.A1 Nontraumatic compartment syndrome of upper extremity**
Nontraumatic compartment syndrome of shoulder, arm, forearm, wrist, hand, and fingers
  M79.A11 Nontraumatic compartment syndrome of right upper extremity
  M79.A12 Nontraumatic compartment syndrome of left upper extremity
  M79.A19 Nontraumatic compartment syndrome of unspecified upper extremity

● **M79.A2 Nontraumatic compartment syndrome of lower extremity**
Nontraumatic compartment syndrome of hip, buttock, thigh, leg, foot, and toes
  M79.A21 Nontraumatic compartment syndrome of right lower extremity
  M79.A22 Nontraumatic compartment syndrome of left lower extremity
  M79.A29 Nontraumatic compartment syndrome of unspecified lower extremity

  M79.A3 Nontraumatic compartment syndrome of abdomen
  M79.A9 Nontraumatic compartment syndrome of other sites

● **M79.8 Other specified soft tissue disorders**
  M79.81 Nontraumatic hematoma of soft tissue
Nontraumatic hematoma of muscle
Nontraumatic seroma of muscle and soft tissue
  M79.89 Other specified soft tissue disorders
Polyalgia

M79.9 Soft tissue disorder, unspecified

OGCR See Section I.C., Chapter 13.d.

Osteoporosis
Osteoporosis is a systemic condition, meaning that all bones of the musculoskeletal system are affected. Therefore, site is not a component of the codes under category M81, Osteoporosis without current pathological fracture. The site codes under category M80, Osteoporosis with current pathological fracture, identify the site of the fracture, not the osteoporosis.

1) Osteoporosis without pathological fracture
Category M81, Osteoporosis without current pathological fracture, is for use for patients with osteoporosis who do not currently have a pathologic fracture due to the osteoporosis, even if they have had a fracture in the past. For patients with a history of osteoporosis fractures, status code Z87.310, Personal history of (healed) osteoporosis fracture, should follow the code from M81.

2) Osteoporosis with current pathological fracture
Category M80, Osteoporosis with current pathological fracture, is for patients who have a current pathologic fracture at the time of an encounter. The codes under M80 identify the site of the fracture. A code from category M80, not a traumatic fracture code, should be used for any patient with known osteoporosis who suffers a fracture, even if the patient had a minor fall or trauma, if that fall or trauma would not usually break a normal, healthy bone.

OSTEOPATHIES AND CHONDROPATHIES (M80-M94)

DISORDERS OF BONE DENSITY AND STRUCTURE (M80-M85)

M80 Osteoporosis with current pathological fracture
Excessive skeletal fragility (porous bone) resulting in bone fractures
Includes   osteoporosis with current fragility fracture
Use additional code to identify major osseous defect, if applicable (M89.7-)
Excludes1   collapsed vertebra NOS (M48.5)
   pathological fracture NOS (M84.4)
   wedging of vertebra NOS (M48.5)
Excludes2   personal history of (healed) osteoporosis fracture (Z87.310)

The appropriate 7th character is to be added to each code from category M80:

A   initial encounter for fracture
  All encounters involving diagnosis and treatment
D   subsequent encounter for fracture with routine healing
G   subsequent encounter for fracture with delayed healing
  Encounters for attention to casting or fixation devices, medication, and follow-up visits during the healing phase
K   subsequent encounter for fracture with nonunion
  Total failure of fracture healing
P   subsequent encounter for fracture with malunion
  Fracture ends do not heal together correctly.
S   sequela

● **M80.0 Age-related osteoporosis with current pathological fracture**
Involutional osteoporosis with current pathological fracture
Osteoporosis NOS with current pathological fracture
Postmenopausal osteoporosis with current pathological fracture
Senile osteoporosis with current pathological fracture
X ● M80.00 Age-related osteoporosis with current pathological fracture, unspecified site
● M80.01 Age-related osteoporosis with current pathological fracture, shoulder
  ● M80.011 Age-related osteoporosis with current pathological fracture, right shoulder
  ● M80.012 Age-related osteoporosis with current pathological fracture, left shoulder
  ● M80.019 Age-related osteoporosis with current pathological fracture, unspecified shoulder

▶ New ⇒ Revised ~~deleted~~ Deleted OGCR Official Guidelines X Assign placeholder X ● Use Additional Character(s)
Excludes 1 Excludes 2 Includes Use additional Code first Code also Key words
1013

● **M80.02** Age-related osteoporosis with current pathological fracture, humerus
- ● **M80.021** Age-related osteoporosis with current pathological fracture, right humerus
- ● **M80.022** Age-related osteoporosis with current pathological fracture, left humerus
- ● **M80.029** Age-related osteoporosis with current pathological fracture, unspecified humerus

● **M80.03** Age-related osteoporosis with current pathological fracture, forearm
  Age-related osteoporosis with current pathological fracture of wrist
- ● **M80.031** Age-related osteoporosis with current pathological fracture, right forearm
- ● **M80.032** Age-related osteoporosis with current pathological fracture, left forearm
- ● **M80.039** Age-related osteoporosis with current pathological fracture, unspecified forearm

● **M80.04** Age-related osteoporosis with current pathological fracture, hand
- ● **M80.041** Age-related osteoporosis with current pathological fracture, right hand
- ● **M80.042** Age-related osteoporosis with current pathological fracture, left hand
- ● **M80.049** Age-related osteoporosis with current pathological fracture, unspecified hand

● **M80.05** Age-related osteoporosis with current pathological fracture, femur
  Age-related osteoporosis with current pathological fracture of hip
- ● **M80.051** Age-related osteoporosis with current pathological fracture, right femur
- ● **M80.052** Age-related osteoporosis with current pathological fracture, left femur
- ● **M80.059** Age-related osteoporosis with current pathological fracture, unspecified femur

● **M80.06** Age-related osteoporosis with current pathological fracture, lower leg
- ● **M80.061** Age-related osteoporosis with current pathological fracture, right lower leg
- ● **M80.062** Age-related osteoporosis with current pathological fracture, left lower leg
- ● **M80.069** Age-related osteoporosis with current pathological fracture, unspecified lower leg

● **M80.07** Age-related osteoporosis with current pathological fracture, ankle and foot
- ● **M80.071** Age-related osteoporosis with current pathological fracture, right ankle and foot
- ● **M80.072** Age-related osteoporosis with current pathological fracture, left ankle and foot
- ● **M80.079** Age-related osteoporosis with current pathological fracture, unspecified ankle and foot

X ● **M80.08** Age-related osteoporosis with current pathological fracture, vertebra(e)

● **M80.8** Other osteoporosis with current pathological fracture
  Drug-induced osteoporosis with current pathological fracture
  Idiopathic osteoporosis with current pathological fracture
  Osteoporosis of disuse with current pathological fracture
  Postoophorectomy osteoporosis with current pathological fracture
  Postsurgical malabsorption osteoporosis with current pathological fracture
  Post-traumatic osteoporosis with current pathological fracture
  Use additional code for adverse effect, if applicable, to identify drug (T36-T50 with fifth or sixth character 5)

X ● **M80.80** Other osteoporosis with current pathological fracture, unspecified site

● **M80.81** Other osteoporosis with pathological fracture, shoulder
- ● **M80.811** Other osteoporosis with current pathological fracture, right shoulder
- ● **M80.812** Other osteoporosis with current pathological fracture, left shoulder
- ● **M80.819** Other osteoporosis with current pathological fracture, unspecified shoulder

● **M80.82** Other osteoporosis with current pathological fracture, humerus
- ● **M80.821** Other osteoporosis with current pathological fracture, right humerus
- ● **M80.822** Other osteoporosis with current pathological fracture, left humerus
- ● **M80.829** Other osteoporosis with current pathological fracture, unspecified humerus

● **M80.83** Other osteoporosis with current pathological fracture, forearm
  Other osteoporosis with current pathological fracture of wrist
- ● **M80.831** Other osteoporosis with current pathological fracture, right forearm
- ● **M80.832** Other osteoporosis with current pathological fracture, left forearm
- ● **M80.839** Other osteoporosis with current pathological fracture, unspecified forearm

● **M80.84** Other osteoporosis with current pathological fracture, hand
- ● **M80.841** Other osteoporosis with current pathological fracture, right hand
- ● **M80.842** Other osteoporosis with current pathological fracture, left hand
- ● **M80.849** Other osteoporosis with current pathological fracture, unspecified hand

● **M80.85** Other osteoporosis with current pathological fracture, femur
  Other osteoporosis with current pathological fracture of hip
- ● **M80.851** Other osteoporosis with current pathological fracture, right femur
- ● **M80.852** Other osteoporosis with current pathological fracture, left femur
- ● **M80.859** Other osteoporosis with current pathological fracture, unspecified femur

▶ New   ⇒ Revised   ~~deleted~~ Deleted   **OGCR** Official Guidelines   X Assign placeholder X   ● Use Additional Character(s)
Excludes 1   Excludes 2   Includes   Use additional   Code first   Code also   Key words

● M80.86　Other osteoporosis with current pathological fracture, lower leg

　　● M80.861　Other osteoporosis with current pathological fracture, right lower leg

　　● M80.862　Other osteoporosis with current pathological fracture, left lower leg

　　● M80.869　Other osteoporosis with current pathological fracture, unspecified lower leg

● M80.87　Other osteoporosis with current pathological fracture, ankle and foot

　　● M80.871　Other osteoporosis with current pathological fracture, right ankle and foot

　　● M80.872　Other osteoporosis with current pathological fracture, left ankle and foot

　　● M80.879　Other osteoporosis with current pathological fracture, unspecified ankle and foot

X ● M80.88　Other osteoporosis with current pathological fracture, vertebra(e)

● M81　Osteoporosis without current pathological fracture

　　Use additional code to identify:
　　major osseous defect, if applicable (M89.7-)
　　personal history of (healed) osteoporosis fracture, if applicable (Z87.310)

　　Excludes1　osteoporosis with current pathological fracture (M80.-)
　　　　　　　　Sudeck's atrophy (M89.0)

M81.0　Age-related osteoporosis without current pathological fracture

　　Involutional osteoporosis without current pathological fracture
　　Osteoporosis NOS
　　Postmenopausal osteoporosis without current pathological fracture
　　Senile osteoporosis without current pathological fracture

M81.6　Localized osteoporosis [Lequesne]

　　Excludes1　Sudeck's atrophy (M89.0)

M81.8　Other osteoporosis without current pathological fracture

　　Drug-induced osteoporosis without current pathological fracture
　　Idiopathic osteoporosis without current pathological fracture
　　Osteoporosis of disuse without current pathological fracture
　　Postoophorectomy osteoporosis without current pathological fracture
　　Postsurgical malabsorption osteoporosis without current pathological fracture
　　Post-traumatic osteoporosis without current pathological fracture

　　Use additional code for adverse effect, if applicable, to identify drug (T36-T50 with fifth or sixth character 5)

● M83　Adult osteomalacia

　　Excludes1　infantile and juvenile osteomalacia (E55.0)
　　　　　　　　renal osteodystrophy (N25.0)
　　　　　　　　rickets (active) (E55.0)
　　　　　　　　rickets (active) sequelae (E64.3)
　　　　　　　　vitamin D-resistant osteomalacia (E83.3)
　　　　　　　　vitamin D-resistant rickets (active) (E83.3)

M83.0　Puerperal osteomalacia

M83.1　Senile osteomalacia

M83.2　Adult osteomalacia due to malabsorption
　　　　Postsurgical malabsorption osteomalacia in adults

M83.3　Adult osteomalacia due to malnutrition

M83.4　Aluminum bone disease

M83.5　Other drug-induced osteomalacia in adults
　　　　Use additional code for adverse effect, if applicable, to identify drug (T36-T50 with fifth or sixth character 5)

M83.8　Other adult osteomalacia

M83.9　Adult osteomalacia, unspecified

● M84　Disorder of continuity of bone

　　Excludes2　traumatic fracture of bone-see fracture, by site

● M84.3　Stress fracture
　　Fatigue fracture
　　March fracture
　　Stress fracture NOS
　　Stress reaction

　　Use additional external cause code(s) to identify the cause of the stress fracture

　　Excludes1　pathological fracture NOS (M84.4.-)
　　　　　　　　pathological fracture due to osteoporosis (M80.-)
　　　　　　　　traumatic fracture (S12.-, S22.-, S32.-, S42.-, S52.-, S62.-, S72.-, S82.-, S92.-)

　　Excludes2　personal history of (healed) stress (fatigue) fracture (Z87.312)
　　　　　　　　stress fracture of vertebra (M48.4-)

　　The appropriate 7th character is to be added to each code from subcategory M84.3:

　　　A　initial encounter for fracture
　　　D　subsequent encounter for fracture with routine healing
　　　G　subsequent encounter for fracture with delayed healing
　　　K　subsequent encounter for fracture with nonunion
　　　P　subsequent encounter for fracture with malunion
　　　S　sequela

X ● M84.30　Stress fracture, unspecified site

● M84.31　Stress fracture, shoulder

　　● M84.311　Stress fracture, right shoulder
　　● M84.312　Stress fracture, left shoulder
　　● M84.319　Stress fracture, unspecified shoulder

● M84.32　Stress fracture, humerus

　　● M84.321　Stress fracture, right humerus
　　● M84.322　Stress fracture, left humerus
　　● M84.329　Stress fracture, unspecified humerus

● M84.33　Stress fracture, ulna and radius

　　● M84.331　Stress fracture, right ulna
　　● M84.332　Stress fracture, left ulna
　　● M84.333　Stress fracture, right radius
　　● M84.334　Stress fracture, left radius
　　● M84.339　Stress fracture, unspecified ulna and radius

● **M84.34** Stress fracture, hand and fingers
- ● M84.341 Stress fracture, right hand
- ● M84.342 Stress fracture, left hand
- ● M84.343 Stress fracture, unspecified hand
- ● M84.344 Stress fracture, right finger(s)
- ● M84.345 Stress fracture, left finger(s)
- ● M84.346 Stress fracture, unspecified finger(s)

● **M84.35** Stress fracture, pelvis and femur
Stress fracture, hip
- ● M84.350 Stress fracture, pelvis
- ● M84.351 Stress fracture, right femur
- ● M84.352 Stress fracture, left femur
- ● M84.353 Stress fracture, unspecified femur
- ● M84.359 Stress fracture, hip, unspecified

● **M84.36** Stress fracture, tibia and fibula
- ● M84.361 Stress fracture, right tibia
- ● M84.362 Stress fracture, left tibia
- ● M84.363 Stress fracture, right fibula
- ● M84.364 Stress fracture, left fibula
- ● M84.369 Stress fracture, unspecified tibia and fibula

● **M84.37** Stress fracture, ankle, foot and toes
- ● M84.371 Stress fracture, right ankle
- ● M84.372 Stress fracture, left ankle
- ● M84.373 Stress fracture, unspecified ankle
- ● M84.374 Stress fracture, right foot
- ● M84.375 Stress fracture, left foot
- ● M84.376 Stress fracture, unspecified foot
- ● M84.377 Stress fracture, right toe(s)
- ● M84.378 Stress fracture, left toe(s)
- ● M84.379 Stress fracture, unspecified toe(s)

X ● **M84.38** Stress fracture, other site

> **Excludes2**   stress fracture of vertebra (M48.4-)

● **M84.4** Pathological fracture, not elsewhere classified
Chronic fracture
Pathological fracture NOS

> **Excludes1**   collapsed vertebra NEC (M48.5)
> pathological fracture in neoplastic disease (M84.5-)
> pathological fracture in osteoporosis (M80.-)
> pathological fracture in other disease (M84.6-)
> stress fracture (M84.3-)
> traumatic fracture (S12.-, S22.-, S32.-, S42.-, S52.-, S62.-, S72.-, S82.-, S92.-)

> **Excludes2**   personal history of (healed) pathological fracture (Z87.311)

The appropriate 7th character is to be added to each code from subcategory M84.4:

A	initial encounter for fracture
D	subsequent encounter for fracture with routine healing
G	subsequent encounter for fracture with delayed healing
K	subsequent encounter for fracture with nonunion
P	subsequent encounter for fracture with malunion
S	sequela

X ● **M84.40** Pathological fracture, unspecified site

● **M84.41** Pathological fracture, shoulder
- ● M84.411 Pathological fracture, right shoulder
- ● M84.412 Pathological fracture, left shoulder
- ● M84.419 Pathological fracture, unspecified shoulder

● **M84.42** Pathological fracture, humerus
- ● M84.421 Pathological fracture, right humerus
- ● M84.422 Pathological fracture, left humerus
- ● M84.429 Pathological fracture, unspecified humerus

● **M84.43** Pathological fracture, ulna and radius
- ● M84.431 Pathological fracture, right ulna
- ● M84.432 Pathological fracture, left ulna
- ● M84.433 Pathological fracture, right radius
- ● M84.434 Pathological fracture, left radius
- ● M84.439 Pathological fracture, unspecified ulna and radius

● **M84.44** Pathological fracture, hand and fingers
- ● M84.441 Pathological fracture, right hand
- ● M84.442 Pathological fracture, left hand
- ● M84.443 Pathological fracture, unspecified hand
- ● M84.444 Pathological fracture, right finger(s)
- ● M84.445 Pathological fracture, left finger(s)
- ● M84.446 Pathological fracture, unspecified finger(s)

● **M84.45** Pathological fracture, femur and pelvis
- ● M84.451 Pathological fracture, right femur
- ● M84.452 Pathological fracture, left femur
- ● M84.453 Pathological fracture, unspecified femur
- ● M84.454 Pathological fracture, pelvis
- ● M84.459 Pathological fracture, hip, unspecified

● **M84.46** Pathological fracture, tibia and fibula
- ● M84.461 Pathological fracture, right tibia
- ● M84.462 Pathological fracture, left tibia
- ● M84.463 Pathological fracture, right fibula
- ● M84.464 Pathological fracture, left fibula
- ● M84.469 Pathological fracture, unspecified tibia and fibula

● **M84.47** Pathological fracture, ankle, foot and toes
- ● M84.471 Pathological fracture, right ankle
- ● M84.472 Pathological fracture, left ankle
- ● M84.473 Pathological fracture, unspecified ankle
- ● M84.474 Pathological fracture, right foot
- ● M84.475 Pathological fracture, left foot
- ● M84.476 Pathological fracture, unspecified foot
- ● M84.477 Pathological fracture, right toe(s)
- ● M84.478 Pathological fracture, left toe(s)
- ● M84.479 Pathological fracture, unspecified toe(s)

X ● **M84.48** Pathological fracture, other site

OGCR Section I.C. 13.C.

Coding of Pathologic Fractures

7th character A is for use as long as the patient is receiving active treatment for the fracture. While the patient may be seen by a new or different provider over the course of treatment for a pathological fracture, assignment of the 7th character is based on whether the patient is undergoing active treatment and not whether the provider is seeing the patient for the first time.

7th character, D is to be used for encounters after the patient has completed active treatment **for the fracture and is receiving routine care for the fracture during the healing or recovery phase**. The other 7th characters, listed under each subcategory in the Tabular List, are to be used for subsequent encounters for treatment of problems associated with the healing, such as malunions, nonunions, and sequelae.

Care for complications of surgical treatment for fracture repairs during the healing or recovery phase should be coded with the appropriate complication codes.

See Section I.C.19. Coding of traumatic fractures.

▶ New   ⇒ Revised   ~~deleted~~ Deleted   **OGCR** Official Guidelines   X Assign placeholder X   ● Use Additional Character(s)

Excludes 1   Excludes 2   Includes   Use additional   Code first   Code also   Key words

● **M84.5   Pathological fracture in neoplastic disease**

> Code also underlying neoplasm
>
> The appropriate 7th character is to be added to each code from subcategory M84.5:

A	initial encounter for fracture
D	subsequent encounter for fracture with routine healing
G	subsequent encounter for fracture with delayed healing
K	subsequent encounter for fracture with nonunion
P	subsequent encounter for fracture with malunion
S	sequela

X ● **M84.50   Pathological fracture in neoplastic disease, unspecified site**

● **M84.51   Pathological fracture in neoplastic disease, shoulder**
- ● M84.511   Pathological fracture in neoplastic disease, right shoulder
- ● M84.512   Pathological fracture in neoplastic disease, left shoulder
- ● M84.519   Pathological fracture in neoplastic disease, unspecified shoulder

● **M84.52   Pathological fracture in neoplastic disease, humerus**
- ● M84.521   Pathological fracture in neoplastic disease, right humerus
- ● M84.522   Pathological fracture in neoplastic disease, left humerus
- ● M84.529   Pathological fracture in neoplastic disease, unspecified humerus

● **M84.53   Pathological fracture in neoplastic disease, ulna and radius**
- ● M84.531   Pathological fracture in neoplastic disease, right ulna
- ● M84.532   Pathological fracture in neoplastic disease, left ulna
- ● M84.533   Pathological fracture in neoplastic disease, right radius
- ● M84.534   Pathological fracture in neoplastic disease, left radius
- ● M84.539   Pathological fracture in neoplastic disease, unspecified ulna and radius

● **M84.54   Pathological fracture in neoplastic disease, hand**
- ● M84.541   Pathological fracture in neoplastic disease, right hand
- ● M84.542   Pathological fracture in neoplastic disease, left hand
- ● M84.549   Pathological fracture in neoplastic disease, unspecified hand

● **M84.55   Pathological fracture in neoplastic disease, pelvis and femur**
- ● M84.550   Pathological fracture in neoplastic disease, pelvis
- ● M84.551   Pathological fracture in neoplastic disease, right femur
- ● M84.552   Pathological fracture in neoplastic disease, left femur
- ● M84.553   Pathological fracture in neoplastic disease, unspecified femur
- ● M84.559   Pathological fracture in neoplastic disease, hip, unspecified

● **M84.56   Pathological fracture in neoplastic disease, tibia and fibula**
- ● M84.561   Pathological fracture in neoplastic disease, right tibia
- ● M84.562   Pathological fracture in neoplastic disease, left tibia
- ● M84.563   Pathological fracture in neoplastic disease, right fibula
- ● M84.564   Pathological fracture in neoplastic disease, left fibula
- ● M84.569   Pathological fracture in neoplastic disease, unspecified tibia and fibula

● **M84.57   Pathological fracture in neoplastic disease, ankle and foot**
- ● M84.571   Pathological fracture in neoplastic disease, right ankle
- ● M84.572   Pathological fracture in neoplastic disease, left ankle
- ● M84.573   Pathological fracture in neoplastic disease, unspecified ankle
- ● M84.574   Pathological fracture in neoplastic disease, right foot
- ● M84.575   Pathological fracture in neoplastic disease, left foot
- ● M84.576   Pathological fracture in neoplastic disease, unspecified foot

X ● **M84.58   Pathological fracture in neoplastic disease, other specified site**
> Pathological fracture in neoplastic disease, vertebrae

● **M84.6   Pathological fracture in other disease**

> Code also underlying condition
>
> **Excludes 1**   pathological fracture in osteoporosis (M80.-)
>
> The appropriate 7th character is to be added to each code from subcategory M84.6:

A	initial encounter for fracture
D	subsequent encounter for fracture with routine healing
G	subsequent encounter for fracture with delayed healing
K	subsequent encounter for fracture with nonunion
P	subsequent encounter for fracture with malunion
S	sequela

X ● **M84.60   Pathological fracture in other disease, unspecified site**

● **M84.61   Pathological fracture in other disease, shoulder**
- ● M84.611   Pathological fracture in other disease, right shoulder
- ● M84.612   Pathological fracture in other disease, left shoulder
- ● M84.619   Pathological fracture in other disease, unspecified shoulder

● **M84.62   Pathological fracture in other disease, humerus**
- ● M84.621   Pathological fracture in other disease, right humerus
- ● M84.622   Pathological fracture in other disease, left humerus
- ● M84.629   Pathological fracture in other disease, unspecified humerus

CHAPTER 13 (M00-M99)

● M84.63   Pathological fracture in other disease, ulna and radius
- ● M84.631   Pathological fracture in other disease, right ulna
- ● M84.632   Pathological fracture in other disease, left ulna
- ● M84.633   Pathological fracture in other disease, right radius
- ● M84.634   Pathological fracture in other disease, left radius
- ● M84.639   Pathological fracture in other disease, unspecified ulna and radius

● M84.64   Pathological fracture in other disease, hand
- ● M84.641   Pathological fracture in other disease, right hand
- ● M84.642   Pathological fracture in other disease, left hand
- ● M84.649   Pathological fracture in other disease, unspecified hand

● M84.65   Pathological fracture in other disease, pelvis and femur
- ● M84.650   Pathological fracture in other disease, pelvis
- ● M84.651   Pathological fracture in other disease, right femur
- ● M84.652   Pathological fracture in other disease, left femur
- ● M84.653   Pathological fracture in other disease, unspecified femur
- ● M84.659   Pathological fracture in other disease, hip, unspecified

● M84.66   Pathological fracture in other disease, tibia and fibula
- ● M84.661   Pathological fracture in other disease, right tibia
- ● M84.662   Pathological fracture in other disease, left tibia
- ● M84.663   Pathological fracture in other disease, right fibula
- ● M84.664   Pathological fracture in other disease, left fibula
- ● M84.669   Pathological fracture in other disease, unspecified tibia and fibula

● M84.67   Pathological fracture in other disease, ankle and foot
- ● M84.671   Pathological fracture in other disease, right ankle
- ● M84.672   Pathological fracture in other disease, left ankle
- ● M84.673   Pathological fracture in other disease, unspecified ankle
- ● M84.674   Pathological fracture in other disease, right foot
- ● M84.675   Pathological fracture in other disease, left foot
- ● M84.676   Pathological fracture in other disease, unspecified foot

X ● M84.68   Pathological fracture in other disease, other site

● M84.7   Nontraumatic fracture, not elsewhere classified

  ● M84.75   Atypical femoral fracture

The appropriate 7th character is to be added to each code from M84.75:

A	initial encounter for fracture
D	subsequent encounter for fracture with routine healing
G	subsequent encounter for fracture with delayed healing
K	subsequent encounter for fracture with nonunion
P	subsequent encounter for fracture with malunion
S	sequela

- ● M84.750   Atypical femoral fracture, unspecified
- ● M84.751   Incomplete atypical femoral fracture, right leg
- ● M84.752   Incomplete atypical femoral fracture, left leg
- ● M84.753   Incomplete atypical femoral fracture, unspecified leg
- ● M84.754   Complete transverse atypical femoral fracture, right leg
- ● M84.755   Complete transverse atypical femoral fracture, left leg
- ● M84.756   Complete transverse atypical femoral fracture, unspecified leg
- ● M84.757   Complete oblique atypical femoral fracture, right leg
- ● M84.758   Complete oblique atypical femoral fracture, left leg
- ● M84.759   Complete oblique atypical femoral fracture, unspecified leg

● M84.8   Other disorders of continuity of bone
- M84.80   Other disorders of continuity of bone, unspecified site
- ● M84.81   Other disorders of continuity of bone, shoulder
  - M84.811   Other disorders of continuity of bone, right shoulder
  - M84.812   Other disorders of continuity of bone, left shoulder
  - M84.819   Other disorders of continuity of bone, unspecified shoulder
- ● M84.82   Other disorders of continuity of bone, humerus
  - M84.821   Other disorders of continuity of bone, right humerus
  - M84.822   Other disorders of continuity of bone, left humerus
  - M84.829   Other disorders of continuity of bone, unspecified humerus
- ● M84.83   Other disorders of continuity of bone, ulna and radius
  - M84.831   Other disorders of continuity of bone, right ulna
  - M84.832   Other disorders of continuity of bone, left ulna
  - M84.833   Other disorders of continuity of bone, right radius
  - M84.834   Other disorders of continuity of bone, left radius
  - M84.839   Other disorders of continuity of bone, unspecified ulna and radius
- ● M84.84   Other disorders of continuity of bone, hand
  - M84.841   Other disorders of continuity of bone, right hand
  - M84.842   Other disorders of continuity of bone, left hand
  - M84.849   Other disorders of continuity of bone, unspecified hand

● M84.85 Other disorders of continuity of bone, pelvic region and thigh
     M84.851 Other disorders of continuity of bone, right pelvic region and thigh
     M84.852 Other disorders of continuity of bone, left pelvic region and thigh
     M84.859 Other disorders of continuity of bone, unspecified pelvic region and thigh
● M84.86 Other disorders of continuity of bone, tibia and fibula
     M84.861 Other disorders of continuity of bone, right tibia
     M84.862 Other disorders of continuity of bone, left tibia
     M84.863 Other disorders of continuity of bone, right fibula
     M84.864 Other disorders of continuity of bone, left fibula
     M84.869 Other disorders of continuity of bone, unspecified tibia and fibula
● M84.87 Other disorders of continuity of bone, ankle and foot
     M84.871 Other disorders of continuity of bone, right ankle and foot
     M84.872 Other disorders of continuity of bone, left ankle and foot
     M84.879 Other disorders of continuity of bone, unspecified ankle and foot
   M84.88 Other disorders of continuity of bone, other site
   M84.9 Disorder of continuity of bone, unspecified

● M85 Other disorders of bone density and structure
     Excludes1   osteogenesis imperfecta (Q78.0)
                   osteopetrosis (Q78.2)
                   osteopoikilosis (Q78.8)
                   polyostotic fibrous dysplasia (Q78.1)
● M85.0 Fibrous dysplasia (monostotic)
     Excludes2   fibrous dysplasia of jaw (M27.8)
   M85.00 Fibrous dysplasia (monostotic), unspecified site
● M85.01 Fibrous dysplasia (monostotic), shoulder
     M85.011 Fibrous dysplasia (monostotic), right shoulder
     M85.012 Fibrous dysplasia (monostotic), left shoulder
     M85.019 Fibrous dysplasia (monostotic), unspecified shoulder
● M85.02 Fibrous dysplasia (monostotic), upper arm
     M85.021 Fibrous dysplasia (monostotic), right upper arm
     M85.022 Fibrous dysplasia (monostotic), left upper arm
     M85.029 Fibrous dysplasia (monostotic), unspecified upper arm
● M85.03 Fibrous dysplasia (monostotic), forearm
     M85.031 Fibrous dysplasia (monostotic), right forearm
     M85.032 Fibrous dysplasia (monostotic), left forearm
     M85.039 Fibrous dysplasia (monostotic), unspecified forearm
● M85.04 Fibrous dysplasia (monostotic), hand
     M85.041 Fibrous dysplasia (monostotic), right hand
     M85.042 Fibrous dysplasia (monostotic), left hand
     M85.049 Fibrous dysplasia (monostotic), unspecified hand

● M85.05 Fibrous dysplasia (monostotic), thigh
     M85.051 Fibrous dysplasia (monostotic), right thigh
     M85.052 Fibrous dysplasia (monostotic), left thigh
     M85.059 Fibrous dysplasia (monostotic), unspecified thigh
● M85.06 Fibrous dysplasia (monostotic), lower leg
     M85.061 Fibrous dysplasia (monostotic), right lower leg
     M85.062 Fibrous dysplasia (monostotic), left lower leg
     M85.069 Fibrous dysplasia (monostotic), unspecified lower leg
● M85.07 Fibrous dysplasia (monostotic), ankle and foot
     M85.071 Fibrous dysplasia (monostotic), right ankle and foot
     M85.072 Fibrous dysplasia (monostotic), left ankle and foot
     M85.079 Fibrous dysplasia (monostotic), unspecified ankle and foot
   M85.08 Fibrous dysplasia (monostotic), other site
   M85.09 Fibrous dysplasia (monostotic), multiple sites
● M85.1 Skeletal fluorosis
   M85.10 Skeletal fluorosis, unspecified site
● M85.11 Skeletal fluorosis, shoulder
     M85.111 Skeletal fluorosis, right shoulder
     M85.112 Skeletal fluorosis, left shoulder
     M85.119 Skeletal fluorosis, unspecified shoulder
● M85.12 Skeletal fluorosis, upper arm
     M85.121 Skeletal fluorosis, right upper arm
     M85.122 Skeletal fluorosis, left upper arm
     M85.129 Skeletal fluorosis, unspecified upper arm
● M85.13 Skeletal fluorosis, forearm
     M85.131 Skeletal fluorosis, right forearm
     M85.132 Skeletal fluorosis, left forearm
     M85.139 Skeletal fluorosis, unspecified forearm
● M85.14 Skeletal fluorosis, hand
     M85.141 Skeletal fluorosis, right hand
     M85.142 Skeletal fluorosis, left hand
     M85.149 Skeletal fluorosis, unspecified hand
● M85.15 Skeletal fluorosis, thigh
     M85.151 Skeletal fluorosis, right thigh
     M85.152 Skeletal fluorosis, left thigh
     M85.159 Skeletal fluorosis, unspecified thigh
● M85.16 Skeletal fluorosis, lower leg
     M85.161 Skeletal fluorosis, right lower leg
     M85.162 Skeletal fluorosis, left lower leg
     M85.169 Skeletal fluorosis, unspecified lower leg
● M85.17 Skeletal fluorosis, ankle and foot
     M85.171 Skeletal fluorosis, right ankle and foot
     M85.172 Skeletal fluorosis, left ankle and foot
     M85.179 Skeletal fluorosis, unspecified ankle and foot
   M85.18 Skeletal fluorosis, other site
   M85.19 Skeletal fluorosis, multiple sites
   M85.2 Hyperostosis of skull

CHAPTER 13 (M00-M99)

● M85.3 Osteitis condensans
  M85.30 Osteitis condensans, unspecified site
  ● M85.31 Osteitis condensans, shoulder
    M85.311 Osteitis condensans, right shoulder
    M85.312 Osteitis condensans, left shoulder
    M85.319 Osteitis condensans, unspecified shoulder
  ● M85.32 Osteitis condensans, upper arm
    M85.321 Osteitis condensans, right upper arm
    M85.322 Osteitis condensans, left upper arm
    M85.329 Osteitis condensans, unspecified upper arm
  ● M85.33 Osteitis condensans, forearm
    M85.331 Osteitis condensans, right forearm
    M85.332 Osteitis condensans, left forearm
    M85.339 Osteitis condensans, unspecified forearm
  ● M85.34 Osteitis condensans, hand
    M85.341 Osteitis condensans, right hand
    M85.342 Osteitis condensans, left hand
    M85.349 Osteitis condensans, unspecified hand
  ● M85.35 Osteitis condensans, thigh
    M85.351 Osteitis condensans, right thigh
    M85.352 Osteitis condensans, left thigh
    M85.359 Osteitis condensans, unspecified thigh
  ● M85.36 Osteitis condensans, lower leg
    M85.361 Osteitis condensans, right lower leg
    M85.362 Osteitis condensans, left lower leg
    M85.369 Osteitis condensans, unspecified lower leg
  ● M85.37 Osteitis condensans, ankle and foot
    M85.371 Osteitis condensans, right ankle and foot
    M85.372 Osteitis condensans, left ankle and foot
    M85.379 Osteitis condensans, unspecified ankle and foot
  M85.38 Osteitis condensans, other site
  M85.39 Osteitis condensans, multiple sites
● M85.4 Solitary bone cyst
  Excludes2   solitary cyst of jaw (M27.4)
  M85.40 Solitary bone cyst, unspecified site
  ● M85.41 Solitary bone cyst, shoulder
    M85.411 Solitary bone cyst, right shoulder
    M85.412 Solitary bone cyst, left shoulder
    M85.419 Solitary bone cyst, unspecified shoulder
  ● M85.42 Solitary bone cyst, humerus
    M85.421 Solitary bone cyst, right humerus
    M85.422 Solitary bone cyst, left humerus
    M85.429 Solitary bone cyst, unspecified humerus
  ● M85.43 Solitary bone cyst, ulna and radius
    M85.431 Solitary bone cyst, right ulna and radius
    M85.432 Solitary bone cyst, left ulna and radius
    M85.439 Solitary bone cyst, unspecified ulna and radius

● M85.44 Solitary bone cyst, hand
  M85.441 Solitary bone cyst, right hand
  M85.442 Solitary bone cyst, left hand
  M85.449 Solitary bone cyst, unspecified hand
● M85.45 Solitary bone cyst, pelvis
  M85.451 Solitary bone cyst, right pelvis
  M85.452 Solitary bone cyst, left pelvis
  M85.459 Solitary bone cyst, unspecified pelvis
● M85.46 Solitary bone cyst, tibia and fibula
  M85.461 Solitary bone cyst, right tibia and fibula
  M85.462 Solitary bone cyst, left tibia and fibula
  M85.469 Solitary bone cyst, unspecified tibia and fibula
● M85.47 Solitary bone cyst, ankle and foot
  M85.471 Solitary bone cyst, right ankle and foot
  M85.472 Solitary bone cyst, left ankle and foot
  M85.479 Solitary bone cyst, unspecified ankle and foot
  M85.48 Solitary bone cyst, other site
● M85.5 Aneurysmal bone cyst
  Excludes2   aneurysmal cyst of jaw (M27.4)
  M85.50 Aneurysmal bone cyst, unspecified site
  ● M85.51 Aneurysmal bone cyst, shoulder
    M85.511 Aneurysmal bone cyst, right shoulder
    M85.512 Aneurysmal bone cyst, left shoulder
    M85.519 Aneurysmal bone cyst, unspecified shoulder
  ● M85.52 Aneurysmal bone cyst, upper arm
    M85.521 Aneurysmal bone cyst, right upper arm
    M85.522 Aneurysmal bone cyst, left upper arm
    M85.529 Aneurysmal bone cyst, unspecified upper arm
  ● M85.53 Aneurysmal bone cyst, forearm
    M85.531 Aneurysmal bone cyst, right forearm
    M85.532 Aneurysmal bone cyst, left forearm
    M85.539 Aneurysmal bone cyst, unspecified forearm
  ● M85.54 Aneurysmal bone cyst, hand
    M85.541 Aneurysmal bone cyst, right hand
    M85.542 Aneurysmal bone cyst, left hand
    M85.549 Aneurysmal bone cyst, unspecified hand
  ● M85.55 Aneurysmal bone cyst, thigh
    M85.551 Aneurysmal bone cyst, right thigh
    M85.552 Aneurysmal bone cyst, left thigh
    M85.559 Aneurysmal bone cyst, unspecified thigh
  ● M85.56 Aneurysmal bone cyst, lower leg
    M85.561 Aneurysmal bone cyst, right lower leg
    M85.562 Aneurysmal bone cyst, left lower leg
    M85.569 Aneurysmal bone cyst, unspecified lower leg
  ● M85.57 Aneurysmal bone cyst, ankle and foot
    M85.571 Aneurysmal bone cyst, right ankle and foot
    M85.572 Aneurysmal bone cyst, left ankle and foot
    M85.579 Aneurysmal bone cyst, unspecified ankle and foot
  M85.58 Aneurysmal bone cyst, other site
  M85.59 Aneurysmal bone cyst, multiple sites

▶ New   ⇒ Revised   ~~deleted~~ Deleted   OGCR Official Guidelines   X Assign placeholder X   ● Use Additional Character(s)

Excludes 1   Excludes 2   Includes   Use additional   Code first   Code also   Key words

● M85.6   Other cyst of bone
   Excludes1   cyst of jaw NEC (M27.4)
                   osteitis fibrosa cystica generalisata [von
                       Recklinghausen's disease of bone]
                       (E21.0)
   M85.60   Other cyst of bone, unspecified site
● M85.61   Other cyst of bone, shoulder
   M85.611   Other cyst of bone, right shoulder
   M85.612   Other cyst of bone, left shoulder
   M85.619   Other cyst of bone, unspecified
             shoulder
● M85.62   Other cyst of bone, upper arm
   M85.621   Other cyst of bone, right upper arm
   M85.622   Other cyst of bone, left upper arm
   M85.629   Other cyst of bone, unspecified upper
             arm
● M85.63   Other cyst of bone, forearm
   M85.631   Other cyst of bone, right forearm
   M85.632   Other cyst of bone, left forearm
   M85.639   Other cyst of bone, unspecified
             forearm
● M85.64   Other cyst of bone, hand
   M85.641   Other cyst of bone, right hand
   M85.642   Other cyst of bone, left hand
   M85.649   Other cyst of bone, unspecified hand
● M85.65   Other cyst of bone, thigh
   M85.651   Other cyst of bone, right thigh
   M85.652   Other cyst of bone, left thigh
   M85.659   Other cyst of bone, unspecified thigh
● M85.66   Other cyst of bone, lower leg
   M85.661   Other cyst of bone, right lower leg
   M85.662   Other cyst of bone, left lower leg
   M85.669   Other cyst of bone, unspecified lower
             leg
● M85.67   Other cyst of bone, ankle and foot
   M85.671   Other cyst of bone, right ankle and
             foot
   M85.672   Other cyst of bone, left ankle and foot
   M85.679   Other cyst of bone, unspecified ankle
             and foot
   M85.68   Other cyst of bone, other site
   M85.69   Other cyst of bone, multiple sites
● M85.8   Other specified disorders of bone density and structure
          Hyperostosis of bones, except skull
          Osteosclerosis, acquired
   Excludes1   diffuse idiopathic skeletal hyperostosis
                   [DISH] (M48.1)
                   osteosclerosis congenita (Q77.4)
                   osteosclerosis fragilitas (generalista)
                       (Q78.2)
                   osteosclerosis myelofibrosis (D75.81)
   M85.80   Other specified disorders of bone density and
            structure, unspecified site
● M85.81   Other specified disorders of bone density and
           structure, shoulder
   M85.811   Other specified disorders of bone
             density and structure, right shoulder
   M85.812   Other specified disorders of bone
             density and structure, left shoulder
   M85.819   Other specified disorders of bone
             density and structure, unspecified
             shoulder

● M85.82   Other specified disorders of bone density and
           structure, upper arm
   M85.821   Other specified disorders of bone
             density and structure, right upper arm
   M85.822   Other specified disorders of bone
             density and structure, left upper arm
   M85.829   Other specified disorders of bone
             density and structure, unspecified
             upper arm
● M85.83   Other specified disorders of bone density and
           structure, forearm
   M85.831   Other specified disorders of bone
             density and structure, right forearm
   M85.832   Other specified disorders of bone
             density and structure, left forearm
   M85.839   Other specified disorders of bone
             density and structure, unspecified
             forearm
● M85.84   Other specified disorders of bone density and
           structure, hand
   M85.841   Other specified disorders of bone
             density and structure, right hand
   M85.842   Other specified disorders of bone
             density and structure, left hand
   M85.849   Other specified disorders of bone
             density and structure, unspecified
             hand
● M85.85   Other specified disorders of bone density and
           structure, thigh
   M85.851   Other specified disorders of bone
             density and structure, right thigh
   M85.852   Other specified disorders of bone
             density and structure, left thigh
   M85.859   Other specified disorders of bone
             density and structure, unspecified
             thigh
● M85.86   Other specified disorders of bone density and
           structure, lower leg
   M85.861   Other specified disorders of bone
             density and structure, right lower leg
   M85.862   Other specified disorders of bone
             density and structure, left lower leg
   M85.869   Other specified disorders of bone
             density and structure, unspecified
             lower leg
● M85.87   Other specified disorders of bone density and
           structure, ankle and foot
   M85.871   Other specified disorders of bone
             density and structure, right ankle and
             foot
   M85.872   Other specified disorders of bone
             density and structure, left ankle and
             foot
   M85.879   Other specified disorders of bone
             density and structure, unspecified
             ankle and foot
   M85.88   Other specified disorders of bone density and
            structure, other site
   M85.89   Other specified disorders of bone density and
            structure, multiple sites
   M85.9   Disorder of bone density and structure, unspecified

CHAPTER 13 (M00-M99)

Figure 13-6 Osteomyelitis of the spine. A lateral view of the lower thoracic spine demonstrates destruction of the disk space *(arrow)* as well as destruction of the adjoining vertebral bodies. (From Mettler: Essentials of Radiology, ed 2, Saunders, An Imprint of Elsevier, 2005)

Item 13–12 Osteomyelitis is an inflammation of the bone. **Acute osteomyelitis** is a rapidly destructive, pus-producing infection capable of causing severe bone destruction. **Chronic osteomyelitis** can remain long after the initial acute episode has passed and may lead to a recurrence of the acute phase. **Brodie's abscess** is an encapsulated focal abscess that must be surgically drained. **Periostitis** is an inflammation of the periosteum, a dense membrane composed of fibrous connective tissue that closely wraps all bone, except those with articulating surfaces in joints, which are covered by synovial membranes.

OTHER OSTEOPATHIES (M86-M90)

Excludes1   postprocedural osteopathies (M96.-)

● M86   **Osteomyelitis**

Use additional code (B95-B97) to identify infectious agent

Use additional code to identify major osseous defect, if applicable (M89.7-)

Excludes1   osteomyelitis due to:
echinococcus (B67.2)
gonococcus (A54.43)
salmonella (A02.24)

Excludes2   ostemyelitis of:
orbit (H05.0-)
petrous bone (H70.2-)
vertebra (M46.2-)

● M86.0   Acute hematogenous osteomyelitis

    M86.00   Acute hematogenous osteomyelitis, unspecified site

   ● M86.01   Acute hematogenous osteomyelitis, shoulder

       M86.011   Acute hematogenous osteomyelitis, right shoulder

       M86.012   Acute hematogenous osteomyelitis, left shoulder

       M86.019   Acute hematogenous osteomyelitis, unspecified shoulder

   ● M86.02   Acute hematogenous osteomyelitis, humerus

       M86.021   Acute hematogenous osteomyelitis, right humerus

       M86.022   Acute hematogenous osteomyelitis, left humerus

       M86.029   Acute hematogenous osteomyelitis, unspecified humerus

   ● M86.03   Acute hematogenous osteomyelitis, radius and ulna

       M86.031   Acute hematogenous osteomyelitis, right radius and ulna

       M86.032   Acute hematogenous osteomyelitis, left radius and ulna

       M86.039   Acute hematogenous osteomyelitis, unspecified radius and ulna

   ● M86.04   Acute hematogenous osteomyelitis, hand

       M86.041   Acute hematogenous osteomyelitis, right hand

       M86.042   Acute hematogenous osteomyelitis, left hand

       M86.049   Acute hematogenous osteomyelitis, unspecified hand

● M86.05   Acute hematogenous osteomyelitis, femur

       M86.051   Acute hematogenous osteomyelitis, right femur

       M86.052   Acute hematogenous osteomyelitis, left femur

       M86.059   Acute hematogenous osteomyelitis, unspecified femur

● M86.06   Acute hematogenous osteomyelitis, tibia and fibula

       M86.061   Acute hematogenous osteomyelitis, right tibia and fibula

       M86.062   Acute hematogenous osteomyelitis, left tibia and fibula

       M86.069   Acute hematogenous osteomyelitis, unspecified tibia and fibula

● M86.07   Acute hematogenous osteomyelitis, ankle and foot

       M86.071   Acute hematogenous osteomyelitis, right ankle and foot

       M86.072   Acute hematogenous osteomyelitis, left ankle and foot

       M86.079   Acute hematogenous osteomyelitis, unspecified ankle and foot

    M86.08   Acute hematogenous osteomyelitis, other sites

    M86.09   Acute hematogenous osteomyelitis, multiple sites

● M86.1   Other acute osteomyelitis

    M86.10   Other acute osteomyelitis, unspecified site

   ● M86.11   Other acute osteomyelitis, shoulder

       M86.111   Other acute osteomyelitis, right shoulder

       M86.112   Other acute osteomyelitis, left shoulder

       M86.119   Other acute osteomyelitis, unspecified shoulder

   ● M86.12   Other acute osteomyelitis, humerus

       M86.121   Other acute osteomyelitis, right humerus

       M86.122   Other acute osteomyelitis, left humerus

       M86.129   Other acute osteomyelitis, unspecified humerus

   ● M86.13   Other acute osteomyelitis, radius and ulna

       M86.131   Other acute osteomyelitis, right radius and ulna

       M86.132   Other acute osteomyelitis, left radius and ulna

       M86.139   Other acute osteomyelitis, unspecified radius and ulna

   ● M86.14   Other acute osteomyelitis, hand

       M86.141   Other acute osteomyelitis, right hand

       M86.142   Other acute osteomyelitis, left hand

       M86.149   Other acute osteomyelitis, unspecified hand

   ● M86.15   Other acute osteomyelitis, femur

       M86.151   Other acute osteomyelitis, right femur

       M86.152   Other acute osteomyelitis, left femur

       M86.159   Other acute osteomyelitis, unspecified femur

   ● M86.16   Other acute osteomyelitis, tibia and fibula

       M86.161   Other acute osteomyelitis, right tibia and fibula

       M86.162   Other acute osteomyelitis, left tibia and fibula

       M86.169   Other acute osteomyelitis, unspecified tibia and fibula

- M86.17   Other acute osteomyelitis, ankle and foot
  - M86.171   Other acute osteomyelitis, right ankle and foot
  - M86.172   Other acute osteomyelitis, left ankle and foot
  - M86.179   Other acute osteomyelitis, unspecified ankle and foot
- M86.18   Other acute osteomyelitis, other site
- M86.19   Other acute osteomyelitis, multiple sites
- M86.2   Subacute osteomyelitis
  - M86.20   Subacute osteomyelitis, unspecified site
  - M86.21   Subacute osteomyelitis, shoulder
    - M86.211   Subacute osteomyelitis, right shoulder
    - M86.212   Subacute osteomyelitis, left shoulder
    - M86.219   Subacute osteomyelitis, unspecified shoulder
  - M86.22   Subacute osteomyelitis, humerus
    - M86.221   Subacute osteomyelitis, right humerus
    - M86.222   Subacute osteomyelitis, left humerus
    - M86.229   Subacute osteomyelitis, unspecified humerus
  - M86.23   Subacute osteomyelitis, radius and ulna
    - M86.231   Subacute osteomyelitis, right radius and ulna
    - M86.232   Subacute osteomyelitis, left radius and ulna
    - M86.239   Subacute osteomyelitis, unspecified radius and ulna
  - M86.24   Subacute osteomyelitis, hand
    - M86.241   Subacute osteomyelitis, right hand
    - M86.242   Subacute osteomyelitis, left hand
    - M86.249   Subacute osteomyelitis, unspecified hand
  - M86.25   Subacute osteomyelitis, femur
    - M86.251   Subacute osteomyelitis, right femur
    - M86.252   Subacute osteomyelitis, left femur
    - M86.259   Subacute osteomyelitis, unspecified femur
  - M86.26   Subacute osteomyelitis, tibia and fibula
    - M86.261   Subacute osteomyelitis, right tibia and fibula
    - M86.262   Subacute osteomyelitis, left tibia and fibula
    - M86.269   Subacute osteomyelitis, unspecified tibia and fibula
  - M86.27   Subacute osteomyelitis, ankle and foot
    - M86.271   Subacute osteomyelitis, right ankle and foot
    - M86.272   Subacute osteomyelitis, left ankle and foot
    - M86.279   Subacute osteomyelitis, unspecified ankle and foot
  - M86.28   Subacute osteomyelitis, other site
  - M86.29   Subacute osteomyelitis, multiple sites
- M86.3   Chronic multifocal osteomyelitis
  - M86.30   Chronic multifocal osteomyelitis, unspecified site
  - M86.31   Chronic multifocal osteomyelitis, shoulder
    - M86.311   Chronic multifocal osteomyelitis, right shoulder
    - M86.312   Chronic multifocal osteomyelitis, left shoulder
    - M86.319   Chronic multifocal osteomyelitis, unspecified shoulder
- M86.32   Chronic multifocal osteomyelitis, humerus
  - M86.321   Chronic multifocal osteomyelitis, right humerus
  - M86.322   Chronic multifocal osteomyelitis, left humerus
  - M86.329   Chronic multifocal osteomyelitis, unspecified humerus
- M86.33   Chronic multifocal osteomyelitis, radius and ulna
  - M86.331   Chronic multifocal osteomyelitis, right radius and ulna
  - M86.332   Chronic multifocal osteomyelitis, left radius and ulna
  - M86.339   Chronic multifocal osteomyelitis, unspecified radius and ulna
- M86.34   Chronic multifocal osteomyelitis, hand
  - M86.341   Chronic multifocal osteomyelitis, right hand
  - M86.342   Chronic multifocal osteomyelitis, left hand
  - M86.349   Chronic multifocal osteomyelitis, unspecified hand
- M86.35   Chronic multifocal osteomyelitis, femur
  - M86.351   Chronic multifocal osteomyelitis, right femur
  - M86.352   Chronic multifocal osteomyelitis, left femur
  - M86.359   Chronic multifocal osteomyelitis, unspecified femur
- M86.36   Chronic multifocal osteomyelitis, tibia and fibula
  - M86.361   Chronic multifocal osteomyelitis, right tibia and fibula
  - M86.362   Chronic multifocal osteomyelitis, left tibia and fibula
  - M86.369   Chronic multifocal osteomyelitis, unspecified tibia and fibula
- M86.37   Chronic multifocal osteomyelitis, ankle and foot
  - M86.371   Chronic multifocal osteomyelitis, right ankle and foot
  - M86.372   Chronic multifocal osteomyelitis, left ankle and foot
  - M86.379   Chronic multifocal osteomyelitis, unspecified ankle and foot
- M86.38   Chronic multifocal osteomyelitis, other site
- M86.39   Chronic multifocal osteomyelitis, multiple sites
- M86.4   Chronic osteomyelitis with draining sinus
  - M86.40   Chronic osteomyelitis with draining sinus, unspecified site
- M86.41   Chronic osteomyelitis with draining sinus, shoulder
  - M86.411   Chronic osteomyelitis with draining sinus, right shoulder
  - M86.412   Chronic osteomyelitis with draining sinus, left shoulder
  - M86.419   Chronic osteomyelitis with draining sinus, unspecified shoulder
- M86.42   Chronic osteomyelitis with draining sinus, humerus
  - M86.421   Chronic osteomyelitis with draining sinus, right humerus
  - M86.422   Chronic osteomyelitis with draining sinus, left humerus
  - M86.429   Chronic osteomyelitis with draining sinus, unspecified humerus

● **M86.43** Chronic osteomyelitis with draining sinus, radius and ulna
    M86.431 Chronic osteomyelitis with draining sinus, right radius and ulna
    M86.432 Chronic osteomyelitis with draining sinus, left radius and ulna
    M86.439 Chronic osteomyelitis with draining sinus, unspecified radius and ulna
● **M86.44** Chronic osteomyelitis with draining sinus, hand
    M86.441 Chronic osteomyelitis with draining sinus, right hand
    M86.442 Chronic osteomyelitis with draining sinus, left hand
    M86.449 Chronic osteomyelitis with draining sinus, unspecified hand
● **M86.45** Chronic osteomyelitis with draining sinus, femur
    M86.451 Chronic osteomyelitis with draining sinus, right femur
    M86.452 Chronic osteomyelitis with draining sinus, left femur
    M86.459 Chronic osteomyelitis with draining sinus, unspecified femur
● **M86.46** Chronic osteomyelitis with draining sinus, tibia and fibula
    M86.461 Chronic osteomyelitis with draining sinus, right tibia and fibula
    M86.462 Chronic osteomyelitis with draining sinus, left tibia and fibula
    M86.469 Chronic osteomyelitis with draining sinus, unspecified tibia and fibula
● **M86.47** Chronic osteomyelitis with draining sinus, ankle and foot
    M86.471 Chronic osteomyelitis with draining sinus, right ankle and foot
    M86.472 Chronic osteomyelitis with draining sinus, left ankle and foot
    M86.479 Chronic osteomyelitis with draining sinus, unspecified ankle and foot
    M86.48 Chronic osteomyelitis with draining sinus, other site
    M86.49 Chronic osteomyelitis with draining sinus, multiple sites
● **M86.5** Other chronic hematogenous osteomyelitis
    M86.50 Other chronic hematogenous osteomyelitis, unspecified site
● **M86.51** Other chronic hematogenous osteomyelitis, shoulder
    M86.511 Other chronic hematogenous osteomyelitis, right shoulder
    M86.512 Other chronic hematogenous osteomyelitis, left shoulder
    M86.519 Other chronic hematogenous osteomyelitis, unspecified shoulder
● **M86.52** Other chronic hematogenous osteomyelitis, humerus
    M86.521 Other chronic hematogenous osteomyelitis, right humerus
    M86.522 Other chronic hematogenous osteomyelitis, left humerus
    M86.529 Other chronic hematogenous osteomyelitis, unspecified humerus

● **M86.53** Other chronic hematogenous osteomyelitis, radius and ulna
    M86.531 Other chronic hematogenous osteomyelitis, right radius and ulna
    M86.532 Other chronic hematogenous osteomyelitis, left radius and ulna
    M86.539 Other chronic hematogenous osteomyelitis, unspecified radius and ulna
● **M86.54** Other chronic hematogenous osteomyelitis, hand
    M86.541 Other chronic hematogenous osteomyelitis, right hand
    M86.542 Other chronic hematogenous osteomyelitis, left hand
    M86.549 Other chronic hematogenous osteomyelitis, unspecified hand
● **M86.55** Other chronic hematogenous osteomyelitis, femur
    M86.551 Other chronic hematogenous osteomyelitis, right femur
    M86.552 Other chronic hematogenous osteomyelitis, left femur
    M86.559 Other chronic hematogenous osteomyelitis, unspecified femur
● **M86.56** Other chronic hematogenous osteomyelitis, tibia and fibula
    M86.561 Other chronic hematogenous osteomyelitis, right tibia and fibula
    M86.562 Other chronic hematogenous osteomyelitis, left tibia and fibula
    M86.569 Other chronic hematogenous osteomyelitis, unspecified tibia and fibula
● **M86.57** Other chronic hematogenous osteomyelitis, ankle and foot
    M86.571 Other chronic hematogenous osteomyelitis, right ankle and foot
    M86.572 Other chronic hematogenous osteomyelitis, left ankle and foot
    M86.579 Other chronic hematogenous osteomyelitis, unspecified ankle and foot
    M86.58 Other chronic hematogenous osteomyelitis, other site
    M86.59 Other chronic hematogenous osteomyelitis, multiple sites
● **M86.6** Other chronic osteomyelitis
    M86.60 Other chronic osteomyelitis, unspecified site
● **M86.61** Other chronic osteomyelitis, shoulder
    M86.611 Other chronic osteomyelitis, right shoulder
    M86.612 Other chronic osteomyelitis, left shoulder
    M86.619 Other chronic osteomyelitis, unspecified shoulder
● **M86.62** Other chronic osteomyelitis, humerus
    M86.621 Other chronic osteomyelitis, right humerus
    M86.622 Other chronic osteomyelitis, left humerus
    M86.629 Other chronic osteomyelitis, unspecified humerus
● **M86.63** Other chronic osteomyelitis, radius and ulna
    M86.631 Other chronic osteomyelitis, right radius and ulna
    M86.632 Other chronic osteomyelitis, left radius and ulna
    M86.639 Other chronic osteomyelitis, unspecified radius and ulna

▶ New   ⇒ Revised   ~~deleted~~ Deleted   **OGCR** Official Guidelines   X Assign placeholder X   ● Use Additional Character(s)

Excludes 1   Excludes 2   Includes   Use additional   Code first   Code also   Key words

● M86.64 Other chronic osteomyelitis, hand
  M86.641 Other chronic osteomyelitis, right hand
  M86.642 Other chronic osteomyelitis, left hand
  M86.649 Other chronic osteomyelitis, unspecified hand

● M86.65 Other chronic osteomyelitis, thigh
  M86.651 Other chronic osteomyelitis, right thigh
  M86.652 Other chronic osteomyelitis, left thigh
  M86.659 Other chronic osteomyelitis, unspecified thigh

● M86.66 Other chronic osteomyelitis, tibia and fibula
  M86.661 Other chronic osteomyelitis, right tibia and fibula
  M86.662 Other chronic osteomyelitis, left tibia and fibula
  M86.669 Other chronic osteomyelitis, unspecified tibia and fibula

● M86.67 Other chronic osteomyelitis, ankle and foot
  M86.671 Other chronic osteomyelitis, right ankle and foot
  M86.672 Other chronic osteomyelitis, left ankle and foot
  M86.679 Other chronic osteomyelitis, unspecified ankle and foot

 M86.68 Other chronic osteomyelitis, other site
 M86.69 Other chronic osteomyelitis, multiple sites

● M86.8 Other osteomyelitis
  Brodie's abscess
 ● M86.8X Other osteomyelitis
  M86.8X0 Other osteomyelitis, multiple sites
  M86.8X1 Other osteomyelitis, shoulder
  M86.8X2 Other osteomyelitis, upper arm
  M86.8X3 Other osteomyelitis, forearm
  M86.8X4 Other osteomyelitis, hand
  M86.8X5 Other osteomyelitis, thigh
  M86.8X6 Other osteomyelitis, lower leg
  M86.8X7 Other osteomyelitis, ankle and foot
  M86.8X8 Other osteomyelitis, other site
  M86.8X9 Other osteomyelitis, unspecified sites

 M86.9 Osteomyelitis, unspecified
  Infection of bone NOS
  Periostitis without osteomyelitis

● M87 Osteonecrosis
  Includes avascular necrosis of bone
  Use additional code to identify major osseous defect, if applicable (M89.7-)
  Excludes1 juvenile osteonecrosis (M91-M92)
     osteochondropathies (M90-M93)

● M87.0 Idiopathic aseptic necrosis of bone
  M87.00 Idiopathic aseptic necrosis of unspecified bone
 ● M87.01 Idiopathic aseptic necrosis of shoulder
  Idiopathic aseptic necrosis of clavicle and scapula
  M87.011 Idiopathic aseptic necrosis of right shoulder
  M87.012 Idiopathic aseptic necrosis of left shoulder
  M87.019 Idiopathic aseptic necrosis of unspecified shoulder

● M87.02 Idiopathic aseptic necrosis of humerus
  M87.021 Idiopathic aseptic necrosis of right humerus
  M87.022 Idiopathic aseptic necrosis of left humerus
  M87.029 Idiopathic aseptic necrosis of unspecified humerus

● M87.03 Idiopathic aseptic necrosis of radius, ulna and carpus
  M87.031 Idiopathic aseptic necrosis of right radius
  M87.032 Idiopathic aseptic necrosis of left radius
  M87.033 Idiopathic aseptic necrosis of unspecified radius
  M87.034 Idiopathic aseptic necrosis of right ulna
  M87.035 Idiopathic aseptic necrosis of left ulna
  M87.036 Idiopathic aseptic necrosis of unspecified ulna
  M87.037 Idiopathic aseptic necrosis of right carpus
  M87.038 Idiopathic aseptic necrosis of left carpus
  M87.039 Idiopathic aseptic necrosis of unspecified carpus

● M87.04 Idiopathic aseptic necrosis of hand and fingers
  Idiopathic aseptic necrosis of metacarpals and phalanges of hands
  M87.041 Idiopathic aseptic necrosis of right hand
  M87.042 Idiopathic aseptic necrosis of left hand
  M87.043 Idiopathic aseptic necrosis of unspecified hand
  M87.044 Idiopathic aseptic necrosis of right finger(s)
  M87.045 Idiopathic aseptic necrosis of left finger(s)
  M87.046 Idiopathic aseptic necrosis of unspecified finger(s)

● M87.05 Idiopathic aseptic necrosis of pelvis and femur
  M87.050 Idiopathic aseptic necrosis of pelvis
  M87.051 Idiopathic aseptic necrosis of right femur
  M87.052 Idiopathic aseptic necrosis of left femur
  M87.059 Idiopathic aseptic necrosis of unspecified femur
    Idiopathic aseptic necrosis of hip NOS

● M87.06 Idiopathic aseptic necrosis of tibia and fibula
  M87.061 Idiopathic aseptic necrosis of right tibia
  M87.062 Idiopathic aseptic necrosis of left tibia
  M87.063 Idiopathic aseptic necrosis of unspecified tibia
  M87.064 Idiopathic aseptic necrosis of right fibula
  M87.065 Idiopathic aseptic necrosis of left fibula
  M87.066 Idiopathic aseptic necrosis of unspecified fibula

CHAPTER 13 (M00-M99)

▶ New ⇒ Revised ~~deleted~~ Deleted **OGCR** Official Guidelines X Assign placeholder X ● Use Additional Character(s)

Excludes 1 Excludes 2 Includes Use additional Code first Code also Key words

1025

● **M87.07** **Idiopathic aseptic necrosis of ankle, foot and toes**
Idiopathic aseptic necrosis of metatarsus, tarsus, and phalanges of toes

     M87.071 **Idiopathic aseptic necrosis of right ankle**

     M87.072 **Idiopathic aseptic necrosis of left ankle**

     M87.073 **Idiopathic aseptic necrosis of unspecified ankle**

     M87.074 **Idiopathic aseptic necrosis of right foot**

     M87.075 **Idiopathic aseptic necrosis of left foot**

     M87.076 **Idiopathic aseptic necrosis of unspecified foot**

     M87.077 **Idiopathic aseptic necrosis of right toe(s)**

     M87.078 **Idiopathic aseptic necrosis of left toe(s)**

     M87.079 **Idiopathic aseptic necrosis of unspecified toe(s)**

M87.08 **Idiopathic aseptic necrosis of bone, other site**

M87.09 **Idiopathic aseptic necrosis of bone, multiple sites**

● **M87.1** **Osteonecrosis due to drugs**
Use additional code for adverse effect, if applicable, to identify drug (T36-T50 with fifth or sixth character 5)

M87.10 **Osteonecrosis due to drugs, unspecified bone**

● **M87.11** **Osteonecrosis due to drugs, shoulder**

     M87.111 **Osteonecrosis due to drugs, right shoulder**

     M87.112 **Osteonecrosis due to drugs, left shoulder**

     M87.119 **Osteonecrosis due to drugs, unspecified shoulder**

● **M87.12** **Osteonecrosis due to drugs, humerus**

     M87.121 **Osteonecrosis due to drugs, right humerus**

     M87.122 **Osteonecrosis due to drugs, left humerus**

     M87.129 **Osteonecrosis due to drugs, unspecified humerus**

● **M87.13** **Osteonecrosis due to drugs of radius, ulna and carpus**

     M87.131 **Osteonecrosis due to drugs of right radius**

     M87.132 **Osteonecrosis due to drugs of left radius**

     M87.133 **Osteonecrosis due to drugs of unspecified radius**

     M87.134 **Osteonecrosis due to drugs of right ulna**

     M87.135 **Osteonecrosis due to drugs of left ulna**

     M87.136 **Osteonecrosis due to drugs of unspecified ulna**

     M87.137 **Osteonecrosis due to drugs of right carpus**

     M87.138 **Osteonecrosis due to drugs of left carpus**

     M87.139 **Osteonecrosis due to drugs of unspecified carpus**

● **M87.14** **Osteonecrosis due to drugs, hand and fingers**

     M87.141 **Osteonecrosis due to drugs, right hand**

     M87.142 **Osteonecrosis due to drugs, left hand**

     M87.143 **Osteonecrosis due to drugs, unspecified hand**

     M87.144 **Osteonecrosis due to drugs, right finger(s)**

     M87.145 **Osteonecrosis due to drugs, left finger(s)**

     M87.146 **Osteonecrosis due to drugs, unspecified finger(s)**

● **M87.15** **Osteonecrosis due to drugs, pelvis and femur**

     M87.150 **Osteonecrosis due to drugs, pelvis**

     M87.151 **Osteonecrosis due to drugs, right femur**

     M87.152 **Osteonecrosis due to drugs, left femur**

     M87.159 **Osteonecrosis due to drugs, unspecified femur**

● **M87.16** **Osteonecrosis due to drugs, tibia and fibula**

     M87.161 **Osteonecrosis due to drugs, right tibia**

     M87.162 **Osteonecrosis due to drugs, left tibia**

     M87.163 **Osteonecrosis due to drugs, unspecified tibia**

     M87.164 **Osteonecrosis due to drugs, right fibula**

     M87.165 **Osteonecrosis due to drugs, left fibula**

     M87.166 **Osteonecrosis due to drugs, unspecified fibula**

● **M87.17** **Osteonecrosis due to drugs, ankle, foot and toes**

     M87.171 **Osteonecrosis due to drugs, right ankle**

     M87.172 **Osteonecrosis due to drugs, left ankle**

     M87.173 **Osteonecrosis due to drugs, unspecified ankle**

     M87.174 **Osteonecrosis due to drugs, right foot**

     M87.175 **Osteonecrosis due to drugs, left foot**

     M87.176 **Osteonecrosis due to drugs, unspecified foot**

     M87.177 **Osteonecrosis due to drugs, right toe(s)**

     M87.178 **Osteonecrosis due to drugs, left toe(s)**

     M87.179 **Osteonecrosis due to drugs, unspecified toe(s)**

● **M87.18** **Osteonecrosis due to drugs, other site**

     M87.180 **Osteonecrosis due to drugs, jaw**

     M87.188 **Osteonecrosis due to drugs, other site**

M87.19 **Osteonecrosis due to drugs, multiple sites**

● **M87.2** **Osteonecrosis due to previous trauma**

M87.20 **Osteonecrosis due to previous trauma, unspecified bone**

● **M87.21** **Osteonecrosis due to previous trauma, shoulder**

     M87.211 **Osteonecrosis due to previous trauma, right shoulder**

     M87.212 **Osteonecrosis due to previous trauma, left shoulder**

     M87.219 **Osteonecrosis due to previous trauma, unspecified shoulder**

● **M87.22** **Osteonecrosis due to previous trauma, humerus**

     M87.221 **Osteonecrosis due to previous trauma, right humerus**

     M87.222 **Osteonecrosis due to previous trauma, left humerus**

     M87.229 **Osteonecrosis due to previous trauma, unspecified humerus**

▶ New   ⇒ Revised   ~~deleted~~ Deleted   **OGCR** Official Guidelines   X Assign placeholder X   ● Use Additional Character(s)

Excludes 1   Excludes 2   Includes   Use additional   Code first   Code also   Key words

● **M87.23** Osteonecrosis due to previous trauma of radius, ulna and carpus

    M87.231   Osteonecrosis due to previous trauma of right radius

    M87.232   Osteonecrosis due to previous trauma of left radius

    M87.233   Osteonecrosis due to previous trauma of unspecified radius

    M87.234   Osteonecrosis due to previous trauma of right ulna

    M87.235   Osteonecrosis due to previous trauma of left ulna

    M87.236   Osteonecrosis due to previous trauma of unspecified ulna

    M87.237   Osteonecrosis due to previous trauma of right carpus

    M87.238   Osteonecrosis due to previous trauma of left carpus

    M87.239   Osteonecrosis due to previous trauma of unspecified carpus

● **M87.24** Osteonecrosis due to previous trauma, hand and fingers

    M87.241   Osteonecrosis due to previous trauma, right hand

    M87.242   Osteonecrosis due to previous trauma, left hand

    M87.243   Osteonecrosis due to previous trauma, unspecified hand

    M87.244   Osteonecrosis due to previous trauma, right finger(s)

    M87.245   Osteonecrosis due to previous trauma, left finger(s)

    M87.246   Osteonecrosis due to previous trauma, unspecified finger(s)

● **M87.25** Osteonecrosis due to previous trauma, pelvis and femur

    M87.250   Osteonecrosis due to previous trauma, pelvis

    M87.251   Osteonecrosis due to previous trauma, right femur

    M87.252   Osteonecrosis due to previous trauma, left femur

    M87.256   Osteonecrosis due to previous trauma, unspecified femur

● **M87.26** Osteonecrosis due to previous trauma, tibia and fibula

    M87.261   Osteonecrosis due to previous trauma, right tibia

    M87.262   Osteonecrosis due to previous trauma, left tibia

    M87.263   Osteonecrosis due to previous trauma, unspecified tibia

    M87.264   Osteonecrosis due to previous trauma, right fibula

    M87.265   Osteonecrosis due to previous trauma, left fibula

    M87.266   Osteonecrosis due to previous trauma, unspecified fibula

● **M87.27** Osteonecrosis due to previous trauma, ankle, foot and toes

    M87.271   Osteonecrosis due to previous trauma, right ankle

    M87.272   Osteonecrosis due to previous trauma, left ankle

    M87.273   Osteonecrosis due to previous trauma, unspecified ankle

    M87.274   Osteonecrosis due to previous trauma, right foot

    M87.275   Osteonecrosis due to previous trauma, left foot

    M87.276   Osteonecrosis due to previous trauma, unspecified foot

    M87.277   Osteonecrosis due to previous trauma, right toe(s)

    M87.278   Osteonecrosis due to previous trauma, left toe(s)

    M87.279   Osteonecrosis due to previous trauma, unspecified toe(s)

    M87.28   Osteonecrosis due to previous trauma, other site

    M87.29   Osteonecrosis due to previous trauma, multiple sites

● **M87.3** Other secondary osteonecrosis

    M87.30   Other secondary osteonecrosis, unspecified bone

  ● **M87.31** Other secondary osteonecrosis, shoulder

    M87.311   Other secondary osteonecrosis, right shoulder

    M87.312   Other secondary osteonecrosis, left shoulder

    M87.319   Other secondary osteonecrosis, unspecified shoulder

  ● **M87.32** Other secondary osteonecrosis, humerus

    M87.321   Other secondary osteonecrosis, right humerus

    M87.322   Other secondary osteonecrosis, left humerus

    M87.329   Other secondary osteonecrosis, unspecified humerus

  ● **M87.33** Other secondary osteonecrosis of radius, ulna and carpus

    M87.331   Other secondary osteonecrosis of right radius

    M87.332   Other secondary osteonecrosis of left radius

    M87.333   Other secondary osteonecrosis of unspecified radius

    M87.334   Other secondary osteonecrosis of right ulna

    M87.335   Other secondary osteonecrosis of left ulna

    M87.336   Other secondary osteonecrosis of unspecified ulna

    M87.337   Other secondary osteonecrosis of right carpus

    M87.338   Other secondary osteonecrosis of left carpus

    M87.339   Other secondary osteonecrosis of unspecified carpus

  ● **M87.34** Other secondary osteonecrosis, hand and fingers

    M87.341   Other secondary osteonecrosis, right hand

    M87.342   Other secondary osteonecrosis, left hand

    M87.343   Other secondary osteonecrosis, unspecified hand

    M87.344   Other secondary osteonecrosis, right finger(s)

    M87.345   Other secondary osteonecrosis, left finger(s)

    M87.346   Other secondary osteonecrosis, unspecified finger(s)

● **M87.35 Other secondary osteonecrosis, pelvis and femur**
    M87.350 Other secondary osteonecrosis, pelvis
    M87.351 Other secondary osteonecrosis, right femur
    M87.352 Other secondary osteonecrosis, left femur
    M87.353 Other secondary osteonecrosis, unspecified femur

● **M87.36 Other secondary osteonecrosis, tibia and fibula**
    M87.361 Other secondary osteonecrosis, right tibia
    M87.362 Other secondary osteonecrosis, left tibia
    M87.363 Other secondary osteonecrosis, unspecified tibia
    M87.364 Other secondary osteonecrosis, right fibula
    M87.365 Other secondary osteonecrosis, left fibula
    M87.366 Other secondary osteonecrosis, unspecified fibula

● **M87.37 Other secondary osteonecrosis, ankle and foot**
    M87.371 Other secondary osteonecrosis, right ankle
    M87.372 Other secondary osteonecrosis, left ankle
    M87.373 Other secondary osteonecrosis, unspecified ankle
    M87.374 Other secondary osteonecrosis, right foot
    M87.375 Other secondary osteonecrosis, left foot
    M87.376 Other secondary osteonecrosis, unspecified foot
    M87.377 Other secondary osteonecrosis, right toe(s)
    M87.378 Other secondary osteonecrosis, left toe(s)
    M87.379 Other secondary osteonecrosis, unspecified toe(s)

    M87.38 Other secondary osteonecrosis, other site
    M87.39 Other secondary osteonecrosis, multiple sites

● **M87.8 Other osteonecrosis**
    M87.80 Other osteonecrosis, unspecified bone

● **M87.81 Other osteonecrosis, shoulder**
    M87.811 Other osteonecrosis, right shoulder
    M87.812 Other osteonecrosis, left shoulder
    M87.819 Other osteonecrosis, unspecified shoulder

● **M87.82 Other osteonecrosis, humerus**
    M87.821 Other osteonecrosis, right humerus
    M87.822 Other osteonecrosis, left humerus
    M87.829 Other osteonecrosis, unspecified humerus

● **M87.83 Other osteonecrosis of radius, ulna and carpus**
    M87.831 Other osteonecrosis of right radius
    M87.832 Other osteonecrosis of left radius
    M87.833 Other osteonecrosis of unspecified radius
    M87.834 Other osteonecrosis of right ulna
    M87.835 Other osteonecrosis of left ulna
    M87.836 Other osteonecrosis of unspecified ulna
    M87.837 Other osteonecrosis of right carpus
    M87.838 Other osteonecrosis of left carpus
    M87.839 Other osteonecrosis of unspecified carpus

● **M87.84 Other osteonecrosis, hand and fingers**
    M87.841 Other osteonecrosis, right hand
    M87.842 Other osteonecrosis, left hand
    M87.843 Other osteonecrosis, unspecified hand
    M87.844 Other osteonecrosis, right finger(s)
    M87.845 Other osteonecrosis, left finger(s)
    M87.849 Other osteonecrosis, unspecified finger(s)

● **M87.85 Other osteonecrosis, pelvis and femur**
    M87.850 Other osteonecrosis, pelvis
    M87.851 Other osteonecrosis, right femur
    M87.852 Other osteonecrosis, left femur
    M87.859 Other osteonecrosis, unspecified femur

● **M87.86 Other osteonecrosis, tibia and fibula**
    M87.861 Other osteonecrosis, right tibia
    M87.862 Other osteonecrosis, left tibia
    M87.863 Other osteonecrosis, unspecified tibia
    M87.864 Other osteonecrosis, right fibula
    M87.865 Other osteonecrosis, left fibula
    M87.869 Other osteonecrosis, unspecified fibula

● **M87.87 Other osteonecrosis, ankle, foot and toes**
    M87.871 Other osteonecrosis, right ankle
    M87.872 Other osteonecrosis, left ankle
    M87.873 Other osteonecrosis, unspecified ankle
    M87.874 Other osteonecrosis, right foot
    M87.875 Other osteonecrosis, left foot
    M87.876 Other osteonecrosis, unspecified foot
    M87.877 Other osteonecrosis, right toe(s)
    M87.878 Other osteonecrosis, left toe(s)
    M87.879 Other osteonecrosis, unspecified toe(s)

    M87.88 Other osteonecrosis, other site
    M87.89 Other osteonecrosis, multiple sites

    M87.9 Osteonecrosis, unspecified
        Necrosis of bone NOS

● **M88 Osteitis deformans [Paget's disease of bone]**
Chronic disorder that results in enlarged and deformed bones. The excessive breakdown and formation of bone tissue causes bones to weaken and results in bone pain, arthritis, deformities, and fractures.

    Excludes1 osteitis deformans in neoplastic disease (M90.6)

    M88.0 Osteitis deformans of skull
    M88.1 Osteitis deformans of vertebrae

● **M88.8 Osteitis deformans of other bones**
  ● **M88.81 Osteitis deformans of shoulder**
    M88.811 Osteitis deformans of right shoulder
    M88.812 Osteitis deformans of left shoulder
    M88.819 Osteitis deformans of unspecified shoulder

  ● **M88.82 Osteitis deformans of upper arm**
    M88.821 Osteitis deformans of right upper arm
    M88.822 Osteitis deformans of left upper arm
    M88.829 Osteitis deformans of unspecified upper arm

  ● **M88.83 Osteitis deformans of forearm**
    M88.831 Osteitis deformans of right forearm
    M88.832 Osteitis deformans of left forearm
    M88.839 Osteitis deformans of unspecified forearm

▶ New   ⇒ Revised   ~~deleted~~ Deleted   **OGCR** Official Guidelines   X Assign placeholder X   ● Use Additional Character(s)

Excludes 1   Excludes 2   Includes   Use additional   Code first   Code also   Key words

- M88.84 Osteitis deformans of hand
  - M88.841 Osteitis deformans of right hand
  - M88.842 Osteitis deformans of left hand
  - M88.849 Osteitis deformans of unspecified hand
- M88.85 Osteitis deformans of thigh
  - M88.851 Osteitis deformans of right thigh
  - M88.852 Osteitis deformans of left thigh
  - M88.859 Osteitis deformans of unspecified thigh
- M88.86 Osteitis deformans of lower leg
  - M88.861 Osteitis deformans of right lower leg
  - M88.862 Osteitis deformans of left lower leg
  - M88.869 Osteitis deformans of unspecified lower leg
- M88.87 Osteitis deformans of ankle and foot
  - M88.871 Osteitis deformans of right ankle and foot
  - M88.872 Osteitis deformans of left ankle and foot
  - M88.879 Osteitis deformans of unspecified ankle and foot
  - M88.88 Osteitis deformans of other bones
    - **Excludes2** osteitis deformans of skull (M88.Ø)
      osteitis deformans of vertebrae (M88.1)
  - M88.89 Osteitis deformans of multiple sites
  - M88.9 Osteitis deformans of unspecified bone
- M89 Other disorders of bone
  - M89.Ø Algoneurodystrophy
    Shoulder-hand syndrome
    Sudeck's atrophy
    - **Excludes1** causalgia, lower limb (G57.7-)
      causalgia, upper limb (G56.4-)
      complex regional pain syndrome II, lower limb (G57.7-)
      complex regional pain syndrome II, upper limb (G56.4-)
      reflex sympathetic dystrophy (G9Ø.5-)
    - M89.ØØ Algoneurodystrophy, unspecified site
  - M89.Ø1 Algoneurodystrophy, shoulder
    - M89.Ø11 Algoneurodystrophy, right shoulder
    - M89.Ø12 Algoneurodystrophy, left shoulder
    - M89.Ø19 Algoneurodystrophy, unspecified shoulder
  - M89.Ø2 Algoneurodystrophy, upper arm
    - M89.Ø21 Algoneurodystrophy, right upper arm
    - M89.Ø22 Algoneurodystrophy, left upper arm
    - M89.Ø29 Algoneurodystrophy, unspecified upper arm
  - M89.Ø3 Algoneurodystrophy, forearm
    - M89.Ø31 Algoneurodystrophy, right forearm
    - M89.Ø32 Algoneurodystrophy, left forearm
    - M89.Ø39 Algoneurodystrophy, unspecified forearm
  - M89.Ø4 Algoneurodystrophy, hand
    - M89.Ø41 Algoneurodystrophy, right hand
    - M89.Ø42 Algoneurodystrophy, left hand
    - M89.Ø49 Algoneurodystrophy, unspecified hand
  - M89.Ø5 Algoneurodystrophy, thigh
    - M89.Ø51 Algoneurodystrophy, right thigh
    - M89.Ø52 Algoneurodystrophy, left thigh
    - M89.Ø59 Algoneurodystrophy, unspecified thigh

- M89.Ø6 Algoneurodystrophy, lower leg
  - M89.Ø61 Algoneurodystrophy, right lower leg
  - M89.Ø62 Algoneurodystrophy, left lower leg
  - M89.Ø69 Algoneurodystrophy, unspecified lower leg
- M89.Ø7 Algoneurodystrophy, ankle and foot
  - M89.Ø71 Algoneurodystrophy, right ankle and foot
  - M89.Ø72 Algoneurodystrophy, left ankle and foot
  - M89.Ø79 Algoneurodystrophy, unspecified ankle and foot
  - M89.Ø8 Algoneurodystrophy, other site
  - M89.Ø9 Algoneurodystrophy, multiple sites
- M89.1 Physeal arrest
  Arrest of growth plate
  Epiphyseal arrest
  Growth plate arrest
  - M89.12 Physeal arrest, humerus
    - M89.121 Complete physeal arrest, right proximal humerus
    - M89.122 Complete physeal arrest, left proximal humerus
    - M89.123 Partial physeal arrest, right proximal humerus
    - M89.124 Partial physeal arrest, left proximal humerus
    - M89.125 Complete physeal arrest, right distal humerus
    - M89.126 Complete physeal arrest, left distal humerus
    - M89.127 Partial physeal arrest, right distal humerus
    - M89.128 Partial physeal arrest, left distal humerus
    - M89.129 Physeal arrest, humerus, unspecified
  - M89.13 Physeal arrest, forearm
    - M89.131 Complete physeal arrest, right distal radius
    - M89.132 Complete physeal arrest, left distal radius
    - M89.133 Partial physeal arrest, right distal radius
    - M89.134 Partial physeal arrest, left distal radius
    - M89.138 Other physeal arrest of forearm
    - M89.139 Physeal arrest, forearm, unspecified
  - M89.15 Physeal arrest, femur
    - M89.151 Complete physeal arrest, right proximal femur
    - M89.152 Complete physeal arrest, left proximal femur
    - M89.153 Partial physeal arrest, right proximal femur
    - M89.154 Partial physeal arrest, left proximal femur
    - M89.155 Complete physeal arrest, right distal femur
    - M89.156 Complete physeal arrest, left distal femur
    - M89.157 Partial physeal arrest, right distal femur
    - M89.158 Partial physeal arrest, left distal femur
    - M89.159 Physeal arrest, femur, unspecified

CHAPTER 13 (M00-M99)

● M89.16 Physeal arrest, lower leg
    M89.160 Complete physeal arrest, right proximal tibia
    M89.161 Complete physeal arrest, left proximal tibia
    M89.162 Partial physeal arrest, right proximal tibia
    M89.163 Partial physeal arrest, left proximal tibia
    M89.164 Complete physeal arrest, right distal tibia
    M89.165 Complete physeal arrest, left distal tibia
    M89.166 Partial physeal arrest, right distal tibia
    M89.167 Partial physeal arrest, left distal tibia
    M89.168 Other physeal arrest of lower leg
    M89.169 Physeal arrest, lower leg, unspecified
  M89.18 Physeal arrest, other site
● M89.2 Other disorders of bone development and growth
  M89.20 Other disorders of bone development and growth, unspecified site
  ● M89.21 Other disorders of bone development and growth, shoulder
    M89.211 Other disorders of bone development and growth, right shoulder
    M89.212 Other disorders of bone development and growth, left shoulder
    M89.219 Other disorders of bone development and growth, unspecified shoulder
  ● M89.22 Other disorders of bone development and growth, humerus
    M89.221 Other disorders of bone development and growth, right humerus
    M89.222 Other disorders of bone development and growth, left humerus
    M89.229 Other disorders of bone development and growth, unspecified humerus
  ● M89.23 Other disorders of bone development and growth, ulna and radius
    M89.231 Other disorders of bone development and growth, right ulna
    M89.232 Other disorders of bone development and growth, left ulna
    M89.233 Other disorders of bone development and growth, right radius
    M89.234 Other disorders of bone development and growth, left radius
    M89.239 Other disorders of bone development and growth, unspecified ulna and radius
  ● M89.24 Other disorders of bone development and growth, hand
    M89.241 Other disorders of bone development and growth, right hand
    M89.242 Other disorders of bone development and growth, left hand
    M89.249 Other disorders of bone development and growth, unspecified hand

● M89.25 Other disorders of bone development and growth, femur
    M89.251 Other disorders of bone development and growth, right femur
    M89.252 Other disorders of bone development and growth, left femur
    M89.259 Other disorders of bone development and growth, unspecified femur
● M89.26 Other disorders of bone development and growth, tibia and fibula
    M89.261 Other disorders of bone development and growth, right tibia
    M89.262 Other disorders of bone development and growth, left tibia
    M89.263 Other disorders of bone development and growth, right fibula
    M89.264 Other disorders of bone development and growth, left fibula
    M89.269 Other disorders of bone development and growth, unspecified lower leg
● M89.27 Other disorders of bone development and growth, ankle and foot
    M89.271 Other disorders of bone development and growth, right ankle and foot
    M89.272 Other disorders of bone development and growth, left ankle and foot
    M89.279 Other disorders of bone development and growth, unspecified ankle and foot
  M89.28 Other disorders of bone development and growth, other site
  M89.29 Other disorders of bone development and growth, multiple sites
● M89.3 Hypertrophy of bone
  M89.30 Hypertrophy of bone, unspecified site
  ● M89.31 Hypertrophy of bone, shoulder
    M89.311 Hypertrophy of bone, right shoulder
    M89.312 Hypertrophy of bone, left shoulder
    M89.319 Hypertrophy of bone, unspecified shoulder
  ● M89.32 Hypertrophy of bone, humerus
    M89.321 Hypertrophy of bone, right humerus
    M89.322 Hypertrophy of bone, left humerus
    M89.329 Hypertrophy of bone, unspecified humerus
  ● M89.33 Hypertrophy of bone, ulna and radius
    M89.331 Hypertrophy of bone, right ulna
    M89.332 Hypertrophy of bone, left ulna
    M89.333 Hypertrophy of bone, right radius
    M89.334 Hypertrophy of bone, left radius
    M89.339 Hypertrophy of bone, unspecified ulna and radius
  ● M89.34 Hypertrophy of bone, hand
    M89.341 Hypertrophy of bone, right hand
    M89.342 Hypertrophy of bone, left hand
    M89.349 Hypertrophy of bone, unspecified hand
  ● M89.35 Hypertrophy of bone, femur
    M89.351 Hypertrophy of bone, right femur
    M89.352 Hypertrophy of bone, left femur
    M89.359 Hypertrophy of bone, unspecified femur

▶ New   ⮕ Revised   ~~deleted~~ Deleted   **OGCR** Official Guidelines   X Assign placeholder X   ● Use Additional Character(s)

Excludes 1   Excludes 2   Includes   Use additional   Code first   Code also   Key words

● M89.36   Hypertrophy of bone, tibia and fibula
     M89.361   Hypertrophy of bone, right tibia
     M89.362   Hypertrophy of bone, left tibia
     M89.363   Hypertrophy of bone, right fibula
     M89.364   Hypertrophy of bone, left fibula
     M89.369   Hypertrophy of bone, unspecified tibia and fibula

● M89.37   Hypertrophy of bone, ankle and foot
     M89.371   Hypertrophy of bone, right ankle and foot
     M89.372   Hypertrophy of bone, left ankle and foot
     M89.379   Hypertrophy of bone, unspecified ankle and foot

   M89.38   Hypertrophy of bone, other site
   M89.39   Hypertrophy of bone, multiple sites

● M89.4   Other hypertrophic osteoarthropathy
     Marie-Bamberger disease
     Pachydermoperiostosis

   M89.40   Other hypertrophic osteoarthropathy, unspecified site
● M89.41   Other hypertrophic osteoarthropathy, shoulder
     M89.411   Other hypertrophic osteoarthropathy, right shoulder
     M89.412   Other hypertrophic osteoarthropathy, left shoulder
     M89.419   Other hypertrophic osteoarthropathy, unspecified shoulder

● M89.42   Other hypertrophic osteoarthropathy, upper arm
     M89.421   Other hypertrophic osteoarthropathy, right upper arm
     M89.422   Other hypertrophic osteoarthropathy, left upper arm
     M89.429   Other hypertrophic osteoarthropathy, unspecified upper arm

● M89.43   Other hypertrophic osteoarthropathy, forearm
     M89.431   Other hypertrophic osteoarthropathy, right forearm
     M89.432   Other hypertrophic osteoarthropathy, left forearm
     M89.439   Other hypertrophic osteoarthropathy, unspecified forearm

● M89.44   Other hypertrophic osteoarthropathy, hand
     M89.441   Other hypertrophic osteoarthropathy, right hand
     M89.442   Other hypertrophic osteoarthropathy, left hand
     M89.449   Other hypertrophic osteoarthropathy, unspecified hand

● M89.45   Other hypertrophic osteoarthropathy, thigh
     M89.451   Other hypertrophic osteoarthropathy, right thigh
     M89.452   Other hypertrophic osteoarthropathy, left thigh
     M89.459   Other hypertrophic osteoarthropathy, unspecified thigh

● M89.46   Other hypertrophic osteoarthropathy, lower leg
     M89.461   Other hypertrophic osteoarthropathy, right lower leg
     M89.462   Other hypertrophic osteoarthropathy, left lower leg
     M89.469   Other hypertrophic osteoarthropathy, unspecified lower leg

● M89.47   Other hypertrophic osteoarthropathy, ankle and foot
     M89.471   Other hypertrophic osteoarthropathy, right ankle and foot
     M89.472   Other hypertrophic osteoarthropathy, left ankle and foot
     M89.479   Other hypertrophic osteoarthropathy, unspecified ankle and foot

   M89.48   Other hypertrophic osteoarthropathy, other site
   M89.49   Other hypertrophic osteoarthropathy, multiple sites

● M89.5   Osteolysis
     Use additional code to identify major osseous defect, if applicable (M89.7-)
     | Excludes2 | periprosthetic osteolysis of internal prosthetic joint (T84.05-)

   M89.50   Osteolysis, unspecified site
● M89.51   Osteolysis, shoulder
     M89.511   Osteolysis, right shoulder
     M89.512   Osteolysis, left shoulder
     M89.519   Osteolysis, unspecified shoulder
● M89.52   Osteolysis, upper arm
     M89.521   Osteolysis, right upper arm
     M89.522   Osteolysis, left upper arm
     M89.529   Osteolysis, unspecified upper arm
● M89.53   Osteolysis, forearm
     M89.531   Osteolysis, right forearm
     M89.532   Osteolysis, left forearm
     M89.539   Osteolysis, unspecified forearm
● M89.54   Osteolysis, hand
     M89.541   Osteolysis, right hand
     M89.542   Osteolysis, left hand
     M89.549   Osteolysis, unspecified hand
● M89.55   Osteolysis, thigh
     M89.551   Osteolysis, right thigh
     M89.552   Osteolysis, left thigh
     M89.559   Osteolysis, unspecified thigh
● M89.56   Osteolysis, lower leg
     M89.561   Osteolysis, right lower leg
     M89.562   Osteolysis, left lower leg
     M89.569   Osteolysis, unspecified lower leg
● M89.57   Osteolysis, ankle and foot
     M89.571   Osteolysis, right ankle and foot
     M89.572   Osteolysis, left ankle and foot
     M89.579   Osteolysis, unspecified ankle and foot
   M89.58   Osteolysis, other site
   M89.59   Osteolysis, multiple sites

● M89.6   Osteopathy after poliomyelitis
     Use additional code (B91) to identify previous poliomyelitis
     | Excludes1 | postpolio syndrome (G14)

   M89.60   Osteopathy after poliomyelitis, unspecified site
● M89.61   Osteopathy after poliomyelitis, shoulder
     M89.611   Osteopathy after poliomyelitis, right shoulder
     M89.612   Osteopathy after poliomyelitis, left shoulder
     M89.619   Osteopathy after poliomyelitis, unspecified shoulder
● M89.62   Osteopathy after poliomyelitis, upper arm
     M89.621   Osteopathy after poliomyelitis, right upper arm
     M89.622   Osteopathy after poliomyelitis, left upper arm
     M89.629   Osteopathy after poliomyelitis, unspecified upper arm

CHAPTER 13 (M00-M99)

● M89.63 Osteopathy after poliomyelitis, forearm
    M89.631 Osteopathy after poliomyelitis, right forearm
    M89.632 Osteopathy after poliomyelitis, left forearm
    M89.639 Osteopathy after poliomyelitis, unspecified forearm
● M89.64 Osteopathy after poliomyelitis, hand
    M89.641 Osteopathy after poliomyelitis, right hand
    M89.642 Osteopathy after poliomyelitis, left hand
    M89.649 Osteopathy after poliomyelitis, unspecified hand
● M89.65 Osteopathy after poliomyelitis, thigh
    M89.651 Osteopathy after poliomyelitis, right thigh
    M89.652 Osteopathy after poliomyelitis, left thigh
    M89.659 Osteopathy after poliomyelitis, unspecified thigh
● M89.66 Osteopathy after poliomyelitis, lower leg
    M89.661 Osteopathy after poliomyelitis, right lower leg
    M89.662 Osteopathy after poliomyelitis, left lower leg
    M89.669 Osteopathy after poliomyelitis, unspecified lower leg
● M89.67 Osteopathy after poliomyelitis, ankle and foot
    M89.671 Osteopathy after poliomyelitis, right ankle and foot
    M89.672 Osteopathy after poliomyelitis, left ankle and foot
    M89.679 Osteopathy after poliomyelitis, unspecified ankle and foot
  M89.68 Osteopathy after poliomyelitis, other site
  M89.69 Osteopathy after poliomyelitis, multiple sites

● M89.7 Major osseous defect
    Code first underlying disease, if known, such as:
      aseptic necrosis of bone (M87.-)
      malignant neoplasm of bone (C40.-)
      osteolysis (M89.5)
      osteomyelitis (M86.-)
      osteonecrosis (M87.-)
      osteoporosis (M80.-, M81.-)
      periprosthetic osteolysis (T84.05-)
  M89.70 Major osseous defect, unspecified site
● M89.71 Major osseous defect, shoulder region
    Major osseous defect clavicle or scapula
    M89.711 Major osseous defect, right shoulder region
    M89.712 Major osseous defect, left shoulder region
    M89.719 Major osseous defect, unspecified shoulder region
● M89.72 Major osseous defect, humerus
    M89.721 Major osseous defect, right humerus
    M89.722 Major osseous defect, left humerus
    M89.729 Major osseous defect, unspecified humerus

● M89.73 Major osseous defect, forearm
    Major osseous defect of radius and ulna
    M89.731 Major osseous defect, right forearm
    M89.732 Major osseous defect, left forearm
    M89.739 Major osseous defect, unspecified forearm
● M89.74 Major osseous defect, hand
    Major osseous defect of carpus, fingers, metacarpus
    M89.741 Major osseous defect, right hand
    M89.742 Major osseous defect, left hand
    M89.749 Major osseous defect, unspecified hand
● M89.75 Major osseous defect, pelvic region and thigh
    Major osseous defect of femur and pelvis
    M89.751 Major osseous defect, right pelvic region and thigh
    M89.752 Major osseous defect, left pelvic region and thigh
    M89.759 Major osseous defect, unspecified pelvic region and thigh
● M89.76 Major osseous defect, lower leg
    Major osseous defect of fibula and tibia
    M89.761 Major osseous defect, right lower leg
    M89.762 Major osseous defect, left lower leg
    M89.769 Major osseous defect, unspecified lower leg
● M89.77 Major osseous defect, ankle and foot
    Major osseous defect of metatarsus, tarsus, toes
    M89.771 Major osseous defect, right ankle and foot
    M89.772 Major osseous defect, left ankle and foot
    M89.779 Major osseous defect, unspecified ankle and foot
  M89.78 Major osseous defect, other site
  M89.79 Major osseous defect, multiple sites

● M89.8 Other specified disorders of bone
    Infantile cortical hyperostoses
    Post-traumatic subperiosteal ossification
  ● M89.8X Other specified disorders of bone
    M89.8X0 Other specified disorders of bone, multiple sites
    M89.8X1 Other specified disorders of bone, shoulder
    M89.8X2 Other specified disorders of bone, upper arm
    M89.8X3 Other specified disorders of bone, forearm
    M89.8X4 Other specified disorders of bone, hand
    M89.8X5 Other specified disorders of bone, thigh
    M89.8X6 Other specified disorders of bone, lower leg
    M89.8X7 Other specified disorders of bone, ankle and foot
    M89.8X8 Other specified disorders of bone, other site
    M89.8X9 Other specified disorders of bone, unspecified site
  M89.9 Disorder of bone, unspecified

▶ New   ⇒ Revised   deleted Deleted   **OGCR** Official Guidelines   X Assign placeholder X   ● Use Additional Character(s)

Excludes 1   Excludes 2   Includes   Use additional   Code first   Code also   Key words

● **M90 Osteopathies in diseases classified elsewhere**

Excludes1	osteochondritis, osteomyelitis, and osteopathy (in):

cryptococcosis (B45.3)
diabetes mellitus (E08-E13 with .69-)
gonococcal (A54.43)
neurogenic syphilis (A52.11)
renal osteodystrophy (N25.0)
salmonellosis (A02.24)
secondary syphilis (A51.46)
syphilis (late) (A52.77)

● **M90.5 Osteonecrosis in diseases classified elsewhere**

Code first underlying disease, such as:
caisson disease (T70.3)
hemoglobinopathy (D50-D64)

M90.50 Osteonecrosis in diseases classified elsewhere, unspecified site

● **M90.51 Osteonecrosis in diseases classified elsewhere, shoulder**

M90.511 Osteonecrosis in diseases classified elsewhere, right shoulder

M90.512 Osteonecrosis in diseases classified elsewhere, left shoulder

M90.519 Osteonecrosis in diseases classified elsewhere, unspecified shoulder

● **M90.52 Osteonecrosis in diseases classified elsewhere, upper arm**

M90.521 Osteonecrosis in diseases classified elsewhere, right upper arm

M90.522 Osteonecrosis in diseases classified elsewhere, left upper arm

M90.529 Osteonecrosis in diseases classified elsewhere, unspecified upper arm

● **M90.53 Osteonecrosis in diseases classified elsewhere, forearm**

M90.531 Osteonecrosis in diseases classified elsewhere, right forearm

M90.532 Osteonecrosis in diseases classified elsewhere, left forearm

M90.539 Osteonecrosis in diseases classified elsewhere, unspecified forearm

● **M90.54 Osteonecrosis in diseases classified elsewhere, hand**

M90.541 Osteonecrosis in diseases classified elsewhere, right hand

M90.542 Osteonecrosis in diseases classified elsewhere, left hand

M90.549 Osteonecrosis in diseases classified elsewhere, unspecified hand

● **M90.55 Osteonecrosis in diseases classified elsewhere, thigh**

M90.551 Osteonecrosis in diseases classified elsewhere, right thigh

M90.552 Osteonecrosis in diseases classified elsewhere, left thigh

M90.559 Osteonecrosis in diseases classified elsewhere, unspecified thigh

● **M90.56 Osteonecrosis in diseases classified elsewhere, lower leg**

M90.561 Osteonecrosis in diseases classified elsewhere, right lower leg

M90.562 Osteonecrosis in diseases classified elsewhere, left lower leg

M90.569 Osteonecrosis in diseases classified elsewhere, unspecified lower leg

● **M90.57 Osteonecrosis in diseases classified elsewhere, ankle and foot**

M90.571 Osteonecrosis in diseases classified elsewhere, right ankle and foot

M90.572 Osteonecrosis in diseases classified elsewhere, left ankle and foot

M90.579 Osteonecrosis in diseases classified elsewhere, unspecified ankle and foot

M90.58 Osteonecrosis in diseases classified elsewhere, other site

M90.59 Osteonecrosis in diseases classified elsewhere, multiple sites

● **M90.6 Osteitis deformans in neoplastic diseases**

Osteitis deformans in malignant neoplasm of bone

Code first the neoplasm (C40.-, C41.-)

Excludes1	osteitis deformans [Paget's disease of bone] (M88.-)

M90.60 Osteitis deformans in neoplastic diseases, unspecified site

● **M90.61 Osteitis deformans in neoplastic diseases, shoulder**

M90.611 Osteitis deformans in neoplastic diseases, right shoulder

M90.612 Osteitis deformans in neoplastic diseases, left shoulder

M90.619 Osteitis deformans in neoplastic diseases, unspecified shoulder

● **M90.62 Osteitis deformans in neoplastic diseases, upper arm**

M90.621 Osteitis deformans in neoplastic diseases, right upper arm

M90.622 Osteitis deformans in neoplastic diseases, left upper arm

M90.629 Osteitis deformans in neoplastic diseases, unspecified upper arm

● **M90.63 Osteitis deformans in neoplastic diseases, forearm**

M90.631 Osteitis deformans in neoplastic diseases, right forearm

M90.632 Osteitis deformans in neoplastic diseases, left forearm

M90.639 Osteitis deformans in neoplastic diseases, unspecified forearm

● **M90.64 Osteitis deformans in neoplastic diseases, hand**

M90.641 Osteitis deformans in neoplastic diseases, right hand

M90.642 Osteitis deformans in neoplastic diseases, left hand

M90.649 Osteitis deformans in neoplastic diseases, unspecified hand

● **M90.65 Osteitis deformans in neoplastic diseases, thigh**

M90.651 Osteitis deformans in neoplastic diseases, right thigh

M90.652 Osteitis deformans in neoplastic diseases, left thigh

M90.659 Osteitis deformans in neoplastic diseases, unspecified thigh

● **M90.66 Osteitis deformans in neoplastic diseases, lower leg**

M90.661 Osteitis deformans in neoplastic diseases, right lower leg

M90.662 Osteitis deformans in neoplastic diseases, left lower leg

M90.669 Osteitis deformans in neoplastic diseases, unspecified lower leg

CHAPTER 13 (M00-M99)

● M90.67 Osteitis deformans in neoplastic diseases, ankle and foot

M90.671 Osteitis deformans in neoplastic diseases, right ankle and foot

M90.672 Osteitis deformans in neoplastic diseases, left ankle and foot

M90.679 Osteitis deformans in neoplastic diseases, unspecified ankle and foot

M90.68 Osteitis deformans in neoplastic diseases, other site

M90.69 Osteitis deformans in neoplastic diseases, multiple sites

● M90.8 Osteopathy in diseases classified elsewhere

Code first underlying disease, such as:
rickets (E55.0)
vitamin-D-resistant rickets (E83.3)

M90.80 Osteopathy in diseases classified elsewhere, unspecified site

● M90.81 Osteopathy in diseases classified elsewhere, shoulder

M90.811 Osteopathy in diseases classified elsewhere, right shoulder

M90.812 Osteopathy in diseases classified elsewhere, left shoulder

M90.819 Osteopathy in diseases classified elsewhere, unspecified shoulder

● M90.82 Osteopathy in diseases classified elsewhere, upper arm

M90.821 Osteopathy in diseases classified elsewhere, right upper arm

M90.822 Osteopathy in diseases classified elsewhere, left upper arm

M90.829 Osteopathy in diseases classified elsewhere, unspecified upper arm

● M90.83 Osteopathy in diseases classified elsewhere, forearm

M90.831 Osteopathy in diseases classified elsewhere, right forearm

M90.832 Osteopathy in diseases classified elsewhere, left forearm

M90.839 Osteopathy in diseases classified elsewhere, unspecified forearm

● M90.84 Osteopathy in diseases classified elsewhere, hand

M90.841 Osteopathy in diseases classified elsewhere, right hand

M90.842 Osteopathy in diseases classified elsewhere, left hand

M90.849 Osteopathy in diseases classified elsewhere, unspecified hand

● M90.85 Osteopathy in diseases classified elsewhere, thigh

M90.851 Osteopathy in diseases classified elsewhere, right thigh

M90.852 Osteopathy in diseases classified elsewhere, left thigh

M90.859 Osteopathy in diseases classified elsewhere, unspecified thigh

● M90.86 Osteopathy in diseases classified elsewhere, lower leg

M90.861 Osteopathy in diseases classified elsewhere, right lower leg

M90.862 Osteopathy in diseases classified elsewhere, left lower leg

M90.869 Osteopathy in diseases classified elsewhere, unspecified lower leg

● M90.87 Osteopathy in diseases classified elsewhere, ankle and foot

M90.871 Osteopathy in diseases classified elsewhere, right ankle and foot

M90.872 Osteopathy in diseases classified elsewhere, left ankle and foot

M90.879 Osteopathy in diseases classified elsewhere, unspecified ankle and foot

M90.88 Osteopathy in diseases classified elsewhere, other site

M90.89 Osteopathy in diseases classified elsewhere, multiple sites

CHONDROPATHIES (M91-M94)

Excludes1   postprocedural chondropathies (M96.-)

● M91 Juvenile osteochondrosis of hip and pelvis

Excludes1   slipped upper femoral epiphysis (nontraumatic) (M93.0)

M91.0 Juvenile osteochondrosis of pelvis

Osteochondrosis (juvenile) of acetabulum
Osteochondrosis (juvenile) of iliac crest [Buchanan]
Osteochondrosis (juvenile) of ischiopubic synchondrosis [van Neck]
Osteochondrosis (juvenile) of symphysis pubis [Pierson]

● M91.1 Juvenile osteochondrosis of head of femur [Legg-Calvé-Perthes]

M91.10 Juvenile osteochondrosis of head of femur [Legg-Calvé-Perthes], unspecified leg

M91.11 Juvenile osteochondrosis of head of femur [Legg-Calvé-Perthes], right leg

M91.12 Juvenile osteochondrosis of head of femur [Legg-Calvé-Perthes], left leg

● M91.2 Coxa plana

Hip deformity due to previous juvenile osteochondrosis

M91.20 Coxa plana, unspecified hip

M91.21 Coxa plana, right hip

M91.22 Coxa plana, left hip

● M91.3 Pseudocoxalgia

M91.30 Pseudocoxalgia, unspecified hip

M91.31 Pseudocoxalgia, right hip

M91.32 Pseudocoxalgia, left hip

● M91.4 Coxa magna

M91.40 Coxa magna, unspecified hip

M91.41 Coxa magna, right hip

M91.42 Coxa magna, left hip

● M91.8 Other juvenile osteochondrosis of hip and pelvis

Juvenile osteochondrosis after reduction of congenital dislocation of hip

M91.80 Other juvenile osteochondrosis of hip and pelvis, unspecified leg

M91.81 Other juvenile osteochondrosis of hip and pelvis, right leg

M91.82 Other juvenile osteochondrosis of hip and pelvis, left leg

● M91.9 Juvenile osteochondrosis of hip and pelvis, unspecified

M91.90 Juvenile osteochondrosis of hip and pelvis, unspecified, unspecified leg

M91.91 Juvenile osteochondrosis of hip and pelvis, unspecified, right leg

M91.92 Juvenile osteochondrosis of hip and pelvis, unspecified, left leg

▶ New   ⇒ Revised   ~~deleted~~ Deleted   **OGCR** Official Guidelines   X Assign placeholder X   ● Use Additional Character(s)

Excludes 1   Excludes 2   Includes   Use additional   Code first   Code also   Key words

● **M92 Other juvenile osteochondrosis**
  ● **M92.0 Juvenile osteochondrosis of humerus**
    Osteochondrosis (juvenile) of capitulum of humerus [Panner]
    Osteochondrosis (juvenile) of head of humerus [Haas]
    M92.00 Juvenile osteochondrosis of humerus, unspecified arm
    M92.01 Juvenile osteochondrosis of humerus, right arm
    M92.02 Juvenile osteochondrosis of humerus, left arm
  ● **M92.1 Juvenile osteochondrosis of radius and ulna**
    Osteochondrosis (juvenile) of lower ulna [Burns]
    Osteochondrosis (juvenile) of radial head [Brailsford]
    M92.10 Juvenile osteochondrosis of radius and ulna, unspecified arm
    M92.11 Juvenile osteochondrosis of radius and ulna, right arm
    M92.12 Juvenile osteochondrosis of radius and ulna, left arm
  ● **M92.2 Juvenile osteochondrosis, hand**
    ● **M92.20 Unspecified juvenile osteochondrosis, hand**
      M92.201 Unspecified juvenile osteochondrosis, right hand
      M92.202 Unspecified juvenile osteochondrosis, left hand
      M92.209 Unspecified juvenile osteochondrosis, unspecified hand
    ● **M92.21 Osteochondrosis (juvenile) of carpal lunate [Kienböck]**
      M92.211 Osteochondrosis (juvenile) of carpal lunate [Kienböck], right hand
      M92.212 Osteochondrosis (juvenile) of carpal lunate [Kienböck], left hand
      M92.219 Osteochondrosis (juvenile) of carpal lunate [Kienböck], unspecified hand
    ● **M92.22 Osteochondrosis (juvenile) of metacarpal heads [Mauclaire]**
      M92.221 Osteochondrosis (juvenile) of metacarpal heads [Mauclaire], right hand
      M92.222 Osteochondrosis (juvenile) of metacarpal heads [Mauclaire], left hand
      M92.229 Osteochondrosis (juvenile) of metacarpal heads [Mauclaire], unspecified hand
    ● **M92.29 Other juvenile osteochondrosis, hand**
      M92.291 Other juvenile osteochondrosis, right hand
      M92.292 Other juvenile osteochondrosis, left hand
      M92.299 Other juvenile osteochondrosis, unspecified hand
  ● **M92.3 Other juvenile osteochondrosis, upper limb**
    M92.30 Other juvenile osteochondrosis, unspecified upper limb
    M92.31 Other juvenile osteochondrosis, right upper limb
    M92.32 Other juvenile osteochondrosis, left upper limb
  ● **M92.4 Juvenile osteochondrosis of patella**
    Osteochondrosis (juvenile) of primary patellar center [Köhler]
    Osteochondrosis (juvenile) of secondary patellar center [Sinding Larsen]
    M92.40 Juvenile osteochondrosis of patella, unspecified knee
    M92.41 Juvenile osteochondrosis of patella, right knee
    M92.42 Juvenile osteochondrosis of patella, left knee

● **M92.5 Juvenile osteochondrosis of tibia and fibula**
  Osteochondrosis (juvenile) of proximal tibia [Blount]
  Osteochondrosis (juvenile) of tibial tubercle [Osgood-Schlatter]
  Tibia vara
  M92.50 Juvenile osteochondrosis of tibia and fibula, unspecified leg
  M92.51 Juvenile osteochondrosis of tibia and fibula, right leg
  M92.52 Juvenile osteochondrosis of tibia and fibula, left leg
● **M92.6 Juvenile osteochondrosis of tarsus**
  Osteochondrosis (juvenile) of calcaneum [Sever]
  Osteochondrosis (juvenile) of os tibiale externum [Haglund]
  Osteochondrosis (juvenile) of talus [Diaz]
  Osteochondrosis (juvenile) of tarsal navicular [Köhler]
  M92.60 Juvenile osteochondrosis of tarsus, unspecified ankle
  M92.61 Juvenile osteochondrosis of tarsus, right ankle
  M92.62 Juvenile osteochondrosis of tarsus, left ankle
● **M92.7 Juvenile osteochondrosis of metatarsus**
  Osteochondrosis (juvenile) of fifth metatarsus [Iselin]
  Osteochondrosis (juvenile) of second metatarsus [Freiberg]
  M92.70 Juvenile osteochondrosis of metatarsus, unspecified foot
  M92.71 Juvenile osteochondrosis of metatarsus, right foot
  M92.72 Juvenile osteochondrosis of metatarsus, left foot
  M92.8 Other specified juvenile osteochondrosis
    Calcaneal apophysitis
  M92.9 Juvenile osteochondrosis, unspecified
    Juvenile apophysitis NOS
    Juvenile epiphysitis NOS
    Juvenile osteochondritis NOS
    Juvenile osteochondrosis NOS
● **M93 Other osteochondropathies**
  Excludes2 osteochondrosis of spine (M42.-)
  ● **M93.0 Slipped upper femoral epiphysis (nontraumatic)**
    Use additional code for associated chondrolysis (M94.3)
    ● **M93.00 Unspecified slipped upper femoral epiphysis (nontraumatic)**
      M93.001 Unspecified slipped upper femoral epiphysis (nontraumatic), right hip
      M93.002 Unspecified slipped upper femoral epiphysis (nontraumatic), left hip
      M93.003 Unspecified slipped upper femoral epiphysis (nontraumatic), unspecified hip
    ● **M93.01 Acute slipped upper femoral epiphysis (nontraumatic)**
      M93.011 Acute slipped upper femoral epiphysis (nontraumatic), right hip
      M93.012 Acute slipped upper femoral epiphysis (nontraumatic), left hip
      M93.013 Acute slipped upper femoral epiphysis (nontraumatic), unspecified hip
    ● **M93.02 Chronic slipped upper femoral epiphysis (nontraumatic)**
      M93.021 Chronic slipped upper femoral epiphysis (nontraumatic), right hip
      M93.022 Chronic slipped upper femoral epiphysis (nontraumatic), left hip
      M93.023 Chronic slipped upper femoral epiphysis (nontraumatic), unspecified hip

● M93.Ø3   Acute on chronic slipped upper femoral epiphysis (nontraumatic)

    M93.Ø31   Acute on chronic slipped upper femoral epiphysis (nontraumatic), right hip

    M93.Ø32   Acute on chronic slipped upper femoral epiphysis (nontraumatic), left hip

    M93.Ø33   Acute on chronic slipped upper femoral epiphysis (nontraumatic), unspecified hip

M93.1   Kienböck's disease of adults
    Adult osteochondrosis of carpal lunates

● M93.2   Osteochondritis dissecans

    M93.2Ø   Osteochondritis dissecans of unspecified site

● M93.21   Osteochondritis dissecans of shoulder

    M93.211   Osteochondritis dissecans, right shoulder

    M93.212   Osteochondritis dissecans, left shoulder

    M93.219   Osteochondritis dissecans, unspecified shoulder

● M93.22   Osteochondritis dissecans of elbow

    M93.221   Osteochondritis dissecans, right elbow

    M93.222   Osteochondritis dissecans, left elbow

    M93.229   Osteochondritis dissecans, unspecified elbow

● M93.23   Osteochondritis dissecans of wrist

    M93.231   Osteochondritis dissecans, right wrist

    M93.232   Osteochondritis dissecans, left wrist

    M93.239   Osteochondritis dissecans, unspecified wrist

● M93.24   Osteochondritis dissecans of joints of hand

    M93.241   Osteochondritis dissecans, joints of right hand

    M93.242   Osteochondritis dissecans, joints of left hand

    M93.249   Osteochondritis dissecans, joints of unspecified hand

● M93.25   Osteochondritis dissecans of hip

    M93.251   Osteochondritis dissecans, right hip

    M93.252   Osteochondritis dissecans, left hip

    M93.259   Osteochondritis dissecans, unspecified hip

● M93.26   Osteochondritis dissecans knee

    M93.261   Osteochondritis dissecans, right knee

    M93.262   Osteochondritis dissecans, left knee

    M93.269   Osteochondritis dissecans, unspecified knee

● M93.27   Osteochondritis dissecans of ankle and joints of foot

    M93.271   Osteochondritis dissecans, right ankle and joints of right foot

    M93.272   Osteochondritis dissecans, left ankle and joints of left foot

    M93.279   Osteochondritis dissecans, unspecified ankle and joints of foot

    M93.28   Osteochondritis dissecans other site

    M93.29   Osteochondritis dissecans multiple sites

● M93.8   Other specified osteochondropathies

    M93.8Ø   Other specified osteochondropathies of unspecified site

● M93.81   Other specified osteochondropathies of shoulder

    M93.811   Other specified osteochondropathies, right shoulder

    M93.812   Other specified osteochondropathies, left shoulder

    M93.819   Other specified osteochondropathies, unspecified shoulder

● M93.82   Other specified osteochondropathies of upper arm

    M93.821   Other specified osteochondropathies, right upper arm

    M93.822   Other specified osteochondropathies, left upper arm

    M93.829   Other specified osteochondropathies, unspecified upper arm

● M93.83   Other specified osteochondropathies of forearm

    M93.831   Other specified osteochondropathies, right forearm

    M93.832   Other specified osteochondropathies, left forearm

    M93.839   Other specified osteochondropathies, unspecified forearm

● M93.84   Other specified osteochondropathies of hand

    M93.841   Other specified osteochondropathies, right hand

    M93.842   Other specified osteochondropathies, left hand

    M93.849   Other specified osteochondropathies, unspecified hand

● M93.85   Other specified osteochondropathies of thigh

    M93.851   Other specified osteochondropathies, right thigh

    M93.852   Other specified osteochondropathies, left thigh

    M93.859   Other specified osteochondropathies, unspecified thigh

● M93.86   Other specified osteochondropathies lower leg

    M93.861   Other specified osteochondropathies, right lower leg

    M93.862   Other specified osteochondropathies, left lower leg

    M93.869   Other specified osteochondropathies, unspecified lower leg

● M93.87   Other specified osteochondropathies of ankle and foot

    M93.871   Other specified osteochondropathies, right ankle and foot

    M93.872   Other specified osteochondropathies, left ankle and foot

    M93.879   Other specified osteochondropathies, unspecified ankle and foot

    M93.88   Other specified osteochondropathies other

    M93.89   Other specified osteochondropathies multiple sites

M93.9 Osteochondropathy, unspecified
    Apophysitis NOS
    Epiphysitis NOS
    Osteochondritis NOS
    Osteochondrosis NOS
    M93.90 Osteochondropathy, unspecified of unspecified site
    ● M93.91 Osteochondropathy, unspecified of shoulder
        M93.911 Osteochondropathy, unspecified, right shoulder
        M93.912 Osteochondropathy, unspecified, left shoulder
        M93.919 Osteochondropathy, unspecified, unspecified shoulder
    ● M93.92 Osteochondropathy, unspecified of upper arm
        M93.921 Osteochondropathy, unspecified, right upper arm
        M93.922 Osteochondropathy, unspecified, left upper arm
        M93.929 Osteochondropathy, unspecified, unspecified upper arm
    ● M93.93 Osteochondropathy, unspecified of forearm
        M93.931 Osteochondropathy, unspecified, right forearm
        M93.932 Osteochondropathy, unspecified, left forearm
        M93.939 Osteochondropathy, unspecified, unspecified forearm
    ● M93.94 Osteochondropathy, unspecified of hand
        M93.941 Osteochondropathy, unspecified, right hand
        M93.942 Osteochondropathy, unspecified, left hand
        M93.949 Osteochondropathy, unspecified, unspecified hand
    ● M93.95 Osteochondropathy, unspecified of thigh
        M93.951 Osteochondropathy, unspecified, right thigh
        M93.952 Osteochondropathy, unspecified, left thigh
        M93.959 Osteochondropathy, unspecified, unspecified thigh
    ● M93.96 Osteochondropathy, unspecified lower leg
        M93.961 Osteochondropathy, unspecified, right lower leg
        M93.962 Osteochondropathy, unspecified, left lower leg
        M93.969 Osteochondropathy, unspecified, unspecified lower leg
    ● M93.97 Osteochondropathy, unspecified of ankle and foot
        M93.971 Osteochondropathy, unspecified, right ankle and foot
        M93.972 Osteochondropathy, unspecified, left ankle and foot
        M93.979 Osteochondropathy, unspecified, unspecified ankle and foot
    M93.98 Osteochondropathy, unspecified other
    M93.99 Osteochondropathy, unspecified multiple sites

● M94 Other disorders of cartilage
    M94.0 Chondrocostal junction syndrome [Tietze]
        Costochondritis
    M94.1 Relapsing polychondritis
    ● M94.2 Chondromalacia
        Excludes1 chondromalacia patellae (M22.4)
        M94.20 Chondromalacia, unspecified site
        ● M94.21 Chondromalacia, shoulder
            M94.211 Chondromalacia, right shoulder
            M94.212 Chondromalacia, left shoulder
            M94.219 Chondromalacia, unspecified shoulder
        ● M94.22 Chondromalacia, elbow
            M94.221 Chondromalacia, right elbow
            M94.222 Chondromalacia, left elbow
            M94.229 Chondromalacia, unspecified elbow
        ● M94.23 Chondromalacia, wrist
            M94.231 Chondromalacia, right wrist
            M94.232 Chondromalacia, left wrist
            M94.239 Chondromalacia, unspecified wrist
        ● M94.24 Chondromalacia, joints of hand
            M94.241 Chondromalacia, joints of right hand
            M94.242 Chondromalacia, joints of left hand
            M94.249 Chondromalacia, joints of unspecified hand
        ● M94.25 Chondromalacia, hip
            M94.251 Chondromalacia, right hip
            M94.252 Chondromalacia, left hip
            M94.259 Chondromalacia, unspecified hip
        ● M94.26 Chondromalacia, knee
            M94.261 Chondromalacia, right knee
            M94.262 Chondromalacia, left knee
            M94.269 Chondromalacia, unspecified knee
        ● M94.27 Chondromalacia, ankle and joints of foot
            M94.271 Chondromalacia, right ankle and joints of right foot
            M94.272 Chondromalacia, left ankle and joints of left foot
            M94.279 Chondromalacia, unspecified ankle and joints of foot
        M94.28 Chondromalacia, other site
        M94.29 Chondromalacia, multiple sites
    ● M94.3 Chondrolysis
        Code first any associated slipped upper femoral epiphysis (nontraumatic) (M93.0-)
        ● M94.35 Chondrolysis, hip
            M94.351 Chondrolysis, right hip
            M94.352 Chondrolysis, left hip
            M94.359 Chondrolysis, unspecified hip

● M94.8 Other specified disorders of cartilage
 ● M94.8X Other specified disorders of cartilage
  M94.8X0 Other specified disorders of cartilage, multiple sites
  M94.8X1 Other specified disorders of cartilage, shoulder
  M94.8X2 Other specified disorders of cartilage, upper arm
  M94.8X3 Other specified disorders of cartilage, forearm
  M94.8X4 Other specified disorders of cartilage, hand
  M94.8X5 Other specified disorders of cartilage, thigh
  M94.8X6 Other specified disorders of cartilage, lower leg
  M94.8X7 Other specified disorders of cartilage, ankle and foot
  M94.8X8 Other specified disorders of cartilage, other site
  M94.8X9 Other specified disorders of cartilage, unspecified sites
 M94.9 Disorder of cartilage, unspecified

OTHER DISORDERS OF THE MUSCULOSKELETAL SYSTEM AND CONNECTIVE TISSUE (M95)

● M95 Other acquired deformities of musculoskeletal system and connective tissue
 Excludes2 acquired absence of limbs and organs (Z89-Z90)
  acquired deformities of limbs (M20-M21)
  congenital malformations and deformations of the musculoskeletal system (Q65-Q79)
  deforming dorsopathies (M40-M43)
  dentofacial anomalies [including malocclusion] (M26.-)
  postprocedural musculoskeletal disorders (M96.-)
 M95.0 Acquired deformity of nose
  Excludes2 deviated nasal septum (J34.2)
 ● M95.1 Cauliflower ear
  Excludes2 other acquired deformities of ear (H61.1)
  M95.10 Cauliflower ear, unspecified ear
  M95.11 Cauliflower ear, right ear
  M95.12 Cauliflower ear, left ear
 M95.2 Other acquired deformity of head
 M95.3 Acquired deformity of neck
 M95.4 Acquired deformity of chest and rib
 M95.5 Acquired deformity of pelvis
  Excludes1 maternal care for known or suspected disproportion (O33.-)
 M95.8 Other specified acquired deformities of musculoskeletal system
 M95.9 Acquired deformity of musculoskeletal system, unspecified

INTRAOPERATIVE AND POSTPROCEDURAL COMPLICATIONS AND DISORDERS OF MUSCULOSKELETAL SYSTEM, NOT ELSEWHERE CLASSIFIED (M96)

● M96 Intraoperative and postprocedural complications and disorders of musculoskeletal system, not elsewhere classified
 Excludes2 arthropathy following intestinal bypass (M02.0-)
  complications of internal orthopedic prosthetic devices, implants and grafts (T84.-)
  disorders associated with osteoporosis (M80)
  periprosthetic fracture around internal prosthetic joint (M97.-)
  presence of functional implants and other devices (Z96-Z97)
 M96.0 Pseudarthrosis after fusion or arthrodesis
 M96.1 Postlaminectomy syndrome, not elsewhere classified
 M96.2 Postradiation kyphosis
 M96.3 Postlaminectomy kyphosis
 M96.4 Postsurgical lordosis
 M96.5 Postradiation scoliosis
 ● M96.6 Fracture of bone following insertion of orthopedic implant, joint prosthesis, or bone plate
  Intraoperative fracture of bone during insertion of orthopedic implant, joint prosthesis, or bone plate
  Excludes2 complication of internal orthopedic devices, implants or grafts (T84.-)
 ● M96.62 Fracture of humerus following insertion of orthopedic implant, joint prosthesis, or bone plate
  M96.621 Fracture of humerus following insertion of orthopedic implant, joint prosthesis, or bone plate, right arm
  M96.622 Fracture of humerus following insertion of orthopedic implant, joint prosthesis, or bone plate, left arm
  M96.629 Fracture of humerus following insertion of orthopedic implant, joint prosthesis, or bone plate, unspecified arm
 ● M96.63 Fracture of radius or ulna following insertion of orthopedic implant, joint prosthesis, or bone plate
  M96.631 Fracture of radius or ulna following insertion of orthopedic implant, joint prosthesis, or bone plate, right arm
  M96.632 Fracture of radius or ulna following insertion of orthopedic implant, joint prosthesis, or bone plate, left arm
  M96.639 Fracture of radius or ulna following insertion of orthopedic implant, joint prosthesis, or bone plate, unspecified arm
 M96.65 Fracture of pelvis following insertion of orthopedic implant, joint prosthesis, or bone plate

● **M96.66** Fracture of femur following insertion of orthopedic implant, joint prosthesis, or bone plate

　　M96.661 Fracture of femur following insertion of orthopedic implant, joint prosthesis, or bone plate, right leg

　　M96.662 Fracture of femur following insertion of orthopedic implant, joint prosthesis, or bone plate, left leg

　　M96.669 Fracture of femur following insertion of orthopedic implant, joint prosthesis, or bone plate, unspecified leg

● **M96.67** Fracture of tibia or fibula following insertion of orthopedic implant, joint prosthesis, or bone plate

　　M96.671 Fracture of tibia or fibula following insertion of orthopedic implant, joint prosthesis, or bone plate, right leg

　　M96.672 Fracture of tibia or fibula following insertion of orthopedic implant, joint prosthesis, or bone plate, left leg

　　M96.679 Fracture of tibia or fibula following insertion of orthopedic implant, joint prosthesis, or bone plate, unspecified leg

　　M96.69 Fracture of other bone following insertion of orthopedic implant, joint prosthesis, or bone plate

● **M96.8** Other intraoperative and postprocedural complications and disorders of musculoskeletal system, not elsewhere classified

● **M96.81** Intraoperative hemorrhage and hematoma of a musculoskeletal structure complicating a procedure

　　　Excludes1 intraoperative hemorrhage and hematoma of a musculoskeletal structure due to accidental puncture and laceration during a procedure (M96.82-)

　　M96.810 Intraoperative hemorrhage and hematoma of a musculoskeletal structure complicating a musculoskeletal system procedure

　　M96.811 Intraoperative hemorrhage and hematoma of a musculoskeletal structure complicating other procedure

● **M96.82** Accidental puncture and laceration of a musculoskeletal structure during a procedure

　　M96.820 Accidental puncture and laceration of a musculoskeletal structure during a musculoskeletal system procedure

　　M96.821 Accidental puncture and laceration of a musculoskeletal structure during other procedure

● **M96.83** Postprocedural hemorrhage of a musculoskeletal structure following a procedure

　　M96.830 Postprocedural hemorrhage of a musculoskeletal structure following a musculoskeletal system procedure

　　M96.831 Postprocedural hemorrhage of a musculoskeletal structure following other procedure

● **M96.84** Postprocedural hematoma and seroma of a musculoskeletal structure following a procedure

　　M96.840 Postprocedural hematoma of a musculoskeletal structure following a musculoskeletal system procedure

　　M96.841 Postprocedural hematoma of a musculoskeletal structure following other procedure

　　M96.842 Postprocedural seroma of a musculoskeletal structure following a musculoskeletal system procedure

　　M96.843 Postprocedural seroma of a musculoskeletal structure following other procedure

　　M96.89 Other intraoperative and postprocedural complications and disorders of the musculoskeletal system

　　　Instability of joint secondary to removal of joint prosthesis

　　　Use additional code, if applicable, to further specify disorder

---

PERIPROSTHETIC FRACTURE AROUND INTERNAL PROSTHETIC JOINT (M97)

● **M97** Periprosthetic fracture around internal prosthetic joint

　　Excludes2 fracture of bone following insertion of orthopedic implant, joint prosthesis or bone plate (M96.6-)

　　　breakage (fracture) of prosthetic joint (T84.01-)

The appropriate 7th character is to be added to each code from category M97:

A	initial encounter
D	subsequent encounter
S	sequela

● **M97.0** Periprosthetic fracture around internal prosthetic hip joint

　X ● **M97.01** Periprosthetic fracture around internal prosthetic right hip joint

　X ● **M97.02** Periprosthetic fracture around internal prosthetic left hip joint

● **M97.1** Periprosthetic fracture around internal prosthetic knee joint

　X ● **M97.11** Periprosthetic fracture around internal prosthetic right knee joint

　X ● **M97.12** Periprosthetic fracture around internal prosthetic left knee joint

● **M97.2** Periprosthetic fracture around internal prosthetic ankle joint

　X ● **M97.21** Periprosthetic fracture around internal prosthetic right ankle joint

　X ● **M97.22** Periprosthetic fracture around internal prosthetic left ankle joint

● **M97.3** Periprosthetic fracture around internal prosthetic shoulder joint

　X ● **M97.31** Periprosthetic fracture around internal prosthetic right shoulder joint

　X ● **M97.32** Periprosthetic fracture around internal prosthetic left shoulder joint

● **M97.4** Periprosthetic fracture around internal prosthetic elbow joint

　X ● **M97.41** Periprosthetic fracture around internal prosthetic right elbow joint

　X ● **M97.42** Periprosthetic fracture around internal prosthetic left elbow joint

CHAPTER 13 (M00-M99)

X ● **M97.8** **Periprosthetic fracture around** other **internal prosthetic joint**

    Periprosthetic fracture around internal prosthetic finger joint

    Periprosthetic fracture around internal prosthetic spinal joint

    Periprosthetic fracture around internal prosthetic toe joint

    Periprosthetic fracture around internal prosthetic wrist joint

    Use additional code to identify the joint (Z96.6-)

X ● **M97.9** **Periprosthetic fracture around** unspecified **internal prosthetic joint**

BIOMECHANICAL LESIONS, NOT ELSEWHERE CLASSIFIED (M99)

● **M99** **Biomechanical lesions, not elsewhere classified**

    Note: This category should not be used if the condition can be classified elsewhere.

● **M99.0** **Segmental and somatic dysfunction**

    M99.00 Segmental and somatic dysfunction of head region

    M99.01 Segmental and somatic dysfunction of cervical region

    M99.02 Segmental and somatic dysfunction of thoracic region

    M99.03 Segmental and somatic dysfunction of lumbar region

    M99.04 Segmental and somatic dysfunction of sacral region

    M99.05 Segmental and somatic dysfunction of pelvic region

    M99.06 Segmental and somatic dysfunction of lower extremity

    M99.07 Segmental and somatic dysfunction of upper extremity

    M99.08 Segmental and somatic dysfunction of rib cage

    M99.09 Segmental and somatic dysfunction of abdomen and other regions

● **M99.1** **Subluxation complex (vertebral)**

    M99.10 Subluxation complex (vertebral) of head region

    M99.11 Subluxation complex (vertebral) of cervical region

    M99.12 Subluxation complex (vertebral) of thoracic region

    M99.13 Subluxation complex (vertebral) of lumbar region

    M99.14 Subluxation complex (vertebral) of sacral region

    M99.15 Subluxation complex (vertebral) of pelvic region

    M99.16 Subluxation complex (vertebral) of lower extremity

    M99.17 Subluxation complex (vertebral) of upper extremity

    M99.18 Subluxation complex (vertebral) of rib cage

    M99.19 Subluxation complex (vertebral) of abdomen and other regions

● **M99.2** **Subluxation stenosis of neural canal**

    M99.20 Subluxation stenosis of neural canal of head region

    M99.21 Subluxation stenosis of neural canal of cervical region

    M99.22 Subluxation stenosis of neural canal of thoracic region

    M99.23 Subluxation stenosis of neural canal of lumbar region

    M99.24 Subluxation stenosis of neural canal of sacral region

    M99.25 Subluxation stenosis of neural canal of pelvic region

    M99.26 Subluxation stenosis of neural canal of lower extremity

    M99.27 Subluxation stenosis of neural canal of upper extremity

    M99.28 Subluxation stenosis of neural canal of rib cage

    M99.29 Subluxation stenosis of neural canal of abdomen and other regions

● **M99.3** **Osseous stenosis of neural canal**

    M99.30 Osseous stenosis of neural canal of head region

    M99.31 Osseous stenosis of neural canal of cervical region

    M99.32 Osseous stenosis of neural canal of thoracic region

    M99.33 Osseous stenosis of neural canal of lumbar region

    M99.34 Osseous stenosis of neural canal of sacral region

    M99.35 Osseous stenosis of neural canal of pelvic region

    M99.36 Osseous stenosis of neural canal of lower extremity

    M99.37 Osseous stenosis of neural canal of upper extremity

    M99.38 Osseous stenosis of neural canal of rib cage

    M99.39 Osseous stenosis of neural canal of abdomen and other regions

● **M99.4** **Connective tissue stenosis of neural canal**

    M99.40 Connective tissue stenosis of neural canal of head region

    M99.41 Connective tissue stenosis of neural canal of cervical region

    M99.42 Connective tissue stenosis of neural canal of thoracic region

    M99.43 Connective tissue stenosis of neural canal of lumbar region

    M99.44 Connective tissue stenosis of neural canal of sacral region

    M99.45 Connective tissue stenosis of neural canal of pelvic region

    M99.46 Connective tissue stenosis of neural canal of lower extremity

    M99.47 Connective tissue stenosis of neural canal of upper extremity

    M99.48 Connective tissue stenosis of neural canal of rib cage

    M99.49 Connective tissue stenosis of neural canal of abdomen and other regions

► New   ⇒ Revised   ~~deleted~~ Deleted   **OGCR** Official Guidelines   X Assign placeholder X   ● Use Additional Character(s)

Excludes 1   Excludes 2   Includes   Use additional   Code first   Code also   Key words

● **M99.5   Intervertebral disc stenosis of neural canal**

     M99.50   Intervertebral disc stenosis of neural canal of head region

     M99.51   Intervertebral disc stenosis of neural canal of cervical region

     M99.52   Intervertebral disc stenosis of neural canal of thoracic region

     M99.53   Intervertebral disc stenosis of neural canal of lumbar region

     M99.54   Intervertebral disc stenosis of neural canal of sacral region

     M99.55   Intervertebral disc stenosis of neural canal of pelvic region

     M99.56   Intervertebral disc stenosis of neural canal of lower extremity

     M99.57   Intervertebral disc stenosis of neural canal of upper extremity

     M99.58   Intervertebral disc stenosis of neural canal of rib cage

     M99.59   Intervertebral disc stenosis of neural canal of abdomen and other regions

● **M99.6   Osseous and subluxation stenosis of intervertebral foramina**

     M99.60   Osseous and subluxation stenosis of intervertebral foramina of head region

     M99.61   Osseous and subluxation stenosis of intervertebral foramina of cervical region

     M99.62   Osseous and subluxation stenosis of intervertebral foramina of thoracic region

     M99.63   Osseous and subluxation stenosis of intervertebral foramina of lumbar region

     M99.64   Osseous and subluxation stenosis of intervertebral foramina of sacral region

     M99.65   Osseous and subluxation stenosis of intervertebral foramina of pelvic region

     M99.66   Osseous and subluxation stenosis of intervertebral foramina of lower extremity

     M99.67   Osseous and subluxation stenosis of intervertebral foramina of upper extremity

     M99.68   Osseous and subluxation stenosis of intervertebral foramina of rib cage

     M99.69   Osseous and subluxation stenosis of intervertebral foramina of abdomen and other regions

● **M99.7   Connective tissue and disc stenosis of intervertebral foramina**

     M99.70   Connective tissue and disc stenosis of intervertebral foramina of head region

     M99.71   Connective tissue and disc stenosis of intervertebral foramina of cervical region

     M99.72   Connective tissue and disc stenosis of intervertebral foramina of thoracic region

     M99.73   Connective tissue and disc stenosis of intervertebral foramina of lumbar region

     M99.74   Connective tissue and disc stenosis of intervertebral foramina of sacral region

     M99.75   Connective tissue and disc stenosis of intervertebral foramina of pelvic region

     M99.76   Connective tissue and disc stenosis of intervertebral foramina of lower extremity

     M99.77   Connective tissue and disc stenosis of intervertebral foramina of upper extremity

     M99.78   Connective tissue and disc stenosis of intervertebral foramina of rib cage

     M99.79   Connective tissue and disc stenosis of intervertebral foramina of abdomen and other regions

● **M99.8   Other biomechanical lesions**

     M99.80   Other biomechanical lesions of head region

     M99.81   Other biomechanical lesions of cervical region

     M99.82   Other biomechanical lesions of thoracic region

     M99.83   Other biomechanical lesions of lumbar region

     M99.84   Other biomechanical lesions of sacral region

     M99.85   Other biomechanical lesions of pelvic region

     M99.86   Other biomechanical lesions of lower extremity

     M99.87   Other biomechanical lesions of upper extremity

     M99.88   Other biomechanical lesions of rib cage

     M99.89   Other biomechanical lesions of abdomen and other regions

     M99.9   Biomechanical lesion, unspecified

CHAPTER 13 (M00-M99)

CHAPTER 14

DISEASES OF THE GENITOURINARY SYSTEM (N00-N99)

OGCR Chapter-Specific Coding Guidelines

> 14. **Chapter 14: Diseases of Genitourinary System (N00-N99)**
>
>   **a. Chronic kidney disease**
>
>   **1) Stages of chronic kidney disease (CKD)**
> The ICD-10-CM classifies CKD based on severity. The severity of CKD is designated by stages 1-5. Stage 2, code N18.2, equates to mild CKD; stage 3, code N18.3, equates to moderate CKD; and stage 4, code N18.4, equates to severe CKD. Code N18.6, End stage renal disease (ESRD), is assigned when the provider has documented end-stage-renal disease (ESRD).
>
>   If both a stage of CKD and ESRD are documented, assign code N18.6 only.
>
>   **2) Chronic kidney disease and kidney transplant status**
> Patients who have undergone kidney transplant may still have some form of chronic kidney disease CKD because the kidney transplant may not fully restore kidney function. Therefore, the presence of CKD alone does not constitute a transplant complication. Assign the appropriate N18 code for the patient's stage of CKD and code Z94.0, Kidney transplant status. If a transplant complication such as failure or rejection or other transplant complication is documented, see section I.C.19.g for information on coding complications of a kidney transplant. If the documentation is unclear as to whether the patient has a complication of the transplant, query the provider.
>
>   **3) Chronic kidney disease with other conditions**
> Patients with CKD may also suffer from other serious conditions, most commonly diabetes mellitus and hypertension. The sequencing of the CKD code in relationship to codes for other contributing conditions is based on the conventions in the Tabular List.
>   *See I.C.9. Hypertensive chronic kidney disease.*
>   *See I.C.19. Chronic kidney disease and kidney transplant complications.*

Item 14–1 Nephritis (inflammation) or **nephropathy** (disease) **with lesion of proliferative glomerulonephritis** results from a streptococcal infection.

   Nephritis (inflammation) or **nephropathy** (disease) **with lesion of membranous glomerulonephritis** is characterized by deposits along the epithelial side of the basement membrane.

   Nephritis (inflammation) or **nephropathy** (disease) **with lesion of membranoproliferative glomerulonephritis** is characterized by alterations in the basement membranes of the kidney and the glomerular cells.

   Nephritis (inflammation) or **nephropathy** (disease) **with lesion of rapidly progressive glomerulonephritis** is characterized by rapid and progressive decline in renal function.

   Nephritis (inflammation) or **nephropathy** (disease) **with lesion of renal cortical necrosis** is characterized by death of the cortical tissues.

   Nephritis (inflammation) or **nephropathy** (disease) **with lesion of renal medullary necrosis** is characterized by death of the tissues that collect urine.

Figure 14-1   Kidneys within the urinary system.

Item 14–2 Glomerulonephritis is nephritis accompanied by inflammation of the glomeruli of the kidney, resulting in the degeneration of the glomeruli and the nephrons.

   Acute glomerulonephritis primarily affects children and young adults and is usually a result of a streptococcal infection.

   Proliferative glomerulonephritis is the acute form of the disease resulting from a streptococcal infection.

   Rapidly progressive glomerulonephritis, also known as **crescentic** or **malignant glomerulonephritis,** is the acute form of the disease, which leads quickly to rapid and progressive decline in renal function.

CHAPTER 14

DISEASES OF THE GENITOURINARY SYSTEM (N00-N99)

Excludes2	certain conditions originating in the perinatal period (P04-P96)
	certain infectious and parasitic diseases (A00-B99)
	complications of pregnancy, childbirth and the puerperium (O00-O9A)
	congenital malformations, deformations and chromosomal abnormalities (Q00-Q99)
	endocrine, nutritional and metabolic diseases (E00-E88)
	injury, poisoning and certain other consequences of external causes (S00-T88)
	neoplasms (C00-D49)
	symptoms, signs and abnormal clinical and laboratory findings, not elsewhere classified (R00-R94)

This chapter contains the following blocks:

N00-N08	Glomerular diseases
N10-N16	Renal tubulo-interstitial diseases
N17-N19	Acute kidney failure and chronic kidney disease
N20-N23	Urolithiasis
N25-N29	Other disorders of kidney and ureter
N30-N39	Other diseases of the urinary system
N40-N53	Diseases of male genital organs
N60-N65	Disorders of breast
N70-N77	Inflammatory diseases of female pelvic organs
N80-N98	Noninflammatory disorders of female genital tract
N99	Intraoperative and postprocedural complications and disorders of genitourinary system, not elsewhere classified

GLOMERULAR DISEASES (N00-N08)

Code also any associated kidney failure (N17-N19)

Excludes1	hypertensive chronic kidney disease (I12.-)

● **N00   Acute nephritic syndrome**

Includes	acute glomerular disease
	acute glomerulonephritis
	acute nephritis

Excludes1	acute tubulo-interstitial nephritis (N10)
	nephritic syndrome NOS (N05.-)

  N00.0   Acute nephritic syndrome with minor glomerular abnormality
        Acute nephritic syndrome with minimal change lesion

  N00.1   Acute nephritic syndrome with focal and segmental glomerular lesions
        Acute nephritic syndrome with focal and segmental hyalinosis
        Acute nephritic syndrome with focal and segmental sclerosis
        Acute nephritic syndrome with focal glomerulonephritis

▶ New   ⇒ Revised   ~~deleted~~ Deleted   **OGCR** Official Guidelines   X Assign placeholder X   ● Use Additional Character(s)

Excludes 1	Excludes 2	Includes	Use additional	Code first	Code also	Key words

N00.2   **Acute nephritic syndrome with** diffuse membranous glomerulonephritis

N00.3   **Acute nephritic syndrome with** diffuse mesangial proliferative glomerulonephritis

N00.4   **Acute nephritic syndrome with** diffuse endocapillary proliferative glomerulonephritis

N00.5   **Acute nephritic syndrome with** diffuse mesangiocapillary glomerulonephritis
> Acute nephritic syndrome with membranoproliferative glomerulonephritis, types 1 and 3, or NOS

N00.6   **Acute nephritic syndrome with** dense deposit disease
> Acute nephritic syndrome with membranoproliferative glomerulonephritis, type 2

N00.7   **Acute nephritic syndrome with** diffuse crescentic glomerulonephritis
> Acute nephritic syndrome with extracapillary glomerulonephritis

N00.8   **Acute nephritic syndrome with** other morphologic changes
> Acute nephritic syndrome with proliferative glomerulonephritis NOS

N00.9   **Acute nephritic syndrome with** unspecified morphologic changes

● **N01   Rapidly progressive nephritic syndrome**
> **Includes**   rapidly progressive glomerular disease
> rapidly progressive glomerulonephritis
> rapidly progressive nephritis
>
> **Excludes1**   nephritic syndrome NOS (N05.-)

N01.0   **Rapidly progressive nephritic syndrome with** minor glomerular abnormality
> Rapidly progressive nephritic syndrome with minimal change lesion

N01.1   **Rapidly progressive nephritic syndrome with** focal and segmental glomerular lesions
> Rapidly progressive nephritic syndrome with focal and segmental hyalinosis
> Rapidly progressive nephritic syndrome with focal and segmental sclerosis
> Rapidly progressive nephritic syndrome with focal glomerulonephritis

N01.2   **Rapidly progressive nephritic syndrome with** diffuse membranous glomerulonephritis

N01.3   **Rapidly progressive nephritic syndrome with** diffuse mesangial proliferative glomerulonephritis

N01.4   **Rapidly progressive nephritic syndrome with** diffuse endocapillary proliferative glomerulonephritis

N01.5   **Rapidly progressive nephritic syndrome with** diffuse mesangiocapillary glomerulonephritis
> Rapidly progressive nephritic syndrome with membranoproliferative glomerulonephritis, types 1 and 3, or NOS

N01.6   **Rapidly progressive nephritic syndrome with** dense deposit disease
> Rapidly progressive nephritic syndrome with membranoproliferative glomerulonephritis, type 2

N01.7   **Rapidly progressive nephritic syndrome with** diffuse crescentic glomerulonephritis
> Rapidly progressive nephritic syndrome with extracapillary glomerulonephritis

N01.8   **Rapidly progressive nephritic syndrome with** other morphologic changes
> Rapidly progressive nephritic syndrome with proliferative glomerulonephritis NOS

N01.9   **Rapidly progressive nephritic syndrome with** unspecified morphologic changes

● **N02   Recurrent and persistent hematuria**
> **Excludes1**   acute cystitis with hematuria (N30.01)
> hematuria NOS (R31.9)
> hematuria not associated with specified morphologic lesions (R31.-)

N02.0   **Recurrent and persistent hematuria with** minor glomerular abnormality
> Recurrent and persistent hematuria with minimal change lesion

N02.1   **Recurrent and persistent hematuria with** focal and segmental glomerular lesions
> Recurrent and persistent hematuria with focal and segmental hyalinosis
> Recurrent and persistent hematuria with focal and segmental sclerosis
> Recurrent and persistent hematuria with focal glomerulonephritis

N02.2   **Recurrent and persistent hematuria with** diffuse membranous glomerulonephritis

N02.3   **Recurrent and persistent hematuria with** diffuse mesangial proliferative glomerulonephritis

N02.4   **Recurrent and persistent hematuria with** diffuse endocapillary proliferative glomerulonephritis

N02.5   **Recurrent and persistent hematuria with** diffuse mesangiocapillary glomerulonephritis
> Recurrent and persistent hematuria with membranoproliferative glomerulonephritis, types 1 and 3, or NOS

N02.6   **Recurrent and persistent hematuria with** dense deposit disease
> Recurrent and persistent hematuria with membranoproliferative glomerulonephritis, type 2

N02.7   **Recurrent and persistent hematuria with** diffuse crescentic glomerulonephritis
> Recurrent and persistent hematuria with extracapillary glomerulonephritis

N02.8   **Recurrent and persistent hematuria with** other morphologic changes
> Recurrent and persistent hematuria with proliferative glomerulonephritis NOS

N02.9   **Recurrent and persistent hematuria with** unspecified morphologic changes

● **N03   Chronic nephritic syndrome**
> **Includes**   chronic glomerular disease
> chronic glomerulonephritis
> chronic nephritis
>
> **Excludes1**   chronic tubulo-interstitial nephritis (N11.-)
> diffuse sclerosing glomerulonephritis (N05.8-)
> nephritic syndrome NOS (N05.-)

N03.0   **Chronic nephritic syndrome with** minor glomerular abnormality
> Chronic nephritic syndrome with minimal change lesion

N03.1   **Chronic nephritic syndrome with** focal and segmental glomerular lesions
> Chronic nephritic syndrome with focal and segmental hyalinosis
> Chronic nephritic syndrome with focal and segmental sclerosis
> Chronic nephritic syndrome with focal glomerulonephritis

N03.2   **Chronic nephritic syndrome with** diffuse membranous glomerulonephritis

N03.3   **Chronic nephritic syndrome with** diffuse mesangial proliferative glomerulonephritis

Item 14–3 Chronic glomerulonephritis (GN) persists over a period of years, with remissions and exacerbation.

Chronic GN with lesion of proliferative glomerulonephritis results from a streptococcal infection.

Chronic GN with lesion of membranous glomerulonephritis, also known as membranous nephropathy, is characterized by deposits along the epithelial side of the basement membrane.

Chronic GN with lesion of membrano-proliferative glomerulonephritis (MPGN) is a group of disorders characterized by alterations in the basement membranes of the kidney and the glomerular cells.

Chronic GN with lesion of rapidly progressive glomerulonephritis is characterized by necrosis, endothelial proliferation, and mesangial proliferation. The condition is marked by rapid and progressive decline in renal function.

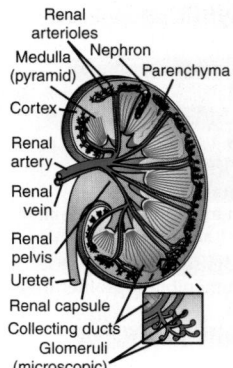

Figure 14-2 Kidney cross section.

N03.4   **Chronic nephritic syndrome with diffuse endocapillary proliferative glomerulonephritis**

N03.5   **Chronic nephritic syndrome with diffuse mesangiocapillary glomerulonephritis**
     Chronic nephritic syndrome with membranoproliferative glomerulonephritis, types 1 and 3, or NOS

N03.6   **Chronic nephritic syndrome with dense deposit disease**
     Chronic nephritic syndrome with membranoproliferative glomerulonephritis, type 2

N03.7   **Chronic nephritic syndrome with diffuse crescentic glomerulonephritis**
     Chronic nephritic syndrome with extracapillary glomerulonephritis

N03.8   **Chronic nephritic syndrome with other morphologic changes**
     Chronic nephritic syndrome with proliferative glomerulonephritis NOS

N03.9   **Chronic nephritic syndrome with unspecified morphologic changes**

● **N04**   **Nephrotic syndrome**
    Includes   congenital nephrotic syndrome
                   lipoid nephrosis

N04.0   **Nephrotic syndrome with minor glomerular abnormality**
     Nephrotic syndrome with minimal change lesion

N04.1   **Nephrotic syndrome with focal and segmental glomerular lesions**
     Nephrotic syndrome with focal and segmental hyalinosis
     Nephrotic syndrome with focal and segmental sclerosis
     Nephrotic syndrome with focal glomerulonephritis

N04.2   **Nephrotic syndrome with diffuse membranous glomerulonephritis**

N04.3   **Nephrotic syndrome with diffuse mesangial proliferative glomerulonephritis**

N04.4   **Nephrotic syndrome with diffuse endocapillary proliferative glomerulonephritis**

N04.5   **Nephrotic syndrome with diffuse mesangiocapillary glomerulonephritis**
     Nephrotic syndrome with membranoproliferative glomerulonephritis, types 1 and 3, or NOS

N04.6   **Nephrotic syndrome with dense deposit disease**
     Nephrotic syndrome with membranoproliferative glomerulonephritis, type 2

N04.7   **Nephrotic syndrome with diffuse crescentic glomerulonephritis**
     Nephrotic syndrome with extracapillary glomerulonephritis

N04.8   **Nephrotic syndrome with other morphologic changes**
     Nephrotic syndrome with proliferative glomerulonephritis NOS

N04.9   **Nephrotic syndrome with unspecified morphologic changes**

Item 14–4 Nephrotic syndrome (NS) is marked by massive proteinuria (protein in the urine) and water retention. Patients with NS are particularly vulnerable to staphylococcal and pneumococcal infections. NS with lesion of proliferative glomerulonephritis results from a streptococcal infection. NS with lesion of membranous glomerulonephritis results in thickening of the capillary walls. NS with lesion of minimal change glomerulonephritis is usually a benign disorder that occurs mostly in children and requires electron microscopy (biopsy) to verify changes in the glomeruli.

● **N05**   **Unspecified nephritic syndrome**
    Includes   glomerular disease NOS
                   glomerulonephritis NOS
                   nephritis NOS
                   nephropathy NOS and renal disease NOS with morphological lesion specified in .0-.8

    Excludes1   nephropathy NOS with no stated morphological lesion (N28.9)
                   renal disease NOS with no stated morphological lesion (N28.9)
                   tubulo-interstitial nephritis NOS (N12)

N05.0   **Unspecified nephritic syndrome with minor glomerular abnormality**
     Unspecified nephritic syndrome with minimal change lesion

N05.1   **Unspecified nephritic syndrome with focal and segmental glomerular lesions**
     Unspecified nephritic syndrome with focal and segmental hyalinosis
     Unspecified nephritic syndrome with focal and segmental sclerosis
     Unspecified nephritic syndrome with focal glomerulonephritis

N05.2   **Unspecified nephritic syndrome with diffuse membranous glomerulonephritis**

N05.3   **Unspecified nephritic syndrome with diffuse mesangial proliferative glomerulonephritis**

N05.4   **Unspecified nephritic syndrome with diffuse endocapillary proliferative glomerulonephritis**

N05.5   **Unspecified nephritic syndrome with diffuse mesangiocapillary glomerulonephritis**
     Unspecified nephritic syndrome with membranoproliferative glomerulonephritis, types 1 and 3, or NOS

N05.6   **Unspecified nephritic syndrome with dense deposit disease**
     Unspecified nephritic syndrome with membranoproliferative glomerulonephritis, type 2

N05.7   **Unspecified nephritic syndrome with diffuse crescentic glomerulonephritis**
     Unspecified nephritic syndrome with extracapillary glomerulonephritis

N05.8   **Unspecified nephritic syndrome with other morphologic changes**
     Unspecified nephritic syndrome with proliferative glomerulonephritis NOS

N05.9   **Unspecified nephritic syndrome with unspecified morphologic changes**

CHAPTER 14 (N00-N99)

● **N06**   **Isolated proteinuria with specified morphological lesion**
> **Excludes1**   proteinuria not associated with specific morphologic lesions (R80.0)

N06.0   **Isolated proteinuria with minor glomerular abnormality**
Isolated proteinuria with minimal change lesion

N06.1   **Isolated proteinuria with focal and segmental glomerular lesions**
Isolated proteinuria with focal and segmental hyalinosis
Isolated proteinuria with focal and segmental sclerosis
Isolated proteinuria with focal glomerulonephritis

N06.2   **Isolated proteinuria with diffuse membranous glomerulonephritis**

N06.3   **Isolated proteinuria with diffuse mesangial proliferative glomerulonephritis**

N06.4   **Isolated proteinuria with diffuse endocapillary proliferative glomerulonephritis**

N06.5   **Isolated proteinuria with diffuse mesangiocapillary glomerulonephritis**
Isolated proteinuria with membranoproliferative glomerulonephritis, types 1 and 3, or NOS

N06.6   **Isolated proteinuria with dense deposit disease**
Isolated proteinuria with membranoproliferative glomerulonephritis, type 2

N06.7   **Isolated proteinuria with diffuse crescentic glomerulonephritis**
Isolated proteinuria with extracapillary glomerulonephritis

N06.8   **Isolated proteinuria with other morphologic lesion**
Isolated proteinuria with proliferative glomerulonephritis NOS

N06.9   **Isolated proteinuria with unspecified morphologic lesion**

● **N07**   **Hereditary nephropathy, not elsewhere classified**
> **Excludes2**   Alport's syndrome (Q87.81-)
> hereditary amyloid nephropathy (E85.-)
> nail patella syndrome (Q87.2)
> non-neuropathic heredofamilial amyloidosis (E85.-)

N07.0   **Hereditary nephropathy, not elsewhere classified with minor glomerular abnormality**
Hereditary nephropathy, not elsewhere classified with minimal change lesion

N07.1   **Hereditary nephropathy, not elsewhere classified with focal and segmental glomerular lesions**
Hereditary nephropathy, not elsewhere classified with focal and segmental hyalinosis
Hereditary nephropathy, not elsewhere classified with focal and segmental sclerosis
Hereditary nephropathy, not elsewhere classified with focal glomerulonephritis

N07.2   **Hereditary nephropathy, not elsewhere classified with diffuse membranous glomerulonephritis**

N07.3   **Hereditary nephropathy, not elsewhere classified with diffuse mesangial proliferative glomerulonephritis**

N07.4   **Hereditary nephropathy, not elsewhere classified with diffuse endocapillary proliferative glomerulonephritis**

N07.5   **Hereditary nephropathy, not elsewhere classified with diffuse mesangiocapillary glomerulonephritis**
Hereditary nephropathy, not elsewhere classified with membranoproliferative glomerulonephritis, types 1 and 3, or NOS

N07.6   **Hereditary nephropathy, not elsewhere classified with dense deposit disease**
Hereditary nephropathy, not elsewhere classified with membranoproliferative glomerulonephritis, type 2

N07.7   **Hereditary nephropathy, not elsewhere classified with diffuse crescentic glomerulonephritis**
Hereditary nephropathy, not elsewhere classified with extracapillary glomerulonephritis

N07.8   **Hereditary nephropathy, not elsewhere classified with other morphologic lesions**
Hereditary nephropathy, not elsewhere classified with proliferative glomerulonephritis NOS

N07.9   **Hereditary nephropathy, not elsewhere classified with unspecified morphologic lesions**

N08   **Glomerular disorders in diseases classified elsewhere**
Glomerulonephritis
Nephritis
Nephropathy
Code first underlying disease, such as:
   amyloidosis (E85.-)
   congenital syphilis (A50.5)
   cryoglobulinemia (D89.1)
   disseminated intravascular coagulation (D65)
   gout (M1A.-, M10.-)
   microscopic polyangiitis (M31.7)
   multiple myeloma (C90.0-)
   sepsis (A40.0-A41.9)
   sickle-cell disease (D57.0-D57.8)
> **Excludes1**   glomerulonephritis, nephritis and nephropathy (in):
> antiglomerular basement membrane disease (M31.0)
> diabetes (E08-E13 with .21)
> gonococcal (A54.21)
> Goodpasture's syndrome (M31.0)
> hemolytic-uremic syndrome (D59.3)
> lupus (M32.14)
> mumps (B26.83)
> syphilis (A52.75)
> systemic lupus erythematosus (M32.14)
> Wegener's granulomatosis (M31.31)
> pyelonephritis in diseases classified elsewhere (N16)
> renal tubulo-interstitial disorders classified elsewhere (N16)

RENAL TUBULO-INTERSTITIAL DISEASES (N10-N16)

> **Includes**   pyelonephritis
> **Excludes1**   pyeloureteritis cystica (N28.85)

N10   **Acute pyelonephritis**
Acute infectious interstitial nephritis
Acute pyelitis
Acute tubulo-interstitial nephritis
Hemoglobin nephrosis
Myoglobin nephrosis
Use additional code (B95-B97), to identify infectious agent

● **N11**   **Chronic tubulo-interstitial nephritis**
> **Includes**   chronic infectious interstitial nephritis
> chronic pyelitis
> chronic pyelonephritis

Use additional code (B95-B97), to identify infectious agent

N11.0   **Nonobstructive reflux-associated chronic pyelonephritis**
Pyelonephritis (chronic) associated with (vesicoureteral) reflux
> **Excludes1**   vesicoureteral reflux NOS (N13.70)

N11.1   **Chronic obstructive pyelonephritis**
Pyelonephritis (chronic) associated with anomaly of pelviureteric junction
Pyelonephritis (chronic) associated with anomaly of pyeloureteric junction
Pyelonephritis (chronic) associated with crossing of vessel
Pyelonephritis (chronic) associated with kinking of ureter
Pyelonephritis (chronic) associated with obstruction of ureter
Pyelonephritis (chronic) associated with stricture of pelviureteric junction
Pyelonephritis (chronic) associated with stricture of ureter
> **Excludes1**   calculous pyelonephritis (N20.9)
> obstructive uropathy (N13.-)

N11.8   **Other chronic tubulo-interstitial nephritis**
Nonobstructive chronic pyelonephritis NOS

N11.9   **Chronic tubulo-interstitial nephritis, unspecified**
Chronic interstitial nephritis NOS
Chronic pyelitis NOS
Chronic pyelonephritis NOS

CHAPTER 14 (N00-N99)

Figure 14-3   Acute pyelonephritis. Cortical surface exhibits grayish white areas of inflammation and abscess formation. (From Frazier MS, Drzymkowski JW: Essentials of Human Diseases and Conditions, St. Louis, Saunders/Elsevier, 2009)

Item 14–5 Pyelonephritis is an infection of the kidneys and ureters and may be chronic or acute in one or both kidneys.

N12   Tubulo-interstitial nephritis, not specified as acute or chronic
Interstitial nephritis NOS
Pyelitis NOS
Pyelonephritis NOS
> **Excludes1**   calculous pyelonephritis (N20.9)

● **N13   Obstructive and reflux uropathy**
> **Excludes2**   calculus of kidney and ureter without hydronephrosis (N20.-)
> congenital obstructive defects of renal pelvis and ureter (Q62.0-Q62.3)
> ⇒ hydronephrosis with ureteropelvic junction obstruction (Q62.11)
> obstructive pyelonephritis (N11.1)

N13.0   Hydronephrosis with ureteropelvic junction obstruction
Hydronephrosis due to acquired occlusion of ureteropelvic junction
> **Excludes2**   Hydronephrosis with ureteropelvic junction obstruction due to calculus (N13.2)

N13.1   Hydronephrosis with ureteral stricture, not elsewhere classified
> **Excludes1**   hydronephrosis with ureteral stricture with infection (N13.6)

N13.2   Hydronephrosis with renal and ureteral calculous obstruction
> **Excludes1**   hydronephrosis with renal and ureteral calculous obstruction with infection (N13.6)

● **N13.3   Other and unspecified hydronephrosis**
> **Excludes1**   hydronephrosis with infection (N13.6)

N13.30   Unspecified hydronephrosis

N13.39   Other hydronephrosis

N13.4   Hydroureter
> **Excludes1**   congenital hydroureter (Q62.3-)
> hydroureter with infection (N13.6)
> vesicoureteral-reflux with hydroureter (N13.73-)

N13.5   Crossing vessel and stricture of ureter without hydronephrosis
Kinking and stricture of ureter without hydronephrosis
> **Excludes1**   crossing vessel and stricture of ureter without hydronephrosis with infection (N13.6)

N13.6   Pyonephrosis
Conditions in N13.0-N13.5 with infection
Obstructive uropathy with infection
> Use additional code (B95-B97), to identify infectious agent

● **N13.7   Vesicoureteral-reflux**
> **Excludes1**   reflux-associated pyelonephritis (N11.0)

N13.70   Vesicoureteral-reflux, unspecified
> *Occurs when urine flows from bladder back into ureters*
> Vesicoureteral-reflux NOS

N13.71   Vesicoureteral-reflux without reflux nephropathy

● **N13.72   Vesicoureteral-reflux with reflux nephropathy without hydroureter**

N13.721   Vesicoureteral-reflux with reflux nephropathy without hydroureter, unilateral

N13.722   Vesicoureteral-reflux with reflux nephropathy without hydroureter, bilateral

N13.729   Vesicoureteral-reflux with reflux nephropathy without hydroureter, unspecified

● **N13.73   Vesicoureteral-reflux with reflux nephropathy with hydroureter**

N13.731   Vesicoureteral-reflux with reflux nephropathy with hydroureter, unilateral

N13.732   Vesicoureteral-reflux with reflux nephropathy with hydroureter, bilateral

N13.739   Vesicoureteral-reflux with reflux nephropathy with hydroureter, unspecified

N13.8   Other obstructive and reflux uropathy
Urinary tract obstruction due to specified cause
> *Code first, if applicable, any causal condition first, such as:* enlarged prostate (N40.1)

N13.9   Obstructive and reflux uropathy, unspecified
Urinary tract obstruction NOS

● **N14   Drug- and heavy-metal-induced tubulo-interstitial and tubular conditions**
> *Code first poisoning due to drug or toxin, if applicable (T36-T65 with fifth or sixth character 1-4 or 6)*
> Use additional code for adverse effect, if applicable, to identify drug (T36-T50 with fifth or sixth character 5)

N14.0   Analgesic nephropathy

N14.1   Nephropathy induced by other drugs, medicaments and biological substances

N14.2   Nephropathy induced by unspecified drug, medicament or biological substance

N14.3   Nephropathy induced by heavy metals

N14.4   Toxic nephropathy, not elsewhere classified

● **N15   Other renal tubulo-interstitial diseases**

N15.0   Balkan nephropathy
Balkan endemic nephropathy

N15.1   Renal and perinephric abscess

N15.8   Other specified renal tubulo-interstitial diseases

N15.9   Renal tubulo-interstitial disease, unspecified
Infection of kidney NOS
> **Excludes1**   urinary tract infection NOS (N39.0)

Figure 14-4   Hydronephrosis of the kidney, with marked dilatation of pelvis and calyces and thinning of renal parenchyma. (From Kumar: Robbins and Cotran: Pathologic Basis of Disease, ed 8, Saunders, An Imprint of Elsevier, 2009)

▶ New   ⇒ Revised   ~~deleted~~ Deleted   **OGCR** Official Guidelines   X Assign placeholder X   ● Use Additional Character(s)
Excludes 1   Excludes 2   Includes   Use additional   Code first   Code also   Key words

N16 **Renal tubulo-interstitial disorders in diseases classified elsewhere**
Pyelonephritis
Tubulo-interstitial nephritis
Code first underlying disease, such as:
brucellosis (A23.0-A23.9)
cryoglobulinemia (D89.1)
glycogen storage disease (E74.0)
leukemia (C91-C95)
lymphoma (C81.0-C85.9, C96.0-C96.9)
multiple myeloma (C90.0-)
sepsis (A40.0-A41.9)
Wilson's disease (E83.0)

Excludes1 diphtheritic pyelonephritis and tubulo-interstitial nephritis (A36.84)
pyelonephritis and tubulo-interstitial nephritis in candidiasis (B37.49)
pyelonephritis and tubulo-interstitial nephritis in cystinosis (E72.04)
pyelonephritis and tubulo-interstitial nephritis in salmonella infection (A02.25)
pyelonephritis and tubulo-interstitial nephritis in sarcoidosis (D86.84)
pyelonephritis and tubulo-interstitial nephritis in sicca syndrome [Sjogren's] (M35.04)
pyelonephritis and tubulo-interstitial nephritis in systemic lupus erythematosus (M32.15)
pyelonephritis and tubulo-interstitial nephritis in toxoplasmosis (B58.83)
renal tubular degeneration in diabetes (E08-E13 with .29)
syphilitic pyelonephritis and tubulo-interstitial nephritis (A52.75)

ACUTE KIDNEY FAILURE AND CHRONIC KIDNEY DISEASE (N17-N19)

Excludes2 congenital renal failure (P96.0)
drug- and heavy-metal-induced tubulo-interstitial and tubular conditions (N14.-)
extrarenal uremia (R39.2)
hemolytic-uremic syndrome (D59.3)
hepatorenal syndrome (K76.7)
postpartum hepatorenal syndrome (O90.4)
posttraumatic renal failure (T79.5)
prerenal uremia (R39.2)
renal failure complicating abortion or ectopic or molar pregnancy (O00-O07, O08.4)
renal failure following labor and delivery (O90.4)
renal failure postprocedural (N99.0)

● N17 **Acute kidney failure**
Code also associated underlying condition
Excludes1 posttraumatic renal failure (T79.5)

N17.0 **Acute kidney failure with tubular necrosis**
Acute tubular necrosis
Renal tubular necrosis
Tubular necrosis NOS

N17.1 **Acute kidney failure with acute cortical necrosis**
Acute cortical necrosis
Cortical necrosis NOS
Renal cortical necrosis

N17.2 **Acute kidney failure with medullary necrosis**
Medullary [papillary] necrosis NOS
Acute medullary [papillary] necrosis
Renal medullary [papillary] necrosis

N17.8 **Other acute kidney failure**

N17.9 **Acute kidney failure, unspecified**
Acute kidney injury (nontraumatic)
Excludes2 traumatic kidney injury (S37.0-)

● N18 **Chronic kidney disease (CKD)**
Code first any associated:
diabetic chronic kidney disease (E08.22, E09.22, E10.22, E11.22, E13.22)
hypertensive chronic kidney disease (I12.-, I13.-)
Use additional code to identify kidney transplant status, if applicable, (Z94.0)

N18.1 **Chronic kidney disease, stage 1**

N18.2 **Chronic kidney disease, stage 2 (mild)**

N18.3 **Chronic kidney disease, stage 3 (moderate)**

N18.4 **Chronic kidney disease, stage 4 (severe)**

N18.5 **Chronic kidney disease, stage 5**
Excludes1 chronic kidney disease, stage 5 requiring chronic dialysis (N18.6)

N18.6 **End stage renal disease**
Chronic kidney disease requiring chronic dialysis
Use additional code to identify dialysis status (Z99.2)

N18.9 **Chronic kidney disease, unspecified**
Chronic renal disease
Chronic renal failure NOS
Chronic renal insufficiency
➡Chronic uremia NOS
▶Diffuse sclerosing glomerulonephritis NOS

N19 **Unspecified kidney failure**
Uremia NOS
Excludes1 acute kidney failure (N17.-)
chronic kidney disease (N18.-)
chronic uremia (N18.9)
extrarenal uremia (R39.2)
prerenal uremia (R39.2)
renal insufficiency (acute) (N28.9)
uremia of newborn (P96.0)

UROLITHIASIS (N20-N23)

● N20 **Calculus of kidney and ureter**
Calculous pyelonephritis
Excludes1 nephrocalcinosis (E83.5)
that with hydronephrosis (N13.2)

N20.0 **Calculus of kidney**
Nephrolithiasis NOS   Staghorn calculus
Renal calculus   Stone in kidney
Renal stone

N20.1 **Calculus of ureter**
Ureteric stone

N20.2 **Calculus of kidney with calculus of ureter**

N20.9 **Urinary calculus, unspecified**

Figure 14-5 Multiple urinary calculi.

Multiple calculi

Item 14-6 Decreased blood flow is the usual cause of **acute renal failure** that offers a good prognosis for recovery.
  Chronic renal failure is usually the result of long-standing kidney disease and is a very serious condition that generally results in death.

▶ New   ➡ Revised   ~~deleted~~ Deleted   **OGCR** Official Guidelines   X Assign placeholder X   ● Use Additional Character(s)

Excludes 1 | Excludes 2 | Includes | Use additional | Code first | Code also | Key words

● N21   Calculus of lower urinary tract

   Includes   calculus of lower urinary tract with cystitis and urethritis

   N21.0   Calculus in bladder
   Calculus in diverticulum of bladder
   Urinary bladder stone
   > **Excludes2**   staghorn calculus (N20.0)

   N21.1   Calculus in urethra
   > **Excludes2**   calculus of prostate (N42.0)

   N21.8   Other lower urinary tract calculus

   N21.9   Calculus of lower urinary tract, unspecified
   > **Excludes1**   calculus of urinary tract NOS (N20.9)

N22   Calculus of urinary tract in diseases classified elsewhere

   Code first underlying disease, such as:
   gout (M1A.-, M10.-)
   schistosomiasis (B65.0-B65.9)

N23   Unspecified renal colic

OTHER DISORDERS OF KIDNEY AND URETER (N25-N29)

> **Excludes2**   disorders of kidney and ureter with urolithiasis (N20-N23)

● N25   Disorders resulting from impaired renal tubular function
   > ~~Excludes1~~   ~~metabolic disorders classifiable to E70-E88~~

   N25.0   Renal osteodystrophy
   Azotemic osteodystrophy
   Phosphate-losing tubular disorders
   Renal rickets
   Renal short stature
   ▶ **Excludes2**   metabolic disorders classifiable to E70-E88

   N25.1   Nephrogenic diabetes insipidus
   > **Excludes1**   diabetes insipidus NOS (E23.2)

   ● N25.8   Other disorders resulting from impaired renal tubular function

      N25.81   Secondary hyperparathyroidism of renal origin
      > **Excludes1**   secondary hyperparathyroidism, non-renal (E21.1)
      ▶ **Excludes2**   metabolic disorders classifiable to E70-E88

      N25.89   Other disorders resulting from impaired renal tubular function
      Hypokalemic nephropathy
      Lightwood-Albright syndrome
      Renal tubular acidosis NOS

   N25.9   Disorder resulting from impaired renal tubular function, unspecified

● N26   Unspecified contracted kidney
   > **Excludes1**   contracted kidney due to hypertension (I12.-)
   diffuse sclerosing glomerulonephritis (N05.8.-)
   hypertensive nephrosclerosis (arteriolar) (arteriosclerotic) (I12.-)
   small kidney of unknown cause (N27.-)

   N26.1   Atrophy of kidney (terminal)
   N26.2   Page kidney
   N26.9   Renal sclerosis, unspecified

● N27   Small kidney of unknown cause
   Includes   oligonephronia
   N27.0   Small kidney, unilateral
   N27.1   Small kidney, bilateral
   N27.9   Small kidney, unspecified

● N28   Other disorders of kidney and ureter, not elsewhere classified

   N28.0   Ischemia and infarction of kidney
   Renal artery embolism
   Renal artery obstruction
   Renal artery occlusion
   Renal artery thrombosis
   Renal infarct
   > **Excludes1**   atherosclerosis of renal artery (extrarenal part) (I70.1)
   congenital stenosis of renal artery (Q27.1)
   Goldblatt's kidney (I70.1)

   N28.1   Cyst of kidney, acquired
   ➡ Cyst (multiple) (solitary) of kidney, (acquired)
   > **Excludes1**   cystic kidney disease (congenital) (Q61.-)

   ● N28.8   Other specified disorders of kidney and ureter
   > **Excludes1**   hydroureter (N13.4)
   ureteric stricture with hydronephrosis (N13.1)
   ureteric stricture without hydronephrosis (N13.5)

      N28.81   Hypertrophy of kidney
      N28.82   Megaloureter
      N28.83   Nephroptosis
      N28.84   Pyelitis cystica
      N28.85   Pyeloureteritis cystica
      N28.86   Ureteritis cystica
      N28.89   Other specified disorders of kidney and ureter

   N28.9   Disorder of kidney and ureter, unspecified
   Nephropathy NOS
   Renal disease (acute) NOS
   Renal insufficiency (acute)
   > **Excludes1**   chronic renal insufficiency (N18.9)
   unspecified nephritic syndrome (N05.-)

N29   Other disorders of kidney and ureter in diseases classified elsewhere

   Code first underlying disease, such as:
   amyloidosis (E85.-)
   nephrocalcinosis (E83.5)
   schistosomiasis (B65.0-B65.9)
   > **Excludes1**   disorders of kidney and ureter in:
   cystinosis (E72.0)
   gonorrhea (A54.21)
   syphilis (A52.75)
   tuberculosis (A18.11)

OTHER DISEASES OF THE URINARY SYSTEM (N30-N39)

> **Excludes1**   urinary infection (complicating):
   abortion or ectopic or molar pregnancy (O00-O07, O08.8)
   pregnancy, childbirth and the puerperium (O23.-, O75.3, O86.2-)

● N30   Cystitis
   Infection of bladder and irritation in lower urinary tract
   Use additional code to identify infectious agent (B95-B97)
   > **Excludes1**   prostatocystitis (N41.3)

   ● N30.0   Acute cystitis
   > **Excludes1**   irradiation cystitis (N30.4-)
   trigonitis (N30.3-)

      N30.00   Acute cystitis without hematuria
      N30.01   Acute cystitis with hematuria

   ● N30.1   Interstitial cystitis (chronic)
   Ongoing infection of kidney glomeruli and tubules
      N30.10   Interstitial cystitis (chronic) without hematuria
      N30.11   Interstitial cystitis (chronic) with hematuria

   ● N30.2   Other chronic cystitis
      N30.20   Other chronic cystitis without hematuria
      N30.21   Other chronic cystitis with hematuria

▶ New   ➡ Revised   ~~deleted~~ Deleted   **OGCR** Official Guidelines   X Assign placeholder X   ● Use Additional Character(s)

Excludes 1   Excludes 2   Includes   Use additional   Code first   Code also   Key words

● **N30.3** Trigonitis
    Inflammation of triangular area of bladder (where the ureters and urethra come together)
    Urethrotrigonitis
    N30.30   Trigonitis without hematuria
    N30.31   Trigonitis with hematuria

● **N30.4** Irradiation cystitis
    N30.40   Irradiation cystitis without hematuria
    N30.41   Irradiation cystitis with hematuria

● **N30.8** Other cystitis
    Abscess of bladder
    N30.80   Other cystitis without hematuria
    N30.81   Other cystitis with hematuria

● **N30.9** Cystitis, unspecified
    N30.90   Cystitis, unspecified without hematuria
    N30.91   Cystitis, unspecified with hematuria

● **N31** **Neuromuscular dysfunction of bladder, not elsewhere classified**
    Use additional code to identify any associated urinary incontinence (N39.3-N39.4-)
    Excludes1   cord bladder NOS (G95.89)
              neurogenic bladder due to cauda equina syndrome (G83.4)
              neuromuscular dysfunction due to spinal cord lesion (G95.89)

    N31.0   Uninhibited neuropathic bladder, not elsewhere classified

    N31.1   Reflex neuropathic bladder, not elsewhere classified

    N31.2   Flaccid neuropathic bladder, not elsewhere classified
         Atonic (motor) (sensory) neuropathic bladder
         Diminished tone of bladder muscle
         Autonomous neuropathic bladder
         Nonreflex neuropathic bladder

    N31.8   Other neuromuscular dysfunction of bladder

    N31.9   Neuromuscular dysfunction of bladder, unspecified
         Neurogenic bladder dysfunction NOS

● **N32** **Other disorders of bladder**
    Excludes2   calculus of bladder (N21.0)
              cystocele (N81.1-)
              hernia or prolapse of bladder, female (N81.1-)

    N32.0   Bladder-neck obstruction
         Bladder-neck stenosis (acquired)
         Excludes1   congenital bladder-neck obstruction (Q64.3-)

    N32.1   Vesicointestinal fistula
         Vesicorectal fistula

    N32.2   Vesical fistula, not elsewhere classified
         Excludes1   fistula between bladder and female genital tract (N82.0-N82.1)

    N32.3   Diverticulum of bladder
         Formation of sac from a herniation of wall of bladder
         Excludes1   congenital diverticulum of bladder (Q64.6)
                   diverticulitis of bladder (N30.8-)

● **N32.8** Other specified disorders of bladder
    N32.81   Overactive bladder
         Detrusor muscle hyperactivity
         Excludes1   frequent urination due to specified bladder condition-code to condition

    N32.89   Other specified disorders of bladder
         Bladder hemorrhage
         Bladder hypertrophy
         Calcified bladder
         Contracted bladder

    N32.9   Bladder disorder, unspecified

N33 **Bladder disorders in diseases classified elsewhere**
    Code first underlying disease, such as:
    schistosomiasis (B65.0-B65.9)
    Excludes1   bladder disorder in syphilis (A52.76)
              bladder disorder in tuberculosis (A18.12)
              candidal cystitis (B37.41)
              chlamydial cystitis (A56.01)
              cystitis in gonorrhea (A54.01)
              cystitis in neurogenic bladder (N31.-)
              diphtheritic cystitis (A36.85)
              syphilitic cystitis (A52.76)
              trichomonal cystitis (A59.03)

● **N34** **Urethritis and urethral syndrome**
    Use additional code (B95-B97), to identify infectious agent
    Excludes2   Reiter's disease (M02.3-)
              urethritis in diseases with a predominantly sexual mode of transmission (A50-A64)
              urethrotrigonitis (N30.3-)

    N34.0   Urethral abscess
         Abscess (of) Cowper's gland
         Abscess (of) Littré's gland
         Abscess (of) urethral (gland)
         Periurethral abscess
         Excludes1   urethral caruncle (N36.2)

    N34.1   Nonspecific urethritis
         Nongonococcal urethritis
         Nonvenereal urethritis

    N34.2   Other urethritis
         Inflammation of urethra
         Meatitis, urethral
         Postmenopausal urethritis
         Ulcer of urethra (meatus)
         Urethritis NOS

    N34.3   Urethral syndrome, unspecified

● **N35** **Urethral stricture**
    Narrowing of lumen of urethra caused by scarring due to infection or injury
    Excludes1   congenital urethral stricture (Q64.3-)
              postprocedural urethral stricture (N99.1-)

● **N35.0** Post-traumatic urethral stricture
    Urethral stricture due to injury
    Excludes1   postprocedural urethral stricture (N99.1-)

    ● **N35.01** Post-traumatic urethral stricture, male
         N35.010   Post-traumatic urethral stricture, male, meatal
         N35.011   Post-traumatic bulbous urethral stricture
         N35.012   Post-traumatic membranous urethral stricture
         N35.013   Post-traumatic anterior urethral stricture
         N35.014   Post-traumatic urethral stricture, male, unspecified

    ● **N35.02** Post-traumatic urethral stricture, female
         N35.021   Urethral stricture due to childbirth
         N35.028   Other post-traumatic urethral stricture, female

CHAPTER 14 (N00-N99)

● **N35.1** **Postinfective** urethral stricture, not elsewhere classified
> **Excludes1**   urethral stricture associated with schistosomiasis (B65.-, N29)
>   gonococcal urethral stricture (A54.01)
>   syphilitic urethral stricture (A52.76)

   ● **N35.11** Postinfective urethral stricture, not elsewhere classified, **male**

       N35.111 Postinfective urethral stricture, not elsewhere classified, male, **meatal**

      ⇒ **N35.112** Postinfective **bulbous** urethral stricture, not elsewhere classified, male

      ⇒ **N35.113** Postinfective **membranous** urethral stricture, not elsewhere classified, male

      ⇒ **N35.114** Postinfective **anterior** urethral stricture, not elsewhere classified, male

      N35.119 Postinfective urethral stricture, not elsewhere classified, male, **unspecified**

   N35.12 Postinfective urethral stricture, not elsewhere classified, **female**

  N35.8 **Other** urethral stricture
> **Excludes1**   postprocedural urethral stricture (N99.1-)

  N35.9 Urethral stricture, **unspecified**

● **N36** Other disorders of urethra
  N36.0 Urethral **fistula**
     Urethroperineal fistula
     Urethrorectal fistula
     Urinary fistula NOS
> **Excludes1**   urethroscrotal fistula (N50.89)
>   urethrovaginal fistula (N82.1)
>   urethrovesicovaginal fistula (N82.1)

  N36.1 Urethral **diverticulum**
  N36.2 Urethral **caruncle**
● **N36.4** Urethral **functional and muscular disorders**
    Use additional code to identify associated urinary stress incontinence (N39.3)

   N36.41 **Hypermobility** of urethra
   N36.42 **Intrinsic sphincter deficiency (ISD)**
   N36.43 **Combined hypermobility** of urethra and intrinsic sphincter deficiency
   N36.44 **Muscular disorders** of urethra
      Bladder sphincter dyssynergy

  N36.5 Urethral **false passage**
  N36.8 **Other** specified disorders of urethra
> **Excludes1**   congenital urethrocele (Q64.7)
>   female urethrocele (N81.0)

  N36.9 Urethral disorder, **unspecified**

N37 Urethral disorders in diseases classified elsewhere
   Code first underlying disease
> **Excludes1**   urethritis (in):
>   candidal infection (B37.41)
>   chlamydial (A56.01)
>   gonorrhea (A54.01)
>   syphilis (A52.76)
>   trichomonal infection (A59.03)
>   tuberculosis (A18.13)

● **N39** Other disorders of urinary system
> **Excludes2**   hematuria NOS (R31.-)
>   recurrent or persistent hematuria (N02.-)
>   recurrent or persistent hematuria with specified morphological lesion (N02.-)
>   proteinuria NOS (R80.-)

  N39.0 Urinary tract infection, site not specified
    Use additional code (B95-B97), to identify infectious agent
> **Excludes1**   candidiasis of urinary tract (B37.4-)
>   neonatal urinary tract infection (P39.3)
>   urinary tract infection of specified site, such as:
>   cystitis (N30.-)
>   urethritis (N34.-)

  N39.3 Stress incontinence (female) (male)
    Code also any associated overactive bladder (N32.81)
> **Excludes1**   mixed incontinence (N39.46)

● **N39.4** Other specified urinary incontinence
    Code also any associated overactive bladder (N32.81)
> **Excludes1**   enuresis NOS (R32)
>   functional urinary incontinence (R39.81)
>   urinary incontinence associated with cognitive impairment (R39.81)
>   urinary incontinence NOS (R32)
>   urinary incontinence of nonorganic origin (F98.0)

  N39.41 Urge incontinence
> **Excludes1**   mixed incontinence (N39.46)

  N39.42 Incontinence without sensory awareness
      Insensible (urinary) incontinence

  N39.43 Post-void dribbling
  N39.44 Nocturnal enuresis
  N39.45 Continuous leakage
  N39.46 Mixed incontinence
      Urge and stress incontinence

  ● **N39.49** Other specified urinary incontinence
    N39.490 Overflow incontinence
    N39.491 Coital incontinence
    N39.492 Postural (urinary) incontinence
    N39.498 Other specified urinary incontinence
       Reflex incontinence
       Total incontinence

N39.8 **Other** specified disorders of urinary system
N39.9 Disorder of urinary system, **unspecified**

▶ New   ⇒ Revised   ~~deleted~~ Deleted   **OGCR** Official Guidelines   X Assign placeholder X   ● Use Additional Character(s)

Excludes 1   Excludes 2   Includes   Use additional   Code first   Code also   Key words

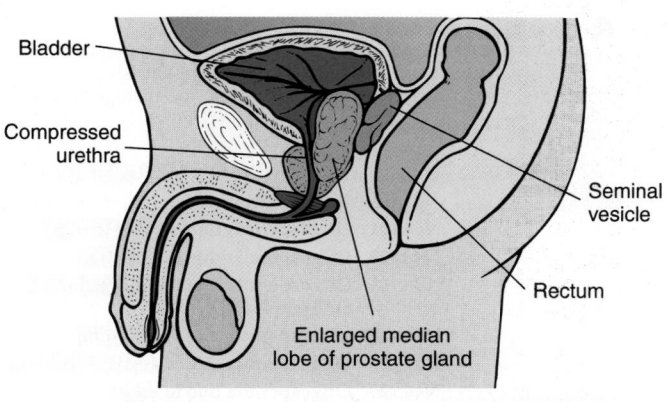

Figure 14-6 Benign prostatic hyperplasia. (From Shiland: Mastering Healthcare Terminology, ed 3, St. Louis, Mosby, 2010)

DISEASES OF MALE GENITAL ORGANS (N40-N53)

★**(See Plate 387 on page 53.)**

● **N40　Benign prostatic hyperplasia**
> **Includes**　adenofibromatous hypertrophy of prostate
> benign hypertrophy of the prostate
> *Enlargement of prostate gland usually occurring with age and causing obstructed urine flow*
> benign prostatic hypertrophy
> BPH
> enlarged prostate
> nodular prostate
> polyp of prostate
>
> **Excludes1**　benign neoplasms of prostate (adenoma, benign) (fibroadenoma) (fibroma) (myoma) (D29.1)
> malignant neoplasm of prostate (C61)

N40.0　Benign prostatic hyperplasia without lower urinary tract symptoms
> Enlarged prostate without LUTS
> Enlarged prostate NOS

N40.1　Benign prostatic hyperplasia with lower urinary tract symptoms
> Enlarged prostate with LUTS
> Use additional code for associated symptoms, when specified:
> incomplete bladder emptying (R39.14)
> nocturia (R35.1)
> straining on urination (R39.16)
> urinary frequency (R35.0)
> urinary hesitancy (R39.11)
> urinary incontinence (N39.4-)
> urinary obstruction (N13.8)
> urinary retention (R33.8)
> urinary urgency (R39.15)
> weak urinary stream (R39.12)

N40.2　Nodular prostate without lower urinary tract symptoms
> Nodular prostate without LUTS

N40.3　Nodular prostate with lower urinary tract symptoms
> Use additional code for associated symptoms, when specified:
> incomplete bladder emptying (R39.14)
> nocturia (R35.1)
> straining on urination (R39.16)
> urinary frequency (R35.0)
> urinary hesitancy (R39.11)
> urinary incontinence (N39.4-)
> urinary obstruction (N13.8)
> urinary retention (R33.8)
> urinary urgency (R39.15)
> weak urinary stream (R39.12)

● **N41　Inflammatory diseases of prostate**
> Use additional code (B95-B97), to identify infectious agent

N41.0　Acute prostatitis
N41.1　Chronic prostatitis
N41.2　Abscess of prostate
N41.3　Prostatocystitis
N41.4　Granulomatous prostatitis
N41.8　Other inflammatory diseases of prostate
N41.9　Inflammatory disease of prostate, unspecified
> Prostatitis NOS

● **N42　Other and unspecified disorders of prostate**

N42.0　Calculus of prostate
> Prostatic stone

N42.1　Congestion and hemorrhage of prostate
> **Excludes1**　enlarged prostate (N40.-)
> hematuria (R31.-)
> hyperplasia of prostate (N40.-)
> inflammatory diseases of prostate (N41.-)

● **N42.3　Dysplasia of prostate**
N42.30　Unspecified dysplasia of prostate
N42.31　Prostatic intraepithelial neoplasia
> PIN
> Prostatic intraepithelial neoplasia I (PIN I)
> Prostatic intraepithelial neoplasia II (PIN II)
>
> **Excludes1**　prostatic intraepithelial neoplasia III (PIN III) (D07.5)

N42.32　Atypical small acinar proliferation of prostate
N42.39　Other dysplasia of prostate

● **N42.8　Other specified disorders of prostate**
N42.81　Prostatodynia syndrome
> Painful prostate syndrome

N42.82　Prostatosis syndrome
N42.83　Cyst of prostate
N42.89　Other specified disorders of prostate
N42.9　Disorder of prostate, unspecified

● **N43　Hydrocele and spermatocele**
> **Includes**　hydrocele of spermatic cord, testis or tunica vaginalis
>
> **Excludes1**　congenital hydrocele (P83.5)

N43.0　Encysted hydrocele
N43.1　Infected hydrocele
> Use additional code (B95-B97), to identify infectious agent

N43.2　Other hydrocele
N43.3　Hydrocele, unspecified

Item 14–7　Hydrocele is a sac of fluid accumulating in the testes membrane.

Figure 14-7　A. Hydrocele. **B.** Newborn with large right hydrocele. (**B** from Nelson WE, Kliegman R: Nelson Textbook of Pediatrics, Philadelphia, Saunders Elsevier, 2011)

▶ New　⇒ Revised　d̶e̶l̶e̶t̶e̶d̶ Deleted　**OGCR** Official Guidelines　X Assign placeholder X　● Use Additional Character(s)

Excludes 1 | Excludes 2 | Includes | Use additional | Code first | Code also | Key words

- **N43.4 Spermatocele of epididymis**
  Spermatic cyst
  - N43.40 Spermatocele of epididymis, unspecified
  - N43.41 Spermatocele of epididymis, single
  - N43.42 Spermatocele of epididymis, multiple

- **N44 Noninflammatory disorders of testis**
  - **N44.0 Torsion of testis**
    - N44.00 Torsion of testis, unspecified
    - N44.01 Extravaginal torsion of spermatic cord
    - N44.02 Intravaginal torsion of spermatic cord
      Torsion of spermatic cord NOS
    - N44.03 Torsion of appendix testis
    - N44.04 Torsion of appendix epididymis
  - N44.1 Cyst of tunica albuginea testis
  - N44.2 Benign cyst of testis
  - N44.8 Other noninflammatory disorders of the testis

- **N45 Orchitis and epididymitis**
  Orchitis is inflammation of one or both of the testes as a result of mumps or other infection, trauma, or metastasis. Epididymitis is inflammation of the tubular structure that connects the testicle with the vas deferens.

  Use additional code (B95-B97), to identify infectious agent
  - N45.1 Epididymitis
  - N45.2 Orchitis
  - N45.3 Epididymo-orchitis
  - N45.4 Abscess of epididymis or testis

- **N46 Male infertility**
  | Excludes1 | vasectomy status (Z98.52) |
  - **N46.0 Azoospermia**
    Absolute male infertility
    Male infertility due to germinal (cell) aplasia
    Male infertility due to spermatogenic arrest (complete)
    - N46.01 Organic azoospermia
      Azoospermia NOS
    - **N46.02 Azoospermia due to extratesticular causes**
      Code also associated cause
      - N46.021 Azoospermia due to drug therapy
      - N46.022 Azoospermia due to infection
      - N46.023 Azoospermia due to obstruction of efferent ducts
      - N46.024 Azoospermia due to radiation
      - N46.025 Azoospermia due to systemic disease
      - N46.029 Azoospermia due to other extratesticular causes

- **N46.1 Oligospermia**
  Male infertility due to germinal cell desquamation
  Male infertility due to hypospermatogenesis
  Male infertility due to incomplete spermatogenic arrest
  - N46.11 Organic oligospermia
    Oligospermia NOS
  - **N46.12 Oligospermia due to extratesticular causes**
    Code also associated cause
    - N46.121 Oligospermia due to drug therapy
    - N46.122 Oligospermia due to infection
    - N46.123 Oligospermia due to obstruction of efferent ducts
    - N46.124 Oligospermia due to radiation
    - N46.125 Oligospermia due to systemic disease
    - N46.129 Oligospermia due to other extratesticular causes
  - N46.8 Other male infertility
  - N46.9 Male infertility, unspecified

- **N47 Disorders of prepuce**
  - N47.0 Adherent prepuce, newborn
  - N47.1 Phimosis
  - N47.2 Paraphimosis
  - N47.3 Deficient foreskin
  - N47.4 Benign cyst of prepuce
  - N47.5 Adhesions of prepuce and glans penis
  - N47.6 Balanoposthitis
    Use additional code (B95-B97), to identify infectious agent
    | Excludes1 | balanitis (N48.1) |
  - N47.7 Other inflammatory diseases of prepuce
    Use additional code (B95-B97), to identify infectious agent
  - N47.8 Other disorders of prepuce

- **N48 Other disorders of penis**
  - N48.0 Leukoplakia of penis
    Balanitis xerotica obliterans
    Kraurosis of penis
    Lichen sclerosus of external male genital organs
    | Excludes1 | carcinoma in situ of penis (D07.4) |
  - N48.1 Balanitis
    Use additional code (B95-B97), to identify infectious agent
    | Excludes1 | amebic balanitis (A06.8) |
    | | balanitis xerotica obliterans (N48.0) |
    | | candidal balanitis (B37.42) |
    | | gonococcal balanitis (A54.23) |
    | | herpesviral [herpes simplex] balanitis (A60.01) |
  - **N48.2 Other inflammatory disorders of penis**
    Use additional code (B95-B97), to identify infectious agent
    | Excludes1 | balanitis (N48.1) |
    | | balanitis xerotica obliterans (N48.0) |
    | | balanoposthitis (N47.6) |
    - N48.21 Abscess of corpus cavernosum and penis
    - N48.22 Cellulitis of corpus cavernosum and penis
    - N48.29 Other inflammatory disorders of penis
  - **N48.3 Priapism**
    Painful erection
    Code first underlying cause
    - N48.30 Priapism, unspecified
    - N48.31 Priapism due to trauma
    - N48.32 Priapism due to disease classified elsewhere
    - N48.33 Priapism, drug-induced
    - N48.39 Other priapism
  - N48.5 Ulcer of penis

Item 14–8 Male infertility is the inability of the female sex partner to conceive after one year of unprotected intercourse.

Azoospermia is no sperm ejaculated and **oligospermia** is few sperm ejaculated—both resulting in infertility. Extratesticular causes such as injury, infections, radiation, and chemotherapy may also cause male infertility.

▶ New   ⟹ Revised   ~~deleted~~ Deleted   **OGCR** Official Guidelines   **X** Assign placeholder X   ● Use Additional Character(s)

| Excludes 1 | | Excludes 2 | | Includes | | Use additional | | Code first | | Code also | | Key words |

N48.6 Induration penis plastica
Peyronie's disease
Plastic induration of penis
● **N48.8 Other specified disorders of penis**
N48.81 Thrombosis of superficial vein of penis
N48.82 Acquired torsion of penis
Acquired torsion of penis NOS
Excludes1   congenital torsion of penis
(Q55.63)
N48.83 Acquired buried penis
Excludes1   congenital hidden penis (Q55.64)
N48.89 Other specified disorders of penis
N48.9 Disorder of penis, unspecified

● **N49 Inflammatory disorders of male genital organs, not elsewhere classified**
Use additional code (B95-B97), to identify infectious agent
Excludes1   inflammation of penis (N48.1, N48.2-)
orchitis and epididymitis (N45.-)
N49.0 Inflammatory disorders of seminal vesicle
Vesiculitis NOS
N49.1 Inflammatory disorders of spermatic cord, tunica vaginalis and vas deferens
Vasitis
N49.2 Inflammatory disorders of scrotum
N49.3 Fournier gangrene
N49.8 Inflammatory disorders of other specified male genital organs
Inflammation of multiple sites in male genital organs
N49.9 Inflammatory disorder of unspecified male genital organ
Abscess of unspecified male genital organ
Boil of unspecified male genital organ
Carbuncle of unspecified male genital organ
Cellulitis of unspecified male genital organ

● **N50 Other and unspecified disorders of male genital organs**
Excludes2   torsion of testis (N44.0-)
N50.0 Atrophy of testis
N50.1 Vascular disorders of male genital organs
Hematocele, NOS, of male genital organs
Hemorrhage of male genital organs
Thrombosis of male genital organs
N50.3 Cyst of epididymis

Item 14–9 Seminal vesiculitis is an inflammation of the seminal vesicle. **Spermatocele** is a benign cystic accumulation of sperm arising from the head of the epididymis. **Torsion of the testis** is a medical emergency occurring most commonly in boys 7 to 12 years of age and results from a congenital abnormality of the covering of the testis allowing the testis to twist within its sac and cutting off the blood supply to the testis.

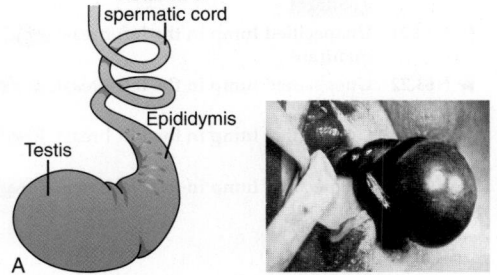

Figure 14-8   A. Torsion of testis. **B.** Torsion of the testis. (**B** from Kliegman R, Nelson WE: Nelson Textbook of Pediatrics, Philadelphia, Saunders, 2007)

● **N50.8 Other specified disorders of male genital organs**
● **N50.81 Testicular pain**
N50.811 Right testicular pain
N50.812 Left testicular pain
N50.819 Testicular pain, unspecified
N50.82 Scrotal pain
N50.89 Other specified disorders of the male genital organs
Atrophy of scrotum, seminal vesicle, spermatic cord, tunica vaginalis and vas deferens
Chylocele, tunica vaginalis (nonfilarial) NOS
Edema of scrotum, seminal vesicle, spermatic cord, tunica vaginalis and vas deferens
Hypertrophy of scrotum, seminal vesicle, spermatic cord, tunica vaginalis and vas deferens
Stricture of spermatic cord, tunica vaginalis, and vas deferens
Ulcer of scrotum, seminal vesicle, spermatic cord, testis, tunica vaginalis and vas deferens
Urethroscrotal fistula
N50.9 Disorder of male genital organs, unspecified

N51 Disorders of male genital organs in diseases classified elsewhere
Code first underlying disease, such as:
filariasis (B74.0-B74.9)
Excludes1   amebic balanitis (A06.8)
candidal balanitis (B37.42)
gonococcal balanitis (A54.23)
gonococcal prostatitis (A54.22)
herpesviral [herpes simplex] balanitis (A60.01)
trichomonal prostatitis (A59.02)
tuberculous prostatitis (A18.14)

● **N52 Male erectile dysfunction**
Excludes1   psychogenic impotence (F52.21)
● **N52.0 Vasculogenic erectile dysfunction**
N52.01 Erectile dysfunction due to arterial insufficiency
N52.02 Corporo-venous occlusive erectile dysfunction
N52.03 Combined arterial insufficiency and corporo-venous occlusive erectile dysfunction
N52.1 Erectile dysfunction due to diseases classified elsewhere
Code first underlying disease
N52.2 Drug-induced erectile dysfunction
● **N52.3 Postprocedural erectile dysfunction**
N52.31 Erectile dysfunction following radical prostatectomy
N52.32 Erectile dysfunction following radical cystectomy
N52.33 Erectile dysfunction following urethral surgery
N52.34 Erectile dysfunction following simple prostatectomy
N52.35 Erectile dysfunction following radiation therapy
N52.36 Erectile dysfunction following interstitial seed therapy
N52.37 Erectile dysfunction following prostate ablative therapy
Erectile dysfunction following cryotherapy
Erectile dysfunction following other prostate ablative therapies
Erectile dysfunction following ultrasound ablative therapies
N52.39 Other and unspecified postprocedural erectile dysfunction
N52.8 Other male erectile dysfunction
N52.9 Male erectile dysfunction, unspecified
Impotence NOS

▶ New   ⇢ Revised   ~~deleted~~ Deleted   **OGCR** Official Guidelines   X Assign placeholder X   ● Use Additional Character(s)
Excludes 1   Excludes 2   Includes   Use additional   Code first   Code also   Key words

CHAPTER 14 (N00-N99)

● **N53   Other male sexual dysfunction**
> **Excludes1**   psychogenic sexual dysfunction (F52.-)

● **N53.1   Ejaculatory dysfunction**
> **Excludes1**   premature ejaculation (F52.4)

    N53.11   **Retarded** ejaculation
    N53.12   **Painful** ejaculation
    N53.13   **Anejaculatory** orgasm
    N53.14   **Retrograde** ejaculation
    N53.19   **Other** ejaculatory dysfunction
           Ejaculatory dysfunction NOS

   N53.8   **Other** male sexual dysfunction
   N53.9   **Unspecified** male sexual dysfunction

DISORDERS OF BREAST (N60-N65)

> **Excludes1**   disorders of breast associated with childbirth (O91-O92)

● **N60   Benign mammary dysplasia**
> *Benign lumpiness of breast*
> **Includes**   fibrocystic mastopathy

● **N60.0   Solitary cyst of breast**
       Cyst of breast
    N60.01   Solitary cyst of **right** breast
    N60.02   Solitary cyst of **left** breast
    N60.09   Solitary cyst of **unspecified** breast

● **N60.1   Diffuse cystic mastopathy**
       Cystic breast
       Fibrocystic disease of breast
> **Excludes1**   diffuse cystic mastopathy with epithelial proliferation (N60.3-)

    N60.11   Diffuse cystic mastopathy of **right** breast
    N60.12   Diffuse cystic mastopathy of **left** breast
    N60.19   Diffuse cystic mastopathy of **unspecified** breast

● **N60.2   Fibroadenosis of breast**
       Adenofibrosis of breast
> **Excludes2**   fibroadenoma of breast (D24.-)

    N60.21   Fibroadenosis of **right** breast
    N60.22   Fibroadenosis of **left** breast
    N60.29   Fibroadenosis of **unspecified** breast

● **N60.3   Fibrosclerosis of breast**
       Cystic mastopathy with epithelial proliferation
    N60.31   Fibrosclerosis of **right** breast
    N60.32   Fibrosclerosis of **left** breast
    N60.39   Fibrosclerosis of **unspecified** breast

● **N60.4   Mammary duct ectasia**
    N60.41   Mammary duct ectasia of **right** breast
    N60.42   Mammary duct ectasia of **left** breast
    N60.49   Mammary duct ectasia of **unspecified** breast

● **N60.8   Other benign mammary dysplasias**
    N60.81   Other benign mammary dysplasias of **right** breast
    N60.82   Other benign mammary dysplasias of **left** breast
    N60.89   Other benign mammary dysplasias of **unspecified** breast

● **N60.9   Unspecified benign mammary dysplasia**
    N60.91   Unspecified benign mammary dysplasia of **right** breast
    N60.92   Unspecified benign mammary dysplasia of **left** breast
    N60.99   Unspecified benign mammary dysplasia of **unspecified** breast

● **N61   Inflammatory disorders of breast**
> **Excludes1**   inflammatory carcinoma of breast (C50.9)
> inflammatory disorder of breast associated with childbirth (O91.-)
> neonatal infective mastitis (P39.0)
> thrombophlebitis of breast [Mondor's disease] (I80.8)

   N61.0   Mastitis without abscess
       Infective mastitis (acute) (nonpuerperal) (subacute)
       Mastitis (acute) (nonpuerperal) (subacute) NOS
       Cellulitis (acute) (nonpuerperal) (subacute) of breast NOS
       Cellulitis (acute) (nonpuerperal) (subacute) of nipple NOS

   N61.1   Abscess of the breast and nipple
       Abscess (acute) (chronic) (nonpuerperal) of areola
       Abscess (acute) (chronic) (nonpuerperal) of breast
       Carbuncle of breast
       Mastitis with abscess

   N62   Hypertrophy of breast
       Gynecomastia
       Hypertrophy of breast NOS
       Massive pubertal hypertrophy of breast
> **Excludes1**   breast engorgement of newborn (P83.4)
> disproportion of reconstructed breast (N65.1)

● **N63   Unspecified lump in breast**
       Nodule(s) NOS in breast
▶   **N63.0   Unspecified lump in unspecified breast**
▶●   **N63.1   Unspecified lump in the right breast**
     ▶   N63.10   Unspecified lump in the right breast, **unspecified quadrant**
     ▶   N63.11   Unspecified lump in the right breast, **upper outer** quadrant
     ▶   N63.12   Unspecified lump in the right breast, **upper inner** quadrant
     ▶   N63.13   Unspecified lump in the right breast, **lower outer** quadrant
     ▶   N63.14   Unspecified lump in the right breast, **lower inner** quadrant
▶●   **N63.2   Unspecified lump in the left breast**
     ▶   N63.20   Unspecified lump in the left breast, **unspecified** quadrant
     ▶   N63.21   Unspecified lump in the left breast, **upper outer** quadrant
     ▶   N63.22   Unspecified lump in the left breast, **upper inner** quadrant
     ▶   N63.23   Unspecified lump in the left breast, **lower outer** quadrant
     ▶   N63.24   Unspecified lump in the left breast, **lower inner** quadrant

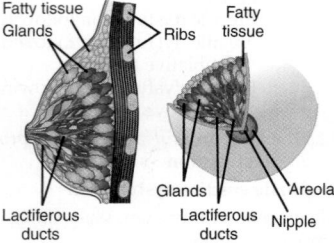

Figure 14-9   Breast.

▶ New   �v Revised   ~~deleted~~ Deleted   **OGCR** Official Guidelines   X Assign placeholder X   ● Use Additional Character(s)

Excludes 1   Excludes 2   Includes   Use additional   Code first   Code also   Key words

▶● **N63.3** **Unspecified lump in axillary tail**
  ▶ **N63.31** **Unspecified lump in axillary tail of the right breast**
  ▶ **N63.32** **Unspecified lump in axillary tail of the left breast**
▶● **N63.4** **Unspecified lump in breast, subareolar**
  ▶ **N63.41** **Unspecified lump in right breast, subareolar**
  ▶ **N63.42** **Unspecified lump in left breast, subareolar**

● **N64** **Other disorders of breast**
  Excludes2 mechanical complication of breast prosthesis and implant (T85.4-)
  N64.0 **Fissure and fistula of nipple**
  N64.1 **Fat necrosis of breast**
    Fat necrosis (segmental) of breast
    Code first breast necrosis due to breast graft (T85.898)
  N64.2 **Atrophy of breast**
  N64.3 **Galactorrhea not associated with childbirth**
    Excessive or spontaneous flow of milk
  N64.4 **Mastodynia**
● **N64.5** **Other signs and symptoms in breast**
    Excludes2 abnormal findings on diagnostic imaging of breast (R92.-)
    N64.51 **Induration of breast**
    N64.52 **Nipple discharge**
      Excludes1 abnormal findings in nipple discharge (R89.-)
    N64.53 **Retraction of nipple**
    N64.59 **Other signs and symptoms in breast**
● **N64.8** **Other specified disorders of breast**
    N64.81 **Ptosis of breast**
      Excludes1 ptosis of native breast in relation to reconstructed breast (N65.1)
    N64.82 **Hypoplasia of breast**
      Micromastia
      Excludes1 congenital absence of breast (Q83.0)
        hypoplasia of native breast in relation to reconstructed breast (N65.1)
    N64.89 **Other specified disorders of breast**
      Galactocele
      Subinvolution of breast (postlactational)
  N64.9 **Disorder of breast, unspecified**

● **N65** **Deformity and disproportion of reconstructed breast**
  N65.0 **Deformity of reconstructed breast**
    Contour irregularity in reconstructed breast
    Excess tissue in reconstructed breast
    Misshapen reconstructed breast
  N65.1 **Disproportion of reconstructed breast**
    Breast asymmetry between native breast and reconstructed breast
    Disproportion between native breast and reconstructed breast

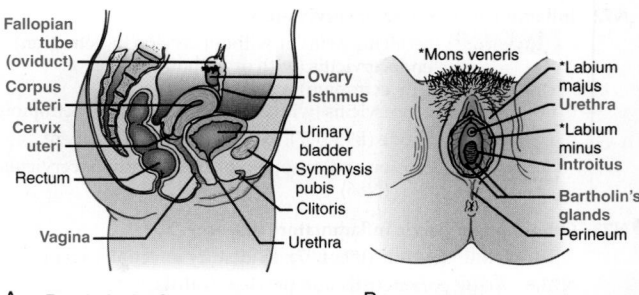

Figure 14-10 A. Female genital system. **B.** External female genital system. (From Buck CJ: Step-by-Step Medical Coding, ed 2016, St. Louis, Elsevier, 2016)

Item 14–10 Salpingitis is an infection of one or both fallopian tubes. **Oophoritis** is an infection of one or both ovaries.

INFLAMMATORY DISEASES OF FEMALE PELVIC ORGANS (N70-N77)
  Excludes1 inflammatory diseases of female pelvic organs complicating:
    abortion or ectopic or molar pregnancy (O00-O07, O08.0)
    pregnancy, childbirth and the puerperium (O23.-, O75.3, O85, O86.-)

★ **(See Plate 360 on page 80.)**

● **N70** **Salpingitis and oophoritis**
    Oophoritis = inflammation of ovary
    Salpingitis = inflammation of fallopian tube
    Includes abscess (of) fallopian tube
      abscess (of) ovary
      pyosalpinx
      salpingo-oophoritis
      tubo-ovarian abscess
      tubo-ovarian inflammatory disease
    Use additional code (B95-B97), to identify infectious agent
    Excludes1 gonococcal infection (A54.24)
      tuberculous infection (A18.17)
  ● **N70.0** **Acute salpingitis and oophoritis**
    N70.01 **Acute salpingitis**
    N70.02 **Acute oophoritis**
    N70.03 **Acute salpingitis and oophoritis**
  ● **N70.1** **Chronic salpingitis and oophoritis**
    Hydrosalpinx
    N70.11 **Chronic salpingitis**
    N70.12 **Chronic oophoritis**
    N70.13 **Chronic salpingitis and oophoritis**
  ● **N70.9** **Salpingitis and oophoritis, unspecified**
    N70.91 **Salpingitis, unspecified**
    N70.92 **Oophoritis, unspecified**
    N70.93 **Salpingitis and oophoritis, unspecified**

● **N71** **Inflammatory disease of uterus, except cervix**
    Includes endo (myo) metritis
      metritis
      myometritis
      pyometra
      uterine abscess
    Use additional code (B95-B97), to identify infectious agent
    Excludes1 hyperplastic endometritis (N85.0-)
      infection of uterus following delivery (O85, O86.-)
  N71.0 **Acute inflammatory disease of uterus**
  N71.1 **Chronic inflammatory disease of uterus**
  N71.9 **Inflammatory disease of uterus, unspecified**

CHAPTER 14 (N00-N99)

N72   **Inflammatory disease of cervix uteri**

     Includes   cervicitis (with or without erosion or ectropion)
             endocervicitis (with or without erosion or
                 ectropion)
             exocervicitis (with or without erosion or ectropion)

     Use additional code (B95-B97), to identify infectious agent

     Excludes1   erosion and ectropion of cervix without cervicitis
                    (N86)

● **N73**   **Other female pelvic inflammatory diseases**

     Use additional code (B95-B97), to identify infectious agent

   N73.0   **Acute parametritis and pelvic cellulitis**
             Abscess of broad ligament
             Abscess of parametrium
             Pelvic cellulitis, female

   N73.1   **Chronic parametritis and pelvic cellulitis**
             Any condition in N73.0 specified as chronic

         Excludes1   tuberculous parametritis and pelvic
                         cellultis (A18.17)

   N73.2   **Unspecified parametritis and pelvic cellulitis**
             Any condition in N73.0 unspecified whether acute or
                 chronic

   N73.3   **Female acute pelvic peritonitis**

   N73.4   **Female chronic pelvic peritonitis**

         Excludes1   tuberculous pelvic (female) peritonitis
                       (A18.17)

   N73.5   **Female pelvic peritonitis, unspecified**

   N73.6   **Female pelvic peritoneal adhesions (postinfective)**

         Excludes2   postprocedural pelvic peritoneal
                       adhesions (N99.4)

   N73.8   **Other specified female pelvic inflammatory diseases**

   N73.9   **Female pelvic inflammatory disease, unspecified**
             Female pelvic infection or inflammation NOS

N74   **Female pelvic inflammatory disorders in diseases classified elsewhere**

     Code first underlying disease

     Excludes1   chlamydial cervicitis (A56.02)
                 chlamydial pelvic inflammatory disease (A56.11)
                 gonococcal cervicitis (A54.03)
                 gonococcal pelvic inflammatory disease (A54.24)
                 herpesviral [herpes simplex] cervicitis (A60.03)
                 herpesviral [herpes simplex] pelvic inflammatory
                     disease (A60.09)
                 syphilitic cervicitis (A52.76)
                 syphilitic pelvic inflammatory disease (A52.76)
                 trichomonal cervicitis (A59.09)
                 tuberculous cervicitis (A18.16)
                 tuberculous pelvic inflammatory disease (A18.17)

● **N75**   **Diseases of Bartholin's gland**

   N75.0   **Cyst of Bartholin's gland**
             Cysts filled with liquid or semisolid material

   N75.1   **Abscess of Bartholin's gland**
             Localized collection of pus

   N75.8   **Other diseases of Bartholin's gland**
             Bartholinitis

   N75.9   **Disease of Bartholin's gland, unspecified**

● **N76**   **Other inflammation of vagina and vulva**

     Use additional code (B95-B97), to identify infectious agent

     Excludes2   senile (atrophic) vaginitis (N95.2)
                    vulvar vestibulitis (N94.810)

   N76.0   **Acute vaginitis**
             Acute vulvovaginitis
             Vaginitis NOS
             Vulvovaginitis NOS

   N76.1   **Subacute and chronic vaginitis**
             Chronic vulvovaginitis
             Subacute vulvovaginitis

   N76.2   **Acute vulvitis**
             Vulvitis NOS

   N76.3   **Subacute and chronic vulvitis**

   N76.4   **Abscess of vulva**
             Furuncle of vulva

   N76.5   **Ulceration of vagina**

   N76.6   **Ulceration of vulva**

●   **N76.8**   **Other specified inflammation of vagina and vulva**

     N76.81   **Mucositis (ulcerative) of vagina and vulva**

         Code also type of associated therapy, such as:
             antineoplastic and immunosuppressive
                 drugs (T45.1X-)
             radiological procedure and radiotherapy
                 (Y84.2)

         Excludes2   gastrointestinal mucositis
                       (ulcerative) (K92.81)
                     nasal mucositis (ulcerative)
                       (J34.81)
                     oral mucositis (ulcerative) (K12.3-)

     N76.89   **Other specified inflammation of vagina and
             vulva**

● **N77**   **Vulvovaginal ulceration and inflammation in diseases classified elsewhere**

   N77.0   **Ulceration of vulva in diseases classified elsewhere**

     Code first underlying disease, such as:
         Behçet's disease (M35.2)

     Excludes1   ulceration of vulva in gonococcal
                    infection (A54.02)
                 ulceration of vulva in herpesviral [herpes
                    simplex] infection (A60.04)
                 ulceration of vulva in syphilis (A51.0)
                 ulceration of vulva in tuberculosis (A18.18)

   N77.1   **Vaginitis, vulvitis and vulvovaginitis in diseases classified elsewhere**

     Code first underlying disease, such as:
         pinworm (B80)

     Excludes1   candidial vulvovaginitis (B37.3)
                 chlamydial vulvovaginitis (A56.02)
                 gonococcal vulvovaginitis (A54.02)
                 herpesviral [herpes simplex]
                    vulvovaginitis (A60.04)
                 trichomonal vulvovaginitis (A59.01)
                 tuberculous vulvovaginitis (A18.18)
                 vulvovaginitis in early syphilis (A51.0)
                 vulvovaginitis in late syphilis (A52.76)

▶ New   ⇒ Revised   ~~deleted~~ Deleted   **OGCR** Official Guidelines   X Assign placeholder X   ● Use Additional Character(s)

Excludes 1   Excludes 2   Includes   Use additional   Code first   Code also   Key words

Item 14–11 Endometriosis is a condition for which no clear cause has been identified. Endometrial tissue is expelled from the uterus into the abdominal cavity and can implant onto a variety of organs. Classification is based on the site of implant of the endometrial tissue.

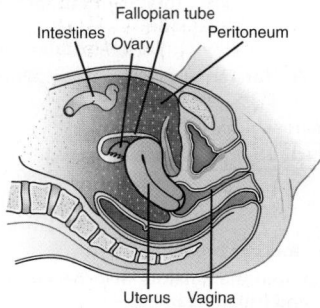

Fallopian tube
Intestines   Ovary   Peritoneum

Uterus   Vagina

Figure 14-11   Sites of potential endometrial implants.

NONINFLAMMATORY DISORDERS OF FEMALE GENITAL TRACT (N80-N98)

● **N80   Endometriosis**
    N80.0   Endometriosis of uterus
        Adenomyosis
        Excludes1   stromal endometriosis (D39.0)
    N80.1   Endometriosis of ovary
    N80.2   Endometriosis of fallopian tube
    N80.3   Endometriosis of pelvic peritoneum
    N80.4   Endometriosis of rectovaginal septum and vagina
    N80.5   Endometriosis of intestine
    N80.6   Endometriosis in cutaneous scar
    N80.8   Other endometriosis
        ▶Endometriosis of thorax
    N80.9   Endometriosis, unspecified

● **N81   Female genital prolapse**
    Excludes1   genital prolapse complicating pregnancy, labor or delivery (O34.5-)
               prolapse and hernia of ovary and fallopian tube (N83.4-)
               prolapse of vaginal vault after hysterectomy (N99.3)
    N81.0   Urethrocele
        Excludes1   urethrocele with cystocele (N81.1-)
                  urethrocele with prolapse of uterus (N81.2-N81.4)
    ● **N81.1   Cystocele**
        Cystocele with urethrocele
        Cystourethrocele
        Excludes1   cystocele with prolapse of uterus (N81.2-N81.4)
        N81.10   Cystocele, unspecified
            Prolapse of (anterior) vaginal wall NOS
        N81.11   Cystocele, midline
        N81.12   Cystocele, lateral
            Paravaginal cystocele

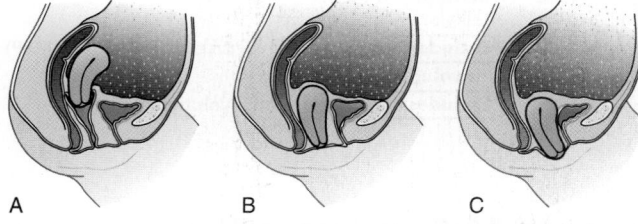

A   B   C

Figure 14-12   Three stages of uterine prolapse. **A.** Uterus is prolapsed. **B.** Vagina and uterus are prolapsed (incomplete uterovaginal prolapse). **C.** Vagina and uterus are completely prolapsed and are exposed through the external genitalia (complete uterovaginal prolapse).

    N81.2   Incomplete uterovaginal prolapse
        First degree uterine prolapse
        Prolapse of cervix NOS
        Second degree uterine prolapse
        ⇒ **Excludes1**   cervical stump prolapse (N81.85)
    N81.3   Complete uterovaginal prolapse
        Procidentia (uteri) NOS
        Third degree uterine prolapse
    N81.4   Uterovaginal prolapse, unspecified
        Prolapse of uterus NOS
    N81.5   Vaginal enterocele
        Excludes1   enterocele with prolapse of uterus (N81.2-N81.4)
    N81.6   Rectocele
        Prolapse of posterior vaginal wall
        Use additional code for any associated fecal incontinence, if applicable (R15.-)
        Excludes2   perineocele (N81.81)
                  rectal prolapse (K62.3)
                  rectocele with prolapse of uterus (N81.2-N81.4)
    ● **N81.8   Other female genital prolapse**
        N81.81   Perineocele
        N81.82   Incompetence or weakening of pubocervical tissue
        N81.83   Incompetence or weakening of rectovaginal tissue
        N81.84   Pelvic muscle wasting
            Disuse atrophy of pelvic muscles and anal sphincter
        N81.85   Cervical stump prolapse
        N81.89   Other female genital prolapse
            Deficient perineum
            Old laceration of muscles of pelvic floor
    N81.9   Female genital prolapse, unspecified

● **N82   Fistulae involving female genital tract**
    Excludes1   vesicointestinal fistulae (N32.1)
    N82.0   Vesicovaginal fistula
    N82.1   Other female urinary-genital tract fistulae
        Cervicovesical fistula
        Ureterovaginal fistula
        Urethrovaginal fistula
        Uteroureteric fistula
        Uterovesical fistula
    N82.2   Fistula of vagina to small intestine
    N82.3   Fistula of vagina to large intestine
        Rectovaginal fistula
    N82.4   Other female intestinal-genital tract fistulae
        Intestinouterine fistula
    N82.5   Female genital tract-skin fistulae
        Uterus to abdominal wall fistula
        Vaginoperineal fistula
    N82.8   Other female genital tract fistulae
    N82.9   Female genital tract fistula, unspecified

● **N83   Noninflammatory disorders of ovary, fallopian tube and broad ligament**
    Excludes2   hydrosalpinx (N70.1-)
    ● **N83.0   Follicular cyst of ovary**
        Cyst of graafian follicle
        Hemorrhagic follicular cyst (of ovary)
        N83.00   Follicular cyst of ovary, unspecified side
        N83.01   Follicular cyst of right ovary
        N83.02   Follicular cyst of left ovary
    ● **N83.1   Corpus luteum cyst**
        Hemorrhagic corpus luteum cyst
        N83.10   Corpus luteum cyst of ovary, unspecified side
        N83.11   Corpus luteum cyst of right ovary
        N83.12   Corpus luteum cyst of left ovary

▶ New   ⇒ Revised   ~~deleted~~ Deleted   **OGCR** Official Guidelines   X Assign placeholder X   ● Use Additional Character(s)

Excludes 1   Excludes 2   Includes   Use additional   Code first   Code also   Key words

● **N83.2 Other and unspecified ovarian cysts**

> Excludes1 developmental ovarian cyst (Q50.1)
> neoplastic ovarian cyst (D27.-)
> polycystic ovarian syndrome (E28.2)
> Stein-Leventhal syndrome (E28.2)

● **N83.20 Unspecified ovarian cysts**

N83.201 Unspecified ovarian cyst, right side

N83.202 Unspecified ovarian cyst, left side

N83.209 Unspecified ovarian cyst, unspecified side
> Ovarian cyst, NOS

● **N83.29 Other ovarian cysts**
> Retention cyst of ovary
> Simple cyst of ovary

N83.291 Other ovarian cyst, right side

N83.292 Other ovarian cyst, left side

N83.299 Other ovarian cyst, unspecified side

● **N83.3 Acquired atrophy of ovary and fallopian tube**

● **N83.31 Acquired atrophy of ovary**

N83.311 Acquired atrophy of right ovary

N83.312 Acquired atrophy of left ovary

N83.319 Acquired atrophy of ovary, unspecified side
> Acquired atrophy of ovary, NOS

● **N83.32 Acquired atrophy of fallopian tube**

N83.321 Acquired atrophy of right fallopian tube

N83.322 Acquired atrophy of left fallopian tube

N83.329 Acquired atrophy of fallopian tube, unspecified side
> Acquired atrophy of fallopian tube, NOS

● **N83.33 Acquired atrophy of ovary and fallopian tube**

N83.331 Acquired atrophy of right ovary and fallopian tube

N83.332 Acquired atrophy of left ovary and fallopian tube

N83.339 Acquired atrophy of ovary and fallopian tube, unspecified side
> Acquired atrophy of ovary and fallopian tube, NOS

● **N83.4 Prolapse and hernia of ovary and fallopian tube**

N83.40 Prolapse and hernia of ovary and fallopian tube, unspecified side
> Prolapse and hernia of ovary and fallopian tube, NOS

N83.41 Prolapse and hernia of right ovary and fallopian tube

N83.42 Prolapse and hernia of left ovary and fallopian tube

● **N83.5 Torsion of ovary, ovarian pedicle and fallopian tube**
> Torsion of accessory tube

● **N83.51 Torsion of ovary and ovarian pedicle**

N83.511 Torsion of right ovary and ovarian pedicle

N83.512 Torsion of left ovary and ovarian pedicle

N83.519 Torsion of ovary and ovarian pedicle, unspecified side
> Torsion of ovary and ovarian pedicle, NOS

● **N83.52 Torsion of fallopian tube**
> Torsion of hydatid of Morgagni

N83.521 Torsion of right fallopian tube

N83.522 Torsion of left fallopian tube

N83.529 Torsion of fallopian tube, unspecified side
> Torsion of fallopian tube, NOS

N83.53 Torsion of ovary, ovarian pedicle and fallopian tube

N83.6 Hematosalpinx

> Excludes1 hematosalpinx (with) (in):
> hematocolpos (N89.7)
> hematometra (N85.7)
> tubal pregnancy (O00.1-)

N83.7 Hematoma of broad ligament

N83.8 Other noninflammatory disorders of ovary, fallopian tube and broad ligament
> Broad ligament laceration syndrome [Allen-Masters]

N83.9 Noninflammatory disorder of ovary, fallopian tube and broad ligament, unspecified

● **N84 Polyp of female genital tract**

> Excludes1 adenomatous polyp (D28.-)
> placental polyp (O90.89)

N84.0 Polyp of corpus uteri
> Polyp of endometrium
> Polyp of uterus NOS

> Excludes1 polypoid endometrial hyperplasia (N85.0-)

N84.1 Polyp of cervix uteri
> Mucous polyp of cervix

N84.2 Polyp of vagina

N84.3 Polyp of vulva
> Polyp of labia

N84.8 Polyp of other parts of female genital tract

N84.9 Polyp of female genital tract, unspecified

● **N85 Other noninflammatory disorders of uterus, except cervix**

> Excludes1 endometriosis (N80.-)
> inflammatory diseases of uterus (N71.-)
> noninflammatory disorders of cervix, except malposition (N86-N88)
> polyp of corpus uteri (N84.0)
> uterine prolapse (N81.-)

● **N85.0 Endometrial hyperplasia**

N85.00 Endometrial hyperplasia, unspecified
> Hyperplasia (adenomatous) (cystic) (glandular) of endometrium
> Hyperplastic endometritis

N85.01 Benign endometrial hyperplasia
> Endometrial hyperplasia (complex) (simple) without atypia

N85.02 Endometrial intraepithelial neoplasia [EIN]
> Endometrial hyperplasia with atypia

> Excludes1 malignant neoplasm of endometrium (with endometrial intraepithelial neoplasia [EIN]) (C54.1)

N85.2 Hypertrophy of uterus
> Bulky or enlarged uterus

> Excludes1 puerperal hypertrophy of uterus (O90.89)

N85.3 Subinvolution of uterus

> Excludes1 puerperal subinvolution of uterus (O90.89)

▶ New   ⇒ Revised   ~~deleted~~ Deleted   **OGCR** Official Guidelines   X Assign placeholder X   ● Use Additional Character(s)

Excludes 1   Excludes 2   Includes   Use additional   Code first   Code also   Key words

N85.4   **Malposition of uterus**
     Anteversion of uterus
     Retroflexion of uterus
     Retroversion of uterus
     Excludes 1   malposition of uterus complicating pregnancy, labor or delivery (O34.5-, O65.5)

N85.5   **Inversion of uterus**
     Excludes 1   current obstetric trauma (O71.2)
                     postpartum inversion of uterus (O71.2)

N85.6   **Intrauterine synechiae**

N85.7   **Hematometra**
     Hematosalpinx with hematometra
     Excludes 1   hematometra with hematocolpos (N89.7)

N85.8   **Other specified noninflammatory disorders of uterus**
     Atrophy of uterus, acquired
     Fibrosis of uterus NOS

N85.9   **Noninflammatory disorder of uterus, unspecified**
     Disorder of uterus NOS

N86   **Erosion and ectropion of cervix uteri**
     Decubitus (trophic) ulcer of cervix
     Eversion of cervix
     Excludes 1   erosion and ectropion of cervix with cervicitis (N72)

● N87   **Dysplasia of cervix uteri**
     Excludes 1   abnormal results from cervical cytologic examination without histologic confirmation (R87.61-)
                     carcinoma in situ of cervix uteri (D06.-)
                     cervical intraepithelial neoplasia III [CIN III] (D06.-)
                     HGSIL of cervix (R87.613)
                     severe dysplasia of cervix uteri (D06.-)

N87.0   **Mild cervical dysplasia**
     Cervical intraepithelial neoplasia I [CIN I]

N87.1   **Moderate cervical dysplasia**
     Cervical intraepithelial neoplasia II [CIN II]

N87.9   **Dysplasia of cervix uteri, unspecified**
     Anaplasia of cervix
     Cervical atypism
     Cervical dysplasia NOS

● N88   **Other noninflammatory disorders of cervix uteri**
     Excludes 2   inflammatory disease of cervix (N72)
                     polyp of cervix (N84.1)

N88.0   **Leukoplakia of cervix uteri**

N88.1   **Old laceration of cervix uteri**
     Adhesions of cervix
     Excludes 1   current obstetric trauma (O71.3)

N88.2   **Stricture and stenosis of cervix uteri**
     Excludes 1   stricture and stenosis of cervix uteri complicating labor (O65.5)

N88.3   **Incompetence of cervix uteri**
     Investigation and management of (suspected) cervical incompetence in a nonpregnant woman
     Excludes 1   cervical incompetence complicating pregnancy (O34.3-)

N88.4   **Hypertrophic elongation of cervix uteri**

N88.8   **Other specified noninflammatory disorders of cervix uteri**
     Excludes 1   current obstetric trauma (O71.3)

N88.9   **Noninflammatory disorder of cervix uteri, unspecified**

● N89   **Other noninflammatory disorders of vagina**
     Excludes 1   abnormal results from vaginal cytologic examination without histologic confirmation (R87.62-)
                     carcinoma in situ of vagina (D07.2)
                     HGSIL of vagina (R87.623)
                     inflammation of vagina (N76.-)
                     senile (atrophic) vaginitis (N95.2)
                     severe dysplasia of vagina (D07.2)
                     trichomonal leukorrhea (A59.00)
                     vaginal intraepithelial neoplasia [VAIN], grade III (D07.2)

N89.0   **Mild vaginal dysplasia**
     Vaginal intraepithelial neoplasia [VAIN], grade I

N89.1   **Moderate vaginal dysplasia**
     Vaginal intraepithelial neoplasia [VAIN], grade II

N89.3   **Dysplasia of vagina, unspecified**

N89.4   **Leukoplakia of vagina**

N89.5   **Stricture and atresia of vagina**
     Vaginal adhesions   Vaginal stenosis
     Excludes 1   congenital atresia or stricture (Q52.4)
                     postprocedural adhesions of vagina (N99.2)

N89.6   **Tight hymenal ring**
     Rigid hymen   Tight introitus
     Excludes 1   imperforate hymen (Q52.3)

N89.7   **Hematocolpos**
     Hematocolpos with hematometra or hematosalpinx

N89.8   **Other specified noninflammatory disorders of vagina**
     Leukorrhea NOS
     Old vaginal laceration
     Pessary ulcer of vagina
     Excludes 1   current obstetric trauma (O70.-, O71.4, O71.7-O71.8)
                     old laceration involving muscles of pelvic floor (N81.8)

N89.9   **Noninflammatory disorder of vagina, unspecified**

● N90   **Other noninflammatory disorders of vulva and perineum**
     Excludes 1   anogenital (venereal) warts (A63.0)
                     carcinoma in situ of vulva (D07.1)
                     condyloma acuminatum (A63.0)
                     current obstetric trauma (O70.-, O71.7-O71.8)
                     inflammation of vulva (N76.-)
                     severe dysplasia of vulva (D07.1)
                     vulvar intraepithelial neoplasm III [VIN III] (D07.1)

N90.0   **Mild vulvar dysplasia**
     Vulvar intraepithelial neoplasia [VIN], grade I

N90.1   **Moderate vulvar dysplasia**
     Vulvar intraepithelial neoplasia [VIN], grade II

N90.3   **Dysplasia of vulva, unspecified**

N90.4   **Leukoplakia of vulva**
     Dystrophy of vulva
     Kraurosis of vulva
     Lichen sclerosus of external female genital organs

N90.5   **Atrophy of vulva**
     Stenosis of vulva

● N90.6   **Hypertrophy of vulva**

N90.60   **Unspecified hypertrophy of vulva**
     Unspecified hypertrophy of labia

N90.61   **Childhood asymmetric labium majus enlargement**
     CALME

N90.69   **Other specified hypertrophy of vulva**
     Other specified hypertrophy of labia

N90.7　Vulvar cyst

● N90.8　Other specified noninflammatory disorders of vulva and perineum

　● N90.81　Female genital mutilation status
　　　　Female genital cutting status

　　　N90.810　Female genital mutilation status, unspecified
　　　　　　Female genital cutting status, unspecified
　　　　　　Female genital mutilation status NOS

　　　N90.811　Female genital mutilation Type I status
　　　　　　Clitorectomy status
　　　　　　Female genital cutting Type I status

　　　N90.812　Female genital mutilation Type II status
　　　　　　Clitorectomy with excision of labia minora status
　　　　　　Female genital cutting Type II status

　　　N90.813　Female genital mutilation Type III status
　　　　　　Female genital cutting Type III status
　　　　　　Infibulation status

　　　N90.818　Other female genital mutilation status
　　　　　　Female genital cutting Type IV status
　　　　　　Female genital mutilation Type IV status
　　　　　　Other female genital cutting status

　　N90.89　Other specified noninflammatory disorders of vulva and perineum
　　　　Adhesions of vulva
　　　　Hypertrophy of clitoris

N90.9　Noninflammatory disorder of vulva and perineum, unspecified

● N91　Absent, scanty and rare menstruation
　　Excludes1　ovarian dysfunction (E28.-)

N91.0　Primary amenorrhea

N91.1　Secondary amenorrhea

N91.2　Amenorrhea, unspecified

N91.3　Primary oligomenorrhea

N91.4　Secondary oligomenorrhea

N91.5　Oligomenorrhea, unspecified
　　　Hypomenorrhea NOS

● N92　Excessive, frequent and irregular menstruation
　　Excludes1　postmenopausal bleeding (N95.0)
　　　　　　precocious puberty (menstruation) (E30.1)

N92.0　Excessive and frequent menstruation with regular cycle
　　　Heavy periods NOS　　　Polymenorrhea
　　　Menorrhagia NOS

N92.1　Excessive and frequent menstruation with irregular cycle
　　　Irregular intermenstrual bleeding
　　　Irregular, shortened intervals between menstrual bleeding
　　　Menometrorrhagia
　　　Metrorrhagia

N92.2　Excessive menstruation at puberty
　　　Excessive bleeding associated with onset of menstrual periods
　　　Pubertal menorrhagia
　　　Puberty bleeding

N92.3　Ovulation bleeding
　　　Regular intermenstrual bleeding

N92.4　Excessive bleeding in the premenopausal period
　　　Climacteric menorrhagia or metrorrhagia
　　　Menopausal menorrhagia or metrorrhagia
　　　Preclimacteric menorrhagia or metrorrhagia
　　　Premenopausal menorrhagia or metrorrhagia

N92.5　Other specified irregular menstruation

N92.6　Irregular menstruation, unspecified
　　　Irregular bleeding NOS
　　　Irregular periods NOS
　　　Excludes1　irregular menstruation with:
　　　　　　lengthened intervals or scanty bleeding (N91.3-N91.5)
　　　　　　shortened intervals or excessive bleeding (N92.1)

● N93　Other abnormal uterine and vaginal bleeding
　　Excludes1　neonatal vaginal hemorrhage (P54.6)
　　　　　　precocious puberty (menstruation) (E30.1)
　　　　　　pseudomenses (P54.6)

N93.0　Postcoital and contact bleeding

N93.1　Pre-pubertal vaginal bleeding

N93.8　Other specified abnormal uterine and vaginal bleeding
　　　Dysfunctional or functional uterine or vaginal bleeding NOS

N93.9　Abnormal uterine and vaginal bleeding, unspecified

● N94　Pain and other conditions associated with female genital organs and menstrual cycle

N94.0　Mittelschmerz
　　　Ovulation pain

● N94.1　Dyspareunia
　　　Painful intercourse/coitus
　　　Excludes1　psychogenic dyspareunia (F52.6)

　　N94.10　Unspecified dyspareunia

　　N94.11　Superficial (introital) dyspareunia

　　N94.12　Deep dyspareunia

　　N94.19　Other specified dyspareunia

N94.2　Vaginismus
　　　Vagina tightness
　　　Excludes1　psychogenic vaginismus (F52.5)

N94.3　Premenstrual tension syndrome
　　　AKA: PMS
　　　~~Premenstrual dysphoric disorder~~
　　　Code also associated menstrual migraine (G43.82-, G43.83-)
　　　Excludes1　Premenstrual dysphoric disorder (F32.81)

N94.4　Primary dysmenorrhea
　　　Lifelong painful menstruation

N94.5　Secondary dysmenorrhea
　　　Later onset of painful menstruation

N94.6　Dysmenorrhea, unspecified
　　　Excludes1　psychogenic dysmenorrhea (F45.8)

● N94.8　Other specified conditions associated with female genital organs and menstrual cycle

　● N94.81　Vulvodynia
　　　N94.810　Vulvar vestibulitis
　　　N94.818　Other vulvodynia
　　　N94.819　Vulvodynia, unspecified
　　　　　　Vulvodynia NOS

　　N94.89　Other specified conditions associated with female genital organs and menstrual cycle

N94.9　Unspecified condition associated with female genital organs and menstrual cycle

---

▶ New　⇒ Revised　~~deleted~~ Deleted　OGCR Official Guidelines　X Assign placeholder X　● Use Additional Character(s)

Excludes 1　Excludes 2　Includes　Use additional　Code first　Code also　Key words

● **N95   Menopausal and other perimenopausal disorders**
Menopausal and other perimenopausal disorders due to naturally occurring (age-related) menopause and perimenopause
> **Excludes1** excessive bleeding in the premenopausal period (N92.4)
> menopausal and perimenopausal disorders due to artificial or premature menopause (E89.4-, E28.31-)
> premature menopause (E28.31-)
> **Excludes2** postmenopausal osteoporosis (M81.0-)
> postmenopausal osteoporosis with current pathological fracture (M80.0-)
> postmenopausal urethritis (N34.2)

N95.0   Postmenopausal bleeding

N95.1   Menopausal and female climacteric states
Symptoms such as flushing, sleeplessness, headache, lack of concentration, associated with natural (age-related) menopause
Use additional code for associated symptoms
> **Excludes1** asymptomatic menopausal state (Z78.0)
> symptoms associated with artificial menopause (E89.41)
> symptoms associated with premature menopause (E28.310)

N95.2   Postmenopausal atrophic vaginitis
Senile (atrophic) vaginitis

N95.8   Other specified menopausal and perimenopausal disorders

N95.9   Unspecified menopausal and perimenopausal disorder

● **N96   Recurrent pregnancy loss**
Investigation or care in a nonpregnant woman with history of recurrent pregnancy loss
> **Excludes1** recurrent pregnancy loss with current pregnancy (O26.2-)

● **N97   Female infertility**
> **Includes** inability to achieve a pregnancy
> sterility, female NOS
> **Excludes1** female infertility associated with:
> hypopituitarism (E23.0)
> Stein-Leventhal syndrome (E28.2)
> **Excludes2** incompetence of cervix uteri (N88.3)

N97.0   Female infertility associated with anovulation

N97.1   Female infertility of tubal origin
Female infertility associated with congenital anomaly of tube
Female infertility due to tubal block
Female infertility due to tubal occlusion
Female infertility due to tubal stenosis

N97.2   Female infertility of uterine origin
Female infertility associated with congenital anomaly of uterus
Female infertility due to nonimplantation of ovum

N97.8   Female infertility of other origin

N97.9   Female infertility, unspecified

● **N98   Complications associated with artificial fertilization**

N98.0   Infection associated with artificial insemination

N98.1   Hyperstimulation of ovaries
Hyperstimulation of ovaries NOS
Hyperstimulation of ovaries associated with induced ovulation

N98.2   Complications of attempted introduction of fertilized ovum following in vitro fertilization

N98.3   Complications of attempted introduction of embryo in embryo transfer

N98.8   Other complications associated with artificial fertilization

N98.9   Complication associated with artificial fertilization, unspecified

INTRAOPERATIVE AND POSTPROCEDURAL COMPLICATIONS AND DISORDERS OF GENITOURINARY SYSTEM, NOT ELSEWHERE CLASSIFIED (N99)

● **N99   Intraoperative and postprocedural complications and disorders of genitourinary system, not elsewhere classified**
> **Excludes2** irradiation cystitis (N30.4-)
> postoophorectomy osteoporosis with current pathological fracture (M80.8-)
> postoophorectomy osteoporosis without current pathological fracture (M81.8)

N99.0   Postprocedural (acute) (chronic) kidney failure
Use additional code to type of kidney disease

● **N99.1   Postprocedural urethral stricture**
Postcatheterization urethral stricture

> ● **N99.11   Postprocedural urethral stricture, male**
> **N99.110   Postprocedural urethral stricture, male, meatal**
> ➡ **N99.111   Postprocedural bulbous urethral stricture, male**
> ➡ **N99.112   Postprocedural membranous urethral stricture, male**
> ➡ **N99.113   Postprocedural anterior bulbous urethral stricture, male**
> **N99.114   Postprocedural urethral stricture, male, unspecified**
> **N99.115   Postprocedural fossa navicularis urethral stricture**

> **N99.12   Postprocedural urethral stricture, female**

N99.2   Postprocedural adhesions of vagina

N99.3   Prolapse of vaginal vault after hysterectomy

N99.4   Postprocedural pelvic peritoneal adhesions
> **Excludes2** pelvic peritoneal adhesions NOS (N73.6)
> postinfective pelvic peritoneal adhesions (N73.6)

● **N99.5   Complications of stoma of urinary tract**
> **Excludes2** mechanical complication of urinary catheter (T83.0-)

> ● **N99.51   Complication of cystostomy**
> **N99.510   Cystostomy hemorrhage**
> **N99.511   Cystostomy infection**
> **N99.512   Cystostomy malfunction**
> **N99.518   Other cystostomy complication**

> ● **N99.52   Complication of incontinent external stoma of urinary tract**
> **N99.520   Hemorrhage of incontinent external stoma of urinary tract**
> **N99.521   Infection of incontinent external stoma of urinary tract**
> **N99.522   Malfunction of incontinent external stoma of urinary tract**
> **N99.523   Herniation of incontinent stoma of urinary tract**
> **N99.524   Stenosis of incontinent stoma of urinary tract**
> **N99.528   Other complication of incontinent external stoma of urinary tract**

CHAPTER 14 (N00-N99)

▶ New   ➡ Revised   ~~deleted~~ Deleted   **OGCR** Official Guidelines   X Assign placeholder X   ● Use Additional Character(s)

Excludes 1   Excludes 2   Includes   Use additional   Code first   Code also   Key words

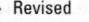

● N99.53 Complication of continent stoma of urinary tract

    N99.530 Hemorrhage of continent stoma of urinary tract

    N99.531 Infection of continent stoma of urinary tract

    N99.532 Malfunction of continent stoma of urinary tract

    N99.533 Herniation of continent stoma of urinary tract

    N99.534 Stenosis of continent stoma of urinary tract

    N99.538 Other complication of continent stoma of urinary tract

● N99.6 Intraoperative hemorrhage and hematoma of a genitourinary system organ or structure complicating a procedure

    Excludes1   intraoperative hemorrhage and hematoma of a genitourinary system organ or structure due to accidental puncture or laceration during a procedure (N99.7-)

    N99.61 Intraoperative hemorrhage and hematoma of a genitourinary system organ or structure complicating a genitourinary system procedure

    N99.62 Intraoperative hemorrhage and hematoma of a genitourinary system organ or structure complicating other procedure

● N99.7 Accidental puncture and laceration of a genitourinary system organ or structure during a procedure

    N99.71 Accidental puncture and laceration of a genitourinary system organ or structure during a genitourinary system procedure

    N99.72 Accidental puncture and laceration of a genitourinary system organ or structure during other procedure

● N99.8 Other intraoperative and postprocedural complications and disorders of genitourinary system

    N99.81 Other intraoperative complications of genitourinary system

● N99.82 Postprocedural hemorrhage of a genitourinary system organ or structure following a procedure

    N99.820 Postprocedural hemorrhage of a genitourinary system organ or structure following a genitourinary system procedure

    N99.821 Postprocedural hemorrhage of a genitourinary system organ or structure following other procedure

    N99.83 Residual ovary syndrome

● N99.84 Postprocedural hematoma and seroma of a genitourinary system organ or structure following a procedure

    N99.840 Postprocedural hematoma of a genitourinary system organ or structure following a genitourinary system procedure

    N99.841 Postprocedural hematoma of a genitourinary system organ or structure following other procedure

    N99.842 Postprocedural seroma of a genitourinary system organ or structure following a genitourinary system procedure

    N99.843 Postprocedural seroma of a genitourinary system organ or structure following other procedure

    N99.89 Other postprocedural complications and disorders of genitourinary system

▶ New   ⇒ Revised   deleted Deleted   **OGCR** Official Guidelines   X Assign placeholder X   ● Use Additional Character(s)

Excludes 1   Excludes 2   Includes   Use additional   Code first   Code also   Key words

CHAPTER 15

PREGNANCY, CHILDBIRTH AND THE PUERPERIUM (O00-O9A)

OGCR Chapter-Specific Coding Guidelines

15. Chapter 15: Pregnancy, Childbirth, and the Puerperium (O00-O9A)

a. General Rules for Obstetric Cases

1) Codes from chapter 15 and sequencing priority

Obstetric cases require codes from chapter 15, codes in the range O00-O9A, Pregnancy, Childbirth, and the Puerperium. Chapter 15 codes have sequencing priority over codes from other chapters. Additional codes from other chapters may be used in conjunction with chapter 15 codes to further specify conditions. Should the provider document that the pregnancy is incidental to the encounter, then code Z33.1, Pregnant state, incidental, should be used in place of any chapter 15 codes. It is the provider's responsibility to state that the condition being treated is not affecting the pregnancy.

2) Chapter 15 codes used only on the maternal record

Chapter 15 codes are to be used only on the maternal record, never on the record of the newborn.

3) Final character for trimester

The majority of codes in Chapter 15 have a final character indicating the trimester of pregnancy. The timeframes for the trimesters are indicated at the beginning of the chapter. If trimester is not a component of a code it is because the condition always occurs in a specific trimester, or the concept of trimester of pregnancy is not applicable. Certain codes have characters for only certain trimesters because the condition does not occur in all trimesters, but it may occur in more than just one.

Assignment of the final character for trimester should be based on the provider's documentation of the trimester (or number of weeks) for the current admission/encounter. This applies to the assignment of trimester for pre-existing conditions as well as those that develop during or are due to the pregnancy. The provider's documentation of the number of weeks may be used to assign the appropriate code identifying the trimester.

Whenever delivery occurs during the current admission, and there is an "in childbirth" option for the obstetric complication being coded, the "in childbirth" code should be assigned.

4) Selection of trimester for inpatient admissions that encompass more than one trimester

In instances when a patient is admitted to a hospital for complications of pregnancy during one trimester and remains in the hospital into a subsequent trimester, the trimester character for the antepartum complication code should be assigned on the basis of the trimester when the complication developed, not the trimester of the discharge. If the condition developed prior to the current admission/encounter or represents a pre-existing condition, the trimester character for the trimester at the time of the admission/encounter should be assigned.

5) Unspecified trimester

Each category that includes codes for trimester has a code for "unspecified trimester." The "unspecified trimester" code should rarely be used, such as when the documentation in the record is insufficient to determine the trimester and it is not possible to obtain clarification.

6) 7th character for Fetus Identification

Where applicable, a 7th character is to be assigned for certain categories (O31, O32, O33.3 - O33.6, O35, O36, O40, O41, O60.1, O60.2, O64, and O69) to identify the fetus for which the complication code applies.

Assign 7th character "0":
- For single gestations
- When the documentation in the record is insufficient to determine the fetus affected and it is not possible to obtain clarification.
- When it is not possible to clinically determine which fetus is affected.

b. Selection of OB Principal or First-listed Diagnosis

1) Routine outpatient prenatal visits

For routine outpatient prenatal visits when no complications are present, a code from category Z34, Encounter for supervision of normal pregnancy, should be used as the first-listed diagnosis. These codes should not be used in conjunction with chapter 15 codes.

2) Supervision of High-Risk Pregnancy

Codes from category O09, Supervision of high-risk pregnancy, are intended for use only during the prenatal period. For complications during the labor or delivery episode as a result of a high-risk pregnancy, assign the applicable complication codes from Chapter 15. If there are no complications during the labor or delivery episode, assign code O80, Encounter for full-term uncomplicated delivery.

For routine prenatal outpatient visits for patients with high-risk pregnancies, a code from category O09, Supervision of high-risk pregnancy, should be used as the first-listed diagnosis. Secondary chapter 15 codes may be used in conjunction with these codes if appropriate.

3) Episodes when no delivery occurs

In episodes when no delivery occurs, the principal diagnosis should correspond to the principal complication of the pregnancy which necessitated the encounter. Should more than one complication exist, all of which are treated or monitored, any of the complications codes may be sequenced first.

4) When a delivery occurs

When an obstetric patient is admitted and delivers during that admission, the condition that prompted the admission should be sequenced as the principal diagnosis. If multiple conditions prompted the admission, sequence the one most related to the delivery as the principal diagnosis. A code for any complication of the delivery should be assigned as an additional diagnosis. In cases of cesarean delivery, if the patient was admitted with a condition that resulted in the performance of a cesarean procedure, that condition should be selected as the principal diagnosis. If the reason for the admission was unrelated to the condition resulting in the cesarean delivery, the condition related to the reason for the admission should be selected as the principal diagnosis.

5) Outcome of delivery

A code from category Z37, Outcome of delivery, should be included on every maternal record when a delivery has occurred. These codes are not to be used on subsequent records or on the newborn record.

c. Pre-existing conditions versus conditions due to the pregnancy

Certain categories in Chapter 15 distinguish between conditions of the mother that existed prior to pregnancy (pre-existing) and those that are a direct result of pregnancy. When assigning codes from Chapter 15, it is important to assess if a condition was pre-existing prior to pregnancy or developed during or due to the pregnancy in order to assign the correct code.

Categories that do not distinguish between pre-existing and pregnancy-related conditions may be used for either. It is acceptable to use codes specifically for the puerperium with codes complicating pregnancy and childbirth if a condition arises postpartum during the delivery encounter.

d. Pre-existing hypertension in pregnancy

Category O10, Pre-existing hypertension complicating pregnancy, childbirth and the puerperium, includes codes for hypertensive heart and hypertensive chronic kidney disease. When assigning one of the O10 codes that includes hypertensive heart disease or hypertensive chronic kidney disease, it is necessary to add a secondary code from the appropriate hypertension category to specify the type of heart failure or chronic kidney disease.

See Section I.C.9. Hypertension.

e. Fetal Conditions Affecting the Management of the Mother

1) Codes from categories O35 and O36

Codes from categories O35, Maternal care for known or suspected fetal abnormality and damage, and O36, Maternal care for other fetal problems, are assigned only when the fetal condition is actually responsible for modifying the management of the mother, i.e., by requiring diagnostic studies, additional observation, special care, or termination of pregnancy. The fact that the fetal condition exists does not justify assigning a code from this series to the mother's record.

2) In utero surgery

In cases when surgery is performed on the fetus, a diagnosis code from category O35, Maternal care for known or suspected fetal abnormality and damage, should be assigned identifying the fetal condition. Assign the appropriate procedure code for the procedure performed.

No code from Chapter 16, the perinatal codes, should be used on the mother's record to identify fetal conditions. Surgery performed in utero on a fetus is still to be coded as an obstetric encounter.

f. HIV Infection in Pregnancy, Childbirth and the Puerperium

During pregnancy, childbirth or the puerperium, a patient admitted because of an HIV-related illness should receive a principal diagnosis from subcategory O98.7-, Human immunodeficiency [HIV] disease complicating pregnancy, childbirth and the puerperium, followed by the code(s) for the HIV-related illness(es).

Patients with asymptomatic HIV infection status admitted during pregnancy, childbirth, or the puerperium should receive codes of O98.7- and Z21, Asymptomatic human immunodeficiency virus [HIV] infection status.

g. Diabetes mellitus in pregnancy

Diabetes mellitus is a significant complicating factor in pregnancy. Pregnant women who are diabetic should be assigned a code from category O24, Diabetes mellitus in pregnancy, childbirth, and the puerperium, first, followed by the appropriate diabetes code(s) (E08-E13) from Chapter 4.

h. Long term use of insulin and oral hypoglycemics
See section I.C.4.a.3 for information on the long term use of insulin and oral hypoglycemic.

i. Gestational (pregnancy induced) diabetes
Gestational (pregnancy induced) diabetes can occur during the second and third trimester of pregnancy in women who were not diabetic prior to pregnancy. Gestational diabetes can cause complications in the pregnancy similar to those of pre-existing diabetes mellitus. It also puts the woman at greater risk of developing diabetes after the pregnancy. Codes for gestational diabetes are in subcategory O24.4, Gestational diabetes mellitus. No other code from category O24, Diabetes mellitus in pregnancy, childbirth, and the puerperium, should be used with a code from O24.4.

The codes under subcategory O24.4 include diet controlled, insulin controlled, and controlled by oral hypoglycemic drugs. If a patient with gestational diabetes is treated with both diet and insulin, only the code for insulin-controlled is required. If a patient with gestational diabetes is treated with both diet and oral hypoglycemic medications, only the code for "controlled by oral hypoglycemic drugs" is required. Code Z79.4, Long-term (current) use of insulin or code Z79.84, Long-term (current) use of oral hypoglycemic drugs, should not be assigned with codes from subcategory O24.4.

An abnormal glucose tolerance in pregnancy is assigned a code from subcategory O99.81, Abnormal glucose complicating pregnancy, childbirth, and the puerperium.

j. Sepsis and septic shock complicating abortion, pregnancy, childbirth and the puerperium
When assigning a chapter 15 code for sepsis complicating abortion, pregnancy, childbirth, and the puerperium, a code for the specific type of infection should be assigned as an additional diagnosis. If severe sepsis is present, a code from subcategory R65.2, Severe sepsis, and code(s) for associated organ dysfunction(s) should also be assigned as additional diagnoses.

k. Puerperal sepsis
Code O85, Puerperal sepsis, should be assigned with a secondary code to identify the causal organism (e.g., for a bacterial infection, assign a code from category B95-B96, Bacterial infections in conditions classified elsewhere). A code from category A40, Streptococcal sepsis, or A41, Other sepsis, should not be used for puerperal sepsis. If applicable, use additional codes to identify severe sepsis (R65.2-) and any associated acute organ dysfunction.

l. Alcohol and tobacco use during pregnancy, childbirth and the puerperium
1) Alcohol use during pregnancy, childbirth and the puerperium
Codes under subcategory O99.31, Alcohol use complicating pregnancy, childbirth, and the puerperium, should be assigned for any pregnancy case when a mother uses alcohol during the pregnancy or postpartum. A secondary code from category F10, Alcohol related disorders, should also be assigned to identify manifestations of the alcohol use.

2) Tobacco use during pregnancy, childbirth and the puerperium
Codes under subcategory O99.33, Smoking (tobacco) complicating pregnancy, childbirth, and the puerperium, should be assigned for any pregnancy case when a mother uses any type of tobacco product during the pregnancy or postpartum. A secondary code from category F17, Nicotine dependence, should also be assigned to identify the type of nicotine dependence.

m. Poisoning, toxic effects, adverse effects and underdosing in a pregnant patient
A code from subcategory O9A.2, Injury, poisoning and certain other consequences of external causes complicating pregnancy, childbirth, and the puerperium, should be sequenced first, followed by the appropriate injury, poisoning, toxic effect, adverse effect or underdosing code, and then the additional code(s) that specifies the condition caused by the poisoning, toxic effect, adverse effect or underdosing.
See Section I.C.19. Adverse effects, poisoning, underdosing and toxic effects.

n. Normal Delivery, Code O80
1) Encounter for full term uncomplicated delivery
Code O80 should be assigned when a woman is admitted for a full-term normal delivery and delivers a single, healthy infant without any complications antepartum, during the delivery, or postpartum during the delivery episode. Code O80 is always a principal diagnosis. It is not to be used if any other code from chapter 15 is needed to describe a current complication of the antenatal, delivery, or perinatal period. Additional codes from other chapters may be used with code O80 if they are not related to or are in any way complicating the pregnancy.

2) Uncomplicated delivery with resolved antepartum complication
Code O80 may be used if the patient had a complication at some point during the pregnancy, but the complication is not present at the time of the admission for delivery.

3) Outcome of delivery for O80
Z37.0, Single live birth, is the only outcome of delivery code appropriate for use with O80.

o. The Peripartum and Postpartum Periods
1) Peripartum and Postpartum periods
The postpartum period begins immediately after delivery and continues for six weeks following delivery. The peripartum period is defined as the last month of pregnancy to five months postpartum.

2) Peripartum and postpartum complication
A postpartum complication is any complication occurring within the six-week period.

3) Pregnancy-related complications after 6 week period
Chapter 15 codes may also be used to describe pregnancy-related complications after the peripartum or postpartum period if the provider documents that a condition is pregnancy related.

4) Admission for routine postpartum care following delivery outside hospital
When the mother delivers outside the hospital prior to admission and is admitted for routine postpartum care and no complications are noted, code Z39.0, Encounter for care and examination of mother immediately after delivery, should be assigned as the principal diagnosis.

5) Pregnancy associated cardiomyopathy
Pregnancy associated cardiomyopathy, code O90.3, is unique in that it may be diagnosed in the third trimester of pregnancy but may continue to progress months after delivery. For this reason, it is referred to as peripartum cardiomyopathy. Code O90.3 is only for use when the cardiomyopathy develops as a result of pregnancy in a woman who did not have pre-existing heart disease.

p. Code O94, Sequelae of complication of pregnancy, childbirth, and the puerperium
1) Code O94
Code O94, Sequelae of complication of pregnancy, childbirth, and the puerperium, is for use in those cases when an initial complication of a pregnancy develops a sequelae requiring care or treatment at a future date.

2) After the initial postpartum period
This code may be used at any time after the initial postpartum period.

3) Sequencing of Code O94
This code, like all sequela codes, is to be sequenced following the code describing the sequelae of the complication.

q. Termination of Pregnancy and Spontaneous abortions
1) Abortion with Liveborn Fetus
When an attempted termination of pregnancy results in a liveborn fetus assign code Z33.2, Encounter for elective termination of pregnancy and a code from category Z37, Outcome of Delivery.

2) Retained Products of Conception following an abortion
Subsequent encounters for retained products of conception following a spontaneous abortion or elective termination of pregnancy, **without complications** are assigned O03.4, **Incomplete spontaneous,** abortion **without complication,** or codes O07.4, Failed attempted termination of pregnancy without complication. This advice is appropriate even when the patient was discharged previously with a discharge diagnosis of complete abortion.
If the patient has a specific complication associated with the spontaneous abortion or elective termination of pregnancy in addition to retained products of conception, assign the appropriate complication in category O03 or O07 instead of code O03.4 or O07.4

3) Complications leading to abortion
Codes from Chapter 15 may be used as additional codes to identify any documented complications of the pregnancy in conjunction with codes in categories in O04, O07 and O08.

r. Abuse in a pregnant patient
For suspected or confirmed cases of abuse of a pregnant patient, a code(s) from subcategories O9A.3, Physical abuse complicating pregnancy, childbirth, and the puerperium, O9A.4, Sexual abuse complicating pregnancy, childbirth, and the puerperium, and O9A.5, Psychological abuse complicating pregnancy, childbirth, and the puerperium, should be sequenced first, followed by the appropriate codes (if applicable) to identify any associated current injury due to physical abuse, sexual abuse, and the perpetrator of abuse.
See Section I.C.19. Adult and child abuse, neglect and other maltreatment.

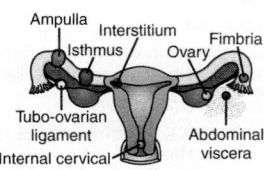

Figure 15-1 Implantation sites of ectopic pregnancy.

Item 15–1 Ectopic pregnancy most often occurs in the fallopian tube. Pregnancy outside the uterus may end in a lifethreatening rupture.

★ **(See Plate 375 on page 52.)**

CHAPTER 15

PREGNANCY, CHILDBIRTH AND THE PUERPERIUM (O00-O9A)

Note: CODES FROM THIS CHAPTER ARE FOR USE ONLY ON MATERNAL RECORDS, NEVER ON NEWBORN RECORDS

Codes from this chapter are for use for conditions related to or aggravated by the pregnancy, childbirth, or by the puerperium (maternal causes or obstetric causes)

Trimesters are counted from the first day of the last menstrual period. They are defined as follows:

1st trimester - less than 14 weeks 0 days

2nd trimester - 14 weeks 0 days to less than 28 weeks 0 days

3rd trimester - 28 weeks 0 days until delivery

Use additional code from category Z3A, Weeks of gestation, to identify the specific week of the pregnancy, if known.

| Excludes1 | supervision of normal pregnancy (Z34.-) |
| Excludes2 | mental and behavioral disorders associated with the puerperium (F53) |

obstetrical tetanus (A34)

postpartum necrosis of pituitary gland (E23.0)

puerperal osteomalacia (M83.0)

This chapter contains the following blocks:

O00-O08	Pregnancy with abortive outcome
O09	Supervision of high risk pregnancy
O10-O16	Edema, proteinuria and hypertensive disorders in pregnancy, childbirth and the puerperium
O20-O29	Other maternal disorders predominantly related to pregnancy
O30-O48	Maternal care related to the fetus and amniotic cavity and possible delivery problems
O60-O77	Complications of labor and delivery
O80, O82	Encounter for delivery
O85-O92	Complications predominantly related to the puerperium
O94-O9A	Other obstetric conditions, not elsewhere classified

PREGNANCY WITH ABORTIVE OUTCOME (O00-O08)

| Excludes1 | continuing pregnancy in multiple gestation after abortion of one fetus or more (O31.1-, O31.3-) |

● **O00 Ectopic pregnancy**

     Includes   ruptured ectopic pregnancy

     Use additional code from category O08 to identify any associated complication

● **O00.0 Abdominal pregnancy**

     | Excludes1 | maternal care for viable fetus in abdominal pregnancy (O36.7-) |

     O00.00 Abdominal pregnancy without intrauterine pregnancy

         Abdominal pregnancy NOS

     O00.01 Abdominal pregnancy with intrauterine pregnancy

● **O00.1 Tubal pregnancy**

     Fallopian pregnancy

     Rupture of (fallopian) tube due to pregnancy

     Tubal abortion

     ● **O00.10 Tubal pregnancy without intrauterine pregnancy**

         Tubal pregnancy NOS

         ▶ **O00.101 Right tubal pregnancy without intrauterine pregnancy**

         ▶ **O00.102 Left tubal pregnancy without intrauterine pregnancy**

         ▶ **O00.109 Unspecified tubal pregnancy without intrauterine pregnancy**

     ● **O00.11 Tubal pregnancy with intrauterine pregnancy**

         ▶ **O00.111 Right tubal pregnancy with intrauterine pregnancy**

         ▶ **O00.112 Left tubal pregnancy with intrauterine pregnancy**

         ▶ **O00.119 Unspecified tubal pregnancy with intrauterine pregnancy**

● **O00.2 Ovarian pregnancy**

     ● **O00.20 Ovarian pregnancy without intrauterine pregnancy**

         Ovarian pregnancy NOS

         ▶ **O00.201 Right ovarian pregnancy without intrauterine pregnancy**

         ▶ **O00.202 Left ovarian pregnancy without intrauterine pregnancy**

         ▶ **O00.209 Unspecified ovarian pregnancy without intrauterine pregnancy**

     ● **O00.21 Ovarian pregnancy with intrauterine pregnancy**

         ▶ **O00.211 Right ovarian pregnancy with intrauterine pregnancy**

         ▶ **O00.212 Left ovarian pregnancy with intrauterine pregnancy**

         ▶ **O00.219 Unspecified ovarian pregnancy with intrauterine pregnancy**

● **O00.8 Other ectopic pregnancy**

     Cervical pregnancy

     Cornual pregnancy

     Intraligamentous pregnancy

     Mural pregnancy

     O00.80 Other ectopic pregnancy without intrauterine pregnancy

         Other ectopic pregnancy NOS

     O00.81 Other ectopic pregnancy with intrauterine pregnancy

● **O00.9 Ectopic pregnancy, unspecified**

     O00.90 Unspecified ectopic pregnancy without intrauterine pregnancy

         Ectopic pregnancy NOS

     O00.91 Unspecified ectopic pregnancy with intrauterine pregnancy

---

▶ New   ⇒ Revised   ~~deleted~~ Deleted   **OGCR** Official Guidelines   X Assign placeholder X   ● Use Additional Character(s)

| Excludes 1 | | Excludes 2 | | Includes | Use additional | | Code first | Code also | Key words |

● **O01   Hydatidiform mole**
    Use additional code from category O08 to identify any
    associated complication
    Excludes1   chorioadenoma (destruens) (D39.2)
                    malignant hydatidiform mole (D39.2)

O01.0   Classical hydatidiform mole
    Complete hydatidiform mole

O01.1   Incomplete and partial hydatidiform mole

O01.9   Hydatidiform mole, unspecified
    Trophoblastic disease NOS
    Vesicular mole NOS

● **O02   Other abnormal products of conception**
    Use additional code from category O08 to identify any
    associated complication
    Excludes1   papyraceous fetus (O31.0-)

O02.0   Blighted ovum and nonhydatidiform mole
    Carneous mole   Molar pregnancy NEC
    Fleshy mole   Pathological ovum
    Intrauterine mole NOS

O02.1   Missed abortion
    Early fetal death, before completion of 20 weeks of
       gestation, with retention of dead fetus
    Excludes1   failed induced abortion (O07.-)
                  fetal death (intrauterine) (late) (O36.4)
                  missed abortion with blighted ovum
                      (O02.0)
                  missed abortion with hydatidiform mole
                      (O01.-)
                  missed abortion with nonhydatidiform
                      (O02.0)
                  missed abortion with other abnormal
                      products of conception (O02.8-)
                  missed delivery (O36.4)
                  stillbirth (P95)

● **O02.8   Other specified abnormal products of conception**
    Excludes1   abnormal products of conception with
                  blighted ovum (O02.0)
                  abnormal products of conception with
                  hydatidiform mole (O01.-)
                  abnormal products of conception with
                  nonhydatidiform mole (O02.0)

**O02.81   Inappropriate change in quantitative human
        chorionic gonadotropin (hCG) in early
        pregnancy**
    Biochemical pregnancy
    Chemical pregnancy
    Inappropriate level of quantitative human
       chorionic gonadotropin (hCG) for
       gestational age in early pregnancy

O02.89   Other abnormal products of conception

O02.9   Abnormal product of conception, unspecified

● **O03   Spontaneous abortion**
    Note: Incomplete abortion includes retained products of
       conception following spontaneous abortion.
    Includes   miscarriage

**O03.0   Genital tract and pelvic infection following incomplete
      spontaneous abortion**
    Endometritis following incomplete spontaneous
       abortion
    Oophoritis following incomplete spontaneous abortion
    Parametritis following incomplete spontaneous
       abortion
    Pelvic peritonitis following incomplete spontaneous
       abortion
    Salpingitis following incomplete spontaneous abortion
    Salpingo-oophoritis following incomplete spontaneous
       abortion
    Excludes1   sepsis following incomplete spontaneous
                  abortion (O03.37)
                  urinary tract infection following
                      incomplete spontaneous abortion
                      (O03.38)

**O03.1   Delayed or excessive hemorrhage following incomplete
      spontaneous abortion**
    Afibrinogenemia following incomplete spontaneous
       abortion
    Defibrination syndrome following incomplete
       spontaneous abortion
    Hemolysis following incomplete spontaneous abortion
    Intravascular coagulation following incomplete
       spontaneous abortion

O03.2   Embolism following incomplete spontaneous abortion
    Air embolism following incomplete spontaneous
       abortion
    Amniotic fluid embolism following incomplete
       spontaneous abortion
    Blood-clot embolism following incomplete spontaneous
       abortion
    Embolism NOS following incomplete spontaneous
       abortion
    Fat embolism following incomplete spontaneous
       abortion
    Pulmonary embolism following incomplete
       spontaneous abortion
    Pyemic embolism following incomplete spontaneous
       abortion
    Septic or septicopyemic embolism following incomplete
       spontaneous abortion
    Soap embolism following incomplete spontaneous
       abortion

● **O03.3   Other and unspecified complications following
      incomplete spontaneous abortion**

**O03.30   Unspecified complication following incomplete
        spontaneous abortion**

**O03.31   Shock following incomplete spontaneous
        abortion**
    Circulatory collapse following incomplete
       spontaneous abortion
    Shock (postprocedural) following incomplete
       spontaneous abortion
    Excludes1   shock due to infection following
                  incomplete spontaneous
                  abortion (O03.37)

**O03.32   Renal failure following incomplete
        spontaneous abortion**
    Kidney failure (acute) following incomplete
       spontaneous abortion
    Oliguria following incomplete spontaneous
       abortion
    Renal shutdown following incomplete
       spontaneous abortion
    Renal tubular necrosis following incomplete
       spontaneous abortion
    Uremia following incomplete spontaneous
       abortion

Item 15–2 A **hydatidiform** mole is an overproduction of placental
tissue. The tumor secretes a hormone, chorionic gonadotropic hormone (CGH),
that indicates a positive pregnancy test. There is no viable fetus. More than
80% of hydatidiform moles are noncancerous.

▶ New   ⇒ Revised   ~~deleted~~ Deleted   **OGCR** Official Guidelines   X Assign placeholder X   ● Use Additional Character(s)
Excludes 1   Excludes 2   Includes   Use additional   Code first   Code also   Key words

O03.33 **Metabolic disorder** following incomplete
spontaneous abortion

O03.34 **Damage to pelvic organs** following incomplete
spontaneous abortion
    Laceration, perforation, tear or chemical
damage of bladder following incomplete
spontaneous abortion
    Laceration, perforation, tear or chemical
damage of bowel following incomplete
spontaneous abortion
    Laceration, perforation, tear or chemical
damage of broad ligament following
incomplete spontaneous abortion
    Laceration, perforation, tear or chemical
damage of cervix following incomplete
spontaneous abortion
    Laceration, perforation, tear or chemical
damage of periurethral tissue following
incomplete spontaneous abortion
    Laceration, perforation, tear or chemical
damage of uterus following incomplete
spontaneous abortion
    Laceration, perforation, tear or chemical
damage of vagina following incomplete
spontaneous abortion

O03.35 **Other venous complications** following
incomplete spontaneous abortion

O03.36 **Cardiac arrest** following incomplete
spontaneous abortion

O03.37 **Sepsis** following incomplete spontaneous
abortion
    Use additional code to identify infectious
agent (B95-B97)
    Use additional code to identify severe sepsis, if
applicable (R65.2-)
    | Excludes1 | septic or septicopyemic
embolism following
incomplete spontaneous
abortion (O03.2)

O03.38 **Urinary tract infection** following incomplete
spontaneous abortion
    Cystitis following incomplete spontaneous
abortion

O03.39 Incomplete spontaneous abortion **with other
complications**

O03.4 Incomplete spontaneous abortion **without complication**

O03.5 **Genital tract and pelvic infection** following **complete or
unspecified** spontaneous abortion
    Endometritis following complete or unspecified
spontaneous abortion
    Oophoritis following complete or unspecified
spontaneous abortion
    Parametritis following complete or unspecified
spontaneous abortion
    Pelvic peritonitis following complete or unspecified
spontaneous abortion
    Salpingitis following complete or unspecified
spontaneous abortion
    Salpingo-oophoritis following complete or unspecified
spontaneous abortion
    | Excludes1 | sepsis following complete or unspecified
spontaneous abortion (O03.87)
urinary tract infection following complete
or unspecified spontaneous abortion
(O03.88)

O03.6 **Delayed or excessive hemorrhage** following **complete or
unspecified** spontaneous abortion
    Afibrinogenemia following complete or unspecified
spontaneous abortion
    Defibrination syndrome following complete or
unspecified spontaneous abortion
    Hemolysis following complete or unspecified
spontaneous abortion
    Intravascular coagulation following complete or
unspecified spontaneous abortion

O03.7 **Embolism** following **complete or unspecified**
spontaneous abortion
    Air embolism following complete or unspecified
spontaneous abortion
    Amniotic fluid embolism following complete or
unspecified spontaneous abortion
    Blood-clot embolism following complete or unspecified
spontaneous abortion
    Embolism NOS following complete or unspecified
spontaneous abortion
    Fat embolism following complete or unspecified
spontaneous abortion
    Pulmonary embolism following complete or
unspecified spontaneous abortion
    Pyemic embolism following complete or unspecified
spontaneous abortion
    Septic or septicopyemic embolism following complete
or unspecified spontaneous abortion
    Soap embolism following complete or unspecified
spontaneous abortion

● O03.8 **Other and unspecified** complications following
complete or unspecified spontaneous abortion

O03.80 **Unspecified** complication following complete
or unspecified spontaneous abortion

O03.81 **Shock** following complete or **unspecified**
spontaneous abortion
    Circulatory collapse following complete or
unspecified spontaneous abortion
    Shock (postprocedural) following complete or
unspecified spontaneous abortion
    | Excludes1 | shock due to infection following
complete or unspecified
spontaneous abortion
(O03.87)

O03.82 **Renal failure** following **complete or unspecified**
spontaneous abortion
    Kidney failure (acute) following complete or
unspecified spontaneous abortion
    Oliguria following complete or unspecified
spontaneous abortion
    Renal shutdown following complete or
unspecified spontaneous abortion
    Renal tubular necrosis following complete or
unspecified spontaneous abortion
    Uremia following complete or unspecified
spontaneous abortion

O03.83 **Metabolic disorder** following **complete** or
unspecified spontaneous abortion

O03.84 **Damage to pelvic organs** following **complete or
unspecified** spontaneous abortion
    Laceration, perforation, tear or chemical
damage of bladder following complete or
unspecified spontaneous abortion
    Laceration, perforation, tear or chemical
damage of bowel following complete or
unspecified spontaneous abortion
    Laceration, perforation, tear or chemical
damage of broad ligament following
complete or unspecified spontaneous
abortion
    Laceration, perforation, tear or chemical
damage of cervix following complete or
unspecified spontaneous abortion
    Laceration, perforation, tear or chemical
damage of periurethral tissue following
complete or unspecified spontaneous
abortion
    Laceration, perforation, tear or chemical
damage of uterus following complete or
unspecified spontaneous abortion
    Laceration, perforation, tear or chemical
damage of vagina following complete or
unspecified spontaneous abortion

O03.85   Other venous complications following complete or unspecified spontaneous abortion

O03.86   Cardiac arrest following complete or unspecified spontaneous abortion

O03.87   Sepsis following complete or unspecified spontaneous abortion

Use additional code to identify infectious agent (B95-B97)

Use additional code to identify severe sepsis, if applicable (R65.2-)

Excludes1   septic or septicopyemic embolism following complete or unspecified spontaneous abortion (O03.7)

O03.88   Urinary tract infection following complete or unspecified spontaneous abortion

Cystitis following complete or unspecified spontaneous abortion

O03.89   Complete or unspecified spontaneous abortion with other complications

O03.9   Complete or unspecified spontaneous abortion without complication

Miscarriage NOS
Spontaneous abortion NOS

● **O04**   Complications following (induced) termination of pregnancy

Includes   complications following (induced) termination of pregnancy

Excludes1   encounter for elective termination of pregnancy, uncomplicated (Z33.2)
failed attempted termination of pregnancy (O07.-)

O04.5   Genital tract and pelvic infection following (induced) termination of pregnancy

Endometritis following (induced) termination of pregnancy
Oophoritis following (induced) termination of pregnancy
Parametritis following (induced) termination of pregnancy
Pelvic peritonitis following (induced) termination of pregnancy
Salpingitis following (induced) termination of pregnancy
Salpingo-oophoritis following (induced) termination of pregnancy

Excludes1   sepsis following (induced) termination of pregnancy (O04.87)
urinary tract infection following (induced) termination of pregnancy (O04.88)

O04.6   Delayed or excessive hemorrhage following (induced) termination of pregnancy

Afibrinogenemia following (induced) termination of pregnancy
Defibrination syndrome following (induced) termination of pregnancy
Hemolysis following (induced) termination of pregnancy
Intravascular coagulation following (induced) termination of pregnancy

O04.7   Embolism following (induced) termination of pregnancy

Air embolism following (induced) termination of pregnancy
Amniotic fluid embolism following (induced) termination of pregnancy
Blood-clot embolism following (induced) termination of pregnancy
Embolism NOS following (induced) termination of pregnancy
Fat embolism following (induced) termination of pregnancy
Pulmonary embolism following (induced) termination of pregnancy
Pyemic embolism following (induced) termination of pregnancy
Septic or septicopyemic embolism following (induced) termination of pregnancy
Soap embolism following (induced) termination of pregnancy

● **O04.8**   (Induced) termination of pregnancy with other and unspecified complications

O04.80   (Induced) termination of pregnancy with unspecified complications

O04.81   Shock following (induced) termination of pregnancy

Circulatory collapse following (induced) termination of pregnancy
Shock (postprocedural) following (induced) termination of pregnancy

Excludes1   shock due to infection following (induced) termination of pregnancy (O04.87)

O04.82   Renal failure following (induced) termination of pregnancy

Kidney failure (acute) following (induced) termination of pregnancy
Oliguria following (induced) termination of pregnancy
Renal shutdown following (induced) termination of pregnancy
Renal tubular necrosis following (induced) termination of pregnancy
Uremia following (induced) termination of pregnancy

O04.83   Metabolic disorder following (induced) termination of pregnancy

O04.84   Damage to pelvic organs following (induced) termination of pregnancy

Laceration, perforation, tear or chemical damage of bladder following (induced) termination of pregnancy
Laceration, perforation, tear or chemical damage of bowel following (induced) termination of pregnancy
Laceration, perforation, tear or chemical damage of broad ligament following (induced) termination of pregnancy
Laceration, perforation, tear or chemical damage of cervix following (induced) termination of pregnancy
Laceration, perforation, tear or chemical damage of periurethral tissue following (induced) termination of pregnancy
Laceration, perforation, tear or chemical damage of uterus following (induced) termination of pregnancy
Laceration, perforation, tear or chemical damage of vagina following (induced) termination of pregnancy

O04.85   Other venous complications following
         (induced) termination of pregnancy

O04.86   Cardiac arrest following (induced) termination
         of pregnancy

O04.87   Sepsis following (induced) termination of
         pregnancy

> Use additional code to identify infectious
> agent (B95-B97)
>
> Use additional code to identify severe sepsis, if
> applicable (R65.2-)
>
> **Excludes 1**   septic or septicopyemic
> embolism following
> (induced) termination of
> pregnancy (O04.7)

O04.88   Urinary tract infection following (induced)
         termination of pregnancy

> Cystitis following (induced) termination of
> pregnancy

O04.89   (Induced) termination of pregnancy with other
         complications

● **O07   Failed attempted termination of pregnancy**

> **Includes**   failure of attempted induction of termination of
> pregnancy
> incomplete elective abortion
>
> **Excludes 1**   incomplete spontaneous abortion (O03.0-)

O07.0   Genital tract and pelvic infection following failed
        attempted termination of pregnancy

> Endometritis following failed attempted termination of
> pregnancy
> Oophoritis following failed attempted termination of
> pregnancy
> Parametritis following failed attempted termination of
> pregnancy
> Pelvic peritonitis following failed attempted
> termination of pregnancy
> Salpingitis following failed attempted termination of
> pregnancy
> Salpingo-oophoritis following failed attempted
> termination of pregnancy
>
> **Excludes 1**   sepsis following failed attempted
> termination of pregnancy (O07.37)
> urinary tract infection following failed
> attempted termination of pregnancy
> (O07.38)

O07.1   Delayed or excessive hemorrhage following failed
        attempted termination of pregnancy

> Afibrinogenemia following failed attempted
> termination of pregnancy
> Defibrination syndrome following failed attempted
> termination of pregnancy
> Hemolysis following failed attempted termination of
> pregnancy
> Intravascular coagulation following failed attempted
> termination of pregnancy

O07.2   Embolism following failed attempted termination of
        pregnancy

> Air embolism following failed attempted termination of
> pregnancy
> Amniotic fluid embolism following failed attempted
> termination of pregnancy
> Blood-clot embolism following failed attempted
> termination of pregnancy
> Embolism NOS following failed attempted termination
> of pregnancy
> Fat embolism following failed attempted termination of
> pregnancy
> Pulmonary embolism following failed attempted
> termination of pregnancy
> Pyemic embolism following failed attempted
> termination of pregnancy
> Septic or septicopyemic embolism following failed
> attempted termination of pregnancy
> Soap embolism following failed attempted termination
> of pregnancy

● O07.3   Failed attempted termination of pregnancy with other
          and unspecified complications

O07.30   Failed attempted termination of pregnancy with
         unspecified complications

O07.31   Shock following failed attempted termination
         of pregnancy

> Circulatory collapse following failed attempted
> termination of pregnancy
> Shock (postprocedural) following failed
> attempted termination of pregnancy
>
> **Excludes 1**   shock due to infection following
> failed attempted termination
> of pregnancy (O07.37)

O07.32   Renal failure following failed attempted
         termination of pregnancy

> Kidney failure (acute) following failed
> attempted termination of pregnancy
> Oliguria following failed attempted
> termination of pregnancy
> Renal shutdown following failed attempted
> termination of pregnancy
> Renal tubular necrosis following failed
> attempted termination of pregnancy
> Uremia following failed attempted termination
> of pregnancy

O07.33   Metabolic disorder following failed attempted
         termination of pregnancy

O07.34   Damage to pelvic organs following failed
         attempted termination of pregnancy

> Laceration, perforation, tear or chemical
> damage of bladder following failed
> attempted termination of pregnancy
> Laceration, perforation, tear or chemical
> damage of bowel following failed
> attempted termination of pregnancy
> Laceration, perforation, tear or chemical
> damage of broad ligament following
> failed attempted termination of pregnancy
> Laceration, perforation, tear or chemical
> damage of cervix following failed
> attempted termination of pregnancy
> Laceration, perforation, tear or chemical
> damage of periurethral tissue following
> failed attempted termination of pregnancy
> Laceration, perforation, tear or chemical
> damage of uterus following failed
> attempted termination of pregnancy
> Laceration, perforation, tear or chemical
> damage of vagina following failed
> attempted termination of pregnancy

O07.35   Other venous complications following failed
         attempted termination of pregnancy

O07.36   Cardiac arrest following failed attempted
         termination of pregnancy

O07.37   Sepsis following failed attempted termination
         of pregnancy

> Use additional code (B95-B97), to identify
> infectious agent
>
> Use additional code (R65.2-) to identify severe
> sepsis, if applicable
>
> **Excludes 1**   septic or septicopyemic
> embolism following failed
> attempted termination of
> pregnancy (O07.2)

O07.38   Urinary tract infection following failed
         attempted termination of pregnancy

> Cystitis following failed attempted termination
> of pregnancy

O07.39   Failed attempted termination of pregnancy with
         other complications

O07.4   Failed attempted termination of pregnancy without
        complication

▶ New   ⇒ Revised   ~~deleted~~ Deleted   **OGCR** Official Guidelines   X Assign placeholder X   ● Use Additional Character(s)

Excludes 1   Excludes 2   Includes   Use additional   Code first   Code also   Key words

● **O08** **Complications following ectopic and molar pregnancy**
This category is for use with categories O00-O02 to identify any associated complications.

O08.0 **Genital tract and pelvic infection** following ectopic and molar pregnancy
Endometritis following ectopic and molar pregnancy
Oophoritis following ectopic and molar pregnancy
Parametritis following ectopic and molar pregnancy
Pelvic peritonitis following ectopic and molar pregnancy
Salpingitis following ectopic and molar pregnancy
Salpingo-oophoritis following ectopic and molar pregnancy
Excludes1   sepsis following ectopic and molar pregnancy (O08.82)
urinary tract infection (O08.83)

O08.1 **Delayed or excessive hemorrhage** following ectopic and molar pregnancy
Afibrinogenemia following ectopic and molar pregnancy
Defibrination syndrome following ectopic and molar pregnancy
Hemolysis following ectopic and molar pregnancy
Intravascular coagulation following ectopic and molar pregnancy
Excludes1   delayed or excessive hemorrhage due to incomplete abortion (O03.1)

O08.2 **Embolism** following ectopic and molar pregnancy
Air embolism following ectopic and molar pregnancy
Amniotic fluid embolism following ectopic and molar pregnancy
Blood-clot embolism following ectopic and molar pregnancy
Embolism NOS following ectopic and molar pregnancy
Fat embolism following ectopic and molar pregnancy
Pulmonary embolism following ectopic and molar pregnancy
Pyemic embolism following ectopic and molar pregnancy
Septic or septicopyemic embolism following ectopic and molar pregnancy
Soap embolism following ectopic and molar pregnancy

O08.3 **Shock** following ectopic and molar pregnancy
Circulatory collapse following ectopic and molar pregnancy
Shock (postprocedural) following ectopic and molar pregnancy
Excludes1   shock due to infection following ectopic and molar pregnancy (O08.82)

O08.4 **Renal failure** following ectopic and molar pregnancy
Kidney failure (acute) following ectopic and molar pregnancy
Oliguria following ectopic and molar pregnancy
Renal shutdown following ectopic and molar pregnancy
Renal tubular necrosis following ectopic and molar pregnancy
Uremia following ectopic and molar pregnancy

O08.5 **Metabolic** disorders following an ectopic and molar pregnancy

O08.6 **Damage to pelvic organs** and tissues following an ectopic and molar pregnancy
Laceration, perforation, tear or chemical damage of bladder following an ectopic and molar pregnancy
Laceration, perforation, tear or chemical damage of bowel following an ectopic and molar pregnancy
Laceration, perforation, tear or chemical damage of broad ligament following an ectopic and molar pregnancy
Laceration, perforation, tear or chemical damage of cervix following an ectopic and molar pregnancy
Laceration, perforation, tear or chemical damage of periurethral tissue following an ectopic and molar pregnancy
Laceration, perforation, tear or chemical damage of uterus following an ectopic and molar pregnancy
Laceration, perforation, tear or chemical damage of vagina following an ectopic and molar pregnancy

O08.7 **Other venous** complications following an ectopic and molar pregnancy

● **O08.8** **Other** complications following an ectopic and molar pregnancy
O08.81 **Cardiac arrest** following an ectopic and molar pregnancy
O08.82 **Sepsis** following ectopic and molar pregnancy
Use additional code (B95-B97), to identify infectious agent
Use additional code (R65.2-) to identify severe sepsis, if applicable
Excludes1   septic or septicopyemic embolism following ectopic and molar pregnancy (O08.2)
O08.83 **Urinary tract infection** following an ectopic and molar pregnancy
Cystitis following an ectopic and molar pregnancy
O08.89 **Other** complications following an ectopic and molar pregnancy

O08.9 **Unspecified** complication following an ectopic and molar pregnancy

SUPERVISION OF HIGH RISK PREGNANCY (O09)

● **O09** Supervision of **high risk** pregnancy
● **O09.0** Supervision of pregnancy with **history of infertility**
O09.00 Supervision of pregnancy with history of infertility, **unspecified trimester**
O09.01 Supervision of pregnancy with history of infertility, **first trimester**
O09.02 Supervision of pregnancy with history of infertility, **second trimester**
O09.03 Supervision of pregnancy with history of infertility, **third trimester**
● **O09.1** Supervision of pregnancy with **history of ectopic pregnancy**
O09.10 Supervision of pregnancy with history of ectopic pregnancy, **unspecified trimester**
O09.11 Supervision of pregnancy with history of ectopic pregnancy, **first trimester**
O09.12 Supervision of pregnancy with history of ectopic pregnancy, **second trimester**
O09.13 Supervision of pregnancy with history of ectopic pregnancy, **third trimester**
● **O09.A** Supervision of pregnancy with **history of molar pregnancy**
O09.A0 Supervision of pregnancy with history of molar pregnancy, **unspecified trimester**
O09.A1 Supervision of pregnancy with history of molar pregnancy, **first trimester**
O09.A2 Supervision of pregnancy with history of molar pregnancy, **second trimester**
O09.A3 Supervision of pregnancy with history of molar pregnancy, **third trimester**

CHAPTER 15 (O00-O9A)

● O09.2   **Supervision of pregnancy with other poor reproductive or obstetric history**

    Excludes2   pregnancy care for patient with history of recurrent pregnancy loss (O26.2-)

● O09.21   **Supervision of pregnancy with history of pre-term labor**

    O09.211   **Supervision of pregnancy with history of pre-term labor, first trimester**

    O09.212   **Supervision of pregnancy with history of pre-term labor, second trimester**

    O09.213   **Supervision of pregnancy with history of pre-term labor, third trimester**

    O09.219   **Supervision of pregnancy with history of pre-term labor, unspecified trimester**

● O09.29   **Supervision of pregnancy with other poor reproductive or obstetric history**

    Supervision of pregnancy with history of neonatal death

    Supervision of pregnancy with history of stillbirth

    O09.291   **Supervision of pregnancy with other poor reproductive or obstetric history, first trimester**

    O09.292   **Supervision of pregnancy with other poor reproductive or obstetric history, second trimester**

    O09.293   **Supervision of pregnancy with other poor reproductive or obstetric history, third trimester**

    O09.299   **Supervision of pregnancy with other poor reproductive or obstetric history, unspecified trimester**

● O09.3   **Supervision of pregnancy with insufficient antenatal care**

    Supervision of concealed pregnancy

    Supervision of hidden pregnancy

    O09.30   **Supervision of pregnancy with insufficient antenatal care, unspecified trimester**

    O09.31   **Supervision of pregnancy with insufficient antenatal care, first trimester**

    O09.32   **Supervision of pregnancy with insufficient antenatal care, second trimester**

    O09.33   **Supervision of pregnancy with insufficient antenatal care, third trimester**

● O09.4   **Supervision of pregnancy with grand multiparity**

    O09.40   **Supervision of pregnancy with grand multiparity, unspecified trimester**

    O09.41   **Supervision of pregnancy with grand multiparity, first trimester**

    O09.42   **Supervision of pregnancy with grand multiparity, second trimester**

    O09.43   **Supervision of pregnancy with grand multiparity, third trimester**

● O09.5   **Supervision of elderly primigravida and multigravida**

    Pregnancy for a female 35 years and older at expected date of delivery

● O09.51   **Supervision of elderly primigravida**

    O09.511   **Supervision of elderly primigravida, first trimester**

    O09.512   **Supervision of elderly primigravida, second trimester**

    O09.513   **Supervision of elderly primigravida, third trimester**

    O09.519   **Supervision of elderly primigravida, unspecified trimester**

● O09.52   **Supervision of elderly multigravida**

    O09.521   **Supervision of elderly multigravida, first trimester**

    O09.522   **Supervision of elderly multigravida, second trimester**

    O09.523   **Supervision of elderly multigravida, third trimester**

    O09.529   **Supervision of elderly multigravida, unspecified trimester**

● O09.6   **Supervision of young primigravida and multigravida**

    Supervision of pregnancy for a female less than 16 years old at expected date of delivery

● O09.61   **Supervision of young primigravida**

    O09.611   **Supervision of young primigravida, first trimester**

    O09.612   **Supervision of young primigravida, second trimester**

    O09.613   **Supervision of young primigravida, third trimester**

    O09.619   **Supervision of young primigravida, unspecified trimester**

● O09.62   **Supervision of young multigravida**

    O09.621   **Supervision of young multigravida, first trimester**

    O09.622   **Supervision of young multigravida, second trimester**

    O09.623   **Supervision of young multigravida, third trimester**

    O09.629   **Supervision of young multigravida, unspecified trimester**

● O09.7   **Supervision of high risk pregnancy due to social problems**

    O09.70   **Supervision of high risk pregnancy due to social problems, unspecified trimester**

    O09.71   **Supervision of high risk pregnancy due to social problems, first trimester**

    O09.72   **Supervision of high risk pregnancy due to social problems, second trimester**

    O09.73   **Supervision of high risk pregnancy due to social problems, third trimester**

● O09.8   **Supervision of other high risk pregnancies**

● O09.81   **Supervision of pregnancy resulting from assisted reproductive technology**

    Supervision of pregnancy resulting from in-vitro fertilization

    Excludes2   gestational carrier status (Z33.3)

    O09.811   **Supervision of pregnancy resulting from assisted reproductive technology, first trimester**

    O09.812   **Supervision of pregnancy resulting from assisted reproductive technology, second trimester**

    O09.813   **Supervision of pregnancy resulting from assisted reproductive technology, third trimester**

    O09.819   **Supervision of pregnancy resulting from assisted reproductive technology, unspecified trimester**

CHAPTER 15 (O00-O9A)

● O09.82   **Supervision of pregnancy with** history of in utero procedure during previous pregnancy

     O09.821   Supervision of pregnancy with history of in utero procedure during previous pregnancy, first trimester

     O09.822   Supervision of pregnancy with history of in utero procedure during previous pregnancy, second trimester

     O09.823   Supervision of pregnancy with history of in utero procedure during previous pregnancy, third trimester

     O09.829   Supervision of pregnancy with history of in utero procedure during previous pregnancy, unspecified trimester

         Excludes1   supervision of pregnancy affected by in utero procedure during current pregnancy (O35.7)

● O09.89   **Supervision of** other high risk pregnancies

     O09.891   Supervision of other high risk pregnancies, first trimester

     O09.892   Supervision of other high risk pregnancies, second trimester

     O09.893   Supervision of other high risk pregnancies, third trimester

     O09.899   Supervision of other high risk pregnancies, unspecified trimester

● O09.9   **Supervision of high risk pregnancy,** unspecified

     O09.90   Supervision of high risk pregnancy, unspecified, unspecified trimester

     O09.91   Supervision of high risk pregnancy, unspecified, first trimester

     O09.92   Supervision of high risk pregnancy, unspecified, second trimester

     O09.93   Supervision of high risk pregnancy, unspecified, third trimester

EDEMA, PROTEINURIA AND HYPERTENSIVE DISORDERS IN PREGNANCY, CHILDBIRTH AND THE PUERPERIUM (O10-O16)

● O10   Pre-existing **hypertension complicating pregnancy, childbirth and the puerperium**

     Includes   pre-existing hypertension with pre-existing proteinuria complicating pregnancy, childbirth and the puerperium

     Excludes2   pre-existing hypertension with superimposed pre-eclampsia complicating pregnancy, childbirth and the puerperium (O11.-)

● O10.0   **Pre-existing** essential **hypertension complicating pregnancy, childbirth and the puerperium**

     Any condition in I10 specified as a reason for obstetric care during pregnancy, childbirth or the puerperium

     ● O10.01   Pre-existing essential hypertension complicating pregnancy

         O10.011   Pre-existing essential hypertension complicating pregnancy, first trimester

         O10.012   Pre-existing essential hypertension complicating pregnancy, second trimester

         O10.013   Pre-existing essential hypertension complicating pregnancy, third trimester

         O10.019   Pre-existing essential hypertension complicating pregnancy, unspecified trimester

     O10.02   Pre-existing essential hypertension complicating childbirth

     O10.03   Pre-existing essential hypertension complicating the puerperium

● O10.1   **Pre-existing hypertensive** heart disease **complicating pregnancy, childbirth and the puerperium**

     Any condition in I11 specified as a reason for obstetric care during pregnancy, childbirth or the puerperium

     Use additional code from I11 to identify the type of hypertensive heart disease

     ● O10.11   Pre-existing hypertensive heart disease complicating pregnancy

         O10.111   Pre-existing hypertensive heart disease complicating pregnancy, first trimester

         O10.112   Pre-existing hypertensive heart disease complicating pregnancy, second trimester

         O10.113   Pre-existing hypertensive heart disease complicating pregnancy, third trimester

         O10.119   Pre-existing hypertensive heart disease complicating pregnancy, unspecified trimester

     O10.12   Pre-existing hypertensive heart disease complicating childbirth

     O10.13   Pre-existing hypertensive heart disease complicating the puerperium

● O10.2   **Pre-existing hypertensive** chronic kidney disease **complicating pregnancy, childbirth and the puerperium**

     Any condition in I12 specified as a reason for obstetric care during pregnancy, childbirth or the puerperium

     Use additional code from I12 to identify the type of hypertensive chronic kidney disease

     ● O10.21   Pre-existing hypertensive chronic kidney disease complicating pregnancy

         O10.211   Pre-existing hypertensive chronic kidney disease complicating pregnancy, first trimester

         O10.212   Pre-existing hypertensive chronic kidney disease complicating pregnancy, second trimester

         O10.213   Pre-existing hypertensive chronic kidney disease complicating pregnancy, third trimester

         O10.219   Pre-existing hypertensive chronic kidney disease complicating pregnancy, unspecified trimester

     O10.22   Pre-existing hypertensive chronic kidney disease complicating childbirth

     O10.23   Pre-existing hypertensive chronic kidney disease complicating the puerperium

● **O10.3**   **Pre-existing hypertensive heart and chronic kidney disease complicating pregnancy, childbirth and the puerperium**
> Any condition in I13 specified as a reason for obstetric care during pregnancy, childbirth or the puerperium
> Use additional code from I13 to identify the type of hypertensive heart and chronic kidney disease

● **O10.31**   **Pre-existing hypertensive heart and chronic kidney disease complicating pregnancy**

    O10.311   Pre-existing hypertensive heart and chronic kidney disease complicating pregnancy, first trimester

    O10.312   Pre-existing hypertensive heart and chronic kidney disease complicating pregnancy, second trimester

    O10.313   Pre-existing hypertensive heart and chronic kidney disease complicating pregnancy, third trimester

    O10.319   Pre-existing hypertensive heart and chronic kidney disease complicating pregnancy, unspecified trimester

   O10.32   Pre-existing hypertensive heart and chronic kidney disease complicating childbirth

   O10.33   Pre-existing hypertensive heart and chronic kidney disease complicating the puerperium

● **O10.4**   **Pre-existing secondary hypertension complicating pregnancy, childbirth and the puerperium**
> Any condition in I15 specified as a reason for obstetric care during pregnancy, childbirth or the puerperium
> Use additional code from I15 to identify the type of secondary hypertension

● **O10.41**   **Pre-existing secondary hypertension complicating pregnancy**

    O10.411   Pre-existing secondary hypertension complicating pregnancy, first trimester

    O10.412   Pre-existing secondary hypertension complicating pregnancy, second trimester

    O10.413   Pre-existing secondary hypertension complicating pregnancy, third trimester

    O10.419   Pre-existing secondary hypertension complicating pregnancy, unspecified trimester

   O10.42   Pre-existing secondary hypertension complicating childbirth

   O10.43   Pre-existing secondary hypertension complicating the puerperium

● **O10.9**   **Unspecified pre-existing hypertension complicating pregnancy, childbirth and the puerperium**

● **O10.91**   **Unspecified pre-existing hypertension complicating pregnancy**

    O10.911   Unspecified pre-existing hypertension complicating pregnancy, first trimester

    O10.912   Unspecified pre-existing hypertension complicating pregnancy, second trimester

    O10.913   Unspecified pre-existing hypertension complicating pregnancy, third trimester

    O10.919   Unspecified pre-existing hypertension complicating pregnancy, unspecified trimester

   O10.92   Unspecified pre-existing hypertension complicating childbirth

   O10.93   Unspecified pre-existing hypertension complicating the puerperium

● **O11**   **Pre-existing hypertension with pre-eclampsia**
> **Includes**   conditions in O10 complicated by pre-eclampsia pre-eclampsia superimposed pre-existing hypertension
> Use additional code from O10 to identify the type of hypertension

   O11.1   Pre-existing hypertension with pre-eclampsia, first trimester

   O11.2   Pre-existing hypertension with pre-eclampsia, second trimester

   O11.3   Pre-existing hypertension with pre-eclampsia, third trimester

   O11.4   Pre-existing hypertension with pre-eclampsia, complicating childbirth

   O11.5   Pre-existing hypertension with pre-eclampsia, complicating the puerperium

   O11.9   Pre-existing hypertension with pre-eclampsia, unspecified trimester

● **O12**   **Gestational [pregnancy-induced] edema and proteinuria without hypertension**

● **O12.0**   **Gestational edema**

   O12.00   Gestational edema, unspecified trimester

   O12.01   Gestational edema, first trimester

   O12.02   Gestational edema, second trimester

   O12.03   Gestational edema, third trimester

   O12.04   Gestational edema, complicating childbirth

   O12.05   Gestational edema, complicating the puerperium

● **O12.1**   **Gestational proteinuria**

   O12.10   Gestational proteinuria, unspecified trimester

   O12.11   Gestational proteinuria, first trimester

   O12.12   Gestational proteinuria, second trimester

   O12.13   Gestational proteinuria, third trimester

   O12.14   Gestational proteinuria, complicating childbirth

   O12.15   Gestational proteinuria, complicating the puerperium

● **O12.2**   **Gestational edema with proteinuria**

   O12.20   Gestational edema with proteinuria, unspecified trimester

   O12.21   Gestational edema with proteinuria, first trimester

   O12.22   Gestational edema with proteinuria, second trimester

   O12.23   Gestational edema with proteinuria, third trimester

   O12.24   Gestational edema with proteinuria, complicating childbirth

   O12.25   Gestational edema with proteinuria, complicating the puerperium

CHAPTER 15 (O00-O9A)

● **O13** Gestational [pregnancy-induced] hypertension without significant proteinuria
> **Includes**   gestational hypertension NOS
> transient hypertension of pregnancy

O13.1   Gestational [pregnancy-induced] hypertension without significant proteinuria, first trimester

O13.2   Gestational [pregnancy-induced] hypertension without significant proteinuria, second trimester

O13.3   Gestational [pregnancy-induced] hypertension without significant proteinuria, third trimester

O13.4   Gestational [pregnancy-induced] hypertension without significant proteinuria, complicating childbirth

O13.5   Gestational [pregnancy-induced] hypertension without significant proteinuria, complicating the puerperium

O13.9   Gestational [pregnancy-induced] hypertension without significant proteinuria, unspecified trimester

● **O14** Pre-eclampsia
> **Excludes1**   pre-existing hypertension with pre-eclampsia (O11)

● O14.0   Mild to moderate pre-eclampsia

O14.00   Mild to moderate pre-eclampsia, unspecified trimester

O14.02   Mild to moderate pre-eclampsia, second trimester

O14.03   Mild to moderate pre-eclampsia, third trimester

O14.04   Mild to moderate pre-eclampsia, complicating childbirth

O14.05   Mild to moderate pre-eclampsia, complicating the puerperium

● O14.1   Severe pre-eclampsia
> **Excludes1**   HELLP syndrome (O14.2-)
>
> *H=hemolysis, EL=elevated liver enzymes, LP=low platelet count*

O14.10   Severe pre-eclampsia, unspecified trimester

O14.12   Severe pre-eclampsia, second trimester

O14.13   Severe pre-eclampsia, third trimester

O14.14   Severe pre-eclampsia complicating childbirth

O14.15   Severe pre-eclampsia, complicating the puerperium

● O14.2   HELLP syndrome
Severe pre-eclampsia with hemolysis, elevated liver enzymes and low platelet count (HELLP)

O14.20   HELLP syndrome (HELLP), unspecified trimester

O14.22   HELLP syndrome (HELLP), second trimester

O14.23   HELLP syndrome (HELLP), third trimester

O14.24   HELLP syndrome, complicating childbirth

O14.25   HELLP syndrome, complicating the puerperium

● O14.9   Unspecified pre-eclampsia

O14.90   Unspecified pre-eclampsia, unspecified trimester

O14.92   Unspecified pre-eclampsia, second trimester

O14.93   Unspecified pre-eclampsia, third trimester

O14.94   Unspecified pre-eclampsia, complicating childbirth

O14.95   Unspecified pre-eclampsia, complicating the puerperium

● **O15** Eclampsia
> **Includes**   convulsions following conditions in O10-O14 and O16

● O15.0   Eclampsia complicating pregnancy

O15.00   Eclampsia complicating pregnancy, unspecified trimester

O15.02   Eclampsia complicating pregnancy, second trimester

O15.03   Eclampsia complicating pregnancy, third trimester

O15.1   Eclampsia complicating labor

O15.2   Eclampsia complicating the puerperium

O15.9   Eclampsia, unspecified as to time period
Eclampsia NOS

● **O16** Unspecified maternal hypertension

O16.1   Unspecified maternal hypertension, first trimester

O16.2   Unspecified maternal hypertension, second trimester

O16.3   Unspecified maternal hypertension, third trimester

O16.4   Unspecified maternal hypertension, complicating childbirth

O16.5   Unspecified maternal hypertension, complicating the puerperium

O16.9   Unspecified maternal hypertension, unspecified trimester

---

OTHER MATERNAL DISORDERS PREDOMINANTLY RELATED TO PREGNANCY (O20-O29)

> **Excludes2**   maternal care related to the fetus and amniotic cavity and possible delivery problems (O30-O48)
> maternal diseases classifiable elsewhere but complicating pregnancy, labor and delivery, and the puerperium (O98-O99)

● **O20** Hemorrhage in early pregnancy
> **Includes**   hemorrhage before completion of 20 weeks gestation
>
> **Excludes1**   pregnancy with abortive outcome (O00-O08)

O20.0   Threatened abortion
Hemorrhage specified as due to threatened abortion

O20.8   Other hemorrhage in early pregnancy

O20.9   Hemorrhage in early pregnancy, unspecified

● **O21** Excessive vomiting in pregnancy

O21.0   Mild hyperemesis gravidarum
Hyperemesis gravidarum, mild or unspecified, starting before the end of the 20th week of gestation

O21.1   Hyperemesis gravidarum with metabolic disturbance
Hyperemesis gravidarum, starting before the end of the 20th week of gestation, with metabolic disturbance such as carbohydrate depletion
Hyperemesis gravidarum, starting before the end of the 20th week of gestation, with metabolic disturbance such as dehydration
Hyperemesis gravidarum, starting before the end of the 20th week of gestation, with metabolic disturbance such as electrolyte imbalance

O21.2   Late vomiting of pregnancy
Excessive vomiting starting after 20 completed weeks of gestation

O21.8   Other vomiting complicating pregnancy
Vomiting due to diseases classified elsewhere, complicating pregnancy
Use additional code, to identify cause

O21.9   Vomiting of pregnancy, unspecified

● **O22** **Venous complications and hemorrhoids in pregnancy**

    Excludes1   venous complications of:
        abortion NOS (O03.9)
        ectopic or molar pregnancy (O08.7)
        failed attempted abortion (O07.35)
        induced abortion (O04.85)
        spontaneous abortion (O03.89)

    Excludes2   obstetric pulmonary embolism (O88.-)
        venous complications and hemorrhoids of
        childbirth and the puerperium (O87.-)

● **O22.0** **Varicose veins of lower extremity in pregnancy**
    Varicose veins NOS in pregnancy

    O22.00 Varicose veins of lower extremity in pregnancy, unspecified trimester

    O22.01 Varicose veins of lower extremity in pregnancy, first trimester

    O22.02 Varicose veins of lower extremity in pregnancy, second trimester

    O22.03 Varicose veins of lower extremity in pregnancy, third trimester

● **O22.1** **Genital varices in pregnancy**
    Perineal varices in pregnancy
    Vaginal varices in pregnancy
    Vulval varices in pregnancy

    O22.10 Genital varices in pregnancy, unspecified trimester

    O22.11 Genital varices in pregnancy, first trimester

    O22.12 Genital varices in pregnancy, second trimester

    O22.13 Genital varices in pregnancy, third trimester

● **O22.2** **Superficial thrombophlebitis in pregnancy**
    Phlebitis in pregnancy NOS
    Thrombophlebitis of legs in pregnancy
    Thrombosis in pregnancy NOS

    Use additional code to identify the superficial
    thrombophlebitis (I80.0-)

    O22.20 Superficial thrombophlebitis in pregnancy, unspecified trimester

    O22.21 Superficial thrombophlebitis in pregnancy, first trimester

    O22.22 Superficial thrombophlebitis in pregnancy, second trimester

    O22.23 Superficial thrombophlebitis in pregnancy, third trimester

● **O22.3** **Deep phlebothrombosis in pregnancy**
    Deep vein thrombosis, antepartum

    Use additional code to identify the deep vein
    thrombosis (I82.4-, I82.5-, I82.62-. I82.72-)

    Use additional code, if applicable, for associated long-
    term (current) use of anticoagulants (Z79.01)

    O22.30 Deep phlebothrombosis in pregnancy, unspecified trimester

    O22.31 Deep phlebothrombosis in pregnancy, first trimester

    O22.32 Deep phlebothrombosis in pregnancy, second trimester

    O22.33 Deep phlebothrombosis in pregnancy, third trimester

● **O22.4** **Hemorrhoids in pregnancy**

    O22.40 Hemorrhoids in pregnancy, unspecified trimester

    O22.41 Hemorrhoids in pregnancy, first trimester

    O22.42 Hemorrhoids in pregnancy, second trimester

    O22.43 Hemorrhoids in pregnancy, third trimester

● **O22.5** **Cerebral venous thrombosis in pregnancy**
    Cerebrovenous sinus thrombosis in pregnancy

    O22.50 Cerebral venous thrombosis in pregnancy, unspecified trimester

    O22.51 Cerebral venous thrombosis in pregnancy, first trimester

    O22.52 Cerebral venous thrombosis in pregnancy, second trimester

    O22.53 Cerebral venous thrombosis in pregnancy, third trimester

● **O22.8** **Other venous complications in pregnancy**

    ● **O22.8X** **Other venous complications in pregnancy**

      O22.8X1 Other venous complications in pregnancy, first trimester

      O22.8X2 Other venous complications in pregnancy, second trimester

      O22.8X3 Other venous complications in pregnancy, third trimester

      O22.8X9 Other venous complications in pregnancy, unspecified trimester

● **O22.9** **Venous complication in pregnancy, unspecified**
    Gestational phlebitis NOS
    Gestational phlebopathy NOS
    Gestational thrombosis NOS

    O22.90 Venous complication in pregnancy, unspecified, unspecified trimester

    O22.91 Venous complication in pregnancy, unspecified, first trimester

    O22.92 Venous complication in pregnancy, unspecified, second trimester

    O22.93 Venous complication in pregnancy, unspecified, third trimester

● **O23** **Infections of genitourinary tract in pregnancy**

    Use additional code to identify organism (B95.-, B96.-)

    Excludes2   gonococcal infections complicating pregnancy,
        childbirth and the puerperium (O98.2)
        infections with a predominantly sexual mode of
        transmission NOS complicating pregnancy,
        childbirth and the puerperium (O98.3)
        syphilis complicating pregnancy, childbirth and
        the puerperium (O98.1)
        tuberculosis of genitourinary system
        complicating pregnancy, childbirth and the
        puerperium (O98.0)
        venereal disease NOS complicating pregnancy,
        childbirth and the puerperium (O98.3)

● **O23.0** **Infections of kidney in pregnancy**
    Pyelonephritis in pregnancy

    O23.00 Infections of kidney in pregnancy, unspecified trimester

    O23.01 Infections of kidney in pregnancy, first trimester

    O23.02 Infections of kidney in pregnancy, second trimester

    O23.03 Infections of kidney in pregnancy, third trimester

● **O23.1** **Infections of bladder in pregnancy**

    O23.10 Infections of bladder in pregnancy, unspecified trimester

    O23.11 Infections of bladder in pregnancy, first trimester

    O23.12 Infections of bladder in pregnancy, second trimester

    O23.13 Infections of bladder in pregnancy, third trimester

CHAPTER 15 (O00-O9A)

● O23.2   Infections of urethra in pregnancy
     O23.20   Infections of urethra in pregnancy, unspecified trimester
     O23.21   Infections of urethra in pregnancy, first trimester
     O23.22   Infections of urethra in pregnancy, second trimester
     O23.23   Infections of urethra in pregnancy, third trimester

● O23.3   Infections of other parts of urinary tract in pregnancy
     O23.30   Infections of other parts of urinary tract in pregnancy, unspecified trimester
     O23.31   Infections of other parts of urinary tract in pregnancy, first trimester
     O23.32   Infections of other parts of urinary tract in pregnancy, second trimester
     O23.33   Infections of other parts of urinary tract in pregnancy, third trimester

● O23.4   Unspecified infection of urinary tract in pregnancy
     O23.40   Unspecified infection of urinary tract in pregnancy, unspecified trimester
     O23.41   Unspecified infection of urinary tract in pregnancy, first trimester
     O23.42   Unspecified infection of urinary tract in pregnancy, second trimester
     O23.43   Unspecified infection of urinary tract in pregnancy, third trimester

● O23.5   Infections of the genital tract in pregnancy
  ● O23.51   Infection of cervix in pregnancy
       O23.511   Infections of cervix in pregnancy, first trimester
       O23.512   Infections of cervix in pregnancy, second trimester
       O23.513   Infections of cervix in pregnancy, third trimester
       O23.519   Infections of cervix in pregnancy, unspecified trimester
  ● O23.52   Salpingo-oophoritis in pregnancy
       Oophoritis = inflammation of ovary
       Salpingitis = inflammation of fallopian tube
       Oophoritis in pregnancy
       Salpingitis in pregnancy
       O23.521   Salpingo-oophoritis in pregnancy, first trimester
       O23.522   Salpingo-oophoritis in pregnancy, second trimester
       O23.523   Salpingo-oophoritis in pregnancy, third trimester
       O23.529   Salpingo-oophoritis in pregnancy, unspecified trimester
  ● O23.59   Infection of other part of genital tract in pregnancy
       O23.591   Infection of other part of genital tract in pregnancy, first trimester
       O23.592   Infection of other part of genital tract in pregnancy, second trimester
       O23.593   Infection of other part of genital tract in pregnancy, third trimester
       O23.599   Infection of other part of genital tract in pregnancy, unspecified trimester

● O23.9   Unspecified genitourinary tract infection in pregnancy
     Genitourinary tract infection in pregnancy NOS
     O23.90   Unspecified genitourinary tract infection in pregnancy, unspecified trimester
     O23.91   Unspecified genitourinary tract infection in pregnancy, first trimester
     O23.92   Unspecified genitourinary tract infection in pregnancy, second trimester
     O23.93   Unspecified genitourinary tract infection in pregnancy, third trimester

OGCR   Section I.C.15.g.

> Diabetes mellitus in pregnancy
> Diabetes mellitus is a significant complicating factor in pregnancy. Pregnant women who are diabetic should be assigned a code from category O24, Diabetes mellitus in pregnancy, childbirth, and the puerperium, first, followed by the appropriate diabetes code(s) (E08-E13) from Chapter 4.

● O24   Diabetes mellitus in pregnancy, childbirth, and the puerperium
  ● O24.0   Pre-existing type 1 diabetes mellitus, in pregnancy, childbirth and the puerperium
       Juvenile onset diabetes mellitus, in pregnancy, childbirth and the puerperium
       Ketosis-prone diabetes mellitus in pregnancy, childbirth and the puerperium
       Use additional code from category E10 to further identify any manifestations
    ● O24.01   Pre-existing type 1 diabetes mellitus, in pregnancy
         O24.011   Pre-existing type 1 diabetes mellitus, in pregnancy, first trimester
         O24.012   Pre-existing type 1 diabetes mellitus, in pregnancy, second trimester
         O24.013   Pre-existing type 1 diabetes mellitus, in pregnancy, third trimester
         O24.019   Pre-existing type 1 diabetes mellitus, in pregnancy, unspecified trimester
     O24.02   Pre-existing type 1 diabetes mellitus, in childbirth
     O24.03   Pre-existing type 1 diabetes mellitus, in the puerperium
  ● O24.1   Pre-existing type 2 diabetes mellitus, in pregnancy, childbirth and the puerperium
       Insulin-resistant diabetes mellitus in pregnancy, childbirth and the puerperium
       Use additional code (for):
         from category E11 to further identify any manifestations
         long-term (current) use of insulin (Z79.4)
    ● O24.11   Pre-existing type 2 diabetes mellitus, in pregnancy
         O24.111   Pre-existing type 2 diabetes mellitus, in pregnancy, first trimester
         O24.112   Pre-existing type 2 diabetes mellitus, in pregnancy, second trimester
         O24.113   Pre-existing type 2 diabetes mellitus, in pregnancy, third trimester
         O24.119   Pre-existing type 2 diabetes mellitus, in pregnancy, unspecified trimester
     O24.12   Pre-existing type 2 diabetes mellitus, in childbirth
     O24.13   Pre-existing type 2 diabetes mellitus, in the puerperium

▶ New   ⇒ Revised   ~~deleted~~ Deleted   **OGCR** Official Guidelines   X Assign placeholder X   ● Use Additional Character(s)
Excludes 1   Excludes 2   Includes   Use additional   Code first   Code also   Key words

● **O24.3** Unspecified pre-existing diabetes mellitus in pregnancy, childbirth and the puerperium

Use additional code (for):
from category E11 to further identify any manifestation
long-term (current) use of insulin (Z79.4)

● **O24.31** Unspecified pre-existing diabetes mellitus in pregnancy

O24.311 Unspecified pre-existing diabetes mellitus in pregnancy, first trimester

O24.312 Unspecified pre-existing diabetes mellitus in pregnancy, second trimester

O24.313 Unspecified pre-existing diabetes mellitus in pregnancy, third trimester

O24.319 Unspecified pre-existing diabetes mellitus in pregnancy, unspecified trimester

O24.32 Unspecified pre-existing diabetes mellitus in childbirth

O24.33 Unspecified pre-existing diabetes mellitus in the puerperium

OGCR Section I.C.15.i.

> Gestational (pregnancy induced) diabetes
>
> Gestational (pregnancy induced) diabetes can occur during the second and third trimester of pregnancy in women who were not diabetic prior to pregnancy. Gestational diabetes can cause complications in the pregnancy similar to those of pre-existing diabetes mellitus. It also puts the woman at greater risk of developing diabetes after the pregnancy. Codes for gestational diabetes are in subcategory O24.4, Gestational diabetes mellitus. No other code from category O24, Diabetes mellitus in pregnancy, childbirth, and the puerperium, should be used with a code from O24.4
>
> The codes under subcategory O24.4 include diet controlled, insulin controlled, **and controlled by oral hypoglycemic drugs.** If a patient with gestational diabetes is treated with both diet and insulin, only the code for insulin-controlled is required. **If a patient with gestational diabetes is treated with both diet and oral hypoglycemic medications, only the code for "controlled by oral hypoglycemic drugs" is required.** Code Z79.4, Long-term (current) use of insulin **or code Z79.84, Long-term (current) use of oral hypoglycemic drugs,** should not be assigned with codes from subcategory O24.4.
>
> An abnormal glucose tolerance in pregnancy is assigned a code from subcategory O99.81, Abnormal glucose complicating pregnancy, childbirth, and the puerperium.

● **O24.4** Gestational diabetes mellitus
Diabetes mellitus arising in pregnancy
Gestational diabetes mellitus NOS

● **O24.41** Gestational diabetes mellitus in pregnancy

O24.410 Gestational diabetes mellitus in pregnancy, diet controlled

O24.414 Gestational diabetes mellitus in pregnancy, insulin controlled

O24.415 Gestational diabetes mellitus in pregnancy, controlled by oral hypoglycemic drugs
Gestational diabetes mellitus in pregnancy, controlled by oral antidiabetic drugs

O24.419 Gestational diabetes mellitus in pregnancy, unspecified control

● **O24.42** Gestational diabetes mellitus in childbirth

O24.420 Gestational diabetes mellitus in childbirth, diet controlled

O24.424 Gestational diabetes mellitus in childbirth, insulin controlled

O24.425 Gestational diabetes mellitus in childbirth, controlled by oral hypoglycemic drugs
Gestational diabetes mellitus in childbirth, controlled by oral antidiabetic drugs

O24.429 Gestational diabetes mellitus in childbirth, unspecified control

● **O24.43** Gestational diabetes mellitus in the puerperium

O24.430 Gestational diabetes mellitus in the puerperium, diet controlled

O24.434 Gestational diabetes mellitus in the puerperium, insulin controlled

O24.435 Gestational diabetes mellitus in puerperium, controlled by oral hypoglycemic drugs
Gestational diabetes mellitus in puerperium, controlled by oral antidiabetic drugs

O24.439 Gestational diabetes mellitus in the puerperium, unspecified control

● **O24.8** Other pre-existing diabetes mellitus in pregnancy, childbirth, and the puerperium

Use additional code (for):
from categories E08, E09 and E13 to further identify any manifestation
long-term (current) use of insulin (Z79.4)

● **O24.81** Other pre-existing diabetes mellitus in pregnancy

O24.811 Other pre-existing diabetes mellitus in pregnancy, first trimester

O24.812 Other pre-existing diabetes mellitus in pregnancy, second trimester

O24.813 Other pre-existing diabetes mellitus in pregnancy, third trimester

O24.819 Other pre-existing diabetes mellitus in pregnancy, unspecified trimester

O24.82 Other pre-existing diabetes mellitus in childbirth

O24.83 Other pre-existing diabetes mellitus in the puerperium

● **O24.9** Unspecified diabetes mellitus in pregnancy, childbirth and the puerperium

Use additional code for long-term (current) use of insulin (Z79.4)

Unknown whether patient was diabetic before pregnancy occurred

● **O24.91** Unspecified diabetes mellitus in pregnancy

O24.911 Unspecified diabetes mellitus in pregnancy, first trimester

O24.912 Unspecified diabetes mellitus in pregnancy, second trimester

O24.913 Unspecified diabetes mellitus in pregnancy, third trimester

O24.919 Unspecified diabetes mellitus in pregnancy, unspecified trimester

O24.92 Unspecified diabetes mellitus in childbirth

O24.93 Unspecified diabetes mellitus in the puerperium

CHAPTER 15 (O00-O9A)

▶ New   ⟹ Revised   ~~deleted~~ Deleted   **OGCR** Official Guidelines   X Assign placeholder X   ● Use Additional Character(s)

Excludes 1   Excludes 2   Includes   Use additional   Code first   Code also   Key words

● **O25** Malnutrition in pregnancy, childbirth and the puerperium
   ● **O25.1** Malnutrition in pregnancy
     O25.10 Malnutrition in pregnancy, unspecified trimester
     O25.11 Malnutrition in pregnancy, first trimester
     O25.12 Malnutrition in pregnancy, second trimester
     O25.13 Malnutrition in pregnancy, third trimester
   O25.2 Malnutrition in childbirth
   O25.3 Malnutrition in the puerperium

● **O26** Maternal care for other conditions predominantly related to pregnancy
   ● **O26.0** Excessive weight gain in pregnancy
     Excludes2   gestational edema (O12.0, O12.2)
     O26.00 Excessive weight gain in pregnancy, unspecified trimester
     O26.01 Excessive weight gain in pregnancy, first trimester
     O26.02 Excessive weight gain in pregnancy, second trimester
     O26.03 Excessive weight gain in pregnancy, third trimester
   ● **O26.1** Low weight gain in pregnancy
     O26.10 Low weight gain in pregnancy, unspecified trimester
     O26.11 Low weight gain in pregnancy, first trimester
     O26.12 Low weight gain in pregnancy, second trimester
     O26.13 Low weight gain in pregnancy, third trimester
   ● **O26.2** Pregnancy care for patient with recurrent pregnancy loss
     O26.20 Pregnancy care for patient with recurrent pregnancy loss, unspecified trimester
     O26.21 Pregnancy care for patient with recurrent pregnancy loss, first trimester
     O26.22 Pregnancy care for patient with recurrent pregnancy loss, second trimester
     O26.23 Pregnancy care for patient with recurrent pregnancy loss, third trimester
   ● **O26.3** Retained intrauterine contraceptive device in pregnancy
     O26.30 Retained intrauterine contraceptive device in pregnancy, unspecified trimester
     O26.31 Retained intrauterine contraceptive device in pregnancy, first trimester
     O26.32 Retained intrauterine contraceptive device in pregnancy, second trimester
     O26.33 Retained intrauterine contraceptive device in pregnancy, third trimester
   ● **O26.4** Herpes gestationis
     O26.40 Herpes gestationis, unspecified trimester
     O26.41 Herpes gestationis, first trimester
     O26.42 Herpes gestationis, second trimester
     O26.43 Herpes gestationis, third trimester
   ● **O26.5** Maternal hypotension syndrome
     Supine hypotensive syndrome
     O26.50 Maternal hypotension syndrome, unspecified trimester
     O26.51 Maternal hypotension syndrome, first trimester
     O26.52 Maternal hypotension syndrome, second trimester
     O26.53 Maternal hypotension syndrome, third trimester

● **O26.6** Liver and biliary tract disorders in pregnancy, childbirth and the puerperium
   Use additional code to identify the specific disorder
   Excludes2   hepatorenal syndrome following labor and delivery (O90.4)
   ● **O26.61** Liver and biliary tract disorders in pregnancy
     O26.611 Liver and biliary tract disorders in pregnancy, first trimester
     O26.612 Liver and biliary tract disorders in pregnancy, second trimester
     O26.613 Liver and biliary tract disorders in pregnancy, third trimester
     O26.619 Liver and biliary tract disorders in pregnancy, unspecified trimester
   O26.62 Liver and biliary tract disorders in childbirth
   O26.63 Liver and biliary tract disorders in the puerperium
   ● **O26.7** Subluxation of symphysis (pubis) in pregnancy, childbirth and the puerperium
     Excludes1   traumatic separation of symphysis (pubis) during childbirth (O71.6)
   ● **O26.71** Subluxation of symphysis (pubis) in pregnancy
     O26.711 Subluxation of symphysis (pubis) in pregnancy, first trimester
     O26.712 Subluxation of symphysis (pubis) in pregnancy, second trimester
     O26.713 Subluxation of symphysis (pubis) in pregnancy, third trimester
     O26.719 Subluxation of symphysis (pubis) in pregnancy, unspecified trimester
   O26.72 Subluxation of symphysis (pubis) in childbirth
   O26.73 Subluxation of symphysis (pubis) in the puerperium
   ● **O26.8** Other specified pregnancy related conditions
   ● **O26.81** Pregnancy related exhaustion and fatigue
     O26.811 Pregnancy related exhaustion and fatigue, first trimester
     O26.812 Pregnancy related exhaustion and fatigue, second trimester
     O26.813 Pregnancy related exhaustion and fatigue, third trimester
     O26.819 Pregnancy related exhaustion and fatigue, unspecified trimester
   ● **O26.82** Pregnancy related peripheral neuritis
     O26.821 Pregnancy related peripheral neuritis, first trimester
     O26.822 Pregnancy related peripheral neuritis, second trimester
     O26.823 Pregnancy related peripheral neuritis, third trimester
     O26.829 Pregnancy related peripheral neuritis, unspecified trimester
   ● **O26.83** Pregnancy related renal disease
     Use additional code to identify the specific disorder
     O26.831 Pregnancy related renal disease, first trimester
     O26.832 Pregnancy related renal disease, second trimester
     O26.833 Pregnancy related renal disease, third trimester
     O26.839 Pregnancy related renal disease, unspecified trimester

▶ New   ⇒ Revised   ~~deleted~~ Deleted   **OGCR** Official Guidelines   X Assign placeholder X   ● Use Additional Character(s)

Excludes 1   Excludes 2   Includes   Use additional   Code first   Code also   Key words

● **O26.84** Uterine size-date discrepancy complicating pregnancy

> | **Excludes1** | encounter for suspected problem with fetal growth ruled out (Z03.74) |

     O26.841 Uterine size-date discrepancy, first trimester

     O26.842 Uterine size-date discrepancy, second trimester

     O26.843 Uterine size-date discrepancy, third trimester

     O26.849 Uterine size-date discrepancy, unspecified trimester

● **O26.85** Spotting complicating pregnancy

     O26.851 Spotting complicating pregnancy, first trimester

     O26.852 Spotting complicating pregnancy, second trimester

     O26.853 Spotting complicating pregnancy, third trimester

     O26.859 Spotting complicating pregnancy, unspecified trimester

     O26.86 Pruritic urticarial papules and plaques of pregnancy (PUPPP)

         Polymorphic eruption of pregnancy

● **O26.87** Cervical shortening

> | **Excludes1** | encounter for suspected cervical shortening ruled out (Z03.75) |

     O26.872 Cervical shortening, second trimester

     O26.873 Cervical shortening, third trimester

     O26.879 Cervical shortening, unspecified trimester

● **O26.89** Other specified pregnancy related conditions

     O26.891 Other specified pregnancy related conditions, first trimester

     O26.892 Other specified pregnancy related conditions, second trimester

     O26.893 Other specified pregnancy related conditions, third trimester

     O26.899 Other specified pregnancy related conditions, unspecified trimester

● **O26.9** Pregnancy related conditions, unspecified

     O26.90 Pregnancy related conditions, unspecified, unspecified trimester

     O26.91 Pregnancy related conditions, unspecified, first trimester

     O26.92 Pregnancy related conditions, unspecified, second trimester

     O26.93 Pregnancy related conditions, unspecified, third trimester

● **O28** Abnormal findings on antenatal screening of mother

> | **Excludes1** | diagnostic findings classified elsewhere - see Alphabetical Index |

     O28.0 Abnormal hematological finding on antenatal screening of mother

     O28.1 Abnormal biochemical finding on antenatal screening of mother

     O28.2 Abnormal cytological finding on antenatal screening of mother

     O28.3 Abnormal ultrasonic finding on antenatal screening of mother

     O28.4 Abnormal radiological finding on antenatal screening of mother

     O28.5 Abnormal chromosomal and genetic finding on antenatal screening of mother

     O28.8 Other abnormal findings on antenatal screening of mother

     O28.9 Unspecified abnormal findings on antenatal screening of mother

● **O29** Complications of anesthesia during pregnancy

> | **Includes** | maternal complications arising from the administration of a general, regional or local anesthetic, analgesic or other sedation during pregnancy |

Use additional code, if necessary, to identify the complication

> | **Excludes2** | complications of anesthesia during labor and delivery (O74.-)
 complications of anesthesia during the puerperium (O89.-) |

● **O29.0** Pulmonary complications of anesthesia during pregnancy

  ● **O29.01** Aspiration pneumonitis due to anesthesia during pregnancy

         Inhalation of stomach contents or secretions NOS due to anesthesia during pregnancy

         Mendelson's syndrome due to anesthesia during pregnancy

     O29.011 Aspiration pneumonitis due to anesthesia during pregnancy, first trimester

     O29.012 Aspiration pneumonitis due to anesthesia during pregnancy, second trimester

     O29.013 Aspiration pneumonitis due to anesthesia during pregnancy, third trimester

     O29.019 Aspiration pneumonitis due to anesthesia during pregnancy, unspecified trimester

  ● **O29.02** Pressure collapse of lung due to anesthesia during pregnancy

     O29.021 Pressure collapse of lung due to anesthesia during pregnancy, first trimester

     O29.022 Pressure collapse of lung due to anesthesia during pregnancy, second trimester

     O29.023 Pressure collapse of lung due to anesthesia during pregnancy, third trimester

     O29.029 Pressure collapse of lung due to anesthesia during pregnancy, unspecified trimester

  ● **O29.09** Other pulmonary complications of anesthesia during pregnancy

     O29.091 Other pulmonary complications of anesthesia during pregnancy, first trimester

     O29.092 Other pulmonary complications of anesthesia during pregnancy, second trimester

     O29.093 Other pulmonary complications of anesthesia during pregnancy, third trimester

     O29.099 Other pulmonary complications of anesthesia during pregnancy, unspecified trimester

CHAPTER 15 (O00-O9A)

● O29.1   **Cardiac** complications of anesthesia during pregnancy
  ● O29.11   **Cardiac arrest** due to anesthesia during pregnancy
     O29.111   Cardiac arrest due to anesthesia during pregnancy, **first trimester**
     O29.112   Cardiac arrest due to anesthesia during pregnancy, **second trimester**
     O29.113   Cardiac arrest due to anesthesia during pregnancy, **third trimester**
     O29.119   Cardiac arrest due to anesthesia during pregnancy, **unspecified trimester**
  ● O29.12   **Cardiac failure** due to anesthesia during pregnancy
     O29.121   Cardiac failure due to anesthesia during pregnancy, **first trimester**
     O29.122   Cardiac failure due to anesthesia during pregnancy, **second trimester**
     O29.123   Cardiac failure due to anesthesia during pregnancy, **third trimester**
     O29.129   Cardiac failure due to anesthesia during pregnancy, **unspecified trimester**
  ● O29.19   **Other** cardiac complications of anesthesia during pregnancy
     O29.191   Other cardiac complications of anesthesia during pregnancy, **first trimester**
     O29.192   Other cardiac complications of anesthesia during pregnancy, **second trimester**
     O29.193   Other cardiac complications of anesthesia during pregnancy, **third trimester**
     O29.199   Other cardiac complications of anesthesia during pregnancy, **unspecified trimester**
● O29.2   **Central nervous** system complications of anesthesia during pregnancy
  ● O29.21   **Cerebral anoxia** due to anesthesia during pregnancy
     O29.211   Cerebral anoxia due to anesthesia during pregnancy, **first trimester**
     O29.212   Cerebral anoxia due to anesthesia during pregnancy, **second trimester**
     O29.213   Cerebral anoxia due to anesthesia during pregnancy, **third trimester**
     O29.219   Cerebral anoxia due to anesthesia during pregnancy, **unspecified trimester**
  ● O29.29   **Other** central nervous system complications of anesthesia during pregnancy
     O29.291   Other central nervous system complications of anesthesia during pregnancy, **first trimester**
     O29.292   Other central nervous system complications of anesthesia during pregnancy, **second trimester**
     O29.293   Other central nervous system complications of anesthesia during pregnancy, **third trimester**
     O29.299   Other central nervous system complications of anesthesia during pregnancy, **unspecified trimester**

● O29.3   **Toxic reaction** to local anesthesia during pregnancy
  ● O29.3X   Toxic reaction to local anesthesia during pregnancy
     O29.3X1   Toxic reaction to local anesthesia during pregnancy, **first trimester**
     O29.3X2   Toxic reaction to local anesthesia during pregnancy, **second trimester**
     O29.3X3   Toxic reaction to local anesthesia during pregnancy, **third trimester**
     O29.3X9   Toxic reaction to local anesthesia during pregnancy, **unspecified trimester**
● O29.4   **Spinal and epidural anesthesia induced headache** during pregnancy
     O29.40   Spinal and epidural anesthesia induced headache during pregnancy, **unspecified trimester**
     O29.41   Spinal and epidural anesthesia induced headache during pregnancy, **first trimester**
     O29.42   Spinal and epidural anesthesia induced headache during pregnancy, **second trimester**
     O29.43   Spinal and epidural anesthesia induced headache during pregnancy, **third trimester**
● O29.5   **Other** complications of spinal and epidural anesthesia during pregnancy
  ● O29.5X   Other complications of spinal and epidural anesthesia during pregnancy
     O29.5X1   Other complications of spinal and epidural anesthesia during pregnancy, **first trimester**
     O29.5X2   Other complications of spinal and epidural anesthesia during pregnancy, **second trimester**
     O29.5X3   Other complications of spinal and epidural anesthesia during pregnancy, **third trimester**
     O29.5X9   Other complications of spinal and epidural anesthesia during pregnancy, **unspecified trimester**
● O29.6   **Failed or difficult intubation** for anesthesia during pregnancy
     O29.60   Failed or difficult intubation for anesthesia during pregnancy, **unspecified trimester**
     O29.61   Failed or difficult intubation for anesthesia during pregnancy, **first trimester**
     O29.62   Failed or difficult intubation for anesthesia during pregnancy, **second trimester**
     O29.63   Failed or difficult intubation for anesthesia during pregnancy, **third trimester**
● O29.8   **Other** complications of anesthesia during pregnancy
  ● O29.8X   Other complications of anesthesia during pregnancy
     O29.8X1   Other complications of anesthesia during pregnancy, **first trimester**
     O29.8X2   Other complications of anesthesia during pregnancy, **second trimester**
     O29.8X3   Other complications of anesthesia during pregnancy, **third trimester**
     O29.8X9   Other complications of anesthesia during pregnancy, **unspecified trimester**

▶ New   ⟾ Revised   ~~deleted~~ Deleted   **OGCR** Official Guidelines   X Assign placeholder X   ● Use Additional Character(s)

Excludes 1   Excludes 2   Includes   Use additional   Code first   Code also   Key words

● **O29.9** **Unspecified** complication of anesthesia during pregnancy

    O29.90   Unspecified complication of anesthesia during pregnancy, **unspecified trimester**

    O29.91   Unspecified complication of anesthesia during pregnancy, **first trimester**

    O29.92   Unspecified complication of anesthesia during pregnancy, **second trimester**

    O29.93   Unspecified complication of anesthesia during pregnancy, **third trimester**

MATERNAL CARE RELATED TO THE FETUS AND AMNIOTIC CAVITY AND POSSIBLE DELIVERY PROBLEMS (O30-O48)

● **O30** **Multiple gestation**

    Code also any complications specific to multiple gestation

● **O30.0** **Twin pregnancy**

  ● **O30.00** Twin pregnancy, **unspecified** number of placenta and **unspecified** number of amniotic sacs

    O30.001   Twin pregnancy, unspecified number of placenta and unspecified number of amniotic sacs, **first trimester**

    O30.002   Twin pregnancy, unspecified number of placenta and unspecified number of amniotic sacs, **second trimester**

    O30.003   Twin pregnancy, unspecified number of placenta and unspecified number of amniotic sacs, **third trimester**

    O30.009   Twin pregnancy, unspecified number of placenta and unspecified number of amniotic sacs, **unspecified trimester**

  ● **O30.01** Twin pregnancy, **monochorionic/monoamniotic**

    Twin pregnancy, one placenta, one amniotic sac

    | **Excludes1** | conjoined twins (O30.02-) |

    O30.011   Twin pregnancy, monochorionic/monoamniotic, **first trimester**

    O30.012   Twin pregnancy, monochorionic/monoamniotic, **second trimester**

    O30.013   Twin pregnancy, monochorionic/monoamniotic, **third trimester**

    O30.019   Twin pregnancy, monochorionic/monoamniotic, **unspecified trimester**

  ● **O30.02** **Conjoined** twin pregnancy

    O30.021   Conjoined twin pregnancy, **first trimester**

    O30.022   Conjoined twin pregnancy, **second trimester**

    O30.023   Conjoined twin pregnancy, **third trimester**

    O30.029   Conjoined twin pregnancy, **unspecified trimester**

  ● **O30.03** Twin pregnancy, **monochorionic/diamniotic**

    Twin pregnancy, one placenta, two amniotic sacs

    O30.031   Twin pregnancy, monochorionic/diamniotic, **first trimester**

    O30.032   Twin pregnancy, monochorionic/diamniotic, **second trimester**

    O30.033   Twin pregnancy, monochorionic/diamniotic, **third trimester**

    O30.039   Twin pregnancy, monochorionic/diamniotic, **unspecified trimester**

  ● **O30.04** Twin pregnancy, **dichorionic/diamniotic**

    Twin pregnancy, two placentae, two amniotic sacs

    O30.041   Twin pregnancy, dichorionic/diamniotic, **first trimester**

    O30.042   Twin pregnancy, dichorionic/diamniotic, **second trimester**

    O30.043   Twin pregnancy, dichorionic/diamniotic, **third trimester**

    O30.049   Twin pregnancy, dichorionic/diamniotic, **unspecified trimester**

  ● **O30.09** Twin pregnancy, **unable to determine** number of placenta and number of amniotic sacs

    O30.091   Twin pregnancy, unable to determine number of placenta and number of amniotic sacs, **first trimester**

    O30.092   Twin pregnancy, unable to determine number of placenta and number of amniotic sacs, **second trimester**

    O30.093   Twin pregnancy, unable to determine number of placenta and number of amniotic sacs, **third trimester**

    O30.099   Twin pregnancy, unable to determine number of placenta and number of amniotic sacs, **unspecified trimester**

● **O30.1** **Triplet pregnancy**

  ● **O30.10** Triplet pregnancy, **unspecified** number of placenta and **unspecified** number of amniotic sacs

    O30.101   Triplet pregnancy, unspecified number of placenta and unspecified number of amniotic sacs, **first trimester**

    O30.102   Triplet pregnancy, unspecified number of placenta and unspecified number of amniotic sacs, **second trimester**

    O30.103   Triplet pregnancy, unspecified number of placenta and unspecified number of amniotic sacs, **third trimester**

    O30.109   Triplet pregnancy, unspecified number of placenta and unspecified number of amniotic sacs, **unspecified trimester**

  ● **O30.11** Triplet pregnancy with **two or more monochorionic fetuses**

    O30.111   Triplet pregnancy with two or more monochorionic fetuses, **first trimester**

    O30.112   Triplet pregnancy with two or more monochorionic fetuses, **second trimester**

    O30.113   Triplet pregnancy with two or more monochorionic fetuses, **third trimester**

    O30.119   Triplet pregnancy with two or more monochorionic fetuses, **unspecified trimester**

  ● **O30.12** Triplet pregnancy with **two or more monoamniotic fetuses**

    O30.121   Triplet pregnancy with two or more monoamniotic fetuses, **first trimester**

    O30.122   Triplet pregnancy with two or more monoamniotic fetuses, **second trimester**

    O30.123   Triplet pregnancy with two or more monoamniotic fetuses, **third trimester**

    O30.129   Triplet pregnancy with two or more monoamniotic fetuses, **unspecified trimester**

● O30.19 Triplet pregnancy, unable to determine number of placenta and number of amniotic sacs

     O30.191   Triplet pregnancy, unable to determine number of placenta and number of amniotic sacs, first trimester

     O30.192   Triplet pregnancy, unable to determine number of placenta and number of amniotic sacs, second trimester

     O30.193   Triplet pregnancy, unable to determine number of placenta and number of amniotic sacs, third trimester

     O30.199   Triplet pregnancy, unable to determine number of placenta and number of amniotic sacs, unspecified trimester

● O30.2 Quadruplet pregnancy

   ● O30.20 Quadruplet pregnancy, unspecified number of placenta and unspecified number of amniotic sacs

     O30.201   Quadruplet pregnancy, unspecified number of placenta and unspecified number of amniotic sacs, first trimester

     O30.202   Quadruplet pregnancy, unspecified number of placenta and unspecified number of amniotic sacs, second trimester

     O30.203   Quadruplet pregnancy, unspecified number of placenta and unspecified number of amniotic sacs, third trimester

     O30.209   Quadruplet pregnancy, unspecified number of placenta and unspecified number of amniotic sacs, unspecified trimester

   ● O30.21 Quadruplet pregnancy with two or more monochorionic fetuses

     O30.211   Quadruplet pregnancy with two or more monochorionic fetuses, first trimester

     O30.212   Quadruplet pregnancy with two or more monochorionic fetuses, second trimester

     O30.213   Quadruplet pregnancy with two or more monochorionic fetuses, third trimester

     O30.219   Quadruplet pregnancy with two or more monochorionic fetuses, unspecified trimester

   ● O30.22 Quadruplet pregnancy with two or more monoamniotic fetuses

     O30.221   Quadruplet pregnancy with two or more monoamniotic fetuses, first trimester

     O30.222   Quadruplet pregnancy with two or more monoamniotic fetuses, second trimester

     O30.223   Quadruplet pregnancy with two or more monoamniotic fetuses, third trimester

     O30.229   Quadruplet pregnancy with two or more monoamniotic fetuses, unspecified trimester

● O30.29 Quadruplet pregnancy, unable to determine number of placenta and number of amniotic sacs

     O30.291   Quadruplet pregnancy, unable to determine number of placenta and number of amniotic sacs, first trimester

     O30.292   Quadruplet pregnancy, unable to determine number of placenta and number of amniotic sacs, second trimester

     O30.293   Quadruplet pregnancy, unable to determine number of placenta and number of amniotic sacs, third trimester

     O30.299   Quadruplet pregnancy, unable to determine number of placenta and number of amniotic sacs, unspecified trimester

● O30.8 Other specified multiple gestation

Multiple gestation pregnancy greater then quadruplets

   ● O30.80 Other specified multiple gestation, unspecified number of placenta and unspecified number of amniotic sacs

     O30.801   Other specified multiple gestation, unspecified number of placenta and unspecified number of amniotic sacs, first trimester

     O30.802   Other specified multiple gestation, unspecified number of placenta and unspecified number of amniotic sacs, second trimester

     O30.803   Other specified multiple gestation, unspecified number of placenta and unspecified number of amniotic sacs, third trimester

     O30.809   Other specified multiple gestation, unspecified number of placenta and unspecified number of amniotic sacs, unspecified trimester

   ● O30.81 Other specified multiple gestation with two or more monochorionic fetuses

     O30.811   Other specified multiple gestation with two or more monochorionic fetuses, first trimester

     O30.812   Other specified multiple gestation with two or more monochorionic fetuses, second trimester

     O30.813   Other specified multiple gestation with two or more monochorionic fetuses, third trimester

     O30.819   Other specified multiple gestation with two or more monochorionic fetuses, unspecified trimester

   ● O30.82 Other specified multiple gestation with two or more monoamniotic fetuses

     O30.821   Other specified multiple gestation with two or more monoamniotic fetuses, first trimester

     O30.822   Other specified multiple gestation with two or more monoamniotic fetuses, second trimester

     O30.823   Other specified multiple gestation with two or more monoamniotic fetuses, third trimester

     O30.829   Other specified multiple gestation with two or more monoamniotic fetuses, unspecified trimester

CHAPTER 15 (O00-O9A)

● **O30.89**   Other specified multiple gestation, unable to determine number of placenta and number of amniotic sacs

     O30.891   Other specified multiple gestation, unable to determine number of placenta and number of amniotic sacs, first trimester

     O30.892   Other specified multiple gestation, unable to determine number of placenta and number of amniotic sacs, second trimester

     O30.893   Other specified multiple gestation, unable to determine number of placenta and number of amniotic sacs, third trimester

     O30.899   Other specified multiple gestation, unable to determine number of placenta and number of amniotic sacs, unspecified trimester

● **O30.9**   Multiple gestation, unspecified
     Multiple pregnancy NOS

     O30.90   Multiple gestation, unspecified, unspecified trimester

     O30.91   Multiple gestation, unspecified, first trimester

     O30.92   Multiple gestation, unspecified, second trimester

     O30.93   Multiple gestation, unspecified, third trimester

● **O31**   **Complications specific to multiple gestation**

   | Excludes2 | delayed delivery of second twin, triplet, etc. (O63.2)
                    malpresentation of one fetus or more (O32.9)
                    placental transfusion syndromes (O43.0-)

One of the following 7th characters is to be assigned to each code under category O31. 7th character Ø is for single gestations and multiple gestations where the fetus is unspecified. 7th characters 1 through 9 are for cases of multiple gestations to identify the fetus for which the code applies. The appropriate code from category O30, Multiple gestation, must also be assigned when assigning a code from category O31 that has a 7th character of 1 through 9.

Ø	not applicable or unspecified
1	fetus 1
2	fetus 2
3	fetus 3
4	fetus 4
5	fetus 5
9	other fetus

● **O31.0**   **Papyraceous fetus**
     Fetus compressus

X ● **O31.00**   Papyraceous fetus, unspecified trimester

X ● **O31.01**   Papyraceous fetus, first trimester

X ● **O31.02**   Papyraceous fetus, second trimester

X ● **O31.03**   Papyraceous fetus, third trimester

● **O31.1**   Continuing pregnancy after spontaneous abortion of one fetus or more

X ● **O31.10**   Continuing pregnancy after spontaneous abortion of one fetus or more, unspecified trimester

X ● **O31.11**   Continuing pregnancy after spontaneous abortion of one fetus or more, first trimester

X ● **O31.12**   Continuing pregnancy after spontaneous abortion of one fetus or more, second trimester

X ● **O31.13**   Continuing pregnancy after spontaneous abortion of one fetus or more, third trimester

● **O31.2**   Continuing pregnancy after intrauterine death of one fetus or more

X ● **O31.20**   Continuing pregnancy after intrauterine death of one fetus or more, unspecified trimester

X ● **O31.21**   Continuing pregnancy after intrauterine death of one fetus or more, first trimester

X ● **O31.22**   Continuing pregnancy after intrauterine death of one fetus or more, second trimester

X ● **O31.23**   Continuing pregnancy after intrauterine death of one fetus or more, third trimester

● **O31.3**   Continuing pregnancy after elective fetal reduction of one fetus or more
     Continuing pregnancy after selective termination of one fetus or more

X ● **O31.30**   Continuing pregnancy after elective fetal reduction of one fetus or more, unspecified trimester

X ● **O31.31**   Continuing pregnancy after elective fetal reduction of one fetus or more, first trimester

X ● **O31.32**   Continuing pregnancy after elective fetal reduction of one fetus or more, second trimester

X ● **O31.33**   Continuing pregnancy after elective fetal reduction of one fetus or more, third trimester

● **O31.8**   Other complications specific to multiple gestation

     O31.8X   Other complications specific to multiple gestation

       ● **O31.8X1**   Other complications specific to multiple gestation, first trimester

       ● **O31.8X2**   Other complications specific to multiple gestation, second trimester

       ● **O31.8X3**   Other complications specific to multiple gestation, third trimester

       ● **O31.8X9**   Other complications specific to multiple gestation, unspecified trimester

● **O32**   **Maternal care for malpresentation of fetus**

   | Includes | the listed conditions as a reason for observation, hospitalization or other obstetric care of the mother, or for cesarean delivery before onset of labor

   | Excludes1 | malpresentation of fetus with obstructed labor (O64.-)

One of the following 7th characters is to be assigned to each code under category O32. 7th character Ø is for single gestations and multiple gestations where the fetus is unspecified. 7th characters 1 through 9 are for cases of multiple gestations to identify the fetus for which the code applies. The appropriate code from category O30, Multiple gestation, must also be assigned when assigning a code from category O32 that has a 7th character of 1 through 9.

Ø	not applicable or unspecified
1	fetus 1
2	fetus 2
3	fetus 3
4	fetus 4
5	fetus 5
9	other fetus

X ● **O32.0**   Maternal care for unstable lie

X ● **O32.1**   Maternal care for breech presentation
     Maternal care for buttocks presentation
     Maternal care for complete breech
     Maternal care for frank breech

     | Excludes1 | footling presentation (O32.8)
                     incomplete breech (O32.8)

X● **O32.2** **Maternal care for transverse and oblique lie**
Maternal care for oblique presentation
Maternal care for transverse presentation

X● **O32.3** **Maternal care for face, brow and chin presentation**

X● **O32.4** **Maternal care for high head at term**
Maternal care for failure of head to enter pelvic brim

X● **O32.6** **Maternal care for compound presentation**

X● **O32.8** **Maternal care for other malpresentation of fetus**
Maternal care for footling presentation
Maternal care for incomplete breech

X● **O32.9** **Maternal care for malpresentation of fetus, unspecified**

● **O33** **Maternal care for disproportion**

> **Includes**   the listed conditions as a reason for observation, hospitalization or other obstetric care of the mother, or for cesarean delivery before onset of labor

> **Excludes1**   disproportion with obstructed labor (O65-O66)

O33.0 **Maternal care for disproportion due to deformity of maternal pelvic bones**
Maternal care for disproportion due to pelvic deformity causing disproportion NOS

O33.1 **Maternal care for disproportion due to generally contracted pelvis**
Maternal care for disproportion due to contracted pelvis NOS causing disproportion

O33.2 **Maternal care for disproportion due to inlet contraction of pelvis**
Maternal care for disproportion due to inlet contraction (pelvis) causing disproportion

X● **O33.3** **Maternal care for disproportion due to outlet contraction of pelvis**
Maternal care for disproportion due to mid-cavity contraction (pelvis)
Maternal care for disproportion due to outlet contraction (pelvis)

One of the following 7th characters is to be assigned to code O33.3. 7th character 0 is for single gestations and multiple gestations where the fetus is unspecified. 7th characters 1 through 9 are for cases of multiple gestations to identify the fetus for which the code applies. The appropriate code from category O30, Multiple gestation, must also be assigned when assigning code O33.3 with a 7th character of 1 through 9.

0	not applicable or unspecified
1	fetus 1
2	fetus 2
3	fetus 3
4	fetus 4
5	fetus 5
9	other fetus

X● **O33.4** **Maternal care for disproportion of mixed maternal and fetal origin**

One of the following 7th characters is to be assigned to code O33.4. 7th character 0 is for single gestations and multiple gestations where the fetus is unspecified. 7th characters 1 through 9 are for cases of multiple gestations to identify the fetus for which the code applies. The appropriate code from category O30, Multiple gestation, must also be assigned when assigning code O33.4 with a 7th character of 1 through 9.

0	not applicable or unspecified
1	fetus 1
2	fetus 2
3	fetus 3
4	fetus 4
5	fetus 5
9	other fetus

X● **O33.5** **Maternal care for disproportion due to unusually large fetus**
Maternal care for disproportion due to disproportion of fetal origin with normally formed fetus
Maternal care for disproportion due to fetal disproportion NOS

One of the following 7th characters is to be assigned to code O33.5. 7th character 0 is for single gestations and multiple gestations where the fetus is unspecified. 7th characters 1 through 9 are for cases of multiple gestations to identify the fetus for which the code applies. The appropriate code from category O30, Multiple gestation, must also be assigned when assigning code O33.5 with a 7th character of 1 through 9.

0	not applicable or unspecified
1	fetus 1
2	fetus 2
3	fetus 3
4	fetus 4
5	fetus 5
9	other fetus

X● **O33.6** **Maternal care for disproportion due to hydrocephalic fetus**

One of the following 7th characters is to be assigned to code O33.6. 7th character 0 is for single gestations and multiple gestations where the fetus is unspecified. 7th characters 1 through 9 are for cases of multiple gestations to identify the fetus for which the code applies. The appropriate code from category O30, Multiple gestation, must also be assigned when assigning code O33.6 with a 7th character of 1 through 9.

0	not applicable or unspecified
1	fetus 1
2	fetus 2
3	fetus 3
4	fetus 4
5	fetus 5
9	other fetus

X● **O33.7** **Maternal care for disproportion due to other fetal deformities**
Maternal care for disproportion due to fetal ascites
Maternal care for disproportion due to fetal hydrops
Maternal care for disproportion due to fetal meningomyelocele
Maternal care for disproportion due to fetal sacral teratoma
Maternal care for disproportion due to fetal tumor

> **Excludes1**   obstructed labor due to other fetal deformities (O66.3)

One of the following 7th characters is to be assigned to code O33.7. 7th character 0 is for single gestations and multiple gestations where the fetus is unspecified. 7th characters 1 through 9 are for cases of multiple gestations to identify the fetus for which the code applies. The appropriate code from category O30, Multiple gestation, must also be assigned when assigning code O33.7 with a 7th character of 1 through 9.

0	not applicable or unspecified
1	fetus 1
2	fetus 2
3	fetus 3
4	fetus 4
5	fetus 5
9	other fetus

O33.8 **Maternal care for disproportion of other origin**

O33.9 **Maternal care for disproportion, unspecified**
Maternal care for disproportion due to cephalopelvic disproportion NOS
Maternal care for disproportion due to fetopelvic disproportion NOS

▶ New   ⇒ Revised   ~~deleted~~ Deleted   **OGCR** Official Guidelines   X Assign placeholder X   ● Use Additional Character(s)

Excludes 1   Excludes 2   Includes   Use additional   Code first   Code also   Key words

● **O34   Maternal care for abnormality of pelvic organs**

> **Includes**   the listed conditions as a reason for hospitalization or other obstetric care of the mother, or for cesarean delivery before onset of labor

> *Code first any associated obstructed labor (O65.5)*
> Use additional code for specific condition

● **O34.0   Maternal care for congenital malformation of uterus**
> Maternal care for double uterus
> Maternal care for uterus bicornis

> **O34.00**   Maternal care for unspecified congenital malformation of uterus, unspecified trimester

> **O34.01**   Maternal care for unspecified congenital malformation of uterus, first trimester

> **O34.02**   Maternal care for unspecified congenital malformation of uterus, second trimester

> **O34.03**   Maternal care for unspecified congenital malformation of uterus, third trimester

● **O34.1   Maternal care for benign tumor of corpus uteri**

> **Excludes2**   maternal care for benign tumor of cervix (O34.4-)
> maternal care for malignant neoplasm of uterus (O9A.1-)

> **O34.10**   Maternal care for benign tumor of corpus uteri, unspecified trimester

> **O34.11**   Maternal care for benign tumor of corpus uteri, first trimester

> **O34.12**   Maternal care for benign tumor of corpus uteri, second trimester

> **O34.13**   Maternal care for benign tumor of corpus uteri, third trimester

● **O34.2   Maternal care due to uterine scar from previous surgery**

> ● **O34.21**   Maternal care for scar from previous cesarean delivery

> > **O34.211**   Maternal care for low transverse scar from previous cesarean delivery

> > **O34.212**   Maternal care for vertical scar from previous cesarean delivery
> > > Maternal care for classical scar from previous cesarean delivery

> > **O34.219**   Maternal care for unspecified type scar from previous cesarean delivery

> **O34.29**   Maternal care due to uterine scar from other previous surgery
> > Maternal care due to uterine scar from other transmural uterine incision

● **O34.3   Maternal care for cervical incompetence**
> Maternal care for cerclage with or without cervical incompetence
> Maternal care for Shirodkar suture with or without cervical incompetence

> **O34.30**   Maternal care for cervical incompetence, unspecified trimester

> **O34.31**   Maternal care for cervical incompetence, first trimester

> **O34.32**   Maternal care for cervical incompetence, second trimester

> **O34.33**   Maternal care for cervical incompetence, third trimester

● **O34.4   Maternal care for other abnormalities of cervix**

> **O34.40**   Maternal care for other abnormalities of cervix, unspecified trimester

> **O34.41**   Maternal care for other abnormalities of cervix, first trimester

> **O34.42**   Maternal care for other abnormalities of cervix, second trimester

> **O34.43**   Maternal care for other abnormalities of cervix, third trimester

● **O34.5   Maternal care for other abnormalities of gravid uterus**

> ● **O34.51**   Maternal care for incarceration of gravid uterus

> > **O34.511**   Maternal care for incarceration of gravid uterus, first trimester

> > **O34.512**   Maternal care for incarceration of gravid uterus, second trimester

> > **O34.513**   Maternal care for incarceration of gravid uterus, third trimester

> > **O34.519**   Maternal care for incarceration of gravid uterus, unspecified trimester

> ● **O34.52**   Maternal care for prolapse of gravid uterus

> > **O34.521**   Maternal care for prolapse of gravid uterus, first trimester

> > **O34.522**   Maternal care for prolapse of gravid uterus, second trimester

> > **O34.523**   Maternal care for prolapse of gravid uterus, third trimester

> > **O34.529**   Maternal care for prolapse of gravid uterus, unspecified trimester

> ● **O34.53**   Maternal care for retroversion of gravid uterus

> > **O34.531**   Maternal care for retroversion of gravid uterus, first trimester

> > **O34.532**   Maternal care for retroversion of gravid uterus, second trimester

> > **O34.533**   Maternal care for retroversion of gravid uterus, third trimester

> > **O34.539**   Maternal care for retroversion of gravid uterus, unspecified trimester

> ● **O34.59**   Maternal care for other abnormalities of gravid uterus

> > **O34.591**   Maternal care for other abnormalities of gravid uterus, first trimester

> > **O34.592**   Maternal care for other abnormalities of gravid uterus, second trimester

> > **O34.593**   Maternal care for other abnormalities of gravid uterus, third trimester

> > **O34.599**   Maternal care for other abnormalities of gravid uterus, unspecified trimester

● **O34.6   Maternal care for abnormality of vagina**

> **Excludes2**   maternal care for vaginal varices in pregnancy (O22.1-)

> **O34.60**   Maternal care for abnormality of vagina, unspecified trimester

> **O34.61**   Maternal care for abnormality of vagina, first trimester

> **O34.62**   Maternal care for abnormality of vagina, second trimester

> **O34.63**   Maternal care for abnormality of vagina, third trimester

● O34.7   Maternal care for abnormality of vulva and perineum

> **Excludes2**   maternal care for perineal and vulval varices in pregnancy (O22.1-)

O34.70   Maternal care for abnormality of vulva and perineum, unspecified trimester

O34.71   Maternal care for abnormality of vulva and perineum, first trimester

O34.72   Maternal care for abnormality of vulva and perineum, second trimester

O34.73   Maternal care for abnormality of vulva and perineum, third trimester

● O34.8   Maternal care for other abnormalities of pelvic organs

O34.80   Maternal care for other abnormalities of pelvic organs, unspecified trimester

O34.81   Maternal care for other abnormalities of pelvic organs, first trimester

O34.82   Maternal care for other abnormalities of pelvic organs, second trimester

O34.83   Maternal care for other abnormalities of pelvic organs, third trimester

● O34.9   Maternal care for abnormality of pelvic organ, unspecified

O34.90   Maternal care for abnormality of pelvic organ, unspecified, unspecified trimester

O34.91   Maternal care for abnormality of pelvic organ, unspecified, first trimester

O34.92   Maternal care for abnormality of pelvic organ, unspecified, second trimester

O34.93   Maternal care for abnormality of pelvic organ, unspecified, third trimester

● O35   Maternal care for known or suspected fetal abnormality and damage

> **Includes**   the listed conditions in the fetus as a reason for hospitalization or other obstetric care to the mother, or for termination of pregnancy

Code also any associated maternal condition

> **Excludes1**   encounter for suspected maternal and fetal conditions ruled out (Z03.7-)

One of the following 7th characters is to be assigned to each code under category O35. 7th character 0 is for single gestations and multiple gestations where the fetus is unspecified. 7th characters 1 through 9 are for cases of multiple gestations to identify the fetus for which the code applies. The appropriate code from category O30, Multiple gestation, must also be assigned when assigning a code from category O35 that has a 7th character of 1 through 9.

0	not applicable or unspecified
1	fetus 1
2	fetus 2
3	fetus 3
4	fetus 4
5	fetus 5
9	other fetus

X● O35.0   Maternal care for (suspected) central nervous system malformation in fetus

Maternal care for fetal anencephaly

Maternal care for fetal hydrocephalus

Maternal care for fetal spina bifida

> **Excludes2**   chromosomal abnormality in fetus (O35.1)

X● O35.1   Maternal care for (suspected) chromosomal abnormality in fetus

X● O35.2   Maternal care for (suspected) hereditary disease in fetus

> **Excludes2**   chromosomal abnormality in fetus (O35.1)

X● O35.3   Maternal care for (suspected) damage to fetus from viral disease in mother

Maternal care for damage to fetus from maternal cytomegalovirus infection

Maternal care for damage to fetus from maternal rubella

X● O35.4   Maternal care for (suspected) damage to fetus from alcohol

X● O35.5   Maternal care for (suspected) damage to fetus by drugs

Maternal care for damage to fetus from drug addiction

X● O35.6   Maternal care for (suspected) damage to fetus by radiation

X● O35.7   Maternal care for (suspected) damage to fetus by other medical procedures

Maternal care for damage to fetus by amniocentesis

Maternal care for damage to fetus by biopsy procedures

Maternal care for damage to fetus by hematological investigation

Maternal care for damage to fetus by intrauterine contraceptive device

Maternal care for damage to fetus by intrauterine surgery

X● O35.8   Maternal care for other (suspected) fetal abnormality and damage

Maternal care for damage to fetus from maternal listeriosis

Maternal care for damage to fetus from maternal toxoplasmosis

X● O35.9   Maternal care for (suspected) fetal abnormality and damage, unspecified

OGCR Section I.C.15.e.l.

Fetal Conditions Affecting the Management of the Mother

1) Code from categories O35 and O36

Codes from categories O35, Maternal care for known or suspected fetal abnormality and damage, and O36, Maternal care for other fetal problems, are assigned only when the fetal condition is actually responsible for modifying the management of the mother, i.e., by requiring diagnostic studies, additional observation, special care, or termination of pregnancy. The fact that the fetal condition exists does not justify assigning a code from this series to the mother's record.

2) In utero surgery

In cases when surgery is performed on the fetus, a diagnosis code from category O35, Maternal care for known or suspected fetal abnormality and damage, should be assigned identifying the fetal condition. Assign the appropriate procedure code for the procedure performed.

No code from Chapter 16, the perinatal codes, should be used on the mother's record to identify fetal conditions. Surgery performed in utero on a fetus is still to be coded as an obstetric encounter.

▶ New   ⇒ Revised   ~~deleted~~ Deleted   **OGCR** Official Guidelines   X Assign placeholder X   ● Use Additional Character(s)

Excludes 1   Excludes 2   Includes   Use additional   Code first   Code also   Key words

● **O36　Maternal care for other fetal problems**

| **Includes** | the listed conditions in the fetus as a reason for hospitalization or other obstetric care of the mother, or for termination of pregnancy |

| **Excludes1** | encounter for suspected maternal and fetal conditions ruled out (Z03.7-) placental transfusion syndromes (O43.0-) |

| **Excludes2** | labor and delivery complicated by fetal stress (O77.-) |

One of the following 7th characters is to be assigned to each code under category O36. 7th character 0 is for single gestations and multiple gestations where the fetus is unspecified. 7th characters 1 through 9 are for cases of multiple gestations to identify the fetus for which the code applies. The appropriate code from category O30, Multiple gestation, must also be assigned when assigning a code from category O36 that has a 7th character of 1 through 9.

> 0　not applicable or unspecified
> 1　fetus 1
> 2　fetus 2
> 3　fetus 3
> 4　fetus 4
> 5　fetus 5
> 9　other fetus

● **O36.0　Maternal care for rhesus isoimmunization**
　　　Maternal care for Rh incompatibility (with hydrops fetalis)

　　● **O36.01　Maternal care for anti-D [Rh] antibodies**
　　　　● **O36.011　Maternal care for anti-D [Rh] antibodies, first trimester**
　　　　● **O36.012　Maternal care for anti-D [Rh] antibodies, second trimester**
　　　　● **O36.013　Maternal care for anti-D [Rh] antibodies, third trimester**
　　　　● **O36.019　Maternal care for anti-D [Rh] antibodies, unspecified trimester**

　　● **O36.09　Maternal care for other rhesus isoimmunization**
　　　　● **O36.091　Maternal care for other rhesus isoimmunization, first trimester**
　　　　● **O36.092　Maternal care for other rhesus isoimmunization, second trimester**
　　　　● **O36.093　Maternal care for other rhesus isoimmunization, third trimester**
　　　　● **O36.099　Maternal care for other rhesus isoimmunization, unspecified trimester**

● **O36.1　Maternal care for other isoimmunization**
　　　Maternal care for ABO isoimmunization

　　● **O36.11　Maternal care for Anti-A sensitization**
　　　　Maternal care for isoimmunization NOS (with hydrops fetalis)
　　　　● **O36.111　Maternal care for Anti-A sensitization, first trimester**
　　　　● **O36.112　Maternal care for Anti-A sensitization, second trimester**
　　　　● **O36.113　Maternal care for Anti-A sensitization, third trimester**
　　　　● **O36.119　Maternal care for Anti-A sensitization, unspecified trimester**

● **O36.19　Maternal care for other isoimmunization**
　　　Maternal care for Anti-B sensitization
　　● **O36.191　Maternal care for other isoimmunization, first trimester**
　　● **O36.192　Maternal care for other isoimmunization, second trimester**
　　● **O36.193　Maternal care for other isoimmunization, third trimester**
　　● **O36.199　Maternal care for other isoimmunization, unspecified trimester**

● **O36.2　Maternal care for hydrops fetalis**
　　　Maternal care for hydrops fetalis NOS
　　　Maternal care for hydrops fetalis not associated with isoimmunization

| **Excludes1** | hydrops fetalis associated with ABO isoimmunization (O36.1-) hydrops fetalis associated with rhesus isoimmunization (O36.0-) |

　　● **O36.20　Maternal care for hydrops fetalis, unspecified trimester**
　　● **O36.21　Maternal care for hydrops fetalis, first trimester**
　　● **O36.22　Maternal care for hydrops fetalis, second trimester**
　　● **O36.23　Maternal care for hydrops fetalis, third trimester**

● **O36.4　Maternal care for intrauterine death**
　　　Maternal care for intrauterine fetal death NOS
　　　Maternal care for intrauterine fetal death after completion of 20 weeks of gestation
　　　Maternal care for late fetal death
　　　Maternal care for missed delivery

| **Excludes1** | missed abortion (O02.1) stillbirth (P95) |

● **O36.5　Maternal care for known or suspected poor fetal growth**

　　● **O36.51　Maternal care for known or suspected placental insufficiency**
　　　　● **O36.511　Maternal care for known or suspected placental insufficiency, first trimester**
　　　　● **O36.512　Maternal care for known or suspected placental insufficiency, second trimester**
　　　　● **O36.513　Maternal care for known or suspected placental insufficiency, third trimester**
　　　　● **O36.519　Maternal care for known or suspected placental insufficiency, unspecified trimester**

　　● **O36.59　Maternal care for other known or suspected poor fetal growth**
　　　　Maternal care for known or suspected light-for-dates NOS
　　　　Maternal care for known or suspected small-for-dates NOS
　　　　● **O36.591　Maternal care for other known or suspected poor fetal growth, first trimester**
　　　　● **O36.592　Maternal care for other known or suspected poor fetal growth, second trimester**
　　　　● **O36.593　Maternal care for other known or suspected poor fetal growth, third trimester**
　　　　● **O36.599　Maternal care for other known or suspected poor fetal growth, unspecified trimester**

● **O36.6 Maternal care for excessive fetal growth**
    Maternal care for known or suspected large-for-dates

X● **O36.60 Maternal care for excessive fetal growth, unspecified trimester**

X● **O36.61 Maternal care for excessive fetal growth, first trimester**

X● **O36.62 Maternal care for excessive fetal growth, second trimester**

X● **O36.63 Maternal care for excessive fetal growth, third trimester**

● **O36.7 Maternal care for viable fetus in abdominal pregnancy**

X● **O36.70 Maternal care for viable fetus in abdominal pregnancy, unspecified trimester**

X● **O36.71 Maternal care for viable fetus in abdominal pregnancy, first trimester**

X● **O36.72 Maternal care for viable fetus in abdominal pregnancy, second trimester**

X● **O36.73 Maternal care for viable fetus in abdominal pregnancy, third trimester**

● **O36.8 Maternal care for other specified fetal problems**

X● **O36.80 Pregnancy with inconclusive fetal viability**
    Encounter to determine fetal viability of pregnancy

● **O36.81 Decreased fetal movements**

● **O36.812 Decreased fetal movements, second trimester**

● **O36.813 Decreased fetal movements, third trimester**

● **O36.819 Decreased fetal movements, unspecified trimester**

● **O36.82 Fetal anemia and thrombocytopenia**

● **O36.821 Fetal anemia and thrombocytopenia, first trimester**

● **O36.822 Fetal anemia and thrombocytopenia, second trimester**

● **O36.823 Fetal anemia and thrombocytopenia, third trimester**

● **O36.829 Fetal anemia and thrombocytopenia, unspecified trimester**

▶● **O36.83 Maternal care for abnormalities of the fetal heart rate or rhythm**

▶● **O36.831 Maternal care for abnormalities of the fetal heart rate or rhythm, first trimester**

▶● **O36.832 Maternal care for abnormalities of the fetal heart rate or rhythm, second trimester**

▶● **O36.833 Maternal care for abnormalities of the fetal heart rate or rhythm, third trimester**

▶● **O36.839 Maternal care for abnormalities of the fetal heart rate or rhythm, unspecified trimester**

● **O36.89 Maternal care for other specified fetal problems**

● **O36.891 Maternal care for other specified fetal problems, first trimester**

● **O36.892 Maternal care for other specified fetal problems, second trimester**

● **O36.893 Maternal care for other specified fetal problems, third trimester**

● **O36.899 Maternal care for other specified fetal problems, unspecified trimester**

● **O36.9 Maternal care for fetal problem, unspecified**

X● **O36.90 Maternal care for fetal problem, unspecified, unspecified trimester**

X● **O36.91 Maternal care for fetal problem, unspecified, first trimester**

X● **O36.92 Maternal care for fetal problem, unspecified, second trimester**

X● **O36.93 Maternal care for fetal problem, unspecified, third trimester**

● **O40 Polyhydramnios**
    Overabundance of amniotic fluid

Includes hydramnios

Excludes1 encounter for suspected maternal and fetal conditions ruled out (Z03.7-)

One of the following 7th characters is to be assigned to each code under category O40. 7th character Ø is for single gestations and multiple gestations where the fetus is unspecified. 7th characters 1 through 9 are for cases of multiple gestations to identify the fetus for which the code applies. The appropriate code from category O30, Multiple gestation, must also be assigned when assigning a code from category O40 that has a 7th character of 1 through 9.

Ø	not applicable or unspecified
1	fetus 1
2	fetus 2
3	fetus 3
4	fetus 4
5	fetus 5
9	other fetus

X● **O40.1 Polyhydramnios, first trimester**

X● **O40.2 Polyhydramnios, second trimester**

X● **O40.3 Polyhydramnios, third trimester**

X● **O40.9 Polyhydramnios, unspecified trimester**

● **O41 Other disorders of amniotic fluid and membranes**

Excludes1 encounter for suspected maternal and fetal conditions ruled out (Z03.7-)

One of the following 7th characters is to be assigned to each code under category O41. 7th character Ø is for single gestations and multiple gestations where the fetus is unspecified. 7th characters 1 through 9 are for cases of multiple gestations to identify the fetus for which the code applies. The appropriate code from category O30, Multiple gestation, must also be assigned when assigning a code from category O41 that has a 7th character of 1 through 9.

Ø	not applicable or unspecified
1	fetus 1
2	fetus 2
3	fetus 3
4	fetus 4
5	fetus 5
9	other fetus

● **O41.0 Oligohydramnios**
    Scant volume of amniotic fluid
    Oligohydramnios without rupture of membranes

X● **O41.00 Oligohydramnios, unspecified trimester**

X● **O41.01 Oligohydramnios, first trimester**

X● **O41.02 Oligohydramnios, second trimester**

X● **O41.03 Oligohydramnios, third trimester**

● **O41.1 Infection of amniotic sac and membranes**

● **O41.10 Infection of amniotic sac and membranes, unspecified**

● **O41.101 Infection of amniotic sac and membranes, unspecified, first trimester**

● **O41.102 Infection of amniotic sac and membranes, unspecified, second trimester**

● **O41.103 Infection of amniotic sac and membranes, unspecified, third trimester**

● **O41.109 Infection of amniotic sac and membranes, unspecified, unspecified trimester**

▶ New   ⇒ Revised   ~~deleted~~ Deleted   **OGCR** Official Guidelines   X Assign placeholder X   ● Use Additional Character(s)

Excludes 1   Excludes 2   Includes   Use additional   Code first   Code also   Key words

● **O41.12   Chorioamnionitis**
  ● **O41.121**   Chorioamnionitis, first trimester
  ● **O41.122**   Chorioamnionitis, second trimester
  ● **O41.123**   Chorioamnionitis, third trimester
  ● **O41.129**   Chorioamnionitis, unspecified trimester
● **O41.14   Placentitis**
  ● **O41.141**   Placentitis, first trimester
  ● **O41.142**   Placentitis, second trimester
  ● **O41.143**   Placentitis, third trimester
  ● **O41.149**   Placentitis, unspecified trimester
● **O41.8   Other specified disorders of amniotic fluid and membranes**
  ● **O41.8X**   Other specified disorders of amniotic fluid and membranes
    ● **O41.8X1**   Other specified disorders of amniotic fluid and membranes, first trimester
    ● **O41.8X2**   Other specified disorders of amniotic fluid and membranes, second trimester
    ● **O41.8X3**   Other specified disorders of amniotic fluid and membranes, third trimester
    ● **O41.8X9**   Other specified disorders of amniotic fluid and membranes, unspecified trimester
● **O41.9   Disorder of amniotic fluid and membranes, unspecified**
  X ● **O41.90**   Disorder of amniotic fluid and membranes, unspecified, unspecified trimester
  X ● **O41.91**   Disorder of amniotic fluid and membranes, unspecified, first trimester
  X ● **O41.92**   Disorder of amniotic fluid and membranes, unspecified, second trimester
  X ● **O41.93**   Disorder of amniotic fluid and membranes, unspecified, third trimester

● **O42   Premature rupture of membranes**
  ● **O42.0   Premature rupture of membranes, onset of labor within 24 hours of rupture**
    O42.00   Premature rupture of membranes, onset of labor within 24 hours of rupture, unspecified weeks of gestation
    ● **O42.01**   Preterm premature rupture of membranes, onset of labor within 24 hours of rupture
      Premature rupture of membranes before 37 completed weeks of gestation
      O42.011   Preterm premature rupture of membranes, onset of labor within 24 hours of rupture, first trimester
      O42.012   Preterm premature rupture of membranes, onset of labor within 24 hours of rupture, second trimester
      O42.013   Preterm premature rupture of membranes, onset of labor within 24 hours of rupture, third trimester
      O42.019   Preterm premature rupture of membranes, onset of labor within 24 hours of rupture, unspecified trimester
    O42.02   Full-term premature rupture of membranes, onset of labor within 24 hours of rupture
      Premature rupture of membranes at or after 37 completed weeks of gestation, onset of labor within 24 hours of rupture

● **O42.1   Premature rupture of membranes, onset of labor more than 24 hours following rupture**
  O42.10   Premature rupture of membranes, onset of labor more than 24 hours following rupture, unspecified weeks of gestation
  ● **O42.11**   Preterm premature rupture of membranes, onset of labor more than 24 hours following rupture
    Premature rupture of membranes before 37 completed weeks of gestation
    O42.111   Preterm premature rupture of membranes, onset of labor more than 24 hours following rupture, first trimester
    O42.112   Preterm premature rupture of membranes, onset of labor more than 24 hours following rupture, second trimester
    O42.113   Preterm premature rupture of membranes, onset of labor more than 24 hours following rupture, third trimester
    O42.119   Preterm premature rupture of membranes, onset of labor more than 24 hours following rupture, unspecified trimester
  O42.12   Full-term premature rupture of membranes, onset of labor more than 24 hours following rupture
    Premature rupture of membranes at or after 37 completed weeks of gestation, onset of labor more than 24 hours following rupture
● **O42.9   Premature rupture of membranes, unspecified as to length of time between rupture and onset of labor**
  O42.90   Premature rupture of membranes, unspecified as to length of time between rupture and onset of labor, unspecified weeks of gestation
  ● **O42.91**   Preterm premature rupture of membranes, unspecified as to length of time between rupture and onset of labor
    Premature rupture of membranes before 37 completed weeks of gestation
    O42.911   Preterm premature rupture of membranes, unspecified as to length of time between rupture and onset of labor, first trimester
    O42.912   Preterm premature rupture of membranes, unspecified as to length of time between rupture and onset of labor, second trimester
    O42.913   Preterm premature rupture of membranes, unspecified as to length of time between rupture and onset of labor, third trimester
    O42.919   Preterm premature rupture of membranes, unspecified as to length of time between rupture and onset of labor, unspecified trimester
  O42.92   Full-term premature rupture of membranes, unspecified as to length of time between rupture and onset of labor
    Premature rupture of membranes at or after 37 completed weeks of gestation, unspecified as to length of time between rupture and onset of labor

---

▶ New   ⇒ Revised   ~~deleted~~ Deleted   **OGCR** Official Guidelines   X Assign placeholder X   ● Use Additional Character(s)

Excludes 1   Excludes 2   Includes   Use additional   Code first   Code also   Key words

● **O43   Placental disorders**

> **Excludes2**   maternal care for poor fetal growth due to placental insufficiency (O36.5-)
> placenta previa (O44.-)
> placental polyp (O90.89)
> placentitis (O41.14-)
> premature separation of placenta [abruptio placentae] (O45.-)

● **O43.0   Placental transfusion syndromes**

   ● **O43.01   Fetomaternal placental transfusion syndrome**
      Maternofetal placental transfusion syndrome

     O43.011   Fetomaternal placental transfusion syndrome, first trimester

     O43.012   Fetomaternal placental transfusion syndrome, second trimester

     O43.013   Fetomaternal placental transfusion syndrome, third trimester

     O43.019   Fetomaternal placental transfusion syndrome, unspecified trimester

   ● **O43.02   Fetus-to-fetus placental transfusion syndrome**

     O43.021   Fetus-to-fetus placental transfusion syndrome, first trimester

     O43.022   Fetus-to-fetus placental transfusion syndrome, second trimester

     O43.023   Fetus-to-fetus placental transfusion syndrome, third trimester

     O43.029   Fetus-to-fetus placental transfusion syndrome, unspecified trimester

● **O43.1   Malformation of placenta**

   ● **O43.10   Malformation of placenta, unspecified**
      Abnormal placenta NOS

     O43.101   Malformation of placenta, unspecified, first trimester

     O43.102   Malformation of placenta, unspecified, second trimester

     O43.103   Malformation of placenta, unspecified, third trimester

     O43.109   Malformation of placenta, unspecified, unspecified trimester

   ● **O43.11   Circumvallate placenta**

     O43.111   Circumvallate placenta, first trimester

     O43.112   Circumvallate placenta, second trimester

     O43.113   Circumvallate placenta, third trimester

     O43.119   Circumvallate placenta, unspecified trimester

   ● **O43.12   Velamentous insertion of umbilical cord**

     O43.121   Velamentous insertion of umbilical cord, first trimester

     O43.122   Velamentous insertion of umbilical cord, second trimester

     O43.123   Velamentous insertion of umbilical cord, third trimester

     O43.129   Velamentous insertion of umbilical cord, unspecified trimester

   ● **O43.19   Other malformation of placenta**

     O43.191   Other malformation of placenta, first trimester

     O43.192   Other malformation of placenta, second trimester

     O43.193   Other malformation of placenta, third trimester

     O43.199   Other malformation of placenta, unspecified trimester

● **O43.2   Morbidly adherent placenta**

> Code also associated third stage postpartum hemorrhage, if applicable (O72.0)
>
> **Excludes1**   retained placenta (O73.-)

   ● **O43.21   Placenta accreta**

     O43.211   Placenta accreta, first trimester

     O43.212   Placenta accreta, second trimester

     O43.213   Placenta accreta, third trimester

     O43.219   Placenta accreta, unspecified trimester

   ● **O43.22   Placenta increta**

     O43.221   Placenta increta, first trimester

     O43.222   Placenta increta, second trimester

     O43.223   Placenta increta, third trimester

     O43.229   Placenta increta, unspecified trimester

   ● **O43.23   Placenta percreta**

     O43.231   Placenta percreta, first trimester

     O43.232   Placenta percreta, second trimester

     O43.233   Placenta percreta, third trimester

     O43.239   Placenta percreta, unspecified trimester

● **O43.8   Other placental disorders**

   ● **O43.81   Placental infarction**

     O43.811   Placental infarction, first trimester

     O43.812   Placental infarction, second trimester

     O43.813   Placental infarction, third trimester

     O43.819   Placental infarction, unspecified trimester

   ● **O43.89   Other placental disorders**
      Placental dysfunction

     O43.891   Other placental disorders, first trimester

     O43.892   Other placental disorders, second trimester

     O43.893   Other placental disorders, third trimester

     O43.899   Other placental disorders, unspecified trimester

● **O43.9   Unspecified placental disorder**

     O43.90   Unspecified placental disorder, unspecified trimester

     O43.91   Unspecified placental disorder, first trimester

     O43.92   Unspecified placental disorder, second trimester

     O43.93   Unspecified placental disorder, third trimester

● **O44   Placenta previa**

   ● **O44.0   Complete placenta previa NOS or without hemorrhage**
      Placenta previa NOS

     O44.00   Complete placenta previa NOS or without hemorrhage, unspecified trimester

     O44.01   Complete placenta previa NOS or without hemorrhage, first trimester

     O44.02   Complete placenta previa NOS or without hemorrhage, second trimester

     O44.03   Complete placenta previa NOS or without hemorrhage, third trimester

▶ New   ⇒ Revised   ~~deleted~~ Deleted   **OGCR** Official Guidelines   X Assign placeholder X   ● Use Additional Character(s)

Excludes 1   Excludes 2   Includes   Use additional   Code first   Code also   Key words

Figure 15-2 **A.** Marginal placento previa. **B.** Partial placenta previa. **C.** Total placento previa.

Item 15–3 Placenta previa is a condition in which the opening of the cervix is obstructed by the displaced placenta. The three types, marginal, partial, and total, are varying degrees of placenta displacement. Placenta abruption is the premature breaking away of the placenta from the site of the uterine implant before the delivery of the fetus.

- O44.1   Complete placenta previa with hemorrhage
  - Excludes1   labor and delivery complicated by hemorrhage from vasa previa (O69.4)
  - O44.10   Complete placenta previa with hemorrhage, unspecified trimester
  - O44.11   Complete placenta previa with hemorrhage, first trimester
  - O44.12   Complete placenta previa with hemorrhage, second trimester
  - O44.13   Complete placenta previa with hemorrhage, third trimester
- O44.2   Partial placenta previa without hemorrhage
  - Marginal placenta previa, NOS or without hemorrhage
  - O44.20   Partial placenta previa NOS or without hemorrhage, unspecified trimester
  - O44.21   Partial placenta previa NOS or without hemorrhage, first trimester
  - O44.22   Partial placenta previa NOS or without hemorrhage, second trimester
  - O44.23   Partial placenta previa NOS or without hemorrhage, third trimester
- O44.3   Partial placenta previa with hemorrhage
  - Marginal placenta previa with hemorrhage
  - O44.30   Partial placenta previa with hemorrhage, unspecified trimester
  - O44.31   Partial placenta previa with hemorrhage, first trimester
  - O44.32   Partial placenta previa with hemorrhage, second trimester
  - O44.33   Partial placenta previa with hemorrhage, third trimester
- O44.4   Low lying placenta NOS or without hemorrhage
  - Low implantation of placenta NOS or without hemorrhage
  - O44.40   Low lying placenta NOS or without hemorrhage, unspecified trimester
  - O44.41   Low lying placenta NOS or without hemorrhage, first trimester
  - O44.42   Low lying placenta NOS or without hemorrhage, second trimester
  - O44.43   Low lying placenta NOS or without hemorrhage, third trimester
- O44.5   Low lying placenta with hemorrhage
  - Low implantation of placenta with hemorrhage
  - O44.50   Low lying placenta with hemorrhage, unspecified trimester
  - O44.51   Low lying placenta with hemorrhage, first trimester
  - O44.52   Low lying placenta with hemorrhage, second trimester
  - O44.53   Low lying placenta with hemorrhage, third trimester

Figure 15-3 Abruptio placentae is classified according to the grade of separation of the placenta from the uterine wall. **A.** Mild separation in which hemorrhage is internal. **B.** Moderate separation in which there is external hemorrhage. **C.** Severe separation in which there is external hemorrhage and extreme separation.

- O45   Premature separation of placenta [abruptio placentae]
  - O45.0   Premature separation of placenta with coagulation defect
    - O45.00   Premature separation of placenta with coagulation defect, unspecified
      - O45.001   Premature separation of placenta with coagulation defect, unspecified, first trimester
      - O45.002   Premature separation of placenta with coagulation defect, unspecified, second trimester
      - O45.003   Premature separation of placenta with coagulation defect, unspecified, third trimester
      - O45.009   Premature separation of placenta with coagulation defect, unspecified, unspecified trimester
    - O45.01   Premature separation of placenta with afibrinogenemia
      - Premature separation of placenta with hypofibrinogenemia
      - O45.011   Premature separation of placenta with afibrinogenemia, first trimester
      - O45.012   Premature separation of placenta with afibrinogenemia, second trimester
      - O45.013   Premature separation of placenta with afibrinogenemia, third trimester
      - O45.019   Premature separation of placenta with afibrinogenemia, unspecified trimester
    - O45.02   Premature separation of placenta with disseminated intravascular coagulation
      - O45.021   Premature separation of placenta with disseminated intravascular coagulation, first trimester
      - O45.022   Premature separation of placenta with disseminated intravascular coagulation, second trimester
      - O45.023   Premature separation of placenta with disseminated intravascular coagulation, third trimester
      - O45.029   Premature separation of placenta with disseminated intravascular coagulation, unspecified trimester

● O45.09 Premature separation of placenta with other coagulation defect

　　　O45.091 Premature separation of placenta with other coagulation defect, first trimester

　　　O45.092 Premature separation of placenta with other coagulation defect, second trimester

　　　O45.093 Premature separation of placenta with other coagulation defect, third trimester

　　　O45.099 Premature separation of placenta with other coagulation defect, unspecified trimester

● O45.8 Other premature separation of placenta

　● O45.8X Other premature separation of placenta

　　　O45.8X1 Other premature separation of placenta, first trimester

　　　O45.8X2 Other premature separation of placenta, second trimester

　　　O45.8X3 Other premature separation of placenta, third trimester

　　　O45.8X9 Other premature separation of placenta, unspecified trimester

● O45.9 Premature separation of placenta, unspecified
　　Abruptio placentae NOS

　　　O45.90 Premature separation of placenta, unspecified, unspecified trimester

　　　O45.91 Premature separation of placenta, unspecified, first trimester

　　　O45.92 Premature separation of placenta, unspecified, second trimester

　　　O45.93 Premature separation of placenta, unspecified, third trimester

● O46 Antepartum hemorrhage, not elsewhere classified

Excludes1	hemorrhage in early pregnancy (O20.-)
	intrapartum hemorrhage NEC (O67.-)
	placenta previa (O44.-)
	premature separation of placenta [abruptio placentae] (O45.-)

　● O46.0 Antepartum hemorrhage with coagulation defect

　　● O46.00 Antepartum hemorrhage with coagulation defect, unspecified

　　　　O46.001 Antepartum hemorrhage with coagulation defect, unspecified, first trimester

　　　　O46.002 Antepartum hemorrhage with coagulation defect, unspecified, second trimester

　　　　O46.003 Antepartum hemorrhage with coagulation defect, unspecified, third trimester

　　　　O46.009 Antepartum hemorrhage with coagulation defect, unspecified, unspecified trimester

　　● O46.01 Antepartum hemorrhage with afibrinogenemia
　　　　Antepartum hemorrhage with hypofibrinogenemia

　　　　O46.011 Antepartum hemorrhage with afibrinogenemia, first trimester

　　　　O46.012 Antepartum hemorrhage with afibrinogenemia, second trimester

　　　　O46.013 Antepartum hemorrhage with afibrinogenemia, third trimester

　　　　O46.019 Antepartum hemorrhage with afibrinogenemia, unspecified trimester

　● O46.02 Antepartum hemorrhage with disseminated intravascular coagulation

　　　O46.021 Antepartum hemorrhage with disseminated intravascular coagulation, first trimester

　　　O46.022 Antepartum hemorrhage with disseminated intravascular coagulation, second trimester

　　　O46.023 Antepartum hemorrhage with disseminated intravascular coagulation, third trimester

　　　O46.029 Antepartum hemorrhage with disseminated intravascular coagulation, unspecified trimester

　● O46.09 Antepartum hemorrhage with other coagulation defect

　　　O46.091 Antepartum hemorrhage with other coagulation defect, first trimester

　　　O46.092 Antepartum hemorrhage with other coagulation defect, second trimester

　　　O46.093 Antepartum hemorrhage with other coagulation defect, third trimester

　　　O46.099 Antepartum hemorrhage with other coagulation defect, unspecified trimester

● O46.8 Other antepartum hemorrhage

　● O46.8x Other antepartum hemorrhage

　　　O46.8x1 Other antepartum hemorrhage, first trimester

　　　O46.8x2 Other antepartum hemorrhage, second trimester

　　　O46.8x3 Other antepartum hemorrhage, third trimester

　　　O46.8x9 Other antepartum hemorrhage, unspecified trimester

● O46.9 Antepartum hemorrhage, unspecified

　　　O46.90 Antepartum hemorrhage, unspecified, unspecified trimester

　　　O46.91 Antepartum hemorrhage, unspecified, first trimester

　　　O46.92 Antepartum hemorrhage, unspecified, second trimester

　　　O46.93 Antepartum hemorrhage, unspecified, third trimester

● O47 False labor

Includes	Braxton Hicks contractions
	threatened labor
Excludes1	preterm labor (O60.-)

　● O47.0 False labor before 37 completed weeks of gestation

　　　O47.00 False labor before 37 completed weeks of gestation, unspecified trimester

　　　O47.02 False labor before 37 completed weeks of gestation, second trimester

　　　O47.03 False labor before 37 completed weeks of gestation, third trimester

　　O47.1 False labor at or after 37 completed weeks of gestation

　　O47.9 False labor, unspecified

● O48 Late pregnancy

　　O48.0 Post-term pregnancy
　　　Pregnancy over 40 completed weeks to 42 completed weeks gestation

　　O48.1 Prolonged pregnancy
　　　Pregnancy which has advanced beyond 42 completed weeks gestation

▶ New　⇒ Revised　deleted Deleted　OGCR Official Guidelines　X Assign placeholder X　● Use Additional Character(s)

| Excludes 1 | Excludes 2 | Includes | Use additional | Code first | Code also | Key words |

COMPLICATIONS OF LABOR AND DELIVERY (O60–O77)

● **O60   Preterm labor**

> **Includes**   onset (spontaneous) of labor before 37 completed weeks of gestation

> **Excludes1**   false labor (O47.0-)
> threatened labor NOS (O47.0-)

● **O60.0   Preterm labor without delivery**

   O60.00   Preterm labor without delivery, unspecified trimester

   O60.02   Preterm labor without delivery, second trimester

   O60.03   Preterm labor without delivery, third trimester

● **O60.1   Preterm labor with preterm delivery**

> One of the following 7th characters is to be assigned to each code under subcategory O60.1. 7th character 0 is for single gestations and multiple gestations where the fetus is unspecified. 7th characters 1 through 9 are for cases of multiple gestations to identify the fetus for which the code applies. The appropriate code from category O30, Multiple gestation, must also be assigned when assigning a code from subcategory O60.1 that has a 7th character of 1 through 9.

> | 0 | not applicable or unspecified |
> |---|---|
> | 1 | fetus 1 |
> | 2 | fetus 2 |
> | 3 | fetus 3 |
> | 4 | fetus 4 |
> | 5 | fetus 5 |
> | 9 | other fetus |

   X● **O60.10**   Preterm labor with preterm delivery, unspecified trimester
   Preterm labor with delivery NOS

   X● **O60.12**   Preterm labor second trimester with preterm delivery second trimester

   X● **O60.13**   Preterm labor second trimester with preterm delivery third trimester

   X● **O60.14**   Preterm labor third trimester with preterm delivery third trimester

● **O60.2   Term delivery with preterm labor**

> One of the following 7th characters is to be assigned to each code under subcategory O60.2. 7th character 0 is for single gestations and multiple gestations where the fetus is unspecified. 7th characters 1 through 9 are for cases of multiple gestations to identify the fetus for which the code applies. The appropriate code from category O30, Multiple gestation, must also be assigned when assigning a code from subcategory O60.2 that has a 7th character of 1 through 9.

> | 0 | not applicable or unspecified |
> |---|---|
> | 1 | fetus 1 |
> | 2 | fetus 2 |
> | 3 | fetus 3 |
> | 4 | fetus 4 |
> | 5 | fetus 5 |
> | 9 | other fetus |

   X● **O60.20**   Term delivery with preterm labor, unspecified trimester

   X● **O60.22**   Term delivery with preterm labor, second trimester

   X● **O60.23**   Term delivery with preterm labor, third trimester

● **O61   Failed induction of labor**

   O61.0   Failed medical induction of labor
   Failed induction (of labor) by oxytocin
   Failed induction (of labor) by prostaglandins

   O61.1   Failed instrumental induction of labor
   Failed mechanical induction (of labor)
   Failed surgical induction (of labor)

   O61.8   Other failed induction of labor

   O61.9   Failed induction of labor, unspecified

● **O62   Abnormalities of forces of labor**

   O62.0   Primary inadequate contractions
   Failure of cervical dilatation
   Primary hypotonic uterine dysfunction
   Uterine inertia during latent phase of labor

   O62.1   Secondary uterine inertia
   Arrested active phase of labor
   Secondary hypotonic uterine dysfunction

   O62.2   Other uterine inertia
   Atony of uterus without hemorrhage
   Atony of uterus NOS
   Desultory labor
   Hypotonic uterine dysfunction NOS
   Irregular labor
   Poor contractions
   Slow slope active phase of labor
   Uterine inertia NOS

> **Excludes1**   atony of uterus with hemorrhage (postpartum) (O72.1)
> postpartum atony of uterus without hemorrhage (O75.89)

   O62.3   Precipitate labor

   O62.4   Hypertonic, incoordinate, and prolonged uterine contractions
   Cervical spasm
   Contraction ring dystocia
   Dyscoordinate labor
   Hour-glass contraction of uterus
   Hypertonic uterine dysfunction
   Incoordinate uterine action
   Tetanic contractions
   Uterine dystocia NOS
   Uterine spasm

> **Excludes1**   dystocia (fetal) (maternal) NOS (O66.9)

   O62.8   Other abnormalities of forces of labor

   O62.9   Abnormality of forces of labor, unspecified

● **O63   Long labor**

   O63.0   Prolonged first stage (of labor)

   O63.1   Prolonged second stage (of labor)

   O63.2   Delayed delivery of second twin, triplet, etc.

   O63.9   Long labor, unspecified
   Prolonged labor NOS

CHAPTER 15 (O00–O9A)

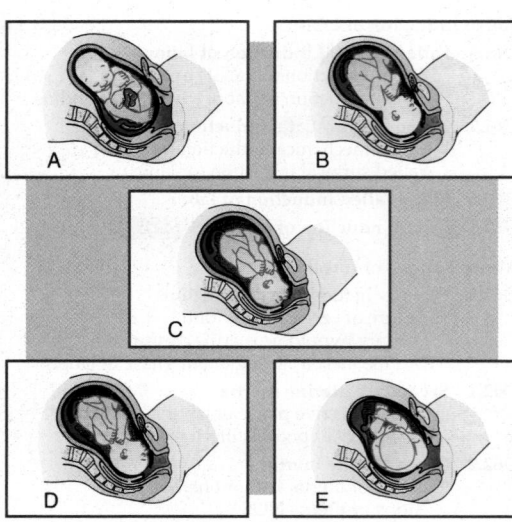

Figure 15-4 Five types of malposition and malpresentation of the fetus: **A.** Breech. **B.** Vertex. **C.** Face. **D.** Brow. **E.** Shoulder.

CHAPTER 15 (O00-O9A)

● **O64 Obstructed labor due to malposition and malpresentation of fetus**

One of the following 7th characters is to be assigned to each code under category O64. 7th character 0 is for single gestations and multiple gestations where the fetus is unspecified. 7th characters 1 through 9 are for cases of multiple gestations to identify the fetus for which the code applies. The appropriate code from category O30, Multiple gestation, must also be assigned when assigning a code from category O64 that has a 7th character of 1 through 9.

0	not applicable or unspecified
1	fetus 1
2	fetus 2
3	fetus 3
4	fetus 4
5	fetus 5
9	other fetus

X● **O64.0 Obstructed labor due to incomplete rotation of fetal head**
Deep transverse arrest
Obstructed labor due to persistent occipitoiliac (position)
Obstructed labor due to persistent occipitoposterior (position)
Obstructed labor due to persistent occipitosacral (position)
Obstructed labor due to persistent occipitotransverse (position)

X● **O64.1 Obstructed labor due to breech presentation**
Obstructed labor due to buttocks presentation
Obstructed labor due to complete breech presentation
Obstructed labor due to frank breech presentation

X● **O64.2 Obstructed labor due to face presentation**
Obstructed labor due to chin presentation

X● **O64.3 Obstructed labor due to brow presentation**

X● **O64.4 Obstructed labor due to shoulder presentation**
Prolapsed arm
Excludes1   impacted shoulders (O66.0)
            shoulder dystocia (O66.0)

X● **O64.5 Obstructed labor due to compound presentation**

X● **O64.8 Obstructed labor due to other malposition and malpresentation**
Obstructed labor due to footling presentation
Obstructed labor due to incomplete breech presentation

X● **O64.9 Obstructed labor due to malposition and malpresentation, unspecified**

● **O65 Obstructed labor due to maternal pelvic abnormality**

O65.0 Obstructed labor due to deformed pelvis

O65.1 Obstructed labor due to generally contracted pelvis

O65.2 Obstructed labor due to pelvic inlet contraction

O65.3 Obstructed labor due to pelvic outlet and mid-cavity contraction

O65.4 Obstructed labor due to fetopelvic disproportion, unspecified
Excludes1   dystocia due to abnormality of fetus (O66.2-O66.3)

O65.5 Obstructed labor due to abnormality of maternal pelvic organs
Obstructed labor due to conditions listed in O34.-
Use additional code to identify abnormality of pelvic organs O34.-

O65.8 Obstructed labor due to other maternal pelvic abnormalities

O65.9 Obstructed labor due to maternal pelvic abnormality, unspecified

● **O66 Other obstructed labor**

O66.0 Obstructed labor due to shoulder dystocia
Impacted shoulders

O66.1 Obstructed labor due to locked twins

O66.2 Obstructed labor due to unusually large fetus

O66.3 Obstructed labor due to other abnormalities of fetus
Dystocia due to fetal ascites
Dystocia due to fetal hydrops
Dystocia due to fetal meningomyelocele
Dystocia due to fetal sacral teratoma
Dystocia due to fetal tumor
Dystocia due to hydrocephalic fetus
Use additional code to identify cause of obstruction

● **O66.4 Failed trial of labor**

O66.40 Failed trial of labor, unspecified

O66.41 Failed attempted vaginal birth after previous cesarean delivery
Code first rupture of uterus, if applicable (O71.0-, O71.1)

O66.5 Attempted application of vacuum extractor and forceps
Attempted application of vacuum or forceps, with subsequent delivery by forceps or cesarean delivery

O66.6 Obstructed labor due to other multiple fetuses

O66.8 Other specified obstructed labor
Use additional code to identify cause of obstruction

O66.9 Obstructed labor, unspecified
Dystocia NOS
Fetal dystocia NOS
Maternal dystocia NOS

Figure 15-5 Hydrocephalic fetus causing disproportion.

▶ New   ⇒ Revised   ~~deleted~~ Deleted   **OGCR** Official Guidelines   X Assign placeholder X   ● Use Additional Character(s)

Excludes 1   Excludes 2   Includes   Use additional   Code first   Code also   Key words

● **O67**   **Labor and delivery complicated by intrapartum hemorrhage, not elsewhere classified**

> | Excludes1 | antepartum hemorrhage NEC (O46.-) |
> |---|---|
> | | placenta previa (O44.-) |
> | | premature separation of placenta [abruptio placentae] (O45.-) |

> | Excludes2 | postpartum hemorrhage (O72.-) |
> |---|---|

    O67.0   **Intrapartum hemorrhage with coagulation defect**
       Intrapartum hemorrhage (excessive) associated with afibrinogenemia
       Intrapartum hemorrhage (excessive) associated with disseminated intravascular coagulation
       Intrapartum hemorrhage (excessive) associated with hyperfibrinolysis
       Intrapartum hemorrhage (excessive) associated with hypofibrinogenemia

    O67.8   **Other intrapartum hemorrhage**
       Excessive intrapartum hemorrhage

    O67.9   **Intrapartum hemorrhage, unspecified**

O68   **Labor and delivery complicated by abnormality of fetal acid-base balance**
       Fetal acidemia complicating labor and delivery
       Fetal acidosis complicating labor and delivery
       Fetal alkalosis complicating labor and delivery
       Fetal metabolic acidemia complicating labor and delivery

> | Excludes1 | fetal stress NOS (O77.9) |
> |---|---|
> | | labor and delivery complicated by electrocardiographic evidence of fetal stress (O77.8) |
> | | labor and delivery complicated by ultrasonic evidence of fetal stress (O77.8) |

> | Excludes2 | abnormality in fetal heart rate or rhythm (O76) |
> |---|---|
> | | labor and delivery complicated by meconium in amniotic fluid (O77.0) |

● **O69**   **Labor and delivery complicated by umbilical cord complications**

    One of the following 7th characters is to be assigned to each code under category O69. 7th character 0 is for single gestations and multiple gestations where the fetus is unspecified. 7th characters 1 through 9 are for cases of multiple gestations to identify the fetus for which the code applies. The appropriate code from category O30, Multiple gestation, must also be assigned when assigning a code from category O69 that has a 7th character of 1 through 9.

> | 0 | not applicable or unspecified |
> |---|---|
> | 1 | fetus 1 |
> | 2 | fetus 2 |
> | 3 | fetus 3 |
> | 4 | fetus 4 |
> | 5 | fetus 5 |
> | 9 | other fetus |

X● **O69.0**   **Labor and delivery complicated by prolapse of cord**

X● **O69.1**   **Labor and delivery complicated by cord around neck, with compression**

> | Excludes1 | labor and delivery complicated by cord around neck, without compression (O69.81) |
> |---|---|

X● **O69.2**   **Labor and delivery complicated by other cord entanglement, with compression**
       Labor and delivery complicated by compression of cord NOS
       Labor and delivery complicated by entanglement of cords of twins in monoamniotic sac
       Labor and delivery complicated by knot in cord

> | Excludes1 | labor and delivery complicated by other cord entanglement, without compression (O69.82) |
> |---|---|

X● **O69.3**   **Labor and delivery complicated by short cord**

X● **O69.4**   **Labor and delivery complicated by vasa previa**
       Labor and delivery complicated by hemorrhage from vasa previa

X● **O69.5**   **Labor and delivery complicated by vascular lesion of cord**
       Labor and delivery complicated by cord bruising
       Labor and delivery complicated by cord hematoma
       Labor and delivery complicated by thrombosis of umbilical vessels

● **O69.8**   **Labor and delivery complicated by other cord complications**

   X● **O69.81**   **Labor and delivery complicated by cord around neck, without compression**

   X● **O69.82**   **Labor and delivery complicated by other cord entanglement, without compression**

   X● **O69.89**   **Labor and delivery complicated by other cord complications**

X● **O69.9**   **Labor and delivery complicated by cord complication, unspecified**

● **O70**   **Perineal laceration during delivery**

> | Includes | episiotomy extended by laceration |
> |---|---|

> | Excludes1 | obstetric high vaginal laceration alone (O71.4) |
> |---|---|

    O70.0   **First degree perineal laceration during delivery**
       Perineal laceration, rupture or tear involving fourchette during delivery
       Perineal laceration, rupture or tear involving labia during delivery
       Perineal laceration, rupture or tear involving skin during delivery
       Perineal laceration, rupture or tear involving vagina during delivery
       Perineal laceration, rupture or tear involving vulva during delivery
       Slight perineal laceration, rupture or tear during delivery

    O70.1   **Second degree perineal laceration during delivery**
       Perineal laceration, rupture or tear during delivery as in O70.0, also involving pelvic floor
       Perineal laceration, rupture or tear during delivery as in O70.0, also involving perineal muscles
       Perineal laceration, rupture or tear during delivery as in O70.0, also involving vaginal muscles

> | Excludes1 | perineal laceration involving anal sphincter (O70.2) |
> |---|---|

CHAPTER 15 (O00-O9A)

Figure 15-6 Perineal lacerations: **A.** First-degree is laceration of superficial tissues. **B.** Second-degree is limited to the pelvic floor and may involve the perineal or vaginal muscles. **C.** Third-degree involves the anal sphincter. **D.** Fourth-degree involves anal or rectal mucosa.

● **O70.2** **Third degree** perineal laceration during delivery
Perineal laceration, rupture or tear during delivery as in O70.1, also involving anal sphincter
Perineal laceration, rupture or tear during delivery as in O70.1, also involving rectovaginal septum
Perineal laceration, rupture or tear during delivery as in O70.1, also involving sphincter NOS

> **Excludes1**   anal sphincter tear during delivery without third degree perineal laceration (O70.4)
> perineal laceration involving anal or rectal mucosa (O70.3)

     O70.20   Third degree perineal laceration during delivery, **unspecified**

     O70.21   Third degree perineal laceration during delivery, **IIIa**
Third degree perineal laceration during delivery with less than 50% of external anal sphincter (EAS) thickness torn

     O70.22   Third degree perineal laceration during delivery, **IIIb**
Third degree perineal laceration during delivery with more than 50% external anal sphincter (EAS) thickness torn

     O70.23   Third degree perineal laceration during delivery, **IIIc**
Third degree perineal laceration during delivery with both external anal sphincter (EAS) and internal anal sphincter (IAS) torn

   O70.3   **Fourth degree** perineal laceration during delivery
Perineal laceration, rupture or tear during delivery as in O70.2, also involving anal mucosa
Perineal laceration, rupture or tear during delivery as in O70.2, also involving rectal mucosa

   O70.4   **Anal sphincter tear** complicating delivery, not associated with third degree laceration

> **Excludes1**   anal sphincter tear with third degree perineal laceration (O70.2)

   O70.9   Perineal laceration during delivery, **unspecified**

● **O71**   Other obstetric trauma

> **Includes**   obstetric damage from instruments

● **O71.0**   Rupture of uterus (spontaneous) **before onset of labor**

> **Excludes1**   disruption of (current) cesarean delivery wound (O90.0)
> laceration of uterus, NEC (O71.81)

     O71.00   Rupture of uterus before onset of labor, **unspecified trimester**

     O71.02   Rupture of uterus before onset of labor, **second trimester**

     O71.03   Rupture of uterus before onset of labor, **third trimester**

   O71.1   Rupture of uterus **during labor**
Rupture of uterus not stated as occurring before onset of labor

> **Excludes1**   disruption of cesarean delivery wound (O90.0)
> laceration of uterus, NEC (O71.81)

   O71.2   Postpartum **inversion of uterus**

   O71.3   Obstetric **laceration of cervix**
Annular detachment of cervix

   O71.4   Obstetric **high vaginal laceration** alone
Laceration of vaginal wall without perineal laceration

> **Excludes1**   obstetric high vaginal laceration with perineal laceration (O70.-)

   O71.5   **Other obstetric injury to pelvic organs**
Obstetric injury to bladder
Obstetric injury to urethra

> **Excludes2**   obstetric periurethral trauma (O71.82)

   O71.6   Obstetric damage to **pelvic joints and ligaments**
Obstetric avulsion of inner symphyseal cartilage
Obstetric damage to coccyx
Obstetric traumatic separation of symphysis (pubis)

   O71.7   Obstetric **hematoma of pelvis**
Obstetric hematoma of perineum
Obstetric hematoma of vagina
Obstetric hematoma of vulva

● **O71.8**   Other specified obstetric trauma

     O71.81   Laceration of uterus, not elsewhere classified

     O71.82   Other specified trauma to perineum and vulva
Obstetric periurethral trauma

     O71.89   Other specified obstetric trauma

   O71.9   Obstetric trauma, **unspecified**

●● **O72**   Postpartum hemorrhage

> **Includes**   hemorrhage after delivery of fetus or infant

   O72.0   **Third-stage** hemorrhage
Hemorrhage associated with retained, trapped or adherent placenta
Retained placenta NOS

> **Code also** type of adherent placenta (O43.2-)

   O72.1   **Other immediate** postpartum hemorrhage
Hemorrhage following delivery of placenta
Postpartum hemorrhage (atonic) NOS
Uterine atony with hemorrhage

> **Excludes1**   uterine atony NOS (O62.2)
> uterine atony without hemorrhage (O62.2)
> postpartum atony of uterus without hemorrhage (O75.89)

   O72.2   **Delayed and secondary** postpartum hemorrhage
Hemorrhage associated with retained portions of placenta or membranes after the first 24 hours following delivery of placenta
Retained products of conception NOS, following delivery

   O72.3   Postpartum **coagulation defects**
Postpartum afibrinogenemia
Postpartum fibrinolysis

●● **O73**   Retained placenta and membranes, **without hemorrhage**

> **Excludes1**   placenta accreta (O43.21-)
> placenta increta (O43.22-)
> placenta percreta (O43.23-)

   O73.0   Retained **placenta** without hemorrhage
Adherent placenta, without hemorrhage
Trapped placenta without hemorrhage

   O73.1   Retained **portions of placenta and membranes**, without hemorrhage
Retained products of conception following delivery, without hemorrhage

▶ New   ⇒ Revised   ~~deleted~~ Deleted   **OGCR** Official Guidelines   X Assign placeholder X   ● Use Additional Character(s)

Excludes 1   Excludes 2   Includes   Use additional   Code first   Code also   Key words

● **O74**   **Complications of anesthesia during labor and delivery**

> **Includes**   maternal complications arising from the administration of a general, regional or local anesthetic, analgesic or other sedation during labor and delivery

> Use additional code, if applicable, to identify specific complication

   O74.0   **Aspiration pneumonitis due to anesthesia during labor and delivery**
> Inhalation of stomach contents or secretions NOS due to anesthesia during labor and delivery
> Mendelson's syndrome due to anesthesia during labor and delivery

   O74.1   **Other pulmonary complications of anesthesia during labor and delivery**

   O74.2   **Cardiac complications of anesthesia during labor and delivery**

   O74.3   **Central nervous system complications of anesthesia during labor and delivery**

   O74.4   **Toxic reaction to local anesthesia during labor and delivery**

   O74.5   **Spinal and epidural anesthesia-induced headache during labor and delivery**

   O74.6   **Other complications of spinal and epidural anesthesia during labor and delivery**

   O74.7   **Failed or difficult intubation for anesthesia during labor and delivery**

   O74.8   **Other complications of anesthesia during labor and delivery**

   O74.9   **Complication of anesthesia during labor and delivery, unspecified**

● **O75**   **Other complications of labor and delivery, not elsewhere classified**

> **Excludes2**   puerperal (postpartum) infection (O86.-)
> puerperal (postpartum) sepsis (O85)

   O75.0   **Maternal distress during labor and delivery**

   O75.1   **Shock during or following labor and delivery**
> Obstetric shock following labor and delivery

   O75.2   **Pyrexia during labor, not elsewhere classified**

   O75.3   **Other infection during labor**
> Sepsis during labor
> Use additional code (B95-B97), to identify infectious agent

   O75.4   **Other complications of obstetric surgery and procedures**
> Cardiac arrest following obstetric surgery or procedures
> Cardiac failure following obstetric surgery or procedures
> Cerebral anoxia following obstetric surgery or procedures
> Pulmonary edema following obstetric surgery or procedures
> Use additional code to identify specific complication
> **Excludes2**   complications of anesthesia during labor and delivery (O74.-)
> disruption of obstetrical (surgical) wound (O90.0-O90.1)
> hematoma of obstetrical (surgical) wound (O90.2)
> infection of obstetrical (surgical) wound (O86.0)

   O75.5   **Delayed delivery after artificial rupture of membranes**

● **O75.8**   **Other specified complications of labor and delivery**

   O75.81   **Maternal exhaustion complicating labor and delivery**

   O75.82   **Onset (spontaneous) of labor after 37 completed weeks of gestation but before 39 completed weeks gestation, with delivery by (planned) cesarean section**
> Delivery by (planned) cesarean section occurring after 37 completed weeks of gestation but before 39 completed weeks gestation due to (spontaneous) onset of labor
> *Code first to specify reason for planned cesarean section such as:*
> cephalopelvic disproportion (normally formed fetus) (O33.9)
> previous cesarean delivery (O34.21)

   O75.89   **Other specified complications of labor and delivery**

   O75.9   **Complication of labor and delivery, unspecified**

O76   **Abnormality in fetal heart rate and rhythm complicating labor and delivery**
> Depressed fetal heart rate tones complicating labor and delivery
> Fetal bradycardia complicating labor and delivery
> Fetal heart rate decelerations complicating labor and delivery
> Fetal heart rate irregularity complicating labor and delivery
> Fetal heart rate abnormal variability complicating labor and delivery
> Fetal tachycardia complicating labor and delivery
> Non-reassuring fetal heart rate or rhythm complicating labor and delivery
> **Excludes1**   fetal stress NOS (O77.9)
> labor and delivery complicated by electrocardiographic evidence of fetal stress (O77.8)
> labor and delivery complicated by ultrasonic evidence of fetal stress (O77.8)
> **Excludes2**   fetal metabolic acidemia (O68)
> other fetal stress (O77.0-O77.1)

● **O77**   **Other fetal stress complicating labor and delivery**

   O77.0   **Labor and delivery complicated by meconium in amniotic fluid**

   O77.1   **Fetal stress in labor or delivery due to drug administration**

   O77.8   **Labor and delivery complicated by other evidence of fetal stress**
> Labor and delivery complicated by electrocardiographic evidence of fetal stress
> Labor and delivery complicated by ultrasonic evidence of fetal stress
> **Excludes1**   abnormality of fetal acid-base balance (O68)
> abnormality in fetal heart rate or rhythm (O76)
> fetal metabolic acidemia (O68)

   O77.9   **Labor and delivery complicated by fetal stress, unspecified**
> **Excludes1**   abnormality of fetal acid-base balance (O68)
> abnormality in fetal heart rate or rhythm (O76)
> fetal metabolic acidemia (O68)

CHAPTER 15 (O00-O9A)

Figure 15-7 The four stages of normal delivery: **I.** Lightening, which occurs 2 to 4 weeks before birth, at which time the fetus turns with head toward the vagina. **II.** Regular contractions begin, the amniotic sac ruptures, and dilation is complete. **III.** Delivery of the head and rotation. **IV.** Expulsion of placenta.

OGCR Section I.C., Chapter 15.n.

Normal Delivery, Code O80

1) Encounter for full term uncomplicated delivery

Code O80 should be assigned when a woman is admitted for a full-term normal delivery and delivers a single, healthy infant without any complications antepartum, during the delivery, or postpartum during the delivery episode. Code O80 is always a principal diagnosis. It is not to be used if any other code from chapter 15 is needed to describe a current complication of the antenatal, delivery, or perinatal period. Additional codes from other chapters may be used with code O80 if they are not related to or are in any way complicating the pregnancy.

2) Uncomplicated delivery with resolved antepartum complication

Code O80 may be used if the patient had a complication at some point during the pregnancy, but the complication is not present at the time of the admission for delivery.

3) Outcome of delivery for O80

Z37.0, Single live brith, is the only outcome of delivery code appropriate for use with O80.

ENCOUNTER FOR DELIVERY (O80-O82)

O80   Encounter for full-term uncomplicated delivery
Delivery requiring minimal or no assistance, with or without episiotomy, without fetal manipulation [e.g., rotation version] or instrumentation [forceps] of a spontaneous, cephalic, vaginal, full-term, single, live-born infant. This code is for use as a single diagnosis code and is not to be used with any other code from chapter 15.

Use additional code to indicate outcome of delivery (Z37.0)

O82   Encounter for cesarean delivery without indication

Use additional code to indicate outcome of delivery (Z37.0)

COMPLICATIONS PREDOMINANTLY RELATED TO THE PUERPERIUM (O85-O92)

Excludes2   mental and behavioral disorders associated with the puerperium (F53)
obstetrical tetanus (A34)
puerperal osteomalacia (M83.0)

O85   Puerperal sepsis
Postpartum sepsis
Puerperal peritonitis
Puerperal pyemia

Use additional code (B95-B97), to identify infectious agent

Use additional code (R65.2-) to identify severe sepsis, if applicable

Excludes1   fever of unknown origin following delivery (O86.4)
genital tract infection following delivery (O86.1-)
obstetric pyemic and septic embolism (O88.3-)
puerperal septic thrombophlebitis (O86.81)
urinary tract infection following delivery (O86.2-)

Excludes2   sepsis during labor (O75.3)

●**O86   Other puerperal infections**
Use additional code (B95-B97), to identify infectious agent
Excludes2   infection during labor (O75.3)
obstetrical tetanus (A34)

O86.0   Infection of obstetric surgical wound
Infected cesarean delivery wound following delivery
Infected perineal repair following delivery

●**O86.1   Other infection of genital tract following delivery**
O86.11   Cervicitis following delivery
O86.12   Endometritis following delivery
O86.13   Vaginitis following delivery
O86.19   Other infection of genital tract following delivery

●**O86.2   Urinary tract infection following delivery**
O86.20   Urinary tract infection following delivery, unspecified
Puerperal urinary tract infection NOS
O86.21   Infection of kidney following delivery
O86.22   Infection of bladder following delivery
Infection of urethra following delivery
O86.29   Other urinary tract infection following delivery

O86.4   Pyrexia of unknown origin following delivery
Puerperal infection NOS following delivery
Puerperal pyrexia NOS following delivery
Excludes2   pyrexia during labor (O75.2)

●**O86.8   Other specified puerperal infections**
O86.81   Puerperal septic thrombophlebitis
O86.89   Other specified puerperal infections

●**O87   Venous complications and hemorrhoids in the puerperium**
Includes   venous complications in labor, delivery and the puerperium
Excludes2   obstetric embolism (O88.-)
puerperal septic thrombophlebitis (O86.81)
venous complications in pregnancy (O22.-)

O87.0   Superficial thrombophlebitis in the puerperium
Puerperal phlebitis NOS
Puerperal thrombosis NOS

O87.1   Deep phlebothrombosis in the puerperium
Deep vein thrombosis, postpartum
Pelvic thrombophlebitis, postpartum
Use additional code to identify the deep vein thrombosis (I82.4-, I82.5-, I82.62-. I82.72-)
Use additional code, if applicable, for associated long-term (current) use of anticoagulants (Z79.01)

O87.2   **Hemorrhoids** in the puerperium

O87.3   **Cerebral venous thrombosis** in the puerperium
     Cerebrovenous sinus thrombosis in the puerperium

O87.4   **Varicose veins of lower extremity** in the puerperium

O87.8   **Other** venous complications in the puerperium
     Genital varices in the puerperium

O87.9   **Venous complication in the puerperium, unspecified**
     Puerperal phlebopathy NOS

O88   **Obstetric embolism**
   Excludes1   embolism complicating abortion NOS (O03.2)
          embolism complicating ectopic or molar
            pregnancy (O08.2)
          embolism complicating failed attempted abortion
            (O07.2)
          embolism complicating induced abortion (O04.7)
          embolism complicating spontaneous abortion
            (O03.2, O03.7)

● O88.0   **Obstetric air embolism**
    ● O88.01   **Obstetric air embolism in pregnancy**
       O88.011   **Air embolism in pregnancy, first trimester**
       O88.012   **Air embolism in pregnancy, second trimester**
       O88.013   **Air embolism in pregnancy, third trimester**
       O88.019   **Air embolism in pregnancy, unspecified trimester**
    O88.02   **Air embolism in childbirth**
    O88.03   **Air embolism in the puerperium**

● O88.1   **Amniotic fluid embolism**
     Anaphylactoid syndrome in pregnancy
    ● O88.11   **Amniotic fluid embolism in pregnancy**
       O88.111   **Amniotic fluid embolism in pregnancy, first trimester**
       O88.112   **Amniotic fluid embolism in pregnancy, second trimester**
       O88.113   **Amniotic fluid embolism in pregnancy, third trimester**
       O88.119   **Amniotic fluid embolism in pregnancy, unspecified trimester**
    O88.12   **Amniotic fluid embolism in childbirth**
    O88.13   **Amniotic fluid embolism in the puerperium**

● O88.2   **Obstetric thromboembolism**
    ● O88.21   **Thromboembolism in pregnancy**
       Obstetric (pulmonary) embolism NOS
       O88.211   **Thromboembolism in pregnancy, first trimester**
       O88.212   **Thromboembolism in pregnancy, second trimester**
       O88.213   **Thromboembolism in pregnancy, third trimester**
       O88.219   **Thromboembolism in pregnancy, unspecified trimester**
    O88.22   **Thromboembolism in childbirth**
    O88.23   **Thromboembolism in the puerperium**
       Puerperal (pulmonary) embolism NOS

● O88.3   **Obstetric pyemic and septic embolism**
    ● O88.31   **Pyemic and septic embolism in pregnancy**
       O88.311   Pyemic and septic embolism in pregnancy, **first trimester**
       O88.312   Pyemic and septic embolism in pregnancy, **second trimester**
       O88.313   Pyemic and septic embolism in pregnancy, **third trimester**
       O88.319   Pyemic and septic embolism in pregnancy, **unspecified trimester**
    O88.32   Pyemic and septic embolism in **childbirth**
    O88.33   Pyemic and septic embolism in the **puerperium**

● O88.8   **Other** obstetric embolism
     Obstetric fat embolism
    ● O88.81   **Other embolism in pregnancy**
       O88.811   **Other embolism in pregnancy, first trimester**
       O88.812   **Other embolism in pregnancy, second trimester**
       O88.813   **Other embolism in pregnancy, third trimester**
       O88.819   **Other embolism in pregnancy, unspecified trimester**
    O88.82   **Other embolism in childbirth**
    O88.83   **Other embolism in the puerperium**

● O89   **Complications of anesthesia during the puerperium**
   Includes   maternal complications arising from the
            administration of a general, regional or
            local anesthetic, analgesic or other sedation
            during the puerperium
   Use additional code, if applicable, to identify specific
     complication
   ● O89.0   **Pulmonary complications of anesthesia during the puerperium**
      O89.01   **Aspiration pneumonitis due to anesthesia during the puerperium**
        Inhalation of stomach contents or secretions
          NOS due to anesthesia during the
          puerperium
        Mendelson's syndrome due to anesthesia
          during the puerperium
      O89.09   **Other pulmonary** complications of anesthesia during the puerperium
   O89.1   **Cardiac** complications of anesthesia during the puerperium
   O89.2   **Central nervous system** complications of anesthesia during the puerperium
   O89.3   **Toxic reaction** to local anesthesia during the puerperium
   O89.4   **Spinal and epidural anesthesia-induced headache** during the puerperium
   O89.5   **Other complications of spinal and epidural** anesthesia during the puerperium
   O89.6   **Failed or difficult intubation** for anesthesia during the puerperium
   O89.8   **Other** complications of anesthesia during the puerperium
   O89.9   **Complication of anesthesia during the puerperium, unspecified**

● **O90 Complications of the puerperium, not elsewhere classified**

O90.0 **Disruption of cesarean delivery wound**
Dehiscence of cesarean delivery wound
> **Excludes1**   rupture of uterus (spontaneous) before
> onset of labor (O71.0-)
> rupture of uterus during labor (O71.1)

O90.1 **Disruption of perineal obstetric wound**
Disruption of wound of episiotomy
Disruption of wound of perineal laceration
Secondary perineal tear

O90.2 **Hematoma of obstetric wound**

O90.3 **Peripartum cardiomyopathy**
Conditions in I42.- arising during pregnancy and the
puerperium
> **Excludes1**   pre-existing heart disease complicating
> pregnancy and the puerperium
> (O99.4-)

O90.4 **Postpartum acute kidney failure**
Hepatorenal syndrome following labor and delivery

O90.5 **Postpartum thyroiditis**

O90.6 **Postpartum mood disturbance**
Postpartum blues   Postpartum sadness
Postpartum dysphoria
> **Excludes1**   postpartum depression (F53)
> puerperal psychosis (F53)

● O90.8 **Other complications of the puerperium, not elsewhere
classified**

O90.81 **Anemia of the puerperium**
Postpartum anemia NOS
> **Excludes1**   pre-existing anemia complicating
> the puerperium (O99.03)

O90.89 **Other complications of the puerperium, not
elsewhere classified**
Placental polyp

O90.9 **Complication of the puerperium, unspecified**

● **O91 Infections of breast associated with pregnancy, the puerperium
and lactation**
Use additional code to identify infection

● O91.0 **Infection of nipple associated with pregnancy, the
puerperium and lactation**

● O91.01 **Infection of nipple associated with pregnancy**
Gestational abscess of nipple

O91.011 **Infection of nipple associated with
pregnancy, first trimester**

O91.012 **Infection of nipple associated with
pregnancy, second trimester**

O91.013 **Infection of nipple associated with
pregnancy, third trimester**

O91.019 **Infection of nipple associated with
pregnancy, unspecified trimester**

O91.02 **Infection of nipple associated with the
puerperium**
Puerperal abscess of nipple

O91.03 **Infection of nipple associated with lactation**
Abscess of nipple associated with lactation

● O91.1 **Abscess of breast associated with pregnancy, the
puerperium and lactation**

● O91.11 **Abscess of breast associated with pregnancy**
Gestational mammary abscess
Gestational purulent mastitis
Gestational subareolar abscess

O91.111 **Abscess of breast associated with
pregnancy, first trimester**

O91.112 **Abscess of breast associated with
pregnancy, second trimester**

O91.113 **Abscess of breast associated with
pregnancy, third trimester**

O91.119 **Abscess of breast associated with
pregnancy, unspecified trimester**

O91.12 **Abscess of breast associated with the
puerperium**
Puerperal mammary abscess
Puerperal purulent mastitis
Puerperal subareolar abscess

O91.13 **Abscess of breast associated with lactation**
Mammary abscess associated with lactation
Purulent mastitis associated with lactation
Subareolar abscess associated with lactation

● O91.2 **Nonpurulent mastitis associated with pregnancy, the
puerperium and lactation**

● O91.21 **Nonpurulent mastitis associated with
pregnancy**
Gestational interstitial mastitis
Gestational lymphangitis of breast
Gestational mastitis NOS
Gestational parenchymatous mastitis

O91.211 **Nonpurulent mastitis associated with
pregnancy, first trimester**

O91.212 **Nonpurulent mastitis associated with
pregnancy, second trimester**

O91.213 **Nonpurulent mastitis associated with
pregnancy, third trimester**

O91.219 **Nonpurulent mastitis associated with
pregnancy, unspecified trimester**

O91.22 **Nonpurulent mastitis associated with the
puerperium**
Puerperal interstitial mastitis
Puerperal lymphangitis of breast
Puerperal mastitis NOS
Puerperal parenchymatous mastitis

O91.23 **Nonpurulent mastitis associated with lactation**
Interstitial mastitis associated with lactation
Lymphangitis of breast associated with
lactation
Mastitis NOS associated with lactation
Parenchymatous mastitis associated with
lactation

● **O92 Other disorders of breast and disorders of lactation associated
with pregnancy and the puerperium**

● O92.0 **Retracted nipple associated with pregnancy, the
puerperium, and lactation**

● O92.01 **Retracted nipple associated with pregnancy**

O92.011 **Retracted nipple associated with
pregnancy, first trimester**

O92.012 **Retracted nipple associated with
pregnancy, second trimester**

O92.013 **Retracted nipple associated with
pregnancy, third trimester**

O92.019 **Retracted nipple associated with
pregnancy, unspecified trimester**

O92.02 **Retracted nipple associated with the
puerperium**

O92.03 **Retracted nipple associated with lactation**

● O92.1 **Cracked nipple associated with pregnancy, the
puerperium, and lactation**
Fissure of nipple, gestational or puerperal

● O92.11 **Cracked nipple associated with pregnancy**

O92.111 **Cracked nipple associated with
pregnancy, first trimester**

O92.112 **Cracked nipple associated with
pregnancy, second trimester**

O92.113 **Cracked nipple associated with
pregnancy, third trimester**

O92.119 **Cracked nipple associated with
pregnancy, unspecified trimester**

O92.12 **Cracked nipple associated with the puerperium**

O92.13 **Cracked nipple associated with lactation**

▶ New   ⇒ Revised   ~~deleted~~ Deleted   **OGCR** Official Guidelines   X Assign placeholder X   ● Use Additional Character(s)

Excludes 1 | Excludes 2 | Includes | Use additional | Code first | Code also | Key words

● **O92.2** **Other and unspecified disorders of breast associated with pregnancy and the puerperium**

     O92.20 Unspecified disorder of breast associated with pregnancy and the puerperium

     O92.29 Other disorders of breast associated with pregnancy and the puerperium

O92.3 **Agalactia**
     Primary agalactia

     | Excludes1 | elective agalactia (O92.5)
     secondary agalactia (O92.5)
     therapeutic agalactia (O92.5)

O92.4 **Hypogalactia**

O92.5 **Suppressed lactation**
     Elective agalactia   Therapeutic agalactia
     Secondary agalactia

     | Excludes1 | primary agalactia (O92.3)

O92.6 **Galactorrhea**

● **O92.7** **Other and unspecified disorders of lactation**

     O92.70 Unspecified disorders of lactation

     O92.79 Other disorders of lactation
         Puerperal galactocele

OTHER OBSTETRIC CONDITIONS, NOT ELSEWHERE CLASSIFIED (O94-O9A)

O94 **Sequelae of complication of pregnancy, childbirth, and the puerperium**

     Note: This category is to be used to indicate conditions in O00-O77.-, O85-O94 and O98-O9A.- as the cause of late effects. The 'sequelae' include conditions specified as such, or as late effects, which may occur at any time after the puerperium.

     Code first condition resulting from (sequela) of complication of pregnancy, childbirth, and the puerperium

O98 **Maternal infectious and parasitic diseases classifiable elsewhere but complicating pregnancy, childbirth and the puerperium**

     | Includes | the listed conditions when complicating the pregnant state, when aggravated by the pregnancy, or as a reason for obstetric care

     Use additional code (Chapter 1), to identify specific infectious or parasitic disease

     | Excludes2 | herpes gestationis (O26.4-)
     infectious carrier state (O99.82-, O99.83-)
     obstetrical tetanus (A34)
     puerperal infection (O86.-)
     puerperal sepsis (O85)
     when the reason for maternal care is that the disease is known or suspected to have affected the fetus (O35-O36)

● **O98.0** **Tuberculosis complicating pregnancy, childbirth and the puerperium**
     Conditions in A15-A19

   ● **O98.01** Tuberculosis complicating pregnancy

       O98.011 Tuberculosis complicating pregnancy, first trimester

       O98.012 Tuberculosis complicating pregnancy, second trimester

       O98.013 Tuberculosis complicating pregnancy, third trimester

       O98.019 Tuberculosis complicating pregnancy, unspecified trimester

     O98.02 Tuberculosis complicating childbirth

     O98.03 Tuberculosis complicating the puerperium

● **O98.1** **Syphilis complicating pregnancy, childbirth and the puerperium**
     Conditions in A50-A53

   ● **O98.11** Syphilis complicating pregnancy

       O98.111 Syphilis complicating pregnancy, first trimester

       O98.112 Syphilis complicating pregnancy, second trimester

       O98.113 Syphilis complicating pregnancy, third trimester

       O98.119 Syphilis complicating pregnancy, unspecified trimester

     O98.12 Syphilis complicating childbirth

     O98.13 Syphilis complicating the puerperium

● **O98.2** **Gonorrhea complicating pregnancy, childbirth and the puerperium**
     Conditions in A54.-

   ● **O98.21** Gonorrhea complicating pregnancy

       O98.211 Gonorrhea complicating pregnancy, first trimester

       O98.212 Gonorrhea complicating pregnancy, second trimester

       O98.213 Gonorrhea complicating pregnancy, third trimester

       O98.219 Gonorrhea complicating pregnancy, unspecified trimester

     O98.22 Gonorrhea complicating childbirth

     O98.23 Gonorrhea complicating the puerperium

● **O98.3** **Other infections with a predominantly sexual mode of transmission complicating pregnancy, childbirth and the puerperium**
     Conditions in A55-A64

   ● **O98.31** Other infections with a predominantly sexual mode of transmission complicating pregnancy

       O98.311 Other infections with a predominantly sexual mode of transmission complicating pregnancy, first trimester

       O98.312 Other infections with a predominantly sexual mode of transmission complicating pregnancy, second trimester

       O98.313 Other infections with a predominantly sexual mode of transmission complicating pregnancy, third trimester

       O98.319 Other infections with a predominantly sexual mode of transmission complicating pregnancy, unspecified trimester

     O98.32 Other infections with a predominantly sexual mode of transmission complicating childbirth

     O98.33 Other infections with a predominantly sexual mode of transmission complicating the puerperium

● **O98.4** **Viral hepatitis complicating pregnancy, childbirth and the puerperium**
     Conditions in B15-B19

   ● **O98.41** Viral hepatitis complicating pregnancy

       O98.411 Viral hepatitis complicating pregnancy, first trimester

       O98.412 Viral hepatitis complicating pregnancy, second trimester

       O98.413 Viral hepatitis complicating pregnancy, third trimester

       O98.419 Viral hepatitis complicating pregnancy, unspecified trimester

     O98.42 Viral hepatitis complicating childbirth

     O98.43 Viral hepatitis complicating the puerperium

CHAPTER 15 (O00-O9A)

● O98.5 Other viral diseases complicating pregnancy, childbirth and the puerperium
Conditions in A80-B09, B25-B34, R87.81-, R87.82-
Excludes:1 human immunodeficiency virus [HIV] disease complicating pregnancy, childbirth and the puerperium (O98.7-)
● O98.51 Other viral diseases complicating pregnancy
O98.511 Other viral diseases complicating pregnancy, first trimester
O98.512 Other viral diseases complicating pregnancy, second trimester
O98.513 Other viral diseases complicating pregnancy, third trimester
O98.519 Other viral diseases complicating pregnancy, unspecified trimester
O98.52 Other viral diseases complicating childbirth
O98.53 Other viral diseases complicating the puerperium
● O98.6 Protozoal diseases complicating pregnancy, childbirth and the puerperium
Conditions in B50-B64
● O98.61 Protozoal diseases complicating pregnancy
O98.611 Protozoal diseases complicating pregnancy, first trimester
O98.612 Protozoal diseases complicating pregnancy, second trimester
O98.613 Protozoal diseases complicating pregnancy, third trimester
O98.619 Protozoal diseases complicating pregnancy, unspecified trimester
O98.62 Protozoal diseases complicating childbirth
O98.63 Protozoal diseases complicating the puerperium
● O98.7 Human immunodeficiency virus [HIV] disease complicating pregnancy, childbirth and the puerperium
Use additional code to identify the type of HIV disease:
Acquired immune deficiency syndrome (AIDS) (B20)
Asymptomatic HIV status (Z21)
HIV positive NOS (Z21)
Symptomatic HIV disease (B20)

OGCR Section I.C.15.f.

HIV Infection in Pregnancy, Childbirth and the Puerperium

During pregnancy, childbirth or the puerperium, a patient admitted because of an HIV-related illness should receive a principal diagnosis from subcategory O98.7-. Human immunodeficiency [HIV] disease complicating pregnancy, childbirth and the puerperium, followed by the code(s) for the HIV-related illness(es).

Patients with asymptomatic HIV infection status admitted during pregnancy, childbirth, or the puerperium should receive codes of O98.7- and Z21, Asymptomatic human immunodeficiency virus [HIV] infection status.

● O98.71 Human immunodeficiency virus [HIV] disease complicating pregnancy
O98.711 Human immunodeficiency virus [HIV] disease complicating pregnancy, first trimester
O98.712 Human immunodeficiency virus [HIV] disease complicating pregnancy, second trimester
O98.713 Human immunodeficiency virus [HIV] disease complicating pregnancy, third trimester
O98.719 Human immunodeficiency virus [HIV] disease complicating pregnancy, unspecified trimester

O98.72 Human immunodeficiency virus [HIV] disease complicating childbirth
O98.73 Human immunodeficiency virus [HIV] disease complicating the puerperium
● O98.8 Other maternal infectious and parasitic diseases complicating pregnancy, childbirth and the puerperium
● O98.81 Other maternal infectious and parasitic diseases complicating pregnancy
O98.811 Other maternal infectious and parasitic diseases complicating pregnancy, first trimester
O98.812 Other maternal infectious and parasitic diseases complicating pregnancy, second trimester
O98.813 Other maternal infectious and parasitic diseases complicating pregnancy, third trimester
O98.819 Other maternal infectious and parasitic diseases complicating pregnancy, unspecified trimester
O98.82 Other maternal infectious and parasitic diseases complicating childbirth
O98.83 Other maternal infectious and parasitic diseases complicating the puerperium
● O98.9 Unspecified maternal infectious and parasitic disease complicating pregnancy, childbirth and the puerperium
● O98.91 Unspecified maternal infectious and parasitic disease complicating pregnancy
O98.911 Unspecified maternal infectious and parasitic disease complicating pregnancy, first trimester
O98.912 Unspecified maternal infectious and parasitic disease complicating pregnancy, second trimester
O98.913 Unspecified maternal infectious and parasitic disease complicating pregnancy, third trimester
O98.919 Unspecified maternal infectious and parasitic disease complicating pregnancy, unspecified trimester
O98.92 Unspecified maternal infectious and parasitic disease complicating childbirth
O98.93 Unspecified maternal infectious and parasitic disease complicating the puerperium

● O99 Other maternal diseases classifiable elsewhere but complicating pregnancy, childbirth and the puerperium
Includes: conditions which complicate the pregnant state, are aggravated by the pregnancy or are a main reason for obstetric care
Use additional code to identify specific condition
Excludes2 when the reason for maternal care is that the condition is known or suspected to have affected the fetus (O35-O36)
● O99.Ø Anemia complicating pregnancy, childbirth and the puerperium
Conditions in D50-D64
Excludes1 anemia arising in the puerperium (O90.81)
postpartum anemia NOS (O90.81)
● O99.Ø1 Anemia complicating pregnancy
O99.Ø11 Anemia complicating pregnancy, first trimester
O99.Ø12 Anemia complicating pregnancy, second trimester
O99.Ø13 Anemia complicating pregnancy, third trimester
O99.Ø19 Anemia complicating pregnancy, unspecified trimester
O99.Ø2 Anemia complicating childbirth
O99.Ø3 Anemia complicating the puerperium
Excludes1 postpartum anemia not pre-existing prior to delivery (O90.81)

● **O99.1**   **Other diseases of the blood and blood-forming organs and certain disorders involving the immune mechanism complicating pregnancy, childbirth and the puerperium**
Conditions in D65-D89

▶ **Excludes1**   hemorrhage with coagulation defects (O45.-, O46.0-, O67.0, O72.3)

Excludes2   ~~hemorrhage with coagulation defects (O45.-, O46.0-, O67.0, O72.3)~~

● **O99.11**   Other diseases of the blood and blood-forming organs and certain disorders involving the immune mechanism complicating pregnancy

     O99.111   Other diseases of the blood and blood-forming organs and certain disorders involving the immune mechanism complicating pregnancy, first trimester

     O99.112   Other diseases of the blood and blood-forming organs and certain disorders involving the immune mechanism complicating pregnancy, second trimester

     O99.113   Other diseases of the blood and blood-forming organs and certain disorders involving the immune mechanism complicating pregnancy, third trimester

     O99.119   Other diseases of the blood and blood-forming organs and certain disorders involving the immune mechanism complicating pregnancy, unspecified trimester

   O99.12   Other diseases of the blood and blood-forming organs and certain disorders involving the immune mechanism complicating childbirth

   O99.13   Other diseases of the blood and blood-forming organs and certain disorders involving the immune mechanism complicating the puerperium

● **O99.2**   **Endocrine, nutritional and metabolic diseases complicating pregnancy, childbirth and the puerperium**
Conditions in E00-E88

Excludes2   diabetes mellitus (O24.-)
malnutrition (O25.-)
postpartum thyroiditis (O90.5)

● **O99.21**   Obesity complicating pregnancy, childbirth, and the puerperium
Use additional code to identify the type of obesity (E66.-)

     O99.210   Obesity complicating pregnancy, unspecified trimester

     O99.211   Obesity complicating pregnancy, first trimester

     O99.212   Obesity complicating pregnancy, second trimester

     O99.213   Obesity complicating pregnancy, third trimester

     O99.214   Obesity complicating childbirth

     O99.215   Obesity complicating the puerperium

● **O99.28**   Other endocrine, nutritional and metabolic diseases complicating pregnancy, childbirth and the puerperium

     O99.280   Endocrine, nutritional and metabolic diseases complicating pregnancy, unspecified trimester

     O99.281   Endocrine, nutritional and metabolic diseases complicating pregnancy, first trimester

     O99.282   Endocrine, nutritional and metabolic diseases complicating pregnancy, second trimester

     O99.283   Endocrine, nutritional and metabolic diseases complicating pregnancy, third trimester

     O99.284   Endocrine, nutritional and metabolic diseases complicating childbirth

     O99.285   Endocrine, nutritional and metabolic diseases complicating the puerperium

● **O99.3**   **Mental disorders and diseases of the nervous system complicating pregnancy, childbirth and the puerperium**

● **O99.31**   Alcohol use complicating pregnancy, childbirth, and the puerperium
Use additional code(s) from F10 to identify manifestations of the alcohol use

     O99.310   Alcohol use complicating pregnancy, unspecified trimester

     O99.311   Alcohol use complicating pregnancy, first trimester

     O99.312   Alcohol use complicating pregnancy, second trimester

     O99.313   Alcohol use complicating pregnancy, third trimester

     O99.314   Alcohol use complicating childbirth

     O99.315   Alcohol use complicating the puerperium

● **O99.32**   Drug use complicating pregnancy, childbirth, and the puerperium
Use additional code(s) from F11-F16 and F18-F19 to identify manifestations of the drug use

     O99.320   Drug use complicating pregnancy, unspecified trimester

     O99.321   Drug use complicating pregnancy, first trimester

     O99.322   Drug use complicating pregnancy, second trimester

     O99.323   Drug use complicating pregnancy, third trimester

     O99.324   Drug use complicating childbirth

     O99.325   Drug use complicating the puerperium

● **O99.33**   Tobacco use disorder complicating pregnancy, childbirth, and the puerperium
Smoking complicating pregnancy, childbirth, and the puerperium
Use additional code from category F17 to identify type of tobacco nicotine dependence

     O99.330   Smoking (tobacco) complicating pregnancy, unspecified trimester

     O99.331   Smoking (tobacco) complicating pregnancy, first trimester

     O99.332   Smoking (tobacco) complicating pregnancy, second trimester

     O99.333   Smoking (tobacco) complicating pregnancy, third trimester

     O99.334   Smoking (tobacco) complicating childbirth

     O99.335   Smoking (tobacco) complicating the puerperium

CHAPTER 15 (O00-O9A)

● **O99.34** Other mental disorders complicating pregnancy, childbirth, and the puerperium
Conditions in F01-F09 and F20-F99

> **Excludes2** postpartum mood disturbance (O90.6)
> postnatal psychosis (F53)
> puerperal psychosis (F53)

O99.340 Other mental disorders complicating pregnancy, unspecified trimester

O99.341 Other mental disorders complicating pregnancy, first trimester

O99.342 Other mental disorders complicating pregnancy, second trimester

O99.343 Other mental disorders complicating pregnancy, third trimester

O99.344 Other mental disorders complicating childbirth

O99.345 Other mental disorders complicating the puerperium

● **O99.35** Diseases of the nervous system complicating pregnancy, childbirth, and the puerperium
Conditions in G00-G99

> **Excludes2** pregnancy related peripheral neuritis (O26.8-)

O99.350 Diseases of the nervous system complicating pregnancy, unspecified trimester

O99.351 Diseases of the nervous system complicating pregnancy, first trimester

O99.352 Diseases of the nervous system complicating pregnancy, second trimester

O99.353 Diseases of the nervous system complicating pregnancy, third trimester

O99.354 Diseases of the nervous system complicating childbirth

O99.355 Diseases of the nervous system complicating the puerperium

● **O99.4** Diseases of the circulatory system complicating pregnancy, childbirth and the puerperium
Conditions in I00-I99

> **Excludes1** peripartum cardiomyopathy (O90.3)
> **Excludes2** hypertensive disorders (O10-O16)
> obstetric embolism (O88.-)
> venous complications and cerebrovenous sinus thrombosis in labor, childbirth and the puerperium (O87.-)
> venous complications and cerebrovenous sinus thrombosis in pregnancy (O22.-)

● **O99.41** Diseases of the circulatory system complicating pregnancy

O99.411 Diseases of the circulatory system complicating pregnancy, first trimester

O99.412 Diseases of the circulatory system complicating pregnancy, second trimester

O99.413 Diseases of the circulatory system complicating pregnancy, third trimester

O99.419 Diseases of the circulatory system complicating pregnancy, unspecified trimester

O99.42 Diseases of the circulatory system complicating childbirth

O99.43 Diseases of the circulatory system complicating the puerperium

● **O99.5** Diseases of the respiratory system complicating pregnancy, childbirth and the puerperium
Conditions in J00-J99

● **O99.51** Diseases of the respiratory system complicating pregnancy

O99.511 Diseases of the respiratory system complicating pregnancy, first trimester

O99.512 Diseases of the respiratory system complicating pregnancy, second trimester

O99.513 Diseases of the respiratory system complicating pregnancy, third trimester

O99.519 Diseases of the respiratory system complicating pregnancy, unspecified trimester

O99.52 Diseases of the respiratory system complicating childbirth

O99.53 Diseases of the respiratory system complicating the puerperium

● **O99.6** Diseases of the digestive system complicating pregnancy, childbirth and the puerperium
Conditions in K00-K93

> **Excludes2** hemorrhoids in pregnancy (O22.4-)
> liver and biliary tract disorders in pregnancy, childbirth and the puerperium (O26.6-)

● **O99.61** Diseases of the digestive system complicating pregnancy

O99.611 Diseases of the digestive system complicating pregnancy, first trimester

O99.612 Diseases of the digestive system complicating pregnancy, second trimester

O99.613 Diseases of the digestive system complicating pregnancy, third trimester

O99.619 Diseases of the digestive system complicating pregnancy, unspecified trimester

O99.62 Diseases of the digestive system complicating childbirth

O99.63 Diseases of the digestive system complicating the puerperium

● **O99.7** Diseases of the skin and subcutaneous tissue complicating pregnancy, childbirth and the puerperium
Conditions in L00-L99

> **Excludes2** herpes gestationis (O26.4)
> pruritic urticarial papules and plaques of pregnancy (PUPPP) (O26.86)

● **O99.71** Diseases of the skin and subcutaneous tissue complicating pregnancy

O99.711 Diseases of the skin and subcutaneous tissue complicating pregnancy, first trimester

O99.712 Diseases of the skin and subcutaneous tissue complicating pregnancy, second trimester

O99.713 Diseases of the skin and subcutaneous tissue complicating pregnancy, third trimester

O99.719 Diseases of the skin and subcutaneous tissue complicating pregnancy, unspecified trimester

O99.72 Diseases of the skin and subcutaneous tissue complicating childbirth

O99.73 Diseases of the skin and subcutaneous tissue complicating the puerperium

▶ New ⇒ Revised ~~deleted~~ Deleted **OGCR** Official Guidelines X Assign placeholder X ● Use Additional Character(s)

Excludes 1 | Excludes 2 | Includes | Use additional | Code first | Code also | Key words

● **O99.8** **Other specified diseases and conditions** complicating **pregnancy, childbirth and the puerperium**
  Conditions in D00-D48, H00-H95, M00-N99, and Q00-Q99
  Use additional code to identify condition
  Excludes2   genitourinary infections in pregnancy (O23.-)
               infection of genitourinary tract following delivery (O86.1-O86.3)
               malignant neoplasm complicating pregnancy, childbirth and the puerperium (O9A.1-)
               maternal care for known or suspected abnormality of maternal pelvic organs (O34.-)
               postpartum acute kidney failure (O90.4)
               traumatic injuries in pregnancy (O9A.2-)

● **O99.81** **Abnormal glucose** complicating pregnancy, childbirth and the puerperium
  Excludes1   gestational diabetes (O24.4-)
  O99.810   Abnormal glucose complicating pregnancy
  O99.814   Abnormal glucose complicating childbirth
  O99.815   Abnormal glucose complicating the puerperium

● **O99.82** **Streptococcus B carrier state** complicating pregnancy, childbirth and the puerperium
  Excludes1   Carrier of streptococcus group B (GBS) in a nonpregnant woman (Z22.330)
  O99.820   Streptococcus B carrier state complicating pregnancy
  O99.824   Streptococcus B carrier state complicating childbirth
  O99.825   Streptococcus B carrier state complicating the puerperium

● **O99.83** **Other infection carrier state** complicating pregnancy, childbirth and the puerperium
  Use additional code to identify the carrier state (Z22.-)
  O99.830   Other infection carrier state complicating pregnancy
  O99.834   Other infection carrier state complicating childbirth
  O99.835   Other infection carrier state complicating the puerperium

● **O99.84** **Bariatric surgery status** complicating pregnancy, childbirth and the puerperium
  Gastric banding status complicating pregnancy, childbirth and the puerperium
  Gastric bypass status for obesity complicating pregnancy, childbirth and the puerperium
  Obesity surgery status complicating pregnancy, childbirth and the puerperium
  O99.840   Bariatric surgery status complicating pregnancy, unspecified trimester
  O99.841   Bariatric surgery status complicating pregnancy, first trimester
  O99.842   Bariatric surgery status complicating pregnancy, second trimester
  O99.843   Bariatric surgery status complicating pregnancy, third trimester
  O99.844   Bariatric surgery status complicating childbirth
  O99.845   Bariatric surgery status complicating the puerperium

  O99.89   **Other specified diseases and conditions** complicating pregnancy, childbirth and the puerperium

OGCR Section I.C.2.I.3.

Malignant neoplasm in a pregnant patient
When a pregnant woman has a malignant neoplasm, a code from subcategory O9A.1-, Malignant neoplasm complicating pregnancy, childbirth, and the puerperium, should be sequenced first, followed by the appropriate code from Chapter 2 to indicate the type of neoplasm.

● **O9A** **Maternal malignant neoplasms, traumatic injuries and abuse** classifiable elsewhere but complicating pregnancy, childbirth and the puerperium

● **O9A.1** **Malignant neoplasm** complicating pregnancy, childbirth and the puerperium
  Conditions in C00-C96
  Use additional code to identify neoplasm
  Excludes2   maternal care for benign tumor of corpus uteri (O34.1-)
               maternal care for benign tumor of cervix (O34.4-)

● **O9A.11** Malignant neoplasm complicating **pregnancy**
  O9A.111   Malignant neoplasm complicating pregnancy, **first trimester**
  O9A.112   Malignant neoplasm complicating pregnancy, **second trimester**
  O9A.113   Malignant neoplasm complicating pregnancy, **third trimester**
  O9A.119   Malignant neoplasm complicating pregnancy, **unspecified trimester**

  O9A.12   Malignant neoplasm complicating **childbirth**
  O9A.13   Malignant neoplasm complicating the **puerperium**

● **O9A.2** **Injury, poisoning and certain other consequences of external causes** complicating pregnancy, childbirth and the puerperium
  Conditions in S00-T88, except T74 and T76
  Use additional code(s) to identify the injury or poisoning
  Excludes2   physical, sexual and psychological abuse complicating pregnancy, childbirth and the puerperium (O9A.3-, O9A.4-, O9A.5-)

● **O9A.21** Injury, poisoning and certain other consequences of external causes complicating **pregnancy**
  O9A.211   Injury, poisoning and certain other consequences of external causes complicating pregnancy, **first trimester**
  O9A.212   Injury, poisoning and certain other consequences of external causes complicating pregnancy, **second trimester**
  O9A.213   Injury, poisoning and certain other consequences of external causes complicating pregnancy, **third trimester**
  O9A.219   Injury, poisoning and certain other consequences of external causes complicating pregnancy, **unspecified trimester**

  O9A.22   Injury, poisoning and certain other consequences of external causes complicating **childbirth**
  O9A.23   Injury, poisoning and certain other consequences of external causes complicating the **puerperium**

CHAPTER 15 (O00-O9A)

● **O9A.3 Physical abuse complicating pregnancy, childbirth and the puerperium**
Conditions in T74.11 or T76.11
Use additional code (if applicable):
    to identify any associated current injury due to physical abuse
    to identify the perpetrator of abuse (Y07.-)
    Excludes2   sexual abuse complicating pregnancy, childbirth and the puerperium (O9A.4)

  ● **O9A.31 Physical abuse complicating pregnancy**
       O9A.311 Physical abuse complicating pregnancy, first trimester
       O9A.312 Physical abuse complicating pregnancy, second trimester
       O9A.313 Physical abuse complicating pregnancy, third trimester
       O9A.319 Physical abuse complicating pregnancy, unspecified trimester
     O9A.32 Physical abuse complicating childbirth
     O9A.33 Physical abuse complicating the puerperium

● **O9A.4 Sexual abuse complicating pregnancy, childbirth and the puerperium**
Conditions in T74.21 or T76.21
Use additional code (if applicable):
    to identify any associated current injury due to sexual abuse
    to identify the perpetrator of abuse (Y07.-)

  ● **O9A.41 Sexual abuse complicating pregnancy**
       O9A.411 Sexual abuse complicating pregnancy, first trimester
       O9A.412 Sexual abuse complicating pregnancy, second trimester
       O9A.413 Sexual abuse complicating pregnancy, third trimester
       O9A.419 Sexual abuse complicating pregnancy, unspecified trimester
     O9A.42 Sexual abuse complicating childbirth
     O9A.43 Sexual abuse complicating the puerperium

● **O9A.5 Psychological abuse complicating pregnancy, childbirth and the puerperium**
Conditions in T74.31 or T76.31
Use additional code to identify the perpetrator of abuse (Y07.-)

  ● **O9A.51 Psychological abuse complicating pregnancy**
       O9A.511 Psychological abuse complicating pregnancy, first trimester
       O9A.512 Psychological abuse complicating pregnancy, second trimester
       O9A.513 Psychological abuse complicating pregnancy, third trimester
       O9A.519 Psychological abuse complicating pregnancy, unspecified trimester
     O9A.52 Psychological abuse complicating childbirth
     O9A.53 Psychological abuse complicating the puerperium

▶ New   ⇒ Revised   ~~deleted~~ Deleted   **OGCR** Official Guidelines   X Assign placeholder X   ● Use Additional Character(s)
Excludes 1   Excludes 2   Includes   Use additional   Code first   Code also   Key words

CHAPTER 16

CERTAIN CONDITIONS ORIGINATING IN THE PERINATAL PERIOD (P00-P96)

OGCR Chapter-Specific Coding Guidelines

16. **Chapter 16: Certain Conditions Originating in the Perinatal Period (P00-P96)**

For coding and reporting purposes the perinatal period is defined as before birth through the 28th day following birth. The following guidelines are provided for reporting purposes

a. General Perinatal Rules

1) Use of Chapter 16 Codes

Codes in this chapter are <u>never</u> for use on the maternal record. Codes from Chapter 15, the obstetric chapter, are never permitted on the newborn record. Chapter 16 codes may be used throughout the life of the patient if the condition is still present.

2) Principal Diagnosis for Birth Record

When coding the birth episode in a newborn record, assign a code from category Z38, Liveborn infants according to place of birth and type of delivery, as the principal diagnosis. A code from category Z38 is assigned only once, to a newborn at the time of birth. If a newborn is transferred to another institution, a code from category Z38 should not be used at the receiving hospital.

A code from category Z38 is used only on the newborn record, not on the mother's record.

3) Use of Codes from other Chapters with Codes from Chapter 16

Codes from other chapters may be used with codes from chapter 16 if the codes from the other chapters provide more specific detail. Codes for signs and symptoms may be assigned when a definitive diagnosis has not been established. If the reason for the encounter is a perinatal condition, the code from chapter 16 should be sequenced first.

4) Use of Chapter 16 Codes after the Perinatal Period

Should a condition originate in the perinatal period, and continue throughout the life of the patient, the perinatal code should continue to be used regardless of the patient's age.

5) Birth process or community acquired conditions

If a newborn has a condition that may be either due to the birth process or community acquired and the documentation does not indicate which it is, the default is due to the birth process and the code from Chapter 16 should be used. If the condition is community-acquired, a code from Chapter 16 should not be assigned.

6) Code all clinically significant conditions

All clinically significant conditions noted on routine newborn examination should be coded. A condition is clinically significant if it requires:

- clinical evaluation; or
- therapeutic treatment; or
- diagnostic procedures; or
- extended length of hospital stay; or
- increased nursing care and/or monitoring; or
- has implications for future health care needs

Note: The perinatal guidelines listed above are the same as the general coding guidelines for "additional diagnoses", except for the final point regarding implications for future health care needs. Codes should be assigned for conditions that have been specified by the provider as having implications for future health care needs.

b. Observation and Evaluation of Newborns for Suspected Conditions not Found

1) Use of Z05 codes

Assign a code from category Z05, Observation and evaluation of newborns and infants for suspected conditions ruled out, to identify those instances when a healthy newborn is evaluated for a suspected condition that is determined after study not to be present. Do not use a code from category Z05 when the patient has identified signs or symptoms of a suspected problem; in such cases code the sign or symptom.

2) Z05 on Other than the Birth Record

A code from category Z05 may also be assigned as a principal or first-listed code for readmissions or encounters when the code from category Z38 code no longer applies. Codes from category Z05 are for use only for healthy newborns and infants for which no condition after study is found to be present.

3) Z05 on a birth record

A code from category Z05 is to be used as a secondary code after the code from category Z38, Liveborn infants according to place of birth and type of delivery.

c. Coding Additional Perinatal Diagnoses

1) Assigning codes for conditions that require treatment

Assign codes for conditions that require treatment or further investigation, prolong the length of stay, or require resource utilization.

2) Codes for conditions specified as having implications for future health care needs

Assign codes for conditions that have been specified by the provider as having implications for future health care needs. **Note:** This guideline should not be used for adult patients.

d. Prematurity and Fetal Growth Retardation

Providers utilize different criteria in determining prematurity. A code for prematurity should not be assigned unless it is documented. Assignment of codes in categories P05, Disorders of newborn related to slow fetal growth and fetal malnutrition, and P07, Disorders of newborn related to short gestation and low birth weight, not elsewhere classified, should be based on the recorded birth weight and estimated gestational age.

When both birth weight and gestational age are available, two codes from category P07 should be assigned, with the code for birth weight sequenced before the code for gestational age.

e. Low birth weight and immaturity status

Codes from category P07, Disorders of newborn related to short gestation and low birth weight, not elsewhere classified, are for use for a child or adult who was premature or had a low birth weight as a newborn and this is affecting the patient's current health status.

See Section I.C.21. Factors influencing health status and contact with health services, Status.

f. Bacterial Sepsis of Newborn

Category P36, Bacterial sepsis of newborn, includes congenital sepsis. If a perinate is documented as having sepsis without documentation of congenital or community acquired, the default is congenital and a code from category P36 should be assigned. If the P36 code includes the causal organism, an additional code from category B95, Streptococcus, Staphylococcus, and Enterococcus as the cause of diseases classified elsewhere, or B96, Other bacterial agents as the cause of diseases classified elsewhere, should not be assigned. If the P36 code does not include the causal organism, assign an additional code from category B96. If applicable, use additional codes to identify severe sepsis (R65.2-) and any associated acute organ dysfunction.

g. Stillbirth

Code P95, Stillbirth, is only for use in institutions that maintain separate records for stillbirths. No other code should be used with P95. Code P95 should not be used on the mother's record.

CHAPTER 16

CERTAIN CONDITIONS ORIGINATING IN THE PERINATAL PERIOD (P00-P96)

Note: Codes from this chapter are for use on newborn records only, never on maternal records.

Includes conditions that have their origin in the fetal or perinatal period (before birth through the first 28 days after birth) even if morbidity occurs later

Excludes2 congenital malformations, deformations and chromosomal abnormalities (Q00-Q99)
endocrine, nutritional and metabolic diseases (E00-E88)
injury, poisoning and certain other consequences of external causes (S00-T88)
neoplasms (C00-D49)
tetanus neonatorum (A33)

This chapter contains the following blocks:

P00-P04	Newborn affected by maternal factors and by complications of pregnancy, labor, and delivery
P05-P08	Disorders of newborns related to length of gestation and fetal growth
P09	Abnormal findings on neonatal screening
P10-P15	Birth trauma
P19-P29	Respiratory and cardiovascular disorders specific to the perinatal period
P35-P39	Infections specific to the perinatal period
P50-P61	Hemorrhagic and hematological disorders of newborn
P70-P74	Transitory endocrine and metabolic disorders specific to newborn
P76-P78	Digestive system disorders of newborn
P80-P83	Conditions involving the integument and temperature regulation of newborn
P84	Other problems with newborn
P90-P96	Other disorders originating in the perinatal period

NEWBORN AFFECTED BY MATERNAL FACTORS AND BY COMPLICATIONS OF PREGNANCY, LABOR, AND DELIVERY (P00–P04)

Note: These codes are for use when the listed maternal conditions are specified as the cause of confirmed morbidity or potential morbidity which have their origin in the perinatal period (before birth through the first 28 days after birth).

● **P00 Newborn affected by maternal conditions that may be unrelated to present pregnancy**
Code first any current condition in newborn
Excludes2 encounter for observation of newborn for suspected diseases and conditions ruled out (Z05.-)
newborn affected by maternal complications of pregnancy (P01.-)
newborn affected by maternal endocrine and metabolic disorders (P70–P74)
newborn affected by noxious substances transmitted via placenta or breast milk (P04.-)

P00.0 Newborn affected by maternal hypertensive disorders
Newborn affected by maternal conditions classifiable to O10-O11, O13-O16

P00.1 Newborn affected by maternal renal and urinary tract diseases
Newborn affected by maternal conditions classifiable to N00-N39

P00.2 Newborn affected by maternal infectious and parasitic diseases
Newborn affected by maternal infectious disease classifiable to A00-B99, J09 and J10
Excludes1 ~~infections specific to the perinatal period (P35-P39)~~
maternal genital tract or other localized infections (P00.8)
▶ **Excludes2** infections specific to the perinatal period (P35-P39)

P00.3 Newborn affected by other maternal circulatory and respiratory diseases
Newborn affected by maternal conditions classifiable to I00-I99, J00-J99, Q20-Q34 and not included in P00.0, P00.2

P00.4 Newborn affected by maternal nutritional disorders
Newborn affected by maternal disorders classifiable to E40-E64
Maternal malnutrition NOS

P00.5 Newborn affected by maternal injury
Newborn affected by maternal conditions classifiable to O9A.2-

P00.6 Newborn affected by surgical procedure on mother
Newborn affected by amniocentesis
Excludes1 Cesarean delivery for present delivery (P03.4)
damage to placenta from amniocentesis, cesarean delivery or surgical induction (P02.1)
previous surgery to uterus or pelvic organs (P03.89)
Excludes2 newborn affected by complication of (fetal) intrauterine procedure (P96.5)

P00.7 Newborn affected by other medical procedures on mother, not elsewhere classified
Newborn affected by radiation to mother
Excludes1 damage to placenta from amniocentesis, cesarean delivery or surgical induction (P02.1)
newborn affected by other complications of labor and delivery (P03.-)

● **P00.8 Newborn affected by other maternal conditions**
P00.81 Newborn affected by periodontal disease in mother
P00.89 Newborn affected by other maternal conditions
Newborn affected by conditions classifiable to T80-T88
Newborn affected by maternal genital tract or other localized infections
Newborn affected by maternal systemic lupus erythematosus

P00.9 Newborn affected by unspecified maternal condition

● **P01 Newborn affected by maternal complications of pregnancy**
Code first any current condition in newborn
Excludes2 encounter for observation of newborn for suspected diseases and conditions ruled out (Z05.-)

P01.0 Newborn affected by incompetent cervix
P01.1 Newborn affected by premature rupture of membranes
P01.2 Newborn affected by oligohydramnios
Excludes1 oligohydramnios due to premature rupture of membranes (P01.1)
P01.3 Newborn affected by polyhydramnios
Excess of amniotic fluid, usually > 2000 mL
Newborn affected by hydramnios

▶ New	⇒ Revised ~~deleted~~ Deleted **OGCR** Official Guidelines X Assign placeholder X ● Use Additional Character(s)

Excludes 1   Excludes 2   Includes   Use additional   Code first   Code also   Key words

P01.4   Newborn affected by ectopic pregnancy
     Newborn affected by abdominal pregnancy

P01.5   Newborn affected by multiple pregnancy
     Newborn affected by triplet (pregnancy)
     Newborn affected by twin (pregnancy)

P01.6   Newborn affected by maternal death

P01.7   Newborn affected by malpresentation before labor
     Newborn affected by breech presentation before labor
     Newborn affected by external version before labor
     Newborn affected by face presentation before labor
     Newborn affected by transverse lie before labor
     Newborn affected by unstable lie before labor

P01.8   Newborn affected by other maternal complications of pregnancy

P01.9   Newborn affected by maternal complication of pregnancy, unspecified

● **P02**   Newborn affected by complications of placenta, cord and membranes

Code first any current condition in newborn

     Excludes2   encounter for observation of newborn for suspected diseases and conditions ruled out (Z05.-)

P02.0   Newborn affected by placenta previa

P02.1   Newborn affected by other forms of placental separation and hemorrhage
     Newborn affected by abruptio placenta
     Newborn affected by accidental hemorrhage
     Newborn affected by antepartum hemorrhage
     Newborn affected by damage to placenta from amniocentesis, cesarean delivery or surgical induction
     Newborn affected by maternal blood loss
     Newborn affected by premature separation of placenta

● **P02.2**   Newborn affected by other and unspecified morphological and functional abnormalities of placenta

     P02.20   Newborn affected by unspecified morphological and functional abnormalities of placenta

     P02.29   Newborn affected by other morphological and functional abnormalities of placenta
         Newborn affected by placental dysfunction
         Newborn affected by placental infarction
         Newborn affected by placental insufficiency

P02.3   Newborn affected by placental transfusion syndromes
     Newborn affected by placental and cord abnormalities resulting in twin-to-twin or other transplacental transfusion

P02.4   Newborn affected by prolapsed cord

P02.5   Newborn affected by other compression of umbilical cord
     Newborn affected by umbilical cord (tightly) around neck
     Newborn affected by entanglement of umbilical cord
     Newborn affected by knot in umbilical cord

● **P02.6**   Newborn affected by other and unspecified conditions of umbilical cord

     P02.60   Newborn affected by unspecified conditions of umbilical cord

     P02.69   Newborn affected by other conditions of umbilical cord
         Newborn affected by short umbilical cord
         Newborn affected by vasa previa
         Excludes1   newborn affected by single umbilical artery (Q27.0)

P02.7   Newborn affected by chorioamnionitis
     Inflammation of chorion and amnion
     Newborn affected by amnionitis
     Newborn affected by membranitis
     Newborn affected by placentitis

P02.8   Newborn affected by other abnormalities of membranes

P02.9   Newborn affected by abnormality of membranes, unspecified

● **P03**   Newborn affected by other complications of labor and delivery

Code first any current condition in newborn

     Excludes2   encounter for observation of newborn for suspected diseases and conditions ruled out (Z05.-)

P03.0   Newborn affected by breech delivery and extraction

P03.1   Newborn affected by other malpresentation, malposition and disproportion during labor and delivery
     Newborn affected by contracted pelvis
     Newborn affected by conditions classifiable to O64-O66
     Newborn affected by persistent occipitoposterior
     Newborn affected by transverse lie

P03.2   Newborn affected by forceps delivery

P03.3   Newborn affected by delivery by vacuum extractor [ventouse]

P03.4   Newborn affected by Cesarean delivery

P03.5   Newborn affected by precipitate delivery
     Newborn affected by rapid second stage

P03.6   Newborn affected by abnormal uterine contractions
     Newborn affected by conditions classifiable to O62.-, except O62.3
     Newborn affected by hypertonic labor
     Newborn affected by uterine inertia

● **P03.8**   Newborn affected by other specified complications of labor and delivery

  ● **P03.81**   Newborn affected by abnormality in fetal (intrauterine) heart rate or rhythm

     Excludes1   neonatal cardiac dysrhythmia (P29.1-)

     P03.810   Newborn affected by abnormality in fetal (intrauterine) heart rate or rhythm before the onset of labor

     P03.811   Newborn affected by abnormality in fetal (intrauterine) heart rate or rhythm during labor

     P03.819   Newborn affected by abnormality in fetal (intrauterine) heart rate or rhythm, unspecified as to time of onset

     P03.82   Meconium passage during delivery
         Excludes1   meconium aspiration (P24.00, P24.01)
             meconium staining (P96.83)

     P03.89   Newborn affected by other specified complications of labor and delivery
         Newborn affected by abnormality of maternal soft tissues
         Newborn affected by conditions classifiable to O60-O75 and by procedures used in labor and delivery not included in P02.- and P03.0-P03.6
         Newborn affected by induction of labor

P03.9   Newborn affected by complication of labor and delivery, unspecified

▶ New   ⇒ Revised   ~~deleted~~ Deleted   **OGCR** Official Guidelines   X Assign placeholder X   ● Use Additional Character(s)

Excludes 1   Excludes 2   Includes   Use additional   Code first   Code also   Key words

● **P04**   **Newborn affected by noxious substances transmitted via placenta or breast milk**

     Includes   nonteratogenic effects of substances transmitted via placenta

     Excludes2   congenital malformations (Q00-Q99)

           encounter for observation of newborn for suspected diseases and conditions ruled out (Z05.-)

           neonatal jaundice from excessive hemolysis due to drugs or toxins transmitted from mother (P58.4)

           newborn in contact with and (suspected) exposures hazardous to health not transmitted via placenta or breast milk (Z77.-)

   P04.0   **Newborn affected by maternal anesthesia and analgesia in pregnancy, labor and delivery**

       Newborn affected by reactions and intoxications from maternal opiates and tranquilizers administered during labor and delivery

   P04.1   **Newborn affected by other maternal medication**

       Newborn affected by cancer chemotherapy

       Newborn affected by cytotoxic drugs

       Excludes1   dysmorphism due to warfarin (Q86.2)

           fetal hydantoin syndrome (Q86.1)

           maternal use of drugs of addiction (P04.4-)

   P04.2   **Newborn affected by maternal use of tobacco**

       Newborn affected by exposure in utero to tobacco smoke

       Excludes2   newborn exposure to environmental tobacco smoke (P96.81)

   P04.3   **Newborn affected by maternal use of alcohol**

       Excludes1   fetal alcohol syndrome (Q86.0)

● **P04.4**   **Newborn affected by maternal use of drugs of addiction**

     P04.41   **Newborn affected by maternal use of cocaine**

         'Crack baby'

     P04.49   **Newborn affected by maternal use of other drugs of addiction**

         Excludes2   newborn affected by maternal anesthesia and analgesia (P04.0)

            withdrawal symptoms from maternal use of drugs of addiction (P96.1)

   P04.5   **Newborn affected by maternal use of nutritional chemical substances**

   P04.6   **Newborn affected by maternal exposure to environmental chemical substances**

   P04.8   **Newborn affected by other maternal noxious substances**

   P04.9   **Newborn affected by maternal noxious substance, unspecified**

OGCR Section I.C.16.d.

Prematurity and Fetal Growth Retardation

Providers utilize different criteria in determining prematurity. A code for prematurity should not be assigned unless it is documented. Assignment of codes in categories P05, Disorders of newborn related to slow fetal growth and fetal malnutrition, and P07, Disorders of newborn related to short gestation and low birth weight, not elsewhere classified, should be based on the recorded birth weight and estimated gestational age.

When both birth weight and gestational age are available, two codes from category P07 should be assigned, with the code for birth weight sequenced before the code for gestational age.

DISORDERS OF NEWBORN RELATED TO LENGTH OF GESTATION AND FETAL GROWTH (P05-P08)

● **P05**   **Disorders of newborn related to slow fetal growth and fetal malnutrition**

   ● **P05.0**   **Newborn light for gestational age**

       Newborn light-for-dates

       Weight below but length above 10th percentile for gestational age

     P05.00   **Newborn light for gestational age, unspecified weight**

     P05.01   **Newborn light for gestational age, less than 500 grams**

     P05.02   **Newborn light for gestational age, 500-749 grams**

     P05.03   **Newborn light for gestational age, 750-999 grams**

     P05.04   **Newborn light for gestational age, 1000-1249 grams**

     P05.05   **Newborn light for gestational age, 1250-1499 grams**

     P05.06   **Newborn light for gestational age, 1500-1749 grams**

     P05.07   **Newborn light for gestational age, 1750-1999 grams**

     P05.08   **Newborn light for gestational age, 2000-2499 grams**

     P05.09   **Newborn light for gestational age, 2500 grams and over**

         Newborn light for gestational age, other

   ● **P05.1**   **Newborn small for gestational age**

       Newborn small-and-light-for-dates

       Newborn small-for-dates

       Weight and length below 10th percentile for gestational age

     P05.10   **Newborn small for gestational age, unspecified weight**

     P05.11   **Newborn small for gestational age, less than 500 grams**

     P05.12   **Newborn small for gestational age, 500-749 grams**

     P05.13   **Newborn small for gestational age, 750-999 grams**

     P05.14   **Newborn small for gestational age, 1000-1249 grams**

     P05.15   **Newborn small for gestational age, 1250-1499 grams**

     P05.16   **Newborn small for gestational age, 1500-1749 grams**

     P05.17   **Newborn small for gestational age, 1750-1999 grams**

     P05.18   **Newborn small for gestational age, 2000-2499 grams**

     P05.19   **Newborn small for gestational age, other**

         Newborn small for gestational age, 2500 grams and over

   P05.2   **Newborn affected by fetal (intrauterine) malnutrition not light or small for gestational age**

       Infant, not light or small for gestational age, showing signs of fetal malnutrition, such as dry, peeling skin and loss of subcutaneous tissue

       Excludes1   newborn affected by fetal malnutrition with light for gestational age (P05.0-)

           newborn affected by fetal malnutrition with small for gestational age (P05.1-)

   P05.9   **Newborn affected by slow intrauterine growth, unspecified**

       Newborn affected by fetal growth retardation NOS

▶ New   ⇒ Revised   ~~deleted~~ Deleted   **OGCR** Official Guidelines   X Assign placeholder X   ● Use Additional Character(s)

Excludes 1   Excludes 2   Includes   Use additional   Code first   Code also   Key words

● **P07** **Disorders of newborn related to short gestation and low birth weight, not elsewhere classified**

> **Note:** When both birth weight and gestational age of the newborn are available, both should be coded with birth weight sequenced before gestational age.

> **Includes** the listed conditions, without further specification, as the cause of morbidity or additional care, in newborn

● **P07.0** **Extremely low birth weight newborn**
> Newborn birth weight 999 g. or less

> > **Excludes1** low birth weight due to slow fetal growth and fetal malnutrition (P05.-)

> **P07.00** **Extremely low birth weight newborn, unspecified weight**

> **P07.01** **Extremely low birth weight newborn, less than 500 grams**

> **P07.02** **Extremely low birth weight newborn, 500-749 grams**

> **P07.03** **Extremely low birth weight newborn, 750-999 grams**

● **P07.1** **Other low birth weight newborn**
> Newborn birth weight 1000-2499 g.

> > **Excludes1** low birth weight due to slow fetal growth and fetal malnutrition (P05.-)

> **P07.10** **Other low birth weight newborn, unspecified weight**

> **P07.14** **Other low birth weight newborn, 1000-1249 grams**

> **P07.15** **Other low birth weight newborn, 1250-1499 grams**

> **P07.16** **Other low birth weight newborn, 1500-1749 grams**

> **P07.17** **Other low birth weight newborn, 1750-1999 grams**

> **P07.18** **Other low birth weight newborn, 2000-2499 grams**

● **P07.2** **Extreme immaturity of newborn**
> Less than 28 completed weeks (less than 196 completed days) of gestation

> **P07.20** **Extreme immaturity of newborn, unspecified weeks of gestation**
> > Gestational age less than 28 completed weeks NOS

> **P07.21** **Extreme immaturity of newborn, gestational age less than 23 completed weeks**
> > Extreme immaturity of newborn, gestational age less than 23 weeks, 0 days

> **P07.22** **Extreme immaturity of newborn, gestational age 23 completed weeks**
> > Extreme immaturity of newborn, gestational age 23 weeks, 0 days through 23 weeks, 6 days

> **P07.23** **Extreme immaturity of newborn, gestational age 24 completed weeks**
> > Extreme immaturity of newborn, gestational age 24 weeks, 0 days through 24 weeks, 6 days

> **P07.24** **Extreme immaturity of newborn, gestational age 25 completed weeks**
> > Extreme immaturity of newborn, gestational age 25 weeks, 0 days through 25 weeks, 6 days

> **P07.25** **Extreme immaturity of newborn, gestational age 26 completed weeks**
> > Extreme immaturity of newborn, gestational age 26 weeks, 0 days through 26 weeks, 6 days

> **P07.26** **Extreme immaturity of newborn, gestational age 27 completed weeks**
> > Extreme immaturity of newborn, gestational age 27 weeks, 0 days through 27 weeks, 6 days

● **P07.3** **Preterm [premature] newborn [other]**
> 28 completed weeks or more but less than 37 completed weeks (196 completed days but less than 259 completed days) of gestation
> Prematurity NOS

> **P07.30** **Preterm newborn, unspecified weeks of gestation**

> **P07.31** **Preterm newborn, gestational age 28 completed weeks**
> > Preterm newborn, gestational age 28 weeks, 0 days through 28 weeks, 6 days

> **P07.32** **Preterm newborn, gestational age 29 completed weeks**
> > Preterm newborn, gestational age 29 weeks, 0 days through 29 weeks, 6 days

> **P07.33** **Preterm newborn, gestational age 30 completed weeks**
> > Preterm newborn, gestational age 30 weeks, 0 days through 30 weeks, 6 days

> **P07.34** **Preterm newborn, gestational age 31 completed weeks**
> > Preterm newborn, gestational age 31 weeks, 0 days through 31 weeks, 6 days

> **P07.35** **Preterm newborn, gestational age 32 completed weeks**
> > Preterm newborn, gestational age 32 weeks, 0 days through 32 weeks, 6 days

> **P07.36** **Preterm newborn, gestational age 33 completed weeks**
> > Preterm newborn, gestational age 33 weeks, 0 days through 33 weeks, 6 days

> **P07.37** **Preterm newborn, gestational age 34 completed weeks**
> > Preterm newborn, gestational age 34 weeks, 0 days through 34 weeks, 6 days

> **P07.38** **Preterm newborn, gestational age 35 completed weeks**
> > Preterm newborn, gestational age 35 weeks, 0 days through 35 weeks, 6 days

> **P07.39** **Preterm newborn, gestational age 36 completed weeks**
> > Preterm newborn, gestational age 36 weeks, 0 days through 36 weeks, 6 days

● **P08** **Disorders of newborn related to long gestation and high birth weight**

> **Note:** When both birth weight and gestational age of the newborn are available, priority of assignment should be given to birth weight.

> **Includes** the listed conditions, without further specification, as causes of morbidity or additional care, in newborn

> **P08.0** **Exceptionally large newborn baby**
> > Usually implies a birth weight of 4500 g. or more

> > > **Excludes1** syndrome of infant of diabetic mother (P70.1)
> > > syndrome of infant of mother with gestational diabetes (P70.0)

> **P08.1** **Other heavy for gestational age newborn**
> > Other newborn heavy- or large-for-dates regardless of period of gestation
> > Usually implies a birth weight of 4000 g. to 4499 g.

> > > **Excludes1** newborn with a birth weight of 4500 or more (P08.0)
> > > syndrome of infant of diabetic mother (P70.1)
> > > syndrome of infant of mother with gestational diabetes (P70.0)

CHAPTER 16 (P00-P96)

● P08.2　Late newborn, not heavy for gestational age
　　P08.21　Post-term newborn
　　　　　Newborn with gestation period over 40 completed weeks to 42 completed weeks
　　P08.22　Prolonged gestation of newborn
　　　　　Newborn with gestation period over 42 completed weeks (294 days or more), not heavy- or large-for-dates
　　　　　Postmaturity NOS

ABNORMAL FINDINGS ON NEONATAL SCREENING (P09)

P09　Abnormal findings on neonatal screening
　　Use additional code to identify signs, symptoms and conditions associated with the screening
　　Excludes2　nonspecific serologic evidence of human immunodeficiency virus [HIV] (R75)

BIRTH TRAUMA (P10-P15)

● P10　Intracranial laceration and hemorrhage due to birth injury
　　Excludes1　intracranial hemorrhage of newborn NOS (P52.9)
　　　　　intracranial hemorrhage of newborn due to anoxia or hypoxia (P52.-)
　　　　　nontraumatic intracranial hemorrhage of newborn (P52.-)
　　P10.0　Subdural hemorrhage due to birth injury
　　　　　Subdural hematoma (localized) due to birth injury
　　　　　Excludes1　subdural hemorrhage accompanying tentorial tear (P10.4)
　　P10.1　Cerebral hemorrhage due to birth injury
　　P10.2　Intraventricular hemorrhage due to birth injury
　　P10.3　Subarachnoid hemorrhage due to birth injury
　　P10.4　Tentorial tear due to birth injury
　　　　　Pertaining to tentorium of cerebellum (extension of dura mater that separates cerebellum from inferior portion of occipital lobes)
　　P10.8　Other intracranial lacerations and hemorrhages due to birth injury
　　P10.9　Unspecified intracranial laceration and hemorrhage due to birth injury

● P11　Other birth injuries to central nervous system
　　P11.0　Cerebral edema due to birth injury
　　P11.1　Other specified brain damage due to birth injury
　　P11.2　Unspecified brain damage due to birth injury
　　P11.3　Birth injury to facial nerve
　　　　　Facial palsy due to birth injury
　　P11.4　Birth injury to other cranial nerves
　　P11.5　Birth injury to spine and spinal cord
　　　　　Fracture of spine due to birth injury
　　P11.9　Birth injury to central nervous system, unspecified

● P12　Birth injury to scalp
　　P12.0　Cephalhematoma due to birth injury
　　P12.1　Chignon (from vacuum extraction) due to birth injury
　　P12.2　Epicranial subaponeurotic hemorrhage due to birth injury
　　　　　Subgaleal hemorrhage
　　P12.3　Bruising of scalp due to birth injury
　　P12.4　Injury of scalp of newborn due to monitoring equipment
　　　　　Sampling incision of scalp of newborn
　　　　　Scalp clip (electrode) injury of newborn
　● P12.8　Other birth injuries to scalp
　　P12.81　Caput succedaneum
　　P12.89　Other birth injuries to scalp
　　P12.9　Birth injury to scalp, unspecified

● P13　Birth injury to skeleton
　　Excludes2　birth injury to spine (P11.5)
　　P13.0　Fracture of skull due to birth injury
　　P13.1　Other birth injuries to skull
　　　　　Excludes1　cephalhematoma (P12.0)
　　P13.2　Birth injury to femur
　　P13.3　Birth injury to other long bones
　　P13.4　Fracture of clavicle due to birth injury
　　P13.8　Birth injuries to other parts of skeleton
　　P13.9　Birth injury to skeleton, unspecified

● P14　Birth injury to peripheral nervous system
　　P14.0　Erb's paralysis due to birth injury
　　P14.1　Klumpke's paralysis due to birth injury
　　P14.2　Phrenic nerve paralysis due to birth injury
　　P14.3　Other brachial plexus birth injuries
　　P14.8　Birth injuries to other parts of peripheral nervous system
　　P14.9　Birth injury to peripheral nervous system, unspecified

Item 16-1 The **peripheral nervous system** consists of 31 pairs of spinal nerves, 12 pairs of cranial nerves, and the autonomic nerves, which are divided into the parasympathetic and sympathetic nerves. The cranial nerves are: olfactory (I), optic (II), oculomotor (III), trochlear (IV), trigeminal (V), abducens (VI), facial (VII), vestibulocochlear (VIII), glossopharyngeal (IX), vagus (X), accessory (XI), and hypoglossal (XII).

Central Nervous System
• Brain
• Spinal cord

Peripheral Nervous System
• Cranial nerves (12)
• Spinal nerves
　cervical (8)
　thoracic (12)
　lumbar (5)
　sacral (5)
　coccyx (1)

Figure 16-1 The central nervous system consists of the brain and spinal cord. The peripheral nervous system consists of nerves that lie outside the skull and spinal cord. (From Stoy: Mosby's EMT-Basic Textbook, ed 2, St. Louis, Mosby, 2007)

▶ New　⇒ Revised　~~deleted~~ Deleted　OGCR Official Guidelines　X Assign placeholder X　● Use Additional Character(s)
Excludes 1　Excludes 2　Includes　Use additional　Code first　Code also　Key words

1112

● **P15   Other birth injuries**

P15.0   Birth injury to liver
Rupture of liver due to birth injury

P15.1   Birth injury to spleen
Rupture of spleen due to birth injury

P15.2   Sternomastoid injury due to birth injury

P15.3   Birth injury to eye
Subconjunctival hemorrhage due to birth injury
Traumatic glaucoma due to birth injury

P15.4   Birth injury to face
Facial congestion due to birth injury

P15.5   Birth injury to external genitalia

P15.6   Subcutaneous fat necrosis due to birth injury

P15.8   Other specified birth injuries

P15.9   Birth injury, unspecified

RESPIRATORY AND CARDIOVASCULAR DISORDERS SPECIFIC TO THE PERINATAL PERIOD (P19-P29)

● **P19   Metabolic acidemia in newborn**
Includes   metabolic acidemia in newborn

P19.0   Metabolic acidemia in newborn first noted before onset of labor

P19.1   Metabolic acidemia in newborn first noted during labor

P19.2   Metabolic acidemia noted at birth

P19.9   Metabolic acidemia, unspecified

● **P22   Respiratory distress of newborn**
Excludes1   respiratory arrest of newborn (P28.81)
respiratory failure of newborn NOS (P28.5)

P22.0   Respiratory distress syndrome of newborn
Cardiorespiratory distress syndrome of newborn
Hyaline membrane disease
Idiopathic respiratory distress syndrome [IRDS or RDS] of newborn
Pulmonary hypoperfusion syndrome
Respiratory distress syndrome, type I

P22.1   Transient tachypnea of newborn
Idiopathic tachypnea of newborn
Respiratory distress syndrome, type II
Wet lung syndrome

P22.8   Other respiratory distress of newborn

P22.9   Respiratory distress of newborn, unspecified

● **P23   Congenital pneumonia**
Includes   infective pneumonia acquired in utero or during birth
Excludes1   neonatal pneumonia resulting from aspiration (P24.-)

P23.0   Congenital pneumonia due to viral agent
Use additional code (B97) to identify organism
Excludes1   congenital rubella pneumonitis (P35.0)

P23.1   Congenital pneumonia due to Chlamydia

P23.2   Congenital pneumonia due to staphylococcus

P23.3   Congenital pneumonia due to streptococcus, group B

P23.4   Congenital pneumonia due to Escherichia coli

P23.5   Congenital pneumonia due to Pseudomonas

P23.6   Congenital pneumonia due to other bacterial agents
Congenital pneumonia due to Hemophilus influenzae
Congenital pneumonia due to Klebsiella pneumoniae
Congenital pneumonia due to Mycoplasma
Congenital pneumonia due to Streptococcus, except group B
Use additional code (B95-B96) to identify organism

P23.8   Congenital pneumonia due to other organisms

P23.9   Congenital pneumonia, unspecified

● **P24   Neonatal aspiration**
Includes   aspiration in utero and during delivery

● **P24.0   Meconium aspiration**
Excludes1   meconium passage (without aspiration) during delivery (P03.82)
meconium staining (P96.83)

P24.00   Meconium aspiration without respiratory symptoms
Meconium aspiration NOS

P24.01   Meconium aspiration with respiratory symptoms
Meconium aspiration pneumonia
Meconium aspiration pneumonitis
Meconium aspiration syndrome NOS
➭ Use additional code to identify any secondary pulmonary hypertension, if applicable (I27.2-)

● **P24.1   Neonatal aspiration of (clear) amniotic fluid and mucus**
Neonatal aspiration of liquor (amnii)

P24.10   Neonatal aspiration of (clear) amniotic fluid and mucus without respiratory symptoms
Neonatal aspiration of amniotic fluid and mucus NOS

P24.11   Neonatal aspiration of (clear) amniotic fluid and mucus with respiratory symptoms
Neonatal aspiration of amniotic fluid and mucus with pneumonia
Neonatal aspiration of amniotic fluid and mucus with pneumonitis
➭ Use additional code to identify any secondary pulmonary hypertension, if applicable (I27.2-)

● **P24.2   Neonatal aspiration of blood**

P24.20   Neonatal aspiration of blood without respiratory symptoms
Neonatal aspiration of blood NOS

P24.21   Neonatal aspiration of blood with respiratory symptoms
Neonatal aspiration of blood with pneumonia
Neonatal aspiration of blood with pneumonitis
➭ Use additional code to identify any secondary pulmonary hypertension, if applicable (I27.2-)

● **P24.3   Neonatal aspiration of milk and regurgitated food**
Neonatal aspiration of stomach contents

P24.30   Neonatal aspiration of milk and regurgitated food without respiratory symptoms
Neonatal aspiration of milk and regurgitated food NOS

P24.31   Neonatal aspiration of milk and regurgitated food with respiratory symptoms
Neonatal aspiration of milk and regurgitated food with pneumonia
Neonatal aspiration of milk and regurgitated food with pneumonitis
➭ Use additional code to identify any secondary pulmonary hypertension, if applicable (I27.2-)

● **P24.8   Other neonatal aspiration**

P24.80   Other neonatal aspiration without respiratory symptoms
Neonatal aspiration NEC

P24.81   Other neonatal aspiration with respiratory symptoms
Neonatal aspiration pneumonia NEC
Neonatal aspiration with pneumonitis NEC
Neonatal aspiration with pneumonia NOS
Neonatal aspiration with pneumonitis NOS
➭ Use additional code to identify any secondary pulmonary hypertension, if applicable (I27.2-)

P24.9   Neonatal aspiration, unspecified

● **P25** Interstitial emphysema and related conditions originating in the perinatal period

     P25.0 Interstitial emphysema originating in the perinatal period

     P25.1 Pneumothorax originating in the perinatal period

     P25.2 Pneumomediastinum originating in the perinatal period

     P25.3 Pneumopericardium originating in the perinatal period

     P25.8 Other conditions related to interstitial emphysema originating in the perinatal period

● **P26** Pulmonary hemorrhage originating in the perinatal period

     | Excludes1 | acute idiopathic hemorrhage in infants over 28 days old (R04.81)

     P26.0 Tracheobronchial hemorrhage originating in the perinatal period

     P26.1 Massive pulmonary hemorrhage originating in the perinatal period

     P26.8 Other pulmonary hemorrhages originating in the perinatal period

     P26.9 Unspecified pulmonary hemorrhage originating in the perinatal period

● **P27** Chronic respiratory disease originating in the perinatal period

     | ~~Excludes1~~ | ~~respiratory distress of newborn (P22.0-P22.9)~~

     ▶ | Excludes2 | respiratory distress of newborn (P22.0-P22.9)

     P27.0 Wilson-Mikity syndrome
           Pulmonary dysmaturity

     P27.1 Bronchopulmonary dysplasia originating in the perinatal period

     P27.8 Other chronic respiratory diseases originating in the perinatal period
           Congenital pulmonary fibrosis
           Ventilator lung in newborn

     P27.9 Unspecified chronic respiratory disease originating in the perinatal period

● **P28** Other respiratory conditions originating in the perinatal period

     | Excludes1 | congenital malformations of the respiratory system (Q30-Q34)

     P28.0 Primary atelectasis of newborn
           Failure of lungs to expand properly at birth
           Primary failure to expand terminal respiratory units
           Pulmonary hypoplasia associated with short gestation
           Pulmonary immaturity NOS

     ● **P28.1** Other and unspecified atelectasis of newborn

         P28.10 Unspecified atelectasis of newborn
             Atelectasis of newborn NOS

         P28.11 Resorption atelectasis without respiratory distress syndrome
             | Excludes1 | resorption atelectasis with respiratory distress syndrome (P22.0)

         P28.19 Other atelectasis of newborn
             Partial atelectasis of newborn
             Secondary atelectasis of newborn

     P28.2 Cyanotic attacks of newborn
           | Excludes1 | apnea of newborn (P28.3-P28.4)

     P28.3 Primary sleep apnea of newborn
           Central sleep apnea of newborn
           Obstructive sleep apnea of newborn
           Sleep apnea of newborn NOS

     P28.4 Other apnea of newborn
           Apnea of prematurity
           Obstructive apnea of newborn
           | Excludes1 | obstructive sleep apnea of newborn (P28.3)

     P28.5 Respiratory failure of newborn
           | Excludes1 | respiratory arrest of newborn (P28.81)
                        respiratory distress of newborn (P22.0-)

● **P28.8** Other specified respiratory conditions of newborn

     P28.81 Respiratory arrest of newborn

     P28.89 Other specified respiratory conditions of newborn
           Congenital laryngeal stridor
           Sniffles in newborn
           Snuffles in newborn
           | Excludes1 | early congenital syphilitic rhinitis (A50.05)

     P28.9 Respiratory condition of newborn, unspecified
           Respiratory depression in newborn

● **P29** Cardiovascular disorders originating in the perinatal period

     | Excludes1 | congenital malformations of the circulatory system (Q20-Q28)

     P29.0 Neonatal cardiac failure

     ● **P29.1** Neonatal cardiac dysrhythmia

         P29.11 Neonatal tachycardia

         P29.12 Neonatal bradycardia

     P29.2 Neonatal hypertension

     ● **P29.3** Persistent fetal circulation
           ~~Delayed closure of ductus arteriosus~~
           ~~(Persistent) pulmonary hypertension of newborn~~

         ▶ **P29.30** Pulmonary hypertension of newborn
             ▶ Persistent pulmonary hypertension of newborn

         ▶ **P29.38** Other persistent fetal circulation
             ▶ Delayed closure of ductus arteriosus

     P29.4 Transient myocardial ischemia in newborn

     ● **P29.8** Other cardiovascular disorders originating in the perinatal period

         P29.81 Cardiac arrest of newborn

         P29.89 Other cardiovascular disorders originating in the perinatal period

     P29.9 Cardiovascular disorder originating in the perinatal period, unspecified

INFECTIONS SPECIFIC TO THE PERINATAL PERIOD (P35-P39)

Infections acquired in utero, during birth via the umbilicus, or during the first 28 days after birth

     | Excludes2 | asymptomatic human immunodeficiency virus [HIV] infection status (Z21)
           congenital gonococcal infection (A54.-)
           congenital pneumonia (P23.-)
           congenital syphilis (A50.-)
           human immunodeficiency virus [HIV] disease (B20)
           infant botulism (A48.51)
           infectious diseases not specific to the perinatal period (A00-B99, J09, J10.-)
           intestinal infectious disease (A00-A09)
           laboratory evidence of human immunodeficiency virus [HIV] (R75)
           tetanus neonatorum (A33)

● **P35** Congenital viral diseases

     | Includes | infections acquired in utero or during birth

     P35.0 Congenital rubella syndrome
           Congenital rubella pneumonitis

     P35.1 Congenital cytomegalovirus infection
           Viruses transmitted by multiple routes that cause mild/ subclinical infection

     P35.2 Congenital herpesviral [herpes simplex] infection

     P35.3 Congenital viral hepatitis

     P35.8 Other congenital viral diseases
           Congenital varicella [chickenpox]

     P35.9 Congenital viral disease, unspecified

● **P36**   **Bacterial sepsis of newborn**
     Includes   congenital sepsis
     Use additional code(s), if applicable, to identify severe sepsis (R65.2-) and associated acute organ dysfunction(s)

   P36.0   Sepsis of newborn due to streptococcus, group B

● **P36.1**   Sepsis of newborn due to other and unspecified streptococci

     P36.10   Sepsis of newborn due to unspecified streptococci

     P36.19   Sepsis of newborn due to other streptococci

   P36.2   Sepsis of newborn due to Staphylococcus aureus

● **P36.3**   Sepsis of newborn due to other and unspecified staphylococci

     P36.30   Sepsis of newborn due to unspecified staphylococci

     P36.39   Sepsis of newborn due to other staphylococci

   P36.4   Sepsis of newborn due to Escherichia coli

   P36.5   Sepsis of newborn due to anaerobes

   P36.8   Other bacterial sepsis of newborn
     Use additional code from category B96 to identify organism

   P36.9   Bacterial sepsis of newborn, unspecified

● **P37**   **Other congenital infectious and parasitic diseases**
     Excludes2   congenital syphilis (A50.-)
         infectious neonatal diarrhea (A00-A09)
         necrotizing enterocolitis in newborn (P77.-)
         noninfectious neonatal diarrhea (P78.3)
         ophthalmia neonatorum due to gonococcus (A54.31)
         tetanus neonatorum (A33)

   P37.0   Congenital tuberculosis

   P37.1   Congenital toxoplasmosis
     Parasitic infection, often causing mild flu-like illness
     Hydrocephalus due to congenital toxoplasmosis

   P37.2   Neonatal (disseminated) listeriosis
     Acquired transplacentally or during/after parturition in which symptoms are those of sepsis

   P37.3   Congenital falciparum malaria

   P37.4   Other congenital malaria

   P37.5   Neonatal candidiasis

   P37.8   Other specified congenital infectious and parasitic diseases

   P37.9   Congenital infectious or parasitic disease, unspecified

● **P38**   **Omphalitis of newborn**
     Inflammation of umbilicus
     Excludes1   omphalitis not of newborn (L08.82)
         tetanus omphalitis (A33)
         umbilical hemorrhage of newborn (P51.-)

   P38.1   Omphalitis with mild hemorrhage

   P38.9   Omphalitis without hemorrhage
     Omphalitis of newborn NOS

● **P39**   **Other infections specific to the perinatal period**
     Use additional code to identify organism or specific infection

   P39.0   Neonatal infective mastitis
     Excludes1   breast engorgement of newborn (P83.4)
         noninfective mastitis of newborn (P83.4)

   P39.1   Neonatal conjunctivitis and dacryocystitis
     Neonatal chlamydial conjunctivitis
     Ophthalmia neonatorum NOS
     Neonate = newborn
     Excludes1   gonococcal conjunctivitis (A54.31)

   P39.2   Intra-amniotic infection affecting newborn, not elsewhere classified

   P39.3   Neonatal urinary tract infection

   P39.4   Neonatal skin infection
     Neonatal pyoderma
     Excludes1   pemphigus neonatorum (L00)
         staphylococcal scalded skin syndrome (L00)

   P39.8   Other specified infections specific to the perinatal period

   P39.9   Infection specific to the perinatal period, unspecified

HEMORRHAGIC AND HEMATOLOGICAL DISORDERS OF NEWBORN (P50-P61)

     Excludes1   congenital stenosis and stricture of bile ducts (Q44.3)
         Crigler-Najjar syndrome (E80.5)
         Dubin-Johnson syndrome (E80.6)
         Gilbert syndrome (E80.4)
         hereditary hemolytic anemias (D55-D58)

● **P50**   **Newborn affected by intrauterine (fetal) blood loss**
     Excludes1   congenital anemia from intrauterine (fetal) blood loss (P61.3)

   P50.0   Newborn affected by intrauterine (fetal) blood loss from vasa previa

   P50.1   Newborn affected by intrauterine (fetal) blood loss from ruptured cord

   P50.2   Newborn affected by intrauterine (fetal) blood loss from placenta

   P50.3   Newborn affected by hemorrhage into co-twin

   P50.4   Newborn affected by hemorrhage into maternal circulation

   P50.5   Newborn affected by intrauterine (fetal) blood loss from cut end of co-twin's cord

   P50.8   Newborn affected by other intrauterine (fetal) blood loss

   P50.9   Newborn affected by intrauterine (fetal) blood loss, unspecified
     Newborn affected by fetal hemorrhage NOS

● **P51**   **Umbilical hemorrhage of newborn**
     Excludes1   omphalitis with mild hemorrhage (P38.1)
         umbilical hemorrhage from cut end of co-twins cord (P50.5)

   P51.0   Massive umbilical hemorrhage of newborn

   P51.8   Other umbilical hemorrhages of newborn
     Slipped umbilical ligature NOS

   P51.9   Umbilical hemorrhage of newborn, unspecified

● **P52**   **Intracranial nontraumatic hemorrhage of newborn**
     Includes   intracranial hemorrhage due to anoxia or hypoxia
     Excludes1   intracranial hemorrhage due to birth injury (P10.-)
         intracranial hemorrhage due to other injury (S06.-)

   P52.0   Intraventricular (nontraumatic) hemorrhage, grade 1, of newborn
     Subependymal hemorrhage (without intraventricular extension)
     Bleeding into germinal matrix

   P52.1   Intraventricular (nontraumatic) hemorrhage, grade 2, of newborn
     Subependymal hemorrhage with intraventricular extension
     Bleeding into ventricle

● **P52.2**   Intraventricular (nontraumatic) hemorrhage, grade 3 and grade 4, of newborn

     P52.21   Intraventricular (nontraumatic) hemorrhage, grade 3, of newborn
         Subependymal hemorrhage with intraventricular extension with enlargement of ventricle

     P52.22   Intraventricular (nontraumatic) hemorrhage, grade 4, of newborn
         Bleeding into cerebral cortex
         Subependymal hemorrhage with intracerebral extension

CHAPTER 16 (P00-P96)

▶ New   ⟹ Revised   ~~deleted~~ Deleted   **OGCR** Official Guidelines   X Assign placeholder X   ● Use Additional Character(s)

| Excludes 1 | Excludes 2 | Includes | Use additional | Code first | Code also | Key words |

P52.3 **Unspecified** intraventricular (nontraumatic) hemorrhage of newborn

P52.4 **Intracerebral** (nontraumatic) hemorrhage of newborn

P52.5 **Subarachnoid** (nontraumatic) hemorrhage of newborn

P52.6 **Cerebellar** (nontraumatic) and posterior fossa hemorrhage of newborn

P52.8 **Other** intracranial (nontraumatic) hemorrhages of newborn

P52.9 Intracranial (nontraumatic) hemorrhage of newborn, **unspecified**

P53 **Hemorrhagic disease** of newborn
Vitamin K deficiency of newborn

● P54 **Other neonatal hemorrhages**
Excludes1 newborn affected by (intrauterine) blood loss (P50.-)
pulmonary hemorrhage originating in the perinatal period (P26.-)

P54.0 Neonatal **hematemesis**
Vomiting of blood
Excludes1 neonatal hematemesis due to swallowed maternal blood (P78.2)

P54.1 Neonatal **melena**
Dark-colored feces stained with blood pigments
Excludes1 neonatal melena due to swallowed maternal blood (P78.2)

P54.2 Neonatal **rectal** hemorrhage

P54.3 Other neonatal **gastrointestinal** hemorrhage

P54.4 Neonatal **adrenal** hemorrhage

P54.5 Neonatal **cutaneous** hemorrhage
Neonatal bruising
Neonatal ecchymoses
Neonatal petechiae
Neonatal superficial hematomata
Excludes2 bruising of scalp due to birth injury (P12.3)
cephalhematoma due to birth injury (P12.0)

P54.6 Neonatal **vaginal** hemorrhage
Neonatal pseudomenses

P54.8 **Other** specified neonatal hemorrhages

P54.9 Neonatal hemorrhage, **unspecified**

● P55 **Hemolytic disease of newborn**
AKA erythroblastosis fetalis and is due to Rh isoimmunization, result of Rh blood factor incompatibilities between mother (Rh negative) and fetus (Rh positive)

P55.0 **Rh** isoimmunization of newborn

P55.1 **ABO** isoimmunization of newborn

P55.8 **Other** hemolytic diseases of newborn

P55.9 Hemolytic disease of newborn, **unspecified**

● P56 **Hydrops fetalis due to hemolytic disease**
Caused by maternal sensitization to fetal blood group antigen
Excludes1 hydrops fetalis NOS (P83.2)

P56.0 Hydrops fetalis due to **isoimmunization**

● P56.9 Hydrops fetalis due to other and unspecified hemolytic disease

P56.90 Hydrops fetalis due to **unspecified** hemolytic disease

P56.99 Hydrops fetalis due to **other** hemolytic disease

● P57 **Kernicterus**
High levels of bilirubin in blood, with severe neural symptoms

P57.0 Kernicterus due to **isoimmunization**

P57.8 **Other** specified kernicterus
Excludes1 Crigler-Najjar syndrome (E80.5)

P57.9 Kernicterus, **unspecified**

● P58 **Neonatal jaundice due to other excessive hemolysis**
Excludes1 jaundice due to isoimmunization (P55-P57)

P58.0 Neonatal jaundice due to **bruising**

P58.1 Neonatal jaundice due to **bleeding**

P58.2 Neonatal jaundice due to **infection**

P58.3 Neonatal jaundice due to **polycythemia**

● P58.4 Neonatal jaundice due to **drugs or toxins** transmitted from mother or given to newborn
Code first poisoning due to drug or toxin, if applicable (T36-T65 with fifth or sixth character 1-4 or 6)
Use additional code for adverse effect, if applicable, to identify drug (T36-T50 with fifth or sixth character 5)

P58.41 Neonatal jaundice due to drugs or toxins **transmitted from mother**

P58.42 Neonatal jaundice due to drugs or toxins **given to newborn**

P58.5 Neonatal jaundice due to **swallowed maternal blood**

P58.8 Neonatal jaundice due to **other** specified excessive hemolysis

P58.9 Neonatal jaundice due to excessive hemolysis, **unspecified**

● P59 **Neonatal jaundice from other and unspecified causes**
Excludes1 jaundice due to inborn errors of metabolism (E70-E88)
kernicterus (P57.-)

P59.0 Neonatal jaundice associated with **preterm delivery**
Hyperbilirubinemia of prematurity
Jaundice due to delayed conjugation associated with preterm delivery

P59.1 **Inspissated bile syndrome**

● P59.2 Neonatal jaundice from other and unspecified **hepatocellular damage**
Excludes1 congenital viral hepatitis (P35.3)

P59.20 Neonatal jaundice from **unspecified** hepatocellular damage

P59.29 Neonatal jaundice from **other** hepatocellular damage
Neonatal giant cell hepatitis
Neonatal (idiopathic) hepatitis

P59.3 Neonatal jaundice from **breast milk inhibitor**

P59.8 Neonatal jaundice from **other** specified causes

P59.9 Neonatal jaundice, **unspecified**
Neonatal physiological jaundice (intense)(prolonged) NOS

P60 **Disseminated intravascular coagulation of newborn**
Defibrination syndrome of newborn

● P61 **Other perinatal hematological disorders**
Excludes1 transient hypogammaglobulinemia of infancy (D80.7)

P61.0 **Transient neonatal thrombocytopenia**
Lack of sufficient numbers of circulating thrombocytes (platelets)
Neonatal thrombocytopenia due to exchange transfusion
Neonatal thrombocytopenia due to idiopathic maternal thrombocytopenia
Neonatal thrombocytopenia due to isoimmunization

P61.1 **Polycythemia neonatorum**
Neonate = newborn

P61.2 **Anemia of prematurity**

P61.3 **Congenital anemia from fetal blood loss**

P61.4 **Other congenital anemias, not elsewhere classified**
Congenital anemia NOS

▶ New   ⇒ Revised   ~~deleted~~ Deleted   **OGCR** Official Guidelines   X Assign placeholder X   ● Use Additional Character(s)
Excludes 1   Excludes 2   Includes   Use additional   Code first   Code also   Key words

P61.5   **Transient neonatal neutropenia**
Low levels of granulocytic neutrophilic white blood cells
> **Excludes1**   congenital neutropenia (nontransient) (D70.0)

P61.6   **Other transient neonatal disorders of coagulation**

P61.8   **Other specified perinatal hematological disorders**

P61.9   **Perinatal hematological disorder, unspecified**

TRANSITORY ENDOCRINE AND METABOLIC DISORDERS SPECIFIC TO NEWBORN (P70-P74)

> **Includes**   transitory endocrine and metabolic disturbances caused by the infant's response to maternal endocrine and metabolic factors, or its adjustment to extrauterine environment

● P70   **Transitory disorders of carbohydrate metabolism specific to newborn**

P70.0   **Syndrome of infant of mother with gestational diabetes**
Newborn (with hypoglycemia) affected by maternal gestational diabetes
> **Excludes1**   newborn (with hypoglycemia) affected by maternal (pre-existing) diabetes mellitus (P70.1)
> syndrome of infant of a diabetic mother (P70.1)

P70.1   **Syndrome of infant of a diabetic mother**
Newborn (with hypoglycemia) affected by maternal (pre-existing) diabetes mellitus
> **Excludes1**   newborn (with hypoglycemia) affected by maternal gestational diabetes (P70.0)
> syndrome of infant of mother with gestational diabetes (P70.0)

P70.2   **Neonatal diabetes mellitus**

P70.3   **Iatrogenic neonatal hypoglycemia**

P70.4   **Other neonatal hypoglycemia**
Transitory neonatal hypoglycemia

P70.8   **Other transitory disorders of carbohydrate metabolism of newborn**

P70.9   **Transitory disorder of carbohydrate metabolism of newborn, unspecified**

● P71   **Transitory neonatal disorders of calcium and magnesium metabolism**

P71.0   **Cow's milk hypocalcemia in newborn**

P71.1   **Other neonatal hypocalcemia**
> **Excludes1**   neonatal hypoparathyroidism (P71.4)

P71.2   **Neonatal hypomagnesemia**

P71.3   **Neonatal tetany without calcium or magnesium deficiency**
Neonatal tetany NOS

P71.4   **Transitory neonatal hypoparathyroidism**

P71.8   **Other transitory neonatal disorders of calcium and magnesium metabolism**

P71.9   **Transitory neonatal disorder of calcium and magnesium metabolism, unspecified**

● P72   **Other transitory neonatal endocrine disorders**
> **Excludes1**   congenital hypothyroidism with or without goiter (E03.0-E03.1)
> dyshormogenetic goiter (E07.1)
> Pendred's syndrome (E07.1)

P72.0   **Neonatal goiter, not elsewhere classified**
Transitory congenital goiter with normal functioning

P72.1   **Transitory neonatal hyperthyroidism**
Neonatal thyrotoxicosis

P72.2   **Other transitory neonatal disorders of thyroid function, not elsewhere classified**
Transitory neonatal hypothyroidism

P72.8   **Other specified transitory neonatal endocrine disorders**

P72.9   **Transitory neonatal endocrine disorder, unspecified**

● P74   **Other transitory neonatal electrolyte and metabolic disturbances**

P74.0   **Late metabolic acidosis of newborn**
> **Excludes1**   (fetal) metabolic acidosis of newborn (P19)

P74.1   **Dehydration of newborn**

P74.2   **Disturbances of sodium balance of newborn**

P74.3   **Disturbances of potassium balance of newborn**

P74.4   **Other transitory electrolyte disturbances of newborn**

P74.5   **Transitory tyrosinemia of newborn**

P74.6   **Transitory hyperammonemia of newborn**

P74.8   **Other transitory metabolic disturbances of newborn**
Amino-acid metabolic disorders described as transitory

P74.9   **Transitory metabolic disturbance of newborn, unspecified**

DIGESTIVE SYSTEM DISORDERS OF NEWBORN (P76-P78)

● P76   **Other intestinal obstruction of newborn**

P76.0   **Meconium plug syndrome**
Fetal stool obstruction in large intestine, present at birth; may be symptom of organic disease.
Meconium ileus NOS
> **Excludes1**   meconium ileus in cystic fibrosis (E84.11)

P76.1   **Transitory ileus of newborn**
Temporary obstruction of ileus (small intestine)
> **Excludes1**   Hirschsprung's disease (Q43.1)

P76.2   **Intestinal obstruction due to inspissated milk**
Being thickened, dried, or made less fluid

P76.8   **Other specified intestinal obstruction of newborn**
> **Excludes1**   intestinal obstruction classifiable to K56.-

P76.9   **Intestinal obstruction of newborn, unspecified**

● P77   **Necrotizing enterocolitis of newborn**

P77.1   **Stage 1 necrotizing enterocolitis in newborn**
Necrotizing enterocolitis without pneumatosis, without perforation

P77.2   **Stage 2 necrotizing enterocolitis in newborn**
Necrotizing enterocolitis with pneumatosis, without perforation

P77.3   **Stage 3 necrotizing enterocolitis in newborn**
Necrotizing enterocolitis with perforation
Necrotizing enterocolitis with pneumatosis and perforation

P77.9   **Necrotizing enterocolitis in newborn, unspecified**
Necrotizing enterocolitis in newborn, NOS

● P78   **Other perinatal digestive system disorders**
> **Excludes1**   cystic fibrosis (E84.0-E84.9)
> neonatal gastrointestinal hemorrhages (P54.0-P54.3)

P78.0   **Perinatal intestinal perforation**
Meconium peritonitis

P78.1   **Other neonatal peritonitis**
Neonatal peritonitis NOS

P78.2   **Neonatal hematemesis and melena due to swallowed maternal blood**

P78.3   **Noninfective neonatal diarrhea**
Neonatal diarrhea NOS

● P78.8   **Other specified perinatal digestive system disorders**

P78.81   **Congenital cirrhosis (of liver)**

P78.82   **Peptic ulcer of newborn**

P78.83   **Newborn esophageal reflux**
Neonatal esophageal reflux

▶ P78.84   **Gestational alloimmune liver disease**
▶ GALD
▶ Neonatal hemochromatosis
> ▶ **Excludes1**   hemochromatosis (E83.11-)

P78.89   **Other specified perinatal digestive system disorders**

P78.9   **Perinatal digestive system disorder, unspecified**

▶ New   ⟱ Revised   ~~deleted~~ Deleted   **OGCR** Official Guidelines   X Assign placeholder X   ● Use Additional Character(s)

| Excludes 1 | Excludes 2 | Includes | Use additional | Code first | Code also | Key words |

CONDITIONS INVOLVING THE INTEGUMENT AND TEMPERATURE REGULATION OF NEWBORN (P80-P83)

● **P80   Hypothermia of newborn**

P80.0   Cold injury syndrome
Severe and usually chronic hypothermia associated with a pink flushed appearance, edema and neurological and biochemical abnormalities.
Excludes1 mild hypothermia of newborn (P80.8)

P80.8   Other hypothermia of newborn
Mild hypothermia of newborn

P80.9   Hypothermia of newborn, unspecified

● **P81   Other disturbances of temperature regulation of newborn**

P81.0   Environmental hyperthermia of newborn

P81.8   Other specified disturbances of temperature regulation of newborn

P81.9   Disturbance of temperature regulation of newborn, unspecified
Fever of newborn NOS

● **P83   Other conditions of integument specific to newborn**
Excludes1 congenital malformations of skin and integument (Q80-Q84)
hydrops fetalis due to hemolytic disease (P56.-)
neonatal skin infection (P39.4)
staphylococcal scalded skin syndrome (L00)
Excludes2 cradle cap (L21.0)
diaper [napkin] dermatitis (L22)

P83.0   Sclerema neonatorum
Neonate = newborn

P83.1   Neonatal erythema toxicum
Benign, generalized, transient pustules that become firm vesicles

P83.2   Hydrops fetalis not due to hemolytic disease
Severe, life-threatening problem of severe edema (swelling) as result of too much fluid leaving blood and entering tissue
Hydrops fetalis NOS

● **P83.3   Other and unspecified edema specific to newborn**

P83.30   Unspecified edema specific to newborn

P83.39   Other edema specific to newborn

P83.4   Breast engorgement of newborn
Noninfective mastitis of newborn

P83.5   Congenital hydrocele

P83.6   Umbilical polyp of newborn

● **P83.8   Other specified conditions of integument specific to newborn**
~~Bronze baby syndrome~~
~~Neonatal scleroderma~~
~~Urticaria neonatorum~~

▶ **P83.81   Umbilical granuloma**
▶ **Excludes2** Granulomatous disorder of the skin and subcutaneous tissue, unspecified (L92.9)

▶ **P83.88   Other specified conditions of integument specific to newborn**
▶Bronze baby syndrome
▶Neonatal scleroderma
▶Urticaria neonatorum

P83.9   Condition of the integument specific to newborn, unspecified

OTHER PROBLEMS WITH NEWBORN (P84)

P84   Other problems with newborn
Acidemia of newborn
Acidosis of newborn
Anoxia of newborn NOS
Asphyxia of newborn NOS
Hypercapnia of newborn
Hypoxemia of newborn
Hypoxia of newborn NOS
Mixed metabolic and respiratory acidosis of newborn
Excludes1 intracranial hemorrhage due to anoxia or hypoxia (P52.-)
hypoxic ischemic encephalopathy [HIE] (P91.6-)
late metabolic acidosis of newborn (P74.0)

OTHER DISORDERS ORIGINATING IN THE PERINATAL PERIOD (P90-P96)

P90   Convulsions of newborn
Excludes1 benign myoclonic epilepsy in infancy (G40.3-)
benign neonatal convulsions (familial) (G40.3-)

● **P91   Other disturbances of cerebral status of newborn**

P91.0   Neonatal cerebral ischemia

P91.1   Acquired periventricular cysts of newborn

P91.2   Neonatal cerebral leukomalacia
Degeneration of white matter adjacent to cerebral ventricles following cerebral hypoxia or brain ischemia in neonates
Periventricular leukomalacia

P91.3   Neonatal cerebral irritability

P91.4   Neonatal cerebral depression

P91.5   Neonatal coma

● **P91.6   Hypoxic ischemic encephalopathy [HIE]**
▶ **Excludes1** Neonatal cerebral depression (P91.4)
▶Neonatal cerebral irritability (P91.3)
▶Neonatal coma (P91.5)

P91.60   Hypoxic ischemic encephalopathy [HIE], unspecified

P91.61   Mild hypoxic ischemic encephalopathy [HIE]

P91.62   Moderate hypoxic ischemic encephalopathy [HIE]

P91.63   Severe hypoxic ischemic encephalopathy [HIE]

● **P91.8   Other specified disturbances of cerebral status of newborn**

▶● **P91.81   Neonatal encephalopathy**

▶ **P91.811   Neonatal encephalopathy in diseases classified elsewhere**
▶*Code first underlying condition, if known, such as:*
▶congenital cirrhosis (of liver) (P78.71)
▶intracranial nontraumatic hemorrhage of newborn (P52.-)
▶kernicterus (P57.-)

▶ **P91.819   Neonatal encephalopathy, unspecified**

▶ **P91.88   Other specified disturbances of cerebral status of newborn**

P91.9   Disturbance of cerebral status of newborn, unspecified

▶ New   ⇒ Revised   ~~deleted~~ Deleted   **OGCR** Official Guidelines   X Assign placeholder X   ● Use Additional Character(s)

Excludes 1   Excludes 2   Includes   Use additional   Code first   Code also   Key words

● **P92** **Feeding problems of newborn**
     Excludes1 ▶ eating disorders (F50.-)
                 feeding problems in child over 28 days old
                      (R63.3)

    ● **P92.0** **Vomiting of newborn**
         Excludes1   vomiting of child over 28 days old (R11.-)

       P92.01 **Bilious vomiting of newborn**
            Excludes1   bilious vomiting in child over
                           28 days old (R11.14)

       P92.09 **Other vomiting of newborn**
            Excludes1   regurgitation of food in newborn
                           (P92.1)

    P92.1 **Regurgitation** and **rumination** of newborn
    P92.2 **Slow feeding** of newborn
    P92.3 **Underfeeding** of newborn
    P92.4 **Overfeeding** of newborn
    P92.5 **Neonatal difficulty in feeding at breast**
    P92.6 **Failure to thrive** in newborn
         Excludes1   failure to thrive in child over 28 days
                       (R62.51)

    P92.8 **Other** feeding problems of newborn
    P92.9 **Feeding problem of newborn, unspecified**

● **P93** **Reactions and intoxications due to drugs administered to newborn**
     Includes   reactions and intoxications due to drugs
                 administered to fetus affecting newborn

     Excludes1   jaundice due to drugs or toxins transmitted from
                 mother or given to newborn (P58.4-)
                 reactions and intoxications from maternal
                      opiates, tranquilizers and other medication
                      (P04.0-P04.1, P04.4)
                 withdrawal symptoms from maternal use of
                      drugs of addiction (P96.1)
                 withdrawal symptoms from therapeutic use of
                      drugs in newborn (P96.2)

    P93.0 **Grey baby syndrome**
         Grey syndrome from chloramphenicol administration
            in newborn

    P93.8 **Other reactions and intoxications due to drugs administered to newborn**
         Use additional code for adverse effect, if applicable,
            to identify drug (T36-T50 with fifth or sixth
            character 5)

● **P94** **Disorders of muscle tone of newborn**
    P94.0 **Transient neonatal myasthenia gravis**
         Excludes1   myasthenia gravis (G70.0)

    P94.1 **Congenital hypertonia**
    P94.2 **Congenital hypotonia**
         Floppy baby syndrome, unspecified
    P94.8 **Other** disorders of muscle tone of newborn
    P94.9 **Disorder of muscle tone of newborn, unspecified**

OGCR   Section I.C.16.g.

Stillbirth
Code P95, Stillbirth, is only for use for institutions that maintain
separate records for stillbirths. No other code should be used with P95.
Code P95 should not be used on the mother's record.

P95 **Stillbirth**
     Deadborn fetus NOS
     Fetal death of unspecified cause
     Stillbirth NOS
     Excludes1   maternal care for intrauterine death (O36.4)
                 missed abortion (O02.1)
                 outcome of delivery, stillbirth (Z37.1, Z37.3,
                      Z37.4, Z37.7)

● **P96** **Other conditions originating in the perinatal period**
    P96.0 **Congenital renal failure**
         Uremia of newborn

    P96.1 **Neonatal withdrawal symptoms from maternal use of drugs of addiction**
         Drug withdrawal syndrome in infant of dependent
            mother
         Neonatal abstinence syndrome
         Excludes1   reactions and intoxications from
                      maternal opiates and tranquilizers
                      administered during labor and
                      delivery (P04.0)

    P96.2 **Withdrawal symptoms from therapeutic use of drugs in newborn**

    P96.3 **Wide cranial sutures of newborn**
         Neonatal craniotabes

    P96.5 **Complication to newborn due to (fetal) intrauterine procedure**
         Excludes2   newborn affected by amniocentesis
                      (P00.6)

   ● **P96.8** **Other specified conditions originating in the perinatal period**
       P96.81 **Exposure to (parental) (environmental) tobacco smoke in the perinatal period**
            Excludes2   newborn affected by in utero
                      exposure to tobacco (P04.2)
                      exposure to environmental
                      tobacco smoke after the
                      perinatal period (Z77.22)

       P96.82 **Delayed separation of umbilical cord**

       P96.83 **Meconium staining**
            Excludes1   meconium aspiration (P24.00,
                      P24.01)
                   meconium passage during
                      delivery (P03.82)

       P96.89 **Other specified conditions originating in the perinatal period**
            Use additional code to specify condition

    P96.9 **Condition originating in the perinatal period, unspecified**
         Congenital debility NOS

CHAPTER 16 (P00-P96)

CHAPTER 17

CONGENITAL MALFORMATIONS, DEFORMATIONS AND CHROMOSOMAL ABNORMALITIES (Q00-Q99)

OGCR Chapter-Specific Coding Guidelines

17. **Chapter 17: Congenital malformations, deformations, and chromosomal abnormalities (Q00-Q99)**
Assign an appropriate code(s) from categories Q00-Q99, Congenital malformations, deformations, and chromosomal abnormalities when a malformation/deformation or chromosomal abnormality is documented. A malformation/deformation/ or chromosomal abnormality may be the principal/first-listed diagnosis on a record or a secondary diagnosis.

When a malformation/deformation/or chromosomal abnormality does not have a unique code assignment, assign additional code(s) for any manifestations that may be present.

When the code assignment specifically identifies the malformation/deformation/or chromosomal abnormality, manifestations that are an inherent component of the anomaly should not be coded separately. Additional codes should be assigned for manifestations that are not an inherent component.

Codes from Chapter 17 may be used throughout the life of the patient. If a congenital malformation or deformity has been corrected, a personal history code should be used to identify the history of the malformation or deformity. Although present at birth, malformation/deformation/or chromosomal abnormality may not be identified until later in life. Whenever the condition is diagnosed by the physician, it is appropriate to assign a code from codes Q00-Q99.

For the birth admission, the appropriate code from category Z38, Liveborn infants, according to place of birth and type of delivery, should be sequenced as the principal diagnosis, followed by any congenital anomaly codes, Q00-Q99.

CHAPTER 17

CONGENITAL MALFORMATIONS, DEFORMATIONS AND CHROMOSOMAL ABNORMALITIES (Q00-Q99)

Note: Codes from this chapter are not for use on maternal or fetal records

> **Excludes2** inborn errors of metabolism (E70-E88)

This chapter contains the following blocks:

Q00-Q07	Congenital malformations of the nervous system
Q10-Q18	Congenital malformations of eye, ear, face and neck
Q20-Q28	Congenital malformations of the circulatory system
Q30-Q34	Congenital malformations of the respiratory system
Q35-Q37	Cleft lip and cleft palate
Q38-Q45	Other congenital malformations of the digestive system
Q50-Q56	Congenital malformations of genital organs
Q60-Q64	Congenital malformations of the urinary system
Q65-Q79	Congenital malformations and deformations of the musculoskeletal system
Q80-Q89	Other congenital malformations
Q90-Q99	Chromosomal abnormalities, not elsewhere classified

Figure 17-1 An infant with a large occipital encephalocele. The large skin-covered encephalocele is visible. (From Swaiman KF, Ashwal S, Ferriero DM: Pediatric Neurology: Principles and Practice, Philadelphia, Saunders, 2012)

CONGENITAL MALFORMATIONS OF THE NERVOUS SYSTEM (Q00–Q07)

● **Q00   Anencephaly and similar malformations**
Q00.0   Anencephaly
Absence of skull with cerebral hemispheres missing or reduced to small masses attached to base of cranium
Acephaly
Acrania
Amyelencephaly
Hemianencephaly
Hemicephaly

Q00.1   Craniorachischisis
Developmental anomaly consisting of fissure of cranium and vertebral column

Q00.2   Iniencephaly
Developmental anomaly characterized by enlargement of foramen magnum and absence of laminae and spinous processes of cervical, dorsal

● **Q01   Encephalocele**
Sac-like protrusions of brain and membranes visible through an opening in skull
> **Includes**   Arnold-Chiari syndrome, type III
encephalocystocele
encephalomyelocele
hydroencephalocele
hydromeningocele, cranial
meningocele, cerebral
meningoencephalocele
> **Excludes1**   Meckel-Gruber syndrome (Q61.9)

Q01.0   Frontal encephalocele
Q01.1   Nasofrontal encephalocele
Q01.2   Occipital encephalocele
Q01.8   Encephalocele of other sites
Q01.9   Encephalocele, unspecified

Q02   Microcephaly
Head size measures significantly below normal based on standardized charts
> **Includes**   hydromicrocephaly
micrencephalon
> **Excludes1**   Meckel-Gruber syndrome (Q61.9)

● **Q03   Congenital hydrocephalus**
Accumulation of cerebrospinal fluid in ventricles resulting in swelling and enlargement
> **Includes**   hydrocephalus in newborn
> **Excludes1**   Arnold-Chiari syndrome, type II (Q07.0-)
acquired hydrocephalus (G91.-)
hydrocephalus due to congenital toxoplasmosis (P37.1)
hydrocephalus with spina bifida (Q05.0-Q05.4)

Q03.0   Malformations of aqueduct of Sylvius
Anomaly of aqueduct of Sylvius
Obstruction of aqueduct of Sylvius, congenital
Stenosis of aqueduct of Sylvius

Q03.1   Atresia of foramina of Magendie and Luschka
Dandy-Walker syndrome

Q03.8   Other congenital hydrocephalus

Q03.9   Congenital hydrocephalus, unspecified

▶ New   ⇒ Revised   ~~deleted~~ Deleted   **OGCR** Official Guidelines   X Assign placeholder X   ● Use Additional Character(s)

Excludes 1   Excludes 2   Includes   Use additional   Code first   Code also   Key words

● **Q04   Other congenital malformations of brain**

> **Excludes1**   cyclopia (Q87.0)
> macrocephaly (Q75.3)

Q04.0   Congenital malformations of corpus callosum
Agenesis of corpus callosum

Q04.1   Arhinencephaly
Congenital absence of olfactory bulbs, tract, or nerves

Q04.2   Holoprosencephaly
Failure of cleavage of forebrain (prosencephalon) resulting in incomplete or absent cortical separation and deficits in midline facial development

Q04.3   Other reduction deformities of brain
Absence of part of brain
Agenesis of part of brain
> *Cerebral cortex are not fully formed, brain surface is smooth*

Agyria
Aplasia of part of brain
Hydranencephaly
Hypoplasia of part of brain
Lissencephaly
> *Congenital malformation or absence of convolutions of cerebral cortex*

Microgyria
> *Malformation of brain characterized by excessive number of small convolutions (gyri) on surface*

Pachygyria
> *Reduction in number of sulci of cerebrum*

> **Excludes1**   congenital malformations of corpus callosum (Q04.0)

Q04.4   Septo-optic dysplasia of brain

Q04.5   Megalencephaly
Abnormally large brain

Q04.6   Congenital cerebral cysts
Porencephaly   Schizencephaly
> **Excludes1**   acquired porencephalic cyst (G93.0)

Q04.8   Other specified congenital malformations of brain
Arnold-Chiari syndrome, type IV
Macrogyria

Q04.9   Congenital malformation of brain, unspecified
Congenital anomaly NOS of brain
Congenital deformity NOS of brain
Congenital disease or lesion NOS of brain
Multiple anomalies NOS of brain, congenital

● **Q05   Spina bifida**
Developmental anomaly characterized by defective closure of vertebral arch, through which spinal cord and meninges may protrude

> **Includes**   hydromeningocele (spinal)
> meningocele (spinal)
> meningomyelocele
> myelocele
> myelomeningocele
> rachischisis
> spina bifida (aperta)(cystica)
> syringomyelocele

Use additional code for any associated paraplegia (paraparesis) (G82.2-)

> **Excludes1**   Arnold-Chiari syndrome, type II (Q07.0-)
> spina bifida occulta (Q76.0)

Q05.0   Cervical spina bifida with hydrocephalus

Q05.1   Thoracic spina bifida with hydrocephalus
Dorsal spina bifida with hydrocephalus
Thoracolumbar spina bifida with hydrocephalus

Q05.2   Lumbar spina bifida with hydrocephalus
Lumbosacral spina bifida with hydrocephalus

Q05.3   Sacral spina bifida with hydrocephalus

Q05.4   Unspecified spina bifida with hydrocephalus

Q05.5   Cervical spina bifida without hydrocephalus

Q05.6   Thoracic spina bifida without hydrocephalus
Dorsal spina bifida NOS
Thoracolumbar spina bifida NOS

Q05.7   Lumbar spina bifida without hydrocephalus
Lumbosacral spina bifida NOS

Q05.8   Sacral spina bifida without hydrocephalus

Q05.9   Spina bifida, unspecified

● **Q06   Other congenital malformations of spinal cord**

Q06.0   Amyelia
Congenital absence of spinal cord

Q06.1   Hypoplasia and dysplasia of spinal cord
Underdevelopment of spinal cord
Atelomyelia
> *Congenitally incomplete development of spinal cord*
Myelatelia
Myelodysplasia of spinal cord
> *Defective development of spinal cord, especially lower segments*

Q06.2   Diastematomyelia
Congenital anomaly, associated with spina bifida, in which spinal cord is split into halves and surrounded by dural sac

Q06.3   Other congenital cauda equina malformations

Q06.4   Hydromyelia
Dilation of central canal of spinal cord with increased fluid accumulation
Hydrorachis

Q06.8   Other specified congenital malformations of spinal cord

Q06.9   Congenital malformation of spinal cord, unspecified
Congenital anomaly NOS of spinal cord
Congenital deformity NOS of spinal cord
Congenital disease or lesion NOS of spinal cord

● **Q07   Other congenital malformations of nervous system**

> **Excludes2**   congenital central alveolar hypoventilation syndrome (G47.35)
> familial dysautonomia [Riley-Day] (G90.1)
> neurofibromatosis (nonmalignant) (Q85.0-)

● **Q07.0   Arnold-Chiari syndrome**
Herniation of cerebellar tonsils and vermis through foramen magnum into spinal canal
Arnold-Chiari syndrome, type II

> **Excludes1**   Arnold-Chiari syndrome, type III (Q01.-)
> Arnold-Chiari syndrome, type IV (Q04.8)

Q07.00   Arnold-Chiari syndrome without spina bifida or hydrocephalus

Q07.01   Arnold-Chiari syndrome with spina bifida

Q07.02   Arnold-Chiari syndrome with hydrocephalus

Q07.03   Arnold-Chiari syndrome with spina bifida and hydrocephalus

Q07.8   Other specified congenital malformations of nervous system
Agenesis of nerve
Displacement of brachial plexus
Jaw-winking syndrome
Marcus Gunn's syndrome

Q07.9   Congenital malformation of nervous system, unspecified
Congenital anomaly NOS of nervous system
Congenital deformity NOS of nervous system
Congenital disease or lesion NOS of nervous system

▶ New   ⮕ Revised   ~~deleted~~ Deleted   **OGCR** Official Guidelines   **X** Assign placeholder X   ● Use Additional Character(s)

Excludes 1   Excludes 2   Includes   Use additional   Code first   Code also   Key words

1121

CHAPTER 17 (Q00-Q99)

CONGENITAL MALFORMATIONS OF EYE, EAR, FACE AND NECK (Q10-Q18)

| Excludes2 | cleft lip and cleft palate (Q35-Q37) |

cleft lip and cleft palate (Q35-Q37)
congenital malformation of cervical spine (Q05.0, Q05.5, Q67.5, Q76.0-Q76.4)
congenital malformation of larynx (Q31.-)
congenital malformation of lip NEC (Q38.0)
congenital malformation of nose (Q30.-)
congenital malformation of parathyroid gland (Q89.2)
congenital malformation of thyroid gland (Q89.2)

● **Q10   Congenital malformations of eyelid, lacrimal apparatus and orbit**

Excludes1   cryptophthalmos NOS (Q11.2)
cryptophthalmos syndrome (Q87.0)

Q10.0   Congenital ptosis
Prolapse or drooping of upper eyelid from paralysis of third nerve or from sympathetic innervations

Q10.1   Congenital ectropion
Outward turning of eyelid

Q10.2   Congenital entropion
Inward turning of eyelid

Q10.3   Other congenital malformations of eyelid
Ablepharon
Blepharophimosis, congenital
Coloboma of eyelid
Congenital absence or agenesis of cilia
Congenital absence or agenesis of eyelid
Congenital accessory eyelid
Congenital accessory eye muscle
Congenital malformation of eyelid NOS

Q10.4   Absence and agenesis of lacrimal apparatus
Congenital absence of punctum lacrimale

Q10.5   Congenital stenosis and stricture of lacrimal duct

Q10.6   Other congenital malformations of lacrimal apparatus
Congenital malformation of lacrimal apparatus NOS

Q10.7   Congenital malformation of orbit

● **Q11   Anophthalmos, microphthalmos and macrophthalmos**
Absence of eye and optic pit

Q11.0   Cystic eyeball

Q11.1   Other anophthalmos
Anophthalmos NOS
Agenesis of eye
Absence of eye
Aplasia of eye

Q11.2   Microphthalmos
Partial absence of eye and optic pit
Cryptophthalmos NOS
Dysplasia of eye
Hypoplasia of eye
Rudimentary eye

Excludes1   cryptophthalmos syndrome (Q87.0)

Q11.3   Macrophthalmos
Congenital enlargement of eyes

Excludes1   macrophthalmos in congenital glaucoma (Q15.0)

● **Q12   Congenital lens malformations**

Q12.0   Congenital cataract

Q12.1   Congenital displaced lens

Q12.2   Coloboma of lens

Q12.3   Congenital aphakia

Q12.4   Spherophakia
Smaller, more spherical optic lens than normal

Q12.8   Other congenital lens malformations
Microphakia

Q12.9   Congenital lens malformation, unspecified

● **Q13   Congenital malformations of anterior segment of eye**

Q13.0   Coloboma of iris
Coloboma NOS

Q13.1   Absence of iris
Aniridia
Use additional code for associated glaucoma (H42)

Q13.2   Other congenital malformations of iris
Anisocoria, congenital
Atresia of pupil
Congenital malformation of iris NOS
Corectopia

Q13.3   Congenital corneal opacity

Q13.4   Other congenital corneal malformations
Congenital malformation of cornea NOS
Microcornea
Peter's anomaly

Q13.5   Blue sclera
Condition of unusual blueness of sclera; not harmful

● **Q13.8   Other congenital malformations of anterior segment of eye**

Q13.81   Rieger's anomaly
Use additional code for associated glaucoma (H42)

Q13.89   Other congenital malformations of anterior segment of eye

Q13.9   Congenital malformation of anterior segment of eye, unspecified

● **Q14   Congenital malformations of posterior segment of eye**

Excludes2   optic nerve hypoplasia (H47.03-)

Q14.0   Congenital malformation of vitreous humor
Congenital vitreous opacity

Q14.1   Congenital malformation of retina
Congenital retinal aneurysm

Q14.2   Congenital malformation of optic disc
Coloboma of optic disc

Q14.3   Congenital malformation of choroid

Q14.8   Other congenital malformations of posterior segment of eye
Coloboma of the fundus

Q14.9   Congenital malformation of posterior segment of eye, unspecified

Figure 17-2   Bilateral congenital **hydrophthalmia,** in which the eyes are very large in comparison to the other facial features due to glaucoma.

▶ New   ⇨ Revised   ~~deleted~~ Deleted   **OGCR** Official Guidelines   X Assign placeholder X   ● Use Additional Character(s)

Excludes 1   Excludes 2   Includes   Use additional   Code first   Code also   Key words

● **Q15　Other congenital malformations of eye**
　　　Excludes1　congenital nystagmus (H55.01)
　　　　　　　　　ocular albinism (E70.31-)
　　　　　　　　　optic nerve hypoplasia (H47.03-)
　　　　　　　　　retinitis pigmentosa (H35.52)
　　Q15.0　Congenital glaucoma
　　　　　Axenfeld's anomaly
　　　　　Buphthalmos
　　　　　　Congenital syndrome characterized by enlargement of the
　　　　　　eye with sympotoms of glaucoma.
　　　　　Glaucoma of childhood
　　　　　Glaucoma of newborn
　　　　　Hydrophthalmos
　　　　　Keratoglobus, congenital, with glaucoma
　　　　　Macrocornea with glaucoma
　　　　　Macrophthalmos in congenital glaucoma
　　　　　Megalocornea with glaucoma
　　Q15.8　Other specified congenital malformations of eye
　　Q15.9　Congenital malformation of eye, unspecified
　　　　　Congenital anomaly of eye
　　　　　Congenital deformity of eye

● **Q16　Congenital malformations of ear causing impairment of hearing**
　　　Excludes1　congenital deafness (H90.-)
　　Q16.0　Congenital absence of (ear) auricle
　　Q16.1　Congenital absence, atresia and stricture of auditory canal (external)
　　　　　Congenital atresia or stricture of osseous meatus
　　Q16.2　Absence of eustachian tube
　　Q16.3　Congenital malformation of ear ossicles
　　　　　Congenital fusion of ear ossicles
　　Q16.4　Other congenital malformations of middle ear
　　　　　Congenital malformation of middle ear NOS
　　Q16.5　Congenital malformation of inner ear
　　　　　Congenital anomaly of membranous labyrinth
　　　　　Congenital anomaly of organ of Corti
　　Q16.9　Congenital malformation of ear causing impairment of hearing, unspecified
　　　　　Congenital absence of ear NOS

● **Q17　Other congenital malformations of ear**
　　　Excludes1　congenital malformations of ear with impairment
　　　　　　　　　of hearing (Q16.0-Q16.9)
　　　　　　　　　preauricular sinus (Q18.1)
　　Q17.0　Accessory auricle
　　　　　Accessory tragus
　　　　　Polyotia
　　　　　Preauricular appendage or tag
　　　　　Supernumerary ear
　　　　　Supernumerary lobule
　　Q17.1　Macrotia
　　　　　Enlarged ears
　　Q17.2　Microtia
　　　　　An abnormally small or underdeveloped external ear
　　Q17.3　Other misshapen ear
　　　　　Pointed ear
　　Q17.4　Misplaced ear
　　　　　Low-set ears
　　　　　Excludes1　cervical auricle (Q18.2)
　　Q17.5　Prominent ear
　　　　　Bat ear
　　Q17.8　Other specified congenital malformations of ear
　　　　　Congenital absence of lobe of ear
　　Q17.9　Congenital malformation of ear, unspecified
　　　　　Congenital anomaly of ear NOS

● **Q18　Other congenital malformations of face and neck**
　　　Excludes1　cleft lip and cleft palate (Q35-Q37)
　　　　　　　　　conditions classified to Q67.0-Q67.4
　　　　　　　　　congenital malformations of skull and face bones
　　　　　　　　　　(Q75.-)
　　　　　　　　　cyclopia (Q87.0)
　　　　　　　　　dentofacial anomalies [including malocclusion]
　　　　　　　　　　(M26.-)
　　　　　　　　　malformation syndromes affecting facial
　　　　　　　　　　appearance (Q87.0)
　　　　　　　　　persistent thyroglossal duct (Q89.2)
　　Q18.0　Sinus, fistula and cyst of branchial cleft
　　　　　Branchial vestige
　　　　　　Brachial remnants (cysts, fistula, skin tags) that are
　　　　　　developmental anomalies
　　Q18.1　Preauricular sinus and cyst
　　　　　Fistula of auricle, congenital
　　　　　Cervicoaural fistula
　　　　　　Abnormal passage in neck originating from first branchial
　　　　　　cleft
　　Q18.2　Other branchial cleft malformations
　　　　　Branchial cleft malformation NOS
　　　　　Cervical auricle
　　　　　Otocephaly
　　Q18.3　Webbing of neck
　　　　　Pterygium colli
　　　　　　Thick fold of skin on side of neck
　　Q18.4　Macrostomia
　　　　　　Results from failure of union of maxillary and mandibular
　　　　　　processes, results in abnormally large mouth
　　Q18.5　Microstomia
　　Q18.6　Macrocheilia
　　　　　　Excessive size of lips
　　　　　Hypertrophy of lip, congenital
　　Q18.7　Microcheilia
　　　　　　Abnormal smallness of lips
　　Q18.8　Other specified congenital malformations of face and neck
　　　　　Medial cyst of face and neck
　　　　　Medial fistula of face and neck
　　　　　Medial sinus of face and neck
　　Q18.9　Congenital malformation of face and neck, unspecified
　　　　　Congenital anomaly NOS of face and neck

CONGENITAL MALFORMATIONS OF THE CIRCULATORY SYSTEM (Q20-Q28)

● **Q20　Congenital malformations of cardiac chambers and connections**
　　　Excludes1　dextrocardia with situs inversus (Q89.3)
　　　　　　　　　mirror-image atrial arrangement with situs
　　　　　　　　　　inversus (Q89.3)
　　Q20.0　Common arterial trunk
　　　　　Persistent truncus arteriosus
　　　　　Excludes1　aortic septal defect (Q21.4)
　　Q20.1　Double outlet right ventricle
　　　　　Taussig-Bing syndrome
　　Q20.2　Double outlet left ventricle
　　Q20.3　Discordant ventriculoarterial connection
　　　　　Dextrotransposition of aorta
　　　　　Transposition of great vessels (complete)
　　Q20.4　Double inlet ventricle
　　　　　Common ventricle
　　　　　Cor triloculare biatriatum
　　　　　Single ventricle
　　Q20.5　Discordant atrioventricular connection
　　　　　Corrected transposition
　　　　　Levotransposition
　　　　　Ventricular inversion
　　Q20.6　Isomerism of atrial appendages
　　　　　Isomerism of atrial appendages with asplenia or
　　　　　　polysplenia
　　Q20.8　Other congenital malformations of cardiac chambers and connections
　　　　　Cor binoculare
　　Q20.9　Congenital malformation of cardiac chambers and connections, unspecified

CHAPTER 17 (Q00-Q99)

● **Q21   Congenital malformations of cardiac septa**

> **Excludes1**   acquired cardiac septal defect (I51.Ø)

     Q21.Ø   Ventricular septal defect
         Roger's disease

     Q21.1   Atrial septal defect
         Coronary sinus defect
         Patent or persistent foramen ovale
         Patent or persistent ostium secundum defect (type II)
         Patent or persistent sinus venosus defect

     Q21.2   Atrioventricular septal defect
         Common atrioventricular canal
         Endocardial cushion defect
         Ostium primum atrial septal defect (type I)

     Q21.3   Tetralogy of Fallot
         Ventricular septal defect with pulmonary stenosis or
         atresia, dextroposition of aorta and hypertrophy of
         right ventricle.

     Q21.4   Aortopulmonary septal defect
         Aortic septal defect
         Aortopulmonary window

     Q21.8   Other congenital malformations of cardiac septa
         Eisenmenger's defect
         Pentalogy of Fallot

> **Excludes1**   ~~Eisenmenger's complex (I27.8)~~
>   ~~Eisenmenger's syndrome (I27.8)~~

         ▶ Code also if applicable:
            ▶ Eisenmenger's complex (I27.83)
            ▶ Eisenmenger's syndrome (I27.83)

     Q21.9   Congenital malformation of cardiac septum, unspecified
         Septal (heart) defect NOS

● **Q22   Congenital malformations of pulmonary and tricuspid valves**

     Q22.Ø   Pulmonary valve atresia

     Q22.1   Congenital pulmonary valve stenosis

     Q22.2   Congenital pulmonary valve insufficiency
         Congenital pulmonary valve regurgitation

     Q22.3   Other congenital malformations of pulmonary valve
         Congenital malformation of pulmonary valve NOS
         Supernumerary cusps of pulmonary valve

     Q22.4   Congenital tricuspid stenosis
         Congenital tricuspid atresia

     Q22.5   Ebstein's anomaly
         Malformation of tricuspid valve

     Q22.6   Hypoplastic right heart syndrome

     Q22.8   Other congenital malformations of tricuspid valve

     Q22.9   Congenital malformation of tricuspid valve, unspecified

● **Q23   Congenital malformations of aortic and mitral valves**

     Q23.Ø   Congenital stenosis of aortic valve
         Congenital aortic atresia
         Congenital aortic stenosis NOS

> **Excludes1**   congenital stenosis of aortic valve in
>   hypoplastic left heart syndrome
>   (Q23.4)
>   congenital subaortic stenosis (Q24.4)
>   supravalvular aortic stenosis (congenital)
>   (Q25.3)

     Q23.1   Congenital insufficiency of aortic valve
         Bicuspid aortic valve
         Congenital aortic insufficiency

     Q23.2   Congenital mitral stenosis
         Congenital mitral atresia

     Q23.3   Congenital mitral insufficiency

     Q23.4   Hypoplastic left heart syndrome

     Q23.8   Other congenital malformations of aortic and mitral valves

     Q23.9   Congenital malformation of aortic and mitral valves, unspecified

● **Q24   Other congenital malformations of heart**

> **Excludes1**   endocardial fibroelastosis (I42.4)

     Q24.Ø   Dextrocardia
         Heart is located in right hemithorax

> **Excludes1**   dextrocardia with situs inversus (Q89.3)
>   isomerism of atrial appendages (with
>   asplenia or polysplenia) (Q2Ø.6)
>   mirror-image atrial arrangement with
>   situs inversus (Q89.3)

     Q24.1   Levocardia
         Normal position of heart but related structures on wrong side

     Q24.2   Cor triatriatum
         Congenital heart defect; left atrium is subdivided

     Q24.3   Pulmonary infundibular stenosis
         Subvalvular pulmonic stenosis

     Q24.4   Congenital subaortic stenosis

     Q24.5   Malformation of coronary vessels
         Congenital coronary (artery) aneurysm

     Q24.6   Congenital heart block

     Q24.8   Other specified congenital malformations of heart
         Congenital diverticulum of left ventricle
         Congenital malformation of myocardium
         Congenital malformation of pericardium
         Malposition of heart
         Uhl's disease

     Q24.9   Congenital malformation of heart, unspecified
         Congenital anomaly of heart
         Congenital disease of heart

● **Q25   Congenital malformations of great arteries**

     Q25.Ø   Patent ductus arteriosus
         Fetal blood vessel connecting left pulmonary artery directly
         *   to descending aorta*
         Patent ductus Botallo
         Persistent ductus arteriosus

     Q25.1   Coarctation of aorta
         Coarctation of aorta (preductal) (postductal)
         Stenosis of aorta

     ● **Q25.2   Atresia of aorta**

         Q25.21   Interruption of aortic arch
               Atresia of aortic arch

         Q25.29   Other atresia of aorta
               Atresia of aorta

     Q25.3   Supravalvular aortic stenosis

> **Excludes1**   congenital aortic stenosis NOS (Q23.Ø)
>   congenital stenosis of aortic valve (Q23.Ø)

     ● **Q25.4   Other congenital malformations of aorta**

> **Excludes1**   hypoplasia of aorta in hypoplastic left
>   heart syndrome (Q23.4)

         Q25.4Ø   Congenital malformation of aorta unspecified

         Q25.41   Absence and aplasia of aorta

         Q25.42   Hypoplasia of aorta

         Q25.43   Congenital aneurysm of aorta
               Congenital aneurysm of aortic root
               Congenital aneurysm of aortic sinus

         Q25.44   Congenital dilation of aorta

         Q25.45   Double aortic arch
               Vascular ring of aorta

         Q25.46   Tortuous aortic arch
               Persistent convolutions of aortic arch

         Q25.47   Right aortic arch
               Persistent right aortic arch

         Q25.48   Anomalous origin of subclavian artery

         Q25.49   Other congenital malformations of aorta
             ▶ Aortic arch
             ▶ Bovine arch

     Q25.5   Atresia of pulmonary artery

     Q25.6   Stenosis of pulmonary artery
         Supravalvular pulmonary stenosis

▶ New   ⇒ Revised   ~~deleted~~ Deleted   **OGCR** Official Guidelines   X Assign placeholder X   ● Use Additional Character(s)

Excludes 1   Excludes 2   Includes   Use additional   Code first   Code also   Key words

● **Q25.7 Other congenital malformations of pulmonary artery**
   Q25.71 Coarctation of pulmonary artery
   Q25.72 Congenital pulmonary arteriovenous malformation
      Congenital pulmonary arteriovenous aneurysm
   Q25.79 Other congenital malformations of pulmonary artery
      Aberrant pulmonary artery
      Agenesis of pulmonary artery
      Congenital aneurysm of pulmonary artery
      Congenital anomaly of pulmonary artery
      Hypoplasia of pulmonary artery
  Q25.8 Other congenital malformations of other great arteries
  Q25.9 Congenital malformation of great arteries, unspecified

● **Q26 Congenital malformations of great veins**
  Q26.0 Congenital stenosis of vena cava
     Congenital stenosis of vena cava (inferior)(superior)
  Q26.1 Persistent left superior vena cava
  Q26.2 Total anomalous pulmonary venous connection
     Total anomalous pulmonary venous return [TAPVR], subdiaphragmatic
     Total anomalous pulmonary venous return [TAPVR], supradiaphragmatic
  Q26.3 Partial anomalous pulmonary venous connection
     Partial anomalous pulmonary venous return
  Q26.4 Anomalous pulmonary venous connection, unspecified
  Q26.5 Anomalous portal venous connection
  Q26.6 Portal vein-hepatic artery fistula
  Q26.8 Other congenital malformations of great veins
     Absence of vena cava (inferior) (superior)
     Azygos continuation of inferior vena cava
     Persistent left posterior cardinal vein
     Scimitar syndrome
  Q26.9 Congenital malformation of great vein, unspecified
     Congenital anomaly of vena cava (inferior) (superior) NOS

● **Q27 Other congenital malformations of peripheral vascular system**
  Excludes2 anomalies of cerebral and precerebral vessels (Q28.0-Q28.3)
     anomalies of coronary vessels (Q24.5)
     anomalies of pulmonary artery (Q25.5-Q25.7)
     congenital retinal aneurysm (Q14.1)
     hemangioma and lymphangioma (D18.-)
  Q27.0 Congenital absence and hypoplasia of umbilical artery
     Single umbilical artery
  Q27.1 Congenital renal artery stenosis
  Q27.2 Other congenital malformations of renal artery
     Congenital malformation of renal artery NOS
     Multiple renal arteries
● **Q27.3 Arteriovenous malformation (peripheral)**
     Arteriovenous aneurysm
    Excludes1 acquired arteriovenous aneurysm (I77.0)
    Excludes2 arteriovenous malformation of cerebral vessels (Q28.2)
     arteriovenous malformation of precerebral vessels (Q28.0)
   Q27.30 Arteriovenous malformation, site unspecified
   Q27.31 Arteriovenous malformation of vessel of upper limb
   Q27.32 Arteriovenous malformation of vessel of lower limb
   Q27.33 Arteriovenous malformation of digestive system vessel
   Q27.34 Arteriovenous malformation of renal vessel
   Q27.39 Arteriovenous malformation, other site

  Q27.4 Congenital phlebectasia
  Q27.8 Other specified congenital malformations of peripheral vascular system
     Absence of peripheral vascular system
     Atresia of peripheral vascular system
     Congenital aneurysm (peripheral)
     Congenital stricture, artery
     Congenital varix
    Excludes1 arteriovenous malformation (Q27.3-)
  Q27.9 Congenital malformation of peripheral vascular system, unspecified
     Anomaly of artery or vein NOS

● **Q28 Other congenital malformations of circulatory system**
  Excludes1 congenital aneurysm NOS (Q27.8)
     congenital coronary aneurysm (Q24.5)
     ruptured cerebral arteriovenous malformation (I60.8)
     ruptured malformation of precerebral vessels (I72.0)
  Excludes2 congenital peripheral aneurysm (Q27.8)
     congenital pulmonary aneurysm (Q25.79)
     congenital retinal aneurysm (Q14.1)
  Q28.0 Arteriovenous malformation of precerebral vessels
     Congenital arteriovenous precerebral aneurysm (nonruptured)
  Q28.1 Other malformations of precerebral vessels
     Congenital malformation of precerebral vessels NOS
     Congenital precerebral aneurysm (nonruptured)
  Q28.2 Arteriovenous malformation of cerebral vessels
     Arteriovenous malformation of brain NOS
     Congenital arteriovenous cerebral aneurysm (nonruptured)
  Q28.3 Other malformations of cerebral vessels
     Congenital cerebral aneurysm (nonruptured)
     Congenital malformation of cerebral vessels NOS
     Developmental venous anomaly
  Q28.8 Other specified congenital malformations of circulatory system
     Congenital aneurysm, specified site NEC
     Spinal vessel anomaly
  Q28.9 Congenital malformation of circulatory system, unspecified

CONGENITAL MALFORMATIONS OF THE RESPIRATORY SYSTEM (Q30-Q34)

● **Q30 Congenital malformations of nose**
  Excludes1 congenital deviation of nasal septum (Q67.4)
  Q30.0 Choanal atresia
     Atresia of nares (anterior) (posterior)
     Congenital stenosis of nares (anterior) (posterior)
  Q30.1 Agenesis and underdevelopment of nose
     Congenital absent of nose
  Q30.2 Fissured, notched and cleft nose
  Q30.3 Congenital perforated nasal septum
  Q30.8 Other congenital malformations of nose
     Accessory nose
     Congenital anomaly of nasal sinus wall
  Q30.9 Congenital malformation of nose, unspecified

● **Q31 Congenital malformations of larynx**
> **Excludes1** congenital laryngeal stridor NOS (P28.89)

Q31.0 Web of larynx
Glottic web of larynx
Subglottic web of larynx
Web of larynx NOS

Q31.1 Congenital subglottic stenosis

Q31.2 Laryngeal hypoplasia

Q31.3 Laryngocele

Q31.5 Congenital laryngomalacia

Q31.8 Other congenital malformations of larynx
Absence of larynx
Agenesis of larynx
Atresia of larynx
Congenital cleft thyroid cartilage
Congenital fissure of epiglottis
Congenital stenosis of larynx NEC
Posterior cleft of cricoid cartilage

Q31.9 Congenital malformation of larynx, unspecified

● **Q32 Congenital malformations of trachea and bronchus**
> **Excludes1** congenital bronchiectasis (Q33.4)

Q32.0 Congenital tracheomalacia

Q32.1 Other congenital malformations of trachea
Atresia of trachea
Congenital anomaly of tracheal cartilage
Congenital dilatation of trachea
Congenital malformation of trachea
Congenital stenosis of trachea
Congenital tracheocele

Q32.2 Congenital bronchomalacia

Q32.3 Congenital stenosis of bronchus

Q32.4 Other congenital malformations of bronchus
Absence of bronchus
Agenesis of bronchus
Atresia of bronchus
Congenital diverticulum of bronchus
Congenital malformation of bronchus NOS

● **Q33 Congenital malformations of lung**

Q33.0 Congenital cystic lung
Congenital cystic lung disease
Congenital honeycomb lung
Congenital polycystic lung disease
> **Excludes1** cystic fibrosis (E84.0)
> cystic lung disease, acquired or
> unspecified (J98.4)

Q33.1 Accessory lobe of lung
Azygos lobe (fissured), lung

Q33.2 Sequestration of lung

Q33.3 Agenesis of lung
Congenital absence of lung (lobe)

Q33.4 Congenital bronchiectasis

Q33.5 Ectopic tissue in lung

Q33.6 Congenital hypoplasia and dysplasia of lung
> **Excludes1** pulmonary hypoplasia associated with
> short gestation (P28.0)

Q33.8 Other congenital malformations of lung

Q33.9 Congenital malformation of lung, unspecified

● **Q34 Other congenital malformations of respiratory system**
> **Excludes2** congenital central alveolar hypoventilation
> syndrome (G47.35)

Q34.0 Anomaly of pleura

Q34.1 Congenital cyst of mediastinum

Q34.8 Other specified congenital malformations of respiratory system
Atresia of nasopharynx

Q34.9 Congenital malformation of respiratory system, unspecified
Congenital absence of respiratory system
Congenital anomaly of respiratory system NOS

Figure 17-3 Cleft palate.

CLEFT LIP AND CLEFT PALATE (Q35-Q37)
Use additional code to identify associated malformation of the nose (Q30.2)
> **Excludes1** Robin's syndrome (Q87.0)

● **Q35 Cleft palate**
> **Includes** fissure of palate
> palatoschisis
> **Excludes1** cleft palate with cleft lip (Q37.-)

Q35.1 Cleft hard palate

Q35.3 Cleft soft palate

Q35.5 Cleft hard palate with cleft soft palate

Q35.7 Cleft uvula

Q35.9 Cleft palate, unspecified
Cleft palate NOS

● **Q36 Cleft lip**
> **Includes** cheiloschisis
> congenital fissure of lip
> harelip
> labium leporinum
> **Excludes1** cleft lip with cleft palate (Q37.-)

Q36.0 Cleft lip, bilateral

Q36.1 Cleft lip, median

Q36.9 Cleft lip, unilateral
Cleft lip NOS

● **Q37 Cleft palate with cleft lip**
> **Includes** cheilopalatoschisis

Q37.0 Cleft hard palate with bilateral cleft lip

Q37.1 Cleft hard palate with unilateral cleft lip
Cleft hard palate with cleft lip NOS

Q37.2 Cleft soft palate with bilateral cleft lip

Q37.3 Cleft soft palate with unilateral cleft lip
Cleft soft palate with cleft lip NOS

Q37.4 Cleft hard and soft palate with bilateral cleft lip

Q37.5 Cleft hard and soft palate with unilateral cleft lip
Cleft hard and soft palate with cleft lip NOS

Q37.8 Unspecified cleft palate with bilateral cleft lip

Q37.9 Unspecified cleft palate with unilateral cleft lip
Cleft palate with cleft lip NOS

OTHER CONGENITAL MALFORMATIONS OF THE DIGESTIVE SYSTEM (Q38-Q45)

● **Q38 Other congenital malformations of tongue, mouth and pharynx**

> **Excludes1** dentofacial anomalies (M26.-)
> macrostomia (Q18.4)
> microstomia (Q18.5)

Q38.0 Congenital malformations of lips, not elsewhere classified
Congenital fistula of lip
Congenital malformation of lip NOS
Van der Woude's syndrome

> **Excludes1** cleft lip (Q36.-)
> cleft lip with cleft palate (Q37.-)
> macrocheilia (Q18.6)
> microcheilia (Q18.7)

Q38.1 Ankyloglossia
Restricted movement of tongue resulting in speech difficulty
Tongue tie

Q38.2 Macroglossia
Excessive size of tongue
Congenital hypertrophy of tongue

Q38.3 Other congenital malformations of tongue
Aglossia
Bifid tongue
Congenital adhesion of tongue
Congenital fissure of tongue
Congenital malformation of tongue NOS
Double tongue
Hypoglossia
Hypoplasia of tongue
Microglossia

Q38.4 Congenital malformations of salivary glands and ducts
Atresia of salivary glands and ducts
Congenital absence of salivary glands and ducts
Congenital accessory salivary glands and ducts
Congenital fistula of salivary gland

Q38.5 Congenital malformations of palate, not elsewhere classified
Congenital absence of uvula
Congenital malformation of palate NOS
Congenital high arched palate

> **Excludes1** cleft palate (Q35.-)
> cleft palate with cleft lip (Q37.-)

Q38.6 Other congenital malformations of mouth
Congenital malformation of mouth NOS

Q38.7 Congenital pharyngeal pouch
Congenital diverticulum of pharynx

> **Excludes1** pharyngeal pouch syndrome (D82.1)

Q38.8 Other congenital malformations of pharynx
Congenital malformation of pharynx NOS
Imperforate pharynx

● **Q39 Congenital malformations of esophagus**

Q39.0 Atresia of esophagus without fistula
Atresia of esophagus NOS

Q39.1 Atresia of esophagus with tracheo-esophageal fistula
Atresia of esophagus with broncho-esophageal fistula

Q39.2 Congenital tracheo-esophageal fistula without atresia
Congenital tracheo-esophageal fistula NOS

Q39.3 Congenital stenosis and stricture of esophagus

Q39.4 Esophageal web

Q39.5 Congenital dilatation of esophagus
Congenital cardiospasm

Q39.6 Congenital diverticulum of esophagus
Congenital esophageal pouch

Q39.8 Other congenital malformations of esophagus
Congenital absence of esophagus
Congenital displacement of esophagus
Congenital duplication of esophagus

Q39.9 Congenital malformation of esophagus, unspecified

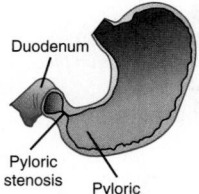

Figure 17-4 Pyloric stenosis.

Duodenum
Pyloric stenosis
Pyloric part of stomach

● **Q40 Other congenital malformations of upper alimentary tract**

Q40.0 Congenital hypertrophic pyloric stenosis
Congenital or infantile constriction
Congenital or infantile hypertrophy
Congenital or infantile spasm
Congenital or infantile stenosis
Congenital or infantile stricture

Q40.1 Congenital hiatus hernia
Congenital displacement of cardia through esophageal hiatus

> **Excludes1** congenital diaphragmatic hernia (Q79.0)

Q40.2 Other specified congenital malformations of stomach
Congenital displacement of stomach
Congenital diverticulum of stomach
Congenital hourglass stomach
Congenital duplication of stomach
Megalogastria
Microgastria

Q40.3 Congenital malformation of stomach, unspecified

Q40.8 Other specified congenital malformations of upper alimentary tract

Q40.9 Congenital malformation of upper alimentary tract, unspecified
Congenital anomaly of upper alimentary tract
Congenital deformity of upper alimentary tract

● **Q41 Congenital absence, atresia and stenosis of small intestine**

> **Includes** congenital obstruction, occlusion or stricture of small intestine or intestine NOS

> **Excludes1** cystic fibrosis with intestinal manifestation (E84.11)
> meconium ileus NOS (without cystic fibrosis) (P76.0)

Q41.0 Congenital absence, atresia and stenosis of duodenum

Q41.1 Congenital absence, atresia and stenosis of jejunum
Apple peel syndrome
Imperforate jejunum

Q41.2 Congenital absence, atresia and stenosis of ileum

Q41.8 Congenital absence, atresia and stenosis of other specified parts of small intestine

Q41.9 Congenital absence, atresia and stenosis of small intestine, part unspecified
Congenital absence, atresia and stenosis of intestine NOS

● **Q42 Congenital absence, atresia and stenosis of large intestine**

> **Includes** congenital obstruction, occlusion and stricture of large intestine

Q42.0 Congenital absence, atresia and stenosis of rectum with fistula

Q42.1 Congenital absence, atresia and stenosis of rectum without fistula
Imperforate rectum

Q42.2 Congenital absence, atresia and stenosis of anus with fistula

Q42.3 Congenital absence, atresia and stenosis of anus without fistula
Imperforate anus

Q42.8 Congenital absence, atresia and stenosis of other parts of large intestine

Q42.9 Congenital absence, atresia and stenosis of large intestine, part unspecified

CHAPTER 17 (Q00-Q99)

● Q43 Other congenital malformations of intestine

Q43.0 Meckel's diverticulum (displaced) (hypertrophic)
Congenital abnormality in which a pouch remains on the lower end of the small intestine
Persistent omphalomesenteric duct
Persistent vitelline duct

Q43.1 Hirschsprung's disease
Developmental disorder of enteric nervous system characterized by absence of ganglion cells in distal colon resulting in functional obstruction
Aganglionosis
Congenital (aganglionic) megacolon

Q43.2 Other congenital functional disorders of colon
Congenital dilatation of colon

Q43.3 Congenital malformations of intestinal fixation
Congenital omental, anomalous adhesions [bands]
Congenital peritoneal adhesions [bands]
Incomplete rotation of cecum and colon
Insufficient rotation of cecum and colon
Jackson's membrane
Malrotation of colon
Rotation failure of cecum and colon
Universal mesentery

Q43.4 Duplication of intestine

Q43.5 Ectopic anus
Anal opening in abnormal location

Q43.6 Congenital fistula of rectum and anus
Excludes1 congenital fistula of anus with absence, atresia and stenosis (Q42.2)
congenital fistula of rectum with absence, atresia and stenosis (Q42.0)
congenital rectovaginal fistula (Q52.2)
congenital urethrorectal fistula (Q64.73)
pilonidal fistula or sinus (L05.-)

Q43.7 Persistent cloaca
Malformation in which rectum, vagina, and urinary tract form one channel AKA congenital cloaca
Cloaca NOS

Q43.8 Other specified congenital malformations of intestine
Congenital blind loop syndrome
Congenital diverticulitis, colon
Congenital diverticulum, intestine
Dolichocolon
Megaloappendix
Megaloduodenum
Microcolon
Transposition of appendix
Transposition of colon
Transposition of intestine

Q43.9 Congenital malformation of intestine, unspecified

● Q44 Congenital malformations of gallbladder, bile ducts and liver

Q44.0 Agenesis, aplasia and hypoplasia of gallbladder
Congenital absence of gallbladder

Q44.1 Other congenital malformations of gallbladder
Congenital malformation of gallbladder NOS
Intrahepatic gallbladder

Q44.2 Atresia of bile ducts

Q44.3 Congenital stenosis and stricture of bile ducts

Q44.4 Choledochal cyst

Q44.5 Other congenital malformations of bile ducts
Accessory hepatic duct
Biliary duct duplication
Congenital malformation of bile duct NOS
Cystic duct duplication

Q44.6 Cystic disease of liver
Fibrocystic disease of liver

Q44.7 Other congenital malformations of liver
Accessory liver
Alagille's syndrome
Congenital absence of liver
Congenital hepatomegaly
Congenital malformation of liver NOS

● Q45 Other congenital malformations of digestive system
Excludes2 congenital diaphragmatic hernia (Q79.0)
congenital hiatus hernia (Q40.1)

Q45.0 Agenesis, aplasia and hypoplasia of pancreas
Congenital absence of pancreas

Q45.1 Annular pancreas

Q45.2 Congenital pancreatic cyst

Q45.3 Other congenital malformations of pancreas and pancreatic duct
Accessory pancreas
Congenital malformation of pancreas or pancreatic duct NOS
Excludes1 congenital diabetes mellitus (E10.-)
cystic fibrosis (E84.0-E84.9)
fibrocystic disease of pancreas (E84.-)
neonatal diabetes mellitus (P70.2)

Q45.8 Other specified congenital malformations of digestive system
Absence (complete) (partial) of alimentary tract NOS
Duplication of digestive system
Malposition, congenital of digestive system

Q45.9 Congenital malformation of digestive system, unspecified
Congenital anomaly of digestive system
Congenital deformity of digestive system

CONGENITAL MALFORMATIONS OF GENITAL ORGANS (Q50-Q56)
Excludes1 androgen insensitivity syndrome (E34.5-)
syndromes associated with anomalies in the number and form of chromosomes (Q90-Q99)

● Q50 Congenital malformations of ovaries, fallopian tubes and broad ligaments

● Q50.0 Congenital absence of ovary
Excludes1 Turner's syndrome (Q96.-)
Q50.01 Congenital absence of ovary, unilateral
Q50.02 Congenital absence of ovary, bilateral

Q50.1 Developmental ovarian cyst

Q50.2 Congenital torsion of ovary

● Q50.3 Other congenital malformations of ovary
Q50.31 Accessory ovary
Q50.32 Ovarian streak
Inadequate ovaries with absent follicular and hormonal function
46, XX with streak gonads
Q50.39 Other congenital malformation of ovary
Congenital malformation of ovary NOS

Q50.4 Embryonic cyst of fallopian tube
Fimbrial cyst

Q50.5 Embryonic cyst of broad ligament
Epoophoron cyst
Parovarian cyst

Q50.6 Other congenital malformations of fallopian tube and broad ligament
Absence of fallopian tube and broad ligament
Accessory fallopian tube and broad ligament
Atresia of fallopian tube and broad ligament
Congenital malformation of fallopian tube or broad ligament NOS

● Q51 Congenital malformations of uterus and cervix
Q51.0 Agenesis and aplasia of uterus
Congenital absence of uterus

● Q51.1 Doubling of uterus with doubling of cervix and vagina
Q51.10 Doubling of uterus with doubling of cervix and vagina without obstruction
Doubling of uterus with doubling of cervix and vagina NOS
Q51.11 Doubling of uterus with doubling of cervix and vagina with obstruction

▶ New ⇒ Revised deleted Deleted **OGCR** Official Guidelines X Assign placeholder X ● Use Additional Character(s)
Excludes 1 Excludes 2 Includes Use additional Code first Code also Key words

Q51.2 **Other doubling of uterus**
Doubling of uterus NOS
Septate uterus, complete or partial

Q51.3 **Bicornate uterus**
Bicornate uterus, complete or partial
Birth defect in which uterus has two separate 'horns' that form top of uterus

Q51.4 **Unicornate uterus**
Unicornate uterus with or without a separate uterine horn
Uterus with only one functioning horn
Uterus with half being undeveloped

Q51.5 **Agenesis and aplasia of cervix**
Congenital absence of cervix

Q51.6 **Embryonic cyst of cervix**

Q51.7 **Congenital fistulae between uterus and digestive and urinary tracts**

● Q51.8 **Other congenital malformations of uterus and cervix**
● Q51.81 Other congenital malformations of uterus
Q51.810 **Arcuate uterus**
Arcuatus uterus
Q51.811 **Hypoplasia of uterus**
Q51.818 **Other congenital malformations of uterus**
Müllerian anomaly of uterus NEC
● Q51.82 Other congenital malformations of cervix
Q51.820 **Cervical duplication**
Q51.821 **Hypoplasia of cervix**
Q51.828 **Other congenital malformations of cervix**

Q51.9 **Congenital malformation of uterus and cervix, unspecified**

● Q52 **Other congenital malformations of female genitalia**
Q52.0 **Congenital absence of vagina**
Vaginal agenesis, total or partial
● Q52.1 **Doubling of vagina**
| Excludes1 | doubling of vagina with doubling of uterus and cervix (Q51.1-) |
Q52.10 **Doubling of vagina, unspecified**
Septate vagina NOS
Q52.11 **Transverse vaginal septum**
● Q52.12 **Longitudinal vaginal septum**
Q52.120 **Longitudinal vaginal septum, nonobstructing**
Q52.121 **Longitudinal vaginal septum, obstructing, right side**
Q52.122 **Longitudinal vaginal septum, obstructing, left side**
Q52.123 **Longitudinal vaginal septum, microperforate, right side**
Q52.124 **Longitudinal vaginal septum, microperforate, left side**
Q52.129 **Other and unspecified longitudinal vaginal septum**

Q52.2 **Congenital rectovaginal fistula**
| Excludes1 | cloaca (Q43.7) |
Q52.3 **Imperforate hymen**
Membrane (hymen) completely closes vaginal orifice
Q52.4 **Other congenital malformations of vagina**
Canal of Nuck cyst, congenital
Congenital malformation of vagina NOS
Embryonic vaginal cyst
Gartner's duct cyst
Q52.5 **Fusion of labia**
Q52.6 **Congenital malformation of clitoris**

● Q52.7 **Other and unspecified congenital malformations of vulva**
Q52.70 **Unspecified congenital malformations of vulva**
Congenital malformation of vulva NOS
Q52.71 **Congenital absence of vulva**
Q52.79 **Other congenital malformations of vulva**
Congenital cyst of vulva

Q52.8 **Other specified congenital malformations of female genitalia**
Q52.9 **Congenital malformation of female genitalia, unspecified**

● Q53 **Undescended and ectopic testicle**
● Q53.0 **Ectopic testis**
Q53.00 Ectopic testis, unspecified
Q53.01 Ectopic testis, unilateral
Q53.02 Ectopic testes, bilateral
● Q53.1 **Undescended testicle, unilateral**
Q53.10 Unspecified undescended testicle, unilateral
● Q53.11 Abdominal testis, unilateral
▶ Q53.111 Unilateral intraabdominal testis
▶ Q53.112 Unilateral inguinal testis
Q53.12 Ectopic perineal testis, unilateral
▶ Q53.13 Unilateral high scrotal testis
● Q53.2 **Undescended testicle, bilateral**
Q53.20 Undescended testicle, unspecified, bilateral
● Q53.21 Abdominal testis, bilateral
▶ Q53.211 Bilateral intraabdominal testes
▶ Q53.212 Bilateral inguinal testes
Q53.22 Ectopic perineal testis, bilateral
▶ Q53.23 Bilateral high scrotal testes
Q53.9 **Undescended testicle, unspecified**
Cryptorchism NOS

● Q54 **Hypospadias**
Birth defect of male; urethra opens in abnormal location on shaft
| Excludes1 | epispadias (Q64.0) |
Q54.0 **Hypospadias, balanic**
Hypospadias, coronal
Hypospadias, glandular
Q54.1 **Hypospadias, penile**
Q54.2 **Hypospadias, penoscrotal**
Q54.3 **Hypospadias, perineal**
Q54.4 **Congenital chordee**
Chordee without hypospadias
Q54.8 **Other hypospadias**
Hypospadias with intersex state
Q54.9 **Hypospadias, unspecified**

Item 17-1 Testes form in the abdomen of the male and only descend into the scrotum during normal embryonic development. "Ectopic" testes are out of their normal place or "retained" (left behind) in the abdomen. Crypto (hidden) orchism (testicle) is a major risk factor for testicular cancer.

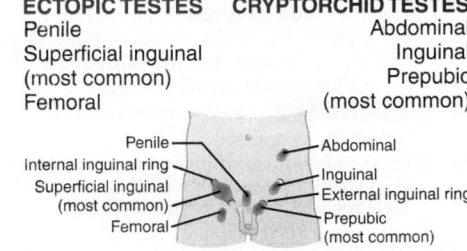

ECTOPIC TESTES	CRYPTORCHID TESTES
Penile	Abdominal
Superficial inguinal	Inguinal
(most common)	Prepubic
Femoral	(most common)

Figure 17-5 Undescended testes and the positions of the testes in various types of cryptorchidism or abnormal paths of descent.

▶ New   ⇒ Revised   ~~deleted~~ Deleted   **OGCR** Official Guidelines   **X** Assign placeholder X   ● Use Additional Character(s)

| Excludes 1 | | Excludes 2 | Includes   Use additional   Code first   Code also   Key words

1129

● **Q55   Other congenital malformations of male genital organs**

     Excludes1   congenital hydrocele (P83.5)
                       hypospadias (Q54.-)

     Q55.0   Absence and aplasia of testis
         Monorchism

     Q55.1   Hypoplasia of testis and scrotum
         Fusion of testes

● **Q55.2   Other and unspecified congenital malformations of testis and scrotum**

         Q55.20   Unspecified congenital malformations of testis and scrotum
                 Congenital malformation of testis or scrotum NOS

         Q55.21   Polyorchism
                 Developmental anomaly characterized by presence of more than two testes

         Q55.22   Retractile testis

         Q55.23   Scrotal transposition

         Q55.29   Other congenital malformations of testis and scrotum

     Q55.3   Atresia of vas deferens
         Code first any associated cystic fibrosis (E84.-)

     Q55.4   Other congenital malformations of vas deferens, epididymis, seminal vesicles and prostate
         Absence or aplasia of prostate
         Absence or aplasia of spermatic cord
         Congenital malformation of vas deferens, epididymis, seminal vesicles or prostate NOS

     Q55.5   Congenital absence and aplasia of penis

● **Q55.6   Other congenital malformations of penis**

         Q55.61   Curvature of penis (lateral)

         Q55.62   Hypoplasia of penis
                 Underdevelopment penis
                 Micropenis

         Q55.63   Congenital torsion of penis
              Excludes1   acquired torsion of penis (N48.82)

         Q55.64   Hidden penis
                 Buried penis
                 Concealed penis
              Excludes1   acquired buried penis (N48.83)

         Q55.69   Other congenital malformation of penis
                 Congenital malformation of penis NOS

     Q55.7   Congenital vasocutaneous fistula
         Abnormal opening between vas deferens and skin

     Q55.8   Other specified congenital malformations of male genital organs

     Q55.9   Congenital malformation of male genital organ, unspecified
         Congenital anomaly of male genital organ
         Congenital deformity of male genital organ

● **Q56   Indeterminate sex and pseudohermaphroditism**
     Internal reproductive organs are opposite external physical characteristics.

     Excludes1   46,XX true hermaphrodite (Q99.1)
                 androgen insensitivity syndrome (E34.5-)
                 chimera 46,XX/46,XY true hermaphrodite (Q99.0)
                 female pseudohermaphroditism with adrenocortical disorder (E25.-)
                 pseudohermaphroditism with specified chromosomal anomaly (Q96-Q99)
                 pure gonadal dysgenesis (Q99.1)

     Q56.0   Hermaphroditism, not elsewhere classified
         Ovotestis

     Q56.1   Male pseudohermaphroditism, not elsewhere classified
         46, XY with streak gonads
         Male pseudohermaphroditism NOS

     Q56.2   Female pseudohermaphroditism, not elsewhere classified
         Female pseudohermaphroditism NOS

     Q56.3   Pseudohermaphroditism, unspecified

     Q56.4   Indeterminate sex, unspecified
         Ambiguous genitalia

CONGENITAL MALFORMATIONS OF THE URINARY SYSTEM (Q60-Q64)

● **Q60   Renal agenesis and other reduction defects of kidney**

     Includes   congenital absence of kidney
               congenital atrophy of kidney
               infantile atrophy of kidney

     Q60.0   Renal agenesis, unilateral

     Q60.1   Renal agenesis, bilateral

     Q60.2   Renal agenesis, unspecified

     Q60.3   Renal hypoplasia, unilateral

     Q60.4   Renal hypoplasia, bilateral

     Q60.5   Renal hypoplasia, unspecified

     Q60.6   Potter's syndrome

● **Q61   Cystic kidney disease**
     Cysts that develop in failing kidney due to end-stage renal disease

     Excludes1   acquired cyst of kidney (N28.1)
                 Potter's syndrome (Q60.6)

● **Q61.0   Congenital renal cyst**

         Q61.00   Congenital renal cyst, unspecified
                 Cyst of kidney NOS (congenital)

         Q61.01   Congenital single renal cyst

         Q61.02   Congenital multiple renal cysts

● **Q61.1   Polycystic kidney, infantile type**
         Polycystic kidney, autosomal recessive

         Q61.11   Cystic dilatation of collecting ducts

         Q61.19   Other polycystic kidney, infantile type

     Q61.2   Polycystic kidney, adult type
         Polycystic kidney, autosomal dominant

     Q61.3   Polycystic kidney, unspecified

     Q61.4   Renal dysplasia
         Multicystic dysplastic kidney
         Multicystic kidney (development)
         Multicystic kidney disease
         Multicystic renal dysplasia
         Excludes1   polycystic kidney disease (Q61.11-Q61.3)

     Q61.5   Medullary cystic kidney
         Nephronopthisis
         Sponge kidney NOS

     Q61.8   Other cystic kidney diseases
         Fibrocystic kidney
         Fibrocystic renal degeneration or disease

     Q61.9   Cystic kidney disease, unspecified
         Meckel-Gruber syndrome

● **Q62   Congenital obstructive defects of renal pelvis and congenital malformations of ureter**

     Q62.0   Congenital hydronephrosis

● **Q62.1   Congenital occlusion of ureter**
         Atresia and stenosis of ureter

         Q62.10   Congenital occlusion of ureter, unspecified

         Q62.11   Congenital occlusion of ureteropelvic junction

         Q62.12   Congenital occlusion of ureterovesical orifice

     Q62.2   Congenital megaureter
         Congenital dilatation of ureter

● **Q62.3   Other obstructive defects of renal pelvis and ureter**

         Q62.31   Congenital ureterocele, orthotopic

         Q62.32   Cecoureterocele
                 Ectopic ureterocele

         Q62.39   Other obstructive defects of renal pelvis and ureter
                 Ureteropelvic junction obstruction NOS

▶ New   ⇥ Revised   ~~deleted~~ Deleted   **OGCR** Official Guidelines   X Assign placeholder X   ● Use Additional Character(s)

Excludes 1   Excludes 2   Includes   Use additional   Code first   Code also   Key words

Q62.4 **Agenesis of ureter**
    Congenital absence ureter

Q62.5 **Duplication of ureter**
    Accessory ureter
    Double ureter

● Q62.6 **Malposition of ureter**
    Q62.60 **Malposition of ureter, unspecified**
    Q62.61 **Deviation of ureter**
    Q62.62 **Displacement of ureter**
    Q62.63 **Anomalous implantation of ureter**
        Ectopia of ureter
        Ectopic ureter
    Q62.69 **Other malposition of ureter**

Q62.7 **Congenital vesico-uretero-renal reflux**

Q62.8 **Other congenital malformations of ureter**
    Anomaly of ureter NOS

● Q63 **Other congenital malformations of kidney**
    Excludes1   congenital nephrotic syndrome (N04.-)

Q63.0 **Accessory kidney**

Q63.1 **Lobulated, fused and horseshoe kidney**

Q63.2 **Ectopic kidney**
    Congenital displaced kidney
    Malrotation of kidney

Q63.3 **Hyperplastic and giant kidney**
    Compensatory hypertrophy of kidney

Q63.8 **Other specified congenital malformations of kidney**
    Congenital renal calculi

Q63.9 **Congenital malformation of kidney, unspecified**

● Q64 **Other congenital malformations of urinary system**

Q64.0 **Epispadias**
    Urethral opening somewhere on dorsum of penis
    Excludes1   hypospadias (Q54.-)

● Q64.1 **Exstrophy of urinary bladder**
    Bladder is exposed, inside out, and protrudes through abdominal wall
    Q64.10 **Exstrophy of urinary bladder, unspecified**
        Ectopia vesicae
    Q64.11 **Supravesical fissure of urinary bladder**
➥   Q64.12 **Cloacal exstrophy of urinary bladder**
    Q64.19 **Other exstrophy of urinary bladder**
        Extroversion of bladder

Q64.2 **Congenital posterior urethral valves**

● Q64.3 **Other atresia and stenosis of urethra and bladder neck**
    Q64.31 **Congenital bladder neck obstruction**
        Congenital obstruction of vesicourethral orifice
    Q64.32 **Congenital stricture of urethra**
    Q64.33 **Congenital stricture of urinary meatus**
    Q64.39 **Other atresia and stenosis of urethra and bladder neck**
        Atresia and stenosis of urethra and bladder neck NOS

Q64.4 **Malformation of urachus**
    Cyst of urachus
    Patent urachus
    Prolapse of urachus

Q64.5 **Congenital absence of bladder and urethra**

Q64.6 **Congenital diverticulum of bladder**

● Q64.7 **Other and unspecified congenital malformations of bladder and urethra**
    Excludes1   congenital prolapse of bladder (mucosa) (Q79.4)
    Q64.70 **Unspecified congenital malformation of bladder and urethra**
        Malformation of bladder or urethra NOS
    Q64.71 **Congenital prolapse of urethra**
    Q64.72 **Congenital prolapse of urinary meatus**
    Q64.73 **Congenital urethrorectal fistula**
    Q64.74 **Double urethra**
    Q64.75 **Double urinary meatus**
    Q64.79 **Other congenital malformations of bladder and urethra**

Q64.8 **Other specified congenital malformations of urinary system**

Q64.9 **Congenital malformation of urinary system, unspecified**
    Congenital anomaly NOS of urinary system
    Congenital deformity NOS of urinary system

CONGENITAL MALFORMATIONS AND DEFORMATIONS OF THE MUSCULOSKELETAL SYSTEM (Q65-Q79)

● Q65 **Congenital deformities of hip**
    Excludes1   clicking hip (R29.4)

● Q65.0 **Congenital dislocation of hip, unilateral**
    Q65.00 **Congenital dislocation of unspecified hip, unilateral**
    Q65.01 **Congenital dislocation of right hip, unilateral**
    Q65.02 **Congenital dislocation of left hip, unilateral**

Q65.1 **Congenital dislocation of hip, bilateral**

Q65.2 **Congenital dislocation of hip, unspecified**

● Q65.3 **Congenital partial dislocation of hip, unilateral**
    Q65.30 **Congenital partial dislocation of unspecified hip, unilateral**
    Q65.31 **Congenital partial dislocation of right hip, unilateral**
    Q65.32 **Congenital partial dislocation of left hip, unilateral**

Q65.4 **Congenital partial dislocation of hip, bilateral**

Q65.5 **Congenital partial dislocation of hip, unspecified**

Q65.6 **Congenital unstable hip**
    Congenital dislocatable hip

● Q65.8 **Other congenital deformities of hip**
    Q65.81 **Congenital coxa valga**
    Q65.82 **Congenital coxa vara**
    Q65.89 **Other specified congenital deformities of hip**
        Anteversion of femoral neck
        Congenital acetabular dysplasia

Q65.9 **Congenital deformity of hip, unspecified**

● Q66 **Congenital deformities of feet**
    Excludes1   reduction defects of feet (Q72.-)
        valgus deformities (acquired) (M21.0-)
        varus deformities (acquired) (M21.1-)

Q66.0 **Congenital talipes equinovarus**
    Heel is turned inward from midline and foot is plantar flexed; AKA clubfoot

Q66.1 **Congenital talipes calcaneovarus**
    Deformity of foot in which heel is turned toward midline of body and anterior of foot is elevated

● Q66.2 **Congenital metatarsus (primus) varus**
    Angulation of first metatarsal bone toward midline of body
    Q66.21 **Congenital metatarsus primus varus**
    Q66.22 **Congenital metatarsus adductus**
        Congenital metatarsus varus

Q66.3 **Other congenital varus deformities of feet**
    Hallux varus, congenital

Q66.4 **Congenital talipes calcaneovalgus**

Item 17–2 **Equinus foot** is a term referring to the hoof of a horse. The deformity is usually congenital or spastic. **Talipes equinovarus** is referred to as clubfoot. The foot tends to be smaller than normal, with the heel pointing downward and the forefoot turning inward. The heel cord (Achilles tendon) is tight, causing the heel to be drawn up toward the leg.

Figure 17-6 Supination and cavus deformity of forefoot. (From Kliegman R, Nelson WE: Nelson Textbook of Pediatrics, Philadelphia, Saunders, 2007)

Talipes cavus   Talipes equinus   Talipes calcaneus

Talipes valgus   Talipes equinovalgus   Talipes calcaneovalgus

Talipes varus   Talipes cavovarus   Talipes equinovarus   Talipes calcaneocavus

Figure 17-7 Talipes. (From Dorland: Dorland's Illustrated Medical Dictionary, ed 31, Saunders, 2007, p 1893)

● **Q66.5** Congenital **pes planus**
       Congenital flat foot
       Congenital rigid flat foot
       Congenital spastic (everted) flat foot
       | Excludes1 | pes planus, acquired (M21.4)

       Q66.50 Congenital pes planus, **unspecified foot**
       Q66.51 Congenital pes planus, **right foot**
       Q66.52 Congenital pes planus, **left foot**
   Q66.6 **Other** congenital valgus deformities of feet
       Inward angulation
       Congenital metatarsus valgus
   Q66.7 Congenital **pes cavus**
● **Q66.8** **Other** congenital deformities of feet
       Q66.80 Congenital vertical talus deformity, **unspecified foot**
       Q66.81 Congenital vertical talus deformity, **right foot**
       Q66.82 Congenital vertical talus deformity, **left foot**
       Q66.89 **Other** specified congenital deformities of feet
          Congenital asymmetric talipes
          Congenital clubfoot NOS
          Congenital talipes NOS
          Congenital tarsal coalition
          Hammer toe, congenital
   Q66.9 Congenital deformity of feet, **unspecified**

● **Q67** Congenital musculoskeletal deformities of **head, face, spine and chest**
       | Excludes1 | congenital malformation syndromes classified to Q87.-
          Potter's syndrome (Q60.6)
   Q67.0 Congenital **facial asymmetry**
   Q67.1 Congenital **compression facies**
   Q67.2 **Dolichocephaly**
       Long head dimension
   Q67.3 **Plagiocephaly**
       Asymmetric shape of head resulting from irregular closure of cranial sutures
   Q67.4 **Other** congenital deformities of **skull, face and jaw**
       Congenital depressions in skull
       Congenital hemifacial atrophy or hypertrophy
       Deviation of nasal septum, congenital
       Squashed or bent nose, congenital
       | Excludes1 | dentofacial anomalies [including malocclusion] (M26.-)
          syphilitic saddle nose (A50.5)
   Q67.5 Congenital deformity of **spine**
       Congenital postural scoliosis
       Congenital scoliosis NOS
       | Excludes1 | infantile idiopathic scoliosis (M41.0)
          scoliosis due to congenital bony malformation (Q76.3)
   Q67.6 Pectus **excavatum**
       Congenital funnel chest
       Funnel-shaped chest depression
   Q67.7 Pectus **carinatum**
       Congenital pigeon chest
   Q67.8 **Other** congenital deformities of **chest**
       Congenital deformity of chest wall NOS
● **Q68** Other congenital **musculoskeletal deformities**
       | Excludes1 | reduction defects of limb(s) (Q71-Q73)
       | Excludes2 | congenital myotonic chondrodystrophy (G71.13)
   Q68.0 Congenital deformity of **sternocleidomastoid muscle**
       Congenital contracture of sternocleidomastoid (muscle)
       Congenital (sternomastoid) torticollis
       Sternomastoid tumor (congenital)
   Q68.1 Congenital deformity of **finger(s) and hand**
       Congenital clubfinger
       Spade-like hand (congenital)
   Q68.2 Congenital deformity of **knee**
       Congenital dislocation of knee
       Congenital genu recurvatum
       Hyperextension of knee resulting from hypermobility
   Q68.3 Congenital bowing of **femur**
       | Excludes1 | anteversion of femur (neck) (Q65.89)
   Q68.4 Congenital bowing of **tibia and fibula**
   Q68.5 Congenital bowing of **long bones of leg, unspecified**
   Q68.6 **Discoid meniscus**

Figure 17-8 Mild to moderate inbowing of the lower leg. (From Lissauer T, Clayden G: Illustrated Textbook of Paediatrics, Edinburgh, Mosby, 2011)

▶ New   ⇒ Revised   ~~deleted~~ Deleted   **OGCR** Official Guidelines   X Assign placeholder X   ● Use Additional Character(s)

| Excludes 1 | | Excludes 2 | Includes   Use additional   Code first   Code also   Key words

Q68.8 **Other** specified congenital musculoskeletal deformities
    Congenital deformity of clavicle
    Congenital deformity of elbow
    Congenital deformity of forearm
    Congenital deformity of scapula
    Congenital deformity of wrist
    Congenital dislocation of elbow
    Congenital dislocation of shoulder
    Congenital dislocation of wrist

● **Q69** **Polydactyly**
    AKA hyperdactyly, consists of supernumerary fingers or toes
    Q69.0 **Accessory finger(s)**
    Q69.1 **Accessory thumb(s)**
    Q69.2 **Accessory toe(s)**
        Accessory hallux
    Q69.9 **Polydactyly, unspecified**
        Supernumerary digit(s) NOS

● **Q70** **Syndactyly**
    Webbing between distal phalanges of adjacent digits
  ● **Q70.0** **Fused fingers**
        Complex syndactyly of fingers with synostosis
    Q70.00 Fused fingers, **unspecified** hand
    Q70.01 Fused fingers, **right** hand
    Q70.02 Fused fingers, **left** hand
    Q70.03 Fused fingers, **bilateral**
  ● **Q70.1** **Webbed fingers**
        Simple syndactyly of fingers without synostosis
    Q70.10 Webbed fingers, **unspecified** hand
    Q70.11 Webbed fingers, **right** hand
    Q70.12 Webbed fingers, **left** hand
    Q70.13 Webbed fingers, **bilateral**
  ● **Q70.2** **Fused toes**
        Complex syndactyly of toes with synostosis
    Q70.20 Fused toes, **unspecified** foot
    Q70.21 Fused toes, **right** foot
    Q70.22 Fused toes, **left** foot
    Q70.23 Fused toes, **bilateral**
  ● **Q70.3** **Webbed toes**
        Simple syndactyly of toes without synostosis
    Q70.30 Webbed toes, **unspecified** foot
    Q70.31 Webbed toes, **right** foot
    Q70.32 Webbed toes, **left** foot
    Q70.33 Webbed toes, **bilateral**
    Q70.4 **Polysyndactyly, unspecified**
        | **Excludes1** | specified syndactyly of hand and feet - code to specified conditions (Q70.0- -Q70.3-) |
        Extra and webbed digits
    Q70.9 **Syndactyly, unspecified**
        Symphalangy NOS

Figure 17-9 Thumb and index finger. (From Chung K: Hand and Upper Extremity Reconstruction, 1e, Saunders, 2008)

● **Q71** **Reduction defects of upper limb**
  ● **Q71.0** Congenital **complete absence** of upper limb
    Q71.00 Congenital complete absence of **unspecified** upper limb
    Q71.01 Congenital complete absence of **right** upper limb
    Q71.02 Congenital complete absence of **left** upper limb
    Q71.03 Congenital complete absence of upper limb, **bilateral**
  ● **Q71.1** Congenital **absence of upper arm and forearm with hand present**
    Q71.10 Congenital absence of **unspecified** upper arm and forearm with hand present
    Q71.11 Congenital absence of **right** upper arm and forearm with hand present
    Q71.12 Congenital absence of **left** upper arm and forearm with hand present
    Q71.13 Congenital absence of upper arm and forearm with hand present, **bilateral**
  ● **Q71.2** Congenital **absence of both forearm and hand**
    Q71.20 Congenital absence of both forearm and hand, **unspecified** upper limb
    Q71.21 Congenital absence of both forearm and hand, **right** upper limb
    Q71.22 Congenital absence of both forearm and hand, **left** upper limb
    Q71.23 Congenital absence of both forearm and hand, **bilateral**
  ● **Q71.3** Congenital **absence of hand and finger**
    Q71.30 Congenital absence of **unspecified** hand and finger
    Q71.31 Congenital absence of **right** hand and finger
    Q71.32 Congenital absence of **left** hand and finger
    Q71.33 Congenital absence of hand and finger, **bilateral**
  ● **Q71.4** Longitudinal reduction defect of **radius**
        Clubhand (congenital)
        Radial clubhand
    Q71.40 Longitudinal reduction defect of **unspecified** radius
    Q71.41 Longitudinal reduction defect of **right** radius
    Q71.42 Longitudinal reduction defect of **left** radius
    Q71.43 Longitudinal reduction defect of radius, **bilateral**
  ● **Q71.5** Longitudinal reduction defect of **ulna**
    Q71.50 Longitudinal reduction defect of **unspecified** ulna
    Q71.51 Longitudinal reduction defect of **right** ulna
    Q71.52 Longitudinal reduction defect of **left** ulna
    Q71.53 Longitudinal reduction defect of ulna, **bilateral**
  ● **Q71.6** **Lobster-claw hand**
    Q71.60 Lobster-claw hand, **unspecified** hand
    Q71.61 Lobster-claw **right** hand
    Q71.62 Lobster-claw **left** hand
    Q71.63 Lobster-claw hand, **bilateral**
  ● **Q71.8** **Other** reduction defects of upper limb
    ● **Q71.81** Congenital **shortening** of upper limb
        Q71.811 Congenital shortening of **right** upper limb
        Q71.812 Congenital shortening of **left** upper limb
        Q71.813 Congenital shortening of upper limb, **bilateral**
        Q71.819 Congenital shortening of **unspecified** upper limb

CHAPTER 17 (Q00-Q99)

● Q71.89   Other reduction defects of upper limb
   Q71.891   Other reduction defects of right upper limb
   Q71.892   Other reduction defects of left upper limb
   Q71.893   Other reduction defects of upper limb, bilateral
   Q71.899   Other reduction defects of unspecified upper limb
● Q71.9   Unspecified reduction defect of upper limb
   Q71.90   Unspecified reduction defect of unspecified upper limb
   Q71.91   Unspecified reduction defect of right upper limb
   Q71.92   Unspecified reduction defect of left upper limb
   Q71.93   Unspecified reduction defect of upper limb, bilateral

● Q72   Reduction defects of lower limb
   ● Q72.0   Congenital complete absence of lower limb
      Q72.00   Congenital complete absence of unspecified lower limb
      Q72.01   Congenital complete absence of right lower limb
      Q72.02   Congenital complete absence of left lower limb
      Q72.03   Congenital complete absence of lower limb, bilateral
   ● Q72.1   Congenital absence of thigh and lower leg with foot present
      Q72.10   Congenital absence of unspecified thigh and lower leg with foot present
      Q72.11   Congenital absence of right thigh and lower leg with foot present
      Q72.12   Congenital absence of left thigh and lower leg with foot present
      Q72.13   Congenital absence of thigh and lower leg with foot present, bilateral
   ● Q72.2   Congenital absence of both lower leg and foot
      Q72.20   Congenital absence of both lower leg and foot, unspecified lower limb
      Q72.21   Congenital absence of both lower leg and foot, right lower limb
      Q72.22   Congenital absence of both left lower leg and foot, left lower limb
      Q72.23   Congenital absence of both lower leg and foot, bilateral
   ● Q72.3   Congenital absence of foot and toe(s)
      Q72.30   Congenital absence of unspecified foot and toe(s)
      Q72.31   Congenital absence of right foot and toe(s)
      Q72.32   Congenital absence of left foot and toe(s)
      Q72.33   Congenital absence of foot and toe(s), bilateral
   ● Q72.4   Longitudinal reduction defect of femur
      Proximal femoral focal deficiency
      Q72.40   Longitudinal reduction defect of unspecified femur
      Q72.41   Longitudinal reduction defect of right femur
      Q72.42   Longitudinal reduction defect of left femur
      Q72.43   Longitudinal reduction defect of femur, bilateral

● Q72.5   Longitudinal reduction defect of tibia
   Q72.50   Longitudinal reduction defect of unspecified tibia
   Q72.51   Longitudinal reduction defect of right tibia
   Q72.52   Longitudinal reduction defect of left tibia
   Q72.53   Longitudinal reduction defect of tibia, bilateral
● Q72.6   Longitudinal reduction defect of fibula
   Q72.60   Longitudinal reduction defect of unspecified fibula
   Q72.61   Longitudinal reduction defect of right fibula
   Q72.62   Longitudinal reduction defect of left fibula
   Q72.63   Longitudinal reduction defect of fibula, bilateral
● Q72.7   Split foot
   Q72.70   Split foot, unspecified lower limb
   Q72.71   Split foot, right lower limb
   Q72.72   Split foot, left lower limb
   Q72.73   Split foot, bilateral
● Q72.8   Other reduction defects of lower limb
   ● Q72.81   Congenital shortening of lower limb
      Q72.811   Congenital shortening of right lower limb
      Q72.812   Congenital shortening of left lower limb
      Q72.813   Congenital shortening of lower limb, bilateral
      Q72.819   Congenital shortening of unspecified lower limb
   ● Q72.89   Other reduction defects of lower limb
      Q72.891   Other reduction defects of right lower limb
      Q72.892   Other reduction defects of left lower limb
      Q72.893   Other reduction defects of lower limb, bilateral
      Q72.899   Other reduction defects of unspecified lower limb
● Q72.9   Unspecified reduction defect of lower limb
   Q72.90   Unspecified reduction defect of unspecified lower limb
   Q72.91   Unspecified reduction defect of right lower limb
   Q72.92   Unspecified reduction defect of left lower limb
   Q72.93   Unspecified reduction defect of lower limb, bilateral

● Q73   Reduction defects of unspecified limb
   Q73.0   Congenital absence of unspecified limb(s)
      Amelia NOS
   Q73.1   Phocomelia, unspecified limb(s)
      Phocomelia NOS
         Absence/shortening of long bones primarily as a result of thalidomide
   Q73.8   Other reduction defects of unspecified limb(s)
      Longitudinal reduction deformity of unspecified limb(s)
      Ectromelia of limb NOS
         Gross hypoplasia or aplasia of one or more long bones of limb(s)
      Hemimelia of limb NOS
         Absence of one-half of long bone
      Reduction defect of limb NOS

▶ New   ⇒ Revised   ~~deleted~~ Deleted   **OGCR** Official Guidelines   X Assign placeholder X   ● Use Additional Character(s)
Excludes 1   Excludes 2   Includes   Use additional   Code first   Code also   Key words

● **Q74 Other congenital malformations of limb(s)**

> **Excludes 1** polydactyly (Q69.-)
> reduction defect of limb (Q71-Q73)
> syndactyly (Q70.-)

Q74.0 Other congenital malformations of upper limb(s), including shoulder girdle
Accessory carpal bones
Cleidocranial dysostosis
Congenital pseudarthrosis of clavicle
Macrodactylia (fingers)
Madelung's deformity
Radioulnar synostosis
Sprengel's deformity
Triphalangeal thumb

Q74.1 Congenital malformation of knee
Congenital absence of patella
Congenital dislocation of patella
Congenital genu valgum
Congenital genu varum
Rudimentary patella

> **Excludes 1** congenital dislocation of knee (Q68.2)
> congenital genu recurvatum (Q68.2)
> nail patella syndrome (Q87.2)

Q74.2 Other congenital malformations of lower limb(s), including pelvic girdle
Congenital fusion of sacroiliac joint
Congenital malformation of ankle joint
Congenital malformation of sacroiliac joint

> **Excludes 1** anteversion of femur (neck) (Q65.89)

Q74.3 Arthrogryposis multiplex congenita

Q74.8 Other specified congenital malformations of limb(s)

Q74.9 Unspecified congenital malformation of limb(s)
Congenital anomaly of limb(s) NOS

● **Q75 Other congenital malformations of skull and face bones**

> **Excludes 1** congenital malformation of face NOS (Q18.-)
> congenital malformation syndromes classified to Q87.-
> dentofacial anomalies [including malocclusion] (M26.-)
> musculoskeletal deformities of head and face (Q67.0-Q67.4)
> skull defects associated with congenital anomalies of brain such as:
> anencephaly (Q00.0)
> encephalocele (Q01.-)
> hydrocephalus (Q03.-)
> microcephaly (Q02)

Q75.0 Craniosynostosis
Premature closure of sutures of skull
Acrocephaly
Imperfect fusion of skull
Oxycephaly
Trigonocephaly

Q75.1 Craniofacial dysostosis
Congenital deformity of head
Crouzon's disease

Q75.2 Hypertelorism

Q75.3 Macrocephaly
Unusually large size of head; AKA megalocephaly

Q75.4 Mandibulofacial dysostosis
Francheschetti syndrome
Treacher Collins syndrome

Q75.5 Oculomandibular dysostosis
Ossification of occular and mandibular bones

Q75.8 Other specified congenital malformations of skull and face bones
Absence of skull bone, congenital
Congenital deformity of forehead
Platybasia

Q75.9 Congenital malformation of skull and face bones, unspecified
Congenital anomaly of face bones NOS
Congenital anomaly of skull NOS

● **Q76 Congenital malformations of spine and bony thorax**

> **Excludes 1** congenital musculoskeletal deformities of spine and chest (Q67.5-Q67.8)

Q76.0 Spina bifida occulta

> **Excludes 1** meningocele (spinal) (Q05.-)
> spina bifida (aperta) (cystica) (Q05.-)

Q76.1 Klippel-Feil syndrome
Cervical fusion syndrome

Q76.2 Congenital spondylolisthesis
Congenital spondylolysis

> **Excludes 1** spondylolisthesis (acquired) (M43.1-)
> spondylolysis (acquired) (M43.0-)

Q76.3 Congenital scoliosis due to congenital bony malformation
Hemivertebra fusion or failure of segmentation with scoliosis

Item 17–3 Anencephalus is a congenital deformity of the cranial vault. **Craniosynostosis,** also known as craniostenosis and stenocephaly, signifies any form of congenital deformity of the skull that results from the premature closing of the sutures of the skull. **Iniencephaly** is a deformity in which the head and neck are flexed backward to a great extent and the head is very large in comparison to the shortened body.

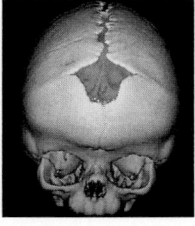

Figure 17-10 Generalized craniosynostosis without symptoms or signs of increased intracranial pressure. (From Goetz C: Textbook of Clinical Neurology, St. Louis, MO, Elsevier, 2007)

Figure 17-11 A. Spina bifida occulta. **B.** Meningocele. **C.** Myelomeningocele. **D.** Myelocystocele (syringomyelocele) or hydromyelia.

Item 17–4 Spina bifida is a midline spinal defect in which one or more vertebrae fail to fuse, leaving an opening in the vertebral canal. When the defect is not visible, it is called spina bifida occulta, and when it is visible, it is called spina bifida cystica.

● Q76.4 **Other** congenital malformations of spine, **not associated with scoliosis**

   ● Q76.41 Congenital **kyphosis**
       Abnormal increase in convexity curvature of thoracic spinal column; AKA humpback

       Q76.411 Congenital kyphosis, **occipito-atlanto-axial region**

       Q76.412 Congenital kyphosis, **cervical** region

       Q76.413 Congenital kyphosis, **cervicothoracic** region

       Q76.414 Congenital kyphosis, **thoracic** region

       Q76.415 Congenital kyphosis, **thoracolumbar** region

       Q76.419 Congenital kyphosis, **unspecified** region

   ● Q76.42 Congenital **lordosis**
       An abnormal increase in curvature of lumbar spine (sway back)

       Q76.425 Congenital lordosis, **thoracolumbar** region

       Q76.426 Congenital lordosis, **lumbar** region

       Q76.427 Congenital lordosis, **lumbosacral** region

       Q76.428 Congenital lordosis, **sacral and sacrococcygeal** region

       Q76.429 Congenital lordosis, **unspecified** region

   Q76.49 **Other** congenital malformations of spine, not associated with scoliosis
       Congenital absence of vertebra NOS
       Congenital fusion of spine NOS
       Congenital malformation of lumbosacral (joint) (region) NOS
       Congenital malformation of spine NOS
       Hemivertebra NOS
       Malformation of spine NOS
       Platyspondylisis NOS
       Supernumerary vertebra NOS

  Q76.5 **Cervical rib**
       Supernumerary rib in cervical region

  Q76.6 **Other** congenital malformations of ribs
       Accessory rib
       Congenital absence of rib
       Congenital fusion of ribs
       Congenital malformation of ribs NOS

    | **Excludes1** | short rib syndrome (Q77.2) |

  Q76.7 **Congenital malformation of sternum**
       Congenital absence of sternum
       Sternum bifidum

  Q76.8 **Other congenital malformations of bony thorax**

  Q76.9 **Congenital malformation of bony thorax, unspecified**

● Q77 **Osteochondrodysplasia with defects of growth of tubular bones and spine**

    | **Excludes1** | mucopolysaccharidosis (E76.0-E76.3) |
    | **Excludes2** | congenital myotonic chondrodystrophy (G71.13) |

  Q77.0 **Achondrogenesis**
       Hypochondrogenesis

  Q77.1 **Thanatophoric short stature**

  Q77.2 **Short rib syndrome**
       Asphyxiating thoracic dysplasia [Jeune]

  Q77.3 **Chondrodysplasia punctata**
       Benign cartilaginous neoplasms

    | **Excludes1** | rhizomelic chondrodysplasia punctata (E71.43) |

  Q77.4 **Achondroplasia**
       Disturbance of epiphyseal chondroblastic growth and maturation, results in dwarfism
       Hypochondroplasia
       Osteosclerosis congenita

  Q77.5 **Diastrophic dysplasia**

  Q77.6 **Chondroectodermal dysplasia**
       Defective development of skin, hair, teeth, with polydactyly and defect of cardiac septum
       Ellis-van Creveld syndrome

  Q77.7 **Spondyloepiphyseal dysplasia**

  Q77.8 **Other osteochondrodysplasia with defects of growth of tubular bones and spine**

  Q77.9 **Osteochondrodysplasia with defects of growth of tubular bones and spine, unspecified**

● Q78 **Other osteochondrodysplasias**
       Disorder of development of bone and cartilage; common cause of dwarfism

    | **Excludes2** | congenital myotonic chondrodystrophy (G71.13) |

  Q78.0 **Osteogenesis imperfecta**
       Fragilitas ossium
       Osteopsathyrosis

  Q78.1 **Polyostotic fibrous dysplasia**
       Albright(-McCune)(-Sternberg) syndrome

  Q78.2 **Osteopetrosis**
       Abnormally dense bone; AKA marble bones disease, ivory bones
       Albers-Schönberg syndrome
       Osteosclerosis NOS

  Q78.3 **Progressive diaphyseal dysplasia**
       Camurati-Engelmann syndrome

  Q78.4 **Enchondromatosis**
       Thinning of overlying cortex of bone and distorted length
       Maffucci's syndrome
       Ollier's disease

  Q78.5 **Metaphyseal dysplasia**
       Disturbance in enchondral bone growth, causing ends of shafts to remain larger than normal in circumference
       Pyle's syndrome

  Q78.6 **Multiple congenital exostoses**
       Diaphyseal aclasis

  Q78.8 **Other specified osteochondrodysplasias**
       Osteopoikilosis

  Q78.9 **Osteochondrodysplasia, unspecified**
       Chondrodystrophy NOS
       AKA skeletal dysplasia (dwarfism) caused by genetic mutations affecting hyaline cartilage capping long bones and vertebrae
       Osteodystrophy NOS

● Q79 **Congenital malformations of musculoskeletal system, not elsewhere classified**

    | **Excludes2** | congenital (sternomastoid) torticollis (Q68.0) |

  Q79.0 **Congenital diaphragmatic hernia**

    | **Excludes1** | congenital hiatus hernia (Q40.1) |

  Q79.1 **Other congenital malformations of diaphragm**
       Absence of diaphragm
       Congenital malformation of diaphragm NOS
       Eventration of diaphragm

  Q79.2 **Exomphalos**
       Abdominal hernia in which part of intestine protrudes at umbilicus; AKA exomphalos and exumbilication
       Omphalocele

    | **Excludes1** | umbilical hernia (K42.-) |

▶ New ➠ Revised ~~deleted~~ Deleted **OGCR** Official Guidelines **X** Assign placeholder X ● Use Additional Character(s)

Excludes 1 Excludes 2 Includes Use additional Code first Code also Key words

Q79.3   **Gastroschisis**
Congenital fissure of anterior abdominal wall often with protrusion of small/large intestine

Q79.4   **Prune belly syndrome**
Congenital prolapse of bladder mucosa
Eagle-Barrett syndrome

● Q79.5   **Other congenital malformations of abdominal wall**
   Excludes1   umbilical hernia (K42.-)

   Q79.51   **Congenital hernia of bladder**

   Q79.59   **Other congenital malformations of abdominal wall**

Q79.6   **Ehlers-Danlos syndrome**
Group of inherited disorders of connective tissue; AKA cutis hyperelastica

Q79.8   **Other congenital malformations of musculoskeletal system**
Absence of muscle
Absence of tendon
Accessory muscle
Amyotrophia congenita
Congenital constricting bands
Congenital shortening of tendon
Poland syndrome

Q79.9   **Congenital malformation of musculoskeletal system, unspecified**
Congenital anomaly of musculoskeletal system NOS
Congenital deformity of musculoskeletal system NOS

OTHER CONGENITAL MALFORMATIONS (Q80-Q89)

● **Q80**   **Congenital ichthyosis**
Characterized by increased keratinization, resulting in noninflammatory scaling of skin
   Excludes1   Refsum's disease (G60.1)

Q80.0   **Ichthyosis vulgaris**

Q80.1   **X-linked ichthyosis**

Q80.2   **Lamellar ichthyosis**
Collodion baby

Q80.3   **Congenital bullous ichthyosiform erythroderma**

Q80.4   **Harlequin fetus**

Q80.8   **Other congenital ichthyosis**

Q80.9   **Congenital ichthyosis, unspecified**

● **Q81**   **Epidermolysis bullosa**
Loosening of epidermis

Q81.0   **Epidermolysis bullosa simplex**
   Excludes1   Cockayne's syndrome (Q87.1)

Q81.1   **Epidermolysis bullosa letalis**
Herlitz' syndrome

Q81.2   **Epidermolysis bullosa dystrophica**

Q81.8   **Other epidermolysis bullosa**

Q81.9   **Epidermolysis bullosa, unspecified**

● **Q82**   **Other congenital malformations of skin**
   Excludes1   acrodermatitis enteropathica (E83.2)
congenital erythropoietic porphyria (E80.0)
pilonidal cyst or sinus (L05.-)
Sturge-Weber (-Dimitri) syndrome (Q85.8)

Q82.0   **Hereditary lymphedema**
Characterized by swelling of subcutaneous tissue caused by obstruction of lymphatic vessels and resulting edema of lymph fluid

Q82.1   **Xeroderma pigmentosum**
Extreme sensitivity to ultraviolet rays that most commonly affects the eyes and skin, but may also involve the nervous system

⟹ Q82.2   **Congenital cutaneous mastocytosis**
Characterized by infiltrates of mast cells in tissues/organs
~~Urticaria pigmentosa~~
▶Congenital diffuse cutaneous mastocytosis
▶Congenital maculopapular cutaneous mastocytosis
▶Congenital urticaria pigmentosa
   Excludes1   ~~malignant mastocytosis (C96.2)~~
▶cutaneous mastocytosis NOS (D47.01)
▶diffuse cutaneous mastocytosis (with onset after newborn period) (D47.01)
▶malignant mastocytosis (C96.2-)
▶systemic mastocytosis (D47.02)
▶urticaria pigmentosa (non-congenital) (with onset after newborn period) (D47.01)

Q82.3   **Incontinentia pigmenti**
Characterized by hypopigmented cutaneous in adults and early childhood

Q82.4   **Ectodermal dysplasia (anhidrotic)**
Absence/deficiency of tissues/structures, including teeth, hair, nails, and certain glands
   Excludes1   Ellis-van Creveld syndrome (Q77.6)

Q82.5   **Congenital non-neoplastic nevus**
Birthmark NOS
Flammeus Nevus
Portwine Nevus
Sanguineous Nevus
Strawberry Nevus
Vascular Nevus NOS
Verrucous Nevus
   Excludes2   Café au lait spots (L81.3)
lentigo (L81.4)
nevus NOS (D22.-)
araneus nevus (I78.1)
melanocytic nevus (D22.-)
pigmented nevus (D22.-)
spider nevus (I78.1)
stellar nevus (I78.1)

Q82.6   **Congenital sacral dimple**
Parasacral dimple
   Excludes2   pilonidal cyst with abscess (L05.01)
pilonidal cyst without abscess (L05.91)

Q82.8   **Other specified congenital malformations of skin**
Abnormal palmar creases
Accessory skin tags
Benign familial pemphigus [Hailey-Hailey]
Congenital poikiloderma
Cutis laxa (hyperelastica)
Dermatoglyphic anomalies
Inherited keratosis palmaris et plantaris
Keratosis follicularis [Darier-White]
   Excludes1   Ehlers-Danlos syndrome (Q79.6)

Q82.9   **Congenital malformation of skin, unspecified**

● **Q83**   **Congenital malformations of breast**
   Excludes2   absence of pectoral muscle (Q79.8)
hypoplasia of breast (N64.82)
micromastia (N64.82)

Q83.0   **Congenital absence of breast with absent nipple**

Q83.1   **Accessory breast**
Supernumerary breast

Q83.2   **Absent nipple**

Q83.3   **Accessory nipple**
Supernumerary nipple

Q83.8   **Other congenital malformations of breast**

Q83.9   **Congenital malformation of breast, unspecified**

CHAPTER 17 (Q00-Q99)

● **Q84 Other congenital malformations of integument**

Q84.0 Congenital alopecia
Congenital atrichosis

Q84.1 Congenital morphological disturbances of hair, not elsewhere classified
Beaded hair
Monilethrix
Pili annulati
>   Excludes1   Menkes' kinky hair syndrome (E83.0)

Q84.2 Other congenital malformations of hair
Congenital hypertrichosis
Congenital malformation of hair NOS
Persistent lanugo

Q84.3 Anonychia
Absence of nail
>   Excludes1   nail patella syndrome (Q87.2)

Q84.4 Congenital leukonychia
Opaque, whitish discoloration of nails; AKA leukopathia unguium

Q84.5 Enlarged and hypertrophic nails
Congenital onychauxis
Pachyonychia

Q84.6 Other congenital malformations of nails
Congenital clubnail
Congenital koilonychia
Congenital malformation of nail NOS

Q84.8 Other specified congenital malformations of integument
Aplasia cutis congenita

Q84.9 Congenital malformation of integument, unspecified
Congenital anomaly of integument NOS
Congenital deformity of integument NOS

● **Q85 Phakomatoses, not elsewhere classified**
>   Excludes1   ataxia telangiectasia [Louis-Bar] (G11.3)
>   familial dysautonomia [Riley-Day] (G90.1)

● **Q85.0 Neurofibromatosis (nonmalignant)**
Developmental changes in nervous system and other structures, with formation of neurofibromas

Q85.00 Neurofibromatosis, unspecified
Q85.01 Neurofibromatosis, type 1
Von Recklinghausen disease
Q85.02 Neurofibromatosis, type 2
Acoustic neurofibromatosis
Q85.03 Schwannomatosis
Q85.09 Other neurofibromatosis

Q85.1 Tuberous sclerosis
Bourneville's disease
Epiloia

Q85.8 Other phakomatoses, not elsewhere classified
Peutz-Jeghers Syndrome
Sturge-Weber(-Dimitri) syndrome
von Hippel-Lindau syndrome
>   Excludes1   Meckel-Gruber syndrome (Q61.9)

Q85.9 Phakomatosis, unspecified
Hamartosis NOS

● **Q86 Congenital malformation syndromes due to known exogenous causes, not elsewhere classified**
>   Excludes2   iodine-deficiency-related hypothyroidism (E00-E02)
>   nonteratogenic effects of substances transmitted via placenta or breast milk (P04.-)

Q86.0 Fetal alcohol syndrome (dysmorphic)

Q86.1 Fetal hydantoin syndrome
Meadow's syndrome

Q86.2 Dysmorphism due to warfarin

Q86.8 Other congenital malformation syndromes due to known exogenous causes

● **Q87 Other specified congenital malformation syndromes affecting multiple systems**
Use additional code(s) to identify all associated manifestations

Q87.0 Congenital malformation syndromes predominantly affecting facial appearance
Acrocephalopolysyndactyly
Acrocephalosyndactyly [Apert]
Cryptophthalmos syndrome
Cyclopia
Goldenhar syndrome
Moebius syndrome
Oro-facial-digital syndrome
Robin syndrome
Whistling face

Q87.1 Congenital malformation syndromes predominantly associated with short stature
Aarskog syndrome
Cockayne syndrome
De Lange syndrome
Dubowitz syndrome
Noonan syndrome
Prader-Willi syndrome
Robinow-Silverman-Smith syndrome
Russell-Silver syndrome
Seckel syndrome
>   Excludes1   Ellis-van Creveld syndrome (Q77.6)
>   Smith-Lemli-Opitz syndrome (E78.72)

Q87.2 Congenital malformation syndromes predominantly involving limbs
Holt-Oram syndrome
Klippel-Trenaunay-Weber syndrome
Nail patella syndrome
Rubinstein-Taybi syndrome
Sirenomelia syndrome
Thrombocytopenia with absent radius [TAR] syndrome
VATER syndrome

Q87.3 Congenital malformation syndromes involving early overgrowth
Beckwith-Wiedemann syndrome
Sotos' syndrome
Weaver syndrome

● **Q87.4 Marfan's syndrome**

Q87.40 Marfan's syndrome, unspecified
● **Q87.41 Marfan's syndrome with cardiovascular manifestations**
Q87.410 Marfan's syndrome with aortic dilation
Q87.418 Marfan's syndrome with other cardiovascular manifestations
Q87.42 Marfan's syndrome with ocular manifestations
Q87.43 Marfan's syndrome with skeletal manifestation

Q87.5 Other congenital malformation syndromes with other skeletal changes

● **Q87.8 Other specified congenital malformation syndromes, not elsewhere classified**
>   Excludes1   Zellweger syndrome (E71.510)

Q87.81 Alport syndrome
Progressive sensorineural hearing loss, progressive pyelonephritis or glomerulonephritis, and ocular defects
Use additional code to identify stage of chronic kidney disease (N18.1-N18.6)

Q87.82 Arterial tortuosity syndrome

Q87.89 Other specified congenital malformation syndromes, not elsewhere classified
Laurence-Moon (-Bardet)-Biedl syndrome

▶ New   ➡ Revised   ~~deleted~~ Deleted   **OGCR** Official Guidelines   X Assign placeholder X   ● Use Additional Character(s)

Excludes 1   Excludes 2   Includes   Use additional   Code first   Code also   Key words

● Q89   Other congenital malformations, not elsewhere classified
  ● Q89.0   Congenital absence and malformations of spleen
            Excludes1   isomerism of atrial appendages (with
                        asplenia or polysplenia) (Q20.6)
    Q89.01   Asplenia (congenital)
    Q89.09   Congenital malformations of spleen
             Congenital splenomegaly
  Q89.1   Congenital malformations of adrenal gland
          Excludes1   adrenogenital disorders (E25.-)
                      congenital adrenal hyperplasia (E25.0)
  Q89.2   Congenital malformations of other endocrine glands
          Congenital malformation of parathyroid or thyroid
             gland
          Persistent thyroglossal duct
          Thyroglossal cyst
          Excludes1   congenital goiter (E03.0)
                      congenital hypothyroidism (E03.1)
  Q89.3   Situs inversus
          Lateral transposition of viscera of thorax and abdomen
          Dextrocardia with situs inversus
          Mirror-image atrial arrangement with situs inversus
          Situs inversus or transversus abdominalis
          Situs inversus or transversus thoracis
          Transposition of abdominal viscera
          Transposition of thoracic viscera
          Excludes1   dextrocardia NOS (Q24.0)
  Q89.4   Conjoined twins
          Craniopagus
          Dicephaly
          Pygopagus
          Thoracopagus
  Q89.7   Multiple congenital malformations, not elsewhere
          classified
          Multiple congenital anomalies NOS
          Multiple congenital deformities NOS
          Excludes1   congenital malformation syndromes
                      affecting multiple systems (Q87.-)
  Q89.8   Other specified congenital malformations
          Use additional code(s) to identify all associated
             manifestations
  Q89.9   Congenital malformation, unspecified
          Congenital anomaly NOS
          Congenital deformity NOS

CHROMOSOMAL ABNORMALITIES, NOT ELSEWHERE CLASSIFIED (Q90-Q99)

          Excludes2   mitochondrial metabolic disorders (E88.4-)

● Q90   Down syndrome
        Use additional code(s) to identify any associated physical
           conditions and degree of intellectual disabilities (F70-F79)
  Q90.0   Trisomy 21, nonmosaicism (meiotic nondisjunction)
          *Trisomy 21, nondisjunction, accounts for 95% of Downs
           syndrome cases*
  Q90.1   Trisomy 21, mosaicism (mitotic nondisjunction)
  Q90.2   Trisomy 21, translocation
  Q90.9   Down syndrome, unspecified
          Trisomy 21 NOS

● Q91   Trisomy 18 and Trisomy 13
  Q91.0   Trisomy 18, nonmosaicism (meiotic nondisjunction)
  Q91.1   Trisomy 18, mosaicism (mitotic nondisjunction)
  Q91.2   Trisomy 18, translocation
  Q91.3   Trisomy 18, unspecified
  Q91.4   Trisomy 13, nonmosaicism (meiotic nondisjunction)
  Q91.5   Trisomy 13, mosaicism (mitotic nondisjunction)
  Q91.6   Trisomy 13, translocation
  Q91.7   Trisomy 13, unspecified

● Q92   Other trisomies and partial trisomies of the autosomes, not
        elsewhere classified
        Includes   unbalanced translocations and insertions
        Excludes1   trisomies of chromosomes 13, 18, 21 (Q90-Q91)
  Q92.0   Whole chromosome trisomy, nonmosaicism (meiotic
          nondisjunction)
  Q92.1   Whole chromosome trisomy, mosaicism (mitotic
          nondisjunction)
  Q92.2   Partial trisomy
          Less than whole arm duplicated
          Whole arm or more duplicated
          Excludes1   partial trisomy due to unbalanced
                      translocation (Q92.5)
  Q92.5   Duplications with other complex rearrangements
          Partial trisomy due to unbalanced translocations
          Code also any associated deletions due to unbalanced
             translocations, inversions and insertions (Q93.7)
  ● Q92.6   Marker chromosomes
          Trisomies due to dicentrics
          Trisomies due to extra rings
          Trisomies due to isochromosomes
          Individual with marker heterochromatin
    Q92.61   Marker chromosomes in normal individual
    Q92.62   Marker chromosomes in abnormal individual
  Q92.7   Triploidy and polyploidy
  Q92.8   Other specified trisomies and partial trisomies of
          autosomes
          Duplications identified by fluorescence in situ
             hybridization (FISH)
          Duplications identified by in situ hybridization (ISH)
          Duplications seen only at prometaphase
  Q92.9   Trisomy and partial trisomy of autosomes, unspecified

● Q93   Monosomies and deletions from the autosomes, not elsewhere
        classified
  Q93.0   Whole chromosome monosomy, nonmosaicism (meiotic
          nondisjunction)
  Q93.1   Whole chromosome monosomy, mosaicism (mitotic
          nondisjunction)
  Q93.2   Chromosome replaced with ring, dicentric or
          isochromosome
  Q93.3   Deletion of short arm of chromosome 4
          Wolff-Hirschorn syndrome
  Q93.4   Deletion of short arm of chromosome 5
          Cri-du-chat syndrome
  Q93.5   Other deletions of part of a chromosome
          Angelman syndrome
  Q93.7   Deletions with other complex rearrangements
          Deletions due to unbalanced translocations, inversions
             and insertions
          Code also any associated duplications due to
             unbalanced translocations, inversions and
             insertions (Q92.5)
  ● Q93.8   Other deletions from the autosomes
    Q93.81   Velo-cardio-facial syndrome
             Deletion 22q11.2
    Q93.88   Other microdeletions Miller-Dieker syndrome
             Smith-Magenis syndrome
    Q93.89   Other deletions from the autosomes
             Deletions identified by fluorescence in situ
                hybridization (FISH)
             Deletions identified by in situ hybridization
                (ISH)
             Deletions seen only at prometaphase
  Q93.9   Deletion from autosomes, unspecified

CHAPTER 17 (Q00-Q99)

▶ New   ⇒ Revised   ~~deleted~~ Deleted   **OGCR** Official Guidelines   **X** Assign placeholder X   ● Use Additional Character(s)
Excludes 1   Excludes 2   Includes   Use additional   Code first   Code also   Key words

● **Q95 Balanced rearrangements and structural markers, not elsewhere classified**

Includes   Robertsonian and balanced reciprocal translocations and insertions

Q95.0 Balanced translocation and insertion in normal individual

Q95.1 Chromosome inversion in normal individual

Q95.2 Balanced autosomal rearrangement in abnormal individual

Q95.3 Balanced sex/autosomal rearrangement in abnormal individual

Q95.5 Individual with autosomal fragile site

Q95.8 Other balanced rearrangements and structural markers

Q95.9 Balanced rearrangement and structural marker, unspecified

● **Q96 Turner's syndrome**

Caused by missing or incomplete X chromosome affecting growth and sexual development

Excludes1   Noonan syndrome (Q87.1)

Q96.0 Karyotype 45, X

Q96.1 Karyotype 46, X iso (Xq)
  Karyotype 46, isochromosome Xq

Q96.2 Karyotype 46, X with abnormal sex chromosome, except iso (Xq)
  Karyotype 46, X with abnormal sex chromosome, except isochromosome Xq

Q96.3 Mosaicism, 45, X/46, XX or XY

Q96.4 Mosaicism, 45, X/other cell line(s) with abnormal sex chromosome

Q96.8 Other variants of Turner's syndrome

Q96.9 Turner's syndrome, unspecified

● **Q97 Other sex chromosome abnormalities, female phenotype, not elsewhere classified**

Excludes1   Turner's syndrome (Q96.-)

Q97.0 Karyotype 47, XXX

Q97.1 Female with more than three X chromosomes

Q97.2 Mosaicism, lines with various numbers of X chromosomes

Q97.3 Female with 46, XY karyotype

Q97.8 Other specified sex chromosome abnormalities, female phenotype

Q97.9 Sex chromosome abnormality, female phenotype, unspecified

● **Q98 Other sex chromosome abnormalities, male phenotype, not elsewhere classified**

Q98.0 Klinefelter syndrome karyotype 47, XXY

Q98.1 Klinefelter syndrome, male with more than two X chromosomes

Q98.3 Other male with 46, XX karyotype

Q98.4 Klinefelter syndrome, unspecified

Q98.5 Karyotype 47, XYY

Q98.6 Male with structurally abnormal sex chromosome

Q98.7 Male with sex chromosome mosaicism

Q98.8 Other specified sex chromosome abnormalities, male phenotype

Q98.9 Sex chromosome abnormality, male phenotype, unspecified

● **Q99 Other chromosome abnormalities, not elsewhere classified**

Q99.0 Chimera 46, XX/46, XY
  Chimera 46, XX/46, XY true hermaphrodite

Q99.1 46, XX true hermaphrodite
  46, XX with streak gonads
  46, XY with streak gonads
  Pure gonadal dysgenesis

Q99.2 Fragile X chromosome
  Fragile X syndrome

Q99.8 Other specified chromosome abnormalities

Q99.9 Chromosomal abnormality, unspecified

▶ New   ⇒ Revised   ~~deleted~~ Deleted   OGCR Official Guidelines   X Assign placeholder X   ● Use Additional Character(s)

Excludes 1   Excludes 2   Includes   Use additional   Code first   Code also   Key words

CHAPTER 18

SYMPTOMS, SIGNS AND ABNORMAL CLINICAL AND LABORATORY FINDINGS, NOT ELSEWHERE CLASSIFIED (R00-R99)

OGCR Chapter-Specific Coding Guidelines

18. **Chapter 18: Symptoms, signs, and abnormal clinical and laboratory findings, not elsewhere classified (R00-R99)**
Chapter 18 includes symptoms, signs, abnormal results of clinical or other investigative procedures, and ill-defined conditions regarding which no diagnosis classifiable elsewhere is recorded. Signs and symptoms that point to a specific diagnosis have been assigned to a category in other chapters of the classification.

a. **Use of symptom codes**
Codes that describe symptoms and signs are acceptable for reporting purposes when a related definitive diagnosis has not been established (confirmed) by the provider.

b. **Use of a symptom code with a definitive diagnosis code**
Codes for signs and symptoms may be reported in addition to a related definitive diagnosis when the sign or symptom is not routinely associated with that diagnosis, such as the various signs and symptoms associated with complex syndromes. The definitive diagnosis code should be sequenced before the symptom code.

Signs or symptoms that are associated routinely with a disease process should not be assigned as additional codes, unless otherwise instructed by the classification.

c. **Combination codes that include symptoms**
ICD-10-CM contains a number of combination codes that identify both the definitive diagnosis and common symptoms of that diagnosis. When using one of these combination codes, an additional code should not be assigned for the symptom.

d. **Repeated falls**
Code R29.6, Repeated falls, is for use for encounters when a patient has recently fallen and the reason for the fall is being investigated.

Code Z91.81, History of falling, is for use when a patient has fallen in the past and is at risk for future falls. When appropriate, both codes R29.6 and Z91.81 may be assigned together.

e. **Coma scale**
The coma scale codes (R40.2-) can be used in conjunction with traumatic brain injury codes, acute cerebrovascular disease or sequelae of cerebrovascular disease codes. These codes are primarily for use by trauma registries, but they may be used in any setting where this information is collected. The coma scale may also be used to assess the status of the central nervous system for other non-trauma conditions, such as monitoring patients in the intensive care unit regardless of medical condition. The coma scale codes should be sequenced after the diagnosis code(s).

These codes, one from each subcategory, are needed to complete the scale. The 7th character indicates when the scale was recorded. The 7th character should match for all three codes.

At a minimum, report the initial score documented on presentation at your facility. This may be a score from the emergency medicine technician (EMT) or in the emergency department. If desired, a facility may choose to capture multiple coma scale scores.

Assign code R40.24, Glasgow coma scale, total score, when only the total score is documented in the medical record and not the individual score(s).

f. **Functional quadriplegia**
GUIDELINE HAS BEEN DELETED EFFECTIVE OCTOBER 1, 2017

g. **SIRS due to Non-Infectious Process**
The systemic inflammatory response syndrome (SIRS) can develop as a result of certain non-infectious disease processes, such as trauma, malignant neoplasm, or pancreatitis. When SIRS is documented with a noninfectious condition, and no subsequent infection is documented, the code for the underlying condition, such as an injury, should be assigned, followed by code R65.10, Systemic inflammatory response syndrome (SIRS) of non-infectious origin without acute organ dysfunction, or code R65.11, Systemic inflammatory response syndrome (SIRS) of non-infectious origin with acute organ dysfunction. If an associated acute organ dysfunction is documented, the appropriate code(s) for the specific type of organ dysfunction(s) should be assigned in addition to code R65.11. If acute organ dysfunction is documented, but it cannot be determined if the acute organ dysfunction is associated with SIRS or due to another condition (e.g., directly due to the trauma), the provider should be queried.

h. **Death NOS**
Code R99, Ill-defined and unknown cause of mortality, is only for use in the very limited circumstance when a patient who has already died is brought into an emergency department or other healthcare facility and is pronounced dead upon arrival. It does not represent the discharge disposition of death.

i. **NIHSS Stroke Scale**
The NIH stroke scale (NIHSS) codes (R29.7- -) can be used in conjunction with acute stroke codes (I63) to identify the patient's neurological status and the severity of the stroke. The stroke scale codes should be sequenced after the acute stroke diagnosis code(s).

At a minimum, report the initial score documented. If desired, a facility may choose to capture multiple stroke scale scores.

See Section I.B.14. for information concerning the medical record documentation that may be used for assignment of the NIHSS codes.

OGCR Section I.B.4.

Signs and symptoms
Codes that describe symptoms and signs, as opposed to diagnoses, are acceptable for reporting purposes when a related definitive diagnosis has not been established (confirmed) by the provider. Chapter 18 of ICD-10-CM, Symptoms, Signs, and Abnormal Clinical and Laboratory Findings, Not Elsewhere Classified (codes R00.0-R99) contains many, but not all codes for symptoms.

CHAPTER 18

SYMPTOMS, SIGNS AND ABNORMAL CLINICAL AND LABORATORY FINDINGS, NOT ELSEWHERE CLASSIFIED (R00-R99)

Note: This chapter includes symptoms, signs, abnormal results of clinical or other investigative procedures, and ill-defined conditions regarding which no diagnosis classifiable elsewhere is recorded.

Signs and symptoms that point rather definitely to a given diagnosis have been assigned to a category in other chapters of the classification. In general, categories in this chapter include the less well-defined conditions and symptoms that, without the necessary study of the case to establish a final diagnosis, point perhaps equally to two or more diseases or to two or more systems of the body. Practically all categories in the chapter could be designated 'not otherwise specified', 'unknown etiology' or 'transient'. The Alphabetical Index should be consulted to determine which symptoms and signs are to be allocated here and which to other chapters. The residual subcategories, numbered .8, are generally provided for other relevant symptoms that cannot be allocated elsewhere in the classification.

The conditions and signs or symptoms included in categories R00-R94 consist of:
(a) cases for which no more specific diagnosis can be made even after all the facts bearing on the case have been investigated;
(b) signs or symptoms existing at the time of initial encounter that proved to be transient and whose causes could not be determined;
(c) provisional diagnosis in a patient who failed to return for further investigation or care;
(d) cases referred elsewhere for investigation or treatment before the diagnosis was made;
(e) cases in which a more precise diagnosis was not available for any other reason;
(f) certain symptoms, for which supplementary information is provided, that represent important problems in medical care in their own right.

Excludes2 abnormal findings on antenatal screening of mother (O28.-)
certain conditions originating in the perinatal period (P04-P96)
signs and symptoms classified in the body system chapters
signs and symptoms of breast (N63, N64.5)

This chapter contains the following blocks:

R00-R09	Symptoms and signs involving the circulatory and respiratory systems
R10-R19	Symptoms and signs involving the digestive system and abdomen
R20-R23	Symptoms and signs involving the skin and subcutaneous tissue
R25-R29	Symptoms and signs involving the nervous and musculoskeletal systems
R30-R39	Symptoms and signs involving the genitourinary system
R40-R46	Symptoms and signs involving cognition, perception, emotional state and behavior
R47-R49	Symptoms and signs involving speech and voice
R50-R69	General symptoms and signs
R70-R79	Abnormal findings on examination of blood, without diagnosis
R80-R82	Abnormal findings on examination of urine, without diagnosis
R83-R89	Abnormal findings on examination of other body fluids, substances and tissues, without diagnosis
R90-R94	Abnormal findings on diagnostic imaging and in function studies, without diagnosis
R97	Abnormal tumor markers
R99	Ill-defined and unknown cause of mortality

SYMPTOMS AND SIGNS INVOLVING THE CIRCULATORY AND RESPIRATORY SYSTEMS (R00-R09)

● **R00 Abnormalities of heart beat**
Excludes1 abnormalities originating in the perinatal period (P29.1-)
Excludes2 specified arrhythmias (I47-I49)

R00.0 Tachycardia, unspecified
Rapid heart rate >100 beats
Rapid heart beat
Sinoauricular tachycardia NOS
Sinus [sinusal] tachycardia NOS
Excludes1 neonatal tachycardia (P29.11)
paroxysmal tachycardia (I47.-)

R00.1 Bradycardia, unspecified
Slow heart rate, <60
Sinoatrial bradycardia
Sinus bradycardia
Slow heart beat
Vagal bradycardia
Use additional code for adverse effect, if applicable, to identify drug (T36-T50 with fifth or sixth character 5)
Excludes1 neonatal bradycardia (P29.12)

R00.2 Palpitations
Awareness of heart beat

R00.8 Other abnormalities of heart beat

R00.9 Unspecified abnormalities of heart beat

● **R01**   **Cardiac murmurs and other cardiac sounds**

> **Excludes1**   cardiac murmurs and sounds originating in the perinatal period (P29.8)

R01.0   **Benign and innocent** cardiac murmurs
> Functional cardiac murmur

R01.1   Cardiac murmur, **unspecified**
> Cardiac bruit NOS
> Heart murmur NOS
> Systolic murmur NOS

R01.2   **Other** cardiac sounds
> Cardiac dullness, increased or decreased
> Precordial friction

OGCR   Section I.C.9.a.7.

> Hypertension, Transient
>
> Assign code R03.0, Elevated blood pressure reading without diagnosis of hypertension, unless patient has an established diagnosis of hypertension. Assign code O13.-, Gestational [pregnancy-induced] hypertension with significant proteinuria, or O14.-, Pre-eclampsia, for transient hypertension of pregnancy.

● **R03**   **Abnormal blood-pressure reading, without diagnosis**

R03.0   **Elevated blood-pressure** reading, without diagnosis of hypertension

> **Note:** This category is to be used to record an episode of elevated blood pressure in a patient in whom no formal diagnosis of hypertension has been made, or as an isolated incidental finding.

R03.1   **Nonspecific low blood-pressure** reading
> **Excludes1**   hypotension (I95.-)
> maternal hypotension syndrome (O26.5-)
> neurogenic orthostatic hypotension (G90.3)

● **R04**   **Hemorrhage from respiratory passages**

R04.0   **Epistaxis**
> Hemorrhage from nose
> Nosebleed

R04.1   **Hemorrhage from throat**
> **Excludes2**   hemoptysis (R04.2)

R04.2   **Hemoptysis**
> Blood-stained sputum
> Cough with hemorrhage

● **R04.8**   **Hemorrhage from other sites in respiratory passages**

R04.81   **Acute idiopathic pulmonary hemorrhage in infants**
> AIPHI
> Acute idiopathic hemorrhage in infants over 28 days old
> **Excludes1**   perinatal pulmonary hemorrhage (P26.-)
> von Willebrand's disease (D68.0)

R04.89   **Hemorrhage from other sites in respiratory passages**
> Pulmonary hemorrhage NOS

R04.9   **Hemorrhage from respiratory passages, unspecified**

● **R05**   **Cough**
> **Excludes1**   cough with hemorrhage (R04.2)
> smoker's cough (J41.0)

● **R06**   **Abnormalities of breathing**
> **Excludes1**   acute respiratory distress syndrome (J80)
> respiratory arrest (R09.2)
> respiratory arrest of newborn (P28.81)
> respiratory distress syndrome of newborn (P22.-)
> respiratory failure (J96.-)
> respiratory failure of newborn (P28.5)

● **R06.0**   **Dyspnea**
> **Excludes1**   tachypnea NOS (R06.82)
> transient tachypnea of newborn (P22.1)

R06.00   **Dyspnea, unspecified**
R06.01   **Orthopnea**
R06.02   **Shortness of breath**
▶ **R06.03**   **Acute respiratory distress**
R06.09   **Other forms of dyspnea**

R06.1   **Stridor**
> *Harsh, high-pitched breath sound*
> **Excludes1**   congenital laryngeal stridor (P28.89)
> laryngismus (stridulus) (J38.5)

R06.2   **Wheezing**
> **Excludes1**   Asthma (J45.-)

R06.3   **Periodic breathing**
> Cheyne-Stokes breathing
> *An abnormal pattern of breathing with gradually increasing and decreasing tidal volume with some periods of apnea*

R06.4   **Hyperventilation**
> **Excludes1**   psychogenic hyperventilation (F45.8)

R06.5   **Mouth breathing**
> **Excludes2**   dry mouth NOS (R68.2)

R06.6   **Hiccough**
> **Excludes1**   psychogenic hiccough (F45.8)

R06.7   **Sneezing**

● **R06.8**   **Other abnormalities of breathing**

R06.81   **Apnea, not elsewhere classified**
> Apnea NOS
> **Excludes1**   apnea (of) newborn (P28.4)
> sleep apnea (G47.3-)
> sleep apnea of newborn (primary) (P28.3)

R06.82   **Tachypnea, not elsewhere classified**
> Tachypnea NOS
> **Excludes1**   transitory tachypnea of newborn (P22.1)

R06.83   **Snoring**
R06.89   **Other abnormalities of breathing**
> Breath-holding (spells)
> Sighing

R06.9   **Unspecified** abnormalities of breathing

● **R07**   **Pain in throat and chest**
> **Excludes1**   epidemic myalgia (B33.0)
> **Excludes2**   jaw pain R68.84
> pain in breast (N64.4)

R07.0   **Pain in throat**
> **Excludes1**   chronic sore throat (J31.2)
> sore throat (acute) NOS (J02.9)
> **Excludes2**   dysphagia (R13.1-)
> pain in neck (M54.2)

R07.1   **Chest** pain on breathing
> Painful respiration

R07.2   **Precordial** pain

● **R07.8**   **Other chest pain**

     R07.81   **Pleurodynia**

         Pleurodynia NOS

         Excludes1   epidemic pleurodynia (B33.0)

     R07.82   **Intercostal pain**

     R07.89   **Other chest pain**

         Anterior chest-wall pain NOS

     R07.9   **Chest pain, unspecified**

● **R09**   **Other symptoms and signs involving the circulatory and respiratory system**

     Excludes1   acute respiratory distress syndrome (J80)

         respiratory arrest of newborn (P28.81)

         respiratory distress syndrome of newborn (P22.0)

         respiratory failure (J96.-)

         respiratory failure of newborn (P28.5)

● **R09.0**   **Asphyxia and hypoxemia**

     Excludes1   asphyxia due to carbon monoxide (T58.-)

         asphyxia due to foreign body in respiratory tract (T17.-)

         birth (intrauterine) asphyxia (P84)

         ~~hypercapnia (R06.4)~~

         hyperventilation (R06.4)

         traumatic asphyxia (T71.-)

     ▶ **Excludes2**   hypercapnia (R06.89)

     R09.01   **Asphyxia**

     R09.02   **Hypoxemia**

     R09.1   **Pleurisy**

         Occurs when double membrane (pleura) lining chest cavity and lung surface becomes inflamed causing sharp pain on inspiration/expiration

         Excludes1   pleurisy with effusion (J90)

     R09.2   **Respiratory arrest**

         Cardiorespiratory failure

         Excludes1   cardiac arrest (I46.-)

         respiratory arrest of newborn (P28.81)

         respiratory distress of newborn (P22.0)

         respiratory failure (J96.-)

         respiratory failure of newborn (P28.5)

         respiratory insufficiency (R06.89)

         respiratory insufficiency of newborn (P28.5)

     R09.3   **Abnormal sputum**

         Abnormal amount of sputum

         Abnormal color of sputum

         Abnormal odor of sputum

         Excessive sputum

         Excludes1   blood-stained sputum (R04.2)

● **R09.8**   **Other specified symptoms and signs involving the circulatory and respiratory systems**

     R09.81   **Nasal congestion**

     R09.82   **Postnasal drip**

     R09.89   **Other specified symptoms and signs involving the circulatory and respiratory systems**

         Bruit (arterial)

         Abnormal chest percussion

         Feeling of foreign body in throat

         Friction sounds in chest

         Chest tympany

         Choking sensation

         Rales

         Wet rattling, clicking, crackling sounds on auscultation

         Weak pulse

         Excludes2   foreign body in throat (T17.2-)

         wheezing (R06.2)

SYMPTOMS AND SIGNS INVOLVING THE DIGESTIVE SYSTEM AND ABDOMEN (R10-R19)

     Excludes2   congenital or infantile pylorospasm (Q40.0)

         gastrointestinal hemorrhage (K92.0-K92.2)

         intestinal obstruction (K56.-)

         newborn gastrointestinal hemorrhage (P54.0-P54.3)

         newborn intestinal obstruction (P76.-)

         pylorospasm (K31.3)

         signs and symptoms involving the urinary system (R30-R39)

         symptoms referable to female genital organs (N94.-)

         symptoms referable to male genital organs (N48-N50)

● **R10**   **Abdominal and pelvic pain**

     Excludes1   renal colic (N23)

     Excludes2   dorsalgia (M54.-)

         flatulence and related conditions (R14.-)

     R10.0   **Acute abdomen**

         Severe abdominal pain (generalized) (with abdominal rigidity)

         Excludes1   abdominal rigidity NOS (R19.3)

         generalized abdominal pain NOS (R10.84)

         localized abdominal pain (R10.1-R10.3-)

● **R10.1**   **Pain localized to upper abdomen**

     R10.10   **Upper abdominal pain, unspecified**

     R10.11   **Right upper quadrant pain**

     R10.12   **Left upper quadrant pain**

     R10.13   **Epigastric pain**

         Dyspepsia

         Excludes1   functional dyspepsia (K30)

     R10.2   **Pelvic and perineal pain**

         Excludes1   vulvodynia (N94.81)

● **R10.3**   **Pain localized to other parts of lower abdomen**

     R10.30   **Lower abdominal pain, unspecified**

     R10.31   **Right lower quadrant pain**

     R10.32   **Left lower quadrant pain**

     R10.33   **Periumbilical pain**

● **R10.8**   **Other abdominal pain**

     ● **R10.81**   **Abdominal tenderness**

         Abdominal tenderness NOS

         R10.811   **Right upper quadrant abdominal tenderness**

         R10.812   **Left upper quadrant abdominal tenderness**

         R10.813   **Right lower quadrant abdominal tenderness**

         R10.814   **Left lower quadrant abdominal tenderness**

         R10.815   **Periumbilic abdominal tenderness**

         R10.816   **Epigastric abdominal tenderness**

         R10.817   **Generalized abdominal tenderness**

         R10.819   **Abdominal tenderness, unspecified site**

● **R10.82** **Rebound** abdominal tenderness

    R10.821 **Right upper** quadrant rebound abdominal tenderness

    R10.822 **Left upper** quadrant rebound abdominal tenderness

    R10.823 **Right lower** quadrant rebound abdominal tenderness

    R10.824 **Left lower** quadrant rebound abdominal tenderness

    R10.825 **Periumbilic** rebound abdominal tenderness

    R10.826 **Epigastric** rebound abdominal tenderness

    R10.827 **Generalized** rebound abdominal tenderness

    R10.829 **Rebound** abdominal tenderness, **unspecified site**

  R10.83 **Colic**

    Colic NOS

    Infantile colic

    | **Excludes1** | colic in adult and child over 12 months old (R10.84) |

  R10.84 **Generalized abdominal pain**

    | **Excludes1** | generalized abdominal pain associated with acute abdomen (R10.0) |

R10.9 **Unspecified** abdominal pain

● **R11** **Nausea and vomiting**

  | **Excludes1** | cyclical vomiting associated with migraine (G43.A-)
excessive vomiting in pregnancy (O21.-)
hematemesis (K92.0)
neonatal hematemesis (P54.0)
newborn vomiting (P92.0-)
psychogenic vomiting (F50.89)
vomiting associated with bulimia nervosa (F50.2)
vomiting following gastrointestinal surgery (K91.0) |

● **R11.0** **Nausea**

    Nausea NOS

    Nausea without vomiting

● **R11.1** **Vomiting**

  R11.10 **Vomiting, unspecified**

    Vomiting NOS

  R11.11 **Vomiting without nausea**

  R11.12 **Projectile** vomiting

  R11.13 **Vomiting of fecal matter**

  R11.14 **Bilious** vomiting

    Bilious emesis

R11.2 **Nausea with vomiting, unspecified**

    Persistent nausea with vomiting NOS

R12 **Heartburn**

  | **Excludes1** | dyspepsia NOS (R10.13)
functional dyspepsia (K30) |

● **R13** **Aphagia and dysphagia**

  R13.0 **Aphagia**

    Inability to swallow

    | **Excludes1** | psychogenic aphagia (F50.9) |

● **R13.1** **Dysphagia**

    Difficulty swallowing

    Code first, if applicable, dysphagia following cerebrovascular disease (I69. with final characters -91)

    | **Excludes1** | psychogenic dysphagia (F45.8) |

  R13.10 **Dysphagia, unspecified**

    Difficulty in swallowing NOS

  R13.11 **Dysphagia, oral phase**

  R13.12 **Dysphagia, oropharyngeal phase**

  R13.13 **Dysphagia, pharyngeal phase**

  R13.14 **Dysphagia, pharyngoesophageal phase**

  R13.19 **Other dysphagia**

    Cervical dysphagia

    Neurogenic dysphagia

● **R14** **Flatulence and related conditions**

  | **Excludes1** | psychogenic aerophagy (F45.8) |

  R14.0 **Abdominal distension (gaseous)**

    Bloating

    Tympanites (abdominal) (intestinal)

  R14.1 **Gas pain**

  R14.2 **Eructation**

    Belching air from stomach through mouth

  R14.3 **Flatulence**

● **R15** **Fecal incontinence**

  | **Includes** | encopresis NOS |

  | **Excludes1** | fecal incontinence of nonorganic origin (F98.1) |

  R15.0 **Incomplete defecation**

    | **Excludes1** | constipation (K59.0-)
fecal impaction (K56.41) |

  R15.1 **Fecal smearing**

    Fecal soiling

  R15.2 **Fecal urgency**

  R15.9 **Full incontinence of feces**

    Fecal incontinence NOS

● **R16** **Hepatomegaly and splenomegaly, not elsewhere classified**

  Enlargement of liver or spleen

  R16.0 **Hepatomegaly, not elsewhere classified**

    Hepatomegaly NOS

  R16.1 **Splenomegaly, not elsewhere classified**

    Splenomegaly NOS

  R16.2 **Hepatomegaly with splenomegaly, not elsewhere classified**

    Hepatosplenomegaly NOS

R17 **Unspecified jaundice**

  | **Excludes1** | neonatal jaundice (P55, P57-P59) |

● **R18** **Ascites**

  | **Includes** | fluid in peritoneal cavity |

  | **Excludes1** | ascites in alcoholic cirrhosis (K70.31)
ascites in alcoholic hepatitis (K70.11)
ascites in toxic liver disease with chronic active hepatitis (K71.51) |

  R18.0 **Malignant ascites**

    Code first malignancy, such as:

      malignant neoplasm of ovary (C56.-)

      secondary malignant neoplasm of retroperitoneum and peritoneum (C78.6)

  R18.8 **Other ascites**

    Ascites NOS

    Peritoneal effusion (chronic)

CHAPTER 18 (R00-R99)

● **R19**   **Other symptoms and signs involving the digestive system and abdomen**
> **Excludes1**   acute abdomen (R10.0)

● **R19.0**   **Intra-abdominal and pelvic swelling, mass and lump**
> **Excludes1**   abdominal distension (gaseous) (R14.-)
> ascites (R18.-)

R19.00   Intra-abdominal and pelvic swelling, mass and lump, unspecified site

R19.01   Right upper quadrant abdominal swelling, mass and lump

R19.02   Left upper quadrant abdominal swelling, mass and lump

R19.03   Right lower quadrant abdominal swelling, mass and lump

R19.04   Left lower quadrant abdominal swelling, mass and lump

R19.05   Periumbilic swelling, mass or lump
> Diffuse or generalized umbilical swelling or mass

R19.06   Epigastric swelling, mass or lump

R19.07   Generalized intra-abdominal and pelvic swelling, mass and lump
> Diffuse or generalized intra-abdominal swelling or mass NOS
> Diffuse or generalized pelvic swelling or mass NOS

R19.09   Other intra-abdominal and pelvic swelling, mass and lump

● **R19.1**   **Abnormal bowel sounds**
R19.11   Absent bowel sounds
R19.12   Hyperactive bowel sounds
R19.15   Other abnormal bowel sounds
> Abnormal bowel sounds NOS

R19.2   **Visible peristalsis**
> Hyperperistalsis

● **R19.3**   **Abdominal rigidity**
> **Excludes1**   abdominal rigidity with severe abdominal pain (R10.0)

R19.30   Abdominal rigidity, unspecified site
R19.31   Right upper quadrant abdominal rigidity
R19.32   Left upper quadrant abdominal rigidity
R19.33   Right lower quadrant abdominal rigidity
R19.34   Left lower quadrant abdominal rigidity
R19.35   Periumbilic abdominal rigidity
R19.36   Epigastric abdominal rigidity
R19.37   Generalized abdominal rigidity

R19.4   **Change in bowel habit**
> **Excludes1**   constipation (K59.0-)
> functional diarrhea (K59.1)

R19.5   **Other fecal abnormalities**
> Abnormal stool color
> Bulky stools
> Mucus in stools
> Occult blood in feces
> Occult blood in stools
> **Excludes1**   melena (K92.1)
> neonatal melena (P54.1)

R19.6   **Halitosis**

R19.7   **Diarrhea, unspecified**
> Diarrhea NOS
> **Excludes1**   functional diarrhea (K59.1)
> neonatal diarrhea (P78.3)
> psychogenic diarrhea (F45.8)

R19.8   **Other specified symptoms and signs involving the digestive system and abdomen**

SYMPTOMS AND SIGNS INVOLVING THE SKIN AND SUBCUTANEOUS TISSUE (R20-R23)
> **Excludes2**   symptoms relating to breast (N64.4-N64.5)

● **R20**   **Disturbances of skin sensation**
> **Excludes1**   dissociative anesthesia and sensory loss (F44.6)
> psychogenic disturbances (F45.8)

R20.0   Anesthesia of skin
> *Loss of sensation*

R20.1   Hypoesthesia of skin
> *Unpleasant abnormal sensation*

R20.2   Paresthesia of skin
> *Abnormal touch sensation, including burning, prickling, often in absence of external stimulus*
> Formication   Tingling skin
> Pins and needles
> **Excludes1**   acroparesthesia (I73.8)

R20.3   Hyperesthesia
R20.8   Other disturbances of skin sensation
R20.9   Unspecified disturbances of skin sensation

R21   **Rash and other nonspecific skin eruption**
> **Includes**   rash NOS
> **Excludes1**   specified type of rash- code to condition
> vesicular eruption (R23.8)

● **R22**   **Localized swelling, mass and lump of skin and subcutaneous tissue**
> **Includes**   subcutaneous nodules (localized) (superficial)
> **Excludes1**   abnormal findings on diagnostic imaging (R90-R93)
> edema (R60.-)
> enlarged lymph nodes (R59.-)
> localized adiposity (E65)
> swelling of joint (M25.4-)

R22.0   Localized swelling, mass and lump, head
R22.1   Localized swelling, mass and lump, neck
R22.2   Localized swelling, mass and lump, trunk
> **Excludes1**   intra-abdominal or pelvic mass and lump (R19.0-)
> intra-abdominal or pelvic swelling (R19.0-)
> **Excludes2**   breast mass and lump (N63)

● **R22.3**   Localized swelling, mass and lump, upper limb
R22.30   Localized swelling, mass and lump, unspecified upper limb
R22.31   Localized swelling, mass and lump, right upper limb
R22.32   Localized swelling, mass and lump, left upper limb
R22.33   Localized swelling, mass and lump, upper limb, bilateral

● **R22.4**   Localized swelling, mass and lump, lower limb
R22.40   Localized swelling, mass and lump, unspecified lower limb
R22.41   Localized swelling, mass and lump, right lower limb
R22.42   Localized swelling, mass and lump, left lower limb
R22.43   Localized swelling, mass and lump, lower limb, bilateral

R22.9   Localized swelling, mass and lump, unspecified

● **R23   Other skin changes**

    R23.0   Cyanosis
> | **Excludes1** | acrocyanosis (I73.8)
> | | cyanotic attacks of newborn (P28.2)

    R23.1   Pallor
         Clammy skin

    R23.2   Flushing
         Excessive blushing
         Code first, if applicable, menopausal and female climacteric states (N95.1)

    R23.3   Spontaneous ecchymoses
         Small hemorrhagic spot of skin; AKA black and blue spot
         Petechiae
> | **Excludes1** | ecchymoses of newborn (P54.5)
> | | purpura (D69.-)

    R23.4   Changes in skin texture
         Desquamation of skin   Scaling of skin
         Induration of skin
> | **Excludes1** | epidermal thickening NOS (L85.9)

    R23.8   Other skin changes

    R23.9   Unspecified skin changes

SYMPTOMS AND SIGNS INVOLVING THE NERVOUS AND MUSCULOSKELETAL SYSTEMS (R25-R29)

● **R25   Abnormal involuntary movements**
> | **Excludes1** | specific movement disorders (G20-G26)
> | | stereotyped movement disorders (F98.4)
> | | tic disorders (F95.-)

    R25.0   Abnormal head movements

    R25.1   Tremor, unspecified
> | **Excludes1** | chorea NOS (G25.5)
> | | essential tremor (G25.0)
> | | hysterical tremor (F44.4)
> | | intention tremor (G25.2)

    R25.2   Cramp and spasm
> | **Excludes2** | carpopedal spasm (R29.0)
> | | charley-horse (M62.831)
> | | infantile spasms (G40.4-)
> | | muscle spasm of back (M62.830)
> | | muscle spasm of calf (M62.831)

    R25.3   Fasciculation
         Twitching NOS

    R25.8   Other abnormal involuntary movements

    R25.9   Unspecified abnormal involuntary movements

● **R26   Abnormalities of gait and mobility**
> | **Excludes1** | ataxia NOS (R27.0)
> | | hereditary ataxia (G11.-)
> | | locomotor (syphilitic) ataxia (A52.11)
> | | immobility syndrome (paraplegic) (M62.3)

    R26.0   Ataxic gait
         Staggering gait

    R26.1   Paralytic gait
         Spastic gait

    R26.2   Difficulty in walking, not elsewhere classified
> | **Excludes1** | falling (R29.6)
> | | unsteadiness on feet (R26.81)

   ● **R26.8   Other abnormalities of gait and mobility**
        R26.81   Unsteadiness on feet
        R26.89   Other abnormalities of gait and mobility

    R26.9   Unspecified abnormalities of gait and mobility

● **R27   Other lack of coordination**
> | **Excludes1** | ataxic gait (R26.0)
> | | hereditary ataxia (G11.-)
> | | vertigo NOS (R42)

    R27.0   Ataxia, unspecified
> | **Excludes1** | ataxia following cerebrovascular disease (I69. with final characters -93)

    R27.8   Other lack of coordination

    R27.9   Unspecified lack of coordination

● **R29   Other symptoms and signs involving the nervous and musculoskeletal systems**

    R29.0   Tetany
         Hyperexcitability of nerves and muscles characterized by spasm, twitching, and cramps
         Carpopedal spasm
> | **Excludes1** | hysterical tetany (F44.5)
> | | neonatal tetany (P71.3)
> | | parathyroid tetany (E20.9)
> | | post-thyroidectomy tetany (E89.2)

    R29.1   Meningismus

    R29.2   Abnormal reflex
> | **Excludes2** | abnormal pupillary reflex (H57.0)
> | | hyperactive gag reflex (J39.2)
> | | vasovagal reaction or syncope (R55)

    R29.3   Abnormal posture

    R29.4   Clicking hip
> | **Excludes1** | congenital deformities of hip (Q65.-)

    R29.5   Transient paralysis
         Code first any associated spinal cord injury (S14.0, S14.1-, S24.0, S24.1-, S34.0-, S34.1-)
> | **Excludes1** | transient ischemic attack (G45.9)

    R29.6   Repeated falls
         Falling
         Tendency to fall
> | **Excludes2** | at risk for falling (Z91.81)
> | | history of falling (Z91.81)

        OGCR   Section I.C.18.d.

> Repeated falls
>
> Code R29.6, Repeated falls, is for use for encounters when a patient has recently fallen and the reason for the fall is being investigated.
>
> Code Z91.81, History of falling, is for use when a patient has fallen in the past and is at risk for future falls. When appropriate, both codes R29.6 and Z91.81 may be assigned together.

● **R29.7   National Institutes of Health Stroke Scale (NIHSS) score**
         Code first the type of cerebral infarction (I63-)

   ● **R29.70   NIHSS score 0-9**
        R29.700   NIHSS score 0
        R29.701   NIHSS score 1
        R29.702   NIHSS score 2
        R29.703   NIHSS score 3
        R29.704   NIHSS score 4
        R29.705   NIHSS score 5
        R29.706   NIHSS score 6
        R29.707   NIHSS score 7
        R29.708   NIHSS score 8
        R29.709   NIHSS score 9

   ● **R29.71   NIHSS score 10-19**
        R29.710   NIHSS score 10
        R29.711   NIHSS score 11
        R29.712   NIHSS score 12
        R29.713   NIHSS score 13
        R29.714   NIHSS score 14
        R29.715   NIHSS score 15
        R29.716   NIHSS score 16
        R29.717   NIHSS score 17
        R29.718   NIHSS score 18
        R29.719   NIHSS score 19

CHAPTER 18 (R00-R99)

OGCR Section I.C.18.i.

> **NIHSS Stroke Scale**
> The NIH stroke scale (NIHSS) codes (R29.7- -) can be used in conjunction with acute stroke codes (I63) to identify the patient's neurological status and the severity of the stroke. The stroke scale codes should be sequenced after the acute stroke diagnosis code(s).
>
> At a minimum, report the initial score documented. If desired, a facility may choose to capture multiple stroke scale scores.

● R29.72   NIHSS score 20-29
    R29.720   NIHSS score 20
    R29.721   NIHSS score 21
    R29.722   NIHSS score 22
    R29.723   NIHSS score 23
    R29.724   NIHSS score 24
    R29.725   NIHSS score 25
    R29.726   NIHSS score 26
    R29.727   NIHSS score 27
    R29.728   NIHSS score 28
    R29.729   NIHSS score 29

● R29.73   NIHSS score 30-39
    R29.730   NIHSS score 30
    R29.731   NIHSS score 31
    R29.732   NIHSS score 32
    R29.733   NIHSS score 33
    R29.734   NIHSS score 34
    R29.735   NIHSS score 35
    R29.736   NIHSS score 36
    R29.737   NIHSS score 37
    R29.738   NIHSS score 38
    R29.739   NIHSS score 39

● R29.74   NIHSS score 40-42
    R29.740   NIHSS score 40
    R29.741   NIHSS score 41
    R29.742   NIHSS score 42

● R29.8   Other symptoms and signs involving the nervous and musculoskeletal systems

● R29.81   Other symptoms and signs involving the nervous system

    R29.810   Facial weakness
      Facial droop
      Excludes1   Bell's palsy (G51.0)
        facial weakness following cerebrovascular disease (I69. with final characters -92)

    R29.818   Other symptoms and signs involving the nervous system

● R29.89   Other symptoms and signs involving the musculoskeletal system
      Excludes2   pain in limb (M79.6-)

    R29.890   Loss of height
      Excludes1   osteoporosis (M80-M81)

    R29.891   Ocular torticollis
      Excludes1   congenital (sterno-mastoid) torticollis Q68.0
        psychogenic torticollis (F45.8)
        spasmodic torticollis (G24.3)
        torticollis due to birth injury (P15.8)
        torticollis NOS M43.6

    R29.898   Other symptoms and signs involving the musculoskeletal system

● R29.9   Unspecified symptoms and signs involving the nervous and musculoskeletal systems

    R29.90   Unspecified symptoms and signs involving the nervous system

    R29.91   Unspecified symptoms and signs involving the musculoskeletal system

SYMPTOMS AND SIGNS INVOLVING THE GENITOURINARY SYSTEM (R30-R39)

● R30   Pain associated with micturition
    Excludes1   psychogenic pain associated with micturition (F45.8)

    R30.0   Dysuria
      Painful urination
      Strangury

    R30.1   Vesical tenesmus
      Straining to urinate, with sensation of a full bladder even when empty

    R30.9   Painful micturition, unspecified
      Painful urination NOS

● R31   Hematuria
    Excludes1   hematuria included with underlying conditions, such as:
      acute cystitis with hematuria (N30.01)
      recurrent and persistent hematuria in glomerular diseases (N02.-)

    R31.0   Gross hematuria
    R31.1   Benign essential microscopic hematuria
   ● R31.2   Other microscopic hematuria
      R31.21   Asymptomatic microscopic hematuria
        AMH
      R31.29   Other microscopic hematuria
    R31.9   Hematuria, unspecified

  R32   Unspecified urinary incontinence
    Enuresis NOS
    Excludes1   functional urinary incontinence (R39.81)
      nonorganic enuresis (F98.0)
      stress incontinence and other specified urinary incontinence (N39.3-N39.4-)
      urinary incontinence associated with cognitive impairment (R39.81)

● R33   Retention of urine
    Excludes1   psychogenic retention of urine (F45.8)

    R33.0   Drug induced retention of urine
      Use additional code for adverse effect, if applicable, to identify drug (T36-T50 with fifth or sixth character 5)

    R33.8   Other retention of urine
      Code first, if applicable, any causal condition, such as:
      enlarged prostate (N40.1)

    R33.9   Retention of urine, unspecified

  R34   Anuria and oliguria
    Excludes1   anuria and oliguria complicating abortion or ectopic or molar pregnancy (O00-O07, O08.4)
      anuria and oliguria complicating pregnancy (O26.83-)
      anuria and oliguria complicating the puerperium (O90.4)

▶ New   ➡ Revised   ~~deleted~~ Deleted   **OGCR** Official Guidelines   **X** Assign placeholder X   ● Use Additional Character(s)

Excludes 1   Excludes 2   Includes   Use additional   Code first   Code also   Key words

● **R35**   **Polyuria**
Passage of excessive volume of urine
Code first, *if applicable, any causal condition, such as:*
     enlarged prostate (N40.1)
     Excludes1   psychogenic polyuria (F45.8)

     R35.0   **Frequency of micturition**
         Discharge or passage of urine; AKA uresis

     R35.1   **Nocturia**
         Urinary frequency at night

     R35.8   **Other polyuria**
         Polyuria NOS

● **R36**   **Urethral discharge**

     R36.0   **Urethral discharge without blood**

     R36.1   **Hematospermia**
         Presence of blood in semen

     R36.9   **Urethral discharge, unspecified**
         Penile discharge NOS
         Urethrorrhea

R37   **Sexual dysfunction, unspecified**

● **R39**   **Other and unspecified symptoms and signs involving the genitourinary system**

     R39.0   **Extravasation of urine**
         Leakage, discharge

     ● **R39.1**   **Other difficulties with micturition**
         Code first, *if applicable, any causal condition, such as:*
           enlarged prostate (N40.1)

         R39.11   **Hesitancy of micturition**

         R39.12   **Poor urinary stream**
              Weak urinary steam

         R39.13   **Splitting of urinary stream**

         R39.14   **Feeling of incomplete bladder emptying**

         R39.15   **Urgency of urination**
              Excludes1   urge incontinence (N39.41, N39.46)

         R39.16   **Straining to void**

         ● **R39.19**   **Other difficulties with micturition**

              R39.191   **Need to immediately re-void**

              R39.192   **Position dependent micturition**

              R39.198   **Other difficulties with micturition**

     R39.2   **Extrarenal uremia**
         Prerenal uremia
         Excludes1   uremia NOS (N19)

     ● **R39.8**   **Other symptoms and signs involving the genitourinary system**

         R39.81   **Functional urinary incontinence**
              Urinary incontinence due to cognitive impairment, or severe physical disability or immobility
              Excludes1   stress incontinence and other specified urinary incontinence (N39.3-N39.4-) urinary incontinence NOS (R32)

         R39.82   **Chronic bladder pain**

         ▶ **R39.83**   **Unilateral non-palpable testicle**

         ▶ **R39.84**   **Bilateral non-palpable testicles**

         R39.89   **Other symptoms and signs involving the genitourinary system**

     R39.9   **Unspecified symptoms and signs involving the genitourinary system**

SYMPTOMS AND SIGNS INVOLVING COGNITION, PERCEPTION, EMOTIONAL STATE AND BEHAVIOR (R40-R46)

     Excludes2   symptoms and signs constituting part of a pattern of mental disorder (F01-F99)

● **R40**   **Somnolence, stupor and coma**
     Excludes1   neonatal coma (P91.5)
              somnolence, stupor and coma in diabetes (E08-E13)
              somnolence, stupor and coma in hepatic failure (K72.-)
              somnolence, stupor and coma in hypoglycemia (nondiabetic) (E15)

     R40.0   **Somnolence**
         Drowsiness
         Excludes1   coma (R40.2-)

     R40.1   **Stupor**
         Lowered level of consciousness
         Catatonic stupor
         Semicoma
         Excludes1   catatonic schizophrenia (F20.2)
              coma (R40.2-)
              depressive stupor (F31-F33)
              dissociative stupor (F44.2)
              manic stupor (F30.2)

OGCR   Section I.C.18.e.

Coma scale

The coma scale codes (R40.2-) can be used in conjunction with traumatic brain injury codes, acute cerebrovascular disease or sequelae of cerebrovascular disease codes. These codes are primarily for use by trauma registries, but they may be used in any setting where this information is collected. **The coma scale may also be used to assess the status of the central nervous system for other non-trauma conditions, such as monitoring patients in the intensive care unit regardless of medical condition.** The coma scale codes should be sequenced after the diagnosis code(s).

These codes, one from each subcategory, are needed to complete the scale. The 7th character indicates when the scale was recorded. The 7th character should match for all three codes.

At a minimum, report the initial score documented on presentation at your facility. This may be a score from the emergency medicine technician (EMT) or in the emergency department. If desired, a facility may choose to capture multiple coma scale scores.

Assign code R40.24, Glasgow coma scale, total score, when only the total score is documented in the medical record and not the individual score(s).

● **R40.2**   **Coma**
     Code first any associated:
         fracture of skull (S02.-)
         intracranial injury (S06.-)
     Note: One code from each subcategory R40.21-R40-23 is required to complete the coma scale

     R40.20   **Unspecified coma**
         Coma NOS
         Unconsciousness NOS

     ● **R40.21**   **Coma scale, eyes open**

         The following appropriate 7th character is to be added to subcategory R40.21-:

         0   unspecified time
         1   in the field [EMT or ambulance]
         2   at arrival to emergency department
         3   at hospital admission
         4   24 hours or more after hospital admission

         ● **R40.211**   **Coma scale, eyes open, never**

         ● **R40.212**   **Coma scale, eyes open, to pain**

         ● **R40.213**   **Coma scale, eyes open, to sound**

         ● **R40.214**   **Coma scale, eyes open, spontaneous**

CHAPTER 18 (R00-R99)

Glasgow Coma Scale

Eye Opening Response	
• Spontaneous--open with blinking at baseline	4 points
• To verbal stimuli, command, speech	3 points
• To pain only (not applied to face)	2 points
• No response	1 point
Verbal Response	
• Oriented	5 points
• Confused conversation, but able to answer questions	4 points
• Inappropriate words	3 points
• Incomprehensible speech	2 points
• No response	1 point
Motor Response	
• Obeys commands for movement	6 points
• Purposeful movement to painful stimulus	5 points
• Withdraws in response to pain	4 points
• Flexion in response to pain (decorticate posturing)	3 points
• Extension response in response to pain (decerebrate posturing)	2 points
• No response	1 point
Categorization: Coma: No eye opening, no ability to follow commands, no word verbalizations (3-8)	
Head Injury Classification: Severe Head Injury--GCS score of 8 or less Moderate Head Injury--GCS score of 9 to 12 Mild head injury--GCS score of 13 to 15	
(Adapted from: Advanced Trauma Life Support: Course for Physicians, American College of Surgeons, 1993). http://www.bt.cdc.gov/masscasulatires/gscale.asp	

Figure 18-1

● R40.22   Coma scale, best verbal response

The following appropriate 7th character is to be added to subcategory R40.22-:

0	unspecified time
1	in the field [EMT or ambulance]
2	at arrival to emergency department
3	at hospital admission
4	24 hours or more after hospital admission

● R40.221   Coma scale, best verbal response, none

● R40.222   Coma scale, best verbal response, incomprehensible words
  ▶Incomprehensible sounds (2-5 years of age)
  ▶Moans/grunts to pain; restless (<2 years old)

● R40.223   Coma scale, best verbal response, inappropriate words
  ▶Inappropriate crying or screaming (< 2 years of age)
  ▶Screaming (2-5 years of age)

● R40.224   Coma scale, best verbal response, confused conversation
  ▶Inappropriate words (2-5 years of age)
  ▶Irritable cries (< 2 years of age)

● R40.225   Coma scale, best verbal response, oriented
  ▶Cooing or babbling or crying appropriately (< 2 years of age)
  ▶Uses appropriate words (2- 5 years of age)

● R40.23   Coma scale, best motor response

The following appropriate 7th character is to be added to subcategory R40.23-:

0	unspecified time
1	in the field [EMT or ambulance]
2	at arrival to emergency department
3	at hospital admission
4	24 hours or more after hospital admission

● R40.231   Coma scale, best motor response, none

● R40.232   Coma scale, best motor response, extension
  ▶Abnormal extensor posturing to pain or noxious stimuli (< 2 years of age)
  ▶Extensor posturing to pain or noxious stimuli (2-5 years of age)

● R40.233   Coma scale, best motor response, abnormal
  ▶Abnormal flexure posturing to pain or noxious stimuli (0-5 years of age)
  ▶Flexion/decorticate posturing (< 2 years of age)

● R40.234   Coma scale, best motor response, flexion withdrawal
  ▶Withdraws from pain or noxious stimuli (0-5 years of age)

● R40.235   Coma scale, best motor response, localizes pain
  ▶Localizes pain (2-5 years of age)
  ▶Withdraws to touch (< 2 years of age)

● R40.236   Coma scale, best motor response, obeys commands
  ▶Normal or spontaneous movement (< 2 years of age)
  ▶Obeys commands (2-5 years of age)

● R40.24   Glasgow coma scale, total score
Note: Assign a code from subcategory R40.24, when only the total coma score is documented
The following appropriate 7th character is to be added to subcategory R40.24-:

0	unspecified time
1	in the field [EMT or ambulance]
2	at arrival to emergency department
3	at hospital admission
4	24 hours or more after hospital admission

● R40.241   Glasgow coma scale score 13-15
● R40.242   Glasgow coma scale score 9-12
● R40.243   Glasgow coma scale score 3-8
● R40.244   Other coma, without documented Glasgow coma scale score, or with partial score reported

R40.3   Persistent vegetative state
R40.4   Transient alteration of awareness

▶ New   ⇨ Revised   deleted Deleted   **OGCR** Official Guidelines   X Assign placeholder X   ● Use Additional Character(s)

Excludes 1   Excludes 2   Includes   Use additional   Code first   Code also   Key words

● R41 **Other symptoms and signs involving cognitive functions and awareness**
> | Excludes1 | dissociative [conversion] disorders (F44.-)
> | | mild cognitive impairment, so stated (G31.84)

R41.0 **Disorientation, unspecified**
  Confusion NOS   Delirium NOS

R41.1 **Anterograde amnesia**

R41.2 **Retrograde amnesia**

R41.3 **Other amnesia**
  Amnesia NOS
  Memory loss NOS
> | Excludes1 | amnestic disorder due to known physiologic condition (F04)
> | | amnestic syndrome due to psychoactive substance use (F10-F19 with 5th character .6)
> | | mild memory disturbance due to known physiological condition (F06.8)
> | | transient global amnesia (G45.4)

R41.4 **Neurologic neglect syndrome**
  Asomatognosia   Left-sided neglect
  Hemi-akinesia   Sensory neglect
  Hemi-inattention   Visuospatial neglect
  Hemispatial neglect
> | Excludes1 | visuospatial deficit (R41.842)

● R41.8 **Other symptoms and signs involving cognitive functions and awareness**

R41.81 **Age-related cognitive decline**
  Senility NOS

R41.82 **Altered mental status, unspecified**
  Change in mental status NOS
> | Excludes1 | altered level of consciousness (R40.-)
> | | altered mental status due to known condition - code to condition
> | | delirium NOS (R41.0)

R41.83 **Borderline intellectual functioning**
  IQ level 71 to 84
> | Excludes1 | intellectual disabilities (F70-F79)

● R41.84 **Other specified cognitive deficit**
> | Excludes1 | cognitive deficits as sequelae of cerebrovascular disease (I69.01-, I69.11-, I69.21-, I69.31-, I69.81-, I69.91-)

R41.840 **Attention and concentration deficit**
> | Excludes1 | attention-deficit hyperactivity disorders (F90.-)

R41.841 **Cognitive communication deficit**

R41.842 **Visuospatial deficit**

R41.843 **Psychomotor deficit**

R41.844 **Frontal lobe and executive function deficit**

R41.89 **Other symptoms and signs involving cognitive functions and awareness**
  Anosognosia

R41.9 **Unspecified symptoms and signs involving cognitive functions and awareness**
  ▶Unspecified neurocognitive disorder

R42 **Dizziness and giddiness**
  Light-headedness
  Vertigo NOS
> | Excludes1 | vertiginous syndromes (H81.-)
> | | vertigo from infrasound (T75.23)

● R43 **Disturbances of smell and taste**

R43.0 **Anosmia**
  Absence of sense of smell; AKA anosphresia and olfactory anesthesia

R43.1 **Parosmia**

R43.2 **Parageusia**
  Perversion of sense of taste or bad taste in mouth; AKA dysgeusia

R43.8 **Other disturbances of smell and taste**
  Mixed disturbance of smell and taste

R43.9 **Unspecified disturbances of smell and taste**

● R44 **Other symptoms and signs involving general sensations and perceptions**
> | Excludes1 | alcoholic hallucinations (F1.5)
> | | hallucinations in drug psychosis (F11-F19 with .5)
> | | hallucinations in mood disorders with psychotic symptoms (F30.2, F31.5, F32.3, F33.3)
> | | hallucinations in schizophrenia, schizotypal and delusional disorders (F20-F29)
> | Excludes2 | disturbances of skin sensation (R20.-)

R44.0 **Auditory hallucinations**

R44.1 **Visual hallucinations**

R44.2 **Other hallucinations**

R44.3 **Hallucinations, unspecified**

R44.8 **Other symptoms and signs involving general sensations and perceptions**

R44.9 **Unspecified symptoms and signs involving general sensations and perceptions**

● R45 **Symptoms and signs involving emotional state**

R45.0 **Nervousness**
  Nervous tension

R45.1 **Restlessness and agitation**

R45.2 **Unhappiness**

R45.3 **Demoralization and apathy**
> | Excludes1 | anhedonia (R45.84)

R45.4 **Irritability and anger**

R45.5 **Hostility**

R45.6 **Violent behavior**

R45.7 **State of emotional shock and stress, unspecified**

● R45.8 **Other symptoms and signs involving emotional state**

R45.81 **Low self-esteem**

R45.82 **Worries**

R45.83 **Excessive crying of child, adolescent or adult**
> | Excludes1 | excessive crying of infant (baby) R68.11

R45.84 **Anhedonia**
  Total loss of feeling of pleasure in pleasurable acts

● R45.85 **Homicidal and suicidal ideations**
> | Excludes1 | suicide attempt (T14.91)

R45.850 **Homicidal ideations**

R45.851 **Suicidal ideations**

R45.86 **Emotional lability**

R45.87 **Impulsiveness**

R45.89 **Other symptoms and signs involving emotional state**

▶ New   ⇒ Revised   ~~deleted~~ Deleted   **OGCR** Official Guidelines   X Assign placeholder X   ● Use Additional Character(s)

| Excludes 1 | Excludes 2 | Includes | Use additional | Code first | Code also | Key words |

● **R46** **Symptoms and signs involving appearance and behavior**

> **Excludes1**   appearance and behavior in schizophrenia, schizotypal and delusional disorders (F20-F29)
> mental and behavioral disorders (F01-F99)

R46.0 **Very low level of personal hygiene**

R46.1 **Bizarre personal appearance**

R46.2 **Strange and inexplicable behavior**

R46.3 **Overactivity**

R46.4 **Slowness and poor responsiveness**

> **Excludes1**   stupor (R40.1)

R46.5 **Suspiciousness and marked evasiveness**

R46.6 **Undue concern and preoccupation with stressful events**

R46.7 **Verbosity and circumstantial detail obscuring reason for contact**

● **R46.8** **Other symptoms and signs involving appearance and behavior**

R46.81 **Obsessive-compulsive behavior**

> **Excludes1**   obsessive-compulsive disorder (F42-)

R46.89 **Other symptoms and signs involving appearance and behavior**

SYMPTOMS AND SIGNS INVOLVING SPEECH AND VOICE (R47-R49)

● **R47** **Speech disturbances, not elsewhere classified**

> **Excludes1**   autism (F84.0)
> cluttering (F80.81)
> specific developmental disorders of speech and language (F80.-)
> stuttering (F80.81)

● **R47.0** **Dysphasia and aphasia**

R47.01 **Aphasia**

> **Excludes1**   aphasia following cerebrovascular disease (I69. with final characters -20)
> progressive isolated aphasia (G31.01)

R47.02 **Dysphasia**

> *Impairment in comprehension of speech, caused by left-sided brain damage*

> **Excludes1**   dysphasia following cerebrovascular disease (I69. with final characters -21)

R47.1 **Dysarthria and anarthria**

> *Motor speech disorder*

> **Excludes1**   dysarthria following cerebrovascular disease (I69. with final characters -22)

● **R47.8** **Other speech disturbances**

> **Excludes1**   dysarthria following cerebrovascular disease (I69. with final characters -28)

R47.81 **Slurred speech**

R47.82 **Fluency disorder in conditions classified elsewhere**

> Stuttering in conditions classified elsewhere

> *Code first underlying disease or condition, such as:*
> Parkinson's disease (G20)

> **Excludes1**   adult onset fluency disorder (F98.5)
> childhood onset fluency disorder (F80.81)
> fluency disorder (stuttering) following cerebrovascular disease (I69. with final characters -23)

R47.89 **Other speech disturbances**

R47.9 **Unspecified speech disturbances**

● **R48** **Dyslexia and other symbolic dysfunctions, not elsewhere classified**

> **Excludes1**   specific developmental disorders of scholastic skills (F81.-)

R48.0 **Dyslexia and alexia**

R48.1 **Agnosia**

> *Loss of ability to recognize objects, persons, sounds, shapes, or smells*
> Astereognosia (astereognosis)
> Autotopagnosia

> **Excludes1**   visual object agnosia (R48.3)

R48.2 **Apraxia**

> *Loss of ability to execute or carry out learned purposeful movements*

> **Excludes1**   apraxia following cerebrovascular disease (I69. with final characters -90)

R48.3 **Visual agnosia**

> Prosopagnosia
> Simultanagnosia (asimultagnosia)

R48.8 **Other symbolic dysfunctions**

> Acalculia
> *Difficulty performing simple mathematical tasks resulting from neurological injury*
> Agraphia

R48.9 **Unspecified symbolic dysfunctions**

● **R49** **Voice and resonance disorders**

> **Excludes1**   psychogenic voice and resonance disorders (F44.4)

R49.0 **Dysphonia**

> Hoarseness

R49.1 **Aphonia**

> Loss of voice

● **R49.2** **Hypernasality and hyponasality**

R49.21 **Hypernasality**

R49.22 **Hyponasality**

R49.8 **Other voice and resonance disorders**

R49.9 **Unspecified voice and resonance disorder**

> Change in voice NOS
> Resonance disorder NOS

GENERAL SYMPTOMS AND SIGNS (R50-R69)

● **R50** **Fever of other and unknown origin**

> **Excludes1**   chills without fever (R68.83)
> febrile convulsions (R56.0-)
> fever of unknown origin during labor (O75.2)
> fever of unknown origin in newborn (P81.9)
> hypothermia due to illness (R68.0)
> malignant hyperthermia due to anesthesia (T88.3)
> puerperal pyrexia NOS (O86.4)

R50.2 **Drug induced fever**

> Use additional code for adverse effect, if applicable, to identify drug (T36-T50 with fifth or sixth character 5)

> **Excludes1**   postvaccination (postimmunization) fever (R50.83)

● **R50.8** **Other specified fever**

R50.81 **Fever presenting with conditions classified elsewhere**

> *Code first underlying condition when associated fever is present, such as with:*
> leukemia (C91-C95)
> neutropenia (D70.-)
> sickle-cell disease (D57.-)

R50.82 **Postprocedural fever**

> **Excludes1**   postprocedural infection (T81.4-)
> posttransfusion fever (R50.84)
> postvaccination (postimmunization) fever (R50.83)

▶ New   ⇒ Revised   ~~deleted~~ Deleted   **OGCR** Official Guidelines   X Assign placeholder X   ● Use Additional Character(s)

Excludes 1   Excludes 2   Includes   Use additional   Code first   Code also   Key words

R50.83   **Postvaccination fever**
     Postimmunization fever

R50.84   **Febrile nonhemolytic transfusion reaction**
     FNHTR
     Posttransfusion fever

R50.9   **Fever, unspecified**
     Fever NOS
     Fever of unknown origin [FUO]
     Fever with chills
     Fever with rigors
     Hyperpyrexia NOS
     Persistent fever
     Pyrexia NOS

R51   **Headache**
     Facial pain NOS
     Excludes1   atypical face pain (G50.1)
           migraine and other headache syndromes (G43-G44)
           trigeminal neuralgia (G50.0)

R52   **Pain, unspecified**
     Acute pain NOS   Pain NOS
     Generalized pain NOS
     Excludes1   acute and chronic pain, not elsewhere classified (G89.-)
           localized pain, unspecified type - code to pain by site, such as:
             abdomen pain (R10.-)
             back pain (M54.9)
             breast pain (N64.4)
             chest pain (R07.1-R07.9)
             ear pain (H92.0-)
             eye pain (H57.1)
             headache (R51)
             joint pain (M25.5-)
             limb pain (M79.6-)
             lumbar region pain (M54.5)
             pelvic and perineal pain (R10.2)
             shoulder pain (M25.51-)
             spine pain (M54.-)
             throat pain (R07.0)
             tongue pain (K14.6)
             tooth pain (K08.8)
             renal colic (N23)
           pain disorders exclusively related to psychological factors (F45.41)

● **R53**   **Malaise and fatigue**

R53.0   **Neoplastic (malignant) related fatigue**
     Code first associated neoplasm

R53.1   **Weakness**
     Asthenia NOS
     Excludes1   age-related weakness (R54)
           muscle weakness (M62.8-)
           sarcopenia (M62.84)
           senile asthenia (R54)

R53.2   **Functional quadriplegia**
     Complete immobility due to severe physical disability or frailty
     Excludes1   frailty NOS (R54)
           hysterical paralysis (F44.4)
           immobility syndrome (M62.3)
           neurologic quadriplegia (G82.5-)
           quadriplegia (G82.50)

● R53.8   **Other malaise and fatigue**
     Excludes1   combat exhaustion and fatigue (F43.0)
           congenital debility (P96.9)
           ~~exhaustion and fatigue due to depressive episode (F32.-)~~
           exhaustion and fatigue due to excessive exertion (T73.3)
           exhaustion and fatigue due to exposure (T73.2)
           exhaustion and fatigue due to heat (T67.-)
           exhaustion and fatigue due to pregnancy (O26.8-)
           exhaustion and fatigue due to recurrent depressive episode (F33)
           exhaustion and fatigue due to senile debility (R54)

R53.81   **Other malaise**
     Chronic debility
     Debility NOS
     General physical deterioration
     Malaise NOS
     Nervous debility
     Excludes1   age-related physical debility (R54)

R53.82   **Chronic fatigue, unspecified**
     Chronic fatigue syndrome NOS
     Excludes1   postviral fatigue syndrome (G93.3)

R53.83   **Other fatigue**
     Fatigue NOS   Lethargy
     Lack of energy   Tiredness
     ▶ **Excludes2**   exhaustion and fatigue due to depressive episode (F32.-)

R54   **Age-related physical debility**
     Frailty   Senile asthenia
     Old age   Senile debility
     Senescence
     Excludes1   age-related cognitive decline (R41.81)
           sarcopenia (M62.84)
           senile psychosis (F03)
           senility NOS (R41.81)

R55   **Syncope and collapse**
     Blackout
     Fainting
     Vasovagal attack
     Excludes1   cardiogenic shock (R57.0)
           carotid sinus syncope (G90.01)
           heat syncope (T67.1)
           neurocirculatory asthenia (F45.8)
           neurogenic orthostatic hypotension (G90.3)
           orthostatic hypotension (I95.1)
           postprocedural shock (T81.1-)
           psychogenic syncope (F48.8)
           shock NOS (R57.9)
           shock complicating or following abortion or ectopic or molar pregnancy (O00-O07, O08.3)
           shock complicating or following labor and delivery (O75.1)
           Stokes-Adams attack (I45.9)
           unconsciousness NOS (R40.2-)

● R56   **Convulsions, not elsewhere classified**
     Excludes1   dissociative convulsions and seizures (F44.5)
           epileptic convulsions and seizures (G40.-)
           newborn convulsions and seizures (P90)

● R56.0   **Febrile convulsions**

R56.00   **Simple febrile convulsions**
     Febrile convulsion NOS
     Febrile seizure NOS

R56.01   **Complex febrile convulsions**
     Atypical febrile seizure
     Complex febrile seizure
     Complicated febrile seizure
     Excludes1   status epilepticus (G40.901)

▶ New   ⇒ Revised   ~~deleted~~ Deleted   **OGCR** Official Guidelines   **X** Assign placeholder X   ● Use Additional Character(s)

Excludes 1   Excludes 2   Includes   Use additional   Code first   Code also   Key words

1153

CHAPTER 18 (R00-R99)

R56.1 **Post traumatic seizures**
    | Excludes1 | post traumatic epilepsy (G40.-)

R56.9 **Unspecified convulsions**
    Convulsion disorder   Recurrent convulsions
    Fit NOS   Seizure(s) (convulsive) NOS

● R57 **Shock, not elsewhere classified**
    | Excludes1 | anaphylactic shock NOS (T78.2)
        anaphylactic reaction or shock due to adverse
            food reaction (T78.0-)
        anaphylactic shock due to adverse effect of
            correct drug or medicament properly
            administered (T88.6)
        anaphylactic shock due to serum (T80.5-)
        anesthetic shock (T88.3)
        electric shock (T75.4)
        obstetric shock (O75.1)
        postprocedural shock (T81.1-)
        psychic shock (F43.0)
        ~~septic shock (R65.21)~~
        shock complicating or following ectopic or molar
            pregnancy (O00-O07, O08.3)
        shock due to lightning (T75.01)
        traumatic shock (T79.4)
        toxic shock syndrome (A48.3)

R57.0 **Cardiogenic shock**
    ▶ | Excludes2 | septic shock (R65.21)

R57.1 **Hypovolemic shock**
    Decreased blood volume (loss)

R57.8 **Other shock**

R57.9 **Shock, unspecified**
    Failure of peripheral circulation NOS
    Resulting in significant blood pressure drop

R58 **Hemorrhage, not elsewhere classified**
    Hemorrhage NOS
    | Excludes1 | hemorrhage included with underlying
            conditions, such as:
            acute duodenal ulcer with hemorrhage (K26.0)
            acute gastritis with bleeding (K29.01)
            ulcerative enterocolitis with rectal bleeding
               (K51.01)

● R59 **Enlarged lymph nodes**
    | Includes | swollen glands
    | Excludes1 | lymphadenitis NOS (I88.9)
        acute lymphadenitis (L04.-)
        chronic lymphadenitis (I88.1)
        mesenteric (acute) (chronic) lymphadenitis (I88.0)

R59.0 **Localized enlarged lymph nodes**

R59.1 **Generalized enlarged lymph nodes**
    Lymphadenopathy NOS

R59.9 **Enlarged lymph nodes, unspecified**

● R60 **Edema, not elsewhere classified**
    | Excludes1 | angioneurotic edema (T78.3)
        ascites (R18.-)
        cerebral edema (G93.6)
        cerebral edema due to birth injury (P11.0)
        edema of larynx (J38.4)
        edema of nasopharynx (J39.2)
        edema of pharynx (J39.2)
        gestational edema (O12.0-)
        hereditary edema (Q82.0)
        hydrops fetalis NOS (P83.2)
        hydrothorax (J94.8)
        ~~nutritional edema (E40-E46)~~
        hydrops fetalis NOS (P83.2)
        newborn edema (P83.3)
        pulmonary edema (J81.-)

R60.0 **Localized edema**

R60.1 **Generalized edema**
    ▶ | Excludes2 | nutritional edema (E40-E46)

R60.9 **Edema, unspecified**
    Fluid retention NOS

R61 **Generalized hyperhidrosis**
    Excessive sweating
    Night sweats
    Secondary hyperhidrosis
    *Code first, if applicable, menopausal and female climacteric states
    (N95.1)*
    | Excludes1 | focal (primary) (secondary) hyperhidrosis (L74.5-)
        Frey's syndrome (L74.52)
        localized (primary) (secondary) hyperhidrosis
            (L74.5-)

● R62 **Lack of expected normal physiological development in
childhood and adults**
    | Excludes1 | delayed puberty (E30.0)
        gonadal dysgenesis (Q99.1)
        hypopituitarism (E23.0)

R62.0 **Delayed milestone in childhood**
    Delayed attainment of expected physiological
        developmental stage
    Late talker
    Late walker

● R62.5 **Other and unspecified lack of expected normal
physiological development in childhood**
    | Excludes1 | HIV disease resulting in failure to thrive
            (B20)
        physical retardation due to malnutrition
            (E45)

R62.50 **Unspecified lack of expected normal
physiological development in childhood**
    Infantilism NOS

R62.51 **Failure to thrive (child)**
    Failure to gain weight
    | Excludes1 | failure to thrive in child under 28
            days old (P92.6)

R62.52 **Short stature (child)**
    Lack of growth   Short stature NOS
    Physical retardation
    | Excludes1 | short stature due to endocrine
            disorder (E34.3)

R62.59 **Other lack of expected normal physiological
development in childhood**

R62.7 **Adult failure to thrive**

● R63 **Symptoms and signs concerning food and fluid intake**
    | Excludes1 | bulimia NOS (F50.2)
        eating disorders of nonorganic origin (F50.-)
        malnutrition (E40-E46)

R63.0 **Anorexia**
    Loss of appetite
    | Excludes1 | anorexia nervosa (F50.0-)
        loss of appetite of nonorganic origin
            (F50.89)

R63.1 **Polydipsia**
    Excessive thirst

R63.2 **Polyphagia**
    Excessive eating   Hyperalimentation NOS

R63.3 **Feeding difficulties**
    Feeding problem (elderly) (infant) NOS
    ▶ Picky eater
    | Excludes1 | ▶ eating disorders (F50.-)
        feeding problems of newborn (P92.-)
        infant feeding disorder of nonorganic
            origin (F98.2-)

R63.4 **Abnormal weight loss**

R63.5 **Abnormal weight gain**
    | Excludes1 | excessive weight gain in pregnancy
        (O26.0-)
        obesity (E66.-)

R63.6   **Underweight**

     Use additional code to identify body mass index (BMI), if known (Z68.-)

     Excludes1   abnormal weight loss (R63.4)
                   anorexia nervosa (F50.0-)
                   malnutrition (E40-E46)

R63.8   **Other symptoms and signs concerning food and fluid intake**

R64   **Cachexia**

     Wasting syndrome

     Code first underlying condition, if known

     Excludes1   abnormal weight loss (R63.4)
                   nutritional marasmus (E41)

● R65   **Symptoms and signs specifically associated with systemic inflammation and infection**

   ● R65.1   **Systemic inflammatory response syndrome (SIRS) of non-infectious origin**

         Code first underlying condition, such as:
           heatstroke (T67.0)
           injury and trauma (S00-T88)

         Excludes1   sepsis - code to infection
                          severe sepsis (R65.2)

         OGCR   Section I.C.18.g.

> SIRS due to Non-Infectious Process
>
> The systemic inflammatory response syndrome (SIRS) can develop as a result of certain non-infectious disease processes, such as trauma, malignant neoplasm, or pancreatitis. When SIRS is documented with a noninfectious condition, and no subsequent infection is documented, the code for the underlying condition, such as an injury, should be assigned, followed by code R65.10, Systemic inflammatory response syndrome (SIRS) of non-infectious origin without acute organ dysfunction, or code R65.11, Systemic inflammatory response syndrome (SIRS) of non-infectious origin with acute organ dysfunction. If an associated acute organ dysfunction is documented, the appropriate code(s) for the specific type of organ dysfunction(s) should be assigned in addition to code R65.11. If acute organ dysfunction is documented, but it cannot be determined if the acute organ dysfunction is associated with SIRS or due to another condition (e.g., directly due to the trauma), the provider should be queried.

     R65.10   **Systemic inflammatory response syndrome (SIRS) of non-infectious origin without acute organ dysfunction**

           Systemic inflammatory response syndrome (SIRS) NOS

     R65.11   **Systemic inflammatory response syndrome (SIRS) of non-infectious origin with acute organ dysfunction**

           Use additional code to identify specific acute organ dysfunction, such as:
           acute kidney failure (N17.-)
           acute respiratory failure (J96.0-)
           critical illness myopathy (G72.81)
           critical illness polyneuropathy (G62.81)
           disseminated intravascular coagulopathy [DIC] (D65)
           encephalopathy (metabolic) (septic) (G93.41)
           hepatic failure (K72.0-)

● R65.2   **Severe sepsis**

     Infection with associated acute organ dysfunction
     Sepsis with acute organ dysfunction
     Sepsis with multiple organ dysfunction
     Systemic inflammatory response syndrome due to infectious process with acute organ dysfunction

     Code first underlying infection, such as:
       infection following a procedure (T81.4-)
       infections following infusion, transfusion and therapeutic injection (T80.2-)
       puerperal sepsis (O85)
       sepsis following complete or unspecified spontaneous abortion (O03.87)
       sepsis following ectopic and molar pregnancy (O08.82)
       sepsis following incomplete spontaneous abortion (O03.37)
       sepsis following (induced) termination of pregnancy (O04.87)
       sepsis NOS (A41.9)

     Use additional code to identify specific acute organ dysfunction, such as:
       acute kidney failure (N17.-)
       acute respiratory failure (J96.0-)
       critical illness myopathy (G72.81)
       critical illness polyneuropathy (G62.81)
       disseminated intravascular coagulopathy [DIC] (D65)
       encephalopathy (metabolic) (septic) (G93.41)
       hepatic failure (K72.0-)

     R65.20   **Severe sepsis without septic shock**
           Severe sepsis NOS

     R65.21   **Severe sepsis with septic shock**

● R68   **Other general symptoms and signs**

   R68.0   **Hypothermia, not associated with low environmental temperature**

         Excludes1   hypothermia NOS (accidental) (T68)
                     hypothermia due to anesthesia (T88.51)
                     hypothermia due to low environmental temperature (T68)
                     newborn hypothermia (P80.-)

   ● R68.1   **Nonspecific symptoms peculiar to infancy**

         Excludes1   colic, infantile (R10.83)
                     neonatal cerebral irritability (P91.3)
                     teething syndrome (K00.7)

     R68.11   **Excessive crying of infant (baby)**

           Excludes1   excessive crying of child, adolescent, or adult (R45.83)

     R68.12   **Fussy infant (baby)**
           Irritable infant

     R68.13   **Apparent life threatening event in infant (ALTE)**

           Apparent life threatening event in newborn
          ▶ Brief resolved unexplained event (BRUE)

           Code first confirmed diagnosis, if known

           Use additional code(s) for associated signs and symptoms if no confirmed diagnosis established, or if signs and symptoms are not associated routinely with confirmed diagnosis, or provide additional information for cause of ALTE

     R68.19   **Other nonspecific symptoms peculiar to infancy**

▶ New   ⇒ Revised   ~~deleted~~ Deleted   **OGCR** Official Guidelines   X Assign placeholder X   ● Use Additional Character(s)

Excludes 1   Excludes 2   Includes   Use additional   Code first   Code also   Key words

R68.2   **Dry mouth, unspecified**

> **Excludes1**   dry mouth due to dehydration (E86.0)
> dry mouth due to sicca syndrome
> [Sjögren] (M35.0-)
> salivary gland hyposecretion (K11.7)

R68.3   **Clubbing of fingers**
Clubbing of nails

> **Excludes1**   congenital clubfinger (Q68.1)

● R68.8   **Other general symptoms and signs**

R68.81   **Early satiety**

R68.82   **Decreased libido**
Decreased sexual desire

R68.83   **Chills (without fever)**
Chills NOS

> **Excludes1**   chills with fever (R50.9)

R68.84   **Jaw pain**
Mandibular pain
Maxilla pain

> **Excludes1**   temporomandibular joint
> arthralgia (M26.62-)

R68.89   **Other general symptoms and signs**

R69   **Illness, unspecified**
Unknown and unspecified cases of morbidity

ABNORMAL FINDINGS ON EXAMINATION OF BLOOD, WITHOUT DIAGNOSIS (R70-R79)

> **Excludes2**   abnormal findings on antenatal screening of
> mother (O28.-)
> abnormalities of lipids (E78.-)
> abnormalities of platelets and thrombocytes
> (D69.-)
> abnormalities of white blood cells classified
> elsewhere (D70-D72)
> coagulation hemorrhagic disorders (D65-D68)
> diagnostic abnormal findings classified
> elsewhere —see Alphabetical Index
> hemorrhagic and hematological disorders of
> newborn (P50-P61)

● R70   **Elevated erythrocyte sedimentation rate and abnormality of plasma viscosity**

R70.0   **Elevated erythrocyte sedimentation rate**

R70.1   **Abnormal plasma viscosity**

● R71   **Abnormality of red blood cells**

> **Excludes1**   anemias (D50-D64)
> anemia of premature infant (P61.2)
> benign (familial) polycythemia (D75.0)
> congenital anemias (P61.2-P61.4)
> newborn anemia due to isoimmunization (P55.-)
> polycythemia neonatorum (P61.1)
> polycythemia NOS (D75.1)
> polycythemia vera (D45)
> secondary polycythemia (D75.1)

R71.0   **Precipitous drop in hematocrit**
Drop (precipitous) in hemoglobin
Drop in hematocrit
Blood volume that has decreased red blood cells

R71.8   **Other abnormality of red blood cells**
Abnormal red-cell morphology NOS
Abnormal red-cell volume NOS
Anisocytosis
Red blood cells of unequal size
Poikilocytosis
Red blood cells of abnormal shape

● R73   **Elevated blood glucose level**

> **Excludes1**   diabetes mellitus (E08-E13)
> diabetes mellitus in pregnancy, childbirth and the
> puerperium (O24.-)
> neonatal disorders (P70.0-P70.2)
> postsurgical hypoinsulinemia (E89.1)

● R73.0   **Abnormal glucose**

> **Excludes1**   abnormal glucose in pregnancy (O99.81-)
> diabetes mellitus (E08-E13)
> dysmetabolic syndrome X (E88.81)
> gestational diabetes (O24.4-)
> glycosuria (R81)
> hypoglycemia (E16.2)

R73.01   **Impaired fasting glucose**
Elevated fasting glucose

R73.02   **Impaired glucose tolerance (oral)**
Elevated glucose tolerance

R73.03   **Prediabetes**
Latent diabetes

R73.09   **Other abnormal glucose**
Abnormal glucose NOS
Abnormal non-fasting glucose tolerance

R73.9   **Hyperglycemia, unspecified**

● R74   **Abnormal serum enzyme levels**

R74.0   **Nonspecific elevation of levels of transaminase and lactic acid dehydrogenase [LDH]**

R74.8   **Abnormal levels of other serum enzymes**
Abnormal level of acid phosphatase
Abnormal level of alkaline phosphatase
Abnormal level of amylase
Abnormal level of lipase [triacylglycerol lipase]

R74.9   **Abnormal serum enzyme level, unspecified**

R75   **Inconclusive laboratory evidence of human immunodeficiency virus [HIV]**
Nonconclusive HIV-test finding in infants

> **Excludes1**   asymptomatic human immunodeficiency virus
> [HIV] infection status (Z21)
> human immunodeficiency virus [HIV] disease (B20)

OGCR Section I.C.1.e and f.

Patients with inconclusive HIV serology

e. Patients with inconclusive HIV serology, but no definitive diagnosis or manifestations of the illness, may be assigned code R75, Inconclusive laboratory evidence of human immunodeficiency virus [HIV].

f. Previously diagnosed HIV-related illness

Patients with any known prior diagnosis of an HIV-related illness should be coded to B20. Once a patient has developed an HIV-related illness, the patient should always be assigned code B20 on every subsequent admission/encounter. Patients previously diagnosed with any HIV illness (B20) should never be assigned to R75 or Z21, Asymptomatic human immunodeficiency virus [HIV] infection status.

▶ New   ⇒ Revised   ~~deleted~~ Deleted   **OGCR** Official Guidelines   X Assign placeholder X   ● Use Additional Character(s)

Excludes 1   Excludes 2   Includes   Use additional   Code first   Code also   Key words

● **R76   Other abnormal immunological findings in serum**

    R76.0   Raised antibody titer
        | Excludes1 | isoimmunization in pregnancy (O36.0-O36.1)
             isoimmunization affecting newborn (P55.-)

● **R76.1   Nonspecific reaction to test for tuberculosis**

    R76.11   Nonspecific reaction to tuberculin skin test without active tuberculosis
        Abnormal result of Mantoux test
        PPD positive
        Tuberculin (skin test) positive
        Tuberculin (skin test) reactor
        | Excludes1 | nonspecific reaction to cell mediated immunity measurement of gamma interferon antigen response without active tuberculosis (R76.12)

    R76.12   Nonspecific reaction to cell mediated immunity measurement of gamma interferon antigen response without active tuberculosis
        Nonspecific reaction to QuantiFERON-TB test (QFT) without active tuberculosis
        | Excludes1 | nonspecific reaction to tuberculin skin test without active tuberculosis (R76.11)
             positive tuberculin skin test (R76.11)

    R76.8   Other specified abnormal immunological findings in serum
        Raised level of immunoglobulins NOS

    R76.9   Abnormal immunological finding in serum, unspecified

● **R77   Other abnormalities of plasma proteins**
    | Excludes1 | disorders of plasma-protein metabolism (E88.0)

    R77.0   Abnormality of albumin

    R77.1   Abnormality of globulin
        Hyperglobulinemia NOS

    R77.2   Abnormality of alphafetoprotein

    R77.8   Other specified abnormalities of plasma proteins

    R77.9   Abnormality of plasma protein, unspecified

● **R78   Findings of drugs and other substances, not normally found in blood**
    Use additional code to identify any retained foreign body, if applicable (Z18.-)
    | Excludes1 | mental or behavioral disorders due to psychoactive substance use (F10-F19)

    R78.0   Finding of alcohol in blood
        Use additional external cause code (Y90.-), for detail regarding alcohol level.

    R78.1   Finding of opiate drug in blood

    R78.2   Finding of cocaine in blood

    R78.3   Finding of hallucinogen in blood

    R78.4   Finding of other drugs of addictive potential in blood

    R78.5   Finding of other psychotropic drug in blood

    R78.6   Finding of steroid agent in blood

● **R78.7   Finding of abnormal level of heavy metals in blood**

    R78.71   Abnormal lead level in blood
        | Excludes1 | lead poisoning (T56.0-)

    R78.79   Finding of abnormal level of heavy metals in blood

● **R78.8   Finding of other specified substances, not normally found in blood**

    R78.81   Bacteremia
        Blood poisoning/bacteremia
        | Excludes1 | sepsis-code to specified infection

    R78.89   Finding of other specified substances, not normally found in blood
        Finding of abnormal level of lithium in blood

    R78.9   Finding of unspecified substance, not normally found in blood

● **R79   Other abnormal findings of blood chemistry**
    Use additional code to identify any retained foreign body, if applicable (Z18.-)
    | Excludes1 | ~~abnormality of fluid, electrolyte or acid-base balance (E86-E87)~~
        asymptomatic hyperuricemia (E79.0)
        hyperglycemia NOS (R73.9)
        hypoglycemia NOS (E16.2)
        neonatal hypoglycemia (P70.3-P70.4)
        specific findings indicating disorder of amino-acid metabolism (E70-E72)
        specific findings indicating disorder of carbohydrate metabolism (E73-E74)
        specific findings indicating disorder of lipid metabolism (E75.-)

    R79.0   Abnormal level of blood mineral
        Abnormal blood level of cobalt
        Abnormal blood level of copper
        Abnormal blood level of iron
        Abnormal blood level of magnesium
        Abnormal blood level of mineral NEC
        Abnormal blood level of zinc
        | Excludes1 | abnormal level of lithium (R78.89)
             disorders of mineral metabolism (E83.-)
             neonatal hypomagnesemia (P71.2)
             nutritional mineral deficiency (E58-E61)

    R79.1   Abnormal coagulation profile
        Abnormal or prolonged bleeding time
        Abnormal or prolonged coagulation time
        Abnormal or prolonged partial thromboplastin time [PTT]
        Abnormal or prolonged prothrombin time [PT]
        | Excludes1 | coagulation defects (D68.-)
        ▶ | Excludes2 | abnormality of fluid, electrolyte or acid-base balance (E86-E87)

● **R79.8   Other specified abnormal findings of blood chemistry**

    R79.81   Abnormal blood-gas level

    R79.82   Elevated C-reactive protein (CRP)

    R79.89   Other specified abnormal findings of blood chemistry

    R79.9   Abnormal finding of blood chemistry, unspecified

ABNORMAL FINDINGS ON EXAMINATION OF URINE, WITHOUT DIAGNOSIS (R80-R82)

    | Excludes1 | abnormal findings on antenatal screening of mother (O28.-)
        diagnostic abnormal findings classified elsewhere - see Alphabetical Index
        specific findings indicating disorder of amino-acid metabolism (E70-E72)
        specific findings indicating disorder of carbohydrate metabolism (E73-E74)

● **R80   Proteinuria**
    | Excludes1 | gestational proteinuria (O12.1-)

    R80.0   Isolated proteinuria
        Idiopathic proteinuria
        | Excludes1 | isolated proteinuria with specific morphological lesion (N06.-)

    R80.1   Persistent proteinuria, unspecified

    R80.2   Orthostatic proteinuria, unspecified
        Postural proteinuria

    R80.3   Bence Jones proteinuria

    R80.8   Other proteinuria

    R80.9   Proteinuria, unspecified
        Albuminuria NOS

R81   Glycosuria
       Excludes1   renal glycosuria (E74.8)

● R82   **Other and unspecified abnormal findings in urine**
       Includes   chromoabnormalities in urine
       Use additional code to identify any retained foreign body, if
            applicable (Z18.-)
       Excludes2   hematuria (R31.-)
       R82.0   **Chyluria**
               White milky urine
               Excludes1   filarial chyluria (B74.-)
       R82.1   **Myoglobinuria**
               Presence of myoglobin (iron containing protein) in urine
       R82.2   **Biliuria**
               Presence of bile pigments/salts in urine
       R82.3   **Hemoglobinuria**
               Presence of hemoglobin in urine
               Excludes1   hemoglobinuria due to hemolysis from
                                external causes NEC (D59.6)
                                hemoglobinuria due to paroxysmal
                                nocturnal [Marchiafava-Micheli]
                                (D59.5)
       R82.4   **Acetonuria**
               Ketonuria
       R82.5   **Elevated urine levels of drugs, medicaments and
               biological substances**
               Elevated urine levels of catecholamines
               Elevated urine levels of indoleacetic acid
               Elevated urine levels of 17-ketosteroids
               Elevated urine levels of steroids
       R82.6   **Abnormal urine levels of substances chiefly
               nonmedicinal as to source**
               Abnormal urine level of heavy metals
     ● R82.7   **Abnormal findings on microbiological examination of
               urine**
               Excludes1   colonization status (Z22.-)
               R82.71   **Bacteriuria**
               R82.79   **Other abnormal findings on microbiological
                        examination of urine**
                        Positive culture findings of urine
       R82.8   **Abnormal findings on cytological and histological
               examination of urine**
     ● R82.9   **Other and unspecified abnormal findings in urine**
               R82.90   **Unspecified abnormal findings in urine**
               R82.91   **Other chromoabnormalities of urine**
                        Chromoconversion (dipstick)
                        Idiopathic dipstick converts positive for blood
                             with no cellular forms in sediment
                        Excludes1   hemoglobinuria (R82.3)
                                         myoglobinuria (R82.1)
               R82.99   **Other abnormal findings in urine**
                        Cells and casts in urine
                        Crystalluria
                        Melanuria

ABNORMAL FINDINGS ON EXAMINATION OF OTHER BODY FLUIDS, SUBSTANCES AND TISSUES, WITHOUT DIAGNOSIS (R83-R89)

       Excludes1   abnormal findings on antenatal screening of
                        mother (O28.-)
                        diagnostic abnormal findings classified elsewhere
                        - see Alphabetical Index
       Excludes2   abnormal findings on examination of blood,
                        without diagnosis (R70-R79)
                        abnormal findings on examination of urine,
                        without diagnosis (R80-R82)
                        abnormal tumor markers (R97.-)

● R83   **Abnormal findings in cerebrospinal fluid**
       R83.0   **Abnormal level of enzymes in cerebrospinal fluid**
       R83.1   **Abnormal level of hormones in cerebrospinal fluid**
       R83.2   **Abnormal level of other drugs, medicaments and
               biological substances in cerebrospinal fluid**
       R83.3   **Abnormal level of substances chiefly nonmedicinal as to
               source in cerebrospinal fluid**
       R83.4   **Abnormal immunological findings in cerebrospinal
               fluid**
       R83.5   **Abnormal microbiological findings in cerebrospinal
               fluid**
               Positive culture findings in cerebrospinal fluid
               Excludes1   colonization status (Z22.-)
       R83.6   **Abnormal cytological findings in cerebrospinal fluid**
       R83.8   **Other abnormal findings in cerebrospinal fluid**
               Abnormal chromosomal findings in cerebrospinal fluid
       R83.9   **Unspecified abnormal finding in cerebrospinal fluid**

● R84   **Abnormal findings in specimens from respiratory organs and
       thorax**
       Includes   abnormal findings in bronchial washings
                       abnormal findings in nasal secretions
                       abnormal findings in pleural fluid
                       abnormal findings in sputum
                       abnormal findings in throat scrapings
       Excludes1   blood-stained sputum (R04.2)
       R84.0   **Abnormal level of enzymes in specimens from
               respiratory organs and thorax**
       R84.1   **Abnormal level of hormones in specimens from
               respiratory organs and thorax**
       R84.2   **Abnormal level of other drugs, medicaments and
               biological substances in specimens from respiratory
               organs and thorax**
       R84.3   **Abnormal level of substances chiefly nonmedicinal as to
               source in specimens from respiratory organs and thorax**
       R84.4   **Abnormal immunological findings in specimens from
               respiratory organs and thorax**
       R84.5   **Abnormal microbiological findings in specimens from
               respiratory organs and thorax**
               Positive culture findings in specimens from respiratory
                    organs and thorax
               Excludes1   colonization status (Z22.-)
       R84.6   **Abnormal cytological findings in specimens from
               respiratory organs and thorax**
       R84.7   **Abnormal histological findings in specimens from
               respiratory organs and thorax**
       R84.8   **Other abnormal findings in specimens from respiratory
               organs and thorax**
               Abnormal chromosomal findings in specimens from
                    respiratory organs and thorax
       R84.9   **Unspecified abnormal finding in specimens from
               respiratory organs and thorax**

▶ New   ⇒ Revised   ~~deleted~~ Deleted   **OGCR** Official Guidelines   X Assign placeholder X   ● Use Additional Character(s)

Excludes 1   Excludes 2   Includes   Use additional   Code first   Code also   Key words

● **R85**   **Abnormal findings in specimens from digestive organs and abdominal cavity**

> **Includes**   abnormal findings in peritoneal fluid
> abnormal findings in saliva

> **Excludes1**   cloudy peritoneal dialysis effluent (R88.Ø)
> fecal abnormalities (R19.5)

R85.Ø   Abnormal level of enzymes in specimens from digestive organs and abdominal cavity

R85.1   Abnormal level of hormones in specimens from digestive organs and abdominal cavity

R85.2   Abnormal level of other drugs, medicaments and biological substances in specimens from digestive organs and abdominal cavity

R85.3   Abnormal level of substances chiefly nonmedicinal as to source in specimens from digestive organs and abdominal cavity

R85.4   Abnormal immunological findings in specimens from digestive organs and abdominal cavity

R85.5   Abnormal microbiological findings in specimens from digestive organs and abdominal cavity

> Positive culture findings in specimens from digestive organs and abdominal cavity

> **Excludes1**   colonization status (Z22.-)

● **R85.6**   Abnormal cytological findings in specimens from digestive organs and abdominal cavity

   ● **R85.61**   Abnormal cytologic smear of anus

> **Excludes1**   abnormal cytological findings in specimens from other digestive organs and abdominal cavity (R85.69)
> carcinoma in situ of anus (histologically confirmed) (DØ1.3)
> anal intraepithelial neoplasia I [AIN I] (K62.82)
> anal intraepithelial neoplasia II [AIN II] (K62.82)
> anal intraepithelial neoplasia III [AIN III] (DØ1.3)
> dysplasia (mild) (moderate) of anus (histologically confirmed) (K62.82)
> severe dysplasia of anus (histologically confirmed) (DØ1.3)

> **Excludes2**   anal high risk human papillomavirus (HPV) DNA test positive (R85.81)
> anal low risk human papillomavirus (HPV) DNA test positive (R85.82)

     R85.61Ø   Atypical squamous cells of undetermined significance on cytologic smear of anus (ASC-US)

     R85.611   Atypical squamous cells cannot exclude high grade squamous intraepithelial lesion on cytologic smear of anus (ASC-H)

     R85.612   Low grade squamous intraepithelial lesion on cytologic smear of anus (LGSIL)

     R85.613   High grade squamous intraepithelial lesion on cytologic smear of anus (HGSIL)

     R85.614   Cytologic evidence of malignancy on smear of anus

     R85.615   Unsatisfactory cytologic smear of anus

> Inadequate sample of cytologic smear of anus

     R85.616   Satisfactory anal smear but lacking transformation zone

     R85.618   Other abnormal cytological findings on specimens from anus

     R85.619   Unspecified abnormal cytological findings in specimens from anus

> Abnormal anal cytology NOS
> Atypical glandular cells of anus NOS

   R85.69   Abnormal cytological findings in specimens from other digestive organs and abdominal cavity

R85.7   Abnormal histological findings in specimens from digestive organs and abdominal cavity

● **R85.8**   Other abnormal findings in specimens from digestive organs and abdominal cavity

   R85.81   Anal high risk human papillomavirus (HPV) DNA test positive

> **Excludes1**   anogenital warts due to human papillomavirus (HPV) (A63.Ø)
> condyloma acuminatum (A63.Ø)

   R85.82   Anal low risk human papillomavirus (HPV) DNA test positive

> Use additional code for associated human papillomavirus (B97.7)

   R85.89   Other abnormal findings in specimens from digestive organs and abdominal cavity

> Abnormal chromosomal findings in specimens from digestive organs and abdominal cavity

R85.9   Unspecified abnormal finding in specimens from digestive organs and abdominal cavity

● **R86**   **Abnormal findings in specimens from male genital organs**

> **Includes**   abnormal findings in prostatic secretions
> abnormal findings in semen, seminal fluid
> abnormal spermatozoa

> **Excludes1**   azoospermia (N46.Ø-)
> oligospermia (N46.1-)

R86.Ø   Abnormal level of enzymes in specimens from male genital organs

R86.1   Abnormal level of hormones in specimens from male genital organs

R86.2   Abnormal level of other drugs, medicaments and biological substances in specimens from male genital organs

R86.3   Abnormal level of substances chiefly nonmedicinal as to source in specimens from male genital organs

R86.4   Abnormal immunological findings in specimens from male genital organs

R86.5   Abnormal microbiological findings in specimens from male genital organs

> Positive culture findings in specimens from male genital organs

> **Excludes1**   colonization status (Z22.-)

R86.6   Abnormal cytological findings in specimens from male genital organs

R86.7   Abnormal histological findings in specimens from male genital organs

R86.8   Other abnormal findings in specimens from male genital organs

> Abnormal chromosomal findings in specimens from male genital organs

R86.9   Unspecified abnormal finding in specimens from male genital organs

CHAPTER 18 (RØØ-R99)

● R87   **Abnormal findings in specimens from** <mark>**female genital organs**</mark>

> **Includes**   abnormal findings in secretion and smears from cervix uteri
>
> abnormal findings in secretion and smears from vagina
>
> abnormal findings in secretion and smears from vulva

R87.0   **Abnormal level of** <mark>**enzymes**</mark> **in specimens from female genital organs**

R87.1   **Abnormal level of** <mark>**hormones**</mark> **in specimens from female genital organs**

R87.2   **Abnormal level of** <mark>**other drugs**</mark>**, medicaments and biological substances in specimens from female genital organs**

R87.3   **Abnormal level of** <mark>**substances chiefly nonmedicinal**</mark> **as to source in specimens from female genital organs**

R87.4   **Abnormal** <mark>**immunological**</mark> **findings in specimens from female genital organs**

R87.5   **Abnormal** <mark>**microbiological**</mark> **findings in specimens from female genital organs**

> Positive culture findings in specimens from female genital organs
>
> **Excludes1**   colonization status (Z22.-)

● R87.6   **Abnormal** <mark>**cytological**</mark> **findings in specimens from female genital organs**

   ● R87.61   **Abnormal cytological findings in specimens from** <mark>**cervix uteri**</mark>

> **Excludes1**   abnormal cytological findings in specimens from other female genital organs (R87.69)
>
> abnormal cytological findings in specimens from vagina (R87.62-)
>
> carcinoma in situ of cervix uteri (histologically confirmed) (D06.-)
>
> cervical intraepithelial neoplasia I [CIN I] (N87.0)
>
> cervical intraepithelial neoplasia II [CIN II] (N87.1)
>
> cervical intraepithelial neoplasia III [CIN III] (D06.-)
>
> dysplasia (mild) (moderate) of cervix uteri (histologically confirmed) (N87.-)
>
> severe dysplasia of cervix uteri (histologically confirmed) (D06.-)
>
> **Excludes2**   cervical high risk human papillomavirus (HPV) DNA test positive (R87.810)
>
> cervical low risk human papillomavirus (HPV) DNA test positive (R87.820)

     R87.610   **Atypical** <mark>**squamous cells of undetermined significance**</mark> **on cytologic smear of cervix (**<mark>**ASC-US**</mark>**)**

     R87.611   **Atypical squamous cells cannot exclude** <mark>**high grade**</mark> **squamous intraepithelial lesion on cytologic smear of cervix (**<mark>**ASC-H**</mark>**)**

     R87.612   <mark>**Low grade**</mark> **squamous intraepithelial lesion on cytologic smear of cervix (LGSIL)**

     R87.613   **High grade squamous intraepithelial lesion on cytologic smear of cervix (HGSIL)**

     R87.614   **Cytologic evidence of** <mark>**malignancy**</mark> **on smear of cervix**

     R87.615   <mark>**Unsatisfactory**</mark> **cytologic smear of cervix**

> Inadequate sample of cytologic smear of cervix

R87.616   <mark>**Satisfactory**</mark> **cervical smear but lacking transformation zone**

R87.618   <mark>**Other**</mark> **abnormal cytological findings on specimens from cervix uteri**

R87.619   <mark>**Unspecified**</mark> **abnormal cytological findings in specimens from cervix uteri**

> Abnormal cervical cytology NOS
>
> Abnormal Papanicolaou smear of cervix NOS
>
> Abnormal thin preparation smear of cervix NOS
>
> Atypical endocervial cells of cervix NOS
>
> Atypical endometrial cells of cervix NOS
>
> Atypical glandular cells of cervix NOS

● R87.62   **Abnormal cytological findings in specimens from vagina**

> **Use additional** code to identify acquired absence of uterus and cervix, if applicable (Z90.71-)
>
> **Excludes1**   abnormal cytological findings in specimens from cervix uteri (R87.61-)
>
> abnormal cytological findings in specimens from other female genital organs (R87.69)
>
> carcinoma in situ of vagina (histologically confirmed) (D07.2)
>
> vaginal intraepithelial neoplasia I [VAIN I] (N89.0)
>
> vaginal intraepithelial neoplasia II [VAIN II] (N89.1)
>
> vaginal intraepithelial neoplasia III [VAIN III] (D07.2)
>
> dysplasia (mild) (moderate) of vagina (histologically confirmed) (N89.-)
>
> severe dysplasia of vagina (histologically confirmed) (D07.2)
>
> **Excludes2**   vaginal high risk human papillomavirus (HPV) DNA test positive (R87.811)
>
> vaginal low risk human papillomavirus (HPV) DNA test positive (R87.821)

R87.620   **Atypical** <mark>**squamous cells of undetermined significance**</mark> **on cytologic smear of vagina (**<mark>**ASC-US**</mark>**)**

R87.621   **Atypical squamous cells cannot exclude** <mark>**high grade**</mark> **squamous intraepithelial lesion on cytologic smear of vagina (**<mark>**ASC-H**</mark>**)**

R87.622   <mark>**Low grade**</mark> **squamous intraepithelial lesion on cytologic smear of vagina (**<mark>**LGSIL**</mark>**)**

R87.623   **High grade squamous intraepithelial lesion on cytologic smear of vagina (HGSIL)**

R87.624   **Cytologic evidence of** <mark>**malignancy**</mark> **on smear of vagina**

R87.625   <mark>**Unsatisfactory**</mark> **cytologic smear of vagina**

> Inadequate sample of cytologic smear of vagina

R87.628   <mark>**Other**</mark> **abnormal cytological findings on specimens from vagina**

▶ New   ⇒ Revised   ~~deleted~~ Deleted   **OGCR** Official Guidelines   X Assign placeholder X   ● Use Additional Character(s)

Excludes 1   Excludes 2   Includes   Use additional   Code first   Code also   Key words

R87.629   **Unspecified** abnormal cytological findings in specimens from vagina
Abnormal Papanicolaou smear of vagina NOS
Abnormal thin preparation smear of vagina NOS
Abnormal vaginal cytology NOS
Atypical endocervical cells of vagina NOS
Atypical endometrial cells of vagina NOS
Atypical glandular cells of vagina NOS

R87.69   Abnormal cytological findings in specimens from other female genital organs
Abnormal cytological findings in specimens from female genital organs NOS
Excludes1   dysplasia of vulva (histologically confirmed) (N90.0-N90.3)

R87.7   Abnormal histological findings in specimens from female genital organs
Excludes1   carcinoma in situ (histologically confirmed) of female genital organs (D06-D07.3)
cervical intraepithelial neoplasia I [CIN I] (N87.0)
cervical intraepithelial neoplasia II [CIN II] (N87.1)
cervical intraepithelial neoplasia III [CIN III] (D06.-)
dysplasia (mild) (moderate) of cervix uteri (histologically confirmed) (N87.-)
dysplasia (mild) (moderate) of vagina (histologically confirmed) (N89.-)
vaginal intraepithelial neoplasia I [VAIN I] (N89.0)
vaginal intraepithelial neoplasia II [VAIN II] (N89.1)
vaginal intraepithelial neoplasia III [VAIN III] (D07.2)
severe dysplasia of cervix uteri (histologically confirmed) (D06.-)
severe dysplasia of vagina (histologically confirmed) (D07.2)

● R87.8   **Other** abnormal findings in specimens from female genital organs

● R87.81   **High risk human papillomavirus (HPV) DNA test positive from female genital organs**
Excludes1   anogenital warts due to human papillomavirus (HPV) (A63.0)
condyloma acuminatum (A63.0)

R87.810   **Cervical** high risk human papillomavirus (HPV) DNA test positive

R87.811   **Vaginal** high risk human papillomavirus (HPV) DNA test positive

● R87.82   **Low risk human papillomavirus (HPV) DNA test positive from female genital organs**
Use additional code for associated human papillomavirus (B97.7)

R87.820   **Cervical** low risk human papillomavirus (HPV) DNA test positive

R87.821   **Vaginal** low risk human papillomavirus (HPV) DNA test positive

R87.89   **Other** abnormal findings in specimens from female genital organs
Abnormal chromosomal findings in specimens from female genital organs

R87.9   **Unspecified** abnormal finding in specimens from female genital organs

● R88   **Abnormal findings in other body fluids and substances**
R88.0   Cloudy (hemodialysis) (peritoneal) dialysis effluent
R88.8   Abnormal findings in other body fluids and substances

● R89   **Abnormal findings in specimens from other organs, systems and tissues**
Includes   abnormal findings in nipple discharge
abnormal findings in synovial fluid
abnormal findings in wound secretions

R89.0   Abnormal level of **enzymes** in specimens from other organs, systems and tissues

R89.1   Abnormal level of **hormones** in specimens from other organs, systems and tissues

R89.2   Abnormal level of **other drugs, medicaments and biological substances** in specimens from other organs, systems and tissues

R89.3   Abnormal level of **substances chiefly nonmedicinal** as to source in specimens from other organs, systems and tissues

R89.4   Abnormal **immunological** findings in specimens from other organs, systems and tissues

R89.5   Abnormal **microbiological** findings in specimens from other organs, systems and tissues
Positive culture findings in specimens from other organs, systems and tissues
Excludes1   colonization status (Z22.-)

R89.6   Abnormal **cytological** findings in specimens from other organs, systems and tissues

R89.7   Abnormal **histological** findings in specimens from other organs, systems and tissues

R89.8   **Other** abnormal findings in specimens from other organs, systems and tissues
Abnormal chromosomal findings in specimens from other organs, systems and tissues

R89.9   **Unspecified** abnormal finding in specimens from other organs, systems and tissues

---

ABNORMAL FINDINGS ON DIAGNOSTIC IMAGING AND IN FUNCTION STUDIES, WITHOUT DIAGNOSIS (R90-R94)

Includes   nonspecific abnormal findings on diagnostic imaging by computerized axial tomography [CAT scan]
nonspecific abnormal findings on diagnostic imaging by magnetic resonance imaging [MRI][NMR]
nonspecific abnormal findings on diagnostic imaging by positron emission tomography [PET scan]
nonspecific abnormal findings on diagnostic imaging by thermography
nonspecific abnormal findings on diagnostic imaging by ultrasound [echogram]
nonspecific abnormal findings on diagnostic imaging by X-ray examination
Excludes1   abnormal findings on antenatal screening of mother (O28.-)
diagnostic abnormal findings classified elsewhere - see Alphabetical Index

● R90   **Abnormal findings on diagnostic imaging of central nervous system**
R90.0   **Intracranial** space-occupying lesion found on diagnostic imaging of central nervous system

● R90.8   Other abnormal findings on diagnostic imaging of central nervous system
R90.81   Abnormal echoencephalogram
R90.82   White matter disease, **unspecified**
R90.89   Other abnormal findings on diagnostic imaging of central nervous system
Other cerebrovascular abnormality found on diagnostic imaging of central nervous system

---

▶ New   ⇒ Revised   ~~deleted~~ Deleted   **OGCR** Official Guidelines   X Assign placeholder X   ● Use Additional Character(s)
Excludes 1   Excludes 2   Includes   Use additional   Code first   Code also   Key words

1161

CHAPTER 18 (R00–R99)

● **R91 Abnormal findings on diagnostic imaging of lung**

    R91.1 Solitary pulmonary nodule
        Coin lesion lung
        Solitary pulmonary nodule, subsegmental branch of the bronchial tree

    R91.8 Other nonspecific abnormal finding of lung field
        Lung mass NOS found on diagnostic imaging of lung
        Pulmonary infiltrate NOS
        Shadow, lung

● **R92 Abnormal and inconclusive findings on diagnostic imaging of breast**

    R92.0 Mammographic microcalcification found on diagnostic imaging of breast
        Excludes2 mammographic calcification (calculus) found on diagnostic imaging of breast (R92.1)

    R92.1 Mammographic calcification found on diagnostic imaging of breast
        Mammographic calculus found on diagnostic imaging of breast

    R92.2 Inconclusive mammogram
        Dense breasts NOS
        Inconclusive mammogram NEC
        Inconclusive mammography due to dense breasts
        Inconclusive mammography NEC

    R92.8 Other abnormal and inconclusive findings on diagnostic imaging of breast

● **R93 Abnormal findings on diagnostic imaging of other body structures**

    R93.0 Abnormal findings on diagnostic imaging of skull and head, not elsewhere classified
        Excludes1 intracranial space-occupying lesion found on diagnostic imaging (R90.0)

    R93.1 Abnormal findings on diagnostic imaging of heart and coronary circulation
        Abnormal echocardiogram NOS
        Abnormal heart shadow

    R93.2 Abnormal findings on diagnostic imaging of liver and biliary tract
        Nonvisualization of gallbladder

    R93.3 Abnormal findings on diagnostic imaging of other parts of digestive tract

    ● **R93.4 Abnormal findings on diagnostic imaging of urinary organs**
        Excludes2 hypertrophy of kidney (N28.81)

        R93.41 Abnormal radiologic findings on diagnostic imaging of renal pelvis, ureter, or bladder
            Filling defect of bladder found on diagnostic imaging
            Filling defect of renal pelvis found on diagnostic imaging
            Filling defect of ureter found on diagnostic imaging

        ● **R93.42 Abnormal radiologic findings on diagnostic imaging of kidney**
            R93.421 Abnormal radiologic findings on diagnostic imaging of right kidney
            R93.422 Abnormal radiologic findings on diagnostic imaging of left kidney
            R93.429 Abnormal radiologic findings on diagnostic imaging of unspecified kidney

        R93.49 Abnormal radiologic findings on diagnostic imaging of other urinary organs

    R93.5 Abnormal findings on diagnostic imaging of other abdominal regions, including retroperitoneum

    R93.6 Abnormal findings on diagnostic imaging of limbs
        Excludes2 abnormal finding in skin and subcutaneous tissue (R93.8)

    R93.7 Abnormal findings on diagnostic imaging of other parts of musculoskeletal system
        Excludes2 abnormal findings on diagnostic imaging of skull (R93.0)

    R93.8 Abnormal findings on diagnostic imaging of other specified body structures
        Abnormal finding by radioisotope localization of placenta
        Abnormal radiological finding in skin and subcutaneous tissue
        Mediastinal shift

    R93.9 Diagnostic imaging inconclusive due to excess body fat of patient

● **R94 Abnormal results of function studies**
    Includes abnormal results of radionuclide [radioisotope] uptake studies
                   abnormal results of scintigraphy

    ● **R94.0 Abnormal results of function studies of central nervous system**
        R94.01 Abnormal electroencephalogram [EEG]
        R94.02 Abnormal brain scan
        R94.09 Abnormal results of other function studies of central nervous system

    ● **R94.1 Abnormal results of function studies of peripheral nervous system and special senses**

        ● **R94.11 Abnormal results of function studies of eye**
            R94.110 Abnormal electro-oculogram [EOG]
            R94.111 Abnormal electroretinogram [ERG]
                Abnormal retinal function study
            R94.112 Abnormal visually evoked potential [VEP]
            R94.113 Abnormal oculomotor study
            R94.118 Abnormal results of other function studies of eye

        ● **R94.12 Abnormal results of function studies of ear and other special senses**
            R94.120 Abnormal auditory function study
            R94.121 Abnormal vestibular function study
            R94.128 Abnormal results of other function studies of ear and other special senses

        ● **R94.13 Abnormal results of function studies of peripheral nervous system**
            R94.130 Abnormal response to nerve stimulation, unspecified
            R94.131 Abnormal electromyogram [EMG]
                Excludes1 electromyogram of eye (R94.113)
            R94.138 Abnormal results of other function studies of peripheral nervous system

---

Item 18–1 The **peripheral nervous system** consists of 31 pairs of spinal nerves, 12 pairs of cranial nerves, and the autonomic nerves, which are divided into the parasympathetic and sympathetic nerves. The cranial nerves are: olfactory (I), optic (II), oculomotor (III), trochlear (IV), trigeminal (V), abducens (VI), facial (VII), vestibulocochlear (VIII), glossopharyngeal (IX), vagus (X), accessory (XI), and hypoglossal (XII).

▶ New   ⇒ Revised   deleted Deleted   **OGCR** Official Guidelines   X Assign placeholder X   ● Use Additional Character(s)

Excludes 1   Excludes 2   Includes   Use additional   Code first   Code also   Key words

Trochlear nerve (IV)

Optic nerve (II)

Olfactory nerve (I)

Abducens nerve (VI)

Oculomotor nerve (III)

Facial nerve (VII)

Trigeminal nerve (V)

Vestibulocochlear nerve (VIII)

Glossopharyngeal nerve (IX)

Vagus nerve (X)

Accessory nerve (XI)

Hypoglossal nerve (XII)

Figure 18-2 Cranial nerves. (From Patton and Thibodeau: Anatomy and physiology, ed 7, St. Louis, Mosby, 2009)

R94.2   **Abnormal results of pulmonary function studies**
Reduced ventilatory capacity
Reduced vital capacity

● R94.3   **Abnormal results of cardiovascular function studies**

     R94.30   **Abnormal result of cardiovascular function study, unspecified**

     R94.31   **Abnormal electrocardiogram [ECG] [EKG]**
       Excludes1   long QT syndrome (I45.81)

     R94.39   **Abnormal result of other cardiovascular function study**
       Abnormal electrophysiological intracardiac studies
       Abnormal phonocardiogram
       Abnormal vectorcardiogram

R94.4   **Abnormal results of kidney function studies**
Abnormal renal function test

R94.5   **Abnormal results of liver function studies**

R94.6   **Abnormal results of thyroid function studies**

R94.7   **Abnormal results of other endocrine function studies**
     Excludes2   abnormal glucose (R73.Ø-)

R94.8   **Abnormal results of function studies of other organs and systems**
Abnormal basal metabolic rate [BMR]
Abnormal bladder function test
Abnormal splenic function test

ABNORMAL TUMOR MARKERS (R97)

● R97   **Abnormal tumor markers**
Elevated tumor associated antigens [TAA]
Elevated tumor specific antigens [TSA]

     R97.Ø   **Elevated carcinoembryonic antigen [CEA]**

     R97.1   **Elevated cancer antigen 125 [CA 125]**

●   R97.2   **Elevated prostate specific antigen [PSA]**

       R97.2Ø   **Elevated prostate specific antigen [PSA]**

       R97.21   **Rising PSA following treatment for malignant neoplasm of prostate**

     R97.8   **Other abnormal tumor markers**

ILL-DEFINED AND UNKNOWN CAUSE OF MORTALITY (R99)

R99   **Ill-defined and unknown cause of mortality**
Death (unexplained) NOS
Unspecified cause of mortality

OGCR   Section I.C.18.h.

Death NOS

Code R99, Ill-defined and unknown cause of mortality, is only for use in the very limited circumstance when a patient who has already died is brought into the emergency department or other healthcare facility and is pronounced dead upon arrival. It does not represent the discharge disposition of death.

CHAPTER 18 (RØØ-R99)

CHAPTER 19

INJURY, POISONING AND CERTAIN OTHER CONSEQUENCES OF EXTERNAL CAUSES (S00-T88)

OGCR Chapter-Specific Coding Guidelines

19. **Chapter 19: Injury, poisoning, and certain other consequences of external causes (S00-T88)**

a. Application of 7th Characters in Chapter 19

Most categories in chapter 19 have a 7th character requirement for each applicable code. Most categories in this chapter have three 7th character values (with the exception of fractures): A, initial encounter, D, subsequent encounter and S, sequela. Categories for traumatic fractures have additional 7th character values. While the patient may be seen by a new or different provider over the course of treatment for an injury, assignment of the 7th character is based on whether the patient is undergoing active treatment and not whether the provider is seeing the patient for the first time.

For complication codes, active treatment refers to treatment for the condition described by the code, even though it may be related to an earlier precipitating problem. For example, code T84.50XA, Infection and inflammatory reaction due to unspecified internal joint prosthesis, initial encounter, is used when active treatment is provided for the infection, even though the condition relates to the prosthetic device, implant or graft that was placed at a previous encounter.

7th character "A", initial encounter is used **for each encounter where** the patient is receiving active treatment for the condition.

7th character "D" subsequent encounter is used for encounters after the patient has **completed** active treatment of the condition and is receiving routine care for the condition during the healing or recovery phase.

The aftercare Z codes should not be used for aftercare for conditions such as injuries or poisonings, where 7th characters are provided to identify subsequent care. For example, for aftercare of an injury, assign the acute injury code with the 7th character "D" (subsequent encounter).

7th character "S", sequela, is for use for complications or conditions that arise as a direct result of a condition, such as scar formation after a burn. The scars are sequelae of the burn. When using 7th character "S", it is necessary to use both the injury code that precipitated the sequela and the code for the sequela itself. The "S" is added only to the injury code, not the sequela code. The 7th character "S" identifies the injury responsible for the sequela. The specific type of sequela (e.g. scar) is sequenced first, followed by the injury code.

See Section I.B.10. Sequelae, (Late Effects)

b. Coding of Injuries

When coding injuries, assign separate codes for each injury unless a combination code is provided, in which case the combination code is assigned. **Codes from category** T07, Unspecified multiple injuries should not be assigned in the inpatient setting unless information for a more specific code is not available. Traumatic injury codes (S00-T14.9) are not to be used for normal, healing surgical wounds or to identify complications of surgical wounds.

The code for the most serious injury, as determined by the provider and the focus of treatment, is sequenced first.

1) Superficial injuries

Superficial injuries such as abrasions or contusions are not coded when associated with more severe injuries of the same site.

2) Primary injury with damage to nerves/blood vessels

When a primary injury results in minor damage to peripheral nerves or blood vessels, the primary injury is sequenced first with additional code(s) for injuries to nerves and spinal cord (such as category S04), and/or injury to blood vessels (such as category S15). When the primary injury is to the blood vessels or nerves, that injury should be sequenced first.

c. Coding of Traumatic Fractures

The principles of multiple coding of injuries should be followed in coding fractures. Fractures of specified sites are coded individually by site in accordance with both the provisions within categories S02, S12, S22, S32, S42, S49, S52, S59, S62, S72, S79, S82, S89, S92 and the level of detail furnished by medical record content.

A fracture not indicated as open or closed should be coded to closed. A fracture not indicated whether displaced or not displaced should be coded to displaced.

More specific guidelines are as follows:

1) Initial vs. Subsequent Encounter for Fractures

Traumatic fractures are coded using the appropriate 7th character for initial encounter (A, B, C) **for each encounter where** the patient is receiving active treatment for the fracture. The appropriate 7th character for initial encounter should also be assigned for a patient who delayed seeking treatment for the fracture or nonunion.

Fractures are coded using the appropriate 7th character for subsequent care for encounters after the patient has completed active treatment of the fracture and is receiving routine care for the fracture during the healing or recovery phase.

Care for complications of surgical treatment for fracture repairs during the healing or recovery phase should be coded with the appropriate complication codes.

Care of complications of fractures, such as malunion and nonunion, should be reported with the appropriate 7th character for subsequent care with nonunion (K, M, N,) or subsequent care with malunion (P, Q, R).

Malunion/nonunion: The appropriate 7th character for initial encounter should also be assigned for a patient who delayed seeking treatment for the fracture or nonunion.

The open fracture designations in the assignment of the 7th character for fractures of the forearm, femur and lower leg, including ankle are based on the Gustilo open fracture classification. When the Gustilo classification type is not specified for an open fracture, the 7th character for open fracture type I or II should be assigned (B, E, H, M, Q).

A code from category M80, not a traumatic fracture code, should be used for any patient with known osteoporosis who suffers a fracture, even if the patient had a minor fall or trauma, if that fall or trauma would not usually break a normal, healthy bone.

See Section I.C.13. Osteoporosis.

The aftercare Z codes should not be used for aftercare for traumatic fractures. For aftercare of a traumatic fracture, assign the acute fracture code with the appropriate 7th character.

2) Multiple fractures sequencing

Multiple fractures are sequenced in accordance with the severity of the fracture.

d. Coding of Burns and Corrosions

The ICD-10-CM makes a distinction between burns and corrosions. The burn codes are for thermal burns, except sunburns, that come from a heat source, such as a fire or hot appliance. The burn codes are also for burns resulting from electricity and radiation. Corrosions are burns due to chemicals. The guidelines are the same for burns and corrosions.

Current burns (T20-T25) are classified by depth, extent and by agent (X code). Burns are classified by depth as first degree (erythema), second degree (blistering), and third degree (full-thickness involvement). Burns of the eye and internal organs (T26-T28) are classified by site, but not by degree.

1) Sequencing of burn and related condition codes

Sequence first the code that reflects the highest degree of burn when more than one burn is present.

  a. When the reason for the admission or encounter is for treatment of external multiple burns, sequence first the code that reflects the burn of the highest degree.

  b. When a patient has both internal and external burns, the circumstances of admission govern the selection of the principal diagnosis or first-listed diagnosis.

  c. When a patient is admitted for burn injuries and other related conditions such as smoke inhalation and/or respiratory failure, the circumstances of admission govern the selection of the principal or first-listed diagnosis.

2) Burns of the same local site

Classify burns of the same local site (three-character category level, T20-T28) but of different degrees to the subcategory identifying the highest degree recorded in the diagnosis.

3) Non-healing burns

Non-healing burns are coded as acute burns.

Necrosis of burned skin should be coded as a non-healed burn.

4) Infected Burn

For any documented infected burn site, use an additional code for the infection.

5) Assign separate codes for each burn site

When coding burns, assign separate codes for each burn site. Category T30, Burn and corrosion, body region unspecified is extremely vague and should rarely be used.

6) Burns and Corrosions Classified According to Extent of Body Surface Involved

Assign codes from category T31, Burns classified according to extent of body surface involved, or T32, Corrosions classified according to extent of body surface involved, when the site of the burn is not specified or when there is a need for additional data. It is advisable to use category T31 as additional coding when needed to provide data for evaluating burn mortality, such as that needed by burn units. It is also advisable to use category T31 as an additional code for reporting purposes when there is mention of a third-degree burn involving 20 percent or more of the body surface.

Categories T31 and T32 are based on the classic "rule of nines" in estimating body surface involved: head and neck are assigned nine percent, each arm nine percent, each leg 18 percent, the anterior trunk 18 percent, posterior trunk 18 percent, and genitalia one percent. Providers may change these percentage assignments where necessary to accommodate infants and children who have proportionately larger heads than adults, and patients who have large buttocks, thighs, or abdomen that involve burns.

7) Encounters for treatment of sequela of burns

Encounters for the treatment of the late effects of burns or corrosions (i.e., scars or joint contractures) should be coded with a burn or corrosion code with the 7th character "S" for sequela.

8) Sequelae with a late effect code and current burn

When appropriate, both a code for a current burn or corrosion with 7th character "A" or "D" and a burn or corrosion code with 7th character "S" may be assigned on the same record (when both a current burn and sequelae of an old burn exist). Burns and corrosions do not heal at the same rate and a current healing wound may still exist with sequela of a healed burn or corrosion.

See Section I.B.10. Sequela, (Late Effects)

9) Use of an external cause code with burns and corrosions

An external cause code should be used with burns and corrosions to identify the source and intent of the burn, as well as the place where it occurred.

e. Adverse Effects, Poisoning , Underdosing and Toxic Effects

Codes in categories T36-T65 are combination codes that include the substance that was taken as well as the intent. No additional external cause code is required for poisonings, toxic effects, adverse effects and underdosing codes.

1) Do not code directly from the Table of Drugs

Do not code directly from the Table of Drugs and Chemicals. Always refer back to the Tabular List.

2) Use as many codes as necessary to describe

Use as many codes as necessary to describe completely all drugs, medicinal or biological substances.

3) If the same code would describe the causative agent

If the same code would describe the causative agent for more than one adverse reaction, poisoning, toxic effect or underdosing, assign the code only once.

4) If two or more drugs, medicinal or biological substances

If two or more drugs, medicinal or biological substances are reported, code each individually unless a combination code is listed in the Table of Drugs and Chemicals.

5) The occurrence of drug toxicity is classified in ICD-10-CM as follows:

(a) Adverse Effect

When coding an adverse effect of a drug that has been correctly prescribed and properly administered, assign the appropriate code for the nature of the adverse effect followed by the appropriate code for the adverse effect of the drug (T36-T50). The code for the drug should have a 5th or 6th character "5" (for example T36.0X5-) Examples of the nature of an adverse effect are tachycardia, delirium, gastrointestinal hemorrhaging, vomiting, hypokalemia, hepatitis, renal failure, or respiratory failure.

(b) Poisoning

When coding a poisoning or reaction to the improper use of a medication (e.g., overdose, wrong substance given or taken in error, wrong route of administration), first assign the appropriate code from categories T36-T50. The poisoning codes have an associated intent as their 5th or 6th character (accidental, intentional self-harm, assault and undetermined). **If the intent of the poisoning is unknown or unspecified, code the intent as accidental intent. The undetermined intent is only for use if the documentation in the record specifies that the intent cannot be determined.** Use additional code(s) for all manifestations of poisonings.

If there is also a diagnosis of abuse or dependence of the substance, the abuse or dependence is assigned as an additional code.

Examples of poisoning include:

(i) Error was made in drug prescription
Errors made in drug prescription or in the administration of the drug by provider, nurse, patient, or other person.

(ii) Overdose of a drug intentionally taken If an overdose of a drug was intentionally taken or administered and resulted in drug toxicity, it would be coded as a poisoning.

(iii) Nonprescribed drug taken with correctly prescribed and properly administered drug. If a nonprescribed drug or medicinal agent was taken in combination with a correctly prescribed and properly administered drug, any drug toxicity or other reaction resulting from the interaction of the two drugs would be classified as a poisoning.

(iv) Interaction of drug(s) and alcohol. When a reaction results from the interaction of a drug(s) and alcohol, this would be classified as poisoning.

See Section I.C.4. if poisoning is the result of insulin pump malfunctions.

(c) Underdosing

Underdosing refers to taking less of a medication than is prescribed by a provider or a manufacturer's instruction. For underdosing, assign the code from categories T36-T50 (fifth or sixth character "6").

Codes for underdosing should never be assigned as principal or first-listed codes. If a patient has a relapse or exacerbation of the medical condition for which the drug is prescribed because of the reduction in dose, then the medical condition itself should be coded.

Noncompliance (Z91.12-, Z91.13-) or complication of care (Y63.6-Y63.9) codes are to be used with an underdosing code to indicate intent, if known.

(d) Toxic Effects

When a harmful substance is ingested or comes in contact with a person, this is classified as a toxic effect. The toxic effect codes are in categories T51-T65.

Toxic effect codes have an associated intent: accidental, intentional self-harm, assault and undetermined.

f. Adult and child abuse, neglect and other maltreatment

Sequence first the appropriate code from categories T74 (Adult and child abuse, neglect and other maltreatment, confirmed) or T76 (Adult and child abuse, neglect and other maltreatment, suspected) for abuse, neglect and other maltreatment, followed by any accompanying mental health or injury code(s).

If the documentation in the medical record states abuse or neglect it is coded as confirmed (T74.-). It is coded as suspected if it is documented as suspected (T76.-).

For cases of confirmed abuse or neglect an external cause code from the assault section (X92-**Y09**) should be added to identify the cause of any physical injuries. A perpetrator code (Y07) should be added when the perpetrator of the abuse is known. For suspected cases of abuse or neglect, do not report external cause or perpetrator code.

If a suspected case of abuse, neglect or mistreatment is ruled out during an encounter code Z04.71, Encounter for examination and observation following alleged physical adult abuse, ruled out, or code Z04.72, Encounter for examination and observation following alleged child physical abuse, ruled out, should be used, not a code from T76.

If a suspected case of alleged rape or sexual abuse is ruled out during an encounter code Z04.41, Encounter for examination and observation following alleged **adult rape** or code Z04.42, Encounter for examination and observation following alleged **child rape**, should be used, not a code from T76.

See Section I.C.15. Abuse in a pregnant patient.

g. Complications of care

1) General guidelines for complications of care

(a) Documentation of complications of care

See Section I.B.16. for information on documentation of complications of care.

2) Pain due to medical devices

Pain associated with devices, implants or grafts left in a surgical site (for example painful hip prosthesis) is assigned to the appropriate code(s) found in Chapter 19, Injury, poisoning, and certain other consequences of external causes. Specific codes for pain due to medical devices are found in the T code section of the ICD-10-CM. Use additional code(s) from category G89 to identify acute or chronic pain due to presence of the device, implant or graft (G89.18 or G89.28).

3) Transplant complications

(a) Transplant complications other than kidney

Codes under category T86, Complications of transplanted organs and tissues, are for use for both complications and rejection of transplanted organs. A transplant complication code is only assigned if the complication affects the function of the transplanted organ. Two codes are required to fully describe a transplant complication: the appropriate code from category T86 and a secondary code that identifies the complication.

Pre-existing conditions or conditions that develop after the transplant are not coded as complications unless they affect the function of the transplanted organs.

See I.C.21. for transplant organ removal status
See I.C.2. for malignant neoplasm associated with transplanted organ.

(b) Kidney transplant complications

Patients who have undergone kidney transplant may still have some form of chronic kidney disease (CKD) because the kidney transplant may not fully restore kidney function. Code T86.1- should be assigned for documented complications of a kidney transplant, such as transplant failure or rejection or other transplant complication. Code T86.1- should not be assigned for post kidney transplant patients who have chronic kidney (CKD) unless a transplant complication such as transplant failure or rejection is documented. If the documentation is unclear as to whether the patient has a complication of the transplant, query the provider.

Conditions that affect the function of the transplanted kidney, other than CKD, should be assigned a code from subcategory T86.1, Complications of transplanted organ, Kidney, and a secondary code that identifies the complication.

For patients with CKD following a kidney transplant, but who do not have a complication such as failure or rejection, *see section I.C.14. Chronic kidney disease and kidney transplant status.*

4) Complication codes that include the external cause

As with certain other T codes, some of the complications of care codes have the external cause included in the code. The code includes the nature of the complication as well as the type of procedure that caused the complication. No external cause code indicating the type of procedure is necessary for these codes.

5) Complications of care codes within the body system chapters

Intraoperative and postprocedural complication codes are found within the body system chapters with codes specific to the organs and structures of that body system. These codes should be sequenced first, followed by a code(s) for the specific complication, if applicable.

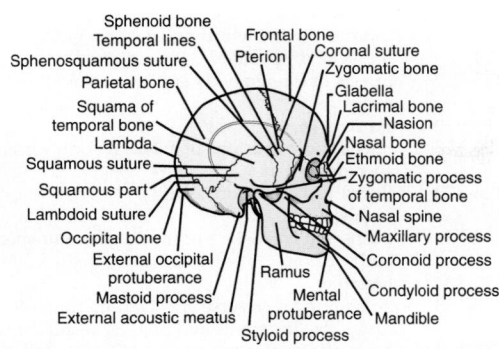

Figure 19-1 Lateral view of skull.

Figure 19-2 Frontal view of skull.

Figure 19-3 Anterior view of vertebral column.

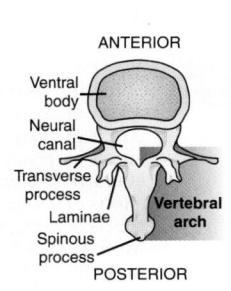

Figure 19-4 Vertebra viewed from above.

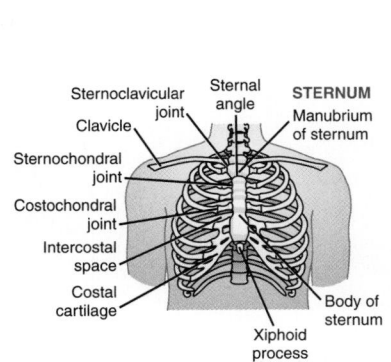

Figure 19-5 Anterior view of rib cage.

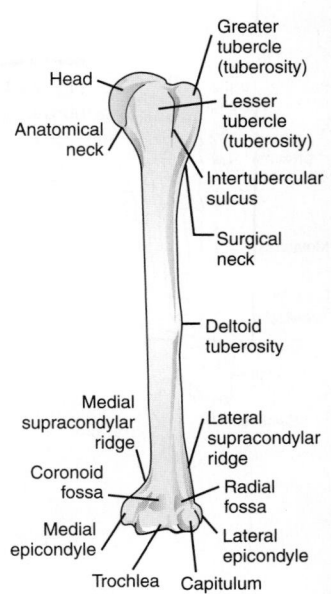

Figure 19-6 Anterior aspect of left humerus.

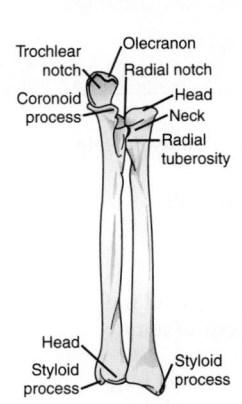

Figure 19-7 Anterior aspect of left radius and ulna.

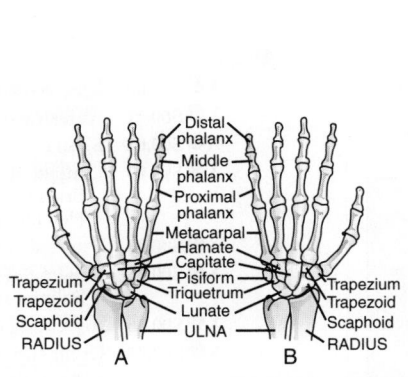

Figure 19-8 Right hand and wrist: **A.** Dorsal surface. **B.** Palmar surface.

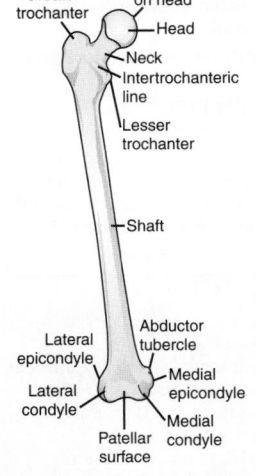

Figure 19-9 Anterior aspect of right femur.

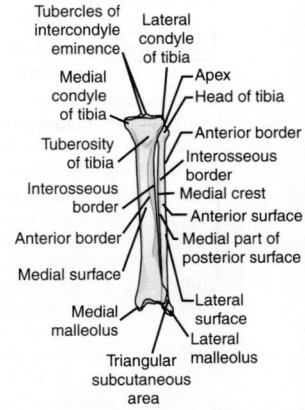

Figure 19-10 Anterior aspect of left tibia and fibula.

CHAPTER 19 (S00-T88)

▶ New　⇒ Revised　~~deleted~~ Deleted　**OGCR** Official Guidelines　X Assign placeholder X　● Use Additional Character(s)

Excludes 1　Excludes 2　Includes　Use additional　Code first　Code also　Key words

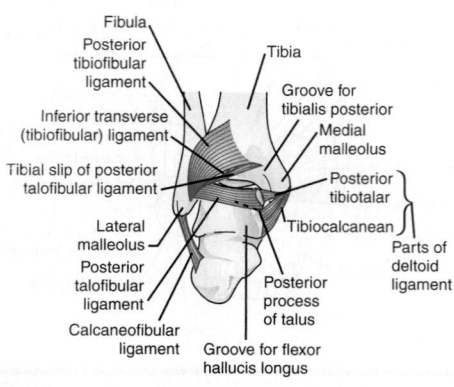

Figure 19-11 Posterior aspect of the left ankle joint.

Figure 19-12 Right foot viewed from above.

CHAPTER 19

INJURY, POISONING AND CERTAIN OTHER CONSEQUENCES OF EXTERNAL CAUSES (S00-T88)

Note: Use secondary code(s) from Chapter 20, External causes of morbidity, to indicate cause of injury. Codes within the T section that include the external cause do not require an additional external cause code.

Use additional code to identify any retained foreign body, if applicable (Z18.-)

Excludes1 birth trauma (P10-P15)
obstetric trauma (O70-O71)

Note: The chapter uses the S-section for coding different types of injuries related to single body regions and the T-section to cover injuries to unspecified body regions as well as poisoning and certain other consequences of external causes.

This chapter contains the following blocks:

S00-S09	Injuries to the head
S10-S19	Injuries to the neck
S20-S29	Injuries to the thorax
S30-S39	Injuries to the abdomen, lower back, lumbar spine, pelvis and external genitals
S40-S49	Injuries to the shoulder and upper arm
S50-S59	Injuries to the elbow and forearm
S60-S69	Injuries to the wrist, hand, and fingers
S70-S79	Injuries to the hip and thigh
S80-S89	Injuries to the knee and lower leg
S90-S99	Injuries to the ankle and foot

T07	Injuries involving multiple body regions
T14	Injury of unspecified body region
T15-T19	Effects of foreign body entering through natural orifice
~~T20-T32~~	~~Burns and corrosions~~
T20-T25	Burns and corrosions of external body surface, specified by site
T26-T28	Burns and corrosions confined to eye and internal organs
T30-T32	Burns and corrosions of multiple and unspecified body regions
T33-T34	Frostbite
T36-T50	Poisoning by, adverse effect of and underdosing of drugs, medicaments and biological substances
T51-T65	Toxic effects of substances chiefly nonmedicinal as to source
T66-T78	Other and unspecified effects of external causes
T79	Certain early complications of trauma
T80-T88	Complications of surgical and medical care, not elsewhere classified

INJURIES TO THE HEAD (S00-S09)

Includes
injuries of ear
injuries of eye
injuries of face [any part]
injuries of gum
injuries of jaw
injuries of oral cavity
injuries of palate
injuries of periocular area
injuries of scalp
injuries of temporomandibular joint area
injuries of tongue
injuries of tooth

Code also for any associated infection

Excludes2 burns and corrosions (T20-T32)
effects of foreign body in ear (T16)
effects of foreign body in larynx (T17.3)
effects of foreign body in mouth NOS (T18.0)
effects of foreign body in nose (T17.0-T17.1)
effects of foreign body in pharynx (T17.2)
effects of foreign body on external eye (T15.-)
frostbite (T33-T34)
insect bite or sting, venomous (T63.4)

● S00   Superficial injury of head
Excludes1 diffuse cerebral contusion (S06.2-)
focal cerebral contusion (S06.3-)
injury of eye and orbit (S05.-)
open wound of head (S01.-)

The appropriate 7th character is to be added to each code from category S00

A	initial encounter
	All encounters involving diagnosis and treatment
D	subsequent encounter
	Encounters during the healing phase
S	sequela

● S00.0   Superficial injury of scalp
X● S00.00   **Unspecified** superficial injury of scalp
X● S00.01   **Abrasion** of scalp
X● S00.02   **Blister** (nonthermal) of scalp
X● S00.03   **Contusion** of scalp
Bruise of scalp
Hematoma of scalp
X● S00.04   **External constriction** of part of scalp
X● S00.05   **Superficial foreign body** of scalp
Splinter in the scalp
X● S00.06   **Insect bite** (nonvenomous) of scalp
X● S00.07   **Other** superficial bite of scalp
Excludes1 open bite of scalp (S01.05)

▶ New   ⇒ Revised   ~~deleted~~ Deleted   **OGCR** Official Guidelines   X Assign placeholder X   ● Use Additional Character(s)

Excludes 1   Excludes 2   Includes   Use additional   Code first   Code also   Key words

- ● **S00.1**   Contusion of eyelid and periocular area
  Black eye
  Excludes2   contusion of eyeball and orbital tissues (S05.1)
  - X ● **S00.10**   Contusion of unspecified eyelid and periocular area
  - X ● **S00.11**   Contusion of right eyelid and periocular area
  - X ● **S00.12**   Contusion of left eyelid and periocular area
- ● **S00.2**   Other and unspecified superficial injuries of eyelid and periocular area
  Excludes2   superficial injury of conjunctiva and cornea (S05.0-)
  - ● **S00.20**   Unspecified superficial injury of eyelid and periocular area
    - ● **S00.201**   Unspecified superficial injury of right eyelid and periocular area
    - ● **S00.202**   Unspecified superficial injury of left eyelid and periocular area
    - ● **S00.209**   Unspecified superficial injury of unspecified eyelid and periocular area
  - ● **S00.21**   Abrasion of eyelid and periocular area
    - ● **S00.211**   Abrasion of right eyelid and periocular area
    - ● **S00.212**   Abrasion of left eyelid and periocular area
    - ● **S00.219**   Abrasion of unspecified eyelid and periocular area
  - ● **S00.22**   Blister (nonthermal) of eyelid and periocular area
    - ● **S00.221**   Blister (nonthermal) of right eyelid and periocular area
    - ● **S00.222**   Blister (nonthermal) of left eyelid and periocular area
    - ● **S00.229**   Blister (nonthermal) of unspecified eyelid and periocular area
  - ● **S00.24**   External constriction of eyelid and periocular area
    - ● **S00.241**   External constriction of right eyelid and periocular area
    - ● **S00.242**   External constriction of left eyelid and periocular area
    - ● **S00.249**   External constriction of unspecified eyelid and periocular area
  - ● **S00.25**   Superficial foreign body of eyelid and periocular area
    Splinter of eyelid and periocular area
    Excludes2   retained foreign body in eyelid (H02.81-)
    - ● **S00.251**   Superficial foreign body of right eyelid and periocular area
    - ● **S00.252**   Superficial foreign body of left eyelid and periocular area
    - ● **S00.259**   Superficial foreign body of unspecified eyelid and periocular area
  - ● **S00.26**   Insect bite (nonvenomous) of eyelid and periocular area
    - ● **S00.261**   Insect bite (nonvenomous) of right eyelid and periocular area
    - ● **S00.262**   Insect bite (nonvenomous) of left eyelid and periocular area
    - ● **S00.269**   Insect bite (nonvenomous) of unspecified eyelid and periocular area

- ● **S00.27**   Other superficial bite of eyelid and periocular area
  Excludes1   open bite of eyelid and periocular area (S01.15)
  - ● **S00.271**   Other superficial bite of right eyelid and periocular area
  - ● **S00.272**   Other superficial bite of left eyelid and periocular area
  - ● **S00.279**   Other superficial bite of unspecified eyelid and periocular area
- ● **S00.3**   Superficial injury of nose
  - X ● **S00.30**   Unspecified superficial injury of nose
  - X ● **S00.31**   Abrasion of nose
  - X ● **S00.32**   Blister (nonthermal) of nose
  - X ● **S00.33**   Contusion of nose
    Bruise of nose
    Hematoma of nose
  - X ● **S00.34**   External constriction of nose
  - X ● **S00.35**   Superficial foreign body of nose
    Splinter in the nose
  - X ● **S00.36**   Insect bite (nonvenomous) of nose
  - X ● **S00.37**   Other superficial bite of nose
    Excludes1   open bite of nose (S01.25)
- ● **S00.4**   Superficial injury of ear
  - ● **S00.40**   Unspecified superficial injury of ear
    - ● **S00.401**   Unspecified superficial injury of right ear
    - ● **S00.402**   Unspecified superficial injury of left ear
    - ● **S00.409**   Unspecified superficial injury of unspecified ear
  - ● **S00.41**   Abrasion of ear
    - ● **S00.411**   Abrasion of right ear
    - ● **S00.412**   Abrasion of left ear
    - ● **S00.419**   Abrasion of unspecified ear
  - ● **S00.42**   Blister (nonthermal) of ear
    - ● **S00.421**   Blister (nonthermal) of right ear
    - ● **S00.422**   Blister (nonthermal) of left ear
    - ● **S00.429**   Blister (nonthermal) of unspecified ear
  - ● **S00.43**   Contusion of ear
    Bruise of ear
    Hematoma of ear
    - ● **S00.431**   Contusion of right ear
    - ● **S00.432**   Contusion of left ear
    - ● **S00.439**   Contusion of unspecified ear
  - ● **S00.44**   External constriction of ear
    - ● **S00.441**   External constriction of right ear
    - ● **S00.442**   External constriction of left ear
    - ● **S00.449**   External constriction of unspecified ear
  - ● **S00.45**   Superficial foreign body of ear
    Splinter in the ear
    - ● **S00.451**   Superficial foreign body of right ear
    - ● **S00.452**   Superficial foreign body of left ear
    - ● **S00.459**   Superficial foreign body of unspecified ear
  - ● **S00.46**   Insect bite (nonvenomous) of ear
    - ● **S00.461**   Insect bite (nonvenomous) of right ear
    - ● **S00.462**   Insect bite (nonvenomous) of left ear
    - ● **S00.469**   Insect bite (nonvenomous) of unspecified ear

CHAPTER 19 (S00–T88)

▶ New   ⮕ Revised   ~~deleted~~ Deleted   **OGCR** Official Guidelines   X Assign placeholder X   ● Use Additional Character(s)

Excludes 1   Excludes 2   Includes   Use additional   Code first   Code also   Key words

● S00.47 **Other superficial bite** of ear
  Excludes1 open bite of ear (S01.35)
  ● S00.471 Other superficial bite of **right** ear
  ● S00.472 Other superficial bite of **left** ear
  ● S00.479 Other superficial bite of **unspecified** ear

● S00.5 **Superficial injury of lip and oral cavity**
  ● S00.50 **Unspecified superficial injury of lip and oral cavity**
    ● S00.501 Unspecified superficial injury of **lip**
    ● S00.502 Unspecified superficial injury of **oral cavity**
  ● S00.51 **Abrasion of lip and oral cavity**
    ● S00.511 Abrasion of **lip**
    ● S00.512 Abrasion of **oral cavity**
  ● S00.52 **Blister (nonthermal) of lip and oral cavity**
    ● S00.521 Blister (nonthermal) of **lip**
    ● S00.522 Blister (nonthermal) of **oral cavity**
  ● S00.53 **Contusion of lip and oral cavity**
    ● S00.531 Contusion of **lip**
      Bruise of lip
      ⇒ Hematoma of lip
    ● S00.532 Contusion of **oral cavity**
      ⇒ Bruise of oral cavity
      Hematoma of oral cavity
  ● S00.54 **External constriction of lip and oral cavity**
    ● S00.541 External constriction of **lip**
    ● S00.542 External constriction of **oral cavity**
  ● S00.55 **Superficial foreign body of lip and oral cavity**
    ● S00.551 Superficial foreign body of **lip**
      Splinter of lip and oral cavity
    ● S00.552 Superficial foreign body of **oral cavity**
      Splinter of lip and oral cavity
  ● S00.56 **Insect bite (nonvenomous) of lip and oral cavity**
    ● S00.561 Insect bite (nonvenomous) of **lip**
    ● S00.562 Insect bite (nonvenomous) of **oral cavity**
  ● S00.57 **Other superficial bite of lip and oral cavity**
    ● S00.571 Other superficial bite of **lip**
      Excludes1 open bite of lip (S01.551)
    ● S00.572 Other superficial bite of **oral cavity**
      Excludes1 open bite of oral cavity (S01.552)

● S00.8 **Superficial injury of other parts of head**
  Superficial injuries of face [any part]
  X● S00.80 **Unspecified** superficial injury of other part of head
  X● S00.81 **Abrasion** of other part of head
  X● S00.82 **Blister (nonthermal)** of other part of head
  X● S00.83 **Contusion** of other part of head
    Bruise of other part of head
    Hematoma of other part of head
  X● S00.84 **External constriction** of other part of head
  X● S00.85 **Superficial foreign body** of other part of head
    Splinter in other part of head
  X● S00.86 **Insect bite (nonvenomous)** of other part of head
  X● S00.87 **Other superficial bite** of other part of head
    Excludes1 open bite of other part of head (S01.85)

● S00.9 **Superficial injury of unspecified part of head**
  X● S00.90 **Unspecified** superficial injury of unspecified part of head
  X● S00.91 **Abrasion** of unspecified part of head
  X● S00.92 **Blister (nonthermal)** of unspecified part of head

X● S00.93 **Contusion** of unspecified part of head
  Bruise of head
  Hematoma of head
X● S00.94 **External constriction** of unspecified part of head
X● S00.95 **Superficial foreign body** of unspecified part of head
  Splinter of head
X● S00.96 **Insect bite (nonvenomous)** of unspecified part of head
X● S00.97 **Other superficial bite** of unspecified part of head
  Excludes1 open bite of head (S01.95)

● S01 **Open wound of head**
  Code also any associated:
    injury of cranial nerve (S04.-)
    injury of muscle and tendon of head (S09.1-)
    intracranial injury (S06.-)
    wound infection
  Excludes1 open skull fracture (S02.- with 7th character B)
  Excludes2 injury of eye and orbit (S05.-)
    traumatic amputation of part of head (S08.-)
  The appropriate 7th character is to be added to each code from category S01
A	initial encounter
D	subsequent encounter
S	sequela

  ● S01.0 **Open wound of scalp**
    Excludes1 avulsion of scalp (S08.0)
    X● S01.00 **Unspecified** open wound of scalp
    X● S01.01 **Laceration without foreign body** of scalp
    X● S01.02 **Laceration with foreign body** of scalp
    X● S01.03 **Puncture wound without foreign body** of scalp
    X● S01.04 **Puncture wound with foreign body** of scalp
    X● S01.05 **Open bite** of scalp
      Bite of scalp NOS
      Excludes1 superficial bite of scalp (S00.06, S00.07-)

  ● S01.1 **Open wound of eyelid and periocular area**
    Open wound of eyelid and periocular area with or without involvement of lacrimal passages
    ● S01.10 **Unspecified** open wound of eyelid and periocular area
      ● S01.101 Unspecified open wound of **right** eyelid and periocular area
      ● S01.102 Unspecified open wound of **left** eyelid and periocular area
      ● S01.109 Unspecified open wound of **unspecified** eyelid and periocular area
    ● S01.11 **Laceration without foreign body** of eyelid and periocular area
      ● S01.111 Laceration without foreign body of **right** eyelid and periocular area
      ● S01.112 Laceration without foreign body of **left** eyelid and periocular area
      ● S01.119 Laceration without foreign body of **unspecified** eyelid and periocular area
    ● S01.12 **Laceration with foreign body** of eyelid and periocular area
      ● S01.121 Laceration with foreign body of **right** eyelid and periocular area
      ● S01.122 Laceration with foreign body of **left** eyelid and periocular area
      ● S01.129 Laceration with foreign body of **unspecified** eyelid and periocular area

● **S01.13**   Puncture wound without foreign body of eyelid and periocular area
- ● **S01.131**   Puncture wound without foreign body of right eyelid and periocular area
- ● **S01.132**   Puncture wound without foreign body of left eyelid and periocular area
- ● **S01.139**   Puncture wound without foreign body of unspecified eyelid and periocular area

● **S01.14**   Puncture wound with foreign body of eyelid and periocular area
- ● **S01.141**   Puncture wound with foreign body of right eyelid and periocular area
- ● **S01.142**   Puncture wound with foreign body of left eyelid and periocular area
- ● **S01.149**   Puncture wound with foreign body of unspecified eyelid and periocular area

● **S01.15**   Open bite of eyelid and periocular area
   Bite of eyelid and periocular area NOS
   Excludes1   superficial bite of eyelid and periocular area (S00.26, S00.27)
- ● **S01.151**   Open bite of right eyelid and periocular area
- ● **S01.152**   Open bite of left eyelid and periocular area
- ● **S01.159**   Open bite of unspecified eyelid and periocular area

● **S01.2**   Open wound of nose
- X ● **S01.20**   Unspecified open wound of nose
- X ● **S01.21**   Laceration without foreign body of nose
- X ● **S01.22**   Laceration with foreign body of nose
- X ● **S01.23**   Puncture wound without foreign body of nose
- X ● **S01.24**   Puncture wound with foreign body of nose
- X ● **S01.25**   Open bite of nose
   Bite of nose NOS
   Excludes1   superficial bite of nose (S00.36, S00.37)

● **S01.3**   Open wound of ear
- ● **S01.30**   Unspecified open wound of ear
  - ● **S01.301**   Unspecified open wound of right ear
  - ● **S01.302**   Unspecified open wound of left ear
  - ● **S01.309**   Unspecified open wound of unspecified ear
- ● **S01.31**   Laceration without foreign body of ear
  - ● **S01.311**   Laceration without foreign body of right ear
  - ● **S01.312**   Laceration without foreign body of left ear
  - ● **S01.319**   Laceration without foreign body of unspecified ear
- ● **S01.32**   Laceration with foreign body of ear
  - ● **S01.321**   Laceration with foreign body of right ear
  - ● **S01.322**   Laceration with foreign body of left ear
  - ● **S01.329**   Laceration with foreign body of unspecified ear

● **S01.33**   Puncture wound without foreign body of ear
- ● **S01.331**   Puncture wound without foreign body of right ear
- ● **S01.332**   Puncture wound without foreign body of left ear
- ● **S01.339**   Puncture wound without foreign body of unspecified ear

● **S01.34**   Puncture wound with foreign body of ear
- ● **S01.341**   Puncture wound with foreign body of right ear
- ● **S01.342**   Puncture wound with foreign body of left ear
- ● **S01.349**   Puncture wound with foreign body of unspecified ear

● **S01.35**   Open bite of ear
   Bite of ear NOS
   Excludes1   superficial bite of ear (S00.46, S00.47)
- ● **S01.351**   Open bite of right ear
- ● **S01.352**   Open bite of left ear
- ● **S01.359**   Open bite of unspecified ear

● **S01.4**   Open wound of cheek and temporomandibular area
- ● **S01.40**   Unspecified open wound of cheek and temporomandibular area
  - ● **S01.401**   Unspecified open wound of right cheek and temporomandibular area
  - ● **S01.402**   Unspecified open wound of left cheek and temporomandibular area
  - ● **S01.409**   Unspecified open wound of unspecified cheek and temporomandibular area
- ● **S01.41**   Laceration without foreign body of cheek and temporomandibular area
  - ● **S01.411**   Laceration without foreign body of right cheek and temporomandibular area
  - ● **S01.412**   Laceration without foreign body of left cheek and temporomandibular area
  - ● **S01.419**   Laceration without foreign body of unspecified cheek and temporomandibular area
- ● **S01.42**   Laceration with foreign body of cheek and temporomandibular area
  - ● **S01.421**   Laceration with foreign body of right cheek and temporomandibular area
  - ● **S01.422**   Laceration with foreign body of left cheek and temporomandibular area
  - ● **S01.429**   Laceration with foreign body of unspecified cheek and temporomandibular area
- ● **S01.43**   Puncture wound without foreign body of cheek and temporomandibular area
  - ● **S01.431**   Puncture wound without foreign body of right cheek and temporomandibular area
  - ● **S01.432**   Puncture wound without foreign body of left cheek and temporomandibular area
  - ● **S01.439**   Puncture wound without foreign body of unspecified cheek and temporomandibular area

● S01.44   Puncture wound with foreign body of cheek and temporomandibular area

   ● S01.441   Puncture wound with foreign body of right cheek and temporomandibular area

   ● S01.442   Puncture wound with foreign body of left cheek and temporomandibular area

   ● S01.449   Puncture wound with foreign body of unspecified cheek and temporomandibular area

● S01.45   Open bite of cheek and temporomandibular area

     Bite of cheek and temporomandibular area NOS

     Excludes2   superficial bite of cheek and temporomandibular area (S00.86, S00.87)

   ● S01.451   Open bite of right cheek and temporomandibular area

   ● S01.452   Open bite of left cheek and temporomandibular area

   ● S01.459   Open bite of unspecified cheek and temporomandibular area

● S01.5   Open wound of lip and oral cavity

    Excludes2   tooth dislocation (S03.2)
                 tooth fracture (S02.5)

● S01.50   Unspecified open wound of lip and oral cavity

   ● S01.501   Unspecified open wound of lip

   ● S01.502   Unspecified open wound of oral cavity

● S01.51   Laceration of lip and oral cavity without foreign body

   ● S01.511   Laceration without foreign body of lip

   ● S01.512   Laceration without foreign body of oral cavity

● S01.52   Laceration of lip and oral cavity with foreign body

   ● S01.521   Laceration with foreign body of lip

   ● S01.522   Laceration with foreign body of oral cavity

● S01.53   Puncture wound of lip and oral cavity without foreign body

   ● S01.531   Puncture wound without foreign body of lip

   ● S01.532   Puncture wound without foreign body of oral cavity

● S01.54   Puncture wound of lip and oral cavity with foreign body

   ● S01.541   Puncture wound with foreign body of lip

   ● S01.542   Puncture wound with foreign body of oral cavity

● S01.55   Open bite of lip and oral cavity

   ● S01.551   Open bite of lip
        Bite of lip NOS
        Excludes1   superficial bite of lip (S00.571)

   ● S01.552   Open bite of oral cavity
        Bite of oral cavity NOS
        Excludes1   superficial bite of oral cavity (S00.572)

● S01.8   Open wound of other parts of head

    X ● S01.80   Unspecified open wound of other part of head

    X ● S01.81   Laceration without foreign body of other part of head

    X ● S01.82   Laceration with foreign body of other part of head

    X ● S01.83   Puncture wound without foreign body of other part of head

    X ● S01.84   Puncture wound with foreign body of other part of head

    X ● S01.85   Open bite of other part of head
        Bite of other part of head NOS
        ➡ Excludes1   superficial bite of other part of head (S00.87)

● S01.9   Open wound of unspecified part of head

    X ● S01.90   Unspecified open wound of unspecified part of head

    X ● S01.91   Laceration without foreign body of unspecified part of head

    X ● S01.92   Laceration with foreign body of unspecified part of head

    X ● S01.93   Puncture wound without foreign body of unspecified part of head

    X ● S01.94   Puncture wound with foreign body of unspecified part of head

    X ● S01.95   Open bite of unspecified part of head
        Bite of head NOS
        Excludes1   superficial bite of head NOS (S00.97)

● S02   Fracture of skull and facial bones

    Note: A fracture not indicated as open or closed should be coded to closed

        The appropriate 7th character is to be added to each code from category S02

     A   initial encounter for closed fracture
     B   initial encounter for open fracture
     D   subsequent encounter for fracture with routine healing
     G   subsequent encounter for fracture with delayed healing
     K   subsequent encounter for fracture with nonunion
     S   sequela

    Code also any associated intracranial injury (S06.-)

   X ● S02.0   Fracture of vault of skull
        Fracture of frontal bone
        Fracture of parietal bone

● S02.1   Fracture of base of skull

    Excludes1   orbit NOS (S02.8)
    Excludes2   orbital floor (S02.3-)

   ● S02.10   Unspecified fracture of base of skull

      ● S02.101   Fracture of base of skull, right side

      ● S02.102   Fracture of base of skull, left side

      ● S02.109   Fracture of base of skull, unspecified side

   ● S02.11   Fracture of occiput

      ● S02.110   Type I occipital condyle fracture, unspecified side

      ● S02.111   Type II occipital condyle fracture, unspecified side

      ● S02.112   Type III occipital condyle fracture, unspecified side

---

▶ New   ➡ Revised   ~~deleted~~ Deleted   OGCR Official Guidelines   X Assign placeholder X   ● Use Additional Character(s)

Excludes 1   Excludes 2   Includes   Use additional   Code first   Code also   Key words

● S02.113　Unspecified occipital condyle fracture
● S02.118　Other fracture of occiput, unspecified side
● S02.119　Unspecified fracture of occiput
● S02.11A　Type I occipital condyle fracture, right side
● S02.11B　Type I occipital condyle fracture, left side
● S02.11C　Type II occipital condyle fracture, right side
● S02.11D　Type II occipital condyle fracture, left side
● S02.11E　Type III occipital condyle fracture, right side
● S02.11F　Type III occipital condyle fracture, left side
● S02.11G　Other fracture of occiput, right side
● S02.11H　Other fracture of occiput, left side
X ● S02.19　Other fracture of base of skull
　　　　Fracture of anterior fossa of base of skull
　　　　Fracture of ethmoid sinus
　　　　Fracture of frontal sinus
　　　　Fracture of middle fossa of base of skull
　　　　Fracture of orbital roof
　　　　Fracture of posterior fossa of base of skull
　　　　Fracture of sphenoid
　　　　Fracture of temporal bone
X ● S02.2　Fracture of nasal bones
● S02.3　Fracture of orbital floor
　　　Excludes1　orbit NOS (S02.8)
　　　Excludes2　orbital roof (S02.1-)
X ● S02.30　Fracture of orbital floor, unspecified side
X ● S02.31　Fracture of orbital floor, right side
X ● S02.32　Fracture of orbital floor, left side
● S02.4　Fracture of malar, maxillary and zygoma bones
　　　Fracture of superior maxilla
　　　Fracture of upper jaw (bone)
　　　Fracture of zygomatic process of temporal bone
● S02.40　Fracture of malar, maxillary and zygoma bones, unspecified
● S02.400　Malar fracture unspecified side
● S02.401　Maxillary fracture, unspecified side
● S02.402　Zygomatic fracture, unspecified side
● S02.40A　Malar fracture, right side
● S02.40B　Malar fracture, left side
● S02.40C　Maxillary fracture, right side
● S02.40D　Maxillary fracture, left side
● S02.40E　Zygomatic fracture, right side
● S02.40F　Zygomatic fracture, left side
● S02.41　LeFort fracture
● S02.411　LeFort I fracture
● S02.412　LeFort II fracture
● S02.413　LeFort III fracture
X ● S02.42　Fracture of alveolus of maxilla
X ● S02.5　Fracture of tooth (traumatic) Broken tooth
　　　Excludes1　cracked tooth (nontraumatic) (K03.81)

● S02.6　Fracture of mandible
　　　Fracture of lower jaw (bone)
● S02.60　Fracture of mandible of unspecified site
● S02.600　Fracture of unspecified part of body of mandible, unspecified side
● S02.601　Fracture of unspecified part of body of right mandible
● S02.602　Fracture of unspecified part of body of left mandible
● S02.609　Fracture of mandible, unspecified
● S02.61　Fracture of condylar process of mandible
● S02.610　Fracture of condylar process of mandible, unspecified side
● S02.611　Fracture of condylar process of right mandible
● S02.612　Fracture of condylar process of left mandible
● S02.62　Fracture of subcondylar process of mandible
● S02.620　Fracture of subcondylar process of mandible, unspecified side
● S02.621　Fracture of subcondylar process of right mandible
● S02.622　Fracture of subcondylar process of left mandible
● S02.63　Fracture of coronoid process of mandible
● S02.630　Fracture of coronoid process of mandible, unspecified side
● S02.631　Fracture of coronoid process of right mandible
● S02.632　Fracture of coronoid process of left mandible
● S02.64　Fracture of ramus of mandible
● S02.640　Fracture of ramus of mandible, unspecified side
● S02.641　Fracture of ramus of right mandible
● S02.642　Fracture of ramus of left mandible
● S02.65　Fracture of angle of mandible
● S02.650　Fracture of angle of mandible, unspecified side
● S02.651　Fracture of angle of right mandible
● S02.652　Fracture of angle of left mandible
X ● S02.66　Fracture of symphysis of mandible
● S02.67　Fracture of alveolus of mandible
● S02.670　Fracture of alveolus of mandible, unspecified side
● S02.671　Fracture of alveolus of right mandible
● S02.672　Fracture of alveolus of left mandible
X ● S02.69　Fracture of mandible of other specified site
● S02.8　Fractures of other specified skull and facial bones
　　　Fracture of orbit NOS
　　　Fracture of palate
　　　Excludes1　fracture of orbital floor (S02.3-)
　　　　　　　　fracture of orbital roof (S02.1-)
X ● S02.80　Fracture of other specified skull and facial bones, unspecified side
X ● S02.81　Fracture of other specified skull and facial bones, right side
X ● S02.82　Fracture of other specified skull and facial bones, left side
● S02.9　Fracture of unspecified skull and facial bones
X ● S02.91　Unspecified fracture of skull
X ● S02.92　Unspecified fracture of facial bones

CHAPTER 19 (S00-T88)

● **S03   Dislocation and sprain of joints and ligaments of head**

Includes   avulsion of joint (capsule) or ligament of head
laceration of cartilage, joint (capsule) or ligament of head
sprain of cartilage, joint (capsule) or ligament of head
traumatic hemarthrosis of joint or ligament of head
traumatic rupture of joint or ligament of head
traumatic subluxation of joint or ligament of head
traumatic tear of joint or ligament of head

Code also any associated open wound

Excludes2   Strain of muscle or tendon of head (S09.1)

The appropriate 7th character is to be added to each code from category S03

A	initial encounter
D	subsequent encounter
S	sequela

● **S03.0   Dislocation of jaw**
Dislocation of jaw (cartilage) (meniscus)
Dislocation of mandible
Dislocation of temporomandibular (joint)

X ● **S03.00   Dislocation of jaw, unspecified side**

X ● **S03.01   Dislocation of jaw, right side**

X ● **S03.02   Dislocation of jaw, left side**

X ● **S03.03   Dislocation of jaw, bilateral side**

X ● **S03.1   Dislocation of septal cartilage of nose**

X ● **S03.2   Dislocation of tooth**

● **S03.4   Sprain of jaw**
Sprain of temporomandibular (joint) (ligament)

X ● **S03.40   Sprain of jaw, unspecified side**

X ● **S03.41   Sprain of jaw, right side**

X ● **S03.42   Sprain of jaw, left side**

X ● **S03.43   Sprain of jaw, bilateral side**

X ● **S03.8   Sprain of joints and ligaments of other parts of head**

X ● **S03.9   Sprain of joints and ligaments of unspecified parts of head**

● **S04   Injury of cranial nerve**
The selection of side should be based on the side of the body being affected

Code first any associated intracranial injury (S06.-)

Code also any associated:
open wound of head (S01.-)
skull fracture (S02.-)

The appropriate 7th character is to be added to each code from category S04

A	initial encounter
D	subsequent encounter
S	sequela

● **S04.0   Injury of optic nerve and pathways**
➡ Use additional code to identify any visual field defect or blindness (H53.4-, H54.-)

● **S04.01   Injury of optic nerve**
Injury of 2nd cranial nerve

● **S04.011   Injury of optic nerve, right eye**

● **S04.012   Injury of optic nerve, left eye**

● **S04.019   Injury of optic nerve, unspecified eye**
Injury of optic nerve NOS

X ● **S04.02   Injury of optic chiasm**

● **S04.03   Injury of optic tract and pathways**
Injury of optic radiation

➡ ● **S04.031   Injury of optic tract and pathways, right side**

➡ ● **S04.032   Injury of optic tract and pathways, left side**

➡ ● **S04.039   Injury of optic tract and pathways, unspecified side**
Injury of optic tract and pathways NOS

Figure 19-13 Cranial nerves. (From Patton and Thibodeau: Anatomy and physiology, ed 7, St. Louis, Mosby, 2009)

Trochlear nerve (IV)
Optic nerve (II)
Olfactory nerve (I)
Abducens nerve (VI)
Oculomotor nerve (III)
Facial nerve (VII)
Trigeminal nerve (V)
Vestibulocochlear nerve (VIII)
Glossopharyngeal nerve (IX)
Vagus nerve (X)
Accessory nerve (XI)
Hypoglossal nerve (XII)

▶ New   ➡ Revised   ~~deleted~~ Deleted   **OGCR** Official Guidelines   X Assign placeholder X   ● Use Additional Character(s)
Excludes 1   Excludes 2   Includes   Use additional   Code first   Code also   Key words

1174

● S04.04   Injury of visual cortex
  ➡● S04.041   Injury of visual cortex, right side
  ➡● S04.042   Injury of visual cortex, left side
  ➡● S04.049   Injury of visual cortex, unspecified side
              Injury of visual cortex NOS
● S04.1   Injury of oculomotor nerve
           Injury of 3rd cranial nerve
  X● S04.10   Injury of oculomotor nerve, unspecified side
  X● S04.11   Injury of oculomotor nerve, right side
  X● S04.12   Injury of oculomotor nerve, left side
● S04.2   Injury of trochlear nerve
           Injury of 4th cranial nerve
  X● S04.20   Injury of trochlear nerve, unspecified side
  X● S04.21   Injury of trochlear nerve, right side
  X● S04.22   Injury of trochlear nerve, left side
● S04.3   Injury of trigeminal nerve
           Injury of 5th cranial nerve
  X● S04.30   Injury of trigeminal nerve, unspecified side
  X● S04.31   Injury of trigeminal nerve, right side
  X● S04.32   Injury of trigeminal nerve, left side
● S04.4   Injury of abducent nerve
           Injury of 6th cranial nerve
  X● S04.40   Injury of abducent nerve, unspecified side
  X● S04.41   Injury of abducent nerve, right side
  X● S04.42   Injury of abducent nerve, left side
● S04.5   Injury of facial nerve
           Injury of 7th cranial nerve
  X● S04.50   Injury of facial nerve, unspecified side
  X● S04.51   Injury of facial nerve, right side
  X● S04.52   Injury of facial nerve, left side
● S04.6   Injury of acoustic nerve
           Injury of auditory nerve
           Injury of 8th cranial nerve
  X● S04.60   Injury of acoustic nerve, unspecified side
  X● S04.61   Injury of acoustic nerve, right side
  X● S04.62   Injury of acoustic nerve, left side
● S04.7   Injury of accessory nerve
           Injury of 11th cranial nerve
  X● S04.70   Injury of accessory nerve, unspecified side
  X● S04.71   Injury of accessory nerve, right side
  X● S04.72   Injury of accessory nerve, left side
● S04.8   Injury of other cranial nerves
  ● S04.81   Injury of olfactory [1st] nerve
    ● S04.811   Injury of olfactory [1st] nerve, right side
    ● S04.812   Injury of olfactory [1st] nerve, left side
    ● S04.819   Injury of olfactory [1st] nerve, unspecified side
  ● S04.89   Injury of other cranial nerves
              Injury of vagus [10th] nerve
    ● S04.891   Injury of other cranial nerves, right side
    ● S04.892   Injury of other cranial nerves, left side
    ● S04.899   Injury of other cranial nerves, unspecified side
X● S04.9   Injury of unspecified cranial nerve

● S05   Injury of eye and orbit
  Includes   open wound of eye and orbit
  Excludes2   2nd cranial [optic] nerve injury (S04.0-)
                   3rd cranial [oculomotor] nerve injury (S04.1-)
                   open wound of eyelid and periocular area (S01.1-)
                   orbital bone fracture (S02.1-, S02.3-, S02.8-)
                   superficial injury of eyelid (S00.1-S00.2)

  The appropriate 7th character is to be added to each code from category S05

A	initial encounter
D	subsequent encounter
S	sequela

● S05.0   Injury of conjunctiva and corneal abrasion without foreign body
  Excludes1   foreign body in conjunctival sac (T15.1)
                   foreign body in cornea (T15.0)
  X● S05.00   Injury of conjunctiva and corneal abrasion without foreign body, unspecified eye
  X● S05.01   Injury of conjunctiva and corneal abrasion without foreign body, right eye
  X● S05.02   Injury of conjunctiva and corneal abrasion without foreign body, left eye
● S05.1   Contusion of eyeball and orbital tissues
           Traumatic hyphema
  Excludes2   black eye NOS (S00.1)
                   contusion of eyelid and periocular area (S00.1)
  X● S05.10   Contusion of eyeball and orbital tissues, unspecified eye
  X● S05.11   Contusion of eyeball and orbital tissues, right eye
  X● S05.12   Contusion of eyeball and orbital tissues, left eye
● S05.2   Ocular laceration and rupture with prolapse or loss of intraocular tissue
  X● S05.20   Ocular laceration and rupture with prolapse or loss of intraocular tissue, unspecified eye
  X● S05.21   Ocular laceration and rupture with prolapse or loss of intraocular tissue, right eye
  X● S05.22   Ocular laceration and rupture with prolapse or loss of intraocular tissue, left eye
● S05.3   Ocular laceration without prolapse or loss of intraocular tissue
           Laceration of eye NOS
  X● S05.30   Ocular laceration without prolapse or loss of intraocular tissue, unspecified eye
  X● S05.31   Ocular laceration without prolapse or loss of intraocular tissue, right eye
  X● S05.32   Ocular laceration without prolapse or loss of intraocular tissue, left eye
● S05.4   Penetrating wound of orbit with or without foreign body
  Excludes2   retained (old) foreign body following penetrating wound in orbit (H05.5-)
  X● S05.40   Penetrating wound of orbit with or without foreign body, unspecified eye
  X● S05.41   Penetrating wound of orbit with or without foreign body, right eye
  X● S05.42   Penetrating wound of orbit with or without foreign body, left eye
● S05.5   Penetrating wound with foreign body of eyeball
  Excludes2   retained (old) intraocular foreign body (H44.6-, H44.7)
  X● S05.50   Penetrating wound with foreign body of unspecified eyeball
  X● S05.51   Penetrating wound with foreign body of right eyeball
  X● S05.52   Penetrating wound with foreign body of left eyeball

▶ New   ➡ Revised   deleted Deleted   **OGCR** Official Guidelines   X Assign placeholder X   ● Use Additional Character(s)
Excludes 1   Excludes 2   Includes   Use additional   Code first   Code also   Key words

1175

CHAPTER 19 (S00-T88)

CHAPTER 19 (S00-T88)

● **S05.6   Penetrating wound without foreign body of eyeball**
         Ocular penetration NOS
   X ● **S05.60   Penetrating wound without foreign body of unspecified eyeball**
   X ● **S05.61   Penetrating wound without foreign body of right eyeball**
   X ● **S05.62   Penetrating wound without foreign body of left eyeball**
● **S05.7   Avulsion of eye**
         Traumatic enucleation
   X ● **S05.70   Avulsion of unspecified eye**
   X ● **S05.71   Avulsion of right eye**
   X ● **S05.72   Avulsion of left eye**
● **S05.8   Other injuries of eye and orbit**
         Lacrimal duct injury
   ● **S05.8X   Other injuries of eye and orbit**
      ● **S05.8X1   Other injuries of right eye and orbit**
      ● **S05.8X2   Other injuries of left eye and orbit**
      ● **S05.8X9   Other injuries of unspecified eye and orbit**
● **S05.9   Unspecified injury of eye and orbit**
         Injury of eye NOS
   X ● **S05.90   Unspecified injury of unspecified eye and orbit**
   X ● **S05.91   Unspecified injury of right eye and orbit**
   X ● **S05.92   Unspecified injury of left eye and orbit**

● **S06   Intracranial injury**

     Includes   traumatic brain injury

     Code also any associated:
         open wound of head (S01.-)
         skull fracture (S02.-)

     Excludes1   head injury NOS (S09.90)

     The appropriate 7th character is to be added to each code from category S06

        | | |
        A   initial encounter
        D   subsequent encounter
        S   sequela

   ▶**Note:** 7th characters D and S do not apply to codes in category S06 with 6th character 7 - death due to brain injury prior to regaining consciousness, or 8 - death due to other cause prior to regaining consciousness.

● **S06.0   Concussion**
         Commotio cerebri
     Excludes1   concussion with other intracranial injuries classified in subcategories S06.1- to S06.6- , S06.81- and S06.82- code to specified intracranial injury
   ● **S06.0X   Concussion**
      ● **S06.0X0   Concussion without loss of consciousness**
      ● **S06.0X1   Concussion with loss of consciousness of 30 minutes or less**
      ● **S06.0X9   Concussion with loss of consciousness of unspecified duration**
           Concussion NOS
● **S06.1   Traumatic cerebral edema**
         Diffuse traumatic cerebral edema
         Focal traumatic cerebral edema

● **S06.1X   Traumatic cerebral edema**
   ● **S06.1X0   Traumatic cerebral edema without loss of consciousness**
   ● **S06.1X1   Traumatic cerebral edema with loss of consciousness of 30 minutes or less**
   ● **S06.1X2   Traumatic cerebral edema with loss of consciousness of 31 minutes to 59 minutes**
   ● **S06.1X3   Traumatic cerebral edema with loss of consciousness of 1 hour to 5 hours 59 minutes**
   ● **S06.1X4   Traumatic cerebral edema with loss of consciousness of 6 hours to 24 hours**
   ● **S06.1X5   Traumatic cerebral edema with loss of consciousness greater than 24 hours with return to pre-existing conscious level**
   ● **S06.1X6   Traumatic cerebral edema with loss of consciousness greater than 24 hours without return to pre-existing conscious level with patient surviving**
   ● **S06.1X7   Traumatic cerebral edema with loss of consciousness of any duration with death due to brain injury prior to regaining consciousness**
   ● **S06.1X8   Traumatic cerebral edema with loss of consciousness of any duration with death due to other cause prior to regaining consciousness**
   ● **S06.1X9   Traumatic cerebral edema with loss of consciousness of unspecified duration**
           Traumatic cerebral edema NOS
● **S06.2   Diffuse traumatic brain injury**
         Diffuse axonal brain injury
     Excludes1   traumatic diffuse cerebral edema (S06.1X-)

● **S06.2X   Diffuse traumatic brain injury**
   ● **S06.2X0   Diffuse traumatic brain injury without loss of consciousness**
   ● **S06.2X1   Diffuse traumatic brain injury with loss of consciousness of 30 minutes or less**
   ● **S06.2X2   Diffuse traumatic brain injury with loss of consciousness of 31 minutes to 59 minutes**
   ● **S06.2X3   Diffuse traumatic brain injury with loss of consciousness of 1 hour to 5 hours 59 minutes**
   ● **S06.2X4   Diffuse traumatic brain injury with loss of consciousness of 6 hours to 24 hours**
   ● **S06.2X5   Diffuse traumatic brain injury with loss of consciousness greater than 24 hours with return to pre-existing conscious levels**
   ● **S06.2X6   Diffuse traumatic brain injury with loss of consciousness greater than 24 hours without return to pre-existing conscious level with patient surviving**
   ● **S06.2X7   Diffuse traumatic brain injury with loss of consciousness of any duration with death due to brain injury prior to regaining consciousness**

● **S06.2X8**   Diffuse traumatic brain injury with loss of consciousness of any duration with death due to other cause prior to regaining consciousness

● **S06.2X9**   Diffuse traumatic brain injury with loss of consciousness of unspecified duration

     Diffuse traumatic brain injury NOS

● **S06.3**   Focal traumatic brain injury

   Excludes1   any condition classifiable to S06.4-S06.6

       focal cerebral edema (S06.1)

● **S06.30**   Unspecified focal traumatic brain injury

   ● **S06.300**   Unspecified focal traumatic brain injury without loss of consciousness

   ● **S06.301**   Unspecified focal traumatic brain injury with loss of consciousness of 30 minutes or less

   ● **S06.302**   Unspecified focal traumatic brain injury with loss of consciousness of 31 minutes to 59 minutes

   ● **S06.303**   Unspecified focal traumatic brain injury with loss of consciousness of 1 hour to 5 hours 59 minutes

   ● **S06.304**   Unspecified focal traumatic brain injury with loss of consciousness of 6 hours to 24 hours

   ● **S06.305**   Unspecified focal traumatic brain injury with loss of consciousness greater than 24 hours with return to pre-existing conscious level

   ● **S06.306**   Unspecified focal traumatic brain injury with loss of consciousness greater than 24 hours without return to pre-existing conscious level with patient surviving

   ● **S06.307**   Unspecified focal traumatic brain injury with loss of consciousness of any duration with death due to brain injury prior to regaining consciousness

   ● **S06.308**   Unspecified focal traumatic brain injury with loss of consciousness of any duration with death due to other cause prior to regaining consciousness

   ● **S06.309**   Unspecified focal traumatic brain injury with loss of consciousness of unspecified duration

      Unspecified focal traumatic brain injury NOS

● **S06.31**   Contusion and laceration of right cerebrum

   ● **S06.310**   Contusion and laceration of right cerebrum without loss of consciousness

   ● **S06.311**   Contusion and laceration of right cerebrum with loss of consciousness of 30 minutes or less

   ● **S06.312**   Contusion and laceration of right cerebrum with loss of consciousness of 31 minutes to 59 minutes

   ● **S06.313**   Contusion and laceration of right cerebrum with loss of consciousness of 1 hour to 5 hours 59 minutes

   ● **S06.314**   Contusion and laceration of right cerebrum with loss of consciousness of 6 hours to 24 hours

● **S06.315**   Contusion and laceration of right cerebrum with loss of consciousness greater than 24 hours with return to pre-existing conscious level

● **S06.316**   Contusion and laceration of right cerebrum with loss of consciousness greater than 24 hours without return to pre-existing conscious level with patient surviving

● **S06.317**   Contusion and laceration of right cerebrum with loss of consciousness of any duration with death due to brain injury prior to regaining consciousness

● **S06.318**   Contusion and laceration of right cerebrum with loss of consciousness of any duration with death due to other cause prior to regaining consciousness

● **S06.319**   Contusion and laceration of right cerebrum with loss of consciousness of unspecified duration

      Contusion and laceration of right cerebrum NOS

● **S06.32**   Contusion and laceration of left cerebrum

   ● **S06.320**   Contusion and laceration of left cerebrum without loss of consciousness

   ● **S06.321**   Contusion and laceration of left cerebrum with loss of consciousness of 30 minutes or less

   ● **S06.322**   Contusion and laceration of left cerebrum with loss of consciousness of 31 minutes to 59 minutes

   ● **S06.323**   Contusion and laceration of left cerebrum with loss of consciousness of 1 hour to 5 hours 59 minutes

   ● **S06.324**   Contusion and laceration of left cerebrum with loss of consciousness of 6 hours to 24 hours

   ● **S06.325**   Contusion and laceration of left cerebrum with loss of consciousness greater than 24 hours with return to pre-existing conscious level

   ● **S06.326**   Contusion and laceration of left cerebrum with loss of consciousness greater than 24 hours without return to pre-existing conscious level with patient surviving

   ● **S06.327**   Contusion and laceration of left cerebrum with loss of consciousness of any duration with death due to brain injury prior to regaining consciousness

   ● **S06.328**   Contusion and laceration of left cerebrum with loss of consciousness of any duration with death due to other cause prior to regaining consciousness

   ● **S06.329**   Contusion and laceration of left cerebrum with loss of consciousness of unspecified duration

      Contusion and laceration of left cerebrum NOS

▶ New   ⇒ Revised   ~~deleted~~ Deleted   **OGCR** Official Guidelines   X Assign placeholder X   ● Use Additional Character(s)

Excludes 1   Excludes 2   Includes   Use additional   Code first   Code also   Key words

● S06.33   Contusion and laceration of cerebrum, unspecified

    ● S06.330   Contusion and laceration of cerebrum, unspecified, without loss of consciousness

    ● S06.331   Contusion and laceration of cerebrum, unspecified, with loss of consciousness of 30 minutes or less

    ● S06.332   Contusion and laceration of cerebrum, unspecified, with loss of consciousness of 31 minutes to 59 minutes

    ● S06.333   Contusion and laceration of cerebrum, unspecified, with loss of consciousness of 1 hour to 5 hours 59 minutes

    ● S06.334   Contusion and laceration of cerebrum, unspecified, with loss of consciousness of 6 hours to 24 hours

    ● S06.335   Contusion and laceration of cerebrum, unspecified, with loss of consciousness greater than 24 hours with return to pre-existing conscious level

    ● S06.336   Contusion and laceration of cerebrum, unspecified, with loss of consciousness greater than 24 hours without return to pre-existing conscious level with patient surviving

    ● S06.337   Contusion and laceration of cerebrum, unspecified, with loss of consciousness of any duration with death due to brain injury prior to regaining consciousness

    ● S06.338   Contusion and laceration of cerebrum, unspecified, with loss of consciousness of any duration with death due to other cause prior to regaining consciousness

    ● S06.339   Contusion and laceration of cerebrum, unspecified, with loss of consciousness of unspecified duration
           Contusion and laceration of cerebrum NOS

● S06.34   Traumatic hemorrhage of right cerebrum
        Traumatic intracerebral hemorrhage and hematoma of right cerebrum

    ● S06.340   Traumatic hemorrhage of right cerebrum without loss of consciousness

    ● S06.341   Traumatic hemorrhage of right cerebrum with loss of consciousness of 30 minutes or less

    ● S06.342   Traumatic hemorrhage of right cerebrum with loss of consciousness of 31 minutes to 59 minutes

    ● S06.343   Traumatic hemorrhage of right cerebrum with loss of consciousness of 1 hours to 5 hours 59 minutes

    ● S06.344   Traumatic hemorrhage of right cerebrum with loss of consciousness of 6 hours to 24 hours

    ● S06.345   Traumatic hemorrhage of right cerebrum with loss of consciousness greater than 24 hours with return to pre-existing conscious level

    ● S06.346   Traumatic hemorrhage of right cerebrum with loss of consciousness greater than 24 hours without return to pre-existing conscious level with patient surviving

    ● S06.347   Traumatic hemorrhage of right cerebrum with loss of consciousness of any duration with death due to brain injury prior to regaining consciousness

    ● S06.348   Traumatic hemorrhage of right cerebrum with loss of consciousness of any duration with death due to other cause prior to regaining consciousness

    ● S06.349   Traumatic hemorrhage of right cerebrum with loss of consciousness of unspecified duration
           Traumatic hemorrhage of right cerebrum NOS

● S06.35   Traumatic hemorrhage of left cerebrum
        Traumatic intracerebral hemorrhage and hematoma of left cerebrum

    ● S06.350   Traumatic hemorrhage of left cerebrum without loss of consciousness

    ● S06.351   Traumatic hemorrhage of left cerebrum with loss of consciousness of 30 minutes or less

    ● S06.352   Traumatic hemorrhage of left cerebrum with loss of consciousness of 31 minutes to 59 minutes

    ● S06.353   Traumatic hemorrhage of left cerebrum with loss of consciousness of 1 hours to 5 hours 59 minutes

    ● S06.354   Traumatic hemorrhage of left cerebrum with loss of consciousness of 6 hours to 24 hours

    ● S06.355   Traumatic hemorrhage of left cerebrum with loss of consciousness greater than 24 hours with return to pre-existing conscious level

    ● S06.356   Traumatic hemorrhage of left cerebrum with loss of consciousness greater than 24 hours without return to pre-existing conscious level with patient surviving

    ● S06.357   Traumatic hemorrhage of left cerebrum with loss of consciousness of any duration with death due to brain injury prior to regaining consciousness

    ● S06.358   Traumatic hemorrhage of left cerebrum with loss of consciousness of any duration with death due to other cause prior to regaining consciousness

    ● S06.359   Traumatic hemorrhage of left cerebrum with loss of consciousness of unspecified duration
           Traumatic hemorrhage of left cerebrum NOS

- S06.36 **Traumatic hemorrhage of cerebrum, unspecified**
  Traumatic intracerebral hemorrhage and hematoma, unspecified
  - S06.360 Traumatic hemorrhage of cerebrum, unspecified, without loss of consciousness
  - S06.361 Traumatic hemorrhage of cerebrum, unspecified, with loss of consciousness of 30 minutes or less
  - S06.362 Traumatic hemorrhage of cerebrum, unspecified, with loss of consciousness of 31 minutes to 59 minutes
  - S06.363 Traumatic hemorrhage of cerebrum, unspecified, with loss of consciousness of 1 hours to 5 hours 59 minutes
  - S06.364 Traumatic hemorrhage of cerebrum, unspecified, with loss of consciousness of 6 hours to 24 hours
  - S06.365 Traumatic hemorrhage of cerebrum, unspecified, with loss of consciousness greater than 24 hours with return to pre-existing conscious level
  - S06.366 Traumatic hemorrhage of cerebrum, unspecified, with loss of consciousness greater than 24 hours without return to pre-existing conscious level with patient surviving
  - S06.367 Traumatic hemorrhage of cerebrum, unspecified, with loss of consciousness of any duration with death due to brain injury prior to regaining consciousness
  - S06.368 Traumatic hemorrhage of cerebrum, unspecified, with loss of consciousness of any duration with death due to other cause prior to regaining consciousness
  - S06.369 Traumatic hemorrhage of cerebrum, unspecified, with loss of consciousness of unspecified duration
    Traumatic hemorrhage of cerebrum NOS

- S06.37 **Contusion, laceration, and hemorrhage of cerebellum**
  - S06.370 Contusion, laceration, and hemorrhage of cerebellum without loss of consciousness
  - S06.371 Contusion, laceration, and hemorrhage of cerebellum with loss of consciousness of 30 minutes or less
  - S06.372 Contusion, laceration, and hemorrhage of cerebellum with loss of consciousness of 31 minutes to 59 minutes
  - S06.373 Contusion, laceration, and hemorrhage of cerebellum with loss of consciousness of 1 hour to 5 hours 59 minutes
  - S06.374 Contusion, laceration, and hemorrhage of cerebellum with loss of consciousness of 6 hours to 24 hours
  - S06.375 Contusion, laceration, and hemorrhage of cerebellum with loss of consciousness greater than 24 hours with return to pre-existing conscious level

  - S06.376 Contusion, laceration, and hemorrhage of cerebellum with loss of consciousness greater than 24 hours without return to pre-existing conscious level with patient surviving
  - S06.377 Contusion, laceration, and hemorrhage of cerebellum with loss of consciousness of any duration with death due to brain injury prior to regaining consciousness
  - S06.378 Contusion, laceration, and hemorrhage of cerebellum with loss of consciousness of any duration with death due to other cause prior to regaining consciousness
  - S06.379 Contusion, laceration, and hemorrhage of cerebellum with loss of consciousness of unspecified duration
    Contusion, laceration, and hemorrhage of cerebellum NOS

- S06.38 **Contusion, laceration, and hemorrhage of brainstem**
  - S06.380 Contusion, laceration, and hemorrhage of brainstem without loss of consciousness
  - S06.381 Contusion, laceration, and hemorrhage of brainstem with loss of consciousness of 30 minutes or less
  - S06.382 Contusion, laceration, and hemorrhage of brainstem with loss of consciousness of 31 minutes to 59 minutes
  - S06.383 Contusion, laceration, and hemorrhage of brainstem with loss of consciousness of 1 hour to 5 hours 59 minutes
  - S06.384 Contusion, laceration, and hemorrhage of brainstem with loss of consciousness of 6 hours to 24 hours
  - S06.385 Contusion, laceration, and hemorrhage of brainstem with loss of consciousness greater than 24 hours with return to pre-existing conscious level
  - S06.386 Contusion, laceration, and hemorrhage of brainstem with loss of consciousness greater than 24 hours without return to pre-existing conscious level with patient surviving
  - S06.387 Contusion, laceration, and hemorrhage of brainstem with loss of consciousness of any duration with death due to brain injury prior to regaining consciousness
  - S06.388 Contusion, laceration, and hemorrhage of brainstem with loss of consciousness of any duration with death due to other cause prior to regaining consciousness
  - S06.389 Contusion, laceration, and hemorrhage of brainstem with loss of consciousness of unspecified duration
    Contusion, laceration, and hemorrhage of brainstem NOS

CHAPTER 19 (S00-T88)

▶ New   ⇒ Revised   ~~deleted~~ Deleted   **OGCR** Official Guidelines   X Assign placeholder X   ● Use Additional Character(s)

| Excludes 1 | Excludes 2 | Includes | Use additional | Code first | Code also | Key words |

● **S06.4** **Epidural hemorrhage**
Situated outside dura mater
Extradural hemorrhage NOS
Intracranial hemorrhage due to trauma
Extradural hemorrhage (traumatic)

● **S06.4X** Epidural hemorrhage

● **S06.4X0** Epidural hemorrhage without loss of consciousness

● **S06.4X1** Epidural hemorrhage with loss of consciousness of 30 minutes or less

● **S06.4X2** Epidural hemorrhage with loss of consciousness of 31 minutes to 59 minutes

● **S06.4X3** Epidural hemorrhage with loss of consciousness of 1 hour to 5 hours 59 minutes

● **S06.4X4** Epidural hemorrhage with loss of consciousness of 6 hours to 24 hours

● **S06.4X5** Epidural hemorrhage with loss of consciousness greater than 24 hours with return to pre-existing conscious level

● **S06.4X6** Epidural hemorrhage with loss of consciousness greater than 24 hours without return to pre-existing conscious level with patient surviving

● **S06.4X7** Epidural hemorrhage with loss of consciousness of any duration with death due to brain injury prior to regaining consciousness

● **S06.4X8** Epidural hemorrhage with loss of consciousness of any duration with death due to other causes prior to regaining consciousness

● **S06.4X9** Epidural hemorrhage with loss of consciousness of unspecified duration
Epidural hemorrhage NOS

● **S06.5** Traumatic subdural hemorrhage

● **S06.5X** Traumatic subdural hemorrhage

● **S06.5X0** Traumatic subdural hemorrhage without loss of consciousness

● **S06.5X1** Traumatic subdural hemorrhage with loss of consciousness of 30 minutes or less

● **S06.5X2** Traumatic subdural hemorrhage with loss of consciousness of 31 minutes to 59 minutes

● **S06.5X3** Traumatic subdural hemorrhage with loss of consciousness of 1 hour to 5 hours 59 minutes

● **S06.5X4** Traumatic subdural hemorrhage with loss of consciousness of 6 hours to 24 hours

● **S06.5X5** Traumatic subdural hemorrhage with loss of consciousness greater than 24 hours with return to pre-existing conscious level

● **S06.5X6** Traumatic subdural hemorrhage with loss of consciousness greater than 24 hours without return to pre-existing conscious level with patient surviving

● **S06.5X7** Traumatic subdural hemorrhage with loss of consciousness of any duration with death due to brain injury before regaining consciousness

● **S06.5X8** Traumatic subdural hemorrhage with loss of consciousness of any duration with death due to other cause before regaining consciousness

● **S06.5X9** Traumatic subdural hemorrhage with loss of consciousness of unspecified duration
Traumatic subdural hemorrhage NOS

● **S06.6** Traumatic subarachnoid hemorrhage
Between arachnoid and pia mater

● **S06.6X** Traumatic subarachnoid hemorrhage

● **S06.6X0** Traumatic subarachnoid hemorrhage without loss of consciousness

● **S06.6X1** Traumatic subarachnoid hemorrhage with loss of consciousness of 30 minutes or less

● **S06.6X2** Traumatic subarachnoid hemorrhage with loss of consciousness of 31 minutes to 59 minutes

● **S06.6X3** Traumatic subarachnoid hemorrhage with loss of consciousness of 1 hour to 5 hours 59 minutes

● **S06.6X4** Traumatic subarachnoid hemorrhage with loss of consciousness of 6 hours to 24 hours

● **S06.6X5** Traumatic subarachnoid hemorrhage with loss of consciousness greater than 24 hours with return to pre-existing conscious level

● **S06.6X6** Traumatic subarachnoid hemorrhage with loss of consciousness greater than 24 hours without return to pre-existing conscious level with patient surviving

● **S06.6X7** Traumatic subarachnoid hemorrhage with loss of consciousness of any duration with death due to brain injury prior to regaining consciousness

● **S06.6X8** Traumatic subarachnoid hemorrhage with loss of consciousness of any duration with death due to other cause prior to regaining consciousness

● **S06.6X9** Traumatic subarachnoid hemorrhage with loss of consciousness of unspecified duration
Traumatic subarachnoid hemorrhage NOS

● **S06.8** Other specified intracranial injuries

● **S06.81** Injury of right internal carotid artery, intracranial portion, not elsewhere classified

● **S06.810** Injury of right internal carotid artery, intracranial portion, not elsewhere classified without loss of consciousness

● **S06.811** Injury of right internal carotid artery, intracranial portion, not elsewhere classified with loss of consciousness of 30 minutes or less

● **S06.812** Injury of right internal carotid artery, intracranial portion, not elsewhere classified with loss of consciousness of 31 minutes to 59 minutes

▶ New ⇒ Revised ~~deleted~~ Deleted **OGCR** Official Guidelines X Assign placeholder X ● Use Additional Character(s)
Excludes 1 Excludes 2 Includes Use additional Code first Code also Key words

● **S06.813** Injury of right internal carotid artery, intracranial portion, not elsewhere classified with loss of consciousness of 1 hour to 5 hours 59 minutes

● **S06.814** Injury of right internal carotid artery, intracranial portion, not elsewhere classified with loss of consciousness of 6 hours to 24 hours

● **S06.815** Injury of right internal carotid artery, intracranial portion, not elsewhere classified with loss of consciousness greater than 24 hours with return to pre-existing conscious level

● **S06.816** Injury of right internal carotid artery, intracranial portion, not elsewhere classified with loss of consciousness greater than 24 hours without return to pre-existing conscious level with patient surviving

● **S06.817** Injury of right internal carotid artery, intracranial portion, not elsewhere classified with loss of consciousness of any duration with death due to brain injury prior to regaining consciousness

● **S06.818** Injury of right internal carotid artery, intracranial portion, not elsewhere classified with loss of consciousness of any duration with death due to other cause prior to regaining consciousness

● **S06.819** Injury of right internal carotid artery, intracranial portion, not elsewhere classified with loss of consciousness of unspecified duration
     Injury of right internal carotid artery, intracranial portion, not elsewhere classified NOS

● **S06.82** Injury of left internal carotid artery, intracranial portion, not elsewhere classified

● **S06.820** Injury of left internal carotid artery, intracranial portion, not elsewhere classified without loss of consciousness

● **S06.821** Injury of left internal carotid artery, intracranial portion, not elsewhere classified with loss of consciousness of 30 minutes or less

● **S06.822** Injury of left internal carotid artery, intracranial portion, not elsewhere classified with loss of consciousness of 31 minutes to 59 minutes

● **S06.823** Injury of left internal carotid artery, intracranial portion, not elsewhere classified with loss of consciousness of 1 hour to 5 hours 59 minutes

● **S06.824** Injury of left internal carotid artery, intracranial portion, not elsewhere classified with loss of consciousness of 6 hours to 24 hours

● **S06.825** Injury of left internal carotid artery, intracranial portion, not elsewhere classified with loss of consciousness greater than 24 hours with return to pre-existing conscious level

● **S06.826** Injury of left internal carotid artery, intracranial portion, not elsewhere classified with loss of consciousness greater than 24 hours without return to pre-existing conscious level with patient surviving

● **S06.827** Injury of left internal carotid artery, intracranial portion, not elsewhere classified with loss of consciousness of any duration with death due to brain injury prior to regaining consciousness

● **S06.828** Injury of left internal carotid artery, intracranial portion, not elsewhere classified with loss of consciousness of any duration with death due to other cause prior to regaining consciousness

● **S06.829** Injury of left internal carotid artery, intracranial portion, not elsewhere classified with loss of consciousness of unspecified duration
     Injury of left internal carotid artery, intracranial portion, not elsewhere classified NOS

● **S06.89** Other specified intracranial injury
   Excludes1   concussion (S06.0X-)

● **S06.890** Other specified intracranial injury without loss of consciousness

● **S06.891** Other specified intracranial injury with loss of consciousness of 30 minutes or less

● **S06.892** Other specified intracranial injury with loss of consciousness of 31 minutes to 59 minutes

● **S06.893** Other specified intracranial injury with loss of consciousness of 1 hour to 5 hours 59 minutes

● **S06.894** Other specified intracranial injury with loss of consciousness of 6 hours to 24 hours

● **S06.895** Other specified intracranial injury with loss of consciousness greater than 24 hours with return to pre-existing conscious level

● **S06.896** Other specified intracranial injury with loss of consciousness greater than 24 hours without return to pre-existing conscious level with patient surviving

● **S06.897** Other specified intracranial injury with loss of consciousness of any duration with death due to brain injury prior to regaining consciousness

● **S06.898** Other specified intracranial injury with loss of consciousness of any duration with death due to other cause prior to regaining consciousness

● **S06.899** Other specified intracranial injury with loss of consciousness of unspecified duration

CHAPTER 19 (S00-T88)

CHAPTER 19 (S00-T88)

● **S06.9** **Unspecified** intracranial injury
　　　Brain injury NOS
　　　Head injury NOS with loss of consciousness
　　　Traumatic brain injury NOS
　　　Excludes1　conditions classifiable to S06.0- to
　　　　　　　　S06.8-code to specified intracranial
　　　　　　　　injury
　　　　　　head injury NOS (S09.90)

　● **S06.9X** **Unspecified** intracranial injury

　　● **S06.9X0** Unspecified intracranial injury
　　　　　　without loss of consciousness

　　● **S06.9X1** Unspecified intracranial injury with
　　　　　　loss of consciousness of 30 minutes or
　　　　　　less

　　● **S06.9X2** Unspecified intracranial injury with
　　　　　　loss of consciousness of 31 minutes to
　　　　　　59 minutes

　　● **S06.9X3** Unspecified intracranial injury with
　　　　　　loss of consciousness of 1 hour to
　　　　　　5 hours 59 minutes

　　● **S06.9X4** Unspecified intracranial injury with
　　　　　　loss of consciousness of 6 hours to
　　　　　　24 hours

　　● **S06.9X5** Unspecified intracranial injury with
　　　　　　loss of consciousness greater than
　　　　　　24 hours with return to pre-existing
　　　　　　conscious level

　　● **S06.9X6** Unspecified intracranial injury with
　　　　　　loss of consciousness greater than
　　　　　　24 hours without return to pre-
　　　　　　existing conscious level with patient
　　　　　　surviving

　　● **S06.9X7** Unspecified intracranial injury with
　　　　　　loss of consciousness of any duration
　　　　　　with death due to brain injury prior
　　　　　　to regaining consciousness

　　● **S06.9X8** Unspecified intracranial injury with
　　　　　　loss of consciousness of any duration
　　　　　　with death due to other cause prior to
　　　　　　regaining consciousness

　　● **S06.9X9** Unspecified intracranial injury with
　　　　　　loss of consciousness of unspecified
　　　　　　duration

● **S07** **Crushing injury of head**
　　Use additional code for all associated injuries, such as:
　　　intracranial injuries (S06.-)
　　　skull fractures (S02.-)

　　The appropriate 7th character is to be added to each code from
　　　category S07

　　　┌─────────────────────────────┐
　　　│ A　initial encounter　　　　　　│
　　　│ D　subsequent encounter　　　　│
　　　│ S　sequela　　　　　　　　　　　│
　　　└─────────────────────────────┘

X● **S07.0** Crushing injury of face
X● **S07.1** Crushing injury of skull
X● **S07.8** Crushing injury of other parts of head
X● **S07.9** Crushing injury of head, part unspecified

● **S08** **Avulsion and traumatic amputation of part of head**
　　An amputation not identified as partial or complete should be
　　　coded to complete
　　The appropriate 7th character is to be added to each code from
　　　category S08

　　　┌─────────────────────────────┐
　　　│ A　initial encounter　　　　　　│
　　　│ D　subsequent encounter　　　　│
　　　│ S　sequela　　　　　　　　　　　│
　　　└─────────────────────────────┘

X● **S08.0** Avulsion of scalp
● **S08.1** Traumatic amputation of ear
　● **S08.11** Complete traumatic amputation of ear
　　● **S08.111** Complete traumatic amputation of
　　　　　　right ear
　　● **S08.112** Complete traumatic amputation of
　　　　　　left ear
　　● **S08.119** Complete traumatic amputation of
　　　　　　unspecified ear
　● **S08.12** Partial traumatic amputation of ear
　　● **S08.121** Partial traumatic amputation of right
　　　　　　ear
　　● **S08.122** Partial traumatic amputation of left
　　　　　　ear
　　● **S08.129** Partial traumatic amputation of
　　　　　　unspecified ear
● **S08.8** Traumatic amputation of other parts of head
　● **S08.81** Traumatic amputation of nose
　　● **S08.811** Complete traumatic amputation of
　　　　　　nose
　　● **S08.812** Partial traumatic amputation of nose
　X● **S08.89** Traumatic amputation of other parts of head

● **S09** **Other and unspecified injuries of head**
　　The appropriate 7th character is to be added to each code from
　　　category S09

　　　┌─────────────────────────────┐
　　　│ A　initial encounter　　　　　　│
　　　│ D　subsequent encounter　　　　│
　　　│ S　sequela　　　　　　　　　　　│
　　　└─────────────────────────────┘

X● **S09.0** Injury of blood vessels of head, not elsewhere classified
　　　Excludes1　injury of cerebral blood vessels (S06.-)
　　　　　　　　injury of precerebral blood vessels (S15.-)
● **S09.1** Injury of muscle and tendon of head
　　Code also any associated open wound (S01.-)
　　Excludes2　sprain to joints and ligament of head
　　　　　　　　(S03.9)
　X● **S09.10** Unspecified injury of muscle and tendon of
　　　　　head
　　　　　Injury of muscle and tendon of head NOS
　X● **S09.11** Strain of muscle and tendon of head
　X● **S09.12** Laceration of muscle and tendon of head
　X● **S09.19** Other specified injury of muscle and tendon of
　　　　　head
● **S09.2** Traumatic rupture of ear drum
　　　Excludes1　traumatic rupture of ear drum due to
　　　　　　　　blast injury (S09.31-)
　X● **S09.20** Traumatic rupture of unspecified ear drum
　X● **S09.21** Traumatic rupture of right ear drum
　X● **S09.22** Traumatic rupture of left ear drum

● S09.3   Other specified and unspecified injury of middle and inner ear

> Excludes1   injury to ear NOS (S09.91-)
>
> Excludes2   injury to external ear (S00.4-, S01.3-, S08.1-)

  ● S09.30   Unspecified injury of middle and inner ear

    ● S09.301   Unspecified injury of right middle and inner ear

    ● S09.302   Unspecified injury of left middle and inner ear

    ● S09.309   Unspecified injury of unspecified middle and inner ear

  ● S09.31   Primary blast injury of ear
    Blast injury of ear NOS

    ● S09.311   Primary blast injury of right ear

    ● S09.312   Primary blast injury of left ear

    ● S09.313   Primary blast injury of ear, bilateral

    ● S09.319   Primary blast injury of unspecified ear

  ● S09.39   Other specified injury of middle and inner ear
    Secondary blast injury to ear

    ● S09.391   Other specified injury of right middle and inner ear

    ● S09.392   Other specified injury of left middle and inner ear

    ● S09.399   Other specified injury of unspecified middle and inner ear

X ● S09.8   Other specified injuries of head

● S09.9   Unspecified injury of face and head

  X ● S09.90   Unspecified injury of head
    Head injury NOS

> Excludes1   brain injury NOS (S06.9-)
> head injury NOS with loss of consciousness (S06.9-)
> intracranial injury NOS (S06.9-)

  X ● S09.91   Unspecified injury of ear
    Injury of ear NOS

  X ● S09.92   Unspecified injury of nose
    Injury of nose NOS

  X ● S09.93   Unspecified injury of face
    Injury of face NOS

INJURIES TO THE NECK (S10-S19)

> Includes   injuries of nape
> injuries of supraclavicular region
> injuries of throat
>
> Excludes2   burns and corrosions (T20-T32)
> effects of foreign body in esophagus (T18.1)
> effects of foreign body in larynx (T17.3)
> effects of foreign body in pharynx (T17.2)
> effects of foreign body in trachea (T17.4)
> frostbite (T33-T34)
> insect bite or sting, venomous (T63.4)

● S10   Superficial injury of neck

The appropriate 7th character is to be added to each code from category S10

A	initial encounter
D	subsequent encounter
S	sequela

X ● S10.0   Contusion of throat
  Contusion of cervical esophagus
  Contusion of larynx
  Contusion of pharynx
  Contusion of trachea

● S10.1   Other and unspecified superficial injuries of throat

  X ● S10.10   Unspecified superficial injuries of throat

  X ● S10.11   Abrasion of throat

  X ● S10.12   Blister (nonthermal) of throat

  X ● S10.14   External constriction of part of throat

  X ● S10.15   Superficial foreign body of throat
    Splinter in the throat

  X ● S10.16   Insect bite (nonvenomous) of throat

  X ● S10.17   Other superficial bite of throat

> Excludes1   open bite of throat (S11.85)

● S10.8   Superficial injury of other specified parts of neck

  X ● S10.80   Unspecified superficial injury of other specified part of neck

  X ● S10.81   Abrasion of other specified part of neck

  X ● S10.82   Blister (nonthermal) of other specified part of neck

  X ● S10.83   Contusion of other specified part of neck

  X ● S10.84   External constriction of other specified part of neck

  X ● S10.85   Superficial foreign body of other specified part of neck
    Splinter in other part of neck

  X ● S10.86   Insect bite of other specified part of neck

  X ● S10.87   Other superficial bite of other specified part of neck

> Excludes1   open bite of other specified parts of neck (S11.85)

● S10.9   Superficial injury of unspecified part of neck

  X ● S10.90   Unspecified superficial injury of unspecified part of neck

  X ● S10.91   Abrasion of unspecified part of neck

  X ● S10.92   Blister (nonthermal) of unspecified part of neck

  X ● S10.93   Contusion of unspecified part of neck

  X ● S10.94   External constriction of unspecified part of neck

  X ● S10.95   Superficial foreign body of unspecified part of neck

  X ● S10.96   Insect bite of unspecified part of neck

  X ● S10.97   Other superficial bite of unspecified part of neck

● S11   Open wound of neck

Code also any associated:
  spinal cord injury (S14.0, S14.1-)
  wound infection

> Excludes2   open fracture of vertebra (S12.- with 7th character B)

The appropriate 7th character is to be added to each code from category S11

A	initial encounter
D	subsequent encounter
S	sequela

● S11.0   Open wound of larynx and trachea

  ● S11.01   Open wound of larynx

> Excludes2   open wound of vocal cord (S11.03)

    ● S11.011   Laceration without foreign body of larynx

    ● S11.012   Laceration with foreign body of larynx

    ● S11.013   Puncture wound without foreign body of larynx

    ● S11.014   Puncture wound with foreign body of larynx

    ● S11.015   Open bite of larynx
      Bite of larynx NOS

    ● S11.019   Unspecified open wound of larynx

● S11.02 Open wound of trachea
            Open wound of cervical trachea
            Open wound of trachea NOS
            | Excludes2 | open wound of thoracic trachea
                                      (S27.5-)
      ● S11.021 Laceration without foreign body of
                    trachea
      ● S11.022 Laceration with foreign body of
                    trachea
      ● S11.023 Puncture wound without foreign
                    body of trachea
      ● S11.024 Puncture wound with foreign body of
                    trachea
      ● S11.025 Open bite of trachea
                    Bite of trachea NOS
      ● S11.029 Unspecified open wound of trachea
● S11.03 Open wound of vocal cord
      ● S11.031 Laceration without foreign body of
                    vocal cord
      ● S11.032 Laceration with foreign body of vocal
                    cord
      ● S11.033 Puncture wound without foreign
                    body of vocal cord
      ● S11.034 Puncture wound with foreign body of
                    vocal cord
      ● S11.035 Open bite of vocal cord
                    Bite of vocal cord NOS
      ● S11.039 Unspecified open wound of vocal
                    cord
● S11.1 Open wound of thyroid gland
   X ● S11.10 Unspecified open wound of thyroid gland
   X ● S11.11 Laceration without foreign body of thyroid
                  gland
   X ● S11.12 Laceration with foreign body of thyroid gland
   X ● S11.13 Puncture wound without foreign body of
                  thyroid gland
   X ● S11.14 Puncture wound with foreign body of thyroid
                  gland
   X ● S11.15 Open bite of thyroid gland
                  Bite of thyroid gland NOS
● S11.2 Open wound of pharynx and cervical esophagus
            | Excludes1 | open wound of esophagus NOS (S27.8-)
   X ● S11.20 Unspecified open wound of pharynx and
                  cervical esophagus
   X ● S11.21 Laceration without foreign body of pharynx
                  and cervical esophagus
   X ● S11.22 Laceration with foreign body of pharynx and
                  cervical esophagus
   X ● S11.23 Puncture wound without foreign body of
                  pharynx and cervical esophagus
   X ● S11.24 Puncture wound with foreign body of pharynx
                  and cervical esophagus
   X ● S11.25 Open bite of pharynx and cervical esophagus
                  Bite of pharynx and cervical esophagus NOS
● S11.8 Open wound of other specified parts of neck
   X ● S11.80 Unspecified open specified wound of other part
                  of neck
   X ● S11.81 Laceration without foreign body of other
                  specified part of neck
   X ● S11.82 Laceration with foreign body of other specified
                  part of neck
   X ● S11.83 Puncture wound without foreign body of other
                  specified part of neck
   X ● S11.84 Puncture wound with foreign body of other
                  specified part of neck
   X ● S11.85 Open bite of other specified part of neck
                  Bite of other part of neck NOS
                  | Excludes1 | superficial bite of other specified
                                            part of neck (S10.87)
   X ● S11.89 Other open wound of other part of neck

● S11.9 Open wound of unspecified part of neck
   X ● S11.90 Unspecified open wound of unspecified part of
                  neck
   X ● S11.91 Laceration without foreign body of unspecified
                  part of neck
   X ● S11.92 Laceration with foreign body of unspecified
                  part of neck
   X ● S11.93 Puncture wound without foreign body of
                  unspecified part of neck
   X ● S11.94 Puncture wound with foreign body of
                  unspecified part of neck
   X ● S11.95 Open bite of unspecified part of neck
                  Bite of neck NOS
                  | Excludes1 | superficial bite of neck (S10.97)

● S12 Fracture of cervical vertebra and other parts of neck
         Note: A fracture not indicated as displaced or nondisplaced
                  should be coded to displaced
                  A fracture not indicated as open or closed should be coded to
                  closed
         | Includes | fracture of cervical neural arch
                              fracture of cervical spine
                              fracture of cervical spinous process
                              fracture of cervical transverse process
                              fracture of cervical vertebral arch
                              fracture of neck

         Code first any associated cervical spinal cord injury (S14.0, S14.1-)
         The appropriate 7th character is to be added to all codes from
         subcategories S12.0-S12.6

         | A   initial encounter for closed fracture
         | B   initial encounter for open fracture
         | D   subsequent encounter for fracture with routine healing
         | G   subsequent encounter for fracture with delayed
         | healing
         | K   subsequent encounter for fracture with nonunion
         | S   sequela

   ● S12.0 Fracture of first cervical vertebra
               Atlas
         ● S12.00 Unspecified fracture of first cervical vertebra
               ● S12.000 Unspecified displaced fracture of first
                             cervical vertebra
               ● S12.001 Unspecified nondisplaced fracture of
                             first cervical vertebra
         X ● S12.01 Stable burst fracture of first cervical vertebra
         X ● S12.02 Unstable burst fracture of first cervical vertebra
         ● S12.03 Posterior arch fracture of first cervical vertebra
               ● S12.030 Displaced posterior arch fracture of
                             first cervical vertebra
               ● S12.031 Nondisplaced posterior arch fracture
                             of first cervical vertebra
         ● S12.04 Lateral mass fracture of first cervical vertebra
               ● S12.040 Displaced lateral mass fracture of first
                             cervical vertebra
               ● S12.041 Nondisplaced lateral mass fracture of
                             first cervical vertebra
         ● S12.09 Other fracture of first cervical vertebra
               ● S12.090 Other displaced fracture of first
                             cervical vertebra
               ● S12.091 Other nondisplaced fracture of first
                             cervical vertebra
   ● S12.1 Fracture of second cervical vertebra
               Axis
         ● S12.10 Unspecified fracture of second cervical vertebra
               ● S12.100 Unspecified displaced fracture of
                             second cervical vertebra
               ● S12.101 Unspecified nondisplaced fracture of
                             second cervical vertebra

▶ New   ⟹ Revised   ~~deleted~~ Deleted   **OGCR** Official Guidelines   X Assign placeholder X   ● Use Additional Character(s)

| Excludes 1 | | Excludes 2 | | Includes | Use additional | Code first | | Code also | | Key words |

● S12.11   Type II dens fracture
  ● S12.110   Anterior displaced Type II dens fracture
  ● S12.111   Posterior displaced Type II dens fracture
  ● S12.112   Nondisplaced Type II dens fracture
● S12.12   Other dens fracture
  ● S12.120   Other displaced dens fracture
  ● S12.121   Other nondisplaced dens fracture
● S12.13   Unspecified traumatic spondylolisthesis of second cervical vertebra
  ● S12.130   Unspecified traumatic displaced spondylolisthesis of second cervical vertebra
  ● S12.131   Unspecified traumatic nondisplaced spondylolisthesis of second cervical vertebra
X ● S12.14   Type III traumatic spondylolisthesis of second cervical vertebra
● S12.15   Other traumatic spondylolisthesis of second cervical vertebra
  ● S12.150   Other traumatic displaced spondylolisthesis of second cervical vertebra
  ● S12.151   Other traumatic nondisplaced spondylolisthesis of second cervical vertebra
● S12.19   Other fracture of second cervical vertebra
  ● S12.190   Other displaced fracture of second cervical vertebra
  ● S12.191   Other nondisplaced fracture of second cervical vertebra
● S12.2   Fracture of third cervical vertebra
  ● S12.20   Unspecified fracture of third cervical vertebra
    ● S12.200   Unspecified displaced fracture of third cervical vertebra
    ● S12.201   Unspecified nondisplaced fracture of third cervical vertebra
  ● S12.23   Unspecified traumatic spondylolisthesis of third cervical vertebra
    ● S12.230   Unspecified traumatic displaced spondylolisthesis of third cervical vertebra
    ● S12.231   Unspecified traumatic nondisplaced spondylolisthesis of third cervical vertebra
X ● S12.24   Type III traumatic spondylolisthesis of third cervical vertebra
  ● S12.25   Other traumatic spondylolisthesis of third cervical vertebra
    ● S12.250   Other traumatic displaced spondylolisthesis of third cervical vertebra
    ● S12.251   Other traumatic nondisplaced spondylolisthesis of third cervical vertebra
  ● S12.29   Other fracture of third cervical vertebra
    ● S12.290   Other displaced fracture of third cervical vertebra
    ● S12.291   Other nondisplaced fracture of third cervical vertebra
● S12.3   Fracture of fourth cervical vertebra
  ● S12.30   Unspecified fracture of fourth cervical vertebra
    ● S12.300   Unspecified displaced fracture of fourth cervical vertebra
    ● S12.301   Unspecified nondisplaced fracture of fourth cervical vertebra

● S12.33   Unspecified traumatic spondylolisthesis of fourth cervical vertebra
  ● S12.330   Unspecified traumatic displaced spondylolisthesis of fourth cervical vertebra
  ● S12.331   Unspecified traumatic nondisplaced spondylolisthesis of fourth cervical vertebra
X ● S12.34   Type III traumatic spondylolisthesis of fourth cervical vertebra
● S12.35   Other traumatic spondylolisthesis of fourth cervical vertebra
  ● S12.350   Other traumatic displaced spondylolisthesis of fourth cervical vertebra
  ● S12.351   Other traumatic nondisplaced spondylolisthesis of fourth cervical vertebra
● S12.39   Other fracture of fourth cervical vertebra
  ● S12.390   Other displaced fracture of fourth cervical vertebra
  ● S12.391   Other nondisplaced fracture of fourth cervical vertebra
● S12.4   Fracture of fifth cervical vertebra
  ● S12.40   Unspecified fracture of fifth cervical vertebra
    ● S12.400   Unspecified displaced fracture of fifth cervical vertebra
    ● S12.401   Unspecified nondisplaced fracture of fifth cervical vertebra
  ● S12.43   Unspecified traumatic spondylolisthesis of fifth cervical vertebra
    ● S12.430   Unspecified traumatic displaced spondylolisthesis of fifth cervical vertebra
    ● S12.431   Unspecified traumatic nondisplaced spondylolisthesis of fifth cervical vertebra
X ● S12.44   Type III traumatic spondylolisthesis of fifth cervical vertebra
  ● S12.45   Other traumatic spondylolisthesis of fifth cervical vertebra
    ● S12.450   Other traumatic displaced spondylolisthesis of fifth cervical vertebra
    ● S12.451   Other traumatic nondisplaced spondylolisthesis of fifth cervical vertebra
  ● S12.49   Other fracture of fifth cervical vertebra
    ● S12.490   Other displaced fracture of fifth cervical vertebra
    ● S12.491   Other nondisplaced fracture of fifth cervical vertebra
● S12.5   Fracture of sixth cervical vertebra
  ● S12.50   Unspecified fracture of sixth cervical vertebra
    ● S12.500   Unspecified displaced fracture of sixth cervical vertebra
    ● S12.501   Unspecified nondisplaced fracture of sixth cervical vertebra
  ● S12.53   Unspecified traumatic spondylolisthesis of sixth cervical vertebra
    ● S12.530   Unspecified traumatic displaced spondylolisthesis of sixth cervical vertebra
    ● S12.531   Unspecified traumatic nondisplaced spondylolisthesis of sixth cervical vertebra

CHAPTER 19 (S00-T88)

▶ New   ⇒ Revised   ~~deleted~~ Deleted   **OGCR** Official Guidelines   X Assign placeholder X   ● Use Additional Character(s)

Excludes 1   Excludes 2   Includes   Use additional   Code first   Code also   Key words

X● **S12.54** Type III traumatic spondylolisthesis of sixth cervical vertebra

● **S12.55** Other traumatic spondylolisthesis of sixth cervical vertebra

● **S12.550** Other traumatic displaced spondylolisthesis of sixth cervical vertebra

● **S12.551** Other traumatic nondisplaced spondylolisthesis of sixth cervical vertebra

● **S12.59** Other fracture of sixth cervical vertebra

● **S12.590** Other displaced fracture of sixth cervical vertebra

● **S12.591** Other nondisplaced fracture of sixth cervical vertebra

● **S12.6** Fracture of seventh cervical vertebra

S12.60 Unspecified fracture of seventh cervical vertebra

● **S12.600** Unspecified displaced fracture of seventh cervical vertebra

● **S12.601** Unspecified nondisplaced fracture of seventh cervical vertebra

● **S12.63** Unspecified traumatic spondylolisthesis of seventh cervical vertebra

● **S12.630** Unspecified traumatic displaced spondylolisthesis of seventh cervical vertebra

● **S12.631** Unspecified traumatic nondisplaced spondylolisthesis of seventh cervical vertebra

X● **S12.64** Type III traumatic spondylolisthesis of seventh cervical vertebra

● **S12.65** Other traumatic spondylolisthesis of seventh cervical vertebra

● **S12.650** Other traumatic displaced spondylolisthesis of seventh cervical vertebra

● **S12.651** Other traumatic nondisplaced spondylolisthesis of seventh cervical vertebra

● **S12.69** Other fracture of seventh cervical vertebra

● **S12.690** Other displaced fracture of seventh cervical vertebra

● **S12.691** Other nondisplaced fracture of seventh cervical vertebra

X● **S12.8** Fracture of other parts of neck

Hyoid bone   Thyroid cartilage
Larynx   Trachea

The appropriate 7th character is to be added to code S12.8

A	initial encounter
D	subsequent encounter
S	sequela

X● **S12.9** Fracture of neck, unspecified

Fracture of neck NOS
Fracture of cervical spine NOS
Fracture of cervical vertebra NOS

The appropriate 7th character is to be added to code S12.9

A	initial encounter
D	subsequent encounter
S	sequela

● **S13** Dislocation and sprain of joints and ligaments at neck level

Includes avulsion of joint or ligament at neck level
laceration of cartilage, joint or ligament at neck level
sprain of cartilage, joint or ligament at neck level
traumatic hemarthrosis of joint or ligament at neck level
traumatic rupture of joint or ligament at neck level
traumatic subluxation of joint or ligament at neck level
traumatic tear of joint or ligament at neck level

Code also any associated open wound

Excludes2 strain of muscle or tendon at neck level (S16.1)

The appropriate 7th character is to be added to each code from category S13

A	initial encounter
D	subsequent encounter
S	sequela

X● **S13.0** Traumatic rupture of cervical intervertebral disc

Excludes1 rupture or displacement (nontraumatic) of cervical intervertebral disc NOS (M50.-)

● **S13.1** Subluxation and dislocation of cervical vertebrae

Code also any associated:
open wound of neck (S11.-)
spinal cord injury (S14.1-)

Excludes2 fracture of cervical vertebrae (S12.0-S12.3-)

● **S13.10** Subluxation and dislocation of unspecified cervical vertebrae

● **S13.100** Subluxation of unspecified cervical vertebrae

● **S13.101** Dislocation of unspecified cervical vertebrae

● **S13.11** Subluxation and dislocation of C0/C1 cervical vertebrae

Subluxation and dislocation of atlantooccipital joint
Subluxation and dislocation of atloidooccipital joint
Subluxation and dislocation of occipitoatloid joint

● **S13.110** Subluxation of C0/C1 cervical vertebrae

● **S13.111** Dislocation of C0/C1 cervical vertebrae

● **S13.12** Subluxation and dislocation of C1/C2 cervical vertebrae

Subluxation and dislocation of atlantoaxial joint

● **S13.120** Subluxation of C1/C2 cervical vertebrae

● **S13.121** Dislocation of C1/C2 cervical vertebrae

● **S13.13** Subluxation and dislocation of C2/C3 cervical vertebrae

● **S13.130** Subluxation of C2/C3 cervical vertebrae

● **S13.131** Dislocation of C2/C3 cervical vertebrae

● **S13.14** Subluxation and dislocation of C3/C4 cervical vertebrae

● **S13.140** Subluxation of C3/C4 cervical vertebrae

● **S13.141** Dislocation of C3/C4 cervical vertebrae

▶ New   ⇒ Revised   ~~deleted~~ Deleted   **OGCR** Official Guidelines   X Assign placeholder X   ● Use Additional Character(s)

Excludes 1   Excludes 2   Includes   Use additional   Code first   Code also   Key words

● S13.15   Subluxation and dislocation of C4/C5 cervical vertebrae
    ● S13.150   Subluxation of C4/C5 cervical vertebrae
    ● S13.151   Dislocation of C4/C5 cervical vertebrae
● S13.16   Subluxation and dislocation of C5/C6 cervical vertebrae
    ● S13.160   Subluxation of C5/C6 cervical vertebrae
    ● S13.161   Dislocation of C5/C6 cervical vertebrae
● S13.17   Subluxation and dislocation of C6/C7 cervical vertebrae
    ● S13.170   Subluxation of C6/C7 cervical vertebrae
    ● S13.171   Dislocation of C6/C7 cervical vertebrae
● S13.18   Subluxation and dislocation of C7/T1 cervical vertebrae
    ● S13.180   Subluxation of C7/T1 cervical vertebrae
    ● S13.181   Dislocation of C7/T1 cervical vertebrae
● S13.2   Dislocation of other and unspecified parts of neck
    X● S13.20   Dislocation of unspecified parts of neck
    X● S13.29   Dislocation of other parts of neck
X● S13.4   Sprain of ligaments of cervical spine
      Sprain of anterior longitudinal (ligament), cervical
      Sprain of atlanto-axial (joints)
      Sprain of atlanto-occipital (joints)
      Whiplash injury of cervical spine
X● S13.5   Sprain of thyroid region
      Sprain of cricoarytenoid (joint) (ligament)
      Sprain of cricothyroid (joint) (ligament)
      Sprain of thyroid cartilage
X● S13.8   Sprain of joints and ligaments of other parts of neck
X● S13.9   Sprain of joints and ligaments of unspecified parts of neck

● **S14**   **Injury of nerves and spinal cord at neck level**
    Note: Code to highest level of cervical cord injury
    Code also any associated:
      fracture of cervical vertebra (S12.0--S12.6.-)
      open wound of neck (S11.-)
      transient paralysis (R29.5)
    The appropriate 7th character is to be added to each code from category S14

A	initial encounter
D	subsequent encounter
S	sequela

X● S14.0   Concussion and edema of cervical spinal cord
● S14.1   Other and unspecified injuries of cervical spinal cord
    ● S14.10   Unspecified injury of cervical spinal cord
      ● S14.101   Unspecified injury at C1 level of cervical spinal cord
      ● S14.102   Unspecified injury at C2 level of cervical spinal cord
      ● S14.103   Unspecified injury at C3 level of cervical spinal cord
      ● S14.104   Unspecified injury at C4 level of cervical spinal cord
      ● S14.105   Unspecified injury at C5 level of cervical spinal cord
      ● S14.106   Unspecified injury at C6 level of cervical spinal cord

● S14.107   Unspecified injury at C7 level of cervical spinal cord
● S14.108   Unspecified injury at C8 level of cervical spinal cord
● S14.109   Unspecified injury at unspecified level of cervical spinal cord
      Injury of cervical spinal cord NOS
● S14.11   Complete lesion of cervical spinal cord
    ● S14.111   Complete lesion at C1 level of cervical spinal cord
    ● S14.112   Complete lesion at C2 level of cervical spinal cord
    ● S14.113   Complete lesion at C3 level of cervical spinal cord
    ● S14.114   Complete lesion at C4 level of cervical spinal cord
    ● S14.115   Complete lesion at C5 level of cervical spinal cord
    ● S14.116   Complete lesion at C6 level of cervical spinal cord
    ● S14.117   Complete lesion at C7 level of cervical spinal cord
    ● S14.118   Complete lesion at C8 level of cervical spinal cord
    ● S14.119   Complete lesion at unspecified level of cervical spinal cord
● S14.12   Central cord syndrome of cervical spinal cord
    ● S14.121   Central cord syndrome at C1 level of cervical spinal cord
    ● S14.122   Central cord syndrome at C2 level of cervical spinal cord
    ● S14.123   Central cord syndrome at C3 level of cervical spinal cord
    ● S14.124   Central cord syndrome at C4 level of cervical spinal cord
    ● S14.125   Central cord syndrome at C5 level of cervical spinal cord
    ● S14.126   Central cord syndrome at C6 level of cervical spinal cord
    ● S14.127   Central cord syndrome at C7 level of cervical spinal cord
    ● S14.128   Central cord syndrome at C8 level of cervical spinal cord
    ● S14.129   Central cord syndrome at unspecified level of cervical spinal cord
● S14.13   Anterior cord syndrome of cervical spinal cord
    ● S14.131   Anterior cord syndrome at C1 level of cervical spinal cord
    ● S14.132   Anterior cord syndrome at C2 level of cervical spinal cord
    ● S14.133   Anterior cord syndrome at C3 level of cervical spinal cord
    ● S14.134   Anterior cord syndrome at C4 level of cervical spinal cord
    ● S14.135   Anterior cord syndrome at C5 level of cervical spinal cord
    ● S14.136   Anterior cord syndrome at C6 level of cervical spinal cord
    ● S14.137   Anterior cord syndrome at C7 level of cervical spinal cord
    ● S14.138   Anterior cord syndrome at C8 level of cervical spinal cord
    ● S14.139   Anterior cord syndrome at unspecified level of cervical spinal cord

● **S14.14** Brown-Séquard syndrome of cervical spinal cord

   ● **S14.141** Brown-Séquard syndrome at C1 level of cervical spinal cord

   ● **S14.142** Brown-Séquard syndrome at C2 level of cervical spinal cord

   ● **S14.143** Brown-Séquard syndrome at C3 level of cervical spinal cord

   ● **S14.144** Brown-Séquard syndrome at C4 level of cervical spinal cord

   ● **S14.145** Brown-Séquard syndrome at C5 level of cervical spinal cord

   ● **S14.146** Brown-Séquard syndrome at C6 level of cervical spinal cord

   ● **S14.147** Brown-Séquard syndrome at C7 level of cervical spinal cord

   ● **S14.148** Brown-Séquard syndrome at C8 level of cervical spinal cord

   ● **S14.149** Brown-Séquard syndrome at unspecified level of cervical spinal cord

● **S14.15** Other incomplete lesions of cervical spinal cord
Incomplete lesion of cervical spinal cord NOS
Posterior cord syndrome of cervical spinal cord

   ● **S14.151** Other incomplete lesion at C1 level of cervical spinal cord

   ● **S14.152** Other incomplete lesion at C2 level of cervical spinal cord

   ● **S14.153** Other incomplete lesion at C3 level of cervical spinal cord

   ● **S14.154** Other incomplete lesion at C4 level of cervical spinal cord

   ● **S14.155** Other incomplete lesion at C5 level of cervical spinal cord

   ● **S14.156** Other incomplete lesion at C6 level of cervical spinal cord

   ● **S14.157** Other incomplete lesion at C7 level of cervical spinal cord

   ● **S14.158** Other incomplete lesion at C8 level of cervical spinal cord

   ● **S14.159** Other incomplete lesion at unspecified level of cervical spinal cord

X● **S14.2** Injury of nerve root of cervical spine

X● **S14.3** Injury of brachial plexus

X● **S14.4** Injury of peripheral nerves of neck

X● **S14.5** Injury of cervical sympathetic nerves

X● **S14.8** Injury of other specified nerves of neck

X● **S14.9** Injury of unspecified nerves of neck

● **S15** Injury of blood vessels at neck level
Code also any associated open wound (S11.-)
The appropriate 7th character is to be added to each code from category S15

> | A | initial encounter |
> | D | subsequent encounter |
> | S | sequela |

● **S15.0** Injury of carotid artery of neck
Injury of carotid artery (common) (external) (internal, extracranial portion)
Injury of carotid artery NOS
Excludes1 injury of internal carotid artery, intracranial portion (S06.8)

 ● **S15.00** Unspecified injury of carotid artery

   ● **S15.001** Unspecified injury of right carotid artery

   ● **S15.002** Unspecified injury of left carotid artery

   ● **S15.009** Unspecified injury of unspecified carotid artery

● **S15.01** Minor laceration of carotid artery
Incomplete transection of carotid artery
Laceration of carotid artery NOS
Superficial laceration of carotid artery

   ● **S15.011** Minor laceration of right carotid artery

   ● **S15.012** Minor laceration of left carotid artery

   ● **S15.019** Minor laceration of unspecified carotid artery

● **S15.02** Major laceration of carotid artery
Complete transection of carotid artery
Traumatic rupture of carotid artery

   ● **S15.021** Major laceration of right carotid artery

   ● **S15.022** Major laceration of left carotid artery

   ● **S15.029** Major laceration of unspecified carotid artery

● **S15.09** Other specified injury of carotid artery

   ● **S15.091** Other specified injury of right carotid artery

   ● **S15.092** Other specified injury of left carotid artery

   ● **S15.099** Other specified injury of unspecified carotid artery

● **S15.1** Injury of vertebral artery

 ● **S15.10** Unspecified injury of vertebral artery

   ● **S15.101** Unspecified injury of right vertebral artery

   ● **S15.102** Unspecified injury of left vertebral artery

   ● **S15.109** Unspecified injury of unspecified vertebral artery

● **S15.11** Minor laceration of vertebral artery
Incomplete transection of vertebral artery
Laceration of vertebral artery NOS
Superficial laceration of vertebral artery

   ● **S15.111** Minor laceration of right vertebral artery

   ● **S15.112** Minor laceration of left vertebral artery

   ● **S15.119** Minor laceration of unspecified vertebral artery

● **S15.12** Major laceration of vertebral artery
Complete transection of vertebral artery
Traumatic rupture of vertebral artery

   ● **S15.121** Major laceration of right vertebral artery

   ● **S15.122** Major laceration of left vertebral artery

   ● **S15.129** Major laceration of unspecified vertebral artery

● **S15.19** Other specified injury of vertebral artery

   ● **S15.191** Other specified injury of right vertebral artery

   ● **S15.192** Other specified injury of left vertebral artery

   ● **S15.199** Other specified injury of unspecified vertebral artery

● **S15.2** Injury of external jugular vein

 ● **S15.20** Unspecified injury of external jugular vein

   ● **S15.201** Unspecified injury of right external jugular vein

   ● **S15.202** Unspecified injury of left external jugular vein

   ● **S15.209** Unspecified injury of unspecified external jugular vein

▶ New   ⇒ Revised   ~~deleted~~ Deleted   **OGCR** Official Guidelines   X Assign placeholder X   ● Use Additional Character(s)

Excludes 1   Excludes 2   Includes   Use additional   Code first   Code also   Key words

● **S15.21** Minor laceration of external jugular vein
     Incomplete transection of external jugular vein
     Laceration of external jugular vein NOS
     Superficial laceration of external jugular vein
     ● **S15.211** Minor laceration of right external jugular vein
     ● **S15.212** Minor laceration of left external jugular vein
     ● **S15.219** Minor laceration of unspecified external jugular vein

● **S15.22** Major laceration of external jugular vein
     Complete transection of external jugular vein
     Traumatic rupture of external jugular vein
     ● **S15.221** Major laceration of right external jugular vein
     ● **S15.222** Major laceration of left external jugular vein
     ● **S15.229** Major laceration of unspecified external jugular vein

● **S15.29** Other specified injury of external jugular vein
     ● **S15.291** Other specified injury of right external jugular vein
     ● **S15.292** Other specified injury of left external jugular vein
     ● **S15.299** Other specified injury of unspecified external jugular vein

● **S15.3** Injury of internal jugular vein
     ● **S15.30** Unspecified injury of internal jugular vein
         ● **S15.301** Unspecified injury of right internal jugular vein
         ● **S15.302** Unspecified injury of left internal jugular vein
         ● **S15.309** Unspecified injury of unspecified internal jugular vein

     ● **S15.31** Minor laceration of internal jugular vein
         Incomplete transection of internal jugular vein
         Laceration of internal jugular vein NOS
         Superficial laceration of internal jugular vein
         ● **S15.311** Minor laceration of right internal jugular vein
         ● **S15.312** Minor laceration of left internal jugular vein
         ● **S15.319** Minor laceration of unspecified internal jugular vein

     ● **S15.32** Major laceration of internal jugular vein
         Complete transection of internal jugular vein
         Traumatic rupture of internal jugular vein
         ● **S15.321** Major laceration of right internal jugular vein
         ● **S15.322** Major laceration of left internal jugular vein
         ● **S15.329** Major laceration of unspecified internal jugular vein

     ● **S15.39** Other specified injury of internal jugular vein
         ● **S15.391** Other specified injury of right internal jugular vein
         ● **S15.392** Other specified injury of left internal jugular vein
         ● **S15.399** Other specified injury of unspecified internal jugular vein

X ● **S15.8** Injury of other specified blood vessels at neck level
X ● **S15.9** Injury of unspecified blood vessel at neck level

● **S16** Injury of muscle, fascia and tendon at neck level
     Code also any associated open wound (S11.-)
     Excludes2 sprain of joint or ligament at neck level (S13.9)
     The appropriate 7th character is to be added to each code from category S16

A	initial encounter
D	subsequent encounter
S	sequela

     X ● **S16.1** Strain of muscle, fascia and tendon at neck level
     X ● **S16.2** Laceration of muscle, fascia and tendon at neck level
     X ● **S16.8** Other specified injury of muscle, fascia and tendon at neck level
     X ● **S16.9** Unspecified injury of muscle, fascia and tendon at neck level

● **S17** Crushing injury of neck
     Use additional code for all associated injuries, such as:
     injury of blood vessels (S15.-)
     open wound of neck (S11.-)
     spinal cord injury (S14.0, S14.1-)
     vertebral fracture (S12.0--S12.3-)

     The appropriate 7th character is to be added to each code from category S17

A	initial encounter
D	subsequent encounter
S	sequela

     X ● **S17.0** Crushing injury of larynx and trachea
     X ● **S17.8** Crushing injury of other specified parts of neck
     X ● **S17.9** Crushing injury of neck, part unspecified

● **S19** Other and unspecified injuries of neck
     The appropriate 7th character is to be added to each code from category S19

A	initial encounter
D	subsequent encounter
S	sequela

     ● **S19.8** Other specified injuries of neck
         X ● **S19.80** Other specified injuries of unspecified part of neck
         X ● **S19.81** Other specified injuries of larynx
         X ● **S19.82** Other specified injuries of cervical trachea
             Excludes2 other specified injury of thoracic trachea (S27.5-)
         X ● **S19.83** Other specified injuries of vocal cord
         X ● **S19.84** Other specified injuries of thyroid gland
         X ● **S19.85** Other specified injuries of pharynx and cervical esophagus
         X ● **S19.89** Other specified injuries of other specified part of neck
     X ● **S19.9** Unspecified injury of neck

INJURIES TO THE THORAX (S20-S29)

Includes	injuries of breast
	injuries of chest (wall)
	injuries of interscapular area
Excludes2	burns and corrosions (T20-T32)
	effects of foreign body in bronchus (T17.5)
	effects of foreign body in esophagus (T18.1)
	effects of foreign body in lung (T17.8)
	effects of foreign body in trachea (T17.4)
	frostbite (T33-T34)
	injuries of axilla
	injuries of clavicle
	injuries of scapular region
	injuries of shoulder
	insect bite or sting, venomous (T63.4)

● S20　Superficial injury of thorax

The appropriate 7th character is to be added to each code from category S20

A	initial encounter
D	subsequent encounter
S	sequela

● S20.0　Contusion of breast
- X ● S20.00　Contusion of breast, unspecified breast
- X ● S20.01　Contusion of right breast
- X ● S20.02　Contusion of left breast

● S20.1　Other and unspecified superficial injuries of breast
- ● S20.10　Unspecified superficial injuries of breast
  - ● S20.101　Unspecified superficial injuries of breast, right breast
  - ● S20.102　Unspecified superficial injuries of breast, left breast
  - ● S20.109　Unspecified superficial injuries of breast, unspecified breast
- ● S20.11　Abrasion of breast
  - ● S20.111　Abrasion of breast, right breast
  - ● S20.112　Abrasion of breast, left breast
  - ● S20.119　Abrasion of breast, unspecified breast
- ● S20.12　Blister (nonthermal) of breast
  - ● S20.121　Blister (nonthermal) of breast, right breast
  - ● S20.122　Blister (nonthermal) of breast, left breast
  - ● S20.129　Blister (nonthermal) of breast, unspecified breast
- ● S20.14　External constriction of part of breast
  - ● S20.141　External constriction of part of breast, right breast
  - ● S20.142　External constriction of part of breast, left breast
  - ● S20.149　External constriction of part of breast, unspecified breast
- ● S20.15　Superficial foreign body of breast
  Splinter in the breast
  - ● S20.151　Superficial foreign body of breast, right breast
  - ● S20.152　Superficial foreign body of breast, left breast
  - ● S20.159　Superficial foreign body of breast, unspecified breast
- ● S20.16　Insect bite (nonvenomous) of breast
  - ● S20.161　Insect bite (nonvenomous) of breast, right breast
  - ● S20.162　Insect bite (nonvenomous) of breast, left breast
  - ● S20.169　Insect bite (nonvenomous) of breast, unspecified breast

- ● S20.17　Other superficial bite of breast
  - Excludes1　open bite of breast (S21.05-)
  - ● S20.171　Other superficial bite of breast, right breast
  - ● S20.172　Other superficial bite of breast, left breast
  - ● S20.179　Other superficial bite of breast, unspecified breast

● S20.2　Contusion of thorax
- X ● S20.20　Contusion of thorax, unspecified
- ● S20.21　Contusion of front wall of thorax
  - ● S20.211　Contusion of right front wall of thorax
  - ● S20.212　Contusion of left front wall of thorax
  - ● S20.219　Contusion of unspecified front wall of thorax
- ● S20.22　Contusion of back wall of thorax
  - ● S20.221　Contusion of right back wall of thorax
  - ● S20.222　Contusion of left back wall of thorax
  - ● S20.229　Contusion of unspecified back wall of thorax

● S20.3　Other and unspecified superficial injuries of front wall of thorax
- ● S20.30　Unspecified superficial injuries of front wall of thorax
  - ● S20.301　Unspecified superficial injuries of right front wall of thorax
  - ● S20.302　Unspecified superficial injuries of left front wall of thorax
  - ● S20.309　Unspecified superficial injuries of unspecified front wall of thorax
- ● S20.31　Abrasion of front wall of thorax
  - ● S20.311　Abrasion of right front wall of thorax
  - ● S20.312　Abrasion of left front wall of thorax
  - ● S20.319　Abrasion of unspecified front wall of thorax
- ● S20.32　Blister (nonthermal) of front wall of thorax
  - ● S20.321　Blister (nonthermal) of right front wall of thorax
  - ● S20.322　Blister (nonthermal) of left front wall of thorax
  - ● S20.329　Blister (nonthermal) of unspecified front wall of thorax
- ● S20.34　External constriction of front wall of thorax
  - ● S20.341　External constriction of right front wall of thorax
  - ● S20.342　External constriction of left front wall of thorax
  - ● S20.349　External constriction of unspecified front wall of thorax
- ● S20.35　Superficial foreign body of front wall of thorax
  Splinter in front wall of thorax
  - ● S20.351　Superficial foreign body of right front wall of thorax
  - ● S20.352　Superficial foreign body of left front wall of thorax
  - ● S20.359　Superficial foreign body of unspecified front wall of thorax
- ● S20.36　Insect bite (nonvenomous) of front wall of thorax
  - ● S20.361　Insect bite (nonvenomous) of right front wall of thorax
  - ● S20.362　Insect bite (nonvenomous) of left front wall of thorax
  - ● S20.369　Insect bite (nonvenomous) of unspecified front wall of thorax

CHAPTER 19 (S00-T88)

● **S20.37** Other superficial bite of front wall of thorax
> **Excludes 1** open bite of front wall of thorax (S21.14)

● **S20.371** Other superficial bite of right front wall of thorax

● **S20.372** Other superficial bite of left front wall of thorax

● **S20.379** Other superficial bite of unspecified front wall of thorax

● **S20.4** Other and unspecified superficial injuries of back wall of thorax

● **S20.40** Unspecified superficial injuries of back wall of thorax

● **S20.401** Unspecified superficial injuries of right back wall of thorax

● **S20.402** Unspecified superficial injuries of left back wall of thorax

● **S20.409** Unspecified superficial injuries of unspecified back wall of thorax

● **S20.41** Abrasion of back wall of thorax

● **S20.411** Abrasion of right back wall of thorax

● **S20.412** Abrasion of left back wall of thorax

● **S20.419** Abrasion of unspecified back wall of thorax

● **S20.42** Blister (nonthermal) of back wall of thorax

● **S20.421** Blister (nonthermal) of right back wall of thorax

● **S20.422** Blister (nonthermal) of left back wall of thorax

● **S20.429** Blister (nonthermal) of unspecified back wall of thorax

● **S20.44** External constriction of back wall of thorax

● **S20.441** External constriction of right back wall of thorax

● **S20.442** External constriction of left back wall of thorax

● **S20.449** External constriction of unspecified back wall of thorax

● **S20.45** Superficial foreign body of back wall of thorax
Splinter of back wall of thorax

● **S20.451** Superficial foreign body of right back wall of thorax

● **S20.452** Superficial foreign body of left back wall of thorax

● **S20.459** Superficial foreign body of unspecified back wall of thorax

● **S20.46** Insect bite (nonvenomous) of back wall of thorax

● **S20.461** Insect bite (nonvenomous) of right back wall of thorax

● **S20.462** Insect bite (nonvenomous) of left back wall of thorax

● **S20.469** Insect bite (nonvenomous) of unspecified back wall of thorax

● **S20.47** Other superficial bite of back wall of thorax
> **Excludes 1** open bite of back wall of thorax (S21.24)

● **S20.471** Other superficial bite of right back wall of thorax

● **S20.472** Other superficial bite of left back wall of thorax

● **S20.479** Other superficial bite of unspecified back wall of thorax

● **S20.9** Superficial injury of unspecified parts of thorax
> **Excludes 1** contusion of thorax NOS (S20.20)

X ● **S20.90** Unspecified superficial injury of unspecified parts of thorax
Superficial injury of thoracic wall NOS

X ● **S20.91** Abrasion of unspecified parts of thorax

X ● **S20.92** Blister (nonthermal) of unspecified parts of thorax

X ● **S20.94** External constriction of unspecified parts of thorax

X ● **S20.95** Superficial foreign body of unspecified parts of thorax
Splinter in thorax NOS

X ● **S20.96** Insect bite (nonvenomous) of unspecified parts of thorax

X ● **S20.97** Other superficial bite of unspecified parts of thorax
> **Excludes 1** open bite of thorax NOS (S21.95)

● **S21** Open wound of thorax
Code also any associated injury such as:
injury of heart (S26.-)
injury of intrathoracic organs (S27.-)
rib fracture (S22.3-, S22.4-)
spinal cord injury (S24.0-, S24.1-)
traumatic hemothorax (S27.1)
traumatic hemopneumothorax (S27.3)
traumatic pneumothorax (S27.0)
wound infection
> **Excludes 1** traumatic amputation (partial) of thorax (S28.1)

The appropriate 7th character is to be added to each code from category S21

A	initial encounter
D	subsequent encounter
S	sequela

● **S21.0** Open wound of breast

● **S21.00** Unspecified open wound of breast

● **S21.001** Unspecified open wound of right breast

● **S21.002** Unspecified open wound of left breast

● **S21.009** Unspecified open wound of unspecified breast

● **S21.01** Laceration without foreign body of breast

● **S21.011** Laceration without foreign body of right breast

● **S21.012** Laceration without foreign body of left breast

● **S21.019** Laceration without foreign body of unspecified breast

● **S21.02** Laceration with foreign body of breast

● **S21.021** Laceration with foreign body of right breast

● **S21.022** Laceration with foreign body of left breast

● **S21.029** Laceration with foreign body of unspecified breast

Item 19-1   Pneumothorax is a collection of gas (positive air pressure) in the pleural space resulting in the lung collapsing. A **tension pneumothorax** is life-threatening and is a result of air in the pleural space causing a displacement in the mediastinal structures and cardiopulmonary function compromise. A **traumatic pneumothorax** results from blunt or penetrating injury that disrupts the parietal/visceral pleura. **Hemothorax** is blood or bloody fluid in the pleural cavity as a result of traumatic blood vessel rupture or inflammation of the lungs from pneumonia.

- S21.03   Puncture wound without foreign body of breast
  - S21.031   Puncture wound without foreign body of right breast
  - S21.032   Puncture wound without foreign body of left breast
  - S21.039   Puncture wound without foreign body of unspecified breast
- S21.04   Puncture wound with foreign body of breast
  - S21.041   Puncture wound with foreign body of right breast
  - S21.042   Puncture wound with foreign body of left breast
  - S21.049   Puncture wound with foreign body of unspecified breast
- S21.05   Open bite of breast
  Bite of breast NOS

  Excludes1   superficial bite of breast (S20.17)

  - S21.051   Open bite of right breast
  - S21.052   Open bite of left breast
  - S21.059   Open bite of unspecified breast
- S21.1   Open wound of front wall of thorax without penetration into thoracic cavity
  Open wound of chest without penetration into thoracic cavity
  - S21.10   Unspecified open wound of front wall of thorax without penetration into thoracic cavity
    - S21.101   Unspecified open wound of right front wall of thorax without penetration into thoracic cavity
    - S21.102   Unspecified open wound of left front wall of thorax without penetration into thoracic cavity
    - S21.109   Unspecified open wound of unspecified front wall of thorax without penetration into thoracic cavity
  - S21.11   Laceration without foreign body of front wall of thorax without penetration into thoracic cavity
    - S21.111   Laceration without foreign body of right front wall of thorax without penetration into thoracic cavity
    - S21.112   Laceration without foreign body of left front wall of thorax without penetration into thoracic cavity
    - S21.119   Laceration without foreign body of unspecified front wall of thorax without penetration into thoracic cavity
  - S21.12   Laceration with foreign body of front wall of thorax without penetration into thoracic cavity
    - S21.121   Laceration with foreign body of right front wall of thorax without penetration into thoracic cavity
    - S21.122   Laceration with foreign body of left front wall of thorax without penetration into thoracic cavity
    - S21.129   Laceration with foreign body of unspecified front wall of thorax without penetration into thoracic cavity

- S21.13   Puncture wound without foreign body of front wall of thorax without penetration into thoracic cavity
  - S21.131   Puncture wound without foreign body of right front wall of thorax without penetration into thoracic cavity
  - S21.132   Puncture wound without foreign body of left front wall of thorax without penetration into thoracic cavity
  - S21.139   Puncture wound without foreign body of unspecified front wall of thorax without penetration into thoracic cavity
- S21.14   Puncture wound with foreign body of front wall of thorax without penetration into thoracic cavity
  - S21.141   Puncture wound with foreign body of right front wall of thorax without penetration into thoracic cavity
  - S21.142   Puncture wound with foreign body of left front wall of thorax without penetration into thoracic cavity
  - S21.149   Puncture wound with foreign body of unspecified front wall of thorax without penetration into thoracic cavity
- S21.15   Open bite of front wall of thorax without penetration into thoracic cavity
  Bite of front wall of thorax NOS

  Excludes1   superficial bite of front wall of thorax (S20.37)

  - S21.151   Open bite of right front wall of thorax without penetration into thoracic cavity
  - S21.152   Open bite of left front wall of thorax without penetration into thoracic cavity
  - S21.159   Open bite of unspecified front wall of thorax without penetration into thoracic cavity
- S21.2   Open wound of back wall of thorax without penetration into thoracic cavity
  - S21.20   Unspecified open wound of back wall of thorax without penetration into thoracic cavity
    - S21.201   Unspecified open wound of right back wall of thorax without penetration into thoracic cavity
    - S21.202   Unspecified open wound of left back wall of thorax without penetration into thoracic cavity
    - S21.209   Unspecified open wound of unspecified back wall of thorax without penetration into thoracic cavity
  - S21.21   Laceration without foreign body of back wall of thorax without penetration into thoracic cavity
    - S21.211   Laceration without foreign body of right back wall of thorax without penetration into thoracic cavity
    - S21.212   Laceration without foreign body of left back wall of thorax without penetration into thoracic cavity
    - S21.219   Laceration without foreign body of unspecified back wall of thorax without penetration into thoracic cavity

● S21.22   Laceration with foreign body of back wall of thorax without penetration into thoracic cavity

    ● S21.221   Laceration with foreign body of right back wall of thorax without penetration into thoracic cavity

    ● S21.222   Laceration with foreign body of left back wall of thorax without penetration into thoracic cavity

    ● S21.229   Laceration with foreign body of unspecified back wall of thorax without penetration into thoracic cavity

● S21.23   Puncture wound without foreign body of back wall of thorax without penetration into thoracic cavity

    ● S21.231   Puncture wound without foreign body of right back wall of thorax without penetration into thoracic cavity

    ● S21.232   Puncture wound without foreign body of left back wall of thorax without penetration into thoracic cavity

    ● S21.239   Puncture wound without foreign body of unspecified back wall of thorax without penetration into thoracic cavity

● S21.24   Puncture wound with foreign body of back wall of thorax without penetration into thoracic cavity

    ● S21.241   Puncture wound with foreign body of right back wall of thorax without penetration into thoracic cavity

    ● S21.242   Puncture wound with foreign body of left back wall of thorax without penetration into thoracic cavity

    ● S21.249   Puncture wound with foreign body of unspecified back wall of thorax without penetration into thoracic cavity

● S21.25   Open bite of back wall of thorax without penetration into thoracic cavity
    Bite of back wall of thorax NOS

    | Excludes1 | superficial bite of back wall of thorax (S20.47) |

    ● S21.251   Open bite of right back wall of thorax without penetration into thoracic cavity

    ● S21.252   Open bite of left back wall of thorax without penetration into thoracic cavity

    ● S21.259   Open bite of unspecified back wall of thorax without penetration into thoracic cavity

● S21.3   Open wound of front wall of thorax with penetration into thoracic cavity
    Open wound of chest with penetration into thoracic cavity

    ● S21.30   Unspecified open wound of front wall of thorax with penetration into thoracic cavity

        ● S21.301   Unspecified open wound of right front wall of thorax with penetration into thoracic cavity

        ● S21.302   Unspecified open wound of left front wall of thorax with penetration into thoracic cavity

        ● S21.309   Unspecified open wound of unspecified front wall of thorax with penetration into thoracic cavity

● S21.31   Laceration without foreign body of front wall of thorax with penetration into thoracic cavity

    ● S21.311   Laceration without foreign body of right front wall of thorax with penetration into thoracic cavity

    ● S21.312   Laceration without foreign body of left front wall of thorax with penetration into thoracic cavity

    ● S21.319   Laceration without foreign body of unspecified front wall of thorax with penetration into thoracic cavity

● S21.32   Laceration with foreign body of front wall of thorax with penetration into thoracic cavity

    ● S21.321   Laceration with foreign body of right front wall of thorax with penetration into thoracic cavity

    ● S21.322   Laceration with foreign body of left front wall of thorax with penetration into thoracic cavity

    ● S21.329   Laceration with foreign body of unspecified front wall of thorax with penetration into thoracic cavity

● S21.33   Puncture wound without foreign body of front wall of thorax with penetration into thoracic cavity

    ● S21.331   Puncture wound without foreign body of right front wall of thorax with penetration into thoracic cavity

    ● S21.332   Puncture wound without foreign body of left front wall of thorax with penetration into thoracic cavity

    ● S21.339   Puncture wound without foreign body of unspecified front wall of thorax with penetration into thoracic cavity

● S21.34   Puncture wound with foreign body of front wall of thorax with penetration into thoracic cavity

    ● S21.341   Puncture wound with foreign body of right front wall of thorax with penetration into thoracic cavity

    ● S21.342   Puncture wound with foreign body of left front wall of thorax with penetration into thoracic cavity

    ● S21.349   Puncture wound with foreign body of unspecified front wall of thorax with penetration into thoracic cavity

● S21.35   Open bite of front wall of thorax with penetration into thoracic cavity

    | Excludes1 | superficial bite of front wall of thorax (S20.37) |

    ● S21.351   Open bite of right front wall of thorax with penetration into thoracic cavity

    ● S21.352   Open bite of left front wall of thorax with penetration into thoracic cavity

    ● S21.359   Open bite of unspecified front wall of thorax with penetration into thoracic cavity

● S21.4   Open wound of back wall of thorax with penetration into thoracic cavity

    ● S21.40   Unspecified open wound of back wall of thorax with penetration into thoracic cavity

        ● S21.401   Unspecified open wound of right back wall of thorax with penetration into thoracic cavity

        ● S21.402   Unspecified open wound of left back wall of thorax with penetration into thoracic cavity

        ● S21.409   Unspecified open wound of unspecified back wall of thorax with penetration into thoracic cavity

---

▶ New   ⇒ Revised   ~~deleted~~ Deleted   OGCR Official Guidelines   X Assign placeholder X   ● Use Additional Character(s)

| Excludes 1 | Excludes 2 | Includes | Use additional | Code first | Code also | Key words |

● **S21.41**   Laceration without foreign body of back wall of thorax with penetration into thoracic cavity

  ● **S21.411**   Laceration without foreign body of right back wall of thorax with penetration into thoracic cavity

  ● **S21.412**   Laceration without foreign body of left back wall of thorax with penetration into thoracic cavity

  ● **S21.419**   Laceration without foreign body of unspecified back wall of thorax with penetration into thoracic cavity

● **S21.42**   Laceration with foreign body of back wall of thorax with penetration into thoracic cavity

  ● **S21.421**   Laceration with foreign body of right back wall of thorax with penetration into thoracic cavity

  ● **S21.422**   Laceration with foreign body of left back wall of thorax with penetration into thoracic cavity

  ● **S21.429**   Laceration with foreign body of unspecified back wall of thorax with penetration into thoracic cavity

● **S21.43**   Puncture wound without foreign body of back wall of thorax with penetration into thoracic cavity

  ● **S21.431**   Puncture wound without foreign body of right back wall of thorax with penetration into thoracic cavity

  ● **S21.432**   Puncture wound without foreign body of left back wall of thorax with penetration into thoracic cavity

  ● **S21.439**   Puncture wound without foreign body of unspecified back wall of thorax with penetration into thoracic cavity

● **S21.44**   Puncture wound with foreign body of back wall of thorax with penetration into thoracic cavity

  ● **S21.441**   Puncture wound with foreign body of right back wall of thorax with penetration into thoracic cavity

  ● **S21.442**   Puncture wound with foreign body of left back wall of thorax with penetration into thoracic cavity

  ● **S21.449**   Puncture wound with foreign body of unspecified back wall of thorax with penetration into thoracic cavity

● **S21.45**   Open bite of back wall of thorax with penetration into thoracic cavity
       Bite of back wall of thorax NOS

    | Excludes1 | superficial bite of back wall of thorax (S20.47) |

  ● **S21.451**   Open bite of right back wall of thorax with penetration into thoracic cavity

  ● **S21.452**   Open bite of left back wall of thorax with penetration into thoracic cavity

  ● **S21.459**   Open bite of unspecified back wall of thorax with penetration into thoracic cavity

● **S21.9**   Open wound of unspecified part of thorax
     Open wound of thoracic wall NOS

X ● **S21.90**   Unspecified open wound of unspecified part of thorax

X ● **S21.91**   Laceration without foreign body of unspecified part of thorax

X ● **S21.92**   Laceration with foreign body of unspecified part of thorax

X ● **S21.93**   Puncture wound without foreign body of unspecified part of thorax

X ● **S21.94**   Puncture wound with foreign body of unspecified part of thorax

X ● **S21.95**   Open bite of unspecified part of thorax

    | Excludes1 | superficial bite of thorax (S20.97) |

● **S22**   Fracture of rib(s), sternum and thoracic spine

Note: A fracture not indicated as displaced or nondisplaced should be coded to displaced

A fracture not indicated as open or closed should be coded to closed

Includes	fracture of thoracic neural arch
	fracture of thoracic spinous process
	fracture of thoracic transverse process
	fracture of thoracic vertebra
	fracture of thoracic vertebral arch

Code first any associated:
injury of intrathoracic organ (S27.-)
spinal cord injury (S24.0-, S24.1-)

Excludes1	transection of thorax (S28.1)
Excludes2	fracture of clavicle (S42.0-)
	fracture of scapula (S42.1-)

The appropriate 7th character is to be added to each code from category S22

A	initial encounter for closed fracture
B	initial encounter for open fracture
D	subsequent encounter for fracture with routine healing
G	subsequent encounter for fracture with delayed healing
K	subsequent encounter for fracture with nonunion
S	sequela

● **S22.0**   Fracture of thoracic vertebra

  ● **S22.00**   Fracture of unspecified thoracic vertebra

    ● **S22.000**   Wedge compression fracture of unspecified thoracic vertebra

    ● **S22.001**   Stable burst fracture of unspecified thoracic vertebra

    ● **S22.002**   Unstable burst fracture of unspecified thoracic vertebra

    ● **S22.008**   Other fracture of unspecified thoracic vertebra

    ● **S22.009**   Unspecified fracture of unspecified thoracic vertebra

  ● **S22.01**   Fracture of first thoracic vertebra

    ● **S22.010**   Wedge compression fracture of first thoracic vertebra

    ● **S22.011**   Stable burst fracture of first thoracic vertebra

    ● **S22.012**   Unstable burst fracture of first thoracic vertebra

    ● **S22.018**   Other fracture of first thoracic vertebra

    ● **S22.019**   Unspecified fracture of first thoracic vertebra

  ● **S22.02**   Fracture of second thoracic vertebra

    ● **S22.020**   Wedge compression fracture of second thoracic vertebra

    ● **S22.021**   Stable burst fracture of second thoracic vertebra

    ● **S22.022**   Unstable burst fracture of second thoracic vertebra

    ● **S22.028**   Other fracture of second thoracic vertebra

    ● **S22.029**   Unspecified fracture of second thoracic vertebra

  ● **S22.03**   Fracture of third thoracic vertebra

    ● **S22.030**   Wedge compression fracture of third thoracic vertebra

    ● **S22.031**   Stable burst fracture of third thoracic vertebra

    ● **S22.032**   Unstable burst fracture of third thoracic vertebra

    ● **S22.038**   Other fracture of third thoracic vertebra

    ● **S22.039**   Unspecified fracture of third thoracic vertebra

● **S22.04**   Fracture of fourth thoracic vertebra
    ● **S22.040**   Wedge compression fracture of fourth thoracic vertebra
    ● **S22.041**   Stable burst fracture of fourth thoracic vertebra
    ● **S22.042**   Unstable burst fracture of fourth thoracic vertebra
    ● **S22.048**   Other fracture of fourth thoracic vertebra
    ● **S22.049**   Unspecified fracture of fourth thoracic vertebra

● **S22.05**   Fracture of T5-T6 vertebra
    ● **S22.050**   Wedge compression fracture of T5-T6 vertebra
    ● **S22.051**   Stable burst fracture of T5-T6 vertebra
    ● **S22.052**   Unstable burst fracture of T5-T6 vertebra
    ● **S22.058**   Other fracture of T5-T6 vertebra
    ● **S22.059**   Unspecified fracture of T5-T6 vertebra

● **S22.06**   Fracture of T7-T8 vertebra
    ● **S22.060**   Wedge compression fracture of T7-T8 vertebra
    ● **S22.061**   Stable burst fracture of T7-T8 vertebra
    ● **S22.062**   Unstable burst fracture of T7-T8 vertebra
    ● **S22.068**   Other fracture of T7-T8 thoracic vertebra
    ● **S22.069**   Unspecified fracture of T7-T8 vertebra

● **S22.07**   Fracture of T9-T10 vertebra
    ● **S22.070**   Wedge compression fracture of T9-T10 vertebra
    ● **S22.071**   Stable burst fracture of T9-T10 vertebra
    ● **S22.072**   Unstable burst fracture of T9-T10 vertebra
    ● **S22.078**   Other fracture of T9-T10 vertebra
    ● **S22.079**   Unspecified fracture of T9-T10 vertebra

● **S22.08**   Fracture of T11-T12 vertebra
    ● **S22.080**   Wedge compression fracture of T11-T12 vertebra
    ● **S22.081**   Stable burst fracture of T11-T12 vertebra
    ● **S22.082**   Unstable burst fracture of T11-T12 vertebra
    ● **S22.088**   Other fracture of T11-T12 vertebra
    ● **S22.089**   Unspecified fracture of T11-T12 vertebra

● **S22.2**   Fracture of sternum
    X ● **S22.20**   Unspecified fracture of sternum
    X ● **S22.21**   Fracture of manubrium
    X ● **S22.22**   Fracture of body of sternum
    X ● **S22.23**   Sternal manubrial dissociation
    X ● **S22.24**   Fracture of xiphoid process

● **S22.3** Fracture of one rib
    X ● **S22.31**   Fracture of one rib, right side
    X ● **S22.32**   Fracture of one rib, left side
    X ● **S22.39**   Fracture of one rib, unspecified side

● **S22.4**   Multiple fractures of ribs
    Fractures of two or more ribs
    Excludes1   flail chest (S22.5-)
    X ● **S22.41**   Multiple fractures of ribs, right side
    X ● **S22.42**   Multiple fractures of ribs, left side
    X ● **S22.43**   Multiple fractures of ribs, bilateral
    X ● **S22.49**   Multiple fractures of ribs, unspecified side

X ● **S22.5**   Flail chest
    Unstable chest due to sternum and/or rib fracture
X ● **S22.9**   Fracture of bony thorax, part unspecified

● **S23**   Dislocation and sprain of joints and ligaments of thorax
    Includes   avulsion of joint or ligament of thorax
         laceration of cartilage, joint or ligament of thorax
         sprain of cartilage, joint or ligament of thorax
         traumatic hemarthrosis of joint or ligament of thorax
         traumatic rupture of joint or ligament of thorax
         traumatic subluxation of joint or ligament of thorax
         traumatic tear of joint or ligament of thorax

Code also any associated open wound
    Excludes2   dislocation, sprain of sternoclavicular joint (S43.2, S43.6)
         strain of muscle or tendon of thorax (S29.01-)

The appropriate 7th character is to be added to each code from category S23

A	initial encounter
D	subsequent encounter
S	sequela

X ● **S23.0**   Traumatic rupture of thoracic intervertebral disc
    Excludes1   rupture or displacement (nontraumatic) of thoracic intervertebral disc NOS (M51.- with fifth character 4)

● **S23.1**   Subluxation and dislocation of thoracic vertebra
    Code also any associated
         open wound of thorax (S21.-)
         spinal cord injury (S24.0-, S24.1-)
    Excludes2   fracture of thoracic vertebrae (S22.0-)
    ● **S23.10**   Subluxation and dislocation of unspecified thoracic vertebra
       ● **S23.100**   Subluxation of unspecified thoracic vertebra
       ● **S23.101**   Dislocation of unspecified thoracic vertebra
    ● **S23.11**   Subluxation and dislocation of T1/T2 thoracic vertebra
       ● **S23.110**   Subluxation of T1/T2 thoracic vertebra
       ● **S23.111**   Dislocation of T1/T2 thoracic vertebra
    ● **S23.12**   Subluxation and dislocation of T2/T3-T3/T4 thoracic vertebra
       ● **S23.120**   Subluxation of T2/T3 thoracic vertebra
       ● **S23.121**   Dislocation of T2/T3 thoracic vertebra
       ● **S23.122**   Subluxation of T3/T4 thoracic vertebra
       ● **S23.123**   Dislocation of T3/T4 thoracic vertebra
    ● **S23.13**   Subluxation and dislocation of T4/T5-T5/T6 thoracic vertebra
       ● **S23.130**   Subluxation of T4/T5 thoracic vertebra
       ● **S23.131**   Dislocation of T4/T5 thoracic vertebra
       ● **S23.132**   Subluxation of T5/T6 thoracic vertebra
       ● **S23.133**   Dislocation of T5/T6 thoracic vertebra
    ● **S23.14**   Subluxation and dislocation of T6/T7-T7/T8 thoracic vertebra
       ● **S23.140**   Subluxation of T6/T7 thoracic vertebra
       ● **S23.141**   Dislocation of T6/T7 thoracic vertebra
       ● **S23.142**   Subluxation of T7/T8 thoracic vertebra
       ● **S23.143**   Dislocation of T7/T8 thoracic vertebra

CHAPTER 19 (S00-T88)

● **S23.15** Subluxation and dislocation of T8/T9-T9/T10 thoracic vertebra
   ● **S23.150** **Subluxation** of T8/T9 thoracic vertebra
   ● **S23.151** **Dislocation** of T8/T9 thoracic vertebra
   ● **S23.152** **Subluxation** of T9/T10 thoracic vertebra
   ● **S23.153** **Dislocation** of T9/T10 thoracic vertebra

● **S23.16** Subluxation and dislocation of T10/T11-T11/T12 thoracic vertebra
   ● **S23.160** **Subluxation** of T10/T11 thoracic vertebra
   ● **S23.161** **Dislocation** of T10/T11 thoracic vertebra
   ● **S23.162** **Subluxation** of T11/T12 thoracic vertebra
   ● **S23.163** **Dislocation** of T11/T12 thoracic vertebra

● **S23.17** Subluxation and dislocation of T12/L1 thoracic vertebra
   ● **S23.170** **Subluxation** of T12/L1 thoracic vertebra
   ● **S23.171** **Dislocation** of T12/L1 thoracic vertebra

● **S23.2** Dislocation of other and unspecified parts of thorax
  X● **S23.20** Dislocation of unspecified part of thorax
  X● **S23.29** Dislocation of other parts of thorax
X● **S23.3** Sprain of ligaments of thoracic spine
● **S23.4** Sprain of ribs and sternum
  X● **S23.41** Sprain of ribs
  ● **S23.42** Sprain of sternum
   ● **S23.420** Sprain of sternoclavicular (joint) (ligament)
   ● **S23.421** Sprain of chondrosternal joint
   ● **S23.428** Other sprain of sternum
   ● **S23.429** **Unspecified** sprain of sternum
X● **S23.8** Sprain of other specified parts of thorax
X● **S23.9** Sprain of unspecified parts of thorax

● **S24** Injury of nerves and spinal cord at thorax level
   Note: Code to highest level of thoracic spinal cord injury.
     Injuries to the spinal cord (S24.0 and S24.1) refer to the cord level and not bone level injury, and can affect nerve roots at and below the level given.
     Code also any associated:
       fracture of thoracic vertebra (S22.0-)
       open wound of thorax (S21.-)
       transient paralysis (R29.5)
     Excludes2 injury of brachial plexus (S14.3)
     The appropriate 7th character is to be added to each code from category S24

> A   initial encounter
> D   subsequent encounter
> S   sequela

X● **S24.0** Concussion and edema of thoracic spinal cord
● **S24.1** Other and unspecified injuries of thoracic spinal cord
  ● **S24.10** Unspecified injury of thoracic spinal cord
   ● **S24.101** Unspecified injury at T1 level of thoracic spinal cord
   ● **S24.102** Unspecified injury at T2-T6 level of thoracic spinal cord
   ● **S24.103** Unspecified injury at T7-T10 level of thoracic spinal cord
   ● **S24.104** Unspecified injury at T11-T12 level of thoracic spinal cord
   ● **S24.109** Unspecified injury at unspecified level of thoracic spinal cord
     Injury of thoracic spinal cord NOS

● **S24.11** Complete lesion of thoracic spinal cord
  ● **S24.111** Complete lesion at T1 level of thoracic spinal cord
  ● **S24.112** Complete lesion at T2-T6 level of thoracic spinal cord
  ● **S24.113** Complete lesion at T7-T10 level of thoracic spinal cord
  ● **S24.114** Complete lesion at T11-T12 level of thoracic spinal cord
  ● **S24.119** Complete lesion at unspecified level of thoracic spinal cord

● **S24.13** Anterior cord syndrome of thoracic spinal cord
  ● **S24.131** Anterior cord syndrome at T1 level of thoracic spinal cord
  ● **S24.132** Anterior cord syndrome at T2-T6 level of thoracic spinal cord
  ● **S24.133** Anterior cord syndrome at T7-T10 level of thoracic spinal cord
  ● **S24.134** Anterior cord syndrome at T11-T12 level of thoracic spinal cord
  ● **S24.139** Anterior cord syndrome at unspecified level of thoracic spinal cord

● **S24.14** Brown-Séquard syndrome of thoracic spinal cord
  ● **S24.141** Brown-Séquard syndrome at T1 level of thoracic spinal cord
  ● **S24.142** Brown-Séquard syndrome at T2-T6 level of thoracic spinal cord
  ● **S24.143** Brown-Séquard syndrome at T7-T10 level of thoracic spinal cord
  ● **S24.144** Brown-Séquard syndrome at T11-T12 level of thoracic spinal cord
  ● **S24.149** Brown-Séquard syndrome at unspecified level of thoracic spinal cord

● **S24.15** Other incomplete lesions of thoracic spinal cord
   Incomplete lesion of thoracic spinal cord NOS
   Posterior cord syndrome of thoracic spinal cord
  ● **S24.151** Other incomplete lesion at T1 level of thoracic spinal cord
  ● **S24.152** Other incomplete lesion at T2-T6 level of thoracic spinal cord
  ● **S24.153** Other incomplete lesion at T7-T10 level of thoracic spinal cord
  ● **S24.154** Other incomplete lesion at T11-T12 level of thoracic spinal cord
  ● **S24.159** Other incomplete lesion at unspecified level of thoracic spinal cord

X● **S24.2** Injury of nerve root of thoracic spine
X● **S24.3** Injury of peripheral nerves of thorax
X● **S24.4** Injury of thoracic sympathetic nervous system
   Injury of cardiac plexus
   Injury of esophageal plexus
   Injury of pulmonary plexus
   Injury of stellate ganglion
   Injury of thoracic sympathetic ganglion
X● **S24.8** Injury of other specified nerves of thorax
X● **S24.9** Injury of unspecified nerve of thorax

▶ New   ⇥ Revised   ~~deleted~~ Deleted   **OGCR** Official Guidelines   X Assign placeholder X   ● Use Additional Character(s)
Excludes 1   Excludes 2   Includes   Use additional   Code first   Code also   Key words

● **S25   Injury of blood vessels of thorax**

The appropriate 7th character is to be added to each code from category S25

> A   initial encounter
> D   subsequent encounter
> S   sequela

Code also any associated open wound (S21.-)

● **S25.0   Injury of thoracic aorta**
     Injury of aorta NOS

   X● **S25.00   Unspecified injury of thoracic aorta**

   X● **S25.01   Minor laceration of thoracic aorta**
       Incomplete transection of thoracic aorta
       Laceration of thoracic aorta NOS
       Superficial laceration of thoracic aorta

   X● **S25.02   Major laceration of thoracic aorta**
       Complete transection of thoracic aorta
       Traumatic rupture of thoracic aorta

   X● **S25.09   Other specified injury of thoracic aorta**

● **S25.1   Injury of innominate or subclavian artery**

   ● **S25.10   Unspecified injury of innominate or subclavian artery**

     ● **S25.101   Unspecified injury of right innominate or subclavian artery**

     ● **S25.102   Unspecified injury of left innominate or subclavian artery**

     ● **S25.109   Unspecified injury of unspecified innominate or subclavian artery**

   ● **S25.11   Minor laceration of innominate or subclavian artery**
       Incomplete transection of innominate or subclavian artery
       Laceration of innominate or subclavian artery NOS
       Superficial laceration of innominate or subclavian artery

     ● **S25.111   Minor laceration of right innominate or subclavian artery**

     ● **S25.112   Minor laceration of left innominate or subclavian artery**

     ● **S25.119   Minor laceration of unspecified innominate or subclavian artery**

   ● **S25.12   Major laceration of innominate or subclavian artery**
       Complete transection of innominate or subclavian artery
       Traumatic rupture of innominate or subclavian artery

     ● **S25.121   Major laceration of right innominate or subclavian artery**

     ● **S25.122   Major laceration of left innominate or subclavian artery**

     ● **S25.129   Major laceration of unspecified innominate or subclavian artery**

   ● **S25.19   Other specified injury of innominate or subclavian artery**

     ● **S25.191   Other specified injury of right innominate or subclavian artery**

     ● **S25.192   Other specified injury of left innominate or subclavian artery**

     ● **S25.199   Other specified injury of unspecified innominate or subclavian artery**

● **S25.2   Injury of superior vena cava**
     Injury of vena cava NOS

   X● **S25.20   Unspecified injury of superior vena cava**

   X● **S25.21   Minor laceration of superior vena cava**
       Incomplete transection of superior vena cava
       Laceration of superior vena cava NOS
       Superficial laceration of superior vena cava

   X● **S25.22   Major laceration of superior vena cava**
       Complete transection of superior vena cava
       Traumatic rupture of superior vena cava

   X● **S25.29   Other specified injury of superior vena cava**

● **S25.3   Injury of innominate or subclavian vein**

   ● **S25.30   Unspecified injury of innominate or subclavian vein**

     ● **S25.301   Unspecified injury of right innominate or subclavian vein**

     ● **S25.302   Unspecified injury of left innominate or subclavian vein**

     ● **S25.309   Unspecified injury of unspecified innominate or subclavian vein**

   ● **S25.31   Minor laceration of innominate or subclavian vein**
       Incomplete transection of innominate or subclavian vein
       Laceration of innominate or subclavian vein NOS
       Superficial laceration of innominate or subclavian vein

     ● **S25.311   Minor laceration of right innominate or subclavian vein**

     ● **S25.312   Minor laceration of left innominate or subclavian vein**

     ● **S25.319   Minor laceration of unspecified innominate or subclavian vein**

   ● **S25.32   Major laceration of innominate or subclavian vein**
       Complete transection of innominate or subclavian vein
       Traumatic rupture of innominate or subclavian vein

     ● **S25.321   Major laceration of right innominate or subclavian vein**

     ● **S25.322   Major laceration of left innominate or subclavian vein**

     ● **S25.329   Major laceration of unspecified innominate or subclavian vein**

   ● **S25.39   Other specified injury of innominate or subclavian vein**

     ● **S25.391   Other specified injury of right innominate or subclavian vein**

     ● **S25.392   Other specified injury of left innominate or subclavian vein**

     ● **S25.399   Other specified injury of unspecified innominate or subclavian vein**

● **S25.4   Injury of pulmonary blood vessels**

   ● **S25.40   Unspecified injury of pulmonary blood vessels**

     ● **S25.401   Unspecified injury of right pulmonary blood vessels**

     ● **S25.402   Unspecified injury of left pulmonary blood vessels**

     ● **S25.409   Unspecified injury of unspecified pulmonary blood vessels**

▶ New   ⇒ Revised   ~~deleted~~ Deleted   **OGCR** Official Guidelines   X Assign placeholder X   ● Use Additional Character(s)

Excludes 1   Excludes 2   Includes   Use additional   Code first   Code also   Key words

● **S25.41**   Minor laceration of pulmonary blood vessels
     Incomplete transection of pulmonary blood vessels
     Laceration of pulmonary blood vessels NOS
     Superficial laceration of pulmonary blood vessels

     ● **S25.411**   Minor laceration of right pulmonary blood vessels

     ● **S25.412**   Minor laceration of left pulmonary blood vessels

     ● **S25.419**   Minor laceration of unspecified pulmonary blood vessels

● **S25.42**   Major laceration of pulmonary blood vessels
     Complete transection of pulmonary blood vessels
     Traumatic rupture of pulmonary blood vessels

     ● **S25.421**   Major laceration of right pulmonary blood vessels

     ● **S25.422**   Major laceration of left pulmonary blood vessels

     ● **S25.429**   Major laceration of unspecified pulmonary blood vessels

● **S25.49**   Other specified injury of pulmonary blood vessels

     ● **S25.491**   Other specified injury of right pulmonary blood vessels

     ● **S25.492**   Other specified injury of left pulmonary blood vessels

     ● **S25.499**   Other specified injury of unspecified pulmonary blood vessels

● **S25.5**   Injury of intercostal blood vessels

     ● **S25.50**   Unspecified injury of intercostal blood vessels

       ● **S25.501**   Unspecified injury of intercostal blood vessels, right side

       ● **S25.502**   Unspecified injury of intercostal blood vessels, left side

       ● **S25.509**   Unspecified injury of intercostal blood vessels, unspecified side

     ● **S25.51**   Laceration of intercostal blood vessels

       ● **S25.511**   Laceration of intercostal blood vessels, right side

       ● **S25.512**   Laceration of intercostal blood vessels, left side

       ● **S25.519**   Laceration of intercostal blood vessels, unspecified side

     ● **S25.59**   Other specified injury of intercostal blood vessels

       ● **S25.591**   Other specified injury of intercostal blood vessels, right side

       ● **S25.592**   Other specified injury of intercostal blood vessels, left side

       ● **S25.599**   Other specified injury of intercostal blood vessels, unspecified side

● **S25.8**   Injury of other blood vessels of thorax
     Injury of azygos vein
     Injury of mammary artery or vein

     ● **S25.80**   Unspecified injury of other blood vessels of thorax

       ● **S25.801**   Unspecified injury of other blood vessels of thorax, right side

       ● **S25.802**   Unspecified injury of other blood vessels of thorax, left side

       ● **S25.809**   Unspecified injury of other blood vessels of thorax, unspecified side

     ● **S25.81**   Laceration of other blood vessels of thorax

       ● **S25.811**   Laceration of other blood vessels of thorax, right side

       ● **S25.812**   Laceration of other blood vessels of thorax, left side

       ● **S25.819**   Laceration of other blood vessels of thorax, unspecified side

● **S25.89**   Other specified injury of other blood vessels of thorax

     ● **S25.891**   Other specified injury of other blood vessels of thorax, right side

     ● **S25.892**   Other specified injury of other blood vessels of thorax, left side

     ● **S25.899**   Other specified injury of other blood vessels of thorax, unspecified side

● **S25.9**   Injury of unspecified blood vessel of thorax

     X ● **S25.90**   Unspecified injury of unspecified blood vessel of thorax

     X ● **S25.91**   Laceration of unspecified blood vessel of thorax

     X ● **S25.99**   Other specified injury of unspecified blood vessel of thorax

● **S26**   **Injury of heart**
     The appropriate 7th character is to be added to each code from category S26

     | A | initial encounter |
     | D | subsequent encounter |
     | S | sequela |

     Code also any associated:
     open wound of thorax (S21.-)
     traumatic hemopneumothorax (S27.2)
     traumatic hemothorax (S27.1)
     traumatic pneumothorax (S27.0)

● **S26.0**   Injury of heart with hemopericardium
     Hemopericardium: effusion of blood within pericardium

     X ● **S26.00**   Unspecified injury of heart with hemopericardium

     X ● **S26.01**   Contusion of heart with hemopericardium

     ● **S26.02**   Laceration of heart with hemopericardium

       ● **S26.020**   Mild laceration of heart with hemopericardium
         Laceration of heart without penetration of heart chamber

       ● **S26.021**   Moderate laceration of heart with hemopericardium
         Laceration of heart with penetration of heart chamber

       ● **S26.022**   Major laceration of heart with hemopericardium
         Laceration of heart with penetration of multiple heart chambers

     X ● **S26.09**   Other injury of heart with hemopericardium

● **S26.1**   Injury of heart without hemopericardium
     Hemopericardium: effusion of blood within pericardium

     X ● **S26.10**   Unspecified injury of heart without hemopericardium

     X ● **S26.11**   Contusion of heart without hemopericardium

     X ● **S26.12**   Laceration of heart without hemopericardium

     X ● **S26.19**   Other injury of heart without hemopericardium

Item 19-2 Pneumothorax is a collection of gas (positive air pressure) in the pleural space resulting in the lung collapsing. A **tension pneumothorax** is life-threatening and is a result of air in the pleural space causing a displacement in the mediastinal structures and cardiopulmonary function compromise. A **traumatic pneumothorax** results from blunt or penetrating injury that disrupts the parietal/visceral pleura. **Hemothorax** is blood or bloody fluid in the pleural cavity as a result of traumatic blood vessel rupture or inflammation of the lungs from pneumonia.

▶ New   ⇒ Revised   ~~deleted~~ Deleted   **OGCR** Official Guidelines   X Assign placeholder X   ● Use Additional Character(s)

| Excludes 1 | Excludes 2 | Includes | Use additional | Code first | Code also | Key words |

- ● S26.9   **Injury of heart, unspecified with or without hemopericardium**
  - *Hemopericardium: effusion of blood within pericardium*
  - X ● S26.90   **Unspecified** injury of heart, unspecified with or without hemopericardium
  - X ● S26.91   **Contusion** of heart, unspecified with or without hemopericardium
  - X ● S26.92   **Laceration** of heart, unspecified with or without hemopericardium
    - Laceration of heart NOS
  - X ● S26.99   **Other** injury of heart, unspecified with or without hemopericardium

- ● S27   **Injury of other and unspecified intrathoracic organs**
  - Code also any associated open wound of thorax (S21.-)
  - **Excludes2**   injury of cervical esophagus (S10-S19)
    - injury of trachea (cervical) (S10-S19)
  - The appropriate 7th character is to be added to each code from category S27
A	initial encounter
D	subsequent encounter
S	sequela
  - X ● S27.0   **Traumatic pneumothorax**
    - **Excludes1**   spontaneous pneumothorax (J93.-)
  - X ● S27.1   **Traumatic hemothorax**
  - X ● S27.2   **Traumatic hemopneumothorax**
  - ● S27.3   **Other and unspecified injuries of lung**
    - ● S27.30   **Unspecified** injury of lung
      - ● S27.301   Unspecified injury of lung, **unilateral**
      - ● S27.302   Unspecified injury of lung, **bilateral**
      - ● S27.309   Unspecified injury of lung, **unspecified**
    - ● S27.31   **Primary blast** injury of lung
      - Blast injury of lung NOS
      - ● S27.311   Primary blast injury of lung, **unilateral**
      - ● S27.312   Primary blast injury of lung, **bilateral**
      - ● S27.319   Primary blast injury of lung, **unspecified**
    - ● S27.32   **Contusion** of lung
      - ● S27.321   Contusion of lung, **unilateral**
      - ● S27.322   Contusion of lung, **bilateral**
      - ● S27.329   Contusion of lung, **unspecified**
    - ● S27.33   **Laceration** of lung
      - ● S27.331   Laceration of lung, **unilateral**
      - ● S27.332   Laceration of lung, **bilateral**
      - ● S27.339   Laceration of lung, **unspecified**
    - ● S27.39   **Other** injuries of lung
      - Secondary blast injury of lung
      - ● S27.391   Other injuries of lung, **unilateral**
      - ● S27.392   Other injuries of lung, **bilateral**
      - ● S27.399   Other injuries of lung, **unspecified**
  - ● S27.4   **Injury of bronchus**
    - ● S27.40   **Unspecified** injury of bronchus
      - ● S27.401   Unspecified injury of bronchus, **unilateral**
      - ● S27.402   Unspecified injury of bronchus, **bilateral**
      - ● S27.409   Unspecified injury of bronchus, **unspecified**

- ● S27.41   **Primary blast** injury of bronchus
  - Blast injury of bronchus NOS
  - ● S27.411   Primary blast injury of bronchus, **unilateral**
  - ● S27.412   Primary blast injury of bronchus, **bilateral**
  - ● S27.419   Primary blast injury of bronchus, **unspecified**
- ● S27.42   **Contusion** of bronchus
  - ● S27.421   Contusion of bronchus, **unilateral**
  - ● S27.422   Contusion of bronchus, **bilateral**
  - ● S27.429   Contusion of bronchus, **unspecified**
- ● S27.43   **Laceration** of bronchus
  - ● S27.431   Laceration of bronchus, **unilateral**
  - ● S27.432   Laceration of bronchus, **bilateral**
  - ● S27.439   Laceration of bronchus, **unspecified**
- ● S27.49   **Other** injury of bronchus
  - Secondary blast injury of bronchus
  - ● S27.491   Other injury of bronchus, **unilateral**
  - ● S27.492   Other injury of bronchus, **bilateral**
  - ● S27.499   Other injury of bronchus, **unspecified**
- ● S27.5   **Injury of thoracic trachea**
  - X ● S27.50   **Unspecified** injury of thoracic trachea
  - X ● S27.51   **Primary blast** injury of thoracic trachea
    - Blast injury of thoracic trachea NOS
  - X ● S27.52   **Contusion** of thoracic trachea
  - X ● S27.53   **Laceration** of thoracic trachea
  - X ● S27.59   **Other** injury of thoracic trachea
    - Secondary blast injury of thoracic trachea
- ● S27.6   **Injury of pleura**
  - X ● S27.60   **Unspecified** injury of pleura
  - X ● S27.63   **Laceration** of pleura
  - X ● S27.69   **Other** injury of pleura
- ● S27.8   **Injury of other specified intrathoracic organs**
  - ● S27.80   **Injury of diaphragm**
    - ● S27.802   **Contusion** of diaphragm
    - ● S27.803   **Laceration** of diaphragm
    - ● S27.808   **Other** injury of diaphragm
    - ● S27.809   **Unspecified** injury of diaphragm
  - ● S27.81   **Injury of esophagus (thoracic part)**
    - ● S27.812   **Contusion** of esophagus (thoracic part)
    - ● S27.813   **Laceration** of esophagus (thoracic part)
    - ● S27.818   **Other** injury of esophagus (thoracic part)
    - ● S27.819   **Unspecified** injury of esophagus (thoracic part)
  - ● S27.89   **Injury of other specified intrathoracic organs**
    - Injury of lymphatic thoracic duct
    - Injury of thymus gland
    - ● S27.892   **Contusion** of other specified intrathoracic organs
    - ● S27.893   **Laceration** of other specified intrathoracic organs
    - ● S27.898   **Other** injury of other specified intrathoracic organs
    - ● S27.899   **Unspecified** injury of other specified intrathoracic organs
  - X ● S27.9   **Injury of unspecified intrathoracic organ**

CHAPTER 19 (S00-T88)

● **S28** **Crushing injury of thorax, and traumatic amputation of part of thorax**

The appropriate 7th character is to be added to each code from category S28

> A   initial encounter
> D   subsequent encounter
> S   sequela

X ● **S28.0** **Crushed chest**
Use additional code for all associated injuries
> Excludes1   flail chest (S22.5)

X ● **S28.1** **Traumatic amputation (partial) of part of thorax, except breast**

● **S28.2** **Traumatic amputation of breast**

● **S28.21** **Complete traumatic amputation of breast**
Traumatic amputation of breast NOS

● **S28.211** **Complete traumatic amputation of right breast**

● **S28.212** **Complete traumatic amputation of left breast**

● **S28.219** **Complete traumatic amputation of unspecified breast**

● **S28.22** **Partial traumatic amputation of breast**

● **S28.221** **Partial traumatic amputation of right breast**

● **S28.222** **Partial traumatic amputation of left breast**

● **S28.229** **Partial traumatic amputation of unspecified breast**

● **S29** **Other and unspecified injuries of thorax**
Code also any associated open wound (S21.-)

The appropriate 7th character is to be added to each code from category S29

> A   initial encounter
> D   subsequent encounter
> S   sequela

● **S29.0** **Injury of muscle and tendon at thorax level**

● **S29.00** **Unspecified injury of muscle and tendon of thorax**

● **S29.001** **Unspecified injury of muscle and tendon of front wall of thorax**

● **S29.002** **Unspecified injury of muscle and tendon of back wall of thorax**

● **S29.009** **Unspecified injury of muscle and tendon of unspecified wall of thorax**

● **S29.01** **Strain of muscle and tendon of thorax**

● **S29.011** **Strain of muscle and tendon of front wall of thorax**

● **S29.012** **Strain of muscle and tendon of back wall of thorax**

● **S29.019** **Strain of muscle and tendon of unspecified wall of thorax**

● **S29.02** **Laceration of muscle and tendon of thorax**

● **S29.021** **Laceration of muscle and tendon of front wall of thorax**

● **S29.022** **Laceration of muscle and tendon of back wall of thorax**

● **S29.029** **Laceration of muscle and tendon of unspecified wall of thorax**

● **S29.09** **Other injury of muscle and tendon of thorax**

● **S29.091** **Other injury of muscle and tendon of front wall of thorax**

● **S29.092** **Other injury of muscle and tendon of back wall of thorax**

● **S29.099** **Other injury of muscle and tendon of unspecified wall of thorax**

X ● **S29.8** **Other specified injuries of thorax**

X ● **S29.9** **Unspecified injury of thorax**

INJURIES TO THE ABDOMEN, LOWER BACK, LUMBAR SPINE PELVIS AND EXTERNAL GENITALS (S30-S39)

> Includes   injuries to the abdominal wall
> injuries to the anus
> injuries to the buttock
> injuries to the external genitalia
> injuries to the flank
> injuries to the groin

> Excludes2   burns and corrosions (T20-T32)
> effects of foreign body in anus and rectum (T18.5)
> effects of foreign body in genitourinary tract (T19.-)
> effects of foreign body in stomach, small intestine and colon (T18.2-T18.4)
> frostbite (T33-T34)
> insect bite or sting, venomous (T63.4)

● **S30** **Superficial injury of abdomen, lower back, pelvis and external genitals**

> Excludes2   superficial injury of hip (S70.-)

The appropriate 7th character is to be added to each code from category S30

> A   initial encounter
> D   subsequent encounter
> S   sequela

X ● **S30.0** **Contusion of lower back and pelvis**
Contusion of buttock

X ● **S30.1** **Contusion of abdominal wall**
Contusion of flank
Contusion of groin

● **S30.2** **Contusion of external genital organs**

● **S30.20** **Contusion of unspecified external genital organ**

● **S30.201** **Contusion of unspecified external genital organ, male**

● **S30.202** **Contusion of unspecified external genital organ, female**

X ● **S30.21** **Contusion of penis**

X ● **S30.22** **Contusion of scrotum and testes**

X ● **S30.23** **Contusion of vagina and vulva**

X ● **S30.3** **Contusion of anus**

● **S30.8** **Other superficial injuries of abdomen, lower back, pelvis and external genitals**

● **S30.81** **Abrasion of abdomen, lower back, pelvis and external genitals**

● **S30.810** **Abrasion of lower back and pelvis**

● **S30.811** **Abrasion of abdominal wall**

● **S30.812** **Abrasion of penis**

● **S30.813** **Abrasion of scrotum and testes**

● **S30.814** **Abrasion of vagina and vulva**

● **S30.815** **Abrasion of unspecified external genital organs, male**

● **S30.816** **Abrasion of unspecified external genital organs, female**

● **S30.817** **Abrasion of anus**

● **S30.82** **Blister (nonthermal) of abdomen, lower back, pelvis and external genitals**

● **S30.820** **Blister (nonthermal) of lower back and pelvis**

● **S30.821** **Blister (nonthermal) of abdominal wall**

● **S30.822** **Blister (nonthermal) of penis**

● **S30.823** **Blister (nonthermal) of scrotum and testes**

● **S30.824** **Blister (nonthermal) of vagina and vulva**

● **S30.825** **Blister (nonthermal) of unspecified external genital organs, male**

● **S30.826** **Blister (nonthermal) of unspecified external genital organs, female**

● **S30.827** **Blister (nonthermal) of anus**

▶ New   ⟹ Revised   deleted Deleted   **OGCR** Official Guidelines   X Assign placeholder X   ● Use Additional Character(s)

Excludes 1   Excludes 2   Includes   Use additional   Code first   Code also   Key words

● S30.84 **External constriction** of abdomen, lower back, pelvis and external genitals

 ● S30.840 External constriction of **lower back and pelvis**

 ● S30.841 External constriction of **abdominal wall**

 ● S30.842 External constriction of **penis**
       Hair tourniquet syndrome of penis
       Use additional cause code to identify the constricting item (W49.0-)

 ● S30.843 External constriction of **scrotum and testes**

 ● S30.844 External constriction of **vagina and vulva**

 ● S30.845 External constriction of **unspecified** external genital organs, **male**

 ● S30.846 External constriction of **unspecified** external genital organs, **female**

● S30.85 **Superficial foreign body** of abdomen, lower back, pelvis and external genitals
   Splinter in the abdomen, lower back, pelvis and external genitals

 ● S30.850 Superficial foreign body of **lower back and pelvis**

 ● S30.851 Superficial foreign body of **abdominal wall**

 ● S30.852 Superficial foreign body of **penis**

 ● S30.853 Superficial foreign body of **scrotum and testes**

 ● S30.854 Superficial foreign body of **vagina and vulva**

 ● S30.855 Superficial foreign body of **unspecified** external genital organs, **male**

 ● S30.856 Superficial foreign body of **unspecified** external genital organs, **female**

 ● S30.857 Superficial foreign body of **anus**

● S30.86 **Insect bite** (nonvenomous) of abdomen, lower back, pelvis and external genitals

 ● S30.860 Insect bite (nonvenomous) of **lower back and pelvis**

 ● S30.861 Insect bite (nonvenomous) of **abdominal wall**

 ● S30.862 Insect bite (nonvenomous) of **penis**

 ● S30.863 Insect bite (nonvenomous) of **scrotum and testes**

 ● S30.864 Insect bite (nonvenomous) of **vagina and vulva**

 ● S30.865 Insect bite (nonvenomous) of **unspecified** external genital organs, **male**

 ● S30.866 Insect bite (nonvenomous) of **unspecified** external genital organs, **female**

 ● S30.867 **Insect** bite (nonvenomous) of **anus**

● S30.87 **Other superficial bite** of abdomen, lower back, pelvis and external genitals

  | Excludes1 | open bite of abdomen, lower back, pelvis and external genitals (S31.05, S31.15, S31.25, S31.35, S31.45, S31.55) |

 ● S30.870 Other superficial bite of **lower back and pelvis**

 ● S30.871 Other superficial bite of **abdominal wall**

● S30.872 Other superficial bite of **penis**

● S30.873 Other superficial bite of **scrotum and testes**

● S30.874 Other superficial bite of **vagina and vulva**

● S30.875 Other superficial bite of **unspecified** external genital organs, **male**

● S30.876 Other superficial bite of **unspecified** external genital organs, **female**

● S30.877 Other superficial bite of **anus**

● S30.9 **Unspecified** superficial injury of abdomen, lower back, pelvis and external genitals

 X ● S30.91 Unspecified superficial injury of **lower back and pelvis**

 X ● S30.92 Unspecified superficial injury of **abdominal wall**

 X ● S30.93 Unspecified superficial injury of **penis**

 X ● S30.94 Unspecified superficial injury of **scrotum and testes**

 X ● S30.95 Unspecified superficial injury of **vagina and vulva**

 X ● S30.96 Unspecified superficial injury of **unspecified** external genital organs, **male**

 X ● S30.97 Unspecified superficial injury of **unspecified** external genital organs, **female**

 X ● S30.98 Unspecified superficial injury of **anus**

● S31 Open wound of abdomen, lower back, pelvis and external genitals

 Code also any associated:
  spinal cord injury (S24.0, S24.1-, S34.0-, S34.1-)
  wound infection

  | Excludes1 | traumatic amputation of part of abdomen, lower back and pelvis (S38.2-, S38.3) |

  | Excludes2 | open wound of hip (S71.00-S71.02) |
  | | open fracture of pelvis (S32.1--S32.9 with 7th character B) |

 The appropriate 7th character is to be added to each code from category S31

  A initial encounter
  D subsequent encounter
  S sequela

● S31.0 Open wound of **lower back and pelvis**

 ● S31.00 **Unspecified** open wound of lower back and pelvis

  ● S31.000 Unspecified open wound of lower back and pelvis **without penetration** into retroperitoneum
      Unspecified open wound of lower back and pelvis NOS

  ● S31.001 Unspecified open wound of lower back and pelvis **with penetration** into retroperitoneum

 ● S31.01 **Laceration without foreign body** of lower back and pelvis

  ● S31.010 Laceration without foreign body of lower back and pelvis **without penetration** into retroperitoneum
      Laceration without foreign body of lower back and pelvis NOS

  ● S31.011 Laceration without foreign body of lower back and pelvis **with penetration** into retroperitoneum

▶ New ⇒ Revised ~~deleted~~ Deleted **OGCR** Official Guidelines X Assign placeholder X ● Use Additional Character(s)

| Excludes 1 | Excludes 2 | Includes | Use additional | Code first | Code also | Key words |

1201

- **S31.02** Laceration with foreign body of lower back and pelvis
  - **S31.020** Laceration with foreign body of lower back and pelvis without penetration into retroperitoneum
    - Laceration with foreign body of lower back and pelvis NOS
  - **S31.021** Laceration with foreign body of lower back and pelvis with penetration into retroperitoneum
- **S31.03** Puncture wound without foreign body of lower back and pelvis
  - **S31.030** Puncture wound without foreign body of lower back and pelvis without penetration into retroperitoneum
    - Puncture wound without foreign body of lower back and pelvis NOS
  - **S31.031** Puncture wound without foreign body of lower back and pelvis with penetration into retroperitoneum
- **S31.04** Puncture wound with foreign body of lower back and pelvis
  - **S31.040** Puncture wound with foreign body of lower back and pelvis without penetration into retroperitoneum
    - Puncture wound with foreign body of lower back and pelvis NOS
  - **S31.041** Puncture wound with foreign body of lower back and pelvis with penetration into retroperitoneum
- **S31.05** Open bite of lower back and pelvis
  - Bite of lower back and pelvis NOS
  - **Excludes1** superficial bite of lower back and pelvis (S30.860, S30.870)
  - **S31.050** Open bite of lower back and pelvis without penetration into retroperitoneum
    - Open bite of lower back and pelvis NOS
  - **S31.051** Open bite of lower back and pelvis with penetration into retroperitoneum
- **S31.1** Open wound of abdominal wall without penetration into peritoneal cavity
  - Open wound of abdominal wall NOS
  - **Excludes2** open wound of abdominal wall with penetration into peritoneal cavity (S31.6-)
  - **S31.10** Unspecified open wound of abdominal wall without penetration into peritoneal cavity
    - **S31.100** Unspecified open wound of abdominal wall, right upper quadrant without penetration into peritoneal cavity
    - **S31.101** Unspecified open wound of abdominal wall, left upper quadrant without penetration into peritoneal cavity
    - **S31.102** Unspecified open wound of abdominal wall, epigastric region without penetration into peritoneal cavity
    - **S31.103** Unspecified open wound of abdominal wall, right lower quadrant without penetration into peritoneal cavity
    - **S31.104** Unspecified open wound of abdominal wall, left lower quadrant without penetration into peritoneal cavity

- **S31.105** Unspecified open wound of abdominal wall, periumbilic region without penetration into peritoneal cavity
- **S31.109** Unspecified open wound of abdominal wall, unspecified quadrant without penetration into peritoneal cavity
  - Unspecified open wound of abdominal wall NOS
- **S31.11** Laceration without foreign body of abdominal wall without penetration into peritoneal cavity
  - **S31.110** Laceration without foreign body of abdominal wall, right upper quadrant without penetration into peritoneal cavity
  - **S31.111** Laceration without foreign body of abdominal wall, left upper quadrant without penetration into peritoneal cavity
  - **S31.112** Laceration without foreign body of abdominal wall, epigastric region without penetration into peritoneal cavity
  - **S31.113** Laceration without foreign body of abdominal wall, right lower quadrant without penetration into peritoneal cavity
  - **S31.114** Laceration without foreign body of abdominal wall, left lower quadrant without penetration into peritoneal cavity
  - **S31.115** Laceration without foreign body of abdominal wall, periumbilic region without penetration into peritoneal cavity
  - **S31.119** Laceration without foreign body of abdominal wall, unspecified quadrant without penetration into peritoneal cavity
- **S31.12** Laceration with foreign body of abdominal wall without penetration into peritoneal cavity
  - **S31.120** Laceration of abdominal wall with foreign body, right upper quadrant without penetration into peritoneal cavity
  - **S31.121** Laceration of abdominal wall with foreign body, left upper quadrant without penetration into peritoneal cavity
  - **S31.122** Laceration of abdominal wall with foreign body, epigastric region without penetration into peritoneal cavity
  - **S31.123** Laceration of abdominal wall with foreign body, right lower quadrant without penetration into peritoneal cavity
  - **S31.124** Laceration of abdominal wall with foreign body, left lower quadrant without penetration into peritoneal cavity
  - **S31.125** Laceration of abdominal wall with foreign body, periumbilic region without penetration into peritoneal cavity
  - **S31.129** Laceration of abdominal wall with foreign body, unspecified quadrant without penetration into peritoneal cavity

● **S31.13**   Puncture wound of abdominal wall without foreign body without penetration into peritoneal cavity

    ● **S31.130**   Puncture wound of abdominal wall without foreign body, right upper quadrant without penetration into peritoneal cavity

    ● **S31.131**   Puncture wound of abdominal wall without foreign body, left upper quadrant without penetration into peritoneal cavity

    ● **S31.132**   Puncture wound of abdominal wall without foreign body, epigastric region without penetration into peritoneal cavity

    ● **S31.133**   Puncture wound of abdominal wall without foreign body, right lower quadrant without penetration into peritoneal cavity

    ● **S31.134**   Puncture wound of abdominal wall without foreign body, left lower quadrant without penetration into peritoneal cavity

    ● **S31.135**   Puncture wound of abdominal wall without foreign body, periumbilic region without penetration into peritoneal cavity

    ● **S31.139**   Puncture wound of abdominal wall without foreign body, unspecified quadrant without penetration into peritoneal cavity

● **S31.14**   Puncture wound of abdominal wall with foreign body without penetration into peritoneal cavity

    ● **S31.140**   Puncture wound of abdominal wall with foreign body, right upper quadrant without penetration into peritoneal cavity

    ● **S31.141**   Puncture wound of abdominal wall with foreign body, left upper quadrant without penetration into peritoneal cavity

    ● **S31.142**   Puncture wound of abdominal wall with foreign body, epigastric region without penetration into peritoneal cavity

    ● **S31.143**   Puncture wound of abdominal wall with foreign body, right lower quadrant without penetration into peritoneal cavity

    ● **S31.144**   Puncture wound of abdominal wall with foreign body, left lower quadrant without penetration into peritoneal cavity

    ● **S31.145**   Puncture wound of abdominal wall with foreign body, periumbilic region without penetration into peritoneal cavity

    ● **S31.149**   Puncture wound of abdominal wall with foreign body, unspecified quadrant without penetration into peritoneal cavity

● **S31.15**   Open bite of abdominal wall without penetration into peritoneal cavity
     Bite of abdominal wall NOS

     Excludes1   superficial bite of abdominal wall (S30.871)

    ● **S31.150**   Open bite of abdominal wall, right upper quadrant without penetration into peritoneal cavity

    ● **S31.151**   Open bite of abdominal wall, left upper quadrant without penetration into peritoneal cavity

    ● **S31.152**   Open bite of abdominal wall, epigastric region without penetration into peritoneal cavity

    ● **S31.153**   Open bite of abdominal wall, right lower quadrant without penetration into peritoneal cavity

    ● **S31.154**   Open bite of abdominal wall, left lower quadrant without penetration into peritoneal cavity

    ● **S31.155**   Open bite of abdominal wall, periumbilic region without penetration into peritoneal cavity

    ● **S31.159**   Open bite of abdominal wall, unspecified quadrant without penetration into peritoneal cavity

● **S31.2**   Open wound of penis

    X ● **S31.20**   Unspecified open wound of penis

    X ● **S31.21**   Laceration without foreign body of penis

    X ● **S31.22**   Laceration with foreign body of penis

    X ● **S31.23**   Puncture wound without foreign body of penis

    X ● **S31.24**   Puncture wound with foreign body of penis

    X ● **S31.25**   Open bite of penis
         Bite of penis NOS

         Excludes1   superficial bite of penis (S30.862, S30.872)

● **S31.3**   Open wound of scrotum and testes

    X ● **S31.30**   Unspecified open wound of scrotum and testes

    X ● **S31.31**   Laceration without foreign body of scrotum and testes

    X ● **S31.32**   Laceration with foreign body of scrotum and testes

    X ● **S31.33**   Puncture wound without foreign body of scrotum and testes

    X ● **S31.34**   Puncture wound with foreign body of scrotum and testes

    X ● **S31.35**   Open bite of scrotum and testes
         Bite of scrotum and testes NOS

         Excludes1   superficial bite of scrotum and testes (S30.863, S30.873)

● **S31.4**   Open wound of vagina and vulva

     Excludes1   injury to vagina and vulva during delivery (O70.-, O71.4)

    X ● **S31.40**   Unspecified open wound of vagina and vulva

    X ● **S31.41**   Laceration without foreign body of vagina and vulva

    X ● **S31.42**   Laceration with foreign body of vagina and vulva

    X ● **S31.43**   Puncture wound without foreign body of vagina and vulva

    X ● **S31.44**   Puncture wound with foreign body of vagina and vulva

    X ● **S31.45**   Open bite of vagina and vulva
         Bite of vagina and vulva NOS

         Excludes1   superficial bite of vagina and vulva (S30.864, S30.874)

CHAPTER 19 (S00-T88)

● **S31.5** Open wound of unspecified external genital organs
> **Excludes1**   traumatic amputation of external genital organs (S38.21, S38.22)

  ● **S31.50** Unspecified open wound of unspecified external genital organs

    ● **S31.501** Unspecified open wound of unspecified external genital organs, male

    ● **S31.502** Unspecified open wound of unspecified external genital organs, female

  ● **S31.51** Laceration without foreign body of unspecified external genital organs

    ● **S31.511** Laceration without foreign body of unspecified external genital organs, male

    ● **S31.512** Laceration without foreign body of unspecified external genital organs, female

  ● **S31.52** Laceration with foreign body of unspecified external genital organs

    ● **S31.521** Laceration with foreign body of unspecified external genital organs, male

    ● **S31.522** Laceration with foreign body of unspecified external genital organs, female

  ● **S31.53** Puncture wound without foreign body of unspecified external genital organs

    ● **S31.531** Puncture wound without foreign body of unspecified external genital organs, male

    ● **S31.532** Puncture wound without foreign body of unspecified external genital organs, female

  ● **S31.54** Puncture wound with foreign body of unspecified external genital organs

    ● **S31.541** Puncture wound with foreign body of unspecified external genital organs, male

    ● **S31.542** Puncture wound with foreign body of unspecified external genital organs, female

  ● **S31.55** Open bite of unspecified external genital organs
> Bite of unspecified external genital organs NOS
>
> **Excludes1**   superficial bite of unspecified external genital organs (S30.865, S30.866, S30.875, S30.876)

    ● **S31.551** Open bite of unspecified external genital organs, male

    ● **S31.552** Open bite of unspecified external genital organs, female

● **S31.6** Open wound of abdominal wall with penetration into peritoneal cavity

  ● **S31.60** Unspecified open wound of abdominal wall with penetration into peritoneal cavity

    ● **S31.600** Unspecified open wound of abdominal wall, right upper quadrant with penetration into peritoneal cavity

    ● **S31.601** Unspecified open wound of abdominal wall, left upper quadrant with penetration into peritoneal cavity

    ● **S31.602** Unspecified open wound of abdominal wall, epigastric region with penetration into peritoneal cavity

    ● **S31.603** Unspecified open wound of abdominal wall, right lower quadrant with penetration into peritoneal cavity

    ● **S31.604** Unspecified open wound of abdominal wall, left lower quadrant with penetration into peritoneal cavity

    ● **S31.605** Unspecified open wound of abdominal wall, periumbilic region with penetration into peritoneal cavity

    ● **S31.609** Unspecified open wound of abdominal wall, unspecified quadrant with penetration into peritoneal cavity

  ● **S31.61** Laceration without foreign body of abdominal wall with penetration into peritoneal cavity

    ● **S31.610** Laceration without foreign body of abdominal wall, right upper quadrant with penetration into peritoneal cavity

    ● **S31.611** Laceration without foreign body of abdominal wall, left upper quadrant with penetration into peritoneal cavity

    ● **S31.612** Laceration without foreign body of abdominal wall, epigastric region with penetration into peritoneal cavity

    ● **S31.613** Laceration without foreign body of abdominal wall, right lower quadrant with penetration into peritoneal cavity

    ● **S31.614** Laceration without foreign body of abdominal wall, left lower quadrant with penetration into peritoneal cavity

    ● **S31.615** Laceration without foreign body of abdominal wall, periumbilic region with penetration into peritoneal cavity

    ● **S31.619** Laceration without foreign body of abdominal wall, unspecified quadrant with penetration into peritoneal cavity

● S31.62   Laceration with foreign body of abdominal
           wall with penetration into peritoneal cavity
   ● S31.620   Laceration with foreign body of
              abdominal wall, right upper quadrant
              with penetration into peritoneal
              cavity
   ● S31.621   Laceration with foreign body of
              abdominal wall, left upper quadrant
              with penetration into peritoneal
              cavity
   ● S31.622   Laceration with foreign body of
              abdominal wall, epigastric region
              with penetration into peritoneal
              cavity
   ● S31.623   Laceration with foreign body of
              abdominal wall, right lower quadrant
              with penetration into peritoneal
              cavity
   ● S31.624   Laceration with foreign body of
              abdominal wall, left lower quadrant
              with penetration into peritoneal
              cavity
   ● S31.625   Laceration with foreign body of
              abdominal wall, periumbilic region
              with penetration into peritoneal
              cavity
   ● S31.629   Laceration with foreign body of
              abdominal wall, unspecified quadrant
              with penetration into peritoneal
              cavity

● S31.63   Puncture wound without foreign body
           of abdominal wall with penetration into
           peritoneal cavity
   ● S31.630   Puncture wound without foreign
              body of abdominal wall, right upper
              quadrant with penetration into
              peritoneal cavity
   ● S31.631   Puncture wound without foreign
              body of abdominal wall, left upper
              quadrant with penetration into
              peritoneal cavity
   ● S31.632   Puncture wound without foreign
              body of abdominal wall, epigastric
              region with penetration into
              peritoneal cavity
   ● S31.633   Puncture wound without foreign
              body of abdominal wall, right lower
              quadrant with penetration into
              peritoneal cavity
   ● S31.634   Puncture wound without foreign
              body of abdominal wall, left lower
              quadrant with penetration into
              peritoneal cavity
   ● S31.635   Puncture wound without foreign
              body of abdominal wall, periumbilic
              region with penetration into
              peritoneal cavity
   ● S31.639   Puncture wound without foreign
              body of abdominal wall, unspecified
              quadrant with penetration into
              peritoneal cavity

● S31.64   Puncture wound with foreign body of
           abdominal wall with penetration into
           peritoneal cavity
   ● S31.640   Puncture wound with foreign body of
              abdominal wall, right upper quadrant
              with penetration into peritoneal
              cavity
   ● S31.641   Puncture wound with foreign body of
              abdominal wall, left upper quadrant
              with penetration into peritoneal
              cavity
   ● S31.642   Puncture wound with foreign body
              of abdominal wall, epigastric region
              with penetration into peritoneal
              cavity
   ● S31.643   Puncture wound with foreign body of
              abdominal wall, right lower quadrant
              with penetration into peritoneal
              cavity
   ● S31.644   Puncture wound with foreign body of
              abdominal wall, left lower quadrant
              with penetration into peritoneal
              cavity
   ● S31.645   Puncture wound with foreign body of
              abdominal wall, periumbilic region
              with penetration into peritoneal
              cavity
   ● S31.649   Puncture wound with foreign body of
              abdominal wall, unspecified quadrant
              with penetration into peritoneal
              cavity

● S31.65   Open bite of abdominal wall with penetration
           into peritoneal cavity
   | Excludes 1 | superficial bite of abdominal
                    wall (S30.861, S30.871)
   ● S31.650   Open bite of abdominal wall, right
              upper quadrant with penetration into
              peritoneal cavity
   ● S31.651   Open bite of abdominal wall, left
              upper quadrant with penetration into
              peritoneal cavity
   ● S31.652   Open bite of abdominal wall,
              epigastric region with penetration
              into peritoneal cavity
   ● S31.653   Open bite of abdominal wall, right
              lower quadrant with penetration into
              peritoneal cavity
   ● S31.654   Open bite of abdominal wall, left
              lower quadrant with penetration into
              peritoneal cavity
   ● S31.655   Open bite of abdominal wall,
              periumbilic region with penetration
              into peritoneal cavity
   ● S31.659   Open bite of abdominal wall,
              unspecified quadrant with penetration
              into peritoneal cavity

CHAPTER 19 (S00-T88)

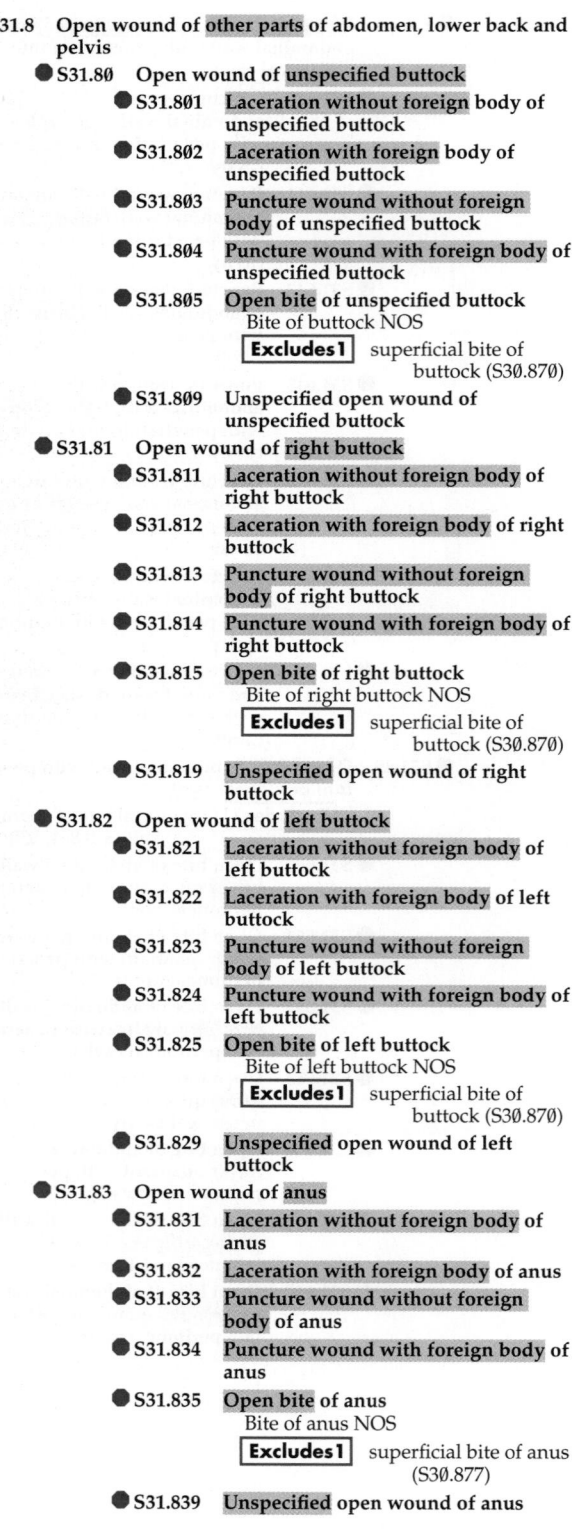

CHAPTER 19 (S00-T88)

● S31.8   Open wound of other parts of abdomen, lower back and pelvis

  ● S31.80   Open wound of unspecified buttock

    ● S31.801   Laceration without foreign body of unspecified buttock

    ● S31.802   Laceration with foreign body of unspecified buttock

    ● S31.803   Puncture wound without foreign body of unspecified buttock

    ● S31.804   Puncture wound with foreign body of unspecified buttock

    ● S31.805   Open bite of unspecified buttock
       Bite of buttock NOS
       Excludes1   superficial bite of buttock (S30.870)

    ● S31.809   Unspecified open wound of unspecified buttock

  ● S31.81   Open wound of right buttock

    ● S31.811   Laceration without foreign body of right buttock

    ● S31.812   Laceration with foreign body of right buttock

    ● S31.813   Puncture wound without foreign body of right buttock

    ● S31.814   Puncture wound with foreign body of right buttock

    ● S31.815   Open bite of right buttock
       Bite of right buttock NOS
       Excludes1   superficial bite of buttock (S30.870)

    ● S31.819   Unspecified open wound of right buttock

  ● S31.82   Open wound of left buttock

    ● S31.821   Laceration without foreign body of left buttock

    ● S31.822   Laceration with foreign body of left buttock

    ● S31.823   Puncture wound without foreign body of left buttock

    ● S31.824   Puncture wound with foreign body of left buttock

    ● S31.825   Open bite of left buttock
       Bite of left buttock NOS
       Excludes1   superficial bite of buttock (S30.870)

    ● S31.829   Unspecified open wound of left buttock

  ● S31.83   Open wound of anus

    ● S31.831   Laceration without foreign body of anus

    ● S31.832   Laceration with foreign body of anus

    ● S31.833   Puncture wound without foreign body of anus

    ● S31.834   Puncture wound with foreign body of anus

    ● S31.835   Open bite of anus
       Bite of anus NOS
       Excludes1   superficial bite of anus (S30.877)

    ● S31.839   Unspecified open wound of anus

● S32   Fracture of lumbar spine and pelvis

   Note: A fracture not indicated as displaced or nondisplaced should be coded to displaced

     A fracture not indicated as opened or closed should be coded to closed

   Includes   fracture of lumbosacral neural arch
          fracture of lumbosacral spinous process
          fracture of lumbosacral transverse process
          fracture of lumbosacral vertebra
          fracture of lumbosacral vertebral arch

   Code first any associated spinal cord and spinal nerve injury (S34.-)

   Excludes1   transection of abdomen (S38.3)

   Excludes2   fracture of hip NOS (S72.0-)

   The appropriate 7th character is to be added to each code from category S32

     | | |
     A   initial encounter for closed fracture
     B   initial encounter for open fracture
     D   subsequent encounter for fracture with routine healing
     G   subsequent encounter for fracture with delayed healing
     K   subsequent encounter for fracture with nonunion
     S   sequela

  ● S32.0   Fracture of lumbar vertebra
     Fracture of lumbar spine NOS

    ● S32.00   Fracture of unspecified lumbar vertebra

      ● S32.000   Wedge compression fracture of unspecified lumbar vertebra

      ● S32.001   Stable burst fracture of unspecified lumbar vertebra

      ● S32.002   Unstable burst fracture of unspecified lumbar vertebra

      ● S32.008   Other fracture of unspecified lumbar vertebra

      ● S32.009   Unspecified fracture of unspecified lumbar vertebra

    ● S32.01   Fracture of first lumbar vertebra

      ● S32.010   Wedge compression fracture of first lumbar vertebra

      ● S32.011   Stable burst fracture of first lumbar vertebra

      ● S32.012   Unstable burst fracture of first lumbar vertebra

      ● S32.018   Other fracture of first lumbar vertebra

      ● S32.019   Unspecified fracture of first lumbar vertebra

    ● S32.02   Fracture of second lumbar vertebra

      ● S32.020   Wedge compression fracture of second lumbar vertebra

      ● S32.021   Stable burst fracture of second lumbar vertebra

      ● S32.022   Unstable burst fracture of second lumbar vertebra

      ● S32.028   Other fracture of second lumbar vertebra

      ● S32.029   Unspecified fracture of second lumbar vertebra

    ● S32.03   Fracture of third lumbar vertebra

      ● S32.030   Wedge compression fracture of third lumbar vertebra

      ● S32.031   Stable burst fracture of third lumbar vertebra

      ● S32.032   Unstable burst fracture of third lumbar vertebra

      ● S32.038   Other fracture of third lumbar vertebra

      ● S32.039   Unspecified fracture of third lumbar vertebra

▶ New   ⇨ Revised   ~~deleted~~ Deleted   **OGCR** Official Guidelines   X Assign placeholder X   ● Use Additional Character(s)

Excludes 1   Excludes 2   Includes   Use additional   Code first   Code also   Key words

● S32.04   Fracture of fourth lumbar vertebra
  ● S32.040   **Wedge compression** fracture of fourth lumbar vertebra
  ● S32.041   **Stable burst** fracture of fourth lumbar vertebra
  ● S32.042   **Unstable burst** fracture of fourth lumbar vertebra
  ● S32.048   **Other** fracture of fourth lumbar vertebra
  ● S32.049   **Unspecified** fracture of fourth lumbar vertebra
● S32.05   Fracture of fifth lumbar vertebra
  ● S32.050   **Wedge compression** fracture of fifth lumbar vertebra
  ● S32.051   **Stable burst** fracture of fifth lumbar vertebra
  ● S32.052   **Unstable burst** fracture of fifth lumbar vertebra
  ● S32.058   **Other** fracture of fifth lumbar vertebra
  ● S32.059   **Unspecified** fracture of fifth lumbar vertebra
● S32.1   Fracture of sacrum
       For vertical fractures, code to most medial fracture extension
       Use two codes if both a vertical and transverse fracture are present
       Code also any associated fracture of pelvic ring (S32.8-)
  X ● S32.10   **Unspecified** fracture of sacrum
  ● S32.11   **Zone I** fracture of sacrum
       Vertical sacral ala fracture of sacrum
    ● S32.110   **Nondisplaced** Zone I fracture of sacrum
    ● S32.111   **Minimally displaced** Zone I fracture of sacrum
    ● S32.112   **Severely displaced** Zone I fracture of sacrum
    ● S32.119   **Unspecified** Zone I fracture of sacrum
  ● S32.12   **Zone II** fracture of sacrum
       Vertical foraminal region fracture of sacrum
    ● S32.120   **Nondisplaced** Zone II fracture of sacrum
    ● S32.121   **Minimally displaced** Zone II fracture of sacrum
    ● S32.122   **Severely displaced** Zone II fracture of sacrum
    ● S32.129   **Unspecified** Zone II fracture of sacrum
  ● S32.13   **Zone III** fracture of sacrum
       Vertical fracture into spinal canal region of sacrum
    ● S32.130   **Nondisplaced** Zone III fracture of sacrum
    ● S32.131   **Minimally displaced** Zone III fracture of sacrum
    ● S32.132   **Severely displaced** Zone III fracture of sacrum
    ● S32.139   **Unspecified** Zone III fracture of sacrum
  X ● S32.14   **Type 1** fracture of sacrum
       Transverse flexion fracture of sacrum without displacement
  X ● S32.15   **Type 2** fracture of sacrum
       Transverse flexion fracture of sacrum with posterior displacement
  X ● S32.16   **Type 3** fracture of sacrum
       Transverse extension fracture of sacrum with anterior displacement
  X ● S32.17   **Type 4** fracture of sacrum
       Transverse segmental comminution of upper sacrum
  X ● S32.19   **Other** fracture of sacrum

X ● S32.2   Fracture of coccyx
● S32.3   Fracture of ilium
       Excludes1   fracture of ilium with associated disruption of pelvic ring (S32.8-)
  ● S32.30   **Unspecified** fracture of ilium
    ● S32.301   Unspecified fracture of **right** ilium
    ● S32.302   Unspecified fracture of **left** ilium
    ● S32.309   Unspecified fracture of **unspecified** ilium
  ● S32.31   **Avulsion** fracture of ilium
    ● S32.311   **Displaced** avulsion fracture of **right** ilium
    ● S32.312   **Displaced** avulsion fracture of **left** ilium
    ● S32.313   **Displaced** avulsion fracture of **unspecified** ilium
    ● S32.314   **Nondisplaced** avulsion fracture of **right** ilium
    ● S32.315   **Nondisplaced** avulsion fracture of **left** ilium
    ● S32.316   **Nondisplaced** avulsion fracture of **unspecified** ilium
  ● S32.39   **Other** fracture of ilium
    ● S32.391   Other fracture of **right** ilium
    ● S32.392   Other fracture of **left** ilium
    ● S32.399   Other fracture of **unspecified** ilium
● S32.4   Fracture of acetabulum
       Code also any associated fracture of pelvic ring (S32.8-)
  ● S32.40   **Unspecified** fracture of acetabulum
    ● S32.401   Unspecified fracture of **right** acetabulum
    ● S32.402   Unspecified fracture of **left** acetabulum
    ● S32.409   Unspecified fracture of **unspecified** acetabulum
  ● S32.41   Fracture of **anterior wall** of acetabulum
    ● S32.411   **Displaced** fracture of anterior wall of **right** acetabulum
    ● S32.412   **Displaced** fracture of anterior wall of **left** acetabulum
    ● S32.413   **Displaced** fracture of anterior wall of **unspecified** acetabulum
    ● S32.414   **Nondisplaced** fracture of anterior wall of **right** acetabulum
    ● S32.415   **Nondisplaced** fracture of anterior wall of **left** acetabulum
    ● S32.416   **Nondisplaced** fracture of anterior wall of **unspecified** acetabulum
  ● S32.42   Fracture of **posterior wall** of acetabulum
    ● S32.421   **Displaced** fracture of posterior wall of **right** acetabulum
    ● S32.422   **Displaced** fracture of posterior wall of **left** acetabulum
    ● S32.423   **Displaced** fracture of posterior wall of **unspecified** acetabulum
    ● S32.424   **Nondisplaced** fracture of posterior wall of **right** acetabulum
    ● S32.425   **Nondisplaced** fracture of posterior wall of **left** acetabulum
    ● S32.426   **Nondisplaced** fracture of posterior wall of **unspecified** acetabulum

CHAPTER 19 (S00-T88)

● **S32.43** Fracture of anterior column [iliopubic] of acetabulum

● **S32.431** Displaced fracture of anterior column [iliopubic] of right acetabulum

● **S32.432** Displaced fracture of anterior column [iliopubic] of left acetabulum

● **S32.433** Displaced fracture of anterior column [iliopubic] of unspecified acetabulum

● **S32.434** Nondisplaced fracture of anterior column [iliopubic] of right acetabulum

● **S32.435** Nondisplaced fracture of anterior column [iliopubic] of left acetabulum

● **S32.436** Nondisplaced fracture of anterior column [iliopubic] of unspecified acetabulum

● **S32.44** Fracture of posterior column [ilioischial] of acetabulum

● **S32.441** Displaced fracture of posterior column [ilioischial] of right acetabulum

● **S32.442** Displaced fracture of posterior column [ilioischial] of left acetabulum

● **S32.443** Displaced fracture of posterior column [ilioischial] of unspecified acetabulum

● **S32.444** Nondisplaced fracture of posterior column [ilioischial] of right acetabulum

● **S32.445** Nondisplaced fracture of posterior column [ilioischial] of left acetabulum

● **S32.446** Nondisplaced fracture of posterior column [ilioischial] of unspecified acetabulum

● **S32.45** Transverse fracture of acetabulum

● **S32.451** Displaced transverse fracture of right acetabulum

● **S32.452** Displaced transverse fracture of left acetabulum

● **S32.453** Displaced transverse fracture of unspecified acetabulum

● **S32.454** Nondisplaced transverse fracture of right acetabulum

● **S32.455** Nondisplaced transverse fracture of left acetabulum

● **S32.456** Nondisplaced transverse fracture of unspecified acetabulum

● **S32.46** Associated transverse-posterior fracture of acetabulum

● **S32.461** Displaced associated transverse-posterior fracture of right acetabulum

● **S32.462** Displaced associated transverse-posterior fracture of left acetabulum

● **S32.463** Displaced associated transverse-posterior fracture of unspecified acetabulum

● **S32.464** Nondisplaced associated transverse-posterior fracture of right acetabulum

● **S32.465** Nondisplaced associated transverse-posterior fracture of left acetabulum

● **S32.466** Nondisplaced associated transverse-posterior fracture of unspecified acetabulum

● **S32.47** Fracture of medial wall of acetabulum

● **S32.471** Displaced fracture of medial wall of right acetabulum

● **S32.472** Displaced fracture of medial wall of left acetabulum

● **S32.473** Displaced fracture of medial wall of unspecified acetabulum

● **S32.474** Nondisplaced fracture of medial wall of right acetabulum

● **S32.475** Nondisplaced fracture of medial wall of left acetabulum

● **S32.476** Nondisplaced fracture of medial wall of unspecified acetabulum

● **S32.48** Dome fracture of acetabulum

● **S32.481** Displaced dome fracture of right acetabulum

● **S32.482** Displaced dome fracture of left acetabulum

● **S32.483** Displaced dome fracture of unspecified acetabulum

● **S32.484** Nondisplaced dome fracture of right acetabulum

● **S32.485** Nondisplaced dome fracture of left acetabulum

● **S32.486** Nondisplaced dome fracture of unspecified acetabulum

● **S32.49** Other fracture of acetabulum

● **S32.491** Other fracture of right acetabulum

● **S32.492** Other fracture of left acetabulum

● **S32.499** Other fracture of unspecified acetabulum

● **S32.5** Fracture of pubis

> **Excludes1**   fracture of pubis with associated disruption of pelvic ring (S32.8-)

● **S32.50** Unspecified fracture of pubis

● **S32.501** Unspecified fracture of right pubis

● **S32.502** Unspecified fracture of left pubis

● **S32.509** Unspecified fracture of unspecified pubis

● **S32.51** Fracture of superior rim of pubis

● **S32.511** Fracture of superior rim of right pubis

● **S32.512** Fracture of superior rim of left pubis

● **S32.519** Fracture of superior rim of unspecified pubis

● **S32.59** Other specified fracture of pubis

● **S32.591** Other specified fracture of right pubis

● **S32.592** Other specified fracture of left pubis

● **S32.599** Other specified fracture of unspecified pubis

● **S32.6** Fracture of ischium

> **Excludes1**   fracture of ischium with associated disruption of pelvic ring (S32.8-)

● **S32.60** Unspecified fracture of ischium

● **S32.601** Unspecified fracture of right ischium

● **S32.602** Unspecified fracture of left ischium

● **S32.609** Unspecified fracture of unspecified ischium

● **S32.61** Avulsion fracture of ischium

● **S32.611** Displaced avulsion fracture of right ischium

● **S32.612** Displaced avulsion fracture of left ischium

● **S32.613** Displaced avulsion fracture of unspecified ischium

● **S32.614** Nondisplaced avulsion fracture of right ischium

● **S32.615** Nondisplaced avulsion fracture of left ischium

● **S32.616** Nondisplaced avulsion fracture of unspecified ischium

● **S32.69** Other specified fracture of ischium

● **S32.691** Other specified fracture of right ischium

● **S32.692** Other specified fracture of left ischium

● **S32.699** Other specified fracture of unspecified ischium

▶ New   ⟹ Revised   ~~deleted~~ Deleted   **OGCR** Official Guidelines   X Assign placeholder X   ● Use Additional Character(s)

Excludes 1   Excludes 2   Includes   Use additional   Code first   Code also   Key words

● **S32.8   Fracture of other parts of pelvis**
   Code also any associated:
      fracture of acetabulum (S32.4-)
      sacral fracture (S32.1-)
   ● **S32.81   Multiple fractures of pelvis with disruption of pelvic ring**
            Multiple pelvic fractures with disruption of pelvic circle
      ● **S32.810   Multiple fractures of pelvis with stable disruption of pelvic ring**
      ● **S32.811   Multiple fractures of pelvis with unstable disruption of pelvic ring**
   X ● **S32.82   Multiple fractures of pelvis without disruption of pelvic ring**
            Multiple pelvic fractures without disruption of pelvic circle
   X ● **S32.89   Fracture of other parts of pelvis**
   X ● **S32.9   Fracture of unspecified parts of lumbosacral spine and pelvis**
            Fracture of lumbosacral spine NOS
            Fracture of pelvis NOS

● **S33   Dislocation and sprain of joints and ligaments of lumbar spine and pelvis**

   | **Includes** | avulsion of joint or ligament of lumbar spine and pelvis |

            laceration of cartilage, joint or ligament of lumbar spine and pelvis
            sprain of cartilage, joint or ligament of lumbar spine and pelvis
            traumatic hemarthrosis of joint or ligament of lumbar spine and pelvis
            traumatic rupture of joint or ligament of lumbar spine and pelvis
            traumatic subluxation of joint or ligament of lumbar spine and pelvis
            traumatic tear of joint or ligament of lumbar spine and pelvis

   Code also any associated open wound

   | **Excludes1** | nontraumatic rupture or displacement of lumbar intervertebral disc NOS (M51.-) |
            obstetric damage to pelvic joints and ligaments (O71.6)

   | **Excludes2** | dislocation and sprain of joints and ligaments of hip (S73.-) |
            strain of muscle of lower back and pelvis (S39.01-)

   The appropriate 7th character is to be added to each code from category S33

A	initial encounter
D	subsequent encounter
S	sequela

   X ● **S33.0   Traumatic rupture of lumbar intervertebral disc**

      | **Excludes1** | rupture or displacement (nontraumatic) of lumbar intervertebral disc NOS (M51.- with fifth character 6) |

   ● **S33.1   Subluxation and dislocation of lumbar vertebra**
         Code also any associated:
            open wound of abdomen, lower back and pelvis (S31)
            spinal cord injury (S24.0, S24.1-, S34.0-, S34.1-)

      | **Excludes2** | fracture of lumbar vertebrae (S32.0-) |

      ● **S33.10   Subluxation and dislocation of unspecified lumbar vertebra**
         ● **S33.100   Subluxation of unspecified lumbar vertebra**
         ● **S33.101   Dislocation of unspecified lumbar vertebra**
      ● **S33.11   Subluxation and dislocation of L1/L2 lumbar vertebra**
         ● **S33.110   Subluxation of L1/L2 lumbar vertebra**
         ● **S33.111   Dislocation of L1/L2 lumbar vertebra**

   ● **S33.12   Subluxation and dislocation of L2/L3 lumbar vertebra**
      ● **S33.120   Subluxation of L2/L3 lumbar vertebra**
      ● **S33.121   Dislocation of L2/L3 lumbar vertebra**
   ● **S33.13   Subluxation and dislocation of L3/L4 lumbar vertebra**
      ● **S33.130   Subluxation of L3/L4 lumbar vertebra**
      ● **S33.131   Dislocation of L3/L4 lumbar vertebra**
   ● **S33.14   Subluxation and dislocation of L4/L5 lumbar vertebra**
      ● **S33.140   Subluxation of L4/L5 lumbar vertebra**
      ● **S33.141   Dislocation of L4/L5 lumbar vertebra**
   X ● **S33.2   Dislocation of sacroiliac and sacrococcygeal joint**
   ● **S33.3   Dislocation of other and unspecified parts of lumbar spine and pelvis**
      X ● **S33.30   Dislocation of unspecified parts of lumbar spine and pelvis**
      X ● **S33.39   Dislocation of other parts of lumbar spine and pelvis**
   X ● **S33.4   Traumatic rupture of symphysis pubis**
   X ● **S33.5   Sprain of ligaments of lumbar spine**
   X ● **S33.6   Sprain of sacroiliac joint**
   X ● **S33.8   Sprain of other parts of lumbar spine and pelvis**
   X ● **S33.9   Sprain of unspecified parts of lumbar spine and pelvis**

● **S34   Injury of lumbar and sacral spinal cord and nerves at abdomen, lower back and pelvis level**
   Note: Code to highest level of lumbar cord injury
      Injuries to the spinal cord (S34.0 and S34.1) refer to the cord level and not bone level injury, and can affect nerve roots at and below the level given.
   The appropriate 7th character is to be added to each code from category S34

A	initial encounter
D	subsequent encounter
S	sequela

   Code also any associated:
      fracture of vertebra (S22.0-, S32.0-)
      open wound of abdomen, lower back and pelvis (S31.-)
      transient paralysis (R29.5)
   ● **S34.0   Concussion and edema of lumbar and sacral spinal cord**
      X ● **S34.01   Concussion and edema of lumbar spinal cord**
      X ● **S34.02   Concussion and edema of sacral spinal cord**
            Concussion and edema of conus medullaris
   ● **S34.1   Other and unspecified injury of lumbar and sacral spinal cord**
      ● **S34.10   Unspecified injury to lumbar spinal cord**
         ● **S34.101   Unspecified injury to L_1 level of lumbar spinal cord**
               Unspecified injury to lumbar spinal cord level 1
         ● **S34.102   Unspecified injury to L_2 level of lumbar spinal cord**
               Unspecified injury to lumbar spinal cord level 2
         ● **S34.103   Unspecified injury to L_3 level of lumbar spinal cord**
               Unspecified injury to lumbar spinal cord level 3
         ● **S34.104   Unspecified injury to L_4 level of lumbar spinal cord**
               Unspecified injury to lumbar spinal cord level 4
         ● **S34.105   Unspecified injury to L_5 level of lumbar spinal cord**
               Unspecified injury to lumbar spinal cord level 5
         ● **S34.109   Unspecified injury to unspecified level of lumbar spinal cord**

CHAPTER 19 (S00-T88)

● **S34.11**   Complete lesion of lumbar spinal cord

    ● **S34.111**   Complete lesion of L_1 level of lumbar spinal cord
            Complete lesion of lumbar spinal cord level 1

    ● **S34.112**   Complete lesion of L_2 level of lumbar spinal cord
            Complete lesion of lumbar spinal cord level 2

    ● **S34.113**   Complete lesion of L_3 level of lumbar spinal cord
            Complete lesion of lumbar spinal cord level 3

    ● **S34.114**   Complete lesion of L_4 level of lumbar spinal cord
            Complete lesion of lumbar spinal cord level 4

    ● **S34.115**   Complete lesion of L_5 level of lumbar spinal cord
            Complete lesion of lumbar spinal cord level 5

    ● **S34.119**   Complete lesion of unspecified level of lumbar spinal cord

● **S34.12**   Incomplete lesion of lumbar spinal cord

    ● **S34.121**   Incomplete lesion of L_1 level of lumbar spinal cord
            Incomplete lesion of lumbar spinal cord level 1

    ● **S34.122**   Incomplete lesion of L_2 level of lumbar spinal cord
            Incomplete lesion of lumbar spinal cord level 2

    ● **S34.123**   Incomplete lesion of L_3 level of lumbar spinal cord
            Incomplete lesion of lumbar spinal cord level 3

    ● **S34.124**   Incomplete lesion of L_4 level of lumbar spinal cord
            Incomplete lesion of lumbar spinal cord level 4

    ● **S34.125**   Incomplete lesion of L_5 level of lumbar spinal cord
            Incomplete lesion of lumbar spinal cord level 5

    ● **S34.129**   Incomplete lesion of unspecified level of lumbar spinal cord

● **S34.13**   Other and unspecified injury to sacral spinal cord
      Other injury to conus medullaris

    ● **S34.131**   Complete lesion of sacral spinal cord
            Complete lesion of conus medullaris

    ● **S34.132**   Incomplete lesion of sacral spinal cord
            Incomplete lesion of conus medullaris

    ● **S34.139**   Unspecified injury to sacral spinal cord
            Unspecified injury of conus medullaris

● **S34.2**   Injury of nerve root of lumbar and sacral spine

  X ● **S34.21**   Injury of nerve root of lumbar spine

  X ● **S34.22**   Injury of nerve root of sacral spine

X ● **S34.3**   Injury of cauda equina

X ● **S34.4**   Injury of lumbosacral plexus

X ● **S34.5**   Injury of lumbar, sacral and pelvic sympathetic nerves
      Injury of celiac ganglion or plexus
      Injury of hypogastric plexus
      Injury of mesenteric plexus (inferior) (superior)
      Injury of splanchnic nerve

X ● **S34.6**   Injury of peripheral nerve(s) at abdomen, lower back and pelvis level

X ● **S34.8**   Injury of other nerves at abdomen, lower back and pelvis level

X ● **S34.9**   Injury of unspecified nerves at abdomen, lower back and pelvis level

● **S35**   Injury of blood vessels at abdomen, lower back and pelvis level
    The appropriate 7th character is to be added to each code from category S35

    | | |
    A   initial encounter
    D   subsequent encounter
    S   sequela

    Code also any associated open wound (S31.-)

   ● **S35.0**   Injury of abdominal aorta
      | Excludes1 | injury of aorta NOS (S25.0)

   X ● **S35.00**   Unspecified injury of abdominal aorta

   X ● **S35.01**   Minor laceration of abdominal aorta
        Incomplete transection of abdominal aorta
        Laceration of abdominal aorta NOS
        Superficial laceration of abdominal aorta

   X ● **S35.02**   Major laceration of abdominal aorta
        Complete transection of abdominal aorta
        Traumatic rupture of abdominal aorta

   X ● **S35.09**   Other injury of abdominal aorta

   ● **S35.1**   Injury of inferior vena cava
      Injury of hepatic vein
      | Excludes1 | injury of vena cava NOS (S25.2)

   X ● **S35.10**   Unspecified injury of inferior vena cava

   X ● **S35.11**   Minor laceration of inferior vena cava
        Incomplete transection of inferior vena cava
        Laceration of inferior vena cava NOS
        Superficial laceration of inferior vena cava

   X ● **S35.12**   Major laceration of inferior vena cava
        Complete transection of inferior vena cava
        Traumatic rupture of inferior vena cava

   X ● **S35.19**   Other injury of inferior vena cava

   ● **S35.2**   Injury of celiac or mesenteric artery and branches

    ● **S35.21**   Injury of celiac artery

      ● **S35.211**   Minor laceration of celiac artery
          Incomplete transection of celiac artery
          Laceration of celiac artery NOS
          Superficial laceration of celiac artery

      ● **S35.212**   Major laceration of celiac artery
          Complete transection of celiac artery
          Traumatic rupture of celiac artery

      ● **S35.218**   Other injury of celiac artery

      ● **S35.219**   Unspecified injury of celiac artery

    ● **S35.22**   Injury of superior mesenteric artery

      ● **S35.221**   Minor laceration of superior mesenteric artery
          Incomplete transection of superior mesenteric artery
          Laceration of superior mesenteric artery NOS
          Superficial laceration of superior mesenteric artery

      ● **S35.222**   Major laceration of superior mesenteric artery
          Complete transection of superior mesenteric artery
          Traumatic rupture of superior mesenteric artery

      ● **S35.228**   Other injury of superior mesenteric artery

      ● **S35.229**   Unspecified injury of superior mesenteric artery

▶ New   ⇒ Revised   ~~deleted~~ Deleted   **OGCR** Official Guidelines   X Assign placeholder X   ● Use Additional Character(s)

| Excludes 1 | | Excludes 2 | | Includes | | Use additional | | Code first | | Code also | | Key words |

● S35.23   Injury of inferior mesenteric artery
  ● S35.231   Minor laceration of inferior mesenteric artery
    Incomplete transection of inferior mesenteric artery
    Laceration of inferior mesenteric artery NOS
    Superficial laceration of inferior mesenteric artery
  ● S35.232   Major laceration of inferior mesenteric artery
    Complete transection of inferior mesenteric artery
    Traumatic rupture of inferior mesenteric artery
  ● S35.238   Other injury of inferior mesenteric artery
  ● S35.239   Unspecified injury of inferior mesenteric artery
● S35.29   Injury of branches of celiac and mesenteric artery
  Injury of gastric artery
  Injury of gastroduodenal artery
  Injury of hepatic artery
  Injury of splenic artery
  ● S35.291   Minor laceration of branches of celiac and mesenteric artery
    Incomplete transection of branches of celiac and mesenteric artery
    Laceration of branches of celiac and mesenteric artery NOS
    Superficial laceration of branches of celiac and mesenteric artery
  ● S35.292   Major laceration of branches of celiac and mesenteric artery
    Complete transection of branches of celiac and mesenteric artery
    Traumatic rupture of branches of celiac and mesenteric artery
  ● S35.298   Other injury of branches of celiac and mesenteric artery
  ● S35.299   Unspecified injury of branches of celiac and mesenteric artery
● S35.3   Injury of portal or splenic vein and branches
  ● S35.31   Injury of portal vein
    ● S35.311   Laceration of portal vein
    ● S35.318   Other specified injury of portal vein
    ● S35.319   Unspecified injury of portal vein
  ● S35.32   Injury of splenic vein
    ● S35.321   Laceration of splenic vein
    ● S35.328   Other specified injury of splenic vein
    ● S35.329   Unspecified injury of splenic vein
  ● S35.33   Injury of superior mesenteric vein
    ● S35.331   Laceration of superior mesenteric vein
    ● S35.338   Other specified injury of superior mesenteric vein
    ● S35.339   Unspecified injury of superior mesenteric vein
  ● S35.34   Injury of inferior mesenteric vein
    ● S35.341   Laceration of inferior mesenteric vein
    ● S35.348   Other specified injury of inferior mesenteric vein
    ● S35.349   Unspecified injury of inferior mesenteric vein

● S35.4   Injury of renal blood vessels
  ● S35.40   Unspecified injury of renal blood vessel
    ● S35.401   Unspecified injury of right renal artery
    ● S35.402   Unspecified injury of left renal artery
    ● S35.403   Unspecified injury of unspecified renal artery
    ● S35.404   Unspecified injury of right renal vein
    ● S35.405   Unspecified injury of left renal vein
    ● S35.406   Unspecified injury of unspecified renal vein
  ● S35.41   Laceration of renal blood vessel
    ● S35.411   Laceration of right renal artery
    ● S35.412   Laceration of left renal artery
    ● S35.413   Laceration of unspecified renal artery
    ● S35.414   Laceration of right renal vein
    ● S35.415   Laceration of left renal vein
    ● S35.416   Laceration of unspecified renal vein
  ● S35.49   Other specified injury of renal blood vessel
    ● S35.491   Other specified injury of right renal artery
    ● S35.492   Other specified injury of left renal artery
    ● S35.493   Other specified injury of unspecified renal artery
    ● S35.494   Other specified injury of right renal vein
    ● S35.495   Other specified injury of left renal vein
    ● S35.496   Other specified injury of unspecified renal vein
● S35.5   Injury of iliac blood vessels
  X ● S35.50   Injury of unspecified iliac blood vessel(s)
  ● S35.51   Injury of iliac artery or vein
    Injury of hypogastric artery or vein
    ● S35.511   Injury of right iliac artery
    ● S35.512   Injury of left iliac artery
    ● S35.513   Injury of unspecified iliac artery
    ● S35.514   Injury of right iliac vein
    ● S35.515   Injury of left iliac vein
    ● S35.516   Injury of unspecified iliac vein
  ● S35.53   Injury of uterine artery or vein
    ● S35.531   Injury of right uterine artery
    ● S35.532   Injury of left uterine artery
    ● S35.533   Injury of unspecified uterine artery
    ● S35.534   Injury of right uterine vein
    ● S35.535   Injury of left uterine vein
    ● S35.536   Injury of unspecified uterine vein
  X ● S35.59   Injury of other iliac blood vessels
● S35.8   Injury of other blood vessels at abdomen, lower back and pelvis level
  Injury of ovarian artery or vein
  ● S35.8X   Injury of other blood vessels at abdomen, lower back and pelvis level
    ● S35.8X1   Laceration of other blood vessels at abdomen, lower back and pelvis level
    ● S35.8X8   Other specified injury of other blood vessels at abdomen, lower back and pelvis level
    ● S35.8X9   Unspecified injury of other blood vessels at abdomen, lower back and pelvis level

● **S35.9**   Injury of unspecified blood vessel at abdomen, lower back and pelvis level

   X ● **S35.90**   Unspecified injury of unspecified blood vessel at abdomen, lower back and pelvis level

   X ● **S35.91**   Laceration of unspecified blood vessel at abdomen, lower back and pelvis level

   X ● **S35.99**   Other specified injury of unspecified blood vessel at abdomen, lower back and pelvis level

● **S36**   Injury of intra-abdominal organs

    The appropriate 7th character is to be added to each code from category S36

> A   initial encounter
> D   subsequent encounter
> S   sequela

    Code also any associated open wound (S31.-)

   ● **S36.0**   Injury of spleen

     X ● **S36.00**   Unspecified injury of spleen

     ● **S36.02**   Contusion of spleen

       ● **S36.020**   Minor contusion of spleen
         Contusion of spleen less than 2 cm

       ● **S36.021**   Major contusion of spleen
         Contusion of spleen greater than 2 cm

       ● **S36.029**   Unspecified contusion of spleen

     ● **S36.03**   Laceration of spleen

       ● **S36.030**   Superficial (capsular) laceration of spleen
         Laceration of spleen less than 1 cm
         Minor laceration of spleen

       ● **S36.031**   Moderate laceration of spleen
         Laceration of spleen 1 to 3 cm

       ● **S36.032**   Major laceration of spleen
         Avulsion of spleen
         Laceration of spleen greater than 3 cm
         Massive laceration of spleen
         Multiple moderate lacerations of spleen
         Stellate laceration of spleen

       ● **S36.039**   Unspecified laceration of spleen

     X ● **S36.09**   Other injury of spleen

   ● **S36.1**   Injury of liver and gallbladder and bile duct

     ● **S36.11**   Injury of liver

       ● **S36.112**   Contusion of liver

       ● **S36.113**   Laceration of liver, unspecified degree

       ● **S36.114**   Minor laceration of liver
         Laceration involving capsule only, or, without significant involvement of hepatic parenchyma [i.e., less than 1 cm deep]

       ● **S36.115**   Moderate laceration of liver
         Laceration involving parenchyma but without major disruption of parenchyma [i.e., less than 10 cm long and less than 3 cm deep]

       ● **S36.116**   Major laceration of liver
         Laceration with significant disruption of hepatic parenchyma [i.e., greater than 10 cm long and 3 cm deep]
         Multiple moderate lacerations, with or without hematoma
         Stellate laceration of liver

       ● **S36.118**   Other injury of liver

       ● **S36.119**   Unspecified injury of liver

   ● **S36.12**   Injury of gallbladder

     ● **S36.122**   Contusion of gallbladder

     ● **S36.123**   Laceration of gallbladder

     ● **S36.128**   Other injury of gallbladder

     ● **S36.129**   Unspecified injury of gallbladder

   X ● **S36.13**   Injury of bile duct

   ● **S36.2**   Injury of pancreas

     ● **S36.20**   Unspecified injury of pancreas

       ● **S36.200**   Unspecified injury of head of pancreas

       ● **S36.201**   Unspecified injury of body of pancreas

       ● **S36.202**   Unspecified injury of tail of pancreas

       ● **S36.209**   Unspecified injury of unspecified part of pancreas

     ● **S36.22**   Contusion of pancreas

       ● **S36.220**   Contusion of head of pancreas

       ● **S36.221**   Contusion of body of pancreas

       ● **S36.222**   Contusion of tail of pancreas

       ● **S36.229**   Contusion of unspecified part of pancreas

     ● **S36.23**   Laceration of pancreas, unspecified degree

       ● **S36.230**   Laceration of head of pancreas, unspecified degree

       ● **S36.231**   Laceration of body of pancreas, unspecified degree

       ● **S36.232**   Laceration of tail of pancreas, unspecified degree

       ● **S36.239**   Laceration of unspecified part of pancreas, unspecified degree

     ● **S36.24**   Minor laceration of pancreas

       ● **S36.240**   Minor laceration of head of pancreas

       ● **S36.241**   Minor laceration of body of pancreas

       ● **S36.242**   Minor laceration of tail of pancreas

       ● **S36.249**   Minor laceration of unspecified part of pancreas

     ● **S36.25**   Moderate laceration of pancreas

       ● **S36.250**   Moderate laceration of head of pancreas

       ● **S36.251**   Moderate laceration of body of pancreas

       ● **S36.252**   Moderate laceration of tail of pancreas

       ● **S36.259**   Moderate laceration of unspecified part of pancreas

     ● **S36.26**   Major laceration of pancreas

       ● **S36.260**   Major laceration of head of pancreas

       ● **S36.261**   Major laceration of body of pancreas

       ● **S36.262**   Major laceration of tail of pancreas

       ● **S36.269**   Major laceration of unspecified part of pancreas

     ● **S36.29**   Other injury of pancreas

       ● **S36.290**   Other injury of head of pancreas

       ● **S36.291**   Other injury of body of pancreas

       ● **S36.292**   Other injury of tail of pancreas

       ● **S36.299**   Other injury of unspecified part of pancreas

   ● **S36.3**   Injury of stomach

     X ● **S36.30**   Unspecified injury of stomach

     X ● **S36.32**   Contusion of stomach

     X ● **S36.33**   Laceration of stomach

     X ● **S36.39**   Other injury of stomach

▶ New   ⇒ Revised   ~~deleted~~ Deleted   **OGCR** Official Guidelines   X Assign placeholder X   ● Use Additional Character(s)

Excludes 1   Excludes 2   Includes   Use additional   Code first   Code also   Key words

CHAPTER 19 (S00-T88)

● **S36.4   Injury of small intestine**
  ● **S36.40   Unspecified** injury of small intestine
    ● **S36.400   Unspecified** injury of **duodenum**
    ● **S36.408   Unspecified** injury of **other** part of small intestine
    ● **S36.409   Unspecified** injury of **unspecified** part of small intestine
  ● **S36.41   Primary blast** injury of small intestine
    Blast injury of small intestine NOS
    ● **S36.410   Primary blast** injury of **duodenum**
    ● **S36.418   Primary blast** injury of **other** part of small intestine
    ● **S36.419   Primary blast** injury of **unspecified** part of small intestine
  ● **S36.42   Contusion** of small intestine
    ● **S36.420   Contusion** of **duodenum**
    ● **S36.428   Contusion** of **other** part of small intestine
    ● **S36.429   Contusion** of **unspecified** part of small intestine
  ● **S36.43   Laceration** of small intestine
    ● **S36.430   Laceration** of **duodenum**
    ● **S36.438   Laceration** of **other** part of small intestine
    ● **S36.439   Laceration** of **unspecified** part of small intestine
  ● **S36.49   Other** injury of small intestine
    ● **S36.490   Other** injury of **duodenum**
    ● **S36.498   Other** injury of **other** part of small intestine
    ● **S36.499   Other** injury of **unspecified** part of small intestine
● **S36.5   Injury of colon**
    Excludes2   injury of rectum (S36.6-)
  ● **S36.50   Unspecified** injury of colon
    ● **S36.500   Unspecified** injury of **ascending** [right] colon
    ● **S36.501   Unspecified** injury of **transverse** colon
    ● **S36.502   Unspecified** injury of **descending** [left] colon
    ● **S36.503   Unspecified** injury of **sigmoid** colon
    ● **S36.508   Unspecified** injury of **other** part of colon
    ● **S36.509   Unspecified** injury of **unspecified** part of colon
  ● **S36.51   Primary blast** injury of colon
    Blast injury of colon NOS
    ● **S36.510   Primary blast** injury of **ascending** [right] colon
    ● **S36.511   Primary blast** injury of **transverse** colon
    ● **S36.512   Primary blast** injury of **descending** [left] colon
    ● **S36.513   Primary blast** injury of **sigmoid** colon
    ● **S36.518   Primary blast** injury of **other** part of colon
    ● **S36.519   Primary blast** injury of **unspecified** part of colon
  ● **S36.52   Contusion** of colon
    ● **S36.520   Contusion** of **ascending** [right] colon
    ● **S36.521   Contusion** of **transverse** colon
    ● **S36.522   Contusion** of **descending** [left] colon
    ● **S36.523   Contusion** of **sigmoid** colon
    ● **S36.528   Contusion** of **other** part of colon
    ● **S36.529   Contusion** of **unspecified** part of colon

● **S36.53   Laceration** of colon
    ● **S36.530   Laceration** of **ascending** [right] colon
    ● **S36.531   Laceration** of **transverse** colon
    ● **S36.532   Laceration** of **descending** [left] colon
    ● **S36.533   Laceration** of **sigmoid** colon
    ● **S36.538   Laceration** of **other** part of colon
      S36.539   Laceration of **unspecified** part of colon
  ● **S36.59   Other** injury of colon
    Secondary blast injury of colon
    ● **S36.590   Other** injury of **ascending** [right] colon
    ● **S36.591   Other** injury of **transverse** colon
    ● **S36.592   Other** injury of **descending** [left] colon
    ● **S36.593   Other** injury of **sigmoid** colon
    ● **S36.598   Other** injury of **other** part of colon
    ● **S36.599   Other** injury of **unspecified** part of colon
● **S36.6   Injury of rectum**
 X ● **S36.60   Unspecified** injury of rectum
 X ● **S36.61   Primary blast** injury of rectum
    Blast injury of rectum NOS
 X ● **S36.62   Contusion** of rectum
 X ● **S36.63   Laceration** of rectum
 X ● **S36.69   Other** injury of rectum
    Secondary blast injury of rectum
● **S36.8   Injury of other intra-abdominal organs**
 X ● **S36.81   Injury of peritoneum**
  ● **S36.89   Injury of other intra-abdominal organs**
    Injury of retroperitoneum
    ● **S36.892   Contusion** of other intra-abdominal organs
    ● **S36.893   Laceration** of other intra-abdominal organs
    ● **S36.898   Other** injury of other intra-abdominal organs
      S36.899   Unspecified injury of other intra-abdominal organs
● **S36.9   Injury of unspecified intra-abdominal organ**
 X ● **S36.90   Unspecified** injury of unspecified intra-abdominal organ
 X ● **S36.92   Contusion** of unspecified intra-abdominal organ
 X ● **S36.93   Laceration** of unspecified intra-abdominal organ
 X ● **S36.99   Other** injury of unspecified intra-abdominal organ

● **S37   Injury of urinary and pelvic organs**
  Code also any associated open wound (S31.-)
  Excludes1   obstetric trauma to pelvic organs (O71.-)
  Excludes2   injury of peritoneum (S36.81)
       injury of retroperitoneum (S36.89-)

  The appropriate 7th character is to be added to each code from category S37

A	initial encounter
D	subsequent encounter
S	sequela

● **S37.0   Injury of kidney**
    Excludes2   acute kidney injury (nontraumatic) (N17.9)
  ● **S37.00   Unspecified** injury of kidney
    ● **S37.001   Unspecified** injury of **right** kidney
    ● **S37.002   Unspecified** injury of **left** kidney
    ● **S37.009   Unspecified** injury of **unspecified** kidney

CHAPTER 19 (S00-T88)

● S37.01   **Minor contusion** of kidney
       Contusion of kidney less than 2 cm
       Contusion of kidney NOS
   ● S37.011   Minor contusion of **right** kidney
   ● S37.012   Minor contusion of **left** kidney
   ● S37.019   Minor contusion of **unspecified** kidney

● S37.02   **Major contusion** of kidney
       Contusion of kidney greater than 2 cm
   ● S37.021   Major contusion of **right** kidney
   ● S37.022   Major contusion of **left** kidney
   ● S37.029   Major contusion of **unspecified** kidney

● S37.03   **Laceration** of kidney, **unspecified degree**
   ● S37.031   Laceration of **right** kidney, unspecified degree
   ● S37.032   Laceration of **left** kidney, unspecified degree
   ● S37.039   Laceration of **unspecified** kidney, unspecified degree

● S37.04   **Minor laceration** of kidney
       Laceration of kidney less than 1 cm
   ● S37.041   Minor laceration of **right** kidney
   ● S37.042   Minor laceration of **left** kidney
   ● S37.049   Minor laceration of **unspecified** kidney

● S37.05   **Moderate laceration** of kidney
       Laceration of kidney 1 to 3 cm
   ● S37.051   Moderate laceration of **right** kidney
   ● S37.052   Moderate laceration of **left** kidney
   ● S37.059   Moderate laceration of **unspecified** kidney

● S37.06   **Major laceration** of kidney
       Avulsion of kidney
       Laceration of kidney greater than 3 cm
       Massive laceration of kidney
       Multiple moderate lacerations of kidney
       Stellate laceration of kidney
   ● S37.061   Major laceration of **right** kidney
   ● S37.062   Major laceration of **left** kidney
   ● S37.069   Major laceration of **unspecified** kidney

● S37.09   **Other injury** of kidney
   ● S37.091   Other injury of **right** kidney
   ● S37.092   Other injury of **left** kidney
   ● S37.099   Other injury of **unspecified** kidney

● S37.1   Injury of **ureter**
   X ● S37.10   **Unspecified** injury of ureter
   X ● S37.12   **Contusion** of ureter
   X ● S37.13   **Laceration** of ureter
   X ● S37.19   **Other** injury of ureter

● S37.2   Injury of **bladder**
   X ● S37.20   **Unspecified** injury of bladder
   X ● S37.22   **Contusion** of bladder
   X ● S37.23   **Laceration** of bladder
   X ● S37.29   **Other** injury of bladder

● S37.3   Injury of **urethra**
   X ● S37.30   **Unspecified** injury of urethra
   X ● S37.32   **Contusion** of urethra
   X ● S37.33   **Laceration** of urethra
   X ● S37.39   **Other** injury of urethra

● S37.4   Injury of **ovary**
   ● S37.40   **Unspecified** injury of ovary
     ● S37.401   Unspecified injury of ovary, **unilateral**
     ● S37.402   Unspecified injury of ovary, **bilateral**
     ● S37.409   Unspecified injury of ovary, **unspecified**

● S37.42   **Contusion** of ovary
   ● S37.421   Contusion of ovary, **unilateral**
   ● S37.422   Contusion of ovary, **bilateral**
   ● S37.429   Contusion of ovary, **unspecified**

● S37.43   **Laceration** of ovary
   ● S37.431   Laceration of ovary, **unilateral**
   ● S37.432   Laceration of ovary, **bilateral**
   ● S37.439   Laceration of ovary, **unspecified**

● S37.49   **Other injury** of ovary
   ● S37.491   Other injury of ovary, **unilateral**
   ● S37.492   Other injury of ovary, **bilateral**
   ● S37.499   Other injury of ovary, **unspecified**

● S37.5   Injury of **fallopian tube**
   ● S37.50   **Unspecified** injury of fallopian tube
     ● S37.501   Unspecified injury of fallopian tube, **unilateral**
     ● S37.502   Unspecified injury of fallopian tube, **bilateral**
     ● S37.509   Unspecified injury of fallopian tube, **unspecified**

   ● S37.51   **Primary blast injury** of fallopian tube
       Blast injury of fallopian tube NOS
     ● S37.511   Primary blast injury of fallopian tube, **unilateral**
     ● S37.512   Primary blast injury of fallopian tube, **bilateral**
     ● S37.519   Primary blast injury of fallopian tube, **unspecified**

   ● S37.52   **Contusion** of fallopian tube
     ● S37.521   Contusion of fallopian tube, **unilateral**
     ● S37.522   Contusion of fallopian tube, **bilateral**
     ● S37.529   Contusion of fallopian tube, **unspecified**

   ● S37.53   **Laceration** of fallopian tube
     ● S37.531   Laceration of fallopian tube, **unilateral**
     ● S37.532   Laceration of fallopian tube, **bilateral**
     ● S37.539   Laceration of fallopian tube, **unspecified**

   ● S37.59   **Other injury** of fallopian tube
       Secondary blast injury of fallopian tube
     ● S37.591   Other injury of fallopian tube, **unilateral**
     ● S37.592   Other injury of fallopian tube, **bilateral**
     ● S37.599   Other injury of fallopian tube, **unspecified**

● S37.6   Injury of **uterus**
   Excludes1   injury to gravid uterus (O9A.2-)
               injury to uterus during delivery (O71.-)
   X ● S37.60   **Unspecified** injury of uterus
   X ● S37.62   **Contusion** of uterus
   X ● S37.63   **Laceration** of uterus
   X ● S37.69   **Other** injury of uterus

● S37.8   Injury of other urinary and pelvic organs
   ● S37.81   Injury of **adrenal gland**
     ● S37.812   **Contusion** of adrenal gland
     ● S37.813   **Laceration** of adrenal gland
     ● S37.818   **Other** injury of adrenal gland
     ● S37.819   **Unspecified** injury of adrenal gland

   ● S37.82   Injury of **prostate**
     ● S37.822   **Contusion** of prostate
     ● S37.823   **Laceration** of prostate
     ● S37.828   **Other** injury of prostate
     ● S37.829   **Unspecified** injury of prostate

▶ New   ⇒ Revised   deleted Deleted   **OGCR** Official Guidelines   X Assign placeholder X   ● Use Additional Character(s)

Excludes 1   Excludes 2   Includes   Use additional   Code first   Code also   Key words

- S37.89   Injury of other urinary and pelvic organ
  - S37.892   Contusion of other urinary and pelvic organ
  - S37.893   Laceration of other urinary and pelvic organ
  - S37.898   Other injury of other urinary and pelvic organ
  - S37.899   Unspecified injury of other urinary and pelvic organ
- S37.9   Injury of unspecified urinary and pelvic organ
  - X● S37.90   Unspecified injury of unspecified urinary and pelvic organ
  - X● S37.92   Contusion of unspecified urinary and pelvic organ
  - X● S37.93   Laceration of unspecified urinary and pelvic organ
  - X● S37.99   Other injury of unspecified urinary and pelvic organ
- S38   Crushing injury and traumatic amputation of abdomen, lower back, pelvis and external genitals

  An amputation not identified as partial or complete should be coded to complete

  The appropriate 7th character is to be added to each code from category S38

A	initial encounter
D	subsequent encounter
S	sequela

  - S38.0   Crushing injury of external genital organs

    Use additional code for any associated injuries
    - S38.00   Crushing injury of unspecified external genital organs
      - S38.001   Crushing injury of unspecified external genital organs, male
      - S38.002   Crushing injury of unspecified external genital organs, female
    - X● S38.01   Crushing injury of penis
    - X● S38.02   Crushing injury of scrotum and testis
    - X● S38.03   Crushing injury of vulva
  - X● S38.1   Crushing injury of abdomen, lower back, and pelvis

    Use additional code for all associated injuries, such as:
      fracture of thoracic or lumbar spine and pelvis (S22.0-, S32.-)
      injury to intra-abdominal organs (S36.-)
      injury to urinary and pelvic organs (S37.-)
      open wound of abdominal wall (S31.-)
      spinal cord injury (S34.0, S34.1-)

    Excludes2   crushing injury of external genital organs (S38.0-)
  - S38.2   Traumatic amputation of external genital organs
    - S38.21   Traumatic amputation of female external genital organs

      Traumatic amputation of clitoris
      Traumatic amputation of labium (majus) (minus)
      Traumatic amputation of vulva
      - S38.211   Complete traumatic amputation of female external genital organs
      - S38.212   Partial traumatic amputation of female external genital organs
    - S38.22   Traumatic amputation of penis
      - S38.221   Complete traumatic amputation of penis
      - S38.222   Partial traumatic amputation of penis

- S38.23   Traumatic amputation of scrotum and testis
  - S38.231   Complete traumatic amputation of scrotum and testis
  - S38.232   Partial traumatic amputation of scrotum and testis
- X● S38.3   Transection (partial) of abdomen
- S39   Other and unspecified injuries of abdomen, lower back, pelvis and external genitals

  Code also any associated open wound (S31.-)

  Excludes2   sprain of joints and ligaments of lumbar spine and pelvis (S33.-)

  The appropriate 7th character is to be added to each code from category S39

A	initial encounter
D	subsequent encounter
S	sequela

  - S39.0   Injury of muscle, fascia and tendon of abdomen, lower back and pelvis
    - S39.00   Unspecified injury of muscle, fascia and tendon of abdomen, lower back and pelvis
      - S39.001   Unspecified injury of muscle, fascia and tendon of abdomen
      - S39.002   Unspecified injury of muscle, fascia and tendon of lower back
      - S39.003   Unspecified injury of muscle, fascia and tendon of pelvis
    - S39.01   Strain of muscle, fascia and tendon of abdomen, lower back and pelvis
      - S39.011   Strain of muscle, fascia and tendon of abdomen
      - S39.012   Strain of muscle, fascia and tendon of lower back
      - S39.013   Strain of muscle, fascia and tendon of pelvis
    - S39.02   Laceration of muscle, fascia and tendon of abdomen, lower back and pelvis
      - S39.021   Laceration of muscle, fascia and tendon of abdomen
      - S39.022   Laceration of muscle, fascia and tendon of lower back
      - S39.023   Laceration of muscle, fascia and tendon of pelvis
    - S39.09   Other injury of muscle, fascia and tendon of abdomen, lower back and pelvis
      - S39.091   Other injury of muscle, fascia and tendon of abdomen
      - S39.092   Other injury of muscle, fascia and tendon of lower back
      - S39.093   Other injury of muscle, fascia and tendon of pelvis
  - S39.8   Other specified injuries of abdomen, lower back, pelvis and external genitals
    - X● S39.81   Other specified injuries of abdomen
    - X● S39.82   Other specified injuries of lower back
    - X● S39.83   Other specified injuries of pelvis
    - S39.84   Other specified injuries of external genitals
      - S39.840   Fracture of corpus cavernosum penis
      - S39.848   Other specified injuries of external genitals
  - S39.9   Unspecified injury of abdomen, lower back, pelvis and external genitals
    - X● S39.91   Unspecified injury of abdomen
    - X● S39.92   Unspecified injury of lower back
    - X● S39.93   Unspecified injury of pelvis
    - X● S39.94   Unspecified injury of external genitals

CHAPTER 19 (S00-T88)

▶ New   ⇒ Revised   ~~deleted~~ Deleted   **OGCR** Official Guidelines   X Assign placeholder X   ● Use Additional Character(s)

| Excludes 1 | Excludes 2 | Includes | Use additional | Code first | Code also | Key words |

INJURIES TO THE SHOULDER AND UPPER ARM (S40-S49)

Includes	injuries of axilla injuries of scapular region
Excludes2	burns and corrosions (T20-T32)
	frostbite (T33-T34)
	injuries of elbow (S50-S59)
	insect bite or sting, venomous (T63.4)

● **S40**   **Superficial injury of shoulder and upper arm**

The appropriate 7th character is to be added to each code from category S40

A	initial encounter
D	subsequent encounter
S	sequela

● **S40.0**   Contusion of shoulder and upper arm
  ● **S40.01**   Contusion of shoulder
    ● S40.011   Contusion of right shoulder
    ● S40.012   Contusion of left shoulder
    ● S40.019   Contusion of unspecified shoulder
  ● **S40.02**   Contusion of upper arm
    ● S40.021   Contusion of right upper arm
    ● S40.022   Contusion of left upper arm
    ● S40.029   Contusion of unspecified upper arm

● **S40.2**   Other superficial injuries of shoulder
  ● **S40.21**   Abrasion of shoulder
    ● S40.211   Abrasion of right shoulder
    ● S40.212   Abrasion of left shoulder
    ● S40.219   Abrasion of unspecified shoulder
  ● **S40.22**   Blister (nonthermal) of shoulder
    ● S40.221   Blister (nonthermal) of right shoulder
    ● S40.222   Blister (nonthermal) of left shoulder
    ● S40.229   Blister (nonthermal) of unspecified shoulder
  ● **S40.24**   External constriction of shoulder
    ● S40.241   External constriction of right shoulder
    ● S40.242   External constriction of left shoulder
    ● S40.249   External constriction of unspecified shoulder
  ● **S40.25**   Superficial foreign body of shoulder
      Splinter in the shoulder
    ● S40.251   Superficial foreign body of right shoulder
    ● S40.252   Superficial foreign body of left shoulder
    ● S40.259   Superficial foreign body of unspecified shoulder
  ● **S40.26**   Insect bite (nonvenomous) of shoulder
    ● S40.261   Insect bite (nonvenomous) of right shoulder
    ● S40.262   Insect bite (nonvenomous) of left shoulder
    ● S40.269   Insect bite (nonvenomous) of unspecified shoulder
  ● **S40.27**   Other superficial bite of shoulder
    Excludes1   open bite of shoulder (S41.05)
    ● S40.271   Other superficial bite of right shoulder
    ● S40.272   Other superficial bite of left shoulder
    ● S40.279   Other superficial bite of unspecified shoulder

● **S40.8**   Other superficial injuries of upper arm
  ● **S40.81**   Abrasion of upper arm
    ● S40.811   Abrasion of right upper arm
    ● S40.812   Abrasion of left upper arm
    ● S40.819   Abrasion of unspecified upper arm
  ● **S40.82**   Blister (nonthermal) of upper arm
    ● S40.821   Blister (nonthermal) of right upper arm
    ● S40.822   Blister (nonthermal) of left upper arm
    ● S40.829   Blister (nonthermal) of unspecified upper arm
  ● **S40.84**   External constriction of upper arm
    ● S40.841   External constriction of right upper arm
    ● S40.842   External constriction of left upper arm
    ● S40.849   External constriction of unspecified upper arm
  ● **S40.85**   Superficial foreign body of upper arm
      Splinter in the upper arm
    ● S40.851   Superficial foreign body of right upper arm
    ● S40.852   Superficial foreign body of left upper arm
    ● S40.859   Superficial foreign body of unspecified upper arm
  ● **S40.86**   Insect bite (nonvenomous) of upper arm
    ● S40.861   Insect bite (nonvenomous) of right upper arm
    ● S40.862   Insect bite (nonvenomous) of left upper arm
    ● S40.869   Insect bite (nonvenomous) of unspecified upper arm
  ● **S40.87**   Other superficial bite of upper arm
    Excludes1   open bite of upper arm (S41.14)
    Excludes2   other superficial bite of shoulder (S40.27-)
    ● S40.871   Other superficial bite of right upper arm
    ● S40.872   Other superficial bite of left upper arm
    ● S40.879   Other superficial bite of unspecified upper arm

● **S40.9**   Unspecified superficial injury of shoulder and upper arm
  ● **S40.91**   Unspecified superficial injury of shoulder
    ● S40.911   Unspecified superficial injury of right shoulder
    ● S40.912   Unspecified superficial injury of left shoulder
    ● S40.919   Unspecified superficial injury of unspecified shoulder
  ● **S40.92**   Unspecified superficial injury of upper arm
    ● S40.921   Unspecified superficial injury of right upper arm
    ● S40.922   Unspecified superficial injury of left upper arm
    ● S40.929   Unspecified superficial injury of unspecified upper arm

▶ New   ⇨ Revised   ~~deleted~~ Deleted   **OGCR** Official Guidelines   X Assign placeholder X   ● Use Additional Character(s)

Excludes 1   Excludes 2   Includes   Use additional   Code first   Code also   Key words

● **S41**   **Open wound of shoulder and upper arm**
Code also any associated wound infection
Excludes1 traumatic amputation of shoulder and upper arm (S48.-)
Excludes2 open fracture of shoulder and upper arm (S42.- with 7th character B or C)

The appropriate 7th character is to be added to each code from category S41

> A   initial encounter
> D   subsequent encounter
> S   sequela

● **S41.0**   **Open wound of shoulder**
   ● **S41.00**   Unspecified open wound of shoulder
     ● **S41.001**   Unspecified open wound of right shoulder
     ● **S41.002**   Unspecified open wound of left shoulder
     ● **S41.009**   Unspecified open wound of unspecified shoulder
   ● **S41.01**   Laceration without foreign body of shoulder
     ● **S41.011**   Laceration without foreign body of right shoulder
     ● **S41.012**   Laceration without foreign body of left shoulder
     ● **S41.019**   Laceration without foreign body of unspecified shoulder
   ● **S41.02**   Laceration with foreign body of shoulder
     ● **S41.021**   Laceration with foreign body of right shoulder
     ● **S41.022**   Laceration with foreign body of left shoulder
     ● **S41.029**   Laceration with foreign body of unspecified shoulder
   ● **S41.03**   Puncture wound without foreign body of shoulder
     ● **S41.031**   Puncture wound without foreign body of right shoulder
     ● **S41.032**   Puncture wound without foreign body of left shoulder
     ● **S41.039**   Puncture wound without foreign body of unspecified shoulder
   ● **S41.04**   Puncture wound with foreign body of shoulder
     ● **S41.041**   Puncture wound with foreign body of right shoulder
     ● **S41.042**   Puncture wound with foreign body of left shoulder
     ● **S41.049**   Puncture wound with foreign body of unspecified shoulder
   ● **S41.05**   Open bite of shoulder
     Bite of shoulder NOS
     Excludes1 superficial bite of shoulder (S40.27)
     ● **S41.051**   Open bite of right shoulder
     ● **S41.052**   Open bite of left shoulder
     ● **S41.059**   Open bite of unspecified shoulder
● **S41.1**   **Open wound of upper arm**
   ● **S41.10**   Unspecified open wound of upper arm
     ● **S41.101**   Unspecified open wound of right upper arm
     ● **S41.102**   Unspecified open wound of left upper arm
     ● **S41.109**   Unspecified open wound of unspecified upper arm

   ● **S41.11**   Laceration without foreign body of upper arm
     ● **S41.111**   Laceration without foreign body of right upper arm
     ● **S41.112**   Laceration without foreign body of left upper arm
     ● **S41.119**   Laceration without foreign body of unspecified upper arm
   ● **S41.12**   Laceration with foreign body of upper arm
     ● **S41.121**   Laceration with foreign body of right upper arm
     ● **S41.122**   Laceration with foreign body of left upper arm
     ● **S41.129**   Laceration with foreign body of unspecified upper arm
   ● **S41.13**   Puncture wound without foreign body of upper arm
     ● **S41.131**   Puncture wound without foreign body of right upper arm
     ● **S41.132**   Puncture wound without foreign body of left upper arm
     ● **S41.139**   Puncture wound without foreign body of unspecified upper arm
   ● **S41.14**   Puncture wound with foreign body of upper arm
     ● **S41.141**   Puncture wound with foreign body of right upper arm
     ● **S41.142**   Puncture wound with foreign body of left upper arm
     ● **S41.149**   Puncture wound with foreign body of unspecified upper arm
   ● **S41.15**   Open bite of upper arm
     Bite of upper arm NOS
     Excludes1 superficial bite of upper arm (S40.87)
     ● **S41.151**   Open bite of right upper arm
     ● **S41.152**   Open bite of left upper arm
     ● **S41.159**   Open bite of unspecified upper arm

● **S42**   **Fracture of shoulder and upper arm**
Note: A fracture not indicated as displaced or nondisplaced should be coded to displaced
A fracture not indicated as open or closed should be coded to closed
Excludes1 traumatic amputation of shoulder and upper arm (S48.-)

The appropriate 7th character is to be added to all codes from category S42

> A   initial encounter for closed fracture
> B   initial encounter for open fracture
> D   subsequent encounter for fracture with routine healing
> G   subsequent encounter for fracture with delayed healing
> K   subsequent encounter for fracture with nonunion
> P   subsequent encounter for fracture with malunion
> S   sequela

● **S42.0**   **Fracture of clavicle**
   ● **S42.00**   Fracture of unspecified part of clavicle
     ● **S42.001**   Fracture of unspecified part of right clavicle
     ● **S42.002**   Fracture of unspecified part of left clavicle
     ● **S42.009**   Fracture of unspecified part of unspecified clavicle

- ● S42.01   Fracture of sternal end of clavicle
  - ● S42.011   Anterior displaced fracture of sternal end of right clavicle
  - ● S42.012   Anterior displaced fracture of sternal end of left clavicle
  - ● S42.013   Anterior displaced fracture of sternal end of unspecified clavicle
    - Displaced fracture of sternal end of clavicle NOS
  - ● S42.014   Posterior displaced fracture of sternal end of right clavicle
  - ● S42.015   Posterior displaced fracture of sternal end of left clavicle
  - ● S42.016   Posterior displaced fracture of sternal end of unspecified clavicle
  - ● S42.017   Nondisplaced fracture of sternal end of right clavicle
  - ● S42.018   Nondisplaced fracture of sternal end of left clavicle
  - ● S42.019   Nondisplaced fracture of sternal end of unspecified clavicle
- ● S42.02   Fracture of shaft of clavicle
  - ● S42.021   Displaced fracture of shaft of right clavicle
  - ● S42.022   Displaced fracture of shaft of left clavicle
  - ● S42.023   Displaced fracture of shaft of unspecified clavicle
  - ● S42.024   Nondisplaced fracture of shaft of right clavicle
  - ● S42.025   Nondisplaced fracture of shaft of left clavicle
  - ● S42.026   Nondisplaced fracture of shaft of unspecified clavicle
- ● S42.03   Fracture of lateral end of clavicle
  - Fracture of acromial end of clavicle
  - ● S42.031   Displaced fracture of lateral end of right clavicle
  - ● S42.032   Displaced fracture of lateral end of left clavicle
  - ● S42.033   Displaced fracture of lateral end of unspecified clavicle
  - ● S42.034   Nondisplaced fracture of lateral end of right clavicle
  - ● S42.035   Nondisplaced fracture of lateral end of left clavicle
  - ● S42.036   Nondisplaced fracture of lateral end of unspecified clavicle
- ● S42.1   Fracture of scapula
  - ● S42.10   Fracture of unspecified part of scapula
    - ● S42.101   Fracture of unspecified part of scapula, right shoulder
    - ● S42.102   Fracture of unspecified part of scapula, left shoulder
    - ● S42.109   Fracture of unspecified part of scapula, unspecified shoulder
  - ● S42.11   Fracture of body of scapula
    - ● S42.111   Displaced fracture of body of scapula, right shoulder
    - ● S42.112   Displaced fracture of body of scapula, left shoulder
    - ● S42.113   Displaced fracture of body of scapula, unspecified shoulder
    - ● S42.114   Nondisplaced fracture of body of scapula, right shoulder
    - ● S42.115   Nondisplaced fracture of body of scapula, left shoulder
    - ● S42.116   Nondisplaced fracture of body of scapula, unspecified shoulder

- ● S42.12   Fracture of acromial process
  - ● S42.121   Displaced fracture of acromial process, right shoulder
  - ● S42.122   Displaced fracture of acromial process, left shoulder
  - ● S42.123   Displaced fracture of acromial process, unspecified shoulder
  - ● S42.124   Nondisplaced fracture of acromial process, right shoulder
  - ● S42.125   Nondisplaced fracture of acromial process, left shoulder
  - ● S42.126   Nondisplaced fracture, of acromial process, unspecified shoulder
- ● S42.13   Fracture of coracoid process
  - ● S42.131   Displaced fracture of coracoid process, right shoulder
  - ● S42.132   Displaced fracture of coracoid process, left shoulder
  - ● S42.133   Displaced fracture of coracoid process, unspecified shoulder
  - ● S42.134   Nondisplaced fracture of coracoid process, right shoulder
  - ● S42.135   Nondisplaced fracture of coracoid process, left shoulder
  - ● S42.136   Nondisplaced fracture of coracoid process, unspecified shoulder
- ● S42.14   Fracture of glenoid cavity of scapula
  - ● S42.141   Displaced fracture of glenoid cavity of scapula, right shoulder
  - ● S42.142   Displaced fracture of glenoid cavity of scapula, left shoulder
  - ● S42.143   Displaced fracture of glenoid cavity of scapula, unspecified shoulder
  - ● S42.144   Nondisplaced fracture of glenoid cavity of scapula, right shoulder
  - ● S42.145   Nondisplaced fracture of glenoid cavity of scapula, left shoulder
  - ● S42.146   Nondisplaced fracture of glenoid cavity of scapula, unspecified shoulder
- ● S42.15   Fracture of neck of scapula
  - ● S42.151   Displaced fracture of neck of scapula, right shoulder
  - ● S42.152   Displaced fracture of neck of scapula, left shoulder
  - ● S42.153   Displaced fracture of neck of scapula, unspecified shoulder
  - ● S42.154   Nondisplaced fracture of neck of scapula, right shoulder
  - ● S42.155   Nondisplaced fracture of neck of scapula, left shoulder
  - ● S42.156   Nondisplaced fracture of neck of scapula, unspecified shoulder
- ● S42.19   Fracture of other part of scapula
  - ● S42.191   Fracture of other part of scapula, right shoulder
  - ● S42.192   Fracture of other part of scapula, left shoulder
  - ● S42.199   Fracture of other part of scapula, unspecified shoulder

▶ New   ⇰ Revised   ~~deleted~~ Deleted   **OGCR** Official Guidelines   X Assign placeholder X   ● Use Additional Character(s)

Excludes 1   Excludes 2   Includes   Use additional   Code first   Code also   Key words

● **S42.2**   Fracture of upper end of humerus
Fracture of proximal end of humerus
| Excludes2 | fracture of shaft of humerus (S42.3-)
physeal fracture of upper end of humerus (S49.0-)

● **S42.20**   Unspecified fracture of upper end of humerus
    ● **S42.201**   Unspecified fracture of upper end of right humerus
    ● **S42.202**   Unspecified fracture of upper end of left humerus
    ● **S42.209**   Unspecified fracture of upper end of unspecified humerus

● **S42.21**   Unspecified fracture of surgical neck of humerus
Fracture of neck of humerus NOS
    ● **S42.211**   Unspecified displaced fracture of surgical neck of right humerus
    ● **S42.212**   Unspecified displaced fracture of surgical neck of left humerus
    ● **S42.213**   Unspecified displaced fracture of surgical neck of unspecified humerus
    ● **S42.214**   Unspecified nondisplaced fracture of surgical neck of right humerus
    ● **S42.215**   Unspecified nondisplaced fracture of surgical neck of left humerus
    ● **S42.216**   Unspecified nondisplaced fracture of surgical neck of unspecified humerus

● **S42.22**   2-part fracture of surgical neck of humerus
    ● **S42.221**   2-part displaced fracture of surgical neck of right humerus
    ● **S42.222**   2-part displaced fracture of surgical neck of left humerus
    ● **S42.223**   2-part displaced fracture of surgical neck of unspecified humerus
    ● **S42.224**   2-part nondisplaced fracture of surgical neck of right humerus
    ● **S42.225**   2-part nondisplaced fracture of surgical neck of left humerus
    ● **S42.226**   2-part nondisplaced fracture of surgical neck of unspecified humerus

● **S42.23**   3-part fracture of surgical neck of humerus
    ● **S42.231**   3-part fracture of surgical neck of right humerus
    ● **S42.232**   3-part fracture of surgical neck of left humerus
    ● **S42.239**   3-part fracture of surgical neck of unspecified humerus

● **S42.24**   4-part fracture of surgical neck of humerus
    ● **S42.241**   4-part fracture of surgical neck of right humerus
    ● **S42.242**   4-part fracture of surgical neck of left humerus
    ● **S42.249**   4-part fracture of surgical neck of unspecified humerus

● **S42.25**   Fracture of greater tuberosity of humerus
    ● **S42.251**   Displaced fracture of greater tuberosity of right humerus
    ● **S42.252**   Displaced fracture of greater tuberosity of left humerus
    ● **S42.253**   Displaced fracture of greater tuberosity of unspecified humerus
    ● **S42.254**   Nondisplaced fracture of greater tuberosity of right humerus
    ● **S42.255**   Nondisplaced fracture of greater tuberosity of left humerus
    ● **S42.256**   Nondisplaced fracture of greater tuberosity of unspecified humerus

● **S42.26**   Fracture of lesser tuberosity of humerus
    ● **S42.261**   Displaced fracture of lesser tuberosity of right humerus
    ● **S42.262**   Displaced fracture of lesser tuberosity of left humerus
    ● **S42.263**   Displaced fracture of lesser tuberosity of unspecified humerus
    ● **S42.264**   Nondisplaced fracture of lesser tuberosity of right humerus
    ● **S42.265**   Nondisplaced fracture of lesser tuberosity of left humerus
    ● **S42.266**   Nondisplaced fracture of lesser tuberosity of unspecified humerus

● **S42.27**   Torus fracture of upper end of humerus
The appropriate 7th character is to be added to all codes in subcategory S42.27

> A   initial encounter for closed fracture
> D   subsequent encounter for fracture with routine healing
> G   subsequent encounter for fracture with delayed healing
> K   subsequent encounter for fracture with nonunion
> P   subsequent encounter for fracture with malunion
> S   sequela

    ● **S42.271**   Torus fracture of upper end of right humerus
    ● **S42.272**   Torus fracture of upper end of left humerus
    ● **S42.279**   Torus fracture of upper end of unspecified humerus

● **S42.29**   Other fracture of upper end of humerus
Fracture of anatomical neck of humerus
Fracture of articular head of humerus
    ● **S42.291**   Other displaced fracture of upper end of right humerus
    ● **S42.292**   Other displaced fracture of upper end of left humerus
    ● **S42.293**   Other displaced fracture of upper end of unspecified humerus
    ● **S42.294**   Other nondisplaced fracture of upper end of right humerus
    ● **S42.295**   Other nondisplaced fracture of upper end of left humerus
    ● **S42.296**   Other nondisplaced fracture of upper end of unspecified humerus

● **S42.3**   Fracture of shaft of humerus
Fracture of humerus NOS
Fracture of upper arm NOS
| Excludes2 | physeal fractures of upper end of humerus (S49.0-)
physeal fractures of lower end of humerus (S49.1-)

● **S42.30**   Unspecified fracture of shaft of humerus
    ● **S42.301**   Unspecified fracture of shaft of humerus, right arm
    ● **S42.302**   Unspecified fracture of shaft of humerus, left arm
    ● **S42.309**   Unspecified fracture of shaft of humerus, unspecified arm

CHAPTER 19 (S00-T88)

● **S42.31**   Greenstick fracture of shaft of humerus

The appropriate 7th character is to be added to all codes in subcategory S42.31

A	initial encounter for closed fracture
D	subsequent encounter for fracture with routine healing
G	subsequent encounter for fracture with delayed healing
K	subsequent encounter for fracture with nonunion
P	subsequent encounter for fracture with malunion
S	sequela

- ● **S42.311**   Greenstick fracture of shaft of humerus, **right** arm
- ● **S42.312**   Greenstick fracture of shaft of humerus, **left** arm
- ● **S42.319**   Greenstick fracture of shaft of humerus, **unspecified** arm

● **S42.32**   Transverse fracture of shaft of humerus

- ● **S42.321**   **Displaced** transverse fracture of shaft of humerus, **right** arm
- ● **S42.322**   **Displaced** transverse fracture of shaft of humerus, **left** arm
- ● **S42.323**   **Displaced** transverse fracture of shaft of humerus, **unspecified** arm
- ● **S42.324**   **Nondisplaced** transverse fracture of shaft of humerus, **right** arm
- ● **S42.325**   **Nondisplaced** transverse fracture of shaft of humerus, **left** arm
- ● **S42.326**   **Nondisplaced** transverse fracture of shaft of humerus, **unspecified** arm

● **S42.33**   Oblique fracture of shaft of humerus

- ● **S42.331**   **Displaced** oblique fracture of shaft of humerus, **right** arm
- ● **S42.332**   **Displaced** oblique fracture of shaft of humerus, **left** arm
- ● **S42.333**   **Displaced** oblique fracture of shaft of humerus, **unspecified** arm
- ● **S42.334**   **Nondisplaced** oblique fracture of shaft of humerus, **right** arm
- ● **S42.335**   **Nondisplaced** oblique fracture of shaft of humerus, **left** arm
- ● **S42.336**   **Nondisplaced** oblique fracture of shaft of humerus, **unspecified** arm

● **S42.34**   Spiral fracture of shaft of humerus

- ● **S42.341**   **Displaced** spiral fracture of shaft of humerus, **right** arm
- ● **S42.342**   **Displaced** spiral fracture of shaft of humerus, **left** arm
- ● **S42.343**   **Displaced** spiral fracture of shaft of humerus, **unspecified** arm
- ● **S42.344**   **Nondisplaced** spiral fracture of shaft of humerus, **right** arm
- ● **S42.345**   **Nondisplaced** spiral fracture of shaft of humerus, **left** arm
- ● **S42.346**   **Nondisplaced** spiral fracture of shaft of humerus, **unspecified** arm

● **S42.35**   Comminuted fracture of shaft of humerus

- ● **S42.351**   **Displaced** comminuted fracture of shaft of humerus, **right** arm
- ● **S42.352**   **Displaced** comminuted fracture of shaft of humerus, **left** arm
- ● **S42.353**   **Displaced** comminuted fracture of shaft of humerus, **unspecified** arm
- ● **S42.354**   **Nondisplaced** comminuted fracture of shaft of humerus, **right** arm
- ● **S42.355**   **Nondisplaced** comminuted fracture of shaft of humerus, **left** arm
- ● **S42.356**   **Nondisplaced** comminuted fracture of shaft of humerus, **unspecified** arm

● **S42.36**   Segmental fracture of shaft of humerus

- ● **S42.361**   **Displaced** segmental fracture of shaft of humerus, **right** arm
- ● **S42.362**   **Displaced** segmental fracture of shaft of humerus, **left** arm
- ● **S42.363**   **Displaced** segmental fracture of shaft of humerus, **unspecified** arm
- ● **S42.364**   **Nondisplaced** segmental fracture of shaft of humerus, **right** arm
- ● **S42.365**   **Nondisplaced** segmental fracture of shaft of humerus, **left** arm
- ● **S42.366**   **Nondisplaced** segmental fracture of shaft of humerus, **unspecified** arm

● **S42.39**   Other fracture of shaft of humerus

- ● **S42.391**   Other fracture of shaft of **right** humerus
- ● **S42.392**   Other fracture of shaft of **left** humerus
- ● **S42.399**   Other fracture of shaft of **unspecified** humerus

● **S42.4**   Fracture of lower end of humerus

Fracture of distal end of humerus

Excludes2	fracture of shaft of humerus (S42.3-)
	physeal fracture of lower end of humerus (S49.1-)

● **S42.40**   Unspecified fracture of lower end of humerus

Fracture of elbow NOS

- ● **S42.401**   Unspecified fracture of lower end of **right** humerus
- ● **S42.402**   Unspecified fracture of lower end of **left** humerus
- ● **S42.409**   Unspecified fracture of lower end of **unspecified** humerus

● **S42.41**   Simple supracondylar fracture without intercondylar fracture of humerus

- ● **S42.411**   **Displaced** simple supracondylar fracture without intercondylar fracture of **right** humerus
- ● **S42.412**   **Displaced** simple supracondylar fracture without intercondylar fracture of **left** humerus
- ● **S42.413**   **Displaced** simple supracondylar fracture without intercondylar fracture of **unspecified** humerus
- ● **S42.414**   **Nondisplaced** simple supracondylar fracture without intercondylar fracture of **right** humerus
- ● **S42.415**   **Nondisplaced** simple supracondylar fracture without intercondylar fracture of **left** humerus
- ● **S42.416**   **Nondisplaced** simple supracondylar fracture without intercondylar fracture of **unspecified** humerus

▶ New   ⇒ Revised   ~~deleted~~ Deleted   **OGCR** Official Guidelines   X Assign placeholder X   ● Use Additional Character(s)

| Excludes 1 | Excludes 2 | Includes | Use additional | Code first | Code also | Key words |

- ● **S42.42** **Comminuted supracondylar** fracture **without intercondylar fracture** of humerus
  - ● **S42.421** **Displaced** comminuted supracondylar fracture without intercondylar fracture of **right** humerus
  - ● **S42.422** **Displaced** comminuted supracondylar fracture without intercondylar fracture of **left** humerus
  - ● **S42.423** **Displaced** comminuted supracondylar fracture without intercondylar fracture of **unspecified** humerus
  - ● **S42.424** **Nondisplaced** comminuted supracondylar fracture without intercondylar fracture of **right** humerus
  - ● **S42.425** **Nondisplaced** comminuted supracondylar fracture without intercondylar fracture of **left** humerus
  - ● **S42.426** **Nondisplaced** comminuted supracondylar fracture without intercondylar fracture of **unspecified** humerus
- ● **S42.43** Fracture (avulsion) of **lateral epicondyle** of humerus
  - ● **S42.431** **Displaced** fracture (avulsion) of lateral epicondyle of **right** humerus
  - ● **S42.432** **Displaced** fracture (avulsion) of lateral epicondyle of **left** humerus
  - ● **S42.433** **Displaced** fracture (avulsion) of lateral epicondyle of **unspecified** humerus
  - ● **S42.434** **Nondisplaced** fracture (avulsion) of lateral epicondyle of **right** humerus
  - ● **S42.435** **Nondisplaced** fracture (avulsion) of lateral epicondyle of **left** humerus
  - ● **S42.436** **Nondisplaced** fracture (avulsion) of lateral epicondyle of **unspecified** humerus
- ● **S42.44** Fracture (avulsion) of **medial epicondyle** of humerus
  - ● **S42.441** **Displaced** fracture (avulsion) of medial epicondyle of **right** humerus
  - ● **S42.442** **Displaced** fracture (avulsion) of medial epicondyle of **left** humerus
  - ● **S42.443** **Displaced** fracture (avulsion) of medial epicondyle of **unspecified** humerus
  - ● **S42.444** **Nondisplaced** fracture (avulsion) of medial epicondyle of **right** humerus
  - ● **S42.445** **Nondisplaced** fracture (avulsion) of medial epicondyle of **left** humerus
  - ● **S42.446** **Nondisplaced** fracture (avulsion) of medial epicondyle of **unspecified** humerus
  - ● **S42.447** **Incarcerated** fracture (avulsion) of medial epicondyle of **right** humerus
  - ● **S42.448** **Incarcerated** fracture (avulsion) of medial epicondyle of **left** humerus
  - ● **S42.449** **Incarcerated** fracture (avulsion) of medial epicondyle of **unspecified** humerus

- ● **S42.45** Fracture of **lateral condyle** of humerus
  Fracture of capitellum of humerus
  - ● **S42.451** **Displaced** fracture of lateral condyle of **right** humerus
  - ● **S42.452** **Displaced** fracture of lateral condyle of **left** humerus
  - ● **S42.453** **Displaced** fracture of lateral condyle of **unspecified** humerus
  - ● **S42.454** **Nondisplaced** fracture of lateral condyle of **right** humerus
  - ● **S42.455** **Nondisplaced** fracture of lateral condyle of **left** humerus
  - ● **S42.456** **Nondisplaced** fracture of lateral condyle of **unspecified** humerus
- ● **S42.46** Fracture of **medial condyle** of humerus
  Trochlea fracture of humerus
  - ● **S42.461** **Displaced** fracture of medial condyle of **right** humerus
  - ● **S42.462** **Displaced** fracture of medial condyle of **left** humerus
  - ● **S42.463** **Displaced** fracture of medial condyle of **unspecified** humerus
  - ● **S42.464** **Nondisplaced** fracture of medial condyle of **right** humerus
  - ● **S42.465** **Nondisplaced** fracture of medial condyle of **left** humerus
  - ● **S42.466** **Nondisplaced** fracture of medial condyle of **unspecified** humerus
- ● **S42.47** **Transcondylar** fracture of humerus
  - ● **S42.471** **Displaced** transcondylar fracture of **right** humerus
  - ● **S42.472** **Displaced** transcondylar fracture of **left** humerus
  - ● **S42.473** **Displaced** transcondylar fracture of **unspecified** humerus
  - ● **S42.474** **Nondisplaced** transcondylar fracture of **right** humerus
  - ● **S42.475** **Nondisplaced** transcondylar fracture of **left** humerus
  - ● **S42.476** **Nondisplaced** transcondylar fracture of **unspecified** humerus
- ● **S42.48** **Torus** fracture of lower end of humerus

  The appropriate 7th character is to be added to all codes in subcategory S42.48

A	initial encounter for closed fracture
D	subsequent encounter for fracture with routine healing
G	subsequent encounter for fracture with delayed healing
K	subsequent encounter for fracture with nonunion
P	subsequent encounter for fracture with malunion
S	sequela

  - ● **S42.481** Torus fracture of lower end of **right** humerus
  - ● **S42.482** Torus fracture of lower end of **left** humerus
  - ● **S42.489** Torus fracture of lower end of **unspecified** humerus

CHAPTER 19 (S00-T88)

- **S42.49**   Other fracture of lower end of humerus
  - **S42.491**   Other displaced fracture of lower end of right humerus
  - **S42.492**   Other displaced fracture of lower end of left humerus
  - **S42.493**   Other displaced fracture of lower end of unspecified humerus
  - **S42.494**   Other nondisplaced fracture of lower end of right humerus
  - **S42.495**   Other nondisplaced fracture of lower end of left humerus
  - **S42.496**   Other nondisplaced fracture of lower end of unspecified humerus
- **S42.9**   Fracture of shoulder girdle, part unspecified
  - Fracture of shoulder NOS
  - X● **S42.90**   Fracture of unspecified shoulder girdle, part unspecified
  - X● **S42.91**   Fracture of right shoulder girdle, part unspecified
  - X● **S42.92**   Fracture of left shoulder girdle, part unspecified

- ● **S43**   Dislocation and sprain of joints and ligaments of shoulder girdle

  Includes   avulsion of joint or ligament of shoulder girdle
  - laceration of cartilage, joint or ligament of shoulder girdle
  - sprain of cartilage, joint or ligament of shoulder girdle
  - traumatic hemarthrosis of joint or ligament of shoulder girdle
  - traumatic rupture of joint or ligament of shoulder girdle
  - traumatic subluxation of joint or ligament of shoulder girdle
  - traumatic tear of joint or ligament of shoulder girdle

  Code also any associated open wound

  Excludes2   strain of muscle, fascia and tendon of shoulder and upper arm (S46.-)

  The appropriate 7th character is to be added to each code from category S43

A	initial encounter
D	subsequent encounter
S	sequela

- ● **S43.0**   Subluxation and dislocation of shoulder joint
  - Dislocation of glenohumeral joint
  - Subluxation of glenohumeral joint
  - ● **S43.00**   Unspecified subluxation and dislocation of shoulder joint
    - Dislocation of humerus NOS
    - Subluxation of humerus NOS
    - ● **S43.001**   Unspecified subluxation of right shoulder joint
    - ● **S43.002**   Unspecified subluxation of left shoulder joint
    - ● **S43.003**   Unspecified subluxation of unspecified shoulder joint
    - ● **S43.004**   Unspecified dislocation of right shoulder joint
    - ● **S43.005**   Unspecified dislocation of left shoulder joint
    - ● **S43.006**   Unspecified dislocation of unspecified shoulder joint

- ● **S43.01**   Anterior subluxation and dislocation of humerus
  - ● **S43.011**   Anterior subluxation of right humerus
  - ● **S43.012**   Anterior subluxation of left humerus
  - ● **S43.013**   Anterior subluxation of unspecified humerus
  - ● **S43.014**   Anterior dislocation of right humerus
  - ● **S43.015**   Anterior dislocation of left humerus
  - ● **S43.016**   Anterior dislocation of unspecified humerus
- ● **S43.02**   Posterior subluxation and dislocation of humerus
  - ● **S43.021**   Posterior subluxation of right humerus
  - ● **S43.022**   Posterior subluxation of left humerus
  - ● **S43.023**   Posterior subluxation of unspecified humerus
  - ● **S43.024**   Posterior dislocation of right humerus
  - ● **S43.025**   Posterior dislocation of left humerus
  - ● **S43.026**   Posterior dislocation of unspecified humerus
- ● **S43.03**   Inferior subluxation and dislocation of humerus
  - ● **S43.031**   Inferior subluxation of right humerus
  - ● **S43.032**   Inferior subluxation of left humerus
  - ● **S43.033**   Inferior subluxation of unspecified humerus
  - ● **S43.034**   Inferior dislocation of right humerus
  - ● **S43.035**   Inferior dislocation of left humerus
  - ● **S43.036**   Inferior dislocation of unspecified humerus
- ● **S43.08**   Other subluxation and dislocation of shoulder joint
  - ● **S43.081**   Other subluxation of right shoulder joint
  - ● **S43.082**   Other subluxation of left shoulder joint
  - ● **S43.083**   Other subluxation of unspecified shoulder joint
  - ● **S43.084**   Other dislocation of right shoulder joint
  - ● **S43.085**   Other dislocation of left shoulder joint
  - ● **S43.086**   Other dislocation of unspecified shoulder joint
- ● **S43.1**   Subluxation and dislocation of acromioclavicular joint
  - ● **S43.10**   Unspecified dislocation of acromioclavicular joint
    - ● **S43.101**   Unspecified dislocation of right acromioclavicular joint
    - ● **S43.102**   Unspecified dislocation of left acromioclavicular joint
    - ● **S43.109**   Unspecified dislocation of unspecified acromioclavicular joint
  - ● **S43.11**   Subluxation of acromioclavicular joint
    - ● **S43.111**   Subluxation of right acromioclavicular joint
    - ● **S43.112**   Subluxation of left acromioclavicular joint
    - ● **S43.119**   Subluxation of unspecified acromioclavicular joint

▶ New   ⇒ Revised   ~~deleted~~ Deleted   **OGCR** Official Guidelines   X Assign placeholder X   ● Use Additional Character(s)

Excludes 1   Excludes 2   Includes   Use additional   Code first   Code also   Key words

- S43.12   Dislocation of acromioclavicular joint, 100%-200% displacement
  - S43.121   Dislocation of right acromioclavicular joint, 100%-200% displacement
  - S43.122   Dislocation of left acromioclavicular joint, 100%-200% displacement
  - S43.129   Dislocation of unspecified acromioclavicular joint, 100%-200% displacement
- S43.13   Dislocation of acromioclavicular joint, greater than 200% displacement
  - S43.131   Dislocation of right acromioclavicular joint, greater than 200% displacement
  - S43.132   Dislocation of left acromioclavicular joint, greater than 200% displacement
  - S43.139   Dislocation of unspecified acromioclavicular joint, greater than 200% displacement
- S43.14   Inferior dislocation of acromioclavicular joint
  - S43.141   Inferior dislocation of right acromioclavicular joint
  - S43.142   Inferior dislocation of left acromioclavicular joint
  - S43.149   Inferior dislocation of unspecified acromioclavicular joint
- S43.15   Posterior dislocation of acromioclavicular joint
  - S43.151   Posterior dislocation of right acromioclavicular joint
  - S43.152   Posterior dislocation of left acromioclavicular joint
  - S43.159   Posterior dislocation of unspecified acromioclavicular joint
- S43.2   Subluxation and dislocation of sternoclavicular joint
  - S43.20   Unspecified subluxation and dislocation of sternoclavicular joint
    - S43.201   Unspecified subluxation of right sternoclavicular joint
    - S43.202   Unspecified subluxation of left sternoclavicular joint
    - S43.203   Unspecified subluxation of unspecified sternoclavicular joint
    - S43.204   Unspecified dislocation of right sternoclavicular joint
    - S43.205   Unspecified dislocation of left sternoclavicular joint
    - S43.206   Unspecified dislocation of unspecified sternoclavicular joint
  - S43.21   Anterior subluxation and dislocation of sternoclavicular joint
    - S43.211   Anterior subluxation of right sternoclavicular joint
    - S43.212   Anterior subluxation of left sternoclavicular joint
    - S43.213   Anterior subluxation of unspecified sternoclavicular joint
    - S43.214   Anterior dislocation of right sternoclavicular joint
    - S43.215   Anterior dislocation of left sternoclavicular joint
    - S43.216   Anterior dislocation of unspecified sternoclavicular joint
- S43.22   Posterior subluxation and dislocation of sternoclavicular joint
  - S43.221   Posterior subluxation of right sternoclavicular joint
  - S43.222   Posterior subluxation of left sternoclavicular joint
  - S43.223   Posterior subluxation of unspecified sternoclavicular joint
  - S43.224   Posterior dislocation of right sternoclavicular joint
  - S43.225   Posterior dislocation of left sternoclavicular joint
  - S43.226   Posterior dislocation of unspecified sternoclavicular joint
- S43.3   Subluxation and dislocation of other and unspecified parts of shoulder girdle
  - S43.30   Subluxation and dislocation of unspecified parts of shoulder girdle
    Dislocation of shoulder girdle NOS
    Subluxation of shoulder girdle NOS
    - S43.301   Subluxation of unspecified parts of right shoulder girdle
    - S43.302   Subluxation of unspecified parts of left shoulder girdle
    - S43.303   Subluxation of unspecified parts of unspecified shoulder girdle
    - S43.304   Dislocation of unspecified parts of right shoulder girdle
    - S43.305   Dislocation of unspecified parts of left shoulder girdle
    - S43.306   Dislocation of unspecified parts of unspecified shoulder girdle
  - S43.31   Subluxation and dislocation of scapula
    - S43.311   Subluxation of right scapula
    - S43.312   Subluxation of left scapula
    - S43.313   Subluxation of unspecified scapula
    - S43.314   Dislocation of right scapula
    - S43.315   Dislocation of left scapula
    - S43.316   Dislocation of unspecified scapula
  - S43.39   Subluxation and dislocation of other parts of shoulder girdle
    - S43.391   Subluxation of other parts of right shoulder girdle
    - S43.392   Subluxation of other parts of left shoulder girdle
    - S43.393   Subluxation of other parts of unspecified shoulder girdle
    - S43.394   Dislocation of other parts of right shoulder girdle
    - S43.395   Dislocation of other parts of left shoulder girdle
    - S43.396   Dislocation of other parts of unspecified shoulder girdle
- S43.4   Sprain of shoulder joint
  - S43.40   Unspecified sprain of shoulder joint
    - S43.401   Unspecified sprain of right shoulder joint
    - S43.402   Unspecified sprain of left shoulder joint
    - S43.409   Unspecified sprain of unspecified shoulder joint

- S43.41   Sprain of coracohumeral (ligament)
  - S43.411   Sprain of right coracohumeral (ligament)
  - S43.412   Sprain of left coracohumeral (ligament)
  - S43.419   Sprain of unspecified coracohumeral (ligament)
- S43.42   Sprain of rotator cuff capsule
  Encounters during the healing phase

  | **Excludes1** | rotator cuff syndrome (complete) (incomplete), not specified as traumatic (M75.1-) |

  | **Excludes2** | injury of tendon of rotator cuff (S46.0-) |

  - S43.421   Sprain of right rotator cuff capsule
  - S43.422   Sprain of left rotator cuff capsule
  - S43.429   Sprain of unspecified rotator cuff capsule
- S43.43   Superior glenoid labrum lesion
  SLAP lesion
  - S43.431   Superior glenoid labrum lesion of right shoulder
  - S43.432   Superior glenoid labrum lesion of left shoulder
  - S43.439   Superior glenoid labrum lesion of unspecified shoulder
- S43.49   Other sprain of shoulder joint
  - S43.491   Other sprain of right shoulder joint
  - S43.492   Other sprain of left shoulder joint
  - S43.499   Other sprain of unspecified shoulder joint
- S43.5   Sprain of acromioclavicular joint
  Sprain of acromioclavicular ligament
  - X● S43.50   Sprain of unspecified acromioclavicular joint
  - X● S43.51   Sprain of right acromioclavicular joint
  - X● S43.52   Sprain of left acromioclavicular joint
- S43.6   Sprain of sternoclavicular joint
  - X● S43.60   Sprain of unspecified sternoclavicular joint
  - X● S43.61   Sprain of right sternoclavicular joint
  - X● S43.62   Sprain of left sternoclavicular joint
- S43.8   Sprain of other specified parts of shoulder girdle
  - X● S43.80   Sprain of other specified parts of unspecified shoulder girdle
  - X● S43.81   Sprain of other specified parts of right shoulder girdle
  - X● S43.82   Sprain of other specified parts of left shoulder girdle
- S43.9   Sprain of unspecified parts of shoulder girdle
  - X● S43.90   Sprain of unspecified parts of unspecified shoulder girdle
    Sprain of shoulder girdle NOS
  - X● S43.91   Sprain of unspecified parts of right shoulder girdle
  - X● S43.92   Sprain of unspecified parts of left shoulder girdle

- S44   Injury of nerves at shoulder and upper arm level
  Code also any associated open wound (S41.-)

  | **Excludes2** | injury of brachial plexus (S14.3-) |

  The appropriate 7th character is to be added to each code from category S44

A	initial encounter
D	subsequent encounter
S	sequela

  - S44.0   Injury of ulnar nerve at upper arm level

    | **Excludes1** | ulnar nerve NOS (S54.0) |

    - X● S44.00   Injury of ulnar nerve at upper arm level, unspecified arm
    - X● S44.01   Injury of ulnar nerve at upper arm level, right arm
    - X● S44.02   Injury of ulnar nerve at upper arm level, left arm
  - S44.1   Injury of median nerve at upper arm level

    | **Excludes1** | median nerve NOS (S54.1) |

    - X● S44.10   Injury of median nerve at upper arm level, unspecified arm
    - X● S44.11   Injury of median nerve at upper arm level, right arm
    - X● S44.12   Injury of median nerve at upper arm level, left arm
  - S44.2   Injury of radial nerve at upper arm level

    | **Excludes1** | radial nerve NOS (S54.2) |

    - X● S44.20   Injury of radial nerve at upper arm level, unspecified arm
    - X● S44.21   Injury of radial nerve at upper arm level, right arm
    - X● S44.22   Injury of radial nerve at upper arm level, left arm
  - S44.3   Injury of axillary nerve
    - X● S44.30   Injury of axillary nerve, unspecified arm
    - X● S44.31   Injury of axillary nerve, right arm
    - X● S44.32   Injury of axillary nerve, left arm
  - S44.4   Injury of musculocutaneous nerve
    - X● S44.40   Injury of musculocutaneous nerve, unspecified arm
    - X● S44.41   Injury of musculocutaneous nerve, right arm
    - X● S44.42   Injury of musculocutaneous nerve, left arm
  - S44.5   Injury of cutaneous sensory nerve at shoulder and upper arm level
    - X● S44.50   Injury of cutaneous sensory nerve at shoulder and upper arm level, unspecified arm
    - X● S44.51   Injury of cutaneous sensory nerve at shoulder and upper arm level, right arm
    - X● S44.52   Injury of cutaneous sensory nerve at shoulder and upper arm level, left arm
  - S44.8   Injury of other nerves at shoulder and upper arm level
    - S44.8X   Injury of other nerves at shoulder and upper arm level
      - S44.8X1   Injury of other nerves at shoulder and upper arm level, right arm
      - S44.8X2   Injury of other nerves at shoulder and upper arm level, left arm
      - S44.8X9   Injury of other nerves at shoulder and upper arm level, unspecified arm
  - S44.9   Injury of unspecified nerve at shoulder and upper arm level
    - X● S44.90   Injury of unspecified nerve at shoulder and upper arm level, unspecified arm
    - X● S44.91   Injury of unspecified nerve at shoulder and upper arm level, right arm
    - X● S44.92   Injury of unspecified nerve at shoulder and upper arm level, left arm

▶ New   ⇒ Revised   ~~deleted~~ Deleted   **OGCR** Official Guidelines   X Assign placeholder X   ● Use Additional Character(s)

Excludes 1   Excludes 2   Includes   Use additional   Code first   Code also   Key words

● **S45   Injury of blood vessels at shoulder and upper arm level**

Code also any associated open wound (S41.-)

Excludes2   injury of subclavian artery (S25.1)
injury of subclavian vein (S25.3)

The appropriate 7th character is to be added to each code from category S45

A   initial encounter
D   subsequent encounter
S   sequela

● **S45.0   Injury of axillary artery**
  ● **S45.00   Unspecified injury of axillary artery**
    ● S45.001   Unspecified injury of axillary artery, right side
    ● S45.002   Unspecified injury of axillary artery, left side
    ● S45.009   Unspecified injury of axillary artery, unspecified side
  ● **S45.01   Laceration of axillary artery**
    ● S45.011   Laceration of axillary artery, right side
    ● S45.012   Laceration of axillary artery, left side
    ● S45.019   Laceration of axillary artery, unspecified side
  ● **S45.09   Other specified injury of axillary artery**
    ● S45.091   Other specified injury of axillary artery, right side
    ● S45.092   Other specified injury of axillary artery, left side
    ● S45.099   Other specified injury of axillary artery, unspecified side

● **S45.1   Injury of brachial artery**
  ● **S45.10   Unspecified injury of brachial artery**
    ● S45.101   Unspecified injury of brachial artery, right side
    ● S45.102   Unspecified injury of brachial artery, left side
    ● S45.109   Unspecified injury of brachial artery, unspecified side
  ● **S45.11   Laceration of brachial artery**
    ● S45.111   Laceration of brachial artery, right side
    ● S45.112   Laceration of brachial artery, left side
    ● S45.119   Laceration of brachial artery, unspecified side
  ● **S45.19   Other specified injury of brachial artery**
    ● S45.191   Other specified injury of brachial artery, right side
    ● S45.192   Other specified injury of brachial artery, left side
    ● S45.199   Other specified injury of brachial artery, unspecified side

● **S45.2   Injury of axillary or brachial vein**
  ● **S45.20   Unspecified injury of axillary or brachial vein**
    ● S45.201   Unspecified injury of axillary or brachial vein, right side
    ● S45.202   Unspecified injury of axillary or brachial vein, left side
    ● S45.209   Unspecified injury of axillary or brachial vein, unspecified side
  ● **S45.21   Laceration of axillary or brachial vein**
    ● S45.211   Laceration of axillary or brachial vein, right side
    ● S45.212   Laceration of axillary or brachial vein, left side
    ● S45.219   Laceration of axillary or brachial vein, unspecified side

  ● **S45.29   Other specified injury of axillary or brachial vein**
    ● S45.291   Other specified injury of axillary or brachial vein, right side
    ● S45.292   Other specified injury of axillary or brachial vein, left side
    ● S45.299   Other specified injury of axillary or brachial vein, unspecified side

● **S45.3   Injury of superficial vein at shoulder and upper arm level**
  ● **S45.30   Unspecified injury of superficial vein at shoulder and upper arm level**
    ● S45.301   Unspecified injury of superficial vein at shoulder and upper arm level, right arm
    ● S45.302   Unspecified injury of superficial vein at shoulder and upper arm level, left arm
    ● S45.309   Unspecified injury of superficial vein at shoulder and upper arm level, unspecified arm
  ● **S45.31   Laceration of superficial vein at shoulder and upper arm level**
    ● S45.311   Laceration of superficial vein at shoulder and upper arm level, right arm
    ● S45.312   Laceration of superficial vein at shoulder and upper arm level, left arm
    ● S45.319   Laceration of superficial vein at shoulder and upper arm level, unspecified arm
  ● **S45.39   Other specified injury of superficial vein at shoulder and upper arm level**
    ● S45.391   Other specified injury of superficial vein at shoulder and upper arm level, right arm
    ● S45.392   Other specified injury of superficial vein at shoulder and upper arm level, left arm
    ● S45.399   Other specified injury of superficial vein at shoulder and upper arm level, unspecified arm

● **S45.8   Injury of other specified blood vessels at shoulder and upper arm level**
  ● **S45.80   Unspecified injury of other specified blood vessels at shoulder and upper arm level**
    ● S45.801   Unspecified injury of other specified blood vessels at shoulder and upper arm level, right arm
    ● S45.802   Unspecified injury of other specified blood vessels at shoulder and upper arm level, left arm
    ● S45.809   Unspecified injury of other specified blood vessels at shoulder and upper arm level, unspecified arm
  ● **S45.81   Laceration of other specified blood vessels at shoulder and upper arm level**
    ● S45.811   Laceration of other specified blood vessels at shoulder and upper arm level, right arm
    ● S45.812   Laceration of other specified blood vessels at shoulder and upper arm level, left arm
    ● S45.819   Laceration of other specified blood vessels at shoulder and upper arm level, unspecified arm

CHAPTER 19 (S00-T88)

● S45.89   **Other** specified injury of other specified blood vessels at shoulder and upper arm level

     ● S45.891   Other specified injury of other specified blood vessels at shoulder and upper arm level, **right** arm

     ● S45.892   Other specified injury of other specified blood vessels at shoulder and upper arm level, **left** arm

     ● S45.899   Other specified injury of other specified blood vessels at shoulder and upper arm level, **unspecified** arm

● S45.9   Injury of **unspecified blood vessel** at shoulder and upper arm level

     ● S45.90   **Unspecified** injury of unspecified blood vessel at shoulder and upper arm level

         ● S45.901   Unspecified injury of unspecified blood vessel at shoulder and upper arm level, **right** arm

         ● S45.902   Unspecified injury of unspecified blood vessel at shoulder and upper arm level, **left** arm

         ● S45.909   Unspecified injury of unspecified blood vessel at shoulder and upper arm level, **unspecified** arm

     ● S45.91   **Laceration** of unspecified blood vessel at shoulder and upper arm level

         ● S45.911   Laceration of unspecified blood vessel at shoulder and upper arm level, **right** arm

         ● S45.912   Laceration of unspecified blood vessel at shoulder and upper arm level, **left** arm

         ● S45.919   Laceration of unspecified blood vessel at shoulder and upper arm level, **unspecified** arm

     ● S45.99   **Other** specified injury of unspecified blood vessel at shoulder and upper arm level

         ● S45.991   Other specified injury of unspecified blood vessel at shoulder and upper arm level, **right** arm

         ● S45.992   Other specified injury of unspecified blood vessel at shoulder and upper arm level, **left** arm

         ● S45.999   Other specified injury of unspecified blood vessel at shoulder and upper arm level, **unspecified** arm

● S46   Injury of muscle, fascia and tendon at shoulder and upper arm level

     Code also any associated open wound (S41.-)

     Excludes2   injury of muscle, fascia and tendon at elbow (S56.-)

         sprain of joints and ligaments of shoulder girdle (S43.9)

     The appropriate 7th character is to be added to each code from category S46

         A   initial encounter
         D   subsequent encounter
         S   sequela

● S46.0   Injury of muscle(s) and tendon(s) of the **rotator cuff** of shoulder

     ● S46.00   **Unspecified** injury of muscle(s) and tendon(s) of the rotator cuff of shoulder

         ● S46.001   Unspecified injury of muscle(s) and tendon(s) of the rotator cuff of **right** shoulder

         ● S46.002   Unspecified injury of muscle(s) and tendon(s) of the rotator cuff of **left** shoulder

         ● S46.009   Unspecified injury of muscle(s) and tendon(s) of the rotator cuff of **unspecified** shoulder

● S46.01   **Strain** of muscle(s) and tendon(s) of the rotator cuff of shoulder

     Acute onset due to trauma to rotator cuff muscle/tendon

     ● S46.011   Strain of muscle(s) and tendon(s) of the rotator cuff of **right** shoulder

     ● S46.012   Strain of muscle(s) and tendon(s) of the rotator cuff of **left** shoulder

     ● S46.019   Strain of muscle(s) and tendon(s) of the rotator cuff of **unspecified** shoulder

● S46.02   **Laceration** of muscle(s) and tendon(s) of the rotator cuff of shoulder

     ● S46.021   Laceration of muscle(s) and tendon(s) of the rotator cuff of **right** shoulder

     ● S46.022   Laceration of muscle(s) and tendon(s) of the rotator cuff of **left** shoulder

     ● S46.029   Laceration of muscle(s) and tendon(s) of the rotator cuff of **unspecified** shoulder

● S46.09   **Other** injury of muscle(s) and tendon(s) of the rotator cuff of shoulder

     ● S46.091   Other injury of muscle(s) and tendon(s) of the rotator cuff of **right** shoulder

     ● S46.092   Other injury of muscle(s) and tendon(s) of the rotator cuff of **left** shoulder

     ● S46.099   Other injury of muscle(s) and tendon(s) of the rotator cuff of **unspecified** shoulder

● S46.1   Injury of muscle, fascia and tendon of long **head of biceps**

     ● S46.10   **Unspecified** injury of muscle, fascia and tendon of long head of biceps

         ● S46.101   Unspecified injury of muscle, fascia and tendon of long head of biceps, **right** arm

         ● S46.102   Unspecified injury of muscle, fascia and tendon of long head of biceps, **left** arm

         ● S46.109   Unspecified injury of muscle, fascia and tendon of long head of biceps, **unspecified** arm

     ● S46.11   Strain of muscle, fascia and tendon of long **head** of biceps

         ● S46.111   Strain of muscle, fascia and tendon of long head of biceps, **right** arm

         ● S46.112   Strain of muscle, fascia and tendon of long head of biceps, **left** arm

         ● S46.119   Strain of muscle, fascia and tendon of long head of biceps, **unspecified** arm

     ● S46.12   **Laceration** of muscle, fascia and tendon of long head of biceps

         ● S46.121   Laceration of muscle, fascia and tendon of long head of biceps, **right** arm

         ● S46.122   Laceration of muscle, fascia and tendon of long head of biceps, **left** arm

         ● S46.129   Laceration of muscle, fascia and tendon of long head of biceps, **unspecified** arm

- S46.19   Other injury of muscle, fascia and tendon of long head of biceps
  - S46.191   Other injury of muscle, fascia and tendon of long head of biceps, right arm
  - S46.192   Other injury of muscle, fascia and tendon of long head of biceps, left arm
  - S46.199   Other injury of muscle, fascia and tendon of long head of biceps, unspecified arm
- S46.2   Injury of muscle, fascia and tendon of other parts of biceps
  - S46.20   Unspecified injury of muscle, fascia and tendon of other parts of biceps
    - S46.201   Unspecified injury of muscle, fascia and tendon of other parts of biceps, right arm
    - S46.202   Unspecified injury of muscle, fascia and tendon of other parts of biceps, left arm
    - S46.209   Unspecified injury of muscle, fascia and tendon of other parts of biceps, unspecified arm
  - S46.21   Strain of muscle, fascia and tendon of other parts of biceps
    - S46.211   Strain of muscle, fascia and tendon of other parts of biceps, right arm
    - S46.212   Strain of muscle, fascia and tendon of other parts of biceps, left arm
    - S46.219   Strain of muscle, fascia and tendon of other parts of biceps, unspecified arm
  - S46.22   Laceration of muscle, fascia and tendon of other parts of biceps
    - S46.221   Laceration of muscle, fascia and tendon of other parts of biceps, right arm
    - S46.222   Laceration of muscle, fascia and tendon of other parts of biceps, left arm
    - S46.229   Laceration of muscle, fascia and tendon of other parts of biceps, unspecified arm
  - S46.29   Other injury of muscle, fascia and tendon of other parts of biceps
    - S46.291   Other injury of muscle, fascia and tendon of other parts of biceps, right arm
    - S46.292   Other injury of muscle, fascia and tendon of other parts of biceps, left arm
    - S46.299   Other injury of muscle, fascia and tendon of other parts of biceps, unspecified arm
- S46.3   Injury of muscle, fascia and tendon of triceps
  - S46.30   Unspecified injury of muscle, fascia and tendon of triceps
    - S46.301   Unspecified injury of muscle, fascia and tendon of triceps, right arm
    - S46.302   Unspecified injury of muscle, fascia and tendon of triceps, left arm
    - S46.309   Unspecified injury of muscle, fascia and tendon of triceps, unspecified arm

- S46.31   Strain of muscle, fascia and tendon of triceps
  - S46.311   Strain of muscle, fascia and tendon of triceps, right arm
  - S46.312   Strain of muscle, fascia and tendon of triceps, left arm
  - S46.319   Strain of muscle, fascia and tendon of triceps, unspecified arm
- S46.32   Laceration of muscle, fascia and tendon of triceps
  - S46.321   Laceration of muscle, fascia and tendon of triceps, right arm
  - S46.322   Laceration of muscle, fascia and tendon of triceps, left arm
  - S46.329   Laceration of muscle, fascia and tendon of triceps, unspecified arm
- S46.39   Other injury of muscle, fascia and tendon of triceps
  - S46.391   Other injury of muscle, fascia and tendon of triceps, right arm
  - S46.392   Other injury of muscle, fascia and tendon of triceps, left arm
  - S46.399   Other injury of muscle, fascia and tendon of triceps, unspecified arm
- S46.8   Injury of other muscles, fascia and tendons at shoulder and upper arm level
  - S46.80   Unspecified injury of other muscles, fascia and tendons at shoulder and upper arm level
    - S46.801   Unspecified injury of other muscles, fascia and tendons at shoulder and upper arm level, right arm
    - S46.802   Unspecified injury of other muscles, fascia and tendons at shoulder and upper arm level, left arm
    - S46.809   Unspecified injury of other muscles, fascia and tendons at shoulder and upper arm level, unspecified arm
  - S46.81   Strain of other muscles, fascia and tendons at shoulder and upper arm level
    - S46.811   Strain of other muscles, fascia and tendons at shoulder and upper arm level, right arm
    - S46.812   Strain of other muscles, fascia and tendons at shoulder and upper arm level, left arm
    - S46.819   Strain of other muscles, fascia and tendons at shoulder and upper arm level, unspecified arm
  - S46.82   Laceration of other muscles, fascia and tendons at shoulder and upper arm level
    - S46.821   Laceration of other muscles, fascia and tendons at shoulder and upper arm level, right arm
    - S46.822   Laceration of other muscles, fascia and tendons at shoulder and upper arm level, left arm
    - S46.829   Laceration of other muscles, fascia and tendons at shoulder and upper arm level, unspecified arm
  - S46.89   Other injury of other muscles, fascia and tendons at shoulder and upper arm level
    - S46.891   Other injury of other muscles, fascia and tendons at shoulder and upper arm level, right arm
    - S46.892   Other injury of other muscles, fascia and tendons at shoulder and upper arm level, left arm
    - S46.899   Other injury of other muscles, fascia and tendons at shoulder and upper arm level, unspecified arm

CHAPTER 19 (S00-T88)

● S46.9   Injury of unspecified muscle, fascia and tendon at shoulder and upper arm level

  ● S46.90   Unspecified injury of unspecified muscle, fascia and tendon at shoulder and upper arm level

    ● S46.901   Unspecified injury of unspecified muscle, fascia and tendon at shoulder and upper arm level, right arm

    ● S46.902   Unspecified injury of unspecified muscle, fascia and tendon at shoulder and upper arm level, left arm

    ● S46.909   Unspecified injury of unspecified muscle, fascia and tendon at shoulder and upper arm level, unspecified arm

  ● S46.91   Strain of unspecified muscle, fascia and tendon at shoulder and upper arm level

    ● S46.911   Strain of unspecified muscle, fascia and tendon at shoulder and upper arm level, right arm

    ● S46.912   Strain of unspecified muscle, fascia and tendon at shoulder and upper arm level, left arm

    ● S46.919   Strain of unspecified muscle, fascia and tendon at shoulder and upper arm level, unspecified arm

  ● S46.92   Laceration of unspecified muscle, fascia and tendon at shoulder and upper arm level

    ● S46.921   Laceration of unspecified muscle, fascia and tendon at shoulder and upper arm level, right arm

    ● S46.922   Laceration of unspecified muscle, fascia and tendon at shoulder and upper arm level, left arm

    ● S46.929   Laceration of unspecified muscle, fascia and tendon at shoulder and upper arm level, unspecified arm

  ● S46.99   Other injury of unspecified muscle, fascia and tendon at shoulder and upper arm level

    ● S46.991   Other injury of unspecified muscle, fascia and tendon at shoulder and upper arm level, right arm

    ● S46.992   Other injury of unspecified muscle, fascia and tendon at shoulder and upper arm level, left arm

    ● S46.999   Other injury of unspecified muscle, fascia and tendon at shoulder and upper arm level, unspecified arm

● S47   Crushing injury of shoulder and upper arm

  Use additional code for all associated injuries

  Excludes2   crushing injury of elbow (S57.0-)

  The appropriate 7th character is to be added to each code from category S47

    A   initial encounter
    D   subsequent encounter
    S   sequela

X ● S47.1   Crushing injury of right shoulder and upper arm

X ● S47.2   Crushing injury of left shoulder and upper arm

X ● S47.9   Crushing injury of shoulder and upper arm, unspecified arm

● S48   Traumatic amputation of shoulder and upper arm

  An amputation not identified as partial or complete should be coded to complete

  Excludes1   traumatic amputation at elbow level (S58.0)

  The appropriate 7th character is to be added to each code from category S48

    A   initial encounter
    D   subsequent encounter
    S   sequela

  ● S48.0   Traumatic amputation at shoulder joint

    ● S48.01   Complete traumatic amputation at shoulder joint

      ● S48.011   Complete traumatic amputation at right shoulder joint

      ● S48.012   Complete traumatic amputation at left shoulder joint

      ● S48.019   Complete traumatic amputation at unspecified shoulder joint

    ● S48.02   Partial traumatic amputation at shoulder joint

      ● S48.021   Partial traumatic amputation at right shoulder joint

      ● S48.022   Partial traumatic amputation at left shoulder joint

      ● S48.029   Partial traumatic amputation at unspecified shoulder joint

  ● S48.1   Traumatic amputation at level between shoulder and elbow

    ● S48.11   Complete traumatic amputation at level between shoulder and elbow

      ● S48.111   Complete traumatic amputation at level between right shoulder and elbow

      ● S48.112   Complete traumatic amputation at level between left shoulder and elbow

      ● S48.119   Complete traumatic amputation at level between unspecified shoulder and elbow

    ● S48.12   Partial traumatic amputation at level between shoulder and elbow

      ● S48.121   Partial traumatic amputation at level between right shoulder and elbow

      ● S48.122   Partial traumatic amputation at level between left shoulder and elbow

      ● S48.129   Partial traumatic amputation at level between unspecified shoulder and elbow

  ● S48.9   Traumatic amputation of shoulder and upper arm, level unspecified

    ● S48.91   Complete traumatic amputation of shoulder and upper arm, level unspecified

      ● S48.911   Complete traumatic amputation of right shoulder and upper arm, level unspecified

      ● S48.912   Complete traumatic amputation of left shoulder and upper arm, level unspecified

      ● S48.919   Complete traumatic amputation of unspecified shoulder and upper arm, level unspecified

▶ New   ⇒ Revised   ~~deleted~~ Deleted   OGCR Official Guidelines   X Assign placeholder X   ● Use Additional Character(s)

Excludes 1   Excludes 2   Includes   Use additional   Code first   Code also   Key words

● S48.92   Partial traumatic amputation of shoulder and upper arm, level unspecified
   ● S48.921   Partial traumatic amputation of right shoulder and upper arm, level unspecified
   ● S48.922   Partial traumatic amputation of left shoulder and upper arm, level unspecified
   ● S48.929   Partial traumatic amputation of unspecified shoulder and upper arm, level unspecified

● S49   Other and unspecified injuries of shoulder and upper arm

The appropriate 7th character is to be added to each code from subcategories S49.0 and S49.1

A	initial encounter for closed fracture
D	subsequent encounter for fracture with routine healing
G	subsequent encounter for fracture with delayed healing
K	subsequent encounter for fracture with nonunion
P	subsequent encounter for fracture with malunion
S	sequela

● S49.0   Physeal fracture of upper end of humerus
  ● S49.00   Unspecified physeal fracture of upper end of humerus
   ● S49.001   Unspecified physeal fracture of upper end of humerus, right arm
   ● S49.002   Unspecified physeal fracture of upper end of humerus, left arm
   ● S49.009   Unspecified physeal fracture of upper end of humerus, unspecified arm
  ● S49.01   Salter-Harris Type I physeal fracture of upper end of humerus
   ● S49.011   Salter-Harris Type I physeal fracture of upper end of humerus, right arm
   ● S49.012   Salter-Harris Type I physeal fracture of upper end of humerus, left arm
   ● S49.019   Salter-Harris Type I physeal fracture of upper end of humerus, unspecified arm
  ● S49.02   Salter-Harris Type II physeal fracture of upper end of humerus
   ● S49.021   Salter-Harris Type II physeal fracture of upper end of humerus, right arm
   ● S49.022   Salter-Harris Type II physeal fracture of upper end of humerus, left arm
   ● S49.029   Salter-Harris Type II physeal fracture of upper end of humerus, unspecified arm
  ● S49.03   Salter-Harris Type III physeal fracture of upper end of humerus
   ● S49.031   Salter-Harris Type III physeal fracture of upper end of humerus, right arm
   ● S49.032   Salter-Harris Type III physeal fracture of upper end of humerus, left arm
   ● S49.039   Salter-Harris Type III physeal fracture of upper end of humerus, unspecified arm

● S49.04   Salter-Harris Type IV physeal fracture of upper end of humerus
   ● S49.041   Salter-Harris Type IV physeal fracture of upper end of humerus, right arm
   ● S49.042   Salter-Harris Type IV physeal fracture of upper end of humerus, left arm
   ● S49.049   Salter-Harris Type IV physeal fracture of upper end of humerus, unspecified arm
  ● S49.09   Other physeal fracture of upper end of humerus
   ● S49.091   Other physeal fracture of upper end of humerus, right arm
   ● S49.092   Other physeal fracture of upper end of humerus, left arm
   ● S49.099   Other physeal fracture of upper end of humerus, unspecified arm

● S49.1   Physeal fracture of lower end of humerus
  ● S49.10   Unspecified physeal fracture of lower end of humerus
   ● S49.101   Unspecified physeal fracture of lower end of humerus, right arm
   ● S49.102   Unspecified physeal fracture of lower end of humerus, left arm
   ● S49.109   Unspecified physeal fracture of lower end of humerus, unspecified arm
  ● S49.11   Salter-Harris Type I physeal fracture of lower end of humerus
   ● S49.111   Salter-Harris Type I physeal fracture of lower end of humerus, right arm
   ● S49.112   Salter-Harris Type I physeal fracture of lower end of humerus, left arm
   ● S49.119   Salter-Harris Type I physeal fracture of lower end of humerus, unspecified arm
  ● S49.12   Salter-Harris Type II physeal fracture of lower end of humerus
   ● S49.121   Salter-Harris Type II physeal fracture of lower end of humerus, right arm
   ● S49.122   Salter-Harris Type II physeal fracture of lower end of humerus, left arm
   ● S49.129   Salter-Harris Type II physeal fracture of lower end of humerus, unspecified arm
  ● S49.13   Salter-Harris Type III physeal fracture of lower end of humerus
   ● S49.131   Salter-Harris Type III physeal fracture of lower end of humerus, right arm
   ● S49.132   Salter-Harris Type III physeal fracture of lower end of humerus, left arm
   ● S49.139   Salter-Harris Type III physeal fracture of lower end of humerus, unspecified arm
  ● S49.14   Salter-Harris Type IV physeal fracture of lower end of humerus
   ● S49.141   Salter-Harris Type IV physeal fracture of lower end of humerus, right arm
   ● S49.142   Salter-Harris Type IV physeal fracture of lower end of humerus, left arm
   ● S49.149   Salter-Harris Type IV physeal fracture of lower end of humerus, unspecified arm
  ● S49.19   Other physeal fracture of lower end of humerus
   ● S49.191   Other physeal fracture of lower end of humerus, right arm
   ● S49.192   Other physeal fracture of lower end of humerus, left arm
   ● S49.199   Other physeal fracture of lower end of humerus, unspecified arm

Item 19–3 SALTER-HARRIS TYPE 1: epiphysis is completely separated from end of bone, or metaphysic growth plate remains attached to epiphysis

SALTER-HARRIS TYPE 2: epiphysis and growth plate are partially separated from metaphysis, which is cracked—most common type

SALTER-HARRIS TYPE 3: fracture occurring through epiphysis and separates part of epiphysis and growth plate from metaphysis fracture, usually at distal end of tibia

SALTER-HARRIS TYPE 4: fracture runs through epiphysis, across growth plate, into metaphysic, surgery is required to restore joint surface to normal and align growth plate

CHAPTER 19 (S00-T88)

▶ New   ⇒ Revised   ~~deleted~~ Deleted   **OGCR** Official Guidelines   X Assign placeholder X   ● Use Additional Character(s)

Excludes 1	Excludes 2	Includes	Use additional	Code first	Code also	Key words

- ● **S49.8** **Other** specified injuries of shoulder and upper arm

  The appropriate 7th character is to be added to each code in subcategory S49.8

A	initial encounter
D	subsequent encounter
S	sequela

  - X● **S49.80** Other specified injuries of shoulder and upper arm, **unspecified** arm
  - X● **S49.81** Other specified injuries of **right** shoulder and upper arm
  - X● **S49.82** Other specified injuries of **left** shoulder and upper arm

- ● **S49.9** **Unspecified** injury of shoulder and upper arm

  The appropriate 7th character is to be added to each code in subcategory S49.9

A	initial encounter
D	subsequent encounter
S	sequela

  - X● **S49.90** Unspecified injury of shoulder and upper arm, **unspecified** arm
  - X● **S49.91** Unspecified injury of **right** shoulder and upper arm
  - X● **S49.92** Unspecified injury of **left** shoulder and upper arm

INJURIES TO THE ELBOW AND FOREARM (S50-S59)

Excludes2   burns and corrosions (T20-T32)
frostbite (T33-T34)
injuries of wrist and hand (S60-S69)
insect bite or sting, venomous (T63.4)

- ● **S50** Superficial injury of elbow and forearm

  Excludes2   superficial injury of wrist and hand (S60.-)

  The appropriate 7th character is to be added to each code from category S50

A	initial encounter
D	subsequent encounter
S	sequela

  - ● **S50.0** Contusion of **elbow**
    - X● **S50.00** Contusion of **unspecified** elbow
    - X● **S50.01** Contusion of **right** elbow
    - X● **S50.02** Contusion of **left** elbow
  - ● **S50.1** Contusion of **forearm**
    - X● **S50.10** Contusion of **unspecified** forearm
    - X● **S50.11** Contusion of **right** forearm
    - X● **S50.12** Contusion of **left** forearm
  - ● **S50.3** Other superficial injuries of **elbow**
    - ● **S50.31** **Abrasion** of elbow
      - ● **S50.311** Abrasion of **right** elbow
      - ● **S50.312** Abrasion of **left** elbow
      - ● **S50.319** Abrasion of **unspecified** elbow
    - ● **S50.32** **Blister** (nonthermal) of elbow
      - ● **S50.321** Blister (nonthermal) of **right** elbow
      - ● **S50.322** Blister (nonthermal) of **left** elbow
      - ● **S50.329** Blister (nonthermal) of **unspecified** elbow
    - ● **S50.34** **External constriction** of elbow
      - ● **S50.341** External constriction of **right** elbow
      - ● **S50.342** External constriction of **left** elbow
      - ● **S50.349** External constriction of **unspecified** elbow

- ● **S50.35** **Superficial foreign body** of elbow
  Splinter in the elbow
  - ● **S50.351** Superficial foreign body of **right** elbow
  - ● **S50.352** Superficial foreign body of **left** elbow
  - ● **S50.359** Superficial foreign body of **unspecified** elbow
- ● **S50.36** **Insect bite** (nonvenomous) of elbow
  - ● **S50.361** Insect bite (nonvenomous) of **right** elbow
  - ● **S50.362** Insect bite (nonvenomous) of **left** elbow
  - ● **S50.369** Insect bite (nonvenomous) of **unspecified** elbow
- ● **S50.37** **Other superficial bite** of elbow
  Excludes1   open bite of elbow (S51.04)
  - ● **S50.371** Other superficial bite of **right** elbow
  - ● **S50.372** Other superficial bite of **left** elbow
  - ● **S50.379** Other superficial bite of **unspecified** elbow
- ● **S50.8** Other superficial injuries of **forearm**
  - ● **S50.81** **Abrasion** of forearm
    - ● **S50.811** Abrasion of **right** forearm
    - ● **S50.812** Abrasion of **left** forearm
    - ● **S50.819** Abrasion of **unspecified** forearm
  - ● **S50.82** **Blister** (nonthermal) of forearm
    - ● **S50.821** Blister (nonthermal) of **right** forearm
    - ● **S50.822** Blister (nonthermal) of **left** forearm
    - ● **S50.829** Blister (nonthermal) of **unspecified** forearm
  - ● **S50.84** **External constriction** of forearm
    - ● **S50.841** External constriction of **right** forearm
    - ● **S50.842** External constriction of **left** forearm
    - ● **S50.849** External constriction of **unspecified** forearm
  - ● **S50.85** **Superficial foreign body** of forearm
    Splinter in the forearm
    - ● **S50.851** Superficial foreign body of **right** forearm
    - ● **S50.852** Superficial foreign body of **left** forearm
    - ● **S50.859** Superficial foreign body of **unspecified** forearm
  - ● **S50.86** **Insect bite** (nonvenomous) of forearm
    - ● **S50.861** Insect bite (nonvenomous) of **right** forearm
    - ● **S50.862** Insect bite (nonvenomous) of **left** forearm
    - ● **S50.869** Insect bite (nonvenomous) of **unspecified** forearm
  - ● **S50.87** **Other superficial bite** of forearm
    Excludes1   open bite of forearm (S51.84)
    - ● **S50.871** Other superficial bite of **right** forearm
    - ● **S50.872** Other superficial bite of **left** forearm
    - ● **S50.879** Other superficial bite of **unspecified** forearm

● **S50.9**   Unspecified superficial injury of elbow and forearm
   ● **S50.90**   Unspecified superficial injury of elbow
     ● **S50.901**   Unspecified superficial injury of right elbow
     ● **S50.902**   Unspecified superficial injury of left elbow
     ● **S50.909**   Unspecified superficial injury of unspecified elbow
   ● **S50.91**   Unspecified superficial injury of forearm
     ● **S50.911**   Unspecified superficial injury of right forearm
     ● **S50.912**   Unspecified superficial injury of left forearm
     ● **S50.919**   Unspecified superficial injury of unspecified forearm

● **S51**   Open wound of elbow and forearm
   Code also any associated wound infection
   Excludes1   open fracture of elbow and forearm (S52.- with open fracture 7th character)
         traumatic amputation of elbow and forearm (S58.-)
   Excludes2   open wound of wrist and hand (S61.-)
   The appropriate 7th character is to be added to each code from category S51

     A   initial encounter
     D   subsequent encounter
     S   sequela

   ● **S51.0**   Open wound of elbow
     ● **S51.00**   Unspecified open wound of elbow
       ● **S51.001**   Unspecified open wound of right elbow
       ● **S51.002**   Unspecified open wound of left elbow
       ● **S51.009**   Unspecified open wound of unspecified elbow
          Open wound of elbow NOS
     ● **S51.01**   Laceration without foreign body of elbow
       ● **S51.011**   Laceration without foreign body of right elbow
       ● **S51.012**   Laceration without foreign body of left elbow
       ● **S51.019**   Laceration without foreign body of unspecified elbow
     ● **S51.02**   Laceration with foreign body of elbow
       ● **S51.021**   Laceration with foreign body of right elbow
       ● **S51.022**   Laceration with foreign body of left elbow
       ● **S51.029**   Laceration with foreign body of unspecified elbow
     ● **S51.03**   Puncture wound without foreign body of elbow
       ● **S51.031**   Puncture wound without foreign body of right elbow
       ● **S51.032**   Puncture wound without foreign body of left elbow
       ● **S51.039**   Puncture wound without foreign body of unspecified elbow

     ● **S51.04**   Puncture wound with foreign body of elbow
       ● **S51.041**   Puncture wound with foreign body of right elbow
       ● **S51.042**   Puncture wound with foreign body of left elbow
       ● **S51.049**   Puncture wound with foreign body of unspecified elbow
     ● **S51.05**   Open bite of elbow
         Bite of elbow NOS
         Excludes1   superficial bite of elbow (S50.36, S50.37)
       ● **S51.051**   Open bite, right elbow
       ● **S51.052**   Open bite, left elbow
       ● **S51.059**   Open bite, unspecified elbow
   ● **S51.8**   Open wound of forearm
     Excludes2   open wound of elbow (S51.0-)
     ● **S51.80**   Unspecified open wound of forearm
       ● **S51.801**   Unspecified open wound of right forearm
       ● **S51.802**   Unspecified open wound of left forearm
       ● **S51.809**   Unspecified open wound of unspecified forearm
          Open wound of forearm NOS
     ● **S51.81**   Laceration without foreign body of forearm
       ● **S51.811**   Laceration without foreign body of right forearm
       ● **S51.812**   Laceration without foreign body of left forearm
       ● **S51.819**   Laceration without foreign body of unspecified forearm
     ● **S51.82**   Laceration with foreign body of forearm
       ● **S51.821**   Laceration with foreign body of right forearm
       ● **S51.822**   Laceration with foreign body of left forearm
       ● **S51.829**   Laceration with foreign body of unspecified forearm
     ● **S51.83**   Puncture wound without foreign body of forearm
       ● **S51.831**   Puncture wound without foreign body of right forearm
       ● **S51.832**   Puncture wound without foreign body of left forearm
       ● **S51.839**   Puncture wound without foreign body of unspecified forearm
     ● **S51.84**   Puncture wound with foreign body of forearm
       ● **S51.841**   Puncture wound with foreign body of right forearm
       ● **S51.842**   Puncture wound with foreign body of left forearm
       ● **S51.849**   Puncture wound with foreign body of unspecified forearm
     ● **S51.85**   Open bite of forearm
         Bite of forearm NOS
         Excludes1   superficial bite of forearm (S50.86, S50.87)
       ● **S51.851**   Open bite of right forearm
       ● **S51.852**   Open bite of left forearm
       ● **S51.859**   Open bite of unspecified forearm

CHAPTER 19 (S00-T88)

● S52   Fracture of forearm

> **Note:** A fracture not identified as displaced or nondisplaced should be coded to displaced
>
> A fracture not designated as open or closed should be coded to closed
>
> The open fracture designations are based on the Gustilo open fracture classification

| Excludes1 | traumatic amputation of forearm (S58.-) |
| Excludes2 | fracture at wrist and hand level (S62.-) |

> The appropriate 7th character is to be added to all codes from category S52

A	initial encounter for closed fracture
B	initial encounter for open fracture type I or II initial encounter for open fracture NOS
C	initial encounter for open fracture type IIIA, IIIB, or IIIC
D	subsequent encounter for closed fracture with routine healing
E	subsequent encounter for open fracture type I or II with routine healing
F	subsequent encounter for open fracture type IIIA, IIIB, or IIIC with routine healing
G	subsequent encounter for closed fracture with delayed healing
H	subsequent encounter for open fracture type I or II with delayed healing
J	subsequent encounter for open fracture type IIIA, IIIB, or IIIC with delayed healing
K	subsequent encounter for closed fracture with nonunion
M	subsequent encounter for open fracture type I or II with nonunion
N	subsequent encounter for open fracture type IIIA, IIIB, or IIIC with nonunion
P	subsequent encounter for closed fracture with malunion
Q	subsequent encounter for open fracture type I or II with malunion
R	subsequent encounter for open fracture type IIIA, IIIB, or IIIC with malunion
S	sequela

● S52.0   Fracture of upper end of ulna
Fracture of proximal end of ulna

| Excludes2 | fracture of elbow NOS (S42.40-)
fractures of shaft of ulna (S52.2-) |

● S52.00   Unspecified fracture of upper end of ulna

● S52.001   Unspecified fracture of upper end of right ulna

● S52.002   Unspecified fracture of upper end of left ulna

● S52.009   Unspecified fracture of upper end of unspecified ulna

● S52.01   Torus fracture of upper end of ulna

> The appropriate 7th character is to be added to all codes in subcategory S52.01

A	initial encounter for closed fracture
D	subsequent encounter for fracture with routine healing
G	subsequent encounter for fracture with delayed healing
K	subsequent encounter for fracture with nonunion
P	subsequent encounter for fracture with malunion
S	sequela

● S52.011   Torus fracture of upper end of right ulna

● S52.012   Torus fracture of upper end of left ulna

● S52.019   Torus fracture of upper end of unspecified ulna

● S52.02   Fracture of olecranon process without intraarticular extension of ulna

● S52.021   Displaced fracture of olecranon process without intraarticular extension of right ulna

● S52.022   Displaced fracture of olecranon process without intraarticular extension of left ulna

● S52.023   Displaced fracture of olecranon process without intraarticular extension of unspecified ulna

● S52.024   Nondisplaced fracture of olecranon process without intraarticular extension of right ulna

● S52.025   Nondisplaced fracture of olecranon process without intraarticular extension of left ulna

● S52.026   Nondisplaced fracture of olecranon process without intraarticular extension of unspecified ulna

● S52.03   Fracture of olecranon process with intraarticular extension of ulna

● S52.031   Displaced fracture of olecranon process with intraarticular extension of right ulna

● S52.032   Displaced fracture of olecranon process with intraarticular extension of left ulna

● S52.033   Displaced fracture of olecranon process with intraarticular extension of unspecified ulna

● S52.034   Nondisplaced fracture of olecranon process with intraarticular extension of right ulna

● S52.035   Nondisplaced fracture of olecranon process with intraarticular extension of left ulna

● S52.036   Nondisplaced fracture of olecranon process with intraarticular extension of unspecified ulna

● S52.04   Fracture of coronoid process of ulna

● S52.041   Displaced fracture of coronoid process of right ulna

● S52.042   Displaced fracture of coronoid process of left ulna

● S52.043   Displaced fracture of coronoid process of unspecified ulna

● S52.044   Nondisplaced fracture of coronoid process of right ulna

● S52.045   Nondisplaced fracture of coronoid process of left ulna

● S52.046   Nondisplaced fracture of coronoid process of unspecified ulna

● S52.09   Other fracture of upper end of ulna

● S52.091   Other fracture of upper end of right ulna

● S52.092   Other fracture of upper end of left ulna

● S52.099   Other fracture of upper end of unspecified ulna

● S52.1   Fracture of upper end of radius
Fracture of proximal end of radius

| Excludes2 | physeal fractures of upper end of radius (S59.2-)
fracture of shaft of radius (S52.3-) |

● S52.10   Unspecified fracture of upper end of radius

● S52.101   Unspecified fracture of upper end of right radius

● S52.102   Unspecified fracture of upper end of left radius

● S52.109   Unspecified fracture of upper end of unspecified radius

● **S52.11**   **Torus** fracture of upper end of radius

The appropriate 7th character is to be added to all codes in subcategory S52.11

A	initial encounter for closed fracture
D	subsequent encounter for fracture with routine healing
G	subsequent encounter for fracture with delayed healing
K	subsequent encounter for fracture with nonunion
P	subsequent encounter for fracture with malunion
S	sequela

  ● **S52.111**   Torus fracture of upper end of **right** radius

  ● **S52.112**   Torus fracture of upper end of **left** radius

  ● **S52.119**   Torus fracture of upper end of **unspecified** radius

● **S52.12**   Fracture of **head** of radius

  ● **S52.121**   **Displaced** fracture of head of **right** radius

  ● **S52.122**   **Displaced** fracture of head of **left** radius

  ● **S52.123**   **Displaced** fracture of head of **unspecified** radius

  ● **S52.124**   **Nondisplaced** fracture of head of **right** radius

  ● **S52.125**   **Nondisplaced** fracture of head of **left** radius

  ● **S52.126**   **Nondisplaced** fracture of head of **unspecified** radius

● **S52.13**   Fracture of **neck** of radius

  ● **S52.131**   **Displaced** fracture of neck of **right** radius

  ● **S52.132**   **Displaced** fracture of neck of **left** radius

  ● **S52.133**   **Displaced** fracture of neck of **unspecified** radius

  ● **S52.134**   **Nondisplaced** fracture of neck of **right** radius

  ● **S52.135**   **Nondisplaced** fracture of neck of **left** radius

  ● **S52.136**   **Nondisplaced** fracture of neck of **unspecified** radius

● **S52.18**   **Other** fracture of upper end of radius

  ● **S52.181**   Other fracture of upper end of **right** radius

  ● **S52.182**   Other fracture of upper end of **left** radius

  ● **S52.189**   Other fracture of upper end of **unspecified** radius

● **S52.2**   Fracture of **shaft of ulna**

  ● **S52.20**   **Unspecified** fracture of shaft of ulna
Fracture of ulna NOS

  ● **S52.201**   Unspecified fracture of shaft of **right** ulna

  ● **S52.202**   Unspecified fracture of shaft of **left** ulna

  ● **S52.209**   Unspecified fracture of shaft of **unspecified** ulna

● **S52.21**   **Greenstick** fracture of shaft of ulna

The appropriate 7th character is to be added to all codes in subcategory S52.21

A	initial encounter for closed fracture
D	subsequent encounter for fracture with routine healing
G	subsequent encounter for fracture with delayed healing
K	subsequent encounter for fracture with nonunion
P	subsequent encounter for fracture with malunion
S	sequela

  ● **S52.211**   Greenstick fracture of shaft of **right** ulna

  ● **S52.212**   Greenstick fracture of shaft of **left** ulna

  ● **S52.219**   Greenstick fracture of shaft of **unspecified** ulna

● **S52.22**   **Transverse** fracture of shaft of ulna

  ● **S52.221**   **Displaced** transverse fracture of shaft of **right** ulna

  ● **S52.222**   **Displaced** transverse fracture of shaft of **left** ulna

  ● **S52.223**   **Displaced** transverse fracture of shaft of **unspecified** ulna

  ● **S52.224**   **Nondisplaced** transverse fracture of shaft of **right** ulna

  ● **S52.225**   **Nondisplaced** transverse fracture of shaft of **left** ulna

  ● **S52.226**   **Nondisplaced** transverse fracture of shaft of **unspecified** ulna

● **S52.23**   **Oblique** fracture of shaft of ulna

  ● **S52.231**   **Displaced** oblique fracture of shaft of **right** ulna

  ● **S52.232**   **Displaced** oblique fracture of shaft of **left** ulna

  ● **S52.233**   **Displaced** oblique fracture of shaft of **unspecified** ulna

  ● **S52.234**   **Nondisplaced** oblique fracture of shaft of **right** ulna

  ● **S52.235**   **Nondisplaced** oblique fracture of shaft of **left** ulna

  ● **S52.236**   **Nondisplaced** oblique fracture of shaft of **unspecified** ulna

● **S52.24**   **Spiral** fracture of shaft of ulna

  ● **S52.241**   **Displaced** spiral fracture of shaft of ulna, **right** arm

  ● **S52.242**   **Displaced** spiral fracture of shaft of ulna, **left** arm

  ● **S52.243**   **Displaced** spiral fracture of shaft of ulna, **unspecified** arm

  ● **S52.244**   **Nondisplaced** spiral fracture of shaft of ulna, **right** arm

  ● **S52.245**   **Nondisplaced** spiral fracture of shaft of ulna, **left** arm

  ● **S52.246**   **Nondisplaced** spiral fracture of shaft of ulna, **unspecified** arm

CHAPTER 19 (S00-T88)

CHAPTER 19 (S00-T88)

● **S52.25**   **Comminuted** fracture of shaft of ulna
  - ● **S52.251**   **Displaced** comminuted fracture of shaft of ulna, **right** arm
  - ● **S52.252**   **Displaced** comminuted fracture of shaft of ulna, **left** arm
  - ● **S52.253**   **Displaced** comminuted fracture of shaft of ulna, **unspecified** arm
  - ● **S52.254**   **Nondisplaced** comminuted fracture of shaft of ulna, **right** arm
  - ● **S52.255**   **Nondisplaced** comminuted fracture of shaft of ulna, **left** arm
  - ● **S52.256**   **Nondisplaced** comminuted fracture of shaft of ulna, **unspecified** arm

● **S52.26**   **Segmental** fracture of shaft of ulna
  - ● **S52.261**   **Displaced** segmental fracture of shaft of ulna, **right** arm
  - ● **S52.262**   **Displaced** segmental fracture of shaft of ulna, **left** arm
  - ● **S52.263**   **Displaced** segmental fracture of shaft of ulna, **unspecified** arm
  - ● **S52.264**   **Nondisplaced** segmental fracture of shaft of ulna, **right** arm
  - ● **S52.265**   **Nondisplaced** segmental fracture of shaft of ulna, **left** arm
  - ● **S52.266**   **Nondisplaced** segmental fracture of shaft of ulna, **unspecified** arm

● **S52.27**   **Monteggia's** fracture of ulna
  Fracture of upper shaft of ulna with dislocation of radial head
  - ● **S52.271**   Monteggia's fracture of **right** ulna
  - ● **S52.272**   Monteggia's fracture of **left** ulna
  - ● **S52.279**   Monteggia's fracture of **unspecified** ulna

● **S52.28**   **Bent bone** of ulna
  - ● **S52.281**   Bent bone of **right** ulna
  - ● **S52.282**   Bent bone of **left** ulna
  - ● **S52.283**   Bent bone of **unspecified** ulna

● **S52.29**   **Other** fracture of shaft of ulna
  - ● **S52.291**   Other fracture of shaft of **right** ulna
  - ● **S52.292**   Other fracture of shaft of **left** ulna
  - ● **S52.299**   Other fracture of shaft of **unspecified** ulna

● **S52.3**   Fracture of **shaft of radius**
  - ● **S52.30**   **Unspecified** fracture of shaft of radius
    - ● **S52.301**   Unspecified fracture of shaft of **right** radius
    - ● **S52.302**   Unspecified fracture of shaft of **left** radius
    - ● **S52.309**   Unspecified fracture of shaft of **unspecified** radius
  - ● **S52.31**   **Greenstick** fracture of shaft of radius

    The appropriate 7th character is to be added to all codes in subcategory S52.31

A	initial encounter for closed fracture
D	subsequent encounter for fracture with routine healing
G	subsequent encounter for fracture with delayed healing
K	subsequent encounter for fracture with nonunion
P	subsequent encounter for fracture with malunion
S	sequela

    - ● **S52.311**   Greenstick fracture of shaft of radius, **right** arm
    - ● **S52.312**   Greenstick fracture of shaft of radius, **left** arm
    - ● **S52.319**   Greenstick fracture of shaft of radius, **unspecified** arm

● **S52.32**   **Transverse** fracture of shaft of radius
  - ● **S52.321**   **Displaced** transverse fracture of shaft of **right** radius
  - ● **S52.322**   **Displaced** transverse fracture of shaft of **left** radius
  - ● **S52.323**   **Displaced** transverse fracture of shaft of **unspecified** radius
  - ● **S52.324**   **Nondisplaced** transverse fracture of shaft of **right** radius
  - ● **S52.325**   **Nondisplaced** transverse fracture of shaft of **left** radius
  - ● **S52.326**   **Nondisplaced** transverse fracture of shaft of **unspecified** radius

● **S52.33**   **Oblique** fracture of shaft of radius
  - ● **S52.331**   **Displaced** oblique fracture of shaft of **right** radius
  - ● **S52.332**   **Displaced** oblique fracture of shaft of **left** radius
  - ● **S52.333**   **Displaced** oblique fracture of shaft of **unspecified** radius
  - ● **S52.334**   **Nondisplaced** oblique fracture of shaft of **right** radius
  - ● **S52.335**   **Nondisplaced** oblique fracture of shaft of **left** radius
  - ● **S52.336**   **Nondisplaced** oblique fracture of shaft of **unspecified** radius

● **S52.34**   **Spiral** fracture of shaft of radius
  - ● **S52.341**   **Displaced** spiral fracture of shaft of radius, **right** arm
  - ● **S52.342**   **Displaced** spiral fracture of shaft of radius, **left** arm
  - ● **S52.343**   **Displaced** spiral fracture of shaft of radius, **unspecified** arm
  - ● **S52.344**   **Nondisplaced** spiral fracture of shaft of radius, **right** arm
  - ● **S52.345**   **Nondisplaced** spiral fracture of shaft of radius, **left** arm
  - ● **S52.346**   **Nondisplaced** spiral fracture of shaft of radius, **unspecified** arm

● **S52.35**   **Comminuted** fracture of shaft of radius
  - ● **S52.351**   **Displaced** comminuted fracture of shaft of radius, **right** arm
  - ● **S52.352**   **Displaced** comminuted fracture of shaft of radius, **left** arm
  - ● **S52.353**   **Displaced** comminuted fracture of shaft of radius, **unspecified** arm
  - ● **S52.354**   **Nondisplaced** comminuted fracture of shaft of radius, **right** arm
  - ● **S52.355**   **Nondisplaced** comminuted fracture of shaft of radius, **left** arm
  - ● **S52.356**   **Nondisplaced** comminuted fracture of shaft of radius, **unspecified** arm

● **S52.36**   **Segmental** fracture of shaft of radius
  - ● **S52.361**   **Displaced** segmental fracture of shaft of radius, **right** arm
  - ● **S52.362**   **Displaced** segmental fracture of shaft of radius, **left** arm
  - ● **S52.363**   **Displaced** segmental fracture of shaft of radius, **unspecified** arm
  - ● **S52.364**   **Nondisplaced** segmental fracture of shaft of radius, **right** arm
  - ● **S52.365**   **Nondisplaced** segmental fracture of shaft of radius, **left** arm
  - ● **S52.366**   **Nondisplaced** segmental fracture of shaft of radius, **unspecified** arm

▶ New   ⟹ Revised   ~~deleted~~ Deleted   **OGCR** Official Guidelines   X Assign placeholder X   ● Use Additional Character(s)

Excludes 1   Excludes 2   Includes   Use additional   Code first   Code also   Key words

- S52.37 Galeazzi's fracture
  Fracture of lower shaft of radius with
  radioulnar joint dislocation
  - S52.371 Galeazzi's fracture of right radius
  - S52.372 Galeazzi's fracture of left radius
  - S52.379 Galeazzi's fracture of unspecified radius
- S52.38 Bent bone of radius
  - S52.381 Bent bone of right radius
  - S52.382 Bent bone of left radius
  - S52.389 Bent bone of unspecified radius
- S52.39 Other fracture of shaft of radius
  - S52.391 Other fracture of shaft of radius, right arm
  - S52.392 Other fracture of shaft of radius, left arm
  - S52.399 Other fracture of shaft of radius, unspecified arm
- S52.5 Fracture of lower end of radius
  Fracture of distal end of radius

  | Excludes2 | physeal fractures of lower end of radius (S59.2-) |

  - S52.50 Unspecified fracture of the lower end of radius
    - S52.501 Unspecified fracture of the lower end of right radius
    - S52.502 Unspecified fracture of the lower end of left radius
    - S52.509 Unspecified fracture of the lower end of unspecified radius
  - S52.51 Fracture of radial styloid process
    - S52.511 Displaced fracture of right radial styloid process
    - S52.512 Displaced fracture of left radial styloid process
    - S52.513 Displaced fracture of unspecified radial styloid process
    - S52.514 Nondisplaced fracture of right radial styloid process
    - S52.515 Nondisplaced fracture of left radial styloid process
    - S52.516 Nondisplaced fracture of unspecified radial styloid process
  - S52.52 Torus fracture of lower end of radius

    The appropriate 7th character is to be added to all codes in subcategory S52.52

A	initial encounter for closed fracture
D	subsequent encounter for fracture with routine healing
G	subsequent encounter for fracture with delayed healing
K	subsequent encounter for fracture with nonunion
P	subsequent encounter for fracture with malunion
S	sequela

    - S52.521 Torus fracture of lower end of right radius
    - S52.522 Torus fracture of lower end of left radius
    - S52.529 Torus fracture of lower end of unspecified radius

- S52.53 Colles' fracture
  - S52.531 Colles' fracture of right radius
  - S52.532 Colles' fracture of left radius
  - S52.539 Colles' fracture of unspecified radius
- S52.54 Smith's fracture
  - S52.541 Smith's fracture of right radius
  - S52.542 Smith's fracture of left radius
  - S52.549 Smith's fracture of unspecified radius
- S52.55 Other extraarticular fracture of lower end of radius
  - S52.551 Other extraarticular fracture of lower end of right radius
  - S52.552 Other extraarticular fracture of lower end of left radius
  - S52.559 Other extraarticular fracture of lower end of unspecified radius
- S52.56 Barton's fracture
  - S52.561 Barton's fracture of right radius
  - S52.562 Barton's fracture of left radius
  - S52.569 Barton's fracture of unspecified radius
- S52.57 Other intraarticular fracture of lower end of radius
  - S52.571 Other intraarticular fracture of lower end of right radius
  - S52.572 Other intraarticular fracture of lower end of left radius
  - S52.579 Other intraarticular fracture of lower end of unspecified radius
- S52.59 Other fractures of lower end of radius
  - S52.591 Other fractures of lower end of right radius
  - S52.592 Other fractures of lower end of left radius
  - S52.599 Other fractures of lower end of unspecified radius
- S52.6 Fracture of lower end of ulna
  - S52.60 Unspecified fracture of lower end of ulna
    - S52.601 Unspecified fracture of lower end of right ulna
    - S52.602 Unspecified fracture of lower end of left ulna
    - S52.609 Unspecified fracture of lower end of unspecified ulna
  - S52.61 Fracture of ulna styloid process
    - S52.611 Displaced fracture of right ulna styloid process
    - S52.612 Displaced fracture of left ulna styloid process
    - S52.613 Displaced fracture of unspecified ulna styloid process
    - S52.614 Nondisplaced fracture of right ulna styloid process
    - S52.615 Nondisplaced fracture of left ulna styloid process
    - S52.616 Nondisplaced fracture of unspecified ulna styloid process

● **S52.62** **Torus** fracture of lower end of ulna

The appropriate 7th character is to be added to all codes in subcategory S52.62

A	initial encounter for closed fracture
D	subsequent encounter for fracture with routine healing
G	subsequent encounter for fracture with delayed healing
K	subsequent encounter for fracture with nonunion
P	subsequent encounter for fracture with malunion
S	sequela

● S52.621　Torus fracture of lower end of **right** ulna

● S52.622　Torus fracture of lower end of **left** ulna

● S52.629　Torus fracture of lower end of **unspecified** ulna

● **S52.69** **Other** fracture of lower end of ulna

● S52.691　Other fracture of lower end of **right** ulna

● S52.692　Other fracture of lower end of **left** ulna

● S52.699　Other fracture of lower end of **unspecified** ulna

● **S52.9** **Unspecified** fracture of **forearm**

X ● **S52.90** Unspecified fracture of **unspecified** forearm

X ● **S52.91** Unspecified fracture of **right** forearm

X ● **S52.92** Unspecified fracture of **left** forearm

● **S53** Dislocation and sprain of joints and ligaments of elbow

Includes　avulsion of joint or ligament of elbow
laceration of cartilage, joint or ligament of elbow
sprain of cartilage, joint or ligament of elbow
traumatic hemarthrosis of joint or ligament of elbow
traumatic rupture of joint or ligament of elbow
traumatic subluxation of joint or ligament of elbow
traumatic tear of joint or ligament of elbow

Code also any associated open wound

Excludes2　strain of muscle, fascia and tendon at forearm level (S56.-)

The appropriate 7th character is to be added to each code from category S53

A	initial encounter
D	subsequent encounter
S	sequela

● **S53.0** Subluxation and dislocation of **radial head**

Dislocation of radiohumeral joint
Subluxation of radiohumeral joint

Excludes1　Monteggia's fracture-dislocation (S52.27-)

● **S53.00** **Unspecified** subluxation and dislocation of radial head

● S53.001　Unspecified **subluxation** of **right** radial head

● S53.002　Unspecified **subluxation** of **left** radial head

● S53.003　Unspecified **subluxation** of **unspecified** radial head

● S53.004　Unspecified **dislocation** of **right** radial head

● S53.005　Unspecified **dislocation** of **left** radial head

● S53.006　Unspecified **dislocation** of **unspecified** radial head

● **S53.01** **Anterior** subluxation and dislocation of radial head

Anteriomedial subluxation and dislocation of radial head

● S53.011　Anterior **subluxation** of **right** radial head

● S53.012　Anterior **subluxation** of **left** radial head

● S53.013　Anterior **subluxation** of **unspecified** radial head

● S53.014　Anterior **dislocation** of **right** radial head

● S53.015　Anterior **dislocation** of **left** radial head

● S53.016　Anterior **dislocation** of **unspecified** radial head

● **S53.02** **Posterior** subluxation and dislocation of radial head

Posteriolateral subluxation and dislocation of radial head

● S53.021　Posterior **subluxation** of **right** radial head

● S53.022　Posterior **subluxation** of **left** radial head

● S53.023　Posterior **subluxation** of **unspecified** radial head

● S53.024　Posterior **dislocation** of **right** radial head

● S53.025　Posterior **dislocation** of **left** radial head

● S53.026　Posterior **dislocation** of **unspecified** radial head

● **S53.03** **Nursemaid's elbow**

● S53.031　Nursemaid's elbow, **right** elbow

● S53.032　Nursemaid's elbow, **left** elbow

● S53.033　Nursemaid's elbow, **unspecified** elbow

● **S53.09** **Other** subluxation and dislocation of radial head

● S53.091　Other **subluxation** of **right** radial head

● S53.092　Other **subluxation** of **left** radial head

● S53.093　Other **subluxation** of **unspecified** radial head

● S53.094　Other **dislocation** of **right** radial head

● S53.095　Other **dislocation** of **left** radial head

● S53.096　Other **dislocation** of **unspecified** radial head

● **S53.1** Subluxation and dislocation of **ulnohumeral** joint

Subluxation and dislocation of elbow NOS

Excludes1　dislocation of radial head alone (S53.0-)

● **S53.10** **Unspecified** subluxation and dislocation of ulnohumeral joint

● S53.101　Unspecified **subluxation** of **right** ulnohumeral joint

● S53.102　Unspecified **subluxation** of **left** ulnohumeral joint

● S53.103　Unspecified **subluxation** of **unspecified** ulnohumeral joint

● S53.104　Unspecified **dislocation** of **right** ulnohumeral joint

● S53.105　Unspecified **dislocation** of **left** ulnohumeral joint

● S53.106　Unspecified **dislocation** of **unspecified** ulnohumeral joint

CHAPTER 19 (S00-T88)

● **S53.11**   Anterior subluxation and dislocation of ulnohumeral joint
- ● **S53.111**   Anterior subluxation of right ulnohumeral joint
- ● **S53.112**   Anterior subluxation of left ulnohumeral joint
- ● **S53.113**   Anterior subluxation of unspecified ulnohumeral joint
- ● **S53.114**   Anterior dislocation of right ulnohumeral joint
- ● **S53.115**   Anterior dislocation of left ulnohumeral joint
- ● **S53.116**   Anterior dislocation of unspecified ulnohumeral joint

● **S53.12**   Posterior subluxation and dislocation of ulnohumeral joint
- ● **S53.121**   Posterior subluxation of right ulnohumeral joint
- ● **S53.122**   Posterior subluxation of left ulnohumeral joint
- ● **S53.123**   Posterior subluxation of unspecified ulnohumeral joint
- ● **S53.124**   Posterior dislocation of right ulnohumeral joint
- ● **S53.125**   Posterior dislocation of left ulnohumeral joint
- ● **S53.126**   Posterior dislocation of unspecified ulnohumeral joint

● **S53.13**   Medial subluxation and dislocation of ulnohumeral joint
- ● **S53.131**   Medial subluxation of right ulnohumeral joint
- ● **S53.132**   Medial subluxation of left ulnohumeral joint
- ● **S53.133**   Medial subluxation of unspecified ulnohumeral joint
- ● **S53.134**   Medial dislocation of right ulnohumeral joint
- ● **S53.135**   Medial dislocation of left ulnohumeral joint
- ● **S53.136**   Medial dislocation of unspecified ulnohumeral joint

● **S53.14**   Lateral subluxation and dislocation of ulnohumeral joint
- ● **S53.141**   Lateral subluxation of right ulnohumeral joint
- ● **S53.142**   Lateral subluxation of left ulnohumeral joint
- ● **S53.143**   Lateral subluxation of unspecified ulnohumeral joint
- ● **S53.144**   Lateral dislocation of right ulnohumeral joint
- ● **S53.145**   Lateral dislocation of left ulnohumeral joint
- ● **S53.146**   Lateral dislocation of unspecified ulnohumeral joint

● **S53.19**   Other subluxation and dislocation of ulnohumeral joint
- ● **S53.191**   Other subluxation of right ulnohumeral joint
- ● **S53.192**   Other subluxation of left ulnohumeral joint
- ● **S53.193**   Other subluxation of unspecified ulnohumeral joint
- ● **S53.194**   Other dislocation of right ulnohumeral joint
- ● **S53.195**   Other dislocation of left ulnohumeral joint
- ● **S53.196**   Other dislocation of unspecified ulnohumeral joint

● **S53.2**   Traumatic rupture of radial collateral ligament
> **Excludes1**   sprain of radial collateral ligament NOS (S53.43-)
- X ● **S53.20**   Traumatic rupture of unspecified radial collateral ligament
- X ● **S53.21**   Traumatic rupture of right radial collateral ligament
- X ● **S53.22**   Traumatic rupture of left radial collateral ligament

● **S53.3**   Traumatic rupture of ulnar collateral ligament
> **Excludes1**   sprain of ulnar collateral ligament (S53.44-)
- X ● **S53.30**   Traumatic rupture of unspecified ulnar collateral ligament
- X ● **S53.31**   Traumatic rupture of right ulnar collateral ligament
- X ● **S53.32**   Traumatic rupture of left ulnar collateral ligament

● **S53.4**   Sprain of elbow
> **Excludes2**   traumatic rupture of radial collateral ligament (S53.2-)
> traumatic rupture of ulnar collateral ligament (S53.3-)
- ● **S53.40**   Unspecified sprain of elbow
  - ● **S53.401**   Unspecified sprain of right elbow
  - ● **S53.402**   Unspecified sprain of left elbow
  - ● **S53.409**   Unspecified sprain of unspecified elbow
    Sprain of elbow NOS
- ● **S53.41**   Radiohumeral (joint) sprain
  - ● **S53.411**   Radiohumeral (joint) sprain of right elbow
  - ● **S53.412**   Radiohumeral (joint) sprain of left elbow
  - ● **S53.419**   Radiohumeral (joint) sprain of unspecified elbow
- ● **S53.42**   Ulnohumeral (joint) sprain
  - ● **S53.421**   Ulnohumeral (joint) sprain of right elbow
  - ● **S53.422**   Ulnohumeral (joint) sprain of left elbow
  - ● **S53.429**   Ulnohumeral (joint) sprain of unspecified elbow
- ● **S53.43**   Radial collateral ligament sprain
  - ● **S53.431**   Radial collateral ligament sprain of right elbow
  - ● **S53.432**   Radial collateral ligament sprain of left elbow
  - ● **S53.439**   Radial collateral ligament sprain of unspecified elbow
- ● **S53.44**   Ulnar collateral ligament sprain
  - ● **S53.441**   Ulnar collateral ligament sprain of right elbow
  - ● **S53.442**   Ulnar collateral ligament sprain of left elbow
  - ● **S53.449**   Ulnar collateral ligament sprain of unspecified elbow
- ● **S53.49**   Other sprain of elbow
  - ● **S53.491**   Other sprain of right elbow
  - ● **S53.492**   Other sprain of left elbow
  - ● **S53.499**   Other sprain of unspecified elbow

S54   Injury of nerves at forearm level

Code also any associated open wound (S51.-)

Excludes2   injury of nerves at wrist and hand level (S64.-)

The appropriate 7th character is to be added to each code from category S54

> A   initial encounter
> D   subsequent encounter
> S   sequela

S54.0   Injury of ulnar nerve at forearm level
Injury of ulnar nerve NOS

X ● **S54.00   Injury of ulnar nerve at forearm level, unspecified arm**

X ● **S54.01   Injury of ulnar nerve at forearm level, right arm**

X ● **S54.02   Injury of ulnar nerve at forearm level, left arm**

S54.1   Injury of median nerve at forearm level
Injury of median nerve NOS

X ● **S54.10   Injury of median nerve at forearm level, unspecified arm**

X ● **S54.11   Injury of median nerve at forearm level, right arm**

X ● **S54.12   Injury of median nerve at forearm level, left arm**

S54.2   Injury of radial nerve at forearm level
Injury of radial nerve NOS

X ● **S54.20   Injury of radial nerve at forearm level, unspecified arm**

X ● **S54.21   Injury of radial nerve at forearm level, right arm**

X ● **S54.22   Injury of radial nerve at forearm level, left arm**

S54.3   Injury of cutaneous sensory nerve at forearm level

X ● **S54.30   Injury of cutaneous sensory nerve at forearm level, unspecified arm**

X ● **S54.31   Injury of cutaneous sensory nerve at forearm level, right arm**

X ● **S54.32   Injury of cutaneous sensory nerve at forearm level, left arm**

S54.8   Injury of other nerves at forearm level

● **S54.8X   Injury of other nerves at forearm level**

● **S54.8X1   Injury of other nerves at forearm level, right arm**

● **S54.8X2   Injury of other nerves at forearm level, left arm**

● **S54.8X9   Injury of other nerves at forearm level, unspecified arm**

S54.9   Injury of unspecified nerve at forearm level

X ● **S54.90   Injury of unspecified nerve at forearm level, unspecified arm**

X ● **S54.91   Injury of unspecified nerve at forearm level, right arm**

X ● **S54.92   Injury of unspecified nerve at forearm level, left arm**

S55   Injury of blood vessels at forearm level

Code also any associated open wound (S51.-)

Excludes2   injury of blood vessels at wrist and hand level (S65.-)
injury of brachial vessels (S45.1-S45.2)

The appropriate 7th character is to be added to each code from category S55

> A   initial encounter
> D   subsequent encounter
> S   sequela

S55.0   Injury of ulnar artery at forearm level

● **S55.00   Unspecified injury of ulnar artery at forearm level**

● **S55.001   Unspecified injury of ulnar artery at forearm level, right arm**

● **S55.002   Unspecified injury of ulnar artery at forearm level, left arm**

● **S55.009   Unspecified injury of ulnar artery at forearm level, unspecified arm**

● **S55.01   Laceration of ulnar artery at forearm level**

● **S55.011   Laceration of ulnar artery at forearm level, right arm**

● **S55.012   Laceration of ulnar artery at forearm level, left arm**

● **S55.019   Laceration of ulnar artery at forearm level, unspecified arm**

● **S55.09   Other specified injury of ulnar artery at forearm level**

● **S55.091   Other specified injury of ulnar artery at forearm level, right arm**

● **S55.092   Other specified injury of ulnar artery at forearm level, left arm**

● **S55.099   Other specified injury of ulnar artery at forearm level, unspecified arm**

S55.1   Injury of radial artery at forearm level

● **S55.10   Unspecified injury of radial artery at forearm level**

● **S55.101   Unspecified injury of radial artery at forearm level, right arm**

● **S55.102   Unspecified injury of radial artery at forearm level, left arm**

● **S55.109   Unspecified injury of radial artery at forearm level, unspecified arm**

● **S55.11   Laceration of radial artery at forearm level**

● **S55.111   Laceration of radial artery at forearm level, right arm**

● **S55.112   Laceration of radial artery at forearm level, left arm**

● **S55.119   Laceration of radial artery at forearm level, unspecified arm**

● **S55.19   Other specified injury of radial artery at forearm level**

● **S55.191   Other specified injury of radial artery at forearm level, right arm**

● **S55.192   Other specified injury of radial artery at forearm level, left arm**

● **S55.199   Other specified injury of radial artery at forearm level, unspecified arm**

▶ New   ⇒ Revised   ~~deleted~~ Deleted   **OGCR** Official Guidelines   X Assign placeholder X   ● Use Additional Character(s)
Excludes 1   Excludes 2   Includes   Use additional   Code first   Code also   Key words

● **S55.2**   Injury of vein at forearm level
   ● **S55.20**   Unspecified injury of vein at forearm level
     ● **S55.201**   Unspecified injury of vein at forearm level, right arm
     ● **S55.202**   Unspecified injury of vein at forearm level, left arm
     ● **S55.209**   Unspecified injury of vein at forearm level, unspecified arm
   ● **S55.21**   Laceration of vein at forearm level
     ● **S55.211**   Laceration of vein at forearm level, right arm
     ● **S55.212**   Laceration of vein at forearm level, left arm
     ● **S55.219**   Laceration of vein at forearm level, unspecified arm
   ● **S55.29**   Other specified injury of vein at forearm level
     ● **S55.291**   Other specified injury of vein at forearm level, right arm
     ● **S55.292**   Other specified injury of vein at forearm level, left arm
     ● **S55.299**   Other specified injury of vein at forearm level, unspecified arm
● **S55.8**   Injury of other blood vessels at forearm level
   ● **S55.80**   Unspecified injury of other blood vessels at forearm level
     ● **S55.801**   Unspecified injury of other blood vessels at forearm level, right arm
     ● **S55.802**   Unspecified injury of other blood vessels at forearm level, left arm
     ● **S55.809**   Unspecified injury of other blood vessels at forearm level, unspecified arm
   ● **S55.81**   Laceration of other blood vessels at forearm level
     ● **S55.811**   Laceration of other blood vessels at forearm level, right arm
     ● **S55.812**   Laceration of other blood vessels at forearm level, left arm
     ● **S55.819**   Laceration of other blood vessels at forearm level, unspecified arm
   ● **S55.89**   Other specified injury of other blood vessels at forearm level
     ● **S55.891**   Other specified injury of other blood vessels at forearm level, right arm
     ● **S55.892**   Other specified injury of other blood vessels at forearm level, left arm
     ● **S55.899**   Other specified injury of other blood vessels at forearm level, unspecified arm
● **S55.9**   Injury of unspecified blood vessel at forearm level
   ● **S55.90**   Unspecified injury of unspecified blood vessel at forearm level
     ● **S55.901**   Unspecified injury of unspecified blood vessel at forearm level, right arm
     ● **S55.902**   Unspecified injury of unspecified blood vessel at forearm level, left arm
     ● **S55.909**   Unspecified injury of unspecified blood vessel at forearm level, unspecified arm

● **S55.91**   Laceration of unspecified blood vessel at forearm level
     ● **S55.911**   Laceration of unspecified blood vessel at forearm level, right arm
     ● **S55.912**   Laceration of unspecified blood vessel at forearm level, left arm
     ● **S55.919**   Laceration of unspecified blood vessel at forearm level, unspecified arm
   ● **S55.99**   Other specified injury of unspecified blood vessel at forearm level
     ● **S55.991**   Other specified injury of unspecified blood vessel at forearm level, right arm
     ● **S55.992**   Other specified injury of unspecified blood vessel at forearm level, left arm
     ● **S55.999**   Other specified injury of unspecified blood vessel at forearm level, unspecified arm

● **S56**   Injury of muscle, fascia and tendon at forearm level
     Code also any associated open wound (S51.-)
     Excludes2   injury of muscle, fascia and tendon at or below wrist (S66.-)
               sprain of joints and ligaments of elbow (S53.4-)
     The appropriate 7th character is to be added to each code from category S56

     | | |
     A   initial encounter
     D   subsequent encounter
     S   sequela

   ● **S56.0**   Injury of flexor muscle, fascia and tendon of thumb at forearm level
     ● **S56.00**   Unspecified injury of flexor muscle, fascia and tendon of thumb at forearm level
       ● **S56.001**   Unspecified injury of flexor muscle, fascia and tendon of right thumb at forearm level
       ● **S56.002**   Unspecified injury of flexor muscle, fascia and tendon of left thumb at forearm level
       ● **S56.009**   Unspecified injury of flexor muscle, fascia and tendon of unspecified thumb at forearm level
     ● **S56.01**   Strain of flexor muscle, fascia and tendon of thumb at forearm level
       ● **S56.011**   Strain of flexor muscle, fascia and tendon of right thumb at forearm level
       ● **S56.012**   Strain of flexor muscle, fascia and tendon of left thumb at forearm level
       ● **S56.019**   Strain of flexor muscle, fascia and tendon of unspecified thumb at forearm level
     ● **S56.02**   Laceration of flexor muscle, fascia and tendon of thumb at forearm level
       ● **S56.021**   Laceration of flexor muscle, fascia and tendon of right thumb at forearm level
       ● **S56.022**   Laceration of flexor muscle, fascia and tendon of left thumb at forearm level
       ● **S56.029**   Laceration of flexor muscle, fascia and tendon of unspecified thumb at forearm level

● S56.Ø9   Other injury of flexor muscle, fascia and tendon of thumb at forearm level
    ● S56.Ø91   Other injury of flexor muscle, fascia and tendon of right thumb at forearm level
    ● S56.Ø92   Other injury of flexor muscle, fascia and tendon of left thumb at forearm level
    ● S56.Ø99   Other injury of flexor muscle, fascia and tendon of unspecified thumb at forearm level

● S56.1   Injury of flexor muscle, fascia and tendon of other and unspecified finger at forearm level
   ● S56.1Ø   Unspecified injury of flexor muscle, fascia and tendon of other and unspecified finger at forearm level
    ● S56.1Ø1   Unspecified injury of flexor muscle, fascia and tendon of right index finger at forearm level
    ● S56.1Ø2   Unspecified injury of flexor muscle, fascia and tendon of left index finger at forearm level
    ● S56.1Ø3   Unspecified injury of flexor muscle, fascia and tendon of right middle finger at forearm level
    ● S56.1Ø4   Unspecified injury of flexor muscle, fascia and tendon of left middle finger at forearm level
    ● S56.1Ø5   Unspecified injury of flexor muscle, fascia and tendon of right ring finger at forearm level
    ● S56.1Ø6   Unspecified injury of flexor muscle, fascia and tendon of left ring finger at forearm level
    ● S56.1Ø7   Unspecified injury of flexor muscle, fascia and tendon of right little finger at forearm level
    ● S56.1Ø8   Unspecified injury of flexor muscle, fascia and tendon of left little finger at forearm level
    ● S56.1Ø9   Unspecified injury of flexor muscle, fascia and tendon of unspecified finger at forearm level

   ● S56.11   Strain of flexor muscle, fascia and tendon of other and unspecified finger at forearm level
    ● S56.111   Strain of flexor muscle, fascia and tendon of right index finger at forearm level
    ● S56.112   Strain of flexor muscle, fascia and tendon of left index finger at forearm level
    ● S56.113   Strain of flexor muscle, fascia and tendon of right middle finger at forearm level
    ● S56.114   Strain of flexor muscle, fascia and tendon of left middle finger at forearm level
    ● S56.115   Strain of flexor muscle, fascia and tendon of right ring finger at forearm level
    ● S56.116   Strain of flexor muscle, fascia and tendon of left ring finger at forearm level
    ● S56.117   Strain of flexor muscle, fascia and tendon of right little finger at forearm level
    ● S56.118   Strain of flexor muscle, fascia and tendon of left little finger at forearm level
    ● S56.119   Strain of flexor muscle, fascia and tendon of finger of unspecified finger at forearm level

● S56.12   Laceration of flexor muscle, fascia and tendon of other and unspecified finger at forearm level
    ● S56.121   Laceration of flexor muscle, fascia and tendon of right index finger at forearm level
    ● S56.122   Laceration of flexor muscle, fascia and tendon of left index finger at forearm level
    ● S56.123   Laceration of flexor muscle, fascia and tendon of right middle finger at forearm level
    ● S56.124   Laceration of flexor muscle, fascia and tendon of left middle finger at forearm level
    ● S56.125   Laceration of flexor muscle, fascia and tendon of right ring finger at forearm level
    ● S56.126   Laceration of flexor muscle, fascia and tendon of left ring finger at forearm level
    ● S56.127   Laceration of flexor muscle, fascia and tendon of right little finger at forearm level
    ● S56.128   Laceration of flexor muscle, fascia and tendon of left little finger at forearm level
    ● S56.129   Laceration of flexor muscle, fascia and tendon of unspecified finger at forearm level

● S56.19   Other injury of flexor muscle, fascia and tendon of other and unspecified finger at forearm level
    ● S56.191   Other injury of flexor muscle, fascia and tendon of right index finger at forearm level
    ● S56.192   Other injury of flexor muscle, fascia and tendon of left index finger at forearm level
    ● S56.193   Other injury of flexor muscle, fascia and tendon of right middle finger at forearm level
    ● S56.194   Other injury of flexor muscle, fascia and tendon of left middle finger at forearm level
    ● S56.195   Other injury of flexor muscle, fascia and tendon of right ring finger at forearm level
    ● S56.196   Other injury of flexor muscle, fascia and tendon of left ring finger at forearm level
    ● S56.197   Other injury of flexor muscle, fascia and tendon of right little finger at forearm level
    ● S56.198   Other injury of flexor muscle, fascia and tendon of left little finger at forearm level
    ● S56.199   Other injury of flexor muscle, fascia and tendon of unspecified finger at forearm level

● S56.2　Injury of other flexor muscle, fascia and tendon at forearm level
　● S56.20　Unspecified injury of other flexor muscle, fascia and tendon at forearm level
　　● S56.201　Unspecified injury of other flexor muscle, fascia and tendon at forearm level, right arm
　　● S56.202　Unspecified injury of other flexor muscle, fascia and tendon at forearm level, left arm
　　● S56.209　Unspecified injury of other flexor muscle, fascia and tendon at forearm level, unspecified arm
　● S56.21　Strain of other flexor muscle, fascia and tendon at forearm level
　　● S56.211　Strain of other flexor muscle, fascia and tendon at forearm level, right arm
　　● S56.212　Strain of other flexor muscle, fascia and tendon at forearm level, left arm
　　● S56.219　Strain of other flexor muscle, fascia and tendon at forearm level, unspecified arm
　● S56.22　Laceration of other flexor muscle, fascia and tendon at forearm level
　　● S56.221　Laceration of other flexor muscle, fascia and tendon at forearm level, right arm
　　● S56.222　Laceration of other flexor muscle, fascia and tendon at forearm level, left arm
　　● S56.229　Laceration of other flexor muscle, fascia and tendon at forearm level, unspecified arm
　● S56.29　Other injury of other flexor muscle, fascia and tendon at forearm level
　　● S56.291　Other injury of other flexor muscle, fascia and tendon at forearm level, right arm
　　● S56.292　Other injury of other flexor muscle, fascia and tendon at forearm level, left arm
　　● S56.299　Other injury of other flexor muscle, fascia and tendon at forearm level, unspecified arm
● S56.3　Injury of extensor or abductor muscles, fascia and tendons of thumb at forearm level
　● S56.30　Unspecified injury of extensor or abductor muscles, fascia and tendons of thumb at forearm level
　　● S56.301　Unspecified injury of extensor or abductor muscles, fascia and tendons of right thumb at forearm level
　　● S56.302　Unspecified injury of extensor or abductor muscles, fascia and tendons of left thumb at forearm level
　　● S56.309　Unspecified injury of extensor or abductor muscles, fascia and tendons of unspecified thumb at forearm level

● S56.31　Strain of extensor or abductor muscles, fascia and tendons of thumb at forearm level
　　● S56.311　Strain of extensor or abductor muscles, fascia and tendons of right thumb at forearm level
　　● S56.312　Strain of extensor or abductor muscles, fascia and tendons of left thumb at forearm level
　　● S56.319　Strain of extensor or abductor muscles, fascia and tendons of unspecified thumb at forearm level
　● S56.32　Laceration of extensor or abductor muscles, fascia and tendons of thumb at forearm level
　　● S56.321　Laceration of extensor or abductor muscles, fascia and tendons of right thumb at forearm level
　　● S56.322　Laceration of extensor or abductor muscles, fascia and tendons of left thumb at forearm level
　　● S56.329　Laceration of extensor or abductor muscles, fascia and tendons of unspecified thumb at forearm level
　● S56.39　Other injury of extensor or abductor muscles, fascia and tendons of thumb at forearm level
　　● S56.391　Other injury of extensor or abductor muscles, fascia and tendons of right thumb at forearm level
　　● S56.392　Other injury of extensor or abductor muscles, fascia and tendons of left thumb at forearm level
　　● S56.399　Other injury of extensor or abductor muscles, fascia and tendons of unspecified thumb at forearm level
● S56.4　Injury of extensor muscle, fascia and tendon of other and unspecified finger at forearm level
　● S56.40　Unspecified injury of extensor muscle, fascia and tendon of other and unspecified finger at forearm level
　　● S56.401　Unspecified injury of extensor muscle, fascia and tendon of right index finger at forearm level
　　● S56.402　Unspecified injury of extensor muscle, fascia and tendon of left index finger at forearm level
　　● S56.403　Unspecified injury of extensor muscle, fascia and tendon of right middle finger at forearm level
　　● S56.404　Unspecified injury of extensor muscle, fascia and tendon of left middle finger at forearm level
　　● S56.405　Unspecified injury of extensor muscle, fascia and tendon of right ring finger at forearm level
　　● S56.406　Unspecified injury of extensor muscle, fascia and tendon of left ring finger at forearm level
　　● S56.407　Unspecified injury of extensor muscle, fascia and tendon of right little finger at forearm level
　　● S56.408　Unspecified injury of extensor muscle, fascia and tendon of left little finger at forearm level
　　● S56.409　Unspecified injury of extensor muscle, fascia and tendon of unspecified finger at forearm level

▶ New　⇒ Revised　deleted Deleted　OGCR Official Guidelines　X Assign placeholder X　● Use Additional Character(s)

Excludes 1　Excludes 2　Includes　Use additional　Code first　Code also　Key words

CHAPTER 19 (S00-T88)

● S56.41 Strain of extensor muscle, fascia and tendon of other and unspecified finger at forearm level
  ● S56.411 Strain of extensor muscle, fascia and tendon of right index finger at forearm level
  ● S56.412 Strain of extensor muscle, fascia and tendon of left index finger at forearm level
  ● S56.413 Strain of extensor muscle, fascia and tendon of right middle finger at forearm level
  ● S56.414 Strain of extensor muscle, fascia and tendon of left middle finger at forearm level
  ● S56.415 Strain of extensor muscle, fascia and tendon of right ring finger at forearm level
  ● S56.416 Strain of extensor muscle, fascia and tendon of left ring finger at forearm level
  ● S56.417 Strain of extensor muscle, fascia and tendon of right little finger at forearm level
  ● S56.418 Strain of extensor muscle, fascia and tendon of left little finger at forearm level
  ● S56.419 Strain of extensor muscle, fascia and tendon of finger, unspecified finger at forearm level
● S56.42 Laceration of extensor muscle, fascia and tendon of other and unspecified finger at forearm level
  ● S56.421 Laceration of extensor muscle, fascia and tendon of right index finger at forearm level
  ● S56.422 Laceration of extensor muscle, fascia and tendon of left index finger at forearm level
  ● S56.423 Laceration of extensor muscle, fascia and tendon of right middle finger at forearm level
  ● S56.424 Laceration of extensor muscle, fascia and tendon of left middle finger at forearm level
  ● S56.425 Laceration of extensor muscle, fascia and tendon of right ring finger at forearm level
  ● S56.426 Laceration of extensor muscle, fascia and tendon of left ring finger at forearm level
  ● S56.427 Laceration of extensor muscle, fascia and tendon of right little finger at forearm level
  ● S56.428 Laceration of extensor muscle, fascia and tendon of left little finger at forearm level
  ● S56.429 Laceration of extensor muscle, fascia and tendon of unspecified finger at forearm level
● S56.49 Other injury of extensor muscle, fascia and tendon of other and unspecified finger at forearm level
  ● S56.491 Other injury of extensor muscle, fascia and tendon of right index finger at forearm level
  ● S56.492 Other injury of extensor muscle, fascia and tendon of left index finger at forearm level

  ● S56.493 Other injury of extensor muscle, fascia and tendon of right middle finger at forearm level
  ● S56.494 Other injury of extensor muscle, fascia and tendon of left middle finger at forearm level
  ● S56.495 Other injury of extensor muscle, fascia and tendon of right ring finger at forearm level
  ● S56.496 Other injury of extensor muscle, fascia and tendon of left ring finger at forearm level
  ● S56.497 Other injury of extensor muscle, fascia and tendon of right little finger at forearm level
  ● S56.498 Other injury of extensor muscle, fascia and tendon of left little finger at forearm level
  ● S56.499 Other injury of extensor muscle, fascia and tendon of unspecified finger at forearm level
● S56.5 Injury of other extensor muscle, fascia and tendon at forearm level
  ● S56.50 Unspecified injury of other extensor muscle, fascia and tendon at forearm level
    ● S56.501 Unspecified injury of other extensor muscle, fascia and tendon at forearm level, right arm
    ● S56.502 Unspecified injury of other extensor muscle, fascia and tendon at forearm level, left arm
    ● S56.509 Unspecified injury of other extensor muscle, fascia and tendon at forearm level, unspecified arm
  ● S56.51 Strain of other extensor muscle, fascia and tendon at forearm level
    ● S56.511 Strain of other extensor muscle, fascia and tendon at forearm level, right arm
    ● S56.512 Strain of other extensor muscle, fascia and tendon at forearm level, left arm
    ● S56.519 Strain of other extensor muscle, fascia and tendon at forearm level, unspecified arm
  ● S56.52 Laceration of other extensor muscle, fascia and tendon at forearm level
    ● S56.521 Laceration of other extensor muscle, fascia and tendon at forearm level, right arm
    ● S56.522 Laceration of other extensor muscle, fascia and tendon at forearm level, left arm
    ● S56.529 Laceration of other extensor muscle, fascia and tendon at forearm level, unspecified arm
  ● S56.59 Other injury of other extensor muscle, fascia and tendon at forearm level
    ● S56.591 Other injury of other extensor muscle, fascia and tendon at forearm level, right arm
    ● S56.592 Other injury of other extensor muscle, fascia and tendon at forearm level, left arm
    ● S56.599 Other injury of other extensor muscle, fascia and tendon at forearm level, unspecified arm

▶ New   ⇒ Revised   ~~deleted~~ Deleted   OGCR Official Guidelines   X Assign placeholder X   ● Use Additional Character(s)
Excludes 1   Excludes 2   Includes   Use additional   Code first   Code also   Key words

● **S56.8**   Injury of other muscles, fascia and tendons at forearm level
- ● **S56.80**   Unspecified injury of other muscles, fascia and tendons at forearm level
  - ● **S56.801**   Unspecified injury of other muscles, fascia and tendons at forearm level, right arm
  - ● **S56.802**   Unspecified injury of other muscles, fascia and tendons at forearm level, left arm
  - ● **S56.809**   Unspecified injury of other muscles, fascia and tendons at forearm level, unspecified arm
- ● **S56.81**   Strain of other muscles, fascia and tendons at forearm level
  - ● **S56.811**   Strain of other muscles, fascia and tendons at forearm level, right arm
  - ● **S56.812**   Strain of other muscles, fascia and tendons at forearm level, left arm
  - ● **S56.819**   Strain of other muscles, fascia and tendons at forearm level, unspecified arm
- ● **S56.82**   Laceration of other muscles, fascia and tendons at forearm level
  - ● **S56.821**   Laceration of other muscles, fascia and tendons at forearm level, right arm
  - ● **S56.822**   Laceration of other muscles, fascia and tendons at forearm level, left arm
  - ● **S56.829**   Laceration of other muscles, fascia and tendons at forearm level, unspecified arm
- ● **S56.89**   Other injury of other muscles, fascia and tendons at forearm level
  - ● **S56.891**   Other injury of other muscles, fascia and tendons at forearm level, right arm
  - ● **S56.892**   Other injury of other muscles, fascia and tendons at forearm level, left arm
  - ● **S56.899**   Other injury of other muscles, fascia and tendons at forearm level, unspecified arm
● **S56.9**   Injury of unspecified muscles, fascia and tendons at forearm level
- ● **S56.90**   Unspecified injury of unspecified muscles, fascia and tendons at forearm level
  - ● **S56.901**   Unspecified injury of unspecified muscles, fascia and tendons at forearm level, right arm
  - ● **S56.902**   Unspecified injury of unspecified muscles, fascia and tendons at forearm level, left arm
  - ● **S56.909**   Unspecified injury of unspecified muscles, fascia and tendons at forearm level, unspecified arm
- ● **S56.91**   Strain of unspecified muscles, fascia and tendons at forearm level
  - ● **S56.911**   Strain of unspecified muscles, fascia and tendons at forearm level, right arm
  - ● **S56.912**   Strain of unspecified muscles, fascia and tendons at forearm level, left arm
  - ● **S56.919**   Strain of unspecified muscles, fascia and tendons at forearm level, unspecified arm

● **S56.92**   Laceration of unspecified muscles, fascia and tendons at forearm level
- ● **S56.921**   Laceration of unspecified muscles, fascia and tendons at forearm level, right arm
- ● **S56.922**   Laceration of unspecified muscles, fascia and tendons at forearm level, left arm
- ● **S56.929**   Laceration of unspecified muscles, fascia and tendons at forearm level, unspecified arm
● **S56.99**   Other injury of unspecified muscles, fascia and tendons at forearm level
- ● **S56.991**   Other injury of unspecified muscles, fascia and tendons at forearm level, right arm
- ● **S56.992**   Other injury of unspecified muscles, fascia and tendons at forearm level, left arm
- ● **S56.999**   Other injury of unspecified muscles, fascia and tendons at forearm level, unspecified arm

● **S57**   **Crushing injury of elbow and forearm**

Use additional code(s) for all associated injuries

Excludes2   crushing injury of wrist and hand (S67.-)

The appropriate 7th character is to be added to each code from category S57

> A   initial encounter
> D   subsequent encounter
> S   sequela

- ● **S57.0**   Crushing injury of elbow
  - X ● **S57.00**   Crushing injury of unspecified elbow
  - X ● **S57.01**   Crushing injury of right elbow
  - X ● **S57.02**   Crushing injury of left elbow
- ● **S57.8**   Crushing injury of forearm
  - X ● **S57.80**   Crushing injury of unspecified forearm
  - X ● **S57.81**   Crushing injury of right forearm
  - X ● **S57.82**   Crushing injury of left forearm

● **S58**   **Traumatic amputation of elbow and forearm**

An amputation not identified as partial or complete should be coded to complete

Excludes1   traumatic amputation of wrist and hand (S68.-)

The appropriate 7th character is to be added to each code from category S58

> A   initial encounter
> D   subsequent encounter
> S   sequela

- ● **S58.0**   Traumatic amputation at elbow level
  - ● **S58.01**   Complete traumatic amputation at elbow level
    - ● **S58.011**   Complete traumatic amputation at elbow level, right arm
    - ● **S58.012**   Complete traumatic amputation at elbow level, left arm
    - ● **S58.019**   Complete traumatic amputation at elbow level, unspecified arm
  - ● **S58.02**   Partial traumatic amputation at elbow level
    - ● **S58.021**   Partial traumatic amputation at elbow level, right arm
    - ● **S58.022**   Partial traumatic amputation at elbow level, left arm
    - ● **S58.029**   Partial traumatic amputation at elbow level, unspecified arm

● **S58.1**   Traumatic amputation at level between elbow and wrist

   ● **S58.11**   **Complete** traumatic amputation at level between elbow and wrist

     ● **S58.111**   Complete traumatic amputation at level between elbow and wrist, **right arm**

     ● **S58.112**   Complete traumatic amputation at level between elbow and wrist, **left arm**

     ● **S58.119**   Complete traumatic amputation at level between elbow and wrist, **unspecified arm**

   ● **S58.12**   **Partial** traumatic amputation at level between elbow and wrist

     ● **S58.121**   Partial traumatic amputation at level between elbow and wrist, **right arm**

     ● **S58.122**   Partial traumatic amputation at level between elbow and wrist, **left arm**

     ● **S58.129**   Partial traumatic amputation at level between elbow and wrist, **unspecified arm**

● **S58.9**   Traumatic amputation of forearm, level unspecified

   | Excludes1 | traumatic amputation of wrist (S68.-)

   ● **S58.91**   **Complete** traumatic amputation of forearm, level unspecified

     ● **S58.911**   Complete traumatic amputation of **right** forearm, level unspecified

     ● **S58.912**   Complete traumatic amputation of **left** forearm, level unspecified

     ● **S58.919**   Complete traumatic amputation of **unspecified** forearm, level unspecified

   ● **S58.92**   **Partial** traumatic amputation of forearm, level unspecified

     ● **S58.921**   Partial traumatic amputation of **right** forearm, level unspecified

     ● **S58.922**   Partial traumatic amputation of **left** forearm, level unspecified

     ● **S58.929**   Partial traumatic amputation of **unspecified** forearm, level unspecified

● **S59**   Other and unspecified injuries of elbow and forearm

   | Excludes2 | other and unspecified injuries of wrist and hand (S69.-)

   The appropriate 7th character is to be added to each code from subcategories S59.Ø, S59.1, and S59.2

A	initial encounter for closed fracture
D	subsequent encounter for fracture with routine healing
G	subsequent encounter for fracture with delayed healing
K	subsequent encounter for fracture with nonunion
P	subsequent encounter for fracture with malunion
S	sequela

● **S59.Ø**   Physeal fracture of lower end of ulna

   ● **S59.ØØ**   **Unspecified** physeal fracture of lower end of ulna

     ● **S59.ØØ1**   Unspecified physeal fracture of lower end of ulna, **right arm**

     ● **S59.ØØ2**   Unspecified physeal fracture of lower end of ulna, **left arm**

     ● **S59.ØØ9**   Unspecified physeal fracture of lower end of ulna, **unspecified arm**

Item 19–4 SALTER-HARRIS TYPE 1: epiphysis is completely separated from end of bone, or metaphysic growth plate remains attached to epiphysis

SALTER-HARRIS TYPE 2: epiphysis and growth plate are partially separated from metaphysis, which is cracked—most common type

SALTER-HARRIS TYPE 3: fracture occurring through epiphysis and separates part of epiphysis and growth plate from metaphysis fracture, usually at distal end of tibia

SALTER-HARRIS TYPE 4: fracture runs through epiphysis, across growth plate, into metaphysic, surgery is required to restore joint surface to normal and align growth plate

   ● **S59.Ø1**   **Salter-Harris Type I** physeal fracture of lower end of ulna

     ● **S59.Ø11**   Salter-Harris Type I physeal fracture of lower end of ulna, **right arm**

     ● **S59.Ø12**   Salter-Harris Type I physeal fracture of lower end of ulna, **left arm**

     ● **S59.Ø19**   Salter-Harris Type I physeal fracture of lower end of ulna, **unspecified arm**

   ● **S59.Ø2**   **Salter-Harris Type II** physeal fracture of lower end of ulna

     ● **S59.Ø21**   Salter-Harris Type II physeal fracture of lower end of ulna, **right arm**

     ● **S59.Ø22**   Salter-Harris Type II physeal fracture of lower end of ulna, **left arm**

     ● **S59.Ø29**   Salter-Harris Type II physeal fracture of lower end of ulna, **unspecified arm**

   ● **S59.Ø3**   **Salter-Harris Type III** physeal fracture of lower end of ulna

     ● **S59.Ø31**   Salter-Harris Type III physeal fracture of lower end of ulna, **right arm**

     ● **S59.Ø32**   Salter-Harris Type III physeal fracture of lower end of ulna, **left arm**

     ● **S59.Ø39**   Salter-Harris Type III physeal fracture of lower end of ulna, **unspecified arm**

   ● **S59.Ø4**   **Salter-Harris Type IV** physeal fracture of lower end of ulna

     ● **S59.Ø41**   Salter-Harris Type IV physeal fracture of lower end of ulna, **right arm**

     ● **S59.Ø42**   Salter-Harris Type IV physeal fracture of lower end of ulna, **left arm**

     ● **S59.Ø49**   Salter-Harris Type IV physeal fracture of lower end of ulna, **unspecified arm**

   ● **S59.Ø9**   **Other** physeal fracture of lower end of ulna

     ● **S59.Ø91**   Other physeal fracture of lower end of ulna, **right arm**

     ● **S59.Ø92**   Other physeal fracture of lower end of ulna, **left arm**

     ● **S59.Ø99**   Other physeal fracture of lower end of ulna, **unspecified arm**

● **S59.1**   Physeal fracture of upper end of radius

   ● **S59.1Ø**   **Unspecified** physeal fracture of upper end of radius

     ● **S59.1Ø1**   Unspecified physeal fracture of upper end of radius, **right arm**

     ● **S59.1Ø2**   Unspecified physeal fracture of upper end of radius, **left arm**

     ● **S59.1Ø9**   Unspecified physeal fracture of upper end of radius, **unspecified arm**

▶ New   ⇒ Revised   ~~deleted~~ Deleted   OGCR Official Guidelines   X Assign placeholder X   ● Use Additional Character(s)

| Excludes 1 | | Excludes 2 | Includes   Use additional   Code first   Code also   Key words

- ● S59.11 Salter-Harris Type I physeal fracture of upper end of radius
  - ● S59.111 Salter-Harris Type I physeal fracture of upper end of radius, right arm
  - ● S59.112 Salter-Harris Type I physeal fracture of upper end of radius, left arm
  - ● S59.119 Salter-Harris Type I physeal fracture of upper end of radius, unspecified arm
- ● S59.12 Salter-Harris Type II physeal fracture of upper end of radius
  - ● S59.121 Salter-Harris Type II physeal fracture of upper end of radius, right arm
  - ● S59.122 Salter-Harris Type II physeal fracture of upper end of radius, left arm
  - ● S59.129 Salter-Harris Type II physeal fracture of upper end of radius, unspecified arm
- ● S59.13 Salter-Harris Type III physeal fracture of upper end of radius
  - ● S59.131 Salter-Harris Type III physeal fracture of upper end of radius, right arm
  - ● S59.132 Salter-Harris Type III physeal fracture of upper end of radius, left arm
  - ● S59.139 Salter-Harris Type III physeal fracture of upper end of radius, unspecified arm
- ● S59.14 Salter-Harris Type IV physeal fracture of upper end of radius
  - ● S59.141 Salter-Harris Type IV physeal fracture of upper end of radius, right arm
  - ● S59.142 Salter-Harris Type IV physeal fracture of upper end of radius, left arm
  - ● S59.149 Salter-Harris Type IV physeal fracture of upper end of radius, unspecified arm
- ● S59.19 Other physeal fracture of upper end of radius
  - ● S59.191 Other physeal fracture of upper end of radius, right arm
  - ● S59.192 Other physeal fracture of upper end of radius, left arm
  - ● S59.199 Other physeal fracture of upper end of radius, unspecified arm
- ● S59.2 Physeal fracture of lower end of radius
  - ● S59.20 Unspecified physeal fracture of lower end of radius
    - ● S59.201 Unspecified physeal fracture of lower end of radius, right arm
    - ● S59.202 Unspecified physeal fracture of lower end of radius, left arm
    - ● S59.209 Unspecified physeal fracture of lower end of radius, unspecified arm
  - ● S59.21 Salter-Harris Type I physeal fracture of lower end of radius
    - ● S59.211 Salter-Harris Type I physeal fracture of lower end of radius, right arm
    - ● S59.212 Salter-Harris Type I physeal fracture of lower end of radius, left arm
    - ● S59.219 Salter-Harris Type I physeal fracture of lower end of radius, unspecified arm
  - ● S59.22 Salter-Harris Type II physeal fracture of lower end of radius
    - ● S59.221 Salter-Harris Type II physeal fracture of lower end of radius, right arm
    - ● S59.222 Salter-Harris Type II physeal fracture of lower end of radius, left arm
    - ● S59.229 Salter-Harris Type II physeal fracture of lower end of radius, unspecified arm

- ● S59.23 Salter-Harris Type III physeal fracture of lower end of radius
  - ● S59.231 Salter-Harris Type III physeal fracture of lower end of radius, right arm
  - ● S59.232 Salter-Harris Type III physeal fracture of lower end of radius, left arm
  - ● S59.239 Salter-Harris Type III physeal fracture of lower end of radius, unspecified arm
- ● S59.24 Salter-Harris Type IV physeal fracture of lower end of radius
  - ● S59.241 Salter-Harris Type IV physeal fracture of lower end of radius, right arm
  - ● S59.242 Salter-Harris Type IV physeal fracture of lower end of radius, left arm
  - ● S59.249 Salter-Harris Type IV physeal fracture of lower end of radius, unspecified arm
- ● S59.29 Other physeal fracture of lower end of radius
  - ● S59.291 Other physeal fracture of lower end of radius, right arm
  - ● S59.292 Other physeal fracture of lower end of radius, left arm
  - ● S59.299 Other physeal fracture of lower end of radius, unspecified arm
- ● S59.8 Other specified injuries of elbow and forearm

  The appropriate 7th character is to be added to each code in subcategory S59.8

A	initial encounter
D	subsequent encounter
S	sequela

  - ● S59.80 Other specified injuries of elbow
    - ● S59.801 Other specified injuries of right elbow
    - ● S59.802 Other specified injuries of left elbow
    - ● S59.809 Other specified injuries of unspecified elbow
  - ● S59.81 Other specified injuries of forearm
    - ● S59.811 Other specified injuries right forearm
    - ● S59.812 Other specified injuries left forearm
    - ● S59.819 Other specified injuries unspecified forearm
- ● S59.9 Unspecified injury of elbow and forearm

  The appropriate 7th character is to be added to each code in subcategory S59.9

A	initial encounter
D	subsequent encounter
S	sequela

  - ● S59.90 Unspecified injury of elbow
    - ● S59.901 Unspecified injury of right elbow
    - ● S59.902 Unspecified injury of left elbow
    - ● S59.909 Unspecified injury of unspecified elbow
  - ● S59.91 Unspecified injury of forearm
    - ● S59.911 Unspecified injury of right forearm
    - ● S59.912 Unspecified injury of left forearm
    - ● S59.919 Unspecified injury of unspecified forearm

CHAPTER 19 (S00-T88)

CHAPTER 19 (S00-T88)

INJURIES TO THE WRIST, HAND AND FINGERS (S60-S69)

> **Excludes2**   burns and corrosions (T20-T32)
> frostbite (T33-T34)
> insect bite or sting, venomous (T63.4)

● **S60**   **Superficial injury of wrist, hand and fingers**

The appropriate 7th character is to be added to each code from category S60

A	initial encounter
D	subsequent encounter
S	sequela

● **S60.0**   Contusion of finger without damage to nail

> **Excludes1**   contusion involving nail (matrix) (S60.1)

X ● **S60.00**   Contusion of unspecified finger without damage to nail
Contusion of finger(s) NOS

● **S60.01**   Contusion of thumb without damage to nail

● **S60.011**   Contusion of right thumb without damage to nail

● **S60.012**   Contusion of left thumb without damage to nail

● **S60.019**   Contusion of unspecified thumb without damage to nail

● **S60.02**   Contusion of index finger without damage to nail

● **S60.021**   Contusion of right index finger without damage to nail

● **S60.022**   Contusion of left index finger without damage to nail

● **S60.029**   Contusion of unspecified index finger without damage to nail

● **S60.03**   Contusion of middle finger without damage to nail

● **S60.031**   Contusion of right middle finger without damage to nail

● **S60.032**   Contusion of left middle finger without damage to nail

● **S60.039**   Contusion of unspecified middle finger without damage to nail

● **S60.04**   Contusion of ring finger without damage to nail

● **S60.041**   Contusion of right ring finger without damage to nail

● **S60.042**   Contusion of left ring finger without damage to nail

● **S60.049**   Contusion of unspecified ring finger without damage to nail

● **S60.05**   Contusion of little finger without damage to nail

● **S60.051**   Contusion of right little finger without damage to nail

● **S60.052**   Contusion of left little finger without damage to nail

● **S60.059**   Contusion of unspecified little finger without damage to nail

● **S60.1**   Contusion of finger with damage to nail

X ● **S60.10**   Contusion of unspecified finger with damage to nail

● **S60.11**   Contusion of thumb with damage to nail

● **S60.111**   Contusion of right thumb with damage to nail

● **S60.112**   Contusion of left thumb with damage to nail

● **S60.119**   Contusion of unspecified thumb with damage to nail

● **S60.12**   Contusion of index finger with damage to nail

● **S60.121**   Contusion of right index finger with damage to nail

● **S60.122**   Contusion of left index finger with damage to nail

● **S60.129**   Contusion of unspecified index finger with damage to nail

● **S60.13**   Contusion of middle finger with damage to nail

● **S60.131**   Contusion of right middle finger with damage to nail

● **S60.132**   Contusion of left middle finger with damage to nail

● **S60.139**   Contusion of unspecified middle finger with damage to nail

● **S60.14**   Contusion of ring finger with damage to nail

● **S60.141**   Contusion of right ring finger with damage to nail

● **S60.142**   Contusion of left ring finger with damage to nail

● **S60.149**   Contusion of unspecified ring finger with damage to nail

● **S60.15**   Contusion of little finger with damage to nail

● **S60.151**   Contusion of right little finger with damage to nail

● **S60.152**   Contusion of left little finger with damage to nail

● **S60.159**   Contusion of unspecified little finger with damage to nail

● **S60.2**   Contusion of wrist and hand

> **Excludes2**   contusion of fingers (S60.0-, S60.1-)

● **S60.21**   Contusion of wrist

● **S60.211**   Contusion of right wrist

● **S60.212**   Contusion of left wrist

● **S60.219**   Contusion of unspecified wrist

● **S60.22**   Contusion of hand

● **S60.221**   Contusion of right hand

● **S60.222**   Contusion of left hand

● **S60.229**   Contusion of unspecified hand

● **S60.3**   Other superficial injuries of thumb

● **S60.31**   Abrasion of thumb

● **S60.311**   Abrasion of right thumb

● **S60.312**   Abrasion of left thumb

● **S60.319**   Abrasion of unspecified thumb

● **S60.32**   Blister (nonthermal) of thumb

● **S60.321**   Blister (nonthermal) of right thumb

● **S60.322**   Blister (nonthermal) of left thumb

● **S60.329**   Blister (nonthermal) of unspecified thumb

● **S60.34**   External constriction of thumb
Hair tourniquet syndrome of thumb
Use additional cause code to identify the constricting item (W49.0-)

● **S60.341**   External constriction of right thumb

● **S60.342**   External constriction of left thumb

● **S60.349**   External constriction of unspecified thumb

● **S60.35**   Superficial foreign body of thumb
Splinter in the thumb

● **S60.351**   Superficial foreign body of right thumb

● **S60.352**   Superficial foreign body of left thumb

● **S60.359**   Superficial foreign body of unspecified thumb

▶ New   ⇒ Revised   ~~deleted~~ Deleted   **OGCR** Official Guidelines   X Assign placeholder X   ● Use Additional Character(s)

Excludes 1   Excludes 2   Includes   Use additional   Code first   Code also   Key words

● S60.36   Insect bite (nonvenomous) of thumb
   ● S60.361   Insect bite (nonvenomous) of right thumb
   ● S60.362   Insect bite (nonvenomous) of left thumb
   ● S60.369   Insect bite (nonvenomous) of unspecified thumb
● S60.37   Other superficial bite of thumb
   Excludes1   open bite of thumb (S61.05-, S61.15-)
   ● S60.371   Other superficial bite of right thumb
   ● S60.372   Other superficial bite of left thumb
   ● S60.379   Other superficial bite of unspecified thumb
● S60.39   Other superficial injuries of thumb
   ● S60.391   Other superficial injuries of right thumb
   ● S60.392   Other superficial injuries of left thumb
   ● S60.399   Other superficial injuries of unspecified thumb
● S60.4   Other superficial injuries of other fingers
  ● S60.41   Abrasion of fingers
   ● S60.410   Abrasion of right index finger
   ● S60.411   Abrasion of left index finger
   ● S60.412   Abrasion of right middle finger
   ● S60.413   Abrasion of left middle finger
   ● S60.414   Abrasion of right ring finger
   ● S60.415   Abrasion of left ring finger
   ● S60.416   Abrasion of right little finger
   ● S60.417   Abrasion of left little finger
   ● S60.418   Abrasion of other finger
     Abrasion of specified finger with unspecified laterality
   ● S60.419   Abrasion of unspecified finger
  ● S60.42   Blister (nonthermal) of fingers
   ● S60.420   Blister (nonthermal) of right index finger
   ● S60.421   Blister (nonthermal) of left index finger
   ● S60.422   Blister (nonthermal) of right middle finger
   ● S60.423   Blister (nonthermal) of left middle finger
   ● S60.424   Blister (nonthermal) of right ring finger
   ● S60.425   Blister (nonthermal) of left ring finger
   ● S60.426   Blister (nonthermal) of right little finger
   ● S60.427   Blister (nonthermal) of left little finger
   ● S60.428   Blister (nonthermal) of other finger
     Blister (nonthermal) of specified finger with unspecified laterality
   ● S60.429   Blister (nonthermal) of unspecified finger
  ● S60.44   External constriction of fingers
     Hair tourniquet syndrome of finger
     Use additional cause code to identify the constricting item (W49.0-)
   ● S60.440   External constriction of right index finger
   ● S60.441   External constriction of left index finger

● S60.442   External constriction of right middle finger
● S60.443   External constriction of left middle finger
● S60.444   External constriction of right ring finger
● S60.445   External constriction of left ring finger
● S60.446   External constriction of right little finger
● S60.447   External constriction of left little finger
● S60.448   External constriction of other finger
   External constriction of specified finger with unspecified laterality
● S60.449   External constriction of unspecified finger
● S60.45   Superficial foreign body of fingers
   Splinter in the finger(s)
  ● S60.450   Superficial foreign body of right index finger
  ● S60.451   Superficial foreign body of left index finger
  ● S60.452   Superficial foreign body of right middle finger
  ● S60.453   Superficial foreign body of left middle finger
  ● S60.454   Superficial foreign body of right ring finger
  ● S60.455   Superficial foreign body of left ring finger
  ● S60.456   Superficial foreign body of right little finger
  ● S60.457   Superficial foreign body of left little finger
  ● S60.458   Superficial foreign body of other finger
     Superficial foreign body of specified finger with unspecified laterality
  ● S60.459   Superficial foreign body of unspecified finger
● S60.46   Insect bite (nonvenomous) of fingers
  ● S60.460   Insect bite (nonvenomous) of right index finger
  ● S60.461   Insect bite (nonvenomous) of left index finger
  ● S60.462   Insect bite (nonvenomous) of right middle finger
  ● S60.463   Insect bite (nonvenomous) of left middle finger
  ● S60.464   Insect bite (nonvenomous) of right ring finger
  ● S60.465   Insect bite (nonvenomous) of left ring finger
  ● S60.466   Insect bite (nonvenomous) of right little finger
  ● S60.467   Insect bite (nonvenomous) of left little finger
  ● S60.468   Insect bite (nonvenomous) of other finger
     Insect bite (nonvenomous) of specified finger with unspecified laterality
  ● S60.469   Insect bite (nonvenomous) of unspecified finger

▶ New   ⇒ Revised   ~~deleted~~ Deleted   **OGCR** Official Guidelines   X Assign placeholder X   ● Use Additional Character(s)

Excludes 1   Excludes 2   Includes   Use additional   Code first   Code also   Key words

CHAPTER 19 (S00-T88)

- S60.47   Other superficial bite of fingers
  - **Excludes1**   open bite of fingers (S61.25-, S61.35-)
  - S60.470   Other superficial bite of right index finger
  - S60.471   Other superficial bite of left index finger
  - S60.472   Other superficial bite of right middle finger
  - S60.473   Other superficial bite of left middle finger
  - S60.474   Other superficial bite of right ring finger
  - S60.475   Other superficial bite of left ring finger
  - S60.476   Other superficial bite of right little finger
  - S60.477   Other superficial bite of left little finger
  - S60.478   Other superficial bite of other finger
    - Other superficial bite of specified finger with unspecified laterality
  - S60.479   Other superficial bite of unspecified finger
- S60.5   Other superficial injuries of hand
  - **Excludes2**   superficial injuries of fingers (S60.3-, S60.4-)
  - S60.51   Abrasion of hand
    - S60.511   Abrasion of right hand
    - S60.512   Abrasion of left hand
    - S60.519   Abrasion of unspecified hand
  - S60.52   Blister (nonthermal) of hand
    - S60.521   Blister (nonthermal) of right hand
    - S60.522   Blister (nonthermal) of left hand
    - S60.529   Blister (nonthermal) of unspecified hand
  - S60.54   External constriction of hand
    - S60.541   External constriction of right hand
    - S60.542   External constriction of left hand
    - S60.549   External constriction of unspecified hand
  - S60.55   Superficial foreign body of hand
    - Splinter in the hand
    - S60.551   Superficial foreign body of right hand
    - S60.552   Superficial foreign body of left hand
    - S60.559   Superficial foreign body of unspecified hand
  - S60.56   Insect bite (nonvenomous) of hand
    - S60.561   Insect bite (nonvenomous) of right hand
    - S60.562   Insect bite (nonvenomous) of left hand
    - S60.569   Insect bite (nonvenomous) of unspecified hand
  - S60.57   Other superficial bite of hand
    - **Excludes1**   open bite of hand (S61.45-)
    - S60.571   Other superficial bite of hand of right hand
    - S60.572   Other superficial bite of hand of left hand
    - S60.579   Other superficial bite of hand of unspecified hand

- S60.8   Other superficial injuries of wrist
  - S60.81   Abrasion of wrist
    - S60.811   Abrasion of right wrist
    - S60.812   Abrasion of left wrist
    - S60.819   Abrasion of unspecified wrist
  - S60.82   Blister (nonthermal) of wrist
    - S60.821   Blister (nonthermal) of right wrist
    - S60.822   Blister (nonthermal) of left wrist
    - S60.829   Blister (nonthermal) of unspecified wrist
  - S60.84   External constriction of wrist
    - S60.841   External constriction of right wrist
    - S60.842   External constriction of left wrist
    - S60.849   External constriction of unspecified wrist
  - S60.85   Superficial foreign body of wrist
    - Splinter in the wrist
    - S60.851   Superficial foreign body of right wrist
    - S60.852   Superficial foreign body of left wrist
    - S60.859   Superficial foreign body of unspecified wrist
  - S60.86   Insect bite (nonvenomous) of wrist
    - S60.861   Insect bite (nonvenomous) of right wrist
    - S60.862   Insect bite (nonvenomous) of left wrist
    - S60.869   Insect bite (nonvenomous) of unspecified wrist
  - S60.87   Other superficial bite of wrist
    - **Excludes1**   open bite of wrist (S61.55)
    - S60.871   Other superficial bite of right wrist
    - S60.872   Other superficial bite of left wrist
    - S60.879   Other superficial bite of unspecified wrist
- S60.9   Unspecified superficial injury of wrist, hand and fingers
  - S60.91   Unspecified superficial injury of wrist
    - S60.911   Unspecified superficial injury of right wrist
    - S60.912   Unspecified superficial injury of left wrist
    - S60.919   Unspecified superficial injury of unspecified wrist
  - S60.92   Unspecified superficial injury of hand
    - S60.921   Unspecified superficial injury of right hand
    - S60.922   Unspecified superficial injury of left hand
    - S60.929   Unspecified superficial injury of unspecified hand
  - S60.93   Unspecified superficial injury of thumb
    - S60.931   Unspecified superficial injury of right thumb
    - S60.932   Unspecified superficial injury of left thumb
    - S60.939   Unspecified superficial injury of unspecified thumb

▶ New   ⮕ Revised   ~~deleted~~ Deleted   **OGCR** Official Guidelines   X Assign placeholder X   ● Use Additional Character(s)

Excludes 1   Excludes 2   Includes   Use additional   Code first   Code also   Key words

● S60.94   Unspecified superficial injury of other fingers
   ● S60.940   Unspecified superficial injury of right index finger
   ● S60.941   Unspecified superficial injury of left index finger
   ● S60.942   Unspecified superficial injury of right middle finger
   ● S60.943   Unspecified superficial injury of left middle finger
   ● S60.944   Unspecified superficial injury of right ring finger
   ● S60.945   Unspecified superficial injury of left ring finger
   ● S60.946   Unspecified superficial injury of right little finger
   ● S60.947   Unspecified superficial injury of left little finger
   ● S60.948   Unspecified superficial injury of other finger
       Unspecified superficial injury of specified finger with unspecified laterality
   ● S60.949   Unspecified superficial injury of unspecified finger

● S61   Open wound of wrist, hand and fingers
   Code also any associated wound infection
   Excludes1   open fracture of wrist, hand and finger (S62.- with 7th character B)
       traumatic amputation of wrist and hand (S68.-)
   The appropriate 7th character is to be added to each code from category S61

     A   initial encounter
     D   subsequent encounter
     S   sequela

 ● S61.0   Open wound of thumb without damage to nail
   Excludes1   open wound of thumb with damage to nail (S61.1-)
  ● S61.00   Unspecified open wound of thumb without damage to nail
   ● S61.001   Unspecified open wound of right thumb without damage to nail
   ● S61.002   Unspecified open wound of left thumb without damage to nail
   ● S61.009   Unspecified open wound of unspecified thumb without damage to nail
  ● S61.01   Laceration without foreign body of thumb without damage to nail
   ● S61.011   Laceration without foreign body of right thumb without damage to nail
   ● S61.012   Laceration without foreign body of left thumb without damage to nail
   ● S61.019   Laceration without foreign body of unspecified thumb without damage to nail
  ● S61.02   Laceration with foreign body of thumb without damage to nail
   ● S61.021   Laceration with foreign body of right thumb without damage to nail
   ● S61.022   Laceration with foreign body of left thumb without damage to nail
   ● S61.029   Laceration with foreign body of unspecified thumb without damage to nail

● S61.03   Puncture wound without foreign body of thumb without damage to nail
   ● S61.031   Puncture wound without foreign body of right thumb without damage to nail
   ● S61.032   Puncture wound without foreign body of left thumb without damage to nail
   ● S61.039   Puncture wound without foreign body of unspecified thumb without damage to nail
● S61.04   Puncture wound with foreign body of thumb without damage to nail
   ● S61.041   Puncture wound with foreign body of right thumb without damage to nail
   ● S61.042   Puncture wound with foreign body of left thumb without damage to nail
   ● S61.049   Puncture wound with foreign body of unspecified thumb without damage to nail
● S61.05   Open bite of thumb without damage to nail
   Bite of thumb NOS
   Excludes1   superficial bite of thumb (S60.36-, S60.37-)
   ● S61.051   Open bite of right thumb without damage to nail
   ● S61.052   Open bite of left thumb without damage to nail
   ● S61.059   Open bite of unspecified thumb without damage to nail
● S61.1   Open wound of thumb with damage to nail
  ● S61.10   Unspecified open wound of thumb with damage to nail
   ● S61.101   Unspecified open wound of right thumb with damage to nail
   ● S61.102   Unspecified open wound of left thumb with damage to nail
   ● S61.109   Unspecified open wound of unspecified thumb with damage to nail
  ● S61.11   Laceration without foreign body of thumb with damage to nail
   ● S61.111   Laceration without foreign body of right thumb with damage to nail
   ● S61.112   Laceration without foreign body of left thumb with damage to nail
   ● S61.119   Laceration without foreign body of unspecified thumb with damage to nail
  ● S61.12   Laceration with foreign body of thumb with damage to nail
   ● S61.121   Laceration with foreign body of right thumb with damage to nail
   ● S61.122   Laceration with foreign body of left thumb with damage to nail
   ● S61.129   Laceration with foreign body of unspecified thumb with damage to nail
  ● S61.13   Puncture wound without foreign body of thumb with damage to nail
   ● S61.131   Puncture wound without foreign body of right thumb with damage to nail
   ● S61.132   Puncture wound without foreign body of left thumb with damage to nail
   ● S61.139   Puncture wound without foreign body of unspecified thumb with damage to nail

CHAPTER 19 (S00-T88)

● **S61.14** Puncture wound with foreign body of thumb with damage to nail
- ● **S61.141** Puncture wound with foreign body of right thumb with damage to nail
- ● **S61.142** Puncture wound with foreign body of left thumb with damage to nail
- ● **S61.149** Puncture wound with foreign body of unspecified thumb with damage to nail

● **S61.15** Open bite of thumb with damage to nail
  Bite of thumb with damage to nail NOS
  Excludes1 superficial bite of thumb (S60.36-, S60.37-)
- ● **S61.151** Open bite of right thumb with damage to nail
- ● **S61.152** Open bite of left thumb with damage to nail
- ● **S61.159** Open bite of unspecified thumb with damage to nail

● **S61.2** Open wound of other finger without damage to nail
  Excludes1 open wound of finger involving nail (matrix) (S61.3-)
  Excludes2 open wound of thumb without damage to nail (S61.0-)
- ● **S61.20** Unspecified open wound of other finger without damage to nail
  - ● **S61.200** Unspecified open wound of right index finger without damage to nail
  - ● **S61.201** Unspecified open wound of left index finger without damage to nail
  - ● **S61.202** Unspecified open wound of right middle finger without damage to nail
  - ● **S61.203** Unspecified open wound of left middle finger without damage to nail
  - ● **S61.204** Unspecified open wound of right ring finger without damage to nail
  - ● **S61.205** Unspecified open wound of left ring finger without damage to nail
  - ● **S61.206** Unspecified open wound of right little finger without damage to nail
  - ● **S61.207** Unspecified open wound of left little finger without damage to nail
  - ● **S61.208** Unspecified open wound of other finger without damage to nail
    Unspecified open wound of specified finger with unspecified laterality without damage to nail
  - ● **S61.209** Unspecified open wound of unspecified finger without damage to nail
- ● **S61.21** Laceration without foreign body of finger without damage to nail
  - ● **S61.210** Laceration without foreign body of right index finger without damage to nail
  - ● **S61.211** Laceration without foreign body of left index finger without damage to nail
  - ● **S61.212** Laceration without foreign body of right middle finger without damage to nail
  - ● **S61.213** Laceration without foreign body of left middle finger without damage to nail
  - ● **S61.214** Laceration without foreign body of right ring finger without damage to nail
  - ● **S61.215** Laceration without foreign body of left ring finger without damage to nail
  - ● **S61.216** Laceration without foreign body of right little finger without damage to nail

- ● **S61.217** Laceration without foreign body of left little finger without damage to nail
- ● **S61.218** Laceration without foreign body of other finger without damage to nail
  Laceration without foreign body of specified finger with unspecified laterality without damage to nail
- ● **S61.219** Laceration without foreign body of unspecified finger without damage to nail

● **S61.22** Laceration with foreign body of finger without damage to nail
- ● **S61.220** Laceration with foreign body of right index finger without damage to nail
- ● **S61.221** Laceration with foreign body of left index finger without damage to nail
- ● **S61.222** Laceration with foreign body of right middle finger without damage to nail
- ● **S61.223** Laceration with foreign body of left middle finger without damage to nail
- ● **S61.224** Laceration with foreign body of right ring finger without damage to nail
- ● **S61.225** Laceration with foreign body of left ring finger without damage to nail
- ● **S61.226** Laceration with foreign body of right little finger without damage to nail
- ● **S61.227** Laceration with foreign body of left little finger without damage to nail
- ● **S61.228** Laceration with foreign body of other finger without damage to nail
  Laceration with foreign body of specified finger with unspecified laterality without damage to nail
- ● **S61.229** Laceration with foreign body of unspecified finger without damage to nail

● **S61.23** Puncture wound without foreign body of finger without damage to nail
- ● **S61.230** Puncture wound without foreign body of right index finger without damage to nail
- ● **S61.231** Puncture wound without foreign body of left index finger without damage to nail
- ● **S61.232** Puncture wound without foreign body of right middle finger without damage to nail
- ● **S61.233** Puncture wound without foreign body of left middle finger without damage to nail
- ● **S61.234** Puncture wound without foreign body of right ring finger without damage to nail
- ● **S61.235** Puncture wound without foreign body of left ring finger without damage to nail
- ● **S61.236** Puncture wound without foreign body of right little finger without damage to nail
- ● **S61.237** Puncture wound without foreign body of left little finger without damage to nail
- ● **S61.238** Puncture wound without foreign body of other finger without damage to nail
  Puncture wound without foreign body of specified finger with unspecified laterality without damage to nail
- ● **S61.239** Puncture wound without foreign body of unspecified finger without damage to nail

▶ New ⇒ Revised ~~deleted~~ Deleted **OGCR** Official Guidelines X Assign placeholder X ● Use Additional Character(s)

Excludes 1 Excludes 2 Includes Use additional Code first Code also Key words

● S61.24　Puncture wound with foreign body of finger
　　　　　without damage to nail

　　● S61.240　Puncture wound with foreign body of
　　　　　　　　right index finger without damage to
　　　　　　　　nail

　　● S61.241　Puncture wound with foreign body
　　　　　　　　of left index finger without damage to
　　　　　　　　nail

　　● S61.242　Puncture wound with foreign body of
　　　　　　　　right middle finger without damage
　　　　　　　　to nail

　　● S61.243　Puncture wound with foreign body of
　　　　　　　　left middle finger without damage to
　　　　　　　　nail

　　● S61.244　Puncture wound with foreign body
　　　　　　　　of right ring finger without damage to
　　　　　　　　nail

　　● S61.245　Puncture wound with foreign body of
　　　　　　　　left ring finger without damage to nail

　　● S61.246　Puncture wound with foreign body of
　　　　　　　　right little finger without damage to
　　　　　　　　nail

　　● S61.247　Puncture wound with foreign body
　　　　　　　　of left little finger without damage to
　　　　　　　　nail

　　● S61.248　Puncture wound with foreign body of
　　　　　　　　other finger without damage to nail
　　　　　　　　　　Puncture wound with foreign
　　　　　　　　　　　　body of specified finger with
　　　　　　　　　　　　unspecified laterality without
　　　　　　　　　　　　damage to nail

　　● S61.249　Puncture wound with foreign body of
　　　　　　　　unspecified finger without damage to
　　　　　　　　nail

● S61.25　Open bite of finger without damage to nail
　　　　　　Bite of finger without damage to nail NOS
　　　　　┌──────────┐
　　　　　│ Excludes1 │　superficial bite of finger (S60.46-,
　　　　　└──────────┘　　S60.47-)

　　● S61.250　Open bite of right index finger
　　　　　　　　without damage to nail

　　● S61.251　Open bite of left index finger without
　　　　　　　　damage to nail

　　● S61.252　Open bite of right middle finger
　　　　　　　　without damage to nail

　　● S61.253　Open bite of left middle finger
　　　　　　　　without damage to nail

　　● S61.254　Open bite of right ring finger without
　　　　　　　　damage to nail

　　● S61.255　Open bite of left ring finger without
　　　　　　　　damage to nail

　　● S61.256　Open bite of right little finger without
　　　　　　　　damage to nail

　　● S61.257　Open bite of left little finger without
　　　　　　　　damage to nail

　　● S61.258　Open bite of other finger without
　　　　　　　　damage to nail
　　　　　　　　　　Open bite of specified finger with
　　　　　　　　　　　　unspecified laterality without
　　　　　　　　　　　　damage to nail

　　● S61.259　Open bite of unspecified finger
　　　　　　　　without damage to nail

● S61.3　Open wound of other finger with damage to nail

　● S61.30　Unspecified open wound of finger with damage
　　　　　　to nail

　　● S61.300　Unspecified open wound of right
　　　　　　　　index finger with damage to nail

　　● S61.301　Unspecified open wound of left index
　　　　　　　　finger with damage to nail

　　● S61.302　Unspecified open wound of right
　　　　　　　　middle finger with damage to nail

　　● S61.303　Unspecified open wound of left
　　　　　　　　middle finger with damage to nail

　　● S61.304　Unspecified open wound of right ring
　　　　　　　　finger with damage to nail

　　● S61.305　Unspecified open wound of left ring
　　　　　　　　finger with damage to nail

　　● S61.306　Unspecified open wound of right little
　　　　　　　　finger with damage to nail

　　● S61.307　Unspecified open wound of left little
　　　　　　　　finger with damage to nail

　　● S61.308　Unspecified open wound of other
　　　　　　　　finger with damage to nail
　　　　　　　　　　Unspecified open wound of
　　　　　　　　　　　　specified finger with
　　　　　　　　　　　　unspecified laterality with
　　　　　　　　　　　　damage to nail

　　● S61.309　Unspecified open wound of
　　　　　　　　unspecified finger with damage to
　　　　　　　　nail

● S61.31　Laceration without foreign body of finger with
　　　　　damage to nail

　　● S61.310　Laceration without foreign body of
　　　　　　　　right index finger with damage to nail

　　● S61.311　Laceration without foreign body of
　　　　　　　　left index finger with damage to nail

　　● S61.312　Laceration without foreign body of
　　　　　　　　right middle finger with damage to
　　　　　　　　nail

　　● S61.313　Laceration without foreign body of
　　　　　　　　left middle finger with damage to nail

　　● S61.314　Laceration without foreign body of
　　　　　　　　right ring finger with damage to nail

　　● S61.315　Laceration without foreign body of
　　　　　　　　left ring finger with damage to nail

　　● S61.316　Laceration without foreign body of
　　　　　　　　right little finger with damage to nail

　　● S61.317　Laceration without foreign body of
　　　　　　　　left little finger with damage to nail

　　● S61.318　Laceration without foreign body of
　　　　　　　　other finger with damage to nail
　　　　　　　　　　Laceration without foreign body
　　　　　　　　　　　　of specified finger with
　　　　　　　　　　　　unspecified laterality with
　　　　　　　　　　　　damage to nail

　　● S61.319　Laceration without foreign body of
　　　　　　　　unspecified finger with damage to
　　　　　　　　nail

● S61.32　Laceration with foreign body of finger with
　　　　　damage to nail

　　● S61.320　Laceration with foreign body of right
　　　　　　　　index finger with damage to nail

　　● S61.321　Laceration with foreign body of left
　　　　　　　　index finger with damage to nail

　　● S61.322　Laceration with foreign body of right
　　　　　　　　middle finger with damage to nail

　　● S61.323　Laceration with foreign body of left
　　　　　　　　middle finger with damage to nail

　　● S61.324　Laceration with foreign body of right
　　　　　　　　ring finger with damage to nail

　　● S61.325　Laceration with foreign body of left
　　　　　　　　ring finger with damage to nail

　　● S61.326　Laceration with foreign body of right
　　　　　　　　little finger with damage to nail

　　● S61.327　Laceration with foreign body of left
　　　　　　　　little finger with damage to nail

　　● S61.328　Laceration with foreign body of other
　　　　　　　　finger with damage to nail
　　　　　　　　　　Laceration with foreign body
　　　　　　　　　　　　of specified finger with
　　　　　　　　　　　　unspecified laterality with
　　　　　　　　　　　　damage to nail

　　● S61.329　Laceration with foreign body of
　　　　　　　　unspecified finger with damage to
　　　　　　　　nail

▶ New　　⇒ Revised　　deleted Deleted　　OGCR Official Guidelines　　X Assign placeholder X　　● Use Additional Character(s)

┌──────────┐ ┌──────────┐ ┌────────┐ ┌────────────┐ ┌──────────┐ ┌─────────┐ ┌──────────┐
│Excludes 1│ │Excludes 2│ │Includes│ │Use additional│ │Code first│ │Code also│ │Key words│
└──────────┘ └──────────┘ └────────┘ └────────────┘ └──────────┘ └─────────┘ └──────────┘

● S61.33 **Puncture wound without foreign body** of finger with damage to nail
  ● S61.330   Puncture wound without foreign body of **right index** finger with damage to nail
  ● S61.331   Puncture wound without foreign body of **left index** finger with damage to nail
  ● S61.332   Puncture wound without foreign body of **right middle** finger with damage to nail
  ● S61.333   Puncture wound without foreign body of **left middle** finger with damage to nail
  ● S61.334   Puncture wound without foreign body of **right ring** finger with damage to nail
  ● S61.335   Puncture wound without foreign body of **left ring** finger with damage to nail
  ● S61.336   Puncture wound without foreign body of **right little** finger with damage to nail
  ● S61.337   Puncture wound without foreign body of **left little** finger with damage to nail
  ● S61.338   Puncture wound without foreign body of **other** finger with damage to nail
           Puncture wound without foreign body of specified finger with unspecified laterality with damage to nail
  ● S61.339   Puncture wound without foreign body of **unspecified** finger with damage to nail

● S61.34 **Puncture wound with foreign body** of finger with damage to nail
  ● S61.340   Puncture wound with foreign body of **right index** finger with damage to nail
  ● S61.341   Puncture wound with foreign body of **left index** finger with damage to nail
  ● S61.342   Puncture wound with foreign body of **right middle** finger with damage to nail
  ● S61.343   Puncture wound with foreign body of **left middle** finger with damage to nail
  ● S61.344   Puncture wound with foreign body of **right ring** finger with damage to nail
  ● S61.345   Puncture wound with foreign body of **left ring** finger with damage to nail
  ● S61.346   Puncture wound with foreign body of **right little** finger with damage to nail
  ● S61.347   Puncture wound with foreign body of **left little** finger with damage to nail
  ● S61.348   Puncture wound with foreign body of **other** finger with damage to nail
           Puncture wound with foreign body of specified finger with unspecified laterality with damage to nail
  ● S61.349   Puncture wound with foreign body of **unspecified** finger with damage to nail

● S61.35 **Open bite** of finger with damage to nail
        Bite of finger with damage to nail NOS
        ┌─────────┐
        │Excludes1│ superficial bite of finger (S60.46-, S60.47-)
        └─────────┘
  ● S61.350   Open bite of **right index** finger with damage to nail
  ● S61.351   Open bite of **left index** finger with damage to nail
  ● S61.352   Open bite of **right middle** finger with damage to nail
  ● S61.353   Open bite of **left middle** finger with damage to nail
  ● S61.354   Open bite of **right ring** finger with damage to nail
  ● S61.355   Open bite of **left ring** finger with damage to nail
  ● S61.356   Open bite of **right little** finger with damage to nail
  ● S61.357   Open bite of **left little** finger with damage to nail
  ● S61.358   Open bite of **other** finger with damage to nail
           Open bite of specified finger with unspecified laterality with damage to nail
  ● S61.359   Open bite of **unspecified** finger with damage to nail

● S61.4 **Open wound of hand**
  ● S61.40 **Unspecified** open wound of hand
    ● S61.401   Unspecified open wound of **right** hand
    ● S61.402   Unspecified open wound of **left** hand
    ● S61.409   Unspecified open wound of **unspecified** hand
  ● S61.41 **Laceration without foreign body** of hand
    ● S61.411   Laceration without foreign body of **right** hand
    ● S61.412   Laceration without foreign body of **left** hand
    ● S61.419   Laceration without foreign body of **unspecified** hand
  ● S61.42 **Laceration with foreign body** of hand
    ● S61.421   Laceration with foreign body of **right** hand
    ● S61.422   Laceration with foreign body of **left** hand
    ● S61.429   Laceration with foreign body of **unspecified** hand
  ● S61.43 **Puncture wound without foreign body** of hand
    ● S61.431   Puncture wound without foreign body of **right** hand
    ● S61.432   Puncture wound without foreign body of **left** hand
    ● S61.439   Puncture wound without foreign body of **unspecified** hand
  ● S61.44 **Puncture wound with foreign body** of hand
    ● S61.441   Puncture wound with foreign body of **right** hand
    ● S61.442   Puncture wound with foreign body of **left** hand
    ● S61.449   Puncture wound with foreign body of **unspecified** hand
  ● S61.45 **Open bite** of hand
        Bite of hand NOS
        ┌─────────┐
        │Excludes1│ superficial bite of hand (S60.56-, S60.57-)
        └─────────┘
    ● S61.451   Open bite of **right** hand
    ● S61.452   Open bite of **left** hand
    ● S61.459   Open bite of **unspecified** hand

▶ New   ➡ Revised   ~~deleted~~ Deleted   **OGCR** Official Guidelines   X Assign placeholder X   ● Use Additional Character(s)

Excludes 1   Excludes 2   Includes   Use additional   Code first   Code also   Key words

● **S61.5**   **Open wound of** wrist
- ● **S61.50**   **Unspecified** open wound of wrist
  - ● **S61.501**   Unspecified open wound of **right** wrist
  - ● **S61.502**   Unspecified open wound of **left** wrist
  - ● **S61.509**   Unspecified open wound of **unspecified** wrist
- ● **S61.51**   **Laceration without foreign body** of wrist
  - ● **S61.511**   Laceration without foreign body of **right** wrist
  - ● **S61.512**   Laceration without foreign body of **left** wrist
  - ● **S61.519**   Laceration without foreign body of **unspecified** wrist
- ● **S61.52**   **Laceration with foreign body** of wrist
  - ● **S61.521**   Laceration with foreign body of **right** wrist
  - ● **S61.522**   Laceration with foreign body of **left** wrist
  - ● **S61.529**   Laceration with foreign body of **unspecified** wrist
- ● **S61.53**   **Puncture wound without foreign** body of wrist
  - ● **S61.531**   Puncture wound without foreign body of **right** wrist
  - ● **S61.532**   Puncture wound without foreign body of **left** wrist
  - ● **S61.539**   Puncture wound without foreign body of **unspecified** wrist
- ● **S61.54**   **Puncture wound with foreign body** of wrist
  - ● **S61.541**   Puncture wound with foreign body of **right** wrist
  - ● **S61.542**   Puncture wound with foreign body of **left** wrist
  - ● **S61.549**   Puncture wound with foreign body of **unspecified** wrist
- ● **S61.55**   **Open bite** of wrist
  Bite of wrist NOS
  > | **Excludes1** | superficial bite of wrist (S60.86-, S60.87-) |
  - ● **S61.551**   Open bite of **right** wrist
  - ● **S61.552**   Open bite of **left** wrist
  - ● **S61.559**   Open bite of **unspecified** wrist

● **S62**   **Fracture at wrist and hand level**
  Note: A fracture not indicated as displaced or nondisplaced should be coded to displaced

  A fracture not indicated as open or closed should be coded to closed

  > | **Excludes1** | traumatic amputation of wrist and hand (S68.-) |
  > | **Excludes2** | fracture of distal parts of ulna and radius (S52.-) |

  The appropriate 7th character is to be added to each code from category S62

A	initial encounter for closed fracture
B	initial encounter for open fracture
D	subsequent encounter for fracture with routine healing
G	subsequent encounter for fracture with delayed healing
K	subsequent encounter for fracture with nonunion
P	subsequent encounter for fracture with malunion
S	sequela

- ● **S62.0**   **Fracture of navicular** [scaphoid] bone of wrist
  - ● **S62.00**   **Unspecified** fracture of navicular [scaphoid] bone of wrist
    - ● **S62.001**   Unspecified fracture of navicular [scaphoid] bone of **right** wrist
    - ● **S62.002**   Unspecified fracture of navicular [scaphoid] bone of **left** wrist
    - ● **S62.009**   Unspecified fracture of navicular [scaphoid] bone of **unspecified** wrist

- ● **S62.01**   Fracture of **distal pole** of navicular [scaphoid] bone of wrist
  Fracture of volar tuberosity of navicular [scaphoid] bone of wrist
  - ● **S62.011**   **Displaced** fracture of distal pole of navicular [scaphoid] bone of **right** wrist
  - ● **S62.012**   **Displaced** fracture of distal pole of navicular [scaphoid] bone of **left** wrist
  - ● **S62.013**   **Displaced** fracture of distal pole of navicular [scaphoid] bone of **unspecified** wrist
  - ● **S62.014**   **Nondisplaced** fracture of distal pole of navicular [scaphoid] bone of **right** wrist
  - ● **S62.015**   **Nondisplaced** fracture of distal pole of navicular [scaphoid] bone of **left** wrist
  - ● **S62.016**   **Nondisplaced** fracture of distal pole of navicular [scaphoid] bone of **unspecified** wrist
- ● **S62.02**   Fracture of **middle third** of navicular [scaphoid] bone of wrist
  - ● **S62.021**   **Displaced** fracture of middle third of navicular [scaphoid] bone of **right** wrist
  - ● **S62.022**   **Displaced** fracture of middle third of navicular [scaphoid] bone of **left** wrist
  - ● **S62.023**   **Displaced** fracture of middle third of navicular [scaphoid] bone of **unspecified** wrist
  - ● **S62.024**   **Nondisplaced** fracture of middle third of navicular [scaphoid] bone of **right** wrist
  - ● **S62.025**   **Nondisplaced** fracture of middle third of navicular [scaphoid] bone of **left** wrist
  - ● **S62.026**   **Nondisplaced** fracture of middle third of navicular [scaphoid] bone of **unspecified** wrist
- ● **S62.03**   Fracture of **proximal third** of navicular [scaphoid] bone of wrist
  - ● **S62.031**   **Displaced** fracture of proximal third of navicular [scaphoid] bone of **right** wrist
  - ● **S62.032**   **Displaced** fracture of proximal third of navicular [scaphoid] bone of **left** wrist
  - ● **S62.033**   **Displaced** fracture of proximal third of navicular [scaphoid] bone of **unspecified** wrist
  - ● **S62.034**   **Nondisplaced** fracture of proximal third of navicular [scaphoid] bone of **right** wrist
  - ● **S62.035**   **Nondisplaced** fracture of proximal third of navicular [scaphoid] bone of **left** wrist
  - ● **S62.036**   **Nondisplaced** fracture of proximal third of navicular [scaphoid] bone of **unspecified** wrist
- ● **S62.1**   Fracture of other and unspecified **carpal bone**(s)
  > | **Excludes2** | fracture of scaphoid of wrist (S62.0-) |
  - ● **S62.10**   Fracture of **unspecified** carpal bone
    Fracture of wrist NOS
    - ● **S62.101**   Fracture of unspecified carpal bone, **right** wrist
    - ● **S62.102**   Fracture of unspecified carpal bone, **left** wrist
    - ● **S62.109**   Fracture of unspecified carpal bone, **unspecified** wrist

● S62.11 Fracture of triquetrum [cuneiform] bone of wrist
 ● S62.111 Displaced fracture of triquetrum [cuneiform] bone, right wrist
 ● S62.112 Displaced fracture of triquetrum [cuneiform] bone, left wrist
 ● S62.113 Displaced fracture of triquetrum [cuneiform] bone, unspecified wrist
 ● S62.114 Nondisplaced fracture of triquetrum [cuneiform] bone, right wrist
 ● S62.115 Nondisplaced fracture of triquetrum [cuneiform] bone, left wrist
 ● S62.116 Nondisplaced fracture of triquetrum [cuneiform] bone, unspecified wrist
● S62.12 Fracture of lunate [semilunar]
 ● S62.121 Displaced fracture of lunate [semilunar], right wrist
 ● S62.122 Displaced fracture of lunate [semilunar], left wrist
 ● S62.123 Displaced fracture of lunate [semilunar], unspecified wrist
 ● S62.124 Nondisplaced fracture of lunate [semilunar], right wrist
 ● S62.125 Nondisplaced fracture of lunate [semilunar], left wrist
 ● S62.126 Nondisplaced fracture of lunate [semilunar], unspecified wrist
● S62.13 Fracture of capitate [os magnum] bone
 ● S62.131 Displaced fracture of capitate [os magnum] bone, right wrist
 ● S62.132 Displaced fracture of capitate [os magnum] bone, left wrist
 ● S62.133 Displaced fracture of capitate [os magnum] bone, unspecified wrist
 ● S62.134 Nondisplaced fracture of capitate [os magnum] bone, right wrist
 ● S62.135 Nondisplaced fracture of capitate [os magnum] bone, left wrist
 ● S62.136 Nondisplaced fracture of capitate [os magnum] bone, unspecified wrist
● S62.14 Fracture of body of hamate [unciform] bone
   Fracture of hamate [unciform] bone NOS
 ● S62.141 Displaced fracture of body of hamate [unciform] bone, right wrist
 ● S62.142 Displaced fracture of body of hamate [unciform] bone, left wrist
 ● S62.143 Displaced fracture of body of hamate [unciform] bone, unspecified wrist
 ● S62.144 Nondisplaced fracture of body of hamate [unciform] bone, right wrist
 ● S62.145 Nondisplaced fracture of body of hamate [unciform] bone, left wrist
 ● S62.146 Nondisplaced fracture of body of hamate [unciform] bone, unspecified wrist
● S62.15 Fracture of hook process of hamate [unciform] bone
   Fracture of unciform process of hamate [unciform] bone
 ● S62.151 Displaced fracture of hook process of hamate [unciform] bone, right wrist
 ● S62.152 Displaced fracture of hook process of hamate [unciform] bone, left wrist
 ● S62.153 Displaced fracture of hook process of hamate [unciform] bone, unspecified wrist
 ● S62.154 Nondisplaced fracture of hook process of hamate [unciform] bone, right wrist
 ● S62.155 Nondisplaced fracture of hook process of hamate [unciform] bone, left wrist
 ● S62.156 Nondisplaced fracture of hook process of hamate [unciform] bone, unspecified wrist

● S62.16 Fracture of pisiform
 ● S62.161 Displaced fracture of pisiform, right wrist
 ● S62.162 Displaced fracture of pisiform, left wrist
 ● S62.163 Displaced fracture of pisiform, unspecified wrist
 ● S62.164 Nondisplaced fracture of pisiform, right wrist
 ● S62.165 Nondisplaced fracture of pisiform, left wrist
 ● S62.166 Nondisplaced fracture of pisiform, unspecified wrist
● S62.17 Fracture of trapezium [larger multangular]
 ● S62.171 Displaced fracture of trapezium [larger multangular], right wrist
 ● S62.172 Displaced fracture of trapezium [larger multangular], left wrist
 ● S62.173 Displaced fracture of trapezium [larger multangular], unspecified wrist
 ● S62.174 Nondisplaced fracture of trapezium [larger multangular], right wrist
 ● S62.175 Nondisplaced fracture of trapezium [larger multangular], left wrist
 ● S62.176 Nondisplaced fracture of trapezium [larger multangular], unspecified wrist
● S62.18 Fracture of trapezoid [smaller multangular]
 ● S62.181 Displaced fracture of trapezoid [smaller multangular], right wrist
 ● S62.182 Displaced fracture of trapezoid [smaller multangular], left wrist
 ● S62.183 Displaced fracture of trapezoid [smaller multangular], unspecified wrist
 ● S62.184 Nondisplaced fracture of trapezoid [smaller multangular], right wrist
 ● S62.185 Nondisplaced fracture of trapezoid [smaller multangular], left wrist
 ● S62.186 Nondisplaced fracture of trapezoid [smaller multangular], unspecified wrist
● S62.2 Fracture of first metacarpal bone
 ● S62.20 Unspecified fracture of first metacarpal bone
  ● S62.201 Unspecified fracture of first metacarpal bone, right hand
  ● S62.202 Unspecified fracture of first metacarpal bone, left hand
  ● S62.209 Unspecified fracture of first metacarpal bone, unspecified hand
 ● S62.21 Bennett's fracture
  ● S62.211 Bennett's fracture, right hand
  ● S62.212 Bennett's fracture, left hand
  ● S62.213 Bennett's fracture, unspecified hand
 ● S62.22 Rolando's fracture
  ● S62.221 Displaced Rolando's fracture, right hand
  ● S62.222 Displaced Rolando's fracture, left hand
  ● S62.223 Displaced Rolando's fracture, unspecified hand
  ● S62.224 Nondisplaced Rolando's fracture, right hand
  ● S62.225 Nondisplaced Rolando's fracture, left hand
  ● S62.226 Nondisplaced Rolando's fracture, unspecified hand

▶ New ⇒ Revised ~~deleted~~ Deleted **OGCR** Official Guidelines X Assign placeholder X ● Use Additional Character(s)
Excludes 1 Excludes 2 Includes Use additional Code first Code also Key words

CHAPTER 19 (S00-T88)

● **S62.23** Other fracture of base of first metacarpal bone

- ● **S62.231** Other displaced fracture of base of first metacarpal bone, right hand
- ● **S62.232** Other displaced fracture of base of first metacarpal bone, left hand
- ● **S62.233** Other displaced fracture of base of first metacarpal bone, unspecified hand
- ● **S62.234** Other nondisplaced fracture of base of first metacarpal bone, right hand
- ● **S62.235** Other nondisplaced fracture of base of first metacarpal bone, left hand
- ● **S62.236** Other nondisplaced fracture of base of first metacarpal bone, unspecified hand

● **S62.24** Fracture of shaft of first metacarpal bone

- ● **S62.241** Displaced fracture of shaft of first metacarpal bone, right hand
- ● **S62.242** Displaced fracture of shaft of first metacarpal bone, left hand
- ● **S62.243** Displaced fracture of shaft of first metacarpal bone, unspecified hand
- ● **S62.244** Nondisplaced fracture of shaft of first metacarpal bone, right hand
- ● **S62.245** Nondisplaced fracture of shaft of first metacarpal bone, left hand
- ● **S62.246** Nondisplaced fracture of shaft of first metacarpal bone, unspecified hand

● **S62.25** Fracture of neck of first metacarpal bone

- ● **S62.251** Displaced fracture of neck of first metacarpal bone, right hand
- ● **S62.252** Displaced fracture of neck of first metacarpal bone, left hand
- ● **S62.253** Displaced fracture of neck of first metacarpal bone, unspecified hand
- ● **S62.254** Nondisplaced fracture of neck of first metacarpal bone, right hand
- ● **S62.255** Nondisplaced fracture of neck of first metacarpal bone, left hand
- ● **S62.256** Nondisplaced fracture of neck of first metacarpal bone, unspecified hand

● **S62.29** Other fracture of first metacarpal bone

- ● **S62.291** Other fracture of first metacarpal bone, right hand
- ● **S62.292** Other fracture of first metacarpal bone, left hand
- ● **S62.299** Other fracture of first metacarpal bone, unspecified hand

● **S62.3** Fracture of other and unspecified metacarpal bone

Excludes2 fracture of first metacarpal bone (S62.2-)

● **S62.30** Unspecified fracture of other metacarpal bone

- ● **S62.300** Unspecified fracture of second metacarpal bone, right hand
- ● **S62.301** Unspecified fracture of second metacarpal bone, left hand
- ● **S62.302** Unspecified fracture of third metacarpal bone, right hand
- ● **S62.303** Unspecified fracture of third metacarpal bone, left hand
- ● **S62.304** Unspecified fracture of fourth metacarpal bone, right hand
- ● **S62.305** Unspecified fracture of fourth metacarpal bone, left hand
- ● **S62.306** Unspecified fracture of fifth metacarpal bone, right hand
- ➡● **S62.307** Unspecified fracture of fifth metacarpal bone, left hand
- ● **S62.308** Unspecified fracture of other metacarpal bone
  Unspecified fracture of specified metacarpal bone with unspecified laterality
- ● **S62.309** Unspecified fracture of unspecified metacarpal bone

● **S62.31** Displaced fracture of base of other metacarpal bone

- ● **S62.310** Displaced fracture of base of second metacarpal bone, right hand
- ➡● **S62.311** Displaced fracture of base of second metacarpal bone, left hand
- ● **S62.312** Displaced fracture of base of third metacarpal bone, right hand
- ● **S62.313** Displaced fracture of base of third metacarpal bone, left hand
- ● **S62.314** Displaced fracture of base of fourth metacarpal bone, right hand
- ● **S62.315** Displaced fracture of base of fourth metacarpal bone, left hand
- ● **S62.316** Displaced fracture of base of fifth metacarpal bone, right hand
- ➡● **S62.317** Displaced fracture of base of fifth metacarpal bone, left hand
- ● **S62.318** Displaced fracture of base of other metacarpal bone
  Displaced fracture of base of specified metacarpal bone with unspecified laterality
- ● **S62.319** Displaced fracture of base of unspecified metacarpal bone

● **S62.32** Displaced fracture of shaft of other metacarpal bone

- ● **S62.320** Displaced fracture of shaft of second metacarpal bone, right hand
- ● **S62.321** Displaced fracture of shaft of second metacarpal bone, left hand
- ● **S62.322** Displaced fracture of shaft of third metacarpal bone, right hand
- ● **S62.323** Displaced fracture of shaft of third metacarpal bone, left hand
- ● **S62.324** Displaced fracture of shaft of fourth metacarpal bone, right hand
- ● **S62.325** Displaced fracture of shaft of fourth metacarpal bone, left hand
- ● **S62.326** Displaced fracture of shaft of fifth metacarpal bone, right hand
- ● **S62.327** Displaced fracture of shaft of fifth metacarpal bone, left hand
- ● **S62.328** Displaced fracture of shaft of other metacarpal bone
  Displaced fracture of shaft of specified metacarpal bone with unspecified laterality
- ● **S62.329** Displaced fracture of shaft of unspecified metacarpal bone

---

▶ New   ➡ Revised   ~~deleted~~ Deleted   **OGCR** Official Guidelines   X Assign placeholder X   ● Use Additional Character(s)

Excludes 1   Excludes 2   Includes   Use additional   Code first   Code also   Key words

● **S62.33** Displaced fracture of neck of other metacarpal bone
- ● **S62.330** Displaced fracture of neck of second metacarpal bone, right hand
- ● **S62.331** Displaced fracture of neck of second metacarpal bone, left hand
- ● **S62.332** Displaced fracture of neck of third metacarpal bone, right hand
- ● **S62.333** Displaced fracture of neck of third metacarpal bone, left hand
- ● **S62.334** Displaced fracture of neck of fourth metacarpal bone, right hand
- ● **S62.335** Displaced fracture of neck of fourth metacarpal bone, left hand
- ● **S62.336** Displaced fracture of neck of fifth metacarpal bone, right hand
- ● **S62.337** Displaced fracture of neck of fifth metacarpal bone, left hand
- ● **S62.338** Displaced fracture of neck of other metacarpal bone
  - Displaced fracture of neck of specified metacarpal bone with unspecified laterality
- ● **S62.339** Displaced fracture of neck of unspecified metacarpal bone

● **S62.34** Nondisplaced fracture of base of other metacarpal bone
- ● **S62.340** Nondisplaced fracture of base of second metacarpal bone, right hand
- ⇒● **S62.341** Nondisplaced fracture of base of second metacarpal bone, left hand
- ● **S62.342** Nondisplaced fracture of base of third metacarpal bone, right hand
- ● **S62.343** Nondisplaced fracture of base of third metacarpal bone, left hand
- ● **S62.344** Nondisplaced fracture of base of fourth metacarpal bone, right hand
- ● **S62.345** Nondisplaced fracture of base of fourth metacarpal bone, left hand
- ● **S62.346** Nondisplaced fracture of base of fifth metacarpal bone, right hand
- ⇒● **S62.347** Nondisplaced fracture of base of fifth metacarpal bone, left hand
- ● **S62.348** Nondisplaced fracture of base of other metacarpal bone
  - Nondisplaced fracture of base of specified metacarpal bone with unspecified laterality
- ● **S62.349** Nondisplaced fracture of base of unspecified metacarpal bone

● **S62.35** Nondisplaced fracture of shaft of other metacarpal bone
- ● **S62.350** Nondisplaced fracture of shaft of second metacarpal bone, right hand
- ● **S62.351** Nondisplaced fracture of shaft of second metacarpal bone, left hand
- ● **S62.352** Nondisplaced fracture of shaft of third metacarpal bone, right hand
- ● **S62.353** Nondisplaced fracture of shaft of third metacarpal bone, left hand
- ● **S62.354** Nondisplaced fracture of shaft of fourth metacarpal bone, right hand
- ● **S62.355** Nondisplaced fracture of shaft of fourth metacarpal bone, left hand
- ● **S62.356** Nondisplaced fracture of shaft of fifth metacarpal bone, right hand

- ● **S62.357** Nondisplaced fracture of shaft of fifth metacarpal bone, left hand
- ● **S62.358** Nondisplaced fracture of shaft of other metacarpal bone
  - Nondisplaced fracture of shaft of specified metacarpal bone with unspecified laterality
- ● **S62.359** Nondisplaced fracture of shaft of unspecified metacarpal bone

● **S62.36** Nondisplaced fracture of neck of other metacarpal bone
- ● **S62.360** Nondisplaced fracture of neck of second metacarpal bone, right hand
- ● **S62.361** Nondisplaced fracture of neck of second metacarpal bone, left hand
- ● **S62.362** Nondisplaced fracture of neck of third metacarpal bone, right hand
- ● **S62.363** Nondisplaced fracture of neck of third metacarpal bone, left hand
- ● **S62.364** Nondisplaced fracture of neck of fourth metacarpal bone, right hand
- ● **S62.365** Nondisplaced fracture of neck of fourth metacarpal bone, left hand
- ● **S62.366** Nondisplaced fracture of neck of fifth metacarpal bone, right hand
- ● **S62.367** Nondisplaced fracture of neck of fifth metacarpal bone, left hand
- ● **S62.368** Nondisplaced fracture of neck of other metacarpal bone
  - Nondisplaced fracture of neck of specified metacarpal bone with unspecified laterality
- ● **S62.369** Nondisplaced fracture of neck of unspecified metacarpal bone

● **S62.39** Other fracture of other metacarpal bone
- ● **S62.390** Other fracture of second metacarpal bone, right hand
- ● **S62.391** Other fracture of second metacarpal bone, left hand
- ● **S62.392** Other fracture of third metacarpal bone, right hand
- ● **S62.393** Other fracture of third metacarpal bone, left hand
- ● **S62.394** Other fracture of fourth metacarpal bone, right hand
- ● **S62.395** Other fracture of fourth metacarpal bone, left hand
- ● **S62.396** Other fracture of fifth metacarpal bone, right hand
- ● **S62.397** Other fracture of fifth metacarpal bone, left hand
- ● **S62.398** Other fracture of other metacarpal bone
  - Other fracture of specified metacarpal bone with unspecified laterality
- ● **S62.399** Other fracture of unspecified metacarpal bone

● **S62.5** Fracture of thumb
- ● **S62.50** Fracture of unspecified phalanx of thumb
  - ● **S62.501** Fracture of unspecified phalanx of right thumb
  - ● **S62.502** Fracture of unspecified phalanx of left thumb
  - ● **S62.509** Fracture of unspecified phalanx of unspecified thumb

▶ New ⇒ Revised ~~deleted~~ Deleted **OGCR** Official Guidelines X Assign placeholder X ● Use Additional Character(s)

Excludes 1 Excludes 2 Includes Use additional Code first Code also Key words

- ● S62.51   Fracture of proximal phalanx of thumb
  - ● S62.511   Displaced fracture of proximal phalanx of right thumb
  - ● S62.512   Displaced fracture of proximal phalanx of left thumb
  - ● S62.513   Displaced fracture of proximal phalanx of unspecified thumb
  - ● S62.514   Nondisplaced fracture of proximal phalanx of right thumb
  - ● S62.515   Nondisplaced fracture of proximal phalanx of left thumb
  - ● S62.516   Nondisplaced fracture of proximal phalanx of unspecified thumb
- ● S62.52   Fracture of distal phalanx of thumb
  - ● S62.521   Displaced fracture of distal phalanx of right thumb
  - ● S62.522   Displaced fracture of distal phalanx of left thumb
  - ● S62.523   Displaced fracture of distal phalanx of unspecified thumb
  - ● S62.524   Nondisplaced fracture of distal phalanx of right thumb
  - ● S62.525   Nondisplaced fracture of distal phalanx of left thumb
  - ● S62.526   Nondisplaced fracture of distal phalanx of unspecified thumb
- ● S62.6   Fracture of other and unspecified finger(s)

  > **Excludes2**   fracture of thumb (S62.5-)

  - ● S62.60   Fracture of unspecified phalanx of finger
    - ● S62.600   Fracture of unspecified phalanx of right index finger
    - ● S62.601   Fracture of unspecified phalanx of left index finger
    - ● S62.602   Fracture of unspecified phalanx of right middle finger
    - ● S62.603   Fracture of unspecified phalanx of left middle finger
    - ● S62.604   Fracture of unspecified phalanx of right ring finger
    - ● S62.605   Fracture of unspecified phalanx of left ring finger
    - ● S62.606   Fracture of unspecified phalanx of right little finger
    - ● S62.607   Fracture of unspecified phalanx of left little finger
    - ● S62.608   Fracture of unspecified phalanx of other finger
      Fracture of unspecified phalanx of specified finger with unspecified laterality
    - ● S62.609   Fracture of unspecified phalanx of unspecified finger
  - ● S62.61   Displaced fracture of proximal phalanx of finger
    - ● S62.610   Displaced fracture of proximal phalanx of right index finger
    - ● S62.611   Displaced fracture of proximal phalanx of left index finger
    - ● S62.612   Displaced fracture of proximal phalanx of right middle finger
    - ● S62.613   Displaced fracture of proximal phalanx of left middle finger
    - ● S62.614   Displaced fracture of proximal phalanx of right ring finger
    - ● S62.615   Displaced fracture of proximal phalanx of left ring finger
    - ● S62.616   Displaced fracture of proximal phalanx of right little finger
    - ● S62.617   Displaced fracture of proximal phalanx of left little finger
    - ● S62.618   Displaced fracture of proximal phalanx of other finger
      Displaced fracture of proximal phalanx of specified finger with unspecified laterality
    - ● S62.619   Displaced fracture of proximal phalanx of unspecified finger
  - ⇒● S62.62   Displaced fracture of middle phalanx of finger
    - ⇒● S62.620   Displaced fracture of middle phalanx of right index finger
    - ⇒● S62.621   Displaced fracture of middle phalanx of left index finger
    - ⇒● S62.622   Displaced fracture of middle phalanx of right middle finger
    - ⇒● S62.623   Displaced fracture of middle phalanx of left middle finger
    - ⇒● S62.624   Displaced fracture of middle phalanx of right ring finger
    - ⇒● S62.625   Displaced fracture of middle phalanx of left ring finger
    - ● S62.626   Displaced fracture of medial phalanx of right little finger
    - ● S62.627   Displaced fracture of medial phalanx of left little finger
    - ● S62.628   Displaced fracture of medial phalanx of other finger
      Displaced fracture of medial phalanx of specified finger with unspecified laterality
    - ● S62.629   Displaced fracture of medial phalanx of unspecified finger
  - ● S62.63   Displaced fracture of distal phalanx of finger
    - ● S62.630   Displaced fracture of distal phalanx of right index finger
    - ● S62.631   Displaced fracture of distal phalanx of left index finger
    - ● S62.632   Displaced fracture of distal phalanx of right middle finger
    - ● S62.633   Displaced fracture of distal phalanx of left middle finger
    - ● S62.634   Displaced fracture of distal phalanx of right ring finger
    - ● S62.635   Displaced fracture of distal phalanx of left ring finger
    - ● S62.636   Displaced fracture of distal phalanx of right little finger
    - ● S62.637   Displaced fracture of distal phalanx of left little finger
    - ● S62.638   Displaced fracture of distal phalanx of other finger
      Displaced fracture of distal phalanx of specified finger with unspecified laterality
    - ● S62.639   Displaced fracture of distal phalanx of unspecified finger

● **S62.64**   Nondisplaced fracture of proximal phalanx of finger

     ● **S62.640**   Nondisplaced fracture of proximal phalanx of right index finger

     ● **S62.641**   Nondisplaced fracture of proximal phalanx of left index finger

     ● **S62.642**   Nondisplaced fracture of proximal phalanx of right middle finger

     ● **S62.643**   Nondisplaced fracture of proximal phalanx of left middle finger

     ● **S62.644**   Nondisplaced fracture of proximal phalanx of right ring finger

     ● **S62.645**   Nondisplaced fracture of proximal phalanx of left ring finger

     ● **S62.646**   Nondisplaced fracture of proximal phalanx of right little finger

     ● **S62.647**   Nondisplaced fracture of proximal phalanx of left little finger

     ● **S62.648**   Nondisplaced fracture of proximal phalanx of other finger
         Nondisplaced fracture of proximal phalanx of specified finger with unspecified laterality

     ● **S62.649**   Nondisplaced fracture of proximal phalanx of unspecified finger

⇒● **S62.65**   Nondisplaced fracture of middle phalanx of finger

     ⇒● **S62.650**   Nondisplaced fracture of middle phalanx of right index finger

     ⇒● **S62.651**   Nondisplaced fracture of middle phalanx of left index finger

     ⇒● **S62.652**   Nondisplaced fracture of middle phalanx of right middle finger

     ⇒● **S62.653**   Nondisplaced fracture of middle phalanx of left middle finger

     ● **S62.654**   Nondisplaced fracture of medial phalanx of right ring finger

     ● **S62.655**   Nondisplaced fracture of medial phalanx of left ring finger

     ● **S62.656**   Nondisplaced fracture of medial phalanx of right little finger

     ● **S62.657**   Nondisplaced fracture of medial phalanx of left little finger

Figure 19-14   Dorsal dislocation of the distal phalanx of the index finger. (From Hardy M, Snaith B: Musculoskeletal Trauma: A Guide to Assessment and Diagnosis, 1e, Elsevier, 2011)

     ● **S62.658**   Nondisplaced fracture of medial phalanx of other finger
         Nondisplaced fracture of medial phalanx of specified finger with unspecified laterality

     ● **S62.659**   Nondisplaced fracture of medial phalanx of unspecified finger

● **S62.66**   Nondisplaced fracture of distal phalanx of finger

     ● **S62.660**   Nondisplaced fracture of distal phalanx of right index finger

     ● **S62.661**   Nondisplaced fracture of distal phalanx of left index finger

     ● **S62.662**   Nondisplaced fracture of distal phalanx of right middle finger

     ● **S62.663**   Nondisplaced fracture of distal phalanx of left middle finger

     ● **S62.664**   Nondisplaced fracture of distal phalanx of right ring finger

     ● **S62.665**   Nondisplaced fracture of distal phalanx of left ring finger

     ● **S62.666**   Nondisplaced fracture of distal phalanx of right little finger

     ● **S62.667**   Nondisplaced fracture of distal phalanx of left little finger

     ● **S62.668**   Nondisplaced fracture of distal phalanx of other finger
         Nondisplaced fracture of distal phalanx of specified finger with unspecified laterality

     ● **S62.669**   Nondisplaced fracture of distal phalanx of unspecified finger

● **S62.9**   Unspecified fracture of wrist and hand

     X ● **S62.90**   Unspecified fracture of unspecified wrist and hand

     X ● **S62.91**   Unspecified fracture of right wrist and hand

     X ● **S62.92**   Unspecified fracture of left wrist and hand

● **S63**   Dislocation and sprain of joints and ligaments at wrist and hand level

     Includes   avulsion of joint or ligament at wrist and hand level

         laceration of cartilage, joint or ligament at wrist and hand level

         sprain of cartilage, joint or ligament at wrist and hand level

         traumatic hemarthrosis of joint or ligament at wrist and hand level

         traumatic rupture of joint or ligament at wrist and hand level

         traumatic subluxation of joint or ligament at wrist and hand level

         traumatic tear of joint or ligament at wrist and hand level

     Code also any associated open wound

     Excludes2   strain of muscle, fascia and tendon of wrist and hand (S66.-)

     The appropriate 7th character is to be added to each code from category S63

     A   initial encounter
     D   subsequent encounter
     S   sequela

● **S63.0**   Subluxation and dislocation of wrist and hand joints

     ● **S63.00**   Unspecified subluxation and dislocation of wrist and hand
         Dislocation of carpal bone NOS
         Dislocation of distal end of radius NOS
         Subluxation of carpal bone NOS
         Subluxation of distal end of radius NOS

     ● **S63.001**   Unspecified subluxation of right wrist and hand

     ● **S63.002**   Unspecified subluxation of left wrist and hand

▶ New   ⇒ Revised   ~~deleted~~ Deleted   **OGCR** Official Guidelines   X Assign placeholder X   ● Use Additional Character(s)

Excludes 1   Excludes 2   Includes   Use additional   Code first   Code also   Key words

- ● S63.003　Unspecified subluxation of unspecified wrist and hand
- ● S63.004　Unspecified dislocation of right wrist and hand
- ● S63.005　Unspecified dislocation of left wrist and hand
- ● S63.006　Unspecified dislocation of unspecified wrist and hand
- ● S63.01　Subluxation and dislocation of distal radioulnar joint
  - ● S63.011　Subluxation of distal radioulnar joint of right wrist
  - ● S63.012　Subluxation of distal radioulnar joint of left wrist
  - ● S63.013　Subluxation of distal radioulnar joint of unspecified wrist
  - ● S63.014　Dislocation of distal radioulnar joint of right wrist
  - ● S63.015　Dislocation of distal radioulnar joint of left wrist
  - ● S63.016　Dislocation of distal radioulnar joint of unspecified wrist
- ● S63.02　Subluxation and dislocation of radiocarpal joint
  - ● S63.021　Subluxation of radiocarpal joint of right wrist
  - ● S63.022　Subluxation of radiocarpal joint of left wrist
  - ● S63.023　Subluxation of radiocarpal joint of unspecified wrist
  - ● S63.024　Dislocation of radiocarpal joint of right wrist
  - ● S63.025　Dislocation of radiocarpal joint of left wrist
  - ● S63.026　Dislocation of radiocarpal joint of unspecified wrist
- ● S63.03　Subluxation and dislocation of midcarpal joint
  - ● S63.031　Subluxation of midcarpal joint of right wrist
  - ● S63.032　Subluxation of midcarpal joint of left wrist
  - ● S63.033　Subluxation of midcarpal joint of unspecified wrist
  - ● S63.034　Dislocation of midcarpal joint of right wrist
  - ● S63.035　Dislocation of midcarpal joint of left wrist
  - ● S63.036　Dislocation of midcarpal joint of unspecified wrist
- ● S63.04　Subluxation and dislocation of carpometacarpal joint of thumb

  | Excludes2 | interphalangeal subluxation and dislocation of thumb (S63.1-) |

  - ● S63.041　Subluxation of carpometacarpal joint of right thumb
  - ● S63.042　Subluxation of carpometacarpal joint of left thumb
  - ● S63.043　Subluxation of carpometacarpal joint of unspecified thumb
  - ● S63.044　Dislocation of carpometacarpal joint of right thumb
  - ● S63.045　Dislocation of carpometacarpal joint of left thumb
  - ● S63.046　Dislocation of carpometacarpal joint of unspecified thumb

- ● S63.05　Subluxation and dislocation of other carpometacarpal joint

  | Excludes2 | subluxation and dislocation of carpometacarpal joint of thumb (S63.04-) |

  - ● S63.051　Subluxation of other carpometacarpal joint of right hand
  - ● S63.052　Subluxation of other carpometacarpal joint of left hand
  - ● S63.053　Subluxation of other carpometacarpal joint of unspecified hand
  - ● S63.054　Dislocation of other carpometacarpal joint of right hand
  - ● S63.055　Dislocation of other carpometacarpal joint of left hand
  - ● S63.056　Dislocation of other carpometacarpal joint of unspecified hand
- ● S63.06　Subluxation and dislocation of metacarpal (bone), proximal end
  - ● S63.061　Subluxation of metacarpal (bone), proximal end of right hand
  - ● S63.062　Subluxation of metacarpal (bone), proximal end of left hand
  - ● S63.063　Subluxation of metacarpal (bone), proximal end of unspecified hand
  - ● S63.064　Dislocation of metacarpal (bone), proximal end of right hand
  - ● S63.065　Dislocation of metacarpal (bone), proximal end of left hand
  - ● S63.066　Dislocation of metacarpal (bone), proximal end of unspecified hand
- ● S63.07　Subluxation and dislocation of distal end of ulna
  - ● S63.071　Subluxation of distal end of right ulna
  - ● S63.072　Subluxation of distal end of left ulna
  - ● S63.073　Subluxation of distal end of unspecified ulna
  - ● S63.074　Dislocation of distal end of right ulna
  - ● S63.075　Dislocation of distal end of left ulna
  - ● S63.076　Dislocation of distal end of unspecified ulna
- ● S63.09　Other subluxation and dislocation of wrist and hand
  - ● S63.091　Other subluxation of right wrist and hand
  - ● S63.092　Other subluxation of left wrist and hand
  - ● S63.093　Other subluxation of unspecified wrist and hand
  - ● S63.094　Other dislocation of right wrist and hand
  - ● S63.095　Other dislocation of left wrist and hand
  - ● S63.096　Other dislocation of unspecified wrist and hand
- ● S63.1　Subluxation and dislocation of thumb
  - ● S63.10　Unspecified subluxation and dislocation of thumb
    - ● S63.101　Unspecified subluxation of right thumb
    - ● S63.102　Unspecified subluxation of left thumb
    - ● S63.103　Unspecified subluxation of unspecified thumb
    - ● S63.104　Unspecified dislocation of right thumb
    - ● S63.105　Unspecified dislocation of left thumb
    - ● S63.106　Unspecified dislocation of unspecified thumb

▶ New　　⮕ Revised　　~~deleted~~ Deleted　　**OGCR** Official Guidelines　　X Assign placeholder X　　● Use Additional Character(s)

| Excludes 1 | | Excludes 2 | | Includes | | Use additional | | Code first | | Code also | | Key words |

● **S63.11**   Subluxation and dislocation of metacarpophalangeal joint of thumb
- ● **S63.111**   Subluxation of metacarpophalangeal joint of right thumb
- ● **S63.112**   Subluxation of metacarpophalangeal joint of left thumb
- ● **S63.113**   Subluxation of metacarpophalangeal joint of unspecified thumb
- ● **S63.114**   Dislocation of metacarpophalangeal joint of right thumb
- ● **S63.115**   Dislocation of metacarpophalangeal joint of left thumb
- ● **S63.116**   Dislocation of metacarpophalangeal joint of unspecified thumb

➡● **S63.12**   Subluxation and dislocation of interphalangeal joint of thumb
- ➡● **S63.121**   Subluxation of interphalangeal joint of right thumb
- ➡● **S63.122**   Subluxation of interphalangeal joint of left thumb
- ➡● **S63.123**   Subluxation of interphalangeal joint of unspecified thumb
- ➡● **S63.124**   Dislocation of interphalangeal joint of right thumb
- ➡● **S63.125**   Dislocation of interphalangeal joint of left thumb
- ➡● **S63.126**   Dislocation of interphalangeal joint of unspecified thumb

~~S63.13~~   ~~Subluxation and dislocation of proximal interphalangeal joint of thumb~~
- ~~S63.131~~   ~~Subluxation of proximal interphalangeal joint of right thumb~~
- ~~S63.132~~   ~~Subluxation of proximal interphalangeal joint of left thumb~~
- ~~S63.133~~   ~~Subluxation of proximal interphalangeal joint of unspecified thumb~~
- ~~S63.134~~   ~~Dislocation of proximal interphalangeal joint of right thumb~~
- ~~S63.135~~   ~~Dislocation of proximal interphalangeal joint of left thumb~~
- ~~S63.136~~   ~~Dislocation of proximal interphalangeal joint of unspecified thumb~~

~~S63.14~~   ~~Subluxation and dislocation of distal interphalangeal joint of thumb~~
- ~~S63.141~~   ~~Subluxation of distal interphalangeal joint of right thumb~~
- ~~S63.142~~   ~~Subluxation of distal interphalangeal joint of left thumb~~
- ~~S63.143~~   ~~Subluxation of distal interphalangeal joint of unspecified thumb~~
- ~~S63.144~~   ~~Dislocation of distal interphalangeal joint of right thumb~~
- ~~S63.145~~   ~~Dislocation of distal interphalangeal joint of left thumb~~
- ~~S63.146~~   ~~Dislocation of distal interphalangeal joint of unspecified thumb~~

● **S63.2**   Subluxation and dislocation of other finger(s)

> **Excludes2**   subluxation and dislocation of thumb (S63.1-)

● **S63.20**   Unspecified subluxation of other finger
- ● **S63.200**   Unspecified subluxation of right index finger
- ● **S63.201**   Unspecified subluxation of left index finger
- ● **S63.202**   Unspecified subluxation of right middle finger
- ● **S63.203**   Unspecified subluxation of left middle finger
- ● **S63.204**   Unspecified subluxation of right ring finger
- ● **S63.205**   Unspecified subluxation of left ring finger
- ● **S63.206**   Unspecified subluxation of right little finger
- ● **S63.207**   Unspecified subluxation of left little finger
- ● **S63.208**   Unspecified subluxation of other finger
  Unspecified subluxation of specified finger with unspecified laterality
- ● **S63.209**   Unspecified subluxation of unspecified finger

● **S63.21**   Subluxation of metacarpophalangeal joint of finger
- ● **S63.210**   Subluxation of metacarpophalangeal joint of right index finger
- ● **S63.211**   Subluxation of metacarpophalangeal joint of left index finger
- ● **S63.212**   Subluxation of metacarpophalangeal joint of right middle finger
- ● **S63.213**   Subluxation of metacarpophalangeal joint of left middle finger
- ● **S63.214**   Subluxation of metacarpophalangeal joint of right ring finger
- ● **S63.215**   Subluxation of metacarpophalangeal joint of left ring finger
- ● **S63.216**   Subluxation of metacarpophalangeal joint of right little finger
- ● **S63.217**   Subluxation of metacarpophalangeal joint of left little finger
- ● **S63.218**   Subluxation of metacarpophalangeal joint of other finger
  Subluxation of metacarpophalangeal joint of specified finger with unspecified laterality
- ● **S63.219**   Subluxation of metacarpophalangeal joint of unspecified finger

● **S63.22**   Subluxation of unspecified interphalangeal joint of finger
- ● **S63.220**   Subluxation of unspecified interphalangeal joint of right index finger
- ● **S63.221**   Subluxation of unspecified interphalangeal joint of left index finger
- ● **S63.222**   Subluxation of unspecified interphalangeal joint of right middle finger
- ● **S63.223**   Subluxation of unspecified interphalangeal joint of left middle finger
- ● **S63.224**   Subluxation of unspecified interphalangeal joint of right ring finger
- ● **S63.225**   Subluxation of unspecified interphalangeal joint of left ring finger
- ● **S63.226**   Subluxation of unspecified interphalangeal joint of right little finger
- ● **S63.227**   Subluxation of unspecified interphalangeal joint of left little finger
- ● **S63.228**   Subluxation of unspecified interphalangeal joint of other finger
  Subluxation of unspecified interphalangeal joint of specified finger with unspecified laterality
- ● **S63.229**   Subluxation of unspecified interphalangeal joint of unspecified finger

▶ New   ➡ Revised   ~~deleted~~ Deleted   **OGCR** Official Guidelines   X Assign placeholder X   ● Use Additional Character(s)

Excludes 1   Excludes 2   Includes   Use additional   Code first   Code also   Key words

● S63.23   Subluxation of proximal interphalangeal joint of finger

  ● S63.230   Subluxation of proximal interphalangeal joint of right index finger

  ● S63.231   Subluxation of proximal interphalangeal joint of left index finger

  ● S63.232   Subluxation of proximal interphalangeal joint of right middle finger

  ● S63.233   Subluxation of proximal interphalangeal joint of left middle finger

  ● S63.234   Subluxation of proximal interphalangeal joint of right ring finger

  ● S63.235   Subluxation of proximal interphalangeal joint of left ring finger

  ● S63.236   Subluxation of proximal interphalangeal joint of right little finger

  ● S63.237   Subluxation of proximal interphalangeal joint of left little finger

  ● S63.238   Subluxation of proximal interphalangeal joint of other finger
       Subluxation of proximal interphalangeal joint of specified finger with unspecified laterality

  ● S63.239   Subluxation of proximal interphalangeal joint of unspecified finger

● S63.24   Subluxation of distal interphalangeal joint of finger

  ● S63.240   Subluxation of distal interphalangeal joint of right index finger

  ● S63.241   Subluxation of distal interphalangeal joint of left index finger

  ● S63.242   Subluxation of distal interphalangeal joint of right middle finger

  ● S63.243   Subluxation of distal interphalangeal joint of left middle finger

  ● S63.244   Subluxation of distal interphalangeal joint of right ring finger

  ● S63.245   Subluxation of distal interphalangeal joint of left ring finger

  ● S63.246   Subluxation of distal interphalangeal joint of right little finger

  ● S63.247   Subluxation of distal interphalangeal joint of left little finger

  ● S63.248   Subluxation of distal interphalangeal joint of other finger
       Subluxation of distal interphalangeal joint of specified finger with unspecified laterality

  ● S63.249   Subluxation of distal interphalangeal joint of unspecified finger

● S63.25   Unspecified dislocation of other finger

  ● S63.250   Unspecified dislocation of right index finger

  ● S63.251   Unspecified dislocation of left index finger

  ● S63.252   Unspecified dislocation of right middle finger

  ● S63.253   Unspecified dislocation of left middle finger

  ● S63.254   Unspecified dislocation of right ring finger

  ● S63.255   Unspecified dislocation of left ring finger

  ● S63.256   Unspecified dislocation of right little finger

  ● S63.257   Unspecified dislocation of left little finger

  ● S63.258   Unspecified dislocation of other finger
       Unspecified dislocation of specified finger with unspecified laterality

  ● S63.259   Unspecified dislocation of unspecified finger
       ⇒ Unspecified dislocation of unspecified finger with unspecified laterality

● S63.26   Dislocation of metacarpophalangeal joint of finger

  ● S63.260   Dislocation of metacarpophalangeal joint of right index finger

  ● S63.261   Dislocation of metacarpophalangeal joint of left index finger

  ● S63.262   Dislocation of metacarpophalangeal joint of right middle finger

  ● S63.263   Dislocation of metacarpophalangeal joint of left middle finger

  ● S63.264   Dislocation of metacarpophalangeal joint of right ring finger

  ● S63.265   Dislocation of metacarpophalangeal joint of left ring finger

  ● S63.266   Dislocation of metacarpophalangeal joint of right little finger

  ● S63.267   Dislocation of metacarpophalangeal joint of left little finger

  ● S63.268   Dislocation of metacarpophalangeal joint of other finger
       Dislocation of metacarpophalangeal joint of specified finger with unspecified laterality

  ● S63.269   Dislocation of metacarpophalangeal joint of unspecified finger

● S63.27   Dislocation of unspecified interphalangeal joint of finger

  ● S63.270   Dislocation of unspecified interphalangeal joint of right index finger

  ● S63.271   Dislocation of unspecified interphalangeal joint of left index finger

CHAPTER 19 (S00-T88)

● S63.272 Dislocation of unspecified interphalangeal joint of right middle finger

● S63.273 Dislocation of unspecified interphalangeal joint of left middle finger

● S63.274 Dislocation of unspecified interphalangeal joint of right ring finger

● S63.275 Dislocation of unspecified interphalangeal joint of left ring finger

● S63.276 Dislocation of unspecified interphalangeal joint of right little finger

● S63.277 Dislocation of unspecified interphalangeal joint of left little finger

● S63.278 Dislocation of unspecified interphalangeal joint of other finger
         Dislocation of unspecified interphalangeal joint of specified finger with unspecified laterality

● S63.279 Dislocation of unspecified interphalangeal joint of unspecified finger
         ⇨ Dislocation of unspecified interphalangeal joint of unspecified finger without specified laterality

● S63.28 Dislocation of proximal interphalangeal joint of finger

● S63.280 Dislocation of proximal interphalangeal joint of right index finger

● S63.281 Dislocation of proximal interphalangeal joint of left index finger

● S63.282 Dislocation of proximal interphalangeal joint of right middle finger

● S63.283 Dislocation of proximal interphalangeal joint of left middle finger

● S63.284 Dislocation of proximal interphalangeal joint of right ring finger

● S63.285 Dislocation of proximal interphalangeal joint of left ring finger

● S63.286 Dislocation of proximal interphalangeal joint of right little finger

● S63.287 Dislocation of proximal interphalangeal joint of left little finger

● S63.288 Dislocation of proximal interphalangeal joint of other finger
         Dislocation of proximal interphalangeal joint of specified finger with unspecified laterality

● S63.289 Dislocation of proximal interphalangeal joint of unspecified finger

● S63.29 Dislocation of distal interphalangeal joint of finger

● S63.290 Dislocation of distal interphalangeal joint of right index finger

● S63.291 Dislocation of distal interphalangeal joint of left index finger

● S63.292 Dislocation of distal interphalangeal joint of right middle finger

● S63.293 Dislocation of distal interphalangeal joint of left middle finger

● S63.294 Dislocation of distal interphalangeal joint of right ring finger

● S63.295 Dislocation of distal interphalangeal joint of left ring finger

● S63.296 Dislocation of distal interphalangeal joint of right little finger

● S63.297 Dislocation of distal interphalangeal joint of left little finger

● S63.298 Dislocation of distal interphalangeal joint of other finger
         Dislocation of distal interphalangeal joint of specified finger with unspecified laterality

● S63.299 Dislocation of distal interphalangeal joint of unspecified finger

● S63.3 Traumatic rupture of ligament of wrist

● S63.30 Traumatic rupture of unspecified ligament of wrist

● S63.301 Traumatic rupture of unspecified ligament of right wrist

● S63.302 Traumatic rupture of unspecified ligament of left wrist

● S63.309 Traumatic rupture of unspecified ligament of unspecified wrist

● S63.31 Traumatic rupture of collateral ligament of wrist

● S63.311 Traumatic rupture of collateral ligament of right wrist

● S63.312 Traumatic rupture of collateral ligament of left wrist

● S63.319 Traumatic rupture of collateral ligament of unspecified wrist

● S63.32 Traumatic rupture of radiocarpal ligament

● S63.321 Traumatic rupture of right radiocarpal ligament

● S63.322 Traumatic rupture of left radiocarpal ligament

● S63.329 Traumatic rupture of unspecified radiocarpal ligament

● S63.33 Traumatic rupture of ulnocarpal (palmar) ligament

● S63.331 Traumatic rupture of right ulnocarpal (palmar) ligament

● S63.332 Traumatic rupture of left ulnocarpal (palmar) ligament

● S63.339 Traumatic rupture of unspecified ulnocarpal (palmar) ligament

● S63.39 Traumatic rupture of other ligament of wrist

● S63.391 Traumatic rupture of other ligament of right wrist

● S63.392 Traumatic rupture of other ligament of left wrist

● S63.399 Traumatic rupture of other ligament of unspecified wrist

▶ New   ⇨ Revised   ~~deleted~~ Deleted   **OGCR** Official Guidelines   X Assign placeholder X   ● Use Additional Character(s)

Excludes 1   Excludes 2   Includes   Use additional   Code first   Code also   Key words

●S63.4　Traumatic rupture of ligament of finger at metacarpophalangeal and interphalangeal joint(s)

　●S63.40　Traumatic rupture of unspecified ligament of finger at metacarpophalangeal and interphalangeal joint

　　●S63.400　Traumatic rupture of unspecified ligament of right index finger at metacarpophalangeal and interphalangeal joint

　　●S63.401　Traumatic rupture of unspecified ligament of left index finger at metacarpophalangeal and interphalangeal joint

　　●S63.402　Traumatic rupture of unspecified ligament of right middle finger at metacarpophalangeal and interphalangeal joint

　　●S63.403　Traumatic rupture of unspecified ligament of left middle finger at metacarpophalangeal and interphalangeal joint

　　●S63.404　Traumatic rupture of unspecified ligament of right ring finger at metacarpophalangeal and interphalangeal joint

　　●S63.405　Traumatic rupture of unspecified ligament of left ring finger at metacarpophalangeal and interphalangeal joint

　　●S63.406　Traumatic rupture of unspecified ligament of right little finger at metacarpophalangeal and interphalangeal joint

　　●S63.407　Traumatic rupture of unspecified ligament of left little finger at metacarpophalangeal and interphalangeal joint

　　●S63.408　Traumatic rupture of unspecified ligament of other finger at metacarpophalangeal and interphalangeal joint
　　　　Traumatic rupture of unspecified ligament of specified finger with unspecified laterality at metacarpophalangeal and interphalangeal joint

　　●S63.409　Traumatic rupture of unspecified ligament of unspecified finger at metacarpophalangeal and interphalangeal joint

　●S63.41　Traumatic rupture of collateral ligament of finger at metacarpophalangeal and interphalangeal joint

　　●S63.410　Traumatic rupture of collateral ligament of right index finger at metacarpophalangeal and interphalangeal joint

　　●S63.411　Traumatic rupture of collateral ligament of left index finger at metacarpophalangeal and interphalangeal joint

　　●S63.412　Traumatic rupture of collateral ligament of right middle finger at metacarpophalangeal and interphalangeal joint

　　●S63.413　Traumatic rupture of collateral ligament of left middle finger at metacarpophalangeal and interphalangeal joint

　　●S63.414　Traumatic rupture of collateral ligament of right ring finger at metacarpophalangeal and interphalangeal joint

　　●S63.415　Traumatic rupture of collateral ligament of left ring finger at metacarpophalangeal and interphalangeal joint

　　●S63.416　Traumatic rupture of collateral ligament of right little finger at metacarpophalangeal and interphalangeal joint

　　●S63.417　Traumatic rupture of collateral ligament of left little finger at metacarpophalangeal and interphalangeal joint

　　●S63.418　Traumatic rupture of collateral ligament of other finger at metacarpophalangeal and interphalangeal joint
　　　　Traumatic rupture of collateral ligament of specified finger with unspecified laterality at metacarpophalangeal and interphalangeal joint

　　●S63.419　Traumatic rupture of collateral ligament of unspecified finger at metacarpophalangeal and interphalangeal joint

　●S63.42　Traumatic rupture of palmar ligament of finger at metacarpophalangeal and interphalangeal joint

　　●S63.420　Traumatic rupture of palmar ligament of right index finger at metacarpophalangeal and interphalangeal joint

　　●S63.421　Traumatic rupture of palmar ligament of left index finger at metacarpophalangeal and interphalangeal joint

　　●S63.422　Traumatic rupture of palmar ligament of right middle finger at metacarpophalangeal and interphalangeal joint

　　●S63.423　Traumatic rupture of palmar ligament of left middle finger at metacarpophalangeal and interphalangeal joint

　　●S63.424　Traumatic rupture of palmar ligament of right ring finger at metacarpophalangeal and interphalangeal joint

　　●S63.425　Traumatic rupture of palmar ligament of left ring finger at metacarpophalangeal and interphalangeal joint

　　●S63.426　Traumatic rupture of palmar ligament of right little finger at metacarpophalangeal and interphalangeal joint

　　●S63.427　Traumatic rupture of palmar ligament of left little finger at metacarpophalangeal and interphalangeal joint

　　●S63.428　Traumatic rupture of palmar ligament of other finger at metacarpophalangeal and interphalangeal joint
　　　　Traumatic rupture of palmar ligament of specified finger with unspecified laterality at metacarpophalangeal and interphalangeal joint

　　●S63.429　Traumatic rupture of palmar ligament of unspecified finger at metacarpophalangeal and interphalangeal joint

▶ New　⇒ Revised　deleted Deleted　OGCR Official Guidelines　X Assign placeholder X　● Use Additional Character(s)

| Excludes 1 | Excludes 2 | Includes | Use additional | Code first | Code also | Key words |

- S63.43　Traumatic rupture of volar plate of finger at metacarpophalangeal and interphalangeal joint
  - S63.430　Traumatic rupture of volar plate of right index finger at metacarpophalangeal and interphalangeal joint
  - S63.431　Traumatic rupture of volar plate of left index finger at metacarpophalangeal and interphalangeal joint
  - S63.432　Traumatic rupture of volar plate of right middle finger at metacarpophalangeal and interphalangeal joint
  - S63.433　Traumatic rupture of volar plate of left middle finger at metacarpophalangeal and interphalangeal joint
  - S63.434　Traumatic rupture of volar plate of right ring finger at metacarpophalangeal and interphalangeal joint
  - S63.435　Traumatic rupture of volar plate of left ring finger at metacarpophalangeal and interphalangeal joint
  - S63.436　Traumatic rupture of volar plate of right little finger at metacarpophalangeal and interphalangeal joint
  - S63.437　Traumatic rupture of volar plate of left little finger at metacarpophalangeal and interphalangeal joint
  - S63.438　Traumatic rupture of volar plate of other finger at metacarpophalangeal and interphalangeal joint
    Traumatic rupture of volar plate of specified finger with unspecified laterality at metacarpophalangeal and interphalangeal joint
  - S63.439　Traumatic rupture of volar plate of unspecified finger at metacarpophalangeal and interphalangeal joint
- S63.49　Traumatic rupture of other ligament of finger at metacarpophalangeal and interphalangeal joint
  - S63.490　Traumatic rupture of other ligament of right index finger at metacarpophalangeal and interphalangeal joint
  - S63.491　Traumatic rupture of other ligament of left index finger at metacarpophalangeal and interphalangeal joint
  - S63.492　Traumatic rupture of other ligament of right middle finger at metacarpophalangeal and interphalangeal joint
  - S63.493　Traumatic rupture of other ligament of left middle finger at metacarpophalangeal and interphalangeal joint
  - S63.494　Traumatic rupture of other ligament of right ring finger at metacarpophalangeal and interphalangeal joint
  - S63.495　Traumatic rupture of other ligament of left ring finger at metacarpophalangeal and interphalangeal joint
  - S63.496　Traumatic rupture of other ligament of right little finger at metacarpophalangeal and interphalangeal joint
  - S63.497　Traumatic rupture of other ligament of left little finger at metacarpophalangeal and interphalangeal joint
  - S63.498　Traumatic rupture of other ligament of other finger at metacarpophalangeal and interphalangeal joint
    Traumatic rupture of ligament of specified finger with unspecified laterality at metacarpophalangeal and interphalangeal joint
  - S63.499　Traumatic rupture of other ligament of unspecified finger at metacarpophalangeal and interphalangeal joint
- S63.5　Other and unspecified sprain of wrist
  - S63.50　Unspecified sprain of wrist
    - S63.501　Unspecified sprain of right wrist
    - S63.502　Unspecified sprain of left wrist
    - S63.509　Unspecified sprain of unspecified wrist
  - S63.51　Sprain of carpal (joint)
    - S63.511　Sprain of carpal joint of right wrist
    - S63.512　Sprain of carpal joint of left wrist
    - S63.519　Sprain of carpal joint of unspecified wrist
  - S63.52　Sprain of radiocarpal joint
    > Excludes1　traumatic rupture of radiocarpal ligament (S63.32-)
    - S63.521　Sprain of radiocarpal joint of right wrist
    - S63.522　Sprain of radiocarpal joint of left wrist
    - S63.529　Sprain of radiocarpal joint of unspecified wrist
  - S63.59　Other specified sprain of wrist
    - S63.591　Other specified sprain of right wrist
    - S63.592　Other specified sprain of left wrist
    - S63.599　Other specified sprain of unspecified wrist
- S63.6　Other and unspecified sprain of finger(s)
  > Excludes1　traumatic rupture of ligament of finger at metacarpophalangeal and interphalangeal joint(s) (S63.4-)
  - S63.60　Unspecified sprain of thumb
    - S63.601　Unspecified sprain of right thumb
    - S63.602　Unspecified sprain of left thumb
    - S63.609　Unspecified sprain of unspecified thumb
  - S63.61　Unspecified sprain of other and unspecified finger(s)
    - S63.610　Unspecified sprain of right index finger
    - S63.611　Unspecified sprain of left index finger
    - S63.612　Unspecified sprain of right middle finger
    - S63.613　Unspecified sprain of left middle finger
    - S63.614　Unspecified sprain of right ring finger
    - S63.615　Unspecified sprain of left ring finger
    - S63.616　Unspecified sprain of right little finger

▶ New　⟹ Revised　~~deleted~~ Deleted　**OGCR** Official Guidelines　X Assign placeholder X　● Use Additional Character(s)

Excludes 1　Excludes 2　Includes　Use additional　Code first　Code also　Key words

● S63.617   Unspecified sprain of left little finger

● S63.618   Unspecified sprain of other finger
     Unspecified sprain of specified finger with unspecified laterality

● S63.619   Unspecified sprain of unspecified finger

● S63.62   Sprain of interphalangeal joint of thumb

   ● S63.621   Sprain of interphalangeal joint of right thumb

   ● S63.622   Sprain of interphalangeal joint of left thumb

   ● S63.629   Sprain of interphalangeal joint of unspecified thumb

● S63.63   Sprain of interphalangeal joint of other and unspecified finger(s)

   ● S63.630   Sprain of interphalangeal joint of right index finger

   ● S63.631   Sprain of interphalangeal joint of left index finger

   ● S63.632   Sprain of interphalangeal joint of right middle finger

   ● S63.633   Sprain of interphalangeal joint of left middle finger

   ● S63.634   Sprain of interphalangeal joint of right ring finger

   ● S63.635   Sprain of interphalangeal joint of left ring finger

   ● S63.636   Sprain of interphalangeal joint of right little finger

   ● S63.637   Sprain of interphalangeal joint of left little finger

   ● S63.638   Sprain of interphalangeal joint of other finger

   ● S63.639   Sprain of interphalangeal joint of unspecified finger

● S63.64   Sprain of metacarpophalangeal joint of thumb

   ● S63.641   Sprain of metacarpophalangeal joint of right thumb

   ● S63.642   Sprain of metacarpophalangeal joint of left thumb

   ● S63.649   Sprain of metacarpophalangeal joint of unspecified thumb

● S63.65   Sprain of metacarpophalangeal joint of other and unspecified finger(s)

   ● S63.650   Sprain of metacarpophalangeal joint of right index finger

   ● S63.651   Sprain of metacarpophalangeal joint of left index finger

   ● S63.652   Sprain of metacarpophalangeal joint of right middle finger

   ● S63.653   Sprain of metacarpophalangeal joint of left middle finger

   ● S63.654   Sprain of metacarpophalangeal joint of right ring finger

   ● S63.655   Sprain of metacarpophalangeal joint of left ring finger

   ● S63.656   Sprain of metacarpophalangeal joint of right little finger

   ● S63.657   Sprain of metacarpophalangeal joint of left little finger

   ● S63.658   Sprain of metacarpophalangeal joint of other finger
     Sprain of metacarpophalangeal joint of specified finger with unspecified laterality

   ● S63.659   Sprain of metacarpophalangeal joint of unspecified finger

● S63.68   Other sprain of thumb

   ● S63.681   Other sprain of right thumb

   ● S63.682   Other sprain of left thumb

   ● S63.689   Other sprain of unspecified thumb

● S63.69   Other sprain of other and unspecified finger(s)

   ● S63.690   Other sprain of right index finger

   ● S63.691   Other sprain of left index finger

   ● S63.692   Other sprain of right middle finger

   ● S63.693   Other sprain of left middle finger

   ● S63.694   Other sprain of right ring finger

   ● S63.695   Other sprain of left ring finger

   ● S63.696   Other sprain of right little finger

   ● S63.697   Other sprain of left little finger

   ● S63.698   Other sprain of other finger
     Other sprain of specified finger with unspecified laterality

   ● S63.699   Other sprain of unspecified finger

● S63.8   Sprain of other part of wrist and hand

   ● S63.8X   Sprain of other part of wrist and hand

     ● S63.8X1   Sprain of other part of right wrist and hand

     ● S63.8X2   Sprain of other part of left wrist and hand

     ● S63.8X9   Sprain of other part of unspecified wrist and hand

● S63.9   Sprain of unspecified part of wrist and hand

   X ● S63.90   Sprain of unspecified part of unspecified wrist and hand

   X ● S63.91   Sprain of unspecified part of right wrist and hand

   X ● S63.92   Sprain of unspecified part of left wrist and hand

● S64   **Injury of nerves at wrist and hand level**

The appropriate 7th character is to be added to each code from category S64

A	initial encounter
D	subsequent encounter
S	sequela

Code also any associated open wound (S61.-)

● S64.0   Injury of ulnar nerve at wrist and hand level

   X ● S64.00   Injury of ulnar nerve at wrist and hand level of unspecified arm

   X ● S64.01   Injury of ulnar nerve at wrist and hand level of right arm

   X ● S64.02   Injury of ulnar nerve at wrist and hand level of left arm

● S64.1   Injury of median nerve at wrist and hand level

   X ● S64.10   Injury of median nerve at wrist and hand level of unspecified arm

   X ● S64.11   Injury of median nerve at wrist and hand level of right arm

   X ● S64.12   Injury of median nerve at wrist and hand level of left arm

● S64.2   Injury of radial nerve at wrist and hand level

   X ● S64.20   Injury of radial nerve at wrist and hand level of unspecified arm

   X ● S64.21   Injury of radial nerve at wrist and hand level of right arm

   X ● S64.22   Injury of radial nerve at wrist and hand level of left arm

● S64.3   Injury of digital nerve of thumb

   X ● S64.30   Injury of digital nerve of unspecified thumb

   X ● S64.31   Injury of digital nerve of right thumb

   X ● S64.32   Injury of digital nerve of left thumb

- S64.4   Injury of digital nerve of other and unspecified finger
  - X● S64.40   Injury of digital nerve of unspecified finger
  - ● S64.49   Injury of digital nerve of other finger
    - ● S64.490   Injury of digital nerve of right index finger
    - ● S64.491   Injury of digital nerve of left index finger
    - ● S64.492   Injury of digital nerve of right middle finger
    - ● S64.493   Injury of digital nerve of left middle finger
    - ● S64.494   Injury of digital nerve of right ring finger
    - ● S64.495   Injury of digital nerve of left ring finger
    - ● S64.496   Injury of digital nerve of right little finger
    - ● S64.497   Injury of digital nerve of left little finger
    - ● S64.498   Injury of digital nerve of other finger
      Injury of digital nerve of specified finger with unspecified laterality
- S64.8   Injury of other nerves at wrist and hand level
  - ● S64.8X   Injury of other nerves at wrist and hand level
    - ● S64.8X1   Injury of other nerves at wrist and hand level of right arm
    - ● S64.8X2   Injury of other nerves at wrist and hand level of left arm
    - ● S64.8X9   Injury of other nerves at wrist and hand level of unspecified arm
- S64.9   Injury of unspecified nerve at wrist and hand level
  - X● S64.90   Injury of unspecified nerve at wrist and hand level of unspecified arm
  - X● S64.91   Injury of unspecified nerve at wrist and hand level of right arm
  - X● S64.92   Injury of unspecified nerve at wrist and hand level of left arm

- S65   Injury of blood vessels at wrist and hand level

  The appropriate 7th character is to be added to each code from category S65

A	initial encounter
D	subsequent encounter
S	sequela

  Code also any associated open wound (S61.-)

- S65.0   Injury of ulnar artery at wrist and hand level
  - ● S65.00   Unspecified injury of ulnar artery at wrist and hand level
    - ● S65.001   Unspecified injury of ulnar artery at wrist and hand level of right arm
    - ● S65.002   Unspecified injury of ulnar artery at wrist and hand level of left arm
    - ● S65.009   Unspecified injury of ulnar artery at wrist and hand level of unspecified arm
  - ● S65.01   Laceration of ulnar artery at wrist and hand level
    - ● S65.011   Laceration of ulnar artery at wrist and hand level of right arm
    - ● S65.012   Laceration of ulnar artery at wrist and hand level of left arm
    - ● S65.019   Laceration of ulnar artery at wrist and hand level of unspecified arm

- ● S65.09   Other specified injury of ulnar artery at wrist and hand level
  - ● S65.091   Other specified injury of ulnar artery at wrist and hand level of right arm
  - ● S65.092   Other specified injury of ulnar artery at wrist and hand level of left arm
  - ● S65.099   Other specified injury of ulnar artery at wrist and hand level of unspecified arm
- ● S65.1   Injury of radial artery at wrist and hand level
  - ● S65.10   Unspecified injury of radial artery at wrist and hand level
    - ● S65.101   Unspecified injury of radial artery at wrist and hand level of right arm
    - ● S65.102   Unspecified injury of radial artery at wrist and hand level of left arm
    - ● S65.109   Unspecified injury of radial artery at wrist and hand level of unspecified arm
  - ● S65.11   Laceration of radial artery at wrist and hand level
    - ● S65.111   Laceration of radial artery at wrist and hand level of right arm
    - ● S65.112   Laceration of radial artery at wrist and hand level of left arm
    - ● S65.119   Laceration of radial artery at wrist and hand level of unspecified arm
  - ● S65.19   Other specified injury of radial artery at wrist and hand level
    - ● S65.191   Other specified injury of radial artery at wrist and hand level of right arm
    - ● S65.192   Other specified injury of radial artery at wrist and hand level of left arm
    - ● S65.199   Other specified injury of radial artery at wrist and hand level of unspecified arm
- ● S65.2   Injury of superficial palmar arch
  - ● S65.20   Unspecified injury of superficial palmar arch
    - ● S65.201   Unspecified injury of superficial palmar arch of right hand
    - ● S65.202   Unspecified injury of superficial palmar arch of left hand
    - ● S65.209   Unspecified injury of superficial palmar arch of unspecified hand
  - ● S65.21   Laceration of superficial palmar arch
    - ● S65.211   Laceration of superficial palmar arch of right hand
    - ● S65.212   Laceration of superficial palmar arch of left hand
    - ● S65.219   Laceration of superficial palmar arch of unspecified hand
  - ● S65.29   Other specified injury of superficial palmar arch
    - ● S65.291   Other specified injury of superficial palmar arch of right hand
    - ● S65.292   Other specified injury of superficial palmar arch of left hand
    - ● S65.299   Other specified injury of superficial palmar arch of unspecified hand
- ● S65.3   Injury of deep palmar arch
  - ● S65.30   Unspecified injury of deep palmar arch
    - ● S65.301   Unspecified injury of deep palmar arch of right hand
    - ● S65.302   Unspecified injury of deep palmar arch of left hand
    - ● S65.309   Unspecified injury of deep palmar arch of unspecified hand

▶ New   ⇒ Revised   ~~deleted~~ Deleted   OGCR Official Guidelines   X Assign placeholder X   ● Use Additional Character(s)

Excludes 1   Excludes 2   Includes   Use additional   Code first   Code also   Key words

- S65.31   Laceration of deep palmar arch
  - S65.311   Laceration of deep palmar arch of right hand
  - S65.312   Laceration of deep palmar arch of left hand
  - S65.319   Laceration of deep palmar arch of unspecified hand
- S65.39   Other specified injury of deep palmar arch
  - S65.391   Other specified injury of deep palmar arch of right hand
  - S65.392   Other specified injury of deep palmar arch of left hand
  - S65.399   Other specified injury of deep palmar arch of unspecified hand
- S65.4   Injury of blood vessel of thumb
  - S65.40   Unspecified injury of blood vessel of thumb
    - S65.401   Unspecified injury of blood vessel of right thumb
    - S65.402   Unspecified injury of blood vessel of left thumb
    - S65.409   Unspecified injury of blood vessel of unspecified thumb
  - S65.41   Laceration of blood vessel of thumb
    - S65.411   Laceration of blood vessel of right thumb
    - S65.412   Laceration of blood vessel of left thumb
    - S65.419   Laceration of blood vessel of unspecified thumb
  - S65.49   Other specified injury of blood vessel of thumb
    - S65.491   Other specified injury of blood vessel of right thumb
    - S65.492   Other specified injury of blood vessel of left thumb
    - S65.499   Other specified injury of blood vessel of unspecified thumb
- S65.5   Injury of blood vessel of other and unspecified finger
  - S65.50   Unspecified injury of blood vessel of other and unspecified finger
    - S65.500   Unspecified injury of blood vessel of right index finger
    - S65.501   Unspecified injury of blood vessel of left index finger
    - S65.502   Unspecified injury of blood vessel of right middle finger
    - S65.503   Unspecified injury of blood vessel of left middle finger
    - S65.504   Unspecified injury of blood vessel of right ring finger
    - S65.505   Unspecified injury of blood vessel of left ring finger
    - S65.506   Unspecified injury of blood vessel of right little finger
    - S65.507   Unspecified injury of blood vessel of left little finger
    - S65.508   Unspecified injury of blood vessel of other finger
      Unspecified injury of blood vessel of specified finger with unspecified laterality
    - S65.509   Unspecified injury of blood vessel of unspecified finger

- S65.51   Laceration of blood vessel of other and unspecified finger
  - S65.510   Laceration of blood vessel of right index finger
  - S65.511   Laceration of blood vessel of left index finger
  - S65.512   Laceration of blood vessel of right middle finger
  - S65.513   Laceration of blood vessel of left middle finger
  - S65.514   Laceration of blood vessel of right ring finger
  - S65.515   Laceration of blood vessel of left ring finger
  - S65.516   Laceration of blood vessel of right little finger
  - S65.517   Laceration of blood vessel of left little finger
  - S65.518   Laceration of blood vessel of other finger
    Laceration of blood vessel of specified finger with unspecified laterality
  - S65.519   Laceration of blood vessel of unspecified finger
- S65.59   Other specified injury of blood vessel of other and unspecified finger
  - S65.590   Other specified injury of blood vessel of right index finger
  - S65.591   Other specified injury of blood vessel of left index finger
  - S65.592   Other specified injury of blood vessel of right middle finger
  - S65.593   Other specified injury of blood vessel of left middle finger
  - S65.594   Other specified injury of blood vessel of right ring finger
  - S65.595   Other specified injury of blood vessel of left ring finger
  - S65.596   Other specified injury of blood vessel of right little finger
  - S65.597   Other specified injury of blood vessel of left little finger
  - S65.598   Other specified injury of blood vessel of other finger
    Other specified injury of blood vessel of specified finger with unspecified laterality
  - S65.599   Other specified injury of blood vessel of unspecified finger
- S65.8   Injury of other blood vessels at wrist and hand level
  - S65.80   Unspecified injury of other blood vessels at wrist and hand level
    - S65.801   Unspecified injury of other blood vessels at wrist and hand level of right arm
    - S65.802   Unspecified injury of other blood vessels at wrist and hand level of left arm
    - S65.809   Unspecified injury of other blood vessels at wrist and hand level of unspecified arm
  - S65.81   Laceration of other blood vessels at wrist and hand level
    - S65.811   Laceration of other blood vessels at wrist and hand level of right arm
    - S65.812   Laceration of other blood vessels at wrist and hand level of left arm
    - S65.819   Laceration of other blood vessels at wrist and hand level of unspecified arm

CHAPTER 19 (S00-T88)

● S65.89   Other specified injury of other blood vessels at wrist and hand level
  ● S65.891   Other specified injury of other blood vessels at wrist and hand level of right arm
  ● S65.892   Other specified injury of other blood vessels at wrist and hand level of left arm
  ● S65.899   Other specified injury of other blood vessels at wrist and hand level of unspecified arm

● S65.9   Injury of unspecified blood vessel at wrist and hand level
  ● S65.90   Unspecified injury of unspecified blood vessel at wrist and hand level
    ● S65.901   Unspecified injury of unspecified blood vessel at wrist and hand level of right arm
    ● S65.902   Unspecified injury of unspecified blood vessel at wrist and hand level of left arm
    ● S65.909   Unspecified injury of unspecified blood vessel at wrist and hand level of unspecified arm
  ● S65.91   Laceration of unspecified blood vessel at wrist and hand level
    ● S65.911   Laceration of unspecified blood vessel at wrist and hand level of right arm
    ● S65.912   Laceration of unspecified blood vessel at wrist and hand level of left arm
    ● S65.919   Laceration of unspecified blood vessel at wrist and hand level of unspecified arm
  ● S65.99   Other specified injury of unspecified blood vessel at wrist and hand level
    ● S65.991   Other specified injury of unspecified blood vessel at wrist and hand of right arm
    ● S65.992   Other specified injury of unspecified blood vessel at wrist and hand of left arm
    ● S65.999   Other specified injury of unspecified blood vessel at wrist and hand of unspecified arm

● S66   Injury of muscle, fascia and tendon at wrist and hand level
      Code also any associated open wound (S61.-)
      Excludes2   sprain of joints and ligaments of wrist and hand (S63.-)

      The appropriate 7th character is to be added to each code from category S66

      | A | initial encounter |
      | D | subsequent encounter |
      | S | sequela |

  ● S66.0   Injury of long flexor muscle, fascia and tendon of thumb at wrist and hand level
    ● S66.00   Unspecified injury of long flexor muscle, fascia and tendon of thumb at wrist and hand level
      ● S66.001   Unspecified injury of long flexor muscle, fascia and tendon of right thumb at wrist and hand level
      ● S66.002   Unspecified injury of long flexor muscle, fascia and tendon of left thumb at wrist and hand level
      ● S66.009   Unspecified injury of long flexor muscle, fascia and tendon of unspecified thumb at wrist and hand level

  ● S66.01   Strain of long flexor muscle, fascia and tendon of thumb at wrist and hand level
    ● S66.011   Strain of long flexor muscle, fascia and tendon of right thumb at wrist and hand level
    ● S66.012   Strain of long flexor muscle, fascia and tendon of left thumb at wrist and hand level
    ● S66.019   Strain of long flexor muscle, fascia and tendon of unspecified thumb at wrist and hand level
  ● S66.02   Laceration of long flexor muscle, fascia and tendon of thumb at wrist and hand level
    ● S66.021   Laceration of long flexor muscle, fascia and tendon of right thumb at wrist and hand level
    ● S66.022   Laceration of long flexor muscle, fascia and tendon of left thumb at wrist and hand level
    ● S66.029   Laceration of long flexor muscle, fascia and tendon of unspecified thumb at wrist and hand level
  ● S66.09   Other specified injury of long flexor muscle, fascia and tendon of thumb at wrist and hand level
    ● S66.091   Other specified injury of long flexor muscle, fascia and tendon of right thumb at wrist and hand level
    ● S66.092   Other specified injury of long flexor muscle, fascia and tendon of left thumb at wrist and hand level
    ● S66.099   Other specified injury of long flexor muscle, fascia and tendon of unspecified thumb at wrist and hand level

● S66.1   Injury of flexor muscle, fascia and tendon of other and unspecified finger at wrist and hand level
      Excludes2   injury of long flexor muscle, fascia and tendon of thumb at wrist and hand level (S66.0-)
  ● S66.10   Unspecified injury of flexor muscle, fascia and tendon of other and unspecified finger at wrist and hand level
    ● S66.100   Unspecified injury of flexor muscle, fascia and tendon of right index finger at wrist and hand level
    ● S66.101   Unspecified injury of flexor muscle, fascia and tendon of left index finger at wrist and hand level
    ● S66.102   Unspecified injury of flexor muscle, fascia and tendon of right middle finger at wrist and hand level
    ● S66.103   Unspecified injury of flexor muscle, fascia and tendon of left middle finger at wrist and hand level
    ● S66.104   Unspecified injury of flexor muscle, fascia and tendon of right ring finger at wrist and hand level
    ● S66.105   Unspecified injury of flexor muscle, fascia and tendon of left ring finger at wrist and hand level
    ● S66.106   Unspecified injury of flexor muscle, fascia and tendon of right little finger at wrist and hand level
    ● S66.107   Unspecified injury of flexor muscle, fascia and tendon of left little finger at wrist and hand level

● **S66.108** **Unspecified injury of flexor muscle, fascia and tendon of other finger at wrist and hand level**

Unspecified injury of flexor muscle, fascia and tendon of specified finger with unspecified laterality at wrist and hand level

● **S66.109** **Unspecified injury of flexor muscle, fascia and tendon of unspecified finger at wrist and hand level**

● **S66.11** **Strain of flexor muscle, fascia and tendon of other and unspecified finger at wrist and hand level**

● **S66.110** **Strain of flexor muscle, fascia and tendon of right index finger at wrist and hand level**

● **S66.111** **Strain of flexor muscle, fascia and tendon of left index finger at wrist and hand level**

● **S66.112** **Strain of flexor muscle, fascia and tendon of right middle finger at wrist and hand level**

● **S66.113** **Strain of flexor muscle, fascia and tendon of left middle finger at wrist and hand level**

● **S66.114** **Strain of flexor muscle, fascia and tendon of right ring finger at wrist and hand level**

● **S66.115** **Strain of flexor muscle, fascia and tendon of left ring finger at wrist and hand level**

● **S66.116** **Strain of flexor muscle, fascia and tendon of right little finger at wrist and hand level**

● **S66.117** **Strain of flexor muscle, fascia and tendon of left little finger at wrist and hand level**

● **S66.118** **Strain of flexor muscle, fascia and tendon of other finger at wrist and hand level**

Strain of flexor muscle, fascia and tendon of specified finger with unspecified laterality at wrist and hand level

● **S66.119** **Strain of flexor muscle, fascia and tendon of unspecified finger at wrist and hand level**

● **S66.12** **Laceration of flexor muscle, fascia and tendon of other and unspecified finger at wrist and hand level**

● **S66.120** **Laceration of flexor muscle, fascia and tendon of right index finger at wrist and hand level**

● **S66.121** **Laceration of flexor muscle, fascia and tendon of left index finger at wrist and hand level**

● **S66.122** **Laceration of flexor muscle, fascia and tendon of right middle finger at wrist and hand level**

● **S66.123** **Laceration of flexor muscle, fascia and tendon of left middle finger at wrist and hand level**

● **S66.124** **Laceration of flexor muscle, fascia and tendon of right ring finger at wrist and hand level**

● **S66.125** **Laceration of flexor muscle, fascia and tendon of left ring finger at wrist and hand level**

● **S66.126** **Laceration of flexor muscle, fascia and tendon of right little finger at wrist and hand level**

● **S66.127** **Laceration of flexor muscle, fascia and tendon of left little finger at wrist and hand level**

● **S66.128** **Laceration of flexor muscle, fascia and tendon of other finger at wrist and hand level**

Laceration of flexor muscle, fascia and tendon of specified finger with unspecified laterality at wrist and hand level

● **S66.129** **Laceration of flexor muscle, fascia and tendon of unspecified finger at wrist and hand level**

● **S66.19** **Other injury of flexor muscle, fascia and tendon of other and unspecified finger at wrist and hand level**

● **S66.190** **Other injury of flexor muscle, fascia and tendon of right index finger at wrist and hand level**

● **S66.191** **Other injury of flexor muscle, fascia and tendon of left index finger at wrist and hand level**

● **S66.192** **Other injury of flexor muscle, fascia and tendon of right middle finger at wrist and hand level**

● **S66.193** **Other injury of flexor muscle, fascia and tendon of left middle finger at wrist and hand level**

● **S66.194** **Other injury of flexor muscle, fascia and tendon of right ring finger at wrist and hand level**

● **S66.195** **Other injury of flexor muscle, fascia and tendon of left ring finger at wrist and hand level**

● **S66.196** **Other injury of flexor muscle, fascia and tendon of right little finger at wrist and hand level**

● **S66.197** **Other injury of flexor muscle, fascia and tendon of left little finger at wrist and hand level**

● **S66.198** **Other injury of flexor muscle, fascia and tendon of other finger at wrist and hand level**

Other injury of flexor muscle, fascia and tendon of specified finger with unspecified laterality at wrist and hand level

● **S66.199** **Other injury of flexor muscle, fascia and tendon of unspecified finger at wrist and hand level**

● **S66.2** **Injury of extensor muscle, fascia and tendon of thumb at wrist and hand level**

● **S66.20** **Unspecified injury of extensor muscle, fascia and tendon of thumb at wrist and hand level**

● **S66.201** **Unspecified injury of extensor muscle, fascia and tendon of right thumb at wrist and hand level**

● **S66.202** **Unspecified injury of extensor muscle, fascia and tendon of left thumb at wrist and hand level**

● **S66.209** **Unspecified injury of extensor muscle, fascia and tendon of unspecified thumb at wrist and hand level**

CHAPTER 19 (S00-T88)

● **S66.21**   Strain of extensor muscle, fascia and tendon of thumb at wrist and hand level

     ● **S66.211**   Strain of extensor muscle, fascia and tendon of right thumb at wrist and hand level

     ● **S66.212**   Strain of extensor muscle, fascia and tendon of left thumb at wrist and hand level

     ● **S66.219**   Strain of extensor muscle, fascia and tendon of unspecified thumb at wrist and hand level

● **S66.22**   Laceration of extensor muscle, fascia and tendon of thumb at wrist and hand level

     ● **S66.221**   Laceration of extensor muscle, fascia and tendon of right thumb at wrist and hand level

     ● **S66.222**   Laceration of extensor muscle, fascia and tendon of left thumb at wrist and hand level

     ● **S66.229**   Laceration of extensor muscle, fascia and tendon of unspecified thumb at wrist and hand level

● **S66.29**   Other specified injury of extensor muscle, fascia and tendon of thumb at wrist and hand level

     ● **S66.291**   Other specified injury of extensor muscle, fascia and tendon of right thumb at wrist and hand level

     ● **S66.292**   Other specified injury of extensor muscle, fascia and tendon of left thumb at wrist and hand level

     ● **S66.299**   Other specified injury of extensor muscle, fascia and tendon of unspecified thumb at wrist and hand level

● **S66.3**   Injury of extensor muscle, fascia and tendon of other and unspecified finger at wrist and hand level

     Excludes2   injury of extensor muscle, fascia and tendon of thumb at wrist and hand level (S66.2-)

   ● **S66.30**   Unspecified injury of extensor muscle, fascia and tendon of other and unspecified finger at wrist and hand level

     ● **S66.300**   Unspecified injury of extensor muscle, fascia and tendon of right index finger at wrist and hand level

     ● **S66.301**   Unspecified injury of extensor muscle, fascia and tendon of left index finger at wrist and hand level

     ● **S66.302**   Unspecified injury of extensor muscle, fascia and tendon of right middle finger at wrist and hand level

     ● **S66.303**   Unspecified injury of extensor muscle, fascia and tendon of left middle finger at wrist and hand level

     ● **S66.304**   Unspecified injury of extensor muscle, fascia and tendon of right ring finger at wrist and hand level

     ● **S66.305**   Unspecified injury of extensor muscle, fascia and tendon of left ring finger at wrist and hand level

     ● **S66.306**   Unspecified injury of extensor muscle, fascia and tendon of right little finger at wrist and hand level

     ● **S66.307**   Unspecified injury of extensor muscle, fascia and tendon of left little finger at wrist and hand level

     ● **S66.308**   Unspecified injury of extensor muscle, fascia and tendon of other finger at wrist and hand level

       Unspecified injury of extensor muscle, fascia and tendon of specified finger with unspecified laterality at wrist and hand level

     ● **S66.309**   Unspecified injury of extensor muscle, fascia and tendon of unspecified finger at wrist and hand level

● **S66.31**   Strain of extensor muscle, fascia and tendon of other and unspecified finger at wrist and hand level

     ● **S66.310**   Strain of extensor muscle, fascia and tendon of right index finger at wrist and hand level

     ● **S66.311**   Strain of extensor muscle, fascia and tendon of left index finger at wrist and hand level

     ● **S66.312**   Strain of extensor muscle, fascia and tendon of right middle finger at wrist and hand level

     ● **S66.313**   Strain of extensor muscle, fascia and tendon of left middle finger at wrist and hand level

     ● **S66.314**   Strain of extensor muscle, fascia and tendon of right ring finger at wrist and hand level

     ● **S66.315**   Strain of extensor muscle, fascia and tendon of left ring finger at wrist and hand level

     ● **S66.316**   Strain of extensor muscle, fascia and tendon of right little finger at wrist and hand level

     ● **S66.317**   Strain of extensor muscle, fascia and tendon of left little finger at wrist and hand level

     ● **S66.318**   Strain of extensor muscle, fascia and tendon of other finger at wrist and hand level

       Strain of extensor muscle, fascia and tendon of specified finger with unspecified laterality at wrist and hand level

     ● **S66.319**   Strain of extensor muscle, fascia and tendon of unspecified finger at wrist and hand level

● **S66.32**   Laceration of extensor muscle, fascia and tendon of other and unspecified finger at wrist and hand level

     ● **S66.320**   Laceration of extensor muscle, fascia and tendon of right index finger at wrist and hand level

     ● **S66.321**   Laceration of extensor muscle, fascia and tendon of left index finger at wrist and hand level

     ● **S66.322**   Laceration of extensor muscle, fascia and tendon of right middle finger at wrist and hand level

     ● **S66.323**   Laceration of extensor muscle, fascia and tendon of left middle finger at wrist and hand level

     ● **S66.324**   Laceration of extensor muscle, fascia and tendon of right ring finger at wrist and hand level

     ● **S66.325**   Laceration of extensor muscle, fascia and tendon of left ring finger at wrist and hand level

     ● **S66.326**   Laceration of extensor muscle, fascia and tendon of right little finger at wrist and hand level

▶ New   ⇒ Revised   ~~deleted~~ Deleted   **OGCR** Official Guidelines   X Assign placeholder X   ● Use Additional Character(s)

Excludes 1   Excludes 2   Includes   Use additional   Code first   Code also   Key words

● S66.327 Laceration of extensor muscle, fascia and tendon of left little finger at wrist and hand level

● S66.328 Laceration of extensor muscle, fascia and tendon of other finger at wrist and hand level

     Laceration of extensor muscle, fascia and tendon of specified finger with unspecified laterality at wrist and hand level

● S66.329 Laceration of extensor muscle, fascia and tendon of unspecified finger at wrist and hand level

● S66.39 Other injury of extensor muscle, fascia and tendon of other and unspecified finger at wrist and hand level

● S66.390 Other injury of extensor muscle, fascia and tendon of right index finger at wrist and hand level

● S66.391 Other injury of extensor muscle, fascia and tendon of left index finger at wrist and hand level

● S66.392 Other injury of extensor muscle, fascia and tendon of right middle finger at wrist and hand level

● S66.393 Other injury of extensor muscle, fascia and tendon of left middle finger at wrist and hand level

● S66.394 Other injury of extensor muscle, fascia and tendon of right ring finger at wrist and hand level

● S66.395 Other injury of extensor muscle, fascia and tendon of left ring finger at wrist and hand level

● S66.396 Other injury of extensor muscle, fascia and tendon of right little finger at wrist and hand level

● S66.397 Other injury of extensor muscle, fascia and tendon of left little finger at wrist and hand level

● S66.398 Other injury of extensor muscle, fascia and tendon of other finger at wrist and hand level

     Other injury of extensor muscle, fascia and tendon of specified finger with unspecified laterality at wrist and hand level

● S66.399 Other injury of extensor muscle, fascia and tendon of unspecified finger at wrist and hand level

● S66.4 Injury of intrinsic muscle, fascia and tendon of thumb at wrist and hand level

● S66.40 Unspecified injury of intrinsic muscle, fascia and tendon of thumb at wrist and hand level

● S66.401 Unspecified injury of intrinsic muscle, fascia and tendon of right thumb at wrist and hand level

● S66.402 Unspecified injury of intrinsic muscle, fascia and tendon of left thumb at wrist and hand level

● S66.409 Unspecified injury of intrinsic muscle, fascia and tendon of unspecified thumb at wrist and hand level

● S66.41 Strain of intrinsic muscle, fascia and tendon of thumb at wrist and hand level

● S66.411 Strain of intrinsic muscle, fascia and tendon of right thumb at wrist and hand level

● S66.412 Strain of intrinsic muscle, fascia and tendon of left thumb at wrist and hand level

● S66.419 Strain of intrinsic muscle, fascia and tendon of unspecified thumb at wrist and hand level

● S66.42 Laceration of intrinsic muscle, fascia and tendon of thumb at wrist and hand level

● S66.421 Laceration of intrinsic muscle, fascia and tendon of right thumb at wrist and hand level

● S66.422 Laceration of intrinsic muscle, fascia and tendon of left thumb at wrist and hand level

● S66.429 Laceration of intrinsic muscle, fascia and tendon of unspecified thumb at wrist and hand level

● S66.49 Other specified injury of intrinsic muscle, fascia and tendon of thumb at wrist and hand level

● S66.491 Other specified injury of intrinsic muscle, fascia and tendon of right thumb at wrist and hand level

● S66.492 Other specified injury of intrinsic muscle, fascia and tendon of left thumb at wrist and hand level

● S66.499 Other specified injury of intrinsic muscle, fascia and tendon of unspecified thumb at wrist and hand level

● S66.5 Injury of intrinsic muscle, fascia and tendon of other and unspecified finger at wrist and hand level

     Excludes2   injury of intrinsic muscle, fascia and tendon of thumb at wrist and hand level (S66.4-)

● S66.50 Unspecified injury of intrinsic muscle, fascia and tendon of other and unspecified finger at wrist and hand level

● S66.500 Unspecified injury of intrinsic muscle, fascia and tendon of right index finger at wrist and hand level

● S66.501 Unspecified injury of intrinsic muscle, fascia and tendon of left index finger at wrist and hand level

● S66.502 Unspecified injury of intrinsic muscle, fascia and tendon of right middle finger at wrist and hand level

● S66.503 Unspecified injury of intrinsic muscle, fascia and tendon of left middle finger at wrist and hand level

● S66.504 Unspecified injury of intrinsic muscle, fascia and tendon of right ring finger at wrist and hand level

● S66.505 Unspecified injury of intrinsic muscle, fascia and tendon of left ring finger at wrist and hand level

● S66.506 Unspecified injury of intrinsic muscle, fascia and tendon of right little finger at wrist and hand level

● S66.507 Unspecified injury of intrinsic muscle, fascia and tendon of left little finger at wrist and hand level

● S66.508 Unspecified injury of intrinsic muscle, fascia and tendon of other finger at wrist and hand level

     Unspecified injury of intrinsic muscle, fascia and tendon of specified finger with unspecified laterality at wrist and hand level

● S66.509 Unspecified injury of intrinsic muscle, fascia and tendon of unspecified finger at wrist and hand level

● **S66.51** **Strain** of intrinsic muscle, fascia and tendon of other and unspecified finger at wrist and hand level

   ● **S66.510** Strain of intrinsic muscle, fascia and tendon of **right index** finger at wrist and hand level

   ● **S66.511** Strain of intrinsic muscle, fascia and tendon of **left index** finger at wrist and hand level

   ● **S66.512** Strain of intrinsic muscle, fascia and tendon of **right middle** finger at wrist and hand level

   ● **S66.513** Strain of intrinsic muscle, fascia and tendon of **left middle** finger at wrist and hand level

   ● **S66.514** Strain of intrinsic muscle, fascia and tendon of **right ring** finger at wrist and hand level

   ● **S66.515** Strain of intrinsic muscle, fascia and tendon of **left ring** finger at wrist and hand level

   ● **S66.516** Strain of intrinsic muscle, fascia and tendon of **right little** finger at wrist and hand level

   ● **S66.517** Strain of intrinsic muscle, fascia and tendon of **left little** finger at wrist and hand level

   ● **S66.518** Strain of intrinsic muscle, fascia and tendon of **other** finger at wrist and hand level

        Strain of intrinsic muscle, fascia and tendon of specified finger with unspecified laterality at wrist and hand level

   ● **S66.519** Strain of intrinsic muscle, fascia and tendon of **unspecified** finger at wrist and hand level

● **S66.52** **Laceration** of intrinsic muscle, fascia and tendon of other and unspecified finger at wrist and hand level

   ● **S66.520** Laceration of intrinsic muscle, fascia and tendon of **right index** finger at wrist and hand level

   ● **S66.521** Laceration of intrinsic muscle, fascia and tendon of **left index** finger at wrist and hand level

   ● **S66.522** Laceration of intrinsic muscle, fascia and tendon of **right middle** finger at wrist and hand level

   ● **S66.523** Laceration of intrinsic muscle, fascia and tendon of **left middle** finger at wrist and hand level

   ● **S66.524** Laceration of intrinsic muscle, fascia and tendon of **right ring** finger at wrist and hand level

   ● **S66.525** Laceration of intrinsic muscle, fascia and tendon of **left ring** finger at wrist and hand level

   ● **S66.526** Laceration of intrinsic muscle, fascia and tendon of **right little** finger at wrist and hand level

   ● **S66.527** Laceration of intrinsic muscle, fascia and tendon of **left little** finger at wrist and hand level

   ● **S66.528** Laceration of intrinsic muscle, fascia and tendon of **other** finger at wrist and hand level

        Laceration of intrinsic muscle, fascia and tendon of specified finger with unspecified laterality at wrist and hand level

   ● **S66.529** Laceration of intrinsic muscle, fascia and tendon of **unspecified** finger at wrist and hand level

● **S66.59** **Other** injury of intrinsic muscle, fascia and tendon of other and unspecified finger at wrist and hand level

   ● **S66.590** Other injury of intrinsic muscle, fascia and tendon of **right index** finger at wrist and hand level

   ● **S66.591** Other injury of intrinsic muscle, fascia and tendon of **left index** finger at wrist and hand level

   ● **S66.592** Other injury of intrinsic muscle, fascia and tendon of **right middle** finger at wrist and hand level

   ● **S66.593** Other injury of intrinsic muscle, fascia and tendon of **left middle** finger at wrist and hand level

   ● **S66.594** Other injury of intrinsic muscle, fascia and tendon of **right ring** finger at wrist and hand level

   ● **S66.595** Other injury of intrinsic muscle, fascia and tendon of **left ring** finger at wrist and hand level

   ● **S66.596** Other injury of intrinsic muscle, fascia and tendon of **right little** finger at wrist and hand level

   ● **S66.597** Other injury of intrinsic muscle, fascia and tendon of **left little** finger at wrist and hand level

   ● **S66.598** Other injury of intrinsic muscle, fascia and tendon of **other** finger at wrist and hand level

        Other injury of intrinsic muscle, fascia and tendon of specified finger with unspecified laterality at wrist and hand level

   ● **S66.599** Other injury of intrinsic muscle, fascia and tendon of **unspecified** finger at wrist and hand level

● **S66.8** Injury of **other specified** muscles, fascia and tendons at wrist and hand level

  ● **S66.80** **Unspecified** injury of other specified muscles, fascia and tendons at wrist and hand level

   ● **S66.801** Unspecified injury of other specified muscles, fascia and tendons at wrist and hand level, **right** hand

   ● **S66.802** Unspecified injury of other specified muscles, fascia and tendons at wrist and hand level, **left** hand

   ● **S66.809** Unspecified injury of other specified muscles, fascia and tendons at wrist and hand level, **unspecified** hand

  ● **S66.81** **Strain** of other specified muscles, fascia and tendons at wrist and hand level

   ● **S66.811** Strain of other specified muscles, fascia and tendons at wrist and hand level, **right** hand

   ● **S66.812** Strain of other specified muscles, fascia and tendons at wrist and hand level, **left** hand

   ● **S66.819** Strain of other specified muscles, fascia and tendons at wrist and hand level, **unspecified** hand

  ● **S66.82** **Laceration** of other specified muscles, fascia and tendons at wrist and hand level

   ● **S66.821** Laceration of other specified muscles, fascia and tendons at wrist and hand level, **right** hand

   ● **S66.822** Laceration of other specified muscles, fascia and tendons at wrist and hand level, **left** hand

   ● **S66.829** Laceration of other specified muscles, fascia and tendons at wrist and hand level, **unspecified** hand

▶ New   ⟹ Revised   ~~deleted~~ Deleted   **OGCR** Official Guidelines   X Assign placeholder X   ● Use Additional Character(s)

Excludes 1   Excludes 2   Includes   Use additional   Code first   Code also   Key words

● **S66.89**   Other injury of other specified muscles, fascia and tendons at wrist and hand level

   ● **S66.891**   Other injury of other specified muscles, fascia and tendons at wrist and hand level, right hand

   ● **S66.892**   Other injury of other specified muscles, fascia and tendons at wrist and hand level, left hand

   ● **S66.899**   Other injury of other specified muscles, fascia and tendons at wrist and hand level, unspecified hand

● **S66.9**   Injury of unspecified muscle, fascia and tendon at wrist and hand level

  ● **S66.90**   Unspecified injury of unspecified muscle, fascia and tendon at wrist and hand level

   ● **S66.901**   Unspecified injury of unspecified muscle, fascia and tendon at wrist and hand level, right hand

   ● **S66.902**   Unspecified injury of unspecified muscle, fascia and tendon at wrist and hand level, left hand

   ● **S66.909**   Unspecified injury of unspecified muscle, fascia and tendon at wrist and hand level, unspecified hand

  ● **S66.91**   Strain of unspecified muscle, fascia and tendon at wrist and hand level

   ● **S66.911**   Strain of unspecified muscle, fascia and tendon at wrist and hand level, right hand

   ● **S66.912**   Strain of unspecified muscle, fascia and tendon at wrist and hand level, left hand

   ● **S66.919**   Strain of unspecified muscle, fascia and tendon at wrist and hand level, unspecified hand

  ● **S66.92**   Laceration of unspecified muscle, fascia and tendon at wrist and hand level

   ● **S66.921**   Laceration of unspecified muscle, fascia and tendon at wrist and hand level, right hand

   ● **S66.922**   Laceration of unspecified muscle, fascia and tendon at wrist and hand level, left hand

   ● **S66.929**   Laceration of unspecified muscle, fascia and tendon at wrist and hand level, unspecified hand

  ● **S66.99**   Other injury of unspecified muscle, fascia and tendon at wrist and hand level

   ● **S66.991**   Other injury of unspecified muscle, fascia and tendon at wrist and hand level, right hand

   ● **S66.992**   Other injury of unspecified muscle, fascia and tendon at wrist and hand level, left hand

   ● **S66.999**   Other injury of unspecified muscle, fascia and tendon at wrist and hand level, unspecified hand

● **S67**   Crushing injury of wrist, hand and fingers

   Use additional code for all associated injuries, such as:
     fracture of wrist and hand (S62.-)
     open wound of wrist and hand (S61.-)

   The appropriate 7th character is to be added to each code from category S67

A	initial encounter
D	subsequent encounter
S	sequela

  ● **S67.0**   Crushing injury of thumb

   X ● **S67.00**   Crushing injury of unspecified thumb

   X ● **S67.01**   Crushing injury of right thumb

   X ● **S67.02**   Crushing injury of left thumb

● **S67.1**   Crushing injury of other and unspecified finger(s)

   Excludes2   crushing injury of thumb (S67.0-)

   X ● **S67.10**   Crushing injury of unspecified finger(s)

  ● **S67.19**   Crushing injury of other finger(s)

   ● **S67.190**   Crushing injury of right index finger

   ● **S67.191**   Crushing injury of left index finger

   ● **S67.192**   Crushing injury of right middle finger

   ● **S67.193**   Crushing injury of left middle finger

   ● **S67.194**   Crushing injury of right ring finger

   ● **S67.195**   Crushing injury of left ring finger

   ● **S67.196**   Crushing injury of right little finger

   ● **S67.197**   Crushing injury of left little finger

   ● **S67.198**   Crushing injury of other finger
     Crushing injury of specified finger with unspecified laterality

● **S67.2**   Crushing injury of hand

   Excludes2   crushing injury of fingers (S67.1-)
               crushing injury of thumb (S67.0-)

   X ● **S67.20**   Crushing injury of unspecified hand

   X ● **S67.21**   Crushing injury of right hand

   X ● **S67.22**   Crushing injury of left hand

● **S67.3**   Crushing injury of wrist

   X ● **S67.30**   Crushing injury of unspecified wrist

   X ● **S67.31**   Crushing injury of right wrist

   X ● **S67.32**   Crushing injury of left wrist

● **S67.4**   Crushing injury of wrist and hand

   Excludes1   crushing injury of hand alone (S67.2-)
               crushing injury of wrist alone (S67.3-)

   Excludes2   crushing injury of fingers (S67.1-)
               crushing injury of thumb (S67.0-)

   X ● **S67.40**   Crushing injury of unspecified wrist and hand

   X ● **S67.41**   Crushing injury of right wrist and hand

   X ● **S67.42**   Crushing injury of left wrist and hand

● **S67.9**   Crushing injury of unspecified part(s) of wrist, hand and fingers

   X ● **S67.90**   Crushing injury of unspecified part(s) of unspecified wrist, hand and fingers

   X ● **S67.91**   Crushing injury of unspecified part(s) of right wrist, hand and fingers

   X ● **S67.92**   Crushing injury of unspecified part(s) of left wrist, hand and fingers

● **S68**   Traumatic amputation of wrist, hand and fingers

   An amputation not identified as partial or complete should be coded to complete

   The appropriate 7th character is to be added to each code from category S68

A	initial encounter
D	subsequent encounter
S	sequela

● **S68.0**   Traumatic metacarpophalangeal amputation of thumb
   Traumatic amputation of thumb NOS

  ● **S68.01**   Complete traumatic metacarpophalangeal amputation of thumb

   ● **S68.011**   Complete traumatic metacarpophalangeal amputation of right thumb

   ● **S68.012**   Complete traumatic metacarpophalangeal amputation of left thumb

   ● **S68.019**   Complete traumatic metacarpophalangeal amputation of unspecified thumb

CHAPTER 19 (S00-T88)

● S68.02   **Partial** traumatic metacarpophalangeal amputation of thumb

  ● S68.021   Partial traumatic metacarpophalangeal amputation of **right** thumb

  ● S68.022   Partial traumatic metacarpophalangeal amputation of **left** thumb

  ● S68.029   Partial traumatic metacarpophalangeal amputation of **unspecified** thumb

● S68.1   Traumatic **metacarpophalangeal** amputation of other and unspecified **finger**

     Traumatic amputation of finger NOS

     | Excludes2 | traumatic metacarpophalangeal amputation of thumb (S68.0-)

  ● S68.11   **Complete** traumatic metacarpophalangeal amputation of other and unspecified finger

    ● S68.110   Complete traumatic metacarpophalangeal amputation of **right index** finger

    ● S68.111   Complete traumatic metacarpophalangeal amputation of **left index** finger

    ● S68.112   Complete traumatic metacarpophalangeal amputation of **right middle** finger

    ● S68.113   Complete traumatic metacarpophalangeal amputation of **left middle** finger

    ● S68.114   Complete traumatic metacarpophalangeal amputation of **right ring** finger

    ● S68.115   Complete traumatic metacarpophalangeal amputation of **left ring** finger

    ● S68.116   Complete traumatic metacarpophalangeal amputation of **right little** finger

    ● S68.117   Complete traumatic metacarpophalangeal amputation of **left little** finger

    ● S68.118   Complete traumatic metacarpophalangeal amputation of **other** finger

        Complete traumatic metacarpophalangeal amputation of specified finger with unspecified laterality

    ● S68.119   Complete traumatic metacarpophalangeal amputation of **unspecified** finger

  ● S68.12   **Partial** traumatic metacarpophalangeal amputation of other and unspecified finger

    ● S68.120   Partial traumatic metacarpophalangeal amputation of **right index** finger

    ● S68.121   Partial traumatic metacarpophalangeal amputation of **left index** finger

    ● S68.122   Partial traumatic metacarpophalangeal amputation of **right middle** finger

    ● S68.123   Partial traumatic metacarpophalangeal amputation of **left middle** finger

    ● S68.124   Partial traumatic metacarpophalangeal amputation of **right ring** finger

    ● S68.125   Partial traumatic metacarpophalangeal amputation of **left ring** finger

    ● S68.126   Partial traumatic metacarpophalangeal amputation of **right little** finger

    ● S68.127   Partial traumatic metacarpophalangeal amputation of **left little** finger

    ● S68.128   Partial traumatic metacarpophalangeal amputation of **other** finger

        Partial traumatic metacarpophalangeal amputation of specified finger with unspecified laterality

    ● S68.129   Partial traumatic metacarpophalangeal amputation of **unspecified** finger

● S68.4   Traumatic amputation of **hand** at wrist level

     Traumatic amputation of hand NOS

     Traumatic amputation of wrist

  ● S68.41   **Complete** traumatic amputation of hand at wrist level

    ● S68.411   Complete traumatic amputation of **right** hand at wrist level

    ● S68.412   Complete traumatic amputation of **left** hand at wrist level

    ● S68.419   Complete traumatic amputation of **unspecified** hand at wrist level

  ● S68.42   **Partial** traumatic amputation of hand at wrist level

    ● S68.421   Partial traumatic amputation of **right** hand at wrist level

    ● S68.422   Partial traumatic amputation of **left** hand at wrist level

    ● S68.429   Partial traumatic amputation of **unspecified** hand at wrist level

● S68.5   Traumatic **transphalangeal** amputation of **thumb**

     Traumatic interphalangeal joint amputation of thumb

  ● S68.51   **Complete** traumatic transphalangeal amputation of thumb

    ● S68.511   Complete traumatic transphalangeal amputation of **right** thumb

    ● S68.512   Complete traumatic transphalangeal amputation of **left** thumb

    ● S68.519   Complete traumatic transphalangeal amputation of **unspecified** thumb

  ● S68.52   **Partial** traumatic transphalangeal amputation of thumb

    ● S68.521   Partial traumatic transphalangeal amputation of **right** thumb

    ● S68.522   Partial traumatic transphalangeal amputation of **left** thumb

    ● S68.529   Partial traumatic transphalangeal amputation of **unspecified** thumb

● S68.6   Traumatic **transphalangeal** amputation of other and unspecified **finger**

  ● S68.61   **Complete** traumatic transphalangeal amputation of other and unspecified finger(s)

    ● S68.610   Complete traumatic transphalangeal amputation of **right index** finger

    ● S68.611   Complete traumatic transphalangeal amputation of **left index** finger

    ● S68.612   Complete traumatic transphalangeal amputation of **right middle** finger

    ● S68.613   Complete traumatic transphalangeal amputation of **left middle** finger

    ● S68.614   Complete traumatic transphalangeal amputation of **right ring** finger

    ● S68.615   Complete traumatic transphalangeal amputation of **left ring** finger

▶ New   ⇒ Revised   ~~deleted~~ Deleted   **OGCR** Official Guidelines   X Assign placeholder X   ● Use Additional Character(s)

| Excludes 1 | | Excludes 2 | Includes   Use additional   Code first   Code also   Key words

● S68.616   Complete traumatic transphalangeal amputation of **right little** finger

● S68.617   Complete traumatic transphalangeal amputation of **left little** finger

● S68.618   Complete traumatic transphalangeal amputation of **other** finger
Complete traumatic transphalangeal amputation of specified finger with unspecified laterality

● S68.619   Complete traumatic transphalangeal amputation of **unspecified** finger

● S68.62   **Partial** traumatic transphalangeal amputation of other and unspecified finger

    ● S68.620   Partial traumatic transphalangeal amputation of **right index** finger

    ● S68.621   Partial traumatic transphalangeal amputation of **left index** finger

    ● S68.622   Partial traumatic transphalangeal amputation of **right middle** finger

    ● S68.623   Partial traumatic transphalangeal amputation of **left middle** finger

    ● S68.624   Partial traumatic transphalangeal amputation of **right ring** finger

    ● S68.625   Partial traumatic transphalangeal amputation of **left ring** finger

    ● S68.626   Partial traumatic transphalangeal amputation of **right little** finger

    ● S68.627   Partial traumatic transphalangeal amputation of **left little** finger

    ● S68.628   Partial traumatic transphalangeal amputation of **other** finger
Partial traumatic transphalangeal amputation of specified finger with unspecified laterality

    ● S68.629   Partial traumatic transphalangeal amputation of **unspecified** finger

● S68.7   Traumatic **transmetacarpal** amputation of **hand**

 ● S68.71   **Complete** traumatic transmetacarpal amputation of hand

    ● S68.711   Complete traumatic transmetacarpal amputation of **right** hand

    ● S68.712   Complete traumatic transmetacarpal amputation of **left** hand

    ● S68.719   Complete traumatic transmetacarpal amputation of **unspecified** hand

 ● S68.72   **Partial** traumatic transmetacarpal amputation of hand

    ● S68.721   Partial traumatic transmetacarpal amputation of **right** hand

    ● S68.722   Partial traumatic transmetacarpal amputation of **left** hand

    ● S68.729   Partial traumatic transmetacarpal amputation of **unspecified** hand

● S69   **Other and unspecified injuries of wrist, hand and finger(s)**
The appropriate 7th character is to be added to each code from category S69

A	initial encounter
D	subsequent encounter
S	sequela

 ● S69.8   **Other** specified injuries of wrist, hand and finger(s)

   X● S69.80   Other specified injuries of **unspecified** wrist, hand and finger(s)

   X● S69.81   Other specified injuries of **right** wrist, hand and finger(s)

   X● S69.82   Other specified injuries of **left** wrist, hand and finger(s)

● S69.9   **Unspecified** injury of wrist, hand and finger(s)

   X● S69.90   Unspecified injury of **unspecified** wrist, hand and finger(s)

   X● S69.91   Unspecified injury of **right** wrist, hand and finger(s)

   X● S69.92   Unspecified injury of **left** wrist, hand and finger(s)

INJURIES TO THE HIP AND THIGH (S70-S79)

Excludes2   burns and corrosions (T20-T32)
frostbite (T33-T34)
snake bite (T63.0-)
venomous insect bite or sting (T63.4-)

● S70   **Superficial injury of hip and thigh**
The appropriate 7th character is to be added to each code from category S70

A	initial encounter
D	subsequent encounter
S	sequela

● S70.0   **Contusion of hip**

   X● S70.00   Contusion of **unspecified** hip

   X● S70.01   Contusion of **right** hip

   X● S70.02   Contusion of **left** hip

● S70.1   **Contusion of thigh**

   X● S70.10   Contusion of **unspecified** thigh

   X● S70.11   Contusion of **right** thigh

   X● S70.12   Contusion of **left** thigh

● S70.2   **Other superficial injuries of hip**

 ● S70.21   **Abrasion** of hip

    ● S70.211   Abrasion, **right** hip

    ● S70.212   Abrasion, **left** hip

    ● S70.219   Abrasion, **unspecified** hip

 ● S70.22   **Blister (nonthermal) of hip**

    ● S70.221   Blister (nonthermal), **right** hip

    ● S70.222   Blister (nonthermal), **left** hip

    ● S70.229   Blister (nonthermal), **unspecified** hip

 ● S70.24   **External constriction** of hip

    ● S70.241   External constriction, **right** hip

    ● S70.242   External constriction, **left** hip

    ● S70.249   External constriction, **unspecified** hip

 ● S70.25   **Superficial foreign** body of hip
Splinter in the hip

    ● S70.251   Superficial foreign body, **right** hip

    ● S70.252   Superficial foreign body, **left** hip

    ● S70.259   Superficial foreign body, **unspecified** hip

 ● S70.26   **Insect bite** (nonvenomous) of hip

    ● S70.261   Insect bite (nonvenomous), **right** hip

    ● S70.262   Insect bite (nonvenomous), **left** hip

    ● S70.269   Insect bite (nonvenomous), **unspecified** hip

 ● S70.27   **Other superficial bite of hip**
Excludes1   open bite of hip (S71.05-)

    ● S70.271   Other superficial bite of hip, **right** hip

    ● S70.272   Other superficial bite of hip, **left** hip

    ● S70.279   Other superficial bite of hip, **unspecified** hip

● S70.3   **Other superficial injuries of thigh**

 ● S70.31   **Abrasion** of thigh

    ● S70.311   Abrasion, **right** thigh

    ● S70.312   Abrasion, **left** thigh

    ● S70.319   Abrasion, **unspecified** thigh

▶ New   ➠ Revised   ~~deleted~~ Deleted   **OGCR** Official Guidelines   X Assign placeholder X   ● Use Additional Character(s)

| Excludes 1 | Excludes 2 | Includes | Use additional | Code first | Code also | Key words |

- ● S70.32   **Blister** (nonthermal) of thigh
  - ● S70.321   Blister (nonthermal), **right** thigh
  - ● S70.322   Blister (nonthermal), **left** thigh
  - ● S70.329   Blister (nonthermal), **unspecified** thigh
- ● S70.34   **External constriction** of thigh
  - ● S70.341   External constriction, **right** thigh
  - ● S70.342   External constriction, **left** thigh
  - ● S70.349   External constriction, **unspecified** thigh
- ● S70.35   **Superficial foreign body** of thigh
  Splinter in the thigh
  - ● S70.351   Superficial foreign body, **right** thigh
  - ● S70.352   Superficial foreign body, **left** thigh
  - ● S70.359   Superficial foreign body, **unspecified** thigh
- ● S70.36   **Insect bite** (nonvenomous) of thigh
  - ● S70.361   Insect bite (nonvenomous), **right** thigh
  - ● S70.362   Insect bite (nonvenomous), **left** thigh
  - ● S70.369   Insect bite (nonvenomous), **unspecified** thigh
- ● S70.37   **Other superficial bite** of thigh
  | **Excludes1** | open bite of thigh (S71.15) |
  - ● S70.371   Other superficial bite of **right** thigh
  - ● S70.372   Other superficial bite of **left** thigh
  - ● S70.379   Other superficial bite of **unspecified** thigh
- ● S70.9   Unspecified superficial injury of hip and thigh
  - ● S70.91   **Unspecified** superficial injury of **hip**
    - ● S70.911   Unspecified superficial injury of **right** hip
    - ● S70.912   Unspecified superficial injury of **left** hip
    - ● S70.919   Unspecified superficial injury of **unspecified** hip
  - ● S70.92   Unspecified superficial injury of **thigh**
    - ● S70.921   Unspecified superficial injury of **right** thigh
    - ● S70.922   Unspecified superficial injury of **left** thigh
    - ● S70.929   Unspecified superficial injury of **unspecified** thigh

- ● S71   Open wound of hip and thigh
  Code also any associated wound infection
Excludes1	open fracture of hip and thigh (S72.-)
	traumatic amputation of hip and thigh (S78.-)
Excludes2	bite of venomous animal (T63.-)
	open wound of ankle, foot and toes (S91.-)
	open wound of knee and lower leg (S81.-)

  The appropriate 7th character is to be added to each code from category S71

A	initial encounter
D	subsequent encounter
S	sequela

  - ● S71.0   Open wound of **hip**
    - ● S71.00   **Unspecified** open wound of hip
      - ● S71.001   Unspecified open wound, **right** hip
      - ● S71.002   Unspecified open wound, **left** hip
      - ● S71.009   Unspecified open wound, **unspecified** hip
    - ● S71.01   **Laceration without foreign body** of hip
      - ● S71.011   Laceration without foreign body, **right** hip
      - ● S71.012   Laceration without foreign body, **left** hip
      - ● S71.019   Laceration without foreign body, **unspecified** hip

- ● S71.02   **Laceration with foreign body** of hip
  - ● S71.021   Laceration with foreign body, **right** hip
  - ● S71.022   Laceration with foreign body, **left** hip
  - ● S71.029   Laceration with foreign body, **unspecified** hip
- ● S71.03   **Puncture wound without foreign** body of hip
  - ● S71.031   Puncture wound without foreign body, **right** hip
  - ● S71.032   Puncture wound without foreign body, **left** hip
  - ● S71.039   Puncture wound without foreign body, **unspecified** hip
- ● S71.04   **Puncture wound with foreign body** of hip
  - ● S71.041   Puncture wound with foreign body, **right** hip
  - ● S71.042   Puncture wound with foreign body, **left** hip
  - ● S71.049   Puncture wound with foreign body, **unspecified** hip
- ● S71.05   **Open bite** of hip
  Bite of hip NOS
  | **Excludes1** | superficial bite of hip (S70.26, S70.27) |
  - ● S71.051   Open bite, **right** hip
  - ● S71.052   Open bite, **left** hip
  - ● S71.059   Open bite, **unspecified** hip
- ● S71.1   Open wound of **thigh**
  - ● S71.10   **Unspecified** open wound of thigh
    - ● S71.101   Unspecified open wound, **right** thigh
    - ● S71.102   Unspecified open wound, **left** thigh
    - ● S71.109   Unspecified open wound, **unspecified** thigh
  - ● S71.11   **Laceration without foreign body** of thigh
    - ● S71.111   Laceration without foreign body, **right** thigh
    - ● S71.112   Laceration without foreign body, **left** thigh
    - ● S71.119   Laceration without foreign body, **unspecified** thigh
  - ● S71.12   **Laceration with foreign body** of thigh
    - ● S71.121   Laceration with foreign body, **right** thigh
    - ● S71.122   Laceration with foreign body, **left** thigh
    - ● S71.129   Laceration with foreign body, **unspecified** thigh
  - ● S71.13   **Puncture wound without foreign** body of thigh
    - ● S71.131   Puncture wound without foreign body, **right** thigh
    - ● S71.132   Puncture wound without foreign body, **left** thigh
    - ● S71.139   Puncture wound without foreign body, **unspecified** thigh
  - ● S71.14   **Puncture wound with foreign body** of thigh
    - ● S71.141   Puncture wound with foreign body, **right** thigh
    - ● S71.142   Puncture wound with foreign body, **left** thigh
    - ● S71.149   Puncture wound with foreign body, **unspecified** thigh
  - ● S71.15   **Open bite** of thigh
    Bite of thigh NOS
    | **Excludes1** | superficial bite of thigh (S70.37-) |
    - ● S71.151   Open bite, **right** thigh
    - ● S71.152   Open bite, **left** thigh
    - ● S71.159   Open bite, **unspecified** thigh

▶ New   ⇒ Revised   ~~deleted~~ Deleted   **OGCR** Official Guidelines   X Assign placeholder X   ● Use Additional Character(s)

| Excludes 1 | Excludes 2 | Includes | Use additional | Code first | Code also | Key words |

● **S72   Fracture of femur**

     Note: A fracture not indicated as displaced or nondisplaced should be coded to displaced

        A fracture not indicated as open or closed should be coded to closed

        The open fracture designations are based on the Gustilo open fracture classification

    Excludes1   traumatic amputation of hip and thigh (S78.-)

    Excludes2   fracture of lower leg and ankle (S82.-)

                fracture of foot (S92.-)

     ⇥ periprosthetic fracture of prosthetic implant of hip (M97.0-)

     The appropriate 7th character is to be added to all codes from category S72

A	initial encounter for closed fracture
B	initial encounter for open fracture type I or II
	initial encounter for open fracture NOS
C	initial encounter for open fracture type IIIA, IIIB, or IIIC
D	subsequent encounter for closed fracture with routine healing
E	subsequent encounter for open fracture type I or II with routine healing
F	subsequent encounter for open fracture type IIIA, IIIB, or IIIC with routine healing
G	subsequent encounter for closed fracture with delayed healing
H	subsequent encounter for open fracture type I or II with delayed healing
J	subsequent encounter for open fracture type IIIA, IIIB, or IIIC with delayed healing
K	subsequent encounter for closed fracture with nonunion
M	subsequent encounter for open fracture type I or II with nonunion
N	subsequent encounter for open fracture type IIIA, IIIB, or IIIC with nonunion
P	subsequent encounter for closed fracture with malunion
Q	subsequent encounter for open fracture type I or II with malunion
R	subsequent encounter for open fracture type IIIA, IIIB, or IIIC with malunion
S	sequela

● **S72.0   Fracture of head and neck of femur**

    Excludes2   physeal fracture of upper end of femur (S79.0-)

   ● **S72.00   Fracture of unspecified part of neck of femur**
                  Fracture of hip NOS
                  Fracture of neck of femur NOS

     ● **S72.001   Fracture of unspecified part of neck of right femur**

     ● **S72.002   Fracture of unspecified part of neck of left femur**

     ● **S72.009   Fracture of unspecified part of neck of unspecified femur**

   ● **S72.01   Unspecified intracapsular fracture of femur**
                  Subcapital fracture of femur

     ● **S72.011   Unspecified intracapsular fracture of right femur**

     ● **S72.012   Unspecified intracapsular fracture of left femur**

     ● **S72.019   Unspecified intracapsular fracture of unspecified femur**

● **S72.02   Fracture of epiphysis (separation) (upper) of femur**
                Transepiphyseal fracture of femur
                Fracture and separation across growth plate

    Excludes1   capital femoral epiphyseal fracture (pediatric) of femur (S79.01-)
                Salter-Harris Type I physeal fracture of upper end of femur (S79.01-)

   ● **S72.021   Displaced fracture of epiphysis (separation) (upper) of right femur**

   ● **S72.022   Displaced fracture of epiphysis (separation) (upper) of left femur**

   ● **S72.023   Displaced fracture of epiphysis (separation) (upper) of unspecified femur**

   ● **S72.024   Nondisplaced fracture of epiphysis (separation) (upper) of right femur**

   ● **S72.025   Nondisplaced fracture of epiphysis (separation) (upper) of left femur**

   ● **S72.026   Nondisplaced fracture of epiphysis (separation) (upper) of unspecified femur**

● **S72.03   Midcervical fracture of femur**
                Transcervical fracture of femur NOS

   ● **S72.031   Displaced midcervical fracture of right femur**

   ● **S72.032   Displaced midcervical fracture of left femur**

   ● **S72.033   Displaced midcervical fracture of unspecified femur**

   ● **S72.034   Nondisplaced midcervical fracture of right femur**

   ● **S72.035   Nondisplaced midcervical fracture of left femur**

   ● **S72.036   Nondisplaced midcervical fracture of unspecified femur**

● **S72.04   Fracture of base of neck of femur**
                Cervicotrochanteric fracture of femur

   ● **S72.041   Displaced fracture of base of neck of right femur**

   ● **S72.042   Displaced fracture of base of neck of left femur**

   ● **S72.043   Displaced fracture of base of neck of unspecified femur**

   ● **S72.044   Nondisplaced fracture of base of neck of right femur**

   ● **S72.045   Nondisplaced fracture of base of neck of left femur**

   ● **S72.046   Nondisplaced fracture of base of neck of unspecified femur**

● **S72.05   Unspecified fracture of head of femur**
                Fracture of head of femur NOS

   ● **S72.051   Unspecified fracture of head of right femur**

   ● **S72.052   Unspecified fracture of head of left femur**

   ● **S72.059   Unspecified fracture of head of unspecified femur**

▶ New   ⇥ Revised   ~~deleted~~ Deleted   **OGCR** Official Guidelines   X Assign placeholder X   ● Use Additional Character(s)

Excludes 1   Excludes 2   Includes   Use additional   Code first   Code also   Key words

- S72.06   Articular fracture of head of femur
  - S72.061   Displaced articular fracture of head of right femur
  - S72.062   Displaced articular fracture of head of left femur
  - S72.063   Displaced articular fracture of head of unspecified femur
  - S72.064   Nondisplaced articular fracture of head of right femur
  - S72.065   Nondisplaced articular fracture of head of left femur
  - S72.066   Nondisplaced articular fracture of head of unspecified femur
- S72.09   Other fracture of head and neck of femur
  - S72.091   Other fracture of head and neck of right femur
  - S72.092   Other fracture of head and neck of left femur
  - S72.099   Other fracture of head and neck of unspecified femur
- S72.1   Pertrochanteric fracture
  Fracture extending close to, but not into, joint
  - S72.10   Unspecified trochanteric fracture of femur
    Fracture of trochanter NOS
    - S72.101   Unspecified trochanteric fracture of right femur
    - S72.102   Unspecified trochanteric fracture of left femur
    - S72.109   Unspecified trochanteric fracture of unspecified femur
  - S72.11   Fracture of greater trochanter of femur
    - S72.111   Displaced fracture of greater trochanter of right femur
    - S72.112   Displaced fracture of greater trochanter of left femur
    - S72.113   Displaced fracture of greater trochanter of unspecified femur
    - S72.114   Nondisplaced fracture of greater trochanter of right femur
    - S72.115   Nondisplaced fracture of greater trochanter of left femur
    - S72.116   Nondisplaced fracture of greater trochanter of unspecified femur
  - S72.12   Fracture of lesser trochanter of femur
    - S72.121   Displaced fracture of lesser trochanter of right femur
    - S72.122   Displaced fracture of lesser trochanter of left femur
    - S72.123   Displaced fracture of lesser trochanter of unspecified femur
    - S72.124   Nondisplaced fracture of lesser trochanter of right femur
    - S72.125   Nondisplaced fracture of lesser trochanter of left femur
    - S72.126   Nondisplaced fracture of lesser trochanter of unspecified femur
  - S72.13   Apophyseal fracture of femur
    Pertaining to articulations between articular facets of adjacent vertebrae

    Excludes1   chronic (nontraumatic) slipped upper femoral epiphysis (M93.0-)
    - S72.131   Displaced apophyseal fracture of right femur
    - S72.132   Displaced apophyseal fracture of left femur
    - S72.133   Displaced apophyseal fracture of unspecified femur

- S72.134   Nondisplaced apophyseal fracture of right femur
- S72.135   Nondisplaced apophyseal fracture of left femur
- S72.136   Nondisplaced apophyseal fracture of unspecified femur
- S72.14   Intertrochanteric fracture of femur
  - S72.141   Displaced intertrochanteric fracture of right femur
  - S72.142   Displaced intertrochanteric fracture of left femur
  - S72.143   Displaced intertrochanteric fracture of unspecified femur
  - S72.144   Nondisplaced intertrochanteric fracture of right femur
  - S72.145   Nondisplaced intertrochanteric fracture of left femur
  - S72.146   Nondisplaced intertrochanteric fracture of unspecified femur
- S72.2   Subtrochanteric fracture of femur
  Subtrochanteric: inferior to trochanter
  - X S72.21   Displaced subtrochanteric fracture of right femur
  - X S72.22   Displaced subtrochanteric fracture of left femur
  - X S72.23   Displaced subtrochanteric fracture of unspecified femur
  - X S72.24   Nondisplaced subtrochanteric fracture of right femur
  - X S72.25   Nondisplaced subtrochanteric fracture of left femur
  - X S72.26   Nondisplaced subtrochanteric fracture of unspecified femur
- S72.3   Fracture of shaft of femur
  - S72.30   Unspecified fracture of shaft of femur
    - S72.301   Unspecified fracture of shaft of right femur
    - S72.302   Unspecified fracture of shaft of left femur
    - S72.309   Unspecified fracture of shaft of unspecified femur
  - S72.32   Transverse fracture of shaft of femur
    - S72.321   Displaced transverse fracture of shaft of right femur
    - S72.322   Displaced transverse fracture of shaft of left femur
    - S72.323   Displaced transverse fracture of shaft of unspecified femur
    - S72.324   Nondisplaced transverse fracture of shaft of right femur
    - S72.325   Nondisplaced transverse fracture of shaft of left femur
    - S72.326   Nondisplaced transverse fracture of shaft of unspecified femur
  - S72.33   Oblique fracture of shaft of femur
    - S72.331   Displaced oblique fracture of shaft of right femur
    - S72.332   Displaced oblique fracture of shaft of left femur
    - S72.333   Displaced oblique fracture of shaft of unspecified femur
    - S72.334   Nondisplaced oblique fracture of shaft of right femur
    - S72.335   Nondisplaced oblique fracture of shaft of left femur
    - S72.336   Nondisplaced oblique fracture of shaft of unspecified femur

▶ New   ⇒ Revised   ~~deleted~~ Deleted   **OGCR** Official Guidelines   X Assign placeholder X   ● Use Additional Character(s)

| Excludes 1 | Excludes 2 | Includes | Use additional | Code first | Code also | Key words |

● S72.34 Spiral fracture of shaft of femur
   ● S72.341 Displaced spiral fracture of shaft of right femur
   ● S72.342 Displaced spiral fracture of shaft of left femur
   ● S72.343 Displaced spiral fracture of shaft of unspecified femur
   ● S72.344 Nondisplaced spiral fracture of shaft of right femur
   ● S72.345 Nondisplaced spiral fracture of shaft of left femur
   ● S72.346 Nondisplaced spiral fracture of shaft of unspecified femur

● S72.35 Comminuted fracture of shaft of femur
   ● S72.351 Displaced comminuted fracture of shaft of right femur
   ● S72.352 Displaced comminuted fracture of shaft of left femur
   ● S72.353 Displaced comminuted fracture of shaft of unspecified femur
   ● S72.354 Nondisplaced comminuted fracture of shaft of right femur
   ● S72.355 Nondisplaced comminuted fracture of shaft of left femur
   ● S72.356 Nondisplaced comminuted fracture of shaft of unspecified femur

● S72.36 Segmental fracture of shaft of femur
   ● S72.361 Displaced segmental fracture of shaft of right femur
   ● S72.362 Displaced segmental fracture of shaft of left femur
   ● S72.363 Displaced segmental fracture of shaft of unspecified femur
   ● S72.364 Nondisplaced segmental fracture of shaft of right femur
   ● S72.365 Nondisplaced segmental fracture of shaft of left femur
   ● S72.366 Nondisplaced segmental fracture of shaft of unspecified femur

● S72.39 Other fracture of shaft of femur
   ● S72.391 Other fracture of shaft of right femur
   ● S72.392 Other fracture of shaft of left femur
   ● S72.399 Other fracture of shaft of unspecified femur

● S72.4 Fracture of lower end of femur
   Fracture of distal end of femur
   Excludes2 fracture of shaft of femur (S72.3-)
          physeal fracture of lower end of femur (S79.1-)

● S72.40 Unspecified fracture of lower end of femur
   ● S72.401 Unspecified fracture of lower end of right femur
   ● S72.402 Unspecified fracture of lower end of left femur
   ● S72.409 Unspecified fracture of lower end of unspecified femur

● S72.41 Unspecified condyle fracture of lower end of femur
   Condyle fracture of femur NOS
   ● S72.411 Displaced unspecified condyle fracture of lower end of right femur
   ● S72.412 Displaced unspecified condyle fracture of lower end of left femur
   ● S72.413 Displaced unspecified condyle fracture of lower end of unspecified femur
   ● S72.414 Nondisplaced unspecified condyle fracture of lower end of right femur
   ● S72.415 Nondisplaced unspecified condyle fracture of lower end of left femur
   ● S72.416 Nondisplaced unspecified condyle fracture of lower end of unspecified femur

● S72.42 Fracture of lateral condyle of femur
   ● S72.421 Displaced fracture of lateral condyle of right femur
   ● S72.422 Displaced fracture of lateral condyle of left femur
   ● S72.423 Displaced fracture of lateral condyle of unspecified femur
   ● S72.424 Nondisplaced fracture of lateral condyle of right femur
   ● S72.425 Nondisplaced fracture of lateral condyle of left femur
   ● S72.426 Nondisplaced fracture of lateral condyle of unspecified femur

● S72.43 Fracture of medial condyle of femur
   ● S72.431 Displaced fracture of medial condyle of right femur
   ● S72.432 Displaced fracture of medial condyle of left femur
   ● S72.433 Displaced fracture of medial condyle of unspecified femur
   ● S72.434 Nondisplaced fracture of medial condyle of right femur
   ● S72.435 Nondisplaced fracture of medial condyle of left femur
   ● S72.436 Nondisplaced fracture of medial condyle of unspecified femur

● S72.44 Fracture of lower epiphysis (separation) of femur
   Excludes1 Salter-Harris Type I physeal fracture of lower end of femur (S79.11-)
   ● S72.441 Displaced fracture of lower epiphysis (separation) of right femur
   ● S72.442 Displaced fracture of lower epiphysis (separation) of left femur
   ● S72.443 Displaced fracture of lower epiphysis (separation) of unspecified femur
   ● S72.444 Nondisplaced fracture of lower epiphysis (separation) of right femur
   ● S72.445 Nondisplaced fracture of lower epiphysis (separation) of left femur
   ● S72.446 Nondisplaced fracture of lower epiphysis (separation) of unspecified femur

CHAPTER 19 (S00-T88)

● **S72.45** **Supracondylar fracture without intracondylar extension of lower end of femur**
    Supracondylar fracture of lower end of femur NOS

> **Excludes1**   supracondylar fracture with intracondylar extension of lower end of femur (S72.46-)

  ● **S72.451** **Displaced** supracondylar fracture without intracondylar extension of lower end of **right** femur
  ● **S72.452** **Displaced** supracondylar fracture without intracondylar extension of lower end of **left** femur
  ● **S72.453** **Displaced** supracondylar fracture without intracondylar extension of lower end of **unspecified** femur
  ● **S72.454** **Nondisplaced** supracondylar fracture without intracondylar extension of lower end of **right** femur
  ● **S72.455** **Nondisplaced** supracondylar fracture without intracondylar extension of lower end of **left** femur
  ● **S72.456** **Nondisplaced** supracondylar fracture without intracondylar extension of lower end of **unspecified** femur

● **S72.46** **Supracondylar fracture with intracondylar extension of lower end of femur**

> **Excludes1**   supracondylar fracture without intracondylar extension of lower end of femur (S72.45-)

  ● **S72.461** **Displaced** supracondylar fracture with intracondylar extension of lower end of **right** femur
  ● **S72.462** **Displaced** supracondylar fracture with intracondylar extension of lower end of **left** femur
  ● **S72.463** **Displaced** supracondylar fracture with intracondylar extension of lower end of **unspecified** femur
  ● **S72.464** **Nondisplaced** supracondylar fracture with intracondylar extension of lower end of **right** femur
  ● **S72.465** **Nondisplaced** supracondylar fracture with intracondylar extension of lower end of **left** femur
  ● **S72.466** **Nondisplaced** supracondylar fracture with intracondylar extension of lower end of **unspecified** femur

● **S72.47** **Torus fracture of lower end of femur**
    The appropriate 7th character is to be added to all codes in subcategory S72.47

A	initial encounter for closed fracture
D	subsequent encounter for fracture with routine healing
G	subsequent encounter for fracture with delayed healing
K	subsequent encounter for fracture with nonunion
P	subsequent encounter for fracture with malunion
S	sequela

  ● **S72.471** **Torus fracture of lower end of right femur**
  ● **S72.472** **Torus fracture of lower end of left femur**
  ● **S72.479** **Torus fracture of lower end of unspecified femur**

● **S72.49** **Other fracture of lower end of femur**
  ● **S72.491** **Other fracture of lower end of right femur**
  ● **S72.492** **Other fracture of lower end of left femur**
  ● **S72.499** **Other fracture of lower end of unspecified femur**

● **S72.8** **Other fracture of femur**
  ● **S72.8X** **Other fracture of femur**
    ● **S72.8X1** **Other fracture of right femur**
    ● **S72.8X2** **Other fracture of left femur**
    ● **S72.8X9** **Other fracture of unspecified femur**

● **S72.9** **Unspecified fracture of femur**
    Fracture of thigh NOS
    Fracture of upper leg NOS

> **Excludes1**   fracture of hip NOS (S72.00-, S72.01-)

  X ● **S72.90** **Unspecified fracture of unspecified femur**
  X ● **S72.91** **Unspecified fracture of right femur**
  X ● **S72.92** **Unspecified fracture of left femur**

● **S73** **Dislocation and sprain of joint and ligaments of hip**

> **Includes**   avulsion of joint or ligament of hip
> laceration of cartilage, joint or ligament of hip
> sprain of cartilage, joint or ligament of hip
> traumatic hemarthrosis of joint or ligament of hip
> traumatic rupture of joint or ligament of hip
> traumatic subluxation of joint or ligament of hip
> traumatic tear of joint or ligament of hip

Code also any associated open wound

> **Excludes2**   strain of muscle, fascia and tendon of hip and thigh (S76.-)

The appropriate 7th character is to be added to each code from category S73

A	initial encounter
D	subsequent encounter
S	sequela

● **S73.0** **Subluxation and dislocation of hip**
    Out of position

> **Excludes2**   dislocation and subluxation of hip prosthesis (T84.020, T84.021)

  ● **S73.00** **Unspecified subluxation and dislocation of hip**
    Dislocation of hip NOS
    Subluxation of hip NOS
    ● **S73.001** **Unspecified subluxation of right hip**
    ● **S73.002** **Unspecified subluxation of left hip**
    ● **S73.003** **Unspecified subluxation of unspecified hip**
    ● **S73.004** **Unspecified dislocation of right hip**
    ● **S73.005** **Unspecified dislocation of left hip**
    ● **S73.006** **Unspecified dislocation of unspecified hip**

  ● **S73.01** **Posterior subluxation and dislocation of hip**
    ● **S73.011** **Posterior subluxation of right hip**
    ● **S73.012** **Posterior subluxation of left hip**
    ● **S73.013** **Posterior subluxation of unspecified hip**
    ● **S73.014** **Posterior dislocation of right hip**
    ● **S73.015** **Posterior dislocation of left hip**
    ● **S73.016** **Posterior dislocation of unspecified hip**

▶ New   ➡ Revised   ~~deleted~~ Deleted   **OGCR** Official Guidelines   X Assign placeholder X   ● Use Additional Character(s)

Excludes 1   Excludes 2   Includes   Use additional   Code first   Code also   Key words

● S73.02   Obturator subluxation and dislocation of hip
   ● S73.021   Obturator subluxation of right hip
   ● S73.022   Obturator subluxation of left hip
   ● S73.023   Obturator subluxation of unspecified hip
   ● S73.024   Obturator dislocation of right hip
   ● S73.025   Obturator dislocation of left hip
   ● S73.026   Obturator dislocation of unspecified hip
⇒● S73.03   Other anterior subluxation and dislocation of hip
   ● S73.031   Other anterior subluxation of right hip
   ● S73.032   Other anterior subluxation of left hip
   ● S73.033   Other anterior subluxation of unspecified hip
   ● S73.034   Other anterior dislocation of right hip
   ● S73.035   Other anterior dislocation of left hip
   ● S73.036   Other anterior dislocation of unspecified hip
⇒● S73.04   Central subluxation and dislocation of hip
   ● S73.041   Central subluxation of right hip
   ● S73.042   Central subluxation of left hip
   ● S73.043   Central subluxation of unspecified hip
   ● S73.044   Central dislocation of right hip
   ● S73.045   Central dislocation of left hip
   ● S73.046   Central dislocation of unspecified hip
● S73.1   Sprain of hip
  ● S73.10   Unspecified sprain of hip
   ● S73.101   Unspecified sprain of right hip
   ● S73.102   Unspecified sprain of left hip
   ● S73.109   Unspecified sprain of unspecified hip
  ● S73.11   Iliofemoral ligament sprain of hip
   ● S73.111   Iliofemoral ligament sprain of right hip
   ● S73.112   Iliofemoral ligament sprain of left hip
   ● S73.119   Iliofemoral ligament sprain of unspecified hip
  ● S73.12   Ischiocapsular (ligament) sprain of hip
   ● S73.121   Ischiocapsular ligament sprain of right hip
   ● S73.122   Ischiocapsular ligament sprain of left hip
   ● S73.129   Ischiocapsular ligament sprain of unspecified hip
  ● S73.19   Other sprain of hip
   ● S73.191   Other sprain of right hip
   ● S73.192   Other sprain of left hip
   ● S73.199   Other sprain of unspecified hip

● S74   Injury of nerves at hip and thigh level

   Code also any associated open wound (S71.-)

   Excludes2   injury of nerves at ankle and foot level (S94.-)
                  injury of nerves at lower leg level (S84.-)

   The appropriate 7th character is to be added to each code from category S74

A	initial encounter
D	subsequent encounter
S	sequela

● S74.0   Injury of sciatic nerve at hip and thigh level
  X● S74.00   Injury of sciatic nerve at hip and thigh level, unspecified leg
  X● S74.01   Injury of sciatic nerve at hip and thigh level, right leg
  X● S74.02   Injury of sciatic nerve at hip and thigh level, left leg

● S74.1   Injury of femoral nerve at hip and thigh level
  X● S74.10   Injury of femoral nerve at hip and thigh level, unspecified leg
  X● S74.11   Injury of femoral nerve at hip and thigh level, right leg
  X● S74.12   Injury of femoral nerve at hip and thigh level, left leg
● S74.2   Injury of cutaneous sensory nerve at hip and thigh level
  X● S74.20   Injury of cutaneous sensory nerve at hip and thigh level, unspecified leg
  X● S74.21   Injury of cutaneous sensory nerve at hip and high level, right leg
  X● S74.22   Injury of cutaneous sensory nerve at hip and thigh level, left leg
● S74.8   Injury of other nerves at hip and thigh level
  ● S74.8X   Injury of other nerves at hip and thigh level
   ● S74.8X1   Injury of other nerves at hip and thigh level, right leg
   ● S74.8X2   Injury of other nerves at hip and thigh level, left leg
   ● S74.8X9   Injury of other nerves at hip and thigh level, unspecified leg
● S74.9   Injury of unspecified nerve at hip and thigh level
  X● S74.90   Injury of unspecified nerve at hip and thigh level, unspecified leg
  X● S74.91   Injury of unspecified nerve at hip and thigh level, right leg
  X● S74.92   Injury of unspecified nerve at hip and thigh level, left leg

● S75   Injury of blood vessels at hip and thigh level

   Code also any associated open wound (S71.-)

   Excludes2   injury of blood vessels at lower leg level (S85.-)
                  injury of popliteal artery (S85.0)

   The appropriate 7th character is to be added to each code from category S75

A	initial encounter
D	subsequent encounter
S	sequela

● S75.0   Injury of femoral artery
  ● S75.00   Unspecified injury of femoral artery
   ● S75.001   Unspecified injury of femoral artery, right leg
   ● S75.002   Unspecified injury of femoral artery, left leg
   ● S75.009   Unspecified injury of femoral artery, unspecified leg
  ● S75.01   Minor laceration of femoral artery
    Incomplete transection of femoral artery
    Laceration of femoral artery NOS
    Superficial laceration of femoral artery
   ● S75.011   Minor laceration of femoral artery, right leg
   ● S75.012   Minor laceration of femoral artery, left leg
   ● S75.019   Minor laceration of femoral artery, unspecified leg
  ● S75.02   Major laceration of femoral artery
    Complete transection of femoral artery
    Traumatic rupture of femoral artery
   ● S75.021   Major laceration of femoral artery, right leg
   ● S75.022   Major laceration of femoral artery, left leg
   ● S75.029   Major laceration of femoral artery, unspecified leg

- S75.09 Other specified injury of femoral artery
  - S75.091 Other specified injury of femoral artery, right leg
  - S75.092 Other specified injury of femoral artery, left leg
  - S75.099 Other specified injury of femoral artery, unspecified leg
- S75.1 Injury of femoral vein at hip and thigh level
  - S75.10 Unspecified injury of femoral vein at hip and thigh level
    - S75.101 Unspecified injury of femoral vein at hip and thigh level, right leg
    - S75.102 Unspecified injury of femoral vein at hip and thigh level, left leg
    - S75.109 Unspecified injury of femoral vein at hip and thigh level, unspecified leg
  - S75.11 Minor laceration of femoral vein at hip and thigh level
    Incomplete transection of femoral vein at hip and thigh level
    Laceration of femoral vein at hip and thigh level NOS
    Superficial laceration of femoral vein at hip and thigh level
    - S75.111 Minor laceration of femoral vein at hip and thigh level, right leg
    - S75.112 Minor laceration of femoral vein at hip and thigh level, left leg
    - S75.119 Minor laceration of femoral vein at hip and thigh level, unspecified leg
  - S75.12 Major laceration of femoral vein at hip and thigh level
    Complete transection of femoral vein at hip and thigh level
    Traumatic rupture of femoral vein at hip and thigh level
    - S75.121 Major laceration of femoral vein at hip and thigh level, right leg
    - S75.122 Major laceration of femoral vein at hip and thigh level, left leg
    - S75.129 Major laceration of femoral vein at hip and thigh level, unspecified leg
  - S75.19 Other specified injury of femoral vein at hip and thigh level
    - S75.191 Other specified injury of femoral vein at hip and thigh level, right leg
    - S75.192 Other specified injury of femoral vein at hip and thigh level, left leg
    - S75.199 Other specified injury of femoral vein at hip and thigh level, unspecified leg
- S75.2 Injury of greater saphenous vein at hip and thigh level
  - **Excludes1** greater saphenous vein NOS (S85.3)
  - S75.20 Unspecified injury of greater saphenous vein at hip and thigh level
    - S75.201 Unspecified injury of greater saphenous vein at hip and thigh level, right leg
    - S75.202 Unspecified injury of greater saphenous vein at hip and thigh level, left leg
    - S75.209 Unspecified injury of greater saphenous vein at hip and thigh level, unspecified leg

- S75.21 Minor laceration of greater saphenous vein at hip and thigh level
  Incomplete transection of greater saphenous vein at hip and thigh level
  Laceration of greater saphenous vein at hip and thigh level NOS
  Superficial laceration of greater saphenous vein at hip and thigh level
  - S75.211 Minor laceration of greater saphenous vein at hip and thigh level, right leg
  - S75.212 Minor laceration of greater saphenous vein at hip and thigh level, left leg
  - S75.219 Minor laceration of greater saphenous vein at hip and thigh level, unspecified leg
- S75.22 Major laceration of greater saphenous vein at hip and thigh level
  Complete transection of greater saphenous vein at hip and thigh level
  Traumatic rupture of greater saphenous vein at hip and thigh level
  - S75.221 Major laceration of greater saphenous vein at hip and thigh level, right leg
  - S75.222 Major laceration of greater saphenous vein at hip and thigh level, left leg
  - S75.229 Major laceration of greater saphenous vein at hip and thigh level, unspecified leg
- S75.29 Other specified injury of greater saphenous vein at hip and thigh level
  - S75.291 Other specified injury of greater saphenous vein at hip and thigh level, right leg
  - S75.292 Other specified injury of greater saphenous vein at hip and thigh level, left leg
  - S75.299 Other specified injury of greater saphenous vein at hip and thigh level, unspecified leg
- S75.8 Injury of other blood vessels at hip and thigh level
  - S75.80 Unspecified injury of other blood vessels at hip and thigh level
    - S75.801 Unspecified injury of other blood vessels at hip and thigh level, right leg
    - S75.802 Unspecified injury of other blood vessels at hip and thigh level, left leg
    - S75.809 Unspecified injury of other blood vessels at hip and thigh level, unspecified leg
  - S75.81 Laceration of other blood vessels at hip and thigh level
    - S75.811 Laceration of other blood vessels at hip and thigh level, right leg
    - S75.812 Laceration of other blood vessels at hip and thigh level, left leg
    - S75.819 Laceration of other blood vessels at hip and thigh level, unspecified leg
  - S75.89 Other specified injury of other blood vessels at hip and thigh level
    - S75.891 Other specified injury of other blood vessels at hip and thigh level, right leg
    - S75.892 Other specified injury of other blood vessels at hip and thigh level, left leg
    - S75.899 Other specified injury of other blood vessels at hip and thigh level, unspecified leg

▶ New ⟹ Revised ~~deleted~~ Deleted **OGCR** Official Guidelines X Assign placeholder X ● Use Additional Character(s)

Excludes 1 Excludes 2 Includes Use additional Code first Code also Key words

- S75.9   Injury of unspecified blood vessel at hip and thigh level
  - S75.90   Unspecified injury of unspecified blood vessel at hip and thigh level
    - S75.901   Unspecified injury of unspecified blood vessel at hip and thigh level, right leg
    - S75.902   Unspecified injury of unspecified blood vessel at hip and thigh level, left leg
    - S75.909   Unspecified injury of unspecified blood vessel at hip and thigh level, unspecified leg
  - S75.91   Laceration of unspecified blood vessel at hip and thigh level
    - S75.911   Laceration of unspecified blood vessel at hip and thigh level, right leg
    - S75.912   Laceration of unspecified blood vessel at hip and thigh level, left leg
    - S75.919   Laceration of unspecified blood vessel at hip and thigh level, unspecified leg
  - S75.99   Other specified injury of unspecified blood vessel at hip and thigh level
    - S75.991   Other specified injury of unspecified blood vessel at hip and thigh level, right leg
    - S75.992   Other specified injury of unspecified blood vessel at hip and thigh level, left leg
    - S75.999   Other specified injury of unspecified blood vessel at hip and thigh level, unspecified leg

- S76   Injury of muscle, fascia and tendon at hip and thigh level

  Code also any associated open wound (S71.-)

  > **Excludes2**   injury of muscle, fascia and tendon at lower leg level (S86)
  >
  > sprain of joint and ligament of hip (S73.1)

  The appropriate 7th character is to be added to each code from category S76

A	initial encounter
D	subsequent encounter
S	sequela

  - S76.0   Injury of muscle, fascia and tendon of hip
    - S76.00   Unspecified injury of muscle, fascia and tendon of hip
      - S76.001   Unspecified injury of muscle, fascia and tendon of right hip
      - S76.002   Unspecified injury of muscle, fascia and tendon of left hip
      - S76.009   Unspecified injury of muscle, fascia and tendon of unspecified hip
    - S76.01   Strain of muscle, fascia and tendon of hip
      - S76.011   Strain of muscle, fascia and tendon of right hip
      - S76.012   Strain of muscle, fascia and tendon of left hip
      - S76.019   Strain of muscle, fascia and tendon of unspecified hip
    - S76.02   Laceration of muscle, fascia and tendon of hip
      - S76.021   Laceration of muscle, fascia and tendon of right hip
      - S76.022   Laceration of muscle, fascia and tendon of left hip
      - S76.029   Laceration of muscle, fascia and tendon of unspecified hip

  - S76.09   Other specified injury of muscle, fascia and tendon of hip
    - S76.091   Other specified injury of muscle, fascia and tendon of right hip
    - S76.092   Other specified injury of muscle, fascia and tendon of left hip
    - S76.099   Other specified injury of muscle, fascia and tendon of unspecified hip
  - S76.1   Injury of quadriceps muscle, fascia and tendon

    Injury of patellar ligament (tendon)
    - S76.10   Unspecified injury of quadriceps muscle, fascia and tendon
      - S76.101   Unspecified injury of right quadriceps muscle, fascia and tendon
      - S76.102   Unspecified injury of left quadriceps muscle, fascia and tendon
      - S76.109   Unspecified injury of unspecified quadriceps muscle, fascia and tendon
    - S76.11   Strain of quadriceps muscle, fascia and tendon
      - S76.111   Strain of right quadriceps muscle, fascia and tendon
      - S76.112   Strain of left quadriceps muscle, fascia and tendon
      - S76.119   Strain of unspecified quadriceps muscle, fascia and tendon
    - S76.12   Laceration of quadriceps muscle, fascia and tendon
      - S76.121   Laceration of right quadriceps muscle, fascia and tendon
      - S76.122   Laceration of left quadriceps muscle, fascia and tendon
      - S76.129   Laceration of unspecified quadriceps muscle, fascia and tendon
    - S76.19   Other specified injury of quadriceps muscle, fascia and tendon
      - S76.191   Other specified injury of right quadriceps muscle, fascia and tendon
      - S76.192   Other specified injury of left quadriceps muscle, fascia and tendon
      - S76.199   Other specified injury of unspecified quadriceps muscle, fascia and tendon
  - S76.2   Injury of adductor muscle, fascia and tendon of thigh
    - S76.20   Unspecified injury of adductor muscle, fascia and tendon of thigh
      - S76.201   Unspecified injury of adductor muscle, fascia and tendon of right thigh
      - S76.202   Unspecified injury of adductor muscle, fascia and tendon of left thigh
      - S76.209   Unspecified injury of adductor muscle, fascia and tendon of unspecified thigh
    - S76.21   Strain of adductor muscle, fascia and tendon of thigh
      - S76.211   Strain of adductor muscle, fascia and tendon of right thigh
      - S76.212   Strain of adductor muscle, fascia and tendon of left thigh
      - S76.219   Strain of adductor muscle, fascia and tendon of unspecified thigh
    - S76.22   Laceration of adductor muscle, fascia and tendon of thigh
      - S76.221   Laceration of adductor muscle, fascia and tendon of right thigh
      - S76.222   Laceration of adductor muscle, fascia and tendon of left thigh
      - S76.229   Laceration of adductor muscle, fascia and tendon of unspecified thigh

● **S76.29**   **Other** injury of adductor muscle, fascia and tendon of thigh
- ● **S76.291**   Other injury of adductor muscle, fascia and tendon of **right** thigh
- ● **S76.292**   Other injury of adductor muscle, fascia and tendon of **left** thigh
- ● **S76.299**   Other injury of adductor muscle, fascia and tendon of **unspecified** thigh

● **S76.3**   Injury of muscle, fascia and tendon of the **posterior muscle group** at thigh level
- ● **S76.30**   **Unspecified** injury of muscle, fascia and tendon of the posterior muscle group at thigh level
  - ● **S76.301**   Unspecified injury of muscle, fascia and tendon of the posterior muscle group at thigh level, **right** thigh
  - ● **S76.302**   Unspecified injury of muscle, fascia and tendon of the posterior muscle group at thigh level, **left** thigh
  - ● **S76.309**   Unspecified injury of muscle, fascia and tendon of the posterior muscle group at thigh level, **unspecified** thigh
- ● **S76.31**   **Strain** of muscle, fascia and tendon of the posterior muscle group at thigh level
  - ● **S76.311**   Strain of muscle, fascia and tendon of the posterior muscle group at thigh level, **right** thigh
  - ● **S76.312**   Strain of muscle, fascia and tendon of the posterior muscle group at thigh level, **left** thigh
  - ● **S76.319**   Strain of muscle, fascia and tendon of the posterior muscle group at thigh level, **unspecified** thigh
- ● **S76.32**   **Laceration** of muscle, fascia and tendon of the posterior muscle group at thigh level
  - ● **S76.321**   Laceration of muscle, fascia and tendon of the posterior muscle group at thigh level, **right** thigh
  - ● **S76.322**   Laceration of muscle, fascia and tendon of the posterior muscle group at thigh level, **left** thigh
  - ● **S76.329**   Laceration of muscle, fascia and tendon of the posterior muscle group at thigh level, **unspecified** thigh
- ● **S76.39**   **Other** specified injury of muscle, fascia and tendon of the posterior muscle group at thigh level
  - ● **S76.391**   Other specified injury of muscle, fascia and tendon of the posterior muscle group at thigh level, **right** thigh
  - ● **S76.392**   Other specified injury of muscle, fascia and tendon of the posterior muscle group at thigh level, **left** thigh
  - ● **S76.399**   Other specified injury of muscle, fascia and tendon of the posterior muscle group at thigh level, **unspecified** thigh

● **S76.8**   Injury of **other specified muscles**, fascia and tendons at thigh level
- ● **S76.80**   **Unspecified** injury of other specified muscles, fascia and tendons at thigh level
  - ● **S76.801**   Unspecified injury of other specified muscles, fascia and tendons at thigh level, **right** thigh
  - ● **S76.802**   Unspecified injury of other specified muscles, fascia and tendons at thigh level, **left** thigh
  - ● **S76.809**   Unspecified injury of other specified muscles, fascia and tendons at thigh level, **unspecified** thigh

● **S76.81**   **Strain** of other specified specified muscles, fascia and tendons at thigh level
- ● **S76.811**   Strain of other specified muscles, fascia and tendons at thigh level, **right** thigh
- ● **S76.812**   Strain of other specified muscles, fascia and tendons at thigh level, **left** thigh
- ● **S76.819**   Strain of other specified muscles, fascia and tendons at thigh level, **unspecified** thigh

● **S76.82**   **Laceration** of other specified muscles, fascia and tendons at thigh level
- ● **S76.821**   Laceration of other specified muscles, fascia and tendons at thigh level, **right** thigh
- ● **S76.822**   Laceration of other specified muscles, fascia and tendons at thigh level, **left** thigh
- ● **S76.829**   Laceration of other specified muscles, fascia and tendons at thigh level, **unspecified** thigh

● **S76.89**   **Other** injury of other specified muscles, fascia and tendons at thigh level
- ● **S76.891**   Other injury of other specified muscles, fascia and tendons at thigh level, **right** thigh
- ● **S76.892**   Other injury of other specified muscles, fascia and tendons at thigh level, **left** thigh
- ● **S76.899**   Other injury of other specified muscles, fascia and tendons at thigh level, **unspecified** thigh

● **S76.9**   Injury of **unspecified muscles**, fascia and tendons at thigh level
- ● **S76.90**   **Unspecified** injury of unspecified muscles, fascia and tendons at thigh level
  - ● **S76.901**   Unspecified injury of unspecified muscles, fascia and tendons at thigh level, **right** thigh
  - ● **S76.902**   Unspecified injury of unspecified muscles, fascia and tendons at thigh level, **left** thigh
  - ● **S76.909**   Unspecified injury of unspecified muscles, fascia and tendons at thigh level, **unspecified** thigh
- ● **S76.91**   **Strain** of unspecified muscles, fascia and tendons at thigh level
  - ● **S76.911**   Strain of unspecified muscles, fascia and tendons at thigh level, **right** thigh
  - ● **S76.912**   Strain of unspecified muscles, fascia and tendons at thigh level, **left** thigh
  - ● **S76.919**   Strain of unspecified muscles fascia and tendons at thigh level, **unspecified** thigh
- ● **S76.92**   **Laceration** of unspecified muscles, fascia and tendons at thigh level
  - ● **S76.921**   Laceration of unspecified muscles, fascia and tendons at thigh level, **right** thigh
  - ● **S76.922**   Laceration of unspecified muscles, fascia and tendons at thigh level, **left** thigh
  - ● **S76.929**   Laceration of unspecified muscles, fascia and tendons at thigh level, **unspecified** thigh

▶ New   ⇒ Revised   ~~deleted~~ Deleted   **OGCR** Official Guidelines   X Assign placeholder X   ● Use Additional Character(s)

Excludes 1   Excludes 2   Includes   Use additional   Code first   Code also   Key words

- S76.99 **Other** specified injury of unspecified muscles, fascia and tendons at thigh level
  - S76.991 Other specified injury of unspecified muscles, fascia and tendons at thigh level, **right** thigh
  - S76.992 Other specified injury of unspecified muscles, fascia and tendons at thigh level, **left** thigh
  - S76.999 Other specified injury of unspecified muscles, fascia and tendons at thigh level, **unspecified** thigh

- S77 **Crushing injury** of hip and thigh

  Use additional code(s) for all associated injuries

  Excludes2   crushing injury of ankle and foot (S97.-)
                crushing injury of lower leg (S87.-)

  The appropriate 7th character is to be added to each code from category S77

  > A   initial encounter
  > D   subsequent encounter
  > S   sequela

  - S77.0   Crushing injury of **hip**
    - X● S77.00   Crushing injury of **unspecified** hip
    - X● S77.01   Crushing injury of **right** hip
    - X● S77.02   Crushing injury of **left** hip
  - S77.1   Crushing injury of **thigh**
    - X● S77.10   Crushing injury of **unspecified** thigh
    - X● S77.11   Crushing injury of **right** thigh
    - X● S77.12   Crushing injury of **left** thigh
  - S77.2   Crushing injury of **hip with thigh**
    - X● S77.20   Crushing injury of **unspecified** hip with thigh
    - X● S77.21   Crushing injury of **right** hip with thigh
    - X● S77.22   Crushing injury of **left** hip with thigh

- S78 **Traumatic amputation** of hip and thigh

  An amputation not identified as partial or complete should be coded to complete

  Excludes1   traumatic amputation of knee (S88.0-)

  The appropriate 7th character is to be added to each code from category S78

  > A   initial encounter
  > D   subsequent encounter
  > S   sequela

  - S78.0   Traumatic amputation at **hip joint**
    - S78.01   **Complete** traumatic amputation at hip joint
      - S78.011   Complete traumatic amputation at **right** hip joint
      - S78.012   Complete traumatic amputation at **left** hip joint
      - S78.019   Complete traumatic amputation at **unspecified** hip joint
    - S78.02   **Partial** traumatic amputation at hip joint
      - S78.021   Partial traumatic amputation at **right** hip joint
      - S78.022   Partial traumatic amputation at **left** hip joint
      - S78.029   Partial traumatic amputation at **unspecified** hip joint

- S78.1   Traumatic amputation at level **between hip and knee**
  - **Excludes1**   traumatic amputation of knee (S88.0-)
  - S78.11   **Complete** traumatic amputation at level between hip and knee
    - S78.111   Complete traumatic amputation at level between **right** hip and knee
    - S78.112   Complete traumatic amputation at level between **left** hip and knee
    - S78.119   Complete traumatic amputation at level between **unspecified** hip and knee
  - S78.12   **Partial** traumatic amputation at level between hip and knee
    - S78.121   Partial traumatic amputation at level between **right** hip and knee
    - S78.122   Partial traumatic amputation at level between **left** hip and knee
    - S78.129   Partial traumatic amputation at level between **unspecified** hip and knee
- S78.9   Traumatic amputation of hip and thigh, **level unspecified**
  - S78.91   **Complete** traumatic amputation of hip and thigh, level unspecified
    - S78.911   Complete traumatic amputation of **right** hip and thigh, level unspecified
    - S78.912   Complete traumatic amputation of **left** hip and thigh, level unspecified
    - S78.919   Complete traumatic amputation of **unspecified** hip and thigh, level unspecified
  - S78.92   **Partial** traumatic amputation of hip and thigh, level unspecified
    - S78.921   Partial traumatic amputation of **right** hip and thigh, level unspecified
    - S78.922   Partial traumatic amputation of **left** hip and thigh, level unspecified
    - S78.929   Partial traumatic amputation of **unspecified** hip and thigh, level unspecified

- S79   Other and unspecified injuries of hip and thigh

  Note: A fracture not indicated as open or closed should be coded to closed

  The appropriate 7th character is to be added to each code from subcategories S79.0 and S79.1

  > A   initial encounter for closed fracture
  > D   subsequent encounter for fracture with routine healing
  > G   subsequent encounter for fracture with delayed healing
  > K   subsequent encounter for fracture with nonunion
  > P   subsequent encounter for fracture with malunion
  > S   sequela

  - S79.0   Physeal fracture of **upper end** of femur
    - **Excludes1**   apophyseal fracture of upper end of femur (S72.13-)
    -                nontraumatic slipped upper femoral epiphysis (M93.0-)
    - S79.00   **Unspecified** physeal fracture of upper end of femur
      - S79.001   Unspecified physeal fracture of upper end of **right** femur
      - S79.002   Unspecified physeal fracture of upper end of **left** femur
      - S79.009   Unspecified physeal fracture of upper end of **unspecified** femur

Item 19–5 SALTER-HARRIS TYPE 1: epiphysis is completely separated from end of bone, or metaphysic growth plate remains attached to epiphysis

SALTER-HARRIS TYPE 2: epiphysis and growth plate are partially separated from metaphysis, which is cracked—most common type

SALTER-HARRIS TYPE 3: fracture occurring through epiphysis and separates part of epiphysis and growth plate from metaphysis fracture, usually at distal end of tibia

SALTER-HARRIS TYPE 4: fracture runs through epiphysis, across growth plate, into metaphysic, surgery is required to restore joint surface to normal and align growth plate

● **S79.01 Salter-Harris Type I** physeal fracture of upper end of femur
     Acute on chronic slipped capital femoral epiphysis (traumatic)
     Acute slipped capital femoral epiphysis (traumatic)
     Capital femoral epiphyseal fracture
     Excludes1 chronic slipped upper femoral epiphysis (nontraumatic) (M93.02-)
   ● **S79.011 Salter-Harris Type I** physeal fracture of upper end of **right** femur
   ● **S79.012 Salter-Harris Type I** physeal fracture of upper end of **left** femur
   ● **S79.019 Salter-Harris Type I** physeal fracture of upper end of **unspecified** femur
● **S79.09 Other** physeal fracture of upper end of femur
   ● **S79.091 Other** physeal fracture of upper end of **right** femur
   ● **S79.092 Other** physeal fracture of upper end of **left** femur
   ● **S79.099 Other** physeal fracture of upper end of **unspecified** femur
● **S79.1 Physeal** fracture of **lower** end of femur
● **S79.10 Unspecified** physeal fracture of lower end of femur
   ● **S79.101 Unspecified** physeal fracture of lower end of **right** femur
   ● **S79.102 Unspecified** physeal fracture of lower end of **left** femur
   ● **S79.109 Unspecified** physeal fracture of lower end of **unspecified** femur
● **S79.11 Salter-Harris Type I** physeal fracture of lower end of femur
   ● **S79.111 Salter-Harris Type I** physeal fracture of lower end of **right** femur
   ● **S79.112 Salter-Harris Type I** physeal fracture of lower end of **left** femur
   ● **S79.119 Salter-Harris Type I** physeal fracture of lower end of **unspecified** femur
● **S79.12 Salter-Harris Type II** physeal fracture of lower end of femur
   ● **S79.121 Salter-Harris Type II** physeal fracture of lower end of **right** femur
   ● **S79.122 Salter-Harris Type II** physeal fracture of lower end of **left** femur
   ● **S79.129 Salter-Harris Type II** physeal fracture of lower end of **unspecified** femur
● **S79.13 Salter-Harris Type III** physeal fracture of lower end of femur
   ● **S79.131 Salter-Harris Type III** physeal fracture of lower end of **right** femur
   ● **S79.132 Salter-Harris Type III** physeal fracture of lower end of **left** femur
   ● **S79.139 Salter-Harris Type III** physeal fracture of lower end of **unspecified** femur

● **S79.14 Salter-Harris Type IV** physeal fracture of lower end of femur
   ● **S79.141 Salter-Harris Type IV** physeal fracture of lower end of **right** femur
   ● **S79.142 Salter-Harris Type IV** physeal fracture of lower end of **left** femur
   ● **S79.149 Salter-Harris Type IV** physeal fracture of lower end of **unspecified** femur
● **S79.19 Other** physeal fracture of lower end of femur
   ● **S79.191 Other** physeal fracture of lower end of **right** femur
   ● **S79.192 Other** physeal fracture of lower end of **left** femur
   ● **S79.199 Other** physeal fracture of lower end of **unspecified** femur
● **S79.8 Other specified injuries of hip and thigh**
     The appropriate 7th character is to be added to each code in subcategory S79.8

A	initial encounter
D	subsequent encounter
S	sequela

   ● **S79.81 Other specified injuries of hip**
     ● **S79.811 Other specified injuries of right** hip
     ● **S79.812 Other specified injuries of left** hip
     ● **S79.819 Other specified injuries of unspecified** hip
   ● **S79.82 Other specified injuries of thigh**
     ● **S79.821 Other specified injuries of right** thigh
     ● **S79.822 Other specified injuries of left** thigh
     ● **S79.829 Other specified injuries of unspecified** thigh
● **S79.9 Unspecified** injury of hip and thigh
     The appropriate 7th character is to be added to each code in subcategory S79.9

A	initial encounter
D	subsequent encounter
S	sequela

   ● **S79.91 Unspecified injury of hip**
     ● **S79.911 Unspecified injury of right** hip
     ● **S79.912 Unspecified injury of left** hip
     ● **S79.919 Unspecified injury of unspecified** hip
   ● **S79.92 Unspecified injury of thigh**
     ● **S79.921 Unspecified injury of right** thigh
     ● **S79.922 Unspecified injury of left** thigh
     ● **S79.929 Unspecified injury of unspecified** thigh

INJURIES TO THE KNEE AND LOWER LEG (S80-S89)

Excludes2 burns and corrosions (T20-T32)
     frostbite (T33-T34)
     injuries of ankle and foot, except fracture of ankle and malleolus (S90-S99)
     insect bite or sting, venomous (T63.4)

● **S80 Superficial injury of knee and lower leg**
     Excludes2 superficial injury of ankle and foot (S90.-)
     The appropriate 7th character is to be added to each code from category S80

A	initial encounter
D	subsequent encounter
S	sequela

   ● **S80.0 Contusion of knee**
   X ● **S80.00 Contusion of unspecified** knee
   X ● **S80.01 Contusion of right** knee
   X ● **S80.02 Contusion of left** knee

▶ New   ⇒ Revised   ~~deleted~~ Deleted   **OGCR** Official Guidelines   X Assign placeholder X   ● Use Additional Character(s)

Excludes 1   Excludes 2   Includes   Use additional   Code first   Code also   Key words

● **S80.1**   **Contusion of lower leg**
   X ● **S80.10**   Contusion of unspecified lower leg
   X ● **S80.11**   Contusion of right lower leg
   X ● **S80.12**   Contusion of left lower leg
● **S80.2**   **Other superficial injuries of knee**
   ● **S80.21**   **Abrasion of knee**
     ● **S80.211**   Abrasion, right knee
     ● **S80.212**   Abrasion, left knee
     ● **S80.219**   Abrasion, unspecified knee
   ● **S80.22**   **Blister (nonthermal) of knee**
     ● **S80.221**   Blister (nonthermal), right knee
     ● **S80.222**   Blister (nonthermal), left knee
     ● **S80.229**   Blister (nonthermal), unspecified knee
   ● **S80.24**   **External constriction of knee**
     ● **S80.241**   External constriction, right knee
     ● **S80.242**   External constriction, left knee
     ● **S80.249**   External constriction, unspecified knee
   ● **S80.25**   **Superficial foreign body of knee**
     Splinter in the knee
     ● **S80.251**   Superficial foreign body, right knee
     ● **S80.252**   Superficial foreign body, left knee
     ● **S80.259**   Superficial foreign body, unspecified knee
   ● **S80.26**   **Insect bite (nonvenomous) of knee**
     ● **S80.261**   Insect bite (nonvenomous), right knee
     ● **S80.262**   Insect bite (nonvenomous), left knee
     ● **S80.269**   Insect bite (nonvenomous), unspecified knee
   ● **S80.27**   **Other superficial bite of knee**
     Excludes1   open bite of knee (S81.05-)
     ● **S80.271**   Other superficial bite of right knee
     ● **S80.272**   Other superficial bite of left knee
     ● **S80.279**   Other superficial bite of unspecified knee
● **S80.8**   **Other superficial injuries of lower leg**
   ● **S80.81**   **Abrasion of lower leg**
     ● **S80.811**   Abrasion, right lower leg
     ● **S80.812**   Abrasion, left lower leg
     ● **S80.819**   Abrasion, unspecified lower leg
   ● **S80.82**   **Blister (nonthermal) of lower leg**
     ● **S80.821**   Blister (nonthermal), right lower leg
     ● **S80.822**   Blister (nonthermal), left lower leg
     ● **S80.829**   Blister (nonthermal), unspecified lower leg
   ● **S80.84**   **External constriction of lower leg**
     ● **S80.841**   External constriction, right lower leg
     ● **S80.842**   External constriction, left lower leg
     ● **S80.849**   External constriction, unspecified lower leg
   ● **S80.85**   **Superficial foreign body of lower leg**
     Splinter in the lower leg
     ● **S80.851**   Superficial foreign body, right lower leg
     ● **S80.852**   Superficial foreign body, left lower leg
     ● **S80.859**   Superficial foreign body, unspecified lower leg

● **S80.86**   **Insect bite (nonvenomous) of lower leg**
   ● **S80.861**   Insect bite (nonvenomous), right lower leg
   ● **S80.862**   Insect bite (nonvenomous), left lower leg
   ● **S80.869**   Insect bite (nonvenomous), unspecified lower leg
● **S80.87**   **Other superficial bite of lower leg**
   Excludes1   open bite of lower leg (S81.85-)
   ● **S80.871**   Other superficial bite, right lower leg
   ● **S80.872**   Other superficial bite, left lower leg
   ● **S80.879**   Other superficial bite, unspecified lower leg
● **S80.9**   **Unspecified superficial injury of knee and lower leg**
   ● **S80.91**   **Unspecified superficial injury of knee**
     ● **S80.911**   Unspecified superficial injury of right knee
     ● **S80.912**   Unspecified superficial injury of left knee
     ● **S80.919**   Unspecified superficial injury of unspecified knee
   ● **S80.92**   **Unspecified superficial injury of lower leg**
     ● **S80.921**   Unspecified superficial injury of right lower leg
     ● **S80.922**   Unspecified superficial injury of left lower leg
     ● **S80.929**   Unspecified superficial injury of unspecified lower leg

● **S81**   **Open wound of knee and lower leg**
   Code also any associated wound infection
   Excludes1   open fracture of knee and lower leg (S82.-)
         traumatic amputation of lower leg (S88.-)
   Excludes2   open wound of ankle and foot (S91.-)
   The appropriate 7th character is to be added to each code from category S81

> A   initial encounter
> D   subsequent encounter
> S   sequela

   ● **S81.0**   **Open wound of knee**
     ● **S81.00**   **Unspecified open wound of knee**
       ● **S81.001**   Unspecified open wound, right knee
       ● **S81.002**   Unspecified open wound, left knee
       ● **S81.009**   Unspecified open wound, unspecified knee
     ● **S81.01**   **Laceration without foreign body of knee**
       ● **S81.011**   Laceration without foreign body, right knee
       ● **S81.012**   Laceration without foreign body, left knee
       ● **S81.019**   Laceration without foreign body, unspecified knee
     ● **S81.02**   **Laceration with foreign body of knee**
       ● **S81.021**   Laceration with foreign body, right knee
       ● **S81.022**   Laceration with foreign body, left knee
       ● **S81.029**   Laceration with foreign body, unspecified knee

---

- S81.03   Puncture wound without foreign body of knee
  - S81.031   Puncture wound without foreign body, right knee
  - S81.032   Puncture wound without foreign body, left knee
  - S81.039   Puncture wound without foreign body, unspecified knee
- S81.04   Puncture wound with foreign body of knee
  - S81.041   Puncture wound with foreign body, right knee
  - S81.042   Puncture wound with foreign body, left knee
  - S81.049   Puncture wound with foreign body, unspecified knee
- S81.05   Open bite of knee
    Bite of knee NOS
    - **Excludes1**   superficial bite of knee (S80.27-)
  - S81.051   Open bite, right knee
  - S81.052   Open bite, left knee
  - S81.059   Open bite, unspecified knee
- S81.8   Open wound of lower leg
  - S81.80   Unspecified open wound of lower leg
    - S81.801   Unspecified open wound, right lower leg
    - S81.802   Unspecified open wound, left lower leg
    - S81.809   Unspecified open wound, unspecified lower leg
  - S81.81   Laceration without foreign body of lower leg
    - S81.811   Laceration without foreign body, right lower leg
    - S81.812   Laceration without foreign body, left lower leg
    - S81.819   Laceration without foreign body, unspecified lower leg
  - S81.82   Laceration with foreign body of lower leg
    - S81.821   Laceration with foreign body, right lower leg
    - S81.822   Laceration with foreign body, left lower leg
    - S81.829   Laceration with foreign body, unspecified lower leg
  - S81.83   Puncture wound without foreign body of lower leg
    - S81.831   Puncture wound without foreign body, right lower leg
    - S81.832   Puncture wound without foreign body, left lower leg
    - S81.839   Puncture wound without foreign body, unspecified lower leg
  - S81.84   Puncture wound with foreign body of lower leg
    - S81.841   Puncture wound with foreign body, right lower leg
    - S81.842   Puncture wound with foreign body, left lower leg
    - S81.849   Puncture wound with foreign body, unspecified lower leg
  - S81.85   Open bite of lower leg
      Bite of lower leg NOS
      - **Excludes1**   superficial bite of lower leg (S80.86-, S80.87-)
    - S81.851   Open bite, right lower leg
    - S81.852   Open bite, left lower leg
    - S81.859   Open bite, unspecified lower leg

- S82   Fracture of lower leg, including ankle
  - **Note:** A fracture not indicated as displaced or nondisplaced should be coded to displaced

    A fracture not indicated as open or closed should be coded to closed

    The open fracture designations are based on the Gustilo open fracture classification
  - **Includes**   fracture of malleolus
  - **Excludes1**   traumatic amputation of lower leg (S88.-)
  - **Excludes2**   fracture of foot, except ankle (S92.-)
    - periprosthetic fracture of prosthetic implant of knee (M97.0-)
  - The appropriate 7th character is to be added to all codes from category S82

A	initial encounter for closed fracture
B	initial encounter for open fracture type I or II initial encounter for open fracture NOS
C	initial encounter for open fracture type IIIA, IIIB, or IIIC
D	subsequent encounter for closed fracture with routine healing
E	subsequent encounter for open fracture type I or II with routine healing
F	subsequent encounter for open fracture type IIIA, IIIB, or IIIC with routine healing
G	subsequent encounter for closed fracture with delayed healing
H	subsequent encounter for open fracture type I or II with delayed healing
J	subsequent encounter for open fracture type IIIA, IIIB, or IIIC with delayed healing
K	subsequent encounter for closed fracture with nonunion
M	subsequent encounter for open fracture type I or II with nonunion
N	subsequent encounter for open fracture type IIIA, IIIB, or IIIC with nonunion
P	subsequent encounter for closed fracture with malunion
Q	subsequent encounter for open fracture type I or II with malunion
R	subsequent encounter for open fracture type IIIA, IIIB, or IIIC with malunion
S	sequela

- S82.0   Fracture of patella
    Knee cap
  - S82.00   Unspecified fracture of patella
    - S82.001   Unspecified fracture of right patella
    - S82.002   Unspecified fracture of left patella
    - S82.009   Unspecified fracture of unspecified patella
  - S82.01   Osteochondral fracture of patella
    - S82.011   Displaced osteochondral fracture of right patella
    - S82.012   Displaced osteochondral fracture of left patella
    - S82.013   Displaced osteochondral fracture of unspecified patella
    - S82.014   Nondisplaced osteochondral fracture of right patella
    - S82.015   Nondisplaced osteochondral fracture of left patella
    - S82.016   Nondisplaced osteochondral fracture of unspecified patella

▶ New   ⇒ Revised   ~~deleted~~ Deleted   **OGCR** Official Guidelines   X Assign placeholder X   ● Use Additional Character(s)

Excludes 1   Excludes 2   Includes   Use additional   Code first   Code also   Key words

- S82.02   Longitudinal fracture of patella
  - S82.021   Displaced longitudinal fracture of right patella
  - S82.022   Displaced longitudinal fracture of left patella
  - S82.023   Displaced longitudinal fracture of unspecified patella
  - S82.024   Nondisplaced longitudinal fracture of right patella
  - S82.025   Nondisplaced longitudinal fracture of left patella
  - S82.026   Nondisplaced longitudinal fracture of unspecified patella
- S82.03   Transverse fracture of patella
  - S82.031   Displaced transverse fracture of right patella
  - S82.032   Displaced transverse fracture of left patella
  - S82.033   Displaced transverse fracture of unspecified patella
  - S82.034   Nondisplaced transverse fracture of right patella
  - S82.035   Nondisplaced transverse fracture of left patella
  - S82.036   Nondisplaced transverse fracture of unspecified patella
- S82.04   Comminuted fracture of patella
  - S82.041   Displaced comminuted fracture of right patella
  - S82.042   Displaced comminuted fracture of left patella
  - S82.043   Displaced comminuted fracture of unspecified patella
  - S82.044   Nondisplaced comminuted fracture of right patella
  - S82.045   Nondisplaced comminuted fracture of left patella
  - S82.046   Nondisplaced comminuted fracture of unspecified patella
- S82.09   Other fracture of patella
  - S82.091   Other fracture of right patella
  - S82.092   Other fracture of left patella
  - S82.099   Other fracture of unspecified patella
- S82.1   Fracture of upper end of tibia
  Fracture of proximal end of tibia

  | Excludes2 | fracture of shaft of tibia (S82.2-) |
  | | physeal fracture of upper end of tibia (S89.0-) |

  - S82.10   Unspecified fracture of upper end of tibia
    - S82.101   Unspecified fracture of upper end of right tibia
    - S82.102   Unspecified fracture of upper end of left tibia
    - S82.109   Unspecified fracture of upper end of unspecified tibia
  - S82.11   Fracture of tibial spine
    - S82.111   Displaced fracture of right tibial spine
    - S82.112   Displaced fracture of left tibial spine
    - S82.113   Displaced fracture of unspecified tibial spine
    - S82.114   Nondisplaced fracture of right tibial spine
    - S82.115   Nondisplaced fracture of left tibial spine
    - S82.116   Nondisplaced fracture of unspecified tibial spine

- S82.12   Fracture of lateral condyle of tibia
  - S82.121   Displaced fracture of lateral condyle of right tibia
  - S82.122   Displaced fracture of lateral condyle of left tibia
  - S82.123   Displaced fracture of lateral condyle of unspecified tibia
  - S82.124   Nondisplaced fracture of lateral condyle of right tibia
  - S82.125   Nondisplaced fracture of lateral condyle of left tibia
  - S82.126   Nondisplaced fracture of lateral condyle of unspecified tibia
- S82.13   Fracture of medial condyle of tibia
  - S82.131   Displaced fracture of medial condyle of right tibia
  - S82.132   Displaced fracture of medial condyle of left tibia
  - S82.133   Displaced fracture of medial condyle of unspecified tibia
  - S82.134   Nondisplaced fracture of medial condyle of right tibia
  - S82.135   Nondisplaced fracture of medial condyle of left tibia
  - S82.136   Nondisplaced fracture of medial condyle of unspecified tibia
- S82.14   Bicondylar fracture of tibia
  Fracture of tibial plateau NOS
  - S82.141   Displaced bicondylar fracture of right tibia
  - S82.142   Displaced bicondylar fracture of left tibia
  - S82.143   Displaced bicondylar fracture of unspecified tibia
  - S82.144   Nondisplaced bicondylar fracture of right tibia
  - S82.145   Nondisplaced bicondylar fracture of left tibia
  - S82.146   Nondisplaced bicondylar fracture of unspecified tibia
- S82.15   Fracture of tibial tuberosity
  - S82.151   Displaced fracture of right tibial tuberosity
  - S82.152   Displaced fracture of left tibial tuberosity
  - S82.153   Displaced fracture of unspecified tibial tuberosity
  - S82.154   Nondisplaced fracture of right tibial tuberosity
  - S82.155   Nondisplaced fracture of left tibial tuberosity
  - S82.156   Nondisplaced fracture of unspecified tibial tuberosity
- S82.16   Torus fracture of upper end of tibia

  The appropriate 7th character is to be added to all codes in subcategory S82.16

A	initial encounter for closed fracture
D	subsequent encounter for fracture with routine healing
G	subsequent encounter for fracture with delayed healing
K	subsequent encounter for fracture with nonunion
P	subsequent encounter for fracture with malunion
S	sequela

  - S82.161   Torus fracture of upper end of right tibia
  - S82.162   Torus fracture of upper end of left tibia
  - S82.169   Torus fracture of upper end of unspecified tibia

- ● S82.19   Other fracture of upper end of tibia
  - ● S82.191   Other fracture of upper end of right tibia
  - ● S82.192   Other fracture of upper end of left tibia
  - ● S82.199   Other fracture of upper end of unspecified tibia
- ● S82.2   Fracture of shaft of tibia
  - ● S82.20   Unspecified fracture of shaft of tibia
    Fracture of tibia NOS
    - ● S82.201   Unspecified fracture of shaft of right tibia
    - ● S82.202   Unspecified fracture of shaft of left tibia
    - ● S82.209   Unspecified fracture of shaft of unspecified tibia
  - ● S82.22   Transverse fracture of shaft of tibia
    - ● S82.221   Displaced transverse fracture of shaft of right tibia
    - ● S82.222   Displaced transverse fracture of shaft of left tibia
    - ● S82.223   Displaced transverse fracture of shaft of unspecified tibia
    - ● S82.224   Nondisplaced transverse fracture of shaft of right tibia
    - ● S82.225   Nondisplaced transverse fracture of shaft of left tibia
    - ● S82.226   Nondisplaced transverse fracture of shaft of unspecified tibia
  - ● S82.23   Oblique fracture of shaft of tibia
    - ● S82.231   Displaced oblique fracture of shaft of right tibia
    - ● S82.232   Displaced oblique fracture of shaft of left tibia
    - ● S82.233   Displaced oblique fracture of shaft of unspecified tibia
    - ● S82.234   Nondisplaced oblique fracture of shaft of right tibia
    - ● S82.235   Nondisplaced oblique fracture of shaft of left tibia
    - ● S82.236   Nondisplaced oblique fracture of shaft of unspecified tibia
  - ● S82.24   Spiral fracture of shaft of tibia
    Toddler fracture
    - ● S82.241   Displaced spiral fracture of shaft of right tibia
    - ● S82.242   Displaced spiral fracture of shaft of left tibia
    - ● S82.243   Displaced spiral fracture of shaft of unspecified tibia
    - ● S82.244   Nondisplaced spiral fracture of shaft of right tibia
    - ● S82.245   Nondisplaced spiral fracture of shaft of left tibia
    - ● S82.246   Nondisplaced spiral fracture of shaft of unspecified tibia
  - ● S82.25   Comminuted fracture of shaft of tibia
    - ● S82.251   Displaced comminuted fracture of shaft of right tibia
    - ● S82.252   Displaced comminuted fracture of shaft of left tibia
    - ● S82.253   Displaced comminuted fracture of shaft of unspecified tibia
    - ● S82.254   Nondisplaced comminuted fracture of shaft of right tibia
    - ● S82.255   Nondisplaced comminuted fracture of shaft of left tibia
    - ● S82.256   Nondisplaced comminuted fracture of shaft of unspecified tibia
  - ● S82.26   Segmental fracture of shaft of tibia
    - ● S82.261   Displaced segmental fracture of shaft of right tibia
    - ● S82.262   Displaced segmental fracture of shaft of left tibia
    - ● S82.263   Displaced segmental fracture of shaft of unspecified tibia
    - ● S82.264   Nondisplaced segmental fracture of shaft of right tibia
    - ● S82.265   Nondisplaced segmental fracture of shaft of left tibia
    - ● S82.266   Nondisplaced segmental fracture of shaft of unspecified tibia
  - ● S82.29   Other fracture of shaft of tibia
    - ● S82.291   Other fracture of shaft of right tibia
    - ● S82.292   Other fracture of shaft of left tibia
    - ● S82.299   Other fracture of shaft of unspecified tibia
- ● S82.3   Fracture of lower end of tibia
  - Excludes1   bimalleolar fracture of lower leg (S82.84-)
    fracture of medial malleolus alone (S82.5-)
    Maisonneuve's fracture (S82.86-)
    pilon fracture of distal tibia (S82.87-)
    trimalleolar fractures of lower leg (S82.85-)
  - ● S82.30   Unspecified fracture of lower end of tibia
    - ● S82.301   Unspecified fracture of lower end of right tibia
    - ● S82.302   Unspecified fracture of lower end of left tibia
    - ● S82.309   Unspecified fracture of lower end of unspecified tibia
  - ● S82.31   Torus fracture of lower end of tibia
    The appropriate 7th character is to be added to all codes in subcategory S82.31

A	initial encounter for closed fracture
D	subsequent encounter for fracture with routine healing
G	subsequent encounter for fracture with delayed healing
K	subsequent encounter for fracture with nonunion
P	subsequent encounter for fracture with malunion
S	sequela

    - ● S82.311   Torus fracture of lower end of right tibia
    - ● S82.312   Torus fracture of lower end of left tibia
    - ● S82.319   Torus fracture of lower end of unspecified tibia
  - ● S82.39   Other fracture of lower end of tibia
    - ● S82.391   Other fracture of lower end of right tibia
    - ● S82.392   Other fracture of lower end of left tibia
    - ● S82.399   Other fracture of lower end of unspecified tibia
- ● S82.4   Fracture of shaft of fibula
  - Excludes2   fracture of lateral malleolus alone (S82.6-)
  - ● S82.40   Unspecified fracture of shaft of fibula
    - ● S82.401   Unspecified fracture of shaft of right fibula
    - ● S82.402   Unspecified fracture of shaft of left fibula
    - ● S82.409   Unspecified fracture of shaft of unspecified fibula

● S82.42 **Transverse** fracture of shaft of fibula
   ● S82.421 Displaced **transverse** fracture of shaft of **right** fibula
   ● S82.422 Displaced **transverse** fracture of shaft of **left** fibula
   ● S82.423 Displaced **transverse** fracture of shaft of **unspecified** fibula
   ● S82.424 Nondisplaced **transverse** fracture of shaft of **right** fibula
   ● S82.425 Nondisplaced **transverse** fracture of shaft of **left** fibula
   ● S82.426 Nondisplaced **transverse** fracture of shaft of **unspecified** fibula

● S82.43 **Oblique** fracture of shaft of fibula
   ● S82.431 Displaced **oblique** fracture of shaft of **right** fibula
   ● S82.432 Displaced **oblique** fracture of shaft of **left** fibula
   ● S82.433 Displaced **oblique** fracture of shaft of **unspecified** fibula
   ● S82.434 Nondisplaced **oblique** fracture of shaft of **right** fibula
   ● S82.435 Nondisplaced **oblique** fracture of shaft of **left** fibula
   ● S82.436 Nondisplaced **oblique** fracture of shaft of **unspecified** fibula

● S82.44 **Spiral** fracture of shaft of fibula
   ● S82.441 Displaced **spiral** fracture of shaft of **right** fibula
   ● S82.442 Displaced **spiral** fracture of shaft of **left** fibula
   ● S82.443 Displaced **spiral** fracture of shaft of **unspecified** fibula
   ● S82.444 Nondisplaced **spiral** fracture of shaft of **right** fibula
   ● S82.445 Nondisplaced **spiral** fracture of shaft of **left** fibula
   ● S82.446 Nondisplaced **spiral** fracture of shaft of **unspecified** fibula

● S82.45 **Comminuted** fracture of shaft of fibula
   ● S82.451 Displaced **comminuted** fracture of shaft of **right** fibula
   ● S82.452 Displaced **comminuted** fracture of shaft of **left** fibula
   ● S82.453 Displaced **comminuted** fracture of shaft of **unspecified** fibula
   ● S82.454 Nondisplaced **comminuted** fracture of shaft of **right** fibula
   ● S82.455 Nondisplaced **comminuted** fracture of shaft of **left** fibula
   ● S82.456 Nondisplaced **comminuted** fracture of shaft of **unspecified** fibula

● S82.46 **Segmental** fracture of shaft of fibula
   ● S82.461 Displaced **segmental** fracture of shaft of **right** fibula
   ● S82.462 Displaced **segmental** fracture of shaft of **left** fibula
   ● S82.463 Displaced **segmental** fracture of shaft of **unspecified** fibula
   ● S82.464 Nondisplaced **segmental** fracture of shaft of **right** fibula
   ● S82.465 Nondisplaced **segmental** fracture of shaft of **left** fibula
   ● S82.466 Nondisplaced **segmental** fracture of shaft of **unspecified** fibula

● S82.49 **Other** fracture of shaft of fibula
   ● S82.491 Other fracture of shaft of **right** fibula
   ● S82.492 Other fracture of shaft of **left** fibula
   ● S82.499 Other fracture of shaft of **unspecified** fibula

● S82.5 Fracture of **medial malleolus**
   Excludes1 pilon fracture of distal tibia (S82.87-)
           Salter-Harris type III of lower end of tibia (S89.13-)
           Salter-Harris type IV of lower end of tibia (S89.14-)
  X ● S82.51 Displaced fracture of medial malleolus of **right** tibia
  X ● S82.52 Displaced fracture of medial malleolus of **left** tibia
  X ● S82.53 Displaced fracture of medial malleolus of **unspecified** tibia
  X ● S82.54 Nondisplaced fracture of medial malleolus of **right** tibia
  X ● S82.55 Nondisplaced fracture of medial malleolus of **left** tibia
  X ● S82.56 Nondisplaced fracture of medial malleolus of **unspecified** tibia

● S82.6 Fracture of **lateral malleolus**
   Excludes1 pilon fracture of distal tibia (S82.87-)
  X ● S82.61 Displaced fracture of lateral malleolus of **right** fibula
  X ● S82.62 Displaced fracture of lateral malleolus of **left** fibula
  X ● S82.63 Displaced fracture of lateral malleolus of **unspecified** fibula
  X ● S82.64 Nondisplaced fracture of lateral malleolus of **right** fibula
  X ● S82.65 Nondisplaced fracture of lateral malleolus of **left** fibula
  X ● S82.66 Nondisplaced fracture of lateral malleolus of **unspecified** fibula

● S82.8 Other fractures of lower leg
   ● S82.81 **Torus** fracture of **upper end** of fibula
       The appropriate 7th character is to be added to all codes in subcategory S82.81

A	initial encounter for closed fracture
D	subsequent encounter for fracture with routine healing
G	subsequent encounter for fracture with delayed healing
K	subsequent encounter for fracture with nonunion
P	subsequent encounter for fracture with malunion
S	sequela

     ● S82.811 Torus fracture of upper end of **right** fibula
     ● S82.812 Torus fracture of upper end of **left** fibula
     ● S82.819 Torus fracture of upper end of **unspecified** fibula

CHAPTER 19 (S00-T88)

● **S82.82** Torus fracture of lower end of fibula

The appropriate 7th character is to be added to all codes in subcategory S82.82

A	initial encounter for closed fracture
D	subsequent encounter for fracture with routine healing
G	subsequent encounter for fracture with delayed healing
K	subsequent encounter for fracture with nonunion
P	subsequent encounter for fracture with malunion
S	sequela

- ● S82.821 Torus fracture of lower end of right fibula
- ● S82.822 Torus fracture of lower end of left fibula
- ● S82.829 Torus fracture of lower end of unspecified fibula

● **S82.83** Other fracture of upper and lower end of fibula
- ● S82.831 Other fracture of upper and lower end of right fibula
- ● S82.832 Other fracture of upper and lower end of left fibula
- ● S82.839 Other fracture of upper and lower end of unspecified fibula

● **S82.84** Bimalleolar fracture of lower leg
- ● S82.841 Displaced bimalleolar fracture of right lower leg
- ● S82.842 Displaced bimalleolar fracture of left lower leg
- ● S82.843 Displaced bimalleolar fracture of unspecified lower leg
- ● S82.844 Nondisplaced bimalleolar fracture of right lower leg
- ● S82.845 Nondisplaced bimalleolar fracture of left lower leg
- ● S82.846 Nondisplaced bimalleolar fracture of unspecified lower leg

● **S82.85** Trimalleolar fracture of lower leg
- ● S82.851 Displaced trimalleolar fracture of right lower leg
- ● S82.852 Displaced trimalleolar fracture of left lower leg
- ● S82.853 Displaced trimalleolar fracture of unspecified lower leg
- ● S82.854 Nondisplaced trimalleolar fracture of right lower leg
- ● S82.855 Nondisplaced trimalleolar fracture of left lower leg
- ● S82.856 Nondisplaced trimalleolar fracture of unspecified lower leg

● **S82.86** Maisonneuve's fracture
- ● S82.861 Displaced Maisonneuve's fracture of right leg
- ● S82.862 Displaced Maisonneuve's fracture of left leg
- ● S82.863 Displaced Maisonneuve's fracture of unspecified leg
- ● S82.864 Nondisplaced Maisonneuve's fracture of right leg
- ● S82.865 Nondisplaced Maisonneuve's fracture of left leg
- ● S82.866 Nondisplaced Maisonneuve's fracture of unspecified leg

● **S82.87** Pilon fracture of tibia
- ● S82.871 Displaced pilon fracture of right tibia
- ● S82.872 Displaced pilon fracture of left tibia
- ● S82.873 Displaced pilon fracture of unspecified tibia
- ● S82.874 Nondisplaced pilon fracture of right tibia
- ● S82.875 Nondisplaced pilon fracture of left tibia
- ● S82.876 Nondisplaced pilon fracture of unspecified tibia

● **S82.89** Other fractures of lower leg
Fracture of ankle NOS
- ● S82.891 Other fracture of right lower leg
- ● S82.892 Other fracture of left lower leg
- ● S82.899 Other fracture of unspecified lower leg

● **S82.9** Unspecified fracture of lower leg
- X● S82.90 Unspecified fracture of unspecified lower leg
- X● S82.91 Unspecified fracture of right lower leg
- X● S82.92 Unspecified fracture of left lower leg

● **S83** Dislocation and sprain of joints and ligaments of knee

Includes avulsion of joint or ligament of knee
laceration of cartilage, joint or ligament of knee
sprain of cartilage, joint or ligament of knee
traumatic hemarthrosis of joint or ligament of knee
traumatic rupture of joint or ligament of knee
traumatic subluxation of joint or ligament of knee
traumatic tear of joint or ligament of knee

Code also any associated open wound

Excludes1 derangement of patella (M22.Ø-M22.3)
injury of patellar ligament (tendon) (S76.1-)
internal derangement of knee (M23.-)
old dislocation of knee (M24.36)
pathological dislocation of knee (M24.36)
recurrent dislocation of knee (M22.Ø)

Excludes2 strain of muscle, fascia and tendon of lower leg (S86.-)

The appropriate 7th character is to be added to each code from category S83

A	initial encounter
D	subsequent encounter
S	sequela

● **S83.Ø** Subluxation and dislocation of patella
- ● S83.ØØ Unspecified subluxation and dislocation of patella
  - ● S83.ØØ1 Unspecified subluxation of right patella
  - ● S83.ØØ2 Unspecified subluxation of left patella
  - ● S83.ØØ3 Unspecified subluxation of unspecified patella
  - ● S83.ØØ4 Unspecified dislocation of right patella
  - ● S83.ØØ5 Unspecified dislocation of left patella
  - ● S83.ØØ6 Unspecified dislocation of unspecified patella
- ● S83.Ø1 Lateral subluxation and dislocation of patella
  - ● S83.Ø11 Lateral subluxation of right patella
  - ● S83.Ø12 Lateral subluxation of left patella
  - ● S83.Ø13 Lateral subluxation of unspecified patella
  - ● S83.Ø14 Lateral dislocation of right patella
  - ● S83.Ø15 Lateral dislocation of left patella
  - ● S83.Ø16 Lateral dislocation of unspecified patella

● S83.09   Other subluxation and dislocation of patella
- ● S83.091   Other subluxation of right patella
- ● S83.092   Other subluxation of left patella
- ● S83.093   Other subluxation of unspecified patella
- ● S83.094   Other dislocation of right patella
- ● S83.095   Other dislocation of left patella
- ● S83.096   Other dislocation of unspecified patella

● S83.1   Subluxation and dislocation of knee

> **Excludes2**   instability of knee prosthesis (T84.022, T84.023)

● S83.10   Unspecified subluxation and dislocation of knee
- ● S83.101   Unspecified subluxation of right knee
- ● S83.102   Unspecified subluxation of left knee
- ● S83.103   Unspecified subluxation of unspecified knee
- ● S83.104   Unspecified dislocation of right knee
- ● S83.105   Unspecified dislocation of left knee
- ● S83.106   Unspecified dislocation of unspecified knee

● S83.11   Anterior subluxation and dislocation of proximal end of tibia
     Posterior subluxation and dislocation of distal end of femur
- ● S83.111   Anterior subluxation of proximal end of tibia, right knee
- ● S83.112   Anterior subluxation of proximal end of tibia, left knee
- ● S83.113   Anterior subluxation of proximal end of tibia, unspecified knee
- ● S83.114   Anterior dislocation of proximal end of tibia, right knee
- ● S83.115   Anterior dislocation of proximal end of tibia, left knee
- ● S83.116   Anterior dislocation of proximal end of tibia, unspecified knee

● S83.12   Posterior subluxation and dislocation of proximal end of tibia
     Anterior dislocation of distal end of femur
- ● S83.121   Posterior subluxation of proximal end of tibia, right knee
- ● S83.122   Posterior subluxation of proximal end of tibia, left knee
- ● S83.123   Posterior subluxation of proximal end of tibia, unspecified knee
- ● S83.124   Posterior dislocation of proximal end of tibia, right knee
- ● S83.125   Posterior dislocation of proximal end of tibia, left knee
- ● S83.126   Posterior dislocation of proximal end of tibia, unspecified knee

● S83.13   Medial subluxation and dislocation of proximal end of tibia
- ● S83.131   Medial subluxation of proximal end of tibia, right knee
- ● S83.132   Medial subluxation of proximal end of tibia, left knee
- ● S83.133   Medial subluxation of proximal end of tibia, unspecified knee
- ● S83.134   Medial dislocation of proximal end of tibia, right knee
- ● S83.135   Medial dislocation of proximal end of tibia, left knee
- ● S83.136   Medial dislocation of proximal end of tibia, unspecified knee

● S83.14   Lateral subluxation and dislocation of proximal end of tibia
- ● S83.141   Lateral subluxation of proximal end of tibia, right knee
- ● S83.142   Lateral subluxation of proximal end of tibia, left knee
- ● S83.143   Lateral subluxation of proximal end of tibia, unspecified knee
- ● S83.144   Lateral dislocation of proximal end of tibia, right knee
- ● S83.145   Lateral dislocation of proximal end of tibia, left knee
- ● S83.146   Lateral dislocation of proximal end of tibia, unspecified knee

● S83.19   Other subluxation and dislocation of knee
- ● S83.191   Other subluxation of right knee
- ● S83.192   Other subluxation of left knee
- ● S83.193   Other subluxation of unspecified knee
- ● S83.194   Other dislocation of right knee
- ● S83.195   Other dislocation of left knee
- ● S83.196   Other dislocation of unspecified knee

● S83.2   Tear of meniscus, current injury

> **Excludes1**   old bucket-handle tear (M23.2)

● S83.20   Tear of unspecified meniscus, current injury
     Tear of meniscus of knee NOS
- ● S83.200   Bucket-handle tear of unspecified meniscus, current injury, right knee
- ● S83.201   Bucket-handle tear of unspecified meniscus, current injury, left knee
- ● S83.202   Bucket-handle tear of unspecified meniscus, current injury, unspecified knee
- ● S83.203   Other tear of unspecified meniscus, current injury, right knee
- ● S83.204   Other tear of unspecified meniscus, current injury, left knee
- ● S83.205   Other tear of unspecified meniscus, current injury, unspecified knee
- ● S83.206   Unspecified tear of unspecified meniscus, current injury, right knee
- ● S83.207   Unspecified tear of unspecified meniscus, current injury, left knee
- ● S83.209   Unspecified tear of unspecified meniscus, current injury, unspecified knee

● S83.21   Bucket-handle tear of medial meniscus, current injury
- ● S83.211   Bucket-handle tear of medial meniscus, current injury, right knee
- ● S83.212   Bucket-handle tear of medial meniscus, current injury, left knee
- ● S83.219   Bucket-handle tear of medial meniscus, current injury, unspecified knee

● S83.22   Peripheral tear of medial meniscus, current injury
- ● S83.221   Peripheral tear of medial meniscus, current injury, right knee
- ● S83.222   Peripheral tear of medial meniscus, current injury, left knee
- ● S83.229   Peripheral tear of medial meniscus, current injury, unspecified knee

CHAPTER 19 (S00–T88)

● S83.23　Complex tear of medial meniscus, current injury
　　● S83.231　Complex tear of medial meniscus, current injury, right knee
　　● S83.232　Complex tear of medial meniscus, current injury, left knee
　　● S83.239　Complex tear of medial meniscus, current injury, unspecified knee

● S83.24　Other tear of medial meniscus, current injury
　　● S83.241　Other tear of medial meniscus, current injury, right knee
　　● S83.242　Other tear of medial meniscus, current injury, left knee
　　● S83.249　Other tear of medial meniscus, current injury, unspecified knee

● S83.25　Bucket-handle tear of lateral meniscus, current injury
　　● S83.251　Bucket-handle tear of lateral meniscus, current injury, right knee
　　● S83.252　Bucket-handle tear of lateral meniscus, current injury, left knee
　　● S83.259　Bucket-handle tear of lateral meniscus, current injury, unspecified knee

● S83.26　Peripheral tear of lateral meniscus, current injury
　　● S83.261　Peripheral tear of lateral meniscus, current injury, right knee
　　● S83.262　Peripheral tear of lateral meniscus, current injury, left knee
　　● S83.269　Peripheral tear of lateral meniscus, current injury, unspecified knee

● S83.27　Complex tear of lateral meniscus, current injury
　　● S83.271　Complex tear of lateral meniscus, current injury, right knee
　　● S83.272　Complex tear of lateral meniscus, current injury, left knee
　　● S83.279　Complex tear of lateral meniscus, current injury, unspecified knee

● S83.28　Other tear of lateral meniscus, current injury
　　● S83.281　Other tear of lateral meniscus, current injury, right knee
　　● S83.282　Other tear of lateral meniscus, current injury, left knee
　　● S83.289　Other tear of lateral meniscus, current injury, unspecified knee

● S83.3　Tear of articular cartilage of knee, current
　X ● S83.30　Tear of articular cartilage of unspecified knee, current
　X ● S83.31　Tear of articular cartilage of right knee, current
　X ● S83.32　Tear of articular cartilage of left knee, current

● S83.4　Sprain of collateral ligament of knee
　● S83.40　Sprain of unspecified collateral ligament of knee
　　● S83.401　Sprain of unspecified collateral ligament of right knee
　　● S83.402　Sprain of unspecified collateral ligament of left knee
　　● S83.409　Sprain of unspecified collateral ligament of unspecified knee
　● S83.41　Sprain of medial collateral ligament of knee
　　　　　Sprain of tibial collateral ligament
　　● S83.411　Sprain of medial collateral ligament of right knee
　　● S83.412　Sprain of medial collateral ligament of left knee
　　● S83.419　Sprain of medial collateral ligament of unspecified knee

● S83.42　Sprain of lateral collateral ligament of knee
　　　　Sprain of fibular collateral ligament
　　● S83.421　Sprain of lateral collateral ligament of right knee
　　● S83.422　Sprain of lateral collateral ligament of left knee
　　● S83.429　Sprain of lateral collateral ligament of unspecified knee

● S83.5　Sprain of cruciate ligament of knee
　● S83.50　Sprain of unspecified cruciate ligament of knee
　　● S83.501　Sprain of unspecified cruciate ligament of right knee
　　● S83.502　Sprain of unspecified cruciate ligament of left knee
　　● S83.509　Sprain of unspecified cruciate ligament of unspecified knee
　● S83.51　Sprain of anterior cruciate ligament of knee
　　● S83.511　Sprain of anterior cruciate ligament of right knee
　　● S83.512　Sprain of anterior cruciate ligament of left knee
　　● S83.519　Sprain of anterior cruciate ligament of unspecified knee
　● S83.52　Sprain of posterior cruciate ligament of knee
　　● S83.521　Sprain of posterior cruciate ligament of right knee
　　● S83.522　Sprain of posterior cruciate ligament of left knee
　　● S83.529　Sprain of posterior cruciate ligament of unspecified knee

● S83.6　Sprain of the superior tibiofibular joint and ligament
　X ● S83.60　Sprain of the superior tibiofibular joint and ligament, unspecified knee
　X ● S83.61　Sprain of the superior tibiofibular joint and ligament, right knee
　X ● S83.62　Sprain of the superior tibiofibular joint and ligament, left knee

● S83.8　Sprain of other specified parts of knee
　● S83.8X　Sprain of other specified parts of knee
　　● S83.8X1　Sprain of other specified parts of right knee
　　● S83.8X2　Sprain of other specified parts of left knee
　　● S83.8X9　Sprain of other specified parts of unspecified knee

● S83.9　Sprain of unspecified site of knee
　X ● S83.90　Sprain of unspecified site of unspecified knee
　X ● S83.91　Sprain of unspecified site of right knee
　X ● S83.92　Sprain of unspecified site of left knee

● S84　Injury of nerves at lower leg level
　　Code also any associated open wound (S81.-)
　　Excludes2　injury of nerves at ankle and foot level (S94.-)
　　The appropriate 7th character is to be added to each code from category S84

A	initial encounter
D	subsequent encounter
S	sequela

● S84.0　Injury of tibial nerve at lower leg level
　X ● S84.00　Injury of tibial nerve at lower leg level, unspecified leg
　X ● S84.01　Injury of tibial nerve at lower leg level, right leg
　X ● S84.02　Injury of tibial nerve at lower leg level, left leg

▶ New　⟹ Revised　̶d̶e̶l̶e̶t̶e̶d̶ Deleted　OGCR Official Guidelines　X Assign placeholder X　● Use Additional Character(s)
Excludes 1　Excludes 2　Includes　Use additional　Code first　Code also　Key words

- S84.1   Injury of peroneal nerve at lower leg level
  - X ● S84.10   Injury of peroneal nerve at lower leg level, unspecified leg
  - X ● S84.11   Injury of peroneal nerve at lower leg level, right leg
  - X ● S84.12   Injury of peroneal nerve at lower leg level, left leg
- S84.2   Injury of cutaneous sensory nerve at lower leg level
  - X ● S84.20   Injury of cutaneous sensory nerve at lower leg level, unspecified leg
  - X ● S84.21   Injury of cutaneous sensory nerve at lower leg level, right leg
  - X ● S84.22   Injury of cutaneous sensory nerve at lower leg level, left leg
- S84.8   Injury of other nerves at lower leg level
  - ● S84.80   Injury of other nerves at lower leg level
    - ● S84.801   Injury of other nerves at lower leg level, right leg
    - ● S84.802   Injury of other nerves at lower leg level, left leg
    - ● S84.809   Injury of other nerves at lower leg level, unspecified leg
- S84.9   Injury of unspecified nerve at lower leg level
  - X ● S84.90   Injury of unspecified nerve at lower leg level, unspecified leg
  - X ● S84.91   Injury of unspecified nerve at lower leg level, right leg
  - X ● S84.92   Injury of unspecified nerve at lower leg level, left leg

- ● S85   **Injury of blood vessels at lower leg level**

  Code also any associated open wound (S81.-)

  | Excludes2 | injury of blood vessels at ankle and foot level (S95.-) |

  The appropriate 7th character is to be added to each code from category S85

A	initial encounter
D	subsequent encounter
S	sequela

- S85.0   Injury of popliteal artery
  - ● S85.00   Unspecified injury of popliteal artery
    - ● S85.001   Unspecified injury of popliteal artery, right leg
    - ● S85.002   Unspecified injury of popliteal artery, left leg
    - ● S85.009   Unspecified injury of popliteal artery, unspecified leg
  - ● S85.01   Laceration of popliteal artery
    - ● S85.011   Laceration of popliteal artery, right leg
    - ● S85.012   Laceration of popliteal artery, left leg
    - ● S85.019   Laceration of popliteal artery, unspecified leg
  - ● S85.09   Other specified injury of popliteal artery
    - ● S85.091   Other specified injury of popliteal artery, right leg
    - ● S85.092   Other specified injury of popliteal artery, left leg
    - ● S85.099   Other specified injury of popliteal artery, unspecified leg

- S85.1   Injury of tibial artery
  - ● S85.10   Unspecified injury of unspecified tibial artery
    Injury of tibial artery NOS
    - ● S85.101   Unspecified injury of unspecified tibial artery, right leg
    - ● S85.102   Unspecified injury of unspecified tibial artery, left leg
    - ● S85.109   Unspecified injury of unspecified tibial artery, unspecified leg
  - ● S85.11   Laceration of unspecified tibial artery
    - ● S85.111   Laceration of unspecified tibial artery, right leg
    - ● S85.112   Laceration of unspecified tibial artery, left leg
    - ● S85.119   Laceration of unspecified tibial artery, unspecified leg
  - ● S85.12   Other specified injury of unspecified tibial artery
    - ● S85.121   Other specified injury of unspecified tibial artery, right leg
    - ● S85.122   Other specified injury of unspecified tibial artery, left leg
    - ● S85.129   Other specified injury of unspecified tibial artery, unspecified leg
  - ● S85.13   Unspecified injury of anterior tibial artery
    - ● S85.131   Unspecified injury of anterior tibial artery, right leg
    - ● S85.132   Unspecified injury of anterior tibial artery, left leg
    - ● S85.139   Unspecified injury of anterior tibial artery, unspecified leg
  - ● S85.14   Laceration of anterior tibial artery
    - ● S85.141   Laceration of anterior tibial artery, right leg
    - ● S85.142   Laceration of anterior tibial artery, left leg
    - ● S85.149   Laceration of anterior tibial artery, unspecified leg
  - ● S85.15   Other specified injury of anterior tibial artery
    - ● S85.151   Other specified injury of anterior tibial artery, right leg
    - ● S85.152   Other specified injury of anterior tibial artery, left leg
    - ● S85.159   Other specified injury of anterior tibial artery, unspecified leg
  - ● S85.16   Unspecified injury of posterior tibial artery
    - ● S85.161   Unspecified injury of posterior tibial artery, right leg
    - ● S85.162   Unspecified injury of posterior tibial artery, left leg
    - ● S85.169   Unspecified injury of posterior tibial artery, unspecified leg
  - ● S85.17   Laceration of posterior tibial artery
    - ● S85.171   Laceration of posterior tibial artery, right leg
    - ● S85.172   Laceration of posterior tibial artery, left leg
    - ● S85.179   Laceration of posterior tibial artery, unspecified leg
  - ● S85.18   Other specified injury of posterior tibial artery
    - ● S85.181   Other specified injury of posterior tibial artery, right leg
    - ● S85.182   Other specified injury of posterior tibial artery, left leg
    - ● S85.189   Other specified injury of posterior tibial artery, unspecified leg

● **S85.2**   Injury of peroneal artery
   ● **S85.20**   Unspecified injury of peroneal artery
     ● **S85.201**   Unspecified injury of peroneal artery, right leg
     ● **S85.202**   Unspecified injury of peroneal artery, left leg
     ● **S85.209**   Unspecified injury of peroneal artery, unspecified leg
   ● **S85.21**   Laceration of peroneal artery
     ● **S85.211**   Laceration of peroneal artery, right leg
     ● **S85.212**   Laceration of peroneal artery, left leg
     ● **S85.219**   Laceration of peroneal artery, unspecified leg
   ● **S85.29**   Other specified injury of peroneal artery
     ● **S85.291**   Other specified injury of peroneal artery, right leg
     ● **S85.292**   Other specified injury of peroneal artery, left leg
     ● **S85.299**   Other specified injury of peroneal artery, unspecified leg

● **S85.3**   Injury of greater saphenous vein at lower leg level
     Injury of greater saphenous vein NOS
     Injury of saphenous vein NOS
   ● **S85.30**   Unspecified injury of greater saphenous vein at lower leg level
     ● **S85.301**   Unspecified injury of greater saphenous vein at lower leg level, right leg
     ● **S85.302**   Unspecified injury of greater saphenous vein at lower leg level, left leg
     ● **S85.309**   Unspecified injury of greater saphenous vein at lower leg level, unspecified leg
   ● **S85.31**   Laceration of greater saphenous vein at lower leg level
     ● **S85.311**   Laceration of greater saphenous vein at lower leg level, right leg
     ● **S85.312**   Laceration of greater saphenous vein at lower leg level, left leg
     ● **S85.319**   Laceration of greater saphenous vein at lower leg level, unspecified leg
   ● **S85.39**   Other specified injury of greater saphenous vein at lower leg level
     ● **S85.391**   Other specified injury of greater saphenous vein at lower leg level, right leg
     ● **S85.392**   Other specified injury of greater saphenous vein at lower leg level, left leg
     ● **S85.399**   Other specified injury of greater saphenous vein at lower leg level, unspecified leg

● **S85.4**   Injury of lesser saphenous vein at lower leg level
   ● **S85.40**   Unspecified injury of lesser saphenous vein at lower leg level
     ● **S85.401**   Unspecified injury of lesser saphenous vein at lower leg level, right leg
     ● **S85.402**   Unspecified injury of lesser saphenous vein at lower leg level, left leg
     ● **S85.409**   Unspecified injury of lesser saphenous vein at lower leg level, unspecified leg

● **S85.41**   Laceration of lesser saphenous vein at lower leg level
     ● **S85.411**   Laceration of lesser saphenous vein at lower leg level, right leg
     ● **S85.412**   Laceration of lesser saphenous vein at lower leg level, left leg
     ● **S85.419**   Laceration of lesser saphenous vein at lower leg level, unspecified leg
   ● **S85.49**   Other specified injury of lesser saphenous vein at lower leg level
     ● **S85.491**   Other specified injury of lesser saphenous vein at lower leg level, right leg
     ● **S85.492**   Other specified injury of lesser saphenous vein at lower leg level, left leg
     ● **S85.499**   Other specified injury of lesser saphenous vein at lower leg level, unspecified leg

● **S85.5**   Injury of popliteal vein
   ● **S85.50**   Unspecified injury of popliteal vein
     ● **S85.501**   Unspecified injury of popliteal vein, right leg
     ● **S85.502**   Unspecified injury of popliteal vein, left leg
     ● **S85.509**   Unspecified injury of popliteal vein, unspecified leg
   ● **S85.51**   Laceration of popliteal vein
     ● **S85.511**   Laceration of popliteal vein, right leg
     ● **S85.512**   Laceration of popliteal vein, left leg
     ● **S85.519**   Laceration of popliteal vein, unspecified leg
   ● **S85.59**   Other specified injury of popliteal vein
     ● **S85.591**   Other specified injury of popliteal vein, right leg
     ● **S85.592**   Other specified injury of popliteal vein, left leg
     ● **S85.599**   Other specified injury of popliteal vein, unspecified leg

● **S85.8**   Injury of other blood vessels at lower leg level
   ● **S85.80**   Unspecified injury of other blood vessels at lower leg level
     ● **S85.801**   Unspecified injury of other blood vessels at lower leg level, right leg
     ● **S85.802**   Unspecified injury of other blood vessels at lower leg level, left leg
     ● **S85.809**   Unspecified injury of other blood vessels at lower leg level, unspecified leg
   ● **S85.81**   Laceration of other blood vessels at lower leg level
     ● **S85.811**   Laceration of other blood vessels at lower leg level, right leg
     ● **S85.812**   Laceration of other blood vessels at lower leg level, left leg
     ● **S85.819**   Laceration of other blood vessels at lower leg level, unspecified leg
   ● **S85.89**   Other specified injury of other blood vessels at lower leg level
     ● **S85.891**   Other specified injury of other blood vessels at lower leg level, right leg
     ● **S85.892**   Other specified injury of other blood vessels at lower leg level, left leg
     ● **S85.899**   Other specified injury of other blood vessels at lower leg level, unspecified leg

▶ New   ⇒ Revised   ~~deleted~~ Deleted   **OGCR** Official Guidelines   X Assign placeholder X   ● Use Additional Character(s)

Excludes 1   Excludes 2   Includes   Use additional   Code first   Code also   Key words

● **S85.9**   Injury of unspecified blood vessel at lower leg level

   ● **S85.90**   Unspecified injury of unspecified blood vessel at lower leg level

     ● **S85.901**   Unspecified injury of unspecified blood vessel at lower leg level, right leg

     ● **S85.902**   Unspecified injury of unspecified blood vessel at lower leg level, left leg

     ● **S85.909**   Unspecified injury of unspecified blood vessel at lower leg level, unspecified leg

   ● **S85.91**   Laceration of unspecified blood vessel at lower leg level

     ● **S85.911**   Laceration of unspecified blood vessel at lower leg level, right leg

     ● **S85.912**   Laceration of unspecified blood vessel at lower leg level, left leg

     ● **S85.919**   Laceration of unspecified blood vessel at lower leg level, unspecified leg

   ● **S85.99**   Other specified injury of unspecified blood vessel at lower leg level

     ● **S85.991**   Other specified injury of unspecified blood vessel at lower leg level, right leg

     ● **S85.992**   Other specified injury of unspecified blood vessel at lower leg level, left leg

     ● **S85.999**   Other specified injury of unspecified blood vessel at lower leg level, unspecified leg

● **S86**   Injury of muscle, fascia and tendon at lower leg level

   Code also any associated open wound (S81.-)

   Excludes2   injury of muscle, fascia and tendon at ankle (S96.-)
       injury of patellar ligament (tendon) (S76.1-)
       sprain of joints and ligaments of knee (S83.-)

   The appropriate 7th character is to be added to each code from category S86

     A   initial encounter
     D   subsequent encounter
     S   sequela

   ● **S86.0**   Injury of Achilles tendon

     ● **S86.00**   Unspecified injury of Achilles tendon

       ● **S86.001**   Unspecified injury of right Achilles tendon

       ● **S86.002**   Unspecified injury of left Achilles tendon

       ● **S86.009**   Unspecified injury of unspecified Achilles tendon

     ● **S86.01**   Strain of Achilles tendon

       ● **S86.011**   Strain of right Achilles tendon

       ● **S86.012**   Strain of left Achilles tendon

       ● **S86.019**   Strain of unspecified Achilles tendon

     ● **S86.02**   Laceration of Achilles tendon

       ● **S86.021**   Laceration of right Achilles tendon

       ● **S86.022**   Laceration of left Achilles tendon

       ● **S86.029**   Laceration of unspecified Achilles tendon

     ● **S86.09**   Other specified injury of Achilles tendon

       ● **S86.091**   Other specified injury of right Achilles tendon

       ● **S86.092**   Other specified injury of left Achilles tendon

       ● **S86.099**   Other specified injury of unspecified Achilles tendon

● **S86.1**   Injury of other muscle(s) and tendon(s) of posterior muscle group at lower leg level

   ● **S86.10**   Unspecified injury of other muscle(s) and tendon(s) of posterior muscle group at lower leg level

     ● **S86.101**   Unspecified injury of other muscle(s) and tendon(s) of posterior muscle group at lower leg level, right leg

     ● **S86.102**   Unspecified injury of other muscle(s) and tendon(s) of posterior muscle group at lower leg level, left leg

     ● **S86.109**   Unspecified injury of other muscle(s) and tendon(s) of posterior muscle group at lower leg level, unspecified leg

   ● **S86.11**   Strain of other muscle(s) and tendon(s) of posterior muscle group at lower leg level

     ● **S86.111**   Strain of other muscle(s) and tendon(s) of posterior muscle group at lower leg level, right leg

     ● **S86.112**   Strain of other muscle(s) and tendon(s) of posterior muscle group at lower leg level, left leg

     ● **S86.119**   Strain of other muscle(s) and tendon(s) of posterior muscle group at lower leg level, unspecified leg

   ● **S86.12**   Laceration of other muscle(s) and tendon(s) of posterior muscle group at lower leg level

     ● **S86.121**   Laceration of other muscle(s) and tendon(s) of posterior muscle group at lower leg level, right leg

     ● **S86.122**   Laceration of other muscle(s) and tendon(s) of posterior muscle group at lower leg level, left leg

     ● **S86.129**   Laceration of other muscle(s) and tendon(s) of posterior muscle group at lower leg level, unspecified leg

   ● **S86.19**   Other injury of other muscle(s) and tendon(s) of posterior muscle group at lower leg level

     ● **S86.191**   Other injury of other muscle(s) and tendon(s) of posterior muscle group at lower leg level, right leg

     ● **S86.192**   Other injury of other muscle(s) and tendon(s) of posterior muscle group at lower leg level, left leg

     ● **S86.199**   Other injury of other muscle(s) and tendon(s) of posterior muscle group at lower leg level, unspecified leg

● **S86.2**   Injury of muscle(s) and tendon(s) of anterior muscle group at lower leg level

   ● **S86.20**   Unspecified injury of muscle(s) and tendon(s) of anterior muscle group at lower leg level

     ● **S86.201**   Unspecified injury of muscle(s) and tendon(s) of anterior muscle group at lower leg level, right leg

     ● **S86.202**   Unspecified injury of muscle(s) and tendon(s) of anterior muscle group at lower leg level, left leg

     ● **S86.209**   Unspecified injury of muscle(s) and tendon(s) of anterior muscle group at lower leg level, unspecified leg

   ● **S86.21**   Strain of muscle(s) and tendon(s) of anterior muscle group at lower leg level

     ● **S86.211**   Strain of muscle(s) and tendon(s) of anterior muscle group at lower leg level, right leg

     ● **S86.212**   Strain of muscle(s) and tendon(s) of anterior muscle group at lower leg level, left leg

     ● **S86.219**   Strain of muscle(s) and tendon(s) of anterior muscle group at lower leg level, unspecified leg

- ● S86.22   Laceration of muscle(s) and tendon(s) of anterior muscle group at lower leg level
  - ● S86.221   Laceration of muscle(s) and tendon(s) of anterior muscle group at lower leg level, right leg
  - ● S86.222   Laceration of muscle(s) and tendon(s) of anterior muscle group at lower leg level, left leg
  - ● S86.229   Laceration of muscle(s) and tendon(s) of anterior muscle group at lower leg level, unspecified leg
- ● S86.29   Other injury of muscle(s) and tendon(s) of anterior muscle group at lower leg level
  - ● S86.291   Other injury of muscle(s) and tendon(s) of anterior muscle group at lower leg level, right leg
  - ● S86.292   Other injury of muscle(s) and tendon(s) of anterior muscle group at lower leg level, left leg
  - ● S86.299   Other injury of muscle(s) and tendon(s) of anterior muscle group at lower leg level, unspecified leg
- ● S86.3   Injury of muscle(s) and tendon(s) of peroneal muscle group at lower leg level
  - ● S86.30   Unspecified injury of muscle(s) and tendon(s) of peroneal muscle group at lower leg level
    - ● S86.301   Unspecified injury of muscle(s) and tendon(s) of peroneal muscle group at lower leg level, right leg
    - ● S86.302   Unspecified injury of muscle(s) and tendon(s) of peroneal muscle group at lower leg level, left leg
    - ● S86.309   Unspecified injury of muscle(s) and tendon(s) of peroneal muscle group at lower leg level, unspecified leg
  - ● S86.31   Strain of muscle(s) and tendon(s) of peroneal muscle group at lower leg level
    - ● S86.311   Strain of muscle(s) and tendon(s) of peroneal muscle group at lower leg level, right leg
    - ● S86.312   Strain of muscle(s) and tendon(s) of peroneal muscle group at lower leg level, left leg
    - ● S86.319   Strain of muscle(s) and tendon(s) of peroneal muscle group at lower leg level, unspecified leg
  - ● S86.32   Laceration of muscle(s) and tendon(s) of peroneal muscle group at lower leg level
    - ● S86.321   Laceration of muscle(s) and tendon(s) of peroneal muscle group at lower leg level, right leg
    - ● S86.322   Laceration of muscle(s) and tendon(s) of peroneal muscle group at lower leg level, left leg
    - ● S86.329   Laceration of muscle(s) and tendon(s) of peroneal muscle group at lower leg level, unspecified leg
  - ● S86.39   Other injury of muscle(s) and tendon(s) of peroneal muscle group at lower leg level
    - ● S86.391   Other injury of muscle(s) and tendon(s) of peroneal muscle group at lower leg level, right leg
    - ● S86.392   Other injury of muscle(s) and tendon(s) of peroneal muscle group at lower leg level, left leg
    - ● S86.399   Other injury of muscle(s) and tendon(s) of peroneal muscle group at lower leg level, unspecified leg

- ● S86.8   Injury of other muscles and tendons at lower leg level
  - ● S86.80   Unspecified injury of other muscles and tendons at lower leg level
    - ● S86.801   Unspecified injury of other muscle(s) and tendon(s) at lower leg level, right leg
    - ● S86.802   Unspecified injury of other muscle(s) and tendon(s) at lower leg level, left leg
    - ● S86.809   Unspecified injury of other muscle(s) and tendon(s) at lower leg level, unspecified leg
  - ● S86.81   Strain of other muscles and tendons at lower leg level
    - ● S86.811   Strain of other muscle(s) and tendon(s) at lower leg level, right leg
    - ● S86.812   Strain of other muscle(s) and tendon(s) at lower leg level, left leg
    - ● S86.819   Strain of other muscle(s) and tendon(s) at lower leg level, unspecified leg
  - ● S86.82   Laceration of other muscles and tendons at lower leg level
    - ● S86.821   Laceration of other muscle(s) and tendon(s) at lower leg level, right leg
    - ● S86.822   Laceration of other muscle(s) and tendon(s) at lower leg level, left leg
    - ● S86.829   Laceration of other muscle(s) and tendon(s) at lower leg level, unspecified leg
  - ● S86.89   Other injury of other muscles and tendons at lower leg level
    - ● S86.891   Other injury of other muscle(s) and tendon(s) at lower leg level, right leg
    - ● S86.892   Other injury of other muscle(s) and tendon(s) at lower leg level, left leg
    - ● S86.899   Other injury of other muscle(s) and tendon(s) at lower leg level, unspecified leg
- ● S86.9   Injury of unspecified muscle and tendon at lower leg level
  - ● S86.90   Unspecified injury of unspecified muscle and tendon at lower leg level
    - ● S86.901   Unspecified injury of unspecified muscle(s) and tendon(s) at lower leg level, right leg
    - ● S86.902   Unspecified injury of unspecified muscle(s) and tendon(s) at lower leg level, left leg
    - ● S86.909   Unspecified injury of unspecified muscle(s) and tendon(s) at lower leg level, unspecified leg
  - ● S86.91   Strain of unspecified muscle and tendon at lower leg level
    - ● S86.911   Strain of unspecified muscle(s) and tendon(s) at lower leg level, right leg
    - ● S86.912   Strain of unspecified muscle(s) and tendon(s) at lower leg level, left leg
    - ● S86.919   Strain of unspecified muscle(s) and tendon(s) at lower leg level, unspecified leg
  - ● S86.92   Laceration of unspecified muscle and tendon at lower leg level
    - ● S86.921   Laceration of unspecified muscle(s) and tendon(s) at lower leg level, right leg
    - ● S86.922   Laceration of unspecified muscle(s) and tendon(s) at lower leg level, left leg
    - ● S86.929   Laceration of unspecified muscle(s) and tendon(s) at lower leg level, unspecified leg

▶ New   ⇒ Revised   ~~deleted~~ Deleted   OGCR Official Guidelines   X Assign placeholder X   ● Use Additional Character(s)

Excludes 1   Excludes 2   Includes   Use additional   Code first   Code also   Key words

● **S86.99** Other injury of unspecified muscle and tendon at lower leg level
   ● **S86.991** Other injury of unspecified muscle(s) and tendon(s) at lower leg level, right leg
   ● **S86.992** Other injury of unspecified muscle(s) and tendon(s) at lower leg level, left leg
   ● **S86.999** Other injury of unspecified muscle(s) and tendon(s) at lower leg level, unspecified leg

● **S87** Crushing injury of lower leg
   Use additional code(s) for all associated injuries
   Excludes2   crushing injury of ankle and foot (S97.-)
   The appropriate 7th character is to be added to each code from category S87

A	initial encounter
D	subsequent encounter
S	sequela

  ● **S87.0** Crushing injury of knee
   X● **S87.00** Crushing injury of unspecified knee
   X● **S87.01** Crushing injury of right knee
   X● **S87.02** Crushing injury of left knee
  ● **S87.8** Crushing injury of lower leg
   X● **S87.80** Crushing injury of unspecified lower leg
   X● **S87.81** Crushing injury of right lower leg
   X● **S87.82** Crushing injury of left lower leg

● **S88** Traumatic amputation of lower leg
   An amputation not identified as partial or complete should be coded to complete
   Excludes1   traumatic amputation of ankle and foot (S98.-)
   The appropriate 7th character is to be added to each code from category S88

A	initial encounter
D	subsequent encounter
S	sequela

  ● **S88.0** Traumatic amputation at knee level
   ● **S88.01** Complete traumatic amputation at knee level
    ● **S88.011** Complete traumatic amputation at knee level, right lower leg
    ● **S88.012** Complete traumatic amputation at knee level, left lower leg
    ● **S88.019** Complete traumatic amputation at knee level, unspecified lower leg
   ● **S88.02** Partial traumatic amputation at knee level
    ● **S88.021** Partial traumatic amputation at knee level, right lower leg
    ● **S88.022** Partial traumatic amputation at knee level, left lower leg
    ● **S88.029** Partial traumatic amputation at knee level, unspecified lower leg
  ● **S88.1** Traumatic amputation at level between knee and ankle
   ● **S88.11** Complete traumatic amputation at level between knee and ankle
    ● **S88.111** Complete traumatic amputation at level between knee and ankle, right lower leg
    ● **S88.112** Complete traumatic amputation at level between knee and ankle, left lower leg
    ● **S88.119** Complete traumatic amputation at level between knee and ankle, unspecified lower leg

   ● **S88.12** Partial traumatic amputation at level between knee and ankle
    ● **S88.121** Partial traumatic amputation at level between knee and ankle, right lower leg
    ● **S88.122** Partial traumatic amputation at level between knee and ankle, left lower leg
    ● **S88.129** Partial traumatic amputation at level between knee and ankle, unspecified lower leg
  ● **S88.9** Traumatic amputation of lower leg, level unspecified
   ● **S88.91** Complete traumatic amputation of lower leg, level unspecified
    ● **S88.911** Complete traumatic amputation of right lower leg, level unspecified
    ● **S88.912** Complete traumatic amputation of left lower leg, level unspecified
    ● **S88.919** Complete traumatic amputation of unspecified lower leg, level unspecified
   ● **S88.92** Partial traumatic amputation of lower leg, level unspecified
    ● **S88.921** Partial traumatic amputation of right lower leg, level unspecified
    ● **S88.922** Partial traumatic amputation of left lower leg, level unspecified
    ● **S88.929** Partial traumatic amputation of unspecified lower leg, level unspecified

● **S89** Other and unspecified injuries of lower leg
   Note: A fracture not indicated as open or closed should be coded to closed
   Excludes2   other and unspecified injuries of ankle and foot (S99.-)
   The appropriate 7th character is to be added to each code from subcategories S89.0, S89.1, S89.2, and S89.3

A	initial encounter for closed fracture
D	subsequent encounter for fracture with routine healing
G	subsequent encounter for fracture with delayed healing
K	subsequent encounter for fracture with nonunion
P	subsequent encounter for fracture with malunion
S	sequela

  ● **S89.0** Physeal fracture of upper end of tibia
   ● **S89.00** Unspecified physeal fracture of upper end of tibia
    ● **S89.001** Unspecified physeal fracture of upper end of right tibia
    ● **S89.002** Unspecified physeal fracture of upper end of left tibia
    ● **S89.009** Unspecified physeal fracture of upper end of unspecified tibia
   ● **S89.01** Salter-Harris Type I physeal fracture of upper end of tibia
    ● **S89.011** Salter-Harris Type I physeal fracture of upper end of right tibia
    ● **S89.012** Salter-Harris Type I physeal fracture of upper end of left tibia
    ● **S89.019** Salter-Harris Type I physeal fracture of upper end of unspecified tibia
   ● **S89.02** Salter-Harris Type II physeal fracture of upper end of tibia
    ● **S89.021** Salter-Harris Type II physeal fracture of upper end of right tibia
    ● **S89.022** Salter-Harris Type II physeal fracture of upper end of left tibia
    ● **S89.029** Salter-Harris Type II physeal fracture of upper end of unspecified tibia

CHAPTER 19 (S00-T88)

● S89.Ø3   **Salter-Harris Type III** physeal fracture of upper end of tibia

  ● S89.Ø31   Salter-Harris Type III physeal fracture of upper end of **right** tibia

  ● S89.Ø32   Salter-Harris Type III physeal fracture of upper end of **left** tibia

  ● S89.Ø39   Salter-Harris Type III physeal fracture of upper end of **unspecified** tibia

● S89.Ø4   **Salter-Harris Type IV** physeal fracture of upper end of tibia

  ● S89.Ø41   Salter-Harris Type IV physeal fracture of upper end of **right** tibia

  ● S89.Ø42   Salter-Harris Type IV physeal fracture of upper end of **left** tibia

  ● S89.Ø49   Salter-Harris Type IV physeal fracture of upper end of **unspecified** tibia

● S89.Ø9   **Other** physeal fracture of upper end of tibia

  ● S89.Ø91   Other physeal fracture of upper end of **right** tibia

  ● S89.Ø92   Other physeal fracture of upper end of **left** tibia

  ● S89.Ø99   Other physeal fracture of upper end of **unspecified** tibia

● S89.1   **Physeal** fracture of **lower end of tibia**

  ● S89.1Ø   **Unspecified** physeal fracture of lower end of tibia

    ● S89.1Ø1   Unspecified physeal fracture of lower end of **right** tibia

    ● S89.1Ø2   Unspecified physeal fracture of lower end of **left** tibia

    ● S89.1Ø9   Unspecified physeal fracture of lower end of **unspecified** tibia

  ● S89.11   **Salter-Harris Type I** physeal fracture of lower end of tibia

    ● S89.111   Salter-Harris Type I physeal fracture of lower end of **right** tibia

    ● S89.112   Salter-Harris Type I physeal fracture of lower end of **left** tibia

    ● S89.119   Salter-Harris Type I physeal fracture of lower end of **unspecified** tibia

  ● S89.12   **Salter-Harris Type II** physeal fracture of lower end of tibia

    ● S89.121   Salter-Harris Type II physeal fracture of lower end of **right** tibia

    ● S89.122   Salter-Harris Type II physeal fracture of lower end of **left** tibia

    ● S89.129   Salter-Harris Type II physeal fracture of lower end of **unspecified** tibia

  ● S89.13   **Salter-Harris Type III** physeal fracture of lower end of tibia

    Excludes1   fracture of medial malleolus (adult) (S82.5-)

    ● S89.131   Salter-Harris Type III physeal fracture of lower end of **right** tibia

    ● S89.132   Salter-Harris Type III physeal fracture of lower end of **left** tibia

    ● S89.139   Salter-Harris Type III physeal fracture of lower end of **unspecified** tibia

  ● S89.14   **Salter-Harris Type IV** physeal fracture of lower end of tibia

    Excludes1   fracture of medial malleolus (adult) (S82.5-)

    ● S89.141   Salter-Harris Type IV physeal fracture of lower end of **right** tibia

    ● S89.142   Salter-Harris Type IV physeal fracture of lower end of **left** tibia

    ● S89.149   Salter-Harris Type IV physeal fracture of lower end of **unspecified** tibia

● S89.19   **Other** physeal fracture of lower end of tibia

  ● S89.191   Other physeal fracture of lower end of **right** tibia

  ● S89.192   Other physeal fracture of lower end of **left** tibia

  ● S89.199   Other physeal fracture of lower end of **unspecified** tibia

● S89.2   **Physeal** fracture of **upper end of fibula**

  ● S89.2Ø   **Unspecified** physeal fracture of upper end of fibula

    ● S89.2Ø1   Unspecified physeal fracture of upper end of **right** fibula

    ● S89.2Ø2   Unspecified physeal fracture of upper end of **left** fibula

    ● S89.2Ø9   Unspecified physeal fracture of upper end of **unspecified** fibula

  ● S89.21   **Salter-Harris Type I** physeal fracture of upper end of fibula

    ● S89.211   Salter-Harris Type I physeal fracture of upper end of **right** fibula

    ● S89.212   Salter-Harris Type I physeal fracture of upper end of **left** fibula

    ● S89.219   Salter-Harris Type I physeal fracture of upper end of **unspecified** fibula

  ● S89.22   **Salter-Harris Type II** physeal fracture of upper end of fibula

    ● S89.221   Salter-Harris Type II physeal fracture of upper end of **right** fibula

    ● S89.222   Salter-Harris Type II physeal fracture of upper end of **left** fibula

    ● S89.229   Salter-Harris Type II physeal fracture of upper end of **unspecified** fibula

  ● S89.29   **Other** physeal fracture of upper end of fibula

    ● S89.291   Other physeal fracture of upper end of **right** fibula

    ● S89.292   Other physeal fracture of upper end of **left** fibula

    ● S89.299   Other physeal fracture of upper end of **unspecified** fibula

● S89.3   **Physeal** fracture of **lower end of fibula**

  ● S89.3Ø   **Unspecified** physeal fracture of lower end of fibula

    ● S89.3Ø1   Unspecified physeal fracture of lower end of **right** fibula

    ● S89.3Ø2   Unspecified physeal fracture of lower end of **left** fibula

    ● S89.3Ø9   Unspecified physeal fracture of lower end of **unspecified** fibula

  ● S89.31   **Salter-Harris Type I** physeal fracture of lower end of fibula

    ● S89.311   Salter-Harris Type I physeal fracture of lower end of **right** fibula

    ● S89.312   Salter-Harris Type I physeal fracture of lower end of **left** fibula

    ● S89.319   Salter-Harris Type I physeal fracture of lower end of **unspecified** fibula

  ● S89.32   **Salter-Harris Type II** physeal fracture of lower end of fibula

    ● S89.321   Salter-Harris Type II physeal fracture of lower end of **right** fibula

    ● S89.322   Salter-Harris Type II physeal fracture of lower end of **left** fibula

    ● S89.329   Salter-Harris Type II physeal fracture of lower end of **unspecified** fibula

▶ New   ⇒ Revised   ~~deleted~~ Deleted   **OGCR** Official Guidelines   X Assign placeholder X   ● Use Additional Character(s)

Excludes 1   Excludes 2   Includes   Use additional   Code first   Code also   Key words

● **S89.39**   Other physeal fracture of lower end of fibula

   ● **S89.391**   Other physeal fracture of lower end of right fibula

   ● **S89.392**   Other physeal fracture of lower end of left fibula

   ● **S89.399**   Other physeal fracture of lower end of unspecified fibula

● **S89.8**   Other specified injuries of lower leg

> The appropriate 7th character is to be added to each code in subcategory S89.8

> | | |
> |---|---|
> | A | initial encounter |
> | D | subsequent encounter |
> | S | sequela |

   X ● **S89.80**   Other specified injuries of unspecified lower leg

   X ● **S89.81**   Other specified injuries of right lower leg

   X ● **S89.82**   Other specified injuries of left lower leg

● **S89.9**   Unspecified injury of lower leg

> The appropriate 7th character is to be added to each code in subcategory S89.9

> | | |
> |---|---|
> | A | initial encounter |
> | D | subsequent encounter |
> | S | sequela |

   X ● **S89.90**   Unspecified injury of unspecified lower leg

   X ● **S89.91**   Unspecified injury of right lower leg

   X ● **S89.92**   Unspecified injury of left lower leg

INJURIES TO THE ANKLE AND FOOT (S90-S99)

Excludes2	burns and corrosions (T20-T32)
	fracture of ankle and malleolus (S82.-)
	frostbite (T33-T34)
	insect bite or sting, venomous (T63.4)

● **S90**   Superficial injury of ankle, foot and toes

> The appropriate 7th character is to be added to each code from category S90

> | | |
> |---|---|
> | A | initial encounter |
> | D | subsequent encounter |
> | S | sequela |

● **S90.0**   Contusion of ankle

   X ● **S90.00**   Contusion of unspecified ankle

   X ● **S90.01**   Contusion of right ankle

   X ● **S90.02**   Contusion of left ankle

● **S90.1**   Contusion of toe without damage to nail

  ● **S90.11**   Contusion of great toe without damage to nail

   ● **S90.111**   Contusion of right great toe without damage to nail

   ● **S90.112**   Contusion of left great toe without damage to nail

   ● **S90.119**   Contusion of unspecified great toe without damage to nail

  ● **S90.12**   Contusion of lesser toe without damage to nail

   ● **S90.121**   Contusion of right lesser toe(s) without damage to nail

   ● **S90.122**   Contusion of left lesser toe(s) without damage to nail

   ● **S90.129**   Contusion of unspecified lesser toe(s) without damage to nail
> Contusion of toe NOS

● **S90.2**   Contusion of toe with damage to nail

  ● **S90.21**   Contusion of great toe with damage to nail

   ● **S90.211**   Contusion of right great toe with damage to nail

   ● **S90.212**   Contusion of left great toe with damage to nail

   ● **S90.219**   Contusion of unspecified great toe with damage to nail

  ● **S90.22**   Contusion of lesser toe with damage to nail

   ● **S90.221**   Contusion of right lesser toe(s) with damage to nail

   ● **S90.222**   Contusion of left lesser toe(s) with damage to nail

   ● **S90.229**   Contusion of unspecified lesser toe(s) with damage to nail

● **S90.3**   Contusion of foot

> | Excludes2 | contusion of toes (S90.1-, S90.2-) |
> |---|---|

   X ● **S90.30**   Contusion of unspecified foot
> Contusion of foot NOS

   X ● **S90.31**   Contusion of right foot

   X ● **S90.32**   Contusion of left foot

● **S90.4**   Other superficial injuries of toe

  ● **S90.41**   Abrasion of toe

   ● **S90.411**   Abrasion, right great toe

   ● **S90.412**   Abrasion, left great toe

   ● **S90.413**   Abrasion, unspecified great toe

   ● **S90.414**   Abrasion, right lesser toe(s)

   ● **S90.415**   Abrasion, left lesser toe(s)

   ● **S90.416**   Abrasion, unspecified lesser toe(s)

  ● **S90.42**   Blister (nonthermal) of toe

   ● **S90.421**   Blister (nonthermal), right great toe

   ● **S90.422**   Blister (nonthermal), left great toe

   ● **S90.423**   Blister (nonthermal), unspecified great toe

   ● **S90.424**   Blister (nonthermal), right lesser toe(s)

   ● **S90.425**   Blister (nonthermal), left lesser toe(s)

   ● **S90.426**   Blister (nonthermal), unspecified lesser toe(s)

  ● **S90.44**   External constriction of toe
> Hair tourniquet syndrome of toe

   ● **S90.441**   External constriction, right great toe

   ● **S90.442**   External constriction, left great toe

   ● **S90.443**   External constriction, unspecified great toe

   ● **S90.444**   External constriction, right lesser toe(s)

   ● **S90.445**   External constriction, left lesser toe(s)

   ● **S90.446**   External constriction, unspecified lesser toe(s)

  ● **S90.45**   Superficial foreign body of toe
> Splinter in the toe

   ● **S90.451**   Superficial foreign body, right great toe

   ● **S90.452**   Superficial foreign body, left great toe

   ● **S90.453**   Superficial foreign body, unspecified great toe

   ● **S90.454**   Superficial foreign body, right lesser toe(s)

   ● **S90.455**   Superficial foreign body, left lesser toe(s)

   ● **S90.456**   Superficial foreign body, unspecified lesser toe(s)

- S90.46 Insect bite (nonvenomous) of toe
  - S90.461 Insect bite (nonvenomous), right great toe
  - S90.462 Insect bite (nonvenomous), left great toe
  - S90.463 Insect bite (nonvenomous), unspecified great toe
  - S90.464 Insect bite (nonvenomous), right lesser toe(s)
  - S90.465 Insect bite (nonvenomous), left lesser toe(s)
  - S90.466 Insect bite (nonvenomous), unspecified lesser toe(s)
- S90.47 Other superficial bite of toe
  - **Excludes1** open bite of toe (S91.15-, S91.25-)
  - S90.471 Other superficial bite of right great toe
  - S90.472 Other superficial bite of left great toe
  - S90.473 Other superficial bite of unspecified great toe
  - S90.474 Other superficial bite of right lesser toe(s)
  - S90.475 Other superficial bite of left lesser toe(s)
  - S90.476 Other superficial bite of unspecified lesser toe(s)
- S90.5 Other superficial injuries of ankle
  - S90.51 Abrasion of ankle
    - S90.511 Abrasion, right ankle
    - S90.512 Abrasion, left ankle
    - S90.519 Abrasion, unspecified ankle
  - S90.52 Blister (nonthermal) of ankle
    - S90.521 Blister (nonthermal), right ankle
    - S90.522 Blister (nonthermal), left ankle
    - S90.529 Blister (nonthermal), unspecified ankle
  - S90.54 External constriction of ankle
    - S90.541 External constriction, right ankle
    - S90.542 External constriction, left ankle
    - S90.549 External constriction, unspecified ankle
  - S90.55 Superficial foreign body of ankle
    Splinter in the ankle
    - S90.551 Superficial foreign body, right ankle
    - S90.552 Superficial foreign body, left ankle
    - S90.559 Superficial foreign body, unspecified ankle
  - S90.56 Insect bite (nonvenomous) of ankle
    - S90.561 Insect bite (nonvenomous), right ankle
    - S90.562 Insect bite (nonvenomous), left ankle
    - S90.569 Insect bite (nonvenomous), unspecified ankle
  - S90.57 Other superficial bite of ankle
    - **Excludes1** open bite of ankle (S91.05-)
    - S90.571 Other superficial bite of ankle, right ankle
    - S90.572 Other superficial bite of ankle, left ankle
    - S90.579 Other superficial bite of ankle, unspecified ankle

- S90.8 Other superficial injuries of foot
  - S90.81 Abrasion of foot
    - S90.811 Abrasion, right foot
    - S90.812 Abrasion, left foot
    - S90.819 Abrasion, unspecified foot
  - S90.82 Blister (nonthermal) of foot
    - S90.821 Blister (nonthermal), right foot
    - S90.822 Blister (nonthermal), left foot
    - S90.829 Blister (nonthermal), unspecified foot
  - S90.84 External constriction of foot
    - S90.841 External constriction, right foot
    - S90.842 External constriction, left foot
    - S90.849 External constriction, unspecified foot
  - S90.85 Superficial foreign body of foot
    Splinter in the foot
    - S90.851 Superficial foreign body, right foot
    - S90.852 Superficial foreign body, left foot
    - S90.859 Superficial foreign body, unspecified foot
  - S90.86 Insect bite (nonvenomous) of foot
    - S90.861 Insect bite (nonvenomous), right foot
    - S90.862 Insect bite (nonvenomous), left foot
    - S90.869 Insect bite (nonvenomous), unspecified foot
  - S90.87 Other superficial bite of foot
    - **Excludes1** open bite of foot (S91.35-)
    - S90.871 Other superficial bite of right foot
    - S90.872 Other superficial bite of left foot
    - S90.879 Other superficial bite of unspecified foot
- S90.9 Unspecified superficial injury of ankle, foot and toe
  - S90.91 Unspecified superficial injury of ankle
    - S90.911 Unspecified superficial injury of right ankle
    - S90.912 Unspecified superficial injury of left ankle
    - S90.919 Unspecified superficial injury of unspecified ankle
  - S90.92 Unspecified superficial injury of foot
    - S90.921 Unspecified superficial injury of right foot
    - S90.922 Unspecified superficial injury of left foot
    - S90.929 Unspecified superficial injury of unspecified foot
  - S90.93 Unspecified superficial injury of toes
    - S90.931 Unspecified superficial injury of right great toe
    - S90.932 Unspecified superficial injury of left great toe
    - S90.933 Unspecified superficial injury of unspecified great toe
    - S90.934 Unspecified superficial injury of right lesser toe(s)
    - S90.935 Unspecified superficial injury of left lesser toe(s)
    - S90.936 Unspecified superficial injury of unspecified lesser toe(s)

▶ New   ⇒ Revised   ~~deleted~~ Deleted   **OGCR** Official Guidelines   X Assign placeholder X   ● Use Additional Character(s)
Excludes 1   Excludes 2   Includes   Use additional   Code first   Code also   Key words

● **S91   Open wound of ankle, foot and toes**

   Code also any associated wound infection

   | Excludes1 | open fracture of ankle, foot and toes (S92.-with 7th character B)
   traumatic amputation of ankle and foot (S98.-)

   The appropriate 7th character is to be added to each code from category S91

   > A   initial encounter
   > D   subsequent encounter
   > S   sequela

● **S91.0   Open wound of ankle**

  ● **S91.00   Unspecified open wound of ankle**
     ● S91.001   Unspecified open wound, right ankle
     ● S91.002   Unspecified open wound, left ankle
     ● S91.009   Unspecified open wound, unspecified ankle

  ● **S91.01   Laceration without foreign body of ankle**
     ● S91.011   Laceration without foreign body, right ankle
     ● S91.012   Laceration without foreign body, left ankle
     ● S91.019   Laceration without foreign body, unspecified ankle

  ● **S91.02   Laceration with foreign body of ankle**
     ● S91.021   Laceration with foreign body, right ankle
     ● S91.022   Laceration with foreign body, left ankle
     ● S91.029   Laceration with foreign body, unspecified ankle

  ● **S91.03   Puncture wound without foreign body of ankle**
     ● S91.031   Puncture wound without foreign body, right ankle
     ● S91.032   Puncture wound without foreign body, left ankle
     ● S91.039   Puncture wound without foreign body, unspecified ankle

  ● **S91.04   Puncture wound with foreign body of ankle**
     ● S91.041   Puncture wound with foreign body, right ankle
     ● S91.042   Puncture wound with foreign body, left ankle
     ● S91.049   Puncture wound with foreign body, unspecified ankle

  ● **S91.05   Open bite of ankle**
        | Excludes1 | superficial bite of ankle (S90.56-, S90.57-)
     ● S91.051   Open bite, right ankle
     ● S91.052   Open bite, left ankle
     ● S91.059   Open bite, unspecified ankle

● **S91.1   Open wound of toe without damage to nail**

  ● **S91.10   Unspecified open wound of toe without damage to nail**
     ● S91.101   Unspecified open wound of right great toe without damage to nail
     ● S91.102   Unspecified open wound of left great toe without damage to nail
     ● S91.103   Unspecified open wound of unspecified great toe without damage to nail
     ● S91.104   Unspecified open wound of right lesser toe(s) without damage to nail
     ● S91.105   Unspecified open wound of left lesser toe(s) without damage to nail
     ● S91.106   Unspecified open wound of unspecified lesser toe(s) without damage to nail
     ● S91.109   Unspecified open wound of unspecified toe(s) without damage to nail

  ● **S91.11   Laceration without foreign body of toe without damage to nail**
     ● S91.111   Laceration without foreign body of right great toe without damage to nail
     ● S91.112   Laceration without foreign body of left great toe without damage to nail
     ● S91.113   Laceration without foreign body of unspecified great toe without damage to nail
     ● S91.114   Laceration without foreign body of right lesser toe(s) without damage to nail
     ● S91.115   Laceration without foreign body of left lesser toe(s) without damage to nail
     ● S91.116   Laceration without foreign body of unspecified lesser toe(s) without damage to nail
     ● S91.119   Laceration without foreign body of unspecified toe without damage to nail

  ● **S91.12   Laceration with foreign body of toe without damage to nail**
     ● S91.121   Laceration with foreign body of right great toe without damage to nail
     ● S91.122   Laceration with foreign body of left great toe without damage to nail
     ● S91.123   Laceration with foreign body of unspecified great toe without damage to nail
     ● S91.124   Laceration with foreign body of right lesser toe(s) without damage to nail
     ● S91.125   Laceration with foreign body of left lesser toe(s) without damage to nail
     ● S91.126   Laceration with foreign body of unspecified lesser toe(s) without damage to nail
     ● S91.129   Laceration with foreign body of unspecified toe(s) without damage to nail

  ● **S91.13   Puncture wound without foreign body of toe without damage to nail**
     ● S91.131   Puncture wound without foreign body of right great toe without damage to nail
     ● S91.132   Puncture wound without foreign body of left great toe without damage to nail
     ● S91.133   Puncture wound without foreign body of unspecified great toe without damage to nail
     ● S91.134   Puncture wound without foreign body of right lesser toe(s) without damage to nail
     ● S91.135   Puncture wound without foreign body of left lesser toe(s) without damage to nail
     ● S91.136   Puncture wound without foreign body of unspecified lesser toe(s) without damage to nail
     ● S91.139   Puncture wound without foreign body of unspecified toe(s) without damage to nail

CHAPTER 19 (S00-T88)

● S91.14   Puncture wound with foreign body of toe without damage to nail

    ● S91.141   Puncture wound with foreign body of right great toe without damage to nail

    ● S91.142   Puncture wound with foreign body of left great toe without damage to nail

    ● S91.143   Puncture wound with foreign body of unspecified great toe without damage to nail

    ● S91.144   Puncture wound with foreign body of right lesser toe(s) without damage to nail

    ● S91.145   Puncture wound with foreign body of left lesser toe(s) without damage to nail

    ● S91.146   Puncture wound with foreign body of unspecified lesser toe(s) without damage to nail

    ● S91.149   Puncture wound with foreign body of unspecified toe(s) without damage to nail

● S91.15   Open bite of toe without damage to nail

    Bite of toe NOS

    Excludes1   superficial bite of toe (S90.46-, S90.47-)

    ● S91.151   Open bite of right great toe without damage to nail

    ● S91.152   Open bite of left great toe without damage to nail

    ● S91.153   Open bite of unspecified great toe without damage to nail

    ● S91.154   Open bite of right lesser toe(s) without damage to nail

    ● S91.155   Open bite of left lesser toe(s) without damage to nail

    ● S91.156   Open bite of unspecified lesser toe(s) without damage to nail

    ● S91.159   Open bite of unspecified toe(s) without damage to nail

● S91.2   Open wound of toe with damage to nail

    ● S91.20   Unspecified open wound of toe with damage to nail

       ● S91.201   Unspecified open wound of right great toe with damage to nail

       ● S91.202   Unspecified open wound of left great toe with damage to nail

       ● S91.203   Unspecified open wound of unspecified great toe with damage to nail

       ● S91.204   Unspecified open wound of right lesser toe(s) with damage to nail

       ● S91.205   Unspecified open wound of left lesser toe(s) with damage to nail

       ● S91.206   Unspecified open wound of unspecified lesser toe(s) with damage to nail

       ● S91.209   Unspecified open wound of unspecified toe(s) with damage to nail

    ● S91.21   Laceration without foreign body of toe with damage to nail

       ● S91.211   Laceration without foreign body of right great toe with damage to nail

       ● S91.212   Laceration without foreign body of left great toe with damage to nail

       ● S91.213   Laceration without foreign body of unspecified great toe with damage to nail

       ● S91.214   Laceration without foreign body of right lesser toe(s) with damage to nail

       ● S91.215   Laceration without foreign body of left lesser toe(s) with damage to nail

       ● S91.216   Laceration without foreign body of unspecified lesser toe(s) with damage to nail

       ● S91.219   Laceration without foreign body of unspecified toe(s) with damage to nail

    ● S91.22   Laceration with foreign body of toe with damage to nail

       ● S91.221   Laceration with foreign body of right great toe with damage to nail

       ● S91.222   Laceration with foreign body of left great toe with damage to nail

       ● S91.223   Laceration with foreign body of unspecified great toe with damage to nail

       ● S91.224   Laceration with foreign body of right lesser toe(s) with damage to nail

       ● S91.225   Laceration with foreign body of left lesser toe(s) with damage to nail

       ● S91.226   Laceration with foreign body of unspecified lesser toe(s) with damage to nail

       ● S91.229   Laceration with foreign body of unspecified toe(s) with damage to nail

    ● S91.23   Puncture wound without foreign body of toe with damage to nail

       ● S91.231   Puncture wound without foreign body of right great toe with damage to nail

       ● S91.232   Puncture wound without foreign body of left great toe with damage to nail

       ● S91.233   Puncture wound without foreign body of unspecified great toe with damage to nail

       ● S91.234   Puncture wound without foreign body of right lesser toe(s) with damage to nail

       ● S91.235   Puncture wound without foreign body of left lesser toe(s) with damage to nail

       ● S91.236   Puncture wound without foreign body of unspecified lesser toe(s) with damage to nail

       ● S91.239   Puncture wound without foreign body of unspecified toe(s) with damage to nail

    ● S91.24   Puncture wound with foreign body of toe with damage to nail

       ● S91.241   Puncture wound with foreign body of right great toe with damage to nail

       ● S91.242   Puncture wound with foreign body of left great toe with damage to nail

       ● S91.243   Puncture wound with foreign body of unspecified great toe with damage to nail

       ● S91.244   Puncture wound with foreign body of right lesser toe(s) with damage to nail

       ● S91.245   Puncture wound with foreign body of left lesser toe(s) with damage to nail

       ● S91.246   Puncture wound with foreign body of unspecified lesser toe(s) with damage to nail

       ● S91.249   Puncture wound with foreign body of unspecified toe(s) with damage to nail

● **S91.25**   Open bite of toe with damage to nail
     Bite of toe with damage to nail NOS
     | **Excludes1** | superficial bite of toe (S90.46-, S90.47-) |

   ● **S91.251**   Open bite of right great toe with damage to nail

   ● **S91.252**   Open bite of left great toe with damage to nail

   ● **S91.253**   Open bite of unspecified great toe with damage to nail

   ● **S91.254**   Open bite of right lesser toe(s) with damage to nail

   ● **S91.255**   Open bite of left lesser toe(s) with damage to nail

   ● **S91.256**   Open bite of unspecified lesser toe(s) with damage to nail

   ● **S91.259**   Open bite of unspecified toe(s) with damage to nail

● **S91.3**   Open wound of foot

   ● **S91.30**   Unspecified open wound of foot

     ● **S91.301**   Unspecified open wound, right foot

     ● **S91.302**   Unspecified open wound, left foot

     ● **S91.309**   Unspecified open wound, unspecified foot

   ● **S91.31**   Laceration without foreign body of foot

     ● **S91.311**   Laceration without foreign body, right foot

     ● **S91.312**   Laceration without foreign body, left foot

     ● **S91.319**   Laceration without foreign body, unspecified foot

   ● **S91.32**   Laceration with foreign body of foot

     ● **S91.321**   Laceration with foreign body, right foot

     ● **S91.322**   Laceration with foreign body, left foot

     ● **S91.329**   Laceration with foreign body, unspecified foot

   ● **S91.33**   Puncture wound without foreign body of foot

     ● **S91.331**   Puncture wound without foreign body, right foot

     ● **S91.332**   Puncture wound without foreign body, left foot

     ● **S91.339**   Puncture wound without foreign body, unspecified foot

   ● **S91.34**   Puncture wound with foreign body of foot

     ● **S91.341**   Puncture wound with foreign body, right foot

     ● **S91.342**   Puncture wound with foreign body, left foot

     ● **S91.349**   Puncture wound with foreign body, unspecified foot

   ● **S91.35**   Open bite of foot
     | **Excludes1** | superficial bite of foot (S90.86-, S90.87-) |

     ● **S91.351**   Open bite, right foot

     ● **S91.352**   Open bite, left foot

     ● **S91.359**   Open bite, unspecified foot

● **S92**   Fracture of foot and toe, except ankle

   Note: A fracture not indicated as displaced or nondisplaced should be coded to displaced

   A fracture not indicated as open or closed should be coded to closed

Excludes1	traumatic amputation of ankle and foot (S98.-)
Excludes2	fracture of ankle (S82.-)
	fracture of malleolus (S82.-)

   The appropriate 7th character is to be added to each code from category S92

A	initial encounter for closed fracture
B	initial encounter for open fracture
D	subsequent encounter for fracture with routine healing
G	subsequent encounter for fracture with delayed healing
K	subsequent encounter for fracture with nonunion
P	subsequent encounter for fracture with malunion
S	sequela

● **S92.0**   Fracture of calcaneus
     Heel bone   Os calcis
     | **Excludes2** | Physeal fracture of calcaneus (S99.0-) |

   ● **S92.00**   Unspecified fracture of calcaneus

     ● **S92.001**   Unspecified fracture of right calcaneus

     ● **S92.002**   Unspecified fracture of left calcaneus

     ● **S92.009**   Unspecified fracture of unspecified calcaneus

   ● **S92.01**   Fracture of body of calcaneus

     ● **S92.011**   Displaced fracture of body of right calcaneus

     ● **S92.012**   Displaced fracture of body of left calcaneus

     ● **S92.013**   Displaced fracture of body of unspecified calcaneus

     ● **S92.014**   Nondisplaced fracture of body of right calcaneus

     ● **S92.015**   Nondisplaced fracture of body of left calcaneus

     ● **S92.016**   Nondisplaced fracture of body of unspecified calcaneus

   ● **S92.02**   Fracture of anterior process of calcaneus

     ● **S92.021**   Displaced fracture of anterior process of right calcaneus

     ● **S92.022**   Displaced fracture of anterior process of left calcaneus

     ● **S92.023**   Displaced fracture of anterior process of unspecified calcaneus

     ● **S92.024**   Nondisplaced fracture of anterior process of right calcaneus

     ● **S92.025**   Nondisplaced fracture of anterior process of left calcaneus

     ● **S92.026**   Nondisplaced fracture of anterior process of unspecified calcaneus

   ● **S92.03**   Avulsion fracture of tuberosity of calcaneus

     ● **S92.031**   Displaced avulsion fracture of tuberosity of right calcaneus

     ● **S92.032**   Displaced avulsion fracture of tuberosity of left calcaneus

     ● **S92.033**   Displaced avulsion fracture of tuberosity of unspecified calcaneus

     ● **S92.034**   Nondisplaced avulsion fracture of tuberosity of right calcaneus

     ● **S92.035**   Nondisplaced avulsion fracture of tuberosity of left calcaneus

     ● **S92.036**   Nondisplaced avulsion fracture of tuberosity of unspecified calcaneus

CHAPTER 19 (S00-T88)

CHAPTER 19 (S00-T88)

- S92.04   Other fracture of tuberosity of calcaneus
  - S92.041   Displaced other fracture of tuberosity of right calcaneus
  - S92.042   Displaced other fracture of tuberosity of left calcaneus
  - S92.043   Displaced other fracture of tuberosity of unspecified calcaneus
  - S92.044   Nondisplaced other fracture of tuberosity of right calcaneus
  - S92.045   Nondisplaced other fracture of tuberosity of left calcaneus
  - S92.046   Nondisplaced other fracture of tuberosity of unspecified calcaneus
- S92.05   Other extraarticular fracture of calcaneus
  - S92.051   Displaced other extraarticular fracture of right calcaneus
  - S92.052   Displaced other extraarticular fracture of left calcaneus
  - S92.053   Displaced other extraarticular fracture of unspecified calcaneus
  - S92.054   Nondisplaced other extraarticular fracture of right calcaneus
  - S92.055   Nondisplaced other extraarticular fracture of left calcaneus
  - S92.056   Nondisplaced other extraarticular fracture of unspecified calcaneus
- S92.06   Intraarticular fracture of calcaneus
  - S92.061   Displaced intraarticular fracture of right calcaneus
  - S92.062   Displaced intraarticular fracture of left calcaneus
  - S92.063   Displaced intraarticular fracture of unspecified calcaneus
  - S92.064   Nondisplaced intraarticular fracture of right calcaneus
  - S92.065   Nondisplaced intraarticular fracture of left calcaneus
  - S92.066   Nondisplaced intraarticular fracture of unspecified calcaneus
- S92.1   Fracture of talus
  Astragalus
  - S92.10   Unspecified fracture of talus
    - S92.101   Unspecified fracture of right talus
    - S92.102   Unspecified fracture of left talus
    - S92.109   Unspecified fracture of unspecified talus
  - S92.11   Fracture of neck of talus
    - S92.111   Displaced fracture of neck of right talus
    - S92.112   Displaced fracture of neck of left talus
    - S92.113   Displaced fracture of neck of unspecified talus
    - S92.114   Nondisplaced fracture of neck of right talus
    - S92.115   Nondisplaced fracture of neck of left talus
    - S92.116   Nondisplaced fracture of neck of unspecified talus
  - S92.12   Fracture of body of talus
    - S92.121   Displaced fracture of body of right talus
    - S92.122   Displaced fracture of body of left talus
    - S92.123   Displaced fracture of body of unspecified talus
    - S92.124   Nondisplaced fracture of body of right talus

- S92.125   Nondisplaced fracture of body of left talus
- S92.126   Nondisplaced fracture of body of unspecified talus
- S92.13   Fracture of posterior process of talus
  - S92.131   Displaced fracture of posterior process of right talus
  - S92.132   Displaced fracture of posterior process of left talus
  - S92.133   Displaced fracture of posterior process of unspecified talus
  - S92.134   Nondisplaced fracture of posterior process of right talus
  - S92.135   Nondisplaced fracture of posterior process of left talus
  - S92.136   Nondisplaced fracture of posterior process of unspecified talus
- S92.14   Dome fracture of talus
  > **Excludes1**   osteochondritis dissecans (M93.2)
  - S92.141   Displaced dome fracture of right talus
  - S92.142   Displaced dome fracture of left talus
  - S92.143   Displaced dome fracture of unspecified talus
  - S92.144   Nondisplaced dome fracture of right talus
  - S92.145   Nondisplaced dome fracture of left talus
  - S92.146   Nondisplaced dome fracture of unspecified talus
- S92.15   Avulsion fracture (chip fracture) of talus
  - S92.151   Displaced avulsion fracture (chip fracture) of right talus
  - S92.152   Displaced avulsion fracture (chip fracture) of left talus
  - S92.153   Displaced avulsion fracture (chip fracture) of unspecified talus
  - S92.154   Nondisplaced avulsion fracture (chip fracture) of right talus
  - S92.155   Nondisplaced avulsion fracture (chip fracture) of left talus
  - S92.156   Nondisplaced avulsion fracture (chip fracture) of unspecified talus
- S92.19   Other fracture of talus
  - S92.191   Other fracture of right talus
  - S92.192   Other fracture of left talus
  - S92.199   Other fracture of unspecified talus
- S92.2   Fracture of other and unspecified tarsal bone(s)
  - S92.20   Fracture of unspecified tarsal bone(s)
    - S92.201   Fracture of unspecified tarsal bone(s) of right foot
    - S92.202   Fracture of unspecified tarsal bone(s) of left foot
    - S92.209   Fracture of unspecified tarsal bone(s) of unspecified foot
  - S92.21   Fracture of cuboid bone
    - S92.211   Displaced fracture of cuboid bone of right foot
    - S92.212   Displaced fracture of cuboid bone of left foot
    - S92.213   Displaced fracture of cuboid bone of unspecified foot
    - S92.214   Nondisplaced fracture of cuboid bone of right foot
    - S92.215   Nondisplaced fracture of cuboid bone of left foot
    - S92.216   Nondisplaced fracture of cuboid bone of unspecified foot

▶ New   ⇒ Revised   ~~deleted~~ Deleted   **OGCR** Official Guidelines   X Assign placeholder X   ● Use Additional Character(s)

Excludes 1   Excludes 2   Includes   Use additional   Code first   Code also   Key words

● S92.22   Fracture of lateral cuneiform
    ● S92.221   Displaced fracture of lateral cuneiform of right foot
    ● S92.222   Displaced fracture of lateral cuneiform of left foot
    ● S92.223   Displaced fracture of lateral cuneiform of unspecified foot
    ● S92.224   Nondisplaced fracture of lateral cuneiform of right foot
    ● S92.225   Nondisplaced fracture of lateral cuneiform of left foot
    ● S92.226   Nondisplaced fracture of lateral cuneiform of unspecified foot

● S92.23   Fracture of intermediate cuneiform
    ● S92.231   Displaced fracture of intermediate cuneiform of right foot
    ● S92.232   Displaced fracture of intermediate cuneiform of left foot
    ● S92.233   Displaced fracture of intermediate cuneiform of unspecified foot
    ● S92.234   Nondisplaced fracture of intermediate cuneiform of right foot
    ● S92.235   Nondisplaced fracture of intermediate cuneiform of left foot
    ● S92.236   Nondisplaced fracture of intermediate cuneiform of unspecified foot

● S92.24   Fracture of medial cuneiform
    ● S92.241   Displaced fracture of medial cuneiform of right foot
    ● S92.242   Displaced fracture of medial cuneiform of left foot
    ● S92.243   Displaced fracture of medial cuneiform of unspecified foot
    ● S92.244   Nondisplaced fracture of medial cuneiform of right foot
    ● S92.245   Nondisplaced fracture of medial cuneiform of left foot
    ● S92.246   Nondisplaced fracture of medial cuneiform of unspecified foot

● S92.25   Fracture of navicular [scaphoid] of foot
    ● S92.251   Displaced fracture of navicular [scaphoid] of right foot
    ● S92.252   Displaced fracture of navicular [scaphoid] of left foot
    ● S92.253   Displaced fracture of navicular [scaphoid] of unspecified foot
    ● S92.254   Nondisplaced fracture of navicular [scaphoid] of right foot
    ● S92.255   Nondisplaced fracture of navicular [scaphoid] of left foot
    ● S92.256   Nondisplaced fracture of navicular [scaphoid] of unspecified foot

● S92.3   Fracture of metatarsal bone(s)
    Excludes2   Physeal fracture of metatarsal (S99.1-)
    ● S92.30   Fracture of unspecified metatarsal bone(s)
        ● S92.301   Fracture of unspecified metatarsal bone(s), right foot
        ● S92.302   Fracture of unspecified metatarsal bone(s), left foot
        ● S92.309   Fracture of unspecified metatarsal bone(s), unspecified foot

● S92.31   Fracture of first metatarsal bone
    ● S92.311   Displaced fracture of first metatarsal bone, right foot
    ● S92.312   Displaced fracture of first metatarsal bone, left foot
    ● S92.313   Displaced fracture of first metatarsal bone, unspecified foot
    ● S92.314   Nondisplaced fracture of first metatarsal bone, right foot
    ● S92.315   Nondisplaced fracture of first metatarsal bone, left foot
    ● S92.316   Nondisplaced fracture of first metatarsal bone, unspecified foot

● S92.32   Fracture of second metatarsal bone
    ● S92.321   Displaced fracture of second metatarsal bone, right foot
    ● S92.322   Displaced fracture of second metatarsal bone, left foot
    ● S92.323   Displaced fracture of second metatarsal bone, unspecified foot
    ● S92.324   Nondisplaced fracture of second metatarsal bone, right foot
    ● S92.325   Nondisplaced fracture of second metatarsal bone, left foot
    ● S92.326   Nondisplaced fracture of second metatarsal bone, unspecified foot

● S92.33   Fracture of third metatarsal bone
    ● S92.331   Displaced fracture of third metatarsal bone, right foot
    ● S92.332   Displaced fracture of third metatarsal bone, left foot
    ● S92.333   Displaced fracture of third metatarsal bone, unspecified foot
    ● S92.334   Nondisplaced fracture of third metatarsal bone, right foot
    ● S92.335   Nondisplaced fracture of third metatarsal bone, left foot
    ● S92.336   Nondisplaced fracture of third metatarsal bone, unspecified foot

● S92.34   Fracture of fourth metatarsal bone
    ● S92.341   Displaced fracture of fourth metatarsal bone, right foot
    ● S92.342   Displaced fracture of fourth metatarsal bone, left foot
    ● S92.343   Displaced fracture of fourth metatarsal bone, unspecified foot
    ● S92.344   Nondisplaced fracture of fourth metatarsal bone, right foot
    ● S92.345   Nondisplaced fracture of fourth metatarsal bone, left foot
    ● S92.346   Nondisplaced fracture of fourth metatarsal bone, unspecified foot

● S92.35   Fracture of fifth metatarsal bone
    ● S92.351   Displaced fracture of fifth metatarsal bone, right foot
    ● S92.352   Displaced fracture of fifth metatarsal bone, left foot
    ● S92.353   Displaced fracture of fifth metatarsal bone, unspecified foot
    ● S92.354   Nondisplaced fracture of fifth metatarsal bone, right foot
    ● S92.355   Nondisplaced fracture of fifth metatarsal bone, left foot
    ● S92.356   Nondisplaced fracture of fifth metatarsal bone, unspecified foot

▶ New   ⇒ Revised   ~~deleted~~ Deleted   OGCR Official Guidelines   X Assign placeholder X   ● Use Additional Character(s)

Excludes 1   Excludes 2   Includes   Use additional   Code first   Code also   Key words

● **S92.4**　Fracture of great toe
　　Excludes2　Physeal fracture of phalanx of toe
　　　　　　　　(S99.2-)

　● **S92.40**　Unspecified fracture of great toe
　　● S92.401　Displaced unspecified fracture of right great toe
　　● S92.402　Displaced unspecified fracture of left great toe
　　● S92.403　Displaced unspecified fracture of unspecified great toe
　　● S92.404　Nondisplaced unspecified fracture of right great toe
　　● S92.405　Nondisplaced unspecified fracture of left great toe
　　● S92.406　Nondisplaced unspecified fracture of unspecified great toe

　● **S92.41**　Fracture of proximal phalanx of great toe
　　● S92.411　Displaced fracture of proximal phalanx of right great toe
　　● S92.412　Displaced fracture of proximal phalanx of left great toe
　　● S92.413　Displaced fracture of proximal phalanx of unspecified great toe
　　● S92.414　Nondisplaced fracture of proximal phalanx of right great toe
　　● S92.415　Nondisplaced fracture of proximal phalanx of left great toe
　　● S92.416　Nondisplaced fracture of proximal phalanx of unspecified great toe

　● **S92.42**　Fracture of distal phalanx of great toe
　　● S92.421　Displaced fracture of distal phalanx of right great toe
　　● S92.422　Displaced fracture of distal phalanx of left great toe
　　● S92.423　Displaced fracture of distal phalanx of unspecified great toe
　　● S92.424　Nondisplaced fracture of distal phalanx of right great toe
　　● S92.425　Nondisplaced fracture of distal phalanx of left great toe
　　● S92.426　Nondisplaced fracture of distal phalanx of unspecified great toe

　● **S92.49**　Other fracture of great toe
　　● S92.491　Other fracture of right great toe
　　● S92.492　Other fracture of left great toe
　　● S92.499　Other fracture of unspecified great toe

● **S92.5**　Fracture of lesser toe(s)
　　Excludes2　Physeal fracture of phalanx of toe
　　　　　　　　(S99.2-)

　● **S92.50**　Unspecified fracture of lesser toe(s)
　　● S92.501　Displaced unspecified fracture of right lesser toe(s)
　　● S92.502　Displaced unspecified fracture of left lesser toe(s)
　　● S92.503　Displaced unspecified fracture of unspecified lesser toe(s)
　　● S92.504　Nondisplaced unspecified fracture of right lesser toe(s)
　　● S92.505　Nondisplaced unspecified fracture of left lesser toe(s)
　　● S92.506　Nondisplaced unspecified fracture of unspecified lesser toe(s)

　● **S92.51**　Fracture of proximal phalanx of lesser toe(s)
　　● S92.511　Displaced fracture of proximal phalanx of right lesser toe(s)
　　● S92.512　Displaced fracture of proximal phalanx of left lesser toe(s)
　　● S92.513　Displaced fracture of proximal phalanx of unspecified lesser toe(s)
　　● S92.514　Nondisplaced fracture of proximal phalanx of right lesser toe(s)
　　● S92.515　Nondisplaced fracture of proximal phalanx of left lesser toe(s)
　　● S92.516　Nondisplaced fracture of proximal phalanx of unspecified lesser toe(s)

　⇨● **S92.52**　Fracture of middle phalanx of lesser toe(s)
　　⇨● S92.521　Displaced fracture of middle phalanx of right lesser toe(s)
　　⇨● S92.522　Displaced fracture of middle phalanx of left lesser toe(s)
　　⇨● S92.523　Displaced fracture of middle phalanx of unspecified lesser toe(s)
　　⇨● S92.524　Nondisplaced fracture of middle phalanx of right lesser toe(s)
　　⇨● S92.525　Nondisplaced fracture of middle phalanx of left lesser toe(s)
　　⇨● S92.526　Nondisplaced fracture of middle phalanx of unspecified lesser toe(s)

　● **S92.53**　Fracture of distal phalanx of lesser toe(s)
　　● S92.531　Displaced fracture of distal phalanx of right lesser toe(s)
　　● S92.532　Displaced fracture of distal phalanx of left lesser toe(s)
　　● S92.533　Displaced fracture of distal phalanx of unspecified lesser toe(s)
　　● S92.534　Nondisplaced fracture of distal phalanx of right lesser toe(s)
　　● S92.535　Nondisplaced fracture of distal phalanx of left lesser toe(s)
　　● S92.536　Nondisplaced fracture of distal phalanx of unspecified lesser toe(s)

　● **S92.59**　Other fracture of lesser toe(s)
　　● S92.591　Other fracture of right lesser toe(s)
　　● S92.592　Other fracture of left lesser toe(s)
　　● S92.599　Other fracture of unspecified lesser toe(s)

● **S92.8**　Other fracture of foot, except ankle
　● **S92.81**　Other fracture of foot
　　　Sesamoid fracture of foot
　　● S92.811　Other fracture of right foot
　　● S92.812　Other fracture of left foot
　　● S92.819　Other fracture of unspecified foot

● **S92.9**　Unspecified fracture of foot and toe
　● **S92.90**　Unspecified fracture of foot
　　● S92.901　Unspecified fracture of right foot
　　● S92.902　Unspecified fracture of left foot
　　● S92.909　Unspecified fracture of unspecified foot
　● **S92.91**　Unspecified fracture of toe
　　● S92.911　Unspecified fracture of right toe(s)
　　● S92.912　Unspecified fracture of left toe(s)
　　● S92.919　Unspecified fracture of unspecified toe(s)

● **S93**   **Dislocation and sprain of joints and ligaments at ankle, foot and toe level**

> **Includes**   avulsion of joint or ligament of ankle, foot and toe
> laceration of cartilage, joint or ligament of ankle, foot and toe
> sprain of cartilage, joint or ligament of ankle, foot and toe
> traumatic hemarthrosis of joint or ligament of ankle, foot and toe
> traumatic rupture of joint or ligament of ankle, foot and toe
> traumatic subluxation of joint or ligament of ankle, foot and toe
> traumatic tear of joint or ligament of ankle, foot and toe

Code also any associated open wound

Excludes2   strain of muscle and tendon of ankle and foot (S96.-)

The appropriate 7th character is to be added to each code from category S93

> A   initial encounter
> D   subsequent encounter
> S   sequela

● **S93.0**   **Subluxation and dislocation of ankle joint**
Subluxation and dislocation of astragalus
Subluxation and dislocation of fibula, lower end
Subluxation and dislocation of talus
Subluxation and dislocation of tibia, lower end

X● **S93.01**   **Subluxation of right ankle joint**
X● **S93.02**   **Subluxation of left ankle joint**
X● **S93.03**   **Subluxation of unspecified ankle joint**
X● **S93.04**   **Dislocation of right ankle joint**
X● **S93.05**   **Dislocation of left ankle joint**
X● **S93.06**   **Dislocation of unspecified ankle joint**

● **S93.1**   **Subluxation and dislocation of toe**

● **S93.10**   **Unspecified subluxation and dislocation of toe**
Dislocation of toe NOS
Subluxation of toe NOS

● **S93.101**   Unspecified **subluxation of right** toe(s)
● **S93.102**   Unspecified **subluxation of left** toe(s)
● **S93.103**   Unspecified **subluxation of unspecified** toe(s)
● **S93.104**   Unspecified **dislocation of right** toe(s)
● **S93.105**   Unspecified **dislocation of left** toe(s)
● **S93.106**   Unspecified **dislocation of unspecified** toe(s)

● **S93.11**   **Dislocation of interphalangeal joint**

● **S93.111**   Dislocation of interphalangeal joint of **right great** toe
● **S93.112**   Dislocation of interphalangeal joint of **left great** toe
● **S93.113**   Dislocation of interphalangeal joint of **unspecified great** toe
● **S93.114**   Dislocation of interphalangeal joint of **right lesser** toe(s)
● **S93.115**   Dislocation of interphalangeal joint of **left lesser** toe(s)
● **S93.116**   Dislocation of interphalangeal joint of **unspecified lesser** toe(s)
● **S93.119**   Dislocation of interphalangeal joint of **unspecified toe(s)**

● **S93.12**   **Dislocation of metatarsophalangeal joint**

● **S93.121**   Dislocation of metatarsophalangeal joint of **right great** toe
● **S93.122**   Dislocation of metatarsophalangeal joint of **left great** toe
● **S93.123**   Dislocation of metatarsophalangeal joint of **unspecified great** toe
● **S93.124**   Dislocation of metatarsophalangeal joint of **right lesser** toe(s)
● **S93.125**   Dislocation of metatarsophalangeal joint of **left lesser** toe(s)
● **S93.126**   Dislocation of metatarsophalangeal joint of **unspecified lesser** toe(s)
● **S93.129**   Dislocation of metatarsophalangeal joint of **unspecified** toe(s)

● **S93.13**   **Subluxation of interphalangeal joint**

● **S93.131**   Subluxation of interphalangeal joint of **right great** toe
● **S93.132**   Subluxation of interphalangeal joint of **left great** toe
● **S93.133**   Subluxation of interphalangeal joint of **unspecified great** toe
● **S93.134**   Subluxation of interphalangeal joint of **right lesser** toe(s)
● **S93.135**   Subluxation of interphalangeal joint of **left lesser** toe(s)
● **S93.136**   Subluxation of interphalangeal joint of **unspecified lesser** toe(s)
● **S93.139**   Subluxation of interphalangeal joint of **unspecified** toe(s)

● **S93.14**   **Subluxation of metatarsophalangeal joint**

● **S93.141**   Subluxation of metatarsophalangeal joint of **right great** toe
● **S93.142**   Subluxation of metatarsophalangeal joint of **left great** toe
● **S93.143**   Subluxation of metatarsophalangeal joint of **unspecified great** toe
● **S93.144**   Subluxation of metatarsophalangeal joint of **right lesser** toe(s)
● **S93.145**   Subluxation of metatarsophalangeal joint of **left lesser** toe(s)
● **S93.146**   Subluxation of metatarsophalangeal joint of **unspecified lesser** toe(s)
● **S93.149**   Subluxation of metatarsophalangeal joint of **unspecified** toe(s)

● **S93.3**   **Subluxation and dislocation of foot**

Excludes2   dislocation of toe (S93.1-)

● **S93.30**   **Unspecified subluxation and dislocation of foot**
Dislocation of foot NOS
Subluxation of foot NOS

● **S93.301**   Unspecified **subluxation of right** foot
● **S93.302**   Unspecified **subluxation of left** foot
● **S93.303**   Unspecified **subluxation of unspecified** foot
● **S93.304**   Unspecified **dislocation of right** foot
● **S93.305**   Unspecified **dislocation of left** foot
● **S93.306**   Unspecified **dislocation of unspecified** foot

● **S93.31**   **Subluxation and dislocation of tarsal joint**

● **S93.311**   **Subluxation** of tarsal joint of **right** foot
● **S93.312**   **Subluxation** of tarsal joint of **left** foot
● **S93.313**   **Subluxation** of tarsal joint of **unspecified** foot
● **S93.314**   **Dislocation** of tarsal joint of **right** foot
● **S93.315**   **Dislocation** of tarsal joint of **left** foot
● **S93.316**   **Dislocation** of tarsal joint of **unspecified** foot

CHAPTER 19 (S00-T88)

- ● S93.32   Subluxation and dislocation of tarsometatarsal joint
  - ● S93.321   Subluxation of tarsometatarsal joint of right foot
  - ● S93.322   Subluxation of tarsometatarsal joint of left foot
  - ● S93.323   Subluxation of tarsometatarsal joint of unspecified foot
  - ● S93.324   Dislocation of tarsometatarsal joint of right foot
  - ● S93.325   Dislocation of tarsometatarsal joint of left foot
  - ● S93.326   Dislocation of tarsometatarsal joint of unspecified foot
- ● S93.33   Other subluxation and dislocation of foot
  - ● S93.331   Other subluxation of right foot
  - ● S93.332   Other subluxation of left foot
  - ● S93.333   Other subluxation of unspecified foot
  - ● S93.334   Other dislocation of right foot
  - ● S93.335   Other dislocation of left foot
  - ● S93.336   Other dislocation of unspecified foot
- ● S93.4   Sprain of ankle
  - *Injury to ligaments when one or more is stretched/torn*
  - Excludes2   injury of Achilles tendon (S86.0-)
  - ● S93.40   Sprain of unspecified ligament of ankle
    - Sprain of ankle NOS
    - Sprained ankle NOS
    - ● S93.401   Sprain of unspecified ligament of right ankle
    - ● S93.402   Sprain of unspecified ligament of left ankle
    - ● S93.409   Sprain of unspecified ligament of unspecified ankle
  - ● S93.41   Sprain of calcaneofibular ligament
    - ● S93.411   Sprain of calcaneofibular ligament of right ankle
    - ● S93.412   Sprain of calcaneofibular ligament of left ankle
    - ● S93.419   Sprain of calcaneofibular ligament of unspecified ankle
  - ● S93.42   Sprain of deltoid ligament
    - ● S93.421   Sprain of deltoid ligament of right ankle
    - ● S93.422   Sprain of deltoid ligament of left ankle
    - ● S93.429   Sprain of deltoid ligament of unspecified ankle
  - ● S93.43   Sprain of tibiofibular ligament
    - ● S93.431   Sprain of tibiofibular ligament of right ankle
    - ● S93.432   Sprain of tibiofibular ligament of left ankle
    - ● S93.439   Sprain of tibiofibular ligament of unspecified ankle
  - ● S93.49   Sprain of other ligament of ankle
    - Sprain of internal collateral ligament
    - Sprain of talofibular ligament
    - ● S93.491   Sprain of other ligament of right ankle
    - ● S93.492   Sprain of other ligament of left ankle
    - ● S93.499   Sprain of other ligament of unspecified ankle

- ● S93.5   Sprain of toe
  - ● S93.50   Unspecified sprain of toe
    - ● S93.501   Unspecified sprain of right great toe
    - ● S93.502   Unspecified sprain of left great toe
    - ● S93.503   Unspecified sprain of unspecified great toe
    - ● S93.504   Unspecified sprain of right lesser toe(s)
    - ● S93.505   Unspecified sprain of left lesser toe(s)
    - ● S93.506   Unspecified sprain of unspecified lesser toe(s)
    - ● S93.509   Unspecified sprain of unspecified toe(s)
  - ● S93.51   Sprain of interphalangeal joint of toe
    - ● S93.511   Sprain of interphalangeal joint of right great toe
    - ● S93.512   Sprain of interphalangeal joint of left great toe
    - ● S93.513   Sprain of interphalangeal joint of unspecified great toe
    - ● S93.514   Sprain of interphalangeal joint of right lesser toe(s)
    - ● S93.515   Sprain of interphalangeal joint of left lesser toe(s)
    - ● S93.516   Sprain of interphalangeal joint of unspecified lesser toe(s)
    - ● S93.519   Sprain of interphalangeal joint of unspecified toe(s)
  - ● S93.52   Sprain of metatarsophalangeal joint of toe
    - ● S93.521   Sprain of metatarsophalangeal joint of right great toe
    - ● S93.522   Sprain of metatarsophalangeal joint of left great toe
    - ● S93.523   Sprain of metatarsophalangeal joint of unspecified great toe
    - ● S93.524   Sprain of metatarsophalangeal joint of right lesser toe(s)
    - ● S93.525   Sprain of metatarsophalangeal joint of left lesser toe(s)
    - ● S93.526   Sprain of metatarsophalangeal joint of unspecified lesser toe(s)
    - ● S93.529   Sprain of metatarsophalangeal joint of unspecified toe(s)
- ● S93.6   Sprain of foot
  - Excludes2   sprain of metatarsophalangeal joint of toe (S93.52-)
  - sprain of toe (S93.5-)
  - ● S93.60   Unspecified sprain of foot
    - ● S93.601   Unspecified sprain of right foot
    - ● S93.602   Unspecified sprain of left foot
    - ● S93.609   Unspecified sprain of unspecified foot
  - ● S93.61   Sprain of tarsal ligament of foot
    - ● S93.611   Sprain of tarsal ligament of right foot
    - ● S93.612   Sprain of tarsal ligament of left foot
    - ● S93.619   Sprain of tarsal ligament of unspecified foot
  - ● S93.62   Sprain of tarsometatarsal ligament of foot
    - ● S93.621   Sprain of tarsometatarsal ligament of right foot
    - ● S93.622   Sprain of tarsometatarsal ligament of left foot
    - ● S93.629   Sprain of tarsometatarsal ligament of unspecified foot
  - ● S93.69   Other sprain of foot
    - ● S93.691   Other sprain of right foot
    - ● S93.692   Other sprain of left foot
    - ● S93.699   Other sprain of unspecified foot

● S94 Injury of nerves at ankle and foot level

   The appropriate 7th character is to be added to each code from category S94

A	initial encounter
D	subsequent encounter
S	sequela

   Code also any associated open wound (S91.-)

● S94.0 Injury of lateral plantar nerve
   X ● S94.00 Injury of lateral plantar nerve, unspecified leg
   X ● S94.01 Injury of lateral plantar nerve, right leg
   X ● S94.02 Injury of lateral plantar nerve, left leg

● S94.1 Injury of medial plantar nerve
   X ● S94.10 Injury of medial plantar nerve, unspecified leg
   X ● S94.11 Injury of medial plantar nerve, right leg
   X ● S94.12 Injury of medial plantar nerve, left leg

● S94.2 Injury of deep peroneal nerve at ankle and foot level
          Injury of terminal, lateral branch of deep peroneal nerve
   X ● S94.20 Injury of deep peroneal nerve at ankle and foot level, unspecified leg
   X ● S94.21 Injury of deep peroneal nerve at ankle and foot level, right leg
   X ● S94.22 Injury of deep peroneal nerve at ankle and foot level, left leg

● S94.3 Injury of cutaneous sensory nerve at ankle and foot level
   X ● S94.30 Injury of cutaneous sensory nerve at ankle and foot level, unspecified leg
   X ● S94.31 Injury of cutaneous sensory nerve at ankle and foot level, right leg
   X ● S94.32 Injury of cutaneous sensory nerve at ankle and foot level, left leg

● S94.8 Injury of other nerves at ankle and foot level
   ● S94.8X Injury of other nerves at ankle and foot level
      ● S94.8X1 Injury of other nerves at ankle and foot level, right leg
      ● S94.8X2 Injury of other nerves at ankle and foot level, left leg
      ● S94.8X9 Injury of other nerves at ankle and foot level, unspecified leg

● S94.9 Injury of unspecified nerve at ankle and foot level
   X ● S94.90 Injury of unspecified nerve at ankle and foot level, unspecified leg
   X ● S94.91 Injury of unspecified nerve at ankle and foot level, right leg
   X ● S94.92 Injury of unspecified nerve at ankle and foot level, left leg

● S95 Injury of blood vessels at ankle and foot level
   Code also any associated open wound (S91.-)
   Excludes2 injury of posterior tibial artery and vein (S85.1-, S85.8-)

   The appropriate 7th character is to be added to each code from category S95

A	initial encounter
D	subsequent encounter
S	sequela

● S95.0 Injury of dorsal artery of foot
   ● S95.00 Unspecified injury of dorsal artery of foot
      ● S95.001 Unspecified injury of dorsal artery of right foot
      ● S95.002 Unspecified injury of dorsal artery of left foot
      ● S95.009 Unspecified injury of dorsal artery of unspecified foot
   ● S95.01 Laceration of dorsal artery of foot
      ● S95.011 Laceration of dorsal artery of right foot
      ● S95.012 Laceration of dorsal artery of left foot
      ● S95.019 Laceration of dorsal artery of unspecified foot

   ● S95.09 Other specified injury of dorsal artery of foot
      ● S95.091 Other specified injury of dorsal artery of right foot
      ● S95.092 Other specified injury of dorsal artery of left foot
      ● S95.099 Other specified injury of dorsal artery of unspecified foot

● S95.1 Injury of plantar artery of foot
   ● S95.10 Unspecified injury of plantar artery of foot
      ● S95.101 Unspecified injury of plantar artery of right foot
      ● S95.102 Unspecified injury of plantar artery of left foot
      ● S95.109 Unspecified injury of plantar artery of unspecified foot
   ● S95.11 Laceration of plantar artery of foot
      ● S95.111 Laceration of plantar artery of right foot
      ● S95.112 Laceration of plantar artery of left foot
      ● S95.119 Laceration of plantar artery of unspecified foot
   ● S95.19 Other specified injury of plantar artery of foot
      ● S95.191 Other specified injury of plantar artery of right foot
      ● S95.192 Other specified injury of plantar artery of left foot
      ● S95.199 Other specified injury of plantar artery of unspecified foot

● S95.2 Injury of dorsal vein of foot
   ● S95.20 Unspecified injury of dorsal vein of foot
      ● S95.201 Unspecified injury of dorsal vein of right foot
      ● S95.202 Unspecified injury of dorsal vein of left foot
      ● S95.209 Unspecified injury of dorsal vein of unspecified foot
   ● S95.21 Laceration of dorsal vein of foot
      ● S95.211 Laceration of dorsal vein of right foot
      ● S95.212 Laceration of dorsal vein of left foot
      ● S95.219 Laceration of dorsal vein of unspecified foot
   ● S95.29 Other specified injury of dorsal vein of foot
      ● S95.291 Other specified injury of dorsal vein of right foot
      ● S95.292 Other specified injury of dorsal vein of left foot
      ● S95.299 Other specified injury of dorsal vein of unspecified foot

● S95.8 Injury of other blood vessels at ankle and foot level
   ● S95.80 Unspecified injury of other blood vessels at ankle and foot level
      ● S95.801 Unspecified injury of other blood vessels at ankle and foot level, right leg
      ● S95.802 Unspecified injury of other blood vessels at ankle and foot level, left leg
      ● S95.809 Unspecified injury of other blood vessels at ankle and foot level, unspecified leg
   ● S95.81 Laceration of other blood vessels at ankle and foot level
      ● S95.811 Laceration of other blood vessels at ankle and foot level, right leg
      ● S95.812 Laceration of other blood vessels at ankle and foot level, left leg
      ● S95.819 Laceration of other blood vessels at ankle and foot level, unspecified leg

- S95.89 Other specified injury of other blood vessels at ankle and foot level
  - S95.891 Other specified injury of other blood vessels at ankle and foot level, right leg
  - S95.892 Other specified injury of other blood vessels at ankle and foot level, left leg
  - S95.899 Other specified injury of other blood vessels at ankle and foot level, unspecified leg
- S95.9 Injury of unspecified blood vessel at ankle and foot level
  - S95.90 Unspecified injury of unspecified blood vessel at ankle and foot level
    - S95.901 Unspecified injury of unspecified blood vessel at ankle and foot level, right leg
    - S95.902 Unspecified injury of unspecified blood vessel at ankle and foot level, left leg
    - S95.909 Unspecified injury of unspecified blood vessel at ankle and foot level, unspecified leg
  - S95.91 Laceration of unspecified blood vessel at ankle and foot level
    - S95.911 Laceration of unspecified blood vessel at ankle and foot level, right leg
    - S95.912 Laceration of unspecified blood vessel at ankle and foot level, left leg
    - S95.919 Laceration of unspecified blood vessel at ankle and foot level, unspecified leg
  - S95.99 Other specified injury of unspecified blood vessel at ankle and foot level
    - S95.991 Other specified injury of unspecified blood vessel at ankle and foot level, right leg
    - S95.992 Other specified injury of unspecified blood vessel at ankle and foot level, left leg
    - S95.999 Other specified injury of unspecified blood vessel at ankle and foot level, unspecified leg

- S96 Injury of muscle and tendon at ankle and foot level

  Code also any associated open wound (S91.-)

  Excludes2   injury of Achilles tendon (S86.0-)
               sprain of joints and ligaments of ankle and foot (S93.-)

  The appropriate 7th character is to be added to each code from category S96

A	initial encounter
D	subsequent encounter
S	sequela

  - S96.0 Injury of muscle and tendon of long flexor muscle of toe at ankle and foot level
    - S96.00 Unspecified injury of muscle and tendon of long flexor muscle of toe at ankle and foot level
      - S96.001 Unspecified injury of muscle and tendon of long flexor muscle of toe at ankle and foot level, right foot
      - S96.002 Unspecified injury of muscle and tendon of long flexor muscle of toe at ankle and foot level, left foot
      - S96.009 Unspecified injury of muscle and tendon of long flexor muscle of toe at ankle and foot level, unspecified foot

  - S96.01 Strain of muscle and tendon of long flexor muscle of toe at ankle and foot level
    - S96.011 Strain of muscle and tendon of long flexor muscle of toe at ankle and foot level, right foot
    - S96.012 Strain of muscle and tendon of long flexor muscle of toe at ankle and foot level, left foot
    - S96.019 Strain of muscle and tendon of long flexor muscle of toe at ankle and foot level, unspecified foot
  - S96.02 Laceration of muscle and tendon of long flexor muscle of toe at ankle and foot level
    - S96.021 Laceration of muscle and tendon of long flexor muscle of toe at ankle and foot level, right foot
    - S96.022 Laceration of muscle and tendon of long flexor muscle of toe at ankle and foot level, left foot
    - S96.029 Laceration of muscle and tendon of long flexor muscle of toe at ankle and foot level, unspecified foot
  - S96.09 Other injury of muscle and tendon of long flexor muscle of toe at ankle and foot level
    - S96.091 Other injury of muscle and tendon of long flexor muscle of toe at ankle and foot level, right foot
    - S96.092 Other injury of muscle and tendon of long flexor muscle of toe at ankle and foot level, left foot
    - S96.099 Other injury of muscle and tendon of long flexor muscle of toe at ankle and foot level, unspecified foot
  - S96.1 Injury of muscle and tendon of long extensor muscle of toe at ankle and foot level
    - S96.10 Unspecified injury of muscle and tendon of long extensor muscle of toe at ankle and foot level
      - S96.101 Unspecified injury of muscle and tendon of long extensor muscle of toe at ankle and foot level, right foot
      - S96.102 Unspecified injury of muscle and tendon of long extensor muscle of toe at ankle and foot level, left foot
      - S96.109 Unspecified injury of muscle and tendon of long extensor muscle of toe at ankle and foot level, unspecified foot
    - S96.11 Strain of muscle and tendon of long extensor muscle of toe at ankle and foot level
      - S96.111 Strain of muscle and tendon of long extensor muscle of toe at ankle and foot level, right foot
      - S96.112 Strain of muscle and tendon of long extensor muscle of toe at ankle and foot level, left foot
      - S96.119 Strain of muscle and tendon of long extensor muscle of toe at ankle and foot level, unspecified foot
    - S96.12 Laceration of muscle and tendon of long extensor muscle of toe at ankle and foot level
      - S96.121 Laceration of muscle and tendon of long extensor muscle of toe at ankle and foot level, right foot
      - S96.122 Laceration of muscle and tendon of long extensor muscle of toe at ankle and foot level, left foot
      - S96.129 Laceration of muscle and tendon of long extensor muscle of toe at ankle and foot level, unspecified foot

- S96.19 Other specified injury of muscle and tendon of long extensor muscle of toe at ankle and foot level
  - S96.191 Other specified injury of muscle and tendon of long extensor muscle of toe at ankle and foot level, right foot
  - S96.192 Other specified injury of muscle and tendon of long extensor muscle of toe at ankle and foot level, left foot
  - S96.199 Other specified injury of muscle and tendon of long extensor muscle of toe at ankle and foot level, unspecified foot
- S96.2 Injury of intrinsic muscle and tendon at ankle and foot level
  - S96.20 Unspecified injury of intrinsic muscle and tendon at ankle and foot level
    - S96.201 Unspecified injury of intrinsic muscle and tendon at ankle and foot level, right foot
    - S96.202 Unspecified injury of intrinsic muscle and tendon at ankle and foot level, left foot
    - S96.209 Unspecified injury of intrinsic muscle and tendon at ankle and foot level, unspecified foot
  - S96.21 Strain of intrinsic muscle and tendon at ankle and foot level
    - S96.211 Strain of intrinsic muscle and tendon at ankle and foot level, right foot
    - S96.212 Strain of intrinsic muscle and tendon at ankle and foot level, left foot
    - S96.219 Strain of intrinsic muscle and tendon at ankle and foot level, unspecified foot
  - S96.22 Laceration of intrinsic muscle and tendon at ankle and foot level
    - S96.221 Laceration of intrinsic muscle and tendon at ankle and foot level, right foot
    - S96.222 Laceration of intrinsic muscle and tendon at left ankle and foot level, left foot
    - S96.229 Laceration of intrinsic muscle and tendon at ankle and foot level, unspecified foot
  - S96.29 Other specified injury of intrinsic muscle and tendon at ankle and foot level
    - S96.291 Other specified injury of intrinsic muscle and tendon at ankle and foot level, right foot
    - S96.292 Other specified injury of intrinsic muscle and tendon at ankle and foot level, left foot
    - S96.299 Other specified injury of intrinsic muscle and tendon at ankle and foot level, unspecified foot
- S96.8 Injury of other specified muscles and tendons at ankle and foot level
  - S96.80 Unspecified injury of other specified muscles and tendons at ankle and foot level
    - S96.801 Unspecified injury of other specified muscles and tendons at ankle and foot level, right foot
    - S96.802 Unspecified injury of other specified muscles and tendons at ankle and foot level, left foot
    - S96.809 Unspecified injury of other specified muscles and tendons at ankle and foot level, unspecified foot

- S96.81 Strain of other specified muscles and tendons at ankle and foot level
  - S96.811 Strain of other specified muscles and tendons at ankle and foot level, right foot
  - S96.812 Strain of other specified muscles and tendons at ankle and foot level, left foot
  - S96.819 Strain of other specified muscles and tendons at ankle and foot level, unspecified foot
- S96.82 Laceration of other specified muscles and tendons at ankle and foot level
  - S96.821 Laceration of other specified muscles and tendons at ankle and foot level, right foot
  - S96.822 Laceration of other specified muscles and tendons at ankle and foot level, left foot
  - S96.829 Laceration of other specified muscles and tendons at ankle and foot level, unspecified foot
- S96.89 Other specified injury of other specified muscles and tendons at ankle and foot level
  - S96.891 Other specified injury of other specified muscles and tendons at ankle and foot level, right foot
  - S96.892 Other specified injury of other specified muscles and tendons at ankle and foot level, left foot
  - S96.899 Other specified injury of other specified muscles and tendons at ankle and foot level, unspecified foot
- S96.9 Injury of unspecified muscle and tendon at ankle and foot level
  - S96.90 Unspecified injury of unspecified muscle and tendon at ankle and foot level
    - S96.901 Unspecified injury of unspecified muscle and tendon at ankle and foot level, right foot
    - S96.902 Unspecified injury of unspecified muscle and tendon at ankle and foot level, left foot
    - S96.909 Unspecified injury of unspecified muscle and tendon at ankle and foot level, unspecified foot
  - S96.91 Strain of unspecified muscle and tendon at ankle and foot level
    - S96.911 Strain of unspecified muscle and tendon at ankle and foot level, right foot
    - S96.912 Strain of unspecified muscle and tendon at ankle and foot level, left foot
    - S96.919 Strain of unspecified muscle and tendon at ankle and foot level, unspecified foot
  - S96.92 Laceration of unspecified muscle and tendon at ankle and foot level
    - S96.921 Laceration of unspecified muscle and tendon at ankle and foot level, right foot
    - S96.922 Laceration of unspecified muscle and tendon at ankle and foot level, left foot
    - S96.929 Laceration of unspecified muscle and tendon at ankle and foot level, unspecified foot

▶ New   ⇒ Revised   ~~deleted~~ Deleted   **OGCR** Official Guidelines   X Assign placeholder X   ● Use Additional Character(s)

Excludes 1   Excludes 2   Includes   Use additional   Code first   Code also   Key words

● S96.99   Other specified injury of unspecified muscle
            and tendon at ankle and foot level
    ● S96.991   Other specified injury of unspecified
                 muscle and tendon at ankle and foot
                 level, right foot
    ● S96.992   Other specified injury of unspecified
                 muscle and tendon at ankle and foot
                 level, left foot
    ● S96.999   Other specified injury of unspecified
                 muscle and tendon at ankle and foot
                 level, unspecified foot

● S97   Crushing injury of ankle and foot
         Use additional code(s) for all associated injuries
         The appropriate 7th character is to be added to each code from
             category S97

         ┌─────────────────────────────────┐
         │ A   initial encounter   │
         │ D   subsequent encounter   │
         │ S   sequela   │
         └─────────────────────────────────┘

    ● S97.0   Crushing injury of ankle
      X ● S97.00   Crushing injury of unspecified ankle
      X ● S97.01   Crushing injury of right ankle
      X ● S97.02   Crushing injury of left ankle
    ● S97.1   Crushing injury of toe
      ● S97.10   Crushing injury of unspecified toe(s)
          ● S97.101   Crushing injury of unspecified right
                       toe(s)
          ● S97.102   Crushing injury of unspecified left
                       toe(s)
          ● S97.109   Crushing injury of unspecified toe(s)
                       Crushing injury of toe NOS
      ● S97.11   Crushing injury of great toe
          ● S97.111   Crushing injury of right great toe
          ● S97.112   Crushing injury of left great toe
          ● S97.119   Crushing injury of unspecified great
                       toe
      ● S97.12   Crushing injury of lesser toe(s)
          ● S97.121   Crushing injury of right lesser toe(s)
          ● S97.122   Crushing injury of left lesser toe(s)
          ● S97.129   Crushing injury of lesser toe(s),
                       unspecified toe(s)
    ● S97.8   Crushing injury of foot
      X ● S97.80   Crushing injury of foot, unspecified side
                    Crushing injury of foot NOS
      X ● S97.81   Crushing injury of right foot
      X ● S97.82   Crushing injury of left foot

● S98   Traumatic amputation of ankle and foot
         An amputation not identified as partial or complete should be
             coded to complete
         The appropriate 7th character is to be added to each code from
             category S98

         ┌─────────────────────────────────┐
         │ A   initial encounter   │
         │ D   subsequent encounter   │
         │ S   sequela   │
         └─────────────────────────────────┘

    ● S98.0   Traumatic amputation of foot at ankle level
      ● S98.01   Complete traumatic amputation of foot at ankle
                  level
          ● S98.011   Complete traumatic amputation of
                       right foot at ankle level
          ● S98.012   Complete traumatic amputation of
                       left foot at ankle level
          ● S98.019   Complete traumatic amputation of
                       unspecified foot at ankle level

● S98.02   Partial traumatic amputation of foot at ankle
            level
    ● S98.021   Partial traumatic amputation of right
                 foot at ankle level
    ● S98.022   Partial traumatic amputation of left
                 foot at ankle level
    ● S98.029   Partial traumatic amputation of
                 unspecified foot at ankle level
● S98.1   Traumatic amputation of one toe
    ● S98.11   Complete traumatic amputation of great toe
        ● S98.111   Complete traumatic amputation of
                     right great toe
        ● S98.112   Complete traumatic amputation of
                     left great toe
        ● S98.119   Complete traumatic amputation of
                     unspecified great toe
    ● S98.12   Partial traumatic amputation of great toe
        ● S98.121   Partial traumatic amputation of right
                     great toe
        ● S98.122   Partial traumatic amputation of left
                     great toe
        ● S98.129   Partial traumatic amputation of
                     unspecified great toe
    ● S98.13   Complete traumatic amputation of one lesser
                toe
                Traumatic amputation of toe NOS
        ● S98.131   Complete traumatic amputation of
                     one right lesser toe
        ● S98.132   Complete traumatic amputation of
                     one left lesser toe
        ● S98.139   Complete traumatic amputation of
                     one unspecified lesser toe
    ● S98.14   Partial traumatic amputation of one lesser toe
        ● S98.141   Partial traumatic amputation of one
                     right lesser toe
        ● S98.142   Partial traumatic amputation of one
                     left lesser toe
        ● S98.149   Partial traumatic amputation of one
                     unspecified lesser toe
● S98.2   Traumatic amputation of two or more lesser toes
    ● S98.21   Complete traumatic amputation of two or more
                lesser toes
        ● S98.211   Complete traumatic amputation of
                     two or more right lesser toes
        ● S98.212   Complete traumatic amputation of
                     two or more left lesser toes
        ● S98.219   Complete traumatic amputation of
                     two or more unspecified lesser toes
    ● S98.22   Partial traumatic amputation of two or more
                lesser toes
        ● S98.221   Partial traumatic amputation of two
                     or more right lesser toes
        ● S98.222   Partial traumatic amputation of two
                     or more left lesser toes
        ● S98.229   Partial traumatic amputation of two
                     or more unspecified lesser toes
● S98.3   Traumatic amputation of midfoot
    ● S98.31   Complete traumatic amputation of midfoot
        ● S98.311   Complete traumatic amputation of
                     right midfoot
        ● S98.312   Complete traumatic amputation of
                     left midfoot
        ● S98.319   Complete traumatic amputation of
                     unspecified midfoot

▶ New   ⇛ Revised   ~~deleted~~ Deleted   **OGCR** Official Guidelines   X Assign placeholder X   ● Use Additional Character(s)

Excludes 1   Excludes 2   Includes   Use additional   Code first   Code also   Key words

● S98.32   Partial traumatic amputation of midfoot
   ● S98.321   Partial traumatic amputation of right midfoot
   ● S98.322   Partial traumatic amputation of left midfoot
   ● S98.329   Partial traumatic amputation of unspecified midfoot

● S98.9   Traumatic amputation of foot, level unspecified
  ● S98.91   Complete traumatic amputation of foot, level unspecified
   ● S98.911   Complete traumatic amputation of right foot, level unspecified
   ● S98.912   Complete traumatic amputation of left foot, level unspecified
   ● S98.919   Complete traumatic amputation of unspecified foot, level unspecified

  ● S98.92   Partial traumatic amputation of foot, level unspecified
   ● S98.921   Partial traumatic amputation of right foot, level unspecified
   ● S98.922   Partial traumatic amputation of left foot, level unspecified
   ● S98.929   Partial traumatic amputation of unspecified foot, level unspecified

● S99   Other and unspecified injuries of ankle and foot
 ● S99.0   Physeal fracture of calcaneus

The appropriate 7th character is to be added to each code from subcategories S99.0

A	initial encounter for closed fracture
B	initial encounter for open fracture
D	subsequent encounter for fracture with routine healing
G	subsequent encounter for fracture with delayed healing
K	subsequent encounter for fracture with nonunion
P	subsequent encounter for fracture with malunion
S	sequela

  ● S99.00   Unspecified physeal fracture of calcaneus
   ● S99.001   Unspecified physeal fracture of right calcaneus
   ● S99.002   Unspecified physeal fracture of left calcaneus
   ● S99.009   Unspecified physeal fracture of unspecified calcaneus

  ● S99.01   Salter-Harris Type I physeal fracture of calcaneus
   ● S99.011   Salter-Harris Type I physeal fracture of right calcaneus
   ● S99.012   Salter-Harris Type I physeal fracture of left calcaneus
   ● S99.019   Salter-Harris Type I physeal fracture of unspecified calcaneus

  ● S99.02   Salter-Harris Type II physeal fracture of calcaneus
   ● S99.021   Salter-Harris Type II physeal fracture of right calcaneus
   ● S99.022   Salter-Harris Type II physeal fracture of left calcaneus
   ● S99.029   Salter-Harris Type II physeal fracture of unspecified calcaneus

  ● S99.03   Salter-Harris Type III physeal fracture of calcaneus
   ● S99.031   Salter-Harris Type III physeal fracture of right calcaneus
   ● S99.032   Salter-Harris Type III physeal fracture of left calcaneus
   ● S99.039   Salter-Harris Type III physeal fracture of unspecified calcaneus

  ● S99.04   Salter-Harris Type IV physeal fracture of calcaneus
   ● S99.041   Salter-Harris Type IV physeal fracture of right calcaneus
   ● S99.042   Salter-Harris Type IV physeal fracture of left calcaneus
   ● S99.049   Salter-Harris Type IV physeal fracture of unspecified calcaneus

  ● S99.09   Other physeal fracture of calcaneus
   ● S99.091   Other physeal fracture of right calcaneus
   ● S99.092   Other physeal fracture of left calcaneus
   ● S99.099   Other physeal fracture of unspecified calcaneus

 ● S99.1   Physeal fracture of metatarsal

The appropriate 7th character is to be added to each code from subcategories S99.1

A	initial encounter for closed fracture
B	initial encounter for open fracture
D	subsequent encounter for fracture with routine healing
G	subsequent encounter for fracture with delayed healing
K	subsequent encounter for fracture with nonunion
P	subsequent encounter for fracture with malunion
S	sequela

  ● S99.10   Unspecified physeal fracture of metatarsal
   ● S99.101   Unspecified physeal fracture of right metatarsal
   ● S99.102   Unspecified physeal fracture of left metatarsal
   ● S99.109   Unspecified physeal fracture of unspecified metatarsal

  ● S99.11   Salter-Harris Type I physeal fracture of metatarsal
   ● S99.111   Salter-Harris Type I physeal fracture of right metatarsal
   ● S99.112   Salter-Harris Type I physeal fracture of left metatarsal
   ● S99.119   Salter-Harris Type I physeal fracture of unspecified metatarsal

  ● S99.12   Salter-Harris Type II physeal fracture of metatarsal
   ● S99.121   Salter-Harris Type II physeal fracture of right metatarsal
   ● S99.122   Salter-Harris Type II physeal fracture of left metatarsal
   ● S99.129   Salter-Harris Type II physeal fracture of unspecified metatarsal

CHAPTER 19 (S00-T88)

CHAPTER 19 (S00-T88)

- ● **S99.13** Salter-Harris Type III physeal fracture of metatarsal
  - ● **S99.131** Salter-Harris Type III physeal fracture of right metatarsal
  - ● **S99.132** Salter-Harris Type III physeal fracture of left metatarsal
  - ● **S99.139** Salter-Harris Type III physeal fracture of unspecified metatarsal
- ● **S99.14** Salter-Harris Type IV physeal fracture of metatarsal
  - ● **S99.141** Salter-Harris Type IV physeal fracture of right metatarsal
  - ● **S99.142** Salter-Harris Type IV physeal fracture of left metatarsal
  - ● **S99.149** Salter-Harris Type IV physeal fracture of unspecified metatarsal
- ● **S99.19** Other physeal fracture of metatarsal
  - ● **S99.191** Other physeal fracture of right metatarsal
  - ● **S99.192** Other physeal fracture of left metatarsal
  - ● **S99.199** Other physeal fracture of unspecified metatarsal
- ● **S99.2** Physeal fracture of phalanx of toe

  The appropriate 7th character is to be added to each code from subcategories S99.2

A	initial encounter for closed fracture
B	initial encounter for open fracture
D	subsequent encounter for fracture with routine healing
G	subsequent encounter for fracture with delayed healing
K	subsequent encounter for fracture with nonunion
P	subsequent encounter for fracture with malunion
S	sequela

  - ● **S99.20** Unspecified physeal fracture of phalanx of toe
    - ● **S99.201** Unspecified physeal fracture of phalanx of right toe
    - ● **S99.202** Unspecified physeal fracture of phalanx of right toe
    - ● **S99.209** Unspecified physeal fracture of phalanx of unspecified toe
  - ● **S99.21** Salter-Harris Type I physeal fracture of phalanx of toe
    - ● **S99.211** Salter-Harris Type I physeal fracture of phalanx of right toe
    - ● **S99.212** Salter-Harris Type I physeal fracture of phalanx of left toe
    - ● **S99.219** Salter-Harris Type I physeal fracture of phalanx of unspecified toe
  - ● **S99.22** Salter-Harris Type II physeal fracture of phalanx of toe
    - ● **S99.221** Salter-Harris Type II physeal fracture of phalanx of right toe
    - ● **S99.222** Salter-Harris Type II physeal fracture of phalanx of left toe
    - ● **S99.229** Salter-Harris Type II physeal fracture of phalanx of unspecified toe

- ● **S99.23** Salter-Harris Type III physeal fracture of phalanx of toe
  - ● **S99.231** Salter-Harris Type III physeal fracture of phalanx of right toe
  - ● **S99.232** Salter-Harris Type III physeal fracture of phalanx of left toe
  - ● **S99.239** Salter-Harris Type III physeal fracture of phalanx of unspecified toe
- ● **S99.24** Salter-Harris Type IV physeal fracture of phalanx of toe
  - ● **S99.241** Salter-Harris Type IV physeal fracture of phalanx of right toe
  - ● **S99.242** Salter-Harris Type IV physeal fracture of phalanx of left toe
  - ● **S99.249** Salter-Harris Type IV physeal fracture of phalanx of unspecified toe
- ● **S99.29** Other physeal fracture of phalanx of toe
  - ● **S99.291** Other physeal fracture of phalanx of right toe
  - ● **S99.292** Other physeal fracture of phalanx of left toe
  - ● **S99.299** Other physeal fracture of phalanx of unspecified toe
- ● **S99.8** Other specified injuries of ankle and foot

  The appropriate 7th character is to be added to each code from subcategory S99.8

A	initial encounter
D	subsequent encounter
S	sequela

  - ● **S99.81** Other specified injuries of ankle
    - ● **S99.811** Other specified injuries of right ankle
    - ● **S99.812** Other specified injuries of left ankle
    - ● **S99.819** Other specified injuries of unspecified ankle
  - ● **S99.82** Other specified injuries of foot
    - ● **S99.821** Other specified injuries of right foot
    - ● **S99.822** Other specified injuries of left foot
    - ● **S99.829** Other specified injuries of unspecified foot
- ● **S99.9** Unspecified injury of ankle and foot

  The appropriate 7th character is to be added to each code from subcategory S99.9

A	initial encounter
D	subsequent encounter
S	sequela

  - ● **S99.91** Unspecified injury of ankle
    - ● **S99.911** Unspecified injury of right ankle
    - ● **S99.912** Unspecified injury of left ankle
    - ● **S99.919** Unspecified injury of unspecified ankle
  - ● **S99.92** Unspecified injury of foot
    - ● **S99.921** Unspecified injury of right foot
    - ● **S99.922** Unspecified injury of left foot
    - ● **S99.929** Unspecified injury of unspecified foot

▶ New   ⇒ Revised   ~~deleted~~ Deleted   **OGCR** Official Guidelines   X Assign placeholder X   ● Use Additional Character(s)

Excludes 1   Excludes 2   Includes   Use additional   Code first   Code also   Key words

INJURY, POISONING AND CERTAIN OTHER CONSEQUENCES OF EXTERNAL CAUSES (T07-T88)

INJURIES INVOLVING MULTIPLE BODY REGIONS (T07)

Excludes1   burns and corrosions (T20-T32)
frostbite (T33-T34)
insect bite or sting, venomous (T63.4)
sunburn (L55.-)

X● **T07**   **Unspecified** multiple injuries

▶ The appropriate 7th character is to be added to code T07

> ▶A   initial encounter
> ▶D   subsequent encounter
> ▶S   sequela

⇒ **Excludes1**   injury NOS (T14.90)

INJURY OF UNSPECIFIED BODY REGION (T14)

● **T14**   **Injury of unspecified body region**

▶ The appropriate 7th character is to be added to each code from category T14

> ▶A   initial encounter
> ▶D   subsequent encounter
> ▶S   sequela

Excludes1   multiple unspecified injuries (T07)

X● **T14.8**   **Other injury of unspecified body region**
Abrasion NOS   Skin injury NOS
Contusion NOS   Vascular injury NOS
Crush injury NOS   ▶Wound NOS
Fracture NOS

● **T14.9**   **Unspecified injury**

X● **T14.90**   **Injury, unspecified**
Injury NOS

X● **T14.91**   **Suicide attempt**
Attempted suicide NOS

EFFECTS OF FOREIGN BODY ENTERING THROUGH NATURAL ORIFICE (T15-T19)

Excludes2   foreign body accidentally left in operation wound (T81.5-)
foreign body in penetrating wound - see open wound by body region
residual foreign body in soft tissue (M79.5)
splinter, without open wound - see superficial injury by body region

● **T15**   **Foreign body on external eye**

Excludes2   foreign body in penetrating wound of orbit and eye ball (S05.4-, S05.5-)
open wound of eyelid and periocular area (S01.1-)
retained foreign body in eyelid (H02.8-)
retained (old) foreign body in penetrating wound of orbit and eye ball (H05.5-, H44.6-, H44.7-)
superficial foreign body of eyelid and periocular area (S00.25-)

The appropriate 7th character is to be added to each code from category T15

> A   initial encounter
> D   subsequent encounter
> S   sequela

● **T15.0**   **Foreign body in cornea**

X● **T15.00**   Foreign body in cornea, **unspecified** eye

X● **T15.01**   Foreign body in cornea, **right** eye

X● **T15.02**   Foreign body in cornea, **left** eye

● **T15.1**   **Foreign body in conjunctival sac**

X● **T15.10**   Foreign body in conjunctival sac, **unspecified** eye

X● **T15.11**   Foreign body in conjunctival sac, **right eye**

X● **T15.12**   Foreign body in conjunctival sac, **left eye**

● **T15.8**   **Foreign body in other and multiple parts of external eye**
Foreign body in lacrimal punctum

X● **T15.80**   Foreign body in other and multiple parts of external eye, **unspecified** eye

X● **T15.81**   Foreign body in other and multiple parts of external eye, **right** eye

X● **T15.82**   Foreign body in other and multiple parts of external eye, **left** eye

● **T15.9**   **Foreign body on external eye, part unspecified**

X● **T15.90**   Foreign body on external eye, part unspecified, **unspecified** eye

X● **T15.91**   Foreign body on external eye, part unspecified, **right eye**

X● **T15.92**   Foreign body on external eye, part unspecified, **left eye**

● **T16**   **Foreign body in ear**

Includes   foreign body in auditory canal

The appropriate 7th character is to be added to each code from category T16

> A   initial encounter
> D   subsequent encounter
> S   sequela

X● **T16.1**   Foreign body in **right ear**

X● **T16.2**   Foreign body in **left ear**

X● **T16.9**   Foreign body in ear, **unspecified** ear

● **T17**   **Foreign body in respiratory tract**

The appropriate 7th character is to be added to each code from category T17

> A   initial encounter
> D   subsequent encounter
> S   sequela

X● **T17.0**   Foreign body in **nasal sinus**

X● **T17.1**   Foreign body in **nostril**
Foreign body in nose NOS

● **T17.2**   **Foreign body in pharynx**
Foreign body in nasopharynx
Foreign body in throat NOS

● **T17.20**   **Unspecified** foreign body in pharynx

● **T17.200**   Unspecified foreign body in pharynx **causing asphyxiation**

● **T17.208**   Unspecified foreign body in pharynx **causing other injury**

● **T17.21**   **Gastric contents** in pharynx
Aspiration of gastric contents into pharynx
Vomitus in pharynx

● **T17.210**   Gastric contents in pharynx **causing asphyxiation**

● **T17.218**   Gastric contents in pharynx **causing other injury**

● **T17.22**   **Food in pharynx**
Bones in pharynx
Seeds in pharynx

● **T17.220**   Food in pharynx **causing asphyxiation**

● **T17.228**   Food in pharynx **causing other injury**

● **T17.29**   **Other** foreign object in pharynx

● **T17.290**   Other foreign object in pharynx **causing asphyxiation**

● **T17.298**   Other foreign object in pharynx **causing other injury**

▶ New   ⇒ Revised   ~~deleted~~ Deleted   **OGCR** Official Guidelines   X Assign placeholder X   ● Use Additional Character(s)

| Excludes 1 | Excludes 2 | Includes | Use additional | Code first | Code also | Key words |

● **T17.3**   Foreign body in larynx
- ● **T17.30**   Unspecified foreign body in larynx
  - ● **T17.300**   Unspecified foreign body in larynx causing asphyxiation
  - ● **T17.308**   Unspecified foreign body in larynx causing other injury
- ● **T17.31**   Gastric contents in larynx
  Aspiration of gastric contents into larynx
  Vomitus in larynx
  - ● **T17.310**   Gastric contents in larynx causing asphyxiation
  - ● **T17.318**   Gastric contents in larynx causing other injury
- ● **T17.32**   Food in larynx
  Bones in larynx
  Seeds in larynx
  - ● **T17.320**   Food in larynx causing asphyxiation
  - ● **T17.328**   Food in larynx causing other injury
- ● **T17.39**   Other foreign object in larynx
  - ● **T17.390**   Other foreign object in larynx causing asphyxiation
  - ● **T17.398**   Other foreign object in larynx causing other injury

● **T17.4**   Foreign body in trachea
- ● **T17.40**   Unspecified foreign body in trachea
  - ● **T17.400**   Unspecified foreign body in trachea causing asphyxiation
  - ● **T17.408**   Unspecified foreign body in trachea causing other injury
- ● **T17.41**   Gastric contents in trachea
  Aspiration of gastric contents into trachea
  Vomitus in trachea
  - ● **T17.410**   Gastric contents in trachea causing asphyxiation
  - ● **T17.418**   Gastric contents in trachea causing other injury
- ● **T17.42**   Food in trachea
  Bones in trachea
  Seeds in trachea
  - ● **T17.420**   Food in trachea causing asphyxiation
  - ● **T17.428**   Food in trachea causing other injury
- ● **T17.49**   Other foreign object in trachea
  - ● **T17.490**   Other foreign object in trachea causing asphyxiation
  - ● **T17.498**   Other foreign object in trachea causing other injury

● **T17.5**   Foreign body in bronchus
- ● **T17.50**   Unspecified foreign body in bronchus
  - ● **T17.500**   Unspecified foreign body in bronchus causing asphyxiation
  - ● **T17.508**   Unspecified foreign body in bronchus causing other injury
- ● **T17.51**   Gastric contents in bronchus
  Aspiration of gastric contents into bronchus
  Vomitus in bronchus
  - ● **T17.510**   Gastric contents in bronchus causing asphyxiation
  - ● **T17.518**   Gastric contents in bronchus causing other injury

● **T17.52**   Food in bronchus
  Bones in bronchus
  Seeds in bronchus
  - ● **T17.520**   Food in bronchus causing asphyxiation
  - ● **T17.528**   Food in bronchus causing other injury
- ● **T17.59**   Other foreign object in bronchus
  - ● **T17.590**   Other foreign object in bronchus causing asphyxiation
  - ● **T17.598**   Other foreign object in bronchus causing other injury

● **T17.8**   Foreign body in other parts of respiratory tract
  Foreign body in bronchioles
  Foreign body in lung
- ● **T17.80**   Unspecified foreign body in other parts of respiratory tract
  - ● **T17.800**   Unspecified foreign body in other parts of respiratory tract causing asphyxiation
  - ● **T17.808**   Unspecified foreign body in other parts of respiratory tract causing other injury
- ● **T17.81**   Gastric contents in other parts of respiratory tract
  Aspiration of gastric contents into other parts of respiratory tract
  Vomitus in other parts of respiratory tract
  - ● **T17.810**   Gastric contents in other parts of respiratory tract causing asphyxiation
  - ● **T17.818**   Gastric contents in other parts of respiratory tract causing other injury
- ● **T17.82**   Food in other parts of respiratory tract
  Bones in other parts of respiratory tract
  Seeds in other parts of respiratory tract
  - ● **T17.820**   Food in other parts of respiratory tract causing asphyxiation
  - ● **T17.828**   Food in other parts of respiratory tract causing other injury
- ● **T17.89**   Other foreign object in other parts of respiratory tract
  - ● **T17.890**   Other foreign object in other parts of respiratory tract causing asphyxiation
  - ● **T17.898**   Other foreign object in other parts of respiratory tract causing other injury

● **T17.9**   Foreign body in respiratory tract, part unspecified
- ● **T17.90**   Unspecified foreign body in respiratory tract, part unspecified
  - ● **T17.900**   Unspecified foreign body in respiratory tract, part unspecified causing asphyxiation
  - ● **T17.908**   Unspecified foreign body in respiratory tract, part unspecified causing other injury
- ● **T17.91**   Gastric contents in respiratory tract, part unspecified
  Aspiration of gastric contents into respiratory tract, part unspecified
  Vomitus in trachea respiratory tract, part unspecified
  - ● **T17.910**   Gastric contents in respiratory tract, part unspecified causing asphyxiation
  - ● **T17.918**   Gastric contents in respiratory tract, part unspecified causing other injury

● **T17.92**   Food in respiratory tract, part unspecified
     Bones in respiratory tract, part unspecified
     Seeds in respiratory tract, part unspecified
   ● **T17.920**   Food in respiratory tract, part unspecified causing asphyxiation
   ● **T17.928**   Food in respiratory tract, part unspecified causing other injury
● **T17.99**   Other foreign object in respiratory tract, part unspecified
   ● **T17.990**   Other foreign object in respiratory tract, part unspecified in causing asphyxiation
   ● **T17.998**   Other foreign object in respiratory tract, part unspecified causing other injury

● **T18**   Foreign body in alimentary tract
   Excludes2   foreign body in pharynx (T17.2-)
   The appropriate 7th character is to be added to each code from category T18

A	initial encounter
D	subsequent encounter
S	sequela

X ● **T18.0**   Foreign body in mouth
X ● **T18.1**   Foreign body in esophagus
     Excludes2   foreign body in respiratory tract (T17.-)
   ● **T18.10**   Unspecified foreign body in esophagus
     ● **T18.100**   Unspecified foreign body in esophagus causing compression of trachea
       Unspecified foreign body in esophagus causing obstruction of respiration
     ● **T18.108**   Unspecified foreign body in esophagus causing other injury
   ● **T18.11**   Gastric contents in esophagus
     Vomitus in esophagus
     ● **T18.110**   Gastric contents in esophagus causing compression of trachea
       Gastric contents in esophagus causing obstruction of respiration
     ● **T18.118**   Gastric contents in esophagus causing other injury
   ● **T18.12**   Food in esophagus
     Bones in esophagus
     Seeds in esophagus
     ● **T18.120**   Food in esophagus causing compression of trachea
       Food in esophagus causing obstruction of respiration
     ● **T18.128**   Food in esophagus causing other injury
   ● **T18.19**   Other foreign object in esophagus
     ● **T18.190**   Other foreign object in esophagus causing compression of trachea
       Other foreign body in esophagus causing obstruction of respiration
     ● **T18.198**   Other foreign object in esophagus causing other injury
X ● **T18.2**   Foreign body in stomach
X ● **T18.3**   Foreign body in small intestine

X ● **T18.4**   Foreign body in colon
X ● **T18.5**   Foreign body in anus and rectum
     Foreign body in rectosigmoid (junction)
X ● **T18.8**   Foreign body in other parts of alimentary tract
X ● **T18.9**   Foreign body of alimentary tract, part unspecified
     Foreign body in digestive system NOS
     Swallowed foreign body NOS

● **T19**   Foreign body in genitourinary tract
   Excludes2   complications due to implanted mesh (T83.7-)
     mechanical complications of contraceptive device (intrauterine) (vaginal) (T83.3-)
     presence of contraceptive device (intrauterine) (vaginal) (Z97.5)
   The appropriate 7th character is to be added to each code from category T19

A	initial encounter
D	subsequent encounter
S	sequela

X ● **T19.0**   Foreign body in urethra
X ● **T19.1**   Foreign body in bladder
X ● **T19.2**   Foreign body in vulva and vagina
X ● **T19.3**   Foreign body in uterus
X ● **T19.4**   Foreign body in penis
X ● **T19.8**   Foreign body in other parts of genitourinary tract
X ● **T19.9**   Foreign body in genitourinary tract, part unspecified

BURNS AND CORROSIONS (T20-T32)

Includes	burns (thermal) from electrical heating appliances
	burns (thermal) from electricity
	burns (thermal) from flame
	burns (thermal) from friction
	burns (thermal) from hot air and hot gases
	burns (thermal) from hot objects
	burns (thermal) from lightning
	burns (thermal) from radiation chemical
	burn [corrosion] (external) (internal) scalds
Excludes2	erythema [dermatitis] ab igne (L59.0)
	radiation-related disorders of the skin and subcutaneous tissue (L55-L59)
	sunburn (L55.-)

OGCR   Section I.C.19.d.

Burns and Corrosions

The ICD-10-CM makes a distinction between burn and corrosions. The burn codes are for thermal burns, except sunburns, that come from a heat source, such as a fire or hot appliance. The burn codes are also for burns resulting from electricity and radiation. Corrosions are burns due to chemicals. The guidelines for burns and corrosions are the same.

Current burns (T20-T25) are classified by depth, extent and by agent (X code). Burns are classified by depth as first degree (erythema), second degree (blistering), and third degree (full-thickness involvement). Burns of the eye and internal organs (T26-T28) are classified by site, but not by degree.

1) Sequencing of burn and related condition codes

Sequence first the code that reflects the highest degree of burn when more than one burn is present.

a. When the reason for the admission or encounter is for treatment of external multiple burns, sequence first the code that reflects the burn of the highest degree.

b. When a patient has both internal and external burns, the circumstances of admission govern the selection of the principal diagnosis or first-listed diagnosis.

c. When a patient is admitted for burn injuries and other related conditions such as smoke inhalation and/or respiratory failure, the circumstances of admission govern the selection of the principal or first-listed diagnosis.

2) Burns of the same local site

Classify burns of the same local site (three-character category level, T20-T28) but of different degrees to the subcategory identifying the highest degree recorded in the diagnosis.

▶ New   ⇒ Revised   ~~deleted~~ Deleted   **OGCR** Official Guidelines   X Assign placeholder X   ● Use Additional Character(s)

Excludes 1	Excludes 2	Includes	Use additional	Code first	Code also	Key words

BURNS AND CORROSIONS OF EXTERNAL BODY SURFACE, SPECIFIED BY SITE (T20-T25)

Includes   burns and corrosions of first degree [erythema]
burns and corrosions of second degree [blisters] [epidermal loss]
burns and corrosions of third degree [deep necrosis of underlying tissue] [full-thickness skin loss]
Use additional code from category T31 or T32 to identify extent of body surface involved

● **T20**   **Burn and corrosion of head, face, and neck**

     Excludes2   burn and corrosion of ear drum (T28.41, T28.91)
                        burn and corrosion of eye and adnexa (T26.-)
                        burn and corrosion of mouth and pharynx (T28.0)

The appropriate 7th character is to be added to each code from category T20

     A   initial encounter
     D   subsequent encounter
     S   sequela

● **T20.0**   **Burn of unspecified degree of head, face, and neck**
Use additional external cause code to identify the source, place and intent of the burn (X00-X19, X75-X77, X96-X98, Y92)

X ● **T20.00**   Burn of unspecified degree of head, face, and neck, **unspecified site**

● **T20.01**   Burn of unspecified degree of **ear** [any part, except ear drum]

     Excludes2   burn of ear drum (T28.41-)

  ● **T20.011**   Burn of unspecified degree of **right** ear [any part, except ear drum]

  ● **T20.012**   Burn of unspecified degree of **left** ear [any part, except ear drum]

  ● **T20.019**   Burn of unspecified degree of **unspecified** ear [any part, except ear drum]

X ● **T20.02**   Burn of unspecified degree of **lip(s)**

X ● **T20.03**   Burn of unspecified degree of **chin**

X ● **T20.04**   Burn of unspecified degree of **nose** (septum)

X ● **T20.05**   Burn of unspecified degree of **scalp** [any part]

X ● **T20.06**   Burn of unspecified degree of **forehead and cheek**

X ● **T20.07**   Burn of unspecified degree of **neck**

X ● **T20.09**   Burn of unspecified degree of **multiple sites** of head, face, and neck

● **T20.1**   **Burn of first degree of head, face, and neck**
Use additional external cause code to identify the source, place and intent of the burn (X00-X19, X75-X77, X96-X98, Y92)

X ● **T20.10**   Burn of first degree of head, face, and neck, **unspecified** site

● **T20.11**   Burn of first degree of ear [any part, except **ear** drum]

     Excludes2   burn of ear drum (T28.41-)

  ● **T20.111**   Burn of first degree of **right** ear [any part, except ear drum]

  ● **T20.112**   Burn of first degree of **left** ear [any part, except ear drum]

  ● **T20.119**   Burn of first degree of **unspecified** ear [any part, except ear drum]

Figure 19-15   **A.** Second-degree burn. **B.** Third-degree burn. (A. From Black J, Hawks J: Medical-Surgical Nursing: Clinical Management for Positive Outcomes, 8e, Saunders, 2008. B. From Marx J, Hockberger R, Walls R: Rosen's Emergency Medicine - Concepts and Clinical Practice, 7e, Mosby, 2009)

X ● **T20.12**   Burn of first degree of **lip(s)**

X ● **T20.13**   Burn of first degree of **chin**

X ● **T20.14**   Burn of first degree of **nose** (septum)

X ● **T20.15**   Burn of first degree of **scalp** [any part]

X ● **T20.16**   Burn of first degree of **forehead and cheek**

X ● **T20.17**   Burn of first degree of **neck**

X ● **T20.19**   Burn of first degree of **multiple sites** of head, face, and neck

● **T20.2**   **Burn of second degree of head, face, and neck**
Use additional external cause code to identify the source, place and intent of the burn (X00-X19, X75-X77, X96-X98, Y92)

X ● **T20.20**   Burn of second degree of head, face, and neck, **unspecified** site

● **T20.21**   Burn of second degree of **ear** [any part, except ear drum]

     Excludes2   burn of ear drum (T28.41-)

  ● **T20.211**   Burn of second degree of **right** ear [any part, except ear drum]

  ● **T20.212**   Burn of second degree of **left** ear [any part, except ear drum]

  ● **T20.219**   Burn of second degree of **unspecified** ear [any part, except ear drum]

X ● **T20.22**   Burn of second degree of **lip(s)**

X ● **T20.23**   Burn of second degree of **chin**

X ● **T20.24**   Burn of second degree of **nose** (septum)

X ● **T20.25**   Burn of second degree of **scalp** [any part]

X ● **T20.26**   Burn of second degree of **forehead and cheek**

X ● **T20.27**   Burn of second degree of **neck**

X ● **T20.29**   Burn of second degree of **multiple sites** of head, face, and neck

● **T20.3**   **Burn of third degree of head, face, and neck**
Use additional external cause code to identify the source, place and intent of the burn (X00-X19, X75-X77, X96-X98, Y92)

X ● **T20.30**   Burn of third degree of head, face, and neck, **unspecified** site

● **T20.31**   Burn of third degree of **ear** [any part, except ear drum]

     Excludes2   burn of ear drum (T28.41-)

  ● **T20.311**   Burn of third degree of **right** ear [any part, except ear drum]

  ● **T20.312**   Burn of third degree of **left** ear [any part, except ear drum]

  ● **T20.319**   Burn of third degree of **unspecified** ear [any part, except ear drum]

▶ New   ⮕ Revised   ~~deleted~~ Deleted   **OGCR** Official Guidelines   X Assign placeholder X   ● Use Additional Character(s)

Excludes 1   Excludes 2   Includes   Use additional   Code first   Code also   Key words

X ● **T20.32**   Burn of third degree of lip(s)

X ● **T20.33**   Burn of third degree of chin

X ● **T20.34**   Burn of third degree of nose (septum)

X ● **T20.35**   Burn of third degree of scalp [any part]

X ● **T20.36**   Burn of third degree of forehead and cheek

X ● **T20.37**   Burn of third degree of neck

X ● **T20.39**   Burn of third degree of multiple sites of head, face, and neck

● **T20.4**   Corrosion of unspecified degree of head, face, and neck

     Code first (T51-T65) to identify chemical and intent

     Use additional external cause code to identify place (Y92)

X ● **T20.40**   Corrosion of unspecified degree of head, face, and neck, unspecified site

● **T20.41**   Corrosion of unspecified degree of ear [any part, except ear drum]

       Excludes2   corrosion of ear drum (T28.91-)

     ● **T20.411**   Corrosion of unspecified degree of right ear [any part, except ear drum]

     ● **T20.412**   Corrosion of unspecified degree of left ear [any part, except ear drum]

     ● **T20.419**   Corrosion of unspecified degree of unspecified ear [any part, except ear drum]

X ● **T20.42**   Corrosion of unspecified degree of lip(s)

X ● **T20.43**   Corrosion of unspecified degree of chin

X ● **T20.44**   Corrosion of unspecified degree of nose (septum)

X ● **T20.45**   Corrosion of unspecified degree of scalp [any part]

X ● **T20.46**   Corrosion of unspecified degree of forehead and cheek

X ● **T20.47**   Corrosion of unspecified degree of neck

X ● **T20.49**   Corrosion of unspecified degree of multiple sites of head, face, and neck

● **T20.5**   Corrosion of first degree of head, face, and neck

     Code first (T51-T65) to identify chemical and intent

     Use additional external cause code to identify place (Y92)

X ● **T20.50**   Corrosion of first degree of head, face, and neck, unspecified site

● **T20.51**   Corrosion of first degree of ear [any part, except ear drum]

       Excludes2   corrosion of ear drum (T28.91-)

     ● **T20.511**   Corrosion of first degree of right ear [any part, except ear drum]

     ● **T20.512**   Corrosion of first degree of left ear [any part, except ear drum]

     ● **T20.519**   Corrosion of first degree of unspecified ear [any part, except ear drum]

X ● **T20.52**   Corrosion of first degree of lip(s)

X ● **T20.53**   Corrosion of first degree of chin

X ● **T20.54**   Corrosion of first degree of nose (septum)

X ● **T20.55**   Corrosion of first degree of scalp [any part]

X ● **T20.56**   Corrosion of first degree of forehead and cheek

X ● **T20.57**   Corrosion of first degree of neck

X ● **T20.59**   Corrosion of first degree of multiple sites of head, face, and neck

● **T20.6**   Corrosion of second degree of head, face, and neck

     Code first (T51-T65) to identify chemical and intent

     Use additional external cause code to identify place (Y92)

X ● **T20.60**   Corrosion of second degree of head, face, and neck, unspecified site

● **T20.61**   Corrosion of second degree of ear [any part, except ear drum]

       Excludes2   corrosion of ear drum (T28.91-)

     ● **T20.611**   Corrosion of second degree of right ear [any part, except ear drum]

     ● **T20.612**   Corrosion of second degree of left ear [any part, except ear drum]

     ● **T20.619**   Corrosion of second degree of unspecified ear [any part, except ear drum]

X ● **T20.62**   Corrosion of second degree of lip(s)

X ● **T20.63**   Corrosion of second degree of chin

X ● **T20.64**   Corrosion of second degree of nose (septum)

X ● **T20.65**   Corrosion of second degree of scalp [any part]

X ● **T20.66**   Corrosion of second degree of forehead and cheek

X ● **T20.67**   Corrosion of second degree of neck

X ● **T20.69**   Corrosion of second degree of multiple sites of head, face, and neck

● **T20.7**   Corrosion of third degree of head, face, and neck

     Code first (T51-T65) to identify chemical and intent

     Use additional external cause code to identify place (Y92)

X ● **T20.70**   Corrosion of third degree of head, face, and neck, unspecified site

● **T20.71**   Corrosion of third degree of ear [any part, except ear drum]

       Excludes2   corrosion of ear drum (T28.91-)

     ● **T20.711**   Corrosion of third degree of right ear [any part, except ear drum]

     ● **T20.712**   Corrosion of third degree of left ear [any part, except ear drum]

     ● **T20.719**   Corrosion of third degree of unspecified ear [any part, except ear drum]

X ● **T20.72**   Corrosion of third degree of lip(s)

X ● **T20.73**   Corrosion of third degree of chin

X ● **T20.74**   Corrosion of third degree of nose (septum)

X ● **T20.75**   Corrosion of third degree of scalp [any part]

X ● **T20.76**   Corrosion of third degree of forehead and cheek

X ● **T20.77**   Corrosion of third degree of neck

X ● **T20.79**   Corrosion of third degree of multiple sites of head, face, and neck

---

▶ New   ⟹ Revised   ~~deleted~~ Deleted   **OGCR** Official Guidelines   X Assign placeholder X   ● Use Additional Character(s)

Excludes 1   Excludes 2   Includes   Use additional   Code first   Code also   Key words

● **T21　Burn and corrosion of trunk**

>　**Includes**　burns and corrosion of hip region
>
>　**Excludes2**　burns and corrosion of axilla (T22.- with fifth character 4)
>　　　　　　　burns and corrosion of scapular region (T22.- with fifth character 6)
>　　　　　　　burns and corrosion of shoulder (T22.- with fifth character 5)
>
>　The appropriate 7th character is to be added to each code from category T21
>
>　　A　initial encounter
>　　D　subsequent encounter
>　　S　sequela

● **T21.0　Burn of unspecified degree of trunk**

>　Use additional external cause code to identify the source, place and intent of the burn (X00-X19, X75-X77, X96-X98, Y92)

　X ● **T21.00　Burn of unspecified degree of trunk, unspecified site**

　X ● **T21.01　Burn of unspecified degree of chest wall**
　　　　　Burn of of unspecified degree of breast

　X ● **T21.02　Burn of unspecified degree of abdominal wall**
　　　　　Burn of unspecified degree of flank
　　　　　Burn of unspecified degree of groin

　X ● **T21.03　Burn of unspecified degree of upper back**
　　　　　Burn of unspecified degree of interscapular region

　X ● **T21.04　Burn of unspecified degree of lower back**

　X ● **T21.05　Burn of unspecified degree of buttock**
　　　　　Burn of unspecified degree of anus

　X ● **T21.06　Burn of unspecified degree of male genital region**
　　　　　Burn of unspecified degree of penis
　　　　　Burn of unspecified degree of scrotum
　　　　　Burn of unspecified degree of testis

　X ● **T21.07　Burn of unspecified degree of female genital region**
　　　　　Burn of unspecified degree of labium (majus) (minus)
　　　　　Burn of unspecified degree of perineum
　　　　　Burn of unspecified degree of vulva
　　　　　Excludes2　burn of vagina (T28.3)

　X ● **T21.09　Burn of unspecified degree of other site of trunk**

● **T21.1　Burn of first degree of trunk**

>　Use additional external cause code to identify the source, place and intent of the burn (X00-X19, X75-X77, X96-X98, Y92)

　X ● **T21.10　Burn of first degree of trunk, unspecified site**

　X ● **T21.11　Burn of first degree of chest wall**
　　　　　Burn of first degree of breast

　X ● **T21.12　Burn of first degree of abdominal wall**
　　　　　Burn of first degree of flank
　　　　　Burn of first degree of groin

　X ● **T21.13　Burn of first degree of upper back**
　　　　　Burn of first degree of interscapular region

　X ● **T21.14　Burn of first degree of lower back**

　X ● **T21.15　Burn of first degree of buttock**
　　　　　Burn of first degree of anus

　X ● **T21.16　Burn of first degree of male genital region**
　　　　　Burn of first degree of penis
　　　　　Burn of first degree of scrotum
　　　　　Burn of first degree of testis

　X ● **T21.17　Burn of first degree of female genital region**
　　　　　Burn of first degree of labium (majus) (minus)
　　　　　Burn of first degree of perineum
　　　　　Burn of first degree of vulva
　　　　　Excludes2　burn of vagina (T28.3)

　X ● **T21.19　Burn of first degree of other site of trunk**

● **T21.2　Burn of second degree of trunk**

>　Use additional external cause code to identify the source, place and intent of the burn (X00-X19, X75-X77, X96-X98, Y92)

　X ● **T21.20　Burn of second degree of trunk, unspecified site**

　X ● **T21.21　Burn of second degree of chest wall**
　　　　　Burn of second degree of breast

　X ● **T21.22　Burn of second degree of abdominal wall**
　　　　　Burn of second degree of flank
　　　　　Burn of second degree of groin

　X ● **T21.23　Burn of second degree of upper back**
　　　　　Burn of second degree of interscapular region

　X ● **T21.24　Burn of second degree of lower back**

　X ● **T21.25　Burn of second degree of buttock**
　　　　　Burn of second degree of anus

　X ● **T21.26　Burn of second degree of male genital region**
　　　　　Burn of second degree of penis
　　　　　Burn of second degree of scrotum
　　　　　Burn of second degree of testis

　X ● **T21.27　Burn of second degree of female genital region**
　　　　　Burn of second degree of labium (majus) (minus)
　　　　　Burn of second degree of perineum
　　　　　Burn of second degree of vulva
　　　　　Excludes2　burn of vagina (T28.3)

　X ● **T21.29　Burn of second degree of other site of trunk**

● **T21.3　Burn of third degree of trunk**

>　Use additional external cause code to identify the source, place and intent of the burn (X00-X19, X75-X77, X96-X98, Y92)

　X ● **T21.30　Burn of third degree of trunk, unspecified site**

　X ● **T21.31　Burn of third degree of chest wall**
　　　　　Burn of third degree of breast

　X ● **T21.32　Burn of third degree of abdominal wall**
　　　　　Burn of third degree of flank
　　　　　Burn of third degree of groin

　X ● **T21.33　Burn of third degree of upper back**
　　　　　Burn of third degree of interscapular region

　X ● **T21.34　Burn of third degree of lower back**

　X ● **T21.35　Burn of third degree of buttock**
　　　　　Burn of third degree of anus

　X ● **T21.36　Burn of third degree of male genital region**
　　　　　Burn of third degree of penis
　　　　　Burn of third degree of scrotum
　　　　　Burn of third degree of testis

　X ● **T21.37　Burn of third degree of female genital region**
　　　　　Burn of third degree of labium (majus) (minus)
　　　　　Burn of third degree of perineum
　　　　　Burn of third degree of vulva
　　　　　Excludes2　burn of vagina (T28.3)

　X ● **T21.39　Burn of third degree of other site of trunk**

▶ New　⇒ Revised　~~deleted~~ Deleted　**OGCR** Official Guidelines　X Assign placeholder X　● Use Additional Character(s)

Excludes 1　Excludes 2　Includes　Use additional　Code first　Code also　Key words

● **T21.4　Corrosion of unspecified degree of trunk**

　　Code first (T51-T65) to identify chemical and intent

　　Use additional external cause code to identify
　　　place (Y92)

X ● **T21.40　Corrosion of unspecified degree of trunk, unspecified site**

X ● **T21.41　Corrosion of unspecified degree of chest wall**
　　　　Corrosion of unspecified degree of breast

X ● **T21.42　Corrosion of unspecified degree of abdominal wall**
　　　　Corrosion of unspecified degree of flank
　　　　Corrosion of unspecified degree of groin

X ● **T21.43　Corrosion of unspecified degree of upper back**
　　　　Corrosion of unspecified degree of interscapular region

X ● **T21.44　Corrosion of unspecified degree of lower back**

X ● **T21.45　Corrosion of unspecified degree of buttock**
　　　　Corrosion of unspecified degree of anus

X ● **T21.46　Corrosion of unspecified degree of male genital region**
　　　　Corrosion of unspecified degree of penis
　　　　Corrosion of unspecified degree of scrotum
　　　　Corrosion of unspecified degree of testis

X ● **T21.47　Corrosion of unspecified degree of female genital region**
　　　　Corrosion of unspecified degree of labium (majus) (minus)
　　　　Corrosion of unspecified degree of perineum
　　　　Corrosion of unspecified degree of vulva
　　　　　Excludes2　corrosion of vagina (T28.8)

X ● **T21.49　Corrosion of unspecified degree of other site of trunk**

● **T21.5　Corrosion of first degree of trunk**

　　Code first (T51-T65) to identify chemical and intent

　　Use additional external cause code to identify
　　　place (Y92)

X ● **T21.50　Corrosion of first degree of trunk, unspecified site**

X ● **T21.51　Corrosion of first degree of chest wall**
　　　　Corrosion of first degree of breast

X ● **T21.52　Corrosion of first degree of abdominal wall**
　　　　Corrosion of first degree of flank
　　　　Corrosion of first degree of groin

X ● **T21.53　Corrosion of first degree of upper back**
　　　　Corrosion of first degree of interscapular region

X ● **T21.54　Corrosion of first degree of lower back**

X ● **T21.55　Corrosion of first degree of buttock**
　　　　Corrosion of first degree of anus

X ● **T21.56　Corrosion of first degree of male genital region**
　　　　Corrosion of first degree of penis
　　　　Corrosion of first degree of scrotum
　　　　Corrosion of first degree of testis

X ● **T21.57　Corrosion of first degree of female genital region**
　　　　Corrosion of first degree of labium (majus) (minus)
　　　　Corrosion of first degree of perineum
　　　　Corrosion of first degree of vulva
　　　　　Excludes2　corrosion of vagina (T28.8)

X ● **T21.59　Corrosion of first degree of other site of trunk**

● **T21.6　Corrosion of second degree of trunk**

　　Code first (T51-T65) to identify chemical and intent

　　Use additional external cause code to identify
　　　place (Y92)

X ● **T21.60　Corrosion of second degree of trunk, unspecified site**

X ● **T21.61　Corrosion of second degree of chest wall**
　　　　Corrosion of second degree of breast

X ● **T21.62　Corrosion of second degree of abdominal wall**
　　　　Corrosion of second degree of flank
　　　　Corrosion of second degree of groin

X ● **T21.63　Corrosion of second degree of upper back**
　　　　Corrosion of second degree of interscapular region

X ● **T21.64　Corrosion of second degree of lower back**

X ● **T21.65　Corrosion of second degree of buttock**
　　　　Corrosion of second degree of anus

X ● **T21.66　Corrosion of second degree of male genital region**
　　　　Corrosion of second degree of penis
　　　　Corrosion of second degree of scrotum
　　　　Corrosion of second degree of testis

X ● **T21.67　Corrosion of second degree of female genital region**
　　　　Corrosion of second degree of labium (majus) (minus)
　　　　Corrosion of second degree of perineum
　　　　Corrosion of second degree of vulva
　　　　　Excludes2　corrosion of vagina (T28.8)

X ● **T21.69　Corrosion of second degree of other site of trunk**

● **T21.7　Corrosion of third degree of trunk**

　　Code first (T51-T65) to identify chemical and intent

　　Use additional external cause code to identify
　　　place (Y92)

X ● **T21.70　Corrosion of third degree of trunk, unspecified site**

X ● **T21.71　Corrosion of third degree of chest wall**
　　　　Corrosion of third degree of breast

X ● **T21.72　Corrosion of third degree of abdominal wall**
　　　　Corrosion of third degree of flank
　　　　Corrosion of third degree of groin

X ● **T21.73　Corrosion of third degree of upper back**
　　　　Corrosion of third degree of interscapular region

X ● **T21.74　Corrosion of third degree of lower back**

X ● **T21.75　Corrosion of third degree of buttock**
　　　　Corrosion of third degree of anus

X ● **T21.76　Corrosion of third degree of male genital region**
　　　　Corrosion of third degree of penis
　　　　Corrosion of third degree of scrotum
　　　　Corrosion of third degree of testis

X ● **T21.77　Corrosion of third degree of female genital region**
　　　　Corrosion of third degree of labium (majus) (minus)
　　　　Corrosion of third degree of perineum
　　　　Corrosion of third degree of vulva
　　　　　Excludes2　corrosion of vagina (T28.8)

X ● **T21.79　Corrosion of third degree of other site of trunk**

CHAPTER 19 (S00-T88)

● **T22** Burn and corrosion of shoulder and upper limb, except wrist and hand

Excludes2: burn and corrosion of interscapular region (T21.-)
burn and corrosion of wrist and hand (T23.-)

The appropriate 7th character is to be added to each code from category T22

A initial encounter
D subsequent encounter
S sequela

● **T22.0** Burn of unspecified degree of shoulder and upper limb, except wrist and hand

Use additional external cause code to identify the source, place and intent of the burn (X00-X19, X75-X77, X96-X98, Y92)

X● **T22.00** Burn of unspecified degree of shoulder and upper limb, except wrist and hand, unspecified site

● **T22.01** Burn of unspecified degree of forearm
- ● T22.011 Burn of unspecified degree of right forearm
- ● T22.012 Burn of unspecified degree of left forearm
- ● T22.019 Burn of unspecified degree of unspecified forearm

● **T22.02** Burn of unspecified degree of elbow
- ● T22.021 Burn of unspecified degree of right elbow
- ● T22.022 Burn of unspecified degree of left elbow
- ● T22.029 Burn of unspecified degree of unspecified elbow

● **T22.03** Burn of unspecified degree of upper arm
- ● T22.031 Burn of unspecified degree of right upper arm
- ● T22.032 Burn of unspecified degree of left upper arm
- ● T22.039 Burn of unspecified degree of unspecified upper arm

● **T22.04** Burn of unspecified degree of axilla
- ● T22.041 Burn of unspecified degree of right axilla
- ● T22.042 Burn of unspecified degree of left axilla
- ● T22.049 Burn of unspecified degree of unspecified axilla

● **T22.05** Burn of unspecified degree of shoulder
- ● T22.051 Burn of unspecified degree of right shoulder
- ● T22.052 Burn of unspecified degree of left shoulder
- ● T22.059 Burn of unspecified degree of unspecified shoulder

● **T22.06** Burn of unspecified degree of scapular region
- ● T22.061 Burn of unspecified degree of right scapular region
- ● T22.062 Burn of unspecified degree of left scapular region
- ● T22.069 Burn of unspecified degree of unspecified scapular region

● **T22.09** Burn of unspecified degree of multiple sites of shoulder and upper limb, except wrist and hand
- ● T22.091 Burn of unspecified degree of multiple sites of right shoulder and upper limb, except wrist and hand
- ● T22.092 Burn of unspecified degree of multiple sites of left shoulder and upper limb, except wrist and hand
- ● T22.099 Burn of unspecified degree of multiple sites of unspecified shoulder and upper limb, except wrist and hand

● **T22.1** Burn of first degree of shoulder and upper limb, except wrist and hand

Use additional external cause code to identify the source, place and intent of the burn (X00-X19, X75-X77, X96-X98, Y92)

X● **T22.10** Burn of first degree of shoulder and upper limb, except wrist and hand, unspecified site

● **T22.11** Burn of first degree of forearm
- ● T22.111 Burn of first degree of right forearm
- ● T22.112 Burn of first degree of left forearm
- ● T22.119 Burn of first degree of unspecified forearm

● **T22.12** Burn of first degree of elbow
- ● T22.121 Burn of first degree of right elbow
- ● T22.122 Burn of first degree of left elbow
- ● T22.129 Burn of first degree of unspecified elbow

● **T22.13** Burn of first degree of upper arm
- ● T22.131 Burn of first degree of right upper arm
- ● T22.132 Burn of first degree of left upper arm
- ● T22.139 Burn of first degree of unspecified upper arm

● **T22.14** Burn of first degree of axilla
- ● T22.141 Burn of first degree of right axilla
- ● T22.142 Burn of first degree of left axilla
- ● T22.149 Burn of first degree of unspecified axilla

● **T22.15** Burn of first degree of shoulder
- ● T22.151 Burn of first degree of right shoulder
- ● T22.152 Burn of first degree of left shoulder
- ● T22.159 Burn of first degree of unspecified shoulder

● **T22.16** Burn of first degree of scapular region
- ● T22.161 Burn of first degree of right scapular region
- ● T22.162 Burn of first degree of left scapular region
- ● T22.169 Burn of first degree of unspecified scapular region

● **T22.19** Burn of first degree of multiple sites of shoulder and upper limb, except wrist and hand
- ● T22.191 Burn of first degree of multiple sites of right shoulder and upper limb, except wrist and hand
- ● T22.192 Burn of first degree of multiple sites of left shoulder and upper limb, except wrist and hand
- ● T22.199 Burn of first degree of multiple sites of unspecified shoulder and upper limb, except wrist and hand

▶ New ⇒ Revised ~~deleted~~ Deleted **OGCR** Official Guidelines X Assign placeholder X ● Use Additional Character(s)
Excludes 1 Excludes 2 Includes Use additional Code first Code also Key words

● **T22.2** Burn of second degree of shoulder and upper limb, except wrist and hand

     Use additional external cause code to identify the source, place and intent of the burn (X00-X19, X75-X77, X96-X98, Y92)

X ● **T22.20**   Burn of second degree of shoulder and upper limb, except wrist and hand, unspecified site

● **T22.21**   Burn of second degree of forearm

    ● **T22.211**   Burn of second degree of right forearm

    ● **T22.212**   Burn of second degree of left forearm

    ● **T22.219**   Burn of second degree of unspecified forearm

● **T22.22**   Burn of second degree of elbow

    ● **T22.221**   Burn of second degree of right elbow

    ● **T22.222**   Burn of second degree of left elbow

    ● **T22.229**   Burn of second degree of unspecified elbow

● **T22.23**   Burn of second degree of upper arm

    ● **T22.231**   Burn of second degree of right upper arm

    ● **T22.232**   Burn of second degree of left upper arm

    ● **T22.239**   Burn of second degree of unspecified upper arm

● **T22.24**   Burn of second degree of axilla

    ● **T22.241**   Burn of second degree of right axilla

    ● **T22.242**   Burn of second degree of left axilla

    ● **T22.249**   Burn of second degree of unspecified axilla

● **T22.25**   Burn of second degree of shoulder

    ● **T22.251**   Burn of second degree of right shoulder

    ● **T22.252**   Burn of second degree of left shoulder

    ● **T22.259**   Burn of second degree of unspecified shoulder

● **T22.26**   Burn of second degree of scapular region

    ● **T22.261**   Burn of second degree of right scapular region

    ● **T22.262**   Burn of second degree of left scapular region

    ● **T22.269**   Burn of second degree of unspecified scapular region

● **T22.29**   Burn of second degree of multiple sites of shoulder and upper limb, except wrist and hand

    ● **T22.291**   Burn of second degree of multiple sites of right shoulder and upper limb, except wrist and hand

    ● **T22.292**   Burn of second degree of multiple sites of left shoulder and upper limb, except wrist and hand

    ● **T22.299**   Burn of second degree of multiple sites of unspecified shoulder and upper limb, except wrist and hand

● **T22.3** Burn of third degree of shoulder and upper limb, except wrist and hand

     Use additional external cause code to identify the source, place and intent of the burn (X00-X19, X75-X77, X96-X98, Y92)

X ● **T22.30**   Burn of third degree of shoulder and upper limb, except wrist and hand, unspecified site

● **T22.31**   Burn of third degree of forearm

    ● **T22.311**   Burn of third degree of right forearm

    ● **T22.312**   Burn of third degree of left forearm

    ● **T22.319**   Burn of third degree of unspecified forearm

● **T22.32**   Burn of third degree of elbow

    ● **T22.321**   Burn of third degree of right elbow

    ● **T22.322**   Burn of third degree of left elbow

    ● **T22.329**   Burn of third degree of unspecified elbow

● **T22.33**   Burn of third degree of upper arm

    ● **T22.331**   Burn of third degree of right upper arm

    ● **T22.332**   Burn of third degree of left upper arm

    ● **T22.339**   Burn of third degree of unspecified upper arm

● **T22.34**   Burn of third degree of axilla

    ● **T22.341**   Burn of third degree of right axilla

    ● **T22.342**   Burn of third degree of left axilla

    ● **T22.349**   Burn of third degree of unspecified axilla

● **T22.35**   Burn of third degree of shoulder

    ● **T22.351**   Burn of third degree of right shoulder

    ● **T22.352**   Burn of third degree of left shoulder

    ● **T22.359**   Burn of third degree of unspecified shoulder

● **T22.36**   Burn of third degree of scapular region

    ● **T22.361**   Burn of third degree of right scapular region

    ● **T22.362**   Burn of third degree of left scapular region

    ● **T22.369**   Burn of third degree of unspecified scapular region

● **T22.39**   Burn of third degree of multiple sites of shoulder and upper limb, except wrist and hand

    ● **T22.391**   Burn of third degree of multiple sites of right shoulder and upper limb, except wrist and hand

    ● **T22.392**   Burn of third degree of multiple sites of left shoulder and upper limb, except wrist and hand

    ● **T22.399**   Burn of third degree of multiple sites of unspecified shoulder and upper limb, except wrist and hand

● **T22.4** Corrosion of unspecified degree of shoulder and upper limb, except wrist and hand

     Code first (T51-T65) to identify chemical and intent

     Use additional external cause code to identify place (Y92)

X ● **T22.40**   Corrosion of unspecified degree of shoulder and upper limb, except wrist and hand, unspecified site

● **T22.41**   Corrosion of unspecified degree of forearm

    ● **T22.411**   Corrosion of unspecified degree of right forearm

    ● **T22.412**   Corrosion of unspecified degree of left forearm

    ● **T22.419**   Corrosion of unspecified degree of unspecified forearm

● **T22.42**   Corrosion of unspecified degree of elbow

    ● **T22.421**   Corrosion of unspecified degree of right elbow

    ● **T22.422**   Corrosion of unspecified degree of left elbow

    ● **T22.429**   Corrosion of unspecified degree of unspecified elbow

● **T22.43**   Corrosion of unspecified degree of upper arm

    ● **T22.431**   Corrosion of unspecified degree of right upper arm

    ● **T22.432**   Corrosion of unspecified degree of left upper arm

    ● **T22.439**   Corrosion of unspecified degree of unspecified upper arm

CHAPTER 19 (S00-T88)

● **T22.44**   Corrosion of unspecified degree of axilla
   ● **T22.441**   Corrosion of unspecified degree of right axilla
   ● **T22.442**   Corrosion of unspecified degree of left axilla
   ● **T22.449**   Corrosion of unspecified degree of unspecified axilla
● **T22.45**   Corrosion of unspecified degree of shoulder
   ● **T22.451**   Corrosion of unspecified degree of right shoulder
   ● **T22.452**   Corrosion of unspecified degree of left shoulder
   ● **T22.459**   Corrosion of unspecified degree of unspecified shoulder
● **T22.46**   Corrosion of unspecified degree of scapular region
   ● **T22.461**   Corrosion of unspecified degree of right scapular region
   ● **T22.462**   Corrosion of unspecified degree of left scapular region
   ● **T22.469**   Corrosion of unspecified degree of unspecified scapular region
● **T22.49**   Corrosion of unspecified degree of multiple sites of shoulder and upper limb, except wrist and hand
   ● **T22.491**   Corrosion of unspecified degree of multiple sites of right shoulder and upper limb, except wrist and hand
   ● **T22.492**   Corrosion of unspecified degree of multiple sites of left shoulder and upper limb, except wrist and hand
   ● **T22.499**   Corrosion of unspecified degree of multiple sites of unspecified shoulder and upper limb, except wrist and hand
● **T22.5**   Corrosion of first degree of shoulder and upper limb, except wrist and hand

    Code first (T51-T65) *to identify chemical and intent*
    Use additional external cause code to identify place (Y92)

X ● **T22.50**   Corrosion of first degree of shoulder and upper limb, except wrist and hand unspecified site
● **T22.51**   Corrosion of first degree of forearm
   ● **T22.511**   Corrosion of first degree of right forearm
   ● **T22.512**   Corrosion of first degree of left forearm
   ● **T22.519**   Corrosion of first degree of unspecified forearm
● **T22.52**   Corrosion of first degree of elbow
   ● **T22.521**   Corrosion of first degree of right elbow
   ● **T22.522**   Corrosion of first degree of left elbow
   ● **T22.529**   Corrosion of first degree of unspecified elbow
● **T22.53**   Corrosion of first degree of upper arm
   ● **T22.531**   Corrosion of first degree of right upper arm
   ● **T22.532**   Corrosion of first degree of left upper arm
   ● **T22.539**   Corrosion of first degree of unspecified upper arm
● **T22.54**   Corrosion of first degree of axilla
   ● **T22.541**   Corrosion of first degree of right axilla
   ● **T22.542**   Corrosion of first degree of left axilla
   ● **T22.549**   Corrosion of first degree of unspecified axilla

● **T22.55**   Corrosion of first degree of shoulder
   ● **T22.551**   Corrosion of first degree of right shoulder
   ● **T22.552**   Corrosion of first degree of left shoulder
   ● **T22.559**   Corrosion of first degree of unspecified shoulder
● **T22.56**   Corrosion of first degree of scapular region
   ● **T22.561**   Corrosion of first degree of right scapular region
   ● **T22.562**   Corrosion of first degree of left scapular region
   ● **T22.569**   Corrosion of first degree of unspecified scapular region
● **T22.59**   Corrosion of first degree of multiple sites of shoulder and upper limb, except wrist and hand
   ● **T22.591**   Corrosion of first degree of multiple sites of right shoulder and upper limb, except wrist and hand
   ● **T22.592**   Corrosion of first degree of multiple sites of left shoulder and upper limb, except wrist and hand
   ● **T22.599**   Corrosion of first degree of multiple sites of unspecified shoulder and upper limb, except wrist and hand
● **T22.6**   Corrosion of second degree of shoulder and upper limb, except wrist and hand

    Code first (T51-T65) *to identify chemical and intent*
    Use additional external cause code to identify place (Y92)

X ● **T22.60**   Corrosion of second degree of shoulder and upper limb, except wrist and hand, unspecified site
● **T22.61**   Corrosion of second degree of forearm
   ● **T22.611**   Corrosion of second degree of right forearm
   ● **T22.612**   Corrosion of second degree of left forearm
   ● **T22.619**   Corrosion of second degree of unspecified forearm
● **T22.62**   Corrosion of second degree of elbow
   ● **T22.621**   Corrosion of second degree of right elbow
   ● **T22.622**   Corrosion of second degree of left elbow
   ● **T22.629**   Corrosion of second degree of unspecified elbow
● **T22.63**   Corrosion of second degree of upper arm
   ● **T22.631**   Corrosion of second degree of right upper arm
   ● **T22.632**   Corrosion of second degree of left upper arm
   ● **T22.639**   Corrosion of second degree of unspecified upper arm
● **T22.64**   Corrosion of second degree of axilla
   ● **T22.641**   Corrosion of second degree of right axilla
   ● **T22.642**   Corrosion of second degree of left axilla
   ● **T22.649**   Corrosion of second degree of unspecified axilla
● **T22.65**   Corrosion of second degree of shoulder
   ● **T22.651**   Corrosion of second degree of right shoulder
   ● **T22.652**   Corrosion of second degree of left shoulder
   ● **T22.659**   Corrosion of second degree of unspecified shoulder

▶ New   ⇒ Revised   ~~deleted~~ Deleted   **OGCR** Official Guidelines   X Assign placeholder X   ● Use Additional Character(s)

Excludes 1   Excludes 2   Includes   Use additional   Code first   Code also   Key words

● **T22.66** Corrosion of second degree of scapular region
  ● **T22.661** Corrosion of second degree of right scapular region
  ● **T22.662** Corrosion of second degree of left scapular region
  ● **T22.669** Corrosion of second degree of unspecified scapular region
● **T22.69** Corrosion of second degree of multiple sites of shoulder and upper limb, except wrist and hand
  ● **T22.691** Corrosion of second degree of multiple sites of right shoulder and upper limb, except wrist and hand
  ● **T22.692** Corrosion of second degree of multiple sites of left shoulder and upper limb, except wrist and hand
  ● **T22.699** Corrosion of second degree of multiple sites of unspecified shoulder and upper limb, except wrist and hand

● **T22.7** Corrosion of third degree of shoulder and upper limb, except wrist and hand
    Code first (T51-T65) to identify chemical and intent
    Use additional external cause code to identify place (Y92)
X ● **T22.70** Corrosion of third degree of shoulder and upper limb, except wrist and hand, unspecified site
● **T22.71** Corrosion of third degree of forearm
  ● **T22.711** Corrosion of third degree of right forearm
  ● **T22.712** Corrosion of third degree of left forearm
  ● **T22.719** Corrosion of third degree of unspecified forearm
● **T22.72** Corrosion of third degree of elbow
  ● **T22.721** Corrosion of third degree of right elbow
  ● **T22.722** Corrosion of third degree of left elbow
  ● **T22.729** Corrosion of third degree of unspecified elbow
● **T22.73** Corrosion of third degree of upper arm
  ● **T22.731** Corrosion of third degree of right upper arm
  ● **T22.732** Corrosion of third degree of left upper arm
  ● **T22.739** Corrosion of third degree of unspecified upper arm
● **T22.74** Corrosion of third degree of axilla
  ● **T22.741** Corrosion of third degree of right axilla
  ● **T22.742** Corrosion of third degree of left axilla
  ● **T22.749** Corrosion of third degree of unspecified axilla
● **T22.75** Corrosion of third degree of shoulder
  ● **T22.751** Corrosion of third degree of right shoulder
  ● **T22.752** Corrosion of third degree of left shoulder
  ● **T22.759** Corrosion of third degree of unspecified shoulder
● **T22.76** Corrosion of third degree of scapular region
  ● **T22.761** Corrosion of third degree of right scapular region
  ● **T22.762** Corrosion of third degree of left scapular region
  ● **T22.769** Corrosion of third degree of unspecified scapular region

● **T22.79** Corrosion of third degree of multiple sites of shoulder and upper limb, except wrist and hand
  ● **T22.791** Corrosion of third degree of multiple sites of right shoulder and upper limb, except wrist and hand
  ● **T22.792** Corrosion of third degree of multiple sites of left shoulder and upper limb, except wrist and hand
  ● **T22.799** Corrosion of third degree of multiple sites of unspecified shoulder and upper limb, except wrist and hand

● **T23** Burn and corrosion of wrist and hand
    The appropriate 7th character is to be added to each code from category T23

A	initial encounter
D	subsequent encounter
S	sequela

● **T23.0** Burn of unspecified degree of wrist and hand
    Use additional external cause code to identify the source, place and intent of the burn (X00-X19, X75-X77, X96-X98, Y92)
● **T23.00** Burn of unspecified degree of hand, unspecified site
  ● **T23.001** Burn of unspecified degree of right hand, unspecified site
  ● **T23.002** Burn of unspecified degree of left hand, unspecified site
  ● **T23.009** Burn of unspecified degree of unspecified hand, unspecified site
● **T23.01** Burn of unspecified degree of thumb (nail)
  ● **T23.011** Burn of unspecified degree of right thumb (nail)
  ● **T23.012** Burn of unspecified degree of left thumb (nail)
  ● **T23.019** Burn of unspecified degree of unspecified thumb (nail)
● **T23.02** Burn of unspecified degree of single finger (nail) except thumb
  ● **T23.021** Burn of unspecified degree of single right finger (nail) except thumb
  ● **T23.022** Burn of unspecified degree of single left finger (nail) except thumb
  ● **T23.029** Burn of unspecified degree of unspecified single finger (nail) except thumb
● **T23.03** Burn of unspecified degree of multiple fingers (nail), not including thumb
  ● **T23.031** Burn of unspecified degree of multiple right fingers (nail), not including thumb
  ● **T23.032** Burn of unspecified degree of multiple left fingers (nail), not including thumb
  ● **T23.039** Burn of unspecified degree of unspecified multiple fingers (nail), not including thumb
● **T23.04** Burn of unspecified degree of multiple fingers (nail), including thumb
  ● **T23.041** Burn of unspecified degree of multiple right fingers (nail), including thumb
  ● **T23.042** Burn of unspecified degree of multiple left fingers (nail), including thumb
  ● **T23.049** Burn of unspecified degree of unspecified multiple fingers (nail), including thumb

CHAPTER 19 (S00-T88)

- **T23.05**   Burn of unspecified degree of palm
  - **T23.051**   Burn of unspecified degree of right palm
  - **T23.052**   Burn of unspecified degree of left palm
  - **T23.059**   Burn of unspecified degree of unspecified palm
- **T23.06**   Burn of unspecified degree of back of hand
  - **T23.061**   Burn of unspecified degree of back of right hand
  - **T23.062**   Burn of unspecified degree of back of left hand
  - **T23.069**   Burn of unspecified degree of back of unspecified hand
- **T23.07**   Burn of unspecified degree of wrist
  - **T23.071**   Burn of unspecified degree of right wrist
  - **T23.072**   Burn of unspecified degree of left wrist
  - **T23.079**   Burn of unspecified degree of unspecified wrist
- **T23.09**   Burn of unspecified degree of multiple sites of wrist and hand
  - **T23.091**   Burn of unspecified degree of multiple sites of right wrist and hand
  - **T23.092**   Burn of unspecified degree of multiple sites of left wrist and hand
  - **T23.099**   Burn of unspecified degree of multiple sites of unspecified wrist and hand
- **T23.1**   Burn of first degree of wrist and hand

  Use additional external cause code to identify the source, place and intent of the burn (X00-X19, X75-X77, X96-X98, Y92)
  - **T23.10**   Burn of first degree of hand, unspecified site
    - **T23.101**   Burn of first degree of right hand, unspecified site
    - **T23.102**   Burn of first degree of left hand, unspecified site
    - **T23.109**   Burn of first degree of unspecified hand, unspecified site
  - **T23.11**   Burn of first degree of thumb (nail)
    - **T23.111**   Burn of first degree of right thumb (nail)
    - **T23.112**   Burn of first degree of left thumb (nail)
    - **T23.119**   Burn of first degree of unspecified thumb (nail)
  - **T23.12**   Burn of first degree of single finger (nail) except thumb
    - **T23.121**   Burn of first degree of single right finger (nail) except thumb
    - **T23.122**   Burn of first degree of single left finger (nail) except thumb
    - **T23.129**   Burn of first degree of unspecified single finger (nail) except thumb
  - **T23.13**   Burn of first degree of multiple fingers (nail), not including thumb
    - **T23.131**   Burn of first degree of multiple right fingers (nail), not including thumb
    - **T23.132**   Burn of first degree of multiple left fingers (nail), not including thumb
    - **T23.139**   Burn of first degree of unspecified multiple fingers (nail), not including thumb

- **T23.14**   Burn of first degree of multiple fingers (nail), including thumb
  - **T23.141**   Burn of first degree of multiple right fingers (nail), including thumb
  - **T23.142**   Burn of first degree of multiple left fingers (nail), including thumb
  - **T23.149**   Burn of first degree of unspecified multiple fingers (nail), including thumb
- **T23.15**   Burn of first degree of palm
  - **T23.151**   Burn of first degree of right palm
  - **T23.152**   Burn of first degree of left palm
  - **T23.159**   Burn of first degree of unspecified palm
- **T23.16**   Burn of first degree of back of hand
  - **T23.161**   Burn of first degree of back of right hand
  - **T23.162**   Burn of first degree of back of left hand
  - **T23.169**   Burn of first degree of back of unspecified hand
- **T23.17**   Burn of first degree of wrist
  - **T23.171**   Burn of first degree of right wrist
  - **T23.172**   Burn of first degree of left wrist
  - **T23.179**   Burn of first degree of unspecified wrist
- **T23.19**   Burn of first degree of multiple sites of wrist and hand
  - **T23.191**   Burn of first degree of multiple sites of right wrist and hand
  - **T23.192**   Burn of first degree of multiple sites of left wrist and hand
  - **T23.199**   Burn of first degree of multiple sites of unspecified wrist and hand
- **T23.2**   Burn of second degree of wrist and hand

  Use additional external cause code to identify the source, place and intent of the burn (X00-X19, X75-X77, X96-X98, Y92)
  - **T23.20**   Burn of second degree of hand, unspecified site
    - **T23.201**   Burn of second degree of right hand, unspecified site
    - **T23.202**   Burn of second degree of left hand, unspecified site
    - **T23.209**   Burn of second degree of unspecified hand, unspecified site
  - **T23.21**   Burn of second degree of thumb (nail)
    - **T23.211**   Burn of second degree of right thumb (nail)
    - **T23.212**   Burn of second degree of left thumb (nail)
    - **T23.219**   Burn of second degree of unspecified thumb (nail)
  - **T23.22**   Burn of second degree of single finger (nail) except thumb
    - **T23.221**   Burn of second degree of single right finger (nail) except thumb
    - **T23.222**   Burn of second degree of single left finger (nail) except thumb
    - **T23.229**   Burn of second degree of unspecified single finger (nail) except thumb
  - **T23.23**   Burn of second degree of multiple fingers (nail), not including thumb
    - **T23.231**   Burn of second degree of multiple right fingers (nail), not including thumb
    - **T23.232**   Burn of second degree of multiple left fingers (nail), not including thumb
    - **T23.239**   Burn of second degree of unspecified multiple fingers (nail), not including thumb

● T23.24   Burn of second degree of multiple fingers (nail), including thumb
- ● T23.241   Burn of second degree of multiple right fingers (nail), including thumb
- ● T23.242   Burn of second degree of multiple left fingers (nail), including thumb
- ● T23.249   Burn of second degree of unspecified multiple fingers (nail), including thumb

● T23.25   Burn of second degree of palm
- ● T23.251   Burn of second degree of right palm
- ● T23.252   Burn of second degree of left palm
- ● T23.259   Burn of second degree of unspecified palm

● T23.26   Burn of second degree of back of hand
- ● T23.261   Burn of second degree of back of right hand
- ● T23.262   Burn of second degree of back of left hand
- ● T23.269   Burn of second degree of back of unspecified hand

● T23.27   Burn of second degree of wrist
- ● T23.271   Burn of second degree of right wrist
- ● T23.272   Burn of second degree of left wrist
- ● T23.279   Burn of second degree of unspecified wrist

● T23.29   Burn of second degree of multiple sites of wrist and hand
- ● T23.291   Burn of second degree of multiple sites of right wrist and hand
- ● T23.292   Burn of second degree of multiple sites of left wrist and hand
- ● T23.299   Burn of second degree of multiple sites of unspecified wrist and hand

● T23.3   Burn of third degree of wrist and hand
> Use additional external cause code to identify the source, place and intent of the burn (X00-X19, X75-X77, X96-X98, Y92)

● T23.30   Burn of third degree of hand, unspecified site
- ● T23.301   Burn of third degree of right hand, unspecified site
- ● T23.302   Burn of third degree of left hand, unspecified site
- ● T23.309   Burn of third degree of unspecified hand, unspecified site

● T23.31   Burn of third degree of thumb (nail)
- ● T23.311   Burn of third degree of right thumb (nail)
- ● T23.312   Burn of third degree of left thumb (nail)
- ● T23.319   Burn of third degree of unspecified thumb (nail)

● T23.32   Burn of third degree of single finger (nail) except thumb
- ● T23.321   Burn of third degree of single right finger (nail) except thumb
- ● T23.322   Burn of third degree of single left finger (nail) except thumb
- ● T23.329   Burn of third degree of unspecified single finger (nail) except thumb

● T23.33   Burn of third degree of multiple fingers (nail), not including thumb
- ● T23.331   Burn of third degree of multiple right fingers (nail), not including thumb
- ● T23.332   Burn of third degree of multiple left fingers (nail), not including thumb
- ● T23.339   Burn of third degree of unspecified multiple fingers (nail), not including thumb

● T23.34   Burn of third degree of multiple fingers (nail), including thumb
- ● T23.341   Burn of third degree of multiple right fingers (nail), including thumb
- ● T23.342   Burn of third degree of multiple left fingers (nail), including thumb
- ● T23.349   Burn of third degree of unspecified multiple fingers (nail), including thumb

● T23.35   Burn of third degree of palm
- ● T23.351   Burn of third degree of right palm
- ● T23.352   Burn of third degree of left palm
- ● T23.359   Burn of third degree of unspecified palm

● T23.36   Burn of third degree of back of hand
- ● T23.361   Burn of third degree of back of right hand
- ● T23.362   Burn of third degree of back of left hand
- ● T23.369   Burn of third degree of back of unspecified hand

● T23.37   Burn of third degree of wrist
- ● T23.371   Burn of third degree of right wrist
- ● T23.372   Burn of third degree of left wrist
- ● T23.379   Burn of third degree of unspecified wrist

● T23.39   Burn of third degree of multiple sites of wrist and hand
- ● T23.391   Burn of third degree of multiple sites of right wrist and hand
- ● T23.392   Burn of third degree of multiple sites of left wrist and hand
- ● T23.399   Burn of third degree of multiple sites of unspecified wrist and hand

● T23.4   Corrosion of unspecified degree of wrist and hand
> *Code first (T51-T65) to identify chemical and intent*
> Use additional external cause code to identify place (Y92)

● T23.40   Corrosion of unspecified degree of hand, unspecified site
- ● T23.401   Corrosion of unspecified degree of right hand, unspecified site
- ● T23.402   Corrosion of unspecified degree of left hand, unspecified site
- ● T23.409   Corrosion of unspecified degree of unspecified hand, unspecified site

● T23.41   Corrosion of unspecified degree of thumb (nail)
- ● T23.411   Corrosion of unspecified degree of right thumb (nail)
- ● T23.412   Corrosion of unspecified degree of left thumb (nail)
- ● T23.419   Corrosion of unspecified degree of unspecified thumb (nail)

CHAPTER 19 (S00-T88)

● **T23.42**   Corrosion of unspecified degree of single finger (nail) except thumb
  - ● **T23.421**   Corrosion of unspecified degree of single right finger (nail) except thumb
  - ● **T23.422**   Corrosion of unspecified degree of single left finger (nail) except thumb
  - ● **T23.429**   Corrosion of unspecified degree of unspecified single finger (nail) except thumb

● **T23.43**   Corrosion of unspecified degree of multiple fingers (nail), not including thumb
  - ● **T23.431**   Corrosion of unspecified degree of multiple right fingers (nail), not including thumb
  - ● **T23.432**   Corrosion of unspecified degree of multiple left fingers (nail), not including thumb
  - ● **T23.439**   Corrosion of unspecified degree of unspecified multiple fingers (nail), not including thumb

● **T23.44**   Corrosion of unspecified degree of multiple fingers (nail), including thumb
  - ● **T23.441**   Corrosion of unspecified degree of multiple right fingers (nail), including thumb
  - ● **T23.442**   Corrosion of unspecified degree of multiple left fingers (nail), including thumb
  - ● **T23.449**   Corrosion of unspecified degree of unspecified multiple fingers (nail), including thumb

● **T23.45**   Corrosion of unspecified degree of palm
  - ● **T23.451**   Corrosion of unspecified degree of right palm
  - ● **T23.452**   Corrosion of unspecified degree of left palm
  - ● **T23.459**   Corrosion of unspecified degree of unspecified palm

● **T23.46**   Corrosion of unspecified degree of back of hand
  - ● **T23.461**   Corrosion of unspecified degree of back of right hand
  - ● **T23.462**   Corrosion of unspecified degree of back of left hand
  - ● **T23.469**   Corrosion of unspecified degree of back of unspecified hand

● **T23.47**   Corrosion of unspecified degree of wrist
  - ● **T23.471**   Corrosion of unspecified degree of right wrist
  - ● **T23.472**   Corrosion of unspecified degree of left wrist
  - ● **T23.479**   Corrosion of unspecified degree of unspecified wrist

● **T23.49**   Corrosion of unspecified degree of multiple sites of wrist and hand
  - ● **T23.491**   Corrosion of unspecified degree of multiple sites of right wrist and hand
  - ● **T23.492**   Corrosion of unspecified degree of multiple sites of left wrist and hand
  - ● **T23.499**   Corrosion of unspecified degree of multiple sites of unspecified wrist and hand

● **T23.5**   Corrosion of first degree of wrist and hand
  Code first (T51-T65) to identify chemical and intent
  Use additional external cause code to identify place (Y92)
  - ● **T23.50**   Corrosion of first degree of hand, unspecified site
    - ● **T23.501**   Corrosion of first degree of right hand, unspecified site
    - ● **T23.502**   Corrosion of first degree of left hand, unspecified site
    - ● **T23.509**   Corrosion of first degree of unspecified hand, unspecified site
  - ● **T23.51**   Corrosion of first degree of thumb (nail)
    - ● **T23.511**   Corrosion of first degree of right thumb (nail)
    - ● **T23.512**   Corrosion of first degree of left thumb (nail)
    - ● **T23.519**   Corrosion of first degree of unspecified thumb (nail)
  - ● **T23.52**   Corrosion of first degree of single finger (nail) except thumb
    - ● **T23.521**   Corrosion of first degree of single right finger (nail) except thumb
    - ● **T23.522**   Corrosion of first degree of single left finger (nail) except thumb
    - ● **T23.529**   Corrosion of first degree of unspecified single finger (nail) except thumb
  - ● **T23.53**   Corrosion of first degree of multiple fingers (nail), not including thumb
    - ● **T23.531**   Corrosion of first degree of multiple right fingers (nail), not including thumb
    - ● **T23.532**   Corrosion of first degree of multiple left fingers (nail), not including thumb
    - ● **T23.539**   Corrosion of first degree of unspecified multiple fingers (nail), not including thumb
  - ● **T23.54**   Corrosion of first degree of multiple fingers (nail), including thumb
    - ● **T23.541**   Corrosion of first degree of multiple right fingers (nail), including thumb
    - ● **T23.542**   Corrosion of first degree of multiple left fingers (nail), including thumb
    - ● **T23.549**   Corrosion of first degree of unspecified multiple fingers (nail), including thumb
  - ● **T23.55**   Corrosion of first degree of palm
    - ● **T23.551**   Corrosion of first degree of right palm
    - ● **T23.552**   Corrosion of first degree of left palm
    - ● **T23.559**   Corrosion of first degree of unspecified palm
  - ● **T23.56**   Corrosion of first degree of back of hand
    - ● **T23.561**   Corrosion of first degree of back of right hand
    - ● **T23.562**   Corrosion of first degree of back of left hand
    - ● **T23.569**   Corrosion of first degree of back of unspecified hand
  - ● **T23.57**   Corrosion of first degree of wrist
    - ● **T23.571**   Corrosion of first degree of right wrist
    - ● **T23.572**   Corrosion of first degree of left wrist
    - ● **T23.579**   Corrosion of first degree of unspecified wrist

▶ New   ⇒ Revised   ~~deleted~~ Deleted   OGCR Official Guidelines   X Assign placeholder X   ● Use Additional Character(s)

Excludes 1   Excludes 2   Includes   Use additional   Code first   Code also   Key words

● **T23.59** Corrosion of first degree of multiple sites of wrist and hand
  ● **T23.591** Corrosion of first degree of multiple sites of right wrist and hand
  ● **T23.592** Corrosion of first degree of multiple sites of left wrist and hand
  ● **T23.599** Corrosion of first degree of multiple sites of unspecified wrist and hand
● **T23.6** Corrosion of second degree of wrist and hand
  Code first (T51-T65) to identify chemical and intent
  Use additional external cause code to identify place (Y92)
  ● **T23.60** Corrosion of second degree of hand, unspecified site
    ● **T23.601** Corrosion of second degree of right hand, unspecified site
    ● **T23.602** Corrosion of second degree of left hand, unspecified site
    ● **T23.609** Corrosion of second degree of unspecified hand, unspecified site
  ● **T23.61** Corrosion of second degree of thumb (nail)
    ● **T23.611** Corrosion of second degree of right thumb (nail)
    ● **T23.612** Corrosion of second degree of left thumb (nail)
    ● **T23.619** Corrosion of second degree of unspecified thumb (nail)
  ● **T23.62** Corrosion of second degree of single finger (nail) except thumb
    ● **T23.621** Corrosion of second degree of single right finger (nail) except thumb
    ● **T23.622** Corrosion of second degree of single left finger (nail) except thumb
    ● **T23.629** Corrosion of second degree of unspecified single finger (nail) except thumb
  ● **T23.63** Corrosion of second degree of multiple fingers (nail), not including thumb
    ● **T23.631** Corrosion of second degree of multiple right fingers (nail), not including thumb
    ● **T23.632** Corrosion of second degree of multiple left fingers (nail), not including thumb
    ● **T23.639** Corrosion of second degree of unspecified multiple fingers (nail), not including thumb
  ● **T23.64** Corrosion of second degree of multiple fingers (nail), including thumb
    ● **T23.641** Corrosion of second degree of multiple right fingers (nail), including thumb
    ● **T23.642** Corrosion of second degree of multiple left fingers (nail), including thumb
    ● **T23.649** Corrosion of second degree of unspecified multiple fingers (nail), including thumb
  ● **T23.65** Corrosion of second degree of palm
    ● **T23.651** Corrosion of second degree of right palm
    ● **T23.652** Corrosion of second degree of left palm
    ● **T23.659** Corrosion of second degree of unspecified palm

● **T23.66** Corrosion of second degree of back of hand
  ● **T23.661** Corrosion of second degree back of right hand
  ● **T23.662** Corrosion of second degree back of left hand
  ● **T23.669** Corrosion of second degree back of unspecified hand
● **T23.67** Corrosion of second degree of wrist
  ● **T23.671** Corrosion of second degree of right wrist
  ● **T23.672** Corrosion of second degree of left wrist
  ● **T23.679** Corrosion of second degree of unspecified wrist
● **T23.69** Corrosion of second degree of multiple sites of wrist and hand
  ● **T23.691** Corrosion of second degree of multiple sites of right wrist and hand
  ● **T23.692** Corrosion of second degree of multiple sites of left wrist and hand
  ● **T23.699** Corrosion of second degree of multiple sites of unspecified wrist and hand
● **T23.7** Corrosion of third degree of wrist and hand
  Code first (T51-T65) to identify chemical and intent
  Use additional external cause code to identify place (Y92)
  ● **T23.70** Corrosion of third degree of hand, unspecified site
    ● **T23.701** Corrosion of third degree of right hand, unspecified site
    ● **T23.702** Corrosion of third degree of left hand, unspecified site
    ● **T23.709** Corrosion of third degree of unspecified hand, unspecified site
  ● **T23.71** Corrosion of third degree of thumb (nail)
    ● **T23.711** Corrosion of third degree of right thumb (nail)
    ● **T23.712** Corrosion of third degree of left thumb (nail)
    ● **T23.719** Corrosion of third degree of unspecified thumb (nail)
  ● **T23.72** Corrosion of third degree of single finger (nail) except thumb
    ● **T23.721** Corrosion of third degree of single right finger (nail) except thumb
    ● **T23.722** Corrosion of third degree of single left finger (nail) except thumb
    ● **T23.729** Corrosion of third degree of unspecified single finger (nail) except thumb
  ● **T23.73** Corrosion of third degree of multiple fingers (nail), not including thumb
    ● **T23.731** Corrosion of third degree of multiple right fingers (nail), not including thumb
    ● **T23.732** Corrosion of third degree of multiple left fingers (nail), not including thumb
    ● **T23.739** Corrosion of third degree of unspecified multiple fingers (nail), not including thumb

● T23.74   Corrosion of third degree of multiple fingers (nail), including thumb

  ● T23.741   Corrosion of third degree of multiple right fingers (nail), including thumb

  ● T23.742   Corrosion of third degree of multiple left fingers (nail), including thumb

  ● T23.749   Corrosion of third degree of unspecified multiple fingers (nail), including thumb

● T23.75   Corrosion of third degree of palm

  ● T23.751   Corrosion of third degree of right palm

  ● T23.752   Corrosion of third degree of left palm

  ● T23.759   Corrosion of third degree of unspecified palm

● T23.76   Corrosion of third degree of back of hand

  ● T23.761   Corrosion of third degree of back of right hand

  ● T23.762   Corrosion of third degree of back of left hand

  ● T23.769   Corrosion of third degree of back of unspecified hand

● T23.77   Corrosion of third degree of wrist

  ● T23.771   Corrosion of third degree of right wrist

  ● T23.772   Corrosion of third degree of left wrist

  ● T23.779   Corrosion of third degree of unspecified wrist

● T23.79   Corrosion of third degree of multiple sites of wrist and hand

  ● T23.791   Corrosion of third degree of multiple sites of right wrist and hand

  ● T23.792   Corrosion of third degree of multiple sites of left wrist and hand

  ● T23.799   Corrosion of third degree of multiple sites of unspecified wrist and hand

● T24   Burn and corrosion of lower limb, except ankle and foot

  Excludes2   burn and corrosion of ankle and foot (T25.-)
             burn and corrosion of hip region (T21.-)

  The appropriate 7th character is to be added to each code from category T24

A	initial encounter
D	subsequent encounter
S	sequela

● T24.0   Burn of unspecified degree of lower limb, except ankle and foot

  Use additional external cause code to identify the source, place and intent of the burn (X00-X19, X75-X77, X96-X98, Y92)

  ● T24.00   Burn of unspecified degree of unspecified site of lower limb, except ankle and foot

    ● T24.001   Burn of unspecified degree of unspecified site of right lower limb, except ankle and foot

    ● T24.002   Burn of unspecified degree of unspecified site of left lower limb, except ankle and foot

    ● T24.009   Burn of unspecified degree of unspecified site of unspecified lower limb, except ankle and foot

  ● T24.01   Burn of unspecified degree of thigh

    ● T24.011   Burn of unspecified degree of right thigh

    ● T24.012   Burn of unspecified degree of left thigh

    ● T24.019   Burn of unspecified degree of unspecified thigh

● T24.02   Burn of unspecified degree of knee

  ● T24.021   Burn of unspecified degree of right knee

  ● T24.022   Burn of unspecified degree of left knee

  ● T24.029   Burn of unspecified degree of unspecified knee

● T24.03   Burn of unspecified degree of lower leg

  ● T24.031   Burn of unspecified degree of right lower leg

  ● T24.032   Burn of unspecified degree of left lower leg

  ● T24.039   Burn of unspecified degree of unspecified lower leg

● T24.09   Burn of unspecified degree of multiple sites of lower limb, except ankle and foot

  ● T24.091   Burn of unspecified degree of multiple sites of right lower limb, except ankle and foot

  ● T24.092   Burn of unspecified degree of multiple sites of left lower limb, except ankle and foot

  ● T24.099   Burn of unspecified degree of multiple sites of unspecified lower limb, except ankle and foot

● T24.1   Burn of first degree of lower limb, except ankle and foot

  Use additional external cause code to identify the source, place and intent of the burn (X00-X19, X75-X77, X96-X98, Y92)

  ● T24.10   Burn of first degree of unspecified site of lower limb, except ankle and foot

    ● T24.101   Burn of first degree of unspecified site of right lower limb, except ankle and foot

    ● T24.102   Burn of first degree of unspecified site of left lower limb, except ankle and foot

    ● T24.109   Burn of first degree of unspecified site of unspecified lower limb, except ankle and foot

  ● T24.11   Burn of first degree of thigh

    ● T24.111   Burn of first degree of right thigh

    ● T24.112   Burn of first degree of left thigh

    ● T24.119   Burn of first degree of unspecified thigh

  ● T24.12   Burn of first degree of knee

    ● T24.121   Burn of first degree of right knee

    ● T24.122   Burn of first degree of left knee

    ● T24.129   Burn of first degree of unspecified knee

  ● T24.13   Burn of first degree of lower leg

    ● T24.131   Burn of first degree of right lower leg

    ● T24.132   Burn of first degree of left lower leg

    ● T24.139   Burn of first degree of unspecified lower leg

  ● T24.19   Burn of first degree of multiple sites of lower limb, except ankle and foot

    ● T24.191   Burn of first degree of multiple sites of right lower limb, except ankle and foot

    ● T24.192   Burn of first degree of multiple sites of left lower limb, except ankle and foot

    ● T24.199   Burn of first degree of multiple sites of unspecified lower limb, except ankle and foot

▶ New   ⇒ Revised   ~~deleted~~ Deleted   **OGCR** Official Guidelines   X Assign placeholder X   ● Use Additional Character(s)

Excludes 1   Excludes 2   Includes   Use additional   Code first   Code also   Key words

● **T24.2**   Burn of second degree of lower limb, except ankle and foot

     Use additional external cause code to identify the source, place and intent of the burn (X00-X19, X75-X77, X96-X98, Y92)

   ● **T24.20**   Burn of second degree of unspecified site of lower limb, except ankle and foot

     ● **T24.201**   Burn of second degree of unspecified site of right lower limb, except ankle and foot

     ● **T24.202**   Burn of second degree of unspecified site of left lower limb, except ankle and foot

     ● **T24.209**   Burn of second degree of unspecified site of unspecified lower limb, except ankle and foot

   ● **T24.21**   Burn of second degree of thigh

     ● **T24.211**   Burn of second degree of right thigh

     ● **T24.212**   Burn of second degree of left thigh

     ● **T24.219**   Burn of second degree of unspecified thigh

   ● **T24.22**   Burn of second degree of knee

     ● **T24.221**   Burn of second degree of right knee

     ● **T24.222**   Burn of second degree of left knee

     ● **T24.229**   Burn of second degree of unspecified knee

   ● **T24.23**   Burn of second degree of lower leg

     ● **T24.231**   Burn of second degree of right lower leg

     ● **T24.232**   Burn of second degree of left lower leg

     ● **T24.239**   Burn of second degree of unspecified lower leg

   ● **T24.29**   Burn of second degree of multiple sites of lower limb, except ankle and foot

     ● **T24.291**   Burn of second degree of multiple sites of right lower limb, except ankle and foot

     ● **T24.292**   Burn of second degree of multiple sites of left lower limb, except ankle and foot

     ● **T24.299**   Burn of second degree of multiple sites of unspecified lower limb, except ankle and foot

● **T24.3**   Burn of third degree of lower limb, except ankle and foot

     Use additional external cause code to identify the source, place and intent of the burn (X00-X19, X75-X77, X96-X98, Y92)

   ● **T24.30**   Burn of third degree of unspecified site of lower limb, except ankle and foot

     ● **T24.301**   Burn of third degree of unspecified site of right lower limb, except ankle and foot

     ● **T24.302**   Burn of third degree of unspecified site of left lower limb, except ankle and foot

     ● **T24.309**   Burn of third degree of unspecified site of unspecified lower limb, except ankle and foot

   ● **T24.31**   Burn of third degree of thigh

     ● **T24.311**   Burn of third degree of right thigh

     ● **T24.312**   Burn of third degree of left thigh

     ● **T24.319**   Burn of third degree of unspecified thigh

   ● **T24.32**   Burn of third degree of knee

     ● **T24.321**   Burn of third degree of right knee

     ● **T24.322**   Burn of third degree of left knee

     ● **T24.329**   Burn of third degree of unspecified knee

   ● **T24.33**   Burn of third degree of lower leg

     ● **T24.331**   Burn of third degree of right lower leg

     ● **T24.332**   Burn of third degree of left lower leg

     ● **T24.339**   Burn of third degree of unspecified lower leg

   ● **T24.39**   Burn of third degree of multiple sites of lower limb, except ankle and foot

     ● **T24.391**   Burn of third degree of multiple sites of right lower limb, except ankle and foot

     ● **T24.392**   Burn of third degree of multiple sites of left lower limb, except ankle and foot

     ● **T24.399**   Burn of third degree of multiple sites of unspecified lower limb, except ankle and foot

● **T24.4**   Corrosion of unspecified degree of lower limb, except ankle and foot

     Code first (T51-T65) to identify chemical and intent

     Use additional external cause code to identify place (Y92)

   ● **T24.40**   Corrosion of unspecified degree of unspecified site of lower limb, except ankle and foot

     ● **T24.401**   Corrosion of unspecified degree of unspecified site of right lower limb, except ankle and foot

     ● **T24.402**   Corrosion of unspecified degree of unspecified site of left lower limb, except ankle and foot

     ● **T24.409**   Corrosion of unspecified degree of unspecified site of unspecified lower limb, except ankle and foot

   ● **T24.41**   Corrosion of unspecified degree of thigh

     ● **T24.411**   Corrosion of unspecified degree of right thigh

     ● **T24.412**   Corrosion of unspecified degree of left thigh

     ● **T24.419**   Corrosion of unspecified degree of unspecified thigh

   ● **T24.42**   Corrosion of unspecified degree of knee

     ● **T24.421**   Corrosion of unspecified degree of right knee

     ● **T24.422**   Corrosion of unspecified degree of left knee

     ● **T24.429**   Corrosion of unspecified degree of unspecified knee

   ● **T24.43**   Corrosion of unspecified degree of lower leg

     ● **T24.431**   Corrosion of unspecified degree of right lower leg

     ● **T24.432**   Corrosion of unspecified degree of left lower leg

     ● **T24.439**   Corrosion of unspecified degree of unspecified lower leg

   ● **T24.49**   Corrosion of unspecified degree of multiple sites of lower limb, except ankle and foot

     ● **T24.491**   Corrosion of unspecified degree of multiple sites of right lower limb, except ankle and foot

     ● **T24.492**   Corrosion of unspecified degree of multiple sites of left lower limb, except ankle and foot

     ● **T24.499**   Corrosion of unspecified degree of multiple sites of unspecified lower limb, except ankle and foot

▶ New   ⮕ Revised   ~~deleted~~ Deleted   **OGCR** Official Guidelines   X Assign placeholder X   ● Use Additional Character(s)

Excludes 1   Excludes 2   Includes   Use additional   Code first   Code also   Key words

● **T24.5**   Corrosion of first degree of lower limb, except ankle and foot

> *Code first* (T51-T65) *to identify chemical and intent*
> Use additional external cause code to identify place (Y92)

● **T24.50**   Corrosion of first degree of unspecified site of lower limb, except ankle and foot

   ● **T24.501**   Corrosion of first degree of unspecified site of right lower limb, except ankle and foot

   ● **T24.502**   Corrosion of first degree of unspecified site of left lower limb, except ankle and foot

   ● **T24.509**   Corrosion of first degree of unspecified site of unspecified lower limb, except ankle and foot

● **T24.51**   Corrosion of first degree of thigh

   ● **T24.511**   Corrosion of first degree of right thigh

   ● **T24.512**   Corrosion of first degree of left thigh

   ● **T24.519**   Corrosion of first degree of unspecified thigh

● **T24.52**   Corrosion of first degree of knee

   ● **T24.521**   Corrosion of first degree of right knee

   ● **T24.522**   Corrosion of first degree of left knee

   ● **T24.529**   Corrosion of first degree of unspecified knee

● **T24.53**   Corrosion of first degree of lower leg

   ● **T24.531**   Corrosion of first degree of right lower leg

   ● **T24.532**   Corrosion of first degree of left lower leg

   ● **T24.539**   Corrosion of first degree of unspecified lower leg

● **T24.59**   Corrosion of first degree of multiple sites of lower limb, except ankle and foot

   ● **T24.591**   Corrosion of first degree of multiple sites of right lower limb, except ankle and foot

   ● **T24.592**   Corrosion of first degree of multiple sites of left lower limb, except ankle and foot

   ● **T24.599**   Corrosion of first degree of multiple sites of unspecified lower limb, except ankle and foot

● **T24.6**   Corrosion of second degree of lower limb, except ankle and foot

> *Code first* (T51-T65) *to identify chemical and intent*
> Use additional external cause code to identify place (Y92)

● **T24.60**   Corrosion of second degree of unspecified site of lower limb, except ankle and foot

   ● **T24.601**   Corrosion of second degree of unspecified site of right lower limb, except ankle and foot

   ● **T24.602**   Corrosion of second degree of unspecified site of left lower limb, except ankle and foot

   ● **T24.609**   Corrosion of second degree of unspecified site of unspecified lower limb, except ankle and foot

● **T24.61**   Corrosion of second degree of thigh

   ● **T24.611**   Corrosion of second degree of right thigh

   ● **T24.612**   Corrosion of second degree of left thigh

   ● **T24.619**   Corrosion of second degree of unspecified thigh

● **T24.62**   Corrosion of second degree of knee

   ● **T24.621**   Corrosion of second degree of right knee

   ● **T24.622**   Corrosion of second degree of left knee

   ● **T24.629**   Corrosion of second degree of unspecified knee

● **T24.63**   Corrosion of second degree of lower leg

   ● **T24.631**   Corrosion of second degree of right lower leg

   ● **T24.632**   Corrosion of second degree of left lower leg

   ● **T24.639**   Corrosion of second degree of unspecified lower leg

● **T24.69**   Corrosion of second degree of multiple sites of lower limb, except ankle and foot

   ● **T24.691**   Corrosion of second degree of multiple sites of right lower limb, except ankle and foot

   ● **T24.692**   Corrosion of second degree of multiple sites of left lower limb, except ankle and foot

   ● **T24.699**   Corrosion of second degree of multiple sites of unspecified lower limb, except ankle and foot

● **T24.7**   Corrosion of third degree of lower limb, except ankle and foot

> *Code first* (T51-T65) *to identify chemical and intent*
> Use additional external cause code to identify place (Y92)

● **T24.70**   Corrosion of third degree of unspecified site of lower limb, except ankle and foot

   ● **T24.701**   Corrosion of third degree of unspecified site of right lower limb, except ankle and foot

   ● **T24.702**   Corrosion of third degree of unspecified site of left lower limb, except ankle and foot

   ● **T24.709**   Corrosion of third degree of unspecified site of unspecified lower limb, except ankle and foot

● **T24.71**   Corrosion of third degree of thigh

   ● **T24.711**   Corrosion of third degree of right thigh

   ● **T24.712**   Corrosion of third degree of left thigh

   ● **T24.719**   Corrosion of third degree of unspecified thigh

● **T24.72**   Corrosion of third degree of knee

   ● **T24.721**   Corrosion of third degree of right knee

   ● **T24.722**   Corrosion of third degree of left knee

   ● **T24.729**   Corrosion of third degree of unspecified knee

● **T24.73**   Corrosion of third degree of lower leg

   ● **T24.731**   Corrosion of third degree of right lower leg

   ● **T24.732**   Corrosion of third degree of left lower leg

   ● **T24.739**   Corrosion of third degree of unspecified lower leg

● **T24.79**   Corrosion of third degree of multiple sites of lower limb, except ankle and foot

   ● **T24.791**   Corrosion of third degree of multiple sites of right lower limb, except ankle and foot

   ● **T24.792**   Corrosion of third degree of multiple sites of left lower limb, except ankle and foot

   ● **T24.799**   Corrosion of third degree of multiple sites of unspecified lower limb, except ankle and foot

► New   ⇒ Revised   ~~deleted~~ Deleted   **OGCR** Official Guidelines   X Assign placeholder X   ● Use Additional Character(s)

Excludes 1   Excludes 2   Includes   Use additional   Code first   Code also   Key words

● **T25**   **Burn and corrosion of ankle and foot**

> The appropriate 7th character is to be added to each code from category T25

> | | |
> |---|---|
> | A | initial encounter |
> | D | subsequent encounter |
> | S | sequela |

● **T25.0**   **Burn of unspecified degree of ankle and foot**

> Use additional external cause code to identify the source, place and intent of the burn (X00-X19, X75-X77, X96-X98, Y92)

  ● **T25.01**   **Burn of unspecified degree of ankle**

    ● **T25.011**   Burn of unspecified degree of **right** ankle

    ● **T25.012**   Burn of unspecified degree of **left** ankle

    ● **T25.019**   Burn of unspecified degree of **unspecified** ankle

  ● **T25.02**   **Burn of unspecified degree of foot**

> **Excludes2**   burn of unspecified degree of toe(s) (nail) (T25.03-)

    ● **T25.021**   Burn of unspecified degree of **right** foot

    ● **T25.022**   Burn of unspecified degree of **left** foot

    ● **T25.029**   Burn of unspecified degree of **unspecified** foot

  ● **T25.03**   **Burn of unspecified degree of toe(s) (nail)**

    ● **T25.031**   Burn of unspecified degree of **right** toe(s) (nail)

    ● **T25.032**   Burn of unspecified degree of **left** toe(s) (nail)

    ● **T25.039**   Burn of unspecified degree of **unspecified** toe(s) (nail)

  ● **T25.09**   **Burn of unspecified degree of multiple sites of ankle and foot**

    ● **T25.091**   Burn of unspecified degree of multiple sites of **right** ankle and foot

    ● **T25.092**   Burn of unspecified degree of multiple sites of **left** ankle and foot

    ● **T25.099**   Burn of unspecified degree of multiple sites of **unspecified** ankle and foot

● **T25.1**   **Burn of first degree of ankle and foot**

> Use additional external cause code to identify the source, place and intent of the burn (X00-X19, X75-X77, X96-X98, Y92)

  ● **T25.11**   **Burn of first degree of ankle**

    ● **T25.111**   Burn of first degree of **right** ankle

    ● **T25.112**   Burn of first degree of **left** ankle

    ● **T25.119**   Burn of first degree of **unspecified** ankle

  ● **T25.12**   **Burn of first degree of foot**

> **Excludes2**   burn of first degree of toe(s) (nail) (T25.13-)

    ● **T25.121**   Burn of first degree of **right** foot

    ● **T25.122**   Burn of first degree of **left** foot

    ● **T25.129**   Burn of first degree of **unspecified** foot

  ● **T25.13**   **Burn of first degree of toe(s) (nail)**

    ● **T25.131**   Burn of first degree of **right** toe(s) (nail)

    ● **T25.132**   Burn of first degree of **left** toe(s) (nail)

    ● **T25.139**   Burn of first degree of **unspecified** toe(s) (nail)

● **T25.19**   **Burn of first degree of multiple sites of ankle and foot**

    ● **T25.191**   Burn of first degree of multiple sites of **right** ankle and foot

    ● **T25.192**   Burn of first degree of multiple sites of **left** ankle and foot

    ● **T25.199**   Burn of first degree of multiple sites of **unspecified** ankle and foot

● **T25.2**   **Burn of second degree of ankle and foot**

> Use additional external cause code to identify the source, place and intent of the burn (X00-X19, X75-X77, X96-X98, Y92)

  ● **T25.21**   **Burn of second degree of ankle**

    ● **T25.211**   Burn of second degree of **right** ankle

    ● **T25.212**   Burn of second degree of **left** ankle

    ● **T25.219**   Burn of second degree of **unspecified** ankle

  ● **T25.22**   **Burn of second degree of foot**

> **Excludes2**   burn of second degree of toe(s) (nail) (T25.23-)

    ● **T25.221**   Burn of second degree of **right** foot

    ● **T25.222**   Burn of second degree of **left** foot

    ● **T25.229**   Burn of second degree of **unspecified** foot

  ● **T25.23**   **Burn of second degree of toe(s) (nail)**

    ● **T25.231**   Burn of second degree of **right** toe(s) (nail)

    ● **T25.232**   Burn of second degree of **left** toe(s) (nail)

    ● **T25.239**   Burn of second degree of **unspecified** toe(s) (nail)

  ● **T25.29**   **Burn of second degree of multiple sites of ankle and foot**

    ● **T25.291**   Burn of second degree of multiple sites of **right** ankle and foot

    ● **T25.292**   Burn of second degree of multiple sites of **left** ankle and foot

    ● **T25.299**   Burn of second degree of multiple sites of **unspecified** ankle and foot

● **T25.3**   **Burn of third degree of ankle and foot**

> Use additional external cause code to identify the source, place and intent of the burn (X00-X19, X75-X77, X96-X98, Y92)

  ● **T25.31**   **Burn of third degree of ankle**

    ● **T25.311**   Burn of third degree of **right** ankle

    ● **T25.312**   Burn of third degree of **left** ankle

    ● **T25.319**   Burn of third degree of **unspecified** ankle

  ● **T25.32**   **Burn of third degree of foot**

> **Excludes2**   burn of third degree of toe(s) (nail) (T25.33-)

    ● **T25.321**   Burn of third degree of **right** foot

    ● **T25.322**   Burn of third degree of **left** foot

    ● **T25.329**   Burn of third degree of **unspecified** foot

  ● **T25.33**   **Burn of third degree of toe(s) (nail)**

    ● **T25.331**   Burn of third degree of **right** toe(s) (nail)

    ● **T25.332**   Burn of third degree of **left** toe(s) (nail)

    ● **T25.339**   Burn of third degree of **unspecified** toe(s) (nail)

CHAPTER 19 (S00-T88)

● T25.39   Burn of third degree of multiple sites of ankle and foot
  ● T25.391   Burn of third degree of multiple sites of right ankle and foot
  ● T25.392   Burn of third degree of multiple sites of left ankle and foot
  ● T25.399   Burn of third degree of multiple sites of unspecified ankle and foot

● T25.4   Corrosion of unspecified degree of ankle and foot
  Code first (T51-T65) to identify chemical and intent
  Use additional external cause code to identify place (Y92)
  ● T25.41   Corrosion of unspecified degree of ankle
    ● T25.411   Corrosion of unspecified degree of right ankle
    ● T25.412   Corrosion of unspecified degree of left ankle
    ● T25.419   Corrosion of unspecified degree of unspecified ankle
  ● T25.42   Corrosion of unspecified degree of foot
    Excludes2   corrosion of unspecified degree of toe(s) (nail) (T25.43-)
    ● T25.421   Corrosion of unspecified degree of right foot
    ● T25.422   Corrosion of unspecified degree of left foot
    ● T25.429   Corrosion of unspecified degree of unspecified foot
  ● T25.43   Corrosion of unspecified degree of toe(s) (nail)
    ● T25.431   Corrosion of unspecified degree of right toe(s) (nail)
    ● T25.432   Corrosion of unspecified degree of left toe(s) (nail)
    ● T25.439   Corrosion of unspecified degree of unspecified toe(s) (nail)
  ● T25.49   Corrosion of unspecified degree of multiple sites of ankle and foot
    ● T25.491   Corrosion of unspecified degree of multiple sites of right ankle and foot
    ● T25.492   Corrosion of unspecified degree of multiple sites of left ankle and foot
    ● T25.499   Corrosion of unspecified degree of multiple sites of unspecified ankle and foot

● T25.5   Corrosion of first degree of ankle and foot
  Code first (T51-T65) to identify chemical and intent
  Use additional external cause code to identify place (Y92)
  ● T25.51   Corrosion of first degree of ankle
    ● T25.511   Corrosion of first degree of right ankle
    ● T25.512   Corrosion of first degree of left ankle
    ● T25.519   Corrosion of first degree of unspecified ankle
  ● T25.52   Corrosion of first degree of foot
    Excludes2   corrosion of first degree of toe(s) (nail) (T25.53-)
    ● T25.521   Corrosion of first degree of right foot
    ● T25.522   Corrosion of first degree of left foot
    ● T25.529   Corrosion of first degree of unspecified foot
  ● T25.53   Corrosion of first degree of toe(s) (nail)
    ● T25.531   Corrosion of first degree of right toe(s) (nail)
    ● T25.532   Corrosion of first degree of left toe(s) (nail)
    ● T25.539   Corrosion of first degree of unspecified toe(s) (nail)

● T25.59   Corrosion of first degree of multiple sites of ankle and foot
  ● T25.591   Corrosion of first degree of multiple sites of right ankle and foot
  ● T25.592   Corrosion of first degree of multiple sites of left ankle and foot
  ● T25.599   Corrosion of first degree of multiple sites of unspecified ankle and foot

● T25.6   Corrosion of second degree of ankle and foot
  Code first (T51-T65) to identify chemical and intent
  Use additional external cause code to identify place (Y92)
  ● T25.61   Corrosion of second degree of ankle
    ● T25.611   Corrosion of second degree of right ankle
    ● T25.612   Corrosion of second degree of left ankle
    ● T25.619   Corrosion of second degree of unspecified ankle
  ● T25.62   Corrosion of second degree of foot
    Excludes2   corrosion of second degree of toe(s) (nail) (T25.63-)
    ● T25.621   Corrosion of second degree of right foot
    ● T25.622   Corrosion of second degree of left foot
    ● T25.629   Corrosion of second degree of unspecified foot
  ● T25.63   Corrosion of second degree of toe(s) (nail)
    ● T25.631   Corrosion of second degree of right toe(s) (nail)
    ● T25.632   Corrosion of second degree of left toe(s) (nail)
    ● T25.639   Corrosion of second degree of unspecified toe(s) (nail)
  ● T25.69   Corrosion of second degree of multiple sites of ankle and foot
    ● T25.691   Corrosion of second degree of right ankle and foot
    ● T25.692   Corrosion of second degree of left ankle and foot
    ● T25.699   Corrosion of second degree of unspecified ankle and foot

● T25.7   Corrosion of third degree of ankle and foot
  Code first (T51-T65) to identify chemical and intent
  Use additional external cause code to identify place (Y92)
  ● T25.71   Corrosion of third degree of ankle
    ● T25.711   Corrosion of third degree of right ankle
    ● T25.712   Corrosion of third degree of left ankle
    ● T25.719   Corrosion of third degree of unspecified ankle
  ● T25.72   Corrosion of third degree of foot
    Excludes2   corrosion of third degree of toe(s) (nail) (T25.73-)
    ● T25.721   Corrosion of third degree of right foot
    ● T25.722   Corrosion of third degree of left foot
    ● T25.729   Corrosion of third degree of unspecified foot
  ● T25.73   Corrosion of third degree of toe(s) (nail)
    ● T25.731   Corrosion of third degree of right toe(s) (nail)
    ● T25.732   Corrosion of third degree of left toe(s) (nail)
    ● T25.739   Corrosion of third degree of unspecified toe(s) (nail)

▶ New   ⟹ Revised   ~~deleted~~ Deleted   **OGCR** Official Guidelines   X Assign placeholder X   ● Use Additional Character(s)

Excludes 1   Excludes 2   Includes   Use additional   Code first   Code also   Key words

● T25.79 Corrosion of third degree of multiple sites of ankle and foot
  ● T25.791 Corrosion of third degree of multiple sites of right ankle and foot
  ● T25.792 Corrosion of third degree of multiple sites of left ankle and foot
  ● T25.799 Corrosion of third degree of multiple sites of unspecified ankle and foot

BURNS AND CORROSIONS CONFINED TO EYE AND INTERNAL ORGANS (T26-T28)

● **T26 Burn and corrosion confined to eye and adnexa**

The appropriate 7th character is to be added to each code from category T26

A	initial encounter
D	subsequent encounter
S	sequela

● **T26.0 Burn of eyelid and periocular area**
  Use additional external cause code to identify the source, place and intent of the burn (X00-X19, X75-X77, X96-X98, Y92)
  X ● T26.00 Burn of unspecified eyelid and periocular area
  X ● T26.01 Burn of right eyelid and periocular area
  X ● T26.02 Burn of left eyelid and periocular area

● **T26.1 Burn of cornea and conjunctival sac**
  Use additional external cause code to identify the source, place and intent of the burn (X00-X19, X75-X77, X96-X98, Y92)
  X ● T26.10 Burn of cornea and conjunctival sac, unspecified eye
  X ● T26.11 Burn of cornea and conjunctival sac, right eye
  X ● T26.12 Burn of cornea and conjunctival sac, left eye

● **T26.2 Burn with resulting rupture and destruction of eyeball**
  Use additional external cause code to identify the source, place and intent of the burn (X00-X19, X75-X77, X96-X98, Y92)
  X ● T26.20 Burn with resulting rupture and destruction of unspecified eyeball
  X ● T26.21 Burn with resulting rupture and destruction of right eyeball
  X ● T26.22 Burn with resulting rupture and destruction of left eyeball

● **T26.3 Burns of other specified parts of eye and adnexa**
  Use additional external cause code to identify the source, place and intent of the burn (X00-X19, X75-X77, X96-X98, Y92)
  X ● T26.30 Burns of other specified parts of unspecified eye and adnexa
  X ● T26.31 Burns of other specified parts of right eye and adnexa
  X ● T26.32 Burns of other specified parts of left eye and adnexa

● **T26.4 Burn of eye and adnexa, part unspecified**
  Use additional external cause code to identify the source, place and intent of the burn (X00-X19, X75-X77, X96-X98, Y92)
  X ● T26.40 Burn of unspecified eye and adnexa, part unspecified
  X ● T26.41 Burn of right eye and adnexa, part unspecified
  X ● T26.42 Burn of left eye and adnexa, part unspecified

● **T26.5 Corrosion of eyelid and periocular area**
  Code first (T51-T65) to identify chemical and intent
  Use additional external cause code to identify place (Y92)
  X ● T26.50 Corrosion of unspecified eyelid and periocular area
  X ● T26.51 Corrosion of right eyelid and periocular area
  X ● T26.52 Corrosion of left eyelid and periocular area

● **T26.6 Corrosion of cornea and conjunctival sac**
  Code first (T51-T65) to identify chemical and intent
  Use additional external cause code to identify place (Y92)
  X ● T26.60 Corrosion of cornea and conjunctival sac, unspecified eye
  X ● T26.61 Corrosion of cornea and conjunctival sac, right eye
  X ● T26.62 Corrosion of cornea and conjunctival sac, left eye

● **T26.7 Corrosion with resulting rupture and destruction of eyeball**
  Code first (T51-T65) to identify chemical and intent
  Use additional external cause code to identify place (Y92)
  X ● T26.70 Corrosion with resulting rupture and destruction of unspecified eyeball
  X ● T26.71 Corrosion with resulting rupture and destruction of right eyeball
  X ● T26.72 Corrosion with resulting rupture and destruction of left eyeball

● **T26.8 Corrosions of other specified parts of eye and adnexa**
  Code first (T51-T65) to identify chemical and intent
  Use additional external cause code to identify place (Y92)
  X ● T26.80 Corrosions of other specified parts of unspecified eye and adnexa
  X ● T26.81 Corrosions of other specified parts of right eye and adnexa
  X ● T26.82 Corrosions of other specified parts of left eye and adnexa

● **T26.9 Corrosion of eye and adnexa, part unspecified**
  Code first (T51-T65) to identify chemical and intent
  Use additional external cause code to identify place (Y92)
  X ● T26.90 Corrosion of unspecified eye and adnexa, part unspecified
  X ● T26.91 Corrosion of right eye and adnexa, part unspecified
  X ● T26.92 Corrosion of left eye and adnexa, part unspecified

● **T27 Burn and corrosion of respiratory tract**
  Use additional external cause code to identify the source and intent of the burn (X00-X19, X75-X77, X96-X98)
  Use additional external cause code to identify place (Y92)
  The appropriate 7th character is to be added to each code from category T27

A	initial encounter
D	subsequent encounter
S	sequela

  X ● **T27.0 Burn of larynx and trachea**
  X ● **T27.1 Burn involving larynx and trachea with lung**
  X ● **T27.2 Burn of other parts of respiratory tract**
    Burn of thoracic cavity
  X ● **T27.3 Burn of respiratory tract, part unspecified**
    Code first (T51-T65) to identify chemical and intent for codes T27.4-T27.7
  X ● **T27.4 Corrosion of larynx and trachea**
    ▶ *Code first (T51-T65) to identify chemical and intent*
  X ● **T27.5 Corrosion involving larynx and trachea with lung**
  X ● **T27.6 Corrosion of other parts of respiratory tract**
    ▶ *Code first (T51-T65) to identify chemical and intent*
  X ● **T27.7 Corrosion of respiratory tract, part unspecified**
    ▶ *Code first (T51-T65) to identify chemical and intent*

CHAPTER 19 (S00-T88)

● **T28**   **Burn and corrosion of other internal organs**

Use additional external cause code to identify the source and intent of the burn (X00-X19, X75-X77, X96-X98)

Use additional external cause code to identify place (Y92)

The appropriate 7th character is to be added to each code from category T28

> A   initial encounter
> D   subsequent encounter
> S   sequela

X ● **T28.0**   **Burn of mouth and pharynx**
X ● **T28.1**   **Burn of esophagus**
X ● **T28.2**   **Burn of other parts of alimentary tract**
X ● **T28.3**   **Burn of internal genitourinary organs**
X ● **T28.4**   **Burns of other and unspecified internal organs**
▶ *Code first (T51-T65) to identify chemical and intent*

X ● **T28.40**   Burn of **unspecified** internal organ
● **T28.41**   Burn of **ear drum**
● **T28.411**   Burn of **right** ear drum
● **T28.412**   Burn of **left** ear drum
● **T28.419**   Burn of **unspecified** ear drum
X ● **T28.49**   Burn of **other** internal organ
> *Code first (T51-T65) to identify chemical and intent for T28.5-T28.9*

X ● **T28.5**   **Corrosion of mouth and pharynx**
▶ *Code first (T51-T65) to identify chemical and intent*
X ● **T28.6**   **Corrosion of esophagus**
▶ *Code first (T51-T65) to identify chemical and intent*
X ● **T28.7**   **Corrosion of other parts of alimentary tract**
▶ *Code first (T51-T65) to identify chemical and intent*
X ● **T28.8**   **Corrosion of internal genitourinary organs**
▶ *Code first (T51-T65) to identify chemical and intent*
● **T28.9**   **Corrosions of other and unspecified internal organs**
▶ *Code first (T51-T65) to identify chemical and intent*

X ● **T28.90**   Corrosions of **unspecified** internal organs
● **T28.91**   Corrosions of **ear drum**
● **T28.911**   Corrosions of **right** ear drum
● **T28.912**   Corrosions of **left** ear drum
● **T28.919**   Corrosions of **unspecified** ear drum
X ● **T28.99**   Corrosions of **other** internal organs

OGCR Section I.C.19.d.5.

Assign separate code for each burn site
When coding burns, assign separate codes for each burn site. Category T30, Burn and corrosion, body region unspecified is extremely vague and should rarely be used.

BURNS AND CORROSIONS OF MULTIPLE AND UNSPECIFIED BODY REGIONS (T30-T32)

● **T30**   **Burn and corrosion, body region unspecified**
T30.0   **Burn of unspecified body region, unspecified degree**
This code is not for inpatient use. Code to specified site and degree of burns
Burn NOS
Multiple burns NOS
T30.4   **Corrosion of unspecified body region, unspecified degree**
This code is not for inpatient use. Code to specified site and degree of corrosion
Corrosion NOS
Multiple corrosion NOS

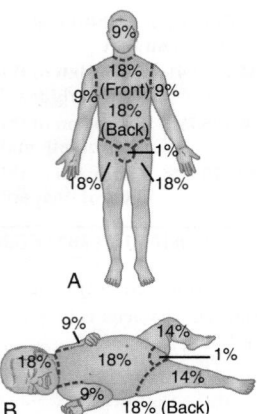

Figure 19-16   Rule of nines: percentages of total body area. (From Marx: Rosen's Emergency Medicine: Concepts and Clinical Practice, ed 6, Mosby, 2006)

● **T31**   **Burns classified according to extent of body surface involved**
Note: This category is to be used as the primary code only when the site of the burn is unspecified. It should be used as a supplementary code with categories T20-T25 when the site is specified.
T31.0   **Burns involving less than 10% of body surface**
● **T31.1**   **Burns involving 10-19% of body surface**
T31.10   **Burns involving 10-19% of body surface with 0% to 9% third degree burns**
Burns involving 10-19% of body surface NOS
T31.11   **Burns involving 10-19% of body surface with 10-19% third degree burns**
● **T31.2**   **Burns involving 20-29% of body surface**
T31.20   **Burns involving 20-29% of body surface with 0% to 9% third degree burns**
Burns involving 20-29% of body surface NOS
T31.21   **Burns involving 20-29% of body surface with 10-19% third degree burns**
T31.22   **Burns involving 20-29% of body surface with 20-29% third degree burns**
● **T31.3**   **Burns involving 30-39% of body surface**
T31.30   **Burns involving 30-39% of body surface with 0% to 9% third degree burns**
Burns involving 30-39% of body surface NOS
T31.31   **Burns involving 30-39% of body surface with 10-19% third degree burns**
T31.32   **Burns involving 30-39% of body surface with 20-29% third degree burns**
T31.33   **Burns involving 30-39% of body surface with 30-39% third degree burns**
● **T31.4**   **Burns involving 40-49% of body surface**
T31.40   **Burns involving 40-49% of body surface with 0% to 9% third degree burns**
Burns involving 40-49% of body surface NOS
T31.41   **Burns involving 40-49% of body surface with 10-19% third degree burns**
T31.42   **Burns involving 40-49% of body surface with 20-29% third degree burns**
T31.43   **Burns involving 40-49% of body surface with 30-39% third degree burns**
T31.44   **Burns involving 40-49% of body surface with 40-49% third degree burns**

▶ New   ⇒ Revised   ~~deleted~~ Deleted   **OGCR** Official Guidelines   X Assign placeholder X   ● Use Additional Character(s)
Excludes 1   Excludes 2   Includes   Use additional   Code first   Code also   Key words

● **T31.5**   **Burns involving 50-59% of body surface**

     T31.50   **Burns involving 50-59% of body surface with 0% to 9% third degree burns**
         Burns involving 50-59% of body surface NOS

     T31.51   **Burns involving 50-59% of body surface with 10-19% third degree burns**

     T31.52   **Burns involving 50-59% of body surface with 20-29% third degree burns**

     T31.53   **Burns involving 50-59% of body surface with 30-39% third degree burns**

     T31.54   **Burns involving 50-59% of body surface with 40-49% third degree burns**

     T31.55   **Burns involving 50-59% of body surface with 50-59% third degree burns**

● **T31.6**   **Burns involving 60-69% of body surface**

     T31.60   **Burns involving 60-69% of body surface with 0% to 9% third degree burns**
         Burns involving 60-69% of body surface NOS

     T31.61   **Burns involving 60-69% of body surface with 10-19% third degree burns**

     T31.62   **Burns involving 60-69% of body surface with 20-29% third degree burns**

     T31.63   **Burns involving 60-69% of body surface with 30-39% third degree burns**

     T31.64   **Burns involving 60-69% of body surface with 40-49% third degree burns**

     T31.65   **Burns involving 60-69% of body surface with 50-59% third degree burns**

     T31.66   **Burns involving 60-69% of body surface with 60-69% third degree burns**

● **T31.7**   **Burns involving 70-79% of body surface**

     T31.70   **Burns involving 70-79% of body surface with 0% to 9% third degree burns**
         Burns involving 70-79% of body surface NOS

     T31.71   **Burns involving 70-79% of body surface with 10-19% third degree burns**

     T31.72   **Burns involving 70-79% of body surface with 20-29% third degree burns**

     T31.73   **Burns involving 70-79% of body surface with 30-39% third degree burns**

     T31.74   **Burns involving 70-79% of body surface with 40-49% third degree burns**

     T31.75   **Burns involving 70-79% of body surface with 50-59% third degree burns**

     T31.76   **Burns involving 70-79% of body surface with 60-69% third degree burns**

     T31.77   **Burns involving 70-79% of body surface with 70-79% third degree burns**

● **T31.8**   **Burns involving 80-89% of body surface**

     T31.80   **Burns involving 80-89% of body surface with 0% to 9% third degree burns**
         Burns involving 80-89% of body surface NOS

     T31.81   **Burns involving 80-89% of body surface with 10-19% third degree burns**

     T31.82   **Burns involving 80-89% of body surface with 20-29% third degree burns**

     T31.83   **Burns involving 80-89% of body surface with 30-39% third degree burns**

     T31.84   **Burns involving 80-89% of body surface with 40-49% third degree burns**

     T31.85   **Burns involving 80-89% of body surface with 50-59% third degree burns**

     T31.86   **Burns involving 80-89% of body surface with 60-69% third degree burns**

     T31.87   **Burns involving 80-89% of body surface with 70-79% third degree burns**

     T31.88   **Burns involving 80-89% of body surface with 80-89% third degree burns**

● **T31.9**   **Burns involving 90% or more of body surface**

     T31.90   **Burns involving 90% or more of body surface with 0% to 9% third degree burns**
         Burns involving 90% or more of body surface NOS

     T31.91   **Burns involving 90% or more of body surface with 10-19% third degree burns**

     T31.92   **Burns involving 90% or more of body surface with 20-29% third degree burns**

     T31.93   **Burns involving 90% or more of body surface with 30-39% third degree burns**

     T31.94   **Burns involving 90% or more of body surface with 40-49% third degree burns**

     T31.95   **Burns involving 90% or more of body surface with 50-59% third degree burns**

     T31.96   **Burns involving 90% or more of body surface with 60-69% third degree burns**

     T31.97   **Burns involving 90% or more of body surface with 70-79% third degree burns**

     T31.98   **Burns involving 90% or more of body surface with 80-89% third degree burns**

     T31.99   **Burns involving 90% or more of body surface with 90% or more third degree burns**

● **T32**   **Corrosions classified according to extent of body surface involved**

     Note: This category is to be used as the primary code only when the site of the corrosion is unspecified. It may be used as a supplementary code with categories T20-T25 when the site is specified.

     T32.0   **Corrosions involving less than 10% of body surface**

● **T32.1**   **Corrosions involving 10-19% of body surface**

     T32.10   **Corrosions involving 10-19% of body surface with 0% to 9% third degree corrosion**
         Corrosions involving 10-19% of body surface NOS

     T32.11   **Corrosions involving 10-19% of body surface with 10-19% third degree corrosion**

● **T32.2**   **Corrosions involving 20-29% of body surface**

     T32.20   **Corrosions involving 20-29% of body surface with 0% to 9% third degree corrosion**

     T32.21   **Corrosions involving 20-29% of body surface with 10-19% third degree corrosion**

     T32.22   **Corrosions involving 20-29% of body surface with 20-29% third degree corrosion**

● **T32.3**   **Corrosions involving 30-39% of body surface**

     T32.30   **Corrosions involving 30-39% of body surface with 0% to 9% third degree corrosion**

     T32.31   **Corrosions involving 30-39% of body surface with 10-19% third degree corrosion**

     T32.32   **Corrosions involving 30-39% of body surface with 20-29% third degree corrosion**

     T32.33   **Corrosions involving 30-39% of body surface with 30-39% third degree corrosion**

● **T32.4**   **Corrosions involving 40-49% of body surface**

     T32.40   **Corrosions involving 40-49% of body surface with 0% to 9% third degree corrosion**

     T32.41   **Corrosions involving 40-49% of body surface with 10-19% third degree corrosion**

     T32.42   **Corrosions involving 40-49% of body surface with 20-29% third degree corrosion**

     T32.43   **Corrosions involving 40-49% of body surface with 30-39% third degree corrosion**

     T32.44   **Corrosions involving 40-49% of body surface with 40-49% third degree corrosion**

● **T32.5**   **Corrosions involving 50-59% of body surface**

    T32.50   Corrosions involving 50-59% of body surface with 0% to 9% third degree corrosion

    T32.51   Corrosions involving 50-59% of body surface with 10-19% third degree corrosion

    T32.52   Corrosions involving 50-59% of body surface with 20-29% third degree corrosion

    T32.53   Corrosions involving 50-59% of body surface with 30-39% third degree corrosion

    T32.54   Corrosions involving 50-59% of body surface with 40-49% third degree corrosion

    T32.55   Corrosions involving 50-59% of body surface with 50-59% third degree corrosion

● **T32.6**   **Corrosions involving 60-69% of body surface**

    T32.60   Corrosions involving 60-69% of body surface with 0% to 9% third degree corrosion

    T32.61   Corrosions involving 60-69% of body surface with 10-19% third degree corrosion

    T32.62   Corrosions involving 60-69% of body surface with 20-29% third degree corrosion

    T32.63   Corrosions involving 60-69% of body surface with 30-39% third degree corrosion

    T32.64   Corrosions involving 60-69% of body surface with 40-49% third degree corrosion

    T32.65   Corrosions involving 60-69% of body surface with 50-59% third degree corrosion

    T32.66   Corrosions involving 60-69% of body surface with 60-69% third degree corrosion

● **T32.7**   **Corrosions involving 70-79% of body surface**

    T32.70   Corrosions involving 70-79% of body surface with 0% to 9% third degree corrosion

    T32.71   Corrosions involving 70-79% of body surface with 10-19% third degree corrosion

    T32.72   Corrosions involving 70-79% of body surface with 20-29% third degree corrosion

    T32.73   Corrosions involving 70-79% of body surface with 30-39% third degree corrosion

    T32.74   Corrosions involving 70-79% of body surface with 40-49% third degree corrosion

    T32.75   Corrosions involving 70-79% of body surface with 50-59% third degree corrosion

    T32.76   Corrosions involving 70-79% of body surface with 60-69% third degree corrosion

    T32.77   Corrosions involving 70-79% of body surface with 70-79% third degree corrosion

● **T32.8**   **Corrosions involving 80-89% of body surface**

    T32.80   Corrosions involving 80-89% of body surface with 0% to 9% third degree corrosion

    T32.81   Corrosions involving 80-89% of body surface with 10-19% third degree corrosion

    T32.82   Corrosions involving 80-89% of body surface with 20-29% third degree corrosion

    T32.83   Corrosions involving 80-89% of body surface with 30-39% third degree corrosion

    T32.84   Corrosions involving 80-89% of body surface with 40-49% third degree corrosion

    T32.85   Corrosions involving 80-89% of body surface with 50-59% third degree corrosion

    T32.86   Corrosions involving 80-89% of body surface with 60-69% third degree corrosion

    T32.87   Corrosions involving 80-89% of body surface with 70-79% third degree corrosion

    T32.88   Corrosions involving 80-89% of body surface with 80-89% third degree corrosion

● **T32.9**   **Corrosions involving 90% or more of body surface**

    T32.90   Corrosions involving 90% or more of body surface with 0% to 9% third degree corrosion

    T32.91   Corrosions involving 90% or more of body surface with 10-19% third degree corrosion

    T32.92   Corrosions involving 90% or more of body surface with 20-29% third degree corrosion

    T32.93   Corrosions involving 90% or more of body surface with 30-39% third degree corrosion

    T32.94   Corrosions involving 90% or more of body surface with 40-49% third degree corrosion

    T32.95   Corrosions involving 90% or more of body surface with 50-59% third degree corrosion

    T32.96   Corrosions involving 90% or more of body surface with 60-69% third degree corrosion

    T32.97   Corrosions involving 90% or more of body surface with 70-79% third degree corrosion

    T32.98   Corrosions involving 90% or more of body surface with 80-89% third degree corrosion

    T32.99   Corrosions involving 90% or more of body surface with 90% or more third degree corrosion

---

FROSTBITE (T33-T34)

Excludes2   hypothermia and other effects of reduced temperature (T68, T69.-)

● **T33**   **Superficial frostbite**

   Includes   frostbite with partial thickness skin loss

   The appropriate 7th character is to be added to each code from category T33

> A   initial encounter
> D   subsequent encounter
> S   sequela

● **T33.0**   **Superficial frostbite of head**

   ● **T33.01**   Superficial frostbite of ear

     ● **T33.011**   Superficial frostbite of right ear

     ● **T33.012**   Superficial frostbite of left ear

     ● **T33.019**   Superficial frostbite of unspecified ear

   X ● **T33.02**   Superficial frostbite of nose

   X ● **T33.09**   Superficial frostbite of other part of head

X ● **T33.1**   **Superficial frostbite of neck**

X ● **T33.2**   **Superficial frostbite of thorax**

X ● **T33.3**   **Superficial frostbite of abdominal wall, lower back and pelvis**

● **T33.4**   **Superficial frostbite of arm**

   Excludes2   superficial frostbite of wrist and hand (T33.5-)

   X ● **T33.40**   Superficial frostbite of unspecified arm

   X ● **T33.41**   Superficial frostbite of right arm

   X ● **T33.42**   Superficial frostbite of left arm

● **T33.5**   **Superficial frostbite of wrist, hand, and fingers**

   ● **T33.51**   Superficial frostbite of wrist

     ● **T33.511**   Superficial frostbite of right wrist

     ● **T33.512**   Superficial frostbite of left wrist

     ● **T33.519**   Superficial frostbite of unspecified wrist

   ● **T33.52**   Superficial frostbite of hand

     Excludes2   superficial frostbite of fingers (T33.53-)

     ● **T33.521**   Superficial frostbite of right hand

     ● **T33.522**   Superficial frostbite of left hand

     ● **T33.529**   Superficial frostbite of unspecified hand

   ● **T33.53**   Superficial frostbite of finger(s)

     ● **T33.531**   Superficial frostbite of right finger(s)

     ● **T33.532**   Superficial frostbite of left finger(s)

     ● **T33.539**   Superficial frostbite of unspecified finger(s)

▶ New   ⇒ Revised   ~~deleted~~ Deleted   OGCR Official Guidelines   X Assign placeholder X   ● Use Additional Character(s)

Excludes 1   Excludes 2   Includes   Use additional   Code first   Code also   Key words

● T33.6   Superficial frostbite of hip and thigh
   X ● T33.60   Superficial frostbite of unspecified hip and thigh
   X ● T33.61   Superficial frostbite of right hip and thigh
   X ● T33.62   Superficial frostbite of left hip and thigh
● T33.7   Superficial frostbite of knee and lower leg
   Excludes2   superficial frostbite of ankle and foot (T33.8-)
   X ● T33.70   Superficial frostbite of unspecified knee and lower leg
   X ● T33.71   Superficial frostbite of right knee and lower leg
   X ● T33.72   Superficial frostbite of left knee and lower leg
● T33.8   Superficial frostbite of ankle, foot, and toe(s)
   ● T33.81   Superficial frostbite of ankle
     ● T33.811   Superficial frostbite of right ankle
     ● T33.812   Superficial frostbite of left ankle
     ● T33.819   Superficial frostbite of unspecified ankle
   ● T33.82   Superficial frostbite of foot
     ● T33.821   Superficial frostbite of right foot
     ● T33.822   Superficial frostbite of left foot
     ● T33.829   Superficial frostbite of unspecified foot
   ● T33.83   Superficial frostbite of toe(s)
     ● T33.831   Superficial frostbite of right toe(s)
     ● T33.832   Superficial frostbite of left toe(s)
     ● T33.839   Superficial frostbite of unspecified toe(s)
● T33.9   Superficial frostbite of other and unspecified sites
   X ● T33.90   Superficial frostbite of unspecified sites
     Superficial frostbite NOS
   X ● T33.99   Superficial frostbite of other sites
     Superficial frostbite of leg NOS
     Superficial frostbite of trunk NOS

● **T34**   Frostbite with tissue necrosis
   The appropriate 7th character is to be added to each code from category T34

A	initial encounter
D	subsequent encounter
S	sequela

  ● T34.0   Frostbite with tissue necrosis of head
   ● T34.01   Frostbite with tissue necrosis of ear
     ● T34.011   Frostbite with tissue necrosis of right ear
     ● T34.012   Frostbite with tissue necrosis of left ear
     ● T34.019   Frostbite with tissue necrosis of unspecified ear
   X ● T34.02   Frostbite with tissue necrosis of nose
   X ● T34.09   Frostbite with tissue necrosis of other part of head
  X ● T34.1   Frostbite with tissue necrosis of neck
  X ● T34.2   Frostbite with tissue necrosis of thorax
  X ● T34.3   Frostbite with tissue necrosis of abdominal wall, lower back and pelvis
  ● T34.4   Frostbite with tissue necrosis of arm
   Excludes2   frostbite with tissue necrosis of wrist and hand (T34.5-)
   X ● T34.40   Frostbite with tissue necrosis of unspecified arm
   X ● T34.41   Frostbite with tissue necrosis of right arm
   X ● T34.42   Frostbite with tissue necrosis of left arm

● T34.5   Frostbite with tissue necrosis of wrist, hand, and finger(s)
   ● T34.51   Frostbite with tissue necrosis of wrist
     ● T34.511   Frostbite with tissue necrosis of right wrist
     ● T34.512   Frostbite with tissue necrosis of left wrist
     ● T34.519   Frostbite with tissue necrosis of unspecified wrist
   ● T34.52   Frostbite with tissue necrosis of hand
     Excludes2   frostbite with tissue necrosis of finger(s) (T34.53-)
     ● T34.521   Frostbite with tissue necrosis of right hand
     ● T34.522   Frostbite with tissue necrosis of left hand
     ● T34.529   Frostbite with tissue necrosis of unspecified hand
   ● T34.53   Frostbite with tissue necrosis of finger(s)
     ● T34.531   Frostbite with tissue necrosis of right finger(s)
     ● T34.532   Frostbite with tissue necrosis of left finger(s)
     ● T34.539   Frostbite with tissue necrosis of unspecified finger(s)
● T34.6   Frostbite with tissue necrosis of hip and thigh
   X ● T34.60   Frostbite with tissue necrosis of unspecified hip and thigh
   X ● T34.61   Frostbite with tissue necrosis of right hip and thigh
   X ● T34.62   Frostbite with tissue necrosis of left hip and thigh
● T34.7   Frostbite with tissue necrosis of knee and lower leg
   Excludes2   frostbite with tissue necrosis of ankle and foot (T34.8-)
   X ● T34.70   Frostbite with tissue necrosis of unspecified knee and lower leg
   X ● T34.71   Frostbite with tissue necrosis of right knee and lower leg
   X ● T34.72   Frostbite with tissue necrosis of left knee and lower leg
● T34.8   Frostbite with tissue necrosis of ankle, foot, and toe(s)
   ● T34.81   Frostbite with tissue necrosis of ankle
     ● T34.811   Frostbite with tissue necrosis of right ankle
     ● T34.812   Frostbite with tissue necrosis of left ankle
     ● T34.819   Frostbite with tissue necrosis of unspecified ankle
   ● T34.82   Frostbite with tissue necrosis of foot
     ● T34.821   Frostbite with tissue necrosis of right foot
     ● T34.822   Frostbite with tissue necrosis of left foot
     ● T34.829   Frostbite with tissue necrosis of unspecified foot
   ● T34.83   Frostbite with tissue necrosis of toe(s)
     ● T34.831   Frostbite with tissue necrosis of right toe(s)
     ● T34.832   Frostbite with tissue necrosis of left toe(s)
     ● T34.839   Frostbite with tissue necrosis of unspecified toe(s)
● T34.9   Frostbite with tissue necrosis of other and unspecified sites
   X ● T34.90   Frostbite with tissue necrosis of unspecified sites
     Frostbite with tissue necrosis NOS
   X ● T34.99   Frostbite with tissue necrosis of other sites
     Frostbite with tissue necrosis of leg NOS
     Frostbite with tissue necrosis of trunk NOS

CHAPTER 19 (S00-T88)

OGCR See Section I.C.19.e.

Adverse Effects, Poisoning , Underdosing and Toxic Effects
Codes in categories T36-T65 are combination codes that include the substance that was taken as well as the intent. No additional external cause code is required for poisonings, toxic effects, adverse effects and underdosing codes.

POISONING BY, ADVERSE EFFECTS OF AND UNDERDOSING OF DRUGS MEDICAMENTS AND BIOLOGICAL SUBSTANCES (T36-T50)

Includes adverse effect of correct substance properly administered
poisoning by overdose of substance
poisoning by wrong substance given or taken in error
underdosing by (inadvertently) (deliberately) taking less substance than prescribed or instructed

Code first, for adverse effects, the nature of the adverse effect, such as:
adverse effect NOS (T88.7)
aspirin gastritis (K29.-)
blood disorders (D56-D76)
contact dermatitis (L23-L25)
dermatitis due to substances taken internally (L27.-)
nephropathy (N14.0-N14.2)

Note: The drug giving rise to the adverse effect should be identified by use of codes from categories T36-T50 with fifth or sixth character 5.

Use additional code(s) to specify:
manifestations of poisoning
underdosing or failure in dosage during medical and surgical care (Y63.6, Y63.8-Y63.9)
underdosing of medication regimen (Z91.12-, Z91.13-)

Excludes1 toxic reaction to local anesthesia in pregnancy (O29.3-)

Excludes2 abuse and dependence of psychoactive substances (F10-F19)
abuse of non-dependence-producing substances (F55.-)
drug reaction and poisoning affecting newborn (P00-P96)
pathological drug intoxication (inebriation) (F10-F19)

● **T36** Poisoning by, adverse effect of and underdosing of systemic antibiotics
Excludes1 antineoplastic antibiotics (T45.1-)
locally applied antibiotic NEC (T49.0)
topically used antibiotic for ear, nose and throat (T49.6)
topically used antibiotic for eye (T49.5)

The appropriate 7th character is to be added to each code from category T36

A initial encounter
D subsequent encounter
S sequela

● **T36.0** Poisoning by, adverse effect of and underdosing of penicillins
● **T36.0X** Poisoning by, adverse effect of and underdosing of penicillins
● **T36.0X1** Poisoning by penicillins, accidental (unintentional)
Poisoning by penicillins NOS
● **T36.0X2** Poisoning by penicillins, intentional self-harm
● **T36.0X3** Poisoning by penicillins, assault
● **T36.0X4** Poisoning by penicillins, undetermined
● **T36.0X5** Adverse effect of penicillins
● **T36.0X6** Underdosing of penicillins

● **T36.1** Poisoning by, adverse effect of and underdosing of cephalosporins and other betalactam antibiotics
● **T36.1X** Poisoning by, adverse effect of and underdosing of cephalosporins and other beta-lactam antibiotics
● **T36.1X1** Poisoning by cephalosporins and other beta-lactam antibiotics, accidental (unintentional)
Poisoning by cephalosporins and other beta-lactam antibiotics NOS
● **T36.1X2** Poisoning by cephalosporins and other beta-lactam antibiotics, intentional self-harm
● **T36.1X3** Poisoning by cephalosporins and other beta-lactam antibiotics, assault
● **T36.1X4** Poisoning by cephalosporins and other beta-lactam antibiotics, undetermined
● **T36.1X5** Adverse effect of cephalosporins and other beta-lactam antibiotics
● **T36.1X6** Underdosing of cephalosporins and other beta-lactam antibiotics

● **T36.2** Poisoning by, adverse effect of and underdosing of chloramphenicol group
● **T36.2X** Poisoning by, adverse effect of and underdosing of chloramphenicol group
● **T36.2X1** Poisoning by chloramphenicol group, accidental (unintentional)
Poisoning by chloramphenicol group NOS
● **T36.2X2** Poisoning by chloramphenicol group, intentional self-harm
● **T36.2X3** Poisoning by chloramphenicol group, assault
● **T36.2X4** Poisoning by chloramphenicol group, undetermined
● **T36.2X5** Adverse effect of chloramphenicol group
● **T36.2X6** Underdosing of chloramphenicol group

● **T36.3** Poisoning by, adverse effect of and underdosing of macrolides
● **T36.3X** Poisoning by, adverse effect of and underdosing of macrolides
● **T36.3X1** Poisoning by macrolides, accidental (unintentional)
Poisoning by macrolides NOS
● **T36.3X2** Poisoning by macrolides, intentional self-harm
● **T36.3X3** Poisoning by macrolides, assault
● **T36.3X4** Poisoning by macrolides, undetermined
● **T36.3X5** Adverse effect of macrolides
● **T36.3X6** Underdosing of macrolides

● **T36.4** Poisoning by, adverse effect of and underdosing of tetracyclines
● **T36.4X** Poisoning by, adverse effect of and underdosing of tetracyclines
● **T36.4X1** Poisoning by tetracyclines, accidental (unintentional)
Poisoning by tetracyclines NOS
● **T36.4X2** Poisoning by tetracyclines, intentional self-harm
● **T36.4X3** Poisoning by tetracyclines, assault
● **T36.4X4** Poisoning by tetracyclines, undetermined
● **T36.4X5** Adverse effect of tetracyclines
● **T36.4X6** Underdosing of tetracyclines

- ● **T36.5**   **Poisoning by, adverse effect of and underdosing of aminoglycosides**
  Poisoning by, adverse effect of and underdosing of streptomycin
  - ● **T36.5X**   **Poisoning by, adverse effect of and underdosing of aminoglycosides**
    - ● **T36.5X1**   **Poisoning by aminoglycosides, accidental (unintentional)**
      Poisoning by aminoglycosides NOS
    - ● **T36.5X2**   **Poisoning by aminoglycosides, intentional self-harm**
    - ● **T36.5X3**   **Poisoning by aminoglycosides, assault**
    - ● **T36.5X4**   **Poisoning by aminoglycosides, undetermined**
    - ● **T36.5X5**   **Adverse effect of aminoglycosides**
    - ● **T36.5X6**   **Underdosing of aminoglycosides**
- ● **T36.6**   **Poisoning by, adverse effect of and underdosing of rifampicins**
  - ● **T36.6X**   **Poisoning by, adverse effect of and underdosing of rifampicins**
    - ● **T36.6X1**   **Poisoning by rifampicins, accidental (unintentional)**
      Poisoning by rifampicins NOS
    - ● **T36.6X2**   **Poisoning by rifampicins, intentional self-harm**
    - ● **T36.6X3**   **Poisoning by rifampicins, assault**
    - ● **T36.6X4**   **Poisoning by rifampicins, undetermined**
    - ● **T36.6X5**   **Adverse effect of rifampicins**
    - ● **T36.6X6**   **Underdosing of rifampicins**
- ● **T36.7**   **Poisoning by, adverse effect of and underdosing of antifungal antibiotics, systemically used**
  - ● **T36.7X**   **Poisoning by, adverse effect of and underdosing of antifungal antibiotics, systemically used**
    - ● **T36.7X1**   **Poisoning by antifungal antibiotics, systemically used, accidental (unintentional)**
      Poisoning by antifungal antibiotics, systemically used NOS
    - ● **T36.7X2**   **Poisoning by antifungal antibiotics, systemically used, intentional self-harm**
    - ● **T36.7X3**   **Poisoning by antifungal antibiotics, systemically used, assault**
    - ● **T36.7X4**   **Poisoning by antifungal antibiotics, systemically used, undetermined**
    - ● **T36.7X5**   **Adverse effect of antifungal antibiotics, systemically used**
    - ● **T36.7X6**   **Underdosing of antifungal antibiotics, systemically used**
- ● **T36.8**   **Poisoning by, adverse effect of and underdosing of other systemic antibiotics**
  - ● **T36.8X**   **Poisoning by, adverse effect of and underdosing of other systemic antibiotics**
    - ● **T36.8X1**   **Poisoning by other systemic antibiotics, accidental (unintentional)**
      Poisoning by other systemic antibiotics NOS
    - ● **T36.8X2**   **Poisoning by other systemic antibiotics, intentional self-harm**
    - ● **T36.8X3**   **Poisoning by other systemic antibiotics, assault**
    - ● **T36.8X4**   **Poisoning by other systemic antibiotics, undetermined**
    - ● **T36.8X5**   **Adverse effect of other systemic antibiotics**
    - ● **T36.8X6**   **Underdosing of other systemic antibiotics**

- ● **T36.9**   **Poisoning by, adverse effect of and underdosing of unspecified systemic antibiotic**
  - X ● **T36.91**   **Poisoning by unspecified systemic antibiotic, accidental (unintentional)**
    Poisoning by systemic antibiotic NOS
  - X ● **T36.92**   **Poisoning by unspecified systemic antibiotic, intentional self-harm**
  - X ● **T36.93**   **Poisoning by unspecified systemic antibiotic, assault**
  - X ● **T36.94**   **Poisoning by unspecified systemic antibiotic, undetermined**
  - X ● **T36.95**   **Adverse effect of unspecified systemic antibiotic**
  - X ● **T36.96**   **Underdosing of unspecified systemic antibiotic**
- ● **T37**   **Poisoning by, adverse effect of and underdosing of other systemic anti-infectives and antiparasitics**

Excludes1	anti-infectives topically used for ear, nose and throat (T49.6-)
	anti-infectives topically used for eye (T49.5-)
	locally applied anti-infectives NEC (T49.0-)

  The appropriate 7th character is to be added to each code from category T37

A	initial encounter
D	subsequent encounter
S	sequela

  - ● **T37.0**   **Poisoning by, adverse effect of and underdosing of sulfonamides**
    - ● **T37.0X**   **Poisoning by, adverse effect of and underdosing of sulfonamides**
      - ● **T37.0X1**   **Poisoning by sulfonamides, accidental (unintentional)**
        Poisoning by sulfonamides NOS
      - ● **T37.0X2**   **Poisoning by sulfonamides, intentional self-harm**
      - ● **T37.0X3**   **Poisoning by sulfonamides, assault**
      - ● **T37.0X4**   **Poisoning by sulfonamides, undetermined**
      - ● **T37.0X5**   **Adverse effect of sulfonamides**
      - ● **T37.0X6**   **Underdosing of sulfonamides**
  - ● **T37.1**   **Poisoning by, adverse effect of and underdosing of antimycobacterial drugs**

Excludes1	rifampicins (T36.6-) streptomycin (T36.5-)

    - ● **T37.1X**   **Poisoning by, adverse effect of and underdosing of antimycobacterial drugs**
      - ● **T37.1X1**   **Poisoning by antimycobacterial drugs, accidental (unintentional)**
        Poisoning by antimycobacterial drugs NOS
      - ● **T37.1X2**   **Poisoning by antimycobacterial drugs, intentional self-harm**
      - ● **T37.1X3**   **Poisoning by antimycobacterial drugs, assault**
      - ● **T37.1X4**   **Poisoning by antimycobacterial drugs, undetermined**
      - ● **T37.1X5**   **Adverse effect of antimycobacterial drugs**
      - ● **T37.1X6**   **Underdosing of antimycobacterial drugs**

CHAPTER 19 (S00-T88)

● **T37.2** Poisoning by, adverse effect of and underdosing of antimalarials and drugs acting on other blood protozoa
> **Excludes1**   hydroxyquinoline derivatives (T37.8-)

  ● **T37.2X** Poisoning by, adverse effect of and underdosing of antimalarials and drugs acting on other blood protozoa

    ● **T37.2X1** Poisoning by antimalarials and drugs acting on other blood protozoa, accidental (unintentional)
> Poisoning by antimalarials and drugs acting on other blood protozoa NOS

    ● **T37.2X2** Poisoning by antimalarials and drugs acting on other blood protozoa, intentional self-harm

    ● **T37.2X3** Poisoning by antimalarials and drugs acting on other blood protozoa, assault

    ● **T37.2X4** Poisoning by antimalarials and drugs acting on other blood protozoa, undetermined

    ● **T37.2X5** Adverse effect of antimalarials and drugs acting on other blood protozoa

    ● **T37.2X6** Underdosing of antimalarials and drugs acting on other blood protozoa

● **T37.3** Poisoning by, adverse effect of and underdosing of other antiprotozoal drugs

  ● **T37.3X** Poisoning by, adverse effect of and underdosing of other antiprotozoal drugs

    ● **T37.3X1** Poisoning by other antiprotozoal drugs, accidental (unintentional)
> Poisoning by other antiprotozoal drugs NOS

    ● **T37.3X2** Poisoning by other antiprotozoal drugs, intentional self-harm

    ● **T37.3X3** Poisoning by other antiprotozoal drugs, assault

    ● **T37.3X4** Poisoning by other antiprotozoal drugs, undetermined

    ● **T37.3X5** Adverse effect of other antiprotozoal drugs

    ● **T37.3X6** Underdosing of other antiprotozoal drugs

● **T37.4** Poisoning by, adverse effect of and underdosing of anthelminthics

  ● **T37.4X** Poisoning by, adverse effect of and underdosing of anthelminthics

    ● **T37.4X1** Poisoning by anthelminthics, accidental (unintentional)
> Poisoning by anthelminthics NOS

    ● **T37.4X2** Poisoning by anthelminthics, intentional self-harm

    ● **T37.4X3** Poisoning by anthelminthics, assault

    ● **T37.4X4** Poisoning by anthelminthics, undetermined

    ● **T37.4X5** Adverse effect of anthelminthics

    ● **T37.4X6** Underdosing of anthelminthics

● **T37.5** Poisoning by, adverse effect of and underdosing of antiviral drugs
> **Excludes1**   amantadine (T42.8-)
> cytarabine (T45.1-)

  ● **T37.5X** Poisoning by, adverse effect of and underdosing of antiviral drugs

    ● **T37.5X1** Poisoning by antiviral drugs, accidental (unintentional)
> Poisoning by antiviral drugs NOS

    ● **T37.5X2** Poisoning by antiviral drugs, intentional self-harm

    ● **T37.5X3** Poisoning by antiviral drugs, assault

    ● **T37.5X4** Poisoning by antiviral drugs, undetermined

    ● **T37.5X5** Adverse effect of antiviral drugs

    ● **T37.5X6** Underdosing of antiviral drugs

● **T37.8** Poisoning by, adverse effect of and underdosing of other specified systemic anti-infectives and antiparasitics
> Poisoning by, adverse effect of and underdosing of hydroxyquinoline derivatives
> **Excludes1**   antimalarial drugs (T37.2-)

  ● **T37.8X** Poisoning by, adverse effect of and underdosing of other specified systemic anti-infectives and antiparasitics

    ● **T37.8X1** Poisoning by other specified systemic anti-infectives and antiparasitics, accidental (unintentional)
> Poisoning by other specified systemic anti-infectives and antiparasitics NOS

    ● **T37.8X2** Poisoning by other specified systemic anti-infectives and antiparasitics, intentional self-harm

    ● **T37.8X3** Poisoning by other specified systemic anti-infectives and antiparasitics, assault

    ● **T37.8X4** Poisoning by other specified systemic anti-infectives and antiparasitics, undetermined

    ● **T37.8X5** Adverse effect of other specified systemic anti-infectives and antiparasitics

    ● **T37.8X6** Underdosing of other specified systemic anti-infectives and antiparasitics

● **T37.9** Poisoning by, adverse effect of and underdosing of unspecified systemic anti-infective and antiparasitics

  X● **T37.91** Poisoning by unspecified systemic anti-infective and antiparasitics, accidental (unintentional)
> Poisoning by, adverse effect of and underdosing of systemic anti-infective and antiparasitics NOS

  X● **T37.92** Poisoning by unspecified systemic anti-infective and antiparasitics, intentional self-harm

  X● **T37.93** Poisoning by unspecified systemic anti-infective and antiparasitics, assault

  X● **T37.94** Poisoning by unspecified systemic anti-infective and antiparasitics, undetermined

  X● **T37.95** Adverse effect of unspecified systemic anti-infective and antiparasitic

  X● **T37.96** Underdosing of unspecified systemic anti-infectives and antiparasitics

▶ New   ⇒ Revised   deleted Deleted   **OGCR** Official Guidelines   X Assign placeholder X   ● Use Additional Character(s)

Excludes 1   Excludes 2   Includes   Use additional   Code first   Code also   Key words

●T38   **Poisoning by, adverse effect of and underdosing of hormones and their synthetic substitutes and antagonists, not elsewhere classified**

> **Excludes1**   mineralocorticoids and their antagonists (T50.0-)
> oxytocic hormones (T48.0-)
> parathyroid hormones and derivatives (T50.9-)

The appropriate 7th character is to be added to each code from category T38

> A   initial encounter
> D   subsequent encounter
> S   sequela

●T38.0   **Poisoning by, adverse effect of and underdosing of glucocorticoids and synthetic analogues**

> **Excludes1**   glucocorticoids, topically used (T49.-)

  ●T38.0X   **Poisoning by, adverse effect of and underdosing of glucocorticoids and synthetic analogues**

    ●T38.0X1   **Poisoning by glucocorticoids and synthetic analogues, accidental (unintentional)**
       Poisoning by glucocorticoids and synthetic analogues NOS

    ●T38.0X2   **Poisoning by glucocorticoids and synthetic analogues, intentional self-harm**

    ●T38.0X3   **Poisoning by glucocorticoids and synthetic analogues, assault**

    ●T38.0X4   **Poisoning by glucocorticoids and synthetic analogues, undetermined**

    ●T38.0X5   **Adverse effect of glucocorticoids and synthetic analogues**

    ●T38.0X6   **Underdosing of glucocorticoids and synthetic analogues**

●T38.1   **Poisoning by, adverse effect of and underdosing of thyroid hormones and substitutes**

  ●T38.1X   **Poisoning by, adverse effect of and underdosing of thyroid hormones and substitutes**

    ●T38.1X1   **Poisoning by thyroid hormones and substitutes, accidental (unintentional)**
       Poisoning by thyroid hormones and substitutes NOS

    ●T38.1X2   **Poisoning by thyroid hormones and substitutes, intentional self-harm**

    ●T38.1X3   **Poisoning by thyroid hormones and substitutes, assault**

    ●T38.1X4   **Poisoning by thyroid hormones and substitutes, undetermined**

    ●T38.1X5   **Adverse effect of thyroid hormones and substitutes**

    ●T38.1X6   **Underdosing of thyroid hormones and substitutes**

●T38.2   **Poisoning by, adverse effect of and underdosing of antithyroid drugs**

  ●T38.2X   **Poisoning by, adverse effect of and underdosing of antithyroid drugs**

    ●T38.2X1   **Poisoning by antithyroid drugs, accidental (unintentional)**
       Poisoning by antithyroid drugs NOS

    ●T38.2X2   **Poisoning by antithyroid drugs, intentional self-harm**

    ●T38.2X3   **Poisoning by antithyroid drugs, assault**

    ●T38.2X4   **Poisoning by antithyroid drugs, undetermined**

    ●T38.2X5   **Adverse effect of antithyroid drugs**

    ●T38.2X6   **Underdosing of antithyroid drugs**

●T38.3   **Poisoning by, adverse effect of and underdosing of insulin and oral hypoglycemic [antidiabetic] drugs**

  ●T38.3X   **Poisoning by, adverse effect of and underdosing of insulin and oral hypoglycemic [antidiabetic] drugs**

    ●T38.3X1   **Poisoning by insulin and oral hypoglycemic [antidiabetic] drugs, accidental (unintentional)**
       Poisoning by insulin and oral hypoglycemic [antidiabetic] drugs NOS

    ●T38.3X2   **Poisoning by insulin and oral hypoglycemic [antidiabetic] drugs, intentional self-harm**

    ●T38.3X3   **Poisoning by insulin and oral hypoglycemic [antidiabetic] drugs, assault**

    ●T38.3X4   **Poisoning by insulin and oral hypoglycemic [antidiabetic] drugs, undetermined**

    ●T38.3X5   **Adverse effect of insulin and oral hypoglycemic [antidiabetic] drugs**

    ●T38.3X6   **Underdosing of insulin and oral hypoglycemic [antidiabetic] drugs**

●T38.4   **Poisoning by, adverse effect of and underdosing of oral contraceptives**
   Poisoning by, adverse effect of and underdosing of multiple- and single-ingredient oral contraceptive preparations

  ●T38.4X   **Poisoning by, adverse effect of and underdosing of oral contraceptives**

    ●T38.4X1   **Poisoning by oral contraceptives, accidental (unintentional)**
       Poisoning by oral contraceptives NOS

    ●T38.4X2   **Poisoning by oral contraceptives, intentional self-harm**

    ●T38.4X3   **Poisoning by oral contraceptives, assault**

    ●T38.4X4   **Poisoning by oral contraceptives, undetermined**

    ●T38.4X5   **Adverse effect of oral contraceptives**

    ●T38.4X6   **Underdosing of oral contraceptives**

●T38.5   **Poisoning by, adverse effect of and underdosing of other estrogens and progestogens**
   Poisoning by, adverse effect of and underdosing of estrogens and progestogens mixtures and substitutes

  ●T38.5X   **Poisoning by, adverse effect of and underdosing of other estrogens and progestogens**

    ●T38.5X1   **Poisoning by other estrogens and progestogens, accidental (unintentional)**
       Poisoning by other estrogens and progestogens NOS

    ●T38.5X2   **Poisoning by other estrogens and progestogens, intentional self-harm**

    ●T38.5X3   **Poisoning by other estrogens and progestogens, assault**

    ●T38.5X4   **Poisoning by other estrogens and progestogens, undetermined**

    ●T38.5X5   **Adverse effect of other estrogens and progestogens**

    ●T38.5X6   **Underdosing of other estrogens and progestogens**

● **T38.6 Poisoning by, adverse effect of and underdosing of antigonadotrophins, antiestrogens, antiandrogens, not elsewhere classified**
Poisoning by, adverse effect of and underdosing of tamoxifen

  ● **T38.6X Poisoning by, adverse effect of and underdosing of antigonadotrophins, antiestrogens, antiandrogens, not elsewhere classified**

    ● **T38.6X1 Poisoning by antigonadotrophins, antiestrogens, antiandrogens, not elsewhere classified, accidental (unintentional)**
Poisoning by antigonadotrophins, antiestrogens, antiandrogens, not elsewhere classified NOS

    ● **T38.6X2 Poisoning by antigonadotrophins, antiestrogens, antiandrogens, not elsewhere classified, intentional self-harm**

    ● **T38.6X3 Poisoning by antigonadotrophins, antiestrogens, antiandrogens, not elsewhere classified, assault**

    ● **T38.6X4 Poisoning by antigonadotrophins, antiestrogens, antiandrogens, not elsewhere classified, undetermined**

    ● **T38.6X5 Adverse effect of antigonadotrophins, antiestrogens, antiandrogens, not elsewhere classified**

    ● **T38.6X6 Underdosing of antigonadotrophins, antiestrogens, antiandrogens, not elsewhere classified**

● **T38.7 Poisoning by, adverse effect of and underdosing of androgens and anabolic congeners**

  ● **T38.7X Poisoning by, adverse effect of and underdosing of androgens and anabolic congeners**

    ● **T38.7X1 Poisoning by androgens and anabolic congeners, accidental (unintentional)**
Poisoning by androgens and anabolic congeners NOS

    ● **T38.7X2 Poisoning by androgens and anabolic congeners, intentional self-harm**

    ● **T38.7X3 Poisoning by androgens and anabolic congeners, assault**

    ● **T38.7X4 Poisoning by androgens and anabolic congeners, undetermined**

    ● **T38.7X5 Adverse effect of androgens and anabolic congeners**

    ● **T38.7X6 Underdosing of androgens and anabolic congeners**

● **T38.8 Poisoning by, adverse effect of and underdosing of other and unspecified hormones and synthetic substitutes**

  ● **T38.80 Poisoning by, adverse effect of and underdosing of unspecified hormones and synthetic substitutes**

    ● **T38.801 Poisoning by unspecified hormones and synthetic substitutes, accidental (unintentional)**
Poisoning by unspecified hormones and synthetic substitutes NOS

    ● **T38.802 Poisoning by unspecified hormones and synthetic substitutes, intentional self-harm**

    ● **T38.803 Poisoning by unspecified hormones and synthetic substitutes, assault**

    ● **T38.804 Poisoning by unspecified hormones and synthetic substitutes, undetermined**

    ● **T38.805 Adverse effect of unspecified hormones and synthetic substitutes**

    ● **T38.806 Underdosing of unspecified hormones and synthetic substitutes**

● **T38.81 Poisoning by, adverse effect of and underdosing of anterior pituitary [adenohypophyseal] hormones**

    ● **T38.811 Poisoning by anterior pituitary [adenohypophyseal] hormones, accidental (unintentional)**
Poisoning by anterior pituitary [adenohypophyseal] hormones NOS

    ● **T38.812 Poisoning by anterior pituitary [adenohypophyseal] hormones, intentional self-harm**

    ● **T38.813 Poisoning by anterior pituitary [adenohypophyseal] hormones, assault**

    ● **T38.814 Poisoning by anterior pituitary [adenohypophyseal] hormones, undetermined**

    ● **T38.815 Adverse effect of anterior pituitary [adenohypophyseal] hormones**

    ● **T38.816 Underdosing of anterior pituitary [adenohypophyseal] hormones**

  ● **T38.89 Poisoning by, adverse effect of and underdosing of other hormones and synthetic substitutes**

    ● **T38.891 Poisoning by other hormones and synthetic substitutes, accidental (unintentional)**
Poisoning by other hormones and synthetic substitutes NOS

    ● **T38.892 Poisoning by other hormones and synthetic substitutes, intentional self-harm**

    ● **T38.893 Poisoning by other hormones and synthetic substitutes, assault**

    ● **T38.894 Poisoning by other hormones and synthetic substitutes, undetermined**

    ● **T38.895 Adverse effect of other hormones and synthetic substitutes**

    ● **T38.896 Underdosing of other hormones and synthetic substitutes**

● **T38.9 Poisoning by, adverse effect of and underdosing of other and unspecified hormone antagonists**

  ● **T38.90 Poisoning by, adverse effect of and underdosing of unspecified hormone antagonists**

    ● **T38.901 Poisoning by unspecified hormone antagonists, accidental (unintentional)**
Poisoning by unspecified hormone antagonists NOS

    ● **T38.902 Poisoning by unspecified hormone antagonists, intentional self-harm**

    ● **T38.903 Poisoning by unspecified hormone antagonists, assault**

    ● **T38.904 Poisoning by unspecified hormone antagonists, undetermined**

    ● **T38.905 Adverse effect of unspecified hormone antagonists**

    ● **T38.906 Underdosing of unspecified hormone antagonists**

▶ New   ⇒ Revised   ~~deleted~~ Deleted   **OGCR** Official Guidelines   X Assign placeholder X   ● Use Additional Character(s)

Excludes 1   Excludes 2   Includes   Use additional   Code first   Code also   Key words

- T38.99　Poisoning by, adverse effect of and underdosing of other hormone antagonists
  - T38.991　Poisoning by other hormone antagonists, accidental (unintentional)
    Poisoning by other hormone antagonists NOS
  - T38.992　Poisoning by other hormone antagonists, intentional self-harm
  - T38.993　Poisoning by other hormone antagonists, assault
  - T38.994　Poisoning by other hormone antagonists, undetermined
  - T38.995　Adverse effect of other hormone antagonists
  - T38.996　Underdosing of other hormone antagonists

- T39　Poisoning by, adverse effect of and underdosing of nonopioid analgesics, antipyretics and antirheumatics

  The appropriate 7th character is to be added to each code from category T39

A	initial encounter
D	subsequent encounter
S	sequela

  - T39.0　Poisoning by, adverse effect of and underdosing of salicylates
    - T39.01　Poisoning by, adverse effect of and underdosing of aspirin
      Poisoning by, adverse effect of and underdosing of acetylsalicylic acid
      - T39.011　Poisoning by aspirin, accidental (unintentional)
      - T39.012　Poisoning by aspirin, intentional self-harm
      - T39.013　Poisoning by aspirin, assault
      - T39.014　Poisoning by aspirin, undetermined
      - T39.015　Adverse effect of aspirin
      - T39.016　Underdosing of aspirin
    - T39.09　Poisoning by, adverse effect of and underdosing of other salicylates
      - T39.091　Poisoning by salicylates, accidental (unintentional)
        Poisoning by salicylates NOS
      - T39.092　Poisoning by salicylates, intentional self-harm
      - T39.093　Poisoning by salicylates, assault
      - T39.094　Poisoning by salicylates, undetermined
      - T39.095　Adverse effect of salicylates
      - T39.096　Underdosing of salicylates
  - T39.1　Poisoning by, adverse effect of and underdosing of 4-Aminophenol derivatives
    - T39.1X　Poisoning by, adverse effect of and underdosing of 4-Aminophenol derivatives
      - T39.1X1　Poisoning by 4-Aminophenol derivatives, accidental (unintentional)
        Poisoning by 4-Aminophenol derivatives NOS
      - T39.1X2　Poisoning by 4-Aminophenol derivatives, intentional self-harm
      - T39.1X3　Poisoning by 4-Aminophenol derivatives, assault
      - T39.1X4　Poisoning by 4-Aminophenol derivatives, undetermined
      - T39.1X5　Adverse effect of 4-Aminophenol derivatives
      - T39.1X6　Underdosing of 4-Aminophenol derivatives

- T39.2　Poisoning by, adverse effect of and underdosing of pyrazolone derivatives
  - T39.2X　Poisoning by, adverse effect of and underdosing of pyrazolone derivatives
    - T39.2X1　Poisoning by pyrazolone derivatives, accidental (unintentional)
      Poisoning by pyrazolone derivatives NOS
    - T39.2X2　Poisoning by pyrazolone derivatives, intentional self-harm
    - T39.2X3　Poisoning by pyrazolone derivatives, assault
    - T39.2X4　Poisoning by pyrazolone derivatives, undetermined
    - T39.2X5　Adverse effect of pyrazolone derivatives
    - T39.2X6　Underdosing of pyrazolone derivatives
- T39.3　Poisoning by, adverse effect of and underdosing of other nonsteroidal anti-inflammatory drugs [NSAID]
  - T39.31　Poisoning by, adverse effect of and underdosing of propionic acid derivatives
    Poisoning by, adverse effect of and underdosing of fenoprofen
    Poisoning by, adverse effect of and underdosing of flurbiprofen
    Poisoning by, adverse effect of and underdosing of ibuprofen
    Poisoning by, adverse effect of and underdosing of ketoprofen
    Poisoning by, adverse effect of and underdosing of naproxen
    Poisoning by, adverse effect of and underdosing of oxaprozin
    - T39.311　Poisoning by propionic acid derivatives, accidental (unintentional)
    - T39.312　Poisoning by propionic acid derivatives, intentional self-harm
    - T39.313　Poisoning by propionic acid derivatives, assault
    - T39.314　Poisoning by propionic acid derivatives, undetermined
    - T39.315　Adverse effect of propionic acid derivatives
    - T39.316　Underdosing of propionic acid derivatives
  - T39.39　Poisoning by, adverse effect of and underdosing of other nonsteroidal anti-inflammatory drugs [NSAID]
    - T39.391　Poisoning by other nonsteroidal anti-inflammatory drugs [NSAID], accidental (unintentional)
      Poisoning by other nonsteroidal anti-inflammatory drugs NOS
    - T39.392　Poisoning by other nonsteroidal anti-inflammatory drugs [NSAID], intentional self-harm
    - T39.393　Poisoning by other nonsteroidal anti-inflammatory drugs [NSAID], assault
    - T39.394　Poisoning by other nonsteroidal anti-inflammatory drugs [NSAID], undetermined
    - T39.395　Adverse effect of other nonsteroidal anti-inflammatory drugs [NSAID]
    - T39.396　Underdosing of other nonsteroidal anti-inflammatory drugs [NSAID]

CHAPTER 19 (S00-T88)

● **T39.4** **Poisoning by, adverse effect of and underdosing of antirheumatics, not elsewhere classified**

> Excludes1   poisoning by, adverse effect of and underdosing of glucocorticoids (T38.0-)
>
> poisoning by, adverse effect of and underdosing of salicylates (T39.0-)

  ● **T39.4X** **Poisoning by, adverse effect of and underdosing of antirheumatics, not elsewhere classified**

    ● **T39.4X1** **Poisoning by antirheumatics, not elsewhere classified, accidental (unintentional)**

       Poisoning by antirheumatics, not elsewhere classified NOS

    ● **T39.4X2** **Poisoning by antirheumatics, not elsewhere classified, intentional self-harm**

    ● **T39.4X3** **Poisoning by antirheumatics, not elsewhere classified, assault**

    ● **T39.4X4** **Poisoning by antirheumatics, not elsewhere classified, undetermined**

    ● **T39.4X5** **Adverse effect of antirheumatics, not elsewhere classified**

    ● **T39.4X6** **Underdosing of antirheumatics, not elsewhere classified**

● **T39.8** **Poisoning by, adverse effect of and underdosing of other nonopioid analgesics and antipyretics, not elsewhere classified**

  ● **T39.8X** **Poisoning by, adverse effect of and underdosing of other nonopioid analgesics and antipyretics, not elsewhere classified**

    ● **T39.8X1** **Poisoning by other nonopioid analgesics and antipyretics, not elsewhere classified, accidental (unintentional)**

       Poisoning by other nonopioid analgesics and antipyretics, not elsewhere classified NOS

    ● **T39.8X2** **Poisoning by other nonopioid analgesics and antipyretics, not elsewhere classified, intentional self-harm**

    ● **T39.8X3** **Poisoning by other nonopioid analgesics and antipyretics, not elsewhere classified, assault**

    ● **T39.8X4** **Poisoning by other nonopioid analgesics and antipyretics, not elsewhere classified, undetermined**

    ● **T39.8X5** **Adverse effect of other nonopioid analgesics and antipyretics, not elsewhere classified**

    ● **T39.8X6** **Underdosing of other nonopioid analgesics and antipyretics, not elsewhere classified**

● **T39.9** **Poisoning by, adverse effect of and underdosing of unspecified nonopioid analgesic, antipyretic and antirheumatic**

  X ● **T39.91** **Poisoning by unspecified nonopioid analgesic, antipyretic and antirheumatic, accidental (unintentional)**

       Poisoning by nonopioid analgesic, antipyretic and antirheumatic NOS

  X ● **T39.92** **Poisoning by unspecified nonopioid analgesic, antipyretic and antirheumatic, intentional self-harm**

  X ● **T39.93** **Poisoning by unspecified nonopioid analgesic, antipyretic and antirheumatic, assault**

  X ● **T39.94** **Poisoning by unspecified nonopioid analgesic, antipyretic and antirheumatic, undetermined**

  X ● **T39.95** **Adverse effect of unspecified nonopioid analgesic, antipyretic and antirheumatic**

  X ● **T39.96** **Underdosing of unspecified nonopioid analgesic, antipyretic and antirheumatic**

● **T40** **Poisoning by, adverse effect of and underdosing of narcotics and psychodysleptics [hallucinogens]**

> Excludes2   drug dependence and related mental and behavioral disorders due to psychoactive substance use (F10.-F19.-)

The appropriate 7th character is to be added to each code from category T40

> A   initial encounter
> D   subsequent encounter
> S   sequela

● **T40.0** **Poisoning by, adverse effect of and underdosing of opium**

  ● **T40.0X** **Poisoning by, adverse effect of and underdosing of opium**

    ● **T40.0X1** **Poisoning by opium, accidental (unintentional)**

       Poisoning by opium NOS

    ● **T40.0X2** **Poisoning by opium, intentional self-harm**

    ● **T40.0X3** **Poisoning by opium, assault**

    ● **T40.0X4** **Poisoning by opium, undetermined**

    ● **T40.0X5** **Adverse effect of opium**

    ● **T40.0X6** **Underdosing of opium**

● **T40.1** **Poisoning by and adverse effect of heroin**

  ● **T40.1X** **Poisoning by and adverse effect of heroin**

    ● **T40.1X1** **Poisoning by heroin, accidental (unintentional)**

       Poisoning by heroin NOS

    ● **T40.1X2** **Poisoning by heroin, intentional self-harm**

    ● **T40.1X3** **Poisoning by heroin, assault**

    ● **T40.1X4** **Poisoning by heroin, undetermined**

● **T40.2** **Poisoning by, adverse effect of and underdosing of other opioids**

  ● **T40.2X** **Poisoning by, adverse effect of and underdosing of other opioids**

    ● **T40.2X1** **Poisoning by other opioids, accidental (unintentional)**

       Poisoning by other opioids NOS

    ● **T40.2X2** **Poisoning by other opioids, intentional self-harm**

    ● **T40.2X3** **Poisoning by other opioids, assault**

    ● **T40.2X4** **Poisoning by other opioids, undetermined**

    ● **T40.2X5** **Adverse effect of other opioids**

    ● **T40.2X6** **Underdosing of other opioids**

● **T40.3** **Poisoning by, adverse effect of and underdosing of methadone**

  ● **T40.3X** **Poisoning by, adverse effect of and underdosing of methadone**

    ● **T40.3X1** **Poisoning by methadone, accidental (unintentional)**

       Poisoning by methadone NOS

    ● **T40.3X2** **Poisoning by methadone, intentional self-harm**

    ● **T40.3X3** **Poisoning by methadone, assault**

    ● **T40.3X4** **Poisoning by methadone, undetermined**

    ● **T40.3X5** **Adverse effect of methadone**

    ● **T40.3X6** **Underdosing of methadone**

▶ New   ⇒ Revised   ~~deleted~~ Deleted   **OGCR** Official Guidelines   X Assign placeholder X   ● Use Additional Character(s)

Excludes 1   Excludes 2   Includes   Use additional   Code first   Code also   Key words

- ● T40.4   Poisoning by, adverse effect of and underdosing of other synthetic narcotics
  - ● T40.4X   Poisoning by, adverse effect of and underdosing of other synthetic narcotics
    - ● T40.4X1   Poisoning by other synthetic narcotics, accidental (unintentional)
      Poisoning by other synthetic narcotics NOS
    - ● T40.4X2   Poisoning by other synthetic narcotics, intentional self-harm
    - ● T40.4X3   Poisoning by other synthetic narcotics, assault
    - ● T40.4X4   Poisoning by other synthetic narcotics, undetermined
    - ● T40.4X5   Adverse effect of other synthetic narcotics
    - ● T40.4X6   Underdosing of other synthetic narcotics
- ● T40.5   Poisoning by, adverse effect of and underdosing of cocaine
  - ● T40.5X   Poisoning by, adverse effect of and underdosing of cocaine
    - ● T40.5X1   Poisoning by cocaine, accidental (unintentional)
      Poisoning by cocaine NOS
    - ● T40.5X2   Poisoning by cocaine, intentional self-harm
    - ● T40.5X3   Poisoning by cocaine, assault
    - ● T40.5X4   Poisoning by cocaine, undetermined
    - ● T40.5X5   Adverse effect of cocaine
    - ● T40.5X6   Underdosing of cocaine
- ● T40.6   Poisoning by, adverse effect of and underdosing of other and unspecified narcotics
  - ● T40.60   Poisoning by, adverse effect of and underdosing of unspecified narcotics
    - ● T40.601   Poisoning by unspecified narcotics, accidental (unintentional)
      Poisoning by narcotics NOS
    - ● T40.602   Poisoning by unspecified narcotics, intentional self-harm
    - ● T40.603   Poisoning by unspecified narcotics, assault
    - ● T40.604   Poisoning by unspecified narcotics, undetermined
    - ● T40.605   Adverse effect of unspecified narcotics
    - ● T40.606   Underdosing of unspecified narcotics
  - ● T40.69   Poisoning by, adverse effect of and underdosing of other narcotics
    - ● T40.691   Poisoning by other narcotics, accidental (unintentional)
      Poisoning by other narcotics NOS
    - ● T40.692   Poisoning by other narcotics, intentional self-harm
    - ● T40.693   Poisoning by other narcotics, assault
    - ● T40.694   Poisoning by other narcotics, undetermined
    - ● T40.695   Adverse effect of other narcotics
    - ● T40.696   Underdosing of other narcotics

- ● T40.7   Poisoning by, adverse effect of and underdosing of cannabis (derivatives)
  - ● T40.7X   Poisoning by, adverse effect of and underdosing of cannabis (derivatives)
    - ● T40.7X1   Poisoning by cannabis (derivatives), accidental (unintentional)
      Poisoning by cannabis NOS
    - ● T40.7X2   Poisoning by cannabis (derivatives), intentional self-harm
    - ● T40.7X3   Poisoning by cannabis (derivatives), assault
    - ● T40.7X4   Poisoning by cannabis (derivatives), undetermined
    - ● T40.7X5   Adverse effect of cannabis (derivatives)
    - ● T40.7X6   Underdosing of cannabis (derivatives)
- ● T40.8   Poisoning by and adverse effect of lysergide [LSD]
  - ● T40.8X   Poisoning by and adverse effect of lysergide [LSD]
    - ● T40.8X1   Poisoning by lysergide [LSD], accidental (unintentional)
      Poisoning by lysergide [LSD] NOS
    - ● T40.8X2   Poisoning by lysergide [LSD], intentional self-harm
    - ● T40.8X3   Poisoning by lysergide [LSD], assault
    - ● T40.8X4   Poisoning by lysergide [LSD], undetermined
- ● T40.9   Poisoning by, adverse effect of and underdosing of other and unspecified psychodysleptics [hallucinogens]
  - ● T40.90   Poisoning by, adverse effect of and underdosing of unspecified psychodysleptics [hallucinogens]
    - ● T40.901   Poisoning by unspecified psychodysleptics [hallucinogens], accidental (unintentional)
    - ● T40.902   Poisoning by unspecified psychodysleptics [hallucinogens], intentional self-harm
    - ● T40.903   Poisoning by unspecified psychodysleptics [hallucinogens], assault
    - ● T40.904   Poisoning by unspecified psychodysleptics [hallucinogens], undetermined
    - ● T40.905   Adverse effect of unspecified psychodysleptics [hallucinogens]
    - ● T40.906   Underdosing of unspecified psychodysleptics
  - ● T40.99   Poisoning by, adverse effect of and underdosing of other psychodysleptics [hallucinogens]
    - ● T40.991   Poisoning by other psychodysleptics [hallucinogens], accidental (unintentional)
      Poisoning by other psychodysleptics [hallucinogens] NOS
    - ● T40.992   Poisoning by other psychodysleptics [hallucinogens], intentional self-harm
    - ● T40.993   Poisoning by other psychodysleptics [hallucinogens], assault
    - ● T40.994   Poisoning by other psychodysleptics [hallucinogens], undetermined
    - ● T40.995   Adverse effect of other psychodysleptics [hallucinogens]
    - ● T40.996   Underdosing of other psychodysleptics

CHAPTER 19 (S00-T88)

● **T41** **Poisoning by, adverse effect of and underdosing of anesthetics and therapeutic gases**

> | **Excludes1** | benzodiazepines (T42.4-) |
> | | cocaine (T40.5-) |
> | | complications of anesthesia during pregnancy (O29.-) |
> | | complications of anesthesia during labor and delivery (O74.-) |
> | | complications of anesthesia during the puerperium (O89.-) opioids (T40.0-T40.2-) |

The appropriate 7th character is to be added to each code from category T41

A	initial encounter
D	subsequent encounter
S	sequela

● **T41.0** **Poisoning by, adverse effect of and underdosing of inhaled anesthetics**

> | **Excludes1** | oxygen (T41.5-) |

- ● **T41.0X** **Poisoning by, adverse effect of and underdosing of inhaled anesthetics**
  - ● **T41.0X1** **Poisoning by inhaled anesthetics, accidental (unintentional)**
    Poisoning by inhaled anesthetics NOS
  - ● **T41.0X2** **Poisoning by inhaled anesthetics, intentional self-harm**
  - ● **T41.0X3** **Poisoning by inhaled anesthetics, assault**
  - ● **T41.0X4** **Poisoning by inhaled anesthetics, undetermined**
  - ● **T41.0X5** **Adverse effect of inhaled anesthetics**
  - ● **T41.0X6** **Underdosing of inhaled anesthetics**

● **T41.1** **Poisoning by, adverse effect of and underdosing of intravenous anesthetics**
  Poisoning by, adverse effect of and underdosing of thiobarbiturates

- ● **T41.1X** **Poisoning by, adverse effect of and underdosing of intravenous anesthetics**
  - ● **T41.1X1** **Poisoning by intravenous anesthetics, accidental (unintentional)**
    Poisoning by intravenous anesthetics NOS
  - ● **T41.1X2** **Poisoning by intravenous anesthetics, intentional self-harm**
  - ● **T41.1X3** **Poisoning by intravenous anesthetics, assault**
  - ● **T41.1X4** **Poisoning by intravenous anesthetics, undetermined**
  - ● **T41.1X5** **Adverse effect of intravenous anesthetics**
  - ● **T41.1X6** **Underdosing of intravenous anesthetics**

● **T41.2** **Poisoning by, adverse effect of and underdosing of other and unspecified general anesthetics**

- ● **T41.20** **Poisoning by, adverse effect of and underdosing of unspecified general anesthetics**
  - ● **T41.201** **Poisoning by unspecified general anesthetics, accidental (unintentional)**
    Poisoning by general anesthetics NOS
  - ● **T41.202** **Poisoning by unspecified general anesthetics, intentional self-harm**
  - ● **T41.203** **Poisoning by unspecified general anesthetics, assault**
  - ● **T41.204** **Poisoning by unspecified general anesthetics, undetermined**
  - ● **T41.205** **Adverse effect of unspecified general anesthetics**
  - ● **T41.206** **Underdosing of unspecified general anesthetics**

- ● **T41.29** **Poisoning by, adverse effect of and underdosing of other general anesthetics**
  - ● **T41.291** **Poisoning by other general anesthetics, accidental (unintentional)**
    Poisoning by other general anesthetics NOS
  - ● **T41.292** **Poisoning by other general anesthetics, intentional self-harm**
  - ● **T41.293** **Poisoning by other general anesthetics, assault**
  - ● **T41.294** **Poisoning by other general anesthetics, undetermined**
  - ● **T41.295** **Adverse effect of other general anesthetics**
  - ● **T41.296** **Underdosing of other general anesthetics**

● **T41.3** **Poisoning by, adverse effect of and underdosing of local anesthetics**
  Cocaine (topical)

> | **Excludes2** | poisoning by cocaine used as a central nervous system stimulant (T40.5X1-T40.5X4) |

- ● **T41.3X** **Poisoning by, adverse effect of and underdosing of local anesthetics**
  - ● **T41.3X1** **Poisoning by local anesthetics, accidental (unintentional)**
    Poisoning by local anesthetics NOS
  - ● **T41.3X2** **Poisoning by local anesthetics, intentional self-harm**
  - ● **T41.3X3** **Poisoning by local anesthetics, assault**
  - ● **T41.3X4** **Poisoning by local anesthetics, undetermined**
  - ● **T41.3X5** **Adverse effect of local anesthetics**
  - ● **T41.3X6** **Underdosing of local anesthetics**

● **T41.4** **Poisoning by, adverse effect of and underdosing of unspecified anesthetic**

- X ● **T41.41** **Poisoning by unspecified anesthetic, accidental (unintentional)**
    Poisoning by anesthetic NOS
- X ● **T41.42** **Poisoning by unspecified anesthetic, intentional self-harm**
- X ● **T41.43** **Poisoning by unspecified anesthetic, assault**
- X ● **T41.44** **Poisoning by unspecified anesthetic, undetermined**
- X ● **T41.45** **Adverse effect of unspecified anesthetic**
- X ● **T41.46** **Underdosing of unspecified anesthetics**

● **T41.5** **Poisoning by, adverse effect of and underdosing of therapeutic gases**

- ● **T41.5X** **Poisoning by, adverse effect of and underdosing of therapeutic gases**
  - ● **T41.5X1** **Poisoning by therapeutic gases, accidental (unintentional)**
    Poisoning by therapeutic gases NOS
  - ● **T41.5X2** **Poisoning by therapeutic gases, intentional self-harm**
  - ● **T41.5X3** **Poisoning by therapeutic gases, assault**
  - ● **T41.5X4** **Poisoning by therapeutic gases, undetermined**
  - ● **T41.5X5** **Adverse effect of therapeutic gases**
  - ● **T41.5X6** **Underdosing of therapeutic gases**

▶ New　⟹ Revised　~~deleted~~ Deleted　**OGCR** Official Guidelines　X Assign placeholder X　● Use Additional Character(s)

Excludes 1　Excludes 2　Includes　Use additional　Code first　Code also　Key words

● **T42**   **Poisoning by, adverse effect of and underdosing of antiepileptic, sedative-hypnotic and antiparkinsonism drugs**

> **Excludes2**   drug dependence and related mental and behavioral disorders due to psychoactive substance use (F10.--F19.-)

> The appropriate 7th character is to be added to each code from category T42

> | | |
> |---|---|
> | A | initial encounter |
> | D | subsequent encounter |
> | S | sequela |

● **T42.0**   Poisoning by, adverse effect of and underdosing of hydantoin derivatives

   ● **T42.0X**   Poisoning by, adverse effect of and underdosing of hydantoin derivatives

     ● **T42.0X1**   Poisoning by hydantoin derivatives, accidental (unintentional)
       Poisoning by hydantoin derivatives NOS

     ● **T42.0X2**   Poisoning by hydantoin derivatives, intentional self-harm

     ● **T42.0X3**   Poisoning by hydantoin derivatives, assault

     ● **T42.0X4**   Poisoning by hydantoin derivatives, undetermined

     ● **T42.0X5**   Adverse effect of hydantoin derivatives

     ● **T42.0X6**   Underdosing of hydantoin derivatives

● **T42.1**   Poisoning by, adverse effect of and underdosing of iminostilbenes
   Poisoning by, adverse effect of and underdosing of carbamazepine

   ● **T42.1X**   Poisoning by, adverse effect of and underdosing of iminostilbenes

     ● **T42.1X1**   Poisoning by iminostilbenes, accidental (unintentional)
       Poisoning by iminostilbenes NOS

     ● **T42.1X2**   Poisoning by iminostilbenes, intentional self-harm

     ● **T42.1X3**   Poisoning by iminostilbenes, assault

     ● **T42.1X4**   Poisoning by iminostilbenes, undetermined

     ● **T42.1X5**   Adverse effect of iminostilbenes

     ● **T42.1X6**   Underdosing of iminostilbenes

● **T42.2**   Poisoning by, adverse effect of and underdosing of succinimides and oxazolidinediones

   ● **T42.2X**   Poisoning by, adverse effect of and underdosing of succinimides and oxazolidinediones

     ● **T42.2X1**   Poisoning by succinimides and oxazolidinediones, accidental (unintentional)
       Poisoning by succinimides and oxazolidinediones NOS

     ● **T42.2X2**   Poisoning by succinimides and oxazolidinediones, intentional self-harm

     ● **T42.2X3**   Poisoning by succinimides and oxazolidinediones, assault

     ● **T42.2X4**   Poisoning by succinimides and oxazolidinediones, undetermined

     ● **T42.2X5**   Adverse effect of succinimides and oxazolidinediones

     ● **T42.2X6**   Underdosing of succinimides and oxazolidinediones

● **T42.3**   Poisoning by, adverse effect of and underdosing of barbiturates

> **Excludes1**   poisoning by, adverse effect of and underdosing of thiobarbiturates (T41.1-)

   ● **T42.3X**   Poisoning by, adverse effect of and underdosing of barbiturates

     ● **T42.3X1**   Poisoning by barbiturates, accidental (unintentional)
       Poisoning by barbiturates NOS

     ● **T42.3X2**   Poisoning by barbiturates, intentional self-harm

     ● **T42.3X3**   Poisoning by barbiturates, assault

     ● **T42.3X4**   Poisoning by barbiturates, undetermined

     ● **T42.3X5**   Adverse effect of barbiturates

     ● **T42.3X6**   Underdosing of barbiturates

● **T42.4**   Poisoning by, adverse effect of and underdosing of benzodiazepines

   ● **T42.4X**   Poisoning by, adverse effect of and underdosing of benzodiazepines

     ● **T42.4X1**   Poisoning by benzodiazepines, accidental (unintentional)
       Poisoning by benzodiazepines NOS

     ● **T42.4X2**   Poisoning by benzodiazepines, intentional self-harm

     ● **T42.4X3**   Poisoning by benzodiazepines, assault

     ● **T42.4X4**   Poisoning by benzodiazepines, undetermined

     ● **T42.4X5**   Adverse effect of benzodiazepines

     ● **T42.4X6**   Underdosing of benzodiazepines

● **T42.5**   Poisoning by, adverse effect of and underdosing of mixed antiepileptics

   ● **T42.5X**   Poisoning by, adverse effect of and underdosing of antiepileptics

     ● **T42.5X1**   Poisoning by mixed antiepileptics, accidental (unintentional)
       Poisoning by mixed antiepileptics NOS

     ● **T42.5X2**   Poisoning by mixed antiepileptics, intentional self-harm

     ● **T42.5X3**   Poisoning by mixed antiepileptics, assault

     ● **T42.5X4**   Poisoning by mixed antiepileptics, undetermined

     ● **T42.5X5**   Adverse effect of mixed antiepileptics

     ● **T42.5X6**   Underdosing of mixed antiepileptics

CHAPTER 19 (S00-T88)

● T42.6   Poisoning by, adverse effect of and underdosing of other antiepileptic and sedative-hypnotic drugs

Poisoning by, adverse effect of and underdosing of methaqualone

Poisoning by, adverse effect of and underdosing of valproic acid

> **Excludes1**   poisoning by, adverse effect of and underdosing of carbamazepine (T42.1-)

   ● T42.6X   Poisoning by, adverse effect of and underdosing of other antiepileptic and sedative-hypnotic drugs

     ● T42.6X1   Poisoning by other antiepileptic and sedative-hypnotic drugs, accidental (unintentional)

       Poisoning by other antiepileptic and sedative-hypnotic drugs NOS

     ● T42.6X2   Poisoning by other antiepileptic and sedative-hypnotic drugs, intentional self-harm

     ● T42.6X3   Poisoning by other antiepileptic and sedative-hypnotic drugs, assault

     ● T42.6X4   Poisoning by other antiepileptic and sedative-hypnotic drugs, undetermined

     ● T42.6X5   Adverse effect of other antiepileptic and sedative-hypnotic drugs

     ● T42.6X6   Underdosing of other antiepileptic and sedative-hypnotic drugs

● T42.7   Poisoning by, adverse effect of and underdosing of unspecified antiepileptic and sedative-hypnotic drugs

   X ● T42.71   Poisoning by unspecified antiepileptic and sedative-hypnotic drugs, accidental (unintentional)

      Poisoning by antiepileptic and sedative-hypnotic drugs NOS

   X ● T42.72   Poisoning by unspecified antiepileptic and sedative-hypnotic drugs, intentional self-harm

   X ● T42.73   Poisoning by unspecified antiepileptic and sedative-hypnotic drugs, assault

   X ● T42.74   Poisoning by unspecified antiepileptic and sedative-hypnotic drugs, undetermined

   X ● T42.75   Adverse effect of unspecified antiepileptic and sedative-hypnotic drugs

   X ● T42.76   Underdosing of unspecified antiepileptic and sedative-hypnotic drugs

● T42.8   Poisoning by, adverse effect of and underdosing of antiparkinsonism drugs and other central muscle-tone depressants

Poisoning by, adverse effect of and underdosing of amantadine

   ● T42.8X   Poisoning by, adverse effect of and underdosing of antiparkinsonism drugs and other central muscle-tone depressants

     ● T42.8X1   Poisoning by antiparkinsonism drugs and other central muscle-tone depressants, accidental (unintentional)

       Poisoning by antiparkinsonism drugs and other central muscle-tone depressants NOS

     ● T42.8X2   Poisoning by antiparkinsonism drugs and other central muscle-tone depressants, intentional self-harm

     ● T42.8X3   Poisoning by antiparkinsonism drugs and other central muscle-tone depressants, assault

     ● T42.8X4   Poisoning by antiparkinsonism drugs and other central muscle-tone depressants, undetermined

     ● T42.8X5   Adverse effect of antiparkinsonism drugs and other central muscle-tone depressants

     ● T42.8X6   Underdosing of antiparkinsonism drugs and other central muscle-tone depressants

● T43   Poisoning by, adverse effect of and underdosing of psychotropic drugs, not elsewhere classified

> **Excludes1**   appetite depressants (T50.5-)
> barbiturates (T42.3-)
> benzodiazepines (T42.4-)
> methaqualone (T42.6-)
> psychodysleptics [hallucinogens] (T40.7-T40.9-)

> **Excludes2**   drug dependence and related mental and behavioral disorders due to psychoactive substance use (F10.--F19.-)

The appropriate 7th character is to be added to each code from category T43

A	initial encounter
D	subsequent encounter
S	sequela

● T43.0   Poisoning by, adverse effect of and underdosing of tricyclic and tetracyclic antidepressants

   ● T43.01   Poisoning by, adverse effect of and underdosing of tricyclic antidepressants

     ● T43.011   Poisoning by tricyclic antidepressants, accidental (unintentional)

       Poisoning by tricyclic antidepressants NOS

     ● T43.012   Poisoning by tricyclic antidepressants, intentional self-harm

     ● T43.013   Poisoning by tricyclic antidepressants, assault

     ● T43.014   Poisoning by tricyclic antidepressants, undetermined

     ● T43.015   Adverse effect of tricyclic antidepressants

     ● T43.016   Underdosing of tricyclic antidepressants

   ● T43.02   Poisoning by, adverse effect of and underdosing of tetracyclic antidepressants

     ● T43.021   Poisoning by tetracyclic antidepressants, accidental (unintentional)

       Poisoning by tetracyclic antidepressants NOS

     ● T43.022   Poisoning by tetracyclic antidepressants, intentional self-harm

     ● T43.023   Poisoning by tetracyclic antidepressants, assault

     ● T43.024   Poisoning by tetracyclic antidepressants, undetermined

     ● T43.025   Adverse effect of tetracyclic antidepressants

     ● T43.026   Underdosing of tetracyclic antidepressants

● T43.1   Poisoning by, adverse effect of and underdosing of monoamine-oxidase-inhibitor antidepressants

   ● T43.1X   Poisoning by, adverse effect of and underdosing of monoamine-oxidase-inhibitor antidepressants

     ● T43.1X1   Poisoning by monoamine-oxidase-inhibitor antidepressants, accidental (unintentional)

       Poisoning by monoamine-oxidase-inhibitor antidepressants NOS

     ● T43.1X2   Poisoning by monoamine-oxidase-inhibitor antidepressants, intentional self-harm

▶ New   ⇒ Revised   ~~deleted~~ Deleted   **OGCR** Official Guidelines   X Assign placeholder X   ● Use Additional Character(s)

| Excludes 1 | Excludes 2 | Includes | Use additional | Code first | Code also | Key words |

● T43.1X3   Poisoning by monoamine-oxidase-inhibitor antidepressants, assault

● T43.1X4   Poisoning by monoamine-oxidase-inhibitor antidepressants, undetermined

● T43.1X5   Adverse effect of monoamine-oxidase-inhibitor antidepressants

● T43.1X6   Underdosing of monoamine-oxidase-inhibitor antidepressants

● T43.2   Poisoning by, adverse effect of and underdosing of other and unspecified antidepressants

   ● T43.20   Poisoning by, adverse effect of and underdosing of unspecified antidepressants

     ● T43.201   Poisoning by unspecified antidepressants, accidental (unintentional)
         Poisoning by antidepressants NOS

     ● T43.202   Poisoning by unspecified antidepressants, intentional self-harm

     ● T43.203   Poisoning by unspecified antidepressants, assault

     ● T43.204   Poisoning by unspecified antidepressants, undetermined

     ● T43.205   Adverse effect of unspecified antidepressants
         ▶ Antidepressant discontinuation syndrome

     ● T43.206   Underdosing of unspecified antidepressants

   ● T43.21   Poisoning by, adverse effect of and underdosing of selective serotonin and norepinephrine reuptake inhibitors
       Poisoning by, adverse effect of and underdosing of SSNRI antidepressants

     ● T43.211   Poisoning by selective serotonin and norepinephrine reuptake inhibitors, accidental (unintentional)

     ● T43.212   Poisoning by selective serotonin and norepinephrine reuptake inhibitors, intentional self-harm

     ● T43.213   Poisoning by selective serotonin and norepinephrine reuptake inhibitors, assault

     ● T43.214   Poisoning by selective serotonin and norepinephrine reuptake inhibitors, undetermined

     ● T43.215   Adverse effect of selective serotonin and norepinephrine reuptake inhibitors

     ● T43.216   Underdosing of selective serotonin and norepinephrine reuptake inhibitors

   ● T43.22   Poisoning by, adverse effect of and underdosing of selective serotonin reuptake inhibitors
       Poisoning by, adverse effect of and underdosing of SSRI antidepressants

     ● T43.221   Poisoning by selective serotonin reuptake inhibitors, accidental (unintentional)

     ● T43.222   Poisoning by selective serotonin reuptake inhibitors, intentional self-harm

     ● T43.223   Poisoning by selective serotonin reuptake inhibitors, assault

     ● T43.224   Poisoning by selective serotonin reuptake inhibitors, undetermined

     ● T43.225   Adverse effect of selective serotonin reuptake inhibitors

     ● T43.226   Underdosing of selective serotonin reuptake inhibitors

   ● T43.29   Poisoning by, adverse effect of and underdosing of other antidepressants

     ● T43.291   Poisoning by other antidepressants, accidental (unintentional)
         Poisoning by other antidepressants NOS

     ● T43.292   Poisoning by other antidepressants, intentional self-harm

     ● T43.293   Poisoning by other antidepressants, assault

     ● T43.294   Poisoning by other antidepressants, undetermined

     ● T43.295   Adverse effect of other antidepressants

     ● T43.296   Underdosing of other antidepressants

● T43.3   Poisoning by, adverse effect of and underdosing of phenothiazine antipsychotics and neuroleptics

   ● T43.3X   Poisoning by, adverse effect of and underdosing of phenothiazine antipsychotics and neuroleptics

     ● T43.3X1   Poisoning by phenothiazine antipsychotics and neuroleptics, accidental (unintentional)
         Poisoning by phenothiazine antipsychotics and neuroleptics NOS

     ● T43.3X2   Poisoning by phenothiazine antipsychotics and neuroleptics, intentional self-harm

     ● T43.3X3   Poisoning by phenothiazine antipsychotics and neuroleptics, assault

     ● T43.3X4   Poisoning by phenothiazine antipsychotics and neuroleptics, undetermined

     ● T43.3X5   Adverse effect of phenothiazine antipsychotics and neuroleptics

     ● T43.3X6   Underdosing of phenothiazine antipsychotics and neuroleptics

● T43.4   Poisoning by, adverse effect of and underdosing of butyrophenone and thiothixene neuroleptics

   ● T43.4X   Poisoning by, adverse effect of and underdosing of butyrophenone and thiothixene neuroleptics

     ● T43.4X1   Poisoning by butyrophenone and thiothixene neuroleptics, accidental (unintentional)
         Poisoning by butyrophenone and thiothixene neuroleptics NOS

     ● T43.4X2   Poisoning by butyrophenone and thiothixene neuroleptics, intentional self-harm

     ● T43.4X3   Poisoning by butyrophenone and thiothixene neuroleptics, assault

     ● T43.4X4   Poisoning by butyrophenone and thiothixene neuroleptics, undetermined

     ● T43.4X5   Adverse effect of butyrophenone and thiothixene neuroleptics

     ● T43.4X6   Underdosing of butyrophenone and thiothixene neuroleptics

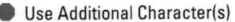

▶ New   ⇒ Revised   ~~deleted~~ Deleted   **OGCR** Official Guidelines   X Assign placeholder X   ● Use Additional Character(s)

Excludes 1   Excludes 2   Includes   Use additional   Code first   Code also   Key words

CHAPTER 19 (S00-T88)

● T43.5   **Poisoning by, adverse effect of and underdosing of other and unspecified antipsychotics and neuroleptics**

   Excludes1   poisoning by, adverse effect of and underdosing of rauwolfia (T46.5-)

   ● T43.50   **Poisoning by, adverse effect of and underdosing of unspecified antipsychotics and neuroleptics**

     ● T43.501   **Poisoning by unspecified antipsychotics and neuroleptics, accidental** (unintentional)

       Poisoning by antipsychotics and neuroleptics NOS

     ● T43.502   **Poisoning by unspecified antipsychotics and neuroleptics, intentional self-harm**

     ● T43.503   **Poisoning by unspecified antipsychotics and neuroleptics, assault**

     ● T43.504   **Poisoning by unspecified antipsychotics and neuroleptics, undetermined**

     ● T43.505   **Adverse effect of unspecified antipsychotics and neuroleptics**

     ● T43.506   **Underdosing of unspecified antipsychotics and neuroleptics**

   ● T43.59   **Poisoning by, adverse effect of and underdosing of other antipsychotics and neuroleptics**

     ● T43.591   **Poisoning by other antipsychotics and neuroleptics, accidental (unintentional)**

       Poisoning by other antipsychotics and neuroleptics NOS

     ● T43.592   **Poisoning by other antipsychotics and neuroleptics, intentional self-harm**

     ● T43.593   **Poisoning by other antipsychotics and neuroleptics, assault**

     ● T43.594   **Poisoning by other antipsychotics and neuroleptics, undetermined**

     ● T43.595   **Adverse effect of other antipsychotics and neuroleptics**

     ● T43.596   **Underdosing of other antipsychotics and neuroleptics**

● T43.6   **Poisoning by, adverse effect of and underdosing of psychostimulants**

   Excludes1   poisoning by, adverse effect of and underdosing of cocaine (T40.5-)

   ● T43.60   **Poisoning by, adverse effect of and underdosing of unspecified psychostimulant**

     ● T43.601   **Poisoning by unspecified psychostimulants, accidental (unintentional)**

       Poisoning by psychostimulants NOS

     ● T43.602   **Poisoning by unspecified psychostimulants, intentional self-harm**

     ● T43.603   **Poisoning by unspecified psychostimulants, assault**

     ● T43.604   **Poisoning by unspecified psychostimulants, undetermined**

     ● T43.605   **Adverse effect of unspecified psychostimulants**

     ● T43.606   **Underdosing of unspecified psychostimulants**

● T43.61   **Poisoning by, adverse effect of and underdosing of caffeine**

     ● T43.611   **Poisoning by caffeine, accidental (unintentional)**

       Poisoning by caffeine NOS

     ● T43.612   **Poisoning by caffeine, intentional self-harm**

     ● T43.613   **Poisoning by caffeine, assault**

     ● T43.614   **Poisoning by caffeine, undetermined**

     ● T43.615   **Adverse effect of caffeine**

     ● T43.616   **Underdosing of caffeine**

● T43.62   **Poisoning by, adverse effect of and underdosing of amphetamines**

   Poisoning by, adverse effect of and underdosing of methamphetamines

     ● T43.621   **Poisoning by amphetamines, accidental (unintentional)**

       Poisoning by amphetamines NOS

     ● T43.622   **Poisoning by amphetamines, intentional self-harm**

     ● T43.623   **Poisoning by amphetamines, assault**

     ● T43.624   **Poisoning by amphetamines, undetermined**

     ● T43.625   **Adverse effect of amphetamines**

     ● T43.626   **Underdosing of amphetamines**

● T43.63   **Poisoning by, adverse effect of and underdosing of methylphenidate**

     ● T43.631   **Poisoning by methylphenidate, accidental (unintentional)**

       Poisoning by methylphenidate NOS

     ● T43.632   **Poisoning by methylphenidate, intentional self-harm**

     ● T43.633   **Poisoning by methylphenidate, assault**

     ● T43.634   **Poisoning by methylphenidate, undetermined**

     ● T43.635   **Adverse effect of methylphenidate**

     ● T43.636   **Underdosing of methylphenidate**

● T43.69   **Poisoning by, adverse effect of and underdosing of other psychostimulants**

     ● T43.691   **Poisoning by other psychostimulants, accidental (unintentional)**

       Poisoning by other psychostimulants NOS

     ● T43.692   **Poisoning by other psychostimulants, intentional self-harm**

     ● T43.693   **Poisoning by other psychostimulants, assault**

     ● T43.694   **Poisoning by other psychostimulants, undetermined**

     ● T43.695   **Adverse effect of other psychostimulants**

     ● T43.696   **Underdosing of other psychostimulants**

● T43.8   **Poisoning by, adverse effect of and underdosing of other psychotropic drugs**

   ● T43.8X   **Poisoning by, adverse effect of and underdosing of other psychotropic drugs**

     ● T43.8X1   **Poisoning by other psychotropic drugs, accidental (unintentional)**

       Poisoning by other psychotropic drugs NOS

     ● T43.8X2   **Poisoning by other psychotropic drugs, intentional self-harm**

▶ New   ⇒ Revised   ~~deleted~~ Deleted   **OGCR** Official Guidelines   X Assign placeholder X   ● Use Additional Character(s)

Excludes 1   Excludes 2   Includes   Use additional   Code first   Code also   Key words

● T43.8X3 Poisoning by other psychotropic drugs, assault

● T43.8X4 Poisoning by other psychotropic drugs, undetermined

● T43.8X5 Adverse effect of other psychotropic drugs

● T43.8X6 Underdosing of other psychotropic drugs

● T43.9 Poisoning by, adverse effect of and underdosing of unspecified psychotropic drug

X ● T43.91 Poisoning by unspecified psychotropic drug, accidental (unintentional)
Poisoning by psychotropic drug NOS

X ● T43.92 Poisoning by unspecified psychotropic drug, intentional self-harm

X ● T43.93 Poisoning by unspecified psychotropic drug, assault

X ● T43.94 Poisoning by unspecified psychotropic drug, undetermined

X ● T43.95 Adverse effect of unspecified psychotropic drug

X ● T43.96 Underdosing of unspecified psychotropic drug

● T44 Poisoning by, adverse effect of and underdosing of drugs primarily affecting the autonomic nervous system

The appropriate 7th character is to be added to each code from category T44

A	initial encounter
D	subsequent encounter
S	sequela

● T44.0 Poisoning by, adverse effect of and underdosing of anticholinesterase agents

● T44.0X Poisoning by, adverse effect of and underdosing of anticholinesterase agents

● T44.0X1 Poisoning by anticholinesterase agents, accidental (unintentional)
Poisoning by anticholinesterase agents NOS

● T44.0X2 Poisoning by anticholinesterase agents, intentional self-harm

● T44.0X3 Poisoning by anticholinesterase agents, assault

● T44.0X4 Poisoning by anticholinesterase agents, undetermined

● T44.0X5 Adverse effect of anticholinesterase agents

● T44.0X6 Underdosing of anticholinesterase agents

● T44.1 Poisoning by, adverse effect of and underdosing of other parasympathomimetics [cholinergics]

● T44.1X Poisoning by, adverse effect of and underdosing of other parasympathomimetics [cholinergics]

● T44.1X1 Poisoning by other parasympathomimetics [cholinergics], accidental (unintentional)
Poisoning by other parasympathomimetics [cholinergics] NOS

● T44.1X2 Poisoning by other parasympathomimetics [cholinergics], intentional self-harm

● T44.1X3 Poisoning by other parasympathomimetics [cholinergics], assault

● T44.1X4 Poisoning by other parasympathomimetics [cholinergics], undetermined

● T44.1X5 Adverse effect of other parasympathomimetics [cholinergics]

● T44.1X6 Underdosing of other parasympathomimetics

● T44.2 Poisoning by, adverse effect of and underdosing of ganglionic blocking drugs

● T44.2X Poisoning by, adverse effect of and underdosing of ganglionic blocking drugs

● T44.2X1 Poisoning by ganglionic blocking drugs, accidental (unintentional)
Poisoning by ganglionic blocking drugs NOS

● T44.2X2 Poisoning by ganglionic blocking drugs, intentional self-harm

● T44.2X3 Poisoning by ganglionic blocking drugs, assault

● T44.2X4 Poisoning by ganglionic blocking drugs, undetermined

● T44.2X5 Adverse effect of ganglionic blocking drugs

● T44.2X6 Underdosing of ganglionic blocking drugs

● T44.3 Poisoning by, adverse effect of and underdosing of other parasympatholytics [anticholinergics and antimuscarinics] and spasmolytics
Poisoning by, adverse effect of and underdosing of papaverine

● T44.3X Poisoning by, adverse effect of and underdosing of other parasympatholytics [anticholinergics and antimuscarinics] and spasmolytics

● T44.3X1 Poisoning by other parasympatholytics [anticholinergics and antimuscarinics] and spasmolytics, accidental (unintentional)
Poisoning by other parasympatholytics [anticholinergics and antimuscarinics] and spasmolytics NOS

● T44.3X2 Poisoning by other parasympatholytics [anticholinergics and antimuscarinics] and spasmolytics, intentional self-harm

● T44.3X3 Poisoning by other parasympatholytics [anticholinergics and antimuscarinics] and spasmolytics, assault

● T44.3X4 Poisoning by other parasympatholytics [anticholinergics and antimuscarinics] and spasmolytics, undetermined

● T44.3X5 Adverse effect of other parasympatholytics [anticholinergics and antimuscarinics] and spasmolytics

● T44.3X6 Underdosing of other parasympatholytics [anticholinergics and antimuscarinics] and spasmolytics

CHAPTER 19 (S00-T88)

● **T44.4 Poisoning by, adverse effect of and underdosing of predominantly alpha-adrenoreceptor agonists**
Poisoning by, adverse effect of and underdosing of metaraminol

  ● **T44.4X Poisoning by, adverse effect of and underdosing of predominantly alpha-adrenoreceptor agonists**

    ● **T44.4X1 Poisoning by predominantly alpha-adrenoreceptor agonists, accidental (unintentional)**
Poisoning by predominantly alpha-adrenoreceptor agonists NOS

    ● **T44.4X2 Poisoning by predominantly alpha-adrenoreceptor agonists, intentional self-harm**

    ● **T44.4X3 Poisoning by predominantly alpha-adrenoreceptor agonists, assault**

    ● **T44.4X4 Poisoning by predominantly alpha-adrenoreceptor agonists, undetermined**

    ● **T44.4X5 Adverse effect of predominantly alpha-adrenoreceptor agonists**

    ● **T44.4X6 Underdosing of predominantly alpha-adrenoreceptor agonists**

● **T44.5 Poisoning by, adverse effect of and underdosing of predominantly beta-adrenoreceptor agonists**

  Excludes1   poisoning by, adverse effect of and underdosing of beta-adrenoreceptor agonists used in asthma therapy (T48.6-)

  ● **T44.5X Poisoning by, adverse effect of and underdosing of predominantly beta-adrenoreceptor agonists**

    ● **T44.5X1 Poisoning by predominantly beta-adrenoreceptor agonists, accidental (unintentional)**
Poisoning by predominantly beta-adrenoreceptor agonists NOS

    ● **T44.5X2 Poisoning by predominantly beta-adrenoreceptor agonists, intentional self-harm**

    ● **T44.5X3 Poisoning by predominantly beta-adrenoreceptor agonists, assault**

    ● **T44.5X4 Poisoning by predominantly beta-adrenoreceptor agonists, undetermined**

    ● **T44.5X5 Adverse effect of predominantly beta-adrenoreceptor agonists**

    ● **T44.5X6 Underdosing of predominantly beta-adrenoreceptor agonists**

● **T44.6 Poisoning by, adverse effect of and underdosing of alpha-adrenoreceptor antagonists**

  Excludes1   poisoning by, adverse effect of and underdosing of ergot alkaloids (T48.0)

  ● **T44.6X Poisoning by, adverse effect of and underdosing of alpha-adrenoreceptor antagonists**

    ● **T44.6X1 Poisoning by alpha-adrenoreceptor antagonists, accidental (unintentional)**
Poisoning by alpha-adrenoreceptor antagonists NOS

    ● **T44.6X2 Poisoning by alpha-adrenoreceptor antagonists, intentional self-harm**

    ● **T44.6X3 Poisoning by alpha-adrenoreceptor antagonists, assault**

    ● **T44.6X4 Poisoning by alpha-adrenoreceptor antagonists, undetermined**

    ● **T44.6X5 Adverse effect of alpha-adrenoreceptor antagonists**

    ● **T44.6X6 Underdosing of alpha-adrenoreceptor antagonists**

● **T44.7 Poisoning by, adverse effect of and underdosing of beta-adrenoreceptor antagonists**

  ● **T44.7X Poisoning by, adverse effect of and underdosing of beta-adrenoreceptor antagonists**

    ● **T44.7X1 Poisoning by beta-adrenoreceptor antagonists, accidental (unintentional)**
Poisoning by beta-adrenoreceptor antagonists NOS

    ● **T44.7X2 Poisoning by beta-adrenoreceptor antagonists, intentional self-harm**

    ● **T44.7X3 Poisoning by beta-adrenoreceptor antagonists, assault**

    ● **T44.7X4 Poisoning by beta-adrenoreceptor antagonists, undetermined**

    ● **T44.7X5 Adverse effect of beta-adrenoreceptor antagonists**

    ● **T44.7X6 Underdosing of beta-adrenoreceptor antagonists**

● **T44.8 Poisoning by, adverse effect of and underdosing of centrally-acting and adrenergic-neuron-blocking agents**

  Excludes1   poisoning by, adverse effect of and underdosing of clonidine (T46.5)
poisoning by, adverse effect of and underdosing of guanethidine (T46.5)

  ● **T44.8X Poisoning by, adverse effect of and underdosing of centrally-acting and adrenergic-neuron-blocking agents**

    ● **T44.8X1 Poisoning by centrally-acting and adrenergic-neuron-blocking agents, accidental (unintentional)**
Poisoning by centrally-acting and adrenergic-neuron-blocking agents NOS

    ● **T44.8X2 Poisoning by centrally-acting and adrenergic-neuron-blocking agents, intentional self-harm**

    ● **T44.8X3 Poisoning by centrally-acting and adrenergic-neuron-blocking agents, assault**

    ● **T44.8X4 Poisoning by centrally-acting and adrenergic-neuron-blocking agents, undetermined**

    ● **T44.8X5 Adverse effect of centrally-acting and adrenergic-neuron-blocking agents**

    ● **T44.8X6 Underdosing of centrally-acting and adrenergic-neuron-blocking agents**

● **T44.9 Poisoning by, adverse effect of and underdosing of other and unspecified drugs primarily affecting the autonomic nervous system**
Poisoning by, adverse effect of and underdosing of drug stimulating both alpha and beta-adrenoreceptors

  ● **T44.90 Poisoning by, adverse effect of and underdosing of unspecified drugs primarily affecting the autonomic nervous system**

    ● **T44.901 Poisoning by unspecified drugs primarily affecting the autonomic nervous system, accidental (unintentional)**
Poisoning by unspecified drugs primarily affecting the autonomic nervous system NOS

    ● **T44.902 Poisoning by unspecified drugs primarily affecting the autonomic nervous system, intentional self-harm**

    ● **T44.903 Poisoning by unspecified drugs primarily affecting the autonomic nervous system, assault**

● T44.904 Poisoning by unspecified drugs
            primarily affecting the autonomic
            nervous system, **undetermined**
● T44.905 **Adverse effect** of unspecified drugs
            primarily affecting the autonomic
            nervous system
● T44.906 **Underdosing** of unspecified drugs
            primarily affecting the autonomic
            nervous system
● T44.99 Poisoning by, adverse effect of and
            underdosing of **other drugs primarily affecting
            the autonomic nervous system**
● T44.991 Poisoning by other drug primarily
            affecting the autonomic nervous
            system, **accidental** (unintentional)
                Poisoning by other drugs primarily
                affecting the autonomic
                nervous system NOS
● T44.992 Poisoning by other drug primarily
            affecting the autonomic nervous
            system, **intentional** self-harm
● T44.993 Poisoning by other drug primarily
            affecting the autonomic nervous
            system, **assault**
● T44.994 Poisoning by other drug primarily
            affecting the autonomic nervous
            system, **undetermined**
● T44.995 **Adverse effect** of other drug primarily
            affecting the autonomic nervous
            system
● T44.996 **Underdosing** of other drug primarily
            affecting the autonomic nervous
            system

● T45 Poisoning by, adverse effect of and underdosing of primarily
        systemic and hematological agents, not elsewhere classified
            The appropriate 7th character is to be added to each code from
            category T45

            A   initial encounter
            D   subsequent encounter
            S   sequela

● T45.0 Poisoning by, adverse effect of and underdosing of
            antiallergic and antiemetic drugs
            Excludes1 poisoning by, adverse effect of and
                        underdosing of phenothiazine-based
                        neuroleptics (T43.3)
● T45.0X Poisoning by, adverse effect of and
            underdosing of **antiallergic and antiemetic
            drugs**
● T45.0X1 Poisoning by antiallergic and
            antiemetic drugs, **accidental**
            (unintentional)
                Poisoning by antiallergic and
                antiemetic drugs NOS
● T45.0X2 Poisoning by antiallergic and
            antiemetic drugs, **intentional**
            self-harm
● T45.0X3 Poisoning by antiallergic and
            antiemetic drugs, **assault**
● T45.0X4 Poisoning by antiallergic and
            antiemetic drugs, **undetermined**
● T45.0X5 **Adverse effect** of antiallergic and
            antiemetic drugs
● T45.0X6 **Underdosing** of antiallergic and
            antiemetic drugs

● T45.1 Poisoning by, adverse effect of and underdosing of
            antineoplastic and immunosuppressive drugs
            Excludes1 poisoning by, adverse effect of and
                        underdosing of tamoxifen (T38.6)
● T45.1X Poisoning by, adverse effect of and underdosing
            of **antineoplastic and immunosuppressive
            drugs**
● T45.1X1 Poisoning by antineoplastic and
            immunosuppressive drugs, **accidental**
            (unintentional)
                Poisoning by antineoplastic and
                immunosuppressive drugs
                NOS
● T45.1X2 Poisoning by antineoplastic
            and immunosuppressive drugs,
            intentional self-harm
● T45.1X3 Poisoning by antineoplastic and
            immunosuppressive drugs, **assault**
● T45.1X4 Poisoning by antineoplastic
            and immunosuppressive drugs,
            undetermined
● T45.1X5 **Adverse effect** of antineoplastic and
            immunosuppressive drugs
● T45.1X6 **Underdosing** of antineoplastic and
            immunosuppressive drugs
● T45.2 Poisoning by, adverse effect of and underdosing of
            vitamins
            Excludes2 poisoning by, adverse effect of and
                        underdosing of nicotinic acid
                        (derivatives) (T46.7)
                        poisoning by, adverse effect of and
                        underdosing of iron (T45.4)
                        poisoning by, adverse effect of and
                        underdosing of vitamin K (T45.7)
● T45.2X Poisoning by, adverse effect of and
            underdosing of **vitamins**
● T45.2X1 Poisoning by vitamins, **accidental**
            (unintentional)
                Poisoning by vitamins NOS
● T45.2X2 Poisoning by vitamins, **intentional**
            self-harm
● T45.2X3 Poisoning by vitamins, **assault**
● T45.2X4 Poisoning by vitamins, **undetermined**
● T45.2X5 **Adverse effect** of vitamins
● T45.2X6 **Underdosing** of vitamins
            Excludes1 vitamin deficiencies
                        (E50-E56)
● T45.3 Poisoning by, adverse effect of and underdosing of
            enzymes
● T45.3X Poisoning by, adverse effect of and
            underdosing of **enzymes**
● T45.3X1 Poisoning by enzymes, **accidental**
            (unintentional)
                Poisoning by enzymes NOS
● T45.3X2 Poisoning by enzymes, **intentional**
            self-harm
● T45.3X3 Poisoning by enzymes, **assault**
● T45.3X4 Poisoning by enzymes, **undetermined**
● T45.3X5 **Adverse effect** of enzymes
● T45.3X6 **Underdosing** of enzymes

- **T45.4 Poisoning by, adverse effect of and underdosing of iron and its compounds**
  - **T45.4X Poisoning by, adverse effect of and underdosing of iron and its compounds**
    - **T45.4X1 Poisoning by iron and its compounds, accidental (unintentional)**
      Poisoning by iron and its compounds NOS
    - **T45.4X2 Poisoning by iron and its compounds, intentional self-harm**
    - **T45.4X3 Poisoning by iron and its compounds, assault**
    - **T45.4X4 Poisoning by iron and its compounds, undetermined**
    - **T45.4X5 Adverse effect of iron and its compounds**
    - **T45.4X6 Underdosing of iron and its compounds**
      Excludes1: iron deficiency (E61.1)
- **T45.5 Poisoning by, adverse effect of and underdosing of anticoagulants and antithrombotic drugs**
  - **T45.51 Poisoning by, adverse effect of and underdosing of anticoagulants**
    - **T45.511 Poisoning by anticoagulants, accidental (unintentional)**
      Poisoning by anticoagulants NOS
    - **T45.512 Poisoning by anticoagulants, intentional self-harm**
    - **T45.513 Poisoning by anticoagulants, assault**
    - **T45.514 Poisoning by anticoagulants, undetermined**
    - **T45.515 Adverse effect of anticoagulants**
    - **T45.516 Underdosing of anticoagulants**
  - **T45.52 Poisoning by, adverse effect of and underdosing of antithrombotic drugs**
    Poisoning by, adverse effect of and underdosing of antiplatelet drugs
    Excludes2: poisoning by, adverse effect of and underdosing of aspirin (T39.01-)
    poisoning by, adverse effect of and underdosing of acetylsalicylic acid (T39.01-)
    - **T45.521 Poisoning by antithrombotic drugs, accidental (unintentional)**
      Poisoning by antithrombotic drug NOS
    - **T45.522 Poisoning by antithrombotic drugs, intentional self-harm**
    - **T45.523 Poisoning by antithrombotic drugs, assault**
    - **T45.524 Poisoning by antithrombotic drugs, undetermined**
    - **T45.525 Adverse effect of antithrombotic drugs**
    - **T45.526 Underdosing of antithrombotic drugs**
- **T45.6 Poisoning by, adverse effect of and underdosing of fibrinolysis-affecting drugs**
  - **T45.60 Poisoning by, adverse effect of and underdosing of unspecified fibrinolysis-affecting drugs**
    - **T45.601 Poisoning by unspecified fibrinolysis-affecting drugs, accidental (unintentional)**
      Poisoning by fibrinolysis-affecting drug NOS
    - **T45.602 Poisoning by unspecified fibrinolysis-affecting drugs, intentional self-harm**

- **T45.603 Poisoning by unspecified fibrinolysis-affecting drugs, assault**
- **T45.604 Poisoning by unspecified fibrinolysis-affecting drugs, undetermined**
- **T45.605 Adverse effect of unspecified fibrinolysis-affecting drugs**
- **T45.606 Underdosing of unspecified fibrinolysis-affecting drugs**
  - **T45.61 Poisoning by, adverse effect of and underdosing of thrombolytic drugs**
    - **T45.611 Poisoning by thrombolytic drug, accidental (unintentional)**
      Poisoning by thrombolytic drug NOS
    - **T45.612 Poisoning by thrombolytic drug, intentional self-harm**
    - **T45.613 Poisoning by thrombolytic drug, assault**
    - **T45.614 Poisoning by thrombolytic drug, undetermined**
    - **T45.615 Adverse effect of thrombolytic drugs**
    - **T45.616 Underdosing of thrombolytic drugs**
  - **T45.62 Poisoning by, adverse effect of and underdosing of hemostatic drugs**
    - **T45.621 Poisoning by hemostatic drug, accidental (unintentional)**
      Poisoning by hemostatic drug NOS
    - **T45.622 Poisoning by hemostatic drug, intentional self-harm**
    - **T45.623 Poisoning by hemostatic drug, assault**
    - **T45.624 Poisoning by hemostatic drug, undetermined**
    - **T45.625 Adverse effect of hemostatic drug**
    - **T45.626 Underdosing of hemostatic drugs**
  - **T45.69 Poisoning by, adverse effect of and underdosing of other fibrinolysis-affecting drugs**
    - **T45.691 Poisoning by other fibrinolysis-affecting drugs, accidental (unintentional)**
      Poisoning by other fibrinolysis-affecting drug NOS
    - **T45.692 Poisoning by other fibrinolysis-affecting drugs, intentional self-harm**
    - **T45.693 Poisoning by other fibrinolysis-affecting drugs, assault**
    - **T45.694 Poisoning by other fibrinolysis-affecting drugs, undetermined**
    - **T45.695 Adverse effect of other fibrinolysis-affecting drugs**
    - **T45.696 Underdosing of other fibrinolysis-affecting drugs**
- **T45.7 Poisoning by, adverse effect of and underdosing of anticoagulant antagonists, vitamin K and other coagulants**
  - **T45.7X Poisoning by, adverse effect of and underdosing of anticoagulant antagonists, vitamin K and other coagulants**
    - **T45.7X1 Poisoning by anticoagulant antagonists, vitamin K and other coagulants, accidental (unintentional)**
      Poisoning by anticoagulant antagonists, vitamin K and other coagulants NOS
    - **T45.7X2 Poisoning by anticoagulant antagonists, vitamin K and other coagulants, intentional self-harm**

▶ New   ⇒ Revised   ~~deleted~~ Deleted   **OGCR** Official Guidelines   X Assign placeholder X   ● Use Additional Character(s)
Excludes 1   Excludes 2   Includes   Use additional   Code first   Code also   Key words

● **T45.7X3** Poisoning by anticoagulant antagonists, vitamin K and other coagulants, assault

● **T45.7X4** Poisoning by anticoagulant antagonists, vitamin K and other coagulants, undetermined

● **T45.7X5** Adverse effect of anticoagulant antagonists, vitamin K and other coagulants

● **T45.7X6** Underdosing of anticoagulant antagonist, vitamin K and other coagulants
  Excludes1 vitamin K deficiency (E56.1)

● **T45.8** Poisoning by, adverse effect of and underdosing of other primarily systemic and hematological agents
  Poisoning by, adverse effect of and underdosing of liver preparations and other antianemic agents
  Poisoning by, adverse effect of and underdosing of natural blood and blood products
  Poisoning by, adverse effect of and underdosing of plasma substitute
  Excludes2 poisoning by, adverse effect of and underdosing of immunoglobulin (T50.Z1)
    poisoning by, adverse effect of and underdosing of iron (T45.4)
    transfusion reactions (T80.-)

● **T45.8X** Poisoning by, adverse effect of and underdosing of other primarily systemic and hematological agents

● **T45.8X1** Poisoning by other primarily systemic and hematological agents, accidental (unintentional)
  Poisoning by other primarily systemic and hematological agents NOS

● **T45.8X2** Poisoning by other primarily systemic and hematological agents, intentional self-harm

● **T45.8X3** Poisoning by other primarily systemic and hematological agents, assault

● **T45.8X4** Poisoning by other primarily systemic and hematological agents, undetermined

● **T45.8X5** Adverse effect of other primarily systemic and hematological agents

● **T45.8X6** Underdosing of other primarily systemic and hematological agents

● **T45.9** Poisoning by, adverse effect of and underdosing of unspecified primarily systemic and hematological agent

X ● **T45.91** Poisoning by unspecified primarily systemic and hematological agent, accidental (unintentional)
  Poisoning by primarily systemic and hematological agent NOS

X ● **T45.92** Poisoning by unspecified primarily systemic and hematological agent, intentional self-harm

X ● **T45.93** Poisoning by unspecified primarily systemic and hematological agent, assault

X ● **T45.94** Poisoning by unspecified primarily systemic and hematological agent, undetermined

X ● **T45.95** Adverse effect of unspecified primarily systemic and hematological agent

X ● **T45.96** Underdosing of unspecified primarily systemic and hematological agent

● **T46** Poisoning by, adverse effect of and underdosing of agents primarily affecting the cardiovascular system
  Excludes1 poisoning by, adverse effect of and underdosing of metaraminol (T44.4)

  The appropriate 7th character is to be added to each code from category T46

A	initial encounter
D	subsequent encounter
S	sequela

● **T46.0** Poisoning by, adverse effect of and underdosing of cardiac-stimulant glycosides and drugs of similar action

● **T46.0X** Poisoning by, adverse effect of and underdosing of cardiac-stimulant glycosides and drugs of similar action

● **T46.0X1** Poisoning by cardiac-stimulant glycosides and drugs of similar action, accidental (unintentional)
  Poisoning by cardiac-stimulant glycosides and drugs of similar action NOS

● **T46.0X2** Poisoning by cardiac-stimulant glycosides and drugs of similar action, intentional self-harm

● **T46.0X3** Poisoning by cardiac-stimulant glycosides and drugs of similar action, assault

● **T46.0X4** Poisoning by cardiac-stimulant glycosides and drugs of similar action, undetermined

● **T46.0X5** Adverse effect of cardiac-stimulant glycosides and drugs of similar action

● **T46.0X6** Underdosing of cardiac-stimulant glycosides and drugs of similar action

● **T46.1** Poisoning by, adverse effect of and underdosing of calcium-channel blockers

● **T46.1X** Poisoning by, adverse effect of and underdosing of calcium-channel blockers

● **T46.1X1** Poisoning by calcium-channel blockers, accidental (unintentional)
  Poisoning by calcium-channel blockers NOS

● **T46.1X2** Poisoning by calcium-channel blockers, intentional self-harm

● **T46.1X3** Poisoning by calcium-channel blockers, assault

● **T46.1X4** Poisoning by calcium-channel blockers, undetermined

● **T46.1X5** Adverse effect of calcium-channel blockers

● **T46.1X6** Underdosing of calcium-channel blockers

● **T46.2** Poisoning by, adverse effect of and underdosing of other antidysrhythmic drugs, not elsewhere classified
  Excludes1 poisoning by, adverse effect of and underdosing of beta-adrenoreceptor antagonists (T44.7-)

● **T46.2X** Poisoning by, adverse effect of and underdosing of other antidysrhythmic drugs

● **T46.2X1** Poisoning by other antidysrhythmic drugs, accidental (unintentional)
  Poisoning by other antidysrhythmic drugs NOS

● **T46.2X2** Poisoning by other antidysrhythmic drugs, intentional self-harm

● **T46.2X3** Poisoning by other antidysrhythmic drugs, assault

● **T46.2X4** Poisoning by other antidysrhythmic drugs, undetermined

● **T46.2X5** Adverse effect of other antidysrhythmic drugs

● **T46.2X6** Underdosing of other antidysrhythmic drugs

CHAPTER 19 (S00-T88)

● **T46.3** **Poisoning by, adverse effect of and underdosing of coronary vasodilators**
     Poisoning by, adverse effect of and underdosing of dipyridamole
     Excludes1   poisoning by, adverse effect of and underdosing of calcium-channel blockers (T46.1)

     ● **T46.3X** **Poisoning by, adverse effect of and underdosing of coronary vasodilators**
         ● **T46.3X1** **Poisoning by coronary vasodilators, accidental (unintentional)**
            Poisoning by coronary vasodilators NOS
         ● **T46.3X2** **Poisoning by coronary vasodilators, intentional self-harm**
         ● **T46.3X3** **Poisoning by coronary vasodilators, assault**
         ● **T46.3X4** **Poisoning by coronary vasodilators, undetermined**
         ● **T46.3X5** **Adverse effect of coronary vasodilators**
         ● **T46.3X6** **Underdosing of coronary vasodilators**

● **T46.4** **Poisoning by, adverse effect of and underdosing of angiotensin-converting-enzyme inhibitors**
     ● **T46.4X** **Poisoning by, adverse effect of and underdosing of angiotensin-converting-enzyme inhibitors**
         ● **T46.4X1** **Poisoning by angiotensin-converting-enzyme inhibitors, accidental (unintentional)**
            Poisoning by angiotensin-converting-enzyme inhibitors NOS
         ● **T46.4X2** **Poisoning by angiotensin-converting-enzyme inhibitors, intentional self-harm**
         ● **T46.4X3** **Poisoning by angiotensin-converting-enzyme inhibitors, assault**
         ● **T46.4X4** **Poisoning by angiotensin-converting-enzyme inhibitors, undetermined**
         ● **T46.4X5** **Adverse effect of angiotensin-converting-enzyme inhibitors**
         ● **T46.4X6** **Underdosing of angiotensin-converting-enzyme inhibitors**

● **T46.5** **Poisoning by, adverse effect of and underdosing of other antihypertensive drugs**
     Excludes2   poisoning by, adverse effect of and underdosing of beta-adrenoreceptor antagonists (T44.7)
            poisoning by, adverse effect of and underdosing of calcium-channel blockers (T46.1)
            poisoning by, adverse effect of and underdosing of diuretics (T50.0-T50.2)

     ● **T46.5X** **Poisoning by, adverse effect of and underdosing of other antihypertensive drugs**
         ● **T46.5X1** **Poisoning by other antihypertensive drugs, accidental (unintentional)**
            Poisoning by other antihypertensive drugs NOS
         ● **T46.5X2** **Poisoning by other antihypertensive drugs, intentional self-harm**
         ● **T46.5X3** **Poisoning by other antihypertensive drugs, assault**
         ● **T46.5X4** **Poisoning by other antihypertensive drugs, undetermined**
         ● **T46.5X5** **Adverse effect of other antihypertensive drugs**
         ● **T46.5X6** **Underdosing of other antihypertensive drugs**

● **T46.6** **Poisoning by, adverse effect of and underdosing of antihyperlipidemic and antiarteriosclerotic drugs**
     ● **T46.6X** **Poisoning by, adverse effect of and underdosing of antihyperlipidemic and antiarteriosclerotic drugs**
         ● **T46.6X1** **Poisoning by antihyperlipidemic and antiarteriosclerotic drugs, accidental (unintentional)**
            Poisoning by antihyperlipidemic and antiarteriosclerotic drugs NOS
         ● **T46.6X2** **Poisoning by antihyperlipidemic and antiarteriosclerotic drugs, intentional self-harm**
         ● **T46.6X3** **Poisoning by antihyperlipidemic and antiarteriosclerotic drugs, assault**
         ● **T46.6X4** **Poisoning by antihyperlipidemic and antiarteriosclerotic drugs, undetermined**
         ● **T46.6X5** **Adverse effect of antihyperlipidemic and antiarteriosclerotic drugs**
         ● **T46.6X6** **Underdosing of antihyperlipidemic and antiarteriosclerotic drugs**

● **T46.7** **Poisoning by, adverse effect of and underdosing of peripheral vasodilators**
     Poisoning by, adverse effect of and underdosing of nicotinic acid (derivatives)
     Excludes1   poisoning by, adverse effect of and underdosing of papaverine (T44.3)

     ● **T46.7X** **Poisoning by, adverse effect of and underdosing of peripheral vasodilators**
         ● **T46.7X1** **Poisoning by peripheral vasodilators, accidental (unintentional)**
            Poisoning by peripheral vasodilators NOS
         ● **T46.7X2** **Poisoning by peripheral vasodilators, intentional self-harm**
         ● **T46.7X3** **Poisoning by peripheral vasodilators, assault**
         ● **T46.7X4** **Poisoning by peripheral vasodilators, undetermined**
         ● **T46.7X5** **Adverse effect of peripheral vasodilators**
         ● **T46.7X6** **Underdosing of peripheral vasodilators**

● **T46.8** **Poisoning by, adverse effect of and underdosing of antivaricose drugs, including sclerosing agents**
     ● **T46.8X** **Poisoning by, adverse effect of and underdosing of antivaricose drugs, including sclerosing agents**
         ● **T46.8X1** **Poisoning by antivaricose drugs, including sclerosing agents, accidental (unintentional)**
            Poisoning by antivaricose drugs, including sclerosing agents NOS
         ● **T46.8X2** **Poisoning by antivaricose drugs, including sclerosing agents, intentional self-harm**
         ● **T46.8X3** **Poisoning by antivaricose drugs, including sclerosing agents, assault**
         ● **T46.8X4** **Poisoning by antivaricose drugs, including sclerosing agents, undetermined**
         ● **T46.8X5** **Adverse effect of antivaricose drugs, including sclerosing agents**
         ● **T46.8X6** **Underdosing of antivaricose drugs, including sclerosing agents**

▶ New   ⇒ Revised   ~~deleted~~ Deleted   **OGCR** Official Guidelines   X Assign placeholder X   ● Use Additional Character(s)

Excludes 1   Excludes 2   Includes   Use additional   Code first   Code also   Key words

● **T46.9** Poisoning by, adverse effect of and underdosing of other and unspecified agents primarily affecting the cardiovascular system

● **T46.90** Poisoning by, adverse effect of and underdosing of unspecified agents primarily affecting the cardiovascular system

● **T46.901** Poisoning by unspecified agents primarily affecting the cardiovascular system, accidental (unintentional)

● **T46.902** Poisoning by unspecified agents primarily affecting the cardiovascular system, intentional self-harm

● **T46.903** Poisoning by unspecified agents primarily affecting the cardiovascular system, assault

● **T46.904** Poisoning by unspecified agents primarily affecting the cardiovascular system, undetermined

● **T46.905** Adverse effect of unspecified agents primarily affecting the cardiovascular system

● **T46.906** Underdosing of unspecified agents primarily affecting the cardiovascular system

● **T46.99** Poisoning by, adverse effect of and underdosing of other agents primarily affecting the cardiovascular system

● **T46.991** Poisoning by other agents primarily affecting the cardiovascular system, accidental (unintentional)

● **T46.992** Poisoning by other agents primarily affecting the cardiovascular system, intentional self-harm

● **T46.993** Poisoning by other agents primarily affecting the cardiovascular system, assault

● **T46.994** Poisoning by other agents primarily affecting the cardiovascular system, undetermined

● **T46.995** Adverse effect of other agents primarily affecting the cardiovascular system

● **T46.996** Underdosing of other agents primarily affecting the cardiovascular system

● **T47** Poisoning by, adverse effect of and underdosing of agents primarily affecting the gastrointestinal system

The appropriate 7th character is to be added to each code from category T47

A	initial encounter
D	subsequent encounter
S	sequela

● **T47.0** Poisoning by, adverse effect of and underdosing of histamine H2-receptor blockers

● **T47.0X** Poisoning by, adverse effect of and underdosing of histamine H2-receptor blockers

● **T47.0X1** Poisoning by histamine H2-receptor blockers, accidental (unintentional)
Poisoning by histamine H2-receptor blockers NOS

● **T47.0X2** Poisoning by histamine H2-receptor blockers, intentional self-harm

● **T47.0X3** Poisoning by histamine H2-receptor blockers, assault

● **T47.0X4** Poisoning by histamine H2-receptor blockers, undetermined

● **T47.0X5** Adverse effect of histamine H2-receptor blockers

● **T47.0X6** Underdosing of histamine H2-receptor blockers

● **T47.1** Poisoning by, adverse effect of and underdosing of other antacids and anti-gastric-secretion drugs

● **T47.1X** Poisoning by, adverse effect of and underdosing of other antacids and anti-gastric-secretion drugs

● **T47.1X1** Poisoning by other antacids and anti-gastric-secretion drugs, accidental (unintentional)
Poisoning by other antacids and anti-gastric-secretion drugs NOS

● **T47.1X2** Poisoning by other antacids and anti-gastric-secretion drugs, intentional self-harm

● **T47.1X3** Poisoning by other antacids and anti-gastric-secretion drugs, assault

● **T47.1X4** Poisoning by other antacids and anti-gastric-secretion drugs, undetermined

● **T47.1X5** Adverse effect of other antacids and anti-gastric-secretion drugs

● **T47.1X6** Underdosing of other antacids and anti-gastric-secretion drugs

● **T47.2** Poisoning by, adverse effect of and underdosing of stimulant laxatives

● **T47.2X** Poisoning by, adverse effect of and underdosing of stimulant laxatives

● **T47.2X1** Poisoning by stimulant laxatives, accidental (unintentional)
Poisoning by stimulant laxatives NOS

● **T47.2X2** Poisoning by stimulant laxatives, intentional self-harm

● **T47.2X3** Poisoning by stimulant laxatives, assault

● **T47.2X4** Poisoning by stimulant laxatives, undetermined

● **T47.2X5** Adverse effect of stimulant laxatives

● **T47.2X6** Underdosing of stimulant laxatives

● **T47.3** Poisoning by, adverse effect of and underdosing of saline and osmotic laxatives

● **T47.3X** Poisoning by and adverse effect of saline and osmotic laxatives

● **T47.3X1** Poisoning by saline and osmotic laxatives, accidental (unintentional)
Poisoning by saline and osmotic laxatives NOS

● **T47.3X2** Poisoning by saline and osmotic laxatives, intentional self-harm

● **T47.3X3** Poisoning by saline and osmotic laxatives, assault

● **T47.3X4** Poisoning by saline and osmotic laxatives, undetermined

● **T47.3X5** Adverse effect of saline and osmotic laxatives

● **T47.3X6** Underdosing of saline and osmotic laxatives

● **T47.4** Poisoning by, adverse effect of and underdosing of other laxatives

● **T47.4X** Poisoning by, adverse effect of and underdosing of other laxatives

● **T47.4X1** Poisoning by other laxatives, accidental (unintentional)
Poisoning by other laxatives NOS

● **T47.4X2** Poisoning by other laxatives, intentional self-harm

● **T47.4X3** Poisoning by other laxatives, assault

● **T47.4X4** Poisoning by other laxatives, undetermined

● **T47.4X5** Adverse effect of other laxatives

● **T47.4X6** Underdosing of other laxatives

CHAPTER 19 (S00-T88)

▶ New ⟹ Revised ~~deleted~~ Deleted **OGCR** Official Guidelines X Assign placeholder X ● Use Additional Character(s)

Excludes 1 | Excludes 2 | Includes | Use additional | Code first | Code also | Key words

● T47.5   Poisoning by, adverse effect of and underdosing of digestants

    ● T47.5X   Poisoning by, adverse effect of and underdosing of digestants

      ● T47.5X1   Poisoning by digestants, accidental (unintentional)
         Poisoning by digestants NOS

      ● T47.5X2   Poisoning by digestants, intentional self-harm

      ● T47.5X3   Poisoning by digestants, assault

      ● T47.5X4   Poisoning by digestants, undetermined

      ● T47.5X5   Adverse effect of digestants

      ● T47.5X6   Underdosing of digestants

● T47.6   Poisoning by, adverse effect of and underdosing of antidiarrheal drugs

    Excludes2   poisoning by, adverse effect of and underdosing of systemic antibiotics and other anti-infectives (T36-T37)

    ● T47.6X   Poisoning by, adverse effect of and underdosing of antidiarrheal drugs

      ● T47.6X1   Poisoning by antidiarrheal drugs, accidental (unintentional)
         Poisoning by antidiarrheal drugs NOS

      ● T47.6X2   Poisoning by antidiarrheal drugs, intentional self-harm

      ● T47.6X3   Poisoning by antidiarrheal drugs, assault

      ● T47.6X4   Poisoning by antidiarrheal drugs, undetermined

      ● T47.6X5   Adverse effect of antidiarrheal drugs

      ● T47.6X6   Underdosing of antidiarrheal drugs

● T47.7   Poisoning by, adverse effect of and underdosing of emetics

    ● T47.7X   Poisoning by, adverse effect of and underdosing of emetics

      ● T47.7X1   Poisoning by emetics, accidental (unintentional)
         Poisoning by emetics NOS

      ● T47.7X2   Poisoning by emetics, intentional self-harm

      ● T47.7X3   Poisoning by emetics, assault

      ● T47.7X4   Poisoning by emetics, undetermined

      ● T47.7X5   Adverse effect of emetics

      ● T47.7X6   Underdosing of emetics

● T47.8   Poisoning by, adverse effect of and underdosing of other agents primarily affecting gastrointestinal system

    ● T47.8X   Poisoning by, adverse effect of and underdosing of other agents primarily affecting gastrointestinal system

      ● T47.8X1   Poisoning by other agents primarily affecting gastrointestinal system, accidental (unintentional)
         Poisoning by other agents primarily affecting gastrointestinal system NOS

      ● T47.8X2   Poisoning by other agents primarily affecting gastrointestinal system, intentional self-harm

      ● T47.8X3   Poisoning by other agents primarily affecting gastrointestinal system, assault

      ● T47.8X4   Poisoning by other agents primarily affecting gastrointestinal system, undetermined

      ● T47.8X5   Adverse effect of other agents primarily affecting gastrointestinal system

      ● T47.8X6   Underdosing of other agents primarily affecting gastrointestinal system

● T47.9   Poisoning by, adverse effect of and underdosing of unspecified agents primarily affecting the gastrointestinal system

    X● T47.91   Poisoning by unspecified agents primarily affecting the gastrointestinal system, accidental (unintentional)
       Poisoning by agents primarily affecting the gastrointestinal system NOS

    X● T47.92   Poisoning by unspecified agents primarily affecting the gastrointestinal system, intentional self-harm

    X● T47.93   Poisoning by unspecified agents primarily affecting the gastrointestinal system, assault

    X● T47.94   Poisoning by unspecified agents primarily affecting the gastrointestinal system, undetermined

    X● T47.95   Adverse effect of unspecified agents primarily affecting the gastrointestinal system

    X● T47.96   Underdosing of unspecified agents primarily affecting the gastrointestinal system

● T48   Poisoning by, adverse effect of and underdosing of agents primarily acting on smooth and skeletal muscles and the respiratory system

    The appropriate 7th character is to be added to each code from category T48

     | | |
     A   initial encounter
     D   subsequent encounter
     S   sequela

    ● T48.0   Poisoning by, adverse effect of and underdosing of oxytocic drugs

      Excludes1   poisoning by, adverse effect of and underdosing of estrogens, progestogens and antagonists (T38.4-T38.6)

     ● T48.0X   Poisoning by, adverse effect of and underdosing of oxytocic drugs

       ● T48.0X1   Poisoning by oxytocic drugs, accidental (unintentional)
         Poisoning by oxytocic drugs NOS

       ● T48.0X2   Poisoning by oxytocic drugs, intentional self-harm

       ● T48.0X3   Poisoning by oxytocic drugs, assault

       ● T48.0X4   Poisoning by oxytocic drugs, undetermined

       ● T48.0X5   Adverse effect of oxytocic drugs

       ● T48.0X6   Underdosing of oxytocic drugs

    ● T48.1   Poisoning by, adverse effect of and underdosing of skeletal muscle relaxants [neuromuscular blocking agents]

     ● T48.1X   Poisoning by, adverse effect of and underdosing of skeletal muscle relaxants [neuromuscular blocking agents]

       ● T48.1X1   Poisoning by skeletal muscle relaxants [neuromuscular blocking agents], accidental (unintentional)
         Poisoning by skeletal muscle relaxants [neuromuscular blocking agents] NOS

       ● T48.1X2   Poisoning by skeletal muscle relaxants [neuromuscular blocking agents], intentional self-harm

       ● T48.1X3   Poisoning by skeletal muscle relaxants [neuromuscular blocking agents], assault

       ● T48.1X4   Poisoning by skeletal muscle relaxants [neuromuscular blocking agents], undetermined

       ● T48.1X5   Adverse effect of skeletal muscle relaxants [neuromuscular blocking agents]

       ● T48.1X6   Underdosing of skeletal muscle relaxants [neuromuscular blocking agents]

▶ New   ⇒ Revised   ~~deleted~~ Deleted   **OGCR** Official Guidelines   X Assign placeholder X   ● Use Additional Character(s)

Excludes 1   Excludes 2   Includes   Use additional   Code first   Code also   Key words

- T48.2   Poisoning by, adverse effect of and underdosing of other and unspecified drugs acting on muscles
  - T48.20   Poisoning by, adverse effect of and underdosing of unspecified drugs acting on muscles
    - T48.201   Poisoning by unspecified drugs acting on muscles, accidental (unintentional)
      Poisoning by unspecified drugs acting on muscles NOS
    - T48.202   Poisoning by unspecified drugs acting on muscles, intentional self-harm
    - T48.203   Poisoning by unspecified drugs acting on muscles, assault
    - T48.204   Poisoning by unspecified drugs acting on muscles, undetermined
    - T48.205   Adverse effect of unspecified drugs acting on muscles
    - T48.206   Underdosing of unspecified drugs acting on muscles
  - T48.29   Poisoning by, adverse effect of and underdosing of other drugs acting on muscles
    - T48.291   Poisoning by other drugs acting on muscles, accidental (unintentional)
      Poisoning by other drugs acting on muscles NOS
    - T48.292   Poisoning by other drugs acting on muscles, intentional self-harm
    - T48.293   Poisoning by other drugs acting on muscles, assault
    - T48.294   Poisoning by other drugs acting on muscles, undetermined
    - T48.295   Adverse effect of other drugs acting on muscles
    - T48.296   Underdosing of other drugs acting on muscles
- T48.3   Poisoning by, adverse effect of and underdosing of antitussives
  - T48.3X   Poisoning by, adverse effect of and underdosing of antitussives
    - T48.3X1   Poisoning by antitussives, accidental (unintentional)
      Poisoning by antitussives NOS
    - T48.3X2   Poisoning by antitussives, intentional self-harm
    - T48.3X3   Poisoning by antitussives, assault
    - T48.3X4   Poisoning by antitussives, undetermined
    - T48.3X5   Adverse effect of antitussives
    - T48.3X6   Underdosing of antitussives
- T48.4   Poisoning by, adverse effect of and underdosing of expectorants
  - T48.4X   Poisoning by, adverse effect of and underdosing of expectorants
    - T48.4X1   Poisoning by expectorants, accidental (unintentional)
      Poisoning by expectorants NOS
    - T48.4X2   Poisoning by expectorants, intentional self-harm
    - T48.4X3   Poisoning by expectorants, assault
    - T48.4X4   Poisoning by expectorants, undetermined
    - T48.4X5   Adverse effect of expectorants
    - T48.4X6   Underdosing of expectorants

- T48.5   Poisoning by, adverse effect of and underdosing of other anti-common-cold drugs
  Poisoning by, adverse effect of and underdosing of decongestants
  > Excludes2   poisoning by, adverse effect of and underdosing of antipyretics, NEC (T39.9-)
  > poisoning by, adverse effect of and underdosing of non-steroidal antiinflammatory drugs (T39.3-)
  > poisoning by, adverse effect of and underdosing of salicylates (T39.0-)
  - T48.5X   Poisoning by, adverse effect of and underdosing of other anti-common-cold drugs
    - T48.5X1   Poisoning by other anti-common-cold drugs, accidental (unintentional)
      Poisoning by other anti-common-cold drugs NOS
    - T48.5X2   Poisoning by other anti-common-cold drugs, intentional self-harm
    - T48.5X3   Poisoning by other anti-common-cold drugs, assault
    - T48.5X4   Poisoning by other anti-common-cold drugs, undetermined
    - T48.5X5   Adverse effect of other anti-common-cold drugs
    - T48.5X6   Underdosing of other anti-common-cold drugs
- T48.6   Poisoning by, adverse effect of and underdosing of antiasthmatics, not elsewhere classified
  Poisoning by, adverse effect of and underdosing of beta-adrenoreceptor agonists used in asthma therapy
  > Excludes1   poisoning by, adverse effect of and underdosing of beta-adrenoreceptor agonists not used in asthma therapy (T44.5)
  > poisoning by, adverse effect of and underdosing of anterior pituitary [adenohypophyseal] hormones (T38.8)
  - T48.6X   Poisoning by, adverse effect of and underdosing of antiasthmatics
    - T48.6X1   Poisoning by antiasthmatics, accidental (unintentional)
      Poisoning by antiasthmatics NOS
    - T48.6X2   Poisoning by antiasthmatics, intentional self-harm
    - T48.6X3   Poisoning by antiasthmatics, assault
    - T48.6X4   Poisoning by antiasthmatics, undetermined
    - T48.6X5   Adverse effect of antiasthmatics
    - T48.6X6   Underdosing of antiasthmatics
- T48.9   Poisoning by, adverse effect of and underdosing of other and unspecified agents primarily acting on the respiratory system
  - T48.90   Poisoning by, adverse effect of and underdosing of unspecified agents primarily acting on the respiratory system
    - T48.901   Poisoning by unspecified agents primarily acting on the respiratory system, accidental (unintentional)
    - T48.902   Poisoning by unspecified agents primarily acting on the respiratory system, intentional self-harm
    - T48.903   Poisoning by unspecified agents primarily acting on the respiratory system, assault
    - T48.904   Poisoning by unspecified agents primarily acting on the respiratory system, undetermined
    - T48.905   Adverse effect of unspecified agents primarily acting on the respiratory system
    - T48.906   Underdosing of unspecified agents primarily acting on the respiratory system

CHAPTER 19 (S00-T88)

● **T48.99**   Poisoning by, adverse effect of and underdosing of other agents primarily acting on the respiratory system

  ● **T48.991**   Poisoning by other agents primarily acting on the respiratory system, accidental (unintentional)

  ● **T48.992**   Poisoning by other agents primarily acting on the respiratory system, intentional self-harm

  ● **T48.993**   Poisoning by other agents primarily acting on the respiratory system, assault

  ● **T48.994**   Poisoning by other agents primarily acting on the respiratory system, undetermined

  ● **T48.995**   Adverse effect of other agents primarily acting on the respiratory system

  ● **T48.996**   Underdosing of other agents primarily acting on the respiratory system

● **T49**   Poisoning by, adverse effect of and underdosing of topical agents primarily affecting skin and mucous membrane and by ophthalmological, otorhinolaryngological and dental drugs

  Includes   poisoning by, adverse effect of and underdosing of glucocorticoids, topically used

  The appropriate 7th character is to be added to each code from category T49

A	initial encounter
D	subsequent encounter
S	sequela

 ● **T49.0**   Poisoning by, adverse effect of and underdosing of local antifungal, anti-infective and anti-inflammatory drugs

  ● **T49.0X**   Poisoning by, adverse effect of and underdosing of local antifungal, anti-infective and anti-inflammatory drugs

   ● **T49.0X1**   Poisoning by local antifungal, anti-infective and anti-inflammatory drugs, accidental (unintentional)
    Poisoning by local antifungal, anti-infective and anti-inflammatory drugs NOS

   ● **T49.0X2**   Poisoning by local antifungal, anti-infective and anti-inflammatory drugs, intentional self-harm

   ● **T49.0X3**   Poisoning by local antifungal, anti-infective and anti-inflammatory drugs, assault

   ● **T49.0X4**   Poisoning by local antifungal, anti-infective and anti-inflammatory drugs, undetermined

   ● **T49.0X5**   Adverse effect of local antifungal, anti-infective and anti-inflammatory drugs

   ● **T49.0X6**   Underdosing of local antifungal, anti-infective and anti-inflammatory drugs

 ● **T49.1**   Poisoning by, adverse effect of and underdosing of antipruritics

  ● **T49.1X**   Poisoning by, adverse effect of and underdosing of antipruritics

   ● **T49.1X1**   Poisoning by antipruritics, accidental (unintentional)
    Poisoning by antipruritics NOS

   ● **T49.1X2**   Poisoning by antipruritics, intentional self-harm

   ● **T49.1X3**   Poisoning by antipruritics, assault

   ● **T49.1X4**   Poisoning by antipruritics, undetermined

   ● **T49.1X5**   Adverse effect of antipruritics

   ● **T49.1X6**   Underdosing of antipruritics

● **T49.2**   Poisoning by, adverse effect of and underdosing of local astringents and local detergents

 ● **T49.2X**   Poisoning by, adverse effect of and underdosing of local astringents and local detergents

  ● **T49.2X1**   Poisoning by local astringents and local detergents, accidental (unintentional)
   Poisoning by local astringents and local detergents NOS

  ● **T49.2X2**   Poisoning by local astringents and local detergents, intentional self-harm

  ● **T49.2X3**   Poisoning by local astringents and local detergents, assault

  ● **T49.2X4**   Poisoning by local astringents and local detergents, undetermined

  ● **T49.2X5**   Adverse effect of local astringents and local detergents

  ● **T49.2X6**   Underdosing of local astringents and local detergents

● **T49.3**   Poisoning by, adverse effect of and underdosing of emollients, demulcents and protectants

 ● **T49.3X**   Poisoning by, adverse effect of and underdosing of emollients, demulcents and protectants

  ● **T49.3X1**   Poisoning by emollients, demulcents and protectants, accidental (unintentional)
   Poisoning by emollients, demulcents and protectants NOS

  ● **T49.3X2**   Poisoning by emollients, demulcents and protectants, intentional self-harm

  ● **T49.3X3**   Poisoning by emollients, demulcents and protectants, assault

  ● **T49.3X4**   Poisoning by emollients, demulcents and protectants, undetermined

  ● **T49.3X5**   Adverse effect of emollients, demulcents and protectants

  ● **T49.3X6**   Underdosing of emollients, demulcents and protectants

● **T49.4**   Poisoning by, adverse effect of and underdosing of keratolytics, keratoplastics, and other hair treatment drugs and preparations

 ● **T49.4X**   Poisoning by, adverse effect of and underdosing of keratolytics, keratoplastics, and other hair treatment drugs and preparations

  ● **T49.4X1**   Poisoning by keratolytics, keratoplastics, and other hair treatment drugs and preparations, accidental (unintentional)
   Poisoning by keratolytics, keratoplastics, and other hair treatment drugs and preparations NOS

  ● **T49.4X2**   Poisoning by keratolytics, keratoplastics, and other hair treatment drugs and preparations, intentional self-harm

  ● **T49.4X3**   Poisoning by keratolytics, keratoplastics, and other hair treatment drugs and preparations, assault

  ● **T49.4X4**   Poisoning by keratolytics, keratoplastics, and other hair treatment drugs and preparations, undetermined

  ● **T49.4X5**   Adverse effect of keratolytics, keratoplastics, and other hair treatment drugs and preparations

  ● **T49.4X6**   Underdosing of keratolytics, keratoplastics, and other hair treatment drugs and preparations

▶ New   ⟹ Revised   ~~deleted~~ Deleted   **OGCR** Official Guidelines   X Assign placeholder X   ● Use Additional Character(s)

Excludes 1   Excludes 2   Includes   Use additional   Code first   Code also   Key words

● **T49.5**   Poisoning by, adverse effect of and underdosing of ophthalmological drugs and preparations

   ● **T49.5X**   Poisoning by, adverse effect of and underdosing of ophthalmological drugs and preparations

     ● **T49.5X1**   Poisoning by ophthalmological drugs and preparations, accidental (unintentional)

       Poisoning by ophthalmological drugs and preparations NOS

     ● **T49.5X2**   Poisoning by ophthalmological drugs and preparations, intentional self-harm

     ● **T49.5X3**   Poisoning by ophthalmological drugs and preparations, assault

     ● **T49.5X4**   Poisoning by ophthalmological drugs and preparations, undetermined

     ● **T49.5X5**   Adverse effect of ophthalmological drugs and preparations

     ● **T49.5X6**   Underdosing of ophthalmological drugs and preparations

● **T49.6**   Poisoning by, adverse effect of and underdosing of otorhinolaryngological drugs and preparations

   ● **T49.6X**   Poisoning by, adverse effect of and underdosing of otorhinolaryngological drugs and preparations

     ● **T49.6X1**   Poisoning by otorhinolaryngological drugs and preparations, accidental (unintentional)

       Poisoning by otorhinolaryngological drugs and preparations NOS

     ● **T49.6X2**   Poisoning by otorhinolaryngological drugs and preparations, intentional self-harm

     ● **T49.6X3**   Poisoning by otorhinolaryngological drugs and preparations, assault

     ● **T49.6X4**   Poisoning by otorhinolaryngological drugs and preparations, undetermined

     ● **T49.6X5**   Adverse effect of otorhinolaryngological drugs and preparations

     ● **T49.6X6**   Underdosing of otorhinolaryngological drugs and preparations

● **T49.7**   Poisoning by, adverse effect of and underdosing of dental drugs, topically applied

   ● **T49.7X**   Poisoning by, adverse effect of and underdosing of dental drugs, topically applied

     ● **T49.7X1**   Poisoning by dental drugs, topically applied, accidental (unintentional)

       Poisoning by dental drugs, topically applied NOS

     ● **T49.7X2**   Poisoning by dental drugs, topically applied, intentional self-harm

     ● **T49.7X3**   Poisoning by dental drugs, topically applied, assault

     ● **T49.7X4**   Poisoning by dental drugs, topically applied, undetermined

     ● **T49.7X5**   Adverse effect of dental drugs, topically applied

     ● **T49.7X6**   Underdosing of dental drugs, topically applied

● **T49.8**   Poisoning by, adverse effect of and underdosing of other topical agents

     Poisoning by, adverse effect of and underdosing of spermicides

   ● **T49.8X**   Poisoning by, adverse effect of and underdosing of other topical agents

     ● **T49.8X1**   Poisoning by other topical agents, accidental (unintentional)

       Poisoning by other topical agents NOS

     ● **T49.8X2**   Poisoning by other topical agents, intentional self-harm

     ● **T49.8X3**   Poisoning by other topical agents, assault

     ● **T49.8X4**   Poisoning by other topical agents, undetermined

     ● **T49.8X5**   Adverse effect of other topical agents

     ● **T49.8X6**   Underdosing of other topical agents

● **T49.9**   Poisoning by, adverse effect of and underdosing of unspecified topical agent

   X ● **T49.91**   Poisoning by unspecified topical agent, accidental (unintentional)

   X ● **T49.92**   Poisoning by unspecified topical agent, intentional self-harm

   X ● **T49.93**   Poisoning by unspecified topical agent, assault

   X ● **T49.94**   Poisoning by unspecified topical agent, undetermined

   X ● **T49.95**   Adverse effect of unspecified topical agent

   X ● **T49.96**   Underdosing of unspecified topical agent

● **T50**   Poisoning by, adverse effect of and underdosing of diuretics and other and unspecified drugs, medicaments and biological substances

     The appropriate 7th character is to be added to each code from category T50

A	initial encounter
D	subsequent encounter
S	sequela

● **T50.0**   Poisoning by, adverse effect of and underdosing of mineralocorticoids and their antagonists

   ● **T50.0X**   Poisoning by, adverse effect of and underdosing of mineralocorticoids and their antagonists

     ● **T50.0X1**   Poisoning by mineralocorticoids and their antagonists, accidental (unintentional)

       Poisoning by mineralocorticoids and their antagonists NOS

     ● **T50.0X2**   Poisoning by mineralocorticoids and their antagonists, intentional self-harm

     ● **T50.0X3**   Poisoning by mineralocorticoids and their antagonists, assault

     ● **T50.0X4**   Poisoning by mineralocorticoids and their antagonists, undetermined

     ● **T50.0X5**   Adverse effect of mineralocorticoids and their antagonists

     ● **T50.0X6**   Underdosing of mineralocorticoids and their antagonists

CHAPTER 19 (S00-T88)

- **T50.1**   Poisoning by, adverse effect of and underdosing of loop [high-ceiling] diuretics
  - **T50.1X**   Poisoning by, adverse effect of and underdosing of loop [high-ceiling] diuretics
    - **T50.1X1**   Poisoning by loop [high-ceiling] diuretics, accidental (unintentional)
      Poisoning by loop [high-ceiling] diuretics NOS
    - **T50.1X2**   Poisoning by loop [high-ceiling] diuretics, intentional self-harm
    - **T50.1X3**   Poisoning by loop [high-ceiling] diuretics, assault
    - **T50.1X4**   Poisoning by loop [high-ceiling] diuretics, undetermined
    - **T50.1X5**   Adverse effect of loop [high-ceiling] diuretics
    - **T50.1X6**   Underdosing of loop [high-ceiling] diuretics
- **T50.2**   Poisoning by, adverse effect of and underdosing of carbonic-anhydrase inhibitors, benzothiadiazides and other diuretics
  Poisoning by, adverse effect of and underdosing of acetazolamide
  - **T50.2X**   Poisoning by, adverse effect of and underdosing of carbonic-anhydrase inhibitors, benzothiadiazides and other diuretics
    - **T50.2X1**   Poisoning by carbonic-anhydrase inhibitors, benzothiadiazides and other diuretics, accidental (unintentional)
      Poisoning by carbonic-anhydrase inhibitors, benzothiadiazides and other diuretics NOS
    - **T50.2X2**   Poisoning by carbonic-anhydrase inhibitors, benzothiadiazides and other diuretics, intentional self-harm
    - **T50.2X3**   Poisoning by carbonic-anhydrase inhibitors, benzothiadiazides and other diuretics, assault
    - **T50.2X4**   Poisoning by carbonic-anhydrase inhibitors, benzothiadiazides and other diuretics, undetermined
    - **T50.2X5**   Adverse effect of carbonic-anhydrase inhibitors, benzothiadiazides and other diuretics
    - **T50.2X6**   Underdosing of carbonic-anhydrase inhibitors, benzothiadiazides and other diuretics
- **T50.3**   Poisoning by, adverse effect of and underdosing of electrolytic, caloric and water-balance agents
  Poisoning by, adverse effect of and underdosing of oral rehydration salts
  - **T50.3X**   Poisoning by, adverse effect of and underdosing of electrolytic, caloric and water-balance agents
    - **T50.3X1**   Poisoning by electrolytic, caloric and water-balance agents, accidental (unintentional)
      Poisoning by electrolytic, caloric and water-balance agents NOS
    - **T50.3X2**   Poisoning by electrolytic, caloric and water-balance agents, intentional self-harm
    - **T50.3X3**   Poisoning by electrolytic, caloric and water-balance agents, assault
    - **T50.3X4**   Poisoning by electrolytic, caloric and water-balance agents, undetermined
    - **T50.3X5**   Adverse effect of electrolytic, caloric and water-balance agents
    - **T50.3X6**   Underdosing of electrolytic, caloric and water-balance agents

- **T50.4**   Poisoning by, adverse effect of and underdosing of drugs affecting uric acid metabolism
  - **T50.4X**   Poisoning by, adverse effect of and underdosing of drugs affecting uric acid metabolism
    - **T50.4X1**   Poisoning by drugs affecting uric acid metabolism, accidental (unintentional)
      Poisoning by drugs affecting uric acid metabolism NOS
    - **T50.4X2**   Poisoning by drugs affecting uric acid metabolism, intentional self-harm
    - **T50.4X3**   Poisoning by drugs affecting uric acid metabolism, assault
    - **T50.4X4**   Poisoning by drugs affecting uric acid metabolism, undetermined
    - **T50.4X5**   Adverse effect of drugs affecting uric acid metabolism
    - **T50.4X6**   Underdosing of drugs affecting uric acid metabolism
- **T50.5**   Poisoning by, adverse effect of and underdosing of appetite depressants
  - **T50.5X**   Poisoning by, adverse effect of and underdosing of appetite depressants
    - **T50.5X1**   Poisoning by appetite depressants, accidental (unintentional)
      Poisoning by appetite depressants NOS
    - **T50.5X2**   Poisoning by appetite depressants, intentional self-harm
    - **T50.5X3**   Poisoning by appetite depressants, assault
    - **T50.5X4**   Poisoning by appetite depressants, undetermined
    - **T50.5X5**   Adverse effect of appetite depressants
    - **T50.5X6**   Underdosing of appetite depressants
- **T50.6**   Poisoning by, adverse effect of and underdosing of antidotes and chelating agents
  Poisoning by, adverse effect of and underdosing of alcohol deterrents
  - **T50.6X**   Poisoning by, adverse effect of and underdosing of antidotes and chelating agents
    - **T50.6X1**   Poisoning by antidotes and chelating agents, accidental (unintentional)
      Poisoning by antidotes and chelating agents NOS
    - **T50.6X2**   Poisoning by antidotes and chelating agents, intentional self-harm
    - **T50.6X3**   Poisoning by antidotes and chelating agents, assault
    - **T50.6X4**   Poisoning by antidotes and chelating agents, undetermined
    - **T50.6X5**   Adverse effect of antidotes and chelating agents
    - **T50.6X6**   Underdosing of antidotes and chelating agents

▶ New   ⮕ Revised   ~~deleted~~ Deleted   **OGCR** Official Guidelines   X Assign placeholder X   ● Use Additional Character(s)

Excludes 1   Excludes 2   Includes   Use additional   Code first   Code also   Key words

● **T50.7**   Poisoning by, adverse effect of and underdosing of analeptics and opioid receptor antagonists

  ● **T50.7X**   Poisoning by, adverse effect of and underdosing of analeptics and opioid receptor antagonists

    ● **T50.7X1**   Poisoning by analeptics and opioid receptor antagonists, accidental (unintentional)

      Poisoning by analeptics and opioid receptor antagonists NOS

    ● **T50.7X2**   Poisoning by analeptics and opioid receptor antagonists, intentional self-harm

    ● **T50.7X3**   Poisoning by analeptics and opioid receptor antagonists, assault

    ● **T50.7X4**   Poisoning by analeptics and opioid receptor antagonists, undetermined

    ● **T50.7X5**   Adverse effect of analeptics and opioid receptor antagonists

    ● **T50.7X6**   Underdosing of analeptics and opioid receptor antagonists

● **T50.8**   Poisoning by, adverse effect of and underdosing of diagnostic agents

  ● **T50.8X**   Poisoning by, adverse effect of and underdosing of diagnostic agents

    ● **T50.8X1**   Poisoning by diagnostic agents, accidental (unintentional)

      Poisoning by diagnostic agents NOS

    ● **T50.8X2**   Poisoning by diagnostic agents, intentional self-harm

    ● **T50.8X3**   Poisoning by diagnostic agents, assault

    ● **T50.8X4**   Poisoning by diagnostic agents, undetermined

    ● **T50.8X5**   Adverse effect of diagnostic agents

    ● **T50.8X6**   Underdosing of diagnostic agents

● **T50.A**   Poisoning by, adverse effect of and underdosing of bacterial vaccines

  ● **T50.A1**   Poisoning by, adverse effect of and underdosing of pertussis vaccine, including combinations with a pertussis component

    ● **T50.A11**   Poisoning by pertussis vaccine, including combinations with a pertussis component, accidental (unintentional)

    ● **T50.A12**   Poisoning by pertussis vaccine, including combinations with a pertussis component, intentional self-harm

    ● **T50.A13**   Poisoning by pertussis vaccine, including combinations with a pertussis component, assault

    ● **T50.A14**   Poisoning by pertussis vaccine, including combinations with a pertussis component, undetermined

    ● **T50.A15**   Adverse effect of pertussis vaccine, including combinations with a pertussis component

    ● **T50.A16**   Underdosing of pertussis vaccine, including combinations with a pertussis component

● **T50.A2**   Poisoning by, adverse effect of and underdosing of mixed bacterial vaccines without a pertussis component

    ● **T50.A21**   Poisoning by mixed bacterial vaccines without a pertussis component, accidental (unintentional)

    ● **T50.A22**   Poisoning by mixed bacterial vaccines without a pertussis component, intentional self-harm

    ● **T50.A23**   Poisoning by mixed bacterial vaccines without a pertussis component, assault

    ● **T50.A24**   Poisoning by mixed bacterial vaccines without a pertussis component, undetermined

    ● **T50.A25**   Adverse effect of mixed bacterial vaccines without a pertussis component

    ● **T50.A26**   Underdosing of mixed bacterial vaccines without a pertussis component

  ● **T50.A9**   Poisoning by, adverse effect of and underdosing of other bacterial vaccines

    ● **T50.A91**   Poisoning by other bacterial vaccines, accidental (unintentional)

    ● **T50.A92**   Poisoning by other bacterial vaccines, intentional self-harm

    ● **T50.A93**   Poisoning by other bacterial vaccines, assault

    ● **T50.A94**   Poisoning by other bacterial vaccines, undetermined

    ● **T50.A95**   Adverse effect of other bacterial vaccines

    ● **T50.A96**   Underdosing of other bacterial vaccines

● **T50.B**   Poisoning by, adverse effect of and underdosing of viral vaccines

  ● **T50.B1**   Poisoning by, adverse effect of and underdosing of smallpox vaccines

    ● **T50.B11**   Poisoning by smallpox vaccines, accidental (unintentional)

    ● **T50.B12**   Poisoning by smallpox vaccines, intentional self-harm

    ● **T50.B13**   Poisoning by smallpox vaccines, assault

    ● **T50.B14**   Poisoning by smallpox vaccines, undetermined

    ● **T50.B15**   Adverse effect of smallpox vaccines

    ● **T50.B16**   Underdosing of smallpox vaccines

  ● **T50.B9**   Poisoning by, adverse effect of and underdosing of other viral vaccines

    ● **T50.B91**   Poisoning by other viral vaccines, accidental (unintentional)

    ● **T50.B92**   Poisoning by other viral vaccines, intentional self-harm

    ● **T50.B93**   Poisoning by other viral vaccines, assault

    ● **T50.B94**   Poisoning by other viral vaccines, undetermined

    ● **T50.B95**   Adverse effect of other viral vaccines

    ● **T50.B96**   Underdosing of other viral vaccines

CHAPTER 19 (S00-T88)

● **T50.Z** Poisoning by, adverse effect of and underdosing of other vaccines and biological substances

   ● **T50.Z1** Poisoning by, adverse effect of and underdosing of immunoglobulin

      ● **T50.Z11** Poisoning by immunoglobulin, accidental (unintentional)

      ● **T50.Z12** Poisoning by immunoglobulin, intentional self-harm

      ● **T50.Z13** Poisoning by immunoglobulin, assault

      ● **T50.Z14** Poisoning by immunoglobulin, undetermined

      ● **T50.Z15** Adverse effect of immunoglobulin

      ● **T50.Z16** Underdosing of immunoglobulin

   ● **T50.Z9** Poisoning by, adverse effect of and underdosing of other vaccines and biological substances

      ● **T50.Z91** Poisoning by other vaccines and biological substances, accidental (unintentional)

      ● **T50.Z92** Poisoning by other vaccines and biological substances, intentional self-harm

      ● **T50.Z93** Poisoning by other vaccines and biological substances, assault

      ● **T50.Z94** Poisoning by other vaccines and biological substances, undetermined

      ● **T50.Z95** Adverse effect of other vaccines and biological substances

      ● **T50.Z96** Underdosing of other vaccines and biological substances

● **T50.9** Poisoning by, adverse effect of and underdosing of other and unspecified drugs, medicaments and biological substances

   ● **T50.90** Poisoning by, adverse effect of and underdosing of unspecified drugs, medicaments and biological substances

      ● **T50.901** Poisoning by unspecified drugs, medicaments and biological substances, accidental (unintentional)

      ● **T50.902** Poisoning by unspecified drugs, medicaments and biological substances, intentional self-harm

      ● **T50.903** Poisoning by unspecified drugs, medicaments and biological substances, assault

      ● **T50.904** Poisoning by unspecified drugs, medicaments and biological substances, undetermined

      ● **T50.905** Adverse effect of unspecified drugs, medicaments and biological substances

      ● **T50.906** Underdosing of unspecified drugs, medicaments and biological substances

   ● **T50.99** Poisoning by, adverse effect of and underdosing of other drugs, medicaments and biological substances

      ● **T50.991** Poisoning by other drugs, medicaments and biological substances, accidental (unintentional)

      ● **T50.992** Poisoning by other drugs, medicaments and biological substances, intentional self-harm

      ● **T50.993** Poisoning by other drugs, medicaments and biological substances, assault

      ● **T50.994** Poisoning by other drugs, medicaments and biological substances, undetermined

      ● **T50.995** Adverse effect of other drugs, medicaments and biological substances

      ● **T50.996** Underdosing of other drugs, medicaments and biological substances

---

TOXIC EFFECTS OF SUBSTANCES CHIEFLY NONMEDICINAL AS TO SOURCE (T51-T65)

Note: When no intent is indicated code to accidental. Undetermined intent is only for use when there is specific documentation in the record that the intent of the toxic effect cannot be determined.

Use additional code(s): for all associated manifestations of toxic effect, such as:
respiratory conditions due to external agents (J60-J70)
personal history of foreign body fully removed (Z87.821)
to identify any retained foreign body, if applicable (Z18.-)

   Excludes1   contact with and (suspected) exposure to toxic substances (Z77.-)

● **T51** Toxic effect of alcohol

The appropriate 7th character is to be added to each code from category T51

> A   initial encounter
> D   subsequent encounter
> S   sequela

   ● **T51.0** Toxic effect of ethanol
       Toxic effect of ethyl alcohol

      Excludes2   acute alcohol intoxication or 'hangover' effects (F10.129, F10.229, F10.929)
                   drunkenness (F10.129, F10.229, F10.929)
                   pathological alcohol intoxication (F10.129, F10.229, F10.929)

     ● **T51.0X** Toxic effect of ethanol

        ● **T51.0X1** Toxic effect of ethanol, accidental (unintentional)
              Toxic effect of ethanol NOS

        ● **T51.0X2** Toxic effect of ethanol, intentional self-harm

        ● **T51.0X3** Toxic effect of ethanol, assault

        ● **T51.0X4** Toxic effect of ethanol, undetermined

   ● **T51.1** Toxic effect of methanol
       Toxic effect of methyl alcohol

     ● **T51.1X** Toxic effect of methanol

        ● **T51.1X1** Toxic effect of methanol, accidental (unintentional)
              Toxic effect of methanol NOS

        ● **T51.1X2** Toxic effect of methanol, intentional self-harm

        ● **T51.1X3** Toxic effect of methanol, assault

        ● **T51.1X4** Toxic effect of methanol, undetermined

   ● **T51.2** Toxic effect of 2-Propanol
       Toxic effect of isopropyl alcohol

     ● **T51.2X** Toxic effect of 2-Propanol

        ● **T51.2X1** Toxic effect of 2-Propanol, accidental (unintentional)
              Toxic effect of 2-Propanol NOS

        ● **T51.2X2** Toxic effect of 2-Propanol, intentional self-harm

        ● **T51.2X3** Toxic effect of 2-Propanol, assault

        ● **T51.2X4** Toxic effect of 2-Propanol, undetermined

---

▶ New   ⇒ Revised   ~~deleted~~ Deleted   **OGCR** Official Guidelines   X Assign placeholder X   ● Use Additional Character(s)

Excludes 1   Excludes 2   Includes   Use additional   Code first   Code also   Key words

● **T51.3** **Toxic effect of fusel oil**
　　Toxic effect of amyl alcohol
　　Toxic effect of butyl [1-butanol] alcohol
　　Toxic effect of propyl [1-propanol] alcohol
　　● **T51.3X** **Toxic effect of fusel oil**
　　　　● **T51.3X1** **Toxic effect of fusel oil, accidental (unintentional)**
　　　　　　Toxic effect of fusel oil NOS
　　　　● **T51.3X2** **Toxic effect of fusel oil, intentional self-harm**
　　　　● **T51.3X3** **Toxic effect of fusel oil, assault**
　　　　● **T51.3X4** **Toxic effect of fusel oil, undetermined**
● **T51.8** **Toxic effect of other alcohols**
　　● **T51.8X** **Toxic effect of other alcohols**
　　　　● **T51.8X1** **Toxic effect of other alcohols, accidental (unintentional)**
　　　　　　Toxic effect of other alcohols NOS
　　　　● **T51.8X2** **Toxic effect of other alcohols, intentional self-harm**
　　　　● **T51.8X3** **Toxic effect of other alcohols, assault**
　　　　● **T51.8X4** **Toxic effect of other alcohols, undetermined**
● **T51.9** **Toxic effect of unspecified alcohol**
　　X ● **T51.91** **Toxic effect of unspecified alcohol, accidental (unintentional)**
　　X ● **T51.92** **Toxic effect of unspecified alcohol, intentional self-harm**
　　X ● **T51.93** **Toxic effect of unspecified alcohol, assault**
　　X ● **T51.94** **Toxic effect of unspecified alcohol, undetermined**

● **T52** **Toxic effect of organic solvents**
　　Excludes1　halogen derivatives of aliphatic and aromatic hydrocarbons (T53.-)
　　The appropriate 7th character is to be added to each code from category T52
　　　　A　initial encounter
　　　　D　subsequent encounter
　　　　S　sequela

● **T52.0** **Toxic effects of petroleum products**
　　Toxic effects of gasoline [petrol]
　　Toxic effects of kerosene [paraffin oil]
　　Toxic effects of paraffin wax
　　Toxic effects of ether petroleum
　　Toxic effects of naphtha petroleum
　　Toxic effects of spirit petroleum
　　● **T52.0X** **Toxic effects of petroleum products**
　　　　● **T52.0X1** **Toxic effect of petroleum products, accidental (unintentional)**
　　　　　　Toxic effects of petroleum products NOS
　　　　● **T52.0X2** **Toxic effect of petroleum products, intentional self-harm**
　　　　● **T52.0X3** **Toxic effect of petroleum products, assault**
　　　　● **T52.0X4** **Toxic effect of petroleum products, undetermined**

● **T52.1** **Toxic effects of benzene**
　　Excludes1　homologues of benzene (T52.2)
　　　　nitroderivatives and aminoderivatives of benzene and its homologues (T65.3)
　　● **T52.1X** **Toxic effects of benzene**
　　　　● **T52.1X1** **Toxic effect of benzene, accidental (unintentional)**
　　　　　　Toxic effects of benzene NOS
　　　　● **T52.1X2** **Toxic effect of benzene, intentional self-harm**
　　　　● **T52.1X3** **Toxic effect of benzene, assault**
　　　　● **T52.1X4** **Toxic effect of benzene, undetermined**
● **T52.2** **Toxic effects of homologues of benzene**
　　Toxic effects of toluene [methylbenzene]
　　Toxic effects of xylene [dimethylbenzene]
　　● **T52.2X** **Toxic effects of homologues of benzene**
　　　　● **T52.2X1** **Toxic effect of homologues of benzene, accidental (unintentional)**
　　　　　　Toxic effects of homologues of benzene NOS
　　　　● **T52.2X2** **Toxic effect of homologues of benzene, intentional self-harm**
　　　　● **T52.2X3** **Toxic effect of homologues of benzene, assault**
　　　　● **T52.2X4** **Toxic effect of homologues of benzene, undetermined**
● **T52.3** **Toxic effects of glycols**
　　● **T52.3X** **Toxic effects of glycols**
　　　　● **T52.3X1** **Toxic effect of glycols, accidental (unintentional)**
　　　　　　Toxic effects of glycols NOS
　　　　● **T52.3X2** **Toxic effect of glycols, intentional self-harm**
　　　　● **T52.3X3** **Toxic effect of glycols, assault**
　　　　● **T52.3X4** **Toxic effect of glycols, undetermined**
● **T52.4** **Toxic effects of ketones**
　　● **T52.4X** **Toxic effects of ketones**
　　　　● **T52.4X1** **Toxic effect of ketones, accidental (unintentional)**
　　　　　　Toxic effects of ketones NOS
　　　　● **T52.4X2** **Toxic effect of ketones, intentional self-harm**
　　　　● **T52.4X3** **Toxic effect of ketones, assault**
　　　　● **T52.4X4** **Toxic effect of ketones, undetermined**
● **T52.8** **Toxic effects of other organic solvents**
　　● **T52.8X** **Toxic effects of other organic solvents**
　　　　● **T52.8X1** **Toxic effect of other organic solvents, accidental (unintentional)**
　　　　　　Toxic effects of other organic solvents NOS
　　　　● **T52.8X2** **Toxic effect of other organic solvents, intentional self-harm**
　　　　● **T52.8X3** **Toxic effect of other organic solvents, assault**
　　　　● **T52.8X4** **Toxic effect of other organic solvents, undetermined**
● **T52.9** **Toxic effects of unspecified organic solvent**
　　X ● **T52.91** **Toxic effect of unspecified organic solvent, accidental (unintentional)**
　　X ● **T52.92** **Toxic effect of unspecified organic solvent, intentional self-harm**
　　X ● **T52.93** **Toxic effect of unspecified organic solvent, assault**
　　X ● **T52.94** **Toxic effect of unspecified organic solvent, undetermined**

CHAPTER 19 (S00-T88)

CHAPTER 19 (S00–T88)

- **T53**   **Toxic effect of halogen derivatives of aliphatic and aromatic hydrocarbons**

  The appropriate 7th character is to be added to each code from category T53

A	initial encounter
D	subsequent encounter
S	sequela

  - **T53.0**   **Toxic effects of carbon tetrachloride**
    Toxic effects of tetrachloromethane
    - **T53.0X**   **Toxic effects of carbon tetrachloride**
      - **T53.0X1**   **Toxic effect of carbon tetrachloride, accidental (unintentional)**
        Toxic effects of carbon tetrachloride NOS
      - **T53.0X2**   **Toxic effect of carbon tetrachloride, intentional self-harm**
      - **T53.0X3**   **Toxic effect of carbon tetrachloride, assault**
      - **T53.0X4**   **Toxic effect of carbon tetrachloride, undetermined**
  - **T53.1**   **Toxic effects of chloroform**
    Toxic effects of trichloromethane
    - **T53.1X**   **Toxic effects of chloroform**
      - **T53.1X1**   **Toxic effect of chloroform, accidental (unintentional)**
        Toxic effects of chloroform NOS
      - **T53.1X2**   **Toxic effect of chloroform, intentional self-harm**
      - **T53.1X3**   **Toxic effect of chloroform, assault**
      - **T53.1X4**   **Toxic effect of chloroform, undetermined**
  - **T53.2**   **Toxic effects of trichloroethylene**
    Toxic effects of trichloroethene
    - **T53.2X**   **Toxic effects of trichloroethylene**
      - **T53.2X1**   **Toxic effect of trichloroethylene, accidental (unintentional)**
        Toxic effects of trichloroethylene NOS
      - **T53.2X2**   **Toxic effect of trichloroethylene, intentional self-harm**
      - **T53.2X3**   **Toxic effect of trichloroethylene, assault**
      - **T53.2X4**   **Toxic effect of trichloroethylene, undetermined**
  - **T53.3**   **Toxic effects of tetrachloroethylene**
    Toxic effects of perchloroethylene
    Toxic effects of tetrachloroethene
    - **T53.3X**   **Toxic effects of tetrachloroethylene**
      - **T53.3X1**   **Toxic effect of tetrachloroethylene, accidental (unintentional)**
        Toxic effects of tetrachloroethylene NOS
      - **T53.3X2**   **Toxic effect of tetrachloroethylene, intentional self-harm**
      - **T53.3X3**   **Toxic effect of tetrachloroethylene, assault**
      - **T53.3X4**   **Toxic effect of tetrachloroethylene, undetermined**

- **T53.4**   **Toxic effects of dichloromethane**
  Toxic effects of methylene chloride
  - **T53.4X**   **Toxic effects of dichloromethane**
    - **T53.4X1**   **Toxic effect of dichloromethane, accidental (unintentional)**
      Toxic effects of dichloromethane NOS
    - **T53.4X2**   **Toxic effect of dichloromethane, intentional self-harm**
    - **T53.4X3**   **Toxic effect of dichloromethane, assault**
    - **T53.4X4**   **Toxic effect of dichloromethane, undetermined**
- **T53.5**   **Toxic effects of chlorofluorocarbons**
  - **T53.5X**   **Toxic effects of chlorofluorocarbons**
    - **T53.5X1**   **Toxic effect of chlorofluorocarbons, accidental (unintentional)**
      Toxic effects of chlorofluorocarbons NOS
    - **T53.5X2**   **Toxic effect of chlorofluorocarbons, intentional self-harm**
    - **T53.5X3**   **Toxic effect of chlorofluorocarbons, assault**
    - **T53.5X4**   **Toxic effect of chlorofluorocarbons, undetermined**
- **T53.6**   **Toxic effects of other halogen derivatives of aliphatic hydrocarbons**
  - **T53.6X**   **Toxic effects of other halogen derivatives of aliphatic hydrocarbons**
    - **T53.6X1**   **Toxic effect of other halogen derivatives of aliphatic hydrocarbons, accidental (unintentional)**
      Toxic effects of other halogen derivatives of aliphatic hydrocarbons NOS
    - **T53.6X2**   **Toxic effect of other halogen derivatives of aliphatic hydrocarbons, intentional self-harm**
    - **T53.6X3**   **Toxic effect of other halogen derivatives of aliphatic hydrocarbons, assault**
    - **T53.6X4**   **Toxic effect of other halogen derivatives of aliphatic hydrocarbons, undetermined**
- **T53.7**   **Toxic effects of other halogen derivatives of aromatic hydrocarbons**
  - **T53.7X**   **Toxic effects of other halogen derivatives of aromatic hydrocarbons**
    - **T53.7X1**   **Toxic effect of other halogen derivatives of aromatic hydrocarbons, accidental (unintentional)**
      Toxic effects of other halogen derivatives of aromatic hydrocarbons NOS
    - **T53.7X2**   **Toxic effect of other halogen derivatives of aromatic hydrocarbons, intentional self-harm**
    - **T53.7X3**   **Toxic effect of other halogen derivatives of aromatic hydrocarbons, assault**
    - **T53.7X4**   **Toxic effect of other halogen derivatives of aromatic hydrocarbons, undetermined**

▶ New   ⇒ Revised   ~~deleted~~ Deleted   **OGCR** Official Guidelines   X Assign placeholder X   ● Use Additional Character(s)

Excludes 1   Excludes 2   Includes   Use additional   Code first   Code also   Key words

● T53.9 Toxic effects of unspecified halogen derivatives of aliphatic and aromatic hydrocarbons

X ● T53.91 Toxic effect of unspecified halogen derivatives of aliphatic and aromatic hydrocarbons, accidental (unintentional)

X ● T53.92 Toxic effect of unspecified halogen derivatives of aliphatic and aromatic hydrocarbons, intentional self-harm

X ● T53.93 Toxic effect of unspecified halogen derivatives of aliphatic and aromatic hydrocarbons, assault

X ● T53.94 Toxic effect of unspecified halogen derivatives of aliphatic and aromatic hydrocarbons, undetermined

● T54 Toxic effect of corrosive substances

The appropriate 7th character is to be added to each code from category T54

A	initial encounter
D	subsequent encounter
S	sequela

● T54.0 Toxic effects of phenol and phenol homologues

● T54.0X Toxic effects of phenol and phenol homologues

● T54.0X1 Toxic effect of phenol and phenol homologues, accidental (unintentional)

Toxic effects of phenol and phenol homologues NOS

● T54.0X2 Toxic effect of phenol and phenol homologues, intentional self-harm

● T54.0X3 Toxic effect of phenol and phenol homologues, assault

● T54.0X4 Toxic effect of phenol and phenol homologues, undetermined

● T54.1 Toxic effects of other corrosive organic compounds

● T54.1X Toxic effects of other corrosive organic compounds

● T54.1X1 Toxic effect of other corrosive organic compounds, accidental (unintentional)

Toxic effects of other corrosive organic compounds NOS

● T54.1X2 Toxic effect of other corrosive organic compounds, intentional self-harm

● T54.1X3 Toxic effect of other corrosive organic compounds, assault

● T54.1X4 Toxic effect of other corrosive organic compounds, undetermined

● T54.2 Toxic effects of corrosive acids and acid-like substances

Toxic effects of hydrochloric acid
Toxic effects of sulfuric acid

● T54.2X Toxic effects of corrosive acids and acid-like substances

● T54.2X1 Toxic effect of corrosive acids and acid-like substances, accidental (unintentional)

Toxic effects of corrosive acids and acid-like substances NOS

● T54.2X2 Toxic effect of corrosive acids and acid-like substances, intentional self-harm

● T54.2X3 Toxic effect of corrosive acids and acid-like substances, assault

● T54.2X4 Toxic effect of corrosive acids and acid-like substances, undetermined

● T54.3 Toxic effects of corrosive alkalis and alkali-like substances

Toxic effects of potassium hydroxide
Toxic effects of sodium hydroxide

● T54.3X Toxic effects of corrosive alkalis and alkali-like substances

● T54.3X1 Toxic effect of corrosive alkalis and alkali-like substances, accidental (unintentional)

Toxic effects of corrosive alkalis and alkali-like substances NOS

● T54.3X2 Toxic effect of corrosive alkalis and alkali-like substances, intentional self-harm

● T54.3X3 Toxic effect of corrosive alkalis and alkali-like substances, assault

● T54.3X4 Toxic effect of corrosive alkalis and alkali-like substances, undetermined

● T54.9 Toxic effects of unspecified corrosive substance

X ● T54.91 Toxic effect of unspecified corrosive substance, accidental (unintentional)

X ● T54.92 Toxic effect of unspecified corrosive substance, intentional self-harm

X ● T54.93 Toxic effect of unspecified corrosive substance, assault

X ● T54.94 Toxic effect of unspecified corrosive substance, undetermined

● T55 Toxic effect of soaps and detergents

The appropriate 7th character is to be added to each code from category T55

A	initial encounter
D	subsequent encounter
S	sequela

● T55.0 Toxic effect of soaps

● T55.0X Toxic effect of soaps

● T55.0X1 Toxic effect of soaps, accidental (unintentional)

Toxic effect of soaps NOS

● T55.0X2 Toxic effect of soaps, intentional self-harm

● T55.0X3 Toxic effect of soaps, assault

● T55.0X4 Toxic effect of soaps, undetermined

● T55.1 Toxic effect of detergents

● T55.1X Toxic effect of detergents

● T55.1X1 Toxic effect of detergents, accidental (unintentional)

Toxic effect of detergents NOS

● T55.1X2 Toxic effect of detergents, intentional self-harm

● T55.1X3 Toxic effect of detergents, assault

● T55.1X4 Toxic effect of detergents, undetermined

CHAPTER 19 (S00-T88)

● **T56   Toxic effect of metals**

    Includes   toxic effects of fumes and vapors of metals
                   toxic effects of metals from all sources, except
                   medicinal substances

    Use additional code to identify any retained metal foreign
           body, if applicable (Z18.0-, T18.1-)

    Excludes1   arsenic and its compounds (T57.0)
                  manganese and its compounds (T57.2)

    The appropriate 7th character is to be added to each code from
      category T56

      | | |
      A   initial encounter
      D   subsequent encounter
      S   sequela

● **T56.0   Toxic effects of lead and its compounds**

   ● **T56.0X   Toxic effects of lead and its compounds**

     ● **T56.0X1   Toxic effect of lead and
               its compounds, accidental
               (unintentional)**
                 Toxic effects of lead and its
                   compounds NOS

     ● **T56.0X2   Toxic effect of lead and its
               compounds, intentional self-harm**

     ● **T56.0X3   Toxic effect of lead and its
               compounds, assault**

     ● **T56.0X4   Toxic effect of lead and its
               compounds, undetermined**

● **T56.1   Toxic effects of mercury and its compounds**

   ● **T56.1X   Toxic effects of mercury and its compounds**

     ● **T56.1X1   Toxic effect of mercury and
               its compounds, accidental
               (unintentional)**
                 Toxic effects of mercury and its
                   compounds NOS

     ● **T56.1X2   Toxic effect of mercury and its
               compounds, intentional self-harm**

     ● **T56.1X3   Toxic effect of mercury and its
               compounds, assault**

     ● **T56.1X4   Toxic effect of mercury and its
               compounds, undetermined**

● **T56.2   Toxic effects of chromium and its compounds**

   ● **T56.2X   Toxic effects of chromium and its compounds**

     ● **T56.2X1   Toxic effect of chromium and
               its compounds, accidental
               (unintentional)**
                 Toxic effects of chromium and its
                   compounds NOS

     ● **T56.2X2   Toxic effect of chromium and its
               compounds, intentional self-harm**

     ● **T56.2X3   Toxic effect of chromium and its
               compounds, assault**

     ● **T56.2X4   Toxic effect of chromium and its
               compounds, undetermined**

● **T56.3   Toxic effects of cadmium and its compounds**

   ● **T56.3X   Toxic effects of cadmium and its compounds**

     ● **T56.3X1   Toxic effect of cadmium and
               its compounds, accidental
               (unintentional)**
                 Toxic effects of cadmium and its
                   compounds NOS

     ● **T56.3X2   Toxic effect of cadmium and its
               compounds, intentional self-harm**

     ● **T56.3X3   Toxic effect of cadmium and its
               compounds, assault**

     ● **T56.3X4   Toxic effect of cadmium and its
               compounds, undetermined**

● **T56.4   Toxic effects of copper and its compounds**

   ● **T56.4X   Toxic effects of copper and its compounds**

     ● **T56.4X1   Toxic effect of copper and
               its compounds, accidental
               (unintentional)**
                 Toxic effects of copper and its
                   compounds NOS

     ● **T56.4X2   Toxic effect of copper and its
               compounds, intentional self-harm**

     ● **T56.4X3   Toxic effect of copper and its
               compounds, assault**

     ● **T56.4X4   Toxic effect of copper and its
               compounds, undetermined**

● **T56.5   Toxic effects of zinc and its compounds**

   ● **T56.5X   Toxic effects of zinc and its compounds**

     ● **T56.5X1   Toxic effect of zinc and
               its compounds, accidental
               (unintentional)**
                 Toxic effects of zinc and its
                   compounds NOS

     ● **T56.5X2   Toxic effect of zinc and its
               compounds, intentional self-harm**

     ● **T56.5X3   Toxic effect of zinc and its
               compounds, assault**

     ● **T56.5X4   Toxic effect of zinc and its
               compounds, undetermined**

● **T56.6   Toxic effects of tin and its compounds**

   ● **T56.6X   Toxic effects of tin and its compounds**

     ● **T56.6X1   Toxic effect of tin and its compounds,
               accidental (unintentional)**
                 Toxic effects of tin and its
                   compounds NOS

     ● **T56.6X2   Toxic effect of tin and its compounds,
               intentional self-harm**

     ● **T56.6X3   Toxic effect of tin and its compounds,
               assault**

     ● **T56.6X4   Toxic effect of tin and its compounds,
               undetermined**

● **T56.7   Toxic effects of beryllium and its compounds**

   ● **T56.7X   Toxic effects of beryllium and its compounds**

     ● **T56.7X1   Toxic effect of beryllium and
               its compounds, accidental
               (unintentional)**
                 Toxic effects of beryllium and its
                   compounds NOS

     ● **T56.7X2   Toxic effect of beryllium and its
               compounds, intentional self-harm**

     ● **T56.7X3   Toxic effect of beryllium and its
               compounds, assault**

     ● **T56.7X4   Toxic effect of beryllium and its
               compounds, undetermined**

● **T56.8   Toxic effects of other metals**

   ● **T56.81   Toxic effect of thallium**

     ● **T56.811   Toxic effect of thallium, accidental
               (unintentional)**
                 Toxic effect of thallium NOS

     ● **T56.812   Toxic effect of thallium, intentional
               self-harm**

     ● **T56.813   Toxic effect of thallium, assault**

     ● **T56.814   Toxic effect of thallium,
               undetermined**

   ● **T56.89   Toxic effects of other metals**

     ● **T56.891   Toxic effect of other metals, accidental
               (unintentional)**
                 Toxic effects of other metals NOS

     ● **T56.892   Toxic effect of other metals,
               intentional self-harm**

     ● **T56.893   Toxic effect of other metals, assault**

     ● **T56.894   Toxic effect of other metals,
               undetermined**

● **T56.9**   Toxic effects of unspecified metal

   X ● **T56.91**   Toxic effect of unspecified metal, accidental (unintentional)

   X ● **T56.92**   Toxic effect of unspecified metal, intentional self-harm

   X ● **T56.93**   Toxic effect of unspecified metal, assault

   X ● **T56.94**   Toxic effect of unspecified metal, undetermined

● **T57**   Toxic effect of other inorganic substances

   The appropriate 7th character is to be added to each code from category T57

> A   initial encounter
> D   subsequent encounter
> S   sequela

   ● **T57.0**   Toxic effect of arsenic and its compounds

     ● **T57.0X**   Toxic effect of arsenic and its compounds

       ● **T57.0X1**   Toxic effect of arsenic and its compounds, accidental (unintentional)

           Toxic effect of arsenic and its compounds NOS

       ● **T57.0X2**   Toxic effect of arsenic and its compounds, intentional self-harm

       ● **T57.0X3**   Toxic effect of arsenic and its compounds, assault

       ● **T57.0X4**   Toxic effect of arsenic and its compounds, undetermined

   ● **T57.1**   Toxic effect of phosphorus and its compounds

     Excludes1   organophosphate insecticides (T60.0)

     ● **T57.1X**   Toxic effect of phosphorus and its compounds

       ● **T57.1X1**   Toxic effect of phosphorus and its compounds, accidental (unintentional)

           Toxic effect of phosphorus and its compounds NOS

       ● **T57.1X2**   Toxic effect of phosphorus and its compounds, intentional self-harm

       ● **T57.1X3**   Toxic effect of phosphorus and its compounds, assault

       ● **T57.1X4**   Toxic effect of phosphorus and its compounds, undetermined

   ● **T57.2**   Toxic effect of manganese and its compounds

     ● **T57.2X**   Toxic effect of manganese and its compounds

       ● **T57.2X1**   Toxic effect of manganese and its compounds, accidental (unintentional)

           Toxic effect of manganese and its compounds NOS

       ● **T57.2X2**   Toxic effect of manganese and its compounds, intentional self-harm

       ● **T57.2X3**   Toxic effect of manganese and its compounds, assault

       ● **T57.2X4**   Toxic effect of manganese and its compounds, undetermined

   ● **T57.3**   Toxic effect of hydrogen cyanide

     ● **T57.3X**   Toxic effect of hydrogen cyanide

       ● **T57.3X1**   Toxic effect of hydrogen cyanide, accidental (unintentional)

           Toxic effect of hydrogen cyanide NOS

       ● **T57.3X2**   Toxic effect of hydrogen cyanide, intentional self-harm

       ● **T57.3X3**   Toxic effect of hydrogen cyanide, assault

       ● **T57.3X4**   Toxic effect of hydrogen cyanide, undetermined

● **T57.8**   Toxic effect of other specified inorganic substances

   ● **T57.8X**   Toxic effect of other specified inorganic substances

     ● **T57.8X1**   Toxic effect of other specified inorganic substances, accidental (unintentional)

       Toxic effect of other specified inorganic substances NOS

     ● **T57.8X2**   Toxic effect of other specified inorganic substances, intentional self-harm

     ● **T57.8X3**   Toxic effect of other specified inorganic substances, assault

     ● **T57.8X4**   Toxic effect of other specified inorganic substances, undetermined

● **T57.9**   Toxic effect of unspecified inorganic substance

   X ● **T57.91**   Toxic effect of unspecified inorganic substance, accidental (unintentional)

   X ● **T57.92**   Toxic effect of unspecified inorganic substance, intentional self-harm

   X ● **T57.93**   Toxic effect of unspecified inorganic substance, assault

   X ● **T57.94**   Toxic effect of unspecified inorganic substance, undetermined

● **T58**   Toxic effect of carbon monoxide

> **Includes**   asphyxiation from carbon monoxide
> toxic effect of carbon monoxide from all sources

   The appropriate 7th character is to be added to each code from category T58

> A   initial encounter
> D   subsequent encounter
> S   sequela

   ● **T58.0**   Toxic effect of carbon monoxide from motor vehicle exhaust

     Toxic effect of exhaust gas from gas engine

     Toxic effect of exhaust gas from motor pump

   X ● **T58.01**   Toxic effect of carbon monoxide from motor vehicle exhaust, accidental (unintentional)

   X ● **T58.02**   Toxic effect of carbon monoxide from motor vehicle exhaust, intentional self-harm

   X ● **T58.03**   Toxic effect of carbon monoxide from motor vehicle exhaust, assault

   X ● **T58.04**   Toxic effect of carbon monoxide from motor vehicle exhaust, undetermined

   ● **T58.1**   Toxic effect of carbon monoxide from utility gas

     Toxic effect of acetylene

     Toxic effect of gas NOS used for lighting, heating, cooking

     Toxic effect of water gas

   X ● **T58.11**   Toxic effect of carbon monoxide from utility gas, accidental (unintentional)

   X ● **T58.12**   Toxic effect of carbon monoxide from utility gas, intentional self-harm

   X ● **T58.13**   Toxic effect of carbon monoxide from utility gas, assault

   X ● **T58.14**   Toxic effect of carbon monoxide from utility gas, undetermined

CHAPTER 19 (S00-T88)

● **T58.2** Toxic effect of carbon monoxide from incomplete combustion of other domestic fuels
Toxic effect of carbon monoxide from incomplete combustion of coal, coke, kerosene, wood

  ● **T58.2X** Toxic effect of carbon monoxide from incomplete combustion of other domestic fuels

    ● **T58.2X1** Toxic effect of carbon monoxide from incomplete combustion of other domestic fuels, accidental (unintentional)

    ● **T58.2X2** Toxic effect of carbon monoxide from incomplete combustion of other domestic fuels, intentional self-harm

    ● **T58.2X3** Toxic effect of carbon monoxide from incomplete combustion of other domestic fuels, assault

    ● **T58.2X4** Toxic effect of carbon monoxide from incomplete combustion of other domestic fuels, undetermined

● **T58.8** Toxic effect of carbon monoxide from other source
Toxic effect of carbon monoxide from blast furnace gas
Toxic effect of carbon monoxide from fuels in industrial use
Toxic effect of carbon monoxide from kiln vapor

  ● **T58.8X** Toxic effect of carbon monoxide from other source

    ● **T58.8X1** Toxic effect of carbon monoxide from other source, accidental (unintentional)

    ● **T58.8X2** Toxic effect of carbon monoxide from other source, intentional self-harm

    ● **T58.8X3** Toxic effect of carbon monoxide from other source, assault

    ● **T58.8X4** Toxic effect of carbon monoxide from other source, undetermined

● **T58.9** Toxic effect of carbon monoxide from unspecified source

  X ● **T58.91** Toxic effect of carbon monoxide from unspecified source, accidental (unintentional)

  X ● **T58.92** Toxic effect of carbon monoxide from unspecified source, intentional self-harm

  X ● **T58.93** Toxic effect of carbon monoxide from unspecified source, assault

  X ● **T58.94** Toxic effect of carbon monoxide from unspecified source, undetermined

● **T59** Toxic effect of other gases, fumes and vapors

  | Includes | aerosol propellants |
  | Excludes1 | chlorofluorocarbons (T53.5) |

  The appropriate 7th character is to be added to each code from category T59

A	initial encounter
D	subsequent encounter
S	sequela

● **T59.0** Toxic effect of nitrogen oxides

  ● **T59.0X** Toxic effect of nitrogen oxides

    ● **T59.0X1** Toxic effect of nitrogen oxides, accidental (unintentional)
Toxic effect of nitrogen oxides NOS

    ● **T59.0X2** Toxic effect of nitrogen oxides, intentional self-harm

    ● **T59.0X3** Toxic effect of nitrogen oxides, assault

    ● **T59.0X4** Toxic effect of nitrogen oxides, undetermined

● **T59.1** Toxic effect of sulfur dioxide

  ● **T59.1X** Toxic effect of sulfur dioxide

    ● **T59.1X1** Toxic effect of sulfur dioxide, accidental (unintentional)
Toxic effect of sulfur dioxide NOS

    ● **T59.1X2** Toxic effect of sulfur dioxide, intentional self-harm

    ● **T59.1X3** Toxic effect of sulfur dioxide, assault

    ● **T59.1X4** Toxic effect of sulfur dioxide, undetermined

● **T59.2** Toxic effect of formaldehyde

  ● **T59.2X** Toxic effect of formaldehyde

    ● **T59.2X1** Toxic effect of formaldehyde, accidental (unintentional)
Toxic effect of formaldehyde NOS

    ● **T59.2X2** Toxic effect of formaldehyde, intentional self-harm

    ● **T59.2X3** Toxic effect of formaldehyde, assault

    ● **T59.2X4** Toxic effect of formaldehyde, undetermined

● **T59.3** Toxic effect of lacrimogenic gas
Toxic effect of tear gas

  ● **T59.3X** Toxic effect of lacrimogenic gas

    ● **T59.3X1** Toxic effect of lacrimogenic gas, accidental (unintentional)
Toxic effect of lacrimogenic gas NOS

    ● **T59.3X2** Toxic effect of lacrimogenic gas, intentional self-harm

    ● **T59.3X3** Toxic effect of lacrimogenic gas, assault

    ● **T59.3X4** Toxic effect of lacrimogenic gas, undetermined

● **T59.4** Toxic effect of chlorine gas

  ● **T59.4X** Toxic effect of chlorine gas

    ● **T59.4X1** Toxic effect of chlorine gas, accidental (unintentional)
Toxic effect of chlorine gas NOS

    ● **T59.4X2** Toxic effect of chlorine gas, intentional self-harm

    ● **T59.4X3** Toxic effect of chlorine gas, assault

    ● **T59.4X4** Toxic effect of chlorine gas, undetermined

● **T59.5** Toxic effect of fluorine gas and hydrogen fluoride

  ● **T59.5X** Toxic effect of fluorine gas and hydrogen fluoride

    ● **T59.5X1** Toxic effect of fluorine gas and hydrogen fluoride, accidental (unintentional)
Toxic effect of fluorine gas and hydrogen fluoride NOS

    ● **T59.5X2** Toxic effect of fluorine gas and hydrogen fluoride, intentional self-harm

    ● **T59.5X3** Toxic effect of fluorine gas and hydrogen fluoride, assault

    ● **T59.5X4** Toxic effect of fluorine gas and hydrogen fluoride, undetermined

● **T59.6** Toxic effect of hydrogen sulfide

  ● **T59.6X** Toxic effect of hydrogen sulfide

    ● **T59.6X1** Toxic effect of hydrogen sulfide, accidental (unintentional)
Toxic effect of hydrogen sulfide NOS

    ● **T59.6X2** Toxic effect of hydrogen sulfide, intentional self-harm

    ● **T59.6X3** Toxic effect of hydrogen sulfide, assault

    ● **T59.6X4** Toxic effect of hydrogen sulfide, undetermined

▶ New   ⟹ Revised   ~~deleted~~ Deleted   **OGCR** Official Guidelines   X Assign placeholder X   ● Use Additional Character(s)

| Excludes 1 | Excludes 2 | Includes | Use additional | Code first | Code also | Key words |

● T59.7   Toxic effect of carbon dioxide
  ● T59.7X   Toxic effect of carbon dioxide
    ● T59.7X1   Toxic effect of carbon dioxide,
      accidental (unintentional)
        Toxic effect of carbon dioxide NOS
    ● T59.7X2   Toxic effect of carbon dioxide,
      intentional self-harm
    ● T59.7X3   Toxic effect of carbon dioxide, assault
    ● T59.7X4   Toxic effect of carbon dioxide,
      undetermined

● T59.8   Toxic effect of other specified gases, fumes and vapors
  ● T59.81   Toxic effect of smoke
    Smoke inhalation
    Excludes2   toxic effect of cigarette (tobacco)
      smoke (T65.22-)
    ● T59.811   Toxic effect of smoke, accidental
      (unintentional)
        Toxic effect of smoke NOS
    ● T59.812   Toxic effect of smoke, intentional
      self-harm
    ● T59.813   Toxic effect of smoke, assault
    ● T59.814   Toxic effect of smoke, undetermined
  ● T59.89   Toxic effect of other specified gases, fumes and vapors
    ● T59.891   Toxic effect of other specified gases, fumes and vapors, accidental (unintentional)
    ● T59.892   Toxic effect of other specified gases, fumes and vapors, intentional self-harm
    ● T59.893   Toxic effect of other specified gases, fumes and vapors, assault
    ● T59.894   Toxic effect of other specified gases, fumes and vapors, undetermined

● T59.9   Toxic effect of unspecified gases, fumes and vapors
  X ● T59.91   Toxic effect of unspecified gases, fumes and vapors, accidental (unintentional)
  X ● T59.92   Toxic effect of unspecified gases, fumes and vapors, intentional self-harm
  X ● T59.93   Toxic effect of unspecified gases, fumes and vapors, assault
  X ● T59.94   Toxic effect of unspecified gases, fumes and vapors, undetermined

● T60   Toxic effect of pesticides
  Includes   toxic effect of wood preservatives
  The appropriate 7th character is to be added to each code from category T60

  A   initial encounter
  D   subsequent encounter
  S   sequela

● T60.0   Toxic effect of organophosphate and carbamate insecticides
  ● T60.0X   Toxic effect of organophosphate and carbamate insecticides
    ● T60.0X1   Toxic effect of organophosphate and carbamate insecticides, accidental (unintentional)
        Toxic effect of organophosphate and carbamate insecticides NOS
    ● T60.0X2   Toxic effect of organophosphate and carbamate insecticides, intentional self-harm
    ● T60.0X3   Toxic effect of organophosphate and carbamate insecticides, assault
    ● T60.0X4   Toxic effect of organophosphate and carbamate insecticides, undetermined

● T60.1   Toxic effect of halogenated insecticides
  Excludes1   chlorinated hydrocarbon (T53.-)
  ● T60.1X   Toxic effect of halogenated insecticides
    ● T60.1X1   Toxic effect of halogenated insecticides, accidental (unintentional)
        Toxic effect of halogenated insecticides NOS
    ● T60.1X2   Toxic effect of halogenated insecticides, intentional self-harm
    ● T60.1X3   Toxic effect of halogenated insecticides, assault
    ● T60.1X4   Toxic effect of halogenated insecticides, undetermined

● T60.2   Toxic effect of other insecticides
  ● T60.2X   Toxic effect of other insecticides
    ● T60.2X1   Toxic effect of other insecticides, accidental (unintentional)
        Toxic effect of other insecticides NOS
    ● T60.2X2   Toxic effect of other insecticides, intentional self-harm
    ● T60.2X3   Toxic effect of other insecticides, assault
    ● T60.2X4   Toxic effect of other insecticides, undetermined

● T60.3   Toxic effect of herbicides and fungicides
  ● T60.3X   Toxic effect of herbicides and fungicides
    ● T60.3X1   Toxic effect of herbicides and fungicides, accidental (unintentional)
        Toxic effect of herbicides and fungicides NOS
    ● T60.3X2   Toxic effect of herbicides and fungicides, intentional self-harm
    ● T60.3X3   Toxic effect of herbicides and fungicides, assault
    ● T60.3X4   Toxic effect of herbicides and fungicides, undetermined

● T60.4   Toxic effect of rodenticides
  Excludes1   strychnine and its salts (T65.1)
    thallium (T56.81-)
  ● T60.4X   Toxic effect of rodenticides
    ● T60.4X1   Toxic effect of rodenticides, accidental (unintentional)
        Toxic effect of rodenticides NOS
    ● T60.4X2   Toxic effect of rodenticides, intentional self-harm
    ● T60.4X3   Toxic effect of rodenticides, assault
    ● T60.4X4   Toxic effect of rodenticides, undetermined

● T60.8   Toxic effect of other pesticides
  ● T60.8X   Toxic effect of other pesticides
    ● T60.8X1   Toxic effect of other pesticides, accidental (unintentional)
        Toxic effect of other pesticides NOS
    ● T60.8X2   Toxic effect of other pesticides, intentional self-harm
    ● T60.8X3   Toxic effect of other pesticides, assault
    ● T60.8X4   Toxic effect of other pesticides, undetermined

● T60.9   Toxic effect of unspecified pesticide
  X ● T60.91   Toxic effect of unspecified pesticide, accidental (unintentional)
  X ● T60.92   Toxic effect of unspecified pesticide, intentional self-harm
  X ● T60.93   Toxic effect of unspecified pesticide, assault
  X ● T60.94   Toxic effect of unspecified pesticide, undetermined

CHAPTER 19 (S00-T88)

● **T61**   **Toxic effect of noxious substances eaten as seafood**

> **Excludes1**   allergic reaction to food, such as:
> > anaphylactic reaction or shock due to adverse food reaction (T78.0-)
> > bacterial foodborne intoxications (A05.-)
> > dermatitis (L23.6, L25.4, L27.2)
> > food protein-induced enterocolitis syndrome (K52.21)
> > food protein-induced enteropathy (K52.22)
> > gastroenteritis (noninfective) (K52.29)
> > toxic effect of aflatoxin and other mycotoxins (T64)
> > toxic effect of cyanides (T65.0-)
> > toxic effect of harmful algae bloom (T65.82-)
> > toxic effect of hydrogen cyanide (T57.3-)
> > toxic effect of mercury (T56.1-)
> > toxic effect of red tide (T65.82-)

> The appropriate 7th character is to be added to each code from category T61
>
> | | |
> |---|---|
> | A | initial encounter |
> | D | subsequent encounter |
> | S | sequela |

● **T61.0**   **Ciguatera fish poisoning**

   X● **T61.01**   Ciguatera fish poisoning, accidental (unintentional)

   X● **T61.02**   Ciguatera fish poisoning, intentional self-harm

   X● **T61.03**   Ciguatera fish poisoning, assault

   X● **T61.04**   Ciguatera fish poisoning, undetermined

● **T61.1**   **Scombroid fish poisoning**
> Histamine-like syndrome

   X● **T61.11**   Scombroid fish poisoning, accidental (unintentional)

   X● **T61.12**   Scombroid fish poisoning, intentional self-harm

   X● **T61.13**   Scombroid fish poisoning, assault

   X● **T61.14**   Scombroid fish poisoning, undetermined

● **T61.7**   **Other fish and shellfish poisoning**

   ● **T61.77**   Other fish poisoning

     ● **T61.771**   Other fish poisoning, accidental (unintentional)

     ● **T61.772**   Other fish poisoning, intentional self-harm

     ● **T61.773**   Other fish poisoning, assault

     ● **T61.774**   Other fish poisoning, undetermined

   ● **T61.78**   Other shellfish poisoning

     ● **T61.781**   Other shellfish poisoning, accidental (unintentional)

     ● **T61.782**   Other shellfish poisoning, intentional self-harm

     ● **T61.783**   Other shellfish poisoning, assault

     ● **T61.784**   Other shellfish poisoning, undetermined

● **T61.8**   **Toxic effect of other seafood**

   ● **T61.8X**   Toxic effect of other seafood

     ● **T61.8X1**   Toxic effect of other seafood, accidental (unintentional)

     ● **T61.8X2**   Toxic effect of other seafood, intentional self-harm

     ● **T61.8X3**   Toxic effect of other seafood, assault

     ● **T61.8X4**   Toxic effect of other seafood, undetermined

● **T61.9**   **Toxic effect of unspecified seafood**

   X● **T61.91**   Toxic effect of unspecified seafood, accidental (unintentional)

   X● **T61.92**   Toxic effect of unspecified seafood, intentional self-harm

   X● **T61.93**   Toxic effect of unspecified seafood, assault

   X● **T61.94**   Toxic effect of unspecified seafood, undetermined

● **T62**   **Toxic effect of other noxious substances eaten as food**

> **Excludes1**   allergic reaction to food, such as:
> > anaphylactic shock (reaction) due to adverse food reaction (T78.0-)
> > dermatitis (L23.6, L25.4, L27.2)
> > food protein-induced enterocolitis syndrome (K52.21)
> > food protein-induced enteropathy (K52.22)
> > gastroenteritis (noninfective) (K52.29)
> > bacterial food borne intoxications (A05.-)
> > toxic effect of aflatoxin and other mycotoxins (T64)
> > toxic effect of cyanides (T65.0-)
> > toxic effect of hydrogen cyanide (T57.3-)
> > toxic effect of mercury (T56.1-)

> The appropriate 7th character is to be added to each code from category T62
>
> | | |
> |---|---|
> | A | initial encounter |
> | D | subsequent encounter |
> | S | sequela |

● **T62.0**   **Toxic effect of ingested mushrooms**

   ● **T62.0X**   Toxic effect of ingested mushrooms

     ● **T62.0X1**   Toxic effect of ingested mushrooms, accidental (unintentional)
> Toxic effect of ingested mushrooms NOS

     ● **T62.0X2**   Toxic effect of ingested mushrooms, intentional self-harm

     ● **T62.0X3**   Toxic effect of ingested mushrooms, assault

     ● **T62.0X4**   Toxic effect of ingested mushrooms, undetermined

● **T62.1**   **Toxic effect of ingested berries**

   ● **T62.1X**   Toxic effect of ingested berries

     ● **T62.1X1**   Toxic effect of ingested berries, accidental (unintentional)
> Toxic effect of ingested berries NOS

     ● **T62.1X2**   Toxic effect of ingested berries, intentional self-harm

     ● **T62.1X3**   Toxic effect of ingested berries, assault

     ● **T62.1X4**   Toxic effect of ingested berries, undetermined

● **T62.2**   **Toxic effect of other ingested (parts of) plant(s)**

   ● **T62.2X**   Toxic effect of other ingested (parts of) plant(s)

     ● **T62.2X1**   Toxic effect of other ingested (parts of) plant(s), accidental (unintentional)
> Toxic effect of other ingested (parts of) plant(s) NOS

     ● **T62.2X2**   Toxic effect of other ingested (parts of) plant(s), intentional self-harm

     ● **T62.2X3**   Toxic effect of other ingested (parts of) plant(s), assault

     ● **T62.2X4**   Toxic effect of other ingested (parts of) plant(s), undetermined

● **T62.8**   **Toxic effect of other specified noxious substances eaten as food**

   ● **T62.8X**   Toxic effect of other specified noxious substances eaten as food

     ● **T62.8X1**   Toxic effect of other specified noxious substances eaten as food, accidental (unintentional)
> Toxic effect of other specified noxious substances eaten as food NOS

     ● **T62.8X2**   Toxic effect of other specified noxious substances eaten as food, intentional self-harm

     ● **T62.8X3**   Toxic effect of other specified noxious substances eaten as food, assault

     ● **T62.8X4**   Toxic effect of other specified noxious substances eaten as food, undetermined

▶ New   ⇒ Revised   ~~deleted~~ Deleted   **OGCR** Official Guidelines   X Assign placeholder X   ● Use Additional Character(s)

Excludes 1   Excludes 2   Includes   Use additional   Code first   Code also   Key words

● **T62.9**   **Toxic effect of unspecified noxious substance eaten as food**

     X● **T62.91**   **Toxic effect of unspecified noxious substance eaten as food, accidental (unintentional)**
         Toxic effect of unspecified noxious substance eaten as food NOS

     X● **T62.92**   **Toxic effect of unspecified noxious substance eaten as food, intentional self-harm**

     X● **T62.93**   **Toxic effect of unspecified noxious substance eaten as food, assault**

     X● **T62.94**   **Toxic effect of unspecified noxious substance eaten as food, undetermined**

● **T63**   **Toxic effect of contact with venomous animals and plants**

     | **Includes** | bite or touch of venomous animal |
                          pricked or stuck by thorn or leaf

     | **Excludes2** | ingestion of toxic animal or plant (T61.-, T62.-) |

     The appropriate 7th character is to be added to each code from category T63

         A   initial encounter
         D   subsequent encounter
         S   sequela

   ● **T63.0**   **Toxic effect of snake venom**

     ● **T63.00**   **Toxic effect of unspecified snake venom**

       ● **T63.001**   **Toxic effect of unspecified snake venom, accidental (unintentional)**
          Toxic effect of unspecified snake venom NOS

       ● **T63.002**   **Toxic effect of unspecified snake venom, intentional self-harm**

       ● **T63.003**   **Toxic effect of unspecified snake venom, assault**

       ● **T63.004**   **Toxic effect of unspecified snake venom, undetermined**

     ● **T63.01**   **Toxic effect of rattlesnake venom**

       ● **T63.011**   **Toxic effect of rattlesnake venom, accidental (unintentional)**
          Toxic effect of rattlesnake venom NOS

       ● **T63.012**   **Toxic effect of rattlesnake venom, intentional self-harm**

       ● **T63.013**   **Toxic effect of rattlesnake venom, assault**

       ● **T63.014**   **Toxic effect of rattlesnake venom, undetermined**

     ● **T63.02**   **Toxic effect of coral snake venom**

       ● **T63.021**   **Toxic effect of coral snake venom, accidental (unintentional)**
          Toxic effect of coral snake venom NOS

       ● **T63.022**   **Toxic effect of coral snake venom, intentional self-harm**

       ● **T63.023**   **Toxic effect of coral snake venom, assault**

       ● **T63.024**   **Toxic effect of coral snake venom, undetermined**

     ● **T63.03**   **Toxic effect of taipan venom**

       ● **T63.031**   **Toxic effect of taipan venom, accidental (unintentional)**
          Toxic effect of taipan venom NOS

       ● **T63.032**   **Toxic effect of taipan venom, intentional self-harm**

       ● **T63.033**   **Toxic effect of taipan venom, assault**

       ● **T63.034**   **Toxic effect of taipan venom, undetermined**

● **T63.04**   **Toxic effect of cobra venom**

     ● **T63.041**   **Toxic effect of cobra venom, accidental (unintentional)**
        Toxic effect of cobra venom NOS

     ● **T63.042**   **Toxic effect of cobra venom, intentional self-harm**

     ● **T63.043**   **Toxic effect of cobra venom, assault**

     ● **T63.044**   **Toxic effect of cobra venom, undetermined**

● **T63.06**   **Toxic effect of venom of other North and South American snake**

     ● **T63.061**   **Toxic effect of venom of other North and South American snake, accidental (unintentional)**
        Toxic effect of venom of other North and South American snake NOS

     ● **T63.062**   **Toxic effect of venom of other North and South American snake, intentional self-harm**

     ● **T63.063**   **Toxic effect of venom of other North and South American snake, assault**

     ● **T63.064**   **Toxic effect of venom of other North and South American snake, undetermined**

● **T63.07**   **Toxic effect of venom of other Australian snake**

     ● **T63.071**   **Toxic effect of venom of other Australian snake, accidental (unintentional)**
        Toxic effect of venom of other Australian snake NOS

     ● **T63.072**   **Toxic effect of venom of other Australian snake, intentional self-harm**

     ● **T63.073**   **Toxic effect of venom of other Australian snake, assault**

     ● **T63.074**   **Toxic effect of venom of other Australian snake, undetermined**

● **T63.08**   **Toxic effect of venom of other African and Asian snake**

     ● **T63.081**   **Toxic effect of venom of other African and Asian snake, accidental (unintentional)**
        Toxic effect of venom of other African and Asian snake NOS

     ● **T63.082**   **Toxic effect of venom of other African and Asian snake, intentional self-harm**

     ● **T63.083**   **Toxic effect of venom of other African and Asian snake, assault**

     ● **T63.084**   **Toxic effect of venom of other African and Asian snake, undetermined**

● **T63.09**   **Toxic effect of venom of other snake**

     ● **T63.091**   **Toxic effect of venom of other snake, accidental (unintentional)**
        Toxic effect of venom of other snake NOS

     ● **T63.092**   **Toxic effect of venom of other snake, intentional self-harm**

     ● **T63.093**   **Toxic effect of venom of other snake, assault**

     ● **T63.094**   **Toxic effect of venom of other snake, undetermined**

CHAPTER 19 (S00-T88)

● T63.1   Toxic effect of venom of other reptiles
  ● T63.11   Toxic effect of venom of gila monster
    ● T63.111   Toxic effect of venom of gila monster, accidental (unintentional)
      Toxic effect of venom of gila monster NOS
    ● T63.112   Toxic effect of venom of gila monster, intentional self-harm
    ● T63.113   Toxic effect of venom of gila monster, assault
    ● T63.114   Toxic effect of venom of gila monster, undetermined
  ● T63.12   Toxic effect of venom of other venomous lizard
    ● T63.121   Toxic effect of venom of other venomous lizard, accidental (unintentional)
      Toxic effect of venom of other venomous lizard NOS
    ● T63.122   Toxic effect of venom of other venomous lizard, intentional self-harm
    ● T63.123   Toxic effect of venom of other venomous lizard, assault
    ● T63.124   Toxic effect of venom of other venomous lizard, undetermined
  ● T63.19   Toxic effect of venom of other reptiles
    ● T63.191   Toxic effect of venom of other reptiles, accidental (unintentional)
      Toxic effect of venom of other reptiles NOS
    ● T63.192   Toxic effect of venom of other reptiles, intentional self-harm
    ● T63.193   Toxic effect of venom of other reptiles, assault
    ● T63.194   Toxic effect of venom of other reptiles, undetermined
● T63.2   Toxic effect of venom of scorpion
  ● T63.2X   Toxic effect of venom of scorpion
    ● T63.2X1   Toxic effect of venom of scorpion, accidental (unintentional)
      Toxic effect of venom of scorpion NOS
    ● T63.2X2   Toxic effect of venom of scorpion, intentional self-harm
    ● T63.2X3   Toxic effect of venom of scorpion, assault
    ● T63.2X4   Toxic effect of venom of scorpion, undetermined
● T63.3   Toxic effect of venom of spider
  ● T63.30   Toxic effect of unspecified spider venom
    ● T63.301   Toxic effect of unspecified spider venom, accidental (unintentional)
    ● T63.302   Toxic effect of unspecified spider venom, intentional self-harm
    ● T63.303   Toxic effect of unspecified spider venom, assault
    ● T63.304   Toxic effect of unspecified spider venom, undetermined
  ● T63.31   Toxic effect of venom of black widow spider
    ● T63.311   Toxic effect of venom of black widow spider, accidental (unintentional)
    ● T63.312   Toxic effect of venom of black widow spider, intentional self-harm
    ● T63.313   Toxic effect of venom of black widow spider, assault
    ● T63.314   Toxic effect of venom of black widow spider, undetermined

● T63.32   Toxic effect of venom of tarantula
    ● T63.321   Toxic effect of venom of tarantula, accidental (unintentional)
    ● T63.322   Toxic effect of venom of tarantula, intentional self-harm
    ● T63.323   Toxic effect of venom of tarantula, assault
    ● T63.324   Toxic effect of venom of tarantula, undetermined
  ● T63.33   Toxic effect of venom of brown recluse spider
    ● T63.331   Toxic effect of venom of brown recluse spider, accidental (unintentional)
    ● T63.332   Toxic effect of venom of brown recluse spider, intentional self-harm
    ● T63.333   Toxic effect of venom of brown recluse spider, assault
    ● T63.334   Toxic effect of venom of brown recluse spider, undetermined
  ● T63.39   Toxic effect of venom of other spider
    ● T63.391   Toxic effect of venom of other spider, accidental (unintentional)
    ● T63.392   Toxic effect of venom of other spider, intentional self-harm
    ● T63.393   Toxic effect of venom of other spider, assault
    ● T63.394   Toxic effect of venom of other spider, undetermined
● T63.4   Toxic effect of venom of other arthropods
  ● T63.41   Toxic effect of venom of centipedes and venomous millipedes
    ● T63.411   Toxic effect of venom of centipedes and venomous millipedes, accidental (unintentional)
    ● T63.412   Toxic effect of venom of centipedes and venomous millipedes, intentional self-harm
    ● T63.413   Toxic effect of venom of centipedes and venomous millipedes, assault
    ● T63.414   Toxic effect of venom of centipedes and venomous millipedes, undetermined
  ● T63.42   Toxic effect of venom of ants
    ● T63.421   Toxic effect of venom of ants, accidental (unintentional)
    ● T63.422   Toxic effect of venom of ants, intentional self-harm
    ● T63.423   Toxic effect of venom of ants, assault
    ● T63.424   Toxic effect of venom of ants, undetermined
  ● T63.43   Toxic effect of venom of caterpillars
    ● T63.431   Toxic effect of venom of caterpillars, accidental (unintentional)
    ● T63.432   Toxic effect of venom of caterpillars, intentional self-harm
    ● T63.433   Toxic effect of venom of caterpillars, assault
    ● T63.434   Toxic effect of venom of caterpillars, undetermined
  ● T63.44   Toxic effect of venom of bees
    ● T63.441   Toxic effect of venom of bees, accidental (unintentional)
    ● T63.442   Toxic effect of venom of bees, intentional self-harm
    ● T63.443   Toxic effect of venom of bees, assault
    ● T63.444   Toxic effect of venom of bees, undetermined

● T63.45　Toxic effect of venom of hornets
　　● T63.451　Toxic effect of venom of hornets, accidental (unintentional)
　　● T63.452　Toxic effect of venom of hornets, intentional self-harm
　　● T63.453　Toxic effect of venom of hornets, assault
　　● T63.454　Toxic effect of venom of hornets, undetermined
● T63.46　Toxic effect of venom of wasps
　　　　　　Toxic effect of yellow jacket
　　● T63.461　Toxic effect of venom of wasps, accidental (unintentional)
　　● T63.462　Toxic effect of venom of wasps, intentional self-harm
　　● T63.463　Toxic effect of venom of wasps, assault
　　● T63.464　Toxic effect of venom of wasps, undetermined
● T63.48　Toxic effect of venom of other arthropod
　　● T63.481　Toxic effect of venom of other arthropod, accidental (unintentional)
　　● T63.482　Toxic effect of venom of other arthropod, intentional self-harm
　　● T63.483　Toxic effect of venom of other arthropod, assault
　　● T63.484　Toxic effect of venom of other arthropod, undetermined
● T63.5　Toxic effect of contact with venomous fish
　　Excludes2　poisoning by ingestion of fish (T61.-)
　● T63.51　Toxic effect of contact with stingray
　　● T63.511　Toxic effect of contact with stingray, accidental (unintentional)
　　● T63.512　Toxic effect of contact with stingray, intentional self-harm
　　● T63.513　Toxic effect of contact with stingray, assault
　　● T63.514　Toxic effect of contact with stingray, undetermined
　● T63.59　Toxic effect of contact with other venomous fish
　　● T63.591　Toxic effect of contact with other venomous fish, accidental (unintentional)
　　● T63.592　Toxic effect of contact with other venomous fish, intentional self-harm
　　● T63.593　Toxic effect of contact with other venomous fish, assault
　　● T63.594　Toxic effect of contact with other venomous fish, undetermined
● T63.6　Toxic effect of contact with other venomous marine animals
　　Excludes1　sea-snake venom (T63.09)
　　Excludes2　poisoning by ingestion of shellfish (T61.78-)
　● T63.61　Toxic effect of contact with Portugese Man-o-war
　　　　　　Toxic effect of contact with bluebottle
　　● T63.611　Toxic effect of contact with Portugese Man-o-war, accidental (unintentional)
　　● T63.612　Toxic effect of contact with Portugese Man-o-war, intentional self-harm
　　● T63.613　Toxic effect of contact with Portugese Man-o-war, assault
　　● T63.614　Toxic effect of contact with Portugese Man-o-war, undetermined

● T63.62　Toxic effect of contact with other jellyfish
　　● T63.621　Toxic effect of contact with other jellyfish, accidental (unintentional)
　　● T63.622　Toxic effect of contact with other jellyfish, intentional self-harm
　　● T63.623　Toxic effect of contact with other jellyfish, assault
　　● T63.624　Toxic effect of contact with other jellyfish, undetermined
● T63.63　Toxic effect of contact with sea anemone
　　● T63.631　Toxic effect of contact with sea anemone, accidental (unintentional)
　　● T63.632　Toxic effect of contact with sea anemone, intentional self-harm
　　● T63.633　Toxic effect of contact with sea anemone, assault
　　● T63.634　Toxic effect of contact with sea anemone, undetermined
● T63.69　Toxic effect of contact with other venomous marine animals
　　● T63.691　Toxic effect of contact with other venomous marine animals, accidental (unintentional)
　　● T63.692　Toxic effect of contact with other venomous marine animals, intentional self-harm
　　● T63.693　Toxic effect of contact with other venomous marine animals, assault
　　● T63.694　Toxic effect of contact with other venomous marine animals, undetermined
● T63.7　Toxic effect of contact with venomous plant
　● T63.71　Toxic effect of contact with venomous marine plant
　　● T63.711　Toxic effect of contact with venomous marine plant, accidental (unintentional)
　　● T63.712　Toxic effect of contact with venomous marine plant, intentional self-harm
　　● T63.713　Toxic effect of contact with venomous marine plant, assault
　　● T63.714　Toxic effect of contact with venomous marine plant, undetermined
　● T63.79　Toxic effect of contact with other venomous plant
　　● T63.791　Toxic effect of contact with other venomous plant, accidental (unintentional)
　　● T63.792　Toxic effect of contact with other venomous plant, intentional self-harm
　　● T63.793　Toxic effect of contact with other venomous plant, assault
　　● T63.794　Toxic effect of contact with other venomous plant, undetermined
● T63.8　Toxic effect of contact with other venomous animals
　● T63.81　Toxic effect of contact with venomous frog
　　　　Excludes1　contact with nonvenomous frog (W62.0)
　　● T63.811　Toxic effect of contact with venomous frog, accidental (unintentional)
　　● T63.812　Toxic effect of contact with venomous frog, intentional self-harm
　　● T63.813　Toxic effect of contact with venomous frog, assault
　　● T63.814　Toxic effect of contact with venomous frog, undetermined

● **T63.82**   Toxic effect of contact with venomous toad
> **Excludes1**   contact with nonvenomous toad (W62.1)

     ● **T63.821**   Toxic effect of contact with venomous toad, accidental (unintentional)

     ● **T63.822**   Toxic effect of contact with venomous toad, intentional self-harm

     ● **T63.823**   Toxic effect of contact with venomous toad, assault

     ● **T63.824**   Toxic effect of contact with venomous toad, undetermined

● **T63.83**   Toxic effect of contact with other venomous amphibian
> **Excludes1**   contact with nonvenomous amphibian (W62.9)

     ● **T63.831**   Toxic effect of contact with other venomous amphibian, accidental (unintentional)

     ● **T63.832**   Toxic effect of contact with other venomous amphibian, intentional self-harm

     ● **T63.833**   Toxic effect of contact with other venomous amphibian, assault

     ● **T63.834**   Toxic effect of contact with other venomous amphibian, undetermined

● **T63.89**   Toxic effect of contact with other venomous animals

     ● **T63.891**   Toxic effect of contact with other venomous animals, accidental (unintentional)

     ● **T63.892**   Toxic effect of contact with other venomous animals, intentional self-harm

     ● **T63.893**   Toxic effect of contact with other venomous animals, assault

     ● **T63.894**   Toxic effect of contact with other venomous animals, undetermined

● **T63.9**   Toxic effect of contact with unspecified venomous animal

     X ● **T63.91**   Toxic effect of contact with unspecified venomous animal, accidental (unintentional)

     X ● **T63.92**   Toxic effect of contact with unspecified venomous animal, intentional self-harm

     X ● **T63.93**   Toxic effect of contact with unspecified venomous animal, assault

     X ● **T63.94**   Toxic effect of contact with unspecified venomous animal, undetermined

● **T64**   Toxic effect of aflatoxin and other mycotoxin food contaminants

The appropriate 7th character is to be added to each code from category T64

A	initial encounter
D	subsequent encounter
S	sequela

● **T64.0**   Toxic effect of aflatoxin

     X ● **T64.01**   Toxic effect of aflatoxin, accidental (unintentional)

     X ● **T64.02**   Toxic effect of aflatoxin, intentional self-harm

     X ● **T64.03**   Toxic effect of aflatoxin, assault

     X ● **T64.04**   Toxic effect of aflatoxin, undetermined

● **T64.8**   Toxic effect of other mycotoxin food contaminants

     X ● **T64.81**   Toxic effect of other mycotoxin food contaminants, accidental (unintentional)

     X ● **T64.82**   Toxic effect of other mycotoxin food contaminants, intentional self-harm

     X ● **T64.83**   Toxic effect of other mycotoxin food contaminants, assault

     X ● **T64.84**   Toxic effect of other mycotoxin food contaminants, undetermined

● **T65**   Toxic effect of other and unspecified substances

The appropriate 7th character is to be added to each code from category T65

A	initial encounter
D	subsequent encounter
S	sequela

● **T65.0**   Toxic effect of cyanides
> **Excludes1**   hydrogen cyanide (T57.3-)

     ● **T65.0X**   Toxic effect of cyanides

        ● **T65.0X1**   Toxic effect of cyanides, accidental (unintentional)
          Toxic effect of cyanides NOS

        ● **T65.0X2**   Toxic effect of cyanides, intentional self-harm

        ● **T65.0X3**   Toxic effect of cyanides, assault

        ● **T65.0X4**   Toxic effect of cyanides, undetermined

● **T65.1**   Toxic effect of strychnine and its salts

     ● **T65.1X**   Toxic effect of strychnine and its salts

        ● **T65.1X1**   Toxic effect of strychnine and its salts, accidental (unintentional)
          Toxic effect of strychnine and its salts NOS

        ● **T65.1X2**   Toxic effect of strychnine and its salts, intentional self-harm

        ● **T65.1X3**   Toxic effect of strychnine and its salts, assault

        ● **T65.1X4**   Toxic effect of strychnine and its salts, undetermined

● **T65.2**   Toxic effect of tobacco and nicotine
> **Excludes2**   nicotine dependence (F17.-)

     ● **T65.21**   Toxic effect of chewing tobacco

        ● **T65.211**   Toxic effect of chewing tobacco, accidental (unintentional)
          Toxic effect of chewing tobacco NOS

        ● **T65.212**   Toxic effect of chewing tobacco, intentional self-harm

        ● **T65.213**   Toxic effect of chewing tobacco, assault

        ● **T65.214**   Toxic effect of chewing tobacco, undetermined

     ● **T65.22**   Toxic effect of tobacco cigarettes
        Toxic effect of tobacco smoke

> Use additional code for exposure to second hand tobacco smoke (Z57.31, Z77.22)

        ● **T65.221**   Toxic effect of tobacco cigarettes, accidental (unintentional)
          Toxic effect of tobacco cigarettes NOS

        ● **T65.222**   Toxic effect of tobacco cigarettes, intentional self-harm

        ● **T65.223**   Toxic effect of tobacco cigarettes, assault

        ● **T65.224**   Toxic effect of tobacco cigarettes, undetermined

     ● **T65.29**   Toxic effect of other tobacco and nicotine

        ● **T65.291**   Toxic effect of other tobacco and nicotine, accidental (unintentional)
          Toxic effect of other tobacco and nicotine NOS

        ● **T65.292**   Toxic effect of other tobacco and nicotine, intentional self-harm

        ● **T65.293**   Toxic effect of other tobacco and nicotine, assault

        ● **T65.294**   Toxic effect of other tobacco and nicotine, undetermined

▶ New   ⟹ Revised   ~~deleted~~ Deleted   **OGCR** Official Guidelines   X Assign placeholder X   ● Use Additional Character(s)

Excludes 1   Excludes 2   Includes   Use additional   Code first   Code also   Key words

● **T65.3** **Toxic effect of nitroderivatives and aminoderivatives of benzene and its homologues**
Toxic effect of anilin [benzenamine]
Toxic effect of nitrobenzene
Toxic effect of trinitrotoluene

   ● **T65.3X** Toxic effect of nitroderivatives and aminoderivatives of benzene and its homologues

      ● **T65.3X1** Toxic effect of nitroderivatives and aminoderivatives of benzene and its homologues, accidental (unintentional)
Toxic effect of nitroderivatives and aminoderivatives of benzene and its homologues NOS

      ● **T65.3X2** Toxic effect of nitroderivatives and aminoderivatives of benzene and its homologues, intentional self-harm

      ● **T65.3X3** Toxic effect of nitroderivatives and aminoderivatives of benzene and its homologues, assault

      ● **T65.3X4** Toxic effect of nitroderivatives and aminoderivatives of benzene and its homologues, undetermined

● **T65.4** **Toxic effect of carbon disulfide**

   ● **T65.4X** Toxic effect of carbon disulfide

      ● **T65.4X1** Toxic effect of carbon disulfide, accidental (unintentional)
Toxic effect of carbon disulfide NOS

      ● **T65.4X2** Toxic effect of carbon disulfide, intentional self-harm

      ● **T65.4X3** Toxic effect of carbon disulfide, assault

      ● **T65.4X4** Toxic effect of carbon disulfide, undetermined

● **T65.5** **Toxic effect of nitroglycerin and other nitric acids and esters**
Toxic effect of 1,2,3-Propanetriol trinitrate

   ● **T65.5X** Toxic effect of nitroglycerin and other nitric acids and esters

      ● **T65.5X1** Toxic effect of nitroglycerin and other nitric acids and esters, accidental (unintentional)
Toxic effect of nitroglycerin and other nitric acids and esters NOS

      ● **T65.5X2** Toxic effect of nitroglycerin and other nitric acids and esters, intentional self-harm

      ● **T65.5X3** Toxic effect of nitroglycerin and other nitric acids and esters, assault

      ● **T65.5X4** Toxic effect of nitroglycerin and other nitric acids and esters, undetermined

● **T65.6** **Toxic effect of paints and dyes, not elsewhere classified**

   ● **T65.6X** Toxic effect of paints and dyes, not elsewhere classified

      ● **T65.6X1** Toxic effect of paints and dyes, not elsewhere classified, accidental (unintentional)
Toxic effect of paints and dyes NOS

      ● **T65.6X2** Toxic effect of paints and dyes, not elsewhere classified, intentional self-harm

      ● **T65.6X3** Toxic effect of paints and dyes, not elsewhere classified, assault

      ● **T65.6X4** Toxic effect of paints and dyes, not elsewhere classified, undetermined

● **T65.8** **Toxic effect of other specified substances**

   ● **T65.81** Toxic effect of latex

      ● **T65.811** Toxic effect of latex, accidental (unintentional)
Toxic effect of latex NOS

      ● **T65.812** Toxic effect of latex, intentional self-harm

      ● **T65.813** Toxic effect of latex, assault

      ● **T65.814** Toxic effect of latex, undetermined

   ● **T65.82** Toxic effect of harmful algae and algae toxins
Toxic effect of (harmful) algae bloom NOS
Toxic effect of blue-green algae bloom
Toxic effect of brown tide
Toxic effect of cyanobacteria bloom
Toxic effect of Florida red tide
Toxic effect of pfiesteria piscicida
Toxic effect of red tide

      ● **T65.821** Toxic effect of harmful algae and algae toxins, accidental (unintentional)
Toxic effect of harmful algae and algae toxins NOS

      ● **T65.822** Toxic effect of harmful algae and algae toxins, intentional self-harm

      ● **T65.823** Toxic effect of harmful algae and algae toxins, assault

      ● **T65.824** Toxic effect of harmful algae and algae toxins, undetermined

   ● **T65.83** Toxic effect of fiberglass

      ● **T65.831** Toxic effect of fiberglass, accidental (unintentional)
Toxic effect of fiberglass NOS

      ● **T65.832** Toxic effect of fiberglass, intentional self-harm

      ● **T65.833** Toxic effect of fiberglass, assault

      ● **T65.834** Toxic effect of fiberglass, undetermined

   ● **T65.89** Toxic effect of other specified substances

      ● **T65.891** Toxic effect of other specified substances, accidental (unintentional)
Toxic effect of other specified substances NOS

      ● **T65.892** Toxic effect of other specified substances, intentional self-harm

      ● **T65.893** Toxic effect of other specified substances, assault

      ● **T65.894** Toxic effect of other specified substances, undetermined

● **T65.9** **Toxic effect of unspecified substance**

   X ● **T65.91** Toxic effect of unspecified substance, accidental (unintentional)
Poisoning NOS

   X ● **T65.92** Toxic effect of unspecified substance, intentional self-harm

   X ● **T65.93** Toxic effect of unspecified substance, assault

   X ● **T65.94** Toxic effect of unspecified substance, undetermined

CHAPTER 19 (S00-T88)

▶ New   ⇒ Revised   ~~deleted~~ Deleted   **OGCR** Official Guidelines   X Assign placeholder X   ● Use Additional Character(s)

Excludes 1   Excludes 2   Includes   Use additional   Code first   Code also   Key words

OTHER AND UNSPECIFIED EFFECTS OF EXTERNAL CAUSES (T66-T78)

● **T66**   **Radiation sickness, unspecified**

> Excludes1   specified adverse effects of radiation, such as:
>> burns (T20-T31)
>> leukemia (C91-C95)
>> radiation gastroenteritis and colitis (K52.0)
>> radiation pneumonitis (J70.0)
>> radiation related disorders of the skin and
>> subcutaneous tissue (L55-L59)
>> sunburn (L55.-)

> The appropriate 7th character is to be added to code T66

>> A   initial encounter
>> D   subsequent encounter
>> S   sequela

● **T67**   **Effects of heat and light**

> Excludes1   erythema [dermatitis] ab igne (L59.0)
>> malignant hyperpyrexia due to anesthesia (T88.3)
>> radiation-related disorders of the skin and
>> subcutaneous tissue (L55-L59)

> Excludes2   burns (T20-T31)
>> sunburn (L55.-)
>> sweat disorder due to heat (L74-L75)

> The appropriate 7th character is to be added to each code from
> category T67

>> A   initial encounter
>> D   subsequent encounter
>> S   sequela

X ● **T67.0**   **Heatstroke and sunstroke**
>> Heat apoplexy
>> Heat pyrexia
>> Siriasis
>> Thermoplegia
>> Use additional code(s) to identify any associated
>> complications of heatstroke, such as:
>>> coma and stupor (R40.-)
>>> systemic inflammatory response syndrome (R65.1-)

X ● **T67.1**   **Heat syncope**
>> Heat collapse

X ● **T67.2**   **Heat cramp**

X ● **T67.3**   **Heat exhaustion, anhydrotic**
>> Heat prostration due to water depletion

>>> Excludes1   heat exhaustion due to salt depletion
>>> (T67.4)

X ● **T67.4**   **Heat exhaustion due to salt depletion**
>> Heat prostration due to salt (and water) depletion

X ● **T67.5**   **Heat exhaustion, unspecified**
>> Heat prostration NOS

X ● **T67.6**   **Heat fatigue, transient**

X ● **T67.7**   **Heat edema**

X ● **T67.8**   **Other effects of heat and light**

X ● **T67.9**   **Effect of heat and light, unspecified**

X ● **T68**   **Hypothermia**
>> Accidental hypothermia
>> Hypothermia NOS
>> Use additional code to identify source of exposure:
>>> Exposure to excessive cold of man-made origin (W93)
>>> Exposure to excessive cold of natural origin (X31)

>> Excludes1   hypothermia following anesthesia (T88.51)
>>> hypothermia not associated with low
>>> environmental temperature (R68.0)
>>> hypothermia of newborn (P80.-)

>> Excludes2   frostbite (T33-T34)

> The appropriate 7th character is to be added to code T68

>> A   initial encounter
>> D   subsequent encounter
>> S   sequela

● **T69**   **Other effects of reduced temperature**

> Use additional code to identify source of exposure:
>> Exposure to excessive cold of man-made origin (W93)
>> Exposure to excessive cold of natural origin (X31)

> Excludes2   frostbite (T33-T34)

> The appropriate 7th character is to be added to each code from
> category T69

>> A   initial encounter
>> D   subsequent encounter
>> S   sequela

● **T69.0**   **Immersion hand and foot**

> ● **T69.01**   **Immersion hand**

>> ● **T69.011**   Immersion hand, right hand
>> ● **T69.012**   Immersion hand, left hand
>> ● **T69.019**   Immersion hand, unspecified hand

> ● **T69.02**   **Immersion foot**
>> Trench foot

>> ● **T69.021**   Immersion foot, right foot
>> ● **T69.022**   Immersion foot, left foot
>> ● **T69.029**   Immersion foot, unspecified foot

X ● **T69.1**   **Chilblains**

X ● **T69.8**   **Other specified effects of reduced temperature**

X ● **T69.9**   **Effect of reduced temperature, unspecified**

● **T70**   **Effects of air pressure and water pressure**

> The appropriate 7th character is to be added to each code from
> category T70

>> A   initial encounter
>> D   subsequent encounter
>> S   sequela

X ● **T70.0**   **Otitic barotrauma**
>> Aero-otitis media
>> Effects of change in ambient atmospheric pressure or
>> water pressure on ears

X ● **T70.1**   **Sinus barotrauma**
>> Aerosinusitis
>> Effects of change in ambient atmospheric pressure on
>> sinuses

● **T70.2**   **Other and unspecified effects of high altitude**

> Excludes2   polycythemia due to high altitude (D75.1)

X ● **T70.20**   **Unspecified effects of high altitude**

X ● **T70.29**   **Other effects of high altitude**
>> Alpine sickness
>> Anoxia due to high altitude
>> Barotrauma NOS
>> Hypobaropathy
>> Mountain sickness

X ● **T70.3**   **Caisson disease [decompression sickness]**
>> Compressed-air disease
>> Diver's palsy or paralysis

X ● **T70.4**   **Effects of high-pressure fluids**
>> Hydraulic jet injection (industrial)
>> Pneumatic jet injection (industrial)
>> Traumatic jet injection (industrial)

X ● **T70.8**   **Other effects of air pressure and water pressure**

X ● **T70.9**   **Effect of air pressure and water pressure, unspecified**

▶ New   ⇒ Revised   ~~deleted~~ Deleted   **OGCR** Official Guidelines   X Assign placeholder X   ● Use Additional Character(s)

| Excludes 1 | Excludes 2 | Includes | Use additional | Code first | Code also | Key words |

● **T71   Asphyxiation**
     Mechanical suffocation
     Traumatic suffocation
     Excludes1   acute respiratory distress (syndrome) (J80)
             anoxia due to high altitude (T70.2)
             asphyxia NOS (R09.01)
             asphyxia from carbon monoxide (T58.-)
             asphyxia from inhalation of food or foreign body
               (T17.-)
             asphyxia from other gases, fumes and vapors
               (T59.-)
             respiratory distress (syndrome) in newborn
               (P22.-)

     The appropriate 7th character is to be added to each code from
       category T71

       A   initial encounter
       D   subsequent encounter
       S   sequela

● **T71.1   Asphyxiation due to mechanical threat to breathing**
     Suffocation due to mechanical threat to breathing
    ● **T71.11   Asphyxiation due to smothering under pillow**
       ● **T71.111   Asphyxiation due to smothering
              under pillow, accidental**
              Asphyxiation due to smothering
                 under pillow NOS
       ● **T71.112   Asphyxiation due to smothering
              under pillow, intentional self-harm**
       ● **T71.113   Asphyxiation due to smothering
              under pillow, assault**
       ● **T71.114   Asphyxiation due to smothering
              under pillow, undetermined**
    ● **T71.12   Asphyxiation due to plastic bag**
       ● **T71.121   Asphyxiation due to plastic bag,
              accidental**
              Asphyxiation due to plastic bag
                 NOS
       ● **T71.122   Asphyxiation due to plastic bag,
              intentional self-harm**
       ● **T71.123   Asphyxiation due to plastic bag,
              assault**
       ● **T71.124   Asphyxiation due to plastic bag,
              undetermined**
    ● **T71.13   Asphyxiation due to being trapped in bed
         linens**
       ● **T71.131   Asphyxiation due to being trapped in
              bed linens, accidental**
              Asphyxiation due to being trapped
                 in bed linens NOS
       ● **T71.132   Asphyxiation due to being trapped in
              bed linens, intentional self-harm**
       ● **T71.133   Asphyxiation due to being trapped in
              bed linens, assault**
       ● **T71.134   Asphyxiation due to being trapped in
              bed linens, undetermined**
    ● **T71.14   Asphyxiation due to smothering under another
         person's body (in bed)**
       ● **T71.141   Asphyxiation due to smothering
              under another person's body (in bed),
              accidental**
              Asphyxiation due to smothering
                 under another person's body
                 (in bed) NOS
       ● **T71.143   Asphyxiation due to smothering
              under another person's body (in bed),
              assault**
       ● **T71.144   Asphyxiation due to smothering
              under another person's body (in bed),
              undetermined**

● **T71.15   Asphyxiation due to smothering in furniture**
       ● **T71.151   Asphyxiation due to smothering in
              furniture, accidental**
              Asphyxiation due to smothering in
                 furniture NOS
       ● **T71.152   Asphyxiation due to smothering in
              furniture, intentional self-harm**
       ● **T71.153   Asphyxiation due to smothering in
              furniture, assault**
       ● **T71.154   Asphyxiation due to smothering in
              furniture, undetermined**
● **T71.16   Asphyxiation due to hanging**
     Hanging by window shade cord
     Use additional code for any associated injuries,
       such as:
       crushing injury of neck (S17.-)
       fracture of cervical vertebrae (S12.0-S12.2-)
       open wound of neck (S11.-)
       ● **T71.161   Asphyxiation due to hanging,
              accidental**
              Asphyxiation due to hanging NOS
              Hanging NOS
       ● **T71.162   Asphyxiation due to hanging,
              intentional self-harm**
       ● **T71.163   Asphyxiation due to hanging, assault**
       ● **T71.164   Asphyxiation due to hanging,
              undetermined**
● **T71.19   Asphyxiation due to mechanical**
     Threat to breathing due to other causes
       ● **T71.191   Asphyxiation due to mechanical
              threat to breathing due to other
              causes, accidental**
              Asphyxiation due to other causes
                 NOS
       ● **T71.192   Asphyxiation due to mechanical
              threat to breathing due to other
              causes, intentional self-harm**
       ● **T71.193   Asphyxiation due to mechanical
              threat to breathing due to other
              causes, assault**
       ● **T71.194   Asphyxiation due to mechanical
              threat to breathing due to other
              causes, undetermined**
● **T71.2   Asphyxiation due to systemic oxygen deficiency due to
     low oxygen content in ambient air**
     Suffocation due to systemic oxygen deficiency due to
       low oxygen content in ambient air
X ● **T71.20   Asphyxiation due to systemic oxygen deficiency
       due to low oxygen content in ambient air due to
       unspecified cause**
X ● **T71.21   Asphyxiation due to cave-in or falling earth**
       Use additional code for any associated
         cataclysm (X34-X38)
    ● **T71.22   Asphyxiation due to being trapped in a car
         trunk**
       ● **T71.221   Asphyxiation due to being trapped in
              a car trunk, accidental**
       ● **T71.222   Asphyxiation due to being trapped in
              a car trunk, intentional self-harm**
       ● **T71.223   Asphyxiation due to being trapped in
              a car trunk, assault**
       ● **T71.224   Asphyxiation due to being trapped in
              a car trunk, undetermined**

● **T71.23**   **Asphyxiation due to being trapped in a (discarded) refrigerator**
     ● **T71.231**   **Asphyxiation due to being trapped in a (discarded) refrigerator, accidental**
     ● **T71.232**   **Asphyxiation due to being trapped in a (discarded) refrigerator, intentional self-harm**
     ● **T71.233**   **Asphyxiation due to being trapped in a (discarded) refrigerator, assault**
     ● **T71.234**   **Asphyxiation due to being trapped in a (discarded) refrigerator, undetermined**
   X ● **T71.29**   **Asphyxiation due to being trapped in other low oxygen environment**
X ● **T71.9**   **Asphyxiation due to unspecified cause**
     Suffocation (by strangulation) due to unspecified cause
     Suffocation NOS
     Systemic oxygen deficiency due to low oxygen content in ambient air due to unspecified cause
     Systemic oxygen deficiency due to mechanical threat to breathing due to unspecified cause
     Traumatic asphyxia NOS

● **T73**   **Effects of other deprivation**
     The appropriate 7th character is to be added to each code from category T73

A	initial encounter
D	subsequent encounter
S	sequela

X ● **T73.0**   **Starvation**
     Deprivation of food
X ● **T73.1**   **Deprivation of water**
X ● **T73.2**   **Exhaustion due to exposure**
X ● **T73.3**   **Exhaustion due to excessive exertion**
     Exhaustion due to overexertion
X ● **T73.8**   **Other effects of deprivation**
X ● **T73.9**   **Effect of deprivation, unspecified**

● **T74**   **Adult and child abuse, neglect and other maltreatment, confirmed**
     Use additional code, if applicable, to identify any associated current injury
     Use additional external cause code to identify perpetrator, if known (Y07.-)
     Excludes1   abuse and maltreatment in pregnancy (O9A.3-, O9A.4-, O9A.5-)
          adult and child maltreatment, suspected (T76.-)
     The appropriate 7th character is to be added to each code from category T74

A	initial encounter
D	subsequent encounter
S	sequela

● **T74.0**   **Neglect or abandonment, confirmed**
   X ● **T74.01**   **Adult neglect or abandonment, confirmed**
   X ● **T74.02**   **Child neglect or abandonment, confirmed**
● **T74.1**   **Physical abuse, confirmed**
     Excludes2   sexual abuse (T74.2-)
   X ● **T74.11**   **Adult physical abuse, confirmed**
   X ● **T74.12**   **Child physical abuse, confirmed**
        Excludes2   shaken infant syndrome (T74.4)

● **T74.2**   **Sexual abuse, confirmed**
     Rape, confirmed
     Sexual assault, confirmed
   X ● **T74.21**   **Adult sexual abuse, confirmed**
   X ● **T74.22**   **Child sexual abuse, confirmed**
● **T74.3**   **Psychological abuse, confirmed**
   X ● **T74.31**   **Adult psychological abuse, confirmed**
   X ● **T74.32**   **Child psychological abuse, confirmed**
X ● **T74.4**   **Shaken infant syndrome**
● **T74.9**   **Unspecified maltreatment, confirmed**
   X ● **T74.91**   **Unspecified adult maltreatment, confirmed**
   X ● **T74.92**   **Unspecified child maltreatment, confirmed**

● **T75**   **Other and unspecified effects of other external causes**
     Excludes1   adverse effects NEC (T78.-)
     Excludes2   burns (electric) (T20-T31)
     The appropriate 7th character is to be added to each code from category T75

A	initial encounter
D	subsequent encounter
S	sequela

● **T75.0**   **Effects of lightning**
     Struck by lightning
   X ● **T75.00**   **Unspecified effects of lightning**
     Struck by lightning NOS
   X ● **T75.01**   **Shock due to being struck by lightning**
   X ● **T75.09**   **Other effects of lightning**
     Use additional code for other effects of lightning
X ● **T75.1**   **Unspecified effects of drowning and nonfatal submersion**
     Immersion
     Excludes1   specified effects of drowning code to effects
● **T75.2**   **Effects of vibration**
   X ● **T75.20**   **Unspecified effects of vibration**
   X ● **T75.21**   **Pneumatic hammer syndrome**
   X ● **T75.22**   **Traumatic vasospastic syndrome**
   X ● **T75.23**   **Vertigo from infrasound**
     Excludes1   vertigo NOS (R42)
   X ● **T75.29**   **Other effects of vibration**
X ● **T75.3**   **Motion sickness**
     Airsickness   Travel sickness
     Seasickness
     Use additional external cause code to identify vehicle or type of motion (Y92.81-, Y93.5-)
X ● **T75.4**   **Electrocution**
     Shock from electric current
     Shock from electroshock gun (taser)
● **T75.8**   **Other specified effects of external causes**
   X ● **T75.81**   **Effects of abnormal gravitation [G] forces**
   X ● **T75.82**   **Effects of weightlessness**
   X ● **T75.89**   **Other specified effects of external causes**

● **T76   Adult and child abuse, neglect and other maltreatment, suspected**

> Use additional code, if applicable, to identify any associated current injury

> **Excludes1**   adult and child maltreatment, confirmed (T74.-)
> suspected abuse and maltreatment in pregnancy (O9A.3-, O9A.4-, O9A.5-)
> suspected adult physical abuse, ruled out (Z04.71)
> suspected adult sexual abuse, ruled out (Z04.41)
> suspected child physical abuse, ruled out (Z04.72)
> suspected child sexual abuse, ruled out (Z04.42)

> The appropriate 7th character is to be added to each code from category T76

> A   initial encounter
> D   subsequent encounter
> S   sequela

● **T76.0   Neglect or abandonment, suspected**
X● **T76.01   Adult neglect or abandonment, suspected**
X● **T76.02   Child neglect or abandonment, suspected**

● **T76.1   Physical abuse, suspected**
X● **T76.11   Adult physical abuse, suspected**
X● **T76.12   Child physical abuse, suspected**

● **T76.2   Sexual abuse, suspected**
> Rape, suspected
> ~~Sexual abuse, suspected~~
> **Excludes1**   alleged abuse, ruled out (Z04.7)
X● **T76.21   Adult sexual abuse, suspected**
X● **T76.22   Child sexual abuse, suspected**

● **T76.3   Psychological abuse, suspected**
X● **T76.31   Adult psychological abuse, suspected**
X● **T76.32   Child psychological abuse, suspected**

● **T76.9   Unspecified maltreatment, suspected**
X● **T76.91   Unspecified adult maltreatment, suspected**
X● **T76.92   Unspecified child maltreatment, suspected**

● **T78   Adverse effects, not elsewhere classified**
> **Excludes2**   complications of surgical and medical care NEC (T80-T88)

> The appropriate 7th character is to be added to each code from category T78

> A   initial encounter
> D   subsequent encounter
> S   sequela

● **T78.0   Anaphylactic reaction due to food**
> Anaphylactic reaction due to adverse food reaction
> Anaphylactic shock or reaction due to nonpoisonous foods
> Anaphylactoid reaction due to food
X● **T78.00   Anaphylactic reaction due to unspecified food**
X● **T78.01   Anaphylactic reaction due to peanuts**
X● **T78.02   Anaphylactic reaction due to shellfish (crustaceans)**
X● **T78.03   Anaphylactic reaction due to other fish**
X● **T78.04   Anaphylactic reaction due to fruits and vegetables**
X● **T78.05   Anaphylactic reaction due to tree nuts and seeds**
> **Excludes2**   anaphylactic reaction due to peanuts (T78.01)
X● **T78.06   Anaphylactic reaction due to food additives**
X● **T78.07   Anaphylactic reaction due to milk and dairy products**
X● **T78.08   Anaphylactic reaction due to eggs**
X● **T78.09   Anaphylactic reaction due to other food products**

X● **T78.1   Other adverse food reactions, not elsewhere classified**
> Use additional code to identify the type of reaction, if applicable
> **Excludes1**   anaphylactic reaction or shock due to adverse food reaction (T78.0-)
> anaphylactic reaction due to food (T78.0-)
> bacterial food borne intoxications (A05.-)
> **Excludes2**   allergic and dietetic gastroenteritis and colitis (K52.29)
> allergic rhinitis due to food (J30.5)
> dermatitis due to food in contact with skin (L23.6, L24.6, L25.4)
> dermatitis due to ingested food (L27.2)
> food protein-induced enterocolitis syndrome (K52.21)
> food protein-induced enteropathy (K52.22)

X● **T78.2   Anaphylactic shock, unspecified**
> *Occurs when allergic response triggers large quantities of histamines, prostaglandins, leukotrienes resulting in systemic vasodilation*
> Allergic shock
> Anaphylactic reaction
> Anaphylaxis
> **Excludes1**   anaphylactic reaction or shock due to adverse effect of correct medicinal substance properly administered (T88.6)
> anaphylactic reaction or shock due to adverse food reaction (T78.0-)
> anaphylactic reaction or shock due to serum (T80.5-)

X● **T78.3   Angioneurotic edema**
> Allergic angioedema
> Giant urticaria
> *Vascular disorder resulting from abnormalities of autonomic nervous system fibers supplying blood vessels*
> Quincke's edema
> **Excludes1**   serum urticaria (T80.6-)
> urticaria (L50.-)

● **T78.4   Other and unspecified allergy**
> **Excludes1**   specified types of allergic reaction such as:
> allergic diarrhea (K52.29)
> allergic gastroenteritis and colitis (K52.29)
> dermatitis (L23-L25, L27.-)
> food protein-induced enterocolitis syndrome (K52.21)
> food protein-induced enteropathy (K52.22)
> hay fever (J30.1)
X● **T78.40   Allergy, unspecified**
> Allergic reaction NOS
> Hypersensitivity NOS
X● **T78.41   Arthus phenomenon**
> Arthus reaction
X● **T78.49   Other allergy**
X● **T78.8   Other adverse effects, not elsewhere classified**

CHAPTER 19 (S00-T88)

CERTAIN EARLY COMPLICATIONS OF TRAUMA (T79)

● **T79** **Certain early complications of trauma, not elsewhere classified**

Excludes2   acute respiratory distress syndrome (J80)
complications occurring during or following medical procedures (T80-T88)
complications of surgical and medical care NEC (T80-T88)
newborn respiratory distress syndrome (P22.0)

The appropriate 7th character is to be added to each code from category T79

> A   initial encounter
> D   subsequent encounter
> S   sequela

X ● **T79.0** **Air embolism (traumatic)**

Excludes1   air embolism complicating abortion or ectopic or molar pregnancy (O00-O07, O08.2)
air embolism complicating pregnancy, childbirth and the puerperium (O88.0)
air embolism following infusion, transfusion, and therapeutic injection (T80.0)
air embolism following procedure NEC (T81.7-)

X ● **T79.1** **Fat embolism (traumatic)**

Excludes1   fat embolism complicating:
abortion or ectopic or molar pregnancy (O00-O07, O08.2)
pregnancy, childbirth and the puerperium (O88.8)

X ● **T79.2** **Traumatic secondary and recurrent hemorrhage and seroma**

X ● **T79.4** **Traumatic shock**
Shock (immediate) (delayed) following injury

Excludes1   anaphylactic shock due to adverse food reaction (T78.0-)
anaphylactic shock due to correct medicinal substance properly administered (T88.6)
anaphylactic shock due to serum (T80.5-)
anaphylactic shock NOS (T78.2)
anesthetic shock (T88.2)
electric shock (T75.4)
nontraumatic shock NEC (R57.-)
obstetric shock (O75.1)
postprocedural shock (T81.1-)
septic shock (R65.21)
shock complicating abortion or ectopic or molar pregnancy (O00-O07, O08.3)
shock due to lightning (T75.01)
shock NOS (R57.9)

X ● **T79.5** **Traumatic anuria**
Crush syndrome
Renal failure following crushing

X ● **T79.6** **Traumatic ischemia of muscle**
Traumatic rhabdomyolysis
Volkmann's ischemic contracture

Excludes2   anterior tibial syndrome (M76.8)
compartment syndrome (traumatic) (T79.A-)
nontraumatic ischemia of muscle (M62.2-)

X ● **T79.7** **Traumatic subcutaneous emphysema**

Excludes1   emphysema NOS (J43)
emphysema (subcutaneous) resulting from a procedure (T81.82)

● **T79.A** **Traumatic compartment syndrome**

Excludes1   fibromyalgia (M79.7)
nontraumatic compartment syndrome (M79.A-)
traumatic ischemic infarction of muscle (T79.6)

X ● **T79.A0** **Compartment syndrome, unspecified**
Compartment syndrome NOS

● **T79.A1** **Traumatic compartment syndrome of upper extremity**
Traumatic compartment syndrome of shoulder, arm, forearm, wrist, hand, and fingers

● **T79.A11** Traumatic compartment syndrome of right upper extremity

● **T79.A12** Traumatic compartment syndrome of left upper extremity

● **T79.A19** Traumatic compartment syndrome of unspecified upper extremity

● **T79.A2** **Traumatic compartment syndrome of lower extremity**
Traumatic compartment syndrome of hip, buttock, thigh, leg, foot, and toes

● **T79.A21** Traumatic compartment syndrome of right lower extremity

● **T79.A22** Traumatic compartment syndrome of left lower extremity

● **T79.A29** Traumatic compartment syndrome of unspecified lower extremity

X ● **T79.A3** **Traumatic compartment syndrome of abdomen**

X ● **T79.A9** **Traumatic compartment syndrome of other sites**

X ● **T79.8** **Other early complications of trauma**

X ● **T79.9** **Unspecified early complication of trauma**

▶ New   ⇒ Revised   deleted Deleted   **OGCR** Official Guidelines   X Assign placeholder X   ● Use Additional Character(s)

Excludes 1   Excludes 2   Includes   Use additional   Code first   Code also   Key words

COMPLICATIONS OF SURGICAL AND MEDICAL CARE NOT ELSEWHERE CLASSIFIED (T80-T88)

Use additional code for adverse effect, if applicable, to identify drug (T36-T50 with fifth or sixth character 5)

Use additional code(s) to identify the specified condition resulting from the complication.

Use additional code to identify devices involved and details of circumstances (Y62-Y82)

Excludes2   any encounters with medical care for postprocedural conditions in which no complications are present, such as:
 artificial opening status (Z93.-)
 closure of external stoma (Z43.-)
 fitting and adjustment of external prosthetic device (Z44.-)
 burns and corrosions from local applications and irradiation (T20-T32)
 complications of surgical procedures during pregnancy, childbirth and the puerperium (O00-O9A)
 mechanical complication of respirator [ventilator] (J95.850)
 poisoning and toxic effects of drugs and chemicals (T36-T65 with fifth or sixth character 1-4 or 6)
 postprocedural fever (R50.82)
 specified complications classified elsewhere, such as:
  cerebrospinal fluid leak from spinal puncture (G97.0)
  colostomy malfunction (K94.0-)
  disorders of fluid and electrolyte imbalance (E86-E87)
  functional disturbances following cardiac surgery (I97.0-I97.1)
  intraoperative and postprocedural complications of specified body systems (D78.-, E36.-, E89.-, G97.3-, G97.4, H59.3-, H59.-, H95.2-, H95.3, I97.4-, I97.5, J95.6-, J95.7, K91.6-, L76.-, M96.-, N99.-)
  ostomy complications (J95.0-, K94.-, N99.5-)
  postgastric surgery syndromes (K91.1)
  postlaminectomy syndrome NEC (M96.1)
  postmastectomy lymphedema syndrome (I97.2)
  postsurgical blind-loop syndrome (K91.2)
  ventilator associated pneumonia (J95.851)

● T80   Complications following infusion, transfusion and therapeutic injection

 Includes   complications following perfusion
 Excludes2   bone marrow transplant rejection (T86.01)
 febrile nonhemolytic transfusion reaction (R50.84)
 fluid overload due to transfusion (E87.71)
 posttransfusion purpura (D69.51)
 transfusion associated circulatory overload (TACO) (E87.71)
 transfusion (red blood cell) associated hemochromatosis (E83.111)
 transfusion related acute lung injury (TRALI) (J95.84)

The appropriate 7th character is to be added to each code from category T80

A	initial encounter
D	subsequent encounter
S	sequela

X ● T80.0   Air embolism following infusion, transfusion and therapeutic injection

X ● T80.1   Vascular complications following infusion, transfusion and therapeutic injection
 Use additional code to identify the vascular complication
 Excludes2   extravasation of vesicant agent (T80.81-)
 infiltration of vesicant agent (T80.81-)
 vascular complications specified as due to prosthetic devices, implants and grafts (T82.8- T83.8-, T84.8-, T85.8-)
 postprocedural vascular complications (T81.7-)

● T80.2   Infections following infusion, transfusion and therapeutic injection
 Use additional code to identify the specific infection, such as:
  sepsis (A41.9)
 Use additional code (R65.2-) to identify severe sepsis, if applicable
 Excludes2   infections specified as due to prosthetic devices, implants and grafts (T82.6-T82.7, T83.5-T83.6, T84.5-T84.7, T85.7)
 postprocedural infections (T81.4-)

● T80.21   Infection due to central venous catheter
 Infection due to pulmonary artery catheter (Swan-Ganz catheter)

● T80.211   Bloodstream infection due to central venous catheter
 Catheter-related bloodstream infection (CRBSI) NOS
 Central line-associated bloodstream infection (CLABSI)
 Bloodstream infection due to Hickman catheter
 Bloodstream infection due to peripherally inserted central catheter (PICC)
 Bloodstream infection due to portacath (port-a-cath)
 Bloodstream infection due to pulmonary artery catheter
 Bloodstream infection due to triple lumen catheter
 Bloodstream infection due to umbilical venous catheter

● T80.212   Local infection due to central venous catheter
 Exit or insertion site infection
 Local infection due to Hickman catheter
 Local infection due to peripherally inserted central catheter (PICC)
 Local infection due to portacath (port-a-cath)
 Local infection due to pulmonary artery catheter
 Local infection due to triple lumen catheter
 Local infection due to umbilical venous catheter
 Port or reservoir infection
 Tunnel infection

● T80.218   Other infection due to central venous catheter
 Other central line-associated infection
 Other infection due to Hickman catheter
 Other infection due to peripherally inserted central catheter (PICC)
 Other infection due to portacath (port-a-cath)
 Other infection due to pulmonary artery catheter
 Other infection due to triple lumen catheter
 Other infection due to umbilical venous catheter

CHAPTER 19 (S00-T88)

● **T80.219**   **Unspecified infection due to central venous catheter**
Central line-associated infection NOS
Unspecified infection due to Hickman catheter
Unspecified infection due to peripherally inserted central catheter (PICC)
Unspecified infection due to portacath (port-a-cath)
Unspecified infection due to pulmonary artery catheter
Unspecified infection due to triple lumen catheter
Unspecified infection due to umbilical venous catheter

X● **T80.22**   **Acute infection following transfusion, infusion, or injection of blood and blood products**

X● **T80.29**   **Infection following other infusion, transfusion and therapeutic injection**

● **T80.3**   **ABO incompatibility reaction due to transfusion of blood or blood products**
> **Excludes1**   minor blood group antigens reactions (Duffy) (E) (K(ell)) (Kidd) (Lewis) (M) (N) (P) (S) (T80.A)

X● **T80.30**   **ABO incompatibility reaction due to transfusion of blood or blood products, unspecified**
ABO incompatibility blood transfusion NOS
Reaction to ABO incompatibility from transfusion NOS

● **T80.31**   **ABO incompatibility with hemolytic transfusion reaction**

● **T80.310**   **ABO incompatibility with acute hemolytic transfusion reaction**
ABO incompatibility with hemolytic transfusion reaction less than 24 hours after transfusion
Acute hemolytic transfusion reaction (AHTR) due to ABO incompatibility

● **T80.311**   **ABO incompatibility with delayed hemolytic transfusion reaction**
ABO incompatibility with hemolytic transfusion reaction 24 hours or more after transfusion
Delayed hemolytic transfusion reaction (DHTR) due to ABO incompatibility

● **T80.319**   **ABO incompatibility with hemolytic transfusion reaction, unspecified**
ABO incompatibility with hemolytic transfusion reaction at unspecified time after transfusion
Hemolytic transfusion reaction (HTR) due to ABO incompatibility NOS

X● **T80.39**   **Other ABO incompatibility reaction due to transfusion of blood or blood products**
Delayed serologic transfusion reaction (DSTR) from ABO incompatibility
Other ABO incompatible blood transfusion
Other reaction to ABO incompatible blood transfusion

● **T80.4**   **Rh incompatibility reaction due to transfusion of blood or blood products**
Reaction due to incompatibility of Rh antigens (C) (c) (D) (E) (e)

X● **T80.40**   **Rh incompatibility reaction due to transfusion of blood or blood products, unspecified**
Reaction due to Rh factor in transfusion NOS
Rh incompatible blood transfusion NOS

● **T80.41**   **Rh incompatibility with hemolytic transfusion reaction**

● **T80.410**   **Rh incompatibility with acute hemolytic transfusion reaction**
Acute hemolytic transfusion reaction (AHTR) due to Rh incompatibility
Rh incompatibility with hemolytic transfusion reaction less than 24 hours after transfusion

● **T80.411**   **Rh incompatibility with delayed hemolytic transfusion reaction**
Delayed hemolytic transfusion reaction (DHTR) due to Rh incompatibility
Rh incompatibility with hemolytic transfusion reaction 24 hours or more after transfusion

● **T80.419**   **Rh incompatibility with hemolytic transfusion reaction, unspecified**
Rh incompatibility with hemolytic transfusion reaction at unspecified time after transfusion
Hemolytic transfusion reaction (HTR) due to Rh incompatibility NOS

X● **T80.49**   **Other Rh incompatibility reaction due to transfusion of blood or blood products**
Delayed serologic transfusion reaction (DSTR) from Rh incompatibility
Other reaction to Rh incompatible blood transfusion

● **T80.A**   **Non-ABO incompatibility reaction due to transfusion of blood or blood products**
Reaction due to incompatibility of minor antigens (Duffy) (Kell) (Kidd) (Lewis) (M) (N) (P) (S)

X● **T80.A0**   **Non-ABO incompatibility reaction due to transfusion of blood or blood products, unspecified**
Non-ABO antigen incompatibility reaction from transfusion NOS

● **T80.A1**   **Non-ABO incompatibility with hemolytic transfusion reaction**

● **T80.A10**   **Non-ABO incompatibility with acute hemolytic transfusion reaction**
Acute hemolytic transfusion reaction (AHTR) due to non-ABO incompatibility
Non-ABO incompatibility with hemolytic transfusion reaction less than 24 hours after transfusion

● **T80.A11**   **Non-ABO incompatibility with delayed hemolytic transfusion reaction**
Delayed hemolytic transfusion reaction (DHTR) due to non-ABO incompatibility
Non-ABO incompatibility with hemolytic transfusion reaction 24 or more hours after transfusion

● **T80.A19**   **Non-ABO incompatibility with hemolytic transfusion reaction, unspecified**
Hemolytic transfusion reaction (HTR) due to non-ABO incompatibility NOS
Non-ABO incompatibility with hemolytic transfusion reaction at unspecified time after transfusion

X● **T80.A9**   **Other non-ABO incompatibility reaction due to transfusion of blood or blood products**
Delayed serologic transfusion reaction (DSTR) from non-ABO incompatibility
Other reaction to non-ABO incompatible blood transfusion

▶ New   ⇒ Revised   ~~deleted~~ Deleted   **OGCR** Official Guidelines   X Assign placeholder X   ● Use Additional Character(s)

Excludes 1   Excludes 2   Includes   Use additional   Code first   Code also   Key words

● **T80.5**   **Anaphylactic reaction due to serum**
    Allergic reaction due to serum
    Anaphylactic shock due to serum
    Anaphylactoid reaction due to serum
    Anaphylaxis due to serum

> **Excludes1**   ABO incompatibility reaction due to
>   transfusion of blood or blood
>   products (T80.3-)
>   allergic reaction or shock NOS (T78.2)
>   anaphylactic reaction or shock NOS
>   (T78.2)
>   anaphylactic reaction or shock due to
>   adverse effect of correct medicinal
>   substance properly administered
>   (T88.6)
>   other serum reaction (T80.6-)

X ● **T80.51**   **Anaphylactic reaction due to administration of blood and blood products**

X ● **T80.52**   **Anaphylactic reaction due to vaccination**

X ● **T80.59**   **Anaphylactic reaction due to other serum**

● **T80.6**   **Other serum reactions**
    Intoxication by serum   Serum sickness
    Protein sickness   Serum urticaria
    Serum rash

> **Excludes2**   serum hepatitis (B16-B19)

X ● **T80.61**   **Other serum reaction due to administration of blood and blood products**

X ● **T80.62**   **Other serum reaction due to vaccination**

X ● **T80.69**   **Other serum reaction due to other serum**

> ▶ Code also, if applicable, arthropathy in
>   hypersensitivity reactions classified
>   elsewhere (M36.4)

● **T80.8**   **Other complications following infusion, transfusion and therapeutic injection**

   ● **T80.81**   **Extravasation of vesicant agent**
      Infiltration of vesicant agent

     ● **T80.810**   **Extravasation of vesicant antineoplastic chemotherapy**
       Infiltration of vesicant antineoplastic chemotherapy

     ● **T80.818**   **Extravasation of other vesicant agent**
       Infiltration of other vesicant agent

X ● **T80.89**   **Other complications following infusion, transfusion and therapeutic injection**
    Delayed serologic transfusion reaction (DSTR), unspecified incompatibility

> Use additional code to identify graft-versus-host reaction, if applicable, (D89.81-)

● **T80.9**   **Unspecified complication following infusion, transfusion and therapeutic injection**

X ● **T80.90**   **Unspecified complication following infusion and therapeutic injection**

   ● **T80.91**   **Hemolytic transfusion reaction, unspecified incompatibility**

> **Excludes1**   ABO incompatibility with
>   hemolytic transfusion
>   reaction (T80.31-)
>   Non-ABO incompatibility with
>   hemolytic transfusion
>   reaction (T80.A1-)
>   Rh incompatibility with
>   hemolytic transfusion
>   reaction (T80.41-)

     ● **T80.910**   **Acute hemolytic transfusion reaction, unspecified incompatibility**

     ● **T80.911**   **Delayed hemolytic transfusion reaction, unspecified incompatibility**

     ● **T80.919**   **Hemolytic transfusion reaction, unspecified incompatibility, unspecified as acute or delayed**
       Hemolytic transfusion reaction NOS

X ● **T80.92**   **Unspecified transfusion reaction**
    Transfusion reaction NOS

● **T81**   **Complications of procedures, not elsewhere classified**

> Use additional code for adverse effect, if applicable, to identify drug (T36-T50 with fifth or sixth character 5)

> **Excludes2**   complications following immunization
>   (T88.0-T88.1)
>   complications following infusion, transfusion and
>   therapeutic injection (T80.-)
>   complications of transplanted organs and tissue
>   (T86.-)
>   poisoning and toxic effects of drugs and
>   chemicals (T36-T65 with fifth or sixth
>   character 1-4 or 6)
>   specified complications classified elsewhere, such
>   as:
>   complication of prosthetic devices, implants
>   and grafts (T82-T85)
>   dermatitis due to drugs and medicaments
>   (L23.3, L24.4, L25.1, L27.0-L27.1)
>   endosseous dental implant failure (M27.6-)
>   floppy iris syndrome (IFIS) (intraoperative)
>   H21.81
>   intraoperative and postprocedural
>   complications of specific body system
>   (D78.-, E36.-, E89.-, G97.3-, G97.4, H59.3-,
>   H59.-, H95.2-, H95.3, I97.4-, I97.5, J95,
>   K91.-, L76.-, M96.-, N99.-)
>   ostomy complications (J95.0-, K94.-, N99.5-)
>   plateau iris syndrome (post-iridectomy)
>   (postprocedural) H21.82

The appropriate 7th character is to be added to each code from category T81

A	initial encounter
D	subsequent encounter
S	sequela

● **T81.1**   **Postprocedural shock**
    Shock during or resulting from a procedure, not elsewhere classified

> **Excludes1**   anaphylactic shock NOS (T78.2)
>   anaphylactic shock due to correct
>   substance properly administered
>   (T88.6)
>   anaphylactic shock due to serum (T80.5-)
>   anesthetic shock (T88.2)
>   electric shock (T75.4)
>   obstetric shock (O75.1)
>   septic shock (R65.21)
>   shock following abortion or ectopic or
>   molar pregnancy (O00-O07, O08.3)
>   traumatic shock (T79.4)

X ● **T81.10**   **Postprocedural shock unspecified**
    Collapse NOS during or resulting from a procedure, not elsewhere classified
    Postprocedural failure of peripheral circulation
    Postprocedural shock NOS

X ● **T81.11**   **Postprocedural cardiogenic shock**

X ● **T81.12**   **Postprocedural septic shock**
    Postprocedural endotoxic shock resulting from a procedure, not elsewhere classified
    Postprocedural gram-negative shock resulting from a procedure, not elsewhere classified

> *Code first underlying infection*

> Use additional code, to identify any associated acute organ dysfunction, if applicable

X ● **T81.19**   **Other postprocedural shock**
    Postprocedural hypovolemic shock

● **T81.3**   **Disruption of wound, not elsewhere classified**
Disruption of any suture materials or other closure methods

> **Excludes1**   breakdown (mechanical) of permanent sutures (T85.612)
> displacement of permanent sutures (T85.622)
> disruption of cesarean delivery wound (O90.0)
> disruption of perineal obstetric wound (O90.1)
> mechanical complication of permanent sutures NEC (T85.692)

X● **T81.30**   **Disruption of wound, unspecified**
Disruption of wound NOS

X● **T81.31**   **Disruption of external operation (surgical) wound, not elsewhere classified**

> **Excludes1**   dehiscence of amputation stump (T87.81)

Dehiscence of operation wound NOS
Disruption of operation wound NOS
Disruption or dehiscence of closure of cornea
Disruption or dehiscence of closure of mucosa
Disruption or dehiscence of closure of skin and subcutaneous tissue
Full-thickness skin disruption or dehiscence
Superficial disruption or dehiscence of operation wound

X● **T81.32**   **Disruption of internal operation (surgical) wound, not elsewhere classified**
Deep disruption or dehiscence of operation wound NOS
Disruption or dehiscence of closure of internal organ or other internal tissue
Disruption or dehiscence of closure of muscle or muscle flap
Disruption or dehiscence of closure of ribs or rib cage
Disruption or dehiscence of closure of skull or craniotomy
Disruption or dehiscence of closure of sternum or sternotomy
Disruption or dehiscence of closure of tendon or ligament
Disruption or dehiscence of closure of superficial or muscular fascia

X● **T81.33**   **Disruption of traumatic injury wound repair**
Disruption or dehiscence of closure of traumatic laceration (external) (internal)

X● **T81.4**   **Infection following a procedure**
Intra-abdominal abscess following a procedure
Postprocedural infection, not elsewhere classified
Sepsis following a procedure
Stitch abscess following a procedure
Subphrenic abscess following a procedure
Wound abscess following a procedure

Use additional code to identify infection
Use additional code (R65.2-) to identify severe sepsis, if applicable

> **Excludes1**   obstetric surgical wound infection (O86.0)
> postprocedural fever NOS (R50.82)
> postprocedural retroperitoneal abscess (K68.11)

> **Excludes2**   bleb associated endophthalmitis (H59.4-)
> infection due to infusion, transfusion and therapeutic injection (T80.2-)
> infection due to prosthetic devices, implants and grafts (T82.6-T82.7, T83.5-T83.6, T84.5-T84.7, T85.7)

● **T81.5**   **Complications of foreign body accidentally left in body following procedure**

● **T81.50**   **Unspecified complication of foreign body accidentally left in body following procedure**

● **T81.500**   Unspecified complication of foreign body accidentally left in body following surgical operation

● **T81.501**   Unspecified complication of foreign body accidentally left in body following infusion or transfusion

● **T81.502**   Unspecified complication of foreign body accidentally left in body following kidney dialysis

● **T81.503**   Unspecified complication of foreign body accidentally left in body following injection or immunization

● **T81.504**   Unspecified complication of foreign body accidentally left in body following endoscopic examination

● **T81.505**   Unspecified complication of foreign body accidentally left in body following heart catheterization

● **T81.506**   Unspecified complication of foreign body accidentally left in body following aspiration, puncture or other catheterization

● **T81.507**   Unspecified complication of foreign body accidentally left in body following removal of catheter or packing

● **T81.508**   Unspecified complication of foreign body accidentally left in body following other procedure

● **T81.509**   Unspecified complication of foreign body accidentally left in body following unspecified procedure

● **T81.51**   **Adhesions due to foreign body accidentally left in body following procedure**

● **T81.510**   Adhesions due to foreign body accidentally left in body following surgical operation

● **T81.511**   Adhesions due to foreign body accidentally left in body following infusion or transfusion

● **T81.512**   Adhesions due to foreign body accidentally left in body following kidney dialysis

● **T81.513**   Adhesions due to foreign body accidentally left in body following injection or immunization

● **T81.514**   Adhesions due to foreign body accidentally left in body following endoscopic examination

● **T81.515**   Adhesions due to foreign body accidentally left in body following heart catheterization

● **T81.516**   Adhesions due to foreign body accidentally left in body following aspiration, puncture or other catheterization

● **T81.517**   Adhesions due to foreign body accidentally left in body following removal of catheter or packing

● **T81.518**   Adhesions due to foreign body accidentally left in body following other procedure

● **T81.519**   Adhesions due to foreign body accidentally left in body following unspecified procedure

● **T81.52** **Obstruction** due to foreign body accidentally left in body following procedure
  ● **T81.520** Obstruction due to foreign body accidentally left in body following surgical operation
  ● **T81.521** Obstruction due to foreign body accidentally left in body following infusion or transfusion
  ● **T81.522** Obstruction due to foreign body accidentally left in body following kidney dialysis
  ● **T81.523** Obstruction due to foreign body accidentally left in body following injection or immunization
  ● **T81.524** Obstruction due to foreign body accidentally left in body following endoscopic examination
  ● **T81.525** Obstruction due to foreign body accidentally left in body following heart catheterization
  ● **T81.526** Obstruction due to foreign body accidentally left in body following aspiration, puncture or other catheterization
  ● **T81.527** Obstruction due to foreign body accidentally left in body following removal of catheter or packing
  ● **T81.528** Obstruction due to foreign body accidentally left in body following other procedure
  ● **T81.529** Obstruction due to foreign body accidentally left in body following unspecified procedure
● **T81.53** **Perforation** due to foreign body accidentally left in body following procedure
  ● **T81.530** Perforation due to foreign body accidentally left in body following surgical operation
  ● **T81.531** Perforation due to foreign body accidentally left in body following infusion or transfusion
  ● **T81.532** Perforation due to foreign body accidentally left in body following kidney dialysis
  ● **T81.533** Perforation due to foreign body accidentally left in body following injection or immunization
  ● **T81.534** Perforation due to foreign body accidentally left in body following endoscopic examination
  ● **T81.535** Perforation due to foreign body accidentally left in body following heart catheterization
  ● **T81.536** Perforation due to foreign body accidentally left in body following aspiration, puncture or other catheterization
  ● **T81.537** Perforation due to foreign body accidentally left in body following removal of catheter or packing
  ● **T81.538** Perforation due to foreign body accidentally left in body following other procedure
  ● **T81.539** Perforation due to foreign body accidentally left in body following unspecified procedure

● **T81.59** **Other** complications of foreign body accidentally left in body following procedure
  Excludes2 obstruction or perforation due to prosthetic devices and implants intentionally left in body (T82.0-T82.5, T83.0-T83.4, T83.7, T84.0-T84.4, T85.0-T85.6)
  ● **T81.590** Other complications of foreign body accidentally left in body following surgical operation
  ● **T81.591** Other complications of foreign body accidentally left in body following infusion or transfusion
  ● **T81.592** Other complications of foreign body accidentally left in body following kidney dialysis
  ● **T81.593** Other complications of foreign body accidentally left in body following injection or immunization
  ● **T81.594** Other complications of foreign body accidentally left in body following endoscopic examination
  ● **T81.595** Other complications of foreign body accidentally left in body following heart catheterization
  ● **T81.596** Other complications of foreign body accidentally left in body following aspiration, puncture or other catheterization
  ● **T81.597** Other complications of foreign body accidentally left in body following removal of catheter or packing
  ● **T81.598** Other complications of foreign body accidentally left in body following other procedure
  ● **T81.599** Other complications of foreign body accidentally left in body following unspecified procedure
● **T81.6** **Acute** reaction to foreign substance accidentally left during a procedure
  Excludes2 complications of foreign body accidentally left in body cavity or operation wound following procedure (T81.5-)
 X ● **T81.60** **Unspecified** acute reaction to foreign substance accidentally left during a procedure
 X ● **T81.61** **Aseptic** peritonitis due to foreign substance accidentally left during a procedure
   Chemical peritonitis
 X ● **T81.69** **Other** acute reaction to foreign substance accidentally left during a procedure

▶ New ⇒ Revised ~~deleted~~ Deleted **OGCR** Official Guidelines X Assign placeholder X ● Use Additional Character(s)

Excludes 1 Excludes 2 Includes Use additional Code first Code also Key words

1391

CHAPTER 19 (S00–T88)

● **T81.7**   **Vascular complications following a procedure, not elsewhere classified**
Air embolism following procedure NEC
Phlebitis or thrombophlebitis resulting from a procedure

> **Excludes1**   embolism complicating abortion or ectopic or molar pregnancy (O00-O07, O08.2)
> embolism complicating pregnancy, childbirth and the puerperium (O88.-)
> traumatic embolism (T79.0)

> **Excludes2**   embolism due to prosthetic devices, implants and grafts (T82.8, T83.81, T84.8-, T85.1-)
> embolism following infusion, transfusion and therapeutic injection (T80.0)

  ● **T81.71**   **Complication of artery following a procedure, not elsewhere classified**

    ● **T81.710**   **Complication of mesenteric artery following a procedure, not elsewhere classified**

    ● **T81.711**   **Complication of renal artery following a procedure, not elsewhere classified**

    ● **T81.718**   **Complication of other artery following a procedure, not elsewhere classified**

    ● **T81.719**   **Complication of unspecified artery following a procedure, not elsewhere classified**

  X● **T81.72**   **Complication of vein following a procedure, not elsewhere classified**

● **T81.8**   **Other complications of procedures, not elsewhere classified**

> **Excludes2**   hypothermia following anesthesia (T88.51)
> malignant hyperpyrexia due to anesthesia (T88.3)

  X● **T81.81**   **Complication of inhalation therapy**

  X● **T81.82**   **Emphysema (subcutaneous) resulting from a procedure**

  X● **T81.83**   **Persistent postprocedural fistula**

  X● **T81.89**   **Other complications of procedures, not elsewhere classified**
Use additional code to specify complication, such as:
postprocedural delirium (F05)

X● **T81.9**   **Unspecified complication of procedure**

● **T82**   **Complications of cardiac and vascular prosthetic devices, implants and grafts**

> **Excludes2**   failure and rejection of transplanted organs and tissue (T86.-)

The appropriate 7th character is to be added to each code from category T82

> A   initial encounter
> D   subsequent encounter
> S   sequela

  ● **T82.0**   **Mechanical complication of heart valve prosthesis**
Mechanical complication of artificial heart valve

> **Excludes1**   mechanical complication of biological heart valve graft (T82.22-)

  X● **T82.01**   **Breakdown (mechanical) of heart valve prosthesis**

  X● **T82.02**   **Displacement of heart valve prosthesis**
Malposition of heart valve prosthesis

  X● **T82.03**   **Leakage of heart valve prosthesis**

  X● **T82.09**   **Other mechanical complication of heart valve prosthesis**
Obstruction (mechanical) of heart valve prosthesis
Perforation of heart valve prosthesis
Protrusion of heart valve prosthesis

● **T82.1**   **Mechanical complication of cardiac electronic device**

  ● **T82.11**   **Breakdown (mechanical) of cardiac electronic device**

    ● **T82.110**   **Breakdown (mechanical) of cardiac electrode**

    ● **T82.111**   **Breakdown (mechanical) of cardiac pulse generator (battery)**

    ● **T82.118**   **Breakdown (mechanical) of other cardiac electronic device**

    ● **T82.119**   **Breakdown (mechanical) of unspecified cardiac electronic device**

  ● **T82.12**   **Displacement of cardiac electronic device**
Malposition of cardiac electronic device

    ● **T82.120**   **Displacement of cardiac electrode**

    ● **T82.121**   **Displacement of cardiac pulse generator (battery)**

    ● **T82.128**   **Displacement of other cardiac electronic device**

    ● **T82.129**   **Displacement of unspecified cardiac electronic device**

  ● **T82.19**   **Other mechanical complication of cardiac electronic device**
Leakage of cardiac electronic device
Obstruction of cardiac electronic device
Perforation of cardiac electronic device
Protrusion of cardiac electronic device

    ● **T82.190**   **Other mechanical complication of cardiac electrode**

    ● **T82.191**   **Other mechanical complication of cardiac pulse generator (battery)**

    ● **T82.198**   **Other mechanical complication of other cardiac electronic device**

    ● **T82.199**   **Other mechanical complication of unspecified cardiac device**

● **T82.2**   **Mechanical complication of coronary artery bypass graft and biological heart valve graft**

> **Excludes1**   mechanical complication of artificial heart valve prosthesis (T82.0-)

  ● **T82.21**   **Mechanical complication of coronary artery bypass graft**

    ● **T82.211**   **Breakdown (mechanical) of coronary artery bypass graft**

    ● **T82.212**   **Displacement of coronary artery bypass graft**
Malposition of coronary artery bypass graft

    ● **T82.213**   **Leakage of coronary artery bypass graft**

    ● **T82.218**   **Other mechanical complication of coronary artery bypass graft**
Obstruction, mechanical of coronary artery bypass graft
Perforation of coronary artery bypass graft
Protrusion of coronary artery bypass graft

  ● **T82.22**   **Mechanical complication of biological heart valve graft**

    ● **T82.221**   **Breakdown (mechanical) of biological heart valve graft**

    ● **T82.222**   **Displacement of biological heart valve graft**
Malposition of biological heart valve graft

    ● **T82.223**   **Leakage of biological heart valve graft**

    ● **T82.228**   **Other mechanical complication of biological heart valve graft**
Obstruction of biological heart valve graft
Perforation of biological heart valve graft
Protrusion of biological heart valve graft

▶ New   ⟹ Revised   ~~deleted~~ Deleted   **OGCR** Official Guidelines   X Assign placeholder X   ● Use Additional Character(s)

Excludes 1   Excludes 2   Includes   Use additional   Code first   Code also   Key words

- ● T82.3   Mechanical complication of other vascular grafts
  - ● T82.31   Breakdown (mechanical) of other vascular grafts
    - ● T82.310   Breakdown (mechanical) of aortic (bifurcation) graft (replacement)
    - ● T82.311   Breakdown (mechanical) of carotid arterial graft (bypass)
    - ● T82.312   Breakdown (mechanical) of femoral arterial graft (bypass)
    - ● T82.318   Breakdown (mechanical) of other vascular grafts
    - ● T82.319   Breakdown (mechanical) of unspecified vascular grafts
  - ● T82.32   Displacement of other vascular grafts
    - Malposition of other vascular grafts
    - ● T82.320   Displacement of aortic (bifurcation) graft (replacement)
    - ● T82.321   Displacement of carotid arterial graft (bypass)
    - ● T82.322   Displacement of femoral arterial graft (bypass)
    - ● T82.328   Displacement of other vascular grafts
    - ● T82.329   Displacement of unspecified vascular grafts
  - ● T82.33   Leakage of other vascular grafts
    - ● T82.330   Leakage of aortic (bifurcation) graft (replacement)
    - ● T82.331   Leakage of carotid arterial graft (bypass)
    - ● T82.332   Leakage of femoral arterial graft (bypass)
    - ● T82.338   Leakage of other vascular grafts
    - ● T82.339   Leakage of unspecified vascular graft
  - ● T82.39   Other mechanical complication of other vascular grafts
    - Obstruction (mechanical) of other vascular grafts
    - Perforation of other vascular grafts
    - Protrusion of other vascular grafts
    - ● T82.390   Other mechanical complication of aortic (bifurcation) graft (replacement)
    - ● T82.391   Other mechanical complication of carotid arterial graft (bypass)
    - ● T82.392   Other mechanical complication of femoral arterial graft (bypass)
    - ● T82.398   Other mechanical complication of other vascular grafts
    - ● T82.399   Other mechanical complication of unspecified vascular grafts
- ● T82.4   Mechanical complication of vascular dialysis catheter
  - Mechanical complication of hemodialysis catheter
  - **Excludes1**   mechanical complication of intraperitoneal dialysis catheter (T85.62)
  - X ● T82.41   Breakdown (mechanical) of vascular dialysis catheter
  - X ● T82.42   Displacement of vascular dialysis catheter
    - Malposition of vascular dialysis catheter
  - X ● T82.43   Leakage of vascular dialysis catheter
  - X ● T82.49   Other complication of vascular dialysis catheter
    - Obstruction (mechanical) of vascular dialysis catheter
    - Perforation of vascular dialysis catheter
    - Protrusion of vascular dialysis catheter

- ● T82.5   Mechanical complication of other cardiac and vascular devices and implants
  - **Excludes2**   mechanical complication of epidural and subdural infusion catheter (T85.61)
  - ● T82.51   Breakdown (mechanical) of other cardiac and vascular devices and implants
    - ● T82.510   Breakdown (mechanical) of surgically created arteriovenous fistula
    - ● T82.511   Breakdown (mechanical) of surgically created arteriovenous shunt
    - ● T82.512   Breakdown (mechanical) of artificial heart
    - ● T82.513   Breakdown (mechanical) of balloon (counterpulsation) device
    - ● T82.514   Breakdown (mechanical) of infusion catheter
    - ● T82.515   Breakdown (mechanical) of umbrella device
    - ● T82.518   Breakdown (mechanical) of other cardiac and vascular devices and implants
    - ● T82.519   Breakdown (mechanical) of unspecified cardiac and vascular devices and implants
  - ● T82.52   Displacement of other cardiac and vascular devices and implants
    - Malposition of other cardiac and vascular devices and implants
    - ● T82.520   Displacement of surgically created arteriovenous fistula
    - ● T82.521   Displacement of surgically created arteriovenous shunt
    - ● T82.522   Displacement of artificial heart
    - ● T82.523   Displacement of balloon (counterpulsation) device
    - ● T82.524   Displacement of infusion catheter
    - ● T82.525   Displacement of umbrella device
    - ● T82.528   Displacement of other cardiac and vascular devices and implants
    - ● T82.529   Displacement of unspecified cardiac and vascular devices and implants
  - ● T82.53   Leakage of other cardiac and vascular devices and implants
    - ● T82.530   Leakage of surgically created arteriovenous fistula
    - ● T82.531   Leakage of surgically created arteriovenous shunt
    - ● T82.532   Leakage of artificial heart
    - ● T82.533   Leakage of balloon (counterpulsation) device
    - ● T82.534   Leakage of infusion catheter
    - ● T82.535   Leakage of umbrella device
    - ● T82.538   Leakage of other cardiac and vascular devices and implants
    - ● T82.539   Leakage of unspecified cardiac and vascular devices and implants

● **T82.59** **Other** mechanical complication of other cardiac and vascular devices and implants

Obstruction (mechanical) of other cardiac and vascular devices and implants

Perforation of other cardiac and vascular devices and implants

Protrusion of other cardiac and vascular devices and implants

  ● **T82.590** **Other mechanical complication of surgically created arteriovenous fistula**

  ● **T82.591** **Other mechanical complication of surgically created arteriovenous shunt**

  ● **T82.592** **Other mechanical complication of artificial heart**

  ● **T82.593** **Other mechanical complication of balloon (counterpulsation) device**

  ● **T82.594** **Other mechanical complication of infusion catheter**

  ● **T82.595** **Other mechanical complication of umbrella device**

  ● **T82.598** **Other mechanical complication of other cardiac and vascular devices and implants**

  ● **T82.599** **Other mechanical complication of unspecified cardiac and vascular devices and implants**

X ● **T82.6** Infection and inflammatory reaction due to **cardiac valve prosthesis**

  Use additional code to identify infection

X ● **T82.7** Infection and inflammatory reaction due to **other cardiac and vascular devices, implants and grafts**

  Use additional code to identify infection

● **T82.8** **Other specified complications** of cardiac and vascular prosthetic devices, implants and grafts

  ● **T82.81** **Embolism** due to cardiac and vascular prosthetic devices, implants and grafts

    ● **T82.817** **Embolism due to cardiac prosthetic devices, implants and grafts**

    ● **T82.818** **Embolism due to vascular prosthetic devices, implants and grafts**

  ● **T82.82** **Fibrosis** due to cardiac and vascular prosthetic devices, implants and grafts

    ● **T82.827** **Fibrosis due to cardiac prosthetic devices, implants and grafts**

    ● **T82.828** **Fibrosis due to vascular prosthetic devices, implants and grafts**

  ● **T82.83** **Hemorrhage** due to cardiac and vascular prosthetic devices, implants and grafts

    ● **T82.837** **Hemorrhage due to cardiac prosthetic devices, implants and grafts**

    ● **T82.838** **Hemorrhage due to vascular prosthetic devices, implants and grafts**

  ● **T82.84** **Pain** due to cardiac and vascular prosthetic devices, implants and grafts

    ● **T82.847** **Pain due to cardiac prosthetic devices, implants and grafts**

    ● **T82.848** **Pain due to vascular prosthetic devices, implants and grafts**

● **T82.85** **Stenosis** due to cardiac and vascular prosthetic devices, implants and grafts

  ● **T82.855** **Stenosis of coronary artery stent**

In-stent stenosis (restenosis) of coronary artery stent

Restenosis of coronary artery stent

  ● **T82.856** **Stenosis of peripheral vascular stent**

In-stent stenosis (restenosis) of peripheral vascular stent

Restenosis of peripheral vascular stent

  ● **T82.857** **Stenosis of other cardiac prosthetic devices, implants and grafts**

  ● **T82.858** **Stenosis of other vascular prosthetic devices, implants and grafts**

● **T82.86** **Thrombosis** of cardiac and vascular prosthetic devices, implants and grafts

  ● **T82.867** **Thrombosis due to cardiac prosthetic devices, implants and grafts**

  ● **T82.868** **Thrombosis due to vascular prosthetic devices, implants and grafts**

● **T82.89** **Other specified complication** of cardiac and vascular prosthetic devices, implants and grafts

  ● **T82.897** **Other specified complication of cardiac prosthetic devices, implants and grafts**

  ● **T82.898** **Other specified complication of vascular prosthetic devices, implants and grafts**

X ● **T82.9** **Unspecified** complication of cardiac and vascular prosthetic device, implant and graft

● **T83** Complications of genitourinary prosthetic devices, implants and grafts

  Excludes2   failure and rejection of transplanted organs and tissue (T86.-)

The appropriate 7th character is to be added to each code from category T83

A	initial encounter
D	subsequent encounter
S	sequela

● **T83.0** Mechanical complication of **urinary catheter**

  Excludes2   complications of stoma of urinary tract (N99.5-)

  ● **T83.01** **Breakdown** (mechanical) of urinary catheter

    ● **T83.010** **Breakdown (mechanical) of cystostomy catheter**

    ● **T83.011** **Breakdown (mechanical) of indwelling urethral catheter**

    ● **T83.012** **Breakdown (mechanical) of nephrostomy catheter**

    ● **T83.018** **Breakdown (mechanical) of other urinary catheter**

Breakdown (mechanical) of Hopkins catheter

Breakdown (mechanical) of ileostomy catheter

Breakdown (mechanical) urostomy catheter

▶ New   ⟹ Revised   ~~deleted~~ Deleted   **OGCR** Official Guidelines   X Assign placeholder X   ● Use Additional Character(s)

Excludes 1   Excludes 2   Includes   Use additional   Code first   Code also   Key words

● **T83.02** Displacement of urinary catheter
  Malposition of urinary catheter
  ● **T83.020** Displacement of cystostomy catheter
  ● **T83.021** Displacement of indwelling urethral catheter
  ● **T83.022** Displacement of nephrostomy catheter
  ● **T83.028** Displacement of other urinary catheter
    Displacement of Hopkins catheter
    Displacement of ileostomy catheter
    Displacement of urostomy catheter
● **T83.03** Leakage of urinary catheter
  ● **T83.030** Leakage of cystostomy catheter
  ● **T83.031** Leakage of indwelling urethral catheter
  ● **T83.032** Leakage of nephrostomy catheter
  ● **T83.038** Leakage of other urinary catheter
    Leakage of Hopkins catheter
    Leakage of ileostomy catheter
    Leakage of urostomy catheter
● **T83.09** Other mechanical complication of urinary catheter
  Obstruction (mechanical) of urinary catheter
  Perforation of urinary catheter
  Protrusion of urinary catheter
  ● **T83.090** Other mechanical complication of cystostomy catheter
  ● **T83.091** Other mechanical complication of indwelling urethral catheter
  ● **T83.092** Other mechanical complication of nephrostomy catheter
  ● **T83.098** Other mechanical complication of other urinary catheter
    Other mechanical complication of Hopkins catheter
    Other mechanical complication of ileostomy catheter
    Other mechanical complication of urostomy catheter
● **T83.1** Mechanical complication of other urinary devices and implants
  ● **T83.11** Breakdown (mechanical) of other urinary devices and implants
    ● **T83.110** Breakdown (mechanical) of urinary electronic stimulator device
      Excludes2 Breakdown (mechanical) of electrode (lead) for sacral nerve neurostimulator (T85.111)
      Breakdown (mechanical) of implanted electronic sacral neurostimulator, pulse generator or receiver (T85.113)
    ● **T83.111** Breakdown (mechanical) of implanted urinary sphincter
    ● **T83.112** Breakdown (mechanical) of indwelling ureteral stent

    ● **T83.113** Breakdown (mechanical) of other urinary stents
      Breakdown (mechanical) of ileal conduit stent
      Breakdown (mechanical) of nephroureteral stent
    ● **T83.118** Breakdown (mechanical) of other urinary devices and implants
  ● **T83.12** Displacement of other urinary devices and implants
    Malposition of other urinary devices and implants
    ● **T83.120** Displacement of urinary electronic stimulator device
      Excludes2 Displacement of electrode (lead) for sacral nerve neurostimulator (T85.121)
      Displacement of implanted electronic sacral neurostimulator, pulse generator or receiver (T85.123)
    ● **T83.121** Displacement of implanted urinary sphincter
    ● **T83.122** Displacement of indwelling ureteral stent
    ● **T83.123** Displacement of other urinary stents
      Displacement of ileal conduit stent
      Displacement of nephroureteral stent
    ● **T83.128** Displacement of other urinary devices and implants
  ● **T83.19** Other mechanical complication of other urinary devices and implants
    Leakage of other urinary devices and implants
    Obstruction (mechanical) of other urinary devices and implants
    Perforation of other urinary devices and implants
    Protrusion of other urinary devices and implants
    ● **T83.190** Other mechanical complication of urinary electronic stimulator device
      Excludes2 Other mechanical complication of electrode (lead) for sacral nerve neurostimulator (T85.191)
      Other mechanical complication of implanted electronic sacral neurostimulator, pulse generator or receiver (T85.193)
    ● **T83.191** Other mechanical complication of implanted urinary sphincter
    ● **T83.192** Other mechanical complication of indwelling ureteral stent
    ● **T83.193** Other mechanical complication of other urinary stent
      Other mechanical complication of ileal conduit stent
      Other mechanical complication of nephroureteral stent
    ● **T83.198** Other mechanical complication of other urinary devices and implants

CHAPTER 19 (S00-T88)

● **T83.2**   Mechanical complication of graft of urinary organ
    X● **T83.21**   **Breakdown** (mechanical) of graft of urinary organ
    X● **T83.22**   **Displacement** of graft of urinary organ
                  Malposition of graft of urinary organ
    X● **T83.23**   **Leakage** of graft of urinary organ
    X● **T83.24**   **Erosion** of graft of urinary organ
    X● **T83.25**   **Exposure** of graft of urinary organ
    X● **T83.29**   **Other** mechanical complication of graft of urinary organ
                  Obstruction (mechanical) of graft of urinary organ
                  Perforation of graft of urinary organ
                  Protrusion of graft of urinary organ

● **T83.3**   Mechanical complication of intrauterine contraceptive device
    X● **T83.31**   **Breakdown** (mechanical) of intrauterine contraceptive device
    X● **T83.32**   **Displacement** of intrauterine contraceptive device
                  Malposition of intrauterine contraceptive device
                  Missing string of intrauterine contraceptive device
    X● **T83.39**   **Other** mechanical complication of intrauterine contraceptive device
                  Leakage of intrauterine contraceptive device
                  Obstruction (mechanical) of intrauterine contraceptive device
                  Perforation of intrauterine contraceptive device
                  Protrusion of intrauterine contraceptive device

● **T83.4**   Mechanical complication of other prosthetic devices, implants and grafts of genital tract
    ● **T83.41**   **Breakdown** (mechanical) of other prosthetic devices, implants and grafts of genital tract
       ● **T83.410**   **Breakdown** (mechanical) of implanted penile prosthesis
             Breakdown (mechanical) of penile prosthesis cylinder
             Breakdown (mechanical) of penile prosthesis pump
             Breakdown (mechanical) of penile prosthesis reservoir
       ● **T83.411**   **Breakdown** (mechanical) of implanted testicular prosthesis
       ● **T83.418**   **Breakdown** (mechanical) of other prosthetic devices, implants and grafts of genital tract
    ● **T83.42**   **Displacement** of other prosthetic devices, implants and grafts of genital tract
             Malposition of other prosthetic devices, implants and grafts of genital tract
       ● **T83.420**   **Displacement** of implanted penile prosthesis
             Displacement of penile prosthesis cylinder
             Displacement of penile prosthesis pump
             Displacement of penile prosthesis reservoir
       ● **T83.421**   **Displacement** of implanted testicular prosthesis
       ● **T83.428**   **Displacement** of other prosthetic devices, implants and grafts of genital tract

● **T83.49**   **Other mechanical complication** of other prosthetic devices, implants and grafts of genital tract
             Leakage of other prosthetic devices, implants and grafts of genital tract
             Obstruction, mechanical of other prosthetic devices, implants and grafts of genital tract
             Perforation of other prosthetic devices, implants and grafts of genital tract
             Protrusion of other prosthetic devices, implants and grafts of genital tract
    ● **T83.490**   **Other mechanical complication of implanted penile prosthesis**
             Other mechanical complication of penile prosthesis cylinder
             Other mechanical complication of penile prosthesis pump
             Other mechanical complication of penile prosthesis reservoir
    ● **T83.491**   **Other mechanical complication of implanted testicular prosthesis**
    ● **T83.498**   **Other mechanical complication of other prosthetic devices, implants and grafts of genital tract**

● **T83.5**   Infection and inflammatory reaction due to prosthetic device, implant and graft in urinary system
       Use additional code to identify infection
    ● **T83.51**   Infection and inflammatory reaction due to urinary catheter
       | Excludes2 | complications of stoma of urinary tract (N99.5-)
       ● **T83.510**   Infection and inflammatory reaction due to cystostomy catheter
       ● **T83.511**   Infection and inflammatory reaction due to indwelling urethral catheter
       ● **T83.512**   Infection and inflammatory reaction due to nephrostomy catheter
       ● **T83.518**   Infection and inflammatory reaction due to other urinary catheter
             Infection and inflammatory reaction due to Hopkins catheter
             Infection and inflammatory reaction due to ileostomy catheter
             Infection and inflammatory reaction due to urostomy catheter
    ● **T83.59**   Infection and inflammatory reaction due to prosthetic device, implant and graft in urinary system
       ● **T83.590**   Infection and inflammatory reaction due to implanted urinary neurostimulation device
          | Excludes2 | Infection and inflammatory reaction due to electrode lead of sacral nerve neurostimulator (T85.732)
             Infection and inflammatory reaction due to pulse generator or receiver of sacral nerve neurostimulator (T85.734)
       ● **T83.591**   Infection and inflammatory reaction due to implanted urinary sphincter
       ● **T83.592**   Infection and inflammatory reaction due to indwelling ureteral stent

CHAPTER 19 (S00-T88)

● **T83.593** **Infection and inflammatory reaction due to other urinary stents**
     Infection and inflammatory reaction due to ileal conduit stents
     Infection and inflammatory reaction due to nephroureteral stent

● **T83.598** **Infection and inflammatory reaction due to other prosthetic device, implant and graft in urinary system**

● **T83.6** **Infection and inflammatory reaction due to prosthetic device, implant and graft in genital tract**
   Use additional code to identify infection

   ● **T83.61** **Infection and inflammatory reaction due to implanted penile prosthesis**
     Infection and inflammatory reaction due to penile prosthesis cylinder
     Infection and inflammatory reaction due to penile prosthesis pump
     Infection and inflammatory reaction due to penile prosthesis reservoir

   ● **T83.62** **Infection and inflammatory reaction due to implanted testicular prosthesis**

   ● **T83.69** **Infection and inflammatory reaction due to other prosthetic device, implant and graft in genital tract**

● **T83.7** **Complications due to implanted mesh and other prosthetic materials**

   ● **T83.71** **Erosion of implanted mesh and other prosthetic materials to surrounding organ or tissue**

     ● **T83.711** **Erosion of implanted vaginal mesh to surrounding organ or tissue**
       Erosion of implanted vaginal mesh into pelvic floor muscles

     ● **T83.712** **Erosion of implanted urethral mesh to surrounding organ or tissue**
       Erosion of implanted female urethral sling
       Erosion of implanted male urethral sling
       Erosion of implanted urethral mesh into pelvic floor muscles

     ● **T83.713** **Erosion of implanted urethral bulking agent to surrounding organ or tissue**

     ● **T83.714** **Erosion of implanted ureteral bulking agent to surrounding organ or tissue**

     ● **T83.718** **Erosion of other implanted mesh to organ or tissue**

     ● **T83.719** **Erosion of other prosthetic materials to surrounding organ or tissue**

   ● **T83.72** **Exposure of implanted mesh and other prosthetic materials into surrounding organ or tissue**
     Extrusion of implanted mesh

     ● **T83.721** **Exposure of implanted vaginal mesh into vagina**
       Exposure of implanted vaginal mesh through vaginal wall

     ● **T83.722** **Exposure of implanted urethral mesh into urethra**
       Exposure of implanted female urethral sling
       Exposure of implanted male urethral sling
       Exposure of implanted urethral mesh through urethral wall

     ● **T83.723** **Exposure of implanted urethral bulking agent into urethra**

     ● **T83.724** **Exposure of implanted ureteral bulking agent into ureter**

● **T83.728** **Exposure of other implanted mesh into organ or tissue**

● **T83.729** **Exposure of other prosthetic materials into organ or tissue**

X ● **T83.79** **Other specified complications due to other genitourinary prosthetic materials**

● **T83.8** **Other specified complications of genitourinary prosthetic devices, implants and grafts**

   X ● **T83.81** **Embolism due to genitourinary prosthetic devices, implants and grafts**

   X ● **T83.82** **Fibrosis due to genitourinary prosthetic devices, implants and grafts**

   X ● **T83.83** **Hemorrhage due to genitourinary prosthetic devices, implants and grafts**

   X ● **T83.84** **Pain due to genitourinary prosthetic devices, implants and grafts**

   X ● **T83.85** **Stenosis due to genitourinary prosthetic devices, implants and grafts**

   X ● **T83.86** **Thrombosis due to genitourinary prosthetic devices, implants and grafts**

   X ● **T83.89** **Other specified complication of genitourinary prosthetic devices, implants and grafts**

X ● **T83.9** **Unspecified complication of genitourinary prosthetic device, implant and graft**

● **T84** **Complications of internal orthopedic prosthetic devices, implants and grafts**

   Excludes2   failure and rejection of transplanted organs and tissues (T86.-)
     fracture of bone following insertion of orthopedic implant, joint prosthesis or bone plate (M96.6)

   The appropriate 7th character is to be added to each code from category T84

A	initial encounter
D	subsequent encounter
S	sequela

   ● **T84.0** **Mechanical complication of internal joint prosthesis**

     ● **T84.01** **Broken internal joint prosthesis**
       Breakage (fracture) of prosthetic joint
       Broken prosthetic joint implant

       ⇒ **Excludes1**   periprosthetic joint implant fracture (M97-)

       ● **T84.010** **Broken internal right hip prosthesis**

       ● **T84.011** **Broken internal left hip prosthesis**

       ● **T84.012** **Broken internal right knee prosthesis**

       ● **T84.013** **Broken internal left knee prosthesis**

       ● **T84.018** **Broken internal joint prosthesis, other site**
         Use additional code to identify the joint (Z96.6-)

       ● **T84.019** **Broken internal joint prosthesis, unspecified site**

     ● **T84.02** **Dislocation of internal joint prosthesis**
       Instability of internal joint prosthesis
       Subluxation of internal joint prosthesis

       ● **T84.020** **Dislocation of internal right hip prosthesis**

       ● **T84.021** **Dislocation of internal left hip prosthesis**

       ● **T84.022** **Instability of internal right knee prosthesis**

       ● **T84.023** **Instability of internal left knee prosthesis**

       ● **T84.028** **Dislocation of other internal joint prosthesis**
         Use additional code to identify the joint (Z96.6-)

       ● **T84.029** **Dislocation of unspecified internal joint prosthesis**

● **T84.03**   **Mechanical loosening of internal prosthetic joint**
Aseptic loosening of prosthetic joint

● **T84.030**   **Mechanical loosening of internal right hip prosthetic joint**

● **T84.031**   **Mechanical loosening of internal left hip prosthetic joint**

● **T84.032**   **Mechanical loosening of internal right knee prosthetic joint**

● **T84.033**   **Mechanical loosening of internal left knee prosthetic joint**

● **T84.038**   **Mechanical loosening of other internal prosthetic joint**
Use additional code to identify the joint (Z96.6-)

● **T84.039**   **Mechanical loosening of unspecified internal prosthetic joint**

● **T84.05**   **Periprosthetic osteolysis of internal prosthetic joint**
Use additional code to identify major osseous defect, if applicable (M89.7-)

● **T84.050**   **Periprosthetic osteolysis of internal prosthetic right hip joint**

● **T84.051**   **Periprosthetic osteolysis of internal prosthetic left hip joint**

● **T84.052**   **Periprosthetic osteolysis of internal prosthetic right knee joint**

● **T84.053**   **Periprosthetic osteolysis of internal prosthetic left knee joint**

● **T84.058**   **Periprosthetic osteolysis of other internal prosthetic joint**
Use additional code to identify the joint (Z96.6-)

● **T84.059**   **Periprosthetic osteolysis of unspecified internal prosthetic joint**

● **T84.06**   **Wear of articular bearing surface of internal prosthetic joint**

● **T84.060**   **Wear of articular bearing surface of internal prosthetic right hip joint**

● **T84.061**   **Wear of articular bearing surface of internal prosthetic left hip joint**

● **T84.062**   **Wear of articular bearing surface of internal prosthetic right knee joint**

● **T84.063**   **Wear of articular bearing surface of internal prosthetic left knee joint**

● **T84.068**   **Wear of articular bearing surface of other internal prosthetic joint**
Use additional code to identify the joint (Z96.6-)

● **T84.069**   **Wear of articular bearing surface of unspecified internal prosthetic joint**

● **T84.09**   **Other mechanical complication of internal joint prosthesis**
Prosthetic joint implant failure NOS

● **T84.090**   **Other mechanical complication of internal right hip prosthesis**

● **T84.091**   **Other mechanical complication of internal left hip prosthesis**

● **T84.092**   **Other mechanical complication of internal right knee prosthesis**

● **T84.093**   **Other mechanical complication of internal left knee prosthesis**

● **T84.098**   **Other mechanical complication of other internal joint prosthesis**
Use additional code to identify the joint (Z96.6-)

● **T84.099**   **Other mechanical complication of unspecified internal joint prosthesis**

● **T84.1**   **Mechanical complication of internal fixation device of bones of limb**

Excludes2   mechanical complication of internal fixation device of bones of feet (T84.2-)
mechanical complication of internal fixation device of bones of fingers (T84.2-)
mechanical complication of internal fixation device of bones of hands (T84.2-)
mechanical complication of internal fixation device of bones of toes (T84.2-)

● **T84.11**   **Breakdown (mechanical) of internal fixation device of bones of limb**

● **T84.110**   **Breakdown (mechanical) of internal fixation device of right humerus**

● **T84.111**   **Breakdown (mechanical) of internal fixation device of left humerus**

● **T84.112**   **Breakdown (mechanical) of internal fixation device of bone of right forearm**

● **T84.113**   **Breakdown (mechanical) of internal fixation device of bone of left forearm**

● **T84.114**   **Breakdown (mechanical) of internal fixation device of right femur**

● **T84.115**   **Breakdown (mechanical) of internal fixation device of left femur**

● **T84.116**   **Breakdown (mechanical) of internal fixation device of bone of right lower leg**

● **T84.117**   **Breakdown (mechanical) of internal fixation device of bone of left lower leg**

● **T84.119**   **Breakdown (mechanical) of internal fixation device of unspecified bone of limb**

● **T84.12**   **Displacement of internal fixation device of bones of limb**
Malposition of internal fixation device of bones of limb

● **T84.120**   **Displacement of internal fixation device of right humerus**

● **T84.121**   **Displacement of internal fixation device of left humerus**

● **T84.122**   **Displacement of internal fixation device of bone of right forearm**

● **T84.123**   **Displacement of internal fixation device of bone of left forearm**

● **T84.124**   **Displacement of internal fixation device of right femur**

● **T84.125**   **Displacement of internal fixation device of left femur**

● **T84.126**   **Displacement of internal fixation device of bone of right lower leg**

● **T84.127**   **Displacement of internal fixation device of bone of left lower leg**

● **T84.129**   **Displacement of internal fixation device of unspecified bone of limb**

▶ New   ⇒ Revised   ~~deleted~~ Deleted   **OGCR** Official Guidelines   X Assign placeholder X   ● Use Additional Character(s)

Excludes 1   Excludes 2   Includes   Use additional   Code first   Code also   Key words

● T84.19 Other mechanical complication of internal
fixation device of bones of limb
    Obstruction (mechanical) of internal fixation
        device of bones of limb
    Perforation of internal fixation device of bones
        of limb
    Protrusion of internal fixation device of bones
        of limb

● T84.190 Other mechanical complication
of internal fixation device of right
humerus

● T84.191 Other mechanical complication
of internal fixation device of left
humerus

● T84.192 Other mechanical complication of
internal fixation device of bone of
right forearm

● T84.193 Other mechanical complication of
internal fixation device of bone of left
forearm

● T84.194 Other mechanical complication of
internal fixation device of right femur

● T84.195 Other mechanical complication of
internal fixation device of left femur

● T84.196 Other mechanical complication of
internal fixation device of bone of
right lower leg

● T84.197 Other mechanical complication of
internal fixation device of bone of left
lower leg

● T84.199 Other mechanical complication of
internal fixation device of unspecified
bone of limb

● T84.2 Mechanical complication of internal fixation device of
other bones

● T84.21 Breakdown (mechanical) of internal fixation
device of other bones

● T84.210 Breakdown (mechanical) of internal
fixation device of bones of hand and
fingers

● T84.213 Breakdown (mechanical) of internal
fixation device of bones of foot and
toes

● T84.216 Breakdown (mechanical) of internal
fixation device of vertebrae

● T84.218 Breakdown (mechanical) of internal
fixation device of other bones

● T84.22 Displacement of internal fixation device of
other bones
    Malposition of internal fixation device of other
        bones

● T84.220 Displacement of internal fixation
device of bones of hand and fingers

● T84.223 Displacement of internal fixation
device of bones of foot and toes

● T84.226 Displacement of internal fixation
device of vertebrae

● T84.228 Displacement of internal fixation
device of other bones

● T84.29 Other mechanical complication of internal
fixation device of other bones
    Obstruction (mechanical) of internal fixation
        device of other bones
    Perforation of internal fixation device of other
        bones
    Protrusion of internal fixation device of other
        bones

● T84.290 Other mechanical complication of
internal fixation device of bones of
hand and fingers

● T84.293 Other mechanical complication of
internal fixation device of bones of
foot and toes

● T84.296 Other mechanical complication of
internal fixation device of vertebrae

● T84.298 Other mechanical complication of
internal fixation device of other bones

● T84.3 Mechanical complication of other bone devices,
implants and grafts

    Excludes2   other complications of bone graft
                 (T86.83-)

● T84.31 Breakdown (mechanical) of other bone devices,
implants and grafts

● T84.310 Breakdown (mechanical) of electronic
bone stimulator

● T84.318 Breakdown (mechanical) of other
bone devices, implants and grafts

● T84.32 Displacement of other bone devices, implants
and grafts
    Malposition of other bone devices, implants
        and grafts

● T84.320 Displacement of electronic bone
stimulator

● T84.328 Displacement of other bone devices,
implants and grafts

● T84.39 Other mechanical complication of other bone
devices, implants and grafts
    Obstruction (mechanical) of other bone
        devices, implants and grafts
    Perforation of other bone devices, implants
        and grafts
    Protrusion of other bone devices, implants and
        grafts

● T84.390 Other mechanical complication of
electronic bone stimulator

● T84.398 Other mechanical complication of
other bone devices, implants and
grafts

● T84.4 Mechanical complication of other internal orthopedic
devices, implants and grafts

● T84.41 Breakdown (mechanical) of other internal
orthopedic devices, implants and grafts

● T84.410 Breakdown (mechanical) of muscle
and tendon graft

● T84.418 Breakdown (mechanical) of other
internal orthopedic devices, implants
and grafts

● T84.42 Displacement of other internal orthopedic
devices, implants and grafts
    Malposition of other internal orthopedic
        devices, implants and grafts

● T84.420 Displacement of muscle and tendon
graft

● T84.428 Displacement of other internal
orthopedic devices, implants and
grafts

● **T84.49** **Other mechanical complication of other internal orthopedic devices, implants and grafts**
Mechanical complication of other internal orthopedic devices, implants and grafts NOS
Obstruction (mechanical) of other internal orthopedic devices, implants and grafts
Perforation of other internal orthopedic devices, implants and grafts
Protrusion of other internal orthopedic devices, implants and grafts

  ● **T84.490** **Other mechanical complication of muscle and tendon graft**

  ● **T84.498** **Other mechanical complication of other internal orthopedic devices, implants and grafts**

● **T84.5** **Infection and inflammatory reaction due to internal joint prosthesis**
Use additional code to identify infection

X● **T84.50** **Infection and inflammatory reaction due to unspecified internal joint prosthesis**

X● **T84.51** **Infection and inflammatory reaction due to internal right hip prosthesis**

X● **T84.52** **Infection and inflammatory reaction due to internal left hip prosthesis**

X● **T84.53** **Infection and inflammatory reaction due to internal right knee prosthesis**

X● **T84.54** **Infection and inflammatory reaction due to internal left knee prosthesis**

X● **T84.59** **Infection and inflammatory reaction due to other internal joint prosthesis**

● **T84.6** **Infection and inflammatory reaction due to internal fixation device**
Use additional code to identify infection

X● **T84.60** **Infection and inflammatory reaction due to internal fixation device of unspecified site**

● **T84.61** **Infection and inflammatory reaction due to internal fixation device of arm**

  ● **T84.610** **Infection and inflammatory reaction due to internal fixation device of right humerus**

  ● **T84.611** **Infection and inflammatory reaction due to internal fixation device of left humerus**

  ● **T84.612** **Infection and inflammatory reaction due to internal fixation device of right radius**

  ● **T84.613** **Infection and inflammatory reaction due to internal fixation device of left radius**

  ● **T84.614** **Infection and inflammatory reaction due to internal fixation device of right ulna**

  ● **T84.615** **Infection and inflammatory reaction due to internal fixation device of left ulna**

  ● **T84.619** **Infection and inflammatory reaction due to internal fixation device of unspecified bone of arm**

● **T84.62** **Infection and inflammatory reaction due to internal fixation device of leg**

  ● **T84.620** **Infection and inflammatory reaction due to internal fixation device of right femur**

  ● **T84.621** **Infection and inflammatory reaction due to internal fixation device of left femur**

  ● **T84.622** **Infection and inflammatory reaction due to internal fixation device of right tibia**

  ● **T84.623** **Infection and inflammatory reaction due to internal fixation device of left tibia**

  ● **T84.624** **Infection and inflammatory reaction due to internal fixation device of right fibula**

  ● **T84.625** **Infection and inflammatory reaction due to internal fixation device of left fibula**

  ● **T84.629** **Infection and inflammatory reaction due to internal fixation device of unspecified bone of leg**

X● **T84.63** **Infection and inflammatory reaction due to internal fixation device of spine**

X● **T84.69** **Infection and inflammatory reaction due to internal fixation device of other site**

● **T84.7** **Infection and inflammatory reaction due to other internal orthopedic prosthetic devices, implants and grafts**
Use additional code to identify infection

● **T84.8** **Other specified complications of internal orthopedic prosthetic devices, implants and grafts**

X● **T84.81** **Embolism due to internal orthopedic prosthetic devices, implants and grafts**

X● **T84.82** **Fibrosis due to internal orthopedic prosthetic devices, implants and grafts**

X● **T84.83** **Hemorrhage due to internal orthopedic prosthetic devices, implants and grafts**

X● **T84.84** **Pain due to internal orthopedic prosthetic devices, implants and grafts**

X● **T84.85** **Stenosis due to internal orthopedic prosthetic devices, implants and grafts**

X● **T84.86** **Thrombosis due to internal orthopedic prosthetic devices, implants and grafts**

X● **T84.89** **Other specified complication of internal orthopedic prosthetic devices, implants and grafts**

X● **T84.9** **Unspecified complication of internal orthopedic prosthetic device, implant and graft**

● **T85** **Complications of other internal prosthetic devices, implants and grafts**

  Excludes2   failure and rejection of transplanted organs and tissue (T86.-)

The appropriate 7th character is to be added to each code from category T85

A	initial encounter
D	subsequent encounter
S	sequela

● **T85.0** **Mechanical complication of ventricular intracranial (communicating) shunt**

X● **T85.01** **Breakdown (mechanical) of ventricular intracranial (communicating) shunt**

X● **T85.02** **Displacement of ventricular intracranial (communicating) shunt**
Malposition of ventricular intracranial (communicating) shunt

X ● **T85.03** Leakage of ventricular intracranial (communicating) shunt

X ● **T85.09** Other mechanical complication of ventricular intracranial (communicating) shunt

Obstruction (mechanical) of ventricular intracranial (communicating) shunt

Perforation of ventricular intracranial (communicating) shunt

Protrusion of ventricular intracranial (communicating) shunt

● **T85.1** Mechanical complication of implanted electronic stimulator of nervous system

● **T85.11** Breakdown (mechanical) of implanted electronic stimulator of nervous system

● **T85.110** Breakdown (mechanical) of implanted electronic neurostimulator of brain electrode (lead)

● **T85.111** Breakdown (mechanical) of implanted electronic neurostimulator of peripheral nerve electrode (lead)

Breakdown of electrode (lead) for cranial nerve neurostimulators

Breakdown of electrode (lead) for gastric neurostimulator

Breakdown of electrode (lead) for sacral nerve neurostimulator

Breakdown of electrode (lead) for vagal nerve neurostimulators

● **T85.112** Breakdown (mechanical) of implanted electronic neurostimulator of spinal cord electrode (lead)

● **T85.113** Breakdown (mechanical) of implanted electronic neurostimulator, generator

Breakdown (mechanical) of implanted electronic neurostimuator generator, brain, peripheral, gastric, spinal

Breakdown (mechanical) of implanted electronic sacral neurostimulator, pulse generator or receiver

● **T85.118** Breakdown (mechanical) of other implanted electronic stimulator of nervous system

● **T85.12** Displacement of implanted electronic stimulator of nervous system

Malposition of implanted electronic stimulator of nervous system

● **T85.120** Displacement of implanted electronic neurostimulator of brain electrode (lead)

● **T85.121** Displacement of implanted electronic neurostimulator of peripheral nerve electrode (lead)

Displacement of electrode (lead) for cranial nerve neurostimulators

Displacement of electrode (lead) for gastric neurostimulator

Displacement of electrode (lead) for sacral nerve neurostimulator

Displacement of electrode (lead) for vagal nerve neurostimulators

● **T85.122** Displacement of implanted electronic neurostimulator of spinal cord electrode (lead)

● **T85.123** Displacement of implanted electronic neurostimulator, generator

Displacement of implanted electronic neurostimulator generator, brain, peripheral, gastric, spinal

Displacement of implanted electronic sacral neurostimulator, pulse generator or receiver

● **T85.128** Displacement of other implanted electronic stimulator of nervous system

● **T85.19** Other mechanical complication of implanted electronic stimulator of nervous system

Leakage of implanted electronic stimulator of nervous system

Obstruction (mechanical) of implanted electronic stimulator of nervous system

Perforation of implanted electronic stimulator of nervous system

Protrusion of implanted electronic stimulator of nervous system

● **T85.190** Other mechanical complication of implanted electronic neurostimulator of brain electrode (lead)

● **T85.191** Other mechanical complication of implanted electronic neurostimulator of peripheral nerve electrode (lead)

Other mechanical complication of electrode (lead) for cranial nerve neurostimulators

Other mechanical complication of electrode (lead) for gastric neurostimulator

Other mechanical complication of electrode (lead) for sacral nerve neurostimulator

Other mechanical complication of electrode (lead) for vagal nerve neurostimulators

● **T85.192** Other mechanical complication of implanted electronic neurostimulator of spinal cord electrode (lead)

● **T85.193** Other mechanical complication of implanted electronic neurostimulator, generator

Other mechanical complication of implanted electronic neurostimulator generator, brain, peripheral, gastric, spinal

Other mechanical complication of implanted electronic sacral neurostimulator, pulse generator or receiver

● **T85.199** Other mechanical complication of other implanted electronic stimulator of nervous system

● **T85.2** Mechanical complication of intraocular lens

X ● **T85.21** Breakdown (mechanical) of intraocular lens

X ● **T85.22** Displacement of intraocular lens

Malposition of intraocular lens

X ● **T85.29** Other mechanical complication of intraocular lens

Obstruction (mechanical) of intraocular lens

Perforation of intraocular lens

Protrusion of intraocular lens

● **T85.3 Mechanical complication of other ocular prosthetic devices, implants and grafts**

> **Excludes2**   other complications of corneal graft (T86.84-)

● **T85.31 Breakdown (mechanical) of other ocular prosthetic devices, implants and grafts**

● **T85.310 Breakdown (mechanical) of prosthetic orbit of right eye**

● **T85.311 Breakdown (mechanical) of prosthetic orbit of left eye**

● **T85.318 Breakdown (mechanical) of other ocular prosthetic devices, implants and grafts**

● **T85.32 Displacement of other ocular prosthetic devices, implants and grafts**

> Malposition of other ocular prosthetic devices, implants and grafts

● **T85.320 Displacement of prosthetic orbit of right eye**

● **T85.321 Displacement of prosthetic orbit of left eye**

● **T85.328 Displacement of other ocular prosthetic devices, implants and grafts**

● **T85.39 Other mechanical complication of other ocular prosthetic devices, implants and grafts**

> Obstruction (mechanical) of other ocular prosthetic devices, implants and grafts
> Perforation of other ocular prosthetic devices, implants and grafts
> Protrusion of other ocular prosthetic devices, implants and grafts

● **T85.390 Other mechanical complication of prosthetic orbit of right eye**

● **T85.391 Other mechanical complication of prosthetic orbit of left eye**

● **T85.398 Other mechanical complication of other ocular prosthetic devices, implants and grafts**

● **T85.4 Mechanical complication of breast prosthesis and implant**

X ● **T85.41 Breakdown (mechanical) of breast prosthesis and implant**

X ● **T85.42 Displacement of breast prosthesis and implant**

> Malposition of breast prosthesis and implant

X ● **T85.43 Leakage of breast prosthesis and implant**

X ● **T85.44 Capsular contracture of breast implant**

X ● **T85.49 Other mechanical complication of breast prosthesis and implant**

> Obstruction (mechanical) of breast prosthesis and implant
> Perforation of breast prosthesis and implant
> Protrusion of breast prosthesis and implant

● **T85.5 Mechanical complication of gastrointestinal prosthetic devices, implants and grafts**

● **T85.51 Breakdown (mechanical) of gastrointestinal prosthetic devices, implants and grafts**

● **T85.510 Breakdown (mechanical) of bile duct prosthesis**

● **T85.511 Breakdown (mechanical) of esophageal anti-reflux device**

● **T85.518 Breakdown (mechanical) of other gastrointestinal prosthetic devices, implants and grafts**

● **T85.52 Displacement of gastrointestinal prosthetic devices, implants and grafts**

> Malposition of gastrointestinal prosthetic devices, implants and grafts

● **T85.520 Displacement of bile duct prosthesis**

● **T85.521 Displacement of esophageal anti-reflux device**

● **T85.528 Displacement of other gastrointestinal prosthetic devices, implants and grafts**

● **T85.59 Other mechanical complication of gastrointestinal prosthetic devices, implants and**

> Obstruction, mechanical of gastrointestinal prosthetic devices, implants and grafts
> Perforation of gastrointestinal prosthetic devices, implants and grafts
> Protrusion of gastrointestinal prosthetic devices, implants and grafts

● **T85.590 Other mechanical complication of bile duct prosthesis**

● **T85.591 Other mechanical complication of esophageal anti-reflux device**

● **T85.598 Other mechanical complication of other gastrointestinal prosthetic devices, implants and grafts**

● **T85.6 Mechanical complication of other specified internal and external prosthetic devices, implants and grafts**

● **T85.61 Breakdown (mechanical) of other specified internal prosthetic devices, implants and grafts**

● **T85.610 Breakdown (mechanical) of cranial or spinal infusion catheter**

> Breakdown (mechanical) of epidural infusion catheter
> Breakdown (mechanical) of intrathecal infusion catheter
> Breakdown (mechanical) of subarachnoid infusion catheter
> Breakdown (mechanical) of subdural infusion catheter

● **T85.611 Breakdown (mechanical) of intraperitoneal dialysis catheter**

> **Excludes1**   mechanical complication of vascular dialysis catheter (T82.4-)

● **T85.612 Breakdown (mechanical) of permanent sutures**

> **Excludes1**   mechanical complication of permanent (wire) suture used in bone repair (T84.1-T84.2)

● **T85.613 Breakdown (mechanical) of artificial skin graft and decellularized allodermis**

> Failure of artificial skin graft and decellularized allodermis
> Non-adherence of artificial skin graft and decellularized allodermis
> Poor incorporation of artificial skin graft and decellularized allodermis
> Shearing of artificial skin graft and decellularized allodermis

● **T85.614 Breakdown (mechanical) of insulin pump**

● **T85.615 Breakdown (mechanical) of other nervous system device, implant or graft**

> Breakdown (mechanical) of intrathecal infusion pump

● **T85.618 Breakdown (mechanical) of other specified internal prosthetic devices, implants and grafts**

● T85.62   **Displacement of other specified internal prosthetic devices, implants and grafts**
Malposition of other specified internal prosthetic devices, implants and grafts

   ● T85.620   **Displacement of cranial or spinal infusion catheter**
Displacement of epidural infusion catheter
Displacement of intrathecal infusion catheter
Displacement of subarachnoid infusion catheter
Displacement of subdural infusion catheter

   ● T85.621   **Displacement of intraperitoneal dialysis catheter**
      Excludes1   mechanical complication of vascular dialysis catheter (T82.4-)

   ● T85.622   **Displacement of permanent sutures**
      Excludes1   mechanical complication of permanent (wire) suture used in bone repair (T84.1-T84.2)

   ● T85.623   **Displacement of artificial skin graft and decellularized allodermis**
Dislodgement of artificial skin graft and decellularized allodermis
~~Displacement of artificial skin graft and decellularized allodermis~~

   ● T85.624   **Displacement of insulin pump**

   ● T85.625   **Displacement of other nervous system device, implant or graft**
Displacement of intrathecal infusion pump

   ● T85.628   **Displacement of other specified internal prosthetic devices, implants and grafts**

● T85.63   **Leakage of other specified internal prosthetic devices, implants and grafts**

   ● T85.630   **Leakage of cranial or spinal infusion catheter**
Leakage of epidural infusion catheter
Leakage of intrathecal infusion catheter
Leakage of subdural infusion catheter
Leakage of subarachnoid infusion catheter

   ● T85.631   **Leakage of intraperitoneal dialysis catheter**
      Excludes1   mechanical complication of vascular dialysis catheter (T82.4)

   ● T85.633   **Leakage of insulin pump**

   ● T85.635   **Leakage of other nervous system device, implant or graft**
Leakage of intrathecal infusion pump

   ● T85.638   **Leakage of other specified internal prosthetic devices, implants and grafts**

● T85.69   **Other mechanical complication of other specified internal prosthetic devices, implants and grafts**
Obstruction, mechanical of other specified internal prosthetic devices, implants and grafts
Perforation of other specified internal prosthetic devices, implants and grafts
Protrusion of other specified internal prosthetic devices, implants and grafts

   ● T85.690   **Other mechanical complication of cranial or spinal infusion catheter**
Other mechanical complication of epidural infusion catheter
Other mechanical complication of intrathecal infusion catheter
Other mechanical complication of subarachnoid infusion catheter
Other mechanical complication of subdural infusion catheter

   ● T85.691   **Other mechanical complication of intraperitoneal dialysis catheter**
      Excludes1   mechanical complication of vascular dialysis catheter (T82.4)

   ● T85.692   **Other mechanical complication of permanent sutures**
      Excludes1   mechanical complication of permanent (wire) suture used in bone repair (T84.1-T84.2)

   ● T85.693   **Other mechanical complication of artificial skin graft and decellularized allodermis**

   ● T85.694   **Other mechanical complication of insulin pump**

   ● T85.695   **Other mechanical complication of other nervous system device, implant or graft**
Other mechanical complication of intrathecal infusion pump

   ● T85.698   **Other mechanical complication of other specified internal prosthetic devices, implants and grafts**
Mechanical complication of nonabsorbable surgical material NOS

● T85.7   **Infection and inflammatory reaction due to other internal prosthetic devices, implants and grafts**
Use additional code to identify infection

X ● T85.71   **Infection and inflammatory reaction due to peritoneal dialysis catheter**

X ● T85.72   **Infection and inflammatory reaction due to insulin pump**

CHAPTER 19 (S00-T88)

● **T85.73** **Infection and inflammatory reaction due to nervous system devices, implants and graft**

  ● **T85.730** **Infection and inflammatory reaction due to ventricular intracranial (communicating) shunt**

  ● **T85.731** **Infection and inflammatory reaction due to implanted electronic neurostimulator of brain, electrode (lead)**

  ● **T85.732** **Infection and inflammatory reaction due to implanted electronic neurostimulator of peripheral nerve, electrode (lead)**

    Infection and inflammatory reaction due to electrode (lead) for cranial nerve neurostimulators

    Infection and inflammatory reaction due to electrode (lead) for gastric neurostimulator

    Infection and inflammatory reaction due to electrode (lead) for sacral nerve neurostimulator

    Infection and inflammatory reaction due to electrode (lead) for vagal nerve neurostimulators

  ● **T85.733** **Infection and inflammatory reaction due to implanted electronic neurostimulator of spinal cord, electrode (lead)**

  ● **T85.734** **Infection and inflammatory reaction due to implanted electronic neurostimulator, generator**

    Generator pocket infection

  ● **T85.735** **Infection and inflammatory reaction due to cranial or spinal infusion catheter**

    Infection and inflammatory reaction due to epidural catheter

    Infection and inflammatory reaction due to intrathecal infusion catheter

    Infection and inflammatory reaction due to subarachnoid catheter

    Infection and inflammatory reaction due to subdural catheter

  ● **T85.738** **Infection and inflammatory reaction due to other nervous system device, implant or graft**

    Infection and inflammatory reaction due to intrathecal infusion pump

X ● **T85.79** **Infection and inflammatory reaction due to other internal prosthetic devices, implants and grafts**

● **T85.8** **Other specified complications of internal prosthetic devices, implants and grafts, not elsewhere classified**

  ● **T85.81** **Embolism due to internal prosthetic devices, implants and grafts, not elsewhere classified**

    ● **T85.810** **Embolism due to nervous system prosthetic devices, implants and grafts**

    ● **T85.818** **Embolism due to other internal prosthetic devices, implants and grafts**

  ● **T85.82** **Fibrosis due to internal prosthetic devices, implants and grafts, not elsewhere classified**

    ● **T85.820** **Fibrosis due to nervous system prosthetic devices, implants and grafts**

    ● **T85.828** **Fibrosis due to other internal prosthetic devices, implants and grafts**

● **T85.83** **Hemorrhage due to internal prosthetic devices, implants and grafts, not elsewhere classified**

  ● **T85.830** **Hemorrhage due to nervous system prosthetic devices, implants and grafts**

  ● **T85.838** **Hemorrhage due to other internal prosthetic devices, implants and grafts**

● **T85.84** **Pain due to internal prosthetic devices, implants and grafts, not elsewhere classified**

  ● **T85.840** **Pain due to nervous system prosthetic devices, implants and grafts**

  ● **T85.848** **Pain due to other internal prosthetic devices, implants and grafts**

● **T85.85** **Stenosis due to internal prosthetic devices, implants and grafts, not elsewhere classified**

  ● **T85.850** **Stenosis due to nervous system prosthetic devices, implants and grafts**

  ● **T85.858** **Stenosis due to other internal prosthetic devices, implants and grafts**

● **T85.86** **Thrombosis due to internal prosthetic devices, implants and grafts, not elsewhere classified**

  ● **T85.860** **Thrombosis due to nervous system prosthetic devices, implants and grafts**

  ● **T85.868** **Thrombosis due to other internal prosthetic devices, implants and grafts**

● **T85.89** **Other specified complication of internal prosthetic devices, implants and grafts, not elsewhere classified**

  ● **T85.890** **Other specified complication of nervous system prosthetic devices, implants and grafts**

  ● **T85.898** **Other specified complication of other internal prosthetic devices, implants and grafts**

X ● **T85.9** **Unspecified complication of internal prosthetic device, implant and graft**

    Complication of internal prosthetic device, implant and graft NOS

OGCR Section I.C.19.g.3.

Organ Transplant Complications

Transplant Complications

(a) Transplant complications other than kidney

Codes under category T86, Complications of transplanted organs and tissues, are for use for both complications and rejection of transplanted organs. A transplant complication code is only assigned if the complication affects the function of the transplanted organ. Two codes are required to fully describe a transplant complication: the appropriate code from category T86 and a secondary code that identifies the complication.

Pre-existing conditions or conditions that develop after the transplant are not coded as complications unless they affect the function of the transplanted organs.

See I.C.21 for transplant organ removal status

See I.C.2 for malignant neoplasm associated with transplanted organ.

● **T86** **Complications of transplanted organs and tissue**

    Use additional code to identify other transplant complications, such as:

    graft-versus-host disease (D89.81-)

    malignancy associated with organ transplant (C80.2)

    post-transplant lymphoproliferative disorders (PTLD) (D47.Z1)

  ● **T86.0** **Complications of bone marrow transplant**

    T86.00 **Unspecified complication of bone marrow transplant**

    T86.01 **Bone marrow transplant rejection**

    T86.02 **Bone marrow transplant failure**

    T86.03 **Bone marrow transplant infection**

    T86.09 **Other complications of bone marrow transplant**

▶ New   ⇒ Revised   ~~deleted~~ Deleted   **OGCR** Official Guidelines   X Assign placeholder X   ● Use Additional Character(s)

Excludes 1   Excludes 2   Includes   Use additional   Code first   Code also   Key words

● **T86.1** **Complications of kidney transplant**

    T86.10 Unspecified complication of kidney transplant

    T86.11 Kidney transplant rejection

    T86.12 Kidney transplant failure

    T86.13 Kidney transplant infection

         Use additional code to specify infection

    T86.19 Other complication of kidney transplant

● **T86.2** **Complications of heart transplant**

     Excludes1   complication of:

         artificial heart device (T82.5)

         heart-lung transplant (T86.3)

    T86.20 Unspecified complication of heart transplant

    T86.21 Heart transplant rejection

    T86.22 Heart transplant failure

    T86.23 Heart transplant infection

         Use additional code to specify infection

  ● **T86.29** Other complications of heart transplant

        T86.290 Cardiac allograft vasculopathy

             Excludes1   atherosclerosis of coronary arteries (I25.75-, I25.76-, I25.81-)

        T86.298 Other complications of heart transplant

● **T86.3** **Complications of heart-lung transplant**

    T86.30 Unspecified complication of heart-lung transplant

    T86.31 Heart-lung transplant rejection

    T86.32 Heart-lung transplant failure

    T86.33 Heart-lung transplant infection

         Use additional code to specify infection

    T86.39 Other complications of heart-lung transplant

● **T86.4** **Complications of liver transplant**

    T86.40 Unspecified complication of liver transplant

    T86.41 Liver transplant rejection

    T86.42 Liver transplant failure

    T86.43 Liver transplant infection

         Use additional code to identify infection, such as:

             Cytomegalovirus (CMV) infection (B25.-)

    T86.49 Other complications of liver transplant

● **T86.5** **Complications of stem cell transplant**

     Complications from stem cells from peripheral blood

     Complications from stem cells from umbilical cord

● **T86.8** **Complications of other transplanted organs and tissues**

  ● **T86.81** Complications of lung transplant

         Excludes1   complication of heart-lung transplant (T86.3-)

        T86.810 Lung transplant rejection

        T86.811 Lung transplant failure

        T86.812 Lung transplant infection

             Use additional code to specify infection

        T86.818 Other complications of lung transplant

        T86.819 Unspecified complication of lung transplant

  ● **T86.82** Complications of skin graft (allograft) (autograft)

         Excludes2   complication of artificial skin graft (T85.693)

        T86.820 Skin graft (allograft) rejection

        T86.821 Skin graft (allograft) (autograft) failure

        T86.822 Skin graft (allograft) (autograft) infection

             Use additional code to specify infection

        T86.828 Other complications of skin graft (allograft) (autograft)

        T86.829 Unspecified complication of skin graft (allograft) (autograft)

  ● **T86.83** Complications of bone graft

         Excludes2   mechanical complications of bone graft (T84.3-)

        T86.830 Bone graft rejection

        T86.831 Bone graft failure

        T86.832 Bone graft infection

             Use additional code to specify infection

        T86.838 Other complications of bone graft

        T86.839 Unspecified complication of bone graft

  ● **T86.84** Complications of corneal transplant

         Excludes2   mechanical complications of corneal graft (T85.3-)

        T86.840 Corneal transplant rejection

        T86.841 Corneal transplant failure

        T86.842 Corneal transplant infection

             Use additional code to specify infection

        T86.848 Other complications of corneal transplant

        T86.849 Unspecified complication of corneal transplant

  ● **T86.85** Complication of intestine transplant

        T86.850 Intestine transplant rejection

        T86.851 Intestine transplant failure

        T86.852 Intestine transplant infection

             Use additional code to specify infection

        T86.858 Other complications of intestine transplant

        T86.859 Unspecified complication of intestine transplant

  ● **T86.89** Complications of other transplanted tissue

         Transplant failure or rejection of pancreas

        T86.890 Other transplanted tissue rejection

        T86.891 Other transplanted tissue failure

        T86.892 Other transplanted tissue infection

             Use additional code to specify infection

        T86.898 Other complications of other transplanted tissue

        T86.899 Unspecified complication of other transplanted tissue

● **T86.9** **Complication of unspecified transplanted organ and tissue**

    T86.90 Unspecified complication of unspecified transplanted organ and tissue

    T86.91 Unspecified transplanted organ and tissue rejection

    T86.92 Unspecified transplanted organ and tissue failure

    T86.93 Unspecified transplanted organ and tissue infection

         Use additional code to specify infection

    T86.99 Other complications of unspecified transplanted organ and tissue

CHAPTER 19 (S00-T88)

▶ New   ⇒ Revised   ~~deleted~~ Deleted   **OGCR** Official Guidelines   X Assign placeholder X   ● Use Additional Character(s)

Excludes 1   Excludes 2   Includes   Use additional   Code first   Code also   Key words

● **T87** **Complications peculiar to reattachment and amputation**
  ● **T87.0** **Complications of reattached (part of) upper extremity**
    ● **T87.0X** **Complications of reattached (part of) upper extremity**
      T87.0X1 **Complications of reattached (part of) right upper extremity**
      T87.0X2 **Complications of reattached (part of) left upper extremity**
      T87.0X9 **Complications of reattached (part of) unspecified upper extremity**
  ● **T87.1** **Complications of reattached (part of) lower extremity**
    ● **T87.1X** **Complications of reattached (part of) lower extremity**
      T87.1X1 **Complications of reattached (part of) right lower extremity**
      T87.1X2 **Complications of reattached (part of) left lower extremity**
      T87.1X9 **Complications of reattached (part of) unspecified lower extremity**
  T87.2 **Complications of other reattached body part**
  ● **T87.3** **Neuroma of amputation stump**
    T87.30 **Neuroma of amputation stump, unspecified extremity**
    T87.31 **Neuroma of amputation stump, right upper extremity**
    T87.32 **Neuroma of amputation stump, left upper extremity**
    T87.33 **Neuroma of amputation stump, right lower extremity**
    T87.34 **Neuroma of amputation stump, left lower extremity**
  ● **T87.4** **Infection of amputation stump**
    T87.40 **Infection of amputation stump, unspecified extremity**
    T87.41 **Infection of amputation stump, right upper extremity**
    T87.42 **Infection of amputation stump, left upper extremity**
    T87.43 **Infection of amputation stump, right lower extremity**
    T87.44 **Infection of amputation stump, left lower extremity**
  ● **T87.5** **Necrosis of amputation stump**
    T87.50 **Necrosis of amputation stump, unspecified extremity**
    T87.51 **Necrosis of amputation stump, right upper extremity**
    T87.52 **Necrosis of amputation stump, left upper extremity**
    T87.53 **Necrosis of amputation stump, right lower extremity**
    T87.54 **Necrosis of amputation stump, left lower extremity**
  ● **T87.8** **Other complications of amputation stump**
    T87.81 **Dehiscence of amputation stump**
    T87.89 **Other complications of amputation stump**
      Amputation stump contracture
      Amputation stump contracture of next proximal joint
      Amputation stump flexion
      Amputation stump edema
      Amputation stump hematoma
      Excludes2 phantom limb syndrome (G54.6-G54.7)
  T87.9 **Unspecified complications of amputation stump**

● **T88** **Other complications of surgical and medical care, not elsewhere classified**
  Excludes2 complication following infusion, transfusion and therapeutic injection (T80.-)
      complication following procedure NEC (T81.-)
      complications of anesthesia in labor and delivery (O74.-)
      complications of anesthesia in pregnancy (O29.-)
      complications of anesthesia in puerperium (O89.-)
      complications of devices, implants and grafts (T82-T85)
      complications of obstetric surgery and procedure (O75.4)
      dermatitis due to drugs and medicaments (L23.3, L24.4, L25.1, L27.0-L27.1)
      poisoning and toxic effects of drugs and chemicals (T36-T65 with fifth or sixth character 1-4 or 6)
      specified complications classified elsewhere
  The appropriate 7th character is to be added to each code from category T88

> A   initial encounter
> D   subsequent encounter
> S   sequela

X● **T88.0** **Infection following immunization**
  Sepsis following immunization
X● **T88.1** **Other complications following immunization, not elsewhere classified**
  Generalized vaccinia
  Rash following immunization
  Excludes1 vaccinia not from vaccine (B08.011)
  Excludes2 anaphylactic shock due to serum (T80.5-)
      other serum reactions (T80.6-)
      postimmunization arthropathy (M02.2)
      postimmunization encephalitis (G04.02)
      postimmunization fever (R50.83)
X● **T88.2** **Shock due to anesthesia**
  Use additional code for adverse effect, if applicable, to identify drug (T41.- with fifth or sixth character 5)
  Excludes1 complications of anesthesia (in):
      labor and delivery (O74.-)
      pregnancy (O29.-)
      puerperium (O89.-)
      postprocedural shock NOS (T81.1-)
X● **T88.3** **Malignant hyperthermia due to anesthesia**
  Use additional code for adverse effect, if applicable, to identify drug (T41.- with fifth or sixth character 5)
X● **T88.4** **Failed or difficult intubation**
● **T88.5** **Other complications of anesthesia**
  Use additional code for adverse effect, if applicable, to identify drug (T41.- with fifth or sixth character 5)
  X● **T88.51** **Hypothermia following anesthesia**
  X● **T88.52** **Failed moderate sedation during procedure**
    Failed conscious sedation during procedure
    Excludes2 personal history of failed moderate sedation (Z92.83)
  X● **T88.53** **Unintended awareness under general anesthesia during procedure**
    Excludes2 personal history of unintended awareness under general anesthesia (Z92.84)
  X● **T88.59** **Other complications of anesthesia**

X ● **T88.6   Anaphylactic reaction due to adverse effect of correct drug or medicament properly administered**

Anaphylactic shock due to adverse effect of correct drug or medicament properly administered

Anaphylactoid reaction NOS

Use additional code for adverse effect, if applicable, to identify drug (T36-T50 with fifth or sixth character 5)

Excludes1	anaphylactic reaction due to serum (T80.5-)
	anaphylactic shock or reaction due to adverse food reaction (T78.0-)

X ● **T88.7   Unspecified adverse effect of drug or medicament**

Drug hypersensitivity NOS

Drug reaction NOS

Use additional code for adverse effect, if applicable, to identify drug (T36-T50 with fifth or sixth character 5)

Excludes1	specified adverse effects of drugs and medicaments (A00-R94 and T80-T88.6, T88.8)

X ● **T88.8   Other specified complications of surgical and medical care, not elsewhere classified**

Use additional code to identify the complication

X ● **T88.9   Complication of surgical and medical care, unspecified**

CHAPTER 20

EXTERNAL CAUSES OF MORBIDITY
(VØØ-Y99)

OGCR Chapter-Specific Coding Guidelines

20. **Chapter 20: External Causes of Morbidity (VØØ-Y99)**
The external causes of morbidity codes should never be sequenced as the first-listed or principal diagnosis.

External cause codes are intended to provide data for injury research and evaluation of injury prevention strategies. These codes capture how the injury or health condition happened (cause), the intent (unintentional or accidental; or intentional, such as suicide or assault), the place where the event occurred the activity of the patient at the time of the event, and the person's status (e.g., civilian, military).

There is no national requirement for mandatory ICD-10-CM external cause code reporting. Unless a provider is subject to a state-based external cause code reporting mandate or these codes are required by a particular payer, reporting of ICD-10-CM codes in Chapter 20, External Causes of Morbidity, is not required. In the absence of a mandatory reporting requirement, providers are encouraged to voluntarily report external cause codes, as they provide valuable data for injury research and evaluation of injury prevention strategies.

a. General External Cause Coding Guidelines

1) Used with any code in the range of AØØ.Ø-T88.9, ZØØ-Z99
An external cause code may be used with any code in the range of AØØ.Ø-T88.9, ZØØ-Z99, classification that **represents** a health condition due to an external cause. Though they are most applicable to injuries, they are also valid for use with such things as infections or diseases due to an external source, and other health conditions, such as a heart attack that occurs during strenuous physical activity.

2) External cause code used for length of treatment
Assign the external cause code, with the appropriate 7th character (initial encounter, subsequent encounter or sequela) for each encounter for which the injury or condition is being treated.

Most categories in chapter 20 have a 7th character requirement for each applicable code. Most categories in this chapter have three 7th character values: A, initial encounter, D, subsequent encounter and S, sequela. While the patient may be seen by a new or different provider over the course of treatment for an injury or condition, assignment of the 7th character for external cause should match the 7th character of the code assigned for the associated injury or condition for the encounter.

3) Use the full range of external cause codes
Use the full range of external cause codes to completely describe the cause, the intent, the place of occurrence and if applicable, the activity of the patient at the time of the event, and the patient's status, for all injuries, and other health conditions due to an external cause.

4) Assign as many external cause codes as necessary
Assign as many external cause codes as necessary to fully explain each cause. If only one external code can be recorded, assign the code most related to the principal diagnosis.

5) The selection of the appropriate external cause code
The selection of the appropriate external cause code is guided by the Alphabetic Index of External Causes and by Inclusion and Exclusion notes in the Tabular List.

6) External cause code can never be a principal diagnosis
An external cause code can never be a principal (first-listed) diagnosis.

7) Combination external cause codes
Certain of the external cause codes are combination codes that identify sequential events that result in an injury, such as a fall which results in striking against an object. The injury may be due to either event or both. The combination external cause code used should correspond to the sequence of events regardless of which caused the most serious injury.

8) No external cause code needed in certain circumstances
No external cause code from Chapter 20 is needed if the external cause and intent are included in a code from another chapter (e.g. T36.ØX1- Poisoning by penicillins, accidental (unintentional)).

b. Place of Occurrence Guideline
Codes from category Y92, Place of occurrence of the external cause, are secondary codes for use after other external cause codes to identify the location of the patient at the time of injury or other condition.

Generally, a place of occurrence code is **assigned** only once, at the initial encounter for treatment. **However, in the rare instance that a new injury occurs during hospitalization, an additional place of occurrence code may be assigned.** No 7th characters are used for Y92. Only one code from Y92 should be recorded on a medical record.

Do not use place of occurrence code Y92.9 if the place is not stated or is not applicable.

c. Activity Code
Assign a code from category Y93, Activity code, to describe the activity of the patient at the time the injury or other health condition occurred.

An activity code is used only once, at the initial encounter for treatment. Only one code from Y93 should be recorded on a medical record.

The activity codes are not applicable to poisonings, adverse effects, misadventures or sequela.

Do not assign Y93.9, Unspecified activity, if the activity is not stated.

A code from category Y93 is appropriate for use with external cause and intent codes if identifying the activity provides additional information about the event.

d. Place of Occurrence, Activity, and Status Codes Used with other External Cause Code
When applicable, place of occurrence, activity, and external cause status codes are sequenced after the main external cause code(s). Regardless of the number of external cause codes assigned, there should be only one place of occurrence code, one activity code, and one external cause status code assigned to an encounter.

e. If the Reporting Format Limits the Number of External Cause Codes

If the reporting format limits the number of external cause codes that can be used in reporting clinical data, report the code for the cause/intent most related to the principal diagnosis. If the format permits capture of additional external cause codes, the cause/intent, including medical misadventures, of the additional events should be reported rather than the codes for place, activity, or external status.

f. Multiple External Cause Coding Guidelines

More than one external cause code is required to fully describe the external cause of an illness or injury. The assignment of external cause codes should be sequenced in the following priority:

If two or more events cause separate injuries, an external cause code should be assigned for each cause. The first-listed external cause code will be selected in the following order:

External codes for child and adult abuse take priority over all other external cause codes.

See Section I.C.19., Child and Adult abuse guidelines.

External codes for terrorism events take priority over all other external cause codes except child and adult abuse.

External cause codes for cataclysmic events take priority over all other external cause codes except child and adult abuse and terrorism.

External cause codes for transport accidents take priority over all other external cause codes except cataclysmic events, child and adult abuse and terrorism.

Activity and external cause status codes are assigned following all causal (intent) external cause codes.

The first-listed external cause code should correspond to the cause of the most serious diagnosis due to an assault, accident, or self-harm, following the order of hierarchy listed above.

g. Child and Adult Abuse Guideline

Adult and child abuse, neglect and maltreatment are classified as assault. Any of the assault codes may be used to indicate the external cause of any injury resulting from the confirmed abuse.

For confirmed cases of abuse, neglect and maltreatment, when the perpetrator is known, a code from Y07, Perpetrator of maltreatment and neglect, should accompany any other assault codes.

See Section I.C.19. Adult and child abuse, neglect and other maltreatment

h. Unknown or Undetermined Intent Guideline

If the intent (accident, self-harm, assault) of the cause of an injury or other condition is unknown or unspecified, code the intent as accidental intent. All transport accident categories assume accidental intent.

1) Use of undetermined intent

External cause codes for events of undetermined intent are only for use if the documentation in the record specifies that the intent cannot be determined.

i. Sequelae (Late Effects) of External Cause Guidelines

1) Sequelae external cause codes

Sequela are reported using the external cause code with the 7th character "S" for sequela. These codes should be used with any report of a late effect or sequela resulting from a previous injury.

See Section I.B.10. Sequela, (Late Effects)

2) Sequela external cause code with a related current injury

A sequela external cause code should never be used with a related current nature of injury code.

3) Use of sequela external cause codes for subsequent visits

Use a late effect external cause code for subsequent visits when a late effect of the initial injury is being treated. Do not use a late effect external cause code for subsequent visits for follow-up care (e.g., to assess healing, to receive rehabilitative therapy) of the injury when no late effect of the injury has been documented.

j. Terrorism Guidelines

1) Cause of injury identified by the Federal Government (FBI) as terrorism

When the cause of an injury is identified by the Federal Government (FBI) as terrorism, the first-listed external cause code should be a code from category Y38, Terrorism. The definition of terrorism employed by the FBI is found at the inclusion note at the beginning of category Y38. Use additional code for place of occurrence (Y92.-). More than one Y38 code may be assigned if the injury is the result of more than one mechanism of terrorism.

2) Cause of an injury is suspected to be the result of terrorism

When the cause of an injury is suspected to be the result of terrorism a code from category Y38 should not be assigned. Suspected cases should be classified as assault.

3) Code Y38.9, Terrorism, secondary effects

Assign code Y38.9, Terrorism, secondary effects, for conditions occurring subsequent to the terrorist event. This code should not be assigned for conditions that are due to the initial terrorist act.

It is acceptable to assign code Y38.9 with another code from Y38 if there is an injury due to the initial terrorist event and an injury that is a subsequent result of the terrorist event.

k. External cause status

A code from category Y99, External cause status, should be assigned whenever any other external cause code is assigned for an encounter, including an Activity code, except for the events noted below. Assign a code from category Y99, External cause status, to indicate the work status of the person at the time the event occurred. The status code indicates whether the event occurred during military activity, whether a non-military person was at work, whether an individual including a student or volunteer was involved in a non-work activity at the time of the causal event.

A code from Y99, External cause status, should be assigned, when applicable, with other external cause codes, such as transport accidents and falls. The external cause status codes are not applicable to poisonings, adverse effects, misadventures or late effects.

Do not assign a code from category Y99 if no other external cause codes (cause, activity) are applicable for the encounter.

An external cause status code is used only once, at the initial encounter for treatment. Only one code from Y99 should be recorded on a medical record.

Do not assign code Y99.9, Unspecified external cause status, if the status is not stated.

CHAPTER 20

EXTERNAL CAUSES OF MORBIDITY (VØØ-Y99)

Note: This chapter permits the classification of environmental events and circumstances as the cause of injury, and other adverse effects. Where a code from this section is applicable, it is intended that it shall be used secondary to a code from another chapter of the Classification indicating the nature of the condition. Most often, the condition will be classifiable to Chapter 19, Injury, poisoning and certain other consequences of external causes (SØØ-T88). Other conditions that may be stated to be due to external causes are classified in Chapters I to XVIII. For these conditions, codes from Chapter 20 should be used to provide additional information as to the cause of the condition.

This chapter contains the following blocks:

VØØ-X58	Accidents
VØØ-V99	Transport accidents
VØØ-VØ9	Pedestrian injured in transport accident
V10-V19	Pedal cycle rider injured in transport accident
V20-V29	Motorcycle rider injured in transport accident
V30-V39	Occupant of three-wheeled motor vehicle injured in transport accident
V40-V49	Car occupant injured in transport accident
V50-V59	Occupant of pick-up truck or van injured in transport accident
V60-V69	Occupant of heavy transport vehicle injured in transport accident
V70-V79	Bus occupant injured in transport accident
V80-V89	Other land transport accidents
V90-V94	Water transport accidents
V95-V97	Air and space transport accidents
V98-V99	Other and unspecified transport accidents
W00-X58	Other external causes of accidental injury
W00-W19	Slipping, tripping, stumbling and falls
W20-W49	Exposure to inanimate mechanical forces
W50-W64	Exposure to animate mechanical forces
W65-W74	Accidental non-transport drowning and submersion
W85-W99	Exposure to electric current, radiation and extreme ambient air temperature and pressure
X00-X08	Exposure to smoke, fire and flames
X10-X19	Contact with heat and hot substances
X30-X39	Exposure to forces of nature
~~X50~~	~~Overexertion and strenuous or repetitive movements~~
X52, X58	Accidental exposure to other specified factors
X71-X83	Intentional self-harm
X92-Y09	Assault
Y21-Y33	Event of undetermined intent
Y35-Y38	Legal intervention, operations of war, military operations, and terrorism
Y62-Y84	Complications of medical and surgical care
Y62-Y69	Misadventures to patients during surgical and medical care
Y70-Y82	Medical devices associated with adverse incidents in diagnostic and therapeutic use
Y83-Y84	Surgical and other medical procedures as the cause of abnormal reaction of the patient, or of later complication, without mention of misadventure at the time of the procedure
Y90-Y99	Supplementary factors related to causes of morbidity classified elsewhere

ACCIDENTS (VØØ-X58)

TRANSPORT ACCIDENTS (VØØ-V99)

Note: This section is structured in 12 groups. Those relating to land transport accidents (VØØ-V89) reflect the victim's mode of transport and are subdivided to identify the victim's 'counterpart' or the type of event. The vehicle of which the injured person is an occupant is identified in the first two characters since it is seen as the most important factor to identify for prevention purposes. A transport accident is one in which the vehicle involved must be moving or running or in use for transport purposes at the time of the accident.

Use additional code to identify:
Airbag injury (W22.1)
Type of street or road (Y92.4-)
Use of cellular telephone and other electronic equipment at the time of the transport accident (Y93.C-)

Excludes1 agricultural vehicles in stationary use or maintenance (W31.-)
assault by crashing of motor vehicle (YØ3.-)
automobile or motor cycle in stationary use or maintenance - code to type of accident
crashing of motor vehicle, undetermined intent (Y32)
intentional self-harm by crashing of motor vehicle (X82)

Excludes2 transport accidents due to cataclysm (X34-X38)

Note: Definitions related to transport accidents:

(a) A transport accident (VØØ-V99) is any accident involving a device designed primarily for, or used at the time primarily for, conveying persons or goods from one place to another.

(b) A public highway [trafficway] or street is the entire width between property lines (or other boundary lines) of land open to the public as a matter of right or custom for purposes of moving persons or property from one place to another. A roadway is that part of the public highway designed, improved and customarily used for vehicular traffic.

(c) A traffic accident is any vehicle accident occurring on the public highway [i.e., originating on, terminating on, or involving a vehicle partially on the highway]. A vehicle accident is assumed to have occurred on the public highway unless another place is specified, except in the case of accidents involving only off-road motor vehicles, which are classified as nontraffic accidents unless the contrary is stated.

(d) A nontraffic accident is any vehicle accident that occurs entirely in any place other than a public highway.

(e) A pedestrian is any person involved in an accident who was not at the time of the accident riding in or on a motor vehicle, railway train, streetcar or animal-drawn or other vehicle, or on a pedal cycle or animal. This includes, a person changing a tire, working on a parked car, or a person on foot. It also includes the user of a pedestrian conveyance such as a baby-stroller, ice-skates, skis, sled, roller skates, a skateboard, nonmotorized or motorized wheelchair, motorized mobility scooter, or nonmotorized scooter.

(f) A driver is an occupant of a transport vehicle who is operating or intending to operate it.

(g) A passenger is any occupant of a transport vehicle other than the driver, except a person traveling on the outside of the vehicle.

(h) A person on the outside of a vehicle is any person being transported by a vehicle but not occupying the space normally reserved for the driver or passengers, or the space intended for the transport of property. This includes a person travelling on the bodywork, bumper, fender, roof, running board or step of a vehicle, as well as, hanging on the outside of the vehicle.

(i) A pedal cycle is any land transport vehicle operated solely by nonmotorized pedals including a bicycle or tricycle.

(j) A pedal cyclist is any person riding a pedal cycle or in a sidecar or trailer attached to a pedal cycle.

(k) A motorcycle is a two-wheeled motor vehicle with one or two riding saddles and sometimes with a third wheel for the support of a sidecar. The sidecar is considered part of the motorcycle. This includes a moped, motor scooter, or motorized bicycle.

(l) A motorcycle rider is any person riding a motorcycle or in a sidecar or trailer attached to the motorcycle.

(m) A three-wheeled motor vehicle is a motorized tricycle designed primarily for on-road use. This includes a motor-driven tricycle, a motorized rickshaw, or a three-wheeled motor car.

(n) A car [automobile] is a four-wheeled motor vehicle designed primarily for carrying up to 7 persons. A trailer being towed by the car is considered part of the car. It does not include a van or minivan—see definition (o)

(o) A pick-up truck or van is a four or six-wheeled motor vehicle designed for carrying passengers as well as property or cargo weighing less than the local limit for classification as a heavy goods vehicle, and not requiring a special driver's license. This includes a minivan and a sport-utility vehicle (SUV).

(p) A heavy transport vehicle is a motor vehicle designed primarily for carrying property, meeting local criteria for classification as a heavy goods vehicle in terms of weight and requiring a special driver's license.

(q) A bus (coach) is a motor vehicle designed or adapted primarily for carrying more than 10 passengers, and requiring a special driver's license.

(r) A railway train or railway vehicle is any device, with or without freight or passenger cars coupled to it, designed for traffic on a railway track. This includes subterranean (subways) or elevated trains.

(s) A streetcar is a device designed and used primarily for transporting passengers within a municipality, running on rails, usually subject to normal traffic control signals, and operated principally on a right-of-way that forms part of the roadway. This includes a tram or trolley that runs on rails. A trailer being towed by a streetcar is considered part of the streetcar.

(t) A special vehicle mainly used on industrial premises is a motor vehicle designed primarily for use within the buildings and premises of industrial or commercial establishments. This includes battery-powered airport passenger vehicles or baggage/mail trucks, forklifts, coal-cars in a coal mine, logging cars and trucks used in mines or quarries.

(u) A special vehicle mainly used in agriculture is a motor vehicle designed specifically for use in farming and agriculture (horticulture), to work the land, tend and harvest crops and transport materials on the farm. This includes harvesters, farm machinery and tractor and trailers.

(v) A special construction vehicle is a motor vehicle designed specifically for use on construction and demolition sites. This includes bulldozers, diggers, earth levellers, dump trucks, backhoes, front-end loaders, pavers, and mechanical shovels.

(w) A special all-terrain vehicle is a motor vehicle of special design to enable it to negotiate over rough or soft terrain, snow or sand. Examples of special design are high construction, special wheels and tires, tracks, and support on a cushion of air. This includes snow mobiles, all-terrain vehicles (ATV), and dune buggies. It does not include passenger vehicle designated as sport utility vehicles (SUV).

(x) A watercraft is any device designed for transporting passengers or goods on water. This includes motor or sail boats, ships, and hovercraft.

(y) An aircraft is any device for transporting passengers or goods in the air. This includes hot-air balloons, gliders, helicopters and airplanes.

(z) A military vehicle is any motorized vehicle operating on a public roadway owned by the military and being operated by a member of the military.

PEDESTRIAN INJURED IN TRANSPORT ACCIDENT (V00-V09)

Includes	person changing tire on transport vehicle
	person examining engine of vehicle broken down in (on side of) road
Excludes1	fall due to non-transport collision with other person (W03)
	pedestrian on foot falling (slipping) on ice and snow (W00.-)
	struck or bumped by another person (W51)

● **V00 Pedestrian conveyance accident**

Use additional place of occurrence and activity external cause codes, if known (Y92.-, Y93.-)

Excludes1   collision with another person without fall (W51)

fall due to person on foot colliding with another person on foot (W03)

fall from non-moving wheelchair, nonmotorized scooter and motorized mobility scooter without collision (W05.-)

pedestrian (conveyance) collision with other land transport vehicle (V01-V09)

pedestrian on foot falling (slipping) on ice and snow (W00.-)

The appropriate 7th character is to be added to each code from category V00

A	initial encounter
D	subsequent encounter
S	sequela

● **V00.0 Pedestrian on foot injured in collision with pedestrian conveyance**

X● **V00.01 Pedestrian on foot injured in collision with roller-skater**

X● **V00.02 Pedestrian on foot injured in collision with skateboarder**

X● **V00.09 Pedestrian on foot injured in collision with other pedestrian conveyance**

● **V00.1 Rolling-type pedestrian conveyance accident**

Excludes1   accident with babystroller (V00.82-)

accident with wheelchair (powered) (V00.81-)

accident with motorized mobility scooter (V00.83-)

● **V00.11 In-line roller-skate accident**

    ● **V00.111 Fall from in-line roller-skates**

    ● **V00.112 In-line roller-skater colliding with stationary object**

    ● **V00.118 Other in-line roller-skate accident**

        Excludes1   roller-skater collision with other land transport vehicle (V01-V09 with 5th character 1)

● **V00.12 Non-in-line roller-skate accident**

    ● **V00.121 Fall from non-in-line roller-skates**

    ● **V00.122 Non-in-line roller-skater colliding with stationary object**

    ● **V00.128 Other non-in-line roller-skating accident**

        Excludes1   roller-skater collision with other land transport vehicle (V01-V09 with 5th character 1)

CHAPTER 20 (V01-Y99)

- ● **V00.13** Skateboard accident
  - ● **V00.131** Fall from skateboard
  - ● **V00.132** Skateboarder colliding with stationary object
  - ● **V00.138** Other skateboard accident
    - **Excludes1** skateboarder collision with other land transport vehicle (V01-V09 with 5th character 2)
- ● **V00.14** Scooter (nonmotorized) accident
  - **Excludes1** motorscooter accident (V20-V29)
  - ● **V00.141** Fall from scooter (nonmotorized)
  - ● **V00.142** Scooter (nonmotorized) colliding with stationary object
  - ● **V00.148** Other scooter (nonmotorized) accident
    - **Excludes1** scooter (non-motorized) collision with other land transport vehicle (V01-V09 with fifth character 9)
- ● **V00.15** Heelies accident
  Rolling shoe
  Wheeled shoe
  Wheelies accident
  - ● **V00.151** Fall from heelies
  - ● **V00.152** Heelies colliding with stationary object
  - ● **V00.158** Other heelies accident
- ● **V00.18** Accident on other rolling-type pedestrian conveyance
  - ● **V00.181** Fall from other rolling-type pedestrian conveyance
  - ● **V00.182** Pedestrian on other rolling-type pedestrian conveyance colliding with stationary object
  - ● **V00.188** Other accident on other rolling-type pedestrian conveyance
- ● **V00.2** Gliding-type pedestrian conveyance accident
  - ● **V00.21** Ice-skates accident
    - ● **V00.211** Fall from ice-skates
    - ● **V00.212** Ice-skater colliding with stationary object
    - ● **V00.218** Other ice-skates accident
      - **Excludes1** ice-skater collision with other land transport vehicle (V01-V09 with 5th digit 9)
  - ● **V00.22** Sled accident
    - ● **V00.221** Fall from sled
    - ● **V00.222** Sledder colliding with stationary object
    - ● **V00.228** Other sled accident
      - **Excludes1** sled collision with other land transport vehicle (V01-V09 with 5th digit 9)

- ● **V00.28** Other gliding-type pedestrian conveyance accident
  - ● **V00.281** Fall from other gliding-type pedestrian conveyance
  - ● **V00.282** Pedestrian on other gliding-type pedestrian conveyance colliding with stationary object
  - ● **V00.288** Other accident on other gliding-type pedestrian conveyance
    - **Excludes1** gliding-type pedestrian conveyance collision with other land transport vehicle (V01-V09 with 5th digit 9)
- ● **V00.3** Flat-bottomed pedestrian conveyance accident
  - ● **V00.31** Snowboard accident
    - ● **V00.311** Fall from snowboard
    - ● **V00.312** Snowboarder colliding with stationary object
    - ● **V00.318** Other snowboard accident
      - **Excludes1** snowboarder collision with other land transport vehicle (V01-V09 with 5th digit 9)
  - ● **V00.32** Snow-ski accident
    - ● **V00.321** Fall from snow-skis
    - ● **V00.322** Snow-skier colliding with stationary object
    - ● **V00.328** Other snow-ski accident
      - **Excludes1** snow-skier collision with other land transport vehicle (V01-V09 with 5th digit 9)
  - ● **V00.38** Other flat-bottomed pedestrian conveyance accident
    - ● **V00.381** Fall from other flat-bottomed pedestrian conveyance
    - ● **V00.382** Pedestrian on other flat-bottomed pedestrian conveyance colliding with stationary object
    - ● **V00.388** Other accident on other flat-bottomed pedestrian conveyance
- ● **V00.8** Accident on other pedestrian conveyance
  - ● **V00.81** Accident with wheelchair (powered)
    - ● **V00.811** Fall from moving wheelchair (powered)
      - **Excludes1** fall from non-moving wheelchair (W05.0)
    - ● **V00.812** Wheelchair (powered) colliding with stationary object
    - ● **V00.818** Other accident with wheelchair (powered)
  - ● **V00.82** Accident with babystroller
    - ● **V00.821** Fall from babystroller
    - ● **V00.822** Babystroller colliding with stationary object
    - ● **V00.828** Other accident with babystroller

▶ New　⇒ Revised　~~deleted~~ Deleted　**OGCR** Official Guidelines　X Assign placeholder X　● Use Additional Character(s)

Excludes 1　Excludes 2　Includes　Use additional　Code first　Code also　Key words

● **V00.83   Accident with motorized mobility scooter**
    ● **V00.831   Fall from motorized mobility scooter**
        | Excludes1 | fall from non-moving motorized mobility scooter (W05.2) |

    ● **V00.832   Motorized mobility scooter colliding with stationary object**
    ● **V00.838   Other accident with motorized mobility scooter**
● **V00.89   Accident on other pedestrian conveyance**
    ● **V00.891   Fall from other pedestrian conveyance**
    ● **V00.892   Pedestrian on other pedestrian conveyance colliding with stationary object**
    ● **V00.898   Other accident on other pedestrian conveyance**
        | Excludes1 | other pedestrian (conveyance) collision with other land transport vehicle (V01-V09 with 5th digit 9) |

● **V01   Pedestrian injured in collision with pedal cycle**
    The appropriate 7th character is to be added to each code from category V01

A	initial encounter
D	subsequent encounter
S	sequela

● **V01.0   Pedestrian injured in collision with pedal cycle in nontraffic accident**
    X ● **V01.00   Pedestrian on foot injured in collision with pedal cycle in nontraffic accident**
        Pedestrian NOS injured in collision with pedal cycle in nontraffic accident
    X ● **V01.01   Pedestrian on roller-skates injured in collision with pedal cycle in nontraffic accident**
    X ● **V01.02   Pedestrian on skateboard injured in collision with pedal cycle in nontraffic accident**
    X ● **V01.09   Pedestrian with other conveyance injured in collision with pedal cycle in nontraffic accident**
        Pedestrian with babystroller injured in collision with pedal cycle in nontraffic accident
        Pedestrian in wheelchair (powered) injured in collision with pedal cycle in nontraffic accident
        Pedestrian in motorized mobility scooter injured in collision with pedal cycle in nontraffic accident
        Pedestrian on ice-skates injured in collision with pedal cycle in nontraffic accident
        Pedestrian on nonmotorized scooter injured in collision with pedal cycle in nontraffic accident
        Pedestrian on sled injured in collision with pedal cycle in nontraffic accident
        Pedestrian on snowboard injured in collision with pedal cycle in nontraffic accident
        Pedestrian on snow-skis injured in collision with pedal cycle in nontraffic accident

● **V01.1   Pedestrian injured in collision with pedal cycle in traffic accident**
    X ● **V01.10   Pedestrian on foot injured in collision with pedal cycle in traffic accident**
        Pedestrian NOS injured in collision with pedal cycle in traffic accident
    X ● **V01.11   Pedestrian on roller-skates injured in collision with pedal cycle in traffic accident**
    X ● **V01.12   Pedestrian on skateboard injured in collision with pedal cycle in traffic accident**
    X ● **V01.19   Pedestrian with other conveyance injured in collision with pedal cycle in traffic accident**
        Pedestrian with babystroller injured in collision with pedal cycle in traffic accident
        Pedestrian in wheelchair (powered) injured in collision with pedal cycle in traffic accident
        Pedestrian in motorized mobility scooter injured in collision with pedal cycle in traffic accident
        Pedestrian on ice-skates injured in collision with pedal cycle in traffic accident
        Pedestrian on nonmotorized scooter injured in collision with pedal cycle in traffic accident
        Pedestrian on sled injured in collision with pedal cycle in traffic accident
        Pedestrian on snowboard injured in collision with pedal cycle in traffic accident
        Pedestrian on snow-skis injured in collision with pedal cycle in traffic accident

● **V01.9   Pedestrian injured in collision with pedal cycle, unspecified whether traffic or nontraffic accident**
    X ● **V01.90   Pedestrian on foot injured in collision with pedal cycle, unspecified whether traffic or nontraffic accident**
        Pedestrian NOS injured in collision with pedal cycle, unspecified whether traffic or nontraffic accident
    X ● **V01.91   Pedestrian on roller-skates injured in collision with pedal cycle, unspecified whether traffic or nontraffic accident**
    X ● **V01.92   Pedestrian on skateboard injured in collision with pedal cycle, unspecified whether traffic or nontraffic accident**
    X ● **V01.99   Pedestrian with other conveyance injured in collision with pedal cycle, unspecified whether traffic or nontraffic accident**
        Pedestrian with babystroller injured in collision with pedal cycle, unspecified whether traffic or nontraffic accident
        Pedestrian in wheelchair (powered) injured in collision with pedal cycle, unspecified whether traffic or nontraffic accident
        Pedestrian in motorized mobility scooter injured in collision with pedal cycle, unspecified whether traffic or nontraffic accident
        Pedestrian on ice-skates injured in collision with pedal cycle unspecified, whether traffic or nontraffic accident
        Pedestrian on nonmotorized scooter injured in collision with pedal cycle, unspecified whether traffic or nontraffic accident
        Pedestrian on sled injured in collision with pedal cycle unspecified, whether traffic or nontraffic accident
        Pedestrian on snowboard injured in collision with pedal cycle, unspecified whether traffic or nontraffic accident
        Pedestrian on snow-skis injured in collision with pedal cycle, unspecified whether traffic or nontraffic accident

CHAPTER 20 (V01-Y99)

● **V02** Pedestrian injured in collision with two- or three-wheeled motor vehicle

The appropriate 7th character is to be added to each code from category V02

> A   initial encounter
> D   subsequent encounter
> S   sequela

● **V02.0** Pedestrian injured in collision with two- or three-wheeled motor vehicle in nontraffic accident

X● **V02.00** Pedestrian on foot injured in collision with two- or three-wheeled motor vehicle in nontraffic accident

Pedestrian NOS injured in collision with two- or three-wheeled motor vehicle in nontraffic accident

X● **V02.01** Pedestrian on roller-skates injured in collision with two- or three-wheeled motor vehicle in nontraffic accident

X● **V02.02** Pedestrian on skateboard injured in collision with two- or three-wheeled motor vehicle in nontraffic accident

X● **V02.09** Pedestrian with other conveyance injured in collision with two- or three-wheeled motor vehicle in nontraffic accident

Pedestrian with babystroller injured in collision with two- or three-wheeled motor vehicle in nontraffic accident

Pedestrian on ice-skates injured in collision with two- or three-wheeled motor vehicle in nontraffic accident

Pedestrian in wheelchair (powered) injured in collision with two- or three-wheeled motor vehicle in nontraffic accident

Pedestrian in motorized mobility scooter injured in collision with two- or three-wheeled motor vehicle in nontraffic accident

Pedestrian on nonmotorized scooter injured in collision with two- or three-wheeled motor vehicle in nontraffic accident

Pedestrian on sled injured in collision with two- or three-wheeled motor vehicle in nontraffic accident

Pedestrian on snowboard injured in collision with two- or three-wheeled motor vehicle in nontraffic accident

Pedestrian on snow-skis injured in collision with two- or three-wheeled motor vehicle in nontraffic accident

● **V02.1** Pedestrian injured in collision with two- or three-wheeled motor vehicle in traffic accident

X● **V02.10** Pedestrian on foot injured in collision with two- or three-wheeled motor vehicle in traffic accident

Pedestrian NOS injured in collision with two- or three-wheeled motor vehicle in traffic accident

X● **V02.11** Pedestrian on roller-skates injured in collision with two- or three-wheeled motor vehicle in traffic accident

X● **V02.12** Pedestrian on skateboard injured in collision with two- or three-wheeled motor vehicle in traffic accident

X● **V02.19** Pedestrian with other conveyance injured in collision with two- or three-wheeled motor vehicle in traffic accident

Pedestrian with babystroller injured in collision with two- or three-wheeled motor vehicle in traffic accident

Pedestrian in wheelchair (powered) injured in collision with two- or three-wheeled motor vehicle in traffic accident

Pedestrian in motorized mobility scooter injured in collision with two- or three-wheeled motor vehicle in traffic accident

Pedestrian on ice-skates injured in collision with two- or three-wheeled motor vehicle in traffic accident

Pedestrian on nonmotorized scooter injured in collision with two- or three-wheeled motor vehicle in traffic accident

Pedestrian on sled injured in collision with two- or three-wheeled motor vehicle in traffic accident

Pedestrian on snowboard injured in collision with two- or three-wheeled motor vehicle in traffic accident

Pedestrian on snow-skis injured in collision with two- or three-wheeled motor vehicle in traffic accident

● **V02.9** Pedestrian injured in collision with two- or three-wheeled motor vehicle, unspecified whether traffic or nontraffic accident

X● **V02.90** Pedestrian on foot injured in collision with two- or three-wheeled motor vehicle, unspecified whether traffic or nontraffic accident

Pedestrian NOS injured in collision with two- or three-wheeled motor vehicle, unspecified whether traffic or nontraffic accident

X● **V02.91** Pedestrian on roller-skates injured in collision with two- or three-wheeled motor vehicle, unspecified whether traffic or nontraffic accident

X● **V02.92** Pedestrian on skateboard injured in collision with two- or three-wheeled motor vehicle, unspecified whether traffic or nontraffic accident

▶ New   ⇒ Revised   ~~deleted~~ Deleted   **OGCR** Official Guidelines   X Assign placeholder X   ● Use Additional Character(s)

Excludes 1   Excludes 2   Includes   Use additional   Code first   Code also   Key words

X● **V02.99** Pedestrian with other conveyance injured in collision with two- or three-wheeled motor vehicle, unspecified whether traffic or nontraffic accident

     Pedestrian with babystroller injured in collision with two- or three-wheeled motor vehicle, unspecified whether traffic or nontraffic accident

     Pedestrian in wheelchair (powered) injured in collision with two- or three-wheeled motor vehicle, unspecified whether traffic or nontraffic accident

     Pedestrian in motorized mobility scooter injured in collision with two- or three-wheeled motor vehicle, unspecified whether traffic or nontraffic accident

     Pedestrian on ice-skates injured in collision with two- or three-wheeled motor vehicle, unspecified whether traffic or nontraffic accident

     Pedestrian on nonmotorized scooter injured in collision with two- or three-wheeled motor vehicle, unspecified whether traffic or nontraffic accident

     Pedestrian on sled injured in collision with two- or three-wheeled motor vehicle, unspecified whether traffic or nontraffic accident

     Pedestrian on snowboard injured in collision with two- or three-wheeled motor vehicle, unspecified whether traffic or nontraffic accident

     Pedestrian on snow-skis injured in collision with two- or three-wheeled motor vehicle, unspecified whether traffic or nontraffic accident

● **V03** Pedestrian injured in collision with car, pick-up truck or van

     The appropriate 7th character is to be added to each code from category V03

A	initial encounter
D	subsequent encounter
S	sequela

● **V03.0** Pedestrian injured in collision with car, pick-up truck or van in nontraffic accident

X● **V03.00** Pedestrian on foot injured in collision with car, pick-up truck or van in nontraffic accident

     Pedestrian NOS injured in collision with car, pick-up truck or van in nontraffic accident

X● **V03.01** Pedestrian on roller-skates injured in collision with car, pick-up truck or van in nontraffic accident

X● **V03.02** Pedestrian on skateboard injured in collision with car, pick-up truck or van in nontraffic accident

X● **V03.09** Pedestrian with other conveyance injured in collision with car, pick-up truck or van in nontraffic accident

     Pedestrian with babystroller injured in collision with car, pick-up truck or van in nontraffic accident

     Pedestrian in wheelchair (powered) injured in collision with car, pick-up truck or van in nontraffic accident

     Pedestrian in motorized mobility scooter injured in collision with car, pick-up truck or van in nontraffic accident

     Pedestrian on ice-skates injured in collision with car, pick-up truck or van in nontraffic accident

     Pedestrian on nonmotorized scooter injured in collision with car, pick-up truck or van in nontraffic accident

     Pedestrian on sled injured in collision with car, pick-up truck or van in nontraffic accident

     Pedestrian on snowboard injured in collision with car, pick-up truck or van in nontraffic accident

     Pedestrian on snow-skis injured in collision with car, pick-up truck or van in nontraffic accident

● **V03.1** Pedestrian injured in collision with car, pick-up truck or van in traffic accident

X● **V03.10** Pedestrian on foot injured in collision with car, pick-up truck or van in traffic accident

     Pedestrian NOS injured in collision with car, pick-up truck or van in traffic accident

X● **V03.11** Pedestrian on roller-skates injured in collision with car, pick-up truck or van in traffic accident

X● **V03.12** Pedestrian on skateboard injured in collision with car, pick-up truck or van in traffic accident

X● **V03.19** Pedestrian with other conveyance injured in collision with car, pick-up truck or van in traffic accident

     Pedestrian with babystroller injured in collision with car, pick-up truck or van in traffic accident

     Pedestrian in wheelchair (powered) injured in collision with car, pick-up truck or van in traffic accident

     Pedestrian in motorized mobility scooter injured in collision with car, pick-up truck or van in traffic accident

     Pedestrian on ice-skates injured in collision with car, pick-up truck or van in traffic accident

     Pedestrian on nonmotorized scooter injured in collision with car, pick-up truck or van in traffic accident

     Pedestrian on sled injured in collision with car, pick-up truck or van in traffic accident

     Pedestrian on snowboard injured in collision with car, pick-up truck or van in traffic accident

     Pedestrian on snow-skis injured in collision with car, pick-up truck or van in traffic accident

CHAPTER 20 (V01-Y99)

● **V03.9** **Pedestrian injured in collision with car, pick-up truck or van, unspecified whether traffic or nontraffic accident**

X● **V03.90** **Pedestrian on foot injured in collision with car, pick-up truck or van, unspecified whether traffic or nontraffic accident**
  Pedestrian NOS injured in collision with car, pick-up truck or van, unspecified whether traffic or nontraffic accident

X● **V03.91** **Pedestrian on roller-skates injured in collision with car, pick-up truck or van, unspecified whether traffic or nontraffic accident**

X● **V03.92** **Pedestrian on skateboard injured in collision with car, pick-up truck or van, unspecified whether traffic or nontraffic accident**

X● **V03.99** **Pedestrian with other conveyance injured in collision with car, pick-up truck or van, unspecified whether traffic or nontraffic accident**
  Pedestrian with babystroller injured in collision with car, pick-up truck or van, unspecified whether traffic or nontraffic accident
  Pedestrian in wheelchair (powered) injured in collision with car, pick-up truck or van, unspecified whether traffic or nontraffic accident
  Pedestrian in motorized mobility scooter injured in collision with car, pick-up truck or van, unspecified whether traffic or nontraffic accident
  Pedestrian on ice-skates injured in collision with car, pick-up truck or van, unspecified whether traffic or nontraffic accident
  Pedestrian on nonmotorized scooter injured in collision with car, pick-up truck or van, unspecified whether traffic or nontraffic accident
  Pedestrian on sled injured in collision with car, pick-up truck or van in nontraffic accident
  Pedestrian on snowboard injured in collision with car, pick-up truck or van, unspecified whether traffic or nontraffic accident
  Pedestrian on snow-skis injured in collision with car, pick-up truck or van, unspecified whether traffic or nontraffic accident

● **V04** **Pedestrian injured in collision with heavy transport vehicle or bus**

  Excludes1   pedestrian injured in collision with military vehicle (V09.01, V09.21)

  The appropriate 7th character is to be added to each code from category V04

A	initial encounter
D	subsequent encounter
S	sequela

● **V04.0** **Pedestrian injured in collision with heavy transport vehicle or bus in nontraffic accident**

X● **V04.00** **Pedestrian on foot injured in collision with heavy transport vehicle or bus in nontraffic accident**
  Pedestrian NOS injured in collision with heavy transport vehicle or bus in nontraffic accident

X● **V04.01** **Pedestrian on roller-skates injured in collision with heavy transport vehicle or bus in nontraffic accident**

X● **V04.02** **Pedestrian on skateboard injured in collision with heavy transport vehicle or bus in nontraffic accident**

X● **V04.09** **Pedestrian with other conveyance injured in collision with heavy transport vehicle or bus in nontraffic accident**
  Pedestrian with babystroller injured in collision with heavy transport vehicle or bus in nontraffic accident
  Pedestrian in wheelchair (powered) injured in collision with heavy transport vehicle or bus in nontraffic accident
  Pedestrian in motorized mobility scooter injured in collision with heavy transport vehicle or bus in nontraffic accident
  Pedestrian on ice-skates injured in collision with heavy transport vehicle or bus in nontraffic accident
  Pedestrian on nonmotorized scooter injured in collision with heavy transport vehicle or bus in nontraffic accident
  Pedestrian on sled injured in collision with heavy transport vehicle or bus in nontraffic accident
  Pedestrian on snowboard injured in collision with heavy transport vehicle or bus in nontraffic accident
  Pedestrian on snow-skis injured in collision with heavy transport vehicle or bus in nontraffic accident

● **V04.1** **Pedestrian injured in collision with heavy transport vehicle or bus in traffic accident**

X● **V04.10** **Pedestrian on foot injured in collision with heavy transport vehicle or bus in traffic accident**
  Pedestrian NOS injured in collision with heavy transport vehicle or bus in traffic accident

X● **V04.11** **Pedestrian on roller-skates injured in collision with heavy transport vehicle or bus in traffic accident**

X● **V04.12** **Pedestrian on skateboard injured in collision with heavy transport vehicle or bus in traffic accident**

X● **V04.19** **Pedestrian with other conveyance injured in collision with heavy transport vehicle or bus in traffic accident**
  Pedestrian with babystroller injured in collision with heavy transport vehicle or bus in traffic accident
  Pedestrian in wheelchair (powered) injured in collision with heavy transport vehicle or bus in traffic accident
  Pedestrian in motorized mobility scooter injured in collision with heavy transport vehicle or bus in traffic accident
  Pedestrian on ice-skates injured in collision with heavy transport vehicle or bus in traffic accident
  Pedestrian on nonmotorized scooter injured in collision with heavy transport vehicle or bus in traffic accident
  Pedestrian on sled injured in collision with heavy transport vehicle or bus in traffic accident
  Pedestrian on snowboard injured in collision with heavy transport vehicle or bus in traffic accident
  Pedestrian on snow-skis injured in collision with heavy transport vehicle or bus in traffic accident

▶ New   ⇒ Revised   ~~deleted~~ Deleted   **OGCR** Official Guidelines   X Assign placeholder X   ● Use Additional Character(s)

Excludes 1   Excludes 2   Includes   Use additional   Code first   Code also   Key words

● **V04.9**   **Pedestrian injured in collision with heavy transport vehicle or bus, unspecified whether traffic or nontraffic accident**

   X● **V04.90**   **Pedestrian on foot injured in collision with heavy transport vehicle or bus, unspecified whether traffic or nontraffic accident**

     Pedestrian NOS injured in collision with heavy transport vehicle or bus, unspecified whether traffic or nontraffic accident

   X● **V04.91**   **Pedestrian on roller-skates injured in collision with heavy transport vehicle or bus, unspecified whether traffic or nontraffic accident**

   X● **V04.92**   **Pedestrian on skateboard injured in collision with heavy transport vehicle or bus, unspecified whether traffic or nontraffic accident**

   X● **V04.99**   **Pedestrian with other conveyance injured in collision with heavy transport vehicle or bus, unspecified whether traffic or nontraffic accident**

     Pedestrian with babystroller injured in collision with heavy transport vehicle or bus, unspecified whether traffic or nontraffic accident

     Pedestrian in wheelchair (powered) injured in collision with heavy transport vehicle or bus, unspecified whether traffic or nontraffic accident

     Pedestrian in motorized mobility scooter injured in collision with heavy transport vehicle or bus, unspecified whether traffic or nontraffic accident

     Pedestrian on ice-skates injured in collision with heavy transport vehicle or bus, unspecified whether traffic or nontraffic accident

     Pedestrian on nonmotorized scooter injured in collision with heavy transport vehicle or bus, unspecified whether traffic or nontraffic accident

     Pedestrian on sled injured in collision with heavy transport vehicle or bus, unspecified whether traffic or nontraffic accident

     Pedestrian on snowboard injured in collision with heavy transport vehicle or bus, unspecified whether traffic or nontraffic accident

     Pedestrian on snow-skis injured in collision with heavy transport vehicle or bus, unspecified whether traffic or nontraffic accident

● **V05**   **Pedestrian injured in collision with railway train or railway vehicle**

   The appropriate 7th character is to be added to each code from category V05

A	initial encounter
D	subsequent encounter
S	sequela

● **V05.0**   **Pedestrian injured in collision with railway train or railway vehicle in nontraffic accident**

   X● **V05.00**   **Pedestrian on foot injured in collision with railway train or railway vehicle in nontraffic accident**

     Pedestrian NOS injured in collision with railway train or railway vehicle in nontraffic accident

   X● **V05.01**   **Pedestrian on roller-skates injured in collision with railway train or railway vehicle in nontraffic accident**

   X● **V05.02**   **Pedestrian on skateboard injured in collision with railway train or railway vehicle in nontraffic accident**

   X● **V05.09**   **Pedestrian with other conveyance injured in collision with railway train or railway vehicle in nontraffic accident**

     Pedestrian with babystroller injured in collision with railway train or railway vehicle in nontraffic accident

     Pedestrian in wheelchair (powered) injured in collision with railway train or railway vehicle in nontraffic accident

     Pedestrian in motorized mobility scooter injured in collision with railway train or railway vehicle in nontraffic accident

     Pedestrian on ice-skates injured in collision with railway train or railway vehicle in nontraffic accident

     Pedestrian on nonmotorized scooter injured in collision with railway train or railway vehicle in nontraffic accident

     Pedestrian on sled injured in collision with railway train or railway vehicle in nontraffic accident

     Pedestrian on snowboard injured in collision with railway train or railway vehicle in nontraffic accident

     Pedestrian on snow-skis injured in collision with railway train or railway vehicle in nontraffic accident

● **V05.1**   **Pedestrian injured in collision with railway train or railway vehicle in traffic accident**

   X● **V05.10**   **Pedestrian on foot injured in collision with railway train or railway vehicle in traffic accident**

     Pedestrian NOS injured in collision with railway train or railway vehicle in traffic accident

   X● **V05.11**   **Pedestrian on roller-skates injured in collision with railway train or railway vehicle in traffic accident**

   X● **V05.12**   **Pedestrian on skateboard injured in collision with railway train or railway vehicle in traffic accident**

   X● **V05.19**   **Pedestrian with other conveyance injured in collision with railway train or railway vehicle in traffic accident**

     Pedestrian with babystroller injured in collision with railway train or railway vehicle in traffic accident

     Pedestrian in wheelchair (powered) injured in collision with railway train or railway vehicle in traffic accident

     Pedestrian in motorized mobility scooter injured in collision with railway train or railway vehicle in traffic accident

     Pedestrian on ice-skates injured in collision with railway train or railway vehicle in traffic accident

     Pedestrian on nonmotorized scooter injured in collision with railway train or railway vehicle in traffic accident

     Pedestrian on sled injured in collision with railway train or railway vehicle in traffic accident

     Pedestrian on snowboard injured in collision with railway train or railway vehicle in traffic accident

     Pedestrian on snow-skis injured in collision with railway train or railway vehicle in traffic accident

CHAPTER 20 (V01-Y99)

▶ New   ⇒ Revised   ~~deleted~~ Deleted   **OGCR** Official Guidelines   X Assign placeholder X   ● Use Additional Character(s)

Excludes 1   Excludes 2   Includes   Use additional   Code first   Code also   Key words

● **V05.9** **Pedestrian injured in collision with railway train or railway vehicle, unspecified whether traffic or nontraffic accident**

   X● **V05.90** **Pedestrian on foot injured in collision with railway train or railway vehicle, unspecified whether traffic or nontraffic accident**

      Pedestrian NOS injured in collision with railway train or railway vehicle, unspecified whether traffic or nontraffic accident

   X● **V05.91** **Pedestrian on roller-skates injured in collision with railway train or railway vehicle, unspecified whether traffic or nontraffic accident**

   X● **V05.92** **Pedestrian on skateboard injured in collision with railway train or railway vehicle, unspecified whether traffic or nontraffic accident**

   X● **V05.99** **Pedestrian with other conveyance injured in collision with railway train or railway vehicle, unspecified whether traffic or nontraffic accident**

      Pedestrian with babystroller injured in collision with railway train or railway vehicle, unspecified whether traffic or nontraffic

      Pedestrian in wheelchair (powered) injured in collision with railway train or railway vehicle, unspecified whether traffic or nontraffic

      Pedestrian in motorized mobility scooter injured in collision with railway train or railway vehicle, unspecified whether traffic or nontraffic

      Pedestrian on ice-skates injured in collision with railway train or railway vehicle, unspecified whether traffic or nontraffic

      Pedestrian on nonmotorized scooter injured in collision with railway train or railway vehicle, unspecified whether traffic or nontraffic

      Pedestrian on sled injured in collision with railway train or railway vehicle, unspecified whether traffic or nontraffic

      Pedestrian on snowboard injured in collision with railway train or railway vehicle, unspecified whether traffic or nontraffic

      Pedestrian on snow-skis injured in collision with railway train or railway vehicle, unspecified whether traffic or nontraffic

● **V06** **Pedestrian injured in collision with other nonmotor vehicle**

   Includes   collision with animal-drawn vehicle, animal being ridden, nonpowered streetcar

   Excludes1   pedestrian injured in collision with pedestrian conveyance (V00.0-)

   The appropriate 7th character is to be added to each code from category V06

     A   initial encounter
     D   subsequent encounter
     S   sequela

● **V06.0** **Pedestrian injured in collision with other nonmotor vehicle in nontraffic accident**

   X● **V06.00** **Pedestrian on foot injured in collision with other nonmotor vehicle in nontraffic accident**

      Pedestrian NOS injured in collision with other nonmotor vehicle in nontraffic accident

   X● **V06.01** **Pedestrian on roller-skates injured in collision with other nonmotor vehicle in nontraffic accident**

   X● **V06.02** **Pedestrian on skateboard injured in collision with other nonmotor vehicle in nontraffic accident**

   X● **V06.09** **Pedestrian with other conveyance injured in collision with other nonmotor vehicle in nontraffic accident**

      Pedestrian with babystroller injured in collision with other nonmotor vehicle in nontraffic accident

      Pedestrian in wheelchair (powered) injured in collision with other nonmotor vehicle in nontraffic accident

      Pedestrian in motorized mobility scooter injured in collision with other nonmotor vehicle in nontraffic accident

      Pedestrian on ice-skates injured in collision with other nonmotor vehicle in nontraffic accident

      Pedestrian on nonmotorized scooter injured in collision with other nonmotor vehicle in nontraffic accident

      Pedestrian on sled injured in collision with other nonmotor vehicle in nontraffic accident

      Pedestrian on snowboard injured in collision with other nonmotor vehicle in nontraffic accident

      Pedestrian on snow-skis injured in collision with other nonmotor vehicle in nontraffic accident

● **V06.1** **Pedestrian injured in collision with other nonmotor vehicle in traffic accident**

   X● **V06.10** **Pedestrian on foot injured in collision with other nonmotor vehicle in traffic accident**

      Pedestrian NOS injured in collision with other nonmotor vehicle in traffic accident

   X● **V06.11** **Pedestrian on roller-skates injured in collision with other nonmotor vehicle in traffic accident**

   X● **V06.12** **Pedestrian on skateboard injured in collision with other nonmotor vehicle in traffic accident**

   X● **V06.19** **Pedestrian with other conveyance injured in collision with other nonmotor vehicle in traffic accident**

      Pedestrian with babystroller injured in collision with other nonmotor vehicle in nontraffic accident

      Pedestrian in wheelchair (powered) injured in collision with other nonmotor vehicle in traffic accident

      Pedestrian in motorized mobility scooter injured in collision with other nonmotor vehicle in traffic accident

      Pedestrian on ice-skates injured in collision with other nonmotor vehicle in traffic accident

      Pedestrian on nonmotorized scooter injured in collision with other nonmotor vehicle in traffic accident

      Pedestrian on sled injured in collision with other nonmotor vehicle in traffic accident

      Pedestrian on snowboard injured in collision with other nonmotor vehicle in traffic accident

      Pedestrian on snow-skis injured in collision with other nonmotor vehicle in traffic accident

● **V06.9** **Pedestrian injured in collision with other nonmotor vehicle, unspecified whether traffic or nontraffic accident**

   X● **V06.90** **Pedestrian on foot injured in collision with other nonmotor vehicle, unspecified whether traffic or nontraffic accident**

      Pedestrian NOS injured in collision with other nonmotor vehicle, unspecified whether traffic or nontraffic accident

   X● **V06.91** **Pedestrian on roller-skates injured in collision with other nonmotor vehicle, unspecified whether traffic or nontraffic accident**

▶ New   ⇒ Revised   ~~deleted~~ Deleted   **OGCR** Official Guidelines   X Assign placeholder X   ● Use Additional Character(s)

Excludes 1   Excludes 2   Includes   Use additional   Code first   Code also   Key words

X● **V06.92** Pedestrian on skateboard injured in collision with other nonmotor vehicle, unspecified whether traffic or nontraffic accident

X● **V06.99** Pedestrian with other conveyance injured in collision with other nonmotor vehicle, unspecified whether traffic or nontraffic accident

Pedestrian with babystroller injured in collision with other nonmotor vehicle, unspecified whether traffic or nontraffic accident

Pedestrian in wheelchair (powered) injured in collision with other nonmotor vehicle, unspecified whether traffic or nontraffic accident

Pedestrian in motorized mobility scooter injured in collision with other nonmotor vehicle, unspecified whether traffic or nontraffic accident

Pedestrian on ice-skates injured in collision with other nonmotor vehicle, unspecified whether traffic or nontraffic accident

Pedestrian on nonmotorized scooter injured in collision with other nonmotor vehicle, unspecified whether traffic or nontraffic accident

Pedestrian on sled injured in collision with other nonmotor vehicle, unspecified whether traffic or nontraffic accident

Pedestrian on snowboard injured in collision with other nonmotor vehicle, unspecified whether traffic or nontraffic accident

Pedestrian on snow-skis injured in collision with other nonmotor vehicle, unspecified whether traffic or nontraffic accident

● **V09** Pedestrian injured in other and unspecified transport accidents

The appropriate 7th character is to be added to each code from category V09

A	initial encounter
D	subsequent encounter
S	sequela

● **V09.0** Pedestrian injured in nontraffic accident involving other and unspecified motor vehicles

X● **V09.00** Pedestrian injured in nontraffic accident involving unspecified motor vehicles

X● **V09.01** Pedestrian injured in nontraffic accident involving military vehicle

X● **V09.09** Pedestrian injured in nontraffic accident involving other motor vehicles

Pedestrian injured in nontraffic accident by special vehicle

X● **V09.1** Pedestrian injured in unspecified nontraffic accident

● **V09.2** Pedestrian injured in traffic accident involving other and unspecified motor vehicles

X● **V09.20** Pedestrian injured in traffic accident involving unspecified motor vehicles

X● **V09.21** Pedestrian injured in traffic accident involving military vehicle

X● **V09.29** Pedestrian injured in traffic accident involving other motor vehicles

X● **V09.3** Pedestrian injured in unspecified traffic accident

X● **V09.9** Pedestrian injured in unspecified transport accident

PEDAL CYCLE RIDER INJURED IN TRANSPORT ACCIDENT (V10-V19)

Includes   any non-motorized vehicle, excluding an animal-drawn vehicle, or a sidecar or trailer attached to the pedal cycle

Excludes2   rupture of pedal cycle tire (W37.0)

● **V10** Pedal cycle rider injured in collision with pedestrian or animal

Excludes1   pedal cycle rider collision with animal-drawn vehicle or animal being ridden (V16.-)

The appropriate 7th character is to be added to each code from category V10

A	initial encounter
D	subsequent encounter
S	sequela

X● **V10.0** Pedal cycle driver injured in collision with pedestrian or animal in nontraffic accident

X● **V10.1** Pedal cycle passenger injured in collision with pedestrian or animal in nontraffic accident

X● **V10.2** Unspecified pedal cyclist injured in collision with pedestrian or animal in nontraffic accident

X● **V10.3** Person boarding or alighting a pedal cycle injured in collision with pedestrian or animal

X● **V10.4** Pedal cycle driver injured in collision with pedestrian or animal in traffic accident

X● **V10.5** Pedal cycle passenger injured in collision with pedestrian or animal in traffic accident

X● **V10.9** Unspecified pedal cyclist injured in collision with pedestrian or animal in traffic accident

● **V11** Pedal cycle rider injured in collision with other pedal cycle

The appropriate 7th character is to be added to each code from category V11

A	initial encounter
D	subsequent encounter
S	sequela

X● **V11.0** Pedal cycle driver injured in collision with other pedal cycle in nontraffic accident

X● **V11.1** Pedal cycle passenger injured in collision with other pedal cycle in nontraffic accident

X● **V11.2** Unspecified pedal cyclist injured in collision with other pedal cycle in nontraffic accident

X● **V11.3** Person boarding or alighting a pedal cycle injured in collision with other pedal cycle

X● **V11.4** Pedal cycle driver injured in collision with other pedal cycle in traffic accident

X● **V11.5** Pedal cycle passenger injured in collision with other pedal cycle in traffic accident

X● **V11.9** Unspecified pedal cyclist injured in collision with other pedal cycle in traffic accident

CHAPTER 20 (VØ1-Y99)

● **V12 Pedal cycle rider injured in collision with two- or three-wheeled motor vehicle**

The appropriate 7th character is to be added to each code from category V12

> A   initial encounter
> D   subsequent encounter
> S   sequela

X ● **V12.Ø Pedal cycle driver injured in collision with two- or three-wheeled motor vehicle in nontraffic accident**

X ● **V12.1 Pedal cycle passenger injured in collision with two- or three-wheeled motor vehicle in nontraffic accident**

X ● **V12.2 Unspecified pedal cyclist injured in collision with two- or three-wheeled motor vehicle in nontraffic accident**

X ● **V12.3 Person boarding or alighting a pedal cycle injured in collision with two- or three-wheeled motor vehicle**

X ● **V12.4 Pedal cycle driver injured in collision with two- or three-wheeled motor vehicle in traffic accident**

X ● **V12.5 Pedal cycle passenger injured in collision with two- or three-wheeled motor vehicle in traffic accident**

X ● **V12.9 Unspecified pedal cyclist injured in collision with two- or three-wheeled motor vehicle in traffic accident**

● **V13 Pedal cycle rider injured in collision with car, pick-up truck or van**

The appropriate 7th character is to be added to each code from category V13

> A   initial encounter
> D   subsequent encounter
> S   sequela

X ● **V13.Ø Pedal cycle driver injured in collision with car, pick-up truck or van in nontraffic accident**

X ● **V13.1 Pedal cycle passenger injured in collision with car, pick-up truck or van in nontraffic accident**

X ● **V13.2 Unspecified pedal cyclist injured in collision with car, pick-up truck or van in nontraffic accident**

X ● **V13.3 Person boarding or alighting a pedal cycle injured in collision with car, pick-up truck or van**

X ● **V13.4 Pedal cycle driver injured in collision with car, pick-up truck or van in traffic accident**

X ● **V13.5 Pedal cycle passenger injured in collision with car, pick-up truck or van in traffic accident**

X ● **V13.9 Unspecified pedal cyclist injured in collision with car, pick-up truck or van in traffic accident**

● **V14 Pedal cycle rider injured in collision with heavy transport vehicle or bus**

> **Excludes1**   pedal cycle rider injured in collision with military vehicle (V19.81)

The appropriate 7th character is to be added to each code from category V14

> A   initial encounter
> D   subsequent encounter
> S   sequela

X ● **V14.Ø Pedal cycle driver injured in collision with heavy transport vehicle or bus in nontraffic accident**

X ● **V14.1 Pedal cycle passenger injured in collision with heavy transport vehicle or bus in nontraffic accident**

X ● **V14.2 Unspecified pedal cyclist injured in collision with heavy transport vehicle or bus in nontraffic accident**

X ● **V14.3 Person boarding or alighting a pedal cycle injured in collision with heavy transport vehicle or bus**

X ● **V14.4 Pedal cycle driver injured in collision with heavy transport vehicle or bus in traffic accident**

X ● **V14.5 Pedal cycle passenger injured in collision with heavy transport vehicle or bus in traffic accident**

X ● **V14.9 Unspecified pedal cyclist injured in collision with heavy transport vehicle or bus in traffic accident**

● **V15 Pedal cycle rider injured in collision with railway train or railway vehicle**

The appropriate 7th character is to be added to each code from category V15

> A   initial encounter
> D   subsequent encounter
> S   sequela

X ● **V15.Ø Pedal cycle driver injured in collision with railway train or railway vehicle in nontraffic accident**

X ● **V15.1 Pedal cycle passenger injured in collision with railway train or railway vehicle in nontraffic accident**

X ● **V15.2 Unspecified pedal cyclist injured in collision with railway train or railway vehicle in nontraffic accident**

X ● **V15.3 Person boarding or alighting a pedal cycle injured in collision with railway train or railway vehicle**

X ● **V15.4 Pedal cycle driver injured in collision with railway train or railway vehicle in traffic accident**

X ● **V15.5 Pedal cycle passenger injured in collision with railway train or railway vehicle in traffic accident**

X ● **V15.9 Unspecified pedal cyclist injured in collision with railway train or railway vehicle in traffic accident**

● **V16 Pedal cycle rider injured in collision with other nonmotor vehicle**

> **Includes**   collision with animal-drawn vehicle, animal being ridden, streetcar

The appropriate 7th character is to be added to each code from category V16

> A   initial encounter
> D   subsequent encounter
> S   sequela

X ● **V16.Ø Pedal cycle driver injured in collision with other nonmotor vehicle in nontraffic accident**

X ● **V16.1 Pedal cycle passenger injured in collision with other nonmotor vehicle in nontraffic accident**

X ● **V16.2 Unspecified pedal cyclist injured in collision with other nonmotor vehicle in nontraffic accident**

X ● **V16.3 Person boarding or alighting a pedal cycle injured in collision with other nonmotor vehicle in nontraffic accident**

X ● **V16.4 Pedal cycle driver injured in collision with other nonmotor vehicle in traffic accident**

X ● **V16.5 Pedal cycle passenger injured in collision with other nonmotor vehicle in traffic accident**

X ● **V16.9 Unspecified pedal cyclist injured in collision with other nonmotor vehicle in traffic accident**

● **V17 Pedal cycle rider injured in collision with fixed or stationary object**

The appropriate 7th character is to be added to each code from category V17

> A   initial encounter
> D   subsequent encounter
> S   sequela

X ● **V17.Ø Pedal cycle driver injured in collision with fixed or stationary object in nontraffic accident**

X ● **V17.1 Pedal cycle passenger injured in collision with fixed or stationary object in nontraffic accident**

X ● **V17.2 Unspecified pedal cyclist injured in collision with fixed or stationary object in nontraffic accident**

X ● **V17.3 Person boarding or alighting a pedal cycle injured in collision with fixed or stationary object**

X ● **V17.4 Pedal cycle driver injured in collision with fixed or stationary object in traffic accident**

X ● **V17.5 Pedal cycle passenger injured in collision with fixed or stationary object in traffic accident**

X ● **V17.9 Unspecified pedal cyclist injured in collision with fixed or stationary object in traffic accident**

● **V18** Pedal cycle rider injured in noncollision transport accident

> **Includes**　　fall or thrown from pedal cycle (without antecedent collision)
> overturning pedal cycle NOS
> overturning pedal cycle without collision

> The appropriate 7th character is to be added to each code from category V18

> | | |
> |---|---|
> | A | initial encounter |
> | D | subsequent encounter |
> | S | sequela |

X● **V18.0** Pedal cycle driver injured in noncollision transport accident in nontraffic accident

X● **V18.1** Pedal cycle passenger injured in noncollision transport accident in nontraffic accident

X● **V18.2** Unspecified pedal cyclist injured in noncollision transport accident in nontraffic accident

X● **V18.3** Person boarding or alighting a pedal cycle injured in noncollision transport accident

X● **V18.4** Pedal cycle driver injured in noncollision transport accident in traffic accident

X● **V18.5** Pedal cycle passenger injured in noncollision transport accident in traffic accident

X● **V18.9** Unspecified pedal cyclist injured in noncollision transport accident in traffic accident

● **V19** Pedal cycle rider injured in other and unspecified transport accidents

> The appropriate 7th character is to be added to each code from category V19

> | | |
> |---|---|
> | A | initial encounter |
> | D | subsequent encounter |
> | S | sequela |

● **V19.0** Pedal cycle driver injured in collision with other and unspecified motor vehicles in nontraffic accident

X● **V19.00** Pedal cycle driver injured in collision with unspecified motor vehicles in nontraffic accident

X● **V19.09** Pedal cycle driver injured in collision with other motor vehicles in nontraffic accident

● **V19.1** Pedal cycle passenger injured in collision with other and unspecified motor vehicles in nontraffic accident

X● **V19.10** Pedal cycle passenger injured in collision with unspecified motor vehicles in nontraffic accident

X● **V19.19** Pedal cycle passenger injured in collision with other motor vehicles in nontraffic accident

● **V19.2** Unspecified pedal cyclist injured in collision with other and unspecified motor vehicles in nontraffic accident

X● **V19.20** Unspecified pedal cyclist injured in collision with unspecified motor vehicles in nontraffic accident
> Pedal cycle collision NOS, nontraffic

X● **V19.29** Unspecified pedal cyclist injured in collision with other motor vehicles in nontraffic accident

X● **V19.3** Pedal cyclist (driver) (passenger) injured in unspecified nontraffic accident
> Pedal cycle accident NOS, nontraffic
> Pedal cyclist injured in nontraffic accident NOS

● **V19.4** Pedal cycle driver injured in collision with other and unspecified motor vehicles in traffic accident

X● **V19.40** Pedal cycle driver injured in collision with unspecified motor vehicles in traffic accident

X● **V19.49** Pedal cycle driver injured in collision with other motor vehicles in traffic accident

● **V19.5** Pedal cycle passenger injured in collision with other and unspecified motor vehicles in traffic accident

X● **V19.50** Pedal cycle passenger injured in collision with unspecified motor vehicles in traffic accident

X● **V19.59** Pedal cycle passenger injured in collision with other motor vehicles in traffic accident

● **V19.6** Unspecified pedal cyclist injured in collision with other and unspecified motor vehicles in traffic accident

X● **V19.60** Unspecified pedal cyclist injured in collision with unspecified motor vehicles in traffic accident
> Pedal cycle collision NOS (traffic)

X● **V19.69** Unspecified pedal cyclist injured in collision with other motor vehicles in traffic accident

● **V19.8** Pedal cyclist (driver) (passenger) injured in other specified transport accidents

X● **V19.81** Pedal cyclist (driver) (passenger) injured in transport accident with military vehicle

X● **V19.88** Pedal cyclist (driver) (passenger) injured in other specified transport accidents

X● **V19.9** Pedal cyclist (driver) (passenger) injured in unspecified traffic accident
> Pedal cycle accident NOS

MOTORCYCLE RIDER INJURED IN TRANSPORT ACCIDENT (V20-V29)

> **Includes**　　moped motorcycle with sidecar motorized bicycle motor scooter

> **Excludes1**　　three-wheeled motor vehicle (V30-V39)

● **V20** Motorcycle rider injured in collision with pedestrian or animal

> **Excludes1**　　motorcycle rider collision with animal-drawn vehicle or animal being ridden (V26.-)

> The appropriate 7th character is to be added to each code from category V20

> | | |
> |---|---|
> | A | initial encounter |
> | D | subsequent encounter |
> | S | sequela |

X● **V20.0** Motorcycle driver injured in collision with pedestrian or animal in nontraffic accident

X● **V20.1** Motorcycle passenger injured in collision with pedestrian or animal in nontraffic accident

X● **V20.2** Unspecified motorcycle rider injured in collision with pedestrian or animal in nontraffic accident

X● **V20.3** Person boarding or alighting a motorcycle injured in collision with pedestrian or animal

X● **V20.4** Motorcycle driver injured in collision with pedestrian or animal in traffic accident

X● **V20.5** Motorcycle passenger injured in collision with pedestrian or animal in traffic accident

X● **V20.9** Unspecified motorcycle rider injured in collision with pedestrian or animal in traffic accident

● **V21** Motorcycle rider injured in collision with pedal cycle

> The appropriate 7th character is to be added to each code from category V21

> | | |
> |---|---|
> | A | initial encounter |
> | D | subsequent encounter |
> | S | sequela |

X● **V21.0** Motorcycle driver injured in collision with pedal cycle in nontraffic accident

X● **V21.1** Motorcycle passenger injured in collision with pedal cycle in nontraffic accident

X● **V21.2** Unspecified motorcycle rider injured in collision with pedal cycle in nontraffic accident

X● **V21.3** Person boarding or alighting a motorcycle injured in collision with pedal cycle

X● **V21.4** Motorcycle driver injured in collision with pedal cycle in traffic accident

X● **V21.5** Motorcycle passenger injured in collision with pedal cycle in traffic accident

X● **V21.9** Unspecified motorcycle rider injured in collision with pedal cycle in traffic accident

---

● **V22** **Motorcycle rider injured in collision with two- or three-wheeled motor vehicle**

The appropriate 7th character is to be added to each code from category V22

> A   initial encounter
> D   subsequent encounter
> S   sequela

X● **V22.0** Motorcycle driver injured in collision with two- or three-wheeled motor vehicle in nontraffic accident

X● **V22.1** Motorcycle passenger injured in collision with two- or three-wheeled motor vehicle in nontraffic accident

X● **V22.2** Unspecified motorcycle rider injured in collision with two- or three-wheeled motor vehicle in nontraffic accident

X● **V22.3** Person boarding or alighting a motorcycle injured in collision with two- or three-wheeled motor vehicle

X● **V22.4** Motorcycle driver injured in collision with two- or three-wheeled motor vehicle in traffic accident

X● **V22.5** Motorcycle passenger injured in collision with two- or three-wheeled motor vehicle in traffic accident

X● **V22.9** Unspecified motorcycle rider injured in collision with two- or three-wheeled motor vehicle in traffic accident

● **V23** **Motorcycle rider injured in collision with car, pick-up truck or van**

The appropriate 7th character is to be added to each code from category V23

> A   initial encounter
> D   subsequent encounter
> S   sequela

X● **V23.0** Motorcycle driver injured in collision with car, pick-up truck or van in nontraffic accident

X● **V23.1** Motorcycle passenger injured in collision with car, pick-up truck or van in nontraffic accident

X● **V23.2** Unspecified motorcycle rider injured in collision with car, pick-up truck or van in nontraffic accident

X● **V23.3** Person boarding or alighting a motorcycle injured in collision with car, pick-up truck or van

X● **V23.4** Motorcycle driver injured in collision with car, pick-up truck or van in traffic accident

X● **V23.5** Motorcycle passenger injured in collision with car, pick-up truck or van in traffic accident

X● **V23.9** Unspecified motorcycle rider injured in collision with car, pick-up truck or van in traffic accident

● **V24** **Motorcycle rider injured in collision with heavy transport vehicle or bus**

> **Excludes1**   motorcycle rider injured in collision with military vehicle (V29.81)

The appropriate 7th character is to be added to each code from category V24

> A   initial encounter
> D   subsequent encounter
> S   sequela

X● **V24.0** Motorcycle driver injured in collision with heavy transport vehicle or bus in nontraffic accident

X● **V24.1** Motorcycle passenger injured in collision with heavy transport vehicle or bus in nontraffic accident

X● **V24.2** Unspecified motorcycle rider injured in collision with heavy transport vehicle or bus in nontraffic accident

X● **V24.3** Person boarding or alighting a motorcycle injured in collision with heavy transport vehicle or bus

X● **V24.4** Motorcycle driver injured in collision with heavy transport vehicle or bus in traffic accident

X● **V24.5** Motorcycle passenger injured in collision with heavy transport vehicle or bus in traffic accident

X● **V24.9** Unspecified motorcycle rider injured in collision with heavy transport vehicle or bus in traffic accident

● **V25** **Motorcycle rider injured in collision with railway train or railway vehicle**

The appropriate 7th character is to be added to each code from category V25

> A   initial encounter
> D   subsequent encounter
> S   sequela

X● **V25.0** Motorcycle driver injured in collision with railway train or railway vehicle in nontraffic accident

X● **V25.1** Motorcycle passenger injured in collision with railway train or railway vehicle in nontraffic accident

X● **V25.2** Unspecified motorcycle rider injured in collision with railway train or railway vehicle in nontraffic accident

X● **V25.3** Person boarding or alighting a motorcycle injured in collision with railway train or railway vehicle

X● **V25.4** Motorcycle driver injured in collision with railway train or railway vehicle in traffic accident

X● **V25.5** Motorcycle passenger injured in collision with railway train or railway vehicle in traffic accident

X● **V25.9** Unspecified motorcycle rider injured in collision with railway train or railway vehicle in traffic accident

● **V26** **Motorcycle rider injured in collision with other nonmotor vehicle**

> **Includes**   collision with animal-drawn vehicle, animal being ridden, streetcar

The appropriate 7th character is to be added to each code from category V26

> A   initial encounter
> D   subsequent encounter
> S   sequela

X● **V26.0** Motorcycle driver injured in collision with other nonmotor vehicle in nontraffic accident

X● **V26.1** Motorcycle passenger injured in collision with other nonmotor vehicle in nontraffic accident

X● **V26.2** Unspecified motorcycle rider injured in collision with other nonmotor vehicle in nontraffic accident

X● **V26.3** Person boarding or alighting a motorcycle injured in collision with other nonmotor vehicle

X● **V26.4** Motorcycle driver injured in collision with other nonmotor vehicle in traffic accident

X● **V26.5** Motorcycle passenger injured in collision with other nonmotor vehicle in traffic accident

X● **V26.9** Unspecified motorcycle rider injured in collision with other nonmotor vehicle in traffic accident

● **V27** **Motorcycle rider injured in collision with fixed or stationary object**

The appropriate 7th character is to be added to each code from category V27

> A   initial encounter
> D   subsequent encounter
> S   sequela

X● **V27.0** Motorcycle driver injured in collision with fixed or stationary object in nontraffic accident

X● **V27.1** Motorcycle passenger injured in collision with fixed or stationary object in nontraffic accident

X● **V27.2** Unspecified motorcycle rider injured in collision with fixed or stationary object in nontraffic accident

X● **V27.3** Person boarding or alighting a motorcycle injured in collision with fixed or stationary object

X● **V27.4** Motorcycle driver injured in collision with fixed or stationary object in traffic accident

X● **V27.5** Motorcycle passenger injured in collision with fixed or stationary object in traffic accident

X● **V27.9** Unspecified motorcycle rider injured in collision with fixed or stationary object in traffic accident

● **V28**   **Motorcycle rider injured in noncollision transport accident**

> | Includes | fall or thrown from motorcycle (without antecedent collision) |
> |---|---|
> | | overturning motorcycle NOS |
> | | overturning motorcycle without collision |

> The appropriate 7th character is to be added to each code from category V28

> | A | initial encounter |
> |---|---|
> | D | subsequent encounter |
> | S | sequela |

X ● **V28.0**   Motorcycle driver injured in noncollision transport accident in nontraffic accident

X ● **V28.1**   Motorcycle passenger injured in noncollision transport accident in nontraffic accident

X ● **V28.2**   Unspecified motorcycle rider injured in noncollision transport accident in nontraffic accident

X ● **V28.3**   Person boarding or alighting a motorcycle injured in noncollision transport accident

X ● **V28.4**   Motorcycle driver injured in noncollision transport accident in traffic accident

X ● **V28.5**   Motorcycle passenger injured in noncollision transport accident in traffic accident

X ● **V28.9**   Unspecified motorcycle rider injured in noncollision transport accident in traffic accident

● **V29**   **Motorcycle rider injured in other and unspecified transport accidents**

> The appropriate 7th character is to be added to each code from category V29

> | A | initial encounter |
> |---|---|
> | D | subsequent encounter |
> | S | sequela |

● **V29.0**   Motorcycle driver injured in collision with other and unspecified motor vehicles in nontraffic accident

   X ● **V29.00**   Motorcycle driver injured in collision with unspecified motor vehicles in nontraffic accident

   X ● **V29.09**   Motorcycle driver injured in collision with other motor vehicles in nontraffic accident

● **V29.1**   Motorcycle passenger injured in collision with other and unspecified motor vehicles in nontraffic accident

   X ● **V29.10**   Motorcycle passenger injured in collision with unspecified motor vehicles in nontraffic accident

   X ● **V29.19**   Motorcycle passenger injured in collision with other motor vehicles in nontraffic accident

● **V29.2**   Unspecified motorcycle rider injured in collision with other and unspecified motor vehicles in nontraffic accident

   X ● **V29.20**   Unspecified motorcycle rider injured in collision with unspecified motor vehicles in nontraffic accident
> Motorcycle collision NOS, nontraffic

   X ● **V29.29**   Unspecified motorcycle rider injured in collision with other motor vehicles in nontraffic accident

X ● **V29.3**   Motorcycle rider (driver) (passenger) injured in unspecified nontraffic accident
> Motorcycle accident NOS, nontraffic
> Motorcycle rider injured in nontraffic accident NOS

● **V29.4**   Motorcycle driver injured in collision with other and unspecified motor vehicles in traffic accident

   X ● **V29.40**   Motorcycle driver injured in collision with unspecified motor vehicles in traffic accident

   X ● **V29.49**   Motorcycle driver injured in collision with other motor vehicles in traffic accident

● **V29.5**   Motorcycle passenger injured in collision with other and unspecified motor vehicles in traffic accident

   X ● **V29.50**   Motorcycle passenger injured in collision with unspecified motor vehicles in traffic accident

   X ● **V29.59**   Motorcycle passenger injured in collision with other motor vehicles in traffic accident

● **V29.6**   Unspecified motorcycle rider injured in collision with other and unspecified motor vehicles in traffic accident

   X ● **V29.60**   Unspecified motorcycle rider injured in collision with unspecified motor vehicles in traffic accident
> Motorcycle collision NOS (traffic)

   X ● **V29.69**   Unspecified motorcycle rider injured in collision with other motor vehicles in traffic accident

● **V29.8**   Motorcycle rider (driver) (passenger) injured in other specified transport accidents

   X ● **V29.81**   Motorcycle rider (driver) (passenger) injured in transport accident with military vehicle

   X ● **V29.88**   Motorcycle rider (driver) (passenger) injured in other specified transport accidents

X ● **V29.9**   Motorcycle rider (driver) (passenger) injured in unspecified traffic accident
> Motorcycle accident NOS

OCCUPANT OF THREE-WHEELED MOTOR VEHICLE INJURED IN TRANSPORT ACCIDENT (V30-V39)

> | Includes | motorized tricycle |
> |---|---|
> | | motorized rickshaw |
> | | three-wheeled motor car |

> | Excludes1 | all-terrain vehicles (V86.-) |
> |---|---|
> | | motorcycle with sidecar (V20-V29) |
> | | vehicle designed primarily for off-road use (V86.-) |

● **V30**   **Occupant of three-wheeled motor vehicle injured in collision with pedestrian or animal**

> | Excludes1 | three-wheeled motor vehicle collision with animal-drawn vehicle or animal being ridden (V36.-) |
> |---|---|

> The appropriate 7th character is to be added to each code from category V30

> | A | initial encounter |
> |---|---|
> | D | subsequent encounter |
> | S | sequela |

X ● **V30.0**   Driver of three-wheeled motor vehicle injured in collision with pedestrian or animal in nontraffic accident

X ● **V30.1**   Passenger in three-wheeled motor vehicle injured in collision with pedestrian or animal in nontraffic accident

X ● **V30.2**   Person on outside of three-wheeled motor vehicle injured in collision with pedestrian or animal in nontraffic accident

X ● **V30.3**   Unspecified occupant of three-wheeled motor vehicle injured in collision with pedestrian or animal in nontraffic accident

X ● **V30.4**   Person boarding or alighting a three-wheeled motor vehicle injured in collision with pedestrian or animal

X ● **V30.5**   Driver of three-wheeled motor vehicle injured in collision with pedestrian or animal in traffic accident

X ● **V30.6**   Passenger in three-wheeled motor vehicle injured in collision with pedestrian or animal in traffic accident

X ● **V30.7**   Person on outside of three-wheeled motor vehicle injured in collision with pedestrian or animal in traffic accident

X ● **V30.9**   Unspecified occupant of three-wheeled motor vehicle injured in collision with pedestrian or animal in traffic accident

---

▶ New   ⇒ Revised   ~~deleted~~ Deleted   **OGCR** Official Guidelines   X Assign placeholder X   ● Use Additional Character(s)

Excludes 1   Excludes 2   Includes   Use additional   Code first   Code also   Key words

● **V31**   **Occupant of three-wheeled motor vehicle injured in collision with pedal cycle**

The appropriate 7th character is to be added to each code from category V31

> A   initial encounter
> D   subsequent encounter
> S   sequela

X ● **V31.0**   Driver of three-wheeled motor vehicle injured in collision with pedal cycle in nontraffic accident

X ● **V31.1**   Passenger in three-wheeled motor vehicle injured in collision with pedal cycle in nontraffic accident

X ● **V31.2**   Person on outside of three-wheeled motor vehicle injured in collision with pedal cycle in nontraffic accident

X ● **V31.3**   Unspecified occupant of three-wheeled motor vehicle injured in collision with pedal cycle in nontraffic accident

X ● **V31.4**   Person boarding or alighting a three-wheeled motor vehicle injured in collision with pedal cycle

X ● **V31.5**   Driver of three-wheeled motor vehicle injured in collision with pedal cycle in traffic accident

X ● **V31.6**   Passenger in three-wheeled motor vehicle injured in collision with pedal cycle in traffic accident

X ● **V31.7**   Person on outside of three-wheeled motor vehicle injured in collision with pedal cycle in traffic accident

X ● **V31.9**   Unspecified occupant of three-wheeled motor vehicle injured in collision with pedal cycle in traffic accident

● **V32**   **Occupant of three-wheeled motor vehicle injured in collision with two- or three-wheeled motor vehicle**

The appropriate 7th character is to be added to each code from category V32

> A   initial encounter
> D   subsequent encounter
> S   sequela

X ● **V32.0**   Driver of three-wheeled motor vehicle injured in collision with two- or three-wheeled motor vehicle in nontraffic accident

X ● **V32.1**   Passenger in three-wheeled motor vehicle injured in collision with two- or three-wheeled motor vehicle in nontraffic accident

X ● **V32.2**   Person on outside of three-wheeled motor vehicle injured in collision with two- or three-wheeled motor vehicle in nontraffic accident

X ● **V32.3**   Unspecified occupant of three-wheeled motor vehicle injured in collision with two- or three-wheeled motor vehicle in nontraffic accident

X ● **V32.4**   Person boarding or alighting a three-wheeled motor vehicle injured in collision with two- or three-wheeled motor vehicle

X ● **V32.5**   Driver of three-wheeled motor vehicle injured in collision with two- or three-wheeled motor vehicle in traffic accident

X ● **V32.6**   Passenger in three-wheeled motor vehicle injured in collision with two- or three-wheeled motor vehicle in traffic accident

X ● **V32.7**   Person on outside of three-wheeled motor vehicle injured in collision with two- or three-wheeled motor vehicle in traffic accident

X ● **V32.9**   Unspecified occupant of three-wheeled motor vehicle injured in collision with two- or three-wheeled motor vehicle in traffic accident

● **V33**   **Occupant of three-wheeled motor vehicle injured in collision with car, pick-up truck or van**

The appropriate 7th character is to be added to each code from category V33

> A   initial encounter
> D   subsequent encounter
> S   sequela

X ● **V33.0**   Driver of three-wheeled motor vehicle injured in collision with car, pick-up truck or van in nontraffic accident

X ● **V33.1**   Passenger in three-wheeled motor vehicle injured in collision with car, pick-up truck or van in nontraffic accident

X ● **V33.2**   Person on outside of three-wheeled motor vehicle injured in collision with car, pick-up truck or van in nontraffic accident

X ● **V33.3**   Unspecified occupant of three-wheeled motor vehicle injured in collision with car, pick-up truck or van in nontraffic accident

X ● **V33.4**   Person boarding or alighting a three-wheeled motor vehicle injured in collision with car, pick-up truck or van

X ● **V33.5**   Driver of three-wheeled motor vehicle injured in collision with car, pick-up truck or van in traffic accident

X ● **V33.6**   Passenger in three-wheeled motor vehicle injured in collision with car, pick-up truck or van in traffic accident

X ● **V33.7**   Person on outside of three-wheeled motor vehicle injured in collision with car, pick-up truck or van in traffic accident

X ● **V33.9**   Unspecified occupant of three-wheeled motor vehicle injured in collision with car, pick-up truck or van in traffic accident

● **V34**   **Occupant of three-wheeled motor vehicle injured in collision with heavy transport vehicle or bus**

> **Excludes1**   occupant of three-wheeled motor vehicle injured in collision with military vehicle (V39.81)

The appropriate 7th character is to be added to each code from category V34

> A   initial encounter
> D   subsequent encounter
> S   sequela

X ● **V34.0**   Driver of three-wheeled motor vehicle injured in collision with heavy transport vehicle or bus in nontraffic accident

X ● **V34.1**   Passenger in three-wheeled motor vehicle injured in collision with heavy transport vehicle or bus in nontraffic accident

X ● **V34.2**   Person on outside of three-wheeled motor vehicle injured in collision with heavy transport vehicle or bus in nontraffic accident

X ● **V34.3**   Unspecified occupant of three-wheeled motor vehicle injured in collision with heavy transport vehicle or bus in nontraffic accident

X ● **V34.4**   Person boarding or alighting a three-wheeled motor vehicle injured in collision with heavy transport vehicle or bus

X ● **V34.5**   Driver of three-wheeled motor vehicle injured in collision with heavy transport vehicle or bus in traffic accident

X ● **V34.6**   Passenger in three-wheeled motor vehicle injured in collision with heavy transport vehicle or bus in traffic accident

X ● **V34.7**   Person on outside of three-wheeled motor vehicle injured in collision with heavy transport vehicle or bus in traffic accident

X ● **V34.9**   Unspecified occupant of three-wheeled motor vehicle injured in collision with heavy transport vehicle or bus in traffic accident

▶ New   ⇒ Revised   ~~deleted~~ Deleted   **OGCR** Official Guidelines   X Assign placeholder X   ● Use Additional Character(s)

Excludes 1   Excludes 2   Includes   Use additional   Code first   Code also   Key words

● **V35**   Occupant of three-wheeled motor vehicle injured in collision with railway train or railway vehicle

> The appropriate 7th character is to be added to each code from category V35
>
> | | |
> |---|---|
> | A | initial encounter |
> | D | subsequent encounter |
> | S | sequela |

X● **V35.0**   Driver of three-wheeled motor vehicle injured in collision with railway train or railway vehicle in nontraffic accident

X● **V35.1**   Passenger in three-wheeled motor vehicle injured in collision with railway train or railway vehicle in nontraffic accident

X● **V35.2**   Person on outside of three-wheeled motor vehicle injured in collision with railway train or railway vehicle in nontraffic accident

X● **V35.3**   Unspecified occupant of three-wheeled motor vehicle injured in collision with railway train or railway vehicle in nontraffic accident

X● **V35.4**   Person boarding or alighting a three-wheeled motor vehicle injured in collision with railway train or railway vehicle

X● **V35.5**   Driver of three-wheeled motor vehicle injured in collision with railway train or railway vehicle in traffic accident

X● **V35.6**   Passenger in three-wheeled motor vehicle injured in collision with railway train or railway vehicle in traffic accident

X● **V35.7**   Person on outside of three-wheeled motor vehicle injured in collision with railway train or railway vehicle in traffic accident

X● **V35.9**   Unspecified occupant of three-wheeled motor vehicle injured in collision with railway train or railway vehicle in traffic accident

● **V36**   Occupant of three-wheeled motor vehicle injured in collision with other nonmotor vehicle

> **Includes**   collision with animal-drawn vehicle, animal being ridden, streetcar
>
> The appropriate 7th character is to be added to each code from category V36
>
> | | |
> |---|---|
> | A | initial encounter |
> | D | subsequent encounter |
> | S | sequela |

X● **V36.0**   Driver of three-wheeled motor vehicle injured in collision with other nonmotor vehicle in nontraffic accident

X● **V36.1**   Passenger in three-wheeled motor vehicle injured in collision with other nonmotor vehicle in nontraffic accident

X● **V36.2**   Person on outside of three-wheeled motor vehicle injured in collision with other nonmotor vehicle in nontraffic accident

X● **V36.3**   Unspecified occupant of three-wheeled motor vehicle injured in collision with other nonmotor vehicle in nontraffic accident

X● **V36.4**   Person boarding or alighting a three-wheeled motor vehicle injured in collision with other nonmotor vehicle

X● **V36.5**   Driver of three-wheeled motor vehicle injured in collision with other nonmotor vehicle in traffic accident

X● **V36.6**   Passenger in three-wheeled motor vehicle injured in collision with other nonmotor vehicle in traffic accident

X● **V36.7**   Person on outside of three-wheeled motor vehicle injured in collision with other nonmotor vehicle in traffic accident

X● **V36.9**   Unspecified occupant of three-wheeled motor vehicle injured in collision with other nonmotor vehicle in traffic accident

● **V37**   Occupant of three-wheeled motor vehicle injured in collision with fixed or stationary object

> The appropriate 7th character is to be added to each code from category V37
>
> | | |
> |---|---|
> | A | initial encounter |
> | D | subsequent encounter |
> | S | sequela |

X● **V37.0**   Driver of three-wheeled motor vehicle injured in collision with fixed or stationary object in nontraffic accident

X● **V37.1**   Passenger in three-wheeled motor vehicle injured in collision with fixed or stationary object in nontraffic accident

X● **V37.2**   Person on outside of three-wheeled motor vehicle injured in collision with fixed or stationary object in nontraffic accident

X● **V37.3**   Unspecified occupant of three-wheeled motor vehicle injured in collision with fixed or stationary object in nontraffic accident

X● **V37.4**   Person boarding or alighting a three-wheeled motor vehicle injured in collision with fixed or stationary object

X● **V37.5**   Driver of three-wheeled motor vehicle injured in collision with fixed or stationary object in traffic accident

X● **V37.6**   Passenger in three-wheeled motor vehicle injured in collision with fixed or stationary object in traffic accident

X● **V37.7**   Person on outside of three-wheeled motor vehicle injured in collision with fixed or stationary object in traffic accident

X● **V37.9**   Unspecified occupant of three-wheeled motor vehicle injured in collision with fixed or stationary object in traffic accident

● **V38**   Occupant of three-wheeled motor vehicle injured in noncollision transport accident

> **Includes**   fall or thrown from three-wheeled motor vehicle
> overturning of three-wheeled motor vehicle NOS
> overturning of three-wheeled motor vehicle without collision
>
> The appropriate 7th character is to be added to each code from category V38
>
> | | |
> |---|---|
> | A | initial encounter |
> | D | subsequent encounter |
> | S | sequela |

X● **V38.0**   Driver of three-wheeled motor vehicle injured in noncollision transport accident in nontraffic accident

X● **V38.1**   Passenger in three-wheeled motor vehicle injured in noncollision transport accident in nontraffic accident

X● **V38.2**   Person on outside of three-wheeled motor vehicle injured in noncollision transport accident in nontraffic accident

X● **V38.3**   Unspecified occupant of three-wheeled motor vehicle injured in noncollision transport accident in nontraffic accident

X● **V38.4**   Person boarding or alighting a three-wheeled motor vehicle injured in noncollision transport accident

X● **V38.5**   Driver of three-wheeled motor vehicle injured in noncollision transport accident in traffic accident

X● **V38.6**   Passenger in three-wheeled motor vehicle injured in noncollision transport accident in traffic accident

X● **V38.7**   Person on outside of three-wheeled motor vehicle injured in noncollision transport accident in traffic accident

X● **V38.9**   Unspecified occupant of three-wheeled motor vehicle injured in noncollision transport accident in traffic accident

CHAPTER 20 (V01-Y99)

● **V39**   **Occupant of three-wheeled motor vehicle injured in other and unspecified transport accidents**

The appropriate 7th character is to be added to each code from category V39

> A   initial encounter
> D   subsequent encounter
> S   sequela

● **V39.0**   **Driver of three-wheeled motor vehicle injured in collision with other and unspecified motor vehicles in nontraffic accident**

   X● **V39.00**   Driver of three-wheeled motor vehicle injured in collision with unspecified motor vehicles in nontraffic accident

   X● **V39.09**   Driver of three-wheeled motor vehicle injured in collision with other motor vehicles in nontraffic accident

● **V39.1**   **Passenger in three-wheeled motor vehicle injured in collision with other and unspecified motor vehicles in nontraffic accident**

   X● **V39.10**   Passenger in three-wheeled motor vehicle injured in collision with unspecified motor vehicles in nontraffic accident

   X● **V39.19**   Passenger in three-wheeled motor vehicle injured in collision with other motor vehicles in nontraffic accident

● **V39.2**   **Unspecified occupant of three-wheeled motor vehicle injured in collision with other and unspecified motor vehicles in nontraffic accident**

   X● **V39.20**   Unspecified occupant of three-wheeled motor vehicle injured in collision with unspecified motor vehicles in nontraffic accident
     Collision NOS involving three-wheeled motor vehicle, nontraffic

   X● **V39.29**   Unspecified occupant of three-wheeled motor vehicle injured in collision with other motor vehicles in nontraffic accident

X● **V39.3**   Occupant (driver) (passenger) of three-wheeled motor vehicle injured in unspecified nontraffic accident
     Accident NOS involving three-wheeled motor vehicle, nontraffic
     Occupant of three-wheeled motor vehicle injured in nontraffic accident NOS

● **V39.4**   **Driver of three-wheeled motor vehicle injured in collision with other and unspecified motor vehicles in traffic accident**

   X● **V39.40**   Driver of three-wheeled motor vehicle injured in collision with unspecified motor vehicles in traffic accident

   X● **V39.49**   Driver of three-wheeled motor vehicle injured in collision with other motor vehicles in traffic accident

● **V39.5**   **Passenger in three-wheeled motor vehicle injured in collision with other and unspecified motor vehicles in traffic accident**

   X● **V39.50**   Passenger in three-wheeled motor vehicle injured in collision with unspecified motor vehicles in traffic accident

   X● **V39.59**   Passenger in three-wheeled motor vehicle injured in collision with other motor vehicles in traffic accident

● **V39.6**   **Unspecified occupant of three-wheeled motor vehicle injured in collision with other and unspecified motor vehicles in traffic accident**

   X● **V39.60**   Unspecified occupant of three-wheeled motor vehicle injured in collision with unspecified motor vehicles in traffic accident
     Collision NOS involving three-wheeled motor vehicle (traffic)

   X● **V39.69**   Unspecified occupant of three-wheeled motor vehicle injured in collision with other motor vehicles in traffic accident

● **V39.8**   **Occupant (driver) (passenger) of three-wheeled motor vehicle injured in other specified transport accidents**

   X● **V39.81**   Occupant (driver) (passenger) of three-wheeled motor vehicle injured in transport accident with military vehicle

   X● **V39.89**   Occupant (driver) (passenger) of three-wheeled motor vehicle injured in other specified transport accidents

X● **V39.9**   Occupant (driver) (passenger) of three-wheeled motor vehicle injured in unspecified traffic accident
     Accident NOS involving three-wheeled motor vehicle

CAR OCCUPANT INJURED IN TRANSPORT ACCIDENT (V40-V49)

Includes	a four-wheeled motor vehicle designed primarily for carrying passengers
	automobile (pulling a trailer or camper)

Excludes1	bus (V50-V59)
	minibus (V50-V59)
	minivan (V50-V59)
	motorcoach (V70-V79)
	pick-up truck (V50-V59)
	sport utility vehicle (SUV) (V50-V59)

● **V40**   **Car occupant injured in collision with pedestrian or animal**

Excludes1	car collision with animal-drawn vehicle or animal being ridden (V46.-)

The appropriate 7th character is to be added to each code from category V40

> A   initial encounter
> D   subsequent encounter
> S   sequela

X● **V40.0**   Car driver injured in collision with pedestrian or animal in nontraffic accident

X● **V40.1**   Car passenger injured in collision with pedestrian or animal in nontraffic accident

X● **V40.2**   Person on outside of car injured in collision with pedestrian or animal in nontraffic accident

X● **V40.3**   Unspecified car occupant injured in collision with pedestrian or animal in nontraffic accident

X● **V40.4**   Person boarding or alighting a car injured in collision with pedestrian or animal

X● **V40.5**   Car driver injured in collision with pedestrian or animal in traffic accident

X● **V40.6**   Car passenger injured in collision with pedestrian or animal in traffic accident

X● **V40.7**   Person on outside of car injured in collision with pedestrian or animal in traffic accident

X● **V40.9**   Unspecified car occupant injured in collision with pedestrian or animal in traffic accident

● **V41**   **Car occupant injured in collision with pedal cycle**

The appropriate 7th character is to be added to each code from category V41

> A   initial encounter
> D   subsequent encounter
> S   sequela

X● **V41.0**   Car driver injured in collision with pedal cycle in nontraffic accident

X● **V41.1**   Car passenger injured in collision with pedal cycle in nontraffic accident

X● **V41.2**   Person on outside of car injured in collision with pedal cycle in nontraffic accident

X● **V41.3**   Unspecified car occupant injured in collision with pedal cycle in nontraffic accident

X● **V41.4**   Person boarding or alighting a car injured in collision with pedal cycle

X● **V41.5**   Car driver injured in collision with pedal cycle in traffic accident

X● **V41.6**   Car passenger injured in collision with pedal cycle in traffic accident

▶ New   ⇨ Revised   ~~deleted~~ Deleted   **OGCR** Official Guidelines   X Assign placeholder X   ● Use Additional Character(s)

Excludes 1   Excludes 2   Includes   Use additional   Code first   Code also   Key words

X● **V41.7** Person on outside of car injured in collision with pedal cycle in traffic accident

X● **V41.9** Unspecified car occupant injured in collision with pedal cycle in traffic accident

● **V42** Car occupant injured in collision with two- or three-wheeled motor vehicle

> The appropriate 7th character is to be added to each code from category V42

> | | |
> |---|---|
> | A | initial encounter |
> | D | subsequent encounter |
> | S | sequela |

X● **V42.0** Car driver injured in collision with two- or three-wheeled motor vehicle in nontraffic accident

X● **V42.1** Car passenger injured in collision with two- or three-wheeled motor vehicle in nontraffic accident

X● **V42.2** Person on outside of car injured in collision with two- or three-wheeled motor vehicle in nontraffic accident

X● **V42.3** Unspecified car occupant injured in collision with two- or three-wheeled motor vehicle in nontraffic accident

X● **V42.4** Person boarding or alighting a car injured in collision with two- or three-wheeled motor vehicle

X● **V42.5** Car driver injured in collision with two- or three-wheeled motor vehicle in traffic accident

X● **V42.6** Car passenger injured in collision with two- or three-wheeled motor vehicle in traffic accident

X● **V42.7** Person on outside of car injured in collision with two- or three-wheeled motor vehicle in traffic accident

X● **V42.9** Unspecified car occupant injured in collision with two- or three-wheeled motor vehicle in traffic accident

● **V43** Car occupant injured in collision with car, pick-up truck or van

> The appropriate 7th character is to be added to each code from category V43

> | | |
> |---|---|
> | A | initial encounter |
> | D | subsequent encounter |
> | S | sequela |

● **V43.0** Car driver injured in collision with car, pick-up truck or van in nontraffic accident

X● **V43.01** Car driver injured in collision with sport utility vehicle in nontraffic accident

X● **V43.02** Car driver injured in collision with other type car in nontraffic accident

X● **V43.03** Car driver injured in collision with pick-up truck in nontraffic accident

X● **V43.04** Car driver injured in collision with van in nontraffic accident

● **V43.1** Car passenger injured in collision with car, pick-up truck or van in nontraffic accident

X● **V43.11** Car passenger injured in collision with sport utility vehicle in nontraffic accident

X● **V43.12** Car passenger injured in collision with other type car in nontraffic accident

X● **V43.13** Car passenger injured in collision with pick-up in nontraffic accident

X● **V43.14** Car passenger injured in collision with van in nontraffic accident

● **V43.2** Person on outside of car injured in collision with car, pick-up truck or van in nontraffic accident

X● **V43.21** Person on outside of car injured in collision with sport utility vehicle in nontraffic accident

X● **V43.22** Person on outside of car injured in collision with other type car in nontraffic accident

X● **V43.23** Person on outside of car injured in collision with pick-up truck in nontraffic accident

X● **V43.24** Person on outside of car injured in collision with van in nontraffic accident

● **V43.3** Unspecified car occupant injured in collision with car, pick-up truck or van in nontraffic accident

X● **V43.31** Unspecified car occupant injured in collision with sport utility vehicle in nontraffic accident

X● **V43.32** Unspecified car occupant injured in collision with other type car in nontraffic accident

X● **V43.33** Unspecified car occupant injured in collision with pick-up truck in nontraffic accident

X● **V43.34** Unspecified car occupant injured in collision with van in nontraffic accident

● **V43.4** Person boarding or alighting a car injured in collision with car, pick-up truck or van

X● **V43.41** Person boarding or alighting a car injured in collision with sport utility vehicle

X● **V43.42** Person boarding or alighting a car injured in collision with other type car

X● **V43.43** Person boarding or alighting a car injured in collision with pick-up truck

X● **V43.44** Person boarding or alighting a car injured in collision with van

● **V43.5** Car driver injured in collision with car, pick-up truck or van in traffic accident

X● **V43.51** Car driver injured in collision with sport utility vehicle in traffic accident

X● **V43.52** Car driver injured in collision with other type car in traffic accident

X● **V43.53** Car driver injured in collision with pick-up truck in traffic accident

X● **V43.54** Car driver injured in collision with van in traffic accident

● **V43.6** Car passenger injured in collision with car, pick-up truck or van in traffic accident

X● **V43.61** Car passenger injured in collision with sport utility vehicle in traffic accident

X● **V43.62** Car passenger injured in collision with other type car in traffic accident

X● **V43.63** Car passenger injured in collision with pick-up truck in traffic accident

X● **V43.64** Car passenger injured in collision with van in traffic accident

● **V43.7** Person on outside of car injured in collision with car, pick-up truck or van in traffic accident

X● **V43.71** Person on outside of car injured in collision with sport utility vehicle in traffic accident

X● **V43.72** Person on outside of car injured in collision with other type car in traffic accident

X● **V43.73** Person on outside of car injured in collision with pick-up truck in traffic accident

X● **V43.74** Person on outside of car injured in collision with van in traffic accident

● **V43.9** Unspecified car occupant injured in collision with car, pick-up truck or van in traffic accident

X● **V43.91** Unspecified car occupant injured in collision with sport utility vehicle in traffic accident

X● **V43.92** Unspecified car occupant injured in collision with other type car in traffic accident

X● **V43.93** Unspecified car occupant injured in collision with pick-up truck in traffic accident

X● **V43.94** Unspecified car occupant injured in collision with van in traffic accident

---

▶ New   ⇒ Revised   ~~deleted~~ Deleted   **OGCR** Official Guidelines   X Assign placeholder X   ● Use Additional Character(s)

Excludes 1   Excludes 2   Includes   Use additional   Code first   Code also   Key words

● **V44** Car occupant injured in collision with heavy transport vehicle or bus

Excludes1   car occupant injured in collision with military vehicle (V49.81)

The appropriate 7th character is to be added to each code from category V44

> A   initial encounter
> D   subsequent encounter
> S   sequela

X● **V44.0** Car driver injured in collision with heavy transport vehicle or bus in nontraffic accident

X● **V44.1** Car passenger injured in collision with heavy transport vehicle or bus in nontraffic accident

X● **V44.2** Person on outside of car injured in collision with heavy transport vehicle or bus in nontraffic accident

X● **V44.3** Unspecified car occupant injured in collision with heavy transport vehicle or bus in nontraffic accident

X● **V44.4** Person boarding or alighting a car injured in collision with heavy transport vehicle or bus

X● **V44.5** Car driver injured in collision with heavy transport vehicle or bus in traffic accident

X● **V44.6** Car passenger injured in collision with heavy transport vehicle or bus in traffic accident

X● **V44.7** Person on outside of car injured in collision with heavy transport vehicle or bus in traffic accident

X● **V44.9** Unspecified car occupant injured in collision with heavy transport vehicle or bus in traffic accident

● **V45** Car occupant injured in collision with railway train or railway vehicle

The appropriate 7th character is to be added to each code from category V45

> A   initial encounter
> D   subsequent encounter
> S   sequela

X● **V45.0** Car driver injured in collision with railway train or railway vehicle in nontraffic accident

X● **V45.1** Car passenger injured in collision with railway train or railway vehicle in nontraffic accident

X● **V45.2** Person on outside of car injured in collision with railway train or railway vehicle in nontraffic accident

X● **V45.3** Unspecified car occupant injured in collision with railway train or railway vehicle in nontraffic accident

X● **V45.4** Person boarding or alighting a car injured in collision with railway train or railway vehicle

X● **V45.5** Car driver injured in collision with railway train or railway vehicle in traffic accident

X● **V45.6** Car passenger injured in collision with railway train or railway vehicle in traffic accident

X● **V45.7** Person on outside of car injured in collision with railway train or railway vehicle in traffic accident

X● **V45.9** Unspecified car occupant injured in collision with railway train or railway vehicle in traffic accident

● **V46** Car occupant injured in collision with other nonmotor vehicle

Includes   collision with animal-drawn vehicle, animal being ridden, streetcar

The appropriate 7th character is to be added to each code from category V46

> A   initial encounter
> D   subsequent encounter
> S   sequela

X● **V46.0** Car driver injured in collision with other nonmotor vehicle in nontraffic accident

X● **V46.1** Car passenger injured in collision with other nonmotor vehicle in nontraffic accident

X● **V46.2** Person on outside of car injured in collision with other nonmotor vehicle in nontraffic accident

X● **V46.3** Unspecified car occupant injured in collision with other nonmotor vehicle in nontraffic accident

X● **V46.4** Person boarding or alighting a car injured in collision with other nonmotor vehicle

X● **V46.5** Car driver injured in collision with other nonmotor vehicle in traffic accident

X● **V46.6** Car passenger injured in collision with other nonmotor vehicle in traffic accident

X● **V46.7** Person on outside of car injured in collision with other nonmotor vehicle in traffic accident

X● **V46.9** Unspecified car occupant injured in collision with other nonmotor vehicle in traffic accident

● **V47** Car occupant injured in collision with fixed or stationary object

The appropriate 7th character is to be added to each code from category V47

> A   initial encounter
> D   subsequent encounter
> S   sequela

X● **V47.0** Car driver injured in collision with fixed or stationary object in nontraffic accident

X● **V47.1** Car passenger injured in collision with fixed or stationary object in nontraffic accident

X● **V47.2** Person on outside of car injured in collision with fixed or stationary object in nontraffic accident

X● **V47.3** Unspecified car occupant injured in collision with fixed or stationary object in nontraffic accident

X● **V47.4** Person boarding or alighting a car injured in collision with fixed or stationary object

X● **V47.5** Car driver injured in collision with fixed or stationary object in traffic accident

X● **V47.6** Car passenger injured in collision with fixed or stationary object in traffic accident

X● **V47.7** Person on outside of car injured in collision with fixed or stationary object in traffic accident

X● **V47.9** Unspecified car occupant injured in collision with fixed or stationary object in traffic accident

● **V48** Car occupant injured in noncollision transport accident

Includes   overturning car NOS
overturning car without collision

The appropriate 7th character is to be added to each code from category V48

> A   initial encounter
> D   subsequent encounter
> S   sequela

X● **V48.0** Car driver injured in noncollision transport accident in nontraffic accident

X● **V48.1** Car passenger injured in noncollision transport accident in nontraffic accident

X● **V48.2** Person on outside of car injured in noncollision transport accident in nontraffic accident

X● **V48.3** Unspecified car occupant injured in noncollision transport accident in nontraffic accident

X● **V48.4** Person boarding or alighting a car injured in noncollision transport accident

X● **V48.5** Car driver injured in noncollision transport accident in traffic accident

X● **V48.6** Car passenger injured in noncollision transport accident in traffic accident

X● **V48.7** Person on outside of car injured in noncollision transport accident in traffic accident

X● **V48.9** Unspecified car occupant injured in noncollision transport accident in traffic accident

▶ New   ⇒ Revised   ~~deleted~~ Deleted   OGCR Official Guidelines   X Assign placeholder X   ● Use Additional Character(s)
Excludes 1   Excludes 2   Includes   Use additional   Code first   Code also   Key words

● **V49**   **Car occupant injured in other and unspecified transport accidents**

> The appropriate 7th character is to be added to each code from category V49

> | | |
> |---|---|
> | A | initial encounter |
> | D | subsequent encounter |
> | S | sequela |

● **V49.0**   Driver injured in collision with other and unspecified motor vehicles in nontraffic accident

   X ● **V49.00**   Driver injured in collision with unspecified motor vehicles in nontraffic accident

   X ● **V49.09**   Driver injured in collision with other motor vehicles in nontraffic accident

● **V49.1**   Passenger injured in collision with other and unspecified motor vehicles in nontraffic accident

   X ● **V49.10**   Passenger injured in collision with unspecified motor vehicles in nontraffic accident

   X ● **V49.19**   Passenger injured in collision with other motor vehicles in nontraffic accident

● **V49.2**   Unspecified car occupant injured in collision with other and unspecified motor vehicles in nontraffic accident

   X ● **V49.20**   Unspecified car occupant injured in collision with unspecified motor vehicles in nontraffic accident
      Car collision NOS, nontraffic

   X ● **V49.29**   Unspecified car occupant injured in collision with other motor vehicles in nontraffic accident

X ● **V49.3**   Car occupant (driver) (passenger) injured in unspecified nontraffic accident
     Car accident NOS, nontraffic
     Car occupant injured in nontraffic accident NOS

● **V49.4**   Driver injured in collision with other and unspecified motor vehicles in traffic accident

   X ● **V49.40**   Driver injured in collision with unspecified motor vehicles in traffic accident

   X ● **V49.49**   Driver injured in collision with other motor vehicles in traffic accident

● **V49.5**   Passenger injured in collision with other and unspecified motor vehicles in traffic accident

   X ● **V49.50**   Passenger injured in collision with unspecified motor vehicles in traffic accident

   X ● **V49.59**   Passenger injured in collision with other motor vehicles in traffic accident

● **V49.6**   Unspecified car occupant injured in collision with other and unspecified motor vehicles in traffic accident

   X ● **V49.60**   Unspecified car occupant injured in collision with unspecified motor vehicles in traffic accident
      Car collision NOS (traffic)

   X ● **V49.69**   Unspecified car occupant injured in collision with other motor vehicles in traffic accident

● **V49.8**   Car occupant (driver) (passenger) injured in other specified transport accidents

   X ● **V49.81**   Car occupant (driver) (passenger) injured in transport accident with military vehicle

   X ● **V49.88**   Car occupant (driver) (passenger) injured in other specified transport accidents

X ● **V49.9**   Car occupant (driver) (passenger) injured in unspecified traffic accident
     Car accident NOS

OCCUPANT OF PICK-UP TRUCK OR VAN INJURED IN TRANSPORT ACCIDENT (V50-V59)

> | **Includes** | a four- or six-wheel motor vehicle designed primarily for carrying passengers and property but weighing less than the local limit for classification as a heavy goods vehicle |
> |---|---|
> | | minibus |
> | | minivan |
> | | sport utility vehicle (SUV) |
> | | truck |
> | | van |

> | **Excludes1** | heavy transport vehicle (V60-V69) |
> |---|---|

● **V50**   **Occupant of pick-up truck or van injured in collision with pedestrian or animal**

> | **Excludes1** | pick-up truck or van collision with animal-drawn vehicle or animal being ridden (V56.-) |
> |---|---|

> The appropriate 7th character is to be added to each code from category V50

> | | |
> |---|---|
> | A | initial encounter |
> | D | subsequent encounter |
> | S | sequela |

   X ● **V50.0**   Driver of pick-up truck or van injured in collision with pedestrian or animal in nontraffic accident

   X ● **V50.1**   Passenger in pick-up truck or van injured in collision with pedestrian or animal in nontraffic accident

   X ● **V50.2**   Person on outside of pick-up truck or van injured in collision with pedestrian or animal in nontraffic accident

   X ● **V50.3**   Unspecified occupant of pick-up truck or van injured in collision with pedestrian or animal in nontraffic accident

   X ● **V50.4**   Person boarding or alighting a pick-up truck or van injured in collision with pedestrian or animal

   X ● **V50.5**   Driver of pick-up truck or van injured in collision with pedestrian or animal in traffic accident

   X ● **V50.6**   Passenger in pick-up truck or van injured in collision with pedestrian or animal in traffic accident

   X ● **V50.7**   Person on outside of pick-up truck or van injured in collision with pedestrian or animal in traffic accident

   X ● **V50.9**   Unspecified occupant of pick-up truck or van injured in collision with pedestrian or animal in traffic accident

● **V51**   **Occupant of pick-up truck or van injured in collision with pedal cycle**

> The appropriate 7th character is to be added to each code from category V51

> | | |
> |---|---|
> | A | initial encounter |
> | D | subsequent encounter |
> | S | sequela |

   X ● **V51.0**   Driver of pick-up truck or van injured in collision with pedal cycle in nontraffic accident

   X ● **V51.1**   Passenger in pick-up truck or van injured in collision with pedal cycle in nontraffic accident

   X ● **V51.2**   Person on outside of pick-up truck or van injured in collision with pedal cycle in nontraffic accident

   X ● **V51.3**   Unspecified occupant of pick-up truck or van injured in collision with pedal cycle in nontraffic accident

   X ● **V51.4**   Person boarding or alighting a pick-up truck or van injured in collision with pedal cycle

   X ● **V51.5**   Driver of pick-up truck or van injured in collision with pedal cycle in traffic accident

   X ● **V51.6**   Passenger in pick-up truck or van injured in collision with pedal cycle in traffic accident

   X ● **V51.7**   Person on outside of pick-up truck or van injured in collision with pedal cycle in traffic accident

   X ● **V51.9**   Unspecified occupant of pick-up truck or van injured in collision with pedal cycle in traffic accident

● **V52 Occupant of pick-up truck or van injured in collision with two- or three-wheeled motor vehicle**

The appropriate 7th character is to be added to each code from category V52

A	initial encounter
D	subsequent encounter
S	sequela

X● **V52.0** Driver of pick-up truck or van injured in collision with two- or three-wheeled motor vehicle in nontraffic accident

X● **V52.1** Passenger in pick-up truck or van injured in collision with two- or three-wheeled motor vehicle in nontraffic accident

X● **V52.2** Person on outside of pick-up truck or van injured in collision with two- or three-wheeled motor vehicle in nontraffic accident

X● **V52.3** Unspecified occupant of pick-up truck or van injured in collision with two- or three-wheeled motor vehicle in nontraffic accident

X● **V52.4** Person boarding or alighting a pick-up truck or van injured in collision with two- or three-wheeled motor vehicle

X● **V52.5** Driver of pick-up truck or van injured in collision with two- or three-wheeled motor vehicle in traffic accident

X● **V52.6** Passenger in pick-up truck or van injured in collision with two- or three-wheeled motor vehicle in traffic accident

X● **V52.7** Person on outside of pick-up truck or van injured in collision with two- or three-wheeled motor vehicle in traffic accident

X● **V52.9** Unspecified occupant of pick-up truck or van injured in collision with two- or three-wheeled motor vehicle in traffic accident

● **V53 Occupant of pick-up truck or van injured in collision with car, pick-up truck or van**

The appropriate 7th character is to be added to each code from category V53

A	initial encounter
D	subsequent encounter
S	sequela

X● **V53.0** Driver of pick-up truck or van injured in collision with car, pick-up truck or van in nontraffic accident

X● **V53.1** Passenger in pick-up truck or van injured in collision with car, pick-up truck or van in nontraffic accident

X● **V53.2** Person on outside of pick-up truck or van injured in collision with car, pick-up truck or van in nontraffic accident

X● **V53.3** Unspecified occupant of pick-up truck or van injured in collision with car, pick-up truck or van in nontraffic accident

X● **V53.4** Person boarding or alighting a pick-up truck or van injured in collision with car, pick-up truck or van

X● **V53.5** Driver of pick-up truck or van injured in collision with car, pick-up truck or van in traffic accident

X● **V53.6** Passenger in pick-up truck or van injured in collision with car, pick-up truck or van in traffic accident

X● **V53.7** Person on outside of pick-up truck or van injured in collision with car, pick-up truck or van in traffic accident

X● **V53.9** Unspecified occupant of pick-up truck or van injured in collision with car, pick-up truck or van in traffic accident

● **V54 Occupant of pick-up truck or van injured in collision with heavy transport vehicle or bus**

Excludes1   occupant of pick-up truck or van injured in collision with military vehicle (V59.81)

The appropriate 7th character is to be added to each code from category V54

A	initial encounter
D	subsequent encounter
S	sequela

X● **V54.0** Driver of pick-up truck or van injured in collision with heavy transport vehicle or bus in nontraffic accident

X● **V54.1** Passenger in pick-up truck or van injured in collision with heavy transport vehicle or bus in nontraffic accident

X● **V54.2** Person on outside of pick-up truck or van injured in collision with heavy transport vehicle or bus in nontraffic accident

X● **V54.3** Unspecified occupant of pick-up truck or van injured in collision with heavy transport vehicle or bus in nontraffic accident

X● **V54.4** Person boarding or alighting a pick-up truck or van injured in collision with heavy transport vehicle or bus

X● **V54.5** Driver of pick-up truck or van injured in collision with heavy transport vehicle or bus in traffic accident

X● **V54.6** Passenger in pick-up truck or van injured in collision with heavy transport vehicle or bus in traffic accident

X● **V54.7** Person on outside of pick-up truck or van injured in collision with heavy transport vehicle or bus in traffic accident

X● **V54.9** Unspecified occupant of pick-up truck or van injured in collision with heavy transport vehicle or bus in traffic accident

● **V55 Occupant of pick-up truck or van injured in collision with railway train or railway vehicle**

The appropriate 7th character is to be added to each code from category V55

A	initial encounter
D	subsequent encounter
S	sequela

X● **V55.0** Driver of pick-up truck or van injured in collision with railway train or railway vehicle in nontraffic accident

X● **V55.1** Passenger in pick-up truck or van injured in collision with railway train or railway vehicle in nontraffic accident

X● **V55.2** Person on outside of pick-up truck or van injured in collision with railway train or railway vehicle in nontraffic accident

X● **V55.3** Unspecified occupant of pick-up truck or van injured in collision with railway train or railway vehicle in nontraffic accident

X● **V55.4** Person boarding or alighting a pick-up truck or van injured in collision with railway train or railway vehicle

X● **V55.5** Driver of pick-up truck or van injured in collision with railway train or railway vehicle in traffic accident

X● **V55.6** Passenger in pick-up truck or van injured in collision with railway train or railway vehicle in traffic accident

X● **V55.7** Person on outside of pick-up truck or van injured in collision with railway train or railway vehicle in traffic accident

X● **V55.9** Unspecified occupant of pick-up truck or van injured in collision with railway train or railway vehicle in traffic accident

▶ New   ⇒ Revised   ~~deleted~~ Deleted   **OGCR** Official Guidelines   X Assign placeholder X   ● Use Additional Character(s)

Excludes 1   Excludes 2   Includes   Use additional   Code first   Code also   Key words

● **V56**   **Occupant of pick-up truck or van injured in collision with other nonmotor vehicle**

> | **Includes** | collision with animal-drawn vehicle, animal being ridden, streetcar |

> The appropriate 7th character is to be added to each code from category V56

> | A | initial encounter |
> | D | subsequent encounter |
> | S | sequela |

X● **V56.0**   Driver of pick-up truck or van injured in collision with other nonmotor vehicle in nontraffic accident

X● **V56.1**   Passenger in pick-up truck or van injured in collision with other nonmotor vehicle in nontraffic accident

X● **V56.2**   Person on outside of pick-up truck or van injured in collision with other nonmotor vehicle in nontraffic accident

X● **V56.3**   Unspecified occupant of pick-up truck or van injured in collision with other nonmotor vehicle in nontraffic accident

X● **V56.4**   Person boarding or alighting a pick-up truck or van injured in collision with other nonmotor vehicle

X● **V56.5**   Driver of pick-up truck or van injured in collision with other nonmotor vehicle in traffic accident

X● **V56.6**   Passenger in pick-up truck or van injured in collision with other nonmotor vehicle in traffic accident

X● **V56.7**   Person on outside of pick-up truck or van injured in collision with other nonmotor vehicle in traffic accident

X● **V56.9**   Unspecified occupant of pick-up truck or van injured in collision with other nonmotor vehicle in traffic accident

● **V57**   **Occupant of pick-up truck or van injured in collision with fixed or stationary object**

> The appropriate 7th character is to be added to each code from category V57

> | A | initial encounter |
> | D | subsequent encounter |
> | S | sequela |

X● **V57.0**   Driver of pick-up truck or van injured in collision with fixed or stationary object in nontraffic accident

X● **V57.1**   Passenger in pick-up truck or van injured in collision with fixed or stationary object in nontraffic accident

X● **V57.2**   Person on outside of pick-up truck or van injured in collision with fixed or stationary object in nontraffic accident

X● **V57.3**   Unspecified occupant of pick-up truck or van injured in collision with fixed or stationary object in nontraffic accident

X● **V57.4**   Person boarding or alighting a pick-up truck or van injured in collision with fixed or stationary object

X● **V57.5**   Driver of pick-up truck or van injured in collision with fixed or stationary object in traffic accident

X● **V57.6**   Passenger in pick-up truck or van injured in collision with fixed or stationary object in traffic accident

X● **V57.7**   Person on outside of pick-up truck or van injured in collision with fixed or stationary object in traffic accident

X● **V57.9**   Unspecified occupant of pick-up truck or van injured in collision with fixed or stationary object in traffic accident

● **V58**   **Occupant of pick-up truck or van injured in noncollision transport accident**

> | **Includes** | overturning pick-up truck or van NOS overturning pick-up truck or van without collision |

> The appropriate 7th character is to be added to each code from category V58

> | A | initial encounter |
> | D | subsequent encounter |
> | S | sequela |

X● **V58.0**   Driver of pick-up truck or van injured in noncollision transport accident in nontraffic accident

X● **V58.1**   Passenger in pick-up truck or van injured in noncollision transport accident in nontraffic accident

X● **V58.2**   Person on outside of pick-up truck or van injured in noncollision transport accident in nontraffic accident

X● **V58.3**   Unspecified occupant of pick-up truck or van injured in noncollision transport accident in nontraffic accident

X● **V58.4**   Person boarding or alighting a pick-up truck or van injured in noncollision transport accident

X● **V58.5**   Driver of pick-up truck or van injured in noncollision transport accident in traffic accident

X● **V58.6**   Passenger in pick-up truck or van injured in noncollision transport accident in traffic accident

X● **V58.7**   Person on outside of pick-up truck or van injured in noncollision transport accident in traffic accident

X● **V58.9**   Unspecified occupant of pick-up truck or van injured in noncollision transport accident in traffic accident

● **V59**   **Occupant of pick-up truck or van injured in other and unspecified transport accidents**

> The appropriate 7th character is to be added to each code from category V59

> | A | initial encounter |
> | D | subsequent encounter |
> | S | sequela |

● **V59.0**   Driver of pick-up truck or van injured in collision with other and unspecified motor vehicles in nontraffic accident

    X● **V59.00**   Driver of pick-up truck or van injured in collision with unspecified motor vehicles in nontraffic accident

    X● **V59.09**   Driver of pick-up truck or van injured in collision with other motor vehicles in nontraffic accident

● **V59.1**   Passenger in pick-up truck or van injured in collision with other and unspecified motor vehicles in nontraffic accident

    X● **V59.10**   Passenger in pick-up truck or van injured in collision with unspecified motor vehicles in nontraffic accident

    X● **V59.19**   Passenger in pick-up truck or van injured in collision with other motor vehicles in nontraffic accident

● **V59.2**   Unspecified occupant of pick-up truck or van injured in collision with other and unspecified motor vehicles in nontraffic accident

    X● **V59.20**   Unspecified occupant of pick-up truck or van injured in collision with unspecified motor vehicles in nontraffic accident
        Collision NOS involving pick-up truck or van, nontraffic

    X● **V59.29**   Unspecified occupant of pick-up truck or van injured in collision with other motor vehicles in nontraffic accident

CHAPTER 20 (V01-Y99)

▶ New   ⇒ Revised   ~~deleted~~ Deleted   **OGCR** Official Guidelines   X Assign placeholder X   ● Use Additional Character(s)

| Excludes 1 | Excludes 2 | Includes | Use additional | Code first | Code also | Key words |

X● **V59.3** Occupant (driver) (passenger) of pick-up truck or van injured in unspecified nontraffic accident
     Accident NOS involving pick-up truck or van, nontraffic
     Occupant of pick-up truck or van injured in nontraffic accident NOS

● **V59.4** Driver of pick-up truck or van injured in collision with other and unspecified motor vehicles in traffic accident

   X● **V59.40** Driver of pick-up truck or van injured in collision with unspecified motor vehicles in traffic accident

   X● **V59.49** Driver of pick-up truck or van injured in collision with other motor vehicles in traffic accident

● **V59.5** Passenger in pick-up truck or van injured in collision with other and unspecified motor vehicles in traffic accident

   X● **V59.50** Passenger in pick-up truck or van injured in collision with unspecified motor vehicles in traffic accident

   X● **V59.59** Passenger in pick-up truck or van injured in collision with other motor vehicles in traffic accident

● **V59.6** Unspecified occupant of pick-up truck or van injured in collision with other and unspecified motor vehicles in traffic accident

   X● **V59.60** Unspecified occupant of pick-up truck or van injured in collision with unspecified motor vehicles in traffic accident
       Collision NOS involving pick-up truck or van (traffic)

   X● **V59.69** Unspecified occupant of pick-up truck or van injured in collision with other motor vehicles in traffic accident

● **V59.8** Occupant (driver) (passenger) of pick-up truck or van injured in other specified transport accidents

   X● **V59.81** Occupant (driver) (passenger) of pick-up truck or van injured in transport accident with military vehicle

   X● **V59.88** Occupant (driver) (passenger) of pick-up truck or van injured in other specified transport accidents

X● **V59.9** Occupant (driver) (passenger) of pick-up truck or van injured in unspecified traffic accident
     Accident NOS involving pick-up truck or van

OCCUPANT OF HEAVY TRANSPORT VEHICLE INJURED IN TRANSPORT ACCIDENT (V60-V69)

Includes	18 wheeler
	armored car
	panel truck
Excludes1	bus
	motorcoach

● **V60** Occupant of heavy transport vehicle injured in collision with pedestrian or animal

   Excludes1 heavy transport vehicle collision with animal-drawn vehicle or animal being ridden (V66.-)

The appropriate 7th character is to be added to each code from category V60

A	initial encounter
D	subsequent encounter
S	sequela

X● **V60.0** Driver of heavy transport vehicle injured in collision with pedestrian or animal in nontraffic accident

X● **V60.1** Passenger in heavy transport vehicle injured in collision with pedestrian or animal in nontraffic accident

X● **V60.2** Person on outside of heavy transport vehicle injured in collision with pedestrian or animal in nontraffic accident

X● **V60.3** Unspecified occupant of heavy transport vehicle injured in collision with pedestrian or animal in nontraffic accident

X● **V60.4** Person boarding or alighting a heavy transport vehicle injured in collision with pedestrian or animal

X● **V60.5** Driver of heavy transport vehicle injured in collision with pedestrian or animal in traffic accident

X● **V60.6** Passenger in heavy transport vehicle injured in collision with pedestrian or animal in traffic accident

X● **V60.7** Person on outside of heavy transport vehicle injured in collision with pedestrian or animal in traffic accident

X● **V60.9** Unspecified occupant of heavy transport vehicle injured in collision with pedestrian or animal in traffic accident

● **V61** Occupant of heavy transport vehicle injured in collision with pedal cycle

The appropriate 7th character is to be added to each code from category V61

A	initial encounter
D	subsequent encounter
S	sequela

X● **V61.0** Driver of heavy transport vehicle injured in collision with pedal cycle in nontraffic accident

X● **V61.1** Passenger in heavy transport vehicle injured in collision with pedal cycle in nontraffic accident

X● **V61.2** Person on outside of heavy transport vehicle injured in collision with pedal cycle in nontraffic accident

X● **V61.3** Unspecified occupant of heavy transport vehicle injured in collision with pedal cycle in nontraffic accident

X● **V61.4** Person boarding or alighting a heavy transport vehicle injured in collision with pedal cycle while boarding or alighting

X● **V61.5** Driver of heavy transport vehicle injured in collision with pedal cycle in traffic accident

X● **V61.6** Passenger in heavy transport vehicle injured in collision with pedal cycle in traffic accident

X● **V61.7** Person on outside of heavy transport vehicle injured in collision with pedal cycle in traffic accident

X● **V61.9** Unspecified occupant of heavy transport vehicle injured in collision with pedal cycle in traffic accident

● **V62** Occupant of heavy transport vehicle injured in collision with two- or three-wheeled motor vehicle

The appropriate 7th character is to be added to each code from category V62

A	initial encounter
D	subsequent encounter
S	sequela

X● **V62.0** Driver of heavy transport vehicle injured in collision with two- or three-wheeled motor vehicle in nontraffic accident

X● **V62.1** Passenger in heavy transport vehicle injured in collision with two- or three-wheeled motor vehicle in nontraffic accident

X● **V62.2** Person on outside of heavy transport vehicle injured in collision with two- or three-wheeled motor vehicle in nontraffic accident

X● **V62.3** Unspecified occupant of heavy transport vehicle injured in collision with two- or three-wheeled motor vehicle in nontraffic accident

X● **V62.4** Person boarding or alighting a heavy transport vehicle injured in collision with two- or three-wheeled motor vehicle

X● **V62.5** Driver of heavy transport vehicle injured in collision with two- or three-wheeled motor vehicle in traffic accident

X● **V62.6** Passenger in heavy transport vehicle injured in collision with two- or three-wheeled motor vehicle in traffic accident

X ● **V62.7** Person on outside of heavy transport vehicle injured in collision with two- or three-wheeled motor vehicle in traffic accident

X ● **V62.9** Unspecified occupant of heavy transport vehicle injured in collision with two- or three-wheeled motor vehicle in traffic accident

● **V63** Occupant of heavy transport vehicle injured in collision with car, pick-up truck or van

The appropriate 7th character is to be added to each code from category V63

A	initial encounter
D	subsequent encounter
S	sequela

X ● **V63.0** Driver of heavy transport vehicle injured in collision with car, pick-up truck or van in nontraffic accident

X ● **V63.1** Passenger in heavy transport vehicle injured in collision with car, pick-up truck or van in nontraffic accident

X ● **V63.2** Person on outside of heavy transport vehicle injured in collision with car, pick-up truck or van in nontraffic accident

X ● **V63.3** Unspecified occupant of heavy transport vehicle injured in collision with car, pick-up truck or van in nontraffic accident

X ● **V63.4** Person boarding or alighting a heavy transport vehicle injured in collision with car, pick-up truck or van

X ● **V63.5** Driver of heavy transport vehicle injured in collision with car, pick-up truck or van in traffic accident

X ● **V63.6** Passenger in heavy transport vehicle injured in collision with car, pick-up truck or van in traffic accident

X ● **V63.7** Person on outside of heavy transport vehicle injured in collision with car, pick-up truck or van in traffic accident

X ● **V63.9** Unspecified occupant of heavy transport vehicle injured in collision with car, pick-up truck or van in traffic accident

● **V64** Occupant of heavy transport vehicle injured in collision with heavy transport vehicle or bus

Excludes1 occupant of heavy transport vehicle injured in collision with military vehicle (V69.81)

The appropriate 7th character is to be added to each code from category V64

A	initial encounter
D	subsequent encounter
S	sequela

X ● **V64.0** Driver of heavy transport vehicle injured in collision with heavy transport vehicle or bus in nontraffic accident

X ● **V64.1** Passenger in heavy transport vehicle injured in collision with heavy transport vehicle or bus in nontraffic accident

X ● **V64.2** Person on outside of heavy transport vehicle injured in collision with heavy transport vehicle or bus in nontraffic accident

X ● **V64.3** Unspecified occupant of heavy transport vehicle injured in collision with heavy transport vehicle or bus in nontraffic accident

X ● **V64.4** Person boarding or alighting a heavy transport vehicle injured in collision with heavy transport vehicle or bus while boarding or alighting

X ● **V64.5** Driver of heavy transport vehicle injured in collision with heavy transport vehicle or bus in traffic accident

X ● **V64.6** Passenger in heavy transport vehicle injured in collision with heavy transport vehicle or bus in traffic accident

X ● **V64.7** Person on outside of heavy transport vehicle injured in collision with heavy transport vehicle or bus in traffic accident

X ● **V64.9** Unspecified occupant of heavy transport vehicle injured in collision with heavy transport vehicle or bus in traffic accident

● **V65** Occupant of heavy transport vehicle injured in collision with railway train or railway vehicle

The appropriate 7th character is to be added to each code from category V65

A	initial encounter
D	subsequent encounter
S	sequela

X ● **V65.0** Driver of heavy transport vehicle injured in collision with railway train or railway vehicle in nontraffic accident

X ● **V65.1** Passenger in heavy transport vehicle injured in collision with railway train or railway vehicle in nontraffic accident

X ● **V65.2** Person on outside of heavy transport vehicle injured in collision with railway train or railway vehicle in nontraffic accident

X ● **V65.3** Unspecified occupant of heavy transport vehicle injured in collision with railway train or railway vehicle in nontraffic accident

X ● **V65.4** Person boarding or alighting a heavy transport vehicle injured in collision with railway train or railway vehicle

X ● **V65.5** Driver of heavy transport vehicle injured in collision with railway train or railway vehicle in traffic accident

X ● **V65.6** Passenger in heavy transport vehicle injured in collision with railway train or railway vehicle in traffic accident

X ● **V65.7** Person on outside of heavy transport vehicle injured in collision with railway train or railway vehicle in traffic accident

X ● **V65.9** Unspecified occupant of heavy transport vehicle injured in collision with railway train or railway vehicle in traffic accident

● **V66** Occupant of heavy transport vehicle injured in collision with other nonmotor vehicle

Includes collision with animal-drawn vehicle, animal being ridden, streetcar

The appropriate 7th character is to be added to each code from category V66

A	initial encounter
D	subsequent encounter
S	sequela

X ● **V66.0** Driver of heavy transport vehicle injured in collision with other nonmotor vehicle in nontraffic accident

X ● **V66.1** Passenger in heavy transport vehicle injured in collision with other nonmotor vehicle in nontraffic accident

X ● **V66.2** Person on outside of heavy transport vehicle injured in collision with other nonmotor vehicle in nontraffic accident

X ● **V66.3** Unspecified occupant of heavy transport vehicle injured in collision with other nonmotor vehicle in nontraffic accident

X ● **V66.4** Person boarding or alighting a heavy transport vehicle injured in collision with other nonmotor vehicle

X ● **V66.5** Driver of heavy transport vehicle injured in collision with other nonmotor vehicle in traffic accident

X ● **V66.6** Passenger in heavy transport vehicle injured in collision with other nonmotor vehicle in traffic accident

X ● **V66.7** Person on outside of heavy transport vehicle injured in collision with other nonmotor vehicle in traffic accident

X ● **V66.9** Unspecified occupant of heavy transport vehicle injured in collision with other nonmotor vehicle in traffic accident

CHAPTER 20 (V01-Y99)

CHAPTER 20 (V01-Y99)

● **V67   Occupant of heavy transport vehicle injured in collision with fixed or stationary object**

The appropriate 7th character is to be added to each code from category V67

A	initial encounter
D	subsequent encounter
S	sequela

X● **V67.0   Driver** of heavy transport vehicle injured in collision with fixed or stationary object in nontraffic accident

X● **V67.1   Passenger** in heavy transport vehicle injured in collision with fixed or stationary object in nontraffic accident

X● **V67.2   Person on outside** of heavy transport vehicle injured in collision with fixed or stationary object in nontraffic accident

X● **V67.3   Unspecified** occupant of heavy transport vehicle injured in collision with fixed or stationary object in nontraffic accident

X● **V67.4   Person boarding or alighting** a heavy transport vehicle injured in collision with fixed or stationary object

X● **V67.5   Driver** of heavy transport vehicle injured in collision with fixed or stationary object in traffic accident

X● **V67.6   Passenger** in heavy transport vehicle injured in collision with fixed or stationary object in traffic accident

X● **V67.7   Person on outside** of heavy transport vehicle injured in collision with fixed or stationary object in traffic accident

X● **V67.9   Unspecified** occupant of heavy transport vehicle injured in collision with fixed or stationary object in traffic accident

● **V68   Occupant of heavy transport vehicle injured in noncollision transport accident**

     Includes   overturning heavy transport vehicle NOS
                            overturning heavy transport vehicle without collision

The appropriate 7th character is to be added to each code from category V68

A	initial encounter
D	subsequent encounter
S	sequela

X● **V68.0   Driver** of heavy transport vehicle injured in noncollision transport accident in nontraffic accident

X● **V68.1   Passenger** in heavy transport vehicle injured in noncollision transport accident in nontraffic accident

X● **V68.2   Person on outside** of heavy transport vehicle injured in noncollision transport accident in nontraffic accident

X● **V68.3   Unspecified** occupant of heavy transport vehicle injured in noncollision transport accident in nontraffic accident

X● **V68.4   Person boarding or alighting** a heavy transport vehicle injured in noncollision transport accident

X● **V68.5   Driver** of heavy transport vehicle injured in noncollision transport accident in traffic accident

X● **V68.6   Passenger** in heavy transport vehicle injured in noncollision transport accident in traffic accident

X● **V68.7   Person on outside** of heavy transport vehicle injured in noncollision transport accident in traffic accident

X● **V68.9   Unspecified** occupant of heavy transport vehicle injured in noncollision transport accident in traffic accident

● **V69   Occupant of heavy transport vehicle injured in other and unspecified transport accidents**

The appropriate 7th character is to be added to each code from category V69

A	initial encounter
D	subsequent encounter
S	sequela

● **V69.0   Driver** of heavy transport vehicle injured in collision with other and unspecified motor vehicles in nontraffic accident

X● **V69.00   Driver** of heavy transport vehicle injured in collision with unspecified motor vehicles in nontraffic accident

X● **V69.09   Driver** of heavy transport vehicle injured in collision with other motor vehicles in nontraffic accident

● **V69.1   Passenger** in heavy transport vehicle injured in collision with other and unspecified motor vehicles in nontraffic accident

X● **V69.10   Passenger** in heavy transport vehicle injured in collision with unspecified motor vehicles in nontraffic accident

X● **V69.19   Passenger** in heavy transport vehicle injured in collision with other motor vehicles in nontraffic accident

● **V69.2   Unspecified** occupant of heavy transport vehicle injured in collision with other and unspecified motor vehicles in nontraffic accident

X● **V69.20   Unspecified** occupant of heavy transport vehicle injured in collision with unspecified motor vehicles in nontraffic accident
           Collision NOS involving heavy transport vehicle, nontraffic

X● **V69.29   Unspecified** occupant of heavy transport vehicle injured in collision with other motor vehicles in nontraffic accident

X● **V69.3   Occupant (driver) (passenger)** of heavy transport vehicle injured in unspecified nontraffic accident
           Accident NOS involving heavy transport vehicle, nontraffic
           Occupant of heavy transport vehicle injured in nontraffic accident NOS

● **V69.4   Driver** of heavy transport vehicle injured in collision with other and unspecified motor vehicles in traffic accident

X● **V69.40   Driver** of heavy transport vehicle injured in collision with unspecified motor vehicles in traffic accident

X● **V69.49   Driver** of heavy transport vehicle injured in collision with other motor vehicles in traffic accident

● **V69.5   Passenger** in heavy transport vehicle injured in collision with other and unspecified motor vehicles in traffic accident

X● **V69.50   Passenger** in heavy transport vehicle injured in collision with unspecified motor vehicles in traffic accident

X● **V69.59   Passenger** in heavy transport vehicle injured in collision with other motor vehicles in traffic accident

▶ New   ⇢ Revised   ~~deleted~~ Deleted   **OGCR** Official Guidelines   X Assign placeholder X   ● Use Additional Character(s)

Excludes 1   Excludes 2   Includes   Use additional   Code first   Code also   Key words

- ● V69.6   Unspecified occupant of heavy transport vehicle injured in collision with other and unspecified motor vehicles in traffic accident
  - X ● V69.60   Unspecified occupant of heavy transport vehicle injured in collision with unspecified motor vehicles in traffic accident
    - Collision NOS involving heavy transport vehicle (traffic)
  - X ● V69.69   Unspecified occupant of heavy transport vehicle injured in collision with other motor vehicles in traffic accident
- ● V69.8   Occupant (driver) (passenger) of heavy transport vehicle injured in other specified transport accidents
  - X ● V69.81   Occupant (driver) (passenger) of heavy transport vehicle injured in transport accidents with military vehicle
  - X ● V69.88   Occupant (driver) (passenger) of heavy transport vehicle injured in other specified transport accidents
- X ● V69.9   Occupant (driver) (passenger) of heavy transport vehicle injured in unspecified traffic accident
  - Accident NOS involving heavy transport vehicle

BUS OCCUPANT INJURED IN TRANSPORT ACCIDENT (V70-V79)

| Includes | motorcoach |
| Excludes1 | minibus (V50-V59) |

- ● V70   Bus occupant injured in collision with pedestrian or animal

  | Excludes1 | bus collision with animal-drawn vehicle or animal being ridden (V76.-) |

  The appropriate 7th character is to be added to each code from category V70

A	initial encounter
D	subsequent encounter
S	sequela

- X ● V70.0   Driver of bus injured in collision with pedestrian or animal in nontraffic accident
- X ● V70.1   Passenger on bus injured in collision with pedestrian or animal in nontraffic accident
- X ● V70.2   Person on outside of bus injured in collision with pedestrian or animal in nontraffic accident
- X ● V70.3   Unspecified occupant of bus injured in collision with pedestrian or animal in nontraffic accident
- X ● V70.4   Person boarding or alighting from bus injured in collision with pedestrian or animal
- X ● V70.5   Driver of bus injured in collision with pedestrian or animal in traffic accident
- X ● V70.6   Passenger on bus injured in collision with pedestrian or animal in traffic accident
- X ● V70.7   Person on outside of bus injured in collision with pedestrian or animal in traffic accident
- X ● V70.9   Unspecified occupant of bus injured in collision with pedestrian or animal in traffic accident

- ● V71   Bus occupant injured in collision with pedal cycle

  The appropriate 7th character is to be added to each code from category V71

A	initial encounter
D	subsequent encounter
S	sequela

- X ● V71.0   Driver of bus injured in collision with pedal cycle in nontraffic accident
- X ● V71.1   Passenger on bus injured in collision with pedal cycle in nontraffic accident
- X ● V71.2   Person on outside of bus injured in collision with pedal cycle in nontraffic accident
- X ● V71.3   Unspecified occupant of bus injured in collision with pedal cycle in nontraffic accident
- X ● V71.4   Person boarding or alighting from bus injured in collision with pedal cycle
- X ● V71.5   Driver of bus injured in collision with pedal cycle in traffic accident
- X ● V71.6   Passenger on bus injured in collision with pedal cycle in traffic accident
- X ● V71.7   Person on outside of bus injured in collision with pedal cycle in traffic accident
- X ● V71.9   Unspecified occupant of bus injured in collision with pedal cycle in traffic accident

- ● V72   Bus occupant injured in collision with two- or three-wheeled motor vehicle

  The appropriate 7th character is to be added to each code from category V72

A	initial encounter
D	subsequent encounter
S	sequela

- X ● V72.0   Driver of bus injured in collision with two- or three-wheeled motor vehicle in nontraffic accident
- X ● V72.1   Passenger on bus injured in collision with two- or three-wheeled motor vehicle in nontraffic accident
- X ● V72.2   Person on outside of bus injured in collision with two- or three-wheeled motor vehicle in nontraffic accident
- X ● V72.3   Unspecified occupant of bus injured in collision with two- or three-wheeled motor vehicle in nontraffic accident
- X ● V72.4   Person boarding or alighting from bus injured in collision with two- or three-wheeled motor vehicle
- X ● V72.5   Driver of bus injured in collision with two- or three-wheeled motor vehicle in traffic accident
- X ● V72.6   Passenger on bus injured in collision with two- or three-wheeled motor vehicle in traffic accident
- X ● V72.7   Person on outside of bus injured in collision with two- or three-wheeled motor vehicle in traffic accident
- X ● V72.9   Unspecified occupant of bus injured in collision with two- or three-wheeled motor vehicle in traffic accident

- ● V73   Bus occupant injured in collision with car, pick-up truck or van

  The appropriate 7th character is to be added to each code from category V73

A	initial encounter
D	subsequent encounter
S	sequela

- X ● V73.0   Driver of bus injured in collision with car, pick-up truck or van in nontraffic accident
- X ● V73.1   Passenger on bus injured in collision with car, pick-up truck or van in nontraffic accident
- X ● V73.2   Person on outside of bus injured in collision with car, pick-up truck or van in nontraffic accident
- X ● V73.3   Unspecified occupant of bus injured in collision with car, pick-up truck or van in nontraffic accident
- X ● V73.4   Person boarding or alighting from bus injured in collision with car, pick-up truck or van
- X ● V73.5   Driver of bus injured in collision with car, pick-up truck or van in traffic accident
- X ● V73.6   Passenger on bus injured in collision with car, pick-up truck or van in traffic accident
- X ● V73.7   Person on outside of bus injured in collision with car, pick-up truck or van in traffic accident
- X ● V73.9   Unspecified occupant of bus injured in collision with car, pick-up truck or van in traffic accident

● **V74**   **Bus occupant injured in collision with heavy transport vehicle or bus**

> **Excludes1**   bus occupant injured in collision with military vehicle (V79.81)

> The appropriate 7th character is to be added to each code from category V74

> | | |
> |---|---|
> | A | initial encounter |
> | D | subsequent encounter |
> | S | sequela |

X ● **V74.0**   Driver of bus injured in collision with heavy transport vehicle or bus in nontraffic accident

X ● **V74.1**   Passenger on bus injured in collision with heavy transport vehicle or bus in nontraffic accident

X ● **V74.2**   Person on outside of bus injured in collision with heavy transport vehicle or bus in nontraffic accident

X ● **V74.3**   Unspecified occupant of bus injured in collision with heavy transport vehicle or bus in nontraffic accident

X ● **V74.4**   Person boarding or alighting from bus injured in collision with heavy transport vehicle or bus

X ● **V74.5**   Driver of bus injured in collision with heavy transport vehicle or bus in traffic accident

X ● **V74.6**   Passenger on bus injured in collision with heavy transport vehicle or bus in traffic accident

X ● **V74.7**   Person on outside of bus injured in collision with heavy transport vehicle or bus in traffic accident

X ● **V74.9**   Unspecified occupant of bus injured in collision with heavy transport vehicle or bus in traffic accident

● **V75**   **Bus occupant injured in collision with railway train or railway vehicle**

> The appropriate 7th character is to be added to each code from category V75

> | | |
> |---|---|
> | A | initial encounter |
> | D | subsequent encounter |
> | S | sequela |

X ● **V75.0**   Driver of bus injured in collision with railway train or railway vehicle in nontraffic accident

X ● **V75.1**   Passenger on bus injured in collision with railway train or railway vehicle in nontraffic accident

X ● **V75.2**   Person on outside of bus injured in collision with railway train or railway vehicle in nontraffic accident

X ● **V75.3**   Unspecified occupant of bus injured in collision with railway train or railway vehicle in nontraffic accident

X ● **V75.4**   Person boarding or alighting from bus injured in collision with railway train or railway vehicle

X ● **V75.5**   Driver of bus injured in collision with railway train or railway vehicle in traffic accident

X ● **V75.6**   Passenger on bus injured in collision with railway train or railway vehicle in traffic accident

X ● **V75.7**   Person on outside of bus injured in collision with railway train or railway vehicle in traffic accident

X ● **V75.9**   Unspecified occupant of bus injured in collision with railway train or railway vehicle in traffic accident

● **V76**   **Bus occupant injured in collision with other nonmotor vehicle**

> **Includes**   collision with animal-drawn vehicle, animal being ridden, streetcar

> The appropriate 7th character is to be added to each code from category V76

> | | |
> |---|---|
> | A | initial encounter |
> | D | subsequent encounter |
> | S | sequela |

X ● **V76.0**   Driver of bus injured in collision with other nonmotor vehicle in nontraffic accident

X ● **V76.1**   Passenger on bus injured in collision with other nonmotor vehicle in nontraffic accident

X ● **V76.2**   Person on outside of bus injured in collision with other nonmotor vehicle in nontraffic accident

X ● **V76.3**   Unspecified occupant of bus injured in collision with other nonmotor vehicle in nontraffic accident

X ● **V76.4**   Person boarding or alighting from bus injured in collision with other nonmotor vehicle

X ● **V76.5**   Driver of bus injured in collision with other nonmotor vehicle in traffic accident

X ● **V76.6**   Passenger on bus injured in collision with other nonmotor vehicle in traffic accident

X ● **V76.7**   Person on outside of bus injured in collision with other nonmotor vehicle in traffic accident

X ● **V76.9**   Unspecified occupant of bus injured in collision with other nonmotor vehicle in traffic accident

● **V77**   **Bus occupant injured in collision with fixed or stationary object**

> The appropriate 7th character is to be added to each code from category V77

> | | |
> |---|---|
> | A | initial encounter |
> | D | subsequent encounter |
> | S | sequela |

X ● **V77.0**   Driver of bus injured in collision with fixed or stationary object in nontraffic accident

X ● **V77.1**   Passenger on bus injured in collision with fixed or stationary object in nontraffic accident

X ● **V77.2**   Person on outside of bus injured in collision with fixed or stationary object in nontraffic accident

X ● **V77.3**   Unspecified occupant of bus injured in collision with fixed or stationary object in nontraffic accident

X ● **V77.4**   Person boarding or alighting from bus injured in collision with fixed or stationary object

X ● **V77.5**   Driver of bus injured in collision with fixed or stationary object in traffic accident

X ● **V77.6**   Passenger on bus injured in collision with fixed or stationary object in traffic accident

X ● **V77.7**   Person on outside of bus injured in collision with fixed or stationary object in traffic accident

X ● **V77.9**   Unspecified occupant of bus injured in collision with fixed or stationary object in traffic accident

● **V78**   **Bus occupant injured in noncollision transport accident**

> **Includes**   overturning bus NOS
> overturning bus without collision

> The appropriate 7th character is to be added to each code from category V78

> | | |
> |---|---|
> | A | initial encounter |
> | D | subsequent encounter |
> | S | sequela |

X ● **V78.0**   Driver of bus injured in noncollision transport accident in nontraffic accident

X ● **V78.1**   Passenger on bus injured in noncollision transport accident in nontraffic accident

X ● **V78.2**   Person on outside of bus injured in noncollision transport accident in nontraffic accident

X ● **V78.3**   Unspecified occupant of bus injured in noncollision transport accident in nontraffic accident

X ● **V78.4**   Person boarding or alighting from bus injured in noncollision transport accident

X ● **V78.5**   Driver of bus injured in noncollision transport accident in traffic accident

X ● **V78.6**   Passenger on bus injured in noncollision transport accident in traffic accident

X ● **V78.7**   Person on outside of bus injured in noncollision transport accident in traffic accident

X ● **V78.9**   Unspecified occupant of bus injured in noncollision transport accident in traffic accident

● **V79**   **Bus occupant injured in other and unspecified transport accidents**

> The appropriate 7th character is to be added to each code from category V79
>
> | | |
> |---|---|
> | A | initial encounter |
> | D | subsequent encounter |
> | S | sequela |

● **V79.0**   Driver of bus injured in collision with other and unspecified motor vehicles in nontraffic accident

   X ● **V79.00**   Driver of bus injured in collision with unspecified motor vehicles in nontraffic accident

   X ● **V79.09**   Driver of bus injured in collision with other motor vehicles in nontraffic accident

● **V79.1**   Passenger on bus injured in collision with other and unspecified motor vehicles in nontraffic accident

   X ● **V79.10**   Passenger on bus injured in collision with unspecified motor vehicles in nontraffic accident

   X ● **V79.19**   Passenger on bus injured in collision with other motor vehicles in nontraffic accident

● **V79.2**   Unspecified bus occupant injured in collision with other and unspecified motor vehicles in nontraffic accident

   X ● **V79.20**   Unspecified bus occupant injured in collision with unspecified motor vehicles in nontraffic accident
> Bus collision NOS, nontraffic

   X ● **V79.29**   Unspecified bus occupant injured in collision with other motor vehicles in nontraffic accident

X ● **V79.3**   Bus occupant (driver) (passenger) injured in unspecified nontraffic accident
> Bus accident NOS, nontraffic
> Bus occupant injured in nontraffic accident NOS

● **V79.4**   Driver of bus injured in collision with other and unspecified motor vehicles in traffic accident

   X ● **V79.40**   Driver of bus injured in collision with unspecified motor vehicles in traffic accident

   X ● **V79.49**   Driver of bus injured in collision with other motor vehicles in traffic accident

● **V79.5**   Passenger on bus injured in collision with other and unspecified motor vehicles in traffic accident

   X ● **V79.50**   Passenger on bus injured in collision with unspecified motor vehicles in traffic accident

   X ● **V79.59**   Passenger on bus injured in collision with other motor vehicles in traffic accident

● **V79.6**   Unspecified bus occupant injured in collision with other and unspecified motor vehicles in traffic accident

   X ● **V79.60**   Unspecified bus occupant injured in collision with unspecified motor vehicles in traffic accident
> Bus collision NOS (traffic)

   X ● **V79.69**   Unspecified bus occupant injured in collision with other motor vehicles in traffic accident

● **V79.8**   Bus occupant (driver) (passenger) injured in other specified transport accidents

   X ● **V79.81**   Bus occupant (driver) (passenger) injured in transport accidents with military vehicle

   X ● **V79.88**   Bus occupant (driver) (passenger) injured in other specified transport accidents

X ● **V79.9**   Bus occupant (driver) (passenger) injured in unspecified traffic accident
> Bus accident NOS

OTHER LAND TRANSPORT ACCIDENTS (V80-V89)

● **V80**   **Animal-rider or occupant of animal-drawn vehicle injured in transport accident**

> The appropriate 7th character is to be added to each code from category V80
>
> | | |
> |---|---|
> | A | initial encounter |
> | D | subsequent encounter |
> | S | sequela |

● **V80.0**   Animal-rider or occupant of animal drawn vehicle injured by fall from or being thrown from animal or animal-drawn vehicle in noncollision accident

   ● **V80.01**   Animal-rider injured by fall from or being thrown from animal in noncollision accident

     ● **V80.010**   Animal-rider injured by fall from or being thrown from horse in noncollision accident

     ● **V80.018**   Animal-rider injured by fall from or being thrown from other animal in noncollision accident

   X ● **V80.02**   Occupant of animal-drawn vehicle injured by fall from or being thrown from animal-drawn vehicle in noncollision accident
> Overturning animal-drawn vehicle NOS
> Overturning animal-drawn vehicle without collision

● **V80.1**   Animal-rider or occupant of animal-drawn vehicle injured in collision with pedestrian or animal

> **Excludes1**   animal-rider or animal-drawn vehicle collision with animal-drawn vehicle or animal being ridden (V80.7)

   X ● **V80.11**   Animal-rider injured in collision with pedestrian or animal

   X ● **V80.12**   Occupant of animal-drawn vehicle injured in collision with pedestrian or animal

● **V80.2**   Animal-rider or occupant of animal-drawn vehicle injured in collision with pedal cycle

   X ● **V80.21**   Animal-rider injured in collision with pedal cycle

   X ● **V80.22**   Occupant of animal-drawn vehicle injured in collision with pedal cycle

● **V80.3**   Animal-rider or occupant of animal-drawn vehicle injured in collision with two- or three-wheeled motor vehicle

   X ● **V80.31**   Animal-rider injured in collision with two- or three-wheeled motor vehicle

   X ● **V80.32**   Occupant of animal-drawn vehicle injured in collision with two- or three-wheeled motor vehicle

● **V80.4**   Animal-rider or occupant of animal-drawn vehicle injured in collision with car, pick-up truck, van, heavy transport vehicle or bus

> **Excludes1**   animal-rider injured in collision with military vehicle (V80.910)
> occupant of animal-drawn vehicle injured in collision with military vehicle (V80.920)

   X ● **V80.41**   Animal-rider injured in collision with car, pick-up truck, van, heavy transport vehicle or bus

   X ● **V80.42**   Occupant of animal-drawn vehicle injured in collision with car, pick-up truck, van, heavy transport vehicle or bus

CHAPTER 20 (V01-Y99)

● **V80.5** Animal-rider or occupant of animal-drawn vehicle injured in collision with other specified motor vehicle

  X ● **V80.51** Animal-rider injured in collision with other specified motor vehicle

  X ● **V80.52** Occupant of animal-drawn vehicle injured in collision with other specified motor vehicle

● **V80.6** Animal-rider or occupant of animal-drawn vehicle injured in collision with railway train or railway vehicle

  X ● **V80.61** Animal-rider injured in collision with railway train or railway vehicle

  X ● **V80.62** Occupant of animal-drawn vehicle injured in collision with railway train or railway vehicle

● **V80.7** Animal-rider or occupant of animal-drawn vehicle injured in collision with other nonmotor vehicles

  ● **V80.71** Animal-rider or occupant of animal-drawn vehicle injured in collision with animal being ridden

    ● **V80.710** Animal-rider injured in collision with other animal being ridden

    ● **V80.711** Occupant of animal-drawn vehicle injured in collision with animal being ridden

  ● **V80.72** Animal-rider or occupant of animal-drawn vehicle injured in collision with other animal-drawn vehicle

    ● **V80.720** Animal-rider injured in collision with animal-drawn vehicle

    ● **V80.721** Occupant of animal-drawn vehicle injured in collision with other animal-drawn vehicle

  ● **V80.73** Animal-rider or occupant of animal-drawn vehicle injured in collision with streetcar

    ● **V80.730** Animal-rider injured in collision with streetcar

    ● **V80.731** Occupant of animal-drawn vehicle injured in collision with streetcar

  ● **V80.79** Animal-rider or occupant of animal-drawn vehicle injured in collision with other nonmotor vehicles

    ● **V80.790** Animal-rider injured in collision with other nonmotor vehicles

    ● **V80.791** Occupant of animal-drawn vehicle injured in collision with other nonmotor vehicles

● **V80.8** Animal-rider or occupant of animal-drawn vehicle injured in collision with fixed or stationary object

  X ● **V80.81** Animal-rider injured in collision with fixed or stationary object

  X ● **V80.82** Occupant of animal-drawn vehicle injured in collision with fixed or stationary object

● **V80.9** Animal-rider or occupant of animal-drawn vehicle injured in other and unspecified transport accidents

  ● **V80.91** Animal-rider injured in other and unspecified transport accidents

    ● **V80.910** Animal-rider injured in transport accident with military vehicle

    ● **V80.918** Animal-rider injured in other transport accident

    ● **V80.919** Animal-rider injured in unspecified transport accident
      Animal rider accident NOS

● **V80.92** Occupant of animal-drawn vehicle injured in other and unspecified transport accidents

  ● **V80.920** Occupant of animal-drawn vehicle injured in transport accident with military vehicle

  ● **V80.928** Occupant of animal-drawn vehicle injured in other transport accident

  ● **V80.929** Occupant of animal-drawn vehicle injured in unspecified transport accident
    Animal-drawn vehicle accident NOS

● **V81** Occupant of railway train or railway vehicle injured in transport accident

  | **Includes** | derailment of railway train or railway vehicle |
  | | person on outside of train |

  Excludes1 streetcar (V82.-)

  The appropriate 7th character is to be added to each code from category V81

A	initial encounter
D	subsequent encounter
S	sequela

  X ● **V81.0** Occupant of railway train or railway vehicle injured in collision with motor vehicle in nontraffic accident

    Excludes1 occupant of railway train or railway vehicle injured due to collision with military vehicle (V81.83)

  X ● **V81.1** Occupant of railway train or railway vehicle injured in collision with motor vehicle in traffic accident

    Excludes1 occupant of railway train or railway vehicle injured due to collision with military vehicle (V81.83)

  X ● **V81.2** Occupant of railway train or railway vehicle injured in collision with or hit by rolling stock

  X ● **V81.3** Occupant of railway train or railway vehicle injured in collision with other object
    Railway collision NOS

  X ● **V81.4** Person injured while boarding or alighting from railway train or railway vehicle

  X ● **V81.5** Occupant of railway train or railway vehicle injured by fall in railway train or railway vehicle

  X ● **V81.6** Occupant of railway train or railway vehicle injured by fall from railway train or railway vehicle

  X ● **V81.7** Occupant of railway train or railway vehicle injured in derailment without antecedent collision

  ● **V81.8** Occupant of railway train or railway vehicle injured in other specified railway accidents

    X ● **V81.81** Occupant of railway train or railway vehicle injured due to explosion or fire on train

    X ● **V81.82** Occupant of railway train or railway vehicle injured due to object falling onto train
      Occupant of railway train or railway vehicle injured due to falling earth onto train
      Occupant of railway train or railway vehicle injured due to falling rocks onto train
      Occupant of railway train or railway vehicle injured due to falling snow onto train
      Occupant of railway train or railway vehicle injured due to falling trees onto train

    X ● **V81.83** Occupant of railway train or railway vehicle injured due to collision with military vehicle

    X ● **V81.89** Occupant of railway train or railway vehicle injured due to other specified railway accident

  X ● **V81.9** Occupant of railway train or railway vehicle injured in unspecified railway accident
    Railway accident NOS

▶ New   ⇒ Revised   ~~deleted~~ Deleted   **OGCR** Official Guidelines   X Assign placeholder X   ● Use Additional Character(s)

Excludes 1   Excludes 2   Includes   Use additional   Code first   Code also   Key words

● **V82 Occupant of powered streetcar injured in transport accident**

> **Includes**   interurban electric car
> person on outside of streetcar
> tram (car)
> trolley (car)
>
> **Excludes1**   bus (V70-V79)
> motorcoach (V70-V79)
> nonpowered streetcar (V76.-)
> train (V81.-)

The appropriate 7th character is to be added to each code from category V82

> A   initial encounter
> D   subsequent encounter
> S   sequela

X ● **V82.0 Occupant of streetcar injured in collision with motor vehicle in nontraffic accident**

X ● **V82.1 Occupant of streetcar injured in collision with motor vehicle in traffic accident**

X ● **V82.2 Occupant of streetcar injured in collision with or hit by rolling stock**

X ● **V82.3 Occupant of streetcar injured in collision with other object**

> **Excludes1**   collision with animal-drawn vehicle or animal being ridden (V82.8)

X ● **V82.4 Person injured while boarding or alighting from streetcar**

X ● **V82.5 Occupant of streetcar injured by fall in streetcar**

> **Excludes1**   fall in streetcar:
> while boarding or alighting (V82.4)
> with antecedent collision (V82.0-V82.3)

X ● **V82.6 Occupant of streetcar injured by fall from streetcar**

> **Excludes1**   fall from streetcar:
> while boarding or alighting (V82.4)
> with antecedent collision (V82.0-V82.3)

X ● **V82.7 Occupant of streetcar injured in derailment without antecedent collision**

> **Excludes1**   occupant of streetcar injured in derailment with antecedent collision (V82.0-V82.3)

X ● **V82.8 Occupant of streetcar injured in other specified transport accidents**
> Streetcar collision with military vehicle
> Streetcar collision with train or nonmotor vehicles

X ● **V82.9 Occupant of streetcar injured in unspecified traffic accident**
> Streetcar accident NOS

● **V83 Occupant of special vehicle mainly used on industrial premises injured in transport accident**

> **Includes**   battery-powered airport passenger vehicle
> battery-powered truck (baggage) (mail)
> coal-car in mine
> forklift (truck)
> logging car
> self-propelled industrial truck
> station baggage truck (powered)
> tram, truck, or tub (powered) in mine or quarry
>
> **Excludes1**   special construction vehicles (V85.-)
> special industrial vehicle in stationary use or maintenance (W31.-)

The appropriate 7th character is to be added to each code from category V83

> A   initial encounter
> D   subsequent encounter
> S   sequela

X ● **V83.0 Driver of special industrial vehicle injured in traffic accident**

X ● **V83.1 Passenger of special industrial vehicle injured in traffic accident**

X ● **V83.2 Person on outside of special industrial vehicle injured in traffic accident**

X ● **V83.3 Unspecified occupant of special industrial vehicle injured in traffic accident**

X ● **V83.4 Person injured while boarding or alighting from special industrial vehicle**

X ● **V83.5 Driver of special industrial vehicle injured in nontraffic accident**

X ● **V83.6 Passenger of special industrial vehicle injured in nontraffic accident**

X ● **V83.7 Person on outside of special industrial vehicle injured in nontraffic accident**

X ● **V83.9 Unspecified occupant of special industrial vehicle injured in nontraffic accident**
> Special-industrial-vehicle accident NOS

● **V84 Occupant of special vehicle mainly used in agriculture injured in transport accident**

> **Includes**   self-propelled farm machinery
> tractor (and trailer)
>
> **Excludes1**   animal-powered farm machinery accident (W30.8-)
> contact with combine harvester (W30.0)
> special agricultural vehicle in stationary use or maintenance (W30.-)

The appropriate 7th character is to be added to each code from category V84

> A   initial encounter
> D   subsequent encounter
> S   sequela

X ● **V84.0 Driver of special agricultural vehicle injured in traffic accident**

X ● **V84.1 Passenger of special agricultural vehicle injured in traffic accident**

X ● **V84.2 Person on outside of special agricultural vehicle injured in traffic accident**

X ● **V84.3 Unspecified occupant of special agricultural vehicle injured in traffic accident**

X ● **V84.4 Person injured while boarding or alighting from special agricultural vehicle**

X ● **V84.5 Driver of special agricultural vehicle injured in nontraffic accident**

X ● **V84.6 Passenger of special agricultural vehicle injured in nontraffic accident**

X ● **V84.7 Person on outside of special agricultural vehicle injured in nontraffic accident**

X ● **V84.9 Unspecified occupant of special agricultural vehicle injured in nontraffic accident**
> Special-agricultural vehicle accident NOS

● **V85 Occupant of special construction vehicle injured in transport accident**

> **Includes**   bulldozer
> digger
> dump truck
> earth-leveller
> mechanical shovel
> road-roller
>
> **Excludes1**   special industrial vehicle (V83.-)
> special construction vehicle in stationary use or maintenance (W31.-)

The appropriate 7th character is to be added to each code from category V85

> A   initial encounter
> D   subsequent encounter
> S   sequela

X ● **V85.0 Driver of special construction vehicle injured in traffic accident**

X ● **V85.1 Passenger of special construction vehicle injured in traffic accident**

X● **V85.2** Person on outside of special construction vehicle injured in traffic accident

X● **V85.3** Unspecified occupant of special construction vehicle injured in traffic accident

X● **V85.4** Person injured while boarding or alighting from special construction vehicle

X● **V85.5** Driver of special construction vehicle injured in nontraffic accident

X● **V85.6** Passenger of special construction vehicle injured in nontraffic accident

X● **V85.7** Person on outside of special construction vehicle injured in nontraffic accident

X● **V85.9** Unspecified occupant of special construction vehicle injured in nontraffic accident

        Special-construction-vehicle accident NOS

● **V86** Occupant of special all-terrain or other off-road motor vehicle, injured in transport accident

    Excludes1   special all-terrain vehicle in stationary use or maintenance (W31.-)

               sport-utility vehicle (V50-V59)

               three-wheeled motor vehicle designed for on-road use (V30-V39)

    The appropriate 7th character is to be added to each code from category V86

       A   initial encounter
       D   subsequent encounter
       S   sequela

● **V86.0** Driver of special all-terrain or other off-road motor vehicle injured in traffic accident

X● **V86.01** Driver of ambulance or fire engine injured in traffic accident

X● **V86.02** Driver of snowmobile injured in traffic accident

X● **V86.03** Driver of dune buggy injured in traffic accident

X● **V86.04** Driver of military vehicle injured in traffic accident

▶X● **V86.05** Driver of 3- or 4-wheeled all-terrain vehicle (ATV) injured in traffic accident

▶X● **V86.06** Driver of dirt bike or motor/cross bike injured in traffic accident

X● **V86.09** Driver of other off-road special all-terrain or other off-road vehicle injured in traffic accident

       Driver of dirt bike injured in traffic accident
       Driver of go cart injured in traffic accident
       Driver of golf cart injured in traffic accident

● **V86.1** Passenger of special all-terrain or other off-road motor vehicle injured in traffic accident

X● **V86.11** Passenger of ambulance or fire engine injured in traffic accident

X● **V86.12** Passenger of snowmobile injured in traffic accident

X● **V86.13** Passenger of dune buggy injured in traffic accident

X● **V86.14** Passenger of military vehicle injured in traffic accident

▶X● **V86.15** Passenger of 3- or 4-wheeled all-terrain vehicle (ATV) injured in traffic accident

▶X● **V86.16** Passenger of dirt bike or motor/cross bike injured in traffic accident

X● **V86.19** Passenger of other off-road special all-terrain or other off-road off-road motor vehicle injured in traffic accident

       Passenger of dirt bike injured in traffic accident
       Passenger of go cart injured in traffic accident
       Passenger of golf cart injured in traffic accident

● **V86.2** Person on outside of special all-terrain or other off-road motor vehicle injured in traffic accident

X● **V86.21** Person on outside of ambulance or fire engine injured in traffic accident

X● **V86.22** Person on outside of snowmobile injured in traffic accident

X● **V86.23** Person on outside of dune buggy injured in traffic accident

X● **V86.24** Person on outside of military vehicle injured in traffic accident

▶X● **V86.25** Person on outside of 3- or 4-wheeled all-terrain vehicle (ATV) injured in traffic accident

▶X● **V86.26** Person on outside of dirt bike or motor/cross bike injured in traffic accident

X● **V86.29** Person on outside of other special all-terrain or other off-road motor vehicle injured in traffic accident

       Person on outside of dirt bike injured in traffic accident
       Person on outside of go cart in traffic accident
       Person on outside of golf cart injured in traffic accident

● **V86.3** Unspecified occupant of special all-terrain or other off-road motor vehicle injured in traffic accident

X● **V86.31** Unspecified occupant of ambulance or fire engine injured in traffic accident

X● **V86.32** Unspecified occupant of snowmobile injured in traffic accident

X● **V86.33** Unspecified occupant of dune buggy injured in traffic accident

X● **V86.34** Unspecified occupant of military vehicle injured in traffic accident

▶X● **V86.35** Unspecified occupant of 3- or 4-wheeled all-terrain vehicle (ATV) injured in traffic accident

▶X● **V86.36** Unspecified occupant of dirt bike or motor/cross bike injured in traffic accident

X● **V86.39** Unspecified occupant of other special all-terrain or other off-road motor vehicle injured in traffic accident

       Unspecified occupant of dirt bike injured in traffic accident
       Unspecified occupant of go cart injured in traffic accident
       Unspecified occupant of golf cart injured in traffic accident

● **V86.4** Person injured while boarding or alighting from special all-terrain or other off-road motor vehicle

X● **V86.41** Person injured while boarding or alighting from ambulance or fire engine

X● **V86.42** Person injured while boarding or alighting from snowmobile

X● **V86.43** Person injured while boarding or alighting from dune buggy

X● **V86.44** Person injured while boarding or alighting from military vehicle

▶X● **V86.45** Person injured while boarding or alighting from a 3- or 4-wheeled all-terrain vehicle (ATV)

▶X● **V86.46** Person injured while boarding or alighting from a dirt bike or motor/cross bike

X● **V86.49** Person injured while boarding or alighting from other special all-terrain or other off-road motor vehicle

       Person injured while boarding or alighting from dirt bike
       Person injured while boarding or alighting from go cart
       Person injured while boarding or alighting from golf cart

▶ New   ➭ Revised   ~~deleted~~ Deleted   **OGCR** Official Guidelines   X Assign placeholder X   ● Use Additional Character(s)

Excludes 1   Excludes 2   Includes   Use additional   Code first   Code also   Key words

● **V86.5**   Driver of special all-terrain or other off-road motor vehicle injured in nontraffic accident

   X ● **V86.51**   Driver of ambulance or fire engine injured in nontraffic accident

   X ● **V86.52**   Driver of snowmobile injured in nontraffic accident

   X ● **V86.53**   Driver of dune buggy injured in nontraffic accident

   X ● **V86.54**   Driver of military vehicle injured in nontraffic accident

▶ X ● **V86.55**   Driver of 3- or 4-wheeled all-terrain vehicle (ATV) injured in nontraffic accident

▶ X ● **V86.56**   Driver of dirt bike or motor/cross bike injured in nontraffic accident

   X ● **V86.59**   Driver of other off-road special all-terrain or other off-road motor vehicle injured in nontraffic accident

      Driver of dirt bike injured in nontraffic accident

      Driver of go cart injured in nontraffic accident

      Driver of golf cart injured in nontraffic accident

● **V86.6**   Passenger of special all-terrain or other off-road motor vehicle injured in nontraffic accident

   X ● **V86.61**   Passenger of ambulance or fire engine injured in nontraffic accident

   X ● **V86.62**   Passenger of snowmobile injured in nontraffic accident

   X ● **V86.63**   Passenger of dune buggy injured in nontraffic accident

   X ● **V86.64**   Passenger of military vehicle injured in nontraffic accident

▶ X ● **V86.65**   Passenger of 3- or 4-wheeled all-terrain vehicle (ATV) injured in nontraffic accident

▶ X ● **V86.66**   Passenger of dirt bike or motor/cross bike injured in nontraffic accident

   X ● **V86.69**   Passenger of other special all-terrain or other off-road vehicle injured in nontraffic accident

      Passenger of dirt bike injured in nontraffic accident

      Passenger of go cart injured in nontraffic accident

      Passenger of golf cart injured in nontraffic accident

● **V86.7**   Person on outside of special all-terrain or other off-road motor vehicle injured in nontraffic accident

   X ● **V86.71**   Person on outside of ambulance or fire engine injured in nontraffic accident

   X ● **V86.72**   Person on outside of snowmobile injured in nontraffic accident

   X ● **V86.73**   Person on outside of dune buggy injured in nontraffic accident

   X ● **V86.74**   Person on outside of military vehicle injured in nontraffic accident

▶ X ● **V86.75**   Person on outside of 3- or 4-wheeled all-terrain vehicle (ATV) injured in nontraffic accident

▶ X ● **V86.76**   Person on outside of dirt bike or motor/cross bike injured in nontraffic accident

   X ● **V86.79**   Person on outside of other special all-terrain or other off-road motor vehicles injured in nontraffic accident

      Person on outside of dirt bike injured in nontraffic accident

      Person on outside of go cart injured in nontraffic accident

      Person on outside of golf cart injured in nontraffic accident

● **V86.9**   Unspecified occupant of special all-terrain or other off-road motor vehicle injured in nontraffic accident

   X ● **V86.91**   Unspecified occupant of ambulance or fire engine injured in nontraffic accident

   X ● **V86.92**   Unspecified occupant of snowmobile injured in nontraffic accident

   X ● **V86.93**   Unspecified occupant of dune buggy injured in nontraffic accident

   X ● **V86.94**   Unspecified occupant of military vehicle injured in nontraffic accident

▶ X ● **V86.95**   Unspecified occupant of 3- or 4-wheeled all-terrain vehicle (ATV) injured in nontraffic accident

▶ X ● **V86.96**   Unspecified occupant of dirt bike or motor/cross bike injured in nontraffic accident

   X ● **V86.99**   Unspecified occupant of other special all-terrain or other off-road motor vehicle injured in nontraffic accident

      ~~All-terrain motor-vehicle accident NOS~~

      Off-road motor-vehicle accident NOS

      Other motor-vehicle accident NOS

      ~~Unspecified occupant of dirt bike injured in nontraffic accident~~

      Unspecified occupant of go cart injured in nontraffic accident

      Unspecified occupant of golf cart injured in nontraffic accident

      Unspecified occupant of race car injured in nontraffic accident

● **V87**   Traffic accident of specified type but victim's mode of transport unknown

   Excludes1   collision involving:

      pedal cycle (V10-V19)

      pedestrian (V01-V09)

   The appropriate 7th character is to be added to each code from category V87

A	initial encounter
D	subsequent encounter
S	sequela

   X ● **V87.0**   Person injured in collision between car and two- or three-wheeled powered vehicle (traffic)

   X ● **V87.1**   Person injured in collision between other motor vehicle and two- or three-wheeled motor vehicle (traffic)

   X ● **V87.2**   Person injured in collision between car and pick-up truck or van (traffic)

   X ● **V87.3**   Person injured in collision between car and bus (traffic)

   X ● **V87.4**   Person injured in collision between car and heavy transport vehicle (traffic)

   X ● **V87.5**   Person injured in collision between heavy transport vehicle and bus (traffic)

   X ● **V87.6**   Person injured in collision between railway train or railway vehicle and car (traffic)

   X ● **V87.7**   Person injured in collision between other specified motor vehicles (traffic)

   X ● **V87.8**   Person injured in other specified noncollision transport accidents involving motor vehicle (traffic)

   X ● **V87.9**   Person injured in other specified (collision) (noncollision) transport accidents involving nonmotor vehicle (traffic)

● **V88**   Nontraffic accident of specified type but victim's mode of transport unknown

   Excludes1   collision involving:

      pedal cycle (V10-V19)

      pedestrian (V01-V09)

   The appropriate 7th character is to be added to each code from category V88

A	initial encounter
D	subsequent encounter
S	sequela

   X ● **V88.0**   Person injured in collision between car and two- or three-wheeled motor vehicle, nontraffic

   X ● **V88.1**   Person injured in collision between other motor vehicle and two- or three-wheeled motor vehicle, nontraffic

   X ● **V88.2**   Person injured in collision between car and pick-up truck or van, nontraffic

---

▶ New   ⇒ Revised   ~~deleted~~ Deleted   **OGCR** Official Guidelines   X Assign placeholder X   ● Use Additional Character(s)

Excludes 1   Excludes 2   Includes   Use additional   Code first   Code also   Key words

X⬤ **V88.3** **Person injured in collision between car and bus, nontraffic**

X⬤ **V88.4** **Person injured in collision between car and heavy transport vehicle, nontraffic**

X⬤ **V88.5** **Person injured in collision between heavy transport vehicle and bus, nontraffic**

X⬤ **V88.6** **Person injured in collision between railway train or railway vehicle and car, nontraffic**

X⬤ **V88.7** **Person injured in collision between other specified motor vehicle, nontraffic**

X⬤ **V88.8** **Person injured in other specified noncollision transport accidents involving motor vehicle, nontraffic**

X⬤ **V88.9** **Person injured in other specified (collision) (noncollision) transport accidents involving nonmotor vehicle, nontraffic**

⬤ **V89** **Motor- or nonmotor-vehicle accident, type of vehicle unspecified**

The appropriate 7th character is to be added to each code from category V89

A	initial encounter
D	subsequent encounter
S	sequela

X⬤ **V89.0** **Person injured in unspecified motor-vehicle accident, nontraffic**
Motor-vehicle accident NOS, nontraffic

X⬤ **V89.1** **Person injured in unspecified nonmotor-vehicle accident, nontraffic**
Nonmotor-vehicle accident NOS (nontraffic)

X⬤ **V89.2** **Person injured in unspecified motor-vehicle accident, traffic**
Motor-vehicle accident [MVA] NOS
Road (traffic) accident [RTA] NOS

X⬤ **V89.3** **Person injured in unspecified nonmotor-vehicle accident, traffic**
Nonmotor-vehicle traffic accident NOS

X⬤ **V89.9** **Person injured in unspecified vehicle accident**
Collision NOS

WATER TRANSPORT ACCIDENTS (V90-V94)

⬤ **V90** **Drowning and submersion due to accident to watercraft**

> **Excludes1** civilian water transport accident involving
> military watercraft (V94.81-)
> fall into water not from watercraft (W16.-)
> military watercraft accident in military or war
> operations (Y36.0-, Y37.0-)
> water-transport–related drowning or submersion
> without accident to watercraft (V92.-)

The appropriate 7th character is to be added to each code from category V90

A	initial encounter
D	subsequent encounter
S	sequela

⬤ **V90.0** **Drowning and submersion due to watercraft overturning**

X⬤ **V90.00** **Drowning and submersion due to merchant ship overturning**

X⬤ **V90.01** **Drowning and submersion due to passenger ship overturning**
Drowning and submersion due to ferry-boat overturning
Drowning and submersion due to liner overturning

X⬤ **V90.02** **Drowning and submersion due to fishing boat overturning**

X⬤ **V90.03** **Drowning and submersion due to other powered watercraft overturning**
Drowning and submersion due to hovercraft (on open water) overturning
Drowning and submersion due to jet ski overturning

X⬤ **V90.04** **Drowning and submersion due to sailboat overturning**

X⬤ **V90.05** **Drowning and submersion due to canoe or kayak overturning**

X⬤ **V90.06** **Drowning and submersion due to (nonpowered) inflatable craft overturning**

X⬤ **V90.08** **Drowning and submersion due to other unpowered watercraft overturning**
Drowning and submersion due to windsurfer overturning

X⬤ **V90.09** **Drowning and submersion due to unspecified watercraft overturning**
Drowning and submersion due to boat NOS overturning
Drowning and submersion due to ship NOS overturning
Drowning and submersion due to watercraft NOS overturning

⬤ **V90.1** **Drowning and submersion due to watercraft sinking**

X⬤ **V90.10** **Drowning and submersion due to merchant ship sinking**

X⬤ **V90.11** **Drowning and submersion due to passenger ship sinking**
Drowning and submersion due to ferry-boat sinking
Drowning and submersion due to liner sinking

X⬤ **V90.12** **Drowning and submersion due to fishing boat sinking**

X⬤ **V90.13** **Drowning and submersion due to other powered watercraft sinking**
Drowning and submersion due to hovercraft (on open water) sinking
Drowning and submersion due to jet ski sinking

X⬤ **V90.14** **Drowning and submersion due to sailboat sinking**

X⬤ **V90.15** **Drowning and submersion due to canoe or kayak sinking**

X⬤ **V90.16** **Drowning and submersion due to (nonpowered) inflatable craft sinking**

X⬤ **V90.18** **Drowning and submersion due to other unpowered watercraft sinking**

X⬤ **V90.19** **Drowning and submersion due to unspecified watercraft sinking**
Drowning and submersion due to boat NOS sinking
Drowning and submersion due to ship NOS sinking
Drowning and submersion due to watercraft NOS sinking

⬤ **V90.2** **Drowning and submersion due to falling or jumping from burning watercraft**

X⬤ **V90.20** **Drowning and submersion due to falling or jumping from burning merchant ship**

X⬤ **V90.21** **Drowning and submersion due to falling or jumping from burning passenger ship**
Drowning and submersion due to falling or jumping from burning ferry-boat
Drowning and submersion due to falling or jumping from burning liner

X⬤ **V90.22** **Drowning and submersion due to falling or jumping from burning fishing boat**

X⬤ **V90.23** **Drowning and submersion due to falling or jumping from other burning powered watercraft**
Drowning and submersion due to falling and jumping from burning hovercraft (on open water)
Drowning and submersion due to falling and jumping from burning jet ski

X⬤ **V90.24** **Drowning and submersion due to falling or jumping from burning sailboat**

▶ New   ⇒ Revised   ~~deleted~~ Deleted   **OGCR** Official Guidelines   X Assign placeholder X   ⬤ Use Additional Character(s)

| Excludes 1 | Excludes 2 | Includes | Use additional | Code first | Code also | Key words |

X● **V90.25** **Drowning and submersion due to falling or jumping from burning canoe or kayak**

X● **V90.26** **Drowning and submersion due to falling or jumping from burning (nonpowered) inflatable craft**

X● **V90.27** **Drowning and submersion due to falling or jumping from burning water-skis**

X● **V90.28** **Drowning and submersion due to falling or jumping from other burning unpowered watercraft**
     Drowning and submersion due to falling and jumping from burning surf-board
     Drowning and submersion due to falling and jumping from burning windsurfer

X● **V90.29** **Drowning and submersion due to falling or jumping from unspecified burning watercraft**
     Drowning and submersion due to falling or jumping from burning boat NOS
     Drowning and submersion due to falling or jumping from burning ship NOS
     Drowning and submersion due to falling or jumping from burning watercraft NOS

● **V90.3** **Drowning and submersion due to falling or jumping from crushed watercraft**

X● **V90.30** **Drowning and submersion due to falling or jumping from crushed merchant ship**

X● **V90.31** **Drowning and submersion due to falling or jumping from crushed passenger ship**
     Drowning and submersion due to falling and jumping from crushed ferry-boat
     Drowning and submersion due to falling and jumping from crushed liner

X● **V90.32** **Drowning and submersion due to falling or jumping from crushed fishing boat**

X● **V90.33** **Drowning and submersion due to falling or jumping from other crushed powered watercraft**
     Drowning and submersion due to falling and jumping from crushed hovercraft
     Drowning and submersion due to falling and jumping from crushed jet ski

X● **V90.34** **Drowning and submersion due to falling or jumping from crushed sailboat**

X● **V90.35** **Drowning and submersion due to falling or jumping from crushed canoe or kayak**

X● **V90.36** **Drowning and submersion due to falling or jumping from crushed (nonpowered) inflatable craft**

X● **V90.37** **Drowning and submersion due to falling or jumping from crushed water-skis**

X● **V90.38** **Drowning and submersion due to falling or jumping from other crushed unpowered watercraft**
     Drowning and submersion due to falling and jumping from crushed surf-board
     Drowning and submersion due to falling and jumping from crushed windsurfer

X● **V90.39** **Drowning and submersion due to falling or jumping from crushed unspecified watercraft**
     Drowning and submersion due to falling and jumping from crushed boat NOS
     Drowning and submersion due to falling and jumping from crushed ship NOS
     Drowning and submersion due to falling and jumping from crushed watercraft NOS

● **V90.8** **Drowning and submersion due to other accident to watercraft**

X● **V90.80** **Drowning and submersion due to other accident to merchant ship**

X● **V90.81** **Drowning and submersion due to other accident to passenger ship**
     Drowning and submersion due to other accident to ferry-boat
     Drowning and submersion due to other accident to liner

X● **V90.82** **Drowning and submersion due to other accident to fishing boat**

X● **V90.83** **Drowning and submersion due to other accident to other powered watercraft**
     Drowning and submersion due to other accident to hovercraft (on open water)
     Drowning and submersion due to other accident to jet ski

X● **V90.84** **Drowning and submersion due to other accident to sailboat**

X● **V90.85** **Drowning and submersion due to other accident to canoe or kayak**

X● **V90.86** **Drowning and submersion due to other accident to (nonpowered) inflatable craft**

X● **V90.87** **Drowning and submersion due to other accident to water-skis**

X● **V90.88** **Drowning and submersion due to other accident to other unpowered watercraft**
     Drowning and submersion due to other accident to surf-board
     Drowning and submersion due to other accident to windsurfer

X● **V90.89** **Drowning and submersion due to other accident to unspecified watercraft**
     Drowning and submersion due to other accident to boat NOS
     Drowning and submersion due to other accident to ship NOS
     Drowning and submersion due to other accident to watercraft NOS

● **V91** **Other injury due to accident to watercraft**

   Includes   any injury except drowning and submersion as a result of an accident to watercraft

   Excludes1   civilian water transport accident involving military watercraft (V94.81-)
       military watercraft accident in military or war operations (Y36, Y37.-)

   Excludes2   drowning and submersion due to accident to watercraft (V90.-)

The appropriate 7th character is to be added to each code from category V91

A	initial encounter
D	subsequent encounter
S	sequela

● **V91.0** **Burn due to watercraft on fire**

   Excludes1   burn from localized fire or explosion on board ship without accident to watercraft (V93.-)

X● **V91.00** **Burn due to merchant ship on fire**

X● **V91.01** **Burn due to passenger ship on fire**
     Burn due to ferry-boat on fire
     Burn due to liner on fire

X● **V91.02** **Burn due to fishing boat on fire**

X● **V91.03** **Burn due to other powered watercraft on fire**
     Burn due to hovercraft (on open water) on fire
     Burn due to jet ski on fire

X● **V91.04** **Burn due to sailboat on fire**

X● **V91.05** **Burn due to canoe or kayak on fire**

X● **V91.06** **Burn due to (nonpowered) inflatable craft on fire**

X● **V91.07** **Burn due to water-skis on fire**

X● **V91.08** **Burn due to other unpowered watercraft on fire**

X● **V91.09** **Burn due to unspecified watercraft on fire**
     Burn due to boat NOS on fire
     Burn due to ship NOS on fire
     Burn due to watercraft NOS on fire

CHAPTER 20 (V01-Y99)

- ● **V91.1** **Crushed between watercraft and other watercraft or other object due to collision**
  Crushed by lifeboat after abandoning ship in a collision
  Note: Select the specified type of watercraft that the victim was on at the time of the collision.
  - X● **V91.10** **Crushed between merchant ship and other watercraft or other object due to collision**
  - X● **V91.11** **Crushed between passenger ship and other watercraft or other object due to collision**
    Crushed between ferry-boat and other watercraft or other object due to collision
    Crushed between liner and other watercraft or other object due to collision
  - X● **V91.12** **Crushed between fishing boat and other watercraft or other object due to collision**
  - X● **V91.13** **Crushed between other powered watercraft and other watercraft or other object due to collision**
    Crushed between hovercraft (on open water) and other watercraft or other object due to collision
    Crushed between jet ski and other watercraft or other object due to collision
  - X● **V91.14** **Crushed between sailboat and other watercraft or other object due to collision**
  - X● **V91.15** **Crushed between canoe or kayak and other watercraft or other object due to collision**
  - X● **V91.16** **Crushed between (nonpowered) inflatable craft and other watercraft or other object due to collision**
  - X● **V91.18** **Crushed between other unpowered watercraft and other watercraft or other object due to collision**
    Crushed between surfboard and other watercraft or other object due to collision
    Crushed between windsurfer and other watercraft or other object due to collision
  - X● **V91.19** **Crushed between unspecified watercraft and other watercraft or other object due to collision**
    Crushed between boat NOS and other watercraft or other object due to collision
    Crushed between ship NOS and other watercraft or other object due to collision
    Crushed between watercraft NOS and other watercraft or other object due to collision
- ● **V91.2** **Fall due to collision between watercraft and other watercraft or other object**
  Fall while remaining on watercraft after collision
  Note: Select the specified type of watercraft that the victim was on at the time of the collision.
  Excludes1 crushed between watercraft and other watercraft and other object due to collision (V91.1-)
  drowning and submersion due to falling from crushed watercraft (V90.3-)
  - X● **V91.20** **Fall due to collision between merchant ship and other watercraft or other object**
  - X● **V91.21** **Fall due to collision between passenger ship and other watercraft or other object**
    Fall due to collision between ferry-boat and other watercraft or other object
    Fall due to collision between liner and other watercraft or other object
  - X● **V91.22** **Fall due to collision between fishing boat and other watercraft or other object**
  - X● **V91.23** **Fall due to collision between other powered watercraft and other watercraft or other object**
    Fall due to collision between hovercraft (on open water) and other watercraft or other object
    Fall due to collision between jet ski and other watercraft or other object

- X● **V91.24** **Fall due to collision between sailboat and other watercraft or other object**
- X● **V91.25** **Fall due to collision between canoe or kayak and other watercraft or other object**
- X● **V91.26** **Fall due to collision between (nonpowered) inflatable craft and other watercraft or other object**
- X● **V91.29** **Fall due to collision between unspecified watercraft and other watercraft or other object**
  Fall due to collision between boat NOS and other watercraft or other object
  Fall due to collision between ship NOS and other watercraft or other object
  Fall due to collision between watercraft NOS and other watercraft or other object
- ● **V91.3** **Hit or struck by falling object due to accident to watercraft**
  Hit or struck by falling object (part of damaged watercraft or other object) after falling or jumping from damaged watercraft
  Excludes2 drowning or submersion due to fall or jumping from damaged watercraft (V90.2-, V90.3-)
  - X● **V91.30** **Hit or struck by falling object due to accident to merchant ship**
  - X● **V91.31** **Hit or struck by falling object due to accident to passenger ship**
    Hit or struck by falling object due to accident to ferry-boat
    Hit or struck by falling object due to accident to liner
  - X● **V91.32** **Hit or struck by falling object due to accident to fishing boat**
  - X● **V91.33** **Hit or struck by falling object due to accident to other powered watercraft**
    Hit or struck by falling object due to accident to hovercraft (on open water)
    Hit or struck by falling object due to accident to jet ski
  - X● **V91.34** **Hit or struck by falling object due to accident to sailboat**
  - X● **V91.35** **Hit or struck by falling object due to accident to canoe or kayak**
  - X● **V91.36** **Hit or struck by falling object due to accident to (nonpowered) inflatable craft**
  - X● **V91.37** **Hit or struck by falling object due to accident to water-skis**
    Hit by water-skis after jumping off of waterskis
  - X● **V91.38** **Hit or struck by falling object due to accident to other unpowered watercraft**
    Hit or struck by surf-board after falling off damaged surf-board
    Hit or struck by object after falling off damaged windsurfer
  - X● **V91.39** **Hit or struck by falling object due to accident to unspecified watercraft**
    Hit or struck by falling object due to accident to boat NOS
    Hit or struck by falling object due to accident to ship NOS
    Hit or struck by falling object due to accident to watercraft NOS

▶ New   ⇒ Revised   ~~deleted~~ Deleted   **OGCR** Official Guidelines   X Assign placeholder X   ● Use Additional Character(s)
Excludes 1   Excludes 2   Includes   Use additional   Code first   Code also   Key words

● V91.8　Other injury due to other accident to watercraft
　X● V91.80　Other injury due to other accident to merchant ship
　X● V91.81　Other injury due to other accident to passenger ship
　　　　　Other injury due to other accident to ferry-boat
　　　　　Other injury due to other accident to liner
　X● V91.82　Other injury due to other accident to fishing boat
　X● V91.83　Other injury due to other accident to other powered watercraft
　　　　　Other injury due to other accident to hovercraft (on open water)
　　　　　Other injury due to other accident to jet ski
　X● V91.84　Other injury due to other accident to sailboat
　X● V91.85　Other injury due to other accident to canoe or kayak
　X● V91.86　Other injury due to other accident to (nonpowered) inflatable craft
　X● V91.87　Other injury due to other accident to water-skis
　X● V91.88　Other injury due to other accident to other unpowered watercraft
　　　　　Other injury due to other accident to surf-board
　　　　　Other injury due to other accident to windsurfer
　X● V91.89　Other injury due to other accident to unspecified watercraft
　　　　　Other injury due to other accident to boat NOS
　　　　　Other injury due to other accident to ship NOS
　　　　　Other injury due to other accident to watercraft NOS

● V92　Drowning and submersion due to accident on board watercraft, without accident to watercraft

> **Excludes1**　civilian water transport accident involving military watercraft (V94.81-)
> drowning or submersion due to accident to watercraft (V90-V91)
> drowning or submersion of diver who voluntarily jumps from boat not involved in an accident (W16.711, W16.721)
> fall into water without watercraft (W16.-)
> military watercraft accident in military or war operations (Y36, Y37)

The appropriate 7th character is to be added to each code from category V92

> A　initial encounter
> D　subsequent encounter
> S　sequela

● V92.0　Drowning and submersion due to fall off watercraft
　　　　Drowning and submersion due to fall from gangplank of watercraft
　　　　Drowning and submersion due to fall overboard watercraft

> **Excludes2**　hitting head on object or bottom of body of water due to fall from watercraft (V94.0-)

　X● V92.00　Drowning and submersion due to fall off merchant ship
　X● V92.01　Drowning and submersion due to fall off passenger ship
　　　　　Drowning and submersion due to fall off ferry-boat
　　　　　Drowning and submersion due to fall off liner
　X● V92.02　Drowning and submersion due to fall off fishing boat

　X● V92.03　Drowning and submersion due to fall off other powered watercraft
　　　　　Drowning and submersion due to fall off hovercraft (on open water)
　　　　　Drowning and submersion due to fall off jet ski
　X● V92.04　Drowning and submersion due to fall off sailboat
　X● V92.05　Drowning and submersion due to fall off canoe or kayak
　X● V92.06　Drowning and submersion due to fall off (nonpowered) inflatable craft
　X● V92.07　Drowning and submersion due to fall off water-skis

> **Excludes1**　drowning and submersion due to falling off burning water-skis (V90.27)
> drowning and submersion due to falling off crushed water-skis (V90.37)
> hit by boat while water-skiing NOS (V94.X)

　X● V92.08　Drowning and submersion due to fall off other unpowered watercraft
　　　　　Drowning and submersion due to fall off surf-board
　　　　　Drowning and submersion due to fall off windsurfer

> **Excludes1**　drowning and submersion due to fall off burning unpowered watercraft (V90.28)
> drowning and submersion due to fall off crushed unpowered watercraft (V90.38)
> drowning and submersion due to fall off damaged unpowered watercraft (V90.88)
> drowning and submersion due to rider of nonpowered watercraft being hit by other watercraft (V94.-)
> other injury due to rider of nonpowered watercraft being hit by other watercraft (V94.-)

　X● V92.09　Drowning and submersion due to fall off unspecified watercraft
　　　　　Drowning and submersion due to fall off boat NOS
　　　　　Drowning and submersion due to fall off ship
　　　　　Drowning and submersion due to fall off watercraft NOS

● V92.1　Drowning and submersion due to being thrown overboard by motion of watercraft

> **Excludes1**　drowning and submersion due to fall off surf-board (V92.08)
> drowning and submersion due to fall off water-skis (V92.07)
> drowning and submersion due to fall off windsurfer (V92.08)

　X● V92.10　Drowning and submersion due to being thrown overboard by motion of merchant ship
　X● V92.11　Drowning and submersion due to being thrown overboard by motion of passenger ship
　　　　　Drowning and submersion due to being thrown overboard by motion of ferry-boat
　　　　　Drowning and submersion due to being thrown overboard by motion of liner

CHAPTER 20 (V01-Y99)

▶ New　⇒ Revised　d̶e̶l̶e̶t̶e̶d̶ Deleted　**OGCR** Official Guidelines　X Assign placeholder X　● Use Additional Character(s)

Excludes 1　Excludes 2　Includes　Use additional　Code first　Code also　Key words

1445

CHAPTER 20 (V01–Y99)

X● **V92.12** **Drowning and submersion due to being thrown overboard by motion of fishing boat**

X● **V92.13** **Drowning and submersion due to being thrown overboard by motion of other powered watercraft**
> Drowning and submersion due to being thrown overboard by motion of hovercraft

X● **V92.14** **Drowning and submersion due to being thrown overboard by motion of sailboat**

X● **V92.15** **Drowning and submersion due to being thrown overboard by motion of canoe or kayak**

X● **V92.16** **Drowning and submersion due to being thrown overboard by motion of (nonpowered) inflatable craft**

X● **V92.19** **Drowning and submersion due to being thrown overboard by motion of unspecified watercraft**
> Drowning and submersion due to being thrown overboard by motion of boat NOS
> Drowning and submersion due to being thrown overboard by motion of ship NOS
> Drowning and submersion due to being thrown overboard by motion of watercraft NOS

● **V92.2** **Drowning and submersion due to being washed overboard from watercraft**
> *Code first any associated cataclysm (X37.0-)*

X● **V92.20** **Drowning and submersion due to being washed overboard from merchant ship**

X● **V92.21** **Drowning and submersion due to being washed overboard from passenger ship**
> Drowning and submersion due to being washed overboard from ferry-boat
> Drowning and submersion due to being washed overboard from liner

X● **V92.22** **Drowning and submersion due to being washed overboard from fishing boat**

X● **V92.23** **Drowning and submersion due to being washed overboard from other powered watercraft**
> Drowning and submersion due to being washed overboard from hovercraft (on open water)
> Drowning and submersion due to being washed overboard from jet ski

X● **V92.24** **Drowning and submersion due to being washed overboard from sailboat**

X● **V92.25** **Drowning and submersion due to being washed overboard from canoe or kayak**

X● **V92.26** **Drowning and submersion due to being washed overboard from (nonpowered) inflatable craft**

X● **V92.27** **Drowning and submersion due to being washed overboard from water-skis**
> **Excludes1**   drowning and submersion due to fall off water-skis (V92.07)

X● **V92.28** **Drowning and submersion due to being washed overboard from other unpowered watercraft**
> Drowning and submersion due to being washed overboard from surf-board
> Drowning and submersion due to being washed overboard from windsurfer

X● **V92.29** **Drowning and submersion due to being washed overboard from unspecified watercraft**
> Drowning and submersion due to being washed overboard from boat NOS
> Drowning and submersion due to being washed overboard from ship NOS
> Drowning and submersion due to being washed overboard from watercraft NOS

● **V93** **Other injury due to accident on board watercraft, without accident to watercraft**
> **Excludes1**   civilian water transport accident involving military watercraft (V94.81-)
> other injury due to accident to watercraft (V91.-)
> military watercraft accident in military or war operations (Y36, Y37.-)
> **Excludes2**   drowning and submersion due to accident on board watercraft, without accident to watercraft (V92.-)

The appropriate 7th character is to be added to each code from category V93

> A   initial encounter
> D   subsequent encounter
> S   sequela

● **V93.0** **Burn due to localized fire on board watercraft**
> **Excludes1**   burn due to watercraft on fire (V91.0-)

X● **V93.00** **Burn due to localized fire on board merchant vessel**

X● **V93.01** **Burn due to localized fire on board passenger vessel**
> Burn due to localized fire on board ferry-boat
> Burn due to localized fire on board liner

X● **V93.02** **Burn due to localized fire on board fishing boat**

X● **V93.03** **Burn due to localized fire on board other powered watercraft**
> Burn due to localized fire on board hovercraft
> Burn due to localized fire on board jet ski

X● **V93.04** **Burn due to localized fire on board sailboat**

X● **V93.09** **Burn due to localized fire on board unspecified watercraft**
> Burn due to localized fire on board boat NOS
> Burn due to localized fire on board ship NOS
> Burn due to localized fire on board watercraft NOS

● **V93.1** **Other burn on board watercraft**
> Burn due to source other than fire on board watercraft
> **Excludes1**   burn due to watercraft on fire (V91.0-)

X● **V93.10** **Other burn on board merchant vessel**

X● **V93.11** **Other burn on board passenger vessel**
> Other burn on board ferry-boat
> Other burn on board liner

X● **V93.12** **Other burn on board fishing boat**

X● **V93.13** **Other burn on board other powered watercraft**
> Other burn on board hovercraft
> Other burn on board jet ski

X● **V93.14** **Other burn on board sailboat**

X● **V93.19** **Other burn on board unspecified watercraft**
> Other burn on board boat NOS
> Other burn on board ship NOS
> Other burn on board watercraft NOS

● **V93.2** **Heat exposure on board watercraft**
> **Excludes1**   exposure to man-made heat not aboard watercraft (W92)
> exposure to natural heat while on board watercraft (X30)
> exposure to sunlight while on board watercraft (X32)
> **Excludes2**   burn due to fire on board watercraft (V93.0-)

X● **V93.20** **Heat exposure on board merchant ship**

X● **V93.21** **Heat exposure on board passenger ship**
> Heat exposure on board ferry-boat
> Heat exposure on board liner

X● **V93.22** **Heat exposure on board fishing boat**

X● **V93.23** **Heat exposure on board other powered watercraft**
> Heat exposure on board hovercraft

X● **V93.24** **Heat exposure on board sailboat**

X● **V93.29** **Heat exposure on board unspecified watercraft**
> Heat exposure on board boat NOS
> Heat exposure on board ship NOS
> Heat exposure on board watercraft NOS

▶ New   ⇒ Revised   ~~deleted~~ Deleted   **OGCR** Official Guidelines   X Assign placeholder X   ● Use Additional Character(s)

Excludes 1   Excludes 2   Includes   Use additional   Code first   Code also   Key words

● V93.3   **Fall on board watercraft**

    Excludes1   fall due to collision of watercraft (V91.2-)

X ● V93.30   **Fall on board merchant ship**

X ● V93.31   **Fall on board passenger ship**
     Fall on board ferry-boat
     Fall on board liner

X ● V93.32   **Fall on board fishing boat**

X ● V93.33   **Fall on board other powered watercraft**
     Fall on board hovercraft (on open water)
     Fall on board jet ski

X ● V93.34   **Fall on board sailboat**

X ● V93.35   **Fall on board canoe or kayak**

X ● V93.36   **Fall on board (nonpowered) inflatable craft**

X ● V93.38   **Fall on board other unpowered watercraft**

X ● V93.39   **Fall on board unspecified watercraft**
     Fall on board boat NOS
     Fall on board ship NOS
     Fall on board watercraft NOS

● V93.4   **Struck by falling object on board watercraft**
     Hit by falling object on board watercraft

    Excludes1   struck by falling object due to accident to watercraft (V91.3)

X ● V93.40   **Struck by falling object on merchant ship**

X ● V93.41   **Struck by falling object on passenger ship**
     Struck by falling object on ferry-boat
     Struck by falling object on liner

X ● V93.42   **Struck by falling object on fishing boat**

X ● V93.43   **Struck by falling object on other powered watercraft**
     Struck by falling object on hovercraft

X ● V93.44   **Struck by falling object on sailboat**

X ● V93.48   **Struck by falling object on other unpowered watercraft**

X ● V93.49   **Struck by falling object on unspecified watercraft**

● V93.5   **Explosion on board watercraft**
     Boiler explosion on steamship

    Excludes2   fire on board watercraft (V93.0-)

X ● V93.50   **Explosion on board merchant ship**

X ● V93.51   **Explosion on board passenger ship**
     Explosion on board ferry-boat
     Explosion on board liner

X ● V93.52   **Explosion on board fishing boat**

X ● V93.53   **Explosion on board other powered watercraft**
     Explosion on board hovercraft
     Explosion on board jet ski

X ● V93.54   **Explosion on board sailboat**

X ● V93.59   **Explosion on board unspecified watercraft**
     Explosion on board boat NOS
     Explosion on board ship NOS
     Explosion on board watercraft NOS

● V93.6   **Machinery accident on board watercraft**

    Excludes1   machinery explosion on board watercraft (V93.4-)
              machinery fire on board watercraft (V93.0-)

X ● V93.60   **Machinery accident on board merchant ship**

X ● V93.61   **Machinery accident on board passenger ship**
     Machinery accident on board ferry-boat
     Machinery accident on board liner

X ● V93.62   **Machinery accident on board fishing boat**

X ● V93.63   **Machinery accident on board other powered watercraft**
     Machinery accident on board hovercraft

X ● V93.64   **Machinery accident on board sailboat**

X ● V93.69   **Machinery accident on board unspecified watercraft**
     Machinery accident on board boat NOS
     Machinery accident on board ship NOS
     Machinery accident on board watercraft NOS

● V93.8   **Other injury due to other accident on board watercraft**
     Accidental poisoning by gases or fumes on watercraft

X ● V93.80   **Other injury due to other accident on board merchant ship**

X ● V93.81   **Other injury due to other accident on board passenger ship**
     Other injury due to other accident on board ferry-boat
     Other injury due to other accident on board liner

X ● V93.82   **Other injury due to other accident on board fishing boat**

X ● V93.83   **Other injury due to other accident on board other powered watercraft**
     Other injury due to other accident on board hovercraft
     Other injury due to other accident on board jet ski

X ● V93.84   **Other injury due to other accident on board sailboat**

X ● V93.85   **Other injury due to other accident on board canoe or kayak**

X ● V93.86   **Other injury due to other accident on board (nonpowered) inflatable craft**

X ● V93.87   **Other injury due to other accident on board water-skis**
     Hit or struck by object while waterskiing

X ● V93.88   **Other injury due to other accident on board other unpowered watercraft**
     Hit or struck by object while surfing
     Hit or struck by object while on board windsurfer

X ● V93.89   **Other injury due to other accident on board unspecified watercraft**
     Other injury due to other accident on board boat NOS
     Other injury due to other accident on board ship NOS
     Other injury due to other accident on board watercraft NOS

● V94   **Other and unspecified water transport accidents**

    Excludes1   military watercraft accidents in military or war operations (Y36, Y37)

    The appropriate 7th character is to be added to each code from category V94

A	initial encounter
D	subsequent encounter
S	sequela

X ● V94.0   **Hitting object or bottom of body of water due to fall from watercraft**

    Excludes2   drowning and submersion due to fall from watercraft (V92.0-)

● V94.1   **Bather struck by watercraft**
     Swimmer hit by watercraft

X ● V94.11   **Bather struck by powered watercraft**

X ● V94.12   **Bather struck by nonpowered watercraft**

● V94.2   **Rider of nonpowered watercraft struck by other watercraft**

X ● V94.21   **Rider of nonpowered watercraft struck by other nonpowered watercraft**
     Canoer hit by other nonpowered watercraft
     Surfer hit by other nonpowered watercraft
     Windsurfer hit by other nonpowered watercraft

X ● V94.22   **Rider of nonpowered watercraft struck by powered watercraft**
     Canoer hit by motorboat
     Surfer hit by motorboat
     Windsurfer hit by motorboat

CHAPTER 20 (V01-Y99)

CHAPTER 20 (V01-Y99)

● **V94.3** Injury to rider of (inflatable) watercraft being pulled behind other watercraft

    X ● **V94.31** Injury to rider of (inflatable) recreational watercraft being pulled behind other watercraft
        Injury to rider of inner-tube pulled behind motor boat

    X ● **V94.32** Injury to rider of non-recreational watercraft being pulled behind other watercraft
        Injury to occupant of dingy being pulled behind boat or ship
        Injury to occupant of life-raft being pulled behind boat or ship

  X ● **V94.4** Injury to barefoot water-skier
        Injury to person being pulled behind boat or ship

  ● **V94.8** Other water transport accident

    ● **V94.81** Water transport accident involving military watercraft

      ● **V94.810** Civilian watercraft involved in water transport accident with military watercraft
        Passenger on civilian watercraft injured due to accident with military watercraft

      ● **V94.811** Civilian in water injured by military watercraft

      ● **V94.818** Other water transport accident involving military watercraft

    X ● **V94.89** Other water transport accident

  X ● **V94.9** Unspecified water transport accident
    Water transport accident NOS

AIR AND SPACE TRANSPORT ACCIDENTS (V95-V97)

> **Excludes1** military aircraft accidents in military or war operations (Y36, Y37)

● **V95** Accident to powered aircraft causing injury to occupant
    The appropriate 7th character is to be added to each code from category V95

> A   initial encounter
> D   subsequent encounter
> S   sequela

  ● **V95.0** Helicopter accident injuring occupant

    X ● **V95.00** Unspecified helicopter accident injuring occupant

    X ● **V95.01** Helicopter crash injuring occupant

    X ● **V95.02** Forced landing of helicopter injuring occupant

    X ● **V95.03** Helicopter collision injuring occupant
        Helicopter collision with any object, fixed, movable or moving

    X ● **V95.04** Helicopter fire injuring occupant

    X ● **V95.05** Helicopter explosion injuring occupant

    X ● **V95.09** Other helicopter accident injuring occupant

  ● **V95.1** Ultralight, microlight or powered-glider accident injuring occupant

    X ● **V95.10** Unspecified ultralight, microlight or powered-glider accident injuring occupant

    X ● **V95.11** Ultralight, microlight or powered-glider crash injuring occupant

    X ● **V95.12** Forced landing of ultralight, microlight or powered-glider injuring occupant

    X ● **V95.13** Ultralight, microlight or powered-glider collision injuring occupant
        Ultralight, microlight or powered-glider collision with any object, fixed, movable or moving

    X ● **V95.14** Ultralight, microlight or powered-glider fire injuring occupant

    X ● **V95.15** Ultralight, microlight or powered-glider explosion injuring occupant

    X ● **V95.19** Other ultralight, microlight or powered-glider accident injuring occupant

  ● **V95.2** Other private fixed-wing aircraft accident injuring occupant

    X ● **V95.20** Unspecified accident to other private fixed-wing aircraft, injuring occupant

    X ● **V95.21** Other private fixed-wing aircraft crash injuring occupant

    X ● **V95.22** Forced landing of other private fixed-wing aircraft injuring occupant

    X ● **V95.23** Other private fixed-wing aircraft collision injuring occupant
        Other private fixed-wing aircraft collision with any object, fixed, movable or moving

    X ● **V95.24** Other private fixed-wing aircraft fire injuring occupant

    X ● **V95.25** Other private fixed-wing aircraft explosion injuring occupant

    X ● **V95.29** Other accident to other private fixed-wing aircraft injuring occupant

  ● **V95.3** Commercial fixed-wing aircraft accident injuring occupant

    X ● **V95.30** Unspecified accident to commercial fixed-wing aircraft injuring occupant

    X ● **V95.31** Commercial fixed-wing aircraft crash injuring occupant

    X ● **V95.32** Forced landing of commercial fixed-wing aircraft injuring occupant

    X ● **V95.33** Commercial fixed-wing aircraft collision injuring occupant
        Commercial fixed-wing aircraft collision with any object, fixed, movable or moving

    X ● **V95.34** Commercial fixed-wing aircraft fire injuring occupant

    X ● **V95.35** Commercial fixed-wing aircraft explosion injuring occupant

    X ● **V95.39** Other accident to commercial fixed-wing aircraft injuring occupant

  ● **V95.4** Spacecraft accident injuring occupant

    X ● **V95.40** Unspecified spacecraft accident injuring occupant

    X ● **V95.41** Spacecraft crash injuring occupant

    X ● **V95.42** Forced landing of spacecraft injuring occupant

    X ● **V95.43** Spacecraft collision injuring occupant
        Spacecraft collision with any object, fixed, moveable or moving

    X ● **V95.44** Spacecraft fire injuring occupant

    X ● **V95.45** Spacecraft explosion injuring occupant

    X ● **V95.49** Other spacecraft accident injuring occupant

  X ● **V95.8** Other powered aircraft accidents injuring occupant

  X ● **V95.9** Unspecified aircraft accident injuring occupant
    Aircraft accident NOS
    Air transport accident NOS

▶ New   ⇒ Revised   ~~deleted~~ Deleted   **OGCR** Official Guidelines   X Assign placeholder X   ● Use Additional Character(s)

Excludes 1   Excludes 2   Includes   Use additional   Code first   Code also   Key words

● **V96**   **Accident to nonpowered aircraft causing injury to occupant**

The appropriate 7th character is to be added to each code from category V96

> A   initial encounter
> D   subsequent encounter
> S   sequela

● **V96.0**   **Balloon accident injuring occupant**

   X ● **V96.00**   **Unspecified balloon accident injuring occupant**

   X ● **V96.01**   **Balloon crash injuring occupant**

   X ● **V96.02**   **Forced landing of balloon injuring occupant**

   X ● **V96.03**   **Balloon collision injuring occupant**
       Balloon collision with any object, fixed, moveable or moving

   X ● **V96.04**   **Balloon fire injuring occupant**

   X ● **V96.05**   **Balloon explosion injuring occupant**

   X ● **V96.09**   **Other balloon accident injuring occupant**

● **V96.1**   **Hang-glider accident injuring occupant**

   X ● **V96.10**   **Unspecified hang-glider accident injuring occupant**

   X ● **V96.11**   **Hang-glider crash injuring occupant**

   X ● **V96.12**   **Forced landing of hang-glider injuring occupant**

   X ● **V96.13**   **Hang-glider collision injuring occupant**
       Hang-glider collision with any object, fixed, moveable or moving

   X ● **V96.14**   **Hang-glider fire injuring occupant**

   X ● **V96.15**   **Hang-glider explosion injuring occupant**

   X ● **V96.19**   **Other hang-glider accident injuring occupant**

● **V96.2**   **Glider (nonpowered) accident injuring occupant**

   X ● **V96.20**   **Unspecified glider (nonpowered) accident injuring occupant**

   X ● **V96.21**   **Glider (nonpowered) crash injuring occupant**

   X ● **V96.22**   **Forced landing of glider (nonpowered) injuring occupant**

   X ● **V96.23**   **Glider (nonpowered) collision injuring occupant**
       Glider (nonpowered) collision with any object, fixed, moveable or moving

   X ● **V96.24**   **Glider (nonpowered) fire injuring occupant**

   X ● **V96.25**   **Glider (nonpowered) explosion injuring occupant**

   X ● **V96.29**   **Other glider (nonpowered) accident injuring occupant**

X ● **V96.8**   **Other nonpowered-aircraft accidents injuring occupant**
       Kite carrying a person accident injuring occupant

X ● **V96.9**   **Unspecified nonpowered-aircraft accident injuring occupant**
       Nonpowered-aircraft accident NOS

● **V97**   **Other specified air transport accidents**

The appropriate 7th character is to be added to each code from category V97

> A   initial encounter
> D   subsequent encounter
> S   sequela

X ● **V97.0**   **Occupant of aircraft injured in other specified air transport accidents**
       Fall in, on or from aircraft in air transport accident

   Excludes1   accident while boarding or alighting aircraft (V97.1)

X ● **V97.1**   **Person injured while boarding or alighting from aircraft**

● **V97.2**   **Parachutist accident**

   X ● **V97.21**   **Parachutist entangled in object**
       Parachutist landing in tree

   X ● **V97.22**   **Parachutist injured on landing**

   X ● **V97.29**   **Other parachutist accident**

● **V97.3**   **Person on ground injured in air transport accident**

   X ● **V97.31**   **Hit by object falling from aircraft**
       Hit by crashing aircraft
       Injured by aircraft hitting house
       Injured by aircraft hitting car

   X ● **V97.32**   **Injured by rotating propeller**

   X ● **V97.33**   **Sucked into jet engine**

   X ● **V97.39**   **Other injury to person on ground due to air transport accident**

● **V97.8**   **Other air transport accidents, not elsewhere classified**

   Excludes1   aircraft accident NOS (V95.9)
       exposure to changes in air pressure during ascent or descent (W94.-)

   ● **V97.81**   **Air transport accident involving military aircraft**

     ● **V97.810**   **Civilian aircraft involved in air transport accident with military aircraft**
       Passenger in civilian aircraft injured due to accident with military aircraft

     ● **V97.811**   **Civilian injured by military aircraft**

     ● **V97.818**   **Other air transport accident involving military aircraft**

   X ● **V97.89**   **Other air transport accidents, not elsewhere classified**
       Injury from machinery on aircraft

OTHER AND UNSPECIFIED TRANSPORT ACCIDENTS (V98-V99)

Excludes1   vehicle accident, type of vehicle unspecified (V89.-)

● **V98**   **Other specified transport accidents**

The appropriate 7th character is to be added to each code from category V98

> A   initial encounter
> D   subsequent encounter
> S   sequela

X ● **V98.0**   **Accident to, on or involving cable-car, not on rails**
       Caught or dragged by cable-car, not on rails
       Fall or jump from cable-car, not on rails
       Object thrown from or in cable-car, not on rails

X ● **V98.1**   **Accident to, on or involving land-yacht**

X ● **V98.2**   **Accident to, on or involving ice yacht**

X ● **V98.3**   **Accident to, on or involving ski lift**
       Accident to, on or involving ski chair-lift
       Accident to, on or involving ski-lift with gondola

X ● **V98.8**   **Other specified transport accidents**

X ● **V99**   **Unspecified transport accident**

The appropriate 7th character is to be added to code V99

> A   initial encounter
> D   subsequent encounter
> S   sequela

CHAPTER 20 (V01-Y99)

OTHER EXTERNAL CAUSES OF ACCIDENTAL INJURY (W00-X58)

SLIPPING, TRIPPING, STUMBLING AND FALLS (W00-W19)

Excludes1	assault involving a fall (Y01-Y02)
	fall from animal (V80.-)
	fall (in) (from) machinery (in operation) (W28-W31)
	fall (in) (from) transport vehicle (V01-V99)
	intentional self-harm involving a fall (X80-X81)

Excludes2	at risk for fall (history of fall) Z91.81
	fall (in) (from) burning building (X00.-)
⇨	fall into fire (X00-X04, X08)

● **W00   Fall due to ice and snow**

Includes	pedestrian on foot falling (slipping) on ice and snow

Excludes1	fall on (from) ice and snow involving pedestrian conveyance (V00.-)
	fall from stairs and steps not due to ice and snow (W10.-)

The appropriate 7th character is to be added to each code from category W00

A	initial encounter
D	subsequent encounter
S	sequela

X● **W00.0   Fall on same level due to ice and snow**
X● **W00.1   Fall from stairs and steps due to ice and snow**
X● **W00.2   Other fall from one level to another due to ice and snow**
X● **W00.9   Unspecified fall due to ice and snow**

● **W01   Fall on same level from slipping, tripping and stumbling**

Includes	fall on moving sidewalk

Excludes1	fall due to bumping (striking) against object (W18.0-)
	fall in shower or bathtub (W18.2-)
	fall on same level NOS (W18.30)
	fall on same level from slipping, tripping and stumbling due to ice or snow (W00.0)
	fall off or from toilet (W18.1-)
	slipping, tripping and stumbling NOS (W18.40)
	slipping, tripping and stumbling without falling (W18.4-)

The appropriate 7th character is to be added to each code from category W01

A	initial encounter
D	subsequent encounter
S	sequela

X● **W01.0   Fall on same level from slipping, tripping and stumbling without subsequent striking against object**
           Falling over animal
● **W01.1   Fall on same level from slipping, tripping and stumbling with subsequent striking against object**
   X● **W01.10   Fall on same level from slipping, tripping and stumbling with subsequent striking against unspecified object**
   ● **W01.11   Fall on same level from slipping, tripping and stumbling with subsequent striking against sharp object**
       ● **W01.110   Fall on same level from slipping, tripping and stumbling with subsequent striking against sharp glass**
       ● **W01.111   Fall on same level from slipping, tripping and stumbling with subsequent striking against power tool or machine**

   ● **W01.118   Fall on same level from slipping, tripping and stumbling with subsequent striking against other sharp object**
   ● **W01.119   Fall on same level from slipping, tripping and stumbling with subsequent striking against unspecified sharp object**
  ● **W01.19   Fall on same level from slipping, tripping and stumbling with subsequent striking against other object**
   ● **W01.190   Fall on same level from slipping, tripping and stumbling with subsequent striking against furniture**
   ● **W01.198   Fall on same level from slipping, tripping and stumbling with subsequent striking against other object**

X● **W03   Other fall on same level due to collision with another person**
        Fall due to non-transport collision with other person

Excludes1	collision with another person without fall (W51)
	crushed or pushed by a crowd or human stampede (W52)
	fall involving pedestrian conveyance (V00-V09)
	fall due to ice or snow (W00)
	fall on same level NOS (W18.30)

The appropriate 7th character is to be added to code W03

A	initial encounter
D	subsequent encounter
S	sequela

X● **W04   Fall while being carried or supported by other persons**
        Accidentally dropped while being carried

The appropriate 7th character is to be added to code W04

A	initial encounter
D	subsequent encounter
S	sequel

● **W05   Fall from non-moving wheelchair, nonmotorized scooter and motorized mobility scooter**

Excludes1	fall from moving wheelchair (powered) (V00.811)
	fall from moving motorized mobility scooter (V00.831)
	fall from nonmotorized scooter (V00.141)

The appropriate 7th character is to be added to each code from category W05

A	initial encounter
D	subsequent encounter
S	sequela

X● **W05.0   Fall from non-moving wheelchair**
X● **W05.1   Fall from non-moving nonmotorized scooter**
X● **W05.2   Fall from non-moving motorized mobility scooter**

X● **W06   Fall from bed**
The appropriate 7th character is to be added to code W06

A	initial encounter
D	subsequent encounter
S	sequela

X● **W07   Fall from chair**
The appropriate 7th character is to be added to code W07

A	initial encounter
D	subsequent encounter
S	sequela

▶ New   ⇨ Revised   ~~deleted~~ Deleted   **OGCR** Official Guidelines   X Assign placeholder X   ● Use Additional Character(s)

Excludes 1   Excludes 2   Includes   Use additional   Code first   Code also   Key words

X● **W08　Fall from other furniture**

>　　The appropriate 7th character is to be added to code W08

>| A | initial encounter |
>|---|---|
>| D | subsequent encounter |
>| S | sequela |

● **W09　Fall on and from playground equipment**

>| **Excludes1** | fall involving recreational machinery (W31) |
>|---|---|

>　　The appropriate 7th character is to be added to each code from category W09

>| A | initial encounter |
>|---|---|
>| D | subsequent encounter |
>| S | sequela |

X● **W09.0　Fall on or from playground slide**

X● **W09.1　Fall from playground swing**

X● **W09.2　Fall on or from jungle gym**

X● **W09.8　Fall on or from other playground equipment**

● **W10　Fall on and from stairs and steps**

>| **Excludes1** | fall from stairs and steps due to ice and snow (W00.1) |
>|---|---|

>　　The appropriate 7th character is to be added to each code from category W10

>| A | initial encounter |
>|---|---|
>| D | subsequent encounter |
>| S | sequela |

X● **W10.0　Fall (on) (from) escalator**

X● **W10.1　Fall (on) (from) sidewalk curb**

X● **W10.2　Fall (on) (from) incline**
>　　Fall (on) (from) ramp

X● **W10.8　Fall (on) (from) other stairs and steps**

X● **W10.9　Fall (on) (from) unspecified stairs and steps**

X● **W11　Fall on and from ladder**

>　　The appropriate 7th character is to be added to code W11

>| A | initial encounter |
>|---|---|
>| D | subsequent encounter |
>| S | sequela |

X● **W12　Fall on and from scaffolding**

>　　The appropriate 7th character is to be added to code W12

>| A | initial encounter |
>|---|---|
>| D | subsequent encounter |
>| S | sequela |

● **W13　Fall from, out of or through building or structure**

>　　The appropriate 7th character is to be added to each code from category W13

>| A | initial encounter |
>|---|---|
>| D | subsequent encounter |
>| S | sequela |

X● **W13.0　Fall from, out of or through balcony**
>　　Fall from, out of or through railing

X● **W13.1　Fall from, out of or through bridge**

X● **W13.2　Fall from, out of or through roof**

X● **W13.3　Fall through floor**

X● **W13.4　Fall from, out of or through window**
>| **Excludes2** | fall with subsequent striking against sharp glass (W01.110) |
>|---|---|

X● **W13.8　Fall from, out of or through other building or structure**
>　　Fall from, out of or through viaduct
>　　Fall from, out of or through wall
>　　Fall from, out of or through flag-pole

X● **W13.9　Fall from, out of or through building, not otherwise specified**
>| **Excludes1** | collapse of a building or structure (W20.-) fall or jump from burning building or structure (X00.-) |
>|---|---|

X● **W14　Fall from tree**

>　　The appropriate 7th character is to be added to code W14

>| A | initial encounter |
>|---|---|
>| D | subsequent encounter |
>| S | sequela |

X● **W15　Fall from cliff**

>　　The appropriate 7th character is to be added to code W15

>| A | initial encounter |
>|---|---|
>| D | subsequent encounter |
>| S | sequela |

● **W16　Fall, jump or diving into water**

>| **Excludes1** | accidental non-watercraft drowning and submersion not involving fall (W65-W74) effects of air pressure from diving (W94.-) fall into water from watercraft (V90-V94) hitting an object or against bottom when falling from watercraft (V94.0) |
>|---|---|
>| **Excludes2** | striking or hitting diving board (W21.4) |

>　　The appropriate 7th character is to be added to each code from category W16

>| A | initial encounter |
>|---|---|
>| D | subsequent encounter |
>| S | sequela |

● **W16.0　Fall into swimming pool**
>　　Fall into swimming pool NOS
>| **Excludes1** | fall into empty swimming pool (W17.3) |
>|---|---|

● **W16.01　Fall into swimming pool striking water surface**

● **W16.011　Fall into swimming pool striking water surface causing drowning and submersion**
>| **Excludes1** | drowning and submersion while in swimming pool without fall (W67) |
>|---|---|

● **W16.012　Fall into swimming pool striking water surface causing other injury**

CHAPTER 20 (V01-Y99)

- ● W16.02   Fall into swimming pool striking bottom
  - ● W16.021   Fall into swimming pool striking bottom causing drowning and submersion
    - **Excludes1**   drowning and submersion while in swimming pool without fall (W67)
  - ● W16.022   Fall into swimming pool striking bottom causing other injury
- ● W16.03   Fall into swimming pool striking wall
  - ● W16.031   Fall into swimming pool striking wall causing drowning and submersion
    - **Excludes1**   drowning and submersion while in swimming pool without fall (W67)
  - ● W16.032   Fall into swimming pool striking wall causing other injury
- ● W16.1   Fall into natural body of water
  - Fall into lake
  - Fall into open sea
  - Fall into river
  - Fall into stream
  - ● W16.11   Fall into natural body of water striking water surface
    - ● W16.111   Fall into natural body of water striking water surface causing drowning and submersion
      - **Excludes1**   drowning and submersion while in natural body of water without fall (W69)
    - ● W16.112   Fall into natural body of water striking water surface causing other injury
  - ● W16.12   Fall into natural body of water striking bottom
    - ● W16.121   Fall into natural body of water striking bottom causing drowning and submersion
      - **Excludes1**   drowning and submersion while in natural body of water without fall (W69)
    - ● W16.122   Fall into natural body of water striking bottom causing other injury
  - ● W16.13   Fall into natural body of water striking side
    - ● W16.131   Fall into natural body of water striking side causing drowning and submersion
      - **Excludes1**   drowning and submersion while in natural body of water without fall (W69)
    - ● W16.132   Fall into natural body of water striking side causing other injury
- ● W16.2   Fall in (into) filled bathtub or bucket of water
  - ● W16.21   Fall in (into) filled bathtub
    - **Excludes1**   fall into empty bathtub (W18.2)
    - ● W16.211   Fall in (into) filled bathtub causing drowning and submersion
      - **Excludes1**   drowning and submersion while in filled bathtub without fall (W65)
    - ● W16.212   Fall in (into) filled bathtub causing other injury

- ● W16.22   Fall in (into) bucket of water
  - ● W16.221   Fall in (into) bucket of water causing drowning and submersion
  - ● W16.222   Fall in (into) bucket of water causing other injury
- ● W16.3   Fall into other water
  - Fall into fountain
  - Fall into reservoir
  - ● W16.31   Fall into other water striking water surface
    - ● W16.311   Fall into other water striking water surface causing drowning and submersion
      - **Excludes1**   drowning and submersion while in other water without fall (W73)
    - ● W16.312   Fall into other water striking water surface causing other injury
  - ● W16.32   Fall into other water striking bottom
    - ● W16.321   Fall into other water striking bottom causing drowning and submersion
      - **Excludes1**   drowning and submersion while in other water without fall (W73)
    - ● W16.322   Fall into other water striking bottom causing other injury
  - ● W16.33   Fall into other water striking wall
    - ● W16.331   Fall into other water striking wall causing drowning and submersion
      - **Excludes1**   drowning and submersion while in other water without fall (W73)
    - ● W16.332   Fall into other water striking wall causing other injury
- ● W16.4   Fall into unspecified water
  - X ● W16.41   Fall into unspecified water causing drowning and submersion
  - X ● W16.42   Fall into unspecified water causing other injury
- ● W16.5   Jumping or diving into swimming pool
  - ● W16.51   Jumping or diving into swimming pool striking water surface
    - ● W16.511   Jumping or diving into swimming pool striking water surface causing drowning and submersion
      - **Excludes1**   drowning and submersion while in swimming pool without jumping or diving (W67)
    - ● W16.512   Jumping or diving into swimming pool striking water surface causing other injury
  - ● W16.52   Jumping or diving into swimming pool striking bottom
    - ● W16.521   Jumping or diving into swimming pool striking bottom causing drowning and submersion
      - **Excludes1**   drowning and submersion while in swimming pool without jumping or diving (W67)
    - ● W16.522   Jumping or diving into swimming pool striking bottom causing other injury

▶ New   ⇒ Revised   ~~deleted~~ Deleted   **OGCR** Official Guidelines   X Assign placeholder X   ● Use Additional Character(s)

Excludes 1   Excludes 2   Includes   Use additional   Code first   Code also   Key words

● **W16.53** Jumping or diving into swimming pool striking wall

  ● **W16.531** Jumping or diving into swimming pool striking wall causing drowning and submersion

       Excludes1   drowning and submersion while in swimming pool without jumping or diving (W67)

  ● **W16.532** Jumping or diving into swimming pool striking wall causing other injury

● **W16.6** Jumping or diving into natural body of water

     Jumping or diving into lake
     Jumping or diving into open sea
     Jumping or diving into river
     Jumping or diving into stream

 ● **W16.61** Jumping or diving into natural body of water striking water surface

  ● **W16.611** Jumping or diving into natural body of water striking water surface causing drowning and submersion

       Excludes1   drowning and submersion while in natural body of water without jumping or diving (W69)

  ● **W16.612** Jumping or diving into natural body of water striking water surface causing other injury

 ● **W16.62** Jumping or diving into natural body of water striking bottom

  ● **W16.621** Jumping or diving into natural body of water striking bottom causing drowning and submersion

       Excludes1   drowning and submersion while in natural body of water without jumping or diving (W69)

  ● **W16.622** Jumping or diving into natural body of water striking bottom causing other injury

● **W16.7** Jumping or diving from boat

     Excludes1   fall from boat into water - see watercraft accident (V90-V94)

 ● **W16.71** Jumping or diving from boat striking water surface

  ● **W16.711** Jumping or diving from boat striking water surface causing drowning and submersion

  ● **W16.712** Jumping or diving from boat striking water surface causing other injury

 ● **W16.72** Jumping or diving from boat striking bottom

  ● **W16.721** Jumping or diving from boat striking bottom causing drowning and submersion

  ● **W16.722** Jumping or diving from boat striking bottom causing other injury

● **W16.8** Jumping or diving into other water

     Jumping or diving into fountain
     Jumping or diving into reservoir

 ● **W16.81** Jumping or diving into other water striking water surface

  ● **W16.811** Jumping or diving into other water striking water surface causing drowning and submersion

       Excludes1   drowning and submersion while in other water without jumping or diving (W73)

  ● **W16.812** Jumping or diving into other water striking water surface causing other injury

 ● **W16.82** Jumping or diving into other water striking bottom

  ● **W16.821** Jumping or diving into other water striking bottom causing drowning and submersion

       Excludes1   drowning and submersion while in other water without jumping or diving (W73)

  ● **W16.822** Jumping or diving into other water striking bottom causing other injury

 ● **W16.83** Jumping or diving into other water striking wall

  ● **W16.831** Jumping or diving into other water striking wall causing drowning and submersion

       Excludes1   drowning and submersion while in other water without jumping or diving (W73)

  ● **W16.832** Jumping or diving into other water striking wall causing other injury

● **W16.9** Jumping or diving into unspecified water

 X ● **W16.91** Jumping or diving into unspecified water causing drowning and submersion

 X ● **W16.92** Jumping or diving into unspecified water causing other injury

● **W17** Other fall from one level to another

     The appropriate 7th character is to be added to each code from category W17

A	initial encounter
D	subsequent encounter
S	sequela

X ● **W17.0** Fall into well

X ● **W17.1** Fall into storm drain or manhole

X ● **W17.2** Fall into hole

     Fall into pit

X ● **W17.3** Fall into empty swimming pool

     Excludes1   fall into filled swimming pool (W16.0-)

X ● **W17.4** Fall from dock

● **W17.8** Other fall from one level to another

 X ● **W17.81** Fall down embankment (hill)

 X ● **W17.82** Fall from (out of) grocery cart

     Fall due to grocery cart tipping over

 X ● **W17.89** Other fall from one level to another

     Fall from cherry picker
     Fall from lifting device
     Fall from mobile elevated work platform [MEWP]
     Fall from sky lift

CHAPTER 20 (V01-Y99)

● **W18**   **Other slipping, tripping and stumbling and falls**

The appropriate 7th character is to be added to each code from category W18

A	initial encounter
D	subsequent encounter
S	sequela

● **W18.0**   **Fall due to bumping against object**

Striking against object with subsequent fall

Excludes1	fall on same level due to slipping, tripping, or stumbling with subsequent striking against object (W01.1-)

X● **W18.00**   **Striking against unspecified object with subsequent fall**

X● **W18.01**   **Striking against sports equipment with subsequent fall**

X● **W18.02**   **Striking against glass with subsequent fall**

X● **W18.09**   **Striking against other object with subsequent fall**

● **W18.1**   **Fall from or off toilet**

X● **W18.11**   **Fall from or off toilet without subsequent striking against object**

Fall from (off) toilet NOS

X● **W18.12**   **Fall from or off toilet with subsequent striking against object**

X● **W18.2**   **Fall in (into) shower or empty bathtub**

Excludes1	fall in full bathtub causing drowning or submersion (W16.21-)

● **W18.3**   **Other and unspecified fall on same level**

X● **W18.30**   **Fall on same level, unspecified**

X● **W18.31**   **Fall on same level due to stepping on an object**

Fall on same level due to stepping on an animal

Excludes1	slipping, tripping and stumbling without fall due to stepping on animal (W18.41)

X● **W18.39**   **Other fall on same level**

● **W18.4**   **Slipping, tripping and stumbling without falling**

Excludes1	collision with another person without fall (W51)

X● **W18.40**   **Slipping, tripping and stumbling without falling, unspecified**

X● **W18.41**   **Slipping, tripping and stumbling without falling due to stepping on object**

Slipping, tripping and stumbling without falling due to stepping on animal

Excludes1	slipping, tripping and stumbling with fall due to stepping on animal (W18.31)

X● **W18.42**   **Slipping, tripping and stumbling without falling due to stepping into hole or opening**

X● **W18.43**   **Slipping, tripping and stumbling without falling due to stepping from one level to another**

X● **W18.49**   **Other slipping, tripping and stumbling without falling**

X● **W19**   **Unspecified fall**

Accidental fall NOS

The appropriate 7th character is to be added to code W19

A	initial encounter
D	subsequent encounter
S	sequela

EXPOSURE TO INANIMATE MECHANICAL FORCES (W20-W49)

Excludes1	assault (X92-Y09)
	contact or collision with animals or persons (W50-W64)
	exposure to inanimate mechanical forces involving military or war operations (Y36.-, Y37.-)
	intentional self-harm (X71-X83)

● **W20**   **Struck by thrown, projected or falling object**

Code first any associated:

cataclysm (X34-X39)

lightning strike (T75.00)

Excludes1	falling object in machinery accident (W24, W28-W31)
	falling object in transport accident (V01-V99)
	object set in motion by explosion (W35-W40)
	object set in motion by firearm (W32-W34)
	struck by thrown sports equipment (W21.-)

The appropriate 7th character is to be added to each code from category W20

A	initial encounter
D	subsequent encounter
S	sequela

X● **W20.0**   **Struck by falling object in cave-in**

Excludes2	asphyxiation due to cave-in (T71.21)

X● **W20.1**   **Struck by object due to collapse of building**

Excludes1	struck by object due to collapse of burning building (X00.2, X02.2)

X● **W20.8**   **Other cause of strike by thrown, projected or falling object**

Excludes1	struck by thrown sports equipment (W21.-)

● **W21**   **Striking against or struck by sports equipment**

Excludes1	assault with sports equipment (Y08.0-)
	striking against or struck by sports equipment with subsequent fall (W18.01)

The appropriate 7th character is to be added to each code from category W21

A	initial encounter
D	subsequent encounter
S	sequela

● **W21.0**   **Struck by hit or thrown ball**

X● **W21.00**   **Struck by hit or thrown ball, unspecified type**

X● **W21.01**   **Struck by football**

X● **W21.02**   **Struck by soccer ball**

X● **W21.03**   **Struck by baseball**

X● **W21.04**   **Struck by golf ball**

X● **W21.05**   **Struck by basketball**

X● **W21.06**   **Struck by volleyball**

X● **W21.07**   **Struck by softball**

X● **W21.09**   **Struck by other hit or thrown ball**

● **W21.1**   **Struck by bat, racquet or club**

X● **W21.11**   **Struck by baseball bat**

X● **W21.12**   **Struck by tennis racquet**

X● **W21.13**   **Struck by golf club**

X● **W21.19**   **Struck by other bat, racquet or club**

● **W21.2**   **Struck by hockey stick or puck**

● **W21.21**   **Struck by hockey stick**

● **W21.210**   **Struck by ice hockey stick**

● **W21.211**   **Struck by field hockey stick**

● **W21.22**   **Struck by hockey puck**

● **W21.220**   **Struck by ice hockey puck**

● **W21.221**   **Struck by field hockey puck**

▶ New   ⇒ Revised   ~~deleted~~ Deleted   **OGCR** Official Guidelines   X Assign placeholder X   ● Use Additional Character(s)

Excludes 1	Excludes 2	Includes	Use additional	Code first	Code also	Key words

● W21.3   **Struck by sports foot wear**
   X ● W21.31   **Struck by shoe cleats**
       Stepped on by shoe cleats
   X ● W21.32   **Struck by skate blades**
       Skated over by skate blades
   X ● W21.39   **Struck by other sports foot wear**
X ● W21.4   **Striking against diving board**
     Use additional code for subsequent falling into water, if applicable (W16.-)
● W21.8   **Striking against or struck by other sports equipment**
   X ● W21.81   **Striking against or struck by football helmet**
   X ● W21.89   **Striking against or struck by other sports equipment**
X ● W21.9   **Striking against or struck by unspecified sports equipment**

● W22   **Striking against or struck by other objects**

Excludes1	striking against or struck by object with subsequent fall (W18.Ø9)

     The appropriate 7th character is to be added to each code from category W22

A	initial encounter
D	subsequent encounter
S	sequela

● W22.Ø   **Striking against stationary object**

Excludes1	striking against stationary sports equipment (W21.8)

   X ● W22.Ø1   **Walked into wall**
   X ● W22.Ø2   **Walked into lamppost**
   X ● W22.Ø3   **Walked into furniture**
   ● W22.Ø4   **Striking against wall of swimming pool**
     ● W22.Ø41   **Striking against wall of swimming pool causing drowning and submersion**

Excludes1	drowning and submersion while swimming without striking against wall (W67)

     ● W22.Ø42   **Striking against wall of swimming pool causing other injury**
   X ● W22.Ø9   **Striking against other stationary object**
● W22.1   **Striking against or struck by automobile airbag**
   X ● W22.10   **Striking against or struck by unspecified automobile airbag**
   X ● W22.11   **Striking against or struck by driver side automobile airbag**
   X ● W22.12   **Striking against or struck by front passenger side automobile airbag**
   X ● W22.19   **Striking against or struck by other automobile airbag**
X ● W22.8   **Striking against or struck by other objects**
     Striking against or struck by object NOS

Excludes1	struck by thrown, projected or falling object (W20.-)

● W23   **Caught, crushed, jammed or pinched in or between objects**

Excludes1	injury caused by cutting or piercing instruments (W25-W27)
	injury caused by firearms malfunction (W32.1, W33.1-, W34.1-)
	injury caused by lifting and transmission devices (W24.-)
	injury caused by machinery (W28-W31)
	injury caused by nonpowered hand tools (W27.-)
	injury caused by transport vehicle being used as a means of transportation (V01-V99)
	injury caused by struck by thrown, projected or falling object (W20.-)

     The appropriate 7th character is to be added to each code from category W23

A	initial encounter
D	subsequent encounter
S	sequela

   X ● W23.Ø   **Caught, crushed, jammed, or pinched between moving objects**
   X ● W23.1   **Caught, crushed, jammed, or pinched between stationary objects**

● W24   **Contact with lifting and transmission devices, not elsewhere classified**

Excludes1	transport accidents (V01-V99)

     The appropriate 7th character is to be added to each code from category W24

A	initial encounter
D	subsequent encounter
S	sequela

   X ● W24.Ø   **Contact with lifting devices, not elsewhere classified**
     Contact with chain hoist
     Contact with drive belt
     Contact with pulley (block)
   X ● W24.1   **Contact with transmission devices, not elsewhere classified**
     Contact with transmission belt or cable

X ● W25   **Contact with sharp glass**
     Code first any associated:
       injury due to flying glass from explosion or firearm discharge (W32-W40)
       transport accident (V00-V99)

Excludes1	fall on same level due to slipping, tripping and stumbling with subsequent striking against sharp glass (W01.10)
	striking against sharp glass with subsequent fall (W18.02)

Excludes2	glass embedded in skin (W45)

     The appropriate 7th character is to be added to code W25

A	initial encounter
D	subsequent encounter
S	sequela

CHAPTER 2Ø (VØ1-Y99)

● **W26**   Contact with other sharp objects

> **Excludes2**   sharp object(s) embedded in skin (W45)

> The appropriate 7th character is to be added to each code from category W26

> | A | initial encounter |
> |---|---|
> | D | subsequent encounter |
> | S | sequela |

X ● **W26.0**   Contact with knife

> **Excludes1**   contact with electric knife (W29.1)

X ● **W26.1**   Contact with sword or dagger

X ● **W26.2**   Contact with edge of stiff paper
> Paper cut

X ● **W26.8**   Contact with other sharp object(s), not elsewhere classified
> Contact with tin can lid

X ● **W26.9**   Contact with unspecified sharp object(s)

● **W27**   Contact with nonpowered hand tool

> The appropriate 7th character is to be added to each code from category W27

> | A | initial encounter |
> |---|---|
> | D | subsequent encounter |
> | S | sequela |

X ● **W27.0**   Contact with workbench tool
> Contact with auger
> Contact with axe
> Contact with chisel
> Contact with handsaw
> Contact with screwdriver

X ● **W27.1**   Contact with garden tool
> Contact with hoe
> Contact with nonpowered lawn mower
> Contact with pitchfork
> Contact with rake

X ● **W27.2**   Contact with scissors

X ● **W27.3**   Contact with needle (sewing)
> **Excludes1**   contact with hypodermic needle (W46.-)

X ● **W27.4**   Contact with kitchen utensil
> Contact with fork
> Contact with ice-pick
> Contact with can-opener NOS

X ● **W27.5**   Contact with paper-cutter

X ● **W27.8**   Contact with other nonpowered hand tool
> Contact with nonpowered sewing machine
> Contact with shovel

X ● **W28**   Contact with powered lawn mower
> Powered lawn mower (commercial) (residential)

> **Excludes1**   contact with nonpowered lawn mower (W27.1)

> **Excludes2**   exposure to electric current (W86.-)

> The appropriate 7th character is to be added to code W28

> | A | initial encounter |
> |---|---|
> | D | subsequent encounter |
> | S | sequela |

● **W29**   Contact with other powered hand tools and household machinery

> **Excludes1**   contact with commercial machinery (W31.82)
> contact with hot household appliance (X15)
> contact with nonpowered hand tool (W27.-)
> exposure to electric current (W86)

> The appropriate 7th character is to be added to each code from category W29

> | A | initial encounter |
> |---|---|
> | D | subsequent encounter |
> | S | sequela |

X ● **W29.0**   Contact with powered kitchen appliance
> Contact with blender
> Contact with can-opener
> Contact with garbage disposal
> Contact with mixer

X ● **W29.1**   Contact with electric knife

X ● **W29.2**   Contact with other powered household machinery
> Contact with electric fan
> Contact with powered dryer (clothes) (powered) (spin)
> Contact with washing-machine
> Contact with sewing machine

X ● **W29.3**   Contact with powered garden and outdoor hand tools and machinery
> Contact with chainsaw
> Contact with edger
> Contact with garden cultivator (tiller)
> Contact with hedge trimmer
> Contact with other powered garden tool
> > **Excludes1**   contact with powered lawn mower (W28)

X ● **W29.4**   Contact with nail gun

➡ X ● **W29.8**   Contact with other powered hand tools and household machinery
> Contact with do-it-yourself tool NOS

● **W30**   Contact with agricultural machinery

> **Includes**   animal-powered farm machine

> **Excludes1**   agricultural transport vehicle accident (V01-V99)
> explosion of grain store (W40.8)
> exposure to electric current (W86.-)

> The appropriate 7th character is to be added to each code from category W30

> | A | initial encounter |
> |---|---|
> | D | subsequent encounter |
> | S | sequela |

X ● **W30.0**   Contact with combine harvester
> Contact with reaper
> Contact with thresher

X ● **W30.1**   Contact with power take-off devices (PTO)

X ● **W30.2**   Contact with hay derrick

X ● **W30.3**   Contact with grain storage elevator
> **Excludes1**   explosion of grain store (W40.8)

● **W30.8**   Contact with other specified agricultural machinery

X ● **W30.81**   Contact with agricultural transport vehicle in stationary use
> Contact with agricultural transport vehicle under repair, not on public roadway
> > **Excludes1**   agricultural transport vehicle accident (V01-V99)

X ● **W30.89**   Contact with other specified agricultural machinery

X ● **W30.9**   Contact with unspecified agricultural machinery
> Contact with farm machinery NOS

● **W31**   **Contact with other and unspecified machinery**

Excludes1	contact with agricultural machinery (W30.-)
	contact with machinery in transport under own power or being towed by a vehicle (V01-V99)
	exposure to electric current (W86)

     The appropriate 7th character is to be added to each code from category W31

A	initial encounter
D	subsequent encounter
S	sequela

X● **W31.0**   **Contact with mining and earth-drilling machinery**
       Contact with bore or drill (land) (seabed)
       Contact with shaft hoist
       Contact with shaft lift
       Contact with undercutter

X● **W31.1**   **Contact with metalworking machines**
       Contact with abrasive wheel
       Contact with forging machine
       Contact with lathe
       Contact with mechanical shears
       Contact with metal drilling machine
       Contact with milling machine
       Contact with power press
       Contact with rolling-mill
       Contact with metal sawing machine

X● **W31.2**   **Contact with powered woodworking and forming machines**
       Contact with band saw
       Contact with bench saw
       Contact with circular saw
       Contact with molding machine
       Contact with overhead plane
       Contact with powered saw
       Contact with radial saw
       Contact with sander

Excludes1	nonpowered woodworking tools (W27.0)

X● **W31.3**   **Contact with prime movers**
       Contact with gas turbine
       Contact with internal combustion engine
       Contact with steam engine
       Contact with water driven turbine

● **W31.8**   **Contact with other specified machinery**

X● **W31.81**   **Contact with recreational machinery**
       Contact with roller-coaster

X● **W31.82**   **Contact with other commercial machinery**
       Contact with commercial electric fan
       Contact with commercial kitchen appliances
       Contact with commercial powered dryer (clothes) (powered) (spin)
       Contact with commercial washing-machine
       Contact with commercial sewing machine

Excludes1	contact with household machinery (W29.-)
	contact with powered lawn mower (W28)

X● **W31.83**   **Contact with special construction vehicle in stationary use**
       Contact with special construction vehicle under repair, not on public roadway

Excludes1	special construction vehicle accident (V01-V99)

X● **W31.89**   **Contact with other specified machinery**

X● **W31.9**   **Contact with unspecified machinery**
       Contact with machinery NOS

● **W32**   **Accidental handgun discharge and malfunction**

Includes	accidental discharge and malfunction of gun for single hand use
	accidental discharge and malfunction of pistol
	accidental discharge and malfunction of revolver
	handgun discharge and malfunction NOS

Excludes1	accidental airgun discharge and malfunction (W34.010, W34.110)
	accidental BB gun discharge and malfunction (W34.010, W34.110)
	accidental pellet gun discharge and malfunction (W34.010, W34.110)
	accidental shotgun discharge and malfunction (W33.01, W33.11)
	assault by handgun discharge (X93)
	handgun discharge involving legal intervention (Y35.0-)
	handgun discharge involving military or war operations (Y36.4-)
	intentional self-harm by handgun discharge (X72)
	Very pistol discharge and malfunction (W34.09, W34.19)

     The appropriate 7th character is to be added to each code from category W32

A	initial encounter
D	subsequent encounter
S	sequela

X● **W32.0**   **Accidental handgun discharge**

X● **W32.1**   **Accidental handgun malfunction**
       Injury due to explosion of handgun (parts)
       Injury due to malfunction of mechanism or component of handgun
       Injury due to recoil of handgun
       Powder burn from handgun

● **W33**   **Accidental rifle, shotgun and larger firearm discharge and malfunction**

Includes	rifle, shotgun and larger firearm discharge and malfunction NOS

Excludes1	accidental airgun discharge and malfunction (W34.010, W34.110)
	accidental BB gun discharge and malfunction (W34.010, W34.110)
	accidental handgun discharge and malfunction (W32.-)
	accidental pellet gun discharge and malfunction (W34.010, W34.110)
	assault by rifle, shotgun and larger firearm discharge (X94)
	firearm discharge involving legal intervention (Y35.0-)
	firearm discharge involving military or war operations (Y36.4-)
	intentional self-harm by rifle, shotgun and larger firearm discharge (X73)

     The appropriate 7th character is to be added to each code from category W33

A	initial encounter
D	subsequent encounter
S	sequela

● **W33.0**   **Accidental rifle, shotgun and larger firearm discharge**

X● **W33.00**   **Accidental discharge of unspecified larger firearm**
       Discharge of unspecified larger firearm NOS

X● **W33.01**   **Accidental discharge of shotgun**
       Discharge of shotgun NOS

X● **W33.02**   **Accidental discharge of hunting rifle**
       Discharge of hunting rifle NOS

X● **W33.03**   **Accidental discharge of machine gun**
       Discharge of machine gun NOS

X● **W33.09**   **Accidental discharge of other larger firearm**
       Discharge of other larger firearm NOS

▶ New   ⇒ Revised   ~~deleted~~ Deleted   **OGCR** Official Guidelines   X Assign placeholder X   ● Use Additional Character(s)

Excludes 1   Excludes 2   Includes   Use additional   Code first   Code also   Key words

● **W33.1** **Accidental rifle, shotgun and larger firearm** malfunction

    Injury due to explosion of rifle, shotgun and larger firearm (parts)

    Injury due to malfunction of mechanism or component of rifle, shotgun and larger firearm

    Injury due to piercing, cutting, crushing or pinching due to (by) slide trigger mechanism, scope or other gun part

    Injury due to recoil of rifle, shotgun and larger firearm

    Powder burn from rifle, shotgun and larger firearm

X● **W33.10** **Accidental malfunction of** unspecified **larger firearm**

    Malfunction of unspecified larger firearm NOS

X● **W33.11** **Accidental malfunction of** shotgun

    Malfunction of shotgun NOS

X● **W33.12** **Accidental malfunction of** hunting rifle

    Malfunction of hunting rifle NOS

X● **W33.13** **Accidental malfunction of** machine gun

    Malfunction of machine gun NOS

X● **W33.19** **Accidental malfunction of** other larger firearm

    Malfunction of other larger firearm NOS

● **W34** **Accidental** discharge **and malfunction from other and unspecified firearms and guns**

    The appropriate 7th character is to be added to each code from category W34

A	initial encounter
D	subsequent encounter
S	sequela

● **W34.0** **Accidental discharge from other and unspecified firearms and guns**

X● **W34.00** **Accidental discharge from** unspecified **firearms or gun**

    Discharge from firearm NOS

    Gunshot wound NOS

    Shot NOS

● **W34.01** **Accidental discharge of gas, air or spring-operated guns**

● **W34.010** **Accidental discharge of** airgun

    Accidental discharge of BB gun

    Accidental discharge of pellet gun

● **W34.011** **Accidental discharge of** paintball gun

    Accidental injury due to paintball discharge

● **W34.018** **Accidental discharge of** other **gas, air or spring-operated gun**

X● **W34.09** **Accidental discharge from** other specified **firearms**

    Accidental discharge from Very pistol [flare]

● **W34.1** **Accidental** malfunction **from other and unspecified firearms and guns**

X● **W34.10** **Accidental malfunction from** unspecified **firearms or gun**

    Firearm malfunction NOS

● **W34.11** **Accidental malfunction of gas, air or spring-operated guns**

● **W34.110** **Accidental malfunction of** airgun

    Accidental malfunction of BB gun

    Accidental malfunction of pellet gun

● **W34.111** **Accidental malfunction of** paintball gun

    Accidental injury due to paintball gun malfunction

● **W34.118** **Accidental malfunction of** other **gas, air or spring-operated gun**

X● **W34.19** **Accidental malfunction from** other specified **firearms**

    Accidental malfunction from Very pistol [flare]

X●**W35** **Explosion and rupture of boiler**

Excludes1 explosion and rupture of boiler on watercraft (V93.4)

    The appropriate 7th character is to be added to code W35

A	initial encounter
D	subsequent encounter
S	sequela

● **W36** **Explosion and rupture of gas cylinder**

    The appropriate 7th character is to be added to each code from category W36

A	initial encounter
D	subsequent encounter
S	sequela

X● **W36.1** **Explosion and rupture of** aerosol can

X● **W36.2** **Explosion and rupture of** air tank

X● **W36.3** **Explosion and rupture of** pressurized-gas tank

X● **W36.8** **Explosion and rupture of** other **gas cylinder**

X● **W36.9** **Explosion and rupture of** unspecified **gas cylinder**

● **W37** **Explosion and rupture of** pressurized tire, pipe or hose

    The appropriate 7th character is to be added to each code from category W37

A	initial encounter
D	subsequent encounter
S	sequela

X● **W37.0** **Explosion of** bicycle tire

X● **W37.8** **Explosion and rupture of** other pressurized tire, **pipe or hose**

X●**W38** **Explosion and rupture of** other specified pressurized devices

    The appropriate 7th character is to be added to code W38

A	initial encounter
D	subsequent encounter
S	sequela

X●**W39** **Discharge of** firework

    The appropriate 7th character is to be added to code W39

A	initial encounter
D	subsequent encounter
S	sequela

● **W40** **Explosion of** other materials

Excludes1 assault by explosive material (X96)

    explosion involving legal intervention (Y35.1-)

    explosion involving military or war operations (Y36.0-, Y36.2-)

    intentional self-harm by explosive material (X75)

    The appropriate 7th character is to be added to each code from category W40

A	initial encounter
D	subsequent encounter
S	sequela

X● **W40.0** **Explosion of** blasting material

    Explosion of blasting cap

    Explosion of detonator

    Explosion of dynamite

    Explosion of explosive (any) used in blasting operations

X● **W40.1** **Explosion of** explosive gases

    Explosion of acetylene

    Explosion of butane

    Explosion of coal gas

    Explosion in mine NOS

    Explosion of explosive gas

    Explosion of fire damp

    Explosion of gasoline fumes

    Explosion of methane

    Explosion of propane

▶ New　　⇒ Revised　　deleted Deleted　　**OGCR** Official Guidelines　　X Assign placeholder X　　● Use Additional Character(s)

Excludes 1　　Excludes 2　　Includes　　Use additional　　Code first　　Code also　　Key words

X ● **W40.8   Explosion of other specified explosive materials**
     Explosion in dump NOS
     Explosion in factory NOS
     Explosion in grain store
     Explosion in munitions

> **Excludes1**   explosion involving legal intervention (Y35.1-)
> explosion involving military or war operations (Y36.0-, Y36.2-)

X ● **W40.9   Explosion of unspecified explosive materials**
     Explosion NOS

● **W42   Exposure to noise**

The appropriate 7th character is to be added to each code from category W42

A	initial encounter
D	subsequent encounter
S	sequela

X ● **W42.0   Exposure to supersonic waves**
X ● **W42.9   Exposure to other noise**
     Exposure to sound waves NOS

● **W45   Foreign body or object entering through skin**

> **Includes**   foreign body or object embedded in skin
> nail embedded in skin

> **Excludes2**   contact with hand tools (nonpowered) (powered) (W27-W29)
> contact with other sharp object(s) (W26.-)
> contact with sharp glass (W25.-)
> struck by objects (W20-W22)

The appropriate 7th character is to be added to each code from category W45

A	initial encounter
D	subsequent encounter
S	sequela

X ● **W45.0   Nail entering through skin**
X ● **W45.8   Other foreign body or object entering through skin**
     Splinter in skin NOS

● **W46   Contact with hypodermic needle**

The appropriate 7th character is to be added to each code from category W46

A	initial encounter
D	subsequent encounter
S	sequela

X ● **W46.0   Contact with hypodermic needle**
     Hypodermic needle stick NOS
X ● **W46.1   Contact with contaminated hypodermic needle**

● **W49   Exposure to other inanimate mechanical forces**

> **Includes**   exposure to abnormal gravitational [G] forces
> exposure to inanimate mechanical forces NEC

> **Excludes1**   exposure to inanimate mechanical forces involving military or war operations (Y36.-, Y37.-)

The appropriate 7th character is to be added to each code from category W49

A	initial encounter
D	subsequent encounter
S	sequela

● **W49.0   Item causing external constriction**
X ● **W49.01   Hair causing external constriction**
X ● **W49.02   String or thread causing external constriction**
X ● **W49.03   Rubber band causing external constriction**
X ● **W49.04   Ring or other jewelry causing external constriction**
X ● **W49.09   Other item causing external constriction**

X ● **W49.9   Exposure to other inanimate mechanical forces**

EXPOSURE TO ANIMATE MECHANICAL FORCES (W50-W64)

> **Excludes1**   toxic effect of contact with venomous animals and plants (T63.-)

● **W50   Accidental hit, strike, kick, twist, bite or scratch by another person**

> **Includes**   hit, strike, kick, twist, bite, or scratch by another person NOS

> **Excludes1**   assault by bodily force (Y04)
> struck by objects (W20-W22)

The appropriate 7th character is to be added to each code from category W50

A	initial encounter
D	subsequent encounter
S	sequela

X ● **W50.0   Accidental hit or strike by another person**
     Hit or strike by another person NOS
X ● **W50.1   Accidental kick by another person**
     Kick by another person NOS
X ● **W50.2   Accidental twist by another person**
     Twist by another person NOS
X ● **W50.3   Accidental bite by another person**
     Human bite
     Bite by another person NOS
X ● **W50.4   Accidental scratch by another person**
     Scratch by another person NOS

X ● **W51   Accidental striking against or bumped into by another person**

> **Excludes1**   assault by striking against or bumping into by another person (Y04.2)
> fall due to collision with another person (W03)

The appropriate 7th character is to be added to code W51

A	initial encounter
D	subsequent encounter
S	sequela

X ● **W52   Crushed, pushed or stepped on by crowd or human stampede**
     Crushed, pushed or stepped on by crowd or human stampede with or without fall

The appropriate 7th character is to be added to code W52

A	initial encounter
D	subsequent encounter
S	sequela

● **W53   Contact with rodent**

> **Includes**   contact with saliva, feces or urine of rodent

The appropriate 7th character is to be added to each code from category W53

A	initial encounter
D	subsequent encounter
S	sequela

● **W53.0   Contact with mouse**
X ● **W53.01   Bitten by mouse**
X ● **W53.09   Other contact with mouse**
● **W53.1   Contact with rat**
X ● **W53.11   Bitten by rat**
X ● **W53.19   Other contact with rat**
● **W53.2   Contact with squirrel**
X ● **W53.21   Bitten by squirrel**
X ● **W53.29   Other contact with squirrel**
● **W53.8   Contact with other rodent**
X ● **W53.81   Bitten by other rodent**
X ● **W53.89   Other contact with other rodent**

CHAPTER 20 (V01-Y99)

CHAPTER 20 (V01-Y99)

● W54   **Contact with dog**

> **Includes**   contact with saliva, feces or urine of dog
>
> The appropriate 7th character is to be added to each code from category W54
>
> | | |
> |---|---|
> | A | initial encounter |
> | D | subsequent encounter |
> | S | sequela |

   X ● **W54.0**   **Bitten by dog**

   X ● **W54.1**   **Struck by dog**
           Knocked over by dog

   X ● **W54.8**   **Other contact with dog**

● W55   **Contact with other mammals**

> **Includes**   contact with saliva, feces or urine of mammal
>
> **Excludes1**   animal being ridden - see transport accidents
> bitten or struck by dog (W54)
> bitten or struck by rodent (W53.-)
> contact with marine mammals (W56.X-)
>
> The appropriate 7th character is to be added to each code from category W55
>
> | | |
> |---|---|
> | A | initial encounter |
> | D | subsequent encounter |
> | S | sequela |

   ● **W55.0**   **Contact with cat**

     X ● **W55.01**   **Bitten by cat**

     X ● **W55.03**   **Scratched by cat**

     X ● **W55.09**   **Other contact with cat**

   ● **W55.1**   **Contact with horse**

     X ● **W55.11**   **Bitten by horse**

     X ● **W55.12**   **Struck by horse**

     X ● **W55.19**   **Other contact with horse**

   ● **W55.2**   **Contact with cow**
           Contact with bull

     X ● **W55.21**   **Bitten by cow**

     X ● **W55.22**   **Struck by cow**
               Gored by bull

     X ● **W55.29**   **Other contact with cow**

   ● **W55.3**   **Contact with other hoof stock**
           Contact with goats
           Contact with sheep

     X ● **W55.31**   **Bitten by other hoof stock**

     X ● **W55.32**   **Struck by other hoof stock**
               Gored by goat
               Gored by ram

     X ● **W55.39**   **Other contact with other hoof stock**

   ● **W55.4**   **Contact with pig**

     X ● **W55.41**   **Bitten by pig**

     X ● **W55.42**   **Struck by pig**

     X ● **W55.49**   **Other contact with pig**

   ● **W55.5**   **Contact with raccoon**

     X ● **W55.51**   **Bitten by raccoon**

     X ● **W55.52**   **Struck by raccoon**

     X ● **W55.59**   **Other contact with raccoon**

   ● **W55.8**   **Contact with other mammals**

     X ● **W55.81**   **Bitten by other mammals**

     X ● **W55.82**   **Struck by other mammals**

     X ● **W55.89**   **Other contact with other mammals**

● W56   **Contact with nonvenomous marine animal**

> **Excludes1**   contact with venomous marine animal (T63.-)
>
> The appropriate 7th character is to be added to each code from category W56
>
> | | |
> |---|---|
> | A | initial encounter |
> | D | subsequent encounter |
> | S | sequela |

   ● **W56.0**   **Contact with dolphin**

     X ● **W56.01**   **Bitten by dolphin**

     X ● **W56.02**   **Struck by dolphin**

     X ● **W56.09**   **Other contact with dolphin**

   ● **W56.1**   **Contact with sea lion**

     X ● **W56.11**   **Bitten by sea lion**

     X ● **W56.12**   **Struck by sea lion**

     X ● **W56.19**   **Other contact with sea lion**

   ● **W56.2**   **Contact with orca**
           Contact with killer whale

     X ● **W56.21**   **Bitten by orca**

     X ● **W56.22**   **Struck by orca**

     X ● **W56.29**   **Other contact with orca**

   ● **W56.3**   **Contact with other marine mammals**

     X ● **W56.31**   **Bitten by other marine mammals**

     X ● **W56.32**   **Struck by other marine mammals**

     X ● **W56.39**   **Other contact with other marine mammals**

   ● **W56.4**   **Contact with shark**

     X ● **W56.41**   **Bitten by shark**

     X ● **W56.42**   **Struck by shark**

     X ● **W56.49**   **Other contact with shark**

   ● **W56.5**   **Contact with other fish**

     X ● **W56.51**   **Bitten by other fish**

     X ● **W56.52**   **Struck by other fish**

     X ● **W56.59**   **Other contact with other fish**

   ● **W56.8**   **Contact with other nonvenomous marine animals**

     X ● **W56.81**   **Bitten by other nonvenomous marine animals**

     X ● **W56.82**   **Struck by other nonvenomous marine animals**

     X ● **W56.89**   **Other contact with other nonvenomous marine animals**

X ● W57   **Bitten or stung by nonvenomous insect and other nonvenomous arthropods**

> **Excludes1**   contact with venomous insects and arthropods (T63.2-, T63.3-, T63.4-)
>
> The appropriate 7th character is to be added to code W57
>
> | | |
> |---|---|
> | A | initial encounter |
> | D | subsequent encounter |
> | S | sequela |

● W58   **Contact with crocodile or alligator**

> The appropriate 7th character is to be added to each code from category W58
>
> | | |
> |---|---|
> | A | initial encounter |
> | D | subsequent encounter |
> | S | sequela |

   ● **W58.0**   **Contact with alligator**

     X ● **W58.01**   **Bitten by alligator**

     X ● **W58.02**   **Struck by alligator**

     X ● **W58.03**   **Crushed by alligator**

     X ● **W58.09**   **Other contact with alligator**

   ● **W58.1**   **Contact with crocodile**

     X ● **W58.11**   **Bitten by crocodile**

     X ● **W58.12**   **Struck by crocodile**

     X ● **W58.13**   **Crushed by crocodile**

     X ● **W58.19**   **Other contact with crocodile**

● **W59   Contact with other nonvenomous reptiles**

> **Excludes1**   contact with venomous reptile (T63.0-, T63.1-)

> The appropriate 7th character is to be added to each code from category W59

> | | |
> |---|---|
> | A | initial encounter |
> | D | subsequent encounter |
> | S | sequela |

   ● **W59.0   Contact with nonvenomous lizards**

     X ● **W59.01   Bitten by nonvenomous lizards**

     X ● **W59.02   Struck by nonvenomous lizards**

     X ● **W59.09   Other contact with nonvenomous lizards**
> Exposure to nonvenomous lizards

   ● **W59.1   Contact with nonvenomous snakes**

     X ● **W59.11   Bitten by nonvenomous snake**

     X ● **W59.12   Struck by nonvenomous snake**

     X ● **W59.13   Crushed by nonvenomous snake**

     X ● **W59.19   Other contact with nonvenomous snake**

   ● **W59.2   Contact with turtles**

> **Excludes1**   contact with tortoises (W59.8-)

     X ● **W59.21   Bitten by turtle**

     X ● **W59.22   Struck by turtle**

     X ● **W59.29   Other contact with turtle**
> Exposure to turtles

   ● **W59.8   Contact with other nonvenomous reptiles**

     X ● **W59.81   Bitten by other nonvenomous reptiles**

     X ● **W59.82   Struck by other nonvenomous reptiles**

     X ● **W59.83   Crushed by other nonvenomous reptiles**

     X ● **W59.89   Other contact with other nonvenomous reptiles**

X ● **W60   Contact with nonvenomous plant thorns and spines and sharp leaves**

> **Excludes1**   contact with venomous plants (T63.X7-)

> The appropriate 7th character is to be added to code W60

> | | |
> |---|---|
> | A | initial encounter |
> | D | subsequent encounter |
> | S | sequela |

● **W61   Contact with birds (domestic) (wild)**

> **Includes**   contact with excreta of birds

> The appropriate 7th character is to be added to each code from category W61

> | | |
> |---|---|
> | A | initial encounter |
> | D | subsequent encounter |
> | S | sequela |

   ● **W61.0   Contact with parrot**

     X ● **W61.01   Bitten by parrot**

     X ● **W61.02   Struck by parrot**

     X ● **W61.09   Other contact with parrot**
> Exposure to parrots

   ● **W61.1   Contact with macaw**

     X ● **W61.11   Bitten by macaw**

     X ● **W61.12   Struck by macaw**

     X ● **W61.19   Other contact with macaw**
> Exposure to macaws

   ● **W61.2   Contact with other psittacines**

     X ● **W61.21   Bitten by other psittacines**

     X ● **W61.22   Struck by other psittacines**

     X ● **W61.29   Other contact with other psittacines**
> Exposure to other psittacines

   ● **W61.3   Contact with chicken**

     X ● **W61.32   Struck by chicken**

     X ● **W61.33   Pecked by chicken**

     X ● **W61.39   Other contact with chicken**
> Exposure to chickens

   ● **W61.4   Contact with turkey**

     X ● **W61.42   Struck by turkey**

     X ● **W61.43   Pecked by turkey**

     X ● **W61.49   Other contact with turkey**

   ● **W61.5   Contact with goose**

     X ● **W61.51   Bitten by goose**

     X ● **W61.52   Struck by goose**

     X ● **W61.59   Other contact with goose**

   ● **W61.6   Contact with duck**

     X ● **W61.61   Bitten by duck**

     X ● **W61.62   Struck by duck**

     X ● **W61.69   Other contact with duck**

   ● **W61.9   Contact with other birds**

     X ● **W61.91   Bitten by other birds**

     X ● **W61.92   Struck by other birds**

     X ● **W61.99   Other contact with other birds**
> Contact with bird NOS

● **W62   Contact with nonvenomous amphibians**

> **Excludes1**   contact with venomous amphibians (T63.81-R63.83)

> The appropriate 7th character is to be added to each code from category W62

> | | |
> |---|---|
> | A | initial encounter |
> | D | subsequent encounter |
> | S | sequela |

X ● **W62.0   Contact with nonvenomous frogs**

X ● **W62.1   Contact with nonvenomous toads**

X ● **W62.9   Contact with other nonvenomous amphibians**

X ● **W64   Exposure to other animate mechanical forces**

> **Includes**   exposure to nonvenomous animal NOS

> **Excludes1**   contact with venomous animal (T63.-)

> The appropriate 7th character is to be added to code W64

> | | |
> |---|---|
> | A | initial encounter |
> | D | subsequent encounter |
> | S | sequela |

ACCIDENTAL NON-TRANSPORT DROWNING AND SUBMERSION (W65-W74)

> **Excludes1**   accidental drowning and submersion due to fall into water (W16.-)
> accidental drowning and submersion due to water transport accident (V90.-, V92.-)

> **Excludes2**   accidental drowning and submersion due to cataclysm (X34-X39)

X ● **W65   Accidental drowning and submersion while in bathtub**

> **Excludes1**   accidental drowning and submersion due to fall in (into) bathtub (W16.211)

> The appropriate 7th character is to be added to code W65

> | | |
> |---|---|
> | A | initial encounter |
> | D | subsequent encounter |
> | S | sequela |

X ● **W67   Accidental drowning and submersion while in swimming pool**

> **Excludes1**   accidental drowning and submersion due to fall into swimming pool (W16.011, W16.021, W16.031)
> accidental drowning and submersion due to striking into wall of swimming pool (W22.041)

> The appropriate 7th character is to be added to code W67

> | | |
> |---|---|
> | A | initial encounter |
> | D | subsequent encounter |
> | S | sequela |

X● **W69** **Accidental drowning and submersion while in natural water**
Accidental drowning and submersion while in lake
Accidental drowning and submersion while in open sea
Accidental drowning and submersion while in river
Accidental drowning and submersion while in stream

> **Excludes1**   accidental drowning and submersion due to fall into natural body of water (W16.111, W16.121, W16.131)

The appropriate 7th character is to be added to code W69

A	initial encounter
D	subsequent encounter
S	sequela

X● **W73** **Other specified cause of accidental non-transport drowning and submersion**
Accidental drowning and submersion while in quenching tank
Accidental drowning and submersion while in reservoir

> **Excludes1**   accidental drowning and submersion due to fall into other water (W16.311, W16.321, W16.331)

The appropriate 7th character is to be added to code W73

A	initial encounter
D	subsequent encounter
S	sequela

X● **W74** **Unspecified cause of accidental drowning and submersion**
Drowning NOS

The appropriate 7th character is to be added to code W74

A	initial encounter
D	subsequent encounter
S	sequela

EXPOSURE TO ELECTRIC CURRENT, RADIATION AND EXTREME AMBIENT AIR TEMPERATURE AND PRESSURE (W85-W99)

> **Excludes1**   exposure to:
> failure in dosage of radiation or temperature during surgical and medical care (Y63.2-Y63.5)
> lightning (T75.Ø-)
> natural cold (X31)
> natural heat (X3Ø)
> natural radiation NOS (X39)
> radiological procedure and radiotherapy (Y84.2)
> sunlight (X32)

X● **W85** **Exposure to electric transmission lines**
Broken power line

The appropriate 7th character is to be added to code W85

A	initial encounter
D	subsequent encounter
S	sequela

● **W86** **Exposure to other specified electric current**

The appropriate 7th character is to be added to each code from category W86

A	initial encounter
D	subsequent encounter
S	sequela

X● **W86.Ø** **Exposure to domestic wiring and appliances**
X● **W86.1** **Exposure to industrial wiring, appliances and electrical machinery**
Exposure to conductors
Exposure to control apparatus
Exposure to electrical equipment and machinery
Exposure to transformers

X● **W86.8** **Exposure to other electric current**
Exposure to wiring and appliances in or on farm (not farmhouse)
Exposure to wiring and appliances outdoors
Exposure to wiring and appliances in or on public building
Exposure to wiring and appliances in or on residential institutions
Exposure to wiring and appliances in or on schools

● **W88** **Exposure to ionizing radiation**

> **Excludes1**   exposure to sunlight (X32)

The appropriate 7th character is to be added to each code from category W88

A	initial encounter
D	subsequent encounter
S	sequela

X● **W88.Ø** **Exposure to X-rays**
X● **W88.1** **Exposure to radioactive isotopes**
X● **W88.8** **Exposure to other ionizing radiation**

● **W89** **Exposure to man-made visible and ultraviolet light**

> **Includes**   exposure to welding light (arc)
> **Excludes1**   exposure to sunlight (X32)

The appropriate 7th character is to be added to each code from category W89

A	initial encounter
D	subsequent encounter
S	sequela

X● **W89.Ø** **Exposure to welding light (arc)**
X● **W89.1** **Exposure to tanning bed**
X● **W89.8** **Exposure to other man-made visible and ultraviolet light**
X● **W89.9** **Exposure to unspecified man-made visible and ultraviolet light**

● **W90** **Exposure to other nonionizing radiation**

> **Excludes1**   exposure to sunlight (X32)

The appropriate 7th character is to be added to each code from category W90

A	initial encounter
D	subsequent encounter
S	sequela

X● **W90.Ø** **Exposure to radiofrequency**
X● **W90.1** **Exposure to infrared radiation**
X● **W90.2** **Exposure to laser radiation**
X● **W90.8** **Exposure to other nonionizing radiation**

X● **W92** **Exposure to excessive heat of man-made origin**

The appropriate 7th character is to be added to code W92

A	initial encounter
D	subsequent encounter
S	sequela

● **W93** **Exposure to excessive cold of man-made origin**

The appropriate 7th character is to be added to each code from category W93

A	initial encounter
D	subsequent encounter
S	sequela

● **W93.Ø** **Contact with or inhalation of dry ice**
X● **W93.Ø1** **Contact with dry ice**
X● **W93.Ø2** **Inhalation of dry ice**

▶ New   ⇒ Revised   ~~deleted~~ Deleted   **OGCR** Official Guidelines   X Assign placeholder X   ● Use Additional Character(s)

Excludes 1   Excludes 2   Includes   Use additional   Code first   Code also   Key words

- W93.1 Contact with or inhalation of liquid air
  - X● W93.11 Contact with liquid air
    - Contact with liquid hydrogen
    - Contact with liquid nitrogen
  - X● W93.12 Inhalation of liquid air
    - Inhalation of liquid hydrogen
    - Inhalation of liquid nitrogen
- X● W93.2 Prolonged exposure in deep freeze unit or refrigerator
- X● W93.8 Exposure to other excessive cold of man-made origin

- W94 Exposure to high and low air pressure and changes in air pressure

  The appropriate 7th character is to be added to each code from category W94

A	initial encounter
D	subsequent encounter
S	sequela

  - X● W94.0 Exposure to prolonged high air pressure
  - W94.1 Exposure to prolonged low air pressure
    - X● W94.11 Exposure to residence or prolonged visit at high altitude
    - X● W94.12 Exposure to other prolonged low air pressure
  - W94.2 Exposure to rapid changes in air pressure during ascent
    - X● W94.21 Exposure to reduction in atmospheric pressure while surfacing from deep-water diving
    - X● W94.22 Exposure to reduction in atmospheric pressure while surfacing from underground
    - X● W94.23 Exposure to sudden change in air pressure in aircraft during ascent
    - X● W94.29 Exposure to other rapid changes in air pressure during ascent
  - W94.3 Exposure to rapid changes in air pressure during descent
    - X● W94.31 Exposure to sudden change in air pressure in aircraft during descent
    - X● W94.32 Exposure to high air pressure from rapid descent in water
    - X● W94.39 Exposure to other rapid changes in air pressure during descent

- X● W99 Exposure to other man-made environmental factors

  The appropriate 7th character is to be added to code W99

A	initial encounter
D	subsequent encounter
S	sequela

EXPOSURE TO SMOKE, FIRE AND FLAMES (X00-X08)

Excludes1   arson (X97)

Excludes2   explosions (W35-W40)
lightning (T75.0-)
transport accident (V01-V99)

- X00 Exposure to uncontrolled fire in building or structure

  Includes   conflagration in building or structure

  Code first any associated cataclysm

  Excludes2   exposure to ignition or melting of nightwear (X05)
  exposure to ignition or melting of other clothing and apparel (X06.-)
  exposure to other specified smoke, fire and flames (X08.-)

  The appropriate 7th character is to be added to each code from category X00

A	initial encounter
D	subsequent encounter
S	sequela

  - X● X00.0 Exposure to flames in uncontrolled fire in building or structure
  - X● X00.1 Exposure to smoke in uncontrolled fire in building or structure

- X● X00.2 Injury due to collapse of burning building or structure in uncontrolled fire

  Excludes1   injury due to collapse of building not on fire (W20.1)

- X● X00.3 Fall from burning building or structure in uncontrolled fire
- X● X00.4 Hit by object from burning building or structure in uncontrolled fire
- X● X00.5 Jump from burning building or structure in uncontrolled fire
- X● X00.8 Other exposure to uncontrolled fire in building or structure

- X01 Exposure to uncontrolled fire, not in building or structure

  Includes   exposure to forest fire

  The appropriate 7th character is to be added to each code from category X01

A	initial encounter
D	subsequent encounter
S	sequela

  - X● X01.0 Exposure to flames in uncontrolled fire, not in building or structure
  - X● X01.1 Exposure to smoke in uncontrolled fire, not in building or structure
  - X● X01.3 Fall due to uncontrolled fire, not in building or structure
  - X● X01.4 Hit by object due to uncontrolled fire, not in building or structure
  - X● X01.8 Other exposure to uncontrolled fire, not in building or structure

- X02 Exposure to controlled fire in building or structure

  Includes   exposure to fire in fireplace exposure to fire in stove

  The appropriate 7th character is to be added to each code from category X02

A	initial encounter
D	subsequent encounter
S	sequela

  - X● X02.0 Exposure to flames in controlled fire in building or structure
  - X● X02.1 Exposure to smoke in controlled fire in building or structure
  - X● X02.2 Injury due to collapse of burning building or structure in controlled fire

    Excludes1   injury due to collapse of building not on fire (W20.1)

  - X● X02.3 Fall from burning building or structure in controlled fire
  - X● X02.4 Hit by object from burning building or structure in controlled fire
  - X● X02.5 Jump from burning building or structure in controlled fire
  - X● X02.8 Other exposure to controlled fire in building or structure

- X03 Exposure to controlled fire, not in building or structure

  Includes   exposure to bon fire exposure to camp fire exposure to trash fire

  The appropriate 7th character is to be added to each code from category X03

A	initial encounter
D	subsequent encounter
S	sequela

  - X● X03.0 Exposure to flames in controlled fire, not in building or structure
  - X● X03.1 Exposure to smoke in controlled fire, not in building or structure
  - X● X03.3 Fall due to controlled fire, not in building or structure
  - X● X03.4 Hit by object due to controlled fire, not in building or structure
  - X● X03.8 Other exposure to controlled fire, not in building or structure

X ● **X04**   **Exposure to ignition of highly flammable material**
     Exposure to ignition of gasoline
     Exposure to ignition of kerosene
     Exposure to ignition of petrol

     | **Excludes2** | exposure to ignition or melting of nightwear (X05)

                exposure to ignition or melting of other clothing and apparel (X06)

     The appropriate 7th character is to be added to code X04

       | A   initial encounter |
       | D   subsequent encounter |
       | S   sequela |

X ● **X05**   **Exposure to ignition or melting of nightwear**

     | **Excludes2** | exposure to uncontrolled fire in building or structure (X00.-)
                exposure to uncontrolled fire, not in building or structure (X01.-)
                exposure to controlled fire in building or structure (X02.-)
                exposure to controlled fire, not in building or structure (X03.-)
                exposure to ignition of highly flammable materials (X04.-)

     The appropriate 7th character is to be added to code X05

       | A   initial encounter |
       | D   subsequent encounter |
       | S   sequela |

● **X06**   **Exposure to ignition or melting of other clothing and apparel**

     | **Excludes2** | exposure to uncontrolled fire in building or structure (X00.-)
                exposure to uncontrolled fire, not in building or structure (X01.-)
                exposure to controlled fire in building or structure (X02.-)
                exposure to controlled fire, not in building or structure (X03.-)
                exposure to ignition of highly flammable materials (X04.-)

     The appropriate 7th character is to be added to each code from category X06

       | A   initial encounter |
       | D   subsequent encounter |
       | S   sequela |

X ● **X06.0**   Exposure to ignition of plastic jewelry
X ● **X06.1**   Exposure to melting of plastic jewelry
X ● **X06.2**   Exposure to ignition of other clothing and apparel
X ● **X06.3**   Exposure to melting of other clothing and apparel

● **X08**   **Exposure to other specified smoke, fire and flames**

     The appropriate 7th character is to be added to each code from category X08

       | A   initial encounter |
       | D   subsequent encounter |
       | S   sequela |

   ● **X08.0**   **Exposure to bed fire**
         Exposure to mattress fire

     X ● **X08.00**   **Exposure to bed fire due to unspecified burning material**
     X ● **X08.01**   **Exposure to bed fire due to burning cigarette**
     X ● **X08.09**   **Exposure to bed fire due to other burning material**

   ● **X08.1**   **Exposure to sofa fire**

     X ● **X08.10**   **Exposure to sofa fire due to unspecified burning material**
     X ● **X08.11**   **Exposure to sofa fire due to burning cigarette**
     X ● **X08.19**   **Exposure to sofa fire due to other burning material**

   ● **X08.2**   **Exposure to other furniture fire**

     X ● **X08.20**   **Exposure to other furniture fire due to unspecified burning material**
     X ● **X08.21**   **Exposure to other furniture fire due to burning cigarette**
     X ● **X08.29**   **Exposure to other furniture fire due to other burning material**

   X ● **X08.8**   **Exposure to other specified smoke, fire and flames**

CONTACT WITH HEAT AND HOT SUBSTANCES (X10-X19)

     | **Excludes1** | exposure to excessive natural heat (X30)
              ⟹ exposure to fire and flames (X00-X08)

● **X10**   **Contact with hot drinks, food, fats and cooking oils**

     The appropriate 7th character is to be added to each code from category X10

       | A   initial encounter |
       | D   subsequent encounter |
       | S   sequela |

X ● **X10.0**   **Contact with hot drinks**
X ● **X10.1**   **Contact with hot food**
X ● **X10.2**   **Contact with fats and cooking oils**

● **X11**   **Contact with hot tap-water**

     | **Includes** | contact with boiling tap-water
               contact with boiling water NOS

     | **Excludes1** | contact with water heated on stove (X12)

     The appropriate 7th character is to be added to each code from category X11

       | A   initial encounter |
       | D   subsequent encounter |
       | S   sequela |

X ● **X11.0**   **Contact with hot water in bath or tub**

     | **Excludes1** | contact with running hot water in bath or tub (X11.1)

X ● **X11.1**   **Contact with running hot water**
     Contact with hot water running out of hose
     Contact with hot water running out of tap

X ● **X11.8**   **Contact with other hot tap-water**
     Contact with hot water in bucket
     Contact with hot tap-water NOS

X ● **X12**   **Contact with other hot fluids**
     Contact with water heated on stove

     | **Excludes1** | hot (liquid) metals (X18)

     The appropriate 7th character is to be added to code X12

       | A   initial encounter |
       | D   subsequent encounter |
       | S   sequela |

● **X13**   **Contact with steam and other hot vapors**

     The appropriate 7th character is to be added to each code from category X13

       | A   initial encounter |
       | D   subsequent encounter |
       | S   sequela |

X ● **X13.0**   **Inhalation of steam and other hot vapors**
X ● **X13.1**   **Other contact with steam and other hot vapors**

▶ New   ⟹ Revised   ~~deleted~~ Deleted   **OGCR** Official Guidelines   X Assign placeholder X   ● Use Additional Character(s)

| Excludes 1 | Excludes 2 | Includes | Use additional | Code first | Code also | Key words |

● **X14**   **Contact with hot air and other hot gases**

The appropriate 7th character is to be added to each code from category X14

A	initial encounter
D	subsequent encounter
S	sequela

X ● **X14.0**   Inhalation of hot air and gases
X ● **X14.1**   Other contact with hot air and other hot gases

● **X15**   **Contact with hot household appliances**

Excludes1	contact with heating appliances (X16)
	contact with powered household appliances (W29.-)
	exposure to controlled fire in building or structure due to household appliance (X02.8)
	exposure to household appliances electrical current (W86.0)

The appropriate 7th character is to be added to each code from category X15

A	initial encounter
D	subsequent encounter
S	sequela

X ● **X15.0**   Contact with hot stove (kitchen)
X ● **X15.1**   Contact with hot toaster
X ● **X15.2**   Contact with hotplate
X ● **X15.3**   Contact with hot saucepan or skillet
X ● **X15.8**   Contact with other hot household appliances
     Contact with cooker
     Contact with kettle
     Contact with light bulbs

X ● **X16**   **Contact with hot heating appliances, radiators and pipes**

Excludes1	contact with powered appliances (W29.-)
	exposure to controlled fire in building or structure due to appliance (X02.8)
	exposure to industrial appliances electrical current (W86.1)

The appropriate 7th character is to be added to code X16

A	initial encounter
D	subsequent encounter
S	sequela

X ● **X17**   **Contact with hot engines, machinery and tools**

Excludes1	contact with hot heating appliances, radiators and pipes (X16)
	contact with hot household appliances (X15)

The appropriate 7th character is to be added to code X17

A	initial encounter
D	subsequent encounter
S	sequela

X ● **X18**   **Contact with other hot metals**

Contact with liquid metal

The appropriate 7th character is to be added to code X18

A	initial encounter
D	subsequent encounter
S	sequela

X ● **X19**   **Contact with other heat and hot substances**

Excludes1	objects that are not normally hot, e.g., an object made hot by a house fire (X00-X08)

The appropriate 7th character is to be added to code X19

A	initial encounter
D	subsequent encounter
S	sequela

EXPOSURE TO FORCES OF NATURE (X30-X39)

X ● **X30**   **Exposure to excessive natural heat**

Exposure to excessive heat as the cause of sunstroke
Exposure to heat NOS

Excludes1	excessive heat of man-made origin (W92)
	exposure to man-made radiation (W89)
	exposure to sunlight (X32)
	exposure to tanning bed (W89)

The appropriate 7th character is to be added to code X30

A	initial encounter
D	subsequent encounter
S	sequela

X ● **X31**   **Exposure to excessive natural cold**

Excessive cold as the cause of chilblains NOS
Excessive cold as the cause of immersion foot or hand
Exposure to cold NOS
Exposure to weather conditions

Excludes1	cold of man-made origin (W93.-)
	contact with or inhalation of dry ice (W93.-)
	contact with or inhalation of liquefied gas (W93.-)

The appropriate 7th character is to be added to code X31

A	initial encounter
D	subsequent encounter
S	sequela

X ● **X32**   **Exposure to sunlight**

Excludes1	man-made radiation (tanning bed) (W89)
▶ Excludes2	radiation-related disorders of the skin and subcutaneous tissue (L55-L59)

The appropriate 7th character is to be added to code X32

A	initial encounter
D	subsequent encounter
S	sequela

X ● **X34**   **Earthquake**

Excludes2	tidal wave (tsunami) due to earthquake (X37.41)

The appropriate 7th character is to be added to code X34

A	initial encounter
D	subsequent encounter
S	sequela

X ● **X35**   **Volcanic eruption**

Excludes2	tidal wave (tsunami) due to volcanic eruption (X37.41)

The appropriate 7th character is to be added to code X35

A	initial encounter
D	subsequent encounter
S	sequela

● **X36**   **Avalanche, landslide and other earth movements**

Includes	victim of mudslide of cataclysmic nature
Excludes1	earthquake (X34)
Excludes2	transport accident involving collision with avalanche or landslide not in motion (V01-V99)

The appropriate 7th character is to be added to each code from category X36

A	initial encounter
D	subsequent encounter
S	sequela

X ● **X36.0**   Collapse of dam or man-made structure causing earth movement
X ● **X36.1**   Avalanche, landslide, or mudslide

▶ New   ⇒ Revised   ~~deleted~~ Deleted   **OGCR** Official Guidelines   X Assign placeholder X   ● Use Additional Character(s)

Excludes 1	Excludes 2	Includes	Use additional	Code first	Code also	Key words

● **X37**   **Cataclysmic storm**

The appropriate 7th character is to be added to each code from category X37

> A   initial encounter
> D   subsequent encounter
> S   sequela

X ● **X37.0**   **Hurricane**
> Storm surge   Typhoon

X ● **X37.1**   **Tornado**
> Cyclone   Twister

X ● **X37.2**   **Blizzard (snow) (ice)**

X ● **X37.3**   **Dust storm**

● **X37.4**   **Tidalwave**

> X ● **X37.41**   **Tidal wave due to earthquake or volcanic eruption**
> > Tidal wave NOS
> > Tsunami

> X ● **X37.42**   **Tidal wave due to storm**

> X ● **X37.43**   **Tidal wave due to landslide**

X ● **X37.8**   **Other cataclysmic storms**
> Cloudburst
> Torrential rain
> > **Excludes2**   flood (X38)

X ● **X37.9**   **Unspecified cataclysmic storm**
> Storm NOS
> > **Excludes1**   collapse of dam or man-made structure causing earth movement (X39.0)

X ● **X38**   **Flood**
> Flood arising from remote storm
> Flood of cataclysmic nature arising from melting snow
> Flood resulting directly from storm
> > **Excludes1**   collapse of dam or man-made structure causing earth movement (X39.0)
> > tidal wave NOS (X37.41)
> > tidal wave caused by storm (X37.2)

> The appropriate 7th character is to be added to code X38

> > A   initial encounter
> > D   subsequent encounter
> > S   sequela

● **X39**   **Exposure to other forces of nature**

The appropriate 7th character is to be added to each code from category X39

> A   initial encounter
> D   subsequent encounter
> S   sequela

● **X39.0**   **Exposure to natural radiation**
> > **Excludes1**   contact with and (suspected) exposure to radon and other naturally occuring radiation (Z77.123)
> > exposure to man-made radiation (W88-W90)
> > exposure to sunlight (X32)

> X ● **X39.01**   **Exposure to radon**

> X ● **X39.08**   **Exposure to other natural radiation**

X ● **X39.8**   **Other exposure to forces of nature**

● **X50**   **Overexertion and strenuous or repetitive movements**

The appropriate 7th character is to be added to each code from category X50

> A   initial encounter
> D   subsequent encounter
> S   sequela

X ● **X50.0**   **Overexertion from strenuous movement or load**
> Lifting heavy objects
> Lifting weights

X ● **X50.1**   **Overexertion from prolonged static or awkward postures**
> Prolonged bending
> Prolonged kneeling
> Prolonged reaching
> Prolonged sitting
> Prolonged standing
> Prolonged twisting
> Static bending
> Static kneeling
> Static reaching
> Static sitting
> Static standing
> Static twisting

X ● **X50.3**   **Overexertion from repetitive movements**
> Use of hand as hammer
> > **Excludes2**   Overuse from prolonged static or awkward postures (X50.1)

X ● **X50.9**   **Other and unspecified overexertion or strenuous movements or postures**
> Contact pressure
> Contact stress

X ● **X52**   **Prolonged stay in weightless environment**
> Weightlessness in spacecraft (simulator)
> The appropriate 7th character is to be added to code X52

> > A   initial encounter
> > D   subsequent encounter
> > S   sequela

X ● **X58**   **Exposure to other specified factors**
> Accident NOS
> Exposure NOS
> The appropriate 7th character is to be added to code X58

> > A   initial encounter
> > D   subsequent encounter
> > S   sequela

Purposely self-inflicted injury
Suicide (attempted)

● **X71**   **Intentional self-harm by drowning and submersion**

The appropriate 7th character is to be added to each code from category X71

> A   initial encounter
> D   subsequent encounter
> S   sequela

X ● **X71.0**   **Intentional self-harm by drowning and submersion while in bathtub**

X ● **X71.1**   **Intentional self-harm by drowning and submersion while in swimming pool**

X ● **X71.2**   **Intentional self-harm by drowning and submersion after jump into swimming pool**

▶ New   ⟹ Revised   ~~deleted~~ Deleted   **OGCR** Official Guidelines   X Assign placeholder X   ● Use Additional Character(s)

Excludes 1   Excludes 2   Includes   Use additional   Code first   Code also   Key words

X ● **X71.3**   **Intentional self-harm by drowning and submersion in** natural water

X ● **X71.8**   Other **intentional self-harm by drowning and** submersion

X ● **X71.9**   **Intentional self-harm by drowning and submersion,** unspecified

X ● **X72**   Intentional self-harm by handgun **discharge**
     Intentional self-harm by gun for single hand use
     Intentional self-harm by pistol
     Intentional self-harm by revolver

    Excludes1   Very pistol (X74.8)

    The appropriate 7th character is to be added to code X72

A	initial encounter
D	subsequent encounter
S	sequela

● **X73**   **Intentional self-harm by rifle, shotgun and larger firearm** discharge

    Excludes1   airgun (X74.01)

    The appropriate 7th character is to be added to each code from category X73

A	initial encounter
D	subsequent encounter
S	sequela

X ● **X73.0**   **Intentional self-harm by** shotgun **discharge**

X ● **X73.1**   **Intentional self-harm by** hunting rifle **discharge**

X ● **X73.2**   **Intentional self-harm by** machine gun **discharge**

X ● **X73.8**   **Intentional self-harm by** other **larger firearm discharge**

X ● **X73.9**   **Intentional self-harm by** unspecified **larger firearm** discharge

● **X74**   **Intentional self-harm by other and unspecified firearm and gun** discharge

    The appropriate 7th character is to be added to each code from category X74

A	initial encounter
D	subsequent encounter
S	sequela

   ● **X74.0**   **Intentional self-harm by gas, air or spring-operated guns**

     X ● **X74.01**   **Intentional self-harm by** airgun
         Intentional self-harm by BB gun discharge
         Intentional self-harm by pellet gun discharge

     X ● **X74.02**   **Intentional self-harm by** paintball gun

     X ● **X74.09**   **Intentional self-harm by** other **gas, air or** spring-operated gun

   X ● **X74.8**   **Intentional self-harm by** other firearm **discharge**
     Intentional self-harm by Very pistol [flare] discharge

   X ● **X74.9**   **Intentional self-harm by** unspecified **firearm discharge**

X ● **X75**   **Intentional self-harm by explosive material**

    The appropriate 7th character is to be added to code X75

A	initial encounter
D	subsequent encounter
S	sequela

X ● **X76**   **Intentional self-harm by smoke, fire and flames**

    The appropriate 7th character is to be added to code X76

A	initial encounter
D	subsequent encounter
S	sequela

● **X77**   **Intentional self-harm by steam, hot vapors and hot objects**

    The appropriate 7th character is to be added to each code from category X77

A	initial encounter
D	subsequent encounter
S	sequela

X ● **X77.0**   **Intentional self-harm by** steam or hot vapors

X ● **X77.1**   **Intentional self-harm by** hot tap water

X ● **X77.2**   **Intentional self-harm by** other hot fluids

X ● **X77.3**   **Intentional self-harm by** hot household appliances

X ● **X77.8**   **Intentional self-harm by** other **hot objects**

X ● **X77.9**   **Intentional self-harm by** unspecified **hot objects**

● **X78**   **Intentional self-harm by sharp object**

    The appropriate 7th character is to be added to each code from category X78

A	initial encounter
D	subsequent encounter
S	sequela

X ● **X78.0**   **Intentional self-harm by sharp** glass

X ● **X78.1**   **Intentional self-harm by** knife

X ● **X78.2**   **Intentional self-harm by** sword or dagger

X ● **X78.8**   **Intentional self-harm by** other **sharp object**

X ● **X78.9**   **Intentional self-harm by** unspecified **sharp object**

X ● **X79**   **Intentional self-harm by blunt object**

    The appropriate 7th character is to be added to code X79

A	initial encounter
D	subsequent encounter
S	sequela

X ● **X80**   **Intentional self-harm by jumping from a high place**
     Intentional fall from one level to another

    The appropriate 7th character is to be added to code X80

A	initial encounter
D	subsequent encounter
S	sequela

● **X81**   **Intentional self-harm by jumping or lying in front of moving** object

    The appropriate 7th character is to be added to each code from category X81

A	initial encounter
D	subsequent encounter
S	sequela

X ● **X81.0**   **Intentional self-harm by jumping or lying in front of** motor vehicle

X ● **X81.1**   **Intentional self-harm by jumping or lying in front of (subway)** train

X ● **X81.8**   **Intentional self-harm by jumping or lying in front of** other moving object

● **X82**   **Intentional self-harm by crashing of motor vehicle**

    The appropriate 7th character is to be added to each code from category X82

A	initial encounter
D	subsequent encounter
S	sequela

X ● **X82.0**   **Intentional collision of motor vehicle with** other motor vehicle

X ● **X82.1**   **Intentional collision of motor vehicle with** train

X ● **X82.2**   **Intentional collision of motor vehicle with** tree

X ● **X82.8**   Other **intentional self-harm by crashing of motor vehicle**

▶ New   ⟹ Revised   ~~deleted~~ Deleted   **OGCR** Official Guidelines   X Assign placeholder X   ● Use Additional Character(s)

| Excludes 1 | Excludes 2 | Includes | Use additional | Code first | Code also | Key words |

● X83   **Intentional self-harm by other specified means**

> **Excludes1**   intentional self-harm by poisoning or contact with toxic substance - see Table of Drugs and Chemicals

> The appropriate 7th character is to be added to each code from category X83

> | A | initial encounter |
> |---|---|
> | D | subsequent encounter |
> | S | sequela |

X● **X83.0**   Intentional self-harm by crashing of aircraft
X● **X83.1**   Intentional self-harm by electrocution
X● **X83.2**   Intentional self-harm by exposure to extremes of cold
X● **X83.8**   Intentional self-harm by other specified means

ASSAULT (X92-Y09)

> **Includes**   homicide injuries inflicted by another person with intent to injure or kill, by any means

> **Excludes1**   injuries due to legal intervention (Y35.-)
> injuries due to operations of war (Y36.-)
> injuries due to terrorism (Y38.-)

● X92   **Assault by drowning and submersion**

> The appropriate 7th character is to be added to each code from category X92

> | A | initial encounter |
> |---|---|
> | D | subsequent encounter |
> | S | sequela |

X● **X92.0**   Assault by drowning and submersion while in bathtub
X● **X92.1**   Assault by drowning and submersion while in swimming pool
X● **X92.2**   Assault by drowning and submersion after push into swimming pool
X● **X92.3**   Assault by drowning and submersion in natural water
X● **X92.8**   Other assault by drowning and submersion
X● **X92.9**   Assault by drowning and submersion, unspecified

X●X93   **Assault by handgun discharge**
> Assault by discharge of gun for single hand use
> Assault by discharge of pistol
> Assault by discharge of revolver

> **Excludes1**   Very pistol (X95.8)

> The appropriate 7th character is to be added to code X93

> | A | initial encounter |
> |---|---|
> | D | subsequent encounter |
> | S | sequela |

● X94   **Assault by rifle, shotgun and larger firearm discharge**

> **Excludes1**   airgun (X95.01)

> The appropriate 7th character is to be added to each code from category X94

> | A | initial encounter |
> |---|---|
> | D | subsequent encounter |
> | S | sequela |

X● **X94.0**   Assault by shotgun
X● **X94.1**   Assault by hunting rifle
X● **X94.2**   Assault by machine gun
X● **X94.8**   Assault by other larger firearm discharge
X● **X94.9**   Assault by unspecified larger firearm discharge

● X95   **Assault by other and unspecified firearm and gun discharge**

> The appropriate 7th character is to be added to each code from category X95

> | A | initial encounter |
> |---|---|
> | D | subsequent encounter |
> | S | sequela |

● **X95.0**   **Assault by gas, air or spring-operated guns**
X● **X95.01**   Assault by airgun discharge
> Assault by BB gun discharge
> Assault by pellet gun discharge
X● **X95.02**   Assault by paintball gun discharge
X● **X95.09**   Assault by other gas, air or spring-operated gun
X● **X95.8**   Assault by other firearm discharge
> Assault by very pistol [flare] discharge
X● **X95.9**   Assault by unspecified firearm discharge

● X96   **Assault by explosive material**

> **Excludes1**   incendiary device (X97)
> terrorism involving explosive material (Y38.2-)

> The appropriate 7th character is to be added to each code from category X96

> | A | initial encounter |
> |---|---|
> | D | subsequent encounter |
> | S | sequela |

X● **X96.0**   Assault by antipersonnel bomb
> **Excludes1**   antipersonnel bomb use in military or war (Y36.2-)
X● **X96.1**   Assault by gasoline bomb
X● **X96.2**   Assault by letter bomb
X● **X96.3**   Assault by fertilizer bomb
X● **X96.4**   Assault by pipe bomb
X● **X96.8**   Assault by other specified explosive
X● **X96.9**   Assault by unspecified explosive

X●X97   **Assault by smoke, fire and flames**
> Assault by arson
> Assault by cigarettes
> Assault by incendiary device

> The appropriate 7th character is to be added to code X97

> | A | initial encounter |
> |---|---|
> | D | subsequent encounter |
> | S | sequela |

● X98   **Assault by steam, hot vapors and hot objects**

> The appropriate 7th character is to be added to each code from category X98

> | A | initial encounter |
> |---|---|
> | D | subsequent encounter |
> | S | sequela |

X● **X98.0**   Assault by steam or hot vapors
X● **X98.1**   Assault by hot tap water
X● **X98.2**   Assault by hot fluids
X● **X98.3**   Assault by hot household appliances
X● **X98.8**   Assault by other hot objects
X● **X98.9**   Assault by unspecified hot objects

▶ New   ⟹ Revised   ~~deleted~~ Deleted   OGCR Official Guidelines   X Assign placeholder X   ● Use Additional Character(s)

Excludes 1   Excludes 2   Includes   Use additional   Code first   Code also   Key words

⬤ **X99**   **Assault by sharp object**

     | **Excludes1** | assault by strike by sports equipment (Y08.0-) |

     The appropriate 7th character is to be added to each code from category X99

        | A | initial encounter |
        | D | subsequent encounter |
        | S | sequela |

X ⬤ **X99.0**   **Assault by sharp glass**
X ⬤ **X99.1**   **Assault by knife**
X ⬤ **X99.2**   **Assault by sword or dagger**
X ⬤ **X99.8**   **Assault by other sharp object**
X ⬤ **X99.9**   **Assault by unspecified sharp object**
         Assault by stabbing NOS

X ⬤ **Y00**   **Assault by blunt object**

     | **Excludes1** | assault by strike by sports equipment (Y08.0) |

     The appropriate 7th character is to be added to code Y00

        | A | initial encounter |
        | D | subsequent encounter |
        | S | sequela |

X ⬤ **Y01**   **Assault by pushing from high place**

     The appropriate 7th character is to be added to code Y01

        | A | initial encounter |
        | D | subsequent encounter |
        | S | sequela |

⬤ **Y02**   **Assault by pushing or placing victim in front of moving object**

     The appropriate 7th character is to be added to each code from category Y02

        | A | initial encounter |
        | D | subsequent encounter |
        | S | sequela |

X ⬤ **Y02.0**   **Assault by pushing or placing victim in front of motor vehicle**
X ⬤ **Y02.1**   **Assault by pushing or placing victim in front of (subway) train**
X ⬤ **Y02.8**   **Assault by pushing or placing victim in front of other moving object**

⬤ **Y03**   **Assault by crashing of motor vehicle**

     The appropriate 7th character is to be added to each code from category Y03

        | A | initial encounter |
        | D | subsequent encounter |
        | S | sequela |

X ⬤ **Y03.0**   **Assault by being hit or run over by motor vehicle**
X ⬤ **Y03.8**   **Other assault by crashing of motor vehicle**

⬤ **Y04**   **Assault by bodily force**

     | **Excludes1** | assault by: |
                   submersion (X92.-)
                   use of weapon (X93-X95, X99, Y00)

     The appropriate 7th character is to be added to each code from category Y04

        | A | initial encounter |
        | D | subsequent encounter |
        | S | sequela |

X ⬤ **Y04.0**   **Assault by unarmed brawl or fight**
X ⬤ **Y04.1**   **Assault by human bite**
X ⬤ **Y04.2**   **Assault by strike against or bumped into by another person**
X ⬤ **Y04.8**   **Assault by other bodily force**
         Assault by bodily force NOS

OGCR Section I.C.19.f.

> Adult and child abuse, neglect and other maltreatment
>
> Sequence first the appropriate code from categories T74 or T76 for abuse, neglect and other maltreatment, followed by any accompanying mental health or injury code(s).
>
> If the documentation in the medical record states abuse or neglect it is coded as confirmed (T74.-). It is coded as suspected if it is documented as suspected (T76.-).
>
> For cases of confirmed abuse or neglect an external cause code from the assault section (X92-Y09) should be added to identify the cause of any physical injuries. A perpetrator code (Y07) should be added when the perpetrator of the abuse is known. For suspected cases of abuse or neglect, do not report external cause or perpetrator code.
>
> If a suspected case of abuse, neglect or mistreatment is ruled out during an encounter code Z04.71, Encounter for examination and observation following alleged physical adult abuse, ruled out, or code Z04.72, Encounter for examination and observation following alleged adult rape, should be used, not a code from T76.
>
> If a suspected case of alleged rape or sexual abuse is ruled out during an encounter code Z04.41, Encounter for examination and observation following alleged adult rape, or code Z04.42, Encounter for examination and observation following alleged child rape should be used, not a code from T76.

⬤ **Y07**   **Perpetrator of assault, maltreatment and neglect**

     Note: Codes from this category are for use only in cases of confirmed abuse (T74.-)

         Selection of the correct perpetrator code is based on the relationship between the perpetrator and the victim

     | **Includes** | perpetrator of abandonment |
                   perpetrator of emotional neglect
                   perpetrator of mental cruelty
                   perpetrator of physical abuse
                   perpetrator of physical neglect
                   perpetrator of sexual abuse
                   perpetrator of torture

⬤ **Y07.0**   **Spouse or partner, perpetrator of maltreatment and neglect**
         Spouse or partner, perpetrator of maltreatment and neglect against spouse or partner

     Y07.01   **Husband, perpetrator of maltreatment and neglect**
     Y07.02   **Wife, perpetrator of maltreatment and neglect**
     Y07.03   **Male partner, perpetrator of maltreatment and neglect**
     Y07.04   **Female partner, perpetrator of maltreatment and neglect**

⬤ **Y07.1**   **Parent (adoptive) (biological), perpetrator of maltreatment and neglect**

     Y07.11   **Biological father, perpetrator of maltreatment and neglect**
     Y07.12   **Biological mother, perpetrator of maltreatment and neglect**
     Y07.13   **Adoptive father, perpetrator of maltreatment and neglect**
     Y07.14   **Adoptive mother, perpetrator of maltreatment and neglect**

⬤ **Y07.4**   **Other family member, perpetrator of maltreatment and neglect**

   ⬤ **Y07.41**   **Sibling, perpetrator of maltreatment and neglect**

     | **Excludes1** | stepsibling, perpetrator of maltreatment and neglect (Y07.435, Y07.436) |

     Y07.410   **Brother, perpetrator of maltreatment and neglect**
     Y07.411   **Sister, perpetrator of maltreatment and neglect**

▶ New   ⇒ Revised   ~~deleted~~ Deleted   **OGCR** Official Guidelines   X Assign placeholder X   ⬤ Use Additional Character(s)

| Excludes 1 | | Excludes 2 | | Includes | Use additional | | Code first | | Code also | | Key words |

● **Y07.42** Foster parent, perpetrator of maltreatment and neglect

    Y07.420 Foster father, perpetrator of maltreatment and neglect

    Y07.421 Foster mother, perpetrator of maltreatment and neglect

● **Y07.43** Stepparent or stepsibling, perpetrator of maltreatment and neglect

    Y07.430 Stepfather, perpetrator of maltreatment and neglect

    Y07.432 Male friend of parent (co-residing in household), perpetrator of maltreatment and neglect

    Y07.433 Stepmother, perpetrator of maltreatment and neglect

    Y07.434 Female friend of parent (co-residing in household), perpetrator of maltreatment and neglect

    Y07.435 Stepbrother, perpetrator or maltreatment and neglect

    Y07.436 Stepsister, perpetrator of maltreatment and neglect

● **Y07.49** Other family member, perpetrator of maltreatment and neglect

    Y07.490 Male cousin, perpetrator of maltreatment and neglect

    Y07.491 Female cousin, perpetrator of maltreatment and neglect

    Y07.499 Other family member, perpetrator of maltreatment and neglect

● **Y07.5** Non-family member, perpetrator of maltreatment and neglect

    Y07.50 Unspecified non-family member, perpetrator of maltreatment and neglect

● **Y07.51** Daycare provider, perpetrator of maltreatment and neglect

    Y07.510 At-home childcare provider, perpetrator of maltreatment and neglect

    Y07.511 Daycare center childcare provider, perpetrator of maltreatment and neglect

    Y07.512 At-home adultcare provider, perpetrator of maltreatment and neglect

    Y07.513 Adultcare center provider, perpetrator of maltreatment and neglect

    Y07.519 Unspecified daycare provider, perpetrator of maltreatment and neglect

● **Y07.52** Healthcare provider, perpetrator of maltreatment and neglect

    Y07.521 Mental health provider, perpetrator of maltreatment and neglect

    Y07.528 Other therapist or healthcare provider, perpetrator of maltreatment and neglect

        Nurse perpetrator of maltreatment and neglect

        Occupational therapist perpetrator of maltreatment and neglect

        Physical therapist perpetrator of maltreatment and neglect

        Speech therapist perpetrator of maltreatment and neglect

    Y07.529 Unspecified healthcare provider, perpetrator of maltreatment and neglect

    Y07.53 Teacher or instructor, perpetrator of maltreatment and neglect

        Coach, perpetrator of maltreatment and neglect

    Y07.59 Other non-family member, perpetrator of maltreatment and neglect

● **Y07.9** Unspecified perpetrator of maltreatment and neglect

● **Y08** Assault by other specified means

The appropriate 7th character is to be added to each code from category Y08

A	initial encounter
D	subsequent encounter
S	sequela

● **Y08.0** Assault by strike by sport equipment

X ● **Y08.01** Assault by strike by hockey stick

X ● **Y08.02** Assault by strike by baseball bat

X ● **Y08.09** Assault by strike by other specified type of sport equipment

● **Y08.8** Assault by other specified means

X ● **Y08.81** Assault by crashing of aircraft

X ● **Y08.89** Assault by other specified means

● **Y09** Assault by unspecified means

Assassination (attempted) NOS

Homicide (attempted) NOS

Manslaughter (attempted) NOS

Murder (attempted) NOS

EVENT OF UNDETERMINED INTENT (Y21-Y33)

Undetermined intent is only for use when there is specific documentation in the record that the intent of the injury cannot be determined. If no such documentation is present, code to accidental (unintentional)

● **Y21** Drowning and submersion, undetermined intent

The appropriate 7th character is to be added to each code from category Y21

A	initial encounter
D	subsequent encounter
S	sequela

X ● **Y21.0** Drowning and submersion while in bathtub, undetermined intent

X ● **Y21.1** Drowning and submersion after fall into bathtub, undetermined intent

X ● **Y21.2** Drowning and submersion while in swimming pool, undetermined intent

X ● **Y21.3** Drowning and submersion after fall into swimming pool, undetermined intent

X ● **Y21.4** Drowning and submersion in natural water, undetermined intent

X ● **Y21.8** Other drowning and submersion, undetermined intent

X ● **Y21.9** Unspecified drowning and submersion, undetermined intent

X ● **Y22** Handgun discharge, undetermined intent

Discharge of gun for single hand use, undetermined intent

Discharge of pistol, undetermined intent

Discharge of revolver, undetermined intent

Excludes2   very pistol (Y24.8)

The appropriate 7th character is to be added to code Y22

A	initial encounter
D	subsequent encounter
S	sequela

▶ New   ⇒ Revised   ~~deleted~~ Deleted   **OGCR** Official Guidelines   X Assign placeholder X   ● Use Additional Character(s)

Excludes 1   Excludes 2   Includes   Use additional   Code first   Code also   Key words

● **Y23**   **Rifle, shotgun and larger firearm** discharge, undetermined intent

     Excludes2   airgun (Y24.Ø)

     The appropriate 7th character is to be added to each code from category Y23

       A   initial encounter
       D   subsequent encounter
       S   sequela

X● **Y23.Ø**   **Shotgun** discharge, undetermined intent
X● **Y23.1**   **Hunting rifle** discharge, undetermined intent
X● **Y23.2**   **Military firearm** discharge, undetermined intent
X● **Y23.3**   **Machine gun** discharge, undetermined intent
X● **Y23.8**   **Other** larger firearm discharge, undetermined intent
X● **Y23.9**   **Unspecified** larger firearm discharge, undetermined intent

● **Y24**   **Other and unspecified firearm discharge, undetermined intent**

     The appropriate 7th character is to be added to each code from category Y24

       A   initial encounter
       D   subsequent encounter
       S   sequela

X● **Y24.Ø**   **Airgun** discharge, undetermined intent
       BB gun discharge, undetermined intent
       Pellet gun discharge, undetermined intent
X● **Y24.8**   **Other firearm** discharge, undetermined intent
       Paintball gun discharge, undetermined intent
       Very pistol [flare] discharge, undetermined intent
X● **Y24.9**   **Unspecified** firearm discharge, undetermined intent

X● **Y25**   **Contact with explosive material, undetermined intent**

     The appropriate 7th character is to be added to code Y25

       A   initial encounter
       D   subsequent encounter
       S   sequela

X● **Y26**   **Exposure to smoke, fire and flames, undetermined intent**

     The appropriate 7th character is to be added to code Y26

       A   initial encounter
       D   subsequent encounter
       S   sequela

● **Y27**   **Contact with steam, hot vapors and hot objects, undetermined intent**

     The appropriate 7th character is to be added to each code from category Y27

       A   initial encounter
       D   subsequent encounter
       S   sequela

X● **Y27.Ø**   Contact with **steam and hot vapors,** undetermined intent
X● **Y27.1**   Contact with **hot tap water,** undetermined intent
X● **Y27.2**   Contact with **hot fluids,** undetermined intent
X● **Y27.3**   Contact with **hot household appliance,** undetermined intent
X● **Y27.8**   Contact with **other hot objects,** undetermined intent
X● **Y27.9**   Contact with **unspecified** hot objects, undetermined intent

● **Y28**   **Contact with sharp object, undetermined intent**

     The appropriate 7th character is to be added to each code from category Y28

       A   initial encounter
       D   subsequent encounter
       S   sequela

X● **Y28.Ø**   Contact with sharp **glass,** undetermined intent
X● **Y28.1**   Contact with **knife,** undetermined intent
X● **Y28.2**   Contact with **sword or dagger,** undetermined intent
X● **Y28.8**   Contact with **other** sharp object, undetermined intent
X● **Y28.9**   Contact with **unspecified** sharp object, undetermined intent

X● **Y29**   **Contact with blunt object, undetermined intent**

     The appropriate 7th character is to be added to code Y29

       A   initial encounter
       D   subsequent encounter
       S   sequela

X● **Y30**   **Falling, jumping or pushed from a high place, undetermined intent**

     Victim falling from one level to another, undetermined intent

     The appropriate 7th character is to be added to code Y30

       A   initial encounter
       D   subsequent encounter
       S   sequela

X● **Y31**   **Falling, lying or running before or into moving object, undetermined intent**

     The appropriate 7th character is to be added to code Y31

       A   initial encounter
       D   subsequent encounter
       S   sequela

X● **Y32**   **Crashing of motor vehicle, undetermined intent**

     The appropriate 7th character is to be added to code Y32

       A   initial encounter
       D   subsequent encounter
       S   sequela

X● **Y33**   **Other specified events, undetermined intent**

     The appropriate 7th character is to be added to code Y33

       A   initial encounter
       D   subsequent encounter
       S   sequela

CHAPTER 2Ø (VØ1-Y99)

▶ New   ⟹ Revised   ~~deleted~~ Deleted   **OGCR** Official Guidelines   X Assign placeholder X   ● Use Additional Character(s)

Excludes 1   Excludes 2   Includes   Use additional   Code first   Code also   Key words

LEGAL INTERVENTION, OPERATIONS OF WAR, MILITARY OPERATIONS, AND TERRORISM (Y35-Y38)

● **Y35   Legal intervention**

Includes   any injury sustained as a result of an encounter with any law enforcement official, serving in any capacity at the time of the encounter, whether on-duty or off-duty. Includes: injury to law enforcement official, suspect and bystander

The appropriate 7th character is to be added to each code from category Y35

> A   initial encounter
> D   subsequent encounter
> S   sequela

● **Y35.0   Legal intervention involving firearm discharge**

  ● **Y35.00   Legal intervention involving unspecified firearm discharge**
    Legal intervention involving gunshot wound
    Legal intervention involving shot NOS

    ● **Y35.001   Legal intervention involving unspecified firearm discharge, law enforcement official injured**

    ● **Y35.002   Legal intervention involving unspecified firearm discharge, bystander injured**

    ● **Y35.003   Legal intervention involving unspecified firearm discharge, suspect injured**

  ● **Y35.01   Legal intervention involving injury by machine gun**

    ● **Y35.011   Legal intervention involving injury by machine gun, law enforcement official injured**

    ● **Y35.012   Legal intervention involving injury by machine gun, bystander injured**

    ● **Y35.013   Legal intervention involving injury by machine gun, suspect injured**

  ● **Y35.02   Legal intervention involving injury by handgun**

    ● **Y35.021   Legal intervention involving injury by handgun, law enforcement official injured**

    ● **Y35.022   Legal intervention involving injury by handgun, bystander injured**

    ● **Y35.023   Legal intervention involving injury by handgun, suspect injured**

  ● **Y35.03   Legal intervention involving injury by rifle pellet**

    ● **Y35.031   Legal intervention involving injury by rifle pellet, law enforcement official injured**

    ● **Y35.032   Legal intervention involving injury by rifle pellet, bystander injured**

    ● **Y35.033   Legal intervention involving injury by rifle pellet, suspect injured**

  ● **Y35.04   Legal intervention involving injury by rubber bullet**

    ● **Y35.041   Legal intervention involving injury by rubber bullet, law enforcement official injured**

    ● **Y35.042   Legal intervention involving injury by rubber bullet, bystander injured**

    ● **Y35.043   Legal intervention involving injury by rubber bullet, suspect injured**

● **Y35.09   Legal intervention involving other firearm discharge**

    ● **Y35.091   Legal intervention involving other firearm discharge, law enforcement official injured**

    ● **Y35.092   Legal intervention involving other firearm discharge, bystander injured**

    ● **Y35.093   Legal intervention involving other firearm discharge, suspect injured**

● **Y35.1   Legal intervention involving explosives**

  ● **Y35.10   Legal intervention involving unspecified explosives**

    ● **Y35.101   Legal intervention involving unspecified explosives, law enforcement official injured**

    ● **Y35.102   Legal intervention involving unspecified explosives, bystander injured**

    ● **Y35.103   Legal intervention involving unspecified explosives, suspect injured**

  ● **Y35.11   Legal intervention involving injury by dynamite**

    ● **Y35.111   Legal intervention involving injury by dynamite, law enforcement official injured**

    ● **Y35.112   Legal intervention involving injury by dynamite, bystander injured**

    ● **Y35.113   Legal intervention involving injury by dynamite, suspect injured**

  ● **Y35.12   Legal intervention involving injury by explosive shell**

    ● **Y35.121   Legal intervention involving injury by explosive shell, law enforcement official injured**

    ● **Y35.122   Legal intervention involving injury by explosive shell, bystander injured**

    ● **Y35.123   Legal intervention involving injury by explosive shell, suspect injured**

  ● **Y35.19   Legal intervention involving other explosives**
    Legal intervention involving injury by grenade
    Legal intervention involving injury by mortar bomb

    ● **Y35.191   Legal intervention involving other explosives, law enforcement official injured**

    ● **Y35.192   Legal intervention involving other explosives, bystander injured**

    ● **Y35.193   Legal intervention involving other explosives, suspect injured**

● **Y35.2   Legal intervention involving gas**
  Legal intervention involving asphyxiation by gas
  Legal intervention involving poisoning by gas

  ● **Y35.20   Legal intervention involving unspecified gas**

    ● **Y35.201   Legal intervention involving unspecified gas, law enforcement official injured**

    ● **Y35.202   Legal intervention involving unspecified gas, bystander injured**

    ● **Y35.203   Legal intervention involving unspecified gas, suspect injured**

▶ New   ⇒ Revised   ~~deleted~~ Deleted   **OGCR** Official Guidelines   X Assign placeholder X   ● Use Additional Character(s)

Excludes 1   Excludes 2   Includes   Use additional   Code first   Code also   Key words

- ● Y35.21   Legal intervention involving injury by tear gas
  - ● Y35.211   Legal intervention involving injury by tear gas, law enforcement official injured
  - ● Y35.212   Legal intervention involving injury by tear gas, bystander injured
  - ● Y35.213   Legal intervention involving injury by tear gas, suspect injured
- ● Y35.29   Legal intervention involving other gas
  - ● Y35.291   Legal intervention involving other gas, law enforcement official injured
  - ● Y35.292   Legal intervention involving other gas, bystander injured
  - ● Y35.293   Legal intervention involving other gas, suspect injured
- ● Y35.3   Legal intervention involving blunt objects
  Legal intervention involving being hit or struck by blunt object
  - ● Y35.30   Legal intervention involving unspecified blunt objects
    - ● Y35.301   Legal intervention involving unspecified blunt objects, law enforcement official injured
    - ● Y35.302   Legal intervention involving unspecified blunt objects, bystander injured
    - ● Y35.303   Legal intervention involving unspecified blunt objects, suspect injured
  - ● Y35.31   Legal intervention involving baton
    - ● Y35.311   Legal intervention involving baton, law enforcement official injured
    - ● Y35.312   Legal intervention involving baton, bystander injured
    - ● Y35.313   Legal intervention involving baton, suspect injured
  - ● Y35.39   Legal intervention involving other blunt objects
    - ● Y35.391   Legal intervention involving other blunt objects, law enforcement official injured
    - ● Y35.392   Legal intervention involving other blunt objects, bystander injured
    - ● Y35.393   Legal intervention involving other blunt objects, suspect injured
- ● Y35.4   Legal intervention involving sharp objects
  Legal intervention involving being cut by sharp objects
  Legal intervention involving being stabbed by sharp objects
  - ● Y35.40   Legal intervention involving unspecified sharp objects
    - ● Y35.401   Legal intervention involving unspecified sharp objects, law enforcement official injured
    - ● Y35.402   Legal intervention involving unspecified sharp objects, bystander injured
    - ● Y35.403   Legal intervention involving unspecified sharp objects, suspect injured
  - ● Y35.41   Legal intervention involving bayonet
    - ● Y35.411   Legal intervention involving bayonet, law enforcement official injured
    - ● Y35.412   Legal intervention involving bayonet, bystander injured
    - ● Y35.413   Legal intervention involving bayonet, suspect injured

- ● Y35.49   Legal intervention involving other sharp objects
  - ● Y35.491   Legal intervention involving other sharp objects, law enforcement official injured
  - ● Y35.492   Legal intervention involving other sharp objects, bystander injured
  - ● Y35.493   Legal intervention involving other sharp objects, suspect injured
- ● Y35.8   Legal intervention involving other specified means
  - ● Y35.81   Legal intervention involving manhandling
    - ● Y35.811   Legal intervention involving manhandling, law enforcement official injured
    - ● Y35.812   Legal intervention involving manhandling, bystander injured
    - ● Y35.813   Legal intervention involving manhandling, suspect injured
  - ● Y35.89   Legal intervention involving other specified means
    - ● Y35.891   Legal intervention involving other specified means, law enforcement official injured
    - ● Y35.892   Legal intervention involving other specified means, bystander injured
    - ● Y35.893   Legal intervention involving other specified means, suspect injured
- ● Y35.9   Legal intervention, means unspecified
  - X ● Y35.91   Legal intervention, means unspecified, law enforcement official injured
  - X ● Y35.92   Legal intervention, means unspecified, bystander injured
  - X ● Y35.93   Legal intervention, means unspecified, suspect injured

- ● Y36   Operations of war

Includes	injuries to military personnel and civilians caused by war, civil insurrection, and peacekeeping missions
Excludes1	injury to military personnel occurring during peacetime military operations (Y37.-) military vehicles involved in transport accidents with non-military vehicle during peacetime (V09.01, V09.21, V19.81, V29.81, V39.81, V49.81, V59.81, V69.81, V79.81)

  The appropriate 7th character is to be added to each code from category Y36

A	initial encounter
D	subsequent encounter
S	sequela

  - ● Y36.0   War operations involving explosion of marine weapons
    Weapons and military watercraft
    - ● Y36.00   War operations involving explosion of unspecified marine weapon
      War operations involving underwater blast NOS
      - ● Y36.000   War operations involving explosion of unspecified marine weapon, military personnel
      - ● Y36.001   War operations involving explosion of unspecified marine weapon, civilian
    - ● Y36.01   War operations involving explosion of depth-charge
      - ● Y36.010   War operations involving explosion of depth-charge, military personnel
      - ● Y36.011   War operations involving explosion of depth-charge, civilian

- Y36.02 **War operations involving explosion of marine mine**
  War operations involving explosion of marine mine, at sea or in harbor
  - Y36.020 War operations involving explosion of marine mine, military personnel
  - Y36.021 War operations involving explosion of marine mine, civilian
- Y36.03 **War operations involving explosion of sea-based artillery shell**
  - Y36.030 War operations involving explosion of sea-based artillery shell, military personnel
  - Y36.031 War operations involving explosion of sea-based artillery shell, civilian
- Y36.04 **War operations involving explosion of torpedo**
  - Y36.040 War operations involving explosion of torpedo, military personnel
  - Y36.041 War operations involving explosion of torpedo, civilian
- Y36.05 **War operations involving accidental detonation of onboard marine weapons**
  - Y36.050 War operations involving accidental detonation of onboard marine weapons, military personnel
  - Y36.051 War operations involving accidental detonation of onboard marine weapons, civilian
- Y36.09 **War operations involving explosion of other marine weapons**
  - Y36.090 War operations involving explosion of other marine weapons, military personnel
  - Y36.091 War operations involving explosion of other marine weapons, civilian
- Y36.1 **War operations involving destruction of aircraft**
  - Y36.10 **War operations involving unspecified destruction of aircraft**
    - Y36.100 War operations involving unspecified destruction of aircraft, military personnel
    - Y36.101 War operations involving unspecified destruction of aircraft, civilian
  - Y36.11 **War operations involving destruction of aircraft due to enemy fire or explosives**
    War operations involving destruction of aircraft due to air to air missile
    War operations involving destruction of aircraft due to explosive placed on aircraft
    War operations involving destruction of aircraft due to rocket propelled grenade [RPG]
    War operations involving destruction of aircraft due to small arms fire
    War operations involving destruction of aircraft due to surface to air missile
    - Y36.110 War operations involving destruction of aircraft due to enemy fire or explosives, military personnel
    - Y36.111 War operations involving destruction of aircraft due to enemy fire or explosives, civilian
  - Y36.12 **War operations involving destruction of aircraft due to collision with other aircraft**
    - Y36.120 War operations involving destruction of aircraft due to collision with other aircraft, military personnel
    - Y36.121 War operations involving destruction of aircraft due to collision with other aircraft, civilian

- Y36.13 **War operations involving destruction of aircraft due to onboard fire**
  - Y36.130 War operations involving destruction of aircraft due to onboard fire, military personnel
  - Y36.131 War operations involving destruction of aircraft due to onboard fire, civilian
- Y36.14 **War operations involving destruction of aircraft due to accidental detonation of onboard munitions and explosives**
  - Y36.140 War operations involving destruction of aircraft due to accidental detonation of onboard munitions and explosives, military personnel
  - Y36.141 War operations involving destruction of aircraft due to accidental detonation of onboard munitions and explosives, civilian
- Y36.19 **War operations involving other destruction of aircraft**
  - Y36.190 War operations involving other destruction of aircraft, military personnel
  - Y36.191 War operations involving other destruction of aircraft, civilian
- Y36.2 **War operations involving other explosions and fragments**

  Excludes1
  war operations involving explosion of aircraft (Y36.1-)
  war operations involving explosion of marine weapons (Y36.0-)
  war operations involving explosion of nuclear weapons (Y36.5-)
  war operations involving explosion occurring after cessation of hostilities (Y36.8-)
  - Y36.20 **War operations involving unspecified explosion and fragments**
    War operations involving air blast NOS
    War operations involving blast NOS
    War operations involving blast fragments NOS
    War operations involving blast wave NOS
    War operations involving blast wind NOS
    War operations involving explosion NOS
    War operations involving explosion of bomb NOS
    - Y36.200 War operations involving unspecified explosion and fragments, military personnel
    - Y36.201 War operations involving unspecified explosion and fragments, civilian
  - Y36.21 **War operations involving explosion of aerial bomb**
    - Y36.210 War operations involving explosion of aerial bomb, military personnel
    - Y36.211 War operations involving explosion of aerial bomb, civilian
  - Y36.22 **War operations involving explosion of guided missile**
    - Y36.220 War operations involving explosion of guided missile, military personnel
    - Y36.221 War operations involving explosion of guided missile, civilian

▶ New   ⟹ Revised   ~~deleted~~ Deleted   **OGCR** Official Guidelines   X Assign placeholder X   ● Use Additional Character(s)

Excludes 1   Excludes 2   Includes   Use additional   Code first   Code also   Key words

● **Y36.23 War operations involving explosion of improvised explosive device [IED]**
War operations involving explosion of person-borne improvised explosive device [IED]
War operations involving explosion of vehicle-borne improvised explosive device [IED]
War operations involving explosion of roadside improvised explosive device [IED]

     ● **Y36.230 War operations involving explosion of improvised explosive device [IED], military personnel**

     ● **Y36.231 War operations involving explosion of improvised explosive device [IED], civilian**

● **Y36.24 War operations involving explosion due to accidental detonation and discharge of own munitions or munitions launch device**

     ● **Y36.240 War operations involving explosion due to accidental detonation and discharge of own munitions or munitions launch device, military personnel**

     ● **Y36.241 War operations involving explosion due to accidental detonation and discharge of own munitions or munitions launch device, civilian**

● **Y36.25 War operations involving fragments from munitions**

     ● **Y36.250 War operations involving fragments from munitions, military personnel**

     ● **Y36.251 War operations involving fragments from munitions, civilian**

● **Y36.26 War operations involving fragments of improvised explosive device [IED]**
War operations involving fragments of person-borne improvised explosive device [IED]
War operations involving fragments of vehicle-borne improvised explosive device [IED]
War operations involving fragments of roadside improvised explosive device [IED]

     ● **Y36.260 War operations involving fragments of improvised explosive device [IED], military personnel**

     ● **Y36.261 War operations involving fragments of improvised explosive device [IED], civilian**

● **Y36.27 War operations involving fragments from weapons**

     ● **Y36.270 War operations involving fragments from weapons, military personnel**

     ● **Y36.271 War operations involving fragments from weapons, civilian**

● **Y36.29 War operations involving other explosions and fragments**
War operations involving explosion of grenade
War operations involving explosions of land mine
War operations involving shrapnel NOS

     ● **Y36.290 War operations involving other explosions and fragments, military personnel**

     ● **Y36.291 War operations involving other explosions and fragments, civilian**

● **Y36.3 War operations involving fires, conflagrations and hot substances**
War operations involving smoke, fumes, and heat from fires, conflagrations and hot substances

     Excludes1   war operations involving fires and conflagrations aboard military aircraft (Y36.1-)
               war operations involving fires and conflagrations aboard military watercraft (Y36.0-)
               war operations involving fires and conflagrations caused indirectly by conventional weapons (Y36.2-)
               war operations involving fires and thermal effects of nuclear weapons (Y36.53-)

     ● **Y36.30 War operations involving unspecified fire, conflagration and hot substance**

         ● **Y36.300 War operations involving unspecified fire, conflagration and hot substance, military personnel**

         ● **Y36.301 War operations involving unspecified fire, conflagration and hot substance, civilian**

     ● **Y36.31 War operations involving gasoline bomb**
War operations involving incendiary bomb
War operations involving petrol bomb

         ● **Y36.310 War operations involving gasoline bomb, military personnel**

         ● **Y36.311 War operations involving gasoline bomb, civilian**

     ● **Y36.32 War operations involving incendiary bullet**

         ● **Y36.320 War operations involving incendiary bullet, military personnel**

         ● **Y36.321 War operations involving incendiary bullet, civilian**

     ● **Y36.33 War operations involving flamethrower**

         ● **Y36.330 War operations involving flamethrower, military personnel**

         ● **Y36.331 War operations involving flamethrower, civilian**

     ● **Y36.39 War operations involving other fires, conflagrations and hot substances**

         ● **Y36.390 War operations involving other fires, conflagrations and hot substances, military personnel**

         ● **Y36.391 War operations involving other fires, conflagrations and hot substances, civilian**

● **Y36.4 War operations involving firearm discharge and other forms of conventional warfare**

     ● **Y36.41 War operations involving rubber bullets**

         ● **Y36.410 War operations involving rubber bullets, military personnel**

         ● **Y36.411 War operations involving rubber bullets, civilian**

     ● **Y36.42 War operations involving firearms pellets**

         ● **Y36.420 War operations involving firearms pellets, military personnel**

         ● **Y36.421 War operations involving firearms pellets, civilian**

● **Y36.43** **War operations involving other firearms discharge**
War operations involving bullets NOS

> Excludes1   war operations involving
> munitions fragments
> (Y36.25-)
> war operations involving
> incendiary bullets (Y36.32-)

   ● **Y36.430** **War operations involving other firearms discharge, military personnel**

   ● **Y36.431** **War operations involving other firearms discharge, civilian**

● **Y36.44** **War operations involving unarmed hand to hand combat**

> Excludes1   war operations involving combat
> using blunt or piercing
> object (Y36.45-)
> war operations involving
> intentional restriction of air
> and airway (Y36.46-)
> war operations involving
> unintentional restriction of
> air and airway (Y36.47-)

   ● **Y36.440** **War operations involving unarmed hand to hand combat, military personnel**

   ● **Y36.441** **War operations involving unarmed hand to hand combat, civilian**

● **Y36.45** **War operations involving combat using blunt or piercing object**

   ● **Y36.450** **War operations involving combat using blunt or piercing object, military personnel**

   ● **Y36.451** **War operations involving combat using blunt or piercing object, civilian**

● **Y36.46** **War operations involving intentional restriction of air and airway**

   ● **Y36.460** **War operations involving intentional restriction of air and airway, military personnel**

   ● **Y36.461** **War operations involving intentional restriction of air and airway, civilian**

● **Y36.47** **War operations involving unintentional restriction of air and airway**

   ● **Y36.470** **War operations involving unintentional restriction of air and airway, military personnel**

   ● **Y36.471** **War operations involving unintentional restriction of air and airway, civilian**

● **Y36.49** **War operations involving other forms of conventional warfare**

   ● **Y36.490** **War operations involving other forms of conventional warfare, military personnel**

   ● **Y36.491** **War operations involving other forms of conventional warfare, civilian**

● **Y36.5** **War operations involving nuclear weapons**
War operations involving dirty bomb NOS

● **Y36.50** **War operations involving unspecified effect of nuclear weapon**

   ● **Y36.500** **War operations involving unspecified effect of nuclear weapon, military personnel**

   ● **Y36.501** **War operations involving unspecified effect of nuclear weapon, civilian**

● **Y36.51** **War operations involving direct blast effect of nuclear weapon**
War operations involving blast pressure of nuclear weapon

   ● **Y36.510** **War operations involving direct blast effect of nuclear weapon, military personnel**

   ● **Y36.511** **War operations involving direct blast effect of nuclear weapon, civilian**

● **Y36.52** **War operations involving indirect blast effect of nuclear weapon**
War operations involving being thrown by blast of nuclear weapon
War operations involving being struck or crushed by blast debris of nuclear weapon

   ● **Y36.520** **War operations involving indirect blast effect of nuclear weapon, military personnel**

   ● **Y36.521** **War operations involving indirect blast effect of nuclear weapon, civilian**

● **Y36.53** **War operations involving thermal radiation effect of nuclear weapon**
War operations involving direct heat from nuclear weapon
War operation involving fireball effects from nuclear weapon

   ● **Y36.530** **War operations involving thermal radiation effect of nuclear weapon, military personnel**

   ● **Y36.531** **War operations involving thermal radiation effect of nuclear weapon, civilian**

● **Y36.54** **War operation involving nuclear radiation effects of nuclear weapon**
War operation involving acute radiation exposure from nuclear weapon
War operation involving exposure to immediate ionizing radiation from nuclear weapon
War operation involving fallout exposure from nuclear weapon
War operation involving secondary effects of nuclear weapons

   ● **Y36.540** **War operation involving nuclear radiation effects of nuclear weapon, military personnel**

   ● **Y36.541** **War operation involving nuclear radiation effects of nuclear weapon, civilian**

● **Y36.59** **War operation involving other effects of nuclear weapons**

   ● **Y36.590** **War operation involving other effects of nuclear weapons, military personnel**

   ● **Y36.591** **War operation involving other effects of nuclear weapons, civilian**

● **Y36.6** **War operations involving biological weapons**

● **Y36.6X** **War operations involving biological weapons**

   ● **Y36.6X0** **War operations involving biological weapons, military personnel**

   ● **Y36.6X1** **War operations involving biological weapons, civilian**

▶ New   ⇒ Revised   ~~deleted~~ Deleted   **OGCR** Official Guidelines   X Assign placeholder X   ● Use Additional Character(s)

Excludes 1   Excludes 2   Includes   Use additional   Code first   Code also   Key words

● **Y36.7 War operations involving chemical weapons and other forms of unconventional warfare**

> **Excludes1**   war operations involving incendiary devices (Y36.3-, Y36.5-)

● **Y36.7X War operations involving chemical weapons and other forms of unconventional warfare**

● **Y36.7X0 War operations involving chemical weapons and other forms of unconventional warfare, military personnel**

● **Y36.7X1 War operations involving chemical weapons and other forms of unconventional warfare, civilian**

● **Y36.8 War operations occurring after cessation of hostilities**

> War operations classifiable to categories Y36.0-Y36.8 but occurring after cessation of hostilities

● **Y36.81 Explosion of mine placed during war operations but exploding after cessation of hostilities**

● **Y36.810 Explosion of mine placed during war operations but exploding after cessation of hostilities, military personnel**

● **Y36.811 Explosion of mine placed during war operations but exploding after cessation of hostilities, civilian**

● **Y36.82 Explosion of bomb placed during war operations but exploding after cessation of hostilities**

● **Y36.820 Explosion of bomb placed during war operations but exploding after cessation of hostilities, military personnel**

● **Y36.821 Explosion of bomb placed during war operations but exploding after cessation of hostilities, civilian**

● **Y36.88 Other war operations occurring after cessation of hostilities**

● **Y36.880 Other war operations occurring after cessation of hostilities, military personnel**

● **Y36.881 Other war operations occurring after cessation of hostilities, civilian**

● **Y36.89 Unspecified war operations occurring after cessation of hostilities**

● **Y36.890 Unspecified war operations occurring after cessation of hostilities, military personnel**

● **Y36.891 Unspecified war operations occurring after cessation of hostilities, civilian**

● **Y36.9 Other and unspecified war operations**

X ● **Y36.90 War operations, unspecified**

X ● **Y36.91 War operations involving unspecified weapon of mass destruction [WMD]**

X ● **Y36.92 War operations involving friendly fire**

● **Y37 Military operations**

> **Includes**   Injuries to military personnel and civilians occurring during peacetime on military property and during routine military exercises and operations

> **Excludes1**   military aircraft involved in aircraft accident with civilian aircraft (V97.81-)
> military vehicles involved in transport accident with civilian vehicle (V09.01, V09.21, V19.81, V29.81, V39.81, V49.81, V59.81, V69.81, V79.81)
> military watercraft involved in water transport accident with civilian watercraft (V94.81-)
> war operations (Y36.-)

The appropriate 7th character is to be added to each code from category Y37

A	initial encounter
D	subsequent encounter
S	sequela

● **Y37.0 Military operations involving explosion of marine weapons**

● **Y37.00 Military operations involving explosion of unspecified marine weapon**

> Military operations involving underwater blast NOS

● **Y37.000 Military operations involving explosion of unspecified marine weapon, military personnel**

● **Y37.001 Military operations involving explosion of unspecified marine weapon, civilian**

● **Y37.01 Military operations involving explosion of depth-charge**

● **Y37.010 Military operations involving explosion of depth-charge, military personnel**

● **Y37.011 Military operations involving explosion of depth-charge, civilian**

● **Y37.02 Military operations involving explosion of marine mine**

> Military operations involving explosion of marine mine, at sea or in harbor

● **Y37.020 Military operations involving explosion of marine mine, military personnel**

● **Y37.021 Military operations involving explosion of marine mine, civilian**

● **Y37.03 Military operations involving explosion of sea-based artillery shell**

● **Y37.030 Military operations involving explosion of sea-based artillery shell, military personnel**

● **Y37.031 Military operations involving explosion of sea-based artillery shell, civilian**

● **Y37.04 Military operations involving explosion of torpedo**

● **Y37.040 Military operations involving explosion of torpedo, military personnel**

● **Y37.041 Military operations involving explosion of torpedo, civilian**

● **Y37.05 Military operations involving accidental detonation of onboard marine weapons**

● **Y37.050 Military operations involving accidental detonation of onboard marine weapons, military personnel**

● **Y37.051 Military operations involving accidental detonation of onboard marine weapons, civilian**

● **Y37.09** Military operations involving explosion of other marine weapons

   ● **Y37.090** Military operations involving explosion of other marine weapons, military personnel

   ● **Y37.091** Military operations involving explosion of other marine weapons, civilian

● **Y37.1** Military operations involving destruction of aircraft

  ● **Y37.10** Military operations involving unspecified destruction of aircraft

   ● **Y37.100** Military operations involving unspecified destruction of aircraft, military personnel

   ● **Y37.101** Military operations involving unspecified destruction of aircraft, civilian

  ● **Y37.11** Military operations involving destruction of aircraft due to enemy fire or explosives

    Military operations involving destruction of aircraft due to air to air missile

    Military operations involving destruction of aircraft due to explosive placed on aircraft

    Military operations involving destruction of aircraft due to rocket propelled grenade [RPG]

    Military operations involving destruction of aircraft due to small arms fire

    Military operations involving destruction of aircraft due to surface to air missile

   ● **Y37.110** Military operations involving destruction of aircraft due to enemy fire or explosives, military personnel

   ● **Y37.111** Military operations involving destruction of aircraft due to enemy fire or explosives, civilian

  ● **Y37.12** Military operations involving destruction of aircraft due to collision with other aircraft

   ● **Y37.120** Military operations involving destruction of aircraft due to collision with other aircraft, military personnel

   ● **Y37.121** Military operations involving destruction of aircraft due to collision with other aircraft, civilian

  ● **Y37.13** Military operations involving destruction of aircraft due to onboard fire

   ● **Y37.130** Military operations involving destruction of aircraft due to onboard fire, military personnel

   ● **Y37.131** Military operations involving destruction of aircraft due to onboard fire, civilian

  ● **Y37.14** Military operations involving destruction of aircraft due to accidental detonation of onboard munitions and explosives

   ● **Y37.140** Military operations involving destruction of aircraft due to accidental detonation of onboard munitions and explosives, military personnel

   ● **Y37.141** Military operations involving destruction of aircraft due to accidental detonation of onboard munitions and explosives, civilian

  ● **Y37.19** Military operations involving other destruction of aircraft

   ● **Y37.190** Military operations involving other destruction of aircraft, military personnel

   ● **Y37.191** Military operations involving other destruction of aircraft, civilian

● **Y37.2** Military operations involving other explosions and fragments

    Excludes1 military operations involving explosion of aircraft (Y37.1-)

            military operations involving explosion of marine weapons (Y37.0-)

            military operations involving explosion of nuclear weapons (Y37.5-)

  ● **Y37.20** Military operations involving unspecified explosion and fragments

    Military operations involving air blast NOS

    Military operations involving blast NOS

    Military operations involving blast fragments NOS

    Military operations involving blast wave NOS

    Military operations involving blast wind NOS

    Military operations involving explosion NOS

    Military operations involving explosion of bomb NOS

   ● **Y37.200** Military operations involving unspecified explosion and fragments, military personnel

   ● **Y37.201** Military operations involving unspecified explosion and fragments, civilian

  ● **Y37.21** Military operations involving explosion of aerial bomb

   ● **Y37.210** Military operations involving explosion of aerial bomb, military personnel

   ● **Y37.211** Military operations involving explosion of aerial bomb, civilian

  ● **Y37.22** Military operations involving explosion of guided missile

   ● **Y37.220** Military operations involving explosion of guided missile, military personnel

   ● **Y37.221** Military operations involving explosion of guided missile, civilian

  ● **Y37.23** Military operations involving explosion of improvised explosive device [IED]

    Military operations involving explosion of person-borne improvised explosive device [IED]

    Military operations involving explosion of vehicle-borne improvised explosive device [IED]

    Military operations involving explosion of roadside improvised explosive device [IED]

   ● **Y37.230** Military operations involving explosion of improvised explosive device [IED], military personnel

   ● **Y37.231** Military operations involving explosion of improvised explosive device [IED], civilian

  ● **Y37.24** Military operations involving explosion due to accidental detonation and discharge of own munitions or munitions launch device

   ● **Y37.240** Military operations involving explosion due to accidental detonation and discharge of own munitions or munitions launch device, military personnel

   ● **Y37.241** Military operations involving explosion due to accidental detonation and discharge of own munitions or munitions launch device, civilian

▶ New   ⇒ Revised   ~~deleted~~ Deleted   **OGCR** Official Guidelines   **X** Assign placeholder X   ● Use Additional Character(s)

Excludes 1   Excludes 2   Includes   Use additional   Code first   Code also   Key words

● **Y37.25**   **Military operations involving fragments from munitions**

   ● **Y37.250**   **Military operations involving fragments from munitions, military personnel**

   ● **Y37.251**   **Military operations involving fragments from munitions, civilian**

● **Y37.26**   **Military operations involving fragments of improvised explosive device [IED]**

   Military operations involving fragments of person-borne improvised explosive device [IED]

   Military operations involving fragments of vehicle-borne improvised explosive device [IED]

   Military operations involving fragments of roadside improvised explosive device [IED]

   ● **Y37.260**   **Military operations involving fragments of improvised explosive device [IED], military personnel**

   ● **Y37.261**   **Military operations involving fragments of improvised explosive device [IED], civilian**

● **Y37.27**   **Military operations involving fragments from weapons**

   ● **Y37.270**   **Military operations involving fragments from weapons, military personnel**

   ● **Y37.271**   **Military operations involving fragments from weapons, civilian**

● **Y37.29**   **Military operations involving other explosions and fragments**

   Military operations involving explosion of grenade

   Military operations involving explosions of land mine

   Military operations involving shrapnel NOS

   ● **Y37.290**   **Military operations involving other explosions and fragments, military personnel**

   ● **Y37.291**   **Military operations involving other explosions and fragments, civilian**

● **Y37.3**   **Military operations involving fires, conflagrations and hot substances**

   Military operations involving smoke, fumes, and heat from fires, conflagrations and hot substances

   | Excludes1 | military operations involving fires and conflagrations aboard military aircraft (Y37.1-)

     military operations involving fires and conflagrations aboard military watercraft (Y37.0-)

     military operations involving fires and conflagrations caused indirectly by conventional weapons (Y37.2-)

     military operations involving fires and thermal effects of nuclear weapons (Y36.53-)

   ● **Y37.30**   **Military operations involving unspecified fire, conflagration and hot substance**

     ● **Y37.300**   **Military operations involving unspecified fire, conflagration and hot substance, military personnel**

     ● **Y37.301**   **Military operations involving unspecified fire, conflagration and hot substance, civilian**

   ● **Y37.31**   **Military operations involving gasoline bomb**

     Military operations involving incendiary bomb

     Military operations involving petrol bomb

     ● **Y37.310**   **Military operations involving gasoline bomb, military personnel**

     ● **Y37.311**   **Military operations involving gasoline bomb, civilian**

● **Y37.32**   **Military operations involving incendiary bullet**

   ● **Y37.320**   **Military operations involving incendiary bullet, military personnel**

   ● **Y37.321**   **Military operations involving incendiary bullet, civilian**

● **Y37.33**   **Military operations involving flamethrower**

   ● **Y37.330**   **Military operations involving flamethrower, military personnel**

   ● **Y37.331**   **Military operations involving flamethrower, civilian**

● **Y37.39**   **Military operations involving other fires, conflagrations and hot substances**

   ● **Y37.390**   **Military operations involving other fires, conflagrations and hot substances, military personnel**

   ● **Y37.391**   **Military operations involving other fires, conflagrations and hot substances, civilian**

● **Y37.4**   **Military operations involving firearm discharge and other forms of conventional warfare**

   ● **Y37.41**   **Military operations involving rubber bullets**

     ● **Y37.410**   **Military operations involving rubber bullets, military personnel**

     ● **Y37.411**   **Military operations involving rubber bullets, civilian**

   ● **Y37.42**   **Military operations involving firearms pellets**

     ● **Y37.420**   **Military operations involving firearms pellets, military personnel**

     ● **Y37.421**   **Military operations involving firearms pellets, civilian**

   ● **Y37.43**   **Military operations involving other firearms discharge**

     Military operations involving bullets NOS

     | Excludes1 | military operations involving munitions fragments (Y37.25-)

       military operations involving incendiary bullets (Y37.32-)

     ● **Y37.430**   **Military operations involving other firearms discharge, military personnel**

     ● **Y37.431**   **Military operations involving other firearms discharge, civilian**

   ● **Y37.44**   **Military operations involving unarmed hand to hand combat**

     | Excludes1 | military operations involving combat using blunt or piercing object (Y37.45-)

       military operations involving intentional restriction of air and airway (Y37.46-)

       military operations involving unintentional restriction of air and airway (Y37.47-)

     ● **Y37.440**   **Military operations involving unarmed hand to hand combat, military personnel**

     ● **Y37.441**   **Military operations involving unarmed hand to hand combat, civilian**

   ● **Y37.45**   **Military operations involving combat using blunt or piercing object**

     ● **Y37.450**   **Military operations involving combat using blunt or piercing object, military personnel**

     ● **Y37.451**   **Military operations involving combat using blunt or piercing object, civilian**

▶ New   ⇒ Revised   ~~deleted~~ Deleted   **OGCR** Official Guidelines   X Assign placeholder X   ● Use Additional Character(s)

| Excludes 1 | | Excludes 2 | Includes   Use additional   Code first   Code also   Key words

● Y37.46　Military operations involving intentional restriction of air and airway
   ● Y37.460　Military operations involving intentional restriction of air and airway, military personnel
   ● Y37.461　Military operations involving intentional restriction of air and airway, civilian

● Y37.47　Military operations involving unintentional restriction of air and airway
   ● Y37.470　Military operations involving unintentional restriction of air and airway, military personnel
   ● Y37.471　Military operations involving unintentional restriction of air and airway, civilian

● Y37.49　Military operations involving other forms of conventional warfare
   ● Y37.490　Military operations involving other forms of conventional warfare, military personnel
   ● Y37.491　Military operations involving other forms of conventional warfare, civilian

● Y37.5　Military operations involving nuclear weapons
   Military operation involving dirty bomb NOS

  ● Y37.50　Military operations involving unspecified effect of nuclear weapon
    ● Y37.500　Military operations involving unspecified effect of nuclear weapon, military personnel
    ● Y37.501　Military operations involving unspecified effect of nuclear weapon, civilian

  ● Y37.51　Military operations involving direct blast effect of nuclear weapon
    Military operations involving blast pressure of nuclear weapon
    ● Y37.510　Military operations involving direct blast effect of nuclear weapon, military personnel
    ● Y37.511　Military operations involving direct blast effect of nuclear weapon, civilian

  ● Y37.52　Military operations involving indirect blast effect of nuclear weapon
    Military operations involving being thrown by blast of nuclear weapon
    Military operations involving being struck or crushed by blast debris of nuclear weapon
    ● Y37.520　Military operations involving indirect blast effect of nuclear weapon, military personnel
    ● Y37.521　Military operations involving indirect blast effect of nuclear weapon, civilian

  ● Y37.53　Military operations involving thermal radiation effect of nuclear weapon
    Military operations involving direct heat from nuclear weapon
    Military operation involving fireball effects from nuclear weapon
    ● Y37.530　Military operations involving thermal radiation effect of nuclear weapon, military personnel
    ● Y37.531　Military operations involving thermal radiation effect of nuclear weapon, civilian

● Y37.54　Military operation involving nuclear radiation effects of nuclear weapon
   Military operation involving acute radiation exposure from nuclear weapon
   Military operation involving exposure to immediate ionizing radiation from nuclear weapon
   Military operation involving fallout exposure from nuclear weapon
   Military operation involving secondary effects of nuclear weapons
   ● Y37.540　Military operation involving nuclear radiation effects of nuclear weapon, military personnel
   ● Y37.541　Military operation involving nuclear radiation effects of nuclear weapon, civilian

● Y37.59　Military operation involving other effects of nuclear weapons
   ● Y37.590　Military operation involving other effects of nuclear weapons, military personnel
   ● Y37.591　Military operation involving other effects of nuclear weapons, civilian

● Y37.6　Military operations involving biological weapons
  ● Y37.6X　Military operations involving biological weapons
    ● Y37.6X0　Military operations involving biological weapons, military personnel
    ● Y37.6X1　Military operations involving biological weapons, civilian

● Y37.7　Military operations involving chemical weapons and other forms of unconventional warfare
   Excludes1　military operations involving incendiary devices (Y36.3-, Y36.5-)
  ● Y37.7X　Military operations involving chemical weapons and other forms of unconventional warfare
    ● Y37.7X0　Military operations involving chemical weapons and other forms of unconventional warfare, military personnel
    ● Y37.7X1　Military operations involving chemical weapons and other forms of unconventional warfare, civilian

● Y37.9　Other and unspecified military operations
  X ● Y37.90　Military operations, unspecified
  X ● Y37.91　Military operations involving unspecified weapon of mass destruction [WMD]
  X ● Y37.92　Military operations involving friendly fire

▶ New　⇒ Revised　~~deleted~~ Deleted　OGCR Official Guidelines　X Assign placeholder X　● Use Additional Character(s)

Excludes 1　Excludes 2　Includes　Use additional　Code first　Code also　Key words

● **Y38 Terrorism**

These codes are for use to identify injuries resulting from the unlawful use of force or violence against persons or property to intimidate or coerce a government, the civilian population, or any segment thereof, in furtherance of political or social objective

Use additional code for place of occurrence (Y92.-)

The appropriate 7th character is to be added to each code from category Y38

A	initial encounter
D	subsequent encounter
S	sequela

● **Y38.0   Terrorism involving explosion of marine weapons**
Terrorism involving depth-charge
Terrorism involving marine mine
Terrorism involving mine NOS, at sea or in harbor
Terrorism involving sea-based artillery shell
Terrorism involving torpedo
Terrorism involving underwater blast

   ● **Y38.0X   Terrorism involving explosion of marine weapons**

      ● **Y38.0X1   Terrorism involving explosion of marine weapons, public safety official injured**

      ● **Y38.0X2   Terrorism involving explosion of marine weapons, civilian injured**

      ● **Y38.0X3   Terrorism involving explosion of marine weapons, terrorist injured**

● **Y38.1   Terrorism involving destruction of aircraft**
Terrorism involving aircraft burned
Terrorism involving aircraft exploded
Terrorism involving aircraft being shot down
Terrorism involving aircraft used as a weapon

   ● **Y38.1X   Terrorism involving destruction of aircraft**

      ● **Y38.1X1   Terrorism involving destruction of aircraft, public safety official injured**

      ● **Y38.1X2   Terrorism involving destruction of aircraft, civilian injured**

      ● **Y38.1X3   Terrorism involving destruction of aircraft, terrorist injured**

● **Y38.2   Terrorism involving other explosions and fragments**
Terrorism involving antipersonnel (fragments) bomb
Terrorism involving blast NOS
Terrorism involving explosion NOS
Terrorism involving explosion of breech block
Terrorism involving explosion of cannon block
Terrorism involving explosion (fragments) of artillery shell
Terrorism involving explosion (fragments) of bomb
Terrorism involving explosion (fragments) of grenade
Terrorism involving explosion (fragments) of guided missile
Terrorism involving explosion (fragments) of land mine
Terrorism involving explosion of mortar bomb
Terrorism involving explosion of munitions
Terrorism involving explosion (fragments) of rocket
Terrorism involving explosion (fragments) of shell
Terrorism involving shrapnel
Terrorism involving mine NOS, on land

    Excludes1   terrorism involving explosion of nuclear weapon (Y38.5)
        terrorism involving suicide bomber (Y38.81)

   ● **Y38.2X   Terrorism involving other explosions and fragments**

      ● **Y38.2X1   Terrorism involving other explosions and fragments, public safety official injured**

      ● **Y38.2X2   Terrorism involving other explosions and fragments, civilian injured**

      ● **Y38.2X3   Terrorism involving other explosions and fragments, terrorist injured**

● **Y38.3   Terrorism involving fires, conflagration and hot substances**
Terrorism involving conflagration NOS
Terrorism involving fire NOS
Terrorism involving petrol bomb

    Excludes1   terrorism involving fire or heat of nuclear weapon (Y38.5)

   ● **Y38.3X   Terrorism involving fires, conflagration and hot substances**

      ● **Y38.3X1   Terrorism involving fires, conflagration and hot substances, public safety official injured**

      ● **Y38.3X2   Terrorism involving fires, conflagration and hot substances, civilian injured**

      ● **Y38.3X3   Terrorism involving fires, conflagration and hot substances, terrorist injured**

● **Y38.4   Terrorism involving firearms**
Terrorism involving carbine bullet
Terrorism involving machine gun bullet
Terrorism involving pellets (shotgun)
Terrorism involving pistol bullet
Terrorism involving rifle bullet
Terrorism involving rubber (rifle) bullet

   ● **Y38.4X   Terrorism involving firearms**

      ● **Y38.4X1   Terrorism involving firearms, public safety official injured**

      ● **Y38.4X2   Terrorism involving firearms, civilian injured**

      ● **Y38.4X3   Terrorism involving firearms, terrorist injured**

● **Y38.5   Terrorism involving nuclear weapons**
Terrorism involving blast effects of nuclear weapon
Terrorism involving exposure to ionizing radiation from nuclear weapon
Terrorism involving fireball effect of nuclear weapon
Terrorism involving heat from nuclear weapon

   ● **Y38.5X   Terrorism involving nuclear weapons**

      ● **Y38.5X1   Terrorism involving nuclear weapons, public safety official injured**

      ● **Y38.5X2   Terrorism involving nuclear weapons, civilian injured**

      ● **Y38.5X3   Terrorism involving nuclear weapons, terrorist injured**

● **Y38.6   Terrorism involving biological weapons**
Terrorism involving anthrax
Terrorism involving cholera
   A serious, often deadly, infectious disease of small intestine
Terrorism involving smallpox

   ● **Y38.6X   Terrorism involving biological weapons**

      ● **Y38.6X1   Terrorism involving biological weapons, public safety official injured**

      ● **Y38.6X2   Terrorism involving biological weapons, civilian injured**

      ● **Y38.6X3   Terrorism involving biological weapons, terrorist injured**

● **Y38.7   Terrorism involving chemical weapons**
Terrorism involving gases, fumes, chemicals
Terrorism involving hydrogen cyanide
Terrorism involving phosgene
Terrorism involving sarin

   ● **Y38.7X   Terrorism involving chemical weapons**

      ● **Y38.7X1   Terrorism involving chemical weapons, public safety official injured**

      ● **Y38.7X2   Terrorism involving chemical weapons, civilian injured**

      ● **Y38.7X3   Terrorism involving chemical weapons, terrorist injured**

CHAPTER 20 (V01-Y99)

▶ New   ➡ Revised   ~~deleted~~ Deleted   **OGCR** Official Guidelines   X Assign placeholder X   ● Use Additional Character(s)

Excludes 1   Excludes 2   Includes   Use additional   Code first   Code also   Key words

● Y38.8   Terrorism involving other and unspecified means
   ● Y38.80   Terrorism involving unspecified means
       Terrorism NOS
   ● Y38.81   Terrorism involving suicide bomber
     ● Y38.811   Terrorism involving suicide bomber, public safety official injured
     ● Y38.812   Terrorism involving suicide bomber, civilian injured
   ● Y38.89   Terrorism involving other means
       Terrorism involving drowning and submersion
       Terrorism involving lasers
       Terrorism involving piercing or stabbing instruments
     ● Y38.891   Terrorism involving other means, public safety official injured
     ● Y38.892   Terrorism involving other means, civilian injured
     ● Y38.893   Terrorism involving other means, terrorist injured
● Y38.9   Terrorism, secondary effects
       Note: This code is for use to identify conditions occurring subsequent to a terrorist attack not those that are due to the initial terrorist attack.
   ● Y38.9X   Terrorism, secondary effects
     ● Y38.9X1   Terrorism, secondary effects, public safety official injured
     ● Y38.9X2   Terrorism, secondary effects, civilian injured categories

COMPLICATIONS OF MEDICAL AND SURGICAL CARE (Y62-Y84)

Includes	complications of medical devices surgical and medical procedures as the cause of abnormal reaction of the patient, or of later complication, without mention of misadventure at the time of the procedure

MISADVENTURES TO PATIENTS DURING SURGICAL AND MEDICAL CARE (Y62-Y69)

Excludes1	surgical and medical procedures as the cause of abnormal reaction of the patient, without mention of misadventure at the time of the procedure (Y83-Y84)
Excludes2	breakdown or malfunctioning of medical device (during procedure) (after implantation) (ongoing use) (Y70-Y82)

● Y62   Failure of sterile precautions during surgical and medical care
   Y62.0   Failure of sterile precautions during surgical operation
   Y62.1   Failure of sterile precautions during infusion or transfusion
   Y62.2   Failure of sterile precautions during kidney dialysis and other perfusion
   Y62.3   Failure of sterile precautions during injection or immunization
   Y62.4   Failure of sterile precautions during endoscopic examination
   Y62.5   Failure of sterile precautions during heart catheterization
   Y62.6   Failure of sterile precautions during aspiration, puncture and other catheterization
   Y62.8   Failure of sterile precautions during other surgical and medical care
   Y62.9   Failure of sterile precautions during unspecified surgical and medical care

● Y63   Failure in dosage during surgical and medical care

Excludes2	accidental overdose of drug or wrong drug given in error (T36-T50)

   Y63.0   Excessive amount of blood or other fluid given during transfusion or infusion
   Y63.1   Incorrect dilution of fluid used during infusion
   Y63.2   Overdose of radiation given during therapy
   Y63.3   Inadvertent exposure of patient to radiation during medical care
   Y63.4   Failure in dosage in electroshock or insulin-shock therapy
   Y63.5   Inappropriate temperature in local application and packing
   Y63.6   Underdosing and nonadministration of necessary drug, medicament or biological substance
   Y63.8   Failure in dosage during other surgical and medical care
   Y63.9   Failure in dosage during unspecified surgical and medical care

● Y64   Contaminated medical or biological substances
   Y64.0   Contaminated medical or biological substance, transfused or infused
   Y64.1   Contaminated medical or biological substance, injected or used for immunization
   Y64.8   Contaminated medical or biological substance administered by other means
   Y64.9   Contaminated medical or biological substance administered by unspecified means
       Administered contaminated medical or biological substance NOS

● Y65   Other misadventures during surgical and medical care
   Y65.0   Mismatched blood in transfusion
   Y65.1   Wrong fluid used in infusion
   Y65.2   Failure in suture or ligature during surgical operation
   Y65.3   Endotracheal tube wrongly placed during anesthetic procedure
   Y65.4   Failure to introduce or to remove other tube or instrument
   ● Y65.5   Performance of wrong procedure (operation)
     ● Y65.51   Performance of wrong procedure (operation) on correct patient
       Wrong device implanted into correct surgical site

Excludes1	performance of correct procedure (operation) on wrong side or body part (Y65.53)

     ● Y65.52   Performance of procedure (operation) on patient not scheduled for surgery
       Performance of procedure (operation) intended for another patient
       Performance of procedure (operation) on wrong patient
     ● Y65.53   Performance of correct procedure (operation) on wrong side or body part
       Performance of correct procedure (operation) on wrong side
       Performance of correct procedure (operation) on wrong site
   Y65.8   Other specified misadventures during surgical and medical care

Y66   Nonadministration of surgical and medical care
       Premature cessation of surgical and medical care

Excludes1	DNR status (Z66) palliative care (Z51.5)

Y69   Unspecified misadventure during surgical and medical care

▶ New   ⇒ Revised   ~~deleted~~ Deleted   **OGCR** Official Guidelines   X Assign placeholder X   ● Use Additional Character(s)

Excludes 1   Excludes 2   Includes   Use additional   Code first   Code also   Key words

MEDICAL DEVICES ASSOCIATED WITH ADVERSE INCIDENTS IN DIAGNOSTIC AND THERAPEUTIC USE (Y70-Y82)

Includes   breakdown or malfunction of medical devices (during use) (after implantation) (ongoing use)

Excludes2   breakdown or malfunctioning of medical device (after implantation) (during procedure) (ongoing use) (Y70-Y82)

later complications following use of medical devices without breakdown or malfunctioning of device (Y83-Y84)

misadventure to patients during surgical and medical care, classifiable to (Y62-Y69)

surgical and other medical procedures as the cause of abnormal reaction of the patient, or of later complication, without mention of misadventure at the time of the procedure (Y83-Y84)

● **Y70**   **Anesthesiology** devices associated with adverse incidents

     Y70.0   **Diagnostic and monitoring** anesthesiology devices associated with adverse incidents

     Y70.1   **Therapeutic (nonsurgical) and rehabilitative** anesthesiology devices associated with adverse incidents

     Y70.2   **Prosthetic and other implants, materials and accessory** anesthesiology devices associated with adverse incidents

     Y70.3   **Surgical instruments, materials and** anesthesiology devices (including sutures) associated with adverse incidents

     Y70.8   **Miscellaneous** anesthesiology devices associated with adverse incidents, not elsewhere classified

● **Y71**   **Cardiovascular** devices associated with adverse incidents

     Y71.0   **Diagnostic and monitoring** cardiovascular devices associated with adverse incidents

     Y71.1   **Therapeutic (nonsurgical) and rehabilitative** cardiovascular devices associated with adverse incidents

     Y71.2   **Prosthetic and other implants, materials and accessory** cardiovascular devices associated with adverse incidents

     Y71.3   **Surgical instruments, materials and** cardiovascular devices (including sutures) associated with adverse incidents

     Y71.8   **Miscellaneous** cardiovascular devices associated with adverse incidents, not elsewhere classified

● **Y72**   **Otorhinolaryngological** devices associated with adverse incidents

     Y72.0   **Diagnostic and monitoring** otorhinolaryngological devices associated with adverse incidents

     Y72.1   **Therapeutic (nonsurgical) and rehabilitative** otorhinolaryngological devices associated with adverse incidents

     Y72.2   **Prosthetic and other implants, materials** and accessory otorhinolaryngological devices associated with adverse incidents

     Y72.3   **Surgical instruments, materials and** otorhinolaryngological devices (including sutures) associated with adverse incidents

     Y72.8   **Miscellaneous** otorhinolaryngological devices associated with adverse incidents, not elsewhere classified

● **Y73**   **Gastroenterology and urology** devices associated with adverse incidents

     Y73.0   **Diagnostic and monitoring** gastroenterology and urology devices associated with adverse incidents

     Y73.1   **Therapeutic (nonsurgical) and rehabilitative** gastroenterology and urology devices associated with adverse incidents

     Y73.2   **Prosthetic and other implants, materials and accessory** gastroenterology and urology devices associated with adverse incidents

     Y73.3   **Surgical instruments, materials and gastroenterology and urology devices (including sutures)** associated with adverse incidents

     Y73.8   **Miscellaneous** gastroenterology and urology devices associated with adverse incidents, not elsewhere classified

● **Y74**   **General hospital and personal-use** devices associated with adverse incidents

     Y74.0   **Diagnostic and monitoring** general hospital and personal-use devices associated with adverse incidents

     Y74.1   **Therapeutic (nonsurgical) and rehabilitative** general hospital and personal-use devices associated with adverse incidents

     Y74.2   **Prosthetic and other implants, materials and accessory** general hospital and personal-use devices associated with adverse incidents

     Y74.3   **Surgical instruments, materials and** general hospital and personal-use devices (including sutures) associated with adverse incidents

     Y74.8   **Miscellaneous** general hospital and personal-use devices associated with adverse incidents, not elsewhere classified

● **Y75**   **Neurological** devices associated with adverse incidents

     Y75.0   **Diagnostic and monitoring** neurological devices associated with adverse incidents

     Y75.1   **Therapeutic (nonsurgical) and rehabilitative** neurological devices associated with adverse incidents

     Y75.2   **Prosthetic and other implants**, materials and neurological devices associated with adverse incidents

     Y75.3   **Surgical instruments, materials and neurological devices** (including sutures) associated with adverse incidents

     Y75.8   **Miscellaneous** neurological devices associated with adverse incidents, not elsewhere classified

● **Y76**   **Obstetric and gynecological** devices associated with adverse incidents

     Y76.0   **Diagnostic and monitoring** obstetric and gynecological devices associated with adverse incidents

     Y76.1   **Therapeutic (nonsurgical) and rehabilitative** obstetric and gynecological devices associated with adverse incidents

     Y76.2   **Prosthetic and other implants, materials and accessory** obstetric and gynecological devices associated with adverse incidents

     Y76.3   **Surgical instruments, materials** and obstetric and gynecological devices (including sutures) associated with adverse incidents

     Y76.8   **Miscellaneous** obstetric and gynecological devices associated with adverse incidents, not elsewhere classified

CHAPTER 20 (V01-Y99)

● **Y77** Ophthalmic devices associated with adverse incidents

Y77.0 Diagnostic and monitoring ophthalmic devices associated with adverse incidents

Y77.1 Therapeutic (nonsurgical) and rehabilitative ophthalmic devices associated with adverse incidents

Y77.2 Prosthetic and other implants, materials and accessory ophthalmic devices associated with adverse incidents

Y77.3 Surgical instruments, materials and ophthalmic devices (including sutures) associated with adverse incidents

Y77.8 Miscellaneous ophthalmic devices associated with adverse incidents, not elsewhere classified

● **Y78** Radiological devices associated with adverse incidents

Y78.0 Diagnostic and monitoring radiological devices associated with adverse incidents

Y78.1 Therapeutic (nonsurgical) and rehabilitative radiological devices associated with adverse incidents

Y78.2 Prosthetic and other implants, materials and accessory radiological devices associated with adverse incidents

Y78.3 Surgical instruments, materials and radiological devices (including sutures) associated with adverse incidents

Y78.8 Miscellaneous radiological devices associated with adverse incidents, not elsewhere classified

● **Y79** Orthopedic devices associated with adverse incidents

Y79.0 Diagnostic and monitoring orthopedic devices associated with adverse incidents

Y79.1 Therapeutic (nonsurgical) and rehabilitative orthopedic devices associated with adverse incidents

Y79.2 Prosthetic and other implants, materials and accessory orthopedic devices associated with adverse incidents

Y79.3 Surgical instruments, materials and orthopedic devices (including sutures) associated with adverse incidents

Y79.8 Miscellaneous orthopedic devices associated with adverse incidents, not elsewhere classified

● **Y80** Physical medicine devices associated with adverse incidents

Y80.0 Diagnostic and monitoring physical medicine devices associated with adverse incidents

Y80.1 Therapeutic (nonsurgical) and rehabilitative physical medicine devices associated with adverse incidents

Y80.2 Prosthetic and other implants, materials and accessory physical medicine devices associated with adverse incidents

Y80.3 Surgical instruments, materials and physical medicine devices (including sutures) associated with adverse incidents

Y80.8 Miscellaneous physical medicine devices associated with adverse incidents, not elsewhere classified

● **Y81** General- and plastic-surgery devices associated with adverse incidents

Y81.0 Diagnostic and monitoring general- and plastic-surgery devices associated with adverse incidents

Y81.1 Therapeutic (nonsurgical) and rehabilitative general- and plastic-surgery devices associated with adverse incidents

Y81.2 Prosthetic and other implants, materials and accessory general- and plastic-surgery devices associated with adverse incidents

Y81.3 Surgical instruments, materials and general- and plastic-surgery devices (including sutures) associated with adverse incidents

Y81.8 Miscellaneous general- and plastic-surgery devices associated with adverse incidents, not elsewhere classified

● **Y82** Other and unspecified medical devices associated with adverse incidents

Y82.8 Other medical devices associated with adverse incidents

Y82.9 Unspecified medical devices associated with adverse incidents

---

SURGICAL AND OTHER MEDICAL PROCEDURES AS THE CAUSE OF ABNORMAL REACTION OF THE PATIENT, OR OF LATER COMPLICATION, WITHOUT MENTION OF MISADVENTURE AT THE TIME OF THE PROCEDURE (Y83-Y84)

Excludes1   misadventures to patients during surgical and medical care, classifiable to (Y62-Y69)

Excludes2   breakdown or malfunctioning of medical device (after implantation) (during procedure) (ongoing use) (Y70-Y82)

● **Y83** Surgical operation and other surgical procedures as the cause of abnormal reaction of the patient, or of later complication, without mention of misadventure at the time of the procedure

Y83.0 Surgical operation with transplant of whole organ as the cause of abnormal reaction of the patient, or of later complication, without mention of misadventure at the time of the procedure

Y83.1 Surgical operation with implant of artificial internal device as the cause of abnormal reaction of the patient, or of later complication, without mention of misadventure at the time of the procedure

Y83.2 Surgical operation with anastomosis, bypass or graft as the cause of abnormal reaction of the patient, or of later complication, without mention of misadventure at the time of the procedure

Y83.3 Surgical operation with formation of external stoma as the cause of abnormal reaction of the patient, or of later complication, without mention of misadventure at the time of the procedure

Y83.4 Other reconstructive surgery as the cause of abnormal reaction of the patient, or of later complication, without mention of misadventure at the time of the procedure

Y83.5 Amputation of limb(s) as the cause of abnormal reaction of the patient, or of later complication, without mention of misadventure at the time of the procedure

Y83.6 Removal of other organ (partial) (total) as the cause of abnormal reaction of the patient, or of later complication, without mention of misadventure at the time of the procedure

Y83.8 Other surgical procedures as the cause of abnormal reaction of the patient, or of later complication, without mention of misadventure at the time of the procedure

Y83.9 Surgical procedure, unspecified as the cause of abnormal reaction of the patient, or of later complication, without mention of misadventure at the time of the procedure

● **Y84** Other medical procedures as the cause of abnormal reaction of the patient, or of later complication, without mention of misadventure at the time of the procedure

Y84.0 Cardiac catheterization as the cause of abnormal reaction of the patient, or of later complication, without mention of misadventure at the time of the procedure

Y84.1 Kidney dialysis as the cause of abnormal reaction of the patient, or of later complication, without mention of misadventure at the time of the procedure

Y84.2 Radiological procedure and radiotherapy as the cause of abnormal reaction of the patient, or of later complication, without mention of misadventure at the time of the procedure

Y84.3 Shock therapy as the cause of abnormal reaction of the patient, or of later complication, without mention of misadventure at the time of the procedure

Y84.4 Aspiration of fluid as the cause of abnormal reaction of the patient, or of later complication, without mention of misadventure at the time of the procedure

Y84.5 Insertion of gastric or duodenal sound as the cause of abnormal reaction of the patient, or of later complication, without mention of misadventure at the time of the procedure

Y84.6 Urinary catheterization as the cause of abnormal reaction of the patient, or of later complication, without mention of misadventure at the time of the procedure

Y84.7 Blood-sampling as the cause of abnormal reaction of the patient, or of later complication, without mention of misadventure at the time of the procedure

---

▶ New   ⇒ Revised   ~~deleted~~ Deleted   **OGCR** Official Guidelines   X Assign placeholder X   ● Use Additional Character(s)

Excludes 1   Excludes 2   Includes   Use additional   Code first   Code also   Key words

Y84.8   **Other medical procedures** as the cause of abnormal reaction of the patient, or of later complication, without mention of misadventure at the time of the procedure

Y84.9   Medical procedure, **unspecified** as the cause of abnormal reaction of the patient, or of later complication, without mention of misadventure at the time of the procedure

SUPPLEMENTARY FACTORS RELATED TO CAUSES OF MORBIDITY CLASSIFIED ELSEWHERE (Y90-Y99)

Note: These categories may be used to provide supplementary information concerning causes of morbidity. They are not to be used for single-condition coding.

● **Y90**   **Evidence of alcohol involvement determined by blood alcohol level**

Code first any associated alcohol related disorders (F10)

Y90.0   Blood alcohol level of **less than 20 mg/100 ml**

Y90.1   Blood alcohol level of **20-39 mg/100 ml**

Y90.2   Blood alcohol level of **40-59 mg/100 ml**

Y90.3   Blood alcohol level of **60-79 mg/100 ml**

Y90.4   Blood alcohol level of **80-99 mg/100 ml**

Y90.5   Blood alcohol level of **100-119 mg/100 ml**

Y90.6   Blood alcohol level of **120-199 mg/100 ml**

Y90.7   Blood alcohol level of **200-239 mg/100 ml**

Y90.8   Blood alcohol level of **240 mg/100 ml or more**

Y90.9   **Presence** of alcohol in blood, **level not specified**

OGCR Section I.C.20.b.

Place of Occurrence Guideline

Codes from category Y92, Place of occurrence of the external cause, are secondary codes for use after other external cause codes to identify the location of the patient at the time of injury or other condition.

Generally, a place of occurrence code is assigned only once, at the initial encounter for treatment. However, in the rare instance that a new injury occurs during hospitalization, an additional place of occurrence code may be assigned. No 7th characters are used for Y92. Only one code from Y92 should be recorded on a medical record.

Do not use place of occurrence code Y92.9 if the place is not stated or is not applicable.

● **Y92**   **Place of occurrence of the external cause**

The following category is for use, when relevant, to identify the place of occurrence of the external cause. Use in conjunction with an activity code.

Place of occurrence should be recorded only at the initial encounter for treatment

● **Y92.0**   **Non-institutional** (private) **residence** as the place of occurrence of the external cause

> **Excludes1**   abandoned or derelict house (Y92.89)
> home under construction but not yet occupied (Y92.6-)
> institutional place of residence (Y92.1-)

● **Y92.00**   **Unspecified** non-institutional (private) residence as the place of occurrence of the external cause

     Y92.000   **Kitchen** of unspecified non-institutional (private) residence as the place of occurrence of the external cause

     Y92.001   **Dining room** of unspecified non-institutional (private) residence as the place of occurrence of the external cause

     Y92.002   **Bathroom** of unspecified non-institutional (private) residence single-family (private) house as the place of occurrence of the external cause

     Y92.003   **Bedroom** of unspecified non-institutional (private) residence as the place of occurrence of the external cause

     Y92.007   **Garden or yard** of unspecified non-institutional (private) residence as the place of occurrence of the external cause

     Y92.008   **Other place** in unspecified non-institutional (private) residence as the place of occurrence of the external cause

     Y92.009   **Unspecified place** in unspecified non-institutional (private) residence as the place of occurrence of the external cause

         Home (NOS) as the place of occurrence of the external cause

● **Y92.01**   **Single-family non-institutional** (private) **house** as the place of occurrence of the external cause

Farmhouse as the place of occurrence of the external cause

> **Excludes1**   barn (Y92.71)
> chicken coop or hen house (Y92.72)
> farm field (Y92.73)
> orchard (Y92.74)
> single family mobile home or trailer (Y92.02-)
> slaughter house (Y92.86)

     Y92.010   **Kitchen** of single-family (private) house as the place of occurrence of the external cause

     Y92.011   **Dining room** of single-family (private) house as the place of occurrence of the external cause

     Y92.012   **Bathroom** of single-family (private) house as the place of occurrence of the external cause

     Y92.013   **Bedroom** of single-family (private) house as the place of occurrence of the external cause

     Y92.014   **Private driveway** to single-family (private) house as the place of occurrence of the external cause

     Y92.015   **Private garage** of single-family (private) house as the place of occurrence of the external cause

     Y92.016   **Swimming pool** in single-family (private) house or garden as the place of occurrence of the external cause

     Y92.017   **Garden or yard** in single-family (private) house as the place of occurrence of the external cause

     Y92.018   **Other place** in single-family (private) house as the place of occurrence of the external cause

     Y92.019   **Unspecified** place in single-family (private) house as the place of occurrence of the external cause

● **Y92.02 Mobile home** as the place of occurrence of the external cause

Y92.020   **Kitchen** in mobile home as the place of occurrence of the external cause

Y92.021   **Dining room** in mobile home as the place of occurrence of the external cause

Y92.022   **Bathroom** in mobile home as the place of occurrence of the external cause

Y92.023   **Bedroom** in mobile home as the place of occurrence of the external cause

Y92.024   **Driveway** of mobile home as the place of occurrence of the external cause

Y92.025   **Garage** of mobile home as the place of occurrence of the external cause

Y92.026   **Swimming pool** of mobile home as the place of occurrence of the external cause

Y92.027   **Garden or yard** of mobile home as the place of occurrence of the external cause

Y92.028   **Other place** in mobile home as the place of occurrence of the external cause

Y92.029   **Unspecified** place in mobile home as the place of occurrence of the external cause

● **Y92.03 Apartment** as the place of occurrence of the external cause

Condominium as the place of occurrence of the external cause

Co-op apartment as the place of occurrence of the external cause

Y92.030   **Kitchen** in apartment as the place of occurrence of the external cause

Y92.031   **Bathroom** in apartment as the place of occurrence of the external cause

Y92.032   **Bedroom** in apartment as the place of occurrence of the external cause

Y92.038   **Other place** in apartment as the place of occurrence of the external cause

Y92.039   **Unspecified** place in apartment as the place of occurrence of the external cause

● **Y92.04 Boarding-house** as the place of occurrence of the external cause

Y92.040   **Kitchen** in boarding-house as the place of occurrence of the external cause

Y92.041   **Bathroom** in boarding-house as the place of occurrence of the external cause

Y92.042   **Bedroom** in boarding-house as the place of occurrence of the external cause

Y92.043   **Driveway** of boarding-house as the place of occurrence of the external cause

Y92.044   **Garage** of boarding-house as the place of occurrence of the external cause

Y92.045   **Swimming pool** of boarding-house as the place of occurrence of the external cause

Y92.046   **Garden or yard** of boarding-house as the place of occurrence of the external cause

Y92.048   **Other place** in boarding-house as the place of occurrence of the external cause

Y92.049   **Unspecified** place in boarding-house as the place of occurrence of the external cause

● **Y92.09 Other non-institutional residence** as the place of occurrence of the external cause

Y92.090   **Kitchen** in other non-institutional residence as the place of occurrence of the external cause

Y92.091   **Bathroom** in other non-institutional residence as the place of occurrence of the external cause

Y92.092   **Bedroom** in other non-institutional residence as the place of occurrence of the external cause

Y92.093   **Driveway** of other non-institutional residence as the place of occurrence of the external cause

Y92.094   **Garage** of other non-institutional residence as the place of occurrence of the external cause

Y92.095   **Swimming pool** of other non-institutional residence as the place of occurrence of the external cause

Y92.096   **Garden or yard** of other non-institutional residence as the place of occurrence of the external cause

Y92.098   **Other place** in other non-institutional residence as the place of occurrence of the external cause

Y92.099   **Unspecified** place in other non-institutional residence as the place of occurrence of the external cause

● **Y92.1 Institutional** (nonprivate) **residence** as the place of occurrence of the external cause

Y92.10   **Unspecified** residential institution as the place of occurrence of the external cause

● **Y92.11 Children's home and orphanage** as the place of occurrence of the external cause

Y92.110   **Kitchen** in children's home and orphanage as the place of occurrence of the external cause

Y92.111   **Bathroom** in children's home and orphanage as the place of occurrence of the external cause

Y92.112   **Bedroom** in children's home and orphanage as the place of occurrence of the external cause

Y92.113   **Driveway** of children's home and orphanage as the place of occurrence of the external cause

Y92.114   **Garage** of children's home and orphanage as the place of occurrence of the external cause

Y92.115   **Swimming pool** of children's home and orphanage as the place of occurrence of the external cause

Y92.116   **Garden or yard** of children's home and orphanage as the place of occurrence of the external cause

Y92.118   **Other place** in children's home and orphanage as the place of occurrence of the external cause

Y92.119   **Unspecified** place in children's home and orphanage as the place of occurrence of the external cause

● **Y92.12**   **Nursing home** as the place of occurrence of the external cause

     Home for the sick as the place of occurrence of the external cause

     Hospice as the place of occurrence of the external cause

   Y92.120   **Kitchen** in nursing home as the place of occurrence of the external cause

   Y92.121   **Bathroom** in nursing home as the place of occurrence of the external cause

   Y92.122   **Bedroom** in nursing home as the place of occurrence of the external cause

   Y92.123   **Driveway** of nursing home as the place of occurrence of the external cause

   Y92.124   **Garage** of nursing home as the place of occurrence of the external cause

   Y92.125   **Swimming pool** of nursing home as the place of occurrence of the external cause

   Y92.126   **Garden or yard** of nursing home as the place of occurrence of the external cause

   Y92.128   **Other place** in nursing home as the place of occurrence of the external cause

   Y92.129   **Unspecified** place in nursing home as the place of occurrence of the external cause

● **Y92.13**   **Military base** as the place of occurrence of the external cause

   | Excludes1 | military training grounds (Y92.83)

   Y92.130   **Kitchen** on military base as the place of occurrence of the external cause

   Y92.131   **Mess hall** on military base as the place of occurrence of the external cause

   Y92.133   **Barracks** on military base as the place of occurrence of the external cause

   Y92.135   **Garage** on military base as the place of occurrence of the external cause

   Y92.136   **Swimming pool** on military base as the place of occurrence of the external cause

   Y92.137   **Garden or yard** on military base as the place of occurrence of the external cause

   Y92.138   **Other place** on military base as the place of occurrence of the external cause

   Y92.139   **Unspecified** place military base as the place of occurrence of the external cause

● **Y92.14**   **Prison** as the place of occurrence of the external cause

   Y92.140   **Kitchen** in prison as the place of occurrence of the external cause

   Y92.141   **Dining room** in prison as the place of occurrence of the external cause

   Y92.142   **Bathroom** in prison as the place of occurrence of the external cause

   Y92.143   **Cell** of prison as the place of occurrence of the external cause

   Y92.146   **Swimming pool** of prison as the place of occurrence of the external cause

   Y92.147   **Courtyard** of prison as the place of occurrence of the external cause

   Y92.148   **Other place** in prison as the place of occurrence of the external cause

   Y92.149   **Unspecified** place in prison as the place of occurrence of the external cause

● **Y92.15**   **Reform school** as the place of occurrence of the external cause

   Y92.150   **Kitchen** in reform school as the place of occurrence of the external cause

   Y92.151   **Dining room** in reform school as the place of occurrence of the external cause

   Y92.152   **Bathroom** in reform school as the place of occurrence of the external cause

   Y92.153   **Bedroom** in reform school as the place of occurrence of the external cause

   Y92.154   **Driveway** of reform school as the place of occurrence of the external cause

   Y92.155   **Garage** of reform school as the place of occurrence of the external cause

   Y92.156   **Swimming pool** of reform school as the place of occurrence of the external cause

   Y92.157   **Garden or yard** of reform school as the place of occurrence of the external cause

   Y92.158   **Other place** in reform school as the place of occurrence of the external cause

   Y92.159   **Unspecified** place in reform school as the place of occurrence of the external cause

● **Y92.16**   **School dormitory** as the place of occurrence of the external cause

   | Excludes1 | reform school as the place of occurrence of the external cause (Y92.15-)

           school buildings and grounds as the place of occurrence of the external cause (Y92.2-)

           school sports and athletic areas as the place of occurrence of the external cause (Y92.3-)

   Y92.160   **Kitchen** in school dormitory as the place of occurrence of the external cause

   Y92.161   **Dining room** in school dormitory as the place of occurrence of the external cause

   Y92.162   **Bathroom** in school dormitory as the place of occurrence of the external cause

   Y92.163   **Bedroom** in school dormitory as the place of occurrence of the external cause

   Y92.168   **Other place** in school dormitory as the place of occurrence of the external cause

   Y92.169   **Unspecified** place in school dormitory as the place of occurrence of the external cause

● **Y92.19** Other specified residential institution as the place of occurrence of the external cause

    Y92.190 Kitchen in other specified residential institution as the place of occurrence of the external cause

    Y92.191 Dining room in other specified residential institution as the place of occurrence of the external cause

    Y92.192 Bathroom in other specified residential institution as the place of occurrence of the external cause

    Y92.193 Bedroom in other specified residential institution as the place of occurrence of the external cause

    Y92.194 Driveway of other specified residential institution as the place of occurrence of the external cause

    Y92.195 Garage of other specified residential institution as the place of occurrence of the external cause

    Y92.196 Pool of other specified residential institution as the place of occurrence of the external cause

    Y92.197 Garden or yard of other specified residential institution as the place of occurrence of the external cause

    Y92.198 Other place in other specified residential institution as the place of occurrence of the external cause

    Y92.199 Unspecified place in other specified residential institution as the place of occurrence of the external cause

● **Y92.2** School, other institution and public administrative area as the place of occurrence of the external cause

    Building and adjacent grounds used by the general public or by a particular group of the public

    Excludes1   building under construction as the place of occurrence of the external cause (Y92.6)

            residential institution as the place of occurrence of the external cause (Y92.1)

            school dormitory as the place of occurrence of the external cause (Y92.16-)

            sports and athletics area of schools as the place of occurrence of the external cause (Y92.3-)

● **Y92.21** School (private) (public) (state) as the place of occurrence of the external cause

    Y92.210 Daycare center as the place of occurrence of the external cause

    Y92.211 Elementary school as the place of occurrence of the external cause

            Kindergarten as the place of occurrence of the external cause

    Y92.212 Middle school as the place of occurrence of the external cause

    Y92.213 High school as the place of occurrence of the external cause

    Y92.214 College as the place of occurrence of the external cause

            University as the place of occurrence of the external cause

    Y92.215 Trade school as the place of occurrence of the external cause

    Y92.218 Other school as the place of occurrence of the external cause

    Y92.219 Unspecified school as the place of occurrence of the external cause

Y92.22 Religious institution as the place of occurrence of the external cause

    Church as the place of occurrence of the external cause

    Mosque as the place of occurrence of the external cause

    Synagogue as the place of occurrence of the external cause

● **Y92.23** Hospital as the place of occurrence of the external cause

    Excludes1   ambulatory (outpatient) health services establishments (Y92.53-)

            home for the sick as the place of occurrence of the external cause (Y92.12-)

            hospice as the place of occurrence of the external cause (Y92.12-)

            nursing home as the place of occurrence of the external cause (Y92.12-)

    Y92.230 Patient room in hospital as the place of occurrence of the external cause

    Y92.231 Patient bathroom in hospital as the place of occurrence of the external cause

    Y92.232 Corridor of hospital as the place of occurrence of the external cause

    Y92.233 Cafeteria of hospital as the place of occurrence of the external cause

    Y92.234 Operating room of hospital as the place of occurrence of the external cause

    Y92.238 Other place in hospital as the place of occurrence of the external cause

    Y92.239 Unspecified place in hospital as the place of occurrence of the external cause

● **Y92.24** Public administrative building as the place of occurrence of the external cause

    Y92.240 Courthouse as the place of occurrence of the external cause

    Y92.241 Library as the place of occurrence of the external cause

    Y92.242 Post office as the place of occurrence of the external cause

    Y92.243 City hall as the place of occurrence of the external cause

    Y92.248 Other public administrative building as the place of occurrence of the external cause

● **Y92.25** Cultural building as the place of occurrence of the external cause

    Y92.250 Art gallery as the place of occurrence of the external cause

    Y92.251 Museum as the place of occurrence of the external cause

    Y92.252 Music hall as the place of occurrence of the external cause

    Y92.253 Opera house as the place of occurrence of the external cause

    Y92.254 Theater (live) as the place of occurrence of the external cause

    Y92.258 Other cultural public building as the place of occurrence of the external cause

Y92.26 Movie house or cinema as the place of occurrence of the external cause

Y92.29 Other specified public building as the place of occurrence of the external cause

    Assembly hall as the place of occurrence of the external cause

    Clubhouse as the place of occurrence of the external cause

▶ New   ⟹ Revised   ~~deleted~~ Deleted   **OGCR** Official Guidelines   X Assign placeholder X   ● Use Additional Character(s)

Excludes 1   Excludes 2   Includes   Use additional   Code first   Code also   Key words

● Y92.3 **Sports and athletics area** as the place of occurrence of the external cause

  ● Y92.31 **Athletic court** as the place of occurrence of the external cause

     Excludes1   tennis court in private home or garden (Y92.09)

     Y92.310 **Basketball** court as the place of occurrence of the external cause

     Y92.311 **Squash** court as the place of occurrence of the external cause

     Y92.312 **Tennis** court as the place of occurrence of the external cause

     Y92.318 **Other** athletic court as the place of occurrence of the external cause

  ● Y92.32 **Athletic field** as the place of occurrence of the external cause

     Y92.320 **Baseball** field as the place of occurrence of the external cause

     Y92.321 **Football** field as the place of occurrence of the external cause

     Y92.322 **Soccer** field as the place of occurrence of the external cause

     Y92.328 **Other** athletic field as the place of occurrence of the external cause
         Cricket field as the place of occurrence of the external cause
         Hockey field as the place of occurrence of the external cause

  ● Y92.33 **Skating rink** as the place of occurrence of the external cause

     Y92.330 **Ice** skating rink (indoor) (outdoor) as the place of occurrence of the external cause

     Y92.331 **Roller** skating rink as the place of occurrence of the external cause

   Y92.34 **Swimming pool (public)** as the place of occurrence of the external cause

     Excludes1   swimming pool in private home or garden (Y92.016)

   Y92.39 **Other specified** sports and athletic area as the place of occurrence of the external cause
     Golf-course as the place of occurrence of the external cause
     Gymnasium as the place of occurrence of the external cause
     Riding-school as the place of occurrence of the external cause
     Stadium as the place of occurrence of the external cause

● Y92.4 **Street, highway and other paved roadways** as the place of occurrence of the external cause

     Excludes1   private driveway of residence (Y92.014, Y92.024, Y92.043, Y92.093, Y92.113, Y92.123, Y92.154, Y92.194)

  ● Y92.41 **Street and highway** as the place of occurrence of the external cause

     Y92.410 **Unspecified** street and highway as the place of occurrence of the external cause
         Road NOS as the place of occurrence of the external cause

     Y92.411 **Interstate** highway as the place of occurrence of the external cause
         Freeway as the place of occurrence of the external cause
         Motorway as the place of occurrence of the external cause

     Y92.412 **Parkway** as the place of occurrence of the external cause

     Y92.413 **State road** as the place of occurrence of the external cause

     Y92.414 **Local residential or business street** as the place of occurrence of the external cause

     Y92.415 **Exit ramp or entrance ramp** of street or highway as the place of occurrence of the external cause

  ● Y92.48 **Other paved roadways** as the place of occurrence of the external cause

     Y92.480 **Sidewalk** as the place of occurrence of the external cause

     Y92.481 **Parking lot** as the place of occurrence of the external cause

     Y92.482 **Bike path** as the place of occurrence of the external cause

     Y92.488 **Other** paved roadways as the place of occurrence of the external cause

● Y92.5 **Trade and service area** as the place of occurrence of the external cause

     Excludes1   garage in private home (Y92.015)
                 schools and other public administration buildings (Y92.2-)

  ● Y92.51 **Private commercial establishments** as the place of occurrence of the external cause

     Y92.510 **Bank** as the place of occurrence of the external cause

     Y92.511 **Restaurant or café** as the place of occurrence of the external cause

     Y92.512 **Supermarket, store or market** as the place of occurrence of the external cause

     Y92.513 **Shop** (commercial) as the place of occurrence of the external cause

  ● Y92.52 **Service areas** as the place of occurrence of the external cause

     Y92.520 **Airport** as the place of occurrence of the external cause

     Y92.521 **Bus station** as the place of occurrence of the external cause

     Y92.522 **Railway station** as the place of occurrence of the external cause

     Y92.523 **Highway rest stop** as the place of occurrence of the external cause

     Y92.524 **Gas station** as the place of occurrence of the external cause
         Petroleum station as the place of occurrence of the external cause
         Service station as the place of occurrence of the external cause

  ● Y92.53 **Ambulatory health services establishments** as the place of occurrence of the external cause

     Y92.530 **Ambulatory surgery center** as the place of occurrence of the external cause
         Outpatient surgery center, including that connected with a hospital as the place of occurrence of the external cause
         Same day surgery center, including that connected with a hospital as the place of occurrence of the external cause

     Y92.531 **Health care provider office** as the place of occurrence of the external cause
         Physician office as the place of occurrence of the external cause

     Y92.532 **Urgent care center** as the place of occurrence of the external cause

     Y92.538 **Other** ambulatory health services establishments as the place of occurrence of the external cause

● New   ⇒ Revised   ~~deleted~~ Deleted   **OGCR** Official Guidelines   X Assign placeholder X   ● Use Additional Character(s)

Excludes 1   Excludes 2   Includes   Use additional   Code first   Code also   Key words

Y92.59   **Other** trade areas as the place of occurrence of the external cause

Office building as the place of occurrence of the external cause

Casino as the place of occurrence of the external cause

Garage (commercial) as the place of occurrence of the external cause

Hotel as the place of occurrence of the external cause

Radio or television station as the place of occurrence of the external cause

Shopping mall as the place of occurrence of the external cause

Warehouse as the place of occurrence of the external cause

● Y92.6   **Industrial and construction area** as the place of occurrence of the external cause

Y92.61   **Building** [any] **under construction** as the place of occurrence of the external cause

Y92.62   **Dock or shipyard** as the place of occurrence of the external cause

Dockyard as the place of occurrence of the external cause

Dry dock as the place of occurrence of the external cause

Shipyard as the place of occurrence of the external cause

Y92.63   **Factory** as the place of occurrence of the external cause

Factory building as the place of occurrence of the external cause

Factory premises as the place of occurrence of the external cause

Industrial yard as the place of occurrence of the external cause

Y92.64   **Mine or pit** as the place of occurrence of the external cause

Mine as the place of occurrence of the external cause

Y92.65   **Oil rig** as the place of occurrence of the external cause

Pit (coal) (gravel) (sand) as the place of occurrence of the external cause

Y92.69   **Other** specified industrial and construction area as the place of occurrence of the external cause

Gasworks as the place of occurrence of the external cause

Power-station (coal) (nuclear) (oil) as the place of occurrence of the external cause

Tunnel under construction as the place of occurrence of the external cause

Workshop as the place of occurrence of the external cause

● Y92.7   **Farm** as the place of occurrence of the external cause

Ranch as the place of occurrence of the external cause

Excludes1   farmhouse and home premises of farm (Y92.01-)

Y92.71   **Barn** as the place of occurrence of the external cause

Y92.72   **Chicken coop** as the place of occurrence of the external cause

Hen house as the place of occurrence of the external cause

Y92.73   Farm **field** as the place of occurrence of the external cause

Y92.74   **Orchard** as the place of occurrence of the external cause

Y92.79   **Other farm location** as the place of occurrence of the external cause

● Y92.8   **Other places** as the place of occurrence of the external cause

● Y92.81   **Transport vehicle** as the place of occurrence of the external cause

Excludes1   transport accidents (V00-V99)

Y92.810   **Car** as the place of occurrence of the external cause

Y92.811   **Bus** as the place of occurrence of the external cause

Y92.812   **Truck** as the place of occurrence of the external cause

Y92.813   **Airplane** as the place of occurrence of the external cause

Y92.814   **Boat** as the place of occurrence of the external cause

Y92.815   **Train** as the place of occurrence of the external cause

Y92.816   **Subway** car as the place of occurrence of the external cause

Y92.818   **Other** transport vehicle as the place of occurrence of the external cause

● Y92.82   **Wilderness area**

Y92.820   **Desert** as the place of occurrence of the external cause

Y92.821   **Forest** as the place of occurrence of the external cause

Y92.828   **Other** wilderness area as the place of occurrence of the external cause

Swamp as the place of occurrence of the external cause

Mountain as the place of occurrence of the external cause

Marsh as the place of occurrence of the external cause

Prairie as the place of occurrence of the external cause

● Y92.83   **Recreation area** as the place of occurrence of the external cause

Y92.830   **Public park** as the place of occurrence of the external cause

Y92.831   **Amusement park** as the place of occurrence of the external cause

Y92.832   **Beach** as the place of occurrence of the external cause

Seashore as the place of occurrence of the external cause

Y92.833   **Campsite** as the place of occurrence of the external cause

Y92.834   **Zoological garden** (zoo) as the place of occurrence of the external cause

Y92.838   **Other** recreation area as the place of occurrence of the external cause

Y92.84   **Military training ground** as the place of occurrence of the external cause

Y92.85   **Railroad track** as the place of occurrence of the external cause

Y92.86   **Slaughter house** as the place of occurrence of the external cause

Y92.89   **Other** specified places as the place of occurrence of the external cause

Derelict house as the place of occurrence of the external cause

OGCR Section I.C.20.b.

Do not use place of occurrence code Y92.9 if the place is not stated or is not applicable.

Y92.9   **Unspecified** place or not applicable

▶ New   ⇒ Revised   ~~deleted~~ Deleted   **OGCR** Official Guidelines   X Assign placeholder X   ● Use Additional Character(s)

Excludes 1   Excludes 2   Includes   Use additional   Code first   Code also   Key words

OGCR See Section I.C.20.c.

Activity Code

Assign a code from category Y93, Activity code, to describe the activity of the patient at the time the injury or other health condition occurred.

An activity code is used only once, at the initial encounter for treatment. Only one code from Y93 should be recorded on a medical record.

The activity codes are not applicable to poisonings, adverse effects, misadventures or sequela.

Do not assign Y93.9, Unspecified activity, if the activity is not stated.

A code from category Y93 is appropriate for use with external cause and intent codes if identifying the activity provides additional information about the event.

● **Y93   Activity codes**

    Note: Category Y93 is provided for use to indicate the activity of the person seeking healthcare for an injury or health condition, such as a heart attack while shoveling snow, which resulted from, or was contributed to, by the activity. These codes are appropriate for use for both acute injuries, such as those from chapter 19, and conditions that are due to the long-term, cumulative effects of an activity, such as those from chapter 13. They are also appropriate for use with external cause codes for cause and intent if identifying the activity provides additional information on the event. These codes should be used in conjunction with codes for external cause status (Y99) and place of occurrence (Y92).

    This section contains the following broad activity categories:

        Y93.0   Activities involving walking and running

        Y93.1   Activities involving water and water craft

        Y93.2   Activities involving ice and snow

        Y93.3   Activities involving climbing, rappelling, and jumping off

        Y93.4   Activities involving dancing and other rhythmic movement

        Y93.5   Activities involving other sports and athletics played individually

        Y93.6   Activities involving other sports and athletics played as a team or group

        Y93.7   Activities involving other specified sports and athletics

        Y93.A   Activities involving other cardiorespiratory exercise

        Y93.B   Activities involving other muscle strengthening exercises

        Y93.C   Activities involving computer technology and electronic devices

        Y93.D   Activities involving arts and handcrafts

        Y93.E   Activities involving personal hygiene and interior property and clothing maintenance

        Y93.F   Activities involving caregiving

        Y93.G   Activities involving food preparation, cooking and grilling

        Y93.H   Activities involving exterior property and land maintenance, building and construction

        Y93.I   Activities involving roller coasters and other types of external motion

        Y93.J   Activities involving playing musical instrument

        Y93.K   Activities involving animal care

        Y93.8   Activities, other specified

        Y93.9   Activity, unspecified

● **Y93.0   Activities involving walking and running**

    | Excludes1 | Activity, walking an animal (Y93.K1)
            Activity, walking or running on a treadmill (Y93.A1)

    Y93.01   Activity, walking, marching and hiking

         Activity, walking, marching and hiking on level or elevated terrain

        | Excludes1 | activity, mountain climbing (Y93.31)

    Y93.02   Activity, running

● **Y93.1   Activities involving water and water craft**

    | Excludes1 | activities involving ice (Y93.2-)

    Y93.11   Activity, swimming

    Y93.12   Activity, springboard and platform diving

    Y93.13   Activity, water polo

    Y93.14   Activity, water aerobics and water exercise

    Y93.15   Activity, underwater diving and snorkeling

         Activity, SCUBA diving

    Y93.16   Activity, rowing, canoeing, kayaking, rafting and tubing

         Activity, canoeing, kayaking, rafting and tubing in calm and turbulent water

    Y93.17   Activity, water skiing and wake boarding

    Y93.18   Activity, surfing, windsurfing and boogie boarding

         Activity, water sliding

    Y93.19   Activity, other involving water and watercraft

         Activity involving water NOS

         Activity, parasailing

         Activity, water survival training and testing

● **Y93.2   Activities involving ice and snow**

    | Excludes1 | activity, shoveling ice and snow (Y93.H1)

    Y93.21   Activity, ice skating

         Activity, figure skating (singles) (pairs)

         Activity, ice dancing

        | Excludes1 | activity, ice hockey (Y93.22)

    Y93.22   Activity, ice hockey

    Y93.23   Activity, snow (alpine) (downhill) skiing, snow boarding, sledding, tobogganing and snow tubing

        | Excludes1 | activity, cross country skiing (Y93.24)

    Y93.24   Activity, cross country skiing

         Activity, nordic skiing

    Y93.29   Activity, other activity involving ice and snow

         Activity, activity involving ice and snow NOS

● **Y93.3   Activities involving climbing, rappelling and jumping off**

    | Excludes1 | activity, hiking on level or elevated terrain (Y93.01)

         activity, jumping rope (Y93.56)

         activity, trampoline jumping (Y93.44)

    Y93.31   Activity, mountain climbing, rock climbing and wall climbing

    Y93.32   Activity, rappelling

    Y93.33   Activity, BASE jumping

         Activity, building, Antenna, Span, Earth jumping

    Y93.34   Activity, bungee jumping

    Y93.35   Activity, hang gliding

    Y93.39   Activity, other activity involving climbing, rappelling and jumping off

● **Y93.4   Activities involving dancing and other rhythmic movement**

    | Excludes1 | activity, martial arts (Y93.75)

    Y93.41   Activity, dancing

    Y93.42   Activity, yoga

    Y93.43   Activity, gymnastics

         Activity, rhythmic gymnastics

        | Excludes1 | activity, trampolining (Y93.44)

    Y93.44   Activity, trampolining

    Y93.45   Activity, cheerleading

    Y93.49   Activity, other involving dancing and other rhythmic movements

---

▶ New   ⇒ Revised   ~~deleted~~ Deleted   **OGCR** Official Guidelines   X Assign placeholder X   ● Use Additional Character(s)

| Excludes 1 | | Excludes 2 | Includes   Use additional   Code first   Code also   Key words

CHAPTER 20 (V01-Y99)

● **Y93.5** **Activities involving other sports and athletics played individually**

Excludes1	activity, dancing (Y93.41)
	activity, gymnastic (Y93.43)
	activity, trampolining (Y93.44)
	activity, yoga (Y93.42)

Y93.51 **Activity, roller skating (inline) and skateboarding**

Y93.52 **Activity, horseback riding**

Y93.53 **Activity, golf**

Y93.54 **Activity, bowling**

Y93.55 **Activity, bike riding**

Y93.56 **Activity, jumping rope**

Y93.57 **Activity, non-running track and field events**

| **Excludes1** | activity, running (any form) (Y93.02) |

Y93.59 **Activity, other involving other sports and athletics played individually**

Excludes1	activities involving climbing, rappelling, and jumping (Y93.3-)
	activities involving ice and snow (Y93.2-)
	activities involving walking and running (Y93.0-)
	activities involving water and watercraft (Y93.1-)

● **Y93.6** **Activities involving other sports and athletics played as a team or group**

| **Excludes1** | activity, ice hockey (Y93.22) |
| | activity, water polo (Y93.13) |

Y93.61 **Activity, American tackle football**
Activity, football NOS

Y93.62 **Activity, American flag or touch football**

Y93.63 **Activity, rugby**

Y93.64 **Activity, baseball**
Activity, softball

Y93.65 **Activity, lacrosse and field hockey**

Y93.66 **Activity, soccer**

Y93.67 **Activity, basketball**

Y93.68 **Activity, volleyball (beach) (court)**

Y93.6A **Activity, physical games generally associated with school recess, summer camp and children**
Activity, capture the flag
Activity, dodge ball
Activity, four square
Activity, kickball

Y93.69 **Activity, other involving other sports and athletics played as a team or group**
Cricket

● **Y93.7** **Activities involving other specified sports and athletics**

Y93.71 **Activity, boxing**

Y93.72 **Activity, wrestling**

Y93.73 **Activity, racquet and hand sports**
Activity, handball
Activity, racquetball
Activity, squash
Activity, tennis

Y93.74 **Activity, frisbee**
Activity, ultimate frisbee

Y93.75 **Activity, martial arts**
Activity, combatives

Y93.79 **Activity, other specified sports and athletics**

| **Excludes1** | sports and athletics activities specified in categories Y93.0-Y93.6 |

● **Y93.A** **Activities involving other cardiorespiratory exercise**
Activities involving physical training

Y93.A1 **Activity, exercise machines primarily for cardiorespiratory conditioning**
Activity, elliptical and stepper machines
Activity, stationary bike
Activity, treadmill

Y93.A2 **Activity, calisthenics**
Activity, jumping jacks
Activity, warm up and cool down

Y93.A3 **Activity, aerobic and step exercise**

Y93.A4 **Activity, circuit training**

Y93.A5 **Activity, obstacle course**
Activity, challenge course
Activity, confidence course

Y93.A6 **Activity, grass drills**
Activity, guerilla drills

Y93.A9 **Activity, other involving other cardiorespiratory exercise**

| **Excludes1** | activities involving cardiorespiratory exercise specified in categories Y93.0-Y93.7 |

● **Y93.B** **Activity involving other muscle strengthening exercises**

Y93.B1 **Activity, exercise machines primarily for muscle strengthening**

Y93.B2 **Activity, push-ups, pull-ups, sit-ups**

Y93.B3 **Activity, free weights**
Activity, barbells
Activity, dumbbells

Y93.B4 **Activity, pilates**

Y93.B9 **Activity, other involving other muscle strengthening exercises**

| **Excludes1** | activities involving muscle strengthening specified in categories Y93.0-Y93.A |

● **Y93.C** **Activities involving computer technology and electronic devices**

| **Excludes1** | activity, electronic musical keyboard or instruments (Y93.J-) |

Y93.C1 **Activity, computer keyboarding**
Activity, electronic game playing using keyboard or other stationary device

Y93.C2 **Activity, hand held interactive electronic device**
Activity, cellular telephone and communication device
Activity, electronic game playing using interactive device

| **Excludes1** | activity, electronic game playing using keyboard or other stationary device (Y93.C1) |

Y93.C9 **Activity, other involving computer technology and electronic devices**

● **Y93.D** **Activities involving arts and handcrafts**

| **Excludes1** | activities involving playing musical instrument (Y93.J-) |

Y93.D1 **Knitting and crocheting**

Y93.D2 **Sewing**

Y93.D3 **Furniture building and finishing**
Furniture repair

Y93.D9 **Activity, other involving arts and handcrafts**

▶ New   ⇒ Revised   ~~deleted~~ Deleted   **OGCR** Official Guidelines   X Assign placeholder X   ● Use Additional Character(s)

| Excludes 1 | Excludes 2 | Includes | Use additional | Code first | Code also | Key words |

● **Y93.E** **Activities involving personal hygiene and interior property and clothing maintenance**

> **Excludes1**   activities involving cooking and grilling (Y93.G-)
> activities involving exterior property and land maintenance, building and construction (Y93.H-)
> activity involving caregiving (Y93.F-)
> activity, dishwashing (Y93.G1)
> activity, food preparation (Y93.G1)
> activity, gardening (Y93.H2)

    Y93.E1   **Activity, personal bathing and showering**

    Y93.E2   **Activity, laundry**

    Y93.E3   **Activity, vacuuming**

    Y93.E4   **Activity, ironing**

    Y93.E5   **Activity, floor mopping and cleaning**

    Y93.E6   **Activity, residential relocation**
        Activity, packing up and unpacking involved in moving to a new residence

    Y93.E8   **Activity, other personal hygiene activity**

    Y93.E9   **Activity, other household maintenance**

● **Y93.F** **Activities involving person providing caregiving**
    Activity involving the provider of caregiving

    Y93.F1   **Activity, caregiving involving bathing**

    Y93.F2   **Activity, caregiving involving lifting**

    Y93.F9   **Activity, other caregiving**

● **Y93.G** **Activities involving food preparation, cooking and grilling**

    Y93.G1   **Activity, food preparation and clean up**
        Activity, dishwashing

    Y93.G2   **Activity, grilling and smoking food**

    Y93.G3   **Activity, cooking and baking**
        Activity, use of stove, oven and microwave oven

    Y93.G9   **Activity, other activity involving cooking and grilling**

● **Y93.H** **Activities involving property and land maintenance, building and construction**

    Y93.H1   **Activity, digging, shoveling and raking**
        Activity, dirt digging
        Activity, raking leaves
        Activity, snow shoveling

    Y93.H2   **Activity, gardening and landscaping**
        Activity, pruning, trimming shrubs, weeding

    Y93.H3   **Activity, building and construction**

    Y93.H9   **Activity, other activity involving property and land maintenance, building and construction**

● **Y93.I** **Activities involving roller coasters and other types of external motion**

    Y93.I1   **Activity, rollercoaster riding**

    Y93.I9   **Activity, other involving external motion**

● **Y93.J** **Activities involving playing musical instrument**
    Activity involving playing electric musical instrument

    Y93.J1   **Activity, piano playing**
        Activity, musical keyboard (electronic) playing

    Y93.J2   **Activity, drum and other percussion instrument playing**

    Y93.J3   **Activity, string instrument playing**

    Y93.J4   **Activity, winds and brass instrument playing**

● **Y93.K** **Activities involving animal care**

> **Excludes1**   activity, horseback riding (Y93.52)

    Y93.K1   **Activity, walking an animal**

    Y93.K2   **Activity, milking an animal**

    Y93.K3   **Activity, grooming and shearing an animal**

    Y93.K9   **Activity, other activity involving animal care**

● **Y93.8** **Other activity**

    Y93.81   **Activity, refereeing a sports activity**

    Y93.82   **Activity, spectator at an event**

    Y93.83   **Activity, rough housing and horseplay**

    Y93.84   **Activity, sleeping**

    Y93.85   **Activity, choking game**
        Activity, blackout game
        Activity, fainting game
        Activity, pass out game

    Y93.89   **Activity, other specified**

OGCR See Section I.C.20.c.

Do not assign Y93.9, Unspecified activity, if the activity is not stated.

● **Y93.9** **Activity, unspecified**

Y95 **Nosocomial condition**

● **Y99** **External cause status**
    Note: A single code from category Y99 should be used in conjunction with the external cause code(s) assigned to a record to indicate the status of the person at the time the event occurred.

    Y99.0   **Civilian activity done for income or pay**
        Civilian activity done for financial or other compensation

> **Excludes1**   military activity (Y99.1)
> volunteer activity (Y99.2)

    Y99.1   **Military activity**

> **Excludes1**   activity of off duty military personnel (Y99.8)

    Y99.2   **Volunteer activity**

> **Excludes1**   activity of child or other family member assisting in compensated work of other family member (Y99.8)

    Y99.8   **Other external cause status**
        Activity NEC
        Activity of child or other family member assisting in compensated work of other family member
        Hobby not done for income
        Leisure activity
        Off-duty activity of military personnel
        Recreation or sport not for income or while a student
        Student activity

> **Excludes1**   civilian activity done for income or compensation (Y99.0)
> military activity (Y99.1)

    Y99.9   **Unspecified external cause status**

CHAPTER 20 (V01-Y99)

CHAPTER 21

FACTORS INFLUENCING HEALTH STATUS AND CONTACT WITH HEALTH SERVICES (Z00-Z99)

OGCR Chapter-Specific Coding Guidelines

21. **Chapter 21: Factors influencing health status and contact with health services (Z00-Z99)**
Note: The chapter specific guidelines provide additional information about the use of Z codes for specified encounters.

a. Use of Z codes in any healthcare setting
Z codes are for use in any healthcare setting. Z codes may be used as either a first-listed (principal diagnosis code in the inpatient setting) or secondary code, depending on the circumstances of the encounter. Certain Z codes may only be used as first-listed or principal diagnosis.

b. Z Codes indicate a reason for an encounter
Z codes are not procedure codes. A corresponding procedure code must accompany a Z code to describe any procedure performed.

c. Categories of Z Codes
1) Contact/Exposure
Category Z20 indicates contact with, and suspected exposure to, communicable diseases. These codes are for patients who do not show any sign or symptom of a disease but are suspected to have been exposed to it by close personal contact with an infected individual or are in an area where a disease is epidemic.

Category Z77, **Other contact with and (suspected) exposures hazardous to health,** indicates contact with and suspected exposures hazardous to health.

Contact/exposure codes may be used as a first-listed code to explain an encounter for testing, or, more commonly, as a secondary code to identify a potential risk.

2) Inoculations and vaccinations
Code Z23 is for encounters for inoculations and vaccinations. It indicates that a patient is being seen to receive a prophylactic inoculation against a disease. Procedure codes are required to identify the actual administration of the injection and the type(s) of immunizations given. Code Z23 may be used as a secondary code if the inoculation is given as a routine part of preventive health care, such as a well-baby visit.

3) Status
Status codes indicate that a patient is either a carrier of a disease or has the sequelae or residual of a past disease or condition. This includes such things as the presence of prosthetic or mechanical devices resulting from past treatment. A status code is informative, because the status may affect the course of treatment and its outcome. A status code is distinct from a history code. The history code indicates that the patient no longer has the condition.

A status code should not be used with a diagnosis code from one of the body system chapters, if the diagnosis code includes the information provided by the status code. For example, code Z94.1, Heart transplant status, should not be used with a code from subcategory T86.2, Complications of heart transplant. The status code does not provide additional information. The complication code indicates that the patient is a heart transplant patient.

For encounters for weaning from a mechanical ventilator, assign a code from subcategory J96.1, Chronic respiratory failure, followed by code Z99.11, Dependence on respirator [ventilator] status.

The status Z codes/categories are:
Z14   Genetic carrier
Genetic carrier status indicates that a person carries a gene, associated with a particular disease, which may be passed to offspring who may develop that disease. The person does not have the disease and is not at risk of developing the disease.
Z15   Genetic susceptibility to disease Genetic susceptibility indicates that a person has a gene that increases the risk of that person developing the disease.

Codes from category Z15 should not be used as principal or first-listed codes. If the patient has the condition to which he/she is susceptible, and that condition is the reason for the encounter, the code for the current condition should be sequenced first. If the patient is being seen for follow-up after completed treatment for this condition, and the condition no longer exists, a follow-up

code should be sequenced first, followed by the appropriate personal history and genetic susceptibility codes. If the purpose of the encounter is genetic counseling associated with procreative management, code Z31.5, Encounter for genetic counseling, should be assigned as the first-listed code, followed by a code from category Z15. Additional codes should be assigned for any applicable family or personal history.

Z16   Resistance to antimicrobial drugs
This code indicates that a patient has a condition that is resistant to antimicrobial drug treatment. Sequence the infection code first.
Z17   Estrogen receptor status
Z18   Retained foreign body fragments
Z19   Hormone sensitivity malignancy status
Z21   Asymptomatic HIV infection status This code indicates that a patient has tested positive for HIV but has manifested no signs or symptoms of the disease.
Z22   Carrier of infectious disease Carrier status indicates that a person harbors the specific organisms of a disease without manifest symptoms and is capable of transmitting the infection.
Z28.3   Underimmunization status
Z33.1   Pregnant state, incidental This code is a secondary code only for use when the pregnancy is in no way complicating the reason for visit. Otherwise, a code from the obstetric chapter is required.
Z66   Do not resuscitate
This code may be used when it is documented by the provider that a patient is on do not resuscitate status at any time during the stay.
Z67   Blood type
Z68   Body mass index (BMI)
As with all other secondary diagnosis codes, the BMI codes should only be assigned when they meet the definition of a reportable diagnosis (see Section III, Reporting Additional Diagnoses).
Z74.01   Bed confinement status
Z76.82   Awaiting organ transplant status
Z78   Other specified health status
Code Z78.1, Physical restraint status, may be used when it is documented by the provider that a patient has been put in restraints during the current encounter. Please note that this code should not be reported when it is documented by the provider that a patient is temporarily restrained during a procedure.
Z79   Long-term (current) drug therapy
Codes from this category indicate a patient's continuous use of a prescribed drug (including such things as aspirin therapy) for the long-term treatment of a condition or for prophylactic use. It is not for use for patients who have addictions to drugs. This subcategory is not for use of medications for detoxification or maintenance programs to prevent withdrawal symptoms in patients with drug dependence (e.g., methadone maintenance for opiate dependence). Assign the appropriate code for the drug dependence instead.

Assign a code from Z79 if the patient is receiving a medication for an extended period as a prophylactic measure (such as for the prevention of deep vein thrombosis) or as treatment of a chronic condition (such as arthritis) or a disease requiring a lengthy course of treatment (such as cancer). Do not assign a code from category Z79 for medication being administered for a brief period of time to treat an acute illness or injury (such as a course of antibiotics to treat acute bronchitis).

Z88   Allergy status to drugs, medicaments and biological substances Except: Z88.9, Allergy status to unspecified drugs, medicaments and biological substances status
Z89   Acquired absence of limb
Z90   Acquired absence of organs, not elsewhere classified
Z91.0-   Allergy status, other than to drugs and biological substances
Z92.82   Status post administration of tPA (rtPA) in a different facility within the last 24 hours prior to admission to a current facility Assign code Z92.82, Status post administration of tPA (rtPA) in a different facility within the last 24 hours prior to admission to current facility, as a secondary diagnosis when a patient is received by transfer into a facility and documentation indicates they were administered tissue plasminogen activator (tPA) within the last 24 hours prior to

admission to the current facility. This guideline applies even if the patient is still receiving the tPA at the time they are received into the current facility. The appropriate code for the condition for which the tPA was administered (such as cerebrovascular disease or myocardial infarction) should be assigned first. Code Z92.82 is only applicable to the receiving facility record and not to the transferring facility record.

Z93	Artificial opening status
Z94	Transplanted organ and tissue status
Z95	Presence of cardiac and vascular implants and grafts
Z96	Presence of other functional implants
Z97	Presence of other devices
Z98	Other postprocedural states

Assign code Z98.85, Transplanted organ removal status, to indicate that a transplanted organ has been previously removed. This code should not be assigned for the encounter in which the transplanted organ is removed. The complication necessitating removal of the transplant organ should be assigned for that encounter.

See section I.C.19. for information on the coding of organ transplant complications.

Z99	Dependence on enabling machines and devices, not elsewhere classified

Note: Categories Z89-Z90 and Z93-Z99 are for use only if there are no complications or malfunctions of the organ or tissue replaced, the amputation site or the equipment on which the patient is dependent.

4) History (of)

There are two types of history Z codes, personal and family. Personal history codes explain a patient's past medical condition that no longer exists and is not receiving any treatment, but that has the potential for recurrence, and therefore may require continued monitoring.

Family history codes are for use when a patient has a family member(s) who has had a particular disease that causes the patient to be at higher risk of also contracting the disease.

Personal history codes may be used in conjunction with follow-up codes and family history codes may be used in conjunction with screening codes to explain the need for a test or procedure. History codes are also acceptable on any medical record regardless of the reason for visit. A history of an illness, even if no longer present, is important information that may alter the type of treatment ordered.

The history Z code categories are:

Z80	Family history of primary malignant neoplasm
Z81	Family history of mental and behavioral disorders
Z82	Family history of certain disabilities and chronic diseases (leading to disablement)
Z83	Family history of other specific disorders
Z84	Family history of other conditions
Z85	Personal history of malignant neoplasm
Z86	Personal history of certain other diseases
Z87	Personal history of other diseases and conditions
Z91.4-	Personal history of psychological trauma, not elsewhere classified
Z91.5	Personal history of self-harm
Z91.81	**History of falling**
Z91.82	**Personal history of military deployment**
Z92	Personal history of medical treatment Except: Z92.0, Personal history of contraception Except: Z92.82, Status post administration of tPA (rtPA) in a different facility within the last 24 hours prior to admission to a current facility

5) Screening

Screening is the testing for disease or disease precursors in seemingly well individuals so that early detection and treatment can be provided for those who test positive for the disease (e.g., screening mammogram).

The testing of a person to rule out or confirm a suspected diagnosis because the patient has some sign or symptom is a diagnostic examination, not a screening. In these cases, the sign or symptom is used to explain the reason for the test.

A screening code may be a first-listed code if the reason for the visit is specifically the screening exam. It may also be used as an additional code if the screening is done during an office visit for other health problems. A screening code is

not necessary if the screening is inherent to a routine examination, such as a pap smear done during a routine pelvic examination.

Should a condition be discovered during the screening then the code for the condition may be assigned as an additional diagnosis.

The Z code indicates that a screening exam is planned. A procedure code is required to confirm that the screening was performed.

The screening Z codes/categories:

Z11	Encounter for screening for infectious and parasitic diseases
Z12	Encounter for screening for malignant neoplasms
Z13	Encounter for screening for other diseases and disorders Except: Z13.9, Encounter for screening, unspecified
Z36	Encounter for antenatal screening for mother

6) Observation

There are **three** observation Z code categories. They are for use in very limited circumstances when a person is being observed for a suspected condition that is ruled out. The observation codes are not for use if an injury or illness or any signs or symptoms related to the suspected condition are present. In such cases the diagnosis/symptom code is used with the corresponding external cause code.

The observation codes are to be used as principal diagnosis only. The only exception to this is when the principal diagnosis is required to be a code from category Z38, Liveborn infants according to place of birth and type of delivery. Then a code from category Z05, Encounter for observation and evaluation of newborn for suspected diseases and conditions ruled out, is sequenced after the Z38 code. Additional codes may be used in addition to the observation code but only if they are unrelated to the suspected condition being observed.

Codes from subcategory Z03.7 Encounter for suspected maternal and fetal conditions ruled out, may either be used as a first-listed or as an additional code assignment depending on the case. They are for use in very limited circumstances on a maternal record when an encounter is for a suspected maternal or fetal condition that is ruled out during that encounter (for example, a maternal or fetal condition may be suspected due to an abnormal test result). These codes should not be used when the condition is confirmed. In those cases, the confirmed condition should be coded. In addition, these codes are not for use if an illness or any signs or symptoms related to the suspected condition or problem are present. In such cases the diagnosis/symptom code is used.

Additional codes may be used in addition to the code from subcategory Z03.7, but only if they are unrelated to the suspected condition being evaluated.

Codes from subcategory Z03.7 may not be used for encounters for antenatal screening of mother. *See Section I.C.21. Screening.*

For encounters for suspected fetal condition that are inconclusive following testing and evaluation, assign the appropriate code from category O35, O36, O40 or O41.

The observation Z code categories:

Z03	Encounter for medical observation for suspected diseases and conditions ruled out
Z04	Encounter for examination and observation for other reasons Except: Z04.9, Encounter for examination and observation for unspecified reason
Z05	Encounter for observation and evaluation of newborn for suspected diseases and conditions ruled out

7) Aftercare

Aftercare visit codes cover situations when the initial treatment of a disease has been performed and the patient requires continued care during the healing or recovery phase, or for the long-term consequences of the disease. The aftercare Z code should not be used if treatment is directed at a current, acute disease. The diagnosis code is to be used in these cases.

Exceptions to this rule are codes Z51.0, Encounter for antineoplastic radiation therapy, and codes from subcategory Z51.1, Encounter for antineoplastic chemotherapy and immunotherapy. These codes are to be first-listed, followed by the diagnosis code when a patient's encounter is solely to receive radiation therapy, chemotherapy, or immunotherapy for the treatment of a neoplasm. If the reason for the encounter is more than one type of antineoplastic therapy, code Z51.0 and a code from subcategory Z51.1 may be assigned together, in which case one of these codes would be reported as a secondary diagnosis.

The aftercare Z codes should also not be used for aftercare for injuries. For aftercare of an injury, assign the acute injury code with the appropriate 7th character (for subsequent encounter).

The aftercare codes are generally first-listed to explain the specific reason for the encounter. An aftercare code may be used as an additional code when some type of aftercare is provided in addition to the reason for admission and no diagnosis code is applicable. An example of this would be the closure of a colostomy during an encounter for treatment of another condition.

Aftercare codes should be used in conjunction with other aftercare codes or diagnosis codes to provide better detail on the specifics of an aftercare encounter visit, unless otherwise directed by the classification. Should a patient receive multiple types of antineoplastic therapy during the same encounter, code Z51.0, Encounter for antineoplastic radiation therapy, and codes from subcategory Z51.1, Encounter for antineoplastic chemotherapy and immunotherapy, may be used together on a record. The sequencing of multiple aftercare codes depends on the circumstances of the encounter.

Certain aftercare Z code categories need a secondary diagnosis code to describe the resolving condition or sequelae. For others, the condition is included in the code title.

Additional Z code aftercare category terms include fitting and adjustment, and attention to artificial openings.

Status Z codes may be used with aftercare Z codes to indicate the nature of the aftercare. For example code Z95.1, Presence of aortocoronary bypass graft, may be used with code Z48.812, Encounter for surgical aftercare following surgery on the circulatory system, to indicate the surgery for which the aftercare is being performed. A status code should not be used when the aftercare code indicates the type of status, such as using Z43.0, Encounter for attention to tracheostomy, with Z93.0, Tracheostomy status.

The aftercare Z category/codes:

Z42	Encounter for plastic and reconstructive surgery following medical procedure or healed injury
Z43	Encounter for attention to artificial openings
Z44	Encounter for fitting and adjustment of external prosthetic device
Z45	Encounter for adjustment and management of implanted device
Z46	Encounter for fitting and adjustment of other devices
Z47	Orthopedic aftercare
Z48	Encounter for other postprocedural aftercare
Z49	Encounter for care involving renal dialysis
Z51	Encounter for other aftercare **and medical care**

8) Follow-up

The follow-up codes are used to explain continuing surveillance following completed treatment of a disease, condition, or injury. They imply that the condition has been fully treated and no longer exists. They should not be confused with aftercare codes, or injury codes with a 7th character for subsequent encounter, that explain ongoing care of a healing condition or its sequelae. Follow-up codes may be used in conjunction with history codes to provide the full picture of the healed condition and its treatment. The follow-up code is sequenced first, followed by the history code.

A follow-up code may be used to explain multiple visits. Should a condition be found to have recurred on the follow-up visit, then the diagnosis code for the condition should be assigned in place of the follow-up code.

The follow-up Z code categories:

Z08	Encounter for follow-up examination after completed treatment for malignant neoplasm
Z09	Encounter for follow-up examination after completed treatment for conditions other than malignant neoplasm
Z39	Encounter for maternal postpartum care and examination

9) Donor

Codes in category Z52, Donors of organs and tissues, are used for living individuals who are donating blood or other body tissue.

These codes are only for individuals donating for others, not for self-donations. They are not used to identify cadaveric donations.

10) Counseling

Counseling Z codes are used when a patient or family member receives assistance in the aftermath of an illness or injury, or when support is required in coping with family or social problems.

The counseling Z codes/categories:

Z30.0-	Encounter for general counseling and advice on contraception
Z31.5	Encounter for **procreative** genetic counseling
Z31.6-	Encounter for general counseling and advice on procreation
Z32.2	Encounter for childbirth instruction
Z32.3	Encounter for childcare instruction
Z69	Encounter for mental health services for victim and perpetrator of abuse
Z70	Counseling related to sexual attitude, behavior and orientation
Z71	Persons encountering health services for other counseling and medical advice, not elsewhere classified
Z76.81	Expectant mother prebirth pediatrician visit

11) Encounters for Obstetrical and Reproductive Services

See Section I.C.15. Pregnancy, Childbirth, and the Puerperium, for further instruction on the use of these codes.

Z codes for pregnancy are for use in those circumstances when none of the problems or complications included in the codes from the Obstetrics chapter exist (a routine prenatal visit or postpartum care). Codes in category Z34, Encounter for supervision of normal pregnancy, are always first listed and are not to be used with any other code from the OB chapter.

Codes in category Z3A, Weeks of gestation, may be assigned to provide additional information about the pregnancy. Category Z3A codes should not be assigned for pregnancies with abortive outcomes (categories O00-O08), elective termination of pregnancy (code Z33.2), nor for postpartum conditions, as category Z3A is not applicable to these conditions. The date of the admission should be used to determine weeks of gestation for inpatient admissions that encompass more than one gestational week.

The outcome of delivery, category Z37, should be included on all maternal delivery records. It is always a secondary code. Codes in category Z37 should not be used on the newborn record.

Z codes for family planning (contraceptive) or procreative management and counseling should be included on an obstetric record either during the pregnancy or the postpartum stage, if applicable.

Z codes/categories for obstetrical and reproductive services:

Z30	Encounter for contraceptive management
Z31	Encounter for procreative management
Z32.2	Encounter for childbirth instruction
Z32.3	Encounter for childcare instruction
Z33	Pregnant state
Z34	Encounter for supervision of normal pregnancy
Z36	Encounter for antenatal screening of mother
Z3A	Weeks of gestation
Z37	Outcome of delivery
Z39	Encounter for maternal postpartum care and examination
Z76.81	Expectant mother prebirth pediatrician visit

12) Newborns and Infants

See Section I.C.16. Newborn (Perinatal) Guidelines, for further instruction on the use of these codes.

Newborn Z codes/categories:

Z76.1	Encounter for health supervision and care of foundling
Z00.1-	Encounter for routine child health examination
Z38	Liveborn infants according to place of birth and type of delivery

13) Routine and administrative examinations

The Z codes allow for the description of encounters for routine examinations, such as, a general check-up, or, examinations for administrative purposes, such as, a pre-employment physical. The codes are not to be used if the examination is for diagnosis of a suspected condition or for treatment purposes. In such cases the diagnosis code is used. During a routine exam, should a diagnosis or condition be discovered, it should be coded as an additional code. Pre-existing and chronic conditions and history codes may also be included as additional codes as long as the examination is for administrative purposes and not focused on any particular condition.

Some of the codes for routine health examinations distinguish between "with" and "without" abnormal findings. Code assignment depends on the information that is known at the time the encounter is being coded. For example, if no abnormal findings were found during the examination, but the encounter is being coded before test results are back, it is acceptable to assign the code for "without abnormal findings." When assigning a code for "with abnormal findings," additional code(s) should be assigned to identify the specific abnormal finding(s).

Pre-operative examination and pre-procedural laboratory examination Z codes are for use only in those situations when a patient is being cleared for a procedure or surgery and no treatment is given.

The Z codes/categories for routine and administrative examinations:

Z00	Encounter for general examination without complaint, suspected or reported diagnosis
Z01	Encounter for other special examination without complaint, suspected or reported diagnosis
Z02	Encounter for administrative examination Except: Z02.9, Encounter for administrative examinations, unspecified
Z32.0-	Encounter for pregnancy test

14) Miscellaneous Z codes

The miscellaneous Z codes capture a number of other health care encounters that do not fall into one of the other categories. Certain of these codes identify the reason for the encounter; others are for use as additional codes that provide useful information on circumstances that may affect a patient's care and treatment.

Prophylactic Organ Removal

For encounters specifically for prophylactic removal of an organ (such as prophylactic removal of breasts due to a genetic susceptibility to cancer or a family history of cancer), the principal or first-listed code should be a code from category Z40, Encounter for prophylactic surgery, followed by the appropriate codes to identify the associated risk factor (such as genetic susceptibility or family history).

If the patient has a malignancy of one site and is having prophylactic removal at another site to prevent either a new primary malignancy or metastatic disease, a code for the malignancy should also be assigned in addition to a code from subcategory Z40.0, Encounter for prophylactic surgery for risk factors related to malignant neoplasms. A Z40.0 code should not be assigned if the patient is having organ removal for treatment of a malignancy, such as the removal of the testes for the treatment of prostate cancer.

Miscellaneous Z codes/categories:

Z28	Immunization not carried out Except: Z28.3, Underimmunization status
Z29	**Encounter for other prophylactic measures**
Z40	Encounter for prophylactic surgery
Z41	Encounter for procedures for purposes other than remedying health state Except: Z41.9, Encounter for procedure for purposes other than remedying health state, unspecified
Z53	Persons encountering health services for specific procedures and treatment, not carried out
Z55	Problems related to education and literacy
Z56	Problems related to employment and unemployment
Z57	Occupational exposure to risk factors
Z58	Problems related to physical environment
Z59	Problems related to housing and economic circumstances
Z60	Problems related to social environment
Z62	Problems related to upbringing
Z63	Other problems related to primary support group, including family circumstances
Z64	Problems related to certain psychosocial circumstances
Z65	Problems related to other psychosocial circumstances
Z72	Problems related to lifestyle Note: These codes should be assigned only when the documentation specifies that the patient has an associated problem

Z73	Problems related to life management difficulty
Z74	Problems related to care provider dependency Except: Z74.01, Bed confinement status
Z75	Problems related to medical facilities and other health care
Z76.0	Encounter for issue of repeat prescription
Z76.3	Healthy person accompanying sick person
Z76.4	Other boarder to healthcare facility
Z76.5	Malingerer [conscious simulation]
Z91.1-	Patient's noncompliance with medical treatment and regimen
Z91.83	Wandering in diseases classified elsewhere
Z91.84-	**Oral health risk factors**
Z91.89	Other specified personal risk factors, not elsewhere classified

15) Nonspecific Z codes

Certain Z codes are so non-specific, or potentially redundant with other codes in the classification, that there can be little justification for their use in the inpatient setting. Their use in the outpatient setting should be limited to those instances when there is no further documentation to permit more precise coding. Otherwise, any sign or symptom or any other reason for visit that is captured in another code should be used.

Nonspecific Z codes/categories:

Z02.9	Encounter for administrative examinations, unspecified
Z04.9	Encounter for examination and observation for unspecified reason
Z13.9	Encounter for screening, unspecified
Z41.9	Encounter for procedure for purposes other than remedying health state, unspecified
Z52.9	Donor of unspecified organ or tissue
Z86.59	Personal history of other mental and behavioral disorders
Z88.9	Allergy status to unspecified drugs, medicaments and biological substances status
Z92.0	Personal history of contraception

16) Z Codes That May Only be Principal/First-Listed Diagnosis

The following Z codes/categories may only be reported as the principal/first-listed diagnosis, except when there are multiple encounters on the same day and the medical records for the encounters are combined:

Z00	Encounter for general examination without complaint, suspected or reported diagnosis Except: Z00.6
Z01	Encounter for other special examination without complaint, suspected or reported diagnosis
Z02	Encounter for administrative examination
Z03	Encounter for medical observation for suspected diseases and conditions ruled out
Z04	Encounter for examination and observation for other reasons
Z33.2	Encounter for elective termination of pregnancy
Z31.81	Encounter for male factor infertility in female patient
Z31.83	Encounter for assisted reproductive fertility procedure cycle
Z31.84	Encounter for fertility preservation procedure
Z34	Encounter for supervision of normal pregnancy
Z39	Encounter for maternal postpartum care and examination
Z38	Liveborn infants according to place of birth and type of delivery
Z40	**Encounter for prophylactic surgery**
Z42	Encounter for plastic and reconstructive surgery following medical procedure or healed injury
Z51.0	Encounter for antineoplastic radiation therapy
Z51.1-	Encounter for antineoplastic chemotherapy and immunotherapy
Z52	Donors of organs and tissues Except: Z52.9, Donor of unspecified organ or tissue
Z76.1	Encounter for health supervision and care of foundling
Z76.2	Encounter for health supervision and care of other healthy infant and child
Z99.12	Encounter for respirator [ventilator] dependence during power failure

CHAPTER 21

FACTORS INFLUENCING HEALTH STATUS AND CONTACT WITH HEALTH SERVICES (Z00-Z99)

Note: Z codes represent reasons for encounters. A corresponding procedure code must accompany a Z code if a procedure is performed. Categories Z00-Z99 are provided for occasions when circumstances other than a disease, injury or external cause classifiable to categories A00-Y89 are recorded as 'diagnoses' or 'problems.' This can arise in two main ways:

(a) When a person who may or may not be sick encounters the health services for some specific purpose, such as to receive limited care or service for a current condition, to donate an organ or tissue, to receive prophylactic vaccination (immunization), or to discuss a problem which is in itself not a disease or injury.

(b) When some circumstance or problem is present which influences the person's health status but is not in itself a current illness or injury.

This chapter contains the following blocks:

Z00-Z13	Persons encountering health services for examination
Z14-Z15	Genetic carrier and genetic susceptibility to disease
Z16	Resistance to antimicrobial drugs
Z17	Estrogen receptor status
Z18	Retained foreign body fragments
~~Z19~~	~~Hormone sensitivity malignancy status~~
Z20-Z29	Persons with potential health hazards related to communicable diseases
Z30-Z39	Persons encountering health services in circumstances related to reproduction
Z40-Z53	Encounters for other specific health care
Z55-Z65	Persons with potential health hazards related to socioeconomic and psychosocial circumstances
Z66	Do not resuscitate status
Z67	Blood type
Z68	Body mass index (BMI)
Z69-Z76	Persons encountering health services in other circumstances
Z77-Z99	Persons with potential health hazards related to family and personal history and certain conditions influencing health status

PERSONS ENCOUNTERING HEALTH SERVICES FOR EXAMINATIONS (Z00-Z13)

Note: Nonspecific abnormal findings disclosed at the time of these examinations are classified to categories R70-R94.

Excludes1   examinations related to pregnancy and reproduction (Z30-Z36, Z39.-)

● **Z00**   **Encounter for general examination without complaint, suspected or reported diagnosis**

Excludes1   encounter for examination for administrative purposes (Z02.-)

Excludes2   encounter for pre-procedural examinations (Z01.81-)
special screening examinations (Z11-Z13)

● **Z00.0**   **Encounter for general adult medical examination**
Encounter for adult periodic examination (annual) (physical) and any associated laboratory and radiologic examinations

Excludes1   encounter for examination of sign or symptom - code to sign or symptom general health check-up of infant or child (Z00.12.-)

Z00.00   **Encounter for general adult medical examination without abnormal findings**
Encounter for adult health check-up NOS

Z00.01   **Encounter for general adult medical examination with abnormal findings**
Use additional code to identify abnormal findings

● **Z00.1**   **Encounter for newborn, infant and child health examinations**

● **Z00.11**   **Newborn health examination**
Health check for child under 29 days old
Use additional code to identify any abnormal findings

Excludes1   health check for child over 28 days old (Z00.12-)

Z00.110   **Health examination for newborn under 8 days old**
Health check for newborn under 8 days old

Z00.111   **Health examination for newborn 8 to 28 days old**
Health check for newborn 8 to 28 days old
Newborn weight check

● **Z00.12**   **Encounter for routine child health examination**
Encounter for development testing of infant or child
Health check (routine) for child over 28 days old

Excludes1   health check for child under 29 days old (Z00.11-)
health supervision of foundling or other healthy infant or child (Z76.1-Z76.2)
newborn health examination (Z00.11-)

Z00.121   **Encounter for routine child health examination with abnormal findings**
Use additional code to identify abnormal findings

Z00.129   **Encounter for routine child health examination without abnormal findings**
Encounter for routine child health examination NOS

Z00.2   **Encounter for examination for period of rapid growth in childhood**

Z00.3   **Encounter for examination for adolescent development state**
Encounter for puberty development state

Z00.5   **Encounter for examination of potential donor of organ and tissue**

Z00.6   **Encounter for examination for normal comparison and control in clinical research program**
Examination of participant or control in clinical research program

● **Z00.7**   **Encounter for examination for period of delayed growth in childhood**

Z00.70   **Encounter for examination for period of delayed growth in childhood without abnormal findings**

Z00.71   **Encounter for examination for period of delayed growth in childhood with abnormal findings**
Use additional code to identify abnormal findings

Z00.8   **Encounter for other general examination**
Encounter for health examination in population surveys

● **Z01**   **Encounter for other special examination without complaint, suspected or reported diagnosis**

     Includes   routine examination of specific system

     Note: Codes from category Z01 represent the reason for the encounter. A separate procedure code is required to identify any examinations or procedures performed.

     Excludes1   encounter for examination for administrative purposes (Z02.-)

           encounter for examination for suspected conditions, proven not to exist (Z03.-)

           encounter for laboratory and radiologic examinations as a component of general medical examinations (Z00.0-)

           encounter for laboratory, radiologic and imaging examinations for sign(s) and symptom(s) - code to the sign(s) or symptom(s)

     Excludes2   screening examinations (Z11-Z13)

● **Z01.0**   **Encounter for examination of eyes and vision**

     Excludes1   examination for driving license (Z02.4)

     Z01.00   **Encounter for examination of eyes and vision without abnormal findings**

           Encounter for examination of eyes and vision NOS

     Z01.01   **Encounter for examination of eyes and vision with abnormal findings**

           Use additional code to identify abnormal findings

● **Z01.1**   **Encounter for examination of ears and hearing**

     Z01.10   **Encounter for examination of ears and hearing without abnormal findings**

           Encounter for examination of ears and hearing NOS

     ● **Z01.11**   **Encounter for examination of ears and hearing with abnormal findings**

         Z01.110   **Encounter for hearing examination following failed hearing screening**

         Z01.118   **Encounter for examination of ears and hearing with other abnormal findings**

             Use additional code to identify abnormal findings

     Z01.12   **Encounter for hearing conservation and treatment**

● **Z01.2**   **Encounter for dental examination and cleaning**

     Z01.20   **Encounter for dental examination and cleaning without abnormal findings**

           Encounter for dental examination and cleaning NOS

     Z01.21   **Encounter for dental examination and cleaning with abnormal findings**

           Use additional code to identify abnormal findings

● **Z01.3**   **Encounter for examination of blood pressure**

     Z01.30   **Encounter for examination of blood pressure without abnormal findings**

           Encounter for examination of blood pressure NOS

     Z01.31   **Encounter for examination of blood pressure with abnormal findings**

           Use additional code to identify abnormal findings

● **Z01.4**   **Encounter for gynecological examination**

     Excludes2   pregnancy examination or test (Z32.0-)

           routine examination for contraceptive maintenance (Z30.4-)

● **Z01.41**   **Encounter for routine gynecological examination**

     Encounter for general gynecological examination with or without cervical smear

     Encounter for gynecological examination (general) (routine) NOS

     Encounter for pelvic examination (annual) (periodic)

     Use additional code:

         for screening for human papillomavirus, if applicable (Z11.51)

         for screening vaginal pap smear, if applicable (Z12.72)

         to identify acquired absence of uterus, if applicable (Z90.71-)

     Excludes1   gynecologic examination status-post hysterectomy for malignant condition (Z08)

           screening cervical pap smear not a part of a routine gynecological examination (Z12.4)

     Z01.411   **Encounter for gynecological examination (general) (routine) with abnormal findings**

           Use additional code to identify any abnormal findings

     Z01.419   **Encounter for gynecological examination (general) (routine) without abnormal findings**

     Z01.42   **Encounter for cervical smear to confirm findings of recent normal smear following initial abnormal smear**

● **Z01.8**   **Encounter for other specified special examinations**

     ● **Z01.81**   **Encounter for preprocedural examinations**

         Encounter for preoperative examinations

         Encounter for radiological and imaging examinations as part of preprocedural examination

         Z01.810   **Encounter for preprocedural cardiovascular examination**

         Z01.811   **Encounter for preprocedural respiratory examination**

         Z01.812   **Encounter for preprocedural laboratory examination**

             Blood and urine tests prior to treatment or procedure

         Z01.818   **Encounter for other preprocedural examination**

             Encounter for preprocedural examination NOS

             Encounter for examinations prior to antineoplastic chemotherapy

     Z01.82   **Encounter for allergy testing**

         Excludes1   encounter for antibody response examination (Z01.84)

     Z01.83   **Encounter for blood typing**

         Encounter for Rh typing

     Z01.84   **Encounter for antibody response examination**

         Encounter for immunity status testing

         Excludes1   encounter for allergy testing (Z01.82)

     Z01.89   **Encounter for other specified special examinations**

CHAPTER 21 (Z00-Z99)

● **Z02   Encounter for administrative examination**

Z02.0   Encounter for examination for admission to educational institution

Encounter for examination for admission to preschool (education)

Encounter for examination for re-admission to school following illness or medical treatment

Z02.1   Encounter for pre-employment examination

Z02.2   Encounter for examination for admission to residential institution

> **Excludes1**   examination for admission to prison (Z02.89)

Z02.3   Encounter for examination for recruitment to armed forces

Z02.4   Encounter for examination for driving license

Z02.5   Encounter for examination for participation in sport

> **Excludes1**   blood-alcohol and blood-drug test (Z02.83)

Z02.6   Encounter for examination for insurance purposes

● **Z02.7   Encounter for issue of medical certificate**

> **Excludes1**   encounter for general medical examination (Z00-Z01, Z02.0-Z02.6, Z02.8-Z02.9)

     Z02.71   Encounter for disability determination

Encounter for issue of medical certificate of incapacity

Encounter for issue of medical certificate of invalidity

     Z02.79   Encounter for issue of other medical certificate

● **Z02.8   Encounter for other administrative examinations**

     Z02.81   Encounter for paternity testing

     Z02.82   Encounter for adoption services

     Z02.83   Encounter for blood-alcohol and blood-drug test

> **Use additional** code for findings of alcohol or drugs in blood (R78.-)

     Z02.89   Encounter for other administrative examinations

Encounter for examination for admission to prison

Encounter for examination for admission to summer camp

Encounter for immigration examination

Encounter for naturalization examination

Encounter for premarital examination

> **Excludes1**   health supervision of foundling or other healthy infant or child (Z76.1-Z76.2)

Z02.9   Encounter for administrative examinations, unspecified

---

OGCR Section II.C.21.c.6.

Observation

There are **three** observation Z code categories. They are for use in very limited circumstances when a person is being observed for a suspected condition that is ruled out. The observation codes are not for use if an injury or illnesses or any signs or symptoms related to the suspected condition are present. In such cases the diagnosis/symptom code is used with the corresponding external cause code.

The observation codes are to be used as principal diagnosis only. **The only exception to this is when the principal diagnosis is required to be a code from category Z38, Liveborn infants according to place of birth and type of delivery. Then a code from category Z05, Encounter for observation and evaluation of newborn for suspected diseases and conditions ruled out, is sequenced after the Z38 code.** Additional codes may be used in addition to the observation code but only if they are unrelated to the suspected condition being observed.

Codes from subcategory Z03.7 Encounter for suspected maternal and fetal conditions ruled out, may either be used as a first listed or as an additional code assignment depending on the case. They are for use in very limited circumstances on a maternal record when an encounter is for a suspected maternal or fetal condition that is ruled out during that encounter (for example, a maternal or fetal condition may be suspected due to an abnormal test result). These codes should not be used when the condition is confirmed. In those cases, the confirmed condition should be coded. In addition, these codes are not for use if an illness or any signs or symptoms related to the suspected condition or problem are present. In such cases the diagnosis/symptom code is used.

Additional codes may be used in addition to the code from subcategory Z03.7, but only if they are unrelated to the suspected condition being evaluated.

Codes from subcategory Z03.7 may not be used for encounters for antenatal screening of mother. *See Section I.C.21. Screening.*

For encounters for suspected fetal condition that are inconclusive following testing and evaluation, assign the appropriate code from category O35, O36, O40 or O41.

The observation Z code categories:

Z03   Encounter for medical observation for suspected diseases and conditions ruled out

Z04   Encounter for examination and observation for other reasons
Except: Z04.9, Encounter for examination and observation for unspecified reason

Z05   Encounter for observation and evaluation of newborn for suspected diseases and conditions ruled out

● **Z03   Encounter for medical observation for suspected diseases and conditions ruled out**

This category is to be used when a person without a diagnosis is suspected of having an abnormal condition, without signs or symptoms, which requires study, but after examination and observation, is ruled out. This category is also for use for administrative and legal observation status.

> **Excludes1**   contact with and (suspected) exposures hazardous to health (Z77.-)
>
> ▶ encounter for observation and evaluation of newborn for suspected diseases and conditions ruled out (Z05.0-)
>
> ~~newborn observation for suspected condition, ruled out (P00-P04)~~
>
> person with feared complaint in whom no diagnosis is made (Z71.1)
>
> signs or symptoms under study - code to signs or symptoms

Z03.6   Encounter for observation for suspected toxic effect from ingested substance ruled out

Encounter for observation for suspected adverse effect from drug

Encounter for observation for suspected poisoning

▶ New   ⇒ Revised   ~~deleted~~ Deleted   **OGCR** Official Guidelines   X Assign placeholder X   ● Use Additional Character(s)

| Excludes 1 | Excludes 2 | Includes | Use additional | Code first | Code also | Key words |

● **Z03.7** **Encounter for suspected maternal and fetal conditions ruled out**
    Encounter for suspected maternal and fetal conditions not found
    | Excludes1 | known or suspected fetal anomalies affecting management of mother, not ruled out (O26.-, O35.-, O36.-, O40.-, O41.-)

    Z03.71 **Encounter for suspected problem with amniotic cavity and membrane ruled out**
        Encounter for suspected oligohydramnios ruled out
        Encounter for suspected polyhydramnios ruled out

    Z03.72 **Encounter for suspected placental problem ruled out**

    Z03.73 **Encounter for suspected fetal anomaly ruled out**

    Z03.74 **Encounter for suspected problem with fetal growth ruled out**

    Z03.75 **Encounter for suspected cervical shortening ruled out**

    Z03.79 **Encounter for other suspected maternal and fetal conditions ruled out**

● **Z03.8** **Encounter for observation for other suspected diseases and conditions ruled out**

  ● **Z03.81** **Encounter for observation for suspected exposure to biological agents ruled out**

    Z03.810 **Encounter for observation for suspected exposure to anthrax ruled out**

    Z03.818 **Encounter for observation for suspected exposure to other biological agents ruled out**

    Z03.89 **Encounter for observation for other suspected diseases and conditions ruled out**

● **Z04** **Encounter for examination and observation for other reasons**
    | Includes | encounter for examination for medicolegal reasons
    This category is to be used when a person without a diagnosis is suspected of having an abnormal condition, without signs or symptoms, which requires study, but after examination and observation, is ruled-out. This category is also for use for administrative and legal observation status.

    Z04.1 **Encounter for examination and observation following transport accident**
      | Excludes1 | encounter for examination and observation following work accident (Z04.2)

    Z04.2 **Encounter for examination and observation following work accident**

    Z04.3 **Encounter for examination and observation following other accident**

  ● **Z04.4** **Encounter for examination and observation following alleged rape**
    Encounter for examination and observation of victim following alleged rape
    Encounter for examination and observation of victim following alleged sexual abuse

    Z04.41 **Encounter for examination and observation following alleged adult rape**
        Suspected adult rape, ruled out
        Suspected adult sexual abuse, ruled out

    Z04.42 **Encounter for examination and observation following alleged child rape**
        Suspected child rape, ruled out
        Suspected child sexual abuse, ruled out

    Z04.6 **Encounter for general psychiatric examination, requested by authority**

● **Z04.7** **Encounter for examination and observation following alleged physical abuse**

    Z04.71 **Encounter for examination and observation following alleged adult physical abuse**
        Suspected adult physical abuse, ruled out
      | Excludes1 | confirmed case of adult physical abuse (T74.-)
        encounter for examination and observation following alleged adult sexual abuse (Z04.41)
        suspected case of adult physical abuse, not ruled out (T76.-)

    Z04.72 **Encounter for examination and observation following alleged child physical abuse**
        Suspected child physical abuse, ruled out
      | Excludes1 | confirmed case of child physical abuse (T74.-)
        encounter for examination and observation following alleged child sexual abuse (Z04.42)
        suspected case of child physical abuse, not ruled out (T76.-)

    Z04.8 **Encounter for examination and observation for other specified reasons**
        Encounter for examination and observation for request for expert evidence

    Z04.9 **Encounter for examination and observation for unspecified reason**
        Encounter for observation NOS

● **Z05** **Encounter for observation and evaluation of newborn for suspected diseases and conditions ruled out**
    ➠ This category is to be used for newborns, within the neonatal period (the first 28 days of life), who are suspected of having an abnormal condition, but without signs or symptoms, and which, after examination and observation, is ruled out.
    | Excludes2 | ~~newborn observation for suspected condition, related to exposure from the mother or birth process (P00-P04)~~

    Z05.0 **Observation and evaluation of newborn for suspected cardiac condition ruled out**

    Z05.1 **Observation and evaluation of newborn for suspected infectious condition ruled out**

    Z05.2 **Observation and evaluation of newborn for suspected neurological condition ruled out**

    Z05.3 **Observation and evaluation of newborn for suspected respiratory condition ruled out**

  ● **Z05.4** **Observation and evaluation of newborn for suspected genetic, metabolic or immunologic condition ruled out**

    Z05.41 **Observation and evaluation of newborn for suspected genetic condition ruled out**

    Z05.42 **Observation and evaluation of newborn for suspected metabolic condition ruled out**

    Z05.43 **Observation and evaluation of newborn for suspected immunologic condition ruled out**

    Z05.5 **Observation and evaluation of newborn for suspected gastrointestinal condition ruled out**

    Z05.6 **Observation and evaluation of newborn for suspected genitourinary condition ruled out**

CHAPTER 21 (Z00-Z99)

● **Z05.7**   **Observation and evaluation of newborn for suspected skin, subcutaneous, musculoskeletal and connective tissue condition ruled out**

     Z05.71   **Observation and evaluation of newborn for suspected skin and subcutaneous tissue condition ruled out**

     Z05.72   **Observation and evaluation of newborn for suspected musculoskeletal condition ruled out**

     Z05.73   **Observation and evaluation of newborn for suspected connective tissue condition ruled out**

Z05.8   **Observation and evaluation of newborn for other specified suspected condition ruled out**

Z05.9   **Observation and evaluation of newborn for unspecified suspected condition ruled out**

OGCR   See Section II.C.21.c.8.

> The follow-up codes are used to explain continuing surveillance following completed treatment of a disease, condition, or injury. They imply that the condition has been fully treated and no longer exists. They should not be confused with aftercare codes, or injury codes with 7th character "D," that explain ongoing care of a healing condition or its sequelae. Follow-up codes may be used in conjunction with history codes to provide the full picture of the healed condition and its treatment. The follow-up code is sequenced first, followed by the history code.
>
> A follow-up code may be used to explain multiple visits. Should a condition be found to have recurred on the follow-up visit, then the diagnosis code for the condition should be assigned in place of the follow-up code.
>
> The follow-up Z code categories:
>
> Z08   Encounter for follow-up examination after completed treatment for malignant neoplasm
>
> Z09   Encounter for follow-up examination after completed treatment for conditions other than malignant neoplasm
>
> Z39   Encounter for maternal postpartum care and examination

Z08   **Encounter for follow-up examination after completed treatment for malignant neoplasm**

     Medical surveillance following completed treatment

     Use additional code to identify any acquired absence of organs (Z90.-)

     Use additional code to identify the personal history of malignant neoplasm (Z85.-)

     Excludes1   aftercare following medical care (Z43-Z49, Z51)

Z09   **Encounter for follow-up examination after completed treatment for conditions other than malignant neoplasm**

     Medical surveillance following completed treatment

     Use additional code to identify any applicable history of disease code (Z86.-. Z87.-)

     Excludes1   aftercare following medical care (Z43-Z49, Z51)
                 surveillance of contraception (Z30.4-)
                 surveillance of prosthetic and other medical devices (Z44-Z46)

OGCR   Section II.C.21.c.5.

> Screening
>
> Screening is the testing for disease or disease precursors in seemingly well individuals so that early detection and treatment can be provided for those who test positive for the disease (e.g., screening mammogram).
>
> The testing of a person to rule out or confirm a suspected diagnosis because the patient has some sign or symptom is a diagnostic examination, not a screening. In these cases, the sign or symptom is used to explain the reason for the test.
>
> A screening code may be a first listed code if the reason for the visit is specifically the screening exam. It may also be used as an additional code if the screening is done during an office visit for other health problems. A screening code is not necessary if the screening is inherent to a routine examination, such as a pap smear done during a routine pelvic examination.
>
> Should a condition be discovered during the screening then the code for the condition may be assigned as an additional diagnosis.
>
> The Z code indicates that a screening exam is planned. A procedure code is required to confirm that the screening was performed.
>
> The screening Z codes /categories:
>
> Z11   Encounter for screening for infectious and parasitic diseases
>
> Z12   Encounter for screening for malignant neoplasms
>
> Z13   Encounter for screening for other diseases and disorders
>   Except: Z13.9, Encounter for screening, unspecified
>
> Z36   Encounter for antenatal screening for mother

● **Z11**   **Encounter for screening for infectious and parasitic diseases**

     Screening is the testing for disease or disease precursors in asymptomatic individuals so that early detection and treatment can be provided for those who test positive for the disease.

     Excludes1   encounter for diagnostic examination - code to sign or symptom

Z11.0   **Encounter for screening for intestinal infectious diseases**

Z11.1   **Encounter for screening for respiratory tuberculosis**

Z11.2   **Encounter for screening for other bacterial diseases**

Z11.3   **Encounter for screening for infections with a predominantly sexual mode of transmission**

     Excludes2   encounter for screening for human immunodeficiency virus [HIV] (Z11.4)
                 encounter for screening for human papillomavirus (Z11.51)

Z11.4   **Encounter for screening for human immunodeficiency virus [HIV]**

● **Z11.5**   **Encounter for screening for other viral diseases**

     Excludes2   encounter for screening for viral intestinal disease (Z11.0)

     Z11.51   **Encounter for screening for human papillomavirus (HPV)**

     Z11.59   **Encounter for screening for other viral diseases**

Z11.6   **Encounter for screening for other protozoal diseases and helminthiases**

     Diseases or infestations caused by parasitic worms

     Excludes2   encounter for screening for protozoal intestinal disease (Z11.0)

Z11.8   **Encounter for screening for other infectious and parasitic diseases**

     Encounter for screening for chlamydia
     Encounter for screening for rickettsial
     Encounter for screening for spirochetal
     Encounter for screening for mycoses

Z11.9   **Encounter for screening for infectious and parasitic diseases, unspecified**

● **Z12   Encounter for screening for malignant neoplasms**

Screening is the testing for disease or disease precursors in asymptomatic individuals so that early detection and treatment can be provided for those who test positive for the disease.

Use additional code to identify any family history of malignant neoplasm (Z80.-)

> Excludes1   encounter for diagnostic examination - code to sign or symptom

Z12.0   Encounter for screening for malignant neoplasm of stomach

● Z12.1   Encounter for screening for malignant neoplasm of intestinal tract

Z12.10   Encounter for screening for malignant neoplasm of intestinal tract, unspecified

Z12.11   Encounter for screening for malignant neoplasm of colon
Encounter for screening colonoscopy NOS

Z12.12   Encounter for screening for malignant neoplasm of rectum

Z12.13   Encounter for screening for malignant neoplasm of small intestine

Z12.2   Encounter for screening for malignant neoplasm of respiratory organs

● Z12.3   Encounter for screening for malignant neoplasm of breast

Z12.31   Encounter for screening mammogram for malignant neoplasm of breast

> Excludes1   inconclusive mammogram (R92.2)

Z12.39   Encounter for other screening for malignant neoplasm of breast

Z12.4   Encounter for screening for malignant neoplasm of cervix
Encounter for screening pap smear for malignant neoplasm of cervix

> Excludes1   when screening is part of general gynecological examination (Z01.4-)

> Excludes2   encounter for screening for human papillomavirus (Z11.51)

Z12.5   Encounter for screening for malignant neoplasm of prostate

Z12.6   Encounter for screening for malignant neoplasm of bladder

● Z12.7   Encounter for screening for malignant neoplasm of other genitourinary organs

Z12.71   Encounter for screening for malignant neoplasm of testis

Z12.72   Encounter for screening for malignant neoplasm of vagina
Vaginal pap smear status - post hysterectomy for non-malignant condition
Use additional code to identify acquired absence of uterus (Z90.71-)

> Excludes1   vaginal pap smear status - post hysterectomy for malignant conditions (Z08)

Z12.73   Encounter for screening for malignant neoplasm of ovary

Z12.79   Encounter for screening for malignant neoplasm of other genitourinary organs

● Z12.8   Encounter for screening for malignant neoplasm of other sites

Z12.81   Encounter for screening for malignant neoplasm of oral cavity

Z12.82   Encounter for screening for malignant neoplasm of nervous system

Z12.83   Encounter for screening for malignant neoplasm of skin

Z12.89   Encounter for screening for malignant neoplasm of other sites

Z12.9   Encounter for screening for malignant neoplasm, site unspecified

● **Z13   Encounter for screening for other diseases and disorders**

Screening is the testing for disease or disease precursors in asymptomatic individuals so that early detection and treatment can be provided for those who test positive for the disease.

> Excludes1   encounter for diagnostic examination - code to sign or symptom

Z13.0   Encounter for screening for diseases of the blood and blood-forming organs and certain disorders involving the immune mechanism

Z13.1   Encounter for screening for diabetes mellitus

● Z13.2   Encounter for screening for nutritional, metabolic and other endocrine disorders

Z13.21   Encounter for screening for nutritional disorder

● Z13.22   Encounter for screening for metabolic disorder

Z13.220   Encounter for screening for lipoid disorders
Encounter for screening for cholesterol level
Encounter for screening for hypercholesterolemia
Encounter for screening for hyperlipidemia

Z13.228   Encounter for screening for other metabolic disorders

Z13.29   Encounter for screening for other suspected endocrine disorder

> Excludes1   encounter for screening for diabetes mellitus (Z13.1)

Z13.4   Encounter for screening for certain developmental disorders in childhood
Encounter for screening for developmental handicaps in early childhood

> Excludes1   routine development testing of infant or child (Z00.1-)

Z13.5   Encounter for screening for eye and ear disorders

> Excludes2   encounter for general hearing examination (Z01.1-)
> encounter for general vision examination (Z01.0-)

Z13.6   Encounter for screening for cardiovascular disorders

● Z13.7   Encounter for screening for genetic and chromosomal anomalies

> Excludes1   genetic testing for procreative management (Z31.4-)

Z13.71   Encounter for nonprocreative screening for genetic disease carrier status

Z13.79   Encounter for other screening for genetic and chromosomal anomalies

CHAPTER 21 (Z00-Z99)

● **Z13.8** Encounter for screening for other specified diseases and disorders

> Excludes2   screening for malignant neoplasms (Z12.-)

● **Z13.81** Encounter for screening for digestive system disorders

    Z13.810 Encounter for screening for upper gastrointestinal disorder

    Z13.811 Encounter for screening for lower gastrointestinal disorder

> Excludes1   encounter for screening for intestinal infectious disease (Z11.0)

    Z13.818 Encounter for screening for other digestive system disorders

● **Z13.82** Encounter for screening for musculoskeletal disorder

    Z13.820 Encounter for screening for osteoporosis

    Z13.828 Encounter for screening for other musculoskeletal disorder

  Z13.83 Encounter for screening for respiratory disorder NEC

> Excludes1   encounter for screening for respiratory tuberculosis (Z11.1)

  Z13.84 Encounter for screening for dental disorders

● **Z13.85** Encounter for screening for nervous system disorders

    Z13.850 Encounter for screening for traumatic brain injury

    Z13.858 Encounter for screening for other nervous system disorders

  Z13.88 Encounter for screening for disorder due to exposure to contaminants

> Excludes1   those exposed to contaminants without suspected disorders (Z57-Z77.-)

  Z13.89 Encounter for screening for other disorder
Encounter for screening for genitourinary disorders

  Z13.9 Encounter for screening, unspecified

GENETIC CARRIER AND GENETIC SUSCEPTIBILITY TO DISEASE (Z14-Z15)

● **Z14** Genetic carrier

● **Z14.0** Hemophilia A carrier

  Z14.01 Asymptomatic hemophilia A carrier

  Z14.02 Symptomatic hemophilia A carrier

  Z14.1 Cystic fibrosis carrier

  Z14.8 Genetic carrier of other disease

● **Z15** Genetic susceptibility to disease

> Excludes1   chromosomal anomalies (Q90-Q99)

> Includes   confirmed abnormal gene

Use additional code, if applicable, for any associated family history of the disease (Z80-Z84)

● **Z15.0** Genetic susceptibility to malignant neoplasm

> *Code first if applicable, any current malignant neoplasm (C00-C75, C81-C96)*

Use additional code, if applicable, for any personal history of malignant neoplasm (Z85.-)

  Z15.01 Genetic susceptibility to malignant neoplasm of breast

  Z15.02 Genetic susceptibility to malignant neoplasm of ovary

  Z15.03 Genetic susceptibility to malignant neoplasm of prostate

  Z15.04 Genetic susceptibility to malignant neoplasm of endometrium

  Z15.09 Genetic susceptibility to other malignant neoplasm

● **Z15.8** Genetic susceptibility to other disease

  Z15.81 Genetic susceptibility to multiple endocrine neoplasia [MEN]

> Excludes1   multiple endocrine neoplasia [MEN] syndromes (E31.2-)

  Z15.89 Genetic susceptibility to other disease

RESISTANCE TO ANTIMICROBIAL DRUGS (Z16)

● **Z16** Resistance to antimicrobial drugs

> **Note:** The codes in this category are provided for use as additional codes to identify the resistance and non-responsiveness of a condition to antimicrobial drugs.

> *Code first the infection*

> Excludes1   Methicillin resistant Staphylococcus aureus infection (A49.02)
> ~~Methicillin resistant Staphylococcus aureus infection in diseases classified elsewhere (B95.62)~~
> Methicillin resistant Staphylococcus aureus pneumonia (J15.212)
> Sepsis due to Methicillin resistant Staphylococcus aureus (A41.02)

● **Z16.1** Resistance to beta lactam antibiotics

  Z16.10 Resistance to unspecified beta lactam antibiotics

  Z16.11 Resistance to penicillins
Resistance to amoxicillin
Resistance to ampicillin

  Z16.12 Extended spectrum beta lactamase (ESBL) resistance

> ▶ Excludes2   Methicillin resistant Staphylococcus aureus infection in diseases classified elsewhere (B95.62)

  Z16.19 Resistance to other specified beta lactam antibiotics
Resistance to cephalosporins

● **Z16.2** Resistance to other antibiotics

  Z16.20 Resistance to unspecified antibiotic
Resistance to antibiotics NOS

  Z16.21 Resistance to vancomycin

  Z16.22 Resistance to vancomycin related antibiotics

  Z16.23 Resistance to quinolones and fluoroquinolones

  Z16.24 Resistance to multiple antibiotics

  Z16.29 Resistance to other single specified antibiotic
Resistance to aminoglycosides
Resistance to macrolides
Resistance to sulfonamides
Resistance to tetracyclines

● **Z16.3** Resistance to other antimicrobial drugs

> Excludes1   resistance to antibiotics (Z16.1-, Z16.2-)

  Z16.30 Resistance to unspecified antimicrobial drugs
Drug resistance NOS

  Z16.31 Resistance to antiparasitic drug(s)
Resistance to quinine and related compounds

  Z16.32 Resistance to antifungal drug(s)

  Z16.33 Resistance to antiviral drug(s)

● **Z16.34** Resistance to antimycobacterial drug(s)
Resistance to tuberculostatics

    Z16.341 Resistance to single antimycobacterial drug
Resistance to antimycobacterial drug NOS

    Z16.342 Resistance to multiple antimycobacterial drugs

▶ New   ⟹ Revised   ~~deleted~~ Deleted   **OGCR** Official Guidelines   X Assign placeholder X   ● Use Additional Character(s)

Excludes 1   Excludes 2   Includes   Use additional   Code first   Code also   Key words

Z16.35   Resistance to multiple antimicrobial drugs

    Excludes1   Resistance to multiple antibiotics only (Z16.24)

Z16.39   Resistance to other specified antimicrobial drug

ESTROGEN RECEPTOR STATUS (Z17)

● **Z17**   Estrogen receptor status

    Code first malignant neoplasm of breast (C50.-)

Z17.0   Estrogen receptor positive status [ER+]

Z17.1   Estrogen receptor negative status [ER-]

RETAINED FOREIGN BODY FRAGMENTS (Z18)

● **Z18**   Retained foreign body fragments

    Includes   embedded fragment (status)
             embedded splinter (status)
             retained foreign body status

    Excludes1   artificial joint prosthesis status (Z96.6-)
             foreign body accidentally left during a procedure (T81.5-)
             foreign body entering through orifice (T15-T19)
             in situ cardiac device (Z95.-)
             organ or tissue replaced by means other than transplant (Z96.-, Z97.-)
             organ or tissue replaced by transplant (Z94.-)
             personal history of retained foreign body fully removed Z87.821
             superficial foreign body (non-embedded splinter) - code to superficial foreign body, by site

● Z18.0   Retained radioactive fragments

Z18.01   Retained depleted uranium fragments

Z18.09   Other retained radioactive fragments
          Other retained depleted isotope fragments
          Retained nontherapeutic radioactive fragments

● Z18.1   Retained metal fragments

    Excludes1   retained radioactive metal fragments (Z18.01-Z18.09)

Z18.10   Retained metal fragments, unspecified
          Retained metal fragment NOS

Z18.11   Retained magnetic metal fragments

Z18.12   Retained nonmagnetic metal fragments

Z18.2   Retained plastic fragments
      Acrylics fragments
      Diethylhexylphthalates fragments
      Isocyanate fragments

● Z18.3   Retained organic fragments

Z18.31   Retained animal quills or spines

Z18.32   Retained tooth

Z18.33   Retained wood fragments

Z18.39   Other retained organic fragments

● Z18.8   Other specified retained foreign body

Z18.81   Retained glass fragments

Z18.83   Retained stone or crystalline fragments
          Retained concrete or cement fragments

Z18.89   Other specified retained foreign body fragments

Z18.9   Retained foreign body fragments, unspecified material

HORMONE SENSITIVITY MALIGNANCY STATUS (Z19)

● **Z19**   Hormone sensitivity malignancy status

    Code first malignant neoplasm —*see* Table of Neoplasms, by site, malignant

Z19.1   Hormone sensitive malignancy status

Z19.2   Hormone resistant malignancy status
      Castrate resistant prostate malignancy status

PERSONS WITH POTENTIAL HEALTH HAZARDS RELATED TO COMMUNICABLE DISEASES (Z20-Z29)

● **Z20**   Contact with and (suspected) exposure to communicable diseases

    Excludes1   carrier of infectious disease (Z22.-)
             diagnosed current infectious or parasitic disease - see Alphabetic Index

    Excludes2   personal history of infectious and parasitic diseases (Z86.1-)

● Z20.0   Contact with and (suspected) exposure to intestinal infectious diseases

Z20.01   Contact with and (suspected) exposure to intestinal infectious diseases due to Escherichia coli (E. coli)

Z20.09   Contact with and (suspected) exposure to other intestinal infectious diseases

Z20.1   Contact with and (suspected) exposure to tuberculosis

Z20.2   Contact with and (suspected) exposure to infections with a predominantly sexual mode of transmission

Z20.3   Contact with and (suspected) exposure to rabies

Z20.4   Contact with and (suspected) exposure to rubella

Z20.5   Contact with and (suspected) exposure to viral hepatitis

Z20.6   Contact with and (suspected) exposure to human immunodeficiency virus [HIV]

    Excludes1   asymptomatic human immunodeficiency virus [HIV]
             HIV infection status (Z21)

Z20.7   Contact with and (suspected) exposure to pediculosis, acariasis and other infestations

● Z20.8   Contact with and (suspected) exposure to other communicable diseases

● Z20.81   Contact with and (suspected) exposure to other bacterial communicable diseases

Z20.810   Contact with and (suspected) exposure to anthrax

Z20.811   Contact with and (suspected) exposure to meningococcus

Z20.818   Contact with and (suspected) exposure to other bacterial communicable diseases

● Z20.82   Contact with and (suspected) exposure to other viral communicable diseases

Z20.820   Contact with and (suspected) exposure to varicella

Z20.828   Contact with and (suspected) exposure to other viral communicable diseases

Z20.89   Contact with and (suspected) exposure to other communicable diseases

Z20.9   Contact with and (suspected) exposure to unspecified communicable disease

Z21   Asymptomatic human immunodeficiency virus [HIV] infection status

    HIV positive NOS

    Code first Human immunodeficiency virus [HIV] disease complicating pregnancy, childbirth and the puerperium, if applicable (O98.7-)

    Excludes1   acquired immunodeficiency syndrome (B20)
             contact with human immunodeficiency virus [HIV] (Z20.6)
             exposure to human immunodeficiency virus [HIV] (Z20.6)
             human immunodeficiency virus [HIV] disease (B20)
             inconclusive laboratory evidence of human immunodeficiency virus [HIV] (R75)

CHAPTER 21 (Z00-Z99)

CHAPTER 21 (Z00-Z99)

● **Z22   Carrier of infectious disease**

> **Includes**   colonization status
> suspected carrier

> **Excludes2**   carrier of viral hepatitis (B18.-)

Z22.0   Carrier of typhoid

Z22.1   Carrier of other intestinal infectious diseases

Z22.2   Carrier of diphtheria

● **Z22.3   Carrier of other specified bacterial diseases**

　Z22.31   Carrier of bacterial disease due to meningococci

　● **Z22.32   Carrier of bacterial disease due to staphylococci**

　　Z22.321   Carrier or suspected carrier of Methicillin susceptible Staphylococcus aureus
　　　MSSA colonization

　　Z22.322   Carrier or suspected carrier of Methicillin resistant Staphylococcus aureus
　　　MRSA colonization

　● **Z22.33   Carrier of bacterial disease due to streptococci**

　　Z22.330   Carrier of Group B streptococcus

> > **Excludes1**   Carrier of streptococcus group B (GBS) complicating pregnancy, childbirth and the puerperium (O99.82-)

　　Z22.338   Carrier of other streptococcus

　Z22.39   Carrier of other specified bacterial diseases

Z22.4   Carrier of infections with a predominantly sexual mode of transmission

Z22.6   Carrier of human T-lymphotropic virus type-1 [HTLV-1] infection

Z22.8   Carrier of other infectious diseases

Z22.9   Carrier of infectious disease, unspecified

Z23   Encounter for immunization

> *Code first any routine childhood examination*

> **Note:** Procedure codes are required to identify the types of immunizations given.

● **Z28   Immunization not carried out and underimmunization status**

> **Includes**   vaccination not carried out

● **Z28.0   Immunization not carried out because of contraindication**

　Z28.01   Immunization not carried out because of acute illness of patient

　Z28.02   Immunization not carried out because of chronic illness or condition of patient

　Z28.03   Immunization not carried out because of immune compromised state of patient

　Z28.04   Immunization not carried out because of patient allergy to vaccine or component

　Z28.09   Immunization not carried out because of other contraindication

Z28.1   Immunization not carried out because of patient decision for reasons of belief or group pressure
　Immunization not carried out because of religious belief

● **Z28.2   Immunization not carried out because of patient decision for other and unspecified reason**

　Z28.20   Immunization not carried out because of patient decision for unspecified reason

　Z28.21   Immunization not carried out because of patient refusal

　Z28.29   Immunization not carried out because of patient decision for other reason

Z28.3   Underimmunization status
> Delinquent immunization status
> Lapsed immunization schedule status

● **Z28.8   Immunization not carried out for other reason**

　Z28.81   Immunization not carried out due to patient having had the disease

　Z28.82   Immunization not carried out because of caregiver refusal
　　Immunization not carried out because of guardian refusal
　　Immunization not carried out because of parent refusal

> > **Excludes1**   immunization not carried out because of caregiver refusal because of religious belief (Z28.1)

　Z28.89   Immunization not carried out for other reason

Z28.9   Immunization not carried out for unspecified reason

● **Z29   Encounter for other prophylactic measures**

> **Excludes1**   desensitization to allergens (Z51.6)
> prophylactic surgery (Z40.-)

● **Z29.1   Encounter for prophylactic immunotherapy**
> Encounter for administration of immunoglobulin

　Z29.11   Encounter for prophylactic immunotherapy for respiratory syncytial virus (RSV)

　Z29.12   Encounter for prophylactic antivenin

　Z29.13   Encounter for prophylactic Rho(D) immune globulin

　Z29.14   Encounter for prophylactic rabies immune globin

Z29.3   Encounter for prophylactic fluoride administration

Z29.8   Encounter for other specified prophylactic measures

Z29.9   Encounter for prophylactic measures, unspecified

PERSONS ENCOUNTERING HEALTH SERVICES IN CIRCUMSTANCES RELATED TO REPRODUCTION (Z30-Z39)

● **Z30   Encounter for contraceptive management**

● **Z30.0   Encounter for general counseling and advice on contraception**

　● **Z30.01   Encounter for initial prescription of contraceptives**

> > **Excludes1**   encounter for surveillance of contraceptives (Z30.4-)

　　Z30.011   Encounter for initial prescription of contraceptive pills

　　Z30.012   Encounter for prescription of emergency contraception
　　　Encounter for postcoital contraception

　　Z30.013   Encounter for initial prescription of injectable contraceptive

　　Z30.014   Encounter for initial prescription of intrauterine contraceptive device

> > > **Excludes1**   encounter for insertion of intrauterine contraceptive device (Z30.430, Z30.432)

　　Z30.015   Encounter for initial prescription of vaginal ring hormonal contraceptive

Z30.016   Encounter for initial prescription of transdermal patch hormonal contraceptive device

Z30.017   Encounter for initial prescription of implantable subdermal contraceptive

Z30.018   Encounter for initial prescription of other contraceptives

Encounter for initial prescription of barrier contraception

Encounter for initial prescription of diaphragm

Z30.019   Encounter for initial prescription of contraceptives, unspecified

Z30.02   Counseling and instruction in natural family planning to avoid pregnancy

Z30.09   Encounter for other general counseling and advice on contraception

Encounter for family planning advice NOS

Z30.2   Encounter for sterilization

● **Z30.4**   Encounter for surveillance of contraceptives

Z30.40   Encounter for surveillance of contraceptives, unspecified

Z30.41   Encounter for surveillance of contraceptive pills

Encounter for repeat prescription for contraceptive pill

Z30.42   Encounter for surveillance of injectable contraceptive

● **Z30.43**   Encounter for surveillance of intrauterine contraceptive device

Z30.430   Encounter for insertion of intrauterine contraceptive device

Z30.431   Encounter for routine checking of intrauterine contraceptive device

Z30.432   Encounter for removal of intrauterine contraceptive device

Z30.433   Encounter for removal and reinsertion of intrauterine contraceptive device

Encounter for replacement of intrauterine contraceptive device

Z30.44   Encounter for surveillance of vaginal ring hormonal contraceptive device

Z30.45   Encounter for surveillance of transdermal patch hormonal contraceptive device

Z30.46   Encounter for surveillance of implantable subdermal contraceptive

Encounter for checking, reinsertion or removal of implantable subdermal contraceptive

Z30.49   Encounter for surveillance of other contraceptives

Encounter for surveillance of barrier contraception

Encounter for surveillance of diaphragm

Z30.8   Encounter for other contraceptive management

Encounter for postvasectomy sperm count

Encounter for routine examination for contraceptive maintenance

Excludes1   sperm count following sterilization reversal (Z31.42)

sperm count for fertility testing (Z31.41)

Z30.9   Encounter for contraceptive management, unspecified

● **Z31**   Encounter for procreative management

Excludes1   complications associated with artificial fertilization (N98.-)

female infertility (N97.-)

male infertility (N46.-)

Z31.0   Encounter for reversal of previous sterilization

● **Z31.4**   Encounter for procreative investigation and testing

Excludes1   postvasectomy sperm count (Z30.8)

Z31.41   Encounter for fertility testing

Encounter for fallopian tube patency testing

Encounter for sperm count for fertility testing

Z31.42   Aftercare following sterilization reversal

Sperm count following sterilization reversal

● **Z31.43**   Encounter for genetic testing of female for procreative management

Use additional code for recurrent pregnancy loss, if applicable (N96, O26.2-)

Excludes1   nonprocreative genetic testing (Z13.7-)

Z31.430   Encounter of female for testing for genetic disease carrier status for procreative management

Z31.438   Encounter for other genetic testing of female for procreative management

● **Z31.44**   Encounter for genetic testing of male for procreative management

Excludes1   nonprocreative genetic testing (Z13.7-)

Z31.440   Encounter of male for testing for genetic disease carrier status for procreative management

Z31.441   Encounter for testing of male partner of patient with recurrent pregnancy loss

Z31.448   Encounter for other genetic testing of male for procreative management

Z31.49   Encounter for other procreative investigation and testing

➠ **Z31.5**   Encounter for procreative genetic counseling

● **Z31.6**   Encounter for general counseling and advice on procreation

Z31.61   Procreative counseling and advice using natural family planning

Z31.62   Encounter for fertility preservation counseling

Encounter for fertility preservation counseling prior to cancer therapy

Encounter for fertility preservation counseling prior to surgical removal of gonads

Z31.69   Encounter for other general counseling and advice on procreation

Z31.7   Encounter for procreative management and counseling for gestational carrier

Excludes1   pregnant state, gestational carrier (Z33.3)

- Z31.8   Encounter for other procreative management
  - Z31.81   Encounter for male factor infertility in female patient
  - Z31.82   Encounter for Rh incompatibility status
  - Z31.83   Encounter for assisted reproductive fertility procedure cycle
    Patient undergoing in vitro fertilization cycle
    Use additional code to identify the type of infertility
    - Excludes1   pre-cycle diagnosis and testing - code to reason for encounter
  - Z31.84   Encounter for fertility preservation procedure
    Encounter for fertility preservation procedure prior to cancer therapy
    Encounter for fertility preservation procedure prior to surgical removal of gonads
  - Z31.89   Encounter for other procreative management
  - Z31.9   Encounter for procreative management, unspecified

- Z32   Encounter for pregnancy test and childbirth and childcare instruction
  - Z32.0   Encounter for pregnancy test
    - Z32.00   Encounter for pregnancy test, result unknown
      Encounter for pregnancy test NOS
    - Z32.01   Encounter for pregnancy test, result positive
    - Z32.02   Encounter for pregnancy test, result negative
  - Z32.2   Encounter for childbirth instruction
  - Z32.3   Encounter for childcare instruction
    Encounter for prenatal or postpartum childcare instruction

- Z33   Pregnant state
  - Z33.1   Pregnant state, incidental
    Pregnant state NOS
    - Excludes1   complications of pregnancy (O00-O9A)
      pregnant state, gestational carrier (Z33.3)
  - Z33.2   Encounter for elective termination of pregnancy
    - Excludes1   early fetal death with retention of dead fetus (O02.1)
      late fetal death (O36.4)
      spontaneous abortion (O03)
  - Z33.3   Pregnant state, gestational carrier
    - Excludes1   encounter for procreative management and counseling for gestational carrier (Z31.7)

- Z34   Encounter for supervision of normal pregnancy
  - Excludes1   any complication of pregnancy (O00-O9A)
    encounter for pregnancy test (Z32.0-)
    encounter for supervision of high risk pregnancy (O09.-)
  - Z34.0   Encounter for supervision of normal first pregnancy
    - Z34.00   Encounter for supervision of normal first pregnancy, unspecified trimester
    - Z34.01   Encounter for supervision of normal first pregnancy, first trimester
    - Z34.02   Encounter for supervision of normal first pregnancy, second trimester
    - Z34.03   Encounter for supervision of normal first pregnancy, third trimester
  - Z34.8   Encounter for supervision of other normal pregnancy
    - Z34.80   Encounter for supervision of other normal pregnancy, unspecified trimester
    - Z34.81   Encounter for supervision of other normal pregnancy, first trimester

| First trimester (0 to 14 weeks) | Second trimester (14 to 28 weeks) | Third trimester (28 weeks to delivery) |

Figure 21-1 Trimesters. (From Shiland, Betsy J. Medical Terminology & Anatomy for ICD-10 Coding, ed 2, Mosby, 2015)

  - Z34.82   Encounter for supervision of other normal pregnancy, second trimester
  - Z34.83   Encounter for supervision of other normal pregnancy, third trimester
  - Z34.9   Encounter for supervision of normal pregnancy, unspecified
    - Z34.90   Encounter for supervision of normal pregnancy, unspecified, unspecified trimester
    - Z34.91   Encounter for supervision of normal pregnancy, unspecified, first trimester
    - Z34.92   Encounter for supervision of normal pregnancy, unspecified, second trimester
    - Z34.93   Encounter for supervision of normal pregnancy, unspecified, third trimester

- Z36   Encounter for antenatal screening of mother
  - Includes   Encounter for placental sample (taken vaginally)
    Screening is the testing for disease or disease precursors in asymptomatic individuals so that early detection and treatment can be provided for those who test positive for the disease.
    - Excludes1   abnormal findings on antenatal screening of mother (O28.-)
      diagnostic examination - code to sign or symptom
      encounter for suspected maternal and fetal conditions ruled out (Z03.7-)
      suspected fetal condition affecting management of pregnancy - code to condition in Chapter 15
    - Excludes2   abnormal findings on antenatal screening of mother (O28.-)
      genetic counseling and testing (Z31.43-, Z31.5)
      routine prenatal care (Z34)
  - Z36.0   Encounter for antenatal screening for chromosomal anomalies
  - Z36.1   Encounter for antenatal screening for raised alphafetoprotein level
    Encounter for antenatal screening for elevated maternal serum alphafetoprotein level
  - Z36.2   Encounter for other antenatal screening follow-up
    Non-visualized anatomy on a previous scan
  - Z36.3   Encounter for antenatal screening for malformations
    Screening for a suspected anomaly
  - Z36.4   Encounter for antenatal screening for fetal growth retardation
    Intrauterine growth restriction (IUGR)/small-for-dates
  - Z36.5   Encounter for antenatal screening for isoimmunization
  - Z36.8   Encounter for other antenatal screening
    - Z36.81   Encounter for antenatal screening for hydrops fetalis
    - Z36.82   Encounter for antenatal screening for nuchal translucency
    - Z36.83   Encounter for fetal screening for congenital cardiac abnormalities
    - Z36.84   Encounter for antenatal screening for fetal lung maturity

▶ **Z36.85 Encounter for antenatal screening for Streptococcus B**

▶ **Z36.86 Encounter for antenatal screening for cervical length**
    ▶Screening for risk of pre-term labor

▶ **Z36.87 Encounter for antenatal screening for uncertain dates**

▶ **Z36.88 Encounter for antenatal screening for fetal macrosomia**
    ▶Screening for large-for-dates

▶ **Z36.89 Encounter for other specified antenatal screening**

▶ **Z36.8A Encounter for antenatal screening for other genetic defects**

▶ **Z36.9 Encounter for antenatal screening, unspecified**

● **Z3A Weeks of gestation**
    Note: Codes from category Z3A are for use, only on the maternal record, to indicate the weeks of gestation of the pregnancy, if known.

    ⇒ *Code first complications of pregnancy, childbirth and the puerperium (O09-O9A)*

● **Z3A.0 Weeks of gestation of pregnancy, unspecified or less than 10 weeks**
    Z3A.00 Weeks of gestation of pregnancy not specified
    Z3A.01 Less than 8 weeks gestation of pregnancy
    Z3A.08 8 weeks gestation of pregnancy
    Z3A.09 9 weeks gestation of pregnancy

● **Z3A.1 Weeks of gestation of pregnancy, weeks 10-19**
    Z3A.10 10 weeks gestation of pregnancy
    Z3A.11 11 weeks gestation of pregnancy
    Z3A.12 12 weeks gestation of pregnancy
    Z3A.13 13 weeks gestation of pregnancy
    Z3A.14 14 weeks gestation of pregnancy
    Z3A.15 15 weeks gestation of pregnancy
    Z3A.16 16 weeks gestation of pregnancy
    Z3A.17 17 weeks gestation of pregnancy
    Z3A.18 18 weeks gestation of pregnancy
    Z3A.19 19 weeks gestation of pregnancy

● **Z3A.2 Weeks of gestation of pregnancy, weeks 20-29**
    Z3A.20 20 weeks gestation of pregnancy
    Z3A.21 21 weeks gestation of pregnancy
    Z3A.22 22 weeks gestation of pregnancy
    Z3A.23 23 weeks gestation of pregnancy
    Z3A.24 24 weeks gestation of pregnancy
    Z3A.25 25 weeks gestation of pregnancy
    Z3A.26 26 weeks gestation of pregnancy
    Z3A.27 27 weeks gestation of pregnancy
    Z3A.28 28 weeks gestation of pregnancy
    Z3A.29 29 weeks gestation of pregnancy

● **Z3A.3 Weeks of gestation of pregnancy, weeks 30-39**
    Z3A.30 30 weeks gestation of pregnancy
    Z3A.31 31 weeks gestation of pregnancy
    Z3A.32 32 weeks gestation of pregnancy
    Z3A.33 33 weeks gestation of pregnancy
    Z3A.34 34 weeks gestation of pregnancy
    Z3A.35 35 weeks gestation of pregnancy
    Z3A.36 36 weeks gestation of pregnancy
    Z3A.37 37 weeks gestation of pregnancy
    Z3A.38 38 weeks gestation of pregnancy
    Z3A.39 39 weeks gestation of pregnancy

● **Z3A.4 Weeks of gestation of pregnancy, weeks 40 or greater**
    Z3A.40 40 weeks gestation of pregnancy
    Z3A.41 41 weeks gestation of pregnancy
    Z3A.42 42 weeks gestation of pregnancy
    Z3A.49 Greater than 42 weeks gestation of pregnancy

● **Z37 Outcome of delivery**
    This category is intended for use as an additional code to identify the outcome of delivery on the mother's record. It is not for use on the newborn record.

    Excludes1 stillbirth (P95)

Z37.0 Single live birth
Z37.1 Single stillbirth
Z37.2 Twins, both liveborn
Z37.3 Twins, one liveborn and one stillborn
Z37.4 Twins, both stillborn
● **Z37.5 Other multiple births, all liveborn**
    Z37.50 Multiple births, unspecified, all liveborn
    Z37.51 Triplets, all liveborn
    Z37.52 Quadruplets, all liveborn
    Z37.53 Quintuplets, all liveborn
    Z37.54 Sextuplets, all liveborn
    Z37.59 Other multiple births, all liveborn
● **Z37.6 Other multiple births, some liveborn**
    Z37.60 Multiple births, unspecified, some liveborn
    Z37.61 Triplets, some liveborn
    Z37.62 Quadruplets, some liveborn
    Z37.63 Quintuplets, some liveborn
    Z37.64 Sextuplets, some liveborn
    Z37.69 Other multiple births, some liveborn
Z37.7 Other multiple births, all stillborn
Z37.9 Outcome of delivery, unspecified
    Multiple birth NOS
    Single birth NOS

● **Z38 Liveborn infants according to place of birth and type of delivery**
    This category is for use as the principal code on the initial record of a newborn baby. It is to be used for the initial birth record only. It is not to be used on the mother's record.

● **Z38.0 Single liveborn infant, born in hospital**
    Single liveborn infant, born in birthing center or other health care facility
    Z38.00 Single liveborn infant, delivered vaginally
    Z38.01 Single liveborn infant, delivered by cesarean
Z38.1 Single liveborn infant, born outside hospital
Z38.2 Single liveborn infant, unspecified as to place of birth
    Single liveborn infant NOS
● **Z38.3 Twin liveborn infant, born in hospital**
    Z38.30 Twin liveborn infant, delivered vaginally
    Z38.31 Twin liveborn infant, delivered by cesarean
Z38.4 Twin liveborn infant, born outside hospital
Z38.5 Twin liveborn infant, unspecified as to place of birth
● **Z38.6 Other multiple liveborn infant, born in hospital**
    Z38.61 Triplet liveborn infant, delivered vaginally
    Z38.62 Triplet liveborn infant, delivered by cesarean
    Z38.63 Quadruplet liveborn infant, delivered vaginally
    Z38.64 Quadruplet liveborn infant, delivered by cesarean
    Z38.65 Quintuplet liveborn infant, delivered vaginally
    Z38.66 Quintuplet liveborn infant, delivered by cesarean
    Z38.68 Other multiple liveborn infant, delivered vaginally
    Z38.69 Other multiple liveborn infant, delivered by cesarean
Z38.7 Other multiple liveborn infant, born outside hospital
Z38.8 Other multiple liveborn infant, unspecified as to place of birth

CHAPTER 21 (Z00-Z99)

CHAPTER 21 (Z00-Z99)

● **Z39** Encounter for maternal postpartum care and examination

  Z39.0 Encounter for care and examination of mother immediately after delivery

    Care and observation in uncomplicated cases when the delivery occurs outside a healthcare facility

    Excludes1 care for postpartum complication - see Alphabetic index

  Z39.1 Encounter for care and examination of lactating mother

    Encounter for supervision of lactation

    Excludes1 disorders of lactation (O92.-)

  Z39.2 Encounter for routine postpartum follow-up

ENCOUNTERS FOR OTHER SPECIFIC HEALTH CARE (Z40-Z53)

Categories Z40-Z53 are intended for use to indicate a reason for care. They may be used for patients who have already been treated for a disease or injury, but who are receiving aftercare or prophylactic care, or care to consolidate the treatment, or to deal with a residual state

  Excludes2 follow-up examination for medical surveillance after treatment (Z08-Z09)

● **Z40** Encounter for prophylactic surgery

  Excludes1 organ donations (Z52.-)

    therapeutic organ removal - code to condition

● **Z40.0** Encounter for prophylactic surgery for risk factors related to malignant neoplasms

    Admission for prophylactic organ removal

    Use additional code to identify risk factor

    Z40.00 Encounter for prophylactic removal of unspecified organ

    Z40.01 Encounter for prophylactic removal of breast

  ➡ **Z40.02** Encounter for prophylactic removal of ovary(s)

    ▶Encounter for prophylactic removal of ovary(s) and fallopian tube(s)

  ▶ **Z40.03** Encounter for prophylactic removal of fallopian tube(s)

    Z40.09 Encounter for prophylactic removal of other organ

  Z40.8 Encounter for other prophylactic surgery

  Z40.9 Encounter for prophylactic surgery, unspecified

● **Z41** Encounter for procedures for purposes other than remedying health state

  Z41.1 Encounter for cosmetic surgery

    Encounter for cosmetic breast implant

    Encounter for cosmetic procedure

    Excludes1 encounter for plastic and reconstructive surgery following medical procedure or healed injury (Z42.-)

      encounter for post-mastectomy breast implantation (Z42.1)

  Z41.2 Encounter for routine and ritual male circumcision

  Z41.3 Encounter for ear piercing

  Z41.8 Encounter for other procedures for purposes other than remedying health state

  Z41.9 Encounter for procedure for purposes other than remedying health state, unspecified

● **Z42** Encounter for plastic and reconstructive surgery following medical procedure or healed injury

  Excludes1 encounter for cosmetic plastic surgery (Z41.1)

    encounter for plastic surgery for treatment of current injury - code to relevent injury

  Z42.1 Encounter for breast reconstruction following mastectomy

    Excludes1 deformity and disproportion of reconstructed breast (N65.1-)

  Z42.8 Encounter for other plastic and reconstructive surgery following medical procedure or healed injury

● **Z43** Encounter for attention to artificial openings

  Includes closure of artificial openings

    passage of sounds or bougies through artificial openings

    reforming artificial openings

    removal of catheter from artificial openings

    toilet or cleansing of artificial openings

  Excludes1 ~~artificial opening status only, without need for care (Z93.-)~~

    complications of external stoma (J95.0-, K94.-, N99.5-)

  Excludes2 fitting and adjustment of prosthetic and other devices (Z44-Z46)

  Z43.0 Encounter for attention to tracheostomy

  Z43.1 Encounter for attention to gastrostomy

    ▶**Excludes2** artificial opening status only, without need for care (Z93.-)

  Z43.2 Encounter for attention to ileostomy

  Z43.3 Encounter for attention to colostomy

  Z43.4 Encounter for attention to other artificial openings of digestive tract

  Z43.5 Encounter for attention to cystostomy

  Z43.6 Encounter for attention to other artificial openings of urinary tract

    Encounter for attention to nephrostomy

    Encounter for attention to ureterostomy

    Encounter for attention to urethrostomy

  Z43.7 Encounter for attention to artificial vagina

  Z43.8 Encounter for attention to other artificial openings

  Z43.9 Encounter for attention to unspecified artificial opening

● **Z44** Encounter for fitting and adjustment of external prosthetic device

  Includes removal or replacement of external prosthetic device

  Excludes1 malfunction or other complications of device - see Alphabetical Index presence of prosthetic device (Z97.-)

● **Z44.0** Encounter for fitting and adjustment of artificial arm

●   **Z44.00** Encounter for fitting and adjustment of unspecified artificial arm

    Z44.001 Encounter for fitting and adjustment of unspecified right artificial arm

    Z44.002 Encounter for fitting and adjustment of unspecified left artificial arm

    Z44.009 Encounter for fitting and adjustment of unspecified artificial arm, unspecified arm

●   **Z44.01** Encounter for fitting and adjustment of complete artificial arm

    Z44.011 Encounter for fitting and adjustment of complete right artificial arm

    Z44.012 Encounter for fitting and adjustment of complete left artificial arm

    Z44.019 Encounter for fitting and adjustment of complete artificial arm, unspecified arm

●   **Z44.02** Encounter for fitting and adjustment of partial artificial arm

    Z44.021 Encounter for fitting and adjustment of partial artificial right arm

    Z44.022 Encounter for fitting and adjustment of partial artificial left arm

    Z44.029 Encounter for fitting and adjustment of partial artificial arm, unspecified arm

▶ New   ⟹ Revised   ~~deleted~~ Deleted   **OGCR** Official Guidelines   X Assign placeholder X   ● Use Additional Character(s)

Excludes 1   Excludes 2   Includes   Use additional   Code first   Code also   Key words

● **Z44.1**   **Encounter for fitting and adjustment of artificial leg**
    ● **Z44.10**   **Encounter for fitting and adjustment of unspecified artificial leg**
       Z44.101   **Encounter for fitting and adjustment of unspecified right artificial leg**
       Z44.102   **Encounter for fitting and adjustment of unspecified left artificial leg**
       Z44.109   **Encounter for fitting and adjustment of unspecified artificial leg, unspecified leg**
    ● **Z44.11**   **Encounter for fitting and adjustment of complete artificial leg**
       Z44.111   **Encounter for fitting and adjustment of complete right artificial leg**
       Z44.112   **Encounter for fitting and adjustment of complete left artificial leg**
       Z44.119   **Encounter for fitting and adjustment of complete artificial leg, unspecified leg**
    ● **Z44.12**   **Encounter for fitting and adjustment of partial artificial leg**
       Z44.121   **Encounter for fitting and adjustment of partial artificial right leg**
       Z44.122   **Encounter for fitting and adjustment of partial artificial left leg**
       Z44.129   **Encounter for fitting and adjustment of partial artificial leg, unspecified leg**

● **Z44.2**   **Encounter for fitting and adjustment of artificial eye**
    | Excludes1 | mechanical complication of ocular prosthesis (T85.3)
       Z44.20   **Encounter for fitting and adjustment of artificial eye, unspecified**
       Z44.21   **Encounter for fitting and adjustment of artificial right eye**
       Z44.22   **Encounter for fitting and adjustment of artificial left eye**

● **Z44.3**   **Encounter for fitting and adjustment of external breast prosthesis**
    | Excludes1 | complications of breast implant (T85.4-)
          encounter for adjustment or removal of breast implant (Z45.81-)
          encounter for initial breast implant insertion for cosmetic breast augmentation (Z41.1)
          encounter for breast reconstruction following mastectomy (Z42.1)
       Z44.30   **Encounter for fitting and adjustment of external breast prosthesis, unspecified breast**
       Z44.31   **Encounter for fitting and adjustment of external right breast prosthesis**
       Z44.32   **Encounter for fitting and adjustment of external left breast prosthesis**

   Z44.8   **Encounter for fitting and adjustment of other external prosthetic devices**

   Z44.9   **Encounter for fitting and adjustment of unspecified external prosthetic device**

● **Z45**   **Encounter for adjustment and management of implanted device**
    | Includes | removal or replacement of implanted device
    | Excludes1 | malfunction or other complications of device - see Alphabetical Index
         ~~presence of prosthetic and other devices (Z95-Z97)~~
    | Excludes2 | encounter for fitting and adjustment of non-implanted device (Z46.-)

● **Z45.0**   **Encounter for adjustment and management of cardiac device**
    ● **Z45.01**   **Encounter for adjustment and management of cardiac pacemaker**
       Encounter for adjustment and management of cardiac resynchronization therapy pacemaker (CRT-P)
       | Excludes1 | encounter for adjustment and management of automatic implantable cardiac defibrillator with synchronous cardiac pacemaker (Z45.02)
       Z45.010   **Encounter for checking and testing of cardiac pacemaker pulse generator [battery]**
          Encounter for replacing cardiac pacemaker pulse generator [battery]
       Z45.018   **Encounter for adjustment and management of other part of cardiac pacemaker**
       ▶ | Excludes2 | presence of prosthetic and other devices (Z95-Z97)
       Z45.02   **Encounter for adjustment and management of automatic implantable cardiac defibrillator**
          Encounter for adjustment and management of automatic implantable cardiac defibrillator with synchronous cardiac pacemaker
          Encounter for adjustment and management of cardiac resynchronization therapy defibrillator (CRT-D)
       Z45.09   **Encounter for adjustment and management of other cardiac device**

   Z45.1   **Encounter for adjustment and management of infusion pump**

   Z45.2   **Encounter for adjustment and management of vascular access device**
       Encounter for adjustment and management of vascular catheters
    | Excludes1 | encounter for adjustment and management of renal dialysis catheter (Z49.01)

● **Z45.3**   **Encounter for adjustment and management of implanted devices of the special senses**
       Z45.31   **Encounter for adjustment and management of implanted visual substitution device**
    ● **Z45.32**   **Encounter for adjustment and management of implanted hearing device**
       | Excludes1 | encounter for fitting and adjustment of hearing aide (Z46.1)
       Z45.320   **Encounter for adjustment and management of bone conduction device**
       Z45.321   **Encounter for adjustment and management of cochlear device**
       Z45.328   **Encounter for adjustment and management of other implanted hearing device**

CHAPTER 21 (Z00-Z99)

● **Z45.4** **Encounter for adjustment and management of implanted nervous system device**

   Z45.41 Encounter for adjustment and management of **cerebrospinal fluid drainage** device

      Encounter for adjustment and management of cerebral ventricular (communicating) shunt

   Z45.42 Encounter for adjustment and management of **neuropacemaker** (brain) (peripheral nerve) (spinal cord)

   Z45.49 Encounter for adjustment and management of **other** implanted nervous system device

● **Z45.8** **Encounter for adjustment and management of other implanted devices**

  ● **Z45.81** Encounter for adjustment or removal of **breast implant**

      Encounter for elective implant exchange (different material) (different size)

      Encounter removal of tissue expander without synchronous insertion of permanent implant

      Excludes1 complications of breast implant (T85.4-)

          encounter for initial breast implant insertion for cosmetic breast augmentation (Z41.1)

          encounter for breast reconstruction following mastectomy (Z42.1)

      Z45.811 Encounter for adjustment or removal of **right** breast implant

      Z45.812 Encounter for adjustment or removal of **left** breast implant

      Z45.819 Encounter for adjustment or removal of **unspecified** breast implant

   Z45.82 Encounter for adjustment or removal of **myringotomy** device (stent) (tube)

   Z45.89 Encounter for adjustment and management of **other** implanted devices

  Z45.9 Encounter for adjustment and management of **unspecified** implanted device

● **Z46** **Encounter for fitting and adjustment of other devices**

   Includes removal or replacement of other device

   Excludes1 malfunction or other complications of device - see Alphabetical Index

   Excludes2 encounter for fitting and management of implanted devices (Z45.-)

      issue of repeat prescription only (Z76.0)

      presence of prosthetic and other devices (Z95-Z97)

  Z46.0 Encounter for fitting and adjustment of **spectacles and contact lenses**

  Z46.1 Encounter for fitting and adjustment of **hearing aid**

    Excludes1 encounter for adjustment and management of implanted hearing device (Z45.32-)

  Z46.2 Encounter for fitting and adjustment of **other devices related to nervous system and special senses**

    Excludes2 encounter for adjustment and management of implanted nervous system device (Z45.4-)

      encounter for adjustment and management of implanted visual substitution device (Z45.31)

  Z46.3 Encounter for fitting and adjustment of **dental prosthetic** device

    Encounter for fitting and adjustment of **dentures**

  Z46.4 Encounter for fitting and adjustment of **orthodontic** device

● **Z46.5** **Encounter for fitting and adjustment of other gastrointestinal appliance and device**

    Excludes1 encounter for attention to artificial openings of digestive tract (Z43.1-Z43.4)

   Z46.51 Encounter for fitting and adjustment of **gastric lap band**

   Z46.59 Encounter for fitting and adjustment of **other** gastrointestinal appliance and device

  Z46.6 Encounter for fitting and adjustment of **urinary device**

    Excludes2 attention to artificial openings of urinary tract (Z43.5, Z43.6)

● **Z46.8** **Encounter for fitting and adjustment of other specified devices**

   Z46.81 Encounter for fitting and adjustment of **insulin pump**

      Encounter for insulin pump instruction and training

      Encounter for insulin pump titration

   Z46.82 Encounter for fitting and adjustment of **non-vascular catheter**

   Z46.89 Encounter for fitting and adjustment of **other** specified devices

      Encounter for fitting and adjustment of wheelchair

  Z46.9 Encounter for fitting and adjustment of **unspecified** device

● **Z47** **Orthopedic aftercare**

   Excludes1 aftercare for healing fracture - code to fracture with 7th character D

  Z47.1 Aftercare following **joint replacement surgery**

    Use additional code to identify the joint (Z96.6-)

  Z47.2 Encounter for removal of **internal fixation device**

    Excludes1 encounter for adjustment of internal fixation device for fracture treatment - code to fracture with appropriate 7th character

      encounter for removal of external fixation device - code to fracture with 7th character D

      infection or inflammatory reaction to internal fixation device (T84.6-)

      mechanical complication of internal fixation device (T84.1-)

● **Z47.3** **Aftercare following explanation of joint prosthesis**

    Aftercare following explantation of joint prosthesis, staged procedure

    Encounter for joint prosthesis insertion following prior explantation of joint prosthesis

   Z47.31 Aftercare following explantation of **shoulder** joint prosthesis

      Excludes1 acquired absence of shoulder joint following prior explantation of shoulder joint prosthesis (Z89.23-)

          shoulder joint prosthesis explantation status (Z89.23-)

   Z47.32 Aftercare following explantation of **hip** joint prosthesis

      Excludes1 acquired absence of hip joint following prior explantation of hip joint prosthesis (Z89.62-)

          hip joint prosthesis explantation status (Z89.62-)

   Z47.33 Aftercare following explantation of **knee** joint prosthesis

      Excludes1 acquired absence of knee joint following prior explantation of knee prosthesis (Z89.52-)

          knee joint prosthesis explantation status (Z89.52-)

● **Z47.8   Encounter for other orthopedic aftercare**

    Z47.81   Encounter for orthopedic aftercare following surgical amputation

        Use additional code to identify the limb amputated (Z89.-)

    Z47.82   Encounter for orthopedic aftercare following scoliosis surgery

    Z47.89   Encounter for other orthopedic aftercare

● **Z48   Encounter for other postprocedural aftercare**

    Excludes1 ▶ encounter for aftercare following injury - code to Injury, by site, with appropriate 7th character for subsequent encounter

        encounter for follow-up examination after completed treatment (Z08-Z09)

    Excludes2   encounter for attention to artificial openings (Z43.-)

        encounter for fitting and adjustment of prosthetic and other devices (Z44-Z46)

● **Z48.0   Encounter for attention to dressings, sutures and drains**

    Excludes1   encounter for planned postprocedural wound closure (Z48.1)

    Z48.00   Encounter for change or removal of nonsurgical wound dressing

        Encounter for change or removal of wound dressing NOS

    Z48.01   Encounter for change or removal of surgical wound dressing

    Z48.02   Encounter for removal of sutures

        Encounter for removal of staples

    Z48.03   Encounter for change or removal of drains

  Z48.1   Encounter for planned postprocedural wound closure

    Excludes1   encounter for attention to dressings and sutures (Z48.0-)

● **Z48.2   Encounter for aftercare following organ transplant**

    Z48.21   Encounter for aftercare following heart transplant

    Z48.22   Encounter for aftercare following kidney transplant

    Z48.23   Encounter for aftercare following liver transplant

    Z48.24   Encounter for aftercare following lung transplant

    ● **Z48.28   Encounter for aftercare following multiple organ transplant**

        Z48.280   Encounter for aftercare following heart-lung transplant

        Z48.288   Encounter for aftercare following multiple organ transplant

    ● **Z48.29   Encounter for aftercare following other organ transplant**

        Z48.290   Encounter for aftercare following bone marrow transplant

        Z48.298   Encounter for aftercare following other organ transplant

  Z48.3   Aftercare following surgery for neoplasm

    Use additional code to identify the neoplasm

● **Z48.8   Encounter for other specified postprocedural aftercare**

    ● **Z48.81   Encounter for surgical aftercare following surgery on specified body systems**

        These codes identify the body system requiring aftercare. They are for use in conjunction with other aftercare codes to fully explain the aftercare encounter. The condition treated should also be coded if still present.

        Excludes1   aftercare for injury - code the injury with 7th character D

            aftercare following surgery for neoplasm (Z48.3)

        Excludes2   aftercare following organ transplant (Z48.2-)

            orthopedic aftercare (Z47.-)

        Z48.810   Encounter for surgical aftercare following surgery on the sense organs

        Z48.811   Encounter for surgical aftercare following surgery on the nervous system

            Excludes2   encounter for surgical aftercare following surgery on the sense organs (Z48.810)

        Z48.812   Encounter for surgical aftercare following surgery on the circulatory system

        Z48.813   Encounter for surgical aftercare following surgery on the respiratory system

        Z48.814   Encounter for surgical aftercare following surgery on the teeth or oral cavity

        Z48.815   Encounter for surgical aftercare following surgery on the digestive system

        Z48.816   Encounter for surgical aftercare following surgery on the genitourinary system

            Excludes1   encounter for aftercare following sterilization reversal (Z31.42)

        Z48.817   Encounter for surgical aftercare following surgery on the skin and subcutaneous tissue

    Z48.89   Encounter for other specified surgical aftercare

● **Z49   Encounter for care involving renal dialysis**

    Code also associated end stage renal disease (N18.6)

  ● **Z49.0   Preparatory care for renal dialysis**

    Encounter for dialysis instruction and training

    Z49.01   Encounter for fitting and adjustment of extracorporeal dialysis catheter

        Removal or replacement of renal dialysis catheter

        Toilet or cleansing of renal dialysis catheter

    Z49.02   Encounter for fitting and adjustment of peritoneal dialysis catheter

  ● **Z49.3   Encounter for adequacy testing for dialysis**

    Z49.31   Encounter for adequacy testing for hemodialysis

    Z49.32   Encounter for adequacy testing for peritoneal dialysis

        Encounter for peritoneal equilibration test

▶ New   ⇒ Revised   ~~deleted~~ Deleted   **OGCR** Official Guidelines   X Assign placeholder X   ● Use Additional Character(s)

| Excludes 1 | Excludes 2 | Includes | Use additional | Code first | Code also | Key words |

● Z51   Encounter for other aftercare and medical care
     Code also condition requiring care
     Excludes1   follow-up examination after treatment (Z08-Z09)

Z51.0   Encounter for antineoplastic radiation therapy

● Z51.1   Encounter for antineoplastic chemotherapy and immunotherapy
     Excludes2   encounter for chemotherapy and immunotherapy for nonneoplastic condition-code to condition

     Z51.11   Encounter for antineoplastic chemotherapy

     Z51.12   Encounter for antineoplastic immunotherapy

Z51.5   Encounter for palliative care

Z51.6   Encounter for desensitization to allergens

● Z51.8   Encounter for other specified aftercare
     Excludes1   holiday relief care (Z75.5)

     Z51.81   Encounter for therapeutic drug level monitoring
         Code also any long-term (current) drug therapy (Z79.-)
         Excludes1   encounter for blood-drug test for administrative or medicolegal reasons (Z02.83)

     Z51.89   Encounter for other specified aftercare

● Z52   Donors of organs and tissues
     Includes   autologous and other living donors
     Excludes1   cadaveric donor - omit code
                  examination of potential donor (Z00.5)

● Z52.0   Blood donor

     ● Z52.00   Unspecified blood donor

         Z52.000   Unspecified donor, whole blood

         Z52.001   Unspecified donor, stem cells

         Z52.008   Unspecified donor, other blood

     ● Z52.01   Autologous blood donor

         Z52.010   Autologous donor, whole blood

         Z52.011   Autologous donor, stem cells

         Z52.018   Autologous donor, other blood

     ● Z52.09   Other blood donor
         Volunteer donor

         Z52.090   Other blood donor, whole blood

         Z52.091   Other blood donor, stem cells

         Z52.098   Other blood donor, other blood

● Z52.1   Skin donor

     Z52.10   Skin donor, unspecified

     Z52.11   Skin donor, autologous

     Z52.19   Skin donor, other

● Z52.2   Bone donor

     Z52.20   Bone donor, unspecified

     Z52.21   Bone donor, autologous

     Z52.29   Bone donor, other

Z52.3   Bone marrow donor

Z52.4   Kidney donor

Z52.5   Cornea donor

Z52.6   Liver donor

● Z52.8   Donor of other specified organs or tissues

     ● Z52.81   Egg (Oocyte) donor

         Z52.810   Egg (Oocyte) donor under age 35, anonymous recipient
            Egg donor under age 35 NOS

         Z52.811   Egg (Oocyte) donor under age 35, designated recipient

         Z52.812   Egg (Oocyte) donor age 35 and over, anonymous recipient
            Egg donor age 35 and over NOS

         Z52.813   Egg (Oocyte) donor age 35 and over, designated recipient

         Z52.819   Egg (Oocyte) donor, unspecified

     Z52.89   Donor of other specified organs or tissues

Z52.9   Donor of unspecified organ or tissue
     Donor NOS

● Z53   Persons encountering health services for specific procedures and treatment, not carried out

● Z53.0   Procedure and treatment not carried out because of contraindication

     Z53.01   Procedure and treatment not carried out due to patient smoking

     Z53.09   Procedure and treatment not carried out because of other contraindication

Z53.1   Procedure and treatment not carried out because of patient's decision for reasons of belief and group pressure

● Z53.2   Procedure and treatment not carried out because of patient's decision for other and unspecified reasons

     Z53.20   Procedure and treatment not carried out because of patient's decision for unspecified reasons

     Z53.21   Procedure and treatment not carried out due to patient leaving prior to being seen by health care provider

     Z53.29   Procedure and treatment not carried out because of patient's decision for other reasons

● Z53.3   Procedure converted to open procedure

     Z53.31   Laparoscopic surgical procedure converted to open procedure

     Z53.32   Thoracoscopic surgical procedure converted to open procedure

     Z53.33   Arthroscopic surgical procedure converted to open procedure

     Z53.39   Other specified procedure converted to open procedure

Z53.8   Procedure and treatment not carried out for other reasons

Z53.9   Procedure and treatment not carried out, unspecified reason

---

PERSONS WITH POTENTIAL HEALTH HAZARDS RELATED TO SOCIOECONOMIC AND PSYCHOSOCIAL CIRCUMSTANCES (Z55-Z65)

● Z55   Problems related to education and literacy
     Excludes1   disorders of psychological development (F80-F89)

Z55.0   Illiteracy and low-level literacy

Z55.1   Schooling unavailable and unattainable

Z55.2   Failed school examinations

Z55.3   Underachievement in school

Z55.4   Educational maladjustment and discord with teachers and classmates

Z55.8   Other problems related to education and literacy
     Problems related to inadequate teaching

Z55.9   Problems related to education and literacy, unspecified
     Academic problems NOS

● **Z56**   **Problems related to employment and unemployment**

> **Excludes2**   occupational exposure to risk factors (Z57.-)
> problems related to housing and economic circumstances (Z59.-)

Z56.0   **Unemployment, unspecified**

Z56.1   **Change of job**

Z56.2   **Threat of job loss**

Z56.3   **Stressful work schedule**

Z56.4   **Discord with boss and workmates**

Z56.5   **Uncongenial work environment**
Difficult conditions at work

Z56.6   **Other physical and mental strain related to work**

● **Z56.8**   **Other problems related to employment**

     Z56.81   **Sexual harassment on the job**

     Z56.82   **Military deployment status**
Individual (civilian or military) currently deployed in theater or in support of military war, peacekeeping and humanitarian operations

     Z56.89   **Other problems related to employment**

Z56.9   **Unspecified problems related to employment**
Occupational problems NOS

● **Z57**   **Occupational exposure to risk factors**

Z57.0   **Occupational exposure to noise**

Z57.1   **Occupational exposure to radiation**

Z57.2   **Occupational exposure to dust**

● **Z57.3**   **Occupational exposure to other air contaminants**

     Z57.31   **Occupational exposure to environmental tobacco smoke**

> **Excludes2**   exposure to environmental tobacco smoke (Z77.22)

     Z57.39   **Occupational exposure to other air contaminants**

Z57.4   **Occupational exposure to toxic agents in agriculture**
Occupational exposure to solids, liquids, gases or vapors in agriculture

Z57.5   **Occupational exposure to toxic agents in other industries**
Occupational exposure to solids, liquids, gases or vapors in other industries

Z57.6   **Occupational exposure to extreme temperature**

Z57.7   **Occupational exposure to vibration**

Z57.8   **Occupational exposure to other risk factors**

Z57.9   **Occupational exposure to unspecified risk factor**

● **Z59**   **Problems related to housing and economic circumstances**

> **Excludes2**   problems related to upbringing (Z62.-)

Z59.0   **Homelessness**

Z59.1   **Inadequate housing**
Lack of heating
Restriction of space
Technical defects in home preventing adequate care
Unsatisfactory surroundings

> **Excludes1**   problems related to the natural and physical environment (Z77.1-)

Z59.2   **Discord with neighbors, lodgers and landlord**

Z59.3   **Problems related to living in residential institution**
Boarding-school resident

> **Excludes1**   institutional upbringing (Z62.2)

Z59.4   **Lack of adequate food and safe drinking water**
Inadequate drinking water supply

> **Excludes1**   effects of hunger (T73.0)
> inappropriate diet or eating habits (Z72.4)
> malnutrition (E40-E46)

Z59.5   **Extreme poverty**

Z59.6   **Low income**

Z59.7   **Insufficient social insurance and welfare support**

Z59.8   **Other problems related to housing and economic circumstances**
Foreclosure on loan
Isolated dwelling
Problems with creditors

Z59.9   **Problem related to housing and economic circumstances, unspecified**

● **Z60**   **Problems related to social environment**

Z60.0   **Problems of adjustment to life-cycle transitions**
Empty nest syndrome
Phase of life problem
Problem with adjustment to retirement [pension]

Z60.2   **Problems related to living alone**

Z60.3   **Acculturation difficulty**
Problem with migration
Problem with social transplantation

Z60.4   **Social exclusion and rejection**
Exclusion and rejection on the basis of personal characteristics, such as unusual physical appearance, illness or behavior.

> **Excludes1**   target of adverse discrimination such as for racial or religious reasons (Z60.5)

Z60.5   **Target of (perceived) adverse discrimination and persecution**

> **Excludes1**   social exclusion and rejection (Z60.4)

Z60.8   **Other problems related to social environment**

Z60.9   **Problem related to social environment, unspecified**

● **Z62**   **Problems related to upbringing**

> **Includes**   current and past negative life events in childhood
> current and past problems of a child related to upbringing

> **Excludes2**   maltreatment syndrome (T74.-)
> problems related to housing and economic circumstances (Z59.-)

Z62.0   **Inadequate parental supervision and control**

Z62.1   **Parental overprotection**

● **Z62.2**   **Upbringing away from parents**

> **Excludes1**   problems with boarding school (Z59.3)

     Z62.21   **Child in welfare custody**
Child in care of non-parental family member
Child in foster care

> **Excludes2**   problem for parent due to child in welfare custody (Z63.5)

     Z62.22   **Institutional upbringing**
Child living in orphanage or group home

     Z62.29   **Other upbringing away from parents**

Z62.3   **Hostility towards and scapegoating of child**

Z62.6   **Inappropriate (excessive) parental pressure**

CHAPTER 21 (Z00-Z99)

- ● Z62.8   **Other specified problems related to upbringing**
  - ● Z62.81   **Personal history of abuse in childhood**
    - Z62.810   **Personal history of physical and sexual abuse in childhood**
      - | Excludes1 | current child physical abuse (T74.12, T76.12)
      - current child sexual abuse (T74.22, T76.22)
    - Z62.811   **Personal history of psychological abuse in childhood**
      - | Excludes1 | current child psychological abuse (T74.32, T76.32)
    - Z62.812   **Personal history of neglect in childhood**
      - | Excludes1 | current child neglect (T74.02, T76.02)
    - Z62.819   **Personal history of unspecified abuse in childhood**
      - | Excludes1 | current child abuse NOS (T74.92, T76.92)
  - ● Z62.82   **Parent-child conflict**
    - Z62.820   **Parent-biological child conflict**
      - Parent-child problem NOS
    - Z62.821   **Parent-adopted child conflict**
    - Z62.822   **Parent-foster child conflict**
  - ● Z62.89   **Other specified problems related to upbringing**
    - Z62.890   **Parent-child estrangement NEC**
    - Z62.891   **Sibling rivalry**
    - Z62.898   **Other specified problems related to upbringing**
- Z62.9   **Problem related to upbringing, unspecified**
- ● Z63   **Other problems related to primary support group, including family circumstances**
  - | Excludes2 | maltreatment syndrome (T74.-, T76)
  - parent-child problems (Z62.-)
  - problems related to negative life events in childhood (Z62.-)
  - problems related to upbringing (Z62.-)
  - Z63.0   **Problems in relationship with spouse or partner**
    - ▶Relationship distress with spouse or intimate partner
    - | Excludes1 | counseling for spousal or partner abuse problems (Z69.1)
    - counseling related to sexual attitude, behavior, and orientation (Z70.-)
  - Z63.1   **Problems in relationship with in-laws**
  - ● Z63.3   **Absence of family member**
    - | Excludes1 | absence of family member due to disappearance and death (Z63.4)
    - absence of family member due to separation and divorce (Z63.5)
    - Z63.31   **Absence of family member due to military deployment**
      - Individual or family affected by other family member being on military deployment
      - | Excludes1 | family disruption due to return of family member from military deployment (Z63.71)
    - Z63.32   **Other absence of family member**

- Z63.4   **Disappearance and death of family member**
  - Assumed death of family member
  - Bereavement
- Z63.5   **Disruption of family by separation and divorce**
  - Marital estrangement
- Z63.6   **Dependent relative needing care at home**
- ● Z63.7   **Other stressful life events affecting family and household**
  - Z63.71   **Stress on family due to return of family member from military deployment**
    - Individual or family affected by family member having returned from military deployment (current or past conflict)
  - Z63.72   **Alcoholism and drug addiction in family**
  - Z63.79   **Other stressful life events affecting family and household**
    - Anxiety (normal) about sick person in family
    - Health problems within family
    - Ill or disturbed family member
    - Isolated family
- Z63.8   **Other specified problems related to primary support group**
  - Family discord NOS
  - Family estrangement NOS
  - High expressed emotional level within family
  - Inadequate family support NOS
  - Inadequate or distorted communication within family
- Z63.9   **Problem related to primary support group, unspecified**
  - Relationship disorder NOS
- ● Z64   **Problems related to certain psychosocial circumstances**
  - Z64.0   **Problems related to unwanted pregnancy**
  - Z64.1   **Problems related to multiparity**
  - Z64.4   **Discord with counselors**
    - Discord with probation officer
    - Discord with social worker
- ● Z65   **Problems related to other psychosocial circumstances**
  - Z65.0   **Conviction in civil and criminal proceedings without imprisonment**
  - Z65.1   **Imprisonment and other incarceration**
  - Z65.2   **Problems related to release from prison**
  - Z65.3   **Problems related to other legal circumstances**
    - Arrest
    - Child custody or support proceedings
    - Litigation
    - Prosecution
  - Z65.4   **Victim of crime and terrorism**
    - Victim of torture
  - Z65.5   **Exposure to disaster, war and other hostilities**
    - | Excludes1 | target of perceived discrimination or persecution (Z60.5)
  - Z65.8   **Other specified problems related to psychosocial circumstances**
    - ▶Religious or spiritual problem
  - Z65.9   **Problem related to unspecified psychosocial circumstances**

DO NOT RESUSCITATE STATUS (Z66)

Z66   **Do not resuscitate**
  - DNR status

BLOOD TYPE (Z67)

● Z67   **Blood type**
- ● Z67.1   Type A blood
  - Z67.10   Type A blood, Rh positive
  - Z67.11   Type A blood, Rh negative
- ● Z67.2   Type B blood
  - Z67.20   Type B blood, Rh positive
  - Z67.21   Type B blood, Rh negative
- ● Z67.3   Type AB blood
  - Z67.30   Type AB blood, Rh positive
  - Z67.31   Type AB blood, Rh negative
- ● Z67.4   Type O blood
  - Z67.40   Type O blood, Rh positive
  - Z67.41   Type O blood, Rh negative
- ● Z67.9   Unspecified blood type
  - Z67.90   Unspecified blood type, Rh positive
  - Z67.91   Unspecified blood type, Rh negative

BODY MASS INDEX [BMI] (Z68)

OGCR   Section I.B.14.

General Coding Guidelines

14. Documentation for BMI, Depth of Non-pressure ulcers, Pressure Ulcer Stages, Coma Scale, and NIH Stroke Scale

For the Body Mass Index (BMI), depth of non-pressure chronic ulcers, pressure ulcer stage, coma scale, and NIH stroke scale (NIHSS) codes, code assignment may be based on medical record documentation from clinicians who are not the patient's provider (i.e., physician or other qualified healthcare practitioner legally accountable for establishing the patient's diagnosis), since this information is typically documented by other clinicians involved in the care of the patient (e.g., a dietitian often documents the BMI, a nurse often documents the pressure ulcer stages, and an emergency medical technician often documents the coma scale). However, the associated diagnosis (such as overweight, obesity, acute stroke, or pressure ulcer) must be documented by the patient's provider. If there is conflicting medical record documentation, either from the same clinician or different clinicians, the patient's attending provider should be queried for clarification.

The BMI, coma scale, and NIHSS codes should only be reported as secondary diagnoses.

● Z68   **Body mass index [BMI]**
  Kilograms per meters squared
  Note: BMI adult codes are for use for persons 21 years of age or older.
  BMI pediatric codes are for use for persons 2-20 years of age. These percentiles are based on the growth charts published by the Centers for Disease Control and Prevention (CDC)
- ⟹ Z68.1   Body mass index (BMI) 19.9 or less, adult
- ● Z68.2   Body mass index (BMI) 20-29, adult
  - Z68.20   Body mass index (BMI) 20.0-20.9, adult
  - Z68.21   Body mass index (BMI) 21.0-21.9, adult
  - Z68.22   Body mass index (BMI) 22.0-22.9, adult
  - Z68.23   Body mass index (BMI) 23.0-23.9, adult
  - Z68.24   Body mass index (BMI) 24.0-24.9, adult
  - Z68.25   Body mass index (BMI) 25.0-25.9, adult
  - Z68.26   Body mass index (BMI) 26.0-26.9, adult
  - Z68.27   Body mass index (BMI) 27.0-27.9, adult
  - Z68.28   Body mass index (BMI) 28.0-28.9, adult
  - Z68.29   Body mass index (BMI) 29.0-29.9, adult

● Z68.3   Body mass index (BMI) 30-39, adult
  - Z68.30   Body mass index (BMI) 30.0-30.9, adult
  - Z68.31   Body mass index (BMI) 31.0-31.9, adult
  - Z68.32   Body mass index (BMI) 32.0-32.9, adult
  - Z68.33   Body mass index (BMI) 33.0-33.9, adult
  - Z68.34   Body mass index (BMI) 34.0-34.9, adult
  - Z68.35   Body mass index (BMI) 35.0-35.9, adult
  - Z68.36   Body mass index (BMI) 36.0-36.9, adult
  - Z68.37   Body mass index (BMI) 37.0-37.9, adult
  - Z68.38   Body mass index (BMI) 38.0-38.9, adult
  - Z68.39   Body mass index (BMI) 39.0-39.9, adult
● Z68.4   Body mass index (BMI) 40 or greater, adult
  - Z68.41   Body mass index (BMI) 40.0-44.9, adult
  - Z68.42   Body mass index (BMI) 45.0-49.9, adult
  - Z68.43   Body mass index (BMI) 50-59.9, adult
  - Z68.44   Body mass index (BMI) 60.0-69.9, adult
  - Z68.45   Body mass index (BMI) 70 or greater, adult
● Z68.5   Body mass index (BMI) pediatric
  - Z68.51   Body mass index (BMI) pediatric, less than 5th percentile for age
  - Z68.52   Body mass index (BMI) pediatric, 5th percentile to less than 85th percentile for age
  - Z68.53   Body mass index (BMI) pediatric, 85th percentile to less than 95th percentile for age
  - Z68.54   Body mass index (BMI) pediatric, greater than or equal to 95th percentile for age

PERSONS ENCOUNTERING HEALTH SERVICES IN OTHER CIRCUMSTANCES (Z69-Z76)

● Z69   **Encounter for mental health services for victim and perpetrator of abuse**
  Includes   counseling for victims and perpetrators of abuse
- ● Z69.0   **Encounter for mental health services for child abuse problems**
  - ● Z69.01   **Encounter for mental health services for parental child abuse**
    - Z69.010   **Encounter for mental health services for victim of parental child abuse**
      - ▶ Encounter for mental health services for victim of child abuse by parent
      - ▶ Encounter for mental health services for victim of child neglect by parent
      - ▶ Encounter for mental health services for victim of child psychological abuse by parent
      - ▶ Encounter for mental health services for victim of child sexual abuse by parent
    - Z69.011   **Encounter for mental health services for perpetrator of parental child abuse**
      - ▶ Encounter for mental health services for perpetrator of parental child neglect
      - ▶ Encounter for mental health services for perpetrator of parental child psychological abuse
      - ▶ Encounter for mental health services for perpetrator of parental child sexual abuse

      Excludes1   encounter for mental health services for non-parental child abuse (Z69.02-)

▶ New   ⟹ Revised   ~~deleted~~ Deleted   **OGCR** Official Guidelines   X Assign placeholder X   ● Use Additional Character(s)

| Excludes 1 | Excludes 2 | Includes | Use additional | Code first | Code also | Key words |

● **Z69.02** **Encounter for mental health services for non-parental child abuse**

Z69.020 **Encounter for mental health services for victim of non-parental child abuse**
▶Encounter for mental health services for victim of non-parental child neglect
▶Encounter for mental health services for victim of non-parental child psychological abuse
▶Encounter for mental health services for victim of non-parental child sexual abuse

Z69.021 **Encounter for mental health services for perpetrator of non- parental child abuse**
▶Encounter for mental health services for perpetrator of non-parental child neglect
▶Encounter for mental health services for perpetrator of non-parental child psychological abuse
▶Encounter for mental health services for perpetrator of non-parental child sexual abuse

● **Z69.1** **Encounter for mental health services for spousal or partner abuse problems**

Z69.11 **Encounter for mental health services for victim of spousal or partner abuse**
▶Encounter for mental health services for victim of spouse or partner neglect
▶Encounter for mental health services for victim of spouse or partner psychological abuse
▶Encounter for mental health services for victim of spouse or partner violence, physical

Z69.12 **Encounter for mental health services for perpetrator of spousal or partner abuse**
▶Encounter for mental health services for perpetrator of spouse or partner neglect
▶Encounter for mental health services for perpetrator of spouse or partner psychological abuse
▶Encounter for mental health services for perpetrator of spouse or partner violence, physical
▶Encounter for mental health services for perpetrator of spouse or partner violence, sexual

● **Z69.8** **Encounter for mental health services for victim or perpetrator of other abuse**

Z69.81 **Encounter for mental health services for victim of other abuse**
▶Encounter for mental health services for perpetrator of non-spousal adult abuse
▶Encounter for mental health services for victim of non-spousal adult abuse
▶Encounter for mental health services for victim of spouse or partner violence, sexual
Encounter for rape victim counseling

Z69.82 **Encounter for mental health services for perpetrator of other abuse**

● **Z70** **Counseling related to sexual attitude, behavior and orientation**

Includes   encounter for mental health services for sexual attitude, behavior and orientation

Excludes2   contraceptive or procreative counseling (Z30-Z31)

Z70.0 **Counseling related to sexual attitude**

Z70.1 **Counseling related to patient's sexual behavior and orientation**
Patient concerned regarding impotence
Patient concerned regarding non-responsiveness
Patient concerned regarding promiscuity
Patient concerned regarding sexual orientation

Z70.2 **Counseling related to sexual behavior and orientation of third party**
Advice sought regarding sexual behavior and orientation of child
Advice sought regarding sexual behavior and orientation of partner
Advice sought regarding sexual behavior and orientation of spouse

Z70.3 **Counseling related to combined concerns regarding sexual attitude, behavior and orientation**

Z70.8 **Other sex counseling**
Encounter for sex education

Z70.9 **Sex counseling, unspecified**

● **Z71** **Persons encountering health services for other counseling and medical advice, not elsewhere classified**

Excludes2   contraceptive or procreation counseling (Z30-Z31)
sex counseling (Z70.-)

Z71.0 **Person encountering health services to consult on behalf of another person**
Person encountering health services to seek advice or treatment for non-attending third party

Excludes2   anxiety (normal) about sick person in family (Z63.7)
expectant (adoptive) parent(s) pre-birth pediatrician visit (Z76.81)

Z71.1 **Person with feared health complaint in whom no diagnosis is made**
Person encountering health services with feared condition which was not demonstrated
Person encountering health services in which problem was normal state
'Worried well'

Excludes1   medical observation for suspected diseases and conditions proven not to exist (Z03.-)

Z71.2 **Person consulting for explanation of examination or test findings**

Z71.3 **Dietary counseling and surveillance**
Use additional code for any associated underlying medical condition
Use additional code to identify body mass index (BMI), if known (Z68.-)

● **Z71.4** **Alcohol abuse counseling and surveillance**
Use additional code for alcohol abuse or dependence (F10.-)

Z71.41 **Alcohol abuse counseling and surveillance of alcoholic**

Z71.42 **Counseling for family member of alcoholic**
Counseling for significant other, partner, or friend of alcoholic

▶ New   ⇒ Revised   ~~deleted~~ Deleted   **OGCR** Official Guidelines   X Assign placeholder X   ● Use Additional Character(s)

Excludes 1   Excludes 2   Includes   Use additional   Code first   Code also   Key words

CHAPTER 21 (Z00-Z99)

● Z71.5   **Drug abuse counseling and surveillance**
     Use additional code for drug abuse or dependence
     (F11-F16, F18-F19)

   Z71.51   **Drug abuse counseling and surveillance of drug abuser**

   Z71.52   **Counseling for family member of drug abuser**
     Counseling for significant other, partner, or friend of drug abuser

  Z71.6   **Tobacco abuse counseling**
     Use additional code for nicotine dependence (F17.-)

  Z71.7   **Human immunodeficiency virus [HIV] counseling**

● Z71.8   **Other specified counseling**
     Excludes2   counseling for contraception (Z30.0-)
       ~~counseling for genetics (Z31.5)~~
       ~~counseling for procreative management (Z31.6-)~~

   Z71.81   **Spiritual or religious counseling**

▶ Z71.82   **Exercise counseling**

▶ Z71.83   **Encounter for nonprocreative genetic counseling**
     Excludes1 ▶ counseling for procreative genetics (Z31.5)
       ▶ counseling for procreative management (Z31.6)

   Z71.89   **Other specified counseling**

  Z71.9   **Counseling, unspecified**
     Encounter for medical advice NOS

● Z72   **Problems related to lifestyle**
     Excludes2   problems related to life-management difficulty (Z73.-)
       problems related to socioeconomic and psychosocial circumstances (Z55-Z65)

  Z72.0   **Tobacco use**
     Tobacco use NOS
     Excludes1   history of tobacco dependence (Z87.891)
       nicotine dependence (F17.2-)
       tobacco dependence (F17.2-)
       tobacco use during pregnancy (O99.33-)

  Z72.3   **Lack of physical exercise**

  Z72.4   **Inappropriate diet and eating habits**
     Excludes1   behavioral eating disorders of infancy or childhood (F98.2-F98.3)
       eating disorders (F50.-)
       lack of adequate food (Z59.4)
       malnutrition and other nutritional deficiencies (E40-E64)

● Z72.5   **High risk sexual behavior**
     Promiscuity
     Excludes1   paraphilias (F65)

   Z72.51   **High risk heterosexual behavior**

   Z72.52   **High risk homosexual behavior**

   Z72.53   **High risk bisexual behavior**

  Z72.6   **Gambling and betting**
     Excludes1   compulsive or pathological gambling (F63.0)

● Z72.8   **Other problems related to lifestyle**

   ● Z72.81   **Antisocial behavior**
     Excludes1   conduct disorders (F91.-)

     Z72.810   **Child and adolescent antisocial behavior**
       Antisocial behavior (child) (adolescent) without manifest psychiatric disorder
       Delinquency NOS
       Group delinquency
       Offenses in the context of gang membership
       Stealing in company with others
       Truancy from school

     Z72.811   **Adult antisocial behavior**
       Adult antisocial behavior without manifest psychiatric disorder

   ● Z72.82   **Problems related to sleep**

     Z72.820   **Sleep deprivation**
       Lack of adequate sleep
       Excludes1   insomnia (G47.0-)

     Z72.821   **Inadequate sleep hygiene**
       Bad sleep habits
       Irregular sleep habits
       Unhealthy sleep wake schedule
       Excludes1   insomnia (F51.0-, G47.0-)

   Z72.89   **Other problems related to lifestyle**
     Self-damaging behavior

  Z72.9   **Problem related to lifestyle, unspecified**

● Z73   **Problems related to life management difficulty**
     Excludes2   problems related to socioeconomic and psychosocial circumstances (Z55-Z65)

  Z73.0   **Burn-out**

  Z73.1   **Type A behavior pattern**

  Z73.2   **Lack of relaxation and leisure**

  Z73.3   **Stress, not elsewhere classified**
     Physical and mental strain NOS
     Excludes1   stress related to employment or unemployment (Z56.-)

  Z73.4   **Inadequate social skills, not elsewhere classified**

  Z73.5   **Social role conflict, not elsewhere classified**

  Z73.6   **Limitation of activities due to disability**
     Excludes1   care-provider dependency (Z74.-)

● Z73.8   **Other problems related to life management difficulty**

   ● Z73.81   **Behavioral insomnia of childhood**

     Z73.810   **Behavioral insomnia of childhood, sleep-onset association type**

     Z73.811   **Behavioral insomnia of childhood, limit setting type**

     Z73.812   **Behavioral insomnia of childhood, combined type**

     Z73.819   **Behavioral insomnia of childhood, unspecified type**

   Z73.82   **Dual sensory impairment**

   Z73.89   **Other problems related to life management difficulty**

  Z73.9   **Problem related to life management difficulty, unspecified**

CHAPTER 21 (Z00-Z99)

●**Z74   Problems related to care provider dependency**
    Excludes2 dependence on enabling machines or devices NEC (Z99.-)

  ●**Z74.0   Reduced mobility**
    Z74.01   Bed confinement status
      Bedridden
    Z74.09   Other reduced mobility
      Chairridden
      Reduced mobility NOS
      Excludes2 wheelchair dependence (Z99.3)

  Z74.1   Need for assistance with personal care
  Z74.2   Need for assistance at home and no other household member able to render care
  Z74.3   Need for continuous supervision
  Z74.8   Other problems related to care provider dependency
  Z74.9   Problem related to care provider dependency, unspecified

●**Z75   Problems related to medical facilities and other health care**
  Z75.0   Medical services not available in home
    Excludes1 no other household member able to render care (Z74.2)
  Z75.1   Person awaiting admission to adequate facility elsewhere
  Z75.2   Other waiting period for investigation and treatment
  Z75.3   Unavailability and inaccessibility of health care facilities
    Excludes1 bed unavailable (Z75.1)
  Z75.4   Unavailability and inaccessibility of other helping agencies
  Z75.5   Holiday relief care
  Z75.8   Other problems related to medical facilities and other health care
  Z75.9   Unspecified problem related to medical facilities and other health care

●**Z76   Persons encountering health services in other circumstances**
  Z76.0   Encounter for issue of repeat prescription
    Encounter for issue of repeat prescription for appliance
    Encounter for issue of repeat prescription for medicaments
    Encounter for issue of repeat prescription for spectacles
    Excludes2 issue of medical certificate (Z02.7)
      repeat prescription for contraceptive (Z30.4-)
  Z76.1   Encounter for health supervision and care of foundling
  Z76.2   Encounter for health supervision and care of other healthy infant and child
    Encounter for medical or nursing care or supervision of healthy infant under circumstances such as adverse socioeconomic conditions at home
    Encounter for medical or nursing care or supervision of healthy infant under circumstances such as awaiting foster or adoptive placement
    Encounter for medical or nursing care or supervision of healthy infant under circumstances such as maternal illness
    Encounter for medical or nursing care or supervision of healthy infant under circumstances such as number of children at home preventing or interfering with normal care
  Z76.3   Healthy person accompanying sick person
  Z76.4   Other boarder to healthcare facility
    Excludes1 homelessness (Z59.0)

  Z76.5   Malingerer [conscious simulation]
    Person feigning illness (with obvious motivation)
    Excludes1 factitious disorder (F68.1-)
      peregrinating patient (F68.1-)

  ●**Z76.8   Persons encountering health services in other specified circumstances**
    Z76.81   Expectant parent(s) prebirth pediatrician visit
      Pre-adoption pediatrician visit for adoptive parent(s)
    Z76.82   Awaiting organ transplant status
      Patient waiting for organ availability
    Z76.89   Persons encountering health services in other specified circumstances
      Persons encountering health services NOS

PERSONS WITH POTENTIAL HEALTH HAZARDS RELATED TO FAMILY AND PERSONAL HISTORY AND CERTAIN CONDITIONS INFLUENCING HEALTH STATUS (Z77-Z99)

  Code also any follow-up examination (Z08-Z09)

●**Z77   Other contact with and (suspected) exposures hazardous to health**
    Includes contact with and (suspected) exposures to potential hazards to health
    Excludes2 contact with and (suspected) exposure to communicable diseases (Z20.-)
      exposure to (parental) (environmental) tobacco smoke in the perinatal period (P96.81)
      newborn affected by noxious substances transmitted via placenta or breast milk (P04.-)
      occupational exposure to risk factors (Z57.-)
      retained foreign body (Z18.-)
      retained foreign body fully removed (Z87.821)
      toxic effects of substances chiefly nonmedicinal as to source (T51-T65)

  ●**Z77.0   Contact with and (suspected) exposure to hazardous, chiefly nonmedicinal, chemicals**
    ●**Z77.01   Contact with and (suspected) exposure to hazardous metals**
      Z77.010   Contact with and (suspected) exposure to arsenic
      Z77.011   Contact with and (suspected) exposure to lead
      Z77.012   Contact with and (suspected) exposure to uranium
        Excludes1 retained depleted uranium fragments (Z18.01)
      Z77.018   Contact with and (suspected) exposure to other hazardous metals
        Contact with and (suspected) exposure to chromium compounds
        Contact with and (suspected) exposure to nickel dust
    ●**Z77.02   Contact with and (suspected) exposure to hazardous aromatic compounds**
      Z77.020   Contact with and (suspected) exposure to aromatic amines
      Z77.021   Contact with and (suspected) exposure to benzene
      Z77.028   Contact with and (suspected) exposure to other hazardous aromatic compounds
        Aromatic dyes NOS
        Polycyclic aromatic hydrocarbons

● **Z77.09** Contact with and (suspected) exposure to other hazardous, chiefly nonmedicinal, chemicals

    Z77.090 Contact with and (suspected) exposure to asbestos

    Z77.098 Contact with and (suspected) exposure to other hazardous, chiefly nonmedicinal, chemicals
        Dyes NOS

● **Z77.1** Contact with and (suspected) exposure to environmental pollution and hazards in the physical environment

  ● **Z77.11** Contact with and (suspected) exposure to environmental pollution

    Z77.110 Contact with and (suspected) exposure to air pollution

    Z77.111 Contact with and (suspected) exposure to water pollution

    Z77.112 Contact with and (suspected) exposure to soil pollution

    Z77.118 Contact with and (suspected) exposure to other environmental pollution

  ● **Z77.12** Contact with and (suspected) exposure to hazards in the physical environment

    Z77.120 Contact with and (suspected) exposure to mold (toxic)

    Z77.121 Contact with and (suspected) exposure to harmful algae and algae toxins
        Contact with and (suspected) exposure to (harmful) algae bloom NOS
        Contact with and (suspected) exposure to blue-green algae bloom
        Contact with and (suspected) exposure to brown tide
        Contact with and (suspected) exposure to cyanobacteria bloom
        Contact with and (suspected) exposure to Florida red tide
        Contact with and (suspected) exposure to pfiesteria piscicida
        Contact with and (suspected) exposure to red tide

    Z77.122 Contact with and (suspected) exposure to noise

    Z77.123 Contact with and (suspected) exposure to radon and other naturally occuring radiation
        Excludes2 radiation exposure as the cause of a confirmed condition (W88-W90, X39.0-)
          radiation sickness NOS (T66)

    Z77.128 Contact with and (suspected) exposure to other hazards in the physical environment

● **Z77.2** Contact with and (suspected) exposure to other hazardous substances

    Z77.21 Contact with and (suspected) exposure to potentially hazardous body fluids

    Z77.22 Contact with and (suspected) exposure to environmental tobacco smoke (acute) (chronic)
        Exposure to second hand tobacco smoke (acute) (chronic)
        Passive smoking (acute) (chronic)
        Excludes1 nicotine dependence (F17.-)
          tobacco use (Z72.0)
        Excludes2 occupational exposure to environmental tobacco smoke (Z57.31)

    Z77.29 Contact with and (suspected) exposure to other hazardous substances

  Z77.9 Other contact with and (suspected) exposures hazardous to health

● **Z78** Other specified health status
    Excludes2 asymptomatic human immunodeficiency virus [HIV] infection status (Z21)
        postprocedural status (Z93-Z99)
        sex reassignment status (Z87.890)

  Z78.0 Asymptomatic menopausal state
    Menopausal state NOS
    Postmenopausal status NOS
    Excludes2 symptomatic menopausal state (N95.1)

  Z78.1 Physical restraint status
    Excludes1 physical restraint due to a procedure - omit code

  Z78.9 Other specified health status

● **Z79** Long term (current) drug therapy
    Includes long term (current) drug use for prophylactic purposes
    Code also any therapeutic drug level monitoring (Z51.81)
    Excludes2 drug abuse and dependence (F11-F19)
        drug use complicating pregnancy, childbirth, and the puerperium (O99.32-)
        long term (current) use of oral antidiabetic drugs (Z79.84)
        long term (current) use of oral hypoglycemic drugs (Z79.84)

  ● **Z79.0** Long term (current) use of anticoagulants and antithrombotics/antiplatelets
    Excludes2 long term (current) use of aspirin (Z79.82)
    Z79.01 Long term (current) use of anticoagulants
    Z79.02 Long term (current) use of antithrombotics/antiplatelets

  Z79.1 Long term (current) use of non-steroidal anti-inflammatories (NSAID)
    Excludes2 long term (current) use of aspirin (Z79.82)

  Z79.2 Long term (current) use of antibiotics

  Z79.3 Long term (current) use of hormonal contraceptives
    Long term (current) use of birth control pill or patch

  Z79.4 Long term (current) use of insulin

  ● **Z79.5** Long term (current) use of steroids
    Z79.51 Long term (current) use of inhaled steroids
    Z79.52 Long term (current) use of systemic steroids

▶ New　　⇒ Revised　　~~deleted~~ Deleted　　**OGCR** Official Guidelines　　**X** Assign placeholder X　　● Use Additional Character(s)

Excludes 1　　Excludes 2　　Includes　　Use additional　　Code first　　Code also　　Key words　　1521

● Z79.8 Other long term (current) drug therapy
- ● Z79.81 Long term (current) use of agents affecting estrogen receptors and estrogen levels
  Code first, if applicable:
  malignant neoplasm of breast (C50.-)
  malignant neoplasm of prostate (C61)

  Use additional code, if applicable, to identify:
  estrogen receptor positive status (Z17.0)
  family history of breast cancer (Z80.3)
  genetic susceptibility to malignant neoplasm (cancer) (Z15.0-)
  personal history of breast cancer (Z85.3)
  personal history of prostate cancer (Z85.46)
  postmenopausal status (Z78.0)

  Excludes1 ➡ hormone replacement therapy (Z79.890)

  - Z79.810 Long term (current) use of selective estrogen receptor modulators (SERMs)
    Long term (current) use of raloxifene (Evista)
    Long term (current) use of tamoxifen (Nolvadex)
    Long term (current) use of toremifene (Fareston)

  - Z79.811 Long term (current) use of aromatase inhibitors
    Long term (current) use of anastrozole (Arimidex)
    Long term (current) use of exemestane (Aromasin)
    Long term (current) use of letrozole (Femara)

  - Z79.818 Long term (current) use of other agents affecting estrogen receptors and estrogen levels
    Long term (current) use of estrogen receptor downregulators
    Long term (current) use of fulvestrant (Faslodex)
    Long term (current) use of gonadotropin-releasing hormone (GnRH) agonist
    Long term (current) use of goserelin acetate (Zoladex)
    Long term (current) use of leuprolide acetate (leuprorelin) (Lupron)
    Long term (current) use of megestrol acetate (Megace)

- Z79.82 Long term (current) use of aspirin
- Z79.83 Long term (current) use of bisphosphonates
- Z79.84 Long term (current) use of oral hypoglycemic drugs
  Long term (current) use of oral antidiabetic drugs

  Excludes2 long term (current) use of insulin (Z79.4)

● Z79.89 Other long term (current) drug therapy
- ➡ Z79.890 Hormone replacement therapy
- Z79.891 Long term (current) use of opiate analgesic
  Long term (current) use of methadone for pain management

  Excludes1 methadone use NOS (F11.9-)
  use of methadone for treatment of heroin addiction (F11.2-)

- Z79.899 Other long term (current) drug therapy

● Z80 Family history of primary malignant neoplasm
- Z80.0 Family history of malignant neoplasm of digestive organs
  Conditions classifiable to C15-C26
- Z80.1 Family history of malignant neoplasm of trachea, bronchus and lung
  Conditions classifiable to C33-C34
- Z80.2 Family history of malignant neoplasm of other respiratory and intrathoracic organs
  Conditions classifiable to C30-C32, C37-C39
- Z80.3 Family history of malignant neoplasm of breast
  Conditions classifiable to C50.-
- ● Z80.4 Family history of malignant neoplasm of genital organs
  Conditions classifiable to C51-C63
  - Z80.41 Family history of malignant neoplasm of ovary
  - Z80.42 Family history of malignant neoplasm of prostate
  - Z80.43 Family history of malignant neoplasm of testis
  - Z80.49 Family history of malignant neoplasm of other genital organs
- ● Z80.5 Family history of malignant neoplasm of urinary tract
  Conditions classifiable to C64-C68
  - Z80.51 Family history of malignant neoplasm of kidney
  - Z80.52 Family history of malignant neoplasm of bladder
  - Z80.59 Family history of malignant neoplasm of other urinary tract organ
- Z80.6 Family history of leukemia
  Conditions classifiable to C91-C95
- Z80.7 Family history of other malignant neoplasms of lymphoid, hematopoietic and related tissues
  Conditions classifiable to C81-C90, C96.-
- Z80.8 Family history of malignant neoplasm of other organs or systems
  Conditions classifiable to C00-C14, C40-C49, C69-C79
- Z80.9 Family history of malignant neoplasm, unspecified
  Conditions classifiable to C80.1

▶ New   ➡ Revised   ~~deleted~~ Deleted   **OGCR** Official Guidelines   X Assign placeholder X   ● Use Additional Character(s)

Excludes 1   Excludes 2   Includes   Use additional   Code first   Code also   Key words

● **Z81 Family history of mental and behavioral disorders**

    Z81.0 Family history of intellectual disabilities
          Conditions classifiable to F70-F79

    Z81.1 Family history of alcohol abuse and dependence
          Conditions classifiable to F10.-

    Z81.2 Family history of tobacco abuse and dependence
          Conditions classifiable to F17.-

    Z81.3 Family history of other psychoactive substance abuse and dependence
          Conditions classifiable to F11-F16, F18-F19

    Z81.4 Family history of other substance abuse and dependence
          Conditions classifiable to F55

    Z81.8 Family history of other mental and behavioral disorders
          Conditions classifiable elsewhere in F01-F99

● **Z82 Family history of certain disabilities and chronic diseases (leading to disablement)**

    Z82.0 Family history of epilepsy and other diseases of the nervous system
          Conditions classifiable to G00-G99

    Z82.1 Family history of blindness and visual loss
          Conditions classifiable to H54.-

    Z82.2 Family history of deafness and hearing loss
          Conditions classifiable to H90-H91

    Z82.3 Family history of stroke
          Conditions classifiable to I60-I64

  ● **Z82.4 Family history of ischemic heart disease and other diseases of the circulatory system**
          Conditions classifiable to I00-I52, I65-I99

        Z82.41 Family history of sudden cardiac death

        Z82.49 Family history of ischemic heart disease and other diseases of the circulatory system

    Z82.5 Family history of asthma and other chronic lower respiratory diseases
          Conditions classifiable to J40-J47

          | Excludes2 | family history of other diseases of the respiratory system (Z83.6) |

  ● **Z82.6 Family history of arthritis and other diseases of the musculoskeletal system and connective tissue**
          Conditions classifiable to M00-M99

        Z82.61 Family history of arthritis

        Z82.62 Family history of osteoporosis

        Z82.69 Family history of other diseases of the musculoskeletal system and connective tissue

  ● **Z82.7 Family history of congenital malformations, deformations and chromosomal abnormalities**
          Conditions classifiable to Q00-Q99

        Z82.71 Family history of polycystic kidney

        Z82.79 Family history of other congenital malformations, deformations and chromosomal abnormalities

    Z82.8 Family history of other disabilities and chronic diseases leading to disablement, not elsewhere classified

● **Z83 Family history of other specific disorders**

    | Excludes2 | contact with and (suspected) exposure to communicable disease in the family (Z20.-) |

    Z83.0 Family history of human immunodeficiency virus [HIV] disease
          Conditions classifiable to B20

    Z83.1 Family history of other infectious and parasitic diseases
          Conditions classifiable to A00-B19, B25-B94, B99

    Z83.2 Family history of diseases of the blood and blood-forming organs and certain disorders involving the immune mechanism
          Conditions classifiable to D50-D89

    Z83.3 Family history of diabetes mellitus
          Conditions classifiable to E08-E13

  ● **Z83.4 Family history of other endocrine, nutritional and metabolic diseases**
          Conditions classifiable to E00-E07, E15-E88

        Z83.41 Family history of multiple endocrine neoplasia [MEN] syndrome

        Z83.42 Family history of familial hypercholesterolemia

        Z83.49 Family history of other endocrine, nutritional and metabolic diseases

  ● **Z83.5 Family history of eye and ear disorders**

    ● **Z83.51 Family history of eye disorders**
          Conditions classifiable to H00-H53, H55-H59

        | Excludes2 | family history of blindness and visual loss (Z82.1) |

        Z83.511 Family history of glaucoma

        Z83.518 Family history of other specified eye disorder

        Z83.52 Family history of ear disorders
          Conditions classifiable to H60-H83, H92-H95

        | Excludes2 | family history of deafness and hearing loss (Z82.2) |

    Z83.6 Family history of other diseases of the respiratory system
          Conditions classifiable to J00-J39, J60-J99

        | Excludes2 | family history of asthma and other chronic lower respiratory diseases (Z82.5) |

  ● **Z83.7 Family history of diseases of the digestive system**
          Conditions classifiable to K00-K93

        Z83.71 Family history of colonic polyps

        | Excludes1 | ~~family history of malignant neoplasm of digestive organs (Z80.0)~~ |

        ▶| Excludes2 | family history of malignant neoplasm of digestive organs (Z80.0) |

        Z83.79 Family history of other diseases of the digestive system

● **Z84 Family history of other conditions**

    Z84.0 Family history of diseases of the skin and subcutaneous tissue
          Conditions classifiable to L00-L99

    Z84.1 Family history of disorders of kidney and ureter
          Conditions classifiable to N00-N29

    Z84.2 Family history of other diseases of the genitourinary system
          Conditions classifiable to N30-N99

    Z84.3 Family history of consanguinity

  ● **Z84.8 Family history of other specified conditions**

        Z84.81 Family history of carrier of genetic disease

        Z84.82 Family history of sudden infant death syndrome
          Family history of SIDS

        Z84.89 Family history of other specified conditions

CHAPTER 21 (Z00-Z99)

● **Z85 Personal history of malignant neoplasm**

Code first any follow-up examination after treatment of malignant neoplasm (Z08)

Use additional code to identify:

alcohol use and dependence (F10.-)

exposure to environmental tobacco smoke (Z77.22)

history of tobacco dependence (Z87.891)

occupational exposure to environmental tobacco smoke (Z57.31)

tobacco dependence (F17.-)

tobacco use (Z72.0)

Excludes2 personal history of benign neoplasm (Z86.01-)

personal history of carcinoma-in-situ (Z86.00-)

● **Z85.0 Personal history of malignant neoplasm of digestive organs**

Z85.00 Personal history of malignant neoplasm of unspecified digestive organ

Z85.01 Personal history of malignant neoplasm of esophagus

Conditions classifiable to C15

● **Z85.02 Personal history of malignant neoplasm of stomach**

Z85.020 Personal history of malignant carcinoid tumor of stomach

Conditions classifiable to C7A.092

Z85.028 Personal history of other malignant neoplasm of stomach

Conditions classifiable to C16

● **Z85.03 Personal history of malignant neoplasm of large intestine**

Z85.030 Personal history of malignant carcinoid tumor of large intestine

Conditions classifiable to C7A.022-C7A.025, C7A.029

Z85.038 Personal history of other malignant neoplasm of large intestine

Conditions classifiable to C18

● **Z85.04 Personal history of malignant neoplasm of rectum, rectosigmoid junction, and anus**

Z85.040 Personal history of malignant carcinoid tumor of rectum

Conditions classifiable to C7A.026

Z85.048 Personal history of other malignant neoplasm of rectum, rectosigmoid junction, and anus

Conditions classifiable to C19-C21

Z85.05 Personal history of malignant neoplasm of liver

Conditions classifiable to C22

● **Z85.06 Personal history of malignant neoplasm of small intestine**

Z85.060 Personal history of malignant carcinoid tumor of small intestine

Conditions classifiable to C7A.01-

Z85.068 Personal history of other malignant neoplasm of small intestine

Conditions classifiable to C17

Z85.07 Personal history of malignant neoplasm of pancreas

Conditions classifiable to C25

Z85.09 Personal history of malignant neoplasm of other digestive organs

● **Z85.1 Personal history of malignant neoplasm of trachea, bronchus and lung**

● **Z85.11 Personal history of malignant neoplasm of bronchus and lung**

Z85.110 Personal history of malignant carcinoid tumor of bronchus and lung

Conditions classifiable to C7A.090

Z85.118 Personal history of other malignant neoplasm of bronchus and lung

Conditions classifiable to C34

Z85.12 Personal history of malignant neoplasm of trachea

Conditions classifiable to C33

● **Z85.2 Personal history of malignant neoplasm of other respiratory and intrathoracic organs**

Z85.20 Personal history of malignant neoplasm of unspecified respiratory organ

Z85.21 Personal history of malignant neoplasm of larynx

Conditions classifiable to C32

Z85.22 Personal history of malignant neoplasm of nasal cavities, middle ear, and accessory sinuses

Conditions classifiable to C30-C31

● **Z85.23 Personal history of malignant neoplasm of thymus**

Z85.230 Personal history of malignant carcinoid tumor of thymus

Conditions classifiable to C7A.091

Z85.238 Personal history of other malignant neoplasm of thymus

Conditions classifiable to C37

Z85.29 Personal history of malignant neoplasm of other respiratory and intrathoracic organs

Z85.3 Personal history of malignant neoplasm of breast

Conditions classifiable to C50.-

● **Z85.4 Personal history of malignant neoplasm of genital organs**

Conditions classifiable to C51-C63

Z85.40 Personal history of malignant neoplasm of unspecified female genital organ

Z85.41 Personal history of malignant neoplasm of cervix uteri

Z85.42 Personal history of malignant neoplasm of other parts of uterus

Z85.43 Personal history of malignant neoplasm of ovary

Z85.44 Personal history of malignant neoplasm of other female genital organs

Z85.45 Personal history of malignant neoplasm of unspecified male genital organ

Z85.46 Personal history of malignant neoplasm of prostate

Z85.47 Personal history of malignant neoplasm of testis

Z85.48 Personal history of malignant neoplasm of epididymis

Z85.49 Personal history of malignant neoplasm of other male genital organs

▶ New ⇒ Revised ~~deleted~~ Deleted **OGCR** Official Guidelines X Assign placeholder X ● Use Additional Character(s)

Excludes 1 Excludes 2 Includes Use additional Code first Code also Key words

● **Z85.5   Personal history of malignant neoplasm of urinary tract**
     Conditions classifiable to C64-C68

     Z85.50   Personal history of malignant neoplasm of unspecified urinary tract organ

     Z85.51   Personal history of malignant neoplasm of bladder

●   **Z85.52   Personal history of malignant neoplasm of kidney**

       Excludes1   personal history of malignant neoplasm of renal pelvis (Z85.53)

       Z85.520   Personal history of malignant carcinoid tumor of kidney
         Conditions classifiable to C7A.093

       Z85.528   Personal history of other malignant neoplasm of kidney
         Conditions classifiable to C64

     Z85.53   Personal history of malignant neoplasm of renal pelvis

     Z85.54   Personal history of malignant neoplasm of ureter

     Z85.59   Personal history of malignant neoplasm of other urinary tract organ

Z85.6   Personal history of leukemia
     Conditions classifiable to C91-C95

     Excludes1   leukemia in remission C91.0-C95.9 with 5th character 1

● **Z85.7   Personal history of other malignant neoplasms of lymphoid, hematopoietic and related tissues**

     Z85.71   Personal history of Hodgkin lymphoma
       Conditions classifiable to C81

     Z85.72   Personal history of non-Hodgkin lymphomas
       Conditions classifiable to C82-C85

     Z85.79   Personal history of other malignant neoplasms of lymphoid, hematopoietic and related tissues
       Conditions classifiable to C88-C90, C96

       Excludes1   multiple myeloma in remission (C90.01)
         plasma cell leukemia in remission (C90.11)
         plasmacytoma in remission (C90.21)

● **Z85.8   Personal history of malignant neoplasms of other organs and systems**
     Conditions classifiable to C00-C14, C40-C49, C69-C75, C7A.098, C76-C79

●   **Z85.81   Personal history of malignant neoplasm of lip, oral cavity, and pharynx**

       Z85.810   Personal history of malignant neoplasm of tongue

       Z85.818   Personal history of malignant neoplasm of other sites of lip, oral cavity, and pharynx

       Z85.819   Personal history of malignant neoplasm of unspecified site of lip, oral cavity, and pharynx

●   **Z85.82   Personal history of malignant neoplasm of skin**

       Z85.820   Personal history of malignant melanoma of skin
         Conditions classifiable to C43

       Z85.821   Personal history of Merkel cell carcinoma
         Conditions classifiable to C4A

       Z85.828   Personal history of other malignant neoplasm of skin
         Conditions classifiable to C44

●   **Z85.83   Personal history of malignant neoplasm of bone and soft tissue**

       Z85.830   Personal history of malignant neoplasm of bone

       Z85.831   Personal history of malignant neoplasm of soft tissue

         Excludes2   personal history of malignant neoplasm of skin (Z85.82-)

●   **Z85.84   Personal history of malignant neoplasm of eye and nervous tissue**

       Z85.840   Personal history of malignant neoplasm of eye

       Z85.841   Personal history of malignant neoplasm of brain

       Z85.848   Personal history of malignant neoplasm of other parts of nervous tissue

●   **Z85.85   Personal history of malignant neoplasm of endocrine glands**

       Z85.850   Personal history of malignant neoplasm of thyroid

       Z85.858   Personal history of malignant neoplasm of other endocrine glands

     Z85.89   Personal history of malignant neoplasm of other organs and systems

Z85.9   Personal history of malignant neoplasm, unspecified
     Conditions classifiable to C7A.00, C80.1

● **Z86   Personal history of certain other diseases**
     Code first any follow-up examination after treatment (Z09)

●   **Z86.0   Personal history of in-situ and benign neoplasms and neoplasms of uncertain behavior**

     Excludes2   personal history of malignant neoplasms (Z85.-)

●   **Z86.00   Personal history of in-situ neoplasm**
       Conditions classifiable to D00-D09

       Z86.000   Personal history of in-situ neoplasm of breast

       Z86.001   Personal history of in-situ neoplasm of cervix uteri
         Personal history of cervical intraepithelial neoplasia III [CIN III]

       Z86.008   Personal history of in-situ neoplasm of other site
         Personal history of vaginal intraepithelial neoplasia III [VAIN III]
         Personal history of vulvar intraepithelial neoplasia III [VIN III]

●   **Z86.01   Personal history of benign neoplasm**

       Z86.010   Personal history of colonic polyps

       Z86.011   Personal history of benign neoplasm of the brain

       Z86.012   Personal history of benign carcinoid tumor

       Z86.018   Personal history of other benign neoplasm

     Z86.03   Personal history of neoplasm of uncertain behavior

● **Z86.1**   Personal history of infectious and parasitic diseases
Conditions classifiable to A00-B89, B99

Excludes1   personal history of infectious diseases specific to a body system sequelae of infectious and parasitic diseases (B90-B94)

Z86.11   Personal history of tuberculosis

Z86.12   Personal history of poliomyelitis

Z86.13   Personal history of malaria

Z86.14   Personal history of Methicillin resistant Staphylococcus aureus infection
Personal history of MRSA infection

Z86.19   Personal history of other infectious and parasitic diseases

Z86.2   Personal history of diseases of the blood and blood-forming organs and certain disorders involving the immune mechanism
Conditions classifiable to D50-D89

● **Z86.3**   Personal history of endocrine, nutritional and metabolic diseases
Conditions classifiable to E00-E88

Z86.31   Personal history of diabetic foot ulcer

Excludes2   current diabetic foot ulcer (E08.621, E09.621, E10.621, E11.621, E13.621)

Z86.32   Personal history of gestational diabetes
Personal history of conditions classifiable to O24.4-

Excludes1   gestational diabetes mellitus in current pregnancy (O24.4-)

Z86.39   Personal history of other endocrine, nutritional and metabolic disease

● **Z86.5**   Personal history of mental and behavioral disorders
Conditions classifiable to F40-F59

Z86.51   Personal history of combat and operational stress reaction

Z86.59   Personal history of other mental and behavioral disorders

● **Z86.6**   Personal history of diseases of the nervous system and sense organs
Conditions classifiable to G00-G99, H00-H95

Z86.61   Personal history of infections of the central nervous system
Personal history of encephalitis
Personal history of meningitis

Z86.69   Personal history of other diseases of the nervous system and sense organs

● **Z86.7**   Personal history of diseases of the circulatory system
Conditions classifiable to I00-I99

Excludes2   old myocardial infarction (I25.2)
personal history of anaphylactic shock (Z87.892)
postmyocardial infarction syndrome (I24.1)

● **Z86.71**   Personal history of venous thrombosis and embolism

Z86.711   Personal history of pulmonary embolism

Z86.718   Personal history of other venous thrombosis and embolism

Z86.72   Personal history of thrombophlebitis

Z86.73   Personal history of transient ischemic attack (TIA), and cerebral infarction without residual deficits
Personal history of prolonged reversible ischemic neurological deficit (PRIND)
Personal history of stroke NOS without residual deficits

Excludes1   personal history of traumatic brain injury (Z87.820)
sequelae of cerebrovascular disease (I69.-)

Z86.74   Personal history of sudden cardiac arrest
Personal history of sudden cardiac death successfully resuscitated

Z86.79   Personal history of other diseases of the circulatory system

● **Z87**   Personal history of other diseases and conditions
Code first any follow-up examination after treatment (Z09)

● **Z87.0**   Personal history of diseases of the respiratory system
Conditions classifiable to J00-J99

Z87.01   Personal history of pneumonia (recurrent)

Z87.09   Personal history of other diseases of the respiratory system

● **Z87.1**   Personal history of diseases of the digestive system
Conditions classifiable to K00-K93

Z87.11   Personal history of peptic ulcer disease

Z87.19   Personal history of other diseases of the digestive system

Z87.2   Personal history of diseases of the skin and subcutaneous tissue
Conditions classifiable to L00-L99

Excludes2   personal history of diabetic foot ulcer (Z86.31)

● **Z87.3**   Personal history of diseases of the musculoskeletal system and connective tissue
Conditions classifiable to M00-M99

Excludes2   personal history of (healed) traumatic fracture (Z87.81)

● **Z87.31**   Personal history of (healed) nontraumatic fracture

Z87.310   Personal history of (healed) osteoporosis fracture
Personal history of (healed) fragility fracture
Personal history of (healed) collapsed vertebra due to osteoporosis

Z87.311   Personal history of (healed) other pathological fracture
Personal history of (healed) collapsed vertebra NOS

Excludes2   personal history of osteoporosis fracture (Z87.310)

Z87.312   Personal history of (healed) stress fracture
Personal history of (healed) fatigue fracture

Z87.39   Personal history of other diseases of the musculoskeletal system and connective tissue

▶ New   ⟹ Revised   ~~deleted~~ Deleted   **OGCR** Official Guidelines   X Assign placeholder X   ● Use Additional Character(s)

Excludes 1   Excludes 2   Includes   Use additional   Code first   Code also   Key words

● Z87.4   Personal history of diseases of genitourinary system
     Conditions classifiable to N00-N99

  ● Z87.41   Personal history of dysplasia of the female genital tract

       Excludes1 ⇨ personal history of intraepithelial neoplasia III of female genital tract (Z86.001, Z86.008)
             personal history of malignant neoplasm of female genital tract (Z85.40-Z85.44)

       Z87.410   Personal history of cervical dysplasia

       Z87.411   Personal history of vaginal dysplasia

       Z87.412   Personal history of vulvar dysplasia

   Z87.42   Personal history of other diseases of the female genital tract

  ● Z87.43   Personal history of diseases of male genital organs

       Z87.430   Personal history of prostatic dysplasia

          Excludes1   personal history of malignant neoplasm of prostate (Z85.46)

       Z87.438   Personal history of other diseases of male genital organs

  ● Z87.44   Personal history of diseases of urinary system

       Excludes1   personal history of malignant neoplasm of cervix uteri (Z85.41)

       Z87.440   Personal history of urinary (tract) infections

       Z87.441   Personal history of nephrotic syndrome

       Z87.442   Personal history of urinary calculi
              Personal history of kidney stones

       Z87.448   Personal history of other diseases of urinary system

● Z87.5   Personal history of complications of pregnancy, childbirth and the puerperium
     Conditions classifiable to O00-O9A

     Excludes2   recurrent pregnancy loss (N96)

   Z87.51   Personal history of pre-term labor

       Excludes1   current pregnancy with history of pre-term labor (O09.21-)

   Z87.59   Personal history of other complications of pregnancy, childbirth and the puerperium
       Personal history of trophoblastic disease

● Z87.7   Personal history of (corrected) congenital malformations
     Conditions classifiable to Q00-Q89 that have been repaired or corrected

     Excludes1   congenital malformations that have been partially corrected or repair but which still require medical treatment - code to condition

     Excludes2   other postprocedural states (Z98.-)
             personal history of medical treatment (Z92.-)
             presence of cardiac and vascular implants and grafts (Z95.-)
             presence of other devices (Z97.-)
             presence of other functional implants (Z96.-)
             transplanted organ and tissue status (Z94.-)

● Z87.71   Personal history of (corrected) congenital malformations of genitourinary system

   Z87.710   Personal history of (corrected) hypospadias

   Z87.718   Personal history of other specified (corrected) congenital malformations of genitourinary system

● Z87.72   Personal history of (corrected) congenital malformations of nervous system and sense organs

   Z87.720   Personal history of (corrected) congenital malformations of eye

   Z87.721   Personal history of (corrected) congenital malformations of ear

   Z87.728   Personal history of other specified (corrected) congenital malformations of nervous system and sense organs

● Z87.73   Personal history of (corrected) congenital malformations of digestive system

   Z87.730   Personal history of (corrected) cleft lip and palate

   Z87.738   Personal history of other specified (corrected) congenital malformations of digestive system

   Z87.74   Personal history of (corrected) congenital malformations of heart and circulatory system

   Z87.75   Personal history of (corrected) congenital malformations of respiratory system

   Z87.76   Personal history of (corrected) congenital malformations of integument, limbs and musculoskeletal system

● Z87.79   Personal history of other (corrected) congenital malformations

   Z87.790   Personal history of (corrected) congenital malformations of face and neck

   Z87.798   Personal history of other (corrected) congenital malformations

● Z87.8   Personal history of other specified conditions

   Excludes2   personal history of self harm (Z91.5)

   Z87.81   Personal history of (healed) traumatic fracture

       Excludes2   personal history of (healed) nontraumatic fracture (Z87.31-)

● Z87.82   Personal history of other (healed) physical injury and trauma
     Conditions classifiable to S00-T88, except traumatic fractures

   Z87.820   Personal history of traumatic brain injury

       Excludes1   personal history of transient ischemic attack (TIA), and cerebral infarction without residual deficits (Z86.73)

   Z87.821   Personal history of retained foreign body fully removed

   Z87.828   Personal history of other (healed) physical injury and trauma

CHAPTER 21 (Z00-Z99)

● Z87.89   Personal history of other specified conditions
     Z87.890   Personal history of sex reassignment
     Z87.891   Personal history of nicotine dependence

> **Excludes1**   current nicotine dependence (F17.2-)

     Z87.892   Personal history of anaphylaxis
         Code also allergy status such as:
           allergy status to drugs, medicaments and biological substances (Z88.-)
           allergy status, other than to drugs and biological substances (Z91.0-)
     Z87.898   Personal history of other specified conditions

● Z88   Allergy status to drugs, medicaments and biological substances

> **Excludes2**   allergy status, other than to drugs and biological substances (Z91.0-)

  Z88.0   Allergy status to penicillin
  Z88.1   Allergy status to other antibiotic agents status
  Z88.2   Allergy status to sulfonamides status
  Z88.3   Allergy status to other anti-infective agents status
  Z88.4   Allergy status to anesthetic agent status
  Z88.5   Allergy status to narcotic agent status
  Z88.6   Allergy status to analgesic agent status
  Z88.7   Allergy status to serum and vaccine status
  Z88.8   Allergy status to other drugs, medicaments and biological substances status
  Z88.9   Allergy status to unspecified drugs, medicaments and biological substances status

● Z89   Acquired absence of limb

> **Includes**   amputation status
> postprocedural loss of limb
> post-traumatic loss of limb

> **Excludes1**   acquired deformities of limbs (M20-M21)
> congenital absence of limbs (Q71-Q73)

● Z89.0   Acquired absence of thumb and other finger(s)
  ● Z89.01   Acquired absence of thumb
     Z89.011   Acquired absence of right thumb
     Z89.012   Acquired absence of left thumb
     Z89.019   Acquired absence of unspecified thumb
  ● Z89.02   Acquired absence of other finger(s)

> **Excludes2**   acquired absence of thumb (Z89.01-)

     Z89.021   Acquired absence of right finger(s)
     Z89.022   Acquired absence of left finger(s)
     Z89.029   Acquired absence of unspecified finger(s)

● Z89.1   Acquired absence of hand and wrist
  ● Z89.11   Acquired absence of hand
     Z89.111   Acquired absence of right hand
     Z89.112   Acquired absence of left hand
     Z89.119   Acquired absence of unspecified hand
  ● Z89.12   Acquired absence of wrist
     Disarticulation at wrist
     Z89.121   Acquired absence of right wrist
     Z89.122   Acquired absence of left wrist
     Z89.129   Acquired absence of unspecified wrist

● Z89.2   Acquired absence of upper limb above wrist
  ● Z89.20   Acquired absence of upper limb, unspecified level
     Z89.201   Acquired absence of right upper limb, unspecified level
     Z89.202   Acquired absence of left upper limb, unspecified level
     Z89.209   Acquired absence of unspecified upper limb, unspecified level
         Acquired absence of arm NOS
  ● Z89.21   Acquired absence of upper limb below elbow
     Z89.211   Acquired absence of right upper limb below elbow
     Z89.212   Acquired absence of left upper limb below elbow
     Z89.219   Acquired absence of unspecified upper limb below elbow
  ● Z89.22   Acquired absence of upper limb above elbow
     Disarticulation at elbow
     Z89.221   Acquired absence of right upper limb above elbow
     Z89.222   Acquired absence of left upper limb above elbow
     Z89.229   Acquired absence of unspecified upper limb above elbow
  ● Z89.23   Acquired absence of shoulder
     Acquired absence of shoulder joint following explantation of shoulder joint prosthesis, with or without presence of antibiotic-impregnated cement spacer
     Z89.231   Acquired absence of right shoulder
     Z89.232   Acquired absence of left shoulder
     Z89.239   Acquired absence of unspecified shoulder

● Z89.4   Acquired absence of toe(s), foot, and ankle
  ● Z89.41   Acquired absence of great toe
     Z89.411   Acquired absence of right great toe
     Z89.412   Acquired absence of left great toe
     Z89.419   Acquired absence of unspecified great toe
  ● Z89.42   Acquired absence of other toe(s)

> **Excludes2**   acquired absence of great toe (Z89.41-)

     Z89.421   Acquired absence of other right toe(s)
     Z89.422   Acquired absence of other left toe(s)
     Z89.429   Acquired absence of other toe(s), unspecified side
  ● Z89.43   Acquired absence of foot
     Z89.431   Acquired absence of right foot
     Z89.432   Acquired absence of left foot
     Z89.439   Acquired absence of unspecified foot
  ● Z89.44   Acquired absence of ankle
     Disarticulation of ankle
     Z89.441   Acquired absence of right ankle
     Z89.442   Acquired absence of left ankle
     Z89.449   Acquired absence of unspecified ankle

▶ New   ⇒ Revised   ~~deleted~~ Deleted   **OGCR** Official Guidelines   X Assign placeholder X   ● Use Additional Character(s)

Excludes 1   Excludes 2   Includes   Use additional   Code first   Code also   Key words

● **Z89.5** Acquired absence of leg below knee

  ● **Z89.51** Acquired absence of leg below knee

    Z89.511 Acquired absence of right leg below knee

    Z89.512 Acquired absence of left leg below knee

    Z89.519 Acquired absence of unspecified leg below knee

  ● **Z89.52** Acquired absence of knee

    Acquired absence of knee joint following explantation of knee joint prosthesis, with or without presence of antibiotic-impregnated cement spacer

    Z89.521 Acquired absence of right knee

    Z89.522 Acquired absence of left knee

    Z89.529 Acquired absence of unspecified knee

● **Z89.6** Acquired absence of leg above knee

  ● **Z89.61** Acquired absence of leg above knee

    Acquired absence of leg NOS
    Disarticulation at knee

    Z89.611 Acquired absence of right leg above knee

    Z89.612 Acquired absence of left leg above knee

    Z89.619 Acquired absence of unspecified leg above knee

  ● **Z89.62** Acquired absence of hip

    Acquired absence of hip joint following explantation of hip joint prosthesis, with or without presence of antibiotic-impregnated cement spacer
    Disarticulation at hip

    Z89.621 Acquired absence of right hip joint

    Z89.622 Acquired absence of left hip joint

    Z89.629 Acquired absence of unspecified hip joint

  Z89.9 Acquired absence of limb, unspecified

● **Z90** Acquired absence of organs, not elsewhere classified

  Includes   postprocedural or post-traumatic loss of body part NEC

  Excludes1 congenital absence - see Alphabetical Index
  Excludes2 postprocedural absence of endocrine glands (E89.-)

  ● **Z90.0** Acquired absence of part of head and neck

    Z90.01 Acquired absence of eye

    Z90.02 Acquired absence of larynx

    Z90.09 Acquired absence of other part of head and neck

      Acquired absence of nose

      Excludes2 teeth (K08.1)

  ● **Z90.1** Acquired absence of breast and nipple

    Z90.10 Acquired absence of unspecified breast and nipple

    Z90.11 Acquired absence of right breast and nipple

    Z90.12 Acquired absence of left breast and nipple

    Z90.13 Acquired absence of bilateral breasts and nipples

  Z90.2 Acquired absence of lung [part of]

  Z90.3 Acquired absence of stomach [part of]

● **Z90.4** Acquired absence of other specified parts of digestive tract

  ● **Z90.41** Acquired absence of pancreas

    Code also exocrine pancreatic insufficiency (K86.81)

    Use additional code to identify any associated:
    insulin use (Z79.4)
    diabetes mellitus, postpancreatectomy (E13.-)

    Z90.410 Acquired total absence of pancreas
      Acquired absence of pancreas NOS

    Z90.411 Acquired partial absence of pancreas

    Z90.49 Acquired absence of other specified parts of digestive tract

  Z90.5 Acquired absence of kidney

  Z90.6 Acquired absence of other parts of urinary tract
    Acquired absence of bladder

  ● **Z90.7** Acquired absence of genital organ(s)

    Excludes1 personal history of sex reassignment (Z87.890)

    Excludes2 female genital mutilation status (N90.81-)

  ● **Z90.71** Acquired absence of cervix and uterus

    Z90.710 Acquired absence of both cervix and uterus
      Acquired absence of uterus NOS
      Status post total hysterectomy

    Z90.711 Acquired absence of uterus with remaining cervical stump
      Status post partial hysterectomy with remaining cervical stump

    Z90.712 Acquired absence of cervix with remaining uterus

  ● **Z90.72** Acquired absence of ovaries

    Z90.721 Acquired absence of ovaries, unilateral

    Z90.722 Acquired absence of ovaries, bilateral

    Z90.79 Acquired absence of other genital organ(s)

  ● **Z90.8** Acquired absence of other organs

    Z90.81 Acquired absence of spleen

    Z90.89 Acquired absence of other organs

● **Z91** Personal risk factors, not elsewhere classified

  Excludes2 contact with and (suspected) exposures hazardous to health (Z77.-)
    exposure to pollution and other problems related to physical environment (Z77.1-)
    ▶female genital mutilation status (N90.81-)
    occupational exposure to risk factors (Z57.-)
    personal history of physical injury and trauma (Z87.81, Z87.82-)

  ● **Z91.0** Allergy status, other than to drugs and biological substances

    Excludes2 allergy status to drugs, medicaments, and biological substances (Z88.-)

  ● **Z91.01** Food allergy status

    Excludes2 food additives allergy status (Z91.02)

    Z91.010 Allergy to peanuts

    Z91.011 Allergy to milk products

      Excludes1 lactose intolerance (E73.-)

    Z91.012 Allergy to eggs

    Z91.013 Allergy to seafood
      Allergy to shellfish
      Allergy to octopus or squid ink

    Z91.018 Allergy to other foods
      Allergy to nuts other than peanuts

CHAPTER 21 (Z00-Z99)

CHAPTER 21 (Z00-Z99)

Z91.02   Food additives allergy status
● Z91.03   Insect allergy status
          Z91.030   Bee allergy status
          Z91.038   Other insect allergy status
● Z91.04   Nonmedicinal substance allergy status
          Z91.040   Latex allergy status
                     Latex sensitivity status
          Z91.041   Radiographic dye allergy status
                     Allergy status to contrast media
                     used for diagnostic X-ray
                     procedure
          Z91.048   Other nonmedicinal substance allergy
                     status
Z91.09   Other allergy status, other than to drugs and
          biological substances
● Z91.1   Patient's noncompliance with medical treatment and
          regimen
Z91.11   Patient's noncompliance with dietary regimen
● Z91.12   Patient's intentional underdosing of medication
          regimen
                Code first underdosing of medication (T36-T50)
                     with fifth or sixth character 6
          Excludes1   adverse effect of prescribed drug
                       taken as directed - code to
                       adverse effect
                       poisoning (overdose) - code to
                       poisoning
          Z91.120   Patient's intentional underdosing of
                     medication regimen due to financial
                     hardship
          Z91.128   Patient's intentional underdosing of
                     medication regimen for other reason
● Z91.13   Patient's unintentional underdosing of
          medication regimen
                Code first underdosing of medication (T36-T50)
                     with fifth or sixth character 6
          Excludes1   adverse effect of prescribed drug
                       taken as directed - code to
                       adverse effect
                       poisoning (overdose) - code to
                       poisoning
          Z91.130   Patient's unintentional underdosing
                     of medication regimen due to age-
                     related debility
          Z91.138   Patient's unintentional underdosing
                     of medication regimen for other
                     reason
Z91.14   Patient's other noncompliance with medication
          regimen
                Patient's underdosing of medication NOS
Z91.15   Patient's noncompliance with renal dialysis
Z91.19   Patient's noncompliance with other medical
          treatment and regimen
          ▶Nonadherence to medical treatment

● Z91.4   Personal history of psychological trauma, not elsewhere
          classified
● Z91.41   Personal history of adult abuse
          Excludes2   personal history of abuse in
                       childhood (Z62.81-)
          Z91.410   Personal history of adult physical and
                     sexual abuse
                     Excludes1   current adult physical
                                  abuse (T74.11,
                                  T76.11)
                                  current adult sexual
                                  abuse (T74.21,
                                  T76.11)
          Z91.411   Personal history of adult
                     psychological abuse
          Z91.412   Personal history of adult neglect
                     Excludes1   current adult neglect
                                  (T74.01, T76.01)
          Z91.419   Personal history of unspecified adult
                     abuse
Z91.49   Other personal history of psychological trauma,
          not elsewhere classified
Z91.5   Personal history of self-harm
          Personal history of parasuicide
          Personal history of self-poisoning
          Personal history of suicide attempt
● Z91.8   Other specified personal risk factors, not elsewhere
          classified
Z91.81   History of falling
          At risk for falling
Z91.82   Personal history of military deployment
          Individual (civilian or military) with past
                history of military war, peacekeeping and
                humanitarian deployment (current or past
                conflict)
          Returned from military deployment
Z91.83   Wandering in diseases classified elsewhere
          Code first underlying disorder such as:
          Alzheimer's disease (G30.-)
          autism or pervasive developmental disorder
                (F84.-)
          intellectual disabilities (F70-F79)
          unspecified dementia with behavioral
                disturbance (F03.9-)
▶● Z91.84   Oral health risk factors
          ▶ Z91.841   Risk for dental caries, low
          ▶ Z91.842   Risk for dental caries, moderate
          ▶ Z91.843   Risk for dental caries, high
          ▶ Z91.849   Unspecified risk for dental caries
Z91.89   Other specified personal risk factors, not
          elsewhere classified

▶ New   ⟹ Revised   ~~deleted~~ Deleted   **OGCR** Official Guidelines   X Assign placeholder X   ● Use Additional Character(s)

Excludes 1   Excludes 2   Includes   Use additional   Code first   Code also   Key words

- ● **Z92 Personal history of medical treatment**
  - Excludes2 postprocedural states (Z98.-)
  - **Z92.0 Personal history of contraception**
    - Excludes1 counseling or management of current contraceptive practices (Z30.-)
      long term (current) use of contraception (Z79.3)
      presence of (intrauterine) contraceptive device (Z97.5)
  - ● **Z92.2 Personal history of drug therapy**
    - Excludes2 long term (current) drug therapy (Z79.-)
    - **Z92.21 Personal history of antineoplastic chemotherapy**
    - **Z92.22 Personal history of monoclonal drug therapy**
    - **Z92.23 Personal history of estrogen therapy**
    - ● **Z92.24 Personal history of steroid therapy**
      - **Z92.240 Personal history of inhaled steroid therapy**
      - **Z92.241 Personal history of systemic steroid therapy**
        Personal history of steroid therapy NOS
    - **Z92.25 Personal history of immunosupression therapy**
      - Excludes2 personal history of steroid therapy (Z92.24)
    - **Z92.29 Personal history of other drug therapy**
  - **Z92.3 Personal history of irradiation**
    Personal history of exposure to therapeutic radiation
    - Excludes1 exposure to radiation in the physical environment (Z77.12)
      occupational exposure to radiation (Z57.1)
  - ● **Z92.8 Personal history of other medical treatment**
    - **Z92.81 Personal history of extracorporeal membrane oxygenation (ECMO)**
    - **Z92.82 Status post administration of tPA (rtPA) in a different facility within the last 24 hours prior to admission to current facility**
      Code first condition requiring tPA administration, such as:
      acute cerebral infarction (I63.-)
      acute myocardial infarction (I21.-, I22.-)
    - **Z92.83 Personal history of failed moderate sedation**
      Personal history of failed conscious sedation
      - Excludes2 failed moderate sedation during procedure (T88.52)
    - **Z92.84 Personal history of unintended awareness under general anesthesia**
      - Excludes2 unintended awareness under general anesthesia during procedure (T88.53)
    - **Z92.89 Personal history of other medical treatment**

- ● **Z93 Artificial opening status**
  - Excludes1 artificial openings requiring attention or management (Z43.-)
    complications of external stoma (J95.0-, K94.-, N99.5-)
  - **Z93.0 Tracheostomy status**
  - **Z93.1 Gastrostomy status**
  - **Z93.2 Ileostomy status**
  - **Z93.3 Colostomy status**
  - **Z93.4 Other artificial openings of gastrointestinal tract status**
  - ● **Z93.5 Cystostomy status**
    - **Z93.50 Unspecified cystostomy status**
    - **Z93.51 Cutaneous-vesicostomy status**
    - **Z93.52 Appendico-vesicostomy status**
    - **Z93.59 Other cystostomy status**
  - **Z93.6 Other artificial openings of urinary tract status**
    Nephrostomy status
    Ureterostomy status
    Urethrostomy status
  - **Z93.8 Other artificial opening status**
  - **Z93.9 Artificial opening status, unspecified**

- ● **Z94 Transplanted organ and tissue status**
  - Includes organ or tissue replaced by heterogenous or homogenous transplant
  - Excludes1 complications of transplanted organ or tissue - see Alphabetical Index
  - Excludes2 presence of vascular grafts (Z95.-)
  - **Z94.0 Kidney transplant status**
  - **Z94.1 Heart transplant status**
    - Excludes1 artificial heart status (Z95.812)
      heart-valve replacement status (Z95.2-Z95.4)
  - **Z94.2 Lung transplant status**
  - **Z94.3 Heart and lungs transplant status**
  - **Z94.4 Liver transplant status**
  - **Z94.5 Skin transplant status**
    Autogenous skin transplant status
  - **Z94.6 Bone transplant status**
  - **Z94.7 Corneal transplant status**
  - ● **Z94.8 Other transplanted organ and tissue status**
    - **Z94.81 Bone marrow transplant status**
    - **Z94.82 Intestine transplant status**
    - **Z94.83 Pancreas transplant status**
    - **Z94.84 Stem cells transplant status**
    - **Z94.89 Other transplanted organ and tissue status**
  - **Z94.9 Transplanted organ and tissue status, unspecified**

▶ New ⟾ Revised deleted Deleted OGCR Official Guidelines X Assign placeholder X ● Use Additional Character(s)
Excludes 1 Excludes 2 Includes Use additional Code first Code also Key words
1531

● **Z95   Presence of cardiac and vascular implants and grafts**

> ~~**Excludes1**~~ ~~complications of cardiac and vascular devices,~~
> ~~implants and grafts (T82.-)~~

> ▶ **Excludes2** complications of cardiac and vascular devices,
> implants and grafts (T82.-)

  Z95.0   Presence of cardiac pacemaker

    Presence of cardiac resynchronization therapy (CRT-P)
pacemaker

> **Excludes1** adjustment or management of cardiac
> device (Z45.0-)
> adjustment or management of cardiac
> pacemaker (Z45.0)
> presence of automatic (implantable)
> cardiac defibrillator with
> synchronous cardiac pacemaker
> (Z95.810)

  Z95.1   Presence of aortocoronary bypass graft

    Presence of coronary artery bypass graft

  Z95.2   Presence of prosthetic heart valve

    Presence of heart valve NOS

  Z95.3   Presence of xenogenic heart valve

  Z95.4   Presence of other heart-valve replacement

  Z95.5   Presence of coronary angioplasty implant and graft

> **Excludes1** coronary angioplasty status without
> implant and graft (Z98.61)

● **Z95.8   Presence of other cardiac and vascular implants and
grafts**

  ● **Z95.81   Presence of other cardiac implants and grafts**

    **Z95.810   Presence of automatic (implantable)
cardiac defibrillator**

      Presence of automatic (implantable)
cardiac defibrillator with
synchronous cardiac pacemaker

      Presence of cardiac
resynchronization therapy
defibrillator (CRT-D)

      Presence of cardioverter-defibrillator
(ICD)

    Z95.811   Presence of heart assist device

    **Z95.812   Presence of fully implantable
artificial heart**

    **Z95.818   Presence of other cardiac implants
and grafts**

  ● **Z95.82   Presence of other vascular implants and grafts**

    **Z95.820   Peripheral vascular angioplasty status
with implants and grafts**

> **Excludes1** peripheral vascular
> angioplasty
> without implant
> and graft (Z98.62)

    **Z95.828   Presence of other vascular implants
and grafts**

      Presence of intravascular prosthesis
NEC

  **Z95.9   Presence of cardiac and vascular implant and graft,
unspecified**

● **Z96   Presence of other functional implants**

> **Excludes2** complications of internal prosthetic devices,
> implants and grafts (T82-T85)
> fitting and adjustment of prosthetic and other
> devices (Z44-Z46)

  Z96.0   Presence of urogenital implants

  Z96.1   Presence of intraocular lens

    Presence of pseudophakia

● **Z96.2   Presence of otological and audiological implants**

  **Z96.20   Presence of otological and audiological
implant, unspecified**

  Z96.21   Cochlear implant status

  Z96.22   Myringotomy tube(s) status

  **Z96.29   Presence of other otological and audiological
implants**

    Presence of bone-conduction hearing device

    Presence of eustachian tube stent

    Stapes replacement

  Z96.3   Presence of artificial larynx

● **Z96.4   Presence of endocrine implants**

  Z96.41   Presence of insulin pump (external) (internal)

  Z96.49   Presence of other endocrine implants

  Z96.5   Presence of tooth-root and mandibular implants

● **Z96.6   Presence of orthopedic joint implants**

  **Z96.60   Presence of unspecified orthopedic joint
implant**

  ● **Z96.61   Presence of artificial shoulder joint**

    **Z96.611   Presence of right artificial shoulder
joint**

    **Z96.612   Presence of left artificial shoulder
joint**

    **Z96.619   Presence of unspecified artificial
shoulder joint**

  ● **Z96.62   Presence of artificial elbow joint**

    Z96.621   Presence of right artificial elbow joint

    Z96.622   Presence of left artificial elbow joint

    **Z96.629   Presence of unspecified artificial
elbow joint**

  ● **Z96.63   Presence of artificial wrist joint**

    Z96.631   Presence of right artificial wrist joint

    Z96.632   Presence of left artificial wrist joint

    **Z96.639   Presence of unspecified artificial wrist
joint**

  ● **Z96.64   Presence of artificial hip joint**

    Hip-joint replacement (partial) (total)

    Z96.641   Presence of right artificial hip joint

    Z96.642   Presence of left artificial hip joint

    **Z96.643   Presence of artificial hip joint,
bilateral**

    **Z96.649   Presence of unspecified artificial hip
joint**

  ● **Z96.65   Presence of artificial knee joint**

    Z96.651   Presence of right artificial knee joint

    Z96.652   Presence of left artificial knee joint

    **Z96.653   Presence of artificial knee joint,
bilateral**

    **Z96.659   Presence of unspecified artificial knee
joint**

  ● **Z96.66   Presence of artificial ankle joint**

    Z96.661   Presence of right artificial ankle joint

    Z96.662   Presence of left artificial ankle joint

    **Z96.669   Presence of unspecified artificial
ankle joint**

  ● **Z96.69   Presence of other orthopedic joint implants**

    **Z96.691   Finger-joint replacement of right
hand**

    Z96.692   Finger-joint replacement of left hand

    Z96.693   Finger-joint replacement, bilateral

    **Z96.698   Presence of other orthopedic joint
implants**

▶ New   ⟹ Revised   ~~deleted~~ Deleted   **OGCR** Official Guidelines   X Assign placeholder X   ● Use Additional Character(s)

Excludes 1   Excludes 2   Includes   Use additional   Code first   Code also   Key words

Z96.7   Presence of other bone and tendon implants
      Presence of skull plate

● Z96.8   Presence of other specified functional implants

     Z96.81   Presence of artificial skin

     Z96.89   Presence of other specified functional implants

Z96.9   Presence of functional implant, unspecified

● **Z97**   **Presence of other devices**

     Excludes1   complications of internal prosthetic devices, implants and grafts (T82-T85)
                 fitting and adjustment of prosthetic and other devices (Z44-Z46)

     Excludes2   presence of cerebrospinal fluid drainage device (Z98.2)

Z97.0   Presence of artificial eye

● Z97.1   Presence of artificial limb (complete) (partial)

     Z97.10   Presence of artificial limb (complete) (partial), unspecified

     Z97.11   Presence of artificial right arm (complete) (partial)

     Z97.12   Presence of artificial left arm (complete) (partial)

     Z97.13   Presence of artificial right leg (complete) (partial)

     Z97.14   Presence of artificial left leg (complete) (partial)

     Z97.15   Presence of artificial arms, bilateral (complete) (partial)

     Z97.16   Presence of artificial legs, bilateral (complete) (partial)

Z97.2   Presence of dental prosthetic device (complete) (partial)
      Presence of dentures (complete) (partial)

Z97.3   Presence of spectacles and contact lenses

Z97.4   Presence of external hearing-aid

Z97.5   Presence of (intrauterine) contraceptive device

     Excludes1   checking, reinsertion or removal of implantable subdermal contraceptive (Z30.46)
                 checking, reinsertion or removal of intrauterine contraceptive device (Z30.43-)

Z97.8   Presence of other specified devices

● **Z98**   **Other postprocedural states**

     Excludes2   aftercare (Z43-Z49, Z51)
                 follow-up medical care (Z08-Z09)
                 postprocedural complication - see Alphabetical Index

Z98.0   Intestinal bypass and anastomosis status

     Excludes2   bariatric surgery status (Z98.84)
                 gastric bypass status (Z98.84)
                 obesity surgery status (Z98.84)

Z98.1   Arthrodesis status

Z98.2   Presence of cerebrospinal fluid drainage device
      Presence of CSF shunt

Z98.3   Post therapeutic collapse of lung status
      Code first underlying disease

● Z98.4   Cataract extraction status
      Use additional code to identify intraocular lens implant status (Z96.1)

     Excludes1   aphakia (H27.0)

     Z98.41   Cataract extraction status, right eye

     Z98.42   Cataract extraction status, left eye

     Z98.49   Cataract extraction status, unspecified eye

● Z98.5   Sterilization status

     Excludes1   female infertility (N97.-)
                 male infertility (N46.-)

     Z98.51   Tubal ligation status

     Z98.52   Vasectomy status

● Z98.6   Angioplasty status

     Z98.61   Coronary angioplasty status

        Excludes1   coronary angioplasty status with implant and graft (Z95.5)

     Z98.62   Peripheral vascular angioplasty status

        Excludes1   peripheral vascular angioplasty status with implant and graft (Z95.820)

● Z98.8   Other specified postprocedural states

   ● Z98.81   Dental procedure status

     Z98.810   Dental sealant status

     Z98.811   Dental restoration status
         Dental crown status
         Dental fillings status

     Z98.818   Other dental procedure status

     Z98.82   Breast implant status

        Excludes1   breast implant removal status (Z98.86)

     Z98.83   Filtering (vitreous) bleb after glaucoma surgery status

        Excludes1   inflammation (infection) of postprocedural bleb (H59.4-)

     Z98.84   Bariatric surgery status
        Gastric banding status
        Gastric bypass status for obesity
        Obesity surgery status

        Excludes1   bariatric surgery status complicating pregnancy, childbirth, or the puerperium (O99.84)

        Excludes2   intestinal bypass and anastomosis status (Z98.0)

     Z98.85   Transplanted organ removal status
        Transplanted organ previously removed due to complication, failure, rejection or infection

        Excludes1   encounter for removal of transplanted organ -code to complication of transplanted organ (T86.-)

     Z98.86   Personal history of breast implant removal

   ● Z98.87   Personal history of in utero procedure

     Z98.870   Personal history of in utero procedure during pregnancy

        Excludes2   complications from in utero procedure for current pregnancy (O35.7)
                 supervision of current pregnancy with history of in utero procedure during previous pregnancy (O09.82-)

     Z98.871   Personal history of in utero procedure while a fetus

CHAPTER 21 (Z00-Z99)

● Z98.89   **Other specified postprocedural states**

    Z98.890   **Other specified postprocedural states**

        Personal history of surgery, not elsewhere classified

    Z98.891   **History of uterine scar from previous surgery**

        Excludes1   Maternal care due to uterine scar from previous surgery (O34.2-)

● **Z99   Dependence on enabling machines and devices, not elsewhere classified**

    Excludes1   cardiac pacemaker status (Z95.0)

Z99.0   Dependence on aspirator

● **Z99.1   Dependence on respirator**

    Dependence on ventilator

    Z99.11   **Dependence on respirator [ventilator] status**

    Z99.12   **Encounter for respirator [ventilator] dependence during power failure**

        Excludes1   mechanical complication of respirator [ventilator] (J95.850)

Z99.2   Dependence on renal dialysis

    Hemodialysis status

    Peritoneal dialysis status

    Presence of arteriovenous shunt for dialysis

    Renal dialysis status NOS

    Excludes1   encounter for fitting and adjustment of dialysis catheter (Z49.0-)

    Excludes2   noncompliance with renal dialysis (Z91.15)

Z99.3   Dependence on wheelchair

    Wheelchair confinement status

    Code first cause of dependence, such as:

    muscular dystrophy (G71.0)

    obesity (E66.-)

● **Z99.8   Dependence on other enabling machines and devices**

    Z99.81   **Dependence on supplemental oxygen**

        Dependence on long-term oxygen

    Z99.89   **Dependence on other enabling machines and devices**

        Dependence on machine or device NOS

▶ New   ⇒ Revised   ~~deleted~~ Deleted   **OGCR** Official Guidelines   X Assign placeholder X   ● Use Additional Character(s)

Excludes 1   Excludes 2   Includes   Use additional   Code first   Code also   Key words

MAKE THE MOST *of your* PHYSICIAN CODING EXAM Review!

ELSEVIER

1. Assess! Take the Pre-Exam

Use the Pre-Exam located on the companion Evolve site to gauge your strengths and weaknesses, develop a plan for focused study, and gain a better understanding of the testing process.

2. Study!

Use the quizzes in this book to sharpen your skills and build competency.

4. Test! Take the Final Exam

Gauge your readiness for the actual physician coding exam with the Final Exam. Boost your test-taking confidence and ensure certification success.

3. Apply! Take the Post-Exam

After studying, apply your knowledge to the Post-Exam located on the companion Evolve site. When finished, you'll receive scores for both the Pre- and Post-Exams and a breakdown of incorrect answers to help you identify areas where you need more detailed study and review.

ISBN: 978-0-323-43078-4

Perfect *your* **understanding** *and* **prepare for certification**
— START YOUR REVIEW NOW!

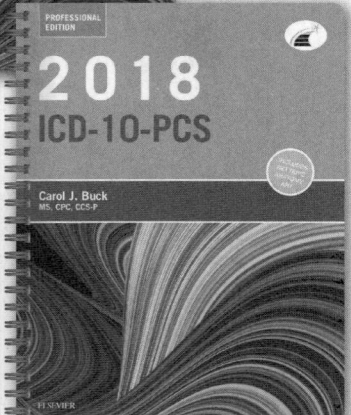